Manual of CLINICAL MICROBIOLOGY

9TH EDITION

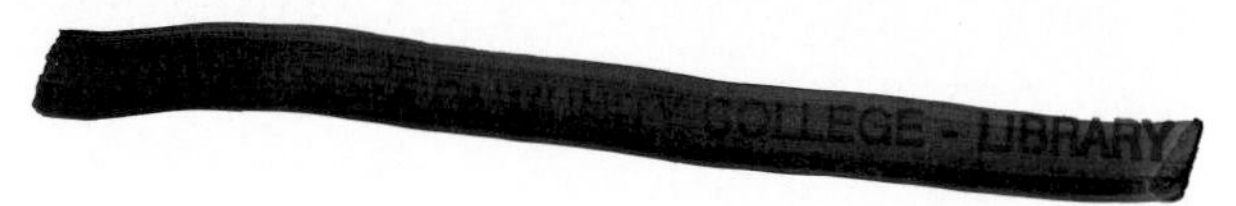

9TH EDITION

Manual of CLINICAL MICROBIOLOGY

EDITOR IN CHIEF

PATRICK R. MURRAY
Department of Laboratory Medicine,
National Institutes of Health Clinical Center, Bethesda, Maryland

EDITORS

ELLEN JO BARON
Department of Pathology, Stanford University
Medical Center, Stanford, California

JAMES H. JORGENSEN
Department of Pathology,
University of Texas Health Science Center,
San Antonio, Texas

MARIE LOUISE LANDRY
Department of Laboratory Medicine,
Yale University School of Medicine,
New Haven, Connecticut

MICHAEL A. PFALLER
Department of Pathology, University of Iowa
College of Medicine, Iowa City, Iowa

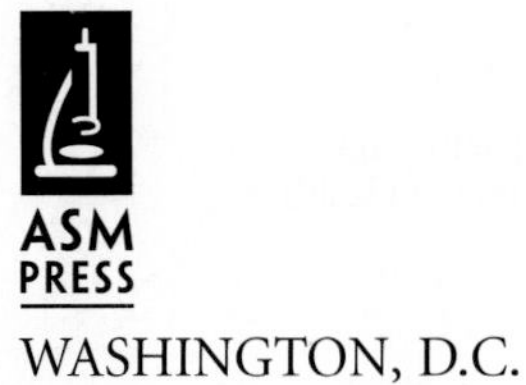

ASM PRESS
WASHINGTON, D.C.

VOLUME 1

Address editorial correspondence to ASM Press, 1752 N St. NW,
Washington, DC 20036-2904, USA

Send orders to ASM Press, P.O. Box 605, Herndon, VA 20172, USA
Phone: 800-546-2416; 703-661-1593
Fax: 703-661-1501
E-mail: books@asmusa.org
Online: estore.asm.org

Library of Congress Cataloging-in-Publication Data

Manual of clinical microbiology/editor in chief, Patrick R. Murray; editors, Ellen Jo Baron . . . [et al.].—9th ed.
p. cm.
Includes bibliographical references and index.
ISBN-10: 1-55581-371-2 (set)
ISBN-13: 978-1-55581-371-0 (set)
1. Medical microbiology—Handbooks, manuals, etc. 2. Diagnostic microbiology—Handbooks, manuals, etc. I. Title: Clinical microbiology.
QR46 .M425 2007
616.9′041—dc22

2006040722

10 9 8 7 6 5 4 3 2 1

Printed in China

Patrick R. Murray's role as editor in chief of this book was carried out in his private capacity and his contribution as an editor does not reflect official support or endorsement by the National Institutes of Health.

Contents

Editorial Board

Contributors

SHARON L. ABBOTT
Microbial Diseases Laboratory, California State Department of Health Services, 850 Marina Bay Parkway, E164, Richmond, CA 94804

MARIA E. AGUERO-ROSENFELD
Clinical Laboratories, Room 1J-04, Westchester Medical Center, Valhalla, NY 10595

ADRIANO AGUZZI
University Hospital Zürich, Institute of Neuropathology, Schmelzbergstrasse 12, CH-8091 Zürich, Switzerland

ABDALLA O. A. AHMED
Department of Pathology and Microbiology, College of Medicine, King Saud University, P.O. Box 2925, Riyadh 11461, Kingdom of Saudi Arabia

AFSAR ALI
Department of Epidemiology and Preventive Medicine, University of Maryland School of Medicine, 10 South Pine Street, MSTF 959, Baltimore, MD 21201

DAVID A. ANDERSON
Macfarlane Burnet Institute for Medical Research and Public Health, AMREP, 85 Commercial Road, Melbourne 3004, Australia

MAX Q. ARENS
Department of Pediatrics, Washington University School of Medicine, One Children's Place, St. Louis, MO 63110

SEVTAP ARIKAN
Department of Microbiology and Clinical Microbiology, Hacettepe University Medical School, 06100 Ankara, Turkey

ROBERT L. ATMAR
Departments of Medicine and Molecular Virology & Microbiology, Baylor College of Medicine, 1 Baylor Plaza, MS BCM280, Houston, TX 77030

TAMMY L. BANNERMAN
Department of Pathology, The Ohio State University, 129 Hamilton Hall, 1645 Neill Avenue, Columbus, OH 43210-1218

ELLEN JO BARON
Department of Pathology, Stanford University Medical College, Stanford University Medical Center, Room H1537-J, MC 5629, 300 Pasteur Drive, Stanford, CA 94305-5250

WILLIAM J. BELLINI
Measles, Mumps, Rubella, and Herpesviruses Branch, Division of Viral Diseases, National Center for Immunizations and Respiratory Diseases, Centers for Disease Control and Prevention, Mail Stop C-22, 1600 Clifton Road, NE, Atlanta, GA 30333

KATHRYN A. BERNARD
National Microbiology Laboratory, Public Health Agency of Canada, Winnipeg, Manitoba, R3E3R2 Canada

BEVERLEY-ANN BIGGS
Victorian Infectious Diseases Service and Department of Medicine, Royal Melbourne Hospital, University of Melbourne, Parkville, Victoria 3050, Australia

JACQUES BILLE
Centre National de Référence Listeria, Institut de Microbiologie, Rue de Bugnon 48, CH-1011 Lausanne, Switzerland

EDITH BLONDEL-HILL
Department of Pathology and Laboratory Medicine, British Columbia Children's Hospital, 2G5, 4500 Oak Street, Vancouver, British Columbia, Canada V6H 3N1

K. D. BOATWRIGHT
Infectious Diseases Division, Medical University of South Carolina, 100 Doughty Street, Room 210BA, Charleston, SC 29425

ROBERT A. BONOMO
Medical Service 111(W), Louis Stokes Cleveland VA Medical Center, 10701 East Boulevard, and Department of Medicine, Case Western Reserve University, Cleveland, OH 44106

CHERYL A. BOPP
Foodborne and Diarrheal Diseases Laboratory Section, Foodborne and Diarrheal Diseases Branch, Division of Bacterial and Mycotic Diseases, National Center for Infectious Diseases, Centers for Disease Control and Prevention, Atlanta, GA 30333

DONALD H. BOUYER
Department of Pathology, University of Texas Medical Branch, 301 University Boulevard, Keiller Building, Galveston, TX 77555-0609

MICHAEL D. BOWEN
Bioterrorism Rapid Response and Advanced Technology Laboratory, Bioterrorism Preparedness and Response Program, Centers for Disease Control and Prevention, MS G42, 1600 Clifton Road, N.E., Atlanta, GA 30333

CLAUDIA BRANDT
Institute of Medical Microbiology, Johann Wolfgang Goethe University, Paul Ehrlich Strasse 40, 60596 Frankfurt, Germany

MARY E. BRANDT
Mycotic Diseases Branch, Division of Bacterial and Mycotic Diseases, National Center for Infectious Diseases, Centers for Disease Control and Prevention, 1600 Clifton Road, N.E., Mailstop G-11, Atlanta, GA 30333

PHILIPPE BROUQUI
Unité des Rickettsies, IFR 48, CNRS UMR 6020, Faculté de Médecine, 27 Boulevard Jean Moulin, 13385 Marseille Cedex 5, and Service des Maladies Infectieuses et Tropicales, CHU Nord, 13015 Marseille, France

BARBARA A. BROWN-ELLIOTT
Department of Microbiology, The University of Texas Health Center at Tyler, 11937 US Highway 271, Tyler, TX 75708

DAVID A. BRUCKNER
Department of Pathology and Laboratory Medicine, David Geffen School of Medicine at UCLA, P.O. Box 951713, Los Angeles, CA 90095-1713

CORNELIA BÜCHEN-OSMOND
Jerome L. and Dawn Greene Infectious Disease Laboratory, Mailman School of Public Health, Department of Epidemiology—Lipkin, 722 W. 168th Street, New York, NY 10032

ANGELA M. CALIENDO
Department of Pathology and Laboratory Medicine, Emory University School of Medicine, 1364 Clifton Road, N.E., Atlanta, GA 30322

VITALIANO CAMA
Division of Parasitic Diseases, Centers for Disease Control and Prevention, 4770 Buford Highway, Atlanta, GA 30341

SHELDON CAMPBELL
Pathology and Laboratory Service, VA Connecticut Healthcare System, 950 Campbell Avenue, West Haven, CT 06516, and Department of Laboratory Medicine, Yale University School of Medicine, New Haven, CT 06520

JOSEPH M. CAMPOS
Department of Laboratory Medicine, Children's National Medical Center, Washington, DC 20010, and Departments of Pediatrics, Pathology, and Microbiology/Tropical Medicine, George Washington University Medical Center, Washington, DC 20037

A. BETTS CARPENTER
Department of Pathology, Joan C. Edwards School of Medicine, Marshall University, 1542 Spring Valley Drive, Huntington, WV 25704

KAREN C. CARROLL
Department of Pathology, The Johns Hopkins University School of Medicine, 600 North Wolfe Street, Baltimore, MD 21287

MARIA DA GLÓRIA SIQUEIRA CARVALHO
Streptococcus Laboratory, Respiratory Diseases Branch, Division of Bacterial Diseases, Centers for Disease Control and Prevention, Mail Stop C0-2, Atlanta, GA 30333

KIMBERLE C. CHAPIN
Department of Pathology and Laboratory Medicine, Rhode Island Hospital, Providence, RI 02903

JINGXIAN CHEN
Department of Pathology, Columbia University College of Physicians & Surgeons, 650 W. 168th Street, New York, NY 10032

BRUNO B. CHOMEL
Department of Population Health and Reproduction, School of Veterinary Medicine, University of California, Davis, CA 95616

SUNWEN CHOU
Department of Medicine, Oregon Health and Sciences University, Portland, OR 97239

MAY C. CHU
Emerging and Dangerous Pathogens Alert and Response Operations, CSR/CDS/WHO, Avenue Appia 20, CH-1211 Geneva, Switzerland

DIANE M. CITRON
R. M. Alden Research Laboratory, 2001 Santa Monica Boulevard, Suite 685W, Santa Monica, CA 90404, and Microbial Research Laboratory, Los Angeles County-University of Southern California Medical Center, 1801 E. Marengo Street, Los Angeles, CA 90033

FRANKLIN COCKERILL
Department of Laboratory Medicine, Mayo Clinic, Rochester, MN 55905

PATRICIA S. CONVILLE
Microbiology Service, Department of Laboratory Medicine, Clinical Center, National Institutes of Health, Building 10, Room 2C-385, 10 Center Drive MSC 1508, Bethesda, MD 20892-1508

ELLIOT P. COWAN
Center for Biologics Evaluation and Research, U.S. Food and Drug Administration, Rockville, MD 20852

FRANCIS E. G. COX
Department of Infectious and Tropical Diseases, London School of Hygiene and Tropical Medicine, London WC1E 7HT, United Kingdom

JAMES E. CROWE, JR.
Departments of Pediatrics and Microbiology and Immunology, Vanderbilt University School of Medicine, T-2220 MCN, 1161 21st Avenue, South, Nashville, TN 37232-2905

BART J. CURRIE
Tropical and Emerging Infectious Diseases Division, Menzies School of Health Research, Charles Darwin University, Darwin 0810, Northern Territory, Australia

MELANIE T. CUSHION
Department of Internal Medicine, Division of Infectious Diseases, University of Cincinnati College of Medicine, 231 Albert Sabin Way, Cincinnati, OH 45267-0560

INGER K. DAMON
Poxvirus Program, Division of Viral and Rickettsial Diseases, National Center for Infectious Diseases, Centers for Disease Control and Prevention, 1600 Clifton Road, Mailstop G43, Atlanta, GA 30333

MARYAM I. DANESHVAR
Centers for Disease Control and Prevention, Atlanta, GA 30333

G. SYBREN DE HOOG
Centraalbureau voor Schimmelcultures, P.O. Box 85167, NL-3508 AD The Netherlands

PETER DEPLAZES
Institute of Parasitology, University of Zurich, Winterthurerstrasse 266a, CH-8057 Zurich, Switzerland

CHARLENE S. DEZZUTTI
Laboratory Branch, Division of HIV/AIDS Prevention, National Center for HIV, STD, and TB Prevention, Centers for Disease Control and Prevention, Atlanta, GA 30333

DANIEL J. DIEKEMA
Division of Medical Microbiology, Department of Pathology, University of Iowa College of Medicine, Iowa City, IA 52242

J. STEPHEN DUMLER
Division of Medical Microbiology, Department of Pathology, The Johns Hopkins University School of Medicine, 720 Rutland Avenue, Ross 624, Baltimore, MD 21205

W. MICHAEL DUNNE, JR.
Departments of Pathology and Immunology, and Molecular Microbiology, Washington University School of Medicine, and Microbiology Laboratory, Barnes-Jewish Hospital, St. Louis, MO 63110

MARCELA ECHAVARRIA
Clinical Virology Laboratory, Center for Medical Education and Clinical Research, University Hospital, Buenos Aires C1431FWO, Argentina

PAUL H. EDELSTEIN
Clinical Microbiology Laboratory, 4th Floor, Gates Building, Hospital of the University of Pennsylvania, 3400 Spruce Street, Philadelphia, PA 19104-4283

SHIRIT EINAV
Department of Medicine, Stanford University, Stanford, CA 94305

HERMES ESCALANTE
Department of Microbiology, School of Biological Sciences, Universidad Nacional de Trujillo, Av. Juan Pablo II S/N, Ciudad Universitaria, Trujillo, Peru

ANA V. ESPINEL-INGROFF
Medical Mycology Research Laboratory, Division of Infectious Diseases, VCU Medical Center, 1101 East Marshall Street, Sanger Hall Room 7-049, Richmond, VA 23298-0049

ANDREAS ESSIG
Department of Medical Microbiology and Hygiene, University Hospital Ulm, D-89081 Ulm, Germany

RICHARD R. FACKLAM
Streptococcus Laboratory, Respiratory Diseases Branch, Division of Bacterial Diseases, Centers for Disease Control and Prevention, Mail Stop C0-2, Atlanta, GA 30333

KERSTIN I. FALK
Centre for Microbiological Preparedness, Swedish Institute for Infectious Disease Control, SE-171 82 Solna, Sweden

TIBOR FARKAS
Division of Infectious Diseases, Department of Pediatrics, Cincinnati Children's Hospital Medical Center, University of Cincinnati College of Medicine, 3333 Burnet Avenue, Cincinnati, OH 45229-3039

J. J. FARMER III
United States Public Health Service (retired), 1781 Silver Hill Road, Stone Mountain, GA 30087-2212

FLORENCE FENOLLAR
Unité des Rickettsies, IFR 48, CNRS UMR 6020, Faculté de Médecine, 27 Boulevard Jean Moulin, 13385 Marseille Cedex 5, France

MARY JANE FERRARO
Clinical Microbiology Laboratory, Massachusetts General Hospital, and Harvard Medical School, Boston, MA 02114

PATRICIA I. FIELDS
Foodborne and Diarrheal Diseases Laboratory Section, Foodborne and Diarrheal Diseases Branch, Division of Bacterial and Mycotic Diseases, National Center for Infectious Diseases, Centers for Disease Control and Prevention, Atlanta, GA 30333

SYDNEY M. FINEGOLD
Infectious Diseases Section, VA Medical Center West Los Angeles, Los Angeles, CA 90073, and Department of Medicine and Department of Microbiology, Immunology, and Molecular Genetics, University of California at Los Angeles School of Medicine, Los Angeles, CA 90025

COLLETTE FITZGERALD
National *Campylobacter* and *Helicobacter* Reference Laboratory, Foodborne and Diarrheal Diseases Branch, Centers for Disease Control and Prevention, Atlanta, GA 30333

MICHAEL S. FORMAN
Department of Pathology, Johns Hopkins Medicine, 600 North Wolfe Street, Meyer B1-193, Baltimore, MD 21287

JAMES G. FOX
Division of Comparative Medicine, Massachusetts Institute of Technology, 77 Massachusetts Avenue, Building 16, Room 825C, Cambridge, MA 02139

RENO FREI
Microbiology Laboratory, University Hospital Basel, Petersgraben 4, 4031 Basel, Switzerland

CHARLES F. FULHORST
Department of Pathology, University of Texas Medical Branch, 301 University Boulevard, Route 0609, Galveston, TX 77555-0609

GUIDO FUNKE
Department of Medical Microbiology and Hygiene, Gärtner & Colleagues Laboratories, D-88212 Ravensburg, Germany

HECTOR H. GARCIA
Department of Microbiology, School of Sciences, Universidad Peruana Cayetano Heredia, Av. Honorio Delgado 430, SMP, Lima 31, Peru, and Cysticercosis Unit, Instituto de Ciencias Neurologicas, Lima, Peru

LYNNE S. GARCIA
LSG & Associates, 512-12th Street, Santa Monica, CA 90402-2908

CHARLOTTE A. GAYDOS
Division of Infectious Diseases and Medicine, Johns Hopkins University, 1159 Ross Building, 720 Rutland Avenue, Baltimore, MD 21205

ANNE A. GERSHON
Department of Pediatrics, Columbia University College of Physicians & Surgeons, 650 W. 168th Street, New York, NY 10032

ANTOINE GESSAIN
EPVO Unit, EEMI Department, Institut Pasteur, Paris 75015, France

MAHMOUD A. GHANNOUM
Center for Medical Mycology, Department of Dermatology, University Hospitals/Case Western Reserve University, 11100 Euclid Avenue, Cleveland, OH 44106

MARKUS GLATZEL
University Hospital Zürich, Institute of Neuropathology, Schmelzbergstrasse 12, CH-8091 Zürich, Switzerland

DAVID R. GRETCH
Viral Hepatitis Laboratory, University of Washington Harborview Medical Center, 325 Ninth Avenue, Box 359690, Seattle, WA 98104

BRIGITTE P. GRIFFITH
Virology Reference Laboratory, VA Connecticut Healthcare System, 950 Campbell Avenue, West Haven, CT 06516, and Department of Laboratory Medicine, Yale University School of Medicine, New Haven, CT 06520

M. CRISTINA GUTIÉRREZ
Reference Laboratory for Mycobacteria, Institut Pasteur, 25 rue du Docteur Roux, 75015 Paris, France

WILLIAM J. HALSALL
Center for Medical Mycology, Department of Dermatology, University Hospitals/Case Western Reserve University, 11100 Euclid Avenue, Cleveland, OH 44106

KEVIN C. HAZEN
Division of Clinical Microbiology, Department of Pathology, University of Virginia Health System, P.O. Box 800255, Charlottesville, VA 22908-0255

DAVID W. HECHT
Department of Medicine, Division of Infectious Diseases, Loyola University Medical Center, 2160 S. First Avenue, Building 54-149, Maywood, IL 60153, and Hines Veterans Administration Hospital, Hines, IL 60141

DEBORAH A. HENRY
Child and Family Research Institute, 950 West 28th Avenue, Room 370, Vancouver, British Columbia, Canada V5Z 4H4

JANET FICK HINDLER
Department of Pathology and Laboratory Medicine, UCLA Medical Center, Los Angeles, CA 90095-1713

RICHARD L. HODINKA
Departments of Pediatrics and Anatomic Pathology and Clinical Laboratories, Clinical Virology Laboratory, Children's Hospital of Philadelphia and University of Pennsylvania School of Medicine, Philadelphia, PA 19104

ALEX HOFFMASTER
Meningitis and Special Pathogens Branch, Division of Bacterial and Mycotic Diseases, National Center for Infectious Diseases, Centers for Disease Control and Prevention, 1600 Clifton Road, MS G34, Atlanta, GA 30333

DANNIE G. HOLLIS
Centers for Disease Control and Prevention, Atlanta, GA 30333

HARVEY T. HOLMES
Laboratory Response Branch, National Center for Infectious Diseases, Centers for Disease Control and Prevention, Atlanta, GA 30333

AMY J. HORNEMAN (formerly Martin-Carnahan)
Department of Epidemiology and Preventive Medicine, University of Maryland School of Medicine, 10 South Pine Street, MSTF 900D, Baltimore, MD 21201

REBECCA T. HORVAT
Department of Pathology and Laboratory Medicine, University of Kansas School of Medicine, 3901 Rainbow Boulevard, Mail Stop 4045, Kansas City, KS 66160

JEAN HOU
Laboratory of Molecular Medicine and Neuroscience, National Institute of Neurological Disorders and Stroke, 10 Center Drive, MSC 1296, Building 10, Room 3B14A, Bethesda, MD 20892-1296

SUSAN A. HOWELL
King's College London, Mycology, St. Johns Institute of Dermatology, Guy's and St. Thomas' NHS Foundation Trust, London SE1 7EH, Great Britain

ROSEMARY HUMES
Association of Public Health Laboratories, 8515 Georgia Avenue, Silver Spring, MD 20910

JOSEPH P. ICENOGLE
Measles, Mumps, Rubella, and Herpesviruses Branch, Division of Viral Diseases, National Center for Immunizations and Respiratory Diseases, Centers for Disease Control and Prevention, Mail Stop C-22, 1600 Clifton Road, NE, Atlanta, GA 30333

CLARK B. INDERLIED
Department of Pathology, Keck School of Medicine, University of Southern California, Los Angeles, CA 90033, and Department of Pathology & Laboratory Medicine, Childrens Hospital Los Angeles, 4650 Sunset Boulevard, Mail Stop #32, Los Angeles, CA 90027

NANCY C. ISHAM
Center for Medical Mycology, Department of Dermatology, University Hospitals/Case Western Reserve University, 11100 Euclid Avenue, Cleveland, OH 44106

J. MICHAEL JANDA
Microbial Diseases Laboratory, California State Department of Health Services, 850 Marina Bay Parkway, Room E164, Richmond, CA 94804

WILLIAM M. JANDA
Clinical Microbiology Laboratory, Department of Pathology, M/C 750, University of Illinois Medical Center, 840 S. Wood Street, Chicago, IL 60612

KEITH R. JEROME
Department of Laboratory Medicine, University of Washington, and Program in Infectious Diseases, Fred Hutchinson Cancer Research Center, 1100 Fairview Avenue N., D3-100, Seattle, WA 98109

XI JIANG
Division of Infectious Diseases, Department of Pediatrics, Cincinnati Children's Hospital Medical Center, University of Cincinnati College of Medicine, 3333 Burnet Avenue, Cincinnati, OH 45229-3039

JUAN A. JIMENEZ
Cysticercosis Unit, Instituto de Ciencias Neurologicas, Jr Ancash 1271, Lima 1, Peru

BARBARA J. B. JOHNSON
Division of Vector-Borne Infectious Diseases, Centers for Disease Control and Prevention, Rampart Road, Foothills Campus, Fort Collins, CO 80522

ERIC A. JOHNSON
Department of Food Microbiology and Toxicology, University of Wisconsin, 1925 Willow Drive, Madison, WI 53706-1187

JUDITH A. JOHNSON
VA Medical Center, 10 North Greene Street, Room 4D-150, Baltimore, MD 21201

ROBERT E. JOHNSON
National Center for HIV, STD, and TB Prevention, E-02, Centers for Disease Control and Prevention, 1600 Clifton Road, NE, Atlanta, GA 30333

JEFFERY L. JONES
Parasitic Diseases Branch, Division of Parasitic Diseases, National Center for Infectious Diseases, Centers for Disease Control and Prevention, MS F-22, 4770 Buford Highway, Atlanta, GA 30341

MALCOLM K. JONES
Molecular Parasitology Laboratory, Queensland Institute of Medical Research, 300 Herston Road, Herston, Queensland 4006, Australia

TIMOTHY F. JONES
Communicable and Environmental Disease Services, Tennessee Department of Health, 4th Floor, Cordell Hull Building, 425 5th Avenue N., Nashville, TN 37247

JEANNE A. JORDAN
Department of Pathology, University of Pittsburgh, Magee-Women's Hospital, 204 Craft Avenue, Pittsburgh, PA 15213

JAMES H. JORGENSEN
Department of Pathology, The University of Texas Health Science Center, 7703 Floyd Curl Drive, San Antonio, TX 78229-3700

JAMES B. KAPER
Center for Vaccine Development and Department of Microbiology & Immunology, University of Maryland School of Medicine, 685 West Baltimore Street, Baltimore, MD 21201

MOGENS KILIAN
Department of Medical Microbiology and Immunology, Bartholin Building, University of Aarhus, DK-8000 Aarhus C, Denmark

EIJA KÖNÖNEN
Anaerobe Reference Laboratory, Department of Bacterial and Inflammatory Diseases, National Public Health Insititute (KTL), FIN-00300 Helsinki, Finland

PIRKKO KOUKILA-KÄHKÖLÄ
HUS Diagnostics, Mycology Laboratory, Helsinki University Central Hospital, Helsinki, Finland

KAREN KRISHER
Detroit Medical Center University Laboratories, 4201 St. Antoine, Detroit, MI 48201

THOMAS G. KSIAZEK
Special Pathogens Branch, MS G-14, Centers for Disease Control and Prevention, 1600 Clifton Road, Atlanta, GA 30333

JAIME A. LABARCA
Department of Medicine, Facultad de Medicine, Pontificia Universidad Catolica de Chile, Lira 44, Santiago, Chile

RENU B. LAL
Epidemiology Branch, Division of HIV/AIDS Prevention, National Center for HIV, STD and TB Prevention, Centers for Disease Control and Prevention, Atlanta, GA 30333

ROBERT S. LANCIOTTI
Diagnostic and Reference Laboratory, Arbovirus Diseases Branch, Centers for Disease Control and Prevention, Fort Collins, CO 80521

MARIE LOUISE LANDRY
Department of Laboratory Medicine, Yale University School of Medicine, P.O. Box 208035, New Haven, CT 06520-8035

MARK T. LAROCCO
Department of Pathology, St. Luke's Episcopal Health System, Houston, TX 77030

PHILIP LARUSSA
Department of Pediatrics, Columbia University College of Physicians & Surgeons, 650 W. 168th Street, New York, NY 10032

TSAI-LING LAUDERDALE
Division of Clinical Research, National Health Research Institutes, Taipei 11529, Taiwan, Republic of China

AMY L. LEBER
Quest Diagnostics, Nichols Institute, 33608 Ortega Highway, San Juan Capistrano, CA 92690

KARIN LEDER
Infectious Disease Epidemiology Unit, Department of Epidemiology and Preventive Medicine, Monash Medical School, Alfred Hospital, Commercial Road, Prahran, Victoria 3181, Australia

DIANE S. LELAND
Indiana University School of Medicine, 350 W. 11th Street, Indianapolis, IN 46202

PAUL N. LEVETT
Provincial Laboratory, Saskatchewan Health, 3211 Albert Street, Regina, Saskatchewan, S4S 5W6 Canada

ANNIKA LINDE
Department of Epidemiology, Swedish Institute for Infectious Disease Control, SE-171 82 Solna, Sweden

DAVID LINDQUIST
Microbial Diseases Laboratory, California Department of Health Services, 850 Marina Bay Parkway, Richmond, CA 94804

DAVID S. LINDSAY
Center for Molecular Medicine and Infectious Diseases, Department of Biomedical Sciences and Pathobiology, Virginia-Maryland Regional College of Veterinary Medicine, Virginia Tech, 1410 Prices Fork Road, Blacksburg, VA 24061-0342

JOHN J. LIPUMA
Department of Pediatrics and Communicable Diseases, University of Michigan Medical School, 1150 W. Medical Center Drive, 8323 MSRB III, 0646, Ann Arbor, MI 48109

SHAWN R. LOCKHART
Department of Biological Sciences, University of Iowa, Iowa City, IA 52242

MICHAEL J. LOEFFELHOLZ
Viromed Laboratories, 6101 Blue Circle Drive, Minnetonka, MN 55343

NIALL A. LOGAN
Department of Biological and Biomedical Sciences, School of Life Sciences, Glasgow Caledonian University, Cowcaddens Road, Glasgow G4 0BA, United Kingdom

GARY D. LUM
Pathology Administration, Northern Territory Government Pathology Service, PO Box 41326, Casuarina NT 0811, Australia

NELL S. LURAIN
Department of Immunology/Microbiology, Rush University Medical Center, 1653 West Congress Parkway, Chicago, IL 60612

JAMES B. MAHONY
Department of Pathology and Molecular Medicine, McMaster University, and Regional Virology and Chlamydiology Laboratory, St. Joseph's Healthcare, 50 Charlton Avenue East, Hamilton, Ontario L8N 4A6, Canada

EUGENE O. MAJOR
Laboratory of Molecular Medicine and Neuroscience, National Institute of Neurological Disorders and Stroke, 10 Center Drive, MSC 1296, Building 10, Room 3B14A, Bethesda, MD 20892-1296

THOMAS MARRIE
Faculty of Medicine and Dentistry, 2J2.01 Walter C. Mackenzie Health Sciences Center, 8440 112th Street, Edmonton, Alberta, Canada T6G 2R7

ALEXANDER MATHIS
Institute of Parasitology, University of Zurich, Winterthurerstrasse 266a, CH-8057 Zurich, Switzerland

DONALD R. MAYO
Virology Reference Laboratory, VA Connecticut Healthcare System, 950 Campbell Avenue, West Haven, CT 06516, and Department of Laboratory Medicine, Yale University School of Medicine, New Haven, CT 06520

JAMES B. McCAULEY
Rush University, 1725 W. Harrison Street, Chicago, IL 60612

MICHAEL R. McGINNIS
Medical Mycology Research Center, Center for Tropic Diseases, University of Texas Medical Branch, 301 University Boulevard, Galveston, TX 77555-0609

DONALD P. McMANUS
Molecular Parasitology Laboratory, Queensland Institute of Medical Research, 300 Herston Road, Herston, Queensland 4006, Australia

TESS McPHERSON
Laboratory of Parasitic Diseases, National Institute of Allergy and Infectious Diseases, National Institutes of Health, 4 Center Drive, Bethesda, MD 20892

FRANCIS MEGRAUD
INSERM ERI 10, Laboratoire de Bactériologie, Université Victor Segalen Bordeaux 2, 33076 Bordeaux Cedex, France

LEONEL MENDOZA
Medical Technology Program, Department of Microbiology and Molecular Genetics, Michigan State University, 322 North Kedzie Hall, East Lansing, MI 48824-1031

J. MICHAEL MILLER
Laboratory Response Branch, National Center for Infectious Diseases, Centers for Disease Control and Prevention, Atlanta, GA 30333

ROBERT C. MOELLERING, JR.
Department of Medicine, Beth Israel Deaconess Medical Center, and Harvard Medical School, Boston, MA 02215

RHODA ASHLEY MORROW
Department of Laboratory Medicine, University of Washington, and Program in Infectious Diseases, Fred Hutchinson Cancer Research Center, 1100 Fairview Avenue N., LE-500, Seattle, WA 98109

PATRICK R. MURRAY
Clinical Center, National Institutes of Health, Bethesda, MD 20892-1508

REINIER MUTTERS
Institute of Medical Microbiology and Hospital Hygiene, Philipps University, D-35037 Marburg, Germany

IRVING NACHAMKIN
Department of Pathology and Laboratory Medicine, University of Pennsylvania School of Medicine, 4th Floor, Gates Building, 3400 Spruce Street, Philadelphia, PA 19104-4283

JAMES P. NATARO
Center for Vaccine Development and Department of Microbiology & Immunology, University of Maryland School of Medicine, 685 West Baltimore Street, Baltimore, MD 21201

RONALD C. NEAFIE
Parasitic Infectious Disease Pathology Branch, The Armed Forces Institute of Pathology, 6825 16th Street, N.W., Washington, DC 20306

PHUC NGUYEN-DINH
Division of Parasitic Diseases, MS F-22, Centers for Disease Control and Prevention, 4770 Buford Highway, N.E., Atlanta, GA 30341

STUART T. NICHOL
Special Pathogens Branch, MS G-14, Centers for Disease Control and Prevention, 1600 Clifton Road, Atlanta, GA 30333

MICHAEL A. NOBLE
Department of Pathology and Laboratory Medicine, University of British Columbia, Room 328A, 2733 Heather Street, Vancouver, British Columbia V5Z 1M9, Canada

FREDERICK S. NOLTE
Department of Pathology and Laboratory Medicine, Emory University School of Medicine, 1364 Clifton Road, N.E., Atlanta, GA 30322

STEVEN J. NORRIS
Department of Pathology and Laboratory Medicine, University of Texas Medical School at Houston, P.O. Box 20708, Houston, TX 77225

SUSAN NOVAK-WEEKLEY
Microbiology Services, Kaiser Permanente Regional Reference Laboratories, 11668 Sherman Way, North Hollywood, CA 91605

THOMAS B. NUTMAN
Laboratory of Parasitic Diseases, National Institute of Allergy and Infectious Diseases, National Institutes of Health, 4 Center Drive, Room B1-03, Bethesda, MD 20892

JUAN P. OLANO
Department of Pathology, University of Texas Medical Branch, Galveston, TX 77555-0609

LILLIAN A. ORCIARI
Poxvirus and Rabies Branch, Division of Viral and Rickettsial Diseases, National Center for Zoonotic, Vector-Borne, and Enteric Diseases, Coordinating Center for Infectious Diseases, Centers for Disease Control and Prevention, Mailstop G-33, Atlanta, GA 30333

ARVIND A. PADHYE
Mycotic Disease Branch, Division of Bacterial and Mycotic Diseases, National Center for Infectious Diseases, Centers

for Disease Control and Prevention, Mail Stop G-11, Atlanta, GA 30333

GRAEME P. PALTRIDGE
Bacteriology and Parasitology Laboratory, Canterbury Health Laboratories, Christchurch, New Zealand

JEAN B. PATEL
Epidemiology and Laboratory Branch, Division of Healthcare Quality Promotion, Centers for Disease Control and Prevention, 1600 Clifton Road, Atlanta, GA 30333

BRUCE K. PATTERSON
Department of Pathology and Medicine, Division of Infectious Diseases and Geographic Medicine, Stanford University Medical School, 300 Pasteur Drive, Room H1537J, M/C 5629, Stanford, CA 94305-5629

SHARON J. PEACOCK
Wellcome Trust-Mahidol University-Oxford Tropical Medicine Research Program, Faculty of Tropical Medicine, Mahidol University, 420/6 Rajvithi Road, Bangkok 10400, Thailand

PHILIP E. PELLETT
Lerner Research Institute, Cleveland Clinic Foundation, 9500 Euclid Avenue, NN10, Cleveland, OH 44106

CATHY A. PETTI
Departments of Pathology and Medicine, University of Utah School of Medicine, Salt Lake City, UT 84132, and Associated Regional and University Pathologists, Salt Lake City, UT 84108

MICHAEL A. PFALLER
Division of Medical Microbiology, Department of Pathology, University of Iowa College of Medicine, Iowa City, IA 52242

GABY E. PFYFFER
Department of Medical Microbiology, Center for Laboratory Medicine, Kantonsspital Luzern, CH-6000 Luzern 16, Switzerland

VICTORIA POPE
National Center for HIV, STD, and TB Prevention, A-12, Centers for Disease Control and Prevention, 1600 Clifton Road, NE, Atlanta, GA 30333 (retired)

TANJA POPOVIC
Centers for Disease Control and Prevention, 1600 Clifton Road, MS D50, Atlanta, GA 30333

IAN R. POXTON
Medical Microbiology, Centre for Infectious Diseases, University of Edinburgh College of Medicine and Veterinary Medicine, The Chancellor's Building, 49, Little France Crescent, Edinburgh EH16 4SB, Scotland

WILL S. PROBERT
Microbial Diseases Laboratory, California Department of Health Services, 850 Marina Bay Parkway, Richmond, CA 94804

GARY W. PROCOP
Miller School of Medicine, The University of Miami, Miami, FL 33136

CLAUDE PUJOL
Department of Biological Sciences, University of Iowa, Iowa City, IA 52242

DIDIER RAOULT
Unité des Rickettsies, IFR 48, CNRS UMR 6020, Faculté de Médecine, 27 Boulevard Jean Moulin, 13385 Marseille Cedex 5, France

J. KAMILE RASHEED
Division of Healthcare Quality Promotion (G-08), National Center for Infectious Diseases, Centers for Disease Control and Prevention, 1600 Clifton Road, Atlanta, GA 30333

LARRY G. REIMER
Departments of Pathology and Medicine, University of Utah School of Medicine, Salt Lake City, UT 84132, and Associated Regional and University Pathologists, Salt Lake City, UT 84108

L. BARTH RELLER
Clinical Microbiology Laboratory, Duke University Medical Center, and Departments of Pathology and Medicine, Duke University School of Medicine, Durham, NC 27710

DAVID RELMAN
Departments of Microbiology & Immunology, and Medicine, Stanford University, and Veterans Affairs Palo Alto Health Care System, Palo Alto, CA 94304

JOHN H. REX
AstraZeneca, Alderley House, Alderley Park, Macclesfield, Cheshire, United Kingdom, and Division of Infectious Diseases, Department of Internal Medicine, Center for the Study of Emerging and Reemerging Pathogens, University of Texas Medical School—Houston, Houston, TX 77030

LOUIS B. RICE
Medical Service 111(W), Louis Stokes Cleveland VA Medical Center, 10701 East Boulevard, and Department of Medicine, Case Western Reserve University, Cleveland, OH 44106

MALCOLM D. RICHARDSON
Mycology Unit, Department of Bacteriology and Immunology, University of Helsinki, Haartman Institute, Haartmaninkatu 3, P.O. Box 21, 00014 Helsinki, Finland

SANDRA S. RICHTER
Medical Microbiology Division, Department of Pathology, C606 GH, University of Iowa College of Medicine, 200 Hawkins Drive, Iowa City, IA 52242-1009

CHRISTINE ROBINSON
Department of Pathology, B120, The Children's Hospital, 1056 E. 19th Avenue, Denver, CO 80218

WILLIAM O. ROGERS
Parasitic Diseases Program, Naval Medical Research Unit 2, American Embassy, Jakarta, Unit 8132 NAMRU-2, FPO AP 96520-8132

JEAN MARC ROLAIN
Unité des Rickettsies, Faculté de Médecine, 27 Boulevard Jean Moulin, 13385 Marseille cedex 05, France

PIERRE E. ROLLIN
Special Pathogens Branch, MS G-14, Centers for Disease Control and Prevention, 1600 Clifton Road, Atlanta, GA 30333

JOSÉ R. ROMERO
Section of Pediatric Infectious Diseases, Departments of Pediatrics, Pathology, and Microbiology, University of Nebraska Medical Center, 982162, Omaha, NE 68198-2162

PAUL ROTA
Measles, Mumps, Rubella and Herpesvirus Branch, MS C-22, Centers for Disease Control and Prevention, 1600 Clifton Road, Atlanta, GA 30333

KATHRYN L. RUOFF
Department of Pathology, Dartmouth Hitchcock Medical Center, One Medical Center Drive, Lebanon, NH 03756-0001

CHARLES E. RUPPRECHT
Poxvirus and Rabies Branch, Division of Viral and Rickettsial Diseases, National Center for Zoonotic, Vector-Borne, and Enteric Diseases, Coordinating Center for Infectious Diseases, Centers for Disease Control and Prevention, Mailstop G-33, Atlanta, GA 30333

CAROLINE RYSCHKEWITSCH
Laboratory of Molecular Medicine and Neuroscience, National Institute of Neurological Disorders and Stroke, 10 Center Drive, MSC 1296, Building 10, Room 3B14A, Bethesda, MD 20892-1296

GARY N. SANDEN
Division of Bacterial and Mycotic Diseases, National Center for Infectious Diseases, Centers for Disease Control and Prevention, MS D-11, 1600 Clifton Road, Atlanta, GA 30333

PAUL C. SCHRECKENBERGER
Department of Pathology, Loyola University Medical Center, 2160 S. First Avenue, Building 103, Room 0021, Maywood, IL 60153

MARTIN E. SCHRIEFER
Division of Vector-Borne Infectious Diseases, Centers for Disease Control and Prevention, Rampart Road, Foothills Campus, Fort Collins, CO 80522

JOHN D. SCOTT
Division of Infectious Diseases, Department of Medicine, University of Washington Harborview Medical Center, 325 Ninth Avenue, Box 359938, Seattle, WA 98104

W. EVAN SECOR
Division of Parasitic Diseases, MS F-13, Centers for Disease Control and Prevention, 4770 Buford Highway, N.E., Atlanta, GA 30341

ROBERT W. SHAFER
Departments of Medicine and Pathology, Stanford University, Stanford, CA 94305

SUSAN E. SHARP
Department of Microbiology, Kaiser Permanente, 13705 N.E. Airport Way, Portland, OR 97230

YVONNE R. SHEA
Microbiology Service, Department of Laboratory Medicine, Clinical Center, National Institutes of Health, Building 10, Room 2C325, 10 Center Drive, Bethesda, MD 20892

HARSHA SHEOREY
Department of Microbiology, St. Vincent's Hospital Melbourne, P.O. Box 2900, Fitzroy, Victoria 3065, Australia

ROBYN Y. SHIMIZU
Department of Pathology and Laboratory Medicine, UCLA Medical Center, Los Angeles, CA 90095-1713

JAMES W. SNYDER
Department of Pathology, Division of Laboratory Medicine, University of Louisville School of Medicine and Hospital, Louisville, KY 40202

DAVID R. SOLL
Department of Biological Sciences, University of Iowa, Iowa City, IA 52242

YULI SONG
Research Service, Wadsworth Anaerobic Bacteriology Laboratory, Room E3-237, Building 304, VA Medical Center West Los Angeles, Los Angeles, CA 90073

DAVID P. SPEERT
Child and Family Research Institute, 950 West 28th Avenue, Room 377, Vancouver, British Columbia, Canada V5Z 4H4

BARBARA SPELLERBERG
Institute of Medical Microbiology and Hygiene, University of Ulm, Robert-Koch-Strasse 8, 89081 Ulm, Germany

SHARON P. STEINBERG
Department of Pediatrics, Columbia University College of Physicians & Surgeons, 650 W. 168th Street, New York, NY 10032

NANCY A. STROCKBINE
Foodborne and Diarrheal Diseases Laboratory Section, Foodborne and Diarrheal Diseases Branch, Division of Bacterial and Mycotic Diseases, National Center for Infectious Diseases, Centers for Disease Control and Prevention, Atlanta, GA 30333

PAULA SUMMANEN
Research Service, VA Medical Center West Los Angeles, Los Angeles, CA 90073

RICHARD C. SUMMERBELL
Fungal Biodiversity Center, Centraalbureau voor Schimmelcultures, Uppsalalaan 8, 3584 CT Utrecht, The Netherlands

DEANNA A. SUTTON
Fungus Testing Laboratory, Department of Pathology, University of Texas Health Science Center at San Antonio, 7703 Floyd Curl Drive, San Antonio, TX 78229-3900

JANA M. SWENSON
Epidemiology and Laboratory Branch, Division of Healthcare Quality Promotion, Centers for Disease Control and Prevention, Mailstop G08, 1600 Clifton Road, Atlanta, GA 30333

ELLA M. SWIERKOSZ
Departments of Pathology and Pediatrics, Saint Louis University School of Medicine, St. Louis, MO 63104

YI-WEI TANG
Departments of Medicine and Pathology, Vanderbilt University School of Medicine, 4605 TVC, 1161 21st Avenue, South, Nashville, TN 37232-5310

DAVID TAYLOR-ROBINSON
Department of Medicine, Imperial College St. Mary's Hospital, Winston Churchill Wing, Paddington, London W2 NY, United Kingdom

GARY E. TEGTMEIER
Viral Testing Laboratories, Community Blood Center of Greater Kansas City, 4040 Main Street, Kansas City, MO 64111

LÚCIA MARTINS TEIXEIRA
Instituto de Microbiologia, Universidade Federal do Rio de Janeiro, Rio de Janeiro, RJ 21941, Brazil

SAM R. TELFORD III
Cummings School of Veterinary Medicine, Tufts University, 200 Westboro Road, North Grafton, MA 01536

FRED C. TENOVER
Division of Healthcare Quality Promotion, National Center for Infectious Diseases, Centers for Disease Control and Prevention, 1600 Clifton Road, Atlanta, GA 30333

KENNETH D. THOMPSON
Department of Pathology, The University of Chicago Medical Center, Chicago, IL 60637

RICHARD B. THOMSON, JR.
Department of Pathology and Laboratory Medicine, Evanston Northwestern Healthcare and Northwestern University Feinberg School of Medicine, Evanston, IL 60201

GRAHAM TIPPLES
National Microbiology Laboratory, Public Health Agency of Canada, 1015 Arlington Street, Winnipeg, Manitoba R3E 3R2, Canada

PETER TRAYNOR
Regulatory Affairs and Technical Support, Oxoid Australia Pty Limited, Thebarton, South Australia 5031, Australia

THEODORE F. TSAI
Novartis Vaccines, Bell Atlantic Tower, 28th Floor, 1717 Arch Street, Philadelphia, PA 19103

JOHN D. TURNIDGE
Microbiology and Infectious Diseases, Women's and Children's Hospital, 72 King William Road, North Adelaide 5006, SA, Australia

STEVE J. UPTON
Division of Biology, Ackert Hall, Kansas State University, Manhattan, KS 66506-4901

ALEXANDRA VALSAMAKIS
Department of Pathology, Johns Hopkins Medicine, 600 North Wolfe Street, Meyer B1-193, Baltimore, MD 21287

PETER A. R. VANDAMME
Laboratorium voor Microbiologie, Faculteit Wetenschappen, Vakgroep Biochemie, Fysiologie en Microbiologie (WE10), Universiteit Gent, Ledeganckstraat 35, B-9000 Gent, Belgium

PAUL E. VERWEIJ
Department of Medical Microbiology, Radboud University Nijmegen Medical Center, PO Box 9101, 6500 HB Nijmegen, The Netherlands

VÉRONIQUE VINCENT
Reference Laboratory for Mycobacteria, Institut Pasteur, 25 rue du Docteur Roux, 75015 Paris, France

GOVINDA S. VISVESVARA
Division of Parasitic Diseases, National Center for Infectious Diseases, Centers for Disease Control and Prevention, 4770 Buford Highway NE, Atlanta, GA 30341-3724

ROXANA G. VITALE
INEI, ANLIS Dr. Carlos Malbrán, Departamento de Micología, Av Velez Sarsfield 563, Capital Federal, Buenos Aires, Argentina 1281

ALEXANDER VON GRAEVENITZ
Institute of Medical Microbiology, University of Zurich, CH 8006 Zurich, Switzerland

WILLIAM G. WADE
King's College London, Department of Microbiology, Guy's Campus, London SE1 9RT, United Kingdom

KEN B. WAITES
Department of Pathology, University of Alabama at Birmingham, WP 230, 619 South 19th Street, Birmingham, AL 35249

DAVID H. WALKER
Department of Pathology, University of Texas Medical Branch, 301 University Boulevard, Keiller Building, Galveston, TX 77555-0609

RICHARD J. WALLACE, JR.
Department of Microbiology, The University of Texas Health Center at Tyler, 11937 US Highway 271, Tyler, TX 75708

AUDREY WANGER
Department of Pathology and Laboratory Medicine, University of Texas Medical School, Houston, TX 77030

DAVID W. WARNOCK
Division of Bacterial and Mycotic Diseases, National Center for Infectious Diseases, Centers for Disease Control and Prevention, 1600 Clifton Road, N.E., Mailstop C-09, Atlanta, GA 30333

NANCY G. WARREN
Bureau of Laboratories, Pennsylvania Department of Health, 110 Pickering Way, Lionville, PA 19353

RAINER WEBER
Division of Infectious Diseases and Hospital Epidemiology, Department of Internal Medicine, University Hospital, CH-8091 Zurich, Switzerland

MELVIN P. WEINSTEIN
Departments of Medicine and Pathology, Robert Wood Johnson Medical School, 1 Robert Wood Johnson Place, MEB 364, New Brunswick, NJ 08903-0019

LOUIS M. WEISS
Albert Einstein College of Medicine, 1300 Morris Park Avenue, Room 504 Forchheimer Building, Bronx, NY 10461

IRENE WEITZMAN
School of Life Sciences, Arizona State University, Tempe, AZ 85287-0002

PETER F. WELLER
Harvard Medical School and Division of Infectious Diseases and Allergy and Inflammation Division, Beth Israel Deaconess Medical Center, Boston, MA 02215

THEODORE C. WHITE
Department of Pathobiology, School of Public Health and Community Medicine, University of Washington, and Seattle Biomedical Research Institute, 307 Westlake Avenue, N., Suite 500, Seattle, WA 98109-5219

ANDREAS F. WIDMER
Department of Infectious Disease and Hospital Epidemiology, Division of Infection Control and Hospital Epidemiology, University Hospital Basel, Petersgraben 4, 4031 Basel, Switzerland

DANNY L. WIEDBRAUK
Virology and Molecular Biology, Warde Medical Laboratory, 300 W. Textile Road, Ann Arbor, MI 48108

BETTINA WILSKE
Max von Pettenkofer-Institute, University of Munich, National Reference Center for Borreliae, Pettenkofer-Strasse 9a, D 80336 Munich, Germany

MARIANNA WILSON
Parasitic Diseases Branch, Division of Parasitic Diseases, National Center for Infectious Diseases, Centers for Disease Control and Prevention, MS F-36, 4770 Buford Highway, Atlanta, GA 30341

MICHAEL L. WILSON
Department of Pathology and Laboratory Services, Denver Medical Health Center, Mail Code #0224, 777 Bannock Street, Denver, CO 80204-4507, and Department of Pathology, University of Colorado School of Medicine, Denver, CO 80262

FRANK G. WITEBSKY
Microbiology Service, Department of Laboratory Medicine, Clinical Center, National Institutes of Health, Building 10, Room 2C-385, 10 Center Drive, Bethesda, MD 20892-1508

GAIL L. WOODS
Department of Pathology and Laboratory Services, University of Arkansas for Medical Sciences, Mail Slot 502, 4301 W. Markham Street, Little Rock, AR 72205

LIHUA XIAO
Division of Parasitic Diseases, Centers for Disease Control and Prevention, 4770 Buford Highway, Atlanta, GA 30341

JOSEPH D. C. YAO
Division of Clinical Microbiology, Department of Laboratory Medicine and Pathology, Mayo Clinic, and Mayo Clinic College of Medicine, Rochester, MN 55905

SHERIF ZAKI
Infectious Disease Pathology Activity, MS G-32, Centers for Disease Control and Prevention, 1600 Clifton Road, Atlanta, GA 30333

REINHARD ZBINDEN
Institute of Medical Microbiology, University of Zurich, CH 8006 Zurich, Switzerland

Acknowledgment of Previous Contributors

The *Manual of Clinical Microbiology* is by its nature a continuously revised work which refines and extends the contributions of previous editions. Since its first edition in 1970, many eminent scientists have contributed to this important reference work. The American Society for Microbiology and its Publications Board gratefully acknowledge the contributions of all of these generous authors over the life of this Manual.

Preface

It seems that much of my professional career has revolved around the *Manual of Clinical Microbiology*, first as an author, then as a section editor, and finally for the last four editions as the editor in chief. I have learned a great deal from this experience, although I must confess that I have forgotten far more science than I have retained. My most valuable lesson has been to rely on my fellow editors. I have been privileged to have worked on all four editions with Ellen Jo Baron and Mike Pfaller, with Jim Jorgensen for the last two editions, and with Marie Landry, who ably filled Bob Yolken's shoes, for this edition. I have also relied on the help of 29 section editors, including 7 new editors for this edition, and hundreds of authors. Almost 40% of the authors of the ninth edition of the *Manual of Clinical Microbiology* (MCM9) are new. For each edition I have purposely selected new editors and authors with the conviction that they will bring a new perspective to their assignment. I have systematically added non-U.S. authors, representing almost 30% of the authors of this edition, so that this Manual will be truly international in scope. These changes have not come without difficulties. My fellow editors and I have frequently had to curtail our authors' "creativity" for the sake of consistency, taught them that eloquence can equate to brevity, and reminded them that deadlines are not the fantasies of publishers. Many unpopular decisions are made in the creation of any work as comprehensive as MCM9, so I must thank the editors and authors for their understanding. If I have offended anyone in the process, it was unintentional.

I am very proud of what we have accomplished with MCM9, and I hope that this feeling is shared by the entire editorial board and all the authors. Although the field of clinical microbiology is undergoing dramatic changes with the confluence of traditional techniques and exciting advances in genomics and proteomics, I believe that the *Manual of Clinical Microbiology* should form the road map for our understanding of this evolving scientific discipline. I hope that the readers share the opinion of the authors and editors that MCM9 successfully meets this goal. An additional feature for the ninth edition is a CD-ROM with close to 500 illustrations from the book. It is available for purchase through ASM Press.

I would be remiss if I did not acknowledge the wisdom and guidance provided by Susan Birch, the ASM Press Production Manager whose name should more appropriately be listed on the cover of MCM9, and Jeff Holtmeier, the director of ASM Press who makes everyone's job a little easier and more pleasant. The entire staff at ASM Press was very supportive and helpful during the process of preparing this edition of the Manual.

PATRICK R. MURRAY

GENERAL ISSUES IN CLINICAL MICROBIOLOGY

I

VOLUME EDITOR
JAMES H. JORGENSEN

SECTION EDITOR
MELVIN P. WEINSTEIN

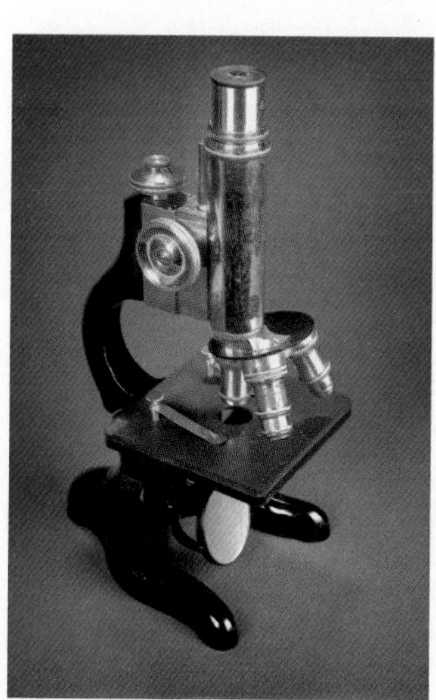

Microscope used during medical school by Joseph W. Mountin, founder of the Communicable Disease Center (from CDC image library).

Introduction to the Ninth Edition of the *Manual of Clinical Microbiology*

PATRICK R. MURRAY

1

The eighth edition of the *Manual of Clinical Microbiology* (MCM8) was a dramatic change from previous editions, growing from one to two volumes and increasing in length by more than 20%. Even though the changes in the ninth edition of the *Manual of Clinical Microbiology* (MCM9) are not as obvious, they are no less substantial. One new volume editor, Marie Louise Landry, and seven new section editors joined the editorial board. Of the 269 authors, almost 40% are new and 28% represent 22 non-U.S. countries. Although we retained the same 11 sections that were introduced in MCM8 and the algorithm chapters that have proved to be practical identification tools, we have expanded the chapters from 141 to 152. The MCM8 chapter "Pathogenic and Indigenous Microorganisms of Humans" was removed in MCM9 because we believed that this topic could not be satisfactorily covered in a limited chapter. To compensate for this deletion, the discussion of the topic was expanded in the individual organism chapters. A new chapter, "Microscopy," was added to section III, Diagnostic Technologies in Clinical Microbiology. This topic was covered in the sixth edition of the Manual but not in subsequent editions, a decision that the editorial board felt should be rectified. Section IV, Bacteriology, was increased by three chapters—coverage of mycobacteria was expanded from two chapters to three; coverage of anaerobes was expanded from three chapters to four; and *Tropheryma* was assigned to a new chapter, chapter 69. The most significant changes in MCM9 occurred in section VI, Virology, reflecting the influence of a new volume editor and three new section editors. The discussion of hepatitis A and hepatitis E viruses was consolidated into one chapter, and three new chapters were added—chapter 91, "Coronaviruses"; chapter 96, "Hendra and Nipah Viruses"; and chapter 98, "Hantaviruses." Coverage in other chapters was expanded to include metapneumoviruses and parechoviruses. Two new chapters were added to section VIII, Mycology—chapter 127, "Mycotoxins"; and chapter 128, "*Lacazia, Pythium*, and *Rhinosporidium*." Finally, section X, Parasitology, was reorganized with the addition of four new chapters. *Cryptosporidium* was transferred to a new chapter, chapter 142, and the coverage of helminths was expanded from two to five chapters.

All chapters in MCM9 were updated with the most current taxonomic and diagnostic information, which is not an insignificant feat in this era of molecular classification and diagnostic tools. Nearly 4,000 of the literature citations in MCM9 were published after the last edition went to press. Despite these efforts, we recognize that by the time that MCM9 will be published, some data will be dated and some statements will be inaccurate. This occurs despite the best efforts of the authors, editors, and ASM staff and is the unfortunate reality of publishing a major reference text. We ask for your understanding, as well as for your help in remedying the inaccuracies. If you discover an error, please contact ASM Press. A system will be established to post both the error and the corrections for the readership. The editorial board hopes that through the efforts of our authors and your careful review of the text, MCM9 will be an accurate, valuable reference source.

Laboratory Management*

W. MICHAEL DUNNE, JR., AND MARK T. LAROCCO

2

The diagnostic microbiology laboratory, regardless of demographics, is a business and needs to be managed with the same basic principles and tenets used by businesses. True, the products provided by microbiology laboratories belong to the service industry, but the day-to-day management of resources, productivity, finances, quality, and clients is no different. Whether the laboratory is for profit, not for profit, academic, or community based, it needs to follow the same financial rules and standards that businesses do. To develop a primer for medical microbiologists on the basics of business theory, economics, financial accounting, organizational behavior, and marketing, etc., within the confines of this chapter is impractical given the wealth of excellent contemporary reference materials currently available (9, 25, 31). Rather, this chapter will highlight four major management issues: operations, finance, personnel, and regulations.

OPERATIONS

The efficient operation of a clinical microbiology laboratory and effective delivery of diagnostic services to clinicians and their patients are vitally dependent on the management and communication skills of laboratory directors, managers, supervisors, and technologists. Quality laboratory services result directly from the performance of competent laboratory scientists, but the key element lies in the delivery of these services, a highly complex management activity. The clinical microbiology manager's task is to integrate and coordinate laboratory resources so that quality laboratory services can be provided as effectively and efficiently as possible. Laboratory management may be described in terms of four basic functions: planning, organization, direction, and control. In practice, the boundaries between these functions are often obscure because of the interdependence of the functions for effective management.

Strategic Planning

Strategic planning is the process of deciding on objectives for the organization that fulfill its mission, selecting and allocating the resources needed to obtain those objectives, and assigning responsibilities and accountabilities to those involved in the process. The microbiology laboratory will likely be included in the strategic plan of the overall department that in turn embraces the plan of the hospital or other parent organization. Nonetheless, the microbiology director or manager should have an appreciation of key features of the hospital's strategic plan.

A mission statement is a concise description of the overall goals and values of the organization. A mission statement may be thought of as the hospital's credo on which all of its actions are based. In a sense, the mission statement serves as the cornerstone of the organization's strategic plan as it represents the highest level of success that the organization hopes to achieve.

Planning at the department level is an essential requirement of laboratory management. Each section of the laboratory should establish a set of goals and objectives, formulate policies to carry out those objectives, develop intermediate and short-range plans to implement policies, and develop detailed procedures for implementing each plan. During the planning process, managers must be aware of any changes that occur in the operational environment because such awareness keeps decisions realistic and expectations achievable (37). An analysis of the operational environment can be accomplished by conducting an objective assessment of the laboratory's strengths, weaknesses, opportunities, and threats (SWOT analysis). Let's say, for example, that the microbiology laboratory is asked to develop a strategic plan to incorporate molecular diagnostic testing into its service offerings. A preliminary SWOT analysis may reveal the following.

Strengths

1. Strong technical leadership in the laboratory facilitates the implementation of new technologies.
2. The hospital supports a solid-organ and stem cell transplant program with patients that will likely produce a high demand for the service.
3. A teaching affiliation with a regional school of medical technology provides recruitment opportunities for trained technologists.

Weaknesses

1. The skill sets of most of the current staff do not include molecular diagnostics.

*This chapter contains information presented in chapter 2 by David L. Sewell and James D. MacLowry in the eighth edition of this Manual.

2. Having no record of performance in molecular diagnostics may place the laboratory at a marketing disadvantage.

3. The lack of experience with managing a molecular diagnostic service in the context of the overall laboratory budget.

Opportunities

1. A new academic affiliation will immediately provide resources (space, personnel, and equipment) for supporting a molecular diagnostic service.

2. There is a paucity of facilities in your geographic area that offer molecular diagnostic testing, and physicians are not happy with the service provided by a regional commercial laboratory. The potential for developing outreach volume is high.

Threats

1. Inappropriate utilization of the technology may create a financial hardship for the laboratory.

2. Competition from other commercial laboratories that call on physicians' offices directly.

Specific goals and objectives provide laboratory management with a clear direction before the planning process begins. When policies are set with these goals and objectives in mind, constraints are in place to guide the planning strategies prior to the major plan development stage. A few examples of goals and objectives for the clinical microbiology laboratory may be as follows.

1. Ensure the quality of diagnostic microbiology services by monitoring key functions and processes to determine improvements for quality and cost.
2. Support research and development by reviewing and testing new methods and equipment.
3. Expand volume by researching new markets for outpatient business.
4. Act as consultants to medical staff and outcomes managers to ensure that the most appropriate diagnostic tests are ordered.
5. Communicate, through results, a philosophy of customer service to patients, physicians, family members, and coworkers.
6. Support the strategic plans of the hospital through the laboratory services provided.
7. Employ personnel who are responsive to the needs of patients, physicians, clients, guests, and coworkers.
8. Provide for the future of laboratory service by participating in educational and training programs for medical technology.

Once a goal is identified, a plan for completion of the project and short-term interim plans are needed. Finally, the details necessary for implementation and the expectations of performance are defined. High performance cannot be achieved, however, without accountability. When there is a lack of accountability, needed information may be missed, decisions are not made when action is required, and people do not receive guidance or support when faced with new challenges. Accountability means that people can count on one another to keep performance commitments and communication agreements. It is the basis for an environment of trust, support, and dedication to excellence (27).

During implementation of any department plan, it is important to periodically measure success. Such an exercise affords management the opportunity to step back and revisit elements of the planning strategy while at the same time providing staff with appropriate feedback and motivation to see a difficult project through to its conclusion.

Organization

Organization in the clinical laboratory refers to both structure and process. Structure exemplifies stated relationships or framework, and process deals with interaction. There are three key elements of organization: the tasks to be performed, the individuals who are to perform the tasks, and the clinical laboratory as a workplace.

A scope of services document provides a detailed list of services provided by the microbiology laboratory. The document should contain general information on the hours of laboratory operation and on staffing. It may also include test-specific information such as specimen collection and transport requirements, reference ranges, locations of testing, (in-house versus reference laboratories), and cutoff times for receipt of specimens. The scope of services provided by the laboratory is often a reflection of the type of hospital or facility it serves.

Organizational charts are common to most business structures as they provide a visualization of who is doing what and the chain of command. Although nobody likes to think of oneself as being below other people, these charts can serve a useful purpose in the clinical laboratory by defining the relationships among tasks, individuals, and the workplace. The organizational chart attempts to show relationships between line and staff. A line position is one in which a superior exercises direct supervision over a subordinate. A staff position is advisory, supportive, or auxiliary. These terms were defined in industry, and health care institutions seldom use the same connotation. When laboratory managers speak of staff, they are usually referring to technologists who are, in fact, serving in line positions.

Written policies and procedures, displayed in printed manuals or made available electronically, are an essential component of the clinical microbiology laboratory. Every procedure should be clear, easy to follow, and consistent in its content and organization. These documents provide direction for the many day-to-day tasks performed by the staff, serve as a teaching tool for students and new employees, and provide information to inspectors from accrediting agencies. The Clinical and Laboratory Standards Institute (formerly NCCLS) has a published guideline, GP2-A4, for writing laboratory procedures (23). The guideline provides instructions and recommendations for writing procedures for the full scope of the laboratory's workflow. The document also contains information about organizing procedure manuals, archiving and managing documents, and using manufacturers' procedures for automated purposes. As a testament to the document's universal acceptance, the College of American Pathologists requires that all written laboratory procedures closely follow the GP2-A4 format.

As defined by Brown (4), process design is a broad plan that is developed to provide a blueprint for completing work or a task at hand. Process design in the clinical microbiology laboratory involves an analysis of size and setting, laboratory design, equipment, test methodology, regulations, and staffing. How the work transitions through the laboratory is defined as workflow, and although workflow analysis is part of process design, it is more detailed. Policies and procedures are developed during workflow analysis (4). Workflow can be divided into three phases of the test cycle: preanalytical, analytical, and postanalytical. The preanalytical phase consists of events that occur prior to actual testing, such as selection, collection, transport, and accessioning of specimens. The analytical phase involves the actual testing. The postanalytical phase consists of events that occur after testing is completed, such as results reporting and interpretation. The preanalytical phase is often the most critical aspect of the test cycle and can be the hardest part of workflow to control.

Strategies to effectively manage and minimize variances associated with the three phases of the test cycle should be included in the clinical laboratory's quality management plan. Quality management is a system for continuously analyzing, improving, and reexamining resources, processes, and services within an organization to produce the best possible outcome (28). Microbiologists have, for many years, concerned themselves with the quality of events that take place within the clinical microbiology laboratory. These events include such things as ensuring the performance of equipment, reagents, stains, and media and monitoring the accuracy of tests performed in the laboratory. These activities fall under the category of quality control (QC). Quality assurance (QA) broadens the scope of traditional QC to encompass processes and events in the preanalytical and postanalytical phases. QA includes such things as determining specimen quality and evaluating the competency and training of personnel. Both QC and QA can be considered aspects of quality management that also includes quality improvement (QI) or quality enhancement. Although applied successfully in industry for many years, QI and quality enhancement are relatively recent concepts in the clinical laboratory setting. Instead of focusing on inspection, identifying poor performance, and taking corrective action, as in traditional QC and QA programs, QI programs emphasize thorough training and prevention and view the system for improvement opportunities rather than the people (8). Continuous QI (CQI), sometimes referred to as total quality management, is an organized, systematic approach to productivity improvement that uses objective methods and a team approach toward improving the quality of all processes, products, and services. The origin of CQI-total quality management is industry based. The approach was promulgated by W. Edwards Deming and grew out of his experience with Japan's industrial reconstruction after World War II. Central to CQI philosophy is the premise that improvement in quality leads to increased productivity, increased customer and employee satisfaction, and decreased cost. The CQI approach is to examine process performance, not people performance, and utilize specific methods of analysis (tools) to better understand and improve those processes. It is a top-down style of QI that requires management commitment and support and involves the participation of all employees. Finally, CQI is viewed as an ongoing initiative.

While these broad definitions may suggest that CQI would be an ideal QI technique for the clinical laboratory, its implementation in clinical laboratories has not been easy. This is due, in part, to the additional time and resource requirements associated with CQI, at least initially, but also relates to an insufficient understanding of how to properly apply CQI to laboratory testing. CQI requires innovative thinking; the traditional internal quality monitors familiar to most laboratories cannot simply be shoehorned into a CQI format. Above all, do not lose sight of the fundamental objective: to improve patient care.

One way for laboratories to avoid this pitfall is to design a CQI program that strives to connect process improvement to clinically relevant patient outcome measures. Outcomes measurement has emerged from the health services research community in response to the changing economic environment in medicine, beginning with the advent of diagnosis-related group (DRG) classifications, and more recently as an important aspect of managed care delivery. Outcomes measurement identifies variations that may adversely affect patient care and can sometimes determine corrective actions for minimizing those variations. Although patient outcomes come in many forms, measurements relevant to laboratory testing generally involve the length of stay, cost, and customer satisfaction, with the customer being both the patient and the physician. Changes in laboratory services and policies that decrease lengths of patient stays, reduce cost, or increase customer satisfaction should be the focus of a laboratory CQI program. Those that have the most impact on outcome measures should be selected for process improvement.

A process is a set of activities that transforms inputs into outputs. Inputs include the needs of patients and physicians, the skill of laboratory personnel, equipment, supplies, and financial resources. Outputs involve laboratory data, diagnoses, and management decisions that are associated with outcomes realized by patients and physicians. Process analysis is often accomplished with techniques such as flowcharting and the use of cause-and-effect diagrams (fishbones), i.e., the tools of CQI, but it is important to remember that the goal of process analysis is to design strategies whereby modifications of the process lead to a measurable improvement in outcome. In clinical microbiology, elements of processes that may be selected for analysis and improvement include specimen rejection criteria, appropriateness of testing, and turnaround times for smear results that acutely affect patient management. Process analysis should include events related to the patient from the time of presentation to the end of an episode of care. For the laboratory, this requires an understanding of how multiple processes related to patient care, including those external to the laboratory, are connected (the output of one process may be the input of another). Failure to understand the interactive dynamic between processes will likely blunt the impact of laboratory improvement initiatives on patient outcomes.

A critical feature of the CQI paradigm is the need to carefully construct and assess any improvement modality before implementing costly changes in policies or procedures on a large scale. Referred to as the Plan-Do-Study-Act cycle for improvement (5, 17), the steps include first stating a specific aim and identifying criteria that will be used to determine if the change represents an improvement. After selection of a change that is practical and most predictive of a positive effect, a plan for evaluating the change in the form of a small pilot study is put forth. The results of the pilot study are assessed for their effect on performance, and then action is taken in the form of process redesign, or if needed, additional pilot studies are conducted. These never-ending cycles of improvement, gradually built into the daily workflow, represent the "meat and potatoes" of a proactive CQI program.

Selection and Implementation of New Equipment and Procedures

As laboratory managers are directly responsible for the quality and productivity of their departments, they must constantly evaluate new technology and equipment for applicability and practicality. Managers must also assess the impact of any new technology on patient care by focusing on attributes such as turnaround time, productivity, and cost. There are several steps involved in this process, including the performance of a needs assessment, research of available technology, and evaluation of performance and cost data gathered before making a decision on implementing a new procedure or making a new instrument purchase (3). This process is discussed in greater detail elsewhere in the Manual (see chapter 15).

FINANCE

Medicare, Medicaid, prospective payment, DRGs, preferred-provider organizations (PPOs), health care maintenance organizations (HMOs), managed care, fixed versus variable costs, return on investment—the financial side of the health care industry possesses a vocabulary that in many cases is as mind-boggling to the clinical microbiologist as real-time PCR is to the hospital financial officer. In order to be successful, however, clinical microbiology laboratory managers must be able to speak both languages and be as concerned about positive cash flow, cost control, and budget variance as they are about QA and procedural controls.

Laboratory Reimbursement

Medicare Part A provides reimbursement for hospital services related to an inpatient stay. Payment is made based on DRG classifications, a prospective payment system (PPS) of reimbursement. The Centers for Medicare and Medicaid Services (CMS) assign a weight to each DRG based on the severity of the diagnosis, the type of procedure, the number of laboratory and other diagnostic tests, the number and types of drugs prescribed, and the presence of complications or comorbid conditions (6).

Based on this method of payment, hospitals are able to determine how much reimbursement they will receive for Medicare patients and will make a profit if they can manage these patients at a cost below the reimbursed amount. This fixed reimbursement system and incentive to reduce the cost of care has put pressure on hospital support services such as the laboratory to lower expenses.

Medicare Part B covers physician services and outpatient ancillary health care services including clinical laboratory testing. In July 2000, Medicare introduced a new PPS for the outpatient setting and developed ambulatory payment classifications as a basis for reimbursement for outpatient services. The ambulatory payment classification system provides payment predictability and promotes efficiency; however, at this time clinical laboratory tests are excluded from the outpatient PPS. Instead, laboratory tests performed on outpatients are paid for from the Medicare Part B laboratory fee schedule. Fees are assigned based on current procedural terminology (CPT-4) or health care common procedure coding system (HCPCS) codes established for each procedure. The actual Medicare payment is the lowest of either the actual charge, the fee schedule amount set by the contractor, or the national fee cap termed the national limitation amount (la).

Private insurers, also affected by increasing health care costs, have also undergone revision in their reimbursement methodologies. Managed care is defined as a means of providing health care services within a network of service providers (6). Although there are a variety of managed care plans, they usually all require that insured individuals see a physician who is part of the plan or else pay a higher copayment. The most common type of managed care plan is the HMO. Reimbursement under managed care plans can occur in several ways. Capitation, usually applied to physician reimbursement, pays a certain amount per patient per month. Payment can cover the cost of all services related to the member's outpatient care, including any necessary diagnostic or therapeutic tests. The physician can make a profit or lose money depending on the numbers of visits with and tests performed on each patient. Inpatient care costs may be reimbursed on a per diem, or per-day, basis. Under this arrangement, the hospital negotiates with insurers a set amount of reimbursement per day during the patient's hospitalization. The hospital staff will use the cost of care per day to help set the per diem rates and can increase the profit margins if they can decrease costs without compromising patient care. Reimbursement per case, similar to the Medicare PPS, is based on a set reimbursement rate for specific diagnoses or procedures. In some instances where hospitals offer specialized procedures or unique types of care, there may be "carve-outs" whereby reimbursement occurs separately from the per diem or per-case rate, usually on a fee-for-service basis.

In all of this discussion, the key message for the laboratory manager is the focus on cost control. In the hospital's financial landscape, the laboratory is considered a cost center. Although it may produce revenue from its outpatient and outreach workload, the reality is that it represents a necessary but significant expense on the hospital's overall balance sheet. Thus, laboratories that focus on providing high-quality service in a cost-effective and efficient manner will be valued by the organization and those that do not will likely be targeted for redesign.

Laboratory Compliance Programs

In 1998 the Office of the Inspector General, in response to costly and at times fraudulent billing errors on the part of some laboratories, issued compliance program guidance for clinical laboratories. Its purpose was to instruct laboratories on how to conduct their business in a lawful and ethical manner. The guidance document requires that every laboratory have a formal compliance program that addresses several essential elements (2). At a minimum, the laboratory compliance program should (i) develop and promote standards of conduct for employees, (ii) promote a commitment to zero tolerance of fraud and abuse, (iii) designate members of a laboratory compliance committee, (iv) identify education and training programs available to employees, (v) promote communication with employees to ensure that the program is effective, (vi) outline monitoring activities to ensure that the program is effective, and (vii) describe the potential disciplinary measures for those violating standards of conduct and compliance procedures.

The laboratory compliance committee has the responsibility to oversee compliance with standards of conduct and other procedures as they relate to lawful and ethical business practices. The membership of the committee should consist of the medical director, the administrative director, section managers or supervisors, a laboratory information systems (LIS) manager, and the manager of outpatient services if one exists. The duties of the compliance committee are to effectively communicate the standards of conduct to all employees and to implement monitoring systems to detect any possible illegal or unethical conduct as it may relate to medical necessity or billing issues. The committee should also be available to employees who believe that they are aware of unethical or illegal activities that violate the standards of conduct and ensure that the enforcement of these standards is consistently done through appropriate disciplinary mechanisms. On a routine basis, the compliance committee should review any appropriate fraud alerts as periodically issued by the Office of the Inspector General and inform and educate employees appropriately as well as keep current with legal and regulatory compliance issues and revise compliance policy as needed.

The laboratory should communicate regularly with the institution's financial services, governmental reporting, and medical records departments regarding coding and billing issues. Laboratory managers are expected to take every reasonable precaution to ensure that the CPT-4 codes for laboratory tests accurately describe the tests that were ordered and performed and to choose the code that most accurately describes the ordered and performed test. Intentional up coding, the selection of a code to maximize reimbursement when such a code is not the most appropriate descriptor of the service, is not allowed. A complete review of CPT-4 codes should be performed at least annually to update codes and descriptions, delete obsolete codes, and validate reference lab coding using the American Medical Association's *Current Procedural Terminology* manual (1) and updates from carrier and fiscal intermediary bulletins.

The laboratory should encourage that physicians order only tests that are medically necessary. Diagnostic information for each test should be submitted by the ordering physician or authorized representative in narrative form or codes provided through the International Classification of Diseases, 9th Revision, Clinical Modification (ICD-9-CM). Laboratory employees should never suggest or supply ICD-9-CM codes. As a means to ensure physician knowledge of compliance issues, the laboratory should disseminate a "notice to physicians" to physician clients on an annual basis. The notice should outline the individual component of every laboratory profile that includes a multichannel test or other automated multiple test result and the CPT-4 codes that the laboratory uses to bill Medicare for each such profile. Physicians should also be told that when ordering tests for which Medicare, Medicaid, or other federally funded reimbursement is sought, they should order only those tests which they believe are medically necessary.

Costs

Operating expenditures in the laboratory may be divided into broad categories of fixed and variable costs. These terms reflect the sensitivity of costs to increases or decreases in test volume. A cost that changes more or less in proportion to the test volume is variable. A cost that remains unchanged for some period of time despite volume fluctuations is fixed. Examples of variable costs include technologist salaries, costs of reagents and supplies, and costs on printed requisition forms. Salaries for nonexempt employees, benefits, and the cost of depreciation of equipment are examples of fixed costs. Costs are also classified as either direct or indirect. Costs that can be specifically linked to a test are considered direct costs. These include technologist salaries, costs of clerical support and overtime, courier fees, and costs of reagents and bacteriological media. Costs that cannot be directly traced to a test but are still part of the laboratory's expenses are indirect costs. Examples of indirect costs include those of depreciation, building and equipment maintenance, and utilities. Laboratory managers are more often concerned about unit costs when making financial decisions because understanding how costs fluctuate in producing a specific unit of service (usually defined as a test) permits measurement of productivity. Unit costs are also divided into fixed and variable categories that behave differently as volume changes. Variable costs remain the same per unit regardless of volume, and fixed costs are reduced per unit when volume increases because the total fixed cost is spread over a larger number of tests. A busy clinical laboratory benefits from economies of scale. In general, variable and direct costs are subject to some degree of management control and fixed and indirect costs are much less so. Regardless of cost classifications, laboratory managers must be continually looking for opportunities to control any and all costs. Accurate cost accounting is an imperative for financial decision making, and in today's managed care environment, correct cost information ensures participation in profitable contracts. The laboratory manager must be efficient in defining and itemizing costs associated with the testing services provided by the laboratory. Moreover, accurate test cost analysis provides the manager with a rational mechanism for selecting the most cost-effective testing method among several new procedures whose suppliers each claim that their test is the least expensive to use. Finally, laboratory budgeting becomes more effective with a reliable cost analysis system in place. A simple test cost analysis worksheet is shown in Appendix 1.

Operating Budgets

The development of an operating budget for the hospital is highly dependent upon clearly stated institutional goals and objectives within which the laboratory has a known role and upon which it can base its own specific objectives. The manager should expect to receive, either directly or indirectly from the hospital administration, budget guidelines that include expected inpatient and outpatient census information for the budget year and any anticipated changes in the total service program of the organization. Clinical service line managers, in particular, should communicate new program plans to support service managers, including laboratory managers, because support services may be impacted by these new programs. If, for example, the hospital has plans to begin performing human stem cell transplants, then the microbiology laboratory needs to budget for the additional volume and specialized testing that patients receiving these transplants will require. In return, managers may be required to provide the laboratory and/or hospital administration with information related to program changes anticipated in their areas that arise because of changes in technology or clinical practice. Examples of such changes include procedures that may diminish in volume because of obsolescence or physician education and increasing volume estimates for newly implemented procedures such as those of molecular diagnostics.

There are several types of operating budgets (18). A fixed budget assumes a single level of output or activity and builds the budget around that level. A fixed budget, however, cannot be used to monitor and control resources during changes in test volumes that the laboratory may experience during the year. A flexible budget reflects expected laboratory revenue and expenses and anticipates the impact of volume changes on both. In this type of budget, some of the expenses are fixed and some are variable. The flexible budget recognizes the difficulty of establishing a flat level of expenditure and provides a tool for controlling costs. Quite simply, a flexible budget allocates dollars for resources based on volumes of tests performed. The accuracy of the flexible budget as a predictive tool, however, is only as good as the test component cost analysis performed during the budget's construction. A program budget is based on a specific program matrix. The matrix includes all proposed services and the resources required to deliver them. The program can include a set of activities, services, staffing, and equipment. It is often used for short-term planning purposes when new programs are launched. A zero-based budget calls for management to reevaluate all activities to decide if they should be re-funded for the next budget cycle. Each manager is required to justify the entire budget for their area of responsibility as if all of its activities were entirely new.

Although there is no single formula for the budgetary process, there are some basic elements that will help ensure success (18). First, establish clear goals and objectives to guide resource allocation. Second, obtain detailed data on existing and potential clients. Third, establish a defined budget period and procedures for development of the budget. Fourth, compile reports with financial and statistical information for comparison with budget information and for variance analysis. Furthermore, when planning a budget, managers should remember the following principles: (i) expenses are charged to the department or cost center that incurs them, (ii) every item of expense must be under the control of someone in the organization, (iii) managers responsible for complying with a budget should participate in the budget's preparation, (iv) managers should not be held accountable for expenditures over which they have no control, and (v) ordinarily, unused funds do not carry over from one budget year to the next.

Variance Analysis

Once the operating budget is established and approved, the extent to which the actual revenues and expenses differ from the budget represents a variance. Controllable variances can be resolved by appropriate management action (32). Salary variances can be addressed by reviewing time cards for excessive overtime. Supply cost variances may prompt an examination of inventory par levels. Suppliers may be approached for deeper discounts, or alternative vendors may be sought. Some variances are not controllable. These often result from unanticipated volume increases due to higher-than-expected numbers of patient admissions, unanticipated (and unbudgeted) price increases, unplanned repair expenses, or an unusual increase in the number of tests requested. A good example of the latter would be an unanticipated epidemic of influenza's producing a large increase in the number of requests for rapid flu testing and the need for the laboratory to purchase an excessive number of kits within a short span of time. As discussed above, a flexible budget should account for month-to-month fluctuations in test volumes and test complexity if properly constructed. Managers may be periodically called upon to communicate their budget performance to the laboratory administration and should be able to accurately record and explain budget variances on a line-by-line basis in their monthly financial statements.

Capital Budgeting

In addition to the operations budget, there must be a process for allocating monies for major investments in facilities and equipment. In accounting terms, a capital item is generally any fixed asset expected to provide service for more than 1 year and has a minimal expense, usually between $500 and $1,000. Items that qualify as capital include new space or renovation of existing space, replacement of equipment, purchase or lease of new equipment, and information technology (hardware, licensing fees, and interfaces, etc.). Capital acquisitions represent a significant investment for the organization and, as such, should be evaluated and justified by a budgetary process. Generally, a fixed amount of funds available for capital is established each fiscal year by the institution. Invariably, the total dollar amount requested for competing capital projects will far exceed the total of funds available. The capital budget process must therefore winnow, select, and prioritize; it is an enormously complex and politically charged task if not handled correctly. But by using a team approach whereby the management maintains focus on the goals and objectives of the organization, the capital budget process can be a successful and rewarding experience.

Prior to the budget process, the pool of total capital dollars available may be divided into smaller pools designed to support different aspects of the institution. For example, a $50 million capital budget may be allocated to allow $5 million for strategic projects, $10 million for information technology, $15 million for patient care, $10 million for facility improvements, and $10 million for ancillary services. If the laboratory is considered part of ancillary services, then the numbers of available dollars is much lower than the overall budget and the laboratory will likely be competing with several other departments for this lesser amount. The evaluation process will seek to classify capital projects in different ways, and managers should be aware of how to appropriately categorize and describe any project submitted for consideration. For example, some projects may represent new or incremental business, some may enhance quality, and some may reduce cost. Finally, capital requests may be prioritized according to need. A nondiscretionary project is a project that must be funded to keep the facility operating. An example would be a renovation project to make the laboratory compliant with regulatory and accreditation mandates. Levels of priority then follow, with level I projects being most critical.

Generally, capital projects of $10,000 or less need minimal analysis. All that is normally required is a brief description of the project and its intended use (new item or replacement, etc.) and the requested dollar amount. Projects with costs exceeding the minimum dollar amount require a higher level of analysis and more detailed documentation supporting the request. In addition to a description of the project and its intended use, proposals for these projects should include an estimate of the life span of the item, an estimate of all costs associated with acquisition, an estimate of yearly incremental cash outflows, and an estimate of yearly incremental cash inflows or savings. Depreciation expense must also be considered. Straight-line depreciation analysis is the most commonly used method of determining the expense of a fixed asset. In this method, the estimated useful life span of the item is divided by the cost of acquisition. A piece of equipment costing $100,000 with a useful life expectancy of 5 years would have a depreciation expense of $20,000 per year.

The financial analysis of large capital projects may have several elements. An illustrative case study follows. Suppose a clinical microbiology laboratory that has historically performed manual bacterial identifications and disk susceptibility tests wishes to purchase an automated system because a new outreach program will significantly increase test volumes. First, a pay-back analysis reveals that with a purchase price of $125,000 and a net cash flow of $137,000 after 3 years, the pay-back period is calculated at 2.68 years. The pay-back method does not take into account the time value of money but serves as a crude measure of risk because it favors projects with a short pay-back horizon. The average rate of return is calculated by dividing the average annual return by the amount of the initial investment. Projects with a higher average rate of return may be rated more favorably, but the method also fails to recognize the impact of time. The concept of present value is very important for capital investment analyses because it takes into account the increase or decrease in the value of a capital investment over time.

The most common method used in the financial analysis of a capital proposal that accounts for the time value of money is the calculation of net present value (NPV). NPV is the present value of all cash flows minus the initial investment. If the NPV is positive or zero, the project is usually considered financially acceptable. This is because all future cash flow has been converted into current dollars, with the use of an expected rate of return (usually set by the institution's financial department), and has been compared with the initial investment. However, projects with a small negative NPV may still be worthwhile since other factors may be considered, such as the size of the initial investment and the benefit to patients. A favorable NPV for any capital proposal may result in a ranking higher than those for projects with similar costs. Laboratory managers would be well advised to support their capital project proposals with sound financial as well as clinical justification. In the end, it may make the difference between getting the equipment the laboratory needs and limping along for another year without it.

Financial Bench Marking

Increasing economic pressures on today's laboratory operations have created the need for managers to be aware of their financial performance in comparison to some internal or external bench mark. Financial bench marking is but one of many tools that the laboratory employs to improve performance, focus on customers, survive, and thrive in an environment with limited resources (39). In selecting indicators for bench marking, the use of ratios is much preferred over the use of raw numbers because the data are viewed in terms of a common denominator, usually some unit of service. The typical unit of service for the laboratory is the billed test because most financial systems are capturing volumes according to CPT codes that have standardized characteristics. A denominator that is often used outside the laboratory is patient-days or patient discharges. Ratios can be used to assess performance in a number of ways. For example, laboratory workload may be measured by calculating the total number of billed tests per calendar day, per patient-day, or per patient discharge, and examining the number of billed tests per full time equivalent reveals service intensity. Labor productivity can be determined from the number of hours worked per 100 billed tests or per patient discharge. Lastly, important cost data may be ascertained from ratios such as labor and supply expenses per 100 billed tests.

The simplest method of bench marking is to use your own laboratory as the standard and measure performance over time. This type of internal bench marking provides consistency of measurement over time and gives managers control over assumptions. In effect, it affords managers a means to continuously monitor performance and make improvements in productivity and cost on an ongoing basis. External bench marking involves a comparison of the laboratory's performance with that of a peer group. The composition of the peer group is critical. Members of the peer group should be alike in as many critical characteristics as possible. Otherwise, whatever performance expectations are placed on an individual laboratory being compared to the peer group may be unreasonable. Sometimes, voluntary agreements are established with other institutions to share productivity and cost information. This arrangement allows control of the size and composition of the peer group and ensures a fair comparison of whatever characteristics are being measured. There are a number of commercial companies that provide bench-marking products, some specific for the laboratory (see http://www.chisolutionsinc.com) and others more broadly applicable to the institution but with drill-down capability for the laboratory (see http://www.solucient.com).

Now that cost efficiency is a watchword in most health care environments, a comprehensive financial management system is an imperative, rather than an option, for laboratory management. Managers who set goals, measure progress, and identify trouble spots will utilize their limited resources more intelligently than those who do not.

PERSONNEL ISSUES

The study of organizational behavior encompasses all of the human factors encountered in the workplace, including motivation, leadership, organizational models, and responsibilities (31). Organizational behavior is defined as the actions and attitudes of people in organizations. When it comes to personnel issues, most diagnostic microbiology laboratories will fall under the auspices of the human resources department (HR) of the parent institution. In that regard, directors, managers, supervisors, technologists, and laboratory assistants alike are obligated to become familiar with and follow institutional policies relative to hiring and firing practices, compensation and benefits, job descriptions, organizational structure, and grievance procedures, etc., and of course to be compliant with federal, state, and local labor laws.

Hiring

Needs Assessment

Before the microbiology manager goes through the expense and time required to hire a full-time employee, he or she should determine whether that position can be eliminated without compromising service and quality expectations. Could the work be redistributed among existing staff? The solution may involve creative management in terms of subdividing assignments among other stations or individuals (or even among different laboratories), but this approach may not be practical in areas such as specimen processing where the workload is constant and could not be easily transferred elsewhere. It may be possible, however, to rearrange schedules such that individuals are transferred into high-volume work areas during times of peak utilization.

A second option may include the use of temporary or part-time employees to fill the shortage. This alternative can be quite attractive from a convenience standpoint but may be more expensive depending on training and agency costs. An excellent source of part-time help may include previous employees who have left the full-time ranks for alternative pursuits and would like to supplement their income. Finally, the hiring process may present an opportune time to examine laboratory productivity. A number of consultant firms are available to perform bench-marking analysis with laboratories having similar workloads and demographics to determine efficiency.

Analysis, Design, and Description

The job description is a summary of two administrative processes: job analysis and job design. Whereas the analytical and design phases involve proactive evaluation and/or reconfiguration of the nature of the work to be performed, the written job description is a document that defines the required skills, functions, conditions, and hierarchy associated with a specific position (35). Poor job analysis and design will lead to a flawed job description.

A job analysis should be comprehensive and detailed such that the nature of the work to be performed is clearly understood. The information required to complete the analysis can be gained through a structured process that measures and documents the number of tasks performed and the time required to complete those tasks, or informally through observation (10). One can also hire consultants to perform job analysis, request input from current staff, or contact laboratory administrators from demographically similar facilities. Job analysis and design should focus on the essential elements of the position, including the array of duties, the workflow and volume, the technological skills required, the degree of employee interaction, the reporting relationships, and the working conditions. This, in turn, will make it easier to define minimum education, experience, and personal attributes appropriate for the job. If done properly, job analysis and design will drive the completion of a formal job description. As an example, consider the following scenario. The microbiology manager is allowed to fill a vacancy for a laboratory assistant on the evening shift. The primary responsibilities of that position are specimen processing and reagent preparation. The manager could use the existing job description to recruit for the position. After careful analysis, however, the manager finds that most laboratory assistants on that shift complete their assigned duties nearly 2 h before the shift ends. At the same time, the volume of *Clostridium difficile* toxin testing by enzyme immunoassay on the day shift has exceeded capacity for months, necessitating overtime for qualified technologists. If the new position was expanded to a technologist level, it would allow for testing of excess *C. difficile* specimens on the evening shift without the loss of sample processing capacity at a fraction of the overtime costs alone.

The job description serves to define the specifics of the position and the requirements for the prospective employee (10). It also provides a tool for communication between the employer and the prospective employee and serves as a recruiting tool (35). It can be used to schedule and set staffing requirements, to assess employee performance and competency, to define wage and salary structure, and to act as a template for future corrective actions (35). It should be flexible to allow for future growth of the position and focus on minimum requirements to prevent the loss of high-end applicants (16). There are no rules to writing a good job description unless institutional guidelines are in place. At the very least, the job description should include the items listed in Table 1 (10, 35). Optional information that can be added includes exempt status (time clock or salaried position), personnel and payroll codes (but not actual dollar ranges), and U.S. Department of Labor (DOL) occupational codes and/or U.S. Employment Service functional job analysis codes (34). Bear in mind that the Clinical Laboratory Improvement Amendments of 1988 (CLIA '88; see below) established only six categories for laboratory personnel; director, technical consultant, clinical consultant, technical or general supervisor, testing personnel, and cytotechnologist. The laboratory can expand on the qualifications required for each of these positions but not reduce them below the minimum requirements as outlined in CLIA '88. All job descriptions on file should be reviewed at least annually in conjunction with the employee's performance review or when the position is vacated and a replacement is sought.

Recruiting, Interviews, and Hiring

Once a job description has been drafted and approved, the recruitment and hiring process can begin. As before, it is best to coordinate activities with the organization's HR personnel, who are more familiar with local, state, and federal regulations pertaining to recruitment and hiring. HR can also provide valuable services such as background checks and validation of a candidate's credentials (14).

The job description should be abstracted to provide the essentials for a classified advertisement. The advertisement should contain the job title, minimum education and licensing requirements, a brief summary of the duties, and if desired, the salary ranges (15, 16, 35, 38). The laboratory has basically two candidate pools to choose from: internal and external. The former is usually an attractive source because current employees have already received system orientation and are familiar with general corporate policies and culture. Mobilization of internal candidates usually takes less time because job listings can be posted in organizational newsletters or on institutional websites. Overall, internal hires are generally less costly, but external candidates can infuse the laboratory with new ideas, experiences, and skills. Generally, external searches take longer and may require the use of recruitment bonuses, employment agencies, the Internet, or advertising in trade magazines such as *ASM News/Microbe* or *Medical Laboratory Observer*. Other possible external recruitment sources include professional schools and organizations such as the American Society for Clinical Pathology, the Canadian College of Microbiologists, and the American College of Microbiology (the certification and training

TABLE 1 Components of a job description

Items	Example[a]
Organization	Central States Medical Center
Department	Microbiology
Position	Microbiologist, day shift
Education	B.S., medical technology or microbiology
Certification	M.T. (ASCP); SM, NRM, or equivalent
Responsibilities	Responsible for processing of specimens, interpretation of culture and susceptibility results, participation in quality management program, and teaching of medical technology students, laboratory medicine residents, and fellows; nonsupervisory position
Competency	Requires semiannual (first year) and annual (thereafter) competency assessment via departmental program
Working conditions/exposure hazards	Modern clinical microbiology laboratory; no heavy lifting; potential exposure to human specimens, including blood and body fluids, and work with BSL 1–3 agents
Pay code	5, Nonexempt

[a] M.T., Medical Technologist; ASCP, American Society for Clinical Pathologists; SM, Specialist Microbiology; NRM, National Registry of Microbiologists; BSL 1–3, biological safety levels 1–3.

branch of the American Society for Microbiology [ASM]). Parent institutions can also use online automated recruitment web pages for both internal and external candidate searches. By logging on to a website, potential candidates can review job openings within the system and create a personal profile that can be used by HR for reviewing qualifications or for matching individuals with future positions as they become available. The ultimate goal is to provide the microbiology administrator with a qualified pool of candidates while trying to maintain workforce diversity according to a U.S. DOL directive (http://www.dol.gov/dol/compliance/comp-eeo.htm). For individuals applying for supervisory or higher positions, a search committee should be convened to expand the sources of potential candidates. Once a candidate pool of qualified individuals has been identified, it is time to begin the interview process.

The interview is a means of allowing the employer and candidate to determine whether they are suited for each other. It is a very important process because a badly conducted interview may scare off a highly qualified candidate. This is also the part of the hiring process in which the unskilled interviewer may pose a liability and one that requires close attention to regulations. There are several questions shown in Table 2 that the Equal Employment Opportunity Commission prevents an employer from asking a potential employee (14, 16, 35, 38). The interview should be organized and standardized to permit a fair evaluation of each candidate. There are three basic formats for an interview: structured, in which the format is predetermined with a list of questions and a review form; unstructured, in which a set panel of questions is not used but the interview consists primarily of a running conversation with the candidate; and pressurized, in which the candidate is asked to provide analysis of various job-related scenarios or to solve a series of hypothetical problems (34). The interview can be a combination of all three and can be conducted individually or by a panel of interviewers. In some organizations, HR conducts a preliminary interview to screen candidates before the microbiology administration conducts final interviews. The ultimate goals are to meet the candidate, check credentials (usually an HR responsibility), collect additional information not provided on the application form, and gather a sense of personality fit. In management, we tend to think of the interview process from one side only. Holland (14) provides an overview of how to prepare for an interview from both the employer's and the employee's perspectives. If there is an evaluation form to be completed, it should be done immediately after the interview so that impressions are not lost with time. Documentation of the search, selection, interview, and orientation processes should be kept on file for at least 4 years should any improprieties be called into question.

Employee-Related Activities

Orientation

Once a candidate is hired, the next phase involves the assimilation of the new employee into the microbiology workforce. The orientation process must be organized and synchronized to keep the new hire active and engaged.

According to Vernadoe (34), there are three basic aspects of employee orientation. The first is at the organizational level to familiarize the new employee with institutional policies, procedures, and benefits. The second focuses on department-specific policies and codes of conduct. The final aspect concentrates on the microbiology laboratory and addresses job responsibilities, reporting structure, and working relationships that exist therein. There are at least four basic approaches to conducting orientation (16, 34). These include (i) formal meetings and training sessions, usually conducted at the institutional level by HR (these cover such topics as risk management, fire and chemical safety, benefits, and infection control); (ii) microbiology supervisor-led sessions to discuss laboratory-specific issues such as competency assessment, biological safety protocols, dress code, telephone conduct, breaks, and scheduling; (iii) a checklist approach; and (iv) a mentor-driven process.

In addition to a systemwide, general orientation program, many microbiology managers choose to develop a stepwise laboratory-specific orientation process that is checklist driven. First is the preorientation checklist, which is preparatory in nature. It allows the microbiology supervisory staff to organize all the materials that the new employee will receive during orientation. The training orientation checklist guides the assigned mentor and trainee through the basic components of orientation. The specific elements of the microbiology laboratory are covered by a series of modules that may include topics such as scheduling orientation, trainer and trainee expectations, supervisor's review procedures, a special shift rotation checklist, and a LIS orientation, to name a few. The entire process is completed with a postorientation checklist to ensure that each component has been covered and entered into the employee's personnel file.

Above all, the orientation period is the process of welcoming. For this reason, the choice of mentors selected to provide training should be carefully considered and limited to individuals with a great deal of experience and respect.

TABLE 2 Topics to be avoided during a hiring interview

Topic	Examples
Age	Date of birth, year of high school graduation
Weight	Waist size, dietary habits
Financial history	Outstanding loans or debts, bankruptcy
Citizenship	Country of origin, immigration status, parental ancestry
Marital status	Maiden name, number of children
Criminal and military records	Military discharge status, court convictions
Organization memberships	Religious or political groups
Mental/medical/physical disabilities	Current medications, therapy, workman's compensation benefits, missed workdays secondary to disabilities

Staffing and Scheduling

The process of adequately staffing a microbiology laboratory and scheduling individuals with widely ranging abilities to provide maximum coverage on each shift is one part science and one part art. It requires advanced planning, and no one strategy works for every facility because peak activity levels, workloads, and the technical complexity of testing differ significantly. Poor planning can lead to low productivity and high labor costs when staffing is excessive. Inadequate staffing may generate high productivity but also lead to increased overtime and employee burnout (21). To avoid these extremes, a number of good guidelines on staffing and scheduling are available for review (4, 36).

Scheduling is simply the process of assigning work responsibilities to a group of individuals and requires the right number of employees and skill levels to complete the work. Most medical laboratories work under the 8/80 rule for full-time employees, i.e., employees work a total of 8 h per day and 10 days over a 2-week pay period. This plan limits the number of hours to be worked in a day but permits the employee to work more consecutive days and is unique to medical facilities. A 40-h work week permits an employee to work any number of hours per day but not to exceed 40 h per week. Other scheduling systems include the use of part- or variable-time help, job sharing, self-directed work teams, and exempted employees (21, 36). In designing a schedule, it is important to choose a plan or combination of plans to provide the greatest degree of flexibility. A mixture of employees on the 8/80 plan and the 40 plan can be used, but a single employee must choose only one option.

The scheduler must know workload patterns and future trends. This is most often done retrospectively by reviewing LIS-generated billing for an estimate of test volume and plotting these data over time for trend analysis for each shift. Recording workload units periodically over time can also provide a helpful bench mark of test volume. However, keeping pace with method advancement is also necessary for projecting future labor needs. The development of molecular and amplification technology has greatly streamlined a number of processes in the microbiology laboratory—most significantly in clinical virology. Armed with this information, the laboratory manager must calculate how many people for each shift and skill set will accommodate the mean test volume, not peak or trough volumes of work (4). From here, the scheduler starts with a rough draft based on ideal staffing levels by using a matrix for each shift where rows correspond with the services to be provided and columns represent the days of the pay period. With the 8/80 plan, a shift is 8 h times 14 days or 112 h per pay period. Full-time employees can cover 80 of these hours (8 h times 10 days), while part-time staff can be used to fill in the balance (generally 24 h per week or less). Once a rough schedule has been outlined, it can be fine tuned by naming the individuals who will fill each slot and the work assigned. From this working draft, the schedule can be modified to accommodate vacations, family leave, illness, earned time off, and shift switching. Schedulers and managers must also remember that work schedules affect employee families and morale (30). Part-time and variable-time employees can be used to fill in gaps, or cross shift coverage can be applied to relieve peak workload stress. A detailed description of this process can be found elsewhere (4, 30, 36). During new employee orientation, a review of the scheduling process should be included so that there are no surprises when the individual is eventually assigned duties.

Winn and Westenfeld (41) provide an excellent summary of scheduling do's and don'ts as follows: (i) define the absolute minimum number of employees required for each situation (weekends, routine, and holidays); (ii) strictly define the duties for each of the positions required for every type of shift, and if a position is open, try to fill it with existing personnel based on the duties assigned to that slot; (iii) allow scheduling to be orchestrated by a coordinator with input from the staff; (iv) solicit vacation requests well in advance (>6 months) and be clear that not all preferences can be accommodated; (v) publish work schedules in advance to allow for personal adjustments; (vi) if allowed, use earned time off instead of overtime; and (vii) fill empty slots with volunteers or part-time help, with a draft as a last resort. In this context, certain laboratories have developed a rotational "hit list" among staff to cover for open slots on the work schedule. The next person up on the list is informed of their standing and allowed one deferral or may switch their obligation with another employee.

In a situation in which the microbiology workload is high or increasing and staffing is static or decreasing, there are a few options left to the administration to relieve the pressure. The first of these is outsourcing, such as finding reference laboratories to perform a variety of low-volume, esoteric, or technically complex testing, e.g., forwarding all mycobacterial identifications with the exception of probe-confirmed identification of *Mycobacterium tuberculosis* and *Mycobacterium avium* complex organisms to a public health mycobacteriology laboratory. Elimination of low-volume testing may not necessarily prove to be cost efficient but maintaining proficiency when the frequency of testing is low should also factor into outsourcing decisions.

Microbiology laboratories can even outsource testing to other laboratories within their own system. For example, automated blood culture systems can be physically located near a rapid-response laboratory. Signal-positive blood cultures can then be removed during all shifts to be subcultured and stained. Gram stains can be read by trained rapid-response technologists, and cultures can be evaluated during the next microbiology shift.

The second option is to examine the extent of evaluation. In many instances, microbiology laboratories can get into the bad habit of providing too much information, such as identifying isolated organisms that are unlikely pathogens in a disease process. This process not only generates an unnecessary workload but may also give the clinician a false sense of importance.

Unfortunately, staffing and scheduling often go hand in hand with absenteeism. As a result, each facility should have a well-defined absentee policy and management plan that are neither onerous to the employee nor subjective and that can be fairly applied. A laboratory policy on absenteeism requires a working definition, equitable and realistic standards (e.g., less than one unscheduled absence per month), and a management plan that uses the same organizational framework for corrective action for issues such as behavioral or performance problems (36). Absenteeism can be chronic, high frequency, and/or patterned (e.g., Mondays, Fridays, or the day after payday). If not addressed and corrected, chronic absenteeism can generate poor morale among other microbiology staff.

Performance Appraisal

A job description defines the duties of an employee and how the employee's success will be measured. The performance appraisal, on the other hand, asks how the employee is succeeding. A performance appraisal has at least five ingredients: (i) an employee with a job description and appropriate qualifications, (ii) a series of clearly defined goals and performance standards, (iii) an objective way of measuring achievements, (iv) someone trained to evaluate the employee's performance, and (v) a feedback loop to gain input from the employee (38). The standards used to judge performance must be outlined in the job description and should be objective and consistent with those used to evaluate other employees. Basically, four markers can be measured either alone or in combination to generate a performance appraisal: results, behavior, skills, and peer comparison (33). However, objectivity in performance appraisal is often difficult to achieve. We all have a tendency to rate individuals we like highly and those we do not like less highly. The actual data recorded in the performance appraisal should include employee information, a list of goals and objectives from the previous and for the next review, a scoring system, a place for the employee to provide his or her own feedback, and a summary section that allows for the appraiser to recommend promotions and salary adjustments and that includes a date for the next appraisal and signatures (11, 33). When complete, the form should become an official part of the employee's personal file (22).

If the parent organization permits, there are a number of alternatives to performance appraisals, including feedback sessions, team or section appraisals, self-appraisal, and process improvement sessions, all of which would require some form of documentation.

Competency Assessment

The directive for competency assessment of laboratory personnel was written into CLIA '88. This legislation was signed into law in 1992 and has been revised five times to provide the final ruling in 2003. It mandates that all laboratories falling under the jurisdiction of the CLIA '88 guidelines must develop a program to document the competency of each laboratory employee in every aspect of the employee's assigned duties. As is the case with many pieces of federal legislation, CLIA '88 did not define how this process is to be accomplished nor did they suggest which core competencies should be monitored. They did, however, place the responsibility for establishing a program and documenting competency assessment squarely on the shoulders of the laboratory director and technical consultant or technical supervisor (11). Fortunately, the Clinical and Laboratory Standards Institute (formerly NCCLS) has published a clear and logical approach to the design of a laboratory-based training and competency assessment program that provides a wealth of sample documents used in the process (22). CLIA '88 clearly define the frequency of personnel assessment: semiannually for new employees and annually thereafter unless changes in procedures and protocols occur. At that point, competency for and familiarity with the new protocol must be documented. All agencies approved by the CMS for the purpose of laboratory accreditation have a competency assessment module included in the review process. These agencies include the College of American Pathologists, the Joint Commission on Accreditation of Healthcare Organizations, and the Commission on Office Laboratory Accreditation. For more details on the history and evolution of competency assessment, please refer to the fine review by Sharp and Elder (29).

The final CLIA rule (2003) consolidates commercially marketed in vitro diagnostic assays into two functional categories, waived and nonwaived. When it comes to competency assessment, however, nonwaived testing is subdivided into moderate- and high-complexity tests for the purpose of defining the educational background and training requirements of those individuals performing the testing (40).

CLIA '88 go so far as to define a choice of methods to be used in the evaluation process (13, 29). These include but are not limited to (i) directly observing an individual performing laboratory functions including testing, plating, culture evaluation, and instrument operation and maintenance; (ii) verifying the accuracy of transcribed test results; (iii) checking the integrity of data entered by the employee for QC records, proficiency tests, preventive maintenance charts, and preliminary patient test results; (iv) challenging the employee with internal and external proficiency series; and (v) evaluating an individual's ability to solve laboratory-related dilemmas. Hundreds of individual skills need to be mastered before a technologist-level employee can be considered a competent microbiologist, and there is no way that each of these can be pinpointed let alone evaluated in a year's time. That being said, there are at least three excellent publications outlining a competency assessment program specifically for the microbiology laboratory, and any of these could be used as a template for design (19, 20, 29). General laboratory-wide plans are also available for review (16, 22). In one model, a database in a spreadsheet format (e.g., an Excel file) is established for each active employee upon hire. All of the potential competencies that the job description encompasses are listed in the first column of the spreadsheet (*y* axis), and the first row (*x* axis) indicates the year of review. Each new employee begins with a series of X's in each competency cell for which training has not yet been conducted or in the cells corresponding to competencies not included in the job description. As training for a particular skill is accomplished, the X is removed and the method of measurement, the date, and the initials of the trainer or observer are recorded in the cell. Methods of measurement can be coded as DO for direct observation, Q for quiz, DR for document review, PT for proficiency test (internal or external), PM for preventive maintenance review, and QC for quality control review, etc. By using the spreadsheet approach, the competency assessment report for each employee is readily available for review and update and can also be used as an orientation tool. A copy of each report can be printed on a yearly basis and added to the employee's personal file.

Continuing Education

The Clinical and Laboratory Standards Institute guidelines on training and competence assessment distinguish between training and education in the following way (22). Education is "schooling for the purposes of gaining knowledge," and training is defined as the acquisition of "a set of skills for the purpose of being able to put the knowledge to a practical use." For the purpose of this chapter, however, continuing education will be defined as the extended process of gaining knowledge and improving skill sets. Continuing education constitutes one of the mandatory requirements for competency assessment and professional development dictated by CLIA '88 and necessary for the maintenance of professional licensure by most accreditation agencies. How can microbiology personnel maintain yearly continuing education requirements under the pressure of reduced operating budgets? A number of opportunities are available to satisfy these requirements, including attendance at local meetings such as branch meetings of the ASM. ASM branches usually sponsor at least one annual educational meeting, and the location and time of each are posted on each branch's website (http://www.asm.org/MemberShip/index.asp?bid=1914). In some cities, local microbiologists have formed clubs that meet during the year and invite guest speakers (usually sponsored) to present topics of interest for continuing education credits. Many medical centers provide weekly opportunities for continuing education purposes such as grand rounds, clinical pathology conferences, infectious diseases case conferences, and microbiology rounds. At one author's facility (W.M.D.), the microbiology laboratory sponsors a weekly case conference open to technologists, infectious diseases staff, and pharmacy personnel. At the organization level, many health centers provide tuition reimbursement for college courses that pertain to the profession of the health care worker.

Other organized microbiological programs for continuing education include teleconferences, workshops, self-assessment materials such as Tech Sample and Check Sample (American Society for Clinical Pathology; http://www.ascp.org/index.asp), and ASM-organized wet laboratory demonstrations, online lectures, and audio lecture series that are available for purchase or subscription (http://www.asm.org).

Termination

Termination refers to the end of a formal business relationship between an employer and employee and can be either voluntary or involuntary (16). The departure of an employee from the workplace can be either amicable or contentious. In any case, procedures are usually developed by HR for employee separation that reflect the situation. For voluntary and amicable termination, the process may include documentation of the date of departure and a forwarding address; discontinuation of payroll, benefits, and parking privileges; and the return of security materials. HR may also wish to conduct an exit interview with the employee to gain insight on laboratory operations and administration (34).

There are good reasons to support the involuntary termination of an employee, including incompetence, chronic absences, violent behavior or verbal abuse, falsification of resume, theft, and insubordination (16). A fair employer will make every reasonable attempt to correct the problem prior to taking disciplinary actions. Detriments to job performance including substance abuse of any kind, stress-related illness, mental illness, or physical disabilities secondary to job activities fall under the auspices of the Americans with Disabilities Act (http://www.usdoj.gov/crt/ada/adahom1.htm) and are not acceptable causes for dismissal (16). A number of variations in the process of progressive disciplinary action have been described for laboratory managers, and each is designed to allow sufficient time for the employee in question to mend his or her ways and for the employer to adequately assess the true nature of the situation (16, 34, 38). The steps generally include (i) verbal counseling, (ii) written counseling, (iii) a penalty phase, and (iv) dismissal. A number of variations on the theme exist. Walters (38) outlines a more creative approach to the resolution or termination process that includes five phases: forewarning, investigation, proof, reflection, and penalty. Importantly, though, employees have the right to representation during any disciplinary process as determined by the National Labor Relations Act (http://www.nlrb.gov/nlrb/legal/manuals/rules/act.asp). If the conclusions of the progressive disciplinary action lead to employee dismissal, the process is usually handled by HR to ensure that all legal steps are followed and documented (16). It is also wise for the employer to retain the personnel file of the departing employee for future reference. Likewise, the departing employee should be informed of the Consolidated Omnibus Budget Reconciliation Act. This act gives workers and their families who lose health benefits the right to continue group health care provided by their current plan for limited periods of time under certain circumstances (http://www.dol.gov/dol/topic/health-plans/cobra.htm).

REGULATIONS

This section will serve as a brief review of those regulations and regulatory agencies that have the most profound effects on the operation of the clinical microbiology laboratory. A more extensive review of laboratory regulations is available in the works of Roseff et al. (26), Walters (38), and Ehrmeyer and Laessig (7).

CLIA '88

CLIA '88 (or simply CLIA) establish baseline performance standards for all U.S. laboratories involved in the testing of human materials for the diagnosis, prevention, or treatment of disease (7). The intention is to ensure the accuracy, reliability, and timeliness of test results no matter which laboratory is performing the testing. They were signed into law in 1988 (12), but five successive final revisions of the initial legislation have been published since, the last of which appeared in the *Federal Register* in 2003 (13, 34). In the first final version of CLIA, laboratory testing was divided into three complexity levels that established the expertise level of personnel performing those tests. Those levels were waived, moderate complexity (including provider-performed microscopy), and high complexity. In the most recent final version of CLIA, testing is now lumped into waived and nonwaived tests (most of the latter were high complexity). However, relative to the qualifications of testing personnel, CLIA still recognize moderate- and high-complexity levels (7, 40).

The administration and implementation of CLIA are under the purview of the CMS (http://www.cms.hhs.gov) in collaboration with the Centers for Disease Control and Prevention (http://www.cdc.gov). The U.S. Food and Drug Administration (http://www.fda.gov) is responsible for classifying the complexity of laboratory testing protocols and the CMS set fee schedules for laboratories providing services to Medicare.

U.S. laboratories wishing to perform and receive compensation for testing of human specimens must apply for a CLIA certificate in one of three complexity categories. If the laboratory meets compliance criteria as judged by the CMS or by one of the recognized professional accreditation agencies, it receives a permanent certificate of compliance or accreditation and becomes subject to the rules, regulations, and inspections of the agency issuing the certification. Organizations that the CMS have deemed suitable for CLIA accreditation of laboratories include the Joint Commission on Accreditation of Healthcare Organizations (http://www.jcaho.org), the Laboratory Accreditation Program of the College of American Pathologists (http://www.cap.org/apps/cap.portal), and the Commission on Office Laboratory Accreditation (http://www.cola.org/).

CLIA lay the foundation for laboratory participation in a proficiency testing program, qualifications of and competency assessment of laboratory personnel, and, establishment of a QC and QA program and ensure the integrity of laboratory testing through all phases of testing. They also call for routine inspection of certified laboratories and the enforcement of penalties for laboratories found to be noncompliant. CLIA dictate that outside or reference laboratories to which specimens are referred from a U.S. health care institution also be CLIA certified or the equivalent. Those wishing to review CLIA '88 in their entirety or to query individual components of the amendments can do so at http://www.phppo.cdc.gov/clia/regs/toc.aspx or http://www.cms.hhs.gov/clia/default.asp. A general description of the program is available at http://www.cms.hhs.gov/clia/progdesc.asp.

HIPAA

Public law 104-191, or the Health Insurance Portability and Accountability Act (HIPAA, Title I) of 1996, was originally written "to improve portability and continuity of health insurance coverage in the group and individual markets, to combat waste, fraud, and abuse in health insurance and health care delivery, to promote the use of medical savings accounts, improve access to long-term care services and coverage, to simplify the administration of health insurance, and for other purposes." However, in 2002, the Department of Health and Human Services issued the HIPAA Privacy Rule (Title II) that set highly restrictive standards on the use and protection of individual demographics and health information (protected health information [PHI]) contained in patient medical records (24). Details are available at http://www.hhs.gov/ocr/hipaa/finalreg.html. The Privacy Rule dictates that all "covered entities" including health insurance plans and health care institutions and providers must obtain written permission from a patient to use or disclose PHI and that the patients must be notified of their right to restrict the use of or disclose PHI (24). Covered entities must also make every attempt to limit PHI disclosure to only that required for any given purpose. From the standpoint of the microbiology laboratory, this means that the release of any PHI attached to bacterial or fungal isolates sent for research or surveillance purposes that can be traced in any way to the patient requires disclosure and consent unless waived by the human studies committee of the institution. The Privacy Rule does not supersede the federal "Common Rule" (see also http://www.hhs.gov/ohrp/humansubjects/guidance/45cfr46.htm) that mandates Institutional Review Board approval of research studies conducted under its auspices (24). As with CLIA '88, the CMS are charged with the responsibility of administering the provisions of HIPAA. For a summary of the HIPAA health insurance reform (Title I) or the HIPAA administrative simplification (Title II), one can access the CMS website at http://www.cms.hhs.gov/hipaa.

Laws Covering Equal Pay and Compensation Discrimination

Several laws have been passed over the past half century to guarantee employees freedom from discrimination in the workplace with regard to wages, compensation, and working conditions. Collectively, these laws are enforced by the U.S. Equal Employment Opportunity Commission and include the Equal Pay Act of 1963, Title VII of the Civil Rights Act of 1964, the Age Discrimination Act of 1967, and Title I of the Americans with Disabilities Act of 1960.

Equal Employment Opportunity Commission

The Equal Employment Opportunity Commission is a federal agency created in 1965 to enforce the Civil Rights Act of 1964 (26). As of 1999, the agency had published new guidelines to further define unlawful harassment in the workplace (including sexual harassment) against the same groups protected by the Civil Rights Act (26, 38; http://www.eeoc.gov). To avoid risk, laboratories and/or HR of the parent institution should have a training module on unlawful harassment in place for employees and supervisory personnel, avenues for rapid reporting and investigation of complaints, and a documentation process for each of these.

Equal Pay Act of 1963

The Equal Pay Act is part of the Fair Labor Standards Act and makes unlawful the practice of wage discrimination between men and women performing the same duties at the same institution in a similar work environment. This act is directed and enforced by the Equal Employment Opportunity Commission and is gender neutral such that it protects males and females equally (38).

Title VII of the Civil Rights Act of 1964

Title VII of the Civil Rights Act of 1964 prohibits the use of race, color, creed, religion, nationality, and sex as a basis for the discharge of or failure to hire an employee, for segregation or classification that would deprive an employee of opportunities or advancement, for the failure or refusal of an employment agency to refer an individual for employment, or for the limitation of training or retraining of an employee.

Age Discrimination in Employment Act of 1967

The Age Discrimination in Employment Act of 1967 applies to individuals 40 years of age and older and, like the Civil Rights Act, prohibits the use of age as a reason for discrimination in the workplace. Interestingly, this law also applies when two candidates over the age of 40 apply for the same job and the younger of the two is hired if the employer has used older age as a negative factor in the selection process (38).

Americans with Disabilities Act

The Americans with Disabilities Act was passed in 1990 and forbids discrimination against an individual who has or has had a disability, is thought to have a disability, or associates with another disabled individual. According to the Americans with Disabilities Act, a disability is a physical or mental deficiency that affects a life function such as walking, talking, employability, and hygiene (38). The Americans with Disabilities Act mandates that an employer reasonably accommodate the needs of any qualified candidate so that he or she can perform the job. For example, the current dimensions of bench tops, shelving, and foot wells in the microbiology laboratory may not be appropriate for wheelchair access by a wheelchair-bound microbiologist and, therefore, require modification. Acceptable dimensions for work-related desk surfaces and shelving are provided in the Americans with Disabilities Act standards for design (http://www.usdoj.gov/crt/ada/stdspdf.htm).

Other Regulations Related to the Workplace

Family and Medical Leave Act

Passed in 1993, the Family and Medical Leave Act provides allowances to eligible employees of an eligible employer to take up to 12 months of unpaid leave during any 12-month period for one or more of the following situations: (i) birth and care of the employee's newborn child, (ii) placement with the employee of a child for adoption or foster care, (iii) care of an immediate family member (spouse, parent, or child) with a serious health problem, and (iv) medical leave secondary to the employee's own serious health problem. The Family and Medical Leave Act falls under the auspices of the U.S. DOL, and definitions of which employers are covered by this act and which employees are eligible can be found at http://www.dol.gov/esa/whd/fmla/.

Fair Labor Standards Act

The DOL also administers the Fair Labor Standards Act, which is legislation that sets basic minimum wage and overtime pay schedules. These regulations are enforced by the

Wage and Hour Division of the DOL, which is a program of the Employment Standards Administration. Pay for overtime (defined as work in excess of 40 h in a work week) is set at a rate of not less than one and one-half times the regular rate of pay. Certain exemptions apply to specific types of businesses or specific types of work. This act does not set requirements for severance pay, sick leave, vacations, or holidays. For more details, one can consult the DOL website at http://www.dol.gov/dol/topic/wages/index.htm.

Affirmative Action

An executive order was issued in 1965 that prohibits contractors engaged in federal contract work exceeding $10,000 from discriminating in hiring decisions against the same protected groups included in the Civil Rights Act. This order has since become known as affirmative action and was updated in 2000 by the Office of Federal Contract Compliance Program of the DOL. In addition, contractors securing more than $50,000 in government business and having more than 50 employees must write and regularly update an affirmative action plan to reflect current guidelines (38). Affirmative action guidelines would apply to many health care institutions and laboratories meeting the criteria defined above because of their participation in federal contracts for care provided to Medicare and Medicaid patients. However, many institutions that do not meet the qualifications outlined in this executive order have chosen to develop a voluntary affirmative action plan. The Office of Federal Contract Compliance Program maintains a website at http://www.dol.gov/esa/regs/compliance/ofccp/faqs/faapfaqs.htm.

APPENDIX 1

Sample test cost analysis form

Test cost analysis worksheet

Test: ______________________________

Patient tests per year ______________________________

Other tests per year (QC, repeats, etc.) ______________________________

Total tests per year ______________________________

Estimated time to perform test ______________________________

Cost analysis

Labor

Direct: __________

Indirect: __________

Supplies

Direct: __________

Indirect: __________

Equipment: __________

Overhead: __________

Cost/Test: __________

Cost/Patient Test: __________ = (cost/test × total test volume)/patient test volume

REFERENCES

1. **American Medical Association.** 2005. *Current Procedural Terminology;* CPT 2006, 4th ed. AMA Press, Chicago, Ill.

1a. **Baselski, V. S., A. S. Weissfeld, and F. Sorrell.** 2004. Charges and fees for laboratory services, p. 574–579. *In* L. S. Garcia, V. S. Baselski, M. D. Burke, D. A. Schwab, D. L. Sewell, J. C. H. Steele, Jr., A. S. Weissfeld, D. S. Wilkinson, and W. C. Winn, Jr. (ed.), *Clinical Laboratory Management.* ASM Press, Washington, D.C.

2. **Baselski, V. S., A. S. Weissfeld, and F. Sorrell.** 2004. Reimbursement compliance, p. 592–602. *In* L. S. Garcia, V. S. Baselski, M. D. Burke, D. A. Schwab, D. L. Sewell, J. C. H. Steele, Jr., A. S. Weissfeld, D. S. Wilkinson, and W. C. Winn, Jr. (ed), *Clinical Laboratory Management.* ASM Press, Washington, D.C.

3. **Beck, C.** 2004. Instrument selection, p. 194–200. *In* J. Hudson (ed.), *Principles of Clinical Laboratory Management.* Prentice-Hall, Inc., Upper Saddle River, N.J.

4. **Brown, S. A.** 2003. Process design—workflow and staffing, p. 244–265. *In* D. M. Harmening (ed.), *Laboratory Management: Principles and Processes.* Prentice-Hall, Inc., Upper Saddle River, N.J.

5. **Curtis, G.** 2004. Quality management, p. 177–183. *In* J. Hudson (ed.). *Principles of Clinical Laboratory Management.* Prentice-Hall, Inc., Upper Saddle River, N.J.

6. **Donnelly, J. M.** 2003. Healthcare reimbursement, p. 209–221. *In* D. M. Harmening (ed.), *Laboratory Management: Principles and Processes.* Prentice-Hall, Inc., Upper Saddle River, N.J.

7. **Ehrmeyer, S. S., and R. H. Laessig.** 2003. Compliance issues—the regulations, p. 225–243. *In* D. M. Harmening (ed.), *Laboratory Management: Principles and Processes.* Prentice-Hall, Inc., Upper Saddle River, N.J.

8. **Englekirk, P. G., J. Duben-Engelkirk, and M. T. LaRocco.** 1993. *Total Quality Management of Clinical Microbiology Services.* Colorado Association for Continuing Medical Laboratory Education Association, Denver, Colo.

9. **Gordon, J. R.** 2002. *Organizational Behavior: a Diagnostic Approach,* 7th ed. Prentice-Hall, Inc., Upper Saddle River, N.J.

10. **Hall, J., and J. O'Malley.** 2003. Job analysis, work descriptions and work groups, p. 106–120. *In* D. M. Harmening (ed.), *Laboratory Management: Principles and Processes.* Prentice-Hall, Inc., Upper Saddle River, N.J.

11. **Halstead, D. C., and D. L. Oblack.** 2004. Performance appraisals and competency assessment, p. 291–325. *In* L. S. Garcia, V. S. Baselski, M. D. Burke, D. A. Schwab, D. L. Sewell, J. C. H. Steele, Jr., A. S. Weissfeld, D. S. Wilkinson, and W. C. Winn, Jr. (ed.), *Clinical Laboratory Management.* ASM Press, Washington, D.C.

12. **Health Care Financing Administration.** 1992. Medicare, Medicaid, and CLIA programs. Regulations implementing the Clinical Laboratory Improvement Amendments of 1988 (CLIA). *Fed. Regist.* **57:**7002–7186.

13. **Health Care Financing Administration.** 2003. Medicare, Medicaid, and CLIA programs; laboratory requirements relating to quality systems and certain personnel qualifications. Final rule. *Fed. Regist.* **68:**3639–3714.

14. **Holland, P.** 2004. Employment interview and selection process, p. 26–32. *In* J. Hudson (ed.), *Principles of Clinical Laboratory Management.* Prentice-Hall, Inc., Upper Saddle River, N.J.

15. **Holland, P.** 2004. Job description and job advertisement, p. 18–25. *In* J. Hudson (ed.), *Principles of Clinical Laboratory Management.* Prentice-Hall, Inc., Upper Saddle River, N.J.

16. **Kurec, A. S.** 2004. Employee selection, p. 277–290. *In* L. S. Garcia, V. S. Baselski, M. D. Burke, D. A. Schwab, D. L. Sewell, J. C. H. Steele, Jr., A. S. Weissfeld, D. S. Wilkinson, and W. C. Winn, Jr. (ed.), *Clinical Laboratory Management.* ASM Press, Washington, D.C.

17. **Langley, G. J., T. W. Nolan, C. Norman, and L. P. Provost.** 1996. *The Improvement Guide: a Practical Approach to Enhancing Organizational Performance.* Jossey-Bass, San Francisco, Calif.

18. **Lutinger, I.** 2003. Effective budgeting in the laboratory: practical tips, p. 196–208. *In* D. M. Harmening (ed.), *Laboratory Management: Principles and Processes.* Prentice-Hall, Inc., Upper Saddle River, N.J.

19. **McCarter, Y. S., and A. Robinson.** 1997. Competency assessment in clinical microbiology. *Clin. Microbiol. Newsl.* **19:**97–101.

20. **McCaskey, L., and M. LaRocco.** 1995. Competency testing in clinical microbiology. *Lab. Med.* **26:**343–349.

21. **Medvescek, P.** 2004. Staffing and scheduling, p. 326–332. *In* L. S. Garcia, V. S. Baselski, M. D. Burke, D. A. Schwab, D. L. Sewell, J. C. H. Steele, Jr., A. S. Weissfeld, D. S. Wilkinson, and W. C. Winn, Jr. (ed.), *Clinical Laboratory Management.* ASM Press, Washington, D.C.

22. **NCCLS.** April 2004. *Training and Competence Assessment; Approved Guideline, GP21-A2,* 2nd ed., vol. 15, no. 21. NCCLS (Clinical and Laboratory Standards Institute), Wayne, Pa.

23. **NCCLS.** 2002. *Clinical Laboratory Technical Procedure Manuals; Approved Guideline, GP2-A4,* 4th ed. NCCLS, Wayne, Pa.

24. **Neale, A. V., and K. L. Schwartz.** 2004. A primer of the HIPAA privacy rule for practice-based researchers. *J. Am. Board Fam. Pract.* **16:**461–465.

25. **Needles, B. E., Jr.** 2005. *Financial Managerial Accounting,* 2005. Houghton Mifflin, Princeton, N.J.

26. **Roseff, S. D., A. L. Harris, and C. H. Rodgers.** 2004. The impact of regulatory requirements, p. 79–134. *In* L. S. Garcia, V. S. Baselski, M. D. Burke, D. A. Schwab, D. L. Sewell, J. C. H. Steele, Jr., A. S. Weissfeld, D. S. Wilkinson, and W. C. Winn, Jr. (ed.), *Clinical Laboratory Management.* ASM Press, Washington, D.C.

27. **Samuel, M.** 2001. *The Accountability Revolution,* p. 5–10. Facts on Demand Press, Tempe, Ariz.

28. **Schifman, R. B., G. Cembrowski, and D. Wolk.** 2004. Quality management, p. 369–390. *In* L. S. Garcia, V. S. Baselski, M. D. Burke, D. A. Schwab, D. L. Sewell, J. C. H. Steele, Jr., A. S. Weissfeld, D. S. Wilkinson, and W. C. Winn, Jr. (ed.), *Clinical Laboratory Management.* ASM Press, Washington, D.C.

29. **Sharp, S. E., and B. L. Elder.** 2004. Competency assessment in the clinical microbiology laboratory. *Clin. Microbiol. Rev.* **17:**681–694.

30. **Shields, K.** 2004. Employee scheduling, p. 148–154. *In* J. Hudson (ed.), *Principles of Clinical Laboratory Management.* Prentice-Hall, Inc., Upper Saddle River, N.J.

31. **Silbiger, S.** 1993. *The Ten Day MBA,* p. 118–156. William Morrow & Company, New York, N.Y.

32. **Tolzmann, G., and R. J. Vincent.** 2004. Costs, budgeting and financial decision making, p. 525–550. *In* L. S. Garcia, V. S. Baselski, M. D. Burke, D. A. Schwab, D. L. Sewell, J. C. H. Steele, Jr., A. S. Weissfeld, D. S. Wilkinson, and W. C. Winn, Jr. (ed.), *Clinical Laboratory Management.* ASM Press, Washington, D.C.

33. **Vernadoe, L. A.** 1996. Appraisal of job performance, p. 94–112. *Medical Laboratory Management and Supervision: Operations, Review and Study Guide.* F. A. Davis Co., Philidelphia, Pa.

34. **Vernadoe, L. A.** 1996. Human resource management: the personnel process, p. 113–142. *Medical Laboratory Management and Supervision: Operations, Review and Study Guide.* F. A. Davis Co., Philidelphia, Pa.

35. **Vernadoe, L. A.** 1996. Job design and job descriptions, p. 81–93. *Medical Laboratory Management and Supervision:*

Operations, Review and Study Guide. F. A. Davis Co., Philidelphia, Pa.

36. **Vernadoe, L. A.** 1996. Staffing and scheduling, p. 218–229. *Medical Laboratory Management and Supervision: Operations, Review and Study Guide.* F. A. Davis Co., Philidelphia, Pa.
37. **Vetter, L. P.** 2004. Management functions, p. 22–40. *In* L. S. Garcia, V. S. Baselski, M. D. Burke, D. A. Schwab, D. L. Sewell, J. C. H. Steele, Jr., A. S. Weissfeld, D. S. Wilkinson, and W. C. Winn, Jr. (ed.), *Clinical Laboratory Management.* ASM Press, Washington, D.C.
38. **Walters, C. V.** 2003. Human resource guidelines and regulations, p. 85–105. *In* D. M. Harmening (ed.), *Laboratory Management: Principles and Processes.* Prentice-Hall, Inc., Upper Saddle River, N.J.
39. **Wells, L. D., and W. C. Winn, Jr.** 2004. Laboratory benchmarking, p. 723–743. *In* L. S. Garcia, V. S. Baselski, M. D. Burke, D. A. Schwab, D. L. Sewell, J. C. H. Steele, Jr., A. S. Weissfeld, D. S. Wilkinson, and W. C. Winn, Jr. (ed.), *Clinical Laboratory Management.* ASM Press, Washington, D.C.
40. **Westgard, J. O.** 4 February 2003, posting date. *Final[5] CLIA Rule, part I. Key Changes.* [Online.] http://www.westgard.com/essay50.htm.
41. **Winn, W. C., Jr. and F. Westenfeld.** 2004. Human resources at the local level: an important component of financial management, p. 513–524. *In* L. S. Garcia, V. S. Baselski, M. D. Burke, D. A. Schwab, D. L. Sewell, J. C. H. Steele, Jr., A. S. Weissfeld, D. S. Wilkinson, and W. C. Winn, Jr. (ed.), *Clinical Laboratory Management.* ASM Press, Washington, D.C.

Laboratory Design

MICHAEL L. WILSON AND L. BARTH RELLER

3

A well-designed laboratory is a safe, pleasant, and efficient place in which to work, as well as an enjoyable place to visit. When a new laboratory is being designed or renovation of an existing one is being planned, the design must meet the needs of laboratory staff who spend all or most of their working time there, the needs of workers who spend part of their time there, and the needs of visitors who have to interact with the staff. Above all other considerations, a clinical laboratory must be a safe place. No other aspect of laboratory design carries a higher priority, both for the staff and for visitors. A pleasant environment improves staff morale and productivity, minimizes unnecessary distractions (thereby reducing laboratory errors), and enhances employee recruitment and retention. An efficient clinical laboratory helps to improve productivity, to reduce errors, and to improve patient care by shortening laboratory test turnaround time (TAT). An efficient laboratory also helps to improve staff morale and contributes significantly to a pleasant work environment.

Good laboratory design is based on the concept that form follows function, so the unique functions of a clinical microbiology laboratory (CML) should be reflected in the laboratory design. When designing a CML, it should be remembered that there are three key differences between a CML and other types of clinical laboratories. First, clinical microbiology involves the isolation, propagation, and handling of pathogenic microorganisms that pose a risk to laboratory personnel. To minimize this risk, the entire CML must have the facilities and processes necessary to meet biosafety level 2 criteria and, depending upon the extent and scope of services provided, all or part of the laboratory must also meet the requirements necessary to meet biosafety level 3 criteria (4, 15). Second, the interpretation of cultures and other microbiologic test results is based on the ability of the laboratory to isolate pathogenic microorganisms while minimizing microbial contaminants. Again, the laboratory design must be such that the necessary precautions can be taken to minimize contaminants. Third, laboratory design must accommodate specialized equipment used only in microbiology laboratories.

This chapter is intended to be an introduction to the processes of laboratory design, construction, and renovation. Reading this chapter should enable the microbiologist who is beginning a construction or renovation project to communicate with all of the parties who are involved. The informed microbiologist not only will understand the terminology of design and construction, but also will be able to make better decisions as the processes unfold. Being well informed also reduces the likelihood of costly mistakes. Not everything can or should be learned by experience.

GENERAL DESIGN PRINCIPLES

The needs of each laboratory will change over time, often many times between the initial construction of the laboratory and any subsequent renovations. Thus, the best approach to designing is to use the most generic design possible, minimizing features that are unique to current circumstances. Not only does a more generic design facilitate the changing needs of the laboratory, but also it reduces the costs of construction, renovations, and ongoing maintenance. Moreover, a generic design is the most flexible one. As stated by Crane and Richmond (5), "the biggest challenge to the laboratory design team is to keep the design simple, not to overdesign the laboratory. . . ." Meeting this challenge requires strong leadership by the laboratory administration and the architect. In particular, leading a design project for either new construction or renovation requires the ability to say "no" to requests for special design features.

Laboratory Location

CMLs providing services for a hospital must be fully integrated with the main hospital laboratory (7, 11, 13). This is a critical factor in providing adequate staffing, ensuring proper specimen processing and handling, reducing errors, and increasing efficiency and productivity. While it is true that off-site reference laboratories serve a useful role in providing esoteric testing and/or routine microbiology services for outpatient clinics and physician offices, we believe that there are important reasons why off-site microbiology laboratories do not serve hospitals well. First, use of off-site laboratories may result in delayed specimen processing, which can adversely affect microbial recovery and timely reporting of results. Second, use of off-site laboratories decreases interaction between microbiologists and clinicians. This is of particular concern when there is a lack of clinician input into specimen processing, which directly affects the clinical interpretation of microbiological tests. Third, as previously mentioned, loss of integration with the rest of the clinical laboratory, particularly specimen receipt and processing areas, increases the risk of incorrect specimen processing and medical errors. Fourth, laboratory staff members in different laboratory sections are unable to interact on a frequent basis, provide coverage for one another, and act as a cohesive unit. Fifth, added complexity and cost are associated with off-site laboratories (e.g., reliable, timely transport of specimens). Sixth, location of the CML close to the main laboratory facilitates access during off-hours and simplifies security. A laboratory that is remote to the main laboratory is unlikely to be visited by clinicians during off-hours, if ever. Last, location of a CML distant to the site of patient care precludes meaningful training of clinical microbiologists, infectious disease physicians, and other health care professionals (7, 11).

Laboratory Size

Only broad generalizations can be made regarding laboratory size. As a general rule, each bench technologist needs a minimum of 50 ft^2 in which to work, excluding space for large pieces of equipment, walls, corridors, storage, lockers, and offices. Areas such as that used for specimen processing require ample space to accommodate the necessary equipment, the specimen receiving bench itself, and foot traffic. Laboratory sections such as mycobacteriology, mycology, and virology require a larger amount of space relative to the number of technologists who work there. Areas such as a dedicated autoclave room or medium preparation room require additional space. If the number of technologists and supervisors is proportional to the test volume and the laboratory is well designed with little wasted space, the space allocated for the laboratory should be between 150 and 200 ft^2 per staff member.

Laboratories should be designed with more space than is needed for current workloads and types of services provided. This serves three purposes. First, an efficient laboratory always has the space needed to accommodate short-term expansion of the types and volumes of services provided by that laboratory. Second, extra space (often referred to as swing space) can be used when part of the laboratory is being renovated or repaired. Third, extra space can be used for future expansion of services. It is unwise to design and build a laboratory to meet current needs only.

Transportation

As with other laboratory sections, an effective transportation system is crucial for providing clinical microbiology services. A variety of transportation systems are in use in hospitals today, including manual transportation, robotic systems, and pneumatic tube systems. Manual systems are notoriously unreliable, particularly in large medical centers, and the associated personnel costs make this approach one of the most expensive. While the capital costs of robotic and pneumatic tube systems are high, over time these costs may be less than those associated with a manual transportation system. Robotic systems are not as widely used as pneumatic tube systems for transportation throughout hospitals. Pneumatic tube systems are widely used in hospitals and have been proven to be an effective method for transporting some types of specimens to clinical laboratories. If they are well designed and maintained, they can play an important role in reducing the costs of transportation, decreasing the number of lost or delayed specimens, and reducing test TAT. In general, however, dedicated pneumatic tube systems are not as useful for CMLs as they are for chemistry and hematology laboratories. This is because most microbiologic tests do not have the same expectation for test TAT, many pneumatic tube systems cannot transport specimens as heavy as full blood culture bottles, and containers used to collect specimens such as urine are prone to leakage when shipped through pneumatic tube systems. Other automated transportation systems are available, but, as with pneumatic tube systems, any benefit to a CML is not as great as it is for other clinical laboratory sections.

Building Codes and Architectural Standards

Laboratorians who have never been involved in the construction or renovation of a laboratory are often unaware of building codes and architectural standards (1). Although it is the responsibility of the architects and engineers to ensure that the plan meets the appropriate codes and standards, laboratory staff members who are involved in a project should understand these issues sufficiently to avoid making requests that are not in compliance with codes and standards. There are definite and specific limits to the way a laboratory can be built.

Interior Design

The design of laboratories that are part of health care systems often involves meeting organization design standards. In some organizations, the types of materials that are used for construction, color schemes, and many other architectural details are specified from the outset. For some organizations this makes a great deal of sense, as a standard interior design lends a sense of continuity throughout the organization. In many instances it also reduces construction and renovation costs, as the organization can purchase materials in large quantities. For other organizations, however, it makes little sense to adopt interior design schemes developed for one part of the organization for a laboratory. Moreover, not all design schemes are successful, so an organization should not be reluctant to abandon one scheme in favor of a better one. At all costs, one should avoid trendy interior design schemes, as they are less likely to please a large number of employees, become dated more quickly than do more traditional design schemes, and tend to be more expensive. It should always be remembered that one might have to live with a laboratory or office for many years.

Technology

Much of the same logic that applies to interior design also applies to the use of advanced technology in a laboratory. Laboratorians, architects, engineers, and designers are all enamored with technology, and there is a strong temptation to use the most advanced technology in a new laboratory or when renovating an existing one (5). Nonetheless, one should assess carefully the cost of advanced technology versus less advanced but proven technology, evidence that advanced technology has been used successfully in comparable laboratories, and any evidence of long-term durability. Advanced technological products may or may not be better than traditional ones, but the newer they are, the less experience there is with them. Moreover, some advanced technology products are trendy and should therefore be avoided for the same reasons that trendy interior design schemes should be avoided. There are reasons why traditional built-in laboratory casework continues to be used widely and why certain commercial products and vendors have been around for decades.

SPECIFIC DESIGN ISSUES

Laboratory Layout

The laboratory layout is crucial for achieving the goals set forth in the introduction to this chapter. The overall layout of a clinical laboratory is determined by the types of services provided, the numbers and types of specimens that are processed, the physical constraints of the building, and the resources that are available for the construction or renovation project. A laboratory that provides only patient care services has needs that are different from those of one engaged in teaching and/or research. Busy clinical laboratories must be efficient to maximize specimen throughput and to minimize test TAT. Laboratories that support teaching and research missions also need to be efficient but must have the space and facilities to support the broader missions. Decisions regarding the overall layout of the laboratory should be made first and should be immutable during the design process.

Most CMLs are divided into sections according to the way that specimens are handled in those laboratories (e.g., a bench devoted to urine cultures, another to blood cultures, and so on) and/or by discipline (e.g., a mycology section). There are obviously many different ways to organize a laboratory. As noted above, the best approach is to use a generic design so that equipment, staff, and processes can be moved as necessary. Areas that require biosafety level 3 conditions cannot be easily moved, so the laboratory staff should take extra care in choosing a location for these areas.

Specimen Preparation Area

All CMLs need an area to receive and process specimens. This area should be located near the laboratory entrance so that other laboratory staff and couriers do not need to enter the rest of the laboratory to drop off specimens. The area should have ample benchtop space for receiving specimens, for any necessary equipment, and for the handling of specimen requisitions. This area should have one or more class II biological safety cabinets (BSC) to accommodate all initial specimen processing. All necessary information technology (IT) infrastructure and telecommunications equipment should be provided. This area should have a sink for handwashing and for performing Gram's stain and other direct examinations. Some laboratories place a microscope in this area for reading stains, whereas others place microscopes in a separate area of the laboratory. A refrigerator should be located in the specimen preparation area to hold specimens and media. Some laboratories do not have separate incubators for the specimen processing area, opting to place inoculated media directly in the main laboratory incubators, but unless specimens can be placed in these incubators quickly, a holding incubator should be located in the processing area.

The specific design of a specimen preparation area needs to be tailored to the number of specimens that are received, as well as to the types of microbiologic tests that are performed. There is no single design that is optimal for all laboratories. For this reason, and because this is often one of the busiest areas of any microbiology laboratory, the specimen preparation area should receive emphasis during the design phase of the project. The perspective and wishes of experienced technologists are especially important here. Function should drive design.

General Laboratory Bench Space

Work Areas

Many laboratories are constructed on the basis of U-shaped modules or linear benches. Modules typically measure 10 by 10 ft and can accommodate two or three persons. Advantages to the modular approach include minimized foot traffic in work areas, generous countertop and storage space, corner space that is available for computer workstations (corners otherwise are wasted space), an increased sense of privacy for workers, and use of less floor space for aisles and corridors. Advantages to the linear bench approach include ease of cleaning, ease of moving about the laboratory, a subjective sense of less clutter, easier location of large pieces of equipment such as incubators and refrigerators, ease of moving modular casework, and lower design, construction, and renovation costs. Some laboratories use a combination of modules and linear benches. In many cases, the physical layout and constraints of the building determine which approach is best for a given laboratory.

The space surrounding workbenches should be sufficient to accommodate ample waste containers, both for paper and for biohazardous waste. It is inefficient for laboratory staff and housekeepers to empty trash containers more often than is necessary. Ample space should be provided so that aisles are unobstructed and free of clutter, yet aisles that are too wide merely waste space.

The laboratory should contain space for storing completed cultures, stock cultures, reference books, and teaching materials (e.g., parasitology slides). It is most efficient for completed cultures and reference materials to be located close to workbenches. The principle applies to frozen, lyophilized, or viable cultures.

Casework

Laboratory casework can be built-in (custom) or modular. The type of casework selected for a laboratory is, to a large degree, determined by the size of the laboratory. It is expensive to install custom built-in casework in a large laboratory; vendors are able to give better pricing for installing modular furniture in larger facilities. Thus, larger laboratories almost always find it to be more economical to buy commercial modular furniture. Smaller laboratories, on the other hand, may find the opposite to be true. Before making a decision, one needs to be familiar with the advantages and disadvantages of each type of casework.

Built-in casework typically is less expensive to install, can be made from a wider variety of building materials to suit individual tastes, can be very strong, and is durable. It is not unusual to see built-in laboratory casework that is decades old but is still functional and aesthetically pleasing. The disadvantages to built-in casework are that it cannot be moved easily, repairs tend to be more difficult and expensive, modifications (e.g., adding additional power and communication lines) also are more difficult and expensive, and, for the most part, it cannot be reused once it is disassembled. From an interior design standpoint, it has the disadvantage of requiring users to live with the aesthetic choices of predecessors and those characteristic of previous eras.

Modular furniture has been, in part, designed to overcome the disadvantages associated with built-in casework. Specifically, some parts of it can be moved easily, repairs and replacements are easy, modifications are easy and less expensive, and entire units can be disassembled and moved to another location. The converse, however, is equally true: many of the advantages associated with built-in casework are not found in modular furniture. Specifically, modular furniture tends to be more expensive (unless one is buying large quantities, decreasing the unit cost), there is a smaller selection of building materials and colors to suit individual aesthetic tastes, and it tends to be less strong and durable.

It should be noted that one of the main advantages to modular furniture, the ability to move it around, tends to be overstated. This is because the stanchions that support the casework are bolted to the floor, plumbing and drains for sinks are not easily moved, and there are practical limits to moving the electrical power supply and IT and telecommunication cables. In fact, with some commercial modular casework systems, only the cabinets, shelves, and countertops can be moved, and even they can be moved only within the confines of the supporting stanchions.

Air, Gas, and Vacuum Supplies

Most modern laboratories have little need for compressed air, gas, and vacuum supplies, except as needed for specific purposes. Use of open flames should be prohibited, so there is no need for a flammable gas supply. Most health care facilities do not have central systems to supply the types of gases used in microbiological incubators. These should be included within the laboratory facility.

A generous amount of space should be allocated for incubators, refrigerators, freezers, floor-model centrifuges, and floor-model diagnostic equipment (e.g., continuous-monitoring blood culture systems). Electrical power, water supply, telecommunications ports, and other features necessary to support such equipment should be part of the design. The load capacity of the facility should be such that it can support the weight of this equipment, particularly if most of it is to be located in one part of the laboratory.

Special Laboratory Bench Space

Anaerobic Bacteriology

The anaerobic bacteriology capacities needed by most hospital-based CMLs can be accommodated by countertop jars. For larger laboratories, or those with a special interest in anaerobic bacteriology, sufficient space should be allocated to accommodate an anaerobic chamber and gas supply. Countertop models have replaced most of the floor-model anaerobic tents that once were common in laboratories. Some gas-liquid chromatographs require a dedicated exhaust system for discharged gases. Most of the other equipment needed for anaerobic bacteriology does not require special design features.

Mycobacteriology, Mycology, and Virology

An important design requirement for many mycobacteriology, mycology, and virology laboratories is that the facility should meet biosafety level 3 criteria, as described in the following section, in order for the staff to safely handle pathogenic microorganisms such as *Mycobacterium tuberculosis*. In addition to biosafety issues, these laboratories require special equipment not used elsewhere in the CML, such as refrigerated centrifuges, special diagnostic equipment, and the incubators required to hold specimens at various temperatures. Equipment for performing tissue cultures may also be needed. Mycology and mycobacteriology laboratories must have a certified class II BSC.

Biosafety Level 2 and 3 Conditions

Most routine clinical microbiology procedures can be performed safely under biosafety level 2 conditions (15). Even though biosafety level 2 conditions can be met without use of a BSC, use of a BSC protects laboratory workers from laboratory-acquired infections and protects specimens from contamination (8, 16). Moreover, laboratory staff do not always receive sufficient information with specimen requisition forms to know which specimens are likely to contain pathogens that are risky to process (3). Therefore, it is strongly recommended that all specimen processing be done in a class II BSC. Isolates or cultures that are known or likely to contain high-risk microorganisms should be processed only in a class II BSC, particularly fungal and mycobacterial cultures (3, 15). If possible, positive blood and cerebrospinal fluid cultures should also be processed in a class II BSC. Adequate space, power, and ventilation should be provided for each BSC.

Biosafety level 2 conditions are met largely via use of standard microbiological practices (15). In addition to these practices, biosafety level 2 conditions require that (i) laboratory personnel have specific training in handling pathogenic agents, (ii) personnel be directed by competent scientists, (iii) laboratory access be limited when work is being conducted, (iv) extreme precautions be taken in handling contaminated sharp items, and (v) procedures likely to generate infectious aerosols or splashes be conducted in either a class II BSC or other physical containment equipment (15).

Biosafety level 3 conditions include all of the requirements for biosafety level 2 conditions plus special facilities, equipment, and procedures for handling "pathogenic and potentially lethal agents" (15). For those CMLs that do not have the facilities specified for biosafety level 3 conditions, routine microbiologic procedures should be done using biosafety level 2 conditions. Biosafety level 3 practices and protective equipment should be used when handling agents that pose a risk of serious or lethal infection. The specific requirements needed to meet biosafety level 3 conditions are given in reference 15. In brief, these include (i) limited laboratory access; (ii) written policies and procedures for handling agents; (iii) adequate training, proficiency, and competency for handling agents; (iv) use of a class II BSC for handling highly infectious agents; (v) use of adequate face and respiratory protection for procedures done outside a BSC; and (vi) written policies and procedures for handling spills. The facility requirements are given in reference 16. In brief, these include (i) a separate area with access through two sets of self-closing doors; (ii) sealed floors, walls, and ceilings to facilitate decontamination; (iii) a waste disposal system that is available within the area; (iv) a ducted air system that draws clean air from outside the area, with all of the exhaust air (i.e., none of the air is recirculated) discharged to the outside; and (v) the use of HEPA filters in the exhaust of BSCs, in vacuum lines, and in equipment or devices that may produce aerosols or splashes (e.g., centrifuges).

Molecular Microbiology

As for the general microbiology laboratory, planning for a molecular diagnostics laboratory should optimize workspace flexibility, since this technology is rapidly changing and new equipment, methods, and applications will be available in the next few years (6, 12, 14). Prior to establishment of molecular testing, thought must be given to the type of services planned. For example, if the laboratory staff plans to perform only Food and Drug Administration-approved and commercially available kit-based assays, then minimal space and equipment may be all that is needed. Alternatively, if the laboratory staff plans to develop and perform in-house assays, then a significantly greater investment in space, equipment, and technical expertise will be required. In addition, consideration must be given to the specific assays that will be performed, as space and equipment needs vary considerably for different types of assays.

If the laboratory staff plans to perform only commercial amplification kit-based assays, bench space will be needed to accommodate a hood-type work enclosure with a UV light source, an amplification and detection apparatus(es), and a few other pieces of equipment, such as a water bath and a microcentrifuge. As little as 15 linear feet of bench space is needed. To reduce the risk of contamination, two geographically separated work areas are needed. Most commercial kit-based assays include methods to prevent carryover amplification, and automated equipment also may reduce the possibility of carryover, both of which minimize the amount of space that is needed. According to the manufacturers of some commercial diagnostic molecular assays, certain assays can now be performed in a single area and with only minimal need for special handling. Experience will show whether this is an acceptable approach, but it is likely that as the technology of molecular diagnosis changes, there will be a decreasing need for separate areas. As this occurs, laboratories will be able to fully integrate diagnostic molecular assays with the rest of the CML.

Development, validation, and performance of in-house methods that involve amplifying nucleic acids require a more elaborate laboratory. A minimum of 500 ft^2 is required for a small molecular diagnostics laboratory, with three separate workspaces. The three work areas include one for reagent preparation, one for specimen preparation, and a third for amplification. General analysis of DNA or RNA requires an assortment of basic laboratory equipment, as well as specialized equipment. Sources of high-grade deionized water, wet ice, and dry ice are needed, as is an autoclave. A fume hood and storage cabinet for solvents and flammables are also needed. Access to a darkroom is advantageous.

The reagent preparation area is the cleanest of the three work areas and can be located in a separate room, in a hood with the fan turned off to minimize aerosolization, or in an enclosed countertop hood or box. This area is used for the preparation of the master mix and other necessary reagents. To minimize contamination, patient samples, prepared DNA, and amplified products must never be brought into this area. Since equipment can become contaminated with DNA, it is imperative that dedicated equipment be used and stored within this area. Reagents should be stored in a refrigerator free of DNA (and especially amplicons), and disposable items such as tubes, tips, and gloves should also be stored in a manner to prevent their contamination. Staff should wear a designated clean laboratory coat along with clean gloves; staff should leave transportable items (e.g., pens, tape, and scissors) in this area.

The second area is the specimen preparation area. In this area, tubes containing the aliquoted master mix should be brought for the addition of nucleic acid; these tubes should not be returned to the reagent preparation area. Specimen preparation activities can be performed in the open laboratory on a bench but might also be performed in an enclosed space such as a benchtop hood or containment box. After nucleic acid is added to the reaction tubes in this area, the tubes are sealed and placed in the thermocycler for amplification. When removed, the tubes should be taken unopened to the third area for product detection.

The third area is the most contaminated of the three work areas. Laboratory staff should take extreme caution to ensure that laboratory coats, gloves, tube racks, and other equipment are never moved back into the reagent or specimen preparation areas. Some laboratories have opted for separate areas for a darkroom/gel electrophoresis room, a room for processing of radioactive samples, and a room for other functions.

Work Flow

Efficient laboratories are designed so that specimens flow in one direction. Traditional microbiologic testing follows a pathway of specimen receipt and plating, incubation, isolate identification, antimicrobial susceptibility testing, and result reporting. Because this sequence is by its nature linear, CMLs benefit from unidirectional work flow. Unidirectional work flow is also important in molecular microbiology laboratories. In this case, the issue is not so much one of efficiency but rather one of minimizing the risk of amplicon carryover and specimen contamination. While much of this can be accomplished by designing unidirectional work processes, the laboratory facility must accommodate the needs of those processes.

Laboratory Storage

Storage space should be adequate but not excessive. Insufficient storage space makes for a cluttered laboratory; unused storage space makes for a dusty one. Short-term storage capacity should meet the daily needs of the staff and no more. Long-term storage of supplies should be in the main laboratory storage room; there is no reason for long-term storage in the CML itself. Storage space, whether on shelves, in overhead cabinets, or in drawers, should be designed so that workers have most of what they need during the day within arm's reach. Storage space should be designed so that it can be cleaned easily.

Incubators, Refrigerators, and Centrifuges

CMLs should have ample space for large floor-model incubators, refrigerators, and centrifuges. Sufficient aisle space should be allocated next to large units so that the aisle remains unobstructed when a door is opened. Adequate electrical power should be incorporated into the area housing these units, as well as any necessary gas or water supplies. The location of these units should help maximize laboratory efficiency and ensure a unidirectional work flow. As a general rule, a refrigerator and centrifuge should be located in the specimen processing area. Although some CMLs have adopted the principle of scattering incubators and refrigerators throughout the laboratory, with the rationale of minimizing the distance from workbenches, a more efficient use of space is to have a separate area in the laboratory for these large pieces of equipment. This is because these units almost always are wider than countertops are deep, so locating them throughout a laboratory requires the aisles to be wider than would otherwise be necessary. Because the additional space in the other parts of the aisle is not needed, a significant amount of floor space will be wasted.

Handwashing, Water Supply, and Plumbing

The CML should have sufficient sinks to accommodate staining, waste disposal, and handwashing. To prevent laboratory-acquired infections (3, 16), handwashing sinks should be designed so that they can be operated with knee or foot controls. One sink should be located near the laboratory entrance to facilitate handwashing by staff and visitors as they leave the laboratory. Drainpipes should be able to handle the types and volumes of liquid waste generated within the laboratory.

Plumbing is expensive to install at any time but especially so once laboratory construction is completed. In addition, the plumbing and water supply cannot be moved easily in modern buildings, as one must drill through a concrete floor and then work in the ceiling space of the floor below. This space typically is filled with heating, ventilating, and air-conditioning (HVAC) systems, lighting, IT and telecommunications cables, and electrical power lines, making it difficult and expensive to work there. Such a project is also disruptive to the occupants of the floor below. Therefore, the water supply and plumbing needs should be assessed carefully during the design phase of the project.

Countertops

Countertops at workbenches should be 24 in. deep, with work areas no more than 4 to 5 ft wide. A working space of these dimensions is the most efficient because the entire space is within arm's length for most workers. There should be additional space to each side for storage and equipment. Some countertops will need to be deeper to accommodate countertop-model equipment. Heavy pieces of equipment should be on freestanding tables designed to accommodate the necessary weight. Centrifuges should also be on freestanding tables to minimize the transfer of vibrational forces to adjacent countertops. Sensitive analytical balances should be on freestanding tables. Most modular casework systems include tables that are of the same length and width as the individual countertop pieces and which can be integrated into the overall laboratory layout.

The height of workbenches can be that of a desk (29 to 30 in.) or a counter (36 in.). While there are advantages to both heights, use of one or the other is largely a matter of personal preference. Modular furniture can be adjusted to either height, whereas built-in casework obviously is fixed at one height.

Countertops should be made of materials that can be cleaned and disinfected easily, are durable, and can be replaced or repaired as needed. Most countertops in CMLs do not need to be acid resistant. Countertops that are stain resistant are desirable. Countertops adjacent to sinks should be constructed of water-resistant materials so that repeated exposure to water does not damage them. Lighter colors tend to show stains more but have the benefit of making the laboratory brighter. Practical issues aside, colors generally are selected on the basis of interior design needs and personal preference.

Electrical Power Supply

Electrical outlets should be liberal in number and in excess of the current need. These are easily installed during construction, but upgrading the electrical power supply can be expensive and difficult once construction is completed. One important task during the design phase of the project is to perform a comprehensive audit of the electrical needs of the laboratory, particularly as related to 110- versus 220-V power supplies. The need for emergency power supplies should also be assessed, as this requires a separate electrical power supply. Only critical pieces of equipment should be on the emergency power supply. Critical equipment should be wired into a central alarm system so that the appropriate persons can be notified of any power failures.

HVAC

The HVAC system in a clinical laboratory must be designed so that the laboratory meets the necessary biosafety level while maintaining a constant ambient temperature within a narrow range. Thus, the design of an HVAC system is a challenging task for architects and mechanical engineers. Moreover, once installed, an HVAC system cannot be easily modified: it is one of the most expensive parts of construction, it resides in a relatively inaccessible space, and changing the HVAC in one area of a building may have effects in other areas of the building.

Installing an HVAC system is one of the more expensive parts of laboratory construction. Because revising an existing HVAC system can be expensive or impractical, it is imperative that the design and installation be done correctly. Balancing the airflow in a CML is challenging: (i) CMLs must have lower air pressure than in adjacent areas; (ii) air temperatures in a CML must be maintained within a narrow range; (iii) exhaust air from a CML cannot recirculate into the building; and (iv) the HVAC system must accommodate special needs for odor control. Although it is desirable to use special plenums that draw off odors from workbenches (which is of particular concern in the specimen processing area, parasitology section, anaerobic bacteriology section, and autoclave room), these can exhaust large amounts of air from the CML and make balancing the airflow difficult. For all these reasons, adjustments to the HVAC system may be necessary after the laboratory has been occupied.

IT and Telecommunications

General Considerations

The modern clinical laboratory is highly dependent upon IT and telecommunications systems. Modern telecommunications systems are complex and need to support telefax units, sophisticated telephone systems, videoconferencing, and other types of telecommunications. In the same way, modern IT systems need to meet both current and anticipated needs such as the introduction of new versions of operating systems, databases, and other applications. The IT infrastructure should accommodate the larger institution's (e.g., hospital's) health care information system, the laboratory information system, the facility intranet, and the Internet. Ideally, the IT infrastructure should be designed for high-speed access, have redundant data storage and processing capacity, and have sufficient types and numbers of workstations to accommodate changing IT needs. Because the most efficient laboratories are paperless, it is important that the IT infrastructure support this type of environment.

For many laboratory staff members, and certainly for clerical and administrative staff, most of the day is spent using a computer. The computer workstation has become the focus of most offices and many laboratories. A robust IT system supports a variety of applications that are of immediate benefit to the laboratory staff. Any modern laboratory should have the infrastructure needed to support a modern IT system. In particular, the cable plant should be generic in design and have a fiber-optic backbone with a fiber-optic cable to each outlet in the laboratory. This cable architecture accommodates current IT needs but will also facilitate future transition to voice and video capability. There should be redundancy in the network infrastructure. IT and telecommunications systems should be designed so that information retrieval is limited to those who are authorized to access patient records. The design and installation of the IT and telecommunications systems in a laboratory should be done in close collaboration with the information services within the institution. Once systems have been installed, it is expensive or impractical to make changes to the IT and telecommunications infrastructure.

Wireless Networks

The increased use of devices such as wireless-capable laptop computers as workstations, personal digital assistants for data storage and retrieval, pen tablets, and "smart" cellular telephone systems makes it necessary for health care facilities to have wireless networks. The primary advantage of wireless systems is that users can receive and transmit data signals from any location rather than from only those locations that are cabled for network access. Wireless systems can also be used for dispatch and communication for employees who, by the nature of their work, need to be contacted at sites removed from traditional workstations. This type of system is often a Voice over Internet Protocol (VoIP) system, which operates much like a cell phone but works only over the wireless network in a facility. Another wireless application is the use of radio frequency identification, which can be used to tag and track items by using a simple web-based interface.

Offices and Administrative Support

Office space should be located close to but not within the laboratory. Offices should be sufficient to support the managerial, administrative, research, and teaching functions of the laboratory. Just as it makes little sense for a clinical laboratory to be located off-site, it makes equally little sense for the office space that ostensibly supports a laboratory to be in a remote location. Successful clinical and faculty recruitment and retention often hinge on adequate office space. Compared with other parts of a health care facility, office space is inexpensive to build, maintain, and renovate. It is in the long-term interests of the institution to make the modest investment needed for this part of the laboratory.

The process of designing offices should follow the same principles as those that guide the design of a clinical laboratory: offices should be private, quiet, efficient, and pleasant places to work or to visit. Although some institutions have opted for an open office plan where low modular barriers separate offices, open offices do not provide the privacy necessary for counseling employees or for discussing confidential matters, nor are they quiet. Offices should be equipped with the office equipment, IT and telecommunications infrastructure, and other features that are necessary to make them efficient. Many offices that are associated with clinical laboratories are too small to be pleasant places to work or to visit. Although offices should be sufficiently large, offices that are too large waste space, which never is in excess. As a general rule, individual offices should be no smaller than 100 ft^2. Traditional furniture is less efficient than modular furniture; office size should be adjusted according to the type of furniture that is used. Laboratory directors and supervisors should have offices that are large enough to accommodate several persons during meetings. Offices of up to 200 ft^2 are not unreasonable for directors.

Work Environment

Ergonomic considerations should receive emphasis in laboratory design. Casework, drawers, shelves, keyboard trays, lighting, and space should all be designed according to ergonomic standards. Both ceiling and task lighting should be abundant and well placed. Signs, bulletin boards, and other means of communication should be placed where laboratory staff and visitors can easily see them. A modest investment in the ergonomic and aesthetic properties in the laboratory will go a long way toward making it a pleasant and efficient workplace.

Safety and Security

As stated in the introduction, above all other considerations, a laboratory should be a safe place. For general safety considerations, this can be achieved by ensuring that the laboratory meets all building codes and architectural standards related to safety. For safety considerations related to the practice of clinical microbiology, this can be achieved by designing the laboratory to meet biosafety level 2 criteria and, where necessary, biosafety level 3 criteria.

Clinical laboratories must meet the safety and security requirements of accrediting and regulatory bodies. Eyewash stations, safety showers, sprinkler systems, fire extinguishers and blankets, fire alarms, spill control kits, and emergency power and lighting should be included as specified by building codes. Water supplies should have either backflow preventers or vacuum breaker devices to prevent the inadvertent contamination of potable water supplies.

The laboratory should be designed so that it can be secured during off-hours, or when staffing is minimal. Institution-specific security concerns will guide the need for more comprehensive security assets such as security cameras, restricted access, or electronic monitoring of access.

Cleaning and Waste Handling

A clinical laboratory should be designed so that it can be cleaned easily. All surfaces should be made of materials that are easily cleaned and disinfected. Carpet should never be used as a floor material in a clinical laboratory. To facilitate cleaning, floors should be kept free of clutter; there is no excuse for using floors in a clinical laboratory for storage space.

The laboratory design should accommodate the handling of the large amounts of biohazardous waste that are generated each day. There should be adequate space for waste containers within the laboratory, for biohazardous waste as well as standard waste. Large bins for both types of waste should be located outside the laboratory but nearby. Large pieces of floor-model equipment should be permanently housed on wheels so that they can be moved easily for cleaning. A housekeeping closet should be located close to the laboratory to facilitate daily cleaning.

Some laboratories maintain an on-site autoclave for medium preparation or decontamination of wastes. Some smaller autoclaves are self-contained, but larger autoclaves require steam lines that must be taken into account early in the design process.

THE DESIGN AND CONSTRUCTION PROCESS

Predesign Phase

Beginning the Process

Architecture, engineering, and construction are complex disciplines. Just as one cannot expect a clinical microbiologist to be familiar with the terminology, processes, and regulations of those disciplines, one should not expect an architect, engineer, or contractor to be familiar with the terminology, processes, and regulations that guide the day-to-day operations of a clinical laboratory. Thus, perhaps the most important skill needed to initiate and complete a design or renovation project is communication. Successful design, construction, and renovation projects are characterized by a commitment to education and communication. This is of particular importance when any of the parties who are involved in the project have little or no prior experience in designing or renovating a laboratory. It is not unusual to meet architects, engineers, or contractors who have no experience with clinical laboratories, just as it is not unusual to meet laboratorians who have never been involved with a laboratory construction or renovation project. It is also not unusual to meet architects, engineers, or contractors who have experience with research or industrial laboratories but not clinical laboratories. Experience with the former does not necessarily translate into expertise in the latter. To facilitate communication and education, it is important to have a clear understanding of the experience and expertise of all the parties who will be involved with the project.

Laboratory Representative

The first step in designing a laboratory is for the laboratory administration to appoint a person who will be the spokesperson throughout the design and construction process. Such an appointment should not be made or taken lightly; this is a significant commitment of time and energy that will extend over one or more years. The laboratory administration must give this person the time needed to meet the commitment, as well as the responsibility and authority to make many decisions, often on short notice. Because so many persons are involved in construction and renovation projects, because projects take so long to complete, and because the staff must live with the outcome for many years, the laboratory representative must have a clear understanding of budget constraints, space allocations, laboratory operations, and hospital and clinic operations. There must be clear lines of communication and authority. The laboratory representative should be selected carefully on the basis of communication skills, experience in laboratory administration, and decision-making ability. This person need not be the laboratory director, although the director generally is in a better position to negotiate for necessary resources than is a senior technologist.

Budget and Space Allocations

The next step in designing a laboratory is to assess, realistically and accurately, the current and future needs of the laboratory, as well as the resources required to meet those needs. Both new and renovated laboratories should be designed to accommodate future expansion of test volume and type. This includes planning for office space, specimen receiving and processing, benches, informatics, communications, and the introduction of automation and future test technologies.

The next step is to obtain realistic design and construction budgets. Hospital laboratory construction is expensive. Nonetheless, fiscal constraints should not interfere with designing and building a safe and efficient laboratory. Along the same lines, realistic allocations of space must be done prior to the design phase. It is expensive and wasteful to design a laboratory and then to be faced with redesigning all or part of it to accommodate changes in the budget or space allocations. An adequate investment to do the project right in the first place is the most economical approach to providing a functional laboratory.

Part of developing a realistic and accurate budget is to decide whether to build a new laboratory or to renovate an older one. This obviously involves decisions about the health care facility as a whole. Estimating the costs of new construction (whether for a new building or expansion of an existing one) is generally straightforward. In contrast, estimating the costs of renovations is challenging. First, original construction drawings may not be available or may no longer be accurate due to changes made after the original construction was completed. Thus, the architect and engineer may have limited knowledge of how the laboratory was constructed or modified. Second, laboratories built according to past architectural standards and building codes may not meet current standards and codes. Third, older facilities are likely to contain asbestos in insulating material and/or floor tiles, as well as lead-based paint. Abating either material is a complex and expensive process. Fourth, older buildings were often built with fixed ceilings and walls, complicating changes in lighting, the HVAC system, IT and telecommunications cabling, plumbing, and the electrical power supply. Fifth, some older buildings do not have the load capacity to support heavy pieces of equipment. Last, construction in older buildings often reveals unexpected issues that must be addressed, adding to the cost and complexity of the project. It is for these and other reasons that it may cost more to renovate an existing building than it would to build a new one.

Design Phase

Several general principles should guide the design phase (10). First, the greater the investment in planning, the more likely a project will be completed on time and under budget. Second, users will be happy with the results of a project only if they believe that they have been able to make significant contributions to it. Third, there need to be clear lines of accountability and communication. Fourth, user expectations should be expressed clearly and unequivocally at the outset; no architect or engineer should be expected to make major changes midway in a project. Last, logic and common sense should guide decisions throughout the process (5).

The first task for the architect, designer, and engineer (the design team) is to understand who the laboratory representative will be, who will have authority to make decisions, and the limits of the budget and space allocations. The next task is for them to learn the needs of the laboratory. These tasks should be undertaken in this order; it is important for the design team to know the constraints of the project before the design phase begins. Once the design team has completed these tasks, the knowledge gained can be used to develop realistic and workable design plans. As the design phase continues, it is for the most part largely one in which the design team works with the laboratory staff to accommodate the needs of the laboratory within the constraints of the project. In many cases, there will be insufficient space or funds to accommodate the needs of the laboratory; in cases such as this, either the laboratory administration must acquire the necessary space or funds or the project will need to be scaled back.

Once preliminary design plans have been drafted and agreed upon, the laboratory staff must address the myriad of details necessary to design a functional laboratory. Every conceivable detail should be thought of and addressed. Nothing should be taken for granted. It is far less expensive and easier to remove features from a design plan than it is to add them at a later point, particularly during the construction phase. The latter process, known as change orders, is one of the most common reasons for construction projects to go over budget. An even thornier problem is the feature that should have been included but cannot be added at any cost once construction has begun.

After final construction documents have been drafted and approved, bids will be requested from general contractors.

Any necessary specifications should be included in the request-for-bids document. Once a general contractor has been selected, that contractor will recruit subcontractors to provide services that the general contractor does not provide. The last step prior to construction is for the institution and general contractor to obtain all necessary building permits and other legal documents needed for the project.

Construction Phase

For new laboratory construction, the construction phase generally proceeds for some time before the laboratory representative needs to be involved. The point at which the laboratory representative needs to work closely with the contractor is when the contractor begins to install walls, electrical power, IT and telecommunications cables, plumbing, and casework. From this point on, the laboratory representative will be called upon to make many unexpected decisions, often on short notice, and to clarify ambiguities in construction documents. It is expensive to make changes at this point in the process, but necessary changes should be made at this time rather than years later, when costs are even higher and the disruption in the laboratory makes the changes impractical.

Renovation projects vary in the amount and types of construction that are needed. Many projects require minimal demolition and few changes to the HVAC, plumbing, electrical power supply, and telecommunications and IT systems. In projects such as these, many of the changes are in casework only, or are more cosmetic in nature, and can be accomplished while the laboratory continues to operate. For more extensive renovations, the required demolition makes it necessary to gut the laboratory, in which case the project more closely resembles that of constructing a new laboratory.

Postconstruction Phase

The postconstruction phase is one of the most important, yet often neglected, phases in the process. Almost all construction projects have a warranty, usually for a short period, and the postconstruction phase provides the opportunity to use the warranty to correct things that were not completed or were done incorrectly. The laboratory staff should monitor carefully everything associated with the project, record their findings, and communicate them to the general contractor at the earliest possible time. The longer one waits, the more difficult it becomes for the contractor to return to the site to correct problems. Once the warranty has expired, then it becomes expensive to fix something that could have been done earlier at no cost.

SUMMARY

The construction of a new clinical laboratory, or the renovation of an existing one, is an excellent opportunity to improve the operations and efficiency of a clinical laboratory. It also offers the laboratory staff an opportunity to assess existing laboratory processes and to modify them. A successful construction or renovation project is characterized by the investment of large amounts of time in planning and designing the new facility, good communication between all of the parties involved in the project, a logical and common-sense approach to the project, and realistic expectations. Done well, a new or renovated laboratory facility will accommodate the needs of the laboratory staff for many years.

RESOURCES

Some general resources are listed in the references (1, 2, 5, 9, 10). The reader who needs additional information should consult The American Institute of Architects (http://www.aia.org/). The Institute can provide additional information, including a list of architects in a given area who have experience in designing laboratories and other health care facilities.

REFERENCES

1. **American Institute of Architects Academy of Architecture for Health and The Facilities Guidelines Institute.** 2001. *Guidelines for Design and Construction of Hospital and Health Care Facilities.* American Institute of Architects, Washington, D.C.
2. **College of American Pathologists.** 1985. *Medical Laboratory Planning and Design.* College of American Pathologists, Skokie, Ill.
3. **Collins, C. H.** 1993. *Laboratory-Acquired Infections,* 3rd ed. Butterworth-Heinemann, Oxford, United Kingdom.
4. **Crane, J. T., and J. F. Riley.** 1997. Design issues in the comprehensive BSL2 and BSL3 laboratory, p. 63–114. *In* J. Y. Richmond (ed.), *Designing a Modern Microbiological/Biomedical Laboratory.* American Public Health Association, Washington, D.C.
5. **Crane, J. T., and J. Y. Richmond.** 2000. Design of biomedical laboratory facilities, p. 283–311. *In* D. O. Fleming and D. L. Hunt (ed.), *Biological Safety: Principles and Practices,* 3rd ed. American Society for Microbiology, Washington, D.C.
6. **Furrows, S. J., and G. L. Ridgway.** 2001. 'Good laboratory practice' in diagnostic laboratories using nucleic acid amplification methods. *Clin. Microbiol. Infect.* **7:**227–229.
7. **Infectious Diseases Society of America.** 2001. Policy statement on consolidation of clinical microbiology laboratories. *Clin. Infect. Dis.* **32:**604.
8. **Kruse, R. H., W. H. Puckett, and J. H. Richardson.** 1991. Biological safety cabinetry. *Clin. Microbiol. Rev.* **4:**207–241.
9. **National Committee for Clinical Laboratory Standards.** 1998. *Laboratory Design. Approved Guideline.* Document GP 18-A. National Committee for Clinical Laboratory Standards, Wayne, Pa.
10. **National Research Council.** 2000. *Laboratory Design, Construction, and Renovation.* National Academy Press, Washington, D.C.
11. **Peterson, L. R., J. D. Hamilton, E. J. Baron, L. S. Tompkins, J. M. Miller, C. M. Wilfert, F. C. Tenover, and R. B. Thomson.** 2001. Role of clinical microbiology laboratories in the management and control of infectious diseases and the delivery of health care. *Clin. Infect. Dis.* **32:** 605–610.
12. **Pfaller, M. A., and L. A. Herwaldt.** 1997. The clinical microbiology laboratory and infection control: emerging pathogens, antimicrobial resistance, and new technology. *Clin. Infect. Dis.* **25:**858–870.
13. **Procop, G. W., and W. Winn; for the Microbiology Resource Committee, College of American Pathologists.** 2003. Outsourcing microbiology and offsite laboratories. Implications on patient care, cost savings, and graduate medical education. *Arch. Pathol. Lab. Med.* **127:**623–624.
14. **Scheckler, W. E., D. Brimhall, A. S. Buck, B. M. Farr, C. Friedman, R. A. Garibaldi, P. A. Gross, J. A. Harris, W. J. Hierholzer, W. J. Martone, L. L. McDonald, and S. L. Solomon.** 1998. Requirements for infrastructure and essential activities of infection control and epidemiology in hospitals: a consensus panel report. *Am. J. Infect. Control* **26:**47–60.
15. **U.S. Department of Health and Human Services, Centers for Disease Control and Prevention, and**

National Institutes of Health. 1999. *Biosafety in Microbiological and Biomedical Laboratories,* 4th ed. J. Y. Richmond and R. W. McKinney (ed.). U.S. Government Printing Office, Washington, D.C.

16. **Wilson, M. L., and L. B. Reller.** 1998. Clinical laboratory-acquired infections, p. 343–355. *In* P. Brachman and J. Bennett (ed.), *Hospital Infections,* 4th ed. Lippincott-Raven, Philadelphia, Pa.

Laboratory Consultation, Communication, and Information Systems

JOSEPH M. CAMPOS

4

The flow of information to and from clinical laboratories was revolutionized more than 30 years ago by the introduction of the first computerized laboratory information system (LIS) (2, 13). The initial rationale for a computerized LIS was purely financial; namely, the LIS enabled more efficient billing for laboratory services. Shortly thereafter, improved reporting of textual and numerical test results was enabled by the evolving feature set. Clinical microbiology laboratories began reaping important benefits when it became possible to issue culture and complex antimicrobial susceptibility reports via the LIS.

LISs continue to thrive in the clinical microbiology laboratory today. These laboratories furnish vital information to health care providers, especially those who manage patients with infectious diseases. Laboratory test results essential for the diagnosis and treatment of infections can be reported in a clear and logically presented manner via the LIS. Additional information that promotes optimum patient management, such as guidance for specimen collection, interpretation of test results, and suggestions for additional testing, can also be added (16). Clinical microbiologists today are brokers of critical information that strongly benefits patient care (20). The goal of this chapter is to review the state of information management in clinical microbiology laboratories today, emphasizing the central role of the LIS.

HEALTH INSURANCE PORTABILITY AND ACCOUNTABILITY ACT OF 1996

A significant event that greatly affects the management of health care information in the United States was the passage of the Health Insurance Portability and Accountability Act of 1996 (HIPAA). HIPAA has had an influence so enormous that it is appropriate to begin this chapter with a description of its impact. One of its primary purposes is to maintain the security and privacy of information found in patient medical records. The standards also address the mechanisms by which information can be coded and exchanged electronically. This exchange includes the distribution of laboratory test data to clinicians, insurers, and patients.

HIPAA governs the manner in which patient-specific health information can be generated, disseminated, and stored in the United States (26). A related regulation intended to assist in the implementation of HIPAA was also promulgated and is entitled *Standards for Privacy of Individually Identifiable Health Information* (the Privacy Rule) (21). It was crafted by the Department of Health and Human Services and became effective on 14 April 2001. Most health care institutions and health care plans were obligated to comply with the Privacy Rule by 14 April 2003. Small health care plans were able to delay compliance until 14 April 2004. Although the provisions of HIPAA and the Privacy Rule do not apply to health care organizations outside of the United States, they establish standards for handling patient information that are relevant to and worthy of consideration by governments in all countries.

The Privacy Rule characterizes the safeguards that health care providers must take to protect the privacy of health information. It establishes standards that protect the medical records and other personal health information of patients. It provides patients more control over their own health data and defines limits on the use and distribution of health records by other entities. It declares that patients are entitled to examine and obtain copies of their own health records and to request that mistaken information be corrected. Patients are also at liberty to find out what disclosures of their health information have been made and to whom. The Privacy Rule holds violators of the standards accountable for their actions by the imposition of civil and criminal penalties. It does, however, permit disclosure of patient-specific health information to public health authorities in order to protect the general public health.

Patient-specific data produced by clinical microbiology laboratories in the United States fall under the jurisdiction of HIPAA. It does not matter whether the information is verbal, written, or electronic. The information may be distributed during the preanalytical, analytical, or postanalytical phase of testing and may be advisory, instructional, results oriented, or interpretive. Clinical microbiologists are expected to deliver this information to health care providers in a timely and comprehensible fashion without violating the tenets of HIPAA.

BUILDING THE MICROBIOLOGY COMPONENTS OF LISs

The LISs in use today offer many tools that support the communication of information between clinical microbiology laboratories and health care providers. In order to capitalize on these tools, the individuals responsible for building the microbiology component of the LIS must thoroughly understand microbiology testing. Ideally, these individuals should be clinical microbiologists with a strong interest in and commitment to building their module of the LIS. If this arrangement is not possible, the builders of the microbiology module should request and receive close guidance from clinical microbiologists during system configuration and validation testing.

In an increasing number of health care facilities, laboratory tests are no longer ordered directly in the LIS by laboratory personnel but instead are requested by clinicians using a computerized order entry system with an electronic interface with the LIS. Under this circumstance, clinical microbiologists must have major input during the selection and formatting of information that will be seen by those ordering microbiology tests in any of these accessory systems. This may require clinical microbiologists to insist that they participate in the order entry information system building and/or validation process. Too often, laboratory personnel are overlooked when teams are assembled for this purpose.

The ordering of microbiology tests and the viewing of microbiology test results are different from those in other laboratory disciplines. Specimens for microbiology testing are collected from a variety of body sites, and there must be a provision in the ordering information system to inform the laboratory from whence specimens were collected. Because the quality of microbiology specimens often deteriorates with time, the time of specimen collection should be documented during the ordering process. Microbiology test results are usually nonnumerical and consist of complex composites of text and tables of antimicrobial susceptibility data. In some instances, initial microbiology test results prompt the automatic ordering of "reflex" tests (e.g., the ordering of antimicrobial susceptibility tests when culture results are positive).

Test Codes

As they are built into the LIS, all laboratory tests are assigned codes (mnemonics) and code translations. It is advantageous if a rigorously applied convention is used during the code assignment process. Logically devised coding conventions promote the remembrance of codes by LIS users. Most systems permit codes of up to six characters in length and allow codes to contain both alphabetical and numerical characters. Although many laboratories depend on alphabetical codes abstracted from actual test names (e.g., URICUL for urine culture and BLOCUL for blood culture), some laboratories use predominantly numerical coding schemes to match codes in other institutional information systems and to eliminate code conflicts among tests with similar names.

A laboratory test may have more than one name in general use (e.g., syphilis serology and the rapid plasma reagin [RPR] test). It is advisable that cross-references to commonly used synonyms for a test be identified during test building so that user-initiated searches for different names for a test will link to the same test code. Otherwise, LIS users will lose patience when they are unable to find a test that they wish to order and they will order it inappropriately as a miscellaneous test.

Entering Results While Ordering Tests

Some LISs allow or even require that results for one or more components of a test or battery be entered during the ordering process. This is often true for microbiology cultures, in which the specimen description is one of the test or battery components. When specimen descriptions are predictable for tests (e.g., a pharyngeal swab for a pharyngeal culture), it is helpful if the LIS can automatically answer the specimen description with a default specimen code. This streamlines the ordering process and eliminates ordering errors. Of course, default specimen description codes should be overridable when appropriate.

TABLE 1 Sample LIS test and battery names and their pending texts[a]

Name	Pending text
Aerobic blood culture	Results in <5 days
CSF culture and Gram stain	Results in <72 h
Fungal culture	Results in <21 days
GC culture	Results in <72 h
Bordetella pertussis culture	Results in <7 days
Urine culture	Results in <24 h
CMV culture	Results in <48 h (M–F)
Res Vir antigen panel	Results in <24 h
Group A *Streptococcus* detection	Results in <2 h
RPR	Results in <24 h

[a] Abbreviations: GC, *Neisseria gonorrhoeae;* CMV, cytomegalovirus; Res Vir, respiratory virus; M–F, Monday through Friday.

Pending Text

Some LISs can be configured to display informative text automatically while test results are pending (Table 1). Examples of "pending text" that might be used with microbiology tests include the expected turnaround time for test results, a telephone number to call if there are questions regarding the test, or a notice that a reflex test will be ordered if the result is positive. The pending text ceases to display once test results have been entered into the LIS.

Text Code Dictionaries

Perhaps the largest effort during the building of the microbiology section of an LIS is in preparing the text code dictionaries. Several dictionaries must be built, including those for microbiology text codes, microbiology method codes, growth medium codes, workload codes, antimicrobial susceptibility codes, specimen description codes, and microorganism name codes.

During the creation of the microbiology dictionaries, an important decision must be made regarding the assignment of microorganism name codes. The use of a consistently applied scheme that is understood by microbiology laboratory personnel simplifies the entry of culture results, since the correct codes for most microorganisms can be determined "on the fly." One coding convention in common use is to take the first letter of the microorganism's genus name and the first several letters of the species name (Table 2). A limitation of this system occurs when codes for different microorganisms turn out to be identical (e.g., ECOLI for both *Escherichia coli* and *Entamoeba coli*). Another system used by some laboratories is to take the first three letters of the genus name and the first three letters of the species name (assuming that the LIS permits six-letter codes). In this case, the mnemonic for *E. coli* the bacterium would be ESCCOL and that for *E. coli* the protozoan would be ENT COL. However, problems still occur in assigning codes for microorganisms like *Oligella ureolytica* and *Oligella urethralis* (OLIURE in both instances). Any coding system utilized will encounter its own set of problems, and thus a secondary

TABLE 2 Sample microorganism name codes and their translations

Microorganism code	Translation
AACTI	*Actinobacillus (Haemophilus) actinomycetemcomitans*
ABAUM	*Acinetobacter baumannii*
ABIOSP	*Abiotrophia (Granulicatella)* sp. (nutritionally variant *Streptococcus*)
ABOVI	*Actinomyces bovis*
ABSISP	*Absidia* sp.
ACANSP	*Acanthamoeba* sp.
ACAVI	*Aeromonas caviae*
ACHRSP	*Achromobacter* sp.
ACIDSP	*Acidiminococcus* sp.
ACINSP	*Acinetobacter* sp.

system should be used when codes specified by the primary convention are ambiguous (e.g., use ECOLI for the bacterium and ENCOLI for the protozoan).

Some LISs permit the creation of group codes for microorganisms that enable users to refer to a group of related microorganisms simultaneously. Generally, group members share a property in common. Examples of group codes might be ANA for anaerobes, GNB for gram-negative bacilli, MOLD for filamentous fungi, and VIRUS for viruses. Rational assignment of microorganisms to groups should be done by individuals with an understanding of both the microbiology laboratory and the planned uses for microorganism group codes in the LIS.

Antimicrobial Susceptibility Batteries

The creation of antimicrobial susceptibility batteries is an essential part of building the microbiology section of an LIS. This undertaking is preceded by defining antimicrobial agent tests that yield numerical results or text codes indicating whether isolates are susceptible, intermediately susceptible, or resistant. Groups of these tests are then assembled to correspond to batteries of antimicrobial agents reflective of the reporting wishes of the laboratory. Separate batteries are usually defined for different categories of microorganisms, like gram-negative bacilli, gram-positive cocci, anaerobes, gram-negative urinary tract isolates, streptococci, and enterococci, among others. In some cases, a separate battery should be created for a single microorganism species (e.g., *Streptococcus pneumoniae*) if that is consistent with accepted local practices (e.g., standards promulgated by the Clinical and Laboratory Standards Institute [CLSI] in the United States) (10). When an isolate belongs to more than one isolate category (e.g., a urine culture isolate of *Escherichia coli* belongs to both the gram-negative bacilli and gram-negative urinary tract isolate categories), then the category that describes the isolate more specifically should take precedence (gram-negative urinary tract isolate battery in this example).

The group of antimicrobial agents assigned to each battery should be based on input from clinicians (particularly infectious diseases physicians), from the microbiology laboratory, and from the recommendations published by the CLSI (10). Many LISs permit the recording and storage of results for a large group of antimicrobial agents but selective reporting of only a limited group of results (e.g., those for agents present in the hospital formulary). As a cost containment initiative, some LISs enable the cascading of results so that a result for an expensive or potentially toxic agent is displayed only if the result for a less expensive or less toxic alternative is resistant (e.g., a ceftriaxone result for *Escherichia coli* is reported only if the cefazolin result is resistant). The decisions of which results to report under different situations should be based on a consensus of the groups mentioned above.

Before antimicrobial susceptibility results can be reported, specific text codes (antimicrobial susceptibility codes) must be defined for the standard designations of susceptible, intermediately susceptible, and resistant (e.g., S for susceptible, I for intermediately susceptible, and R for resistant). Some LISs offer the option of defining additional antimicrobial susceptibility codes that can be used creatively for crafting more functional antimicrobial susceptibility reports. For example, codes can be placed in antimicrobial susceptibility reports to remind technologists to take specific actions. A code like NOINTP can be used to indicate that testing of a particular antimicrobial agent versus a specific microorganism has not been standardized by the CLSI. A code like ESBL can be in place for expressing results for ceftazidime versus *Escherichia coli, Klebsiella pneumoniae, Klebsiella oxytoca,* and *Proteus mirabilis* when the MIC is >1 μg/ml. This code would remind technologists to check isolates for extended-spectrum beta-lactamase production before final reports are issued.

Sophisticated antimicrobial susceptibility reports that include cost information and recommended dosages for antimicrobial agents can be created by some LISs. Reports containing relative or actual cost information reduce pharmacy expenditures by encouraging clinicians to select less expensive antimicrobial agents that still show excellent in vitro activity. Reports with dosage recommendations are particularly helpful in hospitals where medical student, intern, and resident training is taking place.

Billing for Laboratory Tests

The driving force that led to the development of the first LIS was a desire to capture laboratory test billing more efficiently than could be accomplished manually. Because billing transactions could be initiated automatically upon test ordering or upon specimen receipt, it was no longer necessary to complete paper charge tickets that were manually transcribed into ledgers or stand-alone electronic billing systems (23).

Microbiology billing can be more complicated than that in other laboratory sections due to the automatic ordering of follow-up tests (e.g., a laboratory-initiated order for an antimicrobial susceptibility test when a clinically significant microorganism is detected by culture). Such reflex orders may follow initial culture orders by several days, raising the possibility in the United States of difficult-to-reimburse late charges if the billing transactions are handled improperly. Fortunately, most LISs are sophisticated enough to handle billing for laboratory-initiated orders in a manner satisfactory to payers for laboratory services.

Current procedural terminology (CPT) codes were first devised by the American Medical Association in 1966. Among the 8,736 codes in the current 2006 listing is a small group applicable to microbiology testing. Fee-for-service reimbursement for laboratory testing is dependent upon inclusion of the appropriate CPT code(s) in bills for laboratory services rendered. The construction of test and battery billing maintenance in LISs includes indicating the applicable CPT codes so that these critical bits of information can be forwarded electronically to the hospital billing information system. Although significant improvement in the description of microbiology CPT codes has occurred in recent years, enough ambiguity yet remains that individuals with microbiology expertise should be involved in entering CPT codes into the LIS.

Most vendors have fashioned their LIS microbiology modules so that billing for the most frequent reflex test, antimicrobial susceptibility testing, occurs automatically without manual intervention. The billing transaction includes the appropriate CPT code for sending to the hospital billing information system. It is also feasible with some LISs to use the same automatic billing feature to charge for other reflex tests, such as Western blotting for human immunodeficiency virus type 1 (HIV-1) antibody-positive specimens and confirmatory fluorescent treponemal antibody testing for RPR-positive specimens. In these situations, the reflex test can be built in a manner similar to an antimicrobial agent battery. Each band on a Western blot strip, for example, could be defined as an antimicrobial agent test, and unique susceptibility result codes could be defined to indicate the presence or absence of each antibody band. Apart from the automatic billing feature, this approach offers the benefit of querying results from these other reflex tests using LIS microbiology report functionality.

Microbiology laboratories are allowed to bill additionally for specific activities performed during specimen processing or identification of isolates (Table 3). Examples include the grinding of tissue prior to culture inoculation and the performance of three or more biochemical tests to identify a culture isolate. Since these activities apply only to certain specimens or cultures, they need to be billed on an ad hoc basis. This is accomplished via technologist entry of charges into the LIS as the charges are incurred. Alternatively, charges can be entered as a group when final culture results are issued.

LIS Work Sheets

Individual work sheets (or work lists) are used to group similar laboratory tests within the LIS, providing a convenient way to divide the laboratory workload among technologists. Individual work sheets can be printed by technologists at the beginning of a work shift to obtain lists of specimens or cultures that require their attention that day. Work sheets also can be printed at the end of a work shift to double-check that specimens or cultures were not overlooked. The statuses of tests assigned to individual work sheets can be monitored by calling up standard LIS reports. Examples of these reports are those that provide lists of pending test results and overdue test results.

Microbiology tests are usually assigned to work sheets that correspond to laboratory workbenches, such as the blood culture bench, the respiratory culture bench, and the urine culture bench. For this reason, individuals who understand how the microbiology laboratory is organized should have a voice in assigning tests to work sheets.

Some LISs permit the definition of group work sheets, which are groups of individual work sheets that have characteristics in common (Table 4). Group work sheets are of utility to microbiologists with supervisory responsibilities that span more than one workbench. If the microbiology laboratory staff includes separate section supervisors responsible for bacterial testing, fungal testing, and virologic testing, group work sheets can be defined that enable each section supervisor to monitor the statuses of tests in his or her domain. Similarly, an all-encompassing group work sheet can be defined that includes all of the microbiology individual work sheets. By calling up this work sheet, the laboratory supervisor or director can monitor all tests being worked on in the laboratory.

Work sheet maintenance may include the option of defining the number of days following specimen receipt at which results from tests assigned to individual work sheets are considered overdue. For the overdue log to be functional, the results of tests assigned to individual work sheets must become overdue after the same period of time. It would be impractical to place routine blood cultures (incubated for 5 days) and fungal blood cultures (incubated for 21 days) on the same work sheet if the overdue log is going to be used.

LIS Rules

LIS rules enable laboratories to eliminate errors, automate certain tasks, and minimize manual data entry (3, 30). Rules can apply preanalytically to guide the ordering of tests based on the patient's age, the patient's diagnosis, or previous results in the patient's laboratory file. They also can be used to identify unnecessary test orders to eliminate wastage of reagents and technologist time. Rules can be used during the analytical phase of testing to flag questionable antimicrobial susceptibility results or to remind technologists to report critical test results by telephone. Rules can be triggered

TABLE 3 Examples of manually billed microbiology tests[a]

Bill code	Name	CPT code(s)
M8011H	Bacterial ID (aerobic) × 1	87077
M8012H	Bacterial ID (aerobic) × 2	87077 × 2
M8013H	Bacterial ID (aerobic) × 3	87077 × 3
M8016H	Bacterial ID (anaerobic) × 1	87076
M8031H	Yeast ID × 1	87106
M8035H	Mold ID × 1	87107
M8041H	Viral ID × 1	87253
M8056H	ID by gas-liquid chromatography	87143
M8025H	ID by nucleic acid probe	87149
M8058H	ID by pulsed-field gel electrophoresis	87152
M8051H	Serogrouping by agglutination × 1	87147
M8061H	Concn for AFB smear or culture	87015
M8071H	Mycobacterial ID	87118
M8076H	Macroscopic ID (helminth)	87169
M8077H	Macroscopic ID (arthropod)	87168
M8081H	Tissue homogenization	87176

[a] Abbreviations: ID, identification; AFB, acid-fast bacillus.

TABLE 4 Sample group work sheet codes and names

Work sheet code	Work sheet name
BLOOD	Blood cultures
CSF	CSF cultures
MISCEL	Miscellaneous cultures
RESPIR	Respiratory cultures
URINE	Urine cultures
ANA	Anaerobic cultures
MYCOB	Mycobacterial cultures
MYCOL	Mycology cultures
SEROL	Serologic tests
PARA	Parasitology exams
MICRO	Microbiology group
VIROL	Virology group
MICVIR	Microbiology-virology group

postanalytically to provide clinicians with predefined interpretive comments that clarify the clinical significance of test results and recommend additional testing to consider. The creation of LIS rules suitable for microbiology testing requires individuals who understand both the laboratory and the capability of the rules engine.

LIS rules usually are defined as "if-then" statements. An "if" statement specifies the condition that triggers a rule. A "then" statement describes the actions to be taken when an "if" condition is met. An example of a commonly employed microbiology rule is as follows: if a *Staphylococcus aureus* isolate is resistant to oxacillin ("if" statement), then the susceptibility results for all beta-lactam antimicrobial agents should be reported as resistant ("then" statement). Sophisticated rules engines can process more complex "if-then" statements that include multiple conditions linked by operators such as "and," "or," "greater than," "less than," and "equal to."

Rules should be organized into one or more hierarchies. One hierarchy should define the points at which rules should be executed. This is important because when two or more rules apply in temporal proximity to one another, the corresponding actions should be taken in a logical sequence. For example, separate rules that call for ordering a "clean catch" urine culture for patients older than 18 years and then conditionally reporting a fluoroquinolone susceptibility result if the culture result is positive need to be evaluated in the correct order. The execution point for the rule concerning patient age is at the ordering stage and that for the rule regarding susceptibility testing is at the results stage. The logical order for executing these rules is (i) order rule and (ii) results rule, with the results rule being applied only if the order rule has already been executed. This sequence prevents the results rule from causing a fluoroquinolone susceptibility result to be reported for a patient of less than 18 years of age.

A second hierarchy should determine the action sequence when two or more applicable rules have the same execution point. Examples here are (i) a rule that prevents the ordering of duplicate rotavirus antigen tests for the same patient within 24 h and (ii) a rule that adds a rotavirus antigen test to a culture order for stool specimens collected by the emergency department from patients of less than 12 months of age between 1 January and 30 April. Many rules engines in this situation would execute the rules in the order they were created. Logically, the laboratory's intent is for the rule that prevents the ordering of a second rotavirus assay to take precedence over the rule that automatically orders a rotavirus test.

INFORMATION SHARING DURING THE PREANALYTICAL PHASE OF TESTING

During the preanalytical phase of testing, clinicians wish to select tests that are likely to provide diagnostically useful or therapeutically important information. Clinical microbiologists can be extremely helpful during this phase by supplying information that assists in appropriate test selection.

Laboratory Test Catalog

An important way in which clinical microbiologists benefit patient care is by assisting clinicians in selecting tests to order in a rational manner. This assistance can be offered by fielding telephone queries. However, a more effective method that is available at all times is to develop a catalog of tests that is comprehensive, information rich, and easily accessed.

The laboratory test catalog should be a dynamic document. When new diagnostic tests become available, whether they are performed in-house or not, the list of tests available to clinicians should be updated. Strong consideration should be given to supplying more than just the names of tests. Specimen requirements (including minimum quantity, collection container, and transport conditions), expected turnaround times for test results, and charges for tests are among the relevant bits of information that should be included (Table 5).

Many commercial laboratories publish catalogs on paper that are distributed to ordering sites throughout their customer base. Some laboratories prepare catalogs in a looseleaf format that enables easy updating as new tests are added

TABLE 5 Sample catalog information about CSF culture and Gram stain[a]

Category	Information
1. Name of test	CSF culture and Gram stain
2. Synonyms or alternate names	CSF C/S; Culture, CSF
3. Specimen type(s)	CSF, ventricular fluid, or subdural fluid
4. Minimum specimen volume	1 ml
5. Specimen container	Sterile, leak-proof container
6. Transport instructions	Bring to laboratory immediately
7. Information needed	None
8. Special requirements	Send tube no. 2 of 4
9. Test schedule, approx TAT	Daily, 72 h
10. Laboratory section	Microbiology
11. Prior approval or notice	Not needed
12. Requisition	Microbiology
13. Storage instructions	Refrigeration (4°C)
14. Reflexive order conditions	Antimicrobial susceptibility test if pathogen recovered
15. CPT code(s)	87070, 87205
16. Comments	Gram stain automatically performed
17. Price	$x.xx

[a] Abbreviations: C/S, culture and sensitivity; TAT, turnaround time.

and old tests are eliminated. Interactive electronic catalogs offer even more advantages. Electronic catalog contents can be quickly searched by using key words or phrases to locate desired information. They can be modified easily and as often as necessary. They can include links to electronic journal articles, textbooks, and resources found on the Internet that contain more information about the tests.

Laboratory Requisitions

Historically, laboratory requisitions have been sheets of paper containing a list of tests from which clinicians can select their orders. The requisitions are delivered to the laboratory accompanied by appropriately labeled specimens, and laboratory personnel then enter the orders into the LIS (if one is in use). With advances in information system technology, an increasing number of hospitals are now utilizing electronic order entry systems in which caregivers place their own orders and the orders are sent electronically to the LIS. Simultaneously, specimen labels are generated at the ordering location and are placed on specimen containers in the presence of the patient to minimize the likelihood of mislabeled specimens. When the labeled specimens arrive in the laboratory, their receipt is recorded in the LIS. Bar-coding technology enables specimen receipt recording and the subsequent tracking of specimens in the laboratory to be accomplished quickly and accurately by wanding the specimen labels with a bar code scanner.

The use of paper requisitions is decreasing. Their biggest drawback is that these requisitions are inflexible when it comes to the addition or removal of tests from the list of choices. However, when they are necessary they can still be used effectively with a little foresight. They should be printed in small batches that last only a few months. When new batches are ordered, the requisition contents should be reviewed and modified where necessary. There should be a location on the requisition where missing test names can be handwritten, and the date the requisition was printed should be evident to enable efficient removal of outdated requisitions from ordering locations.

Electronic requisitions found in computerized order entry systems are much more flexible than paper requisitions. These requisitions can be accessed through the LIS, the hospital information system, an order entry module with an interface with the LIS, or an Internet-based order entry system. The list of tests can be modified quickly whenever there is a change, and there is no worry of exhausting the supply of requisitions. As with paper requisitions, there must be a capacity for ordering tests that are missing from the electronic list. That is generally accomplished through the use of a "miscellaneous" test category in which test specifics (e.g., test name and specimen description) are entered during the ordering process. When a significant number of requests for the same miscellaneous test are received by the laboratory, a practice should be in place for incorporating the test onto the electronic requisition.

The use of the Internet for ordering laboratory tests has been escalating in frequency because it is possible to order from computer workstations located anywhere in the world (27). All that is needed on the ordering computer are Internet browsing software and authorized access to the password-protected ordering system. A concern over this manner of order communication is the possibility of unauthorized electronic eavesdroppers' acquiring sensitive patient information. Sophisticated means of encrypting the information stream exist to protect patient confidentiality and achieve HIPAA compliance.

INFORMATION MANAGEMENT DURING THE ANALYTICAL PHASE OF TESTING

Although information flows predominantly from clinicians to the laboratory in the preanalytical phase of testing and vice versa during the postanalytical phase of testing, the analytical phase of testing finds the laboratory seeking information from other internal and external sources. The clinical microbiology laboratory, in particular, depends heavily on access to repositories of information during the analytical phase of testing. That is because much of the work is visual or decision table oriented. The information received from these sources is then acted upon by individuals in the laboratory.

Procedure Manuals

Laboratory regulatory agencies require all laboratories to maintain up-to-date procedure manuals that are accessible to workers at all times that testing is in progress. Most laboratories rely on traditional procedure manuals comprising pages of information stored in loose-leaf binders. The loose-leaf format lends itself well to the preparation of photocopies for simultaneous use at multiple workbenches and the replacement of outdated procedures with newer versions. A more modern approach is the conversion of paper procedure manuals into a series of online documents that are stored in a word-processing format (e.g., x.doc), portable document format (e.g., x.pdf), or Internet browser format (e.g., x.htm) (25). Such documents are easily modified and can be printed on paper, if desired. Documentation of annual review can be accomplished efficiently and unequivocally via electronic signature. Color photographs to illustrate procedural steps can be embedded in the documents. Perhaps the greatest advantage is that the entire procedure manual can be searched rapidly by using key words or phrases to quickly locate a particular procedure or group of procedures. The CLSI publishes a frequently revised guideline for the preparation of paper or electronic laboratory procedure manuals (approved guideline GP2-A5) that most laboratories follow (6).

Image Libraries

Photographs are indispensable to the accurate identification of many microorganisms, particularly those in the fungal and parasitic groups. Photographs of gross colonies and microscopic morphologies of a variety of microorganisms can be maintained in image repositories that are useful in differentiating similar microorganisms from one another. Every clinical microbiology laboratory should have a collection of photographs to which technologists can refer during their work. The repository may consist of photographs in a textbook, images in a text atlas, or 35-mm slides maintained in the laboratory.

One of the spin-offs of current information system technology has been a growing reliance in the laboratory on digital images instead of images recorded on film (24, 29). High-resolution images can be stored on inexpensive magnetic and optical media and can easily be manipulated and enhanced with computer software. Many laboratories have taken advantage of the dramatic reductions seen recently in the cost of image-capturing hardware (e.g., scanners and cameras) and are building their own image libraries. Images can be placed on servers located anywhere in the world and be viewed and/or downloaded nearly instantaneously over the Internet (4).

Tables of Microbiological Data

Laboratory identification of many microorganisms is based on a comparison of their physiologic and biochemical test properties with those described in reference databases. This comparison can be accomplished manually with a side-by-side assessment or via flowchart analysis. Many microbiology laboratories still identify microorganisms through analysis of information found in tables and flowcharts in textbooks, journal articles, and government documents. This approach is laborious and time-consuming but has the advantage of including human judgment in the decision-making process.

The use of tables to identify microorganisms relies upon determining the best fit between the properties of an unknown microorganism and those of a group of microorganisms belonging to the same species. The tables usually indicate the percentages of species members that exhibit positive results for particular tests. Although this approach is effective when test results for an unknown microorganism closely match those for an established species, it may yield inaccurate identifications when test results are dissimilar to those for known species.

The same information found in the identification tables described above can be converted into computerized databases and then quickly and accurately compared with the properties of an unknown microorganism. This method has been used for many years in a proprietary fashion by the manufacturers of some commercially available systems for microbial identification. The sophisticated analysis includes weighting of key properties and pattern recognition to derive best-fit identifications. The likelihood of an identification and the degree of a microorganism's dissimilarity from similar microorganisms can also be calculated.

It is also possible for individual clinical microbiologists to convert their own identification tables and those present in the public domain into queriable databases. This can be accomplished by using off-the-shelf database software programs to prepare such databases manually. The same software can then be used to define queries that identify the microorganisms included in the database whose biochemical test results best match those for an unknown microorganism.

Flowchart Algorithms

Flowchart algorithms are another approach to microorganism identification that has been used for many years. This approach differs from the use of tables in that identification test results with the greatest discriminating power are placed at the top of the decision tree and are assigned greater weight than results further down the flowchart. Although the early decisions in the flowchart algorithm are often based on unambiguous test results, the decisions made further down in the flowchart may be based on more ambiguous test results or on test results that have lower discriminating abilities.

Laboratory Work Cards

More than that in any other area of laboratory medicine, accurate microbiology testing depends on a reliable flow of information between technologists assigned to different work shifts or work days. That is because microbiology testing of many specimens (especially cultures) cannot be completed in a single work shift and more than one technologist may be involved in the testing. Accordingly, laboratories must have a mechanism in place for sharing information among technologists that concisely communicates the status of testing. Some form of microbiology work card is the solution for many laboratories. Some microbiology laboratories, even those with an LIS, still employ paper work cards that are maintained at each workstation. Technologists record the work performed daily on individual work cards. Information is documented in the form of handwritten standardized codes, short phrases, or check boxes that are understandable by coworkers. Work cards for completed tests undergo supervisory review and are stored for at least 2 years per regulatory requirement.

Almost all LISs can be configured to record microbiology culture workup information on electronic templates that are accessed by individuals working on the same cultures at later times (Table 6). Information is entered onto the electronic work card in the form of text codes or short strings of free text. Entries on the work card are generally organized by isolate or by culture medium and then by chronological order within each of these categories. The benefits of paperless entry include guaranteed legibility, easy supervisory review of work, and automatic indexing of workup data to simplify data queries later. The electronic work card also can be configured to standardize culture workups and accrue workload data for productivity analyses.

Instrument Interfaces

The proliferation of semiautomated and automated instruments for laboratory testing has greatly increased the volume of data transfer between instruments and LISs. Information transfer can be accomplished through manual transcription or automatic communication of data via electronic interfaces.

Transfer of information to and from instruments that do not have an electronic interface with an LIS is accomplished by manual entry. The number of keystrokes required for this activity can be limited on the LIS side through the use of text codes or keyboard mapping to insert commonly used words, phrases, or even blocks of text. Because of the human component of information entry, transcription errors are an ever-present threat and the fidelity of data entry should be constantly monitored by supervisory review.

Far easier and much more reliable than manual transcription is the automatic transfer of information between instruments and LISs (8, 9). This transfer can be accomplished through the use of scripted or electronic interfaces. A scripted interface is in essence a very fast electronic typist. It transcribes information from an instrument to the LIS in the same manner that a technologist would—but much faster and more accurately. The electronic interface is more complicated in that it converts a stream of data from one system into a format understandable by the other system. Batch

TABLE 6 Sample work card entries for *S. pneumoniae* blood culture isolate

Work card prompt	Response
GRST (Gram stain)	GPCPSM (gram-positive cocci in pairs)
CAT (catalase)	NEG (negative)
PHON (telephone report)	DONE (completed)
OPT (optochin)	POS (positive)
BESC (bile esculin)	NEG (negative)
NACL (6.5% NaCl tolerance)	NEG (negative)
BDIL (broth dilution MIC)	DONE (completed)
PURPLT (purity plate)	AOK (pure culture)
SAVE (save isolate on slant)	DONE (completed)

interfaces send data on demand, and dynamic interfaces send data as soon as they become available. Unidirectional interfaces transfer information in a single direction, either from the LIS to an instrument (download) or from an instrument to the LIS (upload). Bidirectional interfaces are more costly and complicated to set up since data must be able to flow in either direction.

The decision as to which type of interface is more suitable for a microbiology instrument depends on the timeliness with which the data are needed, the traffic capacity (bandwidth) of the interface, and the cost-benefit ratio of having data flow in one or both directions. Interfaces that download specimen demographic information from an LIS to an instrument are almost always desirable because they eliminate the need for transcribing required information from one system to another. Interfaces that upload data from an instrument to an LIS are valuable when the data sets are large and contain information that will be reported directly to clinicians (e.g., microbial identification and antimicrobial susceptibility data). When the instrument data are only preliminary in nature and require follow-up work at the laboratory workbench (e.g., positive blood culture results from an automated blood culture instrument), justifying the expense of a bidirectional interface is more difficult.

Inventory Management

Inventory management modules are available for some LISs and are intended to help organize and monitor the utilization of laboratory supplies (7). Some modules also assist with equipment maintenance activities. These systems generate reports regarding ordering patterns for laboratory supplies and can print equipment maintenance logs. They also provide helpful data for cost analysis studies based on supply utilization. If a record of the usage of supplies can be entered into one of these modules, the module can provide a real-time indication of inventory. Some inventory modules also track expiration dates of supplies by lot number. They alert laboratory personnel when additional supplies should be ordered and may even produce paper or electronic order requisitions for submission to the purchasing department. When new supplies are received, inventory levels can be updated in the module. If supplies are not received when expected, the module can remind laboratory personnel to contact the vendor to determine the reason.

Quality Control

The quality control modules found in many LISs aid clinical microbiology laboratory managers by streamlining the entry and review of quality control data. They provide data entry screens and reports that are customized to the requirements of the laboratory. They offer reminders to the laboratory when scheduled quality control data have not been entered. They also send warnings to the laboratory when quality control results are out of range and require the entry of the remedial action taken. When out-of-range quality control results are entered, the individual entering the results is alerted immediately. The LIS then waits for either replacement of the out-of-range results or acknowledgment that the out-of-range results are correct as entered. Acknowledgment that out-of-range quality control results are correct qualifies the results for an exception report that should be reviewed daily by supervisory personnel.

Most LISs are able to plot numerical quality control data on a LIS-defined Levey-Jennings control chart, evaluate the data, and notify users when results are "out of control." A Levey-Jennings control chart is a graphical display of quality control data that indicates the expected mean, the ±2 standard deviation boundary around the mean, and the ±3 standard deviation boundary around the mean. The assumption is that if the test method is stable and being performed correctly, current quality control results should exhibit a statistical distribution similar to that of past quality control results. Results outside the ±2 standard deviation boundary should be encountered no more than 5% of the time, and results beyond the ±3 standard deviation boundary should be seen no more than 1% of the time. When quality control results fall within the specified boundaries, the test is "in control," the results are acceptable, and patient results can be reported. When quality control results are outside the specified boundaries, the test is out of control, the results are unacceptable, and patient results cannot be reported. The CLSI criteria for evaluating antimicrobial susceptibility quality control data are based on principles similar to those used by Levey-Jennings charts.

Many LISs are also able to evaluate numerical quality control results according to rules developed by Westgard many years ago (31). The data examined may be limited to a single control or may include the results from several controls. An example of a Westgard rule violation that applies to a single control is as follows: a single quality control result falls outside the acceptable range, defined as ±2 standard deviations from the mean. An example of a rule infraction that involves results from several controls is as follows: four consecutive quality control results are more than 1 standard deviation away from the mean in the same direction. The quality control module in most LISs can be set to apply any of the Westgard rules that have been defined within the system. The rules that will be applied usually can be individualized according to the quality control tests being performed.

Quality Assurance

Generic quality assurance rules can be applied automatically to test results to enhance the recognition of potential problems. The rules listed below frequently are "hard coded" in the LIS software used by laboratories. Additional site-specific quality assurance rules can be defined with the aid of the rules engine described earlier in this chapter.

1. Normal-value checking. Most laboratory regulatory agencies mandate that test results be accompanied by the expected values for the test ("normal range"). Expected values for these tests may be expressed as a numerical threshold or a range for quantitative tests (e.g., expected antistreptolysin O titer, <200 IU/ml), or expected results may be expressed as a text code for qualitative tests (e.g., expected HIV-1 antibody result, "negative"). Inclusion of the expected value or result aids clinicians in interpreting the clinical significance of test results. Most LISs provide a mechanism for defining age-specific, gender-specific, and even species-specific expected values for test results. The expected values are incorporated automatically by the LISs into the test report. Results that are outside the normal value range qualify for a daily quality assurance report. In the microbiology laboratory, normal-value checking generally is limited to nonculture testing.

2. Comparison of current results with past results. Virtually all LISs have the capability of comparing current test results for a patient to those from the same test last performed on the same patient within a defined period of time. Sequential results that exhibit a user-defined significant difference trigger a "delta check" flag. It is the laboratory's responsibility to investigate flagged results to confirm that

the sequential specimens were collected from the same patient or that testing irregularities did not occur during the generation of either result. Once confirmation is achieved, the flagged results can be released for viewing by clinicians. Results that elicit a delta check flag qualify for a daily quality assurance report. In the microbiology laboratory, delta checking is limited typically to nonculture testing.

3. Critical-value checking. An unfortunate type of medical error originating in the clinical laboratory is the failure to notify clinicians of critical test results in a timely fashion as mandated by hospital policy. Almost as important as reporting the critical result itself is documenting that prompt clinician notification has occurred. Critical test results usually are defined as results that require immediate medical interventions of a life-saving nature. Examples from the microbiology laboratory include positive cerebrospinal fluid (CSF) Gram stain results and positive blood culture results. Through the use of LIS-defined automatic flagging of critical test results or the use of a rules engine to analyze laboratory data to identify critical results, the LIS can be an important safeguard against these types of medical errors (14, 15, 17). Results that are deemed critical qualify for a daily quality assurance report.

4. Comparison of smear and culture results. Some LISs are able to perform some quality assurance checks that are unique to the clinical microbiology laboratory. One that is often available is comparison of Gram stain and culture results. When Gram stain findings suggest that microorganisms of a particular morphology are present, the LIS will alert users if the culture results do not include a microorganism with that morphology. Deviations between Gram stain and culture results qualify for a daily quality assurance report.

5. Detection of "bug-drug" antimicrobial susceptibility result inconsistencies. Some LISs allow users to define expected antimicrobial susceptibility results for specific antimicrobial agents versus particular microorganisms. When results differ from the expected, a message displays requesting the technologist to review the result and either change it or file it manually. Acceptance of an unexpected result qualifies the result for a daily quality assurance report.

INFORMATION SHARING DURING THE POSTANALYTICAL PHASE OF TESTING

Communication of information to clinicians from the microbiology laboratory is especially vital during the postanalytical phase of testing, for it is this information that is the basis for patient management decisions. The mode of communication may be verbal, written, or electronic, and the information often consists of more than just test results.

Test Results Reporting

The most frequent information passed on to clinicians during the postanalytical phase of testing consists of the test results themselves. When it comes to microbiology testing, some results are released in their entirety all at once and others are issued sequentially as data become available. Examples of the former situation include results from antigen detection tests, nucleic acid probe tests, and certain microscopic assays. Instances of the latter sort include negative antigen detection results that require confirmation by a more sensitive method and culture results accompanied by a Gram stain report and/or antimicrobial susceptibility data. LISs can report initial microbiology results in preliminary reports and then release final reports once all testing is completed.

Some LISs calculate the transport time for microbiology specimens, which is then displayed in the final report. The specimen transport time is the elapsed time between collection and receipt of specimens by the laboratory, although in some external order entry systems the specimen collection time may actually be the test ordering time. Clinical microbiologists should understand the meaning of transport time as calculated by their LISs before relying on these data during investigation of specimen transport problems.

Another important time point in the processing of microbiology specimens for culture is the plating (setup) time—especially when the laboratory inoculating culture media are remote from the specimen collection site. Some LISs now display the plating time in culture reports to identify specimens that may have experienced processing delays. The plating time is also used by these LISs in calculating the elapsed time for "no growth update" reports (e.g., a preliminary blood culture report might read, "No growth after 18 hours of incubation").

Microscopic examination and culture results are usually displayed in separate sections of the LIS report. Stained-smear results typically are found near the top of the report, since they are available first and acted upon more immediately than culture results. Culture findings frequently evolve with time as one or more isolates are detected and then identified in a stepwise process. For example, a culture that is positive for *Haemophilus influenzae* may be reported initially to contain "pleomorphic gram-negative coccobacilli consistent with *Haemophilus* sp.," then to contain "presumptive *Haemophilus* sp.," and finally to contain "*Haemophilus influenzae* not typeable" as more information is learned about the isolate.

Improved taxonomic techniques during the past 30 years have led to the reclassification of many microorganisms into different or newly created genera and species. While microorganism name changes are a nuisance for laboratory personnel as they are forced to adjust to new nomenclature, they can create serious confusion among clinicians trying to interpret the significance of culture results. The LIS can be an effective tool in keeping clinicians up to date with microorganism name changes. By way of illustration, it is no more difficult for an LIS to issue a culture report as "3+ growth of *Rhizobium (Agrobacterium) radiobacter*" than as "3+ growth of *Rhizobium radiobacter*." The former report is helpful to clinicians more familiar with the older taxonomic designation.

Interpretive Reports

One of the more innovative ways that clinical microbiology laboratories can benefit patients is through provision of interpretive reports that accompany test results. This is especially true for tests that yield complex results, like HIV-1 genotyping. Virtually all LISs enable clinical microbiologists to supplement test results with comments that were created and stored previously or with free text comments crafted in real time while test results are being reported. Libraries of prewritten comments can be maintained in the LIS and incorporated into reports individually or strung together as a group of comments when the situation warrants.

Supplementation of Microbiology Test Data with Digital Images

While still an uncommon practice, the potential for enhancement of microbiology reports with digital images is very real. Inclusion of digital photographs of Gram stains, acid-fast stains, ova and parasite preparations, or any other microscopic finding is technologically feasible today. Similarly, photographs of subjectively read test results such as those for group A streptococcal antigen, *Cryptococcus neoformans* antigen, RPR, and many others could also be stored in the LIS for quality assurance purposes. Data from objectively read tests, such as optical density readings from enzyme immunoassays, are commonly stored in the LIS already. It would seem that a more compelling argument could be made for recording visual evidence of subjectively read test results. The precedent for storing digital images has already been set by several commercially available pathology and diagnostic imaging information systems. Many offer optional image storage repositories maintained on separate servers. Pathology and radiology reports can include hypertext links that lead users to photographs stored on the image server. In this way, clinicians have the opportunity to view for themselves the images that led to the pathologist's or radiologist's findings. The same could be true for clinical microbiology results.

Antimicrobial Susceptibility Reports

Antimicrobial susceptibility results, in many circumstances, are more valuable to clinicians postanalytically than are culture results. Hence, these data must be displayed in a fashion that promotes unequivocal understanding of the results so that correct therapeutic decisions can be made. Most LISs enable laboratories to display antimicrobial susceptibility data in a variety of formats, including linear, columnar, and tabular displays. Most enable easy addition or deletion of antimicrobial agents in predefined batteries and also allow the addition of practical information to reports, such as CLSI-recommended comments pertaining to antimicrobial susceptibility test results. In some instances, the report can be customized to show antimicrobial agent dosage information, route of administration, achievable levels of antimicrobial agents in the blood and urine, and the cost of antimicrobial agent therapy.

Virtually all LISs enable the entry of qualitative (S, I, and R) or quantitative (MIC or inhibitory zone diameter) susceptibility data. If quantitative data are entered, the LIS can refer to its own tables of user-entered interpretive criteria (obtained from the CLSI or other official agencies) to convert the data into clinician-friendly qualitative results. The interpretive criteria must be updated frequently by laboratory personnel as important changes are made on an annual basis.

The authors of the CLSI *Performance Standards for Antimicrobial Susceptibility Testing* have recommended carefully worded statements that can be added to susceptibility reports to aid clinicians in the correct interpretation of susceptibility results (10). Such comments can be added via manual insertion of free text, manual insertion of blocks of stored text, or automatic insertion of blocks of stored text after recognition of an appropriate situation by the LIS rules engine.

Nonculture Test Results Reporting

The development of rapid, CLIA-waived, point-of-care assays for diagnosis of infectious diseases has led to an increase in the numbers of nonculture microbiology tests being performed. Most of these tests do not fit into the traditional microbiology battery of microscopic examination, culture findings, and antimicrobial susceptibility results. They are more similar to tests performed in other sections of the clinical laboratory and thus need to be defined in the LIS in a manner different from that for cultures. If such tests are not defined as microbiology tests, it is essential that the report include a description of the specimen, information that is not always part of the test reports from other sections of the clinical laboratory.

Delivery of Test Results to Clinicians

There are many mechanisms by which microbiology test results can be delivered to clinicians. The requirements that all mechanisms have in common are that the results must reach clinicians

1. In a timely manner. Results must be available to clinicians within a time frame that enables appropriate interventions to be made.
2. In a legible and understandable format. Results must be easily read and presented in unambiguous language so that suitable action can be taken.
3. In a form that is free of typographical or transcriptional errors. Systems must be in place that reduce the release of misleading or erroneous laboratory data.

The most frequent means for distributing laboratory test results is still the paper report. Many LISs are set up to print paper reports daily that are then distributed by couriers to clinicians and added to the patient's medical record. Some LISs print the patient's entire up-to-date laboratory file each day with the expectation that reports from previous days will be discarded. Other LISs print only the patient's "new laboratory activity" so that daily reports are added to previously printed reports already in place in the clinician's office or the patient's medical record.

Interim reports show the status of current laboratory activity for each patient selected. Reports can be limited to new activity since the last interim or cumulative report was printed, or they may be printed for all activity that took place over a specified date range. The test results in interim reports are usually displayed in reverse chronological order, with no further sorting available. Some LISs permit interim reports to be called up for groups of patients according to the ordering physician or the patients' location.

Cumulative reports contain results of patient tests grouped by the type of test or the specimen collection site. Examples of cumulative report headers include "Bacterial Cultures," "Fungal Cultures," and "Nucleic Acid Probes" when sorting is by test categorization and "Blood Cultures," "Urine Cultures," and "Genital Nucleic Acid Probes" when sorting is by specimen collection site. It should be the responsibility of the clinical microbiology laboratory leadership, with input from clinicians, to decide the style of cumulative report that is more suitable for a particular hospital. Within each group of tests under a cumulative report header, test results usually are sorted in reverse chronological order. Most LISs can call up cumulative reports by patient, ordering physician, or patient location. Most hospitals depend on postdischarge cumulative reports to serve as the official record of laboratory test results.

Generation of Ad Hoc (User-Defined) Reports

There are occasions in which none of the hard-coded LIS reports available to the laboratory contain the information needed for a specific purpose. Yet, every LIS stores a wealth of useful data elements within tables that may not be accessible via running preset reports (1). Most LISs offer optional modules that enable users to perform user-defined queries of the LIS database. The queries may be made with proprietary LIS-specific tools, or if the LIS data are stored in an open database connectivity (ODBC)-compliant relational database, queries may be made with ODBC-compliant off-the-shelf software (e.g., Microsoft Access or Business Objects

Crystal Reports). Such queries generally are intended to assemble data for a retrospective review of a particular data set. For example, if one wished to obtain a list of all patients during the previous 5 years who had positive blood cultures with simultaneous white blood cell counts of greater than 18,000 per mm^3, an ad hoc query would be the easiest manner to collect the data.

Once the ad hoc query is defined and run, the output report is stored in the LIS or on the user's workstation, usually as a delimited text file, spreadsheet file, or database file. From here the report can be printed on paper or, if resident on the LIS, can be downloaded to a personal computer via a serial port connection to the LIS or via a "file transfer protocol" across the hospital computer network. The ad hoc report file in a personal computer can be opened using standard spreadsheet or database software. Spreadsheet tools (e.g., sorting, filtering, and pivot tables from Microsoft Excel) can be used to analyze the data (22). Database tools (e.g., Microsoft Access and Business Objects Crystal Reports) can be used to perform further queries or configure attractive displays of the data.

Paperless Reports

The trend toward operating clinical laboratories as paperless entities is gathering momentum. Under this paradigm, LIS reports are not printed on paper but instead are printed to files stored on magnetic or optical disk media. Such reports are stored in easily accessible formats, are readily distributed to authorized individuals, and are quickly retrievable for review at any time. If it is necessary to obtain a paper report, the report file can be sent electronically to a printer.

Although an increasing number of hospitals are encouraging clinicians to view laboratory results via a clinician portal rather than in the LIS, all LISs provide on-demand viewing of laboratory test results online. LIS inquiry functions enable the review of test results for specimens collected on a particular date or range of dates or for a single test or group of tests performed in a particular section of the laboratory. Some LISs enable viewing of serial quantitative data in graphical format so that numerical trends are more easily spotted.

For those hospitals that expect clinicians to order laboratory tests and view laboratory results in a clinician order entry-results-viewing portal, an interface must be built between the clinician portal and the LIS. The advantage to this approach is that clinicians can be trained to perform a wide variety of functions (e.g., ordering and viewing laboratory results, ordering and viewing diagnostic imaging results, ordering pharmaceuticals, and viewing patient vital signs and progress notes) on a single information system. This strategy fits in nicely with the tendency in U.S. hospitals toward greater provider interaction with information systems. The major disadvantage is that the format for displaying laboratory test results may not be as feature rich and well organized in a clinician portal as it would be in an LIS.

Electronic Delivery of Reports

When the LIS is a node on the hospital local-area or wide-area computer network, it becomes feasible to transmit report files electronically to workstation nodes and printers on the network. Some LISs possess report scheduling capability by which preset or ad hoc reports can be run at designated daily, weekly, monthly, quarterly, or annual intervals, printed automatically to files, and then sent to workstations or groups of workstations within the network. In fact, a growing number of laboratories no longer print patient discharge cumulative reports on paper. Alternatively, they print the reports to a file and send the file via the hospital local-area network to the health information management department (medical records) for inclusion in the patient's electronic medical record.

Another emerging trend among laboratories is granting access to laboratory test results via the Internet (11). Authorized individuals are able to log in to an Internet information server where an up-to-the-minute copy of the laboratory test result database resides. Users then can view results over a secure, encrypted channel from anywhere in the world.

Another recent technological development is the ability to transmit laboratory test results via a wireless connection to hand-held devices such as alphanumeric pagers, digital telephones, and personal data assistants. Although still in its infancy, this methodology has the potential to replace the telephoning of critical laboratory reports to clinicians, if a means for acknowledging receipt of the report can be implemented. One can also envisage daily downloading of interim reports for a clinician's patient list to a hand-held device. It remains to be seen whether the complex laboratory data found in microbiology reports can be transmitted and viewed effectively on these hand-held devices.

Verbal Delivery of Reports

Verbal delivery of laboratory results, in almost every instance, is an adjunct to conveying results by other means. Verbal reporting very often is the method of choice for initial reporting of critical values. In the microbiology arena these may be preliminary results, such as the Gram stain morphologies of microorganisms growing in blood cultures, or they may be final results such as positive results for a test to detect cryptococcal antigen in CSF. When noncritical laboratory results are delivered verbally, it is often in situations in which clinicians telephone the laboratory because they do not have access to the standard means of results distribution. This method of reporting microbiology results must be carried out with caution since it is very easy for complicated results to be confused or misunderstood. Reading back of verbally communicated critical reports has become the norm in the United States. The other common context for verbal discussion of test results is during the course of a consultation over results released previously in another manner.

Consultations Concerning Laboratory Reports

Passive consultations from the laboratory perspective are those in which clinicians contact the laboratory for advice in interpreting test results. Such consultations concerning microbiology results should be handled by the laboratory director or the supervisor, one of whom should be reachable for this purpose at all times. Active consultations are those in which laboratory directors or supervisors seek out clinicians to discuss the clinical significance of test results and suggest additional tests that should be considered. Although active consultations require commitment and effort on the part of the laboratory staff, the return on the investment is easily appreciated in terms of improved patient care.

An underutilized method of communication between the microbiology laboratory and clinicians is the addition of information signed by the laboratory director to patient medical records. This information can be of great assistance to clinicians in the understanding of test results and can provide valuable suggestions for follow-up testing. The advantages of this route of information sharing are that the clinical microbiologist's observations can be read at the convenience of clinicians and that the information is located in the same place in the medical record as key information from other clinical services.

Most hospitals and regulatory agencies require that the medical staff bylaws specify the individuals who are authorized to place information in patient medical records. It is the responsibility of the microbiology laboratory director and his or her colleagues in laboratory medicine to ensure that they have the necessary authorization if this is a desired practice.

Preparation of Periodic Antibiogram Reports

A much-appreciated service provided by many clinical microbiology laboratories is the distribution of cumulative institutional antimicrobial susceptibility data reports to clinicians (28). These reports generally are prepared on an annual basis but may be offered more frequently if warranted. In an attempt to standardize the contents of antibiogram reports, the CLSI has issued document M39-A2, entitled *Analysis and Presentation of Cumulative Antimicrobial Susceptibility Test Data* (5). This document recommends methods for recording and analyzing antimicrobial susceptibility data for epidemiologically significant microorganisms. To avoid biasing the data, the standard recommends including only the first isolate of a particular species from a patient per analysis period and including only isolates derived from cultures performed for diagnostic purposes. To improve the statistical validity of the data, the standard urges limiting the report to organisms tested 30 or more times during the analysis period.

At the time of this writing, most LIS vendors are still determining how they will help laboratories comply with the recommendations in the CLSI M39-A2 document. In the meantime, clinical microbiologists should consider downloading their antimicrobial susceptibility data to a personal computer and then preparing their cumulative antimicrobial susceptibility reports with the aid of spreadsheet or database software that enables compliance with the CLSI document (Table 7).

TABLE 7 Sample pivot table from Microsoft Excel showing antimicrobial susceptibility data for *S. pneumoniae* tested during calendar year 2005

Culture battery	(All)
Collection month	(All)
Collection year	2005
Order location	(All)
Order physician	(All)
Specimen description	(All)
Gender	(All)

Drug	Result (%)		
	S	I	R
Ceftriaxone (CSF)[a]	68	10	22
Ceftriaxone (other)[a]	81	17	2
Chloramphenicol	100		0
Clindamycin	88	2	10
Erythromycin	59	2	39
Levofloxacin	100	0	0
Penicillin	45	25	30
Trimethoprim-sulfamethoxazole	55	4	41
Vancomycin	100		0

[a] CSF, isolate recovered from cerebrospinal fluid; other, isolate recovered from specimen other than cerebrospinal fluid.

Submission of Laboratory Results to External Repositories

Jurisdictional regulations (e.g., those issued by local, county, state, or national agencies) mandate that hospitals and/or laboratories report positive test results for diagnosis of certain infectious diseases to public health authorities. Traditionally, this reporting has been accomplished via written notification that is either mailed or faxed to the responsible authority. Some LISs are beginning to include software tools that make it easier for clinical microbiology laboratories to comply with reporting regulations (19). Automatic faxing of reports to designated telephone numbers is now a feature of selected LISs. This capability is being extended by some LISs to enable submission of HIPAA-compliant encrypted reports via e-mail and the Internet.

Another emerging phenomenon in some hospitals is a joint venture between clinical microbiology laboratories and infection control departments to export data in a secure fashion to a commercial external data warehouse where the data are analyzed on a fee-for-service basis to detect epidemiologically significant trends. Reported experience has indicated that such a program does enable identification of problem areas in the hospital where infection control intervention might be useful (12).

SUMMARY

LISs have enabled tremendous progress to be made in the dissemination of information from the clinical microbiology laboratory to providers of health care (18). Laboratory test data are delivered more efficiently and accurately than ever before. Other information that is imperative to the ordering of correct tests, the collection of appropriate specimens, and the interpretation of test results can be communicated effectively. The role of these systems in the daily practice of clinical microbiology will only continue to increase in importance. It behooves all clinical microbiologists to become more knowledgeable about and comfortable with information systems, for they are perhaps the most powerful tool available to us in our new role as information brokers.

REFERENCES

1. **Aller, R. D.** 2003. The clinical laboratory data warehouse. An overlooked diamond mine. *Am. J. Clin. Pathol.* **120:** 817–819.
2. **Becich, M. J.** 2000. Information management: moving from test results to clinical information. *Clin. Leadersh. Manag. Rev.* **14:**296–300.
3. **Bissel, M. G.** 2004. Information systems and human error in the lab. *Clin. Leadersh. Manag. Rev.* **18:**349–355.
4. **Cao, F., H. K. Huang, and X. Q. Zhou.** 2003. Medical image security in a HIPAA mandated PACS environment. *Comput. Med. Imaging Graph.* **27:**185–196.
5. **Clinical and Laboratory Standards Institute.** 2005. *Analysis and Presentation of Cumulative Antimicrobial Susceptibility Test Data; Approved Guideline*, 2nd ed. CLSI document M39-A2. Clinical and Laboratory Standards Institute, Wayne, Pa.
6. **Clinical and Laboratory Standards Institute.** 2006. *Laboratory Documents: Development and Control; Approved Guideline*, 5th ed. CLSI document GP2-A5. Clinical and Laboratory Standards Institute, Wayne, Pa.
7. **Clinical and Laboratory Standards Institute.** 1994. *Inventory Control Systems for Laboratory Supplies; Approved Guideline.* CLSI document GP6-A. Clinical and Laboratory Standards Institute, Wayne, Pa.

8. **Clinical and Laboratory Standards Institute.** 2000. *Laboratory Automation: Communications with Automated Clinical Laboratory Systems, Instruments, Devices, and Information Systems; Approved Standard.* CLSI document AUTO3-A. Clinical and Laboratory Standards Institute, Wayne, Pa.
9. **Clinical and Laboratory Standards Institute.** 1995. *Laboratory Instruments and Data Management Systems: Design of Software User Interfaces and End-User Software Systems Validation, Operation, and Monitoring; Approved Guideline.* CLSI document GP19-A. Clinical and Laboratory Standards Institute, Wayne, Pa.
10. **Clinical and Laboratory Standards Institute.** 2006. *Performance Standards for Antimicrobial Susceptibility Testing: 16th Informational Supplement.* CLSI document M100-S16. Clinical and Laboratory Standards Institute, Wayne, Pa.
11. **Friedman, B. A.** 1998. Integrating laboratory processes into clinical processes, Web-based laboratory reporting, and the emergence of the virtual clinical laboratory. *Clin. Lab. Manag. Rev.* **12:**333–338.
12. **Hacek, D. M., R. L. Cordell, G. A. Noskin, and L. R. Peterson.** 2004. Computer-assisted surveillance for detecting clonal outbreaks of nosocomial infection. *J. Clin. Microbiol.* **42:**1170–1175.
13. **Hunter, R. L., Jr.** 1999. The past and future of laboratory information systems. *Ann. Clin. Lab. Sci.* **29:**176–184.
14. **Iordache, S. D., D. Orso, and J. Zelingher.** 2001. A comprehensive computerized critical laboratory results alerting system for ambulatory and hospitalized patients. *Medinfo* **10:**469–473.
15. **Kalra, J.** 2004. Medical errors: impact on clinical laboratories and other critical areas. *Clin. Biochem.* **37:**1052–1062.
16. **Kay, J. D.** 2001. Communicating with clinicians. *Ann. Clin. Biochem.* **38:**103–110.
17. **Kuperman, G. J., J. M. Teich, M. J. Tanasijevic, N. Ma'Luf, E. Rittenberg, A. Jha, J. Fiskio, J. Winkelman, and D. W. Bates.** 1999. Improving response to critical laboratory results with automation: results of a randomized controlled trial. *J. Am. Med. Inf. Assoc.* **6:**512–522.
18. **McPherson, R. A.** 1999. Perspective on the clinical laboratory: new uses for informatics. *J. Clin. Lab. Anal.* **13:**53–58.
19. **M'ikantha, N. M., B. Southwell, and E. Lautenbach.** 2003. Automated laboratory reporting of infectious diseases in a climate of bioterrorism. *Emerg. Infect. Dis.* **9:**1053–1057.
20. **Miller, W. G.** 2000. The changing role of the medical technologist from technologist to information specialist. *Clin. Leadersh. Manag. Rev.* **14:**285–288.
21. **Nosowsky, R., and T. J. Giordano.** 2006. The Health Insurance Portability and Accountability Act of 1996 (HIPAA) Privacy Rule: implications for clinical research. *Annu. Rev. Med.* **57:**575–590.
22. **Oakley, S.** 1999. Data mining, distributed networks, and the laboratory. *Health Manag. Technol.* **20:**26–31.
23. **Park, W. S., S. Y. Yi, S. A. Kim, J. S. Song, and Y. H. Kwak.** 2005. Association between the implementation of a laboratory information system and the revenue of a general hospital. *Arch. Pathol. Lab. Med.* **129:**766–771.
24. **Paxton, A.** 2005. Digging its way in: lab digital imaging. *CAP Today* **19:**1, 46, 48.
25. **Ruby, S. G., and G. Krempel.** 1998. Intranets: virtual procedure manuals for the pathology lab. *MLO Med. Lab. Obs.* **30:**65–75.
26. **Szabo, J.** 2000. HIPAA compliance could cost dearly. *MLO Med. Lab. Obs.* **32:**8–9.
27. **Todebush, C.** 1999. The Internet-linked laboratory: fundamentally changing the delivery of laboratory information and results. *Am. Clin. Lab.* **18:**10.
28. **Trevino, S.** 2000. Antibiotic resistance monitoring: a laboratory perspective. *Mil. Med.* **165:**40–42.
29. **Uehling, M.** 2000. Digital imaging not picture perfect—yet. *CAP Today* **14:**1, 34–38.
30. **Watine, J.** 1999. Are expert systems "more intelligent" than laboratory doctors? *Clin. Biochem.* **32:**485–486.
31. **Westgard, J. O.** 1994. Selecting appropriate quality-control rules. *Clin. Chem.* **40:**499–501.

General Principles of Specimen Collection and Handling

J. MICHAEL MILLER, KAREN KRISHER, AND HARVEY T. HOLMES

5

In terms of the effectiveness of the laboratory, nothing is more important than the appropriate selection, collection, and handling of a specimen for microbiologic diagnosis. When specimen collection and management are not priorities, the laboratory can contribute little to patient care. Consequently, all members of the medical staff involved in this process must understand the critical nature of ensuring specimen quality. It is the responsibility of the laboratory to provide complete and accurate specimen management information in a form that can be easily incorporated into the procedure manual of those health care workers (i.e., nurses and other allied nursing personnel) who have primary responsibility for the collection of specimens. The information provided should address safety, selection, collection, transportation, acceptability, and labeling. This chapter provides an approach for developing a policy for proper collection and handling of specimens destined for analysis in the clinical microbiology laboratory for adult and pediatric patients. Special emphasis is given to and more details are provided for pediatric specimens in this chapter because of the unique character of this patient population and the special procedures often required for obtaining appropriate specimens. Details of specimen management can be found in the relevant chapters for each major group of microorganisms covered in this Manual (bacteriology, chapter 20; virology, chapter 80; mycology, chapter 116; parasitology, chapter 133).

Appropriate specimen management, or the lack of it, affects patient care in several very important ways (19). It is the key to accurate laboratory diagnosis that directly affects patient care and patient outcome; it influences therapeutic decisions; it affects hospital infection control and prevention, patient length of stay, and overall hospital costs; it plays a major role in laboratory costs; and it clearly influences laboratory efficiency. For these reasons, every laboratory should develop a rational, sound, and relevant specimen management policy and enforce it as strictly as possible.

SAFETY

Biosafety at the laboratory bench is of primary concern to laboratorians. Health care workers may be unaware of the potential etiologic agent(s) residing in the specimen being transported to the laboratory. Policies designed to protect laboratory and other personnel from accidental exposure to these agents must be in place. Most microbiology laboratory texts, including chapter 8 of this Manual, have sections on laboratory procedures that should contain safety information related to specimen management. Specific reference material on biosafety should be available in every microbiology laboratory. The reference materials available in the laboratory could include *Biosafety in Microbiological and Biomedical Laboratories*, 4th ed. (69) and *Biosafety in the Laboratory: Prudent Practices for the Handling and Disposal of Infectious Materials* (52).

In general, laboratorians should comply with the following policies for safety in specimen management:

1. Wear gloves, gowns, and, where appropriate, masks and/or goggles when collecting specimens (17).
2. Use leak-proof specimen containers and transport the containers within a sealable, leak-proof plastic bag with a separate compartment for paperwork (18).
3. Never transport syringes with needles to the laboratory. Instead, transfer the contents to a sterile tube or remove the needle with a protective device, recap the syringe, and place it in a sealable, leak-proof plastic bag (60).
4. Do not transport leaking specimen containers to the laboratory or process them. Notify the physician or the responsible nurse of the leaking container and explain the potential compromised nature of the results if processing is continued; ask for a repeat specimen. If a new specimen is submitted, autoclave and discard the leaking one (50). If another specimen cannot be obtained, e.g., needle aspirates, body fluids, or bone marrow, work with the existing specimen container within a biological safety cabinet.

SELECTION AND COLLECTION OF THE SPECIMEN

Before a specimen is collected for analysis, the specimen or the collection site must be selected and must represent a location of active disease. Even careful collection methods will produce a specimen of little clinical value if it is not obtained from a site where the infection is active. Some of the common sites of infection where ready sources of contamination reside include the bladder, where urethral organisms and those from the perineum may easily contaminate the urine specimen; blood, which is not infrequently contaminated by commensal flora from the venipuncture site; the endometrium, which may contain commensal vaginal flora; fistulas, which may contain organisms from the gastrointestinal tract; the middle ear, a specimen from which will be contaminated with flora of the external auditory canal if a swab is used to collect the specimen; the nasal sinus, which may contain nasopharyngeal flora; and sites of subcutaneous infections and superficial wounds, which are commonly contaminated by skin and mucous membrane flora.

General specimen selection and collection guidelines should include the following:

1. Avoid commensal contamination from indigenous flora, whenever possible, to ensure a sample representative of the infectious process (9, 50, 60). Specimens from many sites of infection may contain an etiologic agent that would be considered part of the normal flora in a healthy host. This "background noise" of normal flora (i.e., from skin, membranes, and the respiratory tract) could interfere with the interpretation of culture results as well as overgrow and obscure the true agent of disease.
2. Select the correct anatomic site from which to obtain the specimen and collect the specimen by the proper technique and with the proper supplies, as described in the tables of this and subsequent chapters of this Manual.
3. Optimize the capture of anaerobes from specimens by using the proper precautions, procedures, and supplies; biopsy or needle aspirates are the specimens of choice, while anaerobic swabs are the least desirable (35, 50). Never refrigerate specimens for anaerobic culture but, rather, maintain them at room temperature (32).
4. Collect adequate volumes; insufficient material may yield false-negative results.
5. Place the specimen in a container designed to promote the survival of suspected agents and to eliminate leakage and potential safety hazards.
6. Label each specimen container with the patient's name and identification number, source, specific site, date, time of collection, and initials of the collector (21).

The collection of specimens with swabs may or may not be the method of choice for the collection of a particular specimen for microbiologic analysis (37, 50). It is critical that specimen collectors know the appropriate device and method for the collection of samples. Swab tips for specimen collection are usually made of cotton, Dacron (a polyester), or calcium alginate. Most come with a plastic shaft, although swabs with wooden shafts are available. The swabs with wooden shafts are generally not recommended for routine specimen collection because they may contain toxic products and could inactivate herpes simplex virus and interfere with some *Ureaplasma* identification methods. Cotton-tipped swabs are less popular today because they may contain fatty acids that could interfere with the survival of some bacteria and *Chlamydia* spp. However, most nonfastidious bacteria are not affected if cotton-tipped swabs are used. Cotton-tipped swabs are also suitable for the collection of specimens from the vagina, cervix, or urethra for the detection of *Mycoplasma*. Dacron- and rayon-tipped swabs have a wide range of uses including the collection of specimens for the detection of viruses and can facilitate the survival of *Streptococcus pyogenes*. Calcium alginate-tipped swabs can be toxic for lipid-enveloped viruses and some cell cultures as well as for some strains of *Neisseria gonorrhoeae* and *Ureaplasma urealyticum*. These are useful for the collection of specimens for *Chlamydia* spp. (37). Newer tips of polyurethane foam are finding wide acceptance.

Swabs with flexible wire shafts and small tips are recommended for use for the collection of nasopharyngeal specimens, including sampling for *Bordetella pertussis*, and male urethral specimens for diagnosis of gonorrhoea. Specimens on plastic-shafted swabs that are labeled by the specimen collector as "nasopharyngeal" are not likely to be true representatives of nasopharyngeal flora and may actually contain representatives of the nasal or throat flora (50).

TRANSPORTATION

1. All specimens must be promptly transported to the laboratory, preferably within 2 h (35). If processing is delayed, specimens collected for the detection of bacterial agents may be stored under specified conditions (see chapter 20).
2. In general, do not store specimens for bacterial culture for more than 24 h. Viruses, however, usually remain stable for 2 to 3 days at 4°C (37, 38).
3. Optimal transport of clinical specimens, including specimens for anaerobic culture, depends primarily on the volume of material obtained. Submit small amounts within 15 to 30 min of collection; biopsy tissue may be maintained for up to 20 to 24 h, if stored at 25°C in an anaerobic transport system (35).
4. Otherwise, surgical or biopsy specimens are usually stored at 4°C for up to 1 week or per laboratory policy.
5. Environmentally sensitive organisms include *Shigella* spp. (which should be processed immediately), *Neisseria gonorrhoeae, N. meningitidis,* and *Haemophilus influenzae* (which is sensitive to cold temperatures). Never refrigerate spinal fluid, genital, eye, or internal ear specimens (50). Storage conditions for some specimens and agents are summarized in Table 1.
6. Transportation of clinical specimens and transportation of infectious substances from one health care facility or laboratory to another, regardless of the distance, requires strict attention to specimen packaging and labeling instructions (17, 18, 37). Materials for transport must be labeled properly and packaged and protected during transport. The courier vehicles must also be marked and designated as carrying biologic agents. Any clinical specimen, including swabs, scrapings, body fluids, or tissues, that is known or reasonably expected to contain a pathogen is classified as an *infectious substance*.

For specific packaging and shipping instructions, one can refer to a number of sources; the most comprehensive instructions are described by the Department of Transportation in 49 *Code of Federal Regulations* (http://hazmat.dot.gov/ or http://www.iata.org). Several areas of packaging and shipping are of extreme importance, and one must ensure that everyone involved in packaging and shipping (including courier activities) is current on the specific regulations, including the legal responsibilities of the laboratory as a "shipper"; the proper use of certified packaging (only packaging that has been certified by the United Nations for infectious substances can be used); the proper use of necessary package labeling and markings; and the proper completion of the required documentation. Frequent referral to the appropriate websites is recommended in order to ensure that compliance with the latest recommendations is accomplished.

Bacterial and Fungal Specimen Transport

Containers for specimen transport and directions on how to use them are often available from the laboratory. The potential etiologic agent suspected in the patient dictates the specific collection method and transport system that will support the viability of the agent. Specimens for fungal cultures should not be collected with a swab because of the

TABLE 1 Storage conditions for various transport systems and suspected etiologic agents[a]

Preservative or medium type	Specimens held at 4°C	Specimens held at 25°C
No preservative	Autopsy tissue, bronchial wash, intravenous catheter, CSF (viral agent), lung biopsy, pericardial fluid, sputum, urine (all)	CSF (bacterial agents), synovial fluid
Anaerobic transport media		Abdominal fluid, amniotic fluid, anaerobic cultures, aspirates, bile, cul-de-sac material, deep lesion material, IUD for *Actinomyces* sp., lung aspirate, placenta (delivery by cesarean section), sinus aspirate, tissue (surgery), transtracheal aspirate, urine (suprapubic aspirate)
Direct inoculation of media		Corneal scraping, blood cultures, RL or BG plates for *Bordetella* spp., JEMBEC plates for *Neisseria gonorrhoeae,* vitreous humor
Aerobic transport media[b]	Burn wound biopsy, *Campylobacter* spp., ear (external), *Shigella* spp., *Vibrio* spp., *Yersinia* spp.	Bone marrow, *Bordetella* spp., cervix, conjunctiva, *Corynebacterium* spp., ear (internal), genital cultures, nasopharynx, *Neisseria* spp., *Salmonella* spp., upper respiratory tract specimens

[a]Abbreviations: BG, Bordet-Gengou; IUD, intrauterine device; JEMBEC, John E. Martin biological environmental chamber; RL, Regan-Lowe medium.

[b]Stuart's medium, charcoal-impregnated swabs originally formulated for *N. gonorrhoeae* transport; Amies medium, modified Stuart's medium that incorporates charcoal in medium instead of in the swab; Cary & Blair medium, similar to Stuart's medium but modified for fecal specimens, with the pH increased from 7.4 to 8.4.

potential interference of the swab fibers with direct microscopic examination of the specimen. Swabs are acceptable for use for the collection of specimens for the detection of suspected yeast infections, however. Most specimen containers must be sterile since the presence of contaminating flora from nonsterile containers may lead to errors in culture interpretation. Containers for feces need not be sterile but should be clean containers with tight-fitting lids. If there is a question as to whether a specimen container should be sterile for a specific specimen, assume that it should be sterile.

Other useful products and devices include sterile, screw-capped containers for collecting urine or sputum specimens. The containers should be prepared and packaged for patient use, with directions, including illustrations, that can be understood by patients. Biopsy and tissue specimens may also be placed into these sterile cups, although "biopsy" samples may tend to be smaller than "tissue" samples. To keep these tissues moist, one may add a small amount of nonbacteriostatic saline to the cup rather than wrap the tiny tissue specimen in gauze. Sterile petri dishes or special envelopes can be used to transport hair, skin, or nail scrapings to the mycology laboratory. Commercial transport devices for *N. gonorrhoeae* such as the JEMBEC (John E. Martin biological environmental chamber) system with CO_2 tablets may provide better results than CO_2-containing bottles, especially for transport by courier. The bottles may not have consistent amounts of CO_2, and improper manipulation during inoculation causes a loss of the atmosphere.

As with bacterial specimens, fungal specimens for culture should be placed into sterile containers and transported to the laboratory promptly. For skin and nail scrapings, cleansing of the site with 70% alcohol is required prior to specimen collection. Nail scrapings for submission to the laboratory must be collected from the deeper, infected portion of the nail, and the initial superficial scrapings should be discarded because they will likely be contaminated. A UV lamp (Wood's lamp) is helpful when selecting infected hair since some dermatophytes will fluoresce. Details can be found in chapter 116. Most other specimens, including blood, other sterile body fluids, and urine, respiratory, fecal, and tissue specimens, are collected and submitted as described elsewhere for bacterial or mycobacterial specimens.

Virus, Rickettsia, Chlamydia, and Mycoplasma Transport

The methods and media used for the transport of bacteria are inappropriate for the transport of viruses and chlamydiae. Viral transport media (VTM) prevent drying, maintain viral viability during transport, and prevent the overgrowth of contaminating bacteria. Many of the formulations contain either Eagle's minimum essential medium or Hanks' balanced salt solution, along with fetal bovine serum or bovine serum albumin (BSA). VTM may be prepared in-house or purchased commercially. There is little evidence in the literature that one VTM is better than another. However, in virtually all cases where a specimen is submitted for viral analysis, the specimen should be selected and collected in a manner appropriate for the target organ (37).

Liquid-based transport systems contain a protein (BSA, gelatin, or fetal bovine serum) and a combination of antimicrobial agents in a buffered solution. Tissue for viral analysis may also be placed into this type of medium. A phosphate-buffered sucrose-containing transport system (2SP) may be used for virus and chlamydia transport. The antimicrobial agents present in the 2SP are not inhibitory to *Chlamydia* spp.

A transport system containing human newborn foreskin fibroblasts is commercially available and useful for recovery and early detection of cytomegalovirus and herpes simplex virus. This cell system has a limited shelf life and is useful only for viruses that grow in fibroblasts.

If specimens should arrive in the laboratory having been inappropriately placed into Stuart's or Amies bacterial transport systems, the swabs may be transferred into one of the systems of liquid VTM.

Recovery of rickettsia seems to be enhanced if glutamate is present in a sodium-free, buffered salt solution. A sucrose-phosphate-glutamate transport medium containing BSA is often used to transport rickettsiae, mycoplasmas, and chlamydiae (37). Manufacturers of nucleic acid probes, amplification systems, or enzyme immunoassay (EIA) antigen detection systems often recommend or supply specific transport media and swabs for the collection and transport of specimens to be tested in their systems.

SPECIMEN ACCEPTABILITY OR REJECTION CRITERIA

At times, specimens arriving in the laboratory may have been improperly selected, collected, or transported. This is essentially the equivalent of a specimen being out of control. This out-of-control process must receive the same attention as does an out-of-control identification method or susceptibility test; there must be a corrective action. Processing and reporting results for these specimens to the physicians may provide misleading information that can lead to misdiagnosis and inappropriate therapy. Consequently, the laboratory must adhere to a strict policy of specimen acceptance and rejection.

Listed below are several examples of situations in which specific laboratory policies must be formulated and enforced to ensure specimen quality:

1. No label. Do not process, but immediately contact the submitting physician or nurse. For specimens obtained by noninvasive means (urines, sputums, or throat specimens), have a new specimen submitted. For specimens obtained by invasive procedures (needle aspirates, body fluids, or tissues), process the specimen only after directly consulting with the physician who obtained the specimen and/or the patient's physician. Note the problem on the report, complete with an incident report and documentation of the corrective action taken.
2. Prolonged transport. Do not process, but alert the submitter and request a repeat specimen for specimens obtained by noninvasive means. Note the problem on the patient's report: "Received after prolonged delay." For specimens obtained by invasive procedures (needle aspirates, body fluids, or tissues), directly contact the patient's physician and process as in situation no. 1 above.
3. Improper or leaking container. Do not process. Immediately call the submitter and request a repeat specimen, where appropriate. Note the problem on the patient's report and the corrective action taken. For specimens obtained by invasive procedures (needle aspirates, body fluids, or tissues), directly contact the patient's physician and process as in situation no. 1 above.
4. Specimen unsuitable for request (e.g., request for anaerobic culture for a specimen transported aerobically). Do not process. Contact the submitter, clarify the test request, and indicate the discrepancy. Request a proper specimen for the test requested.
5. Duplicate specimens on the same day for the same test request (except blood and tissue). Do not process. Place the specimen in the proper preservative at the correct storage temperature. Call the submitter and indicate the duplication. Note the problem on the report.

There may be instances in which a given specimen must be processed even though its quality is compromised, e.g., a difficult or unusual case, and then only after a consult between the patient's physician and the laboratory director. Table 2 lists specimens that provide little, if any, clinical information; processing of these specimens should be discouraged.

TABLE 2 Specimens to be discouraged due to questionable microbial information

Specimen type	Alternative or comment
Burn, wounds (swabs)	Submit tissue or aspirate
Colostomy, discharge	Do not process
Decubiti (swabs)	Submit tissue or aspirate
Foley catheter tip	Do not process
Gangrenous lesion (swab)	Submit tissue or aspirate
Gastric aspirates of newborns	Do not process
Lochia	Do not process
Periodontal lesion (swab)	Submit tissue or aspirate
Perirectal abscess (swab)	Submit tissue or aspirate
Varicose ulcer (swab)	Submit tissue or aspirate
Vomitus	Do not process

Sterile body fluids may be submitted from patients with serious or life-threatening illness and must be handled quickly and appropriately. The decision of whether to centrifuge the fluid and culture the specimen on agar media or in blood culture bottles must be incorporated into the laboratory protocol. Table 3 lists some management suggestions for handling sterile body fluids (8).

While the above discussion has focused more on general policy issues surrounding specimen management, the details of specimen management for adults are covered in subsequent and appropriate sections of this Manual. Infants and children represent an important patient population that is often overlooked in specimen management discussions, and there are many instances in which specimens from this patient group require special methods for selection, collection, and transport. The section that follows provides perspective and guidance on these issues.

SPECIMEN MANAGEMENT ISSUES FOR PEDIATRIC PATIENTS

Collection of specimens from pediatric populations may be influenced by factors not encountered when dealing with adults. The types of disease as well as the anatomic areas primarily affected by the infectious agent may differ. Recognition of the critical differences inherent in the collection of specimens for microbiological assays from infants and children aids in optimizing the detection of pathogens from this patient population. Table 4 summarizes the salient features of specimen management in this special population.

The volumes of specimen available for testing vary according to the age and size of the child. Limited volumes are especially pertinent to the collection of blood, urine, cerebrospinal fluid (CSF), other sterile fluids, and tissue samples submitted for culture. Multiple phlebotomies performed for a variety of diagnostic tests can affect the volume of blood collected for culture due to the concern of critical volume depletion in infants and smaller children. The diagnosis of certain types of bacterial meningitis may be hindered by the smaller volumes of CSF available, coupled with the problems inherent in performing lumbar puncture in this age group. The average total volume of CSF in children and

TABLE 3 Specimen management of sterile body fluids other than blood and CSF[a]

Fluid	Collection container	Concentration	Stain	Comment
Amniotic	Anaerobic tube	No	Gram stain	
Culdocentesis	Anaerobic tube	No	Gram stain	
Dialysis effluent	Isolator tube, urine cup, or Bx2	Centrifuge or filter	Gram stain or AO (low detection rate)	<100 leukocytes/ml is normal; use one-third of filter for one of three media
Pericardial	B and/or anaerobic tube	Cytospin from tube	Gram stain from cytospin	Few leukocytes in normal fluid
Peritoneal (ascites)	Bx2 (10 ml) + anaerobic tube	Cytospin from tube	Gram stain from cytospin	<300 leukocytes/ml is normal
Pleural (effusion, transudate, thoracentesis, empyema)	Anaerobic tube	Cytospin from tube	Gram stain from cytospin	>5 ml needed for fungi; none to a few leukocytes is normal; many leukocytes are found with empyema
Synovial	B + anaerobic tube	Cytospin from tube	Gram stain from cytospin	A few leukocytes is normal

[a]The information in this table is from reference 8 and reprinted with permission of Elsevier. Abbreviations: B, blood culture bottle; Bx2, aerobic and anaerobic blood bottles; AO, acridine orange stain. Cultures and stains can be done from any cytospin sediment.

infants is approximately 40 to 90 ml, while the volume range for adults is 90 to 150 ml. Lastly, infants and children not only excrete smaller volumes of urine but are also often unable to void on command. In some cases, <1.0 ml of urine may be available for testing.

The greatest challenge, therefore, for laboratories processing specimens from pediatric patients is making the most of the limited amounts of specimens received for culture. Although the procedures for the collection of many specimen types mirror the protocols used for adult patients, some important differences exist.

Blood Samples for Cultures

Use of proper skin disinfection techniques is even more important in children prior to collection of blood for culture since only one bottle collected during a 24-h period may be available for culture, making the categorization of contaminant versus pathogen difficult to assess. Due to the low incidence of anaerobic bacteremia, routine inoculation of an anaerobic blood culture bottle is not warranted. Although the collection of blood from infants and children by venipuncture is achievable by skilled phlebotomists, venous access in pediatric inpatients is often through peripheral or central venous catheters, which eliminates the need for attempts to gain peripheral venous access. Such lines are used primarily for administration of fluids and therapeutic drugs and are infused with heparin to inhibit clotting when not in use. When the catheter is used to obtain blood cultures, the line must be adequately disinfected and flushed of all inhibitory substances before the specimen is obtained. Since volume depletion in the patient is a concern, the amount of fluid to be discarded, as well as the amount of blood available for testing, is limited. The procedure utilized most often, the discard method, is based on the amount of fluid flushed from the line on the weight and size of the child (39). Minimal discard volumes for infants, for example, are in the range of 0.3 to 1.0 ml (59). In response to the decreased volumes of blood that can be obtained from pediatric patients for culture, blood culture bottles that contain approximately 20 ml of broth and that accommodate an inoculation volume of up to 4 ml are available. The smaller volume of broth allows for a close approximation of the recommended blood-to-broth ratio necessary to diminish the effect of growth inhibitors.

Cerebrospinal Fluid

The primary reason for collection of CSF is for the diagnosis of acute bacterial or viral meningitis or CSF shunt infections. Lumbar puncture is sometimes difficult in an infant or child. A specimen obtained by lumbar puncture that yields only blood is indicative of a failure to access the subarachnoid space (23). If the CSF initially contains a small amount of blood but clears as additional fluid is collected, a repeat lumbar puncture is not required. If only a small amount of fluid is retrieved from the patient due to age and size, CSF containing clotted blood is sometimes sent for culture pending a repeat lumbar puncture. The clot is homogenized prior to plating, and an acridine orange fluorescent stain of a direct smear of a cytospin preparation is recommended to facilitate rapid detection of potential pathogens. Gross blood in the specimen may obscure the visualization of organisms when stained by Gram's method.

Ventricular shunts are used for drainage in patients who overproduce CSF. Ventricular shunt malfunctions in both children and adults are associated with infection and/or disconnection or obstruction of the catheter (26, 54). The majority of shunt infections are acquired at the time of shunt placement and are associated with organisms usually considered skin flora, such as *Staphylococcus epidermidis* or *Propionibacterium acnes* (12, 67).

Specimens for Detection of Otitis and Sinusitis

Acute otitis media is also a common pediatric disease (11, 53). Uncomplicated otitis media does not require confirmation by culture; however, a persistent infection may require retrieval of fluid from the middle ear via tympanocentesis for identification of the specific pathogen causing the infection. A swab specimen of the external auditory canal is unsuitable for diagnosis of acute otitis media or otitis media with effusion. Potential contamination of purulent drainage with resident flora may interfere with accurate analysis of the culture.

Uncomplicated sinusitis is often treated empirically on the basis of the patient's clinical presentation (71). Specimens for culture may be obtained from patients with chronic sinusitis refractory to therapy. Bilateral cultures are recommended (71). Secretions from the region of the maxillary ostium are sampled with a swab under direct vision; however, unless the specimen is obtained very carefully, interpretation of culture

TABLE 4 Requirements for pediatric specimen collection

Specimen type and source	Collection	Comments
Blood for culture		
Peripheral	As for adults. Withdraw a volume of ≥0.5 ml and inoculate into the blood culture bottle.	Collection of larger volumes will aid in retrieval of low concentrations of circulating organisms. Inoculation of one aerobic bottle is usually sufficient.
Peripheral catheter (see comment)	Disinfect the venipuncture site. Insert the catheter and attach a T-connector with syringe to the catheter and withdraw the blood for culture.	A blood culture may be obtained when a peripheral catheter is inserted.
Indwelling central venous catheter	After disinfection, disconnect the extension tubing or cap from the catheter hub. Disinfect the hub. Withdraw a minimum volume of blood and discard. Attach a second sterile syringe and withdraw an additional ≥0.5 ml for culture.	Accidental aspiration of heparin may inhibit the growth of bloodborne pathogens; therefore, flush the catheter with heparin or saline.
Implantable device (for therapy administration)	Disinfect the skin site. Insert a Huber needle through the skin into the apparatus; follow the procedure for collection of blood from a central venous catheter described above.	These devices may rarely be used for vascular access for the retrieval of blood for culture.
CSF		
Lumbar puncture	As for adults.	Difficulties are often encountered in patient positioning and restraint; in addition, there are limitations to the volume of fluid retrievable.
Ventricular shunts	As for adults.	Correct labeling of shunt fluid is important because organisms considered "contaminants" from lumbar punctures may be significant pathogens in ventricular shunt infections.
Dermatologic specimens		
Bacterial and viral cultures		
Pustule or vesicular lesions	Disinfect surface and allow to dry. Unroof the pustule. Aspirate fluid for culture and then insert swab and rotate vigorously to collect fluid and cells from the advancing margin.	Specimens that contain no inflammatory cells are from the superficial areas of the lesion and new specimens must be collected. Viral pathogens are best retrieved from the base of a lesion.
Petechiae, purpura, ecthyma gangrenosa	With a scalpel blade, vigorously scrape the outer margin of the lesion.	A Gram stain of petechiae material may give an indication of meningococcal infection.
Fungi	For a dry lesion, scrape the lesion with a scalpel, glass slide, or toothbrush. For moist lesions, use a Dacron swab. For hair, use scissors and forceps. For nails, scrape with a scalpel. Place scraping directly onto fungal medium or place in a sterile container and send for culture.	A small toothbrush is useful for collection of scrapings.
Specimens for detection of scabies	Disinfect the area and allow to dry. Apply a single drop of mineral oil to the papule and abrade the infested area with a sterile scalpel. Transfer skin scrapings to a sterile container or microscope slide with coverslip for transport to the lab.	Place the microscope slide with coverslip in a secure holder so that the coverslip is not dislodged during transit.
Feces		
Bacterial and viral cultures	As for adults. A rectal swab showing feces is suitable for bacterial or viral culture.	Devices that fit into the toilet bowl or techniques such as lining a diaper with plastic wrap facilitate retrieval of feces for testing.
C. difficile toxin	As for adults.	Toxin-producing strains of *C. difficile* may be normal in some infants <2 years of age. Interpret a positive toxin result for individuals in this age group with caution.

(Continued on next page)

TABLE 4 *(Continued)*

Specimen type and source	Collection	Comments
Ovum and parasite examination	As for adults. Submit feces-coated rectal swabs only for antigen detection EIAs, not routine ovum and parasite examinations.	See bacterial and viral cultures. The volume of preservatives present in commercial ovum and parasite collection and transport tubes should be adjusted to retain the recommended stool-to-fixative ratio of 3:1.
Pinworms	Use a commercial paddle sampling device or place the adhesive side of a cellophane tape strip onto a microscope slide. Peel back the tape to expose the adhesive side of the tape. While holding the slide against an applicator, press the tape firmly against the perianal skin. Replace the tape back over the slide and press the adhesive side onto the slide.	The applicator stick provides a safe backing for the glass slide while gentle pressure is applied to the skin for collection of the specimen with the adhesive. Do not use "invisible" or "magic" tape.
Gastric aspirates (may not provide clinically relevant data)	A premeasured length of lubricated catheter is passed gently into the mouth or nasopharynx and is continued through the esophagus into the stomach. The contents are aspirated and place in a sterile container for immediate transport to the lab. If no gastric secretions are obtained, a lavage of sterile distilled water is collected for specimen processing.	Three consecutive early-morning, fasting specimens are preferred for mycobacterial culture, but infants may not be able to provide such a sample. Collect the aspirate as long after the last feeding as possible. Environmental mycobacterial species may appear in aspirated formula. Neutralization of the specimen must occur upon arrival in the lab.
Genital specimens	Use a small-tipped Dacron swab with a flexible smooth wire. The specimen of choice for a prepubertal female is a vaginal swab or washing. Collect a urethral swab from prepubertal males.	STDs in prepubertal girls involve the vagina as opposed to the cervix. Specimens from adolescents are the same as those collected from adults.
Ear specimens		
Otitis (otitis media)	Cleanse the external auditory canal with an antiseptic. Using an otoscope, insert a 1-ml tuberculin syringe with a 3.5-in 22-gauge spinal needle bent at a 30° angle through the tympanic membrane and aspirate the fluid in the chamber into a sterile vial or syringe.	Needle aspiration of fluid (tympanocentesis) is the recommended method for obtaining a specimen. A purulent discharge from a ruptured membrane can be collected for culture by using a sterile swab.
Respiratory specimens		
Bronchoalveolar lavage specimens	As for adults.	Specimens from unsheathed catheters may contain contaminating oropharyngeal flora. In infants and younger children, <10 ml is often retrieved. If >10 ml is collected, centrifuge the sample prior to plating.
Protected brush specimens	As for adults.	
Nasal specimens	Insert a sterile swab at least 1 cm into the opening of the anterior nares.	Used primarily for surveillance of methicillin-resistant *Staphylococcus aureus* or to assess upper respiratory tract colonization in children with immunologic defects.

(Continued on next page)

TABLE 4 Requirements for pediatric specimen collection *(Continued)*

Specimen type and source	Collection	Comments
Nasal washes	Aspirate approximately 4 ml of sterile saline into a 1-oz tapered rubber bulb. Tip the patient's head back approximately 70 degrees and insert the bulb into the nostril until it is occluded. Squeeze the bulb to dispense the saline, hold for a few seconds and then release to collect the secretions. Dispense the specimen into a sterile container and transport to the lab as soon as possible.	A nasal wash or nasal aspirate (see below) is often cited as the preferred specimen type for collection of respiratory secretions for culture for either viruses or *Bordetella pertussis* and direct smear examination and in pediatric patients. Transport specimens for viral cultures on ice.
Nasopharyngeal aspirate	Attach a sterile suction catheter to a (mucus) trap and introduce the end of the catheter into the nasopharynx until resistance is encountered. Withdraw the catheter 1–2 cm and apply suction to aspirate the sample. Dispense the specimen into a sterile container and immediately transport it to the lab.	See nasal wash. Transport specimens for viral cultures on ice.
Nasopharyngeal swab specimens	Insert the swab into the nasopharyngeal cavity to the point of resistance and then gently rotate it. Place the swab into an appropriate transport medium and send to the lab immediately.	Young children and infants require use of a swab with a small-tip circumference such as a calcium alginate or small-tip Dacron swab. Transport specimens for viral cultures on ice.
Throat swab specimens	Tilt the child's head back and ask the child to open the mouth as wide as possible. Carefully insert the sterile swab(s) into the oral cavity and sample the surfaces of the back of the throat and tonsils.	In children, the major pathogen of bacterial pharyngitis is group A streptococci (GAS). If a rapid screen of a throat swab specimen for GAS is performed, collect two swabs to do a culture to confirm negative screening findings or to rule out a possible false positive caused by a member of the *Streptococcus anginosus* group. Avoid touching other areas of the oral cavity to prevent specimen contamination with oropharyngeal flora.
Tracheal aspirate	After oxygenation of the patient, attach a sterile suction catheter to a (mucus) trap and introduce the end of the catheter into the trachea until resistance is encountered. Withdraw the catheter 1–2 cm and apply suction to aspirate the sample.	Although grading systems for assessment of the quality of pediatric tracheal aspirates have been proposed, careful evaluation is required prior to their implementation.
Transtracheal aspirate	As for adults.	
Sputum specimens	As for adults.	Since children are often unable to produce sputum, tracheal aspirates are more often collected in pediatric populations.
Specimens for detection of viruses	Specimens of choice are similar to others in this table (45).	Rectal swabs are acceptable for detection of rotavirus antigen.
Specimens for detection of *Chlamydia*	Conjunctival and/or nasopharyngeal swabs are appropriate for neonatal screening.	See genital specimens above. Vaginal (females) or urethral (males) swabs are required for chlamydia culture for the determination of sexual abuse.

results may be hindered by the presence of contaminating flora. Needle aspiration of the sinus is recommended for definitive diagnosis of the etiologic agent of infection (49).

Respiratory Specimens

For the diagnosis of group A streptococcal pharyngitis (10, 14), collection of two pharyngeal swabs is optimal for performance of both a rapid antigen detection assay and culture (one swab for each assay). A single swab shared for both methods may reduce the sensitivity of the antigen detection assay due to a reduction in the concentration of organisms available after culture inoculation (10). Although the reported sensitivities of some rapid assays may suggest that a confirmatory culture may be eliminated in the event that the screen is negative, careful consideration must be given to the possible implications of an undetected infection in some children (10). The collection of nasopharyngeal swab specimens, washes, or aspirates for culture and/or detection of antigens of respiratory viruses and *Bordetella pertussis* is satisfactory (4, 47, 48). Again, collection of more than one swab increases the chance of isolate detection. Transport of swabs in a suitable holding medium is necessary to ensure organism viability if delays are anticipated between the time of collection and specimen receipt by the laboratory. Due to the small diameter of the nasal passages in some infants and children, coupled with inflammation of the nasal mucosa during the infection, specimen collection with a swab is sometimes more difficult and thus provides an inadequate sample.

A sputum specimen for diagnosis of pneumonia is difficult to obtain from children. More commonly, a tracheal or endotracheal tube aspirate is sent for microbiological culture. The utility of endotracheal tube aspirates as predictors of pediatric lower respiratory tract infection is influenced by the role that accumulated secretions within the tube play in the promotion of bacterial colonization (30, 62, 75). A bronchoalveolar lavage or the use of a protected brush will provide a superior specimen for intubated children with clinical evidence of pneumonia (44, 46, 74). Although pediatric bronchoscopes are available, the tubing diameter is sometimes too large for certain pediatric patients. In these situations, a small-diameter catheter is useful for performance of the lavage (2, 43). If an unprotected catheter is used, however, commensal oral flora will reduce the chances for recognition of the true etiologic agent. Aspiration of gastric secretions is performed for infants and children with presumed pneumonia caused by *Mycobacterium tuberculosis* (1, 61). After the patient has fasted overnight, the swallowed respiratory secretions are aspirated from the stomach by using gastric intubation and sent for diagnostic testing (1, 64). Problems with this method include the inability of infants on a feeding schedule to maintain a fasting state prior to specimen collection. Lastly, many pediatric centers provide care for children with cystic fibrosis. Specimens from these patients are periodically sent to the laboratory for surveillance of lower respiratory tract colonization by various potentially pathogenic microorganisms. Recommended specimens for culture of these types of organisms include sputum, tracheal aspirates, or throat swabs (6, 29, 56).

Genital Specimens

Genital specimens are usually collected from pediatric patients for (i) investigation of possible sexual abuse or rape or (ii) diagnosis of premenarchal vulvovaginitis and/or urethritis. Since these specimens are often irretrievable, every effort must be made to process pediatric urogenital specimens for culture. Although the cervix is the specimen source for diagnosis of gonorrhea and chlamydia in adolescent and adult females, detection of these sexually transmitted diseases (STDs) in prepubertal females requires sampling of the vaginal vault (5). A urethral swab sample is collected from prepubescent males. Culture is required for confirmation of both types of infections (5). Antigen detection assays are not acceptable due to the high reported rates of false positivity (33, 72). Likewise, the performance of molecular methods has not been adequately assessed for detection of STDs in children and is not considered admissible in the event of legal proceedings (34).

Urine Specimens

Collection of uncontaminated urine specimens from pediatric patients is a challenge. The acquisition of a clean-catch specimen from older children is hindered by the same problems experienced with adult patients. A urine specimen collected by catheterization is used for all pediatric age groups and, if performed properly, can yield a specimen free of urethral contaminants (4). Although suprapubic aspiration is considered the optimum method for urine collection from infants, the technique is frequently unsuccessful in dehydrated patients (4). Specimens must be transported to the lab within 30 min of collection or stored under refrigeration for no longer than 24 h (50). Urine transport systems containing preservatives are available for adult patients, who characteristically excrete larger volumes of urine. For optimum performance, the urine and preservative must be in the ratio recommended by the manufacturer. At present, no transport system is available to accommodate the lower-volume pediatric urine specimens.

Fecal Specimens

The best clinical predictors of a positive stool culture in children are a combination of persistent diarrhea of >24 h in duration, fever, and either blood in the stool or abdominal pain with nausea and vomiting (20, 45, 57, 61, 66). Many cases of endemic diarrhea occur in children <5 years of age and are caused by pathogens that are endemic to an area, such as rotavirus, shigellae, *Giardia lamblia*, and cryptosporidia (20). Since most diarrheal disease is community acquired, a single stool culture obtained during the first 72 h after admission to the hospital can be used for diagnosis for almost 98% of children with bacterial gastroenteritis (15, 16, 55). Depending on the age of the child, nosocomially acquired diarrheal disease is most often attributed to rotavirus or *Clostridium difficile* (13, 28). Interpretation of positive *Clostridium difficile* toxin assay results for children <2 years of age may be difficult due to intestinal colonization of this group with toxin-producing strains (22, 42, 68). A freshly obtained stool sample is preferable for all fecal assays. A rectal swab is less optimal but is acceptable for recovery of bacterial enteric pathogens, surveillance for multidrug-resistant organisms, and performance of certain antigen detection assays. A rectal swab is not recommended for some detection assays for *Clostridium difficile* toxin. If a delay in transport is anticipated, fecal specimens for either bacterial culture or parasite detection should be placed in an appropriate transport medium or preservative, respectively. In order to maintain the 3:1 recommended ratio of stool to preservative for parasite transport vials, the volume of preservative in the vial may require adjustment prior to inoculation of a small pediatric sample.

Pinworm *(Enterobius vermicularis)* infection is a common ailment of children. After establishment of infection in the colon, the female adult pinworm periodically migrates to the perianal area and deposits her eggs on the skin. Commercial sampling paddles are available for sampling, but cellophane or cellulose tape applied to the perianal skin in the morning, before the patient washes or defecates, enables collection of the eggs for identification.

Specimens from Neonates

The neonatal nursery and intensive care unit pose unique challenges for the microbiology laboratory. The problems inherent in decreased sample amounts available from these tiny patients may be compounded by the unpredictable response to infection displayed by neonates (31, 51). For example, isolates retrieved from the mucous membranes, skin, ear canal, nasopharynx, gastric aspirate, or rectum usually do not match the results of blood, CSF, or tissue cultures (31, 51). Differentiation of colonization versus true infection, therefore, may be very difficult. Microorganisms are acquired either through transmission in utero, during delivery, or from nosocomial spread via hospital personnel, various medical devices, or environmental sources (36, 63). Infections reported to occur in neonates include sepsis, meningitis, otitis media, diarrhea, osteomyelitis or septic arthritis, conjunctivitis or orbital cellulitis, pneumonia, and various skin infections (7, 24, 27, 31, 51, 70, 73). Congenital infection is most often caused by agents such as *Toxoplasma gondii* or viruses such as herpes simplex virus, cytomegalovirus, varicella-zoster virus, parvovirus, enterovirus, rubella, or hepatitis B virus (25, 31, 41, 51, 65). Collection methods and appropriate specimen types for neonates are similar to those recommended for older infants and children with the exception of blood for culture. Depending on the age of the newborn, recommended sampling sites include the peripheral vein, umbilical artery, and capillary blood (31). Although a minimum of 0.5 to 1.0 ml is most often cited as the recommended amount of specimen to be collected, larger volumes are recommended for optimal recovery of organisms (40, 58).

Viral Specimens

Since smaller specimen volumes are often received from pediatric patients, newer molecular methods may aid in the detection of pediatric systemic or central nervous system viral infections. The antigenemia assay for detection of cytomegalovirus in blood may be impeded by both the smaller specimen volumes and the smaller polymorphonuclear leukocyte concentrations in neutropenic children undergoing transplantation or therapy for oncological problems. Details regarding diagnosis of viral infections can be found in chapter 80 of this Manual.

Dermatologic Specimens

Rashes are a common manifestation of many childhood illnesses. The same techniques are used to sample skin lesions from children and adults. A small, disposable toothbrush is valuable for obtaining scrapings of certain types of dermatophytic fungal lesions and produces fewer traumas than using a scalpel (3). Retrieval of skin samples for detection of scabies often yields no visible organism; however, the distribution of lesions differs between infants and young children and their older counterparts (3).

REFERENCES

1. **Abadco, D. L., and P. Steiner.** 1992. Gastric lavage is better than bronchoalveolar lavage for isolation of *Mycobacterium tuberculosis* in childhood pulmonary tuberculosis. *Pediatr. Infect. Dis. J.* **11:**735–738.
2. **Alpert, B. E., B. P. O'Sullivan, and H. B. Panitch.** 1992. Nonbronchoscopic approach to bronchoalveolar lavage in children with artificial airways. *Pediatr. Pulmonol.* **13:**38–41.
3. **American Academy of Pediatrics.** 2000. *Red Book.* American Academy of Pediatrics, Elk Grove Village, Ill.
4. **American Academy of Pediatrics.** 1999. Practice parameter:the diagnosis, treatment, and evaluation of the initial urinary tract infection in febrile infants and young children. *Pediatrics* **103:**843–852.
5. **American Academy of Pediatrics.** 1999. Guidelines for the evaluation of sexual abuse of children: subject review. *Pediatrics* **103:**186–191.
6. **Armstrong, D. S., K. Grimwood, J. B. Carlin, R. Carzino, A. Olinsky, and P. D. Phelan.** 1996. Bronchoalveolar lavage or oropharyngeal cultures to identify lower respiratory pathogens in infants with cystic fibrosis. *Pediatr. Pulmonol.* **21:**267–275.
7. **Bale, J. F., and J. R. Murphy.** 1997. Infections of the central nervous system in the newborn. *Clin. Perinatol.* **24:**787–806.
8. **Baron, E. J.** 1994. *Bailey and Scott's Diagnostic Microbiology*, 9th ed. The C. V. Mosby Co., St. Louis, Mo.
9. **Bartlett, R. C.** 1985. Quality control, p. 14–23. *In* E. H. Lennette, A. Balows, W. J. Hausler, Jr., and J. J. Shadomy (ed.), *Manual of Clinical Microbiology,* 4th ed. American Society for Microbiology, Washington, D.C.
10. **Bisno, A.** 2001. Primary care: acute pharyngitis. *N. Engl. J. Med.* **344:**205–211.
11. **Bluestone, C. D., and J. O. Klein (ed.).** 1995. *Otitis Media in Infants and Children,* 2nd ed. W. B. Saunders, Philadelphia, Pa.
12. **Bordes, A., R. Elcuaz, F. J. Noguera, C. Otemin, and G. Egas.** 1997. *Propionibacterium acnes* infections in patients with CSF shunts. *Enferm. Infecc. Microbiol. Clin.* **15:**24–27.
13. **Brady, M. T., D. L. Pacini, C. T. Budde, and M. J. Connell.** 1989. Diagnostic studies of nosocomial diarrhea in children: assessing their use and value. *Am. J. Infect. Control* **17:**77–82.
14. **Carroll, K., and L. Reimer.** 1996. Microbiology and laboratory diagnosis of upper respiratory tract infections. *Clin. Infect. Dis.* **23:**442–448.
15. **Chitkara, Y. K., K. A McCasland, and L. Kenefic.** 1996. Development and implementation of cost-effective guidelines in the laboratory investigation of diarrhea in a community hospital. *Arch. Intern. Med.* **156:**1445–1448.
16. **Church, D. L., G. Cadrain, A. Kabani, T. Jadavji, and C. Trevenen.** 1994. Practice guidelines for ordering stool cultures in a pediatric population. *Am. J. Clin. Pathol.* **103:**149–153.
17. **Clinical and Laboratory Standards Institute/NCCLS.** 2004. *Clinical Laboratory Safety; Approved Guidelines GP17-A2.* Clinical and Laboratory Standards Institute, Wayne, Pa.
18. **Clinical and Laboratory Standards Institute/NCCLS.** 2005. *Protection of Laboratory Workers from Occupationally Acquired Infections; Approved Guidelines M29-A3.* Clinical and Laboratory Standards Institute, Wayne, Pa.
19. **Clinical and Laboratory Standards Institute/NCCLS.** 2003. *Quality Control of Microbiological Transport Systems; Approved Standard M40-A.* Clinical and Laboratory Standards Institute, Wayne, Pa.
20. **Cohen, M. B.** 1991. Etiology and mechanisms of acute infectious diarrhea in infants in the United States. *J. Pediatr.* **118:**S34–S39.
21. **Cook, J. H., and M. Pezzlo.** 1992. Specimen receipt and accessioning. Section 1. Aerobic bacteriology, 1.2.1–1.2.4. *In* H. D. Isenberg (ed. in chief), *Clinical Microbiology Procedures Handbook.* American Society for Microbiology, Washington, D.C.
22. **Craven, D., D. Brick, A. Morrisey, M. A. O'Riordan, V. Petran, and J. R. Schreiber.** 1998. Low yield of bacterial stool culture in children with nosocomial diarrhea. *Pediatr. Infect. Dis. J.* **17:**1040–1044.
23. **Cronan, K. M., and J. F. Wiley.** 1997. Lumbar puncture, p. 541–553. *In* F. M. Henretig and C. King (ed.), *Textbook of Pediatric Emergency Procedures.* Williams and Wilkins, Baltimore, Md.
24. **Dennehy, P. H.** 1987. Respiratory infections in the newborn. *Clin. Perinatol.* **14:**667–682.
25. **Donley, D. K.** 1993. TORCH infections in the newborn. *Semin. Neurol.* **13:**106–115.
26. **Duhaime, A. C., and J. F. Wiley.** 1997. Ventricular shunt and burr hole puncture, p. 553–558. *In* F. M. Henretig and C. King (ed.), *Textbook of Pediatric Emergency Procedures.* Williams and Wilkins, Baltimore, Md.
27. **Eichenwald, E. C.** 1997. Perinatally transmitted neonatal bacterial infections. *Infect. Dis. Clin. N. Am.* **11:**223–239.
28. **Ford-Jones, E. L., C. M. Mindorff, R. Gold, and M. Petric.** 1990. The incidence of viral-associated diarrhea after

admission to a pediatric hospital. *Am. J. Epidemiol.* **131:** 711–718.

29. **Gilligan, P. H.** 1991. Microbiology of airway disease in patients with cystic fibrosis. *Clin. Microbiol. Rev.* **4:**35–51.
30. **Golden, S. E., Z. M. Shehab, J. C. Bjelland, J. R. Kenneth, and C. G. Ray.** 1987. Microbiology of endotracheal aspirates in intubated pediatric intensive care unit patients: correlations with radiographic findings. *Pediatr. Infect. Dis. J.* **6:**665–669.
31. **Gotoff, S. P.** 2000. Infections of the neonatal infant, p. 538–551. *In* R. E. Behrman, R. M. Kleigman, and H. B. Jensen (ed.), *Nelson's Textbook of Pediatrics,* 16th ed. The W. B. Saunders Co., Philadelphia, Pa.
32. **Hagen, J. C., W. S. Wood, and T. Hashimoto.** 1977. Effect of temperature on survival of *Bacteroides fragilis* subsp. *fragilis* and *Escherichia coli* in pus. *J. Clin. Microbiol.* **6:**567–570.
33. **Hammerschlag, M. R.** 1998. Sexually transmitted diseases in sexually abused children: medical and legal implications. *Sex. Transm. Infect.* **74:**167–174.
34. **Hammerschlag, M. R., S. Ajl, and D. Laraque.** 1999. Inappropriate use of nonchlamydia tests for the detection of chlamydia in suspected victims of child sexual abuse: a continuing problem. *Pediatrics* **104:**1137–1139.
35. **Holden, J.** 1992. Collection and transport of clinical specimens for anaerobic culture, 2.2.1–2.2.6. *In* H. D. Isenberg (ed. in chief), *Clinical Microbiology Procedures Handbook.* American Society for Microbiology, Washington, D.C.
36. **Hoogkamp-Korstanje, J. A., B. Cats, R. C. Senders, and I. van Ertgruggen.** 1982. Analysis of bacterial infections in a neonatal intensive care unit. *J. Hosp. Infect.* **393:**275–284.
37. **Isenberg, H. D. (ed. in chief).** 1992. *Clinical Microbiology Procedures Handbook,* vol. 1 and 2. American Society for Microbiology, Washington, D.C.
38. **Johnson, F. B.** 1990. Transport of viral specimens. *Clin. Microbiol. Rev.* **3:**120–131.
39. **Keller, C.** 1994. Methods of drawing blood samples through central venous catheters in pediatric patients undergoing bone marrow transplant: results of a national survey. *Oncol. Nurs. Forum* **21:**879–884.
40. **Kellogg, J. A., F. L. Ferrentino, M. H. Goodstein, S. L. Shapiro, and D. A Bankert.** 1997. Frequency of low level bacteremia in infants from birth to two months of age. *Pediatr. Infect. Dis. J.* **16:**381–385.
41. **Kinney, J. S., and M. L. Kumar.** 1988. Should we expand the TORCH Complex? A description of clinical and diagnostic aspects of selected old and new agents. *Clin. Perinatol.* **15:**727–744.
42. **Knoop, F. C., M. Owens, and I. C. Crocker.** 1993. *Clostridium difficile:* clinical disease and diagnosis. *Clin. Microbiol. Rev.* **6:**251–265.
43. **Koumbourlis, A. C., and G. Kurland.** 1993. Nonbronchoscopic bronchoalveolar lavage in mechanically ventilated infants: technique, efficacy, and applications. *Pediatr. Pulmonol.* **15:**257–262.
44. **Labeene, M., C. Poyart, C. Ranbaud, B. Goldfarb, B. Pron, P. Jouvet, C. Delamare, G. Sebag, and P. Hubert.** 1999. Blind protected specimen brush and bronchoalveolar lavage in ventilated children. *Crit. Care Med.* **27:**2537–2543.
45. **Laney, E. W., and M. B. Cohen.** 1993. Approach to the pediatric patient with diarrhea. *Gastroenterol. Clin. N. Amer.* **22:**499–516.
46. **Linder, J., and S. I. Rennard.** 1988. *Bronchoalveolar Lavage,* p. 1–16. ASCP Press, Chicago, Ill.
47. **Marcon, J. J., A. C. Hamoudi, H. J. Cannon, and M. M. Hribar.** 1987. Comparison of throat and nasopharyngeal swab specimens for culture diagnosis of *Bordetella pertussis* infections. *J. Clin. Microbiol.* **25:**1109–1110.
48. **Masters, H. B., K. O. Weber, J. R. Groothuis, C. G. Wren, and B. A. Lauer.** 1987. Comparisons of nasopharyngeal washings and swab specimens for diagnosis of respiratory syncytial virus by EIA, FAT, and cell culture. *Diagn. Microbiol. Infect. Dis.* **8:**101–105.
49. **McBride, T. P., H. W. Davis, and J. S. Reilly.** 1997. Otolaryngology. *In* B. J. Zitelli and H. W. Davis (ed.), *Atlas of Pediatric Physical Diagnosis.* Mosby-Wolfe, St. Louis, Mo.
50. **Miller, J. M.** 1999. *A Guide to Specimen Management in Clinical Microbiology,* 2nd ed. ASM Press, Washington, D.C.
51. **Mustafa, M. M., and G. H. McCracken.** 1992. Perinatal infections. *In* R. D. Feigin and J. D. Cherry (ed.), *Textbook of Pediatric Infectious Diseases,* 3rd ed. The W. B. Saunders Co., Philadelphia, Pa.
52. **National Research Council.** 1989. *Biosafety in the Laboratory: Prudent Practices for the Handling and Disposal of Infectious Material.* National Academy Press, Washington, D.C.
53. **Pichichero, M. E.** 2000. Acute otitis media. Part I. Improving diagnostic accuracy. *Am. Fam. Physician* **61:**2051–2056.
54. **Renier, D., J. Lacombe, A. Pierre-Kahn, C. Sainte-Rose, and J. F. Hirsch.** 1984. Factors causing acute shunt infection: computer analysis of 1174 operations. *J. Neurosurg.* **61:**1072–1078.
55. **Rohner, P., D. Pittet, B. Pepey, T. Nije-Kinge, and R. Auckenthaler.** 1997. Etiological agents of infectious diarrhea: implications for requests for microbial culture. *J. Clin. Microbiol.* **35:**1427–1432.
56. **Rosenfeld, M., J. Emerson, F. Accurso, D. Armstrong. R. Castile, K. Grimwood, P. Hiatt, K. McCoy, S. McNamara, B. Ramsey, and J. Wagener.** 1999. Diagnostic accuracy of oropharyngeal cultures in infants and young children with cystic fibrosis. *Pediatr. Pulmonol.* **28:**321–328.
57. **Rudolph, J. A., and M. B. Cohen.** 1999. New causes and treatments for infectious diarrhea in children. *Curr. Gastroenterol. Rep.* **1:**238–244.
58. **Schelonka, R. L., M. K. Chai, B. A. Yoder, D. Hensley, R. M. Brockett, and D. P Ascher.** 1996. Volume of blood required to detect common neonatal pathogens. *J. Pediatr.* **129:**275–279.
59. **Schulman, R. J., S. Phillips, L. Laine, P. Gardner, V. Nichols, T. Reed, and E. Hawkins.** 1993. Volume of blood required to obtain central venous catheter blood cultures in infants and children. *JPEN. J. Parenter. Enteral Nutr.* **17:**177–179.
60. **Shea, Y. R.** 1992. Specimen collection and transport. Section 1. Aerobic bacteriology, p. 1.1.1–1.1.30. *In* H. D. Isenberg (ed. in chief), *Clinical Microbiology Procedures Handbook.* American Society for Microbiology, Washington, D.C.
61. **Sherman, P. M., M. Petric, and M. B. Cohen.** 1996. Infectious gastroenterocolitides in children: an update on emerging pathogens. *Pediatr. Clin. N. Am.* **43:**391–407.
62. **Slagle, T. A., E. M. Bifano, J. W. Wolf, and S. J. Gross.** 1989. Routine endotracheal cultures for the prediction of sepsis in ventilated babies. *Arch. Dis. Child.* **64:**34–38.
63. **Smith, D. H.** 1979. Epidemics of infectious diseases in newborn nurseries. *Clin. Obstet. Gynecol.* **22:**409–423.
64. **Somu, N., S. Swaminathan, C. N. Paramasivan, D. Vijayasekaran, A. Chandrabhooshanam, V. K. Vijayan, and R. Prabhakar.** 1995. Value of bronchoalveolar lavage and gastric lavage in the diagnosis of pulmonary tuberculosis in children. *Tuber. Lung Dis.* **76:**295–299.
65. **Strodtbeck, R.** 1995. Viral infections of the newborn. *J. Obstet. Gynecol. Neonatal Nurs.* **24:**659–667.
66. **Stutman, H. R.** 1994. Salmonella, Shigella, and Campylobacter: common bacterial causes of infectious diarrhea. *Pediatr. Ann.* **23:**538–543.
67. **Thompson, T. P., and A. L. Albright.** 1998. *Propionibacterium acnes* infections of cerebrospinal fluid shunts. *Childs Nerv. Sys.* **14:**378–380.

68. **Tullus, K., B. Aronsson, S. Marcus, and R. Mollby.** 1989. Intestinal colonization with *Clostridium difficile* in infants up to 18 months of age. *Eur. J. Clin. Microbiol. Infect. Dis.* **8:**390–393.
69. **U.S. Department of Health and Human Services.** 1999. *Biosafety in Microbiological and Biomedical Laboratories,* 4th ed. HHS publication no. (CDC) 93-8395. U.S. Department of Health and Human Services, Washington, D.C.
70. **Verbov, J.** 2000. Common skin conditions in the newborn. *Semin. Neonatol.* **5:**303–310.
71. **Wald, E. R.** 1995. Chronic sinusitis in children. *J. Pediatr.* **127:**339–347.
72. **Whittington, W. L., R. J. Rice, J. W. Biddle, and J. S. Knapp.** 1988. Incorrect identification of *Neisseria gonorrhoeae* from infants and children. *Pediatr. Infect. Dis. J.* **7:**3–10.
73. **Wright, P. F.** 1998. Infectious diseases in early life in industrialized countries. *Vaccine* **16:**1355–1359.
74. **Yagoda, M. R., J. Stavola, R. Ward, C. Steinberg, and J. Jones.** 1996. Role of bronchoalveolar lavage in hospitalized pediatric patients. *Ann. Otol. Rhinol. Laryngol.* **105:** 863–867.
75. **Zaidi, A. K. M., and L. B. Reller.** 1996. Rejection criteria for endotracheal aspirates from pediatric patients. *J. Clin. Microbiol.* **34:**352–354.

Procedures for the Storage of Microorganisms

CATHY A. PETTI, KAREN C. CARROLL, AND LARRY G. REIMER

6

Long- and short-term preservation of microorganisms for future study has a long tradition in microbiology. Culture collections of microorganisms are valuable resources for scientific research in microbial diversity and evolution, patient care management, epidemiological investigations, and educational purposes. Preserved individual strains of microorganisms serve as permanent records of microorganisms' unique phenotypic profiles and provide the material for further genotypic characterizations. Such reference collections can encompass rare infectious agents unique to an individual or catalog the history of disease caused by common pathogens such as those responsible for community outbreaks.

There are multiple methods for microbial preservation. Effective storage is defined by the ability to maintain an organism in a viable state free of contamination and without changes in its genotypic or phenotypic characteristics. Secondly, the organism must be easily restored to its condition prior to preservation. Microbial preservation methods have been evaluated extensively over the past 50 years, and often, optimal methods for preservation depend on a microorganism's taxonomic classification. Review articles, monographs, and books have been published that provide detailed information about the storage of various types of microorganisms (1, 10, 14, 15, 27). For clinical microbiology laboratories, simple and broadly applied methods are necessary to maintain organisms for short- and long-term recovery. This chapter presents methods that can be used for the storage of bacteria, protozoa, fungi, and viruses.

OVERVIEW OF PRESERVATION METHODS

Short-Term Preservation Methods

Direct Transfer to Subculture

The simplest method for maintaining the short-term viability of microorganisms, most often used for bacteria, is periodic subculture to fresh medium. Although simple, if microorganisms are saved for more than 1 week, this method is potentially labor-intensive, requires extensive laboratory space, and may compromise a microorganism's phenotypic profile. Each transfer to a new subculture increases the likelihood of mutation with undesirable changes in a microorganism's characteristics.

The interval between transfers varies among organisms. Additionally, the rate of mutation is quite variable. Some organisms appear stable indefinitely with repeated transfer, and others may change phenotypic traits after as few as two or three passages. The actual rate of mutation, however, has not been studied using sequencing technology. Issues that must be addressed with direct transfer include the medium to be used, the storage conditions, and the frequency of transfer.

Maintenance Medium

The medium should support the survival of the microorganism but minimize its metabolic processes and slow its rate of growth. Extreme environments should be avoided because microorganisms have the unique ability to adapt through mutation events in order to survive in suboptimal surroundings. A medium with too high a nutrient content will induce rapid replication that requires more frequent transfers. The optimal medium for maintaining microorganisms has not been clearly defined and most likely varies from one genus to another. Media that have been used include distilled water, tryptic soy broth, and nutrient broths (e.g., from Becton Dickinson and Co. and Oxoid Ltd.), all of which may be used with or without cryopreservatives.

Storage Conditions

Many laboratories store organisms, most often bacteria, for short periods on routine agar media at the workbench. Cultures kept in this fashion are subject to drying. A better method is to transfer organisms into screw-top test tubes and to store them in an organized location away from light and significant temperature changes. To prevent drying, caps can include rubber liners, or film can be wrapped over the top of the tube before or after the cap is screwed on. Storage at lower temperatures (5 to 8°C) slows metabolic processes and maintains viability for longer periods.

Frequency of Transfer

There is no set protocol for the frequency of transfer since storage conditions, media used, and types of microorganisms vary among laboratories. Individual laboratories should conduct studies for each category of microorganism to determine acceptable intervals between transfers under their conditions used for storage. Such studies would involve performing subcultures at scheduled times until the laboratory identifies an acceptable interval between transfers at which a microorganism can reliably and reproducibly be recovered. (When transfers are performed, 5 to 10 representative colonies should be used to avoid the possibility of introducing an altered genotypic or phenotypic characteristic.)

Quality Control Procedures

Although it is not necessary with each transfer, the status of the specimen should be assessed periodically. Ongoing viability, stability of phenotype, microorganism identity, and the rate of contamination of specimens should be determined and noted in a log.

Immersion in Oil

An alternative to capping tubes is to add a layer of mineral oil to the top of the specimen. Many bacteria and fungi can be stored for periods of up to 2 to 3 years by this method, and transfers are not needed as frequently. Microorganisms are still metabolically active in this environment, and mutations can still occur. Contamination of the specimen can occur if the mineral oil is not adequately sterilized.

Mineral oil should be medicinal-grade oil with specific gravity of 0.865 to 0.890 (e.g., from Roxane Laboratories or Becton Dickinson and Co.). For sterilization, it should be heated to 170°C for 1 to 2 h in an oven (10). Autoclaving is not considered acceptable.

To prepare the specimen, an inoculum of 5 to 10 colonies of the microorganism should be placed on an agar slant or in tubed broth media. Once growth is identified, a layer of mineral oil at least 1 to 2 cm deep is added, and the agar must not be exposed to air. As with the simple transfer method, tests for viability should be performed to determine the optimal transfer schedule that will ensure microorganism recovery. Transfers will be less frequent than those of microorganisms stored without oil; however, oil is more difficult to add to vials and to clean up in the event of spills.

Freezing at −20°C

Refrigeration or freezing in ordinary freezers at −20°C may be used to preserve microorganisms for periods longer than those that can be accomplished by repeated transfers. Viability may be maintained for as long as 1 to 2 years for specific microorganisms, but overall, damage caused by ice crystal formation (15) and electrolyte fluctuations (10) results in poor long-term survival. The medium used for storage appears to be important, since preservation times vary from a few months to 2 years depending upon which medium is used (12, 15, 17). Modern self-defrosting freezers with freeze-thaw cycles must be avoided because cyclic temperature fluctuation will destroy the microorganism.

Drying

Although most microorganisms do not survive drying, molds and some spore-forming bacteria may be dried and stored for prolonged periods. Soil can be used as a storage medium if it is autoclaved and air dried. Soil should be autoclaved for several hours on two successive days. It is then transferred into sterile glass tubes. A 1-ml suspension of the microorganism is inoculated into the tube, and the tube is left open to air dry before being closed with a sterile stopper. The sample is stored in a refrigerator (10). Although potentially effective, soil is not a standardized, defined, and consistent product for use over long periods. Instead, commercial silica gel can be used in small cotton-plugged tubes after being heated in an oven to 175°C for 1.5 to 2 h (15), with moderately successful recovery of fungi. Alternatively, a suspension of 10^8 microorganisms can be inoculated onto sterile filter paper strips or disks. The paper is dried in air or under a vacuum and is placed in sterile vials. These vials can be stored in the refrigerator for up to 4 years, and then single strips or disks can be removed as needed (10). This method is commonly used for quality control organisms.

Storage in Distilled Water

Most organisms do poorly in distilled water, but some survive for prolonged periods. Many fungi and *Pseudomonas* sp. survive for several years in distilled water at room temperature (15, 21). McGinnis et al. found that with the exception of fungi that do not easily sporulate, 93% of yeasts, mold, and aerobic actinomycetes can be easily and inexpensively preserved this way (20).

Long-Term Preservation Methods

Whereas the methods described above may be used to store microorganisms for periods of up to a few years, ultralow-temperature freezing and freeze-drying (lyophilization) are recommended for long-term storage. Although the initial investment in ultralow-temperature freezers and lyophilization may be costly, these methods are less labor-intensive over time, require less laboratory space (e.g., a cryovial versus broth or agar media), and reduce the chances of mutation events. Of course, mutations may still occur, and this phenonomen was recently observed in *Staphylococcus aureus* strains that lost the *mecA* gene during long-term preservation at −80°C (30). Similar to those with other preservation methods, survival rates after freeze-drying vary with species. Evaluating microorganisms over a 10-year period, Miyamoto-Shinohara et al. found that survival rates after freeze-drying for *Brevibacterium* sp. and *Corynebacterium* sp. approached 80% whereas those for *Streptococcus mutans* decreased to 20% after 10 years (21).

Ultralow-Temperature Freezing

Microorganisms can be maintained at temperatures of −70°C or lower for prolonged periods. Systems for achieving these temperatures include ultralow-temperature electric freezers and liquid nitrogen storage units. With either system, unwanted heating can occur due to the loss of electrical power or liquid nitrogen. Close observation of the system and an adequate alarm mechanism are essential since any increase in temperature will reduce viability. In the event that the temperature does rise, restoring power and returning to the target storage temperature as quickly as possible are essential. The presence of a cryopreservative such as glycerol may reduce the risk to microorganisms upon short exposure to higher temperatures (22). If thawing does occur, there are no guidelines for rapid restoration of the storage condition. Refreezing of the sealed vials as described below may be considered.

Storage Vials

Storage vials must be able to withstand very low temperatures and maintain a seal for their contents. Plastic (polypropylene) or glass (borosilicate) tubes may be used. Plastic vials with screw tops and silicone washers are much easier to use than glass vials that must be sealed with a flame and then scored and broken open. Several commercial suppliers stock acceptable vials (e.g., Fisher Scientific Products, VWR Scientific, Wheaton Science Products, and Becton Dickinson and Co.). Vials come in a variety of sizes. Half-dram vials are available from several suppliers and can be conveniently packaged in a 12-by-12 grid so that 144 vials are stored in one box or layer.

Cryoprotective Agents

To protect microorganisms from damage during the freezing process, during storage, and during thawing, cryoprotective agents are often added to the culture suspension. Whereas most bacteria, fungi, and viruses survive better with such additives, studies have shown that cryoprotective agents will significantly damage others. The reader is referred to detailed references for specifics (Table 1) (1, 15). Rapid freezing without additives may still be acceptable for the long-term survival of protozoa, although freeze-drying may be preferred.

There are two types of cryoprotective agents: those that enter the cell and protect the intracellular environment and others that protect the external milieu of the organism. Glycerol and dimethyl sulfoxide (DMSO) are most often used for the former; sucrose, lactose, glucose, mannitol, sorbitol, dextran, polyvinylpyrrolidone, polyglycol, and skim milk are used for the latter. Combinations of agents as well as detergents (e.g., Tween 80 and Triton WR 1339), other carbohydrates (e.g., honey), and calcium lactobionate have also been used. The most universal cryoprotectant is DMSO; however, the optimal cryoprotectant often varies with the microorganism. For example, glycerol appears to be best suited for the preservation of bacteria. A current and comprehensive review of protectant additives used in the cryopreservation of microorganisms is provided by Hubalek (16).

TABLE 1 Common procedures for preservation of microorganisms

Organism group	Storage method	Cryopreservative	Storage temp (°C)	Storage duration (yr)
Gram-positive bacteria	Transfer	None	Room temp	0.2–0.3
	Immersion in mineral oil	None	4	0.6–2
	Freezing	Sucrose, glycerol	−20	1–3
	Ultralow-temp freezing	Skim milk, sucrose, glycerol	−70 to −196	1–30
	Lyophilization	Skim milk, sucrose	4	30
Streptococci	Freezing	Skim milk	−20	0.2
	Ultralow-temp freezing	Skim milk	−70 to −196	0.2–1
	Lyophilization	Skim milk	4	0.5–30
Mycobacteria	Freezing	Skim milk	−20	3–5
	Ultralow-temp freezing	Skim milk	−70 to −196	3–5
	Lyophilization	Skim milk	4	16–30
Gram-negative bacteria	Transfer	None	Room temp	0.1–0.3
	Immersion in mineral oil	None	4	1–2
	Freezing	Sucrose, lactose	−20	1–2
	Ultralow-temp freezing	Sucrose, lactose, glycerol	−70 to −196	2–30
	Lyophilization	Skim milk, sucrose, lactose	4	30
Spore-forming bacteria	Transfer	None	Room temp	0.2–1
	Immersion in mineral oil	None	4	1
	Drying	None	Room temp	1–2
	Freezing	Glucose	−20	1–2
	Ultralow-temp freezing	Skim milk, glycerol	−70 to −196	2–30
	Lyophilization	Skim milk, lactose	4	30
Filamentous fungi	Transfer	None	4 to 25	2–10
	Immersion in mineral oil	None	Room temp	1–40
	Storage in distilled water	None	Room temp	1–10
	Drying	Soil, silica gel	Room temp	1–4
	Ultralow-temp freezing	Glycerol, DMSO	−70 to −196	2–30
	Lyophilization (sporeformers)	Glycerol, sucrose, DMSO, skim milk	4	2–30
Yeasts	Storage in distilled water	None	Room temp	1–2
	Drying	Nutrient medium	Room temp	1–2
Protozoa	Freezing	Blood, nutrient broth with DMSO or sucrose	−20 to −40	
	Ultralow-temp freezing	Blood, nutrient medium with DMSO or glycerol	−70 to −196	
Viruses	Transfer	Nutrient medium	4	0.5
	Ultralow-temp freezing	SPGA	−70 to −196	1–30
	Lyophilization	SPGA	4	6–10

Glycerol is added at a concentration of 10% (vol/vol), and DMSO is added at 5% (vol/vol). Prior to use, glycerol is sterilized by autoclaving. Once prepared, it can be stocked at room temperature for months. DMSO must be filter sterilized and can be stored in open containers for only 1 month prior to use.

Of the external products, skim milk is the most often used. Dehydrated skim milk is purchased from medical product suppliers (e.g., Becton Dickinson and Co. and Oxoid). It is autoclaved and used in a final concentration of 20% (wt/vol) in distilled water (1). This is double the concentration suggested by the manufacturers if the intent is to make a reconstituted equivalent of regular milk.

Preparation of Microorganisms for Freezing

Microorganisms are inoculated into a medium that adequately supports maximal growth. Cultures are allowed to mature to the late growth or stationary phase before being harvested. Broth specimens are centrifuged to create a pellet of microorganisms. The pellet is withdrawn and resuspended in 2 to 5 ml of broth with the appropriate concentration of cryoprotectant additive. For agar specimens, broth containing the cryoprotectant is placed on the surface of the agar. The surface is scraped with a pipette or sterile loop to suspend microorganisms, and then the broth mixture is pipetted directly into freezer vials. Alternatively, the agar surface can be scraped with a sterile loop. The microorganisms can then be transferred directly into the vial of cryoprotectant and emulsified into a final dense suspension. The volume of the aliquots to be frozen is typically 0.2 to 0.5 ml.

Freezing Method

The American Type Culture Collection (ATCC) recommends slow, controlled-rate freezing at a rate of 1°C per min until the vials cool to a temperature of at least −30°C, followed by more rapid cooling until the final storage temperature is achieved (1). Controlled-rate freezers are required for the initial phase of cooling. Studies in the 1970s showed that uncontrolled-rate freezing may be acceptable for most organisms and is much less expensive or labor-intensive (15). When organisms are stored in liquid nitrogen, however, it is still recommended that vials be placed initially in a −60°C freezer for 1 h and then transferred into the liquid nitrogen. When organisms are stored permanently at −60 to −70°C, the vials can be placed directly into the freezer.

Small glass beads or plastic beads (e.g., from Fisher Scientific Products or Wheaton Science Products) can also be added to storage vials before freezing. The culture suspension will coat the beads, and then individual beads can be removed from storage for reconstitution without thawing the entire sample (8).

Thawing

Damage to microorganisms occurs as they are warmed from the frozen state. Critical temperatures appear to be between −40 and −5°C. Studies suggest that rapid warming through these temperatures improves recovery rates. Stored culture vials should be warmed rapidly in a 35°C water bath until all ice has disappeared (1, 15). Once a vial is thawed, it should be opened and the organism should be transferred to an appropriate growth medium immediately. Great care must be exercised during the thawing phase since rapid temperature changes and resulting air pressure changes inside vials can cause the vials to explode. Protective clothing and eyewear must be worn during this process.

Freeze-Drying (Lyophilization)

Freeze-drying is considered to be the most effective way to provide long-term storage of most bacteria. Better preservation occurs with freeze-drying than with other methods because freeze-drying reduces the risk of intracellular ice crystallization that compromises viability. Removal of water from the specimen effectively prevents this damage. On the other hand, the process of drying causes extensive damage to molds, protozoa, and most viruses. Hence, these microorganisms cannot be stored by this method. Among bacteria, the relative viability with lyophilization is greatest with gram-positive bacteria (sporeformers in particular) and decreases with gram-negative bacteria (15), but overall, the viability of bacteria can be maintained for as long as 30 years. In addition, large numbers of vials of dried microorganisms can be stored with limited space, and organisms can be easily transported long distances at room temperature.

The process combines freezing and dehydration. Organisms are initially frozen and then dried by lowering the atmospheric pressure with a vacuum apparatus. Freeze-drying has been extensively reviewed in the past (14), and the required equipment includes a vacuum pump connected in line to a condenser and to the specimens. Specimens can be connected individually to the condenser (manifold method) or can be placed in a chamber where they are dehydrated in one larger air space (chamber or batch method). Alexander et al. and Heckly have both published detailed descriptions of equipment options (1, 14).

Storage Vials

Glass vials are used for all freeze-dried specimens. When freeze-drying is performed in a chamber, double glass vials are used. In the chamber method, an outer soft-glass vial is added for protection and preservation of the dehydrated specimen. Silica gel granules are placed in the bottom of the outer vial before the inner vial is inserted and cushioned with cotton. For the manifold method, a single glass vial is used. For both methods, the vial containing the actual specimen is lightly plugged with absorbent cotton. The storage vial in the manifold method or the outer vial in the chamber method must be sealed to maintain the vacuum and the dry atmospheric condition. All vials are sterilized prior to use by heating in a hot-air oven.

Cryoprotective Agents

Research concerning cryoprotective agents has been extensively reviewed (14). In general, the two most commonly used agents are skim milk and sucrose. Skim milk is used most often for chamber lyophilization, and sucrose is used most often for manifold lyophilization. Skim milk is prepared by making a 20% (vol/vol) solution of skim milk in distilled water. The solution is divided into 5-ml aliquots and autoclaved at 116°C with care taken to prevent overheating and caramelizaton of the solution. The preparation is then used in smaller volumes as described above for freezing. Sucrose is prepared in an initial mixture of 24% (vol/vol) sucrose in water and added in equal volumes to the microorganism suspension in growth medium to make a final concentration of 12% (vol/vol).

Preparation of Microorganisms for Freezing

As with simple freezing, maximum recovery of organisms is achieved by using microorganisms in the late growth or stationary phase from the growth of an inoculum in an appropriate growth medium. High concentrations of microorganisms are considered to be important. The ATCC recommends a concentration of at least 10^8 CFU/ml (1), and Heckly suggests a concentration of 10^{10} CFU/ml or higher (15).

Freeze-Drying Methods

In the chamber method, inner vials with the microorganism suspension are placed in a single layer inside a stainless steel container. This container is placed in a low-temperature freezer at −60°C for 1 h. The container is then transferred to a chamber containing dry ice and ethyl Cellosolve (Becton Dickinson and Co.) and covered with a sealable vacuum top, which is connected in sequence to a condenser reservoir also filled with dry ice and ethyl Cellosolve and to a vacuum pump. The vacuum is maintained at a minimum of 30 μm Hg for 18 h. At the same time, the outer vials are prepared by being heated in an oven overnight, filled with silica gel granules and cotton, and placed in a dry cabinet with <10% relative humidity. The freeze-dried inner vials are inserted into the outer vials, and the outer vials are heat sealed. Multiple different strains or species should probably not be processed in the same batch. Cross contamination rates vary from 0.8 to 3.3% when two different microorganisms are placed on opposite sides of the same container and are as high as 8.3 to 13.3% when microorganisms are intermingled (3).

In the manifold method, a rack of individual vials is used rather than a single container. The rack is placed in a dry ice-ethyl Cellosolve bath. After the freezing process, the vials are connected by individual rubber tubes in sequence to the condenser container filled with dry ice and ethyl Cellosolve and to the vacuum pump. As in the method described above, the vacuum is maintained at 30 μm Hg for 18 h and then the individual vials are sealed.

Storage

Individual vials need to be appropriately labeled and sorted. Storage at room temperature does not maintain viability and is not recommended. Storage at 4°C in an ordinary refrigerator is acceptable, but survival may be improved at temperatures of −30 to −60°C (1, 14).

Reconstitution

Care must be taken when opening vials for reconstitution because of the vacuum inside the vial. Safety glasses should always be worn, and vials should be covered with gauze to prevent injury if the vial explodes when air rushes in. Reconstitution should also be conducted in a closed hood to avoid dispersal of microorganisms. The surface of the vial should be wiped with 70% alcohol, and then the top of the glass vial can be scored and broken off or punctured with a hot needle. A small amount (0.1 to 0.4 ml) of growth medium is injected into the vial with a needle and syringe or a Pasteur pipette, the contents are stirred until the specimen is dissolved, and then the entire contents are transferred with the same syringe or a pipette to appropriate broth or agar media. A purity check must be done on each specimen because of the possibility of either cross contamination or mutation during the preservation process.

Procedures for Specific Organisms

Procedures for specific organisms are described below and summarized in Table 1.

Bacteria

All of the material presented in this chapter applies primarily to the preservation of bacteria. Simple transfer, storage under mineral oil, drying, or freezing at −20°C can maintain bacteria for short periods; freezing in ultralow-temperature electric freezers at −70°C or in liquid nitrogen at −196°C or freeze-drying can provide long-term preservation. A summary of the studies of bacterial preservation has been published (15). In general, serial transfer will preserve bacteria for up to a few months, storage under mineral oil or with drying will last 1 to 2 years, freezing at −20°C will preserve bacteria for 1 to 3 years, freezing at −70°C will preserve bacteria for 1 to 10 years, and freezing in liquid nitrogen and freeze-drying will preserve bacteria for up to 30 years (10). For fastidious bacteria such as *Streptococcus pneumoniae*, *Neisseria* spp., and *Haemophilus* spp., the optimal methods are lyophilization and freezing at −70°C by using Trypticase soy broth with glycerol as a preservation medium (23, 26, 31). Stock cultures of quality control microorganisms can be maintained in a cryopreservative suspension for up to 1 year at −20°C or indefinitely at −70°C.

Protozoa

Information concerning the preservation of protozoa is limited, in keeping with the infrequent need for such a process in clinical microbiology laboratories. Variable methods for individual genera are described. In general, freezing appears to be preferred to freeze-drying. All of the following procedures are as described by the ATCC (1).

Acanthamoeba sp., *Leishmania* sp., *Naegleria* sp., *Trichomonas* sp., and *Trypansoma* sp. can be handled as described above for ultralow-temperature freezing with 5% (vol/vol) DMSO as the cryoprotecting agent. These organisms should be stored in liquid nitrogen.

Acanthamoeba sp. and *Naegleria* sp. can also be dried at room temperature onto filter paper. Aliquots of a microorganism suspension (0.3 ml) are pipetted onto the paper in a shell vial and dried in air for 14 days at room temperature and then in a vacuum desiccator for an additional week. The vials are sealed and stored in liquid nitrogen.

Entamoeba sp. is stored frozen at −40°C. Specimens should be suspended in a mixture of growth medium containing 12% (vol/vol) DMSO and 6% (vol/vol) sucrose.

Leishmania sp. may also be prepared by inoculation of the organism into an animal host. At the peak of infection, the spleen is harvested and homogenized in half the final volume of ATCC medium 811 salt solution. Freezing is completed with 10% glycerol as the cryoprotectant.

Plasmodium sp. can be stored from infected blood samples. At the height of parasitemia, blood is obtained and anticoagulated with the following preparation: 1.33 g of sodium citrate, 0.47 g of citric acid, 3.00 g of dextrose, 200 mg of heparin (sodium), and 100 ml of distilled water. The final concentration of anticoagulant added to blood is 10%. To this anticoagulated blood, 30% glycerol in 0.0667 M phosphate buffer is added to a final concentration of 10% (vol/vol) glycerol. Freezing should occur in liquid nitrogen.

Trypanosoma sp. must be harvested from an animal host. At the peak of parasitemia, blood is withdrawn into heparinized tubes and diluted 1:1 in Tyrode's solution (8.0 g of NaCl per liter, 0.02 g of KCl per liter, 0.2 g of $CaCl_2$ per liter, 0.1 g of $MgCl_2$ per liter, 0.05 g of NaH_2PO_4 per liter, 1.0 g of $NaHCO_3$ per liter, and 1.0 g of glucose per liter) with 1 to 5% phenol red added. Then 5% DMSO is added as the cryoprotectant, and the specimen is stored in liquid nitrogen.

Yeasts and Filamentous Fungi

All of the techniques described above have been applied to the storage of yeasts and fungi (5, 10, 15, 27). The individual method employed depends upon the species to be preserved and whether or not it sporulates.

Subculturing. Subculturing is the simplest method of maintaining living fungi and involves serial transfer to fresh solid or liquid media. Storage is accomplished usually at room or refrigerator temperature. Fungi may be maintained by subculturing for a number of years. Care must be taken to avoid aerosolization and contamination of the laboratory or other specimens.

Storage under oil. Whereas species of *Aspergillus* and *Penicillium* have remained viable under oil for 40 years (27), many species have shown deterioration after 1 to 2 years and must be transferred periodically. Taddei et al. also reported the successful storage and recovery of actinomycetes stored under paraffin oil for 10 to 30 years (28).

Water storage. Many fungi can be stored successfully for prolonged periods in distilled water (21, 24). A simple method is to pipette 6 to 7 ml of sterile distilled water onto 2-week-old culture slants in screw-cap tubes. The spores and fragments of hyphae are dislodged by scraping with the pipette, and the suspension is transferred to a sterile 1-g vial, which is tightly capped and stored at 25°C. Fungi are revived by subculturing 0.2 to 0.3 ml of the suspension to appropriate media (4).

An alternative method is to cut agar blocks from the growing edge of a fungal colony and place them in sterile distilled water in bottles with screw-cap lids (13). The cultures are stored at 20 to 25°C. The fungi are retrieved by removing a block and placing it mycelium side down on growth medium appropriate for that species (27). Contamination (22.8%) is a significant problem with this method (13).

Drying. Drying as described above has been used for fungi. Only 6 of 16 genera of fungi stored in this fashion survived for 4 years (2). The greatest success is reported for sporulating fungi stored in silica gel or in soil (27).

Freezing. Fungi have been successfully preserved by storage in liquid nitrogen by using glycerol or DMSO as cryopreservatives. Broth cultures containing nonpathogenic fungi are disrupted in a Waring blender and suspended in equal parts of DMSO or glycerol to achieve final concentrations of 5 or 10%, respectively. Pathogens should not be disrupted in a mechanical blender because of the potential biohazard associated with aerosolization. *Histoplasma, Paracoccidioides,* and *Blastomyces* species should be frozen in the yeast phase, and *Coccidioides* species should be frozen in the early mycelial phase to minimize exposure of laboratory personnel. Otherwise, procedures for freezing are as described above.

Freeze-drying. Most spore-forming fungi can be preserved by freeze-drying. Cultures to be stored by freeze-drying should be grown on agar or broth media to the point of maximum sporulation (1) and processed as described above. Survival in storage for many years has been demonstrated (6, 25), but this is true only for sporulating organisms. Young vegetative hyphae of fungi do not survive freeze-drying (27).

Viruses

Viruses tend to be more stable than other microorganisms because of their small size and simple structure and the absence of free water. Many viruses can be stored for months at refrigerator temperatures or for years by ultralow-temperature freezing or freeze-drying. Storage at −20°C is not recommended (15, 18). Larger viruses tend to be less stable than smaller ones (11).

Ultralow-temperature freezing is effective in a number of situations. In addition to cryoprotectants described above, sucrose-phosphate-glutamate containing 1% bovine albumin (SPGA) (15, 18) and hypertonic sucrose are particularly effective, the latter for storing labile viruses such as respiratory syncytial virus (19). If ultralow-temperature freezing is employed, the rate of freezing should be as high as possible, using small-volume suspensions (0.1 to 0.5 ml). In addition to freezing of pure isolates, stool specimens known to contain viral enteric pathogens have been maintained at −70 to −85°C for 6 to 10 years with reasonable recovery and no change in the morphological characteristics of astroviruses, small round structured viruses, enteric adenoviruses, rotaviruses, and caliciviruses (32).

Gallo et al. evaluated five types of media for the storage of human immunodeficiency virus-infected peripheral blood lymphocytes and concluded that freezing peripheral blood lymphocytes in RPMI 1640 containing 10% fetal bovine serum and 10% DMSO and storing them at −60°C is acceptable for human immunodeficiency virus isolation (9).

Freeze-drying is probably the optimum method for preserving viruses for extended periods. A detailed review of acceptable procedures has been published (11). Virus suspensions freeze-dried in medium supported with SPGA appear to survive better (15, 29). Lyophilization of polioviruses and other enteroviruses works best when electrolytes are removed by dialysis or ultrafiltration (15).

Select Agents

In response to the Public Health Security and Bioterrorism Preparedness and Response Act of 2002, federal regulations require laboratories that store select agents to register and comply with the standards established by the act (7). A current and complete list of microorganisms considered to be select agents can be found at www.cdc.gov/od/sap. Regardless of the method for long-term preservation, laboratories must register with the Department of Health and Human Services and Centers for Disease Control and Prevention Select Agent Program. In order to minimize risk to public health and safety, select agents must be stored in a highly secured area with restricted access and appropriate safeguards. Only registered individuals who have completed training for handling select agents can access and retrieve these microorganisms from storage. An accurate and current inventory of select agents held in long-term storage must be maintained.

REFERENCES

1. **Alexander, M., P. M. Daggett, R. Gherna, J. Jong, and F. Simione.** 1980. *American Type Culture Collection Methods,* vol. I. *Laboratory Manual on Preservation, Freezing, and Freeze-Drying as Applied to Algae, Bacteria, Fungi and Protozoa,* p. 1–46. American Type Culture Collection, Rockville, Md.
2. **Antheunisse, J., J. W. DeBruin-Tol, and M. E. Van Der Pol-Van Soest.** 1981. Survival of microorganisms after drying and storage. *Antonie Leeuwenhoek* **47:**539–545.
3. **Barbaree, J. M., and A. Sanchez.** 1982. Cross-contamination during lyophilization. *Cryobiology* **19:**443–447.
4. **Castellani, A.** 1939. Viability of some pathogenic fungi in distilled water. *J. Trop. Med. Hyg.* **42:**225–226.
5. **Crespo, M. J., M. L. Abarca, and F. J. Cabanes.** 2000. Evaluation of different preservation and storage methods for *Malassezia* spp. *J. Clin. Microbiol.* **38:**3872–3875.

6. **Ellis, J. J., and J. A. Roberson.** 1968. Viability of fungus cultures preserved by lyophilization. *Mycologia* **60:**399–404.
7. **Federal Register.** 2005. Possession, use, and transfer of select agents and toxins, final rule. *Fed. Regist.*, vol. 70, no. 52.
8. **Feltham, R. K. A., A. K. Power, P. A. Pell, and P. H. A. Sneath.** 1978. A simple method for storage of bacteria at −76°C. *J. Appl. Bacteriol.* **44:**313–316.
9. **Gallo, D., J. S. Kimpton, and P. J. Johnson.** 1989. Isolation of human immunodeficiency virus from peripheral blood lymphocytes in various transport media and frozen at −60°C. *J. Clin. Microbiol.* **27:**88–90.
10. **Gherna, R. L.** 1981. Preservation, p. 208–217. *In* P. Gerhardt, R. G. E. Murray, R. N. Costilow, E. W. Nester, W. A. Wood, N. R. Krieg, and G. B. Phillips (ed.), *Manual of Methods for General Bacteriology.* ASM Press, Washington, D.C.
11. **Gould, E. A.** 1999. Methods for long-term virus preservation. *Mol. Biotechnol.* **13:**57–66.
12. **Harbec, P. S., and P. Turcotte.** 1996. Preservation of *Neisseria gonorrhoeae* at −20°C. *J. Clin. Microbiol.* **34:**1143–1146.
13. **Hartung de Capriles, C., S. Mata, and M. Middelveen.** 1989. Preservation of fungi in water (Castellani): 20 years. *Mycopathologia* **106:**73–79.
14. **Heckly, R. J.** 1961. Preservation of bacteria by lyophilization. *Adv. Appl. Microbiol.* **3:**1–76.
15. **Heckly, R. J.** 1978. Preservation of microorganisms. *Adv. Appl. Microbiol.* **24:**1–53.
16. **Hubalek, Z.** 2003. Protectants used in the cryopreservation of microorganisms. *Cryobiology* **46:**205–229.
17. **Jackson, H.** 1974. Loss of viability and metabolic injury of *Staphylococcus aureus* resulting from storage at 5°C. *J. Appl. Bacteriol.* **37:**59–64.
18. **Johnson, F. B.** 1990. Transport of viral specimens. *Clin. Microbiol. Rev.* **3:**120–131.
19. **Law, T. J., and R. N. Hull.** 1968. The stabilizing effect of sucrose upon respiratory syncytial virus infectivity. *Proc. Soc. Exp. Biol. Med.* **128:**515–518.
20. **McGinnis, M. R., A. A. Padhye, and L. Ajello.** 1974. Storage of stock cultures of filamentous fungi, yeasts, and some aerobic actinomycetes in sterile distilled water. *Appl. Microbiol.* **28:**218–222.
21. **Miyamoto-Shinohara, Y., T. Imaizumi, J. Sukenobe, Y. Murakami, S. Kawamura, and Y. Komatsu.** 2000. Survival rate of microbes after freeze-drying and long-term storage. *Cryobiology* **41:**251–255.
22. **Pell, P. A., and H. A. Sneath.** 1984. A note on survival of bacteria in cryoprotectant medium at temperatures above 0°C. *J. Appl. Bacteriol.* **57:**165–167.
23. **Popovic, T., G. Ajello, and R. Facklam.** *Laboratory Manual for the Diagnosis of Meningitis Caused by* Neisseria meningitidis, Streptococcus pneumoniae, *and* Haemophilus influenzae. World Health Organization WHO/CDS/EDC/99.7. World Health Organization, Geneva, Switzerland.
24. **Qiangqiang, Z., W. Jiajun, and L. Li.** 1998. Storage of fungi using sterile distilled water or lyophilization: comparison after 12 years. *Mycoses* **41:**255–257.
25. **Rybnikar, A.** 1995. Long-term maintenance of lyophilized fungal cultures of the genera *Epidermophyton*, *Microsporum*, *Paecilomyces* and *Trichophyton*. *Mycoses* **39:**145–147.
26. **Siberry, G., K. N. Brahmadathan, R. Pandian, M. K. Lalitha, M. C. Steinhoff, and T. J. John.** 2001. Comparison of different culture media and storage temperatures for the long-term preservation of *Streptococcus pneumoniae* in the tropics. *Bull. W.H.O.* **79:**43–47.
27. **Smith, D., and A. H. S. Onions.** 1994. *The Preservation and Maintenance of Living Fungi*, 2nd ed., p. 1–122. CAB International, Wallingford Oxon, United Kingdom.
28. **Taddei, A., M. M. Tremarias, and C. Hartung de Capriles.** 1998-1999. Viability studies on actinomycetes. *Mycopathologia* **143:**161–164.
29. **Tannock, G. A., J. C. Hierholzer, D. A. Bryce, C. F. Chee, and J. A. Paul.** 1987. Freeze-drying of respiratory syncytial viruses for transportation and storage. *J. Clin. Microbiol.* **25:**1769–1771.
30. **van Griethuysen, A., I. van Loo, A. van Belkum, C. Vandenbroucke-Grauls, W. Wannet, P. van Keulen, and J. Kluytmans.** 2005. Loss of the *mecA* gene during storage of methicillin-resistant *Staphylococcus aureus* strains. *J. Clin. Microbiol.* **43:**1361–1365.
31. **Votava, M., and M. Stritecka.** 2001. Preservation of *Haemophilus influenzae* and *Haemophilus parainfluenzae* at −70 degrees C. *Cryobiology* **43:**85–87.
32. **Williams, F. P., Jr.** 1989. Electron microscopy of stool-shed viruses: retention of characteristic morphologies after long-term storage at ultralow temperatures. *J. Med. Virol.* **29:**192–195.

THE CLINICAL MICROBIOLOGY LABORATORY IN INFECTION DETECTION, PREVENTION, AND CONTROL

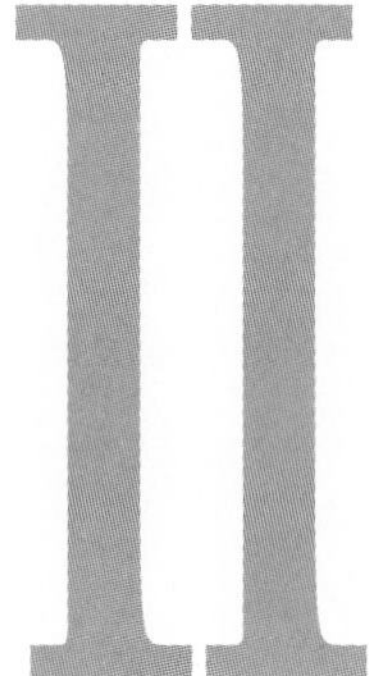

VOLUME EDITOR
MICHAEL A. PFALLER

SECTION EDITOR
LOREEN A. HERWALDT

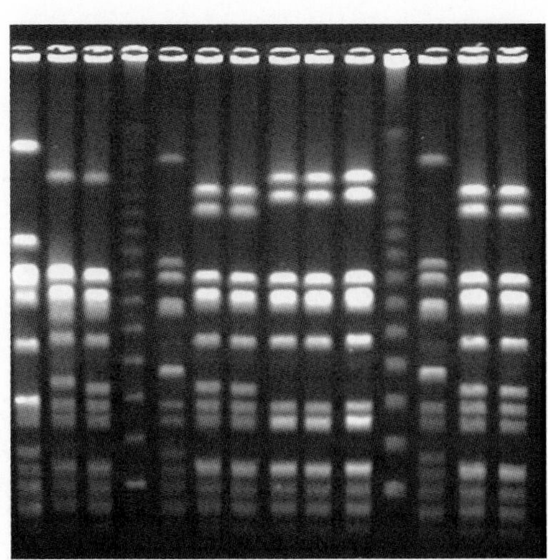

SmaI digest of *Staphylococcus aureus* on PFGE gel (R. Hollis, University of Iowa).

Decontamination, Disinfection, and Sterilization

ANDREAS F. WIDMER AND RENO FREI

7

Decontamination, disinfection, and sterilization are basic components of any infection control program. Patients expect that any reusable instrument or device used for diagnosis or treatment has undergone a process to eliminate any risks for cross-infection. However, the infection control literature documents many reprocessing failures, including numerous reports of transmission of nosocomial pathogens from contaminated endoscopes (30, 102, 224, 231, 234). Before 1990, it was very difficult to prove a causal relationship between a contaminated device and a subsequent nosocomial infection. Today, state-of-the-art clinical epidemiology supported by molecular typing tools such as pulsed-field gel electrophoresis, PCR, and genome sequencing can enable the hospital epidemiologist to prove a causal relationship between the use of a contaminated device and a consequent infection. Molecular epidemiology has, thus, provided scientific tools that can identify the limitations of the available disinfection and sterilization methods and can provide the impetus to improve reprocessing technologies.

Despite those advances, little research has been done that will lead to major breakthroughs in disinfection and sterilization in the near future. Thus, we believe the key issues instead will be to standardize and optimize our applications of current knowledge. Clearly, more research is needed in this field, but resources for such work have been limited. In fact, most disinfectants were introduced to the market more than 20 years ago and little is known about their modes of action and the mechanisms of resistance. Excellent reviews on this topic are published by Block (34), by McDonnell and Russell (169), and by Russell et al. (200). In addition, few basic procedures in decontamination, disinfection, and sterilization have been tested in randomized clinical trials. In this chapter, we have tried to cite the highest level of evidence available. However, given the dearth of studies, we have often had to cite results of observational studies, animal models, in vitro tests, and expert opinion because higher levels of evidence are not available.

Despite the lack of resources, reprocessing techniques, disinfectants, and general infection control practices have garnered more attention recently than in the past. This is due in part to the increasing frequency of multiresistant bacterial pathogens at a time when pharmaceutical companies have shifted from developing antimicrobial agents to designing drugs for chronic diseases (261). Moreover, new pathogens, such as the viruses causing severe acute respiratory syndrome (SARS) and avian influenza (122) and the prions causing Creutzfeldt-Jakob disease (CJD), and variant CJD (vCJD), are emerging for which there are few if any treatments. Consequently, the medical community needs better knowledge on disinfection and sterilization to prevent the spread of these pathogens.

PRINCIPLES OF TERMINOLOGY, DEFINITIONS, AND CLASSIFICATION OF MEDICAL DEVICES

Background

There is no uniform terminology for disinfection and sterilization, and many problems arise as a result. Many terms are ill defined even within the United States and Europe. In addition, the testing procedures for disinfectants are not as far advanced and well defined as those for testing the MIC for an organism based on the recommendations of the Clinical and Laboratory Standards Institute (formerly NCCLS). However, there currently are efforts to standardize and harmonize the terminology on an international level. For example, International Organization for Standardization (ISO) norms for sterilization were published in 2004. Manufacturers now must provide specific data on how to reprocess their medical devices. In the past, such information was frequently missing in the users' manuals.

Classification of Devices for Reprocessing

Background

The principal goal of disinfection and sterilization is to reduce the numbers of microorganisms on a device to a level that is insufficient to transmit infectious organisms, with a considerable safety margin. The most conservative approach would be to reprocess all items and devices with overkill sterilization. Obviously, not all items must undergo the most vigorous process to eliminate any microorganisms. For example, items such as blood pressure cuffs that are used at nonsterile body sites do not need to be sterilized between patients. In contrast, only sterilization will eliminate any risk of infection from devices used in normally sterile body sites. In some cases, the best choice may be to use disposable items instead of reusable devices, because reprocessing may be more expensive or may not provide the desired level of safety. The latter may apply to items in contact with the neural tissue of a patient suffering from any form of CJD or with tonsils and other lymphatic tissues of persons with bovine spongiform encephalopathy (BSE) or vCJD (26, 67, 260). Therefore, devices must be classified to allow staff to define the appropriate method for disinfection and/or sterilization for each item. A classification system should balance the potential risks for transmission of infection (e.g., the infectious dose) and the resources available to achieve the necessary or desired level of antimicrobial killing.

The most commonly used classification was proposed by Earle H. Spaulding in 1968 (232). He proposed three categories that are based on a device's potential for transmitting infectious agents: critical, semicritical, and noncritical (Table 1). The Centers for Disease Control and Prevention (CDC) cites this classification in its *Guidelines for Handwashing and Hospital Environment Control* (http://www.cdc.gov/mmwr/preview/mmwrhtml/rr5116a1.htm), and the U.S. Food and Drug Administration (FDA) cites it in its document *Content and Format of Premarket Notification [510(k)] Submissions for Liquid Chemical Sterilants and High-Level Disinfectants* (see http://www.fda.gov/cdrh/index.html). Most infection control professionals worldwide use this classification as well. However, this simple classification does not work perfectly for all devices. Even the definition of sterilization as the absence of any viable microorganisms must be revised to address the prions responsible for CJD and vCJD (187).

Critical Items

Items that enter normally sterile parts of the human body, such as surgical instruments, implants, and invasive monitoring devices (Table 1), are classified as "critical items." Because items classified as critical carry the highest risk for the patient, sterilization is the preferred method for reprocessing of these items. Autoclaving is the method of choice if the device is not heat labile. Alternative sterilization processes that use ethylene oxide or plasma require prolonged times, and the FDA has not approved them for use with instruments that have small, dead-end lumens, which are difficult to sterilize. Liquid sterilization with a glutaraldehyde-based formulation or peracetic acid is acceptable if sterilization by one of the methods mentioned above is not feasible and the formulation and/or automated device has been cleared by the FDA.

Semicritical Items

Semicritical objects come into contact with mucous membranes or nonintact skin and should be free of microorganisms except spores. Intact mucous membranes generally resist bacterial spores but are susceptible to other microorganisms such as vegetative bacteria (e.g., *Mycobacterium tuberculosis*) and viruses (e.g., human immunodeficiency virus [HIV] and cytomegalovirus). Examples of semicritical equipment include anesthesia equipment, respiratory equipment, and endoscopes. These items should be processed with a high-level disinfectant such as glutaraldehyde, stabilized hydrogen peroxide, peracetic acid, or a chlorine compound. Chlorine compounds corrode items and, therefore, are rarely used to disinfect medical devices.

Noncritical Items

Noncritical items, such as bedside tables, crutches, stethoscopes, furniture, and floors, come into contact with intact skin only. Intact skin is a very effective barrier against microorganisms, and therefore, these items and devices do not need to be sterilized. Such items pose a very low risk for direct transmission of pathogens and can usually be cleaned at the bedside or wherever they have been used with a low-level disinfectant. For example, health care workers can disinfect their stethoscopes by wiping the surfaces with alcohol. However, noncritical devices can contribute to the transmission of pathogens by the indirect route. For instance, up to 60% of cultures of the environments near patients colonized or infected with vancomycin-resistant enterococci are positive for this organism (56). Health care workers can contaminate their hands when they touch these surfaces. If they do not practice hand hygiene, they can spread these pathogens

TABLE 1 Spaulding classification of devices

Clinical device	Definition	Example	Infectious risk	Reprocessing procedure	
				FDA classification	EPA classification
Critical device	Medical device that is intended to enter a normally sterile environment, sterile tissue, or the vasculature	Surgical instruments	High	Sterilization by steam, plasma, or ethylene oxide; liquid sterilization acceptable if no other methods feasible	Sterilant or disinfectant
Semicritical device	Medical device that is intended to come in contact with mucous membranes or minor skin breaches	Flexible endoscope	High, intermediate	Sterilization desirable; high-level disinfection acceptable	Sterilant or disinfectant
Noncritical device	Medical device that comes in contact with intact skin	Blood pressure cuff, electrocardiogram electrodes	Low	Intermediate or low level	Hospital disinfectant with label claim for tuberculocidal activity
Medical equipment	Device or component of a device that does not typically come in direct contact with the patient	Examination table	Low	Low-level disinfection, use of sanitizer	Hospital disinfectant without label claim for tuberculocidal activity but with claim for virucidal activity against HIV

TABLE 2 Principles of medical device classification

Classification	FDA regulation	Premarket requirements by the FDA	Proposed classification by the Global Harmonization Task Force[a]	Examples
Class I	Least regulated, requires fewest regulations	None	A	Band-Aid, tongue depressor
Class II	Must meet federal performance standards	Premarket notification [510(k)]	B	Surgical gowns, drapes, scrub sponges
			C	Orthopedic implants
Class III	Implanted and life-supporting or life-sustaining devices are required to have FDA approval for safety and effectiveness	Premarket approval	D	Artificial hearts

[a] Details available at http://www.ghtf.org/sg1/inventorysg1/pd_sg1_n015r22.pdf.

to devices or directly to other patients. Therefore, noncritical items must be decontaminated if they are likely to be contaminated with pathogenic organisms.

The FDA also has developed a classification based on safety considerations and the regulations manufacturers must meet before marketing a device. Medical products are listed as class I to III products (Table 2). Simple products such as a tongue depressor are classified as class I medical products, which must meet very simple requirements before they can be marketed legally. Class II products, such as autoclaves, require premarket notification [510(k)] demonstrating that the device to be marketed is at least as safe and effective as a legally marketed device. Class III devices are those that support or sustain human life and are of substantial importance in preventing impairment of human health (e.g., a pacemaker). Due to the level of risk associated with class III devices, the FDA requires companies to file a premarket approval (PMA) application to obtain marketing clearance (section 515 of the Federal Food, Drug and Cosmetic Act). The PMA application must contain sufficient valid scientific evidence documenting that the device is safe and effective for its intended use (56).

DECONTAMINATION AND CLEANING

In Europe, decontamination basically means cleaning an item to remove organic material, protein, and fat. In the United States, the term describes a cleaning step and any additional step required to eliminate any risk of infection to health care workers while they handle a device without protective attire. The FDA defines the cleaning process as including all steps necessary to remove, inactivate, or contain contamination, beginning immediately after an item has been used for clinical purposes; continuing with the steps to decontaminate, clean, and package a device up to the first step of the sterilization process; and ending with quality control tests.

Regardless of regulations, cleaning is always the initial step of the decontamination process on both continents. In this chapter, we will use the term decontamination to describe the removal of debris, blood, and proteins and most microorganisms. This process usually, but not necessarily, renders the device "safe to handle" by health care workers who are not wearing protective attire. Basic definitions are outlined in Table 3.

The first step in reprocessing used medical devices is for health care workers to prevent debris from drying on the items. Research on prion diseases demonstrates that removal of debris is seriously impaired if the debris is allowed to dry on a medical device (87). Therefore, the reprocessing cycle should start as soon as possible and items should be kept wet if delays in reprocessing are anticipated (115, 179). Cleaning can be done physically or chemically; it can also be done by hand, by sonication, or by use of washers. In the United States, cleaning is frequently performed manually with water and a detergent. In Europe, many countries rely primarily on washers-disinfectors that rinse items with cold water and then with warm water plus a detergent. The cycle is completed with hot water at >90°C. Items such as bedpans and urinals can be cleaned and disinfected by putting the items into a machine, pushing a button, and removing them after a 2- to 5-min procedure.

All sterilization techniques other than steaming have been shown to fail in 1 to 40% of sterilization cycles if residual proteins and/or salts are not removed by a proper cleaning process (11). Even steam sterilization at 134°C for 18 min, recommended by the World Health Organization (WHO) to inactivate prions, can fail to prevent cross-transmission if the device does not undergo a cleaning process (87, 115, 179).

For floors, surfaces, and noncritical items, cleaning with a detergent is sufficient in most situations and a disinfection process contributes little if any additional effect (76). In addition, residual proteins and debris that escape the cleaning process may interfere with disinfectants and even cause them to lose activity (76). In the United States, routine disinfection of environmental surfaces in patient care areas is recommended as an additional safety precaution in case the environment is contaminated with unrecognized body fluids; in Europe, this practice is restricted to intensive care units and emergency rooms (227).

DISINFECTION

Disinfection is the second critical step in reprocessing of medical devices. To be effective, disinfection must be preceded by thorough cleaning and it must be done properly. Staff must check the disinfectant's concentration regularly if it is diluted at the place of use, even if it is diluted with an electronically monitored dilution device. Failures of the valve or other critical parts of the device can result in an insufficient final concentration, which usually cannot be detected by checking either the appearance or the odor of

TABLE 3 Definitions and terms

Term	Standard[a]	Technical-microbiological log CFU reduction	Comment
Sterilization	(Closely monitored) validated process used to render a product free of all forms of viable microorganisms, including all bacterial endospores	$\geq 10^6$ log CFU reduction of the most resistant spores for the sterilization process studied, achieved at the half-time of the regular cycle (ISO 14937)	Prions require an adapted definition because of their high resistance to any form of sterilization
Disinfection	Elimination of most if not all pathogenic microorganisms, excluding spores	No clear-cut defined reduction level; a minimum estimate is $\geq 10^3$ log CFU reduction of microorganisms, excluding spores; log unit reductions of 4 to 5 commonly achieved for devices; these are estimates, because there is no international standardization	Some high-level disinfectants achieve microbial reduction, including level of reduction of spores similar to sterilization, if long incubation times and/or temperatures of >25°C are applied; this is called liquid sterilization by sterilants
Decontamination	Reduction of pathogenic microorganisms to a level at which items are "safe to handle" without protective attire	Elimination of debris and proteins by cleaning and/or a disinfection or sterilization process; in Europe, the process is restricted to cleaning only, which achieves a minimum reduction of ≥1 log CFU; most cleaning processes achieve ≥ log CFU reductions of 3 to 5; these are estimates, because there is no international standardization	Manual and/or mechanical cleaning with water and detergents or enzymes is a prerequisite before disinfection or sterilization; in Europe, this term is used for cleaning of items; in the United States, it defines the process that makes an item "safe to handle"; it may include a cleaning process but also a disinfection or even a sterilization process; the U.S. term "decontamination" refers to the health care workers' safety; in Europe, the term is used for the item only
Antisepsis	Patient related: disinfection of living tissue or skin Health care worker related: reduction or removal of transient microbiological flora	Preoperative skin preparation with an alcohol-based iodine compound Hand washing: (scrub) reduction of ≥1 log CFU Hand disinfection (rub-in): reduction of ≥2.5 log CFU	Antiseptic agents are handled as drugs by the FDA

[a] Examples for standards are as follows: ethylene oxide sterilization (industrial facility use, ISO 11135; health care facility use, ANSI/AAMI ST 41) and moist-heat sterilization (industrial facility use, ISO 11134; health care facility use, ANSI/AAMI ST 46).

the disinfectant. Many manufacturers provide test strips to check for the appropriate concentration. Of note, numerous outbreaks have occurred when staff members have not followed appropriate protocols. For example, *Klebsiella oxytoca* caused an outbreak after an infection control committee allowed staff members to decrease the concentration of a glutaraldehyde-based surface disinfectant because they did not like the odor. The outbreak stopped after staff members resumed use of the disinfectant to the recommended concentration (190). An outbreak of 58 cases of *Mycobacterium xenopi* infection occurred when instruments used for discovertebral operations were rinsed with tap water after they were disinfected (22).

Principles and Antimicrobial Activities of Compounds

The antimicrobial spectrum of disinfectants varies. Low-level disinfectants destroy lipid-enveloped viruses such as HIV and most vegetative bacteria (Fig. 1) (35), but many disinfectants, including alcohol, are ineffective against nonlipid or small viruses such as poliovirus. For example, isopropyl alcohol has little activity against poliovirus, but >90% ethanol is very active (247). Intermediate-level disinfectants are effective against nonlipid or small viruses, such as poliovirus, and high-level disinfectants are effective against mycobacteria (Table 4).

The antimicrobial spectra of disinfectants are tested differently from those of antimicrobial agents. Microbiology laboratories that test disinfectants must know the special methods needed to accurately assess the activities of disinfectants. In fact, MICs are of little help because the goal of disinfection is to kill rather than inhibit the growth of microorganisms. In contrast to sterilization curves, killing curves for disinfectants are not linear and the rate of log killing decreases as the inoculum concentrations decrease (i.e., as the number of CFU per milliliter decreases). Therefore, a 3-log-unit killing is more easily achieved with disinfectants if the inoculum is large, e.g., 10^8 CFU, than if

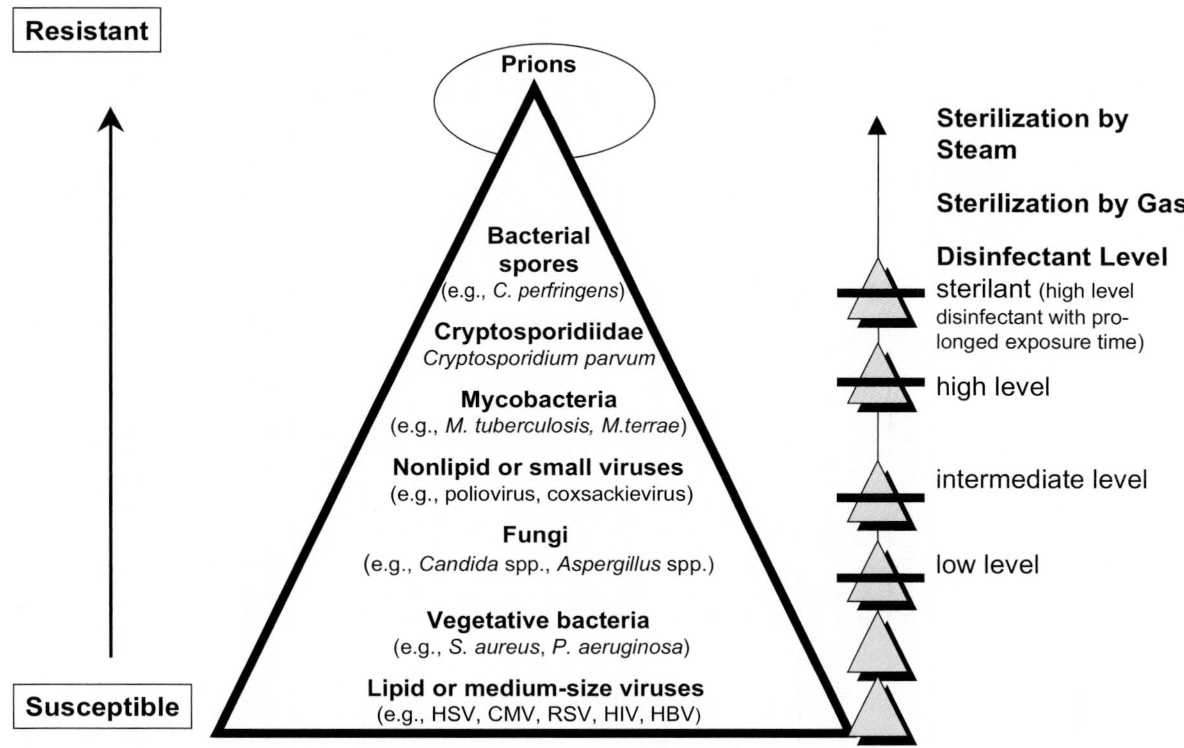

FIGURE 1 Microorganisms' resistance to disinfectants. HSV, herpes simplex virus; CMV, cytomegalovirus; RSV, respiratory syncytial virus; HBV, hepatitis B virus.

the inoculum is 10^4 CFU. Most disinfectants must be inactivated before they are incubated in media or plated because bacteria do not grow in the presence of very low concentrations of a disinfectant (inhibitory effect). However, if the compound is inactivated, bacterial growth can be demonstrated. Like antimicrobial agents, some disinfectants display a postexposure effect on bacterial growth. The postexposure effect has been quantified for a variety of disinfectants. Alcohols in general have little, if any, postexposure effect, but chlorhexidine, octenidine, and chloramine delay regrowth after exposure for several hours (35).

The FDA requires that the microbicidal efficacy of liquid chemical sterilants and high-level disinfectants be assessed in three different types of tests before these products can be legally marketed in the United States.

1. Potency testing incorporates the Environmental Protection Agency (EPA)'s test requirements for registration of germicides, such as the Association of Official Analytical Chemists' (AOAC) sporocidal test, tuberculocidal test, and use dilution tests for *Staphylococcus aureus* ATCC 6538, *Salmonella enterica* serovar Cholerasuis ATCC 10708, and *Pseudomonas aeruginosa;* EPA virucidal tests for viruses including poliovirus type 2 and herpes simplex virus; and FDA-recommended tests, such as total killing and end-point analysis and comparison of survivor and predicted curves. (Note that in Europe, disinfectants should have been tested by the methods defined by established or proposed European Norms [EN] such as EN 1040 [bactericidal activity] and EN 1275 [fungicidal activity]).

2. Simulated-use testing involves testing the disinfectant under artificially created worst-case scenarios to determine how long instruments need to be in contact with the disinfectant if cleaning failed and the instruments are still contaminated with substantial organic matter and microbes. The instruments are contaminated with an organic load and appropriate test microorganisms (the organism depends on the level of disinfection being claimed); the conditions of the artificially contaminated devices represent worst-case postcleaning conditions before exposure to the germicide.

3. "In-use" testing involves cleaning medical devices used for clinical purposes according to a facility's operating procedures.

As noted above, the FDA includes a tuberculocidal test in its test procedures. This test does not account for the effect of cleaning before devices are disinfected. Devices are treated with 2% horse serum (proteinaceous load) and with 10^5 to 10^6 CFU of *Mycobacterium terrae* or equivalent nontuberculous mycobacteria. Under these conditions, a device would need to be immersed in a disinfectant (e.g., 2.4% alkaline glutaraldehyde) for >45 min at >25°C for complete tuberculocidal killing. However, Rutala and Weber demonstrated that proper cleaning eradicates at least 4 log units of microorganisms (209), and Hanson et al. showed that cleaning bronchoscopes before disinfection removes all detectable contaminants, with an up to 8-log-unit reduction in the viral load (114). Therefore, Rutala and Weber recommend that the FDA accept a standardized cleaning protocol followed by a 20-min immersion at 20°C with an FDA-approved disinfectant as adequate to kill mycobacteria (209). The EPA maintains an updated list of registered low-level and intermediate-level disinfectants (http://www.epa.gov/oppad001/chemregindex.htm) and the FDA maintains a list of approved high-level disinfectants and sterilants (http://www.fda.gov/cdrh/ode/germlab.html) on their websites.

TABLE 4 Overview of common disinfectants[a]

Germicide(s)	Use dilution	Level of disinfection	Active against:						Important characteristics									Applications in hospitals
			Bacteria	Lipophilic viruses	Fungi	Small or hydrophilic viruses	*Mycobacterium tuberculosis*	Bacterial spores	Shelf life of >1 wk	Corrosive/ deleterious effect	Residue	Inactivated by organic matter	Skin irritant	Eye irritant	Respiratory irritant	Toxic	Environmental concerns	
Glutaraldehyde	2–3.2%	High/CS	+	+	+	+	+	+	+	−	+	−	+	+	+	+	−	Endoscopes
Hydrogen peroxide	3–25%	High/CS	+	+	+	+	+	±	+	±	−	±	+	+	−	+	−	Contact lenses
Chlorine	100–1,000 ppm free chlorine	High	+	+	+	+	+	±	+	+	+	+	+	+	+	+	±	Selected semicritical devices
Isopropyl alcohol	60–95%	Intermediate	+	+	+	±	+	−	+	±	−	±	±	+	−	+	−	Small-area surfaces
Glucoprotamine	1.5–4%	Intermediate	+	+	+	+	+	−	+	−	−	−	+	+	−	−	−	Diagnostic instruments
Phenolic compounds	0.4–5% aqueous	Intermediate	+	+	+	±	+	−	+	−	+	−	+	+	−	+	+	Surgical instruments
Iodophors	30–50 ppm free iodine	Intermediate	+	+	+	+	±	−	+	±	+	+	±	+	−	+	−	Medical equipment
Quaternary ammonium compounds	0.4–1.6% aqueous	Low	±	+	±	−	−	−	+	−	+	+	+	+	−	+	−	Disinfection in food preparation areas and floors

[a] Data from references 34, 89, 201, and 247 and from the *Laboratory Biosafety Manual*, World Health Organization, Geneva, Switzerland, 1983 (268a). Abbreviations: CS, chemical sterilant; +, yes; −, no; ±, variable results. Efficacy of the disinfectants is based on an exposure time of less than 30 min at room temperature. Spores require prolonged exposure times (up to 10 h) unless used with a washer-disinfector at higher temperatures.

Definitions and Terms (Adapted from FDA and EPA Definitions)

Since the FDA regulates the most critical part of disinfection and sterilization, FDA definitions are used throughout the chapter unless stated otherwise. The most important definitions are given in Table 5.

Guidelines for Choosing a Disinfectant

Rutala published guidelines for the selection and use of disinfectants and recommendations on the preferred method for disinfection and sterilization of patient care items (62, 201, 202). The CDC recently issued guidelines for environmental infection control in health care facilities including recommendations for cleaning and disinfection (227).

When choosing a disinfectant, staff members should review its effectiveness against the expected spectra of pathogens (Tables 4 and 5) to ensure that it is adequate for the intended purpose. In addition, the staff must ensure that the disinfectant is compatible with the devices it is intended to disinfect and that devices that are immersed longer than recommended will not be damaged. The latter factor is important because staff members may forget to remove instruments (e.g., during weekends or night shifts). Prolonged exposure to a disinfectant may damage the instrument. Staff members should also consider the toxicity, odor, compatibility with other compounds, and residual activity of disinfectants (Table 6). It is prudent to contact colleagues already using a disinfectant before introducing it in a health care facility. The experience of health care professionals at different institutions can be helpful, allowing the staff to learn about problems such as interactions with detergents, unexpected coloring and odors, and employees' responses to the change. We have found that employees often complain bitterly after a disinfectant has been changed. Moreover, a new disinfectant used on environmental surfaces may interact with those used in the past and temporarily release unpleasant odors. Written infection control standards describing how to care for environmental surfaces can help staff members avoid combining incompatibile equipment and disinfectants. Once staff members have identified a product that meets a facility's needs, only strong evidence from good studies should lead a facility to replace it with a new product (e.g., one that has improved activity or works faster).

Disinfection by Heat Versus Immersion in Germicides

Disinfection by heat has become much more common than in the past and has replaced disinfection with germicides for many applications in European health care facilities, including our institution, the University Hospital Basel, Basel, Switzerland (225). The advantages of these devices are obvious: (i) the processes are automated and are monitored and documented in a manner similar to that for sterilization, (ii) microogranisms have not developed resistance to the processes, and (iii) the cost per load is probably less than that for germicides. In addition, studies by Gurevich et al. (111) indicate that pasteurization with a germicide is more effective than pasteurization without a germicide. However, washers include a cleaning process with an average reduction of 4 log units, coupled with heat disinfection (5-log-unit killing; washer-disinfectors such as the AMSCO Reliance 430 achieve an inactivation factor of >5 log units [111, 139]), resulting in a total reduction of 8 to 9 log units. This surpasses any international requirements for high-level disinfection.

Thermal disinfection has several disadvantages. First, the cost to purchase and install the equipment is much higher than that for systems using a germicide. Second, considerable power is needed to heat the water. Third, some non-spore-forming microorganisms such as enterococci resist temperatures of up to 71°C for 10 min. Thus, recommendations such as those in the United Kingdom (the Department of Health requires 65°C for 10 min, 71°C for 3 min, or 80°C for 1 min) may not be adequate for these organisms (43).

Medical washer-disinfectors that are intended to clean, low- and intermediate-level disinfectants, and dry surgical instruments, anesthesia equipment, hollowware, and other medical devices are exempt from the premarket notification procedures described by FDA in subpart E of part 807 of the chapter subject to §880.9. The ISO provided standards for these processes in preapproval ISO norm 15883 (prEN ISO 15883), which defines the standards for disinfection of washer-disinfectors by heat with and without the addition of disinfectants (http://www.iso.org). The ISO has not defined a temperature at which these devices must work but rather allows manufacturers to choose a temperature in a given range at which their devices should operate.

In the United States, hot-water pasteurization is generally performed at 77°C for 30 min (36), but few scientific data

TABLE 5 FDA and EPA definitions of important terms

Term	Definition
Germicide	Agent that destroys microorganisms; the prefixes of terms with the suffix "-cide" (e.g., virucide, fungicide, bactericide, sporicide, and tuberculocide) indicate which microorganisms the germicide kills
Sterilant (chemical)	Chemical germicide that achieves sterilization
High-level disinfectant	Germicide that when used according to the labeling kills all microbial pathogens except large numbers of bacterial endospores
Intermediate-level disinfectant	Germicide that when used according to the labeling kills all microbial pathogens except bacterial endospores
Low-level disinfectant	Germicide that when used according to the labeling kills most vegetative bacteria and lipid-enveloped and medium-size viruses; such disinfectants are regulated by the EPA
Minimum effective concentration	Minimum effective concentration of a liquid chemical germicide that achieves the microbicidal activity claimed by the manufacturer
Cleaning (or precleaning)	Removal of foreign material (e.g., organic or inorganic contaminants) from medical devices as part of a decontamination process

TABLE 6 Overview of common antiseptic compounds[a]

Compound(s)	Antiseptic effect on[b]: Gram-positive bacteria	Gram-negative bacteria	Viruses	Fungi	*Mycobacterium tuberculosis*	Rapidity of action	Residual activity[b]	Typical concn(s) (%)	Affected by organic matter	Safety for humans
Alcohols	+++	+++	++[c]	+++	+++	15–30 s	None	70–95	?[e]	Drying, flammable
Chlorhexidine	+++	++	++	+	++	Min	+++	4, 2, 0.5 in alcohol	Minimally	Leads to ototoxicity and keratitis
Iodophors	+++	++	++	++	++	Min	+	10, 7.5, 2, 0.5	Yes	Causes skin irritation
Octenidine[d]	+++	+++	++	++	++	Min	+++	0.1	Minimally	Limited data on safety
PCMX	++	+	+	+	+	Min	++	0.5–3.75	Minimally	Appears to be safe
Triclosan	++	++	++	±	+	Min	++	0.3–1.0	Minimally	Appears to be safe

[a] Data from references 149, 189, and 264.
[b] ± poor; +, fair; ++, good, +++, excellent.
[c] Ethanol at >95% is highly effective against viruses; isopropanol has limited effectiveness against small and nonlipid viruses.
[d] Not available in the United States.
[e] Conflicting data.

support the use of a particular temperature. prEN ISO 15883 introduces the A_0 concept, which is based on the fact that a defined temperature will generate a predictable lethality effect against microorganisms. Corresponding exposure temperatures and time periods that achieve high-level disinfection can be calculated by assuming the presence of particularly heat-resistant microorganisms in numbers in excess of those likely to be encountered on the medical devices to be processed. prEN ISO 15883 introduces the term A_0 for moist-heat disinfection (thermal disinfection). The A_0 value of a moist-heat disinfection process denotes the lethality effects expressed in terms of the equivalent time in seconds at a temperature of 80°C delivered by the process to the medical device with reference to microorganisms possessing a z value of 10. Given a predefined A_0, equivalent killing of microorganisms is achieved if the following formula is followed: $A_0 = \sum 10^{(80-T)/Z} \Delta t$, where T is temperature in Celsius and t is time in seconds. An A_0 value of 600, which can be achieved at 80°C over 10 min, 90°C over 1 min, or 70°C over 100 min, is the minimum requirement for noncritical medical devices (273, 274). An A_0 value of at least 3,000, which can be achieved by exposure to hot water (e.g., at 90°C; the medical device must tolerate this temperature for >5 min), must be employed for medical devices contaminated with heat-resistant viruses such as rotavirus and hepatitis B virus. An A_0 value of at least 3,000 is also appropriate for high-level disinfection of all semicritical devices. The test procedure based on the A_0 concept has been highly reproducible and found to be suitable to test washer-disinfectors (273, 274).

Overview of Commonly Used Disinfectants for Devices

Glutaraldehyde

Among aldehydes that exhibit biocidal activity, including glyoxal, *ortho*-phthalaldehyde (OPA), succinaldehyde, and benzaldehydes, glutaraldehyde and formaldehyde are the most extensively studied aldehydes. In-depth reviews may be found elsewhere (21, 198, 201). Glutaraldehyde is the predominant commercially available aldehyde. Because it has potent and broad-spectrum microbiocidal activity and is compatible with many materials (including metal, rubber, and plastic), glutaraldehyde is often regarded as the high-level disinfectant and chemical sterilant of choice in many health care facilities. Glutaraldehyde-based formulations are most commonly used for high-level disinfection of medical equipment such as endoscopes, transducers, dialysis systems, and anesthesia and respiratory therapy equipment (201).

The mechanism of action is complex and is related to the alkylation of sulfhydryl, hydroxyl, carboxy, and amino groups in the cell wall, cell membrane, nucleic acids, enzymes, and other proteins of microorganisms. The biocidal activities of glutaraldehyde solutions are dependent on a variety of variables, such as pH, temperature, concentration at the time of use, the presence of inorganic ions, and the age of the solution (21). Aqueous solutions of glutaraldehyde are usually acidic and are not sporicidal in this form. Therefore, they need to be activated by adding an alkalinizing agent. These activated solutions, however, rapidly lose their activity because glutaraldehyde molecules polymerize at an alkaline pH. Therefore, the shelf life of such solutions is limited to 14 days unless the manufacturer recommends otherwise. To overcome this problem, some manufacturers have developed novel formulations with longer shelf lives (e.g., activated dialdehyde solutions containing 2.4 to 3.5% glutaraldehyde with a maximum reuse life of 28 days).

The activities of disinfectants increase as the temperature rises. Among eight disinfectants tested, glutaraldehyde was found to be the chemical most strongly affected by temperature (99). Some stable acid glutaraldehydes may be used at temperatures of 35 to 55°C at concentrations below 2%. Glutaraldehyde retains its activity in the presence of organic matter.

A standard 2% aqueous solution of glutaraldehyde buffered to pH 7.5 to 8.5 is bactericidal, tuberculocidal, sporicidal, fungicidal, and virucidal. It rapidly kills both gram-negative and gram-positive vegetative bacteria. Longer exposure times are required to inactivate spores and mycobacteria. Spores of *Bacillus* and *Clostridium* spp. are generally destroyed by 2% glutaraldehyde in 3 h, whereas spores of *Clostridium difficile* are eliminated more rapidly (206). In contrast, *Cryptosporidium parvum* oocysts remain viable and infectious after 10 h in a 2.5% glutaraldehyde solution (268). Several investigators have questioned glutaraldehyde's ability to inactivate mycobacteria. For example, Rubbo et al. (197) demonstrated that glutaraldehyde inactivates *Mycobacterium tuberculosis* more slowly than alcohols, formaldehyde, iodine, and phenol. Ascenzi (21) showed in the quantitative suspension test that 2% glutaraldehyde kills only 2 to 3 log units of *Mycobacterium tuberculosis* in 20 min at 20°C. Similarly, Collins (66) reported that glutaraldehyde cannot completely inactivate a standardized suspension of *Mycobacterium tuberculosis* within 10 min. Nontuberculous mycobacteria such as *Mycobacterium avium*, *Mycobacterium intracellulare*, and *Mycobacterium gordonae* are more resistant to inactivation than *Mycobacterium tuberculosis* (65). These and other data suggest that 20 min (at 20°C) is the minimum exposure time needed to reliably inactivate tuberculous and nontuberculous mycobacteria by using 2% glutaraldehyde, provided that the contaminated item has been thoroughly cleaned before disinfection (131, 201). Glutaraldehyde-resistant mycobacteria have been isolated from endoscope washers-disinfectors (107, 251) (see "Endoscopes" below).

The virucidal activity of glutaraldehyde extends to the nonenveloped (hydrophilic) viruses, which are generally more resistant to disinfectants than are the enveloped (lipophilic) viruses. Numerous viruses were documented to be inactivated, including HIV, hepatitis A virus, hepatitis B virus, poliovirus type 1, coxsackievirus type B, yellow fever virus, and rotavirus (21, 141).

Disadvantages of glutaraldehyde include the fact that it coagulates blood and can fix proteins and tissue to surfaces (167, 201). In addition, glutaraldehyde has a pungent and irritating odor and its vapor at the level of 0.2 ppm irritates the eyes, throat, and nose. Health care workers exposed to glutaraldehyde can develop allergic contact dermatitis, asthma, rhinitis, and epistaxis. Measures that may minimize employee exposure include covering immersion baths with tight-fitting lids, improving ventilation, and using ducted exhaust hoods or ductless fume hoods with vapor absorbents, personal protective equipment, and appropriate automated machines for endoscope disinfection (12, 201). Due to dilution, glutaraldehyde concentrations commonly decline during use in manual and automatic baths used for endoscopes (167). Test strips should be used to ensure that the glutaraldehyde concentration has not fallen below 1 to 1.5%. Equipment disinfected with glutaraldehyde and rinsed inadequately has caused serious clinical complications including proctocolitis (colonoscopes; 79, 262); and keratopathy (ophthalmic instruments; 48). Because the infectivity of prions can be stabilized when instruments are treated with formaldehyde before they are autoclaved (48), aldehydes are no longer recommended for disinfecting endoscopes in some European countries (e.g., France; see "Bovine Spongiform Encephalopathy and Variant Creutzfeldt-Jakob Disease" below).

ortho-Phthalaldehyde

The 0.55% OPA solution has been approved as a high-level disinfectant by the FDA and by agencies in other countries. However, different countries or areas have set different exposure times for a 0.55% solution of OPA at 20°C to achieve high-level disinfection: 12 min in the United States, 10 min in Canada, and 5 min in Europe, Asia, and Latin America.

Compared with glutaraldehyde, OPA has several advantages: (i) it does not require activation, (ii) it is compatible with many materials (i.e., similar to glutaraldehyde), (iii) it is more stable during storage and can be reused as well at a pH range as wide as 3 to 9, (iv) it has low vapor properties, (v) its odor is barely perceptible, and (vi) it is more rapidly mycobactericidal than glutaraldehyde in vitro and has good activity against glutaraldehyde-resistant strains at longer exposure times (93). However, 0.5% OPA is slowly sporicidal and does not inactivate all spores within 270 min of exposure (255). In addition, OPA stains proteins, skin, clothing, and instruments. OPA vapors may irritate the respiratory tract and eyes. At present, the effects of long-term exposure and safe exposure levels are not well defined. Therefore, OPA must be handled with appropriate safety precautions (i.e., by using gloves, fluid-resistant gowns, and eye protection) and it must be stored in containers with tight-fitting lids.

If additional studies corroborate OPA's advantages, this compound may replace glutaraldehyde for many uses, especially endoscope disinfection. The new agent appears to be particularly useful in washer-disinfectors, where glutaraldehyde-resistant mycobacteria have emerged (251, 255).

Formaldehyde

Formaldehyde and its condensates are reviewed in depth elsewhere (192). Formaldehyde in aqueous solutions or as a gas has been used as a disinfectant and sterilant for many decades. Its use in the health care setting, however, has sharply decreased for several reasons. The irritating vapors and pungent odor produced by formaldehyde are apparent at very low levels (<1 ppm). In addition, allergy to formaldehyde is fairly common. Moreover, the Occupational Safety and Health Administration in the United States and the Health and Safety Executive of the United Kingdom indicated that formaldehyde vapors may be carcinogenic. Thus, the Occupational Safety and Health Administration limits the 8-h time-weighted average exposure in the workplace to a concentration of 0.75 ppm. Elevated levels of occupational exposures have been found among workers in dialysis units and gross anatomy laboratories (8). Consequently, formaldehyde and formaldehyde-releasing agents are used infrequently in health care institutions, despite this agent's broad-spectrum microbicidal activity. In fact, formaldehyde has been largely replaced by peracetic acid as an agent for disinfecting hemodialysis equipment and water dialysate tubing systems. Paraformaldehyde vaporized by heat is used to decontaminate biological safety cabinets.

Chlorine and Chlorine-Releasing Compounds

Due to its hazardous nature, chlorine gas is rarely used as a disinfectant. Among the large number of chlorine compounds commercially available, hypochlorites are the most widely used disinfectants. Hypochlorite has been used for more than a century and remains an important disinfectant. Rutala and Weber published an extensive review of uses for inorganic hypochlorite in health care facilities (210), and Karol reviewed the potential hazards and significant benefits of chlorine use (139).

Aqueous solutions of sodium hypochlorite are usually called household bleach. Bleach commonly contains 5.25% sodium hypochlorite, or 52,500 ppm of available chlorine; a 1:10 dilution of bleach provides about 300 to 600 mg of free chlorine per liter. Alternative chlorine-releasing compounds frequently used in health care facilities include chloramine-T, sodium dichloroisocyanurate tablets, and chlorine dioxide. Demand-release chlorine dioxide is an extremely reactive compound and must be prepared at the point of use. It is used primarily to chlorinate potable water, swimming pools, and wastewater. In Europe, commercial chlorine dioxide preparations are available to disinfect instruments.

In aqueous solutions, all chlorine compounds release hypochlorous acid, the most likely active compound. The mechanism of microbicidal action of hypochlorous acid has not been fully elucidated, but it inhibits key enzymatic reactions within cells and denaturates proteins. Lowering the pH or raising the temperature or concentration increases its antimicrobial efficacy. Chlorine compounds have broad antimicrobial spectra including, at higher concentrations, bacterial spores and *Mycobacterium tuberculosis*. Therefore, hypochlorite can be used as a high-level disinfectant for semicritical items.

Concentrations of 100 ppm of available chlorine inactivate vegetative bacteria and viruses in 10 min. Suspension tests document that both enveloped and nonenveloped viruses, including HIV, hepatitis A and B viruses, herpes simplex virus types 1 and 2, poliovirus, coxsackievirus, and rotavirus, are inactivated (210). In one study, a concentration of 100 ppm of chlorine eliminated 99.9% of *Bacillus subtilis* endospores in 5 min (267). However, endospore-forming bacteria, mycobacteria, fungi, and protozoa usually are less susceptible to chlorine than other microorganisms, and high concentrations of chlorine (1,000 ppm) are required to completely destroy them. Despite this limitation, sodium hypochlorite solutions (500 and 1,600 ppm) have been reported to decrease *Clostridium difficile* environmental contamination and to terminate an outbreak of infections caused by this organism (134). *Cryptosporidium* oocysts are particularly resistant to chlorine. These oocysts remain infective for several days in swimming pool water containing recommended chlorine concentrations; because of their small size, they may not be removed efficiently by conventional pool filters. Outbreaks of *Cryptosporidium* infections have been associated with drinking water and swimming pools (16). Of note, chloramine-T and sodium dichloroisocyanurate seem to have lower sporicidal activities than does sodium hypochlorite.

Hypochlorite is fast acting, nonstaining, nonflammable, and inexpensive. However, its use is limited because it is corrosive, inactivated by organic matter, and relatively instable. Sodium hypochlorite can injure tissues; however, such injury occurs rarely in health care facilities (210). Inhalation of chlorine gas may irritate the respiratory tract, resulting in a cough, dyspnea, and pulmonary edema or chemical pneumonitis. The potential carcinogens trihalomethanes have been detected in chlorine-treated water, and high levels of trihalomethanes can be detected when hospitals hyperchlorinate their water systems (118).

Chlorine compounds have other important disadvantages. Blood or other organic matter substantially inactivates hypochlorites and other chlorine compounds. Consequently, items used for patient care and environmental surfaces must be cleaned before hypochlorite is used. In addition, the presence of a biofilm (e.g., in the pipes of a water distribution system) also reduces the efficacy of chlorines significantly. Moreover, the free available chlorine levels in solutions can decay to 40 to 50% of the original concentration after the container has been opened for one month. Therefore, concentrations higher than those established in laboratory experiments should be used in practice. Loss of free chlorine can be minimized if the solutions are dilute and alkaline, kept and used at room temperature, and stored in closed opaque containers.

Depending on the concentrations employed, sodium hypochlorite is used in hospitals as a high-level disinfectant for selected semicritical devices (e.g., dental equipment and mannequins used for cardiopulmonary resuscitation training), as an intermediate-level disinfectant (e.g., hemodialysis equipment), and as a low-level disinfectant for environmental surfaces and hydrotherapy tanks. For example, the CDC recommends that health care workers use a 1:100 dilution (5,000 ppm) of hypochlorite to decontaminate spills of blood and certain other body fluids (53). Because chlorine can be inactivated by blood and other organic material, a full-strength solution or a 1:10 dilution will be safer unless the surface is cleaned before it is disinfected (62, 88, 258). Household bleach also can be used to disinfect table tops and incubators, to clean spills in laboratories, or to disinfect syringes used by drug addicts if sterile disposable syringes are not available (54).

At low concentrations, chlorines (usually about 0.5 ppm of free chlorine) are used to chlorinate the drinking water. Hyperchlorination of institutional water systems has controlled epidemics caused by *Legionella pneumophila* (118) but also corrodes the water distribution system (118). Stabilized solutions of chlorine dioxide appear to be less toxic and more efficacious than chlorine for controlling growth of legionellae (113). A growing number of municipal water treatment plants in the United States are using monochloramine as a residual disinfectant. Chloramination of drinking water has several advantages over the use of free chlorine, including decreasing the risk of Legionnaires' disease at the municipal level or in individual hospitals (144). However, outbreaks of *Cryptosporidium* infections have occurred in cities that use chloramines in their drinking water.

Hydrogen Peroxide

Hydrogen peroxide, a strong oxidizer, is used for high-level disinfection and sterilization. It produces destructive hydroxyl free radicals that attack membrane lipids, DNA, and other essential cell components. Although the catalase produced by anaerobic and some aerobic bacteria may protect cells from hydrogen peroxide, this defense is overwhelmed by the concentrations used for disinfection (154). Generally, a 3% hydrogen peroxide solution is rapidly bactericidal, but it kills organisms with high cellular catalase activity (e.g., *Staphylococcus aureus* and *Serratia marcescens*) less rapidly. Surprisingly, 3% hydrogen peroxide was ineffective against vancomycin-resistant enterococci (164, 223).

Spores are more resistant than vegetative bacteria to hydrogen peroxide. For example, a 3% solution of hydrogen peroxide destroyed 10^6 spores in six of seven exposure trials that were 150 min long; a 10% solution always was successful in 60 min (257). Higher concentrations of hydrogen peroxide (17.7 and 35.4%) killed *Bacillus subtilis* spores in 9.4 and 2.3 min, respectively (152). In a recent investigation,

10% hydrogen peroxide was the most active of the seven chemical disinfectants tested against *Bacillus subtilis* spores (218). However, other investigators found that the sporicidal activity of hydrogen peroxide was lower than those of peracetic acid and chlorine (10). Hydrogen peroxide's sporocidal activity can be enhanced by increasing the concentration or the temperature or by using it in conjunction with ultrasonic energy, ultraviolet radiation, and some chemical agents such as peracetic acid (162, 170, 247).

A 0.3% solution of hydrogen peroxide inactivates HIV in 10 min (162), and a 3% concentration inactivates rhinovirus in 6 to 8 min at 37°C (170). However, a 6% solution did not inactivate poliovirus at 1 min (247).

Hydrogen peroxide does not coagulate blood and does not fix tissues to surfaces. In fact, it may enhance removal of organic material from equipment. Hydrogen peroxide has a low toxicity for humans. It decomposes into oxygen and water, and therefore, it is environmentally safe. It is neither carcinogenic nor mutagenic. Concentrated solutions may irritate the eyes, skin, and mucous membranes. Hydrogen peroxide can be destroyed easily by heat or enzymes (catalase and peroxidases). Stabilized solutions can be used for high-level disinfection of semicritical items. However, one must consider the corrosive effects of hydrogen peroxide on copper, zinc, and brass in using this disinfectant (201). The FDA has approved commercial products containing either 7.5% hydrogen peroxide alone or combinations with peracetic acid as liquid sterilants and high-level disinfectants for processing of reusable medical and dental devices (http://www.fda.gov). Concentrations of 3 to 6% are used to disinfect ventilators, soft contact lenses (3% for 2 to 4 h) (125), and tonometer biprisms (153, 154, 201). Vaporized hydrogen peroxide is also used for plasma sterilization (see below).

Despite its limited toxicity, hydrogen peroxide can damage human tissues. Patients exposed to endoscopes contaminated by residual hydrogen peroxide have developed pseudomembrane-like enterocolitis (pseudolipomatosis) (216). In addition, patients who were exposed to tonometer tips disinfected with hydrogen peroxide and rinsed improperly suffered corneal damage (153). Use of hydrogen peroxide to clean wounds and to develop dental regimens remains controversial (154).

Peracetic Acid

Peracetic acid (or peroxyacetic acid) is a more potent germicidal agent than hydrogen peroxide and was the most active agent in several in vitro studies (9, 219). Concentrations of <1% are sporicidal even at low temperatures. The mechanism of action of peracetic acid has not been fully elucidated, but it is likely to be similar to that of hydrogen peroxide and other oxidizing agents. Peracetic acid remains effective in the presence of organic matter. At low concentrations it is considerably less stable than hydrogen peroxide; preparations with appropriate stabilities have been developed and are commercially available. Peracetic acid corrodes steel, galvanized iron, copper, brass, and bronze, and it attacks natural and synthetic rubbers. In addition, concentrated solutions can seriously damage eyes and skin. Furthermore, some investigators have raised concerns about the potential toxicity of the combination of peracetic and acetic acids (117). Feldman et al. reported that mortality rates in freestanding dialysis facilities that reprocess dialyzers with peracetic and acetic acid are higher than those in facilities that discard dialysis filters or used formaldehyde for reprocessing (86). To date, investigators have not determined whether the higher death rate is caused by the disinfectants or is associated with other practices at the facilities or with patient risk factors.

Nevertheless, because peracetic acid has powerful germicidal activity and does not produce toxic residues, peracetic acid is very attractive for use in health care settings, most frequently in combination with hydrogen peroxide to disinfect hemodialyzers. The FDA lists several commercial products containing a combination of peracetic acid and hydrogen peroxide as high-level disinfectants and chemical sterilants. The use of peracetic acid for chemical sterilization of instruments and endoscopes (STERIS System 1) is discussed below.

Alcohols

For centuries, the alcohols have been appreciated for their antimicrobial properties. Alcohol is defined by the FDA as having one of the following active ingredients: ethyl alcohol, 60 to 95% by volume in an aqueous solution, or isopropyl alcohol, 50 to 91.3% by volume in an aqueous solution. Ethyl alcohol (ethanol) and isopropyl alcohol (isopropanol) are the alcoholic solutions most often used as surface disinfectants and antiseptic agents in health care institutions because they possess many qualities that make them suitable both for disinfection of equipment and for antisepsis of skin. They are fast acting, minimally toxic to the skin, nonstaining, and nonallergenic. Alcohols evaporate readily, which is advantageous for most disinfection and antisepsis procedures. The uptake of alcohol by intact skin and the lungs when alcohol is used topically is negligible. Alcohols have better wetting properties than water due to their lower surface tensions, which along with their cleansing and degreasing actions make alcohols effective skin antiseptics. Alcoholic formulations used to prepare the skin before invasive procedures should be filtered to ensure that they are free of spores, or 0.5% hydrogen peroxide should be added (193). Alcohols are also excellent products for intermediate-level and low-level disinfection of small, clean surfaces, equipment, and the environment (e.g., rubber stoppers of medication vials, stethoscopes, and medication preparation areas).

Alcohols have some disadvantages. If alcoholic antiseptics are used repeatedly, they may dry and irritate the skin. Therefore, preparations for hand disinfection should contain emollients (see "Hygienic Hand Disinfection" below). Moreover, alcohols may damage rubber, certain plastic items, and the shellac mountings of lensed instruments after prolonged and repeated use (201). Moreover, alcohols are flammable (one should consider the flash point) and, thus, must not be used on large surfaces, particularly in closed, poorly ventilated areas. Alcohols cannot penetrate protein-rich materials. Therefore, a spray or a wipe with alcohol may not disinfect a surface contaminated with blood or other body fluids that has not been cleaned first.

The exact mechanism by which alcohols destroy microorganisms is not fully understood. The most plausible explanation for the antimicrobial action is that they coagulate (denaturate) proteins (e.g., enzymatic proteins), impairing specific cellular functions (150). Ethyl and isopropyl alcohols at appropriate concentrations have broad spectra of antimicrobial activities that include vegetative bacteria, fungi, and viruses. In fact, their antimicrobial efficacies are enhanced in the presence of water, with optimal alcohol concentrations being 60 to 90% by volume.

Alcohols (i.e., 70 to 80% ethyl alcohol) rapidly (i.e., 10 to 90 s) kill vegetative bacteria, such as *Staphylococcus aureus*, *Streptococcus pyogenes*, *Enterobacteriaceae*, and *Pseudomonas aeruginosa*, in suspension tests (193). Isopropyl alcohol is slightly more bactericidal than ethyl alcohol (150) and is highly effective against vancomycin-resistant enterococci (223). It also has excellent activity against fungi, such as *Candida* spp., *Cryptococcus neoformans*, *Blastomyces dermatitidis*, *Coccidioides immitis*, *Histoplasma capsulatum*, *Aspergillus niger*, and dermatophytes and mycobacteria, including *Mycobacterium tuberculosis*. However, alcohols generally do not destroy bacterial spores. In fact, fatal infections due to *Clostridium* spp. occurred when alcohol was used to sterilize surgical instruments.

Both ethyl and isopropyl alcohols inactivate most viruses with a lipid envelope (e.g., influenza virus, herpes simplex virus, and adenovirus). However, several investigators found that isopropyl alcohol has lower virucidal activity against naked, nonenveloped viruses (201). In the experiments by Klein and DeForest, 2-propanol, even at 95%, could not inactivate the nonenveloped poliovirus type 1 and coxsackievirus type B in 10 min (141). In contrast, 70% ethanol inactivated these enteroviruses (141). Neither 70% ethanol nor 45% 2-propanol killed hepatitis A virus when their activities were assessed on stainless steel disks contaminated with fecally suspended virus. Among 20 disinfectants tested, only 3 reduced the titer of hepatitis A virus by greater than 99.9% in 1 min (2% glutaraldehyde, sodium hypochlorite with >5,000 ppm of free chlorine, and a quaternary ammonium formulation containing 23% HCl) (166). Bond et al. (35) and Kobayashi et al. (143) demonstrated that 2-propanol (70% for 10 min) or ethanol (80% for 2 min) made human plasma contaminated with hepatitis B virus at high titer noninfectious for susceptible chimpanzees (143). Both 15% ethyl alcohol and 35% isopropyl alcohol (162) readily inactivate HIV, and 70% ethanol rapidly inactivates high titers of HIV in suspension, independent of the protein load. However, the rate of inactivation decreased when virus was dried onto a glass surface and high levels of protein were present (249). In a suspension test, 40% propanol reduced the rotavirus titer by at least 4 logs in 1 min (147) and both 70% propanol and 70% ethanol reduced the release of rotavirus from contaminated fingertips by 2.7 log units. In comparison, the mean reductions obtained with liquid soap and an aqueous solution of chlorhexidine gluconate were 0.9 and 0.7 log units, respectively (17).

Phenolics

Since Lister's pioneering use of phenol (carbolic acid) as an antiseptic, a large number of phenol derivatives (or phenolics) have been developed and marketed. Phenol derivatives originate when one of the hydrogen atoms on an aromatic ring is replaced by a functional group (e.g., an alkyl-, benzyl-, phenyl-, amyl-, or chlorogroup). The three phenolics most commonly used as constituents of disinfectants are *o*-phenylphenol, *o*-benzyl-*p*-chlorophenol, and *p*-*tert*-amylphenol. The addition of detergents to the basic formulation results in products that clean, dissolve proteins, and disinfect in one step. Phenolics at higher concentrations act as gross protoplasmic poisons, penetrating and disrupting the bacterial cell wall and precipitating the cell proteins (180). Lower concentrations of these compounds inactivate cellular enzyme systems and cause essential metabolites to leak from the cell.

Phenol compounds at concentrations of 2 to 5% are generally considered bactericidal, tuberculocidal, fungicidal, and virucidal against lipophilic viruses (180). However, the manufacturers' efficacy claims have generally not been verified by independent laboratories or the EPA (201). A collaborative study by Rutala and Cole documented that randomly selected EPA-registered phenolic detergents or quaternary ammonium compounds do not consistently meet the manufacturers' bactericidal label claims (203). Phenolics tested by the AOAC use dilution method at the recommended use dilution failed to kill *Pseudomonas aeruginosa* in 33 to 78% of laboratories. However, extreme variability of test results has been observed among laboratories testing identical products (203).

Phenolics at in-use dilutions are not lethal to bacterial spores. Terleckyi and Axler found that a 2% phenolic kills a wide spectrum of clinically important fungi except *Aspergillus fumigatus* (242). Although 5% phenol inactivated both lipophilic and hydrophilic viruses, Klein and DeForest found that 12% *o*-phenylphenol was effective only against lipophilic viruses (141). Similarly, other investigators demonstrated little or no virucidal effect of a phenolic against coxsackievirus type B4, echovirus type 11, or poliovirus type 1 (178). Martin et al. showed that a 0.5% commercial phenolic formulation (2.8% *o*-phenylphenol and 2.7% *o*-benzyl-*p*-chlorophenol) inactivated HIV (162) but that another commercial product containing phenolics at a final concentration of 1% did not completely inactivate cell-associated HIV suspended in blood (81). A phenol-based preparation (14.7% phenol diluted 1:256 in tap water) and a bleach dilution (800 ppm of available chlorine) reduced rotavirus numbers similarly and interrupted transfer of virus from disks to fingerpads (222).

Phenolic compounds are relatively tolerant of anionic and organic matter. They are absorbed by rubber and plastics and leave a residual film, which may irritate skin and tissues. *p*-*tert*-butylphenol and *p*-*tert*-amylphenol have been reported to depigment skin. Although differences between the various compounds exist, phenolics are degraded in wastewater at a lower rate than other germicides, which limits their use in Europe.

Phenolic germicidal detergent solutions may be used for intermediate-level and low-level disinfection of surgical instruments and noncritical patient care items. These compounds are also appropriate for decontaminating the hospital environment, including laboratory surfaces. They should not be used to disinfect bassinets and incubators because they can cause hyperbilirubinemia in infants (201).

Quaternary Ammonium Compounds

A wide variety of quaternary ammonium compounds (quats) with antimicrobial activities have been introduced in the past decade. Some of the compounds used in health care settings are benzalkonium chloride, alkyldimethylbenzyl ammonium chloride, and didecyldimethyl ammonium chloride. Quats are cationic surface-active detergents, which appear to kill microorganisms by disrupting cell membranes, inactivating enzymes, and denaturating cell proteins (171). However, they have limited antimicrobial spectra. Products sold as hospital disinfectants are not sporicidal and are generally not tuberculocidal or virucidal against hydrophilic viruses. Scientific investigations using the AOAC use dilution method have not reproduced the bactericidal and tuberculocidal claims made by the manufacturers (204). Consequently, health care workers should be suspicious of the claims on labels and of results from in-house evaluations that have not been verified by an independent laboratory. The germicidal activity may have been overestimated because the compounds tested were incompletely inactivated. In this case, the bacteriostatic (inhibitory) activity rather than the bactericidal activity is measured (171). The antimicrobial spectra of quats may be improved by combining them with amines and biguanides or by using them at higher temperatures in washing machines.

Several outbreaks of infections have been associated with quat solutions contaminated in use by gram-negative bacteria such as *Pseudomonas* spp. or *Serratia marcescens* or by *Mycobacterium abscessus* (90, 177, 244). The contaminated solutions were used as antiseptics on skin and tissue and as disinfectants on patient care supplies and equipment (e.g., cardiac catheters and cystoscopes). In fact, microbiology laboratories use the quat cetrimide in selective media to isolate *Pseudomonas aeruginosa*.

Quats have other disadvantages. Genes conferring resistance to quats have been detected in 6 to 42% of *Staphylococcus aureus* isolates collected in Japan and Europe (165). Organic matter, anionic detergents (soaps), and materials such as cotton and gauze pads can reduce the microbicidal activities of quats. Despite these limitations, quats are nonstaining, odorless, noncorrosive, and relatively nontoxic. They are excellent cleaning agents, but sticky residue may build up on surfaces. On the basis of their limited antimicrobial spectra, they should be used in hospitals only for environmental sanitation of noncritical surfaces such as floors, furniture, and walls (201).

Other Germicides of Interest

Glucoprotamine, the conversion product of L-glutamic acid and cocopropylene-1,3-diamine, possesses a broad antimicrobial spectrum that includes vegetative bacteria, mycobacteria, fungi, and enveloped viruses (77, 173). A clinical study examining used specula from a gynecologic clinic demonstrated that the product killed >6 log units of vegetative bacteria excluding spores (263). The manufacturer's data sheets indicate good compatibility of the compound with humans, the environment, and various materials. A commercial product, available in Europe, can be used to disinfect instruments and endoscopes.

Peroxygen compounds have proven efficacy against bacteria, bacterial spores, fungi, and a broad spectrum of viruses. A 1% concentration of a new commercial formulation containing peroxygen achieved a 10^5-fold increase in killing of *Bacillus subtilis* in 2 to 3 h in the absence of blood, but killing was poor in the presence of blood (64). Moreover, several investigators have found that peroxygen has poor mycobactericidal activity (45, 107). In addition to other applications, these compounds may be suitable for disinfecting laboratory equipment and workbenches.

Superoxidized water is prepared at the point of use by the electrolysis of NaCl solution, which generates hypochlorous acid and a mixture of radicals with strong oxidizing properties (175). Freshly generated solutions rapidly destroy bacteria including spores and mycobacteria, fungi, and viruses in the absence of organic loading (229). A commercial adaption of this process (i.e., Sterilox) has been marketed in Europe since 1999 and recently was approved by the FDA (see "Endoscopes" below) (175). Because Sterilox solutions are unstable, they should be used only once for high-level disinfection. Some investigators have claimed that superoxidized water is compatible with instruments and that it does not damage the environment, irritate the respiratory tract and skin, or corrode metal. However, others have reported that superoxidized water damages flexible endoscopes. Further studies are needed to explore the use of this new disinfectant in clinical settings.

Metals such as copper and silver ions inactivate a wide variety of microorganisms (217). Although further work is required to explore their use in health care, they currently are used to disinfect water and to prevent infections associated with medical devices (e.g., intravascular catheters impregnated with silver sulfadiazine). For example, copper-silver ionization systems are successfully used to minimize legionella colonization in water systems (237).

Surfacine is a new, silver-based surface germicide that may be applied to inanimate or animate surfaces. Surfacine immediately eliminates microorganisms from surfaces and also has long-term residual activity (44, 212). This novel antimicrobial coating might be suitable for a wide range of applications including preventing microbial contamination of medical devices, if further studies confirm the promising preliminary data.

Specific Issues

Cleaning and Disinfecting Surfaces and Floors

In general, the environment is not a primary reservoir for nosocomial pathogens. However, in some cases, such as respiratory syncytial virus (112) and the SARS coronavirus (97), environmental contamination may be important. The CDC's recent guidelines for environmental infection control in health care facilities recommend using an EPA-registered hospital detergent-disinfectant designed for general housekeeping purposes in patient care areas, especially in intensive care units, operating rooms, and emergency rooms, where blood, body fluids, or multidrug-resistant organisms may have contaminated surfaces (227). A one-step process is adequate in most areas, but a rinse step is necessary in nurseries and neonatal intensive care units, especially if a phenolic agent is used (270). Products with quats allow staff members to clean and disinfect in one step, but residual quats may leave surfaces sticky and smeared. Other products may require a two-step approach, a cleaning step and a disinfection step, doubling the human resources needed to do the work. "High-touch" surfaces (e.g., doorknobs, bedrails, and light switches) should be disinfected more frequently than "low-touch" surfaces. A simple detergent is adequate for cleaning surfaces for other patient-care areas and in non-patient-care areas. Cleaning with a detergent is much more important than adding a disinfectant to the solution. In fact, several studies found that adding a disinfectant does not prolong the reduction in bacterial loads on surfaces (76). Routine disinfection of environmental surfaces is necessary in all areas housing patients in contact isolation (e.g., patients infected with methicillin-resistant *Staphylococcus aureus* [MRSA]). A recent study indicates that twice-daily disinfection is necessary to control an outbreak with vancomycin-intermediate *Staphylococcus aureus* (73).

Emergence of Resistance to Biocides

Microorganisms rarely become resistant to disinfectants. However, frequent use of sublethal concentrations of disinfectants can select for resistant strains (19, 37, 253). Mechanisms of resistance include acquisition of resistance plasmids, changes in the cell membrane (e.g., chlorhexidine in *Pseudomonas stutzeri*), capsule formation (*Klebsiella* spp.), and activation of the *norA* efflux pump *(Staphylococcus aureus)*. A large proportion of household soaps now contain antibacterial agents (up to 45% in one study), which may increase the probability that resistant bacteria will emerge (183). Multiple outbreaks have been associated with soaps containing antibacterial agents such as chlorhexidine, hexetidine solution, and chlorxylenol (19, 37, 253). However, the concentrations of biocides used in the health care setting are much higher than the minimum biocidal concentrations in vitro. Therefore, resistance has not become a major problem in the clinical setting to date. Readers desiring more information about disinfectants and antiseptics (34, 89) and resistance to these agents should read several excellent articles (34, 89, 157, 228).

Inactivation of Emerging Pathogens and Antibiotic-Resistant Bacteria

New and emerging pathogens such as vCJD prions, noroviruses, SARS coronavirus, avian influenza virus, hypervirulent *Clostridium difficile*, Panton-Valentine leukocidin-producing *Staphylococcus aureus*, and gram-negative rods producing extended-spectrum β-lactamases or metallo-β-lactamases threaten the public health. Only limited data exist regarding the susceptibility of emerging pathogens to commonly used disinfectants or sterilants. Surrogate microbes have been studied for some pathogens. Examples include feline calicivirus for noroviruses, vaccinia virus for variola virus, and *Bacillus atrophaeus* (formerly *Bacillus subtilis*) for *Bacillus anthracis* (259). Other infectious agents that cannot be evaluated by standard testing procedures (e.g., hepatitis C virus) have been tested by alternative methods, such as PCR. With the exception of prions, there is no evidence that emerging pathogens are less susceptible to approved standard disinfection and sterilization procedures than are comparable classical pathogens. (Inactivation of prions, including those associated with vCJD, is discussed below.) In particular, there are no data demonstrating that disinfectants used at recommended contact conditions and concentrations are less effective against antimicrobial-resistant bacteria than against antimicrobial-susceptible bacteria (213). Standard disinfection and sterilization procedures for patient care equipment as recommended in guidelines and in this chapter are adequate to disinfect or sterilize instruments or devices contaminated with blood and other body fluids (213).

Other than one peroxygen compound, hospital disinfectants registered by the EPA do not have specific claims for activity against noroviruses. Because noroviruses are nonenveloped, most quats do not have significant activity against them. Phenolic-based preparations have been found to be active in vitro against a surrogate virus from this group. However, concentrations two- to fourfold higher than those recommended by the manufacturers for routine use may be required. In the event of a norovirus outbreak, the CDC recommends using a hypochlorite solution (minimum chlorine concentration of 1,000 ppm) to decontaminate hard, nonporous, environmental surfaces (http://www.cdc.gov/ncidod/hip/gastro/norovirus.htm).

SARS coronavirus and avian influenza virus are inactivated by sodium hypochlorite and a commercially available peroxygen compound (148); phenolic compounds and quats are less effective. A sporicidal germicide is required to efficiently eliminate *Clostridium difficile* spores. In a recent study, glutaraldehyde (2%), peracetyl ions (1.6%; equivalent to 0.26% peracetic acid), and acidified nitrite demonstrated biocidal activity against *Clostridium difficile* spores (269). Hypochlorite-based disinfectants have been used, with some success, to disinfect environmental surfaces in areas with ongoing transmission of *Clostridium difficile*. Recent nosocomial outbreaks of *Clostridium difficile* infections caused by virulent strains suggest that hospitals may need to focus more on environmental cleaning and disinfection (168).

Decontamination in the Event of Biological Terrorism

If a biological agent is released, environmental decontamination measures may be necessary to decrease the risk of spreading the disease. A decontamination agent should be effective against possible pathogens and readily available at a reasonable cost. Therefore, sodium hypochlorite (household bleach) is usually recommended, especially if bacterial spores are involved. This agent is well suited for various decontamination procedures in the laboratory and health care settings. In addition, it may be used to decontaminate protective equipment and clothing worn by first responders and decontamination workers.

Smallpox virus does not survive long in the environment but may remain viable for extended periods under favorable conditions. CDC guidelines recommend incinerating items that are not needed or cannot be decontaminated, sterilizing items in an autoclave or an ethylene oxide sterilizer, decontaminating spaces and rooms with vaporized paraformaldehyde (or use of an Amphyl fogger), and soaking equipment or wiping down surfaces with a 5% aqueous solution of a phenolic germicidal detergent (http://www.bt.cdc.gov/DocumentsApp/Smallpox/RPG/GuideF/Guide-F.pdf). Because contaminated clothing can spread the virus to personnel, bed linens and clothes must be autoclaved or laundered in hot water supplemented with bleach (119). Disinfectants that are used for standard hospital infection control, such as sodium hypochlorite and quaternary ammonium compounds, decontaminate surfaces effectively (119). Only vaccinated personnel should perform the decontamination procedures.

Bacillus anthracis spores are extremely stable and can remain viable for decades in the environment (129). The CDC recommends that laboratory staff use a 1:10-diluted hypochlorite solution when addressing spills and items and surfaces contaminated with *Bacillus anthracis* (http://www.bt.cdc.gov/Agent/Anthrax/LevelAProtocol/Anthracis20010417.pdf). Decontamination of a building or of large areas contaminated with anthrax spores is extremely difficult. Spotts Whitney et al. have summarized the literature on the inactivation of *Bacillus anthracis* spores (233). *Clostridium botulinum* and its spores are killed by a 1:10 dilution of sodium hypochlorite. Heat (>85°C for 5 min) or 0.1 M sodium hydroxide (contact time, 20 min) inactivates the toxin (20). Persons with direct exposure to powder or liquid aerosols containing *Franciscella tularensis* should wash their body and clothing with soapy water (74). In the circumstances of a laboratory spill or intentional release, environmental surfaces can be decontaminated with a 1:10-diluted hypochlorite solution. After 10 min, a 70% alcohol solution can be used to further clean the area and reduce the corrosive action of the bleach (74). *Yersinia pestis* does not survive long outside the host. The WHO estimated that a plague aerosol would be effective and infectious for 1 h. Thus, areas exposed to aerosols of *Yersinia pestis* do not need to be decontaminated (128).

Equipment or environmental surfaces contaminated with the agents causing Ebola hemorrhagic fever, Marburg hemorrhagic fever (*Filoviridae*), Lassa fever, and related infections (those with *Arenaviridae* and *Bunyaviridae*) should be disinfected by using a suitable registered hospital disinfectant or a 1:100 dilution of a hypochlorite solution. Surfaces grossly soiled with vomitus or stool should be disinfected with a 1:10 dilution of a hypochlorite solution. If possible, serum samples used for laboratory tests should be pretreated with heat inactivation at 56°C and polyethylene glycol *p-tert*-octylphenyl ether (Triton X-100). Treatment with 10 μl of 10% Triton X-100 per 1 ml of serum for 1 h reduces the titers of hemorrhagic fever viruses in serum samples. If treatment with Triton X-100 is not feasible, heat inactivation alone may reduce infectivity somewhat (52).

Medical, public health, and laboratory responses to the release of organisms and toxins that pose a risk to national security (i.e., variola major virus [smallpox virus], *Bacillus anthracis*, *Clostridium botulinum* toxin, *Francisella tularensis*, *Yersinia pestis*, and certain filoviruses and arenaviruses) are discussed in chapter 9 of this Manual and in numerous publications (20, 74, 119, 128, 129). The CDC published guidelines for the management of patients with suspected viral hemorrhagic fever (52) and recently posted updated guidelines at http://www.cdc.gov/ncidod/hip/BLOOD/VHFinterimGuidance05_19_05.pdf.

Endoscopes

Reprocessing of endoscopes is probably the most challenging reprocessing task in health care. Multiple outbreaks have been associated with insufficient reprocessing techniques or defects in endoscopes (Table 7). However, ample data indicate that a sufficient level of safety can be achieved even with manual disinfection of endoscopes if the guidelines are followed strictly (163). Flexible endoscopes have intricate, sophisticated small parts that are difficult to clean, which must be cleaned before they can be disinfected because organic material such as blood, feces, and respiratory secretions interfere with disinfection (68). A large study of several centers in the United States found that 23.9% of specimens from the internal channels of 71 gastrointestinal reprocessed endoscopes grew ≥10^6 CFU of bacteria and that 78% of the facilities did not sterilize all biopsy forceps (135). Other studies have documented that up to 40% of the institutions do not follow published guidelines for endoscope disinfection (12, 84, 104) and that reuse of disposable endoscopic accessories is common in the United States. These items frequently are not sterilized, and reprocessing protocols are not standardized. Therefore, reused disposable items might be a source of cross-transmission (61, 68).

Currently, most high-level disinfectants approved by the FDA for reprocessing of endoscopes contain >2% aldehyde with or without peracetic acid (http://www.fda.gov/cdrh/ode/germlab.html). However, aldehydes should be used only after completion of the cleaning cycle because they may stain prions to the instruments. Endoscopes, which are semicritical items, must be immersed in ≥2% glutaraldehyde for ≥20 min to achieve the necessary level of disinfection. These parameters are sufficient to kill ≥3 log units of mycobacteria, the most resistant vegetative bacteria. However, glutaraldehyde-resistant mycobacteria have been identified (107). Several authors have raised concerns that *Clostridium difficile* may not be fully inactivated by standard reprocessing procedures, but transmission of *Clostridium difficile* by contaminated endoscopes has not been reported to date. Moreover, cryptosporidia withstand several hours of exposure to glutaraldehyde (268) but do not survive on dry surfaces (191).

The glutaraldehyde concentration in commercial cleaner-disinfectors can decrease by more than 50% after 2 weeks, which may promote the emergence of resistant bacteria (251). Higher concentrations of glutaraldehyde (3.2% instead of 2%) appear to be safe for endoscopes and achieve the required ≥3-log-unit killing with a higher margin of safety than that achieved with the standard concentration (7). OPA and peracetic acid plus hydrogen peroxide can be used to disinfect endoscopes. Because the latter might corrode some endoscopes, reprocessing staff should ensure that the manufacturer of the endoscope approves this disinfectant for reprocessing.

Automated washer-disinfectors specifically for endoscopes were developed, in part, to reduce the work needed to reprocess endoscopes and to decrease the risk of human

TABLE 7 Outbreaks and pseudo-outbreaks associated with contaminated endoscopes or instruments for minimally invasive procedures

Microorganism(s)	No. of cases	No. of deaths	Yr of publication	Problem identified	Type of outbreak	Reference(s)
Klebsiella pneumoniae, *Proteus vulgaris*, *Morganella morganii*	11	0	2005	Loose port of the bronchoscope's biopsy channel	Mixed	57
Pseudomonas aeruginosa	16	0	2005	Defective biopsy forceps	Mixed	68
Pseudomonas aeruginosa	3	0	2004	Probable defective endoscope	Infections	91
Pseudomonas aeruginosa	39	3	2003	Loose biopsy port cap in the bronchoscope	Infections	234
Pseudomonas aeruginosa	18	0	2001	Improper connection to liquid sterilization device	Mixed	230
Mycobacterium xenopi	58	0	2001	Inappropriate disinfection of microsurgical instruments, tap water rinse after disinfection	Infections	22
Pseudomonas aeruginosa	11	2	2000	Failure of washer-disinfector, purchased without expert advice, poor maintenance	Infections	211, 224
Pseudomonas aeruginosa, mycobacteria	29	0	1999	Problems related to the use of STERIS System 1 processor	Mixed	15
Hepatitis C virus	2	0	1997	Cleaning, immersion	Infections	46
Mycobacterium tuberculosis	2	0	1997	Cleaning, immersion	Infections	174
Mycobacterium tuberculosis (multidrug resistant)	5	1	1997	Cleaning, immersion	Infections	3
Pseudomonas aeruginosa	23	0	1996	Failure of washer-disinfector	Pseudo-outbreak	32
Nontuberculous mycobacteria	4	0	1992	Failure of washer-disinfector	Pseudo-outbreak	108
Multiple microorganisms	377	7	1993	Cleaning, immersion, use of tap water, poorly designed washer-disinfector	Infections	231 (review)

errors during manual reprocessing. These machines rinse the endoscopes, clean them in several steps, and run a full-cycle disinfection process. The time endoscopes are exposed to disinfectants is set by the machine and cannot be shortened, as it can be by busy staff members who are manually reprocessing endoscopes.

However, endoscope washers can become contaminated with pathogenic bacteria. For example, one study found gram-negative bacteria and/or mycobacteria in 27% of cultures of specimens obtained before the final alcohol rinse and in 10% of cultures of specimens obtained thereafter. In the same study, 37 and 27% of the manually disinfected endoscopes remained contaminated at the same time points (92). In 1992, Olympus recalled its 835 model endoscope washers because the design allowed the internal tanks and tubing to become colonized by waterborne organisms such as *Pseudomonas* spp. (recall no. Z-039/040-2 by the FDA). In 1999, the CDC reported three outbreaks related to the STERIS System 1 (15). This device is supposed to sterilize the endoscopes, but they must first be cleaned manually (42). Table 7 summarizes outbreaks related to endoscopes, including those related to contaminated washer-disinfectors.

Newer washer-disinfectors should continuously monitor the pressure in all channels to detect debris blocking the channels, provide adapters for all types of endoscopes, use an appropriate disinfection process with an FDA-approved disinfectant, use filtered water or sterile water for rinsing, and have a built-in automatic disinfection process. These washer-disinfectors can help staff members trace problems by monitoring and documenting the disinfecting process in a manner similar to that used by autoclaves.

To avoid problems, knowledgeable staff should review currently marketed machines before purchasing a washer-disinfector to ensure that the one they choose is appropriate for their needs (23). To facilitate this process, the FDA recommends that the manufacturer provide a list of all brands and models of endoscopes that are compatible with the washer-disinfector and highlight limitations associated with processing of certain brands and models of endoscopes and accessories. Preferably, the manufacturer should identify endoscopes and accessories that cannot be reliably reprocessed in the device (negative list). In addition, health care workers should be trained to use the equipment and monitored subsequently to ensure that they follow the protocol exactly. Although not mandatory, it is prudent to regularly culture the rinse water of washer-disinfectors for pathogens such as *Pseudomonas* spp. and *Mycobacterium* spp. to identify problems before clinical cases occur. However, outbreaks may occur despite negative routine culture results (191, 268).

If washer-disinfectors recycle water, residual glutaraldehyde may remain on the endoscopes. Manual reprocessing is more prone to leave residual glutaraldehyde on endoscopes than are automated washer-disinfectors (83). Thus, endoscopes that are manually disinfected should be thoroughly rinsed to remove any residual disinfectant, specifically glutaraldehyde. Patients exposed to residual glutaraldehyde can develop colitis (79, 262).

Reprocessed endoscopes should be stored vertically (to facilitate drying) in a cabinet (to protect them from dust and secondary contamination). Reprocessed endoscopes that are stored for days or weeks probably should be reprocessed again before use or, alternatively, the channels should be rinsed with 70% alcohol that is filtered to remove spores if this agent is compatible with the instrument. However, the necessity of these precautions has not been established.

Guidelines for infection prevention and control in flexible endoscopes have been updated (12) and should be consulted before choosing of a method and/or disinfectant for reprocessing. The following checklist adapted from the FDA recommendations may help staff members reprocessing endoscopes avoid errors (http://www.fda.gov/cdrh/safety/endoreprocess.html).

1. All staff members must comply with the manufacturer's instructions for cleaning endoscopes.
2. Determine whether your endoscope is suitable for reprocessing in an automatic washer-disinfector, which is the preferred method.
3. Compare the reprocessing instructions provided by the endoscope and washer-disinfector manufacturers and resolve any conflicting recommendations.
4. Follow the instructions provided by the manufacturers of the endoscopes and the chemical germicides.
5. Consider drying endoscopes with alcohol.
6. Monitor adherence to the protocols for reprocessing of endoscopes.
7. Provide comprehensive, intensive training for all staff members who reprocess endoscopes; keep records of persons attending training.
8. Label endoscopes sent for repairs as "contaminated equipment for repair."
9. Implement a comprehensive quality control program.

An updated list of sterilants and high-level disinfectants approved by the FDA in a 510(k) with general claims for processing of reusable medical and dental devices can be found on the FDA website (http://www.fda.gov/cdrh/ode/germlab.html). Rutala and Weber have reviewed these substances (211, 212). Of note, more than 20% of all damage to endoscopes is associated with disinfecting agents. Therefore, staff members who reprocess these items must ensure that the instruments and the disinfectant are compatible (61). A new norm (prEN ISO 15883-4) will soon be adapted for washer-disinfectors designed for thermolabile endoscopes.

Dental Equipment

Critical and semicritical dental instruments should be sterilized; if they will not be used immediately, they should be packaged before they are sterilized. All high-speed dental handheld pieces should be sterilized routinely between patients. Handheld pieces that cannot be heat sterilized should be retrofitted to attain heat tolerance; if this is not feasible, they should not be used. The adequacy of sterilization cycles should be verified by periodically (e.g., at least weekly) including a biological indicator with the load. This recommendation is rarely followed in Europe (109). In fact, 33% of British dental practices do not have a policy on general disinfection and sterilization procedures and only 3% own a vacuum autoclave (24).

Environmental contamination can be a problem in dental offices. For example, *Legionella* spp. can contaminate the air-water syringes and high-speed outlets in dental units. Moreover, Piazza et al. found that about 6% of samples from workbenches, air turbine handheld pieces, holders, suction units, forceps, and dental mirrors were positive by PCR for hepatitis C virus (184). Therefore, infection control issues, particularly in regard to hepatitis C and B viruses, may be more important in dentistry than has been appreciated previously.

The CDC and the American Dental Association (ADA) have published guidelines for infection control in dental settings (1, 55). The ADA recommends that metal and porcelain equipment be immersed in glutaraldehyde or exposed to this disinfectant, that removable dentures and acrylic or porcelain be disinfected with iodophors or chlorine compounds, and that wax rims or bite plates be disinfected with a spray containing iodophors. Additional information can be found on the website of the ADA (http://www.ada.org/prof/resources/positions/doc_policies.pdf).

Disinfectants for Living Tissue

Compounds that disinfect living tissue are frequently called antiseptic agents. They must meet many more requirements than compounds used to disinfect inanimate surfaces, e.g., floors. In addition, some of the agents are considered drugs and, thus, are regulated by the FDA. The antimicrobial spectra of commercially available agents are summarized in Table 6. The choice of an agent should not be based only on the desired effect but, like that of antimicrobial agents, on side effects. Antiseptics rarely cause serious side effects, and most agents on the market have excellent safety profiles. Nevertheless, health care workers must remember that these agents can cause side effects such as anaphylactic shock in patients who have contact with chlorhexidine (82, 182).

Hygienic Hand Washing and Hand Disinfection

Hand hygiene is the single most important infection control measure (40). However, it remains difficult to motivate health care workers to perform this simple procedure faithfully (78). The CDC has published detailed guidelines on hand hygiene (40), and in 2006, the WHO launched a global effort to improve hand hygiene in health care facilities (http://www.who.int/patientsafety/events/05/HH_en.pdf). In-depth reviews have been published by several authors (137, 245, 264).

Microorganisms on the hands can be classified into three groups (186): (i) transient flora, which are contaminants taken up from the environment; (ii) resident flora, which are permanent microorganisms on the skin (264); and (iii) infectious flora. Resident bacteria, most of which are on the uppermost level of the stratum corneum, have low pathogenicity and infection rates, and persons with normal immune systems who do not have implants or foreign bodies rarely acquire infections with these organisms. The density of resident bacteria on the skin ranges between 10^2 and 10^3 CFU/cm^2, and these resident bacteria limit colonization with more pathogenic microorganisms (i.e., they contribute to colonization resistance). During their daily work, health care workers can contaminate their hands with pathogens. If they do not practice good hand hygiene, they can transmit these organisms to susceptible patients. Several studies indicated that pathogens such as *Staphylococcus aureus* (127), *Klebsiella pneumoniae* (2), *Acinetobacter* spp., *Enterobacter* spp., and *Candida* spp. can be found on the hands of >20% of health care workers. Moreover, numerous epidemics have been traced to health care workers' contaminated hands (41, 215, 221, 266, 272).

The goal of hand hygiene outside the operating room is to eliminate the transient flora without altering the resident flora. Hand washing for 15 and 30 s kills 0.6 to 1.1 and 1.8 to 2.8 log units, respectively (196). However, health care workers are very busy and frequently wash their hands for less than 10 s, which is insufficient to kill the transient flora (245, 264). One major advantage of the alcohol-based hand rubs is that performing hand hygiene with these products takes about 25% of the time required for hand washing (245, 264). Moreover, compliance with hand-washing procedures does not exceed 40% even under controlled study conditions (40). However, recent studies have shown that compliance with the use of the alcohol-based hand rubs exceeds that with hand washing (185). Furthermore, other studies have demonstrated that rubbing one's hands with an alcohol-based hand rub kills bacteria and most viruses more effectively than hand washing with a medicated soap (27, 194). Of note, investigators have not determined whether the level of killing is associated with the efficacy of preventing nosocomial infections.

Alcohol-based hand rubs have several other practical advantages for hand hygiene over washing with soap and water. Dispensers for the alcohol-based products are less expensive than sinks and can be installed at locations that are more convenient for health care workers. Furthermore, unlike sinks (172), the dispensers have not been associated with outbreaks.

Given the numerous advantages of these products, the CDC's current hand hygiene guidelines recommend that health care facilities consider introducing alcohol-based hand rubs as the primary mode of hand hygiene (40). Most health care institutions in northern Europe now use an alcohol-based hand rub for many indications for which hand washing was previously the standard of care. At the University Hospital Basel, the use of an alcohol-based hand rub has replaced hand washing in >85% of opportunities for hand hygiene, provided that the hands are not visibly soiled (A. Trampuz, N. Lederray, and A. F. Widmer, *Program Abstr. 41st Intersci. Conf. Antimicrob. Agents Chemother.*, abstr. K1335, 2001). Also at the University Hospital Basel, dispensers for alcohol-based hand rub are available between all beds and at each nurse's desk; two dispensers are available at each bed in intensive care units. Among 4,500 health care workers, we have not identified a single case of documented allergy to the alcohol-based hand rub, resulting in an incidence density of <1:45,000 person-years. Dermatitis may occur, most frequently related to insufficient use of emollients and ointments.

In the United States, health care facilities should consult with the fire marshal before installing dispensers because many states have laws that prohibit placing multiple containers in emergency exits and halls. However, there are no published reports of fires caused by these products in Europe and such events are also very rare in the United States (39).

Surgical Hand Washing (Scrub) or Surgical Hand Disinfection (Rub-In)

In contrast to hand hygiene outside of the operating room, the surgical hand scrub aims to eliminate both transient and resident flora so that if the surgeon's gloves are punctured or torn, the bacteria from his or her hands do not contaminate the surgical site. Tiny holes are observed in ≥30% of surgeons' gloves after operations, even when high-quality gloves are used. Cruse and Foord found that the incidence of surgical site infection is three times higher if the surgeon's gloves are punctured than if they are intact after the procedure (5.7 and 1.7%, respectively) (71). An experimental study demonstrated that the level of bacterial leakage through pin holes ranges between 10^3 and 10^4 CFU (94). Moreover, a persistent antimicrobial effect is required after washing or disinfection to limit bacterial regrowth underneath the gloves (96). Thus, antiseptic preparations intended for use as surgical hand preparations are evaluated for their abilities to reduce the number of bacteria released from hands (i) immediately after scrubbing (immediate activity), (ii) after surgical gloves have been worn for 6 h (persistent activity), and (iii) after numerous applications over 5 days (cumulative activity). Immediate and persistent activities are considered the most important. Guidelines in the United States recommend that agents used for surgical hand preparation should significantly reduce the number of microorganisms on intact skin, contain a nonirritating antimicrobial preparation, have broad-spectrum activity, and be fast acting and persistent. Agents such as chlorhexidine that have a prolonged postexposure effect are preferred because of this theoretical advantage, but there are no data from controlled clinical trials proving that the incidence of surgical site infections is lower when chlorhexidine is used.

Alcohol-based surgical rubs have several advantages over traditional surgical scrubs. Alcoholic preparations are more effective than any medicated soap for the surgical scrub, and they do not alter the skin as much as chlorhexidine washes do. Moreover, the water supply in an operating room may harbor *Pseudomonas* spp. that may contaminate the hands of surgical personnel after they perform their surgical scrub (31). Brushes, which are used during a surgical scrub, may do more harm than good, and they should be used only to clean the fingernails, not to clean the skin. Given the advantages of the alcohol-based preparations, the presurgical scrub has been replaced in many European countries by the alcohol-based surgical rubs (245), and the WHO's guidelines recommend the surgical hand rubs (WHO guidelines are available at http://www.who.int). Alcoholic gels are frequently promoted but are significantly less effective than liquids and should not be used in the operating room (146). A very rapid protocol (1.5 min) for the surgical hand rub has been recently proposed and was rapidly accepted by surgeons at the University Hospital Basel (138).

Of note, both routine hand hygiene and surgical hand preparations must balance removing unwanted bacteria from health care workers' hands and maintaining the integrity of the health care workers' skin because damaged skin is more likely than normal skin to become colonized with pathogenic organisms. Therefore, either hand hygiene products should contain emollients or health care facilities should provide moisturizing hand lotions, which do not damage latex, for their staff so their skin does not become dry, cracked, and irritated.

Presurgical Skin Disinfection

The aim of skin disinfection is to remove and kill rapidly the skin flora at the site of a planned surgical incision. However, currently available antiseptics do not eliminate all microorganisms at the incision site. In fact, coagulase-negative staphylococci can be isolated frequently even after three applications of agents such as iodine-alcohol to the skin (98).

The FDA defines a skin disinfectant as a "fast acting, broad-spectrum and persistent antiseptic-containing preparation that significantly reduces the number of microorganisms on intact skin" (14). Spore-free alcohols are well suited for this purpose, but they lack persistent activity; iodine is frequently added for this purpose (100). Povidone-iodine continuously releases free iodine that results in a prolonged antmicrobial effect. However, for a short-term procedure, alcoholic preparations can be sufficient for skin preparation.

Before a patient's skin is prepared for a surgical procedure, the skin should be free of gross contamination (i.e., dirt, soil, or any other debris) (160). Although preoperative showering has not been shown to reduce the incidence of surgical site infections, this practice may decrease bacterial counts and ensure that the skin is clean (195). The antiseptics used to prepare the skin should be applied by using sterile supplies and gloves or a no-touch technique, moving from the incision area to the periphery (160). The person preparing the skin should use pressure because friction increases the antibacterial effect of the antiseptic. For example, alcohol applied without friction reduces bacterial counts by 1.0 to 1.2 log CFU compared with 1.9 to 3.0 log CFU when friction is used. In comparison, alcoholic sprays have little antimicrobial effect and produce potentially explosive vapors (156).

Common Antiseptic Compounds

Alcoholic Compounds

The reader is referred to "Alcohols" above. As outlined above, alcohol is the most important skin disinfectant. Alcohols used for skin disinfection before invasive procedures should generally be free of spores to avoid any contamination. Although the risk of infection is minimal, the low additional cost for a spore-free product is justified. One study indicated that isopropyl alcohol from a commercial hand rub may be absorbed through the dermis, violating religious beliefs of some health care workers (246). However, the WHO resolved this issue in the guidelines that they will publish in 2006.

Chlorhexidine

Chlorhexidine gluconate, a cationic bisbiguanide, has been widely recognized as an effective and safe antiseptic for nearly 40 years (75, 189). Chlorhexidine formulations are extensively used for surgical and hygienic hand disinfection (see the discussion above). Other applications include preoperative showers (or whole-body disinfection), antisepsis in obstetrics and gynecology, management of burns, wound antisepsis, and prevention and treatment of oral disease (e.g., plaque control, pre-and postoperative mouthwash, and oral hygiene) (75, 189). When chlorhexidine is used orally, its bitter taste must be masked and it can stain the teeth. Intravenous catheters coated with chlorhexidine and silver sulfadiazine are used to prevent catheter-associated bloodstream infections (159).

Chlorhexidine is most commonly formulated as a 4% aqueous solution in a detergent base. However, alcoholic preparations have been demonstrated in numerous studies to have better antimicrobial activity than detergent-based formulations (151). Bactericidal concentrations destroy the bacterial cell membrane, causing cellular constituents to leak out of the cell and cell contents to coagulate (75). Chlorhexidine gluconate's bactericidal activity against vegetative gram-positive and gram-negative bacteria is intermediately rapid. In addition, chlorhexidine provides persistent antimicrobial action that prevents the regrowth of microorganisms for up to 6 h. This effect is desirable when a sustained reduction in microbial flora reduces infection risk (e.g., during surgical procedures). Chlorhexidine has little activity against bacterial and fungal spores except at high temperatures. Mycobacteria are inhibited but are not killed by aqueous solutions. Yeasts and dermatophytes are usually susceptible, although the fungicidal action varies with the species (74). Chlorhexidine is effective against lipophilic viruses (e.g., HIV, influenza virus, and herpes simplex virus types 1 and 2), but viruses such as poliovirus, coxsackievirus, and rotavirus are not inactivated (75). Unlike that of povidone-iodine, blood and other organic material do not affect the antimicrobial activity of chlorhexidine significantly (155). However, inorganic anions and organic anions such as soaps are incompatible with chlorhexidine and its activity is reduced at extreme acidic or alkaline pHs and in the presence of anion- and non-ion-based moisturizers and detergents.

Microorganisms can contaminate chlorhexidine solutions (181), and resistant isolates have been identified. For example, Stickler found chlorhexidine-resistant *Proteus mirabilis* after chlorhexidine was used extensively over a long period to prepare patients for bladder catheterization (235). Chlorhexidine resistance among vegetative bacteria was thought to be limited to certain gram-negative bacilli (such as *Pseudomonas aeruginosa*, *Burkholderia* [*Pseudomonas*] *cepacia*, *Proteus mirabilis*, and *Serratia marcescens*) (236). However, genes conferring resistance to various organic cations, including chlorhexidine, have been identified in *Staphylococcus aureus* clinical isolates (165, 176).

Chlorhexidine has several other limitations. When absorbed onto cotton and other fabrics, it usually resists removal by washing. If a hypochlorite (bleach) is used during the washing procedure, a brown stain may develop (75). Long-term experience with the use of chlorhexidine has demonstrated that the incidence of hypersensitivity and skin irritation is low. However, severe allergic reactions including anaphylaxis have been reported previously (82, 271). Although cytotoxicity has been observed with exposed fibroblasts, no deleterious effects on wound healing have been demonstrated in vivo. There is no evidence that chlorhexidine gluconate is toxic if it is absorbed through the skin, but ototoxicity can occur when chlorhexidine is instilled into the middle ear during operative procedures. High concentrations of chlorhexidine and preparations containing other compounds (e.g., alcohols and surfactants) may damage eyes (239).

Iodophors

Iodophors essentially have replaced aqueous iodine and tincture as antiseptics. Iodophors are chemical complexes of iodine bound to a carrier such as polyvinylpyrrolidone (povidone) or ethoxylated nonionic detergents (poloxamers). These complexes gradually release small amounts of free microbicidal iodine. The most commonly used iodophor is povidone-iodine. Its preparations generally contain 1 to 10% povidone-iodine, which is equivalent to 0.1 to 1.0% available iodine. The active component appears to be free molecular iodine (I_2). A paradoxical effect of dilution on the activity of povidone-iodine has been observed. As the dilution increases, bactericidal activity increases up to a maximum and then falls (105). Commercial povidone-iodine solutions at dilutions of 1:2 to 1:100 kill *Staphylococcus aureus* and *Mycobacterium chelonae* more rapidly than do stock solutions (28). *Staphylococcus aureus* can survive a 2-min exposure to full-strength povidone-iodine solution but cannot survive a 15-s exposure to a 1:100 dilution of the iodophor (28). Thus, iodophors must be used at the dilution stated by the manufacturer.

The exact mechanism by which iodine destroys microorganisms is not known. Iodine may react with microorganisms' amino acids and fatty acids, destroying cell structures and enzymes (105). Depending on the concentration of free iodine and other factors, iodophors exhibit a broad range of microbicidal activity. Commercial preparations are bactericidal, mycobactericidal, fungicidal, and virucidal but not sporicidal at the dilutions recommended for use. Prolonged contact times are required to inactivate certain fungi and bacterial spores (201). Despite their bactericidal activities, povidone-iodine and poloxamer-iodine solutions can become contaminated with *Burkholderia (Pseudomonas) cepacia* or *Pseudomonas aeruginosa*, and contaminated solutions have caused outbreaks of pseudobacteremia and peritonitis (29, 69). In fact, *Burkholderia cepacia* survives for up to 68 weeks in a povidone-iodine antiseptic solution (13). The most likely explanation for the prolonged survival of these microorganisms in iodophor solutions is that organic or inorganic material and biofilm may mechanically protect the microorganisms.

Iodophors are widely used for antisepsis of skin, mucous membranes, and wound sites. A 2.5% ophthalmic solution of povidone-iodine is more effective and less toxic than silver nitrate or erythromycin ointment for prophylaxis against neonatal conjunctivitis (ophthalmia neonatorum) (130). In some countries, povidone-iodine alcoholic solutions are used extensively for skin antisepsis before invasive procedures (18). Iodophors containing higher concentrations of free iodine may be used to disinfect medical equipment. Solutions designed for use on the skin should not be used to disinfect hard surfaces because the concentrations of the antiseptic solutions are usually too low for this purpose (201).

The risk of side effects, such as staining, tissue irritation, and resorption, is lower for iodophors than for aqueous iodine. Iodophores do not corrode metal surfaces (105). However, a body surface treated with an iodine or iodophor solution may absorb free iodine. Consequently, increased serum iodine levels (and serum iodide levels) have been found in patients, especially when large areas were treated for a long period (105). For this reason, hyperthyroidism and other disorders of thyroid functions are contraindications for the use of iodine-containing preparations. Likewise, iodophors should not be applied to pregnant and nursing women or to newborns and infants (50). Because severe local and systemic allergic reactions have been observed, iodophors and iodine should not be used for patients with allergies to these preparations (256).

Iodophores have little if any residual effect. However, for a limited time they may have residual bactericidal activity on the skin surface, because free iodine diffuses into deep regions and also back to the skin surface (105). The antimicrobial efficacy of iodophors is reduced in the presence of organic material such as blood.

Triclosan and PCMX

Triclosan (Irgasan DP-300 or Irgacare MP) has been used for more than 30 years in a wide array of skin care products, including hand washes, surgical scrubs, and consumer products. A review of its effectiveness and safety in health care settings has been published previously (132). A concentration of 1% has good activity against gram-positive bacteria, including antibiotic-resistant strains, but less activity against gram-negative organisms, mycobacteria, and fungi. Limited data suggest that triclosan has a relatively broad antiviral spectrum, with high-level activity against enveloped viruses, such as HIV type 1, influenza A virus, and herpes simplex virus type 1. However, the nonenveloped viruses prove more difficult to inactivate. Clinical strains of *Staphylococcus aureus* with low-level resistance to triclosan have been identified, and the clinical significance of this remains unknown (238). Triclosan is added to many soaps, lotions, deodorants, toothpastes, mouthrinses, commonly used household fabrics, plastics, and medical devices. Moreover, the mechanisms of triclosan resistance may be similar to those involved in antimicrobial resistance (6) and some of these mechanisms may account for the observed cross-resistance of laboratory isolates to antimicrobial agents (63). Consequently, concerns have been raised that widespread use of triclosan formulations in non-health care settings and products may select for biocide resistance and even cross-resistance to antibiotics. However, environmental surveys have not demonstrated an association between triclosan usage and antibiotic resistance (199).

Triclosan solutions produce a sustained residual effect against resident and transient microbial flora that is minimally affected by organic matter. Numerous studies have not identified toxic, allergenic, mutagenic, or carcinogenic potential. Triclosan formulations may help control outbreaks of MRSA infections when the formulations are used for hand hygiene and for bathing of patients (132). However, some MRSA isolates have reduced triclosan susceptibility. Triclosan formulations are less effective than 2 to 4% chlorhexidine gluconate when used for surgical scrub solutions; properly formulated triclosan solutions may be used for hygienic hand washing.

PCMX (chloroxylenol) is an antimicrobial used in handwashing products. It is available at concentrations of 0.5 to 3.75%. Its properties are similar to those of triclosan. Nonionic surfactants may neutralize PCMX.

Octenidine

Octenidine dihydrochloride is a novel bispyridine compound, which is an effective and safe antiseptic agent. The 0.1% commercial formulation compares favorably with other antiseptics with respect to antimicrobial activity and toxicologic properties. In vitro and in vivo, it rapidly kills both gram-positive and gram-negative bacteria as well as fungi (101, 226). Octenidine is virucidal against HIV, hepatitis B virus, and herpes simplex virus. Similar to chlorhexidine, it has a marked residual effect. No toxicologic problems have been found when the 0.1% formulation was applied according to the manufacturer's recommendations. The colorless solution is a useful antiseptic for mucous membranes of the female and male genitals and the oral cavity (25), but its bad taste limits its use orally. In a recent observational study, the 0.1% formulation was highly effective and well tolerated for the care of central venous catheter insertion sites (243). The results of this study have also been supported by a randomized controlled clinical trial (M. Dettenkofer and A. F. Widmer, *Abstr. Eur. Congr. Clin. Microbiol. Infect. Dis.*, 2006, Nice, France, abstr. O147). Octenidine is not registered for use in the United States.

STERILIZATION

Principles, Definitions, and Terms

As outlined in Table 3, sterilization is not a relative term but defines the complete absence of any viable microorganisms, including spores. However, this absence cannot be proved by current microbiologic techniques (133). Therefore, sterilization can be defined as a closely monitored, validated process used to render a product free of all forms of viable microorganisms, including all bacterial endospores. To test the ability of sterilization systems to meet the latter definition, manufacturers developed a worst-case scenario that allows the process (log killing) to be quantified and estimates the probability of process failure. Large safety margins were included in this test, which is based on the assumption that items are heavily contaminated with spores, soil, and proteins. Note that although these conditions are used for the testing, in clinical practice items that are heavily soiled should not be sterilized and such a scenario would represent a critical failure of the reprocessing cycle. Any device undergoing sterilization first must undergo an appropriate cleaning process.

A manufacturer must demonstrate that a sterilizer is effective against a wide range of clinically important microorganisms before it can be approved by the FDA. In addition, proof of efficacy must be performed with organisms (usually bacterial spores) that have been shown to be the most resistant to the new technology. A validated and reliable biological indicator must be developed, and studies must establish that sterility will be consistently achieved when critical process parameters operate within a defined range. This assures the operator that as long as there is no operational error or equipment failure, sterility is achieved.

Several guidelines are essential documents for staff members who need to understand reprocessing and sterilization of medical devices. The ISO 14937 document provides general criteria for characterizing a sterilizing agent and for the development, validation, and routine control of a sterilization process for medical devices. ISO 11134 (moist heat) and ISO 11135 (ethylene oxide) documents describe the standards for use of these methods of sterilization in the industrial setting in the United States. The American National Standard Institute/Association for the Advancement of Medical Instrumentation published adaptations of these standards for health care facilities: standard 46 (moist heat) and standard 41 (ethylene oxide) (Table 3). In Europe, EN 550, EN 554, and EN 285 define the standards for steam and ethylene oxide sterilization. ISO 14161 provides guidance that staff can use when selecting and using biological indicators and when interpreting the results of these tests. ISO 17664 specifies which information medical device manufacturers must provide so that the medical device can be processed safely and will continue to function properly. Readers are referred to other references for additional information about sterilization (34, 106, 133).

Monitoring

Any sterilization process must be monitored by mechanical, physical, chemical, and facultatively biological methods. Before routine use, the performance of the machine should be validated with the most difficult load used at the institution to ensure that the process is safe. In addition, a printout of the physical parameters (e.g., temperature and pressure) during sterilization should be kept for documentation purposes. In 1963, Bowie and Dick determined that if residual air remained in a sterilizer after the vacuum phase and there was only one package in the chamber, the air would concentrate in that package (38). They developed the Bowie-Dick test to determine whether steam penetration and air removal occurred successfully. This test does not provide information about the sterilization process.

Chemical indicators placed on items in a sterilizer change color if they are exposed to adequate temperatures and exposure times. They are inexpensive, easy to use, and provide a visual indication that the item has been exposed to the sterilization process. Good clinical indicators are able to identify a sterilizer failure. However, some are too sensitive, giving false-positive results (205, 208), which may cause unnecessary recalls of adequately sterilized items. Less sensitive chemical indicators do not detect small deviations in the process.

Biological indicators are the best monitors of the sterilization process. If the spores in commercially available standard biological indicators do not grow during an appropriate incubation period, the results indicate that the process was able to kill $\geq 10^6$ CFU. For flash sterilization, the Attest Rapid Readout biological indicator detects the presence of a spore-associated enzyme, α-D-glucosidase, and permits the staff to assess the efficacy of sterilization within 60 min (252). Staff members should investigate positive biological indicators because they can provide the only indication that something is wrong with the sterilization process (51).

An important question is whether a load can be distributed before the final results of the biological indicator are available (i.e., parametric release). The Joint Commission on Accreditation of Healthcare Organizations standard allows the use of appropriate chemical indicators without routine use of a biological indicator. A common approach is to use the sterilized items if the physical and chemical parameters of adequate sterilization were met without waiting for the culture results from the biological indicators.

In Europe, routine use of biological indicators is not required if the sterilizer has undergone testing by a validation procedure used for industrial steam sterilization (EN 285, EN 550, EN 554, or EN 556). Most sterilizers in European hospitals probably do not meet these very strict requirements (250), and consequently, biological indicators are used regularly to ensure that they are working properly. These industrial standards for validation of steam sterilization will be implemented in health care organizations, but this change is controversial because of the associated expenses. The future is likely to involve parametric release with regular validation and/or commissions of the equipment. Legal issues will probably determine the outcome of this discussion, and lawyers are likely to accept nothing but a zero risk. However, the goal of a zero risk for contamination in central sterilization services will probably contribute to excessive health care costs. Therefore, standards for sterilization should exclude a risk for contamination after the reprocessing cycle but should avoid steps that are performed only for legal reasons.

Packaging, Loading, and Storage

Items that are clean and dry should be inspected and then wrapped and packaged (or put in containers) before sterilization. Wrappers should allow steam or gas to penetrate into the package but should protect the items from recontamination after sterilization. Items wrapped only in muslin can become contaminated when they are handled after steam sterilization (265). Items should be labeled with information such as expiration date, type of sterilization, and identification code so that items can be traced.

Steam Sterilization

The most reliable method of sterilization is one that uses saturated steam under pressure. It is inexpensive, nontoxic, and very reliable.

Steam penetrates fabrics, and its inherent safety margin is much higher than that of any other sterilization technique. Therefore, it should be used whenever possible. Obviously, other techniques must be used for heat-sensitive items. Steam irreversibly coagulates and denaturates microbial enzymes and proteins. Three parameters are critical to ensuring that steam sterilization is effective: the amount of time the items are exposed to steam, the temperature of the process, and the level of moisture. Unlike time and temperature, the moisture condition in the autoclave cannot be directly determined. The D value determines the time required to kill 10^6 CFU of the spores most resistant to the sterilization process under study. Devices or instruments must reach the desired temperature, which is not necessarily identical to the temperature displayed on the autoclave's gauge. A drop of only 1.7°C (3°F) increases the time required to sterilize an item by 48%. Without moisture, a temperature of 160°C is required for dry-heat sterilization. Dry air does not provide steam for condensation, and the heat transfer to objects is slower than it is when moisture is present. Pressurized steam quickly transfers energy to the sterilizer load and causes more rapid denaturation and coagulation of microbial proteins. In addition, pressurizing the steam allows one to achieve dry 100% saturated steam. Thus, there is no mist that may cause the packaging and/or the items to become wet.

Residual air in the autoclave interferes with the sterilization process. The amount of air within the sterilizer can be estimated by comparing the chamber pressure with the saturated steam pressure calculated from the average chamber temperature. A measured pressure greater than the calculated saturated pressure indicates the presence of residual air in the chamber. Such monitoring devices are common in the United Kingdom.

Several types of autoclaves are available: gravity displacement steam sterilization, prevacuum steam sterilization, and steam flash-pressure pulsing steam sterilization autoclaves. The sterilization process is less consistent in gravity displacement steam sterilizers than in the other sterilizers (70). For example, gravity displacement autoclaves are more likely than the other systems to leave residual air in the chamber before the steam is introduced. Prevacuum sterilizers resolved part of this problem and cut the cycle time in half. However, the effectiveness of sterilization still can be compromised by small leaks (1 to 10 mm Hg/min) in the sterilizer (133). The most current technology is the steam flash-pressure pulsing steam sterilization technique, in which air leaks do not decrease the effectiveness of the process. This method nearly eliminates the problem of air in the chamber and reduces the thermal lag upon heating of the load to the desired exposure temperature (70).

The process of sterilization has several cycles: conditioning, exposure, and drying. Common cycles for steam sterilization in prevacuum or flash-pressure pulsing steam sterilizers are 121°C for 15 min (121°C for 30 min in a gravity displacement sterilizer) and 132°C for 4 min (see the FDA addendum to the sterilizer guidance, issued 19 September 1995 [http://www.cenorm.org]). EN 554 requires steam sterilizers to provide this temperature throughout the entire chamber within a narrow margin (0 to +3°C).

Flash sterilization is an emergency process used, for example, after a surgical instrument, which is needed immediately, is dropped during a procedure (158). Unwrapped devices are placed in a sterilizer (usually in the operating suite and sometimes without a biological indicator) and exposed to pressurized steam for 3 min. The autoclaves employed are gravity displacement sterilizers that have the problems mentioned previously. If health care workers are in a hurry, they may not clean the item properly, which will prevent proper sterilization. In addition, because the items are not wrapped, they can be contaminated easily when they are transported to the operating room. Even properly wrapped sterile items can become contaminated if they are transported several times (265). Moreover, some patients have been injured by items that were flash sterilized (214). Therefore, flash sterilization is controversial, and several investigators have suggested that it should be used only in emergency situations when no other device is available. Flash sterilization should not replace standard sterilization protocols (85) and should not be used to save time in sterilizing items by the standard methods or to avoid purchasing extra instrument sets (160). Because documentation takes time, staff members often do not document appropriately when they use flash sterilization. Consequently, if something goes wrong, tracing the sterilized items may be impossible.

Ethylene Oxide Gas

Temperature- and/or pressure-sensitive items have been sterilized traditionally with ethylene oxide in a standard gas.

Ethylene oxide inactivates all microorganisms, including spores, probably by an alkylation process. *Bacillus subtilis* bacterial spores are among the most resistant, and therefore, these are used as a biological monitor for this process. A new rapid-readout ethylene oxide biological indicator will indicate an ethylene oxide sterilization process failure by producing fluorescence, which is detected in an autoreader within 4 h of incubation at 37°C, and a color change related to a change in the pH of the growth media within 96 h of continued incubation (212).

The process of sterilizing items with ethylene oxide begins by adding nitrogen gas to remove air or by evacuating the chamber. Items are then exposed to ethylene oxide at 55°C (130°F). Six variable but interdependent parameters—gas concentration, vacuum, pressure, temperature, relative humidity, and time of exposure—must be controlled when ethylene oxide is used. The gas concentration cannot be measured on line, limiting the extent of monitoring. Therefore, the concentration should be validated as outlined by ISO 11135.

Ethylene oxide sterilization has several disadvantages; it is useful only as a surface sterilizer because it does not reach blocked-off surfaces. In addition, ethylene oxide is flammable, explosive, and carcinogenic to laboratory animals and it requires special safety precautions. Moreover, items sterilized by ethylene oxide must be aerated for approximately 12 h to remove any traces of the gas. Thus, the entire process takes >16 h, but modern ethylene oxide sterilizers can run at shorter cycles. Furthermore, toxic residues can be trapped in the wrapper or the items. Polyvinyl chloride and polyurethane absorb ethylene oxide readily and require long periods to dissipate the oxide. The wrapper should be a barrier against recontamination after sterilization, but it also can prevent ethylene oxide from reaching the item. Therefore, only materials with documented ethylene oxide penetration and dissipation properties should be used as wrappers.

The future of ethylene oxide in sterilization is limited, mainly due to its toxicity. However, no currently available technology, including plasma sterilization (see below), can replace sterilization with ethylene oxide entirely. In addition, sterilization with ethylene oxide does not fail as frequently as sterilization with plasma when residual proteins and/or salts are present on the items (11).

Plasma Sterilization

Low-temperature plasma is produced in a closed chamber with a deep vacuum, an electromagnetic field, and a chemical precursor (hydrogen peroxide or a mixture of hydrogen peroxide and peracetic acid). The resulting free radicals, the chemical precursors, and the UV radiation are thought to rapidly destroy vegetative microorganisms, including spores.

Sterrad

The Sterrad 100 sterilizer, the first plasma sterilizer for use in health care facilities, has been on the market in Europe since 1990 and in the United States since 1993. In August 1997, the Sterrad 100 system was approved to sterilize certain surgical instruments with long lumens, such as those used in urologic, laparoscopic, and arthroscopic procedures, including instruments with single stainless steel lumens of ≥3 and <400 mm in length. The Sterrad 100S has since replaced the Sterrad 100. The Sterrad 100S adds one sterilization cycle and, thereby, fulfills the requirement to kill 10^6 CFU of spores at the half point of the cycle. A smaller device, the Sterrad 50, has been independently tested for efficacy (207). Other sizes, e.g., the large Sterrad 200, approved by the FDA in 2003, can sterilize small lumens (single stainless steel lumens with an inside diameter of 1 mm or larger and Teflon or polyethylene lumens with an inside diameter of 6 mm or larger). The new Sterrad NX system, approved by the FDA in April 2005, is the fastest low-temperature hydrogen peroxide gas plasma sterilizer yet. This system employs a new vaporization system that removes most of the water from the hydrogen peroxide, improving diffusion of peroxide into lumens. Consequently, a broad range of instruments, including single-channel flexible endoscopes, can be processed within 38 min. In 2001, the FDA cleared biological indicators suitable for plasma sterilization.

Regardless of the model, the basic steps are the same. Medical instruments are placed in the sterilization chamber, a strong vacuum is created in the chamber, and a solution of 59% hydrogen peroxide and water is automatically injected from a cassette into the sterilization chamber. The solution vaporizes and diffuses throughout the chamber, surrounding the items to be sterilized. Radiofrequency energy is applied to create an electric field, which in turn generates the low-temperature plasma, inducing free radicals. The combination of the diffusion pretreatment and plasma phases sterilizes the item while eliminating harmful residuals. At the end of the cycle, the radiofrequency energy is turned off, the vacuum is released, and the chamber is filled with filtered air, returning it to normal atmospheric pressure.

Plasma sterilizers have several disadvantages. First, materials that absorb too much hydrogen peroxide (e.g., cellulosics and some nylons such as those from connectors, cables, and insulators), materials that catalytically decompose hydrogen peroxide (e.g., copper and nickel alloys from electrical wire, solder, and surgical instruments), and materials that react with hydrogen peroxide such as organic dyes (colored anodized aluminum) and organic sulfides of solid lubricants in endoscopic devices cannot be sterilized in a Sterrad. Second, the cassettes required to run the device and the special nonmuslin wrappers are relatively expensive.

Low-Temperature Sterilization by Ozone

The 125L ozone sterilizer uses medical-grade oxygen, water, and electricity to generate ozone within the sterilizer to provide an efficient sterilant without producing toxic chemicals or using high temperatures. (It runs at 25 to 35°C.) Ozone forms when oxygen is submitted to an intense electrical field that separates oxygen molecules into atomic oxygen (O), which in turn combines with other oxygen molecules (O_2) to form triatomic oxygen (O_3), or ozone, providing a sterility assurance level of 10^6 in approximately 4 h. At the end of the cycle, the oxygen and water vapor safely vent directly into the room. The sterilization chamber has a capacity of 125 liters. Processed medical instruments require no aeration at the end of the sterilization cycle. Medical devices are packaged in a TS03 sterilization pouch or in anodized aluminum sterilization containers. The TS03 OZO-TES'P' self-contained biological and chemical indicators should be used to evaluate the machine's performance. An ozone sterilizer can be installed as a free-standing unit or recessed behind a wall. These devices are used primarily in Canada. They are approved by the FDA, but few health care facilities in the United States use them.

Liquid Sterilization

The FDA approved the STERIS System 1 in 1988, but this system is not considered a sterilizer in Europe (72). The machine is designed to sterilize immersible devices, including flexible endoscopes, with 35% liquid peracetic acid (an

FDA-approved sterilant that is sporicidal [123, 126], supplemented with buffering, anticorrosion, wetting, and surface-active agents). Peracetic acid is automatically diluted with sterile filtered water, and the items are exposed for 12 min. The entire sterilization process takes approximately 30 min at ca. 50°C. Items can be used immediately after the process is completed and do not need to be aerated.

Clinical studies of the STERIS System 1 have been performed with bronchoscopes, hysteroscopes, colonoscopes, and rigid endoscopes (42, 254). Independent efficacy tests demonstrated some failures (42). Exposure time and temperature are monitored electronically, and conductivity is used as a surrogate marker for peracetic acid concentration. However, the machine can complete its cycle normally and print a report stating that the concentration of peracetic acid was in the normal range when it was run intentionally without peracetic acid (161). Commercially available spores can be used for monitoring sterilization (145), but false-positive test strips can occur, related to improper use of the clip that attaches the test strips (110). Other disadvantages of this system include the high cost of purchasing and using the equipment, which is considerably greater than the cost of purchasing and using systems for high-level disinfection with glutaraldehyde (95). In addition, the device does not clean the items. Thus, the cleaning step adds to the overall time of reprocessing the items. The STERIS System 1, like all other nonsteam sterilizers, cannot meet the requirements for sterilization if residual debris and/or proteins are present on the items.

Hot Air Sterilization

Hot air sterilization is not a state-of-the-art technology, but it is still used in many countries. However, the distribution of dry heat to the instruments requires long exposure times. Temperatures of >185°C resinify paraffin, destroying instruments' lubrication, and higher temperatures are corrosive, resulting in loss of hardness. Therefore, hot air sterilization has largely been replaced by better, safer, and faster technologies.

REUSE OF SINGLE-USE DEVICES

Current FDA policy states that the responsibility for the safety and performance of reprocessed single-use devices lies with the reprocessor, not the original manufacturer. The FDA considers the hospital to be the manufacturer of a single-use device if the device has been resterilized. Therefore, the reprocessor must ensure that the reprocessed items are sterile and are not contaminated with toxic substances such as endotoxins or residual ethylene oxide and that the product's integrity, composition, and function are essentially identical to those of a new product. Most hospitals cannot afford to generate appropriate data on the quality and performance of reprocessed single-use items. In addition, if a manufacturer changes the product, the reprocessor needs to redo the analyses before the device can legally be marketed after reprocessing (management-of-change guidelines). The FDA published a final guidance (see the website for details: http://www.fda.gov/cdrh/ohip/guidance/1333.html and http://www.fda.gov/cdrh/ohip/guidance/1408.html).

Some institutions resterilize items that have not been used on patients but that, for instance, were dropped and/or had the packages damaged. Even this approach can be problematic. For example, the FDA published an alert documenting that the quality of an implant that was originally sterilized with ethylene oxide and then resterilized with steam was impaired by the reprocessing method (see http://www.fda.gov/cdrh/steamst.html for details). In addition, the quality, product integrity, and performance of many reprocessed plastic or rubber products are unknown. Moreover, the FDA does not allow health care facilities that send equipment and supplies to a reprocessing company to transfer full responsibility to that company (see the full text at http://www.fda.gov/medwatch/safety/1997/device.htm). Furthermore, if a hospital reprocesses a single-use device, the hospital is responsible for ensuring that the device complies with all applicable FDA labeling requirements, even if the device is exempt from the premarket requirements. If the hospital does not ensure that the device complies with FDA labeling requirements, the device is misbranded and the hospital may be considered in violation of section 301(k) of the Food, Drug and Cosmetic Act. As of 14 August 2001 and 14 February 2002, the FDA enforces premarket filing requirements for reprocessed class II devices (i.e., moderate-risk devices such as a cardiac mapping catheter used to map electrical activity of the heart; http://www.fda.gov/cdrh/comp/guidance/1168.pdf) and marketing clearance requirements. Many issues are not yet resolved. The FDA has set a prioritization scheme (http://www.fda.gov/cdrh/reuse/1156.pdf).

In many countries throughout the world, health care facilities reprocess single-use items (sometimes illegally) because resources are limited and this activity may be the only way to provide patients with access to state-of-the-art health care. In fact, a commercial reprocessor in Germany legally reprocessed >4 million single-use items without any serious reported side effects, saving between 30 to 50% of the cost of new items. Thus, we believe that new reprocessing technologies using washer-disinfectors coupled with highly effective low-temperature sterilizers can kill all microorganisms, even in narrow lumens such as cardiac catheters. We also believe that with the expertise of infection control personnel, health care facilities can provide the desired level of microbiological and toxicological safety. However, they probably cannot ensure that the design and function of the devices are still adequate. Thus, in the United States and countries with similar regulations on quality assurance programs, reuse of single-use devices may not be cost-effective. In addition, organizations that sell used single-use devices to patients and/or insurance companies as new devices will encounter legal and ethical issues. Because devices change and new devices are introduced, it is difficult for health care facilities and reprocessing companies to do the studies needed to document that reprocessing is safe, thus making it difficult to reprocess single-use devices on a large scale. However, financial restriction may change the current belief that patients will not accept reprocessed single-use devices. The reader should consult the FDA website and experts in the field before considering reprocessing of single-use devices.

BOVINE SPONGIFORM ENCEPHALOPATHY AND VARIANT CREUTZFELDT-JAKOB DISEASE

CJD has been identified on all continents and is thought to occur worldwide. The incidence of CJD is estimated to be about 1 case per 10^6 persons per year. Most cases of CJD are sporadic; <10% of CJD cases may be related to a genetic autosomal dominant predisposition, and some nosocomial cases are related to the use of contaminated tissue or contaminated human growth hormone. It is generally accepted that eating BSE agent-contaminated meat is the cause of vCJD (121, 188). The vCJD has brought about a major medical and economic crisis in Europe (49, 140, 188).

By 1 January 2006, 154 cases were reported from the United Kingdom. Cases that fulfill the new WHO case definition (21 May 2001) also have been reported from France (14 cases), Canada (1 case), Spain (1 case), Ireland (1 case), and Italy (1 case). The peak of the epidemic was in the year 2000 (28 cases in the United Kingdom), falling to 5 cases in the United Kingdom in December 2005. In the United States, one patient who was a former resident of the United Kingdom has been diagnosed with vCJD and the first case of BSE in cattle was identified in 2003. However, more cases may occur because 37 tons of "meals of meat or offal" that were "unfit for human consumption" was sent from the United Kingdom to the United States in 1997, well after the government banned imports of such risky meat (59). As of 2006, no curative therapy is available for CJD or vCJD; however, several approaches have been investigated with limited success (103).

The agent causing vCJD is not a classic microorganism but an altered prion protein (5, 33, 187, 220). Its origin remains obscure, but the BSE agent from cattle is most probably responsible for the vCJD in humans. In the 1980s a step in tallow extraction from rendered carcasses was eliminated, allowing some tissue infected with scrapie to survive the process and allowing the infectious agent to be recycled as cattle-adapted scrapie or BSE. The animal food was no longer sterilized at 134°C for 20 to 30 min but, rather, was pasteurized before being fed to animals whose carcasses, with encased spinal cords and paraspinal ganglia, were later processed legally into hot dogs, sausages, and precooked meat patties (47). Investigators postulate that a high incidence of scrapie in sheep and a large proportion of sheep in the mix of carcasses that was rendered for livestock feed may explain why the incidence of BSE in British cattle was more than 10 times higher than that in cattle in any other European country. In the United Kingdom, the number of people exposed to potentially infective doses through food may be extremely high.

vCJD has a different clinical presentation and occurs at a much younger age than CJD (60). The mean age at death from vCJD is 28 years; only 6 of 90 patients died at the age of 50 years or older (248). Two hypotheses that may explain why the age group of 50 and under is most affected are that the incubation period is shorter in the young than in the elderly and that the young are more susceptible to infection. In addition, all patients genotyped so far are homozygous for methionine on codon 129 of the prion protein gene. It is postulated that heterozygous individuals may have much longer incubation times before vCJD becomes evident. Therefore, asymptomatic carriers may pose a risk for transmission if they undergo routine surgery and instruments are not reprocessed by a prion-safe program.

Patients suffering from vCJD harbor large numbers of prions in their tonsils and spleens before they have signs, symptoms, and pathological findings from the disease. In contrast, patients with sporadic CJD suffer from spongiform encephalopathy long before the prion spreads into muscles and lymphoid tissue (120). Consequently, France has developed very strict precautions. For example, the United Kingdom required that all tonsillectomies be performed with disposable instruments. In 2002, this practice was discontinued because serious complications arose when disposable instruments were used.

The fact that the vCJD prion agent is found in lymphoid tissue and tonsils indicates that prions are not restricted to neural tissue (103). Studies of sheep naturally infected with scrapie demonstrate that the infectious agent first appears in lymphatic tissue of the tonsils and gastrointestinal tract, suggesting that the oral route may be the principal mode of transmission. In addition, numerous studies underline the importance of B cells in transmission of the BSE agent (142). Lymphatic organs typically show early accumulation of prions and B cells, and follicular dendritic cells are required for efficient neuroinvasion. The actual entry into the central nervous system probably occurs via peripheral nerves, and the prion accumulates in neural tissue once inflammation of the lymphoid tissue is in progress (116).

Experimental evidence from animal models indicates that blood can contain prion infectivity, which suggests a potential risk for transmissible spongiform encephalopathy transmission via proteins isolated from human plasma (124). Three cases of probable transmission by blood transfusion raise more concern about the safety of the blood supply (4). In the United States, beginning in August 1999, persons who resided in or traveled to the United Kingdom for a total of 6 months from 1980 through 1996 have been deferred from blood donation, as have persons who received bovine insulin derived from cattle in the United Kingdom. Recently, both the American Red Cross and the FDA announced new, expanded deferrals for travel and residence in the United Kingdom and other European countries (58) and they are conducting a look back to consider recipients who received potentially contaminated blood. The United Kingdom no longer collects plasma from its inhabitants and, as a further precautionary measure, has instituted leukocyte reduction (removal of white blood cells) for blood transfusions.

Previously, problems with reprocessing of instruments used on patients with CJD were limited to invasive instruments that came into contact with neural tissue, predominantly instruments used in neurosurgery. However, as noted above, vCJD is highly lymphotropic, so that any instruments used on lymphoid tissues may be contaminated with prions (142). As outlined above, appropriate reprocessing of surgical items includes cleaning, disinfection, and sterilization. Aldehydes enhance the resistance of prions and abolish the inactivating effect of autoclaving (48). Therefore, aldehydes are no longer recommended for disinfecting surgical instruments in Europe before they have undergone a thorough cleaning process. In France, aldehydes are no longer used for endoscope reprocessing, despite evidence that peracetic acid may stain prions as well (136). Small resistant subpopulations of infective prions may survive autoclaving at 132 to 138°C. These resistant subpopulations are not inactivated by reautoclaving, and they have biological characteristics that differentiate them from the main population (240). The worst-case scenario is that the agent for vCJD might become self-replicating when it contaminates surgical instruments. Therefore, prions challenge reprocessing techniques like never before.

The minimum requirements for decontamination procedures and precautions for materials potentially contaminated with either the agent that causes CJD or the agent that causes vCJD remain unknown. However, it is clear that dry heat (160°C for 24 h), formaldehyde sterilization, and standard steam sterilization do not sterilize prion-contaminated items (80). The scientific uncertainties and lack of data do not allow agencies like national health departments, the WHO, or the CDC to formulate guidelines that are completely evidence based, and this explains why various countries have taken different approaches to addressing issues of reprocessing of instruments. In January 2001, the British government spent the equivalent of $300 million to improve reprocessing techniques in Central Sterilization Services and required the use of disposable instruments for tonsillectomies. The French Public Health Office published their recommendations on 14 March 2001. They require all surgical instruments with potential exposure to lymphatic tissue, the central nervous system, or the eyes to be soaked in sodium hypochlorite for 1 h or NaOH for 1 h and sterilized at 134°C for 18 min. If instruments do not tolerate this aggressive approach, they must be cleaned twice, treated with various chemicals such as peracetic acid, iodophores, 3% sodium dodecyl sulfate, or 6 M urea, and autoclaved at 121°C for 30 min. Since 2002, Switzerland requires all surgical instruments to be sterilized at 134°C for 18 min. The background of the Swiss recommendation is that the usual rendering process for carcasses, which was discontinued, resulted in only a 1-log-unit reduction of the infectious particles (241). Therefore, a reduction in the number of infectious particles may suffice to stop transmission. The CDC recommends that instruments exposed to potentially prion-contaminated items to be autoclaved for 1 to 1.5 h at 132 to 134°C, immersed in 1 N sodium hydroxide for 1 h at room temperature, or immersed in 0.5% hypochlorite sodium (at least 2% free chlorine) for 2 h at room temperature. (See the CDC website for further information: http://www.cdc.gov/ncidod/dvrd/vcjd/index.htm.) However, these recommendations are not based on what is known about the agent of vCJD.

High-risk patients are patients with suspected CJD and their family members, patients treated with pituitary extracts, and patients who received cornea transplants. In addition, items should be considered contaminated with prions if a brain biopsy for the diagnosis of CJD is requested. Instruments used in such procedures should be discarded or placed under quarantine until the histopathological diagnosis is known. The incidence of vCJD in the United Kingdom is decreasing rapidly, indicating that current reprocessing techniques suffice. However, knowledge about this topic is increasing rapidly over time and our current understanding may be shown to be false in the future (26). In May 2005, British officials published an excellent assessment of the risk for contaminating surgical instruments with prions (http://www.dh.gov.uk/assetRoot/04/11/35/42/04113542.pdf). The key observation in this report is that on average 0.2 mg of protein remains on surgical instruments despite "standard cleaning and disinfection," which is sufficient to cause an experimental case of CJD. Therefore, more research and new methods of cleaning and disinfection are needed for surgical instruments. The reader is referred to the websites of the CDC, the FDA, and the WHO to obtain the most recent updates on this topic.

REFERENCES

1. **ADA Council on Scientific Affairs and ADA Council on Dental Practice.** 1996. Infection control recommendations for the dental office and the dental laboratory. *J. Am. Dent. Assoc.* **127:**672–680.
2. **Adams, B. G., and T. J. Marrie.** 1982. Hand carriage of aerobic gram-negative rods may not be transient. *J. Hyg.* (London) **89:**33–46.
3. **Agerton, T., S. Valway, B. Gore, C. Pozsik, B. Plikaytis, C. Woodley, and I. Onorato.** 1997. Transmission of a highly drug-resistant strain (strain W1) of Mycobacterium tuberculosis. Community outbreak and nosocomial transmission via a contaminated bronchoscope. *JAMA* **278:**1073–1077.
4. **Aguzzi, A., and M. Glatzel.** 2004. vCJD tissue distribution and transmission by transfusion—a worst-case scenario coming true? *Lancet* **363:**411–412.
5. **Aguzzi, A., and C. Weissmann.** 1998. Spongiform encephalopathies. The prion's perplexing persistence. *Nature* **392:**763–764.
6. **Aiello, A. E., and E. Larson.** 2003. Antibacterial cleaning and hygiene products as an emerging risk factor for antibiotic resistance in the community. *Lancet Infect. Dis.* **3:**501–506.
7. **Akamatsu, T., K. Tabata, M. Hironaga, and M. Uyeda.** 1997. Evaluation of the efficacy of a 3.2% glutaraldehyde product for disinfection of fibreoptic endoscopes with an automatic machine. *J. Hosp. Infect.* **35:**47–57.
8. **Akbar-Khanzadeh, F., M. U. Vaquerano, M. Akbar-Khanzadeh, and M. S. Bisesi.** 1994. Formaldehyde exposure, acute pulmonary response, and exposure control options in a gross anatomy laboratory. *Am. J. Ind. Med.* **26:**61–75.
9. **Alasri, A., C. Roques, G. Michel, C. Cabassud, and P. Aptel.** 1992. Bactericidal properties of peracetic acid and hydrogen peroxide, alone and in combination, and chlorine and formaldehyde against bacterial water strains. *Can. J. Microbiol.* **38:**635–642.
10. **Alasri, A., M. Valverde, C. Roques, G. Michel, C. Cabassud, and P. Aptel.** 1993. Sporocidal properties of peracetic acid and hydrogen peroxide, alone and in combination, in comparison with chlorine and formaldehyde for ultrafiltration membrane disinfection. *Can. J. Microbiol.* **39:**52–60.
11. **Alfa, M. J., P. DeGagne, and N. Olson.** 1997. Bacterial killing ability of 10% ethylene oxide plus 90% hydrochlorofluorocarbon sterilizing gas. *Infect. Control Hosp. Epidemiol.* **18:**641–645.
12. **Alvarado, C. J., and M. Reichelderfer.** 2000. APIC guideline for infection prevention and control in flexible endoscopy. Association for Professionals in Infection Control. *Am. J. Infect. Control* **28:**138–155.
13. **Anderson, R. L., R. W. Vess, A. L. Panlilio, and M. S. Favero.** 1990. Prolonged survival of *Pseudomonas cepacia* in commercially manufactured povidone-iodine. *Appl. Environ. Microbiol.* **56:**3598–3600.
14. **Anonymous.** 1994. Tentative final monograph for health-care antiseptic drug products. *Fed. Regist.* **59:**31401–31452.
15. **Anonymous.** 1999. Bronchoscopy-related infections and pseudoinfections—New York, 1996 and 1998. *Morb. Mortal. Wkly. Rep.* **48:**557–560.
16. **Anonymous.** 2001. Protracted outbreaks of cryptosporidiosis associated with swimming pool use—Ohio and Nebraska, 2000. *Morb. Mortal. Wkly. Rep.* **50:**406–410.
17. **Ansari, S. A., S. A. Sattar, V. S. Springthorpe, G. A. Wells, and W. Tostowaryk.** 1989. In vivo protocol for testing efficacy of hand-washing agents against viruses and bacteria: experiments with rotavirus and *Escherichia coli*. *Appl. Environ. Microbiol.* **55:**3113–3118.
18. **Arata, T., T. Murakami, and Y. Hirai.** 1993. Evaluation of povidone-iodine alcoholic solution for operative site disinfection. *Postgrad. Med. J.* **69**(Suppl. 3)**:**S93–S96.
19. **Archibald, L. K., A. Corl, B. Shah, M. Schulte, M. J. Arduino, S. Aguero, D. J. Fisher, B. W. Stechenberg, S. N. Banerjee, and W. R. Jarvis.** 1997. Serratia marcescens outbreak associated with extrinsic contamination of 1% chlorxylenol soap. *Infect. Control Hosp. Epidemiol.* **18:**704–709.
20. **Arnon, S. S., R. Schechter, T. V. Inglesby, D. A. Henderson, J. G. Bartlett, M. S. Ascher, E. Eitzen, A. D. Fine, J. Hauer, M. Layton, S. Lillibridge, M. T. Osterholm, T. O'Toole, G. Parker, T. M. Perl, P. K. Russell, D. L. Swerdlow, and K. Tonat.** 2001. Botulinum toxin as a biological weapon: medical and public health management. *JAMA* **285:**1059–1070.
21. **Ascenzi, J. M.** 1996. Glutaraldehyde-based disinfectants, p. 111–132. In J. P. Ascenzi (ed.), *Handbook of Disinfectants and Antiseptics.* Marcel Dekker, Inc., New York, N.Y.
22. **Astagneau, P., N. Desplaces, V. Vincent, V. Chicheportiche, A. Botherel, S. Maugat, K. Lebascle,**

P. Leonard, J. Desenclos, J. Grosset, J. Ziza, and G. Brucker. 2001. Mycobacterium xenopi spinal infections after discovertebral surgery: investigation and screening of a large outbreak. *Lancet* **358:**747–751.

23. **Axon, A., M. Jung, A. Kruse, T. Ponchon, J. F. Rey, U. Beilenhoff, D. Duforest-Rey, C. Neumann, M. Pietsch, K. Roth, A. Papoz, D. Wilson, I. Kircher-Felgenstreff, M. Stief, R. Blum, K. B. Spencer, J. Mills, E. P. Mart, B. Slowey, H. Biering, and U. Lorenz.** 2000. The European Society of Gastrointestinal Endoscopy (ESGE): check list for the purchase of washer-disinfectors for flexible endoscopes. ESGE Guideline Committee. *Endoscopy* **32:**914–919.
24. **Bagg, J., C. P. Sweeney, K. M. Roy, T. Sharp, and A. Smith.** 2001. Cross infection control measures and the treatment of patients at risk of Creutzfeldt Jakob disease in UK general dental practice. *Br. Dent. J.* **191:**87–90.
25. **Beiswanger, B. B., M. E. Mallatt, M. S. Mau, R. D. Jackson, and D. K. Hennon.** 1990. The clinical effects of a mouthrinse containing 0.1% octenidine. *J. Dent. Res.* **69:**454–457.
26. **Belay, E. D., and L. B. Schonberger.** 2005. The public health impact of prion diseases. *Annu. Rev. Public Health* **26:**191–212.
27. **Bellamy, K., R. Alcock, J. R. Babb, J. G. Davies, and G. A. Ayliffe.** 1993. A test for the assessment of 'hygienic' hand disinfection using rotavirus. *J. Hosp. Infect.* **24:**201–210.
28. **Berkelman, R. L., B. W. Holland, and R. L. Anderson.** 1982. Increased bactericidal activity of dilute preparations of povidone-iodine solutions. *J. Clin. Microbiol.* **15:**635–639.
29. **Berkelman, R. L., S. Lewin, J. R. Allen, R. L. Anderson, L. D. Budnick, S. Shapiro, S. M. Friedman, P. Nicholas, R. S. Holzman, and R. W. Haley.** 1981. Pseudobacteremia attributed to contamination of povidone-iodine with Pseudomonas cepacia. *Ann. Intern. Med.* **95:**32–36.
30. **Biron, F., B. Verrier, and D. Peyramond.** 1997. Transmission of the human immunodeficiency virus and the hepatitis C virus. *N. Engl. J. Med.* **337:**348–349. (Letter and comment.)
31. **Blanc, D. S., I. Nahimana, C. Petignat, A. Wenger, J. Bille, and P. Francioli.** 2004. Faucets as a reservoir of endemic *Pseudomonas aeruginosa* colonization/infections in intensive care units. *Intensive Care Med.* **30:**1964–1968.
32. **Blanc, D. S., T. Parret, B. Janin, P. Raselli, and P. Francioli.** 1997. Nosocomial infections and pseudoinfections from contaminated bronchoscopes: two-year follow up using molecular markers. *Infect. Control Hosp. Epidemiol.* **18:**134–136.
33. **Blattler, T., S. Brandner, A. J. Raeber, M. A. Klein, T. Voigtlander, C. Weissmann, and A. Aguzzi.** 1997. PrP-expressing tissue required for transfer of scrapie infectivity from spleen to brain. *Nature* **389:**69–73.
34. **Block, S. S.** 2001. *Disinfection, Sterilization, and Preservation,* 5th ed. Lippincott Williams & Wilkins, Philadelphia, Pa.
35. **Bond, W. W., M. S. Favero, N. J. Petersen, and J. W. Ebert.** 1983. Inactivation of hepatitis B virus by intermediate-to-high-level disinfectant chemicals. *J. Clin. Microbiol.* **18:**535–538.
36. **Borchardt, M. A., P. D. Bertz, S. K. Spencer, and D. A. Battigelli.** 2003. Incidence of enteric viruses in groundwater from household wells in Wisconsin. *Appl. Environ. Microbiol.* **69:**1172–1180.
37. **Bosi, C., A. Davin-Regli, R. Charrel, B. Rocca, D. Monnet, and C. Bollet.** 1996. Serratia marcescens nosocomial outbreak due to contamination of hexetidine solution. *J. Hosp. Infect.* **33:**217–224.
38. **Bowie, J. H., M. H. Kennedy, and I. Robertson.** 1975. Improved Bowie and Dick test. *Lancet* **i:**1135.
39. **Boyce, J. M., and M. L. Pearson.** 2003. Low frequency of fires from alcohol-based hand rub dispensers in healthcare facilities. *Infect. Control Hosp. Epidemiol.* **24:**618–619.
40. **Boyce, J. M., and D. Pittet.** 2002. Guideline for hand hygiene in health-care settings: recommendations of the Healthcare Infection Control Practices Advisory Committee and the HICPAC/SHEA/APIC/IDSA Hand Hygiene Task Force. *Infect. Control Hosp. Epidemiol.* **23:**S3–S40.
41. **Boyce, J. M., G. Potter-Bynoe, S. M. Opal, L. Dziobek, and A. A. Medeiros.** 1990. A common-source outbreak of Staphylococcus epidermidis infections among patients undergoing cardiac surgery. *J. Infect. Dis.* **161:**493–499.
42. **Bradley, C. R., J. R. Babb, and G. A. Ayliffe.** 1995. Evaluation of the Steris System 1 peracetic acid endoscope processor. *J. Hosp. Infect.* **29:**143–151.
43. **Bradley, C. R., and A. P. Fraise.** 1996. Heat and chemical resistance of enterococci. *J. Hosp. Infect.* **34:**191–196.
44. **Brady, M. J., C. M. Lisay, A. V. Yurkovetskiy, and S. P. Sawan.** 2003. Persistent silver disinfectant for the environmental control of pathogenic bacteria. *Am. J. Infect. Control* **31:**208–214.
45. **Broadley, S. J., J. R. Furr, P. A. Jenkins, and A. D. Russell.** 1993. Antimycobacterial activity of 'Virkon.' *J. Hosp. Infect.* **23:**189–197.
46. **Bronowicki, J. P., V. Venard, C. Botte, N. Monhoven, I. Gastin, L. Chone, H. Hudziak, B. Rhin, C. Delanoe, A. LeFaou, M. A. Bigard, and P. Gaucher.** 1997. Patient-to-patient transmission of hepatitis C virus during colonoscopy. *N. Engl. J. Med.* **337:**237–240.
47. **Brown, P.** 2001. Bovine spongiform encephalopathy and variant Creutzfeldt-Jakob disease. *BMJ* **322:**841–844.
48. **Brown, P., P. P. Liberski, A. Wolff, and D. C. Gajdusek.** 1990. Resistance of scrapie infectivity to steam autoclaving after formaldehyde fixation and limited survival after ashing at 360 degrees C: practical and theoretical implications. *J. Infect. Dis.* **161:**467–472.
49. **Bruce, M. E., R. G. Will, J. W. Ironside, I. McConnell, D. Drummond, A. Suttie, L. McCardle, A. Chree, J. Hope, C. Birkett, S. Cousens, H. Fraser, and C. J. Bostock.** 1997. Transmissions to mice indicate that 'new variant' CJD is caused by the BSE agent. *Nature* **389:**498–501.
50. **Bryant, W. P., and D. Zimmerman.** 1995. Iodine-induced hyperthyroidism in a newborn. *Pediatrics* **95:**434–436. (Erratum, **96:**779.)
51. **Bryce, E. A., F. J. Roberts, B. Clements, and S. MacLean.** 1997. When the biological indicator is positive: investigating autoclave failures. *Infect. Control Hosp. Epidemiol.* **18:**654–656.
52. **Centers for Disease Control.** 1995. Management of patients with suspected viral hemorrhagic fever—United States. *Morb. Mortal. Wkly. Rep.* **44:**475–479.
53. **Centers for Disease Control.** 1989. Guidelines for prevention of transmission of human immunodeficiency virus and hepatitis B virus to health-care and public-safety workers. *Morb. Mortal. Wkly. Rep.* **38**(Suppl. 6)**:**1–37.
54. **Centers for Disease Control and Prevention.** 1996. Community-level prevention of human immunodeficiency virus infection among high-risk populations: the AIDS community demonstration projects. *Morb. Mortal. Wkly. Rep.* **45**(RR6)**:**1–31.
55. **Centers for Disease Control and Prevention.** 1993. Recommended infection-control practices for dentistry. *Morb. Mortal. Wkly. Rep.* **42:**1–12.
56. **Cetinkaya, Y., P. Falk, and C. G. Mayhall.** 2000. Vancomycin-resistant enterococci. *Clin. Microbiol. Rev.* **13:**686–707.
57. **Cetre, J. C., M. C. Nicolle, H. Salord, M. Perol, S. Tigaud, G. David, M. Bourjault, and P. Vanhems.** 2005. Outbreaks of contaminated broncho-alveolar lavage related to intrinsically defective bronchoscopes. *J. Hosp. Infect.* **61:**39–45.
58. **Chamberland, M. E.** 2002. Emerging infectious agents: do they pose a risk to the safety of transfused blood and blood products? *Clin. Infect. Dis.* **34:**797–805.
59. **Charatan, F. 2001.** United States takes precautions against BSE. *West J. Med.* **174:**235.
60. **Chazot, G., E. Broussolle, C. Lapras, T. Blattler, A. Aguzzi, and N. Kopp.** 1996. New variant of Creutzfeldt-Jakob disease

in a 26-year-old French man. *Lancet* **347**:1181. (Letter and comment.)

61. **Cheung, R. J., D. Ortiz, and A. J. DiMarino, Jr.** 1999. GI endoscopic reprocessing practices in the United States. *Gastrointest. Endosc.* **50**:362–368.
62. **Chitnis, V., S. Chitnis, S. Patil, and D. Chitnis.** 2004. Practical limitations of disinfection of body fluid spills with 10,000 ppm sodium hypochlorite (NaOCl). *Am. J. Infect. Control* **32**:306–308.
63. **Chuanchuen, R., K. Beinlich, T. T. Hoang, A. Becher, R. R. Karkhoff-Schweizer, and H. P. Schweizer.** 2001. Cross-resistance between triclosan and antibiotics in *Pseudomonas aeruginosa* is mediated by multidrug efflux pumps: exposure of a susceptible mutant strain to triclosan selects *nfxB* mutants overexpressing MexCD-OprJ. *Antimicrob. Agents Chemother.* **45**:428–432.
64. **Coates, D.** 1996. Sporicidal activity of sodium dichloroisocyanurate, peroxygen and glutaraldehyde disinfectants against Bacillus subtilis. *J. Hosp. Infect.* **32**:283–294.
65. **Collins, F. M.** 1986. Bactericidal activity of alkaline glutaraldehyde solution against a number of atypical mycobacterial species. *J. Appl. Bacteriol.* **61**:247–251.
66. **Collins, F. M.** 1986. Kinetics of the tuberculocidal response by alkaline glutaraldehyde in solution and on an inert surface. *J. Appl. Bacteriol.* **61**:87–93.
67. **Collins, S. J., V. A. Lawson, and C. L. Masters.** 2004. Transmissible spongiform encephalopathies. *Lancet* **363**:51–61.
68. **Corne, P., S. Godreuil, H. Jean-Pierre, O. Jonquet, J. Campos, E. Jumas-Bilak, S. Parer, and H. Marchandin.** 2005. Unusual implication of biopsy forceps in outbreaks of Pseudomonas aeruginosa infections and pseudo-infections related to bronchoscopy. *J. Hosp. Infect.* **61**:20–26.
69. **Craven, D. E., B. Moody, M. G. Connolly, N. R. Kollisch, K. D. Stottmeier, and W. R. McCabe.** 1981. Pseudobacteremia caused by povidone-iodine solution contaminated with Pseudomonas cepacia. *N. Engl. J. Med.* **305**:621–623.
70. **Crow, S.** 1993. Steam sterilizers: an evolution in design. *Infect. Control Hosp. Epidemiol.* **14**:488–490.
71. **Cruse, P. J., and R. Foord.** 1973. A five-year prospective study of 23,649 surgical wounds. *Arch. Surg.* **107**:206–210.
72. **Daschner, F.** 1994. STERIS SYSTEM 1 in Germany. *Infect. Control Hosp. Epidemiol.* **15**:294, 296. (Letter and comment.)
73. **de Lassence, A., N. Hidri, J. F. Timsit, M. L. Joly-Guillou, G. Thiery, A. Boyer, P. Lable, A. Blivet, H. Kalinowski, Y. Martin, J. P. Lajonchere, and D. Dreyfuss.** 2006. Control and outcome of a large outbreak of colonization and infection with glycopeptide-intermediate Staphylococcus aureus in an intensive care unit. *Clin. Infect. Dis.* **42**:170–178.
74. **Dennis, D. T., T. V. Inglesby, D. A. Henderson, J. G. Bartlett, M. S. Ascher, E. Eitzen, A. D. Fine, A. M. Friedlander, J. Hauer, M. Layton, S. R. Lillibridge, J. E. McDade, M. T. Osterholm, T. O'Toole, G. Parker, T. M. Perl, P. K. Russell, and K. Tonat.** 2001. Tularemia as a biological weapon: medical and public health management. *JAMA* **285**:2763–2773.
75. **Denton, G. E.** 2001. Chlorhexidine, p. 321–336. *In* S. S. Block (ed.), *Disinfection, Sterilization and Preservation,* 5th ed. Lippincott Williams & Wilkins, Philadelphia, Pa.
76. **Dharan, S., P. Mourouga, P. Copin, G. Bessmer, B. Tschanz, and D. Pittet.** 1999. Routine disinfection of patients' environmental surfaces. Myth or reality? *J. Hosp. Infect.* **42**:113–117.
77. **Disch, K.** 1994. Glucoprotamine—a new antimicrobial substance. *Zentbl. Hyg. Umweltmed.* **195**:357–365.
78. **Doebbeling, B. N., G. L. Stanley, C. T. Sheetz, M. A. Pfaller, A. K. Houston, L. Annis, N. Li, and R. P. Wenzel.** 1992. Comparative efficacy of alternative hand-washing agents in reducing nosocomial infections in intensive care units. *N. Engl. J. Med.* **327**:88–93.
79. **Dolce, P., M. Gourdeau, N. April, and P. M. Bernard.** 1995. Outbreak of glutaraldehyde-induced proctocolitis. *Am. J. Infect. Control.* **23**:34–39.
80. **Dormont, D.** 1996. How to limit the spread of Creutzfeldt-Jakob disease. *Infect. Control Hosp. Epidemiol.* **17**:521–528.
81. **Druce, J. D., D. Jardine, S. A. Locarnini, and C. J. Birch.** 1995. Susceptibility of HIV to inactivation by disinfectants and ultraviolet light. *J. Hosp. Infect.* **30**:167–180.
82. **Evans, R. J.** 1992. Acute anaphylaxis due to topical chlorhexidine acetate. *BMJ* **304**:686. (Letter.)
83. **Farina, A., M. H. Fievet, F. Plassart, M. C. Menet, and A. Thuillier.** 1999. Residual glutaraldehyde levels in fiberoptic endoscopes: measurement and implications for patient toxicity. *J. Hosp. Infect.* **43**:293–297.
84. **Favero, M. S.** 1991. Strategies for disinfection and sterilization of endoscopes: the gap between basic principles and actual practice. *Infect. Control Hosp. Epidemiol.* **12**: 279–281.
85. **Favero, M. S., and F. A. Manian.** 1993. Is eliminating flash sterilization practical? *Infect. Control Hosp. Epidemiol.* **14**:479–480.
86. **Feldman, H. I., M. Kinosian, W. B. Bilker, C. Simmons, J. H. Holmes, M. V. Pauly, and J. J. Escarce.** 1996. Effect of dialyzer reuse on survival of patients treated with hemodialysis. *JAMA* **276**:1724.
87. **Fichet, G., E. Comoy, C. Duval, K. Antloga, C. Dehen, A. Charbonnier, G. McDonnell, P. Brown, C. I. Lasmezas, and J. P. Deslys.** 2004. Novel methods for disinfection of prion-contaminated medical devices. *Lancet* **364**:521–526.
88. **Flynn, N., S. Jain, E. M. Keddie, J. R. Carlson, M. B. Jennings, H. W. Haverkos, N. Nassar, R. Anderson, S. Cohen, and D. Goldberg.** 1994. In vitro activity of readily available household materials against HIV-1: is bleach enough? *J. Acquir. Immune Defic. Syndr.* **7**:747–753.
89. **Fraise, A. P., P. A. Lambert, and J. Y. Maillard.** 2004. *Russell, Hugo and Ayliffe's Principles and Practice of Disinfections, Preservation and Sterilization.* Blackwell Publishing, Malden, Mass.
90. **Frank, M. J., and W. Schaffner.** 1976. Contaminated aqueous benzalkonium chloride. An unnecessary hospital infection hazard. *JAMA* **236**:2418–2419.
91. **Fraser, T. G., S. Reiner, M. Malczynski, P. R. Yarnold, J. Warren, and G. A. Noskin.** 2004. Multidrug-resistant Pseudomonas aeruginosa cholangitis after endoscopic retrograde cholangiopancreatography: failure of routine endoscope cultures to prevent an outbreak. *Infect. Control Hosp. Epidemiol.* **25**:856–859.
92. **Fraser, V. J., G. Zuckerman, R. E. Clouse, S. O'Rourke, M. Jones, J. Klasner, and P. Murray.** 1993. A prospective randomized trial comparing manual and automated endoscope disinfection methods. *Infect. Control Hosp. Epidemiol.* **14**:383–389.
93. **Fraud, S., J. Y. Maillard, and A. D. Russell.** 2001. Comparison of the mycobactericidal activity of ortho-phthalaldehyde, glutaraldehyde and other dialdehydes by a quantitative suspension test. *J. Hosp. Infect.* **48**:214–221.
94. **Furuhashi, M., and T. Miyamae.** 1979. Effect of pre-operative hand scrubbing and influence of pinholes appearing in surgical rubber gloves during operation. *Bull. Tokyo. Med. Dent. Univ.* **26**:73–80.
95. **Fuselier, H. A. J., and C. Mason.** 1997. Liquid sterilization versus high level disinfection in the urologic office. *Urology* **50**:337–340.
96. **Fuursted, K., A. Hjort, and L. Knudsen.** 1997. Evaluation of bactericidal activity and lag of regrowth (postantibiotic effect) of five antiseptics on nine bacterial pathogens. *J. Antimicrob. Chemother.* **40**:221–226.
97. **Gamage, B., D. Moore, R. Copes, A. Yassi, and E. Bryce.** 2005. Protecting health care workers from SARS and other

respiratory pathogens: a review of the infection control literature. *Am. J. Infect. Control* **33**:114–121.

98. **Garibaldi, R. A., D. Skolnick, T. Lerer, A. Poirot, J. Graham, E. Krisuinas, and R. Lyons.** 1988. The impact of preoperative skin disinfection on preventing intraoperative wound contamination. *Infect. Control Hosp. Epidemiol.* **9**:109–113.
99. **Gelinas, P., J. Goulet, G. M. Tastayre, and G. A. Picard.** 1991. Effect of temperature and contact time on the activity of eight disinfectants—a classification. *J. Food Prot.* **47**:841–847.
100. **Georgiade, G., R. Riefkohl, N. Georgiade, R. Georgiade, and M. F. Wildman.** 1985. Efficacy of povidone-iodine in pre-operative skin preparation. *J. Hosp. Infect.* **6**(Suppl. A):67–71.
101. **Ghannoum, M. A., K. A. Elteen, M. Ellabib, and P. A. Whittaker.** 1990. Antimycotic effects of octenidine and pirtenidine. *J. Antimicrob. Chemother.* **25**:237–245.
102. **Gillespie, T. G., L. Hogg, E. Budge, A. Duncan, and J. E. Coia.** 2000. Mycobacterium chelonae isolated from rinse water within an endoscope washer-disinfector. *J. Hosp. Infect.* **45**:332–334.
103. **Glatzel, M., K. Stoeck, H. Seeger, T. Luhrs, and A. Aguzzi.** 2005. Human prion diseases: molecular and clinical aspects. *Arch. Neurol.* **62**:545–552.
104. **Gorse, G. J., and R. L. Messner.** 1991. Infection control practices in gastrointestinal endoscopy in the United States: a national survey. *Infect. Control Hosp. Epidemiol.* **12**:289–296.
105. **Gottardi, W.** 2001. Iodine and iodine compounds, p. 159–183. *In* S. S. Block (ed.), *Disinfection, Sterilization and Preservation*, 5th ed. Lippincott Williams & Wilkins, Philadelphia, Pa.
106. **Graham, G. S.** 1997. Decontamination: scientific principles, p. 1–9. *In* M. Reichert and J. H. Young (ed.), *Sterilization Technology*. Aspen Publication, Gaithterburg, Md.
107. **Griffiths, P. A., J. R. Babb, C. R. Bradley, and A. P. Fraise.** 1997. Glutaraldehyde-resistant Mycobacterium chelonae from endoscope washer disinfectors. *J. Appl. Microbiol.* **82**:519–526.
108. **Gubler, J. G., M. Salfinger, and A. von Graevenitz.** 1992. Pseudoepidemic of nontuberculous mycobacteria due to a contaminated bronchoscope cleaning machine. Report of an outbreak and review of the literature. *Chest* **101**:1245–1249.
109. **Gurevich, I., R. Dubin, and B. A. Cunha.** 1996. Dental instrument and device sterilization and disinfection practices. *J. Hosp. Infect.* **32**:295–304.
110. **Gurevich, I., S. M. Qadri, and B. A. Cunha.** 1993. False-positive results of spore tests from improper clip use with the STERIS chemical sterilant system. *Am. J. Infect. Control* **21**:42–43. (Letter.)
111. **Gurevich, I., P. Tafuro, P. Ristuccia, J. Herrmann, A. R. Young, and B. A. Cunha.** 1983. Disinfection of respirator tubing: a comparison of chemical versus hot water machine-assisted processing. *J. Hosp. Infect.* **4**:199–208.
112. **Hall, C. B., and R. G. Douglas, Jr.** 1981. Modes of transmission of respiratory syncytial virus. *J. Pediatr.* **99**:100–103.
113. **Hamilton, E., D. V. Seal, and J. Hay.** 1996. Comparison of chlorine and chlorine dioxide disinfection for control of Legionella in a hospital potable water supply. *J. Hosp. Infect.* **32**:156–160. (Letter.)
114. **Hanson, P. J., D. Gor, J. R. Clarke, M. V. Chadwick, B. Gazzard, D. J. Jeffries, H. Gaya, and J. V. Collins.** 1991. Recovery of the human immunodeficiency virus from fibreoptic bronchoscopes. *Thorax* **46**:410–412.
115. **Hanson, P. J., D. J. Jeffries, and J. V. Collins.** 1991. Viral transmission and fibreoptic endoscopy. *J. Hosp. Infect.* **18**(Suppl. A):136–140.
116. **Heikenwalder, M., N. Zeller, H. Seeger, M. Prinz, P. C. Klohn, P. Schwarz, N. H. Ruddle, C. Weissmann, and A. Aguzzi.** 2005. Chronic lymphocytic inflammation specifies the organ tropism of prions. *Science* **307**:1107–1110.
117. **Held, P. J., R. A. Wolfe, D. S. Gaylin, F. K. Port, N. W. Levin, and M. N. Turenne.** 1994. Analysis of the association of dialyzer reuse practices and patient outcomes. *Am. J. Kidney Dis.* **23**:692–708.
118. **Helms, C. M., R. M. Massanari, R. P. Wenzel, M. A. Pfaller, N. P. Moyer, and N. Hall.** 1988. Legionnaires' disease associated with a hospital water system. A five-year progress report on continuous hyperchlorination. *JAMA* **259**:2423–2427.
119. **Henderson, D. A., T. V. Inglesby, J. G. Bartlett, M. S. Ascher, E. Eitzen, P. B. Jahrling, J. Hauer, M. Layton, J. McDade, M. T. Osterholm, T. O'Toole, G. Parker, T. Perl, P. K. Russell, and K. Tonat.** 1999. Smallpox as a biological weapon: medical and public health management. Working Group on Civilian Biodefense. *JAMA* **281**:2127–2137.
120. **Herzog, C., N. Sales, N. Etchegaray, A. Charbonnier, S. Freire, D. Dormont, J. P. Deslys, and C. I. Lasmezas.** 2004. Tissue distribution of bovine spongiform encephalopathy agent in primates after intravenous or oral infection. *Lancet* **363**:422–428.
121. **Hill, A. F., M. Desbruslais, S. Joiner, K. C. Sidle, I. Gowland, J. Collinge, L. J. Doey, and P. Lantos.** 1997. The same prion strain causes vCJD and BSE. *Nature* **389**:448–450.
122. **Holmes, K. V.** 2003. SARS-associated coronavirus. *N. Engl. J. Med.* **348**:1948–1951.
123. **Holton, J., and N. Shetty.** 1997. In-use stability of Nu-Cidex. *J. Hosp. Infect.* **35**:245–248.
124. **Houston, F., J. D. Foster, A. Chong, N. Hunter, and C. J. Bostock.** 2000. Transmission of BSE by blood transfusion in sheep. *Lancet* **356**:999–1000.
125. **Hughes, R., and S. Kilvington.** 2001. Comparison of hydrogen peroxide contact lens disinfection systems and solutions against *Acanthamoeba polyphaga*. *Antimicrob. Agents Chemother.* **45**:2038–2043.
126. **Hussaini, S. N., and K. R. Ruby.** 1976. Sporicidal activity of peracetic acid against B. anthracis spores. *Vet. Rec.* **98**:257–259.
127. **Im, S. W., J. P. Fung, S. Y. So, and D. Y. Yu.** 1982. Unusual dissemination of pseudomonads by ventilators. *Anaesthesia* **37**:1074–1077.
128. **Inglesby, T. V., D. T. Dennis, D. A. Henderson, J. G. Bartlett, M. S. Ascher, E. Eitzen, A. D. Fine, A. M. Friedlander, J. Hauer, J. F. Koerner, M. Layton, J. McDade, M. T. Osterholm, T. O'Toole, G. Parker, T. M. Perl, P. K. Russell, M. Schoch-Spana, and K. Tonat.** 2000. Plague as a biological weapon: medical and public health management. Working Group on Civilian Biodefense. *JAMA* **283**:2281–2290.
129. **Inglesby, T. V., D. A. Henderson, J. G. Bartlett, M. S. Ascher, E. Eitzen, A. M. Friedlander, J. Hauer, J. McDade, M. T. Osterholm, T. O'Toole, G. Parker, T. M. Perl, P. K. Russell, and K. Tonat.** 1999. Anthrax as a biological weapon: medical and public health management. Working Group on Civilian Biodefense. *JAMA* **281**:1735–1745.
130. **Isenberg, S. J., L. Apt, and M. Wood.** 1995. A controlled trial of povidone-iodine as prophylaxis against ophthalmia neonatorum. *N. Engl. J. Med.* **332**:562–566.
131. **Jackson, J., J. E. Leggett, D. A. Wilson, and D. N. Gilbert.** 1996. Mycobacterium gordonae in fiberoptic bronchoscopes. *Am. J. Infect. Control* **24**:19–23.
132. **Jones, R. D., H. B. Jampani, J. L. Newman, and A. S. Lee.** 2000. Triclosan: a review of effectiveness and safety in health care settings. *Am. J. Infect. Control* **28**:184–196.
133. **Joslyn, L. J.** 2001. Sterilization by heat, p. 695–728. *In* S. S. Block (ed.), *Disinfection, Sterilization and Preservation*, 5th ed. Lippincott Williams & Wilkins, Philadelphia, Pa.

134. **Kaatz, G. W., S. D. Gitlin, D. R. Schaberg, K. H. Wilson, C. A. Kauffman, S. M. Seo, and R. Fekety.** 1988. Acquisition of Clostridium difficile from the hospital environment. *Am. J. Epidemiol.* **127:**1289–1293.
135. **Kaczmarek, R. G., R. M. J. Moore, J. McCrohan, D. A. Goldmann, C. Reynolds, C. Caquelin, and E. Israel.** 1992. Multi-state investigation of the actual disinfection/sterilization of endoscopes in health care facilities. *Am. J. Med.* **92:**257–261.
136. **Kampf, G., R. Bloss, and H. Martiny.** 2004. Surface fixation of dried blood by glutaraldehyde and peracetic acid. *J. Hosp. Infect.* **57:**139–143.
137. **Kampf, G., and A. Kramer.** 2004. Epidemiologic background of hand hygiene and evaluation of the most important agents for scrubs and rubs. *Clin. Microbiol. Rev.* **17:**863–893, table.
138. **Kampf, G., C. Ostermeyer, and P. Heeg.** 2005. Surgical hand disinfection with a propanol-based hand rub: equivalence of shorter application times. *J. Hosp. Infect.* **59:**304–310.
139. **Karol, M. H.** 1995. Toxicologic principles do not support the banning of chlorine. A Society of Toxicology position paper. *Fundam. Appl. Toxicol.* **24:**1–2.
140. **Kawashima, T., H. Furukawa, K. Doh-ura, and T. Iwaki.** 1997. Diagnosis of new variant Creutzfeldt-Jakob disease by tonsil biopsy. *Lancet* **350:**68–69. (Letter and comment.)
141. **Klein, M., and A. DeForest.** 1963. The inactivation of viruses by germicides. *Chem. Spec. Manuf. Assoc. Proc.* **49:**116–118.
142. **Klein, M. A., R. Frigg, E. Flechsig, A. J. Raeber, U. Kalinke, H. Bluethman, F. Bootz, J. Suter, R. M. Zinkernagel, and A. Aguzzi.** 1997. A crucial role for B cells in neuroinvasive scrapie. *Nature* **390:**687.
143. **Kobayashi, H., M. Tsuzuki, K. Koshimizu, H. Toyama, N. Yoshihara, T. Shikata, K. Abe, K. Mizuno, N. Otomo, and T. Oda.** 1984. Susceptibility of hepatitis B virus to disinfectants or heat. *J. Clin. Microbiol.* **20:**214–216.
144. **Kool, J. L., J. C. Carpenter, and B. S. Fields.** 1999. Effect of monochloramine disinfection of municipal drinking water on risk of nosocomial Legionnaires' disease. *Lancet* **353:**272–277.
145. **Kralovic, R. C.** 1993. Use of biological indicators designed for steam or ethylene oxide to monitor a liquid chemical sterilization process. *Infect. Control Hosp. Epidemiol.* **14:**313–319. (Erratum, **15:**296, 1994.)
146. **Kramer, A., P. Rudolph, G. Kampf, and D. Pittet.** 2002. Limited efficacy of alcohol-based hand gels. *Lancet* **359:**1489–1490.
147. **Kurtz, J. B., T. W. Lee, and A. J. Parsons.** 1980. The action of alcohols on rotavirus, astrovirus and enterovirus. *J. Hosp. Infect.* **1:**321–325.
148. **Lai, M. Y., P. K. Cheng, and W. W. Lim.** 2005. Survival of severe acute respiratory syndrome coronavirus. *Clin. Infect. Dis.* **41:**e67–e71.
149. **Larson, E.** 1988. Guideline for use of topical antimicrobial agents. *Am. J. Infect. Control* **16:**253–266.
150. **Larson, E. L.** 1991. Alcohols, p. 191–203. *In* S. S. Block (ed.), *Disinfection, Sterilization and Preservation.* Lea & Febiger, Philadelphia, Pa.
151. **Larson, E. L., A. M. Butz, D. L. Gullette, and B. A. Laughon.** 1990. Alcohol for surgical scrubbing? *Infect. Control Hosp. Epidemiol.* **11:**139–143.
152. **Leaper, S.** 1984. Influence of temperature on the synergistic sporicidal effect of peracetic acid plus hydrogen peroxide in Bacillus subtilis SA22 (NCA 72–52). *Food Microbiol.* **1:**199–203.
153. **Levenson, J. E.** 1989. Corneal damage from improperly cleaned tonometer tips. *Arch. Ophthalmol.* **107:**1117.
154. **Lever, A. M., and S. V. W. Sutton.** 1996. Antimicrobial effects of hydrogen peroxide as an antiseptic and disinfectant, p. 159–176. *In* J. P. Ascenzi (ed.), *Handbook of Disinfectants and Antiseptics.* Marcel Dekker, Inc., New York, N.Y.
155. **Lowbury, E. J., and H. A. Lilly.** 1974. The effect of blood on disinfection of surgeons' hands. *Br. J. Surg.* **61:**19–21.
156. **Lowbury, E. J., H. A. Lilly, and J. P. Bull.** 1964. Methods for disinfection of operation sites. *Br. Med. J.* **2:**531–533.
157. **Maillard, J. Y.** 2002. Bacterial target sites for biocide action. *J. Appl. Microbiol.* **92**(Suppl.)**:**16S–27S.
158. **Maki, D. G., and C. A. Hassemer.** 1987. Flash sterilization: carefully measured haste. *Infect. Control* **8:**307–310.
159. **Maki, D. G., S. M. Stolz, S. Wheeler, and L. A. Mermel.** 1997. Prevention of central venous catheter-related bloodstream infection by use of an antiseptic-impregnated catheter. A randomized, controlled trial. *Ann. Intern. Med.* **127:**257–266.
160. **Mangram, A. J., T. C. Horan, M. L. Pearson, L. C. Silver, and W. R. Jarvis.** 1999. Guideline for prevention of surgical site infection, 1999. Hospital Infection Control Practices Advisory Committee. *Infect. Control Hosp. Epidemiol.* **20:**250–278.
161. **Mannion, P. T.** 1995. The use of peracetic acid for the reprocessing of flexible endoscopes and rigid cystoscopes and laparoscopes. *J. Hosp. Infect.* **29:**313–315. (Letter.)
162. **Martin, L. S., J. S. McDougal, and S. L. Loskoski.** 1985. Disinfection and inactivation of the human T lymphotropic virus type III/lymphadenopathy-associated virus. *J. Infect. Dis.* **152:**400–403.
163. **Martin, M. A., and M. Reichelderfer.** 1994. APIC guidelines for infection prevention and control in flexible endoscopy. Association for Professionals in Infection Control and Epidemiology, Inc. 1991, 1992, and 1993 APIC Guidelines Committee. *Am. J. Infect. Control* **22:**19–38.
164. **Mathers, W. D., J. E. Sutphin, R. Folberg, P. A. Meier, R. P. Wenzel, and R. G. Elgin.** 1996. Outbreak of keratitis presumed to be caused by Acanthamoeba. *Am. J. Ophthalmol.* **121:**129–142.
165. **Mayer, S., M. Boos, A. Beyer, A. C. Fluit, and F. J. Schmitz.** 2001. Distribution of the antiseptic resistance genes qacA, qacB and qacC in 497 methicillin-resistant and -susceptible European isolates of Staphylococcus aureus. *J. Antimicrob. Chemother.* **47:**896–897.
166. **Mbithi, J. N., V. S. Springthorpe, and S. A. Sattar.** 1990. Chemical disinfection of hepatitis A virus on environmental surfaces. *Appl. Environ. Microbiol.* **56:**3601–3604.
167. **Mbithi, J. N., V. S. Springthorpe, S. A. Sattar, and M. Pacquette.** 1993. Bactericidal, virucidal, and mycobactericidal activities of reused alkaline glutaraldehyde in an endoscopy unit. *J. Clin. Microbiol.* **31:**2988–2995.
168. **McDonald, L. C., G. E. Killgore, A. Thompson, R. C. Owens, Jr., S. V. Kazakova, S. P. Sambol, S. Johnson, and D. N. Gerding.** 2005. An epidemic, toxin gene-variant strain of Clostridium difficile. *N. Engl. J. Med.* **353:**2433–2441.
169. **McDonnell, G., and A. D. Russell.** 1999. Antiseptics and disinfectants: activity, action, and resistance. *Clin. Microbiol. Rev.* **12:**147–179.
170. **Mentel, R., and J. Schmidt.** 1973. Investigations on rhinovirus inactivation by hydrogen peroxide. *Acta Virol.* **17:**351–354.
171. **Merianos, J. J.** 2001. Surface-active agents, p. 283–320. *In* S. S. Block (ed.), *Disinfection, Sterilization and Preservation,* 5th ed. Lippincott Williams & Wilkins, Philadelphia, Pa.
172. **Mermel, L. A., S. L. Josephson, J. Dempsey, S. Parenteau, C. Perry, and N. Magill.** 1997. Outbreak of *Shigella sonnei* in a clinical microbiology laboratory. *J. Clin. Microbiol.* **35:**3163–3165.
173. **Meyer, B., and C. Kluin.** 1999. Efficacy of glucoprotamin containing disinfectants against different species of atypical mycobacteria. *J. Hosp. Infect.* **42:**151–154.
174. **Michele, T. M., W. A. Cronin, N. M. Graham, D. M. Dwyer, D. S. Pope, S. Harrington, R. E. Chaisson, and**

W. R. Bishai. 1997. Transmission of Mycobacterium tuberculosis by a fiberoptic bronchoscope. Identification by DNA fingerprinting. *JAMA* **278:**1093–1095.

175. **Middleton, A. M., M. V. Chadwick, J. L. Sanderson, and H. Gaya.** 2000. Comparison of a solution of superoxidized water (Sterilox) with glutaraldehyde for the disinfection of bronchoscopes, contaminated. *J. Hosp. Infect.* **45:**278–282.
176. **Mitchell, B. A., M. H. Brown, and R. A. Skurray.** 1998. QacA multidrug efflux pump from *Staphylococcus aureus:* comparative analysis of resistance to diamidines, biguanidines, and guanylhydrazones. *Antimicrob. Agents Chemother.* **42:**475–477.
177. **Nakashima, A. K., A. K. Highsmith, and W. J. Martone.** 1987. Survival of *Serratia marcescens* in benzalkonium chloride and in multiple-dose medication vials: relationship to epidemic septic arthritis. *J. Clin. Microbiol.* **25:**1019–1021.
178. **Narang, H. K., and A. A. Codd.** 1983. Action of commonly used disinfectants against enteroviruses. *J. Hosp. Infect.* **4:**209–212.
179. **Nelson, D. B., W. R. Jarvis, W. A. Rutala, A. E. Foxx-Orenstein, G. Isenberg, G. R. Dash, C. J. Alvarado, M. Ball, J. Griffin-Sobel, C. Petersen, K. A. Ball, J. Henderson, and R. L. Stricof.** 2003. Multi-society guideline for reprocessing flexible gastrointestinal endoscopes. Society for Healthcare Epidemiology of America. *Infect. Control Hosp. Epidemiol.* **24:**532–537.
180. **O'Connor, D. O., and J. R. Rubino.** 1991. Phenolic compounds, p. 204–224. *In* S. S. Block (ed.), *Disinfection, Sterilization and Preservation.* Lea & Febiger, Philadelphia, Pa.
181. **Oie, S., and A. Kamiya.** 1996. Microbial contamination of antiseptics and disinfectants. *Am. J. Infect. Control* **24:**389–395.
182. **Parker, F., and S. Foran.** 1995. Chlorhexidine catheter lubricant anaphylaxis. *Anaesth. Intensive Care* **23:**126. (Letter and comments.)
183. **Perencevich, E. N., M. T. Wong, and A. D. Harris.** 2001. National and regional assessment of the antibacterial soap market: a step toward determining the impact of prevalent antibacterial soaps. *Am. J. Infect. Control* **29:**281–283.
184. **Piazza, M., G. Borgia, L. Picciotto, S. Nappa, S. Cicciarello, and R. Orlando.** 1995. Detection of hepatitis C virus-RNA by polymerase chain reaction in dental surgeries. *J. Med. Virol.* **45:**40–42.
185. **Pittet, D., S. Hugonnet, S. Harbarth, P. Mourouga, V. Sauvan, S. Touveneau, and T. V. Perneger.** 2000. Effectiveness of a hospital-wide programme to improve compliance with hand hygiene. Infection Control Programme. *Lancet* **356:**1307–1312.
186. **Price, P. B.** 1938. The bacteriology of normal skin; a new quantitative test applied to a study of the bacterial flora and the disinfectant action of mechanical cleansing. *J. Infect. Dis.* **63:**301–318.
187. **Prusiner, S. B.** 1982. Novel proteinaceous infectious particles cause scrapie. *Science* **216:**136–144.
188. **Prusiner, S. B.** 1997. Prion diseases and the BSE crisis. *Science* **278:**245–251.
189. **Ranganathan, N. S.** 1996. Chlorhexidine, p. 235–264. *In* J. P. Ascenzi (ed.), *Handbook of Disinfectants and Antiseptics.* Marcel Dekker, Inc., New York, N.Y.
190. **Reiss, I., A. Borkhardt, R. Fussle, A. Sziegoleit, and L. Gortner.** 2000. Disinfectant contaminated with *Klebsiella oxytoca* as a source of sepsis in babies. *Lancet* **356:**310.
191. **Robertson, L. J., A. T. Campbell, and H. V. Smith.** 1992. Survival of *Cryptosporidium parvum* oocysts under various environmental pressures. *Appl. Environ. Microbiol.* **58:**3494–3500.
192. **Rossmoore, H. W., and M. Sondossi.** 1988. Applications and mode of action of formaldehyde condensate biocides. *Adv. Appl. Microbiol.* **33:**223–277.
193. **Rotter, M. A.** 1996. Alcohols for antisepsis of hands and skin, p. 177–234. *In* J. P. Ascenzi (ed.), *Handbook of Disinfectants and Antiseptics.* Marcel Dekker, Inc., New York, N.Y.
194. **Rotter, M. L., W. Koller, G. Wewalka, H. P. Werner, G. A. Ayliffe, and J. R. Babb.** 1986. Evaluation of procedures for hygienic hand-disinfection: controlled parallel experiments on the Vienna test model. *J. Hyg.* (London) **96:**27–37.
195. **Rotter, M. L., S. O. Larsen, E. M. Cooke, J. Dankert, F. Daschner, D. Greco, P. Gronross, O. B. Jepsen, A. Lystad, and B. Nystrom.** 1988. A comparison of the effects of preoperative whole-body bathing with detergent alone and with detergent containing chlorhexidine gluconate on the frequency of wound infections after clean surgery. The European Working Party on Control of Hospital Infections. *J. Hosp. Infect.* **11:**310–320.
196. **Rotter, M. L., R. A. Simpson, and W. Koller.** 1998. Surgical hand disinfection with alcohols at various concentrations: parallel experiments using the new proposed European standards method. *Infect. Control Hosp. Epidemiol.* **19:**778–781.
197. **Rubbo, S. D., J. F. Gardner, and R. L. Webb.** 1967. Biocidal activities of glutaraldehyde and related compounds. *J. Appl. Bacteriol.* **30:**78–87.
198. **Russell, A. D.** 1994. Glutaraldehyde: current status and uses. *Infect. Control Hosp. Epidemiol.* **15:**724–733.
199. **Russell, A. D.** 2004. Whither triclosan? *J. Antimicrob. Chemother.* **53:**693–695.
200. **Russell, A. D., W. B. Hugo, and G. A. J. Ayliffe.** 1999. *Principles and Practice of Disinfection, Preservation and Sterilization* 3rd ed. Blackwell Science, London, England.
201. **Rutala, W. A.** 1996. APIC guideline for selection and use of disinfectants. 1994, 1995, and 1996 APIC Guidelines Committee. Association for Professionals in Infection Control and Epidemiology, Inc. *Am. J. Infect. Control* **24:**313–342.
202. **Rutala, W. A.** 1996. Disinfection and sterilization of patient-care items. *Infect. Control Hosp. Epidemiol.* **17:**377–384.
203. **Rutala, W. A., and E. C. Cole.** 1987. Ineffectiveness of hospital disinfectants against bacteria: a collaborative study. *Infect. Control* **8:**501–506.
204. **Rutala, W. A., E. C. Cole, N. S. Wannamaker, and D. J. Weber.** 1991. Inactivation of Mycobacterium tuberculosis and Mycobacterium bovis by 14 hospital disinfectants. *Am. J. Med.* **91:**267S-271S.
205. **Rutala, W. A., M. F. Gergen, and D. J. Weber.** 1993. Evaluation of a rapid readout biological indicator for flash sterilization with three biological indicators and three chemical indicators. *Infect. Control Hosp. Epidemiol.* **14:**390–394.
206. **Rutala, W. A., M. F. Gergen, and D. J. Weber.** 1993. Inactivation of Clostridium difficile spores by disinfectants. *Infect. Control Hosp. Epidemiol.* **14:**36–39.
207. **Rutala, W. A., M. F. Gergen, and D. J. Weber.** 1999. Sporicidal activity of a new low-temperature sterilization technology: the Sterrad 50 sterilizer. *Infect. Control Hosp. Epidemiol.* **20:**514–516.
208. **Rutala, W. A., S. M. Jones, and D. J. Weber.** 1996. Comparison of a rapid readout biological indicator for steam sterilization with four conventional biological indicators and five chemical indicators. *Infect. Control Hosp. Epidemiol.* **17:**423–428.
209. **Rutala, W. A., and D. J. Weber.** 1995. FDA labeling requirements for disinfection of endoscopes: a counterpoint. *Infect. Control Hosp. Epidemiol.* **16:**231–235.

210. **Rutala, W. A., and D. J. Weber.** 1997. Uses of inorganic hypochlorite (bleach) in health-care facilities. *Clin. Microbiol. Rev.* **10:**597–610.
211. **Rutala, W. A., and D. J. Weber.** 1999. Disinfection of endoscopes: review of new chemical sterilants used for high-level disinfection. *Infect. Control Hosp. Epidemiol.* **20:**69–76.
212. **Rutala, W. A., and D. J. Weber.** 2001. New disinfection and sterilization methods. *Emerg. Infect. Dis.* **7:**348–353.
213. **Rutala, W. A., and D. J. Weber.** 2004. Disinfection and sterilization in health care facilities: what clinicians need to know. *Clin. Infect. Dis.* **39:**702–709.
214. **Rutala, W. A., D. J. Weber, and K. J. Chappell.** 1999. Patient injury from flash-sterilized instruments. *Infect. Control Hosp. Epidemiol.* **20:**458.
215. **Rutala, W. A., D. J. Weber, C. A. Thomann, J. F. John, S. M. Saviteer, and F. A. Sarubbi.** 1988. An outbreak of Pseudomonas cepacia bacteremia associated with a contaminated intra-aortic balloon pump. *J. Thorac. Cardiovasc. Surg.* **96:**157–161.
216. **Ryan, C. K., and G. D. Potter.** 1995. Disinfectant colitis. Rinse as well as you wash. *J. Clin. Gastroenterol.* **21:**6–9.
217. **Sagripanti, J. L.** 1992. Metal-based formulations with high microbicidal activity. *Appl. Environ. Microbiol.* **58:** 3157–3162.
218. **Sagripanti, J. L., and A. Bonifacino.** 1996. Comparative sporicidal effect of liquid chemical germicides on three medical devices contaminated with spores of Bacillus subtilis. *Am. J. Infect. Control* **24:**364–371.
219. **Sagripanti, J. L., C. A. Eklund, P. A. Trost, K. C. Jinneman, C. J. Abeyta, C. A. Kaysner, and W. E. Hill.** 1997. Comparative sensitivity of 13 species of pathogenic bacteria to seven chemical germicides. *Am. J. Infect. Control* **25:**335–339.
220. **Sailer, A., H. Bueler, M. Fischer, A. Aguzzi, and C. Weissmann.** 1994. No propagation of prions in mice devoid of PrP. *Cell* **77:**967–968.
221. **Samore, M. H., L. Venkataraman, P. C. DeGirolami, R. D. Arbeit, and A. W. Karchmer.** 1996. Clinical and molecular epidemiology of sporadic and clustered cases of nosocomial Clostridium difficile diarrhea. *Am. J. Med.* **100:**32–40.
222. **Sattar, S. A., H. Jacobsen, H. Rahman, T. M. Cusack, and J. R. Rubino.** 1994. Interruption of rotavirus spread through chemical disinfection. *Infect. Control Hosp. Epidemiol.* **15:**751–756.
223. **Saurina, G., D. Landman, and J. M. Quale.** 1997. Activity of disinfectants against vancomycin-resistant Enterococcus faecium. *Infect. Control Hosp. Epidemiol.* **18:**345–347.
224. **Schelenz, S., and G. French.** 2000. An outbreak of multidrug-resistant Pseudomonas aeruginosa infection associated with contamination of bronchoscopes and an endoscope washer-disinfector. *J. Hosp. Infect.* **46:**23–30.
225. **Scherrer, M., and K. Kümmerer.** 1997. Manual and automated processing of medical instruments—environmental and economic aspects. *Cent. Serv.* **5:**183–194.
226. **Sedlock, D. M., and D. M. Bailey.** 1985. Microbicidal activity of octenidine hydrochloride, a new alkanediylbis[pyridine] germicidal agent. *Antimicrob. Agents Chemother.* **28:**786–790.
227. **Sehulster, L., and R. Y. Chinn.** 2003. Guidelines for environmental infection control in health-care facilities. Recommendations of CDC and the Healthcare Infection Control Practices Advisory Committee (HICPAC). *MMWR Recomm. Rep.* **52:**1–42.
228. **Sheldon, A. T., Jr.** 2005. Antiseptic "resistance": real or perceived threat? *Clin. Infect. Dis.* **40:**1650–1656.
229. **Shetty, N., S. Srinivasan, J. Holton, and G. L. Ridgway.** 1999. Evaluation of microbicidal activity of a new disinfectant: Sterilox 2500 against Clostridium difficile spores, Helicobacter pylori, vancomycin resistant Enterococcus species, Candida albicans and several Mycobacterium species. *J. Hosp. Infect.* **41:**101–105.
230. **Sorin, M., S. Segal-Maurer, N. Mariano, C. Urban, A. Combest, and J. J. Rahal.** 2001. Nosocomial transmission of imipenem-resistant Pseudomonas aeruginosa following bronchoscopy associated with improper connection to the Steris System 1 processor. *Infect. Control Hosp. Epidemiol.* **22:**409–413.
231. **Spach, D. H., F. E. Silverstein, and W. E. Stamm.** 1993. Transmission of infection by gastrointestinal endoscopy and bronchoscopy. *Ann. Intern. Med.* **118:**117–128.
232. **Spaulding, E. H.** 1968. Chemical disinfection of medical and surgical materials, p. 517–531. *In* S. Block (ed.), *Disinfection, Sterilization and Preservation.* Lea & Febiger, Philadelphia, Pa.
233. **Spotts Whitney, E. A., M. E. Beatty, T. H. Taylor, Jr., R. Weyant, J. Sobel, M. J. Arduino, and D. A. Ashford.** 2003. Inactivation of Bacillus anthracis spores. *Emerg. Infect. Dis.* **9:**623–627.
234. **Srinivasan, A., L. L. Wolfenden, X. Song, K. Mackie, T. L. Hartsell, H. D. Jones, G. B. Diette, J. B. Orens, R. C. Yung, T. L. Ross, W. Merz, P. J. Scheel, E. F. Haponik, and T. M. Perl.** 2003. An outbreak of Pseudomonas aeruginosa infections associated with flexible bronchoscopes. *N. Engl. J. Med.* **348:**221–227.
235. **Stickler, D. J.** 1974. Chlorhexidine resistance in Proteus mirabilis. *J. Clin. Pathol.* **27:**284–287.
236. **Stickler, D. J., and B. Thomas.** 1980. Antiseptic and antibiotic resistance in Gram-negative bacteria causing urinary tract infection. *J. Clin. Pathol.* **33:**288–296.
237. **Stout, J. E., Y. S. Lin, A. M. Goetz, and R. R. Muder.** 1998. Controlling Legionella in hospital water systems: experience with the superheat-and-flush method and copper-silver ionization. *Infect. Control Hosp. Epidemiol.* **19:**911–914.
238. **Suller, M. T., and A. D. Russell.** 2000. Triclosan and antibiotic resistance in Staphylococcus aureus. *J. Antimicrob. Chemother.* **46:**11–18.
239. **Tabor, E., D. C. Bostwick, and C. C. Evans.** 1989. Corneal damage due to eye contact with chlorhexidine gluconate. *JAMA* **261:**557–558. (Letter.)
240. **Taylor, D. M.** 1999. Inactivation of prions by physical and chemical means. *J. Hosp. Infect.* **43**(Suppl.)**:**S69–S76.
241. **Taylor, D. M., S. L. Woodgate, A. J. Fleetwood, and R. J. Cawthorne.** 1997. Effect of rendering procedures on the scrapie agent. *Vet. Rec.* **141:**643–649.
242. **Terleckyi, B., and D. A. Axler.** 1987. Quantitative neutralization assay of fungicidal activity of disinfectants. *Antimicrob. Agents Chemother.* **31:**794–798.
243. **Tietz, A., R. Frei, M. Dangel, D. Bolliger, J. R. Passweg, A. Gratwohl, and A. E. Widmer.** 2005. Octenidine hydrochloride for the care of central venous catheter insertion sites in severely immunocompromised patients. *Infect. Control Hosp. Epidemiol.* **26:**703–707.
244. **Tiwari, T. S., B. Ray, K. C. Jost, Jr., M. K. Rathod, Y. Zhang, B. A. Brown-Elliott, K. Hendricks, and R. J. Wallace, Jr.** 2003. Forty years of disinfectant failure: outbreak of postinjection Mycobacterium abscessus infection caused by contamination of benzalkonium chloride. *Clin. Infect. Dis.* **36:**954–962.
245. **Trampuz, A., and A. F. Widmer.** 2004. Hand hygiene: a frequently missed lifesaving opportunity during patient care. *Mayo Clin. Proc.* **79:**109–116.
246. **Turner, P., B. Saeed, and M. C. Kelsey.** 2004. Dermal absorption of isopropyl alcohol from a commercial hand rub: implications for its use in hand decontamination. *J. Hosp. Infect.* **56:**287–290.

247. **Tyler, R., G. A. Ayliffe, and C. Bradley.** 1990. Virucidal activity of disinfectants: studies with the poliovirus. *J. Hosp. Infect.* **15:**339–345.
248. **Valleron, A. J., P. Y. Boelle, R. Will, and J. Y. Cesbron.** 2001. Estimation of epidemic size and incubation time based on age characteristics of vCJD in the United Kingdom. *Science* **294:**1726–1728.
249. **van Bueren, J., D. P. Larkin, and R. A. Simpson.** 1994. Inactivation of human immunodeficiency virus type 1 by alcohols. *J. Hosp. Infect.* **28:**137–148.
250. **van Doornmalen, J. P., and J. Dankert.** 2005. A validation survey of 197 hospital steam sterilizers in The Netherlands in 2001 and 2002. *J. Hosp. Infect.* **59:**126–130.
251. **Van Klingeren, B., and W. Pullen.** 1993. Glutaraldehyde resistant mycobacteria from endoscope washers. *J. Hosp. Infect.* **25:**147–149.
252. **Vesley, D., M. A. Nellis, and P. B. Allwood.** 1995. Evaluation of a rapid readout biological indicator for 121 degrees C gravity and 132 degrees C vacuum-assisted steam sterilization cycles. *Infect. Control Hosp. Epidemiol.* **16:**281–286. (Erratum, **16:**381.)
253. **Vigeant, P., V. G. Loo, C. Bertrand, C. Dixon, R. Hollis, M. A. Pfaller, A. P. McLean, D. J. Briedis, T. M. Perl, and H. G. Robson.** 1998. An outbreak of Serratia marcescens infections related to contaminated chlorhexidine. *Infect. Control Hosp. Epidemiol.* **19:**791–794.
254. **Wallace, J., P. M. Agee, and D. M. Demicco.** 1995. Liquid chemical sterilization using peracetic acid. An alternative approach to endoscope processing. *ASAIO J.* **41:**151–154.
255. **Walsh, S. E., J. Y. Maillard, and A. D. Russell.** 1999. Ortho-phthalaldehyde: a possible alternative to glutaraldehyde for high level disinfection. *J. Appl. Microbiol.* **86:**1039–1046.
256. **Waran, K. D., and R. A. Munsick.** 1995. Anaphylaxis from povidone-iodine. *Lancet* **345:**1506. (Letter.)
257. **Wardle, M. D., and G. M. Renninger.** 1975. Bactericidal effect of hydrogen peroxide on spacecraft isolates. *Appl. Microbiol.* **30:**710–711.
258. **Weber, D. J., S. L. Barbee, M. D. Sobsey, and W. A. Rutala.** 1999. The effect of blood on the antiviral activity of sodium hypochlorite, a phenolic, and a quaternary ammonium compound. *Infect. Control Hosp. Epidemiol.* **20:**821–827.
259. **Weber, D. J., E. Sickbert-Bennett, M. F. Gergen, and W. A. Rutala.** 2003. Efficacy of selected hand hygiene agents used to remove Bacillus atrophaeus (a surrogate of Bacillus anthracis) from contaminated hands. *JAMA* **289:**1274–1277.
260. **Weissmann, C.** 2005. Birth of a prion: spontaneous generation revisited. *Cell* **122:**165–168.
261. **Wenzel, R. P.** 2004. The antibiotic pipeline—challenges, costs, and values. *N. Engl. J. Med.* **351:**523–526.
262. **West, A. B., S. F. Kuan, M. Bennick, and S. Lagarde.** 1995. Glutaraldehyde colitis following endoscopy: clinical and pathological features and investigation of an outbreak. *Gastroenterology* **108:**1250–1255.
263. **Widmer, A. E., and R. Frei.** 2003. Antimicrobial activity of glucoprotamin: a clinical study of a new disinfectant for instruments. *Infect. Control Hosp. Epidemiol.* **24:**762–764.
264. **Widmer, A. F.** 2000. Replace hand washing with use of a waterless alcohol hand rub? *Clin. Infect. Dis.* **31:**136–143.
265. **Widmer, A. F., A. Houston, E. Bollinger, and R. P. Wenzel.** 1992. A new standard for sterility testing for autoclaved surgical trays. *J. Hosp. Infect.* **21:**253–260.
266. **Widmer, A. F., R. P. Wenzel, A. Trilla, M. J. Bale, R. N. Jones, and B. N. Doebbeling. 1993.** Outbreak of Pseudomonas aeruginosa infections in a surgical intensive care unit: probable transmission via hands of a health care worker. *Clin. Infect. Dis.* **16:**372–376.
267. **Williams, N. D., and A. D. Russell.** 1991. The effects of some halogen-containing compounds on Bacillus subtilis endospores. *J. Appl. Bacteriol.* **70:**427–436.
268. **Wilson, J. A., and A. B. Margolin.** 1999. The efficacy of three common hospital liquid germicides to inactivate Cryptosporidium parvum oocysts. *J. Hosp. Infect.* **42:**231–237.
268a. **World Health Organization.** 1983. *Laboratory Biosafety Manual.* World Health Organization, Geneva, Switzerland.
269. **Wullt, M., I. Odenholt, and M. Walder.** 2003. Activity of three disinfectants and acidified nitrite against Clostridium difficile spores. *Infect. Control Hosp. Epidemiol.* **24:**765–768.
270. **Wysowski, D. K., J. W. J. Flynt, M. Goldfield, R. Altman, and A. T. Davis.** 1978. Epidemic neonatal hyperbilirubinemia and use of a phenolic disinfectant detergent. *Pediatrics* **61:**165–170.
271. **Yong, D., F. C. Parker, and S. M. Foran.** 1995. Severe allergic reactions and intra-urethral chlorhexidine gluconate. *Med. J. Aust.* **162:**257–258.
272. **Zaidi, M., J. Sifuentes, M. Bobadilla, D. Moncada, and S. Ponce de León.** 1989. Epidemic of Serratia marcescens bacteremia and meningitis in a neonatal unit in Mexico City. *Infect. Control Hosp. Epidemiol.* **10:**14–20.
273. **Zuhlsdorf, B., G. Kampf, H. Floss, and H. Martiny.** 2005. Suitability of the German test method for cleaning efficacy in washer-disinfectors for flexible endoscopes according to prEN ISO 15883. *J. Hosp. Infect.* **61:**46–52.
274. **Zuhlsdorf, B., and H. Martiny.** 2005. Intralaboratory reproducibility of the German test method of prEN ISO 15883–1 for determination of the cleaning efficacy of washer-disinfectors for flexible endoscopes. *J. Hosp. Infect.* **59:** 286–291.

Prevention and Control of Laboratory-Acquired Infections*

MICHAEL A. NOBLE

8

Laboratory biosafety describes the active, assertive, evidence-based process that laboratorians use to prevent microbial contamination, infection, or toxic reaction as they actively manipulate live microorganisms or their products, thereby protecting themselves, other laboratory workers, the public, and the environment (43). The goals of a laboratory safety program are to prevent laboratory-acquired infections in workers and to prevent accidental releases of live agents that may endanger humans, animals, and plants. Laboratory safety programs involve all aspects of the laboratory cycle, starting before the specimens or microorganisms arrive in the facility, including the processes used to handle specimens or organisms in the laboratory (e.g., the proper use of reagents, materials, and equipment and the safe storage and transport of specimens and organisms), and culminating when specimens or cultures are terminally sterilized or pathogenic microorganisms are destroyed. Laboratories must train their personnel to use safe practices and must develop methods for monitoring work practices.

EPIDEMIOLOGY

Infections are usually characterized as laboratory acquired in retrospect, and these assessments are often based on the assumption that the only likely exposure occurred while the person was in a laboratory or on the finding that a source of exposure outside the laboratory cannot be identified. Consequently, trivial laboratory events may be considered possible exposures (30, 37). However, one must appreciate that the total laboratory testing cycle begins well before the sample actually reaches the laboratory (the preanalytic phase of laboratory testing) and that personnel can be exposed while they collect and transport samples. In the past, infections acquired while personnel collected samples were considered to be laboratory acquired if the samples were collected solely for a laboratory investigation. Currently, infections acquired by phlebotomists through needle stick injuries are routinely considered to be laboratory-acquired infections (24), but infections acquired by phlebotomists when they inhale droplet nuclei (e.g., those from chicken pox) as they collect samples in patients' rooms are not included in this category (23).

Microbiology laboratories run by pioneers including Pasteur and Koch were active by 1840 to 1860. The first known laboratory-acquired infection, Mediterranean fever, was reported in 1899 (11). Sulkin and Pike conducted the first systematic study of laboratory-acquired infections when they surveyed 5,000 American laboratories in 1951 (22). Sulkin extended this study in 1961 and 1965, and Pike extended it further in 1976. In total, Sulkin and Pike cited 3,921 laboratory infections between 1930 and 1974, with a mortality of 164 (4.1%). These infections were reported from research facilities (2,307; 58.8%), diagnostic facilities (677; 17.3%), industries producing biological products (134; 3.4%), and teaching facilities (106; 2.7%); 697 (17.8%) did not have a source specified.

The results of four surveys performed in the United Kingdom between 1971 and 1991 indicated that within clinical facilities, the most infections were identified among workers in the microbiology laboratory, followed by those in the autopsy service (23). Over the 20-year period, the number of infections reported each year dropped more than 80%, from 104 to only 17. It would be tempting to conclude that this decline indicates that laboratories are becoming safer; however, there are no active monitoring or surveillance programs that capture the true number of accidents and infections. Thus, even comprehensive listings of laboratory-acquired infections are incomplete (52).

LABORATORY SAFETY AND PERSONAL ATTRIBUTES

Phillips conducted a matched-case control study of 33 laboratory workers who experienced laboratory-associated injuries over a 2-year period and found no differences in ages, lengths of employment, years of formal education, use of glasses, use of prescription medications, off-the-job accidents, or driving records for person with injuries and those without injuries (45). However, persons in the group who had accidents were significantly more likely to have had a laboratory accident or a laboratory infection before the 2-year study period and were significantly more likely to have a low opinion of laboratory safety programs. When the conditions surrounding the accidents were examined, 36% of accidents were found to occur when the employee was working too quickly, either just before lunch or at the end of the day. In 30% of accidents, the employee acknowledged breeching safety regulations. In summary, in this study attitudes and work habits were important

*This chapter contains information presented in chapter 9 by Andreas Voss and Eric Nulens in the eighth edition of this Manual.

contributing factors to laboratory accidents. Similar results linking attitudes and behaviors with poor safety practices continue to be found.

Over time, laboratorians have learned that even conventionally accepted practices can result in serious infection. Mouth pipetting, marking blood spots, transporting samples to the laboratory in corked or sheathed sharps, recapping needles, and eating or smoking in the laboratory were at one time common practices in properly run medical laboratories. All of these practices are now known to be risky and are prohibited. Other common practices, such as examining bacterial culture plates with an eyeglass or sniffing plates to help identify organisms, are now controversial (9). Thus, to maintain and improve laboratory safety, staff members must review and critique current practices diligently and be open to changing their procedures as appropriate.

RISK-BASED CLASSIFICATION OF MICROORGANISMS

The international community has developed a common risk classification scheme for microorganisms that can help laboratories determine the best laboratory practices and environmental requirements . Group 1 biological agents are unlikely to cause human disease. Group 2 biological agents can cause human disease and may be a hazard to workers but are unlikely to spread to the community; effective prophylaxis or treatment is usually available. Group 3 biological agents cause severe human disease and are a serious hazard to workers; they may spread to the community, but effective prophylaxis or treatment is usually available. Group 4 biological agents cause severe human disease and are a serious hazard to workers; they may present a high risk of spreading to the community, and effective prophylaxis or treatment is usually not available. A partial list of microorganisms by category is provided in Table 1.

Different countries usually classify organisms consistently. However, there are some organisms that are classified differently by different countries. These differences can affect a laboratory's certification, and laboratories that send agents domestically or internationally must know the local and international requirements.

Conventionally, laboratory behavior and practices have been matched to the level of risk associated with expected hazards. (See Table 2 for practices considered to be appropriate for handling of samples with group 2 agents.) Recently, microbiologists have begun to rely less on a rigid classification of organisms when designing laboratory practices and rather to mix different levels of containment and safety practices to match the risk posed by each organism. Thus, in working with a particular organism, the best laboratory practice may be to use biosafety level 2 containment with a higher level of safety practices. Moreover, laboratorians should not treat all situations as equal. Rather, they must consider biosafety to be a

TABLE 1 Risk-based classification of microorganisms[a]

Group	Bacterium(a)	Virus	Fungus(i)	Parasites
1	No clinical organisms			
2	*Bacillus* species (not *Bacillus anthracis*)	Adenovirus	*Cryptococcus* species	All clinically important parasites
	Clostridium species	Calicivirus	*Candida* species	
	Corynebacterium diphtheriae	Coronavirus (not Co-V)	All dermatophytes	
	Escherichia coli	Herpesvirus	*Aspergillus* species	
	Enterobacteriaceae	Influenza virus		
	Mycobacteria other than *Mycobacterium tuberculosis*			
	Staphylococcus species			
	Streptococcus species			
3	*Bacillus anthracis*	Lymphocytic choriomeningitis	*Coccidioides immitis*	
		Hantaan virus		
	Brucella species	St. Louis encephalitis virus	*Blastomyces dermatitidis*	
	Coxiella burnetii	Japanese encephalitis virus	*Histoplasma capsulatum*	
	Francisella tularensis	Western equine encephalitis virus	*Paracoccidioides braziliensis*	
	Mycobacterium tuberculosis	West Nile encephalitis virus		
	Mycobacterium avium	SARS coronavirus		
		Prions		
4		Lassa virus		
		Marburg virus		
		Ebola virus		
		Herpes simiae virus		

[a]Based on reference 29a. This table is presented as a guide only. It should not be considered to be either complete or consistent with all jurisdictions. Specific national requirements may differ from the information presented in this table.

TABLE 2 Standard microbiology practices for all laboratories (biosafety level 2 and higher)[a]

1. A documented safety manual must be available for all staff.
2. Personnel must receive training on the potential hazards associated with the work involved and the necessary precautions to prevent exposure to infectious agents.
3. Eating, drinking, smoking, storing either food or personal belongings, and applying cosmetics are not permitted.
4. Mouth pipetting is prohibited.
5. Long hair is to be tied back or restrained.
6. Access to laboratory and support areas is limited to authorized personnel.
7. Doors to working areas in laboratories must not be left open.
8. Open wounds and cuts should be covered with waterproof dressings.
9. Laboratories are to be kept clean and tidy.
10. Protective laboratory clothing, properly fastened, and footwear with closed toes and heels must be worn by all personnel, visitors, trainees, and others working in the laboratory.
11. Eye and face protection must be used where there is a known or potential risk of exposure to splashes or flying objects.
12. Gloves must be worn for all procedures that may involve direct skin contact with biohazardous material. Gloves are to be removed when a laboratory task is completed and before leaving the laboratory.
13. Protective laboratory clothing must not be worn in nonlaboratory areas.
14. If known or suspected exposure occurs, contaminated clothing must be decontaminated before laundering.
15. The use of needles, syringes, and other sharp objects should be limited strictly. Needles should not be bent, sheared, recapped, or removed from the syringe; they should be promptly placed in a puncture-resistant sharps container for disposal.
16. Hands must be washed with an appropriate antiseptic soap or rubbed with an alcohol-based hand gel after gloves have been removed, before leaving the laboratory, and at any time after handling materials known or suspected to be contaminated.
17. Work surfaces must be cleaned and decontaminated with a suitable disinfectant at the end of the day and after any spill of potentially biohazardous material.
18. Contaminated materials and equipment that are removed from the laboratory for servicing or disposal must be appropriately decontaminated.
19. Autoclaves used for decontamination should be regularly monitored with biological indicators.
20. All contaminated materials must be decontaminated before disposal or reuse.
21. Leak-proof containers are to be used to transport infectious materials.
22. Spills, accidents, breaches of containment, or exposures to infectious materials must be reported immediately to the laboratory supervisor.
23. An effective rodent and insect control program must be maintained.

[a] Adapted from references 29a and 56a.

dynamic rather than a static interaction. Factors that influence risk include the specific biohazardous agents, the sample volumes, the concentrations of the agents in the samples, the most likely routes of exposure, the workload, host factors (e.g., immunosuppression or pregnancy), the complexity of the task, and the knowledge and experience of the worker.

ASSESSING RISK AND HAZARDS

To plan strategies for improving safety, the staff first must recognize risk factors, potential weak points in processes, and possible solutions. Regular laboratory audits can also help the staff recognize specific problems, and sometimes these problems can be solved by implementing or reactivating established guidelines. A failure modes and effects analysis can help the staff assess current approaches and plan improvements.

BIOSAFETY AND CLINICAL LABORATORY DESIGN

Persons designing laboratories, including the containment equipment and facilities, must know the classifications of microorganisms flowing into a laboratory. For research laboratories, where the microorganism load is known, the process of matching risk and containment is straightforward. However, in clinical laboratories, the contents of samples are usually unknown and specimens may contain microorganisms across the spectrum of classification. That being said, most isolates recovered from clinical samples are classified as biosafety level 1 or 2; thus, most clinical laboratories must be able to provide containment level 2 (Table 3). Laboratories that process viral cultures or investigate mycobacterial cultures should be designed to accommodate level 3. Laboratories that may handle exotic pathogens in risk group 4 must have high-containment level 4 facilities.

In the wake of the 2001 terrorist attacks in New York and the anthrax mail scares that happened shortly afterwards, microbiologists have become aware that laboratory biosafety measures are a component of bioterrorism defense (18, 35, 49, 53). Specific funding has been allocated for the construction of new national and regional biocontainment laboratories. Laboratories with increased levels of containment and security are useful not only for addressing possible bioterrorism and biosecurity issues but also for handling specimens from epidemics of emerging infections, such as severe acute respiratory syndrome (SARS) and pandemic influenza. These laboratories must control access to their facilities, systematize procedures for specimen receiving and disposal, develop incident reporting and emergency response plans, provide security for stored agents, and if appropriate, track specimens accurately and develop trace-back systems (40, 48, 49). Caution needs to be taken to ensure that the needs for confidentiality and information containment do not interfere with the open communications necessary for laboratory safety and public health (37).

TABLE 3 Laboratory design requirements for biosafety level 2 laboratories[a]

1. A space separated from public areas by lockable doors
2. Laboratory doors with appropriate signage
3. Door openings of sufficient size to allow safe passage of equipment
4. Work surfaces that are nonabsorptive and scratch, stain, chemical, and heat resistant
5. A means of treating waste before disposal must be readily available.
6. Windows designed to prevent ingress of flying insects
7. Separate spaces for street and laboratory clothing
8. Ready access to hand-washing sinks
9. Emergency showers and eye-washing stations
10. Biosafety cabinets and other primary containment equipment (recommended)
11. Hand-washing sinks that can be operated without hands (recommended)
12. An air supply of 100% outside air with no recirculation (recommended)

[a] Adapted from references 29a and 56a.

SAFETY EQUIPMENT AND THE CLINICAL LABORATORY

Splashguards

Splashguards, the minimum level of safety equipment, should be made of cleanable, clear glass or plastic and should be large enough to protect workers from gross splashes. Memos and procedure descriptions should not be taped onto splashguards because they prevent workers from seeing what they are doing. Splashguards can be effective barriers provided that they are appropriately placed with respect to both workflow and the workers' heights. Staff members can use splashguards as an appropriate alternative to biosafety cabinets when opening vacuum blood tubes.

Biosafety Cabinets

Biosafety cabinets can protect the laboratory worker and the laboratory environment from splashes and aerosols and also protect samples from becoming contaminated (55, 56). Class 1 cabinets have an open front and are under negative pressure with respect to the laboratory; these cabinets exhaust their air through a HEPA filter, and the exhausted air usually is returned to the work area. Class 2 cabinets increase the level of safety by including a HEPA-filtered downward-flow air curtain, which increases the degree of separation between the air in the room and the air in the cabinet. Class 2 cabinets may exhaust air back to room air (Class 2A) or through an exhaust system to the air outside the building (Class 2B). Class 2B cabinets can be further subclassified based on additional features. Class 3 cabinets are completely enclosed and provide gas-tight containment. They are accessible only through glove ports. Class 3 cabinets provide the most suitable containment for working with exotic pathogens. Because class 1 and class 2A units exhaust air into the laboratory, they should not be used to handle volatile chemicals and reagents. Because biological safety cabinets often have open heating elements or flames and may not have anticorrosive ductwork, they should not be used as alternatives to chemical fume hoods.

All safety cabinets must be tested and certified by a qualified person on a regular basis to ensure that they maintain their required face velocity and negative pressure. That being said, even properly maintained and certified cabinets can malfunction and put staff members at risk if equipment and materials are improperly placed inside the cabinet. If the cabinet is overcrowded or equipment is stacked against the front or back grill, airflow will be disrupted and contaminated air may backwash out the front of the unit.

Chemical Fume Protection

A fume hood is a mechanically ventilated, partially enclosed workspace where harmful volatile chemicals and reagents can be handled safely. The primary function of a fume hood is to contain and remove gases and vapors. Most fume hoods use ducts and a fan to capture heat and airborne chemical contaminants, transport them out of the work area, and discharge them into the atmosphere outside the building. Chemical fume hoods differ from biosafety cabinets in that they are usually ducted, must be constructed of noncombustible materials, and must be explosion proof. Nonducted, or recirculating, fume hoods cannot be used in the laboratory to contain volatile chemicals (17). Laboratories that work with specific highly corrosive reagents or chemicals such as perchloric acid or with radioisotopes need fume hoods designed to accommodate these agents.

Fume hoods must be placed in rooms with sufficient airflow that is properly balanced so that the air entering the fume hood is replaced and backwash into the room is prevented (17). Chemical fume hoods should be tested regularly for face velocity and for containment with the ASHRAE 110 tracer gas test. Face velocity alone is not a valid indication of containment (17).

Centrifuges

The safety centrifuge was first described in 1975 (28). However, accidental contamination of laboratories and personnel continues to occur because staff members do not use centrifuges properly (19, 27). Rotors can become contaminated if plastic centrifuge tubes crack or distort while being spun (27). If the O-ring seals on containers and rotors do not create a good seal, organisms can be aerosolized (29). Thus, centrifuges must be maintained properly (2) and must be used properly. Laboratories should maintain a log for each centrifuge that includes the rotor serial number, the speed in revolutions per minute, the spin duration, the time of use, and the operator's name for each use (2). Basic safety procedures for centrifuges include having workers (i) keep a centrifuge's lid closed while the centrifuge is operating, (ii) stay with a centrifuge until the full operating speed is attained and the machine is running without vibrating, (iii) stop immediately and check the load balances if the centrifuge vibrates, (iv) check swing-out buckets for clearance and support, (v) use a noncorrosive product to clean and disinfect rotors and cups after each use, (vi) report all spills and breakage to the laboratory safety officer, and (vii) clean spills as soon as aerosols have settled.

Sharps Protection

Scalpels, needles, broken glass, and other sharps commonly cause injuries and laboratory-2 acquired infections (7). To the extent possible, staff members either should not use sharps by hand or should use safety barriers (25). Because sharps may be contaminated with infectious or cytotoxic agents or both, they should be discarded in sharps containers.

Sharps containers minimize injuries and transmission of potentially harmful agents if they are readily accessible and appropriately used. Sharps containers used in medical laboratories should be designed specifically for sharps such as needles, syringes with needles, blades, clinical glass, and other items capable of causing cuts or punctures (25). Sharps containers should be leak proof and puncture resistant and should not degrade in autoclaves, either require no assembly or be easy to assemble, have a designated fill line, be appropriately labeled, and be available in a variety of sizes. Within this framework, manufacturers can implement a variety of designs. Sharps containers should resist toppling over and should be durable enough to withstand being dropped onto a hard surface (6). Containers that are not resistant to penetration or compression put staff members at risk. Tin cans or other containers should not be used in lieu of containers designed specifically for sharps.

Sharps containers must be labeled prominently with the universal biohazard symbol. In addition, sharps containers for sharps contaminated with cytotoxics must display the cytotoxic hazard symbol. The international color code is yellow for biohazardous medical sharps and red for cytotoxic medical waste including contaminated sharps.

Staff members should never force sharps into a container, and they should not fill containers to more than three-quarters of their maximum capacity to avoid accidents from overfilling. Once filled, sharps containers should be securely and irreversibly closed for containment. The containers should be sterilized in an autoclave and then disposed of in accordance with local requirements. Containers with sharps contaminated with cytotoxic or prion proteins must be incinerated.

Most sharps containers are designed for single use only. However, some commercial units that can be reused are now available. These containers must be transported to a central disposal unit where they can be opened safely, emptied, decontaminated, and redistributed.

REQUIREMENTS OF THE INTERNATIONAL ORGANIZATION FOR STANDARDIZATION

The International Organization for Standardization Technical Committee 212 has developed documents that medical laboratories should use to improve their performance, including ISO 15189:2003, *Medical Laboratories—Particular Requirements for Quality and Competence* (32c), and ISO 15190:2003, *Medical Laboratories—Requirements for Safety* (32d). In those countries where laboratories are certified or accredited according to International Organization for Standardization requirements, these documents are considered essential standards.

ISO 15190:2003 states that the laboratory's management is responsible for the safety of all employees and visitors to the laboratory and that ultimate responsibility rests with the laboratory director. The laboratory must identify an appropriately trained and experienced laboratory safety officer to assist the laboratory director and managers with safety issues. The laboratory safety officer must have the authority to stop activities that are deemed unsafe. The laboratory safety officer is responsible for designing and maintaining the laboratory safety program and for monitoring its effectiveness. The International Organization for Standardization requires that a laboratory safety program include a laboratory safety manual, safety audits (see Table 4 for audits required by ISO 15190:2003), inspections, risk assessments, and safety records. For further details, ISO 15190:2003 is available through the International Organization for Standardization website (www.iso.ch) or the Clinical and Laboratory Standards Institute (www.clsi.org).

TABLE 4 Laboratory safety audits required by ISO 15190:2003 (32d)

Health and safety policy
Written procedures that include safe work practices
Safety-oriented education and training of staff
Safety-oriented supervision
Use and maintenance of hazardous materials and substances
Health surveillance
First-aid equipment and services
Accident and illness investigations
Health and safety committee review
Records and statistics on accidents and near misses
Review of safety program
Regular site safety inspections

SAFETY PREPAREDNESS AND THE MATERIAL SAFETY DATA SHEET

Every laboratory should have a readily accessible written plan that staff members can use in case of emergencies or accidents. Laboratories can use published guidelines (25) as they prepare their own plan. In addition, up-to-date Material Safety Data Sheets (MSDS) for all chemicals and microorganisms; equipment and materials for containment of spills, including personal protective equipment, absorbent, and disinfectant (bleach or accelerated hydrogen peroxide); and personnel trained in first aid should be readily available, and their locations should be known by all staff members. Moreover, staff members should know the location of emergency equipment, including showers and eye-washing stations; should know routes for evacuation in case of a fire or a spill; and should practice evacuating regularly. Showers and eye-washing stations should be tested regularly to ensure that they will function when needed. A regular internal safety audit program should assess whether staff members are prepared to deal with accidents.

MSDS for chemicals should be obtained from the supplier, or may be available from a variety of commercial and free Internet sites. A list of MSDS for microorganisms is available through the Public Health Agency of Canada website (http://www.phac-aspc.gc.ca/msds-ftss/).

It is beyond the scope of this chapter to address the specifics of the medical management following accidents that involve infectious agents. That being said, laboratories should follow several steps if exposures occur. Staff members should (i) report every accident or injury, including those that are seemingly trivial (30), to the appropriate safety officer or supervisor; (ii) clean scratches and puncture wounds immediately; (iii) seek medical attention quickly, especially if it is recommended by first-aid attenders or occupational health advisors (5); and (iv) give the microorganism's MSDS to the clinician evaluating the injury if the likely or probable agent is known. In addition, staff members should investigate each incident to learn the details of the accident and to identify its root causes and recommend preventive measures. Subsequently, staff members should audit compliance with the recommendations to ensure that they have been incorporated into practice in a timely manner.

HAND HYGIENE AND THE USE OF PERSONAL PROTECTIVE EQUIPMENT

Hand Hygiene

Hand washing and hand antisepsis are the most useful techniques for preventing transmission of microorganisms and for protecting staff from laboratory-acquired infections (14). Hands can become contaminated when staff members collect samples, handle sample containers, handle contaminated equipment, or touch sample storage units.

Nonmedicated detergent-based soap products and water do not disrupt normal skin flora but can reduce the number of transient hand flora, including both bacteria and viruses (14, 54). The efficacy of hand washing with such products is directly related to the duration of the procedure. Plain soaps can dry and irritate skin. Plain soaps may be appropriate in public washrooms but are not appropriate in the clinical laboratory. A variety of antimicrobial products are available, including products containing chlorhexidine, triclosan, iodophors, and others. Staff members should consider issues such as the types of organisms processed by the laboratory and also characteristics of each product (e.g., the fragrance, consistency, and propensity to irritate and dry skin) when selecting products for use in the laboratory.

Waterless, alcohol-based hand hygiene products can be rapid and convenient alternatives to hand washing with water and antimicrobial soap products, especially when a sink with running water is not immediately accessible (38, 54). The efficacy of alcohol-based products may be reduced when staff members' hands are soiled or are contaminated with spore-forming organisms or nonenveloped viruses (54). Staff members should wash their hands with an antimicrobial soap and with water when their hands are visibly soiled or are contaminated with proteinaceous materials or with materials that have a high microbial load.

Gloves

Gloves can be an important barrier within the laboratory, provided that they are used appropriately (25). Clearly, gloves prevent damage when hands are exposed to heat, cold, and toxic materials. For example, staff members should use insulated gloves when they take materials out of −70°C freezers, when they work with liquid nitrogen, and when they remove materials from autoclaves. General purpose utility gloves (kitchen or rubber gloves) provide ample protection for cleaning of biological spills and for decontamination. Utility gloves can be cleaned and reused. They should be examined regularly for cracks, tears, and peeling, and damaged utility gloves should be discarded. Staff members handling chemical solvents, toxic chemicals, and dyes should not use utility gloves but rather should use chemical-resistant gloves that should be available in all laboratories that handle chemical solvents. Disposable gloves of latex, vinyl, or nitrile can effectively reduce exposure risk, especially for handling blood, body fluids, and excrement. These gloves are particularly important because staff members may be unaware of the abrasions on their hands (36). In specific settings, staff members may need gloves that are elbow or shoulder length.

Disposable gloves do not prevent needle stick injuries, but double gloving can reduce the volume of blood or body fluids carried by a needle. Cotton undergloves may provide more protection from sharps injuries than a second vinyl or latex glove. In the morgue, staff members may need to wear chain mail gloves. Gloves provide an important protective barrier; however, they may also be a source of harm. Vinyl, latex, or cotton undergloves can reduce contact irritation that some staff members note when using rubber gloves. If staff members wear gloves for long periods, moisture can damage the skin on their hands (16, 20, 47). Surveys of dentists who wear gloves for 6 h daily indicate that many, especially young women with preexisting eczema, develop glove intolerance including glove-related mucous membrane irritation such as conjunctivitis, rhinitis, and asthma (57).

Gloves are easily torn. In-use durability studies indicate that vinyl gloves may tear as often as 40% of the times they are used, depending upon the presence of powder and the length of the user's fingernails (36). Latex gloves are more durable but may cause atopic reactions.

Staff members must remove their gloves at the end of a task or when the task is interrupted to prevent environmental contamination and transmission of pathogenic organisms. Indeed, persons wearing contaminated gloves can contaminate the equipment (42) and can also transmit organisms that cause serious infections (46). Moreover, gloves reduce microbial contamination of the hands but do not prevent it entirely. Therefore, staff members must still use hand hygiene when they remove gloves. Phlebotomists often wear gloves while collecting specimens, but this may not be essential if the risk of exposure to blood and body fluids is sufficiently low or if gloves of an appropriate size or material are not readily available. Regardless of whether phlebotomists do or do not wear gloves while collecting specimens, they should always remove their gloves between patients and wash their hands or use an alcohol-based hand gel.

IMMUNIZATION

Mental alertness and good laboratory practices are the most important aspects of laboratory safety, but immunizations are also an important source of protection. Immunizations may not prevent infections, but usually they protect persons against serious illness. All laboratory staff, including pregnant women, should have a complete primary immunization with tetanus and diphtheria toxoids and should receive a booster every 10 years (4). Laboratory workers who have direct contact with patients and those with chronic pulmonary or cardiovascular disease or other chronic illnesses including diabetes mellitus and renal dysfunction or who are immunocompromised should receive the influenza immunization annually. All staff members with possible occupational exposure to human blood and body fluids should receive the hepatitis B vaccine.

Cases of meningococcal illness possibly linked to laboratory exposure have been identified (3, 13, 21). Thus, microbiologists who are routinely exposed to meningococci, especially if these organisms may be aerosolized, should consider receiving meningococcal immunization. Laboratorians working with specific pathogens and in specific situations should consider additional immunizations such as a human diploid cell rabies vaccine, typhoid vaccine, and vaccinia vaccine (39, 41). In the past, *Mycobacterium bovis* BCG vaccination was considered of value for health care workers; however, it is no longer recommended as a primary strategy for controlling tuberculosis because the protective efficacy of the vaccine in health care workers is uncertain (8). Prior immunization with BCG may cause difficulty in the interpretation of tuberculin skin test responses following true infection with *Mycobacterium tuberculosis* (15).

LABORATORY-ACQUIRED HIV INFECTION, HEPATITIS B, AND HEPATITIS C

Laboratory workers are at risk for exposure to hepatitis C virus (HCV), hepatitis B virus (HBV), and human immunodeficiency virus (HIV). However, safeguards introduced into medical laboratories have decreased the risk. For example, after the hepatitis B vaccine was introduced in 1982, the incidence of hepatitis B infection was decreased by more than 95% (25).

According to the Division of Health Care Quality Promotion of the Centers for Disease Control and Prevention (http://www.cdc.gov/ncidod/hip/BLOOD/hivpersonnel.htm), between 1978 and December 2001, only 16 clinical laboratory workers acquired HIV infection occupationally; 17 other persons may have acquired their infections in laboratories. We have no information on the prevalence of hepatitis C in health care workers. However, the National Center for Infectious Diseases estimates that about 2 health care workers out of 100 (1.8%) will become infected with HCV (range, 0 to 10%) after injuries with needles or sharps contaminated with HCV-positive blood (http://www.cdc.gov/ncidod/diseases/hepatitis/c/faq.htm#1h).

Given the publicity about bloodborne pathogens, laboratory directors may assume that their employees understand the epidemiology of these organisms and will take steps to protect themselves. However, recent surveys of health care workers demonstrate that existing and new staff members need to be educated frequently (51).

LABORATORY-ACQUIRED PARASITIC INFECTIONS

In her extensive review, Herwaldt has described 200 cases of laboratory-acquired parasitic infections occurring between 1929 and 1999 (30). Although the distribution of infection-associated pathogens changed from decade to decade, the number of cases identified in each decade (19 to 28) remained relatively constant. Sharps (needle and glass) injuries were common factors, often occurring when workers manipulated research animals or produced blood smears for malaria.

PRIONS

Samples from patients with Creutzfeldt-Jakob disease (CJD) may be submitted to the laboratory for investigation. To date there are no known cases of laboratory-acquired CJD and there is no evidence that laboratorians are at increased risk of developing CJD. That being said, staff members who handle samples should wear gloves and should discard samples as medical waste. No special precautions are required for disposal of body fluids (50).

Prions are extremely difficult to inactivate. Therefore, equipment that has been exposed to tissues, especially those of neurological origin, from patients with CJD should either be disposed of if they do not tolerate heat or autoclaved at 134°C for 18 min (prevacuum sterilizer) or at 121 to 132°C for 1 h (gravity displacement sterilizer). Autoclaving in water may be more effective than autoclaving in its absence (26). Equipment may also be soaked in 1N NaOH for 1 h (26, 34). Work surfaces that may have been contaminated by the tissue should be cleaned with a 1:10 dilution of sodium hypochlorite. Other chemical treatments that have been described as milder alternatives include a combination of proteinase K and sodium dodecyl sulfate (34), proteinase K followed by an alkaline cleaner, and proteinase K followed by treatment in vaporized hydrogen peroxide (26).

Variant CJD is unique among human prion disease because the prion protein accumulates in follicular dentritic cells of lymphoid tissue (31, 33). In the United kingdom, studies of lymphoid tissue have identified the presence of prion protein (PrP) in appendices and tonsils (32). This has led to concern of possible contamination of blood, transplant tissues, and surgical instruments. The presence of long-term asymptomatic carriage and the absence of readily available diagnostic tests and a definitive significance of the findings make it difficult to implement new specific policies and procedures for processing routine samples and cleaning surgical and pathology equipment.

SARS CORONAVIRUS

The outbreak of SARS caused by a coronavirus raised international concern among the infection control and laboratory communities about the hazards of aerosol spread of communicable viruses. Information collected during the epidemic demonstrated that staff members in microbiology laboratories and those who receive and accession respiratory samples, especially via vacuum tube delivery systems, may have been at risk (44). However, the virus could be readily contained (10). In fact, laboratory workers had one of the lowest rates of illness or serological conversion and only one death was suspected to result from a laboratory accident, which occurred in a level 4 facility (44).

To ensure that laboratory workers are safe while working with the SARS coronavirus, guidelines developed in Singapore recommend that staff members in laboratories equipped and designed at biosafety level 2 use practices more consistent with biosafety level 3, such as opening specimen containers and handling the samples only in biosafety cabinets (10). In addition, samples should be centrifuged only in sealed safety buckets that are opened within a cabinet. Finally, N95 respirators should be considered for additional protection.

LABORATORY-ACQUIRED INFECTIONS AND EXTERNAL QUALITY ASSESSMENT

Infections acquired in clinical laboratories are not always associated with clinical samples. Documented clusters of bacterial infections have been associated with samples sent to laboratories for proficiency testing (12), and quality control organisms have contaminated other samples in laboratories (1). Regardless of the source of the specimens, staff members in clinical microbiology laboratories must use appropriate biosafety practices when handling any and all viable microorganisms.

SAFETY AND POINT OF CARE

Medical laboratories are responsible for all laboratory tests, even those performed outside of the laboratory itself. Increasingly, medical laboratories are responsible for point-of-care testing for monitoring of blood glucose, coagulation, and oxygenation. Despite the improved equipment and hygiene protocols, patients continue to acquire hepatitis B and C from

TABLE 5 Electronic information sources and resources

Organization or Publication	Abbreviation	Website
Occupational Safety and Health Administration	OSHA	http://www.osha.gov
Clinical Laboratory Improvement Act	CLIA	http://www.cms.hhs.gov/clia
Code of *Federal Register*	CFR	http://www.gpoaccess.gov/cfr/
Department of Transportation	DOT	http://www.dot.gov
Nonregulatory International Organization for Standardization	ISO	http://www.iso.org
Clinical and Laboratory Standards Institute	CLSI	http://www.clsi.org
American Biosafety Association	ABSA	http://www.absa.org
International Air Transport Association	IATA	http://www.iata.org
Public Health Agency of Canada's MSDS "Infectious Substances"	PHAC	http://www.phac-aspc.gc.ca/msds-ftss/msds12e.html

contaminated point-of-care devices. To prevent transmission of bloodborne pathogens when staff members use these devices, they must adhere strictly to infection control protocols for use and cleaning of this equipment. The International Organization for Standardization final draft international standard ISO/FDIS 22870, *Point-of-Care Testing (POCT) Requirements for Quality and Competence* (32b), provides guidance on quality management for point-of-care testing.

TRANSPORTATION OF SAMPLES

Laboratories are responsible to prevent, to the extent possible, people from being exposed to infectious agents that are present in laboratory samples, including samples being transported to and from the laboratory. The laboratory should ensure that leak-proof containers are available for transporting specimens within a clinic or hospital and that the containers are transported in a secure outer package such as a sealable plastic bag, preferably emblazoned with the international biohazard label. Samples that are transported outside of the facility should be packaged in a secure, firm outer container. The sample container itself should be surrounded with materials that protect it and that also could absorb a spill if the container was damaged. Specimens transported outside the facility, especially by road, rail, water, or air, must be packaged and shipped according to local and federal regulations. Most jurisdictions prohibit transporting samples of infectious agents through the postal service.

Air transport of microorganisms is governed by federal regulations that must comply with the requirements of the International Civil Aviation Organization (ICAO) as adopted by the International Air Transport Association. The ICAO specifies the requirements for packaging and labeling, including the proper shipping name and appropriate UN number, for samples known to contain infectious agents based on the sources of the samples and the likely pathogens contained. Every laboratory that transports samples is required to have at least one person who is certified in knowing the requirements for packaging and transport, including how to complete the shipping documents.

For additional information, staff members can refer to the ICAO's *Technical Instructions for the Safe Transport of Dangerous Goods by Air* (32a) or to federal requirements (http://hazmat.dot.gov/regs/rules.htm).

ELECTRONIC INFORMATION SOURCES AND RESOURCES

Laboratory safety is a primary focus of interest for many organizations. Some of the agencies have the authority to regulate laboratory practices in their specific nation or area of jurisdiction. Nonregulatory sites, including international organizations, can provide instructive materials that aid laboratory staff in improving their safety programs. Table 5 contains a list of sites that provide important current safety information.

REFERENCES

1. **Anonymous.** 13 April 2005, posting date. CAP *Laboratories Alerted to Destroy an Influenza A Specimen Included in Some Proficiency Testing Kits.* [Online.] College of American Pathologists, Northfield, Ill. http://www.cap.org/apps/docs/statements/statement_ptinfluenza.html.
2. **Anonymous.** 2004. *General Safety and Laboratory Policies: Centrifuge Safety.* [Online.] National Institute of Environmental Health Sciences. http://www.niehs.nih.gov/odhsb/manual/man4a.htm.
3. **Anonymous.** 2002. Laboratory-acquired meningococcal disease—United States, 2000. *Morb. Mortal. Wkly. Rep.* **51:**141–144.
4. **Anonymous.** 2003. Recommended adult immunization schedule—United States, 2003–2004. *Morb. Mortal. Wkly. Rep.* **52:**965–969.
5. **Anonymous.** 2001. Updated U.S. Public Health Service guidelines for the management of occupational exposures to HBV, HCV, and HIV and recommendations for postexposure prophylaxis. *Morb. Mortal. Wkly. Rep.* **50:**1–42.
6. **Anonymous.** 2002. *Evaluation of Single-Use Medical Sharps Containers for Biohazardous and Cytotoxic Waste,* vol. Z316.6-02. Canadian Standards Association, Missisauga, Ontario, Canada.
7. **Ansa, V. O., E. J. Udoma, M. S. Umoh, and M. U. Anah.** 2002. Occupational risk of infection by human immunodeficiency and hepatitis B viruses among health workers in south-eastern Nigeria. *East Afr. Med. J.* **79:**254–256.
8. **Aronson, N. E., M. Santosham, G. W. Comstock, R. S. Howard, L. H. Moulton, E. R. Rhoades, and L. H. Harrison.** 2004. Long-term efficacy of BCG vaccine in American Indians and Alaska Natives: a 60-year follow-up study. *JAMA* **291:**2086–2091.
9. **Ashdown, L. R.** 1992. Melioidosis and safety in the clinical laboratory. *J. Hosp. Infect.* **21:**301–306.
10. **Barkham, T. M.** 2004. Laboratory safety aspects of SARS at Biosafety Level 2. *Ann. Acad. Med. Singapore* **33:**252–256.
11. **Birt, C., and C. Lamb.** 1899. Mediterranean or Malta fever. *Lancet* **i:**701–710.
12. **Blaser, M. J., and J. P. Lofgren.** 1981. Fatal salmonellosis originating in a clinical microbiology laboratory. *J. Clin. Microbiol.* **13:**855–858.
13. **Boutet, R., J. M. Stuart, E. B. Kaczmarski, S. J. Gray, D. M. Jones, and N. Andrews.** 2001. Risk of laboratory-acquired meningococcal disease. *J. Hosp. Infect.* **49:**282–284.

14. **Boyce, J. M., and D. Pittet.** 2002. Guideline for hand hygiene in health-care settings. Recommendations of the Healthcare Infection Control Practices Advisory Committee and the HIPAC/SHEA/APIC/IDSA Hand Hygiene Task Force. *Am. J. Infect. Control* **30:**S1–S46.
15. **Bugiani, M., A. Borraccino, E. Migliore, A. Carosso, P. Piccioni, M. Cavallero, E. Caria, G. Salamina, and W. Arossa.** 2003. Tuberculin reactivity in adult BCG-vaccinated subjects: a cross-sectional study. *Int. J. Tuberc. Lung Dis.* **7:**320–326.
16. **Burke, F. J., N. H. Wilson, and S. W. Cheung.** 1995. Factors associated with skin irritation of the hands experienced by general dental practitioners. *Contact Dermatitis* **32:**35–38.
17. **Canadian Standards Association.** 2004. *Fume Hoods and Associated Exhaust Systems,* vol. Z316.5. Canadian Standards Association, Toronto, Canada.
18. **Canton, R.** 2005. Role of the microbiology laboratory in infectious disease surveillance, alert and response. *Clin. Microbiol. Infect.* **11**(Suppl. 1):3–8.
19. **Chang, C. L., H. H. Kim, H. C. Son, S. S. Park, M. K. Lee, S. K. Park, W. W. Park, and C. H. Jeon.** 2001. False-positive growth of *Mycobacterium tuberculosis* attributable to laboratory contamination confirmed by restriction fragment length polymorphism analysis. *Int. J. Tuberc. Lung Dis.* **5:**861–867.
20. **Checchi, L., M. R. Gatto, P. Legnani, G. A. Pelliccioni, and P. Bisbini.** 1999. Use of gloves and prevalence of glove-related reactions in a sample of general dental practitioners in Italy. *Quintessence Int.* **30:**633–636.
21. **Christen, G., and D. Tagan.** 2004. Laboratory-acquired *Neisseria meningitidis* infection. *Med. Mal. Infect.* **34:** 137–138. (In French.)
22. **Collins, C.** 1983. *Laboratory Acquired Infections: History, Incidence, Causes and Preventions.* Butterworth's, London, England.
23. **Collins, C. H., and D. A. Kennedy.** 1999. *Laboratory Acquired Infections,* 4th ed. Butterworth-Heinemann, Oxford, England.
24. **Dale, J. C., S. K. Pruett, and M. D. Maker.** 1998. Accidental needlesticks in the phlebotomy service of the Department of Laboratory Medicine and Pathology at Mayo Clinic Rochester. *Mayo Clin. Proc.* **73:**611–615.
25. **David, L., and P. Sewell (ed.).** 2005. *Protection of Laboratory Workers from Occupationally Acquired Infections; Approved Guideline,* 3rd ed., vol. 21. Clinical and Laboratory Standards Institute, Wayne, Pa.
26. **Fichet, G., E. Comoy, C. Duval, K. Antloga, C. Dehen, A. Charbonnier, G. McDonnell, P. Brown, C. I. Lasmezas, and J. P. Deslys.** 2004. Novel methods for disinfection of prion-contaminated medical devices. *Lancet* **364:**521–526.
27. **Fiori, P. L., S. Mastrandrea, P. Rappelli, and P. Cappuccinelli.** 2000. *Brucella abortus* infection acquired in microbiology laboratories. *J. Clin. Microbiol.* **38:**2005–2006.
28. **Hall, C. V.** 1975. A biological safety centrifuge. *Health Lab. Sci.* **12:**104–106.
29. **Hambleton, P., and G. Dedonato.** 1992. Protecting researchers from instrument biohazards. *BioTechniques* **13:**450–453.

29a. **Health Canada.** 2004. *Laboratory Biosafety Guidelines,* 3rd ed. Health Canada, Ottawa, Canada.

30. **Herwaldt, B. L.** 2001. Laboratory-acquired parasitic infections from accidental exposures. *Clin. Microbiol. Rev.* **14:**659–688.
31. **Hilton, D. A.** 2006. Pathogenesis and prevalence of variant Creutzfeldt-Jakob disease. *J. Pathol.* **208:**134–141.
32. **Hilton, D. A., A. C. Ghani, L. Conyers, P. Edwards, L. McCardle, D. Ritchie, M. Penney, D. Hegazy, and J. W. Ironside.** 2004. Prevalence of lymphoreticular prion protein accumulation in UK tissue samples. *J. Pathol.* **203:**733–739.

32a. **International Civil Aviation Organization.** *Technical Instructions for the Safe Transport of Dangerous Goods by Air.* International Civil Aviation Organization.

32b. **International Organization for Standardization.** *Point-of-Care Testing (POCT) Requirements for Quality and Competence; Final Draft.* International standard ISO/FDIS 22870. International Organization for Standardization, Geneva, Switzerland.

32c. **International Organization for Standardization Technical Committee 212.** 2003. *Medical Laboratories—Particular Requirements for Quality and Competence.* ISO 15189:2003. International Organization for Standardization, Geneva, Switzerland.

32d. **International Organization for Standardization Technical Committee 212.** 2003. *Medical Laboratories—Requirements for Safety.* ISO 15190:2003. International Organization for Standardization, Geneva, Switzerland.

33. **Ironside, J. W.** 2000. Pathology of variant Creutzfeldt-Jakob disease. *Arch. Virol. Suppl.* **2000:**143–151.
34. **Jackson, G. S., E. McKintosh, E. Flechsig, K. Prodromidou, P. Hirsch, J. Linehan, S. Brandner, A. R. Clarke, C. Weissmann, and J. Collinge.** 2005. An enzyme-detergent method for effective prion decontamination of surgical steel. *J. Gen. Virol.* **86:**869–878.
35. **James, G., M. Yuen, and L. Gilbert.** 2003. Laboratory investigation of suspected bioterrorism incidents, New South Wales, October 2001 to February 2002. *N. S. W. Public Health Bull.* **14:**221-223.
36. **Jungbauer, F. H., J. J. van der Harst, J. W. Groothoff, and P. J. Coenraads.** 2004. Skin protection in nursing work: promoting the use of gloves and hand alcohol. *Contact Dermatitis* **51:**135–140.
37. **Kahn, L. H.** 2004. Biodefense research: can secrecy and safety coexist? *Biosecur. Bioterror.* **2:**81–85.
38. **Kampf, G., and A. Kramer.** 2004. Epidemiologic background of hand hygiene and evaluation of the most important agents for scrubs and rubs. *Clin. Microbiol. Rev.* **17:**863–893.
39. **Loeb, M., I. Zando, M. C. Orvidas, A. Bialachowski, D. Groves, and J. Mahoney.** 2003. Laboratory-acquired vaccinia infection. *Can. Commun. Dis. Rep.* **29:**134–136.
40. **Logan-Henfrey, L.** 2000. Mitigation of bioterrorist threats in the 21st century. *Ann. N. Y. Acad. Sci.* **916:**121–133.
41. **Mempel, M., G. Isa, N. Klugbauer, H. Meyer, G. Wildi, J. Ring, F. Hofmann, and H. Hofmann.** 2003. Laboratory acquired infection with recombinant vaccinia virus containing an immunomodulating construct. *J. Investig. Dermatol.* **120:**356–358.
42. **Neely, A. N., and D. F. Sittig.** 2002. Basic microbiologic and infection control information to reduce the potential transmission of pathogens to patients via computer hardware. *J. Am. Med. Inform. Assoc.* **9:**500–508.
43. **Noble, M.** 2005. Biological safety for the clinical laboratory, p. 760–768. *In* S. P. Borriello, P. R. Murray, and G. Funke (ed.), *Topley and Wilson's Microbiology & Microbial Infections,* 10th ed., vol. 1. *Bacteriology.* Hodder Arnold, London, England.
44. **Orellana, C.** 2004. Laboratory-acquired SARS raises worries on biosafety. *Lancet Infect. Dis.* **4:**64.
45. **Phillips, G. B.** 1986. Human factors in microbiological laboratory accidents, p. 43–48. *In* B. M. Miller (ed.), *Laboratory Safety: Principles and Practices.* American Society for Microbiology, Washington, D.C.
46. **Piro, S., M. Sammud, S. Badi, and L. Al Ssabi.** 2001. Hospital-acquired malaria transmitted by contaminated gloves. *J. Hosp. Infect.* **47:**156–158.
47. **Ramsing, D. W., and T. Agner.** 1996. Effect of glove occlusion on human skin. I. Short-term experimental exposure. *Contact Dermatitis* **34:**1–5.
48. **Richmond, J. Y., and S. L. Nesby-O'Dell.** 2002. Laboratory security and emergency response guidance for

laboratories working with select agents. *Morb. Mortal. Wkly. Rep.* **51**(RR-19):1–6.

49. **Robinson-Dunn, B.** 2002. The microbiology laboratory's role in response to bioterrorism. *Arch. Pathol. Lab. Med.* **126**:291–294.
50. **Rutala, W. A., and D. J. Weber.** 2001. Creutzfeldt-Jakob disease: recommendations for disinfection and sterilization. *Clin. Infect. Dis.* **32**:1348–1356.
51. **Scoular, A., A. D. Watt, M. Watson, and B. Kelly.** 2000. Knowledge and attitudes of hospital staff to occupational exposure to bloodborne viruses. *Commun. Dis. Public Health* **3**:247–249.
52. **Sewell, D.** 1995. Laboratory-associated infections and biosafety. *Clin. Microbiol. Rev.* **8**:389–405.
53. **Sewell, D. L.** 2003. Laboratory safety practices associated with potential agents of biocrime or bioterrorism. *J. Clin. Microbiol.* **41**:2801–2809.
54. **Sickbert-Bennett, E. E., D. J. Weber, M. F. Gergen-Teague, M. D. Sobsey, G. P. Samsa, and W. A. Rutala.** 2005. Comparative efficacy of hand hygiene agents in the reduction of bacteria and viruses. *Am. J. Infect. Control* **33**:67–77.
55. **Simhon, A., G. Rahav, M. Shapiro, and C. Block.** 2001. Skin disease presenting as an outbreak of pseudobacteremia in a laboratory worker. *J. Clin. Microbiol.* **39**:392–393.
56. **Thomson, R. B., Jr., S. J. Vanzo, N. K. Henry, K. L. Guenther, and J. A. Washington II.** 1984. Contamination of cultures processed with the isolator lysis-centrifugation blood culture tube. *J. Clin. Microbiol.* **19**:97–99.

56a. **U.S. Department of Health and Human Services.** 1999. *Biosafety in Microbiological and Biomedical Laboratories*, 4th ed. U.S. Department of Health and Human Services, Washington, D.C.

57. **Wrangsjo, K., L. M. Wallenhammar, U. Ortengren, L. Barregard, H. Andreasson, B. Bjorkner, S. Karlsson, and B. Meding.** 2001. Protective gloves in Swedish dentistry: use and side-effects. *Br. J. Dermatol.* **145**:32–37.

Laboratory Detection of Potential Agents of Bioterrorism*

ROSEMARY HUMES AND JAMES W. SNYDER

9

Since the events of 11 September 2001 and the anthrax release in October 2001, bioterrorism preparedness and response have remained a high priority for the nation. Clinical microbiology laboratories serve as sentinels with the major responsibility to raise suspicion of a possible bioterrorism-associated agent based on the information gleaned from the recovery of a suspicious microbial agent. Consequently, clinical microbiologists must be familiar, through education and training, with the targeted agents of bioterrorism and the application of standardized diagnostic procedures designed to rule out or refer such agents for confirmatory testing. Clinical and public health laboratories must enhance their partnerships and communication to ensure that potential bioterrorism events are detected early. This chapter provides an overview of the most important issues. Other American Society for Microbiology (ASM) publications on this subject include references 15 and 21, the second edition of the *Clinical Microbiology Procedures Handbook* (18), and the ASM website (http://www.asm.org). The Centers for Disease Control and Prevention (CDC) also provides extensive information on bioterrorism preparedness and the agents of concern on its website (http://www.bt.cdc.gov).

HISTORY

There is evidence of germ warfare dating back to the ancient Greeks and Romans, long before individuals understood the germ theory of disease or deliberately tried to produce biological weapons of mass destruction. The U.S. Army and Air Force had an offensive biological weapons research program at Fort Detrick, Md., from 1942 to 1969. The Biological and Toxic Weapon Convention in 1972 resulted in an agreement that development of biological weapons should be stopped worldwide (9, 28). Most Western governments ceased their offensive programs; however, the former Soviet Union activated a clandestine program that was called Biopreparat. Following his defection from the Soviet Union in 1992, Ken Alibeck, Deputy Director of Biopreparat, revealed important details about the program's development of a variety of bioterrorist agents (1, 11).

Immediately following the Gulf War of 1991, the United Nations' inspectors in Iraq found evidence that Saddam Hussein had been building a bioweapons program, and they destroyed all biologic material that was found. Concerned that Iraq had reestablished a program to create weapons of mass destruction, the U.S. government developed extensive smallpox response plans and vaccinated health care workers, first responders, and soldiers in 2003, before the second Gulf War (2). However, UN inspectors did not find any evidence of an active bioweapons program when the regime fell.

Prior to 2001, the most well-known example of bioterrorism in the United States occurred in 1984, when followers of Bhagwan Shree Rajneesh sprayed an aerosolized form of *Salmonella enterica* serovar Typhimurium on salad bars at two local restaurants in Dalles, Oreg., to prevent local citizens from voting in an upcoming election. The resulting outbreak affected 750 people (35).

The threat posed by bioterrorism and the panic caused by such events were demonstrated in the fall of 2001, when 23 cases of anthrax (12 cases of inhalational anthrax and 7 confirmed and 4 suspected cases of cutaneous anthrax) occurred among persons in the District of Columbia, Florida, New Jersey, New York, and Connecticut after an unidentified perpetrator mailed *Bacillus anthracis* spores in letters (5–7, 19, 20, 23, 24, 36). Law enforcement personnel, public health officials, and community health care providers, including clinical laboratories, were inundated by citizens who found powdery substances, letters, packages, and other materials which they were certain contained anthrax spores. More than 125,000 samples were tested, many in areas where there was no evidence of anthrax contamination (27). This outbreak and its aftermath demonstrated that federal, state, community, and institutional bioterrorism readiness plans needed to be updated. Clinical microbiologists have an essential role in these plans; they will likely be the first to detect the etiologic agent(s) and must promptly report their results to the proper authorities. Consequently, clinical microbiologists should have a general understanding of biological terrorism, including the technical and administrative principles that will help them recognize and manage such an event.

GENERAL FEATURES OF BIOTERRORISM

Definitions

Biological terrorism (bioterrorism) is defined as "the intentional use of microorganisms or toxins derived from living organisms to produce death or disease in humans, animals,

* This chapter contains information presented in chapter 10 by James W. Snyder and Alice S. Weissfeld in the eighth edition of this Manual.

or plants." From the public and private health perspective, bioterrorism can be defined as the deliberate release of pathogens or toxins into a civilian population with the intent to cause illness or death (17, 19, 21). Humans, agricultural animals, and plants could be targets of bioterrorism (17, 39).

Biological warfare refers to using biological agents (i.e., microbial pathogens and/or toxins) indiscriminately against masses of people including either military personnel or civilians. The terms biocrime or biothreat are used when a bioterrorist, which may be an individual or a state- or nonstate-sponsored group, targets a specific group or individual. A biocrime is a criminal act in which biological agents are used as weapons, and a biothreat is characterized as a suspected but unconfirmed release of a biological agent(s) (15). The bioterrorism-associated cases of anthrax that occurred in the United States in October and November 2001 are examples of a biocrime.

Bioterrorism events are categorized as either overt or covert. A covert event or attack will not be recognized immediately because of the delay between exposure and onset of illness (i.e., the incubation period). For example, the case of inhalational anthrax in the journalist from Florida in 2001 represented a *covert* event because the etiology was unknown until gram-positive bacilli were seen in the patient's cerebral spinal fluid, but the subsequent anthrax cases were *overt* events because the contaminated letters contained a note announcing the threat. As exemplified in the Florida case, emergency medicine physicians and other primary health care providers, including clinical microbiologists, will most likely identify the first cases in a covert event (8).

Characteristics Suggesting Biological Attacks

Covert attacks pose the greatest challenge to early detection; thus, microbiologists should be aware of the epidemiological and microbiological clues that suggest that an act of bioterrorism or a biocrime has occurred (21; U.S. Army Medical Research Institute of Infectious Diseases (USAMRIID): Biological Warfare and Terrorism Medical Issues and Response Satellite Broadcast, 26 to 28 September 2000). Some key indicators are as follows:

- A single case of a disease is caused by an uncommon agent (e.g., *Burkholderia mallei*, *Burkholderia pseudomallei*, or hemorrhagic fever virus)
- Large numbers of people have unexplained diseases or die unexpectedly
- A disease does not occur naturally in a given geographic area
- The illness is unusual (or atypical) for a given population or age group, or presents in an unusual fashion
- The incidence of a disease (e.g., tularemia or plague) increases substantially above its stable endemic rate
- Unusual deaths or illness among animals precedes or accompanies illness or death in humans
- Isolates from distinct sources at different times or locations have a similar genetic type
- The agent is transmitted in an atypical manner through aerosols, food, or water, suggesting deliberate sabotage

CATEGORIZATION OF BIOLOGICAL AGENTS

Biological agents are classified as pathogens or toxins. The CDC and its affiliated partners developed a targeted (critical) agent list (Table 1) based on (i) the agent's ability to cause mass casualties, be widely disseminated, and be transmitted from person to person and (ii) the public's likely perceptions of a potential intentional release of particular agents. Although few individuals or terrorist groups possess the scientific and

TABLE 1 Critical biological agent categories for public health preparedness

Biological agent(s)	Disease
Category A[a]	
Bacillus anthracis	Anthrax
Clostridium botulinum (botulinum toxins)	Botulism
Francisella tularensis	Tularemia
Yersinia pestis	Plague
Variola major	Smallpox
Filoviruses and Arenaviruses (e.g., Ebola virus, Lassa virus)	Viral hemorrhagic fevers
Category B[b]	
Coxiella burnetii	Q fever
Brucella spp.	Brucellosis
Burkholderia mallei	Glanders
Burkholderia pseudomallei	Melioidosis
Alphaviruses (VEE, EEE, WEE)[c]	Viral encephalitis
Rickettsia prowazekii	Epidemic typhus
Toxins (e.g., ricin, staphylococcal enterotoxin B, *Clostridium perfringens* epsilon toxin)	Toxic syndromes
Chlamydia psittaci	Psittacosis
Food safety threats (e.g., *Salmonella* spp., *Escherichia coli* O157:H7, *Shigella* spp.)	Gastroenteritis, hemolytic uremic syndrome
Water safety threats (e.g., *Vibrio cholerae*, *Cryptosporidium parvum*)	Gastroenteritis
Category C	
Emerging pathogens and potential risks for the future	
Emerging threat agents (e.g., Nipah virus, hantavirus)	

[a] Agents that pose the greatest threat due to their infectiousness relative, ease of transmission, or high mortality.
[b] Agents having a moderate ease of transmission and morbidity with a low rate of mortality.
[c] VEE, Venezuelan equine virus; EEE, eastern equine encephalomyelitis virus; WEE, western equine encephalomyelitis virus.

technical resources needed to weaponize and successfully disperse an agent via aerosol (the most likely mode of dispersal), the targeted agents possess unique advantages that make them suitable for bioterrorism or biocrimes.

The CDC has defined biothreat levels (A to C) to categorize the critical agents on the basis of their threat to national security, their ability to cause morbidity and mortality, and their potential for genetic engineering. Category A organisms are considered to pose the greatest threat to national security because they (i) can be easily disseminated or transmitted from person to person; (ii) cause high mortality; (iii) may afflict large numbers of people, overwhelming the health care and public health systems; (iv) may cause public panic and social disruption; and (v) require special preparations such as enhanced surveillance, enhanced diagnostic capabilities in microbiology laboratories, and stockpiles of medicines and equipment to protect the public's health. Category B agents are moderately easy to disseminate, cause moderate morbidity and low mortality, and challenge the national capacity for surveillance and diagnosis. This category includes pathogens that are foodborne or waterborne (e.g., *Salmonella* species, *Shigella dysenteriae, Escherichia coli* O157:H7, *Vibrio cholerae,* and *Cryptosporidium parvum*). Category C agents are primarily emerging pathogens that could be engineered for mass dissemination in the future (8, 25, 30).

PREPAREDNESS AND RESPONSE TO BIOTERRORISM

The U.S. Department of Homeland Security (DHS) was created in 2002 to prevent and deter terrorist attacks, protect citizens from threats and hazards, and respond to possible attacks. As defined in the 2003 Homeland Security Presidential Directive/HSPD-5, DHS serves as the lead agency in managing and coordinating the national response to acts of terrorism, natural disasters, or other emergencies (http://www.dhs.gov, www.fema.gov/pdf/reg-ii/hspd_5.pdf). The Federal Emergency Management Agency (FEMA), responsible for planning for and responding to disasters and for helping communities mitigate and recover from catastrophes, became part of DHS in March 2003.

A National Response Plan (NRP), National Incident Management System (NIMS), and Interim National Preparedness Goal (NPG) have been developed to provide standards for planning and response. Bioterrorism preparedness has been integrated into all-hazards—chemical, biologic, radiologic, nuclear, explosive (CBRNE)—emergency response planning. Several Homeland Security Presidential Directives establish roles for other federal agencies, including the Department of Health and Human Services (HHS) and the Environmental Protection Agency, in prevention of and response to CBRNE. The Federal Bureau of Investigation (FBI) is the federal agency that leads criminal investigations.

The Department of Defense has created over 32 "weapons of mass destruction civil support teams" (WMD-CST) that help local and state authorities respond to CBRNE domestic incidents of terrorism. The WMD-CSTs identify agents and substances, assess consequences, advise local and state authorities about how to respond, and assist with requests for additional military support. Additional CST teams are being added to provide coverage in every state (http://www.globalsecurity.org/military/agency/army/wmd-cst.htm; http://www.defenselink.mil/news/Jan2004/n01202004_200401201.html).

Professional organizations for the first responder and medical communities have developed numerous training programs and online resources. The Association of Professionals in Infection Control and Epidemiology and the CDC developed a Bioterrorism Preparedness and Response Program for hospitals to use in creating institutional plans for disease surveillance, epidemiologic investigation, rapid laboratory diagnosis, communication, and assessing readiness (12; http://www.apic.org/Content/NavigationMenu/PracticeGuidance/Topics/Bioterrorism/APIC_BTWG_BTRSugg.pdf). In addition, ASM has included on its website a template that clinical microbiology laboratories can use to create a bioterrorism response plan.

Since 2000, HHS, through the CDC, has provided funding to state and city health departments to enhance local emergency preparedness. Public health laboratories have received funding to rebuild infrastructure and to improve their molecular detection capabilities and the biosafety and biosecurity in existing facilities (38). The CDC has also established a strategic national stockpile of supplies necessary for treating persons affected by bioemergencies, including therapeutics (e.g., chemical antidotes, antimicrobical agents, antitoxins, life support medications, and supplies and equipment for intravenous fluids, airway maintenance, and surgical procedures), vaccines, and personal protective equipment. Since 2002, the Health Resources and Services Administration (HRSA) has awarded funds that hospitals and communities have used to improve their capacity to care for mass casualties. Funds from CDC and HRSA have been used to provide training and reference materials for clinical sentinel laboratories and to strengthen communication and partnerships between clinical and public health laboratories (APHL Public Health Laboratory Issues in Brief: Bioterrorism Capacity; http://www.aphl.org/docs/bt_issue_brief_2005_final.pdf).

LRN

In 1999, the CDC, in collaboration with the Association of Public Health Laboratories (APHL) and the FBI, established a model in which clinical and public health laboratories would be linked and integrated into a network called the Laboratory Response Network (LRN). The goal of the LRN is to facilitate rapid detection and confirmatory testing of suspected agents of bioterrorism. As shown in Fig. 1, all laboratories have a defined role and level of responsibility (8, 14, 21, 26). Although the LRN was initially structured to test only

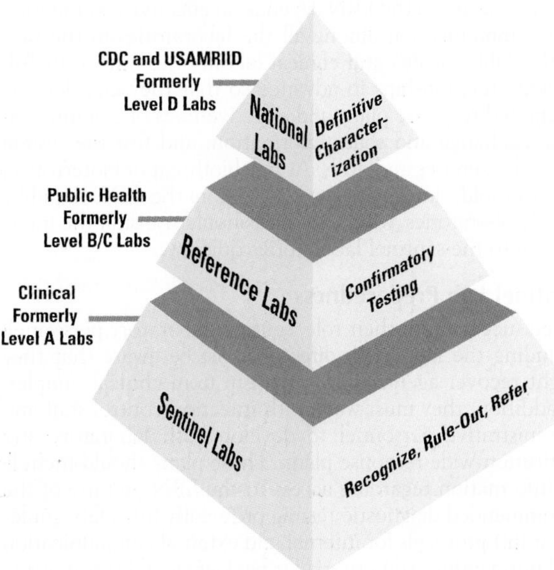

FIGURE 1 Laboratory Response Network (LRN).

clinical specimens for biologic agents, during the anthrax events of 2001, the LRN performed more than one million tests on clinical and environmental samples.

Most hospital and commercial reference laboratories have been classified as sentinel (formerly level A) laboratories. The primary role of sentinel laboratories is to "raise suspicion" when rule-out testing indicates that a targeted agent may be present in a clinical sample and to promptly refer suspicious isolates and specimens to an LRN reference laboratory for confirmatory testing (26, 34). For example, the microbiologists who initially isolated *B. anthracis* from the journalist in Florida were suspicious that the organism was the etiologic agent for anthrax but they could not confirm the species identification or definitively prove that this organism did not cause the infection. Thus, they referred the isolate to the Florida State Department of Health Laboratory, which confirmed the isolate to be *B. anthracis*. Sentinel laboratories are restricted to testing human specimens only and *must* forward or refer all other samples, e.g., environmental and animal, to a reference level (formerly level B/C; also known as confirmatory laboratories) laboratory (31, 34).

The nationwide network of LRN reference laboratories comprises local, state, and federal public health laboratories; food testing, veterinary diagnostic, and environmental testing laboratories affiliated with state and local public health departments and federal agencies; laboratories on military installations; and selected international laboratories. In general, these laboratories have biosafety level 3 (BSL-3) facilities, federally approved equipment, and standardized validated reagents for clinical and environmental testing so that they can respond to biological terrorism and other public health emergencies. Reference laboratories have established functional linkages with law enforcement, including the FBI, and employ chain-of-custody and LRN-approved testing protocols that are consistent with legal evidentiary requirements (4). Reference level laboratories perform rapid tests, such as PCR and fluorescent-antibody tests, to presumptively identify microorganisms or toxins; biochemical tests to confirm the identification of suspect isolates; and antimicrobial susceptibility tests of these isolates. National (formerly level D) laboratories, located at the CDC and USAMRIID, perform definitive characterization of biologic agents and have BSL-4 facilities in which highly infectious agents can be handled safely.

The success of the LRN depends on effective coordination and communication among all the laboratories in the network. Public health and clinical laboratories must establish working relationships in advance so that they can develop integrated response plans and effective lines of communication, exchange and share information, and test the system through exercises and drills. As any biothreat or bioterrorism event unfolds, information will flow from the CDC to public health laboratories, which, in turn, should transmit the information to the sentinel laboratories quickly.

Sentinel Lab Preparedness

To be successful in their role, sentinel laboratory personnel, including the laboratory director, must be aware that they might recover agents of bioterrorism from clinical samples. In addition, they must work with infection control staff and administrative personnel to develop both laboratory and institution-wide response plans. These plans should include (i) information regarding access to the LRN and use of the recommended diagnostic testing protocols; (ii) safety guidelines; (iii) protocols for internal and external communication and notification; (iv) criteria for packaging and transporting infectious substances safely; (v) measures to increase laboratory security; and (vi) telephone numbers for the local and state public health laboratories and the CDC (21, 34). A template for a laboratory response plan is available on the ASM website. If a bioterrorism event exposes a large number of people, clinical and public health laboratories will be overwhelmed with specimens. Thus, laboratory response plans should consider surge capacity needs for personnel and supplies (32).

Because most likely agents of bioterrorism are encountered rarely in clinical settings, laboratory personnel should be trained to recognize the targeted agents and apply the sentinel laboratory standardized testing protocols for ruling out these agents and for referring suspicious isolates (14). These protocols are available at the ASM website (http://www.asm.org/Policy/index.asp?bid=6342). In addition, because any clinical microbiology laboratory could have a sentinel role in detecting potential agents of bioterrorism, CDC, ASM, and APHL jointly recommend that, at a minimum, all sentinel clinical microbiology laboratories (i) meet facility and operational criteria for BSL-2, including the availability and use of a certified Class II biological safety cabinet (37); (ii) have appropriate Clinical Laboratory Improvement Amendments certification; (iii) enroll in proficiency testing (or an equivalent measurement) for Comprehensive Bacteriology and Laboratory Preparedness; and (iv) participate in training and exercises for bioterrorism agent rule-out testing sponsored by a state public health laboratory or other appropriate agency. Laboratories whose physical facilities do not meet these criteria must recognize that they may receive samples containing agents of concern, and thus, their staff should be trained and be familiar with rule-out and referral procedures and biosafety issues. In February 2006, ASM, CDC, and APHL approved a formal definition of sentinel laboratories; it can be found at http://www.asm.org/Policy/index.asp?bid=6342.

It is essential that clinical microbiology laboratories develop a relationship with their local and state health laboratories, many of which provide formal training in laboratory safety, procedures for ruling out targeted biological agents, characteristics of diseases produced by these agents, and packaging and shipping of infectious substances.

Safety

Laboratory personnel must be vigilant in case they isolate one of the targeted agents from what appears to be a routine specimen. Category A and B agents have caused laboratory-acquired infections (29, 31). To reduce the risk that laboratory personnel will be exposed to these agents, flowcharts for LRN sentinel laboratory procedures should be incorporated into standard operating procedures, and physicians should be taught to inform the laboratory when highly infectious agents are in the differential diagnosis (31, 33). If laboratory personnel suspect that a specimen or culture may contain a biothreat-related agent, they should conduct all manipulations in a biosafety cabinet to prevent transmission of the organism. Additional information regarding biosafety is available in chapter 8.

Environmental samples and "unknown packages" may contain very high concentrations of disease-causing agents or toxins, a volatile, toxic chemical, or a radioactive substance; such packages could even be explosive. Powders, in particular, may be highly contaminated and can be aerosolized easily. *Thus, to ensure that personnel and patients are not endangered, sentinel laboratories should not accept or process nonhuman specimens (animal or environmental) but should forward such specimens directly to the state public health laboratory as directed by law enforcement or public health authorities* (31, 34). Public health laboratories have worked with law enforcement and first responders to develop procedures for evaluating the level of threat posed by environmental samples and to screen these samples for safety (http://www.bt.cdc.gov/planning/pdf/suspicious-package-biothreat.pdf).

Sentinel Laboratory Protocols

A partnership of subject matter experts from CDC, ASM, and APHL developed protocols for LRN sentinel laboratories, which describe a number of the targeted Category A and B agents of bioterrorism (Table 2) and provide standardized methods for ruling out critical agents and referring specimens to LRN reference laboratories. These detailed protocols are published on the ASM website (http://www.asm.org/Policy/index.asp?bid=6342). If sentinel laboratory testing fails to rule out an agent of bioterrorism, all suspicious specimens and isolates should be immediately sent to an LRN reference laboratory, where the specialized tests necessary to definitively identify these organisms (e.g., molecular detection methods, enzyme immunoassays, and direct and indirect fluorescent-antibody assays) are available. Clinical laboratories should maintain a subculture of all suspicious isolates that are forwarded for LRN reference testing until the reference laboratory has completed the definitive identification. Sentinel laboratories do not routinely process specimens following law enforcement chain-of-custody guidelines. However, they may be instructed by law enforcement or public health officials to implement specific procedures if a biocrime is suspected.

To simplify matters for hospital laboratories, the procedures provide practical conventional microbiological methods to rule out four of the most likely agents, *B. anthracis*, *Francisella tularensis*, *Brucella* species, and *Yersinia pestis*, using only eight simple procedures: oxidase, catalase, hemolysis, motility, satelliting, β-lactamase, Gram stain, and urease. The flowcharts from these procedures are reproduced here (Fig. 2 to 5). ASM, CDC, and APHL, as partners in the LRN, recommend that all sentinel laboratories use the LRN sentinel protocols to rule out bioterrorism agents, including *B. anthracis*, rather than using newly described molecular detection assays, new commercial detection and rule-out assays, or tests that will be developed in the near future. If personnel from sentinel laboratories choose to use the latter set of tests, they first must understand the limitations of the assays and the necessary quality control measures and the validation requirements.

TABLE 2 Sentinel laboratory protocols available at ASM website

Bacillus anthracis (anthrax)
Botulinum toxin
Brucella spp.
Burkholderia mallei and *B. pseudomallei*
Coxiella burnetii
Francisella tularensis (tularemia)
Staphylococcal enterotoxin B
Yersinia pestis (plague)
Unknown viruses
Packaging and shipping
Bioterrorism readiness plan for laboratories

Bacillus anthracis

Humans can become infected with *B. anthracis* by handling contaminated materials or consuming undercooked contaminated meat. Infection may also result from inhalation of *B. anthracis* spores from contaminated animal products, or following the intentional release of spores. Human-to-human transmission has not been reported. Three forms of anthrax occur in humans: cutaneous, gastrointestinal, and inhalational. Appropriate specimen types will depend on the disease

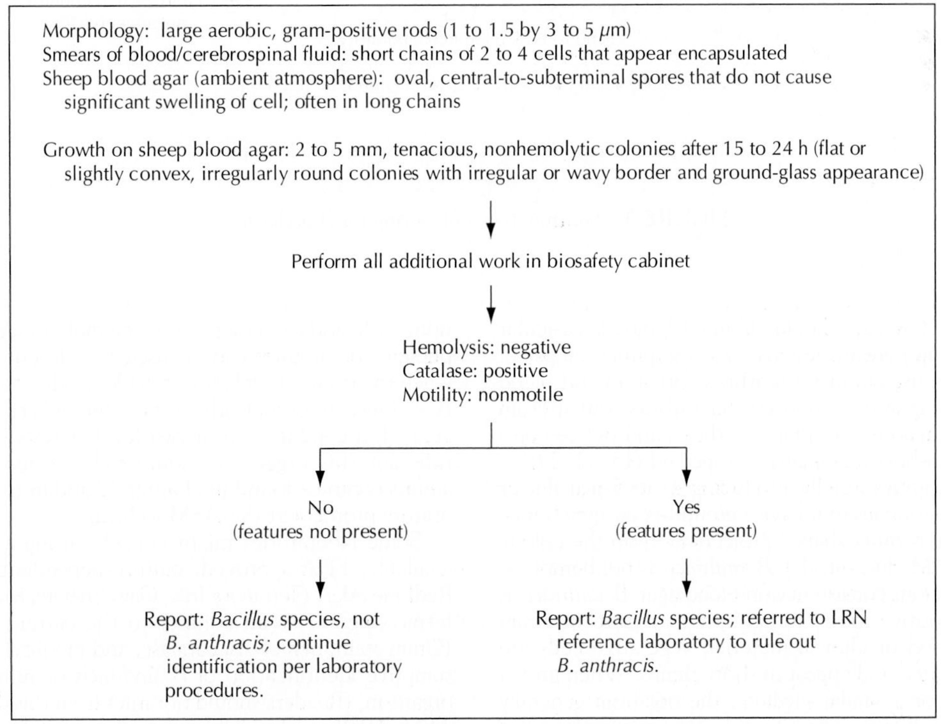

FIGURE 2 Sentinel rule-out testing for *B. anthracis*.

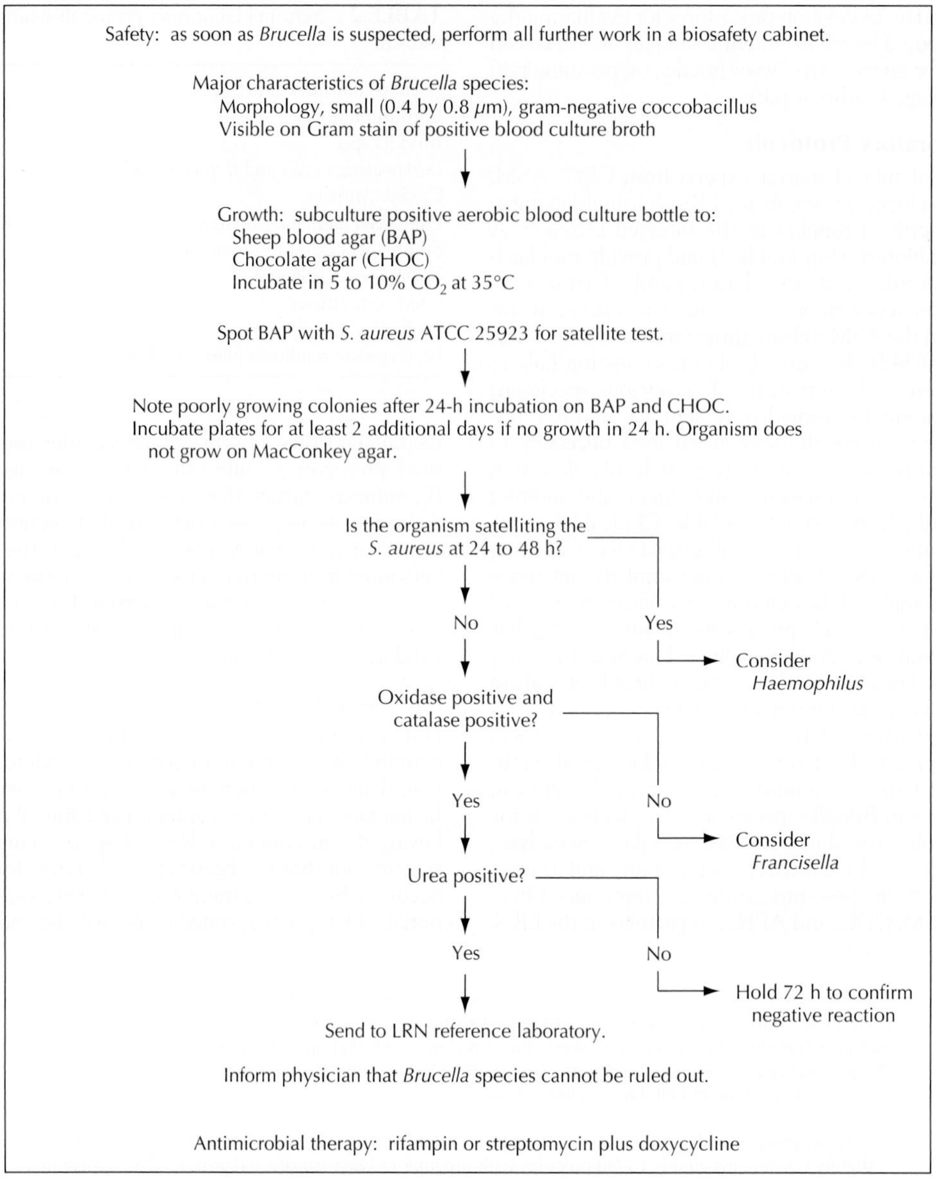

Safety: as soon as *Brucella* is suspected, perform all further work in a biosafety cabinet.

Major characteristics of *Brucella* species:
Morphology, small (0.4 by 0.8 μm), gram-negative coccobacillus
Visible on Gram stain of positive blood culture broth

↓

Growth: subculture positive aerobic blood culture bottle to:
Sheep blood agar (BAP)
Chocolate agar (CHOC)
Incubate in 5 to 10% CO_2 at 35°C

Spot BAP with *S. aureus* ATCC 25923 for satellite test.

↓

Note poorly growing colonies after 24-h incubation on BAP and CHOC.
Incubate plates for at least 2 additional days if no growth in 24 h. Organism does not grow on MacConkey agar.

↓

Is the organism satelliting the *S. aureus* at 24 to 48 h?

No ↓ — Yes → Consider *Haemophilus*

Oxidase positive and catalase positive?

Yes ↓ — No → Consider *Francisella*

Urea positive?

Yes ↓ — No → Hold 72 h to confirm negative reaction

Send to LRN reference laboratory.

Inform physician that *Brucella* species cannot be ruled out.

Antimicrobial therapy: rifampin or streptomycin plus doxycycline

FIGURE 3 Sentinel rule-out testing for *Brucella* spp.

presentation. Clinicians should submit (i) blood, vesicular fluid, swabs from beneath lesions, or tissue/punch biopsy of eschars to diagnose cutaneous anthrax; (ii) stool and blood specimens to diagnose gastrointestinal anthrax; (iii) sputum and blood to diagnose inhalational anthrax; and (iv) cerebrospinal fluid if anthrax meningitis is suspected (15, 22, 29).

B. anthracis grows rapidly, producing 2- to 5-μm flat or slightly convex colonies that have a ground-glass appearance and often have comma-shaped projections from the colony edge (i.e., the "Medusa-head"). *B. anthracis* is nonhemolytic and has a tenacious consistency on blood agar. *B. anthracis* is a large gram-positive rod (1 to 1.5 by 3 to 5 μm). In Gram stains from blood or clinical material, vegetative cells are often encapsulated and appear in short chains. When grown on blood agar or a similar medium, the organism generally appears as long chains of bacilli; it is not encapsulated but may form oval, central-to-subterminal spores. *B. anthracis* is nonmotile and catalase positive. Hemolysis, Gram stain morphology, or motility can be used to rule out this organism when the result provides clear evidence that the isolate is not *B. anthracis* (e.g., a clearly visible zone of beta-hemolysis). In general, a combination of two level A tests is necessary to rule out this organism. Additional information about *B. anthracis* can be found in chapter 32 and in the sentinel laboratory protocol at the ASM website.

Some laboratories might consider using a commercially available, FDA-approved, culture-dependent method, the RedLine Alert (Tetracore Inc., Gaithersburg, Md.; http://www.tetracore.com) as an adjunct to the current sentinel tests (Gram stain, hemolysis, catalase, and motility) for rapid, presumptive identification of *B. anthracis* or ruling out of this organism. (Readers should not infer from this discussion that ASM, APHL, or the CDC endorse this test.) The test, a lateral-flow immunoassay housed in a plastic cassette, was designed

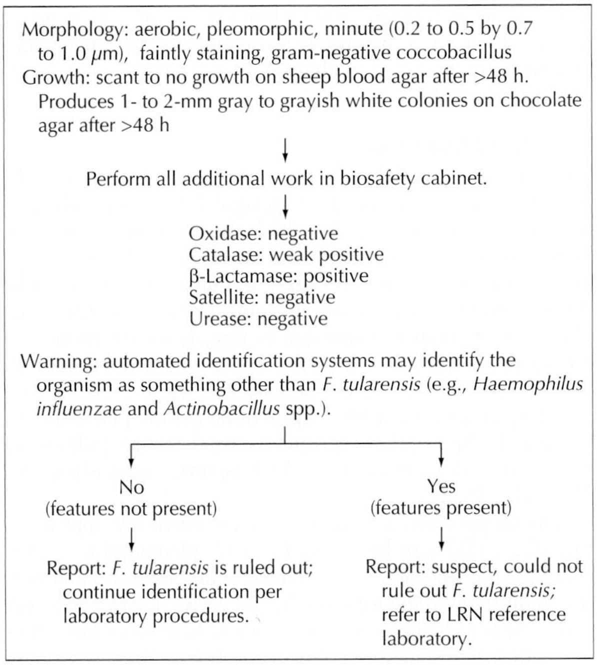

Morphology: aerobic, pleomorphic, minute (0.2 to 0.5 by 0.7 to 1.0 μm), faintly staining, gram-negative coccobacillus
Growth: scant to no growth on sheep blood agar after >48 h. Produces 1- to 2-mm gray to grayish white colonies on chocolate agar after >48 h

↓

Perform all additional work in biosafety cabinet.

↓

Oxidase: negative
Catalase: weak positive
β-Lactamase: positive
Satellite: negative
Urease: negative

Warning: automated identification systems may identify the organism as something other than *F. tularensis* (e.g., *Haemophilus influenzae* and *Actinobacillus* spp.).

No (features not present) → Report: *F. tularensis* is ruled out; continue identification per laboratory procedures.

Yes (features present) → Report: suspect, could not rule out *F. tularensis;* refer to LRN reference laboratory.

FIGURE 4 Sentinel rule-out testing for *F. tularensis.*

primarily to screen nonhemolytic *Bacillus* colonies cultured on sheep blood agar. The principal target of the test is a cell surface protein commonly found in *B. anthracis* vegetative cells, and the presence or absence of this protein can be used to differentiate *B. anthracis* from other nonhemolytic *Bacillus* colonies. A positive control (lyophilized antigen derived from the nonpathogenic Sterne strain of *B. anthracis*) and reconstitution buffer (Colony Isolation Buffer) are provided in the test kit. A non-*Bacillus* species, such as *Staphylococcus aureus*, or a nonhemolytic *Bacillus* species, such as *B. megaterium*, can be used as external negative controls. The Sterne strain (avirulent; devoid of plasmid pXO2) of *B. anthracis* has been excluded from the Select Agent Rule and can be used as an additional external positive control. Test results are available within 15 min. If the test is positive and the bacterial colony is nonhemolytic, *B. anthracis* cannot be ruled out and the sample must be sent to an LRN reference laboratory for confirmation. To ensure that the test is accurate and performs appropriately, external controls should be performed with each new test lot.

According to the manufacturer, the RedLine Alert test has been extensively evaluated against many strains of *B. anthracis*, non-*anthracis Bacillus* species, and non-*Bacillus* pathogens. The test's limitations include the following: (i) only colonies grown on sheep blood agar should be tested; (ii) hemolytic colonies, including *Bacillus* species, should not be tested; (iii) suspicious powders, other environmental samples, or spore preparations should not be tested; (iv) false-negative results may occur if the amount of specific antigen is below the sensitivity of the test; (v) the test cassette cannot be reused; and (vi) isolates that produce negative results but are suspected of being *B. anthracis* by other criteria (e.g., colonies that are flat or slightly convex and irregularly rounded, with edges that are slightly undulate, have a ground-glass appearance, or exhibit a tenacious consistency) should be forwarded to an LRN reference laboratory for confirmatory testing.

Brucella spp.

Brucellosis is a zoonotic infection; there are four species recognized as causing infection in humans: *Brucella abortus* (cattle), *Brucella melitensis* (goats, sheep, and camels), *Brucella suis* (pigs), and *Brucella canis* (dogs). Infection may occur via enteric, percutaneous, or respiratory exposure. The infective dose for these organisms is very low if acquired via the inhalation route, which makes them a potentially effective bioterrorism agent and also makes them hazardous in the clinical microbiology laboratory. Specimens suspected or known to contain *Brucella* spp. and *Brucella* spp. isolates should be handled in a biologic safety cabinet, and all culture plates

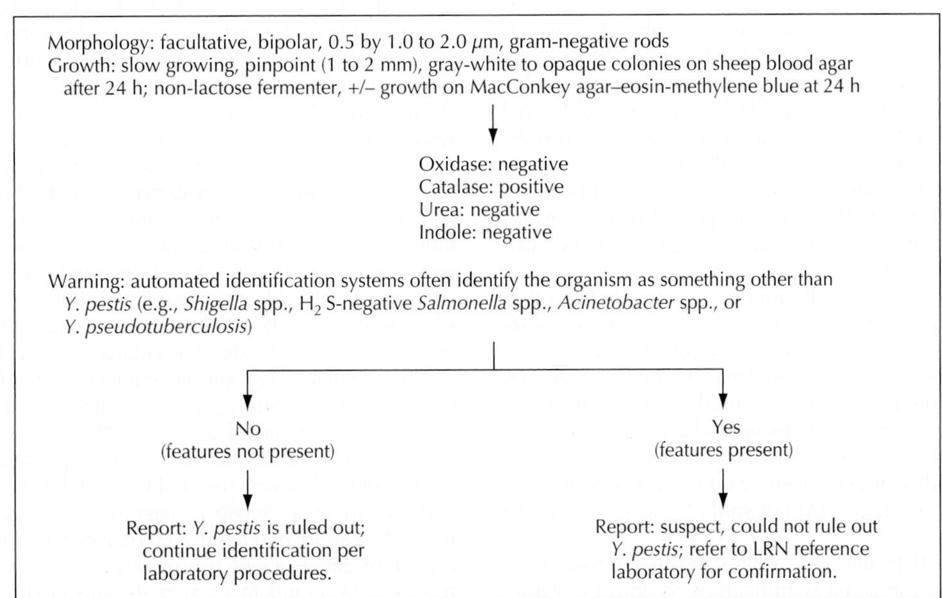

FIGURE 5 Sentinel rule-out testing for *Y. pestis.*

should be sealed. Blood and bone marrow are the best specimens for diagnostic cultures, but spleen, liver, joint fluid, samples from abscesses, and cerebrospinal fluid occasionally yield *Brucella* spp. Serologic studies are available; both acute- and convalescent-phase (>14 days after acute phase) serum samples should be collected (10, 15, 29).

Brucella spp. are tiny (0.5 to 0.7 μm by 1.5 μm), faintly staining gram-negative coccobacilli. Isolation of *Brucella* spp. in blood culture is often delayed, and incubation should be extended for 10 to 21 days if infection with this organism is suspected. On blood or chocolate agar, these organisms produce pinpoint, nonhemolytic, convex, smooth colonies after 48 h. To rule out these organisms, sentinel laboratories should perform the oxidase, catalase, and urea tests, all of which are positive for *Brucella* spp. With the Christensen's tube test, urea hydrolysis can be observed in as early as 15 min of incubation with *B. suis* strains, 1 day for most strains of *B. abortus* and *B. melitensis*, and more than 1 day for some *B. melitensis* strains. Refer to chapter 52 of this Manual and to the sentinel laboratory protocol for additional information.

Burkholderia mallei and *Burkholderia pseudomallei*

Burkholderia mallei is the etiologic agent of glanders, a febrile illness typically seen in horses, mules, and donkeys. Naturally occurring human infection, most often the result of exposure to an infected animal, presents as cutaneous nodules with lymphadenitis or as systemic disease with pneumonia and bacteremia. *Burkholderia pseudomallei* is an environmental organism found in soil and water and is most likely acquired by direct contact with or aerosols from environmental sources. This organism can cause melioidosis, a disease endemic to the tropical regions of the world, which can manifest as an asymptomatic, acute, subacute, or chronic process. Appropriate specimens for diagnosis of glanders and melioidois include blood or bone marrow, sputum or bronchoscopy specimens, material from abscesses, wound swabs, and urine. Acute- and convalescent-phase serum specimens should be collected for serologic diagnosis of *B. pseudomallei*. Currently, no serology test for *B. mallei* is available in the United States. All cultures suspected of containing *B. mallei* or *B. pseudomallei* should be handled in a biological safety cabinet (16).

B. mallei is a small gram-negative coccobacillus, which typically grows in 2 days on sheep blood agar as smooth, gray, translucent colonies, without pigment or distinctive odor. Colonies may or may not grow on MacConkey agar. Additional presumptive identification criteria include these test results: oxidase variable and indole and motility negative; catalase, arginine dihydrolase, and nitrate positive; and resistance to colistin and polymyxin B. Isolates suspected to be *B. mallei* based on colony and Gram stain morphology should be evaluated with these tests.

B. pseudomallei is a small gram-negative rod that often appears on sheep blood agar as small, smooth, creamy colonies in 1 to 2 days, which gradually change after a few days to dry, wrinkled colonies similar to *Pseudomonas stutzeri*. Colonies are neither yellow nor violet pigmented. The organism also grows on MacConkey agar. *B. pseudomallei* often produces a distinctive musty or earthy odor that is very pronounced on opening a petri dish or even opening an incubator door when a positive plate is present. Do not sniff plates, as this can be very dangerous.

B. mallei and *B. pseudomallei* are not in the databases used by some of the commercial identification systems; laboratory staff should consult with the manufacturer to determine whether the system they use includes this information. More details about these agents and their disease spectrum and diagnosis are discussed in chapter 49 and in the sentinel laboratory protocol.

Francisella tularensis

Tularemia is caused by the zoonotic agent *F. tularensis*. In humans, disease can occur in several forms, depending to some extent on the route by which the bacterium enters the body. If used for bioterrorism, the organism would most likely be dispersed via aerosol, resulting in pulmonary or typhoidal disease. Symptoms for both syndromes are often nonspecific. Human-to-human transmission is rare; however, numerous laboratory-acquired infections have been documented. Laboratory staff should manipulate suspicious cultures in a biosafety cabinet using BSL-3 practices; culture plates should be sealed. Appropriate specimens to diagnose pulmonary disease include sputum, bronchial aspirates or washes, and blood (10, 15, 31).

On Gram stain, *F. tularensis* characteristically appears as tiny (0.2 to 0.7 μm by 0.7 to 1.0 μm), pleomorphic, poorly staining, gram-negative coccobacilli. The organism is fastidious, requires cysteine for growth, and grows slowly, producing tiny grayish white colonies after 48 to 72 h. Isolates with characteristic Gram stain and culture morphology that are oxidase negative, catalase weakly positive, beta-lactamase positive, satellite or XV test negative, and urease test negative could be *F. tularensis* (cannot be ruled out) and should be immediately referred to the nearest LRN reference laboratory.

Additional information about other clinical manifestations of tularemia, the modes of transmission, and the organism's characteristics are discussed in chapter 52 as well as the sentinel laboratory protocol.

Yersinia pestis

Plague is a zoonotic disease caused by *Y. pestis*. Humans can acquire plague through the bite of infected fleas, direct contact with contaminated tissue, or inhalation of aerosolized bacteria. Plague presents in one of three clinical syndromes: bubonic, septicemic, or pneumonic. In a bioterrorism event, the agent would most likely be aerosolized, resulting in pneumonic disease, which has a high mortality rate and is highly transmissible from person to person. Appropriate specimens include tracheal or bronchial washes, sputum, blood, and aspirates or biopsy specimens of affected tissues (bubos). Acute- and, if necessary, convalescent-phase sera can be tested for antibodies to *Y. pestis* (3, 15, 29).

Gram stains of specimens and cultures containing *Y. pestis* often reveal plump, gram-negative rods (1 to 2 μm by 0.5 μm) with a bipolar or safety pin appearance. Bipolar staining may be more apparent with Wright stain. This appearance should trigger suspicion of *Y. pestis*. On routine media, pinpoint colonies can appear after 24 h. After incubation for 48 h, the small gray-white to slightly yellow colonies are opaque and produce little or no hemolysis. Under ×4 enlargement, colonies have a raised, irregular "fried egg" appearance, which becomes more prominent as the culture ages. Colonies also can be described as having a "hammered copper" shiny surface. *Y. pestis* grows best at 28°C. Isolates that are catalase positive and oxidase, urease, and indole negative and that exhibit classic Gram stain and growth characteristics suggestive of *Y. pestis* should be referred to an LRN reference laboratory for confirmatory testing. More details about this organism and disease manifestations can be found in chapter 44 and in the LRN sentinel laboratory protocol.

Smallpox (Variola Virus)

The CDC has developed an extensive smallpox response plan and a clinical algorithm to assist physicians as they assess patients and develop differential diagnoses. Varicella (chickenpox) is the infection most likely to be confused with smallpox. Guidelines for specimen collection and laboratory testing for variola, the causative agent of smallpox, and other look-alike diseases are also provided on the CDC website (http://www.bt.cdc.gov/agent/smallpox). If clinicians suspect that a patient has smallpox, the person designated by the facility should contact the public health laboratory and state health officials immediately.

Variola virus can grow and amplify easily in most routine cell lines used for cultivating herpesviruses such as varicella-zoster virus and herpes simplex virus (21, 29). While clinical microbiology/virology laboratories should never attempt to isolate this virus, which requires BSL-4, technologists may neither suspect nor recognize the potential hazard. If technologists manipulate a culture in the routine manner or passage the culture while trying to confirm the etiology of the cytopathic effects, they may increase the risk that personnel will be exposed to smallpox virus. Therefore, laboratory personnel should be familiar with the risks from the most likely viral agents of bioterrorism and understand appropriate safety practices (see the "Unknown Virus" protocol for sentinel laboratories on the ASM website for helpful materials). If a laboratory inadvertently isolates the smallpox virus, the laboratory director should notify both the state health laboratory and the CDC immediately.

Reporting

The sentinel laboratory staff should inform infection control personnel promptly if they identify suspicious isolates. Infection control staff should follow internal chain of command and communication policies for notifying local and state health officials, who are responsible to communicate with law enforcement. The chain of command should be clearly described in each institution's bioterrorism preparedness program (34). There are several reasons why sentinel laboratories should not report possible bioterrorism events externally. First, many potential agents of bioterrorism are found naturally in certain geographic areas and cause sporadic infections. Second, incorrect characterization of a suspect agent can cause public panic, placing undue burdens on public health and law enforcement agencies.

Regulatory Issues

Packaging and Shipping

Sentinel laboratories must refer suspicious isolates to reference laboratories. Therefore, proper packaging and shipping of infectious agents is one of their important functions (refer to chapter 5, "General Principles of Specimen Collection and Handling"). Cultures and clinical specimens known or suspected to contain infectious substances must be packaged according to domestic and international regulations on dangerous goods and infectious substances promulgated by the U.S. Department of Transportation (DOT), the International Air Transport Association, and the Canadian Transportation of Dangerous Goods Regulations. Recently various regulatory authorities have attempted to harmonize the requirements; updated regulations are published periodically. Anyone, including microbiologists, who ships infectious substances is required to complete formal training, become certified in the application of these regulations, and be familiar with current regulations. Formal training is available through the U.S. DOT and most commercial suppliers of approved packaging containers (see the DOT's and the commercial suppliers' websites).

Select Agent Program

In accordance with provisions of Public Law 107-188, the "Public Health Security and Bioterrorism Preparedness Response Act of 2002," the CDC and the U.S. Department of Agriculture Animal and Plant Health Inspection Service (USDA-APHIS) regulate the possession, use, and transfer of biological agents and toxins that could pose a severe threat to public health and safety (13). The CDC maintains a list of select agents that threaten humans, and the USDA-APHIS maintains a list of organisms that threaten animals; together they maintain a shared (overlap) list of organisms, primarily "high consequence" zoonotic agents that threaten humans and animals (42 CFR Part 73, 7 CFR Part 331, and 9 CFR Part 121). The Select Agent regulation requires all entities, including individuals, government agencies, universities, research institutions, and commercial facilities that possess, use, or transfer biologic agents and toxins that pose a significant threat to public health, to register with either CDC or USDA depending on the agents they possess. As a condition of registration, each entity must designate a Responsible Official to ensure that staff members comply with the regulation and to develop and implement a written security plan. Persons with access to select agents must submit required forms for a security risk assessment through the U.S. Attorney General, Department of Justice.

As described in 42 CFR Part 73.5, clinical or diagnostic laboratories that acquire a select agent from a specimen presented for diagnosis or verification are exempt from the regulation, provided that (i) laboratory personnel transfer or destroy the select agent within 7 days after the organism's identification has been confirmed; (ii) the agent is secured against theft, loss, or release during the period between identification and transfer or destruction; and (iii) laboratory personnel report the select agent to the CDC or USDA as defined in the regulation (usually within 7 days; viral hemorrhagic fever viruses, variola virus, and *Y. pestis* must be reported immediately). The laboratory must document that the organism was transferred or, if the organism was destroyed, the method of destruction and must maintain these records for 3 years. Additional exemptions apply to clinical and diagnostic laboratories that acquire a select agent as part of a proficiency testing exercise, provided that the agent is transferred or destroyed within 90 days; that the agent is properly secured against theft, loss, or release; and that the CDC or USDA is notified within 90 days.

Sources for Additional and Updated Information

Information and guidelines on bioterrorism continue to change and may be updated if a bioterrorism event is detected. Microbiologists are encouraged to remain current with local, state, and federal guidelines and should contact the local health department regarding emergencies and to report suspected or confirmed exposures to biological agents. In addition, laboratory personnel and clinicians can use the CDC Emergency Response Hotline (phone: 770-488-7100) at all hours to receive emergency consultation from subject matter experts in bioterrorism, chemical exposure, and natural disasters. Check http://www.bt.cdc.gov/emcontact/ for updated contact information.

Other current information on terrorism preparedness can be obtained from a variety of Internet sites, including the following.

1. Federal agencies and preparedness
CDC—http://www.cdc.gov
CDC Bioterrorism Preparedness and Response Program—http://www.bt.cdc.gov
Department of Health and Human Services—http://www.hhs.gov
Department of Homeland Security—http://www.dhs.gov
Federal Emergency Management Agency—http://www.fema.gov
National Response Plan—http://www.dhs.gov/interweb/assetlibrary/ NRP_FullText.pdf
National Incident Management System—http://www.fema.gov/nims/
Interim National Preparedness Goal—http://www.ojp.usdoj.gov/odp/docs/InterimNationalPreparednessGoal_03-31-05_1.pdf
Interim Public Health and Healthcare Supplement to the National Preparedness Goal—http://www.hhs.gov/ophep/npgs.html

2. General information
ASM—http://www.asm.org
Center for Biosecurity of the University of Pittsburgh Medical Center (UPMC)—http://www.upmc-biosecurity.org/
Center for Infectious Disease Research and Preparedness—http://www.cidrap.umn.edu/index.html

3. Sentinel laboratory testing protocols
ASM—http://www.asm.org/Policy/index.asp?bid=6342
CDC—http://www.bt.cdc.gov

4. Bioterrorism readiness plans and templates for health care facilities
Association of Professionals in Infection Control—http://www.apic.org/Content/NavigationMenu/PracticeGuidance/Topics/Bioterrorism/Bioterrorism.htm
CDC—http://www.bt.cdc.gov/planning/#healthcare
ASM—http://www.asm.org/Policy/index.asp?bid=520
DHS—National Disaster Medical System (NDMS)—http://www.oep-ndms.dhhs.gov

5. Packaging and shipping regulations
Department of Transportation Hazardous Materials Regulations (49 CFR parts 171 to 180, shipment of biological and clinical specimens)—http://hazmat.dot.gov/
IATA—http://www.iata.org
World Health Organization—http://www.who.org
International Civil Aviation Organization—http://www.icao.org
TDGR—http://www.cftcanada.com/c203547.2.html

6. Select agent regulations
CDC—http://www.cdc.gov/od/sap/
USDA-APHIS—http://www.aphis.usda.gov/programs/ag_selectagent/

REFERENCES

1. **Alibek, K., and S. Handelman.** 1999. *Biohazard: the Chilling True Story of the Largest Covert Biological Weapons Program in the World—Told from the Inside by the Man Who Ran It*, 1st ed. Random House, New York, N.Y.
2. **Baciu, A., A. P. Anason, K. Stratton, and B. Strom (ed.).** 2005. *The Smallpox Vaccination Program: Public Health in an Age of Terrorism.* National Academies Press, Washington, D.C.
3. **Bockemuhl, J., and J. D. Wong.** 2003. *Yersinia*, p. 672–683. *In* P. R. Murray, E. J. Baron, M. A. Pfaller, F. C. Tenover, and R. H. Yolken (ed.), *Manual of Clinical Microbiology*, 8th ed. American Society for Microbiology, Washington, D.C.
4. **Butler, J. C., M. L. Cohen, C. R. Friedman, R. M. Scripp, and C. G. Watz.** 2002. Collaboration between public health and law enforcement: new paradigms and partnerships for bioterrorism planning and response. *Emerg. Infect. Dis.* **8:** 1152–1156.
5. **Centers for Disease Control and Prevention.** 2001. Update: investigation of bioterrorism-related anthrax—Connecticut. *Morb. Mortal. Wkly. Rep.* **50:**1077–1079.
6. **Centers for Disease Control and Prevention.** 2001. Notice to readers: considerations for distinguishing influenza-like illness from inhalational anthrax. *Morb. Mortal. Wkly. Rep.* **50:**984–986.
7. **Centers for Disease Control and Prevention.** 2001. Update: investigation of bioterrorism-related anthrax and interim guidelines for clinical evaluation of persons with possible anthrax. *Morb. Mortal. Wkly. Rep.* **50:**941–948.
8. **Centers for Disease Control and Prevention.** 2000. Biological and chemical terrorism: strategic plan for preparedness and response. *Morb. Mortal. Wkly. Rep.* **49**(RR04)**:** 1–14.
9. **Christopher, G. W., T. J. Cieslak, J. A. Pavlin, and E. M. Eitzen, Jr.** 1997. Biological warfare: a historical perspective. *JAMA* **278:**412–417.
10. **Chu, M. C., and R. S. Weyant.** 2003. *Francisella* and *Brucella*, p. 789–808. *In* P. R. Murray, E. J. Baron, J. H. Jorgensen, M. A. Pfaller, and R. H. Yolken (ed.), *Manual of Clinical Microbiology*, 8th ed. American Society for Microbiology, Washington, D.C.
11. **Davis, C. J.** 1999. Nuclear blindness: an overview of the biological weapons programs of the former Soviet Union and Iraq. *Emerg. Infect. Dis.* **5:**509–512.
12. **English, J. F.** 1999. Overview of bioterrorism readiness plan: a template for health care facilities. *Am. J. Infect. Control* **27:**468–469.
13. **Federal Register.** 2005. Possession, use and transfer of select agents and toxins; final rule. *Fed. Regist.* **70:**13294–13325.
14. **Gilchrist, M. J. R.** 2000. A national laboratory network for bioterrorism: evolution from a prototype network of laboratories performing routine surveillance. *Mil. Med.* **156** (Suppl.)**:**28–34.
15. **Gilchrist, M. J. R., W. P. McKinney, J. M. Miller, and A. S. Weissfeld.** 2000. *Cumitech 33, Laboratory Safety, Management, and Diagnosis of Biological Agents Associated with Bioterrorism.* Coordinating ed., J. W. Snyder. ASM Press, Washington, D.C.
16. **Gilligan, P. H., G. Lum, P. Vandamme, and S. Whittier.** 2003. *Burkholderia, Stenotrophomonas, Ralstonia, Brevundimonas, Comamonas,* and *Acidovorax*, p. 729–748. *In* P. R. Murray, E. J. Baron, M. A. Pfaller, F. C. Tenover, and R. H. Yolken (ed.), *Manual of Clinical Microbiology*, 8th ed. American Society for Microbiology, Washington, D.C.
17. **Horn, F.** 2000. Agricultural bioterrorism, p. 109–115. *In* B. Roberts (ed.), *Hype or Reality? The "New Terrorism" and Mass Casualty Attacks.* The Chemical and Biological Arms Control Institute, Alexandria, Va.
18. **Isenberg, H. D. (ed.).** 2004. *Clinical Microbiology Procedures Handbook*, 2nd ed. ASM Press, Washington, D.C.
19. **Jernigan, J. A., D. S. Stephens, D. A. Ashford, C. Omenaca, M. S. Topiel, M. Galbraith, M. Tapper, T. L. Fisk, S. Zaki, T. Popovic, R. F. Meyer, C. P. Quinn, S. A. Harper, S. K. Fridkin, J. J. Sejvar, C. W. Shepard, M. McConnell, J. Guarner, W. J. Shieh, J. M. Malecki, J. L. Gerberding, J. M. Hughes, B. A. Perkins, and members of the Anthrax Bioterrorism Investigation Team.** 2001. Bioterrorism-related inhalational anthrax: the first 10 cases reported in the United States. *Emerg. Infect. Dis.* **7:**933–944.

20. **Jernigan, D. B., P. L. Raghunathan, B. P. Bell, R. Brechner, E. A. Bresnitz, J. C. Butler, M. Cetron, M. Cohen, T. Doyle, M. Fischer, C. Greene, K. S. Griffith, J. Guarner, J. L. Hadler, J. A. Hayslett, R. Meyer, L. R. Petersen, M. Phillips, R. Pinner, T. Popovic, C. P. Quinn, J. Reefhuis, D. Reissman, N. Rosenstein, A. Schuchat, W. Shieh, L. Siegal, D. L. Swerdlow, F. C. Tenover, M. Traeger, J. W. Ward, I. Weisfuse, S. Wiersma, K. Yeskey, S. Zaki, D. A. Ashford, B. A. Perkins, S. Ostroff, J. Hughes, D. Fleming, J. P. Koplan, J. L. Gerberding, and the National Anthrax Epidemiologic Investigation Team.** 2002. Investigation of bioterrorism related anthrax, United States, 2001: epidemiologic findings. *Emerg. Infect. Dis.* **8:**1019–1028.
21. **Klietmann, W. F., and K. L. Ruoff.** 2001. Bioterrorism: implications for the clinical microbiologist. *Clin. Microbiol. Rev.* **14:**364–381.
22. **Logan, N. A., and P. C. Turnbull.** 2003. *Bacillus* and other aerobic endospore-forming bacteria, p. 445–460. *In* P. R. Murray, E. J. Baron, J. H. Jorgensen, M. A. Pfaller, and R. H. Yolken (ed.), *Manual of Clinical Microbiology*, 8th ed. American Society for Microbiology, Washington, D.C.
23. **Luciana, B., D. Frank, M. Venkat, V. Mani, C. Chirboga, M. Pollanen, M. Ripple, S. Ali, C. DiAngelo, J. Lee, J. Arden, J. Titus, D. Fowler, T. O'Toole, H. Masur, J. Bartlett, and T. Inglesby.** 2001. Death due to bioterrorism-related inhalational anthrax: report of 2 patients. *JAMA* **286:**2554–2559.
24. **Mayer, T. A., S. Bersoof-Matcha, C. Murphy, J. Earls, S. Harper, D. Pauze, M. Nguyen, J. Rosenthall, D. Cerva, Jr., G. Druckenbrod, D. Hanfling, N. Fatteh, A. Napoli, A. Nayyar, and E. L. Berman.** 2001. Clinical presentation of inhalational anthrax following bioterrorism exposure: report of 2 surviving patients. *JAMA* **286:**2549–2553.
25. **Morse, S. A.** 2001. Bioterrorism: laboratory security. *Lab. Med.* **32:**303–306.
26. **Morse, S. A., R. B. Kellogg, S. Perry, R. F. Meyer, D. Bray, D. Nichelson, and J. M. Miller.** 2003. Detecting biothreat agents: the laboratory response network. *ASM News* **69:**433–437.
27. **Perkins, B. A., T. Popovic, and K. Yeskey.** 2002. Public health in the time of bioterrorism. *Emerg. Infect. Dis.* **8:**1015–1018.
28. **Poupard, J. A., and L. A. Miller.** 1992. History of biological warfare: catapults to capsomeres. *Ann. N.Y. Acad. Sci.* **666:**9–20.
29. **Robinson-Dunn, B.** 2002. Microbiology laboratory's role in response to bioterrorism. *Arch. Pathol. Lab. Med.* **126:** 291–294.
30. **Rotz, L. D., A. S. Khan, S. R. Lillibridge, S. M. Ostroff, and J. M. Hughes.** 2002. Public health assessment of potential biological terrorism agents. *Emerg. Infect. Dis.* **8:**225–230.
31. **Sewell, D. L.** 2003. Laboratory safety practices associated with potential agents of biocrime or bioterrroism. *J. Clin. Microbiol.* **41:**2801–2809.
32. **Shapiro, D. S.** 2003. Surge capacity for response to bioterrorism in hospital clinical microbiology laboratories. *J. Clin. Microbiol.* **41:**5372–5376.
33. **Shapiro, D. S., and D. R. Schwartz.** 2002. Exposure of laboratory workers to *Francisella tularensis* despite a bioterrorism procedure. *J. Clin. Microbiol.* **40:**2278–2281.
34. **Snyder, J. W.** 2003. Role of the hospital-based microbiology laboratory in preparation for and response to a bioterrorism event. *J. Clin. Microbiol.* **41:**1–4.
35. **Torok, T. J., R. V. Tauxe, R. P. Wise, J. R. Livengood, R. Sokolow, S. Mauvais, K. A. Birkness, M. R. Skeels, J. M. Horan, and L. R. Foster.** 1997. A large community outbreak of salmonellosis caused by intentional contamination of restaurant salad bars. *JAMA* **278:**389–395.
36. **Traeger, M. S., S. T. Wiersma, N. E. Rosenstein, J. M. Malecki, C. W. Shepard, and P. L. Raghunathan.** 2002. First case of bioterrorism-related inhalational anthrax in the United States, Palm Beach County, Florida, 2001. *Emerg. Infect. Dis.* **8:**1029–1034.
37. **U.S. Department of Health and Human Services.** 1999. *Biosafety in Microbiological and Biomedical Laboratories*, 4th ed. U.S. Government Printing Office, Washington, D.C.
38. **U.S. General Accountability Office.** 2003. *Bioterrorism: Preparedness varied Across State and Local Jurisdictions.* GAO-03-373 (April 2003). [Online.] http://www.gao.gov/new.items/d03373.pdf.
39. **Wilkening, D. A.** 1999. BCW attack scenarios, p. 76114. *In* S. D. Drell, A. D. Sofaer, and G. D. Wilson (ed.), *The New Terror: Facing the Threat of Biological and Chemical Weapons*. Hoover Institution Press, Stanford, Calif.

Infection Control Epidemiology and Clinical Microbiology

DANIEL J. DIEKEMA AND MICHAEL A. PFALLER

10

In 2000, the Institute of Medicine issued a landmark report on medical errors, estimating that between 44,000 and 98,000 deaths per year in U.S. hospitals are a result of injuries or complications sustained during the delivery of health care (44). Health care-associated (or nosocomial) infections represent one of the most common complications of care, affecting approximately 2 million persons admitted to acute-care hospitals each year (8). For this reason, every health care facility should have an infection control program charged with monitoring, preventing, and controlling the spread of infections in the health care environment. Because infection control requires the ability to detect infections when they occur, the clinical microbiology laboratory is inextricably linked to any comprehensive infection control program. In this chapter we will discuss the impact of nosocomial infections, outline the organization of the hospital infection control program, and describe the important role of the clinical microbiology laboratory in the prevention and control of health care-associated infections.

NOSOCOMIAL INFECTION

Definition

A nosocomial infection is one that is acquired in a hospital or health care facility (i.e., the infection was not present or incubating at the time of admission). For most bacterial infections, an onset of symptoms more than 48 h after admission is evidence of nosocomial acquisition. To determine whether some infections such as legionellosis are hospital acquired, one must consider the usual incubation periods and determine whether the patient was hospitalized during that time period. Because hospital stays are getting shorter and more patients are treated in the outpatient setting, many health care-associated infections are not recognized during hospitalization. Infection control programs must therefore devise strategies for effective outpatient surveillance in order to accurately monitor nosocomial infection rates (38).

Infection Rates and Predominant Pathogens

At least 5% of patients may acquire an infection during hospitalization (6, 34). The urinary tract is the most commonly involved site, with 30 to 40% of all nosocomial infections occurring at this site. Surgical wound and lower respiratory tract infections are the next most frequent, with each accounting for about 15 to 20% of nosocomial infections, followed by bloodstream infections (5 to 15%). The vast majority of nosocomial infections are related to devices (e.g., urinary tract catheters, endotracheal tubes in ventilated patients, and central venous catheters). For this reason, and as a way to adjust for risk when comparing rates over time or between similar units in different facilities, the Centers for Disease Control and Prevention (CDC) recommends calculating nosocomial infection rates in the intensive care unit (ICU) by using device days as the denominator (Table 1 gives definitions of common epidemiology terms).

Table 2 lists the five most common bacterial pathogens isolated from various sites of nosocomial infection in U.S. hospital ICUs (17, 80). Over the past 3 decades, the spectrum of nosocomial pathogens has shifted from gram-negative to gram-positive organisms and *Candida* spp. have emerged as a major problem (55). The incidence of nosocomial infections caused by staphylococci and enterococci has increased, in part because these organisms are becoming increasingly resistant to antimicrobial agents (21).

Morbidity, Mortality, and Cost

Nosocomial infections cause or contribute to thousands of deaths annually (6, 76). Because patients with the most severe underlying illnesses are also those most vulnerable to nosocomial infections, it is very difficult to estimate the proportion of crude or overall mortality that is directly attributable to nosocomial infections. Studies that attempt to address this question by carefully controlling for many potentially confounding variables are called attributable mortality studies. Estimates of the attributable mortality associated with nosocomial bloodstream infections have ranged from 14% for infections caused by coagulase-negative staphylococci (49), 31 and 37% for infections caused by vancomycin-susceptible and vancomycin-resistant enterococci (26, 46), respectively, and 38 to 49% for infections caused by *Candida* spp. (32, 78) (Table 3).

Nosocomial infections also increase hospital costs and lengths of stay (LOS), thereby costing the health care system billions of dollars annually. At the University of Iowa, the median excess LOS for nosocomial bloodstream infections caused by coagulase-negative staphylococci and *Candida* spp. were 8 and 30 days, respectively (49, 78). Nosocomial bloodstream infections in the ICU were associated with an excess LOS of 24 days and excess hospital costs of $40,000

TABLE 1 Commonly used terms in health care epidemiology[a]

Term	Definition or Summary
Epidemiology	Study of the occurrence, distribution, and determinants of health and disease in a population. Hospital or health care epidemiology is the study of disease occurrence and distribution in the hospital or health care system.
Nosocomial infection	An infection acquired in a hospital or other health care facility.
Endemic infections	Infections occurring as part of the background or usual rate of infection in a specified population.
Epidemic infections	Infections occurring as part of an outbreak (or epidemic) of infection—defined as a significant increase in the usual rate of that infection in the specified population.
Incidence rate	Ratio of the number of new cases of infection in a specified population at risk during a defined time period to the overall number of people in the population at risk (the denominator).
Device-associated incidence rate	Ratio of the number of new cases of device-related infection in a specified population at risk during a defined time period to the number of days of device utilization in the population at risk.
Prevalence rate	Total number of cases of infection in the defined population at risk at one point in time (point prevalence) or in a given time period (period prevalence).
Observational or descriptive study	Study of the natural course of events, without an intervention in the process.
Case control study	Study frequently done as part of an outbreak investigation: a group of patients with the outcome of interest (e.g., cases of nosocomial infection) is compared to a control group of patients without the outcome. A comparison of specific factors between groups (e.g., exposures of interest) may suggest why infection occurred.
Crude or overall mortality rate	Ratio of the number of patients who die to the overall number of patients in a specified population.
Attributable mortality	Ratio of the number of patients who die as a direct result of the disease of interest to the overall population with the disease.

[a] Adapted from reference 50.

per survivor (60). Kirkland et al. found that surgical site infections increased LOS by more than 6 days and increased hospital costs by more than $3,000 per infection (42).

The premise upon which infection control programs operate is that many of these life-threatening and costly nosocomial infections are preventable. The Study of the Efficacy of Nosocomial Infection Control indicated that the presence of an active surveillance and infection control program was associated with a 32% decrease in nosocomial infection rates and that the absence of such a program was associated with an 18% increase in nosocomial infection rates (35). More recently, the CDC National Nosocomial Infection Surveillance (NNIS) system of hospitals reported a reduction in risk-adjusted infection rates in ICUs for all monitored infection sites (urinary tract, bloodstream, and lung) during the 1990s. The elements that were critical for reducing rates included targeted surveillance of high-risk populations (using standard definitions); adequate numbers of trained infection control professionals (ICPs), who inform health care providers of infection rates; and prevention efforts designed to address issues identified during evaluation of infection rates (18). Clearly, an effective infection control program improves patient care, saves lives, and decreases health care costs.

TABLE 2 Distribution of the five most common nosocomial pathogens isolated from major infection sites in the ICU

Pathogen	% of total at each infection site
Bloodstream infection[a]	
CoNS[b]	35.9
S. aureus	16.8
Candida spp.	10.1
Enterococcus spp.	9.8
Pseudomonas aeruginosa	4.7
Pneumonia[c]	
S. aureus	18.1
Pseudomonas aeruginosa	17.0
Enterobacter spp.	11.2
Klebsiella pneumoniae	7.2
Haemophilus influenzae	4.3
Urinary tract infection[c]	
Escherichia coli	17.5
Candida albicans	15.8
Enterococcus spp.	13.8
Pseudomonas aeruginosa	11.0
Klebsiella pneumoniae	6.2

[a] Data from SCOPE (80); collected between March 1995 and September 2002.
[b] CoNS, coagulase-negative *Staphylococcus* spp.
[c] Data from NNIS (17); collected between January 1990 and May 1999.

TABLE 3 Attributable mortality of nosocomial bloodstream infection due to selected pathogens[a]

Organism	Mortality among cases (%)	Mortality among matched controls (%)	Attributable mortality (%)	Reference(s)
CoNS[b]	31	17	14	49
Enterococcus spp.	43	12	31	46
VRE	67	30	37	26
Candida spp.	57–61	12–19	38–49	32, 78

[a] Adapted from reference 23, with permission.
[b] CoNS, coagulase-negative *Staphylococcus* spp.

THE HOSPITAL INFECTION CONTROL PROGRAM

The hospital infection control program should include surveillance and prevention of nosocomial infections, continuing education of medical staff, control of infectious disease outbreaks, protection of employees from infection, and advice on new products and procedures. The program is generally directed by a physician-epidemiologist and enforced by the infection control committee. Every hospital must also have a working infection control staff, comprising one or more ICPs. The ICPs should collect data on nosocomial infections and provide the data to the infection control committee.

Infection Control Committee

The infection control committee is responsible for reporting and evaluating nosocomial infection data and for drafting and implementing policies, procedures, and guidelines pertinent to the practice of infection control. Of note, in some hospitals the infection control program staff performs the functions just described and the infection control committee approves the reports, policies, procedures, and guidelines. The committee should be multidisciplinary, with representatives from all departments, including clinical microbiology, and should meet every 1 to 3 months to review hospital-specific nosocomial infection data and to formulate policy. The members bring the needs and perspectives of their departments to the committee and, in turn, take back important information about infection control initiatives and policies, etc. Other responsibilities of the committee include reviewing technical information about new products, devices, or procedures pertinent to infection control and instituting all necessary control measures in the event of an outbreak or other infection control emergency.

A clinical microbiologist must be on the infection control committee in order to provide expertise in the interpretation of culture results, advice about the appropriateness and feasibility of microbiological approaches to an infection control problem, and input regarding the laboratory resources necessary to accomplish the goals of the committee. One of the most important contributions of the clinical microbiologist is to inform the infection control committee of the strengths and limitations of methods employed to detect and characterize nosocomial pathogens. He or she should describe how changes in the methods used for detection, identification, and susceptibility testing of nosocomial pathogens would affect the infection control program. For example, if the laboratory introduces a urinary antigen detection test for diagnosis of legionellosis, the clinical microbiologist must inform the committee that the test is sensitive and specific only for detection of *Legionella pneumophila* serogroup 1 and that culture is required to evaluate for nosocomial legionellosis due to other species or serogroups. The committee should also be made aware of the budgetary and personnel constraints under which the laboratory operates to ensure that they do not expend valuable laboratory resources unless there is a clear epidemiologic indication to do so.

Nosocomial Infection Surveillance

Active nosocomial infection surveillance programs are associated with a reduction in infection rates and their consequent morbidity and mortality (22, 35), and national and state accrediting agencies require hospitals to do surveillance for nosocomial infections. Thus, systematic surveillance of nosocomial infections is the infection control program's most important activity. Surveillance is also the infection control program's most costly and time-consuming activity. Surveillance allows the infection control program staff to monitor the frequency and types of nosocomial infections, detect outbreaks, evaluate compliance with infection control guidelines, provide data for policy development, and monitor the effect of infection control interventions on nosocomial infection rates. To accomplish the overall goal of decreasing infection rates, the infection control program personnel must give the surveillance data and suggestions for improvement, including reminders to staff of existing infection control practices, back to the clinicians as soon as possible. Infection control programs that follow the CDC's advice about using device days as the denominator for calculating rates of nosocomial infection in ICUs can compare their rates with national benchmarks compiled and reported by the CDC NNIS system (17, 18). Figure 1 is a sample format for comparing infection rates in an ICU of a tertiary-care center with national benchmark data. The infection control program should provide infection rates, recommendations for improving rates, and assistance in

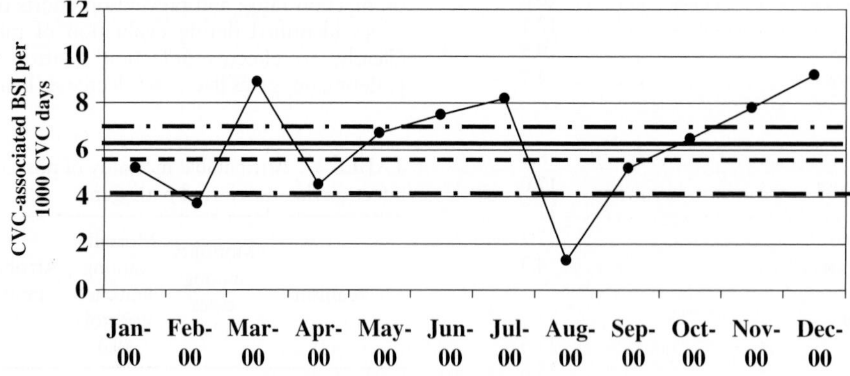

FIGURE 1 Medical ICU catheter-associated bloodstream infection rates. •———•, central venous catheter (CVC)-associated bloodstream infection rate per 1,000 catheter-days; ———, mean CVC-associated bloodstream infection rate in Hospital A medical ICU; – – – –, pooled mean CVC-associated bloodstream infection rate for the CDC NNIS hospital medical ICUs (n = 131); —▪—, 25th and 75th percentiles for CVC-associated bloodstream infection rate in NNIS hospitals.

implementing interventions to unit personnel such as medical directors, nurse managers, and clinicians.

The infection control program staff should design a surveillance system that is appropriate for the specific needs of the hospital and feasible based on the hospital's budget. For example, program personnel wishing to use device days as a denominator must develop a system for counting or accurately estimating device utilization in their ICUs. Because surveillance consumes more resources than any other infection control activity (27), infection control programs must devise the most efficient surveillance system possible. The most complete and accurate surveillance program might require an ICP to review charts of all hospitalized patients daily, but this approach obviously is not practical in any but the smallest of hospitals. Infection control programs should focus their limited resources on the highest-risk areas (e.g., intensive care, hematology-oncology, burn, and organ transplant wards) and use various screening techniques to increase surveillance efficiency. ICPs can use microbiology reports, nursing care plans, antibiotic orders, radiology reports, vital signs, and discharge diagnoses to determine which charts should be further reviewed.

Review of microbiology reports is probably the most common method for case finding, and it compares favorably in some circumstances with more comprehensive ward-based surveillance (31, 77). For example, Yokoe and colleagues reported that review of microbiology data alone was both more resource efficient and as effective as applying the CDC's definition of nosocomial bloodstream infection (85). Such laboratory-based surveillance allows the ICP to efficiently review a large amount of data. Moreover, medical information systems can enhance laboratory-based surveillance further by linking laboratory data with data from many sources (71), including pharmacies (e.g., antimicrobial use), radiology departments, billing departments (e.g., diagnostic codes), and nursing notes (e.g., vital signs and care plans).

Although reviewing microbiology reports is an essential part of surveillance, these data alone may not detect all nosocomial infections or all outbreaks. The sensitivity and specificity of laboratory-based surveillance depend upon both the frequency at which clinicians obtain cultures and the quality of the culture specimens received by the laboratory. In addition, while laboratory-based surveillance may quickly detect outbreaks due to unusual pathogens, or infections at unusual sites, outbreaks or clusters due to common pathogens at common sites (e.g., *Escherichia coli* urinary tract infection) may go undetected for longer periods of time. An optimal surveillance program will include data from more than one source (e.g., nursing care plans and microbiology reports) to help ICPs determine which charts deserve further review. The University of Iowa, Iowa City, previously validated a surveillance strategy using primarily microbiology reports and nursing care plans and found the sensitivity and specificity to be 81 and 98%, respectively (5). More recently, we introduced a computer-based screening algorithm that provides a list for each ICP each day of all patients in their units that had positive cultures or that had a *Clostridium difficile* toxin test or a respiratory syncytial virus antigen test ordered or one of the following combinations of tests ordered within a 24-h period: chest radiograph and culture of respiratory secretions or cultures from two or more body sites. After reviewing this information, the ICPs review the medical records of a small percentage of patients, thereby reducing the amount of time required for surveillance.

The frequency of surveillance of specific hospital units should be determined by the infection control committee based on the types of patients hospitalized, the procedures and treatments done in the facility, the resources available for surveillance, prevailing infection rates, and other factors. In addition, the infection control committee, in consultation with clinical microbiology personnel, should decide the mechanism by which the laboratory provides specific information needed for surveillance (e.g., all positive results or selected or sorted reports, etc.).

The recent movement toward public disclosure of nosocomial infection rates (16, 75, 81) has important implications for surveillance. If interhospital comparisons of nosocomial infection rates are to have any meaning, all hospitals must use the same methods for surveillance and risk adjustment (16, 75). Unfortunately, at the time this chapter was written, methods for nosocomial infection surveillance varied widely among hospitals and validated methods for risk adjustment rates were not available (40). Thus, although public disclosure of nosocomial infection rates is a laudable goal and the policy is being introduced by law in many states, much work needs to be done to ensure that such reporting improves, rather than hinders, efforts to prevent nosocomial infections.

Process Surveillance

Several recent studies clearly demonstrate that implementing evidence-based infection control practices, such as good hand hygiene (61) and guidelines for the placement and care of central venous catheters (4, 10), can dramatically reduce nosocomial infection rates (4, 61, 86). The obvious implication of these studies is that health care workers do not routinely adhere to the safest processes of care. For this reason, ICPs must now perform surveillance not only for important outcomes (infections) but also for important processes (e.g., rates of hand hygiene performance, use of maximal sterile barriers during central venous catheter placement, and elevation of the heads of beds to 30° for ventilated patients, etc.). Process measures can help infection control personnel understand some of the variation in nosocomial infection rates. In addition, reporting compliance rates to personnel may improve practices and reduce nosocomial infection rates.

ROLE OF THE MICROBIOLOGY LABORATORY IN INFECTION CONTROL

With this overview of the structure and activities of the hospital infection control program in mind, we will now focus on the most important specific roles played by the microbiology laboratory in the day-to-day practice of infection control.

Specimen Collection

Many nosocomial pathogens (e.g., coagulase-negative staphylococci) also commonly colonize patients' skin or mucous membranes and can easily contaminate cultures if specimens are not collected or handled properly. If contaminants are mistakenly considered to be infecting organisms, ICPs may inadvertently count these as representatives of nosocomial infections, thereby inflating the infection rates (2). Consequently, microbiologists must monitor specimen quality carefully and also set and enforce strict criteria for acceptable clinical specimens (see chapter 5).

Accurate Identification and Susceptibility Testing of Nosocomial Pathogens

Commercial identification and susceptibility testing systems allow most laboratories to identify microorganisms to the species level and perform antimicrobial susceptibility testing (AST). However, the expanding spectrum of organisms that colonize and infect seriously ill patients challenges the ability of the clinical microbiology laboratory to identify and characterize nosocomial pathogens accurately (56). For example, while many nosocomial pathogens (e.g., *Staphylococcus* spp. and the *Enterobacteriaceae*) are easily detected and identified with commonly used automated systems, many nonfermentative gram-negative organisms that cause nosocomial infections can be much more difficult to identify. Laboratories that identify nosocomial pathogens to the species level may find outbreaks that would otherwise have been undetected because clusters of unusual organisms or unusual clusters of common organisms may be clues to outbreaks. Thus, laboratories should establish a system for sending unusual nosocomial pathogens to a reference laboratory for definitive identification. In addition, viral, fungal, and mycobacterial pathogens can cause nosocomial infections and also can be difficult to identify to a level appropriate for infection control needs.

New antimicrobial resistances continue to emerge, and existing resistances are increasing in frequency. To guard against significant AST errors for some organism-antimicrobial combinations, laboratories must supplement automated systems with additional methods. AST errors are most likely for organisms that display heteroresistance or inducible resistance mechanisms or for newly emerging resistances. For example, some systems previously underestimated oxacillin resistance among *Staphylococcus* species (82) and did not adequately detect extended-spectrum beta-lactamase (ESBL) production by certain *Enterobacteriaceae* (3, 29, 70). Some automated systems have not detected all enterococci with certain vancomycin resistance phenotypes (68). More recently, investigators have found that automated systems were not adequate to detect vancomycin-resistant *Staphylococcus aureus* (VRSA), and therefore, laboratories must use new screening methods to detect this organism (67). If the laboratory uses methods that do not accurately identify organisms or particular resistance patterns, the infection control program may not identify serious problems or even outbreaks. Conversely, infection control personnel may investigate spurious problems, thereby diverting and wasting precious resources.

Laboratories that recognize such problems should bring them to the manufacturers' attention so that manufacturers can improve the instrumentation, panels, or software programs and, thereby, improve accuracy. This process of ongoing independent evaluation of automated systems and feedback to responsive industry representatives is extremely important. Unfortunately, in the era of managed care and shrinking laboratory resources, fewer laboratories have the ability to perform rigorous internal evaluations of new technology. The most important resistances emerging in nosocomial pathogens include ESBL production among *Enterobacteriaceae* (58, 64), glycopeptide resistance among enterococci (21) and staphylococci (9, 11, 12, 14, 19, 51, 65), and methicillin resistance among *S. aureus* strains (25). Moreover, four patients are known to have been infected with VRSA (11, 12, 14, 51), which is particularly concerning because *S. aureus* is a virulent organism and options for bactericidal therapy for infections caused by multiply resistant methicillin-resistant *S. aureus* (MRSA) are limited. The infection control program must implement control measures to prevent the spread of these important antimicrobial-resistant pathogens. However, the success of the program depends upon the ability of the laboratory to detect these organisms. Laboratory directors must read current literature regarding automated systems' ability to detect emerging resistances and implement, if necessary, additional methods to detect or confirm particular resistance patterns. The CDC website provides fact sheets summarizing current recommendations for detecting these resistances (http://www.cdc.gov/ncidod/hip/lab/lab.htm). Antimicrobial resistance detection is also reviewed in chapters 17, 74, and 78 of this Manual.

Laboratory Information Systems

An information system that can do prospective data mining and interface with other parts of the computerized patient record could help ICPs do surveillance, monitor patient-to-patient spread of pathogens, and detect outbreaks early (54, 59). Thus, persons choosing a laboratory information system must consult with both laboratory and infection control personnel before purchasing the best system for the hospital. Chapters 4 and 17 include more complete discussions of laboratory information systems and expert systems for data analysis.

Rapid Diagnostic Testing

During the past decade, numerous rapid diagnostic tests have been developed that use molecular or immunologic methods. For example, a variety of methods are now available for rapid detection of respiratory syncytial virus (41), *Clostridium difficile* (30), *Mycobacterium tuberculosis* (36, 39), and *Legionella pneumophila* serogroup 1 (62). Rapid methods for detecting important antimicrobial resistances are also being developed. Latex agglutination testing for the altered penicillin binding protein 2a (84)—or real-time molecular detection of the *mecA* gene coding for this protein (7, 73, 87)—detects MRSA more rapidly than traditional methods. Some hospitals, including that at the University of Iowa, are using methods that detect the *vanA* and *vanB* genes in real time to identify patients who carry vancomycin-resistant *Enterococcus* spp. (VRE) (24). A positive result from any of these tests will allow clinicians to implement appropriate isolation precautions quickly in order to prevent the spread of the organisms. Thus, such tests can help infection control programs control the spread of important pathogens. Of course, if clinicians order the tests indiscriminately or the laboratory has poor quality control, rapid diagnostic tests can lead to errors, including falsely positive tests that lead to inappropriate treatment and isolation of patients. Erroneous results may also cause the infection control program staff to waste time investigating a pseudo-outbreak (48). The clinical microbiologist must also assess the negative predictive value of any rapid tests provided by the laboratory. If the negative predictive value is not high enough, decisions to discontinue isolation precautions should not be based on the results of the rapid test.

Reporting of Laboratory Data

Culture and AST results are an important data source for infection control and are usually reviewed daily by ICPs. Thus, routine microbiology laboratory results should be readily accessible to ICPs. In most cases, results are stored in a computer database, facilitating retrieval and analysis. The laboratory should store the following information: specimen type, date of collection, patient name, hospital number, hospital service, ward location, organisms identified, AST results, and the results of any specialized testing performed (e.g., typing). Both clinicians and ICPs benefit from periodic summaries of selected microbiology results such as an antibiogram specifically for nosocomial pathogens. These results can be presented in a table that includes the antibiograms of the most common nosocomial pathogens organized by anatomical site and hospital service and that also includes cost information for the most commonly used antimicrobials. This information will help clinicians choose empiric antimicrobial therapy for patients with nosocomial infections. The Clinical and Laboratory Standards Institute has developed guidelines for antibiogram preparation, which are discussed in chapter 4 (20).

Laboratory personnel should call the ICP directly to report some culture results to ensure that appropriate control measures are implemented. Examples include sterile-site cultures positive for *Neisseria meningitidis* and *Legionella pneumophila* and smears or cultures positive for acid-fast bacilli, enteric pathogens such as *Salmonella* and *Shigella* spp., and certain antimicrobial-resistant pathogens such as MRSA, VRSA, and VRE. In addition, new or unusual pathogens and potential agents of bioterrorism (e.g., *Bacillus anthracis*, *Yersinia pestis*, and orthopox viruses) should be reported promptly to the ICP.

In addition to providing printed and verbal reports, laboratory staff should meet regularly with infection control staff to ensure that their communication is direct and clear. They can discuss areas of mutual concern, such as the status of epidemiological and microbiological investigations of clusters or outbreaks. Together they can determine whether supplementary studies such as molecular typing or environmental cultures will be necessary. If these studies are necessary, they can determine exactly what needs to be done, who will perform these procedures, and when they will be carried out.

Outbreak Recognition and Investigation: Epidemic versus Endemic Infections

Most nosocomial infections are not associated with outbreaks, that is, they are endemic rather than epidemic infections. If rates of nosocomial infections are consistently defined by prospective surveillance, infection control personnel may occasionally identify outbreaks of nosocomial infections—an increase in infection rate beyond that expected during a defined time period—by reviewing these rates. However, more often infection control personnel learn about potential outbreaks while interacting with personnel in the ward, in clinics, or in the laboratory.

When the infection control team detects a cluster or outbreak of nosocomial infections, they must act promptly to identify the etiologic agent if it is not known, define the extent of the outbreak, learn the mode of transmission of the pathogen, and institute appropriate control measures. The clinical microbiology laboratory must provide appropriate laboratory support during this time. Table 4 outlines recommended steps in an outbreak investigation and points out the important role of the clinical microbiology laboratory at each step.

TABLE 4 Steps in nosocomial outbreak investigation, and the role of the laboratory at each step[a]

Investigative step	Role of the clinical microbiology laboratory
Recognize problem	Maintain surveillance and early-warning system—ideally part of the laboratory information system; notify infection control personnel of clusters of infections, unusual resistance patterns, and possible patient-to-patient transmission
Establish case definition	Assist and advise regarding inclusion of laboratory diagnosis in case definition
Confirm cases	Perform laboratory confirmation of diagnosis
Complete case finding	Characterize isolates with accuracy; store all sterile-site isolates and epidemiologically important isolates; search laboratory database for new cases
Establish background rate of disease, compare to attack rate during suspected outbreak	Provide data for use in ongoing surveillance, which provide baseline rates for selected units and infection sites; search laboratory database for all prior cases of the entity if baseline rate is not prospectively monitored
Characterize outbreak (descriptive epidemiology)	Perform typing of involved strains and compare to previously isolated endemic strains to determine if the outbreak involves a single strain (see chapter 11); this can be done only if selected pathogens are routinely stored (see above)
Generate hypotheses about causation: Identify potential reservoirs Identify potential modes of spread Identify potential vectors Perform case control study or cohort study	Perform supplementary studies or cultures as needed, but only if justified by epidemiologic link to transmission: personnel, patients, environment
Institute control measures	Adjust laboratory procedures as necessary
Perform ongoing surveillance to document efficacy of control measures	Maintain surveillance and early-warning function of the laboratory

[a] Adapted from reference 50.

Because the demands on the laboratory may be great during outbreaks, the laboratory staff should prepare in advance. Laboratory personnel periodically should ask ICPs what types of outbreaks have occurred in the past or may be anticipated in the future and what laboratory resources would be required should similar outbreaks occur. Laboratory staff should also anticipate the extra costs associated with outbreak investigations so that they can work with hospital administrators to include funds for these efforts in annual budgets. Costs should not be borne by the laboratory or charged to individual patients involved in the outbreak.

Some problems and potential pitfalls of outbreak investigation are pertinent to the clinical microbiology laboratory and bear specific mention. Foremost among these is the problem of determining when to proceed with an outbreak investigation in the first place. The number of cases necessary to constitute an outbreak depends upon the organism, the patient population, and the institution involved. For example, while numerous cases of *Escherichia coli* urinary tract infection in a long-term-care facility may not constitute an outbreak, even a single nosocomial case of group A streptococcal surgical wound infection or VRSA infection merits an outbreak investigation. Laboratories should consider instituting a computerized program that recognizes clusters of pathogens within the hospital. Organisms that appear to be part of a cluster could be further characterized to evaluate whether they are genetically related (see chapter 11), which would suggest patient-to-patient spread or exposure to a contaminated common source. Investigators at Northwestern University hospital implemented such a system and noted that their rates of nosocomial infections decreased in temporal association with this intervention (33).

A second important problem is that of a pseudo-outbreak. A pseudo-outbreak has occurred when an apparent outbreak turns out not to be an outbreak after all. The usual cause of a pseudo-outbreak is either misdiagnosis (e.g., infection has not actually occurred) or misinterpretation of epidemiologic data (e.g., infections have occurred, but clustering or epidemic transmission has not). The microbiology laboratory can be the source of pseudo-outbreaks (1, 28, 37, 45, 47, 66, 72, 83). Problems in the laboratory that lead to pseudo-outbreaks include contamination of reagents for stains (37), false AST results (28), and contamination of culture specimens (often from construction or renovation projects [47] or cross-contamination during specimen processing [83]). Careful attention to quality control, use of sterile techniques for specimen processing, and preventive measures during construction and renovation projects can decrease the likelihood of pseudo-outbreaks that originate in the laboratory.

Molecular Typing To Support Infection Control Activities

Outbreaks of nosocomial infection often result when a number of hospitalized patients are exposed to a contaminated common source or a reservoir of a pathogenic agent (e.g., water from a hot water tank colonized with *Legionella* spp.). The organisms causing such outbreaks would all derive from a single strain (i.e., they are clonally related). The infection control program team may, therefore, request that the microbiology laboratory characterize isolates that may be associated with outbreaks to determine whether they are genetically related. In the appropriate clinical setting, species-level identification and AST results (antibiogram) may provide strong evidence for an epidemiologic link. However, more sensitive methods of strain delineation are often necessary. In this setting, genotypic or DNA-based typing methods have essentially replaced phenotypic typing methods (e.g., AST, biochemical profiles, and bacteriophage susceptibility patterns), which discriminate poorly among isolates (52, 63, 74).

Genotypic typing methods provide meaningful data and are cost-effective only when they are used for well-defined epidemiologic objectives. These objectives include (i) determining the source and extent of an outbreak, (ii) determining the mode of transmission of a nosocomial pathogen, (iii) evaluating the efficacy of preventative measures, and (iv) monitoring transmission of pathogens in high-risk areas (e.g., ICUs), where cross-infection is a recognized hazard.

The ideal genotypic typing system should be standardized, reproducible, stable, sensitive, broadly applicable, readily available, and inexpensive. The typing method should also have proven value in previous epidemiologic investigations. Further discussion of the relative advantages and disadvantages of the many available typing systems is beyond the scope of this chapter and has been summarized in several reviews (52, 63, 69, 74) and in chapter 11 of this text.

Organism Storage

Of course, the laboratory cannot provide the infection control program with supplemental testing such as molecular typing if the appropriate isolates have not been saved. The laboratory should plan ahead and be sure to save all epidemiologically important isolates (see chapter 6). Laboratory and infection control personnel should decide which isolates should be banked and how long they should be stored based upon their epidemiological importance and the available resources. We recommend that all isolates from normally sterile sites (e.g., blood and cerebrospinal fluid), important antibiotic-resistant organisms (MRSA, VRE, and ESBL-producing *Enterobacteriaceae*) from any site, and other epidemiologically important pathogens (e.g., *Mycobacterium tuberculosis*) be saved for a period of 3 to 5 years.

Cultures of Specimens from Hospital Personnel and the Environment

The laboratory should perform cultures of specimens from hospital personnel and the environment (surfaces, air, and water) rarely and only when the epidemiologic evidence suggests that personnel or the environment was associated with transmission of a nosocomial pathogen. Various potential sources and appropriate culture methods are outlined in Table 5. Although infection control staff frequently consider obtaining such cultures, these cultures are labor-intensive, nonstandardized, and difficult to interpret and rarely provide useful information.

Because health care workers' hands can transmit nosocomial pathogens from patient to patient, hand cultures are sometimes useful in confirming the mechanism of cross-infection during an outbreak investigation (79). Similarly, because the anterior nares represent the usual reservoir for *S. aureus* (including MRSA) colonization in humans (43), nares cultures from patients and health care personnel are sometimes appropriate during an *S. aureus* infection outbreak.

Laboratory and infection control personnel should weigh two important factors before deciding to culture specimens from hospital personnel during an outbreak investigation: (i) finding the outbreak strain on the hands or in the nares of a health care worker does not establish the direction of transmission or definitively implicate a health care worker as the source or reservoir for the outbreak, and (ii) culturing specimens from hospital personnel indiscriminately can lead

TABLE 5 Cultures of personnel or environmental sources of infection in the hospital[a,b]

Source	Culture method	Comment
Blood products	Broth culture incubated aerobically and anaerobically at 30–32°C for 10 days	Following transfusion reaction; obtain simultaneous blood cultures by venipuncture
Environmental surfaces	Swab-rinse or impression plate	No evidence that any particular level of contamination correlates with nosocomial infection
Disinfectants and antiseptics	Plating of serial dilutions of the product with and without specific neutralizers	Organisms usually nonfermenting gram-negative aerobic bacilli
Air	Mechanical air sampler (preferred); settling plates (poor)	No uniform agreement on acceptable levels of contamination; lack of correlation with infection
Water (for *Legionella* spp.)	Membrane filter for water samples, swab of faucets and showerheads	Number of sites positive for *Legionella* spp. may correlate with risk for nosocomial cases; culture after confirmed case of nosocomial legionellosis; no consensus on performance of routine water cultures for *Legionella* (see text)
Hands of personnel	Broth-bag: 10–20 ml nutrient broth in sterile plastic bag; wash hands in broth and plate semiquantitatively	May confirm the mechanism of cross-infection; impress the importance of hand washing
Anterior nares of personnel	Swab culture	Carriage of outbreak strain may be eradicated by application of topical agent (e.g., mupirocin for *S. aureus*); recolonization with the same strain is frequent

[a] Cultures to be performed only if clearly indicated by epidemiologic data.
[b] Adapted from references 23 and 57, with permission.

to confusing results and can generate ill will toward the infection control program. In general, only specimens from health care workers epidemiologically linked to cases should be cultured. We recommend that infection control programs obtain cultures of specimens from hospital personnel only after consulting with a hospital epidemiologist experienced in outbreak investigation.

As a general rule, routine cultures of specimens from hospital personnel and the environment should not be performed. Exceptions include routine monitoring of sterilized items, infant formula, products prepared in the hospital, blood components (e.g., platelets) prepared in an open system, and hemodialysis fluid. The CDC and other experts have not reached a consensus about the utility of routine water cultures for the presence of *Legionella* spp. While the CDC suggests that such culturing may be an important aspect of preventing nosocomial legionellosis among very high risk patients (e.g., transplant recipients), the CDC has not made a recommendation about obtaining routine water cultures in health care settings other than transplant units if cases of nosocomial legionellosis have not been identified (13, 15). A complete discussion of this issue is beyond the scope of this chapter but can be found in the CDC guidelines (13, 15) and in a recent review by O'Neill and Humphreys (53).

Routine surveillance cultures should not be obtained from the following persons or items because the cost is high and the cultures rarely provide useful clinical or epidemiologic information: patients and hospital personnel, commercial patient care items, antiseptics and disinfectants that are in use, random blood units, respiratory therapy equipment, peritoneal dialysate, and air. Routine cultures from these sources are a burden to the laboratory and seldom, if ever, provide useful information or lead to specific interventions (13).

CONCLUSION

The clinical microbiology laboratory is an essential component of any effective infection control program. The development and application of new technologies in the clinical laboratory can greatly enhance infection control efforts. A good working relationship between clinical laboratory and infection control personnel will greatly facilitate the investigation and control of health care-associated infections.

REFERENCES

1. **Ashford, D. A., S. Kellerman, M. Yakrus, S. Brim, R. C. Good, L. Finelli, W. R. Jarvis, and M. M. McNeil.** 1997. Pseudo-outbreak of septicemia due to rapidly growing mycobacteria associated with extrinsic contamination of culture supplement. *J. Clin. Microbiol.* **35:**2040–2042.
2. **Beekmann, S. E., D. J. Diekema, and G. V. Doern.** 2005. Determining the clinical significance of coagulase-negative staphylococci isolated from blood cultures. *Infect. Control Hosp. Epidemiol.* **26:**559–566.

3. **Beidenbach, D. J., and R. N. Jones.** 1995. Interpretive errors using an automated system for the susceptibility testing of imipenem and aztreonam. *Diagn. Microbiol. Infect. Dis.* **21:**57–60.
4. **Berenholtz, S. M., P. J. Pronovost, P. A. Lipsett, D. Hobson, K. Earsing, J. E. Farley, S. Milanovich, E. Garrett-Mayer, B. D. Winters, H. R. Rubin, T. Dorman, and T. M. Perl.** 2004. Eliminating catheter-related bloodstream infections in the intensive care unit. *Crit. Care Med.* **32:**2014–2020.
5. **Broderick, A., M. Mori, M. D. Nettleman, S. A. Streed, and R. P. Wenzel.** 1990. Nosocomial infections: validation of surveillance and computer modeling to identify patients at risk. *Am. J. Epidemiol.* **131:**734–742.
6. **Burke, J. P.** 2003. Infection control—a problem for patient safety. *N. Engl. J. Med.* **348:**651–656.
7. **Carroll, K. C., R. B. Leonard, P. L. Newdomb-Gayman, and D. R. Hillyard.** 1996. Rapid detection of the staphylococcal *mecA* gene from BACTEC blood culture bottles by PCR. *Am. J. Clin. Pathol.* **106:**600–605.
8. **Centers for Disease Control.** 1992. Public health focus: surveillance, prevention and control of nosocomial infections. *Morb. Mortal. Wkly. Rep.* **41:**783–787.
9. **Centers for Disease Control and Prevention.** 1997. Update: *Staphylococcus aureus* with reduced susceptibility to vancomycin—United States, 1997. *Morb. Mortal. Wkly. Rep.* **46:**813–815.
10. **Centers for Disease Control and Prevention.** 2002. Guidelines for the prevention of intravascular catheter-related infections. *Morb. Mortal. Wkly. Rep.* **51**(RR-10):1–32.
11. **Centers for Disease Control and Prevention.** 2002. Public health dispatch: vancomycin-resistant *Staphylococcus aureus*—Pennsylvania, 2002. *Morb. Mortal. Wkly. Rep.* **51:**902.
12. **Centers for Disease Control and Prevention.** 2002. *Staphylococcus aureus* resistant to vancomycin. *Morb. Mortal. Wkly. Rep.* **51:**565–567.
13. **Centers for Disease Control and Prevention.** 2003. Guidelines for the environmental infection control in healthcare facilities. *Morb. Mortal. Wkly. Rep.* **52:**1–42.
14. **Centers for Disease Control and Prevention.** 2004. Brief report: vancomycin-resistant *Staphylococcus aureus*—New York, 2004. *Morb. Mortal. Wkly. Rep.* **53:**322–323.
15. **Centers for Disease Control and Prevention.** 2004. Guidelines for preventing health-care associated pneumonia, 2003. *Morb. Mortal. Wkly. Rep.* 53(RR-03):1–36.
16. **Centers for Disease Control and Prevention.** 28 February 2005, posting date. *Guidance on Public Reporting of Healthcare-Associated Infections: recommendations of the Healthcare Infection Control Practices Advisory Committee.* [Online.] Centers for Disease Control and Prevention, Atlanta, Ga. http://www.cdc.gov/ncidod/hip/PublicReportingGuide.pdf.
17. **Centers for Disease Control and Prevention NNIS System.** 1999. National Nosocomial Infections Surveillance (NNIS) report, data summary from January 1990–May 1999, issued June 1999. *Am. J. Infect. Control* **27:**520–532.
18. **Centers for Disease Control and Prevention NNIS System.** 2000. Monitoring hospital-acquired infections to promote patient safety—United States, 1990–1999. *Morb. Mortal. Wkly. Rep.* **49**(08)**:**149–153.
19. **Chang, S., D. M. Sievert, J. C. Hageman, et al.** 2003. Brief report: infection with vancomycin-resistant *Staphylococcus aureus* containing the *vanA* resistance gene. *N. Engl. J. Med.* **348:**1342–1347.
20. **Clinical and Laboratory Standards Institute.** 2002. *Analysis and Presentation of Cumulative Antimicrobial Susceptibility Test Data.* Document M39-A. Clinical and Laboratory Standards Institute, Wayne, Pa.
21. **Cormican, M. G., and R. N. Jones.** 1996. Emerging resistance to antimicrobial agents in gram-positive bacteria: enterococci, staphylococci, and non-pneumococcal streptococci. *Drugs* **51**(Suppl. 1):6–12.
22. **Cruse, P. J. E.** 1970. Surgical wound sepsis. *Can. Med. Assoc. J.* **102:**251–258.
23. **Diekema, D. J., and M. A. Pfaller.** 2001. Role of the clinical microbiology laboratory in hospital epidemiology and infection control, p. 1247–1255. *In* K. McClatchey (ed.), *Clinical Laboratory Medicine*, 2nd ed. Lippincott Williams and Wilkins, New York, N.Y.
24. **Diekema, D. J., K. J. Dodgson, B. Sigurdardottir, and M. A. Pfaller.** 2004. Rapid detection of antimicrobial-resistant organism carriage: an unmet clinical need. *J. Clin. Microbiol.* **42:**2879–2883.
25. **Diekema, D. J., M. A. Pfaller, F. J. Schmitz, J. Smayevsky, J. Bell, R. N. Jones, M. L. Beach, and the SENTRY Participants Group.** 2001. Survey of infections due to *Staphylococcus* species: frequency of occurrence and antimicrobial susceptibility of isolates collected in the US, Canada and Latin America for the SENTRY program, 1997–1999. *Clin. Infect. Dis.* **32**(Suppl. 2)**:**S114–S132.
26. **Edmond, M. B., J. F. Ober, J. D. Dawson, D. L. Weinbaum, and R. P. Wenzel.** 1996. Vancomycin-resistant enterococcal bacteremia: natural history and attributable mortality. *Clin. Infect. Dis.* **23:**1234–1239.
27. **Emori, T. G., R. W. Haley, and J. S. Garner.** 1981. Technique and use of nosocomial infection surveillance in U. S. hospitals. *Am. J. Med.* **70:**933–940.
28. **Ender, P. T., S. J. Durning, W. K. Woelk, R. M. Brockett, A. Astorga, R. Reddy, and P. A. Meier.** 1999. Pseudo-outbreak of methicillin-resistant *Staphylococcus aureus*. *Mayo Clin. Proc.* **74:**885–889.
29. **Ferraro, M. J., and J. H. Jorgensen.** 1995. Instrument-based antibacterial susceptibility testing, p. 1379–1384. In P. R. Murray, E. J. Baron, M. A. Pfaller, F. C. Tenover, and R. H. Yolken (ed.), *Manual of Clinical Microbiology*, 6th ed. American Society for Microbiology, Washington, D.C.
30. **Gerding, D. N., and J. S. Brazier.** 1993. Optimal methods for identifying *Clostridium difficile* infections. *Clin. Infect. Dis.* **16**(Suppl. 4)**:**S439–S442.
31. **Gross, P. A., A. Beaugard, and C. Van Antwerpen.** 1980. Surveillance for nosocomial infections: can the sources of data be reduced? *Infect. Control* **1:**233–236.
32. **Gudlaugsson, O., S. Gillespie, K. Lee, J. Vande Berg, J. Hu, S. Messer, L. Herwaldt, M. Pfaller, and D. Diekema.** 2003. Attributable mortality of nosocomial candidemia, revisited. *Clin. Infect. Dis.* **37:**1172–1177.
33. **Hacek, D. M., T. Suriano, G. A. Noskin, J. Kruszynsky, B. Reisberg, and L. R. Peterson.** 1999. Medical and economic benefit of a comprehensive infection control program that includes routine determination of microbial clonality. *Am. J. Clin. Pathol.* **111:**647–654.
34. **Haley, R. W., D. H. Culver, J. W. White, W. M. Morgan, and T. G. Emori.** 1985. The nationwide nosocomial infection rate. A new need for vital statistics. *Am. J. Epidemiol.* **121:**159–167.
35. **Haley, R. W., D. H. Culver, J. W. White, W. M. Morgan, T. G. Emori, V. P. Munn, and T. M. Hooten.** 1985. The efficacy of infection control surveillance and control programs in preventing nosocomial infections in U.S. hospitals. *Am. J. Epidemiol.* **121:**182–205.
36. **Hazbon, M. H.** 2004. Recent advances in molecular methods for early diagnosis of tuberculosis and drug-resistant tuberculosis. *Biomedica* **24:**163–164.
37. **Hopfer, R. L., R. L. Katz, and V. Fainstein.** 1982. Pseudooutbreak of cryptococcal meningitis. *J. Clin. Microbiol.* **15:**1141–1143.
38. **Jarvis, W. R.** 2001. Infection control and changing health-care delivery systems. *Emerg. Infect. Dis.* **7:**170–173.
39. **Kearns, A. M., R. Freeman, M. Steward, and J. G. Magee.** 1998. A rapid PCR technique for detecting

M. *tuberculosis* in a variety of clinical specimens. *J. Clin. Pathol.* **51:**922–924.
40. **Keita-Perse, O., and R. P. Gaynes.** 1996. Severity of illness scoring systems to adjust nosocomial infection rates: a review and commentary. *Am. J. Infect. Control* **24:**429–434.
41. **Kellog, J. A.** 1991. Culture versus direct antigen assays for detection of microbial pathogens from lower respiratory tract specimens suspected of containing the respiratory syncytial virus. *Arch. Pathol. Lab. Med.* **115:**451–458.
42. **Kirkland, K. B., J. P. Briggs, S. L. Trivette, W. E. Wilkinson, and D. J. Sexton.** 1999. The impact of surgical-site infections in the 1990s: attributable mortality, excess length of hospitalization, and extra costs. *Infect. Control Hosp. Epidemiol.* **20:**725–730.
43. **Kluytmans, J., A. van Belkum, and H. Verbrugh.** 1997. Nasal carriage of *Staphylococcus aureus:* epidemiology, underlying mechanisms, and associated risks. *Clin. Microbiol. Rev.* **10:**505–520.
44. **Kohn, L. T., J. M. Corrigan, and M. S. Donaldson (ed.).** 2000. *To Err Is Human: Building a Safer Health System.* National Academy Press, Washington, D.C.
45. **Lai, K. K., B. A. Brown, J. A. Westerling, S. A. Fontecchio, Y. Zhang, and R. J. Wallace.** 1998. Long-term laboratory contamination by *Mycobacterium abscessus* resulting in two pseudo-outbreaks: recognition with use of RAPD PCR. *Clin. Infect. Dis.* **27:**169–175.
46. **Landry, S. L., D. L. Kaiser, and R. P. Wenzel.** 1989. Hospital stay and mortality attributed to nosocomial enterococcal bacteremia: a controlled study. *Am. J. Infect. Control* **17:**323–329.
47. **Laurel, V. L., P. A. Meier, A. Astorga, D. Dolan, R. Brockett, and M. G. Rinaldi.** 1999. Pseudoepidemic of *Aspergillus niger* infections traced to specimen contamination in the microbiology laboratory. *J. Clin. Microbiol.* **37:**1612–1615.
48. **Laussucq, S., D. Schuster, W. J. Alexander, W. L. Thacker, H. W. Wilkinson, and J. S. Spika.** 1988. False-positive DNA probe test for *Legionella* species associated with a cluster of respiratory illnesses. *J. Clin. Microbiol.* **26:**1442–1444.
49. **Martin, M. A., M. A. Pfaller, and R. P. Wenzel.** 1989. Mortality and hospital stay attributable to coagulase-negative staphylococcal bacteremia. *Ann. Intern. Med.* **110:**9–16.
50. **McGowan, J. E., and B. G. Metchock.** 1999. Infection control epidemiology and clinical microbiology, p. 107–115. *In* P. R. Murray, E. J. Baron, M. A. Pfaller, F. C. Tenover, and R. H. Yolken (ed.), *Manual of Clinical Microbiology*, 7th ed. ASM Press, Washington, D.C.
51. **Michigan Department of Community Health.** February 2005, posting date. *Bureau of Laboratory Broadcast Fax: Second Michigan VRSA Case.* [Online.] Michigan Department of Community Health, Lansing, Mich. http://www.michigan.gov/ documents/VRSA_Feb05_HAN_118391_7.pdf.
52. **Olive, D. M., and P. Bean.** 1999. Principles and applications of methods for DNA-based typing of microbial organisms. *J. Clin. Microbiol.* **37:**1661–1669.
53. **O'Neill, E., and H. Humphreys.** 2005. Surveillance of hospital water and primary prevention of nosocomial legionellosis: what is the evidence? *J. Hosp. Infect.* **59:** 273–279.
54. **Peterson, L. R., and S. E. Brossette.** 2002. Hunting health care-associated infections from the clinical microbiology laboratory: passive, active and virtual surveillance. *J. Clin. Microbiol.* **40:**1–4.
55. **Pfaller, M. A.** 1996. Nosocomial candidiasis: emerging species, reservoirs, and modes of transmission. *Clin. Infect. Dis.* **22**(S-2):S89–S94.
56. **Pfaller, M. A., and L. A. Herwaldt.** 1997. The clinical microbiology laboratory and infection control: emerging pathogens, antimicrobial resistance, and new technology. *Clin. Infect. Dis.* **25:**858–870.
57. **Pfaller, M. A., and M. G. Cormican.** 1997. Microbiology: the role of the clinical laboratory, p. 95–118. *In* R. P. Wenzel (ed.), *Prevention and Control of Nosocomial Infections.* Williams & Wilkins, Baltimore, Md.
58. **Philippon, A., G. Arlet, and P. H. Lagrange.** 1994. Origin and impact of plasmid-mediated extended spectrum beta-lactamases. *Eur. J. Clin. Microbiol. Infect. Dis.* **13**(S1)**:**17–29.
59. **Pittet, D.** 2005. Infection control and quality health care in the new millennium. *Am. J. Infect. Control* **33:**258–267.
60. **Pittet, D., D. Tarara, and R. P. Wenzel.** 1994. Nosocomial bloodstream infection in critically ill patients: excess length of stay, extra costs, and attributable mortality. *JAMA* **271:**1598–1601.
61. **Pittet, D., S. Hugonnet, S. Harbarth, P. Mourouga, V. Sauvan, S. Touveneau, and T. V. Perneger.** 2000. Effectiveness of a hospital-wide programme to improve compliance with hand hygiene. *Lancet* **356:**1307–1312.
62. **Plouffe, J. F., T. M. File, Jr., R. F. Breiman, B. A. Hackman, S. J. Salstrom, B. J. Marston, B. S. Fields, et al.** 1995. Reevaluation of the definition of Legionnaires' disease: use of the urinary antigen assay. *Clin. Infect. Dis.* **20:**1286–1291.
63. **Sader, H. S., R. J. Hollis, and M. A. Pfaller.** 1995. The use of molecular techniques in the epidemiology and control of infectious diseases. *Clin. Lab. Med.* **15:**407–431.
64. **Sanders, C. C., and W. E. Sanders.** 1992. Beta-lactam resistance in gram-negative bacteria: global trends and clinical impact. *Clin. Infect. Dis.* **15:**824–839.
65. **Schwalbe, R. S., J. T. Stapleton, and P. H. Gilligan.** 1987. Emergence of vancomycin resistance in coagulase-negative staphylococci. *N. Engl. J. Med.* **316:**927–931.
66. **Segal-Maurer, S., B. N. Kreiswirth, J. M. Burns, S. Lavie, M. Lim, C. Urban, and J. J. Rahal.** 1998. *Mycobacterium tuberculosis* specimen contamination revisited: the role of laboratory environmental control in a pseudo-outbreak. *Infect. Control Hosp. Epidemiol.* **19:**101–105.
67. **Tenover, F. C., and L. C. McDonald.** 2005. Vancomycin-resistant staphylococci and enterococci: epidemiology and control. *Curr. Opin. Infect. Dis.* **18:**300–305.
68. **Tenover, F. C., J. M. Swenson, C. M. O'Hara, and S. A. Stocker.** 1995. Ability of commercial and reference antimicrobial susceptibility testing methods to detect vancomycin resistance in enterococci. *J. Clin. Microbiol.* **33:**1524–1527.
69. **Tenover, F. C., R. D. Arbeit, R. V. Goering, and the Molecular Working Group of the Society for Healthcare Epidemiology of America.** 1997. How to select and interpret molecular strain typing methods for epidemiological studies of bacterial infections: a review for healthcare epidemiologists. *Infect. Control Hosp. Epidemiol.* **18:** 426–439.
70. **Thompson, K. S., and C. C. Sanders.** 1992. Detection of extended-spectrum beta-lactamases in members of the family *Enterobacteriaceae:* comparison of the double-disk and three-dimensional tests. *Antimicrob. Agents Chemother.* **36:**1877–1882.
71. **Trick, W. E., B. M. Zagorski, J. I. Tokars, M. O. Vernon, S. F. Welbel, M. F. Wisniewski, C. Richards, and R. A. Weinstein.** 2004. Computer algorithms to detect bloodstream infections. *Emerg. Infect. Dis.* **10:**1612–1620.
72. **Tsakris, A., A. Pantazi, S. Pournaras, A. Maniatis, A. Polyzou, and D. Sofianou.** 2000. Pseudo-outbreak of imipenem-resistant *Acinetobacter baumanii* resulting from false susceptibility testing by a rapid automated system. *J. Clin. Microbiol.* **38:**3505–3507.
73. **Warren, D. K., R. S. Liao, L. R. Merz, M. Eveland, and W. M. Dunne, Jr.** 2004. Detection of methicillin-resistant *Staphylococcus aureus* directly from nasal swab specimens by a real-time PCR assay. *J. Clin. Microbiol.* **42:**5578–5581.

74. **Weber, S., M. A. Pfaller, and L. A. Herwaldt.** 1997. Role of molecular epidemiology in infection control. *Infect. Dis. Clin. N. Am.* **11**:257–278.
75. **Weinstein, R. A., J. D. Siegel, and P. J. Brennan.** 2005. Infection control report cards—securing patient safety. *N. Engl. J. Med.* **353**:225–227.
76. **Wenzel, R. P., and M. B. Edmond.** 2001. The impact of hospital-acquired bloodstream infections. *Emerg. Infect. Dis.* **7**:174–177.
77. **Wenzel, R. P., C. A. Osterman, K. J. Hunting, and J. M. Gwaltney, Jr.** 1976. Hospital-acquired infections. I. Surveillance in a university hospital. *Am. J. Epidemiol.* **103**:251–260.
78. **Wey, S. B., M. Mori, M. A. Pfaller, R. F. Woolson, and R. P. Wenzel.** 1988. Hospital acquired candidemia: attributable mortality and excess length of stay. *Arch. Intern. Med.* **148**:2642–2645.
79. **Widmer, A. F., R. P. Wenzel, A. Trilla, M. J. Bale, R. N. Jones, and B. N. Doebbeling.** 1993. Outbreak of *Pseudomonas aeruginosa* infections in a surgical intensive care unit: probable transmission via hands of a healthcare worker. *Clin. Infect. Dis.* **16**:372–376.
80. **Wisplinghoff, H., T. Bischoff, S. M. Tallent, H. Seifert, R. P. Wenzel, and M. B. Edmond.** 2004. Nosocomial bloodstream infections in US hospitals: analysis of 24,179 cases from a prospective nationwide surveillance study. *Clin. Infect. Dis.* **39**:309–317.
81. **Wong, E. S., M. E. Rupp, L. Mermel, T. M. Perl, S. Bradley, K. M. Ramsey, B. Ostrowsky, A. J. Valenti, J. A. Jernigan, A. Voss, and M. L. Tapper.** 2005. Public disclosure of healthcare-associated infections. *Infect. Control Hosp. Epidemiol.* **26**:210–212.
82. **Woods, G. L., D. LaTemple, and C. Cruz.** 1994. Evaluation of Microscan rapid gram-positive panels for detection of oxacillin-resistant staphylococci. *J. Clin. Microbiol.* **32**:1058–1059.
83. **Wurtz, R., P. Demarais, W. Trainor, J. McAuley, F. Kocka, L. Mosher, and S. Dietrich.** 1996. Specimen contamination in mycobacteriology laboratory detected by pseudo-outbreak of multidrug-resistant tuberculosis: analysis by routine epidemiology and confirmation by molecular technique. *J. Clin. Microbiol.* **34**:1017–1019.
84. **Yamazumi, T., S. A. Marshall, W. W. Wilke, D. J. Diekema, M. A. Pfaller, and R. N. Jones.** 2001. Comparison of the Vitek Gram-Positive Susceptibility 106 card and the MRSA-screen latex agglutination test for determining oxacillin resistance in clinical bloodstream isolates of *Staphylococcus aureus*. *J. Clin. Microbiol.* **39**:53–56.
85. **Yokoe, D. S., J. Anderson, R. Chambers, M. Connor, R. Finberg, C. Hopkins, D. Lichtenberg, S. Marino, D. McGlaughlin, E. O'Rourke, M. Samore, K. Sands, J. Strymish, E. Yamplin, N. Vallonde, and R. Platt.** 1998. Simplified surveillance for nosocomial bloodstream infections. *Infect. Control Hosp. Epidemiol.* **19**:657–660.
86. **Zack, J. E., T. Garrison, E. Trovillion, D. Clinkscale, C. M. Coopersmith, V. J. Fraser, and M. H. Kollef.** 2002. Effect of an education program aimed at reducing the occurrence of ventilator-associated pneumonia. *Crit. Care Med.* **30**:2407–2412.
87. **Zheng, X., C. P. Kolbert, P. Varga-Delmore, J. Arruda, M. Lewis, J. Kolberg, F. R. Cockerill, and D. H. Persing.** 1999. Direct *mecA* detection from blood culture bottles by branched-DNA signal amplification. *J. Clin. Microbiol.* **37**:4192–4193.

Laboratory Procedures for the Epidemiological Analysis of Microorganisms

DAVID R. SOLL, CLAUDE PUJOL, AND SHAWN R. LOCKHART

11

In dealing with an infection, one often is faced with the need for species identification in order to prescribe effective treatment. In some clinical cases, however, one must pursue the identity of the infecting organism to the subspecies level. The typing techniques that have evolved for such discrimination at both of these levels of relatedness must be as rapid as possible. These techniques, therefore, usually focus on phenotypic characteristics and rarely provide the resolution necessary to obtain measurements of genetic relatedness among isolates of the same species or the same subspecies. Such resolution is essential for a number of epidemiological questions. In order to accurately identify the origin of a nosocomial infection, track the transmission of a disease, the emergence of a new hypervirulent or drug-resistant strain, or the microevolution of a commensal or infecting strain, and examine the general population structure of a pathogen, one must move from species typing to strain and substrain typing. Methods must be selected that provide information on the level of genetic relatedness. Methods have evolved that indeed provide such information, but researchers rarely validate the method they select for characterizing relatedness (135) or ask if the method they have selected has the resolving power for the question posed. Their results may, therefore, suggest stability when in fact the infecting organism is undergoing rapid microevolution. Alternatively, researchers may ask a question related to strain grouping that requires the genesis of deep-rooted dendrograms and then apply a method that relies mainly on hypervariable changes. Again, their results may not provide them with a valid answer, in this case because hypervariable changes will affect clustering due to homoplasy, which is the presence of identical characteristics in distinct phylogenetic lineages that are acquired not through descent, but rather through convergence, parallelism, or reversion. It is, therefore, imperative that one accurately formulate the question to be answered, define the level of genetic relatedness that must be assessed, and select a genetic fingerprinting method with the resolution necessary to answer that question (135).

BIOTYPING AND GENETIC FINGERPRINTING TECHNIQUES

Prior to the development of DNA-based techniques for assessing genetic relatedness, scientists relied on biotyping techniques, which measure phenotypic differences. The logic behind this approach was that phenotype reflects genotype, and so if one employs a number of phenotypic parameters, one can obtain a measure of genetic relatedness. In discriminating between genuses and species in both bacteria and fungi, biotyping still provides us with fast and reliable diagnostic methods. Kits measuring assimilation patterns (biochemical profiles) are still a mainstay for discriminating among a variety of bacterial and fungal species (25, 76, 78, 82, 106, 139, 163), antibody-based tests (serotyping) continue to be used to discriminate among groups within bacterial species and fungi like *Cryptococcus neoformans* (7, 132, 138, 174), and phage typing continues to be used to discriminate among groups within bacterial species (9, 70). However, these types of methods in general do not provide the kind of genetic discrimination usually necessary for addressing epidemiological questions. First, most of these tests do not provide enough unrelated parameters to obtain a good reflection of genotype. Usually they discriminate among only a limited number of groups, as in the case of serotyping. Second, and more important, the expression of many genes is affected by environmental changes and by developmental programs or reversible phenotypic switching (11, 54, 134, 143). In addition, phage and plasmids can be transmitted horizontally (23, 173). Most biotyping methods, therefore, fall short as genetic fingerprinting techniques. There is, however, one major exception, multilocus enzyme electrophoresis (MLEE) (105, 115). MLEE represents a robust genetic fingerprinting method that exhibits performance parity with many of the most effective DNA fingerprinting methods (111, 156).

DNA fingerprinting techniques, by virtue of the fact that they assess differences in genetic material, have been assumed to be the most accurate methods for genetic fingerprinting. This is not necessarily the case (135). As noted, some are as effective as MLEE and others fall short. Some are poor indicators of microevolution, and others are good indicators of microevolution but measure DNA sequences that are too hypervariable for deep-rooted cluster analyses (111). Some techniques are effective for analyzing bacteria but less effective for analyzing eukaryotes, and vice versa, because of inherent genomic differences. Finally, while some DNA fingerprinting techniques are excellent for cluster analyses of large collections of isolates, they are not favored by evolutionary biologists because they do not provide codominant markers (150), although this requirement has been challenged quite effectively (154, 155).

What, then, are the general methods of DNA fingerprinting? The methods that will be reviewed in this chapter have, for the most part, been used for bacteria, fungi, and parasites. One of the earliest methods applied to bacteria and fungi took advantage of the fact that in the divergence of strains within a species, restriction sites identified by restriction enzymes, or endonucleases, change, leading to changes in the lengths of DNA sequences between sites. These changes accumulate as strains diverge during evolution, and the sum of the changes provides an indicator of evolutionary distance. The pattern of restriction fragments is referred to as the restriction fragment length polymorphism (RFLP) pattern. The comparison of the RFLP patterns between different isolates is referred to as RFLP analysis. This method has proved to be effective in DNA fingerprinting of bacteria, especially with the use of infrequent cutters in combination with pulsed-field gel electrophoresis (PFGE) (151), but less effective in fingerprinting of eukaryotic pathogens like the infectious fungi (10, 123). To obtain a more limited and more specific pattern, Southern blots can be hybridized with a DNA probe. Although this method is also referred to as RFLP analysis in the literature, we will distinguish it by calling it RFLP with a probe. The probes in this case must distinguish more than one fragment and, therefore, usually contain a repetitive sequence (124, 141, 145) or a combination of unique and repetitive sequences (41, 72, 91). The former are referred to as repetitive-element probes, and the latter are referred to as complex probes (135). A second approach to DNA fingerprinting takes advantage of PCR to amplify a variety of sequence fragments from the genome by utilizing sequences identified by the primers used in the PCR. The use of arbitrary primers for amplification has been referred to as random amplification of polymorphic DNA (RAPD) analysis (165, 167). This method has been used for DNA fingerprinting of a number of prokaryotic and eukaryotic pathogens (35, 77, 109, 156, 165). In recent years, PCR-based methods have been developed that employ primers that recognize identified sequences and in some cases these methods have been used in combination with RFLP analysis. Some of these methods are preferred by evolutionary biologists since the data they generate represent identified alleles (150). A third DNA fingerprinting method that has evolved in the last decade is based on PFGE methods for separating chromosome-sized DNA fragments (26, 126). This method has been successfully used to karyotype many fungi (14, 36, 79) and other eukaryotic microorganisms (69, 133) and, in the case of prokaryotes, to separate large fragments generated by endonucleases that identify infrequent restriction sites (3, 15, 35). Finally, sequencing of portions of one or several genes is a basic tool for answering evolutionary questions and a rapidly emerging tool for assessing epidemiological questions (42, 75, 95). Multilocus sequence typing (MLST) (95) has evolved rapidly in the past 5 years for DNA fingerprinting of both bacteria and lower eukaryotes (20, 37, 46, 149, 157). Finally, microarray typing based on probing oligonucleotides representing alleles of loci with PCR products provides a very new and potentially powerful method of discrimination (51, 56, 86, 140). Since MLEE and the variety of DNA fingerprinting methods outlined above are all tools for epidemiological studies of the genetic relatedness of isolates, we will refer to them as genetic fingerprinting methods.

GENERAL REQUIREMENTS OF AN EFFECTIVE GENETIC FINGERPRINTING METHOD

Before considering in detail each DNA fingerprinting method, a consideration of the general requirements of fingerprinting methods is in order. Although a list of requirements will be formulated, it should be realized that each epidemiological question posed will require different levels of resolution or stringency.

A Method Should Provide Data That Reflect Genetic Distance at the Level Necessary for Answering the Question Posed

An effective genetic fingerprinting system should do more than demonstrate that two isolates are nonidentical or that a collection of isolates differ. In many cases, a researcher must know how unrelated (or related) two or more isolates are. If one does not know the resolving power of the genetic fingerprinting method applied, one may conclude that because there are differences in the fingerprinting data, two isolates are unrelated or that because the fingerprinting patterns are identical, the isolates represent the same strain. However, if in the former case the method identifies hypervariable changes in the genome that can occur as frequently as 1 in every 200 cell divisions, the isolates may in fact be highly related, and in the latter case, if the method measures only rare changes, the isolates may in fact be quite unrelated. With this in mind, what are the levels of relatedness that we must consider? Because few methods provide a true measure of genetic relatedness, with some functioning better at discriminating one level than another, and since evolutionary time can only be estimated, we will categorize the levels rather than consider them as a continuum. The categories, diagrammed in Fig. 1, are "identical," "highly related but nonidentical," "moderately related," and "unrelated." The utility of using these categories will become evident in considering the effectiveness of the separate methods.

A Genetic Fingerprinting Method Should Be Resistant to Environmental Perturbations and High-Frequency Genomic Reorganization

As in the case of MLEE, the targeted sequences for a DNA fingerprinting method must be carefully selected. For instance, plasmid DNA and minichromosomal DNA may in

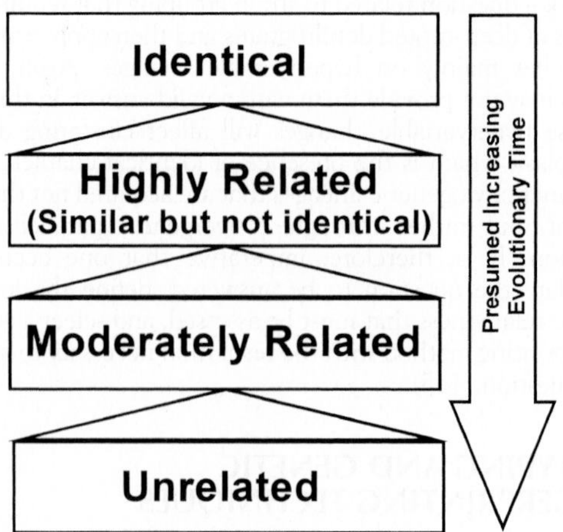

FIGURE 1 Categories of genetic relatedness for isolates within a species.

some cases be bad choices since growth rate and cellular phenotype may affect the maintenance of the genetic markers and the rate of reorganization (22, 27). Sequences involved in phase transitions in such bacteria as *Salmonella enterica* serovar Typhimurium and *Escherichia coli* undergo reversible transitions (61), as is also the case for the expressed mating type locus in *Saccharomyces cerevisiae* (65). In addition, some genomic reorganization events are repressed by silencing genes (58) and derepressed in mutants (63) and the frequencies of other reorganizational events are affected by the expressed phase in phenotypic switching systems (113).

In Most Cases, a Genetic Fingerprinting Method Should Be Fast, Feasible, Affordable, and Amenable to Computer-Assisted Analysis

In many instances, a genetic fingerprinting study involves few isolates and limited goals. If a study, however, involves large numbers of isolates requiring complex measurements of relatedness, and if retrospective use of the data in the future is entertained, one must select a method amenable to automatic computer-assisted analysis and storage. One must also select a method that is within one's technical abilities, that is affordable, that can be accomplished in a reasonable amount of time, and that will answer the question posed.

COMMON GENETIC FINGERPRINTING METHODS

There are several basic genetic fingerprinting methods that have been used repeatedly for prokaryotic and eukaryotic pathogens to answer a variety of epidemiological questions. In the sections that follow, the most commonly used methods are described and evaluated.

Multilocus Enzyme Electrophoresis

It is immediately obvious that a method based on enzyme electrophoresis is not DNA based. However, MLEE fulfills the requirements set forth for DNA-based fingerprinting systems (135) and has been demonstrated to attain resolution at all of the levels categorized in Fig. 1 (105, 111, 115, 156). The MLEE method relies on phenotypic polymorphisms, but these polymorphisms are rooted in protein structures that are reflections of the sequences of the structural genes that encode them. The MLEE method resolves polymorphisms through differences in the electrophoretic mobilities of the gene products of different alleles of the same gene. Electrophoretic mobility depends primarily on the net charge of the protein, which is a consequence of the primary protein structure but which is also influenced by secondary, tertiary, and quaternary structures. The latter levels of structure can conceal or reveal charged amino acid residues that contribute to the total charge of a protein and therefore to its exact electrophoretic mobility. In addition, MLEE detects polymorphisms only within the coding region of a gene. Even in coding regions, many mutations do not cause a polymorphism. It is, therefore, difficult to estimate what proportion of base changes leading to amino acid substitutions or other mutations in a protein is detected by the MLEE method, but it is generally accepted that only approximately 15% of the amino acid changes in an average protein can be resolved by MLEE (115). This level of sensitivity is sufficient for assessing the various levels of genetic relationships outlined in Fig. 1.

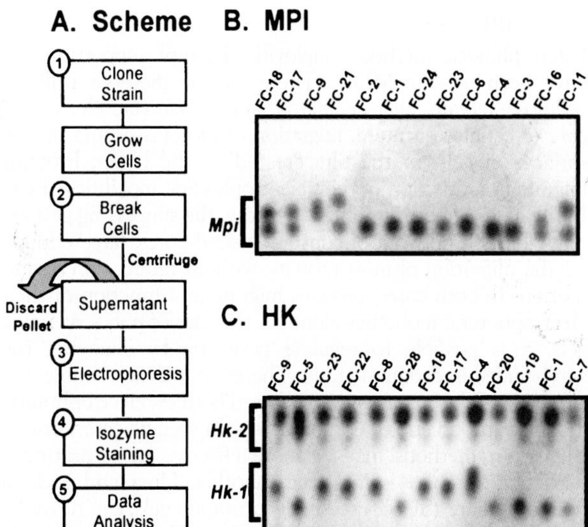

FIGURE 2 MLEE. (A) Generic version of the steps in the MLEE method. (B and C) Examples of enzyme phenotypes using starch gel electrophoresis for mannose-6-phosphate isomerase (MPI) (B) and hexokinase (HK) (C) in 13 *C. albicans* isolates (111). Note that there are two different HK genes, *Hk-1* and *Hk-2*.

In Fig. 2A, a generic version of the MLEE method is presented.

Preparation of Cells

One must begin with a clone. Primary isolates must be cloned, and each clone must be individually grown for protein extraction. For most infectious microorganisms, homogeneous cell populations can be grown in culture to the levels necessary for standard assays. Precaution must be taken, however, in the growth of the different isolates in a test set. Growth conditions for isolates must be uniform, which is not as stringent a requirement for DNA-based methods. If some isolates grow at different rates, reach stationary phase at different times, or express different general phenotypes under the same culture conditions, there may be effects on the isozyme patterns that would not represent changes in DNA sequence.

Preparation of Protein Extracts

Cells are harvested (e.g., pelleted by centrifugation) and washed (e.g., with distilled water). The cell sample (e.g., 200 μl of wet cells) is mixed with glass beads (e.g., 200 μl) and distilled water (e.g., 200 μl) in a 1.5-ml microcentrifuge tube and vortexed. The extraction solution must be appropriate for the maintenance of enzyme activity. Distilled water is in many cases appropriate for large, concentrated biological samples. In some cases, proteinase inhibitors must be employed. Bead friction during vortexing will produce heat that can denature proteins. To avoid this, cooling intervals (e.g., placing the tube in ice water) are interspersed with vortexing pulses. A number of different lysis methods are available, each with different attributes. Immediately after disruption, samples are centrifuged to remove insoluble materials. The supernatant containing the soluble enzymes of interest can then be divided into small aliquots (e.g., 50-μl aliquots) and immediately used or stored at ≤20°C. Enzymes must be selected that retain activity through the extraction procedure.

Electrophoresis

Electrophoretic methods employing different supporting gels have been used in MLEE. These include methods utilizing cellulose acetate, agarose, starch, and polyacrylamide. In the case of cellulose acetate, migration of proteins occurs on the surfaces of gels, in the film created by the buffer. Proteins migrate as a function of their electrophoretic mobilities alone. In the cases of both starch and agarose, the supporting gels are made up of a network of constantly sized pores, large enough for the migration of most proteins without retardation due to friction. In both cases, proteins migrate as a function of their electrophoretic mobilities alone. In the case of polyacrylamide gels, it is possible to regulate pore size by changing the acrylamide/bisacrylamide ratio. Therefore, polyacrylamide gels can be used to separate proteins based both on electrophoretic mobility and on size or conformation. In specific cases, one of these four methods may be more effective in separating a particular set of isozymes than another. Urea and sodium dodecyl sulfate (SDS), used in denaturation gels, can never be included in the electrophoresis procedure. The electrophoretic temperature usually must be maintained at close to 4°C in order to avoid thermal denaturation of the protein. The composition of the electrophoresis buffer must be optimized empirically by the enzymes selected for analysis. Buffer characteristics that affect both activity and separation include pH, ionic strength, and the specific concentrations of cations and anions.

Staining of Enzymes for Visualization of Specific Activities

Once enzymes are separated, enzyme positions must be visualized. This is achieved by using the specific activities of the isozymes. This basic approach requires that the mutations that affect mobility do not affect enzyme activity. In visualizing enzyme activity, one of the enzyme products is usually stained by a second reaction. Examples of stained isozymes are presented in Fig. 2B and C.

Application and Analysis

If the patterns of a single set of isozymes for a particular gene are used to assess genetic relatedness, the information level is too meager. For a haploid organism, one band is obtained per sample, and for diploids, one or two bands are usually obtained. Electrophoretic patterns may be more complex if the enzyme is active in multimeric forms, but this does not increase the information that can be used to assess genetic relatedness. In the patterns generated by MLEE (Fig. 2B and C), the alleles are codominant, which means that for heterozygous loci in diploid organisms, both alleles are expressed. Electrophoretic conditions should, therefore, be developed that provide the best separation of the different isozymes of each gene. For monomeric enzymes (composed of a single polypeptide), a homozygote will exhibit one band and a heterozygote will exhibit two bands. For a dimeric enzyme (composed of two polypeptides) in diploid organisms, heterozygotes could show three bands. Similarly, a heterozygote for a tetrameric enzyme should show up to five bands. Such patterns are sometimes difficult to resolve. On rare occasions, enzymes are composed of two or more polypeptides encoded by independent genes, and even greater complications then arise. To generate complex enough data to assess relatedness at all levels (Fig. 1), several genes must be analyzed. On average, 10 to 20 genes should make up the data set for each microorganism (see, e.g., Table 1). The selected genes must exhibit variability between independent isolates. Therefore, for each organism, a set of enzymes must be established empirically. For well-studied organisms, this job usually has already been performed, so scrutiny of the literature should provide one with a list of enzymes and references to the chemical reactions for visualization. The general approach for selecting enzymes was recently described by Pujol et al. (110, 111) in developing an MLEE method for *Candida albicans*. In two independent studies, 21 enzyme loci were tested with collections of 55 and 29 isolates of *C. albicans*. In both studies, 13 loci (62%) exhibited variability among the test strains and their products were selected as the set of analytical enzymes. In MLEE studies of bacterial collections, 9 polymorphic enzymes were used to analyze *Campylobacter jejuni* isolates (103) and 16 were used to analyze the genetic diversity of *Helicobacter pylori* (66). In MLEE studies of fungal collections, 7 polymorphic enzymes were used to analyze *Aspergillus fumigatus* (17) and 12 were used to analyze *Cryptococcus neoformans* (16). In MLEE studies of parasite collections, 22 polymorphic enzyme loci were used to analyze *Trypanosoma cruzi* isolates (12) and 16 were used to analyze *Leishmania* spp. (8). Examples of sets of enzymes used effectively in an MLEE study of a bacterium (13), a fungus (111), and a parasite (2) are presented in Table 1.

The result of an MLEE analysis involving, for example, 10 analyzed genes is a phenotype composed of 10 sets of values for each isolate. Each analyzed test isolate must then be compared with every other isolate at every locus in order to obtain a summed similarity coefficient. The method for doing this will be dealt with later in this chapter.

Restriction Fragment Length Polymorphism without Hybridization

As previously noted, one of the earliest methods for DNA fingerprinting of infectious microorganisms was restriction enzyme analysis, more commonly referred to as RFLP analysis. RFLP has been useful in answering limited epidemiological questions posed for a number of lower eukaryotic pathogens, but because of the composition of eukaryotic genomes, RFLP as presently applied presents limitations as a DNA fingerprinting method. For this reason, the application of RFLP to eukaryotic microorganisms will first be described and discussed and a discussion of its application to bacteria, which has been far more effective, will follow separately. The basic method of RFLP has also been incorporated into a number of additional, more complex fingerprinting methods, usually involving repetitive-hybridization probes.

Use of RFLP To Analyze Lower Eukaryotic Pathogens

The general method of RFLP analysis is relatively straightforward (Fig. 3A). Total cellular DNA is extracted from cells, digested usually with one endonuclease, separated by agarose gel electrophoresis, and stained usually with ethidium bromide. The final banding pattern represents differences in the sizes of the digestion fragments. Differences between patterns are assumed to represent differences in genetic relatedness. Fragment polymorphisms are determined by the positions of restriction sites identified by the particular endonuclease(s) employed. Differences in the banding patterns of two isolates of the same species are due to differences in fragment sizes that can occur as a result of changes in restriction site sequences, secondary modifications of restriction sites, deletion or insertion of restriction sites, or deletion or insertion of sequences between

TABLE 1 Examples of enzyme sets used to perform MLEE analyses of an infectious bacterium, an infectious fungus, and a protozoan parasite

Enzyme sets used for analysis of:		
Neisseria meningitidis[a,d]	*Candida albicans*[b,d]	*Plasmodium falciparum*[c,d]
ADH (EC 1.1.1.1)	ADH (EC 1.1.1.1)	LDH (EC 1.1.1.27)
ME (EC 1.1.1.40)	SDH (EC 1.1.1.14)	IDH (EC 1.1.1.42)
IDH (EC 1.1.1.42)	MDH (EC 1.1.1.37)	6PGD (EC 1.1.1.44)
G6PD (EC 1.1.1.49)	IDH (EC 1.1.1.42)	NAD-GDH (EC 1.4.1.2)
UDH (EC 1.1.1)	G6PD (EC 1.1.1.49)	GSR (EC 1.6.4.2)
NAD-GDH (EC 1.4.1.2)	SOD (EC 1.15.1.1)	HK (EC 2.7.1.1)
NADP-GDH (EC 1.4.1.4)	AAT (EC 2.6.1.1)	NH-i (EC 3.2.2)
IPO (EC 1.9.3.1)	HK (EC 2.7.1.1)	LAP (EC 3.4.11.1)
AK (EC 2.7.4.3)	PK (EC 2.7.1.40)	PEP1 (EC 3.4.11; Leu-Leu-Leu)
AKP (EC 3.1.3.1)	EST (EC 3.1.1.1)	PEP2 (EC 3.4.11; Leu-Ala)
PEP (EC 3.4)	LAP (EC 3.4.11.1)	ADA (EC 3.5.4.4)
ACO (EC 4.2.1.3)	PEP1 (EC 3.4.13.18; Val-Leu)	GPI (5.3.1.9)
FUM (EC 4.2.1.2)	PEP2 (EC 3.4.11.4; Leu-Gly-Gly)	
	PEP3 (EC 3.4.13.9; Phe-Pro)	
	MPI (EC 3.5.1.8)	
	ALD (EC 4.1.2.13)	
	FUM (4.2.1.2)	
	GPI (EC 5.3.1.9)	
	PGM (EC 5.4.2.2)	

[a] Data from Bart et al. (13).
[b] Data from Pujol et al. (111).
[c] Data from Abderrazak et al. (2).
[d] Enzyme activities are indicated (with Enzyme Commission numbers). ADH, alcohol dehydrogenase; ME, malic enzyme; IDH, isocitrate dehydrogenase; G6PD, glucose-6-phosphate dehydrogenase; UDH, unidentified dehydrogenase; NAD-GDH, glutamate dehydrogenase (NAD$^+$ dependent); NADP-GDH, glutamate dehydrogenase (NADP$^+$ dependent); IPO, indophenol oxydase; AK, adenylate kinase; AKP, alkaline phosphatase; PEP, peptidase (the substrates are indicated for the different peptidases used with *C. albicans* and *P. falciparum*); ACO, aconitase; FUM, fumarase; SDH, sorbitol dehydrogenase; MDH, malate dehydrogenase; SOD, superoxide dismutase; AAT, aspartate aminotransferase; HK, hexokinase; PK, pyruvate kinase; EST, esterase; LAP, leucine aminopeptidase; MPI, mannose-6-phosphate isomerase; ALD, aldolase; GPI, glucose-6-phosphate isomerase; PGM, phosphoglucomutase; LDH, lactate dehydrogenase; 6PGD, 6-phosphogluconate dehydrogenase; GSR, glutathione reductase; NH-i, nucleoside hydrolase (substrate inosine); ADA, adenosine deaminase.

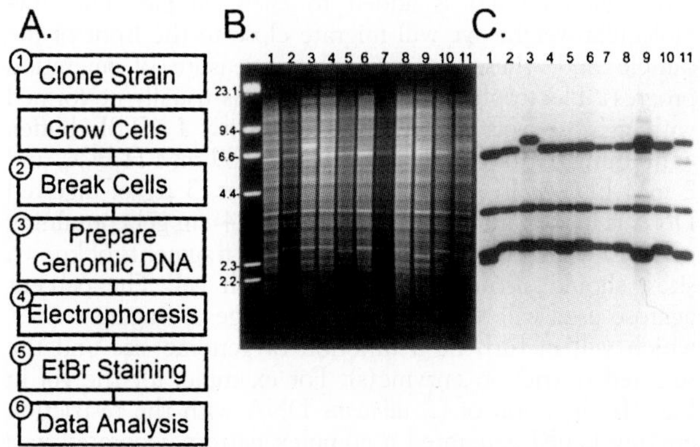

FIGURE 3 RFLP. (A) Generic version of the steps in the RFLP method as it is commonly applied to lower eukaryotic pathogens. EtBr, ethidium bromide. (B) Example of an ethidium bromide-stained gel of EcoRI-digested DNA from 10 test isolates of *C. albicans* (lanes 2 to 11) and a control isolate (lane 1). The first lane, not numbered, contains molecular mass standards. Molecular sizes (in kilobases) are indicated to the left. (C) The gel in panel B Southern blotted and hybridized with a ribosomal probe that identifies 28, 17, and 5S rRNA genes.

restriction sites. Therefore, selection of the most effective endonuclease for generating a pattern must be empirical. A good example of an RFLP pattern for isolates of the yeast pathogen *C. albicans* is presented in Fig. 3B. One should immediately recognize first that not all bands are easily resolvable. Because of the complexity of the eukaryotic genome, the number of digestion fragments is greater than that in prokaryotes. This reduces resolution between bands in an agarose gel and leads to the normally smeared nature of an average RFLP profile. The dominant bands are resolvable, but unfortunately, these bands represent primarily the repetitive ribosomal cistrons and to a lesser extent mitochondrial DNA sequences. Unlike those of prokaryotes, the ribosomal cistrons of eukaryotes are clustered on one or two chromosomes (62, 128). The cistrons are in tandem with interspersed spacer regions and are structurally quite homogeneous. Therefore, endonuclease digestion that results in a complex RFLP pattern results in a relatively simple rRNA gene pattern. To demonstrate this point, the ethidium bromide-stained gel with *C. albicans* whole-cell DNA in Fig. 3B was destained, Southern blotted, and hybridized with an rRNA gene probe containing the high-molecular-mass (28S), low-molecular-mass (17S), and 5S rRNA gene sequences (Fig. 3C). Only three intense bands and a few minor bands were resolved with a reasonable degree of resolution in each pattern. The number and variability of the major RFLP bands among independent *C. albicans* isolates, therefore, do not provide enough complexity for resolving differences between moderately or highly related isolates and in some cases may not even be able to distinguish between unrelated isolates. In contrast, the complexity of the pattern of unique-sequence DNA, which should be great enough for assessing genetic distance, is blurred by the congestion of bands in a normal gel. Even so, the use of RFLP patterns for distinguishing between unrelated isolates or identifying different isolates of the same strains of eukaryotic pathogens continues and can sometimes be reasonably effective, if one does not demand resolution at the levels of moderate relatedness (Fig. 1).

In Fig. 3A, a generic version of the RFLP method (121) as applied to eukaryotic pathogens is presented. The major steps are dealt with individually below.

Preparation of Cells

As in the case of the MLEE method, one must begin with a clone. Each clone must be individually grown for DNA extraction. In contrast to MLEE, however, RFLP analysis does not require one to worry about uniform growth conditions since genotypes should be stable under different conditions.

Preparation of DNA

Many lower eukaryotic pathogens are encased in cell walls, and the walls must be removed prior to cell lysis. Here, a general protocol is described for infectious yeast. Cells from agar cultures are grown to stationary phase in a rich liquid growth medium. Cells are pelleted, washed, and resuspended in medium that removes cell walls and osmotically maintains the integrity of the resulting spheroplasts (cells that have had their walls removed). For generation of spheroplasts, cells are first suspended in the medium SPP, containing 1 M sorbitol and 50 mM potassium phosphate, pH 7.4. To remove the cell wall, a variety of enzymes are used, depending on the nature of the wall. To remove yeast cell walls, the snail enzyme Zymolyase can be used. For *C. albicans*, which has a very tough wall, 15 μl of a solution containing 100 mg of Zymolyase 20 T (Seikagaku America, Ijamsville, Md.) in 800 μl of 50 mM sodium phosphate (pH 6.5)–50% glycerol is added to 0.7 ml of SPP containing 10^8 cells. Cells are then incubated in suspension for 30 to 90 min at 37°C. The time for wall removal varies, even between strains of the same species. A preparation is assessed microscopically for spheroplast formation and is usually terminated when the proportion of spheroplasts in the population is >80%. The percentage of spheroplasts can be assessed by adding 1 μl of 10% KOH to a droplet of spheroplasts on a microscope slide and counting the proportion of lysed cells. At the time of 80% lysis, the spheroplasts are pelleted at 2,500 × *g* for 10 min at room temperature, washed in SPP, and finally resuspended in 500 μl of a lysis buffer containing 50 mM Tris-HCl, pH 7.4, and 20 mM EDTA. Fifty microliters of 10% SDS is added to the preparation, which is then incubated for 30 min at 65°C. Two hundred microliters of 5 M potassium acetate is then added, and the preparation is incubated in an ice bath for 1 h. The lysate is centrifuged at 10,000 × *g* for 10 min at 4°C, and the supernatant, containing DNA, is extracted with an equal volume of a 1:1 solution of phenol-chloroform. The DNA in the supernatant is precipitated with an equal volume of cold isopropanol. The DNA is then washed twice with 750 μl of 75% ethanol, dried, and resuspended in 100 μl of a solution containing 10 mM Tris-HCl, pH 7.5, and 1 mM EDTA. Contaminating RNA can be removed by adding 2 μl of a 10-mg/ml solution of RNase A and incubating for 1 h at 37°C. This solution is again extracted with phenol-chloroform and precipitated, as in earlier steps. The final precipitate is then resuspended in 100 μl of the Tris-HCl–EDTA solution and may be stored at 4°C. This solution should not be frozen.

Endonuclease Digestion

Three micrograms of DNA extracted from each test isolate is incubated in 25 μl of reaction buffer containing one or more selected endonucleases according to the manufacturer's instructions. The units of endonuclease should be threefold over the recommended value to ensure complete digestion, a necessary prerequisite for obtaining reproducible, well-separated RFLP patterns. Endonucleases, or restriction enzymes, identify precise sequences throughout the genome. For example, EcoRI identifies and cleaves (cuts) at sites with the sequence 5′GAATTC3′, BamHI cleaves at 5′GGATCC3′, and HinfI cleaves at 5′GANTC3′, where N is any nucleotide. Restriction sites vary in abundance. An infrequent cutter is an enzyme that identifies infrequent sites in a particular genome and is the basis for the RFLP method combined with PFGE that is frequently applied to prokaryotes. Two examples of infrequent cutters used in fungal studies are NotI, which cleaves sites with the sequence 5′GCGGCCGC3′, and SfiI, which cleaves sites with the sequence 5′GGCCNNNNNGGCC3′, where N is any nucleotide. In bacteria, SmaI is an infrequent cutter which cleaves sites with the sequence 5′CCCGGG3′. An infrequent cutter will generate a limited number of genomic fragments. These fragments may be too large to be separated by standard gel electrophoresis. On the other hand, some restriction sites are too common, resulting in patterns containing too many bands for good pattern resolution. It should be clear from this brief discussion that one must carefully choose the endonuclease or combination of endonucleases to be used in an RFLP analysis.

Electrophoresis

After digestion is complete and prior to electrophoresis, 3 μl of DNA loading dye (e.g., 40% Ficoll and 0.01% bromophenol blue) is added to each sample. The low-molecular-weight dye will migrate close to the front of the sample and, therefore, provide a measure of migration progress. Electrophoresis, in this case, is usually performed with agarose gels cast in and run with 1× TBE buffer, containing 89 mM Tris-HCl (pH 8.1), 89 mM H_3BO_3, and 2 mM EDTA. In a standard experiment, 3 μg of digested DNA is loaded into a well of a 13- by 24-cm gel containing 12 to 15 wells. A set of standards, DNA fragments of known sizes, should also be loaded onto each gel. The percent agarose used will depend upon the range of fragment sizes, which will in turn be a function of genome size and the selected restriction enzyme(s). For example, for the gel in Fig. 3B, digestion of *C. albicans* DNA with the restriction enzyme EcoRI generated a complex pattern separated in a 0.8% agarose gel. For these gel specifications, the dye front should migrate 16 cm from the loading well.

Staining

To visualize the banding patterns of RFLPs, the gel is soaked for 1 h in a solution of 0.2 μg of ethidium bromide/ml. The pattern is then viewed and photographed with a UV light source. It is suggested that a ruler be placed next to the gel when the gel is photographed so that migration distances can be assigned.

Analysis

The standard RFLP method for eukaryotic pathogens generates patterns that are sometimes difficult to compare. Because of band crowding, automatic computer-assisted analyses are difficult and too much information is lost due to the lack of discrimination. The positions of the major bands in RFLP patterns can be manually digitized into a database, but as noted above, the major bands represent primarily rRNA gene fragments. However, when RFLP studies involve small numbers of isolates, and all that is demanded from the data is an assessment of identity and nonidentity, qualitative interpretations can be sufficient. The problems of RFLP analyses of eukaryotic pathogens are resolved to some extent by applying hybridization probes, the subject of a later section of this chapter.

Use of RFLP To Analyze Prokaryotes

The bacterial genome is usually composed of a single DNA molecule (i.e., a single chromosome). These genomes can vary significantly in size and complexity, but in the majority of cases, bacterial genomes are less complex than lower eukaryotic genomes. One, therefore, may expect greater resolution in an RFLP pattern generated with a prokaryotic genome, but that is really not the case. When a frequent cutter is used, the ethidium bromide-stained pattern is still crowded. Standard RFLP analysis without probes has, therefore, not been a popular epidemiological tool for bacteria. Instead, bacterial epidemiologists have used infrequent cutters to generate a limited number of DNA fragments, which are then separated by an electrophoretic method customized for large fragments (33). In Fig. 4A, a generic version of this method is presented. A clone is grown to stationary phase in medium recommended for the particular species. In many cases, this represents an overnight growth culture. Cells are usually pelleted by centrifugation and resuspended in a medium customized for the species under analysis. For instance, in a procedure applied to *Staphylococcus aureus* (68), cells are washed in a solution containing 0.15 M NaCl and 10 mM EDTA, pH 8.0, and resuspended in a solution containing 1 M NaCl and 10 mM EDTA, pH 8.0. This cell suspension is then mixed with an equal volume of 1.2% low-melting-temperature agarose, and the mixture is allowed to solidify in 100-μl molds. The blocks are then incubated in lysis solution containing 1 M NaCl, 10 mM EDTA, 10 mM Tris-HCl (pH 8.0), and a lysis cocktail that includes 0.5% (wt/vol) Brij 58, 0.2% (wt/vol) deoxycholate, 0.5% (wt/vol) Sarkosyl, 1 mg of lysozyme/ml, and 4 mg of acromopeptidase/ml. The blocks are next incubated in a solution containing 0.25 M EDTA, 1% (wt/vol) Sarkosyl, and 0.1 mg of proteinase K/ml at 50°C, followed by a solution containing 10 mM Tris-HCl (pH 8.0), 1 mM EDTA, and 1 mM phenylmethylsulfonyl fluoride. Sections of blocks are then incubated with restriction enzyme and electrophoresed in a 0.9% agarose gel by using contour-clamped homogeneous electric field electrophoresis (29), the PFGE system of choice for this form of fingerprinting. Staining and data analysis are as described for RFLP analysis of lower eukaryotes. An example of the application of RFLP-PFGE to *Staphylococcus aureus* is presented in Fig. 4B. A standardized protocol for the refined preparation of DNA for PFGE analysis has been described by Chang and Chui (28) and should serve as a good starting point for individuals interested in an RFLP method for fingerprinting of bacteria. Chung et al. (30) give a protocol for PFGE analysis of *Staphylococcus aureus* with specific details on troubleshooting.

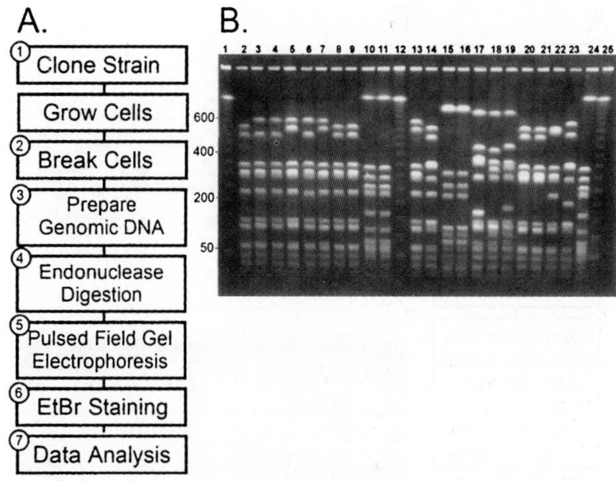

FIGURE 4 RFLP as it is commonly applied to prokaryotic pathogens, using PFGE to separate large DNA fragments. (A) Generic version of the steps in the RFLP-PFGE method. EtBr, ethidium bromide. (B) Example of RFLP-PFGE as it was applied to 22 *Staphylococcus aureus* isolates (provided by M. Pfaller, University of Iowa). Standards were run in lanes 1, 12, and 25. Molecular sizes are given in kilobases.

Restriction Fragment End Labeling

Restriction fragment end labeling was developed as a fingerprinting method for bacteria because of the compact size of the bacterial genome. In this method, total genomic DNA is digested with a restriction endonuclease and all of the fragments are end labeled using the Klenow fragment of DNA polymerase I. Following labeling, the fragments are separated by electrophoresis through a polyacrylamide-urea gel, such as what would be used for DNA sequencing. The number of bands will depend upon the species and isolates of the bacteria that will be analyzed and on the characteristics of the gel. van Steenbergen et al. (161) found that of the 11 species of bacteria that they analyzed, they could distinguish between 30 and 50 bands per isolate in the 100- to 400-bp size range. This method has been successfully applied to the molecular epidemiology of several bacterial species, including *Streptococcus pneumoniae* (19) and *Helicobacter pylori* (159).

Application of Hybridization Probes to RFLPs

Because hybridization probes allow visualization of a subset of fragments in an RFLP pattern, the resolution of the pattern increases over that with RFLP without a probe. The increase in resolution is evident in the comparison between the RFLP pattern (Fig. 3B) and the Southern blot pattern of the same gel hybridized with an rRNA gene probe (Fig. 3C). The success of this fingerprinting strategy has been mixed and depends upon the selected hybridization probe. Therefore, after a description of the general method, the caveats of the method will be reviewed. In Fig. 5A, a generic version of the RFLP method with a hybridization probe is presented.

Steps i to vi

Steps i through vi are identical to those already described for the RFLP method without a probe, and a description of them will not be repeated.

Steps vii and viii

To hybridize with a probe, the ethidium bromide-stained DNA is transferred onto a nitrocellulose or nylon membrane,

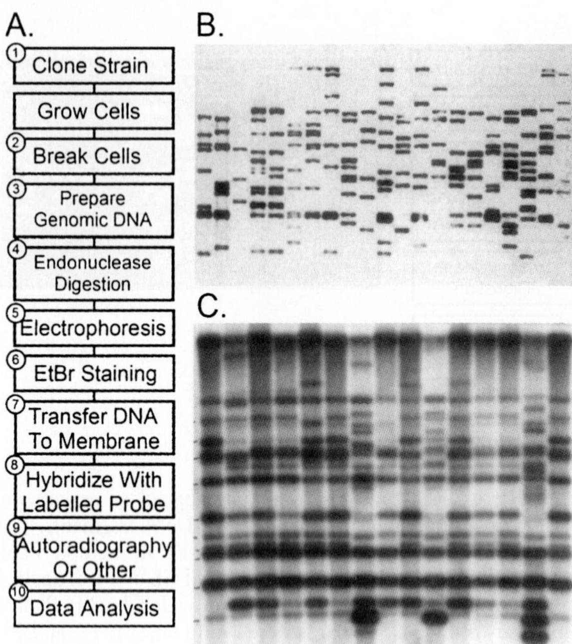

FIGURE 5 RFLP with probe. (A) Generic version of the steps in the RFLP-with-probe method. EtBr, ethidium bromide. (B) Example of RFLP with probe applied to a bacterium, in this case an IS probe applied to PvuII-digested *Mycobacterium tuberculosis* DNA (160). Molecular sizes are presented in kilobases to the left of the gel. (C) Example of RFLP with probe applied to a yeast, in this case the complex probe Ca3 applied to EcoRI-digested *C. albicans* DNA (S. Joly and D. R. Soll, unpublished results).

a process referred to as Southern blotting. The method for this process can be found in *Current Protocols in Molecular Biology*, volume 1 (6), or in *Molecular Cloning: a Laboratory Manual* (121). In brief, the gel is first treated with 0.25 M HCl. This step results in partial depurination and strand cleavage of DNA. The gel is rinsed in water and soaked in a solution containing 0.5 M NaOH and 1.5 M NaCl. This treatment denatures the DNA, a necessary step prior to hybridization. If a nitrocellulose membrane is used, the gel must then be neutralized to a pH below 9.0. The transfer to a membrane can then be achieved by a number of protocols, the most common ones based on upward or downward capillary transfer (60, 121). The Southern blot is then ready for the hybridization step. The probe must be labeled. The most common method is random priming with [α-^{32}P]dCTP or [α-^{32}P]dATP. A nonradioactive method employs a digoxigenin label (67), which can generate sharper banding patterns than radioactive probes but is usually less sensitive. For both methods, the gel must first be treated with hybridization buffer containing 150 μg of sheared, denatured salmon sperm, calf thymus, or other DNA per ml for approximately 4 h at 65°C to block nonspecific binding of the probe. Hybridization is then performed with the same prehybridization buffer containing the labeled probe. One standard hybridization buffer contains 50 mM NaH_2PO_4 (pH 7.5), 50 mM EDTA, 0.9 M NaCl, 5% dextran sulfate, and 0.3% SDS. The hybridization reaction is performed for 16 to 24 h at 65°C. Hybridization is terminated by washing the membrane at 45°C with a solution containing 0.3 M NaCl, 0.03 M sodium citrate (pH 7.0), and 2% SDS.

Step ix

The hybridization pattern generated by a radioactive probe is visualized by exposing the blot to X-ray film with the aid of intensifying screens. Examples of Southern blot hybridization patterns for bacteria and yeast are presented in Fig. 5B and C, respectively. To visualize digoxigenin-labeled patterns, one can treat the gel with anti-digoxigenin antibody conjugated to horseradish peroxidase (39). The antibody binds to digoxygenin. Next, one adds the substrate luminol under alkaline conditions. Horseradish peroxide and hydrogen peroxide catalyze luminol oxidation. Oxidized luminol decays, releasing light, which can be visualized with X-ray film.

Step x

Because hybridization is a result of ionic rather than covalent bonding, one can strip a Southern blot of a probe and rehybridize with additional probes.

Selection of a Hybridization Probe

Selection of a probe for a study should be based on a firm understanding of the exact information a particular probe will provide. Some of the first probes used for DNA fingerprinting of the infectious fungi included single gene sequences, rRNA genes, and mitochrondrial DNA. It should be evident that a single-gene probe will usually hybridize to only one band in a haploid organism and one or two bands in a diploid organism. Although differences in the sizes of the fragments carrying the gene may exist between isolates, the data are never sufficient for epidemiological studies that require measurements of moderate relatedness.

The use of rRNA genes as a fingerprinting probe for both prokaryotic and eukaryotic pathogens was predicated on the idea that single-copy DNA probes would not provide adequate data complexity. In bacteria, rRNA gene probes, which are the basis of the most popular automatic typing systems such as the Riboprinter microbial characterization system (Qualicon, Wilmington, Del.), are effective because rRNA cistrons are dispersed throughout the single chromosome (104). Variability in banding patterns results from changes in bordering sequences (34, 43, 97, 107, 169).

In contrast, the rRNA cistrons of eukaryotes are clustered, usually in only one chromosome (62, 128). These cistrons are separated by spacers. Endonuclease digestion usually results in a very limited number of bands, generating unexpectedly simple patterns (Fig. 3C) that are not much more complex than those generated by single-copy probes. Therefore, other repetitive sequences were sought that provided more complex patterns. In particular, repetitive sequences were sought that were dispersed throughout the genome. The expectation was that changes in the flanking sequences would generate differences in the patterns of different isolates that could be interpreted in terms of genetic distance. In some bacteria, transposable elements have been used as DNA fingerprinting probes. For instance, in *Mycobacterium tuberculosis*, insertion sequences such as IS*6110* (also known as IS986) have been used as probes (83). The copy number of IS*6110* per strain varies between 1 and 19, but the majority of strains carry between 8 and 15 copies dispersed throughout the chromosome (114). Therefore, patterns generated with the IS*6110* probe and PvuII-digested *Mycobacterium tuberculosis* DNA are relatively complex and vary between unrelated isolates (Fig. 5B).

For the fungi, a variety of moderately repetitive sequences have been used. For instance, poly(GT) and several oligonucleotides, such as $(GGAT)_4$, $(GTG)_5$, $(GATA)_4$, and

$(GACA)_4$, have been used for DNA fingerprinting of *Candida* species (142). These sequences, which identify microsatellite regions, generate complex patterns that may prove to be effective fingerprinting probes, but none have been fully verified. In *C. albicans*, the repeat sequence CARE2 (84), which is represented 10 to 14 times in the genome, generates a relatively complex Southern blot hybridization pattern. However, CARE2 and other repetitive sequences that reorganize at a rapid evolutionary rate are sometimes ineffective in identifying clusters of moderately related isolates of a species, a problem to which we will return.

For fungi, complex probes have been cloned that have proven effective at all levels of relatedness. Complex probes are genomic fragments between 10 and 20 kb in length that contain and therefore identify highly variable repetitive sequences, moderately variable sequences, and monomorphic sequences. These probes hybridize in a species-specific fashion and generate patterns that are complex but distinct enough for automatic computer-assisted methods of analysis. They have been cloned from every fungal species so far tested, including *C. albicans* (4, 89, 119), *C. tropicalis* (71), *C. glabrata* (91), *C. dubliniensis* (72), *C. parapsilosis* (41), *C. lusitaniae* (S. Lockhart and D. R. Soll, unpublished results), and *Aspergillus fumigatus* (60). The methods for cloning and characterizing complex probes have been recently reviewed by Lockhart et al. (88). An example of patterns obtained with the Ca3 probe for *C. albicans* is presented in Fig. 5C.

Random Amplification of Polymorphic DNA

RAPD is one of the most frequently used methods for DNA fingerprinting of eukaryotic organisms (24, 165, 167). As we shall see in a following section dealing with verification, this method, when developed correctly, is highly effective for assessing relatedness at all levels of resolution. However, in contrast to RFLP, RFLP-PFGE, and RFLP with a hybridization probe, the RAPD method is compromised by problems of reproducibility among laboratories. The method, presented in a generic form in Fig. 6A and B, is straightforward. With the use of random primers of approximately 10 bases in length, amplicons throughout the genome are amplified by PCR as described in Fig. 6A. The amplification products are separated on an agarose gel and visualized by ethidium bromide staining. Polymorphisms arise when the distances between primer hybridization sites change or when primer sites appear, disappear, or change location due to insertion, deletion, or recombination. If a primer hybridizes to a large number of sites on opposing Crick and Watson strands (i.e., identifies a significant number of amplicons), that primer will generate a complex pattern. Usually, however, each 10-bp primer will generate one or a few major bands and a few minor bands (Fig. 7). Because some minor bands may not be highly reproducible in repeat experiments in the same laboratory, only the major bands are usually used for analysis. This irreproducibility is probably the result of low annealing temperatures and short primer sequences, which result in mispairing. Several primers must be used and the data must be pooled to obtain the necessary level of complexity for epidemiological studies. As a general guideline, it is recommended that one use approximately eight primers, each generating at least two reproducible, strong bands, resulting in at least 16 polymorphic bands. Too low a degree of polymorphism will bias a study. Based on our experience with the RAPD method, we recommend the selection of polymorphic bands present in between 10 and 90% of isolates (41, 91, 111). To obtain an effective collection of primers, one should begin with 30 or 40 primers and test each with a representative collection of isolates if one is setting up one's own RAPD protocol. Primer collections can be readily obtained commercially. The test sequences can usually be obtained from collections used for studies of related organisms. In an analysis of *C. glabrata*, Lockhart et al. (91) selected the following nine primers: GGACTGCAGA, GTGACATGCC, CAGGCCCTTA, TGCCGAGCTG, AATCGGGCTG, GTGATCGCAG, TCGGCGATAG, AGCCAGCGAA, and AGGTGACCGT. In an analysis of *C. albicans*, Pujol et al. (111) selected the following eight primers: CCAGATGCAC, GTGACATGCC, TTATCGCCCC, GGACTGCAGA, ACGGCGTATG, AACGGTGACC, GGAAGCTTGG, and ACGGTACCAG. In an analysis of *Salmonella enterica* serovar Typhimurium isolates, Malorny et al. (96) selected 13 primers, and in an analysis of *Burkholderia pseudomallei* (85), 30 primers were tested for their efficacy in RAPD analysis. In contrast, in several studies, isolates have been grouped using a single primer (31). In some cases, a single primer can in fact provide enough data to generate a dendrogram (see, e.g., reference 112).

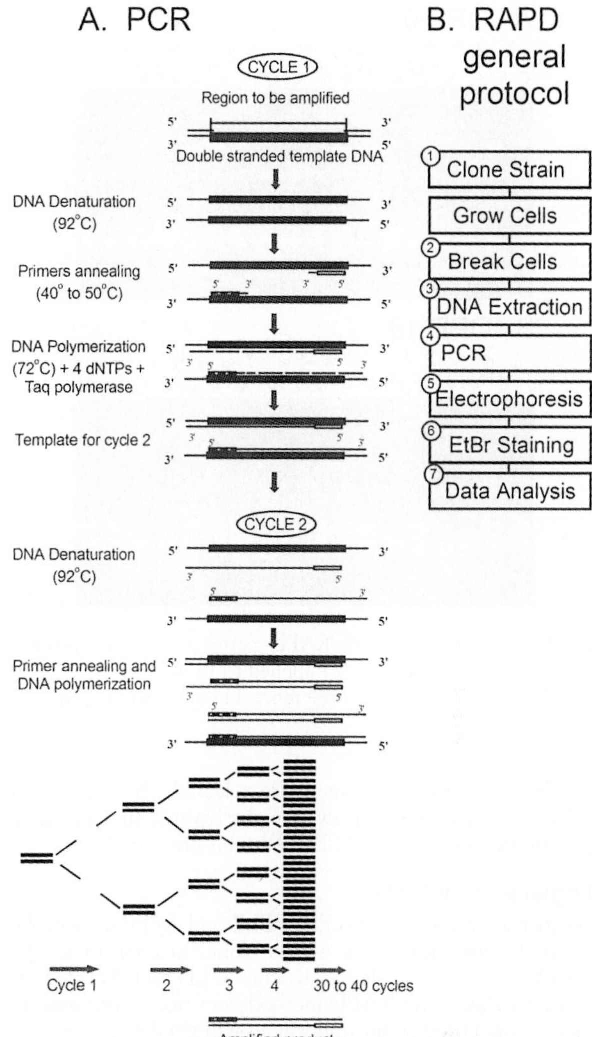

FIGURE 6 RAPD. (A) Description of PCR. (B) Generic version of the steps in the RAPD method. EtBr, ethidium bromide.

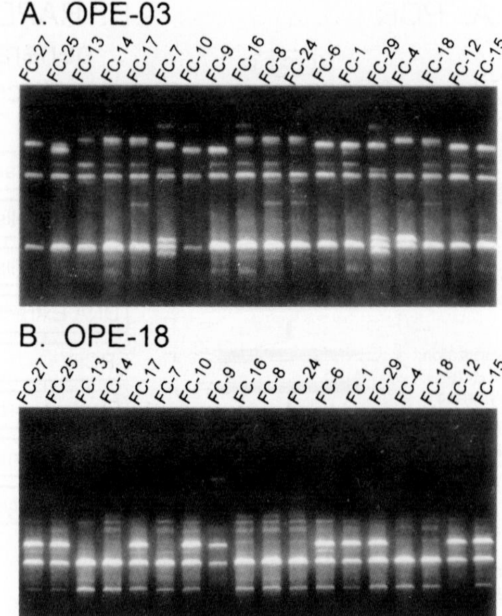

FIGURE 7 Examples of RAPD patterns with the primers OPE-03 (A) and OPE-18 (B) applied to 18 isolates of the yeast *C. albicans*. Reprinted from reference 111 with permission.

Once a primer or primers are selected, the method of RAPD analysis is relatively straightforward. In Fig. 6B, a generic version of the RAPD method is presented.

Preparation of Cells

As in the case of the MLEE, RFLP, and RFLP-with-probe methods, one must begin with a clone. In contrast to the MLEE method, but similar to the RFLP and RFLP-with-probe methods, the RAPD method does not require one to be too concerned about uniform growth conditions.

Preparation of DNA

The preparation of DNA is similar to that for RFLP, with some modifications. First, since the DNA has to be pure to facilitate the PCR, several chloroform extractions are necessary. To prevent DNA degradation, EDTA can be added during extraction, but EDTA should be absent from the final DNA suspension solution since 0.1 μM EDTA can affect the efficiency of *Taq* polymerase in the PCR. The following protocol is relatively simple, has been successfully used for the analysis of several fungal species, and can be adapted for other organisms. A 500-μl suspension of cells (5×10^9 cells per ml) in a solution of 10 mM Tris-HCl (pH 8.0)–1 mM EDTA is mixed with an equal volume of glass beads (0.45 mm in diameter) in a 1.5-ml microcentrifuge tube and disrupted in a bead beater. SDS is then added to a final concentration of 2% (wt/vol), and the suspension is mixed by repeatedly inverting the tube. DNA is then purified by two rounds of phenol extraction followed by three rounds of chloroform extraction. DNA is precipitated in 0.3 M sodium acetate (pH 4.5) and 2 volumes of 100% ethanol. The final DNA precipitate is resuspended in distilled water.

PCR Amplification

The following is a simple version of PCR amplification. To a 0.5-ml microcentrifuge tube is added 25 μl of a reaction mixture containing 5 ng of genomic DNA, 2.5 μl of 10× buffer provided by the manufacturer with purchased *Taq* DNA polymerase, 1.5 mM $MgCl_2$, 0.5 to 1.5 U of *Taq* DNA polymerase, 250 μM (each) dATP, dCTP, dGTP, and dTTP, and 0.2 mM selected 10-bp primers. Amplification is performed in a thermal cycler programmed for 45 cycles of 1-min duration at 94°C, 2 min at 36°C, and 2 min at 73°C. Amplification products are separated by electrophoresis in a 1.5% agarose gel run for 4 h at 110 V so that the bromophenol blue marker dye migrates approximately 10 cm. For the separation of low-molecular-mass (<500 bp) amplification products, acrylamide gels can be used.

Visualization of Bands

The gel is stained with ethidium bromide as described for RFLP gels and viewed with a UV light box.

Problems Inherent in the RAPD Method and Controls That Must Be Applied

Because there is a problem of reproducibility not only between laboratories but also within the same laboratory over time, one must be cognizant of the pitfalls in the procedure. Most aspects of PCR affect reproducibility, including small differences in the primer-to-template ratios, the concentrations of magnesium, and temperatures (40, 94, 99). Second, variation can occur as a result of the source of *Taq* enzyme (94, 99).

The following steps should, therefore, be taken to obtain reproducible banding patterns. First, DNA from different strains should be tested at a variety of dilutions to assess the impact of dilution on pattern stability. Second, the DNA of a single strain should be extracted several times to test whether minor variations in the preparation of DNA affect patterns. Finally, the amplification reaction should be performed in parallel and in sequence for a single DNA preparation that will be used as a control to test intralaboratory reproducibility.

Other PCR-Based Methods for DNA Fingerprinting

A variety of additional DNA fingerprinting methods have been developed that are PCR based. One modification to RAPD is the amplified fragment length polymorphism method, in which restriction fragments are selected for amplification (130, 158, 164). In this method, DNA is first digested with a restriction enzyme and random restriction fragments are singled out by using a specific base sequence at the 3′ ends of the primers. While the amplified fragment length polymorphism method has been developed to target restriction sites, PCR methods have also been developed to target other known sequences distributed throughout the genome, such as microsatellite sequences and spacer regions between tRNAs or rRNAs. In interrepeat PCR, the variable-length segments found between consecutive repeat elements, rather than the repeat elements themselves, are amplified. Oligonucleotide primers are designed such that they hybridize to the 5′ and/or 3′ ends of repetitive elements, but instead of amplifying the elements, they face outward from the elements and amplify the internal spacer sequences. PCR fragments are separated by agarose gel electrophoresis following amplification and are viewed by staining with ethidium bromide. The number of bands produced is dependent upon the number of repetitive elements within the genome as well as the number that are adjacent and close enough for *Taq* DNA polymerase to amplify the sequences between them (usually around 5,000 bp). Single-primer interrepeat PCR using the M13 core sequence or the microsatellite primers

$(GTG)_5$ and $(GACA)_4$ has been successfully used for a number of fungal species, including *Candida* spp. (101) and *Cryptococcus neoformans* (100), and the parasite *Leishmania* spp. (125). In bacteria, there are at least two commonly used inverted-repeat elements, BOX and the enterobacterial repetitive intergenic consensus (ERIC) sequence. These elements have been successfully used for typing of *Streptococcus pneumoniae* with the single BOXA primer (80) and *Pseudomonas aeruginosa* with both BOXA and primers ERIC1 and ERIC2 (146). A specific protocol for fingerprinting of *Mycobacterium tuberculosis* strains called double repetitive element PCR utilizes two sets of primers, two of which amplify out from the repetitive element IS*6110* and two of which amplify out from the polymorphic GC-rich repetitive sequence PGRS element, in order to generate patterns for isolates with small numbers of IS*6110* repetitive elements (53). Another typing method that has been applied to *Mycobacterium* is spoligotyping. This method uses interrepeat PCR to amplify the regions between a repetitive element known as DR. Rather than separating the interrepeat regions on a gel, one of the primers is end labeled and the products are hybridized to an array of oligonucleotides corresponding to 43 known inter-DR regions (38, 73, 81).

Variable-number-of-tandem-repeat elements (VNTRs) or microsatellites are very short tandem repetitive elements found within the genomes of both prokaryotes and eukaryotes. The VNTR fingerprinting method is PCR based and relies on the amplification of specific VNTRs by using primers specific to the outside flanking regions of the elements. The bands that are generated are distinguished by size following gel electrophoresis. In an article by Lott et al. (93), VNTR profiles were generated for one dimorphic and three polymorphic loci from 114 isolates of *C. albicans* and the methodology was verified by comparing the deduced phylogeny to that which was found using some of the same strains in a previously verified fingerprinting system (111). Mazars et al. (98) identified 12 VNTR regions within the *Mycobacterium tuberculosis* genome that had from two to eight alleles each in the 72 isolates that were tested. This corresponds to a potential for more than 16 million combinations of alleles. VNTR typing has also been successfully applied to the parasite *Plasmodium falciparum*. Anderson et al. (5) described 12 variable-length microsatellite loci and were able to do a population structure analysis of isolates from 465 cases of infection.

Because some evolutionary biologists believe that patterns must account for identified alleles (i.e., a change in a band size in a pattern must be attributed to a change in the size or another aspect of a known sequence), PCR-based methods have been developed that employ genetic markers, either identified or anonymous. Karl and Avise (74) have devised a method that has been applied to a number of lower eukaryotic pathogens, in which arbitrary primers are used to identify monomorphic amplicons, which are then partially sequenced. Customized pairs of primers are then developed for specific bands. Changes in these identifiable bands are then assessed through either RFLP or single-strand conformational polymorphism (SSCP) analysis, which involves the identification of single base pair changes in a sequence through nonhomologous renaturation of DNA and separation on a sequencing gel. For the use of these markers in fungi, see the review by Taylor et al. (150). For *C. albicans*, both PCR-SSCP (52, 64) and PCR-RFLP (171, 172) have been used with equally good results. PCR and the use of specific allelic probes have also been applied to *C. albicans* (32). Similar approaches have also been developed that target the noncoding regions of loci. Development of primer pairs is based on published sequences, and polymorphisms can again be identified by SSCP or RFLP. In these types of PCR-based methods, several pairs of primers must be employed and the pairs must be selected not only because they identify a known sequence but also because they produce the necessary levels of variation between strains. Although these methods have been argued to be superior to standard RFLP because one knows the identity of bands in different strains, analyses of the efficacy of RAPDs in band identification have demonstrated levels of identity between patterns that far exceed those required for effective analysis. Reiseberg (116) tested the homology of 220 pairs of comigrating RAPD fragments from three closely related species (not strains!) of sunflower and found that 91% exhibited homology. Thormann and coworkers (152) demonstrated an extremely high degree of similarity of hybridization patterns of RAPD bands within several plant species. Both these interspecies and intraspecies analyses support the conclusion that RAPD fragment size within a plant species is a strong indicator of homology, and by inference, this should be true for microbial pathogens. More important, verification of the RAPD method through comparison of its clustering abilities with those of unrelated methods has demonstrated its efficacy, as will be discussed in a later section of this chapter. The bottom line is that it is not necessary to identify the RAPD bands being analyzed to use the RAPD method in genetic fingerprinting, as has been amply argued by Tibayrenc (154–156).

Electrophoretic Karyotyping

Since lower eukaryotes possess multiple chromosomes within the size separation range of PFGE technology, this method (26, 126) has been used as a way of fingerprinting eukaryotic pathogens (Fig. 8). If the cell possesses a wall, the wall must be removed. The resulting spheroplasts are embedded in an agarose plug. Detergent and proteinase are added, which removes membrane, digests protein, and releases nucleic acid. The agarose matrix reduces shear forces and thus protects the large chromosomal DNAs from fragmenting. The agarose plug is placed in a well of an agarose slab gel, and electrophoresis is

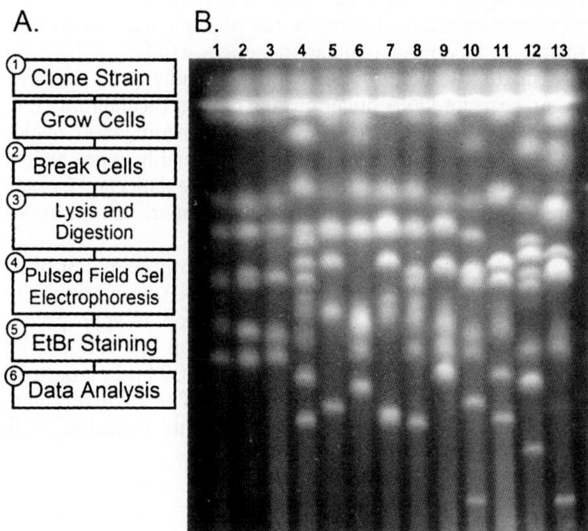

FIGURE 8 PFGE. (A) Generic version of the steps in the PFGE method. EtBr, ethidium bromide. (B) Example of ethidium bromide-stained chromosomes of isolates of the yeasts *C. albicans* (lanes 1 to 3) and *C. dubliniensis* (lanes 4 to 13).

carried out according to the protocol for the specific system used (e.g., orthogonal-field-alternation gel electrophoresis [127], contour-clamped homogeneous electric field electrophoresis [29], or transverse alternating-field electrophoresis [57]). After electrophoresis, chromosomal DNAs are visualized by ethidium bromide staining. Chromosomes can then be identified by Southern blot hybridization with chromosome-specific probes. For infectious yeast, Sangeorzan et al. (122) demonstrated that patterns were reproducible among experiments and relatively insensitive to the method of preparation. However, there have been other studies that demonstrate pattern variability due to reagents, sample preparation, and eletrophoretic conditions. Thrash-Bingham and Gorman (153) demonstrated that in spite of karyotypic variability between strains, the general organization of the genome was maintained, although some chromosomal translocations contributed to karyotypic variability between strains of *C. albicans*. In addition, it has been demonstrated that the frequency of changes in electrophoretic karyotypes can be dramatically influenced by high-frequency phenotypic switching (113). In a sequence of high-frequency switching, the electrophoretic karyotype of a strain diverged from and then reverted to the original pattern, a process that would invalidate the use of this method for assessing moderate levels of relatedness (113). There are reasons to believe that the majority of changes in the chromosome harboring rRNA cistrons in *C. albicans* were due to a release from silencing (113), a process involving *SIR* genes in *Saccharomyces cerevisiae* (58, 63). Whatever the mechanism proves to be, the problem that arises from these observations is that the rate of change identified by PFGE methods may not always reflect genetic distance.

Multilocus Sequence Typing

Although nucleotide sequencing provides the most exact data for assessing polymorphisms within a species, until recently it has been used primarily to analyze mutations associated with phenotypic change and to generate single-locus phylogenetic trees at the interspecies level. At the intraspecies level, multiple loci must be sequenced and the combined data must be analyzed. Recent advances in automated sequencing and the complete sequence data of genomes of select microorganisms have led to the use of sequence data to type isolates and perform population genetic studies of bacteria and fungi. MLST (95) has evolved rapidly over the past several years for DNA fingerprinting of bacteria and fungi (20, 21, 37, 45, 49, 157). It replaces MLEE, providing more alleles per locus and resulting data that are highly reproducible between laboratories. In addition, sequence data can be easily stored and shared via the Internet for comparison and use in large-scale epidemiology studies (1).

A general protocol for MLST has recently been described by Lockhart et al. (90). For template DNA extraction, the protocol proposed for the RAPD method is appropriate. Alternatively, commercial DNA extraction kits can also be used. PCR fragments should be around 500 bp in length to be easily sequenced in both directions. The PCR products must be purified by using any commonly available PCR cleanup kit before sequencing.

Choice of Loci

A selection of six to seven genes is commonly used. These are usually selected among core metabolic genes (housekeeping genes) that are believed to be unaffected by selection. Their use, therefore, precludes microevolutionary analysis. In a few studies, microevolutionary changes have been assessed by using hypervariable genes or genes that are known to be affected by selection. Morelli et al. (102) have analyzed the microevolution of a clonal lineage of *Neisseria meningitidis* by sequencing multiple DNA fragments, including genes encoding cell surface antigens and intergenic regions. Similarly, Feavers et al. (44) used antigen sequences to analyze an outbreak of *Neisseria meningitidis* infection. More recently, Robinson and Enright (117) have used surface-associated genes to supplement their MLST data in order to document the emergence of methicillin-resistant *Staphylococcus aureus* isolates. While MLST schemes have been used to fingerprint fungi (21, 37, 55, 149), the MLST approach was originally designed for bacterial analyses. The use of coding sequences is appropriate for the majority of bacteria because many bacterial species present a high number of polymorphisms. If noncoding sequences were to be used, homoplasy may render interpretations difficult. However, for some microorganisms, and fungi in particular, this approach may not be optimum due to lower genetic variability than that in bacteria. For instance, in the yeast *C. parapsilosis*, three distinct genetic groups can be distinguished (41, 87, 147). Group I strains are the most pervasive and account for between 60 and 90% of isolates (41, 87). Groups II and III are less frequently found and have recently been considered distinct species (147). Tavanti et al. (147) have sequenced a total of 7.5 kb over 11 genes for 21 *C. parapsilosis* group I isolates. They found limited genetic variability, with only two polymorphic nucleotide positions in their entire collection.

MLST and Heterozygosity

The MLST method has been used primarily for fingerprinting of species with haploid genomes. MLST has been successfully used for at least one diploid species, the yeast *C. albicans* (20, 21, 148). While direct sequencing of PCR products identifies single alleles in haploid species, in diploid species, the sequences obtained reflect the combination of two homologous alleles. Heterozygosities are revealed by double peaks in the sequencing traces. Thus, where heterozygosities exist at multiple nucleotide sites in any particular locus, assignment of individual alleles is not possible. This issue may be overcome by cloning the PCR product into a suitable plasmid vector and sequencing one cloned allele. The remaining allele may then be inferred. In diploid genomes, loci containing insertion or deletion polymorphisms need to be avoided. Where such polymorphisms are present, the sequences of the two alleles will be out of phase and the sequencing traces will be unreadable.

Microarray Typing

The latest development in typing techniques has evolved from advances in genome sequencing and DNA microarray technology. Microarray typing methods are rapidly emerging as powerful high-throughput typing strategies. The general method is based on the use of oligonucleotides of around 30 bp in length. These oligonucleotides are selected to target variable single nucleotide polymorphism sequences based on the presence of known polymorphisms. A set of specific oligonuclotides representing each allele of a given locus is used to detect polymorphisms in PCR products of the respective loci. It is a multilocus-based method with which several loci can be analyzed simultaneously. This approach has been used to fingerprint several bacteria (56, 129, 144, 168), viruses (59, 86), parasites (140), and fungi (51). The method has been shown to be effective in detecting heterozygosities in diploid organisms (51).

VERIFYING THE EFFICACY OF A GENETIC FINGERPRINTING METHOD

As noted earlier, one must be sure that a fingerprinting method provides the correct level of genetic resolution for the question posed. Therefore, one must select a method that has already been verified or perform tests to verify the method. The most straightforward test is comparison with an unrelated method by using a set of test isolates with known or implied relatedness. The levels to be tested are (i) identical, (ii) highly similar but nonidentical, (iii) moderately related, and (iv) unrelated (Fig. 1). The test collection is fingerprinted by the individual methods, and similarity coefficients are computed by the same analytical method for every pair of isolates. Dendrograms based on the independent sets of data are then generated and compared. If the unrelated methods both identify known identical isolates as identical, presumed highly related isolates as similar but nonidentical, and presumed unrelated isolates as dissimilar and if the independent methods group isolates into the same clusters, they in essence cross-verify each other's efficacy at every level of relatedness. If they identify as identical presumably identical isolates and identify as similar but nonidentical highly related isolates but do not cluster in a similar fashion moderately related to unrelated isolates, then one or both methods may be ineffective in assessing lower levels of relatedness. This general method of cross-verification has been used to assess the efficiency of a variety of fingerprinting methods for bacterial, fungal, and parasitic pathogens (see, e.g., references 81, 111, and 156). It should be emphasized that without cross-verification, a genetic fingerprinting method is always suspect for the different levels of relatedness (Fig. 1), no matter how valid the system seems to be. One must realize, however, that such cross-verification is possible only for microorganisms with clonal population structures (111, 154–156).

DATA ANALYSIS

Computing Similarity Coefficients

Genetic fingerprinting data come in different forms. MLEE provides multiple spot patterns, RAPD provides single or multiple banding patterns, RFLP, RFLP with a probe, and PFGE provide single or multiple banding patterns, and MLST provides sequence data. Regardless of the data form, the goal of a genetic fingerprinting method is to compute similarity coefficients (S_{AB}s) for every pair of isolates in order to generate a dendrogram, or tree. The formula for computing S_{AB}s and the formula for generating a tree from the S_{AB}s must be carefully selected, and excellent reviews of these computations are available (47, 131, 166). Here, we will review only the most common of these. For a detailed description of these methods, the reader is referred specifically to Sneath and Sokal's *Numerical Taxonomy: the Principles and Practice of Numerical Classification* (131). The challenges of MLST data analysis will be dealt with in a separate section.

Band Positions Alone

For methods that produce patterns of bands, the presence or absence of a band is described by the binary value 1 or 0, respectively, n_{AB} is the number of common bands in the two patterns A and B (coded 1, 1), a is the number of bands in A with no counterpart in B (coded 1, 0), b is the number of bands in B with no counterpart in A (coded 0, 1), and c is the number of bands absent in A and B (coded 0, 0). The sample size x represents the total number of bands, described by the following formula: $x = n_{AB} + a + b + c$. The number of matches (m) is, therefore, $m = n_{AB} + c$, and the number of mismatches (u) is $u = a + b$. Using this basic logic, a number of formulas for S_{AB}s based on band position alone have been developed, most notably those for the coefficient of Jaccard (S_j):

$$S_j = \frac{n_{AB}}{n_{AB} + a + b}$$

the coefficient of Dice (S_D):

$$S_D = \frac{2n_{AB}}{2n_{AB} + a + b}$$

the sample-matching coefficient (S_m):

$$S_m = \frac{n_{AB} + c}{n_{AB} + a + b + c}$$

the Pearson coefficient (S_Ψ):

$$S_\Psi = \frac{(n_{AB}c - ab)}{\sqrt{[(n_{AB} + a)(n_{AB} + b)(b + c)(a + c)]}}$$

and others such as mean square difference/total bands. It should also be noted that data such as those obtained by MLEE or RAPDs, in which a series of primers provide binomial data, can be converted into binary values to generate a matrix similar to that obtained with banding data that can then be used to compute S_{AB}s for every pair of isolates. The same formulas for S_{AB}s can then be considered.

Band Position and Intensity

In many cases, the information garnered from band intensity is added to that of band position. In these formulas, X_{iA} and X_{iB} represent the intensities of bands in patterns A and B, respectively, $\bar{X}_{iA}$ and $\bar{X}_{iB}$ represent the respective means of all intensities, and n represents the total number of bands. A number of formulas for S_{AB}s based on band position and intensity have been developed, most notably those for Pearson's product-moment correlation coefficient (S_r):

$$S_r = \frac{\sum_{i=1}^{n}[(X_{iA} - \bar{X}_{iA})(X_{iB} - \bar{X}_{iB})]}{\sum_{i=1}^{n}(X_{iA} - \bar{X}_{iA})^2\sum_{i=1}^{n}(X_{iB} - \bar{X}_{iB})^2}$$

absolute difference/total area (S_{AB}):

$$S_{AB} = 1.0 - \frac{\sum_{i=1}^{n}|X_{iA} - X_{iB}|}{\sum_{i=1}^{n}|X_{iA} + X_{iB}|}$$

and others such as absolute difference/maximum intensity similarity coefficient, mean square difference/intensity similarity coefficient, and mean square difference/maximum intensity similarity coefficient.

In selecting a method for computing S_{AB}s, several points should be kept in mind. First, if the reproducibility of band intensities is not good, then an S_{AB} based on band positions alone is obviously more accurate. Second, if a method involves the presence or absence of bands as if they were alleles, S_{AB}s based on band position alone are used. One must realize, however, that in most of the DNA fingerprinting methods employed, allelism is not always verified. Third, it must be realized that in methods based on repeat sequences, band intensities may provide as much or more information on relatedness as position, and a method based on both may, therefore, be preferable.

The different similarity coefficients described above do not require the identification of alleles at given loci. For this reason, they are favored when cross-verifying methods are applied since one or more of the methods may rely on dominant markers. Genetic similarity can also be assessed by using genetic distances based on the frequencies of codominant markers (see references 47, 131, and 166).

Generating Dendrograms

The computation of S_{AB}s leads to a matrix of values generated for every pair of isolates in an epidemiological study. These values are the basis for generation of a dendrogram. The most commonly used method for connecting isolates into a tree is the unweighted-pair group method using arithmetic averages (UPGMA) first employed by Rohlf (118). This method generates a rooted tree. The Fitch-Margoliash method with evolutionary clock (50) also generates a rooted dendrogram, with the additional feature that it tests alternative topologies for the tree by rearranging nodes to minimize the sum of squares computed between genetic distances and branch lengths, making it more time-consuming to perform. There are also methods that do not assume a common molecular clock for all strains and, therefore, generate unrooted trees. These methods, which include the neighbor-joining method (120) and the Fitch-Margoliash method without evolutionary clock (50), generate unrooted trees that in fact should have more exact topographies. Because the neighbor-joining method and more particularly the UPGMA are faster than the other methods, they may be preferable for large experimental samples. There are, therefore, tradeoffs among methods. It should be realized that these methods were developed for generating trees at the species level rather than subspecies levels of relatedness, but they still result in interpretable trees at the subspecies and strain levels. If the data are robust, similar dendrograms should be generated no matter which method is applied. Dendrograms generated for intraspecies analysis should not be considered a purely phylogenetic representation of lineages but rather a practical tool that provides a visual description of genetic similarities and divergence between strains and that may be useful in identifying groups, or clades. The derived dendrograms represent true phylogenies only when each strain is derived through a purely clonal lineage (i.e., with no genetic exchange) and homoplasy is negligible. These conditions are rarely verified for the markers used in epidemiological studies.

Let us consider how the UPGMA is performed. The S_{AB} matrix is scanned for the most similar isolates. If more than one group (two or more) are identified, the first is arbitrarily taken as group one. The isolates are joined at the appropriate position along the S_{AB} axis. The matrix is scanned once again for the next most similar isolate or group of isolates, which is then connected along the S_{AB} matrix to the first group, and this function is repeated over and over again until all isolates are incorporated into the tree. A sample dendrogram that includes 67 *C. albicans* isolates is presented in Fig. 9. In this dendrogram, thresholds and

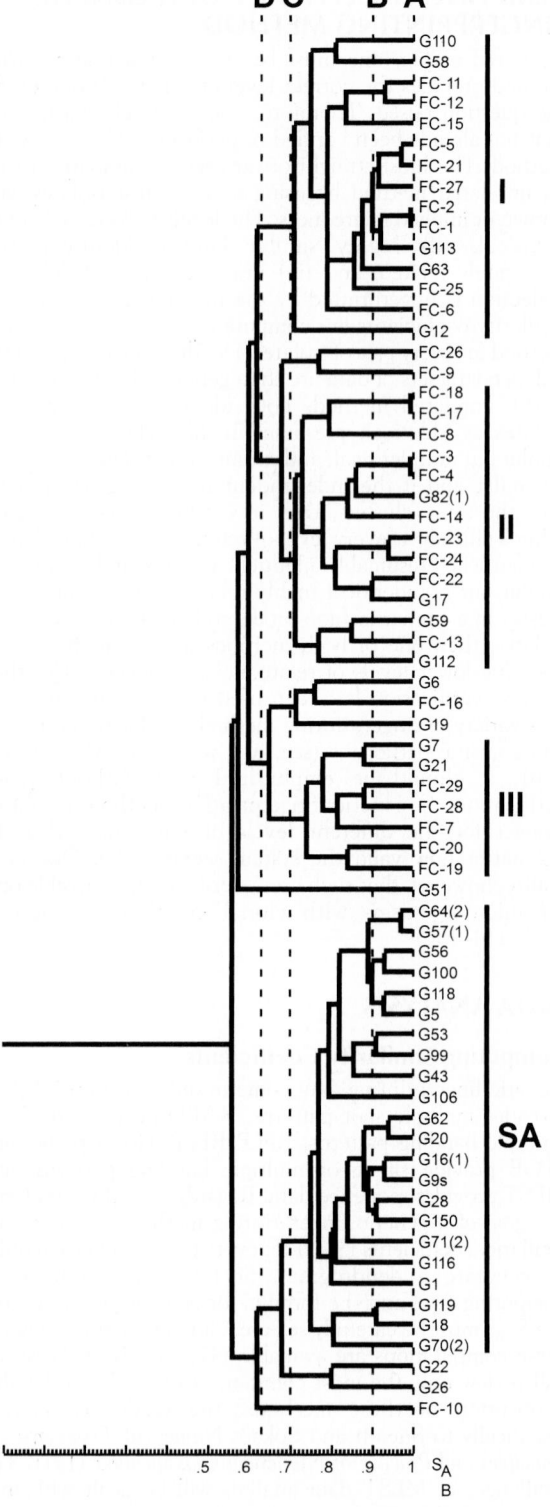

FIGURE 9 Example of a dendrogram. The similarity coefficients (S_{AB}s) were generated from the patterns of 67 isolates of *C. albicans* fingerprinted with the complex Ca3 probe. The value A represents identicalness, at an S_{AB} of 1.00; threshold B demarcates highly related isolates at an S_{AB} of 0.90; threshold C demarcates clades at an S_{AB} of 0.70; and the value D represents the average S_{AB} at 0.63. In this example, a South African-specific clade of *C. albicans* (SA) was identified in addition to the three clades (I, II, and III) present in U.S. collections (18).

landmarks are noted, one (A) which represents identity, at an S_{AB} of 1.00; one (B) which demarcates highly related isolates, at an S_{AB} of 0.90; one (C) which demarcates moderately related groups, in this example at an S_{AB} of 0.70; and one (D) which denotes the average S_{AB} for all strains in the dendrogram, in this example at an S_{AB} of 0.63. The C threshold is the one which best demarcates clades. The selection of thresholds and landmarks in a dendrogram is sometimes somewhat arbitrary (135) but extremely important in interpreting a tree. Confidence in these values comes with increased familiarity with the origins of isolates and assumptions of relatedness based on those origins.

Testing the Integrity of Clusters and Statistical Analyses

Although the selection of a threshold for defining clusters may be somewhat arbitrary, one can demonstrate that the content of a cluster is stable and that the identity of the cluster is in fact valid. First, the order in which isolates are chosen in the generation of a dendrogram can be randomized (2), an important control when the UPGMA is used since this method is prone to mistakes in higher-order clusters. For instance, one can apply 10 random starts to assess whether a cluster remains intact. Second, "noise" can be introduced by adding or subtracting a set percentage of the S_{AB}s in every pairwise comparison (108). Noise can affect and, therefore, be used to assess the stability of second-tier groupings. Third, one can use the comparison of clustering patterns generated by two independent genetic fingerprinting methods to assess the stability of a cluster (81, 111, 156).

The most common method used by evolutionary biologists to analyze the integrity of clusters is bootstrapping (48). In this process, one generates deletions and duplications by random sampling. This process is normally performed 1,000 times. A consensus tree of all dendrograms is then generated, and a "majority rule consensus" algorithm is used to compute the percentage of occurrence of each node. A percentage above 80% suggests a stable node. In a second common method called jackknifing (170), subsets of the collection are randomly selected approximately 100 times, a consensus dendrogram is generated, and the percentage of occurrence at each node is computed. These methods, however, were developed for DNA fingerprinting methods in which the data represent alleles of identified loci, not for patterns like those generated by RFLP or RAPD. They are, therefore, not commonly used in general epidemiological studies. They can, however, be used for RAPD data if each primer is considered an independent gene.

For comparing the relatedness of different populations of isolates, it is often the case that the mean S_{AB} of an entire collection is not informative, although comparisons of mean S_{AB}s of different collections may be informative. The Student *t* test can assess whether mean S_{AB}s are significantly different. In applying the Student *t* test, a probability value of 0.05 (i.e., less than 5%) usually represents significance.

Challenges of MLST Data Analysis

MLST data have also been typically represented by dendrogram-based methods. In addition to that approach, an increasingly popular method, called eBURST (for "based upon related sequence types"), has been developed to accommodate the specific needs associated with the analysis of large MLST data sets (46, 137). The eBURST approach was developed to provide a simple representation of relationships between closely related isolates. As such, eBURST does not try to represent relationships among all analyzed isolates. The development of eBURST was warranted by the fact that dendrograms based on the bifurcating of lineages cannot correctly represent patterns of evolutionary descent within closely related strains from a clonal group. In addition, dendrograms of thousands of strains are hard to display and to analyze. The solution proposed by Feil et al. (46) and Spratt et al. (137) is based on a simple evolutionary model in which clonal lineages are assumed to be founded by a parental clone that, as it increases in frequency, will diversify by accumulation of mutations or by recombination. The eBURST algorithm identifies clonal lineages, predicts their founding genotypes, and displays the most parsimonious pattern of descent for the isolates of each clonal group from the putative founding genotype.

The eBURST algorithm first divides the collection analyzed into groups of closely related strains. The level of relatedness used is user defined. As a general rule, members assigned to the same group share identical alleles at a minimum of one locus with at least one other member of the group. This is the most stringent definition for clonal groups. A threshold of two (or fewer) loci can also be used, but the outcome may be harder to interpret. This step results in a set of nonoverlapping groups of related strains. Then, based on the number of single-locus variants, strains that differ at a single locus, observed for each strain, the algorithm predicts which genotype is the founder for each group. The strain with the highest number of single-locus variants will be defined as having the founder genotype. This process can be supplemented by bootstrap analysis in troublesome cases. The descent from the founder genotype to all of the other genotypes of a given group is then inferred and represented as a radial diagram. The eBURST approach can be used to analyze large samples of thousands of isolates (46, 137).

While the eBURST method is becoming very popular in bacterial MLST studies due to its attractive and convenient representation of evolutionary descent in clonal groups, users should be aware of a few limitations. The eBURST analysis will perform better on large samples. In small samples, clonal groups may not be correctly inferred due to the absence of intermediary genotypes that may have connected groups otherwise deemed independent. Even in larger samples, however, this problem may persist if the missing link has become extinct. Because the founder genotype is inferred from the genotypes present in the sample, predictions of the founder genotype may be affected by sampling biases. Again, this problem should be more limited in large samples. The eBURST method, therefore, offers a useful representation that complements the more commonly used dendrogram-based methods.

ROLE OF COMPUTERS IN GENETIC FINGERPRINTING

For epidemiological studies in which only a few isolates are compared or in which qualitative comparisons are sufficient to obtain an answer, it is simple enough to interpret results, including the computation of similarity coefficients, without the use of computers. However, when dealing with bigger collections, one must recruit a customized computer program. Computer programs are available that can assist in virtually every step in a cluster analysis. For fingerprinting methods that create complex patterns, the systems will automatically acquire the original image and with the assistance of the user will remove distortion, identify lanes, normalize to a universal standard, identify bands, measure the intensity of bands, compute similarity coefficients, generate dendrograms, identify clusters, and perform statistical tests (135). Computer systems will also store data at any or all levels of analysis for retrospective studies and future comparisons with new collections. An automatic genetic fingerprint analysis system can perform searches based on any aspect of the fingerprinting data (e.g., a particular band length), any characteristic of a patient (e.g., human immunodeficiency virus positivity), or any characteristic of the infecting organism (e.g., drug susceptibility). An outline of the steps for computer-assisted analysis of generic complex RFLP, RFLP-with-probe, and select PCR-based patterns follows. The generic software will be referred to simply as the Program.

Digitizing the Pattern

The pattern of an autoradiogram or its equivalent is digitized into the computer's hard drive (Fig. 10A) by using a scanner with software that supports grayscale scanning that saves the image in the correct format (e.g., bitmap or tiff). The scanner should be sensitive to a reasonable range of grayscales (e.g., around 256 grayscales).

Local Standard

In order to straighten a pattern for automatic analysis and compare patterns obtained on different gels, landmark bands must exist in a set of standards either run in lanes alongside test samples, added to the test samples, or incorporated as components of the pattern (e.g., monomorphic bands). In all three cases, standards must include bands that span the entire molecular-weight range of bands in test patterns.

Global Standard

For studies in which the patterns of multiple gels are compared, each test pattern must be normalized to a global standard in the database. The global standard must share bands in the local standard.

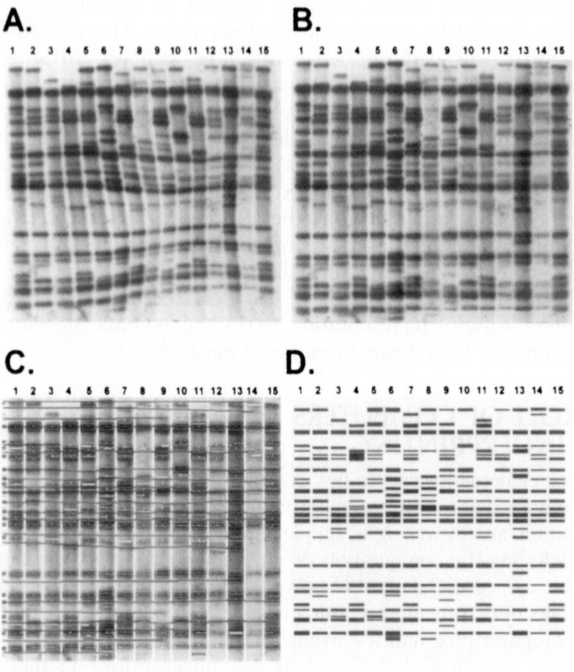

FIGURE 10 Computer-assisted processing and analysis of DNA fingerprint patterns generated with the complex Ca3 probe of 15 isolates of *C. albicans*. (A) Original digitized image with inherent distortions; (B) straightened patterns; (C) correlations of bands with universal standards; (D) model generated from data.

Initial Image Processing

The need for processing stems from artifacts that distort the pattern. First, because of uneven polymerization or electrophoresis, the entire gel pattern may contain "smiles," "frowns," skews, and other linear or nonlinear distortions (Fig. 10A). Unwarping is the process of pattern straightening. Local standards are essential for unwarping. Horizontal lines are drawn between common bands for horizontal distortions, and vertical lines are drawn through spaces for vertical distortions. Once lines are drawn, the Program reconstructs the processed pattern (Fig. 10B). Second, because of unequal loading, the pattern in a single lane can be intensified or deintensified.

Automatic Lane and Band Detection

The Program scans and automatically detects lanes and separates them by spaces to facilitate band identification. At this point, the Program should allow editing for final band alignment that includes lane sliding, stretching, or compressing. This may be necessary if lanes were loaded unequally, which can result in slightly different migration rates for bands of the same molecular weight. Next, the Program should perform a densitometric analysis of grayscales along the lane, subtracting background intensity. Integration at peaks or an intensity threshold can be used for band identification, and band intensity can be categorized (e.g., from 0 to 5), directly measured, or converted according to a normalization curve. Models of the gel can then be generated from band position and intensity (Fig. 10D).

Calibrating to the Global Standard and Linking

The local standard is calibrated to the global standard (Fig. 10C), providing molecular weights of the standard bands. The Program then automatically links bands in test lanes to bands in the local standard. The user must specify a degree of tolerance for considering bands to be the same size. Bands with no correlate in the standard can be linked, and the option should exist for adding new bands to the global standard, if desired.

Creating the Basic Data File

The preceding data provide a text map in which the band number, molecular size, or pixel distance of each band is listed in descending order along the vertical axis for each labeled isolate. At each position, either the binary value 0 or 1 for position alone or the band intensity is listed. If one has collected binary data by using MLEE, RAPD, MLST, or other multilocus methods, one can manually generate the data file at this point in the computer program, or the software can combine the data automatically.

Computing Similarity Coefficients and Generating Dendrograms

The Program must provide the user with a choice of formulas for computing S_{AB}s. Once a particular formula is selected, the Program generates a matrix of S_{AB}s for all pairs of isolates. The Program must then provide the user with a choice of algorithms for generating a dendrogram from the S_{AB} matrix and software for separating groups by thresholding, testing of the stability of clusters, and statistical analyses (Fig. 9).

Other Useful Functions

The Program should provide accessible storage and comparative capabilities so that every new set of genetically fingerprinted isolates can be compared with previously fingerprinted isolates in the database. It must also allow searches based on other elements such as patient and isolate characteristics. The former include disease state, treatment, geographical location, anatomical origin of the isolate, age, sex, weight, and predisposing conditions. The latter include growth characteristics, sugar assimilation patterns, antigenicity, drug susceptibility, switching repertoire, and other phenotypic traits, most notably those involved in virulence and pathogenicity. One must also be able to mine the genetic fingerprint database for particular characteristics, such as the presence of a particular MLEE allele or RFLP fragment.

THE COLLECTION

Because genetic fingerprinting is time-consuming, one must carefully consider the original collection. Yet, this first step is often the most poorly conceived. This problem stems no doubt in part from the assumption that colonizing populations of pathogens are genetically homogenous. It has become increasingly apparent that in many cases, infecting populations, especially in immunocompromised patients, may consist of multiple species, multiple strains of the same species, or diverging substrains. Species heterogeneity has been demonstrated in recurrent infections and commensals (92, 162). In each case in which heterogeneity was demonstrated, care was taken in obtaining the original collection.

In most standard methods of collection, the primary samples are aspirates, tissue, blood, other fluids, or swabs. These materials may be transported to a microbiology laboratory for anaerobic or aerobic culturing. In some cases, the microorganism must be released from the material. Blood cells may be lysed, tissue may be minced, and fluids may be filtered or centrifuged. The problem is clonality. If the sampled colonizing population is homogeneous (i.e., consists of one genetically homogenous strain), there is no problem. However, if the population is heterogeneous (consists of multiple species, strains, or substrains), several problematic scenarios can arise. First, if the culture is genetically heterogeneous at the time of genetic fingerprinting, a mixed fingerprint will arise. Second, if the primary culture contains mixed strains or substrains and is mass cultured, the strain or substrain that grows fastest under the culture conditions employed will enrich. Finally, a problem arises when a primary culture containing mixed strains or substrains is cultured and only one clone is picked for analysis. The single clone may not represent the majority genotype of the infecting population. The solutions to these problems are straightforward. First, the primary sample should be clonally plated, which may entail assessment of concentration, serial dilution, or knowledge of approximate density. Second, indicator agars can be used for initial screening of species. Third, more than one colony can be picked for genetic fingerprinting. The number picked and analyzed will depend on the size of the collection and the objectives of the study. These considerations apply mainly to bacteria and fungi. The problems may be harder to resolve for many parasites that cannot be grown as isolated colonies on agar media.

In addition to sample homogeneity, a second problem arises in some cases that is related to space and time. There is growing evidence of body location specificity in commensalism, geographical specificity of strains, and rapid microevolution (88, 89, 108, 135). It is prudent to consider what body location is sampled, since a pathogen like *C. albicans* can colonize multiple sites (136). It is also important to realize that if one is testing strain specificity for a particular disease, geographical differences may outweigh disease specialization. For instance, within a geographical region, one might find that isolates from a particular disease state are genetically similar, but when isolates from that disease state are collected from different geographical regions and compared, they may prove to be genetically dissimilar (108). One must, therefore, consider restricting the geographical boundaries of the collection or choosing distinct multiple populations. Finally, one must consider the speed of microevolution and the timing of sampling. If one is analyzing substrain specialization, the linear rate of microevolution may outweigh substrain differences related to different disease states or antibiotic resistance. One must, therefore, consider restricting the time window of collection.

CONCLUDING REMARKS

The preceding survey of methods used to fingerprint microbial pathogens should demonstrate that there is no dominant method that has emerged for all of the pathogen categories (bacteria, fungi, and parasites) or even for all species within a category. For instance, in bacteria, although RFLP-PFGE is the most commonly used method for *Streptococcus pneumoniae* and *Staphylococcus aureus*, RFLP with a probe is the most commonly used method for *Mycobacterium tuberculosis* (Table 2). The same variability holds true between fungal and parasite species (Table 2). The reason is twofold. First, differences between the genomes of different species warrant in some cases different methods. Second, different methods are effective for measuring different levels of relatedness. Third, and maybe

TABLE 2 Rough estimates of the use of the most common genetic fingerprinting methods[a]

Pathogen category	Genus or species	Most common genetic fingerprinting methods
Bacteria	*Streptococcus pneumoniae*	42% RFLP-PFGE; 17% RepE1 PCR; 10% restriction fragment end labeling
	Mycobacterium tuberculosis	54% RFLP + probe: 23% spoligotyping
	Staphylococcus aureus	56% RFLP-PFGE; 13% PCR-RFLP; 11% RAPD
Fungi	*Candida*	30% RAPD; 29% karyotyping; 22% RFLP + probe; 12% RFLP
	Aspergillus	71% RAPD; 18% MLEE; 11% RFLP + probe
	Cryptococcus	53% RAPD; 21% karyotyping; 18% RFLP + probe
Parasites	*Trypanosoma*	47% MLEE; 30% RAPD
	Leishmania	69% MLEE; 16% RAPD
	Plasmodium	81% PCR-RFLP; 11% RAPD

[a] Estimates were made from a literature search beginning in 1996.

not as scientific, a particular method may take hold for a particular species due to a consensus of the scientists working in that area and the history of the methods first applied. Fourth, selections may be based on expediency. Whatever the reason, the take-home message of this chapter should be clear. Select a fingerprinting method that will answer the question posed. Make sure that the method has been verified for efficacy at the level of genetic relatedness necessary. Use computer-assisted systems, and save data in a format accessible for retrospective analyses and comparisons with new data. Finally, carefully consider the methods used for obtaining the collection.

REFERENCES

1. **Aanensen, D. M., and B. G. Spratt.** 1 July 2005, posting date. The multilocus sequence typing network: mlst.net. *Nucleic Acids Res.* **33**(Web server issue):W728–W733. [On line.] DOI: 10.1093/nar/gki415.
2. **Abderrazak, S. B., B. Oury, A. A. Lal, M. F. Bosseno, P. Force-Barge, J. P. Dujardin, T. Fandeur, J. F. Molez, F. Kjellberg, F. J. Ayala, and M. Tibayrenc.** 1999. *Plasmodium falciparum:* population genetic analysis by multilocus enzyme electrophoresis and other molecular markers. *Exp. Parasitol.* **92:**232–238.
3. **Agodi, A., F. Campanile, G. Basile, F. Viglianisi, and S. Stefani.** 1999. Phylogenetic analysis of macrorestriction fragments as a measure of genetic relatedness in *Staphylococcus aureus:* the epidemiological impact of methicillin resistance. *Eur. J. Epidemiol.* **15:**637–642.
4. **Anderson, J. M., T. Srikantha, B. Morrow, S. H. Miyasaki, T. C. White, N. Agabian, J. Schmid, and D. R. Soll.** 1993. Characterization and partial nucleotide sequence of the DNA fingerprinting probe Ca3 of *Candida albicans*. *J. Clin. Microbiol.* **31:**1472–1480.
5. **Anderson, T. J., B. Haubold, J. T. Williams, J. G. Estrada-Franco, L. Richardson, R. Mollinedo, M. Bockarie, J. Molkili, S. Mharakurwa, N. French, J. Whitworth, I. D. Velez, A. H. Brockman, F. Nosten, M. U. Ferreira, and K. P. Day.** 2000. Microsatellite markers reveal a spectrum of population structures in the malaria parasite *Plasmodium falciparum*. *Mol. Biol. Evol.* **17:**1467–1482.
6. **Ausbel, F. M., R. Brent, R. E. Kingston, D. D. Moore, J. G. Seidman, J. A. Smith, and K. Struhl (ed.).** 1994. *Current Protocols in Molecular Biology*, vol. 1. John Wiley & Sons, Inc., New York, N.Y.
7. **Babl, F. E., S. I. Pelton, S. Theodore, and J. O. Klein.** 2001. Constancy of distribution of serogroups of invasive pneumococcal isolates among children: experience during 4 decades. *Clin. Infect. Dis.* **32:**1155–1161.
8. **Banuls, A. L., J. C. Dujardin, F. Guerrini, S. de Doncker, D. Jacquet, J. Arevalo, S. Noel, D. Le Ray, and M. Tibayrenc.** 2000. Is *Leishmania* (Viannia) *peruviana* a distinct species? A MLEE/RAPD evolutionary genetics answer. *J. Eukaryot. Microbiol.* **47:**197–207.
9. **Barakate, M. S., Y. X. Yang, S. H. Foo, A. M. Vickery, C. A. Sharp, L. D. Fowler, J. P. Harris, R. H. West, C. Mcleod, and R. A. Benn.** 2000. An epidemiological survey of methicillin-resistant *Staphylococcus aureus* in a tertiary referral hospital. *J. Hosp. Infect.* **44:**19–26.
10. **Barberio, C., R. Fani, A. Raso, A. Carli, and M. Polsinelli.** 1994. DNA fingerprinting of yeast strains by restriction enzyme analysis. *Res. Microbiol.* **145:**659–666.
11. **Barbour, A.** 1989. Antigenic variation in relapsing fever *Borrelia* species: genetic aspects, p. 783–790. *In* D. E. Berg and M. M. Howe (ed.), *Mobile DNA*. American Society for Microbiology, Washington, D.C.
12. **Barnabe, C., K. Neubauer, A. Solari, and M. Tibayrenc.** 2001. *Trypanosoma cruzi:* presence of the two major phylogenetic lineages and of several lesser discrete typing units (DTUs) in Chile and Paraguay. *Acta Trop.* **78:**127–137.
13. **Bart, A., I. G. Schuurman, M. Achtman, D. A. Caugant, J. Dankert, and A. van der Ende.** 1998. Randomly amplified polymorphic DNA genotyping of serogroup A meningococci yields results similar to those obtained by multilocus enzyme electrophoresis and reveals new genotypes. *J. Clin. Microbiol.* **36:**1746–1749.
14. **Bart-Delabesse, E., H. van Deventer, W. Goessens, J. L. Poirot, N. Lioret, A. van Belkum, and F. Dromer.** 1995. Contribution of molecular typing methods and antifungal susceptibility testing to the study of a candidemia cluster in a burn care unit. *J. Clin. Microbiol.* **33:**3278–3283.
15. **Bartie, K. L., M. J. Wilson, D. W. Williams, and M. A. Lewis.** 2000. Macrorestriction fingerprinting of "*Streptococcus milleri*" group bacteria by pulsed-field gel electrophoresis. *J. Clin. Microbiol.* **38:**2141–2149.
16. **Bertout, S., F. Renaud, D. Swinne, M. Mallie, and J. M. Bastide.** 1999. Genetic multilocus studies of different strains of *Cryptococcus neoformans:* taxonomy and genetic structure. *J. Clin. Microbiol.* **37:**715–720.
17. **Bertout, S., F. Renaud, T. De Meeus, M. A. Piens, B. Lebeau, M. A. Viviani, M. Mallie, and J. M. Bastide.** 2000. Multilocus enzyme electrophoresis analysis of *Aspergillus fumigatus* strains isolated from the first clinical sample from patients with invasive aspergillosis. *J. Med. Microbiol.* **49:**375–381.
18. **Blignaut, E., C. Pujol, S. Lockhart, S. Joly, and D. R. Soll.** 2002. Ca3 fingerprinting of *Candida albicans* isolates from human immunodeficiency virus-positive individuals reveals a new clade in South Africa. *J. Clin. Microbiol.* **40:**826–836.
19. **Bogaert D., P. W. Hermans, I. N. Grivea, G. S. Katopodis, T. J. Mitchell, M. Sluijter, R. De Groot, N. G. Beratis, and G. A. Syrogiannopoulos.** 2003. Molecular epidemiology of penicillin-susceptible non-beta-lactam-resistant *Streptococcus pneumoniae* isolates from Greek children. *J. Clin. Microbiol.* **41:**5633–5639.
20. **Bougnoux, M. E., D. M. Aanensen, S. Morand, M. Theraud, B. G. Spratt, and C. d'Enfert.** 2004. Multilocus sequence typing of *Candida albicans:* strategies, data exchange and applications. *Infect. Genet. Evol.* **4:**243–252.
21. **Bougnoux, M. E., S. Morand, and C. d'Enfert.** 2002. Usefulness of multilocus sequence typing for characterization of clinical isolates of *Candida albicans*. *J. Clin. Microbiol.* **40:**1290–1297.
22. **Brownlie, L., J. R. Stephenson, and J. A. Cole.** 1990. Effect of growth rate on plasmid maintenance by *Escherichia coli* HB101(pAT153). *J. Gen. Microbiol.* **136:**2471–2480.
23. **Brunder, W., and H. Karch.** 2000. Genome plasticity in Enterobacteriaceae. *Int. J. Med. Microbiol.* **290:**153–165.
24. **Caetano-Anolles, G.** 1993. Amplifying DNA with arbitrary oligonucleotide primers. *Genome Res.* **3:**85–94.
25. **Canton, R., M. Perez-Vazquez, A. Oliver, B. Sanchez Del Saz, M. O. Gutierrez, M. Martinez-Ferrer, and F. Baquero.** 2000. Evaluation of the Wider system, a new computer-assisted image-processing device for bacterial identification and susceptibility testing. *J. Clin. Microbiol.* **38:**1339–1346.
26. **Carle, G. F., and M. V. Olson.** 1985. An electrophoretic karyotype for yeast. *Proc. Natl. Acad. Sci. USA* **82:** 3756–3760.
27. **Caulcott, C. A., A. Dunn, H.A. Robertson, N. S. Cooper, M. E. Brown, and P. M. Rhodes.** 1987. Investigation of the effect of growth environment on the stability of low-copy-number plasmids in *Escherichia coli*. *J. Gen. Microbiol.* **133:**1881–1889.
28. **Chang, N., and L. Chui.** 1998. A standardized protocol for the rapid preparation of bacterial DNA for pulsed-field gel electrophoresis. *Diagn. Microbiol. Infect. Dis.* **31:**275–279.

29. **Chu, G., D. Vollrath, and R. W. Davis.** 1986. Separation of large DNA molecules by contour-clamped homogeneous electric fields. *Science* **234:**1582–1585.
30. **Chung, M., H. de Lencastre, P. Matthews, A. Tomasz, I. Adamsson, M. Aries de Sousa, T. Camou, C. Cocuzza, A. Corso, I. Couto, A. Dominguez, M. Gniadkowski, R. Goering, A. Gomes, K. Kikuchi, A. Marchese, R. Mato, O. Melter, D. Oliveira, R. Palacio, R. Sa-Leao, I. Santos Sanches, J. H. Song, P. T. Tassios, P. Villari, et al.** 2000. Molecular typing of methicillin-resistant *Staphylococcus aureus* by pulsed-field gel electrophoresis: comparison of results obtained in a multilaboratory effort using identical protocols and MRSA strains. *Microb. Drug Resist.* **6:**189–198.
31. **Clode, F. E., M. E. Kaufmann, H. Malnick, and T. L. Pitt.** 2000. Distribution of genes encoding putative transmissibility factors among epidemic and nonepidemic strains of *Burkholderia cepacia* from cystic fibrosis patients in the United Kingdom. *J. Clin. Microbiol.* **38:**1763–1766.
32. **Cowen, L. E., C. Sirjusingh, R. C. Summerbell, S. Walmsley, S. Richardson, L. M. Kohn, and J. B. Anderson.** 1999. Multilocus genotypes and DNA fingerprinting do not predict variation in azole resistance among clinical isolates of *Candida albicans*. *Antimicrob. Agents Chemother.* **43:**2930–2938.
33. **del Campo, R., M. I. Morosini, E. G. de la Pedrosa, A. Fenoll, C. Munoz-Almagro, L. Maiz, F. Baquero, R. Canton, and the Spanish Pneumococcal Infection Study Network.** 2005. Population structure, antimicrobial resistance, and mutation frequencies of *Streptococcus pneumoniae* isolates from cystic fibrosis patients. *J. Clin. Microbiol.* **43:**2207–2214.
34. **Demarta, A., M. Tonolla, A. Caminada, M. Beretta, and R. Peduzzi.** 2000. Epidemiological relationships between *Aeromonas* strains isolated from symptomatic children and household environments as determined by ribotyping. *Eur. J. Epidemiol.* **16:**447–453.
35. **de Souza Lopes, A. C., J. Falcao Rodrigues, and M. A. de Morais, Jr.** 2005. Molecular typing of *Klebsiella pneumoniae* isolates from public hospitals in Recife, Brazil. *Microbiol. Res.* **160:**37–46.
36. **Dib, J. C., M. Dube, C. Kelly, M. G. Rinaldi, and J. E. Patterson.** 1996. Evaluation of pulsed-field gel electrophoresis as a typing system for *Candida rugosa:* comparison of karyotype and restriction fragment length polymorphisms. *J. Clin. Microbiol.* **34:**1494–1496.
37. **Dodgson, A. R., C. Pujol, D. W. Denning, D. R. Soll, and A. J. Fox.** 2003. Multilocus sequence typing of *Candida glabrata* reveals geographically enriched clades. *J. Clin. Microbiol.* **41:**5709–5717.
38. **Drobniewski, F., Y. Balabanova, V. Nikolayevsky, M. Ruddy, S. Kuznetzov, S. Zakharova, A. Melentyev, and I. Fedorin.** 2005. Drug-resistant tuberculosis, clinical virulence, and the dominance of the Beijing strain family in Russia. *JAMA* **293:**2726–2731.
39. **During, K.** 1993. Non-radioactive detection methods for nucleic acids separated by electrophoresis. *J. Chromatogr.* **618:**105–131.
40. **Ellsworth, D. L., K. D. Rittenhouse, and R. L. Honeycutt.** 1993. Artifactual variation in randomly amplified polymorphic DNA banding patterns. *BioTechniques* **14:**214–217.
41. **Enger, L., S. Joly, C. Pujol, P. Simonson, M. A. Pfaller, and D. R. Soll.** 2001. Cloning and characterization of a complex DNA fingerprinting probe for *Candida parapsilosis*. *J. Clin Microbiol.* **39:**658–669.
42. **Enright, M. C., and B. G. Spratt.** 1999. Multilocus sequence typing. *Trends Microbiol.* **7:**482–487.
43. **Eribe, E. R., and I. Olsen.** 2000. Strain differentiation in *Bacteroides fragilis* by ribotyping and computer-assisted gel analysis. *APMIS* **108:**429–438.
44. **Feavers, I. M., S. J. Gray, R. Urwin, J. E. Russell, J. A. Bygraves, E. B. Kaczmarski, and M. C. Maiden.** 1999. Multilocus sequence typing and antigen gene sequencing in the investigation of a meningococcal disease outbreak. *J. Clin. Microbiol.* **37:**3883–3887.
45. **Feil, E. J., and M. C. Enright.** 2004. Analyses of clonality and the evolution of bacterial pathogens. *Curr. Opin. Microbiol.* **7:**308–313.
46. **Feil, E. J., B. C. Li, D. M. Aanensen, W. P. Hanage, and B. G. Spratt.** 2004. eBURST: inferring patterns of evolutionary descent among clusters of related bacterial genotypes from multilocus sequence typing data. *J. Bacteriol.* **186:**1518–1530.
47. **Felsenstein, J.** 1984. Distance methods for inferring phylogenies: a justification. *Evolution* **38:**16–24.
48. **Felsenstein, J.** 1985. Confidence limits on phylogenies: an approach using the bootstrap. *Evolution* **39:**783–791.
49. **Feng, X., S. M. Rich, D. Akiyoshi, J. K. Tumwine, A. Kekitiinwa, N. Nabukeera, S. Tzipori, and G. Widmer.** 2000. Extensive polymorphism in *Cryptosporidium parvum* identified by multilocus microsatellite analysis. *Appl. Environ. Microbiol.* **66:**3344–3349.
50. **Fitch, W. M., and E. Margoliash.** 1967. Construction of phylogenetic trees. *Science* **155:**279–284.
51. **Forche, A., G. May, and P. T. Magee.** 2005. Demonstration of loss of heterozygosity by single-nucleotide polymorphism microarray analysis and alterations in strain morphology in *Candida albicans* strains during infection. *Eukaryot. Cell* **4:**156–165.
52. **Forche, A., G. Schönian, Y. Gräser, R. Vilgalys, and T. G. Mitchell.** 1999. Genetic structure of typical and atypical populations of *Candida albicans* from Africa. *Fungal Genet. Biol.* **28:**107–125.
53. **Friedman, C. R., M. Y. Stoeckle, W. D. Johnson, Jr., and L. W. Riley.** 1995. Double-repetitive-element PCR method for subtyping *Mycobacterium tuberculosis* clinical isolates. *J. Clin. Microbiol.* **33:**1383–1384.
54. **Fries, B. C., D. L. Goldman, and A. Casadevall.** 2002. Phenotypic switching in *Cryptococcus neoformans*. *Microbes Infect.* **4:**1345–1352.
55. **Fundyga, R. E., R. J. Kuykendall, W. Lee-Yang, and T. J. Lott.** 2004. Evidence for aneuploidy and recombination in the human commensal yeast *Candida parapsilosis*. *Infect. Genet. Evol.* **4:**37–43.
56. **Garaizar, J., S. Porwollik, A. Echeita, A. Rementeria, S. Herrera, R. M. Wong, J. Frye, M. A. Usera, and M. McClelland.** 2002. DNA microarray-based typing of an atypical monophasic *Salmonella enterica* serovar. *J. Clin. Microbiol.* **40:**2074–2078.
57. **Gardiner, K., and D. Patterson.** 1989. Transverse alternating field electrophoresis and applications to mammalian genome mapping. *Electrophoresis* **10:**296–302.
58. **Gartenberg, M. R.** 2000. The Sir proteins of *Saccharomyces cerevisiae:* mediators of transcriptional silencing and much more. *Curr. Opin. Microbiol.* **3:**132–137.
59. **Gharizadeh, B., M. Kaller, P. Nyren, A. Andersson, M. Uhlen, J. Lundeberg, and A. Ahmadian.** 15 November 2003, posting date. Viral and microbial genotyping by a combination of multiplex competitive hybridization and specific extension followed by hybridization to generic tag arrays. *Nucleic Acids Res.* **31:**e146. DOI: 10.1093/nar/gng147.
60. **Girardin, H., J. P. Latge, T. Srikantha., B. Morrow, and D. R. Soll.** 1993. Development of DNA probes for fingerprinting *Aspergillus fumigatus*. *J. Clin. Microbiol.* **31:**1547–1554.
61. **Glasgow, A. C., K. T. Hughes, and M. I. Simon.** 1989. Bacterial DNA inversion systems, p. 637–660. *In* D. E. Berg and M. M. Howe (ed.), *Mobile DNA*. American Society for Microbiology, Washington, D.C.
62. **Glover, D. M.** 1983. Genes for ribosomal DNA, p. 207–224. *In* M. Maclean, S. P. Gregory, and R. A. Flavell (ed.),

Eukaryotic Genes: Their Structure and Regulation. Butterworth & Co., Cambridge, United Kingdom.
63. **Gottlieb, S., and R. E. Esposito.** 1989. A new role for a yeast transcriptional silencer gene, *SIR2*, in regulation of recombination in ribosomal DNA. *Cell* **56:**771–776.
64. **Gräser, Y., M. Volovsek, J. Arrington, G. Schönian, W. Presber, T. G. Mitchell, and R. Vilgalys.** 1996. Molecular markers reveal that population structure of the human pathogen *Candida albicans* exhibits both clonality and recombination. *Proc. Natl. Acad. Sci. USA* **93:** 12473–12477.
65. **Haber, J. E.** 1998. A locus control region regulates yeast recombination. *Trends Genet.* **14:**317–321.
66. **Hazell, S. L., R. H. Andrews, H. M. Mitchell, and G. Daskalopoulous.** 1997. Genetic relationship among isolates of *Helicobacter pylori:* evidence for the existence of a *Helicobacter pylori* species-complex. *FEMS Microbiol. Lett.* **150:**27–32.
67. **Holtke, H. J., W. Ankebauer, K. Muhlegger, R. Rein, G. Sagner, R. Seibl, and T. Walter.** 1995. The digoxigenin (DIG) system for non-radioactive labelling and detection of nucleic acids—an overview. *Cell. Mol. Biol.* **41:**883–905.
68. **Ichiyama, S. M., M. Ohta, K. Shimokata, N. Kato, and J. Takeuchi.** 1991. Genomic DNA fingerprinting by pulsed-field gel electrophoresis as an epidemiological marker for study of nosocomial infections caused by methicillin-resistant *Staphylococcus aureus. J. Clin. Microbiol.* **29:**2690–2695.
69. **Isaac-Renton, J. L., C. Cordeiro, K. Sarafis, and H. Shahriari.** 1993. Characterization of *Giardia duodenalis* isolates from a waterborne outbreak. *J. Infect. Dis.* **167:**431–440.
70. **Isaacs, S., J. Aramini, B. Ciebin, J. A. Farrar, R. Ahmed, D. Middleton, A. U. Chandran, L. J. Harris, M. Howes, E. Chan, A. S. Pichette, K. Campbell, A. Gupta, L. Y. Lior, M. Pearce, C. Clark, F. Rodgers, F. Jamieson, I. Brophy, A. Ellis, and the *Salmonella enteritidis* PT30 Outbreak Investigation Working Group.** 2005. An international outbreak of salmonellosis associated with raw almonds contaminated with a rare phage type of *Salmonella enteritidis. J. Food Prot.* **68:**191–198.
71. **Joly, S., C. Pujol, K. Schroppel, and D. R. Soll.** 1996. Development of two species-specific fingerprinting probes for broad computer-assisted epidemiological studies of *Candida tropicalis. J. Clin. Microbiol.* **34:**3063–3071.
72. **Joly, S., C. Pujol, M. Rysz, K. Vargas, and D. R. Soll.** 1999. Development and characterization of complex DNA fingerprinting probes for the infectious yeast *Candida dubliniensis. J. Clin. Microbiol.* **37:**1035–1044.
73. **Kamerbeek, J., L. Schouls, A. Kolk, M. van Agterveld, D. van Soolingen, S. Kuigper, A. Bunschoten, H. Molhuizen, R. Shaw, M. Goyal, and J. van Embden.** 1997. Simultaneous detection and strain differentiation of *Mycobacterium tuberculosis* for diagnosis and epidemiology. *J. Clin. Microbiol.* **35:**907–914.
74. **Karl, S. A., and J. C. Avise.** 1993. PCR-based assays of Mendelian polymorphisms from anonymous single-copy nuclear DNA: techniques and applications for population genetics. *Mol. Biol. Evol.* **10:**342–361.
75. **Kasuga, T., J. W. Taylor, and T. J. White.** 1999. Phylogenetic relationships of varieties and geographical groups of the human pathogenic fungus *Histoplasma capsulatum* Darling. *J. Clin. Microbiol.* **37:**653–663.
76. **Kenchappa, P., and B. Sreenivasmurthy.** 2003. Simplified panel of assimilation tests for identification of *Acinetobacter* species. *Indian J. Pathol. Microbiol.* **46:**700–706.
77. **Khatib, R., J. Ramanathan, K. M. Riederer, D. DePoister, Jr., and J. Baran, Jr.** 2002. Limited genetic diversity of *Candida albicans* in fecal flora of healthy volunteers and inpatients: a proposed basis for strain homogeneity in clinical isolates. *Mycoses* **45:**393–398.
78. **Kiska, D. L., K. Hicks, and D. J. Pettit.** 2002. Identification of medically relevant *Nocardia* species with an abbreviated battery of tests. *J. Clin. Microbiol.* **40:**1346–1351.
79. **Klepser, M. E., and M. A. Pfaller.** 1998. Variation in electrophoretic karyotype and antifungal susceptibility of clinical isolates of *Cryptococcus neoformans* at a university-affiliated teaching hospital from 1987 to 1994. *J. Clin. Microbiol.* **36:**3653–3656.
80. **Ko, A. I., J. N. Reis, S. J. Coppola, E. L. Gouveia, S. M. Cordeiro, R. S. Lobo, R. M. Pinheiro, K. Salgado, C. M. Ribeiro Dourado, J. Tavares-Neto, H. Rocha, M. Galvao Reis, W. D. Johnson, Jr., and L. W. Riley.** 2000. Clonally related penicillin-nonsusceptible *Streptococcus pneumoniae* serotype 14 from cases of meningitis in Salvador, Brazil. *Clin. Infect. Dis.* **30:**78–86.
81. **Kremer, K., D. van Soolingen, R. Frothingham, W. H. Hass, P. W. M. Hermans, C. Martin, P. Palittapongarnpim, B. B. Plikaytis, L. W. Riley, M. A. Yakrus, J. M. Musser, and J. D. A. van Embden.** 1999. Comparison of methods based on different molecular epidemiological markers for typing of *Mycobacterium tuberculosis* complex strains: interlaboratory study of discriminatory power and reproducibility. *J. Clin. Microbiol.* **37:**2607–2618.
82. **Krieg, N. R. (ed.).** 1984. *Bergey's Manual of Systematic Bacteriology,* vol. 1. Williams & Wilkins, Baltimore, Md.
83. **Kurepina, N., E. Likhoshvay, E. Shashkina, B. Mathema, K. Kremer, D. van Soolingen, P. Bifani, and B. N. Kreiswirth.** 2005. Targeted hybridization of IS6110 fingerprints identifies the W-Beijing *Mycobacterium tuberculosis* strains among clinical isolates. *J. Clin. Microbiol.* **43:**2148–2154.
84. **Lasker, B. A., L. S. Page, T. J. Lott, and G. S. Kobayashi.** 1992. Isolation, characterization, and sequencing of *Candida albicans* repetitive element 2. *Gene* **116:**51–57.
85. **Leelayuwat, C., A. Romphruk, A. Lulitanond, S. Trakulsomboon, and V. Thamlikitkul.** 2000. Genotype analysis of *Burkholderia pseudomallei* using randomly amplified polymorphic DNA (RAPD): indicative of genetic differences amongst environmental and clinical isolates. *Acta Trop.* **77:**229–237.
86. **Li, J., S. Chen, and D. H. Evans.** 2001. Typing and subtyping influenza virus using DNA microarrays and multiplex reverse transcriptase PCR. *J. Clin. Microbiol.* **39:**696–704.
87. **Lin, D., L. C. Wu, M. G. Rinaldi, and P. F. Lehmann.** 1995. Three distinct genotypes within *Candida parapsilosis* from clinical sources. *J. Clin. Microbiol.* **33:**1815–1821.
88. **Lockhart, S., C. Pujol, S. Joly, and D. R. Soll.** 2001. Development and use of complex probes for DNA fingerprinting the infectious fungi. *J. Med. Mycol.* **39:**1–8.
89. **Lockhart, S., J. J. Fritch, S. Meier, K. Schroppel, R. Srikantha, R. Galask, and D. R. Soll.** 1995. Colonizing populations of *Candida albicans* are clonal in origin but undergo microevolution through C1 fragment reorganization as demonstrated by DNA fingerprinting and Cl sequencing. *J. Clin. Microbiol.* **33:**1501–1509.
90. **Lockhart, S. R., C. Pujol, A. R. Dodgson, and D. R. Soll.** 2005. Deoxyribonucleic acid fingerprinting methods for *Candida* species. *Methods Mol. Med.* **118:**15–25.
91. **Lockhart, S. R., S. Joly, C. Pujol, J. D. Sobel, M. A. Pfaller, and D. R. Soll.** 1997. Development and verification of fingerprinting probes for *Candida glabrata. Microbiology* **143:**3733–3746.
92. **Lockhart, S. R., S. Joly, K. Vargas, J. Swails-Wenger, L. Enger, and D. R. Soll.** 1999. Barriers against oral *Candida* colonization break down in the elderly. *J. Dent. Res.* **78:**857–868.
93. **Lott, T. J., B. P. Holloway, D. A. Logan, R. Fundyga, and J. Arnold.** 1999. Towards understanding the evolution of the human commensal yeast *Candida albicans. Microbiology* **145:**1137–1143.

94. **Loudon, K. W., A. P. Coke, and J. P. Burnie.** 1995. "Pseudoclusters" and typing by random amplification of polymorphic DNA of *Aspergillus fumigatus. J. Clin. Pathol.* **48:**183–184.
95. **Maiden, M. C., J. A. Bygraves, E. Feil, G. Morelli, J. E. Russell, R. Urwin, Q. Zhang, J. Zhou, K. Zurth, D. A. Caugant, I. M. Feavers, M. Achtman, and B. G. Spratt.** 1998. Multilocus sequence typing: a portable approach to the identification of clones within populations of pathogenic microorganisms. *Proc. Natl. Acad. Sci. USA* **95:** 3140–3145.
96. **Malorny, B., A. Schroeter, C. Bunge, B. Hoog, A. Steinbeck, and R. Helmuth.** 2001. Evaluation of molecular typing methods for *Salmonella enterica* serovar Typhimurium DT104 isolated in Germany from healthy pigs. *Vet. Res.* **32:**119–129.
97. **Masseret, E., J. Boudeau, J. F. Colombel, C. Neut, P. Desreumaux, B. Joly, A. Cortot, and A. Darfeuille-Michaud.** 2001. Genetically related *Escherichia coli* strains associated with Crohn's disease. *Gut* **48:**320–325.
98. **Mazars, E., S. Lesjean, A. Banuls, M. Gilbert, V. Vincent, B. Gicquel, M. Tibayrenc, C. Locht, and P. Supply.** 2001. High-resolution minisatellite-based typing as a portable approach to global analysis of *Mycobacterium tuberculosis* molecular epidemiology. *Proc. Natl. Acad. Sci. USA* **98:**1901–1906.
99. **Meunier, J. R., and P. A. Grimont.** 1993. Factors affecting reproducibility of random amplified polymorphic DNA fingerprinting. *Res. Microbiol.* **144:**373–379.
100. **Meyer, W., and T. G. Mitchell.** 1995. Polymerase chain reaction fingerprinting in fungi using single primers specific to minisatellites and simple repetitive DNA sequences strain variation in *Cryptococcus neoformans. Electrophoresis* **16:**1648–1656.
101. **Meyer, W., G. N. Latouche, H. M. Daniel, M. Thanos, T. G. Mitchell, D. Yarrow, G. Schonian, and T. C. Sorrell.** 1997. Identification of pathogenic yeasts of the imperfect genus *Candida* by polymerase chain reaction fingerprinting. *Electrophoresis* **18:**1548–1559.
102. **Morelli, G., B. Malorny, K. Muller, A. Seiler, J. F. Wang, J. del Valle, and M. Achtman.** 1997. Clonal descent and microevolution of *Neisseria meningitidis* during 30 years of epidemic spread. *Mol. Microbiol.* **25:**1047–1064.
103. **Nachamkin, I., J. Engberg, M. Gutacker, R. J. Meinersman, C. Y. Li, P. Arzate, E. Teeple, V. Fussing, T. W. Ho, A. K. Asbury, J. W. Griffin, G. M. McKhann, and J. C. Piffaretti.** 2001. Molecular population genetic analysis of *Campylobacter jejuni* HS:19 associated with Guillain-Barre syndrome and gastroenteritis. *J. Infect. Dis.* **184:**221–226.
104. **Nomura, M., and E. A. Morgan.** 1977. Genetics of bacterial ribosomes. *Annu. Rev. Genet.* **11:**297–347.
105. **Pasteur, N., G. Pasteur, F. Bonhomme, J. Catalan, and J. Britton-Davidian.** 1988. *Practical Isozyme Genetics.* Halsted Press, New York, N.Y.
106. **Paugam, A., M. Benchetrit, A. Fiacre, C. Tourte-Schaefer, and J. Dupouy-Camet.** 1999. Comparison of four commercialized biochemical systems for clinical yeast identification by colour-producing reactions. *Med. Mycol.* **37:**11–17.
107. **Pfaller, M. A., I. Mujeeb, R. J. Hollis, R. N. Jones, and G. V. Doern.** 2000. Evaluation of the discriminatory powers of the Dienes test and ribotyping as typing methods for *Proteus mirabilis. J. Clin. Microbiol.* **38:**1077–1080.
108. **Pfaller, M. A., S. R. Lockhart, C. Pujol, J. A. Swails-Wenger, S. A. Messer, M. B. Edmund, R. N. Jones, R. P. Wenzel, and D. R. Soll.** 1998. Hospital specificity, region specificity, and fluconazole-resistance of *Candida albicans* bloodstream isolates. *J. Clin. Microbiol.* **36:**1518–1529.
109. **Pinto, B., E. Chenoll, and R. Aznar.** 2005. Identification and typing of food-borne *Staphylococcus aureus* by PCR-based techniques. *Syst. Appl. Microbiol.* **28:**340–352.
110. **Pujol, C., J. Reynes, F. Renaud, M. Raymond, M. Tibayrenc, F. J. Ayala, F. Janbon, M. Mallie, and J. M. Bastide.** 1993. The yeast *Candida albicans* has a clonal mode of reproduction in a population of infected human immunodeficiency virus-positive patients. *Proc. Natl. Acad. Sci. USA* **90:**9456–9459.
111. **Pujol, C., S. Joly, S. R. Lockhart, S. Noel, M. Tibayrenc, and D. R. Soll.** 1997. Parity among the randomly amplified polymorphic DNA method, multilocus enzyme electrophoresis, and Southern blot hybridization with the moderately repetitive DNA probe Ca3 for fingerprinting *Candida albicans. J. Clin. Microbiol.* **35:**2348–2358.
112. **Radua, S., O. W. Ling, S. Srimontree, A. Lulitanond, W. F. Hin, Yuherman, S. Lihan, G. Rusul, and A. R. Mutalib.** 2000. Characterization of *Burkholderia pseudomallei* isolated in Thailand and Malaysia. *Diagn. Microbiol. Infect. Dis.* **38:**141–145.
113. **Ramsey, H., B. Morrow, and D. R. Soll.** 1994. An increase in switching frequency correlates with an increase in recombination of the ribosomal chromosomes of *Candida albicans* strain 3153A. *Microbiology* **140:**1525–1531.
114. **Ravins, M., H. Bercovier, D. Chemtob, Y. Fishman, and G. Rahav.** 2001. Molecular epidemiology of *Mycobacterium tuberculosis* infection in Israel. *J. Clin. Microbiol.* **39:**1175–1177.
115. **Richardson, B. J., P. R. Baverstock, and M. Adams.** 1986. *Allozyme Electrophoresis, a Handbook for Animal Systematics and Population Studies.* Academic Press, Inc., Orlando, Fla.
116. **Rieseberg, L. H.** 1996. Homology among RAPD fragments in interspecific comparisons. *Mol. Ecol.* **5:**99–105.
117. **Robinson, D. A., and M. C. Enright.** 2003. Evolutionary models of the emergence of methicillin-resistant *Staphylococcus aureus. Antimicrob. Agents Chemother.* **47:**3926–3934.
118. **Rohlf, F. J.** 1963. Classification of *Aedes* by numerical taxonomic methods (Diptera: Culcidae). *Ann. Entomol. Soc. Am.* **56:**798–804.
119. **Sadhu, C., M. J. McEachern, E. P. Rustchenko-Bulgac, J. Schmid, D. R. Soll, and J. B. Hicks.** 1991. Telomeric and dispersed repeat sequences in *Candida* yeasts and their use in strain identification. *J. Bacteriol.* **173:**842–850.
120. **Saitou, N., and M. Nei.** 1987. The neighbor-joining method: a new method for reconstructing phylogenetic trees. *Mol. Biol. Evol.* **4:**406–425.
121. **Sambrook, J., E. F. Fritsch, and T. Maniatis.** 1989. *Molecular Cloning: a Laboratory Manual.* Cold Spring Harbor Laboratory Press, Cold Spring Harbor, N.Y.
122. **Sangeorzan, J. A., M. J. Zervos, S. Donabedian, and C. A. Kauffman.** 1995. Validity of contour-clamped homogeneous electric field electrophoresis as a typing system for *Candida albicans. Mycoses* **38:**29–36.
123. **Scherer, S., and D. A. Stevens.** 1987. Application of DNA typing methods to epidemiology and taxonomy of *Candida* species. *J. Clin. Microbiol.* **25:**675–679.
124. **Scherer, S., and D. A. Stevens.** 1988. A *Candida albicans* dispersed, repeated gene family and its epidemiological applications. *Proc. Natl. Acad. Sci. USA* **85:**1452–1456.
125. **Schonian, G., C. Schweynoch, K. Zlateva, L. Oskam, N. Kroon, Y. Graser, and W. Presber.** 1996. Identification and determination of the relationships of species and strains within the genus *Leishmania* using single primers in the polymerase chain reaction. *Mol. Biochem. Parasitol.* **77:**19–29.

126. **Schwartz, D. C., W. Saffran, J. Welsh, R. Haas, M. Goldenberg, and C. R. Cantor.** 1983. New techniques for purifying large DNAs and studying their properties and packaging. *Cold Spring Harbor Symp. Quant. Biol.* **47:**189–195.

127. **Schwartz, D. C., and C. R. Cantor.** 1984. Separation of yeast chromosome-sized DNAs by pulsed field gradient gel electrophoresis. *Cell* **37:**67–75.

128. **Schweizer, E., C. MacKechnie, and H. D. Halvorson.** 1969. The redundancy of ribosomal and transfer DNA genes in *Saccharomyces cerevisiae*. *J. Mol. Biol.* **40:**261–278.

129. **Shepard, J. R., Y. Danin-Poleg, Y. Kashi, and D. R. Walt.** 2005. Array-based binary analysis for bacterial typing. *Anal. Chem.* **77:**319–326.

130. **Singh, D. V., M. H. Matte, G. R. Matte, S. Jiang, F. Sabeena, B. N. Shukla, S. C. Sanyal, A. Huq, and R. R. Colwell.** 2001. Molecular analysis of *Vibrio cholerae* O1, O139, non-O1, and non-O139 strains: clonal relationships between clinical and environmental isolates. *Appl. Environ. Microbiol.* **67:**910–921.

131. **Sneath, P. H., and R. R. Sokal.** 1973. *Numerical Taxonomy: the Principles and Practice of Numerical Classsification.* W. H. Freeman and Co., San Francisco, Calif.

132. **Soewignjo S., B. D. Gessner, A. Sutanto, M. Steinhoff, M. Prijanto, C. Nelson, A. Widjaya, and S. Arjoso.** 2001. *Streptococcus pneumoniae* nasopharyngeal carriage prevalence, serotype distribution, and resistance patterns among children on Lombok Island, Indonesia. *Clin. Infect. Dis.* **32:**1039–1043.

133. **Solari, A., R. Campillay, S. Ortiz, and A. Wallace.** 2001. Identification of *Trypanosoma cruzi* genotypes circulating in Chilean chagasic patients. *Exp. Parasitol.* **97:**226–233.

134. **Soll, D. R.** 1992. High frequency switching in *Candida albicans*. *Clin. Microbiol. Rev.* **5:**183–203.

135. **Soll, D. R.** 2000. The ins and outs of DNA fingerprinting the infectious fungi. *Clin. Microbiol. Rev.* **13:**332–370.

136. **Soll, D. R., R. Galask, J. Schmid, C. Hanna, K. Mac, and B. Morrow.** 1991. Genetic dissimilarity of commensal strains of *Candida* spp. carried in different anatomical locations of the same healthy women. *J. Clin. Microbiol.* **29:**1702–1710.

137. **Spratt, B. G., W. P. Hanage, B. Li, D. M. Aanensen, and E. J. Feil.** 2004. Displaying the relatedness among isolates of bacterial species—the eBURST approach. *FEMS Microbiol. Lett.* **241:**129–134.

138. **Sriburee, P., S. Khayhan, C. Khamwan, S. Panjaisee, and P. Tharavichitkul.** 2004. Serotype and PCR-fingerprints of clinical and environmental isolates of *Cryptococcus neoformans* in Chiang Mai, Thailand. *Mycopathologia* **158:**25–31.

139. **Stock, I., S. Burak, and B. Wiedemann.** 2004. Natural antimicrobial susceptibility patterns and biochemical profiles of *Leclercia adecarboxylata* strains. *Clin. Microbiol. Infect.* **10:**724–733.

140. **Su, C., C. Hott, B. H. Brownstein, and L. D. Sibley.** 2004. Typing single-nucleotide polymorphisms in *Toxoplasma gondii* by allele-specific primer extension and microarray detection. *Methods Mol. Biol.* **270:**249–262.

141. **Suffys, P. N., M. E. Ivens de Araujo, M. L. Rossetti, A. Zahab, E. W. Barroso, A. M. Barreto, E. Campos, D. van Soolingen, K. Kremer, H. Heersma, and W. M. Degrave.** 2000. Usefulness of IS6110-restriction fragment length polymorphism typing of Brazilian strains of *Mycobacterium tuberculosis* and comparison with an international fingerprint database. *Res. Microbiol.* **151:**343–351.

142. **Sullivan, D., D. Bennett, M. Henman, P. Harwood, S. Flint, F. Mulcahy, D. Shanley, and D. Coleman.** 1993. Oligonucleotide fingerprinting of isolates of *Candida* species other than *C. albicans* and of atypical *Candida* species from human immunodeficiency virus-positive and AIDS patients. *J. Clin. Microbiol.* **31:**2124–2133.

143. **Swanson, J., and J. M. Koomey.** 1989. Mechanisms for variation of pili and outer membrane protein II in *Neisseria gonorrhoeae*, p. 743–762. *In* D. E. Berg and M. M. Howe (ed.), *Mobile DNA*. American Society for Microbiology, Washington, D.C.

144. **Swiderek, H., H. Claus, M. Frosch, and U. Vogel.** 2005. Evaluation of custom-made DNA microarrays for multilocus sequence typing of *Neisseria meningitidis*. *Int. J. Med. Microbiol.* **295:**39–45.

145. **Symms, C., B. Cookson, J. Stanley, and J. V. Hookey.** 1998. Analysis of methicillin-resistant *Staphylococcus aureus* by IS1181 profiling. *Epidemiol. Infect.* **120:**271–279.

146. **Syrmis, M. W., M. R. O'Carroll, T. P. Sloots, C. Coulter, C. E. Wainwright, S. C. Bell, and M. D. Nissen.** 2004. Rapid genotyping of *Pseudomonas aeruginosa* isolates harboured by adult and paediatric patients with cystic fibrosis using repetitive-element-based PCR assays. *J. Med. Microbiol.* **53:**1089–1096.

147. **Tavanti, A., A. D. Davidson, N. A. Gow, M. C. Maiden, and F. C. Odds.** 2005. *Candida orthopsilosis* and *Candida metapsilosis* spp. nov. to replace *Candida parapsilosis* groups II and III. *J. Clin. Microbiol.* **43:**284–292.

148. **Tavanti, A., N. A. Gow, S. Senesi, M. C. Maiden, and F. C. Odds.** 2003. Optimization and validation of multilocus sequence typing for *Candida albicans*. *J. Clin. Microbiol.* **41:**3765–3776.

149. **Taylor, J. W., and M. C. Fisher.** 2003. Fungal multilocus sequence typing—it's not just for bacteria. *Curr. Opin. Microbiol.* **6:**351–356.

150. **Taylor, J. W., D. M. Geiser, A. Burt, and V. Koufopanou.** 1999. The evolutionary biology and population genetics underlying fungal strain typing. *Clin. Microbiol. Rev.* **12:**126–146.

151. **Tenover, F. C., R. D. Arbeit, R. V. Goering, P. A. Mickelsen, B. E. Murray, D. H. Persing, and B. Swaminathan.** 1995. Interpreting chromosomal DNA restriction patterns produced by pulsed-field gel electrophoresis: criteria for bacterial strain typing. *J. Clin. Microbiol.* **33:**2233–2239.

152. **Thormann, C. E., M. E. Ferreira, L. E. Camargo, J. G. Tivang, and T. C. Osborn.** 1994. Comparison of RFLP and RAPD markers to estimate the genetic relationships within and among cruciferous species. *Theor. Appl. Genet.* **88:**973–980.

153. **Thrash-Bingham, C., and J. A. Gorman.** 1992. DNA translocations contribute to chromosome length polymorphisms in *Candida albicans*. *Curr. Genet.* **22:**93–100.

154. **Tibayrenc, M.** 1995. Population genetics and strain typing of microorganisms: how to detect departures from panmixia without individualizing alleles and loci. *C. R. Acad. Sci. Ser. III* **318:**135–139.

155. **Tibayrenc, M.** 1996. Towards a unified evolutionary genetics of microorganisms. *Ann. Rev. Microbiol.* **50:**401–429.

156. **Tibayrenc, M., K. Neubauer, C. Barnabe, F. Guerrini, D. Skarecky, and F. J. Ayala.** 1993. Genetic characterization of six parasitic protozoa: parity between random-primer DNA typing and multilocus enzyme electrophoresis. *Proc. Natl. Acad. Sci. USA* **90:**1335–1339.

157. **Urwin, R., and M. C. Maiden.** 2003. Multi-locus sequence typing: a tool for global epidemiology. *Trends Microbiol.* **11:**479–487.

158. **van Der Zwet, W. C., G. A. Parlevliet, P. H. Savelkoul, J. Stoof, A. M. Kaiser, A. M. Van Furth, and C. M. Vandenbroucke-Grauls.** 2000. Outbreak of *Bacillus cereus* infections in a neonatal intensive care unit traced to balloons used in manual ventilation. *J. Clin. Microbiol.* **38:**4131–4136.

159. **van Doorn, N. E., F. Namavar, J. G. Kusters, E. P. van Rees, E. J. Kulipers, and J. de Graaff.** 1998. Genomic DNA fingerprinting of clinical isolates of *Helicobacter*

pylori by REP-PCR and restriction fragment end-labeling. *FEMS Microbiol. Lett.* **160:**145–150.

160. **van Soolingen, D., P. W. M. Hermans, P. E. W. de Hans, D. R. Soll, and J. D. A. van Enbden.** 1991. Occurrence and stability of insertion sequences in *Mycobacterium tuberculosis* complex strains: evaluation of an insertion sequence-dependent DNA polymorphism as a tool in the epidemiology of tuberculosis. *J. Clin. Microbiol.* **29:** 2578–2586.
161. **van Steenbergen, T. J., S. D. Colloms, P. W. Hermans, J. de Graaff, and R. H. Plasterk.** 1995. Genomic DNA fingerprinting by restriction fragment end-labeling. *Proc. Natl. Acad. Sci. USA* **92:**5572–5576.
162. **Vargas, K., S. A. Messer, M. Pfaller, S. R. Lockhart, J. Stapleton, J. Hellstein, and D. R. Soll.** 2000. Elevated switching and drug resistance of *Candida* from human immunodeficiency virus-positive individuals prior to thrush. *J. Clin. Microbiol.* **38:**3995–3607.
163. **Verweij, P. E., I. M. Breuker, A. J. Rijs, and J. F. Meis.** 1999. Comparative study of seven commercial yeast identification systems. *J. Clin. Pathol.* **52:**271–273.
164. **Vos, P., R. Hogers, M. Bleeker, M. Reijans, T. van de Lee, M. Hornes, A. Frijters, J. Pot, J. Peleman, and M. Kuiper.** 1995. AFLP: a new technique for DNA fingerprinting. *Nucleic Acids Res.* **23:**4407–4414.
165. **Welsch, J., and M. McClelland.** 1990. Fingerprinting genomes using PCR with arbitrary primers. *Nucleic Acids Res.* **18:**7213–7224.
166. **Wiley, E. O.** 1981. *Phylogenetics: the Theory and Practice of Phylogenetic Systematics.* Wiley & Sons, New York, N.Y.
167. **Williams, J. G., A. R. Kubelik, K. J. Livak and S. V. Tingey.** 1990. DNA polymorphisms amplified by arbitrary primers are useful as genetic markers. *Nucleic Acids Res.* **18:**6531–6535.
168. **Willse, A., T. M. Straub, S. C. Wunschel, J. A. Small, D. R. Call, D. S. Daly, and D. P. Chandler.** 2004. Quantitative oligonucleotide microarray fingerprinting of *Salmonella enterica* isolates. *Nucleic Acids Res.* **32:**1848–1856.
169. **Wolf, B., L. C. Rey, S. Brisse, L. B. Moreira, D. Milatovic, A. Fleer, J. J. Roord, and J. Verhoef.** 2000. Molecular epidemiology of penicillin-resistant *Streptococcus pneumoniae* colonizing children with community-acquired pneumonia and children attending day-care centres in Fortaleza, Brazil. *J. Antimicrob. Chemother.* **46:**757–765.
170. **Wu, C. F. J.** 1986. Jacknife, bootstrap and other resampling plans in regression analysis. *Ann. Stat.* **14:** 1261–1295.
171. **Xu, J., R. Vilgalys, and T. G. Mitchell.** 1999. Lack of genetic differentiation between two geographically diverse samples of *Candida albicans* isolated from patients infected with human immunodeficiency virus. *J. Bacteriol.* **181:**1369–1373.
172. **Xu, J., T. G. Mitchell, and R. Vilgalys.** 1999. PCR-restriction fragment length polymorphism (RFLP) analyses reveal both extensive clonality and local genetic differences in *Candida albicans*. *Mol. Ecol.* **8:**59–73.
173. **Yan, J. J., J. J. Wu, W. C. Ko, S. H. Tsai, C. L. Chuang, H. M. Wu, Y. J. Lu, and J. D. Li.** 2004. Plasmid-mediated 16S rRNA methylases conferring high-level aminoglycoside resistance in *Escherichia coli* and *Klebsiella pneumoniae* isolates from two Taiwanese hospitals. *J. Antimicrob. Chemother.* **54:**1007–1012.
174. **Yu, J., J. Lin, W. H. Benjamin, Jr., K. B. Waites, C. H. Lee, and M. H. Nahm.** 2005. Rapid multiplex assay for serotyping pneumococci with monoclonal and polyclonal antibodies. *J. Clin. Microbiol.* **43:**156–162.

Investigation of Foodborne and Waterborne Disease Outbreaks*

TIMOTHY F. JONES

12

Each year approximately 4 billion cases of diarrhea occur worldwide (26). In 2002, foodborne and waterborne diarrheal diseases were estimated to have killed 1.8 million people, most of whom were under 5 years of age. In the United States alone, foodborne diseases are estimated to cause 76 million illnesses, 325,000 hospitalizations, and 5,000 deaths each year (21). Food and water safety issues are complex, and foodborne and waterborne diseases can have a myriad of potential causes. Because outbreaks can affect large numbers of persons, prompt and thorough investigations of potential outbreaks can prevent substantial morbidity. In addition, outbreak investigations provide information that increases our understanding of the epidemiology of these diseases and allows us to develop preventive measures.

Foodborne and waterborne disease outbreaks are generally defined as clusters of two or more persons with a similar illness resulting from ingestion of a common food (6) or epidemiologically linked to recreational or drinking water (10). Foodborne and waterborne disease outbreaks may be caused by bacteria, viruses, protozoa, fungi, helminths, prions, and biologic or environmental toxins. Viral agents cause two-thirds of foodborne disease outbreaks in the United States, bacteria cause approximately one-third, and parasites are relatively uncommon etiologic agents. Of viruses, noroviruses are by far the most common cause of foodborne disease outbreaks. The most common bacterial causes are *Salmonella* and *Campylobacter* (21).

Many foodborne and waterborne diseases are self-limited and characterized by gastrointestinal symptoms such as vomiting and diarrhea. Others, however, may manifest as systemic or neurological disease and result in substantial morbidity and mortality. Examples include infection with *Escherichia coli* O157:H7, which can be associated with hemolytic-uremic syndrome; *Helicobacter pylori,* which has been linked to gastric cancers; *Listeria,* which can cause meningitis and miscarriage; *Salmonella,* which can cause reactive arthritis; and prions, which cause invariably fatal new-variant Creutzfeldt-Jakob disease.

Improved basic sanitation, medical care, and diagnostic capabilities have helped substantially reduce both the risks for foodborne and waterborne diseases and the frequency of complications. However, other factors have allowed old scourges to persist and new threats to emerge. Noroviruses, rotaviruses, astroviruses, *Cryptosporidium parvum, Campylobacter* spp., *E. coli* O157:H7, hepatitis E, and the prion associated with bovine-spongiform encephalopathy are among foodborne and waterborne pathogens identified since 1972. The population of vulnerable persons is growing, and new populations are being exposed to potential pathogens because more people are living longer, are living with immunosuppressive conditions, or are traveling internationally. Moreover, the food supply has been globalized so that people are eating at home foods that travel medicine physicians tell them not to eat when they are traveling abroad. Outbreaks of cryptosporidiosis in Milwaukee, Wis., in 1993, which sickened 400,000 persons and led to 100 deaths, primarily in human immunodeficiency virus-infected persons (20), and *E. coli* O157:H7 in Japan, which caused over 6,000 illnesses among persons who ate radish sprouts from a single supplier (24), are examples demonstrating the large and dramatic sequelae of such social changes.

It is important to investigate foodborne outbreaks so that the etiology, vehicle, and mechanisms associated with disease can be identified and similar outbreaks can be prevented in the future. This chapter provides a framework for understanding the general principles and strategies of outbreak investigations. Details on the clinical and epidemiologic characteristics of specific pathogens can be found in other chapters of this Manual. Additional information on outbreak investigation and testing of environmental and food specimens is available from other published sources (http://www.cdc.gov/foodborneoutbreaks/, http://www.cdc.gov/ncidod/dpd/healthywater/professional.htm, and http://www.cdc.gov/healthyswimming/outbreak.htm) (5, 12–14, 16–18).

EPIDEMIOLOGY OF FOODBORNE AND WATERBORNE DISEASE OUTBREAKS

Beginning in 1938, the U.S. Public Health Service has maintained and reported data on foodborne and waterborne disease outbreaks (6). Between 2001 and 2003, the Centers for Disease Control and Prevention (CDC) received an annual mean of 1,214 reports of outbreaks from federal, state, and local epidemiologists throughout the United States who conducted outbreak investigations (http://www.cdc.gov/foodborneoutbreaks/report_pub.htm) (11). These outbreaks involved approximately 24,000 persons. Of reported

*This chapter contains information presented in chapter 13 by John Besser, James Beebe, and Bala Swaminathan in the eighth edition of this Manual.

outbreaks during this period, approximately one-fifth were due to bacterial pathogens, about one-eighth were due to viruses, and less than one-twentieth were due to chemicals and parasitic agents. It is noteworthy that the etiology of two-thirds of the outbreaks was not identified. The pathogens most commonly identified in outbreaks reported in 2003 are shown in Fig. 1.

In the United States over one-half of the outbreaks of foodborne and waterborne disease are associated with restaurants. In contrast, nearly 90% of the global burden of diarrheal disease is attributable to unsafe water supplies (25). In 2001–2002, 96 waterborne disease outbreaks in the United States were reported to the CDC, of which 31 were associated with drinking water and 65 were associated with recreational water (10). Figure 2 illustrates the etiologic agents causing outbreaks associated with drinking water, and Fig. 3 describes the clinical syndromes seen in outbreaks related to recreational water.

The response to preventive measures and the treatment of clinical infections vary markedly depending on the etiologic agent involved. It is therefore of concern that the etiologic agents were not identified for nearly two-thirds of foodborne disease outbreaks reported to the CDC in 2001–2003 and for one-fourth of drinking-water-associated outbreaks reported in 2001–2002. This deficit is due in part to the fact that stool specimens are rarely tested in such outbreaks. In fact, stool specimens were tested for only one of seven waterborne outbreaks of acute gastrointestinal illness for which the etiology was unknown (10) and stool specimens were not collected for laboratory testing in two-thirds of foodborne disease outbreaks of unknown etiology occurring at seven sites in 1998 and 1999 (19). While many factors can impede investigators as they work up outbreaks, laboratory testing is usually necessary to confirm an etiology.

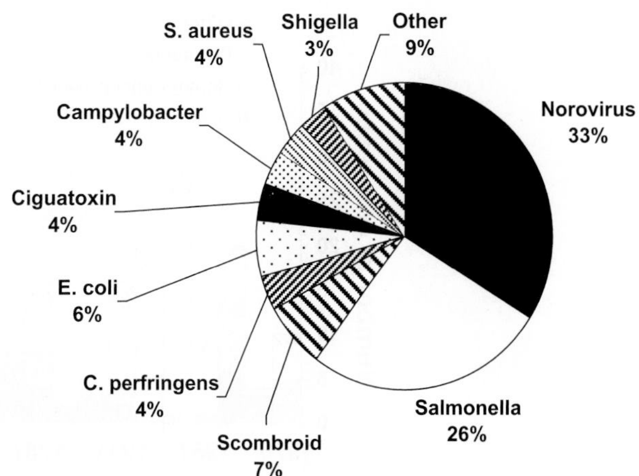

FIGURE 1 Causes of foodborne disease outbreaks with a confirmed etiology, among those reported to the Centers for Disease Control and Prevention, 2003.

GENERAL APPROACH TO AN OUTBREAK INVESTIGATION

Standard steps in an outbreak investigation are outlined in Table 1. Potential foodborne and waterborne disease outbreaks may come to the attention of health authorities through a number of mechanisms. Laboratorians, clinicians, or public health agencies may recognize unusual numbers or types of illness and report them, or patients may report illnesses to public health agencies directly. Foodborne and waterborne disease outbreaks must be reported to public health departments in most jurisdictions, and public health personnel frequently coordinate community-wide investigations, although clinicians, laboratorians, environmentalists, and institutional representatives all may play important roles in outbreak investigations. Local and state public health authorities generally have legal responsibility for outbreak investigations and may involve the CDC or other local, state, and federal agencies as appropriate. The roles of various government agencies in outbreak investigations are outlined in Table 2.

One of the first steps in responding to a possible foodborne or waterborne disease outbreak is confirming whether an "outbreak" has actually occurred. The CDC defines a foodborne disease outbreak as "the occurrence of two or

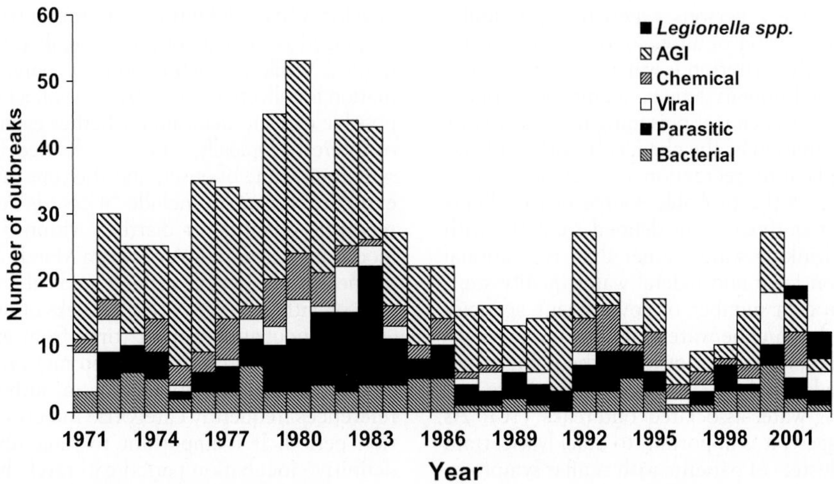

FIGURE 2 Drinking-water-associated outbreaks, by year and etiologic agent—United States, 1971–2001 (n = 764). AGI, acute gastrointestinal illness of unknown etiology. For *Legionella* spp., Legionnaires' disease was added to the surveillance system (and *Legionella* spp. were classified separately) beginning with 2001. Adapted from reference 10.

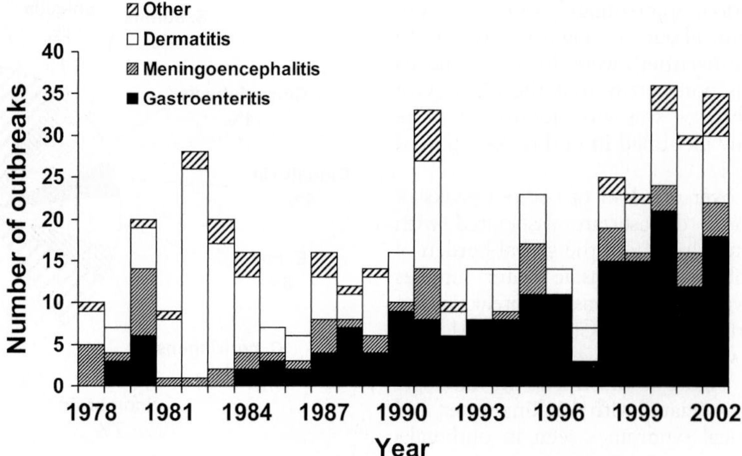

FIGURE 3 Waterborne-disease outbreaks ($n = 65$) associated with recreational water, by etiologic agent—United States, 1978–2002. "Other" includes keratitis, conjunctivitis, otitis, bronchitis, meningitis, hepatitis, leptospirosis, Pontiac fever, and acute respiratory illness. "Meningoencephalitis" also includes data from report of ameba infections (28). Adapted from reference 10.

TABLE 1 Steps of an outbreak investigation[a]

1. Establish the existence of an outbreak.
2. Verify the diagnosis.
3. Define and count cases.
4. Determine the population at risk.
5. Describe epidemiology.
6. Develop hypotheses.
7. Evaluate hypotheses.
8. Perform additional epidemiologic, environmental, and laboratory studies, as necessary.
9. Implement control and prevention measures.
10. Communicate findings.

[a]Adapted from references 5 and 14, with permission.

more cases of a similar illness resulting from ingestion of a common food" (6). The CDC defines a recreational water-associated outbreak as ≥2 persons experiencing a similar illness after exposure to water or air encountered in a recreational water setting (this criterion is waived for single cases of laboratory-confirmed primary amebic meningoencephalitis, wound infections, or chemical poisoning if water quality data indicate contamination by the chemical), with epidemiologic evidence implicating recreational water or a recreational water setting as the probable source of the illness (10). Drinking-water outbreaks are defined similarly, with the implication of drinking water rather than recreational water. Information on local and federal water quality standards is available from a number of government agencies (http://www.cdc.gov/nceh/ehhe/water/data.htm). Outbreaks caused by contamination of water or ice at the point of use (e.g., a contaminated faucet or serving container) are not classified as drinking-water-associated outbreaks (10). As these definitions suggest, it is important to quickly ascertain whether apparent clusters of patients with similar symptoms or laboratory-confirmed disease are linked epidemiologically by exposure to a common food or water source. In practical terms, many outbreaks are recognized through routine surveillance for diseases that must be reported (Table 3). If public health officials identify unusual numbers of cases clustered by time or place, they often investigate further and identify a previously unrecognized epidemiologic link between cases. To recognize unusual clusters of illness, public health officials obviously must have knowledge of what "normal" or baseline rates of a disease are in the affected community. This important information may be available from routine disease surveillance performed by public health authorities and institutional infection control personnel. To decide whether a potential cluster of disease warrants further investigation, one needs basic epidemiologic data about the potential cluster and one must consider other factors such as the resources available for an investigation, the severity of the disease, the community affected, and the likelihood that useful data can be obtained from an investigation.

To recognize and characterize a potential outbreak, one must identify the persons affected by the outbreak ("cases") and organize data about these cases by time, place, exposure history, and other characteristics. Investigators should develop a "case definition," or criteria by which a person will be judged to be part of an outbreak (or not), early in their inquiry. While this definition may change as additional information is collected, it is critical to collect sufficient data on all possible cases to determine whether each is part of the group of interest. Typically, cases are defined by criteria including symptoms, time of onset, and the time and place of potential exposure. Examples include "a case is defined as any person reporting vomiting or diarrhea within 5 days of consuming food from Restaurant A between March 2 and 5" or "a case is defined as any person seeking medical care for a rash illness, with or without fever, within 2 weeks of swimming at Lake X."

The incubation period (time from exposure to an etiologic agent until onset of symptoms) provides an important clue to the possible etiology of an outbreak. Textbooks and references frequently categorize infectious agents by incubation period. It is important to remember, however, that a definitive incubation period can rarely be determined based on a single patient's history. Typical signs and symptoms and the mean incubation period and duration of illness are most useful when evaluated in aggregate, for a number of ill patients. In addition, patients often assume that recent meals or particular events caused their illnesses, when

TABLE 2 Roles of selected government agencies in responding to possible foodborne or waterborne disease outbreaks in the United States[a]

Agency	Responsibilities	Product or situation of interest
Local and state health departments	Generally authorized under state laws to be responsible for surveillance for notifiable diseases and investigation of most foodborne and waterborne outbreaks in their jurisdiction. Often responsible to inspect and regulate restaurants within jurisdiction. State health laboratories support outbreak investigations.	Any legally notifiable disease or outbreak of public health importance.
Local and state water regulatory agencies	Generally authorized under state laws to have oversight of surface water, municipal water systems, wells, and other water supplies. Responsibility may be under the jurisdiction of different agencies, including health, agriculture, or environmental safety departments.	Regulation of recreational and drinking water supplies including surface water, wells, source water protection, and public water systems.
State department of agriculture	Enforce state food safety laws and perform investigations associated with facilities or products they regulate.	Farms, food production facilities and warehouses, milk production facilities, water bottling facilities, grocery stores, and many retail food establishments within the state.
Federal Centers for Disease Control and Prevention (CDC)	Assists state and local authorities in outbreak investigations, by invitation. May provide extensive laboratory and epidemiology support. Frequently participates in multistate and international outbreaks.	Any disease or outbreak of public health importance.
U.S. Food and Drug Administration (FDA)	May assist local authorities in investigations associated with products they regulate, perform interstate or international product tracebacks, and provide laboratory and regulatory support.	Manufacturers, processors, and distributors of human and animal foods (except meat, poultry, and processed egg products); potable water, bottled water, and dietary supplements shipped in interstate commerce.
U.S. Department of Agriculture, Food Safety and Inspection Service (FSIS)	May assist local authorities in investigations associated with products they regulate, perform interstate or international product tracebacks, and provide laboratory and regulatory support.	Domestic and imported meat, poultry, and egg products, including soups, stews, pizzas, and frozen foods which contain meat or poultry.
Environmental Protection Agency (EPA)	Works with other agencies in responding to outbreaks associated with contaminated water or environmental contaminants.	Drinking water, toxic substances, and wastes to prevent their entry into the environment and food chain.
Law enforcement	Federal Bureau of Investigation (FBI) has the authority to lead the investigation of any outbreak suspected of being associated with terrorism. Works with other health and regulatory agencies on the investigation.	Outbreaks involving criminal actions, including acts of terrorism.

[a]This table provides a general outline of typical responsibilities for different agencies involved in investigation of food- and waterborne outbreaks. All states have unique food and water safety laws, policies, and organizational structures that will affect investigations, and many other agencies and organizations may play important roles in certain situations. Additional information is available at the Gateway to Government Food Safety Information website (http://www.foodsafety.gov/) and the EPA website (http://www.epa.gov/ebtpages/water.html).

further epidemiologic investigation implicates earlier exposures. Moreover, many foodborne and waterborne infections present with clinical signs and symptoms that are indistinguishable from those of other common diseases, and few have pathognomonic clinical features. Thus, clinicians evaluating individual patients may have difficulty identifying the source of the infection, and persons investigating an outbreak should not jump to conclusions regarding the source of infection. In any epidemiologic study of a potential outbreak, the investigators must systematically and completely assess the population of affected persons and systematically identify the involved cohort or well controls, which may be challenging. Laboratories can assist the investigators by reporting all laboratory-confirmed cases of the disease of

TABLE 3 Foodborne and waterborne diseases and conditions designated as notifiable at the national level in the United States, 2003[a]

Bacterial diseases and conditions
Anthrax
Botulism
Brucellosis
Cholera
Enterohemorrhagic *E. coli*
Hemolytic-uremic syndrome, postdiarrheal
Listeriosis
Salmonellosis
Shigellosis
Typhoid fever (*S. enterica* serovars Typhi and Paratyphi infections)
Viral diseases
Hepatitis A
Parasitic diseases
Cryptosporidiosis
Cyclosporiasis
Giardiasis
Trichinellosis

[a]Adapted from reference 9. Additional diseases and conditions may be reportable at the state level, and outbreaks of public health importance are reportable regardless of etiology.

interest within a specific geographic area or time period. Public health authorities may augment routine surveillance for notifiable diseases by contacting medical providers, hospitals, and laboratories directly or by pursuing other means of active surveillance. Media reports can encourage ill persons to report their illnesses directly to public health authorities, and known cases may be able to identify other ill persons or well persons with similar exposures who could be controls for epidemiologic studies.

To identify the entire exposed group, investigators may need to collect information on all persons who attended a large function, residents of an institution, patrons of a restaurant, or other potentially exposed groups. Public health authorities have substantial legal authority to gather data from individuals, groups, and institutions when investigating outbreaks that threaten the public health. For example, they may at times review credit card receipts to identify patrons of a restaurant, use records generated by grocery stores' frequent-shopper discount cards, or make public announcements to identify enough cases or controls for an investigation. However, epidemiologists must assess potential biases introduced into a study by the mechanisms through which they identify the cases or controls.

EPIDEMIOLOGIC INTERVIEWS

After confirming the existence of an outbreak, investigators must interview affected persons to identify demographic characteristics of cases, the nature and timing of symptoms, and potential causative exposures. As noted previously, interviews can also help investigators identify other ill persons or well persons with similar characteristics who may be enrolled in the epidemiologic studies. The initial broad-based and open-ended interviews provide data that allow investigators to generate hypotheses about the suspected etiologic agents and exposures (e.g., particular foods, restaurants, water sources, etc.) in order to efficiently focus subsequent investigations.

Standardized written questionnaires can help investigators collect data consistently and completely from all study participants. The CDC and others maintain sample templates of questionnaires, which can be modified, for preliminary outbreak investigations (http://www.cdc.gov/foodborneoutbreaks/standard_questionnaire.htm). While standard templates are a useful starting point, a "one-size-fits-all" approach is rarely optimal, and questionnaires likely will need to be modified depending on the suspected etiology, affected population, and particular details surrounding a specific outbreak. Moreover, investigators inevitably want to be comprehensive, but this desire must be balanced by practical considerations including the ease with which support staff can use the questionnaire and its acceptability to study participants. Complete answers to reasonably limited questions are generally preferred over incomplete answers to an unreasonable number. The design of a questionnaire should be tailored for the population to whom it is directed, the mode of administration, and the sophistication of those collecting the data. Collection of data via telephone, face-to-face interview, written survey, self-administered questionnaire, and electronic data capture all have associated advantages and disadvantages that must be considered in the planning stages of a study. Before the study begins, all persons who will collect data must be taught how to introduce the study to participants and answer questions. Data collectors must also be given guidelines for obtaining data and standard definitions so that the data are elicited consistently and completely, thereby minimizing bias and erroneous information.

Data on cases can be organized in various formats for different purposes. Basic information about cases is frequently entered on a "line-listing" or spreadsheet. The distribution of cases over time (frequently categorized by date or time of symptom onset) can be represented graphically as an "epidemic curve" (Fig. 4), and the geographic distribution of cases can be plotted on a map. The line-list, the epidemic curve, and the map can give the investigator clues about the source of an outbreak. For example, if these representations suggest that the outbreak is acute and associated with an exposure at a single time and place ("point source outbreak"), such as all patrons of a single restaurant on a single day, the outbreak may have been caused by a contamination event that is relatively easy to identify and correct. In contrast, if the line-list, epidemic curve, and map indicate that the outbreak has occurred over a large area or over a prolonged time period, the investigators may need to search for contaminated food or water products distributed over a wide area, a source of intermittent or low-level contamination, a means by which products are recurrently contaminated during production, storage, or serving, or a component of person-to-person spread (i.e., secondary cases) following an initial food or water-related source, and a potential ongoing threat to the public health.

The intensity of an investigation may vary widely, depending on the nature of an outbreak, the population involved, the etiologic agent, and available resources. In some cases, basic laboratory testing and interviews of a limited number of ill persons may provide investigators with sufficient information to identify the source of the outbreak and institute adequate interventions and preventive measures. In many cases, more extensive epidemiologic investigation is required. If the population affected by the outbreak is well defined, such as attendees of a church picnic or patrons of a single restaurant within a 3-day period, a retrospective cohort study can be performed. In this situation, all members or a representative sample of the affected group (the "cohort")

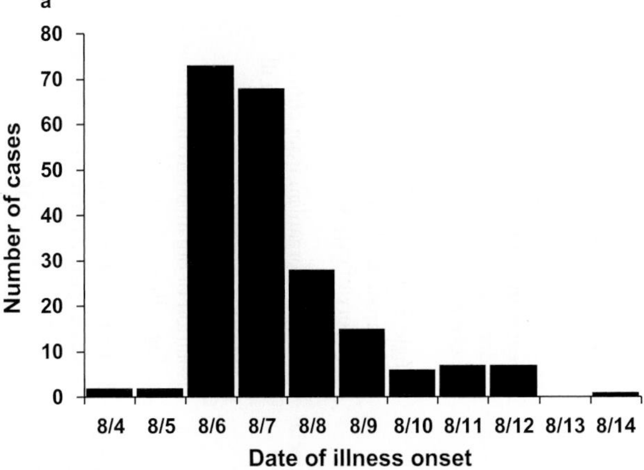

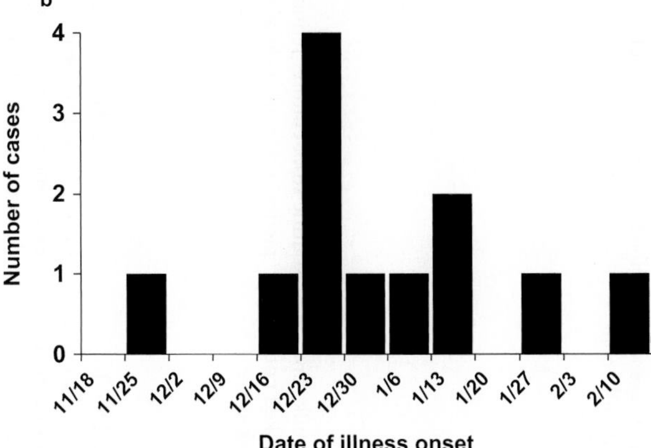

FIGURE 4 (a) Epidemic curve, point-source outbreak of *Salmonella* associated with a restaurant in Tennessee. All ill patrons ate at the establishment on the same day, and the distribution of illness onset times reflects natural variation in incubation period. (b) Epidemic curve, continuing common-source outbreak of *Yersinia* associated with chitterlings in Tennessee. The distribution of dates of illness onset suggests that the source of infection was a contaminated product handled over several weeks. Under different conditions, a similar epidemic curve might reflect a propagated outbreak, in which earlier cases were the source of infection for subsequent cases.

are interviewed to assess whether they were ill and what foods or water they consumed. Rates of illness among persons who did or did not consume particular foods (or among persons who were or were not exposed to other factors of interest) are compared by appropriate statistical methods to help investigators identify likely causes of an outbreak (5, 14). If the affected population is not well defined or a cohort study is not practical, a case-control study may be performed. In such outbreaks, persons with the illness of interest (cases) are compared to those without it (controls).

Statistical analyses can help investigators summarize their findings from the epidemiologic investigation and help them draw conclusions from data that may be complicated. Basic descriptive statistics should include the number of ill persons, a summary of the characteristics of cases and the population at risk, the proportion of ill persons experiencing particular symptoms, mean and/or median incubation period (time between exposure and onset of symptoms), and mean and/or median duration of illness. Data from cohort studies may be used to calculate the attack rate (proportion of persons exposed to an etiologic agent who subsequently developed disease). Data from cohort and case-control studies can be used to estimate the risk (using "risk ratios" and "odds ratios," respectively) of developing disease after exposure to particular foods, water sources, or other risk factors. Basic two-by-two tables or comparisons of relative risks of illness among those exposed to and those not exposed to particular foods frequently suffice to support the most imperative decisions during an outbreak investigation. More advanced statistical techniques, such as stratified analyses, regression modeling, and sensitivity analyses, may also be appropriate. Detailed information on doing and interpreting statistical analyses of epidemiologic data is available from multiple sources (5, 14, 22, 23). While statistical analytic techniques can be powerful tools, investigators must remember that all statistics must be interpreted cautiously and with a component of judgment. The obvious cause of a foodborne or waterborne disease outbreak should not be discounted simply because its associated "P value" (a commonly cited measure of statistical significance) is greater than 0.05, and likewise measures of statistical significance (particularly in larger studies) do not necessarily prove that a result is biologically plausible or meaningful in a given situation.

LABORATORY INVESTIGATION

Laboratory testing is usually needed to confirm the etiology of an outbreak. In most foodborne or waterborne outbreaks, the etiologic agent should be isolated from the stool specimens of two or more ill persons or from the epidemiologically implicated food (Table 4). In a few situations, such as mushroom poisoning, ciguatera fish poisoning, or other chemical intoxications, it is sufficient to document the clinical syndrome among affected persons. *Staphylococcus* can also be problematic because the organism may not be viable in stool or food samples and most laboratories cannot test for enterotoxin. Thus, investigators must collect sufficient numbers of specimens (potentially including stool and other clinical specimens and also food, water, or environmental specimens) and handle them appropriately to ensure that laboratory testing identifies the etiologic agent.

Epidemiologists, environmentalists, or others participating in outbreak investigations should communicate early and openly with laboratorians to ensure that the specimens collected can be tested for all suspected etiologic agents and that appropriate specimens are collected. Many organisms (including most bacterial causes of foodborne and waterborne diseases) can be isolated from both clinical and environmental specimens. In such cases, molecular methods (such as pulsed-field gel electrophoresis [PFGE]) can be used to demonstrate similarities between isolates from affected persons and the putative source, thereby confirming the epidemiological studies. Other common agents, such as norovirus, are not recovered easily from food or water, whereas many toxins are more readily identified in food than in clinical specimens. Moreover, if the laboratory needs to identify or quantify pathogens in food, the epidemiologic investigators must tell the laboratory which pathogens are suspected so that resources are not wasted.

Most clinical laboratories currently cannot test specimens for norovirus, which is the most common cause of foodborne disease in the United States. Most state health department laboratories offer reverse transcriptase (RT)-PCR testing for norovirus and can help coordinate appropriate testing of

TABLE 4 Typical characteristics of foodborne and waterborne disease outbreaks and guidelines for confirmation[a]

Etiologic agent	Incubation period	Clinical syndrome	Typical vehicle	Diagnostic testing	Confirmation of outbreak etiology
Bacterial					
Bacillus cereus					
Preformed toxin	1–6 h	Vomiting; some patients with diarrhea; fever uncommon	Improperly stored cooked or fried rice, meats	Clinical diagnosis; clinical laboratories do not routinely identify; stool and food specimens may be tested at a reference laboratory for culture and toxin identification	Isolation of organism from stool of two or more ill persons and not from stool of control patients OR Isolation of 10^5 organisms/g from epidemiologically implicated food, provided specimen is properly handled
Diarrheal toxin	10–16 h	Diarrhea, abdominal cramps, and vomiting in some patients; fever uncommon	Cereal products, soups, custards and sauces, meatloaf, sausage, cooked vegetables, reconstituted dried potatoes, refried beans	Stool and food specimens may be tested at a reference laboratory for culture and toxin identification	Isolation of organism from stool of two or more ill persons and not from stool of control patients OR Isolation of 10^5 organisms/g from epidemiologically implicated food, provided specimen is properly handled
Brucella	7–21 days	Weakness, fever, headache, sweats, chills, arthralgia, weight loss, splenomegaly, bloody stools	Raw milk, goat cheese from unpasteurized milk, contaminated meats	Blood cultures and serology	Two or more ill persons and isolation of organism in culture of blood or bone marrow OR Greater-than-fourfold increase in standard agglutination titer (SAT) over several weeks OR Single SAT of 1:160 in person who has compatible clinical symptoms and history of exposure
Campylobacter jejuni/coli	2–10 days; usually 2–5 days	Diarrhea (often bloody), abdominal pain, fever, vomiting	Unpasteurized milk, raw and undercooked poultry, contaminated water	Routine stool culture; requires special media and incubation at 42°C	Isolation of organism from clinical specimens from two or more ill persons OR Isolation of organism from epidemiologically implicated food
Clostridium botulinum (toxin)	12–72 h	Vomiting, diarrhea, blurred vision, diplopia, dysphagia, descending muscle weakness	Canned low-acid foods, smoked fish, cooked potatoes in foil, garlic in oil, fish, marine mammals	Stool, serum, and food tested for toxin; stool and food cultured for organism; testing available at state health department or CDC laboratories	Detection of botulinum toxin in serum, stool, gastric contents, or implicated food OR

					Isolation of organism from stool or intestine
Clostridium perfringens (toxin)	8–16 h	Watery diarrhea, nausea, abdominal cramps; vomiting and fever uncommon	Meats, poultry, gravy, dried or precooked foods, time- and/or temperature-abused foods	Stools tested for enterotoxin and cultured; because *C. perfringens* can normally be found in stool, quantitative cultures must be done	Isolation of 10^6 organisms/g from stool of two or more ill persons, provided specimen is properly handled OR Demonstration of enterotoxin in the stool of two or more ill persons OR Isolation of 10^5 organisms/g from epidemiologically implicated food, provided specimen is properly handled
Escherichia coli					
Enterohemorrhagic *E. coli* (EHEC) including *E. coli* O157:H7 and other Shiga toxin-producing *E. coli* (STEC)	1–8 days	Diarrhea (often bloody), abdominal pain, vomiting; fever is rare	Undercooked beef (especially hamburger), unpasteurized milk and juice, raw fruits and vegetables (e.g., sprouts), contaminated water	Stool culture; Shiga toxin may be detected using commercial kits; positive isolates should be forwarded to public health laboratories for confirmation and serotyping	Isolation of *E. coli* O157:H7 or other Shiga-like toxin-producing *E. coli* strains from clinical specimen from two or more ill persons or from epidemiologically implicated food
Enterotoxigenic *E. coli* (ETEC)	1–3 days	Watery diarrhea, abdominal cramps; vomiting and fever less common	Water or foods contaminated with human feces	Stool culture; special laboratory techniques are required to identify ETEC; if suspected, request specific testing	Isolation of organism of same serotype that produces heat-stable and/or heat-labile enterotoxin from stool of two or more ill persons
Enteropathogenic *E. coli* (EPEC)	Variable	Diarrhea, fever, abdominal cramps	Water, fecal-oral contamination	Stool culture; special laboratory techniques are required to identify EPEC; if suspected, request specific testing	Isolation of organism of same enteropathogenic serotype from stool of two or more ill persons
Enteroinvasive *E. coli* (EIEC)	Variable	Diarrhea (might be bloody), fever, abdominal cramps	Salads and other foods not subsequently heated, water	Stool culture; special laboratory techniques are required to identify EIEC; if suspected, request specific testing	Isolation of same enteroinvasive serotype from stool of two or more ill persons
Listeria monocytogenes					
Invasive disease	2–6 weeks	Meningitis, neonatal sepsis, fever	Coleslaw, milk, soft cheese, pâté, turkey franks, processed meats	Blood or cerebrospinal fluid cultures; asymptomatic fecal carriage occurs; antibody to listerolysin O	Isolation of organism from normally sterile site
Diarrheal disease	Unknown	Diarrhea, abdominal cramps, fever	Corn salad, chocolate milk	Stool culture	Isolation of organism of same serotype from stool of two or more ill persons exposed to food that is epidemiologically implicated or from which organism of same serotype has been isolated

(Continued on next page)

TABLE 4 Typical characteristics of foodborne and waterborne disease outbreaks and guidelines for confirmation[a] *(Continued)*

Etiologic agent	Incubation period	Clinical syndrome	Typical vehicle	Diagnostic testing	Confirmation of outbreak etiology
Salmonella Non-Typhi	1–3 days	Diarrhea, often with fever and abdominal cramps	Poultry, eggs, meat products, raw milk or juice, cheese, contaminated raw fruits and vegetables (sprouts, melons)	Stool culture	Isolation of organism of same serotype from clinical specimens from two or more ill persons OR Isolation of organism from epidemiologically implicated food
Serovar Typhi	3–60 days; usually 7–14 days	Fever, anorexia, malaise, headache, and myalgia; sometimes diarrhea or constipation	Shellfish, any food contaminated by infected person, raw milk, meat contaminated after processing, cheese, watercress, water	Stool culture, blood culture.	Isolation of organism from clinical specimens from two or more ill persons OR Isolation of organism from epidemiologically implicated food
Shigella spp.	24–48 h	Diarrhea (often bloody), often accompanied by fever and abdominal cramps	Any food contaminated by infected person; frequently salads, poi, water	Stool culture	Isolation of organism of same serotype from clinical specimens from two or more ill persons OR Isolation of organism from epidemiologically implicated food
Staphylococcus aureus (preformed toxin)	1–6 h	Sudden onset of severe nausea and vomiting, diarrhea; fever may be present	Unrefrigerated or improperly stored meats, potato and egg salads, cream pastries	Normally a clinical diagnosis; stool, vomitus, and food can be tested for toxin	Isolation of organism of same phage type from stool or vomitus of two or more ill persons OR Detection of enterotoxin in epidemiologically implicated food OR Isolation of 10^5 organisms/g from epidemiologically implicated food, provided specimen is properly handled
Streptococcus, group A	1–4 days	Fever, pharyngitis, scarlet fever, upper respiratory infection	Raw milk, egg-containing salads	Throat culture, culture of food	Isolation of organism of same M- or T-type from throats of two or more ill persons OR Isolation of organism of same M- or T-type from epidemiologically implicated food
Vibrio cholerae O1 or O139	24–72 h	Profuse watery diarrhea and vomiting; dehydration and death can occur within hours	Raw fish, shellfish, crustaceans, contaminated water	Stool culture; special media required to isolate the organism; request specific testing if suspected	Isolation of toxigenic organism from stool or vomitus of two or more ill persons OR Significant rise in vibriocidal, bacterial agglutinating, or antitoxin antibodies in acute- and early

					convalescent-phase sera among persons not recently immunized OR Isolation of toxigenic organism from epidemiologically implicated food
Non-O1 and non-O139	1–5 days	Watery diarrhea	Shellfish, fish	Stool culture; special media required to isolate the organism; request specific testing if suspected	Isolation of organism of same serotype from stool of two or more ill persons
Vibrio parahaemolyticus	2–48 h	Watery diarrhea, cramps, nausea, vomiting	Undercooked or raw seafood or cooked seafood contaminated with seawater or by utensils used on raw seafood	Stool culture; special media required to isolate the organism; request specific testing if suspected	Isolation of Kanagawa-positive organism from stool of two or more ill persons OR Isolation of 10^5 Kanagawa-positive organisms/g from epidemiologically implicated food, provided specimen is properly handled
Yersinia enterocolitica and *Y. pseudotuberculosis*	24–48 h	Diarrhea, abdominal pain (often severe), appendicitis-like symptoms	Undercooked pork, unpasteurized milk, tofu, contaminated water, chitterlings	Stool, vomitus or blood culture; special media required to isolate the organism; request specific testing if suspected; serology available in reference laboratories	Isolation of organism from clinical specimen from two or more ill persons OR Isolation of pathogenic strain of organism from epidemiologically implicated food
Chemical					
Marine toxins					
Ciguatera toxin	1–48 h; usually 2–8 h	Usually gastrointestinal symptoms followed by neurologic symptoms (including paresthesia of lips, tongue, throat, or extremities) and reversal of hot and cold sensation	Numerous varieties of tropical fish, e.g., barracuda, grouper, red snapper, amberjack, goatfish, skipjack, parrotfish	Radioassay for toxin in fish or a consistent history	Demonstration of ciguatoxin in epidemiologically implicated fish OR Clinical syndrome among persons who have eaten a type of fish previously associated with ciguatera fish poisoning (e.g., snapper, grouper, or barracuda)
Scombroid toxin (histamine)	1 min–3 h; usually <1 h	Flushing, dizziness, burning of mouth and throat, headache, gastrointestinal symptoms, urticaria, and generalized pruritis	Fish: tuna, mackerel, Pacific dolphin (mahi mahi), bluefin, marlin, escolar	Detect histamine in food or clinical diagnosis	Demonstration of histamine in epidemiologically implicated fish OR Clinical syndrome among persons who have eaten a type of fish previously associated with histamine fish poisoning (e.g., mahimahi or fish of order Scombroidei)

(Continued on next page)

TABLE 4 Typical characteristics of foodborne and waterborne disease outbreaks and guidelines for confirmation[a] *(Continued)*

Etiologic agent	Incubation period	Clinical syndrome	Typical vehicle	Diagnostic testing	Confirmation of outbreak etiology
Paralytic or neurotoxic shellfish poison	30 min–3 h	Paresthesia of lips, mouth, or face and extremities; intestinal symptoms or weakness, including respiratory difficulty	Mussels, clams, scallops	High-pressure liquid chromatography to detect toxin in food or water where fish are located	Detection of toxin in epidemiologically implicated food OR Detection of large numbers of a dinoflagellate species associated with shellfish poisoning in water from which epidemiologically implicated mollusks are gathered
Puffer fish, tetrodotoxin	10 min–3 h; usually 10–45 min	Paresthesia of lips, tongue, face, or extremities, often following numbness; loss of proprioception or floating sensations	Puffer-type fish	Toxin testing of fish	Demonstration of tetrodotoxin in epidemiologically implicated fish OR Clinical syndrome among persons who have eaten puffer fish
Heavy metals: antimony, cadmium, copper, iron, tin, zinc	5 min–8 h; usually <1 h	Vomiting, often metallic taste	High-acid foods and beverages, metal-colored cake decorations	Testing foods	Demonstration of high concentration of metal in epidemiologically implicated food
Monosodium glutamate (MSG)	3 min–2 h; usually <1 h	Burning sensation in chest, neck, abdomen, or extremities; sensation of lightness and pressure over face or heavy feeling in chest	Foods seasoned with MSG	Clinical diagnosis; testing food	Clinical syndrome among persons who have eaten food containing MSG (e.g., usually 1.5 g of MSG)
Mushroom toxins					
Shorter-acting toxins	2 h	Vomiting and diarrhea; other symptoms differ with toxin	Many species of wild mushrooms	Typical syndrome, identify mushroom, detect toxin	Clinical syndrome among persons who have eaten mushroom identified as toxic type OR Demonstration of toxin in epidemiologically implicated mushroom or food containing mushroom
Muscimol		Confusion, visual disturbance			
Muscarine		Salivation, diaphoresis			
Psilocybin		Hallucinations			
Coprinus artrementaris		Disulfiram-like reaction			
Ibotenic acid		Confusion, visual disturbance			

Longer-acting toxins (e.g., *Amanita* spp.)	6–24 h	Diarrhea and abdominal cramps for 24 h followed by hepatic and renal failure	Wild mushrooms	Typical syndrome, identify mushroom, detect toxin	Clinical syndrome among persons who have eaten mushroom identified as toxic type OR Demonstration of toxin in epidemiologically implicated mushroom or food containing mushrooms
Parasitic					
Cryptosporidium parvum	2–28 days; median, 7 days	Diarrhea, nausea, vomiting, fever	Water, any uncooked food or food contaminated after cooking	Request specific examination of stool, food, or water for *Cryptosporidium*	Demonstration of organism or antigen in stool or in small-bowel biopsy specimens of two or more ill persons OR Demonstration of organism in epidemiologically implicated food
Cyclospora cayetanensis	1–11 days; median, 7 days	Fatigue, protracted diarrhea, often relapsing	Produce including raspberries, lettuce, basil; water	Request specific examination of stool, food, or water for *Cyclospora*	Demonstration of organism in stool of two or more ill persons
Giardia lamblia	3–25 days; median, 7 days	Diarrhea, gas, cramps, nausea, fatigue	Any uncooked food or food contaminated by ill food-handler, water	Stool examination for ova and parasites; may require at least 3 specimens	Two or more ill persons and detection of antigen in stool or demonstration of organism in stool, duodenal contents, or small-bowel biopsy specimen
Trichinella spp.	1–2 days for intestinal phase; 2–4 weeks for systemic phase	Fever, myalgia, periorbital edema, high eosinophil count	Pork, bear meat, walrus flesh, cross-contaminated ground beef, lamb	Positive serology, demonstration of larvae in muscle biopsy specimen, increase in eosinophils	Two or more ill persons and positive serologic test or demonstration of larvae in muscle biopsy OR Demonstration of larvae in epidemiologically implicated meat
Viral					
Hepatitis A	15–50 days; median, 28 days	Jaundice, dark urine, fatigue, anorexia, nausea	Water, raw shellfish, any food contaminated by infected person	Increase in ALT, bilirubin; positive IgM and anti-hepatitis A antibodies	Detection of immunoglobulin M anti-hepatitis A virus in serum from two or more persons who consumed epidemiologically implicated food
Noroviruses (and other caliciviruses)	12–48 h	Vomiting, cramps, diarrhea, headache, fever	Shellfish, any food contaminated by infected person	Routine RT-PCR and electron microscopy on fresh unpreserved stool samples; negative bacterial cultures; stool negative for white blood cells	Detection of viral RNA in stool or vomitus by RT-PCR OR Visualization of small, round-structured viruses that react with patient's convalescent-phase sera but not

(Continued on next page)

TABLE 4 Typical characteristics of foodborne and waterborne disease outbreaks and guidelines for confirmation[a] *(Continued)*

Etiologic agent	Incubation period	Clinical syndrome	Typical vehicle	Diagnostic testing	Confirmation of outbreak etiology
					acute-phase sera by immune-electron microscopy OR More than fourfold rise in antibody titer to Norwalk virus or Norwalk-like virus in acute and convalescent sera in most serum pairs
Astrovirus	15–77 h; usually 24–48 h	Vomiting, cramps, diarrhea, headache	Ready-to-eat foods contaminated by infected food-handler	Identification of virus in early acute-phase stool specimen, serology; commercial enzyme-linked immunosorbent assay kits available	Detection of virus antigen by enzyme immunoassay OR Detection of viral RNA in stool or vomitus by RT-PCR OR Visualization of viruses with characteristic surface morphology by electron microscopy

[a] Adapted from references 6 and 18.

specimens if this agent is suspected as the cause of an outbreak. Likewise, many laboratories do not serotype *Salmonella,* and few can definitively identify enterotoxigenic *E. coli,* non-O157:H7 enterohemorrhagic *E. coli* strains, or staphylococcal enterotoxin. Consequently, investigators should notify the appropriate health departments early in the course of an outbreak investigation if such laboratory services are necessary.

Guidelines for collecting appropriate specimens during an outbreak investigation are listed in Table 5. It can be difficult to collect adequate specimens for laboratory testing. If the outbreak is not reported promptly or the investigation is delayed, affected persons may have recovered and appropriate clinical specimens may not be available for testing. Investigators may need to expend substantial effort convincing patients to provide stool specimens and may need to provide transportation for the patients or the specimens, convenient collection materials, and free testing so that sufficient specimens are obtained. Investigators should promptly contact laboratories that may have received previous specimens from outbreak-associated patients to ask that the original specimens be held for possible additional testing. Suspected "vehicles," such as water or food samples, should be collected as soon as possible after an outbreak is recognized. If possible, investigators should collect specimens from the batches or lots of food or water that cases actually ate or drank. If this is not possible (as is often the case in outbreaks caused by pathogens with long incubation periods), the investigators should collect food or water from stored products, leftovers, suppliers, or other sources that represent as closely as possible what was consumed by the cases. If investigators suspect that the source of an outbreak is contaminated packaged food, they should collect unopened packages from the implicated lot. In such cases, investigators should work with the appropriate regulatory authorities to ensure that specimens are handled and tested properly because the specimens might provide important evidence for product tracebacks or other regulatory interventions. If specimens, such as leftovers from an implicated meal, have been handled and stored by ill persons, investigators must interpret the results cautiously, because the case may have contaminated the products after becoming infected.

Molecular microbiology technology has markedly changed the nature of many acute-disease epidemiology investigations. For example, PFGE can provide DNA fingerprints of bacterial isolates from clinical and food specimens. If the PFGE patterns are the same, the investigators have evidence that the suspected food item is implicated in the event. PFGE can also help investigators include related cases and exclude concurrent cases that are epidemiologically unrelated to the outbreak. PulseNet, a CDC-sponsored program that allows PFGE patterns to be shared nationally, has greatly helped public health officials recognize multistate outbreaks affecting small numbers of persons scattered over time or large geographic areas. In the absence of this technology, the epidemiologic link between cases is often missed.

Bender et al. evaluated the PFGE patterns of *E. coli* O157:H7 isolates obtained during a 2-year period in Minnesota (2). These investigators identified 10 outbreaks, of which 40% were identified solely based on subtype-specific surveillance. In addition, 8 of 11 (73%) "apparent outbreaks" (i.e., increases in numbers of reported cases) were not associated with clonal outbreaks, and 2 of the remaining 3 outbreaks were actually multiple clonal outbreaks occurring within the same time period. The same group studied the molecular epidemiology of *Salmonella enterica* serovar Typhimurium and identified 16 outbreaks over a 5-year period, including 10

TABLE 5 Guidelines for collection and handling of stool specimens during a foodborne or waterborne disease outbreak investigation[a]

Procedure	Instructions regarding specimens to be tested for:			
	Bacteria	Parasites[c]	Viruses[d]	Chemicals
Collection[b]				
When to collect	During period of active diarrhea (preferably as soon as possible after onset of illness).	Anytime after onset of illness (preferably as soon as possible).	Within 48–72 h after onset of illness.	Soon after onset of illness (preferably within 48 h of exposure to contaminant).
How much to collect	Two rectal swabs or swabs of fresh stool from 10 ill persons; whole stool is preferred if testing for nonbacterial pathogens is considered.	A fresh stool sample from 10 ill persons; to enhance detection, 3 stool specimens per patient can be collected >48 h apart.	As much stool sample as possible from 10 ill persons (a minimum of 10 ml of stool from each).	A fresh urine sample (50 ml) from 10 ill persons; samples from 10 controls also can be submitted; collect vomitus, if vomiting occurs within 12 h of exposure; collect 5–10 ml of whole blood if a toxin/poison that is not excreted in urine is suspected.
Method of collection	For rectal swabs, moisten 2 swabs in an appropriate transport medium (e.g., Cary-Blair, Stuart, Amies; buffered glycerol-saline is suitable for *E. coli*, *Salmonella*, *Shigella*, and *Y. enterocolitica* but not for *Campylobacter* and *Vibrio*); insert swabs 1–1.5 inches into rectum and gently rotate; place both swabs into the same tube deep enough that medium covers the cotton tips; break off top portion of sticks and discard; alternatively, swab whole stools and put the swabs into Cary-Blair medium.	Collect bulk stool specimen, unmixed with urine, in a clean container; place a portion of each stool sample into 10% formalin and polyvinyl alcohol preservative at a ratio of one part stool to three parts preservative; mix well; save portion of the unpreserved stool placed into a leakproof container for antigen or PCR testing.	Place fresh stool specimens (liquid preferable), unmixed with urine, in clean, dry containers, e.g., urine specimen cups.	Collect urine, blood, or vomitus in prescreened containers[e]; if prescreened containers are not available, submit field blanks with samples[f]; most analyses from blood require separation of serum from red cells; cyanide, lead, and mercury analyses require whole blood collected in prescreened EDTA tubes; volatile organic compounds require whole blood collected in a specially prepared gray-top tube.
Storage	Refrigerate swabs in transport media at 4°C; when possible, test within 48 h after collection; otherwise, freeze samples at −70°C; refrigerate whole stool, process it within 2 h after collection; store portion of each stool specimen frozen at less than −15°C for antigen or PCR testing.	Store specimen in fixative at room temperature or refrigerate unpreserved specimen at 4°C; a portion of unpreserved stool specimen may be frozen at less than −15°C for antigen or PCR testing.	Immediately refrigerate at 4°C; store portion of each stool specimen frozen at less than −15°C for antigen or PCR testing.	Immediately refrigerate at 4°C and if possible freeze urine, serum, and vomitus specimens at less than −15°C; refrigerate whole blood for volatile organic compounds and metals at 4°C.

(*Continued on next page*)

TABLE 5 Guidelines for collection and handling of stool specimens during a foodborne or waterborne disease outbreak investigation[a] (*Continued*)

Procedure	Instructions regarding specimens to be tested for:			
	Bacteria	Parasites[c]	Viruses[d]	Chemicals
Transportation	For refrigeration, follow instructions for viral samples. For frozen samples, place bagged and sealed samples on dry ice. Mail in insulated box by overnight mail.	For refrigeration, follow instructions for viral samples. For room-temperature samples, mail in waterproof container.	Keep refrigerated; place bagged and sealed specimens on ice or with frozen refrigerant packs in an insulated box; send by overnight mail. Send frozen specimens on dry ice for antigen or PCR testing.	Place double-bagged and sealed urine, serum, and vomitus specimens on dry ice; mail in an insulated box by overnight mail. Ship whole blood in an insulated container with prefrozen ice packs. Avoid placing specimens directly on ice packs.

[a] Adapted from reference 7.
[b] Put the samples in sealed, waterproof containers (i.e., plastic bags). Label each specimen container in a waterproof manner. Batch the collection and send by overnight mail to arrive at the testing laboratory on a weekday during business hours unless other arrangements have been made in advance with the testing laboratory. Contact the testing laboratory before shipping, and give the testing laboratory as much advance notice as possible so that testing can begin as soon as samples arrive. When etiology is unclear and syndrome is nonspecific, consider collecting all four types of specimens.
[c] For more detailed instructions on how to collect specimens for specific parasites, please see the CDC DPDx website (http://www.dpd.cdc.gov/dpdx/).
[d] For more detailed instructions on how to collect specimens for viral testing, please see http://www.cdc.gov/mmwr/PDF/RR/RR5009.pdf.
[e] The containers must be tested for the presence of the chemical of interest prior to use.
[f] Unused specimen collection containers that have been brought to the field and subjected to the same field conditions as the used containers. These containers are then tested for trace amounts of the chemical of interest.

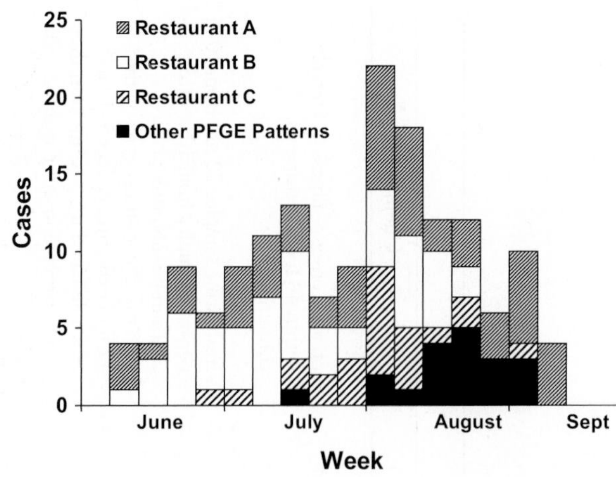

FIGURE 5 Patterns of PFGE of isolates of *Salmonella enterica* serovar Typhimurium collected in Minnesota during 4 months in 1995. Molecular subtyping allowed investigators to recognize three concurrent outbreaks caused by different strains and associated with different restaurants and to associate particular strains with particular outbreaks or document that particular strains are not associated with particular outbreaks. Adapted from reference 3, with permission.

institutional outbreaks with small numbers of cases. Four of six larger community outbreaks would not have been recognized without molecular subtyping (Fig. 5) (3).

Genetic sequencing technology has become more readily available and has been useful for assessing the relatedness of various pathogens involved in food- and waterborne outbreaks. For example, sequencing of hepatitis A viruses collected during three large outbreaks associated with green onions demonstrated that similar virus strains caused all three outbreaks and that this strain was related to hepatitis A strains commonly isolated from patients living in the region of Mexico where the green onions were grown (8). Sequencing of noroviruses is also becoming increasingly useful in identifying relatedness among potential outbreak-associated viruses.

CONTROL AND PREVENTION

The most immediate priorities for anyone investigating outbreaks of foodborne or waterborne disease are to implement appropriate measures to control the outbreak, mitigate associated morbidity, and prevent recurrences. While the steps of an outbreak investigation (Table 1) are listed sequentially, in practice many of those steps will be addressed concurrently. Not infrequently, public health officials must institute substantial and occasionally controversial control measures before the investigation is complete and before all desired data are available because there appears to be considerable potential for continued transmission of infection and thus continued morbidity or mortality. Control measures may include confiscating food products from markets, excluding foodhandlers or ill cases from work, closing retail food establishments or implicated venues, and publicly notifying persons who may have been exposed. Because such interventions can have important medical, emotional, and economic implications for all parties involved, investigators, laboratorians, regulatory partners, and other involved groups must assimilate available data rapidly and communicate effectively with each other and the public. Such collaboration is imperative to ensure that ongoing transmission is eliminated while minimizing the adverse consequences associated with control measures.

The causes of foodborne and waterborne disease outbreaks can be multifactorial and complex. A single incident or event, such as an ill foodhandler with poor hygiene who prepared cake frosting barehanded or chlorination that was not adequate to disinfect well water contaminated by agricultural runoff, may be identified as the proximate cause of an outbreak. Frequently, however, seemingly simple explanations may belie complex underlying factors that contributed to the final outcome. For example, foodhandlers may be poorly educated regarding proper techniques for preparing food, may not understand English, or may lose their jobs if they miss work because they are ill. In addition, food may be prepared at temperatures inadequate to kill organisms, food may be stored at temperatures that encourage microbial growth, or equipment for preparing or storing food may fail to reach the appropriate temperature. These and other such factors can contribute to the immediate cause of an outbreak. The CDC attempts to capture some data on "contributing factors" on the standard reports it uses for foodborne disease outbreaks (http://www.cdc.gov/foodborneoutbreaks/report_f.htm). To ensure that similar incidents do not recur after an outbreak, investigators should identify modifiable contributing factors and recommend measures to correct them.

INTENTIONAL OUTBREAKS

Most foodborne and waterborne disease outbreaks have resulted from unintentional contamination of food or water sources at any of innumerable points in the long food production and service chain. In recent years public health officials and the public have become concerned that the food supply system is a potential target of intentional acts of contamination, sabotage, or terrorism. In fact, the food and water supply is considered a high-risk target for potential terrorist activity because it is difficult to protect the myriad stages from "farm-to-fork," tremendous volumes of product are rapidly distributed worldwide, and techniques for detecting intentional events are inadequate. Virtually all governmental agencies associated with food safety are increasing efforts to improve security at all stages of the food supply chain (http://www.foodsafety.gov).

Given the existence of active terrorist groups, persons investigating outbreaks of foodborne or waterborne disease must consider intentional contamination as a possible cause. Several outbreaks related to intentional contamination of food have been identified in the United States (1). In 1984, a religious group deliberately contaminated food at salad bars in Oregon with *S. enterica* serovar Typhimurium in an attempt to influence a local election. In total, 751 persons became ill. In 1996, a disgruntled laboratory employee in Texas deliberately contaminated doughnuts with a laboratory strain of *Shigella*, leading to illness in 12 coworkers. In 2003, a Michigan supermarket employee intentionally contaminated 200 pounds of ground beef with a nicotine-containing pesticide, causing illness in 92 persons (http://www.fda.gov/ora/training/orau/FoodSecurity/). In another incident that year, a parishioner put arsenic in coffee served at a church in Maine, causing 12 persons to become ill; one person died (15). While these have been isolated incidents, they demonstrate the range of agents and modes by which persons could deliberately cause an outbreak.

In some instances of intentional contamination, the perpetrators may claim responsibility for the subsequent outbreak. In general, however, these outbreaks are likely to be identified and reported in the same way that unintentional foodborne and waterborne disease outbreaks are reported. Thus, continued surveillance is necessary and standard epidemiologic methods remain essential to the investigations. Potential clues that might suggest bioterrorism or intentionally caused outbreaks are described in Table 6. If purposeful contamination is suspected as a cause, investigators must include law enforcement officials in the investigation. In any instance involving food- or water-related terrorism, the Federal Bureau of Investigation will lead the investigation and will coordinate the response.

TABLE 6 Potential clues that might increase suspicion that intentional contamination is the cause of a foodborne or waterborne disease outbreak

Occurrence of a rare or novel disease
Outbreak due to a disease occurring outside its normal range of endemicity
Disease occurring during unusual season
Unusual drug resistance
Unusual epidemiologic characteristics
Unusual demographic population affected
Unusual clinical presentation of disease
Widespread contamination without apparent explanation
Claims or social context suggesting intentional contamination

REPORTING AND SUMMARIZING OUTBREAKS

Under the law in most states, all suspected foodborne and waterborne disease outbreaks must be reported to the public health department. Public health authorities will work with other involved parties to determine whether further investigation is warranted and who will perform those investigations. Whether public health authorities or other agencies or institutions perform the investigation, health departments have the authority and obligation to ensure that the response to a potential outbreak protects the public's health. By mutual agreement, state or local departments of health collect basic descriptive data on all foodborne and waterborne disease outbreaks in their jurisdictions and share reports with the CDC, which periodically summarizes those data. Examples of the forms, the electronic database used for foodborne disease outbreaks, and recent data are accessible online (http://www.cdc.gov/foodborneoutbreaks/info_healthprofessional.htm). Organizations other than the CDC regularly monitor outbreaks reported via public health agencies and other venues (4).

Public health and regulatory agencies and most other institutions involved in outbreak investigations adhere to strict guidelines protecting the confidentiality of data collected during those investigations. Although confidentiality laws may vary by jurisdiction and agency, personally identifiable medical information regarding involved case patients is strictly protected in all cases. In the absence of a court subpoena or permission from the patient, personally identifiable information cannot be released to other parties. Such assurances of confidentiality are necessary to ensure that persons involved in the outbreak trust the investigators and provide critical information during investigations. In many cases, proprietary information and the names of institutions involved in outbreaks are also protected from public dissemination. Occasionally, such information may be disseminated publicly if it is necessary to protect people from infection.

TABLE 7 Recommended components of an outbreak investigation summary report

List of participants in the investigation and contact information for lead investigator
Dates of outbreak and investigation
Description of process by which outbreak was recognized and reported
Description of the epidemiologic steps followed in the investigation
Definition of cases included in the outbreak
Summary of total number of affected persons and description of the population exposed
Description of clinical syndrome, including proportion of persons experiencing common symptoms, summary of incubation period, duration of illness, and indicators of morbidity such as proportion seeking medical care or mortality rates
Description of results from epidemiologic studies, including numbers of cases or controls enrolled in cohort or case-control studies, and results of analyses assessing possible sources
Summary of supporting laboratory data obtained by testing clinical, food, or environmental specimens
Summary of findings of various groups contributing to the investigation, including epidemiologists, environmentalists/sanitarians, regulatory agencies, institutional representatives, medical providers, or others not primarily writing report
Conclusions about the etiology, vehicle, cause, and underlying contributing factors leading to the outbreak
Lessons learned during the investigation, which may benefit others in similar situations in the future
Limitations of the investigation
Specific recommendations made and control measures implemented (including dates and how and when communicated)
Results of intervention, if known
Recommendations for preventing similar incidents in the future

For example, media announcements may be used to notify restaurant patrons potentially exposed to hepatitis A from a foodhandler that they should get prophylactic immune globulin. In such cases, public health authorities and regulators work closely with other involved parties to ensure that appropriate measures are taken to avoid an inappropriate breach of confidentiality.

Investigators frequently summarize the results of outbreak investigations in narrative reports, which are maintained locally and disseminated based on institutional policy. These reports are an important medical, legal, and scientific resource for documenting the process of an investigation, nature of an outbreak, conclusions about its causes and control, and preventive measures instituted. Sufficient detail is required in those reports to ensure that the audience understands the outbreak and investigation, while maintaining confidentiality of protected information. An example of the components that should be in an outbreak investigation report is shown in Table 7. Summary reports should be shared with appropriate persons and agencies, and outbreak descriptions should be published in peer-reviewed literature when the information can contribute to improving future investigations or the general understanding of diseases, epidemiology, laboratory methods, or other aspects of outbreak response.

REFERENCES

1. **Ashford, D. A., R. M. Kaiser, M. E. Bales, K. Shitt, A. Patrawalla, A. McShan, J. W. Tappero, B. A. Perkins, and A. L. Dannenberg.** 2003. Planning against biological terrorism: lessons from outbreak investigations. *Emerg. Infect. Dis.* **9:**515–519.
2. **Bender, J. B., C. W. Hedberg, J. M. Besser, D. J. Boxrud, K. L. MacDonald, and M. T. Osterholm.** 1997. Surveillance for *Escherichia coli* O157:H7 infections in Minnesota by molecular subtyping. *N. Engl. J. Med.* **337:** 388–394.
3. **Bender, J. B., C. W. Hedberg, D. J. Boxrud, J. M. Besser, J. H. Wicklund, K. E. Smith, and M. T. Osterholm.** 2001. Use of molecular subtyping in surveillance for *Salmonella enterica* serotype typhimurium. *N. Engl. J. Med.* **344:** 189–195.
4. **Center for Science in the Public Interest.** *Outbreak Alert! Closing the Gaps in Our Federal Food-Safety Net.* 6th ed., March 2004. Washington, D.C. Center for Science in the Public Interest. [Online.] http://www.cspinet.org.
5. **Centers for Disease Control and Prevention.** 1992. *Principles of Epidemiology. An Introduction to Applied Epidemiology and Biostatistics.* U.S. Department of Health and Human Services, Atlanta, Ga.
6. **Centers for Disease Control and Prevention.** 2000. Surveillance for foodborne-disease outbreaks—United States, 1993-1997. *Morb. Mortal. Wkly. Rep.* **49**(SS-1): 1–62.
7. **Centers for Disease Control and Prevention.** 2001. Diagnosis and management of foodborne illnesses. A primer for physicians. *Morb. Mortal. Wkly. Rep.* **50:**1–70.
8. **Centers for Disease Control and Prevention.** 2003. Hepatitis A outbreak associated with green onions at a restaurant—Monaca, Pennsylvania, 2003. *Morb. Mortal. Wkly. Rep.* **52:**1155–1157.
9. **Centers for Disease Control and Prevention.** 2004. Diagnosis and management of foodborne illnesses. A primer for physicians. *Morb. Mortal. Wkly. Rep.* **53:**1–33.
10. **Centers for Disease Control and Prevention.** 2004. Surveillance for waterborne-disease outbreaks associated with recreational water—United States, 2001–2002 and surveillance for waterborne-disease outbreaks associated with drinking water—United States, 2001–2002. *Morb. Mortal. Wkly. Rep.* **53**(SS-8)**:**1–45.
11. **Centers for Disease Control and Prevention.** 2005. *US Foodborne Disease Outbreaks.* Centers for Disease Control and Prevention. Atlanta, Ga.
12. **Clesceri, L. S., A. E. Greenberg, and A. E. Eaton (ed.).** 2005. *Standard Methods for the Examination of Water and Wastewater.* American Public Health Association, Washington, D.C.
13. **Downes, F. P., and K. Ito (ed.).** 2001. *Compendium of Methods for the Microbiological Examination of Foods.* American Public Health Association, Washington, D.C.
14. **Gregg, M. B. (ed.).** 2002. *Field Epidemiology.* Oxford University Press, New York, N.Y.
15. **Hamson, R.** 2003. Town goes from shock to shock. *USA Today* May 22, 2003.
16. **Hui, Y. H., J. R. Gorham, D. Kitts, K. D. Murrell, W. K. Nip, M. D. Pierson, S. A. Sattar, R. A. Smith, D. G.**

Spoerke, and P. S. Stanfield (ed.). 2001. *Foodborne Disease Handbook.* Marcel Dekker, Inc., New York, N.Y.

17. **International Association of Milk Food and Environmental Sanitarians.** 1996. *Procedures to Investigate Waterborne Illness.* IAMFES, Inc., Des Moines, Iowa.
18. **International Association of Milk Food and Environmental Sanitarians.** 1999. *Procedures to Investigate Foodborne Illness.* IAMFES, Inc., Des Moines, Iowa.
19. **Jones, T. F., B. Imhoff, M. Samuel, P. Mshar, K. Gibbs McCombs, M. Hawkins, V. Deneen, M. Cambridge, and S. J. Olsen.** 2004. Limitations to successful investigation and reporting of foodborne outbreaks: an analysis of foodborne disease outbreaks in FoodNet catchment areas, 1998-1999. *Clin. Infect. Dis.* **38:**S297–S302.
20. **MacKenzie, W. R., N. J. Hoxie, M. E. Proctor, M. S. Gradus, K. A. Blair, D. E. Peterso, J. J. Kazmierzak, D. G. Addiss, K. R. Fox, J. B. Rose, et al.** 1994. A massive outbreak in Milwaukee of cryptosporidium infection transmitted through the public water supply. *N. Engl. J. Med.* **331:**161–167.
21. **Mead, P. S., L. Slutsker, V. Dietz, L. F. McCaig, J. S. Bresee, C. Shapiro, P. M. Griffin, and R. V. Tauxe.** 1999. Food-related illness and death in the United States. *Emerg. Infect. Dis.* **5:**607–625.
22. **Rothman, K. J., and K. Greenland (ed.).** 1998. *Modern Epidemiology.* Lippincott-Raven, Philadelphia, Pa.
23. **Selvin, S.** 2004. *Statistical Analysis of Epidemiologic Data.* Oxford University Press, New York, N.Y.
24. **Watanabe, Y., K. Ozasa, J. H. Mermin, P. M. Griffin, K. Masuda, S. Imashuku, and T. Sawada.** 1999. Factory outbreak of *Escherichia coli* O157:H7 infection in Japan. *Emerg. Infect. Dis.* **5:**424–428.
25. **World Health Organization.** 2005. *Burden of Disease and Cost-Effectiveness Estimates.* WHO, Geneva, Switzerland.
26. **World Health Organization.** 2005. *Water-Related Diseases.* WHO, Geneva, Switzerland.

DIAGNOSTIC TECHNOLOGIES IN CLINICAL MICROBIOLOGY

VOLUME EDITOR
JAMES H. JORGENSEN

SECTION EDITOR
MELVIN P. WEINSTEIN

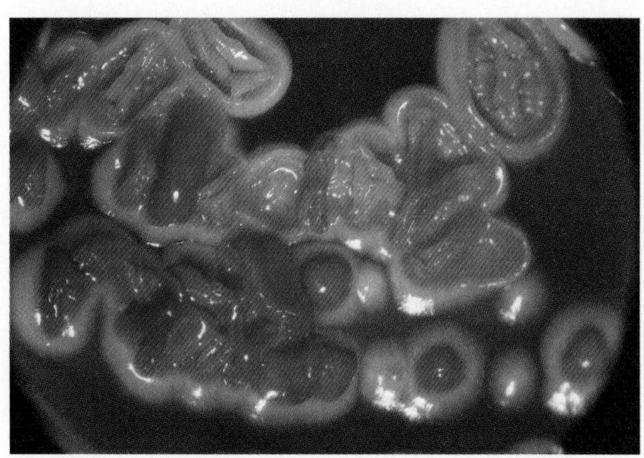

Actinomadura madurae (P. Conville, NIH).

Microscopy

DANNY L. WIEDBRAUK

13

The history of microscopy is closely linked to the beginning of microbiology; Hooke, Divini, Kircher, and van Leeuwenhoek were among the first individuals to describe microscopic lifeforms (7). Hooke, in his 1665 treatise, "*Micrographica*," included illustrations of mold forms and the anatomy of the flea (7). Antonie van Leeuwenhoek provided detailed descriptions of protozoa and bacteria in his letters to the Royal Society in London. His descriptions of "very small animalcules" included drawings of basic organism shapes and movement (7). Today, light microscopy is used not only in microbiology and cell biology but also in metallurgy, computer chip design, and microsurgical applications. This chapter attempts to describe the basic concepts of light microscopy as they are practiced in the microbiology laboratory.

TECHNICAL BACKGROUND AND DEFINITION OF TERMS

Aberration

Aberrations are unwanted artifacts in the microscopic image that are caused by elements in the optical path. Aberration can be caused by physical objects such as dust or oils on the optical surfaces, by alterations in the light path caused by improper alignment or aperture settings, and by imperfections in the lens systems. Two main types of optical aberrations can occur when white light passes through a convex lens: spherical aberration and chromatic aberration. Spherical aberration is hallmarked by images that appear to be in focus in the center of the field and out of focus at the periphery (5). Chromatic aberration occurs because shorter light wavelengths are refracted to a greater extent than longer wavelengths (5). This wavelength separation (also called dispersion) produces color fringes within the image field. Chromatic aberration is reduced or eliminated in optical systems by combining two lenses with different color dispersion characteristics (5).

Contrast

Contrast is a measure of the differences in image luminance that provides gray-scale or color information. Contrast is expressed as the ratio of the difference in luminance between two points divided by the average luminance in the field (1). Under optimum conditions, the human eye can detect the presence of 2% contrast (1).

Depth of Field and Depth of Focus

Depth of field is a subjective measure of the vertical distance between the nearest and farthest objects in the specimen that appear to be in sharp focus. Depth of field decreases as the numerical aperture (NA) of the lens increases (3). Depth of focus is the area around the image plane where the image appears to be sharply focused. The image plane is formed within the microscope tube at or near the level of the ocular lenses. Microscopes with greater depth of focus allow the user to employ ocular lenses with different working distances, magnification factors, and visual compensation systems without losing image sharpness. Like depth of field, depth of focus depends on the NA of the objective. However, depth of focus increases as the NA increases (3).

Immersion Fluid (Immersion Oil)

Immersion fluid is a term used to describe any liquid that occupies the space between the object and microscope objective lens. Immersion fluids are usually required for objectives that have working distances of 3 mm or less (5). Many microscopy applications employ immersion fluids that possess the same refractive index as the glass slide (refractive index = 1.515) (3, 5). This procedure produces a homogeneous optical path which minimizes light refraction and maximizes the effective NA of the objective lens. Immersion fluids are also used between the condenser and the microscope slide in transmitted light fluorescence microscopy and in dark-field microscopy to minimize refraction, increase the NA of the objective, and improve optical resolution (3, 5).

Köhler Illumination

Köhler illumination was first introduced in 1893 by August Köhler of the Carl Zeiss corporation as a method of providing the optimum specimen illumination (5). In this procedure, the collector lens projects an enlarged and focused image of the lamp filament onto the plane of the aperture diaphragm. Because the light source is not focused at the specimen, the specimen is bathed in a uniformly bright, glare-free light that is not seriously affected by dust or imperfections on the glass surfaces of the condenser. Köhler illumination is required to produce the maximum optical resolution and high-quality photomicrographs (4, 5).

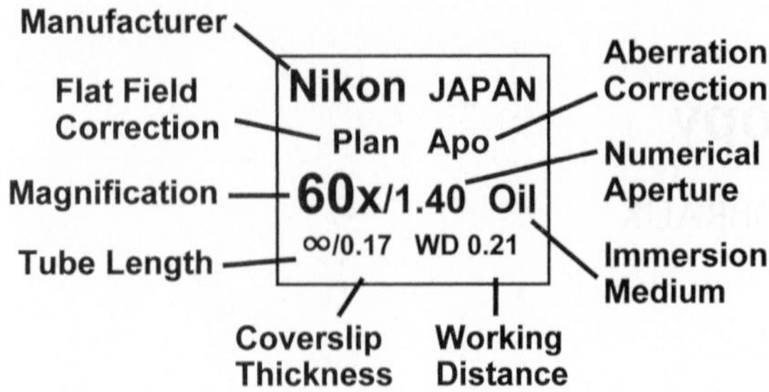

FIGURE 1 Objective lens labeling. Objective lenses are labeled with information on the manufacturer, correction factors, NA, tube length, coverslip thickness, working distance, and expected immersion medium. Objectives without a listed aberration correction are considered achromats. Objectives without a listed immersion medium (Oil, Oel, W, Gly) are considered dry objectives and are meant to operate with air between the lens and the specimen.

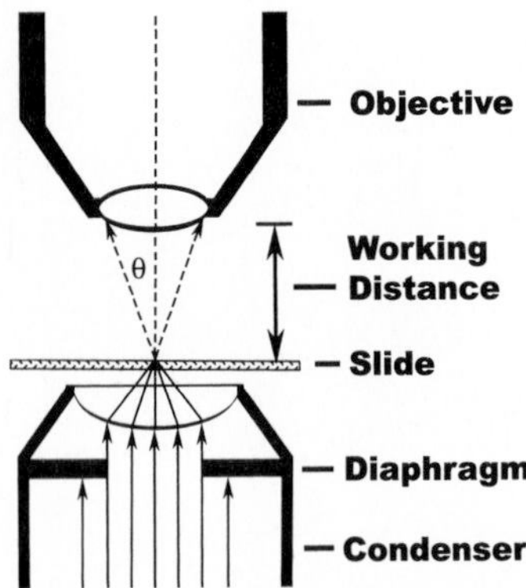

FIGURE 2 Typical configuration for bright-field microscopy. The column of light generated by the field lens and the field diaphragm enters the bottom of the condenser and is focused on the slide by the condenser lens. The condenser diaphragm controls the angle of the light, the NA of the condenser, and the amount of contrast in the image. The working distance is the vertical distance from the top of the specimen to the leading edge of the objective lens. The semiangle of the objective aperture (θ) is used to calculate the NA. Modified from reference 7.

Mechanical Tube Length

Mechanical tube length describes the light path distance within the microscope body tube. Tube length is measured from the objective opening in the nosepiece to the top edge of the observation tube. Tube length is usually inscribed on the barrel of the objective as the length in millimeters (e.g., 160, 170, 210, etc.) for fixed lengths, or the infinity symbol (∞) for infinity-corrected tube lengths (Fig. 1). Many of the newer objectives are infinity corrected, whereas older objectives are corrected for 160-mm (Nikon, Olympus, Zeiss) or 170-mm (Leica) tube lengths (5).

Numerical Aperture

NA is a measure of the light-gathering capability of a lens or condenser. Higher NA objectives have better resolving power and brighter images than lower NA objectives. Higher NA objectives also have shallower depth of field. The equation for determining NA is as follows: $NA = n \cdot \sin(\theta)$, where n is the refractive index of the imaging medium between the objective and the specimen and θ is one-half the angular aperture of the objective (Fig. 2) (3, 5, 7, 12).

Refractive Index (Index of Refraction)

Index of refraction is the ratio of the velocity of light in a vacuum to its velocity in a transparent or translucent medium (3, 5, 7, 11, 12). As the refractive index of a material increases, light beams entering or leaving a material are deflected (refracted) to a greater extent. The refractive index of a medium depends upon the wavelength of light passing through it. Light beams containing multiple wavelengths (e.g., white light) are dispersed when they move into a different medium because each wavelength in the beam is refracted to a slightly different degree. Light dispersion causes chromatic aberration in microscope objectives (5). Refractive index is also an important variable in calculating NA (see "Numerical Aperture" above). Moving from a high-dry microscope objective that uses air as the imaging medium (refractive index of air = 1.003) to an oil immersion objective of the same power (refractive index of immersion oil = 1.515) increases the maximum theoretical NA of a given lens from 1.0 to 1.5, producing a 50% increase in light-gathering capability (3, 5).

Resolution (Resolving Power)

The resolution of an optical microscope is defined as the shortest distance between two points that can be distinguished by the observer or camera system as separate entities (3, 7, 12). The resolving power of a microscope is the most important feature of the optical system because it defines our ability to distinguish fine details in a specimen. The theoretical limit of resolution for a given lens is defined mathematically as $r = \lambda/(2NA)$, where r is the resolution, λ is the imaging wavelength, and NA is the numerical aperture of the lens (3, 7, 12). From this equation it is obvious that only the light wavelength and NA directly affect the resolving power. Thus, a 40× oil objective with an NA of 1.30 can have the same resolving power as a 100× oil objective (Table 1). In the same manner, the resolving power of a 100× oil objective is higher when using UV wavelengths than it is when using visible light (Table 1).

TABLE 1 Resolving power of selected lenses with different NAs

Lens system	NA	Light color	Avg wavelength (nm)	Medium	Resolution (μm)
Eye		White	550	Air	700
Hand magnifier	0.03	White	550	Air	10
10× objective	0.30	White	550	Air	0.92
40× objective	0.75	White	550	Air	0.37
40× objective (oil)	1.30	White	550	Oil	0.21
100× objective	1.30	White	550	Oil	0.21
100× objective	1.30	UV	400	Oil	0.15

Working Distance

Working distance is the distance between the objective front lens and the top of the cover glass when the specimen is in focus (Fig. 2). The working distance of an objective generally decreases as magnification increases (3). The working distance of an objective may not be inscribed on the barrel of older objectives, but newer objectives often contain the working distance in millimeters (Fig. 1). Longer working distance objectives are important when examining the inside surface of glass tubes (tube cultures) and cell culture flasks.

SIMPLE MICROSCOPE

Common objects such as jewelers' loupes, photographic slide viewers, and simple magnifying or reading glasses are all examples of simple microscopes in routine use today. A simple microscope is composed of a single biconvex magnifying lens which is thicker in the center than at the periphery. In contrast with compound microscopes, simple microscopes produce a magnified image that is in the same orientation as the original object. Because of their low NA, simple microscopes have limited resolution and magnifying power. Most commercial magnifiers are able to produce a magnification of ×2 to ×30, and the better lenses have a resolution of about 10 μm. Simple magnifiers are useful for dissection, examination of bacterial colonies, and interpretation of agglutination reactions.

COMPOUND MICROSCOPE

The first compound microscopes were constructed around 1590 by Dutch spectacle makers Zaccharias Janssen and Hans Janssen. The Janssen microscope consisted of an object lens (objective) that was placed close to the specimen and an eye or ocular lens that was placed close to the eye. The lenses were separated by a body tube. In this microscope, the objective lens projected a magnified image into the body tube and the eyepiece magnified the projected image, thereby producing a two-stage magnification. Modern compound microscopes still use this general design and have two separate lens systems mounted at opposite ends of a body tube.

The stereoscopic microscope combines two compound microscopes which produce separate images for each eye. Stereoscopic microscopes may have one or two separate objectives, and many have a zoom magnification function. These microscopes are used for reflected or transmitted illumination, but the absence of a substage condenser limits their NA and resolution. Stereomicroscopes are useful in examining colonial morphology of bacteria, fungi, and cell cultures (12).

The modern light microscope is composed of optical and mechanical components that, together with the mounted specimen, make up the optical train. The optical train of a typical bright-field microscope consists of an illuminator (light source and collector lens), a substage condenser, a specimen, an objective, an eyepiece, and a detector. The detector can be a camera or the observer's eye.

Specimen illumination is one of the most critical elements in optical microscopy. Inadequate or improper sample illumination can reduce contrast in the specimen and significantly decrease the resolving power of any microscope. There are numerous commercially available illuminators for microscopes, but 50- or 100-W tungsten halogen lamp systems are frequently used due to their low cost and long life. Light generated by the light source is passed through a collector and a field lens (Fig. 3) before being directed into the substage condenser and onto the specimen. Image-forming light rays are captured by the microscope objective and passed into the eyepieces or a camera port. Alignment of the optical components of a microscope is critical to produce a good image.

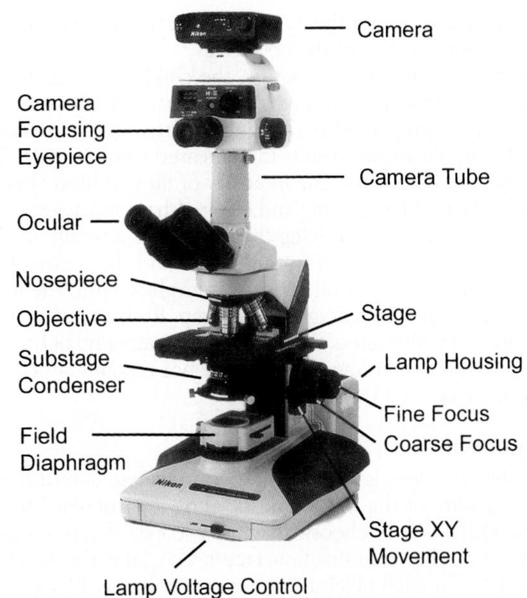

FIGURE 3 Anatomy of a typical clinical microscope with an integral camera.

Field Diaphragm

The field diaphragm is located in the light path between the light source and the substage condenser (Fig. 3). This iris-like mechanism controls the width of the light beam that enters the substage condenser. The field diaphragm does not affect the optical resolution, NA, or the intensity of illumination. However, the field diaphragm should be centered in the optical path and opened far enough that it just overfills the field of view. This adjustment is important for preventing glare and loss of contrast in the observed image. When the field diaphragm is opened too far, scattered light and reflections can degrade image quality.

Substage Condenser

The substage condenser is typically mounted beneath the microscope stage in a bracket that can be raised or lowered independently of the stage (Fig. 3). The substage condenser gathers light from the field diaphragm and concentrates it into a cone of light that illuminates the specimen with uniform intensity over the entire field of view. Adjustment of the substage condenser is probably the most critical element for achieving proper illumination, and it is the main source of image degradation and poor-quality photomicrography. The condenser light cone must be properly adjusted to optimize the intensity and angle of light entering the objective. Because each objective has different light-gathering capabilities (NA), the substage condenser should be adjusted to provide a light cone that matches the NA of the new objective. This is done by adjusting the aperture (or condenser) diaphragm control. Substage condensers on newer microscopes have a scale embossed on the condenser and an index mark on the aperture control that allows the user to quickly switch from one NA range to another. Many manufacturers are now synchronizing the NA gradations to correspond with the approximate NA of the objectives.

In clinical laboratory practice, the condenser aperture is often made smaller to improve the contrast of wet mounts of some stained preparations (7). This practice, while effective for some applications, results in decreased resolution (1, 7). It should be noted that the intensity of illumination should not be adjusted by opening and closing the condenser aperture diaphragm or by moving the condenser laterally in the light path. Illumination intensity should be controlled through the use of neutral density filters placed into the light path or by reducing voltage to the lamp. Reducing the voltage, however, also alters the color of the incoming light. For this reason, lamp voltage changes are not recommended for photomicroscopy (4).

Objectives

The objective lens is the most important single determinant of the quality of the image produced by a particular microscope (12). When choosing a microscope, the purchaser must select the magnification factor, NA, and the level of correction for each objective. Lenses with higher NA values have higher resolution and produce a brighter field of view. The level of optical correction in the objective depends on the ultimate use of the microscope. Achromatic (achromat) objectives are the least expensive objectives found on laboratory microscopes. Achromat objectives are corrected for axial chromatic aberration in two wavelengths (red and blue), and they are corrected for spherical aberration in one color (green) (5). The limited correction of achromatic objectives can cause a number of optical artifacts when specimens are examined and photographed in color (e.g., green images often have a reddish magenta halo) (5). Achromat objectives produce the best results with light passed through a green filter and when performing black and white photomicroscopy. Flatness of field is also a problem when using straight achromat objectives because the center of the field is in focus while the edges are out of focus (5). In the past few years, most manufacturers have begun providing flat-field corrections for achromat objectives. These objectives are called plan-achromats.

The next higher level of correction and cost is found in objectives called fluorites or semiapochromats. Fluorite objectives are produced from advanced glass formulations that allow for greatly improved correction of optical aberration. Like the achromat objectives, the fluorite objectives are also corrected chromatically for red and blue light (5). Fluorites are also corrected spherically for two or three colors instead of a single color, like achromats (5). The superior correction of fluorite objectives compared to achromats enables these objectives to be made with a higher NA. Fluorite lenses therefore produce brighter images than achromats. Fluorite objectives also have better resolving power than achromats and provide a higher degree of contrast, making them better suited for color photomicrography in white light (3, 5).

Apochromats

Apochromats are the most highly corrected microscope lenses and the most costly. Apochromats are corrected chromatically for three colors (red, green, and blue), almost eliminating chromatic aberration, and are corrected spherically for either two or three wavelengths (5). Apochromat objectives are the best choice for color photomicrography in white light. Because of their high level of correction, apochromat objectives usually have, for a given magnification, higher numerical apertures than do achromats or fluorites (3, 5).

Fluorescence Objectives

Fluorescence objectives are designed with quartz and other special glasses that have high transmission rates of UV, visible, and infrared light. These objectives are extremely low in autofluorescence and use specialized optical cements and antireflection coatings that protect the lens and allow it to operate with a wide variety of excitation wavelengths. The correction for optical aberration and NA values in UV fluor objectives usually approaches that of apochromats, which contributes to image brightness and enhanced image resolution (2, 5). The primary drawback of high-performance fluorescence objectives is that many are not corrected for field curvature and produce images that do not have uniform focus throughout the entire field of view. This is not a large problem when performing direct or indirect fluorescent-antibody testing, but it can be troublesome if you have to use the same objectives to do bright-field and phase-contrast microscopy.

Microscope objectives that use air as the medium between the coverslip and the objective lens are considered dry objectives. The maximum working NA of a dry-objective system is limited to 0.95, and greater values can be achieved only by using optics designed for immersion media. Immersion media have the same refractive index and dispersion values as glass (refractive index = 1.51). The use of immersion media produces a homogeneous light path from the coverslip to the lens so that light is not refracted away from the objective. The use of immersion fluids and lenses significantly increases the NA and the optical resolution of the system. In addition to "oil" lenses, specially corrected objective lenses designed for glycerin and water immersion are available commercially. The proper immersion fluid type is always stamped on the side of the objective. The advantages of oil immersion objectives are severely compromised if the wrong immersion fluid is utilized. Microscope manufacturers produce immersion objectives with tight refractive index and dispersion tolerances (5). It is therefore advisable to use only the immersion fluid recommended by the objective manufacturer. Mixing of immersion fluids from different manufacturers should be avoided because mixing can produce unexpected crystallization artifacts or phase separations that compromise image quality.

Many high-power (NA, ≥0.8) dry objectives are engineered to operate through 0.17-mm coverslips (designated as number 1½). In practice, however, the total thickness of the specimen-coverslip sandwich can be greater or less than 0.17 mm due to variations in coverslip and/or mounting fluid thickness (3, 5). Under these conditions, there will be noticeable spherical aberration in the microscopic image (3, 5). A 0.2-mm deviation in coverslip thickness produces an 8% decrease in image intensity when using a 0.79 NA objective and 57% with a 0.85 NA high-dry objective (5). Therefore, some of the more advanced dry objectives are engineered with a coverslip correction collar that adjusts the objective lens elements to compensate for coverslip thickness variations. Objectives with a coverslip correction collar are labeled Corr, w/Corr, or CR. However, this labeling is usually unnecessary because the objective has a distinctive knurled ring and graduated scale on the side. The expected coverslip thickness for an objective is etched on the barrel of the objective (Fig. 1).

The eyepiece or ocular objective contains the final lens system in the optical train. The purpose of the ocular objective is to magnify and focus the projected image onto the eye of the viewer. Ocular lenses generally have a magnification factor of ×10 to ×20 and the total magnification of the microscope is the product of the objective magnification and the ocular magnification. (5, 7, 11, 12). Thus, a microscope with a 40× objective and a 10× ocular lens would have a magnification value of ×400. Many eyepieces have a shelf at the level of the fixed eyepiece diaphragm that allows for the insertion of ocular micrometers, pointers, or crosshairs. This shelf is located at the focal plane of the image projected by the objective lens so that the inserted element is in focus when the specimen image is in focus.

DARK-FIELD MICROSCOPY

Dark-field microscopy is a specialized illumination technique that is used in the clinical laboratory to detect thin organisms such as spirochetes and *Leptospira* (refer to chapters 61 and 63). High-resolution dark-field microscopy utilizes a specialized high-NA cardioid dark-field condenser that blocks the central light path light and produces a hollow cone of illumination that is directed away from the objective lens at an oblique angle (Fig. 4). Bacteria on the slide have a refractive index slightly different from that of the surrounding medium, and light rays passing through the organism are refracted into the objective lens. Light rays that do not pass through an organism do not enter the lens. This type of illumination produces bright organism profiles against a dark background. Dark-field microscopy requires careful alignment of the condenser and the placement of immersion oil between the slide and the substage condenser. Dark-field microscopy, when done correctly, increases the resolution of the microscope to 0.1 μm or less (1, 7). The resolution of bright-field microscopy is 0.2 μm (7, 12).

PHASE-CONTRAST MICROSCOPY

Many unstained biological specimens are virtually transparent when observed under bright-field illumination. To improve visibility in wet mounts and cell cultures, microscopists often reduce the opening size of the substage condenser iris diaphragm (7), but this maneuver is accompanied by a serious loss of resolution and the introduction of diffraction artifacts (1, 5). Phase-contrast microscopy significantly improves the contrast in these specimens without significant loss in resolution (1).

In phase-contrast microscopy, a ring annulus is placed directly under the lower lens of the condenser to produce a hollow cylinder of light. This light is essentially unchanged as it passes into the objective, and it arrives at the rear focal plane of the objective in the shape of a ring. Light that goes through the specimen is refracted and slowed slightly so that it is out of phase with the unchanged light by about one-quater wavelength. This light is spread over the entire focal plane. Light passing through the rear focal plane of the objective interacts with a ring-shaped phase plate that alters the direct light path by one-quarter wavelength (1). When the direct light and the refracted light arrive at the image plane, they are out of phase by one-half wavelength. This out-of-phase light interacts destructively so that specimen details appear as dark areas against a lighter background (1). Because the phase-shifting calculations are based upon on a one-quarter wavelength of green light, the phase image has the best resolution when a green filter is placed in the light path (1). Green filters also allow the microscopist to use less expensive achromat lenses that are spherically corrected for green light. Phase microscopy is an important tool for examining living and/or unstained material in wet mounts and cell cultures. However, phase-contrast microscopy has lower resolution than bright-field microscopy of stained specimens (1). In addition, viewed objects are often surrounded by halos that can obscure boundary details. Phase-contrast microscopy does not work well with thick specimens because the phase shift may be greater than the expected one-quarter wavelength.

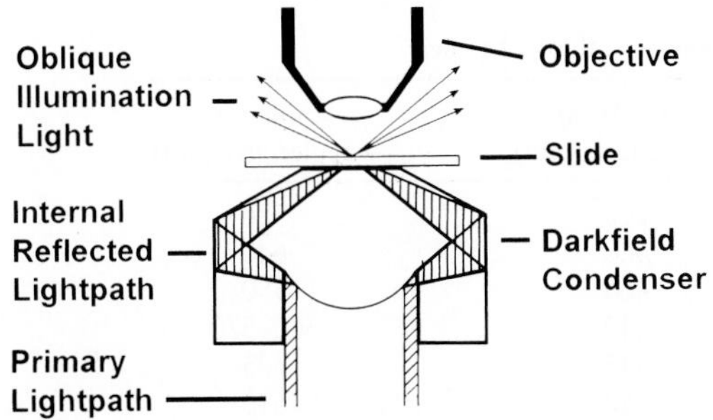

FIGURE 4 Dark-field illumination. The central light path interacts with the silvered dome located at the bottom of the condenser and is reflected away from the specimen. Peripheral light is reflected into the condenser and is reflected again by the internal condenser surfaces to produce a cone of light that is directed obliquely away from the objective.

FLUORESCENCE MICROSCOPY

The fluorescence microscope was developed in the early 1900s, and many of the initial microscopic studies involved identification and localization of compounds that autofluoresced when irradiated with UV light. In the 1930s a number of investigators began using fluorescent compounds to identify specific tissue components and infectious agents that did not autofluoresce (2). These stains are not organism specific, but rather, they bind to and stain specific structures within the organism. Examples of this type of staining include acridine orange (intercalcates into DNA and RNA), auramine-rhodamine (mycolic acids), calcofluor white (fungal cell wall polysaccharides), Evans blue (cytoplasm of fixed cells), and Hoechst 33258 (minor groove of AT-rich double-stranded DNA).

The use of fluorochrome-antibody conjugates (immunofluorescence) was first described in the 1940s when Coons et al. (8, 9) used fluorescein-labeled antibodies to detect pneumococcal polysaccharide antigens in tissue sections of infected mice. Fluorescent antibody staining expanded significantly with the development of fluorescein isocyanate in 1950 (10) and the more stable fluorescein isothiocyanate (FITC) derivative in 1958 (13, 15, 16, 22, 24). Today fluorescence microscopy is also used in conjunction with nucleic acid hybridization to visualize the location of fluorescent in situ hybridization (FISH) and multicolor FISH probes (23, 26).

Fluorescence microscopy is dependent on the ability of fluorescent substances to absorb near-UV light energy and reemit that energy (light) at a lower wavelength (2). To work properly, the fluorescence microscope must irradiate the specimen with UV excitation light and separate the much weaker emitted light from the brighter excitation light so that only the emitted light reaches the eye. The resulting image consists of brightly shining areas against a dark background (2). Older fluorescent microscopes are configured for dark-field illumination. In these instruments, UV excitation light enters a dark-field condenser and the light is directed onto the specimen at an oblique angle (Fig. 4). Fluorescent compounds in the specimen absorb the excitation light, and the emitted light is collected by the objective lens. The emitted light then passes through a barrier filter to remove any excitation light that may enter the objective. These microscopes are difficult to use for routine diagnostics because the condenser and the objective must be carefully oiled. The dark-field condenser also reduces the effective NA of the objectives, thereby producing dim images that lack resolution (2). Most modern fluorescence microscopes use reflected light (epifluorescence). In these instruments, the excitation light is directed downward through the objective and onto the specimen. The emitted light and the reflected excitation light are collected by the objective, and they pass through a dichroic mirror which removes the excitation light and allows the longer-wavelength emitted light to form an image. With epifluorescence, the objective acts as a condenser and the alignment and oiling issues associated with a dark-field condenser are eliminated (2). The visual field is brighter with epifluorescence, the resolution is higher, and fluorescence quenching occurs only in the field of view (2).

Fluorescence microscopy requires high levels of illumination because the quantum yield of most fluorochromes is low. The most common lamps are mercury vapor (HBO) lamps, ranging in wattage from 50 to 200 W, or xenon vapor (XBO) lamps, which range from 75 to 200 W. It should be noted that lamp wattage is not necessarily a measure of usable brightness in a fluorescence lamp. The HBO 100-W lamp is 4 times brighter than the 200-W HBO lamp and 11 times brighter than the XBO 150-W lamp (2). When purchasing a fluorescence microscope, it is also important to determine whether the emission spectrum of the lamp is compatible with the fluorochromes used in the laboratory. HBO and XBO lamps are under high pressure, and care must be taken to prevent the lamps from exploding. One should never touch these lamps with bare hands because oils on the fingers can etch or discolor the glass.

Fluorochromes must be excited by specific light wavelengths in order to generate the maximum amount of emitted light. Therefore, specific exciter and barrier filter combinations are used to maximize the quantum yield of the fluorophore. Exciter filters are used to select the required light wavelengths from the spectrum of light generated by the lamp (2). Excitation filters are provided in narrow, medium, and wide bandpass configurations that pass a narrower and wider range of light frequencies, respectively. Barrier filters block shorter light wavelengths and allow longer wavelengths to pass through the filter. Barrier filters are important because they remove the high-intensity excitation light that could overwhelm the low-intensity emitted light. Barrier filters also prevent UV light from entering the eye, where it can cause cataracts and retinal damage. Wide bandpass barrier filters generally produce brighter images, but care must be taken to prevent the introduction of background light that could overwhelm the emitted light. Epifluorescence microscopes also have a dichromatic mirror (beam splitter) that reflects the incoming excitation light to the objective and allows the emitted light to pass to the barrier filter and on to the objectives. In most modern epifluorescence microscopes, the barrier filter, the excitation mirror, and the beam splitter are housed in removable optical blocks and several of these blocks can be installed in the microscope at one time. This configuration allows the user to quickly change the excitation and barrier filters to accommodate different fluorochromes. Care must be exercised when selecting optical blocks. The excitation filter should match the excitation wavelength of the fluorophore (Table 2), and the emission barrier should allow the emitted light to pass through. For example, direct fluorescent-antibody testing for viral antigens in cell smears typically employs FITC-labeled antibodies and an Evans blue counterstain. Choosing an optical block with a 450- to 490-nm excitation filter and a 515-nm-wide bandpass barrier filter produces a bright field of view, and the counterstained cells will appear orange-red. By selecting a more restricted bandpass barrier filter (520 to 560 nm), the field of view will be darker and the red emitted light from the Evans blue counterstain will not be visible. The images produced by this optical block have more contrast because the background is darker. Both filter combinations are appropriate for this task, but the final choice depends on user preference.

One of the major problems in the use and examination of fluorescent microscopic images is the tendency of fluorophores to lose fluorescence when exposed to excitation light for several minutes. This loss of fluorescence is caused by two mechanisms, photobleaching and quenching. Photobleaching (fading) is a permanent loss of fluorescence that is caused by chemical damage to the fluorophore (2). Quenching is caused by the presence of free radicals, salts of heavy metals, or halogen compounds (2). Quenching can also be caused by transfer of emission light energy to other fluorescent molecules in close proximity to the fluorophore in a process called fluorescent resonance energy transfer. To lessen the effect of quenching, slides should be stored in the dark at 2 to 8°C. In addition, the user should block the excitation light path when not viewing or photographing the specimen. Most epifluorescence microscopes have a shutter in the light path for this purpose. Quenching can be a significant problem when photographing fluorescent images because the shutter may be open for 1 min or more. Quenching can be reduced somewhat

TABLE 2 Excitation and emission wavelengths of commonly used fluorochromes[a]

Fluorescent compound	Excitation wavelength (nm)	Emission wavelength (nm)
Acridine orange (single-stranded nucleic acid)	500	526
Acridine orange (double-stranded nucleic acid)	460	640
Auramine O	460	550
Calcofluor white	440	500–520
Ethidium bromide	545	605
Evans blue	550	610
FITC	490	525
Hoechst 33258	352	461
Rhodamine B	540	625
TRITC[b]	555	580

[a] Excitation and emission wavelengths can vary depending on the solvent and the pH of the solution.
[b] TRITC, tetramethylrhodamine isothiocyanate.

by adding free-radical scavengers such as *p*-phenylenediamine (16), 1,4-diazabicyclo(2,2,2)-octane (DABCO) (17), or *n*-propylgallate (14) to the mounting fluid. *P*-Phenylenediamine and *n*-propylgallate can be used to reduce quenching in FITC and rhodamine. DABCO is slightly less effective than *p*-phenylenediamine for FITC fluorescence, but unlike *p*-phenylenediamine, DABCO does not darken when exposed to light and it is safer to use. Quench-resistant mounting media are also available from Vector Laboratories (Burlingame, Calif.), Molecular Probes Inc. (Carslbad, Calif.), and Bio-Rad Laboratories (Hercules, Calif.).

LINEAR MEASUREMENTS (MICROMETRY)

The first reported micrometric procedures were credited to Antonie van Leeuwenhoek, who used fine grains of sand as a gauge to determine the size of human erythrocytes. Since then, a variety of methods have been used to determine the dimensions of microscopic organisms. The crudest method for determining size in the clinical laboratory involves comparing the object size to the measured or calculated view field size. Other micrometric techniques include the addition of polystyrene beads of known size into the specimen. Comparative measurements are then performed utilizing a photomicrograph or digital image. The accuracy of this method is variable and depends on the homogeneity of the comparison objects. Direct measurements of microorganisms can be done by placing them on calibrated microscope slides or counting chambers. The accuracy of this method depends on the separation distance between ruled lines but averages between 10 and 50 μm. The most common procedure used in the clinical laboratory utilizes a graduated scale (reticle) located within one of the eyepieces (21). Reticles must be calibrated against a stage micrometer for each objective (21). The accuracy of this type of measurement is approximately 2 to 10 μm (3 to 5%), depending on magnification and the resolution of the stage micrometer (21).

PHOTOMICROSCOPY

Microscopists began capturing microscopic images on film shortly after the photographic process was invented (4). Micrographic images have long been used for investigations of morphology, in scientific publications and lectures, and in teaching. Modern film technologies have high resolution and clarity, but the use of photomicrographs in day-to-day microscopy has been hampered by long turnaround times associated with film development and printing. Reacquiring fluorescence images is a particular concern because the fluorescence can fade (2). The availability of high-quality digital cameras has significantly changed how photomicrographs are used in the microbiology laboratory. Today it is not unusual for digital photomicrographs to be shared with experts via the Internet. This process significantly extends the capabilities of the on-site microbiologist and can enhance patient care. Microscope-based digital cameras and video systems are also used to perform "plate rounds" in remote hospitals and clinics within a multihospital system. Newer Internet technologies involving robotic microscopes and high-resolution video systems now allow microbiologists to change the focus and the slide positioning of a microscope located anywhere in the world and view the resulting images on a monitor in their office. The availability of digital photomicroscopy has significantly enhanced the microbial identification process and has helped to standardize microbe identification.

A wide variety of microscopes that have integrated camera systems and sophisticated light metering and exposure controls are currently available. Accessory cameras are also available from a large number of aftermarket manufacturers. The performance and optical characteristics of these systems are too diverse to discuss in a single chapter. Photographs are a stern judge of microscopic quality (4), and the purchase of an expensive camera system does not automatically confer the ability to produce high-quality images. High-quality photomicrographs require proper specimen illumination and optical train alignment to achieve its ultimate potential (4). Color photography can be very demanding because specimens may appear yellow or blue under tungsten halogen (3200K color temperature) light depending on whether the lamp voltage is above or below the recommended 9-V setting. Photographs will also appear blue if the daylight blue filter is not removed from the light path. Photographs can also appear yellow when tungsten halogen (3200K) illumination is used in conjunction with daylight (5500K) film or digital cameras designed for daylight photography. Under these conditions, a Kodak 80A (3200K to 5500K) color conversion filter should be placed in the light path to achieve the proper 5500K color temperature (4).

Not all microbiologists can afford a microscope with an integrated camera system. Simple eyepiece cameras can also be used to capture bright-field images. The simplest configuration for eyepiece photography involves the use of a point-and-shoot digital camera. Some improvisation may be necessary with this method because few adapters are available for coupling a fixed-lens camera to the microscope eyepiece. Instead, the microscopist can use a camera tripod or some other support bracket to hold the camera in its proper position. Entry of stray light can be minimized by using a piece of black polyvinyl chloride pipe with an appropriate diameter and a black camera cloth. During photography, the camera lens system should be set to infinity focus (the default in fixed-lens cameras) and the lens should be positioned so that it is at the eyepoint (focal point) of the eyepiece. Location of the eyepoint can be determined by holding a piece of white paper just above the objective with the microscope turned on and focused (4). A bright circle of light will be projected onto the paper. The eyepoint is the position where the light circle is smallest (4). Photographs produced under these conditions are often acceptable, but they may be dark. Cameras with adjustable aperture settings should be set to the largest aperture value (smallest f-stop number) to maximize the amount of light entering the camera. This method also produces some chromatic aberration (due to different lens correction factors) and vignetting (pipe view effect).

Another method for photomicroscopy is to use the camera port on microscopes fitted with a trinocular head. Olympus and Nikon have introduced adapters that allow their digital cameras to attach to the camera tube of their microscopes. In addition, camera tube and eyepiece adapters for a number of digital cameras are available from Microscope Depot (Tracy, Calif.). Photography under these conditions is best done using a camera with through-the-lens exposure metering. These devices work well if the exposure is not longer than several seconds or shorter than one-third of a second (4). Many of these cameras have built-in flashes that should be turned off during photomicroscopy. These cameras may have problems with fluorescence microscopy due to the extreme contrast of fluorescent images and the tendency of metering systems to average exposure values over the entire field (4).

CARE AND USE OF THE MICROSCOPE

Proper care and maintenance of the microscope will prolong the usable life of the instrument and allow for more accurate interpretation of microbiological images. The microscope should be kept in a low-vibration, low-dust environment to facilitate viewing and decrease damage to the optical systems. The optical elements should be kept completely free of dust, dirt, oil, solvents, and any other contaminants (21). Ideally, the microscope should be covered and the lamp should be turned off when the microscope is not in use. Do not touch the optical surfaces with your fingers (21). Keep the lenses clean and be sure to remove oil or mounting fluid from the objectives, condenser, and mechanical stage after each session. Avoid dragging the high-dry objective through oil or fluorescence mounting fluid. One way to avoid accidental contact with these fluids is to place the high-dry objective and the oil immersion objective in the nosepiece on opposite sides of the low-power objective (4). Lenses should be dusted with residue-free compressed air and cleaned with lens paper and a commercial lens cleaner that is approved by the microscope manufacturer. Organic solvents such as alcohols and acetone should not be used on the lenses because the solvent may dissolve the optical mounting cement (7). Unused spaces in the nosepiece (Fig. 3) should be plugged, and the eyepieces should remain installed at all times to prevent introduction of dust into the body tube. The stage should be cleaned regularly and any spilled immersion oil must be removed or else slides will stick when they are moved across the stage. Spilled immersion oil also collects dust and grit that can damage the optical and mechanical parts. Microscopists should not attempt to remove or disassemble the objectives, as this increases the potential for damage (7, 21). This is a job that is best left to professionals (21). The gears and rackwork should be cleaned and treated with new grease at intervals specified by the manufacturer. Do not use light oil on the gears or bearing surfaces because this may cause the condenser and stage to sink from their own weight (21). Periodic cleaning and adjustment by a professional microscope repair person also help to extend the usable life of the microscope.

ERGONOMICS

Peering into a microscope eyepiece for long periods is not an activity for which the body is well adapted. Microscope work requires the head and arms to be locked in a forward position and inclined toward the microscope with rounded shoulders. This unusual positioning is further exaggerated when the feet are placed on the ring-style footrests that are common to many laboratory stools. Poor posture and awkward positioning during microscopy can cause pain or injury to the neck, wrists, back, shoulders, and arms. In one regional survey of cytotechnologists, Kalavar and Hunting (18) found that 70.5% of respondents reported neck, shoulder, or upper back pain during microscopy and 56% had an increased prevalence of hand and wrist symptoms. Eyestrain and leg and foot discomfort have also been documented with long-term microscope use (6). When using older microscopes, users often have their heads inclined up to 45° from vertical and their upper backs may be inclined by as much as 30°. Even 30° inclinations of the head can produce significant muscle contractions, fatigue, and pain (6). For this reason, microscopists should be taught to sit upright and hold their head in a neutral position (25).

During microscopy, the laboratorian should sit erect and maintain the natural curve of the spine (25). The lower back and shoulder blades should be supported by the chair and a lumbar support cushion should be used if necessary. The legs and feet should rest firmly on the floor or a footrest. The chair should have a pneumatic height adjustment (21), and the seat should have a sloping front edge to prevent undue pressure on the thighs. The backrest should be adjustable for both height and angle, and the chair should have a five-pointed star base with caster wheels. Knee spaces, which are often used for laboratory storage, should be free from obstructions, and there should be a minimum of 2 in. of clearance between the thigh and the bottom of the desk or counter (18). Obstructions that prevent the microscopists from holding their shoulders perpendicular to the ocular axis of the microscope should be removed (27). The upper arms should be perpendicular to the floor with the elbows close to the body. The forearms should be parallel with the floor, and the wrists should be straight. The head should be upright and the neck should bend as little as possible, preferably no more than 10 to 15°. The eyepieces should be just below the eyes, and the eyes should look downward at a 30 to 45° angle. The use of tilting microscope heads can significantly improve the comfort of the microscopist (18, 19, 27). Repetitive motions of the hands and the contact stress of arms resting on (the edge of) a hard surface can cause pain and nerve injury, leading to repetitive stress injuries and/or carpal tunnel syndrome. The use of padded arm rests can moderate some of these problems. In addition, microscopes should not be placed under an air vent in order to prevent stiffening of the muscles during microscopy.

Most laboratory microscopes are used by multiple individuals, and it is often a challenge to find conditions or microscope configurations that satisfy everyone. Some laboratories place microscopes on books or heavy blocks of wood to accommodate taller microscopists (21). This configuration creates a number of problems. If the microscope is raised to a sufficient height to prevent neck flexion, users may be forced to bend their wrists into an unnatural position. If the microscope is lowered to allow the forearms to remain parallel to the floor, the neck is forced to bend. Lowering the chair to its lowest position causes leg discomfort. Vertically challenged individuals may have to raise the chair to a level where their feet no longer touch the floor. Foot rests can ameliorate this problem, but some individuals may have insufficient space under the bench top to accommodate their legs. In practice, most laboratories will elect to use a suboptimum but workable microscope configuration that all users can employ. Under these conditions, microscopists can reduce stress and fatigue by taking 1-min "microbreaks" every 10 to 15 min during which they can stand, stretch, and allow the eyes to focus at a distance.

Eye fatigue can be a major problem for microscope users, especially if they have poor vision. The diopter adjustment provided on most microscope eyepieces can be adjusted to compensate for minor near- and far-sightedness, thereby allowing the users to remove their glasses during microscope use. The diopter adjustments do not adjust for astigmatism, and users with moderate to severe astigmatism should wear glasses when using the microscope. Most microscope manufacturers now produce high-eyepoint eyepieces that move the visual observation point further from the eyepiece, thereby facilitating the use of glasses during microscopy. Ensuring that the microscope images are as bright, sharp, and crisp as possible will also help to reduce eye fatigue and associated headaches. The importance of proper alignment of the microscope and optical components cannot be overstressed. Proper optical alignment and the use of newer objectives with higher NA values will produce brighter images and better resolution, which eases the strain of searching for tiny specimen details. The use of a neutral blue (daylight) filter during bright-field microscopy can also help to lessen eyestrain when examining microbiological specimens. In the future, many new microscopes will display the specimen image on a computer monitor. This innovation could alleviate many of the eyestrain problems that develop during extended microscope use (27).

Microscopes are as different as the people who use them, and the previous comments should not be construed as a prescription for alleviating strain or repetitive motion injuries in every situation. When purchasing a microscope, every effort should be made to allow microscopists to evaluate the new microscope under their normal working conditions. Some microscopes will be comfortable for some users and uncomfortable for others. In the long run, the feel and fit of the microscope are just as important as the optical characteristics.

CONCLUSION

Advances in the design, resolution, and ergonomics of modern microscopes have greatly enhanced our ability to study and identify microorganisms. Microscopy still has a central role in the detection of infectious agents despite highly publicized advances in DNA and RNA detection systems. Microscopic examination of clinical specimens provides a rapid and inexpensive "first pass" in the detection and identification of infectious agents. Thus, clinical microscopy will continue to be a core competency in clinical microbiology laboratories for the foreseeable future.

REFERENCES

1. **Abramowitz, M.** 1988. *Contrast Methods in Microscopy: Transmitted Light,* vol. 2. Olympus America, Inc., Melville, N.Y.
2. **Abramowitz, M.** 1993. *Fluorescence Microscopy: The Essentials,* vol. 4. Olympus America, Inc., Melville, N.Y.
3. **Abramowitz, M.** 1994. *Optics: a Primer*. Olympus America, Inc., Melville, N.Y.
4. **Abramowitz, M.** 1998. *Photomicrography: a Practical Guide,* vol. 5. Olympus America, Inc., Melville, N.Y.
5. **Abramowitz, M.** 2003. *Microscope: Basics and Beyond,* vol. 1. Olympus America, Inc., Melville: N.Y.
6. **Chaffin, D., and G. Andersson.** 1991. *Occupational Biomechanics.* John Wiley & Sons, Inc., New York, N.Y.
7. **Chapin, K.** 1995. Clinical microscopy, p. 33–51. *In* P. R. Murray, E. J. Baron, M. A. Pfaller, F. C. Tenover, and R. H. Yolken (ed.), *Manual of Clinical Microbiology,* 6th ed. American Society for Microbiology, Washington, D.C.
8. **Coons, A. H., H. J. Creech, and R. N. Jones.** 1941. Immunological properties of an antibody containing a fluorescent group. *Proc. Soc. Exp. Biol. Med.* **47:**200–202.
9. **Coons, A. H., H. J. Creech, R. N. Jones, and E. Berliner.** 1942. The demonstration of a pneumococcal antigen in tissues by use of fluorescent antibody. *J. Immunol.* **45:**159–170.
10. **Coons, A. H. and M. M. Kaplan.** 1950. Localization of antigen in tissue cells. II. Improvements in a method for the detection of antigen by means of fluorescent antibody. *J. Exp. Med.* **91:**1–13.
11. **Delost, M. D.** 1997. *Introduction to Diagnostic Microbiology: A Text and Workbook,* p. 37–41. Mosby-Year Book, Inc., St. Louis, Mo.
12. **Douglas, S. D.** 1985. Microscopy, p. 8–13. *In* E. H. Lennette, A. Balows, W. J. Hausler, Jr., and H. J. Shadomy (ed.), *Manual of Clinical Microbiology,* 4th ed. American Society for Microbiology, Washington, D.C.
13. **Gardner, P. S., and J. McQuillin.** 1974. *Rapid Virus Diagnosis: Application of Immunofluorescence,* 2nd ed. Butterworth, London, United Kingdom.
14. **Giloh, H., and J. W. Sedat.** 1982. Fluorescence microscopy: reduced photobleaching of rhodamine and fluorescein protein conjugates by n-propyl gallate. *Science* **217:**1252–1255.
15. **Goldman, M.** 1968. *Fluorescent Antibody Methods.* Academic Press, New York, N.Y.
16. **Johnson, G. D., and G. M. de C. Nogueira Araujo.** 1981. A simple method of reducing the fading of immunofluorescence during microscopy. *J. Immunol. Methods* **43:**349–350.
17. **Johnson, G. D., R. S. Davidson, K. C. McNamee, G. Russell, D. Goodwin, and E. J. Holborow.** 1982. Fading of immunofluorescence during microscopy: a study of the phenomenon and its remedy. *J. Immunol. Methods* **55:**213–242.
18. **Kalavar, S. S., and K. L. Hunting.** 1996. Musculoskeletal symptoms among cytotechnologists. *Lab. Med.* **27:**765–769.
19. **Kofler, M., A. Kreczy, and A. Gschwendtner.** 1999. Underestimated health hazard: proposal for an ergonomic microscope workstation. *Lancet* **354:**1701–1702.
20. **Kofler, M., A. Kreczy, and A. Gschwendtner.** 2002. "Occupational backache"—surface electromyography demonstrates the advantage of an ergonomic versus a standard microscope workstation. *Eur. J. Appl. Physiol.* **86:**492–497.
21. **Murray, R. G. E.** 1999. Introduction to morphology. p. 5–20. *In* P. Gerhardt, R. G. E. Murray, W. A. Wood, and N. R. Kreig (ed.), *Methods for General and Molecular Bacteriology.* American Society for Microbiology, Washington, D.C.
22. **Nairn, R. C.** 1976. *Fluorescent Protein Tracing,* 4th ed. Livingstone, London, United Kingdom.
23. **Reid, T., A. Baldini, T. C. Rand, and D. C. Ward.** 1992. Simultaneous visualization of seven different DNA probes by *in situ* hybridization using combinatorial fluorescence and digital imaging microscopy. *Proc. Natl. Acad. Sci. USA* **89:**1388–1392.
24. **Riggs, J. L., R. J. Seiwald, J. Burckhalter, C. M. Downs, and T. G. Metcalf.** 1958. Isothiocyanate compounds as fluorescent labeling agents for immune serum. *Am. J. Pathol.* **34:**1081–1097.
25. **Thompson, S. K., E. Mason, and S. Dukes.** 2003. Ergonomics and cytotechnologists: reported musculoskeletal discomfort. *Diagn. Cytopathol.* **29:**364–367.
26. **Tkachuk, D. C., D. Pinkel, W. L. Kuo, H. U. Weier, and J. W. Gray.** 1991. Clinical applications of fluorescence *in situ* hybridization. *Genet. Anal. Tech. Appl.* **8:**67–74.
27. **Vratney, M.** 1999. Considerations in microscope design to avoid cumulative trauma disorder in clinical laboratory applications. *Am. Clin. Lab.* **18:**8.

Principles of Stains and Media*

KIMBERLE C. CHAPIN

14

DIRECT EXAMINATION OF SPECIMENS

The first step in the processing of most clinical material is the microscopic examination of the specimen. Direct examination is a rapid and cost-effective diagnostic aid developed to reveal and enumerate microorganisms and eukaryotic cells. Visible microorganisms or the lack thereof may denote the presumptive etiologic agent, guiding the laboratory in the selection of the appropriate isolation media and the physician in the selection of the appropriate empirical antibiotic therapy. The quality of the specimen and the measure of the inflammatory response can also be evaluated. In addition, the direct smear serves as a quality control indicator for attempts to cultivate observed organisms (18). The first part of this chapter discusses the principles of staining methods used in the direct examination of specimens. Tables 1 to 3 give a brief overview of all commonly performed staining methods noted in this Manual. Procedures for performance of the stains are available in the chapters on reagents, stains, and media for bacteriology (chapter 21), virology (chapter 81), mycology (chapter 117), and parasitology (chapter 134). Technical aspects of microscopy are described in chapter 13. An excellent website with exquisite detail containing all aspects of microscopy is available at http://www.zeiss.com.

CHEMICAL BASIS OF STAINING

Simple wet mounts, consisting of clinical material in a drop of saline, allow determination of cellular composition, morphology, and motility. However, cellular material and organisms are usually transparent and best distinguished by the use of dyes or biological stains. Antonie van Leeuwenhoek was the first to attempt the differentiation of bacteria with the use of natural colored agents such as beet juice in 1719 (16). Staining procedures and the understanding of the chemical basis of staining developed extensively in the area of histology, where cellular constituents were desired to be more clearly demarcated. The specific chemical basis of many stains used in clinical microbiology is described in detail in histology texts (10, 12, 13, 21). Additionally, websites pertaining to the basic properties of stains for histology are helpful, including the following site that lists stains alphabetically, http://focosi.immunesig.org/histochemistry.html.

Metachromasia is a characteristic color change which natural dyes (aniline dyes or products of such natural products) exhibit when bound to certain substances either in tissue or in aqueous solution. With the exception of hematoxylin, natural dyes have for the most part been replaced by artificial dyes. Artificial dyes are products of chemical derivatives from substances in coal tar, especially benzene. Two other important chemical groups, the chromophore and auxochrome, complete the dye compound (12, 13).

A chromophoric group is the group of atoms within a dye molecule responsible for its color. Benzene, an aromatic organic compound, undergoes substitution reactions with radicals to form these new compounds, which constitute the dye resonance system. Some of the molecular changes result in a colored product. The most important chromophoric groups are C=C, C=O, C=S, C=N, N=N, N=O, and NO_2. The number of chromophores in a compound determines the intensity of the compound color. Benzene plus a chromophore group is a chromogen. Although the chromogen is colored and typically ionic, it does not have great affinity for bacteria or tissues, and washing or mechanical processes will readily remove the compound. Thus, this group does not in itself constitute a dye. The molecule must also possess an ionizing group called an auxochrome, which allows the dye molecule as a unit to have affinity (cationic or anionic) for a compound and to function as a dye. The auxochrome group gives the compound the property of electrostatic dissociation, or the ability to form salt linkages with the ionizable radicals on proteins, glycoproteins, and lipoproteins on tissue or organism cellular components. This process can occur either directly or through a chelating action of a mordant (13). Commonly occurring auxochromes are amino groups ($-NH_2^+$), hydroxyl groups (–OH), sulfates ($-SO_3^-$), and carboxyl groups (–COOH). With the exception of the amino groups, which ionize to produce a positive charge and are considered basic (cationic), all of these auxochromes ionize to produce negative charges and are acidic (anionic). Some dyes have more than one auxochrome. Even in combinations with basic and acid auxochromes, the negative charge typically predominates (10, 12, 21).

Dyes are usually sold as salts; thus, it is the auxochrome group that usually determines whether a dye is classified as cationic (basic) or anionic (acidic). Most dyes will retain their cationic or anionic properties throughout the pH range of

*This chapter contains information presented in chapter 18 by Kimberle C. Chapin and Patrick R. Murray in the eighth edition of this Manual.

staining (pH 3 to 9) and thus reliably stain those structures that are oppositely charged. For example, DNA phosphate groups and mucopolysaccharides, which are negatively charged and acidic, will be stained with a basic dye. Basic (positively charged) components in cytoplasm will stain with an acid dye. Crystal violet, methylene blue, and safranin are typical cationic (basic) dyes, and eosin, acid fuchsin, and picric acid are typical anionic (acid) dyes.

WET MOUNTS AND SINGLE-STAIN METHODS

Wet-mount preparations are used to determine the cellular composition of a specimen as well as the morphology of organisms, their gross structure, and their biological activity, including motility (Table 1). The specimens can be examined by bright-field, phase-contrast, or dark-field microscopy. True wet mounts do not involve fixation of the clinical material and are viewed immediately upon preparation. Single-stain methods, such as methylene blue or iodine, enhance visualization of organisms by increasing the contrast of structures and can be performed either as a wet mount or with fixed material (e.g., M'Faydean stain) (3, 4). All organisms and cellular components stain shades of a similar color.

DIFFERENTIAL STAINING

While direct visualization of specimens in various wet mounts is useful, differentially stained specimens are the most helpful for presumptive grouping of the majority of pathogens. The

TABLE 1 Wet mounts and single-stain methods

Direct-examination method	Applications	Principle	Time required (min)	Advantages	Disadvantages
Wet mount	Direct clinical examination of stool, vaginal discharge, urine sediment, aspirates	Used to detect organism motility and morphology of parasitic forms and fungi	1	Rapid	Limited contrast and resolution; Brownian movement may be confused with motility; experienced microscopist required
10% KOH	Direct examinations of specimens for fungi, e.g., skin scrapings, fluid aspirates	Proteinaceous host cell components are partially digested by alkali; fungal cell walls stay intact	5–10	Rapid detection of fungi	Background material may cause confusion; experienced microscopist required
10% KOH with lactophenol cotton blue	Direct examination of specimens for fungi, e.g., skin scrapings, fluid aspirates	Adds contrast for detection of fungi	5–10	Dye enhances detection of fungi	Background material may cause confusion; experienced microscopist required
Colloidal carbon (India ink, nigrosin)	Direct examination of CSF[a] and other body fluids for *Cryptococcus neoformans*	Polysaccharide capsule excludes ink particles producing a halo appearance	1	Rapid; diagnostic in CSF when present	Not as sensitive as cryptococcal antigen; cells and artifacts may cause confusion; experienced microscopist required
Lugol's iodine	Direct examination of stool	Nonspecific contrast dye to help differentiate parasitic cysts from leukocytes; cysts retain dye and appear light brown	1	Rapid; enhances differentiation	Background material may cause confusion; experienced microscopist required
Methylene blue staining	Direct examination of stool for leukocytes; detection of bacteria, particularly poorly staining gram-negative organisms, spirochetes, and *Corynebacterium diphtheriae*	Leukocytes and bacteria stain blue	1; up to 10 min if *C. diphtheriae*	Rapid; enhances differentiation	Leukocytes may disintegrate if stool is not examined promptly; overstaining may mask granules
M'Fadyean staining	Fixed examination of clinical specimens from patients suspected to have anthrax	Methylene blue dye stains *Bacillus anthracis* deep blue and demarcated pink capsule zone	4	Rapid; enhances differentiation of capsule	Stain rarely performed

[a] CSF, cerebrospinal fluid.

Gram stain and acid-fast stain are examples of differential stains. In addition, fluorescent stains (see below) may aid in the identification of organisms when specific attachment of fluorochromes occurs with organism components: auramine, calcofluor white, and fluorescein isothiocyanate (FITC) bound to monoclonal antibodies or synthetic protein nucleic acids (PNAs) (19).

In fixed differential smear preparations, four components are typically used in a progressive manner: the primary stain, a mordant, a decolorizing agent(s), and a secondary stain or a counterstain. The primary stain usually stains all cellular components and organisms in the specimen the same color, as seen in simple procedures with a single stain (e.g., methylene blue). The mordant aids in the attachment of a dye to cellular components. Heat, phenol, and iodine are examples of mordants. Decolorizing agents are typically acids and alcohols, such as the acetone and alcohol mixture used in the Gram stain and sulfuric acid used in the modified Kinyoun (modified acid-fast) stain. Removal of the primary stain with the decolorizing agent allows a secondary stain (counterstain) to be taken up by any decolorized organisms and background material. The secondary stain differentiates between those cells that retain the primary stain and those that do not. Examples include the purple (primary stain) and pink (counterstain) organisms seen with the Gram staining procedure or the organism and the background, as seen with a pink acid-fast organism (primary stain) in a blue-counterstained background.

Gram Stains

The Gram stain is the most commonly performed differential fixed stain in microbiology. The Gram reaction, morphology, and arrangement of the organisms give the physician clues to the preliminary identification and significance of the organisms. Gram-positive organisms are thought to retain the crystal violet dye because of the increased number of cross-linked teichoic acids and the decreased permeabilities of their cell walls to organic solvents because they contain little lipid. While the gram-positive organisms take up the counterstain, their color is not altered. The cell walls of gram-negative organisms, because of the higher lipid content associated with the cell wall, show increased permeability to decolorizer, and these organisms lose the crystal violet dye and take up the counterstain dye, safranin (6).

Some enhancement techniques are basic modifications of more standard differential or single-stain methods. These include the use of tartrazine and light green (enhanced Gram stain [Remel]) in place of safranin in the Gram stain and the addition of basic fuchsin to methylene blue (Wayson stain). Many other combinations and manipulations exist (Table 2). The main purpose of these stains is to make organisms that are normally difficult to detect by the Gram staining method stand out more prominently. Typically, these enhancement techniques are used for the better visualization of gram-negative organisms. This is done by two methods. One method is to simply use a stain that will make the organism a darker color so that the normally weakly staining gram-negative organisms are visible (4, 9, 17). The second method is to make the background inflammatory cells and mucus, which often masks gram-negative organisms, a different color than the usual red-pink. This method is used with the tartrazine-light green stain, which makes the background gray or green and the organism easily visible. In this staining method the Gram reaction of the organisms is preserved (J. Kee, A. Hill, and K. Chapin, *Abstr. 94th Gen. Meet. Am Soc. Microbiol. 1994*, abstr. C-242, 1994).

Acid-Fast Stains

The cells of certain organisms contain long-chain (34- to 90-carbon) fatty acids (mycolic acids) that give them a coat impervious to crystal violet and other basic dyes. Heat or detergent must be used to allow penetration of the primary dye fuchsin into the bacterium. Once the dye has been forced into the cell, it forms a stable complex and the usual acid-alcohol solvent cannot decolorize the organism. The acid-fast stain is useful for identification of a specific group of bacteria (e.g., *Mycobacterium, Nocardia, Rhodococcus, Tsukamurella, Gordonia, and Legionella micdadei*) and the oocysts of *Cryptosporidium, Isopora, Sarcocystis*, and *Cyclospora*. A number of modifications have been developed from the original acid-fast stains described by Ziehl in 1882 and Neelsen in 1883. The modifications most commonly used are the Kinyoun and modified Kinyoun (modified acid-fast). Age of the organisms or slight differences in the fatty acids between species can also alter the stain choice (1, 14; J. Brown, CDC, personal communication).

FLUORESCENT MICROSCOPY

See Table 3 and chapter 13 for technical aspects of fluorescent microscopy.

ANTIBODY STAINING METHODS

See chapter 18 on immunoassays.

HISTOLOGICAL TISSUE SPECIMEN INTERPRETATION

The clinical microbiologist is often asked to consult on smear interpretation of blood and body fluid specimens and histologically stained sections of tissue. The differences between organisms stained directly from blood and those stained in fixed tissues need to be noted. In general, it should be remembered that most fungi, parasites, viral inclusions, and bacteria in histological preparations cannot be identified definitively. For instance, the stain typically used in the hematology laboratory for blood and body fluids is the Wright-Giemsa preparation, which uniformly stains all bacteria blue. Thus, one must not call a blue coccus a gram-positive coccus until Gram staining can be done to help in differentiation. In addition, in stained tissue preparations, pathogens may be significantly different in appearance owing to the staining and fixative practices used in the histology laboratory. For instance, vacuolated areas may give the appearance of a capsule in a nonencapsulated organism. However, some organisms, such as *Borrelia, Anaplasma*, and *Ehrlichia*, are best visualized in direct blood smears of buffy coats with Wright-Giemsa.

Histological preparations often stain organisms similarly to the stains used in microbiology but have been modified for tissue. The Brown-Brenn (Gram) stain and Fite-Faraco (acid-fast) stain are examples of tissue stains with which the organisms retain the color appearance seen with their microbiology counterpart (2, 15). Other common tissue stains often viewed by microbiologists include silver stains, such as Warthin-Starry or Dieterle, and the Wright-Giemsa stain. The Wright-Giemsa stain does not stain bacteria or fungi reliably in tissue, with the important exception of *Histoplasma capsulatum*, which will stain by Wright staining of bone marrow and peripheral blood. These histological preparations, as well as others, can also be used to stain infected cell culture monolayers and aid in the visualization of viral and

TABLE 2 Differential fixed staining methods

Differential fixed staining method	Application	Principle	Time required	Advantages	Disadvantages
Gram staining (conventional or Atkins' modification)	Differential bacterial and yeast stains; used to assess suitability of specimen for bacterial culture	Gram-positive organisms retain crystal violet and stain blue; gram-negative organisms do not retain crystal violet and stain pink due to the counterstain safranin	3 min	Rapid; commonly performed; can aid in choice of antibiotic therapy; used to assess specimen for culture and compare smear result to culture result	Organisms with damaged cell walls will stain unpredictably; *Nocardia* and fungi may not take up crystal violet completely; background and cellular elements stain pink, often masking gram-negative organisms
Anaerobic Gram staining variation	Differential stain used to detect anaerobic organisms (especially gram-negative bacteria) not easily seen with regular Gram stain	0.1–0.5% basic carbol fuchsin used as counterstain instead of safranin; enhances detection of gram-negative organisms	3 min	Darker staining of gram-negative anaerobes such as *Fusobacterium* as well as other slender gram-negative organisms, such as *Helicobacter* and *Campylobacter*	
Tartrazine-fast green Gram staining variation	Differential bacterial stain that enhances detection of organisms because cellular background is green	Use of fast green and tartrazine before safranin counterstain allows significant suppression of red-pink color of the background material; organisms still stain purple (gram positive) or pink (gram negative)	3 min	Allows excellent enhancement of small gram-negative organisms and detection of mixed cultures	Slight change in color appearance of organisms compared with regular Gram stain may be confusing
Spore staining (Wirtz-Conklin)	Differential stain for detection of bacterial spores	Spores take up the malachite green stain and the cellular debris, and bacteria appear pink from the safranin counterstain.	Slides can be stained for 45 min or gently heated to steaming for 3–6 min.	Facilitates detection of bacterial spores which may otherwise be difficult to observe. While a heating step is more cumbersome, it enhances uptake of the stain into the spore.	Gentle heating of slide may be difficult to control
Wayson staining	Direct examination of CSF[a] and other specimens for bacteria and amebae	A mixture of the dyes basic fuchsin and methylene blue that results in contrast staining between bacteria that stain deep blue and other material that stains light blue or purple	3 min	Rapid; enhances differentiation	Staining reagents unstable; slides cannot be restained with Gram stain
Acid-fast staining (Ziehl-Neelsen, Kinyoun, modified Kinyoun)	Detection of acid-fast and weakly acid-fast organisms (e.g., *Mycobacterium*, *Nocardia*, *L. micdadei*, *Rhodococcus*, *Tsukamurella*, *Gordonia*, *Cryptosporidium*, *Isospora*, *Cyclospora*, and *Sarcocystis*)	Presence of long-chain fatty acids (mycolic acids) in cell wall or cystic forms makes organisms resistant to decolorization; organisms retain the carbol fuchsin dye and appear pink	2 h	Used to detect acid-fast and partially acid-fast organisms; presence generally significant from direct specimens	Low organism number makes slide examination tedious; tissue homogenates often mask presence of organisms because of deeply staining background

(Continued on next page)

TABLE 2 Differential fixed staining methods *(Continued)*

Differential fixed staining method	Application	Principle	Time required	Advantages	Disadvantages
Periodic acid-Schiff staining	Detection of fungi, specifically yeast cells and hyphae, in tissue specimens. *Tropheryma whipplei* bacilli appear as inclusions in macrophages.	Combination of acid hydrolysis and staining of cell wall carbohydrates; fungi stain pink-magenta or purple, and background appears orange or green if picric acid or light green, respectively, is used as the counterstain. Diastase-resistant, magenta-stained inclusions within macrophages are pathognomic of Whipple's disease.	1 h	Most fungi stain	Time-consuming; respiratory specimens must be digested or mucin will also stain pink-magenta. Inclusion staining pattern seen in diseases other than Whipple's disease.
Toluidine blue O staining	Rapid examinations of lung biopsy imprints and respiratory specimens for *P. jiroveci*	Background material removed by sulfation reagent and appears light blue; *P. jiroveci* cysts stain reddish blue or dark purple against the lighter background	20 min	Rapid method for detection of *P. jiroveci* cysts from appropriate specimen, such as bronchoalveolar lavage specimen	Differentiation of *P. jiroveci* from yeast may be difficult; cysts often appear crescent shaped; trophozoites are not discernible
Wright-Giemsa staining	Detection of parasites from blood smears, viral and chlamydial inclusions, toxoplasmosis, *Pneumocystis carinii* trophozoites, *Histoplasma* yeast forms in tissue, *Yersinia, Helicobacter, Ehrlichia,* and *Rickettsia*	Differential staining of basophilic and acidophilic material. Combination of stains allows uptake by multiple structures.	10 min–1 h	Detection of multiple organisms and cellular inclusions	Not specific for inclusions (*Chlamydia* is the exception); cannot determine bacterial Gram reaction
Gimenez staining	Intracellular organisms, especially *Coxiella, Rickettsia* from cell cultures, and *Legionella pneumophila*	Gram-negative organisms take up the carbol fuchsin and appear red against a green background with the counterstain that contains malachite and fast green.	3 min	Provides enhanced contrast of the gram-negative cell wall not able to be achieved with the Gram stain	Stain needs to be heated to 37°C 48 h prior to use and then filtered. Not commonly available in microbiology laboratories. Not specific.
Trichrome staining, Wheatley	Detection of intestinal protozoan cysts and trophozoites	Provides contrast between parasite cytoplasm (blue-green tinged) and internal structures (red or purplish red) and background debris (green to blue-green) by using chromotrope 2R and light green combination	1 h	Permits detection of diagnostic internal structures of protozoa	Helminth eggs are generally stained very dark; human cells, yeast, and artifacts may also stain.

(Continued on next page)

TABLE 2 *(Continued)*

Differential fixed staining method	Application	Principle	Time required	Advantages	Disadvantages
Trichrome staining, modified (Weber-Green) (Ryan-Blue)	Detection of microsporidial spores	Increase in chromotrope 2R stain concentration and staining time permits detection of pink microsporidial spores.	2 h	Permits detection of pink microsporidial spores against a green (Weber) or blue (Ryan) background	Time-consuming stain
Iron hematoxylin staining (Delafield's)	Detection of microfilariae	Provides contrast so internal filarial structures can be visualized. Hematein, an amphoteric dye, when combined with iron that acts as a mordant, creates an ionically charged dye lake that has affinity for cellular components.	45 min	Permits greater detection of nuclei and sheath of microfilaria compared to Giemsa or Wright's stains	Stain not available commercially and involves extensive aging process
Iron hematoxylin staining	Detection of intestinal protozoan cysts, inclusions, nuclei, and trophozoites	Provides contrast between parasites and background debris. Cytoplasm will have a blue-gray color, sometimes with a tinge of black; cysts tend to be slightly darker; nuclei and inclusions have a dark gray-blue color. Background is pale gray or blue.	60 min	Permits detection of diagnostic structures of protozoa	Helminth eggs are generally stained too dark to discern specific structural differences.

Chlamydia inclusion bodies, *Coxiella, Ehrlichia,* and *Toxoplasma* in tissue. Silver stains provide a differential stain that is best for detection of fungi and *Pneumocystis jiroveci* cyst walls in tissue (20). However, the stain also can detect bacteria and parasites. Differentiation of various yeast forms of *P. jiroveci* as well as other yeasts such as *Cryptococcus* is difficult, and interpretation should be done with caution and in conjunction with the use of other specific stains, such as Fontana-Mason (melanin) and mucicarmine (mucopolysaccharide). Thus, for the best outcome in the histological diagnosis of infectious etiologies, good communication among the surgical pathologist, hematologist, microbiologist, and primary physician will result in the securing of tissue for staining as well as for culture.

PRINCIPLES OF MEDIA

The purposes and descriptions of media for bacteriology, virology, mycology, and parasitology are provided in chapters 21, 81, 117, and 134, respectively. This chapter focuses on the principles of media used mainly for the isolation of bacteria.

General Considerations

Many components optimize the growth of microorganisms on media. The basic requirements for a medium include a nutrient source, a solidifying agent (for solid media), a specific pH, and any number of specific additives. The nutritional requirements of most microorganisms are complex. Most utilize an array of nutrient sources including nitrogen, carbon, inorganic salts, minerals, and other diverse substances. While some organisms can utilize a very simple medium such as nitrate or ammonia, most require protein hydrolysates or peptones. Peptones are the most common nutrient additives in media and are water-soluble materials prepared by enzymatic or acid hydrolysis of animal tissues or products and vegetable substances. Meat infusions were the initial growth-supporting components in media, but because they are cumbersome to prepare and lack batch-to-batch consistency, they are not truly defined. However, meat infusions are still used in some media. Agar serves as the solidifying agent and is derived from red seaweed. The acidity or alkalinity (pH) of a medium is important because microorganisms have strict pH requirements, with most growing in the range of pH neutrality. Components may be added to a medium for purposes of evaluating the pH. These include dyes that change color at a specific pH secondary to the production of acid or alkaline by-products by the organism and buffers that allow determination of the hydrogen ion concentration. Other selective agents, such as antibiotics, dyes, and other nutrients, can be incorporated

TABLE 3 Fluorescent staining methods

Fluorescent stain	Application	Principle	Time required	Advantages	Disadvantages
Acridine orange stain (8, 11)	Detection of bacteria in blood cultures, CSF,[a] buffy coats, and corneal scrapings; detection of fungi	Fluorochrome intercalates nucleic acid in both native and denatured states; bacterial and fungal DNA fluoresces orange and mammalian DNA fluoresces green with UV excitation	3 min	Sensitive method of detection in blood, CSF, and tissues; detects organisms difficult to see with Gram stain and low numbers of organisms such as *Bartonella* and *Helicobacter;* thick or bloody smears can be used; can Gram stain same slide to confirm result	Cellular specimens with an abundance of DNA may be difficult to interpret; interobserver variability seen with some specimens (e.g., buffy coat smears)
Auramine-rhodamine stain	Detection of mycobacteria and other acid-fast organisms	Nonspecific fluorochromes that bind to mycolic acids and resist decolorization by acid-alcohol (identical to acid-fast stains); organisms fluoresce orange-yellow with UV excitation and use of the secondary potassium permanganate stain	30 min	Allows rapid screening of specimens at lower magnification; is more sensitive than other acid-fast stains; can use other acid-fast stains on the same slide to confirm suspicious organisms	Low numbers of organisms may be difficult to confirm with routine acid-fast procedures
Calcofluor white stain (7)	Detection of fungi, *P. jiroveci* cysts, and parasites, such as microsporidia and cysts of free-living amebae in clinical specimens	Nonspecific fluorochrome that binds to cellulose and chitin. Organisms fluoresce blue-white or green if a barrier filter is used. Optimal fluorescence occurs with UV and blue-violet excitation. For eye protection, barrier filters of 510–530 nm are recommended.	KOH clearing if necessary, and then immediate viewing after adding stain	Can be mixed with KOH to clear specimens such as hair, skin, and nails for dermatophytes; rapid, sensitive, and inexpensive screening test. Smears can be restained with conventional stains such as Gram stain.	Difficulty in interpretation with cellular specimens that contain fluorescing collagen and elastic fibers. Variable fluorescence is seen with darkly pigmented fungi. Use with Evans blue helps to suppress green background fluorescence and imparts a red color when blue-violet excitation is used.
Fluorescein-conjugated antibodies and PNA probes	Identification of specific organisms in clinical material; used to confirm specific organism identification from cultures (CMV,[b] *Erhlichia, Francisella*) and growth from blood culture broth (yeast and bacteria)	Monoclonal antibodies or probes bound to the fluorochrome FITC to detect antigens or nucleic acids for specific pathogens in clinical specimens; pathogens fluoresce apple green or red depending on barrier filters used	1–3 h	Rapid and specific organism identification; especially useful for commonly occurring blood culture isolates, specifically staphylococci, *Candida albicans,* enterococci, *Bordetella, Legionella, Pneumocystis,* and viruses.	Adequate clinical specimen must be submitted if done with direct specimen

[a] CSF, cerebrospinal fluid.
[b] CMV, cytomegalovirus.

into media for the isolation of a particular organism. Other considerations that allow optimal microorganism growth include the incubation temperature and the gas in the growth environment. Most clinically significant organisms are mesophiles, which means that they will grow optimally at temperatures of between 25 and 40°C. In addition, most species grow in ambient air, but others require CO_2 or the total removal of O_2. Liquid media require all of the ingredients and conditions described above but lack a solidifying agent (e.g., agar).

Medium Types

Transport Media and Preservatives

Transport media are used in the collection and transport of specimens and were devised initially because fastidious organisms would not survive transport from the bedside to inoculation in the laboratory. Now transport media are even more crucial in providing an appropriate environment for specimens as more and more specimens are transported from distant sites and for long periods.

Generally, bacterial transport media come packaged in a plastic tube sleeve or in tubes with a small amount of liquid medium. A single or a double swab attached to a cap is used for collection of the specimen, which is then placed into the tube and secured. The cap allows the swab(s) to be easily removed from the transport medium for inoculation. The swab component and shaft material, such as Dacron versus rayon and aluminum versus calcium alginate, respectively, may be significant depending on the organism targeted for isolation or the assay system used. Generally, transport media provide a nonnutrient source that sustains the viability of both aerobic and anaerobic organisms without allowing significant growth. Most transport media have specific ingredients that accomplish these goals. These include a small amount of agar or sponge to allow a solid base to which the organisms can attach and to reduce desiccation, an indicator oxidation-reduction agent which shows when oxidation has occurred, and reagents that maintain the pH. Other additives allow the survival of specific organisms, such as sodium thioglycolate for anaerobes or charcoal, which reduce the effects of toxic metabolic products and which subsequently enhance the growth of the pathogens. Other ingredients are added for specific purposes and are noted below. Transport media generally allow stability of specimens for 6 to 12 h at ambient temperatures and should not be refrigerated because some organisms do not survive at colder temperatures. When the specimen arrives in the laboratory, it should be plated as soon as possible. The material in the swab is extracted and placed onto the medium of choice. Care should be taken to inoculate the material from the swab itself when it is extracted from the tube and not the material that may have been in the swab system, such as the gel.

Viruses and chlamydiae have different transport requirements. Viral and *Chlamydia* transport media are designed to provide an isotonic solution containing protein, antibiotics to control bacteria, and a buffer to control pH. The media come in polypropylene centrifuge tubes that contain approximately 1 to 3 ml of medium, 1-dram freezer vials with up to 2 ml of medium, and a tube and swab form with a gel base. While separate transport media for viral pathogens and *Chlamydia* exist, more often laboratories use systems that can accomplish the culture of both of these types of pathogens as well as the *Ureaplasma* and *Mycoplasma* groups. The antibiotics used in these media are not inhibitory to the bacterial pathogens desired or viruses.

Parasitology transport media are actually preservatives meant to maintain the integrity of the parasite and not to maintain viability.

General-Purpose, Enriched, Selective, Differential, and Specialized Media

General purpose, enriched, selective, differential, and specialized are the general categories of media that are used for growth and cultivation of microorganisms. Each type of medium is not exclusive; e.g., many selective media are also differential media. An example is MacConkey agar, which is selective for gram-negative organisms but which is also differential in that it is used to identify lactose-fermenting organisms. Descriptions of each type of medium follow.

General Purpose

General-purpose media are those media capable of detecting most aerobic and facultatively anaerobic organisms. An example of a medium in this category is sheep blood agar, which is commonly used for the general isolation of organisms directly from primary specimens inoculated onto the agar.

Enriched

Enriched media are media that allow fastidious organisms to grow. These organisms may not grow well on general media. An example in this category is the growth of *Francisella* on chocolate agar because the agar is supplemented with cysteine.

Selective

Selective media are media that contain additives that enhance the detection of the desired organism by inhibiting other organisms. Most commonly, selection is attained with a dye or with the addition of an antibiotic. Examples include MacConkey agar that contains crystal violet, which inhibits most gram-positive organisms, and colistin-nalidixic acid agar, which contains antibiotics that inhibit most gram-negative organisms. The effectiveness of selective media varies and is not always complete. Thus, small colonies of partially inhibited organisms may be present on the media. In addition, the ingredients that make media highly selective may actually inhibit the desired pathogen, e.g., a vancomycin-supplemented medium that is selective for *Neisseria gonorrhoeae* (gonococci [GC]) may inhibit some strains of GC.

Differential

Differential media aid in the presumptive identification of organisms based on the organisms' appearance on the media. This can be demonstrated by colony color or a precipitate that forms on or around the colony. Examples include the agars used for the isolation of enteric pathogens (e.g., MacConkey, Hektoen enteric, and xylose-lactose-desoxycholate agars). In the case of MacConkey agar, lactose fermentation by the organism and exhibition of a bright pink magenta color by the colony mean that the organism is utilizing lactose. Further enhancements of differential media exist, such as specific chromogenic media that are also very selective, and allow groups of organisms within a genus to be more clearly recognized than with use of the usual primary media alone. See chromogenic media in chapter 21 for specific descriptions.

Specialized

Specialized media are those media developed with additives for the purpose of isolating a specific pathogen. Such media include buffered charcoal yeast extract medium (BCYE), which is designed for the purpose of isolating *Legionella* species. Specialized media typically include nutrients that the specific pathogen requires but that are not found in general-purpose or enriched media. In the case of BCYE, cysteine and ferric pyrophosphate are provided. Other examples include virology culture media with essential amino acids that are required for the maintenance of cell lines and growth of viruses and anaerobic media that typically include vitamin K, hemin, and reducing agents.

Susceptibility Media

Susceptibility testing media have well-defined formulations designed to support the growth of the most common bacterial and fungal isolates. Hydrolysates of casein and beef extract with low concentrations of thymidine and thymine are used because excess amounts of thymine and thymidine can make organisms appear to be more susceptible to sulfonamides and trimethoprim. Adjustment of small ion concentrations may be necessary for correct susceptibility reporting. Calcium and magnesium ion concentrations are adjusted to allow correct interpretations of *Pseudomonas* susceptibility results with the aminoglycosides, colistin, and tetracycline.

Mycobacteriology Media

Most of the nonselective media used for the isolation and cultivation of mycobacteria are enriched media that are egg based or agar based and that contain additives with fatty acids essential for growth of the organism. Common additives include albumin, which protects the tubercle bacilli from toxic agents; inorganic salts essential for growth; glycerol as a carbon and an energy source; and malachite green, which partially inhibits contaminating bacteria other than mycobacteria and acts as a pH indicator. Because malachite green is a photosensitive dye, a medium with this ingredient should be stored in the dark. Mycobacteria prefer moisture, and tubes of media should be tightly sealed before inoculation. Liquid media are used for the optimum recovery of mycobacteria and for decreasing the time to detection of the organisms. The broths are also used to subculture stock strains and for other tests, such as susceptibility testing and tests with DNA probes.

Anaerobic Media

All general-purpose nonselective anaerobic blood agar media have similar formulations and include peptones, yeast extract, vitamin K (which is required for some *Porphyromonas* spp.), hemin (which enhances the growth of some *Bacteroides* spp.), 5% sheep blood (which allows for the detection of hemolysis), and reducing agents. All allow the isolation and cultivation of both strictly anaerobic and fastidiously anaerobic organisms. The difference in each of the media is the small variation in the peptones used and the inclusion of dextrose in some media as an energy source. These differences may make some of the media better for gram-negative or gram-positive organisms with slight variations in colonial characteristics. Additives used with some of these media allow the media to have both selective and differential properties. Enrichment broths are available in a number of formulations but are increasingly less commonly used for the routine isolation of anaerobes. It should be noted that media are available that are prepared and stored in a prereduced atmosphere specifically for optimization of anaerobic isolation (prereduced anaerobically sterile [PRAS] media).

Preparation of Media

When preparing media from dehydrated materials, the manufacturers' instructions should be followed closely. Chemically cleaned glassware and distilled and/or demineralized water should always be used unless specified otherwise. Care in terms of accuracy should be taken when measuring liquid and dry ingredients. Mixing and solubilization of ingredients are typically done on hot plates, with magnetic stir bars placed in the bottom of the flask or beaker. Excessive heating should be avoided. Autoclaving or filtration sterilizes the media. Autoclaving of volumes of up to 500 ml at 121°C for 15 min is adequate. Larger volumes may require up to 20 to 30 min. The stir bars should be removed before sterilization. For quality control of autoclaving, specialized tape or paper is placed on the medium flask at the time of autoclaving. Enrichments such as blood and other labile additives such as filter-sterilized antibiotics should be added aseptically after the base medium has cooled.

Quality Control

The Clinical and Laboratory Standards Institute has specific requirements for quality assurance of commercially prepared media, which have been updated and documented in standard M22-A3 (3). However, these recommendations do not apply to all media. In addition, any medium that is prepared by the user requires its own specific quality control. Storage of media should be in the dark at 2 to 8°C. Storage in the dark is preferred because additives, such as dyes, will deteriorate faster in the light. This is especially true for chromogenic media that rely heavily on color differentiation between organisms in the same genus. The date that the medium was received in the laboratory and the medium expiration date should be marked and easily visible when stored. Media should be in use only up to the expiration date. Prolonged or incorrect storage of media, including transport media, can lead to desiccation of the medium and to changes in the composition of nutrients and selective agents, and it can compromise organism isolation.

REFERENCES

1. **Balows, A., and W. Hausler.** 1988. *Diagnostic Procedures for Bacterial, Mycotic and Parasitic Infection*, 7th ed. American Public Health Association, Washington, D.C.
2. **Cherukian, C. J., and E. A. Schenk.** 1982. A method of demonstrating gram-positive and gram-negative bacteria. *J. Histotechnol.* 5:127–128.
3. **Clinical and Laboratory Standards Institute.** 2004. *Quality Assurance for Commercially Prepared Microbiological Culture Media.* Standard M22-A3. Clinical and Laboratory Standards Institute, Wayne, Pa.
4. **Daly, J. A., W. M. Gooch III, and J. M. Matsen.** 1985. Evaluation of the Wayson variation of a methylene blue staining procedure for the detection of microorganisms in cerebrospinal fluid. *J. Clin. Microbiol.* **21:**919–921.
5. **Fawcett, D. W.** 1997. *Bloom and Fawcett: a Textbook of Histology*, 12th ed. Hodder Arnold Publishers, London, United Kingdom.
6. **Forbes, B. A., D. Sahm, and A. Weissfeld.** 1999. Role of microscopy in the diagnosis of infectious disease, p.134–146. *In Bailey and Scott's Diagnostic Microbiology*, 10th ed. The C. V. Mosby Co., St. Louis, Mo.
7. **Harrington, B. J., and G. J. Hague.** 1991. Calcofluor white: tips for improving its use. *Clin. Microbiol. Newsl.* **13:**3–5.
8. **Henrickson, K. J., K. R. Powell, and D. H. Ryan.** 1988. Evaluation of acridine orange-stained buffy coat smears for identification of bacteremia in children. *J. Pediatr.* **112:**65–86.
9. **Jousimies-Somer, H., P. E. Summanen, D. M. Citron, E. J. Baron, H. M. Wexler, and S. M. Finegold.** 2002. *Wadsworth Anaerobic Bacteriology Manual*, 6th ed. Star Publishing Co., Belmont, Calif.
10. **Kiernan, J. A.** 1999. *Histological and Histochemical Methods: Theory and Practice*, 3rd ed. Butterworth-Heineman Medical, Elsevier Publishers, Philadelphia, Pa.
11. **Kronvall, G., and E. Myhre.** 1979. Differential staining of bacteria in clinical specimens using acridine orange, buffered at low pH. *Acta Pathol. Microbiol. Scand. Sect. B* **85:**249–254.
12. **Lillie, R. D.** 1977. The general nature of dyes and their classification, p. 19–39. *In* E. H. Stotz and V. M. Emmel (ed.), *H. J. Conn's Biological Stains*, 9th ed. The Williams & Wilkins Co., Baltimore, Md.
13. **Lillie, R. D.** 1977. The mechanism of staining, p. 40–59. *In* E. H. Stotz and V. M. Emmel (ed.), *H. J. Conn's Biological Stains*, 9th ed. The Williams & Wilkins Co., Baltimore, Md.

14. **Luna, J. G.** 1968. *Manual of Histologic Staining Methods of the Armed Forces Institute of Pathology*, 3rd ed., p. 102. McGraw Hill, New York, N.Y.
15. **Luna, J. G.** 1968. *Manual of Histologic Staining Methods of the Armed Forces Institute of Pathology*, 3rd ed., p. 217–218. McGraw Hill, New York, N.Y.
16. **Marti-Ibanez, F.** 1962. Baroque medicine, p. 185–195. *In* F. Marti-Ibanez (ed.), *The Epic of Medicine*. Clarkson N. Potter, Inc., New York, N.Y.
17. **Mirrett, S., B. A. Lauer, G. A. Miller, and L. B. Reller.** 1982. Comparison of acridine orange, methylene blue, and Gram stains for blood cultures. *J. Clin. Microbiol.* **15:**562–566.
18. **Murray, P. R., and J. A. Washington, II** 1975. Microscopic and bacteriologic analysis of expectorated sputum. *Mayo Clin. Proc.* **50:**339–344.
19. **Oliveira, K., G. W. Procop, D. Wilson, J. Coull, and H. Stender.** 2002. Rapid identification of *Staphylococcus aureus* directly from blood cultures by fluorescence in situ hybridization with peptide nucleic acids. *J. Clin. Microbiol.* **40:**247–251.
20. **Paradis, I. L., C. Ross, A. Dekker, and J. Dauber.** 1990. A comparison of modified methenamine silver and toluidine blue stains for the detection of *Pneumocystis carinii* in bronchoalveolar lavage specimens from immunosuppressed patients. *Acta Cytol.* **34:**511–518.
21. **Thompson, S. W.** 1966. *Selected Histochemical and Histopathological Methods*. Charles C Thomas, Springfield, Ill.
22. **Woods, G. L., and D. H. Walker.** 1996. Detection of infection or infectious agents by use of cytologic and histologic stains. *Clin. Microbiol. Rev.* **9:**382–404.

Manual and Automated Systems for Detection and Identification of Microorganisms*

KAREN C. CARROLL AND MELVIN P. WEINSTEIN

15

The last two decades have seen a trend away from the use of conventional, tube-based methods for the detection and identification of microorganisms and toward the use of instrument-based methods. Automation in microbiology first occurred in the early 1970s with the introduction of the first semiautomated blood culture instruments, followed by the early instrumented systems for identification and susceptibility testing of bacteria. In the 1980s, an instrumented screening device for the detection of bacteriuria was introduced. The trend toward automation has accelerated with the introduction and development of automated continuous-monitoring blood culture systems (CMBCSs) and more rapid systems for antimicrobial identification and susceptibility testing. Improvements to these instruments have included expansion of databases, implementation of combinations of technologies to decrease time to detection, and significant improvements in expert computer systems that provide laboratories with the ability to interpret, store, and manipulate data. Commercially available platforms have made improvements in their databases to incorporate or improve identification of category A and B potential agents of bioterrorism. Since the last edition of this manual, few publications have appeared evaluating these conventional methods, with the exception of the literature on a new automated identification and susceptibility testing instrument (Phoenix; BD Diagnostics, Sparks, Md.) (16, 50, 66). More has been published on susceptibility testing performance of some of these instruments (reviewed in chapter 17).

Progress has been made in the development of molecular platforms that provide real-time and simultaneous detection of multiple pathogens, most of which target viruses and agents of sexually transmitted diseases. However, it is unlikely that molecular technologies will completely replace the less expensive phenotypic methods in the short term. Regardless of whether a laboratory is using manual, automated, or molecular methods, the fundamental principles that provide the scientific bases for both detection and identification of microorganisms remain important.

This chapter reviews the systems used for the detection of microorganisms in clinical specimens, with primary emphasis on the underlying principles and systems for blood cultures, systems for microorganism identification, and criteria for assessing and selecting a system. For an expanded review and discussion of the blood culture issues, the reader is referred to more detailed reviews (5, 48, 63, 67). Discussions relevant to systems for antimicrobial susceptibility testing (chapter 17), immunoassays (chapter 18), molecular diagnostics (chapter 16), and rapid detection of mycobacteria (chapter 36) are found elsewhere in this Manual.

BLOOD CULTURE DETECTION SYSTEMS

Development and introduction of automated CMBCSs during the 1990s accelerated the trend away from conventional manual methods. However, the fundamental principles that provide the scientific basis for modern blood culture methods remain important, even with the new, automated technologies. The key variables will be reviewed briefly. For expanded review and discussion of these issues, the reader is referred to more detailed treatises (5, 55, 74).

Technical Variables That Affect Blood Cultures

Volume of Blood Cultured

The volume of blood obtained for culture is one of the most important variables in the detection of bloodstream infections (BSIs) (12, 56, 87). It has been well documented that BSIs in adults may be characterized by fewer than a single microorganism per 10 ml of blood. Studies have shown a direct relationship between the diagnostic yield of blood cultures and the volume of blood obtained for culture (12, 23, 30, 52, 69). Consensus guidelines recommend obtaining 20 to 30 ml per culture from adults (5). This cannot be accomplished with the use of a single blood culture set, and laboratories that accept single sets should discourage this practice (see discussion below). The importance of volume for detecting BSIs in infants and small children has become evident in recent years as well. Isaacman et al. (31) showed that the detection rate with 6 ml of blood was double that with 2 ml of blood from the same blood sample. Kellogg et al. (32) documented that low-level bacteremia occurs in children and recommended that

* This chapter contains information presented in chapter 14 by Caroline Mohr O'Hara, Melvin P. Weinstein, and J. Michael Miller in the eighth edition of this Manual.

4 to 4.5% of a child's blood volume be obtained for optimal detection of BSIs in this patient population. With tiny, premature infants, however, it may be impossible to obtain the volumes recommended by Kellogg et al. (32).

Culture Medium

No one medium or commercial product is capable of optimally detecting all microorganisms. Decisions by microbiologists as to medium formulations should be based on data from well-controlled field trials in which large numbers of cultures were assessed. The most widely used medium for blood cultures is soybean casein digest broth; brain heart infusion (BHI) broth may be equivalent or even superior for the recovery of yeasts and some bacteria (88).

Ratio of Blood to Broth

A number of substances in human blood are capable of inhibiting microbial growth, including leukocytes, complement, and lysozyme. Moreover, nearly one-third of patients from whom blood samples were obtained in a recent study (84) already were receiving antimicrobials at the time the blood samples were obtained. Dilution of blood in broth by a ratio of at least 1:5 has been shown to enhance detection (3, 58), probably by reducing the concentrations of the natural inhibitory substances and antimicrobial agents to subinhibitory levels. Some commercial media, notably those containing resins, may have blood-to-broth ratios of less than 1:5; however, these media have been shown to have sufficiently improved recovery rates such that the suboptimal blood-to-broth ratios are overcome.

Some manufacturers have marketed "pediatric" blood culture bottles with decreased volumes of broth medium designed to maintain a blood-to-broth ratio of 1:5 to 1:10 when only small volumes of blood can be obtained from young children. The broth media in these bottles are supplemented with X and V factors to enhance the yield of *Haemophilus influenzae* and have reduced concentrations of sodium polyanetholsulfonate (SPS) for improved detection of *Neisseria* species. Although these bottles have become popular, there are few objective data to indicate that they provide higher yields or detect microorganisms earlier than conventional blood culture bottles. Moreover, with the availability of the *H. influenzae* type b vaccine, *H. influenzae* bacteremia in children is now rare. Thus, whether the use of pediatric blood culture bottles is truly necessary remains an unanswered question for clinical microbiology laboratories.

Anticoagulants

The yield from blood cultures may be reduced if the blood clots. Therefore, all broth-based blood culture medium formulations contain anticoagulants, the most common being SPS in concentrations of 0.025 to 0.050%. In addition to inhibiting clotting, SPS inhibits lysozyme, inactivates aminoglycoside antibiotics, and inhibits parts of the complement cascade and phagocytosis. SPS has some negative attributes, albeit fewer than some other anticoagulants used in blood culture media over the years. SPS has been shown to inhibit the growth of *Neisseria gonorrhoeae, Neisseria meningitidis, Gardnerella vaginalis, Streptobacillus moniliformis, Peptostreptococcus anaerobius, Francisella tularensis,* and *Moraxella catarrhalis* (19, 54, 55, 65). In general, higher concentrations of SPS have enhanced the growth of gram-positive cocci but inhibited the growth of gram-negative bacteria. Although SPS has its limitations, no other anticoagulant has been shown to be superior.

Neutralization and Inactivation of Antimicrobials

Because many patients are already being treated with antimicrobials before blood samples are obtained (84), potentially reducing test sensitivity, some manufacturers market media designed to bind, absorb, or inactivate these agents. Some medium formulations include additives designed to bind or absorb antimicrobial agents, thereby enhancing the yield of microorganisms. The BACTEC blood culture system (BD Diagnostics) utilizes antibiotic-binding resins on tiny glass beads, whereas the BacT/Alert blood culture system (bioMerieux Inc., Durham, N.C.) uses activated charcoal. In both systems, culture media containing these additives have been shown to have improved abilities to detect microorganisms overall, especially staphylococci and yeasts, and improved yields for patients receiving theoretically effective antimicrobial therapy (41) compared to medium formulations without the additives (15, 63, 77, 88). More coagulase-negative staphylococcal contaminants may be detected in the media containing the resins and activated charcoal than in the media without these additives (77, 88).

Atmosphere of Incubation

Traditional blood cultures have consisted of two blood culture bottles, one designed to support the growth of aerobes and facultative anaerobic bacteria and the other designed to support obligate anaerobes as well as facultative microorganisms. Aerobic blood culture bottles usually contain an ambient atmosphere in the bottle headspace to which various amounts of carbon dioxide have been added to support the growth of certain microorganisms. Anaerobic blood culture bottles usually contain carbon dioxide and nitrogen but no oxygen in the bottle headspace. With the decrease in the proportion of bacteremias caused by obligate anaerobes in recent decades (5, 17, 38, 48), some investigators have concluded that the routine use of anaerobic blood culture bottles in a culture set is not necessary (46, 48, 61, 91). Rather, use of a second aerobic bottle is recommended to enhance the detection of the more common aerobic and facultative organisms and yeasts and to ensure that at least 20 ml of blood from adults will be cultured. An anaerobic bottle would be used only selectively for patients deemed at high risk for anaerobic bacteremia. However, a recent study using media with activated charcoal that compared two aerobic bottles with an aerobic and anaerobic pair of bottles found improved overall detection of microorganisms with the aerobic-anaerobic pair (57). A potential limitation of the study was the presence of few fungemias in the study population. Whether to use only aerobic bottles or to use a more traditional aerobic and anaerobic pair of bottles remains controversial (5, 74).

Bottle Agitation

Several studies have assessed the value of bottle agitation, documenting an enhanced yield and improved speed of detection of positive blood cultures from aerobic bottles (27, 53, 75). All of the commercially available CMBCSs agitate aerobic bottles, and most agitate anaerobic bottles as well.

Subcultures

The processing of conventional manual blood cultures includes Gram staining and blind subculturing of the aerobic culture bottles, usually after the first overnight incubation and, if the cultures remain negative, at the end of the incubation period. Blind subcultures of the anaerobic culture bottles in manual systems and of all bottles in instrumented systems are unnecessary (5).

Length of Incubation

In routine situations, manual blood cultures need not be incubated for more than 7 days. Studies of the instrumented blood culture systems have shown that 5 days of incubation is sufficient for the detection of most pathogens (12, 20, 25, 39, 86). Some investigators have suggested that incubation periods of 4 days (14) and even 3 days (8, 24) may be sufficient for certain systems and media. However, the current standard remains a 5-day duration of incubation. Although it has been common to extend the incubation period when infective endocarditis is suspected, Washington (71) noted that this practice rarely increases the ability to detect the etiologic agent. A recent study from the Mayo Clinic, using a CMBCS, demonstrated that 99.5% of nonendocarditis BSIs and 100% of endocarditis episodes were detected within the standard 5-day incubation period (12). Similarly, in the best medium formulations of the modern CMBCSs, extended incubation periods appear not to be necessary for the detection of the most common *Candida* species. However, published data for *Candida glabrata* and *Cryptococcus neoformans* are lacking.

Clinical Practices That Affect Blood Cultures

Skin Antisepsis and Prevention of Contamination

The probability that a positive blood culture represents infection rather than contamination is a function of the effectiveness of skin antisepsis at the time of the venipuncture or, when blood is obtained from an indwelling device, a function of the effectiveness of antisepsis of that device. Growth of blood culture contaminants, especially coagulase-negative staphylococci, which are the most common etiologic agents of catheter-associated bacteremia as well as the most common blood culture contaminants, not only may be confusing to clinicians but also is associated with substantial expense (6). Thus, reducing contamination is a key issue for both the microbiology laboratory and the health care system in general. For many years, contamination rates (number of contaminated blood culture sets/total number of blood culture sets obtained) of <3% were considered the benchmark for good blood culture practices. A 1998 report from the College of American Pathologists of 640 institutions determined that the median contamination rate was 2.5% (60). In that study, the contamination rate for laboratories in the 10th percentile was 5.4% and that for laboratories in the 90th percentile was 0.9%.

The traditional recommendation for skin preparation has been the application of 70% alcohol followed by either povidone-iodine or 2% iodine tincture. Povidone-iodine preparations require 1.5 to 2 min of contact time for maximum antiseptic effect (74), whereas iodine tincture requires 0.5 min (34). Two studies have documented lower contamination rates with the use of iodine tincture rather than with an iodophor (37, 68). Recently, chlorhexidine has been recommended for use prior to venipuncture. One study demonstrated lower contamination rates with this preparation than with an iodophor (43). Another report compared chlorhexidine tincture with iodine tincture and found equivalent contamination rates (4).

Regardless of the type of skin preparation used, meticulous care and an aseptic technique are required to reduce contamination. Studies have demonstrated that a dedicated blood culture team and/or phlebotomists are less likely than other health care workers to contaminate blood cultures (73; R. B. Sivadas, B. Vazirani, S. Mirrett, and M. P. Weinstein, *Abstr. 101st Gen. Meet. Am. Soc. Microbiol.*, abstr. C10, 2001). Lastly, blood samples for culture obtained by peripheral venipuncture are less likely than those obtained from indwelling catheters to grow contaminating microorganisms (11, 90; Sivadas et al., *Abstr. 101st Gen. Meet. Am. Soc. Microbiol.*).

Number of Blood Samples Cultured

Studies with manual blood culture systems into which 20 ml of blood was inoculated for culture provided good evidence that culture of two or three blood samples will detect virtually all (≥99%) BSIs in adults (70, 83). A recent study using the same volume of blood obtained from adults and inoculated into one of the CMBCSs reported a nonendocarditis BSI detection rate of 96% with culture of three blood samples (12).

Culture of a single blood sample should be discouraged if not forbidden altogether (2). A single sample will provide insufficient blood volume for detection of some infections. Moreover, the growth of a coagulase-negative staphylococcus, a viridans group streptococcus, or a diphtheroid in a single blood culture most often represents contamination but may represent a clinically important infection (84). Interpretation of the positive result under these circumstances is very difficult.

Timing of Blood Cultures

Few studies have systematically addressed the timing of collection of blood for culture. Although bacteremia is associated with rigors (7), this physiologic event usually precedes fever, and it is the latter that most often triggers the request for a blood culture. Some authorities have recommended that blood for culture be drawn at arbitrary intervals (67). However, in a retrospective study, Li et al. (35) showed no difference in yields whether blood samples obtained during a 24-h period were drawn simultaneously or at spaced intervals. The clinician and microbiologist should be guided by the patient's clinical status and suspected diagnosis. With a septic, unstable patient, blood samples should be cultured promptly so that therapy can be instituted. Conversely, if subacute infective endocarditis is suspected in an otherwise stable patient, several blood samples can be obtained at spaced intervals.

BLOOD CULTURE SYSTEMS

Manual Systems

Only three manual blood culture systems are currently marketed in the United States: Septi-Chek (BD Diagnostics), Signal (Remel Inc., Lenexa, Kans.), and Isolator (Wampole Laboratories, Cranbury, N.J.). The Septi-Chek system originally was developed as a labor-saving alternative to conventional blood cultures, which had to be subcultured manually. It consists of a conventional aerobic broth blood culture bottle to which is attached an agar-coated paddle in a clear plastic cylinder, creating a biphasic system similar to that of the classic Castaneda bottle. After blood is inoculated into the bottle, the paddle is attached and the blood-broth mixture is inverted to flood the agar, inoculating onto the agar any microorganisms that may be present. A companion anaerobic bottle that does not use the paddle attachment, which is permeable to oxygen, can be used as well and processed manually. The bottles are incubated with or without agitation and inspected macroscopically for evidence of microbial growth once or twice daily. The agar paddle can be removed from its cylinder for better inspection. Following each examination of the agar paddle, the bottle is inverted, in effect repeating the subculture. There are several Septi-Chek broth medium formulations. The paddles contain three agars: chocolate, MacConkey, and malt. The Septi-Chek system performed well in published clinical trials (10, 51, 80–82).

The Signal is a one-bottle manual blood culture system that also was developed as a labor-saving alternative to conventional manual blood cultures. After blood is inoculated into the bottle in a conventional fashion, a clear plastic signal device is attached to the top of the bottle. An outer plastic sleeve that slides over the neck of the bottle anchors this signal device. Within the device is a long needle that extends beneath the level of the blood-broth mixture. If microbial growth occurs in the bottle, gases are produced in the bottle headspace. This creates increased atmospheric pressure, which forces some of the blood-broth mixture through the needle and into the clear plastic signal cylinder, where it can be detected visually by the microbiologist who inspects the bottles daily. Only one medium formulation has been marketed. In published controlled clinical trials done in the United States, the Signal system performed less well than its competitors (47, 75, 76, 78).

The Isolator blood culture system is unique as the only commercial system that does not utilize a broth culture medium. Rather, it is based on the principle of lysis-centrifugation. Blood is inoculated into an Isolator tube that contains a lysing solution consisting of saponin, the anticoagulant EDTA, and a fluorocarbon that acts as a cushion during the centrifugation step of blood processing. After the blood is lysed and centrifuged, the tube is placed into the Isostat system, which applies a disposable cap that penetrates the rubber stopper, permitting access to the contents of the tube. The disposable supernatant pipette is used to remove the supernatant, and the concentrate pipette is used to transfer the sediment from the tube directly to culture media that will support the growth of the pathogens of which detection is desired. The Isolator can be used for detection of routine bacterial pathogens; however, it has been reported to have a reduced ability to detect anaerobes, *Haemophilus* species, and pneumococci if specimens are not processed within 8 h (28, 29, 33, 72). The Isolator is an excellent system for detecting yeasts and dimorphic fungi, mycobacteria, and *Bartonella* species (9). The system is labor-intensive compared to the newer automated CMBCSs, especially during the initial processing of specimens in the laboratory.

Instrumented Systems

All of the commercially available CMBCSs have a number of characteristics in common. Some of the relevant information pertaining to these systems is shown in Table 1.

The CMBCSs have been adapted or modified so that they can be used to detect the growth of mycobacteria; additional information is provided in chapter 36 of this Manual. The CMBCSs have also been used, as have manual and earlier automated systems, to detect the growth of microorganisms from other normally sterile body fluids, for example, peritoneal fluid (22, 62).

The BacT/Alert system (bioMerieux Inc.) was the first CMBCS and was marketed in 1990; the system was updated in 1999 as the BacT/Alert 3D, which has a smaller instrument footprint than the original and a computer touch screen to ease technologist manipulations. Each incubator module has a capacity of 240 culture bottles. At the base of each bottle is a colorimetric CO_2 sensor that is separated from the blood-broth mixture by a CO_2-semipermeable membrane that monitors the amount of CO_2 in the bottle. At the base of each bottle's holding cell in the incubator unit are light-emitting and light-sensing diodes. With microbial

TABLE 1 Commercially available continuous-monitoring blood culture systems[a]

System (manufacturer)	Method for detecting growth	Capacity per module (no. of bottles)	Maximum no. of modules (no. of bottles) per system	Test cycle (min)	Agitation type/speed (no. of back-and-forth strokes/min)	Dimensions (cm)
BacT/Alert 240 (bioMerieux Inc.)	CO_2, colorimetric	240	6 (1,440)	10	Rocking/34	175 by 87 by 66
BacT/Alert 120	CO_2, colorimetric	120	6 (720)	10	Rocking/34	87 by 87 by 55
BacT/Alert 3D	CO_2, colorimetric	240	12 (2,880)	10	Rocking/34	90 by 49 by 61
BACTEC 9240 (BD Diagnostics)	CO_2, O_2,[b] fluorescence	240	5 (1,200)/20 (4,800)/ 50 (12,000)[c]	10	Rocking/30	93 by 128 by 55
BACTEC 9120	CO_2, O_2,[b] fluorescence	120	5 (600)/20 (2,400)/ 50 (6,000)[c]	10	Rocking/30	61 by 129 by 56
BACTEC 9050	CO_2, O_2,[b] fluorescence	50	1 (50)	10	Continuous rotation	61 by 72 by 65
VersaTREK (TREK Diagnostic Systems)	Manometric	96–240	6 (1,440)	12 (aerobic), 24 (anaerobic)	Vortexing, aerobic only	40 by 52 by 36
VersaTREK	Manometric	528	6 (3,168)	12 (aerobic), 24 (anaerobic)	Vortexing, aerobic only	76 by 52 by 31

[a] Adapted from Reimer et al. (55) and Wilson and Weinstein (87) and modified by Weinstein and Reller (79).
[b] O_2 detection is for Myco/F-Lytic medium only.
[c] Maximum number of bottles accommodated depends on data management system selected (core, Vision, or Epicenter).

growth and production of CO_2, the bottle's sensor changes color, altering the amount of light reflected. The change in reflectance is measured by the instrument, and the information is transmitted to the instrument's computer. The computer has several algorithms to report the detection of a positive culture that is noted when (i) the reflectance exceeds an arbitrary threshold, (ii) the instrument recognizes a linear increase in the CO_2 level, or (iii) there is a change in the rate of CO_2 production. Several medium formulations are available: (i) standard aerobic (SA) and anaerobic (SN) media that contain 40 ml of supplemented tryptic soy broth (TSB) and accept up to 10 ml of blood; (ii) aerobic FAN (FA) and anaerobic FAN (FN) media that contain 30 and 40 ml, respectively, of peptone-enriched TSB, supplemented with BHI solids, and activated charcoal designed to inactivate or bind antimicrobial agents and other inhibitory substances in the blood; and (iii) a FAN medium with a lower volume (20 ml) of peptone-enriched TSB, supplemented with BHI solids, and activated charcoal marketed for use with pediatric patients and those elderly patients from whom it is difficult to obtain larger volumes of blood. A detailed review of published comparative clinical trials is beyond the scope of this chapter, and more comprehensive reviews can be found elsewhere (57, 79, 89). Overall, the system is equivalent to the other commercially available CMBCSs with regard to the yield and speed of detection of microorganisms (79, 89). BacT/Alert media now are available in clear, shatter-resistant, plastic bottles that have performance characteristics equivalent to those of glass bottles.

The BACTEC 9000 (BD Diagnostics) CMBCS offers three instrument formats. The incubator module for the 9240 instrument holds 240 bottles, versus 120 bottles per module in the 9120 instrument. For small laboratories, the company markets the bench-top 9050 instrument that holds 50 bottles. Similar to the BacT/Alert system, the BACTEC system features a CO_2 sensor at the base of each culture bottle, but unlike BacT/Alert, the BACTEC instrument uses a fluorescence-sensing mechanism to detect the growth of microorganisms. When the amount of CO_2 increases, the concomitant increase in fluorescence is detected by the instrument; the principal detection criteria are a linear increase in fluorescence and an increase in the rate of fluorescence. The BACTEC system has multiple medium formulations: (i) standard aerobic and anaerobic media that contain 40 ml of soybean casein digest broth, (ii) aerobic and anaerobic Plus media that contain 25 ml of soybean casein digest broth plus antibiotic-binding resins on glass beads, (iii) an anaerobic lytic medium that contains 40 ml of soybean casein digest broth plus a lysing agent, (iv) a resin medium formulated for pediatric patients, and (v) a medium designated Myco/F-Lytic designed for improved detection of fungi and mycobacteria but which also supports the growth of bacterial pathogens. All BACTEC bottles accept up to 10 ml of blood, except the pediatric bottle, which accepts up to 5 ml. Published comparative clinical evaluations of the BACTEC 9000 system versus other CMBCSs have demonstrated that the system performs in a fashion relatively equivalent to those of its competitors in terms of both sensitivity and speed of detection of positive cultures (79).

The VersaTREK (TREK Diagnostic Systems) blood culture system uses the same technology as its commercial predecessor, the ESP system, and differs from BacT/Alert and BACTEC 9000 in several ways. In this system, bottles are placed into the instrument and monitored with a transducer for pressure changes within the bottle headspaces as gases (oxygen, hydrogen, nitrogen, and carbon dioxide) are either produced or consumed by metabolizing microorganisms. Aerobic (REDOX 1) bottles are monitored every 12 min, and anaerobic (REDOX 2) bottles are monitored every 24 min. Pressure is plotted against time to yield growth curves, and positive cultures are signaled according to the instrument's proprietary algorithms. Aerobic bottles are agitated by vortexing of the blood-broth mixture with a small, stainless-steel stir bar within each bottle, whereas agitation is accomplished by gentle rocking in the other two systems. Anaerobic bottles are not agitated, whereas anaerobic bottles in the other two systems are agitated in the same manner as their aerobic counterparts. In the VersaTREK system, the basal culture medium is supplemented soy casein-peptone broth in the aerobic bottle and modified proteose-peptone broth in the anaerobic bottle. As of this writing, there are no published comparative clinical evaluations of the VersaTREK system versus either the BacT/Alert or BACTEC 9000 system. The ESP blood culture system, which was marketed by the same manufacturer and which preceded VersaTREK, was shown to compare favorably with BacT/Alert and earlier BACTEC instrument systems in studies where the latter two systems utilized their standard medium formulations (45, 79, 92). However, fewer staphylococci and enteric gram-negative rods were detected by using ESP aerobic bottles than by using BacT/Alert aerobic FAN bottles (14, 45, 92).

Interpretation of Positive Blood Cultures

In most general hospitals, 8 to 14% of blood samples obtained will be positive by culture. Of the isolates in these positive blood cultures, one-half to two-thirds will be isolates that are the causes of bacteremia or fungemia and the remainder will be contaminants or isolates of unknown clinical significance. Thus, interpretation of the clinical significance of positive blood cultures is sometimes a vexing clinical problem. Misinterpretation of positive results can be expensive for both the patient and the institution (6). Several useful criteria may assist in interpretation. These include the identity of the microorganism itself, the presence of more than a single blood culture positive for the same microorganism, and growth of the same microorganism as that found in the blood from another normally sterile site.

Microorganisms that almost always represent true infection when isolated from blood include *Staphylococcus aureus*, *Escherichia coli*, and other members of the family *Enterobacteriaceae*, *Pseudomonas aeruginosa*, *Streptococcus pneumoniae*, and *Candida albicans* (84). Isolates from blood that rarely represent true bacteremia include *Corynebacterium* species, *Bacillus* species, and *Propionibacterium* species (84). Coagulase-negative staphylococci are perhaps the most problematic group with regard to interpreting clinical significance, in part because of their ubiquity and also because 12 to 15% of blood isolates are pathogens rather than contaminants (84). The number of positive culture bottles in a blood culture set is not a reliable criterion for decisions regarding the clinical significance of coagulase-negative staphylococci (44; S. J. Peacock, I. C. J. W. Bowler, and D. W. M. Crook, Letter, *Lancet* **346:**191–192, 1995).

A useful interpretive factor is the number of culture sets that are positive relative to the number of sets obtained. If most or all sets are positive for the same microorganism(s), clinical significance is virtually assured (83). Although, ultimately, it is the physician who must make the final judgment, the microbiologist may provide important guidance regarding the clinical significance of blood isolates.

ORGANISM IDENTIFICATION SYSTEMS

Overview of Methods and Mechanisms of Identification

From the early years of diagnostic methods in microbiology until the 1960s, when advances in microbial identification began to emerge, skill in interpretive judgment and the use of tubed and plated media were the bases of microbial identification. Organisms were identified by what we now refer to as "conventional procedures," which include reactions in tubed media and observation of physical characteristics, such as colony morphology and odor, coupled with the results of Gram staining, agglutination tests, and antimicrobial susceptibility profiles. These conventional procedures eventually defined the genera and species of bacteria and yeasts and became the reference methods by which we confirm the identities of isolates.

The next step in the evolution of identification methods simply miniaturized commonly used biochemical reactions into a more convenient format (26). A system-dependent approach became the industry standard, and it remains the approach upon which most currently used substrate profile systems rely. In a system-dependent methodology, a set of substrates that will allow positive and negative reaction patterns to emerge is carefully selected. These patterns create a metabolic profile that can be compared with an established database profile. In many systems, it is necessary to use different sets of substrates to identify rapidly growing members of the family *Enterobacteriaceae*, slower-growing gram-negative non-*Enterobacteriaceae*, gram-positive cocci, gram-negative cocci, and anaerobes. Yeasts require yet another profile set.

Biochemical profiles are determined by the reactions of individual organisms with each of the substrates in the system. The accuracy of the reactions is dependent upon the users' following the directions of the manufacturer regarding inoculum preparation, inoculum density, incubation conditions, and test interpretation. Most systems rely upon one or a combination of several indicators. These include (i) pH changes resulting from utilization of the substrate, (ii) enzymatic reactions that allow the release of a chromogenic or fluorogenic compound, (iii) tetrazolium-based indicators of metabolic activity in the presence of a variety of carbon sources, (iv) detection of volatile or nonvolatile acids, and (v) recognition of visible growth (Table 2). Additional tests for microbial identification that use other means of detecting a positive response for a given substrate may also be included.

Although no formal definition of "rapid" exists for describing the time required for results to be generated, most microbiologists expect rapid systems to provide usable results within 2 to 4 h of incubation. Clearly, the generation times of microbes (usually 30 min or longer) will not allow growth-dependent methods to generate detectable biochemical responses within this time. To overcome the problem of generation times, manufacturers of rapid systems use novel substrates with which preformed enzymes, produced by the organisms to be tested, may react to elicit responses detectable within 2 to 4 h.

Most recently, molecular methods that amplify particular gene targets novel enough to distinguish among genera and species and automated sequencing technology have

TABLE 2 Basis of identification system reactivity

System reactivity	Need for growth	Analyte	Indicator of positive result	Examples of system
pH-based reactions (mostly 15–24 h)	Yes	Carbohydrate utilization	Color change due to pH indicator; carbohydrate utilization = acid pH; protein utilization or release of nitrogen-containing products = alkaline pH	API panels, Crystal panels, Vitek cards, MicroScan conventional panels, Phoenix panels, Sensititre panels
Enzyme profile (mostly 2–4 h)	No	Preformed enzymes	Color change due to chromogen or fluorogen release when colorless complex is hydrolyzed by an appropriate enzyme	MicroScan rapid panels, IDS panels, Crystal panels, Vitek cards, Phoenix panels, Sensititre panels
Carbon source utilization	Yes	Organic products	Color change as a result of metabolic activity transferring electrons to colorless tetrazolium-labeled carbon sources and converting the dye to purple	Biolog
Volatile or nonvolatile acid detection	Yes	Cellular fatty acids	Chromatographic tracing based on detection of end products, which are then compared to a library of known patterns	MIDI
Visual detection of growth	Yes	Various substrates	Turbidity due to growth of organism in the presence of a substrate	API 20C AUX panels

supplanted phenotypic methods for microbial identification for difficult-to-identify microorganisms. These methods have expanded our knowledge of pathogenesis and have expanded and resolved erroneous taxonomic classifications in some cases. Where appropriate throughout this text, more detailed descriptions of molecular methods for detection and identification of pathogens are provided in discussions of particular organism groups. The future will likely see more widespread implementation of these platforms as costs decrease and technologies improve.

System Construction

Microbial identification systems are either manual or automated. Manual methods offer the advantage of using the analytical skills of the technologists for reading and interpreting the tests, whereas automated systems offer a hands-off approach, allowing more technologist time for other duties. For all systems, the backbone of accuracy is the strength and utility of the database. Databases are constructed by using known, clinically relevant strains and include the type strains of most taxa. In some cases, before an organism is added to the database, it is evaluated to confirm its relationship to other strains in the same taxon by using the likelihood fraction. This compares the biochemical characteristics of the new strain to those of a typical culture of the same species.

The number of species included in a database may vary from just a few for some manual assays to over 1,900 for some of the automated systems, particularly if the system is to be used not only in clinical laboratory settings but also in environmental and research settings. For most commercial systems, database maintenance is a continuous process and software upgrades incorporating major taxonomic changes are provided by the manufacturer at intervals of up to every 4 years. Some systems may allow users to make minor changes at the local workstation.

System identifications are supported by algorithm-based decision making that is generally available through a computer. Occasionally, these identifications are compiled into a preprinted index, which is used to manually convert the organism's biochemical profile number into an identification. Bayes's theorem, or modifications of it, is often the basis of algorithm construction from data matrices.

Bayes's theorem is one of the statistical methods that manufacturers use to arrive at an identification of a certain taxon based on the reaction profile produced by the unknown clinical isolate (85). Bayes's theorem considers two important issues in order to arrive at an accurate conclusion: (i) $P(t_i/R)$ is the probability that an organism exhibiting test pattern R belongs to taxon t_i, and (ii) $P(R/t_i)$ is the probability that members of taxon t_i will exhibit test pattern R. Before testing, we make the assumption that an unknown isolate has an equal chance of being any taxon and that each test used to identify the isolate is independent of all other tests. In this case, Bayes's theorem can be written as

$$P\left(t_i / R\right) = \frac{P\left(R / t_i\right)}{\sum_i P\left(R / t_i\right)}$$

By observing reference identification charts derived by conventional biochemical tests, we know the expected pattern of the population of taxon t_i (e.g., *Escherichia coli* is indole positive and citrate negative). R in the formula is the test pattern composed of R_1, R_2, . . . R_n, where R_1 is the result for test 1 and R_2 is the result for test 2, etc., for a given taxon. We can then incorporate the percentages (likelihoods that t_i will exhibit R_1, etc.) into Bayes's theorem to arrive at an accurate taxon.

Clinical microbiologists must not, however, become dependent upon these likelihoods and percentages when interpretive judgment would suggest an alternative taxonomic conclusion. Bacteria often tend to stretch the rules of nomenclature when isolated from clinical specimens, and they may not react as expected in a commercial system, even though a legitimate result is produced (e.g., lactose-positive *Salmonella* spp. or H_2S-positive *Escherichia coli*). The result from the most reliable system can be misleading. In these cases, an alternative method of identification must be used. D'Amato et al. (13) have described how the systems use the database profiles and probability matrices to arrive at an identification of an unknown taxon.

The manufacturers of commercial identification systems rely heavily on input from their customers. Laboratories are encouraged to communicate with the product manufacturer about problems such as unusual organism identifications that develop when a method or system is being used. Manufacturers depend on customer satisfaction, and most are willing to assist in problem solving or in projects that could add strength to their systems. These companies, like their users, are clearly interested in the highest quality of cost-effective patient care. Tables 3 to 8 provide a detailed summary of the available identification systems and compare the features offered by the automated and nonautomated organism identification methods.

CRITERIA FOR SELECTING INSTRUMENTED SYSTEMS

Whether selecting a blood culture system or a method for identification and susceptibility testing, the laboratorian must consider several important issues. Criteria for determining the need for an instrument-based system and its selection are provided in detail in the chapter on laboratory management (chapter 2). Supervisors and managers in the laboratory should make such major decisions carefully and with expert consultation. The process begins by answering key questions about the needs for a new system in the context of laboratory versus patient benefits.

Once these questions are answered, the next step is to begin the search for the right instrument or system to meet the needs of the laboratory and the medical staff. As a general rule, it is best not to be the first to purchase a new system without having seen in the peer-reviewed literature the results of evaluations performed by reputable clinical laboratories. If microbiology journals are unavailable, the manufacturer's representative can be asked to supply peer-reviewed articles about the ability of the system to correctly identify the range of isolates usually seen in your laboratory in the case of identification and susceptibility testing instruments or the results of well-designed, controlled comparative clinical evaluations with large numbers of observations (e.g., more than 5,000 comparisons and more than 500 positive cultures) in the case of blood culture systems. This phase requires demonstrations and conversations regarding space requirements, technical applications, manufacturer issues such as interface capabilities and service contracts, and personnel-related concerns such as sample preparation and throughput.

It is often helpful to visit other laboratories similar to one's own that are using the system under consideration to

TABLE 3 Summary of identification systems available in 2005

System	Manufacturer	Organisms targeted	Storage temp (°C)	No. of tests	Incubation	Automated
Systems for anaerobe identification						
AN Microplate	Biolog	Anaerobes	2–8	95	20–24 h	Yes
ANI Card	bioMerieux	Anaerobes	2–8	28	4 h; aerobic	Fill only[a]
API 20A	bioMerieux	Anaerobes	2–8	21	24–48 h; anaerobic	No
BBL Crystal Anaerobe	BD[b]	Anaerobes	2–8	29	4 h; aerobic	No
RapID ANA II	Remel	Anaerobes	2–8	18	4–6 h; aerobic	No
Rapid Anaerobe	Dade MicroScan	Anaerobes	2–8	24	4 h; aerobic	Yes
Rapid ID 32A	bioMerieux	Anaerobes	2–8	29	4 h; aerobic	No
Systems for *Enterobacteriaceae* and other gram-negative bacilli						
API 20E	bioMerieux	*Enterobacteriaceae* and nonfermenting gram-negative bacteria	2–8	21	18–24 h; 48 h; aerobic	No
API Rapid 20E	bioMerieux	*Enterobacteriaceae*	2–8	20	4 h	No
BBL Crystal E/NF	BD	*Enterobacteriaceae*, and some gram-negative nonfermenters	2–25	30	18–20 h	Reader only
Enterotube II	BD	*Enterobacteriaceae*	2–8	15	18–24 h	No
EPS (Enteric Pathogen Screen)	bioMerieux	*Edwardsiella, Salmonella, Shigella,* and *Yersinia* spp.	2–8	10	4–6 h	Yes
GN2 Microplate	Biolog	Aerobic gram-negative bacteria	2–8	95	4–24 h	Yes
Microbact 12A[c], 12E	Oxoid	*Enterobacteriaceae* and miscellaneous gram-negative bacilli	2–8	12	18–48 h	No
Microbact 12B[c]	Oxoid	Gram-negative bacilli not detected by Microbact 12A	2–8	12	24–48 h	No
Microbact 24E[c]	Oxoid	*Enterobacteriaceae* and other gram-negative bacilli	2–8	24	24–48 h	No
Micro-ID	Remel	*Enterobacteriaceae*	2–8	15	4 h	No
NEG ID Type 2	Dade MicroScan	*Enterobacteriaceae* and other fermenting and nonfermenting bacteria	2–25	32	16-18 h	Yes
PASCO Gram-NEG MIC/ID	BD	*Enterobacteriaceae* and other gram-negative bacilli	−70 – −20	27	16–20 h	Reader only
PASCO Tri-Panel	BD	Gram-negative and gram-positive bacteria	−70 – −20	27	16–20 h	Reader only
Phoenix NID[d]	BD	*Enterobacteriaceae* and other gram-negative bacilli	RT[e]	45	2–12 h	Yes
Rapid NEG ID Type 3	Dade MicroScan	*Enterobacteriaceae* and other fermenting and nonfermenting bacteria	2–8	36	2.5 h	Yes
RapID ONE	Remel	*Enterobacteriaceae* and other oxidase-negative bacteria	2–8	19	4 h	No
RapID SS/u	Remel	Common urinary tract pathogens and *Enterobacteriaceae*	2–8	12	2 h	No
r/b Enteric Differential System	Remel	*Enterobacteriaceae*	2–8	15	18–24 h	No
Sensititre GNID	TREK Diagnostic Systems, Inc.	*Enterobacteriaceae* and nonfermenting gram-negative bacteria	RT	32	5 h (Aris); 18–24 h off-line	Yes
UID-1/UID-3[f]	bioMerieux	Urinary tract pathogens directly from urine	2–8	9	1–13 h	Yes
ID-GNB Vitek 2	bioMerieux	Gram-negative fermenting and nonfermenting bacilli	2–8	41	3 h	Yes
Vitek GNI+	bioMerieux	*Enterobacteriaceae*, vibrios, and nonfermenting bacteria	2–8	28	2–12 h	Yes
Vitek 2 GN	bioMerieux	Fermenting and nonfermenting gram-negative bacilli	2–8	47	≤10 h (3–10 h)	Yes
Systems for identification of gram-negative non-*Enterobacteriaceae*						
API 20 NE	bioMerieux	Gram-negative non-*Enterobacteriaceae*	2–8	20	24–48 h; aerobic	No
Oxi-Ferm II	BD	Gram-negative, oxidase-positive glucose fermenters and nonfermenters	2–8	14	48 h	No
RapID NF Plus	Remel	Nonfermenting and selected fermenting gram-negative bacteria	2–8	17	4 h	No
Uni-N/F Tek plate[g]	Remel	Gram-negative nonfermenting bacteria	2–8	13	18–48 h	No

(Continued on next page)

TABLE 3 Summary of identification systems available in 2005 *(Continued)*

System	Manufacturer	Organisms targeted	Storage temp (°C)	No. of tests	Incubation	Automated
Systems for identification of fastidious gram-negative organisms						
API NH	bioMerieux	*Neisseria* and *Haemophilus* spp. and *Moraxella catarrhalis*	2–8	12	2 h; aerobic	No
BBL Crystal *Neisseria/ Haemophilus*	BD	*Neisseria, Haemophilus, Moraxella,* and *Gardnerella* spp. and other fastidious pathogens	2–8	29	4 h	No
HNID	Dade MicroScan	*Neisseria* and *Haemophilus* spp., *Moraxella catarrhalis,* and *Gardnerella vaginalis*	2–8	18	4 h	Yes
Neisseria Enzyme Test	Remel	Three *Neisseria* species and *Moraxella catarrhalis*	2–8	3	30 min	No
NHI	bioMerieux	*Neisseria* and *Haemophilus* spp. and other fastidious bacteria	2–8	15	4 h	No
RapID NH	Remel	*Neisseriaceae, Haemophilus* spp., and other gram-negative bacteria	2–8	13	4 h; 1 h for gonococci	No
Systems for identification of gram-positive cocci						
API 20 Strep	bioMerieux	Streptococci and enterococci	2–8	20	4–24 h; aerobic	No
API Staph	bioMerieux	Staphylococci and micrococci	2–8	20	18–24 h	No
BBL Crystal Gram-Positive	BD	Gram-positive cocci and bacilli	2–8	29	18–24 h	Reader only
BBL Crystal Rapid Gram-Positive	BD	Gram-positive cocci and bacilli	2–8	29	4 h	No
GP2 Microplate	Biolog	Aerobic gram-positive bacteria	2–8	95	4–24 h	Yes
GPI	bioMerieux	Gram-positive cocci and bacilli	2–8	29	2–15 h	Yes
ID-GPC Vitek 2	bioMerieux	Gram-positive cocci	2–8	46	2–6 h	Yes
Microbact Staph 12S	Oxoid	Staphylococci	2–8	12	24 h	No
PASCO Gram-Pos MIC/ID	BD	Gram-positive bacteria	−70 – −20	27	16–20 h	Reader only
Phoenix PID[d]	BD	Gram-positive bacteria	RT	45	2–16 h	Yes
Pos ID 2	Dade MicroScan	Gram-positive cocci and *Listeria* spp.	2–25	27	16–18 h	Yes
RAPIDEC STAPH	bioMerieux	Staphylococci	2–8	4	2 h	No
Rapid POS ID	Dade MicroScan	Gram-positive cocci and *Listeria* spp.	2–8	34	2.5 h	Yes
RapID STR	Remel	Streptococci and related organisms	2–8	14	4 h	No
Sensititre GPID	TREK Diagnostic Systems, Inc.	Gram-positive bacteria	RT	32	24 h	Yes
Vitek 2 GP	bioMerieux	Gram-positive cocci and bacilli	2–8	43	≤8 h(3–8 h)	Yes
Systems for identification of gram-positive bacilli						
API Coryne	bioMerieux	*Corynebacteria* and corynebacterium-like organisms	2–8	20	24 h; aerobic	No
Microbact Listeria 12L	Oxoid	*Listeria* spp.	2–8	12	4 h; 18–24 h	No
Micro-ID Listeria	Remel	*Listeria* spp.	2–8	15	24 h	No
RapID CB Plus	Remel	Coryneform bacilli	2–8	18	4 h	No
Systems for identification of yeasts and fungi						
API 20C AUX	bioMerieux	Yeasts	2–8	19	48–72 h	No
FF Microplate	Biolog	Filamentous fungi and selected yeasts	2–8	95	1–4 h; 7 days	Yes
ID-YST Vitek 2	bioMerieux	Yeasts	2–8	46	15 h	Yes
Rapid Yeast ID	Dade MicroScan	Yeasts	2–8	27	4 h	Yes
RapID Yeast Plus	Remel	Yeasts and yeast-like organisms	2–8	18	4 h	No
Uni-Yeast Tek[h]	Remel	Yeasts	2–8	11	24 h–7 days	No
YBC	bioMerieux	Yeasts	2–8	26	24–48 h[i]	Yes
YT Microplate	Biolog	Yeasts	2–8	94	24–72 h	Yes
Vitek 2 Yeast	bioMerieux	Yeasts and yeast-like organisms	2–8	46	18 h	Yes

[a] Cards are filled automatically but read visually.

[b] BD, BD Diagnostics.

[c] Microbact 12A and 12B are in a strip format; the 12E and 24E have microplate formats.

[d] Also available are combination identification and susceptibility panels: NMIC/ID and PMIC/ID for gram-negative and gram-positive organisms, respectively.

[e] RT, room temperature.

[f] For one sample and three samples, respectively.

[g] Part of the N/F system which also includes the N/F Screen 42P and the N/F GNF screen which are tubed media that are used for the identification of pigmented strains of *Pseudomonas aeruginosa* and the *Pseudomonas fluorescens-Pseudomonas putida* group.

[h] Part of the yeast system which also contains the C/N screen for *Cryptococcus neoformans*; GBE tube for presumptive identification of *Candida albicans* and *C. stellatoidea*, and the SAM tube for differentiation of *Candida albicans* and *Candida stellatoidea*.

[i] Off-line incubation required.

TABLE 4 Comparison of features of automated identification systems[a]

Feature	Values for automated identification systems							
	Vitek Legacy[b]	Vitek 2[b,c]	autoSCAN-4[d]	WalkAway SI[d]	Phoenix[e]	Sensititre Aris 2X[f]	Biolog[g]	MIDI[h]
Capacity of system	60/240/480	60/120	Unlimited	40/96	100	64	50	200+[i]
No. of species in database[j] (no. of substrates)								
Gram-negative organisms	116 (30)	130 (47)	142 (24)	142 (24),[k] 149 (44)[l]	167 (45)	128 (32)	524 (95)	482 (NA)[m]
Gram-positive organisms	52 (30)	54 (49)	49 (27)	49 (27),[k] (42)[l]	140 (45)	70 (32)[n]	351 (95)	451 (NA)
Anaerobes	85 (29)[o]	No	54 (24)	54 (24)	NA	No	361 (95)	732 (NA)
Fastidious organisms	9 (30)[o]	Expected release in 2006	21 (18)	20 (18)	Included in tests for gram-negative and gram-positive organisms	No	Included in tests for gram-negative and gram-positive organisms	50 (NA)
Environmental organisms	No	No	No	No	No	No	Included in tests for gram-negative and gram-positive organisms	Included in tests for gram-negative and gram-positive organisms
Yeasts	36 (30)[o]	54 (46)	44 (27)	44 (27)	No	No	267 (95)	196 (NA)
Mycobacteria	No	No	No	No	No	No	No	31 (NA)
Inoculation	Automated	Automated	Manual	Manual	Manual	Automated	Manual	Automated
Type of incubation, incubation time	On-line	On-line	Off-line	On-line	On-line	On-line	On-line	On-line
Gram-negative organisms	2–18 h	3 h	16–18 h	2.5 or 16–18 h	2–16 h	5 h	4–6 or 16–24 h	9–30 min
Gram-positive organisms	2–15 h	2–6 h	16–18 h	2.5 or 16–18 h	2–16 h	24 h	4–6 or 16–24 h	9–30 min
Anaerobes	4 h	NA	4 h	4 h	NA	NA	20–24 h	30 min
Fastidious organisms	4 h	NA	4 h	4 h	NA	NA	4–6 or 16–24 h	9–30 min
Environmental organisms	NA	NA	NA	NA	NA	NA	NA	9–30 min
Yeasts	24–48 h	15 h	4 h	4 h	NA	NA	24, 48, 72 h	30 min
Mycobacteria	NA	NA	NA	NA	NA	NA	NA	30 min
Manual reagent addition	No	No	Yes	No	No	No	No	No
Additional tests required before incubation	Yes	No	Yes	Yes	No	No	Yes	No
Storage temp	2–8°C[p]	2–8°C	RT[q]	RT, 4°C	RT	RT	4°C	RT
Other features								
Susceptibility testing	Yes	Yes	Yes	Yes	Yes	Yes	No	No
Urine screen or identification	Yes	No	No	No	No	No	No	No
DMS[r]	Yes	Yes	Yes	Yes	Yes	Yes	Yes	Yes

(Continued on next page)

TABLE 4 Comparison of features of automated identification systems[a] *(Continued)*

Feature	Values for automated identification systems							
	Vitek Legacy[b]	Vitek 2[b,c]	autoSCAN-4[d]	WalkAway SI[d]	Phoenix[e]	Sensititre Aris 2X[f]	Biolog[g]	MIDI[h]
Computer interface	Yes	Yes	Yes	Yes	Yes	No	Yes	Yes

[a] Modified from O'Hara (50) and Stager and Davis (64) and updated in 2005.
[b] Manufacturer: bioMerieux Inc., 100 Rodolphe St., Durham, NC 27712. Phone: (800) 682-2666. http://www.bioMerieux.com.
[c] A compact model of this instrument (capacity 30/60) was released in 2005. It uses the same cards as Vitek 2.
[d] Manufacturer: Dade Behring, MicroScan, Inc., 1717 Deerfield Rd., Deerfield, IL 60015. Phone: (847) 267-5300. http://www.dadebehring.com.
[e] Manufacturer: BD Diagnostics, Inc., 1 Becton Drive, Franklin Lakes, NJ 07417. Phone: (201) 847-6800. http://www.bd-com/us/.
[f] Manufacturer: TREK Diagnostic Systems, Inc., 982 Keynote Circle, Suite 6, Cleveland, OH 44131. Phone: (800) 871-8909. http://www.trek.com.
[g] Manufacturer: Biolog, Inc., 21124 Cabot Blvd., Hayward, CA 94545. Phone: (510) 785-2564. E-mail: info@biolog.com.
[h] Manufacturer: MIDI, 125 Sandy Dr., Newark, DE 19713. Phone: (800) 276-8068.
[i] Based upon whether the rapid or standard method is used.
[j] Species in database indicates the groups, genera, or species identified.
[k] Conventional identification panel.
[l] Fluorogenic identification panel.
[m] NA, not applicable.
[n] U.S. clinical database (veterinary database not included).
[o] Although these panels have off-line incubation, they use the Vitek filling module for inoculation and the data management system for generation of identification.
[p] RT, room temperature.
[q] All rapid identification panels.
[r] DMS, data management system.

ask if they like the system, whether they would buy it again, how much downtime they have experienced, whether the service from the manufacturer has been acceptable, and whether the system has been mechanically reliable.

The laboratory should select a system that has been fully evaluated and whose accuracy exceeds 90% in its overall ability to identify common and uncommon bacteria normally seen in your hospital or laboratory. The system should be able to identify commonly isolated organisms with at least 95% accuracy compared with conventional methods.

The accuracy of antimicrobial susceptibility testing for combination panels is as important as the accuracy of identification, perhaps more so. Chapter 17 of this Manual discusses the issues involved in instrument susceptibility test methods.

EVALUATING AN INSTRUMENT OR SYSTEM

Several references provide useful information on the approach to evaluation, verification, and validation of kits, assays, and instruments in the clinical laboratory (18, 40, 42, 49, 64). Anytime an identification system is added to the laboratory, it is necessary to document that the system performs as described by the manufacturer. The first evidence of acceptable performance should be found in published reports by other laboratories that have evaluated the system in a sound, scientific manner (64). The next evidence of acceptable performance by a new identification instrument should be in-laboratory verification of performance by the purchasing laboratory. Verification is the documentation of test accuracy in the laboratory where the instrument will be used (40). The Clinical Laboratory Improvement Amendments of 1988 (21) specify the conditions for systems placed into service (see chapter 2).

Smaller laboratories will have fewer resources than larger laboratories for verification of the accuracy of an identification system. Laboratory size, however, has no bearing on the need to ensure the accuracies of laboratory identification methods and of the work performed by a laboratory in support of patient care. The role of verification by the purchasing laboratory should be to ensure that the personnel using the system can make it perform at the levels of accuracy already documented by the manufacturer and published in the literature. The laboratorian should expect a level of 95% agreement with the existing system or reference method and accept, in the final analysis, no less than 90% agreement. This takes into account the fact that the new system may be more accurate than the old one.

As of early 1998, the Food and Drug Administration (FDA) no longer does premarket [510(K)] evaluations to "clear" automated or manual phenotypic identification systems, nor does it receive or approve quality control protocols from these devices to meet the 1988 Clinical Laboratory Improvement Amendment requirements. Laboratorians must be aware that the identification component of the new or modified system that they are using is not cleared by the FDA because this approval is no longer required. This makes it even more important for laboratorians to search the literature for valid evaluations of their chosen instrument and to conduct their own in-house validation to make sure that the instrument meets the claims of the manufacturer regarding identification.

TABLE 5 Database entries of the *Enterobacteriaceae* (human isolates) manual systems

Organism	API 20E, version 4.0	BBL Crystal E/NF, version 4.0	RapID ONE, version 1.93	Microbact 24E[e]	MIDI, version 5.0
Budvicia aquatica				×	
Buttiauxella agrestis	×			×	
Cedecea davisae	×	×	×	×	
Cedecea lapagei	×	×	×	×	
Cedecea neteri		×	×	×	
Cedecea sp. 3			×	×	
Cedecea sp. 5			×	×	
Citrobacter amalonaticus	× (*Citrobacter koseri*)[a]	×	×	×	×
Citrobacter braakii	×			×	×
Citrobacter farmeri	× (*Citrobacter koseri*)			×	×
Citrobacter freundii	×	×	×	×	×
Citrobacter gillenii					
Citrobacter koseri	× (*Citrobacter amalonaticus*)	×	×	×	×
Citrobacter murliniae					
Citrobacter sedlakii				×	
Citrobacter werkmanii				×	
Citrobacter youngae	×			×	
Edwardsiella hoshinae	×	×	×	×	
Edwardsiella ictaluri				×	
Edwardsiella tarda	×	×	×	×	×
Enterobacter aerogenes	×	×	×	×	×
Enterobacter amnigenus group 1	×		×		
Enterobacter amnigenus group 2	×				
Enterobacter asburiae	×	×	×		
Enterobacter cancerogenus	×	× (*Enterobacter taylorae*)[c]	×		×
Enterobacter cloacae	×	×	×	×	×
Enterobacter gergoviae	×	×	×	×	×
Enterobacter hormaechei					
Enterobacter intermedius	×		×		×
Enterobacter sakazakii	×	×	×	×	×
Escherichia coli	×	×[d] (O111, O157)	×	×	×
Escherichia fergusonii	×	×	×		
Escherichia hermannii	×	×	×		×
Escherichia vulneris	×	×	×	×	×
Ewingella americana	×	×	×	×	
Hafnia alvei	×	×	×	×	×
Klebsiella oxytoca	×	×	×	×	×
Klebsiella planticola			×	×	
Klebsiella pneumoniae subsp. *ozaenae*	×	×	×	×	×
Klebsiella pneumoniae subsp. *pneumoniae*	×	×	×	×	×
Klebsiella pneumoniae subsp. *rhinoscleromatis*	×	×	×	×	×
Klebsiella terrigena	×			×	×
Kluyvera ascorbata	#[b]	×	×	×	×

(*Continued on next page*)

TABLE 5 Database entries of the *Enterobacteriaceae* (human isolates) manual systems *(Continued)*

Organism	API 20E, version 4.0	BBL Crystal E/NF, version 4.0	RapID ONE, version 1.93	Microbact 24E[e]	MIDI, version 5.0
Kluyvera cryocrescens	#[b]	×	×	×	×
Leclercia adecarboxylata	×	×	×	×	×
Leminorella grimontii			×	×	
Leminorella richardii			×	×	
Moellerella wisconsensis	×	×	×	×	
Morganella morganii	×	×	×	×	×
Pantoea agglomerans	#[b]	×	×		×
Pantoea dispersa	#[b]				
Proteus mirabilis	×	×		×	×
Proteus penneri	×	×	×	×	×
Proteus vulgaris	×	×	×	×	×
Providencia alcalifaciens	× (*Providencia rustigianii*)	×	×	×	×
Providencia heimbachae				×	×
Providencia rettgeri	×	×	×	×	×
Providencia rustigianii	× (*Providencia alcalifaciens*)	×	×	×	×
Providencia stuartii	×	×	×	×	×
Rahnella aquatilis	×	×	×	×	×
Raoultella ornithinolytica	× (*Klebsiella*)[c]	× (*Klebsiella*)[c]	× (*Klebsiella*)[c]	× (*Klebsiella*)[c]	
Salmonella	× (six groups)	× (four groups)	× (seven groups)	× (eight groups)	× (four groups)
Serratia ficaria	×	×		×	
Serratia fonticola	×	×		×	×
Serratia liquefaciens	×	×	×	×	×
Serratia marcescens	×	×	×	×	×
Serratia odorifera group 1	×	×	×	×	×
Serratia odorifera group 2	×	×	×	×	
Serratia plymuthica	×	×	×	×	×
Serratia rubidaea	×	×	×	×	×
Shigella sp.	× (*Shigella sonnei*)	× (two groups)	#[b] (*Shigella sonnei*)	× (two groups)	× (six groups)
Tatumella ptyseos		×	×	×	
Yersinia enterocolitica	×	× (group)[f]	×	×	×
Yersinia frederiksenii	× (*Yersinia intermedia*)		×	×	×
Yersinia intermedia	× (*Yersinia frederiksenii*)		×	×	×
Yersinia kristensenii	×		×	×	×
Yersinia pestis	×			×	×
Yersinia pseudotuberculosis	×	×	×	×	×
Yersinia ruckeri				×	
Yokenella regensburgei		×	×	×	

[a] Some products give a choice between two species; the alternate species is indicated in parentheses.
[b] #, genus-level identification only.
[c] Previous taxonomic designation.
[d] Able to differentiate O111 from O157.
[e] Also contains 10 unnamed enteric groups in the database.
[f] "Group" indicates *Yersinia* group.

TABLE 6 Database entries of the *Enterobacteriaceae* (human isolates) for automated systems[a]

Organism	Vitek GNI+, version 10.01	Vitek 2 GN, version 4.01	Dade Behring MicroScan		MicroLog, version 6.01/6.02	Sensititre, version 2.6	Phoenix
			Conventional LabPro, version 1.6	Rapid LabPro, version 1.6			
Budvicia aquatica	×				×		
Buttiauxella agrestis		×			×		
Cedecea davisae	×	×	×	×	×	×	×
Cedecea lapagei	×	×	×	×	×	×	×
Cedecea neteri			×	×	×	×	×
Cedecea sp. 3			×	"3/5"			
Cedecea sp. 5			×	"3/5"			
Citrobacter amalonaticus	×	×	×	×	×	×	×
Citrobacter braakii	×	×		× (*Citrobacter braaki/ freundii/sedlakii*)	×		×
Citrobacter farmeri		×		×	×		×
Citrobacter freundii	×	×	×	× (*Citrobacter braaki/ freundii/sedlakii*)	×	×	×
Citrobacter gillenii					×		
Citrobacter koseri	×	×	×	×	×	×	×
Citrobacter murliniae					×		
Citrobacter sedlakii		×		× (*Citrobacter braaki/ freundii/sedlakii*)	×		×
Citrobacter werkmanii				× (*Citrobacter werkmanii/ C. youngae*)	×		×
Citrobacter youngae		×		× (*Citrobacter werkmanii/ C. youngae*)	×		×
Edwardsiella hoshinae	×	×		×	×	×	×
Edwardsiella ictaluri					×	×	×
Edwardsiella tarda	×	×	×	×	×	×	×
Enterobacter aerogenes	×	×	×	×	×	×	×
Enterobacter amnigenus group 1	×	×	×	×	×	×	×
Enterobacter amnigenus group 2	×	×	×	×			×
Enterobacter asburiae		×	×	×	×	×	×
Enterobacter cancerogenus	×	×	×	×	×	×	×
Enterobacter cloacae	×	×	×	×	×	×	×
Enterobacter gergoviae	×	×	×	×	×	×	×
Enterobacter hormaechei	×			×	×		×
Enterobacter intermedius	×	×	×	×	×	×	×
Enterobacter sakazakii	×	×	×	×	×	×	×
Escherichia coli	×	× (O157)[b]	×	× (O157:H7)[b]	×	×	×
Escherichia fergusonii	×	×	×	×	×		×
Escherichia hermannii	×	×	×	×	×	×	×
Escherichia vulneris	×	×	×	×	×	×	×
Ewingella americana	×	×	×	×	×	×	×
Hafnia alvei	×	×	×	×	×	×	×

(*Continued on next page*)

TABLE 6 Database entries of the *Enterobacteriaceae* (human isolates) for automated systems[a] *(Continued)*

Organism	Vitek GNI+, version 10.01	Vitek 2 GN, version 4.01	Dade Behring MicroScan		MicroLog, version 6.01/6.02	Sensititre, version 2.6	Phoenix
			Conventional LabPro, version 1.6	Rapid LabPro, version 1.6			
Klebsiella oxytoca	× (*Klebsiella pneumoniae*)	×	×	×	×	×	×
Klebsiella pneumoniae subsp. *ozaenae*	×	×	×	×	×	×	×
Klebsiella pneumoniae subsp. *pneumoniae*		×	×	×	×	×	×
Klebsiella pneumoniae subsp. *rhinoscleromatis*	×	×	×	×	×	×	×
Kluyvera ascorbata	#[c]	×	×	#	×	×	×
Kluyvera cryocrescens	#	×	×	#	×	×	×
Leclercia adecarboxylata	×	×	×	×	×	×	×
Leminorella grimontii			#	#	×	#	×
Leminorella richardii			#	#	×	#	×
Moellerella wisconsensis	×	×	×	×	×	×	×
Morganella morganii		×	×	×	×	×	×
Pantoea agglomerans	×	×	× (*Enterobacter agglomerans*)	× (*Enterobacter agglomerans*)	×	×	×
Pantoea dispersa					×		
Pragia fontium					×		×
Proteus mirabilis	×	×	×	×	×	×	×
Proteus penneri	× (*Proteus vulgaris*)	× (*Proteus vulgaris*)	×	×	× (*Proteus vulgaris*)	×	×
Proteus vulgaris	× (*Proteus penneri*)	× (*Proteus penneri*)	×	×	× (*Proteus penneri*)	×	×
Providencia alcalifaciens	×	×	×	×	×	×	×
Providencia heimbachae					×		
Providencia rettgeri	×	×	×	×	×	×	×
Providencia rustigianii		×	×	×	×		×
Providencia stuartii	×	×	×	×	×	×	×
Rahnella aquatilis	×	×			×		×
Raoultella ornithinolytica	×	×	×	×	× (*Raoultella planticola*)		×
Raoultella planticola					× (*Raoultella ornithinolytica*)	×	
Raoultella terrigena					×	×	
Salmonella	#[a] and *Salmonella enterica* serovar Typhi	× (five groups)	× (four groups)	× (four groups)	× (twelve groups)	× (thirteen groups)	× (seven groups)
Serratia ficaria		×		×	×		×
Serratia fonticola	×	×	×	×	×	×	×
Serratia liquefaciens	×	×	×	×	× (*Serratia grimesii*)	×	×
Serratia marcescens	×	×	×	×	×	×	×
Serratia odorifera group 1	×	×	×	×	×	×	×
Serratia odorifera group 2			×	×			×

Serratia plymuthica	×	×	×	×	×	×	×
Serratia rubidaea	×	×	×	×	×	×	×
Shigella sp.	× (four groups)	× (two groups)	× (*Shigella sonnei*), #	× (*Shigella sonnei*) #	× (four groups)	× (four groups)	× (four groups)
Tatumella ptyseos			×	×	×	×	×
Trabulsiella guamensis					×		
Yersinia enterocolitica	×	×	× (group)[d]	× (group)	×	×	×
Yersinia frederiksenii	×		× (group)	× (group)	×	×	×
Yersinia intermedia	×		× (group)	× (group)	×	×	×
Yersinia kristensenii	×		× (group)	× (group)	×	×	×
Yersinia pestis	×	×	×	×	×	×	
Yersinia pseudotuberculosis	×	×	×	×	×	×	×
Yersinia ruckeri		×	×	×	×		×
Yokenella regensburgi	×	×	×	×	×	×	×

[a] Some products give a choice between two or more species; the alternate species is in parentheses.
[b] Includes the ability to differentiate between serogroups O111 and O157.
[c] #, genus designation only.
[d] "Group" indicates *Yersinia* group.

Devices and methods incorporating probes, nucleic acid amplification, and other genetic methods, as well as the susceptibility test component of commercial instruments, will continue to be reviewed by the FDA for clearance.

LIMITATIONS OF MICROORGANISM IDENTIFICATION SYSTEMS

The databases of microbial identification systems must be revised frequently to accommodate newly named species. For example, had *Enterobacter sakazakii* (the yellow-pigmented variant of *Enterobacter cloacae*) not been added to the databases of these instruments, the clinical correlation of *E. sakazakii* with neonatal meningitis would likely be obscured if only *E. cloacae* was reported. Laboratorians must be aware that the accuracy of a system is limited to the claims of the manufacturer for the version of the database currently in the instrument and that the database may be outdated.

The laboratory procedure manual must stipulate the action to be taken when a result is questionable either because of the unusual biochemical profile of the organism or because of the appearance of an unexpected susceptibility profile. A backup method must be used to achieve an accurate identification profile. Otherwise the isolate should be sent to a reference laboratory for analysis.

The biochemical properties of closely related species may make it difficult or impossible for the algorithms of the identification process to separate these organisms accurately; however, the inability to distinguish all species within a genus does not always have a negative effect on patient outcome. For example, accurate identification of all of the newly recognized *Citrobacter* species may not be possible for some of the systems. In this case, the effect on patient outcome because of the inability of a system to recognize *Citrobacter werkmanii* may be negligible, and a simple report of "*Citrobacter* species" may provide adequate data for patient management. Where such distinctions may be critical is in the recognition of a potential agent of bioterrorism. This has implications not only for the individual patient, but also for public health. Although some commercial systems have these organisms in their databases (Table 9), the inability to identify members of some of the genera to the species level (e.g., *Yersinia* spp.) makes these systems unreliable for identification (36). Users of these systems should be aware of the limitations of commercial products with respect to their biopreparedness plans and substitute other tests for presumptive diagnosis per recommended guidelines (1). Suspicious pathogens should be referred to a public health or other reference laboratory for definitive identification. Table 9 summarizes the agents of bioterrorism included in the databases of the more frequently used identification systems.

As pathogens continue to evolve and taxonomic classifications are revised, laboratorians must pay attention to the manufacturer's communications about products, such as letters, notices, or test exclusions regarding the accuracy of their methods, as well as the published literature describing the potential problems encountered by others using these identification systems. Likewise, the user has a responsibility to report continued problems with a system or product where poor performance may lead to adverse patient outcomes.

TABLE 7 Database entries of the gram-positive organisms (human isolates) for bioMerieux and Dade MicroScan products[b]

Organism	API		VITEK GPI, version 10.01	VITEK 2 GP, version 4.01	MicroScan	
	Staph, version 4.0	20 Strep, version 6.0			Conventional Pos ID, LabPro version 1.6	Rapid Pos ID, LabPro version 1.6
Listeria monocytogenes		×	#[a]	×	×	×
Micrococcaceae						
Kocuria (Micrococcus) kristinae	×			×	×	×
Micrococcus luteus	*Micrococcus* species			× (*Micrococcus lylae*)	*Micrococcus* species	*Micrococcus* species
Micrococcus lylae				× (*Micrococcus luteus*)	*Micrococcus* species	*Micrococcus* species
Kocuria (Micrococcus) rosea	× (*Micrococcus varians*)			×	*Micrococcus* species	×
Kocuria varians	× (*Micrococcus rosea*)			×	*Micrococcus* species	*Micrococcus* species
Micrococcus sedentarius					*Micrococcus* species	*Micrococcus* species
Rothia dentocariosa						
Rothia mucilaginosa				×		
Staphylococcus arlettae				×		×
Staphylococcus aureus	×		×	×	×	×
Staphylococcus auricularis	×		×	×	×	×
Staphylococcus capitis subsp. *capitis*	×		×	×	×	×
Staphylococcus capitis subsp. *ureolyticus*					×	
Staphylococcus caprae	×			×		×
Staphylococcus carnosus	×			×		×
Staphylococcus caseolyticus						
Staphylococcus chromogenes	×					× (*Staphylococcus hyicus*)
Staphylococcus cohnii subsp. *cohnii*	×		×	×	×	×
Staphylococcus cohnii subsp. *urealyticum*	×			×	×	
Staphylococcus epidermidis	×		×	×	×	×
Staphylococcus equorum				×		×
Staphylococcus felis						
Staphylococcus gallinarum				×		×
Staphylococcus haemolyticus	×		×	×	×	×
Staphylococcus hominis subsp. *hominis*	×		×	×	×	×
Staphylococcus hominis subsp. *novobiosepticus*					×	
Staphylococcus hyicus	×		×	×	×	× (*Staphylococcus chromogenes*)
Staphylococcus intermedius			×	×	×	×
Staphylococcus kloosii				×		×
Staphylococcus lentus	×		×	×		×
Staphylococcus lugdunensis	×			×	×	×
Staphylococcus pasteuri						
Staphylococcus saccharolyticus						

Staphylococcus saprophyticus	×		×	×	×	×
Staphylococcus schleiferi	×			×	×	×
Staphylococcus sciuri	×		×	×	×	×
Staphylococcus simulans	×		×	×	×	×
Staphylococcus vitulinus				×		
Staphylococcus warneri	×		×	×	×	×
Staphylococcus xylosus	×		×	×	×	×
Streptococcaceae						
Abiotrophia adiacens		×				
Abiotrophis defectiva		×	×	×		
Aerococcus urinae			×	×		
Aerococcus viridans		×	×	×	×	×
Alloiococcus otitidis			×	×		
Dermacoccus nishinomiyaensis			×	×		
Enterococcus avium		×	×	×	×	×
Enterococcus casseliflavus			×	×	×	×
Enterococcus durans		×	×	×	× (*Enterococcus hirae*)	×
Enterococcus faecalis		×	×	×	×	×
Enterococcus faecium		×	×	×	×	×
Enterococcus gallinarum		×	×	×	×	
Enterococcus hirae				×	× (*Enterococcus durans*)	
Enterococcus malodoratus						
Enterococcus raffinosus					×	
Facklamia hominis						
Gemella haemolysans		×		×		
Gemella morbillorum		×	×	×		×
Globicatella sanguinis				×		
Granulicatella sp.						
Helcoccus kunzii				×		
Lactococcus species		×		×		
Leuconostoc species		×		×	×	
Pediococcus species				×	×	
Streptococcus acidominimus		×	×			
Streptococcus agalactiae		×	×	×	×	×
Streptococcus anginosus			×	×		
Streptococcus β-hemolytic non-A, non-B					×	
Streptococcus bovis		×	×		×	×
Streptococcus constellatus			×	×		
Streptococcus criceti						
Streptococcus cremoris/thermophilus						
Streptococcus cristatus			×			
Streptococcus dysgalactiae/subsp. *dysgalactiae*/subsp. *equisimilis equisimilis*		×	×	×		

(*Continued on next page*)

TABLE 7 Database entries of the gram-positive organisms (human isolates) for bioMerieux and Dade MicroScan products[b] *(Continued)*

Organism	API		VITEK GPI, version 10.01	VITEK 2 GP, version 4.01	MicroScan	
	Staph, version 4.0	20 Strep, version 6.0			Conventional Pos ID, LabPro version 1.6	Rapid Pos ID, LabPro version 1.6
Streptococcus equi subsp. *equi*		×	×	×		× (*Streptococcus equisimilis*)
Streptococcus equi subsp. *zooepidemicus*						×
Streptococcus equinus		×	×	×		×
Streptococcus gordonii			× (*Streptococcus sanguis*)			
Streptococcus groups E, G, L, P, and U		×	× Group G			
Streptococcus intermedius		×	×	×		
Streptococcus lactis/diacetylacis						
Streptococcus milleri group			×		×	×
Streptococcus mitis group		×	×	×	×	×
Streptococcus mutans		×	×	×	×	×
Streptococcus oralis		×	×	× (*Streptococcus mitis*)		
Streptococcus parasanguis				×		
Streptococcus pneumoniae		×	×	×	×	×
Streptococcus porcinus		×		×		
Streptococcus pyogenes		×	×	×	×	×
Streptococcus salivarius		×	×	×	×	×
Streptococcus sanguinis			×	×		
Streptococcus sanguis		×	×		×	×
Streptococcus sobrinus				×		
Streptococcus uberis		×	×	×		
Streptococcus vestibularis				×		
Vagococcus fluvialis				×		
Weissella confusus						

[a] #, genus identification only.
[b] Some products give a choice between two species; the alternate species is in parentheses.

TABLE 8 Database entries of the gram-positive organisms for BD Diagnostics, Remel, TREK, Biolog, and MIDI products[c]

Organism	BBL Crystal		Remel RapID STR	Oxoid Microbact Staph 12S	TREK Sensititre GPID	Biolog GP2 version 6.11/6.12	MIDI version 5.0	BD Diagnostics Phoenix-100 GPID PMIC/II-100
	Gram-Pos ID	Rapid Gram-Pos ID						
Listeria species	× (four species)	× (three species)	× (*Listeria monocytogenes*)	*[a]	× (four species)	× (seven species)	× (five species)	× (five species)
Micrococcaceae								
Kocuria (Micrococcus) kristinae	#[b]	× (*Micrococcus*)			×	×	×	×
Kocuria (Micrococcus) rosea	#	× (*Micrococcus*)			×	×	×	×
Kocuria varians						×	×	×
Kytococcus sedentarius	#				×	×		×
Macrococcus (Staphylococcus) caseolyticus						×	×	×
Micrococcus luteus	#	×			×	×	×	×
Micrococcus lylae	#				×	×	×	×
Rothia dentocariosa	×					×	×	
Rothia mucilaginosus	× (*Stomatococcus*)	× (*Stomatococcus*)				×	×	×
Staphylococcus arlettae						×	×	
Staphylococcus aureus	×	×		×	×	×	×	×
Staphylococcus auricularis	×			×		×	×	×
Staphylococcus capitis subsp. *capitis*	×			×	×	×	×	×
Staphylococcus capitis subsp. *ureolyticus*	×			×				×
Staphylococcus caprae	×			×		×		×
Staphylococcus carnosus	×			×		×	×	×
Staphylococcus chromogenes				×		×	×	×
Staphylococcus cohnii subsp. *cohnii*	×			×		×	×	×
Staphylococcus cohnii subsp. *urealyticum*	×			×				×
Staphylococcus epidermidis	×	×		×	×	×	×	×
Staphylococcus equorum	×					×	×	×
Staphylococcus felis	×					×		×
Staphylococcus gallinarum	×	×				×	×	×
Staphylococcus haemolyticus	×	×		×	×	×	×	×
Staphylococcus hominis subsp. *hominis*	×	×		×	×	×	×	×
Staphylococcus hominis subsp. *novobiosepticus*						×		×
Staphylococcus hyicus				×	×	×	×	×
Staphylococcus intermedius	×	×		×	×	×	×	×
Staphylococcus kloosii	×					×	×	×

(Continued on next page)

TABLE 8 Database entries of the gram-positive organisms for BD Dianostics, Remel, TREK, Biolog, and MIDI products[c] *(Continued)*

Organism	BBL Crystal		Remel RapID STR	Oxoid Microbact Staph 12S	TREK Sensititre GPID	Biolog CP2 version 6.11/6.12	MIDI version 5.0	BD Diagnostics Phoenix-100 GPID PMIC/II-100
	Gram-Pos ID	Rapid Gram-Pos ID						
Staphylococcus lentus	×	×		×		×	×	×
Staphylococcus lugdunensis	×	×		×		×	×	×
Staphylococcus pasteuri	×					×		×
Staphylococcus saccharolyticus	×	×						×
Staphylococcus saprophyticus	×	×		×	×	×	×	×
Staphylococcus schleiferi	× (two subspecies)					×	×	× (two subspecies)
Staphylococcus sciuri	×	×		×		×	×	×
Staphylococcus simulans	×	×		×		×	×	×
Staphylococcus vitulinus	×							×
Staphylococcus warneri	×	×		×	×	×	×	×
Staphylococcus xylosus	×	×		×	×	×	×	×
Streptococcaceae								
Abiotrophia species								
Aerococcus urinae	×					×		×
Aerococcus viridans	×	×	#		×	×	×	×
Alloiococcus otitidis	×					×		×
Dermacoccus nishinomiyaensis						×		×
Enterococcus avium	×	×	×		×	×	×	×
Enterococcus casseliflavus	× (*Enterococcus gallinarum*)	× (*Enterococcus gallinarum*)	× (*Enterococcus mundtii*)			×	×	×
Enterococcus cecorum						×	×	
Enterococcus columbae						×	×	
Enterococcus durans	×	×	× (*Enterococcus hirae*)		×	×	×	×
Enterococcus faecalis	×	×	×		×	×	×	×
Enterococcus faecium	×	×	×		×	×	×	×
Enterococcus gallinarum	× (*Enterococcus casseliflavus*)	× (*Enterococcus casseliflavus*)	×			×	×	×
Enterococcus hirae	×		× (*Enterococcus durans*)			×	×	×
Enterococcus malodoratus			×			×	×	
Enterococcus mundtii						×	×	
Enterococcus raffinosus	×	×	×			×		×
Enterococcus solitarius	×					×		
Gemella haemolysans	×	×			×	× (*Gemella morbillorum*)	×	×
Gemella morbillorum	×	×	×			× (*Gemella haemolysans*)		×
Globicatella sanguinis	×					×		×

Helcoccus kunzii	×				×		×
Lactococcus species	× (five species)	× (four species)			× (seven species)		× (six species)
Leuconostoc species	× (four species)	× (three species)	× (three species)		× (eight species)		× (five species)
Pediococcus species	× (three species)	× (three species)	× (two species)		× (five species)	× (one species)	× (five species)
Streptococcus acidominimus	×	×	×		×		×
Streptococcus agalactiae	×	×	×	×	×	×	×
Streptococcus anginosus	×	×	×	×	×	×	×
Streptococcus bovis	× (bovis I and II)	× (bovis I and II)	×	×	×	×	
Streptococcus constellatus	×	×	×	×	×		×
Streptococcus cricetus	×	×			×		
Streptococcus cristatus	×				×		×
Streptococcus crista	× (included in *Streptococcus sanguis* group)	×					×
Streptococcus dysgalactiae/ subsp. *dysgalactiae*/ subsp. *equisimilis*				×	×		×
Streptococcus equi subsp. *equi*/ subsp. *zooepidemicus*	×	×	Group C streptococcus	×	×	×	×
Streptococcus equinus	×	×	×		×	×	×
Streptococcus gordonii	×	×	× (*Streptococcus sanguis*)		×	×	×
Streptococcus intermedius	×	×	×		×	×	×
Streptococcus milleri group	×	×		×			
Streptococcus mitis	×	×	×	×	×	×	×
Streptococcus mutans	×	×	×	×	× (*Streptococcus ratti*)	×	×
Streptococcus oralis	×	×			×	×	×
Streptococcus parasanguis	×				×	×	×
Streptococcus pneumoniae	×	×		×	×	×	×
Streptococcus porcinus	×				×	×	×
Streptococcus pyogenes	×	×	×	×	×	×	×
Streptococcus salivarius	×	×	× (*Streptococcus vestibularis*)	×	×	×	×
Streptococcus sanguinis					×		×
Streptococcus sanguis	×	×	× (*Streptococcus gordonii*)	×		×	
Streptococcus sobrinus	×	×			×	×	×
Streptococcus uberis	×	×		×	×	×	×
Streptococcus vestibularis	×	×	× (*Streptococcus salivarius*)		×	×	×
Weisella confusus			×				

[a] Oxoid has a similar product for *Listeria* identification called the Listeria Identification System 12 S. It identifies six species.
[b] #, Genus-level identification only.
[c] Some products give a choice between two species; the alternate species is indicated in parentheses.

TABLE 9 Database entries for highly pathogenic organisms for select assays or systems

System	Category A agents				Category B agents					
	Bacillus anthracis	*Yersinia pestis*	*Francisella tularensis*	*Brucella* sp.	*Salmonella*	*Shigella*	Shiga toxin-producing *Escherichia coli*	*Burkholderia mallei*	*Burkholderia pseudomallei*	*Vibrio cholerae*
API 20 E and NE		×			×	×				×
BBL Crystal E/NF					×	×	× (O157, O111)[c]		×	×
GNI+ (Vitek)		×			×	×		×	×	×
GN (Vitek 2)		×	×	×	×	×	× (O157)[c]	×	×	×
MicroLog[a]	×	×	×	×	×	×	× (O157)[c]	×	×	×
Microbact 24E		×			×	×			×	×
MicroScan Conventional		×			×	×			×	×
MicroScan Rapid		×			×	×				×
MIDI (BTR2.0)[a,b]	×	×	×	×	×	×		×	×	×
Phoenix GNID					×	×				×
Sensititre		×			×	×				×

[a] This commercial system has a dangerous-pathogens database.
[b] The MIDI system has been awarded "official methods status" for confirmatory identification of *Bacillus anthracis* (59).
[c] Systems are able to presumptively identify these serotypes.

We thank the various companies that provided current and detailed information about their products.

REFERENCES

1. **American Society for Microbiology.** 11 December 2003, posting date. *Sentinel Laboratory Guidelines for Suspected Agents of Bioterrorism: Clinical Laboratory Bioterrorism Readiness Plan.* [Online.] American Society for Microbiology, Washington, D.C. http://www.asm.org/ASM/ files/LEFTMARGINHEADERLIST/downloadfilename/0000001204/BTtemplate.pdf.
2. **Aronson, M. D., and D. F. Bor.** 1987. Blood cultures. *Ann. Intern. Med.* **106:**246–253.
3. **Auckenthaler, R., D. M. Ilstrup, and J. A. Washington II.** 1982. Comparison of recovery of organisms from blood cultures diluted 10% (volume/volume) and 20% (volume/volume). *J. Clin. Microbiol.* **15:**860–864.
4. **Barenfanger, J., C. Drake, J. Lawhorn, and S. J. Verhuist.** 2004. Comparison of chlorhexidine and tincture of iodine for skin antisepsis in preparation for blood sample collection. *J. Clin. Microbiol.* **37:**1415–1418.
5. **Baron, E. J., M. P. Weinstein, W. M. Dunne, Jr., P. Yagupsky, D. F. Welch, and D. M. Wilson.** 2005. *Cumitech 1C, Blood Cultures IV*. Coordinating ed., E. J. Baron. ASM Press, Washington, D.C.
6. **Bates, D. W., L. Goldman, and T. H. Lee.** 1991. Contaminant blood cultures and resources utilization: the true consequences of false-positive results. *JAMA* **265:**365–369.
7. **Bennett, I. L., Jr., and P. B. Beeson.** 1954. Bacteremia: a consideration of some experimental and clinical aspects. *Yale J. Biol. Med.* **26:**241–262.
8. **Bourbeau, P. P., and J. K. Pohlman.** 2001. Three days of incubation may be sufficient for routine blood cultures with BacT/ALERT FAN blood culture bottles. *J. Clin. Microbiol.* **39:**2079–2082.
9. **Brenner, S. A., J. A. Rooney, P. Manzewitsch, and R. L. Regnery.** 1997. Isolation of *Bartonella* (*Rochalimaea*) *henselae*: effects of methods of blood collection and handling. *J. Clin. Microbiol.* **35:**544–547.
10. **Bryan, L. E.** 1981. Comparison of a slide blood culture system with a supplemented peptone broth culture method. *J. Clin. Microbiol.* **14:**389–392.
11. **Bryant, J. K., and C. L. Strand.** 1987. Reliability of blood cultures collected from intravascular catheter versus venipuncture. *Am. J. Clin. Pathol.* **88:**113–116.
12. **Cockerill, F. R., J. W. Wilson, E. A. Vetter, K. M. Goodman, C. A. Torgerson, W. S. Harmsen, C. D. Schleck, D. M. Ilstrup, J. A. Washington II, and W. R. Wilson.** 2004. Optimal testing parameters for blood cultures. *Clin. Infect. Dis.* **38:**1724–1730.
13. **D'Amato, R. F., B. Holmes, and E. J. Bottone.** 1981. The systems approach to diagnostic microbiology. *Crit. Rev. Microbiol.* **9:**1–44.
14. **Doern, G. V., A. B. Brueggemann, W. M. Dunne, S. G. Jenkins, D. C. Halstead, and J. C. McLaughlin.** 1997. Four-day incubation period for blood culture bottles processed with the Difco ESP blood culture system. *J. Clin. Microbiol.* **35:**1290–1292.
15. **Doern, G. V., A. Barton, and S. Rao.** 1998. Controlled comparative evaluation of BacT/ALERT FAN and ESP 80A aerobic media as means for detecting bacteremia and fungemia. *J. Clin. Microbiol.* **36:**2686–2689.
16. **Donay, J. L., D. Mathieu, P. Fernandes, C. Pregermain, P. Bruel, A. Wargnier, I. Casin, F. X. Weill, P. H. Lagrange, and J. L. Herrmann.** 2004. Evaluation of the automated Phoenix system for potential routine use in the clininical microbiology laboratory. *J. Clin. Microbiol.* **42:**1542–1546.

17. **Dorsher, C. W., J. E. Rosenblatt, W. R. Wilson, and D. M. Ilstrup.** 1991. Anaerobic bacteremia: decreasing rate over a 15 year period. *Rev. Infect. Dis.* **13:**633–636.
18. **Edberg, S. C., and L. S. Konowe.** 1982. A systematic means to conduct a microbiology evaluation, p. 268–299. *In* V. Lorian (ed.), *Significance of Medical Microbiology in the Care of Patients*, 2nd ed. The Williams & Wilkins Co., Baltimore, Md.
19. **Eng, J.** 1975. Effect of sodium polyanethol sulfonate in blood cultures. *J. Clin. Microbiol.* **1:**119–123.
20. **Evans, M. R., A. L. Truant, J. Kostman, and L. Locke.** 1991. The detection of positive blood cultures by the BACTEC NR660: the clinical importance of four-day versus seven-day testing. *Diagn. Microbiol. Infect. Dis.* **14:** 107–110.
21. **Federal Register.** 1992. Clinical Laboratory Improvement Amendments of 1988, final rule. *Fed. Regist.* **57:**7164.
22. **Fuller, D. D., and T. E. Davis.** 1997. Comparison of BACTEC Plus Aerobic/F, Anaerobic/F, Peds Plus/F, and Lytic/F media with and without fastidious organism supplement to conventional methods for culture of sterile body fluids. *Diagn. Microbiol. Infect. Dis.* **29:**219–225.
23. **Hall, M. M., D. M. Ilstrup, and J. A. Washington II.** 1976. Effect of volume of blood cultured on detection of bacteremia. *J. Clin. Microbiol.* **3:**643–645.
24. **Han, X. Y., and A. L. Truant.** 1999. The detection of positive blood cultures by the AccuMed ESP-384 system: the clinical significance of three-day testing. *Diagn. Microbiol. Infect. Dis.* **33:**1–6.
25. **Hardy, D. J., B. B. Hulbert, and P. C. Migneault.** 1992. Time to detection of positive BacT/ALERT blood cultures and lack of need for routine subculture of 5- to 7-day negative cultures. *J. Clin. Microbiol.* **30:**2743–2745.
26. **Hartman, P. A.** 1968. *Miniaturized Microbiological Methods.* Academic Press, Inc., New York, N.Y.
27. **Hawkins, B. L., E. M. Peterson, and L. M. de la Maza.** 1986. Improvement of positive blood culture detection by agitation. *Diagn. Microbiol. Infect. Dis.* **5:**207–213.
28. **Henry, N. K., C. M. Grewell, P. E. Van Grevenhof, D. M. Ilstrup, and J. A. Washington II.** 1984. Comparison of lysis-centrifugation with a biphasic blood culture medium for the recovery of aerobic and facultatively anaerobic bacteria. *J. Clin. Microbiol.* **20:**413–416.
29. **Henry, N. K., C. A. McLimans, A. J. Wright, R. L. Thompson, W. R. Wilson, and J. A. Washington II.** 1983. Microbiological and clinical evaluation of the Isolator lysis-centrifugation blood culture tube. *J. Clin. Microbiol.* **17:** 864–869.
30. **Ilstrup, D. M., and J. A. Washington II.** 1983. The importance of volume of blood cultures in the detection of bacteremia and fungemia. *Diagn. Microbiol. Infect. Dis.* **1:**107–110.
31. **Isaacman, D. J., R. B. Karasic, E. A. Reynolds, and S. I. Kost.** 1996. Effect of number of blood cultures and volume of blood on detection of bacteremia in children. *J. Pediatr.* **128:**190–195.
32. **Kellogg, J. A., J. P. Manzella, and D. A. Bankert.** 2000. Frequency of low-level bacteremia in children from birth to fifteen years of age. *J. Clin. Microbiol.* **38:**2181–2185.
33. **Kiehn, T. E., B. Wong, F. F. Edwards, and D. Armstrong.** 1983. Comparative recovery of bacteria and yeasts from lysis-centrifugation and a conventional blood culture system. *J. Clin. Microbiol.* **18:**300–304.
34. **King, T. C., and P. B. Price.** 1963. An evaluation of iodophors as skin antiseptics. *Surg. Gynecol. Obstet.* **116:**361–365.
35. **Li, J., J. J. Plorde, and L. G. Carlson.** 1994. Effects of volume and periodicity on blood cultures. *J. Clin. Microbiol.* **32:**2829–2831.
36. **Linde, H. J., H. Neubauer, H. Meyer, S. Aleksic, and N. Lehn.** 1999. Identification of *Yersinia* species by the Vitek GNI card. *J. Clin. Microbiol.* **37:**211–214.
37. **Little, J. R., P. R. Murray, P. Traynor, and E. Spitznagel.** 1999. A randomized trial of povidone-iodine compared with iodine tincture for venipuncture site disinfection: effects on rates of blood culture contamination. *Am. J. Med.* **107:**119–125.
38. **Lombardi, D. P., and N. C. Engleberg.** 1992. Anaerobic bacteremia: incidence, patient characteristics, and clinical significance. *Am. J. Med.* **92:**53–60.
39. **Masterson, K. C., and J. E. McGowan, Jr.** 1988. Detection of positive blood cultures by the BACTEC NR660: the clinical importance of five versus seven days of testing. *Am. J. Clin. Pathol.* **90:**91–94.
40. **McCurdy, B. W., B. L. Elder, S. A. Hansen, J. A. Kellogg, F. J. Marsik, and R. J. Zabransky.** 1997. *Cumitech 31, Verification and Validation of Procedures in the Clinical Microbiology Laboratory.* Coordinating ed., B. W. McCurdy. American Society for Microbiology, Washington, D.C.
41. **McDonald, L. C., J. Fune, L. D. Guido, M. P. Weinstein, L. G. Reimer, T. M. Flynn, M. L. Wilson, S. Mirrett, and L. B. Reller.** 1996. Clinical importance of the increased sensitivity of BacT/Alert FAN aerobic and anaerobic blood culture bottles. *J. Clin. Microbiol.* **34:**2180–2184.
42. **Miller, J. M.** 1991. Evaluating biochemical identification systems. *J. Clin. Microbiol.* **29:**1559–1561.
43. **Mimoz, O., A. Karim, A. Mercat, M. Cosseron, B. Falissard, F. Parker, C. Richard, K. Samii, and P. Nordmann.** 1999. Chlorhexidine compared with povidone-iodine as skin preparation before blood culture: a randomized, controlled trial. *Ann. Intern. Med.* **131:**834–837.
44. **Mirrett, S., M. P. Weinstein, L. G. Reimer, M. L. Wilson, and L. B. Reller.** 2001. Relevance of the number of positive bottles in determining clinical significance of coagulase-negative staphylococci in blood cultures. *J. Clin. Microbiol.* **39:**3279–3281.
45. **Morello, J. A., C. Leitsh, S. Nitz, J. W. Dyke, M. Andruszewski, G. Maier, W. Landau, and M. A. Beard.** 1994. Detection of bacteremia by Difco ESP blood culture system. *J. Clin. Microbiol.* **32:**811–818.
46. **Morris, A. J., M. L. Wilson, S. Mirrett, and L. B. Reller.** 1993. Rationale for selective use of anaerobic blood cultures. *J. Clin. Microbiol.* **31:**2110–2113.
47. **Murray, P. R., A. C. Niles, R. L. Heeren, M. M. Curren, L. E. James, and J. E. Hoppe-Bauer.** 1988. Comparative evaluation of the Oxoid Signal and Roche Septi-Chek blood culture systems. *J. Clin. Microbiol.* **26:**2526–2530.
48. **Murray, P. R., P. Traynor, and D. Hopson.** 1992. Critical assessment of blood culture techniques: analysis of recovery of obligate and facultative anaerobes, strict aerobic bacteria, and fungi in aerobic and anaerobic blood culture bottles. *J. Clin. Microbiol.* **30:**1462–1468.
49. **NCCLS.** 2002. *Evaluation of Qualitative Test Performance EP-12A.* NCCLS, Wayne, Pa.
50. **O'Hara, C. M.** 2005. Manual and automated instrumentation for identification of *Enterobacteriaceae* and other aerobic gram-negative bacilli. *Clin. Microbiol. Rev.* **18:** 147–162.
51. **Pfaller, M. A., T. K. Sibley, L. M. Westfall, J. E. Hoppe-Bauer, M. A. Keating, and P. R. Murray.** 1982. Clinical laboratory comparison of a slide blood culture system with a conventional broth system. *J. Clin. Microbiol.* **16:**525–530.
52. **Plorde, J. J., F. C. Tenover, and L. G. Carlson.** 1985. Specimen volume versus yield in the BACTEC blood culture system. *J. Clin. Microbiol.* **22:**292–295.
53. **Prag, J., M. Nir, J. Jensen, and M. Arpi.** 1991. Should aerobic blood cultures be shaken intermittently or continuously? *APMIS* **99:**1078–1082.

54. **Reimer, L. G., and L. B. Reller.** 1985. Effect of sodium polyanetholesulfate on the recovery of *Gardnerella vaginalis* from blood culture media. *J. Clin. Microbiol.* **21:** 686–688.
55. **Reimer, L. G., M. L. Wilson, and M. P. Weinstein.** 1997. Update on detection of bacteremia and fungemia. *Clin. Microbiol. Rev.* **10:**444–465.
56. **Reller, L. B., P. R. Murray, and J. D. MacLowry.** 1982. *Cumitech 1A, Blood Cultures II.* Coordinating ed., J. A. Washington II. American Society for Microbiology, Washington, D.C.
57. **Riley, J. A., B. J. Heiter, and P. P. Bourbeau.** 2003. Comparison of recovery of blood culture isolates from two BacT/ALERT FAN aerobic blood culture bottles with recovery from one FAN aerobic bottle and one FAN anaerobic bottle. *J. Clin. Microbiol.* **41:**1399–1403.
58. **Salventi, J. F., T. A. Davies, E. L. Randall, S. Whitaker, and J. R. Waters.** 1979. Effect of blood dilution on recovery of organisms from clinical blood cultures in medium containing sodium polyanethol sulfonate. *J. Clin. Microbiol.* **9:**248–252.
59. **Sasser, M., C. Kunitsky, G. Jackoway, et al.** 2005. Identification of *Bacillus anthracis* from culture using gas chromatographic analysis of fatty acid methyl esters. *J. AOAC Int.* **88:**178–181.
60. **Schiffman, R. B., C. L. Strand, F. A. Meier, and P. J. Howantiz.** 1998. Blood culture contamination: a College of American Pathologists Q-Probes study involving 640 institutions and 497,134 specimens from adults. *Arch. Pathol. Lab. Med.* **122:**216–221.
61. **Sharp, S. E., J. C. McLaughlin, J. M. Goodman, J. Moore, S. M. Spanes, D. W. Keller III, and R. J. Poppiti, Jr.** 1993. Clinical assessment of anaerobic isolates from blood cultures. *Diagn. Microbiol. Infect. Dis.* **17:**19–22.
62. **Simor, A. E., K. Scythes, H. Meaney, and M. Louie.** 2000. Evaluation of the Bac-T/ALERT microbial detection system with FAN aerobic and FAN anaerobic bottles for culturing normally sterile body fluids other than blood. *Diagn. Microbiol. Infect. Dis.* **37:**5–9.
63. **Smith, J. A., E. A. Bryce, J. H. Ngui-Yen, and F. J. Roberts.** 1995. Comparison of BACTEC 9240 and BacT/ALERT blood culture systems in an adult hospital. *J. Clin. Microbiol.* **33:**1905–1908.
64. **Stager, C. E., and J. R. Davis.** 1992. Automated systems for identification of microorganisms. *Clin. Microbiol. Rev.* **5:**302–327.
65. **Staneck, J. L., and S. Vincent.** 1981. Inhibition of *Neisseria gonorrhoeae* by sodium polyanetholesulfonate. *J. Clin. Microbiol.* **13:**463–467.
66. **Stefaniuk, E., A. Baraniak, M. Gniadkowski, and W. Hryniewicz.** 2003. Evaluation of the BD Phoenix automated identification and susceptibility testing system in clinical microbiology practice. *Eur. J. Clin. Microbiol.* **22:**479–485.
67. **Strand, C. L.** 1988. *Blood Cultures: Consensus Recommendations in 1988.* Microbiology no. MB 88-1 (MB-172). American Society for Clinical Pathologists Check Sample Continuing Education Program, American Society for Clinical Pathologists, Chicago, Ill.
68. **Strand, C. L., R. R. Wajsbort, and K. Sturmann.** 1993. Effect of iodophor vs. iodine tincture skin preparation on blood culture contamination rate. *JAMA* **269:** 1004–1006.
69. **Tenney, J. H., L. B. Reller, S. Mirrett, and W.-L. L. Wang.** 1982. Controlled evaluation of the volume of blood cultured in detection of bacteremia and fungemia. *J. Clin. Microbiol.* **15:**558–561.
70. **Washington, J. A., II.** 1975. Blood cultures: principles and techniques. *Mayo Clin. Proc.* **50:**91–98.
71. **Washington, J. A., II.** 1994. Collection, transport, and processing of blood cultures. *Clin. Lab. Med.* **14:**59–68.
72. **Washington, J. A., II, and D. M. Ilstrup.** 1986. Blood cultures: issues and controversies. *Rev. Infect. Dis.* **8:** 792–802.
73. **Weinbaum, F. I., S. Lavie, M. Danek, D. Sixsmith, G. F. Heinrich, and S. S. Mills.** 1997. Doing it right the first time: quality improvement and the contaminant blood culture. *J. Clin. Microbiol.* **35:**53–55.
74. **Weinstein, M. P.** 1996. Current blood culture methods and systems: clinical concepts, technology, and interpretation of results. *Clin. Infect. Dis.* **23:**40–46.
75. **Weinstein, M. P., S. Mirrett, L. G. Reimer, and L. B. Reller.** 1989. Effect of agitation and terminal subcultures on yield and speed of detection of the Oxoid Signal blood culture system versus the BACTEC radiometric system. *J. Clin. Microbiol.* **27:**427–430.
76. **Weinstein, M. P., S. Mirrett, L. G. Reimer, and L. B. Reller.** 1990. Effect of altered headspace atmosphere on yield and speed of detection of the Oxoid Signal blood culture system versus the BACTEC radiometric system. *J. Clin. Microbiol.* **28:**795–797.
77. **Weinstein, M. P., S. Mirrett, L. G. Reimer, M. L. Wilson, S. Smith-Elekes, C. R. Chuard, K. L. Joho, and L. B. Reller.** 1995. Controlled evaluation of BacT/ALERT standard aerobic and FAN aerobic blood culture bottles for detection of bacteremia and fungemia. *J. Clin. Microbiol.* **33:**978–981.
78. **Weinstein, M. P., S. Mirrett, and L. B. Reller.** 1988. Comparative evaluation of the Oxoid Signal and BACTEC radiometric blood culture systems for the detection of bacteremia and fungemia. *J. Clin. Microbiol.* **26:**962–964.
79. **Weinstein, M. P., and L. B. Reller.** 2001. Commercial blood culture systems and methods, p. 12–21. *In* A. Truant (ed.), *Manual of Commercial Methods in Clinical Microbiology.* American Society for Microbiology, Washington, D.C.
80. **Weinstein, M. P., L. B. Reller, S. Mirrett, C. W. Stratton, L. G. Reimer, and W.-L. L. Wang.** 1986. Controlled evaluation of the agar slide and radiometric blood culture systems for the detection of bacteremia and fungemia. *J. Clin. Microbiol.* **23:**221–225.
81. **Weinstein, M. P., L. B. Reller, S. Mirrett, W.-L. L. Wang, and D. V. Alcid.** 1985. Controlled evaluation of Trypticase soy broth in agar slide and conventional blood culture systems. *J. Clin. Microbiol.* **21:**626–629.
82. **Weinstein, M. P., L. B. Reller, S. Mirrett, W.-L. L. Wang, and D. V. Alcid.** 1985. Clinical comparison of an agar slide blood culture system with Trypticase soy broth and a conventional blood culture bottle with supplemented peptone broth. *J. Clin. Microbiol.* **21:**815–818.
83. **Weinstein, M. P., L. B. Reller, J. R. Murphy, and K. A. Lichtenstein.** 1983. The clinical significance of positive blood cultures: a comprehensive analysis of 500 episodes of bacteremia and fungemia in adults. I. Laboratory and epidemiologic observations. *Rev. Infect. Dis.* **5:**35–53.
84. **Weinstein, M. P., M. L. Towns, S. M. Quartey, S. Mirrett, L. G. Reimer, G. Parmagiani, and L. B. Reller.** 1997. The clinical significance of positive blood cultures in the 1990s: a prospective comprehensive evaluation of the microbiology, epidemiology, and outcome of bacteremia and fungemia in adults. *Clin. Infect. Dis.* **24:**584–602.
85. **Willcox, W. R., S. P. Lapage, S. Bascomb, and M. A. Curtis.** 1973. Identification of bacteria by computer: theory and programming. *J. Gen. Microbiol.* **77:**317–330.
86. **Wilson, M. L., S. Mirrett, L. B. Reller, M. P. Weinstein, and L. G. Reimer.** 1993. Recovery of clinically important microorganisms from the BacT/ALERT blood culture

system does not require testing for 7 days. *Diagn. Microbiol. Infect. Dis.* **16:**31–34.

87. **Wilson, M. L., and M. P. Weinstein.** 1994. General principles in the laboratory detection of bacteremia and fungemia. *Clin. Lab. Med.* **14:**69–82.
88. **Wilson, M. L., M. P. Weinstein, S. Mirrett, L. G. Reimer, S. Smith-Elekes, C. R. Chuard, and L. B. Reller.** 1995. Controlled evaluation of BacT/ALERT standard anaerobic and FAN anaerobic blood culture bottles for the detection of bacteremia and fungemia. *J. Clin. Microbiol.* **33:** 2265–2270.
89. **Wilson, M. L., M. P. Weinstein, L. G. Reimer, S. Mirrett, and L. B. Reller.** 1992. Controlled comparison of the BacT/ALERT and BACTEC 660/730 nonradiometric blood culture systems. *J. Clin. Microbiol.* **30:** 323–329.
90. **Wormser, G., I. M. Onorato, T. J. Preminger, D. Culver, and W. J. Martone.** 1990. Sensitivity and specificity of blood cultures obtained through intravascular catheters. *Crit. Care Med.* **18:**152–156.
91. **Zaidi, A. K. M., A. L. Knaut, S. Mirrett, and L. B. Reller.** 1995. Value of routine anaerobic blood cultures for pediatric patients. *J. Pediatr.* **127:**263–268.
92. **Zwadyk, P., Jr., C. L. Pierson, and C. Young.** 1994. Comparison of Difco ESP and Organon Teknika BacT/Alert continuous-monitoring blood culture systems. *J. Clin. Microbiol.* **32:**1273–1279.

Molecular Detection and Identification of Microorganisms

FREDERICK S. NOLTE AND ANGELA M. CALIENDO

16

Since the publication of the eighth edition of this Manual, significant changes have occurred in the practice of diagnostic molecular microbiology. Nucleic acid amplification techniques are now commonly used to diagnose infectious diseases and manage patients with infectious diseases. The growth in the number of commercially available test kits and analyte-specific reagents (ASRs) has facilitated the use of this technology in the clinical laboratory. Technological advances in real-time PCR techniques, nucleic acid sequencing, DNA microarrays, and proteomics have invigorated the field and created new opportunities for growth.

Molecular microbiology is the leading area in molecular pathology in terms of both the numbers of tests performed and clinical relevance. This technology has reduced the dependency of the clinical microbiology laboratory on culture-based methods and created new opportunities for the clinical laboratory to affect patient care. This chapter covers amplified and nonamplified probe techniques, postamplification detection and analysis, clinical applications of these techniques, and the special challenges and opportunities that these techniques provide for the clinical laboratory. Molecular methods used in epidemiological investigations are covered in chapter 11. A more comprehensive discussion of many of the topics covered in this chapter is found in Persing et al., *Molecular Microbiology: Diagnostic Principles and Practice* (96).

NONAMPLIFIED NUCLEIC ACID PROBES

Nucleic acid probes are segments of DNA or RNA labeled with radioisotopes, enzymes, or chemiluminescent reporter molecules that can bind to complementary nucleic acid sequences with high degrees of specificity. Although probes can range from 15 to thousands of nucleotides in size, synthetic oligonucleotides of <50 nucleotides are most commonly incorporated into commercial kits. The probes can be designed to identify microorganisms at any taxonomic level. A number of commercially available DNA probes have been developed for direct detection of pathogens in clinical specimens and identification of pathogens after isolation by culture.

The commonly used formats for probe hybridization include liquid-phase, solid-phase, and in situ hybridization. The leading method used in clinical microbiology laboratories is a liquid-phase hybridization protection assay (Gen-Probe, Inc., San Diego, Calif.). In this method, a single-stranded DNA probe labeled with an acridinium ester is incubated with the target nucleic acid. Alkaline hydrolysis follows the hybridization step, and probe binding is measured in a luminometer after the addition of peroxides. For a positive sample, the acridinium ester on the bound probe is protected from hydrolysis and, upon the addition of peroxides, emits light. The hybridization protection assay can be completed in several hours and does not require removal of unbound single-stranded probe or isolation of probe-bound double-stranded sequences (3).

In solid-phase hybridization, target nucleic acids are bound to nylon or nitrocellulose and are hybridized with a probe in solution (122). The unbound probe is washed away, and the bound probe is detected by means of fluorescence, luminescence, radioactivity, or color development. Although solid-phase hybridization is a powerful research tool, the length of time required and the complexity of the procedure limit its application in clinical practice.

In situ hybridization is another type of solid-phase hybridization in which the nucleic acid is contained in tissues or cells which are affixed to microscope slides and is governed by the same basic principles described previously (44). In most clinical applications, formalin-fixed, paraffin-embedded tissue sections are used. The sensitivity of in situ hybridization is often limited by the accessibility of the target nucleic acid in the cells.

In general, due to the poor analytical sensitivities of nonamplified probe techniques, the application of these techniques to direct detection of pathogens in clinical specimens is limited to those situations in which the number of organisms is large. Such situations include cases of group A streptococcal pharyngitis and genital tract infections with *Neisseria gonorrhoeae* and *Chlamydia trachomatis*. These techniques are used most effectively in culture confirmation assays for mycobacteria and systemic dimorphic fungi. These culture confirmation tests have a positive effect on patient management by providing rapid and accurate detection of these slowly growing, often difficult to identify pathogens.

Nucleic acid probes for direct detection of group A streptococci, *C. trachomatis*, and *N. gonorrhoeae* are available from Gen-Probe. Probes for identification of *Blastomyces dermatitidis*, *Coccidioides immitis*, *Histoplasma capsulatum*, *Campylobacter* spp., enterococci, group A streptococci, group B streptococci, *Haemophilus influenzae*, *Listeria monocytogenes*, mycobacteria, *N. gonorrhoeae*, *Staphylococcus aureus*, and

Streptococcus pneumoniae isolated in culture are also available from Gen-Probe.

Peptide nucleic acid (PNA) probes are DNA mimics in which the negatively charged sugar phosphate backbone of DNA is replaced with a noncharged polyamide or "peptide" backbone. PNA probes contain the same nucleotide bases as DNA and follow standard Watson-Crick base pairing rules when hybridizing to complementary nucleic acid sequences (115). Because PNA probes are noncharged, they do not have to overcome the destabilizing electrostatic repulsion that occurs when two negatively charged DNA molecules hybridize. As a result, PNA probes bind more rapidly and tightly to nucleic acid targets. In addition, the relatively hydrophobic character of the PNA probes enables them to penetrate the hydrophobic cell membrane following preparation of a standard smear.

PNA probes have been used for identification of *S. aureus*, *Escherichia coli*, *Pseudomonas aeruginosa*, and *Candida albicans* directly from positive blood culture bottles (90, 102, 112) and direct detection of *Mycobacterium tuberculosis* in smear-positive sputum samples (116). PNA probes for direct identification of *S. aureus*, *Enterococcus faecalis*, and *C. albicans* from positive blood culture bottles are available from AdvanDx, Woburn, Mass.

AMPLIFIED NUCLEIC ACID TECHNIQUES

The development of the PCR by Saiki et al. (108) was a milestone in biotechnology and heralded the beginning of molecular diagnostics. PCR had its 20th birthday in 2005 and has stood the test of time. Although PCR is the best-developed and most widely used nucleic acid amplification strategy, other strategies have been developed, and several have clinical utility. These strategies are based on signal, target, or probe amplification. Examples of each category will be discussed in the sections that follow. These techniques have sensitivity unparalleled in laboratory medicine, have created new opportunities for the clinical laboratory to have an effect on patient care, and have become the new "gold standards" for laboratory diagnosis of several infectious diseases.

SIGNAL AMPLIFICATION TECHNIQUES

In signal amplification methods, the concentration of the probe or target does not increase. The increased analytical sensitivity comes from increasing the concentration of labeled molecules attached to the target nucleic acid. Multiple enzymes, multiple probes, multiple layers of probes, and reduction of background noise have all been used to enhance target detection (59). Target amplification systems generally have greater analytical sensitivity than signal amplification methods, but technological developments, particularly in branched DNA (bDNA) assays, have lowered the limits of detection to levels that may rival those of target amplification assays in some applications (57).

Signal amplification assays have several advantages over target amplification assays. In signal amplification systems, the number of target molecules is not altered, and as a result, the signal is directly proportional to the amount of the target sequence present in the clinical specimen. This reduces concerns about false-positive results due to cross contamination and simplifies the development of quantitative assays. Since signal amplification systems are not dependent on enzymatic processes to amplify the target sequence, they are not affected by the presence of enzyme inhibitors in clinical specimens. Consequently, less cumbersome nucleic acid extraction methods may be used. Typically, signal amplification systems use either larger probes or more probes than target amplification systems and, consequently, are less susceptible to errors resulting from target sequence heterogeneity. Finally, RNA levels can be measured directly without the synthesis of a cDNA intermediate.

bDNA Assays

The bDNA signal amplification system is a solid-phase, sandwich hybridization assay incorporating multiple sets of synthetic oligonucleotide probes (86). The key to this technology is the amplifier molecule, a bDNA molecule with 15 identical branches, each of which can bind to three labeled probes.

The bDNA signal amplification system is illustrated in Fig. 1. Multiple target-specific probes are used to capture the target nucleic acid onto the surface of a microtiter well. A second set of target-specific probes also binds to the target. Preamplifier molecules bind to the second set of target probes and up to eight bDNA amplifiers. Three alkaline phosphatase-labeled probes hybridize to each branch of the amplifier. Detection of bound labeled probes is achieved by incubating the complex with dioxetane, an enzyme-triggerable substrate, and measuring the light emission in a luminometer. The resulting signal is directly proportional to the quantity of the target in the sample. The quantity of the target in the sample is determined from an external standard curve.

Nonspecific hybridization of any of the amplification probes and nontarget nucleic acids leads to amplification of the background signal. In order to reduce potential hybridization to nontarget nucleic acids, isocytidine (isoC) and isoguanosine (isoG) were incorporated into the preamplifier and labeled probes were used in the third-generation bDNA assays (21). IsoC and isoG form base pairs with each other but not with any of the four naturally occurring bases (97). The use of isoC- and isoG-containing probes in bDNA assays increases target-specific signal amplification without a concomitant increase in the background signal, thereby greatly enhancing the detection limits without loss of specificity. The detection limit of the third-generation bDNA assay for human immunodeficiency virus type 1 (HIV-1) RNA is 75 copies/ml. bDNA assays for the quantitation of hepatitis B virus (HBV) DNA, hepatitis C virus (HCV) RNA, and HIV-1 RNA are commercially available (Bayer HealthCare, Diagnostics Division, Tarrytown, N.Y.). The System 340 analyzer for bDNA assays automates the incubation, washing, reading, and data-processing steps.

Hybrid Capture Assays

The hybrid capture system is a solution hybridization-antibody capture assay that uses chemiluminescence detection of the hybrid molecules. The target DNA in the specimen is denatured and then hybridized with a specific RNA probe. The DNA-RNA hybrids are captured by antihybrid antibodies that are used to coat the surface of a tube. Alkaline phosphatase-conjugated antihybrid antibodies bind to the immobilized hybrids. The bound antibody conjugate is detected with a chemiluminescent substrate, and the light emitted is measured in a luminometer. Multiple alkaline phosphatase conjugates bind to each hybrid molecule, amplifying the signal. The intensity of the emitted light is proportional to the amount of target DNA in the specimen. Hybrid capture assays for detection of *N. gonorrhoeae, C. trachomatis,* human papillomavirus (HPV) (23), and cytomegalovirus (CMV) (76) in clinical specimens are commercially available (Digene Corp., Gaithersburg, Md.).

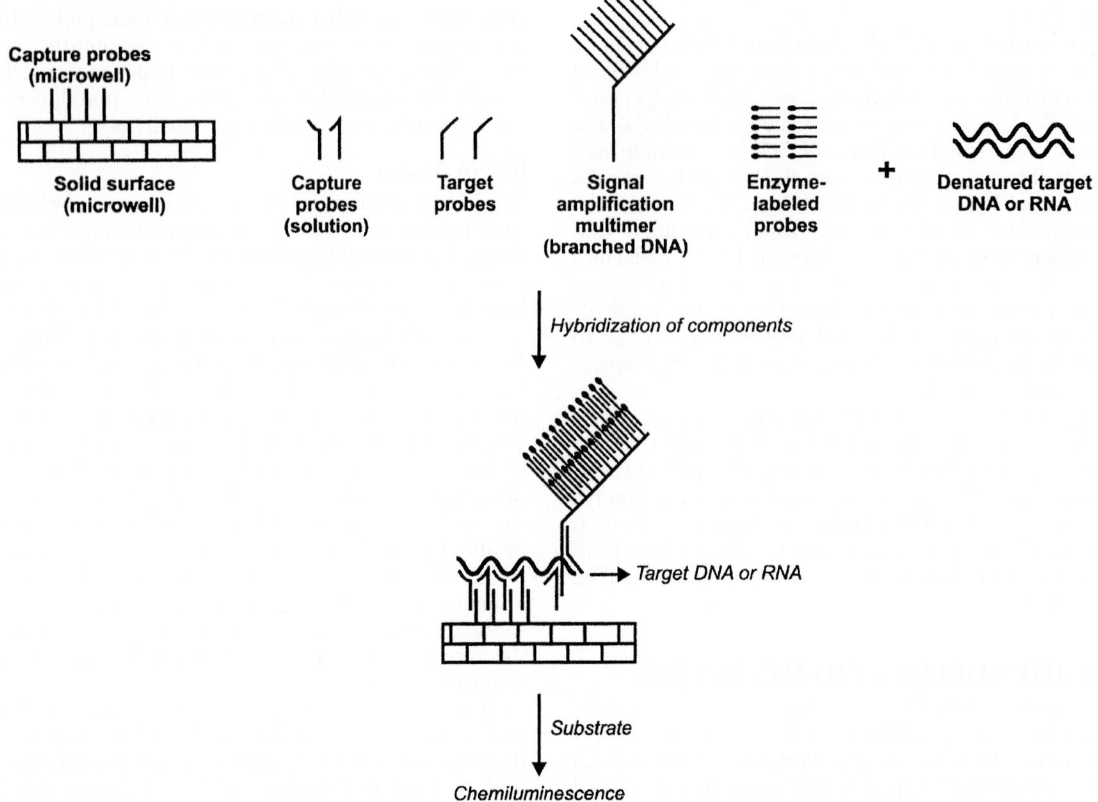

FIGURE 1 bDNA signal amplification (reprinted with permission of Elsevier from reference 134).

TARGET AMPLIFICATION TECHNIQUES

All of the target amplification systems share certain fundamental characteristics. They use enzyme-mediated processes, in which a single enzyme or multiple enzymes synthesize copies of target nucleic acid. In all of these techniques, the amplification products are detected by two oligonucleotide primers that bind to complementary sequences on opposite strands of double-stranded targets. All the techniques result in the production of millions to billions of copies of the targeted sequence in a matter of hours, and in each case, the amplification products can serve as templates for subsequent rounds of amplification. Because of this, all of the techniques are sensitive to contamination with product molecules that can lead to false-positive reactions. The potential for cross contamination is real and should be adequately addressed before any of these techniques are used in the clinical laboratory. However, the occurrence of false-positive reactions can be reduced through special laboratory design, practices, and workflow.

PCR

PCR is a simple, in vitro, chemical reaction that permits the synthesis of essentially limitless quantities of a targeted nucleic acid sequence. This is accomplished through the action of a DNA polymerase that, under the proper conditions, can copy a DNA strand (Fig. 2). At its simplest, a PCR consists of target DNA, a molar excess of two oligonucleotide primers, a heat-stable DNA polymerase, an equimolar mixture of deoxyribonucleotide triphosphates (dNTPs; dATP, dCTP, dGTP, and dTTP), $MgCl_2$, KCl, and a Tris-HCl buffer. The two primers flank the double-stranded DNA sequence to be amplified, typically <100 to several hundred bases, and are complementary to opposite strands of the target.

To initiate a PCR, the reaction mixture is heated to separate the two strands of target DNA and is then cooled to permit the primers to anneal to the target DNA in a sequence-specific manner. The DNA polymerase then initiates extension of the primers at their 3′ ends toward one another. The primer extension products are dissociated from the target DNA by heating. Each extension product, as well as the original target, can serve as a template for subsequent rounds of primer annealing and extension.

At the end of each cycle, the PCR products are theoretically doubled. Thus, after n PCR cycles the target sequence can be amplified 2^n-fold. The whole procedure is carried out in a programmable thermal cycler that precisely controls the temperature at which the steps occur, the lengths of time that the reaction mixture is held at the different temperatures, and the number of cycles. Ideally, after 20 cycles of PCR a 10^6-fold amplification is achieved and after 30 cycles a 10^9-fold amplification occurs. In practice, the amplification may not be completely efficient due to failure to optimize the reaction conditions or the presence of inhibitors of the DNA polymerase. In such cases, the total amplification is best described by the expression $(1 + e)^n$, where e is the amplification efficiency ($0 \leq e \leq 1$) and n is the total number of cycles.

RT-PCR

As it was originally described, PCR was a technique for DNA amplification. Reverse transcriptase PCR (RT-PCR) was

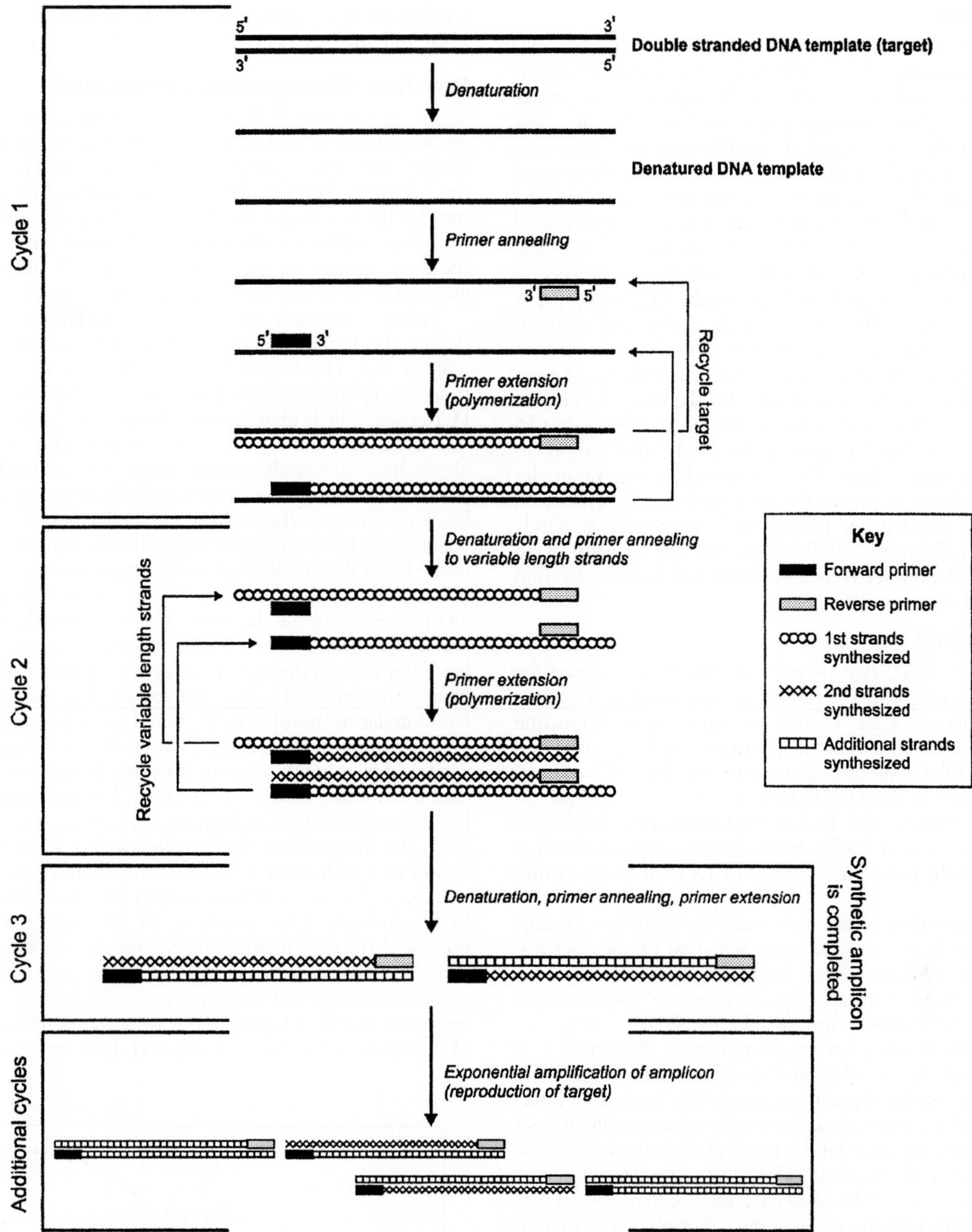

FIGURE 2 PCR target amplification (reprinted with permission of Elsevier from reference 134).

developed to amplify RNA targets. In this process, cDNA is first produced from RNA targets by reverse transcription and then the cDNA is amplified by PCR. As it was originally described, RT-PCR used two enzymes, a heat-labile RT such as avian myeloblastosis virus RT and a thermostable DNA polymerase. Because of the temperature requirements of the heat-labile enzyme, cDNA synthesis had to occur at temperatures below the optimal annealing temperatures of the primers. This presented problems in terms of both nonspecific primer annealing and inefficient primer extension due to the formation of RNA secondary structures. These problems have largely been overcome by the development of a thermostable DNA polymerase derived from *Thermus thermophilus* that under the proper conditions can function efficiently as both an RT and a DNA polymerase (82). RT-PCRs with this enzyme are more specific and efficient than previous protocols with conventional, heat-labile RT enzymes. Commercially available kits (Roche Diagnostics, Indianapolis, Ind.) that use this single-enzyme technology are available for detection of HCV RNA and for quantitation of HIV-1 and HCV RNA in clinical specimens.

Nested PCR

Nested PCR was developed to increase both the sensitivity and the specificity of PCR (45). It uses two pairs of amplification primers and two rounds of PCR. Typically, one primer pair is used in the first round of PCR for 15 to 30 cycles. The products of the first round of amplification are then subjected to a second round of amplification with the second set of primers that anneal to a sequence internal to the sequence amplified by the first primer set. The increased sensitivity arises from the high total cycle number, and the increased specificity arises from the annealing of the second primer set to sequences found only in the first-round products, thus verifying the identity of the first-round product. The major disadvantage of nested PCR is the high rates of contamination that can occur during the transfer of first-round products to the second tube for the second round of amplification. This contamination can be avoided either by physically separating the first- and second-round amplification mixtures with a layer of wax or oil or by designing single-tube amplification protocols. In practice, the enhanced sensitivity afforded by nested PCR protocols is rarely required in diagnostic applications, and the identity of an amplification product is usually confirmed by hybridization with a nucleic acid probe.

Multiplex PCR

In multiplex PCR, two or more primer sets designed for amplification of different targets are included in the same reaction mixture (12). By this technique, more than one target sequence in a clinical specimen can be coamplified in a single tube. The primers used in multiplexed reactions must be carefully selected so that they have similar annealing temperatures and lack complementarity. Multiplex PCRs have proved to be more complicated to develop and are usually less sensitive than PCRs with single primer sets.

Many multiplex assays have been developed, especially for the detection of central nervous system (9, 24) and respiratory (58, 121) pathogens. Multiplex PCR assays for bacterial and viral respiratory pathogens are commercially available from Prodesse, Inc., Waukesha, Wis.

A promising new platform for multiplex PCR analysis is the LabMAP system (Luminex Corp., Austin, Tex.). The LabMAP system incorporates a proprietary process to internally dye polystyrene microspheres with two spectrally distinct fluorochromes. By using precise ratios of these fluorochromes, an array is created consisting of 100 different microsphere sets with specific spectral addresses. Each microsphere set can possess a different reactant on its surface. For nucleic acid analysis, oligonucleotide probes would be covalently bound to the microsphere surface by carbodiimide coupling. Since each microsphere set can be distinguished by its spectral address, the sets can be combined, allowing up to 100 different analytes to be measured simultaneously in a single reaction vessel. A third fluorochrome coupled to a reporter molecule quantifies the biomolecular interaction that occurs at the microsphere surface.

Microspheres are investigated individually in a rapidly flowing liquid stream as they pass by two separate lasers in the Luminex 100 flow cytometer. High-speed digital signal processing classifies each microsphere based on its spectral address and quantifies the reaction on its surface. Thousands of microspheres are investigated per second, resulting in an analysis system capable of analyzing and reporting up to 100 different reactions in a single reaction vessel in a few seconds. The technology has been adapted to a wide variety of applications in bacteriology (27), mycology (25), and virology (111, 129).

Real-Time (Homogeneous, Kinetic) PCR

The term real-time PCR describes methods in which the target amplification and detection steps occur simultaneously in the same tube (homogeneous). These methods require special thermal cyclers with precision optics that can monitor the fluorescence emission from the sample wells. The computer software supporting the thermal cycler monitors the data throughout the PCR at every cycle and generates an amplification plot for each reaction (kinetic).

Figure 3 shows a representative amplification plot and defines the terms used in real-time PCR quantitation. The amplification plot shows the normalized fluorescence signal from the reporter at each cycle number. In the initial cycles of PCR, there is little change in the fluorescence signal. This initial signal level defines the baseline for the plot. An increase above the baseline indicates the detection of accumulated PCR product. A fixed fluorescence threshold can be set above the baseline. The cycle threshold (C_T) is defined as the cycle number at which the fluorescence passes the fixed threshold. A plot of the log of the initial target concentration versus C_T for a set of standards is a straight line (49). The amount of the target in an unknown sample is determined by measuring the sample C_T and using a standard curve to determine the starting copy number. Alternatively, the cycle number corresponding to the maximal change in fluorescence, the second derivative maximum, has a similar relationship to the initial target concentration.

In its simplest format, the PCR product is detected as it is produced by using fluorescent dyes that preferentially bind to double-stranded DNA. SYBR Green I is one such dye that has been used in this application (81). In the dye's unbound state, the fluorescence is relatively low, but when the dye is bound to double-stranded DNA, the fluorescence is greatly enhanced. The dye will bind to both specific and nonspecific PCR products. The specificity of the detection can be improved through melting curve analysis. As the temperature is slowly raised, the two strands of the amplicon will melt apart and the amount of fluorescence will decrease. The data are transformed and analyzed by plotting the first derivative of the fluorescence on the *y* axis and the temperature on the

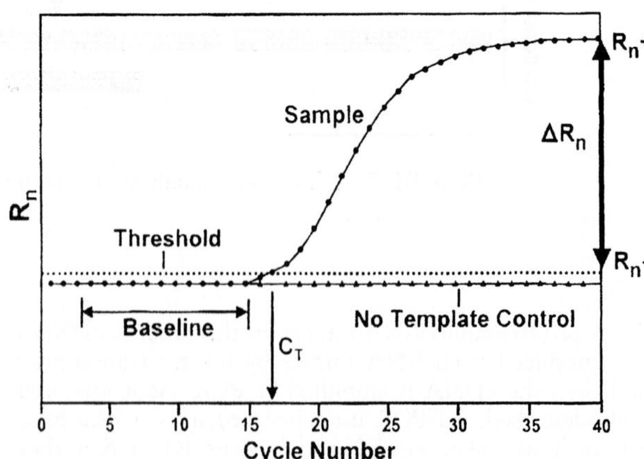

FIGURE 3 Real-time PCR amplification plot with commonly used terms and abbreviations. R_n, normalized fluorescent signal from reporter dye. (From *TaqMan Universal PCR Master Mix Protocol*, Foster City, Calif.: Applied Biosystems; 2002:5–94. Reprinted with permission.)

x axis. The specific amplified product will have a characteristic melting peak at its predicted melting temperature (T_m), whereas the primer dimers and other nonspecific products should have different T_ms or give broader peaks (103).

The specificity of real-time PCR can also be increased by including fluorescent resonance energy transfer (FRET) probes in the reaction mixture. These probes are labeled with fluorescent dyes or with combinations of fluorescent and quencher dyes. In 5′ exonuclease PCR (TaqMan) assays, the 5′ to 3′ exonuclease activity of *Taq* DNA polymerase is used to cleave a nonextendable hybridization probe during the primer extension phase of PCR (50). This approach uses dual-labeled fluorogenic hybridization probes and is illustrated in Fig. 4. One fluorescent dye serves as a reporter, and its emission spectrum is quenched by the second fluorescent dye. The nuclease degradation of the hybridization probe releases the

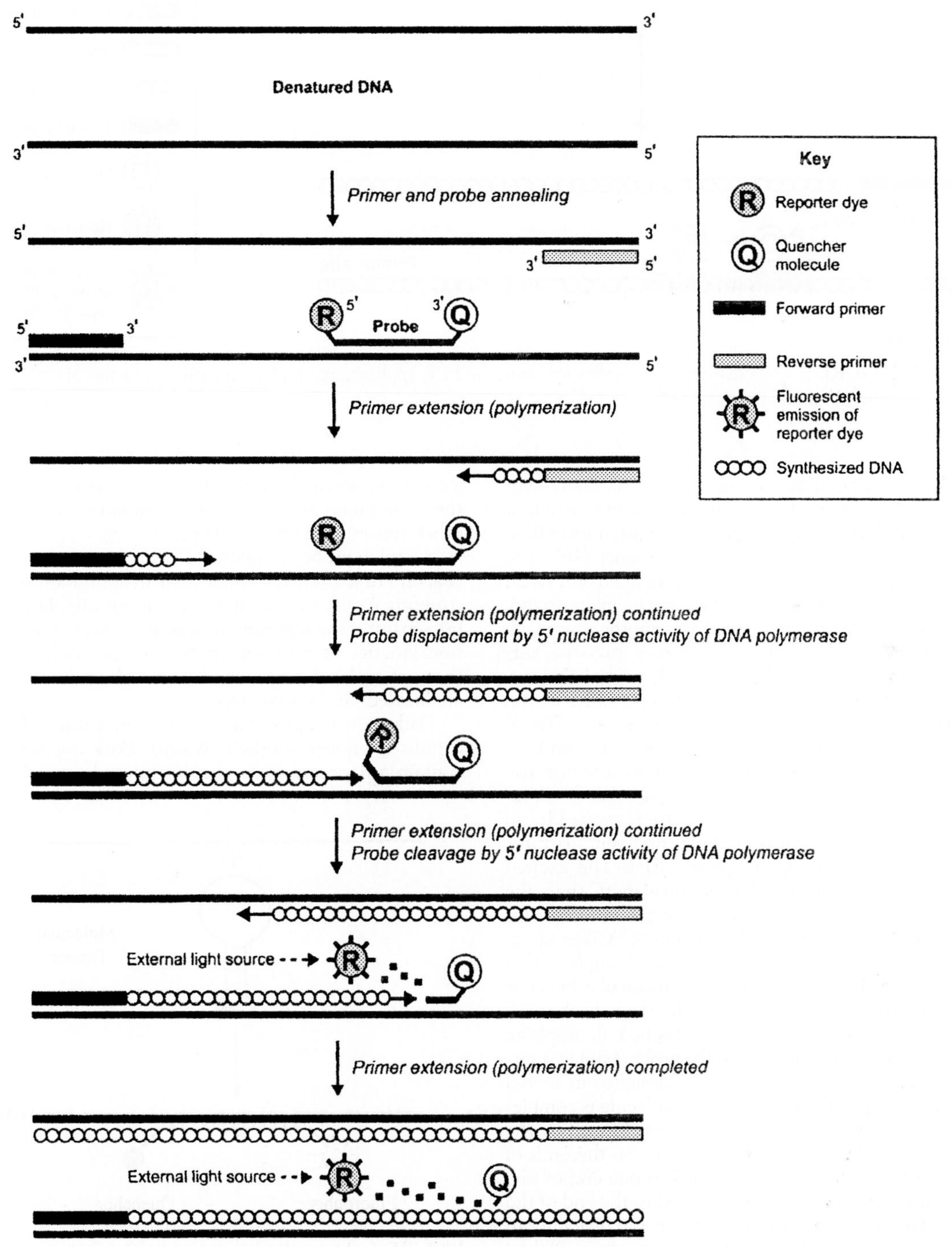

FIGURE 4 5′ exonuclease chemistry for real-time PCR applications (reprinted with permission of Elsevier from reference 134).

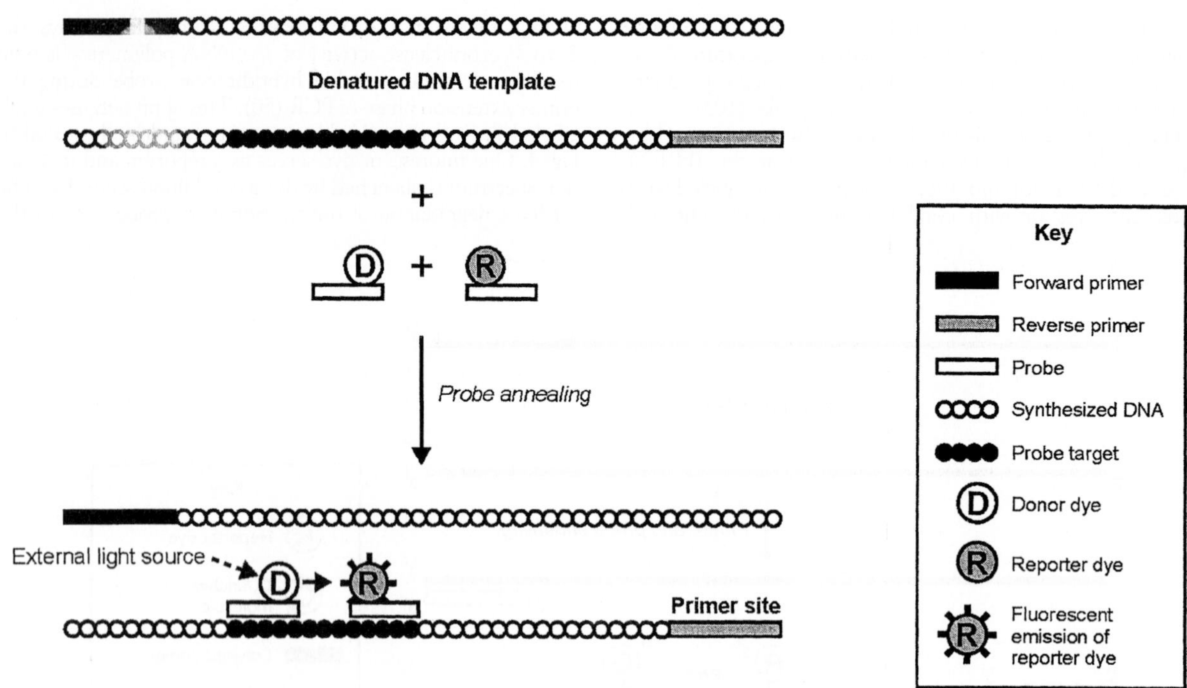

FIGURE 5 Dual hybridization probes for real-time PCR applications (reprinted with permission of Elsevier from reference 134).

reporter dye, resulting in an increase in the peak fluorescent emission. The increase in fluorescent emission indicates that specific PCR product has been made, and the intensity of fluorescence is related to the amount of the product (46). The specificity is increased because a signal is generated only when the primer and probe are bound to the same template strand.

The use of dual hybridization probes is another approach to real-time PCR (65). This method uses two specially designed sequence-specific oligonucleotide probes (Fig. 5). These hybridization probes are designed to hybridize within 1 to 5 nucleotides apart on the product molecule. The 3′ end of the anchor probe is labeled with a donor dye, and the 5′ end of the reporter probe is labeled with an acceptor dye. The 3′ end of the reporter probe is phosphorylated to prevent extension during PCR. The donor dye is excited by an external light source, and instead of emitting light, it transfers its energy to the acceptor dye by FRET. The excited acceptor dye emits light at a longer wavelength than the unbound donor dye, and the intensity of the acceptor dye light emission is proportional to the amount of PCR product.

Real-time detection and quantitation of amplification products can also be accomplished with molecular beacons (126). Molecular beacons are hairpin-shaped oligonucleotide probes with an internally quenched fluorophore whose fluorescence is restored when the probes bind to a target nucleic acid (Fig. 6). The probes are designed in such a way that the loop portion of each probe molecule is complementary to the target sequence. The stem is formed by the annealing of complementary arm sequences on the ends of the probe. A fluorescent dye is attached to one end of one arm, and a quenching molecule is attached to the end of the other arm. The stem keeps the fluorophore and quencher in close proximity such that no light emission occurs. When the probe encounters a target molecule, it forms a hybrid that is longer and more stable than the stem and undergoes a conformational change that forces the stem apart, causing the fluorophore and the quencher to move away from each other, restoring the fluorescence.

Scorpion probes combine a PCR primer with a molecular beacon (124, 131). Intramolecular hybridization of the loop structure to a downstream portion of the amplification product separates the reporter and quencher dyes. The hybridization kinetics of Scorpion probes are generally faster than those of molecular beacons because the primer and probe are located on the same molecule.

Dark quencher probes are also used in real-time PCR applications (Nanogen, Bothell, Wash.). Dark quencher probes contain a fluorophore on the 5′ end and a nonfluorescent

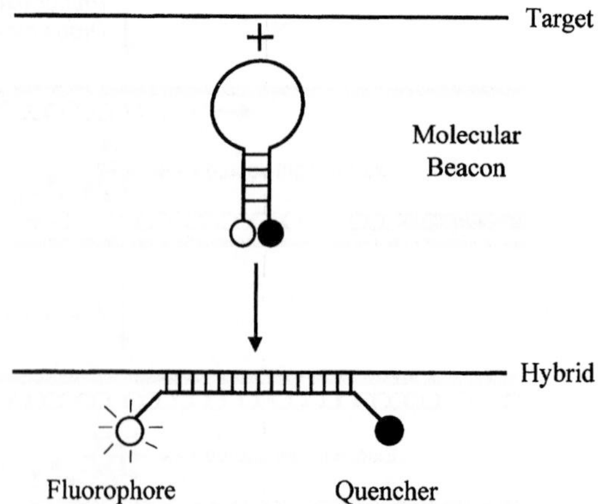

FIGURE 6 Molecular beacon probes for real-time amplification applications (reprinted with permission of Elsevier from reference 134).

quencher molecule on the 3′ end (62). The fluorescence is quenched when the probe is a random coil and emitted when the probe anneals to the target sequence. Unlike fluorogenic 5′ nuclease probes, these probes are not degraded by the DNA polymerase during target amplification. Since the dark quencher is not fluorescent, it does not contribute to the background signal. This trait has the advantage of improving the signal-to-noise ratio for the detection system, which may improve sensitivity. These probes also incorporate a hybridization-stabilizing compound, known as a minor groove binder. It is a small, crescent-shaped molecule that is covalently linked to the 3′ end of the probe that spans about 3 to 4 nucleotides and snugly fits into the minor groove of DNA, where it forms hydrogen bonds with the template. Minor groove binders will increase the T_m of the probe. The minor groove binder allows for the use of shorter probes because of the increased T_ms and enables improved T_m leveling, which increases the specificity of the detection reaction.

Real-time PCR methods decrease the time required to perform nucleic acid assays because there are no post-PCR processing steps. Also, since amplification and detection occur in the same closed tube, these methods eliminate the postamplification manipulations that can lead to laboratory contamination with the amplicon. In addition, real-time PCR methods lend themselves well to quantitative applications because analysis is performed early in the log phase of product accumulation and, as a result, is less prone to error resulting from differences in sample-to-sample amplification efficiency.

Transcription-Based Amplification Methods

Nucleic acid sequence-based amplification (NASBA) and transcription-mediated amplification (TMA) are both isothermal RNA amplification methods modeled after retroviral replication (22, 39, 63). The methods are similar in that the RNA target is reverse transcribed into cDNA and then RNA copies are synthesized with an RNA polymerase. NASBA uses avian myeloblastosis virus RT, RNase H, and T7 bacteriophage RNA polymerase, whereas TMA uses an RT enzyme with endogenous RNase H activity and T7 RNA polymerase.

Amplification involves the synthesis of cDNA from the RNA target with a primer containing the T7 RNA polymerase promoter sequence (Fig. 7). The RNase H then degrades the initial strand of target RNA in the RNA-cDNA hybrid. The second primer then binds to the cDNA and is extended by the DNA polymerase activity of the RT, resulting in the formation of double-stranded DNA containing the T7 RNA polymerase promoter. The RNA polymerase then generates multiple copies of single-stranded, antisense RNA. These RNA product molecules reenter the cycle, with subsequent formation of more double-stranded cDNA molecules that can serve as templates for more RNA synthesis. A 10^9-fold amplification of the target RNA can be achieved in less than 2 h by this method.

The single-stranded RNA products of TMA in the Gen-Probe tests are detected by modification of the hybridization protection assay. Oligonucleotide probes are labeled with modified acridinium esters with either fast or slow chemiluminescence kinetics so that signals from two hybridization reactions can be analyzed simultaneously in the same tube. The NASBA products in the bioMérieux (Durham, N.C.) tests are detected by hybridization with probes labeled with tris(2,2′-bispyridine)ruthenium and electrochemiluminescence. NASBA has also been used with molecular beacons to create a homogeneous, kinetic amplification system similar to real-time PCR (68).

Transcription-based amplification systems have several strengths, including no requirement for a thermal cycler, rapid kinetics, and a single-stranded RNA product that does not require denaturation prior to detection. Also, single-tube clinical assays and a labile RNA product may help minimize contamination risks. Limitations include the poor performance with DNA targets and concerns about the stability of complex multienzyme systems. Gen-Probe has developed TMA-based assays for detection of *Mycobacterium tuberculosis*, *C. trachomatis*, *N. gonorrhoeae*, HCV, and HIV-1. NASBA-based kits (bioMérieux) for the detection and quantitation of HIV-1 RNA and CMV RNA transcripts and detection of enterovirus and respiratory syncytial virus RNA are commercially available. A basic NASBA kit is also available for the development of other applications defined by the user.

Strand Displacement Amplification

Strand displacement amplification (SDA) is an isothermal template amplification technique that can be used to detect trace amounts of DNA or RNA of a particular sequence. SDA, as it was first described, was a conceptually straightforward amplification process with some technical limitations (128). Since its initial description, however, it has evolved into a highly versatile tool that is technically simple to perform but conceptually complex. SDA is the intellectual property of Becton Dickinson and Company, Sparks, Md.

In its current iteration, SDA occurs in two discrete phases, target generation and exponential target amplification (70). Both are illustrated in Fig. 8. In the target generation phase, a double-stranded DNA target is denatured and hybridized to two different primer pairs, designated as bumper and amplification primers. The amplification primers include the single-stranded restriction endonuclease enzyme sequence for BsoB1 located at the 5′ end of the target binding sequence. The bumper primers are shorter and anneal to the target DNA just upstream of the region to be amplified. In the presence of BsoB1, an exonuclease-free DNA polymerase, and a dNTP mixture consisting of dUTP, dATP, dGTP, and thiolated dCTP (C_s), simultaneous extension products of both the bumper and amplification primers are generated. This process displaces the amplification primer products, which are available for hybridization with the opposite-strand products with the opposite-strand bumper and amplification primers.

The simultaneous extension of opposite-strand primers produces strands complementary to the product formed by extension of the first amplification primer with C_s incorporated into the BsoB1 cleavage site. This product enters the exponential target amplification phase of the reaction. The BsoB1 enzyme recognizes the double-stranded site, but because one strand contains C_s, it is nicked rather than cleaved by the enzyme. The DNA polymerase then binds to the nicked site and begins synthesis of a new strand while simultaneously displacing the downstream strand. This step re-creates the double-stranded species with the hemimodified restriction endonuclease recognition sequence, and the iterative nicking and displacement process repeats. The displaced strands are capable of binding to opposite-strand primers, which produces exponential amplification of the target sequences.

These single-stranded products also bind to detector probes for real-time detection. The detector probes are single-stranded DNA molecules with fluorescein and rhodamine labels. The region between the labels includes a stem-loop structure. The loop contains the recognition site for the BsoB1 enzyme. The target-specific sequences are located 3′ of

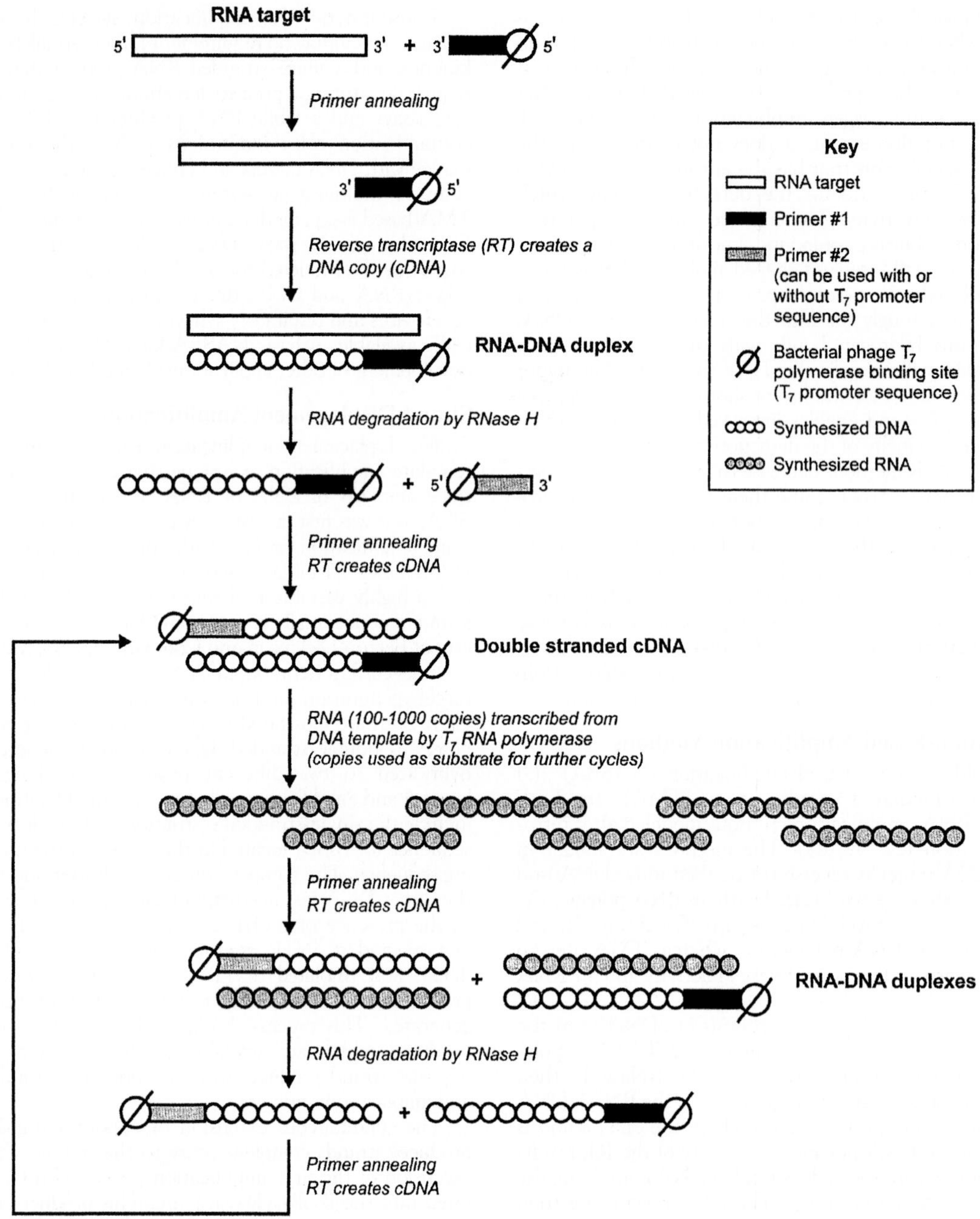

FIGURE 7 Transcription-based target amplification. NASBA and TMA are examples of transcription-based amplification systems (reprinted with permission of Elsevier from reference 134).

the rhodamine label. In the absence of a specific target, the stem-loop structure is maintained with the fluorescein and rhodamine labels in close proximity. The net effect is that very little emission for the fluorescein is detected after excitation. After SDA, the probe is converted to a double-stranded species, which is cleaved by BsoB1. The cleavage causes physical separation of the fluorescein and rhodamine labels, which results in an increase in emission from the flourescein label.

The diagnostic applications of SDA include the direct detection of *M. tuberculosis*, *C. trachomatis*, and *N. gonorrhoeae* in clinical specimens. SDA has a reported sensitivity high enough to detect as few as 10 to 50 copies of a target molecule (128). By using a primer set designed to amplify a repetitive sequence with 10 copies in the *M. tuberculosis* genome, the assay is sensitive enough to detect 1 to 5 genome copies from the bacterium. Recently, SDA has been adapted to quantitate RNA by adding an RT step (RT-SDA). In this case, a primer hybridizes to the target RNA and an RT synthesizes a cDNA molecule. This cDNA can then serve as a template for primer incorporation and strand displacement. The products of this strand displacement then feed into the amplification scheme described above. RT-SDA has been used for the determination of HIV viral load (88).

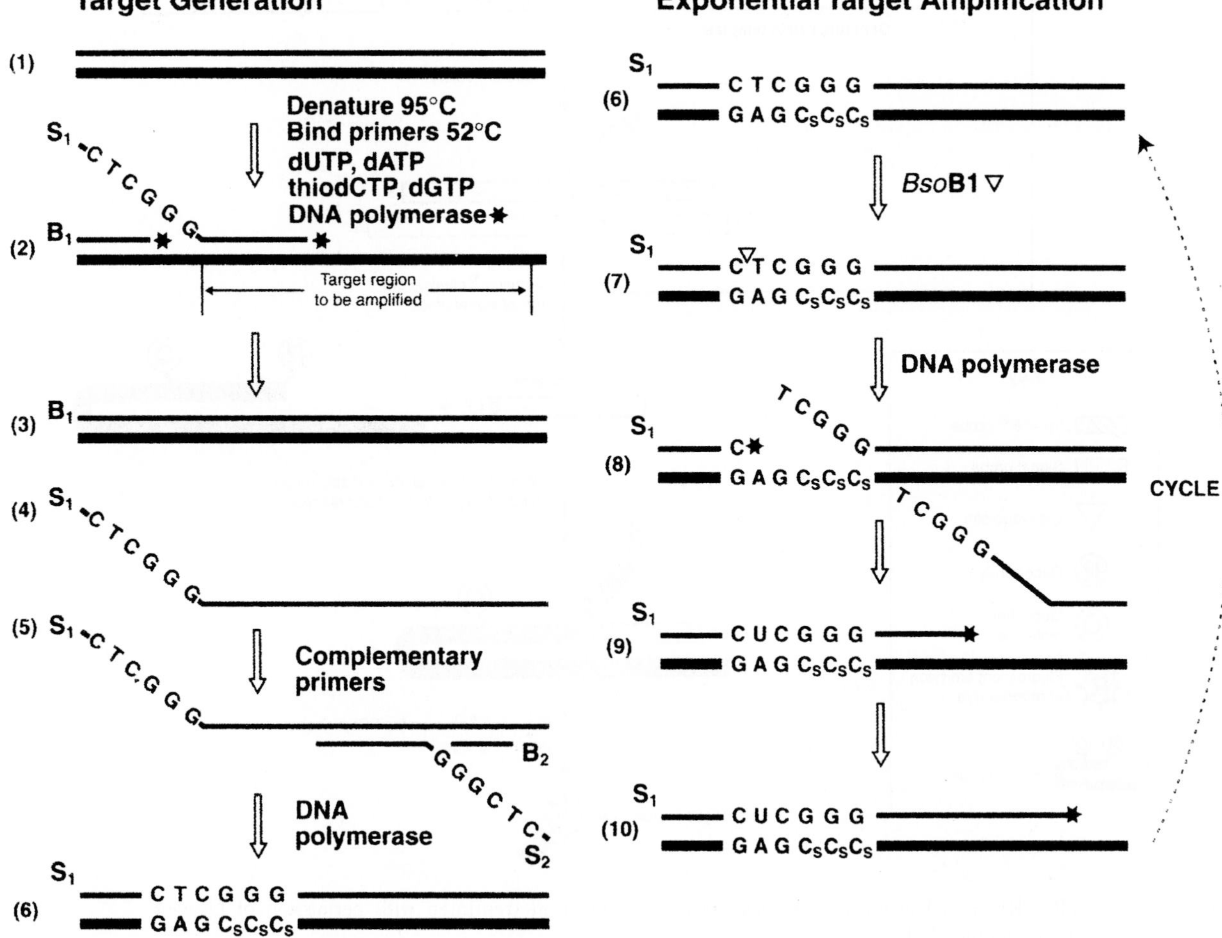

FIGURE 8 Strand displacement target amplification. The process is shown for only one strand of a double-stranded DNA target, but amplification occurs on both strands simultaneously. B_1 and B_2, bumper primers; S_1 and S_2, amplification primers. (Modified from reference 70.)

The main advantage of SDA is that it is an isothermal process that, unlike PCR, can be performed at a single temperature after initial target denaturation. This eliminates the need for expensive thermal cyclers. Furthermore, samples can be subjected to SDA in a single tube, with amplification times varying from 30 min to 2 h. The main disadvantage of SDA lies in the fact that, unlike those at which PCR is performed, the relatively low temperature at which SDA is carried out (52.5°C) can result in nonspecific primer hybridization to sequences found in complex mixtures such as genomic DNA. Hence, when the target is in low abundance compared to background DNA, nonspecific amplification products can swamp the system, decreasing the sensitivity of the technique. However, the use of organic solvents to increase stringency at low temperatures and the recent introduction of more thermostable polymerases capable of strand displacement have alleviated much of this problem.

PROBE AMPLIFICATION TECHNIQUES

Probe amplification methods differ from target amplification methods in that the amplification products contain only a sequence present in the initial probes. Ligase chain reaction (136), cycling probe technology (31), and cleavase-invader technology (73) are all examples of probe amplification methods for which diagnostic applications have been developed. However, diagnostic tests based on ligase chain reaction and cycling probe technology are no longer available in the United States.

Cleavase-Invader Technology

Invader assays (Third Wave Technologies, Madison, Wis.) are based on a probe amplification method that relies upon the specific recognition and cleavage of particular DNA structures by cleavase, a member of the FEN-1 family of DNA polymerases. These polymerases will cleave the 5′ single-stranded flap of a branched base-paired duplex. This enzymatic activity likely plays an essential role in the elimination of the complex nucleic acid structures that arise during DNA replication and repair. Since these structures may occur anywhere in a replicating genome, the enzyme recognizes the molecular structure of the substrate without regard to the sequence of the nucleic acids making up the DNA complex (69).

In the invader assays, two primers are designed which hybridize to the target sequence in an overlapping fashion

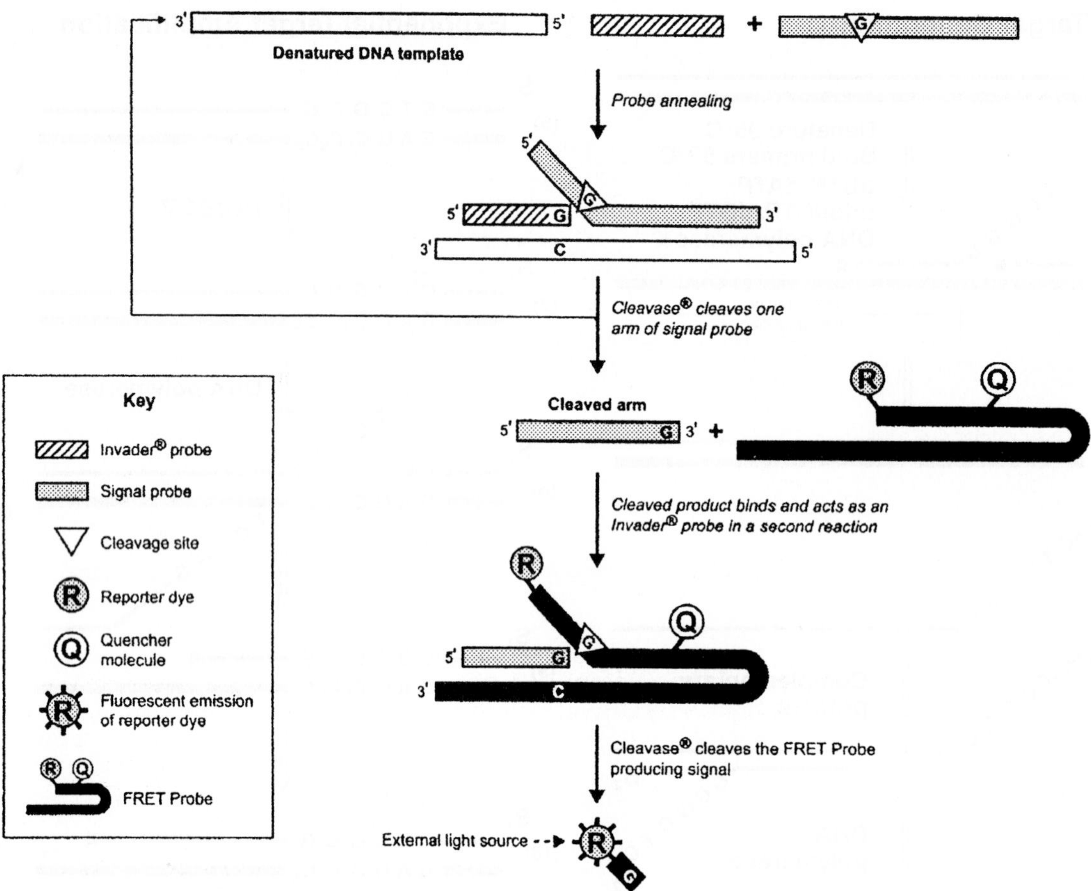

FIGURE 9 Cleavase-invader probe-based amplification (reprinted with permission of Elsevier from reference 134).

(Fig. 9). Under the proper annealing conditions, the probe oligonucleotide binds to the target sequence. The invader oligonucleotide is designed such that it hybridizes upstream of the probe with a region of overlap between the 3′ end of the invader and the 5′ end of the probe. Cleavase cleaves the 5′ end of the probe and releases it. It is in this way that the target sequence acts as a scaffold upon which the proper DNA structure can form. Since the DNA structure necessary to serve as a cleavase substrate will occur only in the presence of the target sequence, the generation of cleavage products indicates the presence of the target. Use of a thermostable cleavase enzyme allows reactions to be run at temperatures high enough for a primer exchange equilibrium to exist. This allows multiple cleavase products to form off of a single target molecule.

Various methods can be used to detect the cleavage products. Third Wave Technologies uses FRET probes and a second invasive cleavage reaction to detect the target-specific products. Invader technology can be used for genotyping, detection of mutations, and viral load testing. An ASR for HCV genotyping is currently available from Third Wave Technologies. ASRs are described in detail in the "Regulatory and Reimbursement Issues" section of this chapter.

The invader assay has several inherent advantages. Because the overlap in the invader probe need be only 1 bp, this technology can easily be adapted to detect point mutations of interest by designing the overlap region to encompass the mutation to be detected (74). The detection of these point mutations would not require postreaction restriction digestion, since the primers would be differentially cleaved on the basis of the presence or the absence of the mutation in question. This feature could be exploited to track mutations in pathogens associated with drug resistance or virulence. In addition, unlike amplification techniques such as PCR, SDA, and TMA, in which the target sequence itself is amplified, the invader assay does not increase the amount of the target sequence. As a consequence, invader assays are less prone to problems of false-positive results due to amplicon cross contamination.

POSTAMPLIFICATION DETECTION AND ANALYSIS

Gel Analysis

Visualization of amplification products in agarose gels after electrophoresis and ethidium bromide staining was the earliest detection method. After gel electrophoresis, DNA is often transferred onto a nitrocellulose or nylon membrane and hybridized to a specific probe to increase both the sensitivity and the specificity of detection. Membranes with bound radiolabeled probes are placed in proximity to X-ray film, and the hybrids are visualized as dark bands. Enzyme-labeled probes can be visualized through either light or color production after the addition of the appropriate chemiluminescent or chromogenic substrates. Many of these nonisotopic approaches are at least as sensitive as isotopic methods and are faster. In addition, the enzyme-labeled probes are more stable. Although gel electrophoresis and blotting remain important research tools, these techniques are being replaced by faster and simpler methods in the clinical laboratory.

Single-strand conformation polymorphism (SSCP) analysis and restriction fragment length polymorphism (RFLP) analysis have been used to ascertain information about the base compositions of the amplification products visualized in a gel. In SSCP analysis, the PCR product is denatured and then subjected to electrophoresis in a nondenaturing gel (92). Variations in the physical conformations of the PCR products are related to the base compositions and are detected by differential gel migration. This technique has successfully been used to detect mutations causing rifampin resistance in *M. tuberculosis* (120).

RFLP analysis uses restriction endonucleases to cleave amplification products at specific recognition sites. The fragments are separated by electrophoresis, and the resulting banding pattern provides information about the nucleic acid sequence. When coupled with a hybridization reaction, RFLP analysis can also provide information about the location and number of loci homologous to the probe. Both SSCP analysis and RFLP analysis of short products have largely been replaced by direct DNA sequencing as this technology has improved and the costs have decreased.

Colorimetric Microtiter Plate Systems

Colorimetric microtiter plate (CMP) systems are convenient alternatives to traditional gel and blotting techniques for detection of amplified products. In these systems, the amplified product is captured in microtiter plate wells by specific oligonucleotide probes coating the plastic surface. Bound product is detected by a color change that takes place after addition of an enzyme conjugate and the appropriate substrate. These systems resemble enzyme immunoassays and use microtiter plate washers and readers commonly found in clinical laboratories. CMP systems are more practical and faster than the traditional membrane hybridization techniques described above.

Several variations of CMP systems are commercially available. In one popular approach, biotinylated primers are used to amplify the target, and the biotin-containing PCR product is denatured and added to the microtiter well. After hybridization with a capture probe, the bound product is detected with a streptavidin-enzyme conjugate and a chromogenic substrate (71). Enzyme-conjugated antibodies directed against double-stranded DNA have also been used to detect PCR products in CMP systems (75). Another approach uses digoxigenin-dUTP to label the PCR product and enzyme-conjugated antidigoxigenin antibodies to detect the captured product (98).

Allele-Specific Hybridization

Line probe assays are manufactured by Innogenetics (Ghent, Belgium) for genotyping of HCV and HBV, identification of mycobacteria, and analysis for drug resistance mutations in HIV-1, HBV, *M. tuberculosis*, and *Helicobacter pylori* (105, 117, 118). The HCV line probe assays are distributed by Bayer. In these assays, a series of probes with poly(T) tails are attached to nitrocellulose strips. Biotin-labeled PCR product is then hybridized to the immobilized probes on the strip. The labeled PCR product hybridizes only to the probes that give a perfect sequence match under the stringent hybridization conditions used. After hybridization, streptavidin labeled with alkaline phosphatase is added and binds to the biotinylated hybrids. Incubation with a chromogen results in a purple precipitate. The pattern of hybridization provides information about the nucleic acid sequence of the amplicon. This method is capable of detecting single-nucleotide polymorphisms.

Direct Sequencing

The combination of PCR and dideoxynucleotide chain termination methods can be used to determine DNA sequences in clinical samples (52). The use of fluorescent dye terminator chemistry and laser scanning in a polyacrylamide gel electrophoresis format has been the standard in electrophoretic separation technology. However, the recent application of capillary electrophoresis techniques to the separation of PCR and dideoxy chain termination products has streamlined the sequencing process by eliminating some of the labor-intensive steps, which makes the technology a better fit for diagnostic applications (30). The Clinical and Laboratory Standards Institute (CLSI) has recently developed guidelines for nucleic acid sequencing in clinical laboratories (19, 85).

CLIP (a coupled amplification and sequencing method) uses oligonucleotide primers labeled with different fluorescent dyes, standard dideoxynucleotide termination reagents, and PCR to produce extension products that end with a chain-terminating nucleotide. The nucleic acid sequence is deduced from the electrophoretic mobilities of the different extension products from a set of four reactions, each product containing a different chain-terminating nucleotide. A unique feature of CLIP sequencing is that one reaction produces sequence information for both nucleic acid strands. CLIP sequencing serves as the basis for commercially available assays for HIV-1 drug resistance and HCV genotyping (Bayer).

The ViroSeq HIV-1 genotyping assays (Celera Diagnostics, Alameda, Calif.; distributed by Abbott Molecular Diagnostics, Des Plains, Ill.) also use dideoxy chain-terminating sequencing, but each dideoxynucleotide is labeled with a different fluorescent dye. Each reaction mixture contains one primer but all four uniquely labeled dideoxynucleotides. Separation of the terminated PCR products is done by capillary electrophoresis.

Although direct sequencing of PCR products by electrophoresis is a powerful research tool, its routine use in the clinical laboratory depends upon the development of high-throughput systems with integrated databases and data analysis software. Such systems are available for HIV-1 and HCV genotyping and for identification of bacteria and fungi by rRNA gene sequence analysis.

Pyrosequencing (Biotage, Uppsala, Sweden) represents an alternative approach to conventional sequencing and is useful for genotyping and short-read-length sequencing (26). Pyrosequencing is based on the luminometric detection of pyrophosphate that is generated during DNA synthesis.

A sequencing primer is hybridized to a single-stranded PCR amplicon and incubated with the enzymes DNA polymerase, ATP sulfurylase, luciferase, and apyrase and the substrates adenosine 5′ phosphosulfate and luciferin. The first of four dNTPs is added to the reaction mixture. DNA polymerase catalyzes the incorporation of the dNTP into the DNA strand. Each incorporation event is accompanied by release of pyrophosphate (PP_i) in a quantity equimolar to the amount of incorporated nucleotide. The ATP sulfurylase quantitatively converts PP_i to ATP in the presence of adenosine 5′ phosphosulfate. This ATP drives the luciferase-mediated conversion of luciferin to oxyluciferin that generates light in amounts that are proportional to the amount of ATP. The light produced in the reaction is detected by a charge-coupled device camera.

A program is produced in which the height of each peak is proportional to the number of nucleotides incorporated. Apyrase, a nucleotide-degrading enzyme, continuously degrades ATP and unincorporated dNTPs. This degradation switches off the light and regenerates the reaction solution. The next dNTP is added, and the process is repeated.

Pyrosequencing has been used in microbiology to detect drug resistance mutations and to identify and type bacteria, viruses, and fungi (2, 37, 40, 91). Unlike conventional sequencing strategies, pyrosequencing provides reliable data for sequences adjacent to the sequencing primer termini. Pyrosequencing provides a simple-to-use and robust platform for short-read-length sequencing.

Hybridization Arrays

DNA hybridization arrays are produced by attaching or synthesizing hundreds or thousands of oligonucleotides on a solid support in precise patterns. A labeled amplification product is hybridized to the probes, and hybridization signals are mapped to various positions within the array. If the number of probes is sufficiently large, the sequence of the PCR product can be deduced from the pattern of hybridization. A number of manufacturers are developing DNA microarrays and the instrumentation required to acquire and analyze the data. Hybridization arrays have a number of applications in microbiology, including microbial and host gene expression profiling and diagnostic sequencing. The CLSI has published a guideline for the use of diagnostic nucleic acid microarrays (18).

One of the most developed approaches brings together advances in synthetic nucleic acid chemistry with photolithography, a process used in the manufacture of semiconductors for the computer industry. This approach uses light to direct the synthesis of short oligonucleotides on a silica wafer (94). On a 15-mm-square chip, thousands of individual sites or features can be established. At each feature, specific oligonucleotides are assembled one nucleotide at a time by light-activated chemistry.

The DNA chip is incubated in a flow cell with DNA product that has been fragmented and labeled with a fluorophore. After hybridization, a scanning laser confocal microscope evaluates the surface fluorescence intensity of the chip. Automated scanning by the microscope takes only a few minutes to acquire an image of the entire surface of the chip, and computer software analyzes the fluorescent image and determines the nucleic acid sequence of the PCR product. A DNA chip based on this technology for the detection of HIV-1 drug resistance mutations is commercially available (Affymetrix, Santa Clara, Calif.).

Another method of producing DNA hybridization arrays involves the precise micropipetting of premade double-stranded DNA probes (typically 200 to 2,000 bp in length) onto glass slides with a robotic device (110). These arrays are not suitable for mutation detection due to the size and density of the arrayed DNA probes but have facilitated gene expression profiling. DNA arrays of this type can be used to determine the activation states (mRNA levels) of thousands of genes simultaneously. Gene expression profiling of pathogens by use of arrays may provide new insights into pathogenic mechanisms and help identify new therapeutic and vaccine targets.

Nanogen (San Diego, Calif.) has developed a bioelectronic chip with 100 individually addressable electrodes. The silicon chip is manufactured by using the same type of photolithographic and deposition techniques used in the microelectronics industry. The technology uses electrical fields to move biological samples through the chip and direct the samples to the electrodes. Cheng and colleagues (13) used a microelectrode array to separate *E. coli* cells from a whole-blood sample and then to lyse the isolated *E. coli* cells on the chip. The lysate was then transferred to another bioelectronic chip for an electronically enhanced hybridization assay developed previously (114). The development of fully integrated analytical systems that function as a laboratory, the so-called "lab on a chip," is the ultimate goal of microchip designers.

DNA microarrays and bioelectronics hold much promise for molecular diagnostics. However, the current technology has several limitations, including the complexity of fabricating the microarrays, limited availability, and high test cost.

QUANTITATIVE METHODS

Many of the methods discussed above can be used to quantify the amount of RNA or DNA in a clinical sample. The most commonly used methods include PCR and RT-PCR, transcription-based amplification, bDNA assays, and hybrid capture. The principle of quantitative molecular methods is that there is a linear relationship between the quantity of the input template and the amount of the product or signal generated. Competitive PCR (cPCR) is a reliable and robust method that is commonly used in commercial and laboratory-developed assays. The basic concept behind cPCR is the coamplification in the same reaction tube of target and calibrator templates with equal or similar lengths and with the same primer binding sequences. Since both templates are amplified with the same primer pair, identical thermodynamics and amplification efficiencies are ensured. The amount of the calibrator must be known, and after amplification, products from both templates must be distinguishable from each other. Different types of calibrators have been used in cPCR, but in general those calibrators similar in size and base composition to the target work most effectively. RNA competitors should be used in quantitative RT-PCRs to address the problem of variable RT efficiency. This competitive amplification approach has also been used effectively with transcription-based amplification methods using RNA targets and RNA calibrators.

For cPCR, the concentration of the target template in the clinical sample can be determined by a simple calculation. The yield of the PCR product is described by the equation $Y = I(1 + e)^n$, where Y is the quantity of the PCR product, I is the quantity of the template at the beginning of the reaction, e is the efficiency of the reaction, and n is the number of cycles. In cPCR, this equation is written for both templates, as follows: competitor, $Y_c = I_c(1 + e)^n$; target, $Y_t = I_t(1 + e)^n$. Since e and n are the same for both the competitor and the target, the relative product ratio Y_c/Y_t directly depends on the initial concentration ratio I_c/I_t and the function $Y_c/Y_t = I_c/I_t$ is linear.

An alternative method of quantification is to run multiple concentrations of the calibrator in parallel with the reaction mixtures containing the target molecules. The signal generated from these external calibrators is used to generate a calibration curve, and the amount of the target in the original specimen is calculated based on comparison to the curve. The use of external calibration with the target amplification methods offers the advantage that the calibrators do not compete with the target for assay components. However, since the final amount of the amplified product depends on exponential amplification of the initial quantity of the template, minor differences in amplification efficiency may lead to very large and unpredictable differences in the final product yield (16). The sample-to-sample differences may depend on sample preparation, nucleic acid purification procedures, the presence of inhibitors, and thermal cycler performance. For these reasons, simple quantitation of the amplified product and the use of external standard reference curves may not provide reliable quantitation of the template initially present in the sample.

Real-time amplification and detection methods are particularly well suited for quantification of nucleic acid because the amount of the fluorescent signal generated is proportional to the concentration of the target DNA or RNA in the original sample. Real-time PCR and transcription-based amplification methods are the most commonly used quantitative methods. For real-time PCR, the fluorescent signal is measured during the exponential phase of amplification, which is where the amplification plot crosses the threshold (Fig. 3). This is in contrast to standard PCR methods that measure the end point signal. There are advantages to measuring the fluorescent signal during the exponential phase of amplification; the reaction components are not limiting, and the assay is less sensitive to the effects of inhibitors. As a result, real-time PCR assays are more reproducible than standard PCR assays. Both internal and external calibrators can be used with real-time assays, but the improved precision of real-time assays allows more reliable results to be obtained with an external calibration curve than would be obtained with standard PCR. When external calibrators are used, a calibration curve is generated by plotting the $\log_{10}$ concentration of the external calibrator versus the C_T and this plot is used to calculate the concentration of nucleic acid in the sample. The concentration of nucleic acid in the sample is inversely related to the C_T: the higher the concentration of the nucleic acid, the lower the C_T (49). In general, quantitative real-time PCR assays are not more sensitive than standard PCR assays; however, they have a much broader linear range, typically 6 to 7 orders of magnitude.

The CLSI has published guidelines for quantitative molecular methods for infectious diseases that address the development and application of quantitative PCR assays and other nucleic acid amplification methods (84).

AUTOMATION AND INSTRUMENTATION

Molecular assays consist of three major steps: specimen processing, nucleic acid amplification, and product detection. Sample processing is usually the most labor-intensive step and has represented the biggest challenge for manufacturers of automated test systems. However, in the past several years there have been considerable advances in this area with the availability of both semiautomated and fully automated systems. Automation of the nucleic acid extraction process offers laboratories several advantages, including ease of use, limited handling of the sample, improved reproducibility, reduced opportunity for cross contamination, and for some systems, postelution functions such as adding samples into the master mix. These advantages need to be weighed against the costs of automated systems, the inflexibility of batch size, and the large sizes of many of the automated instruments. The systems vary in the types of nucleic acid extraction methods that they provide and include total nucleic acid, DNA-only, and RNA-only protocols. Other features of automated extraction systems to consider are the availability of protocols for various specimen types and volumes, variable elution volumes, the availability of target-specific and/or generic target extraction methods, and specimen throughput. The available automated systems range from fully automated high-throughput systems such as the MagNA Pure system (Roche) and *m*2000 generic extractor (Abbott) to those designed for a small number of specimens with random access capabilities, such as BioRobot EZ1 (Qiagen).

There are a few automated systems available for the conventional amplification methods, such the COBAS system (Roche) for PCR and the System 340 platform for bDNA assays (Bayer). Considerable advances in automation have been made with the availability of real-time amplification and detection systems.

Several instruments are commercially available for real-time PCR testing. These instruments vary as to speed, capacity of samples per test run, reaction volume, optics, and support for different fluorescence probe types. The time required for analysis depends to a great extent on the time required for thermocycling, and the speed of thermocycling depends on how quickly the instrument can change temperature over time. For example, some instruments can change the temperature at 20°C per s, permitting instrument analysis of up to 32 samples in as little as 30 min. Capacity may offset thermocycling speed. Although a higher-capacity instrument may have a longer thermocycling time than a lower-capacity instrument, potentially more samples may be analyzed by the high-capacity instrument in a specific time period than by the low-capacity instrument.

The reaction mixture volume assayed may also vary from one system to another. If target nucleic acid is present in extremely small amounts in a sample, an instrument that permits higher-volume analysis may be preferred.

Real-time PCR instruments utilize a variety of optics for fluorescence detection. A tungsten source lamp for excitation and selectable filters for excitation and emission wavelength detection are used in a number of instruments. Light-emitting diodes or laser excitation devices coupled with emission wavelength detection may also be used. The new real-time PCR instruments allow up to five different fluorogenic dyes to be used simultaneously in one reaction. Until recently, real-time PCR instruments were designed for research applications. The ABI Prism series of sequence detection systems (Celera), LightCycler (Roche), and SmartCycler (Cepheid, Sunnyvale, Calif.) are examples of research instruments that find widespread use in molecular diagnostics laboratories. The COBAS TaqMan analyzer (Roche) and the *m*2000 system (Abbott) are the first real-time instruments designed specifically for use in clinical laboratories (5).

Many manufacturers are coupling automated nucleic acid extraction instruments with amplification and detection systems to create high-throughput, fully automated nucleic acid analyzers. The TIGRIS system (Gen-Probe) (77), the AmpliPrep-COBAS TaqMan system (Roche), and the *m*2000 system (Abbott) are examples of fully automated and integrated systems designed to perform sample processing, nucleic acid amplification, and product detection. The TIGRIS system was developed for screening the blood supply for HCV and HIV RNA and can process up to 500 nucleic acid detection tests in 8 h. The GeneXpert system (Cepheid) represents the other end of the automation spectrum in which a single sample is added to a disposable fluidic cartridge that fully automates and integrates sample preparation, amplification, and real-time detection. The instrument is a random access design, raising the possibility of on-demand molecular testing.

PROTEOMICS

The term proteome was coined in 1994 to describe the set of proteins encoded by the genome (132). Proteomics, the study of the proteome, has come to encompass the identification, characterization, and quantification of the complete set of proteins expressed by the entire genome in the lifetime of a given cell, tissue, or organism. Development of vaccines, therapeutics, and diagnostics directed at a particular infectious disease commonly requires analysis of organisms at the protein level. Genome level analysis of an organism, as valuable as that has been, is incomplete because only a fraction of the genome is translated into mRNA. Similarly, analysis of an organism at the mRNA level (transcriptome) may also be misleading because proteins translated from mRNA can undergo posttranslational modifications.

Two-dimensional gel electrophoresis and mass spectrometry are the tools used to define an organism's proteomic signature. Comparison of the proteomic signature of a reference state to a proteomic signature derived under experimental conditions or a disease state can reveal important information about the biology of the pathogen and the host's immune response to it (11, 54, 56, 127). Proteomic approaches have been used successfully to identify diagnostic markers for gastric disease caused by *Helicobacter pylori* (41), Lyme disease (55), severe acute respiratory disease (101), and tuberculosis (4).

The same approaches that are used to find biomarkers can also be used to develop rapid, sensitive, and high-throughput multimarker assays. The premise is to first establish composite fingerprint profiles for both disease and nondisease states and then use the composite profiles to make a diagnosis with an unknown patient sample. The development of chip-based protein differential display systems will facilitate the development of diagnostics based on protein expression analysis (33).

CURRENT APPLICATIONS

Molecular methods have created new opportunities for the clinical microbiology laboratory to impact patient care in the areas of initial diagnosis, disease prognosis, and monitoring of response to therapy. Over time the methods have become more automated, the cost of testing has decreased, and clinical utility has been proven for the diagnosis and management of a variety of infectious diseases. As a result, molecular testing is now routinely performed in many clinical microbiology laboratories and clinical applications will continue to expand in the future.

Initial Diagnosis

With the development of molecular methods, the clinical microbiology laboratory is no longer reliant solely on the traditional culture methods for detection of pathogens in clinical specimens. Culture-based methods have long been the gold standard for infectious disease diagnosis, but for several diseases, nucleic acid-based tests have replaced culture as the gold standard. Hepatitis C infection, enteroviral meningitis, pertussis, herpes simplex virus (HSV) encephalitis, and genital infections due to *C. trachomatis* are some examples of infectious diseases in which nucleic acid-based tests are the new gold standards for diagnosis. This technology has been used to best advantage in situations in which traditional methods are slow, insensitive, expensive, or not available. These techniques work particularly well with fragile or fastidious microorganisms that may die in transit or be overgrown by contaminating flora when cultured. *N. gonorrhoeae* is an example in which the nucleic acid can be detected under circumstances in which the organism cannot be cultured. The use of improper collection media, inappropriate transport conditions, or delays in transport can reduce the viability of the pathogen but may leave the nucleic acid still detectable. It is beyond the scope of this chapter to review all of the possible applications or to provide a compendium of methods for detection of various pathogens. The reader is directed to another excellent resource for this information (96).

Opportunities to actually replace culture for bacterial pathogens in routine practice are limited by the need to isolate the organisms for antibiotic susceptibility testing. In those applications in which culture has actually been replaced by nucleic acid testing, the pathogens are of predictable susceptibilities and, consequently, routine susceptibility testing is not performed, or the genetics of resistance are well defined and simple to detect, such as methicillin resistance in *S. aureus*.

Molecular methods have had the biggest impact in clinical virology in which the molecular approaches are often faster, more sensitive, and more cost-effective than the traditional methods. The diagnoses of enteroviral meningitis, HSV encephalitis, and CMV infections in immunocompromised patients are examples of clinically relevant and cost-effective applications of nucleic acid-based tests. There are greater opportunities to replace the conventional methods in virology than in bacteriology because the culture-based methods are costly and antiviral susceptibility testing is not routinely performed. In those situations in which antiviral susceptibility testing is required, such as identification of ganciclovir-resistant CMV, it may also be more amenable to molecular approaches. A limitation of molecular tests for viral diagnostics is the clinical need for simultaneous identification of multiple pathogens, for example, respiratory viruses. Multiplex PCR can be difficult to optimize, so detection of common respiratory pathogens may require multiple tests.

Perhaps the greatest impact of molecular methods has been in the discovery of previously unrecognized or uncultivable pathogens. During the past 15 years, a number of infectious agents were first identified directly from clinical material by using molecular methods. HCV, the principal etiologic agent of what was once known as non-A, non-B hepatitis, was discovered in 1989 through the application of molecular cloning techniques by investigators from the Centers for Disease Control and the Chiron Corporation (15). Cloning and analysis of the HCV genome led to production of viral antigens that now serve as the basis of the specific serological tests used to screen the blood supply and to diagnose hepatitis C. To date, HCV has resisted all attempts at sustained in vitro propagation. As a result, RT-PCR is used to detect, quantitate, and genotype HCV in infected individuals.

Tropheryma whippelii, the causative agent of Whipple's disease, is another example of an uncultivable microorganism which was initially identified by molecular methods (100). It was discovered by the use of broad-range PCR, in which primers are directed against conserved sequences in the bacterial 16S rRNA gene. Sequence analysis of the PCR product and comparison with known 16S rRNA gene sequences were used to characterize the organism and establish its disease association. This approach provides a new paradigm for discovery of unrecognized pathogens that is of value in other diseases with features that suggest an infectious etiology.

Recently, molecular methods were used to rapidly identify the etiologic agent of severe acute respiratory syndrome as a coronavirus (60, 95). Within a few months of the recognized outbreak, the virus was identified and sequenced and the molecular assays were developed that played an essential role in diagnosing the infection and defining the epidemiology of the infection.

Identification of Bacteria and Fungi by Nucleic Acid Sequencing

Nucleotide sequence analysis of the 16S bacterial rRNA gene has expanded our knowledge of the phylogenetic relationships among bacteria and is the new standard for bacterial identification. rRNA contains several functionally different regions, with some regions having highly conserved and others having highly varied nucleic acid sequences (133). The sequence of the 16S rRNA gene is a stable genotypic signature that can be used to identify an organism at a genus or species level. The 16S gene sequence can be determined rapidly and provides objective results independent of phenotypic characteristics. As discussed in the preceding section, it can also be used to characterize previously unrecognized species. A similar approach that targets the nuclear large subunit of the rRNA gene can be used for the identification of fungi (61). This gene is universally found in all fungi and contains sufficient variation to identify most fungi accurately to the species level.

The DNA sequencing approach to microbial identification involves extraction of the nucleic acids, amplification of the target sequence by PCR, sequence determination, and a computer software-aided search of an appropriate sequence database. The major limitations of this approach to microbial identification include the high cost of automated nucleic acid sequencers, the lack of appropriate analysis software, and limited databases.

Applied Biosystems (Foster City, Calif.) has developed ribosomal gene sequencing kits for bacteria and fungi. A sequence from an unknown bacterium is compared with either full or partial 16S rRNA sequences from over 1,000 type strains by using the MicroSeq analysis software (119). The software analysis provides percent base pair differences between the unknown bacterium and the 20 most closely related bacteria, alignment tools to show differences between the related sequences, and phylogenetic tree tools to verify that the unknown bacterium actually clusters with the 20 closest bacteria in the database. The MicroSeq fungal identification system is similar to the bacterial identification system but targets D2 large-subunit rRNA (42, 43). Continued improvements in automation, refinements of analysis software, and decreases in cost should lead to more widespread use of nucleic acid sequence-based approaches to microbial identification.

Disease Prognosis

Molecular techniques have created opportunities for the laboratory to provide important information that may predict disease progression. Probably the best example is HIV-1 viral load as a predictor of progression to AIDS and death in infected individuals. This predictive value was first demonstrated in 1996 as part of a multicenter AIDS cohort study (79). The investigators showed that the risk of progression to AIDS and death was directly related to the magnitude of the viral load in plasma at study entry. The viral load in plasma was a better predictor of disease progression than the number of $CD4^+$ lymphocytes. Subsequent studies have confirmed that baseline viral load critically influences disease progression.

Subtyping of certain viruses by molecular methods may also have prognostic value. Subtyping of respiratory syncytial viruses may provide information about the severity of infection in hospitalized infants, with those infected with group A viruses having poorer outcomes (130). HPV causes dysplasia, intraepithelial neoplasia, and carcinoma of the cervix in women. HPV types 16 and 18 are associated with a high risk of progression to neoplasia, and types 6 and 11 are associated with a low risk of progression (99). The clinical utility of molecular testing for high-risk HPV DNA has been established for managing women with the cervical cytologic diagnosis of atypical squamous cells of undetermined significance. Women with this condition can be referred for colposcopy based on the detection of high-risk HPV DNA (113). HPV DNA testing was recently approved by the Food and Drug Administration (FDA) for use as an adjunct to cytology for cervical cancer screening in women aged 30 years or more (135).

CMV viral load testing has recently been shown to be useful for deciding when to initiate preemptive therapy in organ transplant recipients and distinguishing active disease from asymptomatic infection. Qualitative CMV DNA PCR assays have been unable to distinguish patients with asymptomatic CMV infection from those with active CMV disease (36, 89). Recently, studies have shown that the level of CMV DNA can predict the development of active CMV disease. With the availability of standardized commercial assays, it is possible to establish viral load cutoffs for predicting the development of CMV disease and initiating preemptive therapy (1, 51). It is likely that quantitative assays will be useful in distinguishing disease from infection with other herpesviruses such as Epstein-Barr virus and human herpesvirus type 6.

Response to Therapy

Molecular methods have been developed to detect the genes responsible for resistance to single antibiotics or classes of antibiotics in bacteria and in many cases are superior to the phenotypic, growth-based methods. The detection of methicillin resistance in staphylococci, vancomycin resistance in enterococci, and rifampin resistance in *M. tuberculosis* provide examples of where molecular methods are used to supplement the growth-based methods (123). However, it is difficult to imagine, given our current state of knowledge of the molecular genetics of antimicrobial resistance and the technological limitations, that a genotypic approach to routine antimicrobial susceptibility testing of bacteria could rival the phenotypic methods in terms of information content and cost.

Molecular techniques are playing an increasing role in predicting and monitoring patient response to antiviral therapy. The laboratory may have a role in predicting response to therapy by detecting specific drug resistance mutations, determining viral load, and genotyping. Both viral load and genotype are independent predictors of response to combination therapy with pegylated interferon and ribavirin in chronic HCV infections (32, 78). Those patients with high pretreatment viral loads of >2 million copies/ml or with genotype 1 infections have poor sustained response rates. Both of these virological parameters are used in conjunction with other factors to determine the duration of therapy (83).

Quantitative tests for HIV-1 RNA are the standard of practice for guiding clinicians in initiating, monitoring, and changing antiretroviral therapy. Several commercially available HIV-1 viral load assays have been FDA approved, and guidelines for their use in clinical practice have been published (107). Viral load assays have also been used in monitoring response to therapy in patients chronically infected with HBV and HCV (32, 47, 67). In organ transplant recipients, the persistence of CMV viral load after several weeks of antiviral therapy is associated with the development of resistant virus (10).

LABORATORY PRACTICE

The unparalleled analytical sensitivity of nucleic acid amplification techniques coupled with their susceptibility to cross contamination presents unique challenges to the routine application of these techniques in the clinical laboratory. There are special concerns in the areas of specimen processing, workflow, quality assurance, and interpretation of test results. Additional information can be found in the CLSI documents MM3-A2, *Molecular Diagnostic Methods for Infectious Diseases; Approved Guideline,* 2nd ed. (20), and MM13-A, *Collection, Transport, Preparation, and Storage of Specimens and Samples for Molecular Methods; Approved Guideline* (17).

Specimen Collection, Transport, and Processing

Proper collection, transport, and processing of clinical specimens are essential to ensure reliable results from molecular assays. Nucleic acid integrity must be maintained throughout these processes. Important issues to consider in specimen collection are the timing of specimen collection in relationship to disease state and the proper specimen type. Other factors that come into play include the use of the proper anticoagulant, transport and storage temperatures, and time to processing of the specimen. HIV-1 viral load testing is an example in which the proper conditions for specimen collection, transport, and processing have been well described and has provided insight into the importance of these factors. For HIV-1 viral load testing, the plasma needs to be separated from the cells within 6 h of collection to minimize degradation of RNA. Once the plasma has been separated, it can be stored at 4°C for several days, but −70°C is recommended for long-term storage (107). Most types of specimens are best stored at −20 to −70°C prior to processing.

Molecular methods have several advantages over conventional culture with regard to specimen collection. It may be easier to maintain the integrity of nucleic acid than the viability of an organism. Molecular tests for the detection of *C. trachomatis* and *N. gonorrhoeae* are an example in which DNA is stable on dry cervical swabs for a week at room temperature or refrigeration temperatures, which is in stark contrast to the conditions required to maintain organism viability for culture. Nucleic acid persists in specimens after initiation of treatment (35, 66), thus allowing detection of a pathogen even though the organism can no longer be cultured. Also, due to the increased sensitivity of molecular assays, it may be possible to test a smaller volume of specimen or use a specimen that is collected using a less invasive method.

The major goals of specimen processing are to release nucleic acid from the organism, maintain the integrity of the nucleic acid, render the sample noninfectious, remove inhibiting substances, and in some instances concentrate the specimen. These processes need to be balanced with minimizing manipulation of the specimen. Complex specimen processing methods are time-consuming and may lead to the loss of target nucleic acid or result in contamination between specimens. Care must be taken to avoid carrying over inhibitory substances, such as phenol or alcohol, from the nucleic acid isolation step to the amplification reaction.

There are several general methods for nucleic acid extraction. Different methods may be used depending on whether the desire is to purify RNA or DNA or both. Another factor to consider when deciding on a nucleic acid extraction method is the type of pathogen sought. Some pathogens, such as viruses, can be very easy to lyse, and mycobacteria, staphylococci, and fungi can be very difficult to lyse. Enzyme digestion or harsh lysis conditions may be required to disrupt the cell walls of these organisms.

DNA isolation methods often use detergents to solubilize the cell wall or membranes, a proteolytic enzyme, such as proteinase K, to digest proteins, and EDTA to chelate divalent cations needed for nuclease activity (7, 38). The lysate can be used directly in amplification assays, or additional steps may follow to purify the nucleic acid. These additional steps remove proteins and traces of organic solvents and concentrate the specimen. In order to successfully use a crude lysate, the target DNA must be present in a relatively high concentration and there must be minimal inhibitors of amplification in the sample. If these criteria are not met, additional purification steps should be used.

Another commonly used method of nucleic acid isolation involves disruption of cells or organisms with the chaotropic agent guanidinium thiocyanate and a detergent (14). After a short incubation, the nucleic acid can be precipitated with isopropanol. Guanidinium thiocyanate denatures proteins and is also a strong inhibitor of ribonucleases, making it a very useful method of RNA isolation, although it is also used for purification of DNA. The Boom extraction method is also based on the lysing and nuclease-inactivating properties of guanidinium thiocyanate but utilizes the acid-binding properties of silica or glass particles to purify nucleic acid (8). Over the past several years, various manufacturers have developed commercially available reagents using one of these basic methods or a modification of these methods. Many of these methods rely on the use of spin column technology, are easy to use, and provide a rapid, reproducible method for purification of nucleic acid from a wide variety of clinical specimens. In recent years, further advances have been made with the introduction of magnetic silica particles which are coupled with instruments providing various degrees of automation, thus further simplifying nucleic acid extraction and purification. These reagents tend to be expensive, but the additional cost can be offset by labor savings.

Tissue samples need to be disrupted prior to the nucleic acid extraction process. This can be accomplished by cutting the tissue into small pieces or mechanically homogenizing the tissue prior to proceeding with one of the above-described extraction methods. Preserved tissue specimens require removal of the paraffin with solvents and slicing into fine sections prior to processing.

Removing inhibitors of amplification is a key function of the nucleic acid extraction process. Simple methods of nucleic acid extraction that involve boiling of the specimen have been used for relatively acellular specimens such as cerebrospinal fluid (CSF). Though the boiling method is fast and easy, there are problems with inhibitors of amplification in CSF that are not inactivated by boiling (80). The inhibition rate can be reduced to <1% by using a silica-based extraction method. Similarly, crude lysates of urine and cervical swab specimens are commonly used for the detection of *C. trachomatis* and *N. gonorrhoeae*. Specimens containing amplification inhibitors have been reported to range from 1 to 5% for urine to as much as 20% for cervical swabs (104). Common inhibitory substances include hemoglobin, crystals, β-human chorionic gonadotropin, and nitrates. Blood samples are used commonly for detection and/or quantification of a variety of viral pathogens including HIV-1, HCV, and CMV. HIV-1 viral load testing is an example in which the effects of different anticoagulants have been well studied. HIV-1 viral RNA is most stable when collected in EDTA, and heparin has been shown to be inhibitory to amplification and should be avoided (6, 53). In addition, very small volumes of whole blood (1%) can be inhibitory to *Taq* DNA polymerase (48). Other compounds such as acidic polysaccharides, which are components of glycoproteins present in sputum and cervical specimens and bile salts found in stool, can also inhibit polymerase (34). With the recognition of such a wide array of inhibitors of amplification and the availability of simple, reliable, semiautomated and automated nucleic acid extraction methods, the use of crude lysates for testing becomes more difficult to justify. Regardless of the nucleic acid extraction method employed, the laboratory should monitor inhibition rates for different specimen types and nucleic acid extraction methods (see "Quality Control and Assurance").

Contamination Control

Several types of contamination can occur with molecular testing: cross contamination of specimens during the nucleic acid extraction step, contamination of specimens with positive control material, and carryover contamination of amplified products. Contamination with amplified products can occur with DNA or RNA target amplification and with probe amplification methods. It does not occur with signal amplification assays since no nucleic acid molecules are synthesized with these methods. Cross contamination that occurs during specimen processing or handling of positive control material can occur with all amplification methods. The approach to the control of contamination due to amplified products has changed dramatically with the widespread use of real-time amplification and detection methods. Since the reaction tube is not opened after amplification, there is minimal risk of contamination from the amplified product. Many laboratories using real-time methods continue to use a variety of good laboratory practices to control for contamination, but the focus is on minimizing cross contamination between specimens rather than contamination from the amplified product. Refer to CLSI document MM3-P2, *Molecular Diagnostic Methods for Infectious Diseases; Proposed Guideline,* 2nd ed. (20), for a detailed description of good laboratory practices to minimize contamination.

Clinical microbiologists have long been concerned about minimizing contamination between samples with microorganisms during specimen processing. Molecular methods have raised the level of concern considerably, and for good reason, as current methods can detect a few molecules. The previously undetected low levels of contamination that occurred in processing specimens for routine culture can lead to false-positive results in molecular assays. Prevention of contamination due to target DNA is best done by careful handling of specimens to avoid splashing, opening only one specimen tube at a time, pulse-spinning tubes prior to opening, using screw-top tubes rather than snap-cap tubes to minimize aerosolization, bleaching work surfaces, and using plugged pipette tips. Some of these approaches can be difficult for high-volume laboratories, which is why automated extraction systems can be very useful. Care must be taken with these systems to ensure that there is no cross contamination during the automated process. This is often done by alternating negative and high-titer specimens in a checkerboard arrangement and monitoring for carryover of sample into the negative specimens. These experiments should be designed with an understanding of the concentration of the organism in the clinical specimen. For example, the concentration of HSV in CSF from patients with meningitis is quite low compared to the concentration of BK virus in the urine of a patient with nephropathy.

Preventing contamination of the laboratory with DNA from a clinical specimen or positive control material is very important, because eliminating contamination with target DNA once it occurs can be very difficult. This is why care should be taken to use a positive control at the lowest concentration that consistently amplifies. The enzymatic and photochemical inactivation methods used to control carryover contamination of amplified products are not effective in preventing contamination with target DNA.

Enzymatic inactivation of amplified product can be accomplished with uracil-*N*-glycosylase (UNG), a DNA repair enzyme found in a variety of bacterial species. During the PCR, dTTP is replaced with dUTP so that dUTP is incorporated into the newly synthesized DNA products. This allows for a distinction between starting template DNA and amplified products; only newly synthesized PCR products will contain deoxyuracil. If UTP-containing amplification products are present as contaminants, the addition of UNG to the reaction mixture will result in the cleavage of deoxyuracil residues, thus destroying the contaminating DNA (72). The use of UNG increases the amount of carryover DNA needed to contaminate the reaction mixture by several orders of magnitude (93). When UNG is used, it is important to keep the annealing temperature above 55°C so that the UNG remains inactive, thus avoiding degradation of newly synthesized product. For the same reason, after completion of amplification, the reaction mixture should be held at 72°C (125). UNG can be inactivated at 94°C, but prolonged inactivation at 94°C may also affect the activity of the polymerase enzyme. UNG will not remove uracil from RNA molecules and is therefore ineffective in controlling contamination in RNA amplification assays, such as TMA and NASBA.

When UTP and UNG are used, the PCR reaction conditions should be reoptimized as the magnesium requirement may increase. The efficiency of amplification may be reduced when UTP is substituted for TTP. This can be overcome by adding a mixture of dUTP and dTTP into the master mix. The efficiency of inactivation using UNG depends on the size of the amplified product and its G+C content. Inactivation may not be effective with amplified products of fewer than 100 bp, as maximum UNG efficiency requires the DNA molecule to be 150 bp (28).

Quality Control and Assurance

Verification and validation are terms that are often used interchangeably; however, they are very different processes. Verification is the process by which assay performance is determined; parameters such as sensitivity, specificity, positive and negative predictive value, and accuracy are established. The verification of an assay is completed before the assay is used for patient testing. Validation is the ongoing process of proving that the assay is performing as expected and achieves the intended results.

The verification of an assay includes analytical verification and clinical verification. The analytical verification provides information on the performance characteristics of the assay, and the clinical verification determines the clinical utility of the assay. Determining the clinical utility of a molecular assay can be difficult when the molecular assay is more sensitive than the gold standard. This situation was seen with the commercial assays designed to detect *C. trachomatis* in genital specimens. Molecular assays proved to be much more sensitive than the gold standard method of culture. An insensitive gold standard can make a molecular assay appear to have a falsely low specificity. In this situation, an expanded gold standard can be used. For *C. trachomatis,* this included direct fluorescent-antibody testing and/or another molecular method (35, 66, 109). There are additional challenges in determining the clinical utility of molecular assays that detect rare pathogens. These assays are usually laboratory developed, and any given medical center may see very few cases of the disease, making clinical verification difficult. Moreover, standards and control material can be difficult to obtain for rare pathogens. Several companies now provide control material for the more common molecular assays such as those for *C. trachomatis*, *N. gonorrhoeae*, HIV-1, HCV, and CMV.

A positive control is designed to ensure that the test can consistently detect a concentration of target nucleic acid at or near the limit of detection of the assay. The positive control should be at the lowest concentration that can be reproducibly amplified. A positive control that is significantly greater than the cutoff of the assay may not detect small decreases in amplification efficiency. In addition, large amounts of target DNA can increase problems with contamination in the laboratory. Depending on the availability of material, the positive control may be purified nucleic acid or lysed or intact organisms. An extraction control tests the ability of the nucleic acid extraction or purification method to successfully free nucleic acid from the organism. The extraction control, which should be intact organisms, can also serve as a positive control if it is used at the appropriate concentration.

Monitoring for the presence of inhibitors in a specimen is important, particularly for complex specimens such as blood or sputum. Several methods can be used to control for inhibition. A commonly used method is to amplify two aliquots of a clinical specimen, one directly and the second spiked with an aliquot of positive control DNA. For a specimen to be considered negative for the target analyte, testing results for the direct specimen must be negative and those for the spiked specimen must be positive. If an inhibitor of amplification was present, the spiked specimen would be negative. The concentration of positive control used for the spike must be near the limit of detection of the assay to ensure that low-level inhibition of amplification is detected.

Another approach to monitoring for inhibition of amplification is adding an internal control to the clinical specimen prior to nucleic acid extraction. As discussed in "Quantitative Methods," the internal control molecule may be designed with the same primer binding sites as the target molecule but modified in some manner so as to allow detection separate from the target based on size or sequence. An internal control is an effective way to monitor for inhibition, but it may decrease the sensitivity of the assay due to competition for assay components. Amplification of a human housekeeping gene such as that for β-globin may also be used as an internal control, but the gene should not be present in vast excess of the target molecule or inhibition of amplification of the target molecule can occur without evidence of inhibition of the housekeeping gene. Inhibition controls should be included in assays that use a new specimen extraction method or specimen type. However, a cost-effective approach is to discontinue these controls once the inhibition rate is determined to be less than 1 to 2%.

Under certain conditions, there may be a need to determine if there is adequate nucleic acid in a specimen, for example, when using paraffin-embedded tissue or when evaluating the quality of a specimen. In these situations, amplification of housekeeping genes can be used to determine if the specimen contains human DNA. The absence of amplifiable human DNA from the specimen raises concern about whether the specimen quality is adequate.

Negative controls should be included in all assays and processed in a manner similar to the processing of the clinical specimens. The negative control should be taken through all steps of the assay, including the nucleic acid extraction process. However, no amplification in the negative control does not ensure that there is not contamination in the run, as contamination is often low level and sporadic. Including multiple negative controls in the run may provide additional assurance that there is no contamination, but this approach may be cost prohibitive. Ideally, the negative control should be a clinical specimen that does not contain the analyte of interest. These types of controls may be difficult to obtain, so water or buffer is often substituted.

Currently, the College of American Pathologists is the only Centers for Medicare and Medicaid Services-approved proficiency program for molecular testing for infectious diseases. The College of American Pathologists provides proficiency testing for many common pathogens for which routine testing is done in the clinical laboratory. The Quality Control for Molecular Diagnostics proficiency program, which is jointly sponsored by the European Society for Clinical Virology and the European Society for Clinical Microbiology and Infectious Diseases (Glasgow, Scotland, United Kingdom), also provides testing for a variety of pathogens. The Centers for Disease Control and Prevention also offer a model performance evaluation program for HIV-1 twice per year. When formal external proficiency testing programs are not available, laboratories may split sample testing with other laboratories, split samples between a new method and an established laboratory-developed method, or clinically validate the test result by clinical diagnosis. When exchanging specimens between laboratories for proficiency testing, it is important that both laboratories use the same method, particularly for quantitative methods, as viral load values will differ among the various assays.

Reporting and Interpretation of Results

The interpretation of molecular assays requires a basic understanding of the strengths and limitations of these technologies. There are unique problems in interpreting molecular testing results that are not routinely encountered with traditional microbiologic assays, such as culture and serology. Some of the problems that may occur in interpreting molecular assays include recognizing false-positive results, distinguishing viable from nonviable organisms, and correlating nucleic acid detection with the presence of disease.

For interpretation of a positive test result, the issues that need to be considered are assay specificity and contamination. The specificities of most molecular assays are established by the primers and probes used during amplification and detection steps; if they cross-react with other pathogens, then false-positive results are possible. For example, primers designed to detect *Mycobacterium pneumoniae* from respiratory specimens must not cross-react with organisms that are part of normal oral flora or other common respiratory pathogens, such as *Streptococcus pneumoniae*. Although uncommon, problems with primer specificity do occur; the primers designed to amplify the 5′ untranslated region of enteroviruses have been reported to cross-react with rhinoviruses (106). This would not be a problem for testing of CSF specimens but would preclude using the assay on respiratory specimens. Problems with primer specificity have also been reported for a commercially available PCR assay designed to detect *N. gonorrhoeae*. The primers used in this assay cross-react with *Neisseria subflava*, a nonpathogenic organism found in the oropharynx (29). False-positive results can also be due to contamination, which may occur during specimen processing or as a result of carryover contamination of previously amplified products.

The interpretation of a negative result requires consideration of assay sensitivity, specimen quality, nucleic acid extraction efficacy, and amplification efficiency. Problems with any of these factors can lead to a false-negative result, which is why measures to control for each of these parameters should be included in assays whenever feasible. Another source of false-positive results is sequence variation, which may prevent binding of either primers or probes. To minimize this problem, one should perform a thorough search of known sequences before designing the assay and occasionally reexamine the available databases after the assay is put into clinical use.

Molecular assays detect pathogen nucleic acid but cannot determine whether that nucleic acid is found in a viable or nonviable organism. Pathogen nucleic acid can be detected for long periods of time after appropriate treatment is initiated. For example, *C. trachomatis* DNA can be found in the urine of patients for up to 3 weeks after completion of a course of therapy (35). Similar results have been reported for the detection of HSV DNA in the CSF of patients with encephalitis. DNA can persist for 2 weeks or longer after the initiation of acyclovir therapy (64). Due to the persistence of pathogen DNA after initiation of therapy, qualitative molecular assays should not be used to monitor response to therapy. One notable exception is the use of a qualitative HCV RNA RT-PCR assay to monitor the response to therapy with pegylated interferon and ribavirin. In this instance, the absence of detectable viral RNA from plasma is used to define treatment response (32).

The detection of pathogen nucleic acid does not ensure that the organism is the cause of disease. The organism may be present as part of the normal flora, as a colonizer of a particular area, or as a cause of infection. Distinguishing between colonization and infection may be more difficult when molecular techniques that are more sensitive than culture are used. Organisms present in very low concentrations, which may have gone undetected by routine culture methods, may be detected by using molecular techniques.

Distinguishing colonization from infection is easier when testing a specimen from a normally sterile site such as CSF or blood; however, this factor alone does not ensure that the organism is a true pathogen. This distinction is a concern with the detection of herpesviruses, which cause lifelong latent infections. An important example of distinguishing these two states is monitoring transplant recipients for CMV disease using molecular methods. Initial studies used very sensitive qualitative PCR assays (36, 87), and it was clear that CMV DNA could be detected in the blood of patients that never went on to develop symptomatic disease.

Reporting the results of a qualitative molecular assay is usually straightforward; results are often reported as DNA detected or not detected. Several key parameters that may also be reported are the limit of detection of the assay, data pertaining to the rate of inhibition for a given sample type, the gene target, and the amplification method used for testing. Reporting results from quantitative assays is more complex and requires consideration of several parameters including dynamic range, units, and precision. Results of quantitative assays can be expressed as copies, weight (nanograms or picograms), or international units of the target nucleic acid in a defined volume, such as milliliters of plasma or blood, grams of tissue, or number of leukocytes. When the results of quantitative assays are reported, the precision of the assays needs to be considered. For the currently available HIV-1 viral load assays, the assay and biological variability are approximately 0.5 $\log_{10}$ (107). Therefore, changes in viral load must exceed 0.5 $\log_{10}$ (threefold) in order to represent a biologically significant change in viral replication. For these assays, values should be reported as $\log_{10}$ rather than integers to avoid the overinterpretation of small changes in viral load. Quantitative assays have a defined linear or dynamic range. Values below the lower limit of quantification should be reported as less than the lower limit of the linear range, rather than as negative. Values above the upper limit of quantification should be reported as greater than the upper limit of the linear range. For values above the limit of detection but below the limit of quantitation, results may be reported as detectable, less than the lower limit of the linear range. For example, if the lower limit of quantitation of an HIV-1 viral load assay is 400 copies/ml, a value of 250 copies/ml could be reported as detectable, <400 copies/ml. Inclusion of the amplification method and specimen type in the report is particularly important for quantitative assays, as values from different assay types are not always comparable.

Regulatory and Reimbursement Issues

The medical needs for new molecular microbiology tests have exceeded the capacity of the diagnostic industry to provide FDA-cleared test kits to fill these needs. Table 1 lists the FDA-cleared nucleic acid-based tests for infectious diseases. Notably absent from the list are tests that have become a standard of care in a variety of diseases such as HSV encephalitis, enteroviral meningitis, and pertussis. Many laboratories have developed tests to fill these unmet needs. These laboratory-developed tests must be appropriately verified and validated as specified in the Centers for Medicare and Medicaid Services final rule for laboratory requirements, 42 CFR part 493 (88a). Such tests are eligible for reimbursement by Medicare and other payers if they are determined to be part of a standard of care or to be of proven clinical benefit.

Laboratory-developed tests often utilize a combination of reagents from different manufacturers, some of which are ASRs. ASRs are chemical substances, for example, antibodies or nucleic acid sequences, that are used in diagnostic tests to detect another specific substance in a specimen and are purchased from manufacturers under this label. ASRs do not include a protocol for use or information on analytical performance or clinical indication. The FDA requires a disclaimer on reports for laboratory-developed tests using ASRs, and it reads: "This test result was developed and its performance characteristics determined by [laboratory name]. It has not been cleared or approved by the U.S. Food and Drug Administration." This disclaimer was not intended to cover laboratory-developed tests not using ASRs or the off-label uses of FDA-cleared products.

A laboratory may want to include clarifying statements in the reports of results from laboratory-developed tests employing ASRs. These statements may point out that FDA clearance is not necessary for these tests and that they are used for clinical purposes. Additional information may include that the laboratory is certified under the Clinical Laboratory Improvement Amendments of 1988 to perform high-complexity testing and that pursuant to the requirements of the amendments the laboratory has established and verified the test's accuracy and precision.

Correct current procedural terminology (CPT) coding of molecular microbiology tests is essential to coverage and reimbursement by payers. In 1998, many analyte-specific codes for tests using direct probes, amplified probes, and amplified probes with quantification were established in the microbiology section of the CPT coding manual, and this list of available codes continues to expand (1a). Prior to 1998, molecular microbiology tests were billed using multiple-component CPT codes selected from the molecular pathology section of the manual. The introduction of analyte-specific codes has simplified the coding process and in many cases

TABLE 1 FDA-cleared or -approved molecular diagnostic tests for infectious diseases[a]

Test objective	Manufacturer (distributor)	Test name	Method[b]
C. trachomatis detection (single organism)	Digene Corp., Gaithersburg, Md.	HC2 CT ID	HC
	Gen-Probe, Inc., San Diego, Calif.	APTIMA CT assay	TMA
	Gen-Probe, Inc.	PACE 2 CT and PACE 2 CT probe competition assay	HPA
	Roche Diagnostics, Indianapolis, Ind.	AMPLICOR CT/NG test for *C. trachomatis*	PCR
	Roche Diagnostics	COBAS AMPLICOR CT/NG test for *C. trachomatis*	PCR
N. gonorrhoeae detection (single organism)	Digene Corp.	HC2 GC ID	HC
	Gen-Probe, Inc.	APTIMA GC assay	TMA
	Gen-Probe, Inc.	PACE 2 GC and PACE 2 GC probe competition assay	HPA
	Roche Diagnostics	AMPLICOR CT/NG test for *N. gonorrhoeae*	PCR
	Roche Diagnostics	COBAS AMPLICOR CT/NG test for *N. gonorrhoeae*	PCR
C. trachomatis and *N. gonorrhoeae* detection	Becton Dickinson and Company, Sparks, Md.	BD ProbeTec ET *C. trachomatis* and *N. gonorrhoeae* amplified DNA assay	SDA
	Digene Corp.	HC2 CT/GC combo test	HC
	Gen-Probe, Inc.	APTIMA combo 2 assay	TMA
	Gen-Probe, Inc.	PACE 2C CT/GC	HPA
	Roche Diagnostics	AMPLICOR CT/NG test	PCR
	Roche Diagnostics	COBAS AMPLICOR CT/NG test	PCR
Gardnerella spp. *Trichomonas vaginalis*, and *Candida* spp. detection	Becton Dickinson and Company	BD Affirm VPIII microbial identification test	Hybridization
Group A *Streptococcus* detection	Gen-Probe, Inc.	GASDirect	HPA
Group B *Streptococcus* detection	GeneOhm Sciences, Inc., San Diego, Calif. (Cepheid, Sunnyvale, Calif.)	IDI-Strep B assay	Real-time PCR
Legionella pneumophila detection	Becton Dickinson and Company	BD ProbeTec ET *Legionella pneumophila* amplified DNA assay	SDA
Methicillin-resistant *S. aureus detection*	GeneOhm Sciences, Inc. (Cepheid)	IDI-MRSA assay	Real-time PCR
M. tuberculosis detection	Gen-Probe, Inc.	AMPLIFIED *M. tuberculosis* direct test	TMA
	Roche Diagnostics	AMPLICOR *M. tuberculosis* test	PCR
Culture confirmation of *Mycobacterium* spp., various fungi, and other bacteria[c]	Gen-Probe, Inc	AccuProbe culture identification tests	HPA
CMV detection	Digene Corp.	HC1 CMV DNA test	HC
	bioMérieux, Inc., Durham, N.C.	CMV pp67 mRNA	NASBA
HCV detection	Gen-Probe, Inc. (Bayer HealthCare, Diagnostics Division, Tarrytown, N.Y.)	VERSANT HCV RNA	TMA
	Roche Diagnostics	AMPLICOR HCV test, version 2.0	RT-PCR
	Roche Diagnostics	COBAS AMPLICOR HCV test, version 2.0	RT-PCR
HCV quantitation	Bayer HealthCare, Diagnostics Division	VERSANT HCV RNA 3.0 bDNA assay	bDNA assay
HIV-1 drug resistance detection	Celera Diagnostics, Alameda, Calif. (Abbott Molecular Diagnostics, Des Plains, Ill.)	ViroSeq HIV-1 genotyping system	Sequencing
	Bayer HealthCare, Diagnostics Division	TruGene HIV-1 genotyping system	Sequencing

(Continued on next page)

TABLE 1 *(Continued)*

Test objective	Manufacturer (distributor)	Test name	Method[b]
HIV-1 quantitation	Bayer HealthCare, Diagnostics Division	VERSANT HIV-1 RNA 3.0 bDNA assay	bDNA assay
	bioMérieux, Inc.	NucliSens HIV-1 QT	NASBA
	Roche Diagnostics	AMPLICOR HIV-1 MONITOR test, version 1.5	RT-PCR
	Roche Diagnostics	COBAS AMPLICOR HIV-1 MONITOR test, version 1.5	RT-PCR
HBV, HCV, and HIV-1 screening for blood donations	Gen-Probe, Inc. (Chiron, Emeryville, Calif.)	Procleix HIV-1/HCV assay	TMA
	National Genetics Institute, Los Angeles, Calif.	UltraQual HCV RT-PCR assay	RT-PCR
	National Genetics Institute	UltraQual HIV-1 RT-PCR assay	RT-PCR
	Roche Diagnostics	COBAS AmpliScreen HBV test	PCR
	Roche Diagnostics	COBAS AmpliScreen HCV test, version 2.0	RT-PCR
	Roche Diagnostics	COBAS AmpliScreen HIV-1 test, version 1.5	RT-PCR
HPV detection	Digene Corp.	HC2 HR and LR	HC
	Digene Corp.	HC2 HPV HR	HC
	Digene Corp.	HC2 DNA with Pap	HC

[a] Information was current as of 15 August 2005. Modified from www.ampweb.org.
[b] HC, hybrid capture; HPA, hybridization protection assay.
[c] Mycobacteria include *M. avium*, *M. intracellulare*, the *M. avium* complex, *M. gordonae*, *M. kansasii*, and the *M. tuberculosis* complex. Fungi include *Blastomyces dermatitidis*, *Coccidioides immitis*, *Cryptococcus neoformans*, and *Histoplasma capsulatum*. Other bacteria include *Campylobacter* spp., *Enterococcus* spp., group A *Streptococcus*, group B *Streptococcus*, *Haemophilus influenzae*, *Listeria monocytogenes*, *N. gonorrhoeae*, *Streptococcus pneumoniae*, and *S. aureus*.

increased the reimbursement for molecular microbiology procedures, although there continues to be considerable regional variation in reimbursement rates for the codes. The analyte-specific codes cover all aspects of testing, including the interpretation of the test result, and the use of these specific codes precludes the use of the component codes.

Credentials

Staffing a molecular diagnostics laboratory with individuals who have an appropriate knowledge base and skill set remains a challenge. Until recently, molecular diagnostics was not part of the core curriculum in medical technology programs. However, the situation is changing, and the acquisition of credentials in this area is now available for medical technologists and technicians from the American Board of Bioanalysts, the National Credentialing Agency, and the American Society for Clinical Pathology. Laboratory directors may receive credentials in molecular diagnostics through the American Board of Bioanalysts (physicians and clinical laboratory scientists), the American Board of Clinical Chemistry (physicians and clinical laboratory scientists), and jointly through the American Boards of Pathology and Medical Genetics (physicians only).

FUTURE DIRECTIONS

Nucleic acid testing will continue to be one of the leading growth areas in laboratory medicine. The number of applications of this technology in diagnostic microbiology will continue to increase, and the technology will increasingly be incorporated into routine clinical microbiology laboratories as it becomes less technically complex and more accessible. More clinical and financial outcome data will be needed to justify the use of this expensive technology in an era of declining reimbursement and increased cost consciousness.

Despite its growth, molecular diagnostics largely remains a cottage industry, with the proliferation of tests developed by individual laboratories to satisfy new medical needs not met by the diagnostic test industry. As a result, one of the biggest concerns for the future is the development of effective proficiency testing programs that will help ensure that the results of these tests are reliable and reproducible among laboratories.

To a great extent, the future of molecular microbiology depends on automation. Many of the available tests are labor-intensive, with much of the labor devoted to tedious sample processing methods. Sample processing remains the greatest challenge to automation, but the recent development of fully automated systems for molecular diagnostics offers hope for the future. Perhaps the most exciting prospects for automation come from the biochip and microfluidics sectors. With the currently available technology, it is not difficult to imagine the development in the near future of a small chip that could automate several functions of the microbiology laboratory.

The use of multiplex nucleic acid-based assays to screen at-risk patients for panels of probable pathogens remains a goal for molecular microbiology. Success to date has been limited by technical difficulties, but the development of such assays is key to providing molecular tests with the same broad diagnostic range provided by culture and other conventional methods.

Advances in human genomics will be exploited in the future to develop tests for immunogenetic factors that may influence the risk of becoming infected with certain pathogens or the progression of disease. Human gene expression profiling with microarrays may be important in defining patterns of host gene expression associated with different pathogens or disease states. Better understanding of pathogen genomics, gene expression, and proteomics will lead to the discovery of new diagnostic and therapeutic targets.

REFERENCES

1. **Aitken, C., W. Barrett-Muir, C. Millar, K. Templeton, J. Thomas, F. Sheridan, D. Jeffries, M. Yaqoob, and J. Breuer.** 1999. Use of molecular assays in diagnosis and monitoring of cytomegalovirus disease following renal transplantation. *J. Clin. Microbiol.* **37:**2804–2807.

1a. **American Medical Association.** 2006. *CPT 2006, Current Procedural Terminology.* AMA Press, Chicago, Ill.
2. **Arnold, C., L. Westland, G. Mowat, A. Underwood, J. Magee, and S. Gharbia.** 2005. Single-nucleotide polymorphism-based differentiation and drug resistance detection in *Mycobacterium tuberculosis* from isolates or directly from sputum. *Clin. Microbiol. Infect.* **11:**122–130.
3. **Arnold, L. J., Jr., P. W. Hammond, W. A. Wiese, and N. C. Nelson.** 1989. Assay formats involving acridinium ester-labeled DNA probes. *Clin. Chem.* **35:**1588–1594.
4. **Bahk, Y. Y., S. A. Kim, J. S. Kim, H. J. Euh, G. H. Bai, S. N. Cho, and Y. S. Kim.** 2004. Antigens secreted from *Mycobacterium tuberculosis:* identification by proteomics approach and test for diagnostic marker. *Proteomics* **4:** 3299–3307.
5. **Barbeau, J. M., J. Goforth, A. M. Caliendo, and F. S. Nolte.** 2004. Performance characteristics of a quantitative TaqMan hepatitis C virus RNA analyte-specific reagent. *J. Clin. Microbiol.* **42:**3739–3746.
6. **Beutler, E., T. Gelbart, and W. Kuhl.** 1990. Interference of heparin with the polymerase chain reaction. *BioTechniques* **9:**166.
7. **Blin, N., and D. W. Stafford.** 1976. A general method for isolation of high molecular weight DNA from eukaryotes. *Nucleic Acids Res.* **3:**2303–2308.
8. **Boom, R., C. Sol, M. Salimans, C. Jansen, P. M. Wertheim-van Dillen, and J. van derNoordaa.** 1990. Rapid and simple method for purification of nucleic acids. *J. Clin. Microbiol.* **28:**495–503.
9. **Boriskin, Y. S., P. S. Rice, R. A. Stabler, J. Hinds, H. Al-Ghusein, K. Vass, and P. D. Butcher.** 2004. DNA microarrays for virus detection in cases of central nervous system infection. *J. Clin. Microbiol.* **42:**5811–5818.
10. **Caliendo, A. M., K. St. George, S. Y. Kao, J. Allega, B. H. Tan, R. LaFontaine, L. Bui, and C. R. Rinaldo.** 2000. Comparison of quantitative cytomegalovirus (CMV) PCR in plasma and CMV antigenemia assay: clinical utility of the prototype AMPLICOR CMV MONITOR test in transplant recipients. *J. Clin. Microbiol.* **38:**2122–2127.
11. **Cash, P., E. Argo, L. Ford, L. Lawrie, and H. McKenzie.** 1999. A proteomic analysis of erythromycin resistance in *Streptococcus pneumoniae*. *Electrophoresis* **20:**2259–2268.
12. **Chamberlain, J. S., R. A. Gibbs, J. E. Rainer, P. N. Nguyen, and C. T. Caskey.** 1988. Deletion screening of the Duchenne muscular dystrophy locus via multiplex DNA amplification. *Nucleic Acids Res.* **16:**11141–11156.
13. **Cheng, J., E. L. Sheldon, L. Wu, A. Uribe, L. O. Gerrue, J. Carrino, M. J. Heller, and J. P. O'Connell.** 1998. Preparation and hybridization analysis of DNA/RNA from *E. coli* on microfabricated bioelectronic chips. *Nat. Biotechnol.* **16:**541–546.
14. **Chomczynski, P., and N. Sacchi.** 1987. Single-step method of RNA isolation by acid guanidinium thiocyanate-phenol-chloroform extraction. *Anal. Biochem.* **62:**156–159.
15. **Choo, Q. L., G. Kuo, A. J. Weiner, L. R. Overby, D. W. Bradley, and M. Houghton.** 1989. Isolation of a cDNA clone derived from a blood-borne non-A, non-B viral hepatitis genome. *Science* **244:**359–362.
16. **Clementi, M., S. Menzo, P. Bagnarelli, A. Manzin, A. Valenza, and P. E. Varaldo.** 1993. Quantitative PCR and RT-PCR in virology. *PCR Methods Appl.* **2:**191–196.
17. **Clinical and Laboratory Standards Institute.** 2006. *Collection, Transport, Preparation, and Storage of Specimens and Samples for Molecular Methods; Approved Guideline.* CLSI document MM13-A. Clinical and Laboratory Standards Institute, Wayne, Pa.
18. **Clinical and Laboratory Standards Institute.** 2005. *Diagnostic Nucleic Acid Microarrays; Proposed Guideline.* CLSI document MMP12-P. Clinical and Laboratory Standards Institute, Wayne, Pa.
19. **Clinical and Laboratory Standards Institute.** 2006. *Genotyping for Infectious Diseases: Identification and Characterizations; Approved Guideline.* CLSI document MM10-A. Clinical and Laboratory Standards Institute, Wayne, Pa.
20. **Clinical and Laboratory Standards Institute.** 2006. *Molecular Diagnostic Methods for Infectious Diseases; Approved Guideline*, 2nd ed. CLSI document MM3-A2. Clinical and Laboratory Standards Institute, Wayne, Pa.
21. **Collins, M. L., C. Zayati, J. J. Detmer, B. Daly, J. A. Kolberg, T. Cha, B. D. Irvine, J. Tucker, and M. S. Urdea.** 1995. Preparation and characterization of RNA standards for use in quantitative branched-DNA hybridization assays. *Anal. Biochem.* **226:**120–129.
22. **Compton, J.** 1991. Nucleic acid sequence-based amplification. *Nature* **350:**91–92.
23. **Cope, J. J., A. Hildesheim, M. H. Schiffman, M. M. Manos, A. T. Lorincz, R. D. Burk, A. G. Glass, C. Greer, J. Burkland, K. Helgesen, D. R. Scott, M. E. Sherman, R. J. Kurman, and K.-L. Liaw.** 1997. Comparison of the hybrid capture tube test and PCR for detection of human papillomavirus DNA in cervical specimens. *J. Clin. Microbiol.* **35:**2262–2265.
24. **Corless, C. E., M. Guiver, R. Borrow, V. Edwards-Jones, A. J. Fox, and E. B. Kaczmarski.** 2001. Simultaneous detection of *Neisseria meningitidis, Haemophilus influenzae*, and *Streptococcus pneumoniae* in suspected cases of meningitis and septicemia using real-time PCR. *J. Clin. Microbiol.* **39:**1553–1558.
25. **Diaz, M. R., and J. W. Fell.** 2004. High-throughput detection of pathogenic yeasts of the genus trichosporon. *J. Clin. Microbiol.* **42:**3696–3706.
26. **Diggle, M. A., and S. C. Clarke.** 2004. Pyrosequencing: sequence typing at the speed of light. *Mol. Biotechnol.* **28:** 129–137.
27. **Dunbar, S. A., C. A. Vander Zee, K. G. Oliver, K. L. Karem, and J. W. Jacobson.** 2003. Quantitative, multiplexed detection of bacterial pathogens: DNA and protein applications of the Luminex LabMAP system. *J. Microbiol. Methods* **53:**245–252.
28. **Espy, M. J., T. F. Smith, and D. H. Persing.** 1993. Dependence of polymerase chain reaction product inactivation protocols on amplicon length and sequence composition. *J. Clin. Microbiol.* **31:**2361–2365.
29. **Farrell, D. J.** 1999. Evaluation of AMPLICOR *Neisseria gonorrhoeae* PCR using *cppB* nested PCR and 16S rRNA PCR. *J. Clin. Microbiol.* **37:**386–390.
30. **Felmlee, T. A., R. P. Oda, D. A. Persing, and J. P. Landers.** 1995. Capillary electrophoresis of DNA potential utility for clinical diagnoses. *J. Chromatogr.* **A717:**127–137.
31. **Fong, W. K., Z. Modrusan, J. P. McNevin, J. Marostenmaki, B. Zin, and F. Bekkaoui.** 2000. Rapid solid-phase immunoassay for detection of methicillin-resistant *Staphylococcus aureus* using cycling probe technology. *J. Clin. Microbiol.* **38:** 2525–2529.
32. **Fried, M. W., M. L. Shiffman, K. R. Reddy, C. Smith, G. Marinos, F. L. Goncales, Jr., D. Haussinger, M. Diago, G. Carosi, D. Dhumeaux, A. Craxi, A. Lin, J. Hoffman, and J. Yu.** 2002. Peginterferon alfa-2a plus ribavirin for chronic hepatitis C virus infection. *N. Engl. J. Med.* **347:** 975–982.
33. **Fung, E. T., V. Thulasiraman, S. R. Weinberger, and E. A. Dalmasso.** 2001. Protein biochips for differential profiling. *Curr. Opin. Biotechnol.* **12:**65–69.
34. **Furukawa, K., and V. P. Bhavanandan.** 1983. Influences of anionic polysaccharides on DNA synthesis in isolated nuclei and by DNA polymerase alpha: correlation of observed effects with properties of the polysaccharides. *Biochim. Biophys. Acta* **740:**466–475.
35. **Gaydos, C. A., K. A. Crotchfelt, M. R. Howell, S. Kralian, P. Hauptman, and T. C. Quinn.** 1998. Molecular

amplification assays to detect chlamydial infections in urine specimens from high school female students and to monitor the persistence of chlamydial DNA after therapy. *J. Infect. Dis.* **177:**417–424.

36. **Gerna, G., D. Zipeto, M. Parea, M. G. Revello, E. Silini, E. Percivalle, M. Zavattoni, P. Grossi, and G. Milanesi.** 1991. Monitoring of human cytomegalovirus infections and ganciclovir treatment in heart transplant recipients by determination of viremia, antigenemia, and DNAemia. *J. Infect. Dis.* **164:**488–498.
37. **Gharizadeh, B., E. Norberg, J. Loffler, S. Jalal, J. Tollemar, H. Einsele, L. Klingspor, and P. Nyren.** 2004. Identification of medically important fungi by the Pyrosequencing technology. *Mycoses* **47:**29–33.
38. **Gross-Bellard, M., P. Oudet, and P. Chambon.** 1973. Isolation of high-molecular-weight DNA from mammalian cells. *Eur. J. Biochem.* **36:**32–38.
39. **Guatelli, J. C., K. M. Whitfield, D. Y. Kwoh, K. J. Barringer, D. D. Richman, and T. R. Gingeras.** 1990. Isothermal *in vitro* amplification of nucleic acids by multienzyme reaction modeled after retroviral replication. *Proc. Natl. Acad. Sci. USA* **87:**1874–1878.
40. **Haanpera, M., P. Huovinen, and J. Jalava.** 2005. Detection and quantification of macrolide resistance mutations at positions 2058 and 2059 of the 23S rRNA gene by pyrosequencing. *Antimicrob. Agents Chemother.* **49:**457–460.
41. **Haas, G., G. Karaali, K. Ebermayer, W. G. Metzger, S. Lamer, U. Zimny-Arndt, S. Diescher, U. B. Goebel, K. Vogt, A. B. Roznowski, B. J. Wiedenmann, T. F. Meyer, T. Aebischer, and P. R. Jungblut.** 2002. Immunoproteomics of *Helicobacter pylori* infection and relation to gastric disease. *Proteomics* **2:**313–324.
42. **Hall, L., S. Wohlfiel, and G. D. Roberts.** 2003. Experience with the MicroSeq D2 large-subunit ribosomal DNA sequencing kit for identification of commonly encountered, clinically important yeast species. *J. Clin. Microbiol.* **41:** 5099–5102.
43. **Hall, L., S. Wohlfiel, and G. D. Roberts.** 2004. Experience with the MicroSeq D2 large-subunit ribosomal DNA sequencing kit for identification of filamentous fungi encountered in the clinical laboratory. *J. Clin. Microbiol.* **42:**622–626.
44. **Hankin, R. C.** 1992. In situ hybridization: principles and applications. *Lab. Med.* **23:**764–770.
45. **Haqqi, T. M., G. Sarkar, C. S. David, and S. S. Sommer.** 1988. Specific amplification with PCR of a refractory segment of genomic DNA. *Nucleic Acids Res.* **16:**11844.
46. **Heid, C., J. Stevens, K. J. Livak, and P. Mickey Williams.** 1996. Real time quantitative PCR. *Genome Res.* **6:**986–994.
47. **Hendricks, D. A., B. J. Stowe, B. S. Hoo, J. Kolberg, B. D. Irvine, P. D. Neuwald, M. S. Urdea, and R. P. Perrillo.** 1995. Quantitation of HBV DNA in human serum using a branched DNA (bDNA) signal amplification assay. *Am. J. Clin. Pathol.* **104:**537–546.
48. **Higuchi, R.** 1989. *Simple and Rapid Preparation of Samples for PCR.* Stockton Press, New York, N.Y.
49. **Higuchi, R., C. Fockler, G. Dollinger, and R. Watson.** 1993. Kinetic PCR analysis: real-time monitoring of DNA amplification reactions. *Bio/Technology* **11:**1026–1030.
50. **Holland, P. M., R. D. Abramson, R. Watson, and D. H. Gelfand.** 1991. Detection of specific polymerase chain reaction product by utilizing the 5′ → 3′ exonuclease activity of *Thermus aquaticus* DNA polymerase. *Proc. Natl. Acad. Sci. USA* **88:**7276–7280.
51. **Humar, A., D. Gregson, A. M. Caliendo, A. McGeer, G. Malkan, M. Krajden, P. Corey, P. Greig, S. Walmsley, G. Levy, and T. Mazzulli.** 1999. Clinical utility of quantitative cytomegalovirus viral load determination for predicting cytomegalovirus disease in liver transplant recipients. *Transplantation* **68:**1305–1311.
52. **Innis, M. A., K. B. Myambo, D. H. Gelfand, and M. A. Brow.** 1998. DNA sequencing with *Thermus aquaticus* DNA polymerase and direct sequencing of polymerase chain reaction-amplified DNA. *Proc. Natl. Acad. Sci. USA* **85:**9436–9440.
53. **Izreli, S., C. Pfleiderer, and T. Lion.** 1991. Detection of gene expression by PCR amplification of RNA derived from frozen heparinized whole blood. *Nucleic Acids Res.* **19:**6051.
54. **Jungblut, P. R., D. Bumann, G. Haas, U. Zimny-Arndt, P. Holland, S. Lamer, F. Siejak, A. Aebischer, and T. F. Meyer.** 2000. Comparative proteome analysis of *Helicobacter pylori*. *Mol. Microbiol.* **36:**710–725.
55. **Jungblut, P. R., G. Grabher, and G. Stoffler.** 1999. Comprehensive detection of immunorelevant *Borrelia garinii* antigens by two-dimensional electrophoresis. *Electrophoresis* **20:**3611–3622.
56. **Jungblut, P. R., U. E. Schaible, H. J. Mollenkopf, U. Zimny-Arndt, B. Raupach, J. Mattow, P. Halada, S. Lamer, K. Hagens, and S. H. Kaufmann.** 1999. Comparative proteome analysis of *Mycobacterium tuberculosis* and *Mycobacterium bovis* BCG strains: towards functional genomics of microbial pathogens. *Mol. Microbiol.* **33:**1103–1117.
57. **Kern, D., M. Collins, T. Fultz, J. Detmer, S. Hamren, J. J. Peterkin, P. Sheridan, M. Urdea, R. White, T. Yeghiazarian, and J. Todd.** 1996. An enhanced-sensitivity branched-DNA assay for quantification of human immunodeficiency virus type 1 RNA in plasma. *J. Clin. Microbiol.* **34:** 3196–3202.
58. **Khanna, M., J. Fan, K. Pehler-Harrington, C. Waters, P. Douglass, J. Stallock, S. Kehl, and K. J. Henrickson.** 2005. The pneumoplex assays, a multiplex PCR-enzyme hybridization assay that allows simultaneous detection of five organisms, *Mycoplasma pneumoniae*, *Chlamydia* (Chlamydophila) *pneumoniae*, *Legionella pneumophila*, *Legionella micdadei*, and *Bordetella pertussis*, and its real-time counterpart. *J. Clin. Microbiol.* **43:**565–571.
59. **Kricka, L. J.** 1999. Nucleic acid detection technologies—labels, strategies, and formats. *Clin. Chem.* **45:**453–458.
60. **Ksiazek, T. G., D. Erdman, C. S. Goldsmith, S. R. Zaki, T. Peret, S. Emery, S. Tong, C. Urbani, J. A. Comer, W. Lim, P. E. Rollin, S. F. Dowell, A. E. Ling, C. D. Humphrey, W. J. Shieh, J. Guarner, C. D. Paddock, P. Rota, B. Fields, J. DeRisi, J. Y. Yang, N. Cox, J. M. Hughes, J. W. LeDuc, W. J. Bellini, L. J. Anderson, and the SARS Working Group.** 2003. A novel coronavirus associated with severe acute respiratory syndrome. *N. Engl. J. Med.* **348:**1953–1966.
61. **Kurtzman, C. P., and C. J. Robnett.** 1997. Identification of clinically important ascomycetous yeasts based on nucleotide divergence in the 5′ end of the large-subunit (26S) ribosomal DNA gene. *J. Clin. Microbiol.* **35:**1216–1223.
62. **Kutyavin, I. V., I. A. Afonina, A. Mills, V. V. Gorn, E. A. Lukhtanov, E. S. Belousov, M. J. Singer, D. K. Walburger, S. G. Lokhov, A. A. Gall, R. Dempcy, M. W. Reed, R. B. Meyer, and J. Hedgpeth.** 2000. 3′-Minor groove binder-DNA probes increase sequence specificity at PCR extension temperatures. *Nucleic Acids Res.* **28:**655–661.
63. **Kwoh, D. Y., G. R. David, K. M. Whitfield, H. L. Chapelle, L. J. DiMichele, and T. R. Gingeras.** 1989. Transcription-based amplification system and detection of amplified human immunodeficiency virus type 1 with a bead-based sandwich hybridization format. *Proc. Natl. Acad. Sci. USA* **86:**1173–1177.
64. **Lakeman, F. D., R. J. Whitley, and the National Institute of Allergy and Infectious Diseases Collaborative Antiviral Study Group.** 1995. Diagnosis of herpes simplex encephalitis: application of polymerase chain reaction to cerebrospinal fluid from brain-biopsied patients and correlation with disease. *J. Infect. Dis.* **171:**857–863.

65. **Lay, M. J., and C. T. Wittwer.** 1997. Real-time fluorescence genotyping of factor V leiden during rapid cycle PCR. *Clin. Chem.* **43:**2262–2267.

66. **Lee, H. H., M. A. Chernesky, J. Schachter, J. D. Burczak, W. W. Andrews, S. Muldoon, G. Leckie, and W. E. Stamm.** 1995. Diagnosis of *Chlamydia trachomatis* genitourinary infection in women by ligase chain reaction assay of urine. *Lancet* **345:**213–216.

67. **Lee, S. S., E. J. Heathcote, K. R. Reddy, S. Zeuzem, M. W. Fried, T. L. Wright, P. J. Pockros, D. Haussinger, C. I. Smith, A. Lin, and S. C. Pappas.** 2002. Prognostic factors and early predictability of sustained viral response with peginterferon alfa-2a (40KD). *J. Hepatol.* **37:**500–506.

68. **Leone, G., H. van Schijndel, B. van Gemen, F. R. Kramer, and C. D. Schoen.** 1998. Molecular beacon probes combined with amplification by NASBA enable homogeneous, real-time detection of RNA. *Nucleic Acids Res.* **26:**2150–2155.

69. **Lieber, M. R.** 1997. The FEN-1 family of structure-specific nucleases in eukaryotic DNA replication, recombination and repair. *Bioessays* **19:**233–240.

70. **Little, M. C., J. Andrews, R. Moore, S. Bustos, L. Jones, C. Embres, G. Durmowicz, J. Harris, D. Berger, K. Yanson, C. Rostkowski, D. Yursis, J. Price, T. Fort, A. Walters, M. Collis, O. Llorin, J. Wood, F. Failing, C. O'Keefe, B. Scrivens, B. Pope, T. Hansen, K. Marino, and K. Williams.** 1999. Strand displacement amplification and homogeneous real-time detection incorporated in a second-generation DNA probe system, BDProbeTecET. *Clin. Chem.* **45:**777–784.

71. **Loeffelholz, M. J., C. A. Lewinski, S. R. Silver, A. Purohit, S. A. Herman, D. A. Buonagurio, and E. A. Dragon.** 1992. Detection of *Chlamydia trachomatis* in endocervical specimens by polymerase chain reaction. *J. Clin. Microbiol.* **30:**2847–2851.

72. **Longo, M. C., M. S. Berninger, and J. L. Hartley.** 1990. Use of uracil DNA glycosylase to control carry-over contamination in polymerase chain reactions. *Gene* **93:**125–128.

73. **Lyamichev, V., A. Mast, J. G. Hall, J. R. Prudent, M. W. Kaiser, T. Takova, et al.** 1999. Polymorphism identification and quantitative detection from genomic DNA by invasive cleavage of oligonucleotide probes. *Nat. Biotechnol.* **17:** 292–296.

74. **Lyamichev, V., and B. Neri.** 2003. Invader assay for SNP genotyping. *Methods Mol. Biol.* **212:**229–240.

75. **Mantero, G., A. Zonaro, A. Albertini, P. Bertolo, and D. Primi.** 1991. DNA enzyme immunoassay: general method for detecting products of polymerase chain reaction. *Clin. Chem.* **37:**422–429.

76. **Mazzulli, T., L. W. Drew, B. Yen-Lieberman, D. Jekic-McMullen, D. J. Kohn, C. Isada, G. Moussa, R. Chua, and S. Walmsley.** 1999. Multicenter comparison of the Digene hybrid capture CMV DNA assay (version 2.0), the pp65 antigenemia assay, and cell culture for detection of cytomegalovirus viremia. *J. Clin. Microbiol.* **37:**958–963.

77. **McDonough, S. H., C. Giachetti, Y. Yang, D. P. Kolk, E. Billyard, and L. Mimms.** 1998. High throughput assay for the simultaneous or separate detection of human immunodeficiency virus (HIV) and hepatitis type C virus (HCV). *Infusther. Transfusmed.* **25:**164–169. [Online.] doi:10.1159/000053415.

78. **McHutchinson, J. G., S. C. Gordon, E. R. Schiff, M. L. Shiffman, W. M. Lee, V. K. Rustgi, Z. D. Goodman, M.-H. Ling, S. Cort, J. K. Albrecht, et al.** 1998. Interferon alfa-2b alone or in combination with ribavirin as initial treatment for chronic hepatitis C. *N. Engl. J. Med.* **339:** 1485–1492.

79. **Mellors, J. W., C. R. Rinaldo, Jr., P. Gupta, R. M. White, J. A. Todd, and L. A. Kingsley.** 1996. Prognosis in HIV-1 infection predicted by the quantity of virus in plasma. *Science* **272:**1167–1170.

80. **Mitchell, P. S., M. J. Espy, T. F. Smith, D. R. Toal, P. N. Rys, E. F. Berbari, D. R. Osmon, and D. H. Persing.** 1997. Laboratory diagnosis of central nervous system infections with herpes simplex virus by PCR performed with cerebrospinal fluid specimens. *J. Clin. Microbiol.* **35:** 2873–2877.

81. **Morrison, T., J. J. Weiss, and C. T. Wittwer.** 1998. Quantification of low copy transcripts by continuous SYBR green I dye monitoring during amplification. *BioTechniques* **24:**954–958.

82. **Myers, T. W., and D. H. Gelfand.** 1991. Reverse transcription and DNA amplification by a *Thermus thermophilus* DNA polymerase. *Biochemistry* **30:**7661–7666.

83. **National Institutes of Health.** 2002. *NIH Consensus and State of the Science Statements*, vol. 19, p. 1–46. National Institutes of Health, Bethesda, Md.

84. **NCCLS.** 2001. *Quantitative Molecular Methods for Infectious Diseases.* NCCLS document MM6-A. NCCLS, Wayne, Pa.

85. **NCCLS.** 2004. *Nucleic Acid Sequencing Methods in Diagnostic Laboratory Medicine.* NCCLS document MM9-A. NCCLS, Wayne, Pa.

86. **Nolte, F. S.** 1999. Branched DNA signal amplification for direct quantitation of nucleic acid sequences in clinical specimens. *Adv. Clin. Chem.* **33:**201–235.

87. **Nolte, F. S., R. K. Emmens, C. Thurmond, P. S. Mitchell, C. Pascuzzi, S. M. Devine, R. Saral, and J. R. Wingard.** 1995. Early detection of human cytomegalovirus viremia in bone marrow transplant recipients by DNA amplification. *J. Clin. Microbiol.* **33:**1263–1266.

88. **Nycz, C. M., C. H. Dean, P. D. Haaland, C. A. Spargo, and G. T. Walker.** 1998. Quantitative reverse transcription strand displacement amplification; quantitation of nucleic acids using an isothermal amplification technique. *Anal. Biochem.* **259:**226–234.

88a. **Office of the Federal Register.** 2004. *Code of Federal Regulations. Clinical Laboratory Improvement Act Regulations*, part 493, subpart K, section 1253. U.S. Government Printing Office and Office of the Federal Register, Washington, D.C. [Online.] http://www.phppo.cdc.gov/clia/regs/subpart_k.aspx.

89. **Oldenburg, N., K. M. Lam, M. A. Khan, B. Top, N. M. Tacken, A. McKie, G. W. Mikhail, J. M. Middeldorp, A. Wright, N. R. Banner, and M. Yacoub.** 2000. Evaluation of human cytomegalovirus gene expression in thoracic organ transplant recipients using nucleic acid sequence-based amplification. *Transplantation* **70:** 1209–1215.

90. **Oliveira, K., S. M. Brecher, A. Durbin, D. S. Shapiro, D. R. Schwartz, P. C. De Girolami, J. Dakos, G. W. Procop, D. Wilson, C. S. Hanna, G. Haase, H. Peltroche-Llacsahuanga, K. C. Chapin, M. C. Musgnug, M. H. Levi, C. Shoemaker, and H. Stender.** 2003. Direct identification of *Staphylococcus aureus* from positive blood culture bottles. *J. Clin. Microbiol.* **41:**889–891.

91. **O'Meara, D., K. Wilbe, T. Leitner, B. Hejdeman, J. Albert, and J. Lundeberg.** 2001. Monitoring resistance to human immunodeficiency virus type 1 protease inhibitors by pyrosequencing. *J. Clin. Microbiol.* **39:**464–473.

92. **Orita, M., H. Iwahana, H. Kanazawa, K. Hayashi, and T. Sekiya.** 1989. Detection of polymorphism of human DNA by gel electrophoresis as single-strand conformation polymorphisms. *Proc. Natl. Acad. Sci. USA* **86:**2766–2770.

93. **Pang, J., J. Modlin, and R. Yolken.** 1992. Use of modified nucleotides and uracil-DNA glycosylase (UNG) for the control of contamination in the PCR-based amplification of RNA. *Mol. Cell. Probes* **6:**251–256.

94. **Pease, A. C., D. Solas, E. J. Sullivan, M. T. Cronin, C. P. Holmes, and S. P. Fodor.** 1994. Light-generated oligonucleotide arrays for rapid DNA sequence analysis. *Proc. Natl. Acad. Sci. USA* **91:**5022–5026.

95. **Peiris, J. S., S. T. Lai, L. L. Poon, Y. Guan, L. Y. Yam, W. Lim, J. Nicholls, W. K. Yee, W. W. Yan, M. T. Cheung, V. C. Cheng, K. H. Chan, D. N. Tsang, R. W. Yung, T. K. Ng, K. Y. Yuen, et al.** 2003. Coronavirus as a possible cause of severe acute respiratory syndrome. *Lancet* **361:**1319–1325.
96. **Persing, D. H., F. C. Tenover, J. Versalovic, Y.-W. Tang, E. Unger, D. A. Relman, and T. J. White (ed.).** 2004. *Molecular Microbiology: Diagnostic Principles and Practice.* ASM Press, Washington, D.C.
97. **Piccirilli, J. A., T. Krauch, S. E. Moroney, and S. A. Benner.** 1990. Enzymatic incorporation of a new base pair into DNA and RNA extends the genetic alphabet. *Nature* **343:**33–37.
98. **Poljak, M., and K. Seme.** 1996. Rapid detection and typing of human papillomaviruses by consensus polymerase chain reaction and enzyme-linked immunosorbent assay. *J. Virol. Methods* **56:**231–238.
99. **Reid, R., M. Greenberg, A. B. Jensen, M. Husain, J. Willett, Y. Daoud, G. Temple, C. R. Stanhope, A. Sherman, and D. G. Phibbs.** 1987. Sexually transmitted papillomaviral infections. I. The anatomic distribution and pathologic grade of neoplastic lesions associated with different viral types. *Am. J. Obstet. Gynecol.* **156:**212–222.
100. **Relman, D. A., T. M. Schmidt, R. P. MacDermott, and S. Falkow.** 1992. Identification of the uncultured bacillus of Whipple's disease. *N. Engl. J. Med.* **327:**293–301.
101. **Ren, Y., Q. Y. He, J. Fan, B. Jones, Y. Zhou, Y. Xie, C. Y. Cheung, A. Wu, J. F. Chiu, J. S. Peiris, and P. K. Tam.** 2004. The use of proteomics in the discovery of serum biomarkers from patients with severe acute respiratory syndrome. *Proteomics* **4:**3477–3484.
102. **Rigby, S., G. W. Procop, G. Haase, D. Wilson, G. Hall, C. Kurtzman, K. Oliveira, S. Von Oy, J. J. Hyldig-Nielsen, J. Coull, and H. Stender.** 2002. Fluorescence in situ hybridization with peptide nucleic acid probes for rapid identification of *Candida albicans* directly from blood culture bottles. *J. Clin. Microbiol.* **40:**2182–2186.
103. **Ririe, K., R. P. Rasmussen, and C. T. Wittwer.** 1997. Product differentiation by analysis of DNA melting curves during the polymerase chain reaction. *Anal. Biochem.* **245:**154–160.
104. **Rosenstraus, M., Z. Wang, S. Y. Chang, D. DeBonville, and J. P. Spadoro.** 1998. An internal control for routine diagnostic PCR: design, properties, and effect on clinical performance. *J. Clin. Microbiol.* **36:**191–197.
105. **Rossau, R., H. Traore, H. De Beenhouwer, W. Mijs, G. Jannes, P. De Rijk, and F. Portaels.** 1997. Evaluation of the INNO-LiPA Rif. TB assay, a reverse hybridization assay for the simultaneous detection of *Mycobacterium tuberculosis* complex and its resistance to rifampin. *Antimicrob. Agents Chemother.* **41:**2093–2098.
106. **Rotbart, H. A.** 1991. Nucleic acid detection systems for enteroviruses. *Clin. Microbiol. Rev.* **4:**156–168.
107. **Saag, M. S., M. Holodniy, D. R. Kuritzkes, W. A. O'Brien, R. Coombs, M. E. Poscher, D. M. Jacobsen, G. M. Shaw, D. D. Richman, and P. A. Volberding.** 1996. HIV viral load markers in clinical practice. *Nat. Med.* **2:**625–629.
108. **Saiki, R. K., D. H. Gelfand, S. Stoffel, S. J. Scharf, R. Higuchi, K. B. Mullis, G. Horn, and H. A. Ehrlich.** 1988. Primer-directed enzymatic amplification of DNA with a thermostable DNA polymerase. *Science* **239:**487–491.
109. **Schachter, J., W. E. Stamm, T. C. Quinn, W. W. Andrews, J. D. Burczak, and H. H. Lee.** 1994. Ligase chain reaction to detect *Chlamydia trachomatis* infection of the cervix. *J. Clin. Microbiol.* **32:**2540–2543.
110. **Schena, M., D. Shalon, R. Heller, A. Chai, P. O. Brown, and R. W. Davis.** 1996. Parallel human genome analysis: microarray-based expression monitoring of 1000 genes. *Proc. Natl. Acad. Sci. USA* **93:**10614–10619.
111. **Smith, P. L., C. R. WalkerPeach, R. J. Fulton, and D. B. DuBois.** 1998. A rapid, sensitive, multiplexed assay for detection of viral nucleic acids using the FlowMetrix system. *Clin. Chem.* **44:**2054–2056.
112. **Sogaard, M., H. Stender, and H. C. Schonheyder.** 2005. Direct identification of major blood culture pathogens, including *Pseudomonas aeruginosa* and *Escherichia coli,* by a panel of fluorescence in situ hybridization assays using peptide nucleic acid probes. *J. Clin. Microbiol.* **43:** 1947–1949.
113. **Solomon, D., M. Schiffman, R. Tarone, et al.** 2001. Comparison of three management strategies for patients with atypical squamous cells of undetermined significance: baseline results from a randomized trial. *J. Natl. Cancer Inst.* **93:**293–299.
114. **Sosnowski, R. G., E. Tu, W. F. Butler, J. P. O'Connell, and M. J. Heller.** 1997. Rapid determination of single base mismatch mutations in DNA hybrids by direct electric field control. *Proc. Natl. Acad. Sci. USA* **94:**1119–1123.
115. **Stender, H., M. Fiandaca, J. J. Hyldig-Nielsen, and J. Coull.** 2002. PNA for rapid microbiology. *J. Microbiol. Methods* **48:**1–17.
116. **Stender, H., T. A. Mollerup, K. Lund, K. H. Petersen, P. Hongmanee, and S. E. Godtfredsen.** 1999. Direct detection and identification of Mycobacterium tuberculosis in smear-positive sputum samples by fluorescence in situ hybridization (FISH) using peptide nucleic acid (PNA) probes. *Int. J. Tuberc. Lung Dis.* **3:**830–837.
117. **Stuyver, L., A. Wyseur, A. Rombout, J. Louwagie, T. Scarcez, C. Verhofstede, D. Rimland, R. F. Schinazi, and R. Rossau.** 1997. Line probe assay for rapid detection of drug-selected mutations in the human immunodeficiency virus type 1 reverse transcriptase gene. *Antimicrob. Agents Chemother.* **41:**284–291.
118. **Stuyver, L., A. Wyseur, W. van Arnhem, F. Hernandez, and G. Maertens.** 1996. Second-generation line probe assay for hepatitis C virus genotyping. *J. Clin. Microbiol.* **34:**2259–2266.
119. **Tang, Y. W., N. M. Ellis, M. K. Hopkins, D. H. Smith, D. E. Dodge, and D. H. Persing.** 1998. Comparison of phenotypic and genotypic techniques for identification of unusual aerobic pathogenic gram-negative bacilli. *J. Clin. Microbiol.* **36:**3674–3679.
120. **Telenti, A., P. Imboden, F. Marchesi, T. Schmidheini, and T. Bodmer.** 1993. Direct, automated detection of rifampin-resistant *Mycobacterium tuberculosis* by polymerase chain reaction and single-strand conformation polymorphism analysis. *Antimicrob. Agents Chemother.* **37:** 2054–2058.
121. **Templeton, K. E., S. A. Scheltinga, M. F. Beersma, A. C. Kroes, and E. C. Claas.** 2004. Rapid and sensitive method using multiplex real-time PCR for diagnosis of infections by influenza A and influenza B viruses, respiratory syncytial virus, and parainfluenza viruses 1, 2, 3, and 4. *J. Clin. Microbiol.* **42:**1564–1569.
122. **Tenover, F. C.** 1988. Diagnostic deoxyribonucleic acid probes for infectious diseases. *Clin. Microbiol. Rev.* **1:**82–101.
123. **Tenover, F. C., and J. Kamile.** 2004. Detection of antimicrobial resistance genes and mutations associated with antimicrobial resistance in microorganism, p. 391–406. *In* D. H. Persing, F. C. Tenover, J. Versalovic, Y.-W. Tang, E. Unger, D. A. Relman, and T. J. White (ed.), *Molecular Microbiology: Diagnostic Principles and Practice.* ASM Press, Washington, D.C.
124. **Thelwell, N., S. Millington, A. Solinas, J. Booth, and T. Brown.** 2000. Mode of action and application of Scorpion primers to mutation detection. *Nucleic Acids Res.* **28:**3752–3761.
125. **Thornton, C. G., J. L. Hartley, and A. Rashtchian.** 1992. Utilizing uracil DNA glycosylase to control carryover

contamination in PCR: characterization of residual UDG activity following thermal cycling. *BioTechniques* **13:**180–184.

126. **Tyagi, S., D. P. Bratu, and F. R. Kramer.** 1998. Multicolor molecular beacons for allele discrimination. *Nat. Biotechnol.* **16:**49–53.
127. **Walduck, A., T. Rudel, and T. F. Meyer.** 2004. Proteomic and gene profiling approaches to study host responses to bacterial infection. *Curr. Opin. Microbiol.* **7:**33–38.
128. **Walker, G. T., M. S. Fraiser, J. L. Schram, M. C. Little, J. G. Nadeau, and D. P. Malinowski.** 1992. Strand displacement amplification—an isothermal, in vitro DNA amplification technique. *Nucleic Acids Res.* **20:**1691–1696.
129. **Wallace, J., B. A. Woda, and G. Pihan.** 2005. Facile, comprehensive, high-throughput genotyping of human genital papillomaviruses using spectrally addressable liquid bead microarrays. *J. Mol. Diagn.* **7:**72–80.
130. **Walsh, E. E., K. M. McConnochie, C. E. Long, and C. B. Hall.** 1997. Severity of respiratory syncytial virus infection is related to virus strain. *J. Infect. Dis.* **175:**814–820.
131. **Whitcombe, D., J. Theaker, S. P. Guy, T. Brown, and S. Little.** 1999. Detection of PCR products using self-probing amplicons and fluorescence. *Nat. Biotechnol.* **17:**804–807.
132. **Wilkins, M. R., C. Pasquali, R. D. Appel, K. Ou, O. Golaz, J. C. Sanchez, J. X. Yan, A. A. Gooley, G. Hughes, I. Humphery-Smith, K. L. Williams, and D. F. Hochstrasser.** 1996. From proteins to proteomes: large scale protein identification by two-dimensional electrophoresis and amino acid analysis. *Bio/Technology* **14:**61–65.
133. **Woese, C. R.** 1987. Bacterial evolution. *Microbiol. Rev.* **51:**221–271.
134. **Wolk, D., S. Mitchell, and R. Patel.** 2001. Principles of molecular microbiology testing methods. *Infect. Dis. Clin. N. Am.* **15:**1157–1204.
135. **Wright, T. C., Jr., M. Schiffman, D. Solomon, J. T. Cox, F. Garcia, S. Goldie, K. Hatch, K. L. Noller, N. Roach, C. Runowicz, and D. Saslow.** 2004. Interim guidance for the use of human papillomavirus DNA testing as an adjunct to cervical cytology for screening. *Obstet. Gynecol.* **103:**304–309.
136. **Wu, D. Y., and R. B. Wallace.** 1989. The ligation amplification reaction (LAR)—amplification of specific DNA sequences using sequential rounds of template-dependent ligation. *Genomics* **4:**560–569.

Susceptibility Testing Instrumentation and Computerized Expert Systems for Data Analysis and Interpretation*

SANDRA S. RICHTER AND MARY JANE FERRARO

17

Commercial antimicrobial susceptibility testing (AST) systems were introduced into clinical microbiology laboratories during the 1980s and have been used in the majority of laboratories since the 1990s (46). Manual and semiautomated broth microdilution systems are utilized for small volumes of susceptibility testing, while larger laboratories often choose an automated broth microdilution system. Most AST systems also perform organism identification as described in chapter 15. Semiautomated systems available for the disk diffusion method are marketed primarily outside the United States. The AST systems include data management software that may be interfaced with a laboratory information system (LIS) and offer various levels of expert system analysis. Epidemiology and pharmacy software packages are also available.

The U.S. Food and Drug Administration (FDA) provides regulatory oversight for AST systems marketed in the United States. Susceptibility test systems are classified as class II medical devices (subject to general and special controls) and require premarket notification with a 510(k) submission for FDA clearance (30, 31). A 510(k) submission must demonstrate that a device is substantially equivalent to other devices marketed in the United States. The FDA recommends a multicenter comparison of an AST system to the Clinical and Laboratory Standards Institute (CLSI, formerly NCCLS) reference method (16, 17). The level of performance considered acceptable for each antimicrobial agent-organism combination is >89.9% categorical agreement (same susceptible, intermediate, or resistant classification), >89.9% essential agreement (MIC results within 1 dilution of the reference method), ≤1.5% very major errors (VME, false susceptibility based on the number of resistant organisms), and ≤3% major errors (ME, false resistance based on the number of susceptible isolates) (31). Any antimicrobial agent-organism combination not meeting these standards must be listed as a limitation in the package insert with a recommendation to use an alternative method. Limitation statements are also required if the evaluation did not include a sufficient number of resistant organisms, showed unacceptable (<95%) reproducibility, or showed an elevated "no growth" rate (>10%) for an organism group (31). The FDA allows reporting of AST results only if the antimicrobial agent has known clinical efficacy against the organism (31). Current information describing FDA regulations and a list of approved devices can be found online (http://www.fda.gov/cdrh/consumer/mda/index.html).

This chapter will focus primarily on commercial susceptibility testing systems currently available in the United States. The broth microdilution AST systems are manufactured by four companies: bioMerieux (Durham, N.C.; http://www.biomerieux-usa.com), Dade Behring, Inc. (Sacramento, Calif.; http://www.dadebehring.com), Becton Dickinson Diagnostics (Sparks, Md.; http://www.bd.com), and TREK Diagnostic Systems (Cleveland, Ohio; http://www.trekds.com). Only one disk diffusion system, manufactured by Giles Scientific (Santa Barbara, Calif.; http://www.biomic.com), has FDA clearance. Readers should be aware that susceptibility testing system components are constantly changing in response to new technology and problems that are discovered.

SEMIAUTOMATED INSTRUMENTATION FOR DISK DIFFUSION TESTING

The advantages of the disk diffusion method of susceptibility testing include simplicity, reliability, low cost, and a high degree of flexibility in the selection of agents tested (46). Semiautomated systems available for reading and interpreting disk diffusion inhibition zones are listed in Table 1. For all systems, agar plates are manually inserted into an instrument after incubation for image acquisition and measurement of the zone of inhibition. Despite advances in imaging technology, a visual review of plates for faint growth or pinpoint colonies within the zone is recommended to assess the need for manual adjustment of the diameter measurement. Data management software determines the categorical interpretation (susceptible, intermediate, or resistant) and may be interfaced with an LIS. Although linear regression may be used to generate an MIC from a zone measurement, the validity of this method for some antimicrobial agent-organism combinations has been questioned (93). Expert system analysis and epidemiology software are available for the systems. The primary advantages of these instruments are (i) less variability in zone measurement (in comparison to caliper readings by different technologists), (ii) reduced transcription errors,

*This chapter contains information presented in chapter 15 by Mary Jane Ferraro and James H. Jorgensen in the eighth edition of this Manual.

TABLE 1 Overview of manual and semiautomated susceptibility testing instrumentation

Type	Features	Manufacturer(s)[a]	System	Reference(s)
Semiautomated disk diffusion	Assistance in reading, recording, and interpreting zones of inhibition; data management with expert and epidemiology software.	Giles Scientific	BIOMIC V3	4, 33, 54
		i2a	SIRSCAN[b]	63, 66
		Oxoid	Aura Image[b]	1
		Mast	Mastacan Elite[b]	97
		Bio-Rad	Osiris[b]	5, 6, 52, 66, 74
Manual broth microdilution	Devices to facilitate visual interpretation, recording, and reporting.	Dade Behring	MicroScan LabPro	
		Becton Dickinson	PASCO data management	
		TREK Diagnostics	Sensititre SensiTouch	
Semiautomated broth microdilution	Automated devices read and report results after off-line incubation of tray or strip.	Dade Behring	Microscan AutoSCAN-4	
		TREK Diagnostics	Sensititre AutoReader	
		bioMerieux	Mini API[b]	

[a] Bio-Rad, Hercules, Calif., http://bio-rad.com; i2a, Montleier, France; Mast, Bootle, United Kingdom, http://www.mastascan.com; Oxoid, Basingstoke, United Kingdom, http://www.oxoid.com; see text for other manufacturers.

[b] These systems are not currently available in the United States.

(iii) labor savings, (iv) improved data management capabilities, and (v) expert review to ensure correct reporting of results that are consistent with known resistance phenotypes. In general, these instruments provide reproducible and accurate results. In evaluations of the systems, organisms with faint growth accounted for most discrepancies (33, 63, 66).

MANUAL BROTH MICRODILUTION SYSTEMS

The manual broth microdilution systems listed in Table 1 facilitate the visual reading and recording of MICs. The panels are frozen (Pasco system, TREK custom plates) or dehydrated microwell trays (MicroScan, Sensititre). Devices for rehydration and inoculation of dehydrated trays include the manual RENOK device (MicroScan), the microprocessor-controlled Sensititre Autoinoculator, and the Sensititre multichannel electronic pipette.

After off-line incubation, results are recorded on the Pasco Reader with a light pen and transferred to a data management system. The MicroScan data management system (LabPro) displays an image of the tray configuration for recording manual results directly on the computer. The Sensititre SensiTouch reader sequentially illuminates a liquid crystal display superimposed on the tray to guide the reading of endpoints that are recorded via a keypad and transferred to the data management system (SWIN, Sensititre Windows software) with expert analysis. The SWIN data management system is also available for recording of manual results without the SensiTouch reader.

Most manufacturers offer standard gram-positive, gram-negative, *Streptococcus pneumoniae*, and extended-spectrum β-lactamase (ESBL) confirmatory panels. TREK Diagnostic Systems also offers FDA-cleared yeast panels (Sensititre YeastOne) and "research use only" Sensititre panels for mycobacteria (rapid and slow growers) and anaerobes that can be read manually or on the SensiTouch.

SEMIAUTOMATED BROTH MICRODILUTION SYSTEMS

The semiautomated broth microdilution systems listed in Table 1 utilize automated devices to read endpoints after overnight off-line incubation. The results are transferred to a data management system that may include expert system analysis using the same software available for the automated systems. The Sensititre AutoReader and miniAPI read susceptibility and identification tests, while the MicroScan AutoSCAN-4 reads only susceptibility results from overnight panels. Further information regarding MicroScan and Sensititre panels is presented in the section on automated systems.

AUTOMATED BROTH MICRODILUTION SYSTEMS

Automated AST systems do not require further manual intervention to obtain results after placement of the test panel in an instrument where incubation and reading of endpoints occur. An overview of the automated systems currently available in the United States is presented in Table 2. The VITEK 1, VITEK 2, MicroScan WalkAway, and Phoenix systems provide AST results after short-term incubation (<16 h); the currently available Sensititre ARIS panels and some MicroScan WalkAway panels require overnight incubation. Manufacturers should be consulted regarding the current antimicrobial agents available for each system.

VITEK 1

The first VITEK instrument developed for the provision of rapid MIC results was introduced in the 1980s. The identification of common gram-positive and gram-negative bacteria may be determined simultaneously by running a separate ID card. The AST panels are thin plastic 45-well cards with one to five concentrations of 15 to 19 antimicrobial agents. After manual preparation of the inoculum, cards are placed in a vacuum module for card inoculation. Cards are then manually lifted to a sealing device and placed in a carousel within the incubator-reader unit. A robotic system moves cards to a photometer every 15 min for turbidimetric measurement of growth. Linear regression analysis is used to determine algorithm-derived MICs that are reported in 4 to 16 h. The system includes a computer with monitor and printer, an expert system, and a data management system (DataTrac) to archive test data and generate reports.

TABLE 2 Overview of automated broth microdilution susceptibility testing instrumentation[a]

Manufacturer	System	Panel capacity	Panels	Types of panels (no.)	Instrument features	Software
Becton Dickinson	BD Phoenix	100	Two-sided polystyrene tray: 85-well AST/ 51-well ID	Gram pos (2), gram neg (8), *S. pneumoniae* (1)	AST panels available as MIC +/− ID substrates. Turbidimetric and redox indicator readings every 20 min up to 16 h. Full-range MICs.	BDXpert, BD EpiCenter
bioMerieux	VITEK 1	32, 60, 120, 240, 480	45-Well cards	Gram pos (6), gram neg (36)	Turbidimetric reading every 15 min. MICs derived from 1–5 antimicrobial agent dilutions.	DataTrac, Expert System, Stellara
	VITEK 2 VITEK 2 XL	60 120	64-Well cards	Gram pos (2), gram neg (9), *S. pneumoniae* (1)	Most automated system with reduced time for initial setup. Also automated AST dilution and filling/ sealing of cards. Turbidimetric readings every 15 min. MICs derived from 1–6 antimicrobial agent dilutions.	DataTrac, AES, Stellara
	VITEK 2 Compact	30 or 60	Same as VITEK 2	Same as VITEK 2	Less automated, more affordable than VITEK 2. Windows-based DMS and expert system has improved visual aesthetics.	Observa, AES, Stellara
Dade Behring	MicroScan WalkAway SI	40 or 96	Standard 96-microwell trays	Overnight (23), *S. pneumoniae* (1) Rapid (7), Synergies Plus (6)	Panels available as full-range MIC or breakpoint. Combo panels include ID substrates. MIC readings: ON, turbidimetric; "read when ready," colorimetric; rapid panels (4.5–15 h), fluorometric.	LabPro, LabPro Alert, PharmLink
TREK	Sensititre ARIS 2x	64	Standard 96-microwell trays	Gram pos (4), gram neg (6), *S. pneumoniae* (1)	Fluorometric readings after ON incubation of full-range MIC trays. Nonfermenter, *Haemophilus*/ *S. pneumoniae*, custom MIC panels also available.	SWIN

[a] Abbreviations: DMS, data management system; ID, identification; neg, negative; ON, overnight; pos, positive.

VITEK 2

The VITEK 2 received FDA clearance in 2000 and is the most automated AST instrument currently available. The cards are slightly thicker than VITEK 1 cards, with 64 wells that contain one to six concentrations of 9 to 20 antimicrobial agents. An identification card for common gram-positive or gram-negative bacteria may be run simultaneously with each AST card. The Smart Carrier Station includes a bar code scanner and base unit with microprocessor that holds a cassette with a capacity of 15 cards. A memory chip on the cassette allows the transfer of scanned information to the reader-incubator unit. The workflow for large laboratories can be optimized by placement of Smart Carrier Stations at multiple locations. After placement of a cassette into the VITEK 2 loading station, it is automatically moved through stations for bar code reading, AST dilution preparation, card inoculation, and card sealing. The transport system then places cards on a carousel with a 60-card capacity for incubation. The VITEK 2XL instrument has a capacity of 120 cards. Each card is moved to an optic station every 15 min for measurement of light transmittance that is proportional to growth. The Advanced Expert System (AES) is discussed in a later section.

The VITEK 2 Compact was introduced in 2005 for smaller labs and uses the same cards as the VITEK 2 system. The instrument is available in two sizes that accommodate 30 or 60 cards. The VITEK 2 Compact is less automated and more affordable than the VITEK 2. The initial inoculum and dilution preparation is manual, but a bar code reader replaces the hand labeling required with VITEK 1. Cards are initially placed into the vacuum unit (on the left side of the instrument) for filling followed by manual transfer to the right side of the instrument for automated sealing and transfer to the incubator-reader unit. The VITEK 2 Compact data management system (Observa) is PC Windows-based with better visual aesthetics and a more layered presentation of the same expert system (AES) analysis originally offered with the VITEK 2. Observa software may be used for preparing epidemiologic reports with data from VITEK 2 Compact and the manufacturer's blood culture instrument, BacT/ALERT. Observa software is expected to become available for VITEK 2 in 2006.

All of the VITEK systems connect to Stellara, a new system component launched in 2005 utilizing wireless technology to allow Health Insurance Portability and Accountability Act-compliant real-time communication of lab results to pharmacists and clinicians. The results are compared to patient records, allowing clinicians to be notified via a personal digital assistant of inappropriate antimicrobial therapy with suggested changes. Other lab results (chemistry or hematology) may also be reported with Stellara.

MicroScan WalkAway

The MicroScan WalkAway system was developed in the late 1980s and until recently offered two major types of AST panels: conventional panels read turbidimetrically after overnight incubation and rapid panels read fluorometrically after 4.5 to 15 h of incubation. These panels, all conventional 96-well microdilution trays, include (i) MIC panels (a broad range of antimicrobial agent dilutions); (ii) MIC combo panels (some wells used for identification); and (iii) breakpoint combo panels (identification with a limited range of antimicrobial agent dilutions for a categorical result of susceptible, intermediate, or resistant). A third type of MicroScan panel, Synergies plus, became available in 2005. Synergies plus combines three methods in one panel: "read-when-ready" AST results available as quickly as 4.5 h (colorimetric reading), overnight results for drugs requiring longer incubation (turbidimetric reading), and identification (fluorometric results within 2.5 h). Synergies plus gram-negative panels contain 19 to 25 antimicrobial agents; FDA clearance for the gram-positive panel is pending.

The WalkAway system includes an incubator-reader unit, a personal computer with an LIS interface, and a printer. "Prompt" is available for preparation of the inoculum for overnight panels without measurement of turbidity and is stable for 4 h. A manual device (RENOK) rehydrates and inoculates panels. The humidified incubator-reader unit has a bar code scanner, rotating carousel, and robotics to position panels under a central photometer or fluorometer for readings. An updated data management system, LabPro, interprets results, generates patient reports, and archives data to allow production of user-defined reports (antibiograms, trend analysis, and epidemiology reports). Since 2002, the data management system may be coupled with an expert system (LabPro Alert) that incorporates >100 rules that may be customized. Two instrument sizes accommodate 40 or 96 panels. A new SI version of the WalkAway instrument available since 1999 has eliminated the need for manual addition of identification reagents; older instruments may be upgraded to SI capability.

BD Phoenix

The BD Phoenix System was launched in Europe in 2001 and the United States in 2004. The instrument holds up to 100 test panels. The panels are polystyrene trays containing 136 wells divided into a 51-well identification (ID) side and an 85-well AST side with 16 to 22 antimicrobial agents. After preparation of the AST inoculum, a drop of redox indicator is added. The suspension is manually poured into the AST side of the panel, sealed with a plastic cap, and bar coded prior to placement on the instrument. The instrument reads panels every 20 min using both the colorimetric change in the redox indicator and turbidity to determine organism growth. Growth (metabolic activity) causes the redox indicator to change from an oxidized (blue) state to a reduced (pink) form. A full range of antimicrobial agent concentrations and a "growth" or "no growth" reading for each well allow the system to provide direct rather than calculated MICs.

The BDXpert system applies rules based on CLSI guidelines to analyze AST results. AST results will not be reported for an organism-antimicrobial agent combination if clinical efficacy is unknown, there are no approved MIC interpretive criteria, or the organism has intrinsic resistance. The BD EpiCenter is data management software for analyzing epidemiologic trends and generating reports using information from multiple BD instruments (Phoenix, BACTEC blood culture, and MGIT 960 systems). Features of BD EpiCenter include an LIS interface, reporting of inferred results for antimicrobial agents not on panels, and the capability to apply BDXpert system analysis to manual off-line AST results.

Sensititre ARIS 2x

The Sensititre ARIS (Automated Reading and Incubation System) was introduced in the United States in 1992 and provides overnight AST results (13, 14). The latest ARIS 2x version with hardware and software upgrades was released in 2004. The ARIS 2x instrument fits on the Sensititre

AutoReader and holds up to 64 plates (standard 96-microwell trays) available as MIC panels or separate identification plates. Plates are rehydrated and inoculated with the Sensititre AutoInoculator or a handheld multichannel electronic pipette before placement in the instrument's carousel. An internal bar code scanner identifies the plate type to assign the appropriate time of incubation. After 16 to 24 h of incubation, each AST plate is transported to the AutoReader for fluorometric reading of endpoints. The data management software (SWIN) provides expert analysis of results.

ADVANTAGES OF AUTOMATED SYSTEMS

Advantages of automated AST systems include labor savings, reproducibility, data management with expert system analysis, and the opportunity to generate results more rapidly. A workflow and performance evaluation of the VITEK 2 and Phoenix systems reported a longer mean setup time per isolate for Phoenix (3 min) than for VITEK 2 (1.5 min) but more monthly maintenance time for VITEK 2 (63.2 min) than for Phoenix (21.2 min) (24). The mean time to generate AST results for *Enterobacteriaceae* isolates was higher for Phoenix (11.7 ± 2.6 h) than for VITEK 2 (7.5 ± 1.3 h) (24). Ligozzi et al. reported that the time required for VITEK 2 AST for gram-positive cocci was 6 to 17 h, with 90% of results available as follows: 8 h, *S. aureus;* 11 h, coagulase-negative staphylococci (CoNS); 9 h, enterococci; 7 h, *Streptococcus agalactiae;* 9 h, *S. pneumoniae* (56). The average times required for AST results in a Phoenix study were as follows: for *Enterococcus* spp., 5.5 h; for *Staphylococcus* spp., 7 h; for *Enterobacteriaceae*, 6.5 h; and for nonfermenting gram-negative bacilli, 12 h (T. Wiles, D. Turner, W. B. Brasso, J. Hong, and J. Reuben, Abstr. 99th Gen. Meet. Am. Soc. Microbiol., abstr. C-94, p. 123, 1999). There are limited data showing financial and clinical benefits in association with the rapid provision of AST results. Doern et al. reported lower mortality rates and cost savings (fewer diagnostic tests and days in intensive care) associated with the rapid reporting of AST results (22). Barenfanger et al. also demonstrated reduced lengths of stay and cost savings for patients with rapid reporting of AST results that were attributed to earlier adjustments in antimicrobial therapy (2). Effective communication of the results to clinicians and pharmacists is essential to realizing the potential benefits of rapid testing. Communication may be enhanced by software packages that interface with medication records and alert clinicians or pharmacists when adjustments in antimicrobial therapy are needed.

DISADVANTAGES OF AUTOMATED SYSTEMS

Disadvantages of automated systems include a higher cost for equipment and consumables than manual methods, predetermined antimicrobial panels, an inability to test all clinically relevant organisms, and problems with detection of some resistance phenotypes (47). Reports of AST performance for detecting problematic resistance phenotypes are discussed below. The current performance of a system may not be accurately reflected by studies utilizing panels and software that are no longer available. A higher error rate should be accepted for evaluations using challenge strains with difficult to detect phenotypes than for studies that test populations of isolates usually encountered in the clinical laboratory.

Vancomycin Resistance in Enterococci

Problems with the detection of low-level vancomycin resistance (*vanB* and *vanC)* among enterococci by automated systems have been demonstrated in multiple studies (72, 89). The change from a 30-well to a 45-well VITEK 1 card in 1999 increased the testing of vancomycin from 3 wells to 4 wells and improved sensitivity for *vanB* isolates (26, 41, 67). A VITEK 2 evaluation reported difficulty detecting only *vanC2 (Enterococcus casseliflavus)* strains (94). Other VITEK 2 and Phoenix studies have demonstrated accurate detection of vancomycin-resistant enterococci, but rigorous studies comparing systems are lacking (27, 32). MicroScan overnight panel studies reported detection of all isolates except those containing *vanC*, which are difficult to detect for all AST systems since their MICs (4 to 16 μg/ml) span susceptible and intermediate categories (15, 19).

HLAR in *Enterococcus* spp.

The detection of high-level aminoglycoside resistance (HLAR) in enterococci by overnight and short-incubation AST systems has been improved by changes in growth medium and extended incubation (95, 98). Initial problems detecting high-level streptomycin resistance (HLSR) in MicroScan overnight panels appear to have been resolved after a broth reformulation, since two subsequent studies have demonstrated detection of HLAR that compared favorably to that obtained with reference and molecular methods (15, 65). A study reporting a higher VME rate for MicroScan detection of HLSR (19) may not have performed the recommended read at 48 h for isolates that appear streptomycin susceptible after overnight incubation; in one study that read improved detection of HLSR by 6.2% (15). Separate VITEK 2 and Phoenix evaluations testing different strains reported VME rates of 0 to 5.2% and ME rates of 0.9 to 7.3% for the detection of high-level streptomycin or gentamicin resistance (27, 32).

Oxacillin Resistance in Staphylococci

Most of the studies discussed below used *mecA* PCR as the "gold standard" when evaluating the accuracy of a system for detection of oxacillin resistance in staphylococci. Multiple studies have demonstrated excellent sensitivity and specificity of automated systems for detecting methicillin-resistant *Staphylococcus aureus* (MRSA) (27, 56, 73, 100). However, an evaluation focusing on low-level MRSA isolates reported problems detecting heterogeneous MRSA strains that are often undetected by routine oxacillin testing (29). After assessing the detection of heterogeneous oxacillin-resistant strains among *S. aureus* challenge organisms by eight methods including VITEK 1, MicroScan conventional, and MicroScan rapid panels, Swenson et al. concluded that no phenotypic system was totally reliable and suggested using several methods (86).

For the detection of oxacillin resistance among CoNS, VITEK 1, VITEK 2, and Phoenix evaluations have demonstrated excellent sensitivities (95.7 to 99.4%) with lower specificities (64.9 to 95.5%) (27, 37–39, 56, 61, 62, 80, 99). Isolates with false-resistant results often have MICs of 0.5 to 2 μg/ml that would have been considered susceptible under previous CLSI CoNS oxacillin breakpoints, which were lowered to ≤0.25 μg/ml in 1999 (38). Some of the major errors involved *Staphylococcus lugdunensis* isolates with oxacillin MICs now considered susceptible based on the CLSI 2005 decision to apply *S. aureus* breakpoints (≤2 μg/ml) to this species of CoNS (37, 38).

The lower CoNS oxacillin breakpoint is most accurate for detecting *mecA* carriage in *Staphylococcus hominis*, *Staphylococcus haemolyticus*, and *Staphylococcus epidermidis* isolates but may overcall oxacillin resistance for other CoNS species (40, 62, 69, 99). Current CLSI guidelines promote *mecA* or PBP 2a assays as the most accurate means of detecting oxacillin resistance and suggest the use of these assays for testing CoNS isolates (not *S. epidermidis*) with oxacillin MICs of 0.5 to 2 μg/ml causing serious infections (18).

Reduced Glycopeptide Susceptibility in Staphylococci

The inability of automated AST systems or disk diffusion to reliably detect vancomycin-intermediate and vancomycin-resistant *S. aureus* (11, 70, 90, 91) led to the current CLSI recommendation to supplement those methods with a 6-μg/ml vancomycin agar screening plate incubated 24 h (18). AST system detection of CoNS with reduced glycopeptide susceptibility is also unreliable (20, 70). Any staphylococcal isolate with a reproducible vancomycin MIC ≥4 μg/ml requires confirmation at a reference laboratory (18, 70).

Inducible Clindamycin Resistance

Routine testing of macrolide-resistant staphylococci and nonpneumococcal streptococci to detect inducible clindamycin resistance by use of a disk approximation test is recommended by CLSI (18). The inoculum purity plates from an automated broth AST system may be used for the induction test and should replace the practice of reporting all macrolide-resistant staphylococci or streptococci as resistant to clindamycin (49). An investigation of *S. aureus* isolates with VITEK 1 erythromycin-intermediate results showed that all were resistant by broth microdilution (87). VITEK 2 and Phoenix revealed accurate results (erythromycin resistant) for 96 to 100% of the isolates (87). Disk diffusion testing found that 95% of the isolates had inducible clindamycin resistance, but expert rules did not override the clindamycin-susceptible results for any of the systems (87). Use of the disk approximation test in nonpneumococcal streptococci is supported by the inability of VITEK 1 and VITEK 2 to accurately detect macrolide resistance phenotypes among group B streptococci (88).

Pneumococcal Resistance

The VITEK 2 *S. pneumoniae* panel represents the first commercial method for rapid AST of pneumococci. Initial testing of the VITEK 2 *S. pneumoniae* panel demonstrated provision of reliable results in a mean time of 8.1 h, with most errors classified as minor (35, 45). VITEK 2 detected 86.7% of 60 gatifloxacin-resistant and 95.6% of 23 moxifloxacin-resistant pneumococci without any major errors (48). A Phoenix pneumococcal panel recently received FDA approval. Overnight *S. pneumoniae* trays are available from MicroScan and Sensititre, with accurate results reported for antimicrobial agents other than trimethoprim-sulfamethoxazole (TMP/SMX), for which the discrepancies were attributed to trailing endpoints (36).

ESBL-Producing *Enterobacteriaceae*

Confirmatory ESBL tests that typically measure the inhibitory effect of clavulanate on ceftazidime and cefotaxime are available for all of the automated systems listed in Table 2. The first automated ESBL test was available for VITEK 1 and demonstrated reliable performance (99.5% sensitivity and 100% specificity) for organisms that are the most common ESBL producers (*Escherichia coli*, *Klebsiella oxytoca*, and *Klebsiella pneumoniae*) (75). A comparative evaluation of ESBL detection among multiresistant *E. coli* and *Klebsiella* spp., using three AST systems, revealed sensitivities of 83% (VITEK 1), 74% (VITEK 2), and 92% (Phoenix) with specificities of 82 to 85% (55). Evaluations of a single AST system (VITEK 2 or Phoenix) have reported sensitivities of 95.8 to 100% and specificities of 96.2 to 99.3% for ESBL detection (78, 79, 81). A recent evaluation of VITEK 1 and MicroScan ESBL confirmation tests reported sensitivities of 99 and 100%, respectively, and a specificity of 98% for both systems (58). The MicroScan ESBL confirmation overnight panels accurately detected ESBL-positive strains of *Proteus mirabilis*, *E. coli*, and *Klebsiella* spp. (53, 85). False-positive ESBL results for K1-hyperproducing *K. oxytoca* isolates have been reported for MicroScan (85) and Phoenix systems (78, 84).

Pseudomonas Resistance

Automated commercial AST systems are contraindicated for testing isolates of *Pseudomonas aeruginosa* from cystic fibrosis patients due to high VME rates and poor correlation with reference methods attributed to slow growth and mucoid strains (10). Problems with false-intermediate and false-resistant results for cefepime-susceptible *P. aeruginosa* isolates tested on VITEK 1 and MicroScan WalkAway systems have been reported (7). Problems with the VITEK 1 system overcalling *P. aeruginosa* resistance to piperacillin, ticarcillin-clavulanic acid, and cefepime led to software adjustments; a subsequent study reported acceptable piperacillin results, but elevated VME and ME rates for ticarcillin-clavulanic acid and increased minor errors with cefepime (12). Susceptibility testing of *P. aeruginosa* isolates by use of VITEK 2 identified only a small number of agents with categorical agreement <90% (cefepime, cefotaxime, and gentamicin) that were predominantly minor errors (50). A Phoenix study reported low categorical agreement for *P. aeruginosa* isolates primarily due to minor and major errors with β-lactams (23).

Other Gram-Negative Resistance

An assessment of ciprofloxacin resistance detection using a challenge set of *Enterobacteriaceae* isolates revealed elevated error rates for both MicroScan WalkAway and VITEK 1 systems (83). In evaluations testing different collections of gram-negative isolates with a single system (VITEK 2 or Phoenix), antimicrobial agents with low essential or categorical agreement reported by at least one study were aztreonam, cefotaxime, ceftazidime, cefepime, imipenem, piperacillin, piperacillin-tazobactam, ciprofloxacin, and TMP/SMX (25, 57, 81).

Outbreaks reported in New York City of infections by ESBL-positive *K. pneumoniae* organisms that also possess the carbapenem-hydrolyzing β-lactamase KPC-2 are cause for concern (9). A surveillance study identified three clinical labs that each failed to detect an ESBL/KPC-positive isolate with MicroScan WalkAway or VITEK systems; thus, an alternative method to confirm carbapenem susceptibility in *Enterobacteriaceae* that are resistant to third-generation cephalosporins may become necessary (9).

More common is the problem of false resistance when determining carbapenem susceptibility. The CDC could confirm only 8.9% of 123 *Enterobacteriaceae* and 74.2% of 325 *P. aeruginosa* isolates initially reported as imipenem nonsusceptible by 44 U.S. hospital laboratories during 1996–99 (82). Most isolates had been tested locally using VITEK or MicroScan, but retesting at CDC using the systems showed minimal errors except for a 20% ME rate for VITEK 1 testing of imipenem against *P. aeruginosa* (82). The lack of a clear explanation for this overdetection of carbapenem resistance (82) emphasizes the need for confirmation of any unusual AST results. Testing of five *K. pneumoniae* VIM-1-producing challenge isolates by using VITEK 2, Phoenix, and MicroScan Autoscan-4 resulted in false carbapenem resistance determinations by VITEK 2 and Phoenix (34). Tsakris et al. reported a problem with VITEK 1 overcalling imipenem resistance for *Acinetobacter baumannii* isolates in Greece (92). Antimicrobial agent deterioration in test panels (96) and technical errors are factors that may contribute to the overdetection of carbapenem resistance by AST systems (82, 92). Results of false resistance obtained by VITEK 1 for *P. aeruginosa* and *Enterobacteriaceae* have been attributed to heavy inoculum density—particularly for agents active against the cell wall (piperacillin, mezlocillin, aztreonam, ticarcillin, ticarcillin-clavulanic acid, ampicillin-sulbactam, and imipenem) (21, 43).

COMPUTERIZED EXPERT SYSTEMS

Expert systems to assist in the critical review of AST results are available for all commercial susceptibility systems currently marketed in the United States. Expert systems can enhance workflow by identifying the subset of results that require human expert attention and may also improve the quality of AST results reported from smaller labs that may lack a human expert (77). By continuous monitoring, the algorithms allow more rapid recognition of incorrect results and more uniform reporting. However, the software must be frequently updated to reflect the emergence of new resistance and changes in reporting guidelines recommended by national organizations such as CLSI. Users must be aware of what rules and comments are activated in their system and work closely with manufacturer-provided specialists to customize the expert system for their laboratory. Ideally an expert system will report actual MICs with categorical interpretation before and after recommended changes.

Most expert systems use a rules-based approach focusing on AST results for only one drug at a time without considering results for other agents tested simultaneously. The VITEK 2 AES differs from rules-based expert systems by performing an "interpretive reading" that compares the MICs for multiple agents to a large database of known resistance phenotypes and MIC distributions for different species (59). The rationale for interpretative reading with phenotype assignment is that a single mechanism typically mediates resistance to multiple agents (60). An evaluation of the VITEK 2 AES assignment of β-lactam phenotypes for *Enterobacteriaceae* and *P. aeruginosa* provides insight into the process of phenotype analysis (76). The VITEK 2 AES also deduces the susceptibility of an isolate to agents not tested and detects inconsistencies between organism identification and AST results (77).

Excellent concordance of VITEK 2 AES interpretive reading with resistance genotypes has been reported in multicenter studies (3, 59). When AES was compared to human expert analysis of VITEK 2 results for 259 consecutive clinical isolates in a university-based microbiology laboratory, there was disagreement for only 5 of the 65 isolates (7.7%) with AES corrections (77). A limitation that has been noted for the AES is an inability to interpret multiple inconsistent results as being caused by a single problem (8, 77).

CRITICAL REVIEW OF AST RESULTS

Regardless of whether a laboratory is using a commercial expert system, it is important to be aware of unusual "resistant" (Table 3) and "susceptible" (Table 4) results that require verification of the organism's identification and repeat of the susceptibility test by the same or a different method (18, 60). An example of an unprecedented phenotype that should prompt retesting is an *Enterobacteriaceae* or *P. aeruginosa* isolate that appears more resistant to piperacillin-tazobactam than to piperacillin (51). There are a number of antimicrobial agents that may appear active in vitro but lack clinical efficacy (Table 5) and to which the organisms should be reported as resistant. The most recent CLSI M100 document should be consulted for current recommendations regarding agents to test for specific organisms, methodology, interpretive criteria, results that may be inferred without testing a specific agent, antimicrobial agents to report based on the site of infection, and unusual results requiring verification.

SELECTING AN AST SYSTEM

Factors to consider when selecting an AST system include cost, performance, workflow, data management capabilities, and manufacturer technical support (44, 64). Performance may be assessed by comparing dilutions of FDA-cleared antimicrobial agents and limitations (antimicrobial agent/organisms listed in package inserts that require an alternative method) of panels from different manufacturers.

TABLE 3 Resistance phenotypes that are rare or have not been detected

Organism	Antimicrobial agent(s) to which resistance requires verification
Gram positive	
Enterococcus faecalis	Linezolid, daptomycin, ampicillin
Enterococcus faecium	Linezolid, daptomycin, quinupristin-dalfopristin
S. pneumoniae	Vancomycin, linezolid, fluoroquinolone
Viridans group streptococci	Vancomycin, linezolid, daptomycin
Beta-hemolytic streptococci	Vancomycin, linezolid, daptomycin, ampicillin, penicillin, cephalosporins
Coagulase-negative staphylococci	Vancomycin, linezolid, daptomycin, quinupristin-dalfopristin
S. aureus	Vancomycin, linezolid, daptomycin, quinupristin-dalfopristin
Gram negative	
Enterobacteriaceae (all)	Carbapenem
Neisseria gonorrhoeae, N. meningitidis	Extended-spectrum cephalosporin
Haemophilus influenzae	Third-generation cephalosporin, aztreonam, carbapenem, fluoroquinolone

TABLE 4 Gram-negative organisms with expected resistance to commonly tested antimicrobial agents

Organism	Agent(s) to which organism is usually resistant
Enterobacteriaceae	
Citrobacter, Enterobacter, Klebsiella, Morganella, Proteus penneri, Proteus vulgaris, Providencia, Serratia, Yersinia	Ampicillin
Citrobacter freundii, Enterobacter, Morganella, Proteus penneri, Proteus vulgaris, Providencia, Serratia, Yersinia	Cefazolin, cephalothin
Klebsiella	Ticarcillin
C. freundii, Enterobacter, Serratia	Cefoxitin, cefotetan
C. freundii, Enterobacter, Proteus vulgaris, Serratia	Cefuroxime
Citrobacter, Enterobacter, Serratia	Amoxicillin-clavulanic acid, ampicillin-sulbactam
Non-*Enterobacteriaceae*	
Acinetobacter, Burkholderia cepacia, Pseudomonas aeruginosa, Stenotrophomonas maltophilia	Ampicillin, 1st- and 2nd-generation cephalosporins
Burkholderia cepacia, Stenotrophomonas maltophilia	Aminoglycosides
Stenotrophomonas maltophilia	Carbapenems
P. aeruginosa	Trimethoprim-sulfamethoxazole

TABLE 5 Antimicrobial agents that may appear active in vitro but lack clinical efficacy

Organism	Antimicrobial agents to which the organisms should be reported as resistant
Oxacillin-resistant staphylococci	All β-lactam agents including β-lactam/β-lactamase inhibitor combinations, cephems, and carbapenems
Enterococcus spp.	Aminoglycosides (other than high-level), cephalosporins, clindamycin, trimethoprim-sulfamethoxazole
ESBL-producing *E. coli*, *Klebsiella* spp., and *Proteus mirabilis*	Aztreonam, cephalosporins (except cephamycins), penicillins
Listeria spp.	Cephalosporins
Salmonella and *Shigella* spp.	Aminoglycosides, 1st- and 2nd-generation cephalosporins
Yersinia pestis	All β-lactam agents

Current users of systems should be consulted, and publications in peer-reviewed journals should be reviewed. Manufacturers should be asked if problems reported for particular antimicrobial agent-organism combinations have been resolved and what is under development. Extensive exhibits at the annual American Society for Microbiology general meeting provide demonstrations of systems and a convenient venue for interaction with manufacturer representatives. Poster presentations at national meetings may provide new information and the opportunity to interact with recent users of systems.

Another method of assessing the performance of AST systems is participation in proficiency testing surveys such as that of the College of American Pathology (42, 68), whose final critiques of susceptibility testing challenges provide information regarding AST methods used and problem antimicrobial agent-organism combinations with high error rates.

An AST system's ability to perform identification is also important because expert rules are linked to organism identity. Additional information regarding the selection of an AST system and laboratory verification of performance as required by the Clinical Laboratory Improvement Amendments of 1988 (28) is in the *Clinical Microbiology Procedures Handbook* (64).

SUMMARY

AST systems provide accurate and reproducible results for many antimicrobial agent-organism combinations. Expert analysis may improve workflow as well as the quality of reported results. The labor savings attributed to automated AST systems is particularly important for laboratories in regions with current or projected technologist shortages. In addition, the provision of more rapid AST results with a short incubation system may improve patient care and lower health care costs. Future advances in AST system development will likely increase their clinical impact with the incorporation of real-time PCR growth detection (71) or gene arrays for common resistance determinants that dramatically shorten the time required for results.

REFERENCES

1. **Andrew, J. M., F. J. Boswell, and R. Wise.** 2000. Evaluation of the Oxoid Aura image system for measuring zones of inhibition with the disc diffusion technique. *J. Antimicrob. Chemother.* **46:**535–540.
2. **Barenfanger, J., C. Drake, and G. Kacich.** 1999. Clinical and financial benefits of rapid bacterial identification and antimicrobial susceptibility testing. *J. Clin. Microbiol.* **37:**1415–1418.
3. **Barry, J., A. Brown, V. Ensor, U. Lakhani, D. Petts, C. Warren, and T. Winstanley.** 2003. Comparative evaluation of the VITEK 2 Advanced Expert System (AES) in five UK hospitals. *J. Antimicrob. Chemother.* **51:**1191–1202.
4. **Berke, I., and P. M. Tierno, Jr.** 1996. Comparison of efficacy and cost-effectiveness of BIOMIC VIDEO and VITEK antimicrobial susceptibility test systems for use in

the clinical microbiology laboratory. *J. Clin. Microbiol.* **34:**1980–1984.

5. **Bert, F., M. Juvin, Z. Ould-Hocine, G. Clarebout, E. Keller, N. Lambert, and G. Arlet.** 2005. Evaluation and updating of the Osiris expert system for identification of *Escherichia coli* β-lactam resistance phenotypes. *J. Clin. Microbiol.* **43:**1846–1850.
6. **Bert, F., Z. Ould-Hocine, M. Juvin, V. Dubois, V. Loncle-Provot, V. LeFranc, C. Quentin, N. Lambert, and G. Arlet.** 2003. Evaluation of the Osiris expert system for identification of β-lactam phenotypes in isolates of *Pseudomonas aeruginosa*. *J. Clin. Microbiol.* **41:**3712–3718.
7. **Biedenbach, D. J., S. A. Marshall, and R. N. Jones.** 1999. Accuracy of cefepime antimicrobial susceptibility testing results for *Pseudomonas aeruginosa* tested on the MicroScan WalkAway system. *Diagn. Microbiol. Infect. Dis.* **33:**305–307. (Letter.)
8. **Blondel-Hill, E., C. Hetchler, D. Andrews, and L. Lapointe.** 2003. Evaluation of VITEK 2 for analysis of *Enterobacteriaceae* using the Advanced Expert System (AES) versus interpretive susceptibility guidelines used at Dynacare Kasper Medical Laboratories, Edmonton, Alberta. *Clin. Microbiol. Infect.* **9:**1091–1103.
9. **Bratu, S., D. Landman, R. Haag, R. Recco, A. Eramo, M. Alam, and J. Quale.** 2005. Rapid spread of carbapenem-resistant *Klebsiella pneumoniae* in New York City. *Arch. Intern. Med.* **165:**1430–1435.
10. **Burns, J. L., L. Saiman, S. Whittier, J. Krzewinski, Z. Liu, D. Larone, S. A. Marshall, and R. N. Jones.** 2001. Comparison of two commercial systems (VITEK and MicroScan-WalkAway) for antimicrobial susceptibility testing of *Pseudomonas aeruginosa* isolates from cystic fibrosis patients. *Diagn. Microbiol. Infect. Dis.* **39:**257–260.
11. **Centers for Disease Control and Prevention.** 2004. Vancomycin-resistant *Staphylococcus aureus*—New York, 2004. *Morb. Mortal. Wkly. Rep.* **53:**322–323.
12. **Chandler, L. J., M. Poulter, B. Reisner, and G. Woods.** 2002. Clinical evaluation of the VITEK automated system with cards GNS 122 and 127 and VTK-R07.01 software for antimicrobial susceptibility testing of *Pseudomonas aeruginosa*. *Diagn. Microbiol. Infect. Dis.* **42:**71–73.
13. **Chapin, K. C., and M. C. Musgnug.** 2003. Validation of the automated reading and incubation system with Sensititre plates for antimicrobial susceptibility testing. *J. Clin. Microbiol.* **41:**1951–1956.
14. **Chapin, K. C., and M. C. Musgnug.** 2004. Evaluation of Sensititre automated system for automated reading of Sensititre broth microdilution susceptibility plates. *J. Clin. Microbiol.* **42:**909–911.
15. **Chen, Y.-S., S. A. Marshall, P. L. Winokur, S. L. Coffman, W. W. Wilkie, P. R. Murray, C. A. Spiegel, M. A. Pfaller, G. V. Doern, and R. N. Jones.** 1998. Use of molecular and reference susceptibility testing methods in a multicenter evaluation of MicroScan dried overnight gram-positive MIC panels for detection of vancomycin and high-level aminoglycoside resistances in enterococci. *J. Clin. Microbiol.* **36:**2996–3001.
16. **Clinical and Laboratory Standards Institute/NCCLS.** 2001. *Development of* In Vitro *Susceptibility Testing Criteria and Quality Control Parameters; Approved Guideline,* 2nd ed. M23-A2. Clinical and Laboratory Standards Institute, Wayne, Pa.
17. **Clinical and Laboratory Standards Institute/NCCLS.** 2003. *Methods for Dilution Antimicrobial Susceptibility Tests for Bacteria that Grow Aerobically*, 6th ed. Approved Standard M7-A6. Clinical and Laboratory Standards Institute, Wayne, Pa.
18. **Clinical and Laboratory Standards Institute/NCCLS.** 2005. *Performance Standards for Antimicrobial Susceptibility Testing;* 15th Informational Supplement M100-S15. Clinical and Laboratory Standards Institute, Wayne, Pa.
19. **d'Azevedo, P. A., C. A. G. Dias, A. L. Goncalves, F. Rowe, and L. M. Teixeira.** 2001. Evaluation of an automated system for the identification and antimicrobial susceptibility testing of enterococci. *Diagn. Microbiol. Infect. Dis.* **40:**157–161.
20. **Del' Alamo, L., R. F. Cereda, I. Tosin, E. A. Miranda, and H. S. Sader.** 1999. Antimicrobial susceptibility of coagulase-negative staphylococci and characterization of isolates with reduced susceptibility to glycopeptides. *Diagn. Microbiol. Infect. Dis.* **34:**185–191.
21. **Doern, G. V., A. B. Brueggemann, R. Perla, J. Daly, D. Halkias, R. N. Jones, and M. A. Saubolle.** 1997. Multicenter laboratory evaluation of the bioMerieux VITEK antimicrobial susceptibility testing system with 11 antimicrobial agents versus members of the family *Enterobacteriaceae* and *Pseudomonas aeruginosa*. *J. Clin. Microbiol.* **35:**2115–2119.
22. **Doern, G. V., R. Vautour, M. Gaudet, and B. Levy.** 1994. Clinical impact of rapid in vitro susceptibility testing and bacterial identification. *J. Clin. Microbiol.* **32:**1757–1762.
23. **Donay, J.-L., D. Mathieu, P. Fernandes, C. Pregermain, P. Bruel, A. Wargnier, I. Casin, F. X. Weill, P. H. Lagrange, and J. L. Herrmann.** 2004. Evaluation of the automated Phoenix system for potential routine use in the clinical microbiology laboratory. *J. Clin. Microbiol.* **42:**1542–1546.
24. **Eigner, U., A. Schmid, U. Wild, D. Bertsch, and A.-M. Fahr.** 2005. Analysis of the comparative workflow and performance characteristics of the VITEK 2 and Phoenix systems. *J. Clin. Microbiol.* **43:**3829–3834.
25. **Endimiani, A., F. Luzzaro, A. Tamborini, G. Lombardi, V. Elia, R. Belloni, and A. Toniolo.** 2002. Identification and antimicrobial susceptibility testing of clinical isolates of nonfermenting gram-negative bacteria by the Phoenix automated microbiology system. *Microbiologica* **25:**323–329.
26. **Endtz, H. P., N. Van den Braak, A. Van Belkum, W. H. Goessens, D. Kreft, A. B. Stroebel, and H. A. Verbrugh.** 1998. Comparison of eight methods to detect vancomycin resistance in enterococci. *J. Clin. Microbiol.* **36:**592–594.
27. **Fahr, A. M., U. Eigner, M. Armbrust, A. Caganic, G. Dettori, C. Chezzi, L. Bertoncini, M. Benecchi, and M. G. Menozzi.** 2003. Two-center collaborative evaluation of the performance of the BD Phoenix automated microbiology system for identification and antimicrobial susceptibility testing of *Enterococcus* spp. and *Staphylococcus* spp. *J. Clin. Microbiol.* **41:**1135–1142.
28. **Federal Register.** 1992. *Clinical Laboratory Improvement Amendments of 1988; Final Rule. Fed. Regist.* **57:**7164.
29. **Felten, A., B. Grandry, P. H. Lagrange, and I. Casin.** 2002. Evaluation of three techniques for detection of low-level methicillin-resistant *Staphylococcus aureus* (MRSA): a disk diffusion method with cefoxitin and moxalactam, the VITEK 2 system, and the MRSA-screen latex agglutination test. *J. Clin. Microbiol.* **40:**2766–2771.
30. **Food and Drug Administration.** 2003. *Establishment Registration and Device Listing for Manufacturers and Initial Importers of Devices.* 21 CFR 807. Food and Drug Administration, Department of Health and Human Services, Rockville, Md.
31. **Food and Drug Administration.** February 5, 2003. *Class II Special Controls Guidance Document: Antimicrobial Susceptibility Test (AST) Systems; Guidance for Industry and FDA.* Food and Drug Administration, Rockville, Md.
32. **Garcia-Garrote, F., E. Cercenado, and E. Bouza.** 2000. Evaluation of a new system, VITEK 2, for identification and antimicrobial susceptibility testing of enterococci. *J. Clin. Microbiol.* **38:**2108–2111.
33. **Geiss, H. K., and U. E. Klar.** 2000. Evaluation of the BIOMIC video reader system for routine use in the clinical microbiology laboratory. *Diagn. Microbiol. Infect. Dis.* **37:**151–155.

34. **Giakkoupi, P., L. S. Tzouvelekis, G. L. Daikos, V. Miriagou, G. Petrikkos, N. J. Legakis, and A. C. Vatopoulos.** 2005. Discrepancies and interpretation problems in susceptibility testing of VIM-1-producing *Klebsiella pneumoniae* isolates. *J. Clin. Microbiol.* **43:**494–496.
35. **Goessens, W. H. F., N. Lemmens-den Toom, J. Hageman, P. W. M. Hermans, M. Sluijter, R. de Groot, and H. A. Verbrugh.** 2000. Evaluation of the VITEK 2 system for susceptibility testing of *Streptococcus pneumoniae* isolates. *Eur. J. Clin. Microbiol. Infect. Dis.* **19:**618–622.
36. **Guthrie, L. L., S. Banks, W. Setiawan, and K. B. Waites.** 1999. Comparison of MicroScan MICroSTREP, Pasco, and Sensititre MIC panels for determining antimicrobial susceptibilities of *Streptococcus pneumoniae*. *Diagn. Microbiol. Infect. Dis.* **33:**267–273.
37. **Horstkotte, M. A., J. K.-M. Knobloch, H. Rohde, S. Dobinsky, and D. Mack.** 2002. Rapid detection of methicillin resistance in coagulase-negative staphylococci with the VITEK 2 system. *J. Clin. Microbiol.* **40:**3291–3295.
38. **Horstkotte, M. A., J. K.-M. Knobloch, H. Rohde, S. Dobinsky, and D. Mack.** 2004. Evaluation of the BD PHOENIX automated system for detection of methicillin resistance in coagulase-negative staphylococci. *J. Clin. Microbiol.* **42:**5041–5046.
39. **Hussain, Z., L. Stoakes, M. A. John, S. Garrow, and V. Fitzgerald.** 2002. Detection of methicillin resistance in primary blood culture isolates of coagulase-negative staphylococci by PCR, slide agglutination, disk diffusion, and a commercial method. *J. Clin. Microbiol.* **40:**2251–2253.
40. **Hussain, Z., L. Stoakes, V. Massey, D. Diagre, V. Fitzgerald, S. El Sayed, and R. Lannigan.** 2000. Correlation of oxacillin MIC with *mecA* gene carriage in coagulase-negative staphylococci. *J. Clin. Microbiol.* **38:**752–754.
41. **Jett, B., L. Free, and D. F. Sahm.** 1996. Factors influencing the VITEK gram-positive susceptibility system's detection of *vanB*-encoded vancomycin resistance among enterococci. *J. Clin. Microbiol.* **34:**701–706.
42. **Jones, R. N.** 2001. Methods preferences and test accuracy of antimicrobial susceptibility testing: updates from the College of American Pathologists Microbiology Survey Program (2000). *Arch. Pathol. Lab. Med.* **125:**1285–1289.
43. **Jones, R. N., S. A. Marshall, and L. Zerva.** 1997. Critical evaluation of the VITEK GNS F6 card results compared to standardized, reference susceptibility test methods. *Diagn. Microbiol. Infect. Dis.* **28:**35–40.
44. **Jorgensen, J. H.** 1993. Selection criteria for an antimicrobial susceptibility testing system. *J. Clin. Microbiol.* **31:** 2841–2844.
45. **Jorgensen, J. H., A. L. Barry, M. M. Traczewski, D. F. Sahm, M. L. McElmeel, and S. A. Crawford.** 2000. Rapid automated antimicrobial susceptibility testing of *Streptococcus pneumoniae* by use of the bioMerieux VITEK 2. *J. Clin. Microbiol.* **38:**2814–2818.
46. **Jorgensen, J. H., and M. J. Ferraro.** 1998. Antimicrobial susceptibility testing: general principles and contemporary practices. *Clin. Infect. Dis.* **26:**973–980.
47. **Jorgensen, J. H., and M. J. Ferraro.** 2000. Antimicrobial susceptibility testing: special needs for fastidious organisms and difficult-to-detect resistance mechanisms. *Clin. Infect. Dis.* **30:**799–808.
48. **Jorgensen, J. H., S. A. Crawford, L. M. McElmeel, and C. G. Whitney.** 2004. Detection of resistance to gatifloxacin and moxifloxacin in *Streptococcus pneumoniae* with the VITEK 2 instrument. *J. Clin. Microbiol.* **42:**5928–5930.
49. **Jorgensen, J. H., S. A. Crawford, M. L. McElmeel, and K. R. Fiebelkorn.** 2004. Detection of inducible clindamycin resistance in conjunction with performance of automated broth susceptibility testing. *J. Clin. Microbiol.* **42:**1800–1802.
50. **Joyanes, P., M. D. C. Conejo, L. Martinez-Martinez, and E. J. Perea.** 2001. Evaluation of the VITEK 2 system for the identification and susceptibility testing of three species of nonfermenting gram-negative rods frequently isolated from clinical samples. *J. Clin. Microbiol.* **39:**3247–3253.
51. **Karlowsky, J. A., M. K. Weaver, C. Thornsberry, M. J. Dowzicky, M. E. Jones, and D. F. Sahm.** 2003. Comparison of four antimicrobial susceptibility testing methods to determine the in vitro activities of piperacillin and piperacillin-tazobactam against clinical isolates of *Enterobacteriaceae* and *Pseudomonas aeruginosa*. *J. Clin. Microbiol.* **41:**3339–3343.
52. **Kolbert, M., F. Chegrani, and P. M. Shah.** 2004. Evaluation of the OSIRIS video reader as an automated measurement system for the agar disk diffusion technique. *Clin. Microbiol. Infect.* **10:**416–420.
53. **Komatsu, M., M. Aihara, K. Shimakawa, M. Iwasaki, Y. Nagasaka, S. Fukuda, S. Matsuo, and Y. Iwatani.** 2003. Evaluation of MicroScan ESBL confirmation panel for *Enterobacteriaceae*-producing, extended-spectrum β-lactamases isolated in Japan. *Diagn. Microbiol. Infect. Dis.* **46:**125–130.
54. **Korgenski, E. K., and J. A. Daly.** 1998. Evaluation of the BIOMIC video reader system for determining interpretive categories of isolates on the basis of disk diffusion susceptibility results. *J. Clin. Microbiol.* **36:**302–304.
55. **Leverstein-van Hall, M., A. C. Fluit, A. Paauw, A. T. A. Box, S. Brisse, and J. Verhoef.** 2002. Evaluation of the Etest ESBL and the BD Phoenix, VITEK 1, and VITEK 2 automated instruments for detection of extended-spectrum beta-lactamases in multiresistant *Escherichia coli* and *Klebsiella* spp. *J. Clin. Microbiol.* **40:**3703–3711.
56. **Ligozzi, M., C. Bernini, M. G. Bonora, M. de Fatima, J. Zuliani, and R. Fontana.** 2002. Evaluation of the VITEK 2 system for identification and antimicrobial susceptibility testing of medically relevant gram-positive cocci. *J. Clin. Microbiol.* **40:**1681–1686.
57. **Ling, T. K. W., P. C. Tam, Z. K. Liu, and A. F. B. Cheng.** 2001. Evaluation of VITEK 2 rapid identification and susceptibility testing system against gram-negative clinical isolates. *J. Clin. Microbiol.* **39:**2964–2966.
58. **Linscott, A. J., and W. J. Brown.** 2005. Evaluation of four commercially available extended-spectrum beta-lactamase phenotypic confirmation tests. *J. Clin. Microbiol.* **43:** 1081–1085.
59. **Livermore, D. M., M. Struelens, J. Amorin, F. Baquero, J. Bille, R. Canton, S. Henning, S. Gatermann, A. Marchese, H. Mittermayer, C. Nonhoff, K. J. Oakton, F. Praplan, H. Ramos, G. C. Schito, J. Van Eldere, J. Verhaegen, J. Verhoef, and M. R. Visser.** 2002. Multicentre evaluation of the VITEK 2 Advanced Expert System for interpretive reading of antimicrobial resistance tests. *J. Antimicrob. Chemother.* **49:**289–300.
60. **Livermore, D. M., T. G. Winstanley, and K. P. Shannon.** 2001. Interpretative reading: recognizing the unusual and inferring resistance mechanisms from resistance phenotypes. *J. Antimicrob. Chemother.* **47**(Suppl. l)**:**87–102.
61. **Marshall, S. A., M. A. Pfaller, and R. N. Jones.** 1999. Ability of the modified VITEK card to detect coagulase-negative staphylococci with *mecA* and oxacillin-resistant phenotypes. *J. Clin. Microbiol.* **37:**2122–2123.
62. **Martinez, F., L. J. Chandler, B. S. Reisner, and G. L. Woods.** 2001. Evaluation of the VITEK card GPS105 and VTK-R07.01 software for detection of oxacillin resistance in clinically relevant coagulase-negative staphylococci. *J. Clin. Microbiol.* **39:**3733–3735.
63. **Medeiros, A. A., and J. Crellin.** 2000. Evaluation of the Sirscan automated zone reader in a clinical microbiology laboratory. *J. Clin. Microbiol.* **38:**1688–1693.

64. **Munro, S., R. M. Mulder, S. M. Farnham, and B. Grinius.** 2004. Evaluating antimicrobial susceptibility test systems. p. 5.17.1–5.17.9. *In* H. D. Isenberg (ed.), *Clinical Microbiology Procedures Handbook,* 2nd ed. ASM Press, Washington, D.C.
65. **Murdoch, D. R., S. Mirrett, L. J. Harrell, S. M. Donabedian, M. J. Zervos, and L. B. Reller.** 2003. Comparison of MicroScan broth microdilution, synergy quad plate agar dilution, and disk diffusion screening methods for detection of high-level aminoglycoside resistance in *Enterococcus* species. *J. Clin. Microbiol.* **41:**2703–2705.
66. **Nijs, A., R. Cartuyvels, A. Mewis, V. Peeters, J. L. Rummens, and K. Magerman.** 2003. Comparison and evaluation of Osiris and Sirscan 2000 antimicrobial susceptibility systems in the clinical microbiology laboratory. *J. Clin. Microbiol.* **41:**3627–3630.
67. **Okabe, T., K. Oana, Y. Kawakami, M. Yamaguchi, Y. Takahashi, Y. Okimura, T. Honda, and T. Katsuyama.** 2000. Limitations of VITEK GPS-418 cards in exact detection of vancomycin-resistant enterococci with the *vanB* genotype. *J. Clin. Microbiol.* **38:**2409–2411.
68. **Pfaller, M. A., and R. N. Jones.** Performance accuracy of antibacterial and antifungal susceptibility test methods: report from the College of American Pathologists (CAP) Microbiology Surveys program (2001–2003). Submitted for publication.
69. **Ramotar, K., W. Woods, and B. Toye.** 2001. Oxacillin susceptibility testing of *Staphylococcus saprophyticus* using disk diffusion, agar dilution, broth microdilution, and the VITEK GPS-10 card. *Diagn. Microbiol. Infect. Dis.* **40:**203–205.
70. **Raney, P. M., P. P. Williams, J. E. McGowan, and F. C. Tenover.** 2002. Validation of VITEK version 7.01 software for testing staphylococci against vancomycin. *Diagn. Microbiol. Infect. Dis.* **43:**135–140.
71. **Rolain, J. M., M. N. Mallet, P. E. Fournier, and D. Raoult.** 2004. Real-time PCR for universal antibiotic susceptibility testing. *J. Antimicrob. Chemother.* **54:**538–541.
72. **Rosenberg, J., F. C. Tenover, J. Wong, W. Jarvis, and D. J. Vugia.** 1997. Are clinical laboratories in California accurately reporting vancomycin-resistant enterococci? *J. Clin. Microbiol.* **35:**2526–2530.
73. **Sakoulas, G., H. S. Gold, L. Venkataraman, P. C. Degirolami, G. M. Eliopoulos, and Q. Qian.** 2001. Methicillin-resistant *Staphylococcus aureus:* comparison of susceptibility testing methods and analysis of *mecA* positive susceptible strains. *J. Clin. Microbiol.* **39:**3946–3951.
74. **Sanchez, M. A., B. Sanchez del Saz, E. Loza, F. Baquero, and R. Canton.** 2001. Evaluation of the OSIRIS video reader for disk diffusion susceptibility test reading. *Clin. Microbiol. Infect.* **7:**352–357.
75. **Sanders, C. C., A. L. Barry, J. A. Washington, C. Shubert, E. S. Moland, M. M. Traczewski, C. Knapp, and R. Mulder.** 1996. Detection of extended-spectrum beta-lactamase-producing members of the family *Enterobacteriaceae* with the VITEK ESBL test. *J. Clin. Microbiol.* **34:**2997–3001.
76. **Sanders, C. C., M. Peyret, E. S. Moland, C. Shubert, K. S. Thomson, J.-M. Boeufgras, and W. E. Sanders.** 2000. Ability of the VITEK 2 Advanced Expert System to identify β-lactam phenotypes in isolates of *Enterobacteriaceae* and *Pseudomonas aeruginosa. J. Clin. Microbiol.* **38:**570–574.
77. **Sanders, C. C., M. Peyret, E. S. Moland, S. J. Cavalieri, C. Shubert, K. S. Thomson, J.-M. Boeufgras, and W. E. Sanders.** 2001. Potential impact of the VITEK 2 System and the Advanced Expert System on the clinical laboratory of a university-based hospital. *J. Clin. Microbiol.* **39:**2379–2385.
78. **Sanguinetti, M., B. Posteraro, T. Spanu, D. Ciccaglione, L. Romano, B. Fiori, G. Nicoletti, S. Zanetti, and G. Fadda.** 2003. Characterization of clinical isolates of *Enterobacteriaceae* from Italy by the Phoenix extended-spectrum β-lactamase detection method. *J. Clin. Microbiol.* **41:** 1463–1468.
79. **Sorlozano, A., J. Gutierrez, G. Piedrola, and M. J. Soto.** 2005. Acceptable performance of VITEK 2 system to detect extended-spectrum β-lactamases in clinical isolates of *Escherichia coli:* a comparative study of phenotypic commercial methods and NCCLS guidelines. *Diagn. Microbiol. Infect. Dis.* **51:**191–193.
80. **Spanu, T., M. Sanguinetti, T. D'Inzeo, D. Ciccaglione, L. Romano, F. Leone, P. Mazzella, and G. Fadda.** 2004. Identification of methicillin-resistant isolates of *Staphylococcus aureus* and coagulase-negative staphylococci responsible for bloodstream infections with the Phoenix system. *Diagn. Microb. Infect. Dis.* **48:**221–227.
81. **Stefaniuk, E., A. Baraniak, M. Gniadkowski, and W. Hryniewicz.** 2003. Evaluation of the BD Phoenix automated identification and susceptibility testing system in clinical microbiology laboratory practice. *Eur. J. Clin. Microbiol. Infect. Dis.* **22:**479–485.
82. **Steward, C. D., J. M. Mohammed, J. M. Swenson, S. A. Stocker, P. P. Williams, R. P. Gaynes, J. E. McGowan, and F. C. Tenover.** 2003. Antimicrobial susceptibility testing of carbapenems: multicenter validity and accuracy levels of five antimicrobial test methods for detecting resistance in *Enterobacteriaceae* and *Pseudomonas aeruginosa* isolates. *J. Clin. Microbiol.* **41:**351–358.
83. **Steward, C. D., S. A. Stocker, J. M. Swensen, C. M. O'Hara, J. R. Edwards, R. P. Gaynes, J. E. McGowan, and F. C. Tenover.** 1999. Comparison of agar dilution, disk diffusion, MicroScan, and VITEK antimicrobial susceptibility testing methods to broth microdilution for detection of fluoroquinolone-resistant isolates of the family *Enterobacteriaceae. J. Clin. Microbiol.* **37:**544–547.
84. **Sturenburg, E., I. Sobottka, H.-H. Feucht, D. Mack, and R. Laufs.** 2003. Comparison of BD Phoenix and VITEK 2 automated antimicrobial susceptibility test systems for extended-spectrum beta-lactamase detection in *Escherichia coli* and *Klebsiella* species clinical isolates. *Diagn. Microbiol. Infect. Dis.* **45:**29–34.
85. **Sturenburg, E., M. Lang, M. A. Horstkotte, R. Laufs, and D. Mack.** 2004. Evaluation of the MicroScan ESBL plus confirmation panel for detection of extended-spectrum β-lactamases in clinical isolates of oxyimino-cephalosporin-resistant gram-negative bacteria. *J. Antimicrob. Chemother.* **54:**870–875.
86. **Swenson, J. M., P. P. Williams, G. Killgore, C. M. O'Hara, and F. C. Tenover.** 2001. Performance of eight methods, including two new rapid methods, for detection of oxacillin resistance in a challenge set of *Staphylococcus aureus* organisms. *J. Clin. Microbiol.* **39:**3785–3788.
87. **Tang, P., D. E. Low, S. Atkinson, K. Pike, A. Ashi-Sulaiman, A. Simor, S. Richardson, and B. M. Wiley.** 2003. Investigation of *Staphylococcus aureus* isolates identified as erythromycin intermediate by the VITEK-1 system: comparison with results obtained with the VITEK-2 and Phoenix systems. *J. Clin. Microbiol.* **41:**4823–4825.
88. **Tang, P., P. Ng, M. Lum, M. Skulnick, G. W. Small, D. E. Low, A. Sarabia, T. Mazzulli, K. Wong, A. E. Simor, and B. M. Willey.** 2004. Use of the VITEK-1 and VITEK-2 systems for detection of constitutive and inducible macrolide resistance in group B streptococci. *J. Clin. Microbiol.* **42:**2282–2284.
89. **Tenover, F. C., J. M. Swensen, C. M. O'Hara, and S. A. Stocker.** 1995. Ability of commercial and reference antimicrobial susceptibility testing methods to detect vancomycin resistance in enterococci. *J. Clin. Microbiol.* **33:**1524–1527.

90. **Tenover, F. C., L. M. Weigel, P. C. Appelbaum, L. K. McDougal, J. Chaitram, S. McAllister, N. Clark, G. Killgore, C. M. O'Hara, L. Jevitt, J. B. Patel, and B. Bozdogan.** 2004. Vancomycin-resistant *Staphylococcus aureus* isolate from a patient in Pennsylvania. *Antimicrob. Agents Chemother.* **48:**275–280.

91. **Tenover, F. C., M. V. Lancaster, B. C. Hill, C. D. Steward, S. A. Stocker, G. A. Hancock, C. M. O'Hara, N. C. Clark, and K. Hiramatsu.** 1998. Characterization of staphylococci with reduced susceptibilities to vancomycin and other glycopeptides. *J. Clin. Microbiol.* **36:**1020–1027.

92. **Tsakris, A., A. Pantazi, S. Pournaras, A. Maniatis, A. Polyzou, and D. Sofianou.** 2000. Pseudo-outbreak of imipenem-resistant *Acinetobacter baumannii* resulting from false susceptibility testing by a rapid automated system. *J. Clin. Microbiol.* **38:**3505–3507.

93. **Turnidge, J. D., and J. M. Bell.** 2005. Antimicrobial susceptibility on solid media, p. 8–60. *In* V. Lorin (ed.), *Antibiotics in Laboratory Medicine*, 5th ed. The Williams & Wilkins Co., Baltimore, Md.

94. **Van Den Braak, N., W. Goessens, A. van Belkum, H. A. Verbrugh, and H. P. Endtz.** 2001. Accuracy of the VITEK 2 system to detect glycopeptide resistance in enterococci. *J. Clin. Microbiol.* **39:**351–353.

95. **Weissmann, D., J. Spargo, C. Wennersten, and M. J. Ferrarro.** 1991. Detection of enterococcal high-level aminoglycoside resistance with MicroScan freeze-dried panels containing newly modified medium and VITEK gram-positive susceptibility cards. *J. Clin. Microbiol.* **29:**1232–1235.

96. **White, R. L., M. B. Kays, L. V. Friedrich, E. W. Brown, and J. R. Koonce.** 1991. Pseudoresistance of *Pseudomonas aeruginosa* resulting from degradation of imipenem in an automated susceptibility testing system with predried panels. *J. Clin. Microbiol.* **29:**398–400.

97. **Winstanley, T. G., H. K. Parsons, M. A. Horstkotte, I. Sobottka, and E. Sturenburg.** 2005. Phenotypic detection of β-lactamase-mediated resistance to oxyimino-cephalosporins in Enterobacteriaceae: evaluation of the Mastacan Elite Expert System. *J. Antimicrob. Chemother.* **56:**292–296.

98. **Woods, G. L., B. DiGiovanni, M. Levison, P. Pitsakis, and D. LaTemple.** 1993. Evaluation of MicroScan rapid panels for detection of high-level aminoglycoside resistance in enterococci. *J. Clin. Microbiol.* **31:**2786–2787.

99. **Yamazumi, T., I. Furuta, D. J. Diekema, M. A. Pfaller, and R. N. Jones.** 2001. Comparison of the VITEK gram-positive susceptibility 106 card, the MRSA-screen latex agglutination test, and *mecA* analysis for detecting oxacillin resistance in a geographically diverse collection of clinical isolates of coagulase-negative staphylococci. *J. Clin. Microbiol.* **39:**3633–3636.

100. **Yamazumi, T., S. A. Marshall, W. W. Wilke, D. J. Diekema, M. A. Pfaller, and R. N. Jones.** 2001. Comparison of the VITEK gram-positive susceptibility 106 card and the MRSA-screen latex agglutination test for determining oxacillin resistance in clinical bloodstream isolates of *Staphylococcus aureus*. *J. Clin. Microbiol.* **39:**53–56.

Immunoassays for the Diagnosis of Infectious Diseases*

A. BETTS CARPENTER

18

Immunoassays are laboratory tests that employ antibodies as analytical reagents (8, 22, 24, 29, 30, 48). They have become increasingly used in the diagnosis of infectious diseases either as a primary means of diagnosis or as a confirmation of culture results. Overall immunoassays are specific, sensitive, and relatively inexpensive. They are used in all parts of the clinical laboratory. Due to the high specificity of the antigen-antibody reaction and the ease of use, immunoassays are leading the way for an increasing number of laboratory tests that are available at the patient bedside (point-of-care testing), in doctors' offices, and even in at-home testing. This chapter summarizes the variety of different assays available and their particular application in the field of infectious disease. The discussion emphasizes general assay design with important caveats relevant to test interpretation and development. Relevant examples are given as they relate to testing for particular infectious disease agents; however, for in-depth discussions, the reader is directed to the particular chapters on the specific agents.

HISTORY OF DEVELOPMENT OF IMMUNOASSAYS

Immunoassays have changed significantly over time with improvements in the types of antibodies and antigens available as well as improved detection systems (8, 22, 24, 27, 30, 48). With immunoassays, any analyte can be measured if an antibody can be raised to it or an antigenic form is available. The first immunoassays available measured milligram to microgram quantities of antibodies and relied primarily upon precipitation reactions between antigen and antibody. In the 1960s, the advent of radioimmunoassay (RIA) heralded techniques with greater sensitivity and greatly expanded the repertoire of analytes available for testing. By use of RIA, previously undetectable analytes were now easily available for testing in the clinical laboratory. The discovery of monoclonal antibodies led to assays with greater specificities and further expanded the repertoire of analytes available for measurement. Concerns about utilization of radioactivity and the desire for greater sensitivities led to the development of chemiluminescence (CL) immunoassays and use of the avidin-biotin detection system. Increasing automation of laboratory testing has expanded into the area of immunoassays, with many tests requiring only limited technologist input. As immunoassays have evolved, there has been increased utilization of various solid-phase matrices for adherence of either antigens or antibodies. Initially polypropylene test tubes were used. This has evolved to microtiter plates, and with the increased use of automated systems, smaller solid phases such as tiny disks or spheres are being increasingly used. Thus, immunoassays have significantly advanced in both the level of sensitivity detected and the breadth of their utilization, so they are now some of the most popular and most widely used of all laboratory tests.

DEFINITION OF TERMS

The array of terms used for immunoassays can be a confusing alphabet soup. This chapter discusses some widely used conventions in terminology; however, the reader may find some references in which the terms are used differently. Overall, most assays utilize the term "immuno" coupled with a second term which describes the type of assay or label used. For example, immunoprecipitation is an immunoassay utilizing a precipitation reaction. RIA is an immunoassay that utilizes radioactivity as the label. The term enzyme immunoassay (EIA) is a more general term that can be applied to any immunoassay which uses an enzyme label, although often EIA is used to refer to reagent-limited competitive type assays. The term enzyme-linked immunosorbent assay (ELISA) can also be used as a general term for any assay utilizing an enzyme label; however, it is most often used to refer to assays in which the antigen or antibody is adsorbed to a solid-phase matrix, often then employing a second enzyme labeled antibody, the so-called "sandwich" assay format. Immunometric is an additional term used and generally refers to any reagent excess assay. For the purposes of this chapter, the term EIA is used to refer to any assay using an enzyme, while ELISA refers only to solid-phase "sandwich"-type assays.

GENERAL CONCEPTS OF ASSAY DESIGN

There are a number of ways to characterize immunoassays. One useful classification scheme looks at the amount of label and reagent available (18). There are three major

*This chapter contains information presented in chapter 16 by Niel T. Constantine and Dolores P. Lana in the eighth edition of this Manual.

groups of immunoassays: label free, reagent excess, and reagent limited. The assays which are label free rely upon the ability of antigen and antibodies to bind and form a detectable agglutination or precipitation. There are many classic agglutination assays used in the diagnosis of infectious disease such as the Widal test for typhoid fever. The reagent excess methods require an excess of labeled antigen or antibody, use either one or two sites, and include immunoblotting and solid-phase ELISA. These are commonly employed immunoassays in microbiology today. Reagent-limited assays are competitive-based tests and employ a limited amount of either antigen or antibody and either require separation or are separation free. These include classic RIA and EIA and are less often used in diagnosis of infectious disease.

Another commonly used classification scheme looks at immunoassays as either heterogeneous (solid phase) or homogeneous (free-solution assays) (8, 24). Heterogeneous assays are ones in which the bound and free components must be separated, whereas homogeneous assays do not require a separation step. In addition, heterogeneous assays involve some type of solid phase to which the immunoreactants are attached. Homogeneous assays generally are free-solution methods. While this is a useful and commonly employed classification scheme, there are assays that do not strictly fit into this classification scheme. For example, agglutination assays and particle-enhanced light-scattering methods are considered homogeneous assays; however, the antibody is bound to a solid phase, and there is no required separation of the bound from the free components.

ASSAY INTERPRETATION

When choosing an assay for the laboratory and in-patient diagnosis, it is critical to understand the concepts of sensitivity, specificity, and predictive values (48). Sensitivity is the proportion of individuals *with* a disease that are correctly identified with a particular test. Sensitivity defines the true positives (TP), which are the number of patients with disease detected by the assay. Conversely, false negatives (FN) are the patients with disease who are not detected by the test. The formula for sensitivity is as follows: Sensitivity = [TP/(TP + FN)] × 100. Specificity is the proportion of those *without* the disease that are correctly classified. Conversely, specificity is a measure of the true negatives (TN), which are the number of patients without disease not detected by the assay. False positives (FP) are the proportion of patients without disease who test positive. The formula for specificity is as follows: Specificity = [TN/(TN + FP)] × 100. With a highly sensitive test, the majority of diseased individuals are picked up, and thus the number of false-negative results is very low. In contrast, with a highly specific test, the majority of individuals without the disease test negative, so the number of false-positive results is very low. When an assay is developed, the diagnostic cutoffs can be modified to alter both the sensitivity and the specificity. For example, if one moves the cutoff to a lower level, the assay sensitivity is increased with a resulting decrease in specificity. The optimal balance of these two components must be evaluated for each laboratory test and depends on multiple factors such as the utility of the test and the prevalence of the disease in the population.

The probability of having the disease, given the results of a test, is called the predictive value of the test. Positive predictive value (PPV) determines the percentage of patients with positive results who are diseased: PPV = [TP/(TP + FP)] × 100; the negative predictive value (NPV) calculates the percentage of patients with negative test results who do not have the disease: NPV = [TN/(TN + FN)] × 100. The predictive value of a test combines the prevalence of disease in a particular population with the sensitivity and specificity. Positive and negative predictive values are important because they assess the ability of a test to predict the presence or absence of disease in a patient from a particular population. In this context, the disease prevalence is a critical component. Prevalence is the proportion of the population with the disease in question. If a disease state has a low prevalence in the target population, a positive result will most likely be a false-positive result, whereas the opposite is true in a high prevalence population. A potential use of a high negative predictive value is that a negative test can exclude disease. In addition to the values discussed above, there are a variety of other statistical methods that can be used to evaluate laboratory tests such as odds ratio, receiver-operator curve analysis, and likelihood ratios, among others. It is beyond the scope of this chapter to discuss these, and the reader is referred to other sources for a more complete discussion (43).

SCREENING VERSUS DIAGNOSTIC ASSAYS

An important component of assay design is based upon the ultimate use of the test, i.e., whether it will be used as a screening or diagnostic test (37, 45). Screening tests are designed to pick up disease in asymptomatic individuals who may have early disease or precursors of disease, whereas diagnostic tests are performed for persons with specific indications of possible disease. However, the screening procedure itself does not diagnose the illness; those individuals with a positive result from the screening test need further evaluation with additional diagnostic tests. If the individual has a previous positive screening test, the diagnostic test acts as a confirmatory test. The ideal screening test should be both highly specific and sensitive; however, this may be difficult to achieve. As there is such a variety of screening tests available, there is not a particular sensitivity target value which is suggested; nevertheless, the sensitivity should be as high as possible without sacrificing specificity. It is not advisable to use a test with low specificity as a screening test, since many people without the disease will screen positive and potentially receive unnecessary diagnostic procedures. Moreover, for an effective screening test, the prevalence of disease in the population should be high; for if the prevalence of the disease is low, then a positive test will most likely be a false positive, leading to further unnecessary testing. Other considerations in regard to screening tests include weighing the cost of the test versus the impact of early detection. Overall, good screening tests should be easy to perform, inexpensive, and performed in high disease prevalence populations. In addition, early detection of disease should have a measurable impact on patient outcomes.

SEROLOGICAL ASSAYS

Traditionally, serological assays referred to the use of serum or plasma samples for the detection of antibodies to a variety of antigens. This concept has been broadened to refer to a variety of patient samples such as cerebrospinal fluid, urine, and other body fluids. In addition, it refers to the detection of both antibodies and antigen. There are a variety of clinical scenarios in which serological assessment is the test of choice. For the identification of organisms for which culture is difficult or requires prolonged incubation, the determination of antibody titers or antigen detection can often give a quick answer. Although molecular techniques have sometimes supplanted serology in these situations, often cost issues make serology a more viable technique. There are frequent clinical situations where it is unnecessary to perform a culture if an antigen test is positive. One of the most common situations is the diagnosis of group A beta-hemolytic streptococcal throat infection. A rapid immunoassay for the detection of the group A streptococcal antigen is performed. If this is positive, then treatment can be instituted. Only when this quick test is negative is it necessary to perform a culture.

Basic Immunologic Reactions

In order to facilitate understanding of antibody titers, a brief review of basic immunologic reactions is provided (1, 2). Upon initial exposure to an infectious disease (primary antibody response), there are four phases in the subsequent response: an initial lag (or window) phase, when there is no antibody detected; a log phase, when the antibody titer increases in a logarithmic fashion; a plateau phase, in which the amount of antibody stabilizes; and a decline phase, during which the antibody is cleared or catabolized. The actual time course and ultimate maximum antibody titer depend on the antigen and the host. In the primary response, the initial antibody response is the production of immunoglobulin M (IgM), which usually appears after 10 days. The period after initial exposure, but before antibody is produced or is at sufficient levels to be detected, is called the "window period." This can vary, depending on the infectious agent, from as short as 10 days to as long as 6 months. IgG antibody production usually begins 10 days after exposure but is much less than the IgM response. As the IgM antibody level decreases, the IgG level increases, so that usually by the end of the first month, only IgG antibody is detectable. If there is a repeat infection with the same infectious agent, the kinetics of the response are different, with a lag phase of only 1 to 3 days, and IgG antibody is the primary isotype produced. In the months following antigen exposure, the IgG level reaches a plateau, and the antibody may remain detectable for life, even if there is no further exposure to the antigen. B lymphocytes utilize membrane-bound antibodies to recognize a wide array of antigens. In the case of infectious disease agents, the antigens are often expressed on the microbial surfaces. The particular parts of the expressed antigens that are bound by antibodies are referred to as epitopes; the strength of the binding of one epitope to one antibody is called the affinity. Upon repeated infection with a microbe, there is an increase in the strength of the antigen-antibody binding, a phenomenon called affinity maturation. However, depending upon the immunoglobulin molecule present, there are more than one antigen binding sites on each immunoglobulin (IgG, 2 sites; polymerized IgA, 4 sites; IgM, 10 sites); therefore, the total strength of the antigen-antibody binding is much greater than the affinity of a single interaction. This is called the avidity. Just as with affinity maturation, there is an increase in avidity with additional exposure to an antigen. Upon initial exposure to an antigen, the avidity of the IgG is low; upon secondary exposure, there is an increase in IgG avidity. Although there is exquisite specificity in the antigen-antibody reaction, there can be a spectrum of antibodies produced in response to a particular antigen; they can have differing affinities and avidities with a particular antigen and thus can be responsible for cross-reactions. Recognizing cross-reacting antibodies can be critical to assay specificity. Often, initial screening assays are set up with crude antigen preparations in which false-positive reactions can occur. Secondary confirmatory or diagnostic assays utilize purified and more expensive antigen preparations which confer greater specificity. Recognition of cross-reactivity is critical in tests used in infectious disease, because often organisms within the same genus and species share multiple antigenic determinants, making cross-reactivity a common problem. Although assays are designed to obviate these problems, laboratorians and clinicians should just be cognizant of the potential for cross-reactions.

Caveats in Serologic Interpretation

In general, a positive IgG titer means only that an individual has been exposed to a particular infectious agent and thus is "immune." For each infectious agent, the laboratory result is usually set up so that a positive result is the minimum amount of IgG antibody present which makes the individual "immune." For purposes of this discussion, the term "immune" is used; however, this does not necessarily mean that the level of antibody is protective against reinfection. The actual amount of antigen-specific antibody present in the serum of a particular individual is host determined and is controlled by immune-response genes which are products of the human histocompatibility system. The level of the IgG titer from a single serum sample to a particular infectious agent may not be used to determine if the infection is recent or remote. For example, person A may be a high responder to certain antigens and a low responder to others. Therefore, if a high titer of IgG is obtained for an individual, it may be tempting to think that this may represent a more recent exposure; however, this may indicate only that the individual is a high responder to that particular antigen. Therefore, a positive IgG titer establishes only that the individual has been exposed to a particular agent at some time in the past and has detectable IgG. In addition, the nature of the antigen is important, as some antigens are more effective than others in stimulating the immune system. Moreover, the ability of the immune system to respond to antigens can be affected by a variety of factors, such as age. For example, the very young may be unable to respond to certain types of antigens (e.g., carbohydrates) (1, 2).

Using serologic methods, there are several ways to determine if the infection is recent. The most useful and frequently used method is assessment of IgM antibody to a particular infectious disease agent. In general, a positive IgM titer to a particular organism is evidence of an active (i.e., recently acquired) infection with that agent. However, there are several considerations to keep in mind in the interpretation of this test. First of all, a positive IgM titer does not always mean that the infection is recent. There have been reports of persistent elevations of IgM antibody for a year or more. This has been seen with multiple organisms, including cytomegalovirus, *Mycoplasma pneumoniae,* hepatitis A virus, and *Toxoplasma gondii,* among others (9, 33, 45). Conversely, a negative IgM titer does not exclude a recent exposure. The amount of IgM may have been small and resolved quickly; thus, it was not detected at the time of the assay. The second way to establish a primary infection is to determine acute- and convalescent-phase titers. This requires drawing two sets of antibody titers: one set early in the exposure to the infectious agent and a second set 2 to 3 weeks later. Evidence of an acute infection can be confirmed if there is a fourfold increase in antibody titer between the first and second titers.

While this can sometimes provide information on the pathogenesis of a disease state, it requires at least 2 to 3 weeks for definitive results, thus obviating its use for early clinical management. Also, a false-negative reaction is not uncommon due to the fact that it requires drawing the specimen at a point low enough on the log part of the antibody response curve to obtain the required fourfold increase in antibody titer. Therefore, the lack of a fourfold increase does not rule out a primary infection.

At present, many assays report results as absorbance values or international units, making it problematic to apply the concept of a fourfold increase in titer. While it is possible to develop an approximate equivalency between titers and absorbance values, this has to be individually developed for each assay. One method to do this involves collecting multiple pairs of acute- and convalescent-phase sera to use as reference sera. They must demonstrate a fourfold increase in titer on traditional assays. They are then run on the EIA for the agent in question, and reference ranges are reported in optical density units. Assuming that the EIA provides distinctly different absorbance ranges to adequately separate acute- and convalescent-phase sera, pairs of test sera can then be run on the EIA, and the values can be compared to the reference ranges. While this can theoretically provide an adequate way to evaluate acute- and convalescent-phase titers by using the newer assay formats, it can have multiple problems. First of all, establishment of the reference range has to be performed separately on assays for each infectious agent, which can be expensive and time-consuming. Secondly, the lab has to have multiple sets of positive acute- and convalescent-phase paired sera for each organism tested, which can be quite difficult to obtain. In addition, depending on the EIA used and the range of the standard curve, titer values may not be easily converted into equivalent and meaningful absorbance values. Considering the cost and difficulties associated with this type of analysis, it is not generally recommended. Instead, it is preferable to test for the presence of an acute infection by using an IgM assay or an IgG avidity test (see below) or to directly test for the organism by using one of the increasingly available molecular techniques.

An additional test to perform, which can address some of the concerns with IgM testing and acute- and convalescent-phase titers, is an IgG avidity test (28, 33, 39). IgG antibodies produced early in infection have a low avidity, but a much greater avidity is seen with a secondary exposure. Using an avidity assay, in conjunction with the assessment of IgG and IgM antibody levels to a pathogen, can provide a much clearer indication of acute infection. Avidity tests are performed with a modification of the standard IgG EIA, in which IgG antibodies are exposed to a dissociating agent (usually high concentrations of urea). The serum IgG avidity is estimated by comparing the treated sample with one untreated. While this test can be quite useful, there are several caveats with its use. First of all, low avidity does not always mean that the infection is recent because low avidity antibodies can persist for months to years. In addition, there can be quality control issues in this testing with variability in test results related to the type of assay plates used, the antigens employed, and the type of dissociating agent used. This test has special utility in testing for some of the pathogens associated with pre- and perinatal infections (toxoplasmosis, rubella, and cytomegalovirus) (28, 33). For example, one algorithm suggested for prenatal toxoplasmosis testing follows all positive IgG antibody assays with an avidity test. If the avidity test is high, an acute infection is ruled out; however, if the avidity test is low, an IgM test is then performed. If the IgM test is positive, then a recent IgM infection is highly suspected. However, considering the implications for pregnancy, the FDA recommends that sera with positive IgM results obtained at a nonreference laboratory should then be sent to a toxoplasma reference laboratory for confirmatory testing.

SPECIFIC IMMUNOASSAYS

The spectrum of immunologic assays is discussed in detail in the following sections. Table 1 lists selected assays in order of relative sensitivities and provides approximate levels of detection.

Precipitation Reactions

When soluble antigens and antibodies are in equimolar concentrations, they bind and form insoluble antigen-antibody complexes which form a visible precipitate (24, 29). There are a number of laboratory tests available that utilize this reaction. Immunodiffusion is the simplest of the precipitation assays and involves putting the immune reactants in an inert semisolid material and then viewing the visible precipitation line. There are several variants of immunodiffusion. Radial immunodiffusion is designed to provide protein quantitation, whereas double immunodiffusion (Ouchterlony analysis) allows characterization of the relationship between different antigens. Overall, immunodiffusion reactions are simple to perform, easy to evaluate, and inexpensive and can be adapted to a variety of health care settings. The drawbacks include low sensitivity, as the level of detection is microgram quantities of antibody or antigen; requirements for relatively large amounts of antigens and antibody; and long assay times. Immunodiffusion is also routinely used for determination of antibody titers to a variety of agents, most commonly antifungal antibodies (*Coccidioides*, *Aspergillus*, *Histoplasma*, and *Entamoeba histolytica*).

Agglutination Reactions

Agglutination reactions require a particulate antigen and its antibody with the resultant visible clumping as evidence of a positive reaction (21, 24, 29, 30). A test involving the particulate antigen which agglutinates the antibody present in the patient sample is termed a direct agglutination assay. To enhance the visibility of the agglutination reaction, an indirect assay format can be used, in which the antigen is coupled with a variety of particles that serve as an inert matrix. Various materials which have been employed include gelatin, latex, erythrocytes, polypeptides, and silicates. In addition, soluble antigen can be detected in a patient sample by absorption of a specific antibody to a particle; this is termed

TABLE 1 Sensitivity of immunoassays (34, 41)

Technique	Approximate sensitivity (per ml)
Precipitation, tube	100 mg
Immunodiffusion	1–3 mg
Agglutination	1 mg
Hemagglutination, passive	15–30 mg
Complement fixation	0.001 mg
Particle immunoassay	30–50 ng
EIA	<1 ng

reverse agglutination. Due to the large IgM molecule with its pentameric structure, IgM antibodies are several hundred times more efficient at agglutination than IgG and thus give more consistent and stable agglutination reactions. If the immune response involves primarily IgG antibody, the reaction may require some type of chemical enhancement or an antiglobulin reagent. Flocculation assays are another variant of agglutination assays, in which the particles are suspended. The most frequently used assays are the Venereal Disease Research Laboratory and rapid plasma reagin tests for syphilis.

Many agglutination assays, called hemagglutination assays, employ red blood cells (RBC) and use either a direct or an indirect assay format. Direct agglutination of RBC is commonly used in the blood bank for ABO typing. For infectious disease diagnosis, one of the most frequently ordered direct hemagglutination assays is the monospot test. This test detects the presence of a heterophile antibody which is produced in infectious mononucleosis and happens to spontaneously agglutinate equine RBC. The indirect hemagglutination assay is a commonly used format in which antigen is adsorbed to RBC, thus testing for the presence of specific antibody in the patient serum. Alternatively, the assay can be modified to test for antigen, in which case it is called reverse agglutination assay. For infectious disease testing, hemagglutination (especially indirect) is a popular assay format, as it is sensitive and simple to perform and does not require sophisticated equipment. For these reasons, it has been used in many third world countries for testing of a variety of infectious disease agents such as human immunodeficency virus (HIV), hepatitis virus (A, B, and C), and *Treponema pallidum.* There is a unique type of hemagglutination assay format used primarily in viral serology called hemagglutination inhibition. It is most commonly used for detection and quantitation of anti-influenza antibodies. It is based on the principle that some viruses have surface proteins that will agglutinate RBC, so the assay uses the ability of antiviral antibodies in the patient sample to inhibit the spontaneous agglutination of the test RBC. The titer of antiviral antibodies is reported as the last dilution of the patient serum still able to inhibit the agglutination reaction.

Specialized types of agglutination assays that require optical counting are called particle immunoassays (8, 15, 16, 26). They involve primarily the measurement of scattered light which occurs upon the antigen-antibody reaction, and this is measured by either turbidimetry or nephelometry. They can be used for testing a wide range of proteins and analytes. Particle immunoassays are 3 orders of magnitude more sensitive than standard agglutination. One additional assay is the particle-counting immunoassay, which is used for quantitating haptens, antigens, and antibody. It is also available in a fully automated immunoassay format. In this assay, optical cell counting is employed, and there is an assessment of the decrease in agglutination following the immunoreaction. These assays are sensitive to a level of nanograms per milliliter. The patient sample is mixed with latex beads coated with antibody. As the antigen-antibody reaction occurs, the antigen particles are no longer dispersed in the solution; therefore, the antigen concentration is inversely proportional to the amount of antigen particles remaining in solution. Antibody can also be quantitated in this assay. The use of a particle-counting immunoassay has been reported for quantitation of hepatitis B virus surface antigen, along with quantitation of antibodies to hepatitis C virus, *T. pallidum,* and *T. gondii* (15, 16, 20).

Overall, basic agglutination assays are easy to perform and inexpensive and can be done in a variety of clinical settings such as the doctor's office, the emergency room, and the hospital bedside and in the field. They are performed either on a card, in tubes, or in microtiter plates. Often they provide only qualitative results, although an antibody or antigen titer can be obtained through serial dilutions of the sample. Direct assays continue to be performed for rare pathogens such as *Francisella* and *Brucella.* They utilize an inactivated source of the whole organism mixed with the patient sera. Although agglutination assays suffer from both limited sensitivity and limited specificity, they continue to be utilized because they are easy to perform and relatively inexpensive. If a more quantitative assay is needed, the assay can be adapted to light-scattering equipment such as a nephelometer to provide more quantitative and sensitive results. Overall the major drawback to direct agglutination assays is their limited sensitivity. They detect only to a level of microgram to milligram quantities of analytes per ml. However, greater sensitivities can be achieved with many of the variants of direct agglutination. For example, microtiter passive hemagglutination assays for infectious agents can achieve a sensitivity equivalent to that of a conventional EIA. The more sensitive hemagglutination assays for measuring antigen can measure as low as 15 to 30 μg/ml. If an agglutination assay is read visually, it is reported as a titer value. While these are fairly sensitive assays, titer values are always plus or minus one tube dilution, so that a titer of 16 could actually represent a titer of either 8 or 32. With latex-enhanced nephelometry or turbidimetry, sensitivity ranges in the area of 30 to 50 ng/ml.

There are several problems that can affect both sensitivity and specificity. The first problem affecting sensitivity is called the prozone effect (8, 24, 29). This refers to a lack of agglutination due to an excessive amount of antibodies in the patient sample. The high concentration of antibody inhibits agglutination, giving a false-negative result. This can be easily overcome by simply diluting the sample. In regard to specificity, the major concern is false-positive reactions from IgM rheumatoid factor (RF) (8, 11, 24, 29, 32). This occurs most commonly in assays in which the latex beads are coated with IgG antibody. This has been commonly reported for the latex agglutination test for cryptococcal antigen (24, 46). IgM RF, which is specific for the Fc portion of the IgG molecule, binds and gives a false-positive reaction. RF has also been reported to bind to other serum proteins nonspecifically, also giving a false-positive reaction. It is crucial that the clinician notify the laboratory if the patient has a known RF. There are several measures that could be taken. First of all, if a false-positive reaction is suspected, the sample result can be compared to the reaction using control particles coated with normal IgG. If this indicates that there is a false-positive reaction, the sample can be treated with a reducing agent such as 2-mercaptoethanol or it can be treated with pronase. Both of these treatments have been shown to reduce the majority of false-positive reactions due to IgM RF. Alternatively, the sample could be pretreated with aggregated IgG to remove the IgM RF; however, this can result in loss of antigen or specific antibodies and give a false-negative result. Also, an alternate test method could be used for assessment of the ordered analyte. Most importantly, communication of pertinent clinical information to the laboratory is critical to ensure the most accurate diagnostic information.

CF Test

Another traditional immunoassay is the complement fixation (CF) test, which is based upon the interaction of immune complexes with complement (29). As antigen-antibody complexes form, the complement cascade is activated and complement components are "fixed" or consumed. Conversely, if there is no antigen-antibody complex formation, there will be no activation of the complement cascade. This two-step test is primarily used to determine the titer of antibodies to specific antigens. For example, to set up a CF test for anti-*Mycoplasma pneumoniae* antibodies, patient serum would be incubated with M. *pneumoniae* antigen and a defined quantity of guinea pig complement. If the patient sample contains M. *pneumoniae* antibody, immune complexes will form and fix the complement. RBC coated with antierythrocyte antibodies are then added to the tube. The final readout for the assay is the release of hemoglobin from any lysed RBC. If the patient sample is positive for M. *pneumoniae,* then there will be no complement remaining, so there will be no release of hemoglobulin. The opposite will occur if the patient sample is negative for anti-M. *pneumoniae* antibody. Although CF assays are relatively sensitive and inexpensive, they can be technically demanding and time-consuming. Therefore, many of these assays have been converted to ELISA formats. However, a number of laboratories still use them as a confirmatory test for the presence of antibodies to a variety of infectious agents such as *Coccidioides, Histoplasma capsulatum,* adenovirus, herpesvirus, influenza virus, M. *pneumoniae,* and rickettsias.

Neutralization Assays

Neutralization assays are traditional laboratory tests used to determine if an antibody which can neutralize the infectivity of a particular virus is present (29). The classic assay involves mixing patient serum antibody samples with virus and then using this mix to inoculate either a cell line or a preparation of peripheral blood mononuclear cells. The readout involves either the assessment of viral cytopathic effect in the cell line or some other measure of viral replication, such as that obtained by a classic immunoassay of viral protein. For example, in the case of HIV testing, one can perform a p24 antigen test or reverse transcriptase assay and look for lower values. Evidence of decreased viral replication confirms the presence of neutralizing antibody. Although these assays are relatively simple, they can be expensive and can take days to complete. In addition, they can be difficult to standardize, especially when comparing results from different laboratories. To decrease the assay length, the quantitation of viral products can be assessed using PCR; however, this technique can be expensive and also difficult to standardize between laboratories. A blocking ELISA can also be performed, in which viral antigen and serum are mixed, after which a standard ELISA for virus is performed and the decrease in the amount of antibody detected is assessed. An additional traditional neutralization assay is a reverse passive hemagglutination, as previously discussed. In the field of HIV vaccine development, there is interest in developing new and better assays for neutralization, since it is crucial in the assessment of vaccine efficacy to demonstrate that a putative virus can initiate antibody production to prevent infection (35).

IFAs

The immunofluorescence assay (IFA) uses a histochemical technique to detect either antigen or serum antibody, utilizing a fluorescent-compound-labeled detector antibody (24, 29, 30). There are two types of IFA, direct and indirect (Fig. 1). Direct assays are used to detect the presence of antigens in tissue or body fluids. For example, to detect the presence of influenza virus in a nasal wash specimen, it is applied to a slide, and then it is overlaid with a fluorescent-compound-labeled anti-influenza antibody. If there is influenza antigen present, there is emission of fluorescent light, which is evaluated with a fluorescent microscope. Indirect assays are two-step tests used primarily for the detection of antibodies in serum or a body fluid. The patient sample is applied to a slide containing the target antigen; this is allowed to incubate, and specific antibody in the patient sample forms immune complexes with the antigen present on the slide. Any unbound reagent is then washed away, and the slide is overlaid with a fluorescent-compound-labeled anti-immunoglobulin. Positive staining is the emission of fluorescent light. Overall, IFAs are useful tests that are relatively easy to perform and inexpensive. In addition, they allow the localization of the antibody to a specific antigen location in the tissue. For example, the IFA for antibody to Epstein-Barr virus early antigen allows visualization of a specific pattern of staining of the virus-infected cell line. The disadvantages of this assay are that it is relatively time-consuming and requires both the purchase of an expensive fluorescence microscope and the presence of trained and experienced personnel for interpretation.

EIAs

EIAs are taking on increasingly more prominent roles in laboratory medicine (7, 8, 22, 24, 30, 47, 48). They are found in all areas of the clinical laboratory, in physicians' offices, and in at-home testing and are being increasingly used in molecular pathology laboratories. EIAs have taken the place of the RIAs in many laboratories, as they offer comparable sensitivity without the problems of disposal and the short half-life associated with radioactive materials. They are also replacing a variety of other techniques in the laboratory such as immunofluorescence and agglutination because EIAs provide greater objectivity, the potential to automate, and the ability to process large numbers of samples with less hands-on technician time. As a single unit of enzyme label can amplify a reaction product manyfold, many EIAs are optimized for detection at the pico- or attomole level. EIAs can be broadly classified as either homogeneous or heterogeneous assays. In homogeneous assays, the enzyme activity is altered as part of the immunologic reaction itself. In these assays, there is no requirement to separate the bound from the free immunoreactants. Although this technique is especially suited for the measurement of drugs and haptens, homogeneous assays

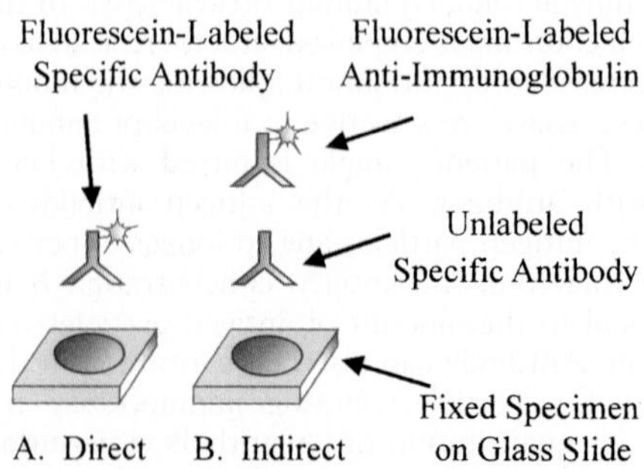

FIGURE 1 Direct and indirect immunofluorescence assays.

have not achieved widespread use in microbiology laboratories. In contrast, heterogeneous immunoassays are widely used in microbiology. In these assays, the enzyme activity of the labeled immunoreactant is not directly involved in the immunologic reaction itself.

The basic principle of the heterogeneous EIA is the use of an antibody or antigen conjugated with an enzyme which, upon reacting with its substrate, forms a measurable reaction product. Often a color reaction product is produced. The color change is monitored visually or with the use of a spectrophotometer to determine the proportionality between the amount of color and the amount of analyte present. An essential component of these assays is the separation of the bound enzyme-labeled component from the free labeled reagent. Assays can be competitive or noncompetitive and can be used to measure antigens or antibodies. The presence of all antibody isotypes can be quantitated depending on the specificity of the antibodies used. Whenever antibody or antigen is absorbed to the solid phase, the assay is referred to as an ELISA and also as a "sandwich" assay.

EIAs can be set up primarily as competitive or noncompetitive (7). Competitive assays most commonly measure antigens and are set up with either antibody or antigen on the solid phase. They are often termed "limited reagent" methods because the antigens and antibodies are used in measured and limited amounts. When the assay design uses specific antibody with which the solid phase is coated, the patient sample containing the putative antigen and the labeled antigen are added simultaneously and compete for binding to this matrix (Fig. 2). It is critical that the avidity of the antibody for both the labeled and unlabeled antigens be the same. In addition, a separate reaction is set up using enzyme-labeled antigen and buffer alone, which are added to the antibody-adsorbed solid phase. The substrate for the enzyme is added, and the color reaction is assessed. If the patient sample contains the antigen in question, it will effectively compete for binding to the solid phase, thus preventing any enzyme-labeled antigen from binding, thus giving no or minimal color. This reaction is compared to a reaction well to which buffer alone is substituted for the patient sample. The separation of the bound reactant from the free reactant is achieved through the washing steps. As is true with all competitive assays, the amount of labeled immunoreactant detected through the enzymatic reaction is inversely proportional to the amount of antigen present in the sample.

Antigens present in a patient sample can also be measured by using the coating of the solid phase with antigen. For this technique, the test sample containing the antigen in question is mixed with a limited amount of enzyme-labeled antibody. If the patient's sample contains the antigen, it will bind the labeled antigen, thus preventing this antibody from binding to the antigen with which the solid phase is coated. Following the washing step, the color reaction is developed and again, no color is seen if the sample contains the antigen. This technique can be modified by using unlabeled antibody in the first step and then adding a secondary enzyme-labeled anti-Ig.

Another variant of a competitive technique uses a two-step procedure. In the first step, test antigen is preincubated with its specific antibody. Any antigen-antibody complexes that have formed are removed during a wash step. Enzyme-labeled antigen (ag*) is then added to bind any remaining free antibody not bound by test antigen in the initial reaction. In the second step, beads coated with anti-immunoglobulin are added. These beads will bind any ag*-antibody complexes which formed in the previous step, and they can be quantitated in the pellet following centrifugation.

Compared to noncompetitive assays, competitive tests often provide greater specificity with less sensitivity; however, this is dependent on the affinity and purity of the immunological reagents and the design of the particular system. Competitive assays are ideal for measuring relatively small molecules which can be obtained in relative purity and in large enough amounts to be labeled with an enzyme. As they generally require small amounts of antibody, competitive assays are ideal for use in systems which have a limited amount of antibody available.

Noncompetitive ELISAs

The next major type of assay is the noncompetitive indirect solid-phase ELISA. This method is one of the most frequently employed immunoassays in the clinical laboratory. As with competitive assays, the two major variants involve using either antigen or antibody on the solid phase. When antigen is used for coating, specific antibodies in the sample bind to the solid phase and are detected with an enzyme-labeled anti-immunoglobulin secondary antibody (Fig. 3). Isotype-specific, enzyme-labeled anti-Ig antibodies can be used to determine the specific Ig class present. This type of assay is commonly used in the measurement of immune status to infectious agents and for autoantibody testing. A variety of solid-phase supports are used, including microtiter plates, nitrocellulose, and beads. One common variant, which uses nitrocellulose membranes, is the dot blot assay (12, 29, 40). In this system, the antigen or antibody is coupled to the membrane, and usually the reaction is assessed

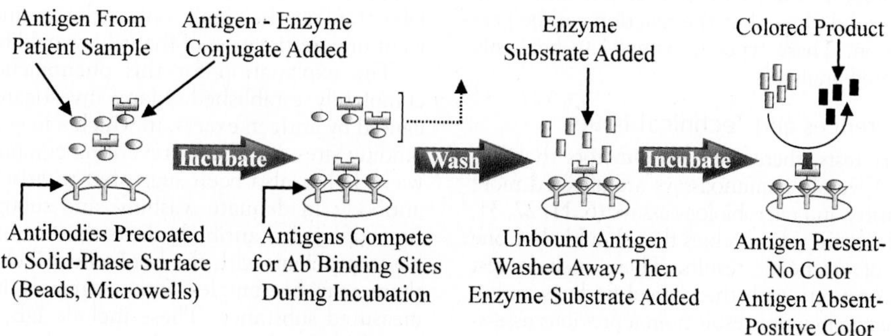

FIGURE 2 Competitive EIA.

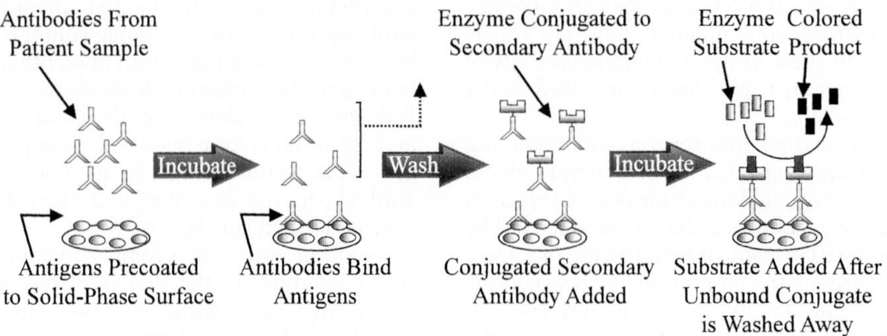

FIGURE 3 Noncompetitive indirect solid-phase ELISA.

visually by a colored reaction production, providing a qualitative assay. Many of the at-home testing kits (e.g., pregnancy kits) use a variant of this technique. This assay can be modified for increased sensitivity with such variants as can be made semiquantitative by using a densitometer for reading the color reaction.

When the antibody is coupled to the solid phase, these assays are often termed "capture" or "sandwich" assays, because the antigen in the sample is captured by an antibody-coated matrix. An enzyme-labeled secondary antibody directed to a different antigenic epitope is then added, completing the sandwich. There are numerous variations of this type of assay. The antigen captured can be an immunoglobulin, a viral protein, or any antigen that has at least two epitopes.

Noncompetitive ELISAs can also be modified by incorporating additional layers of immune reactants. This increases the sensitivity of the assay, but it also increases both the cost and time requirements. The most frequent application is the so-called avidin-biotin-peroxidase complex (ABC method) which can significantly improve the level of detectability. Biotinylated anti-Ig is generally used as the second antibody of the sandwich. This is then reacted with a preformed mixture of avidin and biotinylated peroxidase (ABC). The peroxidase can be developed with chemiluminescent reagents for increased sensitivity. Other variants include peroxidase anti-peroxidase methods and the incorporation of lectins as bridging molecules.

Microparticle Enzyme Immunoassay

The microparticle enzyme immunoassay is a variant of the ELISA that utilizes tiny beads (1-mm-diameter or less) that can be coupled with antibody or antigens (24, 28). The small size leads to a greater surface area for binding of antibody or antigen, which results in a decrease in reaction time. The particles act as the solid phase, but the reaction can be performed in suspension. These types of assays can be easily adapted to automated analyzers.

Analytical Interferences and Technical Issues

As in all laboratory tests, there are always factors that can affect test validity. Overall, immunoassays are affected more than routine chemistry and microbiology assays (6, 11, 22, 31, 32, 42, 47, 48). There are various clues that should alert one to the possibility of erroneous results. These include test results that are inconsistent with the clinical findings and/or an unexplained change in a test result from a previous assessment. These findings should prompt consideration of the possibility of technical issues or some type of test interference.

Plate Variability

There are several issues to consider with solid-phase microtiter plates that are often used for reagent excess sandwich-type ELISA (7, 47, 48). First, there can be variability between readings on adjacent wells of a microtiter plate. This variability is expressed as the well coefficient of variation, which should not be greater than 3 to 5% between wells. Secondly, there is the "edge effect," which refers to the variability between the readings on the outer wells of a microtiter plate and the readings on the inside wells. Although manufacturing variability in the plates must be evaluated as a possible cause, this occurs primarily due to differences in temperature between outer wells and interior ones. This can affect both the antigen-antibody and enzyme-substrate reactions. There are several ways to deal with the edge effect. One easy solution is to use smaller break-apart wells that can be placed in a larger plate. Simply being careful to protect the plate from exposure to light can also easily solve this problem. It is crucial that different plates from several manufacturers be screened for this effect when initially setting up an assay. In addition, when the lot of a plate is changed, the plates should be reevaluated to ensure that it is not necessary to modify any of the assay parameters.

Hook Effect

The hook effect refers to an unexpected fall in the amount of an analyte at the high end of the dose-response curve, resulting in a gross underestimation of the analyte (6, 11, 22, 31, 32, 42, 47, 48). This is particularly a problem in sandwich immunoassays with patient samples which contain an extremely high level of an analyte. The patient sample gives a low to moderately high result when using the standard assay dilution. However, upon further dilution of the sample, either the result is out-of-range high or, if it is diluted far enough, the sample gives an extremely elevated value. Therefore, if the laboratory ran the sample only at the routine dilution, a significant underestimation of the value would be reported.

The explanation for this phenomenon has not been completely established. Many investigators feel that it is caused by antigen excess, in which a majority of the antigen binding sites are filled, preventing completion of the sandwich. It has also been suggested to arise from low-affinity antibody, inadequate washing, and suboptimal concentrations of labeled antibody. Tests that are especially susceptible to problems with the hook effect include ones in which there may be samples with extremely high levels of the measured substance. These include IgE, human chorionic gonadotropin, tumor markers, ferritin, infectious antigens, and antibodies.

Numerous suggestions have been made regarding ways that laboratories can deal with the hook effect. One obvious strategy is to run all patient samples at 2 dilutions to screen for this problem. If the sample provides an answer with the first dilution, while the more dilute sample is out-of-range high, then the laboratory is alerted to the possibility of the hook effect. Although this is an effective approach, many laboratories are concerned about the time, cost, and labor involved in running 2 dilutions for every sample to avoid problems with only a small minority of patients. Thus, there are other strategies which can lessen the probability of the hook effect occurring.

First of all, always ensure that adequate washing is performed between all steps of the ELISA, especially between the steps following the addition of each antibody. Automatic plate washers are relatively inexpensive and can simplify this task. In addition, good communication with the kit manufacturers can also lessen the frequency of this problem. A number of companies have established the level at which the hook effect occurs and will readily share this information. Also, when completing new kit evaluations, testing specimens with high levels of the analyte is also crucial, as the frequency of the hook effect with different kits may be variable. Lastly, good communication with the clinician is also important; include discussion of the hook effect with a suggestion of notifying the laboratory when patients are expected to have very high levels of the analyte ordered.

Antibody Interference

There are a number of endogenous antibodies in patients' sera that may cause either positive or negative interferences in immunoassays (6, 11, 22, 31, 32, 42, 47, 48). There are multiple types of antibody interferences; they can be caused by antibodies binding to the actual analyte (e.g., antiviral antibodies), binding to components of the detection system (e.g., anti-alkaline phosphatase), and binding to reagent antibodies (e.g., anti-immunoglobulin antibodies). The last category is the most common and involves three types of antibodies. First, there are heterophile antibodies, which are weak antibodies to immunoglobulins from multiple species with no known or obvious identifiable immunogen. Secondly, RF can have a known effect on a variety of immunoassays and is most often found in patients with connective tissue diseases. Thirdly, there are various types of anti-animal antibodies; the most commonly reported are human anti-mouse antibodies (HAMA). Estimates of the prevalence of anti-mouse antibodies in normal sera vary greatly, from 0.5% to as high as 40%, depending on the sensitivity of the testing assay. There are both iatrogenic and noniatrogenic causes for the development of HAMA. In regard to iatrogenic causes, the culprit appears to be the increasing use of mouse monoclonal antibodies for therapeutic and imaging purposes. In regard to noniatrogenic causes, there are a number of suggested etiologies including environmental exposure to mice, maternal transfer across the placenta, passage of dietary antigens across the gut wall in inflammatory conditions, such as celiac disease, and association with a number of disease states, such as cardiomyopathy (25). While mouse anti-human antibodies can affect a variety of immunoassays, they are most often reported in two-site murine monoclonal antibody assays which often require only a small serum dilution. The presence of these antibodies can have a variable effect on immunoassays. If the analyte is present, they may cause either an over- or an underestimation. However, if the analyte is not present, a false-positive result may arise from the anti-mouse antibody cross-linking the two mouse monoclonal antibodies of the sandwich (the coating and conjugate antibodies). There have been a number of techniques advocated for decreasing the interference caused by heterophile antibodies and HAMA. These include heating the sample to 70°C, precipitating with polyethylene glycol, blocking with mouse IgG, and blocking with solid-phase anti-human IgG or mouse IgG. Caution should be observed in using heat treatment. The most popular method is the addition of nonimmune mouse immunoglobulin; however, the amount and source of the mouse serum may be crucial. Some studies with interfering anti-mouse antibodies demonstrated that the serum had to be from the same strain of mouse as the monoclonal antibody used in the assay. Therefore, it is recommended that a pool of mouse immunoglobulin from various strains be used to increase the probability of blocking as many patients' samples as possible. Most studies use approximately 10% mouse serum added to the reaction buffer; however, a few patient samples required a high concentration (>20%) of normal serum coupled with a long incubation time to correct the interference. To obviate problems with the majority of samples, laboratorians should consider routinely adding normal pooled heterologous sera to the dilution buffer of sandwich assays. In addition, special attention should be given to any sample for which the lab result is discordant with the clinical presentation, as this may represent a heterophile antibody resistant to the standard protocols.

Measurement of IgM

Quantitation of the IgM isotype of specific antibody poses special technical problems (7, 24, 28, 48). False positivity is common due to the presence of IgM RF in the patient sample. In addition, false negativity can occur from competitive inhibition of IgM binding in the presence of high levels of specific IgG. Previously, assays for IgM used a standard indirect solid-phase ELISA with the antigen immobilized and an IgM-specific secondary antibody. However, these assays were frought with the problems of false positivity and negativity. To obviate these problems, an IgM capture assay was developed (Fig. 4). In this procedure, a polyclonal anti-IgM antibody is bound to the solid phase. Upon incubation of the patient sample, all IgM is captured on the plate. The test antigen is then added, binding any specific IgM present on the plate. An enzyme-labeled secondary antibody is then added, and the reaction is completed. This assay obviates the problems with false-negative results due to competitive inhibition with IgM, as all the IgG in the patient sample is washed away in the first step. False-positive results, however, may still occur due to bound IgM RF reacting with either the IgG conjugate or binding any antigen-specific IgG in the sample. One way to avoid the problem with conjugate binding is to use $F(ab')_2$-conjugated capture antibodies. Alternatively, the assay can be modified to a direct technique by employing enzyme-labeled antigen in the second step, thus eliminating any Ig which could bind RF. Even with these modifications, problems can still occur with borderline and low positive IgM results. For this reason, all IgM-specific antibody results should be evaluated cautiously. As mentioned above, often running an IgG avidity assay can help in the evaluation of IgM results.

RIA

RIA was the original immunoassay technique and ushered in the area of improved and more sensitive immunoassays. Basically, all principles of assay design for EIA were based upon the experience gleaned from the RIA. Although RIA

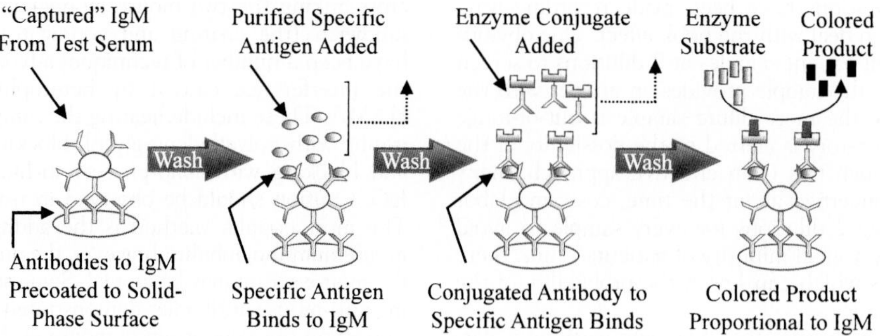

FIGURE 4 IgM capture assay.

is still a viable technique, it has largely been replaced by CL and EIA in most clinical laboratories. A variety of radioisotopes are utilized, most commonly ^{125}I, ^{3}H, and ^{14}C. Both CL and EIA offer more stable reagents and comparable to more sensitive detection limits, and they present no problems with hazardous waste disposal.

FIAs

The fluorescence immunoassay (FIA) uses fluorescence as the detection end point, and this method can be used in either homogeneous or heterogeneous assays (8, 24, 29). Fluorescence is the emission of photons of light as electrons go from an excited singlet state to the original ground state. The system requires a light source, excitation and emission filters, and a detection system utilizing photo multiplier tubes. A mercury lamp is the most frequently used light source, although xenon, halogen, and laser can also be used as excitation light. Fluorescein isothiocyanate and rhodamine are two of the most popular fluorochromes; however, there are a variety of other compounds used which have unique properties making them especially suited to a particular assay design.

There are numerous homogeneous assays which are performed in the liquid phase and do not require a separation of the bound from the free components. One popular homogeneous technique is the fluorescence polarization immunoassay. Some popular clinical analyzers utilize this methodology. This technique gives a measure of the bound/free ratio of the analyte without requiring a separation step. Polarization of light is measured by illuminating a sample with two polarizers in the same plane as the incident light and then at 90° to each other. The assay is based on an increase in light polarization which occurs when a fluorescent-tag antigen binds antibody and forms an immune complex. The labeled antigen is small and thus can rotate rapidly, causing depolarization of light. When the antigen-antibody complex forms, the increase in molecular weight causes a slower rotation and an increased emission of highly polarized light. This technique is primarily utilized for measurement of drugs and some hormones; however, it has utility for the detection of infectious disease. Its use has been described for the detection of antibodies to a variety of organisms such as gram-negative bacteria (*Brucella* spp. and *Salmonella* spp.) and equine infectious anemia virus (20, 44). There are a number of variants of both homogeneous and heterogeneous assays; however, it is beyond the scope of this chapter to discuss these and the reader is referred to other sources (24). FIAs have a number of advantages including high sensitivity and speed, and they are at least as sensitive as RIA. In addition, the reagents are stable and the assays are easily performed. For the fluorescence polarization immunoassay, one limitation is that the antigen used must be relatively small (i.e., with an MW no greater than 2,000) to allow a significant difference in the polarization when it forms an immune complex. Another important drawback in the use of fluorescent assays is the problem of autofluorescent compounds both in the patient sample and in the reaction mixture. This can be a significant problem in homogeneous assays where no washing steps occur and sample components are present during the entire assay. To circumvent this problem, samples can be treated with proteolytic enzymes, oxidizing agents, or denaturing reagents which will limit the amount of autofluorescence. In solid-phase assays, the majority of inferring substance will be washed away.

CL Immunoassays

The chemiluminescence (CL) immunoassay is a very popular technique which is widely utilized in many different assay formats (8, 24). Chemiluminescence is the emission of light which occurs when a substrate decays from an excited state to a ground state. In contrast to the fluorescence reaction which utilizes incident radiation for energy, chemiluminescence derives energy from the chemical reaction itself, which most often is an oxidation reaction. It is one of the most sensitive of all immunoassays, with detection limits down to the attomole (10^{18}) or zeptomole (10^{21}) level. CL substrates are used as the end point in both homogeneous and heterogeneous assays, in addition to their use in immunoblotting and multianalyte detection. Either chemiluminescence is used as a direct label on an antigen or antibody in a reaction which is catalyzed by adding a substrate, or a chemiluminescence compound is used as the substrate for an enzyme-labeled immunoreactant. The acridinium ester labels most commonly employed are derivatives of isoluminol and acridinium esters. The latter is a popular label which is the most sensitive and widely used. It can be conjugated to antigen and antibody by using standard techniques. Detection is relatively simple with the addition of sodium hydroxide and hydrogen peroxide. This reaction results in a flash of light which is read using a luminometer. In addition, the light signal can be captured on photographic film.

Western Blot and Immunoblot

Western blot and immunoblot are two solid-phase assays which combine the separation of proteins, using separation by denaturing gel electrophoresis followed by transfer to a filter (Fig. 5), and the determination of reactivity of the patient sera with the individually separated proteins, using a

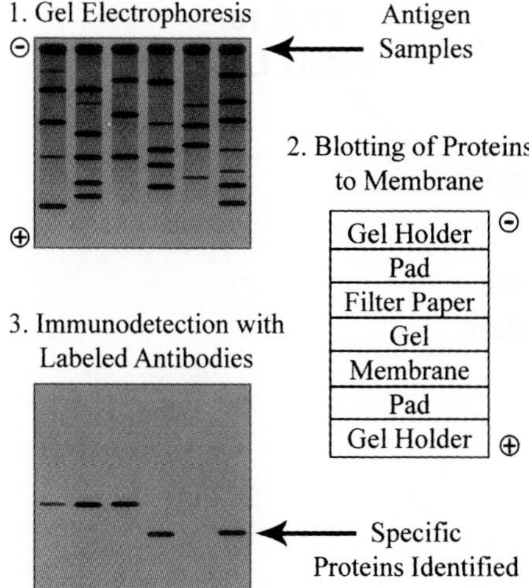

FIGURE 5 Western blot procedure.

typical sandwich-type ELISA. Immunoblotting utilizes a solid-support membrane filter containing antigens which are identified by a specific reaction with antibody. Most commonly, this technique is utilized for identifying the specific pattern of antibody to various infectious disease agents. One common application is for confirmation of antibody to HIV. Immunoblotting patterns can be read visually, using radiolabeled isotopes or using a CL substrate which is then developed on X-ray or photographic film or a charged-coupled device camera.

IPCR

The immuno-PCR (IPCR) is a novel technique that combines traditional ELISA with PCR (3, 4, 5, 11, 13, 27, 36). It uses antibodies labeled directly with nucleic acids (Fig. 6). It is an ultrasensitive technique which has been used for the detection of a variety of viruses. It has the advantage of being able to detect prion proteins where there is no nucleic acid present. In addition, it can detect viral proteins not associated with nucleic acids. This technique has been reported for ultrasensitive detection of a variety of infectious agents such as *Streptococcus*, HIV, and rotavirus, among others. In the case of rotavirus, it has been reported to detect as few as 100 viral particles/ml (versus 100,000 particles detected by ELISA). For detection of p24 HIV antigen, IPCR is a very sensitive test for determination of HIV type 1 viral load for p24 antigen. Although IPCR is a powerful technique, there can be technical issues when combining nucleic acids to proteins, and there can be problems with high assay backgrounds. An alternative approach which uses an indirect double-stranded DNA substrate for alkaline phosphatase has also been published (4). Overall, these highly sensitive methodologies represent the wave of the future, and there will be an increasing number of applications in infectious disease testing.

Rapid Immunoassays

The development of a multitude of rapid immunoassays has revolutionized diagnostic testing, for many tests that were previously available only in specialized or reference laboratories are now easily performed and can usually be completed in less than 30 min (10, 17, 29, 37, 38). There are a variety of formats utilized for these assays which can detect both antigens and antibodies along with products of nucleic acid amplification tests. One of the most popular formats is the lateral-flow immunoassay or immunochromatography. This has the advantage of being a one-step assay. One common format uses a chromatographic pad with three zones: sample application area, conjugate pad, and capture line (Fig. 7). The conjugate pad can use a variety of types of conjugates to generate a signal including colloidal gold, dye, or latex beads. The sample is applied to the sample pad and flows laterally by capillary action. Upon reaching the conjugate pad, if the analyte is present, it binds to the conjugate, forming an immune complex. The complex then continues to flow laterally along the pad by capillary action and is captured by the second antibody or antigen impregnated in the capture line. The presence of a colored line is a positive reaction. There is a positive control line also included in the test to make sure that the test was properly performed. There are variations to this assay format with systems which require no separate venipuncture, combining collection of fingerstick samples with testing in a one-step lateral-flow assay. Another frequently used type of rapid test is the dot blot immunoassay, which has been previously discussed. These rapid assay formats have been especially useful for HIV testing and have been used extensively in testing for HIV in underdeveloped countries. Overall, rapid assays are simple and easy to perform, can be used in field conditions, and can be performed by individuals with little training. While many are not as sensitive as conventional EIAs, there are reports of some with sensitivities approaching the traditional assays (10). Problems with rapid assays include the facts that they cannot be automated, that interpretation can be subjective, and that performance by individuals with no formal laboratory training can result in erroneous results. However, considering their overall advantages and low cost, their use will continue and be expanded as more analytes are adapted to this type of testing.

Automated Technologies

With the expansion of EIAs available, the immunoassay market of automated analyzers and the repertoire of tests available have exploded. Recently, 36 immunoassay analyzers that can run a wide spectrum of tests important in infectious disease testing were profiled (14). The machines run the gamut of serological assays (both antigen and antibody determinations) for infectious disease including HIV infection, hepatitis (A, B, and C), *T. gondii* infection, cytomegalovirus infection, rubella, and *Chlamydia trachomatis* infection, among others. Many of the systems listed are walk-away machines, requiring only limited technologist input. There are also robotic systems available which are cost-effective for even moderate-size hospital laboratories. For detailed information about each analyzer, the complete table can be downloaded from the Internet (http://www.cap.org).

An exciting new area is the development of multiplex immunoassay systems (19, 23). These are laboratory instruments which combine several technologies and allow rapid and simultaneous tests of multiple analytes in a single sample. There are many different assay designs which combine an array of technologies including CL, FIA, flow cytometry, and molecular diagnostics (PCR and use of oligonucleotides and nanoparticles). As these assays provide rapid results and can be performed with very small sample sizes, they have wide applicability to epidemiological studies and vaccine trials. These assays are also especially suited to the assessment of multiple biological agents in a variety of samples.

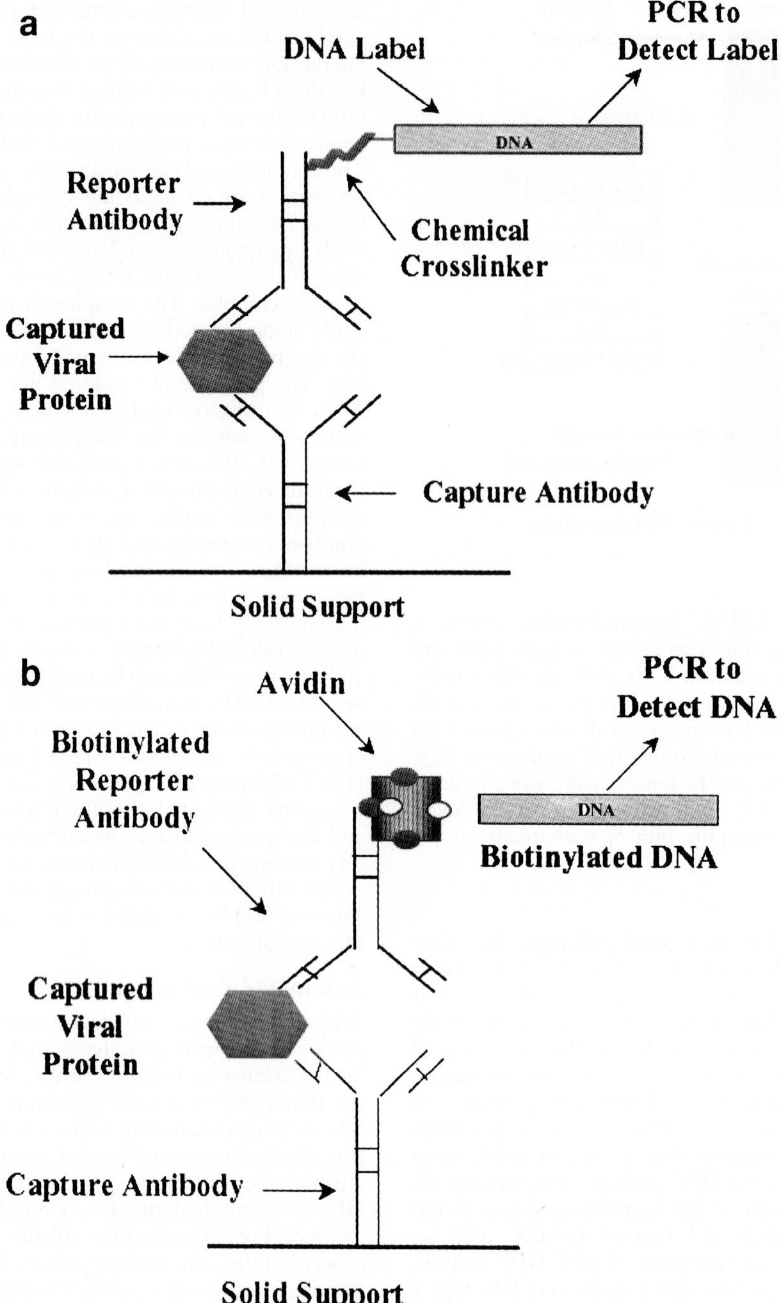

FIGURE 6 Principle of immuno-PCR. (a) DNA directly conjugated to reporter antibody; (b) DNA conjugated via an avidin-biotin reaction.

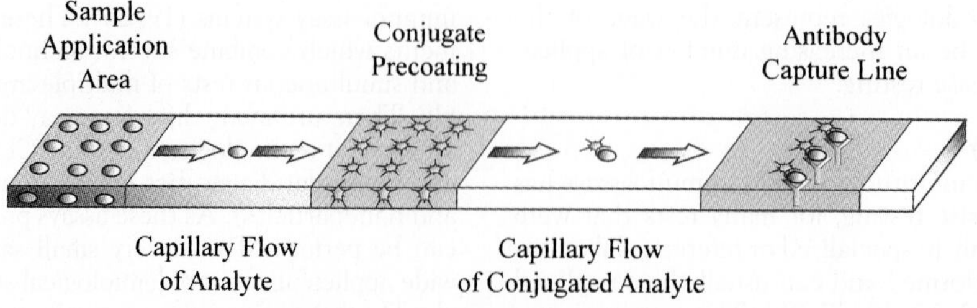

FIGURE 7 Lateral-flow immunoassay.

With this advent of extensive tests easily performed by automated systems, the potential for both improper test utilization and incorrect interpretation of results will increase. This results in even greater pressure on laboratorians and infectious disease specialists to provide information to both their colleagues and patients about the proper use and interpretation of laboratory tests for diagnosis of infectious disease agents.

Special recognition goes to Ryan Morrison, Ph.D., for his expertise and creativity in preparing the figures for this chapter.

REFERENCES

1. **Abbas, A. K., and A. H. Lichtman.** 2005. *Cellular and Molecular Immunology,* 5th ed. Elsevier Saunders, Philadelphia, Pa.
2. **Abbas, A. K., and A. H. Lichtman.** 2001. *Basic Immunology.* W. B. Saunders, Philadelphia, Pa.
3. **Adler, M., S. Schulz, R. Fischer, and C. M. Niemeyer.** 2005. Detection of rotavirus from stool samples using standardized immuno-PCR ("Imperacer") method with endpoint and real-time detection. *Biochem. Biophys. Res. Commun.* **12:**333.
4. **Banin, S., S. M. Wilson, and C. J. Stanley.** 2004. Demonstration of an alternative approach to immuno-PCR. *Clin. Chem.* **50:**1932–1934.
5. **Barletta, J. M., D. C. Edelman, and N. T. Constantine.** 2004. Lowering the detection limits of HIV-1 viral load using real-time immuno-PCR for HIV-1 p24 antigen. *Am. J. Clin. Pathol.* **122:**20–27.
6. **Bjerner, J., K. Nustaf, L. F. Norum, K. H. Olsen, and O. P. Bermer.** 2002. Immunometric assay interference. *Clin. Chem.* **48:**613–621.
7. **Carpenter, A. B.** 1997. Enzyme-linked immunoassays, p. 20–29. *In* N. R. Rose, E. Conway de Macario, J. D. Folds, H. C. Lane, and R. M. Nakamura (ed.), *Manual of Clinical Immunology,* 5th ed. ASM Press, Washington, D.C.
8. **Carpenter, A. B.** 2002. Antibody-based methods, p. 20–30. *In* N. R. Rose., E. Conway de Macario, J. D. Folds, H. C. Lane, and R. M. Nakamura (ed.), *Manual of Clinical Immunology,* 5th ed. ASM Press, Washington, D.C.
9. **Centers for Disease Control and Prevention.** 2005. Positive test results for acute hepatitis A virus infection among persons with no recent history of acute hepatitis—United States, 2002–2004. *Morb. Mortal. Wkly. Rep.* **54:**453–456.
10. **Constantine, N. T., and H. Zink.** 2005. HIV testing technologies after two decades of evolution. *Indian J. Med. Res.* **121:**519–538.
11. **Demers, L. M., and J. J. Miller.** 2003. Immunoassay testing: interferences, technology and future direction. [CD-ROM.] AACC Press, Washington, D.C.
12. **Deodhar, L., A. Gogate, R. C. Padhi, and C. R. Desai.** 1998. Standardization of a dot blot immunoassay for antigen detection in cases of pulmonary tuberculosis and its evaluation with respect to the conventional techniques. *Indian J. Med. Res.* **108:**75–79.
13. **Ezan, E., and J. Grassi.** 2000. Optimization, p. 187–210. *In* J. P. Gosling (ed.), *Immunoassays. Practical Approach.* Oxford University Press, Oxford, United Kingdom.
14. **Ford, A.** 2005. Immunoassay market overflowing with change. *CAP Today* **19:**18–56.
15. **Galanti, L. M., J. Dell'Omo, B. Wanet, J. L. Guarin, J. Jamart, M. G. Garrino, P. L. Masson, and C. L. Cambiaso.** 1997. Particle counting assay for anti-toxoplasma IgG antibodies. Comparison with four automated commercial enzyme-linked immunoassays. *J. Immunol. Methods* **207:**195–201.
16. **Galanti, L. M., C. L. Cambiaso, C. J. Cornu, M. E. Lamy, and P. L. Masson.** 1987. Immunoassay of hepatitis B surface antigen by particle counting after pepsin digestion. *J. Virol. Methods* **18:**215–223.
17. **Garcia-de-Lomas, J., and D. Navarro.** 1997. New directions in diagnostics. *Pediatr. Infect. Dis. J.* **16:**S43–S48.
18. **Gosling, J. P.** 2000. Analysis by specific binding, p. 1–18. *In* J. P. Gosling (ed.), *Immunoassays. Practical Approach.* Oxford University Press, Oxford, United Kingdom.
19. **Hindson, B. J., M. T. McBride, A. J. Makarewicz, B. D. Henderer, U. Setlur, S. M. Smith, D. M. Gutierrez, T. R. Metz, S. L. Nasarabadi, K. S. Venkateswaran, S. W. Farrow, B. W. Colston, Jr., and J. M. Dzenitis.** 2005. Autonomous detection of aerosolized biological agents by multiplexed immunoassay with polymerase chain reaction confirmation. *Anal. Chem.* **77:**284–289.
20. **Jolley, M. E., and M. S. Nasir.** 2003. The use of fluorescence polarization assays for the detection of infectious diseases. *Comb. Chem. High Throughput Screen.* **6:**235–244.
21. **Kasahara, Y.** 1997. Agglutination immunoassays, p. 7–12. *In* N. R. Rose, E. Conway de Macario, J. D. Folds, H. C. Lane, and R. M. Nakamura (ed.), *Manual of Clinical Immunology,* 5th ed. ASM Press, Washington, D.C.
22. **Kemeny, D. M., and S. J. Challacombe.** 1988. *ELISA and Other Solid Phase Immunoassays. Theoretical and Practical Aspects.* John Wiley & Sons, Chichester, United Kingdom.
23. **Kim, K. S., and J. K. Park.** 2005. Magnetic force-based multiplexed immunoassay using superparamagnetic nanoparticles in microfluidic channel. *Lab Chip* **5:**657–664.
24. **Kricka, L. J.** 2006. Principles of immunochemical techniques, p. 219–244. *In* C. A. Burtis, E. R. Ashwood, and D. E. Bruns (ed.), *Tietz Textbook of Clinical Chemistry and Molecular Diagnostics,* 4th ed. Elsevier Saunders, St. Louis, Mo.
25. **Kricka, L. J.** 1999. Human anti-animal antibody interferences in immunological assays. *Clin. Chem.* **45:**942–956.
26. **Kudo, T., A. Kido, Y. Nishiyama, H. Koganeya, M. Nabeshima, Y. Iinuma, and S. Ichiyama.** 2004. Whole-blood counting immunoassay as a short-turnaround detection of hepatitis B surface antigen, anti-hepatitis C virus antibodies and anti-*Treponema pallidum* antibodies. *J. Clin. Microbiol.* **42:**4250–4252.
27. **Liang, H., S. E. Cordova, T. L. Kieft, and S. Rogelj.** 2003. A highly sensitive immuno-PCR assay for detecting Group A Streptococcus. *J. Immunol. Methods* **279:**101–110.
28. **Liesenfeld, Q., J. G. Montoya, S. Kinney, C. Press, and J. S. Remington.** 2001. Effect of testing for IgG avidity in the diagnosis of *Toxoplasma gondii* infection in pregnant women: experience in a US reference laboratory. *J. Infect. Dis.* **183:**1248–1253.
29. **Lowell, C.** 2001. Clinical laboratory methods for detection of antigens and antibodies, p. 215–233. *In* T. G. Parslow, D. P. Stites, A. I. Terr, and J. B. Imboden (ed.), *Medical Immunology,* 10th ed. Lange Medical Books/McGraw-Hill, New York, N.Y.
30. **Mahony, J. B., and M. A. Chernesky.** 2000. Immunoassays for the diagnosis of infectious diseases, p. 202–214. In P. R. Murray, E. J. Baron, M. A. Pfaller, F. C. Tenover, and R. H. Yolken (ed.), *Manual of Clinical Microbiology,* 7th ed. ASM Press, Washington, D.C.
31. **Marks, V.** 2002. False-positive immunoassay results: a multicenter survey of erroneous immunoassay results from assays of 74 analytes in 10 donors from 66 laboratories in seven countries. *Clin. Chem.* **48:**2008–2016.
32. **Miller, J. J., and S. S. Levinson.** 1996. Interferences in immunoassays, p. 165–190. *In* E. P. Diamandis and T. K. Christopoulous (ed.), *Immunoassay.* Academic Press, San Diego, Calif.
33. **Montoya, J., O. Liesenfeld, S. Kinney, C. Press, and J. S. Remington.** 2002. VIDAS test for avidity of *Toxoplasma*-specific immunoglobulin. Confirmatory testing of pregnant women. *J. Clin. Microbiol.* **40:**2504–2508.

34. **Nakamura, R. M., E. S. Tucker III, and I. H. Carlson.** 1991. Immunoassays in the clinical laboratory, p. 848–884. *In* John Bernard Henry (ed.), *Diagnosis and Management by Laboratory Methods*, 18th ed. W. B. Saunders, Philadelphia, Pa.

35. **Nara, P. L., and G. Lin.** 2005. HIV-1: the confounding variables of virus neutralization. *Curr. Drug Targets Infect. Disord.* **5:**157–170.

36. **Niemeyer, C. M., M. Adler, and R. Wacker.** 2005. Immuno-PCR: high sensitivity detection of proteins by nucleic acid amplification. *Trends Biotechnol.* **23:**208–216.

37. **Percival, D. A.** 1996. The measurement of hormones and bacterial antigens using rapid particle-based immunoassays. *Pure & Appl. Chem.* **68:**1893–1895.

38. **Pezzlo, M.** 1986. Role of screening tests in rapid testing. *Diagn. Microbiol. Infect. Dis.* **4:**121S–134S.

39. **Prince, H. E., and A. L. Leber.** 2002. Validation of an in-house assay for cytomegalovirus immunoglobulin G (CMV IgG) avidity and relationship of avidity to CMV IgM levels. *Clin. Diagn. Lab. Immunol.* **9:**824–827.

40. **Reina, J., M. Munar, and I. Blanco.** 1996. Evaluation of a direct immunofluorescence assay dot-blot enzyme immunoassay, and shell vial culture in the diagnosis of lower respiratory infections caused by influenza A virus. *Diagn. Microbiol. Infect. Dis.* **25:**143–145.

41. **Rodgers Channing, R. P.** 1994. Clinical laboratory methods for detection of antigens and antibodies, p. 151–194. *In* D. A. Stites, A. I. Terr, and T. G. Parslow (ed.), *Basic and Clinical Immunology*, 8th ed. Appleton and Lange, Norwalk, Conn.

42. **Ryall, R. G., C. J. Story, and D. R. Turner.** 1982. Reappraisal of the causes of the "hook effect" in two site immunoradiometric assays. *Anal. Biochem.* **127:**308–315.

43. **Shultz, E. K., C. Aliferis, and D. Aronsky.** 2006. Clinical evaluation of methods, p. 409–424. *In* C. A. Burtis, E. R. Ashwood, and D. E. Bruns (ed.), *Tietz Textbook of Clinical Chemistry and Molecular Diagnostics,* 4th ed. Elsevier Saunders, St. Louis, Mo.

44. **Tencza, S. B., K. R Islam, V. Kalia, M. S. Nasir, E. Jolley, and R. C. Montelaro.** 2000. Development of a fluorescence polarization-based diagnostic assay for equine infectious anemia virus. *J. Clin. Microbiol.* **38:**1854–1859.

45. **Thacker, W. L., and D. F. Talkington.** 2000. Analysis of complement fixation and commercial enzyme immunoassays for detection of antibodies to mycoplasma pneumoniae in human serum. *Clin. Diagn. Lab. Immunol.* **7:**778–780.

46. **Thomson, R. B., Jr., and H. Bertram.** 2001. Laboratory diagnosis of central nervous system infections. *Infect. Dis. Clin. N. Am.* **15:**1047–1071.

47. **Tijssen, P.** 1985. *Practice and Theory of Enzyme Immunoassays.* Elsevier Science Publishers, Amsterdam, The Netherlands.

48. **Wu, J. T.** 2000. *Quantitative Immunoassay; a Practical Guide for Assay Establishment, Troubleshooting and Clinical Application.* AACC Press, Washington, D.C.

BACTERIOLOGY

VOLUME EDITOR
ELLEN JO BARON

SECTION EDITORS
J. STEPHEN DUMLER, GUIDO FUNKE,
J. MICHAEL JANDA, IRVING NACHAMKIN,
AND JAMES VERSALOVIC

GENERAL

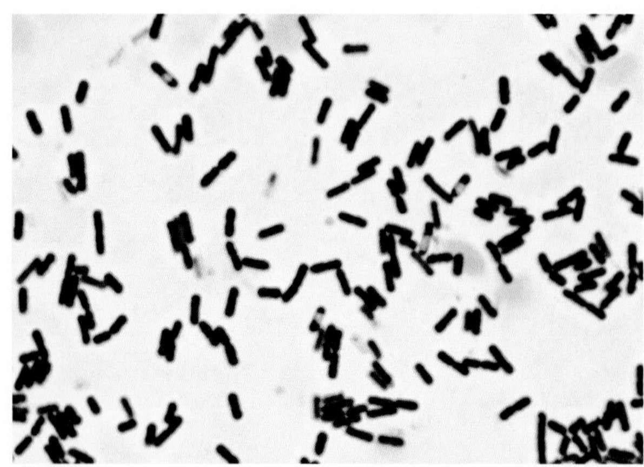

Bacillus cereus, Gram stain (D. Fedorko, NIH).

GRAM-POSITIVE COCCI

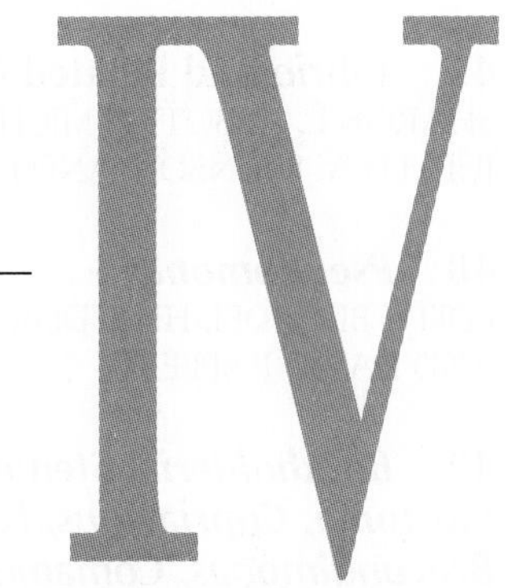

(continued)

GENERAL

Taxonomy and Classification of Bacteria

PETER A. R. VANDAMME

19

Taxonomy is written by taxonomists for taxonomists; in this form the subject is so dull that few, if any, non-taxonomists are tempted to read it and presumably even fewer try their hand at it. It is the most subjective branch of any biological discipline, and in many ways is more of an art than a science.

With these words, S. T. Cowan introduced a sparkling essay on the sense and nonsense in bacterial taxonomy in 1971 (18). His contributions to the practice of bacterial taxonomy, written in the 1960s and 1970s (15–18), should be read by everyone interested in this field. Taxonomy is generally considered a synonym of systematics and is traditionally divided into classification (the orderly arrangement of organisms into taxonomic groups on the basis of similarity), nomenclature (the labeling of the units), and identification (the process of determining whether an unknown belongs to one of the units defined) (16). During the past decade, it became generally accepted that bacterial classification should reflect as much as possible the natural relationships between bacteria, which are considered the phylogenetic relationships as encoded in highly conserved macromolecules such as 16S or 23S rRNA genes (68, 132). Nowadays, whole-genome comparisons offer new and exciting opportunities for the study of these natural relationships.

It is nevertheless true that every classification is artificial and that boundaries are made by humans. However, classification serves very practical purposes, i.e., the recognition of organisms that were encountered previously and the categorization of new ones into a logical and tractable system. In this era of whole-genome sequence analysis, it is more than ever obvious that the genomes of microbes undergo change, sometimes considerably. Although the extent of lateral gene transfer is controversial, it does not alter our need to identify organisms, particularly in the context of epidemiological studies and surveillance, as identification bears a tremendous amount of accompanying information. Science indeed has a way of making itself useful, and the useful application of classification is identification (15).

CLASSIFICATION OF BACTERIA

The process of species delineation in bacterial systematics underwent drastic modifications as the species concept evolved in parallel with technical progress. Early classification systems used mainly morphological and biochemical criteria to delineate the species of bacteria. This type of classification was monothetic, as it was based on a unique set of characteristics necessary and sufficient to delineate groups. This early classification concept was replaced by theories of so-called natural concepts, which were the phenetic and phylogenetic classifications (36). In the former, relationships between bacteria were based on the overall similarity of both phenotypic and genotypic characteristics. Phenetic classifications demonstrate the relationships between organisms as they exist, without reference to ancestry or evolution. In phylogenetic classifications, relationships are described by ancestry, not according to their present properties.

Special-purpose and general-purpose classification systems are the main categories of classification systems. Special-purpose classification systems are objectively determined and do not fit a preconceived idea. For instance, the separation between the very closely related species *Escherichia coli* and *Shigella dysenteriae* or between *Bordetella pertussis* and *Bordetella bronchiseptica* does not conform to the general ideas of present-day species delineation (see below) but fits primarily a practical and historical purpose (36). Yet, nowadays, most taxonomists favor a general-purpose classification system that is stable, objective, and predictive and that can be applied to all bacteria. The classifications obtained with a general-purpose classification system do not fit a single purpose but attempt to reflect the natural diversity among bacteria. The best way to generate such general-purpose classifications is by combining the strengths of both phenetic and phylogenetic studies, a practice now often referred to as polyphasic taxonomy (118).

Criteria for Species Delineation

The criteria used to delineate species have developed in parallel with technology. The early classifications were based on morphology and biochemical data. When evaluated by means of our present views, many of these early phenotype-based classifications generated extremely heterogeneous assemblages of bacteria. Individual species were characterized by a common set of phenotypic characters and differed from other species in one or a few characters which were considered important. The introduction of computer technology allowed comparison of large sets of characteristics for large numbers of strains, forming the basis for phenetic taxonomy (96, 98). Such numerical analyses of phenotypic characters yielded superior classifications in terms of objectivity and stability. Gradually, chemotaxonomic and genotypic methods were introduced into classification systems. Numerous different chemical compounds were extracted from bacterial cells, and their suitability for use in the classification of bacteria and the definition of species has been analyzed.

In 1987, the Ad Hoc Committee on Reconciliation of Approaches to Bacterial Systematics (125) stated that taxonomy should be determined phylogenetically and that the complete genome sequence should therefore be the standard for species delineation. In present-day practice, whole-genome DNA-DNA hybridization analysis approaches the sequence standard and represents the best applicable procedure. A bacterial species was therefore defined as a group of strains, including the type strain, that share 70% or greater DNA-DNA relatedness with a ΔT_m of 5°C or less (T_m is the melting temperature of the hybrid, as determined by stepwise denaturation; ΔT_m is the difference in T_m [in degrees Celsius] between the homologous hybrid and the heterologous hybrid formed under standard conditions [135]). This species definition was based on a large amount of empirical data including both DNA-DNA hybridization data and other characteristics. The designated type strain of a species serves as the name bearer of the species and as the reference specimen (104). It was also recommended that phenotypic and chemotaxonomic features should agree with this definition. Preferentially, several simple and straightforward tests should endorse the species delineation based on DNA-DNA hybridization values. Groups of strains which were delineated by means of DNA-DNA hybridization studies as distinct species but which could not be distinguished by phenotypic characteristics should not be named. The term "genomovar" was subsequently introduced for such phenotypically similar genomic species (110); however, this term may be somewhat misleading, as these taxa are given an infraspecific rank, whereas by definition they are to be considered species that cannot be reliably differentiated by phenotypic tests.

The level of DNA-DNA hybridization thus plays a key role in our present species concept as defined by Wayne et al. (125). Although that seems to suggest that the species definition has become less vague, the practice of DNA-DNA hybridization is very complex (see below).

The Polyphasic Species Concept

A wide variety of cellular components have been used to study relationships between bacteria and to design classifications. The information present at the DNA level has been analyzed by estimations of the DNA base composition and the genome size, whole-genome DNA-DNA hybridization, restriction enzyme analysis, and, increasingly more, by direct sequence analysis of various genes. rRNA fractions have been studied intensively, particularly because they serve as phylogenetic markers (68). Various chemical compounds including fatty acids, mycolic acids, polar lipids, polysaccharides, sugars, polyamines, and respiratory quinones, as well as, again, a tremendous number of expressed features (data derived from, e.g., morphologic, serologic, and enzymologic studies), were all used to characterize bacteria. Several of these approaches have been applied to taxonomic analyses of virtually all bacteria. Others, such as amino acid sequencing, were performed with a limited number of organisms because they are laborious, time-consuming, or technically demanding or because they were relevant only for a particular group.

The term "polyphasic taxonomy" was coined by Colwell (12) in 1970 and described the integration of all available genotypic, phenotypic, and phylogenetic information into a consensus type of general-purpose classification. It departs from the assumption that the overall biological diversity cannot be encoded in a single molecule and that the variability of characters is group dependent. Therefore, it integrates several generally accepted ideas for the classification and reclassification of bacteria. Polyphasic taxonomy is phylogeny based and uses sequence analysis and signature features of rRNA for the deduction of a phylogenetic framework for the classification of bacteria (43, 118, 121). Several other macromolecules such as the beta subunit of ATPase, elongation factor Tu, chaperonin, various ribosomal proteins, RNA polymerases, and tRNAs (43, 68) have similar potential. The next step in the process of classification is the delineation of individual species—and other taxa—within these phylogenetic branches. Despite its drawbacks, DNA-DNA hybridization forms the cornerstone of species delineation. However, the threshold value for species delineation should be allowed considerable variation. This polyphasic approach is pragmatic; for instance, *B. pertussis*, *Bordetella parapertussis*, and *B. bronchiseptica*, which share DNA-DNA hybridization levels of over 80%, are considered three distinct species because they differ in many phenotypic and chemotaxonomic aspects (114). In other genera which are phenotypically more homogeneous, such as *Acidovorax* (131), species are defined as groups of strains that have DNA-DNA hybridization levels of at least 40%. It is essential that the boundaries of species demarcation be flexible in order to achieve a classification scheme that facilitates identification.

The application of numerous other types of analyses of genotypic, chemotaxonomic, and phenotypic characteristics of bacteria to the delineation of bacteria at various hierarchical levels represents the third component of polyphasic taxonomy (118). The goal is to collect as much information as possible and to evaluate all results in relation to each other in order to draw useful conclusions. An additional advantage is that, once the taxonomic resolution of these approaches has been established for a particular group of bacteria through the analysis of a set of taxonomically well-characterized strains, they may be used as alternative tools to classify new isolates at different taxonomic levels. A typical example is the application of one-dimensional whole-cell protein electrophoresis to replace DNA-DNA hybridization experiments for identification to the species level of *Helicobacter* species (117). It should be noted that the resolution of these alternative methods is often group dependent. For instance, cellular fatty acid analysis is useful for the accurate identification of strains of many bacterial species to the species level. In certain bacterial groups, however, the cellular fatty acid profile may be indicative of the genus or a group of phylogenetically related genera but not of a particular species within one of these genera (118). Within the group of the gram-negative nonfermenting bacteria, this is nicely illustrated by the characteristic fatty acid profiles of members of the genera *Chryseobacterium*, *Empedobacter*, *Ornithobacterium*, and *Riemerella* (the last two genera are of veterinary interest), which are characterized by extremely high percentages (80 to 90% of the total fatty acid content) of saturated branched-chain fatty acids in the *iso* and *anteiso* configurations (119, 120).

The contours of a polyphasic bacterial species are obviously less clear than the ones defined by Wayne et al.

(125), and this lack of a rigid definition has been contested as it allows too many interpretations (135). Polyphasic classification is empirical and contains elements from both phenetic and phylogenetic classifications. There are no strict rules or guidelines, and the approach integrates any significant information on the organisms, resulting in a consensus type of classification. Its main weakness is indeed that it relies on common sense to draw its conclusions. The bacterial species appears as a group of isolates in which a steady generation of genetic diversity resulted in clones characterized by a certain degree of phenotypic consistency, by a significant degree of DNA-DNA hybridization, and by a high level of 16S rRNA sequence similarity (118).

Obviously, the species is the most important and, at the same time, the central element of bacterial taxonomy. There are at present no rules for the delineation of higher hierarchical ranks such as genus, family, and order. Although there is an expectation that at the generic level taxa should be supported by phenotypic descriptions (76), in practice higher ranks are mostly delineated on the basis of 16S rRNA sequence comparison and stability analyses of the clusters that are obtained. Undoubtedly, the latter has weakened the emphasis on phenotypic descriptions of taxa (135). In polyphasic taxonomy, attempts are made to endorse these phylogeny-driven demarcations by other data. An example is the subdivision of the former genus *Campylobacter* into the revised genus *Campylobacter* and the novel genera *Arcobacter* and *Helicobacter* (38, 116). Although this subdivision was mainly phylogeny based, it was supported by differences in respiratory quinone components and ultrastructural properties.

A New Species Concept?

In 2002, a new Ad Hoc Committee for the reevaluation of the species definition in bacteriology made various recommendations regarding the species definition in light of developments in methodologies available to systematists (99). As stated by the Ad Hoc Committee, the introduction of innovative methods is providing new opportunities for prokaryotic systematics. One of the particularly interesting developments includes the analysis of complete genome sequences. There is a growing interest in using these genome sequence data to assess evolutionary relationships among prokaryotic species. It has become clear that, in addition to nucleotide substitutions, other genetic forces such as gene loss, gene duplication, horizontal (or lateral) gene transfer, and chromosomal rearrangements shape the genome and that considerable fractions of the genome of any particular strain may be unique to that strain (9, 59). With an increasing number of species for which multiple whole-genome sequences are available, a range of novel approaches for assessing taxonomic relationships within and between closely related species become available. These novel approaches include analysis of gene content and gene order, comparative sequence analysis of conserved and other macromolecules or of complete genomes, presence-absence analyses, nucleotide signature composition analyses, and even metabolic pathway reaction content analyses (reviewed in reference 9). Despite the documented enormous strain-to-strain variation in genome content, these novel taxonomic analytical tools generally substantiate that bacterial species delineated by DNA-DNA hybridization experiments and ordered in a phylogenetic backbone through comparative 16S rRNA sequence analysis represent coherent biological entities, although, in terms of population genetics, they still encompass considerable ecological and genetic heterogeneity (10).

Studies by Konstantinidis and Tiedje (59) revealed the average nucleotide identity of the shared genes between two strains to be a robust means to compare genetic relatedness among strains and that average nucleotide identity values of approximately 94% corresponded to the traditional 70% DNA-DNA reassociation standard of the current species definition. At the 94% average nucleotide identity cutoff, current species included only moderately homogeneous strains, apparently as a result of the strains having evolved in different ecological settings. A large fraction of the differences in gene content within species was associated with bacteriophage and transposase elements, revealing an important role of these elements during bacterial speciation. These findings were consistent with a definition for species that would include a more homogeneous set of strains than that provided by the current definition and one that considers the ecology of the strains in addition to their evolutionary distance (10).

Multilocus sequence analysis (MLSA) is another novel approach that holds great promise. In contrast to multilocus sequence typing, a specific tool designed for molecular epidemiology and for defining strains within named species, whereby similarities and differences are usually measured as differences in allelic profiles, MLSA aims to amplify and sequence gene fragments of strains representing different species within and between genera. Gene sequences are subsequently studied by traditional software used for phylogenetic analyses. Examples of such studies have recently been published for two groups of *Burkholderia* species, i.e., *Burkholderia mallei*, *Burkholderia pseudomallei*, and *Burkholderia thailandensis* (34) and the *Burkholderia cepacia* complex (2), and for *Yersinia* species (61). Especially for depicting relationships within and between closely related species, this approach promises a resolution superior to the traditional 16S rRNA gene sequence analysis. The deduced phylogenetic trees not only provide a phylogenetic backbone but also reveal intraspecies relationships at a level where comparative 16S rRNA sequence analysis is no longer discriminatory. It is for instance noteworthy that the DNA-DNA hybridization results which demonstrated that *Yersinia pestis* and *Yersinia pseudotuberculosis* on the one hand and *B. mallei* and *B. pseudomallei* on the other hand represented a single species each were mirrored in the MLSA trees where *Y. pestis* clusters among *Y. pseudotuberculosis* strains and *B. mallei* clusters among *B. pseudomallei* strains. Two studies of complete genomes have suggested a universal set of protein-coding genes that may be useful for such an MLSA-based approach to microbial taxonomy (91, 138).

Major Groups of Bacteria

The tree of life based on comparative small subunit rRNA studies comprises three lines of descent that are nowadays referred to as the domains *Bacteria*, *Archaea*, and *Eucarya* (132). The *Bacteria* have been grouped into 23 phyla, which are further subdivided into 28 classes (62). Three phyla, the *Proteobacteria*, the *Firmicutes* (gram-positive organisms with low G+C contents, including *Bacillus*, *Clostridium*, *Staphylococcus*, *Mycoplasma*, and the classical lactic acid bacteria such as *Enterococcus*, *Streptococcus*, and *Lactobacillus*), and the *Actinobacteria* (gram-positive organisms with high G+C contents, including *Bifidobacterium*, *Mycobacterium*, and *Corynebacterium*), comprise the large majority of the clinically relevant species. The *Bacteroidetes* (*Bacteroides*, flavobacteria, and sphingobacteria), the *Spirochaetes* (spirochetes and leptospiras), and the *Chlamydiae* (chlamydias) represent some of the other phyla. A detailed overview is given by Krieg and Garrity (62) and Ludwig and Klenk (66) in their introductory chapters to the second edition of *Bergey's Manual of Systematic Bacteriology*. That edition is structured in an order based on the topology of the 16S rRNA phylogenetic tree.

The largest phylum by far is the *Proteobacteria*, which contains five main clusters (classes) of genera that are referred to with the Greek letters alpha, beta, gamma, delta, and epsilon (102). The *Proteobacteria* comprise the majority of the known gram-negative bacteria of medical, industrial, and agricultural significance. This phylum includes *Brucella*, *Ehrlichia*, and *Rickettsia* (*Alphaproteobacteria*); *Burkholderia*, *Bordetella*, and *Neisseria* (*Betaproteobacteria*); *Aeromonas*, *Legionella*, and *Vibrio* and the family *Enterobacteriaceae* (*Gammaproteobacteria*); and *Campylobacter* and *Helicobacter* (*Epsilonproteobacteria*). The *Deltaproteobacteria* comprise a variety of mainly sulfate-reducing bacteria that have little clinical relevance.

Unculturable Bacteria

The classification and nomenclature of unculturable bacteria that are only minimally characterized by morphological characteristics or by differences in a molecular sequence (77) are outstanding challenges in bacterial classification. The members of the International Committee on Systematic Bacteriology have agreed to recognize a category that formally classifies incompletely described prokaryotes (78). This action was useful and timely because of the increasing involvement of sequencing technology in the characterization of prokaryotes that are difficult to cultivate. *Candidatus* is considered a taxonomic status for uncultured "candidate" species for which relatedness has been determined (for instance, for which phylogenetic relatedness has been determined by amplification and sequence analysis of prokaryotic RNA genes by use of universal prokaryotic primers) and authenticity has been verified by in situ probing or a similar technique for cell identification. In addition, it is also mandatory that information concerning phenotypic, metabolic, or physiological features be made available. The latter data may serve as a starting point for further investigation and eventual description and naming. A detailed list of items for inclusion in the codified record of a *Candidatus* taxon is provided elsewhere (78). With the increasing application of molecular methods to the assessment of the diversity of prokaryotic populations in nature and to the study of complex symbioses, it was anticipated that numerous *Candidatus* organisms would be recorded (78). There are several caveats. Information derived from 16S rRNA gene sequence analysis may not be sufficient to ensure that the uncultured organism represents a novel species (see below). Also, 16S rRNA gene sequences are not available for all known bacteria for comparison. Alternatively, morphological characteristics, for example, may not be sufficiently reliable to conclude that uncultured cells represent a novel organism (118).

CLASSIFICATION METHODS

In principle, all genotypic, phenotypic, and phylogenetic information can be used to classify bacteria. Genotypic information is derived from the nucleic acids (DNA and RNA) present in the cell, whereas phenotypic information is derived from proteins and their functions, different chemotaxonomic markers, and a wide range of other expressed features.

When working one's way through lists of methods, it is of primary interest to understand at which level these methods carry information and to realize their technical complexity, i.e., the amount of time and work required to analyze a certain number of isolates. The list of methods given below is not meant to be complete or to describe all of their aspects. It comprises the major categories of taxonomic techniques required to study bacteria at different taxonomic levels and roughly describes general concepts and applications of those techniques, as well as some other considerations. Detailed descriptions of such methods can be found in handbooks such as those by Goodfellow and O'Donnell (36) or Priest and Austin (89).

Genotypic Methods

DNA-DNA Hybridization Studies

At present, DNA-DNA hybridization is acknowledged as the reference method to establish relationships within and between species. Different DNA-DNA hybridization procedures have been described: the hydroxyapatite method (4), the optical renaturation method (20), and the S1 nuclease method (19, 41) have mostly been used. These classical techniques, however, need considerable amounts of DNA and are time-consuming. New quick methods that consume less DNA have been described (6, 24, 51) and have partially replaced the classical methodologies.

Many DNA-DNA hybridization protocols have been described, and it is often not clear if hybridizations were performed under optimal, stringent, or suboptimal conditions. The stringency of the reaction is determined by the salt and formamide concentration and by the temperature and the mol percent G+C contents of the DNAs used. DNA-DNA hybridizations are often performed under standard conditions that are not necessarily optimal or stringent for all bacterial DNAs. As a standard, optimal conditions for hybridizations should be preferred because the optimal temperature curve for hybridization is rather broad (about 5°C) (118).

Obviously, quantitative comparisons of DNA hybridization values generated with different techniques should be handled with caution. When different methodologies are used, it is safer to distinguish categories of DNA-DNA relatedness, such as "high DNA-DNA relatedness" (denoting relationships between strains of a single species), "low but significant DNA-DNA relatedness" (comprising the significant hybridization levels below the cutoff for a separate species; the depth of this range depends primarily on the technique used), and finally, "non-significant DNA-DNA relatedness" (denoting that the degree of DNA hybridization is too low to be measured by the method used).

rRNA Similarity Studies

It is now generally accepted that rRNA is the best target for studying phylogenetic relationships because it is present in all bacteria, it is functionally constant, and it is composed of highly conserved as well as more variable domains (43, 62, 66, 93, 100, 132). The components of the ribosome (rRNA and ribosomal proteins) have been the subjects of phylogenetic studies for several decades. The gradual development of molecular techniques enabled microbiologists to focus on the comparative study of the rRNA molecules, and direct sequencing of parts of, or nearly entire, 16S or 23S rRNA molecules by the PCR technique with a selection of appropriate primers has become common practice. These sequences provide a phylogenetic framework that serves as the backbone for modern microbial taxonomy (62, 66). The larger the conserved elements examined, the more information they bear and the more reliable the conclusions become. International databases comprising published and unpublished partial or complete sequences have been constructed (82, 121). The presence of universal sequence motifs in the bacterial rRNA genes allowed taxonomists to classify unculturable organisms and to perform phylogenetic identifications and in situ detection of individual cells without cultivation (1).

More recently, however, it has been found that rRNA sequence analysis is no longer exclusively used to determine relationships between genera, families, and other higher ranks but often replaces DNA-DNA hybridization studies for the delineation of species in taxonomic practice. In many cases, such application of rRNA similarity data is not appropriate. In 1992, Fox et al. (28) reported that 16S rRNA sequence identity is not always sufficient to guarantee species identity. Indeed, three phenotypically similar *Bacillus* strains exhibited more than 99.5% rRNA sequence similarity, while DNA-DNA hybridization experiments indicated that they belonged to two distinct species. Stackebrandt and Goebel (100) reported on the place for 16S rRNA gene sequence analysis and DNA-DNA reassociation in the present species definition in bacteriology. Their extensive literature review revealed that organisms sharing more than 97% rRNA similarity may or may not belong to a single species and that the resolution of 16S rRNA sequence analysis for determination of the degree of relatedness between closely related organisms is generally low. There is obviously no threshold value of 16S rRNA similarity for species recognition (100). However, they reported that organisms with less than 97% 16S rRNA sequence similarity do not give a DNA-DNA reassociation level of more than 60%, no matter which DNA-DNA hybridization method is used. In fact, rRNA sequence analysis seemed to rightfully replace DNA-DNA hybridization studies as part of the description of new species, provided that the rRNA similarity level was below 97% and provided that rRNA sequence data for all relevant taxa were available for comparison. However, more recent studies extended the observations on intraspecies 16S rRNA divergence considerably, as differences in 16S rRNA gene sequence of up to 4.5% were reported among strains of several species belonging to the *Epsilonproteobacteria* (46, 117).

Clearly, one should be prudent in drawing conclusions based on analysis of a single sequence. In 1995, Clayton and colleagues (8) presented a detailed comparison of duplicate rRNA sequences present in the GenBank database with remarkable results. Unexpectedly high levels of intraspecies variation (within and between strains) of 16S rRNA sequences were found. The variability was thought to represent interoperon variation within a single strain, strain-to-strain variation within a species, misidentification of strains, sequencing error, or other laboratory errors. Critical selection and the use of sequences from databases are required. More recently, studies by Jaspers and Overmann (53) and Gonzales-Escalona et al. (35) provided new examples of diversity among 16S rRNA genes within single organisms and sequence identity in bacteria with highly divergent genomes and ecophysiologies. Alternatively, numerous other macromolecules have been examined for their potential as microbiological clocks. Among others, various ribosomal proteins (81), the beta subunit of ATPase (66, 67), elongation factor Tu (66, 67), chaperonin (123), RNA polymerases (58, 140), and manganese-dependent superoxide dismutase (29) were shown to be valuable molecular chronometers in bacterial systematics. These alternative macromolecules should be universally distributed among bacteria, they should not be transmitted horizontally, and their molecular evolution rate should be comparable to, or somewhat higher than, that of 16S rRNA, which would render them more suitable for differentiation of closely related organisms (for example, see reference 29).

Other Applications of rRNA in Taxonomy

The interesting taxonomic properties of rRNA or rRNA gene molecules have been exploited in several alternative ways (5, 40, 44, 48, 128). An rRNA operon typically consists of the following components (5′ to 3′): 16S, spacer, 23S, spacer, and 5S rRNA sequences. Amplification of part of this operon by means of PCR assays, followed by digestion of the amplicon by means of restriction enzymes and the electrophoretic separation of the resulting array of DNA fragments, is referred to as amplified rRNA restriction analysis or rRNA restriction fragment length polymorphism analysis (44). Depending on the target selected, the banding pattern is useful for species level discrimination (for target sequences that are highly conserved) or for strain typing (for target sequences that are variable). The technique has most of the advantages inherent in the rRNA approach; in addition, it is clearly less expensive and more rapid than direct sequence analysis and large numbers of strains can easily be examined. This not only renders the method a useful screening tool but also provides a better view on the intraspecies variability of the rRNA operon.

Another rRNA-based approach for the identification and classification of bacteria is ribotyping (3, 40). By this procedure, genomic DNA is digested with a restriction enzyme (or with a set of restriction enzymes). The digest is separated by electrophoresis, and the bands are transferred to a membrane and hybridized with a labeled rRNA probe. This probe may be based on 16S rRNA, 23S rRNA, or both, with or without the spacer region, or on a conserved fragment of one of the rRNA genes. Although designed and mostly used to determine interstrain relationships (40), a fully automated procedure for identification of bacteria to the species level is commercially available (RiboPrinter; Dupont Qualicon Inc., Wilmington, Del.).

Finally, terminal restriction fragment length polymorphism analysis of 16S rRNA genes has been used in several studies for the characterization of microbial diversity in natural specimens and for identification of the members therein (65, 90). The technique employs a PCR assay in which one of the two primers used is fluorescently labeled at the 5′ end and is used to amplify a selected region of bacterial genes encoding 16S rRNA from total community DNA. The PCR product is digested with restriction enzymes, and the fluorescently labeled terminal restriction fragment is precisely measured by using an automated DNA sequencer. Computer-simulated analysis of terminal restriction fragment length polymorphisms for 1,002 bacterial sequences showed that with proper selection of PCR primers and restriction enzymes, 686 sequences could be PCR amplified and classified into 233 unique terminal restriction fragment lengths or “ribotypes” (65).

Other Genotypic Methods for Bacterial Classification

A range of different genotypic techniques has been used to characterize bacteria at various taxonomic levels. The molar percentage of guanosine plus cytosine (the DNA base ratio or percent G+C value) is one of the classical genotypic characteristics and is part of the standard description of bacterial taxa. Generally, the range observed within a species should not be more than 3%, and within a genus it should not be more than 10% (101). It varies between 24 and 76% in the bacterial world.

During the past decade, a tremendous number of molecular diagnostic methods, most of which are PCR based, have been developed. Most of these generate arrays of DNA fragments that are separated and detected in various ways, and appropriate software has been developed for pattern recognition and analysis and for database construction.

One of these DNA fingerprinting methods, amplified-fragment length polymorphism (AFLP) analysis (136), was shown to be very useful for the classification of strains at the species and genus levels. The basic principle of AFLP is restriction fragment length polymorphism analysis, modified by using a PCR-mediated amplification to select particular DNA fragments from the pool of restriction fragments. AFLP analysis screens for AFLPs by selective amplification of restriction fragments. The restriction is performed with two restriction enzymes, which yield DNA fragments with two different types of sticky ends that are randomly combined. To these ends, short oligonucleotides (adapters) are ligated to form templates for the PCR. The selective amplification reaction is performed by using two different primers that contain the same sequence as the adapters but whose sequences are extended to include one or more selective bases next to the restriction site of the primer. Only those fragments that completely match the primer sequence are amplified. The amplification process results in an array of about 30 to 40 DNA fragments, some of which are group specific, while others are strain specific (52).

PCR-based typing methods that use random or repetitive elements as primers have been applied to strain characterization of a wide variety of bacteria (47, 70, 112, 127, 128). In several of these studies, species-specific DNA fragments or patterns have been generated (e.g., for species belonging to the genera *Campylobacter*, *Capnocytophaga*, *Enterococcus*, and *Naegleria* [21, 31]). These specific DNA fragments may be useful as probes to rapidly screen and identify other isolates. Although primarily applied for infraspecies strain comparisons, these techniques are useful in classification as well.

Phenotypic Methods

Phenotypic methods comprise all those that are not directed toward DNA or RNA and therefore also include the chemical or chemotaxonomic techniques. As the introduction of chemotaxonomy is generally considered one of the essential milestones in the development of modern bacterial classification, it is often treated as a separate unit in taxonomic reviews. The classical phenotypic tests traditionally constituted the basis for the formal description of bacterial species, subspecies, genera, and families. While genotypic data are used to allocate taxa on a phylogenetic tree and to draw the major borderlines in classification systems, phenotypic consistency is required to generate useful classification systems and may therefore influence the depth of a hierarchical line (118, 125). The paucity or variability of phenotypic characteristics for certain bacterial groups regularly causes problems in describing or differentiating taxa. For such bacteria, alternative chemotaxonomic or genotypic methods are often required to reliably characterize strains.

The classical phenotypic characteristics of bacteria comprise morphological, physiological, and biochemical features. Individually, many of these characteristics were shown to be poor parameters for genetic relatedness, yet as a whole, they provide descriptive information for the recognition of taxa. The morphology of a bacterium comprises both cellular (shape; the presence of an endospore, flagella, and inclusion bodies; and Gram staining characteristics) and colonial (color, dimensions, and form) characteristics. The physiological and biochemical features comprise data on growth at different temperatures; growth in the presence of different pH values, salt concentrations, or atmospheric conditions; and growth in the presence of various substances such as antimicrobial agents and data on the presence or activities of various enzymes, utilization of compounds, etc. Very often, highly standardized procedures are required to obtain reproducible results within and between laboratories (for examples, see references 83 and 84).

In taxonomic practice, phenotypic characterization became compromised and sometimes more of a burden than a useful taxonomic activity. Frequently, phenotypic data are compared with literature data, which were obtained using other conditions or methods. The need for continued phenotypic characterization at every taxonomic level not only to delineate taxa and appreciate their phenotypic coherence but also to evaluate their physiological and ecological functions cannot be denied. A minimal phenotypic description is not only the identity card of a taxon but also a key to its biology. Although accepted as necessary, differential phenotypic characters are often hard to find with a reasonable amount of effort and time.

Numerical Analysis

Phenotypic data were the first to be analyzed by means of computer-assisted numerical comparison. In the 1950s, numerical taxonomy arose in parallel with the development of computers (96, 98) and allowed comparison of large numbers of phenotypic traits for large numbers of strains. Data matrices showing the degree of similarity between each pair of strains and cluster analyses resulting in dendrograms revealed a general picture of the phenotypic consistency of a particular group of strains. As such large numbers of characteristics reflect a considerable amount of genotypic information, it soon became evident that numerical analysis of large numbers of phenotypic characteristics was indeed taxonomically relevant.

Semiautomated Systems

A large number of miniaturized semiautomated phenotypic test systems are commercially available and partially replace classical phenotypic analyses. These microtest galleries can be used for both classification and identification (see chapter 15). It should be noted that the outcomes of a particular test obtained with a commercial system and by a classical procedure may be different. This, however, may occur with two classical procedures of the same test as well.

Chemical Methods

The term "chemotaxonomy" refers to the application of analytical methods to the collection of information on various chemical constituents of the cell to classify bacteria. As for the other phenotypic and genotypic techniques, some of the chemotaxonomic methods have been widely applied on vast numbers of bacteria, whereas others were so specific that their application was restricted to particular taxa. Similarly, a high degree of automation was introduced with the development of novel technologies such as matrix-assisted laser desorption ionization time-of-flight mass spectrometry (MALDI-TOF [MS]) or Fourier transform infrared (FTIR) spectroscopy.

Apart from the chemical markers discussed in more detail below, a range of other chemical markers have been examined in bacterial classification. They include cytochromes, polyamines, pigments, particular enzymes, sterols, and hopanoids (37, 107). Very often, analytical difficulties have been the main restrictions to their wide-scale application.

Cellular Fatty Acid Analysis

Over 300 fatty acids and related compounds are present in bacterial cells. Polar lipids are the constituents of the lipid bilayer of bacterial membranes and have been frequently studied for classification and identification purposes. Other types of lipids, such as sphingophospholipids, occur in only a restricted number of taxa and were shown to have taxonomic value within these groups (54). Fatty acids are the major constituents of lipids and lipopolysaccharides and have been used extensively for taxonomic purposes. Variabilities in chain lengths, double-bond positions, and substituent groups are very useful for the characterization of bacterial taxa (105). Mostly, the total cellular fatty acid fraction is extracted, but particular fractions, such as the polar lipids, have also been analyzed.

The cellular fatty acid methyl ester composition is a stable parameter, provided highly standardized culture conditions are used. The methylated fatty acids are typically separated by gas-liquid chromatography, and both the occurrence and the relative amounts of methylated fatty acids characterize bacterial fatty acid profiles.

Cellular fatty acid analysis offers many advantages over other phenotype-based identification systems; however, it has several limitations as well. First, the result of the analysis is culture dependent. Strains must be grown under identical conditions so that their fatty acid compositions can be compared. Although the conditions recommended by the manufacturer allow cultivation of a large number of bacteria, different sets of conditions and databases are used for different groups of bacteria (e.g., the aerobic bacteria, anaerobic bacteria, and mycobacteria). In addition, the level of resolution is organism dependent. Many bacteria may be adequately characterized and identified at the species level by means of their cellular fatty acid profile. However, others are not, and often species of the same genus or even different genera have highly similar fatty acid compositions. Whole-cell fatty acid analysis is widely used both in taxonomic studies and in identification analyses. The applications and restraints of the technique were extensively discussed and documented by Welch (126). In the framework of polyphasic taxonomy, cellular fatty acid analysis is often very useful as a rapid and fairly inexpensive screening method. The method allows the comparison and clustering of large numbers of strains with a minimal effort and yields descriptive information to characterize the organisms.

MALDI-TOF (MS)

The first reports involving the use of MALDI-TOF (MS) were published in the late 1980s, and its application increased exponentially during the past 15 years. The two main research areas are the field of proteomics, where it is used as an instrument to identify proteins, and the detection of biomarkers of several diseases including cancer, Alzheimer's disease, arthritis, and allergy (72, 137). In MALDI-TOF (MS), the sample is mixed with a matrix that is chosen such that it specifically absorbs a laser beam. The resulting high-energy impact is followed by the formation of ions that are extracted through an electric field and that are subsequently focused and detected as an m/z (mass/charge) spectrum. The potential to desorb high-molecular-weight thermolabile molecules, the extremely high precision and sensitivity, and the large mass range (1 to 300 kDa) indicate that MALDI-TOF (MS) is a promising tool for the study of biomolecules in complex biological samples. The simplicity and speed of analysis represent part of its strength. Sample processing is potentially restricted to adding matrix to a bacterial sample, and all measurements can be performed within a few minutes. The whole process can be highly automatized. These features make the approach particularly attractive to research laboratories that routinely deal with the analysis and identification of large numbers of bacterial isolates. In microbiology, MALDI-TOF (MS) has been used to distinguish antimicrobial-resistant isolates from susceptible ones and to differentiate strains within a single species, thus highlighting its potential as a tool for strain quality control and identity check (57, 111). The most challenging diagnostic problem, i.e., the differentiation of closely related species through the analysis of an appropriate number of reference strains of multiple closely related species, is gradually being explored (23, 57, 103, 111).

Surface enhanced laser desorption ionization (SELDI) is distinguished from MALDI in its use of an active sample probe—the ProteinChip array—which has an adsorptive surface that allows bacterial lysates to be subjected directly, without prior treatments, to on-chip sample preparation steps, such as selective washing and desalting. This procedure minimizes sample losses, while speeding up and simplifying sample preparation, compared to the standard methods normally employed prior to the use of MALDI. Furthermore, the active capture of the proteins by the ProteinChip array ensures nondiscriminatory binding of target proteins, which in turn improves the reproducibility and allows both peak mass-to-charge (m/z) ratios and intensity to be used in sample characterization. SELDI-TOF-MS was used by Lundquist et al. (69) to discriminate between the four subspecies of *Francisella tularensis*.

FTIR Spectroscopy

FTIR spectroscopy is used for the identification of substances in chemical analyses. In general, the wave number, the reciprocal of the wavelength, is used as the physical unit. FTIR spectroscopy involves the observation of vibrations of molecules that are excited by an infrared beam. Molecules are able to absorb the energy of distinct light quanta and start a rocking or rotation movement. The FTIR spectrum uses only vibrations that lead to a change in the dipole moment. An infrared spectrum represents a fingerprint which is characteristic for any chemical substance. The composition of biological material and thus of its FTIR spectrum is exceedingly complex, representing a characteristic fingerprint. Naumann and coworkers suggested identifying microorganisms by FTIR spectroscopy (79). In principle, a reference spectrum library is assembled based on well-characterized strains and species. The FTIR spectrum of any unidentified isolate is then measured under the same conditions as those used for the reference spectra and is compared to spectra in the reference spectrum library. The application of FTIR spectroscopy has been reported for a limited number of strains of some species of the genera *Lactobacillus*, *Actinomyces*, *Listeria*, *Streptococcus*, and *Clostridium* (63). More extensive studies have been published for yeasts (63, 130) and coryneform bacteria (80); these organisms display a certain degree of overlapping distribution of different taxonomical markers, leading to a limited differentiation capacity of nongenotypical identification methods. The easy handling, rapid identification (within 25 h starting from a single colony), satisfactory differentiation capacity, and low cost have shown FTIR technology to be superior to routine methods for the identification of coryneform bacteria and related taxa.

Whole-Cell Protein Analysis

The comparison of whole-cell protein patterns obtained by a highly standardized procedure, sodium dodecyl sulfate polyacrylamide gel electrophoresis, has proved to be extremely reliable for comparison and grouping of large numbers of closely related strains, and numerous studies document the application of this procedure in taxonomic studies (14, 56, 88). Bacterial strains cultivated under highly standardized conditions have characteristic protein compositions that can be separated and visualized by electrophoretic techniques. Mostly, a high similarity in whole-cell protein content is an indication of extensive DNA-DNA hybridization (14, 56, 88). Therefore, an obvious advantage of this technique is that, once the correlation between percentage similarity in whole-cell protein composition and DNA-DNA relatedness for a particular group has been established, it can replace DNA-DNA hybridization experiments. Provided highly standardized conditions are used throughout the procedures of cultivation and electrophoresis, computer-assisted numerical comparisons of protein patterns are feasible, and databases can be created for identification purposes. This allows comparison of large numbers of strains and grouping of the strains in clusters of closely related strains (14, 56, 88). For some bacteria, numerical analysis is strongly hindered by the presence of distorted protein profiles or hypervariable (often immunogenic) dense protein bands. In these cases, visual comparison is essential to interpret the similarity of protein patterns.

Cell Wall Composition

The distinction between gram-negative and gram-positive types of bacteria is still one of the characteristics that is first analyzed in order to guide subsequent characterization and identification steps. The determination of the cell wall composition has traditionally been important for gram-positive bacteria. The peptidoglycan type of cell wall of gram-negative bacteria is rather uniform and provides little information. The cell walls of gram-positive bacteria, in contrast, contain various peptidoglycan types which may be genus or species specific (92, 105). The most valuable information is derived from the type and composition of the peptide cross-link between adjacent chains in the polymer network. A variable that received little attention is the degree of N and O acetylation of the amino sugars of the glycan chain. The analytical procedure is time-consuming, although a rapid screening method has been proposed. Membrane-bound teichoic acid is present in all gram-positive species, but cell wall-bound teichoic acid is present in only some gram-positive species. Teichoic acids can easily be extracted and purified and can be analyzed by gas-liquid chromatography (25).

Isoprenoid Quinones

Isoprenoid quinones occur in the cytoplasmic membranes of most prokaryotes and play important roles in electron transport, oxidative phosphorylation, and, possibly, active transport (11, 105). Two major structural groups, the naphthoquinones and the benzoquinones, are distinguished. The former can be further subdivided into two main types, the phylloquinones, which occur less commonly in bacteria, and the menaquinones. The large variability of the side chains (e.g., differences in length, saturation, and hydrogenation) can be used to characterize bacteria at different taxonomic levels (11).

IDENTIFICATION

Identification is part of taxonomy. It is the process whereby an organism is recognized as belonging to a known taxon (species, genus) and designated accordingly. It relies on a comparison of the characters of an unknown with those of established units in order to name it appropriately. This implies that identification depends on adequate characterization.

Identification Strategy

In routine diagnostic laboratories, the majority of isolates are identified using classical biochemical tests and a combination of intuition and stepwise analysis of results that are obtained. However, if an organism is not readily identified in a minimal amount of time and at minimal expense, it often remains unidentified. Such strains must be identified without a clue to their phylogenetic affiliation. Comparison of (nearly) entire 16S rRNA gene sequences is arguably one of the most powerful tools for establishment of the phylogenetic neighborhood of an unknown organism, and commercial identification systems based on analysis of rRNA gene sequences have become available (e.g., MicroSeq 500 and 16S rDNA Bacterial Sequencing Kit [Perkin-Elmer Applied Biosystems, Foster City, Calif.]). A fraction of the 5′-terminal region of the 16S rRNA gene (positions 60 to 110 of the *Escherichia coli* numbering system) is one of the most informative or discriminating regions for closely related organisms (66). Similar variable regions (flanked by highly conserved regions) occur in the 23S rRNA gene (113). A review by Clarridge recently covered this topic in detail (7) but struggled with the rRNA sequence similarity level as a limit for species delineation. As outlined above, use of the DNA-DNA hybridization level as a threshold for species delineation is more than just a mere "proposal" (7) and is now supported by a range of whole-genome-based analyses. Comparison of 16S rRNA gene sequences will lead to correct identification to the species level in many bacterial genera, but it is equally true that many taxonomic studies have revealed that comparative rRNA sequence analysis is often not sensitive enough to identify strains to the species level. There is clearly a lack of knowledge not only of the strain-to-strain variation within a species but also of the interoperon variation within a single strain. Therefore, concluding that an unidentified isolate belongs to a particular species because it shares a high percentage of its 16S rRNA gene sequence with particular species or concluding that it represents a novel species because it occupies a unique position in the phylogenetic tree or because it shares only 97% of its 16S rRNA sequence with its closest neighbor is premature in the absence of appropriate complementary data. This is even more true for partial sequence data, as partial rRNA gene sequences carry only limited information of the molecule and different parts of the gene may carry information for different taxonomic levels (66, 68). Nevertheless, erroneous claims that 16S rRNA gene sequencing represents the general "gold standard" for identification of new isolates appear regularly in medical (and other) microbiological literature (27).

Alternative Approaches

As part of identification strategies, dichotomous keys based on morphological and biochemical characteristics have only partly been replaced by other methods. As described above, taxonomic analyses provided an impressive array of alternative techniques derived from analytical biochemistry and molecular biology for examination of numerous cellular compounds (36, 37, 89). Each of these parameters is useful for characterization and hence identification of bacteria. Databases of rRNA sequences, whole-cell fatty acid components, ribotyping profiles, MALDI-TOF mass spectra and FTIR spectra, or miniaturized series of phenotypic characteristics are available (see above and chapter 15) and allow identification of many isolates. Yet, the success of these databases also depends on the exactness of the methods and how carefully the individual entries have been delineated. The classification of new or unusual isolates will, however, often require a polyphasic approach, whereby an unknown is allocated to a certain phylogenetic neighborhood (typically by using 16S rRNA gene sequence analysis), followed by a comparison of characteristics of the unknown with those of its closest phylogenetic neighbors by using appropriate taxonomic tools in order to assign it a particular species rank.

Molecular Diagnostics

The information content of the rRNA cistrons and other genomic information have been used in several alternative ways for the identification of bacteria by the development of a range of DNA or RNA probes and amplification assays. Although the overall rRNA sequence similarity may be very high, the presence of variable regions in 16S or 23S RNA genes can provide the basis for specific and sensitive targets for identification purposes (for examples, see references 68, 94, and 113). During the last 20 years, DNA technology has emerged, and the tools of molecular biology are now used for the detection, characterization, and identification of bacteria. The first applications were labeled probes intended to hybridize with specific nucleic acid fragments. Later, in vitro nucleic acid amplification procedures were developed. It was thought that this enzymatic duplication and amplification of specific nucleic acid sequences would gradually replace culture-based approaches. However, it became rapidly clear that the molecular diagnostic approach has its own difficulties in terms of sensitivity, specificity, turn-around time, and cost. As a consequence, its application was restricted to the solution of these problems in cases in which it is superior to the conventional approach (50). Molecular diagnostic techniques are indicated for the detection of organisms that cannot be grown in vitro, for which current culture techniques are too insensitive, or that require sophisticated media or cell cultures and/or prolonged incubation times.

The basic principle of any molecular diagnostic test is the detection of a specific nucleic acid sequence by hybridization to a complementary sequence of DNA or RNA, a probe, followed by detection of the hybrid (68). There are two types of molecular diagnostic techniques: those in which the hybrids are not amplified prior to detection and those in which they are. With the probe technology not involving amplification, the probes used for the detection of complementary nucleic acid sequences are labeled with enzymes, chemiluminiscent moieties, radioisotopes, or antigenic substrates (49). This technology was first applied in the field of infectious diseases for the detection of enterotoxigenic *E. coli* in stool samples by DNA hybridization after growth on MacConkey agar plates (74). This application illustrated the major advantage of the technology: in a mixture of pathogenic and nonpathogenic bacteria belonging to the same species, present in the same specimen, and difficult to distinguish by traditional culture and identification techniques, the former bacteria were easily detected and identified (49).

Alternatively, any DNA fragment can be copied by using a DNA polymerase, provided that some sequence data are known for the design of appropriate primers. In vitro DNA replication was made possible in 1959 when Kornberg (60) discovered DNA polymerase I, but only in 1986 did Mullis and coworkers (75) introduce the idea of PCR, i.e., reiteration of the process of DNA polymerization, leading to an exponential increase of the nucleic acid. Alternative nucleic acid amplification techniques have been developed by using different enzymes and strategies, but they are all based on reiterative reactions. In most of these the target nucleic acid is amplified; in some the probe is multiplied (13, 33, 42, 64, 124). The advantages of these amplification systems are obvious: they can be highly specific and rapid, and they have very high sensitivities. However, there are many practical problems as well (chapter 16; see also references 49 and 50).

Immunological Techniques

Immunoassays are procedures which measure antigen or antibody levels to determine whether patients are infected or are immunologically responding to infection or immunization. Two general approaches are distinguished: testing for specific microbial antigens and testing for specific microbial antigen-specific antibodies. These immunological techniques are described in detail in chapter 18. An important advantage of immunoassay tests is that they provide information even when culture and Gram staining results are negative for patients who received antimicrobial therapy.

Conclusion

At present, the scientifically and economically ideal identification technique remains beyond reach. Cowan's (15) intuitive approach (which is used when the identity of the unknown is anticipated) and the stepwise method (which involves the use of dichotomous keys) suffice for numerous isolates and require only simple, rapid, and cheap biochemical tests. Cowan's views are easily adapted to modern methodology. If this first-line approach fails, alternative procedures are required and available. At present, complete 16S rRNA gene sequence analysis is the most straightforward and obvious choice to establish a rough identity of an isolate, although in the present species concept with DNA-DNA hybridization levels as the cornerstones, it often fails to differentiate closely related species. Much of its superiority is based on its capacity to reveal the phylogenetic neighborhood of the organism studied, which is information not provided by any of the other current identification protocols. This information will direct the additional analyses required for final identification to the species level.

NOMENCLATURE

Valid Publication of Bacterial Names

The *International Code of Nomenclature of Bacteria* (97) includes rules on how to name bacteria at different taxonomic ranks. The aim of nomenclature is to ensure that an organism is tagged with a unique name that carries valuable information. Prior to 1980, a proposal of a new bacterial taxon could be validly published in any microbiological book or journal, and the authors of the relevant sections of the successive editions of *Bergey's Manual of Determinative Bacteriology* had to attempt to give a complete list of the members of any particular genus or group of genera. The unavailability of type strains and the fact that microbiologists from different disciplines were not always familiar with one another's work caused great difficulty. All too often a worker would discover several years later that "his" or "her" organism had in fact been described earlier under a different name.

To overcome such problems and others, 1 January 1980 was chosen as a new starting date for bacterial nomenclature. At that time, Approved Lists of Bacterial Names were published on behalf of the Judicial Commission of the International Committee on Systematic Bacteriology (95). Only those names included on these lists had standing in bacterial nomenclature, and names of taxa were to be included only if they were adequately described and if a type strain was available. From then onward, all new names were validly published only in the *International Journal of Systematic Bacteriology* (now the *International Journal of Systematic and Evolutionary Microbiology*). Names could effectively be published in other journals and then validated subsequently by announcement in Validation Lists in the *International Journal of Systematic and Evolutionary Microbiology*. A number of organisms were involuntarily omitted from the Approved Lists and were revived later (for instance, see reference 72). After 1980 several updates of these lists were published in the form of Validation Lists, and in 1989, an update of all names validly published between 1 January 1980 and 1 January 1989 was published by Moore and Moore (73). Nowadays, complete overviews of validly published names can easily be obtained through Internet sites such as http://www.bacterio.cict.fr/ or http://www.dsmz.de/bactnom/genera1.htm. Proposals of new taxa can continue to be made in any journal, but their names are only validated the moment that they are included in one of the Validation Lists, published regularly in the *International Journal of Systematic and Evolutionary Microbiology*. In case different names for the same organism are validly published, nomenclatural priority goes to the name that was validated first. As a result of this practice, all validly named species in any particular group can easily be traced and reference strains are available.

Why Do Names Change?

There are more important causes for the modification of bacterial names than the occasional detection of synonymy. As described above, our present view on bacterial classification is phylogeny based. With the advent of rRNA-DNA hybridization and, subsequently, the various rRNA gene sequencing methods, taxonomists had a new framework in which they could revise classification schemes. The classical—and extreme—example is the revision of the taxonomy and nomenclature of the genus *Pseudomonas*, which has been proceeding painstakingly slowly during the past 3 decades. The most important reason for this slow progress is that, through the work of De Vos and De Ley (22), it became clear not only that the genus *Pseudomonas* consisted of five major species clusters (87) but also that these clusters formed a polyphyletic part of a major group of bacteria now known as the *Proteobacteria*. Revision of the taxonomy of the pseudomonads had to consider the relationships of the various subbranches toward their numerous respective neighbors (55).

The modification of our view on classification is by far the most important reason for name changes. However, various forms of poor taxonomic practice also invoke a lot of changes, and hence irritation. As observed long ago (18), nomenclature often is "the generator of heat, bad temper and ill-will among taxonomists and every kind of microbiologists." The classification (and identification) of *Helicobacter* species represents a fine example of the difficulties encountered in our present-day view on taxonomy. Although this view is often challenged, it is the level of DNA-DNA hybridization and not the level of 16S rRNA gene sequence similarity that is the most critical parameter for species delineation. Relatively few laboratories have the experience required to perform DNA-DNA hybridization experiments in a highly standardized way. Yet, because of the tremendous clinical relevance of these bacteria, numerous investigators study all sorts of *Helicobacter*-like organisms from human and animal hosts. The biodiversity within *Helicobacter* is very high, and there is a need for many DNA-DNA hybridization data to delineate the species. Regrettably, helicobacters mostly are fastidious organisms, and many are difficult (and some nearly impossible) to culture in vitro; in addition, the preparation of sufficient DNA for the hybridization experiments is a hardy, if not impossible, task. In practice, new species have often been described on the basis of 16S rRNA gene sequence data and a limited number of differential phenotypic characteristics. A recent study that involved various taxonomic approaches, including DNA-DNA hybridization experiments, demonstrated that comparison of nearly complete 16S rRNA gene sequences combined with minimal biochemical characterization does not provide conclusive evidence for identification to the species level and may prove highly misleading (117).

Another example is the ongoing revision of the classification and nomenclature of group II pseudomonads. In 1992, Yabuuchi et al. (133) reclassified several rRNA group II pseudomonads as *Burkholderia* species. However, in this study only some of the rRNA group II pseudomonads were examined and the conclusions were based on data for only a limited set of strains. As a consequence, several additional rounds of name changes were required to reclassify the remaining rRNA group II pseudomonads as *Burkholderia* species (32, 109, 134, 139). This group of bacteria also serves as an example to illustrate other causes for name changes: the lack of criteria for genus delineation (two of the *Burkholderia* species [*B. solanacearum* and *B. pickettii*] were again reclassified into the new genus *Ralstonia* [32, 134], and some of the *Ralstonia* species were then further reclassified into the novel genus *Wautersia* [122]) and the intrinsically inadequate description of species that comprise only a single isolate. The lack of precise guidelines for genus level delineation was discussed recently by Young (135), who argued strongly that phenotypic coherence at the genus level should have priority over phylogenetic information.

The *Ralstonia* example also illustrates a tedious problem raised by Clarridge (7), namely, the challenges in the nomenclature for organisms named before their correct taxonomy was revealed by 16S rRNA gene sequence comparisons. Shortly after the reclassification of several *Ralstonia* species into the novel genus *Wautersia* (122), Vandamme and Coenye (115) reported that *Wautersia eutropha*, the type species of the genus *Wautersia*, is a junior synonym of *Cupriavidus necator,* the type (and only) species of the genus *Cupriavidus,* which was validly named in 1987, i.e., long before 16S rRNA gene sequence studies were performed routinely (71). The only possible consequence—if one does not decide to bend the rules each time they turn out to be inconvenient—was to replace the name *Wautersia* by *Cupriavidus* and to consider all species of the genus *Wautersia* species of the genus *Cupriavidus*. While renaming and subsequent further renaming of bacterial species cause confusion and—not the least—irritation in the wider microbiological community, adhering to the rules of nomenclature is essential for establishing a truly systematic taxonomy.

The so-called "one strain taxa" (species or genera that are proposed on the basis of data for only one strain) have probably caused more problems than they have solved, and this is definitely the case in the context of diagnostic microbiology. It is not possible to estimate the variability of the phenotype in the case of a species with one strain or in the case of a genus with one species and one strain, for which many recent examples exist. The question of whether such strains can be validly named has been the subject of many debates. There are different views, each with advantages and disadvantages. In diagnostic microbiology, it is well known that a species is characterized by a certain degree of variability. This variability can be measured by both phenotypic and genotypic criteria and may be revealed by simple biochemical testing or sophisticated genomic fingerprinting techniques. In the absence of sufficient strains for quantitation of the range of divergence within a species, it will be difficult or impossible to identify new isolates of this organism without DNA-DNA hybridization experiments. A classification based on results obtained with a single strain cannot be stable. Indeed, the detection of a second strain will inevitably necessitate revision of the original species description.

Clearly, some of the instances of nomenclatural modifications described above could have been avoided, and that is the main reason why they jeopardize the credibility of taxonomists in the microbiology community. As a concluding remark, it should be mentioned that there is no "undo" function in bacterial nomenclature. A name that was validly published remains valid regardless of the number of modifications it undergoes thereafter. For instance, the changes of the name *Pseudomonas maltophilia* to *Xanthomonas maltophilia* (106) and finally to *Stenotrophomonas maltophilia* (85) or the changes of the name *Pseudomonas acidovorans* to *Comamonas acidovorans* (108) and finally to *Delftia acidovorans* (129) may be reasonable to some taxonomists, but the changes, particularly the most recent, have been refuted by many clinical microbiologists. As these six names were all proposed according to the rules of bacterial nomenclature, they were all validated, and the use of each of them is correct and valid. Use of the original *Pseudomonas* names could imply that the user disagrees with the phylogenetic rationale for present-day genus level classification. Use of the names *X. maltophilia* or *C. acidovorans* may simply indicate that one disagrees with the most recent modification, whether the reason is scientific or practical, or it may be a simple statement of discord with successive and excessive name changes.

CONCLUSION

A much broader range of taxonomic studies of bacteria has gradually replaced the former reliance upon morphological, physiological, and biochemical characterization. This polyphasic taxonomy takes into account all available phenotypic and genotypic information and integrates it in a consensus type of classification, framed in a general phylogeny derived from 16S rRNA gene sequence analysis. The bacterial species appears as a group of isolates which originated from a common ancestor population in which a steady generation of genetic diversity resulted in clones that had different degrees of recombination and that were characterized by a certain degree of phenotypic consistency, a significant degree of DNA-DNA hybridization, and a high degree of 16S rRNA gene sequence similarity (118).

The majority of bacteria in routine diagnostic laboratories will continue to be identified by classical methods, as these methods are adequate, cheap, readily available, and easy to handle. In the case of new or atypical isolates, or for many research groups in which, for example, bacteria are isolated from new sources, a straightforward means of identification of microorganisms by a single method is often not possible, and several methods are needed. The most direct approach is first to allocate such isolates in the phylogenetic framework and then to determine the finer relationships by means of an appropriate approach, which may be polyphasic. This tendency of identification to become polyphasic is an unavoidable reality.

In some cases, the consensus classification is a compromise that contains a minimum of contradictions. It is thought that the more parameters that become available in the future, the more polyphasic classification will gain stability. Although the idea is purely speculative at present, insight into the vast amount of data that are potentially available could be the basis for a perfectly reliable and stable classification system. However, already with our present data, it is sometimes unclear if it makes sense to order bacteria into a classification system. Undoubtedly, there is a huge amount of biodiversity, which can be handled in a practical manner only if it is arrayed in an ordered structure, artificial or not, with appropriate terms for communication.

Our present view on classification reflects the best science of this time. The same was true in the past, when only data from morphological and biochemical analyses were available. The main perspective in bacterial taxonomy is that technological progress will dominate and drastically influence methodology, as it always has. More data will become available, more bacteria will be detected (whether they can be cultivated or not), there will be more automation, and bioinformatics will have to address the combination and linking of databases. Most important, the increasing access to whole-genome sequences will generate proposals for novel species concepts. These future concepts may be based on whole-genome sequences, on a shared core of genes, on a certain type of genes such as housekeeping or informational genes (26, 45), or on a well-balanced selection of genes included in an MLSA type of analysis (9, 30). It will be a formidable challenge to translate such information into classification and identification schemes and to evaluate classifications that have been carefully designed.

REFERENCES

1. **Amann, R. I., W. Ludwig, and K.-H. Schleifer.** 1995. Phylogenetic identification and in situ detection of individual microbial cells without cultivation. *Microbiol. Rev.* **59:**143–169.
2. **Baldwin, A., E. Mahenthiralingam, K. M. Thickett, D. Honeybourne, M. C. Maiden, J. R. Govan, D. P. Speert, J. J. LiPuma, P. Vandamme, and C. G. Dowson.** 2005.

Multilocus sequence typing scheme that provides both species and strain differentiation for the *Burkholderia cepacia* complex. *J. Clin. Microbiol.* **43:**4665–4673.
3. **Bingen, E. H., E. Denamur, and J. Elion.** 1994. Use of ribotyping in epidemiological surveillance of nosocomial outbreaks. *Clin. Microbiol. Rev.* **7:**311–327.
4. **Brenner, D. J., G. R. Fanning, A. V. Rake, and K. E. Johnson.** 1969. Batch procedure for thermal elution of DNA from hydroxyapatite. *Anal. Biochem.* **28:**447–459.
5. **Chen, C. C., L. J. Teng, S. Kaiung, and T. C. Chang.** 2005. Identification of clinically relevant viridans streptococci by an oligonucleotide array. *J. Clin. Microbiol.* **43:** 1515–1521.
6. **Christensen, H., O. Angen, R. Mutters, J. E. Olsen, and M. Bisgaard.** 2000. DNA-DNA hybridization determined in micro-wells using covalent attachment of DNA. *Int. J. Syst. Evol. Microbiol.* **50:**1095–1102.
7. **Clarridge, J. E.** 2004. Impact of 16S rRNA gene sequence analysis for identification of bacteria on clinical microbiology and infectious diseases. *Clin. Microbiol. Rev.* **17:**840–862.
8. **Clayton, R. A., G. Sutton, P. S. Hinkle, C. Bult, and C. Fields.** 1995. Intraspecific variation in small-subunit rRNA sequences in GenBank: why single sequences may not adequately represent prokaryotic taxa. *Int. J. Syst. Bacteriol.* **45:**595–599.
9. **Coenye, T., D. Gevers, Y. Van de Peer, P. Vandamme, and J. Swings.** 2005. Towards a prokaryotic genomic taxonomy. *FEMS Microbiol. Rev.* **29:**147–167.
10. **Cohan, F. M.** 2002. What are bacterial species? *Annu. Rev. Microbiol.* **56:**457–487.
11. **Collins, M. D.** 1994. Isoprenoid quinones, p. 265–311. *In* M. Goodfellow and A. G. O'Donnell (ed.), *Modern Microbial Methods. Chemical Methods in Prokaryotic Systematics.* J. Wiley and Sons, Chichester, United Kingdom.
12. **Colwell, R. R.** 1970. Polyphasic taxonomy of the genus *Vibrio:* numerical taxonomy of *Vibrio cholerae, Vibrio parahaemolyticus,* and related *Vibrio* species. *J. Bacteriol.* **104:**410–433.
13. **Compton, J.** 1991. Nucleic acid sequence-based amplification. *Nature* (London) **350:**91–92.
14. **Costas, M.** 1992. Classification, identification, and typing of bacteria by the analysis of their one-dimensional polyacrylamide gel electrophoretic protein patterns, p. 351–408. *In* A. Chambrach, M. J. Dunn, and B. J. Radola (ed.), *Advances in Electrophoresis,* vol. 5. VCH Verlagsgesellschaft, Weinheim, Germany.
15. **Cowan, S. T.** 1965. Principles and practice of bacterial taxonomy—a forward look. *J. Gen. Microbiol.* **39:**143–153.
16. **Cowan, S. T.** 1968. *A Dictionary of Microbial Taxonomic Usage.* Oliver & Boyd, Edinburgh, United Kingdom.
17. **Cowan, S. T.** 1970. Heretical taxonomy for bacteriologists. *J. Gen. Microbiol.* **61:**145–154.
18. **Cowan, S. T.** 1971. Sense and nonsense in bacterial taxonomy. *J. Gen. Microbiol.* **67:**1–8.
19. **Crosa, J. H., D. J. Brenner, and S. Falkow.** 1973. Use of a single-strand specific nuclease for analysis of bacterial and plasmid deoxyribonucleic acid homo- and heteroduplexes. *J. Bacteriol.* **115:**904–911.
20. **De Ley, J., H. Cattoir, and A. Reynaerts.** 1970. The quantitative measurement of DNA hybridization from renaturation rates. *Eur. J. Biochem.* **12:**133–142.
21. **Descheemaeker, P., C. Lammens, B. Pot, P. Vandamme, and H. Goossens.** 1997. Evaluation of arbitrarily primed PCR analysis and pulsed-field gel electrophoresis of large genomic DNA fragments for identification of enterococci important in human medicine. *Int. J. Syst. Bacteriol.* **47:**555–561.
22. **De Vos, P., and J. De Ley.** 1983. Intra- and intergeneric similarities of *Pseudomonas* and *Xanthomonas* ribosomal ribonucleic acid cistrons. *Int. J. Syst. Bacteriol.* **33:**487–509.
23. **Dickinson, D. N., M. T. La Duc, M. Satomi, J. D. Winefordner, D. H. Powell, and K. Venkateswaran.** 2004. MALDI-TOFMS compared with other polyphasic taxonomy approaches for the identification and classification of *Bacillus pumilus* spores. *J. Microbiol. Methods* **58:**1–12.
24. **Ezaki, T., Y. Hashimoto, and E. Yabuuchi.** 1989. Fluorometric deoxyribonucleic acid-deoxyribonucleic acid hybridization in microdilution wells as an alternative to membrane filter hybridization in which radioisotopes are used to determine genetic relatedness among bacterial strains. *Int. J. Syst. Bacteriol.* **39:**224–229.
25. **Fischer, W., P. Rösel, and H. U. Koch.** 1981. Effect of alanine ester substitution and other structural features of lipoteichoic acids on their inhibitory activity against autolysins of *Staphylococcus aureus*. *J. Bacteriol.* **146:** 467–475.
26. **Fitz-Gibbon, S. T., and C. H. House.** 1999. Whole-genome based phylogenetic analysis of free-living microorganisms. *Nucleic Acids Res.* **27:**4218–4222.
27. **Fontana, C., M. Favaro, M. Pelliccioni, E. S. Pistoia, and C. Favalli.** 2005. Use of the MicroSeq 500 16S rRNA gene-based sequencing for identification of bacterial isolates that commercial automated systems failed to identify correctly. *J. Clin. Microbiol.* **43:**615–619.
28. **Fox, G. E., J. D. Wisotzkey, and P. Jurtshuk.** 1992. How close is close: 16S rRNA sequence identity may not be sufficient to guarantee species identity. *Int. J. Syst. Bacteriol.* **42:**166–170.
29. **Gautier, A.-L., D. Dubois, F. Escande, J.-L. Avril, P. Trieu-Cuot, and O. Gaillot.** 2005. Rapid and accurate identification of human isolates of *Pasteurella* and related species by sequencing the *sodA* gene. *J. Clin. Microbiol.* **43:**2307–2314.
30. **Gevers, D., F. M. Cohan, J. G. Lawrence, B. G. Spratt, T. Coenye, E. J. Feil, E. Stackebrandt, Y. Van de Peer, P. Vandamme, F. L. Thompson, and J. Swings.** 2005. Reevaluating prokaryotic species. *Nat. Rev. Microbiol.* **3:**733–739.
31. **Giesendorf, B. A., W. G. Quint, P. Vandamme, and A. van Belkum.** 1996. Generation of DNA probes for detection of microorganisms by polymerase chain reaction fingerprinting. *Zentbl. Bakteriol.* **283:**417–430.
32. **Gillis, M., T. V. Van, R. Bardin, M. Goor, P. Hebbar, A. Willems, P. Segers, K. Kersters, T. Heulin, and M. P. Fernandez.** 1995. Polyphasic taxonomy in the genus *Burkholderia* leading to an emended description of the genus and proposition of *Burkholderia vietnamiensis* sp. nov. for N_2-fixing isolates from rice in Vietnam. *Int. J. Syst. Bacteriol.* **45:**274–289.
33. **Gingeras, T. R., P. Prodanovich, T. Latimer, J. C. Guatelli, and D. D. Richman.** 1991. Use of self-sustained sequence replication amplification reaction to analyze and detect mutations in zidovudine-resistant human immunodeficiency virus. *J. Infect. Dis.* **164:**1066–1074.
34. **Godoy, D., G. Randle, A. J. Simpson, D. M. Aanensen, T. L. Pitt, R. Kinoshita, and B. G. Spratt.** 2003. Multilocus sequence typing and evolutionary relationships among the causative agents of melioidosis and glanders, *Burkholderia pseudomallei* and *Burkholderia mallei*. *J. Clin. Microbiol.* **41:**2068–2079.
35. **Gonzalez-Escalona, N., J. Romero, and R. T. Espejo.** 2005. Polymorphism and gene conversion of the 16S rRNA genes in the multiple rRNA operons of *Vibrio parahaemolyticus*. *FEMS Microbiol. Lett.* **246:**213–219.
36. **Goodfellow, M., and A. G. O'Donnell.** 1993. *Handbook of New Bacterial Systematics.* Academic Press, London, United Kingdom.
37. **Goodfellow, M., and A. G. O'Donnell.** 1994. *Modern Microbial Methods. Chemical Methods in Prokaryotic*

Systematics. J. Wiley and Sons, Ltd., Chichester, United Kingdom.

38. **Goodwin, C. S., J. A. Armstrong, T. Chilvers, M. Peters, M. D. Collins, L. Sly, W. McConnell, and W. E. S. Harper.** 1989. Transfer of *Campylobacter pylori* and *Campylobacter mustelae* to *Helicobacter* gen. nov. as *Helicobacter pylori* comb. nov. and *Helicobacter mustelae* comb. nov., respectively. *Int. J. Syst. Bacteriol.* **39:**397–405.
39. **Goris, J., K. Suzuki, P. De Vos, T. Nakase, and K. Kersters.** 1998. Evaluation of a microplate DNA-DNA hybridization method compared with the initial renaturation method. *Can. J. Microbiol.* **44:**1148–1153.
40. **Grimont, F., and P. Grimont.** 1986. Ribosomal ribonucleic acid gene restriction patterns as possible taxonomic tools. *Ann. Inst. Pasteur/Microbiol. (Paris)* **137B:**165–175.
41. **Grimont, P. A. D., M. Y. Popoff, F. Grimont, C. Coynault, and M. Lemelin.** 1980. Reproducibility and correlation study of three deoxyribonucleic acid hybridization procedures. *Curr. Microbiol.* **4:**325–330.
42. **Guatelli, J. C., K. M. Whitfield, D. Y. Kwoh, K. J. Barringer, D. D. Richman, and T. R. Gingeras.** 1990. Isothermal, *in vitro* amplification of nucleic acids by a multienzyme reaction modeled after retroviral replication. *Proc. Natl. Acad. Sci. USA* **87:**1874–1878.
43. **Gupta, R. S.** 1998. Protein phylogenies and signature sequences: a reappraisal of evolutionary relationships among Archaebacteria, Eubacteria, and Eukaryotes. *Microbiol. Mol. Biol. Rev.* **62:**1435–1491.
44. **Gürtler, V., and V. A. Stanisich.** 1996. New approaches to typing and identification of bacteria using the 16S-23S rDNA spacer region. *Microbiology* **142:**3–16.
45. **Gürtler, V., and B. C. Mayal.** 2001. Genomic approaches to typing, taxonomy and evolution of bacterial isolates. *Int. J. Syst. Evol. Microbiol.* **51:**3–16.
46. **Harrington, C. S., and S. L. On.** 1999. Extensive 16S ribosomal RNA gene sequence diversity in *Campylobacter hyointestinalis* strains: taxonomic and applied implications. *Int. J. Syst. Bacteriol.* **49:**1171–1175.
47. **Healy, M., J. Huong, T. Bittner, M. Lising, S. Frye, S. Raza, R. Schrock, J. Manry, A. Renwick, R. Nieto, C. Woods, J. Versalovic, and J. R. Lupski.** 2005. Microbial DNA typing by automated repetitive-sequence-based PCR. *J. Clin. Microbiol.* **43:**199–207.
48. **Höfle, M. G.** 1990. Transfer RNAs as genotypic fingerprints of eubacteria. *Arch. Microbiol.* **153:**299–304.
49. **Ieven, M.** 1998. Bacterial pathogenesis. Detection, speciation, and identification. 3.2 Detection. *Methods Microbiol.* **27:**40–50.
50. **Ieven, M., and H. Goossens.** 1997. Relevance of nucleic acid amplification techniques for diagnosis of respiratory tract infections in the clinical laboratory. *Clin. Microbiol. Rev.* **10:**242–256.
51. **Jahnke, K.-D.** 1994. A modified method of quantitative colorimetric DNA-DNA hybridization on membrane filters for bacterial identification. *J. Microbiol. Methods* **20:**273–288.
52. **Janssen, P., R. Coopman, G. Huys, J. Swings, M. Bleeker, P. Vos, M. Zabeau, and K. Kersters.** 1996. Evaluation of the DNA fingerprinting method AFLP as a new tool in bacterial taxonomy. *Microbiology* **142:**1881–1893.
53. **Jaspers, E., and J. Overmann.** 2004. Ecological significance of microdiversity: identical 16S rRNA gene sequences can be found in bacteria with highly divergent genomes and ecophysiologies. *Appl. Environ. Microbiol.* **70:**4831–4839.
54. **Jones, D., and N. R. Krieg.** 1984. Serology and chemotaxonomy, p. 15–18. *In* N. R. Krieg and J. G. Holt (ed.), *Bergey's Manual of Systematic Bacteriology*, vol. 1. The Williams & Wilkins Co., Baltimore, Md.
55. **Kersters, K., W. Ludwig, M. Vancanneyt, P. De Vos, M. Gillis, and K.-H. Schleifer.** 1996. Recent changes in the classification of the pseudomonads: an overview. *Syst. Appl. Microbiol.* **19:**465–477.
56. **Kersters, K., B. Pot, D. Dewettinck, U. Torck, M. Vancanneyt, L. Vauterin, and P. Vandamme.** 1994. Identification and typing of bacteria by protein electrophoresis, p. 51–66. *In* F. G. Priest, A. Ramos-Cormenzana, and B. Tyndall (ed.), *Bacterial Diversity and Systematics.* Plenum Press, New York, N.Y.
57. **Keys, C. J., D. J. Dare, H. Sutton, G. Wells, M. Lunt, T. McKenna, M. McDowall, and H. N. Shah.** 2004. Compilation of a MALDI-TOF mass spectral database for the rapid screening and characterisation of bacteria implicated in human infectious diseases. *Infect. Genet. Evol.* **4:**221–242.
58. **Khamis, A., D. Raoult, and B. La Scola.** 2005. Comparison between *rpoB* and 16S rRNA gene sequencing for molecular identification of 168 clinical isolates of *Corynebacterium. J. Clin. Microbiol.* **43:**1934–1936.
59. **Konstantinidis, K. T., and J. M. Tiedje.** 2005. Genomic insights that advance the species definition for prokaryotes. *Proc. Natl. Acad. Sci. USA* **102:**2567–2572.
60. **Kornberg, A.** 1959. Enzymic synthesis of desoxyribonucleic acid. *Harvey Lect.* **53:**83–112.
61. **Kotetishvili, M., A. Kreger, G. Wauters, J. G. Morris, Jr., A. Sulakvelidze, and O. C. Stine.** 2005. Multilocus sequence typing for studying genetic relationships among *Yersinia* species. *J. Clin. Microbiol.* **43:**2674–2684.
62. **Krieg, N. R., and G. M. Garrity.** 2001. On using the manual, p. 15–19. *In* D. R. Boone, R. W. Castenholz, and G. M. Garrity (ed.), *Bergey's Manual of Systematic Bacteriology*, vol. 2. Springer-Verlag, New York, N.Y.
63. **Kümmerle, M., S. Scherer, and H. Seiler.** 1998. Rapid and reliable identification of food-borne yeasts by Fourier-transform infrared spectroscopy. *Appl. Environ. Microbiol.* **64:**2207–2214.
64. **Kwoh, D. Y., G. R. Davis, K. M. Whitfield, H. L. Chapelle, L. J. DiMichele, and T. R. Gingeras.** 1989. Transcription based amplification system and detection of amplified human immunodeficiency virus type 1 with a bead-based sandwich hybridization format. *Proc. Natl. Acad. Sci. USA* **86:**1173–1177.
65. **Liu, W., T. L. Marsh, H. Cheng, and L. J. Forney.** 1997. Characterization of microbial diversity by determining terminal restriction fragment length polymorphism of genes encoding 16S rRNA. *Appl. Environ. Microbiol.* **63:** 4516–4522.
66. **Ludwig, J., and H.-P. Klenk.** 2001. Overview: a phylogenetic backbone and taxonomic framework for procaryotic systematics, p. 49–65. *In* D. R. Boone, R. W. Castenholz, and G. M. Garrity (ed.), *Bergey's Manual of Systematic Bacteriology*, vol. 2. Springer-Verlag, New York, N.Y.
67. **Ludwig, J., W. Neumann, N. Klugbauer, E. Brockmann, C. Roller, S. Jilg, K. Reetz, I. Schchtner, A. Ludvigsen, G. Wallner, M. Bachleitner, U. Fisher, and K. H. Schleifer.** 1993. Phylogenetic relationships of bacteria based on comparative sequence analysis of elongation factor Tu and ATP-synthase beta subunit genes. *Antonie Leeuwenhoek J. Microbiol. Serol.* **64:**285–305.
68. **Ludwig, J., O. Strunk, S. Klugbauer, N. Klugbauer, M. Weienegger, J. Neumaier, M. Bachleitner, and K. H. Schleifer.** 1998. Bacterial phylogeny based on comparative sequence analysis. *Electrophoresis* **19:**554–568.
69. **Lundquist, M., M. B. Caspersen, P. Wikström, and M. Forsman.** 2005. Discrimination of *Francisella tularensis* subspecies using surface enhanced laser desorption ionization mass spectrometry and multivariate data analysis. *FEMS Microbiol. Lett.* **243:**303–310.

70. **Lupski, J. R., and G. E. Weinstock.** 1992. Short, interspersed repetitive DNA sequences in prokaryotic genomes. *J. Bacteriol.* **174:**4525–4529.
71. **Makkar, N. S., and L. E. Casida.** 1987. *Cupriavidus necator* gen. nov., sp. nov.: a nonobligate bacterial predator of bacteria in soil. *Int. J. Syst. Bacteriol.* **37:**323–326.
72. **Marvin, L. F., M. A. Roberts, and L. B. Fay.** 2003. Matrix-assisted laser desorption/ionization time-of-flight mass spectrometry in clinical chemistry. *Clin. Chim. Acta* **337:**11–21.
73. **Moore, W. E. C., and L. V. H. Moore (ed.).** 1989. *Index of the Bacterial and Yeast Nomenclatural Changes Published in the* International Journal of Systematic Bacteriology *since the 1980 Approved Lists of Bacterial Names (1 January 1980 to 1 January 1989).* American Society for Microbiology, Washington, D.C.
74. **Moseley, S. L., I. Huq, A. R. Alim, M. So, M. Samadpour-Motalebi, and S. Falkow.** 1980. Detection of enterotoxigenic *Escherichia coli* by DNA colony hybridization. *J. Infect. Dis.* **142:**892–898.
75. **Mullis, K., F. Faloona, S. Scharf, R. Saiki, G. Horn, and H. Erlich.** 1986. Specific enzymatic amplification of DNA in vitro: the polymerase chain reaction. *Cold Spring Harbor Symp. Quant. Biol.* **51**(Pt. 1):263–273.
76. **Murray, R. G. E., D. J. Brenner, R. R. Colwell, P. De Vos, M. Goodfellow, P. A. D. Grimont, N. Pfennig, E. Stackebrandt, and G. A. Zavarzin.** 1990. Report of the ad hoc committee on approaches to taxonomy within the *Proteobacteria. Int. J. Syst. Bacteriol.* **40:**213–215.
77. **Murray, R. G. E., and K. H. Schleifer.** 1994. Taxonomic notes: a proposal for recording the properties of putative taxa of procaryotes. *Int. J. Syst. Bacteriol.* **44:**174–176.
78. **Murray, R. G. E., and E. Stackebrandt.** 1995. Taxonomic note: implementation of the provisional status *Candidatus* for incompletely described procaryotes. *Int. J. Syst. Bacteriol.* **45:**186–187.
79. **Naumann, D., D. Helm, and H. Labischinski.** 1991. Microbiological characterizations by FT-IR spectroscopy. *Nature* **351:**81–82.
80. **Oberreuter, H., H. Seiler, and S. Scherer.** 2002. Identification of coryneform bacteria and related taxa by Fourier-transform infrared (FT-IR) spectroscopy. *Int. J. Syst. Evol. Microbiol.* **52:**91–100.
81. **Ochi, K.** 1995. Comparative ribosomal protein sequence analyses of a phylogenetically defined genus, *Pseudomonas*, and its relatives. *Int. J. Syst. Bacteriol.* **45:**268–273.
82. **Olsen, G. J., G. Larsen, and C. R. Woese.** 1991. The ribosomal RNA database project. *Nucleic Acids Res.* **19** (Suppl.):2017–2021.
83. **On, S. L. W., and B. Holmes.** 1991. Reproducibility of tolerance tests that are useful in the identification of campylobacteria. *J. Clin. Microbiol.* **29:**1785–1788.
84. **On, S. L. W., and B. Holmes.** 1992. Assessment of enzyme detection tests useful in identification of campylobacteria. *J. Clin. Microbiol.* **30:**746–749.
85. **Palleroni, N. J., and J. F. Bradbury.** 1993. *Stenotrophomonas*, a new bacterial genus for *Xanthomonas maltophilia* (Hugh 1980) Swings et al. 1983. *Int. J. Syst. Bacteriol.* **43:**606–609.
86. **Palleroni, N. J., and B. Holmes.** 1981. *Pseudomonas cepacia* sp. nov., nom. rev. *Int. J. Syst. Bacteriol.* **31:**479–481.
87. **Palleroni, N. J., R. Kunisawa, R. Contopoulou, and M. Doudoroff.** 1973. Nucleic acid homologies in the genus *Pseudomonas. Int. J. Syst. Bacteriol.* **23:**333–339.
88. **Pot, B., P. Vandamme, and K. Kersters.** 1994. Analysis of electrophoretic whole-organism protein fingerprints, p. 493–521. *In* M. Goodfellow and A. G. O'Donnell (ed.), *Modern Microbial Methods. Chemical Methods in Prokaryotic Systematics.* J. Wiley and Sons Ltd., Chichester, United Kingdom.
89. **Priest, F., and B. Austin.** 1993. *Modern Bacterial Taxonomy.* Chapman & Hall, London, United Kingdom.
90. **Rogers, G. B., M. P. Carroll, D. J. Serisier, P. M. Hockey, G. Jones, and K. D. Bruce.** 2004. Characterization of bacterial community diversity in cystic fibrosis lung infections by use of 16S ribosomal DNA terminal restriction fragment length polymorphism profiling. *J. Clin. Microbiol.* **42:**5176–5183.
91. **Santos, S. R., and H. Ochman.** 2004. Identification and phylogenetic sorting of bacterial lineages with universally conserved genes and proteins. *Environ. Microbiol.* **6:**754–759.
92. **Schleifer, K. H., and O. Kandler.** 1972. Peptidoglycan types of bacterial cell walls and their taxonomic implications. *Bacteriol. Rev.* **36:**407–477.
93. **Schleifer, K. H., and W. Ludwig.** 1989. Phylogenetic relationships of bacteria, p. 103–117. *In* B. Fernholm, K. Bremer, and H. Jörnvall (ed.), *The Hierarchy of Life.* Elsevier Science Publishers B.V., Amsterdam, The Netherlands.
94. **Schleifer, K. H., W. Ludwig, and R. Amann.** 1993. Nucleic acid probes, p. 463–510. *In* M. Goodfellow. and A. G. O'Donnell (ed.), *Handbook of New Bacterial Systematics.* Academic Press, London, United Kingdom.
95. **Skerman, V. B. D., V. McGowan, and P. H. A. Sneath (ed.).** 1980. Approved lists of bacterial names. *Int. J. Syst. Bacteriol.* **30:**225–420.
96. **Sneath, P. H. A.** 1984. Numerical taxonomy, p. 111–118. *In* N. R. Krieg and J. G. Holt (ed.), *Bergey's Manual of Systematic Bacteriology*, vol. 1. The Williams & Wilkins Co., Baltimore, Md.
97. **Sneath, P. H. A. (ed).** 1992. *International Code of Nomenclature of Bacteria,* 1990 revision. American Society for Microbiology, Washington, D.C.
98. **Sokal, R. R., and P. H. A. Sneath.** 1963. *Principles of Numerical Taxonomy.* W. H. Freeman and Co., San Francisco, Calif.
99. **Stackebrandt, E., W. Frederiksen, G. M. Garrity, P. A. Grimont, P. Kampfer, M. C. Maiden, X. Nesme, R. Rossello-Mora, J. Swings, H. G. Truper, L. Vauterin, A. C. Ward, and W. B. Whitman.** 2002. Report of the ad hoc committee for the re-evaluation of the species definition in bacteriology. *Int. J. Syst. Evol. Microbiol.* **52:**1043–1047.
100. **Stackebrandt, E., and B. M. Goebel.** 1994. Taxonomic note: a place for DNA-DNA reassociation and 16S rRNA sequence analysis in the present species definition in bacteriology. *Int. J. Syst. Bacteriol.* **44:**846–849.
101. **Stackebrandt, E., and W. Liesack.** 1993. Nucleic acids and classification, p. 151–194. *In* M. Goodfellow and A. G. O'Donnell (ed.), *Handbook of New Bacterial Systematics.* Academic Press, London, United Kingdom.
102. **Stackebrandt, E., R. G. E. Murray, and G. H. Trüper.** 1988. *Proteobacteria* classis nov., a name for the phylogenetic taxon that includes the "purple bacteria and their relatives." *Int. J. Syst. Bacteriol.* **38:**321–325.
103. **Stackebrandt, E., O. Pauker, and M. Erhard.** 2005. Grouping myxococci *(Corallococcus)* strains by matrix-assisted laser desorption ionization time-of-flight (MALDI TOF) mass spectrometry: comparison with gene sequence phylogenies. *Curr. Microbiol.* **50:**71–77.
104. **Staley, J. T., and N. J. Krieg.** 1984. Classification of prokaryotic organisms: an overview, p. 1–3. *In* N. R. Krieg and J. G. Holt (ed.), *Bergey's Manual of Systematic Bacteriology,* vol. 1. The Williams & Wilkins Co., Baltimore, Md.
105. **Suzuki, K., M. Goodfellow, and A. G. O'Donnell.** 1993. Cell envelopes and classification, p. 195–250 *In* M. Goodfellow and A. G. O'Donnell (ed.), *Handbook of New Bacterial Systematics.* Academic Press, London, United Kingdom.
106. **Swings, J., P. De Vos, M. Van den Mooter, and J. De Ley.** 1983. Transfer of *Pseudomonas maltophilia* Hugh 1981

to the genus *Xanthomonas* as *Xanthomonas maltophilia* (Hugh 1981) comb. nov. *Int. J. Syst. Bacteriol.* **33:**409–413.

107. **Tabor, C. W., and H. Tabor.** 1985. Polyamines in microorganisms. *Microbiol. Rev.* **49:** 81–99.
108. **Tamaoka, J., D.-M. Ha, and K. Komagata.** 1987. Reclassification of *Pseudomonas acidovorans* den Dooren de Jong 1926 and *Pseudomonas testosteroni* Marcus and Talalay 1956 as *Comamonas acidovorans* comb. nov. and *Comamonas testosteroni* comb. nov. with an emended description of the genus *Comamonas*. *Int. J. Syst. Bacteriol.* **37:**52–59.
109. **Urakami, T., C. Ito-Yoshida, H. Araki, T. Kijima, K.-I. Suzuki, and K. Komagata.** 1994. Transfer of *Pseudomonas plantarii* and *Pseudomonas glumae* to *Burkholderia* as *Burkholderia* spp. and description of *Burkholderia vandii* sp. nov. *Int. J. Syst. Bacteriol.* **44:**235–245.
110. **Ursing, J. B., R. A. Rossello-Mora, E. Garcia-Valdes, and J. Lalucat.** 1995. Taxonomic note: a pragmatic approach to the nomenclature of phenotypically similar genomic groups. *Int. J. Syst. Bacteriol.* **45:**604.
111. **van Baar, B. L.** 2000. Characterisation of bacteria by matrix-assisted laser desorption/ionisation and electrospray mass spectrometry. *FEMS Microbiol. Rev.* **24:**193–219.
112. **Van Belkum, A.** 1994. DNA fingerprinting of medically important microorganisms by use of PCR. *Clin. Microbiol. Rev.* **7:**174–184.
113. **Van Camp, G., S. Chapelle, and R. De Wachter.** 1993. Amplification and sequencing of variable regions in bacterial 23S ribosomal RNA genes with conserved primer sequences. *Curr. Microbiol.* **27:**147–151.
114. **Vancanneyt, M., P. Vandamme, and K. Kersters.** 1995. Differentiation of *Bordetella pertussis*, *B. parapertussis*, and *B. bronchiseptica* by whole-cell protein electrophoresis and fatty acid analysis. *Int. J. Syst. Bacteriol.* **45:**843–847.
115. **Vandamme, P., and T. Coenye.** 2004. Taxonomy of the genus *Cupriavidus*: a tale of lost and found. *Int. J. Syst. Evol. Microbiol.* **54:**2285–2289.
116. **Vandamme, P., E. Falsen, R. Rossau, B. Hoste, P. Segers, R. Tytgat, and J. De Ley.** 1991. Revision of *Campylobacter*, *Helicobacter*, and *Wolinella* taxonomy: emendation of generic descriptions and proposal of *Arcobacter* gen. nov. *Int. J. Syst. Bacteriol.* **41:**88–103.
117. **Vandamme, P., C. S. Harrington, K. Jalava, and S. L. W. On.** 2000. Misidentifying helicobacters: the *Helicobacter cinaedi* example. *J. Clin. Microbiol.* **38:**2261–2266.
118. **Vandamme, P., B. Pot, M. Gillis, P. De Vos, K. Kersters, and J. Swings.** 1996. Polyphasic taxonomy, a consensus approach to bacterial classification. *Microbiol. Rev.* **60:**407–438.
119. **Vandamme, P., P. Segers, M. Vancanneyt, K. Van Hove, R. Mutters, J. Hommez, F. E. Dewhirst, B. J. Paster, K. Kersters, E. Falsen, L. A. Devriese, M. Bisgaard, K.-H. Hinz, and W. Mannheim.** 1994. *Ornithobacterium rhinotracheale* gen. nov., sp. nov., isolated from the avian respiratory tract. *Int. J. Syst. Bacteriol.* **44:**24–37.
120. **Vandamme, P., M. Vancanneyt, P. Segers, M. Ryll, B. Köhler, W. Ludwig, and K. H. Hinz.** 1999. *Coenonia anatina* gen. nov., sp. nov., a novel bacterium associated with respiratory disease in ducks and geese. *Int. J. Syst. Bacteriol.* **49:**867–874.
121. **Van de Peer, Y., J. Jansen, P. De Rijk, and R. De Wachter.** 1997. Database on the structure of small ribosomal subunit RNA sequences. *Nucleic Acids Res.* **25:**111–116.
122. **Vaneechoutte, M., P. Kaempfer, T. De Baere, E. Falsen, and G. Verschraegen.** 2004. *Wautersia* gen. nov., a novel genus accommodating the phylogenetic lineage including *Ralstonia eutropha* and related species, and proposal of *Ralstonia* [*Pseudomonas*] *syzygii* (Roberts et al. 1990) comb. nov. *Int. J. Syst. Evol. Microbiol.* **54:**317–327.
123. **Viale, A. M., A. K. Arakaki, F. C. Soncini, and R. G. Ferreyra.** 1994. Evolutionary relationships among eubacterial groups as inferred from GroEL (chaperonin) sequence comparisons. *Int. J. Syst. Bacteriol.* **44:**527–533.
124. **Walker, G. T., M. C. Little, J. G. Nadeau, and D. D. Shank.** 1992. Isothermal *in vitro* amplification of DNA by a restriction enzyme DNA polymerase system. *Proc. Natl. Acad. Sci. USA* **89:**392–396.
125. **Wayne, L. G., D. J. Brenner, R. R. Colwell, P. A. D. Grimont, P. Kandler, M. I. Krichevsky, L. H. Moore, W. E. C. Moore, R. G. E. Murray, E. Stackebrandt, M. P. Starr, and H. G. Trüper.** 1987. Report of the ad hoc committee on reconciliation of approaches to bacterial systematics. *Int. J. Syst. Bacteriol.* **37:**463–464.
126. **Welch, D. F.** 1991. Applications of cellular fatty acid analysis. *Clin. Microbiol. Rev.* **4:**422–438.
127. **Welsh, J., and M. McClelland.** 1990. Fingerprinting genomes using PCR with arbitrary primers. *Nucleic Acids Res.* **18:**7213–7218.
128. **Welsh, J., and M. McClelland.** 1992. PCR-amplified length polymorphisms in tRNA intergenic spacers for categorizing staphylococci. *Mol. Microbiol.* **6:**1673–1680.
129. **Wen, A., M. Fegan, C. Hayward, S. Chakraborty, and L. I. Sly.** 1999. Phylogenetic relationships among members of the *Comamonadaceae*, and description of *Delftia acidovorans* (den Dooren de Jong 1926 and Tamaoka *et al.* 1987) gen. nov., comb. nov. *Int. J. Syst. Bacteriol.* **49:**567–576.
130. **Wenning, M., H. Seiler, and S. Scherer.** 2002. Fourier-transform infrared microspectroscopy, a novel and rapid tool for identification of yeasts. *Appl. Environ. Microbiol.* **68:**4717–4721.
131. **Willems, A., E. Falsen, B. Pot, E. Jantzen, B. Hoste, P. Vandamme, M. Gillis, K. Kersters, and J. De Ley.** 1990. *Acidovorax*, a new genus for *Pseudomonas facilis*, *Pseudomonas delafieldii*, E. Falsen (EF) Group 13, EF Group 16, and several clinical isolates, with the species *Acidovorax facilis* comb. nov., *Acidovorax delafieldii* comb. nov., and *Acidovorax temperans* sp. nov. *Int. J. Syst. Bacteriol.* **40:**384–398.
132. **Woese, C. R.** 1987. Bacterial evolution. *Microbiol. Rev.* **51:**221–271.
133. **Yabuuchi, E., Y. Kosako, H. Oyaizu, I. Yano, H. Hotta, Y. Hashimoto, T. Ezaki, and M. Arakawa.** 1992. Proposal of *Burkholderia* gen. nov. and transfer of seven species of the genus *Pseudomonas* homology group II to the new genus, with the type species *Burkholderia cepacia* (Palleroni and Holmes 1981) comb. nov. *Microbiol. Immunol.* **36:**1251–1275.
134. **Yabuuchi, E., Y. Kosako, I. Yano, H. Hotta, and Y. Nishiuchi.** 1995. Transfer of two *Burkholderia* and an *Alcaligenes* species to *Ralstonia* gen. nov.: proposal of *Ralstonia pickettii* (Ralston, Palleroni and Doudoroff 1973) comb. nov., *Ralstonia solanacearum* (Smith 1896) comb. nov. and *Ralstonia eutropha* (Davis 1969) comb. nov. *Microbiol. Immunol.* **39:**897–904.
135. **Young, J. M.** 2001. Implications of alternative classifications and horizontal gene transfer for bacterial taxonomy. *Int. J. Syst. Evol. Microbiol.* **51:**945–953.
136. **Zabeau, M., and P. Vos.** 1993. *Selective Restriction Fragment Amplification: a General Method for DNA Fingerprinting*. Publication 0534858 A1. European Patent Office, Munich, Germany.
137. **Zaluzec, E. J., D. A. Gage, and J. T. Watson.** 1995. Matrix-assisted laser desorption ionization mass spectrometry: applications in peptide and protein characterization. *Protein Expr. Purif.* **6:**109–123.
138. **Zeigler, D. R.** 2003. Gene sequences useful for predicting relatedness of whole genomes in bacteria. *Int. J. Syst. Evol. Microbiol.* **53:**1893–1900.

139. **Zhao, N., C. Qu, E. Wang, and W. Chen.** 1995. Phylogenetic evidence for the transfer of *Pseudomonas cocovenenans* (van Damme et al. 1960) to the genus *Burkholderia* as *Burkholderia cocovenenans* (van Damme et al. 1960) comb. nov. *Int. J. Syst. Bacteriol.* **45:**600–603.

140. **Zillig, W., H.-P. Klenk, P. Palm, G. Pühler, F. Gropp, R. A. Garret, and H. Leffers.** 1989. The phylogenetic relations of DNA-dependent RNA polymerases of archaebacteria, eukaryotes, and eubacteria. *Can. J. Microbiol.* **35:**73–80.

Specimen Collection, Transport, and Processing: Bacteriology*

RICHARD B. THOMSON, JR.

20

The use of specimens for bacteriological analysis requires that specific clinical material be collected, stabilized, and transported according to exacting specifications to ensure valid results. Poor specimen quality contributes to misdiagnosis and inappropriate antimicrobial therapy. Communication between the laboratory representative and clinician is essential to the proper selection of bacteriology tests and interpretation of their results. Laboratory personnel are responsible for monitoring and educating those collecting and transporting specimens. The use of professional journals is an excellent approach to the continuing education of all who work in and use the laboratory. Laboratories are required by accrediting agencies to provide specimen collection and transport manuals. A useful alternative to printed manuals is an electronic version available over a local area network (13, 100).

Specimens for bacteriological culture should be collected as soon as possible after the onset of disease and before the initiation of antimicrobial therapy. A second specimen may be necessary because of poor specimen quality or inadequate transport conditions that affected the first specimen, but is otherwise rarely required for diagnosis of an acute infectious disease. Exceptions include the collection of multiple blood specimens for culture and those obtained for the detection of fastidious or unusual pathogens not originally suspected.

SELECTION AND COLLECTION OF SPECIMENS

Material for bacteriological testing should be collected from a site representative of the active disease process. Sites of an inflammatory process and free of contaminating flora are optimal. In practice, most specimen collection sites are contaminated with various quantities of commensal bacteria. As examples, urethral floras contaminate urine collected by micturition, skin floras contaminate blood collected by percutaneous venipuncture, vaginal and cervical floras contaminate endometrial specimens collected through the endocervix, skin and environmental floras contaminate cutaneous fistulas and deep wounds that are open to skin or mucous membrane surfaces, floras in the external ear canal contaminate middle ear fluid following rupture of the tympanic membrane, floras in the nasopharynx and nasal passages contaminate specimens from the nasal sinuses, and the floras in the upper respiratory tract contaminate sputum and other lower respiratory tract specimens. Table 1 lists common diseases with appropriate and inappropriate clinical specimens (11, 224). General specimen selection and collection guidelines include the following (122).

1. Select the proper anatomic site from which to collect the specimen.
2. Avoid contamination with indigenous flora. Growth and reporting of normal flora can be mistaken by the physician or caregiver as the cause of the infectious process. In addition, the flora can overgrow and obscure the true etiology.
3. Surface disinfection followed by aspiration and biopsy of tissue are appropriate methods for specimen collection when anaerobic bacteria are suspected (Table 2). Collection with a swab is not recommended because of the relatively small amount of specimen sampled, difficulty of actually obtaining anaerobes on the swab, aeration of swabs, and the ease with which the swab can be contaminated with adjacent members of the normal flora. Unless they are in a completely airtight container, specimens for anaerobic culture should be stored at room, not refrigeration, temperature, since oxygen diffuses into cold specimens more readily.
4. Collect sufficient volume of material to enable all test requests to be performed satisfactorily. Insufficient material may yield false-negative results.
5. Label each specimen with the patient's name and identification number, source of specimen, date and time of collection, and initials of the collector.
6. Use a specimen container designed to promote survival of pathogenic bacteria, eliminate leakage of specimen, and allow safe handling during transport and processing. Do not transport specimens in syringes.

Specific specimen collection guidelines are summarized in Table 3.

TRANSPORT OF SPECIMENS

Specimens for bacterial culture should be transported to the laboratory immediately. Excessive delay or exposure to temperature extremes compromises results and must be avoided.

* This chapter contains information presented in chapter 20 by Richard B. Thomson, Jr., and J. Michael Miller in the eighth edition of this Manual.

TABLE 1 Selection of common clinical specimens for bacterial culture[a]

Anatomic site	Clinical specimen(s)	
	Appropriate	Inappropriate
Lower respiratory tract	Freshly expectorated mucus and inflammatory cells (pus), sputum	Saliva, oropharyngeal secretions, sinus drainage from nasopharynx
Sinus	Secretions collected by direct sinus aspiration, or washes, curettage, and biopsy material collected during endoscopy	Nasal or nasopharyngeal swab, nasopharyngeal secretions, sputum, and saliva
Urinary tract	Midstream urine, urine collected by "straight" catheterization, urine collected by suprapubic aspiration, urine collected during cystoscopy or other surgical procedure	Urine from Foley catheter collection bag, "bagged" urine from infants
Superficial wound	Aspirations of pus or local irrigation fluid (nonbacteriostatic saline), swab of purulence originating from beneath the dermis	Swab of surface material or specimen contaminated with surface material, irrigation with saline containing preservative
Deep wound	Purulence, necrosis, or tissue from deep subcutaneous site	Specimen contaminated with surface material
Gastrointestinal tract	Freshly passed stool, washes, or feces collected during endoscopy; rectal swab (in selected cases)	Rectal swab, specimen for bacterial culture if diarrhea developed after patient was in hospital for >3 days
Venous blood	Two or three blood specimens collected from separate venipunctures, before initiation of antibiotics, each containing approx 20 ml of blood for patients >90 lb (see Table 7 for pediatric volumes); antisepsis with iodine-containing compound or chlorhexidine	Clotted blood; one or more than three blood specimens collected within a 24-h period; vol of blood <20 ml per culture (i.e., per venipuncture); antisepsis with alcohol only (adults)

[a] Reprinted from reference 195 with permission.

TABLE 2 Suitability of various specimens for anaerobic culture

Acceptable material (method of collection)	Unacceptable material
Aspirate (by needle and syringe)	Bronchoalveolar lavage washing
Bartholin's gland inflammation/secretions	Cervical secretions
Blood (venipuncture)	Endotracheal secretions (aspirate)
Bone marrow (aspirate)	Lochia secretions
Bronchoscopic secretions (protected specimen brush)	Nasopharyngeal swab
Culdocentesis fluid (aspirate)	Perineal swab
Fallopian tube fluid or tissue (aspirate/biopsy)	Prostatic or seminal fluid
IUD, for *Actinomyces* spp.	Sinus washings or swabs
Nasal sinus (aspirate)	Sputum (expectorated or induced)
Placenta tissue (via cesarean delivery)	Stool or rectal swab samples
Stool, for *C. difficile*	Tracheostomy secretions
Surgical site (aspirate, tissue)	Urethral secretions
Transtracheal aspirate	Urine (voided or from catheter)
Urine (suprapubic aspirate)	Vaginal or vulvar secretions (swab)

TABLE 3 Bacteriology collection, transport, and storage guidelines[a]

Specimen type (reference)	Collection guidelines	Transport device and/or minimum vol	Transport[b] time and temp	Storage time and temp	Replica limits	Comments
Abscess (17)						
General	Remove surface exudate by wiping with sterile saline or 70% alcohol.					Tissue or aspirate is always superior to a swab specimen. If swabs must be used (aerobic culture only), collect two, one for culture and one for Gram staining. Preserve swab material by placing in Stuart's or Amies medium.
Open	Aspirate if possible or pass a swab deep into the lesion to firmly sample the lesion's "fresh border."	Swab transport system	≤2 h, RT	≤24 h, RT	1/day/source	Samples of the base of the lesion and abscess wall are most productive.
Closed	Aspirate abscess material with needle and syringe. Aseptically transfer *all* material into anaerobic transport device.	Anaerobic transport system, ≥1 ml	≤2 h, RT	≤24 h, RT	1/day/source	Contamination with surface material will introduce colonizing bacteria not involved in the infectious process. Do not use syringe for transport.
Bite wound	See Abscess					Do not culture animal bite wounds ≤12 h old (agents are usually not recovered) unless signs of infection are present.
Blood (15, 160)	Disinfect culture bottle; apply 70% isopropyl alcohol or phenolic disinfectant to rubber stoppers and wait 1 min. Palpate vein before disinfection of venipuncture site. Disinfection of venipuncture site: 1. Cleanse site with 70% alcohol. 2. Swab concentrically, starting at the center, with tincture of iodine or chlorhexidine. 3. Allow the disinfectant to dry. 4. *Do not palpate vein at this point without sterile glove.*	Blood culture bottles for bacteria; adult, 20 ml/set (higher vol most productive); infant and child, 1–20 ml/set depending on wt of patient (see Table 7)	≤2 h, RT	≤2 h, RT or per instructions	3 sets in 24 h	Acute febrile episode: 2 sets[c] from separate sites, all within 10 min (before antimicrobials) Nonacute disease, antimicrobials will not be started or changed immediately: 2 or 3 sets from separate sites, all within 24 h at intervals no closer than 3 h (before antimicrobials) Endocarditis, acute: 3 sets from 3 separate sites, within 1–2 h, before antimicrobials if possible Fever of unknown origin: 2 or 3 sets from separate sites ≥1 h apart during 24-h period. If negative at 24–48 h, obtain 2 or 3 more sets. Some data indicate that an additional aerobic or fungal bottle is more productive than the anaerobic bottle.

(Continued on next page)

TABLE 3 Bacteriology collection, transport, and storage guidelines[a] *(Continued)*

Specimen type (reference)	Collection guidelines	Transport device and/or minimum vol	Transport[b] time and temp	Storage time and temp	Replica limits	Comments
	5. Collect blood. 6. After venipuncture, remove iodine from the skin with alcohol.					Pediatric: collect immediately; rarely necessary to document ccontinuous bacteremia with hours between cultures.
Bone marrow aspirate	Prepare puncture site as for surgical incision.	Inoculate blood culture bottle or a 1.5-ml lysis centrifugation tube.	≤24 h, RT, if in culture bottle or tube	≤24 h, RT	1/day	Small volumes of bone marrow may be inoculated directly onto culture media. Routine bacterial culture of bone marrow is rarely useful.
Burn	Clean and debride the burn.	Tissue is placed into a sterile screw-cap container; aspirate or swab exudates; transport in sterile container or swab transport system	≤24 h, RT	≤24 h, RT	1/day/source	A 3- to 4-mm punch biopsy specimen is optimum when quantitative cultures are ordered. Process for aerobic culture only. Quantitative culture may or may not be valuable. Cultures of surface samples of burns may be misleading.
Catheter						
i.v. (109)	1. Cleanse the skin around the catheter site with alcohol. 2. Aseptically remove catheter and clip 5 cm of distal tip directly into a sterile tube. Some elect to culture the 5-cm intracutaneous portion to evaluate for soft tissue infection. 3. Transport immediately to microbiology laboratory to prevent drying.	Sterile screw-cap tube or cup	≤15 min, RT	≤2 h, 4°C	None	Acceptable i.v. catheters for semiquantitative culture (Maki method): central, CVP, Hickman, Broviac, peripheral, arterial, umbilical, hyperalimentation, Swan-Ganz
Foley	Do *not* culture, since growth represents distal urethral flora.					Not acceptable for culture.
Cellulitis, aspirate from area of (17)	1. Cleanse site by wiping with sterile saline or 70% alcohol.	Sterile tube (syringe transport not recommended)	≤15 min, RT	≤24 h, RT	None	Yield of potential pathogens in minority of specimens cultured

	2. Aspirate the area of maximum inflammation (commonly the center rather than the leading edge) with a needle and syringe. Irrigation with a small amount of sterile saline may be necessary. 3. Aspirate saline into syringe and expel into sterile screw-cap tube.					
CSF	1. Disinfect site with iodine preparation. 2. Insert a needle with stylet at L3-L4, L4-L5, or L5-S1 interspace. 3. Upon reaching the subarachnoid space, remove the stylet and collect 1–2 ml of fluid into each of 3 leakproof tubes.	Sterile screw-cap tubes Minimum amt required: bacteria, ≥1 ml	Bacteria: never refrigerate; ≤15 min, RT	≤24 h, RT	None	Obtain blood for culture also. If only 1 tube of CSF is collected, it should be submitted to microbiology first; otherwise submit tube 2 to microbiology. Aspirate of brain abscess or a biopsy sample may be necessary to detect anaerobic bacteria or parasites.
Decubitus ulcer (17)	A swab is not the specimen of choice (see comments). 1. Cleanse surface with sterile saline. 2. If a biopsy sample is not available, aspirate inflammatory material from the base of the ulcer.	Sterile tube/container (aerobic) or anaerobic system (for tissue)	≤2 h, RT	≤24 h, RT	1/day/source	Since a swab specimen of a decubitus ulcer provides no clinical information, it should not be submitted. A tissue biopsy sample or needle aspirate is the specimen of choice.
Dental culture: gingival, periodontal, periapical, Vincent's stomatitis	1. Carefully cleanse gingival margin and supragingival tooth surface to remove saliva, debris, and plaque. 2. Using a periodontal scaler, carefully remove subgingival lesion material and transfer it to an anaerobic transport system. 3. Prepare smear for staining with specimen collected in the same fashion.	Anaerobic transport system	≤2 h, RT	≤24 h, RT	1/day	Periodontal lesions should be processed only by laboratories equipped to provide specialized techniques for the detection and enumeration of recognized pathogens.

(Continued on next page)

TABLE 3 Bacteriology collection, transport, and storage guidelines[a] *(Continued)*

Specimen type (reference)	Collection guidelines	Transport device and/or minimum vol	Transport[b] time and temp	Storage time and temp	Replica limits	Comments
Ear						
Inner (25)	Tympanocentesis reserved for complicated, recurrent, or chronic persistent otitis media 1. For intact eardrum, clean ear canal with soap solution and collect fluid via syringe aspiration technique (tympanocentesis). 2. For ruptured eardrum, collect fluid on flexible shaft swab via an auditory speculum (aerobic culture only).	Sterile tube, swab transport medium, or anaerobic system	≤2 h, RT	≤24 h, RT	1/day/source	Results of throat or nasopharyngeal swab cultures are not predictive of agents responsible for otitis media and should not be submitted for that purpose.
Outer (168)	1. Use moistened swab to remove any debris or crust from the ear canal. 2. Obtain a sample by firmly rotating swab in the outer canal.	Swab transport	≤2 h, RT	≤24 h, 4°C	1/day/source	For otitis externa, *vigorous* swabbing is required since surface swabbing may miss streptococcal cellulitis.
Eye						
Conjunctiva (4, 86)	1. Sample both eyes with separate swabs (premoistened with sterile saline) by rolling them over each conjunctiva. 2. Medium may be inoculated at time of collection. 3. Smear may be prepared at time of collection. Roll swab over 1- to 2-cm area of slide.	Direct culture inoculation: BAP and CHOC Laboratory inoculation: swab transport	Plates: ≤15 min, RT Swabs: ≤2 h, RT	≤24 h, RT	None	If possible, sample both conjunctivas, even if only one is infected, to determine indigenous microflora. The uninfected eye can serve as a control with which to compare the agents isolated from the infected eye. If cost prohibits this approach, rely on the Gram stain to assist in interpretation of culture.
Corneal scrapings (4, 86)	1. Specimen collected by ophthalmologist 2. Using sterile spatula, scrape ulcers or lesions, and inoculate scraping directly onto medium. 3. Prepare 2 smears by rubbing material from spatula onto 1- to 2-cm area of slide.	Direct culture inoculations: BHI with 10% sheep blood, CHOC, and inhibitory mold agar	≤15 min, RT	≤24 h, RT	None	If conjunctival specimen is collected, do so before anesthetic application, which may inhibit some bacteria. Corneal scrapings are obtained after anesthesia. Include fungal media.

Vitreous fluid aspirates	Prepare eye for needle aspiration of fluid.	Sterile screw-cap tube or direct inoculation of small amount of fluid onto media	≤15 min, RT	≤24 h, RT	1/day	Include fungal media. Anesthetics may be inhibitory to some etiologic agents.
Feces						
Routine culture (63)	Pass specimen directly into a clean, dry container. Transport to microbiology laboratory within 1 h of collection or transfer to Cary-Blair holding medium.	Clean, leakproof, widemouthed container or use Cary-Blair holding medium (>2 g)	Unpreserved: ≤1 h, RT Holding medium: ≤24 h, RT	≤24 h, 4°C ≤48 h, RT or 4°C	1/day	Do not perform routine stool cultures for patients whose length of hospital stay is >3 days and the admitting diagnosis was not gastroenteritis without consultation with physician. Tests for C. *difficile* should be considered for these patients. Swabs for routine pathogens are not recommended except for infants (see Rectal swabs).
C. *difficile* (84)	Pass liquid or soft stool directly into a clean, dry container. Soft stool is defined as stool assuming the shape of its container. Swab specimens are not recommended for toxin testing.	Sterile, leakproof, widemouthed container, >5 ml	≤1 h, RT; 1–24 h, 4°C; >24 h, −20°C or colder	2 days, 4°C, for culture; 3 days at 4°C or longer at −70°C for toxin test	1 or 2 specimens may be necessary to detect low toxin levels.	Patients should be passing ≥5 liquid or soft stools per 24 h. Testing of formed or hard stool is not recommended. Freezing at −20°C or above results in rapid loss of cytotoxin activity.
E. coli (O157:H7) and other Shiga toxin-producing serotypes (5, 50)	Pass liquid or bloody stool into a clean, dry container.	Sterile, leakproof, widemouthed container, or Cary-Blair holding medium (>2 g)	Unpreserved. ≤1 h, RT Swab transport system: ≤24 h, RT or 4°C	≤24 h, 4°C ≤24 h, RT	1/day	Bloody or liquid stools collected within 6 days of onset from patients with abdominal cramps have the highest yield. Shiga toxin assay for all EHEC serotypes is better than sorbitol MacConkey or chromogenic agar culture for O157:H7 only.
Leukocyte detection (68) (not recommended for use with patients who have acute infectious diarrhea)						This procedure should be discouraged because it provides results of little clinical value.

(Continued on next page)

TABLE 3 Bacteriology collection, transport, and storage guidelines[a] *(Continued)*

Specimen type (reference)	Collection guidelines	Transport device and/or minimum vol	Transport[b] time and temp	Storage time and temp	Replica limits	Comments
Rectal swab	1. Carefully insert a swab approx 1 in. beyond the anal sphincter. 2. Gently rotate the swab to sample the anal crypts. 3. Feces should be visible on the swab for detection of diarrheal pathogens.	Swab transport	≤2 h, RT	≤24 h, RT	1/day	Reserved for detecting *N. gonorrhoeae, Shigella, Campylobacter,* herpes simplex virus, and anal carriage of group B *Streptococcus* and other beta-hemolytic streptococci, or for patients unable to pass a specimen.
Fistula	See Abscess					
Fluids: abdominal, amniotic, ascites, bile, joint, paracentesis, pericardial, peritoneal, pleural, synovial, thoracentesis (17)	1. Disinfect overlying skin with iodine preparation. 2. Obtain specimen via percutaneous needle aspiration or surgery. 3. Always submit as much fluid as possible; *never* submit a swab dipped in fluid.	Anaerobic transport system, sterile screw-cap tube, or blood culture bottle for bacteria; transport immediately to laboratory Bacteria, >1 ml	≤15 min, RT	≤24 h, RT; pericardial fluid and fluids for fungal cultures, ≤24 h, 4°C	None	Amniotic and culdocentesis fluids should be transported in an anaerobic system and need not be centrifuged prior to Gram staining. Other fluids are best examined by Gram staining of a cytocentrifuged preparation. One aerobic blood culture bottle inoculated at bedside is highly recommended.
Gangrenous tissue	See Abscess					Discourage sampling of surface or superficial tissue. Tissue biopsy or aspirates should be collected.
Gastric						
Wash or lavage for mycobacteria (24)	Collect in early morning before patients eat and while they are still in bed. 1. Introduce a nasogastric tube to the stomach. 2. Perform lavage with 25–50 ml of chilled sterile, distilled water. 3. Recover sample and place in a leakproof, sterile container.	Sterile, leakproof container	≤15 min, RT, or neutralize within 1 h of collection	≤24 h, 4°C	1/day	The specimen must be processed promptly, since mycobacteria die rapidly in gastric washings. Neutralize with sodium bicarbonate when holding for > 1 h.
Biopsy for *H. pylori*	Collected by gastroenterologist during endoscopy.	Sterile tube with transport medium	<1 h, RT	≤24 h, 4°C	None	Culture may be needed for antimicrobial testing.
Genital, female						
Amniotic fluid (209)	Aspirate via amniocentesis, or collect during cesarean delivery.	Anaerobic transport system, ≥1 ml	≤2 h, RT	≤24 h, RT	None	Swabbing or aspiration of vaginal secretions is *not* acceptable because of the potential for contamination with commensal vaginal flora.

Bartholin gland secretions	1. Disinfect skin with iodine preparation. 2. Aspirate fluid from ducts.	Anaerobic transport system, ≥1 ml	≤2 h, RT	≤24 h, RT	1/day	
Cervical secretions (6)	1. Visualize the cervix using a speculum without lubricant. 2. Remove mucus and secretions from the cervical os with swab and discard the swab. 3. Firmly yet gently sample the endocervical canal with a new sterile swab.	Swab transport	≤2 h, RT	≤24 h, RT	1/day	See text for collection and transport need for *C. trachomatis* and *N. gonorrhoeae*.
Cul-de-sac fluid	Submit aspirate or fluid.	Anaerobic transport system, >1 ml	≤2 h, RT	≤24 h, RT	1/day	
Endometrial tissue and secretions	1. Collect transcervical aspirate via a telescoping catheter. 2. Transfer entire amount to anaerobic transport system.	Anaerobic transport system, ≥1 ml	≤2 h, RT	≤24 h, RT	1/day	
Products of conception	1. Submit a portion of tissue in a sterile container. 2. If obtained by cesarean delivery, immediately transfer to an anaerobic transport system.	Sterile tube or anaerobic transport system	≤2 h, RT	≤24 h, RT	1/day	Do not process lochia, culture of which may give misleading results.
Urethral secretions (6)	Collect at least 1 h after patient has urinated. 1. Remove old exudate from the urethral orifice. 2. Collect discharge material on a swab by massaging the urethra against the pubic symphysis through the vagina.	Swab transport	≤2 h, RT	≤24 h, RT	1/day	If no discharge can be obtained, wash the periurethral area with Betadine soap and rinse with water. Insert a small swab 2–4 cm into the urethra, rotate swab, and leave swab in place for at least 2 s to facilitate absorption.
Vaginal secretions (6)	1. Wipe away old secretions/discharge. 2. Obtain secretions from the mucosal membrane of the vaginal wall with a sterile swab or pipette. 3. If a smear is also needed, use a second swab.	Swab transport	≤2 h, RT	≤24 h, RT	1/day	For IUDs, place entire device into a sterile container and submit at RT. Gram stain, not culture, is recommended for diagnosis of BV.

(Continued on next page)

TABLE 3 Bacteriology collection, transport, and storage guidelines[a] *(Continued)*

Specimen type (reference)	Collection guidelines	Transport device and/or minimum vol	Transport[b] time and temp	Storage time and temp	Replica limits	Comments
Genital, female or male lesion	1. Clean with sterile saline and remove lesion's surface with a sterile scalped blade. 2. Allow transudate to accumulate. 3. While pressing the base of the lesion, *firmly* rub base with a sterile swab to collect fluid.	Swab transport	≤2 h, RT	≤24 h, RT	1/day	For dark-field examination to detect *T. pallidum*, touch a glass slide to the transudate, add coverslip, and transport immediately to the laboratory in a humidified chamber (petri dish with moist gauze). *T. pallidum* cannot be cultured on artificial media.
Genital, male						
Prostate	1. Cleanse urethral meatus with soap and water. 2. Massage prostate through rectum. 3. Collect fluid expressed from urethra on a sterile swab.	Swab transport or sterile tube for >1 ml of specimen	≤2 h, RT	≤24 h, RT	1/day	Pathogens in prostatic secretions may be identified by quantitative culture of urine before and after massage. Ejaculate may also be cultured.
Urethra	Insert a small swab 2–4 cm into the urethral lumen, rotate swab, and leave it in place for at least 2 s to facilitate absorption.	Swab transport	≤2 h, RT	≤24 h, RT	1/day	
Pilonidal cyst	See Abscess					
Respiratory, lower						
Bronchoalveolar lavage, brush or wash, endotracheal aspirate	1. Collect washing or aspirate in a sputum trap. 2. Place brush in sterile container with 1 ml of saline.	Sterile container, >1 ml	≤2 h, RT	≤24 h, 4°C	1/day	A total of 40–80 ml of fluid is needed for quantitative analysis. For quantitative analysis of brushings, place brush into 1.0 ml of saline.
Sputum, expectorated (10)	1. Collect specimen under the direct supervision of a nurse or physician. 2. Have patient rinse or gargle with water to remove excess oral flora. 3. Instruct patient to cough deeply to produce a lower respiratory specimen (not postnasal fluid). 4. Collect in a sterile container.	Sterile container, >1 ml Minimum amt: bacteria, >1 ml	≤2 h, RT	≤24 h, 4°C	1/day	For pediatric patients unable to produce a sputum specimen, a respiratory therapist should collect a specimen via suction. The best specimen from all patients should have ≤10 squamous cells/100× field (10× objective and 10× ocular).

Sputum, induced (10)	1. Have patient rinse mouth with water after brushing gums and tongue. 2. With the aid of a nebulizer, have patients inhale approx 25 ml of 3–10% sterile saline. 3. Collect in a sterile container.	Sterile container, >1 ml	≤2 h, RT	≤24 h, RT	1/day	Same as above for sputum, expectorated.
Respiratory, upper						
Oral	1. Remove oral secretions and debris from the surface of the lesion with a swab. Discard this swab. 2. Using a second swab, vigorously sample the lesion, avoiding any areas of normal tissue.	Swab transport	≤2 h, RT	≤24 h, RT	1/day	Discourage sampling of superficial tissue for bacterial evaluation. Tissue biopsy specimens or needle aspirates are the specimens of choice.
Nasal	1. Insert a swab, premoistened with sterile saline, approx 1–2 cm into the nares. 2. Rotate the swab against the nasal mucosa.	Swab transport	≤2 h, RT	≤24 h, RT	1/day	Anterior nose cultures are reserved for identifying staphylococcal carriers or for nasal lesions.
Nasopharynx (25)	1. Gently insert a small swab (e.g., calcium alginate) into the posterior nasopharynx via the nose. 2. Rotate swab slowly for 5 s to absorb secretions.	Direct medium inoculation at bedside or examination table, swab transport	Plates: ≤15 min, RT Swabs: ≤2 h, RT	≤24 h, RT	1/day	
Throat or pharynx	1. Depress tongue with a tongue depressor. 2. Sample the posterior pharynx, tonsils, and inflamed areas with a sterile swab.	Swab transport (dry swab with or without silica gel is good for *S. pyogenes* and *C. diphtheriae*)	≤2 h, RT	≤24 h, RT	1/day	Throat swab cultures are contraindicated for patients with epiglottitis. Swabs for *N. gonorrhoeae* should be placed in charcoal-containing transport medium and plated ≤12 h after collection. JEMBEC, Bio-Bags, and the GonoPak are better for transport at RT.
Tissue	Collected during surgery or cutaneous biopsy procedure	Anaerobic transport system or sterile, screw-cap container. Add several drops of sterile saline to keep small pieces of tissue moist.	≤15 min, RT	≤24 h, RT	None	Always submit as much tissue as possible. If excess tissue is available, save a portion of surgical tissue at −70°C in case further studies are needed. Never submit a swab that has been rubbed over the surface of a tissue. For quantitative study, a sample of 1 cm^3 is appropriate.

(*Continued on next page*)

TABLE 3 Bacteriology collection, transport, and storage guidelines[a] *(Continued)*

Specimen type (reference)	Collection guidelines	Transport device and/or minimum vol	Transport[b] time and temp	Storage time and temp	Replica limits	Comments
Urine						
Female, midstream (29)	1. While holding the labia apart, begin voiding. 2. After several milliliters has passed, collect a midstream portion without stopping the flow of urine. 3. The midstream portion is used for bacterial culture.	Sterile, widemouthed container, ≥1 ml, or urine transport tube with boric acid preservative	Unpreserved: ≤2 h, RT Preserved: ≤24 h, RT	≤24 h, 4°C	1/day	Chlamydial DNA detection in urine from women is less sensitive than in urine from men. Urine is toxic to cell lines and is therefore not the specimen of choice for chlamydial culture. Cleansing before voiding does not improve urine specimen quality; i.e., midstream urine samples are equivalent to clean-catch midstream urine samples.
Male, midstream (29)	1. While holding the foreskin retracted, begin voiding. 2. After several milliliters has passed, collect a midstream portion without stopping the flow of urine. 3. The midstream portion is used for culture.	Sterile, widemouthed container, ≥1 ml, or urine transport tube with boric acid preservative	Unpreserved: ≤2 h, RT	≤24 h, 4°C	1/day	First part of urine stream is used for probe and DNA amplification tests for *Chlamydia*. Collect urine for probe and DNA amplification tests at least 2 h after previous urination.
Straight catheter (29)	1. Thoroughly cleanse the urethral opening with soap and water. 2. Rinse area with wet gauze pads. 3. Aseptically, insert catheter into the bladder. 4. After allowing approx 15 ml to pass, collect urine to be submitted in a sterile container.	Sterile, leakproof container or urine transport tube with boric acid preservative	Unpreserved: ≤2 h, RT Preserved: ≤24 h, RT	≤24 h, 4°C	1/day	Catheterization may introduce urethral flora into the bladder and increase the risk of iatrogenic infection.
Indwelling catheter	1. Disinfect the catheter collection port with 70% alcohol. Clamp catheter below port and allow urine to collect in tubing for 10–20 min. 2. Use needle and syringe to aseptically collect 5 to 10 ml of urine. 3. Transfer to a sterile tube or container.	Sterile leakproof container or urine transport tube with boric acid preservative	Unpreserved: ≤2 h, RT Preserved: ≤24 h, RT	≤24 h, 4°C	1/day	Patients with indwelling catheters always have bacteria in their bladders. Do not collect urine from these patients unless they are symptomatic.
Wound	See Abscess					

[a] Abbreviations: AFB, acid-fast bacilli; BAP, blood agar plate; BHI, brain heart infusion; CHOC, chocolate agar; CVP, central venous pressure; i.v., intravenous; PVA, polyvinyl alcohol fixative; RT, room temperature.
[b] All specimen containers are to be transported in leakproof plastic bags having a separate compartment for the requisition.
[c] One set refers to one culture with both aerobic and anaerobic broths.

General specimen transport guidelines include the following (11, 122).

1. Specimens must be transported promptly to the laboratory. If transport will require more than 2 h, a special holding medium or refrigeration temperature is required (Table 3).

2. Do not store specimens for bacterial culture for more than 24 h even with appropriate holding medium or refrigeration temperature.

3. Optimal transport times of clinical specimens for bacteriological culture depend on the volume of material obtained. Small volumes of fluid (<1 ml) or tissue (<1 cm^3) should be submitted within 15 to 30 min to avoid evaporation, drying, and exposure to ambient conditions. Larger volumes and those specimens in holding medium may be stored as long as 24 h.

4. Bacteria that are especially sensitive to ambient conditions include *Shigella* spp., *Neisseria gonorrhoeae, Neisseria meningitidis, Haemophilus influenzae, Streptococcus pneumoniae,* and anaerobes. Reliable detection of these species requires immediate processing. Delays of up to 6 h result in minimal loss of CFU when transport media are used. Longer delays, even with the use of transport media, result in significant losses of organisms. For delays beyond 6 h, refrigeration improves recovery; however, specimens containing anaerobes should be stored at ambient temperatures (2, 42).

5. Transport of clinical specimens and infectious substances from one laboratory to another, regardless of the distance, requires strict attention to specimen packaging and labeling instructions. Materials for transport must be labeled properly, packaged, and protected during transport. Refer to the Centers for Disease Control and Prevention (CDC) website (http://www.phppo.cdc.gov/nltn/nphtcs/ps2005.aspx) for a complete description of packaging and shipping regulations mandated by the U.S. Department of Transportation.

Specific specimen transport guidelines are summarized in Table 3.

SPECIMENS FOR INFREQUENTLY ENCOUNTERED BACTERIA

Some bacteria cause infections that are infrequently encountered and require special transport conditions or holding medium. In many instances, these specimens will be shipped to reference laboratories; this necessitates relatively long transport times. Table 4 is a list of specimens and transport conditions for these bacteria (39).

PROCESSING OF SPECIMENS

Specimen processing includes detection of bacteria by staining and culturing, performing immunologic assays for microbial antigen, and the use of molecular techniques that identify specific nucleic acid sequences. The recommendations that follow are neither all-inclusive nor applicable to all laboratory settings (Table 5). Gram-stained smears are recommended whenever (i) rapid stain results are necessary for patient care, (ii) analysis of cellularity is used to determine adequacy of specimen, or (iii) results are needed to help interpret culture findings by the laboratory technologist. Anaerobic culture should be included only when ordered with an appropriate specimen source (Table 2) and when the specimen was transported in an oxygen-free container free of contamination with normal skin and mucosal anaerobic flora. Gram-stained smear and culture interpretation may require the intervention and opinion of a laboratory director trained in medical microbiology or pathology, and capable of reviewing clinical information with the patient's physician prior to report generation.

General Considerations

Safety

Refer to chapters 5, 8, and 9 for a complete description of safety issues.

Processing

Specimens for detection of bacteria by methods which include culture, staining, and antigen or nucleic acid detection must be processed in a timely manner. The lability of microorganisms, and their antigens and nucleic acids, mandates holding conditions and processing time limits. Improper handling prior to processing can result in death of pathogenic bacteria or overgrowth of contaminating bacteria. In addition, correct interpretations of culture results generally require a rough quantitation of bacterial densities in the clinical specimen. Allowing bacteria to multiply out of proportion to their original numbers may result in erroneous, sometimes detrimental, interpretations. General considerations for holding specimens and acceptable processing delays are summarized in Table 3 (122).

Processing at a Remote Site

Consolidation of laboratory services results in centralized microbiology laboratories located miles from the sites of specimen collection. Adhering to transport and processing time limits developed for laboratories located within or adjacent to the specimen collection site (e.g., hospital) is impossible for remote laboratories. The best approach to location of a core laboratory and the amount of local processing that should be performed can be determined on the basis of guidelines proposed by the Infectious Disease Society of America (149).

Specimen Labeling and Test Ordering Requirements

Upon arrival of specimens in the laboratory, the time and date of receipt should be recorded. Subsequently, the time of plating, which may differ substantially from the time of receipt, should be recorded. At the time of receipt, all specimens and requisitions should be carefully inspected. Specimens must be labeled and accompanied by a requisition reflecting the physician's order. Specimens are labeled with the patient's name and a description of the specimen source. The requisition must include the following information: patient name, age, sex, identifying number (such as social security number or unique registration/billing number), and location (hospital room, physician's office address, etc.); ordering physician's name; specimen source; date and time of collection; and test ordered. If the information is incomplete, laboratory personnel must call the collecting location and request the missing information. If a specimen is mislabeled or no patient name is provided, another specimen should be collected. Relabeling of a specimen is allowed only if the specimen cannot be recollected, such as tissue collected during a surgical procedure. Laboratory procedures must clearly state the exceptions that are allowed, the steps needed to verify and document exceptions, and the individuals responsible for relabeling. When relabeling has occurred, the course of events must be outlined in the laboratory report so the physician interpreting the results is aware of potential errors.

TABLE 4 Specimen management for infrequently encountered organisms[a]

Organism	Specimen(s) of choice	Transport issues	Comment
Bartonella sp. (cat scratch fever)	Blood, tissue, lymph node aspirate	1 wk at 4°C; indefinitely at −70°C	May see organisms in or on erythrocytes with Giemsa stain. Use Warthin-Starry silver stain for tissue. SPS is toxic.
Borrelia burgdorferi (Lyme disease)	Skin biopsy sample at lesion periphery, blood, CSF	Keep tissue moist and sterile; hand carry to laboratory if possible.	Consider PCR in addition to culture. Culture yield is low. Warthin-Starry silver stain for tissue. AO and Giemsa for blood and CSF.
Borrelia sp. (relapsing fever)	Blood smear (blood)	Hand carry to laboratory if possible.	Use direct wet mount in saline for dark-field microscopy. Stain with Wright's or Giemsa stain. Blood culture is unreliable.
Coxiella (Q fever),[b] *Rickettsia* (spotted fevers; typhus)	Serum, tissue (blood)	Blood and tissue are frozen at −70°C until shipped.	Refer isolation to reference laboratory. Serologic diagnosis is preferred.
Ehrlichia sp.	Blood smear, skin biopsy sample, blood (with heparin or EDTA anticoagulant), CSF, serum	Material for culture sent on ice; keep tissue moist and sterile; hold at 4–20°C until tested or at −70°C for shipment; transport on ice or frozen for PCR test.	Serologic diagnosis preferred. Fix smear in methanol. Tissue stained with FA or Gimenez stain. Refer isolation to reference laboratory. CSF for direct examination and PCR.
Francisella sp. (tularemia)[b]	Lymph node aspirate, scrapings, lesion biopsy sample, blood, sputum	Rapid transport to laboratory or freeze; ship on dry ice.	Send to reference laboratory. Serology helpful. Gram stain of tissue is not productive. IFA available. Culture effective 10% of the time.
Leptospira sp.	Serum, blood (citrate-containing anticoagulants should not be used), CSF (1st wk), urine (after 1st wk)	Blood, <1 h; urine, <1 h or dilute 1:10 in 1% bovine serum albumin and store at 4–20°C.	Serology most helpful. Acidic urine is detrimental. Dark-field microscopy and direct FA available. Warthin-Starry silver stain for tissue.
Streptobacillus sp. (rat-bite fever, Haverhill fever)	Blood, aspirates of joint fluid	High-vol bottle preferred	Do not refrigerate. Requires blood, serum, or ascitic fluid for growth. SPS is inhibitory. AO staining is helpful.

[a] Abbreviations: AO, acridine-orange; FA, fluorescent antibody; IFA, indirect fluorescent antibody.
[b] Laboratory safety hazard. Class II biological safety cabinet required. Also see chapter 9.

Laws governing specimen labeling can be reviewed at the Centers for Medicare and Medicaid Services website (http://www.hcfa.gov). Specimens from outpatient facilities require additional information for Medicare and Medicaid billing. Patient diagnosis, in the form of an ICD-9 code, is needed to confirm the need for a particular test. If a test is not deemed necessary for a specific diagnosis, the patient must sign an advanced beneficiary notice documenting that the test is not considered necessary and, if performed, the patient will be required to pay the test charge. Medicare and Medicaid compliance rules also can be reviewed at the Centers for Medicare and Medicaid Services website.

Specimen Rejection

In spite of acceptable labeling, some specimen collection sites, transport containers, or transport conditions render the specimen unacceptable for processing (164). Table 3 lists acceptable criteria for specimen management based on collection or transport conditions and times. When specimens fall outside these limits, new specimens should be collected whenever possible. In addition, specimens may be rejected because of the quality of specimen material collected rather than the conditions of transport (Table 6). Specimen quality is evaluated by examining the quantity and cellular composition. Although the quantity of many specimens is limited by the collection method or physical size of the infected area, some specimens, such as urine, stool, and sputum, are available in abundance. If another specimen can be collected easily with a larger volume, it is appropriate and necessary to request new or additional material. If the specimen volume must be limited, small volumes of liquid specimens can be extended by adding 1 to 2 ml of sterile saline or a

TABLE 5 Recommendations for Gram stain and plating media for bacteriology specimens or organisms

Specimen or organism	Gram stain	Aerobic media[a]	Anaerobic media[a,b]	Comments
Body cavity fluids	x (separate fluid specimen needed)			Blood culture bottles should be used to incubate large volumes of specimens for all body cavity fluids.
CSF (routine)	x	B C		
CSF (shunt)	x	B C Th		
Pericardial	x	B C	BBA	
Pleural	x	B C	BBA	
Peritoneal	x	B C Mac CNA	BBA LKV BBE CNA	
CAPD	x	B C Th	BBA	
Synovial	x	B C		
Bone marrow	x	B C	BBA	
Catheter tip		B		
Ear external fluid/swab	x	B C Mac		
Ear internal fluid	x	B C	BBA	
Eye	x	B C		
Gastrointestinal tract				
Feces		B Mac HE Ca EB (Sorbitol Mac/ chromogenic agar/Shiga toxin testing optional)		*C. jejuni/coli* in 5% O_2, 10% CO_2, and 85% N_2 at 42°C for all gastrointestinal tract specimens
Rectal swab		B Mac HE Ca EB		
Genitourinary tract				
Vaginal/cervix		B TM		
Urethra/penis	x	TM		
Other	x	B C Mac TM	BBA LKV BBE CNA	
Group B streptococcal screen (vaginal/anal screen)		Selective broth, subculture to B		
Lower respiratory tract				
Sputum	x	B C Mac (PC OFPBL for cystic fibrosis)		
Tracheal aspirate	x	B C Mac CNA		
Bronchoalveolar lavage fluid	x	B C Mac CNA	BBA LKV CNA	Protected bronchoscope brushing (in anaerobic transport) required for anaerobic culture
Bronchoalveolar brushing, washing	x	B C Mac		
Tissue	x	B C Mac Th	BBA LKV BBE CNA	
Upper respiratory tract				
Nasopharynx		B C		
Nose		B chromogenic agar		
Throat		B or SSA		
Urine		B Mac or chromogenic agar		
Wound or abscess				
Swab	x	B C Mac		
Aspirate	x	B C Mac CNA	BBA LKV BBE CNA	
B. pertussis and *B. parapertussis*		Regan Lowe		
Brucella spp.		B C		

(Continued on next page)

TABLE 5 Recommendations for Gram stain and plating media for bacteriology specimens or organisms *(Continued)*

Specimen or organism	Gram stain	Aerobic media[a]	Anaerobic media[a,b]	Comments
C. diphtheriae		Cystine-tellurite or Loeffler's serum		
C. difficile		CCFA		
E. coli O157:H7 (EHEC)		Sorbitol-Mac or chromogenic agar		Shiga toxin EIA more sensitive
F. tularensis		C or BCYE		
H. ducreyi		C + vancomycin (3 μg/ml)		Gram stain resembling "school of fish"
H. pylori	x	B		*Campylobacter* gaseous atmosphere at 35–37°C
Legionella		BCYE		
Leptospira		Fletcher's medium or EMJH		30°C for up to 13 wk
N. gonorrhoeae		TM		
Vibrio		TCBS		
Yersinia		CIN		

[a] B, blood agar; C, chocolate blood agar; Mac, MacConkey agar; Th, thioglycolate broth; Ca, *Campylobacter* agar; HE, Hektoen enteric; EB, enrichment broth; SSA, group A *Streptococcus* selective agar; TM, Thayer-Martin; BCYE, buffered charcoal yeast extract; TCBS, thiosulfate citrate bile salts sucrose; CIN, cefsulodin-Irgasan-novobiocin; BBA, brucella blood agar; LKV, laked blood with kanamycin and vancomycin; BBE, *Bacteroides* bile-esculin; CNA, anaerobic colistin-nalidixic acid; CCFA, cycloserine-cefoxitin-fructose agar; EMJH, Ellinghausen-McCullough-Johnson-Harris medium; CAPD, fluid from chronic ambulatory peritoneal dialysis; PC, *P. cepacia* agar; OFPBL, oxidative-fermentative-polymyxin B-bacitracin-lactose.

[b] Set up anaerobic culture upon request, if specimen is collected and transported appropriately. Call physician if appropriate specimen does not have request for anaerobic culture.

nutrient broth. It is important to add just enough liquid to provide specimen for all tests requested.

Examining the cellular composition of clinical material first requires a gross examination of the specimen. Infection gives rise to purulence (abundant polymorphonuclear cells), blood, necrosis, and mucus (mucous membrane specimens). In general, gross examination should identify yellow to tan purulence, red to rust-colored blood, clear and tenacious mucus, and brown to black discoloration of tissue denoting necrosis. Portions for smear and inoculation to culture media should be taken from these areas. It may be beneficial to ask the assistance of a surgical pathologist when choosing the best portion of excised tissue for examination (197). Ideally, microscopic examination of smears, using a 10× microscope objective, should demonstrate many polymorphonuclear cells and few or no squamous epithelial cells indicating the absence of cutaneous or mucocutaneous contamination with normal bacterial flora. Specimens in which tissue necrosis is present also may show elastin fibers in stained smears. Lower respiratory tract specimens are likely to show alveolar macrophages and Curschmann's spirals, indicating that secretions have originated from the distal airways. Curschmann's spirals are casts of bronchioles found in patients with chronic lung disease caused most commonly by asthma and cigarette smoking. Figures 1 and 2 illustrate elastin fibers and Curschmann's spirals, respectively. Although elastin fibers are present in noninfected surgical wounds and specimens from areas of tissue damage, they are also found in infected tissue where necrosis has occurred. Specimens determined to have gross bacterial contamination from normal flora, indicated by an abundance of squamous epithelial cells, should be rejected. Specimens are rejected by contacting the patient's caregiver, explaining the reason for rejection, and requesting a replacement specimen of acceptable quality. Timely notification and collection of a replacement are necessary, especially in instances where antimicrobial therapy has been initiated. Specimen rejection criteria should be reviewed by appropriate laboratory and medical staff representatives before becoming policy. Examples of acceptable and unacceptable specimens are listed in Table 6.

Culture Interpretation

Following examination of the stained smear and culture incubation, agar culture plates are interpreted for bacterial growth by attempting to differentiate potential pathogens, requiring identification and antimicrobial testing, from contamination by colonizing members of the normal bacterial flora. This is accomplished by examining the relative quantities of each isolate, correlating culture results with Gram-stained smear results, and recognizing usual contaminants and pathogens from respective specimen sites. In general, in cultures of specimens from sites likely to be contaminated (e.g., sputum, urine, and superficial wounds), potential pathogens should outnumber indigenous flora and should be seen in the direct Gram stain. In cultures of specimens from presumably sterile sites (e.g., cerebrospinal fluid [CSF], joint

TABLE 6 Screening specimens requested for routine bacterial culture to ensure quality[a]

Specimen (reference)	Screening method	Results of screen[b]	
		Acceptable	Unacceptable
Sputum (135)	Microscopic examination of Gram-stained smear	<10 SEC/average 10× field	>10 SEC/average 10× field
Endotracheal aspirate (129)	Microscopic examination of Gram-stained smear	<10 SEC/average 10× field and bacteria detected in at least 1 of 20 fields (100×)	>10 SEC/average 10× field and no bacteria detected in 20 fields (100×)
Bronchoalveolar lavage fluid (200)	Microscopic examination of Gram-stained smear	<1% of cells present are SEC	>1% of cells present are SEC
Urine (213)	Urinalysis, Gram stain of urine sediment	<3+ SEC on urinalysis. Positive LE[b] test result with >10 polymorphonuclear leukocytes/mm^3 from symptomatic patient (patients with asymptomatic bacteriuria may not have increased number of leukocytes)	≥3+ SEC on urinalysis or more than 3 potential pathogens by Gram stain implies gross contamination
Superficial wound (178)	Microscopic examination of Gram-stained smear	<2+ SEC, polymorphonuclear leukocytes present	>2+ SEC and no polymorphonuclear neutrophils
Stool for bacterial pathogens (127)	Location of patient? Duration of hospitalization?	Outpatient or inpatient for ≤3 days	In hospital >3 days, or diarrhea developed while in hospital
Other specimens	Screening methods unavailable or unproven		

[a] Reprinted from reference 195 with permission.
[b] LE, leukocyte esterase; SEC, squamous epithelial cells.

fluids, other body fluids, and deep tissue), potential pathogens occur in any quantity and may or may not be seen in the direct Gram-stained smear. Specific criteria for identifying potentially significant isolates and contaminating members of the normal flora are addressed in the following sections of this chapter. It is a useful policy to save the culture plates for 1 week, allowing physicians the opportunity to call to request further identification or antimicrobial testing when clinically indicated.

Critical Values in Microbiology

Many results in clinical microbiology can have an immediate impact on patient care. Although cultures require days to weeks to become positive, stained-smear results, results of antigen or nucleic acid detection, and culture results from presumably sterile specimen sources may contain information necessitating important changes in therapy or care. Examples of medical emergencies that require immediate notification of the patient's health care provider include a positive blood culture; positive CSF Gram stain or culture; group A streptococcus detected in a surgical wound specimen; Gram stain suggesting gas gangrene, necrotizing fasciitis, or other systemic toxemia; and positive blood smear for malaria. Examples of results that require notification of the physician or health care provider during a day shift, but not so immediate that calls are necessary during evening or overnight hours, include a positive acid-fast stain, new or unusual antimicrobial resistance, and the detection of highly significant or unusual microorganisms such as *Listeria*, *Legionella*, or *Brucella*. Most critical values are unique to individual medical centers and require laboratories to consult with medical staff representatives before compiling a call list for critical values (95, 108).

Blood and Intravascular Catheter Specimens

Blood is one of the most important specimens received by the laboratory for culture. In most cases, bacteria present in blood (bacteremia) indicate an infection that has spread from a primary site such as the lungs (pneumonia). Such a bacteremia is referred to as a secondary bacteremia. In the absence of an identifiable infected source, the bacteremia is referred to as a primary bacteremia. Primary bacteremia can also result from "silent," subclinical passage of bacteria from contaminated areas of the body, such as mucous membranes, into the blood. Consequences of a clinically apparent primary or secondary bacteremia are sepsis, septic shock, or severe sepsis. Sepsis implies a bacteremia with signs and symptoms, such as fever, chills, and tachycardia. Septic shock indicates the presence of hypotension with sepsis. Severe sepsis is characterized by septic shock with organ system failure and is associated with a 20 to 40% mortality rate (15).

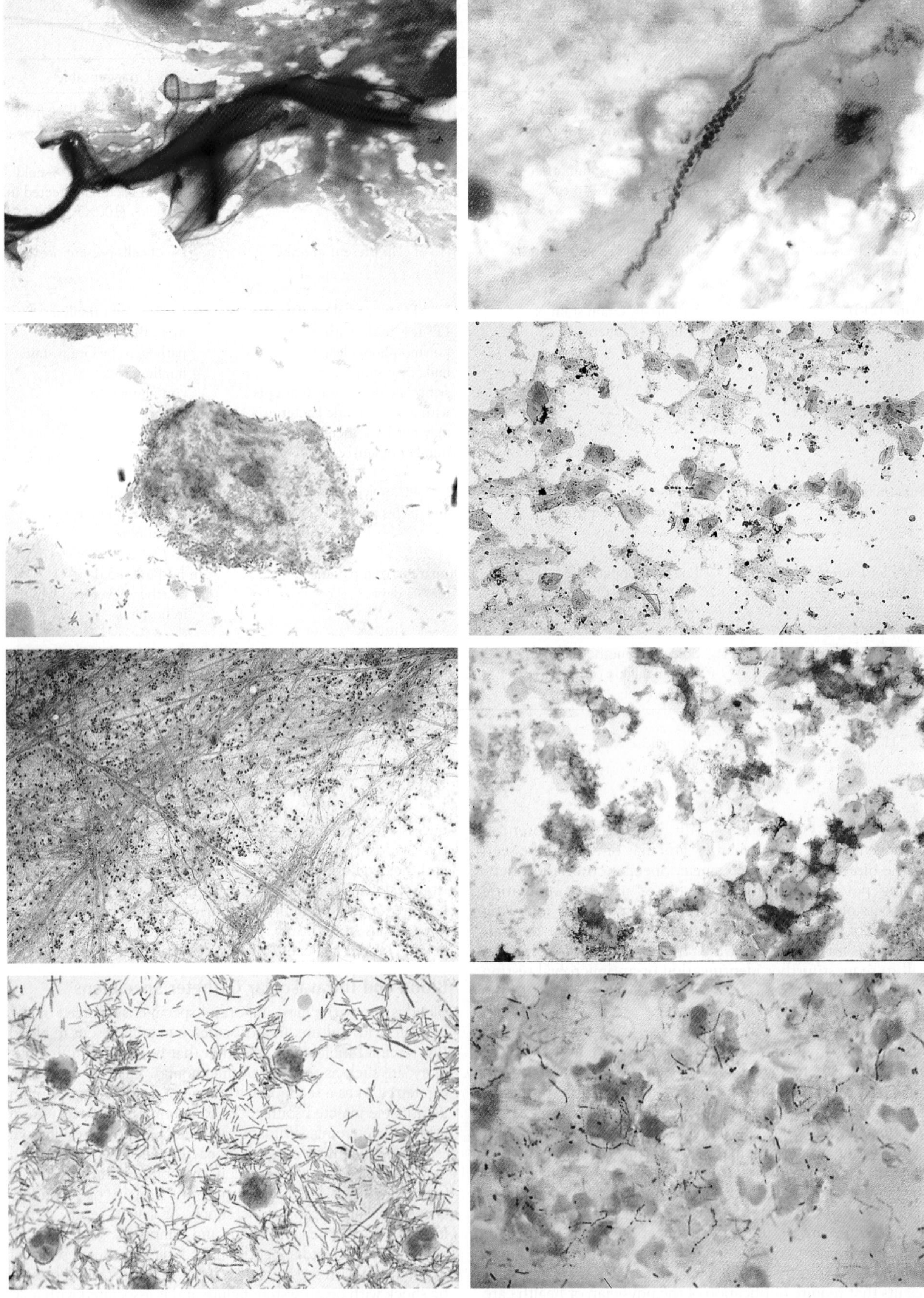

A wide variety of bacteria are involved in bloodstream infections, the majority belonging to groups of bacteria, such as the streptococci/enterococci, staphylococci, or *Enterobacteriaceae,* that grow rapidly in culture (8, 220). It is important to recognize potential contaminants that grow, since treating contaminants as significant isolates is associated with unnecessary expense and dangers of antimicrobial misuse (12). Common contaminants include coagulase-negative staphylococci, corynebacteria, *Bacillus* spp., and propionibacteria. In general, single cultures positive for these bacteria represent contamination. Multiple, separate cultures growing one of these isolates are more likely to indicate a clinically significant bacteremia (90, 125, 219). Contamination is controlled by proper skin antisepsis before venipuncture. Iodine-containing antiseptics, including iodophors (iodine with a detergent) and tincture of iodine (iodine with alcohol, considered more effective than iodophors), or chlorhexidine is needed to reduce the number of viable bacteria at the venipuncture site (106, 124). Contamination rates of less than 3% are desired (172). Higher rates should be investigated and corrected by educational efforts (161).

Bacteremic patients fall into many patterns that determine specimen collection methods. Most patients are intermittently bacteremic, implying that bacteria are present in the blood for periods of time followed by nonbacteremic periods. Other patients who have intravascular sites of primary infection (such as endocarditis) are continuously bacteremic. All patients are likely to have very low quantities of bacteria in the blood, in spite of severe clinical symptoms. For these reasons, multiple blood cultures, each containing large volumes of blood, are required to detect bacteremia. As a rule for adults, two or three separate blood cultures, each inoculated with at least 20 ml of blood, are recommended per 24-h period (8, 219). Pediatric recommendations are similar, except for the volumes of blood recommended (8, 87). Adult and pediatric requirements for blood collection for culture are summarized in Tables 3 and 7.

It is best to collect blood directly into culture bottles during the venipuncture procedure, rather than into transport tubes that are sent to the laboratory for subsequent transfer of blood into the culture bottles. Collection directly into culture bottles enables bacteria to begin growing immediately, decreases the amount of anticoagulant to which bacteria are exposed, and decreases the chances of needlestick accidents for health care personnel. The anticoagulant used in all blood culture systems is sodium polyanethanolsulfonate (SPS) and is known to be inhibitory to meningococci, gonococci, *Peptostreptococcus anaerobius, Streptobacillus moniliformis,* and *Gardnerella vaginalis* (159). Although few practical methods are available to avoid exposure of these bacteria in blood to SPS, it is advisable to diminish the total amount of SPS used by avoiding transport tubes that also include SPS.

Culture of blood is the most sensitive method available for the detection of bacteremia. Semiautomated blood culture systems are present in nearly every clinical laboratory. Refer to chapter 15 for a complete discussion of manual and automated blood culture systems. Occasionally, direct staining of blood collected by venipuncture can provide rapid, nearly immediate, detection of bacteria in blood (157, 163). Gram staining a smear of peripheral blood or buffy coat layer may detect bacterial cells in the blood of patients with meningococcemia, *S. pneumoniae* infection, or overwhelming sepsis caused by other bacteria when the bacterial concentration in blood is very high (approaching 10,000 bacterial cells per ml of blood). In spite of published reports documenting the occasional use of direct staining of blood, the likelihood of results impacting patient management does not warrant use as a routine laboratory procedure.

Some bacteria, such as *Legionella* spp., mycobacteria, some *N. meningitidis* strains, and *N. gonorrhoeae,* fail to grow in routine commercial media and should be sought by using another method, such as lysis centrifugation. Other bacteria may require the addition of adsorbents to bind antimicrobials or inhibitory substances, or more specialized methods such as tissue culture. Prolonged incubation beyond the usual 5-day protocols for automated instruments is not necessary; however, blind subculture may be needed if the patient is receiving antimicrobials at the time of blood collection (7, 150).

Positive blood culture bottles are evaluated initially by examining a Gram-stained smear of the broth. The report should include a description of the bacterial morphology and the Gram reaction. If a presumptive identification of the microorganism can be made, it may be added to the report. For example, a blood culture Gram stain report might state "gram positive in clusters suggesting staphylococci." Specimens in positive blood culture bottles should be subcultured to media based on the organism seen in the Gram-stained smear. In addition, since 5 to 10% of all bacteremias

---

FIGURE 1 (row 1, left) Gram stain (×100) of surgical wound showing elastin fibers.

FIGURE 2 (row 1, right) Gram stain (×1,000) of sputum showing Curschmann's spirals.

FIGURE 3 (row 2, left) Gram stain (×1,000) of vaginal secretions showing clue cells.

FIGURE 4 (row 2, right) Gram stain (×100) of unacceptable sputum specimen (grossly contaminated with oropharyngeal flora) showing >10 squamous epithelial cells per low-power field.

FIGURE 5 (row 3, left) Gram stain (×100) of acceptable sputum specimen showing <10 squamous epithelial cells per low-power field.

FIGURE 6 (row 3, right) Gram stain (×100) of urine showing 4+ squamous epithelial cells, indicating gross contamination with vaginal or periurethral secretions and bacteria.

FIGURE 7 (row 4, left) Gram stain (×1,000) of urine showing polymorphonuclear leukocytes and 4+ gram-negative bacilli.

FIGURE 8 (row 4, right) Gram stain (×1,000) of a wound showing polymorphonuclear leukocytes, mixed bacterial morphotypes suggesting aerobic and anaerobic bacteria, and both intra- and extracellular bacteria. This appearance suggests a mixed aerobic and anaerobic abscess or closed-space infection.

TABLE 7 Pediatric bacterial blood cultures: recommended blood volume[a]

Patient wt (lb)	Recommended blood vol per culture (ml)	Total blood vol for 2 cultures (ml)	Vol of blood equal to 1% of patient's total blood vol (ml)[b]
<19	1	2	2
18–30	3	6	6–10
30–60	5	10	10–20
60–90	10	20	20–30
90–120	15	30	30–40
>120	20	40	>40

[a] Data from reference 87.

[b] Blood volume calculated by assuming 85 ml/kg in newborns and 73 ml/kg in other patients. Two 20-ml blood specimens collected from an 80-kg adult (40 ml total) represent approximately 0.7% of the patient's total blood volume.

are polymicrobial (contain more than one bacterial type), the addition of a Columbia-colistin-nalidixic acid, or other agar medium inhibitory to gram-negative organisms, to cultures showing gram-negative bacilli in the Gram stain, or the addition of a MacConkey or related selective agar plate to cultures showing gram-positive bacteria, is recommended. Anaerobic media and culture conditions should be used if the morphology of the organism seen in the Gram-stained smear is suggestive of an anaerobic bacterium or if the organism is recovered from an anaerobic culture bottle only.

Special Considerations for Blood Cultures

Anaerobes

Anaerobes have always accounted for a relatively small percentage of organisms recovered from blood. Over the past several years, some investigators have noted a decline in bloodstream infections by anaerobes (134). However, this is not the case in all hospitals (30). Therefore, laboratories should review their own data when deciding whether to include an anaerobic culture bottle as part of the routine setup of blood specimens. Anaerobic media available for use with the automated systems appear to perform adequately. It is important to note that if the anaerobic component of a blood culture is dropped, the inoculum should be added to an additional aerobic bottle to ensure that the full volume of blood is cultured.

Lysis Centrifugation

The Isolator lysis centrifugation system (Wampole Laboratories, Cranbury, N.J.) is a commercially available manual blood culture method (219). The system consists of a tube containing anticoagulant (SPS), EDTA, and saponin. After the tube is filled with blood during phlebotomy, the contents are mixed and centrifuged, and the resulting pellet is inoculated onto agar media. The system effectively recovers aerobic and facultative bacteria and fungi. The Isolator system does not perform as well as other systems when recovering *S. pneumoniae,* other streptococci, *Pseudomonas aeruginosa,* or anaerobes (219). Advantages of the Isolator system are the ability to inoculate the pellet to specific agar media when attempting to detect unusual etiologies of bacteremia, such as those caused by *Legionella pneumophila, Franciscella tularensis,* and *Bartonella* spp., and to provide colony counts, reported as CFU per milliliter of blood (38, 219). Disadvantages of the system are the labor involved with initial processing and the potential for increased contamination that accompanies manipulation during processing (199).

Intravascular Catheter Tips

Culture of intravascular catheter tips is performed to determine the source of a bacteremia and should be performed only when concurrent blood cultures are obtained. Soft tissue infections around a catheter insertion site are cultured as a wound specimen using freshly expressed purulence that can be aspirated. The most common technique used to culture the intravascular portion of a catheter is the semiquantitative method, in which the 5-cm distal portion of the catheter is rolled across a blood agar plate four times (109). The catheter tip is discarded. Growth of more than 15 colonies is considered to be significant; i.e., it implicates the catheter tip as the likely source of a bacteremia if a similar isolate is detected in a blood culture.

Other techniques have been described for the identification of catheter-related infections. A meta-analysis of data was reported concerning the use of three types of catheter segment culture and three blood culture methods to determine the sensitivity and specificity of each method (182). The three catheter segment cultures included qualitative, semiquantitative (e.g., catheter roll method), and quantitative (dilutions to determine bacterial quantities used), while the three blood culture methods included qualitative catheter blood culture (reported as positive or negative), quantitative catheter blood culture, and paired quantitative catheter and peripheral venipuncture blood cultures. Based on this analysis, quantitative catheter segment culture was the most accurate method, with pooled sensitivity and specificity both >90%. The optimal method in all clinical settings for determining that an intravascular catheter is the source of a bacteremia has not been determined. Because the most serious manifestation of catheter infections is bacteremia, ordinary blood cultures may be the best way to determine which patients require therapy (158).

Sterile Body Fluid Specimens

CSF

CSF is collected for the diagnosis of meningitis (67). Bacterial meningitis can be divided into acute and chronic clinical presentations (196). Acute meningitis with onset of symptoms within the previous 24 h is usually caused by pyogenic bacteria. Specific etiologies are related to the age of the patient and whether the disease is community or nosocomially acquired. Chronic meningitis, with symptoms lasting at least 4 weeks, can have a wide variety of causes (Table 8). As with all clinical specimens, even those collected from a presumably sterile site, growth of contaminants occasionally does occur.

CSF is usually obtained by lumbar spinal puncture. Although bacterial staining and culture can be performed with as little as 0.5 ml of fluid, larger volumes are preferred since culture methods are more sensitive when low numbers of bacteria are concentrated by centrifugation before culture. A minimum of 5.0 ml and high-speed (3,000 × *g*) centrifugation are recommended for recovery of *Mycobacterium tuberculosis,* although the yield may still be low. Filtration through a 0.45-μm-pore-size filter results in better concentration of *M. tuberculosis* in CSF. Specimens should be transported to the laboratory immediately in a sterile container maintained at room temperature. All smears should be prepared by cytocentrifugation (176), and cultures should be inoculated with

TABLE 8 Usual etiologies of infectious disease syndromes

Disease	Etiologies
Central nervous system infection	
Acute meningitis, neutrophilic pleocytosis	*S. pneumoniae*
	N. meningitidis
	Listeria monocytogenes
	Streptococcus agalactiae
	H. influenzae
	S. aureus
	Gram-negative rods[a]
	Bacillus anthracis
Acute meningitis, CSF shunt related	Coagulase-negative staphylococci
	S. aureus
	Propionibacterium spp.
	Gram-negative enteric rods (e.g., *E. coli* and *Klebsiella* spp.)
	Gram-negative nonfermenting rods (e.g., *P. aeruginosa* and *Acinetobacter* spp.)
Chronic meningitis, predominantly lymphocytic pleocytosis	*Nocardia* species
	Brucella species
	L. interrogans
	M. tuberculosis
	T. pallidum
	Borrelia burgdorferi
Gastrointestinal tract infection	
Infectious diarrhea[b]	*Salmonella* serotypes
	Shigella spp.
	C. jejuni/coli
	Campylobacter spp. (other)
	EHEC serotypes
	C. difficile
	Vibrio spp.
	Aeromonas spp.
	P. shigelloides
	Y. enterocolitica
	E. coli toxigenic, invasive, and effacing strains
	Listeria monocytogenes (rare)
	Clostridium perfringens
	B. cereus
Ingestion of preformed toxin[c]	S. aureus
	B. cereus
	C. botulinum
Gastritis/gastric and duodenal ulcers	*H. pylori*
Genital tract infection	
Ulcers	*T. pallidum*
	H. ducreyi
	C. trachomatis (LGV)
	Klebsiella granulomatis
Urethritis	*N. gonorrhoeae*
	C. trachomatis
Vulvovaginitis	*N. gonorrhoeae* and *C. trachomatis* in prepubescent girls
BV	Overgrowth of vaginal flora with anaerobic bacteria
Cervicitis	*N. gonorrhoeae*
	C. trachomatis
Endometritis	*Enterobacteriaceae*
	Streptococci (groups A and B)
	Enterococci
	Mixed anaerobic genera
Salpingitis/oophoritis	*N. gonorrhoeae*
	C. trachomatis
	Mixed aerobic and anaerobic flora
Pelvic abscess	Mixed aerobic and anaerobic flora

(Continued on next page)

TABLE 8 Usual etiologies of infectious disease syndromes *(Continued)*

Disease	Etiologies
Epididymitis	*N. gonorrhoeae*
	C. trachomatis
	Enterobacteriaceae
	P. aeruginosa
	Various gram-positive cocci
Ocular infections	
Conjunctivitis	*S. pneumoniae*
	S. aureus
	H. influenzae
	N. meningitidis
	N. gonorrhoeae
	C. trachomatis (inclusion conjunctivitis)
	C. trachomatis (trachoma)
	Others[d]
Keratitis	*S. aureus*
	S. pneumoniae
	P. aeruginosa
	Enterococci
	S. pyogenes (group A)
	Enterobacteriaceae
	Pasteurella multocida
	Others[e]
Endophthalmitis	*S. aureus*
	P. aeruginosa
	Propionibacterium acnes
	S. pneumoniae
	N. meningitidis
Periorbital cellulitis	*S. aureus*
	S. pyogenes (group A)
	S. pneumoniae
	H. influenzae
	Clostridium spp.
Otitis	
Otitis externa	*S. aureus*
	S. pyogenes (group A)
	P. aeruginosa
	Vibrio alginolyticus
Otitis media	*S. pneumoniae*
	H. influenzae
	Moraxella catarrhalis
	S. aureus
	Rare pathogens
	Gram-negative rods
	Anaerobes
Respiratory tract infection	
Tracheitis, intubated patient	*Enterobacteriaceae*
	S. aureus
	P. aeruginosa
	Other nonfermenting gram-negative rods
Bronchitis, community acquired	*S. pneumoniae*
	H. influenzae (rarely, other *Haemophilus* species)
	M. catarrhalis
	S. aureus
	C. pneumoniae
	M. pneumoniae
	B. pertussis
	S. pyogenes (group A)
	Less commonly, same as hospital acquired

(Continued on next page)

TABLE 8 *(Continued)*

Disease	Etiologies
Bronchitis, hospital acquired	*Enterobacteriaceae* *S. aureus* *P. aeruginosa* Other nonfermenting gram-negative rods Less commonly, same as community acquired
Pneumonia, community acquired	*S. pneumoniae* *H. influenzae* *M. catarrhalis* *C. pneumoniae* *M. pneumoniae* *L. pneumophila* *Nocardia* species *P. multocida* Aspiration (anaerobes) Less commonly, same as hospital acquired
Pneumonia, hospital acquired	*Enterobacteriaceae* *S. aureus* *P. aeruginosa* *L. pneumophila* Other nonfermenting gram-negative rods Aspiration (anaerobes) Less commonly, same as community acquired
Lung abscess	*S. aureus* *Klebsiella pneumoniae* *P. aeruginosa* *S. pyogenes* (group A) Anaerobes (aspiration pneumonia) *Nocardia* species
Empyema	*S. pneumoniae* Anaerobes Viridans group streptococci, especially *Streptococcus anginosus* group *S. aureus* *S. pyogenes* (group A) Gram-negative rods
Urinary tract infection	
Prostatitis	*Enterobacteriaceae* *P. aeruginosa* Enterococci
Urethral syndrome	Same us cystitis, but in lower numbers *C. trachomatis/N. gonorrhoeae* Unknown—negative culture (about 15% of this disease group)
Cystitis	*Enterobacteriaceae*, especially *E. coli* Enterococci *Staphylococcus saprophyticus* (women of childbearing age) Nonfermenting gram-negative rods *Corynebacterium urealyticum* (patients with underlying urinary tract pathology)
Pyelonephritis	*Enterobacteriaceae* Enterococci Agents of bacteremia (descending infection), e.g., *S. aureus*

[a] Gram-negative rods, including *Enterobacteriaceae*, *P. aeruginosa*, and other nonfermenting gram-negative rods.
[b] Disease caused by ingestion of bacterium followed by tissue invasion, toxin production, or other pathogenic mechanism.
[c] Disease caused by ingestion of preformed toxin.
[d] *C. diphtheriae*, *M. tuberculosis*, *F. tularensis*, *T. pallidum*, *B. henselae* (cat scratch disease), *P. multocida*, *Bacillus thuringiensis*, and *M. lacunata*.
[e] *T. pallidum*, *N. gonorrhoeae*, *Moraxella* sp., *C. diphtheriae*, *Bacillus* spp., anaerobes, and nontuberculous mycobacteria.

0.5 ml of CSF or sediment resuspended in 0.5 ml of CSF following centrifugation (1,500 × *g* for 15 min) when >1 ml of fluid is received. Recently, PCR has emerged as a potentially useful test for the diagnosis of tuberculous meningitis (27).

Smears should be Gram stained, and the results should be reported to the physician immediately. Results should include a description and semiquantitative enumeration of polymorphonuclear inflammatory cells and bacterial morphology. If the results are suggestive of a bacterial group, this too can be communicated. Because of their low sensitivity and lack of effect on the care and management of patients, and because the cost of antigen testing is much higher than the cost of the Gram stain, direct antigen tests should be considered only when direct communication with the clinical service documents a specific need, such as prior antimicrobial therapy (67, 91, 118, 145, 187). Media are inoculated in accordance with recommendations in Table 5. Broth culture media are not necessary unless CSF is cultured from patients with a CSF shunt or external reservoir (119, 194).

Special Considerations for Sterile Body Fluid Specimens

Anaerobic Bacteria

Anaerobic culture of CSF is very rarely necessary and should be performed only when consultation with the clinical service provides evidence of risk factors for anaerobic etiology such as chronic otitis media with mastoiditis, chronic sinusitis, mixed aerobic-anaerobic soft tissue infection overlying the spine, or the possibility of anaerobic brain abscess, subdural empyema, or epidural abscess (74, 76). Even when a parameningeal abscess contains anaerobes, detection of anaerobes by culture of CSF is unlikely to be helpful, since diagnosis and management are based on microbiological evaluation of the abscess.

Leptospira spp.

Leptospires can be detected in CSF during the first 10 days of acute illness. CSF should be collected before initiation of antimicrobial therapy and while the patient is febrile. Direct detection of leptospires by dark-field examination of CSF has been used in the past but is no longer recommended. Culture should be performed using 1 or 2 drops of CSF inoculated into Ellinghausen-McCullough-Johnson-Harris medium. Cultures should be incubated at room temperature for up to 13 weeks (39) (see chapter 61).

Other Body Fluids

Specimens include pericardial, pleural, peritoneal, peritoneal dialysis, and synovial fluids. A volume of 1 to 5 ml is adequate for the isolation of most bacteria. Fluid submitted on a swab is not optimal. Educational efforts should address the habits of physicians and caregivers who use swabs rather than adding aspirated fluid to an appropriate transport tube. Specimens for anaerobic culture should be transported in an oxygen-free tube. Specimens for the diagnosis of peritonitis associated with chronic ambulatory peritoneal dialysis should include at least 10 ml of fluid (212). All body fluids should be inoculated directly into blood culture bottles in the laboratory or at bedside. For the latter, 0.5 ml should be left in a separate sterile tube for preparation of a smear (14). Body fluids that may clot during transport should be transported in tubes containing anticoagulant. Because heparin, sodium citrate, and EDTA are inhibitory to some bacteria, SPS-containing tubes are recommended. Physicians should be made aware that SPS is inhibitory also and affects the growth of *N. meningitidis*, *N. gonorrhoeae*, *P. anaerobius*, *S. moniliformis*, and *G. vaginalis* (160).

In the laboratory, volumes greater than 1.0 ml for culture should be centrifuged at 1,500 × *g* for 15 min. The supernatant is removed, leaving about 0.5 ml in which to resuspend the sediment. The resuspended sediment is used to inoculate culture media. Cytocentrifugation of 0.5 ml or less (depending on the turbidity of the specimen) should be used to prepare smears for Gram staining before centrifugation to concentrate for culture. Alternatively, smears can be prepared from the same sediment as used to inoculate media; however, this method is less sensitive than cytocentrifugation (176).

Solid media used for culture of body fluid specimens should include chocolate and blood agar, and selective agars for gram-positive and gram-negative organisms if mixed infections are expected (e.g., abdominal fluids from patients with appendicitis) (Table 5). The inoculation of aerobic blood culture bottles with excess fluid is suggested for pericardial, pleural, and synovial fluids, in addition to peritoneal fluids from chronic ambulatory peritoneal dialysis patients, to enhance detection of low numbers of bacteria that may be intracellular or inhibited by prior antimicrobial therapy (16). Cultures should be incubated at 35 to 37°C in the presence of 3 to 5% CO_2 for a minimum of 3 days before being discarded as negative. Blood culture bottles should be incubated for the usual 5- or 7-day protocol.

Some experts question the need to culture abdominal fluid or purulence from patients with intestinal tract perforation, since surgical drainage and broad-spectrum antimicrobials are effective in the majority of cases (137, 185). Complications occur in this clinical setting when microorganisms other than the expected *Enterobacteriaceae*, anaerobes, and enterococci are involved. Standard empirical therapy may not adequately treat *Staphylococcus aureus*, *P. aeruginosa*, *Candida* spp., or bacteria more resistant to antimicrobial agents than expected (66). A policy to refuse culture requests or limit identification of isolates that do grow to an arbitrary number (such as 3 or fewer) may not apply uniformly to all patients.

Ear Specimens

Two types of ear specimens are received most commonly by the laboratory, swab specimens for the diagnosis of otitis externa and middle ear fluid specimens for the diagnosis of otitis media (Table 5). Potential pathogens at these two sites differ (Table 8) (20, 25, 168). Since anaerobic bacteria may be involved in middle ear infections, anaerobic culture should be performed on properly collected and transported specimens when requested. Direct examination of Gram-stained smears of middle ear fluid is helpful and is recommended with all culture requests.

External ear specimens may be contaminated with normal flora from the skin or ear canal. Isolates of coagulase-negative staphylococci, diphtheroids, and viridans group streptococci may be listed as presumptive identifications without including results of antimicrobial testing. It is a useful policy to save the culture plates for 1 week, allowing physicians the opportunity to call to request further identification or antimicrobial testing when clinically indicated. Middle ear fluid is less likely to be contaminated. All isolates should be reported, and if requested, antimicrobial testing should be performed on strains with unpredictable susceptibility to antimicrobials.

Eye Specimens

Several types of specimens may be collected for the microbioloigcal analysis of eye infections, including conjunctival scrapings obtained with a swab or sterile spatula for the diagnosis of conjunctivitis, corneal scrapings collected with a sterile spatula for the diagnosis of keratitis, vitreous fluid collected by aspiration for the diagnosis of endophthalmitis, and fluid material collected by aspiration or tissue biopsy for the diagnosis of periorbital cellulitis (223). Pathogenic bacteria potentially present in these anatomic sites are listed in Table 8. Because the volume of specimen collected from corneal scrapings and vitreous fluid aspiration is very small, direct inoculation of agar culture plates and preparation of smears in the clinic or at the bedside are recommended (223). A close working association is needed between the laboratory and ophthalmologist to ensure a supply of appropriate culture media, the correct technique for inoculation of media, and rapid transport of plates and smears to the laboratory. Media should be inoculated by rubbing the specimen onto a small area of the agar plates. Plates are placed directly into the incubator without cross-streaking by laboratory personnel. This allows the plate reader to detect more easily airborne contaminants that settle on the plate during inoculation procedures that occur outside controlled laboratory conditions.

Media needed for the detection of usual pathogens should include chocolate agar for fastidious bacteria (Table 5). Media for other microorganisms (fungi, viruses, mycobacteria, etc.) should be inoculated if deemed appropriate by the ophthalmologist and microbiologist, and specifically ordered. Incubation at 35 to 37°C in 3 to 5% CO_2 is necessary.

Special Considerations for Eye Specimens

Chlamydia trachomatis

Direct examination of conjunctival smears and detection of chamydial antigen in conjunctival scrapings are useful in the diagnosis of inclusion conjunctivitis or trachoma (45). Diagnosis of chlamydial infection is accomplished using direct fluorescent-antibody (DFA) staining with fluorescein-conjugated monoclonal antibodies or enzyme immunoassays (EIAs) (191). A less sensitive but readily available method is examination of Giemsa-stained conjunctival smears for intracytoplasmic, perinuclear inclusions within epithelial cells. Cell culture for the isolation of *C. trachomatis* is sensitive but more time-consuming and technically demanding than DFA or EIA. Conjunctival scrapings and secretions for culture should be transported in 2SP medium (sucrose phosphate or sucrose phosphate glutamate) with bovine serum and antimicrobials (usually gentamicin, vancomycin, and nystatin or amphotericin B). Swabs with wooden shafts should be avoided since constituents of the wood are toxic to chlamydiae. Specimens for culture should be refrigerated during short delays or stored at −70°C for delays longer than 48 h. Molecular probes and PCR methods are available for the detection of *C. trachomatis* but are not FDA approved at this time for eye specimens (71, 96).

Gastrointestinal Tract Specimens

Feces and, in some cases, rectal swab specimens are submitted to the microbiology laboratory to determine the etiologic agent of infectious diarrhea or food poisoning. Feces should be collected in a clean container with a tight lid and should not be contaminated with urine, barium, or toilet paper. Because intestinal pathogens can be killed by the metabolism of members of the fecal flora rapidly acidifying the specimen, specimens should be transferred to Cary-Blair transport medium soon after collection. Rectal swabs should be placed in a transport system containing an all-purpose medium such as Stuart's.

It should be standard practice in all laboratories to evaluate the appropriateness of stool culture requests. It is well established that hospitalized patients who did not enter the hospital with diarrhea are unlikely to develop enterocolitis caused by bacterial agents other than *Clostridium difficile* (68, 127). For this reason, stool for routine bacterial culture from patients who have been hospitalized for more than 3 days should not be processed without consultation and justification by the patient's physician or caregiver. Diarrhea that develops during hospitalization is likely to be caused by *C. difficile* or occur for noninfectious reasons (60). A simple policy of rejecting stool for routine bacterial culture from patients hospitalized for more than 3 days and offering *C. difficile* testing for nosocomial diarrhea is recommended. On the other hand, *C. difficile* colitis does occur as a community-acquired disease following hospital discharge or the use of outpatient antimicrobial therapy, and requests for diagnostic testing should not be rejected when ordered in the outpatient setting.

Fecal leukocyte examinations have been recommended for the differentiation of inflammatory diarrheas (fecal leukocyte positive) from secretory diarrheas (fecal leukocyte negative). Infectious, inflammatory diarrheas are caused by invasive bacteria, while secretory diarrheas result from toxin-producing bacteria, viruses, and protozoan pathogens (68, 170, 192). Unfortunately, fecal leukocyte morphology degrades in feces during transport and processing delays, making accurate recognition and quantitation difficult. This problem can be solved by using lactoferrin as a surrogate marker for fecal leukocytes (Leuko-Test; TechLab, Blacksburg, Va.), since lactoferrin is not degraded during normal transport and processing times. Lactoferrin-positive stool specimens are considered positive for fecal leukocytes. In addition, invasive pathogens may result in fecal leukocytes being intermittently present or unevenly distributed in stool specimens. Algorithms have been proposed depicting schemes for stool processing based on the use of a lactoferrin assay (63), but they are not commonly used or recommended for the diagnosis of acute, infectious diarrhea (68). The lactoferrin assay is used in the evaluation of patients with inflammatory bowel disease (52).

Usual gastrointestinal pathogens are listed in Table 8 (63). Inclusion of less frequently encountered pathogens should be considered when epidemiological factors suggest an increased likelihood. This may require periodic surveys of one's community to establish which pathogens are most common, especially when considering the addition of selective media or toxin assay for the routine detection of enterohemorrhagic *Escherichia coli* (EHEC), non-*jejuni*/*coli Campylobacter*, *Vibrio* spp., and *Yersinia enterocolitica*.

Selective and differential media are used to detect *Salmonella* and *Shigella* spp. (Table 5). These should include one that is differential but not selective for these pathogens, such as MacConkey agar, and one that is a mildly selective medium, such as Hektoen enteric or xylose-lysine desoxycholate agar. In some settings, a highly selective medium such as salmonella-shigella agar is also included. In addition, enrichment broth, such as gram-negative broth or Selenite-F broth, may increase detection of *Salmonella* and is recommended for testing sensitive populations such as food handlers. Subculture of gram-negative and Selenite-F broths to a mildly selective and differential medium after 6 to 8 h and 12 to 18 h of incubation, respectively, is necessary to prevent overgrowth of normal flora and decreased usefulness of the broth (116). All agar plates should be incubated in air at 35 to 37°C for 2 days before being reported as negative. The decision of whether to use a highly selective agar medium and an enrichment broth will vary from one laboratory to another.

Optimally, additional media are used for a trial period to determine their value, which is measured by the detection of strains not present on the two standard media. In settings where such a trial is not possible, the use of MacConkey, Hektoen enteric, or xylose-lysine desoxycholate agar and an enrichment broth is recommended (63).

Campylobacter jejuni and *Campylobacter coli* are detected with a medium such as campylobacter agar with 10% sheep blood and selective antimicrobial agents (Table 5). Media are incubated at 42°C in a microaerophilic atmosphere of nitrogen (85%), carbon dioxide (10%), and oxygen (5%) for up to 3 days. Special enrichment broths are available for the recovery of *Campylobacter;* however, their routine use does not increase the number of campylobacter-positive cultures significantly (1). Detection of other *Campylobacter* species may require media without antibiotics and 37°C incubation (33).

Special Considerations for Gastrointestinal Tract Specimens

Other Enteric Pathogens

A physician order for testing for *Vibrio* spp., *Y. enterocolitica, Aeromonas* spp., and *Plesiomonas shigelloides* may be needed in some geographic locations or epidemiological situations, since incidence is so low in most parts of the United States that the routine use of selective media is not justified. Media used for these enteric pathogens include thiosulfate citrate bile salts sucrose agar for vibrios, cefsulodin-Irgasan-novobiocin agar for *Y. enterocolitica,* and blood agar or selective blood agar to demonstrate hemolysis and provide a medium for oxidase testing for *Aeromonas* spp. and *P. shigelloides* (both oxidase positive) (63). All of these enteric pathogens grow on usual media, but detection is enhanced and simplified using specific selective media.

EHEC

The prevalence of EHEC varies in different parts of the United States and the rest of the world. It has been established that in addition to *E. coli* O157:H7, other serotypes are implicated as enterohemorrhagic strains. In fact, in the United States approximately 50% of Shiga toxin-producing strains, those capable of causing hemorrhagic colitis and hemolytic uremic syndrome, are not serotype O157:H7 (5, 50). For this reason, many laboratories have chosen to perform a Shiga toxin assay by EIA to detect all serotypes, rather than culture or antigen detection for O157:H7 strains only. Some Shiga toxin-producing strains may not harbor all the mechanisms needed to be fully pathogenic in humans. Strategies include testing all specimens year-round, testing all specimens only during summer months (when incidence is highest), testing only specimens containing gross blood, testing only when specifically ordered, testing only specimens from pediatric patients, or testing based on a combination of these factors (58). The best approach for a specific laboratory can be determined by a culture survey of all stool specimens during summer months. Alternatively, one can contact neighboring hospital laboratories or local health departments, which may be able to provide prevalence data. Laboratories should check with public health authorities to see if EHEC-containing stools need to be forwarded for serotyping of toxin-producing *E. coli* strains.

C. difficile

Approximately 15% of people who develop diarrhea following antimicrobial use have antibiotic-associated diarrhea caused by *C. difficile.* If use of the offending antimicrobial continues and disease remains undiagnosed and untreated, pathology may progress to more severe colitis, pseudomembranous colitis, and, possibly, death (9, 60). Nearly 100% of cases of pseudomembranous colitis are caused by *C. difficile.* Disease is caused by toxins (toxin A and toxin B) produced by *C. difficile.* The disease is diagnosed by detecting the organism or its toxins in stool, in conjunction with clinical criteria (84). Cell culture cytotoxicity assay for the detection of toxin B, EIA for the detection of toxin A or toxins A and B, latex agglutination or EIA for the detection of glutamate dehydrogenase (an antigen associated with *C. difficile* and occasionally other bacterial species), and culture of *C. difficile* from stool followed by toxin testing of the isolate are all methods used for diagnosis (9, 110). In practice, an EIA for toxin A or one that detects both toxins A and B is most practical since it requires minutes to hours to complete, compared to 24 to 48 h for the cell culture cytotoxicity assay or 2 to 4 days for culture and toxin testing of the isolate. A single specimen tested by EIA identifies 85 to 100% of specimens eventually proven to be toxin positive, whereas a single specimen tested by cell culture identifies nearly 100% of specimens eventually proven to be positive (110, 201). Testing of a second specimen, after a single negative EIA result, may be needed if symptoms persist and an alternative diagnosis has not been made (110), but testing a second specimen following a single cell culture negative result is not recommended (201).

Although *C. difficile*-associated gastrointestinal disease is most common in hospitalized patients, it can occur in any patient treated with antimicrobials, whether institutionalized or in the community. Testing should not be performed on formed stool (no diarrhea), or as a follow-up to therapy to confirm cure. Repeat testing is appropriate only if symptoms persist or recur (110). Symptoms in those successfully treated will resolve over a few days, in spite of the fact that patients may continue to carry *C. difficile* and even remain toxin positive for days or weeks (181). It is a faulty practice to require negative toxin or culture for *C. difficile* before allowing patients admission to long-term care facilities. Patients who do not have diarrhea and are not incontinent of stool are not an increased risk to other patients, even if carrying *C. difficile* and its toxins, when usual infection control measures are followed (9).

Rare and even fatal disease can be caused by toxin A-deficient strains (toxin B only produced), necessitating occasional use of a toxin A-plus-B immunoassay or cell culture. It is estimated that 2.4% of strains causing human disease are toxin A deficient (85). For epidemiological purposes, stool or rectal swabs placed in anaerobic transport medium may be cultured anaerobically to isolate *C. difficile.* The sample is inoculated to a selective medium such as cycloserine-cefoxitin-fructose agar and incubated anaerobically for 48 h (60).

Since 2002, outbreaks of severe *C. difficile* disease in North America and Europe have been reported. The strains involved are reported to be hyperproducers of toxins A and B. The putative cause is mutation of the regulator controlling production of both toxins. Peak average toxin levels were 16 to 32 times higher than normal in strains without regulator mutations (215). In addition, a third toxin, named the binary toxin, which is found in approximately 5% of all *C. difficile* strains, is reported to be present in nearly two-thirds of strains causing severe disease. Further investigation is needed to establish whether this newly detected toxin is an additional factor in the pathogenicity of *C. difficile* (3, 115).

S. aureus, Methicillin-Resistant *S. aureus* (MRSA), and *Bacillus cereus*

Stool specimens or gastric contents collected from persons with short-incubation food poisoning (2 to 6 h) can be evaluated for *S. aureus* and *B. cereus*. In general, investigation is beneficial for general public health, rather than a sick individual who recovers quickly, and is best performed by public health laboratories rather than hospital clinical microbiology laboratories. Specimens should be examined by Gram stain, and, because both of these organisms may be present normally in food, quantitative cultures must be performed. A series of dilutions (10^{-1} to 10^{-5}) of the specimen are prepared in buffered gelatin diluent, and 0.1-ml samples of the undiluted specimen and each of the dilutions are plated onto colistin-nalidixic acid or phenylethyl alcohol blood agar. The presence of 10^5 CFU or more of *S. aureus* or *B. cereus* per g of specimen is of potential significance (22, 120).

S. aureus is a possible cause of antibiotic-associated diarrhea (18). The incidence is controversial but receiving more attention. Gram stain of smears of nonformed stool showing sheets of staphylococcal clusters in combination with appropriate clinical findings suggests the diagnosis.

MRSA may be a cause of nosocomial antibiotic-associated diarrhea (18). The overall incidence is unknown. Diagnosis consists of the detection of heavy growth of MRSA in combination with the detection of staphylococcal enterotoxin in stool. Greater recognition of this disease should confirm its significance and result in rapid diagnostic methods and appropriate treatment.

Clostridium botulinum

The clinical diagnosis of foodborne and infant botulism may be confirmed by detecting botulinal toxin, *C. botulinum*, or both in feces (121). Optimally, 25 to 50 g of stool, 15 to 20 ml of serum, and a sample of suspect food should be collected. Most clinical laboratories are not properly equipped to process specimens from persons with suspected botulism. In the United States, when a case of botulism is suspected, investigators at the CDC should be notified to ensure appropriate diagnosis, treatment, and investigation of the potential outbreak. Botulinal toxin could be used as a biological weapon (see chapter 9). Unexpected numbers of cases or unusual presentations should be investigated.

Helicobacter pylori

H. pylori is an important cause of gastritis and peptic ulcer disease (206). The organism can be observed in tissue sections by using hematoxylin and eosin, Giemsa, or Warthin-Starry silver staining. In addition, organisms can be visualized in touch preparations of dissected tissue stained with the Gram stain. The presence of *H. pylori* in stomach or small bowel lesions can be confirmed by culture, antigen detection, urease detection, or the detection of exhaled bacterial metabolite (*H. pylori* breath test) (101, 205, 206). Tissue biopsy specimens collected during endoscopy are used for culture and urease detection. Specimens for culture should be placed in transport medium (medium containing 20% glycerol, such as brucella broth, are best for transport and storage) and transported to the laboratory immediately, or refrigerated during delays (72). Lightly minced tissue is inoculated to freshly prepared blood agar and incubated in a humid, microaerophilic atmosphere (5 to 10% carbon dioxide, 80 to 90% nitrogen, and 5 to 10% oxygen) at 37°C for 7 days (Table 5). The addition of 5% hydrogen should improve the yield of *H. pylori*. Tissue for urease detection is placed as soon as possible into the detection system and processed as specified by the manufacturer. Stool for antigen detection should be collected and handled according to instructions included with the Premier Platinum HpSA test (Meridian Biosciences, Inc., Cincinnati, Ohio) (64, 205). In some clinical situations serologic testing for *H. pylori* antibody may be necessary. Serum should be collected and stored at refrigeration temperature for short periods (up to 1 week) or frozen at –70°C for longer periods (101).

Screening for VRE or Beta-Hemolytic Streptococci

Identifying Carriers of Vancomycin-Resistant Enterococci (VRE) for infection control purposes, detecting group B streptococci in pregnant patients, and detecting group A streptococci during investigations of outbreaks of necrotizing fasciitis or streptococcal toxic shock require collection of a rectal swab specimen. Carriers of VRE can be identified by culturing rectal swab or perirectal swab material (218). Specimens are inoculated to selective enrichment broth, such as Enterococcosel broth with 6 μg of vancomycin per ml, or agar media, such as colistin-nalidixic acid blood agar containing 6 μg of vancomycin per ml (see chapter 30). Carriers of group A streptococci can be identified by culturing rectal swab specimens on sheep blood agar or selective streptococcal agars used to identify patients with streptococcal pharyngitis. Carriers of group B streptococci are identified by culturing vaginal secretions and rectal swab material as discussed below (28).

Genital Tract Specimens

Genital tract specimens are sent to the microbiology laboratory to determine the etiology of various clinical syndromes, including vulvovaginitis, bacterial vaginosis (BV), genital ulcers, urethritis, cervicitis, endometritis, salpingitis, and ovarian abscess in females and urethritis, epididymitis, prostatitis, and genital ulcers in males. These diseases and their etiologies are listed in Table 8 (6).

Many specimens are contaminated with normal skin or mucous membrane flora. Pathogens such as *Haemophilus ducreyi*, *N. gonorrhoeae*, *Trichomonas vaginalis*, *Treponema pallidum*, and *C. trachomatis* are always significant. Other organisms, such as *S. aureus*, beta-hemolytic streptococci, *Enterobacteriaceae*, and anaerobes, are pathogenic only in certain clinical situations. The specimen source, relative quantity of potential pathogen compared to normal flora, and Gram stain interpretation help the technologist determine which isolates require identification and antimicrobial testing. At a minimum, isolates from presumably sterile specimens and pure or predominant potential pathogens from specimens likely to be contaminated with normal flora and containing polymorphonuclear neutrophils should be identified and reported. Mixtures of anaerobes do not require individual identification and listing in most cases. Laboratories should avoid isolating, identifying, and performing antimicrobial testing on every bacterial isolate from all specimens (6). In addition to the excessive cost of this approach, unnecessary reporting of bacterial species contributes to excessive treatment of patients. Exact protocols for workup and reporting may require discussion and mutual agreement with knowledgeable clinicians in each practice environment.

Special Considerations for Genital Tract Specimens

Detection of *N. gonorrhoeae* and *C. trachomatis*

Nucleic acid probe and amplification methods are commercially available for direct detection of *N. gonorrhoeae* and *C. trachomatis* in endocervical, urethral, and urine specimens. Users must pay close attention to the types of specimens approved for use with each kit. Specimens should be collected using the procedures and collection kits recommended by the manufacturer. In addition, false-positive reactions have been reported with some kits, necessitating confirmation of positive results (208).

Although not as sensitive as molecular methods, both EIA and DFA tests are commercially available for the direct detection of *C. trachomatis* in endocervical, urethral, and, with some EIA kits, urine specimens (171). If these kits are used, collection and processing must follow instructions provided by the manufacturer. Cell culture for *C. trachomatis* is recommended for use with specimens not approved for molecular or EIA kits. These are likely to include eye, rectal, and abscess specimens collected during surgery. In addition, culture is the only acceptable diagnostic procedure in some jurisdictions for medical-legal cases.

Culture for *N. gonorrhoeae* is optimal when the specimen is directly inoculated to a selective medium, such as modified Thayer-Martin medium, and incubated immediately (48). Transport of inoculated media to the laboratory must be in an increased CO_2-containing environment. Swab specimens (cotton swabs should be avoided because they may be toxic) should be placed in a transport system containing Stuart's or Amies medium and delivered to the laboratory as quickly as possible. Specimens for *N. gonorrhoeae* culture should be held at refrigeration temperature during transport. As transport time increases, recovery by culture decreases. Specimens requiring more than 24 h for transport are unacceptable. Detection by nonculture methods is recommended in most settings where the additional cost of testing by molecular technique or immunoasssay is not prohibitive (204).

BV and Vaginitis

BV occurs when conditions result in overgrowth of usual vaginal flora with various anaerobic genera, including *Mobiluncus* and *Bacteroides* (184). Although not characterized by a polymorphonuclear response, BV results in an increase in vaginal secretions that are relatively alkaline ($pH > 4.5$) compared to normal, the usual predominant flora of lactobacilli being replaced by anaerobes, and the presence of aromatic amines which are detected by adding 10% potassium hydroxide and noting a pungent, fishy odor. In addition, excessive growth of a facultative bacterium called *G. vaginalis* generally coincides with BV. Although *G. vaginalis* commonly is a member of the normal vaginal flora, the presence of increased concentrations that adhere to vaginal squamous epithelial cells, called clue cells, is pathognomonic of BV. Clue cells are squamous epithelial cells peppered with anaerobic coccobacilli and *G. vaginalis* bacteria, frequently showing heavier adherence toward the periphery of the cell and appearing like a donut (Fig. 3). As a result of these characteristic changes, BV is diagnosed best without culture (140). Wet-mount or Gram-stained smears should be examined and interpreted according to Table 9. In summary, BV should be diagnosed by performing a "bedside" pH and KOH "whiff test" and a laboratory Gram stain.

Candida and *Trichomonas* infections of the vulvovaginal areas are inflammatory conditions referred to as vaginitis rather than vaginosis. *Candida* spp. and *T. vaginalis* can be detected using microscopic examination of a saline wet-mount preparation. Low-power examination (×10 to ×20) will detect budding yeasts and pseudohyphae of *Candida* spp. or motile trophozoites of *Trichomonas*. Cultures are much more sensitive than direct wet preparations. Alternatively, a combination probe assay (Affirm VPIII identification test; Becton Dickinson, Sparks, Md.) is commercially available for the simultaneous detection of *Candida* spp., *G. vaginalis*, and *T. vaginalis* in vaginal secretions (21). Specimens must be collected using procedures recommended by the manufacturer.

Screening for Group B Streptococcus

Group B streptococcus carriers are identified by culturing vaginal secretions and rectal swab material. Swabs of the vaginal introitus and anorectum are collected and inoculated into a single enrichment broth such as LIM broth. This broth is incubated at 35°C overnight and subcultured to a blood agar plate the following day (173). A rapid molecular assay is available for the detection of group B streptococcus colonization in pregnant women (35). The performance of this test allows for rapid intrapartum detection of group B streptococci.

Dark-Field Examination for *T. pallidum*

Dark-field examination of tissues, tissue exudates, and material collected from chancres can be used to confirm the diagnosis of syphilis. For dark-field microscopy, the specimen should be examined within 20 min of collection to ensure motility of treponemes and should not be exposed to temperature extremes during transport to a dark-field microscope. The test requires a microscope equipped with a dark-field condenser and experienced personnel who are able to recognize *T. pallidum* spirochetes based on the tightness and regularity of the spirals and on their characteristic corkscrew movement (98). A DFA stain can be used and is performed on air-dried smears. The stability of the smear during transport and the easily identified, fluorescing treponemes make the DFA an attractive alternative to dark-field microscopy (98). Unfortunately, reagents for the DFA test are not commercially or widely available; it may be performed at some public health laboratories.

H. ducreyi

If infection with *H. ducreyi* is suspected, material from the base of the ulcer is collected and held at room temperature until needed for processing (102). One swab is used to prepare a smear for Gram staining. The presence of many small, pleomorphic, gram-negative bacilli and coccobacilli arranged

TABLE 9 Diagnosis of BV using a Gram-stained smear of vaginal secretions, by the Vaginal Infection and Prematurity Study Group criteria[a]

Morphotype	Score for indicated no. of morphotypes seen per oil power field				
	None	≤1	1–5	5–30	>30
Lactobacillus	4	3	2	1	0
Gardnerella/Bacteroides spp.	0	1	2	3	4
Curved gram-variable rods (*Mobiluncus* spp.)	0	1	2	3	4

[a] Adapted from reference 140. Total score = *Lactobacillus* morphotypes + *Gardnerella/Bacteroides* morphotypes + *Mobiluncus* morphotypes. A score of 0 to 3 is considered normal, 4 to 6 is intermediate, and 7 to 10 indicates BV.

in chains and groups (school of fish) suggests *H. ducreyi* but is rarely seen (see chapter 41). Recovery of the organisms by culturing on an enriched medium such as GC agar containing 3 μg of vancomycin per ml, 1% hemoglobin, 5% fetal bovine serum, and 1% IsoVitaleX, or Mueller-Hinton agar with 5% horse blood, 1% IsoVitaleX, and 3 μg of vancomycin per ml, is necessary to confirm the diagnosis; culturing at 33°C yields better recovery than does culturing at 35°C (see chapter 41).

Actinomyces spp.

Actinomyces spp. may cause pelvic inflammatory disease in women who use intrauterine contraceptive devices (IUD) (104). An IUD submitted for culture should be placed in a sterile liquid medium (preferably reduced, such as thioglycolate) and vortexed, and the liquid medium should be used to inoculate aerobic and anaerobic culture media. Inflammatory debris and tissue attached to the IUD should be removed and cultured aerobically and anaerobically. *Actinomyces* spp. produce small knots of intertwined bacterial filaments called grains or granules, which may be 1 mm or more in diameter. These grains should be crushed on a slide for staining (Gram stain is acceptable) and transferred to media for culture. The presence of branching gram-positive filaments suggests *Actinomyces,* which characteristically occurs in mixed infections with other aerobic and anaerobic bacteria. Culture confirms the diagnosis.

Lower Respiratory Tract Specimens

Specimens from the lower respiratory tract are submitted to determine the etiology of airway disease (tracheitis and bronchitis), pneumonia, lung abscess, and empyema (10, 138, 179). Table 8 gives a list of lower respiratory tract diseases and their common etiologies. Usual specimens submitted consist of lower respiratory tract secretions and inflammation in the form of expectorated sputum, induced sputum, endotracheal tube aspirations (intubated patients), bronchial brushings, washes or alveolar lavage samples collected during bronchoscopy, and pleural fluid (198). Specimens should be delivered to the laboratory promptly and processed without delay (within 1 h of collection). If delays are unavoidable, the specimen should be refrigerated.

Usual pathogens detected in lower respiratory tract secretions are present in specimens containing acute inflammatory cells (polymorphonuclear leukocytes) and in quantities greater than contaminating respiratory flora. Frequently, pathogenic bacteria are present within the polymorphonuclear leukocytes. There are many ways to assess the quality of respiratory tract specimens. A simple screening method involves assessment of squamous epithelial cells only (128, 129, 135). Squamous epithelial cells are found in the oropharynx but not in the lower respiratory tract. Increased numbers (defined as >10 per 10× objective microscopic field) indicate gross contamination with oropharyngeal contents, which include usual oral bacterial flora (Fig. 4 and 5). Most bacterial lower respiratory tract disease is caused by inapparent aspiration of oropharyngeal contents. It follows that oropharyngeal floras include the bacteria that cause lower respiratory tract disease. Detection of a potential pathogen in a grossly contaminated specimen may represent contamination with oropharyngeal flora. The lack of usefulness of data from contaminated specimens has resulted in policies for screening and rejecting grossly contaminated respiratory tract specimens. Table 6 lists respiratory tract specimens and usual screening policies. Respiratory tract specimens for the detection of *Mycoplasma pneumoniae, Legionella* spp., dimorphic fungi, and *M. tuberculosis* should not be screened for adequacy. All specimens are considered acceptable for the detection of these microorganisms (34).

Once respiratory tract specimens have been deemed acceptable, Gram-stained smears should be examined further for inflammatory cells, bacteria, and other indicators of lower respiratory tract pathology, such as mucus, necrosis, intracellular bacteria, alveolar macrophages, and Curschmann's spirals (Fig. 2) (231). Tracheal and bronchial mucopurulence can be trapped behind an airway obstruction or within a lung abscess cavity or may pool in the bronchi or trachea, resulting in the death and disintegration of cells, reflected as necrosis and cell debris in stained smears. Intracellular bacteria can be differentiated from bacteria "lying" on top of polymorphonuclear leukocytes by their greater concentration within the phagocytic cell than in nearby extracellular areas. Phagocytosis is an active uptake process resulting in concentration of bacteria within the cell. Alveolar macrophages are identified by their vacuolated cytoplasm and round eccentric nucleus, which is difficult to see in Gram-stained smears. Alveolar macrophages and Curschmann's spirals indicate areas within the smear that originated within the alveoli and distal airways (Fig. 2). Occasionally elastin fibers are seen in respiratory tract specimens (Fig. 1).

Bacteria should be reported when detected in Gram-stained smears if they are potential pathogens. Bacteria not in sufficient quantity or not representative of morphotypes resembling potential pathogens should be lumped together and reported as normal respiratory flora. It is important to differentiate contaminating respiratory flora from respiratory flora causing aspiration pneumonia. Aspiration of relatively large amounts of oropharyngeal contents following loss of consciousness, paralysis of muscles involved with swallowing and breathing, or medical procedures such as intubation can result in infection of the airways with mixed respiratory flora leading to lung abscess and empyema (111). Gram stain of sputum from patients with aspiration pneumonia can be highly suggestive of the diagnosis. Stained smears show many polymorphonuclear leukocytes and many mixed respiratory flora morphotypes, especially those suggesting streptococci and anaerobes. Much of the flora is intracellular. Aspiration pneumonia can be detected in hospitalized patients and those admitted directly from the community (10, 138).

Cultures of respiratory tract material should include a medium selective for gram-negative organisms, such as MacConkey's agar, sheep blood agar, and chocolate agar for the detection of *Haemophilus* spp. (Table 5). Culture plates should be incubated at 35°C in 3 to 5% CO_2 for 48 h before being reported as negative. Cultures are interpreted by examining the relative numbers and types of bacteria that grow. Table 10 summarizes interpretative criteria used with respiratory tract specimens (200).

Special Considerations for Lower Respiratory Tract Specimens

Specimens Collected During Bronchoscopy

Bronchoalveolar lavage fluid and bronchial brush specimens from patients with suspected pneumonia should be cultured quantitatively to evaluate the significance of potential pathogens recovered (23). Bronchial brush specimens, which contain approximately 0.01 to 0.001 ml of secretions, should be placed in 1 ml of sterile nonbacteriostatic saline after collection. The specimen should be delivered to the laboratory immediately. In the laboratory, the specimen is agitated on a vortex mixer, a smear is prepared by cytocentrifugation for staining with the Gram stain, and 0.01 ml of specimen is inoculated to appropriate media by using a pipette or calibrated loop. Colony counts of more than 1,000 CFU of potential pathogens per ml (corresponding to 10^6 CFU of original specimen per ml) appear to correlate with disease. Bronchoalveolar lavage results in collection of 50 ml or more of saline from a larger lung volume. In the laboratory, a smear is prepared by cytocentrifugation and Gram stained (155). The Gram stain report should include a comment about the presence of squamous epithelial cells and intracellular bacteria. Grossly contaminated fluid (>1% of all cells are squamous epithelial cells) may have falsely elevated counts of potential pathogens. Intracellular bacteria are more likely to be potential pathogens. A 0.01- or 0.001-ml aliquot of bronchoalveolar lavage fluid should be inoculated to agar media (Table 5). The recovery of <10,000 bacteria/ml suggests contamination. The recovery of >100,000 bacteria/ml suggests that the isolate is a potential pathogen. Detection of 10,000 to 100,000 bacteria per ml represents a "gray" zone (200). Counts of pathogens may be reduced by prior antimicrobial therapy or variations in "return" of lavage fluid during the bronchoscopy procedure (Table 10).

Legionella spp.

Legionella spp., especially *L. pneumophila,* are important causes of community- and hospital-acquired pneumonia (51). Legionellosis can be diagnosed by culture, DFA staining of smears of respiratory secretions, detection of antigens in urine, or serologic testing. Culture is preferred because, unlike other methods, it is not limited to detection of certain species or serotypes. Before culture, respiratory samples should be diluted 10-fold in a bacteriological broth, such as tryptic soy, or sterile water to dilute inhibitory substances that may be present in the specimen. Because legionellae grow slowly, optimal isolation from highly contaminated specimens, such as sputum, is achieved by decontaminating the specimens with acid before plating (214). The specimen is diluted 1:10 in KCl-HCl buffer (pH 2.2) and incubated for 4 min at room temperature. It is important not to incubate the specimen for longer than 4 min because legionellae may themselves be killed by acid exposure. Specimens are inoculated onto buffered charcoal yeast extract agar with and without antimicrobial agents (e.g., vancomycin, polymyxin B, and anisomycin). The cultures are incubated in humidfied air at 35°C for a minimum of 5 days. Using a dissecting microscope, small colonies with a ground-glass appearance, typical of *Legionella* spp., can be detected after 3 days of incubation.

M. pneumoniae

Mycoplasma pneumoniae is a common cause of pneumonia, referred to as primary atypical pneumonia. Because *M. pneumoniae* is fastidious and grows very slowly, a definitive diagnosis is often based on the results of serologic tests. When culture is required, the specimen of choice is a throat swab; however, sputum or other respiratory specimens are also acceptable. The specimen should be placed immediately into a transport medium containing protein, such as albumin, and penicillin to reduce the growth of contaminating bacteria. Specimens may be stored in the transport medium for up to 48 h at 4°C or frozen for longer periods at –70°C. PCR methods have been used successfully to detect *M. pneumoniae* directly in respiratory tract specimens. Molecular detection by PCR or a related technique may be the most sensitive method for the detection of *M. pneumoniae* (156).

Specimens from Patients with Cystic Fibrosis

Burkholderia cepacia is an important respiratory pathogen in persons with cystic fibrosis (31, 62). This organism grows well on routine media; however, selective media such as *B. cepacia* selective agar, *Pseudomonas cepacia* agar, and oxidative-fermentative-polymyxin B-bacitracin-lactose agar are useful for optimal recovery from respiratory secretions (79, 80). Comparative studies show *B. cepacia* selective agar to be superior (79) (also see chapter 49).

Chlamydia and *Chlamydophila* spp.

Chlamydiae are important causes of respiratory illnesses in children and adults (143). *C. trachomatis* can cause serious respiratory disease in newborn infants. *Chlamydophila pneumoniae*

TABLE 10 Interpretation of bacterial lower respiratory tract culture results[a]

Specimen	Likely to be significant	Not likely to be significant	Additional data suggesting that isolate is significant
Sputum—coughed or induced	Predominant potential pathogen in Gram stain and culture. Neutrophils abundant.	Potential pathogen not present in Gram stain and only 1–2+ growth in culture. Neutrophils not abundant in Gram stain.	Potential pathogen within neutrophils (intracellular bacteria)
Endotracheal tube aspirate (112)	Predominant potential pathogen in Gram stain and culture. Neutrophils abundant.	Potential pathogen only 1–2+ growth in culture. Neutrophils not abundant in Gram stain.	Potential pathogen in quantities $>10^6$ CFU/ml. Potential pathogen within neutrophils (intracellular bacteria)
Bronchoalveolar lavage fluid	Predominant potential pathogen seen in every 100× field of Gram stain. Quantitative culture detects $>10^5$ CFU of potential pathogen/ml.	Potential pathogen not seen in Gram stain. Quantitative culture detects $<10^4$ CFU of potential pathogen/ml.	Potential pathogen within neutrophils (intracellular bacteria)

[a] Reprinted from reference 195 with permission.

causes illness in all age groups, but most disease occurs in adolescents and young adults. *Chlamydophila psittaci* is primarily an animal pathogen but occasionally causes disease in humans exposed to sick animals. Lower respiratory tract secretions, in addition to nasopharyngeal washes, for the detection of chlamydiae are collected and transported to the laboratory immediately in a medium containing antimicrobial agents (e.g., gentamicin and nystatin). If delays in transport or processing occur, the specimen should be stored at 4°C for up to 48 h. Longer storage should be at –70°C or colder. Chlamydiae are detected by rapid cell culture techniques (shell vial) using McCoy cells for *C. trachomatis* and *C. psittaci* and HEp-2 cells for *C. pneumoniae.* As with *M. pneumoniae,* PCR may prove to be the most sensitive method for the detection of respiratory chlamydiae (156).

Nocardia Species

Respiratory specimens for the detection of *Nocardia* species should be transported to the laboratory as soon as they are collected. For short delays, storage at 4°C is acceptable. Direct examination of a Gram-stained smear containing a *Nocardia* species shows thin, beaded gram-positive branching filaments. The filaments are also partially acid fast when stained by the modified Kinyoun method. There are no media used routinely for the specific recovery of *Nocardia* spp. since they grow readily on many common media such as sheep blood and chocolate agar plates, Sabouraud agar for fungi, Lowenstein-Jensen medium for mycobacteria, and charcoal yeast extract agar for legionellae. Mycobacterial decontamination procedures reduce the recovery of *Nocardia.* Selective charcoal yeast extract agar is optimal for culture from contaminated specimens (210). Although *Nocardia* spp. are detected commonly following 1 week of incubation, cultures are incubated for a total of 3 weeks at 35°C.

Upper Respiratory Tract Specimens

Upper respiratory tract specimens include the external nares, nasopharynx, throat, oral ulcerations, and inflammatory material from the nasal sinuses. Although few serious diseases involve these areas, many pathogens colonize or persist in these sites while causing symptomatic infection in deeper, less accessible sites (147).

Throat specimens are collected to diagnose pharyngitis caused by *Streptococcus pyogenes.* Swab specimens should be placed in a standard transport carrier containing Amies or modified Stuart's medium. Refrigeration is preferred if transport requires more than a few hours. Many rapid direct tests for group A streptococci are commercially available, including EIA, optical immunoassay, and nucleic acid-based probe assays (59, 190). The reported sensitivities of EIAs and an optical immunoassay vary between 60 and 95% but can be as low as 31% (25, 217). The nucleic acid-based assay has a sensitivity of >90% (75, 78). When a rapid test is requested, two throat swabs should be collected. If only one swab is received, the culture plate should be inoculated first. Material remaining on the swab is used for the direct test. If the rapid test is positive, the second swab can be discarded, but if the rapid test is negative, the second swab must be used for culture to confirm the negative direct test. The nucleic acid-based probe test is considered sensitive and specific enough by many to obviate confirmatory culture (78). A position paper by representatives of the American Academy of Family Physicians, the American College of Physicians-American Society of Internal Medicine, and the CDC states that rapid tests do not require confirmatory culture when used with adult patients (32). This recommendation does not hold for specimens from children.

To culture group A streptococci, either sheep blood agar or selective blood agar may be used. Selective agar makes the organism easier to visualize by inhibiting accompanying flora but may delay the appearance of colonies of *S. pyogenes.* Cultures should be incubated for 48 h at 35°C in an environment of reduced oxygen achieved by incubating them anaerobically, in 5% CO_2, or in air with multiple "stabs" through the agar surface. Stabbing the agar surface with the inoculating loop pushes inoculum containing streptococci below the surface, where the oxygen concentration is reduced compared to ambient (25, 89). These culture conditions allow the recovery of group C and G streptococci, organisms which may cause pharyngitis but do not cause the serious sequelae associated with group A streptococci (203, 232).

Throat specimens also are used to identify patients infected with *N. gonorrhoeae.* For best results, the specimen should be inoculated immediately to a selective medium, such as modified Thayer-Martin agar. Cultures are incubated at 35°C in the presence of 5% CO_2 for 72 h.

The external nares can be cultured to identify carriers of *S. aureus* by using a single swab to collect secretions from both the left and right nares. The usual carrier systems used for swab transport containing Amies or Stuart's medium are acceptable. In the laboratory, the specimen can be inoculated to a sheep blood agar plate; however, use of selective media such as colistin-nalidixic acid agar, or a selective and differential medium such as BBL CHROMagar *Staph aureus* (BD Diagnostics, Sparks, Md.), BBL CHROMagar MRSA (BD Diagnostics), or mannitol salt agar is helpful in differentiating *S. aureus* or MRSA from other floras and useful when interpreting large numbers of specimens (53, 54, 57, 221). Published comparisons show the CHROMagar formulations to be superior (53, 54). Cultures should be incubated at 35°C for 2 days. Molecular testing by PCR for the detection of *S. aureus* in swabs from the external nares has been shown to be as sensitive as culture but much more rapid (142). A commercially available, FDA-approved molecular test (IDI-MRSA; Infectio Diagnostic, Inc., Sainte-Foy, Quebec, Canada) for the detection of MRSA in nasal swabs is also an option for those seeking a rapid test (216).

Nasopharyngeal secretions and cells are used to identify patients infected with *Bordetella* spp. and carriers of *N. meningitidis* (113). Specimens for the recovery of *Bordetella pertussis* and *Bordetella parapertussis* should be collected with a small-tipped Dacron swab. Cotton may be toxic to the organism. Swabs should be transported to the laboratory in special media. For delays of up to 24 h, Amies medium with charcoal can be used. If the transport time will exceed 24 h, Regan-Lowe transport medium should be used (82, 126). Culture, DFA staining, and PCR can be used for detection. PCR is the most sensitive method for detecting *B. pertussis* and *B. parapertussis* (Dacron swabs are preferred for PCR tests) (107). Culture is performed using Regan-Lowe charcoal agar containing 10% horse blood and cephalexin. Because a few strains of *B. pertussis* do not grow in the presence of cephalexin, the use of Regan-Lowe medium with and without cephalexin is recommended for optimal recovery (77, 183). Cultures are incubated at 35°C for 5 to 7 days in a humid atmosphere. The DFA test has a lower sensitivity and specificity than PCR for *Bordetella* but offers rapid results (107). Depending on the reagents used, either *B. pertussis* or *B. parapertussis* is detected.

Nasopharyngeal swab specimens are used to identify carriers of *N. meningitidis.* Transport in a swab container with Amies or Stuart's medium is acceptable. Specimens should be inoculated as quickly as possible to sheep blood or chocolate agar; however, selective agars for pathogenic *Neisseria* spp., such as modified Thayer-Martin, are necessary if interference by normal flora is expected. Culture plates are incubated for 72 h in a humidified atmosphere at 35°C in the presence of 5% CO_2.

Vincent's angina is an oral infection characterized by pharyngitis, membranous exudate, fetid breath, and oral ulcerations. Sometimes referred to as fusospirochetal disease or necrotizing ulcerative gingivitis, it is caused by *Fusobacterium* spp., *Borrelia* spp., and other anaerobes. Diagnosis is made by direct examination of a smear of a swab specimen collected from the ulcerated lesions and stained with the Gram stain (147). The presence of many spirochetes, fusiform bacilli, and polymorphonuclear leukocytes is presumptive evidence of this disease. Culture is not helpful. It should be noted that canker sores do not have a microbial etiology and should not be cultured.

Inflammatory material from the nasal sinuses should be cultured to detect the etiologies of sinusitis. Nearly all cases of bacterial sinusitis follow a primary, upper respiratory tract viral infection. Bacteria are trapped in the sinus as a result of damage to the epithelial lining cells of the sinus and inflammation and swelling that narrows or closes the nasal ostium, preventing normal drainage (69). Specimens collected during endoscopic procedures by physicians specializing in otorhinolaryngology are optimal, since they are sampled directly from the infected sinus, avoiding contamination by normal flora in the nasal passages. Aspirates, washes, scrapings or debridements, and biopsy material should be kept moist and sent in a sterile container to the laboratory (69). Examination of Gram-stained smears can provide a rapid, presumptive identification of likely pathogens. Aerobic culture is needed in all cases; anaerobic transport and culture may be needed in cases of chronic sinisitis. Ventilator-associated sinusitis occurs in fewer than 10% of patients with nasotracheal intubation. Members of the nosocomial flora are implicated. Endoscopic inspection is needed to obtain acceptable specimen for culture (222).

Special Considerations for Upper Respiratory Tract Specimens

Arcanobacterium haemolyticum

A. haemolyticum can cause pharyngitis and peritonsillar abscess (88). The organism can be recovered on media used to detect *S. pyogenes.* Colonies of *A. haemolyticum* are beta-hemolytic and easily confused with those of beta-hemolytic streptococci. Rapid differentiation can be accomplished with the Gram stain. *A. haemolyticum* is a diphtheroid-shaped gram-positive rod (see chapter 34). Incubation of plates at 35°C for up to 72 h may be required for optimal detection.

Corynebacterium diphtheriae

Cultures of both throat and nasopharyngeal specimens are used in the diagnosis of diphtheria. When specimens are processed for culture without delay, no special transport medium or conditions are required. For transport to a reference laboratory, specimens should be sent dry in a container with desiccant (44). Alternatively, specimens collected on swabs may be placed in Stuart's or Amies medium for transport to the laboratory. Smears of specimens for *C. diphtheriae* can be stained with the Gram stain and examined for pleomorphic (diphtheroid morphology) gram-positive rods. In addition, smears can be stained with Loeffler's methylene blue stain and examined for pleomorphic, beaded rods with swollen (club-shaped) ends and reddish purple metachromatic granules. Bacteria with these characteristics are suggestive of but not specific for *C. diphtheriae.* Specimens should be inoculated to Loeffler's serum and potassium tellurite media for the recovery of *C. diphtheriae.* Cultures are incubated for 2 days at 35°C in 5% CO_2 before being reported as negative.

Epiglottitis

A throat swab specimen may be helpful in determining the etiology of epiglottitis, a rapidly progressing cellulitis of the epiglottis and adjacent structures with the potential for swollen tissues to cause airway obstruction. Epiglottitis is almost always caused by *H. influenzae* serotype b but occasionally by other bacteria such as *S. pneumoniae* and *S. pyogenes* (202). The specimen should be collected by a physician only in a setting where emergency intubation can be performed immediately to secure a patent airway. Specimens should be inoculated onto enriched medium, such as chocolate agar, and incubated at 35°C in an atmosphere of 5% CO_2 for 72 h. Nearly 100% of patients with epiglottitis caused by *H. influenzae* have a blood culture positive for the same bacterium.

Tissue Specimens

Tissue specimens are obtained during surgical procedures at significant risk and expense to the patient. Therefore, it is mandatory for the laboratory to receive sufficient specimen for both histopathologic and microbiological examination, bearing in mind that many microbiological tests and cultures may have been ordered. Histopathologic examination of the lesion serves to differentiate between infection and malignancy, and also to distinguish between acute and chronic infectious processes (227). Swabs provide too little specimen and should be discouraged and eliminated through educational efforts. For complete setup of routine, anaerobic, fungal, and acid-fast bacillus cultures and smears, one needs approximately 1 cm^3 of tissue.

Tissue should be transported in a sterile container that maintains moisture. To avoid drying, small pieces of tissue can be moistened with a few drops of sterile, nonbacteriostatic saline. Alternatively, very small pieces of tissue can be placed on a square of moistened sterile gauze. This serves to maintain moisture and allow easy identification by those receiving and processing the specimen. Tissue should be gently minced or ground during processing to release microorganisms and to provide equal specimen for all media and smears. This can be accomplished by cutting with a sterile scalpel, grinding with a mortar and pestle or tissue grinder, or using a stomacher (Seward Co., London, United Kingdom) or masticator (available from several suppliers) (180). The resulting homogenate is used to prepare smears for staining and to inoculate culture media. The Gram stain should be examined for the presence of polymorphonuclear leukocytes and bacteria. Grinding renders most cell morphology and tissue architecture difficult to recognize and often renders fungal hyphae nonviable. A small piece of intact tissue should be retained for inoculation into fungal media. Smears should be examined closely for intracellular bacteria, especially common with staphylococci and streptococci. For bacterial culture, processed tissue should be inoculated to enriched agar media. The use of a broth medium is controversial (128, 130). Anaerobic culture should be included when ordered and when tissue is transported in an oxygen-free environment. Large pieces of tissue, approximately 1 cm^3 or greater, maintain a reduced atmosphere in spite of brief aerobic transport. Oxygen-free transport may not be necessary in this circumstance, and the absence of anaerobic transport should not disqualify large pieces of tissue from anaerobic culture. Routine, aerobic cultures are incubated at 35°C in the presence of 5% CO_2 for 72 h.

Collecting and processing tissue offers an opportunity for exogenous contamination. Cultures growing small numbers of bacteria not commonly associated with infection, such as coagulase-negative staphylococci, corynebacteria, propionibacteria, and saprophytic *Neisseria* spp., may represent contamination rather than true "pathogens." In general, growth of these bacterial groups in broth culture only represents contamination (128, 130). One or two bacterial colonies growing on a single plate, of multiple plates inoculated, and not growing in broth culture, if used, generally represent contamination. Growth of one or two bacterial colonies on agar media not in the area of specimen inoculation or on streak lines in the second through fourth plate quadrants also is likely to represent contamination. In addition, it is assumed that bacteria considered contaminants were not detected in Gram-stained smears prepared from the original specimen. On the other hand, detection of the bacteria listed above as unlikely pathogens should always be reported when seen in the original Gram-stained smear, when present in quantities above a few colonies, and when detected on or in multiple media (41).

Special Circumstances for Tissue Specimens

Bone Marrow

Bone marrow aspirates can be submitted for culture in lysis centrifugation tubes (Isolator; Wampole Laboratories). The "pediatric" tube holds a maximum of 1.5 ml of specimen. One or more of the 1.5-ml tubes can be used. Aspirates may also be submitted in a sterile container containing anticoagulant. Sterile tubes with anticoagulant are less desirable since they use heparin, sodium citrate, or EDTA as anticoagulant, all of which are more inhibitory than SPS (49, 166). Although SPS inhibits meningococci, gonococci, *G. vaginalis,* anaerobic cocci, and *S. moniliformis,* these bacteria are unlikely to be detected in bone marrow aspirate specimens (159).

Although bone marrow aspirate cultures may be helpful in identifying disseminated fungal and mycobacterial diseases, they are unlikely to assist in the identification of usual bacterial diseases (211). Patients infected with human immunodeficiency virus may benefit from bone marrow culture when other specimen cultures have been unsuccessful (47). It is policy in some laboratories to consult with the ordering physician and suggest that routine bacterial culture is not necessary. In most cases, blood or other organ system culture is preferred for the identification of disseminated bacterial infections. Even if bone marrow culture is performed, direct Gram stain of bone marrow aspirates is not helpful and should not be a routine component of bacterial culture.

Lymph Nodes

Lymph node cultures from immunocompetent patients are positive only when there is a granuloma or acute inflammatory lesion, in which case etiologies detected are limited to mycobacteria and fungi. Bacterial culture of lymph nodes from immunocompetent patients may not be necessary without specific clinical or epidemiological findings, such as suspected tularemia *(F. tularensis)* (56).

Quantitative Tissue Culture

Tissue from traumatic wound or burn injury may be submitted for quantitative culture, with results of $\geq 10^3$ CFU/ml being used to predict the likelihood of the development of wound-related sepsis (117, 228). Limitations include the lack of reproducible results and the low predictive value compared to histologic examination of tissue. To perform a quantitative culture, a portion of the specimen is weighed and homogenized in saline. The saline suspension is used to prepare serial dilutions for culture. Detailed procedures for quantitative tissue culture are given elsewhere (230).

Bartonella

Bartonella henselae is the agent of cat scratch disease in healthy hosts and causes bacteremia, endocarditis, bacillary angiomatosis, and bacillary peliosis primarily in immunocompromised hosts. Optimal detection of the organism requires PCR (186). Culture is very difficult but can be attempted using Isolator tubes (Wampole Laboratories) and freshly prepared rabbit blood agar plates incubated in a moist environment for an extended period (19). Tissue culture may have a better yield than agar (see chapter 54). Lymph node tissue is macerated and inoculated into media directly. Because the detection of *B. henselae* is time-consuming and expensive, the diagnosis of cat scratch disease is most often made by clinical criteria and exclusion of other diseases. *B. henselae* can be observed in sections of fixed tissue stained with Warthin-Starry or Diederle's silver stain (94, 123).

Urinary Tract Specimens

Diseases of the urinary tract include prostatitis, urethral syndrome, cystitis, and pyelonephritis. Etiologies are summarized in Table 8. Urine, prostatic secretion, or urethral cells or secretion specimens are needed to diagnose these diseases. Urine can be collected by midstream collection, catheterization (straight/in-out or indwelling), cystoscopic collection, or suprapubic aspiration. Foley catheter tips should not be submitted or accepted for culture since they are always contaminated with urethral flora and quantitation is not possible. A first-voided morning urine is optimal, since in most cases bacteria have been sitting in the bladder multiplying for a number of hours. Clean-catch urine, implying cleansing of periurethral areas, has not been shown to improve the quality of urine culture and is not recommended (103, 154).

Urine specimens should be transported to the laboratory immediately and processed within 2 h of collection. If a delay occurs, specimens may be refrigerated for up to 24 h. Transport tubes containing boric acid are available to stabilize the bacterial population at room temperature for 24 h, if refrigeration is not available (99). Boric acid-preserved urines are acceptable for dipstick leukocyte esterase testing (229).

Urine culture is the most common test performed by most microbiology laboratories, and most urine cultures are negative; i.e., no specific potential pathogen is detected. Screening methods are available that attempt to rapidly separate those specimens containing significant counts of bacteria from negative specimens. In general, screening methods compare well with specimens containing 10^5 CFU of bacteria per ml or greater but perform poorly when colony counts are lower. Screening urine specimens by staining with the Gram stain is rapid and economical with regard to reagents but is labor-intensive and requires a trained technologist. The presence of 1 or 2 bacteria of similar morphotype, or more, in each oil immersion field (100× objective lens) correlates with a count of 100,000 or greater by culture (162, 226). Commercially available dipstick tests that detect leukocyte esterase (an enzyme produced by neutrophils) and nitrite (the result of bacterial nitrate reductase acting on nitrate in the urine) are rapid, inexpensive, and simple to perform, but their sensitivity is low in some patient populations (144, 153, 175). False-negative dipstick screening occurs because frequent voiding dilutes the concentration of leukocyte esterase and nitrite in urine, enterococci and other less common urinary tract pathogens do not produce nitrate reductase, and many patients with asymptomatic bacteriuria do not have significant numbers of leukocytes in their urine. In spite of this, outpatient screening algorithms have been proposed that incorporate enzyme screening in a "reflexive" urine test; i.e., urinalysis is performed, and if positive for leukocyte esterase or nitrate reductase, a culture will be set up, and if negative, a culture will not be done (29). Such screening works best in symptomatic patients, diabetics, and women older than 60 years (144, 153, 175).

In addition to the Gram stain and dipstick tests for leukocyte esterase and nitrite, several urine screening systems have been marketed (151). Notable among these are the FiltraCheck-UTI and a semiautomated version called the Bac-T-Screen, the UTI screen Bacterial ATP Assay, and the Cellenium automated urine screening system (133, 141, 151, 152, 162, 188). Currently, all are no longer available or not actively marketed, and they are not discussed further here.

The standard for quantitative bacterial culture of urine is the inoculation of 0.01 or 0.001 ml of specimen using a calibrated plastic or wire loop to appropriate media, usually sheep blood and MacConkey agars. The loop is dipped vertically into the well-mixed urine, just far enough to cover the loop, and the loopful of urine is spread over the surface of the agar plate by streaking from top to bottom in a vertical line and again from top to bottom perpendicular to this line in a back-and-forth fashion. Prior to plate inoculation, it is necessary to ensure that a film of urine fills the loop with no bubbles to alter the calibrated volume. The inoculum of urine is spread over the entire agar surface to simplify counting of colonies after growth. Urine cultures are incubated at 35°C for 24 to 48 h. Although most urinary tract pathogens grow readily on usual agar media, slowly growing pathogens and those inhibited by the presence of antimicrobials in the patient specimen may not appear after overnight incubation (16 h). One approach uses the results of the leukocyte esterase and nitrite tests to determine which cultures get incubated for a full 48 h. Urine cultures that are negative after overnight incubation but had one or both positive enzyme tests are incubated for an additional day. Those that had negative enzyme tests are reported as "no growth" in the final report (26, 132).

Contamination of urine is detected in approximately 5 to 40% of cultures. Contamination is not reduced by the use of central processing areas, refrigeration, urine screening systems, specimen preservatives, or insulated specimen transport (207).

Agar paddles are available for urine culture in settings where inoculation and incubation of conventional agar plates are not convenient or possible (165). A standard film of urine is distributed over the agar-covered paddle, usually by dipping the paddle into a jar of urine. The paddle is then reinserted into its plastic container for incubation. Following incubation, the density of growth is estimated by comparison to photographs or drawings. A preliminary identification of gram positive or gram negative can be determined by colony color and morphology, and, when appropriate, the entire paddle can be forwarded to a reference laboratory for complete identification and antimicrobial testing of the isolate. Agar paddle culture of urine with approximate colony counts compares favorably with standard culture (165).

The urinary tract above the urethra is sterile in healthy humans, but the urethra is colonized normally with many different bacteria. Because of this, urine collected by midstream voiding techniques becomes contaminated during passage. Commensal bacteria are differentiated from potential pathogens by quantitative culture. Bacterial counts indicating "significant" bacteriuria (isolate is a likely pathogen) vary with the host and type of infection. Table 11 summarizes significant counts for common clinical situations (189).

TABLE 11 Interpretation of urine culture results[a]

Urine specimen and patient[b]	Likely to be significant[b]	Not likely to be significant[b]	Additional data suggesting that isolate is significant
Midstream, female with cystitis	$>10^2$ CFU of potential pathogen/ml, urine LE is positive	Quantity of potential pathogen ≤ quantity of contaminating flora.	
Midstream, female with pyelonephritis	$>10^5$ CFU of potential pathogen/ml, urine LE is positive	Quantity of potential pathogen ≤ quantity of contaminating flora.	Gram stain demonstrates potential pathogen in neutrophils and/or casts.
Midstream, asymptomatic bacteriuria	$>10^5$ CFU of potential pathogen/ml, LE is usually negative	$<10^5$ CFU of potential pathogen/ml; quantity of potential pathogen ≤ quantity of contaminating flora.	Confirm by repeating urine when clinically indicated.
Midstream, male with UTI	$>10^3$ CFU of potential pathogen/ml, urine LE is positive	$<10^3$ CFU of potential pathogen/ml; quantity of potential pathogen ≤ quantity of contaminating flora.	Gram stain demonstrates potential pathogen in neutrophils and/or casts.
Straight catheter, all patients	$>10^2$ CFU of potential pathogen/ml, urine LE positive for symptomatic patients	$<10^2$ CFU of potential pathogen/ml; urine LE is negative.	Gram stain demonstrates potential pathogen in neutrophils and/or casts.
Indwelling catheter, all patients	$>10^3$ CFU of potential pathogens/ml (multiple pathogens may be present)	Bacteriuria detected in asymptomatic patients; urine LE positive or negative.	No reason to culture unless patient is symptomatic.

[a] Reprinted from reference 195 with permission.
[b] LE, leukocyte esterase; UTI, urinary tract infection.

Severe urinary tract infection generally involves the kidneys (pyelonephritis) and results in bacteremia. Rapid diagnosis and administration of appropriate antimicrobial therapy are necessary. In this clinical setting, blood cultures are needed and a stat Gram stain of the urine can be useful. The Gram stain provides an immediate indication of the quality of the urine and a preliminary identification of the likely pathogen. Specimens containing high numbers of squamous epithelial cells are likely to be grossly contaminated with periurethral or vaginal flora and new specimens should be collected immediately, before antimicrobials inhibit growth of the true pathogen (Fig. 6) (195). Gram stain identification of a potential pathogen confirms that empirical therapy is correct or may suggest a change based on an unexpected pathogen, such as *S. aureus* (Fig. 7).

Special Considerations for Urinary Tract Specimens

Leptospires

Leptospira interrogans can be recovered from blood and CSF during the acute stages of disease and from urine after the first week of illness and for several months thereafter. Urine should be processed as soon as possible after collection, because the acidity of urine harms the organisms. If a delay in processing is expected, urine should be neutralized with sodium bicarbonate, centrifuged (1,500 × *g* for 30 min), and resuspended in buffered saline before being used to inoculate media (see chapter 61). Alternatively, the urine may be diluted 1:10 in 1% bovine serum albumin and stored at 5 to 20°C. Undiluted urine and urine diluted 1:10, 1:100, and 1:1,000 in sterile buffered saline should be inoculated to Ellinghausen-McCullough-Johnson-Harris or equivalent medium, with and without neomycin (39). Cultures should be incubated at 30°C for at least 13 weeks (Table 5).

Bacterial Antigen Testing

Bacterial antigen testing kits, for the purpose of diagnosing bacterial meningitis, include procedures for use with urine specimens. In general, these kits should not be used with urine specimens for the diagnosis of bacterial meningitis. In addition, the FDA issued a product alert specifically cautioning against the use of the group B streptococcus antigen kits with urine specimens because of the risk of both false-positive and false-negative results (55).

An EIA is commercially available for the detection of *L. pneumophila* serogroup 1 antigen in urine. The antigen may be detectable in urine for months following an infection. The assay has a sensitivity of 80% when performed on unconcentrated urine (70, 73). Sensitivity is increased when urine is concentrated. The drawback of this assay is that only disease caused by *L. pneumophila* serogroup 1 is detected. A new EIA has been evaluated that detects all *L. pneumophila* serogroup antigens in urine (40).

S. pneumoniae antigen can be detected in urine using a commercially available EIA (NOW *S. pneumoniae* urinary antigen test; Binax, Portland, Maine) (83, 131, 167). Although the sensitivity for detecting urine antigen is 80% for patients with positive blood cultures and 52% for patients with positive sputum cultures, the specificity is high. This test may prove to be useful in settings where culture is not available, but at present it should be used in addition to, not in place of, culture.

Wound and Abscess Specimens

Abscess specimens should be collected by aspiration. Small amounts of purulence or wounds with nothing to aspirate can be irrigated with sterile, nonbacteriostatic saline to facilitate aspiration. In addition, wounds can be sampled by dissecting a small portion of infected tissue. Purulent specimens and wound specimens characterized by ulceration or necrosis, but with little moisture, can be collected with a swab, but this is generally inferior to aspiration or biopsy. Swab specimens contain less material, are more likely to be contaminated with adjacent flora, and are not amenable to optimal anaerobic transport. When swabs are used for collection, two swabs should be used, one for culture and one for preparation of a smear. Deep lesions that communicate with the surface are most problematic. The cutaneous portion and sinus tract are contaminated with bacteria found at the surface. Surgical debridement and sampling are recommended. If surgery is not performed, effort should be made to aspirate a "pocket" of infected material that is not open to the surface. As a last option, fresh specimen should be expressed from deep within the wound. A swab used to collect specimen from the surface overlying the draining wound is not acceptable. This is of particular importance when evaluating diabetic foot ulcers or infected pressure sores (169). Only deep specimens collected by aspiration or during debridement offer useful culture information (17, 105).

Gram staining of wound and abscess specimens is very important. The Gram stain result provides rapid presumptive identification of etiology, it can be used to evaluate the quality of the specimen submitted, and it guides the workup of culture results. Examination of a Gram-stained smear reveals bacterial morphotypes, acute inflammatory cells (polymorphonuclear neutrophils), intracellular bacteria, cell necrosis, and elastin fibers resulting from tissue necrosis. The quality of the wound specimen can be evaluated by comparing the number of polymorphonuclear cells and squamous epithelial cells (Table 12) (178). Excess numbers of squamous epithelial cells suggest gross contamination with cutaneous flora. It is acceptable to limit workup of bacterial isolates when the specimen shows gross contamination. An example of a limited workup would be to list by Gram stain morphology the isolates encountered, with a comment explaining that the physician must call if a replacement specimen cannot be collected and further identification and antimicrobial testing are clinically warranted.

Special Circumstances for Wound and Abscess Specimens

Cellulitis

Specimens from patients with cellulitis but without abscess are very difficult to collect. Recommendations have been made to inject a small volume of sterile, nonbacteriostatic saline into the infected tissue. The few drops that one can aspirate back should be sent for Gram stain and culture. Under the best of conditions, these specimens are unlikely to be positive (65, 81). Blood cultures from patients with cellulitis also are unlikely to be positive (146). In spite of the shortcomings of microbiology testing for patients with cellulitis, seriously ill patients may require biopsy and all should have blood collected for culture.

Necrotizing Fasciitis and Gas Gangrene

Necrotizing fasciitis and gas gangrene (myonecrosis) are medical emergencies requiring immediate diagnosis and therapy that may include antimicrobials, surgical debridement, and the use of immune globulin and immune mediators to combat the fatal complications of severe septic shock (177, 193). Necrotizing fasciitis and gas gangrene are caused most commonly by toxin-producing *S. pyogenes*, other beta-hemolytic

TABLE 12 Screening wound specimens to ensure quality[a]

Quantity of cells per 10× (objective lens) microscopic field					
No. of neutrophils	Q-value for neutrophils	Q-value for squamous epithelial cells present in the following no.[b]:			
		0	1–9	10–24	≥25
		0	−1	−2	−3
0	0	(1)	0	0	0
1–9	+1	1	0	−1	−2
10–24	+2	+2	+1	0	−1
≥25	+3	+3	+2	+1	0

[a] Attach Q-values to squamous cell and neutrophil quantities. Add the two Q-values together. Specimens with positive Q-values (+1 to +3) are more likely to contain increased numbers of potential pathogens and decreased numbers of potential contaminants. Specimens with negative Q-values (or a Q-value of zero) are likely to be contaminated with local flora. Specimens with no squamous cells or neutrophils are scored as one (1), allowing samples from neutropenic patients or those with necrotic or serous secretions to be processed as acceptable.

[b] The first row of numbers in the table is the Q-value for squamous epithelial cells only. The following four rows are the Q-values for the sum of the neutrophils and squamous epithelial cells.

streptococci, *S. aureus, Clostridium* spp., and mixed aerobic and anaerobic bacteria (46). The diagnosis is made by clinical examination of the patient and is confirmed by Gram stain and culture. Gram-stained smears generally show proteinaceous fluid, necrotic cell debris, rare or few polymorphonuclear leukocytes (because of cell lysis), and the bacterial etiology. Culture should confirm the etiology and provide antimicrobial testing results where appropriate.

Anaerobic Abscess

Anaerobes characteristically produce purulent infections in areas adjacent to mucous membranes containing anaerobes from the normal flora. Specimens must be transported to the laboratory in sterile, oxygen-free containers (148). As reviewed above, aspirated fluid or excised tissue is the recommended specimen. Specimens should be stored at room temperature (not refrigerated) during transport and processing delays. Infections of the mouth and gums (and adjacent areas), aspiration pneumonia, empyema, intra-abdominal infections, deep tissue abscesses, infections of the female genital tract, infected pressure sores, and diabetic foot ulcers are caused generally by a mixture of aerobes and anaerobes. Because of the usual microscopic appearance of mixed aerobic-anaerobic abscesses, the Gram stain can rapidly identify these infectious processes (Fig. 8). The presence of many polymorphonuclear leukocytes, many bacteria with anaerobic morphotypes (thin gram-negative bacilli, thin and poorly staining gram-positive bacilli, and boxcar-shaped gram-positive bacilli suggesting *Clostridium* spp.), and many intracellular bacteria suggests the presence of a mixed aerobic-anaerobic infectious process. Culture can determine the exact etiologies, characteristically a mixture of aerobes and anaerobes. However, the identification of most anaerobic bacteria and their susceptibility results are not necessary for the management of mixed infections. Aerobic and facultative bacteria present need full identification and antimicrobial testing results for proper therapeutic selection.

Specimens for anaerobic culture should be processed as soon as possible after arrival in the laboratory. Usual media include an anaerobic blood agar plate (CDC blood agar or brucella blood agar), a medium that inhibits gram-positive and facultative gram-negative bacilli such as blood agar with kanamycin and vancomycin, a differential or selective medium such as *Bacteroides* bile-esculin, and a gram-positive selective medium such as colistin-nalidixic acid blood agar or phenylethyl alcohol blood agar (Table 5). Media should be incubated in an anaerobic environment immediately after inoculation. Incubation in anaerobic containers, such as GasPak jars (Becton Dickinson Microbiology Systems, Cockeysville, Md.), AnaeroPack (Mitsubishi Gas Chemical America, Inc., New York, N.Y.), or Bio-Bag Anaerobic Culture Set (Becton Dickinson Microbiology Systems), or in an anaerobic chamber is acceptable (36, 37). Anaerobes grow more slowly than aerobic or facultative bacteria, necessitating a full 48 h of incubation before colony size is large enough to interpret accurately. Negative anaerobic cultures should be held for 3 to 5 days before being reported as negative. Longer incubation is necessary for isolation of *Actinomyces* and some other fastidious anaerobes.

Autopsy Specimens

Microbiology testing as a component of the autopsy examination has been and continues to be controversial (114, 174, 225). Postmortem and agonal invasion of sterile tissues confuses the significance of positive culture results, prompting some to argue against microbiology testing. Others have found that postmortem examination continues to uncover a significant number of infectious diagnoses, whether in the community or university hospital setting, which were missed by modern high-technology medicine (97). In addition, an important portion of missed diagnoses represents treatable diseases (136). The value of autopsy microbiology is further enhanced by its use to identify emerging diseases, etiologies of biological warfare, community outbreaks, nosocomial infections, and antimicrobial resistance and to uncover the cause of death in organ transplant patients and others with immunocompromising conditions. Safety precautions designed to protect the pathologist and dissection assistants during autopsy procedures have been thoroughly reviewed (139).

To minimize contamination of postmortem specimens, the body should be moved to a refrigerated locker (4 to 6°C) as soon as possible after death. Limited movement of the body has been shown to decrease the incidence of false-positive postmortem cultures (43). Although it has been shown that cultures collected within 48 h of death from a refrigerated cadaver did not show an increase in false-positive results, tissue and fluid specimens, as a rule, should be taken from refrigerated bodies within 15 h of death (93). This serves to diminish the likelihood of postmortem overgrowth of contaminants and improve detection of true pathogens.

Specimens should be obtained by sterilizing the surface of the organ with a hot spatula or iron surface until the surface is thoroughly dry (43). Body fluids, including blood, should be collected first. For blood collection, the wall of the heart and large vessel should be seared and a sterile needle (18 to 20 gauge) should be inserted. A 20-ml volume, or as close to 20 ml as possible, should be collected and injected directly into aerobic and anaerobic blood culture bottles. Blood culture results obtained before opening the chest cavity by percutaneous subxyphoid aspiration have been shown to have greater interpretive value (less contamination but detection of relevant organisms). Most conclude that postmortem blood cultures rarely provide information that is not already known. Solid viscera should be sampled by immediately cutting blocks of tissue from the center of the seared area. Samples should be submitted to microbiology with a requisition providing a full explanation of the studies needed. Postmortem cultures can be very useful for detecting pathogens that are not considered normal human flora, such as *M. tuberculosis*, *Brucella* spp., *B. pertussis*, some systemic fungi (*Histoplasma capsulatum*, *Coccidiodes immitis*, etc.), parasitic helminths, and agents of biological warfare. Tissue samples should be transported to the microbiology laboratory immediately in sterile tubes. The use of transport media and laboratory processing methods should follow recommendations for premortem specimens. An efficient way to avoid unnecessary workup of contaminating microorganisms is to issue a preliminary report to the pathologist who performed the autopsy listing organisms detected by colony or Gram stain morphology, such as "lactose-fermenting gram-negative rod" or "gram-positive cocci in clusters." This is accompanied with a notation that further identification and antimicrobial testing will not be performed unless there is consultation with the laboratory director or technologist conducting the culture investigation. Plates can be held for 1 week and discarded if no additional information is requested.

Specimens for the Detection of Agents of Biological Warfare

An excellent review of the potential agents of biological warfare and their management in the clinical microbiology laboratory can be found in Cumitech 33 and chapter 9 of this Manual (61, 92).

REFERENCES

1. **Agulla, A., F. J. Merino, P. A. Villasante, J. V. Saz, A. Diaz, and A. C. Velasco.** 1987. Evaluation of four enrichment media for isolation of *Campylobacter jejuni*. *J. Clin. Microbiol.* **25:**174–175.
2. **Arbique, J. C., K. R. Forward, and J. LeBlanc.** 2000. Evaluation of four commercial transport media for the survival of *Neisseria gonorrhoeae*. *Diagn. Microbiol. Infect. Dis.* **36:**163–168.
3. **Aslam, S., R. J. Hamill, and D. M. Musher.** 2005. Treatment of *Clostridium difficile*-associated disease: old therapies and new strategies. *Lancet Infect. Dis.* **5:**549–557.
4. **Baker, A. S., B. Paton, and J. Haaf.** 1989. Ocular infections: clinical and laboratory considerations. *Clin. Microbiol. Newsl.* **11:**97–101.
5. **Banatvala, N., P. M. Griffin, K. D. Greene, T. J. Barrett, W. F. Bibb, J. H. Green, and J. G. Wells.** 2001. The United States National Prospective Hemolytic Uremic Syndrome Study: microbiologic, serologic, clinical, and epidemiologic findings. *J. Infect. Dis.* **183:**1063–1070.
6. **Baron, E., G. Cassell, L. Duffy, D. Eschenbach, J. R. Greenwood, S. Harvey, N. Madinger, E. Peterson, and K. Waites.** 1993. Cumitech 17 A, *Laboratory Diagnosis of Female Genital Tract Infections*. Coordinating ed., E. J. Baron. American Society for Microbiology, Washington, D.C.
7. **Baron, E. J., J. D. Scott, and L. S. Tompkins.** 2005. Prolonged incubation and extensive subculturing do not increase recovery of clinically significant microorganisms from standard automated blood cultures. *Clin. Infect. Dis.* **41:**1677–1680.
8. **Baron, E. J., M. P. Weinstein, W. M. Dunne, P. Yagupsky, D. F. Welch, and D. M. Wilson.** 2005. Cumitech 1C, *Blood Cultures IV.* Coordinating ed., E. J. Baron. ASM Press, Washington, D.C.
9. **Bartlett, J. G.** 2002. Clinical practice. Antibiotic-associated diarrhea. *N. Engl. J. Med.* **346:**334–339.
10. **Bartlett, J. G., S. F. Dowell, L. A. Mandell, T. M. File, Jr. D. M. Musher, and M. J. Fine.** 2000. Practice guidelines for the management of community-acquired pneumonia in adults. Infectious Diseases Society of America. *Clin. Infect. Dis.* **31:**347–382.
11. **Bartlett, R. C., M. Mazens-Sullivan, J. Z. Tetreault, S. Lobel, and J. Nivard.** 1994. Evolving approaches to management of quality in clinical microbiology. *Clin. Microbiol. Rev.* **7:**55–88.
12. **Bates, D. W., L. Goldman, and T. H. Lee.** 1991. Contaminant blood cultures and resource utilization. The true consequences of false-positive results. *JAMA* **265:**365–369.
13. **Bennett, S. T., and D. A. Kern.** 2002. Automated production of an on-line laboratory reference manual from a laboratory information system. *J. Med. Syst.* **26:**145–149.
14. **Blondeau, J. M., G. B. Pylypchuk, J. E. Kappel, B. Pilkey, and C. Lawler.** 1998. Comparison of bedside- and laboratory-inoculated Bactec high- and low-volume resin bottles for the recovery of microorganisms causing peritonitis in CAPD patients. *Diagn. Microbiol. Infect. Dis.* **31:**281–287.
15. **Bone, R. C.** 1991. The pathogenesis of sepsis. *Ann. Intern. Med.* **115:**457–469.
16. **Bourbeau, P., J. Riley, B. J. Heiter, R. Master, C. Young, and C. Pierson.** 1998. Use of the BacT/Alert blood culture system for culture of sterile body fluids other than blood. *J. Clin. Microbiol.* **36:**3273–3277.
17. **Bowler, P. G., B. I. Duerden, and D. G. Armstrong.** 2001. Wound microbiology and associated approaches to wound management. *Clin. Microbiol. Rev.* **14:**244–269.
18. **Boyce, J. M., and N. L. Havill.** 2005. Nosocomial antibiotic-associated diarrhea associated with enterotoxin-producing strains of methicillin-resistant *Staphylococcus aureus*. *Am. J. Gastroenterol.* **100:**1828–1834.
19. **Brenner, S. A., J. A. Rooney, P. Manzewitsch, and R. L. Regnery.** 1997. Isolation of *Bartonella (Rochalimaea) henselae*: effects of methods of blood collection and handling. *J. Clin. Microbiol.* **35:**544–547.
20. **Brook, I.** 1998. Microbiology of common infections in the upper respiratory tract. *Prim. Care* **25:**633–648.
21. **Brown, H. L., D. A. Fuller, T. E. Davis, J. R. Schwebke, and S. L. Hillier.** 2001. Evaluation of the Affirm Ambient Temperature Transport System for the detection and identification of *Trichomonas vaginalis*, *Gardnerella vaginalis*, and *Candida* species from vaginal fluid specimens. *J. Clin. Microbiol.* **39:**3197–3199.
22. **Bryan, F. L.** 1995. Procedures to use during outbreaks of food-borne disease, p. 209–226. *In* P. R. Murray, E. J. Baron, M. A. Pfaller, F. C. Tenover, and R. H. Yolken, (ed.), *Manual of Clinical Microbiology*, 6th ed. ASM Press, Washington, D.C.

23. **Cantral, D. E., T. G. Tape, E. C. Reed, J. R. Spurzem, S. I. Rennard, and A. B. Thompson.** 1993. Quantitative culture of bronchoalveolar lavage fluid for the diagnosis of bacterial pneumonia. *Am. J. Med.* **95:**601–607.
24. **Carr, D. T., A. G. Karlson, and G. G. Stillwell.** 1967. A comparison of cultures of induced sputum and gastric washings in the diagnosis of tuberculosis. *Mayo Clin. Proc.* **42:** 23–25.
25. **Carroll, K., and L. Reimer.** 1996. Microbiology and laboratory diagnosis of upper respiratory tract infections. *Clin. Infect. Dis.* **23:**442–448.
26. **Cavagnolo, R.** 1995. Evaluation of incubation times for urine cultures. *J. Clin. Microbiol.* **33:**1954–1956.
27. **Caws, M., S. M. Wilson, C. Clough, and F. Drobniewski.** 2000. Role of IS*6110*- targeted PCR, culture, biochemical, clinical, and immunological criteria for diagnosis of tuberculous meningitis. *J. Clin. Microbiol.* **38:**3150–3155.
28. **Centers for Disease Control and Prevention.** 2000. Early-onset group B streptococcal disease—United States, 1998–1999. *JAMA* **284:**1508–1510.
29. **Clarridge, J. E., M. T. Pezzlo, and K. L. Vosti.** 1987. Cumitech 2A, *Laboratory Diagnosis of Urinary Tract Infections.* Coordinating ed., A. S. Weissfeld. American Society for Microbiology, Washington, D.C.
30. **Cockerill, F. R., III, J. G. Hughes, E. A. Vetter, R. A. Mueller, A. L. Weaver, D. M. Ilstrup, J. E. Rosenblatt, and W. R. Wilson.** 1997. Analysis of 281,797 consecutive blood cultures performed over an eight-year period: trends in microorganisms isolated and the value of anaerobic culture of blood. *Clin. Infect. Dis.* **24:**403–418.
31. **Coenye, T., P. Vandamme, J. R. Govan, and J. J. LiPuma.** 2001. Taxonomy and identification of the *Burkholderia cepacia* complex. *J. Clin. Microbiol.* **39:**3427–3436.
32. **Cooper, R. J., J. R. Hoffman, J. G. Bartlett, R. E. Besser, R. Gonzales, J. M. Hickner, and M. A. Sande.** 2001. Principles of appropriate antibiotic use for acute pharyngitis in adults: background. *Ann. Emerg. Med.* **37:**711–719.
33. **Cornick, N. A., and S. L. Gorbach.** 1988. Campylobacter. *Infect. Dis. Clin. N. Am.* **2:**643–654.
34. **Curione, C. J., Jr., G. S. Kaneko, J. L. Voss, F. Hesse, and R. F. Smith.** 1977. Gram stain evaluation of the quality of sputum specimens for mycobacterial culture. *J. Clin. Microbiol.* **5:**381–382.
35. **Davies, H. D., M. A. Miller, S. Faro, D. Gregson, S. C. Kehl, and J. A. Jordan.** 2004. Multicenter study of a rapid molecular-based assay for the diagnosis of group B *Streptococcus* colonization in pregnant women. *Clin. Infect. Dis.* **39:**1129–1135.
36. **Delaney, M. L., and A. B. Onderdonk.** 1997. Evaluation of the AnaeroPack system for growth of clinically significant anaerobes. *J. Clin. Microbiol.* **35:**558–562.
37. **Doan, N., A. Contreras, J. Flynn, J. Morrison, and J. Slots.** 1999. Proficiencies of three anaerobic culture systems for recovering periodontal pathogenic bacteria. *J. Clin. Microbiol.* **37:**171–174.
38. **Doern, G. V.** 1994. Manual blood culture systems and the antimicrobial removal device. *Clin. Lab. Med.* **14:**133–147.
39. **Doern, G. V.** 2000. Detection of selected fastidious bacteria. *Clin. Infect. Dis.* **30:**166–173.
40. **Domi, J., N. Gali, S. Blanco, P. Pedroso, C. Prat, L. Matas, and V. Ausina.** 2001. Assessment of a new test to detect *Legionella* urinary antigen for the diagnosis of Legionnaires' disease. *Diagn. Microbiol. Infect. Dis.* **41:** 199–203.
41. **Dow, G., A. Browne, and R. G. Sibbald.** 1999. Infection in chronic wounds: controversies in diagnosis and treatment. *Ostomy Wound Manag.* **45:**23–27, 29–40; quiz, 41–42.
42. **Drake, C., J. Barenfanger, J. Lawhorn, and S. Verhulst.** 2005. Comparison of Easy-Flow Copan liquid Stuart's and Starplex Swab Transport Systems for recovery of fastidious aerobic bacteria. *J. Clin. Microbiol.* **43:**1301–1303.
43. **du Moulin, G. C., and W. Love.** 1988. The value of autopsy microbiology. *Clin. Microbiol. Newsl.* **10:**165–167.
44. **Efstratiou, A., K. H. Engler, I. K. Mazurova, T. Glushkevich, J. Vuopio-Varkila, and T. Popovic.** 2000. Current approaches to the laboratory diagnosis of diphtheria. *J. Infect. Dis.* **181**(Suppl. 1):S138–S145.
45. **Elbagir, A., and P. A. Mardh.** 1990. Evaluation of chlamydial tests in early trachoma. *APMIS* **98:**276–280.
46. **Elliott, D., J. A. Kufera, and R. A. Myers.** 2000. The microbiology of necrotizing soft tissue infections. *Am. J. Surg.* **179:**361–366.
47. **Engels, E., P. W. Marks, and P. Kazanjian.** 1995. Usefulness of bone marrow examination in the evaluation of unexplained fevers in patients infected with human immunodeficiency virus. *Clin. Infect. Dis.* **21:**427–428.
48. **Evangelista, A., and H. Beilstein.** 1993. Cumitech 4A, *Laboratory Diagnosis of Gonorrhea.* Coordinating ed., C. Abramson. American Society for Microbiology, Washington, D.C.
49. **Evans, G. L., T. Cekoric, Jr., and R. L. Searcy.** 1968. Comparative effects of anticoagulants on bacterial growth in experimental blood cultures. *Am. J. Med. Technol.* **34:**103–112.
50. **Fey, P. D., R. S. Wickert, M. E. Rupp, T. J. Safranek, and S. H. Hinrichs.** 2000. Prevalence of non-O157:H7 shiga toxin-producing *Escherichia coli* in diarrheal stool samples from Nebraska. *Emerg. Infect. Dis.* **6:**530–533.
51. **File, T. M.** 2000. The epidemiology of respiratory tract infections. *Semin. Respir. Infect.* **15:**184–194.
52. **Fine, K. D., F. Ogunji, J. George, M. D. Niehaus, and R. L. Guerrant.** 1998. Utility of a rapid fecal latex agglutination test detecting the neutrophil protein, lactoferrin, for diagnosing inflammatory causes of chronic diarrhea. *Am. J. Gastroenterol.* **93:**1300–1305.
53. **Flayhart, D., J. F. Hindler, D. A. Bruckner, G. Hall, R. K. Shrestha, S. A. Vogel, S. S. Richter, W. Howard, R. Walther, and K. C. Carroll.** 2005. Multicenter evaluation of BBL CHROMagar MRSA medium for direct detection of methicillin-resistant *Staphylococcus aureus* from surveillance cultures of the anterior nares. *J. Clin. Microbiol.* **43:** 5536–5540.
54. **Flayhart, D., C. Lema, A. Borek, and K. C. Carroll.** 2004. Comparison of the BBL CHROMagar Staph aureus agar medium to conventional media for detection of *Staphylococcus aureus* in respiratory samples. *J. Clin. Microbiol.* **42:**3566–3569.
55. **Food and Drug Administration.** 1997. *FDA Safety Alert: Risks of Devices for Direct Detection of Group B Streptococcal Antigen.* Food and Drug Administration, Washington, D.C.
56. **Freidig, E. E., S. P. McClure, W. R. Wilson, P. M. Banks, and J. A. Washington II.** 1986. Clinical-histologic-microbiologic analysis of 419 lymph node biopsy specimens. *Rev. Infect. Dis.* **8:**322–328.
57. **Gardam, M., J. Brunton, B. Willey, A. McGeer, D. Low, and J. Conly.** 2001. A blinded comparison of three laboratory protocols for the identification of patients colonized with methicillin-resistant *Staphylococcus aureus. Infect. Control Hosp. Epidemiol.* **22:**152–156.
58. **Gavin, P. J., L. R. Peterson, A. C. Pasquariello, J. Blackburn, M. G. Hamming, K. J. Kuo, and R. B. Thomson, Jr.** 2004. Evaluation of performance and potential clinical impact of ProSpecT Shiga toxin *Escherichia coli* Microplate assay for detection of Shiga toxin-producing *E. coli* in stool samples. *J. Clin. Microbiol.* **42:**1652–1656.
59. **Gerber, M. A.** 1986. Diagnosis of group A beta-hemolytic streptococcal pharyngitis. Use of antigen detection tests. *Diagn. Microbiol. Infect. Dis.* **4:**5S–15S.

60. **Gerding, D. N., S. Johnson, L. R. Peterson, M. E. Mulligan, and J. Silva, Jr.** 1995. *Clostridium difficile*-associated diarrhea and colitis. *Infect. Control Hosp. Epidemiol.* **16:**459–477.
61. **Gilchrist, M., W. P. McKinney, J. M. Miller, and A. Weissfeld.** 2000. Cumitech 33, *Biological Agents Associated with Bioterrorism.* Coordinating ed., J. Snyder. ASM Press, Washington, D.C.
62. **Gilligan, P. H.** 1991. Microbiology of airway disease in patients with cystic fibrosis. *Clin. Microbiol. Rev.* **4:**35–51.
63. **Gilligan, P. H., J. M. Janda, M. A. Karmali, and J. M. Miller.** 1992. Cumitech 12A, *Laboratory Diagnosis of Bacterial Diarrhea.* Coordinating ed., F. Nolte. American Society for Microbiology, Washington, D.C.
64. **Gisbert, J. P., and J. M. Pajares.** 2001. Diagnosis of *Helicobacter pylori* infection by stool antigen determination: a systematic review. *Am. J. Gastroenterol.* **96:**2829–2838.
65. **Goldgeier, M. H.** 1983. The microbial evaluation of acute cellulitis. *Cutis* **31:**649–650, 653–654, 656.
66. **Gorbach, S. L.** 1993. Treatment of intra-abdominal infections. *J. Antimicrob. Chemother.* **31**(Suppl. A)**:**67–78.
67. **Gray, L. D., and D. P. Fedorko.** 1992. Laboratory diagnosis of bacterial meningitis. *Clin. Microbiol. Rev.* **5:**130–145.
68. **Guerrant, R. L., T. Van Gilder, T. S. Steiner, N. M. Thielman, L. Slutsker, R. V. Tauxe, T. Hennessy, P. M. Griffin, H. DuPont, R. B. Sack, P. Tarr, M. Neill, I. Nachamkin, L. B. Reller, M. T. Osterholm, M. L. Bennish, and L. K. Pickering.** 2001. Practice guidelines for the management of infectious diarrhea. *Clin. Infect. Dis.* **32:**331–351.
69. **Gwaltney, J. M., Jr.** 1996. Acute community-acquired sinusitis. *Clin. Infect. Dis.* **23:**1209–1223; quiz, 1224–1225.
70. **Hackman, B. A., J. F. Plouffe, R. F. Benson, B. S. Fields, and R. F. Breiman.** 1996. Comparison of Binax Legionella Urinary Antigen EIA kit with Binax RIA Urinary Antigen kit for detection of *Legionella pneumophila* serogroup 1 antigen. *J. Clin. Microbiol.* **34:**1579–1580.
71. **Hammerschlag, M. R., P. M. Roblin, M. Gelling, N. Tsumura, J. E. Jule, and A. Kutlin.** 1997. Use of polymerase chain reaction for the detection of *Chlamydia trachomatis* in ocular and nasopharyngeal specimens from infants with conjunctivitis. *Pediatr. Infect. Dis. J.* **16:**293–297.
72. **Han, S. W., R. Flamm, C. Y. Hachem, H. Y. Kim, J. E. Clarridge, D. G. Evans, J. Beyer, J. Drnec, and D. Y. Graham.** 1995. Transport and storage of *Helicobacter pylori* from gastric mucosal biopsies and clinical isolates. *Eur. J. Clin. Microbiol. Infect. Dis.* **14:**349–352.
73. **Harrison, T., S. Uldum, S. Alexiou-Daniel, J. Bangsborg, S. Bernander, V. Drashrevear, J. Etienne, J. Helbig, D. Lindsay, I. Lochman, T. Marques, F. de Ory, I. Tartakovskii, G. Wewalka, and F. Fehrenbach.** 1998. A multicenter evaluation of the Biotest *Legionella* urinary antigen EIA. *Clin. Microbiol. Infect.* **4:**359–365.
74. **Hawkey, P. M., and L. A. Jewes.** 1985. How common is meningitis caused by anaerobic bacteria? *J. Clin. Microbiol.* **22:**325.
75. **Heelan, J. S., S. Wilbur, G. Depetris, and C. Letourneau.** 1996. Rapid antigen testing for group A *Streptococcus* by DNA probe. *Diagn. Microbiol. Infect. Dis.* **24:**65–69.
76. **Heerema, M. S., M. E. Ein, D. M. Musher, M. W. Bradshaw, and T. W. Williams, Jr.** 1979. Anaerobic bacterial meningitis. *Am. J. Med.* **67:**219–227.
77. **Heininger, U., G. Schmidt-Schlapfer, J. D. Cherry, and K. Stehr.** 2000. Clinical validation of a polymerase chain reaction assay for the diagnosis of pertussis by comparison with serology, culture, and symptoms during a large pertussis vaccine efficacy trial. *Pediatrics* **105:**E31.
78. **Heiter, B. J., and P. P. Bourbeau.** 1993. Comparison of the Gen-Probe Group A Streptococcus Direct Test with culture and a rapid streptococcal antigen detection assay for diagnosis of streptococcal pharyngitis. *J. Clin. Microbiol.* **31:**2070–2073.
79. **Henry, D., M. Campbell, C. McGimpsey, A. Clarke, L. Louden, J. L. Burns, M. H. Roe, P. Vandamme, and D. Speert.** 1999. Comparison of isolation media for recovery of *Burkholderia cepacia* complex from respiratory secretions of patients with cystic fibrosis. *J. Clin. Microbiol.* **37:**1004–1007.
80. **Henry, D. A., M. E. Campbell, J. J. LiPuma, and D. P. Speert.** 1997. Identification of *Burkholderia cepacia* isolates from patients with cystic fibrosis and use of a simple new selective medium. *J. Clin. Microbiol.* **35:**614–619. (Erratum, *J. Clin. Microbiol.* **37:**1237, 1999.)
81. **Ho, P. W., F. D. Pien, and D. Hamburg.** 1979. Value of cultures in patients with acute cellulitis. *South. Med. J.* **72:**1402–1403.
82. **Hoppe, J. E., and A. Weiss.** 1987. Recovery of *Bordetella pertussis* from four kinds of swabs. *Eur. J. Clin. Microbiol.* **6:**203–205.
83. **Ishida, T., T. Hashimoto, M. Arita, Y. Tojo, H. Tachibana, and M. Jinnai.** 2004. A 3-year prospective study of a urinary antigen-detection test for *Streptococcus pneumoniae* in community-acquired pneumonia: utility and clinical impact on the reported etiology. *J. Infect. Chemother.* **10:**359–363.
84. **Johnson, S., and D. Gerding.** 1998. *Clostridium difficile*-associated diarrhea. *Clin. Infect. Dis.* **26:**1027–1036.
85. **Johnson, S., S. A. Kent, K. J. O'Leary, M. M. Merrigan, S. P. Sambol, L. R. Peterson, and D. N. Gerding.** 2001. Fatal pseudomembranous colitis associated with a variant *Clostridium difficile* strain not detected by toxin A immunoassay. *Ann. Intern. Med.* **135:**434–438.
86. **Jones, D. B., T. J. Lisegang, and N. M. Robinson.** 1981. Cumitech 13, *Laboratory Diagnosis of Ocular Infections.* Coordinating ed., J. A. Washington II. American Society for Microbiology, Washington, D.C.
87. **Kaditis, A. G., A. S. O'Marcaigh, K. H. Rhodes, A. L. Weaver, and N. K. Henry.** 1996. Yield of positive blood cultures in pediatric oncology patients by a new method of blood culture collection. *Pediatr. Infect. Dis. J.* **15:**615–620.
88. **Kain, K. C., M. A. Noble, R. L. Barteluk, and R. H. Tubbesing.** 1991. *Arcanobacterium hemolyticum* infection: confused with scarlet fever and diphtheria. *J. Emerg. Med.* **9:**33–35.
89. **Kellogg, J. A.** 1990. Suitability of throat culture procedures for detection of group A streptococci and as reference standards for evaluation of streptococcal antigen detection kits. *J. Clin. Microbiol.* **28:**165–169.
90. **Kim, S. D., L. C. McDonald, W. R. Jarvis, S. K. McAllister, R. Jerris, L. A. Carson, and J. M. Miller.** 2000. Determining the significance of coagulase-negative staphylococci isolated from blood cultures at a community hospital: a role for species and strain identification. *Infect. Control Hosp. Epidemiol.* **21:**213–217.
91. **Kiska, D. L., M. C. Jones, M. E. Mangum, D. Orkiszewski, and P. H. Gilligan.** 1995. Quality assurance study of bacterial antigen testing of cerebrospinal fluid. *J. Clin. Microbiol.* **33:**1141–1144.
92. **Klietmann, W. F., and K. L. Ruoff.** 2001. Bioterrorism: implications for the clinical microbiologist. *Clin. Microbiol. Rev.* **14:**364–381.
93. **Koneman, E. W., T. M. Minckler, D. B. Shires, and D. S. De Jongh.** 1971. Postmortem bacteriology. II. Selection of cases for culture. *Am. J. Clin. Pathol.* **55:**17–23.
94. **Korbi, S., M. F. Toccanier, G. Leyvraz, J. Stalder, and Y. Kapanci.** 1986. Use of silver staining (Dieterle's stain) in the diagnosis of cat scratch disease. *Histopathology* **10:**1015–1021.
95. **Kost, G. J.** 1990. Critical limits for urgent clinician notification at U.S. medical centers. *JAMA* **263:**704–707.
96. **Kowalski, R. P., M. Uhrin, L. M. Karenchak, R. L. Sweet, and Y. J. Gordon.** 1995. Evaluation of the polymerase chain

reaction test for detecting chlamydial DNA in adult chlamydial conjunctivitis. *Ophthalmology* **102:**1016–1019.

97. **Landefeld, C. S., M. M. Chren, A. Myers, R. Geller, S. Robbins, and L. Goldman.** 1988. Diagnostic yield of the autopsy in a university hospital and a community hospital. *N. Engl. J. Med.* **318:**1249–1254.
98. **Larsen, S. A.** 1989. Syphilis. *Clin. Lab. Med.* **9:**545–557.
99. **Lauer, B. A., L. B. Reller, and S. Mirrett.** 1979. Evaluation of preservative fluid for urine collected for culture. *J. Clin. Microbiol.* **10:**42–45.
100. **Lazinger, B., J. Steif, and E. Granit.** 1989. An online tests catalog for clinical laboratories. *J. Med. Syst.* **13:**187–192.
101. **Leodolter, A., K. Wolle, and P. Malfertheiner.** 2001. Current standards in the diagnosis of *Helicobacter pylori* infection. *Dig. Dis.* **19:**116–122.
102. **Lewis, D. A.** 2000. Diagnostic tests for chancroid. *Sex Transm. Infect.* **76:**137–141.
103. **Lifshitz, E., and L. Kramer.** 2000. Outpatient urine culture: does collection technique matter? *Arch. Intern. Med.* **160:**2537–2540.
104. **Lippes, J.** 1999. Pelvic actinomycosis: a review and preliminary look at prevalence. *Am. J. Obstet. Gynecol.* **180:**265–269.
105. **Lipsky, B., A. Berendt, H. Gunner Deery, J. Embil, W. Joseph, A. Karchmer, J. LeFrock, D. Lew, J. Mader, C. Norden, and J. Tan.** 2004. Diagnosis and treatment of diabetic foot infections. *Clin. Infect. Dis.* **39:**885–910.
106. **Little, J. R., P. R. Murray, P. S. Traynor, and E. Spitznagel.** 1999. A randomized trial of povidone-iodine compared with iodine tincture for venipuncture site disinfection: effects on rates of blood culture contamination. *Am. J. Med.* **107:**119–125.
107. **Loeffelholz, M. J., C. J. Thompson, K. S. Long, and M. J. Gilchrist.** 1999. Comparison of PCR, culture, and direct fluorescent-antibody testing for detection of *Bordetella pertussis*. *J. Clin. Microbiol.* **37:**2872–2876.
108. **Lum, G.** 1998. Critical limits (alert values) for physician notification: universal or medical center specific limits? *Ann. Clin. Lab. Sci.* **28:**261–271.
109. **Maki, D. G., C. E. Weise, and H. W. Sarafin.** 1977. A semiquantitative culture method for identifying intravenous-catheter-related infection. *N. Engl. J. Med.* **296:**1305–1309.
110. **Manabe, Y. C., J. M. Vinetz, R. D. Moore, C. Merz, P. Charache, and J. G. Bartlett.** 1995. *Clostridium difficile* colitis: an efficient clinical approach to diagnosis. *Ann. Intern. Med.* **123:**835–840.
111. **Marik, P. E.** 2001. Aspiration pneumonitis and aspiration pneumonia. *N. Engl. J. Med.* **344:**665–671.
112. **Marquette, C. H., H. Georges, F. Wallet, P. Ramon, F. Saulnier, R. Neviere, D. Mathieu, A. Rime, and A. B. Tonnel.** 1993. Diagnostic efficiency of endotracheal aspirates with quantitative bacterial cultures in intubated patients with suspected pneumonia. Comparison with the protected specimen brush. *Am. Rev. Respir. Dis.* **148:** 138–144.
113. **Matoo, S., and J. D. Cherry.** 2005. Molecular pathogeneis, epidemiology, and clinical manifestations of respiratory infections due to *Bordetella pertussis* and other *Bordetella* subspecies. *Clin. Microbiol. Rev.* **18:**326–382.
114. **McCurdy, B.** 2001. Cumitech 35, *Postmortem Microbiology*. Coordinating ed., B. McCurdy. ASM Press, Washington, D.C.
115. **McEllistrem, M. C., R. J. Carman, D. N. Gerding, C. W. Genheimer, and L. Zheng.** 2005. A hospital outbreak of *Clostridium difficile* disease associated with isolates carrying binary toxin genes. *Clin. Infect. Dis.* **40:**265–272.
116. **McGowan, K. L., and M. T. Rubenstein.** 1989. Use of a rapid latex agglutination test to detect *Salmonella* and *Shigella* antigens from gram-negative enrichment broth. *Am. J. Clin. Pathol.* **92:**679–682.
117. **McManus, A. T., S. H. Kim, W. F. McManus, A. D. Mason, Jr., and B. A. Pruitt, Jr.** 1987. Comparison of quantitative microbiology and histopathology in divided burn-wound biopsy specimens. *Arch. Surg.* **122:**74–76.
118. **Mein, J., and G. Lum.** 1999. CSF bacterial antigen detection tests offer no advantage over Gram's stain in the diagnosis of bacterial meningitis. *Pathology* **31:**67–69.
119. **Meredith, F. T., H. K. Phillips, and L. B. Reller.** 1997. Clinical utility of broth cultures of cerebrospinal fluid from patients at risk for shunt infections. *J. Clin. Microbiol.* **35:**3109–3111.
120. **Messer, J. W., T. F. Midura, and J. T. Peeler.** 1993. Sampling plans, sample collection, shipment, and preparation for analysis, p. 25–49. *In* C. Vanderzaant and D. Splittstoesser (ed.), *Compendium of Methods for the Microbiological Examination of Foods*, 3rd ed. American Public Health Association, Washington, D.C.
121. **Midura, T. F.** 1996. Update: infant botulism. *Clin. Microbiol. Rev.* **9:**119–125.
122. **Miller, J. M.** 1998. *A Guide to Specimen Management in Clinical Microbiology*, 2nd ed. ASM Press, Washington, D.C.
123. **Miller-Catchpole, R., D. Variakojis, J. W. Vardiman, J. M. Loew, and J. Carter.** 1986. Cat scratch disease. Identification of bacteria in seven cases of lymphadenitis. *Am. J. Surg. Pathol.* **10:**276–281.
124. **Mimoz, O., A. Karim, A. Mercat, M. Cosseron, B. Falissard, F. Parker, C. Richard, K. Samii, and P. Nordmann.** 1999. Chlorhexidine compared with povidone-iodine as skin preparation before blood culture. A randomized, controlled trial. *Ann. Intern. Med.* **131:**834–837.
125. **Mirrett, S., M. P. Weinstein, L. G. Reimer, M. L. Wilson, and L. B. Reller.** 2001. Relevance of the number of positive bottles in determining clinical significance of coagulase-negative staphylococci in blood cultures. *J. Clin. Microbiol.* **39:**3279–3281.
126. **Morrill, W. E., J. M. Barbaree, B. S. Fields, G. N. Sanden, and W. T. Martin.** 1988. Effects of transport temperature and medium on recovery of *Bordetella pertussis* from nasopharyngeal swabs. *J. Clin. Microbiol.* **26:**1814–1817.
127. **Morris, A. J., P. R. Murray, and L. B. Reller.** 1996. Contemporary testing for enteric pathogens: the potential for cost, time, and health care savings. *J. Clin. Microbiol.* **34:**1776–1778.
128. **Morris, A. J., L. K. Smith, S. Mirrett, and L. B. Reller.** 1996. Cost and time savings following introduction of rejection criteria for clinical specimens. *J. Clin. Microbiol.* **34:**355–357.
129. **Morris, A. J., D. C. Tanner, and L. B. Reller.** 1993. Rejection criteria for endotracheal aspirates from adults. *J. Clin. Microbiol.* **31:**1027–1028.
130. **Morris, A. J., S. J. Wilson, C. E. Marx, M. L. Wilson, S. Mirett, and L. B. Reller.** 1995. Clinical impact of bacteria and fungi recovered only from broth cultures. *J. Clin. Microbiol.* **33:**161–165.
131. **Murdoch, D. R., R. T. Laing, G. D. Mills, N. C. Karalus, G. I. Town, S. Mirrett, and L. B. Reller.** 2001. Evaluation of a rapid immunochromatographic test for detection of *Streptococcus pneumoniae* antigen in urine samples from adults with community-acquired pneumonia. *J. Clin. Microbiol.* **39:**3495–3498.
132. **Murray, P., P. Traynor, and D. Hopson.** 1992. Evaluation of microbiological processing of urine specimens: comparison of overnight versus two-day incubation. *J. Clin. Microbiol.* **30:**1600–1601.
133. **Murray, P. R., A. C. Niles, R. L. Heeren, and F. Pikul.** 1988. Evaluation of the modified Bac-T-Screen and FiltraCheck-UTI urine screening systems for detection of

clinically significant bacteriuria. *J. Clin. Microbiol.* **26:** 2347–2350.

134. **Murray, P. R., P. Traynor, and D. Hopson.** 1992. Critical assessment of blood culture techniques: analysis of recovery of obligate and facultative anaerobes, strict aerobic bacteria, and fungi in aerobic and anaerobic blood culture bottles. *J. Clin. Microbiol.* **30:**1462–1468.
135. **Murray, P. R., and J. A. Washington.** 1975. Microscopic and bacteriologic analysis of expectorated sputum. *Mayo Clin. Proc.* **50:**339–344.
136. **Nichols, L., P. Aronica, and C. Babe.** 1998. Are autopsies obsolete? *Am. J. Clin. Pathol.* **110:**210–218.
137. **Nichols, R. L.** 1985. Intraabdominal infections: an overview. *Rev. Infect. Dis.* **7**(Suppl. 4):S709–S715.
138. **Niederman, M. S., and D. E. Craven.** 2005. Guidelines for the management of adults with hospital-acquired, ventilator-associated, and healthcare-associated pneumonia. *Am. J. Respir. Crit. Care Med.* **171:**388–416.
139. **Nolte, K. B., D. G. Taylor, and J. Y. Richmond.** 2002. Biosafety considerations for autopsy. *Am. J. Forensic Med. Pathol.* **23**(2):107–122.
140. **Nugent, R. P., M. A. Krohn, and S. L. Hillier.** 1991. Reliability of diagnosing bacterial vaginosis is improved by a standardized method of Gram stain interpretation. *J. Clin. Microbiol.* **29:**297–301.
141. **Pancholi, P., K. Pavletich, and P. Della-Latta.** 2005. Rapid screening of urine specimens for bacteriuria by the Cellenium system. *J. Clin. Microbiol.* **43:**5288–5290.
142. **Paule, S. M., A. C., Pasquariello, D. M. Hacek, A. G. Fisher, R. B. Thomson, Jr., K. L. Kaul, and L. R. Peterson.** 2004. Direct detection of *Staphylococcus aureus* from adult and neonate nasal swab specimens using real-time polymerase chain reaction. *J. Mol. Diagn.* **6:** 191–196.
143. **Peeling, R. W., and R. C. Brunham.** 1996. Chlamydiae as pathogens: new species and new issues. *Emerg. Infect. Dis.* **2:**307–319.
144. **Pels, R. J., D. H. Bor, S. Woolhandler, D. U. Himmelstein, and R. S. Lawrence.** 1989. Dipstick urinalysis screening of asymptomatic adults for urinary tract disorders. II. Bacteriuria. *JAMA* **262:**1221–1224.
145. **Perkins, M. D., S. Mirrett, and L. B. Reller.** 1995. Rapid bacterial antigen detection is not clinically useful. *J. Clin. Microbiol.* **33:**1486–1491.
146. **Perl, B., N. P. Gottehrer, D. Raveh, Y. Schlesinger, B. Rudensky, and A. M. Yinnon.** 1999. Cost-effectiveness of blood cultures for adult patients with cellulitis. *Clin. Infect. Dis.* **29:**1483–1488.
147. **Peterson, L., and R. B. Thomson, Jr.** 1999. Use of the clinical microbiology laboratory for the diagnosis and management of infectious diseases related to the oral cavity. *Infect. Dis. Clin. N. Am.* **13:**775–795.
148. **Peterson, L. R.** 1997. Effect of media on transport and recovery of anaerobic bacteria. *Clin. Infect. Dis.* **25**(Suppl. 2):S134–S136.
149. **Peterson, L. R., J. D. Hamilton, E. J. Baron, L. S. Tompkins, J. M. Miller, C. M. Wilfert, F. C. Tenover, and R. B. Thomson, Jr.** 2001. Role of clinical microbiology laboratories in the management and control of infectious diseases and the delivery of health care. *Clin. Infect. Dis.* **32:**605–611.
150. **Petti, C. A., H. S. Bhally, M. P. Weinstein, K. Joho, T. Wakefield. L. B. Reller, and K. C. Carroll.** 2006. Utility of extended blood culture incubation for isolation of *Haemophilus, Actinobacillus, Cardiobacterium, Eikenella,* and *Kingella* organisms: a retrospective multicenter evaluation. *J. Clin. Microbiol.* **44:**257–259.
151. **Pezzlo, M.** 1988. Detection of urinary tract infections by rapid methods. *Clin. Microbiol. Rev.* **1:**268–280.
152. **Pezzlo, M. T., V. Ige, A. P. Woolard, E. M. Peterson, and L. M. de la Maza.** 1989. Rapid bioluminescence method for bacteriuria screening. *J. Clin. Microbiol.* **27:**716–720.
153. **Pfaller, M. A., and F. P. Koontz.** 1985. Laboratory evaluation of leukocyte esterase and nitrite tests for the detection of bacteriuria. *J. Clin. Microbiol.* **21:**840–842.
154. **Prandoni, D., M. H. Boone, E. Larson, C. G. Blane, and H. Fitzpatrick.** 1996. Assessment of urine collection technique for microbial culture. *Am. J. Infect. Control* **24:**219–221.
155. **Prekates, A., S. Nanas, A. Argyropoulou, G. Margariti, T. Kyprianou, E. Papagalos, O. Paniara, and C. Roussos.** 1998. The diagnostic value of gram stain of bronchoalveolar lavage samples in patients with suspected ventilator-associated pneumonia. *Scand. J. Infect. Dis.* **30:**43–47.
156. **Ramirez, J. A., S. Ahkee, A. Tolentino, R. D. Miller, and J. T. Summersgill.** 1996. Diagnosis of *Legionella pneumophila, Mycoplasma pneumoniae,* or *Chlamydia pneumoniae* lower respiratory infection using the polymerase chain reaction on a single throat swab specimen. *Diagn. Microbiol. Infect. Dis.* **24:**7–14.
157. **Reik, H., and S. J. Rubin.** 1981. Evaluation of the buffy-coat smear for rapid detection of bacteremia. *JAMA* **245:**357–359.
158. **Reimer, L. G.** 1994. Catheter-related infections and blood cultures. *Clin. Lab. Med.* **14:**51–58.
159. **Reimer, L. G., and L. B. Reller.** 1985. Effect of sodium polyanetholesulfonate and gelatin on the recovery of *Gardnerella vaginalis* from blood culture media. *J. Clin. Microbiol.* **21:**686–688.
160. **Reimer, L. G., M. L. Wilson, and M. P. Weinstein.** 1997. Update on detection of bacteremia and fungemia. *Clin. Microbiol. Rev.* **10:**444–465.
161. **Richter, S. S., S. E. Beekmann, J. L. Croco, D. J. Dickema, F. P. Koontz, M. A. Pfaller, and G. V. Doern.** 2002. Minimizing the workup of blood culture contaminants: implementation and evaluation of a laboratory-based algorithm. *J. Clin. Microbiol.* **40:**2437–2444.
162. **Rippin, K. P., W. C. Stinson, J. Eisenstadt, and J. A. Washington.** 1995. Clinical evaluation of the slide centrifuge (cytospin) Gram's stained smear for the detection of bacteriuria and comparison with the FiltraCheck-UTI and UTIscreen. *Am. J. Clin. Pathol.* **103:**316–319.
163. **Ristuccia, P. A., R. A. Hoeffner, M. Digamon-Beltran, and B. A. Cunha.** 1987. Detection of bacteremia by buffy coat smears. *Scand. J. Infect. Dis.* **19:**215–217.
164. **Robinson, A.** 1994. Rationale for cost-effective laboratory medicine. *Clin. Microbiol. Rev.* **7:**185–199.
165. **Rosenberg, M., S. A. Berger, M. Barki, S. Goldberg, A. Fink, and A. Miskin.** 1992. Initial testing of a novel urine culture device. *J. Clin. Microbiol.* **30:**2686–2691.
166. **Rosett, W., and G. R. Hodges.** 1980. Antimicrobial activity of heparin. *J. Clin. Microbiol.* **11:**30–34.
167. **Roson, B., N. Fernandez-Sabe, J. Carratala, R. Verdaguer, J. Dorca, F. Manresa, and F. Gudiol.** 2004. Contribution of a urinary antigen assay (Binax NOW) to the early diagnosis of pneumococcal pneumonia. *Clin. Infect. Dis.* **38:**222–226.
168. **Sander, R.** 2001. Otitis externa: a practical guide to treatment and prevention. *Am. Fam. Physician* **63:**927–936, 941–942.
169. **Sapico, F. L., H. N. Canawati, J. L. Witte, J. Z. Montgomerie, F. W. Wagner, Jr., and A. N. Bessman.** 1980. Quantitative aerobic and anaerobic bacteriology of infected diabetic feet. *J. Clin. Microbiol.* **12:**413–420.
170. **Savola, K. L., E. J. Baron, L. S. Tompkins, and D. J. Passaro.** 2001. Fecal leukocyte stain has diagnostic value for outpatients but not inpatients. *J. Clin. Microbiol.* **39:**266–269.

171. **Schachter, J.** 1997. DFA, EIA, PCR, LCR and other technologies: what tests should be used for diagnosis of chlamydia infections? *Immunol. Investig.* **26:**157–161.

172. **Schifman, R. B., C. L. Strand, F. A. Meier, and P. J. Howanitz.** 1998. Blood culture contamination: a College of American Pathologists Q-Probes study involving 640 institutions and 497,134 specimens from adult patients. *Arch. Pathol. Lab. Med.* **122:**216–221.

173. **Schrag, S., R. Gorwitz, K. Fultz-Butts, and A. Schuchat.** 2002. Prevention of perinatal group B streptococcal disease. Revised guidelines from CDC. *Morb. Mortal. Wkly.* Rep. **15**(RR–11):1–22.

174. **Schwartz, D. A., and C. J. Herman.** 1996. The importance of the autopsy in emerging and reemerging infectious diseases. *Clin. Infect. Dis.* **23:**248–254.

175. **Semeniuk, H., and D. Church.** 1999. Evaluation of the leukocyte esterase and nitrite urine dipstick screening tests for detection of bacteriuria in women with suspected uncomplicated urinary tract infections. *J. Clin. Microbiol.* **37:**3051–3052.

176. **Shanholtzer, C. J., P. J. Schaper, and L. R. Peterson.** 1982. Concentrated gram stain smears prepared with a cytospin centrifuge. *J. Clin. Microbiol.* **16:**1052–1056.

177. **Sharkawy, A., D. E. Low, R. Saginur, D. Gregson, B. Schwartz, P. Jessamine, K. Green, and A. McGeer.** 2002. Severe group A streptococcal soft-tissue infections in Ontario: 1992–1996. *Clin. Infect. Dis.* **34:**454–460.

178. **Sharp, S.** 1999. Algorithms for wound specimens. *Clin. Microbiol. Newsl.* **21:**118–120.

179. **Sharp, S. E., A. Robinson, M. Saubolle, M. Santa Cruz, K. Carroll, and V. Baselski.** 2004. Cumitech 7B, *Lower Respiratory Tract Infections*. Coordinating ed., S. E. Sharp. ASM Press, Washington, D.C.

180. **Sharpe, A. N., and A. K. Johnson.** 1972. Stomaching: a new concept in bacteriological sample preparation. *Appl. Microbiol.* **24:**175–178.

181. **Shim, J. K., S. Johnson, M. H. Samore, D. Z. Bliss, and D. N. Gerding.** 1998. Primary symptomless colonisation by *Clostridium difficile* and decreased risk of subsequent diarrhoea. *Lancet* **351:**633–636.

182. **Siegman-Igra, Y., A. M. Anglim, D. E. Shapiro, K. A. Adal, B. A. Strain, and B. M. Farr.** 1997. Diagnosis of vascular catheter-related bloodstream infection: a meta-analysis. *J. Clin. Microbiol.* **35:**928–936.

183. **Sloan, L. M., M. K. Hopkins, P. S. Mitchell, E. A. Vetter, J. E. Rosenblatt, W. S. Harmsen, F. R. Cockerill, and R. Patel.** 2002. Multiplex LightCycler PCR assay for detection and differentiation of *Bordetella pertussis* and *Bordetella parapertussis* in nasopharyngeal specimens. *J. Clin. Microbiol.* **40:**96–100.

184. **Sobel, J. D.** 2000. Bacterial vaginosis. *Annu. Rev. Med.* **51:**349–356.

185. **Solomkin, J. S., J. E. Mazuski, E. J. Baron, R. G. Sawyer, A. B. Nathens, J. T. DiPiro, T. Buchman, E. P. Delinger, J. Jernigan, S. Gorbach, A. W. Chow, and J. Bartlett.** 2003. Guidelines for the selection of anti-infective agents for complicated intra-abdominal infections. *Clin. Infect. Dis.* **37:**997–1005.

186. **Spach, D. H., and J. E. Koehler.** 1998. *Bartonella*-associated infections. *Infect. Dis. Clin. N. Am.* **12:**137–155.

187. **Sridharan, G., T. J. John, M. K. Lalitha, L. H. Harrison, and M. C. Steinhoff.** 1994. Serotypes of *Streptococcus pneumoniae* causing meningitis in southern India. Use of new direct latex agglutination antigen detection tests in cerebrospinal fluid. *Diagn. Microbiol. Infect. Dis.* **18:** 211–214.

188. **Stager, C. E., and J. R. Davis.** 1990. Evaluation of the FiltraCheck-UTI for detection of bacteriuria. *Diagn. Microbiol. Infect. Dis.* **13:**289–295.

189. **Stamm, W. E., and T. M. Hooton.** 1993. Management of urinary tract infections in adults. *N. Engl. J. Med.* **329:**1328–1334.

190. **Steed, L. L., E. K. Korgenski, and J. A. Daly.** 1993. Rapid detection of *Streptococcus pyogenes* in pediatric patient specimens by DNA probe. *J. Clin. Microbiol.* **31:**2996–3000.

191. **Stenberg, K., B. Herrmann, L. Dannevig, A. N. Elbagir, and P. A. Mardh.** 1990. Culture, ELISA and immunofluorescence tests for the diagnosis of conjunctivitis caused by *Chlamydia trachomatis* in neonates and adults. *APMIS* **98:**514–520.

192. **Stephen, J.** 2001. Pathogenesis of infectious diarrhea. *Can. J. Gastroenterol.* **15:**669–683.

193. **Stevens, D. L.** 2000. Streptococcal toxic shock syndrome associated with necrotizing fasciitis. *Annu. Rev. Med.* **51:**271–288.

194. **Sturgis, C. D., L. R. Peterson, and J. R. Warren.** 1997. Cerebrospinal fluid broth culture isolates: their significance for antibiotic treatment. *Am. J. Clin. Pathol.* **108:**217–221.

195. **Thomson, R. B., Jr.** 2002. Use of microbiology laboratory tests in the diagnosis of infectious diseases, p. 1–41. *In* J. S. Tan (ed.), *Expert Guide to Infectious Diseases*. American College of Physicians, Philadelphia, Pa.

196. **Thomson, R. B., Jr., and H. Bertram.** 2001. Laboratory diagnosis of central nervous system infections. *Infect. Dis. Clin. N. Am.* **15:**1047–1071.

197. **Thomson, R. B., Jr., and R. Clarke.** 1988. Interaction between the clinical microbiology and anatomic pathology services. *Clin. Microbiol. Newsl.* **10:**45–47.

198. **Thomson, R. B., Jr., and L. Peterson.** 2001. Microbiology laboratory diagnosis of pulmonary infections, p. 541–559. *In* M. S. Niederman, G. A. Sarosi, and J. Glassroth (ed.), *Respiratory Infections*, 2nd ed. Lippincott Williams & Wilkins, Philadelphia, Pa.

199. **Thomson, R. B., Jr., S. J. Vanzo, N. K. Henry, K. L. Guenther, and J. A. Washington II.** 1984. Contamination of cultures processed with the Isolator lysis-centrifugation blood culture tube. *J. Clin. Microbiol.* **19:**97–99.

200. **Thorpe, J. E., R. P. Baughman, P. T. Frame, T. A. Wesseler, and J. L. Staneck.** 1987. Bronchoalveolar lavage for diagnosing acute bacterial pneumonia. *J. Infect. Dis.* **155:**855–861.

201. **Ticehurst, J. R., D. Z. Aird, L. M. Dam, A. P. Borek, J. T. Hargrove, and K. C. Carroll.** 2006. Effective detection of *Clostridium difficile* by a two-step algorithm including tests for antigen and cytotoxin. *J. Clin. Microbiol.* **44:**1145–1149.

202. **Trollfors, B., O. Nylen, C. Carenfelt, M. Fogle-Hansson, A. Freijd, A. Geterud, S. Hugosson, K. Prellner, E. Neovius, H. Nordell, A. Backman, B. Kaijser, T. Lagergard, M. Leinonen, P. Olcen, and J. Pilichowska-Paszkiet.** 1998. Aetiology of acute epiglottitis in adults. *Scand. J. Infect. Dis.* **30:**49–51.

203. **Turner, J. C., F. G. Hayden, M. C. Lobo, C. E. Ramirez, and D. Murren.** 1997. Epidemiologic evidence for Lancefield group C beta-hemolytic streptococci as a cause of exudative pharyngitis in college students. *J. Clin. Microbiol.* **35:**1–4.

204. **Uhrin, M.** 1997. Molecular diagnostics. The polymerase chain reaction and its use in the diagnosis of *Chlamydia trachomatis* and *Neisseria gonorrhoeae*. *Gac. Med. Mex.* **133:**133–137.

205. **Vaira, D., N. Vakil, M. Menegatti, B. van't Hoff, C. Ricci, L. Gatta, G. Gasbarrini, M. Quina, J. M. Pajares Garcia, A. van Der Ende, R. van Der Hulst, M. Anti, C. Duarte, J. P. Gisbert, M. Miglioli, and G. Tytgat.** 2002. The stool antigen test for detection of *Helicobacter pylori* after eradication therapy. *Ann. Intern. Med.* **136:**280–287.

206. **Vakil, N., D. Rhew, A. Soll, and J. J. Ofman.** 2000. The cost-effectiveness of diagnostic testing strategies for *Helicobacter pylori*. *Am. J. Gastroenterol.* **95:**1691–1698.
207. **Valenstein, P., and F. Meier.** 1998. Urine culture contamination: a College of American Pathologists Q-Probes study of contaminated urine cultures in 906 institutions. *Arch. Pathol. Lab. Med.* **122:**123–129.
208. **Van Der Pol, B., D. H. Martin, J. Schachter, T. C. Quinn, C. A. Gaydos, R. B. Jones, K. Crotchfelt, J. Moncada, D. Jungkind, B. Turner, C. Peyton, J. F. Kelly, J. B. Weiss, and M. Rosenstraus.** 2001. Enhancing the specificity of the COBAS AMPLICOR CT/NG test for *Neisseria gonorrhoeae* by retesting specimens with equivocal results. *J. Clin. Microbiol.* **39:**3092–3098.
209. **Van Enk, R. A., and K. D. Thompson.** 1990. Microbiologic analysis of amniotic fluid. *Clin. Microbiol. Newsl.* **12:**169–172.
210. **Vickers, R. M., J. D. Rihs, and V. L. Yu.** 1992. Clinical demonstration of isolation of *Nocardia asteroides* on buffered charcoal-yeast extract media. *J. Clin. Microbiol.* **30:**227–228.
211. **Volk, E. E., M. L. Miller, B. A. Kirkley, and J. A. Washington.** 1998. The diagnostic usefulness of bone marrow cultures in patients with fever of unknown origin. *Am. J. Clin. Pathol.* **110:**150–153.
212. **von Graevenitz, A., and D. Amsterdam.** 1992. Microbiological aspects of peritonitis associated with continuous ambulatory peritoneal dialysis. *Clin. Microbiol. Rev.* **5:**36–48.
213. **Walter, F. G., R. L. Gibly, R. K. Knopp, and D. J. Roe.** 1998. Squamous cells as predictors of bacterial contamination in urine samples. *Ann. Emerg. Med.* **31:**455–458.
214. **Ward, K. W.** 1992. Processing and interpretation of specimens for *Legionella* spp. l. *Legionella* specimen processing, p. 1.12.1–1.12.8. *In* H. D. Isenberg (ed.), *Clinical Microbiology Procedures Handbook.* American Society for Microbiology, Washington, D.C.
215. **Warny, M., J. Pepin, A. Fang, G. Killgore, A. Thompson, J. Brazier, E. Frost, and L. C. McDonald.** 2005. Toxin production by an emerging strain of *Clostridium difficile* associated with outbreaks of severe disease in North America and Europe. *Lancet* **366:**1079–1084.
216. **Warren, D. K., R. S. Liao, L. R. Merz, M. Eveland, and W. M. Dunne, Jr.** 2004. Detection of methicillin-resistant *Staphylococcus aureus* directly from nasal swab specimens by a real-time PCR assay. *J. Clin. Microbiol.* **42:**5578–5581.
217. **Wegner, D. L., D. L. Witte, and R. D. Schrantz.** 1992. Insensitivity of rapid antigen detection methods and single blood agar plate culture for diagnosing streptococcal pharyngitis. *JAMA* **267:**695–697.
218. **Weinstein, J. W., S. Tallapragada, P. Farrel, and L. M. Dembry.** 1996. Comparison of rectal and perirectal swabs for detection of colonization with vancomycin-resistant enterococci. *J. Clin. Microbiol.* **34:**210–212.
219. **Weinstein, M. P.** 1996. Current blood culture methods and systems: clinical concepts, technology, and interpretation of results. *Clin. Infect. Dis.* **23:**40–46.
220. **Weinstein, M. P., M. L. Towns, S. M. Quartey, S. Mirrett, L. G. Reimer, G. Parmigiani, and L. B. Reller.** 1997. The clinical significance of positive blood cultures in the 1990s: a prospective comprehensive evaluation of the microbiology, epidemiology, and outcome of bacteremia and fungemia in adults. *Clin. Infect. Dis.* **24:**584–602.
221. **Wenzel, R. P., D. R. Reagan, J. S. Bertino, Jr., E. J. Baron, and K. Arias.** 1998. Methicillin-resistant *Staphylococcus aureus* outbreak; a consensus panel's definition and management guidelines. *Am. J. Infect. Control* **26:**102–110.
222. **Westergren, V., L. Lundblad, H. B. Hellquist, and U. Forsum.** 1998. Ventilator-associated sinusitis: a review. *Clin. Infect. Dis.* **27:**851–864.
223. **Wilhelmus, K., T. Liesagang, M. Osato, and D. Jones.** 1994. Cumitech 13A, *Laboratory Diagnosis of Ocular Infections*. Coordinating ed., S. C. Spector. ASM Press, Washington, D.C.
224. **Wilson, M. L.** 1997. Clinically relevant, cost-effective clinical microbiology. Strategies to decrease unnecessary testing. *Am. J. Clin. Pathol.* **107:**154–167.
225. **Wilson, S. J., M. L. Wilson, and L. B. Reller.** 1993. Diagnostic utility of postmortem blood cultures. *Arch. Pathol. Lab. Med.* **117:**986–988.
226. **Winquist, A. G., M. A. Orrico, and L. R. Peterson.** 1997. Evaluation of the cytocentrifuge Gram stain as a screening test for bacteriuria in specimens from specific patient populations. *Am. J. Clin. Pathol.* **108:**515–524.
227. **Woods, G. L., and D. H. Walker.** 1996. Detection of infection or infectious agents by use of cytologic and histologic stains. *Clin. Microbiol. Rev.* **9:**382–404.
228. **Woolfrey, B. F., J. M. Fox, and C. O. Quall.** 1981. An evaluation of burn wound quantitative microbiology. I. Quantitative eschar cultures. *Am. J. Clin. Pathol.* **75:**532–537.
229. **Wright, D. N., R. Boshard, P. Ahlin, B. Saxon, and J. M. Matsen.** 1985. Effect of urine preservation on urine screening and organism identification. *Arch. Pathol. Lab. Med.* **109:**819–822.
230. **York, M. K.** 2004. Quantitative cultures of wound tissues, p. 3.13.2.1–3.13.2.4. *In* H. D. Isenberg (ed.), *Clinical Microbiology Procedures Handbook*, 2nd ed. American Society for Microbiology, Washington, D.C.
231. **Yungbluth, M.** 1995. The laboratory diagnosis of pneumonia. The role of the community hospital pathologist. *Clin. Lab. Med.* **15:**209–234.
232. **Zwart, S., G. J. Ruijs, A. P. Sachs, W. J. van Leeuwen, J. W. Gubbels, and R. A. de Melker.** 2000. Beta-haemolytic streptococci isolated from acute sore-throat patients: cause or coincidence? A case-control study in general practice. *Scand. J. Infect. Dis.* **32:**377–384.

Reagents, Stains, and Media: Bacteriology

KIMBERLE C. CHAPIN AND TSAI-LING LAUDERDALE

21

REAGENTS

The reagents listed in this chapter include those in common use and a few highly specialized ones. For information on specific reagents not included here, refer to literature cited in the chapter in which the reagent is mentioned or the general references listed at the end of this chapter (11, 49). Reagents are listed in alphabetical order, with brief descriptions of their intended uses and ingredients. The test protocol is included where appropriate. A fresh 18- to 24-h pure broth culture or well-isolated colonies from nonselective medium are most often appropriate to use for testing. Many of these reagents and tests are available commercially either individually or incorporated into commercial identification systems. The reader should be aware that commercial preparations in which two reagents are already combined may not contain the traditional percentage of each reagent and may require adjustment of laboratory protocols. Mycobacterial mucolytic and decontamination preparations from a number of manufacturers are an example. Unless stated otherwise, the reagents listed in this section should be prepared by dissolving the reagent components in the stated liquid with a magnetic stirring bar. The standard sterilization technique of autoclaving at 121°C at 15 lb/in^2 for 15 min followed by a slow exhaust cycle should be used when needed. However, certain solutions, such as those containing antibiotics or carbohydrates, cannot be autoclaved because the supplements will be denatured. These solutions are sterilized by filtration through a 0.22-μm-pore-size filter. Additionally, certain reagents require different heat sterilization times. Instructions for reagents that require special preparation or sterilization protocols are included in the discussion of the reagent.

It is critical that distilled, deionized water be used in the preparation of all components. Removal of contaminating pyrogens and minerals from water used for culture reagents is imperative, especially for the success of cell culture systems.

Storage of prepared reagents in sterile, airtight, screw-cap containers is recommended. Some reagents require storage in dark containers, and some need to be stored refrigerated (2 to 8°C) instead of at room temperature. Special storage instructions are given when appropriate. Standard safety precautions should be taken when preparing the reagents. Follow the safety guidelines for the chemicals being used, in addition to the laboratory safety protocols. For reagents that are prepared in-house, proper quality control measures must be taken with appropriate positive and negative controls.

■ Acetoin (acetyl-methyl-carbinol)

See Voges-Proskauer (VP) test.

■ *N*-Acetyl-L-cysteine-sodium hydroxide (NALC-NaOH)

NALC is a mucolytic agent used for digestion, and NaOH is a decontamination agent used in the processing of specimens for mycobacteriology. Sodium citrate is included in the mixture to exert a stabilizing effect on the acetylcysteine.

4% NaOH, sterile	50 ml
2.9% Sodium citrate, sterile	50 ml
NALC powder	0.5 g

Mix well in a sterile container. Use within 24 h of preparation.

■ L-Alanine-7-amido-4-methycoumarin (Gram-Sure; Remel)

Gram-Sure is a reagent-impregnated disk with the fluorogenic compound L-alanine-7-amido-4-methycoumarin. This is a rapid disk test that is used as an adjunct to the Gram stain to distinguish between gram-negative and gram-positive aerobic rods or coccobacilli and is used most commonly with gram-positive organisms that may appear gram variable or gram negative, such as *Bacillus* or *Lactobacillus*. The mechanism of the test is dependent on the presence of aminopeptidase in the cell walls of gram-negative organisms, which will hydrolyze the reagent L-alanine-7-amido-4-methycoumarin in the disk from a nonfluorescent substrate to a blue fluorescent compound. A pure colony growth is inoculated into demineralized water and then inoculated onto the disk. The disk is incubated at room temperature for 5 to 10 min and then observed under long-wave UV light for blue fluorescence. Blue fluorescence is gram negative, and the absence of blue fluorescence is gram positive. Obligate anaerobes may fail to give expected results (50).

■ Bile solubility (10% sodium deoxycholate)

The bile solubility test is used as a presumptive identification test for *Streptococcus pneumoniae*. Sodium deoxycholate is a surface-active bile salt. It acts upon the cell wall of pneumococci, resulting in cell lysis. The test is performed with alpha-hemolytic streptococcal colonies. Oxgall is a dehydrated bile that can be used, but sodium deoxycholate is preferred.

Sodium deoxycholate	1.0 g
Sterile distilled water	9.0 ml

The pH should be 7.0. Store refrigerated in a sterile dark bottle.

Tube method

Prepare a heavy suspension of the organism in 2 ml of buffered broth (pH 7.4) or physiological saline (pH 7.0). The pH of the solution should not be below 6.8. Divide the organism suspension into two tubes. To one tube add a few drops of the 10% sodium deoxycholate solution. To the other tube add the same amount of sterile physiological saline. Incubate at 35°C. If the organism is bile soluble, the tube containing the bile salt will lose its turbidity in 5 to 15 min and show an increase in viscosity concomitant with clearing.

Agar colony test

Put a couple of drops of sodium deoxycholate on the suspected colonies. Incubate the plate right side up for 30 min at 35°C. Pneumococcal colonies will be lysed, but viridans group streptococci will not.

■ Bovine albumin fraction V, 0.2%

The 0.2% bovine albumin solution is used to buffer specimens for mycobacterial culture following decontamination with NALC-NaOH.

Bovine albumin solution, 5%	40.0 ml
Sodium chloride	8.5 g
Distilled water	960.0 ml

Adjust to pH 6.8 ± 0.2 with 4% NaOH. Sterilize by filtration. Aliquot into sterile screw-cap tubes. Store refrigerated.

Following decontamination and concentration by centrifugation, the sedimented specimen is resuspended in 1 to 2 ml of sterile 0.2% bovine albumin fraction V. This suspension is then used to inoculate media and prepare microscopic smears.

■ Catalase

Hydrogen peroxide (H_2O_2) is used to determine if bacteria produce the enzyme catalase. H_2O_2 (3%) is commercially available. Superoxol is a 30% H_2O_2 that is used for identification of *Neisseria* spp. (see chapter 39), and a 15% concentration is often used for differentiation and identification of anaerobes.

Slide method

Transfer a test colony to a clean glass slide and add 1 drop of 3% H_2O_2. Development of bubbles is considered a positive result. Extreme care should be taken to avoid picking up any media from a blood-containing agar plate because catalase is present in erythrocytes and any carryover of blood cells can cause a false-positive reaction. Hydrogen peroxide solution for detection of catalase in anaerobes is typically 15%.

Tube method

Add 1.0 ml of 3% H_2O_2 to an overnight pure culture slant. (Do not use blood agar medium.) Observe for immediate bubbling.

■ Cetylpyridinium chloride-sodium chloride (CPC-NaCl)

CPC-NaCl is used for decontamination of transported sputum specimens for mycobacteriology culture.

CPC	1 g
Sodium chloride	2 g
Distilled water	100 ml

Mix and store in a sealed brown bottle at room temperature. If crystals form, the solution should be gently heated before use.

An equal amount of sputum and CPC-NaCl is mixed until the specimen is liquefied, and then the specimen can be shipped to the testing site. Specimens treated with CPC-NaCl must be cultured on egg-based media or else residual CPC will inhibit mycobacterial growth.

■ Coagulase

The coagulase test is used to detect free coagulase or bound coagulase (clumping factor) and differentiate coagulase-producing *Staphylococcus* from other *Staphylococcus* spp. Dehydrated rabbit plasma reagent with EDTA is commercially available. Rehydrate and perform the test according to the manufacturer's directions. While human plasma is preferred for detection of clumping factor with *Staphylococcus lugdunensis* and *Staphylococcus schleiferi*, it is not recommended for routine testing because it may contain antibodies against staphylococci.

Slide test

The slide test detects bound coagulase (clumping factor). Emulsify a heavy suspension of staphylococci in a small drop of water on a clean glass slide. If autoagglutination occurs, do not continue; instead, perform a tube test. Add 1 small drop of rabbit plasma reagent to the suspension. Mix with a continuous circular motion while observing for the formation of visible white clumps. Known positive and negative controls should be set up in parallel. Negative or delayed positive (20 to 60 s) results should be confirmed by the tube test.

Tube coagulase test

The tube coagulase test detects bound and free coagulase. Dispense 0.5 ml of rabbit plasma into a sterile tube. Inoculate a loopful of the test organism into the tube. Incubate the tube at 35°C for 4 h. Observe for clotting at intervals during the first 4 h because some staphylococci produce fibrolysin, which could lyse the clot. Do not shake or agitate the tube while checking for clotting. The formation of a clot is considered positive. The majority of coagulase-positive *Staphylococcus aureus* isolates will form a clot within 4 h. Incubate the tube at room temperature overnight if no visible clot is observed after 4 h. However, a clot may have formed and subsequently dissolved over the 24 h, so overnight incubation is not always specific. Some investigators have recommended incubation at 35°C.

■ Dyes and pH indicators

A variety of dyes and pH indicators are used in media and reagents. The most common are given in Table 1.

■ Efrotomycin

Efrotomycin is used to separate *Enterococcus casseliflavus* and *Enterococcus gallinarum* (resistant) from *Enterococcus faecium* (susceptible). Dissolve 100 mg of efrotomycin (Merck

TABLE 1 Dyes and pH indicators

Indicator	pH and color
Acid fuchsin (Andrade's)	5.0, pink 8.0, pale yellow
Bromcresol green	3.8, yellow 5.4, blue
Bromcresol purple	5.2, yellow 6.8, purple
Bromphenol blue	3.0, yellow 4.6, blue
Bromthymol blue	6.0, yellow 7.6, dark blue
Chlorcresol green	4.0, yellow 5.6, blue
Chlorphenol red	5.0, yellow 6.6, red
Cresolphthalein	8.2, colorless 9.8, red
m-Cresol purple	7.4, yellow 9.0, purple
Cresol red	7.2, yellow 8.8, red
Methyl red	4.4, red 6.2, yellow
Neutral red	6.8, red 8.0, yellow
Phenolphthalein	8.3, colorless 10.0, red
Phenol red	6.8, yellow 8.4, red
Resazurin	Oxidized: blue, nonfluorescent Reduced: red, fluorescent
Thymol blue	8.0, yellow 9.6, blue
Triphenyl-tetrazolium chloride	Oxidized: colorless Reduced: red

Sharpe & Dohme) in 0.1 ml of dimethyl sulfoxide and dilute in 9.9 ml of sterile distilled water. Dispense 10 μl of this solution onto filter paper disks and dry in the dark at room temperature for 5 to 6 h. A heavy inoculum of bacteria is spread with a loop or swab over half of a Trypticase soy blood agar plate, the efrotomycin disk is then placed on the heavy inoculum, and the plate is incubated for 18 to 24 h at 35°C. Organisms with any growth inhibition are considered efrotomycin susceptible. The availability of this antibiotic may be limited. An alternative test is the 1-O-methyl-α-D-glucopyranoside test (see below).

■ Ehrlich reagent

See Indole test.

■ Ferric ammonium citrate, 1%

Hydrolysis of esculin to esculetin is detected when the product reacts with ferric ammonium citrate to form a brown or black complex.

Dissolve 1.0 g of ferric ammonium citrate in 100 ml of distilled water. Store in a dark bottle, refrigerated, for up to 1 year.

After esculin broth is inoculated with the test organism and incubated for 1 to 2 days, a few drops of ferric ammonium citrate are added. A brown-black color develops immediately in positive tests. This test can also be performed by incorporating an iron salt into esculin agar medium.

■ Ferric chloride reagent

Ferric chloride reagent is used in both the phenylalanine deaminase test and the sodium hippurate hydrolysis test.

Ferric chloride ($FeCl_3 \cdot 6H_2O$) . . . . 12 g
Hydrochloric acid, 2% . . . . 100 ml

Hydrochloric acid (2%) is prepared by adding 5.4 ml of concentrated hydrochloric acid (37%) to 94.6 ml of distilled water.

Test procedure. Adding 4 or 5 drops of ferric chloride reagent onto overnight growth on phenylalanine agar or broth performs the phenylalanine deaminase test. If phenylpyruvic acid has formed, a brown color develops in the medium (positive reaction). Ferric chloride reagent can also be added to inoculated broths (e.g., heart infusion broth or Todd-Hewitt broth) supplemented with hippurate. Hydrolysis of hippurate produces benzoic acid and glycine. An insoluble brown ferric benzoate precipitate will form in a positive hydrolysis reaction.

■ Fildes enrichment

Fildes enrichment is a source of growth factors used to supplement media for the isolation of fastidious organisms. Commercial preparations are available and include the following ingredients.

Pepsin . . . . 4.0 g
Sodium chloride . . . . 5.4 g
Sodium hydroxide. . . . . 70.0 ml
Hydrochloride acid, concentrated . . . . 24.0 ml
Sheep blood . . . . 200 ml
Deionized water . . . . 600 ml

The pH should be 7.0 ± 0.2. Media should be supplemented to a final concentration of 5.0%.

■ Formate-fumarate

Supplementation of media with formate and fumarate has been used to characterize selected anaerobes (e.g., *Bacteroides ureolyticus*).

Sodium formate . . . . 3.0 g
Fumaric acid . . . . 3.0 g
Distilled water . . . . 50.0 ml

To adjust the pH, add 20 pellets of NaOH, stirring until the pellets are dissolved and the fumaric acid is in solution. Bring the final pH to 7.0 with 4 N NaOH. Sterilize by filtration. Store refrigerated for up to 6 months. Add 0.5 ml of this solution to 10 ml of thioglycolate broth. Anaerobic growth in supplemented broth is then compared with the growth in unsupplemented broth.

■ β-Galactosidase

See *o*-Nitrophenyl-β-D-galactopyranoside (ONPG).

■ β-Glucuronidase (see also β-Methylumbelliferyl-β-D-glucuronidase [MUG] test)

Detection of β-glucuronidase activity is useful for the rapid identification of *Escherichia coli,* members of the *Streptococcus anginosus* group, and other bacteria. A solution of 0.1% (wt/vol) *p*-nitrophenyl-β-D-glucopyranoside (colorimetric substrate) in 0.067 M Sorensen phosphate buffer (pH 8.0) is prepared. Tubes containing 0.5 ml of the substrate solution are inoculated with a loopful of bacteria from an overnight culture. The tubes are incubated at 35°C and examined after 4 h for the appearance of a yellow color (liberated *p*-nitrophenol). The fluorometric substrate 4-methylumbelliferyl-β-D-glucuronide is commercially available and yields a fluorescent product when hydrolyzed by β-glucuronidase.

■ Glycine-buffered saline

Glycine-buffered saline (0.043 M glycine, 0.15 M NaCl [pH 9.0]) is used in some serological procedures and is also used as a transport medium for enteric organisms.

Glycine	3.23 g
NaCl	8.77 g
Distilled water	1,000 ml

■ Hemin solution, 5-mg/ml stock

Hemin solution is one of the additives in thioglycolate and *Brucella* base medium that makes them enriched for fastidious organisms. Dissolve 0.5 g of hemin in 10 ml of 1 N NaOH. Bring the volume up to 100 ml with distilled water (final concentration of stock solution, 5 mg/ml). Sterilize by autoclaving. Store refrigerated for up to 1 month. It is used at a final concentration of 5μg/ml of medium.

■ Hippurate test

The hippurate test measures the hydrolysis of sodium hippurate. Hippurate is hydrolyzed to benzoic acid and glycine by the enzyme hippurate hydrolase (hippuricase), which is produced by some bacteria, including group B streptococci (GBS), some *Listeria* spp., *Gardnerella vaginalis, Campylobacter jejuni,* and *Legionella pneumophila*. The procedure described here detects the presence of glycine with the ninhydrin reagent. Ferric chloride reagents can also be used (see above).

Test procedure. A 1% (wt/vol) solution of sodium hippurate is prepared in 0.067 M Sorensen phosphate buffer (pH 6.4). Tubes containing 0.5 ml of this solution are inoculated and incubated at 35°C for 2 h, after which 0.2 ml of the ninhydrin reagent is added. Development of a deep blue-purple color within 5 min is a positive reaction.

For *L. pneumophila,* inoculate a 0.5-ml aliquot of 1% sodium hippurate solution with a loopful of organism and incubate at 35°C in ambient air for 18 to 20 h. Add 0.2 ml of ninhydrin reagent, mix well, and incubate for an additional 10 min at 35°C. Observe for 20 min for blue-purple color development.

Ninhydrin reagent, 3.5%

Ninhydrin	3.5 g
Acetone	50 ml
1-Butanol	50 ml

Mix acetone and butanol in a sterile dark container. Add ninhydrin, mix, and store at room temperature.

■ Indole test

The indole test is used for the determination of the organism's ability to produce indole from deamination of tryptophan by tryptophanase. Both the Ehrlich and Kovàcs reagents should be stored refrigerated away from light. For the Ehrlich and Kovàcs reagents, dissolve the aldehyde in alcohol and then slowly add acid to the mixture.

Ehrlich reagent

Ethyl alcohol, 95%	95 ml
p-Dimethylaminobenzaldehyde	1 g
Hydrochloric acid, concentrated	20 ml

Test procedure. Indole is first extracted with xylene. Add 1 ml of xylene to a 48-h tryptone broth or other tryptophan-containing broth medium. Shake the tube vigorously for 20 s and let stand for 1 to 2 min to allow the xylene extract to come to the top of the broth. Gently add 0.5 ml of the Ehrlich reagent down the side of the tube. Do not shake the tube. A red ring at the interface of the medium and the reagent phase within 5 min represents a positive test. Ehrlich's reagent is preferred for organisms that produce small amounts of indole such as nonfermenters and anaerobes.

Kovàcs indole reagent

Pure amyl or isoamyl alcohol	150 ml
p-Dimethylaminobenzaldehyde	10 g
Hydrochloric acid, concentrated	50 ml

Test procedure. Add 5 drops of Kovàcs reagent to either 48-h-old 2% tryptone broth or an 18- to 24-h-old tryptophan broth culture. Do not shake the tube after the addition of reagent. A red color at the surface of the medium is a positive test.

Spot indole test

p-Dimethylaminocinnamaldehyde (DMACA)	200 mg
Hydrochloric acid, concentrated	2 ml
Distilled water	18 ml

Add the acid to the water, and let it cool before adding DMACA.

Test procedure. Moisten a piece of Whatman no. 3 paper with a couple drops of the reagent. Remove a well-isolated colony from an 18- to 24-h-old culture onto a blood agar plate with a sterile inoculating loop or a wooden stick and smear it onto the moistened filter paper. Observe for a blue to blue-green color within 2 min, which is a positive reaction. No color change or a pinkish tinge is considered negative. This test should be used only on colonies from media containing sufficient tryptophan and no glucose. Colonies from media containing dyes (e.g., MacConkey or eosin-methylene blue [EMB] agar) may cause misleading results and should not be used. Colonies from mixed cultures should not be used, as indole-positive colonies can cause indole-negative colonies to appear weakly positive.

■ LAP (leucine aminopeptidase or leucine arylamidase) test

The LAP test detects the presence of leucine aminopeptidase (LAP). The substrate leucine-α-naphthylamide is hydrolyzed by LAP to leucine and free α-naphthylamine. a-Naphthylamine reacts with DMACA to form a red color. The LAP test, along with pyrrolidonyl-α-naphthylamide (PYR) hydrolysis, is helpful in the presumptive characterization of catalase-negative, gram-positive cocci (streptococci, enterococci, and streptococcus-like organisms). Some commercial identification kits include an assay for this enzyme, and commercial rapid disk tests are also available.

■ Lysozyme solution

Lysozyme .... 50 mg
Hydrochloric acid, 0.01 N .... 50 ml

Mix and sterilize by filtration. Store refrigerated. It may be stored for only 1 week.

Test procedure. Add 5 ml of lysozyme solution to 95 ml of basal glycerol broth, dispense in 5-ml aliquots, and keep refrigerated. Growth of the test organism in the lysozyme-supplemented glycerol broth is compared with the growth in the unsupplemented glycerol broth.

■ Lysozyme test

The lysozyme test measures the ability of organisms, such as *Nocardia*, to grow in the presence of lysozyme.

Basal glycerol broth

Peptone .... 1.0 g
Beef extract .... 0.6 g
Glycerol .... 14.0 ml
Distilled water .... 200 ml

Mix well and autoclave to sterilize. Store refrigerated. It may be stored for up to 3 months.

■ McFarland standard

For different McFarland standards, mix the designated amounts of 1% anhydrous barium chloride ($BaCl_2$) and 1% (vol/vol) cold pure sulfuric acid (H_2SO_4) as shown in Table 2 in screw-cap tubes. Tightly seal the tubes. When the barium sulfate is shaken up well, the density in each tube corresponds approximately to the bacterial suspension listed in Table 2. Store the prepared standard tubes in the dark at room temperature. The absorbance of the 0.5 McFarland standard should be 0.08 to 0.10 at 625 nm using a spectrophotometer with a 1-cm light path. The standard should be checked regularly to make sure the density is still accurate.

■ 1-*o*-Methyl-α-D-glucopyranoside (MGP) (α-methyl-D-glucoside)

The MGP test is used to separate *E. casseliflavus* and *E. gallinarum* (positive) from *Enterococcus faecalis* and *E. faecium* (negative). Heart infusion broth is prepared with 1% MGP and 0.006% bromcresol purple indicator, distributed into 2-ml aliquots, and autoclaved for 10 min. The broth is inoculated with a drop of an overnight broth culture or several colonies from a blood agar plate and incubated for 1 day at 35°C. Prolonged incubation (for up to 7 days) may be necessary. Development of a yellow color indicates a positive reaction.

TABLE 2 McFarland standards protocol

Standard	Vol (ml)		Corresponding bacterial suspension (10^8 CFU/ml)
	1% $BaCl_2$	1% H_2SO_4	
0.5	0.05	9.95	1.5
1	0.1	9.9	3
2	0.2	9.8	6
3	0.3	9.7	9
4	0.4	9.6	12
5	0.5	9.5	15
6	0.6	9.4	18
7	0.7	9.3	21
8	0.8	9.2	24
9	0.9	9.1	27
10	1.0	9.0	30

■ Methylumbelliferyl-β-D-glucuronidase (MUG) test (see also β-Glucuronidase)

The MUG test is the fluorogenic assay for β-glucuronidase. The enzyme hydrolyzes the substrate 4-methylumbelliferyl-β-D-glucuronide to yield 4-methylumbelliferyl, which fluoresces blue under long-wave UV light. The test is normally used for the presumptive identification of *E. coli* and more recently for streptococcal strains. The colorimetric test method is described under β-Glucuronidase.

Dissolve 50 mg of 4-methylumbelliferyl-β-D-glucuronide in 10 ml of 0.05 M Sorensen phosphate buffer, pH 7.5. Dilute 1:16 of the stock 4-methylumbelliferyl-β-D-glucuronide and add 1.25 ml to a vial containing 50 sterile paper disks. Allow the disks to be thoroughly saturated until no liquid remains in the vial. Spread the saturated disks out and allow to dry completely. The disks can be stored in a dark bottle at −20°C for 1 year or at 4°C for 1 month.

Test procedure. Wet disk with 1 drop of sterile water. Apply the organism to the disk using a wooden stick or loop and then incubate the disk for up to 2 h at 35°C. Shine a long-wave UV light on the disk. A positive reaction is indicated by blue fluorescence. A negative reaction is indicated by the lack of fluorescence.

■ Middlebrook enrichment (oleic acid-albumin-dextrose-catalase [OADC] and albumin-dextrose-catalase [ADC])

The Middlebrook enrichment is added to various Middlebrook media. The OADC and enrichment contain oleic acid as a carbon source, and both supplements contain dextrose as a carbon source and bovine albumin fraction V and catalase as growth factors. WR 1339 Triton encourages cording in *Mycobacterium tuberculosis*. All the enrichments described below are prepared in 100 ml and added to 900 ml of preautoclaved medium that has been cooled to 50 to 55°C.

OADC enrichment

Bovine albumin fraction V .... 5.0 g
Dextrose .... 2.0 g
Sodium chloride .... 0.85 g
Oleic acid .... 0.05 g
Catalase........................ 4.0 mg (0.004 g)

Add all components to distilled and deionized water and bring the volume to 100 ml. Mix thoroughly and filter sterilize.

OADC enrichment with WR 1339

Add 0.25 g of WR 1339 Triton to the above OADC ingredients. Prepare as described above.

ADC enrichment

Bovine albumin fraction V .... 5.0 g
Dextrose .... 2.0 g
Catalase........................ 4.0 mg (0.004 g)

Add all components to distilled and deionized water and bring the volume to 100 ml. Mix thoroughly and filter sterilize.

■ Modified oxidase

The test is used for differentiation of *Micrococcus* and related organisms from most other aerobic gram-positive cocci. Six percent tetramethyl-*p*-phenylenediamine dihydrochloride (the same chemical used in Kovàcs oxidase reagent) dissolved in dimethyl sulfoxide is used as the reagent. Keep the reagent away from light. A loopful of colonies from blood agar plates is smeared onto filter paper, and the reagent is dropped onto the bacterial growth. Development of a blue to purple-blue color in 2 min indicates a positive reaction. Commercially prepared disks are available (26).

■ Nessler reagent

The Nessler reagent is used in the determination of acetamide hydrolysis by some gram-negative bacteria.

Nessler reagent

Solution A
Dissolve 1 g of mercuric chloride in 6 ml of distilled water. Add 2 or 3 drops of concentrated hydrochloric acid (HCl) to dissolve the sediment.

Solution B
Dissolve 2.5 g of potassium iodide in 6 ml of distilled water completely. Add to solution A.

Solution C
Dissolve 6 g of potassium hydroxide in 6 ml of distilled water completely. Add to the mixture of solutions A and B. Add 13 ml of distilled water. Mix well. Filter using a sintered-glass funnel before use and store in a dark bottle. Note: do not use a Nalgene filter. The Nessler reagent solution may decompose at room temperature after several weeks and should therefore be checked with each use.

Test procedure. Inoculate 1 ml of mineral-based broth medium (carbon assimilation medium) supplemented with 0.1% acetamide. After incubation for 24 h at 30°C, 1 drop of Nessler reagent is added. A positive reaction is indicated by a red-brown sediment due to the presence of ammonia from the action of acylamidase. Acetamide agar is available commercially.

■ Nitrate reduction

The nitrate reduction test is used to determine the ability of an organism to reduce nitrate to nitrite or free nitrogen gas.

Reagent A

N,N-Dimethyl-naphthylamine	0.6 ml
Acetic acid (5 N), 30%	100 ml

Reagent B

Sulfanilic acid	0.8 g
Acetic acid (5 N), 30%	100 ml

Store each reagent in a brown glass bottle in the refrigerator. Store away from light.

Test procedure. At the time of testing, mix equal portions of the reagents and then add 10 drops to the overnight growth from the nitrate broth culture. A positive reaction is indicated by the development of a red color within 1 to 2 min, which means that nitrate has been reduced to nitrite. Negative reactions are confirmed by adding a pinch (approximately 20 mg) of zinc dust with development of red color within 5 to 10 min, which indicates that nitrate has not been reduced by the organism. If the tube remains clear, nitrate has been reduced to free nitrogen gas, and a clear tube is considered a positive reaction.

■ *o*-Nitrophenyl-β-D-galactopyranoside (ONPG)

The ONPG test is used to determine the ability of an organism to ferment lactose. It is especially useful for identification of members of the family *Enterobacteriaceae*. ONPG-impregnated tablets can be purchased commercially. Commercially prepared reagents are recommended because it is tedious and difficult to prepare the reagent in-house.

■ Oxalic acid, 5%

Oxalic acid is used as a decontamination agent for specimens that contain *Pseudomonas* spp. when culturing for mycobacteria. The reagent is especially helpful when processing respiratory specimens from cystic fibrosis patients.

Oxalic acid	50 g
Distilled water	1,000 ml

Autoclave to sterilize and store at room temperature. The solution has an expiration date of 1 year.

■ Oxidase test

The oxidase test detects the presence of a cytochrome oxidase system. Production of a dark blue-purple color on either a filter paper strip or disk indicates a positive test. A number of reagents can be used for this test.

Kovàcs oxidase reagent:
  1% tetramethyl-*p*-phenylenediamine dihydrochloride (in water)
Gordon and McLeod's reagent:
  1% dimethyl-*p*-phenylenediamine dihydrochloride (in water)
Gaby and Hadley (indolphenol oxidase) reagents:
  1% α-naphthol in 95% ethanol
  1% *p*-aminodimethylaniline HCl

Kovàcs reagent is less toxic and more sensitive than the other reagents. Add a few drops of the reagent to a strip of filter paper (Whatman no. 2 or equivalent) and then smear a loopful of the organism on the paper using a platinum loop or wooden stick. A wire loop containing iron may give a false-positive reaction. The oxidase test should not be performed on colonies growing on medium containing a high concentration of glucose because the fermentation of glucose may inhibit oxidase activity. Only colonies from nonselective, nondifferential media should be used to detect oxidase. A positive reaction with the Kovàcs reagent develops within 10 to 15 s and is characterized by a dark purple-black color. If the Kovàcs solution becomes blue due to autoxidation, it should be discarded. The dimethyl compound in Gordon and McLeod's reagent is more stable than the tetramethyl compound (Kovàcs reagent). A positive reaction is characterized by a blue color and develops within 10 to 30 min.

■ Oxidase, modified.

See Modified oxidase test.

■ Phosphate-buffered saline (PBS)

10× stock solutions

1. 0.1 M NaH_2PO_4 (sodium phosphate, monobasic). Dissolve 13.9 g of NaH_2PO_4 in 1,000 ml of deionized water.
2. 0.1 M Na_2HPO_4 (sodium phosphate, dibasic). Dissolve 26.8 g of $Na_2HPO_4 \cdot 7H_2O$ in 1,000 ml of deionized water.
3. 8.5% NaCl (sodium chloride). Dissolve 85.0 g of NaCl in 1,000 ml of deionized water. Sterilize by autoclaving for 20 min or by filtration. Store refrigerated.

Working PBS

Prepare a solution of the desired pH by combining the 10× stocks.

0.1 M NaH_2PO_4	See Table 3
0.1 M Na_2HPO_4	See Table 3
8.5% NaCl	100 ml
Deionized water	to 1,000 ml

■ Polysorbate 80

See Tween 80.

■ Potassium chloride solution (0.2 M, pH 2.2)

Potassium chloride is used to treat respiratory specimens for the recovery of *Legionella*.

For 100 ml of potassium chloride, 0.2 M (pH 2.2), solution

Potassium chloride, 0.2 M (solution A): place 1.49 g of potassium chloride into a volumetric flask and dilute to 100 ml with deionized water

Hydrochloric acid, 0.2 M (solution B): add 1.67 ml of concentrated hydrochloric acid to 75 ml of deionized water in a volumetric flask and QS to 100 ml. Add 13.5 ml of solution B to 86.5 ml of solution A and mix.

Potassium hydroxide (0.1 N), used for neutralizing the specimen after mixing with potassium chloride solution: add 0.56 g of potassium hydroxide to a volumetric flask and dilute to 100 ml with deionized water.

Test procedure. Approximately 0.5 ml of specimen is mixed thoroughly with 4.5 ml of the 0.2 M potassium chloride (pH 2.2) solution, and the mixture is allowed to stand for 15 min at room temperature. The mixture is then neutralized to pH 7.0 with 0.1 N KOH and is inoculated onto isolation media.

TABLE 3 Preparation of pH-specific 0.1 M sodium phosphate buffer[a]

pH	Vol (ml) A	Vol (ml) B	pH	Vol (ml) A	Vol (ml) B
5.7	93.5	6.5	6.9	45.0	55.0
5.8	92.0	8.0	7.0	39.0	61.0
5.9	90.0	10.0	7.1	33.0	67.0
6.0	87.7	12.3	7.2	28.0	72.0
6.1	85.0	15.0	7.3	23.0	77.0
6.2	81.5	18.5	7.4	19.0	81.0
6.3	77.5	22.5	7.5	16.0	84.0
6.4	73.5	26.5	7.6	13.0	87.0
6.5	68.5	31.5	7.7	10.5	89.5
6.6	62.5	37.5	7.8	8.5	91.5
6.7	56.5	43.5	7.9	7.0	93.0
6.8	51.0	49.0	8.0	5.3	94.7

[a] A, 0.1 M NaH_2PO_4; B, 0.1 M Na_2HPO_4.

■ Pyrrolidonyl-α-naphthylamide (PYR) hydrolysis

PYR is hydrolyzed by organisms that possess the enzyme pyrrolidonyl arylamidase (56). The PYR test is used for rapid presumptive identification of group A alpha-hemolytic streptococci (*Streptococcus pyogenes*), *Enterococcus* spp., and other gram-positive cocci that grow aerobically and form cells arranged in pairs and chains. A pure culture or isolated colony for testing is critical given the number of PYR-positive organisms with similar Gram stain morphology and hemolytic characteristics.

PYR substrate (L-pyrrolidonyl-α-naphthylamide)

Dissolve L-pyrrolidonyl-α-naphthylamide in methyl alcohol first and then dilute with sterile distilled water. Adjust pH to 5.7 to 6.0. It is used at 0.01% in broth or agar media and at 0.02% in filter paper strips.

PYR reagent (DMACA)

DMACA	200 mg
Hydrochloric acid, concentrated	2 ml
Distilled water	18 ml

Add the acid to the water, and let it cool before adding DMACA.

Tube method. Prepare PYR broth (Todd-Hewitt broth containing 0.01% PYR substrate). Autoclave to sterilize. Dispense 0.15 ml per tube. Emulsify colonies from a blood agar plate in the PYR broth to a turbidity of McFarland no. 2 standard (milky suspension). Incubate at 35°C for 2 h. Add 1 drop of the PYR reagent to each tube, with gentle shaking. Observe for development of a cherry red color after 2 min. Yellow, orange, or orange-pink color is considered negative.

Spot paper strip method. Cut Whatman no. 3 filter paper into strips. Saturate the strips with 0.02% PYR substrate. Dry at room temperature and store desiccated at 2 to 6°C. Prior to testing, moisten the strip with sterile distilled water. Using an inoculating loop or wooden stick, rub colonies onto strip. Incubate for 10 min at 35°C. Then add PYR reagent to the strip and observe for development of a red color change. Yellow, orange, or pink is considered negative. For both methods, a positive reaction is indicated by cherry red to dark purple-red color. A negative reaction is indicated by orange or yellow (no change) color. PYR media, disks, and strips are available commercially.

■ Saline

Saline is used as a diluent in a variety of procedures. Normal or physiological saline is 0.85%.

Sodium chloride	8.5 g
Distilled water	1,000 ml

Other concentrations (e.g., 0.45%) are also used.

■ Skim milk, 20%

Skim milk is used to stabilize bacterial suspensions, particularly those containing anaerobes, for freezing.

Skim milk powder .... 20 g
Distilled water .... 100 ml

After the skim milk is dissolved in the water, dispense 0.25 to 0.5 ml into 2-ml vials. Autoclave at 110°C for 10 min. The vials can be refrigerated for up to 6 months.

■ Sodium bicarbonate ($NaHCO_3$), 20 mg/ml

Sodium bicarbonate is added to thioglycolate broth to enrich it for the recovery of anaerobes. Dissolve 2 g of $NaHCO_3$ in 100 ml of distilled water. Filter sterilize and store refrigerated for up to 6 months. Add 0.5 ml to 10 ml of thioglycolate broth.

■ Sodium citrate (0.1 M), 2.9%

Sodium citrate, dihydrate .... 29.4 g
Distilled water .... 1,000 ml

Dissolve and autoclave. Store at room temperature. If a precipitate forms, discard and prepare a fresh solution.

■ Sodium hydroxide (1 N), 4%

Sodium hydroxide .... 40 g
Distilled water .... 1,000 ml

Dissolve and autoclave. Store at room temperature. If a precipitate forms, discard and prepare a fresh solution.

■ Sodium polyanetholesulfonate (SPS) disks

SPS disks are used to differentiate *Peptostreptococcus anaerobius* (which is inhibited by SPS) from other anaerobic cocci. Dissolve 5 g of SPS in 100 ml of distilled water, filter sterilize, and then dispense 2 μl onto 6-mm-diameter sterile filter paper disks. Allow the disks to dry at room temperature for 72 h. The dried disks are stable at room temperature for up to 6 months. A zone of inhibition of 12 mm indicates that the organism is susceptible.

■ Sorensen pH buffer solutions (M/15 phosphate buffer solutions)

Solution A

M/15 (0.067 M) sodium phosphate, dibasic. Dissolve 9.464 g of anhydrous Na_2HPO_4 in 1 liter of distilled water.

Solution B

M/15 (0.067 M) potassium phosphate, monobasic. Dissolve 9.073 g of anhydrous KH_2PO_4 in 1 liter of distilled water. Mix *x* ml of solution A and solution B as indicated in Table 4 for a buffer of the desired pH.

TABLE 4 Sorensen pH buffer solutions

pH	Vol (ml)	
	Solution A	Solution B
5.29	0.25	9.75
5.59	0.5	9.5
5.91	1.0	9.0
6.24	2.0	8.0
6.47	3.0	7.0
6.64	4.0	6.0
6.81	5.0	5.0
6.98	6.0	4.0
7.17	7.0	3.0
7.38	8.0	2.0
7.73	9.0	1.0
8.04	9.5	0.5

■ Tween 80 (polysorbate 80), 10%

Tween 80 (polysorbate 80) .... 10 ml
Distilled water .... 90 ml

Mix Tween 80 with water until dissolved. Autoclave at 121°C at 15 lb/in^2 for 10 min. Swirl the solution immediately after autoclaving and during cooling to resolubilize the Tween 80. Store refrigerated. The solution can be used for 6 months. Add 0.5 ml of 10% Tween 80 to 10 ml of broth medium when it is used as a medium supplement.

■ Urease test

Rapid enzymatic test used for identification purposes for a number of organisms. The procedure for identifying *Haemophilus* spp. is described.

KH_2PO_4 .... 0.1 g
K_2HPO_4 .... 0.1 g
NaCl .... 0.5 g
Phenol red, 1:500 .... 0.5 ml

Add all ingredients into 100 ml of distilled water. Adjust the pH to 7.0 with NaOH, and add 10.4 ml of a 20% (wt/vol) aqueous solution of urea. To make 1:500 phenol red, dissolve 0.2 g of phenol red in NaOH and add distilled water to 100 ml. Red color developing within 4 h after inoculation indicates urease activity.

■ Vitamin K_1, 10-mg/ml stock

Vitamin K_1 (3-phytylmenadione) is added to enrich media for the recovery of anaerobes. Mix 0.2 g of vitamin K_1 in 20 ml of 95% ethanol by aseptic technique. Vitamin K_1 is a viscous liquid, and it may be hard to measure the exact amount. Adjust the amount of 95% ethanol accordingly to obtain a 10-mg/ml stock. Store refrigerated in a sterile dark bottle. The stock solution can be further diluted in sterile distilled water to obtain a 1-mg/ml working solution, which can be stored refrigerated in a dark bottle for up to 30 days.

■ Voges-Proskauer (VP) test

The VP test is used to detect acetoin (acetyl-methylcarbinol), which is produced by certain microorganisms during growth in a buffered peptone-glucose broth (MR-VP broth). The VP test is commonly used to aid in the differentiation between genera (such as *E. coli* from the *Klebsiella* and *Enterobacter* groups) and other species of the *Enterobacteriaceae* family. The test can be used as a differential test for other organism groups (viridans group streptococci).

Reagent A: 5%-α-naphthol

Dissolve 5 g of α-naphthol in 100 ml of absolute ethanol. Store refrigerated in a brown glass bottle away from light.

Reagent B: 40% KOH
Dissolve 40 g of potassium hydroxide in 100 ml of distilled water.

Test procedure. Inoculate MR-VP broth and incubate until good growth is obtained. Add 0.6 ml of the α-naphthol solution and 0.2 ml of the 40% KOH to 2.5 ml of culture broth. Shake well after the addition of each reagent. A positive reaction, indicated by the formation of a pink-red product, occurs within 5 min. However, allow 15 min for color development before considering the test negative.

STAINS

Direct Examination of Specimens

The first step in the processing of most clinical material is microscopic examination of the specimen. Direct examination is a rapid, cost-effective diagnostic aid. Methods for direct examination are designed to reveal and enumerate microorganisms and eukaryotic cells. Visible microorganisms may denote the presumptive etiologic agent, guiding the laboratory in the selection of the appropriate isolation media and the physician in the selection of the appropriate empirical antibiotic therapy. The quality of the specimen and the measure of the inflammatory response can also be evaluated. In addition, the direct smear serves as a quality control indicator for attempts to isolate observed organisms (1, 27, 28, 33, 54, 55).

Smear Preparation

Smears may be made from clinical material, culture broths, or isolated colonies. These smears should be prepared on clean glass slides, since dirt and grease may interfere with adhesion of the sample to the slide and with the staining process. The best smears are prepared after thoughtful selection of those portions of the sample most likely to reveal the etiologic agent (e.g., a purulent portion of sputum). Smears should contain enough material for an adequate survey of the specimen but should not be overly thick because thick smears may peel or flake off the slide during staining procedures. Thick smears also make the timing of decolorization harder to judge. Smears from swabs should be prepared by rolling the swab over the slide. This method of application helps to preserve host cell morphology and microorganism cell arrangements. Tissue smears may be prepared either by touching freshly exposed cut surfaces directly onto a slide or by first using a tissue grinder or stomacher to homogenize the sample. However, tissue grinding may distort cellular morphology. Smears from aspirates or body fluids may be prepared in several different ways, depending upon the amount of material and equipment available. When the quantity of a liquid sample is limited, a single drop placed on a slide will suffice. If more sample is available, the material should be centrifuged (1,500 × g for 15 min) to concentrate any cells, and the sediment can then be used to prepare the smear. An additional option for the preparation of smears from liquid samples is the use of cytocentrifugation. The cytocentrifuge method uses specimen funnels that are mounted with a slide and filter card and placed in the centrifuge. During centrifugation, the filter card absorbs the supernatant, while cells and microorganisms are centrifuged through a hole in the filter paper strip and are deposited in a continuous layering fashion onto a 6-mm-diameter circular area of the slide. The method is sensitive for the detection of pathogens from sterile body fluids, particularly cerebrospinal fluid (CSF) and peritoneal fluids (10, 62). The method has also been used for detection of acid-fast organisms and *Pneumocystis jiroveci* from respiratory specimens (8, 29). The deposition of specimen in a discrete area and the ability to lyse erythrocytes during centrifugation are particularly advantageous characteristics that allow more rapid and enhanced resolution in a smear examination.

Samples are fixed to the slides with either heat or methanol. Methanol fixation is preferred since heating may produce artifacts, may create aerosols, and may not adhere the specimen adequately to the slide (51). Once dry, the fixed smear is ready for staining.

Smear Preparations and Staining Methods

The following staining methods and techniques are individual methods used most often in the clinical bacteriology laboratory. They are presented in the following categories: wet mounts and single-stain methods, differential, acid-fast, and fluorescent. The stain method and significant characteristics are described. The principles of stains used for all microorganisms are described in chapter 14. Readers are referred to chapters 81, 117, and 134 for those staining procedures most commonly performed in the specialties of virology, mycology, and parasitology, respectively, and to other specific references (6, 23, 39, 47, 51, 58, 66).

Wet Mounts and Single-Stain Methods

■ Colloidal carbon wet mounts (India ink, nigrosin)

See chapter 117.

■ KOH with and without lactophenol cotton blue

See chapter 117.

■ Lugol's iodine

See chapter 134.

■ Methylene blue stain

Methylene blue is a simple direct stain used for a variety of purposes. The stain reveals the morphology of fusiform bacteria and spirochetes from oral infections (Vincent's angina). It may also establish the intracellular location of microorganisms such as *Neisseria.* Methylene blue is the stain of choice for identification of the metachromatic granules of diphtheria; however, one should be careful about overstaining, because this will lessen the contrast between the bacteria and the granules. Methylene blue stains organisms or leukocytes a deep blue in a light gray background. *Corynebacterium diphtheriae* appears as a blue bacillus with prominent darker blue metachromatic granules.

Basic procedure
Fix the prepared slide in absolute methanol for 1 to 3 min or heat fix. Air dry the slide and then stain with 0.5 to 1.0% aqueous methylene blue for 30 to 60 s and up to 10 min for possible *C. diphtheriae* granules. Rinse in water, blot dry, and examine at ×100 to ×1,000 magnification.

■ M'Fadyean stain

The M'Fadyean stain is a modification of the methylene blue stain developed originally for detecting *Bacillus anthracis* in clinical specimens. The rectangular bacteria stain black-deep blue in chains of two to a few cells. Virulent *B. anthracis* rods will be surrounded by a clearly demarcated zone giving the appearance of a reddish-pink capsule ("M'Fadyean reaction").

Basic procedure

As *B. anthracis* is suspected, safety precautions must be taken throughout the procedure. All materials, including spent staining washes, should be discarded into disinfectant effective against endospores or autoclaved. See chapter 7. The staining reagent is prepared by dissolving 0.05 mg of methylene blue solution per ml in 20 mM potassium phosphate adjusted to pH 7.3. After the prepared slide is air dried, it is fixed in absolute methanol for 2 to 3 min. The slide is then dried and a large drop of the methylene blue solution is placed on the slide for 1 min. Rinse the slide under water into a 10% hypochlorite solution, blot, and allow to dry. Examine at ×100 to ×1,000 magnification.

Differential Staining Methods

■ Gram staining

Gram staining is the single most useful test in the clinical microbiology laboratory. It is the differential staining procedure most commonly used for direct microscopic examination of specimens and bacterial colonies because it has a broad staining spectrum. First devised by Hans Christian Joachim Gram late in the 19th century, it has remained basically the same procedure and serves in dividing bacteria into two main groups: gram-positive organisms, which retain the primary crystal violet dye and which appear deep blue or purple, and gram-negative organisms, which can be decolorized, thereby losing the primary stain and subsequently taking up the counterstain safranin and appearing red or pink. The staining spectrum includes almost all bacteria, many fungi, and parasites such as *Trichomonas, Strongyloides,* and miscellaneous protozoan cysts. The significant exceptions include organisms such as *Treponema, Mycoplasma, Chlamydia,* and *Rickettsia,* which are too small to visualize by light microscopy or which lack a cell wall. Mycobacteria are generally not seen by Gram staining; however, in smears illustrating heavy infections, the organisms may give a beaded appearance that is somewhat similar to that of *Nocardia* spp. or may exhibit organism "ghosts" (27). Gram staining can also be used to differentiate epithelial and inflammatory cells, thus providing information about the state of infection and the quality of the specimen (34, 54, 55, 63).

The Gram reaction, morphology, and arrangement of the organisms give the physician clues to the preliminary identification and significance of the organisms. Problems with analysis of the Gram staining generally result from errors in preparation of the slide, such as a smear that is too thick, excessive heat fixing (which can distort organisms), improper decolorization, and inexperience. Overdecolorization results in an abundance of bacteria that appear to be gram negative, while underdecolorizing results in too many bacteria that appear to be gram positive. If a chain of cocci resembling streptococci (normally gram positive) and epithelial cells appears to be gram negative, the slide is overdecolorized. Slides stained by Atkins' Gram staining method are less sensitive to decolorization because the mordant is more effective in retaining crystal violet. This allows better visualization of gram-positive organisms, especially those very sensitive to decolorization such as *S. pneumoniae* and *Bacillus* spp. Atkins' method does not offer a significant advantage over the conventional Gram staining procedure in visualizing gram-negative organisms, and in fact, such visualization may be more difficult with some specimens, such as blood cultures.

Other variations of the Gram stain exist in which the counterstain components may be different, specifically for the purpose of enhancing the appearance of gram-negative organisms. An example is the use of basic carbol fuchsin instead of safranin for easier identification of gram-negative anaerobic organisms (Table 2).

Laboratorians should note that organisms may not always stain true to their cell wall. Anaerobic organisms, older cultures, and organisms that are exhibiting the effects of antibiotics may be especially difficult to interpret. Two methods that may help in the cell wall identification include a string test noted to help distinguish gram-negative anaerobes. Another test is a simple fluorogenic disk test, Gram-Sure (Remel), that helps to differentiate aerobic gram-negative organisms (fluoresce blue with long-wavelength UV light) and gram-positive organisms (no fluorescence). See the reagent section for a full description (50).

Laboratories should evaluate various Gram staining procedure and then institute one as the routine procedure. Two methods of Gram staining are presented here. The first method is the conventional Gram staining method used by most laboratories. The second is an altered Gram staining method devised by Atkins (3) in 1920 that uses gentian violet, a different mordant, and acetone as the decolorizing agent. Each of the staining components is readily available commercially from a number of manufacturers (see Appendix 1).

Basic procedure—conventional Gram staining

The prepared slide is fixed in 95% methanol for 2 min. After air drying, the slide is flooded with crystal violet (10 g of 90% dye in 500 ml of absolute methanol). After at least 15 s, the slide is washed with water and flooded with iodine (6 g of I_2 and 12 g of KI in 1,800 ml of H_2O). The slide is washed with water after 15 s, decolorized with acetone-alcohol (400 ml of acetone in 1,200 ml of 95% ethanol), washed immediately, and counterstained for at least 15 s with safranin (10 g of dye in 1,000 ml of H_2O). This slide is then washed, blotted dry, and examined at ×100 to ×1,000 magnification.

Basic procedure—Atkins' Gram staining

The primary stain is gentian violet (20 g of crystal violet is dissolved in 200 ml of 95% methanol, 8 g of ammonium oxalate is dissolved in 800 ml of distilled water, and the solutions are mixed together and filtered after 24 h). The mordant is Atkins' iodine (20 g of crystals is dissolved in 100 ml of 1 N NaOH; the mixture is then combined with 900 ml of distilled water and stored in a brown bottle at room temperature). Acetone is the decolorizer, and safranin is the counterstain. The staining procedure is the same as that used for conventional Gram staining. The two dyes and the mordant should each be allowed to remain on the slide for at least 15 s. More time has little effect. The most critical aspect of this stain is the amount of time that the decolorizer is used. Unfortunately, the amount of decolorizer is directly related to the thickness of the specimen on the slide. The old benchmark that the slide should continue to receive decolorizer until no more crystal violet is seen to be washing away is still true but is difficult to attain in practice.

■ Spore stain (Wirtz-Conklin)

The Wirtz-Conklin spore stain is a differential stain for detection of spores. Spore-forming bacteria and cell debris will appear pink-red with green-staining spores.

Basic procedure

After the prepared slide is air dried and heat fixed, it is flooded with 5 to 10% aqueous malachite green. Stain is left on the slide for 45 min. Alternatively, the slide can be heated gently to steaming for 3 to 6 min. Heating to steaming enhances the uptake of the stain into the spores. The slide is then rinsed with tap water. Aqueous safranin (0.5%) is used as a counterstain for 30 s. Rinse in water, blot dry, and examine at ×400 to ×1,000 magnification.

■ Wayson stain

The Wayson stain is a modification of the methylene blue stain and is actually a mix of two stains. It has been used for screening CSF for bacteria and amoebae and for demonstrating bipolar staining and examining tissue specimens for *Yersinia pestis* (15). The advantage of this stain is that the contrast between organisms and proteinaceous background is good. Organisms stain dark blue, leukocytes stain light blue and purple, and the background is light blue. However, slides stained by this method cannot be restained with the Gram stain, and the tinctorial qualities of the stain deteriorate over time.

Basic procedure

The staining reagents are prepared by dissolving 0.2 g of basic fuchsin in 10 ml of 95% ethyl alcohol and 0.75 g of methylene blue in 10 ml of 95% ethyl alcohol. The two solutions are added together slowly into 200 ml of 5% phenol in distilled water. The stain is then filtered and stored in an opaque bottle at room temperature. After the prepared slide is air dried, it is fixed in methanol for 2 min and stained for 1 min. Rinse in water, blot dry, and examine at ×100 to ×1,000 magnification.

■ Gimenez stain

The Gimenez stain formula and full description are in chapter 68 and Table 2 in chapter 14. This differential stain is used for the visualization of *Rickettsia* and *Coxiella* from cell cultures and *L. pneumophila*. Carbol fuchsin is the primary stain and fast green and Malachite green are the counterstains, allowing greater contrast with the organisms and background for easier visualization of the organisms. The stain must be heated 48 h prior to use and filtered.

Acid-Fast Staining Methods

The cells of certain organisms contain long-chain (30- to 90-carbon) fatty acids (mycolic acids) that give them a coat impervious to crystal violet and other basic dyes. Heat or detergent must be used to allow penetration of the primary dye into the bacterium. Once the dye has been forced into the cell, it cannot be decolorized by the usual solvent process. The acid-fast stains are useful for identification of a specific group of bacteria (e.g., *Mycobacterium, Nocardia, Rhodococcus, Tsukamurella, Gordonia,* and *Legionella micdadei*) and the oocysts of *Cryptosporidium, Isospora, Sarcocystis,* and *Cyclospora*. The Ziehl-Neelsen (Z-N) stain is one of the original acid-fast stains described. A number of modifications of the Z-N staining procedure have been made to differentiate various acid-fast organisms as well as to simplify the staining process (7, 41, 48, 66).

■ Ziehl-Neelsen (Z-N)

Basic procedure

The prepared slide is heat fixed for 2 h at 70°C. The slide is then flooded with carbol fuchsin (0.3 g of basic fuchsin is dissolved in 10 ml of 95% ethanol, 5 ml of phenol, and 95 ml of water; the solution is filtered before use). Heat the slide slowly to steaming and maintain for 3 to 5 min at 60°C. After cooling, wash with water and decolorize the slide with acid-alcohol (97 ml of 95% ethanol in 3 ml of HCl). Wash and counterstain for 20 to 30 s with methylene blue (0.3 g of dye in 100 ml of H_2O). Wash, blot dry, and examine at ×400 to ×1,000 magnification. An acid-fast organism will stain red, and the background of cellular elements and other bacteria will be blue, the color of the counterstain.

■ Kinyoun stain (Kinyoun modification of Z-N stain)

The basic difference between the Z-N and Kinyoun stains is the replacement of heating with the use of a higher concentration of phenol in the primary stain. The primary stain consists of 4 g of basic fuchsin in 20 ml of 95% alcohol, 8 g of phenol, and 100 ml of distilled water. The Z-N and Kinyoun stains have the same sensitivity and specificity; however, the Kinyoun (cold) staining procedure is less time-consuming and is easier to perform.

■ Modified Kinyoun stain (modified acid-fast stain)

Another modification of the acid-fast staining procedure has been the use of a weaker decolorizing agent (0.5 to 1.0% sulfuric acid) in place of the 3% acid-alcohol. This particular stain helps differentiate those organisms known to be partially or weakly acid-fast, particularly *Nocardia, Rhodococcus, Tsukamurella, Gordonia,* and *Diezia*. These organisms do not stain well with the Z-N or Kinyoun stain.

The acid-fast stains are important clinically and are relatively simple to use. Definitive identification of an acid-fast organism from a clinical specimen cannot be made by staining alone, but certain clues may be helpful. Mycobacteria often appear as slender, slightly curved rods and may show darker granules that give the impression of beading. *M. tuberculosis* can appear as beaded rods arranged in parallel strands or "cords"; *Mycobacterium kansasii* may form long, often broad and banded cells; and *Mycobacterium avium* complex cells appear as short, uniformly staining coccobacilli. *Nocardia* spp. often branch and almost always show a speckled appearance.

Difficulty in interpretation can result from smears that are too thick or insufficiently decolorized, yielding an acid-fast artifact. As a quality control measure, a known acid-fast organism such as nonpathogenic *M. tuberculosis* HRV 37 and a non-acid-fast organism such as *Streptomyces* can be stained in parallel with the clinical specimen.

Factors such as age, exposure to drugs, and a particular acid-fast organism itself may vary the acid-fast presentation. For example, while *M. tuberculosis* is consistently acid fast (with the Z-N or Kinyoun stain), rapidly growing mycobacteria and *Nocardia* are not. Therefore, use of the modified Kinyoun stain may be necessary for these organisms (41, 48, 66). Other modifications used in tissue preparations, such as the Fite-Faraco stain and Pottz stain, may be preferred for unusual isolates such as *Mycobacterium leprae* (66).

Detection of small numbers of acid-fast organisms in clinical specimens is generally significant. However, the use of acid-fast stains for gastric aspirates in the interpretation of pulmonary disease in adults or for stool specimens from human immunodeficiency virus-positive patients in diagnosing *Mycobacterium avium-Mycobacterium intracellulare* infection yields very poor specificity (false-positive smears with saprophytic organisms) as well as poor sensitivity (65). In addition, patients receiving adequate therapy may still have positive smears without positive cultures for a number of weeks. Rarely, small numbers of acid-fast organisms in a smear may represent transferred contamination or the use of reagents contaminated with nonviable saprophytic mycobacteria (e.g., *Mycobacterium gordonae*). All smear-positive but culture-negative specimens should be investigated carefully.

Fluorescent Staining Procedures

See chapter 13 for fluorochrome filter recommendations.

■ Acridine orange

Acridine orange is a fluorochrome that can be intercalated into nucleic acid in both the native and the denatured states (61). The staining procedure is rapid and is more sensitive than the Gram staining procedure in the detection of organisms in blood culture broths, CSF, and buffy coat preparations (34, 44, 45, 52). Acridine orange is also useful in a number of miscellaneous infections, such as *Acanthamoeba* infections, infectious keratitis, and *Helicobacter pylori* gastritis (31). Bacterial and fungal DNAs fluoresce orange under UV light, and mammalian DNA fluoresces green. Results for cellular specimens or heavily laden bacterial specimens may be difficult to interpret owing to excessive fluorescence, and some interobserver variability may be noted.

Basic procedure

After the prepared slide is air dried and fixed in methanol, it is flooded with the acridine orange solution (stock solution, 1 g of dye in 100 ml of H_2O; working solution, 0.5 ml of stock added to 5 ml of 0.2 M acetate buffer [pH 4.0]). After 2 min, rinse the slide with tap water, air dry, and examine with UV light at ×100 to ×1,000 magnification.

■ Auramine-rhodamine

Auramine and rhodamine are nonspecific fluorochromes that bind to mycolic acids and that are resistant to decolorization with acid-alcohol (28). Staining procedures with these fluorochromes are thus equivalent to the fuchsin-based acid-fast procedures. The stain has become commonplace in laboratories that routinely perform acid-fast examinations because it allows rapid screening of specimens and because the procedure is more sensitive than the traditional acid-fast procedures. Acid-fast organisms fluoresce orange-yellow in a black background. If the secondary stain is not used, the organisms will fluoresce a yellow-green color. Smears with suspicious organisms may be confirmed directly with a Kinyoun stain. However, a single organism or a small number of organisms may be difficult to confirm.

Basic procedure

The prepared slide is fixed at 65°C for at least 2 h. It is then stained for 15 min with the auramine-rhodamine solution (1.5 g of auramine O, 0.75 g of rhodamine B, 75 ml of glycerol, 10 ml of phenol, and 50 ml of H_2O) and rinsed with water, followed by decolorization for 2 to 3 min with 0.5% HCl in 70% ethanol. After being rinsed, the slide is counterstained with 0.5% potassium permanganate for 2 to 4 min. The slide is rinsed, dried, and examined under UV light at ×100 to ×400 magnification.

Antibody Staining Methods

See chapter 18 on immunoassays.

MEDIA

This section reviews the basic components necessary in media for the growth and identification of organisms isolated in the clinical microbiology laboratory, specifically bacteriology. Media for the major groups of microorganisms are listed alphabetically. Refer to chapter 14 for discussion of principles of different media. The specific intended use and significant components are provided for each medium. Because media may be purchased from a number of suppliers and minor formulation variations exist for each medium, formulas as well as inoculation and incubation conditions, quality control, and limitations to the use of the media are not specifically mentioned except in rare instances. Readers are referred to comprehensive references on microbiological media (4, 7, 12, 20, 24, 25, 38, 40, 60, 70), including the *Handbook of Media for Clinical Microbiology*, 2nd edition (5), by R. M. Atlas and J. W. Snyder. In addition, the package inserts or websites from each company with purchased and/or specialized media offer excellent and specific descriptions. Recently, the first edition of a combined manual of both Difco and BBL products has been published as *The Difco and BBL Manual* (9). This manual includes numerous color photographs that depict colony morphology and color reactions as well as extensive descriptions of media and relevant references. *The Difco Manual*, 10th (18) and 11th (19) editions, from BD Biosciences, and other media supplier manuals continue to be good references because of historical media, as are other supplier manuals that may contain their own unique products. The formulations of a given medium from different manufacturers do vary slightly and may have been modified from the original description of the medium. A typical comment from the manufacturer is that the "classical" formula has been adjusted to meet performance standards. Again, the package insert or the formula being prepared from a reference should be followed closely. Chapters in this Manual are noted when appropriate to describe a referenced method cited by the authors for a specific organism. These referenced methods and media are found in the Isolation Procedures section within the chapter cited. Appendix 1 describes additives commonly added to media. Refer to Appendix 2 for suppliers of media and reagents as mentioned throughout this Manual. Media are available as prepared plates, tubes, bottles, or dehydrated products.

Preparation of Media

When preparing media from dehydrated materials, the manufacturers' instructions should be followed closely. Chemically cleaned glassware and distilled and/or demineralized water should always be used unless specified otherwise. Care in terms of accuracy should be taken when measuring liquid and dry ingredients. Mixing and solubilization of ingredients are typically done on hot plates, with magnetic stir bars placed in the bottom of the flask or beaker. Excessive heating should be avoided. Autoclaving or filtration sterilizes the media. Autoclaving of volumes of up to 500 ml at 121°C for 15 min is adequate. Larger volumes may require up to 20 to 30 min. The stir bars should be removed before sterilization. For quality control of autoclaving, specialized tape or paper is placed on the medium flask at the time of autoclaving. Enrichments such as blood and other labile additives such as filter-sterilized antibiotics should be added aseptically after the base medium has cooled.

While many dehydrated media are available, most clinical laboratories rely on prepared media from a commercial manufacturer because of convenience and lack of appropriate medium preparation facilities. In addition, overnight shipping even for small-volume purchases is often available for specialized media from the laboratory's routine medium distributor.

Quality Control

The Clinical and Laboratory Standards Institute (CLSI) has specific requirements for quality assurance of commercially prepared media, as documented in standard M22-A3 (13). However, these recommendations do not apply to all media. In addition, any medium that is prepared by the user requires its own specific quality control. Storage of media should be in the dark at 2 to 8°C. Storage in the dark is preferred because additives, such as dyes, will deteriorate faster in the light. The date that the medium was received in the laboratory and the medium expiration date should be marked and easily visible when stored. Media should be in use only up to the expiration date. Prolonged or incorrect storage of media, including transport media, can lead to desiccation of the media, changing the composition of nutrients and selective agents.

Plating of Specimens on Media and Incubation

Media should be warmed to room temperature before inoculation of specimens. In addition, a medium that has obvious contamination, such as colony growth or turbidity in broth medium, or that looks damaged in any way should not be used. Damage may include such things as a cracked petri dish and agar that has changed color, demonstrates precipitates, or is dehydrated.

Finally, it is important that the appropriate atmospheric incubation and temperature of media be used to optimize those pathogens likely to be in specimens submitted. Examples would include those conditions optimal for *Enterobacteriaceae* and *Campylobacter*. Isolation of *Enterobacteriaceae* from MacConkey agar may not be optimal if the agar is placed in CO_2, since the acidity with increased CO_2 may inhibit some of these organisms (S. M. Kircher, R. J. Cote, N. J. Dick, and W. F. Seip, *Abstr. 2000 Gen. Meet. Am. Soc. Microbiol.*, abstr. C-242, 2000), and *Campylobacter* should always be in a microaerophilic environment and at 42°C.

Bacteriology Media

■ A7 and A8 agars

A7 and A8 agars are selective and differential media used for the cultivation, identification, and differentiation of *Ureaplasma* spp. and *Mycoplasma hominis*. Both media contain soy and casein digests in an agar base and a supplement solution that contains yeast extract, horse serum, cysteine enrichment solution, and penicillin. Incorporation of urea aids in the identification of urease production to differentiate the organisms on the basis of the appearance of golden to dark brown colonies. There are two main differences between the agars: the use of manganous sulfate in A7 agar and putrescine dihydrochloride and calcium chloride in A8 agar for the detection and enhancement of growth of urease-positive colonies. *Ureaplasma* colonies are small golden brown colonies that are usually identified at 72 h. *Mycoplasma* colonies have a fried egg appearance and may have a golden or amber color. See also Mycotrim GU and Mycotrim RS.

■ Alkaline peptone water

Alkaline peptone water is an enrichment broth used for the isolation of small numbers of *Vibrio* and *Aeromonas* organisms from stool specimens. Adjustment of the broth to pH 8.4 and inclusion of sodium chloride at a concentration of 0.5 to 1.0% make it selective for *Vibrio* species.

■ American Trudeau Society medium

American Trudeau Society medium is a nonselective enriched medium used for the isolation and cultivation of mycobacteria. It is an egg-based medium. The coagulated egg provides fatty acids essential for support of mycobacterial growth. Glycerol and potato flour provide other nutrients. Malachite green is a partially selective agent that inhibits bacteria. The concentration of malachite green is low, and no other antibiotics are present in this medium; thus, it is very susceptible to proteolytic damage caused by contaminating organisms. This medium is best for specimens not usually contaminated with other microorganisms, e.g., tissue biopsy specimens or CSF. See also Lowenstein-Jensen and Middlebrook media.

■ Amies transport medium with and without charcoal

Amies transport medium is a modification of Stuart's medium. The glycerol phosphate used to maintain the pH in Stuart's medium has been found to enhance the growth of certain organisms that utilize this as a nutrient and to allow overgrowth of potential contaminants. In Amies medium, phosphate buffer replaced the glycerol phosphate ingredient and other salts were added to control the permeability of bacterial cells. Amies medium with charcoal is preferred for the isolation of *Neisseria* spp. because the charcoal neutralizes metabolic products toxic to the organisms.

■ Anaerobic blood agar (CDC)

The Centers for Disease Control and Prevention (CDC) formulation of anaerobic blood agar is a general-purpose medium used for the isolation and cultivation of anaerobic bacteria. The nutritive base is tryptic soy agar supplemented with yeast extract, vitamin K, hemin, and sheep blood. This medium is best for the isolation of anaerobic gram-positive cocci. See chapter 55 for other selective anaerobic medium recommendations for gram-positive bacteria.

■ 10B arginine broth; Shepard's broth

10B arginine broth is a medium used for the transport and growth of *M. hominis* and *Ureaplasma urealyticum*. The medium contains nitrogenous components, amino acids, and other components necessary for growth, and penicillin G or a semisynthetic penicillin is added to reduce bacterial contamination. Shepard's broth contains cefoperazone. Two primary compounds, namely, urea and arginine, as well as the phenol red indicator, aid in the identification of the organisms. *Ureaplasma* hydrolyzes urea and releases ammonia; *Mycoplasma* deaminates the arginine. Both reactions result in an alkaline pH shift and change the color of the medium from yellow to pink. *Ureaplasma* depletes urea in the medium quickly (<12 h), with subsequent death of the culture. Thus, after the color changes, the cultures need to be subcultured quickly to a medium such as A8 or A7 agar that supports the organisms. Limitations of the medium are that other species of *Mycoplasma* and other bacteria may also change the color of the medium.

■ Ashdown agar

Ashdown agar is a selective and differential medium consisting of Trypticase soy agar with 4% glycerol, 0.005 mg of crystal violet per ml, 0.05 mg of neutral red per ml, and 0.004 mg of gentamicin per ml, specifically designed for the isolation of *Pseudomonas pseudomallei*, the causative agent of melioidosis. Glycerol and neutral red allow differentiation from other pseudomonads since *P. pseudomallei* appears flat, with rough wrinkled colonies due to the glycerol, and absorbs the neutral red dye, whereas other pseudomonads do not. The medium is made selective by the addition of crystal violet, which inhibits gram-positive organisms, and gentamicin, which inhibits gram-negative organisms. Ashdown broth with 50 mg of colistin per liter enhances recovery over direct plating by 25% (2, 68).

■ *Bacillus cereus* medium

B. cereus medium is an enriched medium used for the isolation of *B. cereus*. The base includes agar, yeast extract, and buffers. Mannitol combined with bromcresol purple as the indicator dye makes the medium differential. An egg yolk emulsion is added for the detection of the lecithinase activity seen with *B. cereus*.

■ BACTEC 12B radiometric medium

BACTEC 12B medium (BD Biosciences) is a liquid nonselective medium used for the isolation and identification of *Mycobacterium* species in conjunction with the BACTEC system. The medium consists of a 7H9 broth base. The radiometric BACTEC system incorporates ^{14}C-labeled palmitic acid and detects radioactive carbon dioxide; the medium is referred to as 7H12 or BACTEC 12B medium. An antibiotic enrichment supplement is added to the medium to make it selective for mycobacteria. This supplement includes the antibiotics polymyxin B, amphotericin B, nalidixic acid, trimethoprim, and azlocillin, with polyoxylene stearate as a *Mycobacterium* growth enhancer. A total of 0.5 ml of processed specimen may be accommodated in the vial. The BACTEC 12B medium is most commonly used for susceptibility testing. Newer nonradiometric systems are available for monitoring for mycobacterial growth and/or used for susceptibility testing. These include the 9200 series (BD Biosciences), MGIT (BD Biosciences), ESPII (TREK Diagnostic Systems), and MB/BacT ALERT 3D (bioMérieux, Inc.). Manual medium systems also exist for the detection of mycobacteria, such as the Isolator (Wampole Laboratories) and Septi-Chek AFB (BD Biosciences). The reader is referred to chapters 36 and 77 for specifics on medium formulations and antibiotic supplements for each system.

■ *Bacteroides* bile esculin agar

Bacteroides bile esculin agar is an enriched, selective, and differential medium used for the isolation and presumptive identification of members of the *Bacteroides fragilis* group and *Bilophila wadsworthia*. The nutritive base includes casein and soybean peptones, hemin, and vitamin K. The differential characteristic of esculin hydrolysis is identified by the product, esculetin, which reacts with the ferric ammonium citrate to form a complex and produce brown-black coloration around the colony. The selective agents include bile, which inhibits most gram-positive bacteria and anaerobic organisms other than members of the *B. fragilis* group, and gentamicin, which inhibits facultative anaerobes. Bile esculin agar with kanamycin and enriched with vitamin K and hemin is a formulation that is more enriched and selective than *Bacteroides* bile esculin agar for isolation of the *B. fragilis* group. This medium includes beef extract and pancreatic digest of gelatin, vitamin K, and hemin as the nutritive base. Bile inhibits the same organisms as described above, and kanamycin is inhibitory for facultatively anaerobic and aerobic gram-negative bacilli.

■ Baird-Parker agar base

Baird-Parker agar base is a beef extract, peptone, and yeast extract base used to prepare egg-tellurite-glycine-pyruvate agar (ETGPA). ETGPA is an enriched, selective, and differential agar used for the detection of coagulase-positive staphylococci (*S. aureus*) from food and other nonclinical sources. Glycerol and lithium make the medium selective by inhibiting many bacteria. Tellurite is also inhibitory to bacteria. The egg yolk emulsion is an enrichment. Tellurite and the egg yolk emulsion also act as differential determinants. When *S. aureus* reduces tellurite, it imparts a black color to the colony, and lecithinase activity is demonstrated by a clearing around the colony. *S. aureus* appears as black-brown colonies with clear zones around them.

■ Barbour-Stoenner-Kelly medium (Sigma-Aldrich Co., St. Louis, Mo.)

Barbour-Stoenner-Kelly medium is a complicated medium for the isolation of *Borrelia burgdorferi*. Bovine serum albumin, rabbit serum, and sodium bicarbonate are significant components. While a defined medium has been described, variability in components makes for differences in the ability to isolate the organism (59).

■ Bile esculin agar

Bile esculin agar is a selective and differential medium used for the isolation and differentiation of *Enterococcus* and *Streptococcus bovis* (group D *Streptococcus*) from non-group D *Streptococcus*. The nutritive base includes peptone and beef extract. The selective agent is bile (oxgall), which inhibits gram-positive organisms and most strains of streptococci except *S. bovis* and *Enterococcus*. Esculin hydrolysis is a characteristic to differentiate enterococci and *S. bovis* from other organisms. Esculin in the medium is hydrolyzed to esculetin and dextrose. A black-brown pigment forms when the iron salt (ferric citrate) is used as the color indicator of esculin hydrolysis and subsequent esculetin formation. *S. bovis* and *E. faecalis* grow on the medium and exhibit blackening around the colony.

■ Bile esculin agar plus vancomycin at 6 μg/ml

Bile esculin agar plus vancomycin is a selective and differential medium used to identify vancomycin-resistant streptococci and enterococci. Colonies appear the same as they do on bile esculin agar. Growth of group D streptococci and enterococci occurs with esculin hydrolysis in the presence of bile, appearing as blackening of the medium.

■ Bile esculin azide agar and broth (Enterococcosel)

Bile esculin azide agar or broth is a selective and differential medium for *S. bovis* (group D streptococcus) and enterococci. As with bile esculin agar, esculin is incorporated into the medium, and precipitation with ferric ions forms a brown-black pigment, which identifies these species. Bile esculin azide medium has a reduced percentage of bile and makes the medium less inhibitory to non-group D streptococci.

Sodium azide is incorporated to inhibit gram-negative organisms. The addition of 6 μg of vancomycin per ml makes the medium selective for vancomycin-resistant enterococci. Incorporation of aztreonam subsequently increases the selectivity by inhibiting other organsims, especially gram-negative organisms, contaminating specimens.

■ Bismuth sulfite agar

Bismuth sulfite agar is a highly selective and differential medium used for the isolation of *Salmonella enterica* serovar Typhi and other enteric bacilli. Beef extract, peptones, and dextrose are the nutritive base. Bismuth sulfite, a heavy metal, and brilliant green are selective agents which inhibit most commensal gram-positive and gram-negative organisms. Ferrous sulfate is an indicator for hydrogen sulfide production, which occurs when the hydrogen sulfide produced by *Salmonella* reacts with the iron salt. This reaction causes a black or green metallic colony and a black or brown precipitate. Colony morphology and color help differentiate *Salmonella* species. This medium may be inhibitory for some species of *Shigella*. Readers are referred to chapter 42 for other selective media for enteric organisms.

■ Blood agar

See Columbia agar with 5% sheep blood.

■ Blood culture media

All blood culture medium formulations are based on a nutrient peptone broth with variations due to hydrolysis or digestion of the source protein. Additives for neutralization of serum components and/or inactivation of antibiotics, such as SPS, chelators, or resins, vary with the manufacturer. The reader is referred to chapter 15 for formulations for specific blood culture media and various commercial systems.

■ Bordet-Gengou medium

Bordet-Gengou medium is an enriched medium used for the isolation and cultivation of *Bordetella pertussis* from clinical specimens. The medium contains potato infusion, glycerol, and peptones as the nutritive base. Sheep blood allows detection of hemolytic reactions and provides other nutrients for *Bordetella*. The medium can be supplemented with methicillin, which inhibits some of the normal oral flora that is obtained upon collection of the specimen. Culture plates should be held for at least 7 days. Incubation up to 12 days identifies *Bordetella parapertussis*. Bordet-Gengou medium is not as effective for the recovery of *Bordetella* as Regan-Lowe medium, and freshly prepared medium must be used for optimum recovery.

■ Brain heart infusion agar

Brain heart infusion agar is a general-purpose medium used for the isolation of a wide variety of pathogens, including yeasts, molds, and bacteria. The basic formula includes brain heart infusion from solids as well as meat peptones, yeast extract, and dextrose. One variation that exists is brain heart infusion agar with vitamin K and hemin for the enrichment of anaerobes. The anaerobic formulation may be optimal for the isolation of *Eubacterium* spp. but inferior for the isolation of anaerobic gram-negative organisms, especially those that produce pigment.

■ Brain heart infusion agar with 7% horse blood and brain heart infusion agar with 1% serum (see Brain heart infusion agar)

Brain heart infusion agar with horse blood or serum enriches the medium for isolation of *Helicobacter* spp.

■ Brain heart infusion broth

Brain heart infusion broth is a general-purpose clear liquid medium that is used to cultivate a wide variety of organisms. It is also used for the preparation of inocula for susceptibility tests and identification. The medium is especially useful as a blood culture medium. The main nutritive base includes infusion from brains and beef heart. Peptones, glucose, sodium chloride, and buffers are other additives. Sodium chloride acts as an osmotic agent, and disodium phosphate acts as a buffer. Formulations with 6.5% NaCl are used for the isolation of salt-tolerant streptococci, formulations with 0.1% agar that reduce O_2 tension favor anaerobes, and formulations with Fildes enrichment are used for the isolation of fastidious organisms such as *Haemophilus* and *Neisseria*. Brain heart infusion broth is also used for the preparation of inocula for antimicrobial susceptibility testing and broth dilution MIC testing procedures. The medium contains infusions of brain, casein, and meat peptones.

■ Brain heart infusion-vancomycin agar (see Brain heart infusion agar)

Brain heart infusion-vancomycin agar is a selective medium used for the isolation of vancomycin-resistant enterococci. The base is brain heart infusion agar. Vancomycin (6 μg/ml) is added to select for vancomycin-resistant enterococci.

■ Brilliant green agar

Brilliant green agar is a highly selective and differential medium used for the isolation of *Salmonella* species except for serovar Typhi. The nutritive base contains meat and casein peptones. Brilliant green dye at a high concentration is the selective agent and inhibits most gram-positive and gram-negative bacteria, including *Shigella* species and serovar Typhi. Phenol red is the pH indicator. Yeast extract provides additional nutrients. Sugars included in the medium are sucrose and lactose. Acid production in the fermentation of these sugars produces yellow-green colonies with a yellow-green zone. Nonfermenters of sucrose and lactose may range in color from white to reddish pink with a red zone around the colony (*Salmonella*).

■ Brucella agar

Brucella agar is a medium designed originally for the purpose of isolating *Brucella* spp. from dairy products. Brucella agar with 5% horse blood can be used as a general-purpose medium for the isolation of both fastidious aerobic and anaerobic organisms. The nutritive base includes a peptone mix, including meat peptones, dextrose, and yeast extract.

■ Brucella agar with cefoxitin and cycloserine

Brucella agar with cefoxitin and cycloserine is a selective and differential sheep blood medium used for the isolation of *Clostridium difficile*. Brucella agar is the nutritive base. Vitamin K and sheep blood provide other growth enhancers. Cefoxitin and cycloserine inhibit most gram-positive and gram-negative organisms, respectively. *Enterococcus* is not inhibited. Another differential characteristic is that *C. difficile* colonies fluoresce yellow-green under UV light.

■ Brucella agar with hemin and vitamin K

Brucella agar with hemin and vitamin K is a general-purpose nonselective and enriched medium used for the isolation and cultivation of anaerobic bacteria. Casein peptones, dextrose, and yeast extract are the nutritive base. Hemin and vitamin K provide further enrichments. Defibrinated sheep blood allows determination of hemolytic reactions. Because of the high carbohydrate content, colonies with beta-hemolytic reactions may have a greenish hue. The medium is better for gram-negative organisms.

■ Brucella agar with 5% horse blood

Horse blood enriches brucella agar for fastidious organisms, such as *H. pylori*, by providing both hemin (factor X) and NAD (factor V) factors. The use of horse blood also allows determination of hemolytic reactions. However, hemolytic reactions for *Streptococcus* and *Haemophilus* on horse blood differ from those on media with sheep blood.

■ Brucella broth

Brucella broth is a liquid medium that is used to cultivate *Campylobacter* species and to identify the organisms to the species level. Brucella base that contains peptones, dextrose, and yeast extract is the nutritive base.

■ Buffered charcoal yeast extract (BCYE) (selective and nonselective)

BCYE is a specialized enriched agar medium used for the isolation and cultivation of *Legionella* species from environmental and clinical specimens. *Legionella* species, especially *L. pneumophila*, require specific nutrients for growth. One is iron and the other is the amino acid L-cysteine. These are provided in BCYE by ferric pyrophosphate and L-cysteine hydrochloride. The nutritive base is yeast extract and α-ketoglutarate. *N*-(2-Acetamido)-2-aminoethanesulfonic acid buffer maintains the pH of the medium. Charcoal acts as a detoxifying agent and surface tension modifier. Antibiotics may also be added to the medium. Typically, manufacturers provide the medium in two combinations of three antibiotics. One is polymyxin B, anisomycin, and vancomycin, and the other is polymyxin B, anisomycin, and cefamandole (PAC). In these combinations polymyxin B inhibits gram-negative rods, anisomycin inhibits yeasts, vancomycin inhibits gram-positive organisms, and cefamandole inhibits both gram-positive and gram-negative organisms. BCYE with PAC may be inhibitory to some strains of *L. micdadei*. Nonselective BCYE can support the growth of other fastidious organisms such as *Nocardia* and *Francisella*. BCYE can also be a differential medium with the addition of the dyes bromcresol purple and bromthymol blue. *L. pneumophila* produces light blue colonies with a pale green tint. This differential medium is also called Wadowsky-Lee medium and can be used for isolation of actinomycetes.

■ Buffered glycerol saline

Buffered glycerol saline is a multipurpose transport medium. The transport medium has been used for the isolation of bacteria, such as *Aeromonas* spp., as well as viruses. In addition, glycerol-containing media may also be used for long-term storage of isolates and for transport and storage of biopsy specimens.

■ *Burkholderia cepacia* selective agar

B. cepacia selective agar is an enriched and selective medium used for the isolation of *B. cepacia*. Trypticase peptone, yeast extract, sodium chloride, sucrose, and lactose are the nutritive base. The medium is made selective by the addition of polymyxin B, gentamicin, vancomycin, and crystal violet. The medium supports the growth of *B. cepacia* and inhibits >90% of other isolates. This agar is more sensitive and more selective than *Pseudomonas cepacia* (PC) agar, oxidative-fermentative polymyxin B-bacitracin-lactose medium, and other selective media for isolation of *B. cepacia* from patients with cystic fibrosis (35). See chapter 49.

■ *Campylobacter* blood agar

Campylobacter blood agar is an enriched selective blood agar medium used for the isolation of *Campylobacter* species. The nutritive base is brucella agar. Sheep blood provides heme and other growth factors. The selectivity of the medium comes from the incorporation of five antimicrobial agents: trimethoprim, vancomycin, amphotericin B, polymyxin B, and cephalothin. These agents inhibit normal stool flora such as members of the family *Enterobacteriaceae*, staphylococci, and yeasts. Plates should be incubated in a microaerophilic environment. Due to the dextrose content of the brucella base, weak oxidase reactions may be exhibited. Some species of *Campylobacter* (e.g., *Campylobacter fetus* subsp. *fetus* and *Campylobacter upsaliensis*) are inhibited by cephalosporins. Media with cephalothin have been shown to be more inhibitory to *C. jejuni* and *Campylobacter coli* than those with cefoperazone. See chapter 59 for additional selective media.

■ *Campylobacter* charcoal differential (CCD) agar

CCD agar is a blood-free selective medium used for the isolation of *Campylobacter* from stool specimens. Cefoperazone replaces cefazolin in other selective agars. The nutritive base is Preston agar, which consists of beef extract and peptones. This agar has been shown to be less inhibitory than other *Campylobacter* agars for all *Campylobacter* species as well as more inhibitory to contaminating organisms (36).

■ *Campylobacter* thioglycolate medium

Campylobacter thioglycolate medium is a selective holding medium used for the isolation of *Campylobacter* species. The low concentration of agar in thioglycolate broth provides a reduced oxygen content. The selective agents include the same as those in *Campylobacter* agar: trimethoprim, vancomycin, polymyxin B, cephalothin, and amphotericin B.

■ Cary-Blair transport medium

Cary-Blair transport medium was specifically designed to enhance the survival of enteric bacterial pathogens. The medium has a low nutrient content, which allows organism survival without replication; sodium thioglycolate, which allows a low oxidation-reduction potential; and a high pH, which minimizes the destruction of bacteria when acid is produced.

■ Cefoperazone-vancomycin-amphotericin B (CVA) medium

CVA medium is a selective and enriched blood agar medium used for the isolation of *Campylobacter* species. The nutritive agar base is brucella agar. Sheep blood provides hemin and other growth nutrients. The antibiotics in this medium are vancomycin, amphotericin B, and cefoperazone, which inhibit gram-positive organisms, fungi, and anaerobic gram-negative organisms. The limitations of this medium are that some campylobacters (e.g., *C. fetus* subsp. *fetus*) are inhibited and that weak oxidase reactions may occur due to the dextrose in the brucella agar base. CVA is a good medium to use if only a single selective medium for *Campylobacter* can be used.

■ Cefsulodin-Irgasan-novobiocin (CIN) medium (*Yersinia* selective agar)

CIN, or *Yersinia* selective agar, is a selective and differential medium used for the isolation and differentiation of *Yersinia enterocolitica* from clinical specimens and food sources. The nutritive base includes peptones and beef and yeast extracts. The selective agents are sodium desoxycholate, crystal violet, cefsulodin, Irgasan (triclosan), and novobiocin. The medium is available with various concentrations of cefsulodin (4, 8, or 15 μg/ml). The lower concentration is recommended for better growth of clinically significant *Yersinia* spp. as well as growth of *Aeromonas* spp. Mannitol is the sugar, and neutral red is the indicator. Organisms that ferment mannitol in the presence of the neutral red dye cause a pH drop around the colony. The colony becomes transparent, with the absorption of the red dye to form a red bulls-eye appearance in the center with *Yersinia*, and *Aeromonas* will have a pink center with an uneven clear apron. Most other bacteria, including other enteric mannitol fermenters, are inhibited. Some yersiniae may require cold enrichment at 4°C and subsequent subculture to CIN medium. See also chapters 44 and 46.

■ Cetrimide agar

Cetrimide agar is a selective and differential medium used for the identification of *Pseudomonas aeruginosa*. Cetrimide is the selective agent and inhibits most bacteria by acting as a detergent. *Pseudomonas* produces a number of pigments. Two pigments can be detected with this medium. The magnesium chloride and potassium sulfate stimulate the blue-green pyocyanin pigment, and the fluorescent yellow-green pigment can be seen with a UV light. The low iron content of the medium also stimulates pigment production.

■ Charcoal selective medium

Charcoal selective medium is an enriched selective medium used for the isolation of *Campylobacter* species. In this medium the nutritive base is a Columbia agar base, and charcoal is used to effectively replace blood components. The selective agents used in this medium include vancomycin, cefoperazone, and cycloheximide. Vancomycin and cefoperazone effectively inhibit gram-positive and gram-negative organisms, including *Pseudomonas*. Fungi are inhibited by cycloheximide. The limitation of this medium is that some *Campylobacter* species, e.g., *C. fetus* subsp. *fetus*, are inhibited by cephalosporins.

■ Chocolate agar

Chocolate agar is a general-purpose medium used for the isolation and detection of a wide variety of microorganisms, including fastidious species such as *Neisseria* and *Haemophilus*. Chocolate agar originated as a GC agar base which includes meat and casein peptones, phosphate buffer to maintain pH, and cornstarch to detoxify fatty acids in the medium. Hemoglobin is added to the medium to provide hemin (X factor). The appearance of hemin in dry powdered form is reddish brown. When hemoglobin is hydrated and added to the medium, it gives the agar base the "chocolate" appearance. Other enrichments added include defined supplements, such as IsoVitaleX or Vitox, which provides NAD (V factor). Both of these components added to the GC agar base make the enriched chocolate agar. Levinthal agar is a variation on chocolate agar. The medium is a selective and differential medium used for the isolation and identification of *Haemophilus influenzae* type b. The medium is a chocolate agar base that is made transparent by the removal of particulate matter by either centrifugation or filtration through sterile filter paper. The medium contains bacitracin to inhibit respiratory flora and *H. influenzae* type b antiserum, allowing detection of an immunoprecipitation reaction. Colonies of encapsulated strains show a bright iridescence (red-blue-green-yellow) when light is transmitted from behind the clear medium.

■ Chopped meat glucose broth

Chopped meat glucose broth is an enriched medium that supports the growth of most anaerobes. It is most commonly used to isolate *Clostridium botulinum* from mixed bacterial growth. Beef heart, peptones, and dextrose supply the essential nutrients. The −SH groups from cooked and denatured muscle protein are the reducing agents in the medium. Vitamin K and hemin are additives used to maximize the growth of specific anaerobes. The medium helps to induce sporulation of *Clostridium* spp.

■ CHROMagar (Rambach agar)

CHROMagar is a microorganism-specific, chromogenic culture medium used for isolation and identification for a variety of organisms. CHROMagar was developed by Alain Rambach, who first formulated agars that were monochromogenic for the detection of *E. coli* and *Salmonella* spp. Second-generation agars are multicolor. Both types are differential and selective. The nutritive agar base includes peptone and glucose. Different additives, proprietary chromogenic mixtures, and antibiotics have resulted in a series of media specific for such organisms as *Listeria*, *S. aureus*, methicillin-resistant *S. aureus* (MRSA), *E. coli* O157, yeasts, and other organisms. BD Biosciences has a licensing agreement for development of the CHROMagar media. Many other chromogenic media with proprietary components are also now available through a number of manufacturers. Most commonly evaluated are chromogenic media for the detection of MRSA. These include MRSA ID (bioMérieux), MSA-CFOX (Oxoid), and MRSA*Select* (Bio-Rad) (17, 64). Greater recovery of organisms, increased specificity, and elimination of nonselective media are benefits of chromogenic agar use. Cost per plate compared to those of standard media and limited shelf life need to be considered before implementation.

■ Columbia agar with 5% sheep blood

Columbia agar with 5% sheep blood is a general-purpose medium used for the isolation of a variety of microorganisms, including fastidious organisms. This medium contains meat and casein peptones and beef extract, yeast extract, and cornstarch as the nutritive base. Sheep blood allows determination of hemolytic reactions and provides X factor. However, the substantial carbohydrate content may make beta-hemolytic streptococci appear to be alpha-hemolytic or take on a greenish hue. NADase enzyme in sheep blood destroys the V factor (NAD); thus, organisms that require this factor do not grow. Incorporation of horse or rabbit blood allows beta-hemolysis to be seen better. Addition of 20 μg of ampicillin per ml is helpful in isolation of *Aeromonas*.

■ Columbia broth

Columbia broth is a general-purpose clear liquid medium used especially for blood culture medium. The broth supports the growth of a wide range of microorganisms. The base is similar to Columbia agar, with meat peptones, casein, and yeast extract. Salt and Tris buffers have been added to enhance the growth of microorganisms and increase the buffering capacity, respectively. For the purpose of blood culture medium, additional ingredients include carbon dioxide, which is stimulatory for many organisms; cysteine, which improves isolation of anaerobic and aerobic organisms from blood; SPS, a polyanionic anticoagulant which inactivates aminoglycosides and which interferes with the complement, lysozyme activity, and the phagocytic activity inherent in a blood specimen; and glucose, which provides a hypertonic medium for the isolation of cell wall-deficient forms.

■ Columbia-colistin-nalidixic acid agar with 5% sheep blood

Columbia-colistin-nalidixic acid agar with 5% sheep blood is a selective and differential medium commonly used in the isolation of gram-positive aerobic and anaerobic organisms from mixed clinical specimens. The base is Columbia agar with 5% sheep blood, which allows the detection of hemolytic reactions and provides additional enrichment and X factor (heme). The medium is made selective by the inclusion of the antibiotics colistin and nalidixic acid, which inhibit gram-negative organisms. Swarming *Proteus* spp. are inhibited. Supplementation with glutathione and lead acetate allows a selective and differential medium for anaerobic gram-positive cocci.

■ Cycloserine-cefoxitin-fructose agar

Cycloserine-cefoxitin-fructose agar is a selective and differential agar medium used for the isolation of *C. difficile*. The nutritive base includes animal peptones and fructose. The selective agents include cycloserine and cefoxitin. Cycloserine inhibits gram-negative organisms, especially *E. coli*, and cefoxitin is a broad-spectrum antibiotic that is active against both gram-positive and gram-negative organisms. *Enterococcus* is not inhibited. The medium is made differential by the addition of neutral red. *Clostridium* raises the pH of the medium and allows the neutral red indicator to change to yellow. Both the colony and the surrounding medium turn yellow. In addition, *C. difficile* colonies yield a gold-yellow fluorescence when viewed under long-wave UV light.

■ Cysteine-albumin broth with 20% glycerol

Cysteine-albumin broth with 20% glycerol is used for transport and storage of gastric biopsy specimens for the recovery of *H. pylori* (37).

■ Cystine glucose blood agar

Cystine glucose blood agar is an enriched medium used for the isolation of *Francisella* spp. The nutritive base is beef heart infusion, peptones, and glucose. *Francisella* requires cystine for growth. Rabbit blood provides hemoglobin enrichment.

■ Cystine-tellurite blood agar

Cystine-tellurite blood agar is a modification of Tinsdale agar and is both a selective and differential medium used for the detection of *C. diphtheriae*. Casein peptones, beef infusion, and yeast extract are the nutritive base. Potassium tellurite is both the selective and differential agent. Gram-negative organisms and most organisms of the upper respiratory flora are inhibited; *Corynebacterium* spp. are the exception. The potassium tellurite also allows differentiation of *C. diphtheriae* from other biotypes by the dull metal gray or black colony appearance indicative of tellurite reductase activity and the brown halo around the colony consistent with cystinase activity. Other organisms, such as staphylococci, may reduce tellurite and produce black colonies. These are easily differentiated by Gram staining.

■ Cystine tryptic agar

Cystine tryptic agar is a pancreatic digest of casein-enriched medium that is most commonly used for cultivation and maintenance of fastidious organisms. Addition of 1% carbohydrates and phenol red for determination of fermentation reactions is especially helpful for differentiating *Neisseria* spp.

■ Diagnostic sensitivity agar

Diagnostic sensitivity agar is a medium used in the cultivation of organisms for susceptibility testing. The base is proteose peptone, veal infusion solids, agar, and glucose, with other additives. The medium is available as a premixed powder from Oxoid.

■ DNA-toluidine blue agar

DNA-toluidine blue agar is a differential medium used most commonly for the detection and differentiation of *Staphylococcus* spp. The nutritive base is tryptic soy agar. Supplementation with DNA permits detection of DNase activity (or heat-stable staphylococcal nuclease) that has endo- and exonucleolytic properties and can cleave DNA or RNA produced in most coagulase-positive staphylococci. The medium is blue due to the toluidine blue O, and DNase activity is detected by a pink zone around the colony secondary to the metachromatic property of the dye.

■ Dubos Tween-albumin broth

Dubos Tween-albumin broth is a nonselective medium used for the isolation and cultivation of mycobacteria. Polysorbate 80 (Tween 80) is an oleic acid ester and acts as an essential fatty acid necessary for the growth of mycobacteria. In addition, Tween 80 acts as a dispersal agent and allows a small inoculum to grow more homogeneously. Casein peptone and asparagine provide other nutrients. Phosphates provide a buffering system, and albumin, a source of protein, provides protection from toxic substances in the medium. Cultures of *M. tuberculosis* may form cords in the medium, and other mycobacteria grow more diffusely. See also Middlebrook 7H9 broth.

■ Egg yolk agar (modified McClung-Toabe agar)

Egg yolk agar medium (modified McClung-Toabe agar) is a selective and differential medium used for the isolation and differentiation of *Clostridium* spp. McClung and Toabe (51a) reported on the use of egg yolk medium for the identification of species of clostridia by the detection of lecithinase and lipase activities. Degradation of lecithin results in an opaque precipitate around the colony, and lipase destroys fats in the egg yolk, which results in an iridescent sheen on the colony surface. Proteolysis can also be determined with egg yolk agar, as indicated by a translucent clearing of the medium around the colony. The medium should be incubated anaerobically for a minimum of 48 h. It should be held for up to 7 days for the detection of lipase activity. Addition of neomycin makes the egg yolk agar moderately selective by inhibiting some facultative anaerobic gram-negative rods. Lecithinase positivity is also seen with some *Bacillus* spp. Lipase and proteolytic activity can also be demonstated with some anaerobes.

■ Ellinghausen-McCullough/Johnson-Harris medium

Ellinghausen-McCullough/Johnson-Harris medium is an enriched semisolid medium used for the isolation and cultivation of *Leptospira*. Stuart's medium is the base to which multiple modifications for optimization of the recovery of *Leptospira* have been made since the original description. Bovine albumin and Tween provide lipids and long-chain fatty acids. B vitamins and ammonium ion provide essential vitamins and a nitrogen source. Lysed erythrocytes provide other essential supplements, such as iron. The medium is made selective by adding 5-fluorouracil either alone or with fosfomycin and nalidixic acid (21). This medium is available as a dehydrated medium base and supplement from BD Biosciences.

■ Enterococcosel agar

See Bile esculin azide agar and broth.

■ Eosin-methylene blue (EMB) agar

EMB agar is a selective and differential medium used for the isolation and differentiation of enteric pathogens from contaminated clinical specimens. Pancreatic digest makes up the nutritive base. Eosin and methylene blue are the selective agents and inhibit gram-positive organisms. The sugars are lactose and, in certain modifications, sucrose. Organisms that ferment lactose bind to the dyes under acidic conditions and appear as blue-black colonies with a metallic sheen. Under less acidic conditions, other coliforms appear as mucoid and brown-pink colonies. Nonfermenters such as *Salmonella*, *Shigella*, and *Proteus* will appear amber or transparent (colorless). EMB agar should be stored in the dark because of the loss of support of growth when it is exposed to visible light.

■ ESP Culture System II

ESP Myco medium is used with ESP Culture System II (TREK Diagnostic Systems) for the detection of mycobacterial growth. The medium is a Middlebrook 7H9 broth enriched with glycerol, Casitone, and cellulose sponge disks. OADC enrichment is added prior to use.

■ ETGPA

See Baird-Parker agar base.

■ Fastidious anaerobic agar (*Fusobacterium* selective agar)

Fastidious anaerobic agar is an enriched sheep blood medium used for the isolation and cultivation of anaerobic organisms. Peptone, glucose, agar, and starch make up the solid base. Sheep blood, vitamin K, and hemin are enrichments for anaerobes. A greater amount of hemin is used in fastidious anaerobic agar than in other anaerobic media. This medium is used for the isolation of *Fusobacterium* spp. and formate-fumarate-requiring species.

■ Fletcher's medium

Fletcher's medium is an enriched semisolid medium used for the isolation and growth of *Leptospira*. The medium is a peptone and beef extract base with a 1.5% agar concentration. Rabbit serum supplies long-chain fatty acids and albumin and has been found to be superior to other serum sources for the isolation of *Leptospira*. 5-Fluorouracil may be added to select for *Leptospira*. Cultures should be incubated in air and at 28 to 30°C. See Ellinghausen-McCullough/Johnson-Harris medium.

■ FlexTrans viral and chlamydia transport medium

FlexTrans viral and chlamydia transport medium (Trinity Biotech) is intended to be used as a transport medium for viruses and/or chlamydiae. The medium consists of minimal essential medium, bovine serum albumin, glutamine, and sucrose, with a phenol red indicator. Microbial growth is inhibited by the incorporation of the antibiotics amphotericin B, gentamicin, and streptomycin.

■ GC agar base

GC agar base is a chocolate agar base used with various additives for the purpose of isolating *Neisseria gonorrhoeae* and other fastidious organisms, such as *Haemophilus* spp., including *Haemophilus ducreyi*, and for susceptibility testing of *N. gonorrhoeae*. GC agar base includes digest of casein, animal peptones, cornstarch, NaCl, and buffers. A 1% defined growth supplement with yeast and X (hemin) and V (NAD) factors is added. The supplement contains a low concentration of cysteine to avoid activation of various beta-lactam antibiotics such as penems, carbapenems, and clavulanic acid. GC agar base with 5% fetal bovine serum and 10% CVA enrichment allows for isolation of *H. ducreyi* (53).

■ GN broth

GN broth is an enriched selective broth medium used for the isolation of gram-negative rods. Specifically, *Salmonella* and *Shigella* are isolated more effectively in GN broth than on solid medium alone. The nutritive base includes casein and meat peptones as well as mannitol and dextrose. The concentration of mannitol limits the growth of some other contaminating enteric organisms. Sodium deoxycholate and sodium citrate inhibit gram-positive and some gram-negative organisms. Enteric organisms do not overgrow the pathogens in the first 6 h of incubation, at which time the broth should be subcultured.

■ Haemophilus test medium (HTM) and broth

HTM is an enriched medium used for susceptibility testing of *Haemophilus* species. The medium contains beef and casein extracts. Yeast extract, hematin, and nicotinamide (NAD) provide necessary growth factors and enrichments. Antagonists to sulfonamides and trimethoprim are removed by thymidine phosphorylase. The calcium and magnesium concentrations are adjusted to the concentrations recommended by the CLSI. Although the agar medium is a clear agar base and should exhibit clear endpoint interpretations, some investigators have reported difficulties with interpreting zone sizes and poor growth with some strains. Broth microdilution methods also use HTM, which consists of cation-adjusted Mueller-Hinton broth and the supplements described above. Broth dilution methods with HTM provide clearer endpoints. See chapter 75 for specific formulations and references.

■ Heart infusion agar and broth

Heart infusion agar and broth are general-purpose media used for the isolation of a variety of microorganisms. Heart muscle infusion, casein peptones, and yeast extract are the nutritive base. Fastidious organisms do not grow well on or in this medium because no additional enrichments or sheep blood is incorporated. Incorporation with 5% rabbit blood allows detection of the more fastidious *Actinomyces*.

■ Hektoen enteric agar

Hektoen enteric agar is a selective and differential medium used for the isolation and differentiation of enteric pathogens from contaminated clinical specimens. Animal peptones and yeast extract provide the nutritive base. Bile salts and the indicator dyes (bromthymol blue and acid fuchsin) in the medium are the selective agents and inhibit gram-positive organisms. Lactose, sucrose, and salicin are the carbohydrates incorporated to differentiate fermenters from nonfermenters. In addition, differentiation of species occurs with the use of sodium thiosulfate and ferric ammonium citrate, which allow detection of hydrogen sulfide production. Organisms that produce hydrogen sulfide appear with the formation of a black precipitate on the colony. Fermenters such as *E. coli* produce colonies which are yellow-pink, *Shigella* spp. are green or transparent, and *Salmonella* spp. are green or transparent with black centers.

■ Hemin-supplemented egg yolk agar

See Neomycin egg yolk agar.

■ Isolator or lysis-centrifugation tube (Wampole Laboratories)

The Isolator is a unique system for the purpose of recovering organisms from blood through a simultaneous process of lysis and centrifugation. The tubes contain saponin, a lysing agent, and EDTA, an anticoagulant as well as a fluorocarbon that acts as a cushioning agent during centrifugation. The system creates a layer that is subsequently plated onto media appropriate for organism recovery. The system is especially good for the recovery of dimorphic fungi, yeasts, mycobacteria, and *Bartonella* spp. Recovery of anaerobes, *Haemophilus* spp., and pneumococci may be reduced.

■ Iso-Sensitest agar and broth

Iso-Sensitest agar and broth are media used for susceptibility testing in countries outside the United States. The base includes hydrolyzed casein, peptones, and glucose, with other additives. The medium is available as a premixed powder from Oxoid Unipath. See chapter 70 for specific uses.

■ John E. Martin Biological Enrichment Chamber (JEMBEC) (BBL) and InTray GC System transport medium (Biotest)

The JEMBEC and InTray GC devices are transport/inoculation media for direct plating of specimens for the detection of *N. gonorrhoeae*. JEMBEC contains GC-Lect agar, and InTray GC contains modified Thayer-Martin medium, both of which are a chocolate agar base. Each system is self-contained with a tablet that allows production of a CO_2 atmosphere and enhances recovery of the pathogen. The InTray GC system can be stored and transported at room temperature. GC-Lect helps to specifically inhibit *Capnocytophaga* spp. See chapter 39 for specific antibiotic components for various media used for the purpose of isolating *Neisseria* spp.

■ Kanamycin-vancomycin laked sheep blood agar

Kanamycin-vancomycin laked sheep blood agar is an enriched, selective, and differential medium used for the isolation and cultivation of anaerobic bacteria, especially slowly growing and fastidious anaerobes from clinical specimens, such as *Bacteroides* spp. and *Prevotella* spp. The base is CDC anaerobic blood agar. The selective agents are kanamycin and vancomycin (7.5 μg/ml) to prevent growth of obligate facultative gram-negative and gram-positive bacteria and facultative anaerobic bacteria, respectively. Use of a medium with 2 μg of vancomycin per ml allows better growth of *Porphyromonas* spp. Laked blood is used to allow optimal pigmentation of anaerobes such as the pigmented *Prevotella* spp.

■ Lactobacillus MRS broth

Lactobacillus MRS (deMan, Rogosa, and Sharpe) broth is a nonselective liquid medium used for the isolation and cultivation of lactobacilli from clinical specimens and dairy and food products. The nutritive base includes peptones, yeast extract with buffers, and glucose. Polysorbate 80 (Tween 80) supplies fatty acids and magnesium for additional growth requirements. Sodium acetate and ammonium citrate may inhibit normal flora, including gram-negative bacteria, oral flora, and fungi, and improve the growth of lactobacilli. The growth of lactobacilli is favored when the pH is adjusted to 6.1 to 6.6. Gas production can help identify *Leuconostoc* from *Pediococcus* in conjunction with arginine degradation to differentiate these organisms from *Lactobacillus* (16). See chapter 31.

■ Levinthal agar with bacitracin and *H. influenzae* antiserum

See Chocolate agar.

■ Lim broth

Lim broth is a modification of Todd-Hewitt broth and is an enriched selective liquid medium used for the isolation and cultivation of *Streptococcus agalactiae*. Peptones, salts, and dextrose provide the nutritive base. Yeast extract provides B vitamins and additional enrichment. The antibiotics colistin and nalidixic acid inhibit gram-negative organisms. Lim broth has shown better recovery of GBS than Todd-Hewitt broth with gentamicin and nalidixic acid (22). See also StrepB carrot broth and GBS broth.

■ Lithium chloride-phenylethanol-moxalactam agar

Lithium chloride-phenylethanol-moxalactam agar is an enriched and selective agar used for the isolation and cultivation of *Listeria monocytogenes*. Peptones and beef extract are the nutritive base. Phenylethyl alcohol, glycine anhydride, and lithium chloride suppress the growth of gram-positive and gram-negative organisms. Moxalactam makes the agar more selective by inhibiting gram-negative organisms such as *Pseudomonas* and additional gram-positive organisms. Enrichment of *Listeria* in a broth for 24 h is subsequently subcultured onto the selective medium for isolation when trying to isolate the organisms from contaminated sites. The medium is not differential, but use of oblique lighting may show *Listeria* colonies to be blue, while other colonies appear yellow or orange (14, 46, 67).

■ Loeffler's medium

Loeffler's medium is an enriched nonselective medium used for the cultivation of corynebacteria, especially *C. diphtheriae*. The nutritive base is heart infusion and peptones with dextrose. Horse serum and egg cause the medium to coagulate during sterilization and provide other nutritive proteins. The medium enhances the production of metachromatic granules within the cells of the organisms. These granules are seen when smears of the organism are viewed with the methylene blue stain.

■ Lombard-Dowell egg yolk agar

See Neomycin egg yolk agar.

■ Lowenstein-Jensen medium

Lowenstein-Jensen medium is an enriched nonselective medium used for the isolation and cultivation of mycobacteria. It is similar to American Trudeau Society medium in its content and its ability to grow mycobacteria. Lowenstein-Jensen medium is an egg-based medium with glycerol and potato flour and, as with all egg-based media, is susceptible to liquefying when specimens are contaminated with other bacteria. The concentration of malachite green is twice that in American Trudeau Society medium, and thus, the malachite green is somewhat more inhibitory for contaminating organisms. Inorganic salts may make the medium more enriched for mycobacteria.

■ Lowenstein-Jensen medium (Gruft modification)

The Gruft modification of Lowenstein-Jensen medium is an enriched selective medium used for the isolation of mycobacteria. Penicillin and nalidixic acid are added to the medium and inhibit gram-positive and gram-negative organisms, respectively. RNA is added as a growth stimulant.

■ Lowenstein-Jensen medium (Mycobactosel modification)

The Mycobactosel modification of Lowenstein-Jensen medium is an enriched selective medium for the isolation of mycobacteria. Different antibiotics from the Gruft modification are added to make the medium more selective against bacteria. Cycloheximide, lincomycin, and nalidixic acid inhibit saprophytic fungi, gram-positive organisms, and gram-negative organisms, respectively. No RNA is added.

■ Lowenstein-Jensen medium with 1% ferric ammonium citrate

Lowenstein-Jensen medium with 1% ferric ammonium citrate is an enriched and selective egg-based medium used for the recovery of *Mycobacterium haemophilum*. Ferric ammonium citrate is the additive which allows this organism to grow.

■ Lowenstein-Jensen medium with 5% NaCl

Lowenstein-Jensen medium with 5% NaCl is an enriched selective medium used to differentiate sodium chloride-tolerant strains of *Mycobacterium*. Most rapid growers, e.g., the *Mycobacterium fortuitum* complex, as well as the more slowly growing organism *Mycobacterium triviale*, will grow on this medium. The exception is the more resistant organism *Mycobacterium chelonae*, which will not grow on this medium.

■ Lysis-centrifugation tube

See Isolator.

■ MacConkey agar

MacConkey agar is a selective and differential medium used for the isolation of gram-negative organisms. The nutritive base includes a variety of peptones. The medium is made selective by the incorporation of bile (although at levels less than those used in other enteric media) and crystal violet, which inhibit gram-positive organisms, especially enterococci and staphylococci. An agar concentration greater than that described in the original reference helps to inhibit swarming *Proteus*. The medium is made differential by use of the combination of neutral red and lactose. When an organism ferments lactose, the drop in pH causes the colony to take on a pink-red appearance.

■ MacConkey agar with sorbitol (SMAC)

SMAC is a selective and differential medium used for the isolation and differentiation of sorbitol-negative *E. coli*. Shiga toxin-producing strains of *E. coli*, such as *E. coli* O157:H7, which may cause hemorrhagic colitis, are indistinguishable from other *E. coli* serotypes on routine stool isolation media such as MacConkey agar because they all ferment lactose. SMAC has D-sorbitol instead of the lactose in the MacConkey agar formulation. Shiga toxin-producing strains of *E. coli* do not ferment sorbitol and appear as colorless colonies. Sorbitol-fermenting strains are pink. The medium inhibits enterococci with crystal violet and other gram-positive organisms with bile salts. SMAC with cefixime and tellurite may be more selective for detection of *E. coli*. However, some strains may be inhibited. SMAC does not identify all Shiga toxin-producing strains of *E. coli*.

■ MacConkey broth

MacConkey broth is a differential medium containing the indicator bromcresol purple used for the detection of coliform organisms from contaminated food, water, or stools. The broth contains peptone, lactose, bile salts, and sodium chloride. Bromcresol purple is less inhibitory than neutral red for coliforms. The color change from purple to yellow is a more sensitive and definitive indication of acid formation.

■ Mannitol-egg yolk-polymyxin B agar

Mannitol-egg yolk-polymyxin B agar is an enriched, selective, and differential medium used for the isolation of *B. cereus* from mixed clinical specimens. The nutritive base includes peptone and beef extract. Egg yolk emulsion is added for the detection of lecithinase activity, which is usually limited to *B. cereus*. Phenol red and mannitol are combined to make the medium differential. Contaminating gram-negative organisms are inhibited by the polymyxin B.

■ Mannitol salt agar

Mannitol salt agar is a selective and differential medium used for the isolation of *S. aureus*. The nutritive base includes peptones, beef extract, and mannitol. Phenol red is the indicator. The selective nature of the medium is the high salt content (7.5% NaCl), which inhibits most organisms except staphylococci. The differential component for identification of *S. aureus* is the combination of mannitol and phenol red. The color change around the colony from red to yellow upon the fermentation of mannitol and the subsequent drop in the pH of the medium identify staphylococci.

■ Martin-Lewis agar

Martin-Lewis agar is an enriched and selective medium for the isolation of *N. gonorrhoeae*. Martin-Lewis agar is a modification of the modified Thayer-Martin formulation. The nutritive base is chocolate agar. The specific differences from the modified Thayer-Martin formulation are the use of a greater concentration of vancomycin (4.0 versus 3.0 μg/ml), which inhibits more gram-positive organisms, and the replacement of nystatin with anisomycin, which improves the inhibition of *Candida* species. Trimethoprim and colistin are incorporated as well for inhibition of other commensal organisms. Some strains of pathogenic *Neisseria* have been reported to be inhibited by vancomycin and trimethoprim. See also JEMBEC and Thayer-Martin agar. Chapter 39, Table 3, lists antimicrobial agent amounts for each *Neisseria* selective medium.

■ MB/BacT ALERT (bioMèrieux)

MB/BacT ALERT contains a modified Middlebrook 7H9 medium supplemented with casein, bovine serum albumin, and catalase. It is used with MB/BacT ALERT 3D (bioMérieux, Inc.) for the cultivation and detection of mycobacterial growth.

■ MGIT (mycobacteria growth indicator tube) (BD Diagnostic Systems)

MGIT is a Middlebrook 7H9-based broth system that contains a fluorescence indicator, which is used for the detection of mycobacterial growth. The 7H9 broth is supplemented with multiple growth enrichments prior to use. Chapter 36, on *Mycobacterium*, describes and compares this system with the BACTEC system in more detail.

■ Middlebrook 7H10 agar

Middlebrook 7H10 agar is an enriched nonselective agar-based medium used for the isolation and cultivation of mycobacterial species. Essential ingredients include inorganic salts, glycerol, and OADC enrichment. The OADC enrichment includes oleic acid, which is a fatty acid used in the metabolism of mycobacteria; albumin, which protects against toxic agents and which is a source of protein; dextrose, which is used as a source of energy; and catalase, which destroys toxic peroxides in the medium. This is the recommended medium for mycobacterial susceptibility testing. However, because standard formulations of the agar and especially the OADC supplement may vary, quality control is critical. Middlebrook medium allows visualization of mycobacterial colonies 1 to 2 weeks earlier than Lowenstein-Jensen formulations.

■ Middlebrook 7H11 agar

Middlebrook 7H11 agar is a nonselective agar-based medium used for the isolation and cultivation of *Mycobacterium* species. The formulation is identical to that of Middlebrook 7H10 medium except for the addition of casein hydrolysate. Casein hydrolysate is added as a growth stimulant for drug-resistant strains of *M. tuberculosis*. The formulation of Middlebrook 7H11 thin-pour agar is identical to that of Middlebrook 7H11 agar except that the agar plate has a reduced volume. The plates are sealed and every 2 days are examined along the isolation streak lines for evidence of microcolonies. This technique allows for faster detection on solid medium than in standard tube media or on thick media on plates.

■ Middlebrook 7H9 broth with glycerol

Middlebrook 7H9 broth with glycerol is an enriched nonselective broth for the isolation of *Mycobacterium* species. Glycerol, inorganic compounds, and cations supply essential nutrients and stimulate growth. ADC enrichment is added to the broth. ADC enrichment includes albumin, which binds to free fatty acids that are toxic to *Mycobacterium* species; dextrose, which supplies energy; and catalase, which destroys toxic peroxides that may be present in the medium.

■ Mitchison 7H11 selective agar

Mitchison 7H11 selective agar is an enriched selective agar-based medium used for the isolation of *Mycobacterium* species. The basic formulation is Middlebrook 7H11 agar: glycerol, inorganic salts, casein hydrolysate, malachite green, and OADC enrichment. Antibiotics are added to make the medium very selective for mycobacteria. Carbenicillin and polymyxin B, amphotericin B, and trimethoprim are active against most members of the family *Enterobacteriaceae*, yeasts, and *Proteus* species, respectively.

■ Modified Irgasan-ticarcillin-potassium chromate broth

Modified Irgasan-ticarcillin-potassium chromate broth is a selective broth used for the isolation of *Y. enterocolitica*. The base is the modified Rappaport-Vassiliadis enrichment broth with minor alterations. Irgasan and ticarcillin replace the carbenicillin. The chromate makes the medium more selective by inhibiting members of the family *Enterobacteriaceae*. *Enterobacteriaceae* have A nitrase activity, which splits chlorate to toxic by-products. *Yersinia* spp. have B nitrase activity, which cannot split the chlorate.

■ Modified Thayer-Martin agar

Modified Thayer-Martin agar is an enriched and selective agar for the isolation of pathogenic *Neisseria* species from clinical specimens with mixed flora. The nutritive base is chocolate agar. Modified Thayer-Martin agar has three significant changes from the original Thayer-Martin medium. The medium has less agar and less dextrose, and these characteristics improve the growth of *Neisseria*. The third change is the addition of trimethoprim, which inhibits swarming *Proteus* spp. Vancomycin and colistin inhibit gram-positive and gram-negative bacteria, respectively. This medium is recommended over the original formulation for the isolation of pathogenic *Neisseria*. Some strains of pathogenic *Neisseria* have been reported to be inhibited by vancomycin and trimethoprim. See also Martin-Lewis agar.

■ Mueller-Hinton agar with and without 5% sheep blood

Mueller-Hinton agar is the agar recommended by the CLSI for routine susceptibility testing of nonfastidious microorganisms by the Kirby-Bauer disk diffusion susceptibility method. Mueller-Hinton agar with 5% sheep blood is used for susceptibility testing of *S. pneumoniae*. Beef and casein extracts and soluble starch in an agar base make up the nutritive base of the medium. Starch protects the organism from toxic materials that may be in the medium. Calcium and magnesium concentrations are controlled. Mueller-Hinton agar with 5% chocolatized blood plus 1% IsoVitaleX and 3 μg of vancomycin per ml is used for the isolation of *H. ducreyi*. See GC agar and chapter 41.

■ Mueller-Hinton agar with 2% NaCl

Mueller-Hinton agar with 2% NaCl is a selective medium used for testing the susceptibility of *Staphylococcus* to the penicillinase-resistant penicillins methicillin, nafcillin, and oxacillin by agar dilution or with the gradient-based system (E test). The sodium chloride added to the medium enhances the growth of staphylococci. Heteroresistant methicillin-resistant strains are more easily detected with this medium by increasing the incubation time to 24 h and by incubation at cooler temperatures (30 to 35°C).

■ Mueller-Hinton agar with 4% NaCl and 6 μg of oxacillin per ml

Mueller-Hinton agar with 4% NaCl and 6 μg of oxacillin per ml is the selective, differential medium used to screen *S. aureus* (not coagulase-negative staphylococci) for resistance to penicillinase-resistant penicillins (e.g., nafcillin, methicillin, and oxacillin). A sample from overnight growth on nonselective medium is used. Incubation for a full 24 h at 35°C in ambient air is recommended before interpretation of growth.

■ Mueller-Hinton broth

Mueller-Hinton broth is a magnesium and calcium cation-adjusted liquid medium used in procedures for susceptibility testing of aerobic gram-positive and gram-negative organisms by both macrodilution and microdilution methods. The nutritive base includes beef extract and peptones. Starch is a detoxifying agent.

■ Multiprobe media (M4-3, M5, and M4-RT) (Remel)

M4-3 contains vancomycin, amphotericin B, and colistin and is suitable for transport of viruses, chlamydiae, *Mycoplasma*, and *Ureaplasma*. M5 is similar to M4-3, but it does not contain gelatin. M5 is suitable for transport of viruses, chlamydiae, *Mycoplasma*, and *Ureaplasma*. M4-RT contains gentamicin and amphotericin B and is suitable only for transport of viruses and chlamydiae. All the media are supplemented Hanks' balanced salt solution buffered with HEPES buffer, with phenol red as the pH indicator. The antibiotics are added to inhibit bacterial organisms, and therefore, the medium cannot be used for bacterial culture.

■ Mycobactosel agar

Mycobactosel is a BBL trade name for an enriched selective agar-based medium used for isolation of *Mycobacterium* species. The medium is called by other names, depending on the manufacturer. The basic formulation is a Middlebrook 7H11 base, glycerol, inorganic salts, casein hydrolysate, malachite green, and OADC enrichment. Antibiotics are added to make the medium selective. The principle used for the Middlebrook 7H11 formulation to which antibiotics are added is the same as that used for Mitchison 7H11 medium. The antibiotics differ between Mycobactosel agar and Mitchison 7H11 medium. The antibiotics in Mycobactosel agar are cycloheximide, lincomycin, and nalidixic acid, which inhibit saprophytic fungi, gram-positive organisms, and gram-negative organisms, respectively.

■ MycoTrim GU and MycoTrim RS (Irvine Scientific)

The MycoTrim GU and MycoTrim RS culture systems are unique triphasic flask systems specifically designed for the isolation and identification of *M. hominis*, *U. urealyticum* (GU), and *Mycoplasma pneumoniae* (RS). The flask systems contain both agar and an enriched broth formulated for growth of these organisms that contain PPLO broth, containing meat digests, peptones, beef extracts, glucose, arginine, urea, horse serum, yeast extract, phenol red indicator, calcium, phosphate, and agar at a concentration that allows spreading growth of the colonies. The specimen is inoculated into the flask, and antibiotic disks (cefoperazone and nystatin) are added to prevent bacterial contamination. The system is incubated agar side up. Growth of the organism results in a pH change and is indicated by a color change in the media from red to orange and/or yellow. If no color change occurs in the first 24 h, the agar surface is reinoculated with the growth media. Because mycoplasmas do not cause turbidity, the color change is crucial. Colonial growth is confirmed by visualizing colonies using a light microscope and the 10× objective. The color change and colony morphology, including size and appearance, distinguish between *M. hominis*, *U. urealyticum*, and *M. pneumoniae*.

■ NAG medium

NAG medium is an enriched and selective medium used for the isolation and cultivation of *Haemophilus* species from clinical specimens with mixed flora. The agar base is blood agar with *N*-acetyl-D-glucosamine (NAG), hemin, and NAD. NAG medium allows spheroblastic *H. influenzae* to revert morphologically. Spheroblastic forms may be seen in specimens from patients receiving beta-lactam antibiotics. Bacitracin makes the medium selective by inhibiting gram-positive organisms that occur as normal respiratory flora. This medium has been found to be especially helpful in isolating *H. influenzae* from respiratory specimens from cystic fibrosis patients. Placement of cefsulodin disks on the primary streak helps to inhibit *Pseudomonas* spp. to make the medium more selective.

■ Neomycin egg yolk agar

Neomycin egg yolk agar is a selective and differential medium used for the differentiation of anaerobic organisms that are lipase positive, including *Clostridium* spp., *Prevotella intermedia, Fusobacterium necrophorum*, and some strains of *Prevotella loescheii*. The nutritive base includes peptones and yeast extract. Vitamin K and L-cystine make the medium optimal for the isolation of anaerobes. Egg emulsion adds enrichment and makes the medium differential by detecting lipase activity. Neomycin makes the medium selective by inhibiting both gram-positive and gram-negative organisms and differential by the fermentation of lactose.

■ Neomycin-vancomycin agar

Neomycin-vancomycin agar is an enriched and selective medium that is particularly good for the isolation and cultivation of *Fusobacterium* from clinical specimens. The nutritive base is fastidious anaerobe agar with 5% sheep blood. The selective agents include neomycin and vancomycin, which inhibit gram-negative and gram-positive organisms, respectively.

■ New York City medium

New York City medium is an enriched and selective medium for the isolation of pathogenic *Neisseria* from clinical specimens. It also supports the growth of large-colony mycoplasmas and *U. urealyticum*. The medium is a clear peptone-cornstarch agar base with lysed horse erythrocytes, horse plasma, and yeast dialysate, which are used instead of the hemoglobin and the supplements used for the other enriched and selective media for *Neisseria*. The antibiotics that make the medium selective include vancomycin, colistin, and amphotericin B, which inhibit gram-positive bacteria, gram-negative bacteria, and fungi, respectively. While human blood products can replace the horse blood products, sheep blood cannot be used.

■ Nucleic acid transport (NAT) (Medical Packaging Corporation)

NAT is a nucleic acid transport device that is FDA cleared for use with multiple amplification and hybridization testing formats.

■ Oxford agar

Oxford agar is an enriched and selective medium used for the isolation of *L. monocytogenes*. Columbia agar is the base, and it is supplemented with esculin and ferric ammonium citrate for the detection of esculin hydrolysis by listeriae. Suppression of contaminants is accomplished by the addition of lithium, cycloheximide, colistin, acriflavine, cefotetan, and fosfomycin. A modified Oxford agar replaces cycloheximide, acriflavine, cefotetan, and fosfomycin with moxalactam. *Listeria* spp. appear black with a black halo.

■ Oxidative-fermentative polymyxin B-bacitracin-lactose agar

Oxidative-fermentative polymyxin B-bacitracin-lactose medium is a selective and differential medium used for the isolation of *B. cepacia* from respiratory specimens from patients with cystic fibrosis. The nutritive base is an oxidative-fermentative medium with peptones. When acid is produced from the utilization of the lactose sugar, as occurs with *B. cepacia*, the bromthymol blue indicator changes the colony from green to yellow. Polymyxin B and bacitracin are the selective agents and inhibit some gram-negative and gram-positive organisms, respectively. Other organisms seen in cystic fibrosis patients may grow on this medium and are differentiated by the inability to produce acid from lactose. See also *Burkholderia cepacia* selective agar and *Pseudomonas cepacia* (PC) agar.

■ P agar

P agar is an enriched medium used for cultivation and isolation of staphylococci. The agar base includes peptone, yeast extract, NaCl, and glucose.

■ Peptone yeast extract broth

Peptone yeast extract broth is used in the analysis of metabolic products by gas-liquid chromatography because there is negligible acid volatility within the medium.

■ Petragnani medium

Petragnani medium is an egg-based medium. It contains more than twice the concentration of malachite green in Lowenstein-Jensen medium and is most commonly used for the isolation and cultivation of mycobacteria from heavily contaminated specimens. It is also used for the cultivation and maintenance of *Mycobacterium smegmatis*.

■ Phenylethyl alcohol agar

Phenylethyl alcohol agar is an enriched and selective blood agar medium used for the detection and isolation of anaerobic organisms, particularly fastidious and slowly growing bacteria, from clinical specimens with mixed flora. The base is Trypticase soy agar with yeast extract, vitamin K, cystine, and hemin. The medium is selective as a result of the incorporation of phenylethyl alcohol, which reversibly inhibits DNA synthesis and thus inhibits facultative anaerobic gram-negative bacteria, such as members of the family *Enterobacteriaceae*. Phenylethyl alcohol agar inhibits swarming by *Proteus* spp. and *Clostridium septicum*.

■ PLM-5 TM

PLM-5 TM is a proprietary medium formulation (Intergen Co., Purchase, N.Y.) similar to Ellinghausen-McCullough/Johnson-Harris medium that is used for the isolation and cultivation of *Leptospira*. It has less agar and 5-fluorouracil.

■ Polymyxin B-acriflavine-lithium chloride-ceftazidime-esculin-mannitol (PALCAM) agar

PALCAM agar is an enriched, differential, and selective agar medium used for the isolation of *L. monocytogenes*. Columbia agar supplemented with glucose, mannitol, and yeast extract is the nutritive base. Esculin and ferric ammonium citrate are added to detect esculin hydrolysis by listeriae. Fermentation of mannitol is detected with the indicator dye phenol red. Lithium, acriflavine, ceftazidime, and polymyxin B are added as selective agents. For contaminated specimens an enriched broth is inoculated and incubated for 24 h. Subsequently 0.1 ml is subcultured onto PALCAM agar. Listeria colonies appear gray-green with a sunken black center.

■ Polymyxin B-lysozyme-EDTA-thallous acetate agar

Polymyxin B-lysozyme-EDTA-thallous acetate agar is a selective agar used for the isolation of *B. anthracis* from environmental specimens. Heart infusion agar is the base. Thallous acetate and EDTA are additional additives speculated to have advantages for the recovery of *B. anthracis*. Lysozyme is an additive which inhibits *Bacillus* spp. other than *B. cereus* and *B. anthracis*. The addition of thallous acetate, EDTA, and lysozyme together has an additive effect which results in the inhibition of most non-*B. anthracis* species. Polymyxin B inhibits gram-negative organisms. Colonies of *B. anthracis* grown on polymyxin B-lysozyme-EDTA-thallous acetate agar are smaller and smoother than those grown on plain heart infusion agar and are creamy white with a ground-glass texture. *B. cereus* is usually inhibited (43).

■ Polymyxin B-pyruvate-egg yolk-mannitol-bromthymol blue agar

Polymyxin B-pyruvate-egg yolk-mannitol-bromthymol blue agar is an enriched, selective, and differential medium used for the isolation of *B. cereus*. The nutritive agar base includes peptones, agar, and buffers. Egg yolk emulsion allows detection of lecithinase activity, which is unique to *B. cereus*. Sodium pyruvate is added to reduce the size of the colonies, which may be important when performing plate counts. Bromthymol blue and mannitol combine to make the medium differential. *B. cereus* does not produce acid from mannitol and has a distinctive bright blue color. Polymyxin B inhibits contaminating gram-negative organisms from clinical specimens with mixed flora, such as stool specimens. Mannitol-egg yolk-polymyxin B agar and *B. cereus* medium are similarly used for the isolation of *B. cereus*.

■ Polysorbate 80 medium

See Ellinghausen-McCullough/Johnson-Harris medium.

■ PRAS media

Prereduced anaerobically sterilized (PRAS) media are specifically manufactured (Anaerobe Systems) and packaged to eliminate oxygen to enhance growth of anaerobic organisms. Systems come with and without swabs and are available in various collection formats: tubes, widemouthed collection containers for surgical specimens, and prepackaged plates.

■ *Pseudomonas cepacia* (PC) agar

PC agar is a selective medium used for the isolation of *B. cepacia* (formerly *Pseudomonas cepacia*) from respiratory specimens from cystic fibrosis patients. The medium was originally derived from a holding medium containing salts, phenol red, and agar in a phosphate buffer. Selective agents include crystal violet, ticarcillin, and polymyxin B, which inhibit many gram-positive and gram-negative organisms. PC agar may inhibit *B. cepacia* as well (30, 35, 69). See also *Burkholderia cepacia* selective agar and oxidative-fermentative polymyxin B-bacitracin-lactose agar.

■ Rambach agar

See CHROMagar.

■ Rappaport-Vassiliadis enrichment broth

Rappaport-Vassiliadis enrichment broth is a selective and enriched broth used for the isolation and cultivation of *Salmonella* spp. from food and environmental specimens. A modified Rappaport-Vassiliadis broth is a more selective broth used for the isolation and cultivation of *Y. enterocolitica* from foods. Basic Rappaport-Vassiliadis medium contains soybean peptone digest with salts and malachite green. Malachite green suppresses the growth of contaminating bacteria. The modified Rappaport-Vassiliadis broth uses pancreatic digest of casein with salts, malachite green, and carbenicillin.

■ Regan-Lowe medium

Regan-Lowe medium is an enriched and selective medium used for the isolation of *B. pertussis*. Beef extract pancreatic digest, horse blood, and niacin are the nutritional base. Starch and charcoal neutralize substances, such as fatty acids and peroxides, that are toxic to *Bordetella*. Cephalexin is added to inhibit the normal flora in the nasopharynx. Regan-Lowe transport medium contains half-strength charcoal and horse blood, provides better isolation of *Bordetella* than Bordet-Gengou medium, and has a longer shelf life.

■ Salmonella-shigella agar

Salmonella-shigella agar is a selective and differential medium used for the isolation and differentiation of *Salmonella* and *Shigella* from clinical specimens and other sources. The nutritive base contains animal and casein peptones and beef extract. The selective agents are bile salts, citrates, and brilliant green dye, which inhibit gram-positive organisms. The high degree of selectivity of the medium inhibits some strains of *Shigella*, and the medium is not recommended as a primary medium for isolation of this species. The medium contains only lactose and thus differentiates organisms on the basis of lactose fermentation. The formation of acid on fermentation of lactose causes the neutral red indicator to make red colonies. Non-lactose-fermenting organisms are clear on the medium. As with Hektoen enteric agar, sodium thiosulfate and ferric ammonium citrate allow the differentiation of organisms that produce hydrogen sulfide. Lactose fermenters, such as *E. coli*, have colonies which are pink with a precipitate, *Shigella* appears transparent or amber, and *Salmonella* appears transparent or amber with black centers. Some strains of *Shigella dysenteriae* are inhibited.

■ Schaedler's agar

Schaedler's agar is a general-purpose medium used for the isolation and cultivation of anaerobic bacteria. The nutritive base includes vegetable and meat peptones, dextrose, and yeast extract. Sheep blood, vitamin K, and hemin provide other additives that stimulate the growth of fastidious anaerobes. Because of the high carbohydrate content, colonies with beta-hemolytic reactions may have a greenish hue. This medium may be better than other nonselective anaerobic media for the isolation of fastidious anaerobic organisms.

■ Schleifer-Kramer agar

Schleifer-Kramer agar is a selective medium used for the isolation of *Staphylococcus* from heavily contaminated specimens such as feces. The nutritional base includes casein peptones with beef and yeast extracts, glycine, and sodium pyruvate. Sodium azide at 0.45% makes the medium selective for staphylococci and some other gram-positive organisms by inhibiting gram-negative organisms.

■ Selenite broth

Selenite broth is an enrichment broth medium used for the isolation of *Salmonella* and *Shigella* species. Casein and meat peptones provide nutrients. Selenite inhibits enterococci and coliforms that are part of the normal flora if the broth medium is subcultured within 12 to 18 h. However, reduction of selenite produces an alkaline condition that may also inhibit the recovery of *Salmonella*. Lactose and phosphate buffers are added to allow stability of the pH. When fermenting organisms produce acid, the acid neutralizes the effect of the selenite reduction and subsequent alkalinization. Cystine added to selenite broth enhances the recovery of *Salmonella*.

■ Sensitest agar

Sensitest agar is a medium used in susceptibility testing outside of the United States. The base is pancreatic digest of casein, peptones, and glucose with other additives. The medium is available as a premixed powder from Oxoid Unipath. See chapter 70 for specific uses.

■ Septic-Chek biphasic mycobacterial media

The Septic-Chek system (Becton Dickinson Microbiology Systems) is a mycobacterial culture system which contains modified 7H9 broth and three types of solid media, modified Lowenstein-Jensen, Middlebrook 7H11, and chocolate agars, with various supplements.

■ Skirrow medium

Skirrow medium is an enriched selective blood agar medium used for the isolation of *Campylobacter* spp. from specimens with mixed flora. The nutritive base is a blood-based agar. Hematin is provided by sheep blood. The selective agents are trimethoprim, vancomycin, and polymyxin B, which inhibit the normal flora found in fecal specimens.

■ STGG

STGG medium (skim milk, tryptone, glucose, and glycerin) is a transport medium that has been used for collection of nasopharyngeal swabs for the purposes of isolation and preservation of *S. pneumoniae*. Collection and storage of nasopharyngeal swabs on STGG at −70 or −20°C were shown to be equal to direct plating of nasopharyngeal swabs onto selective medium (57).

■ Storage media

See chapter 6.

■ StrepB carrot broth kit (Hardy Diagnostics) and GBS broth (Northeast Laboratory Services)

Carrot broth and GBS broth are media that allow for the detection of red, red-orange, or orange pigment production by beta-hemolytic *S. agalactiae* (GBS) due to the hemolytic reaction with substrates such as starch, protease, peptone, and serum. There is a direct genetic linkage identified with the hemolytic activity and pigment production, with about 95% of GBS strains demonstrating hemolysis. The medium is supplemented with growth-promoting components that are added in the form of a disk (antibiotics). Generation of a bright orange or red color occurs within 6 to 24 h. These media have shown to be very specific, with more rapid turnaround time to detection of GBS than subculture to Lim broth (32). Also see Lim broth.

■ Streptococcus selective agar

Streptococcus selective agar is a selective medium for detection of streptococci. The agar base is Columbia agar. Various antibiotic supplements have been used to make the medium selective for streptococci and reduce the numbers of gram-negative organisms. Colistin and oxolinic acid are one combination less detrimental to *Streptococcus* spp. (42).

■ Stuart's transport media with and without charcoal

Stuart's transport medium is an early transport medium first described in 1948. This medium uses glycerol phosphate to maintain the specimen as well as maintain the pH, agar, methylene blue as a redox indicator, and sodium thioglycolate to allow the survival of anaerobes. The glycerol phosphate has also been found to be used as an energy source by certain contaminants which may overgrow the desired pathogen. Charcoal may be added as a detoxifying agent.

■ Sucrose-phosphate-glutamate transport medium

Sucrose-phosphate-glutamate transport medium is used for the maintenance and transport of *Chlamydia* species and viruses. Sucrose and two buffer solutions are the base. Bovine serum and glutamic acid are additives. Glutamic acid is a stabilizing agent that is especially useful for enveloped viruses. The antibiotic combination may be the same as or slightly different from that in 2-sucrose-phosphate. Most commonly the antibiotic combination is vancomycin, streptomycin, and nystatin, which inhibit both gram-positive and gram-negative organisms, as well as yeasts.

■ 2-Sucrose-phosphate transport media

2-Sucrose-phosphate medium is used for transport of specimens for the purpose of culturing *Chlamydia trachomatis* and *Mycoplasma* spp. Sucrose (0.2 M) and two potassium phosphate buffers are the base. Fetal bovine serum allows *Chlamydia* to maintain infectivity, and nystatin and gentamicin are added to inhibit yeasts and bacteria. 4-Sucrose-phosphate agar and broth (Remel) with a higher concentration of sucrose are also used for the isolation of *Mycoplasma* spp.

■ Tetrathionate broth base

Tetrathionate broth base is an enriched liquid medium used for the isolation of *Salmonella* species in contaminated clinical specimens and other products. The nutritive base includes pancreatic digest of casein and peptic digest of animal tissue with sodium thiosulfate. Bile salts inhibit gram-positive organisms and tetrathionate, which is formed when an iodine-potassium iodide solution is added and which is inhibitory to other normal intestinal flora. Addition of brilliant green inhibits gram-positive and gram-negative organisms, including some *Salmonella* spp.

■ Thayer-Martin agar

Thayer-Martin agar is an enriched and selective medium used for the isolation of *Neisseria* from clinical specimens with mixed flora. The nutritive base is chocolate agar, which is a GC agar base with casein and meat peptones, cornstarch for the neutralization of fatty acids, and phosphate buffer for control of the pH. The chocolate agar occurs with the addition of hemoglobin, which provides hemin or X factor, and IsoVitaleX enrichment, which provides NAD, vitamins, and other nutrients, to improve the growth of pathogenic *Neisseria*. The medium is made selective by the addition of vancomycin, colistin, and nystatin, which inhibit the normal flora of gram-positive bacteria, gram-negative bacteria, and fungi, respectively. Some strains of pathogenic *Neisseria* have been reported to be inhibited by vancomycin and trimethoprim. See also Modified Thayer-Martin agar and Martin-Lewis agar.

■ Thioglycolate with hemin and vitamin K

Thioglycolate broth with hemin and vitamin K is an enriched liquid medium used to support the growth of microaerophilic and anaerobic organisms, including fastidious organisms. Casein and soy peptones supply the basic nutrients. Sodium thioglycolate and L-cystine are the reducing agents in the medium, while hemin and vitamin K are additional additives that allow more fastidious anaerobes to thrive. A small amount of agar helps to slow the diffusion of oxygen and is more suitable for anaerobic organisms.

■ Thiosulfate citrate bile salt sucrose (TCBS)

TCBS is a highly selective and differential medium for the recovery of *Vibrio* spp. except *Vibrio hollisae* and *Vibrio cincinnatiensis*. The medium is inhibitory to gram-positive organisms by incorporation of oxgall, a naturally occurring substance containing a mixture of bile salts and sodium cholate, a pure bile salt. Peptic and casein digests are the nutritive base, and sucrose is a fermentable carbohydrate for the metabolism of *Vibrio*. Sodium thiosulfate provides a sulfur source, and ferric citrate detects hydrogen sulfide production. Bromthymol blue and thymol blue are the pH indicators. Alkaline pH enhances the recovery of *Vibrio cholerae*. Color appearance on the agar is dependent on the species. See chapter 47.

■ Tinsdale agar

See Cystine-tellurite blood agar.

■ Todd-Hewitt broth with gentamicin and nalidixic acid

Todd-Hewitt broth is used for the isolation of beta-hemolytic streptococci from mixed flora, especially vaginal specimens for GBS. Beef heart infusion and peptone are the nutritive base, with dextrose as the energy source and sodium-based buffers to protect the hemolysin from inactivation. The antibiotics make the medium selective by inhibiting gram-negative rods.

■ Tryptic or Trypticase soy agar base with 5% sheep blood

Tryptic or Trypticase soy agar base with 5% sheep blood is a general-purpose medium used for the isolation of a wide variety of organisms. The medium contains soybean and casein peptones as the nutritive base. The addition of sheep blood enriches the medium, and the sheep blood allows the growth of more fastidious organisms by providing hemin (X factor). V factor (NAD) is inactivated by enzymes in the sheep blood and thus does not allow the growth of organisms that require the NAD additive, such as *H. influenzae*. The use of sheep blood provides an excellent means of interpretation of hemolytic reactions, especially those of *Streptococcus* spp.

■ Tryptic or Trypticase soy broth

Tryptic or Trypticase soy broth is a general-purpose clear liquid medium used for the cultivation of a wide variety of organisms. It is also recommended by the CLSI for preparation of an inoculum for Kirby-Bauer disk diffusion susceptibility testing and is the CLSI's choice as a sterility testing medium. The base includes digests of casein and soybean, with additional additives of glucose, sodium chloride to maintain osmotic equilibrium, and buffers. For the purpose of a blood culture medium, additional additives include carbon dioxide to enhance the growth of microorganisms and SPS, an anticoagulant, to inactivate blood components and aminoglycosides. Formulations with 6.5% NaCl exist for the purposes of differentiating enterococcal species or salt-tolerant streptococci. Fildes enrichment is added to cultivate fastidious organisms such as *Haemophilus* spp.

■ Trypticase soy agar with horse or rabbit blood

Trypticase soy agar with horse or rabbit blood medium is used for the isolation of *Haemophilus* species. The nutritive base is a combination of soy and casein peptones. The medium provides smaller but adequate amounts of X (hemin) and V (NAD) factors compared to the amounts in sheep blood and is used for the isolation of *Haemophilus* species. In addition, the medium with horse or rabbit blood allows determination of hemolytic reactions.

■ University of Vermont modified listeria enrichment broth

University of Vermont modified listeria enrichment broth is an enriched and selective liquid medium used for the isolation of *L. monocytogenes*. The nutritive base contains pancreatic digest of casein and animal tissue and beef and yeast extract and is supplemented with esculin, acriflavine, and nalidixic acid.

■ V agar

V agar is an enriched and selective medium used for the isolation of *G. vaginalis* from clinical specimens. The nutritive base is GC agar. The addition of 2% hemoglobin, 5% fetal bovine serum, and a supplement containing NAD enhances the recovery of the organism. Vancomycin (3 μg/ml) is added to the medium to inhibit contaminating bacteria. Many formulations with the GC agar base, the enrichments, and vancomycin exist.

■ VMGA III medium

VMGA III (viability medium, Göteborg, anaerobic) is a transport and collection medium specifically designed to maintain viability of mixed anaerobes from peridontal and endodontal sites. The medium is particularly useful for transport of paper points that are placed in gingival crevices to soak up secretions. A total of 0.5 to 2.0 ml of prereduced, buffered salt suspension is placed into a tube of similar total volume (2 ml) with or without six to eight glass beads (0.1 to 1.5 mm in diameter). The beads aid in dispersing polysaccharide matrices that occur within gingival plaques and granular aggregates (39).

■ Wadowsky-Yee medium

See Buffered charcoal yeast extract (BCYE).

■ Wilkins-Chalgren broth and agar

Wilkins-Chalgren medium is recommended for susceptibility testing with anaerobic organisms. The medium contains specific nutrients that support the growth of anaerobes such as yeast extract, vitamin K, hemin, and arginine. The use of peptones allows a more standardized medium.

■ Xylose-lysine-desoxycholate agar

Xylose-lysine-desoxycholate agar is a selective and differential medium used for the isolation and differentiation of enteric pathogens from clinical specimens. The nutritive base includes carbohydrates and yeast extract. This medium is more supportive of fastidious enteric organisms such as *Shigella*. The selective agent is desoxycholate, which inhibits gram-positive organisms. Phenol red is the color indicator. As with Hektoen enteric and salmonella-shigella agars, ferric ammonium citrate (indicator) and sodium thiosulfate (sulfur source) allow identification of organisms that produce H_2S with the appearance of colonies with a black center. The medium contains xylose, which most enteric organisms ferment. The most important exception is *Shigella*, the colonies of which appear to be transparent or the color of the red media. The enteric organisms that contain the lysine decarboxylase enzyme utilize the lysine in the medium. For *Salmonella*, which contains the lysine enzyme, this reaction reverts the pH to an alkaline state and the colony appears to be transparent or red with a black center. The lactose and sucrose in the medium help to differentiate other enteric organisms. When other enteric organisms ferment these sugars, they maintain the pH at an acidic condition and the colonies appear yellow or yellow-red. A number of other similar media for isolation of enteric pathogens exist, including xylose-galactosidase medium, which is more specific for *Aeromonas* spp. See chapters 43 and 46, which give specific references for performance of the various xylose-containing media.

■ Yersinia selective agar

See Cefsulodin-Irgasan-novobiocin medium.

APPENDIX 1
Medium Additives

N-(2-Acetamido)-2-aminoethanesulfonic acid (ACES): allows optimal pH buffering capacity without inhibition of bacteria as seen with other inorganic buffers

Acriflavine: selective agent; suppresses gram-positive organisms

ADC enrichment: a supplement added to mycobacteriology media that includes albumin, dextrose, catalase, and sodium chloride; catalase destroys peroxides that may be in the medium

Agar used in broth medium (0.05 to 0.1%): used to reduce O_2 tension

Albumin: protects against toxic by-products in medium; binds free fatty acids

Antibiotics: one or many may be added to make a medium selective; inhibitory capacity may vary depending on the concentration used

Bicarbonate-citric acid pellet: used to generate CO_2 gas within closed environment after exposure to moistures; used in transport devices for isolating *Neisseria gonorrhoeae*

Bismuth sulfite: heavy metal that is inhibitory to commensal organisms

Carbohydrates: energy source; used to make medium differential when combined with an indicator

Cetrimide: acts as a quaternary ammonium cationic detergent that causes nitrogen and phosphorus to be released from bacterial cells other than *Pseudomonas aeruginosa*

Charcoal: detoxifying agent, surface tension modifier, scavenger of radicals and peroxides

Cornstarch: works as a detoxifying agent; may provide additional nutrients as an energy source

Dent's supplement (Oxoid): vancomycin, trimethoprim, cefsulodin, and amphotericin B added to Columbia blood agar and laked horse blood for isolation of *Helicobacter*

Dextrose: makes the medium hypertonic; energy source

Egg yolk: used to demonstrate lecithinase, lipase, and proteolytic activities and fatty acids

Ferric ammonium citrate: iron salt used in combination with other agents (esculin, sodium thiosulfate) to make medium differential by producing a black precipitate

Fildes enrichment: peptic digest of sheep blood that provides a rich source of nutrients, including X (hemin) and V (NAD) factors; X originally stood for unknown and V originally stood for vitamin

Glycerol: a purified alcohol and an abundant source of carbon; used in culture, transport, and storage medium and reagent preparation

Glycine: a selective agent that is inhibitory to organisms

Horse serum: an enrichment used in growth media for such organisms as *Mycoplasma* and *Ureaplasma*

IsoVitaleX (BBL): provides V factor (NAD) and additional nutritive ingredients, such as vitamins, amino acids, ferric ion, and dextrose, to stimulate growth of fastidious organisms

Laked blood or laked horse blood: created by freeze-thaw cycles of blood; enhances pigment production of anaerobes and used in susceptibility testing of fastidious organisms

Lithium chloride: a selective agent that inhibits organisms

Malachite green: a dye that partially inhibits bacteria

NAD (V factor): necessary for growth of some fastidious organisms

OADC enrichment: a supplement added to mycobacteriology media that includes oleic acid, albumin, dextrose, catalase, and sodium chloride; the oleic acid provides fatty acids utilized by mycobacteria, and the catalase destroys peroxides that may be in the medium

Oxgall (bile): inhibits specific organisms; allows medium to be selective

Peptones: carbohydrate-free source of nutrients

Phenylethyl alcohol: reversibly inhibits DNA synthesis; results in inhibition of facultative anaerobic gram-negative organisms

Pyridoxal: liquid supplement added to media for isolation of fastidious organisms; also comes in the form of a disk to be used in satelliting tests

Rabbit blood: enhances pigment production of anaerobes; hemolytic reactions of streptococci are "correct"; additive to heart infusion agar for isolation of *Bartonella* spp.

Serum: albumin, fatty acids

Sheep blood and human blood: provide hemin and other nutrients; allow true hemolytic reactions of streptococci; NADase enzyme inactivates the NAD in the sheep blood and is not available for organisms

Skirrow's supplement: vancomycin, trimethoprim, and polymyxin B added to Columbia agar and laked horse blood for isolation of *Helicobacter*

Sodium azide: a selective agent that inhibits gram-negative organisms

Sodium bicarbonate: neutralization agent used with gastric wash or lavage specimens for recovery of acid-fast organisms
Sodium bisulfite: disinfectant, antioxidant, or reducing agent
Sodium chloride: maintains osmotic equilibrium; when added at a high concentration it may be a selective agent
Sodium citrate: a selective agent inhibitory to organisms
Sodium desoxycholate: a salt of bile acid and a selective agent that inhibits gram-positive and spore-forming organisms
Sodium polyanetholesulfonate (SPS): a polyanionic anticoagulant that inactivates aminoglycosides and interferes with the complement cascade, lysozyme activity, and phagocytic activity inherent in blood. May be inhibitory to *Neisseria, Gardnerella, Streptobacillus, Peptostreptococcus, Francisella,* and *Moraxella* spp.
Sodium pyruvate: growth stimulant
Sodium selenite: a selective agent that inhibits coliforms
Sodium thioglycolate: a reducing agent
Starch: a polysaccharide and detoxifying agent incorporated into some media as a differential agent
Tellurite: is toxic to egg-clearing strains of bacteria; imparts black color to colony
Tween 80 (polysorbate 80): an oleic acid ester that stimulates growth and provides fatty acids as well as acts as a dispersal agent
Vitamin K: ingredient required for optimal growth of certain obligate anaerobes, such as the *Bacteroides* group
Vitox (Oxoid): provides V factor (NAD) and other essential growth factors to stimulate growth of fastidious organisms; see IsoVitaleX.
Yeast extract: water-soluble product that provides B vitamins and protein

APPENDIX 2
Product Suppliers and Manufacturers of Reagents, Stains, Microscopes, and Media

1. American Type Culture Collection
   P.O. Box 1549
   Manassas, VA 20108
   http://www.atcc.org
2. AdvanDx, Incorporated
   10A Roessler Road
   Woburn, MA 01801
   http://www.advandx.com
3. Anaerobe Systems
   15906 Concord Circle
   Morgan Hill, CA 95037
   http://www.anaerobesystems.com
4. Applied Biosystems
   850 Lincoln Centre Drive
   Foster City, CA 94404
   http://www.appliedbiosystems.com
5. BBL/Difco (see BD Biosciences)
6. BD Diagnostic Systems
   7 Loveton Circle
   Sparks, MD 21152
   http://www.bd.com/ds
7. BD Biosciences
   1 Becton Drive
   Franklin Lakes, NJ 07417
   and
   2350 Qume Drive
   San Jose, CA 95131
   http://www.bdbiosciences.com
8. BioMed Diagnostics Inc.
   1388 Antelope Road
   White City, OR 97503-1619
   http://www.biomed1.com
9. Carl Zeiss, Microimaging, Incorporated
   1 Zeiss Drive
   Thorwood, NY 10594
   http://www.zeiss.com/micro
10. Chromager
    4, place du 18 Juin 1940
    Paris, F-75006
    France
    http://www.chromager.com
11. Copan Diagnostics, Incorporated
    2175 Sampson Avenue, Suite 124
    Corona, CA 92879
    http://www.copanusa.com
12. Fisher Scientific International Inc.
    Liberty Lane
    Hampton, NH 03842
    http://www.fisherscientific.com
13. Hardy Diagnostics
    1430 West McCoy Lane
    Santa Monica, CA 93455
    http://www.hardydiagnostics.com
14. Heipha Diagnostica Biotest
    Lilienthalstrasse 16
    D-69214 Eppelheim
    Germany
    http://www.heipha.de
15. Intergen Company
    2 Manhattanville Road
    Purchase, NY 10577
    http://www.intergenco.com
16. Invitrogen (Gibco)
    1600 Faraday Avenue
    P.O. Box 6482
    Carlsbad, CA 92008
    http://www.invitrogen.com
17. Irvine Scientific
    2511 Daimler Street
    Santa Ana, CA 92705-5588
    http://www.nucleus@irvinesci.com
18. Key Scientific Products
    1402 Chisholm Trail
    Round Rock, TX 78681
    http://www.keyscientific.com
19. Marcor Development Corporation
    341 Michele Place
    Carlstadt, NJ 07072-2304
    http://www.marcordev.com
20. Medical Chemical Corporation
    19430 Van Ness Avenue
    Torrance, CA 90501
    http://www.med-chem.com
21. Medical Packaging Corporation
    941 Avenido Acaso
    Camarillo, CA 93012
    http://www.devicelink.com
22. Medical Wire & Equipment-MWE
    29 Leafield Way
    Corsham
    Wiltshire
    SN13 9RT
    United Kingdom
    http://www.mwe.co.uk
23. Nikon Instruments, Incorporated
    1300 Walt Whitman Road
    Melville, NY 11747
    http://www.nikonusa.com
24. Northeast Laboratory Services
    Rt. 137 China Rd.
    Winslow, ME 04901
    http://www.nelabservices.com
25. Olympus America, Incorporated
    2 Corporate Center Drive
    Melville, NY 11747
    http://www.olympusamerica.com
26. Oxoid Limited (Remel distributor in the United States)
    Wade Road
    Basingstoke
    Hampshire

RG24 8PW
United Kingdom
http://www.oxoid.com

27. PML Microbiologicals
27120 SW 95th Avenue
Wilsonville, OR 97070
http://www.pmlmicro.com
28. Remel, Incorporated
12076 Santa Fe Drive
Lenexa, KS 66215
http://www.remelinc.com
29. Sigma-Aldrich Company
P.O. Box 14508
St. Louis, MO 63178
http://www.sigma-aldrich.com
30. Starplex Scientific, Incorporated
50A Steinway Boulevard
Etobicoke, Ontario M9W 6Y3
Canada
http://www.starplexscientific.com
31. Wampole Laboratories
Half Acre Road
Cranbury, NJ 0851

REFERENCES

1. **Ash, L., and T. Orihel.** 1997. *Atlas of Human Parasitology*, 4th ed. American Society of Clinical Pathologists, Chicago, Ill.
2. **Ashdown, L. R.** 1979. An improved screening technique for isolation of Pseudomonas pseudomallei from clinical specimens. *Pathology* **11:**293–297.
3. **Atkins, K. N.** 1920. Report of committee on descriptive chart. Part III. A modification of the Gram stain. *J. Bacteriol.* **5:**321–324.
4. **Atlas, R. M., and L. C. Parks.** 1997. *Microbiological Media.* CRC Press, Inc., Boca Raton, Fla.
5. **Atlas, R. M., and J. W. Snyder.** 1995. *Handbook of Media for Clinical Microbiology*, 2nd ed. CRC Press, Inc., Boca Raton, Fla.
6. **Balows, A., and W. Hausler.** 1988. *Diagnostic Procedures for Bacterial, Mycotic and Parasitic Infection*, 7th ed. American Public Health Association, Washington, D.C.
7. **Balows, A., W. J. Hausler, Jr., K. L. Herrmann, H. D. Isenberg, and H. J. Shadomy (ed.).** 1991. *Manual of Clinical Microbiology*, 5th ed. American Society for Microbiology, Washington, D.C.
8. **Baselski, V. S., M. K. Robison, L. W. Pifer, and D. R. Woods.** 1990. Rapid detection of *Pneumocystis cariniii* in bronchoalveolar lavage samples by using calcofluor staining. *J. Clin. Microbiol.* **28:**393–394.
9. **BD Biosciences.** 2005. *The Difco and BBL Manual.* BD Biosciences, Sparks, Md.
10. **Chapin-Robertson, K., S. E. Dahlberg, and S. C. Edberg.** 1992. Clinical and laboratory analyses of cytospin-prepared Gram stains for recovery and diagnosis of bacteria from sterile body fluids. *J. Clin. Microbiol.* **30:**377–380.
11. **Clinical and Laboratory Standards Institute.** 2002. *Abbreviated Identification of Bacteria and Yeast.* Approved guideline M35-A. Clinical and Laboratory Standards Institute, Wayne, Pa.
12. **Clinical and Laboratory Standards Institute.** 2004. *Methods for Antimicrobial Susceptibility Testing of Anaerobic Bacteria.* Approved standard, 6th ed. M11-A6. Clinical and Laboratory Standards Institute, Wayne, Pa.
13. **Clinical and Laboratory Standards Institute.** 2004. *Quality Assurance for Commercially Prepared Microbiological Culture Media.* Standard M22-A3. Clinical and Laboratory Standards Institute, Wayne, Pa.
14. **Curis, G. D. W., R. Mitchell, A. F. King, and E. J. Griffin.** 1989. A selective differential medium for the isolation of *Listeria monocytogenes*. *Lett. Appl. Microbiol.* **8:**95–98.
15. **Daly, J. A., W. M. Gooch III, and J. M. Matsen.** 1985. Evaluation of the Wayson variation of a methylene blue staining procedure for the detection of microorganisms in cerebrospinal fluid. *J. Clin. Microbiol.* **21:**919–921.
16. **deMan, J. C., M. Rogosa, and M. E. Sharpe.** 1960. A medium for the cultivation of lactobacilli. *J. Appl. Bacteriol.* **23:**130–135.
17. **Diederen, B. M. W., M. van Leest, I. Van Duijn, P. Willemse, P. H. J. van Keulen, and J. A. J. Kluytmans.** 2006. Performance of MRSA ID, a new chromogenic medium for detection of methicillin-resistant *Staphylococcus aureus*. *J. Clin. Microbiol.* **44:**586–588.
18. **Difco Laboratories.** 1985. Dehydrated culture media and reagents for microbiology, p. 9–25. *In The Difco Manual*, 10th ed. Difco Laboratories, Detroit, Mich.
19. **Difco Laboratories.** 1998. *The Difco Manual*, 11th ed. Difco Laboratories, Division of Becton Dickinson, Sparks, Md.
20. **Doern, G. V., and R. N. Jones.** 1991. Antimicrobial susceptibility test: fastidious and unusual bacteria, p. 1130. *In* A. Balows, W. J. Hausler, Jr., K. L. Herrmann, H. D. Isenberg, and H. J. Shadomy (ed.), *Manual of Clinical Microbiology*, 5th ed. American Society for Microbiology, Washington, D.C.
21. **Ellinghausen, H. C.** 1960. Some observations on cultural and biochemical characteristics of *Leptospira pomona*. *J. Infect. Dis.* **106:**237–244.
22. **Elsayed, S., D. Gregson, and D. Church.** 2003. Comparison of direct selective versus nonselective agar media plus LIM broth enrichment for determination of Group B Streptococcus colonization status in pregnant women. *Arch. Pathol. Lab. Med.* **127:**718–720.
23. **Emmons, C., C. Binford, K. J. Kwon-Chung, and J. Utz.** 1977. *Medical Mycology*, 3rd ed. Lea & Febiger, Philadelphia, Pa.
24. **Engelkirk, P. G., J. Duben-Engelkirk, and V. R. Dowell.** 1992. *Principles and Practice of Clinical Anaerobic Bacteriology.* Star Publishing Co., Belmont, Calif.
25. **Ewing, W. H.** 1986. *Edwards and Ewing's Identification of* Enterobacteriaceae, 4th ed. Elsevier, New York, N.Y.
26. **Faller, A., and K.-H. Schleifer.** 1981. Modified oxidase and benzidine tests for separation of staphylococci from micrococci. *J. Clin. Microbiol.* **13:**1031–1035.
27. **Fisher, J. F., M. Ganapathy, B. H. Edwards, and C. L. Newman.** 1990. Utility of Gram's and Giemsa stains in the diagnosis of pulmonary tuberculosis. *Am. Rev. Respir. Dis.* **141:**511–513.
28. **Forbes, B. A., D. F. Sahm, and A. S. Weissfeld.** 1998. Role of microscopy in the diagnosis of infectious disease, p. 134–149. *In Bailey and Scott's Diagnostic Microbiology*, 10th ed. Mosby, Inc., St. Louis, Mo.
29. **Gill, V. J., N. A. Nelson, F. Stock, and G. Evans.** 1988. Optimal use of the cytocentrifuge for recovery and diagnosis of *Pneumocystis jiroveci* in bronchoalveolar lavage and sputum specimens. *J. Clin. Microbiol.* **26:**1641–1644.
30. **Gilligan, P. H., P. A. Gage, L. M. Bradshaw, D. V. Schidlow, and B. T. DeCicco.** 1985. Isolation medium for the recovery of *Pseudomonas cepacia* from respiratory secretions of patients with cystic fibrosis. *J. Clin. Microbiol.* **22:**5–8.
31. **Groden, L. R., J. Rodnite, J. H. Brinser, and G. I. Genvert.** 1990. Acridine orange and Gram stains in infectious keratitis. *Cornea* **9:**122–124.
32. **Heelan, J. S., J. Struminsky, P. Lauro, and C. J. Sung.** 2005. Evaluation of a new selective enrichment broth for detection of group B streptococci in pregnant women. *J. Clin. Microbiol.* **43:**896–897.
33. **Heineman, H. S., J. K. Chawla, and W. M. Lofton.** 1977. Misinformation from sputum cultures without microscopic examination. *J. Clin. Microbiol.* **6:**518–527.
34. **Henrickson, K. J., K. R. Powell, and D. H. Ryan.** 1988. Evaluation of acridine orange-stained buffy coat smears for

identification of bacteremia in children. *J. Pediatr.* **112:**65–86.
35. **Henry, D., M. Campbell, C. McGimpsey, A. L. Clarke, L. Louden, J. L. Burns, M. H. Roe, P. Vandamme, and D. Speert.** 1999. Comparison of isolation media for recovery of *Burkholderia cepacia* complex from respiratory secretions of patients with cystic fibrosis. *J. Clin. Microbiol.* **37:**1004–1007.
36. **Hutchinson, D. N., and F. J. Bolton.** 1984. Improved blood free selective medium for the isolation of Campylobacter jejuni from faecal specimens. *J. Clin. Pathol.* **37:**956–957.
37. **Ian, S. W., R. Flamm, C. Y. Hachem, H. Y. Kim, J. E. Clarridge, D. G. Evans, J. Beyer, J. Drnec, and D. Y. Graham.** 1995. Transport and storage of *Helicobacter pylori* from gastric mucosal biopsies and clinical isolates. *Eur. J. Clin. Microbiol. Infect. Dis.* **14:**349–352.
38. **Isenberg, H. D. (ed.).** 2004. *Clinical Microbiology Procedures Handbook,* 2nd ed. American Society for Microbiology, Washington, D.C.
39. **Jousimies-Somer, H., P. E. Summanen, D. M. Citron, E. J. Baron, H. M. Wexler, and S. M. Finegold.** 2002. *Wadsworth Anaerobic Bacteriology Manual,* 6th ed. Star Publishing Co., Belmont, Calif.
40. **Kent, P. T., and G. P. Kubica.** 1985. *Public Health Mycobacteriology—a Guide for the Level III Laboratory.* Centers for Disease Control, Atlanta, Ga.
41. **Kiernan, J. A.** 1999. *Histological and Histochemical Methods: Theory and Practice,* 3rd ed. Butterworth-Heineman Medical, Elsevier Publishers, Philadelphia, Pa.
42. **Kirby, R., and K. L. Ruoff.** 1995. Cost-effective, clinically relevant method for rapid identification of beta-hemolytic streptococci and enterococci. *J. Clin. Microbiol.* **33:** 1154–1157.
43. **Knisely, R. F.** 1966. Selective medium for *Bacillus anthracis. J. Bacteriol.* **92:**784–786.
44. **Kronvall, G., and E. Myhre.** 1979. Differential staining of bacteria in clinical specimens using acridine orange, buffered at low pH. *Acta Pathol. Microbiol. Scand. Sect. B* **85:**249–254.
45. **Lauer, B. A., L. B. Reller, and S. Mirrett.** 1981. Comparison of acridine orange and Gram stains for detection of microorganisms in cerebrospinal fluid and other clinical specimens. *J. Clin. Microbiol.* **14:**201–205.
46. **Lee, W. H., and D. McClain.** 1986. Improved *Listeria monocytogenes* selective agar. *Appl. Environ. Microbiol.* **52:**1215–1217.
47. **Lillie, R. D.** 1977. The general nature of dyes and their classification, p. 19–39. *In* E. H. Stotz and V. M. Emmel (ed.), *H. J. Conn's Biological Stains,* 9th ed. The Williams & Wilkins Co., Baltimore, Md.
48. **Luna, J. G. 1968.** *Manual of Histologic Staining Methods of the Armed Forces Institute of Pathology,* 3rd ed., p. 102. McGraw-Hill, New York, N.Y.
49. **MacFaddin, J. F.** 2000. *Biochemical Tests for Identification of Medical Bacteria,* 3rd ed. Lippincott Williams & Wilkins, Philadelphia, Pa.
50. **Manafi, M., and W. Kneifel.** 1990. Rapid methods for differentiating gram-positive from gram-negative aerobic and facultative anaerobic bacteria. *J. Appl. Bacteriol.* **69:**822–827.
51. **Mangels, J. I., M. E. Cox, and L. H. Lindberg.** 1984. Methanol fixation: an alternative to heat fixation of smears before staining. *Diagn. Microbiol. Infect. Dis.* **2:**129.
51a. **McClung, L. S., and R. Toabe.** 1947. The egg yolk plate reaction for the presumptive diagnosis of Clostridium sporogenes and certain species of the gangrene and botulinum groups. *J. Bacteriol.* **53:**139–147.
52. **Mirrett, S., B. A. Lauer, G. A. Miller, and L. B. Rfeller.** 1982. Comparison of acridine orange, methylene blue, and Gram stains for blood cultures. *J. Clin. Microbiol.* **15:**562–566.
53. **Morse, S.** 1989. Chancroid and *Haemophilus ducreyi. Clin. Microbiol. Rev.* **2:**137–157.
54. **Murray, P. R., and J. A. Washington II.** 1975. Microscopic and bacteriologic analysis of expectorated sputum. *Mayo Clin. Proc.* **50:**339–344.
55. **Nugent, P. P., N. A. Krohn, and S. L. Hillier.** 1991. Reliability of diagnosing bacterial vaginosis is improved by a standardized method of Gram stain interpretation. *J. Clin. Microbiol.* **29:**297–301.
56. **Oberhofer, T. R.** 1986. Value of the L-pyrrolidonyl-α-naphthylamide hydrolysis test for identification of select Gram-positive cocci. *Diagn. Microbiol. Infect. Dis.* **4:**43–47.
57. **O'Brien, K. L., M. A. Bronsdon, R. Dagan, P. Yagupsky, J. Janco, J. Elliott, C. G. Whitney, Y.-H. Yang, L. E. Robinson, B. Schwartz, and G. M. Carlone.** 2001. Evaluation of a medium (STGG) for transport and optimal recovery of *Streptococcus pneumoniae* from nasopharyngeal secretions collected during field studies. *J. Clin. Microbiol.* **39:**1020–1024.
58. **Paradis, I. L., C. Ross, A. Dekker, and J. Dauber.** 1990. A comparison of modified methenamine silver and toluidine blue stains for the detection of *Pneumocystis carinii* in bronchoalveolar lavage specimens from immunosuppressed patients. *Acta Cytol.* **34:**511–518.
59. **Pollack, R. J., S. R. Telford III, and A. Spielman.** 1993. Standardization of medium for culturing Lyme disease spirochetes. *J. Clin. Microbiol.* **31:**1251–1255.
60. **Power, D. A., and P. J. McCuen.** 1988. *Manual of BBL Products and Laboratory Procedures,* 6th ed. Becton Dickinson Microbiology Systems, Cockeysville, Md.
61. **Rose, R. A.** 1982. Light microscopy, p. 1–19. *In* J. D. Bancroft and A. Stevens (ed.), *Theory and Practice of Histological Techniques,* 2nd ed. Churchill Livingstone, New York, N.Y.
62. **Shanholtzer, C. J., P. J. Schaper, and L. R. Peterson.** 1982. Concentrated Gram stain smears prepared with a cytospin centrifuge. *J. Clin. Microbiol.* **16:**1052–1056.
63. **Sharp, S. E., A. Robinson, M. Saubolle, M. Santa Cruz, K. Carroll, and V. Baselski.** 2004. *Cumitech 7B, Lower Respiratory Tract Infections.* Coordinating ed., S. E. Sharp. ASM Press, Washington, D.C.
64. **Stoakes, L., R. Reyes, J. Daniel, G. Lennox, M. A. John, R. Lannigan, and Z. Hussain.** 2006. Prospective comparison of a new chromogen medium, MRSASelect, to CHROMagar MRSA and mannitol-salt medium supplemented with oxacillin or cefoxitin for detection of methicillin-resistant *Staphylococcus aureus. J. Clin. Microbiol.* **44:**637–639.
65. **Strumpf, I. J., A. Y. Tsang, M. A. Schork, and J. G. Weg.** 1976. The reliability of gastric smears by auramine-rhodamine staining technique for the diagnosis of tuberculosis. *Am. Rev. Respir. Dis.* **114:**971–976.
66. **Thompson, S. W.** 1960. *Selected Histochemical and Histopathological Methods.* Charles C Thomas, Springfield, Ill.
67. **Van Netten, P., I. Perales, A. van de Moosdijk, D. W. Curtis, and D. A. A. Mossel.** 1989. Liquid and solid differentiation media for enumeration of *L. moncytogenes* and other *Listeria* spp. *J. Food Microbiol.* **8:**299–316.
68. **Walsh, A. L., V. Wuthiekanun, M. D. Smith, Y. Supputtamongkol, and N. J. White.** 1995. Selective broths for the isolation of *Pseudomonas pseudomallei* from clinical samples. *Trans. R. Soc. Trop. Med. Hyg.* **89:**124.
69. **Welch, D. F., M. J. Muszynski, H. P. Chik, M. J. Marcon, M. M. Hribar, P. H. Gilligan, J. M. Matsen, P. A. Ahlin, B. C. Hilman, and S. A. Chartrand.** 1987. Selective and differential medium for recovery of *Pseudomonas cepacia* from the respiratory tracts of patients with cystic fibrosis. *J. Clin. Microbiol.* **25:**1730–1734.
70. **Weyant, R. S., C. W. Moss, R. E. Weaver, D. G. Hollis, J. G. Jordan, E. C. Cook, and M. I. Daneshvar.** 1995. *Identification of Unusual Pathogenic Gram-Negative Aerobic and Facultative Anaerobic Bacteria,* 2nd ed. The Williams & Wilkins Co., Baltimore, Md.

Algorithm for Identification of Aerobic Gram-Positive Cocci

KATHRYN L. RUOFF

22

Most gram-positive cocci recovered from aerobic cultures can be differentiated with the tests shown in Tables 1 and 2. These organisms include "aerotolerant anaerobes," facultative anaerobes, microaerophiles, and obligate aerobes. The genera display various colony morphologies and hemolytic and catalase reactions (Tables 1 and 2). Their cellular morphologies as revealed by Gram staining of broth cultures are generally either streptococcal, in which gram-positive cocci or coccobacilli are arranged in pairs and/or chains, or staphylococcal, in which cells appear as cocci arranged in pairs, tetrads, clusters, and irregular groups. No taxonomic kinship is implied by division of these bacteria into two groups based on cellular morphology. As new genera and species are described and characterized, it becomes increasingly difficult to identify some of the less frequently isolated organisms solely on the basis of phenotypic traits. The reader is referred to the chapters noted in the tables for more detailed descriptions of these organisms.

TABLE 1 Characteristics of catalase-negative gram-positive cocci that grow aerobically and form cells arranged in pairs and chains[a]

PYR	LAP	6.5% NaCl	BE	Motility	45°C	Probe	HIP	Satellitism	10°C	Vancomycin resistance	Organism(s) (chapter)
+	+	+	+	+	+						*Enterococcus* (30)
					−						*Vagococcus* (31)
				−		+					*Enterococcus* (30)
						−					*Lactococcus* (31)
			−				+	−			*Facklamia* spp.[b] (31)
							−	V			*Ignavigranum* (31)
		−	+	+							*Vagococcus* (31)
				−							*Lactococcus* (31)
			−					+			*Abiotrophia*, *Granulicatella* (31)
								−			*Gemella* spp.[c] (31)
	−	+									*Globicatella* (31)
		−									*Dolosicoccus* (31)
−	−									+	*Leuconostoc*[d] (31)
										−	*Globicatella* (31)
	+								+		*Lactococcus* (31)
									−		*Streptococcus*[e] (29)

[a] See chapters 21 and 29 to 31 for descriptions of the methods for performing the tests referred to in this table. Reactions shown are typical, but exceptions may occur. Abbreviations, terms, and symbols: PYR, production of pyrrolidonyl arylamidase; LAP, production of leucine aminopeptidase; 6.5% NaCl, growth in 6.5% NaCl; BE, hydrolysis of esculin in the presence of 40% bile; 45°C, growth at 45°C; probe, reaction with commercially available nucleic acid probe for the genus *Enterococcus*; HIP, hydrolysis of hippurate; satellitism, satelliting growth behavior; 10°C, growth at 10°C; +, most strains positive; −, most strains negative; V, variable reactions are observed.

[b] The reactions listed in this table are typical for *F. hominis*, *F. sourekii*, and *F. ignava*. *F. languida* cells tend to be arranged in clusters, and isolates are hippurate hydrolysis negative (Table 2).

[c] *G. morbillorum*, *G. bergeri*, and *G. sanguinis* cells tend to be arranged in pairs and chains, in contrast to the cells of *G. haemolysans*, which are arranged in pairs, tetrads, and clusters (Table 2).

[d] *Leuconostoc* is distinguished from the other catalase-negative organisms in Table 1 by its ability to produce gas as an end product of glucose metabolism and by its intrinsic resistance to vancomycin. The phenotypically similar genus *Weissella* contains organisms formerly classified as leuconostocs and the species formerly named *Lactobacillus confusus* (see chapter 31).

[e] Most streptococci are PYR negative, with the exception of *S. pyogenes* isolates and some strains of *S. pneumoniae*, which are PYR positive.

TABLE 2 Differentiating features of gram-positive cocci that grow aerobically and form cells arranged in clusters or irregular groups[a]

Catalase	Obligate aerobe	Oxidase	PYR	LAP	NaCl	ESC	Hemolysis	Vancomycin resistance	BGUR	Organism (chapter)
+	+	+			+[b]					*Micrococcus* (28)
		−			+[c]					*Alloiococcus* (28)
	−	−			+[b]					*Staphylococcus* (28)
					−[b]					*Rothia mucilaginosa*[d] (28, 34)
−	−		+	+	+[c]	+			−	*Dolosigranulum* (31)
									+	*Aerococcus sanguinicola* (31)
						−			−	*Facklamia languida*[e] (31)
					−[c]	+				*Rothia mucilaginosa*[d] (28, 34)
						−				*Gemella haemolysans*[f] (31)
				−			α			*Aerococcus viridans*[g] (31)
							γ			*Helcococcus kunzii*[g] (31)
			−	+				R		*Pediococcus*[h] (31)
								S	+	*Aerococcus urinae* (31)
				−					+	*Aerococcus urinaehominis* (31)
									−	*Aerococcus christensenii* (31)

[a] See chapters 21, 28, and 31 for descriptions of methods for performing the phenotypic tests referred to in this table. Reactions shown are typical; exceptions may occur. Abbreviations and symbols: PYR, production of pyrrolidonyl arylamidase; LAP, production of leucine aminopeptidase; NaCl, growth in the presence of either 5 or 6.5% NaCl (see footnotes *b* and *c*); ESC, esculin hydrolysis; BGUR, production of β-glucuronidase; +, most strains positive; −, most strains negative; V, variable reactions are observed; α, alpha-hemolysis on sheep blood agar; γ, nonhemolytic reaction on sheep blood agar; S, susceptible; R, resistant.

[b] Growth in the presence of 5% sodium chloride.

[c] Growth in the presence of 6.5% sodium chloride.

[d] *R. mucilaginosa* isolates are usually catalase negative or weakly positive but may be strongly catalase positive.

[e] *Ignavigranum ruoffiae* (Table 1) exhibits reactions identical to those of *F. languida* in the PYR, ESC, and NaCl tests. However, *I. ruoffiae* cells are arranged primarily in chains and *F. languida* cells usually form clusters. Other *Facklamia* species form cells arranged in pairs and chains (Table 1).

[f] *G. haemolysans* cells tend to be arranged in pairs, tetrads, and groups, in contrast to the cells of other *Gemella* species, which usually occur in pairs and short chains (Table 1).

[g] *H. kunzii* strains form tiny, pinpoint, nonhemolytic colonies on blood agar after 24 h of aerobic incubation at 35°C, and *A. viridans* isolates form larger, alpha-hemolytic colonies under similar incubation conditions. In contrast to *H. kunzii, A. viridans* prefers aerobic incubation atmospheres. Two additional species of *Helcococcus* isolated from human sources have been described, each based on a single isolate. In contrast to *H. kunzii*, the new species *H. sueciensis* and the proposed species "*H. pyogenes*" are PYR negative (see chapter 31).

[h] The genera *Pediococcus* and *Tetragenococcus* have similar phenotypic characteristics, except that tetragenococci are vancomycin susceptible. The bile esculin test can differentiate between tetragenococci (positive) and *Aerococcus urinae* (negative); see chapter 31.

Algorithm for Identification of Aerobic Gram-Positive Rods

GUIDO FUNKE

23

The aim of the algorithm for the identification of aerobic gram-positive rods described in this chapter is simply to guide the reader to the appropriate chapter of this Manual for further information. The algorithm emphasizes that Gram stain (performed on 24- to 48-h-old colonies from rich media) and macroscopic morphologies are the initial key features for the differentiation of aerobic gram-positive rods. All strains of aerobic gram-positive rods (except the non-rapidly growing mycobacteria) are initially grown on blood agar plates.

Regular rods are organisms with cells whose longitudinal edges are usually not curved but are parallel. If spore formation is not observed initially, it can be tested for on a nutritionally depleted medium. Catalase activity should be tested with colonies from media lacking heme groups. The type of metabolism can be checked in oxidative-fermentative media or in cystine Trypticase agar medium. Irregular rods are organisms with cells whose longitudinal edges are curved and not parallel. Diagnostic end products of glucose metabolism are detected by chromatographic methods. Slight beta-hemolysis is best observed when cells are incubated in a CO_2-enriched atmosphere. Yellow- or orange-pigmented colonies are always composed of irregular rods. Some genera that stain partially acid-fast (e.g., *Gordonia* and *Rhodococcus*) may also show a yellow-orange pigment. Rods exhibiting vegetative substrate filaments may show branched hyphae, which either form spores or reproduce by fragmentation. It is obvious that vegetative substrate filaments might not be present initially (i.e., within 48 h), and so these organisms are prone to initial misidentification.

For the yellow-orange genera (e.g., *Microbacterium*, *Curtobacterium*, and *Leifsonia*), as well as the rods exhibiting vegetative substrate filaments, chemotaxonomic methods must very often be used for definitive identification to the genus level; for example, partially acid-fast bacteria can be identified to the genus level by analysis of mycolic acids.

Genera which contain strict anaerobic gram-positive rods may also contain aerobically growing species. This is particularly true for the genus *Actinomyces* (as it is presently defined). *Clostridium tertium* (a strong gas producer) may also grow aerobically. Furthermore, some aerobic gram-positive cocci (e.g., *Leuconostoc* spp. or *Streptococcus mutans*) might initially be misidentified as gram-positive rods because of their initial Gram stain appearance. Likewise, but less frequently, some gram-positive rods (e.g., *Rhodococcus* spp.) might be initially misidentified as gram-positive cocci because of their initial Gram stain appearance.

This algorithm should serve only as the basis of a preliminary identification of an unknown aerobic gram-positive rod, and the reader is referred to the chapters given in Table 1 for further information.

TABLE 1 Algorithm for identification of aerobic gram-positive rods

Cellular morphology	Yellow-orange pigment	Vegetative substrate filaments	Spore formation	Catalase	Metabolism[a]	H_2S in TSI	Other unusual Gram stain feature	Diagnostic end product of glucose metabolism[b]	Slight beta-hemolysis	Slow acid production	Acid-fast stain	Partially acid-fast stain	Aerial vegetative filaments	Motility	Growth at 50°C	Organism (chapter)
Regular			+													*Bacillus*, including *Paeni-*, *Brevi-*, *Aneurini-*, and *Virgibacillus* (32)
			−	+	O											*Kurthia*
					F											*Listeria* (33)
				−		+										*Erysipelothrix* (33)
						−										*Lactobacillus* (56)
Irregular	−			+			Club-shaped rods									*Corynebacterium* (34)
							Slim, long rods									*Turicella* (34)
							Very coccoid rods									*Dermabacter* (34)
							May show jointed rods									*Arthrobacter* (34)
							May show short rods									*Brevibacterium* (34)
							May show branching									*Actinomyces* (56), *Propionibacterium* (56), *Rothia* (28, 34)
				−			Coccoid rods, Gram variable									*Gardnerella* (34)
								S	+ −							*Arcanobacterium* (34) *Actinomyces* (56)
								A								*Bifidobacterium* (56)
								L								*Rothia* (28, 34)
	+	+														*Oerskovia*, *Cellulosimicrobium* (both 34)

(*Continued on next page*)

TABLE 1 Algorithm for identification of aerobic gram-positive rods (*Continued*)

Cellular morphology	Yellow-orange pigment	Vegetative substrate filaments	Spore formation	Catalase	Metabolism[a]	H_2S in TSI	Other unusual Gram stain feature	Diagnostic end product of glucose metabolism[b]	Slight beta-hemolysis	Slow acid production	Acid-fast stain	Partially acid-fast stain	Aerial vegetative filaments	Motility	Growth at 50°C	Organism (chapter)
		−		+	O					+						*Curtobacterium* (34)
										−						*Microbacterium*, *Leifsonia* (both 34)
					F											*Microbacterium*, *Cellulomonas*, *Exiguobacterium* (all 34)
				−												*Microbacterium* (34)
	−	+									+					*Mycobacterium* (36, 38)
											−	+	+			*Nocardia* (35)
													−			*Tsukamurella*, *Gordonia*, *Rhodococcus*, *Dietzia* (all 35)
												−		+		*Dermatophilus* (35)
														−		*Actinomadura* (both 35)
													+		+	*Saccharomonospora*, *Saccharopolyspora*, *Thermoactinomyces* (all 35)
															−	*Actinomadura*, *Amycolatopsis*, *Nocardiopsis*, *Pseudonocardia*, *Streptomyces* (all 35)

[a] O, oxidative; F, fermentative.
[b] S, succinic acid; A, acetic acid; L, lactic acid.

Algorithms for Identification of Aerobic Gram-Negative Bacteria*

PAUL C. SCHRECKENBERGER AND DAVID LINDQUIST

24

These algorithms are meant to assist in the identification of organisms that are not readily identified by methods in place in most clinical laboratories. Microbiologists planning to identify an unknown gram-negative rod begin with colonies on an agar plate. Our definition of "good growth on blood agar plate (BAP)" is the presence of distinct colonies (approximately 1 mm) on Trypticase soy agar with 5% sheep blood after 24 h of incubation at 35°C in room atmosphere. Poor growth indicates that more than 24 h of incubation is necessary for the development of distinct colonies. If an organism fails to grow on BAP after 72 h, it is considered to show "no growth." Morphological and phenotypic criteria were chosen not only for their discriminatory value but also because the methods are available in most laboratories. Cellular morphology is determined by using a Gram stain from a young colony on a BAP. The description of "tiny coccobacilli" used for *Brucella* and *Francisella* in Table 2 implies almost indiscernible cells resembling grains of sand. For many organisms with pleomorphic morphologies, we chose to represent the dominant shape.

The urea test refers to conventional Christensen's urea reaction after 24 h of incubation, whereas the rapid urea result is read after 4 h. Glucose fermentation refers to an acid reaction in the butt of a Kligler iron agar (KIA) or triple sugar iron agar (TSI) tube. "Glucose oxidized" refers to acid production in the upper portion of oxidative-fermentative (OF) media. "BHI+serum" refers to brain heart infusion agar with 10% (vol/vol) serum added. The oxidase test refers to results obtained with the *N*,*N*,*N*,*N*-tetramethyl-*p*-phenylenediamine dihydrochloride reagent. Motility is best observed by preparing a wet preparation from a young colony on a BAP. Decarboxylase reactions are determined by using an extremely turbid inoculum in Moeller's media (heavier than usual inoculum). Polymyxin B sensitivity is indicated by any zone of inhibition surrounding a 300-U disk on a BAP. For glucose-nonfermenting rods and other fastidious organisms, the indole test is performed using the Ehrlich's extraction method (see chapter 50). "Esculin" refers to hydrolysis of esculin in media without bile.

These algorithms are dichotomous, since many organisms may fall into more than one group due to phenotypic variability of a given trait. The presence of two or more atypical traits or a major variation from the ideal phenotype depicted in an algorithm, due to antibiotic use, auxotrophy, or other reasons, may limit the algorithm's utility. These algorithms are intended as a guide to presumptive identification of an unknown isolate. The reference chapter describing the organism should be consulted to determine the definitive identification. To use the algorithms, start with Table 1 for gram-negative bacteria that grow well on blood agar in 24 h at room atmosphere and Table 2 for fastidious gram-negative bacteria. Note that Table 1 consists of three parts, which we have designated Table 1a, Table 1b, and Table 1c. In each case begin in the upper left-hand column of the table; if the test organism matches the given characteristic, then continue horizontally to the right to the next reaction. If the reaction in the box matches your test organism, continue moving horizontally until you reach the organisms listed in the right-hand column. When the reaction in the box does not match your test organism, then move down the column vertically to find the reaction that matches. Repeat the process until you reach the right-hand column. Be sure to check all your reactions with the organism characteristics given in the referenced chapter.

*This chapter contains information presented in chapter 23 by Paul C. Schreckenberger and Jane D. Wong in the eighth edition of this Manual.

TABLE 1a Identification algorithm for gram-negative bacteria that grow well on blood agar (part 1)

Cell morphology	Glucose fermented	Pigmented colonies	Oxidase	6% NaCl	Motility	Sucrose fermented	H_2S in TSI	Indole	Glucose oxidized	Fluorescent pigment	Yellow-pigmented colonies	Polymyxin B	ONPG[a]	Lysine decarboxylase	Arginine decarboxylase	Urea	Esculin	OF mannitol	OF maltose	Growth on MacConkey	Lactose, trehalose, or xylose fermented	Phenylalanine deaminase	H_2S in TSI	ONPG	Nitrate to gas	Organism group (chapter)
Rod	+	Purple																								*Chromobacterium* (40)
		Other	+	+																						*Vibrio* (47)
				−	+																					*Aeromonas* (46), *Plesiomonas* (45)
					−	+																				*Pasteurella* (40), *Actinobacillus* (40)
						−		+																		*Pasteurella bettyae* (40)
								−							+											EF4a (40)
															−											*Pasteurella avium* (40), *Actinobacillus actinomycetemcomitans* (40)
			−	+																						*Vibrio metschnikovii* (47)
				−																+	+					*Enterobacteriaceae* (42–45)
																					−	+				*Providencia, Morganella* (42, 45)
																						−	+			*Edwardsiella* (42, 45)
																							−			*Pasteurella bettyae* (40)
																				−						*P. bettyae* (40)
	−	Pink																								*Asaia, Azospirillum, Methylobacterium, Roseomonas* (50)
		Not pink	+		+		+																			*Shewanella* spp. (50)

		– +						*Balneatrix alpica* (50)
		–	+ +					*Pseudomonas aeruginosa, P. fluorescens, P. putida* (48)
			– +					*Agrobacterium* Yellow Grp, O-1, O-2, *Sphingomonas* spp. (50)
			–	R +		+		*Pseudomonas*-like group 2 (50)
						–		*Burkholderia cepacia* complex (49)
				– +				*B. stabilis* (49)
				– +				*B. pseudomallei* (49)
				–	+			*Ralstonia mannolilytica* (49)
					–			*Pandoraea* spp., *Ralstonia* spp. (49)
				S +	+			*Ochrobactrum anthropi, Achromobacter* groups B and E (50)
					– + +			CDC Vb-3 (48), OFBA-1, *Ochrobactrum* spp. (50)
					–			*Ochrobactrum* spp. (50), *Acidovorax* spp. (49), *Pseudomonas*-like group 2 (50)
					–			*P. mendocina* (48), CDC Ic , *Ochrobactrum* spp. (50)
				–	+ +		+	*Rhizobium radiobacter* (50)
							–	*Ochrobactrum anthropi, Achromobacter* Group F, *Halomonas venusta, Inquilinus limosus* (50)
					–		+	*P. stutzeri* (48), *Ochrobactrum anthropi* (50)
							–	*Pseudomonas*-like group 2, *Herbaspirillum*, CDC halophilic nonfermenter group 1 (50)
					– +			CDC group O-3, *Inquilinus limosus, Massilia timonae* (50), *Brevundimonas vesicularis* (49)
					–		+	*P. stutzeri* (48), *Achromobacter xylosoxidans* (50)
							–	*A. xylosoxidans* (50), *Brevundimonas diminuta* (49)

[a]ONPG, *O*-nitrophenyl-beta-D-galactopyranoside.

TABLE 1b Identification algorithm for gram-negative bacteria that grow well on blood agar (part 2)

Cell morphology	Glucose fermented	Pigmented colonies	Oxidase	Motility	H_2S in TSI	Indole	Glucose oxidized	Yellow-pigmented colonies	Polymyxin B	Arginine decarboxylase	Rapid urea	NO_2 reduction	Acetamide	Esculin	OF mannitol	Urea	Growth in 6.5% NaCl	Gelatin	NO_3 to NO_2	Curved rods	Organism group (chapter)
Rod	−	Not pink	+	+	−	−	−		R												*Pandoraea* spp. (49)
									S	+										+	*Laribacter hongkongensis* (50)
																				−	*P. pseudoalcaligenes, P. alcaligenes, Pseudomonas* species group 1 (48)
										−	+										*Bordetella bronchiseptica, Oligella ureolytica, Cupriavidus pauculus* (50)
											−	+							+		*Pseudomonas* species group 1 (48), *Achromobacter denitrificans* (50)
																			−		*Alcaligenes faecalis* (50)
												−	+		+						*Delftia acidovorans* (49)
															−				+		*Achromobacter piechaudii* (50)
																			−		*Bordetella avium* (50, 51)
													−				+				CDC halophilic group 1 (50)
																	−		+		*P. pseudoalcaligenes, P. alcaligenes* (48), *Comamonas terrigena, C. testosteroni* (49), *Achromobacter piechaudii, Cupriavidus taiwanensis* (50)
																			−		*Brevundimonas diminuta, Brevundimonas vesicularis* (49), *Bordetella hinzii* (50, 51), *P. alcaligenes* (48), *Cupriavidus gilardii, Cupriavidus respiraculi* (50)
				−		+		+													*Chryseobacterium indologenes/gleum, Empedobacter brevis*, CDC group IIi (50)
								−			+										*Bergeyella zoohelcum* (50)
											−			+	+						*Elizabethkingia meningoseptica* (50)
															−						CDC group IIc, IIh, IIi (50)
														−				+			*Weeksella virosa, Empedobacter brevis* (50)
																		−			CDC group IIe, IIg (50)
						−	+							+	+						*Sphingobacterium spiritivorum, Inquilinus limosus* (50)
															−	+			+		*Sphingobacterium thalpophilum* (50)
																			−		*Sphingobacterium multivorum* (50)
																−					*Sphingomonas paucimobilis, Flavobacterium mizutaii* (50)
														−					+		EF-4b, *Paracoccus yeei, Psychrobacter immobilis* (50)
																			−		EO-3, EO-4 (50)
							−				+							+			*Myroides* spp. (50)
																		−			*Oligella ureolytica* (50)
											−			+							*Alishewanella fetalis* (50)
														−							*Neisseria weaveri, N. elongata*, Gilardi rod group 1 (39, 50)

TABLE 1c Identification algorithm for gram-negative bacteria that grow well on blood agar (part 3)

Cell morphology	Glucose fermented	Pigmented colonies	Oxidase	Motility	Glucose oxidized	DNase	Urea	Mannitol	Lysine decarboxylase or OF lactose	Lysine decarboxylase	OF maltose	Esculin	Gelatin	NO_2 reduced	NO_3 reduced	Brown diffusible pigment	Growth at 42°C	Organism group (chapter)
Rod	–	Not pink	–	+	+			+	+									*Burkholderia cepacia* complex (48)
									Both negative		+	+						*Pseudomonas luteola* (47)
												–						*P. oryzihabitans* (47)
											–							*Burkholderia gladioli* (48)
								–		+								*Stenotrophomonas maltophilia* (48)
										–								*Sphingomonas paucimobilis* (49)
					–								+					*Bordetella ansorpii* (50, 51)
													–				+	*Kerstersia gyiorum* (50)
																	–	*Bordetella trematum* (50, 51)
				–	+													*Acinetobacter baumannii*, EO-5 (50)
					–		+											*Bordetella parapertussis* (50, 51)
							–								+			CDC NO-1 (50)
															–	+		*Bordetella holmesii* (50, 51)
																–		*Acinetobacter lwoffii* (50)
Diplococci			+															*Neisseria* (39), *Moraxella catarrhalis* (50)
			–															*Acinetobacter* (50)
Coccobacilli			+	+														*Oligella ureolytica* (50)
				–	+										+			EF-4b, *Paracoccus yeei*, *Psychrobacter immobilis* (saccharolytic) (50)
															–			EO-3, EO-4 (50)
					–	+												*Moraxella canis*, *M. catarrhalis* (50)
						–	+											*Psychrobacter phenylpyruvica* (50), *Brucella* spp. (52)
							–							+				*Oligella urethralis* (50)
														–	+			*Moraxella lacunata*, *M. nonliquefaciens*, *M. osloensis*, *P. immobilis* (asaccharolytic) (50)
															–			*M. atlantae*, *M. lincolnii*, *M. osloensis*, *P. immobilis* (asaccharolytic) (50)
			–	–	+													*Acinetobacter baumannii*, EO-5 (50)
					–		+											*Bordetella parapertussis* (50, 51)
							–								+			CDC NO-1 (50)
															–	+		*Bordetella holmesii* (50, 51)
																–		*Acinetobacter lwoffii* (50)

TABLE 2 Identification algorithm for gram-negative bacteria with poor or no growth on blood agar[a]

Growth on BAP	Growth only on:	Cellular morphology	Urea	Pigmented colonies	Oxidase	6% NaCl	H_2S in TSI	Cauliflower-like colonies	O-shaped cells	Require X ± V	Organism group (chapter)
Poor		Tiny coccobacilli	+								*Brucella* (52)
			−		+		+				*Francisella philomiragia* (52)
							−				*Bordetella* (50)
					−						*Francisella* (52)
		Rods		Pink							*Asaia, Azospirillum, Methylobacterium, Roseomonas* (50)
				Other				+			*Bartonella* (54)
								−			*Haemophilus aphrophilus* (41), *Cardiobacterium, Dysgonomonas, Eikenella, Kingella, Simonsiella, Suttonella* (40)
		Diplococci or coccobacilli							+		*Paracoccus yeei* (50)
									−		*Neisseria* (39), *Moraxella* (50)
None	Chocolate	Diplococci or coccobacilli									*Neisseria* (39)
		Fusiform rod									*Capnocytophaga* (40)
		Rod						+			*Bartonella, Afipia* (54)
								−		+	*Haemophilus* (41)
										−	*Francisella* (52)
	BCYE	Long gram-negative rods									*Legionella* (53)
		Regular rods			+						*Bordetella* (51)
					−						*Francisella* (52)
	BHI+ serum	Pleomorphic, beaded filamentous rods									*Streptobacillus* (40)
		Small rods									*Bartonella, Afipia* (54)

[a] Abbreviations: BCYE, buffered charcoal yeast extract agar; X, hemin; V, nicotinamide adenine dinucleotide.

Algorithm for Identification of Anaerobic Bacteria

DIANE M. CITRON

25

Anaerobic bacteria are defined for the purposes of this algorithm as organisms displaying better growth when incubated in an anaerobic environment than in the presence of oxygen. The use of selective and differential agars for the primary setup of clinical specimens and prompt incubation in an anaerobic environment can provide rapid presumptive identification of important groups of anaerobes based on distinctive characteristics, such as bile resistance, pigmented colonies, a double zone of beta-hemolysis, or the presence of fusiform cells on Gram stain. Examples of such agars include Bacteroides-bile-esculin (BBE) for isolation and presumptive identification of the *Bacteroides fragilis* group and *Bilophila wadsworthia*. Brucella agar supplemented with laked blood, kanamycin, and vancomycin inhibits enteric and gram-positive organisms and is thus useful for isolation and characterization of *Bacteroides, Prevotella,* and some strains of fusobacteria. Pigmented *Prevotella* spp. produce pigment more rapidly and intensely on laked blood agar. Phenylethyl alcohol blood agar (PEA) and colistin nalidixic acid blood agar inhibit enteric organisms and swarming *Proteus* spp. but allow for growth and isolation of many gram-positive and gram-negative anaerobes. PEA also inhibits the swarming by *Clostridium septicum,* which can completely overgrow and contaminate other anaerobic organisms in a mixed culture. All media for culture of anaerobes should be supplemented with vitamin K_1 and hemin.

Simple tests, such as tests for susceptibility (inhibition zone diameters, $\geq$10 mm) to the special potency disks with 1,000 μg of kanamycin, 5 μg of vancomycin, and 10 μg of colistin; tests for growth in the presence of 20% bile; the spot indole test; and tests for nitrate reduction, catalase and urease production, and lecithinase and lipase production on egg yolk medium are rapid and useful for initial grouping of many anaerobes (1).

The gram-positive non-spore-forming rods are difficult to group by simple tests. Nitrate-reducing strains include *Actinomyces, Propionibacterium,* and some of the *Eubacterium*-like group members. Most *Propionibacterium* spp. and some species of *Actinomyces* are catalase positive. Lactobacilli and bifidobacteria do not reduce nitrate and are catalase, urease, and indole negative.

The genus *Clostridium* includes the gram-positive spore-forming rods; however, many members of this group appear to be gram negative, and spores can be difficult to see under routine conditions. While many species require extensive testing for complete identification, some very clinically important species can be recognized by easily observable characteristics.

Anaerobic bacteria are a diverse group of organisms and include members that often exhibit seemingly contradictory characteristics, such as gram-negative rods sensitive to vancomycin (certain clostridia, *Porphyromonas* spp.), gram-positive rods resistant to vancomycin (some lactobacilli), or rods that appear as cocci (some *Prevotella* and *Porphyromonas* spp.). The algorithm in Table 1 includes characteristics that should be helpful for suggesting the correct category for anaerobes encountered in clinical specimens.

REFERENCE

1. **Jousimies-Somer, H., P. Summanen, D. M. Citron, E. J. Baron, H. M. Wexler, and S. M. Finegold.** 2002. *Wadsworth-KTL Anaerobic Bacteriology Manual,* 6th ed. Star Publishing Co., Belmont, Calif.

TABLE 1 Algorithm for identification of bacteria that grow better anaerobically than aerobically

Cellular morphology	Gram reaction	Growth on BBE	Pattern on kanamycin and vancomycin disk[a]	Pigment or red fluorescence	Nitrate	Catalase	Spores	Spreading, irregular, peaked, or large colony	Large boxcar-shaped cells, beta-hemolysis	Organism (chapter)
Rod or coccobacillus	–	+	R/R							*B. fragilis* group (58)
			S/R		–	–				*Fusobacterium mortiferum/varium* group (58)
					+	+				*Bilophila wadsworthia* (58)
		–	R/S	+/–	–	–/+				*Porphyromonas* (58)
			R/R	+/–	–	–				*Prevotella* (58)
				–			rare	+		*Clostridium innocuum* (57)
			S/S	+			rare	–		*Clostridium ramosum* (57)
				–			rare	–		*Clostridium clostridioforme* group (57)
			S/R		+	–				*Bacteroides ureolyticus*, *B. ureolyticus*-like, or *Campylobacter*-like spp. (58, 59)
					–					*Fusobacterium* (58)
	+/variable		S/R							*Lactobacillus* (56)
			S/S	–	–	–				*Lactobacillus*, *Bifidobacterium*, or "*Eubacterium*-like" group (56)
				+/–	+	+/–				*Actinomyces*, *Propionibacterium*, "*Eubacterium*-like" group (56)
				+	–	–	rare			*Clostridium ramosum* (57)
				–	+/–	–	+	+		*Clostridium* spp. (57)
							–	+	+	*Clostridium perfringens* (57)
Coccus	+		S/S							Anaerobic gram-positive cocci (55)
	–		S/R							*Veillonella*, *Acidaminococcus*, or *Megasphaera* (55)

[a] R, resistant; S, susceptible.

Algorithms for Identification of Curved and Spiral-Shaped Gram-Negative Rods*

IRVING NACHAMKIN

26

Curved and spiral-shaped bacteria have a common microscopic morphology but represent diverse bacterial pathogens (Table 1). These organisms are curved, helical, or spiral-shaped gram-negative rods. Specific detection of these organisms may require a combination of tests including microscopy, histologic staining of tissue, biochemical tests, antigen tests, serologic tests, bacteriologic culture, and molecular approaches (Fig. 1).

Most bacteria in this group of organisms are isolated from patients with gastrointestinal and related infections. *Campylobacter jejuni* subsp. *jejuni* is the most frequently isolated curved gram-negative rod associated with diarrheal illness, but under proper culture conditions, other *Campylobacter* spp., *Helicobacter* spp., and *Vibrio* species may be detected in routine stool cultures. *Helicobacter pylori* is the most common curved gram-negative rod isolated from gastric tissue, but other *Helicobacter* species have also been reported in this site.

Other less commonly isolated curved gram-negative rods include the anaerobes *Desulfovibrio* spp., *Sutterella wadsworthensis, Wolinella succinogenes,* and *Anaerobiospirillum succiniciproducens,* which may be isolated from blood, abscess material, or other clinical samples. Several oxidase-positive nonfermenters may also have a curved appearance, including *Laribacter hongkongensis, Herbaspirillum* species 3, and CDC O-3 (see chapter 50).

The spirochetes *Borrelia* spp. and *Leptospira* spp. cause systemic infections and are infrequently isolated in clinical laboratories, usually only with specialized media. These bacteria are strictly aerobic and have optimal growth temperatures at 28 to 30°C (*Leptospira* spp.) and 30 to 33°C (*Borrelia* spp.). *Treponema* spp. of clinical importance are identified based on clinical and epidemiologic findings, as well as microscopic, serologic, and molecular test procedures.

* This chapter contains information presented in chapter 25 by James Versalovic in the eighth edition of this Manual.

TABLE 1 Curved gram-negative bacilli that may be encountered in clinical specimens[a]

Clinical finding	Specimen type(s)	Curved gram-negative organisms encountered: Genus or group	Curved gram-negative organisms encountered: Species	Microscopic appearance in specimen	Culture conditions and media	Chapter
Gastroenteritis	Stool; intestinal biopsy specimen	*Arcobacter*	*A. butzleri, A. cryaerophilus, A. skirrowii*	Slightly curved, curved, S-shaped, or helical	Microaerobic, may grow aerobically or anaerobically, nonhemolytic, grows on nonselective blood agar (with filtration method), may grow on Campy-CVA	59
		Brachyspira	*B. aalborgi, B. pilosicoli*	Spirochete	Anaerobic, prolonged incubation (1–2 weeks) on anaerobic media, selective media may be required	58
		Campylobacter	*C. jejuni* subsp. *jejuni, C. jejuni* subsp. *doylei, C. coli, C. upsaliensis, C. fetus* subsp. *fetus, C. lari, C. curvus, C. rectus, C. hominis, C. lanienae, C. hyointestinalis, C. sputorum*	Curved, spiral, gull, S-shaped GNR	Microaerobic, 37 or 42°C, increased H_2 required for some non-*C. jejuni/C. coli* species, selective media required such as Campy-CVA, charcoal-based media such as CCDA; filtration method for less common species and H_2-requiring species	59
		Helicobacter (Gastric) (Intestinal)	*H. pylori, H. bizzozeronii, H. canis, H. canadensis, H. cinaedi, H. fennelliae, H. pullorum, Helicobacter* spp. and flexispira taxon 8	Curved, spiral, gull, S-shaped GNR	Microaerobic, 37°C, increased H_2 required for intestinal species, nonselective blood agar for *H. pylori*, selective supplements (Skirrows, Dents) may be needed for contaminated gastric samples	60
		Laribacter	*L. hongkongensis*	Gull or spiral-shaped	Asaccharolytic nonfermenter, aerobic growth on blood agar, MacConkey agar	50
		Vibrio	*V. cholerae, V. parahaemolyticus, V. fluvialis, V. alginolyticus, V. cincinnatiensis, V. damsela, V. furnissii, V. hollisae, V. metschnikovii, V. mimicus*	Comma-shaped or plain rods, larger than *Campylobacter*	Aerobic conditions, 37°C, grows on routine laboratory media, blood agar, MacConkey agar; use selective medium such as TCBS for primary isolation from stool samples	47
Bacteremia	Blood	*Borrelia* Lyme group	*B. afzelii, B. burgdorferi, B. garinii*	Not seen in routine BC bottles	Difficult to isolate, special media required for isolation; BSK, MKP	62
		Relapsing fever group	*B. recurrentis, B. miyamotoi, B. lonestari, B. hermsii*			

(Continued on next page)

TABLE 1 *(Continued)*

Clinical finding	Specimen type(s)	Curved gram-negative organisms encountered		Microscopic appearance in specimen	Culture conditions and media	Chapter
		Genus or group	Species			
		Campylobacter	*C. jejuni* subsp. *jejuni*, *C. fetus* subsp. *fetus*, *C. upsaliensis*, *C. lari*, *C. concisus*	Curved, spiral, gull, S-shaped GNR	Microaerobic, incubate subcultures at 37°C, increased H_2 required for some non-*C. jejuni*/*C. coli* species	59
		Herbaspirillum	*Herbaspirillum* species 3 (formerly EF-1)	Curved or helical GNR	Growth properties not described	50
		Helicobacter	*H. cinaedi*, *H. fennelliae*	Curved, spiral, gull, S-shaped GNR	Microaerobic, incubate subcultures at 37°C, increased H_2 required	60
		Leptospira	*L. biflexa*, *L. interrogans*	Not seen in routine BC bottles but may be seen in direct wet preparations of anticoagulated blood	Aerobic growth, 28–30°C, specialized media required for isolation such as EMJH, PLM-5	61
		Vibrio	*V. vulnificus*, *V. damsela*, *V. metschnikovii*, *V. cincinnatiensis*	Comma-shaped or straight rods	Aerobic growth, 37°C, grows on routine blood agar, MacConkey agar	47
		CDC O-3		Thin, medium to slightly long curved rods with tapered ends	Saccharolytic nonfermenter, no growth or poor growth on MacConkey agar, grows on Campy-CVA medium	50
		Spirillum	"Spirillum minus"	Not seen in routine BC bottles	Cannot be cultured in vitro	
Tissue infection, oral	Tissue biopsy specimen, abscess fluid	*Campylobacter*	*C. concisus*, *C. curvus*, *C. rectus*, *C. gracilis*, *C. showae*	Curved, spiral, gull, S-shaped GNR	Microaerobic, incubate cultures at 37°C, increased H_2 required for oral species, use nonselective blood agar or CCDA with filtration method	59
Tissue infection, skin, wound, other	Skin biopsy specimen, lesion fluid	*Borrelia*	Lyme group spp.	Histologic stains required	Difficult to isolate, special media required for isolation; BSK, MKP	62
		Treponema	*T. pallidum* subsp. *pallidum* (syphilis), *T. carateum* (pinta), *T. pallidum* subsp. *pertenue* (yaws), *T. pallidum* subsp. *endemicum* (endemic)	Spirochetes; silver stain; dark-field; DFA	Has not been isolated in vitro	63
		Vibrio	*V. vulnificus*, *V. damsela*, *V. alginolyticus*, *V. harveyi*	Comma-shaped or straight rods, larger than *Campylobacter* spp.	Aerobic, grows on routine laboratory media, blood agar, MacConkey agar	47

(Continued on next page)

TABLE 1 Curved gram-negative bacilli that may be encountered in clinical specimens[a] *(Continued)*

Clinical finding	Specimen type(s)	Curved gram-negative organisms encountered: Genus or group	Curved gram-negative organisms encountered: Species	Microscopic appearance in specimen	Culture conditions and media	Chapter
		Anaerobes	*Desulfovibrio, Sutterella wadsworthensis, Wolinella succinogenes, Anaerobiospirillum, succiniciproducens*	Curved rods	Growth under anaerobic conditions, use anaerobe media	58
		CDC O-3		Thin, medium to slightly long curved rods with tapered ends	Saccharolytic nonfermenter, no growth or poor growth on MacConkey agar, grows on Campy-CVA medium	50
		Herbaspirillum	*Herbaspirillum* species 3	Curved or helical GNR	Growth properties not described	50
		Spirillum	"Spirillum minus"	Short, tightly coiled GNR	Unable to isolate in vitro	
	Urine	*Leptospira*	*L. biflexa, L. interrogans*	Spirochete with curved ends observed by darkfield	Aerobic growth, 28–30°C, specialized media required for isolation such as EMJH, PLM-5	61

[a]Not all species listed have been shown to cause human diseases; they are listed if they have been isolated from human clinical specimens. BC, blood culture; GNR, gram-negative rod; DFA, direct fluorescent antibody; Campy CVA, Campy-cefoperazone, vancomycin, amphotericin; CCDA, charcoal cefoperazone deoxycholate agar; TCBS, thiosulfate-citrate-bile salts-sucrose agar; BSK, Barbour-Stoenner-Kelly medium; MKP, modified Kelley medium; EMJH, Ellinghausen-McCullough-Johnson-Harris medium.

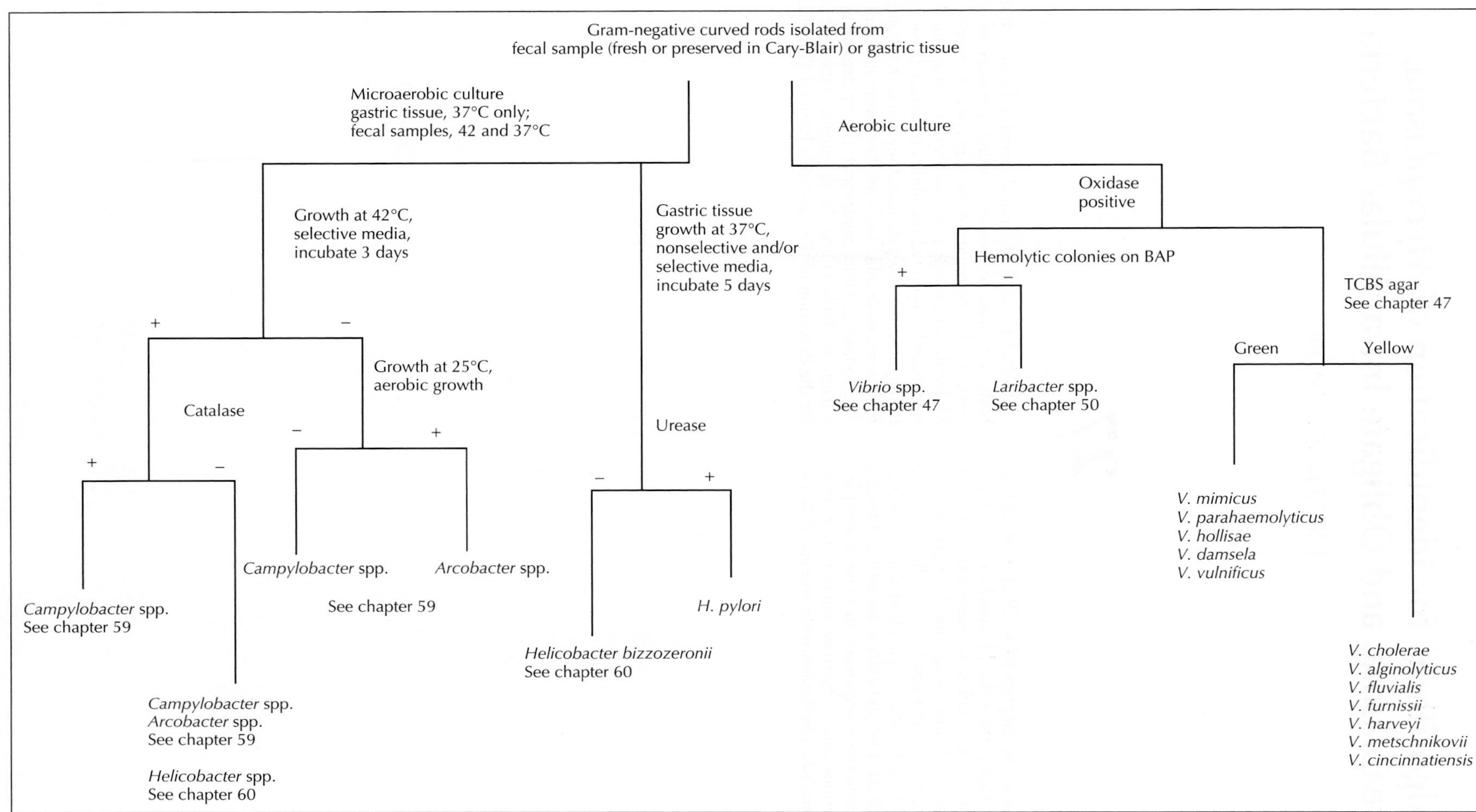

FIGURE 1 Algorithm for identification of curved gram-negative bacilli from fecal and gastric clinical samples. BAP, blood agar plate; TCBS, thiosulfate-citrate-bile salts-sucrose.

Algorithms for Identification of *Mycoplasma, Ureaplasma,* and Obligate Intracellular Bacteria

J. STEPHEN DUMLER

27

The bacteria discussed in chapters 64 to 69 differ from bacteria described in other parts of this Manual by several characteristics, including lack of efficient characterization with the Gram stain method and except for *Mycoplasma* and *Ureaplasma* species, the requirement for intracellular growth. Thus, the most frequently used tests in clinical microbiology laboratories, the Gram stain and culture on artificial media, are unable to detect these organisms in clinical samples. Diagnosis of infections caused by these bacteria has traditionally been accomplished by Romanowsky staining (Giemsa and Wright stains) of clinical samples, by detection of antibody responses to infection using a variety of serological tests, or by histopathologic analysis of biopsy samples. Molecular diagnostic tools and better culture methods have significantly improved the ability to detect these agents and to diagnose the diseases that they cause. For some of these infections, molecular tools are becoming standard practice. The following tables summarize the epidemiology of these infections (Table 1) and the diagnostic tests most often used for the detection of the causative bacteria (Table 2).

TABLE 1 Epidemiology and clinical disease associated with *Anaplasma, Chlamydia, Chlamydophila, Coxiella, Ehrlichia, Mycoplasma, Rickettsia, Tropheryma,* and *Ureaplasma* infections

Organism	Disease	Reservoir	Vector and mode of transmission
Anaplasma phagocytophilum	Human granulocytotropic anaplasmosis (HGA); fever, headache, myalgia, systemic involvement except for central nervous system	White-footed mouse, other small mammals, ruminants, deer	*Ixodes scapularis* (deer or black-legged tick), *I. pacificus* (western black-legged tick), *I. ricinus* (rabbit tick), and *I. persulcatus* tick bites
Chlamydia trachomatis	Endemic trachoma, inclusion keratoconjunctivitis, urethritis, epididymitis, endometritis, salpingitis, perihepatitis, pneumonia, lymphogranuloma venereum	Humans	Sexual contact, hand-eye contact, insect fomites, infected birth canal
Chlamydophila pneumoniae	Pneumonia, bronchitis, sinusitis, pharyngitis	Humans	Inhalation of infected aerosols
Chlamydophila psittaci	Psittacosis (pneumonia), systemic infections	Birds, domestic animals	Inhalation of infected aerosols
Coxiella burnetii	Acute Q fever (self-limited febrile illness ± pneumonia, hepatitis); chronic Q fever (endocarditis, endovascular infections)	Cattle, sheep, goats, cats, rabbits, dogs, ticks	Inhalation of infected aerosols; ingestion of nonpasteurized dairy products
Ehrlichia chaffeensis	Human monocytotropic ehrlichiosis (HME): fever, headache, myalgia, systemic involvement including central nervous system	White-tailed deer, dogs and other canids, raccoons	*Amblyomma americanum* (Lone Star tick) and potentially *Dermacentor variabilis* (American dog tick) tick bites
Ehrlichia ewingii	"Ewingii" ehrlichiosis: fever, headache, myalgia, predominantly in immunocompromised individuals	Dogs and other canids	*Amblyomma americanum* (Lone Star tick) tick bites
Mycoplasma genitalium	Urethritis, cervicitis, endometritis, conjunctivitis	Humans	Sexual contact, vertical transmission in utero or intrapartum
Mycoplasma hominis	Acute pyelonephritis, bacterial vaginosis, pelvic inflammatory disease, postabortion bacteremia	Humans	Sexual contact, vertical transmission in utero or intrapartum
Mycoplasma pneumoniae	Tracheobronchitis, pneumonia, pharyngitis, extrapulmonary complications (meningoencephalitis, arthritis, etc.)	Humans	Contact with infectious aerosols or fomites
Orientia tsutsugamushi	Scrub typhus	Chiggers (larval mites)	*Leptotrombidium* spp. (chigger) bites
Rickettsia africae	African tick-bite fever	Not established	*Amblyomma* spp. tick bites
Rickettsia akari	Rickettsialpox	Mice and other small mammals	*Allodermanyssus sanguineus* (mouse mite) bites
Rickettsia conorii	Boutonneuse fever or Mediterranean spotted fever	Small mammals and ticks	*Rhipicephalus sanguineus* (Brown dog) tick bites
Rickettsia felis	Murine typhus-like illness	Fleas, opossums, cats, dogs	*Ctenocephalides felis* (cat fleas); contamination of infected flea feces into flea bite
Rickettsia prowazekii	Epidemic typhus	Humans, lice, flying squirrels	*Pediculus humanus* subsp. *corporis* (body louse); contamination of infected louse feces into louse bite
Rickettsia rickettsii	Rocky Mountain spotted fever	Ticks, small and medium-size mammals	*Dermacentor variabilis* (American dog tick), *Dermacentor andersoni* (wood tick), *Rhipicephalus sanguineus* (North and Central America), *Amblyomma cajennense* (Central and South America) tick bites
Rickettsia typhi	Murine typhus	Rats and other rodents, opossums	*Xenopsylla cheopis* (rat fleas) and *Ctenocephalides felis* (cat fleas); contamination of flea bite wound with infected flea feces
Tropheryma whipplei	Malabsorption, arthralgias, lymphadenopathy, culture-negative endocarditis, encephalitis	Humans	Environmental contacts (sewage, human stool, saliva); genetic predispositions
Ureaplasma urealyticum	Urethritis, epididymo-orchitis, urinary calculi, abortion, chorioamnionitis	Humans	Sexual contact, in utero or peripartum vertical transmission

TABLE 2 Diagnostic tests for *Anaplasma, Chlamydia, Chlamydophila, Coxiella, Ehrlichia, Mycoplasma, Rickettsia,* and *Ureaplasma*

Organism	Diagnostic test[a]
Anaplasma phagocytophilum	**Microscopy:** Giemsa or Wright stain of peripheral blood or buffy coat smears is positive in approximately 60% of infected persons. **Antigen tests:** None available. **Molecular tests:** EDTA-anticoagulated blood collected during the pretreatment acute phase of illness is used for PCR amplification. Species- and genus-specific tests are available. Current test of choice for diagnosis during active infection. **Culture:** EDTA-anticoagulated peripheral blood is inoculated onto HL-60, THP1, or other myelocytic cell lines. Positive cultures may be obtained between 3 and 30 days from many samples if inoculated within 24 h and if obtained before antimicrobial therapy. Lack of timely results precludes frequent use. **Serologic tests:** IFA is the most frequently used test. A fourfold or greater rise in titer or a single peak titer of ≥80 in a patient with typical clinical features of HGA confirms infection. Test sensitivity is between 90 and 100%; specificity is approximately 95%.
Chlamydia trachomatis	**Microscopy:** Organisms may be detected by Giemsa stain or DFA test. DFA is more sensitive, but neither test should be used alone. **Antigen tests:** Commercial EIAs vary in sensitivity but may cross-react with other bacterial LPS and used alone are not suitable for screening. EIA using blocking antibodies may increase specificity to 99.5%. Point-of-care tests are only 62–72% sensitive compared to culture and less sensitive compared to molecular tests. **Molecular tests:** Commercial NAATs (PCR, transcription-mediated amplification, strand-displacement amplification) are available and are tests of choice for confirmation of *C. trachomatis* infections. **Culture:** Recovered in many different cell cultures commonly including McCoy and HeLa cells. Test sensitivity is dependent on the quality of the submitted specimen. **Serologic tests:** MIF test is most sensitive and specific (test of choice). Diagnosis for acute *C. trachomatis* infection is confirmed by fourfold or greater rise in titer. Rising antibody titers may not be observed with chronic, repeated, or systemic infections. A single IgM titer of ≥32 supports a diagnosis of neonatal pneumonia.
Chlamydophila pneumoniae	**Microscopy:** Organisms may be detected by Giemsa stain or DFA test directed against LPS, but both tests are relatively insensitive. **Antigen tests:** Available EIA tests directed against LPS detect all *Chlamydia* and *Chlamydophila* species but are licensed only for *C. trachomatis*. **Molecular tests:** None commercially available. **Culture:** Recovered best if inoculated onto HL cells or Hep-2 cells. **Serologic tests:** MIF test is the test of choice. Diagnosis is confirmed by fourfold or greater rise in titer or single samples with IgM titer of ≥16 and/or IgG titer of ≥512.
Chlamydophila psittacii	**Microscopy:** Organisms may be detected by Giemsa stain or DFA test directed against LPS, but both tests are relatively insensitive. **Antigen tests:** Available EIA tests directed against LPS detect all *Chlamydia* and *Chlamydophila* species but are licensed only for *C. trachomatis*. **Molecular tests:** None commercially available. **Culture:** Recovered in many different cell cultures commonly including McCoy and HeLa cells. **Serologic tests:** MIF test is most sensitive and specific (test of choice).
Coxiella burnetii	**Microscopy:** DFA or immunohistochemistry tests may be performed but are insensitive and not widely available. **Antigen tests:** None commercially available. **Molecular tests:** PCR available only through reference laboratories; more sensitive than culture from frozen tissue, blood, or for chronic disease; less useful for serum, especially if stored frozen. **Culture:** May be cultivated in a variety of cell lines, especially Vero cells and HEL cells, or by inoculation into embryonated chicken yolk sacs or laboratory animals. **Serologic tests:** Most frequently used diagnostic test. The IFA test is recommended. Acute Q fever is confirmed by a fourfold or greater rise in titer to phase II antigens, or a single IgM titer of ≥50 and IgG titer of ≥200. Chronic Q fever is confirmed in a single serum sample with a ≥800 IgG titer to phase I antigen. A decreasing antibody titer suggests successful therapy.
Ehrlichia chaffeensis	**Microscopy:** Giemsa or Wright stain of peripheral blood or buffy coat smears is positive in up to 29% of infected persons. **Antigen tests:** None available. **Molecular tests:** EDTA-anticoagulated blood collected during the pretreatment acute phase of illness is used for PCR amplification. Species- and genus-specific tests are available. Current test of choice for diagnosis during active infection. Sensitivity ranges from 56 to 100%. **Culture:** EDTA-anticoagulated peripheral blood or CSF is inoculated onto DH82, THP1, HEL-22, Vero, HL-60, or other cell lines. Positive cultures may be obtained between 5 and >30 days from most samples if inoculated within 12 h and if obtained before antimicrobial therapy. Lack of timely results precludes frequent use.

(Continued on next page)

TABLE 2 *(Continued)*

Organism	Diagnostic test[a]
	Serologic tests: IFA is the most frequently used test. A fourfold or greater rise in titer or a single peak titer of ≥64 in a patient with a clinically compatible illness is considered evidence of infection. Test sensitivity is believed to be high.
Ehrlichia ewingii	**Microscopy:** Giemsa or Wright stain of peripheral blood or buffy coat smears occasionally reveals bacterial clusters (morulae) in neutrophils of infected persons. **Antigen tests:** None available. **Molecular tests:** EDTA-anticoagulated blood collected during the pretreatment acute phase of illness is used for PCR amplification. Species- and genus-specific tests are available in some reference and public health laboratories. Current test of choice for diagnosis during active infection. Sensitivity is not currently known but is suspected to be high. **Culture:** No method of in vitro culture has been developed. **Serologic tests:** No specific antibody test is available. Antibody tests are based largely on cross-reactivity with *E. chaffeensis* and alone are not diagnostic.
Mycoplasma genitalium	**Microscopy:** May be detected in genital fluids using DNA fluorochrome stains (Hoechst 33258 or acridine orange), but these are not specific. **Antigen tests:** Not recommended for diagnostic purposes. **Molecular tests:** PCR amplification tests are highly sensitive and have unknown specificity, but clinical studies have yielded variable results when compared with culture and serology. May be the only practical means for detection of the pathogen. Commercial kits are not currently available in the United States. **Culture:** Organisms are isolated from a variety of genital fluids. Wood-shafted cotton swabs should be avoided. Mycoplasmas are extremely labile, and appropriate transport medium should be used. Can be recovered on SP4 glucose broth supplemented with arginine. Growth conditions are not well established. Widely considered insensitive for diagnosis confirmation. **Serologic tests:** MIF and Western immunoblot methods have been described, although none are commercially available.
Mycoplasma hominis	**Microscopy:** May be detected in body fluids using DNA fluorochrome stains (Hoechst 33258 or acridine orange), but these are not specific. **Antigen tests:** None commercially available. **Molecular tests:** PCR tests have been developed but are less useful than culture. **Culture:** Organisms are isolated from a variety of clinical samples. Wood-shafted cotton swabs should be avoided. Mycoplasmas are extremely labile, and appropriate transport medium should be used. Can be recovered on SP4 glucose broth supplemented with arginine, on Shepard's 10B broth, or A8 agar. Growth occurs within 2 to 4 days. **Serologic tests:** Not recommended for routine use.
Mycoplasma pneumoniae	**Microscopy:** May be detected in body fluids by using DNA fluorochrome stains (Hoechst 33258 or acridine orange), but these are not specific. **Antigen tests:** Not recommended for diagnostic purposes. **Molecular tests:** PCR amplification tests are highly sensitive and have unknown specificity, but clinical studies have yielded variable results when compared with culture and serology. Commercial kits are not currently available in the United States. **Culture:** Organisms are isolated from a variety of clinical samples. Wood-shafted cotton swabs should be avoided. Mycoplasmas are extremely labile, and appropriate transport medium should be used. Can be recovered on SP4 glucose broth supplemented with arginine. Growth occurs after 21 days. Widely considered insensitive for diagnosis confirmation. **Serologic tests:** EIA tests are more sensitive and specific than CF and IFA; detection of seroconversion by demonstration of a fourfold increase in antibody titer is preferred, but detection of IgM antibodies in single serum samples may be useful. The cold agglutinin test is not recommended for diagnosis of *M. pneumoniae* infection.
Orientia tsutsugamushi	**Microscopy:** DFA or immunohistochemistry on skin or other tissues may be performed, but tests are not widely available. **Antigen tests:** Not available. **Molecular tests:** PCR amplification performed on EDTA-anticoagulated blood, buffy coat leukocytes, plasma, or tissue samples obtained during the acute phase of illness; available only through reference laboratories. **Culture:** Isolation is performed by intraperitoneal inoculation of mice. Performed only in reference and research laboratories. **Serologic tests:** With the IFA test in a region of endemicity, a titer of ≥400 is 98% specific and 48% sensitive. Lower cutoffs are used for populations in which the infection is not endemic. Indirect immunoperoxidase is also sensitive and specific with diagnostic cutoffs of ≥128 for IgG and ≥32 for IgM. Dot EIA kits are available and have lower sensitivity and specificity than IFA. Weil-Felix (*Proteus*) febrile agglutinins test is insensitive and nonspecific.

(Continued on next page)

TABLE 2 Diagnostic tests for *Anaplasma, Chlamydia, Chlamydophila, Coxiella, Ehrlichia, Mycoplasma, Rickettsia,* and *Ureaplasma* (Continued)

Organism	Diagnostic test[a]
Rickettsia africae and *Rickettsia conorii*	**Microscopy:** DFA or immunohistochemistry on skin biopsy of rash or eschar is sensitive and specific for spotted fever group rickettsiae. Antibodies are not commercially available. **Antigen tests:** Not available. **Molecular tests:** PCR amplification performed on EDTA-anticoagulated blood, buffy coat leukocytes, plasma, skin biopsy, or tissue samples obtained during acute phase of illness; available only through reference laboratories. **Culture:** Heparin-anticoagulated plasma or buffy coat cells or triturated skin biopsy specimens are inoculated into shell vials seeded with cell lines such as Vero, L-929, HEL, or MRC5. Infected cells are detected by immunofluorescence or PCR after 48 to 72 h; sensitivity is up to 59%. **Serologic tests:** IFA is sensitive using *R. africae, R. conorii,* or other spotted fever group rickettsial antigens (e.g., *R. rickettsii*) but is low during the acute phase of illness. A fourfold increase in titer is generally considered most specific, but single titers of ≥128 for IgG and ≥32 for IgM are considered diagnostically significant. A Dot EIA test that is modestly less sensitive and specific is available for *R. conorii*.
Rickettsia akari	**Microscopy:** DFA or immunohistochemistry on skin biopsy of rash or eschar is sensitive and specific for spotted fever group rickettsiae. Antibodies are not commercially available. **Antigen tests:** Not available. **Molecular tests:** PCR amplification performed on skin biopsy specimens of eschars obtained during acute phase of illness; available only through reference laboratories. **Culture:** Heparin-anticoagulated blood plasma or buffy coat cells are inoculated into shell vials seeded with cell lines such as Vero, L-929, HEL, or MRC-5. Infected cells are detected by Giemsa, Gimenez, or fluorescent antibody staining after 48 to 72 h. Sensitivity is not known. **Serologic tests:** IFA is sensitive using either *R. akari* or other spotted fever group rickettsial antigens (e.g., *R. rickettsii*) but is low during the acute phase of illness. A fourfold increase in titer is generally considered most specific, but single titers of ≥128 for IgG and ≥32 for IgM are considered diagnostically significant. *R. akari*-specific testing can be obtained in reference or public health laboratories.
Rickettsia felis	**Microscopy:** Not available. **Antigen tests:** Not available. **Molecular tests:** PCR amplification performed on EDTA-anticoagulated blood, buffy coat leukocytes, plasma, or tissue samples obtained during the acute phase of illness; available only through reference laboratories. **Culture:** Not available except through research laboratories. **Serologic tests:** IFA is sensitive using either *R. felis* or other spotted fever or typhus group rickettsial antigens but is low during the acute phase of illness. A fourfold increase in titer is generally considered most specific; diagnostic titers have not been established. *R. felis*-specific testing can be obtained in reference or public health laboratories.
Rickettsia prowazekii	**Microscopy:** Not available. **Antigen tests:** Not available. **Molecular tests:** PCR amplification performed on EDTA-anticoagulated blood, buffy coat leukocytes, plasma, or tissue samples obtained during the acute phase of illness; available only through reference laboratories. **Culture:** Heparin-anticoagulated blood plasma or buffy coat cells are inoculated into shell vials seeded with cell lines such as Vero, L-929, HEL, or MRC-5. Infected cells are detected by Giemsa, Gimenez, or fluorescent-antibody staining after 48 to 72 h. Sensitivity is not known. **Serologic tests:** IFA is sensitive using either *R. prowazekii* or *R. typhi* as antigen. A fourfold increase in titer is generally considered most specific, but single titers of ≥128 for IgG and ≥32 for IgM are considered diagnostically significant.
Rickettsia rickettsii	**Microscopy:** DFA or immunohistochemistry on skin biopsy of rash is 70% sensitive and 100% specific. Antibodies are not commercially available. **Antigen tests:** Not available. **Molecular tests:** PCR amplification performed on EDTA-anticoagulated blood, buffy coat leukocytes, plasma, or tissue samples obtained during the acute phase of illness; available only through reference laboratories. **Culture:** Heparin-anticoagulated blood plasma or buffy coat cells are inoculated into shell vials seeded with cell lines such as Vero, L-929, HEL, or MRC-5. Infected cells are detected by Giemsa, Gimenez, or fluorescent-antibody staining after 48 to 72 h. Sensitivity is not known. **Serologic tests:** IFA is sensitive using *R. rickettsii* or other spotted fever group rickettsial antigens (for example) but is low during the acute phase of illness. A fourfold increase in titer is generally considered most specific, but single titers of ≥128 for IgG and ≥32 for IgM are considered diagnostically significant.
Rickettsia typhi	**Microscopy:** DFA or immunohistochemistry on skin biopsy of rash is sensitive and specific. Antibodies are not commercially available.

(Continued on next page)

TABLE 2 *(Continued)*

Organism	Diagnostic test[a]
	Antigen tests: Not available. **Molecular tests:** PCR amplification performed on EDTA-anticoagulated blood, buffy coat leukocytes, plasma, or tissue samples obtained during the acute phase of illness; available only through reference laboratories. **Culture:** Heparin-anticoagulated blood plasma or buffy coat cells are inoculated into shell vials seeded with cell lines such as Vero, L-929, HEL, or MRC-5. Infected cells are detected by Giemsa, Gimenez, or fluorescent-antibody staining after 48 to 72 h. Sensitivity is not known. **Serologic tests:** IFA is sensitive using either *R. prowazekii* or *R. typhi* as antigen. A fourfold increase in titer is generally considered most specific, but single titers of ≥128 for IgG and ≥32 for IgM are considered diagnostically significant. A Dot EIA test that is modestly less sensitive and specific is available for *R. typhi*.
Tropheryma whipplei	**Microscopy:** Tissue biopsy with periodic acid-Schiff stain or immunohistochemistry. **Antigen tests:** None available. **Molecular tests:** PCR tests are currently the preferred method for specific diagnosis; performed with small intestinal biopsy specimens, blood, cardiac valve tissues; available through reference laboratories. **Culture:** Blood, small intestine tissue, cardiac valves, CSF, aqueous humor, and synovial fluid can be inoculated onto human fibroblast cell culture. Sensitivity of culture is not known, and at least 30 days are required before detection. **Serologic tests:** Not currently available.
Ureaplasma urealyticum	**Microscopy:** May be detected in body fluids using DNA fluorochrome stains (Hoechst 33258 or acridine orange), but these are not specific. **Antigen tests:** None commercially available. **Molecular tests:** PCR tests have been developed but are less useful than culture. **Culture:** Organisms are isolated from a variety of clinical samples. Wood-shafted cotton swabs should be avoided. Ureaplasmas are extremely labile, and appropriate transport medium should be used. Can be recovered on Shepard's 10B urea broth and A8 urea agar. Growth occurs within 2 to 4 days. **Serologic tests:** Not recommended for routine use.

[a]Abbreviations: CF, complement fixation; CIE, counterimmunoelectrophoresis; CSF, cerebrospinal fluid; DFA, direct fluorescent antibody; EIA, enzyme immunoassay; IFA, indirect fluorescent antibody; Ig, immunoglobulin; MIF, microimmunofluorescence; NAAT, nucleic acid amplification tests.

GRAM-POSITIVE COCCI

Staphylococcus, Micrococcus, and Other Catalase-Positive Cocci

TAMMY L. BANNERMAN AND SHARON J. PEACOCK

28

TAXONOMY

Members of the genera *Staphylococcus* and *Micrococcus* are gram-positive, catalase-positive cocci that were placed together with *Stomatococcus* and *Planococcus* in the family *Micrococcaceae* (162). However, the results of DNA base composition testing (155a), DNA-rRNA hybridization (86), and comparative oligonucleotide cataloguing of 16S rRNA (117, 179) indicate that the genera *Staphylococcus* and *Micrococcus* are not closely related. The genus *Staphylococcus* is most closely related to the newly described genus *Macrococcus* (100), but it also has a relatively close relationship to the genera *Bacillus, Brochothrix, Gemella, Listeria,* and *Planococcus*. These genera have been tentatively arranged together with staphylococci and several other genera in the family *Bacillaceae* (22) of the broad *Bacillus-Lactobacillus-Streptococcus* cluster (118, 178) or the order *Bacillales* (22). The genus *Micrococcus* is most closely related to the genus *Arthrobacter* of the coryneform or actinomycete group (177, 179). The genus *Micrococcus* has been dissected into the six genera, *Micrococcus* (comprising the species *Micrococcus luteus*, *Micrococcus lylae*, and *Micrococcus antarcticus*), *Kocuria* (comprising the species formerly known as *Micrococcus roseus, Micrococcus varians,* and *Micrococcus kristinae*), *Kytococcus* (formerly *Micrococcus sedentarius*), *Nesterenkonia* (formerly *Micrococcus halobius*), *Dermacoccus* (formerly *Micrococcus nishinomiyaensis*), and *Arthrobacter* (formerly *Micrococcus agilis*, a member of the "*Arthrobacter globiformis-Arthrobacter citreus* group") (95, 110, 176). The genus *Kocuria* is more closely related to the genus *Rothia* than to other actinomycetes and the genus *Kytococcus* is most closely related to the genus *Dermacoccus* (176). Additional gram-positive, catalase-positive cocci include *Alloiococcus otitis* (1, 49), *Rothia mucilaginosa* (formerly *Stomatococcus mucilaginosus*) (8, 37), and on occasion *Aerococcus* species. *Aerococcus* will be discussed in chapter 31.

DESCRIPTION OF THE GENERA

Members of the genus *Staphylococcus* are gram-positive cocci (0.5 to 1.5 μm in diameter) that occur in irregular grape-like clusters and, less often, singly and in pairs, tetrads, and short chains (three or four cells). They are nonmotile, non-spore forming, and usually catalase positive and are typically unencapsulated or have limited capsule formation under laboratory conditions. The species do not form gas from carbohydrates and are facultative anaerobes with the exception of *Staphylococcus saccharolyticus* and *S. aureus* subsp. *anaerobius*, which initially grow anaerobically but may become more aerotolerant on subculture (Table 1). The genus *Staphylococcus* is currently composed of 37 species (readers are referred to http://www.bacterio.cict.fr/, which provides a list of validly published names of species). Some uncommon strains of staphylococci require the presence of CO_2 or factors such as hemin or menadione for growth. Small-colony variants (SCVs) of *S. aureus* have been described which grow as small, nonpigmented, and nonhemolytic colonies on routine media such as blood agar. SCVs are often auxotrophic for menadione or hemin, have a reduced range of carbohydrate utilization, may fail to express several putative virulence factors, and are resistant to gentamicin owing to poor drug uptake. SCVs are proposed to have a defect in the electron transport chain.

The genome of *S. aureus* has a guanine-plus-cytosine (G+C) content of approximately 32% and is composed of a single chromosome of around 2.8 Mb predicted to carry approximately 2,500 genes. Several sequenced strains also contain a plasmid. Whole genome sequencing is in progress or has been completed for eight *S. aureus* isolates. Published sequences are available for strains N315, Mu50, MW2, COL, MRSA252, and MSSA476 (6, 59, 76, 99); sequencing of strains NCTC 8325 and Michigan vancomycin-resistant *S. aureus* (VRSA) is ongoing. Whole genome sequences have been published for *S. epidermidis* ATCC 12228 and RP62A (59, 206). The whole genome sequence of *S. epidermidis* consists of a single chromosome plus various numbers of plasmids (*S. epidermidis* ATCC 12228 contains six plasmids and strain RP62A contains one) totalling approximately 2.5 Mb. This species has a G+C content of 32% and contains around 2,400 to 2,500 coding sequences. Both *S. epidermidis* genomes contain fewer putative virulence determinants than that of *S. aureus*.

Members of the genus *Micrococcus* are gram-positive cocci (1 to 1.8 μm in diameter) occurring mostly in irregular clusters, tetrads, and pairs. Micrococci and staphylococci have been confused with one another for more than a century on the basis of similar cellular morphologies and Gram-stained appearances and positive catalase activities. Both genera are commonly found on mammalian skin and may be present in various human and veterinary clinical specimens, although micrococci are found less frequently

TABLE 1 Differentiation of members of the genus *Staphylococcus* from other gram-positive cocci[a]

Genus and exceptional species	G+C content (molecular %) of DNA	Strict aerobe	Facultative anaerobe or microaerophile	Strict anaerobe	Tetrad cell arrangement	Strong adherence on agar	Motility	Growth on:					Catalase reaction result[d]	Benzidine test result[e]	Modified oxidase test result[f]	Anaerobic acid production from glucose[g]	Aerobic acid production from glycerol	Resistance to:			
								5% NaCl agar	6.5% NaCl agar	12% NaCl agar	P agar in 18 h[b]	Schleifer-Kramer agar[c]						Lysostaphin (200 μg/ml)	Erythromycin (0.4 μg/ml)	Bacitracin (0.04 U)[h]	Furazolidone (100 μg)[i]
Staphylococcus spp.	30–39	−	*d*	−	*d*	−[j]	−	+	+	*d*	+	+	+	+	−	*d*	+	−	+	+	−
S. aureus subsp. *anaerobius*		−	±	±	−	−	−	+	+	*d*	−	ND	−	−	−	+	+	−	+	ND	−
S. saccharolyticus		−	±	±	+	−	−	+	+	±	−	ND	−	±	−	+	+	−	+	ND	−
S. hominis		±[k]	±	−	+	−	−	+	+	±	+	+	+	+	−	+	+	−	+	+	−
S. auricularis		−	+	−	+	−	−	+	+	±	−	ND	+	+	−	+	+	−	+	+	−
S. saprophyticus, *S. cohnii*, *S. xylosus*		*d*	*d*	−	−	−	−	+	+	±	+	+	+	+	−	−	+	−	+	+	−
S. kloosii, *S. equorum*, *S. arlettae*		±	±	−	−	−	−	+	+	±	*d*	+	+	+	−	−	+	−	+	+	−
S. intermedius		−	+	−	−	−	−	+	+	+	+	±	+	+	−	+	+	−	+	+	−
S. sciuri, *S. lentus*, *S. vitulinus*		±	±	−	*d*	−	−	+	+	*d*	*d*	+	+	+	+	−	+	−	+	+	−
Macrococcus[l]	38–45	±	±	−	*d*	−	−	+	+	±	*d*	ND	+	+	+	−	*d*	−	+	+	−
Enterococcus	34–42	−	+	−	−	−	*d*	+	+	(±)	±	(±)	−	−	−	+	*d*	+	+	+	−
Streptococcus	34–46	−	+	*d*	−	−	−	*d*	*d*	−	−	−	−	−	−	+	*d*	+	−	*d*	−
Aerococcus	35–40	−	+	−	+	−	−	+	+	+	−	ND	−	−	−	(+)	ND	+	ND	−	−
Planococcus	39–52	+	−	−	*d*	−	+	+	+	+	−	ND	+	+	ND	−	−	+	ND	ND	−
Alloiococcus	44–45	+	−	−	−	−	−	+	+	ND	ND	ND	±	−	−	ND	−	ND	ND	ND	ND
R. mucilaginosa	56–60	−	+	−	*d*	+	−	−	−	−	−	ND	±	+	−	+	*d*	+	ND	−	*d*
Micrococcus	66–75	+	−	−	+	−	−	+	+	*d*	−	−	+	+	+	−	−	+	−[m]	−	+
Kocuria kristinae	67	±	±	−	+	−	−	+	+	±	−	(±)	+	+	+	(+)	+	+	−	−	+

[a] Symbols and abbreviations: +, 90% or more species or strains positive; ±, 90% or more species or strains weakly positive; −, 90% or more species or strains negative; *d*, 11 to 89% of species or strains positive; ND, not determined. Parentheses indicate a delayed reaction.

[b] Growth on P agar is under aerobic conditions at 35 to 37°C. Positive growth is indicated for detectable formation of colonies of at least 1 mm in diameter; ± indicates detectable formation of colonies of between 0.5 and 1 mm in diameter. Growth on sheep or bovine blood agar is slightly greater but less discriminative between staphylococci and other genera.

[c] Growth is under aerobic conditions at 35 to 37°C for 24 to 48 h. Positive growth is indicated for a number of CFU on selective medium comparable to that on plate count agar and a colony of 0.5 mm in diameter; ± indicates a significant reduction in the number of CFU on the selective medium compared to that on plate count agar, and parentheses indicate a colony of pinpoint size to 0.5 mm in diameter.

[d] Sometimes a weak catalase or pseudocatalase reaction can be observed with certain strains of species designated as catalase negative. In some species, catalase activity may be activated by hemin supplementation.

[e] Detects the presence of cytochromes. Some strains of benzidine test-negative species can synthesize cytochromes on aerobic media supplemented with hemin (50).

[f] See reference 163.

[g] Standard oxidation/fermentation test (163).

[h] A disk is used. Positive indicates resistance and no zone of inhibition. *Micrococcus, Kocuria, Kytococcus, Stomatococcus*, and *Aerococcus* spp. are susceptible and have an inhibition zone of 10 to 25 mm in diameter.

[i] A disk is used. Positive indicates resistance and no zone of inhibition or a zone of up to 9 mm in diameter. Susceptible species have an inhibition zone of 15 to 35 mm in diameter.

[j] Some strains of *S. epidermidis* adhere tenaciously to the surface of agar, and this property is correlated with heavy slime production.

[k] *S. hominis* does not demonstrate growth in the anaerobic portion of a thioglycolate medium within 24 h and may produce only very poor growth in this portion following 3 to 5 days of incubation. However, it will grow and ferment glucose anaerobically (standard oxidation-fermentation test). Failure to grow anaerobically in thioglycolate may be due in part to inhibition by the ingredients.

[l] *Macrococcus* species can also be differentiated from *Staphylococcus* species on the basis of their generally larger Gram-stained cell size (≥2 μm) and larger number of chromosome fragments produced by digestion with NotI (12 to 36 fragments).

[m] A few *Micrococcus* strains demonstrate high-level (MIC, ≥50 μg/ml) erythromycin resistance.

than staphylococci and are generally regarded as saprophytic rather than as opportunistic pathogens. By the mid-1960s, a clear distinction could be made between staphylococci and micrococci on the basis of DNA base composition (155a). Members of the genus *Staphylococcus* have a G+C content of 30 to 39%, whereas members of the *Micrococcus* and related genera have G+C contents within the range of 66 to 75%. The genus *Micrococcus* is currently composed of three species (110, 176). *Micrococcus luteus* is the most common micrococcal species found in nature and in clinical specimens. In the diagnostic laboratory, staphylococci can be distinguished from micrococci on the basis of the former's resistance to bacitracin and susceptibility to furazolidone. Micrococci are oxidase positive, and staphylococci are oxidase negative, with the exception of *S. lentus*, *S. sciuri*, *S. vitulus*, and *S. fleurettii*. The more distantly related species *Kocuria varians*, *Kocuria kristinae*, and *Kytococcus sedentarius* are occasionally found in clinical specimens and can be distinguished from micrococci on the basis of their cellular fatty acid compositions and results of several simple tests listed below in the section on the identification of *Micrococcus* species.

Alloiococci are aerobic, gram-positive cocci, weakly catalase positive, occurring mostly in clusters and pairs. The G+C content is 44 to 45%. These organisms can be easily distinguished from the aerobic micrococci by their negative oxidase reaction.

R. mucilaginosa is a gram-positive coccus occurring mostly in clusters, is a facultative anaerobe, and is catalase variable. The G+C content is 56 to 60.4%. *R. mucilaginosa* can easily be distinguished from staphylococci and micrococci by its inability to grow on 5% NaCl agar.

Members of the genus *Macrococcus* (including the species *Macrococcus caseolyticus* [formerly *Staphylococcus caseolyticus*], *Macrococcus equipercicus*, *Macrococcus bovicus*, and *Macrococcus carouselicus*) can be distinguished from staphylococci on the basis of their higher G+C contents (38 to 45%), absence of cell wall teichoic acid (with the possible exception of *Macrococcus caseolyticus*), smaller genome size of approximately 1.5 to 1.8 Mb, and larger Gram-stained cell size of 1.3 to 2.5 μm in diameter. They can also be distinguished from most species of staphylococci by their oxidase activity. They are susceptible to a wide range of antibiotics and do not exhibit the antibiotic resistance profiles characteristic of many staphylococcal species. However, like staphylococci, macrococci have a cell wall peptidoglycan that has L-lysine as the diamino acid with an interpeptide bridge that is susceptible to the action of lysostaphin. Since the clinical significance of macrococci has yet to be established and the genus has a rather restricted host range including only whales and related aquatic mammals and hoofed animals, they will not be described further in this chapter.

NATURAL HABITATS

Staphylococci are widespread in nature, their major habitat being the skin and mucous membranes of mammals and birds. They may be found in the mouth, mammary glands, and intestinal, genitourinary, and upper respiratory tracts of these hosts. Staphylococci generally have a benign or symbiotic relationship with their hosts but can become pathogenic after gaining entry into the host tissue through trauma of the cutaneous barrier, inoculation by needles, or direct implantation of medical devices. Staphylococci found on humans and other primates include *S. aureus*, *S. epidermidis*, *S. capitis*, *S. caprae*, *S. saccharolyticus*, *S. warneri*, *S. pasteuri*, *S. haemolyticus*, *S. hominis*, *S. lugdunensis*, *S. schleiferi*, *S. auricularis*, *S. saprophyticus*, *S. cohnii*, *S. xylosus*, and *S. simulans* (88, 141). Most of these species produce resident populations on humans, although *S. xylosus* and *S. simulans* are usually transient residents on humans and are acquired primarily from domestic animals and their products. Some of the human staphylococcal species are transient or temporary residents on domestic animals. *S. aureus* is a major (resident and transient) species for primates, while specific ecovars or biotypes can be found occasionally living on different domestic animals or birds (41, 87). *S. schleiferi*, *S. intermedius*, and *S. felis* are commonly found living on carnivora (141). *S. lutrae* has been isolated from the European otter (53). *S. xylosus*, *S. kloosii*, and *S. sciuri* are common residents on a variety of rodents (141). *S. hyicus*, *S. chromogenes*, *S. sciuri*, *S. lentus*, and *S. vitulus* are common residents of ungulates and, in addition, may be isolated from their food products (42). The last three species are also common residents of whales and related aquatic mammals. Other staphylococci associated with food products include *S. fleurettii*, *S. condimenti*, *S. carnosus*, and *S. piscifermentans* (150, 183, 193). *S. nepalensis* has been isolated from goats of the Himalayas (173), and *S. pseudointermedius* has been isolated from a range of mammals (43).

Some *Staphylococcus* species demonstrate habitat or niche preferences on their particular hosts (88). For example, *S. capitis* subsp. *capitis* is found in large populations on the adult human head, especially the scalp and forehead, where sebaceous glands are numerous and well developed. *S. capitis* subsp. *ureolyticus* is also found on the head but may produce relatively large populations in the axillae of some individuals. *S. auricularis* has a strong preference for the external auditory meatus. *S. hominis* and *S. haemolyticus* generally produce larger populations on areas of the skin where apocrine glands are numerous, such as the axillae and pubic areas (88). *S. aureus* prefers the anterior nares as a habitat (93). The novobiocin-resistant staphylococci, particularly *S. cohnii*, are found in large populations on the human feet. *S. saprophyticus* appears in high numbers in the female genitourinary tract (154).

Micrococci are widespread in nature and are commonly found on the skin of humans and other mammals (91). They are generally believed to be temporary residents and are most frequently found on the exposed skin of the face, arms, hands, and legs. Alloiococci have been isolated from human middle ear fluid (1, 49), and *R. mucilaginosa* is probably a normal inhabitant of the mouth and upper respiratory tract (8).

CLINICAL SIGNIFICANCE

Staphylococcus

S. aureus is an important cause of community-acquired sepsis and is a leading nosocomial pathogen. Disease manifestations can be broadly divided into toxin-mediated diseases (such as food poisoning, scalded skin syndrome, and toxic shock syndrome [TSS]), infection of the skin and soft tissues (furuncles or boils, cellulitis, and impetigo), infection of deep sites (such as bone and joints and the heart valve, spleen, and liver [almost any organ can be involved]), and infection of the lung and urinary tract. An important complication of *S. aureus* bacteremia is dissemination of the organism to one or more distant sites. Additional manifestations of hospital-acquired infection include surgical wound infection, ventilator-associated pneumonia, bacteremia associated with intravenous devices, and infection associated with other types of prosthetic material such as cerebrospinal fluid shunts, prosthetic joints, and vascular grafts.

S. aureus toxin-mediated diseases range in severity from self-limiting to life threatening. TSS is associated with colonization by or infection with a strain of *S. aureus* that is positive for one of the superantigens, most commonly TSS toxin-1 (TSST-1; around 75% of all TSS cases). TSST-1 is a member of a superantigen family that has the ability to stimulate T cells and induce tumor necrosis factor and the cytokine interleukin-1. Gaining notoriety in the 1980s in association with the use of high-absorbancy tampons (45), TSS is now also recognized to occur in nonmenstrual settings including invasive disease and *S. aureus* colonization of sites such as postoperative wounds. Those affected present with severe disease with high fever, hypotension, an erythematous rash that becomes desquamating 1 to 2 weeks later, and involvement of three or more organs (45). Diagnosis is made on clinical grounds. A clinical case definition devised by the Centers for Disease Control and Prevention is useful (26), although not all cases of suspected TSS have sufficient criteria to fulfill this definition. In such cases, circumstantial evidence for the diagnosis includes the isolation of an *S. aureus* strain that is capable of producing TSST-1 or another superantigen (the remainder being positive for staphylococcal enterotoxin B or C). Methods for detecting TSST-1 and enterotoxin production include enzyme-linked immunosorbent assay (128), reverse passive latex agglutination (Oxoid, Ogdensburg, N.Y.), and PCR (7, 125, 129, 164).

Staphylococcal scalded skin syndrome affects primarily neonates and young children and results from the action of *S. aureus* exfoliative toxins on skin epidermidis. Fragile blisters form which rupture and lead to skin loss associated with poor temperature control, fluid loss, and secondary infection (102). Diagnosis is made on the basis of clinical features, including Nikolsky's sign, in which the skin wrinkles on gentle pressure. *S. aureus* may be isolated from a site of localized infection, such as the umbilical stump, but blister fluid is usually culture negative for *S. aureus*.

Staphylococcal food poisoning results from ingestion of preformed staphylococcal enterotoxins (45). Nausea and vomiting occur after an incubation period of 2 and 6 h. Abdominal pain and diarrhea are also common features. Diagnosis is made on clinical grounds; suspected food can be cultured for the presence of *S. aureus*.

S. aureus bacteremia is a major scourge of modern medical care. Around two-thirds of all cases are related to nosocomial infection, much of which is associated with the use of intravenous devices. One of the greatest challenges faced in caring for individuals with *S. aureus* bacteremia is to determine whether the disease is uncomplicated or complicated (that is, associated with bacterial spread to one or more distant sites). A study of clinical identifiers for complicated disease represents significant progress (55). The most common deep-site infections involve bones, joints, and heart valves. Rates of *S. aureus* endocarditis have increased, with the use of intravenous catheters potentially contributing to this rise. A rare but important syndrome of rapidly progressive *S. aureus* necrotizing pneumonia and other invasive diseases affecting previously healthy children and young adults have recently been described (17, 60, 160). The strains responsible were positive for Panton-Valentine leukocidin, and pneumonia was often preceded by influenza-like symptoms. The increase in community-associated methicillin-resistant *S. aureus* (MRSA) infections is further discussed later in "Antimicrobial Susceptibilities."

The role of coagulase-negative staphylococci (CoNS) as nosocomial pathogens has been recognized and well documented over the last 2 decades, especially for the species *S. epidermidis* (147). An increase in the number of infections involving CoNS has paralleled the increasing use of prosthetic and in-dwelling devices and the growing number of immunocompromised patients in hospitals. *S. epidermidis* has been documented as a pathogen in numerous cases of bacteremia; native and prosthetic valve endocarditis; surgical (particularly sternal) wounds, urinary tract, and ophthalmologic infections; and prosthetic joint-, ventricular shunt-, peritoneal dialysis-, and intravascular catheter-related infections (158, 197). *S. saprophyticus* is an important opportunistic pathogen in human urinary tract infections, especially in young, sexually active females. It has been proposed as an agent of nongonococcal urethritis in males and as a cause of other sexually transmitted diseases, prostatitis, wound infections, and septicemia (158). *S. haemolyticus*, the second most frequently encountered CoNS species associated with human infections, has been implicated in native valve endocarditis, septicemia, peritonitis, urinary tract infections, and wound, bone, and joint infections (89, 158). *S. lugdunensis* has been reported as a cause of endocarditis (189). The aggressive nature of *S. lugdunensis* endocarditis, as reflected by the frequent need for valve replacement and the high mortality rate, indicates that rapid recognition of *S. lugdunensis* is needed. *S. lugdunensis* has also been implicated in arthritis, bacteremia, urinary tract infection, and prosthetic material-associated infection (89).

Other CoNS have been implicated in a variety of infections. For example, *S. capitis, S. caprae, S. saccharolyticus, S. simulans,* and *S. warneri* have been implicated in endocarditis; *S. capitis, S. cohnii, S. hominis, S. schleiferi, S. simulans,* and *S. warneri* have been implicated in bacteremia; *S. epidermidis* and *S. haemolyticus* have been implicated in meningitis (79); *S. warneri* and *S. simulans* have been implicated in osteomyelitis; *S. cohnii* has been implicated in native valve endocarditis and pneumonia; *S. cohnii, S. xylosus, S. schleiferi, S. hominis,* and *S. caprae* have been implicated in urinary tract infections; *S. caprae* and *S. cohnii* have been implicated in arthritis; *S. schleiferi* and *S. caprae* have been implicated in wound and joint infections and osteomyelitis (20); *S. warneri* has been implicated in multifocal discitis; and *S. capitis, S. schleiferi,* and *S. warneri* have been implicated in catheter-related infections (89, 158). *S. schleiferi* may cause wound infections in humans and has been implicated in infections related to pacemaker insertion (25, 75). *S. hominis* subsp. *novobiosepticus* has been isolated from human blood cultures and has been associated with clinically significant septicemia (90). *S. sciuri* has been isolated from wounds and from individuals with skin and soft tissue infections (123).

The coagulase-positive species *S. intermedius* and the coagulase-variable species *S. hyicus* are of particular importance in veterinary infections. *S. aureus* and these two coagulase-positive species are serious opportunistic pathogens of animals. *S. intermedius* has been associated with a variety of canine infections including cellulitis, otitis externa, pyoderma, abscesses, reproductive tract infections, mastitis, and wound infections (61). *S. intermedius* infections in humans are usually associated with animal bites. This species has been implicated in a food-poisoning outbreak involving butter blend products (85). *S. hyicus* has been implicated in infectious exudative epidermitis and septic polyarthritis in pigs and mastitis in cows. *S. schleiferi* subsp. *schleiferi* and *S. schleiferi* subsp. *coagulans* have been isolated from dogs with pyoderma, and *S. schleiferi* subsp. *coagulans* has been isolated from dogs with external otitis (81).

Micrococcus, Alloiococcus, and *R. mucilaginosa*

Members of the genus *Micrococcus* and the related coccal genera *Kocuria* and *Kytococcus* are generally harmless saprophytes that inhabit or contaminate the skin, mucosa, and perhaps also the oropharynx; however, they can be opportunistic pathogens for the immunocompromised. *Micrococcus luteus* has been implicated as the causative agent in cases of intracranial abscesses, pneumonia, septic arthritis, endocarditis, and meningitis (165). *Kytococcus sedentarius* has been associated with prosthetic valve endocarditis. Other infections associated with micrococci and their relatives include bacteremia, continuous ambulatory peritoneal dialysis peritonitis, and infection associated with ventricular shunts and central venous catheters (3, 139).

Significant levels of inflammatory cells along with the observation of intracellular *Alloiococcus* led Faden and Dryja to suggest that this organism plays a pathogenic role in persistent otitis media (49). Additional studies employing either culture (65) or PCR (11, 74) support the role of alloiococci in chronic otitis media, but its pathogenic potential should be the subject of further investigation since it has also been found as an inhabitant of the external outer ear in healthy individuals (57).

R. mucilaginosa has been implicated in numerous reports of infection since the mid to late 1980s. This organism has been isolated in cases of bacteremia, endocarditis, endophthalmitis, intravascular catheter-related and central nervous system infections, pneumonia, peritonitis, and septicemia (64, 66, 103) and from a patient with cervical necrotizing fasciitis arising from an infected parotid cyst (116).

PREVENTION OF STAPHYLOCOCCAL INFECTION

There are no licensed vaccines available for the prevention of staphylococcal disease. Data on the efficacy of passive vaccination using hyperimmune antistaphylococcal immunoglobulin for the prevention of staphylococcal disease in high-risk groups have not been published to date. Hospital infection control measures are central to the prevention of nosocomial infection. Guidelines for the prevention of nosocomial transmission of MRSA are available (132). The recommendations continue to include the use of contact precautions for patients colonized by or infected with MRSA but also suggest that hospitals implement a program of active surveillance cultures to identify possible reservoirs in patients at high risk for carriage of MRSA at the time of hospital admission. A full discourse is outside the scope of this chapter; readers are referred to standard texts. Nasal carriage of *S. aureus* has been suggested as a risk factor for the development of infection (196). Infection rates are higher in carriers than in noncarriers, and patients with *S. aureus* sepsis are often infected with their own strain. Multiple studies have been conducted to determine the effect of temporary eradication of *S. aureus* carriage. This is usually achieved by the topical application of mupirocin to the anterior nose. Most studies have been conducted with the dialysis population. Several studies have shown a reduction in the rate of *S. aureus* infection in those receiving hemodialysis (14, 77, 94). Topical mupirocin applied to the peritoneal dialysis catheter exit site reduces *S. aureus* exit site infection and peritonitis (9, 185, 187). The effect of routine decolonization using mupirocin on the rate at which drug resistance will emerge is unclear. A double-blind, placebo-controlled trial of intranasal mupirocin treatment of patients undergoing surgery did not result in a significantly reduced rate of *S. aureus* surgical site infections overall, but the treatment did decrease the rate of all nosocomial *S. aureus* infections among patients who were *S. aureus* carriers (144). An evidence-based review of intranasal mupirocin treatment concluded that this was highly effective at eradication of nasal carriage in the short term, but this did not convert into clinical benefit overall (104). However, this review also reported that subgroup analyses and several small studies revealed lower rates of *S. aureus* infection among selected populations (such as the dialysis population) (104). A systematic review of the effect of mupirocin on rates of *S. aureus* infection in the peritoneal dialysis and hemodialysis populations provided further support for nasal eradication in these patients (182). A Cochrane review of the effects of topical and systemic antimicrobial agents on nasal and extranasal MRSA carriage, adverse events, and the incidence of subsequent MRSA infections concluded that there is insufficient evidence to support the use of topical or systemic antimicrobial therapy for eradicating nasal or extranasal MRSA (112). In summary, the strongest evidence for the efficacy of interrupting nasal *S. aureus* carriage rests with the renal dialysis population; the optimal use of nasal decolonization in other patient groups is less well defined. Despite the use of mupirocin for several decades, little resistance has been observed to date (16, 24, 111, 204). Rectal carriage may represent a reservoir for *S. aureus* for patients in the intensive care unit and liver transplant recipients (174); it is unclear whether nasal decolonization would interrupt gut or rectal carriage.

COLLECTION, TRANSPORT, AND STORAGE OF SPECIMENS

The general principles of collection, transport, and storage of specimens as described in chapters 5, 6, and 20 of this Manual are applicable to the organisms listed in this chapter. No special methods or precautions are usually required for these organisms because they are easily obtained from clinical material of most infection sites and are relatively resistant to drying and to moderate temperature changes. Some strains of staphylococci may require anaerobic conditions or CO_2 supplementation for satisfactory growth, but these survive transport and limited storage in air.

DIRECT EXAMINATION

The direct microscopic examination of normally sterile fluids such as cerebrospinal fluid and joint aspirates may be useful. Direct examination of certain nonsterile fluids may also be useful if the microscopist evaluates the specimen by noting the presence of inflammatory cells versus epithelial cells. Even if large numbers of gram-positive cocci are present, only a presumptive report of "gram-positive cocci resembling staphylococci (or micrococci)" should be made. Culture and appropriate identification techniques must confirm this report; microscopy alone cannot adequately differentiate various species of staphylococci or micrococci from one another or from planococci, some streptococci, aerococci, various anaerobic cocci, and other cocci related to micrococci.

ISOLATION PROCEDURES

Considering the widespread distribution of staphylococci and micrococci over the body surface, careful procedures should be used to isolate organisms from the focus or foci of infection without collecting surrounding normal flora (89). Distinguishing contaminants from the infecting staphylococci and micrococci continues to be an important clinical challenge.

The basic procedures for culture and isolation described in chapter 20 of this Manual should be followed. Every specimen should be plated onto blood agar (preferably sheep blood agar) and other media as indicated. On blood agar, abundant growth of most staphylococcal species occurs within 18 to 24 h, and abundant growth of micrococci occurs within 36 to 48 h. Although most CoNS colony morphologies cannot be distinguished from one another, preliminary identification testing should begin after overnight incubation. Further incubation of the primary isolation plate for 2 to 3 days allows the colony morphology to develop and helps to determine if the culture is mixed or pure. Failure to hold plates for 72 h can result in (i) selection of more than one species or strain if two or more colonies are sampled to produce an inoculum, (ii) selection of an organism(s) not producing the infection if the specimen contains two or more different species or strains, and (iii) incorrect labeling of a mixed culture as a pure culture. Colonies should be Gram stained, subcultured, and tested for genus, species, and when applicable, strain properties. The degree to which staphylococci are identified is discussed in more detail below. Most staphylococci of major medical interest produce growth in the upper as well as the lower anaerobic portions of the thioglycolate broth or semisolid agar.

Specimens from heavily contaminated sources such as feces should be streaked onto a selective medium such as mannitol-salt agar, Columbia colistin-nalidixic acid agar, lipase-salt-mannitol agar (Remel, Lenexa, Kans.), or phenylethyl alcohol agar. These media inhibit the growth of gram-negative organisms but allow staphylococci and certain other gram-positive cocci to grow. In addition, two chromogenic agars, CHROMagar Staph aureus (BD, Sparks, Md.) and *S. aureus* ID (bioMérieux, Hazelwood, Mo.), have been evaluated for their ability to isolate *S. aureus* from clinical specimens (46, 52, 58, 127, 146, 161). CHROMagar Staph aureus medium has been shown to inhibit *Pseudomonas* strains from cystic fibrosis patients as well as provide a better means to recover SCVs.

PCR methodology has been described that can detect MRSA directly from clinical samples. Most reports describe the use of a selective preenrichment step in overnight broth prior to PCR (51, 70, 82). One report described PCR using nasal swab material following an enrichment step for *S. aureus* with the use of immunomagnetic separation (56). Direct PCR has also been applied to a small number of nasal swabs without an enrichment step (80) and to clinical blood culture specimens (140). Detection of *S. aureus* directly from blood cultures using peptide nucleic acid fluorescence in situ hybridization (AdvanDx, Woburn, Mass.) has also been described (33).

IDENTIFICATION

Staphylococcus Species

Laboratory tests that differentiate members of the genus *Staphylococcus* from other gram-positive cocci are listed in Table 1. *Staphylococcus* species can be identified on the basis of a variety of conventional phenotypic characteristics, as shown in Table 2. The most clinically significant species can be identified on the basis of several key characteristics; these are shown in Table 3. In more specialized settings, species can be identified on the basis of molecular constituents such as cellular fatty acids (97) and further identified or characterized using genotypic tests such as analysis of macrorestriction patterns, ribotyping (21), amplification of DNA regions (62, 119, 126, 203), gene sequencing of loci including the 16s RNA gene, *hsp*, *sodA*, and *tuf* (73, 101, 170), and use of a PCR-enzyme-linked immunosorbent assay system (201). Most molecular methods pertaining to species-level identification are confined to the reference or research laboratory. Further discussion of the role of bacterial typing in clinical microbiology and the methods available is provided later in this chapter.

Colony Morphological Appearance

On nonselective blood agar, nutrient agar, tryptic soy agar, or brain heart infusion agar, isolated colonies of most staphylococci are 1 to 3 mm in diameter within 24 h and 3 to 8 mm in diameter after 3 days of incubation in air at 34 to 37°C, depending on the species. Exceptions are *S. aureus* subsp. *anaerobius*, *S. saccharolyticus*, *S. auricularis*, *S. equorum*, *S. vitulus*, and *S. lentus*, which grow more slowly and usually require 24 to 36 h for detectable colony development. Colony morphology can be a useful supplementary characteristic in the identification of species. In order for morphology differences among species to be observed, isolated colonies need to develop for several days at 34 to 37°C (and should be further augmented by 2 days of growth at room temperature).

The typical 24-h *S. aureus* colony is pigmented (cream yellow to orange), smooth, entire, slightly raised, and hemolytic on routine blood agar. Rare strains that produce abundant capsule material may have a glistening, wet appearance. Colonies reach 6 to 8 mm in diameter by 3 days of incubation. SCVs of *S. aureus* may require at least 48 h of incubation to become visible. Colony size is usually about 1/10 that of the wild type, and the colony lacks pigment. SCVs are often auxotrophic for menadione or hemin, have a reduced range of carbohydrate utilization, and are resistant to gentamicin (152). They may be isolated in purity or mixed with colonies with normal morphotypes, giving the appearance of a mixed culture, and may remain stable upon subculture or may rapidly revert to the wild type. They are most commonly isolated from patient populations with unusually persistent infections such as cystic fibrosis or chronic osteomyelitis and/or from patients who have prolonged exposure to aminoglycosides and trimethoprim-sulfamethoxazole (113, 152). Normal growth may be restored if the isolate is grown in the presence of menadione, hemin, and/or CO_2 supplementation (153).

The typical 24-h CoNS colony is nonpigmented, smooth, entire, glistening, slightly raised to convex, and opaque. Rare strong slime producers develop a mucoid colony morphology. Colony diameter reaches 2.5 to 6 mm by 3 days of incubation. Colonies of *S. haemolyticus* are smooth, butyrous, and opaque and are usually larger than those of *S. epidermidis* and *S. hominis*. *S. haemolyticus* and *S. hominis* may be nonpigmented or cream to yellow-orange. Colonies of *S. lugdunensis* are usually 4 to 7 mm in diameter by 3 days of incubation, smooth and glossy and may be nonpigmented or cream to yellow-orange. The edges are entire and rather flat, and the centers are slightly domed. *S. schleiferi* colonies are usually 3 to 5 mm in diameter by 3 days of incubation and are nonpigmented. They are smooth and glossy and are slightly convex, with entire edges. Colonies of *S. saprophyticus* are large (5 to 8 mm in diameter by day 3), entire, very glossy, opaque, smooth, butyrous, and more convex than the colonies of the aforementioned species. Approximately one-half of the strains are pigmented, ranging from cream to yellow-orange. Colonies of *S. intermedius* and *S. hyicus* are relatively large, usually 5 to 8 mm in diameter. They are slightly convex, entire, smooth, glossy, and usually nonpigmented. Colonies of *S. intermedius* are translucent. Those of *S. hyicus* are more opaque, becoming translucent with prolonged incubation.

Colonies of the same strain generally exhibit similar features of size, consistency, edge, profile, luster, and color on nonselective media commonly used for the culture of staphylococci or micrococci. Certain strains may exhibit variant morphotypes, and in these situations, chromosomal analyses can be used to clarify the relationship of each morphotype. At least one colony of each morphotype should be selected from the primary isolation plate for subsequent analyses. Members of the same strain usually have the same biotype profile. However, further differentiation may be necessary if the strain has a common biotype profile.

Coagulase Production

The ability to clot plasma continues to be widely used as a criterion for the identification of pathogenic staphylococci associated with acute infections, i.e., *S. aureus* in humans and animals and *S. intermedius* and *S. hyicus* in animals. This activity is due to the action of coagulase which is secreted during bacterial growth. The test is performed by mixing 0.1 ml of an overnight culture in brain heart infusion broth with 0.5 ml of reconstituted plasma, incubating the mixture at 37°C in a water bath or heat block for 4 h, and observing the tube for clot formation by slowly tilting the tube 90° from the vertical. Alternatively, a large, well-isolated colony on a noninhibitory agar can be transferred into 0.5 ml of reconstituted plasma and incubated as described above. Any degree of clotting constitutes a positive test result. A flocculent or fibrous precipitate is not a true clot and should be recorded as negative. If no clot is formed by 4 h, the tube should be reincubated overnight at 35 to 37°C. Some strains of *S. intermedius* and most coagulase-producing strains of *S. hyicus* require more than 4 h for a positive coagulase test. If incubation exceeds 4 h, the following points must be considered: (i) staphylokinase produced by some strains may lyse the clot after prolonged incubation, yielding false-negative results; (ii) false-positive or false-negative results may occur if the plasma used is not sterile; and (iii) an inoculum from an agar-grown colony may not be pure and a contaminant may produce false results after prolonged incubation. For uncommon *S. aureus* strains requiring a longer clotting period, other characteristics (Table 3) should also be tested to confirm identity. Additional characteristics are required to identify rare coagulase-negative *S. aureus* strains.

Slide Agglutination Test

The slide agglutination test detects bacterial aggregation of *S. aureus* in the presence of plasma through the action of a cell wall-associated protein termed clumping factor A, which is an adhesin for fibrinogen. A positive slide test may also aid in the identification of *S. lugdunensis* and *S. schleiferi* (Table 3). It is performed by making a heavy uniform suspension of growth in distilled water, stirring the mixture to a homogeneous composition so as not to confuse clumping with autoagglutination, adding 1 drop of plasma, and observing for clumping within 10 s. Slide tests must be read quickly because false-positive results may appear with reaction times of longer than 10 s. In addition, colonies for testing must not be picked from media containing high concentrations of salt (e.g., mannitol-salt agar) because autoagglutination and false-positive results may occur. Some uncommon strains of *S. intermedius* may give a positive slide test result. Alternative methods include commercial kits that detect one or more of the following: clumping factor, protein A, and other surface antigens. Latex agglutination tests often have a higher specificity and sensitivity than the conventional slide test for the identification of *S. aureus*, although they are generally less reliable for the identification of *S. lugdunensis*. Some members of the *S. saprophyticus* and *S. sciuri* species groups and *Macrococcus* species may produce positive results with latex agglutination tests, but they are usually negative in the slide test. Due to the low levels of bound coagulase and protein A in MRSA strains, the detection of MRSA by rapid agglutination tests requires the incorporation of antibodies against staphylococcal capsular polysaccharide. Latex agglutination tests that detect both serotype 5 and serotype 8 capsular polysaccharides of methicillin-susceptible *S. aureus* and MRSA strains are available (54); however, false-positive reactions can occur (13, 68, 191). When the test organism is suspected to be *S. aureus*, negative slide tests should be confirmed by the coagulase test. Various manufacturers provide commercial latex agglutination kits, including the Slidex Staph (bioMérieux), BBL Staphyloslide (BD), Staphaurex (Murex Diagnostics Inc., Norcross, Ga.), Staphaurex and Staphaurex Plus (Remel), Mastastaph (Mast, Merseyside, United Kingdom), and Staphytect Plus and Dry Spot Staphytect Plus (Oxoid). A variety of plasmas may be used for the coagulase or slide agglutination tests. Dehydrated rabbit plasma containing EDTA is commercially available. Human plasma should not be used unless it has been tested for clotting capability and lack of infectious agents.

Heat-Stable Nuclease Production

A heat-stable staphylococcal nuclease (thermonuclease [TNase]) that has endo- and exonucleolytic properties and can cleave DNA or RNA is produced by most strains of *S. aureus*, *S. schleiferi*, *S. intermedius*, and *S. hyicus*. Some strains of *S. epidermidis*, *S. simulans*, and *S. carnosus* demonstrate weak TNase activity. TNase can be detected by a metachromatic-agar diffusion procedure and DNA-toluidine blue agar. A commercial TNase test with toluidine blue agar is available (Remel), and results can be interpreted in 4 h. Regular DNase agar such as that used for differentiation of *Enterobacteriaceae* should not be used for TNase detection.

Phosphatase Activity

Detection of phosphatase activity is based on the hydrolysis of *p*-nitrophenylphosphate into phosphate and *p*-nitrophenol by alkaline phosphatase. This process has been incorporated into several commercial biochemical test systems for staphylococcal species identification. Phosphatase activity is indicated by the release of yellow *p*-nitrophenol from the colorless substrate. Strains of *S. aureus*, *S. schleiferi*, *S. intermedius*, and *S. hyicus* and most strains of *S. epidermidis* are alkaline phosphatase positive. Phosphatase-negative strains of *S. epidermidis* can be distinguished from the related species *S. hominis* on the basis of their strong anaerobic growth in thioglycolate within 18 to 24 h or resistance to polymyxin B on a 300-U disk (BD).

Pyrrolidonyl Arylamidase Activity

Pyrrolidonyl arylamidase (pyrrolidonase) activity can be determined by the hydrolysis of pyroglutamyl-ß-naphthylamide (L-pyrrolidonyl-ß-naphthylamide [PYR]) into L-pyrrolidone and ß-naphthylamine, which combines with a PYR reagent (*p*-dimethylaminocinnamaldehyde) to produce a red color.

TABLE 2 Differentiation of *Staphylococcus* species

Species	Characteristic[a]																																			
						Expression of:																		Acid production (aerobically) from:												
	Large colonies[b]	Colony pigmentation[c]	Anaerobic growth[d]	Aerobic growth[e]	Coagulase test result	Clumping factor[f]	Heat-stable nuclease	Hemolysins[g]	Catalase[h]	Oxidase[i]	Alkaline phosphatase	Arginine arylamidase	Pyrrolidonyl arylamidase[j]	Ornithine decarboxylase	Urease[j]	β-Glucosidase[j]	β-Glucuronidase[j]	β-Galactosidase[j]	Arginine utilization[j]	Acetoin production	Nitrate reduction	Esculin hydrolysis	Novobiocin resistance[k]	Polymyxin B resistance[l]	D-Trehalose	D-Mannitol	D-Mannose	D-Turanose	D-Xylose	D-Cellobiose	L-Arabinose	Maltose	α-Lactose	Sucrose	*N*-Acetylglucosamine	Raffinose
S. aureus subsp. *aureus*	+	+	+	+	+	+	+	+	+	−	+	−	−	−	*d*	+	−	−	+	+	+	−	−	+	+	+	+	+	−	−	−	+	+	+	+	−
S. aureus subsp. *anaerobius*	−	−	(+)	(±)	+	−	+	+	−	−	+	ND	ND	ND	ND	−	−	−	ND	−	−	−	−	ND	−	ND	−	ND	−	−	−	+	−	+	−	−
S. epidermidis	−	−	+	+	−	−	−	(*d*)	+	−	+[m]	−	−	(*d*)	+	(*d*)	−	−	*d*	+	+	−	−	+	−	−	(+)	(*d*)	−	−	−	+	*d*	+	−	−
S. capitis subsp. *capitis*	−	−	(+)	+	−	−	−	(*d*)	+	−	−	−	−	−	−	−	−	−	*d*	*d*	*d*	−	−	−	−	+	+	−	−	−	−	−	−	(+)	−	−
S. capitis subsp. *urealyticus*	−	(*d*)	(+)	+	−	−	−	(*d*)	+	−	−	−	(*d*)	−	+	−	−	−	+	*d*	+	−	−	ND	−	+	+	−	−	−	−	+	(*d*)	+	−	−
S. caprae	*d*	−	(+)	+	−	−	−	(*d*)	+	−	(+)	−	*d*	−	+	−	−	−	+	+	+	−	−	−	(+)	*d*	+	−	−	−	−	(*d*)	+	−	−	−
S. saccharolyticus	−	−	+	(±)	−	−	−	−	−	−	*d*	−	ND	ND	ND	ND	ND	ND	+	ND	+	ND	−	ND	−	−	(+)	ND	−	−	−	−	−	−	ND	−
S. warneri	*d*	*d*	+	+	−	−	−	(*d*)	+	−	−	−	−	−	+	+	*d*	−	*d*	+	*d*	−	−	−	+	*d*	−	(*d*)	−	−	−	(+)	*d*	+	−	−
S. pasteuri[n]	*d*	*d*	+	+	−	−	−	(*d*)	+	−	−	−	−	−	+	+	+	−	*d*	*d*	*d*	−	−	ND	+	*d*	−	(*d*)	−	−	−	(*d*)	*d*	+	ND	−
S. haemolyticus	+	*d*	(+)	+	−	−	−	(+)	+	−	−	−	+	−	−	*d*	*d*	−	+	+	+	−	−	−	+	*d*	−	(*d*)	−	−	−	+	*d*	+	+	−
S. hominis subsp. *hominis*	−	*d*	−	+	−	−	−	−	+	−	−	−	−	−	+	−	−	−	*d*	*d*	*d*	−	−	−	*d*	−	−	+	−	−	−	+	*d*	(+)	*d*	−
S. hominis subsp. *novobiosepticus*[o]	−	−	−	+	−	−	−	−	+	−	−	ND	−	−	+	−	−	−	−	*d*	*d*	−	+	ND	−	−	−	ND	−	−	−	+	*d*	(+)	−	−
S. lugdunensis	*d*	*d*	+	+	−	(+)	−	(+)	+	−	−	−	+	+	*d*	+	−	−	−	+	+	−	−	*d*	+	−	+	(*d*)	−	−	−	+	+	+	+	−
S. schleiferi subsp. *schleiferi*	−	−	+	+	−	+	+	(+)	+	−	+	−	+	−	−	−	−	(+)	+	+	+	−	−	−	*d*	−	+	−	−	−	−	−	−	−	(+)	−
S. schleiferi subsp. *coagulans*	*d*	−	+	+	+	−	+	(+)	+	−	+	ND	ND	ND	+	ND	ND	ND	+	+	+	ND	−	ND	−	*d*	+	ND	−	−	−	−	*d*	*d*	ND	−
S. muscae	*d*	−	+	+	−	−	−	(+)	+	−	+	ND	ND	−	−	ND	ND	−	−	−	ND	ND	−	ND	+	−	−	+	+	−	−	−	−	+	ND	−
S. auricularis	−	−	(±)	(+)	−	−	−	−	+	−	−	+	*d*	−	−	−	−	(*d*)	*d*	−	(*d*)	−	−	−	(+)	−	−	(*d*)	−	−	−	(+)	−	*d*	−	−
S. saprophyticus subsp. *saprophyticus*	+	*d*	(+)	+	−	−	−	−	+	−	−	−	−	−	+	*d*	−	+	−	+	−	−	+	−	+	*d*	−	+	−	−	−	+	*d*	+	*d*	−
S. saprophyticus subsp. *bovis*	−	+	+	+	−	−	−	−	+	−	−	−	+	−	+	*d*	−	*d*	−	*d*	+	−	+	ND	+	+	−	+	−	−	−	+	−	+	+	−
S. cohnii subsp. *cohnii*	*d*	−	*d*	+	−	−	−	(*d*)	+	−	−	−	−	−	−	−	−	−	−	*d*	−	−	+	−	+	*d*	(*d*)	−	−	−	−	(*d*)	−	−	−	−

(Continued on next page)

TABLE 2 Differentiation of *Staphylococcus* species *(Continued)*

Species	Characteristic[a]				Expression of:													
	Large colonies[b]	Colony pigmentation[c]	Anaerobic growth[d]	Aerobic growth[e]	Coagulase test result	Clumping factor[f]	Heat-stable nuclease	Hemolysins[g]	Catalase[h]	Oxidase[i]	Alkaline phosphatase	Arginine arylamidase	Pyrrolidonyl arylamidase[j]	Ornithine decarboxylase	Urease[j]	β-Glucosidase[j]	β-Glucuronidase[j]	β-Galactosidase[j]
S. cohnii subsp. *urealyticus*	+	*d*	(+)	+	–	–	–	(*d*)	+	–	+	–	*d*	–	+	–	+	+
S. xylosus	+	*d*	*d*	+	–	–	–	–	+	–	*d*	–	*d*	–	+	+	+	+
S. kloosii	*d*	*d*	–	+	–	–	–	(*d*)	+	–	*d*	–	*d*	–	*d*	*d*	*d*	*d*
S. equorum	–	–	–	(+)	–	–	–	(*d*)	+	–	(+)	–	–	–	+	ND	+	*d*
S. arlettae	*d*	+	–	+	–	–	–	–	+	–	(+)	–	–	–	–	ND	+	*d*
S. gallinarum	+	*d*	(+)	+	–	–	–	(*d*)	+	–	(+)	–	–	–	+	+	*d*	*d*
S. succinus	ND	–	–	+	ND	ND	ND	ND	+	–	+	ND	–	ND	+	ND	ND	ND
S. simulans	+	–	+	+	–	–	–	(*d*)	+	–	(*d*)	–	+	–	+	–	*d*	+
S. carnosus subsp. *carnosus*	+	–	+	+	–	–	–	–	+	–	+	–	+	–	–	–	–	+
S. carnosus subsp. *utilis*	–	–	+	+	–	ND	ND	ND	+	ND	–	ND	ND	ND	–	ND	–	–
S. piscifermentans	ND	*d*	+	+	–	ND	–	–	+	–	+	ND	ND	ND	+	+	–	–
S. condimenti	ND	*d*	+	+	–	ND	ND	ND	+	ND	+	ND	ND	ND	+	ND	–	+
S. felis	+	–	+	+	–	–	–	(*d*)	+	–	+	ND	ND	ND	+	–	–	+
S. lutrae	–	–	+	+	+	–	(±)	+	+	–	+	ND	ND	ND	+	ND	ND	+
S. intermedius	+	–	(+)	+	+	*d*	+	*d*	+	–	+	–	+	–	+	*d*	–	+
S. delphini	+	–	(+)	+	+	–	–	+	+	–	+	ND	ND	ND	+	ND	ND	ND
S. hyicus	+	–	+	+	*d*	–	+	–	+	–	+	–	–	–	*d*	d	+	–
S. chromogenes	+	+	+	+	–	–	–	–	+	–	+	–	*d*	–	+	*d*	–	–
S. sciuri subsp. *sciuri*	+	*d*	(+)	+	–	–	–	(±)	+	+	+	–	–	–	–	+	–	–
S. sciuri subsp. *carnaticus*	–	*d*	(*d*)	+	–	*d*[p]	–	(±)	+	+	*d*	–	–	–	–	+	–	–
S. sciuri subsp. *rodentium*	*d*	*d*	(*d*)	+	–	+[p]	–	(±)	+	+	*d*	–	–	–	–	+	–	–
S. lentus	–	*d*	(±)	(+)	–	–	–	–	+	+	(±)	–	–	–	–	+	–	–
S. fleurettii	–	–	+	+	–	–	–	ND	+	+	*d*	–	–	–	–	ND	–	–
S. nepalensis	–	–	+	+	–	–	–	–	+	–	+	–	+	–	+	ND	+	+
S. pseudointermedius	+	–	ND	+	+	–	+	+	+	ND	+[q]	ND	+	ND	+	+	–	+

Species	Arginine utilization[j]	Acetoin production	Nitrate reduction	Esculin hydrolysis	Novobiocin resistance[k]	Polymyxin B resistance[l]	Acid production (aerobically) from:											
							D-Trehalose	D-Mannitol	D-Mannose	D-Turanose	D-Xylose	D-Cellobiose	L-Arabinose	Maltose	α-Lactose	Sucrose	*N*-Acetylglucosamine	Raffinose
S. cohnii subsp. *urealyticus*	–	*d*	–	–	+	–	+	+	+	–	–	–	–	(+)	+	–	*d*	–
S. xylosus	–	*d*	*d*	*d*	+	–	+	+	+	*d*	+	–	*d*	+	*d*	+	+	–
S. kloosii	–	*d*	–	d	+	–	+	+	–	–	(*d*)	–	*d*	*d*	(*d*)	(±)	–	–
S. equorum	–	–	+	*d*	+	ND	+	+	+	*d*	+	(*d*)	+	*d*	*d*	+	*d*	–
S. arlettae	–	ND	–	–	+	ND	+	+	+	+	+	–	+	+	+	+	–	+
S. gallinarum	–	–	+	+	+	–	+	+	+	+	+	+	+	+	*d*	+	+	+
S. succinus	–	–	–	ND	ND	ND	+	ND	+	ND	ND	ND	ND	ND	+	ND	ND	(*d*)
S. simulans	+	*d*	+	–	–	–	*d*	+	*d*	–	–	–	–	(±)	+	+	+	–
S. carnosus subsp. *carnosus*	+	+	+	–	–	–	*d*	+	+	–	–	–	–	–	*d*	–	ND	–
S. carnosus subsp. *utilis*	+	ND	*d*	–	ND	ND	*d*	–	–	–	ND	–	–	–	–	–	ND	–
S. piscifermentans	+	–	+	+	–	ND	+	*d*	–	–	–	–	–	*d*	*d*	*d*	ND	–
S. condimenti	+	ND	+	–	ND	ND	+	+	+	–	ND	–	–	–	+	±	ND	–
S. felis	+	–	+	ND	–	ND	+	+	+	ND	–	–	–	–	+	*d*	+	–
S. lutrae	–	–	+	ND	–	ND	+	*d*	+	ND	+	ND	ND	+	+	ND	ND	ND
S. intermedius	*d*	–	+	–	–	–	+	(*d*)	+	*d*	–	–	–	(±)	*d*	+	+	–
S. delphini	+	–	+	ND	–	ND	–	(+)	+	ND	–	ND	–	+	+	+	ND	ND
S. hyicus	+	–	+	–	–	+	+	–	+	–	–	–	–	–	+	+	+	–
S. chromogenes	+	–	+	–	–	+	+	*d*	+	*d*	–	–	–	*d*	+	+	*d*	–
S. sciuri subsp. *sciuri*	–	–	+	+	+	–	+	+	(*d*)	(±)	(*d*)	+	*d*	(*d*)	(*d*)	+	–	–
S. sciuri subsp. *carnaticus*	–	–	+	+	+	–	+	+	(*d*)	ND	+	(*d*)	*d*	(*d*)	(*d*)	+	–	–
S. sciuri subsp. *rodentium*	–	–	+	+	+	–	(+)	+	(+)	ND	(*d*)	*d*	(*d*)	(*d*)	–	+	–	–
S. lentus	–	–	+	+	+	–	+	+	(+)	(±)	(±)	+	*d*	*d*	*d*	+	*d*	+
S. fleurettii	–	*d*	+	*d*	+	ND	+	ND	+	+	*d*	–	*d*	+	–	+	ND	–
S. nepalensis	–	–	+	+	+	–	+	+	+	*d*	+	–	+	+	+	+	+	–
S. pseudointermedius	ND	+	+	ND	–	ND	+	(+)	+	(+)	–	–	–	+	+	+	+	–

S. vitulinus	−	+	−	(+)	−	−	−	−	+	+	−	ND	−	−	−	*d*	−	−	−	−	+	*d*	+	ND	(*d*)	+	−	−	*d*	*d*	−	−	−	+	−	−

[a] Symbols and abbreviations (unless otherwise indicated): +, 90% or more strains positive; ±, 90% or more strains weakly positive; −, 90% or more strains negative; *d*, 11 to 89% of strains positive; ND, not determined. Parentheses indicate a delayed reaction.

[b] Positive is defined as a colony diameter of ≥ 6 mm after incubation on P agar at 34 to 35°C for 3 days and at room temperature (ca. 25°C) for an additional 2 days; exceptions are *S. succinus* (4 to 6 mm on tryptic soy agar) and *S. fleuretti* (8 to 12 mm on tryptic soy agar).

[c] Positive is defined by the visual detection of carotenoid pigments (e.g., yellow, yellow-orange, or orange) during colony development at normal incubation or room temperatures. Pigments may be enhanced by the addition of milk, fat, glycerol monoacetate, or soaps to P agar.

[d] Growth is in a semisolid thioglycolate medium. Symbols: +, moderate or heavy growth down the tube within 18 to 24 h; ±, heavier growth in the upper portion of the tube and weaker growth in the lower, anaerobic portion of tube; −, no visible growth within 48 h but very weak diffuse growth or a few scattered, small colonies may be observed in the lower portion of the tube by 72 to 96 h. Parentheses indicate delayed growth appearing within 24 to 72 h, sometimes noted as large, discrete colonies in the lower portion of the tube.

[e] Growth is on P agar or bovine, sheep, or human blood agar at 34 to 37°C. *S. equorum* grows slowly at 35 to 37°C; its optimum growth temperature is 30°C. Anaerobic species *S. saccharolyticus* and *S. aureus* subsp. *anaerobius* grow very slowly in the presence of air. *S. aureus* subsp. *anaerobius* requires the addition of blood, serum, or egg yolk for growth on primary isolation medium. *S. auricularis, S. lentus*, and *S. vitulus* produce just-detectable colonies on P agar in 24 to 36 h, and these colonies remain very small (1 to 2 mm in diameter).

[f] The slide agglutination test using rabbit or human plasma detects the expression of clumping factor. Use human plasma for *S. lugdunensis* and *S. schleiferi*. Latex agglutination is less reliable for the detection of clumping factor in *S. lugdunensis*.

[g] Hemolysis on bovine blood agar. Symbols and abbreviations: +, wide zone of hemolysis within 24 to 36 h; (+), delayed moderate to wide zone of hemolysis within 48 to 72 h; (*d*), no or delayed hemolysis; −, no or only very narrow (1 mm) zone of hemolysis within 72 h. Some strains designated as negative may produce a slight greening or browning of blood agar.

[h] Catalase and cytochrome synthesis cannot be induced in *S. aureus* subsp. *anaerobius* by the addition of H_2O_2 or hemin to the culture medium. Catalase activity can be induced in *S. saccharolyticus* by hemin supplementation. In this species, cytochromes *a* and *b* are present in small quantities.

[i] Determined by the modified oxidase test to detect the presence of cytochrome *c* (50).

[j] Determined primarily by commercial rapid identification tests (see the text).

[k] Positive (resistant) is defined by an MIC of ≥1.6 μg/ml or a growth inhibition zone diameter of ≤16 mm with a 5-μg novobiocin disk.

[l] Positive is defined by a growth inhibition zone diameter of <10 mm with a 300-U polymyxin B disk.

[m] Approximately 6 to 15% of strains of *S. epidermidis* are negative for alkaline phosphatase activity, depending on the population sampled. A low but significant number of clinical isolates are phosphatase negative.

[n] rRNA gene restriction site polymorphism using pBA2 as a probe can distinguish this species from other staphylococcal species, including *S. warneri* (34).

[o] All strains tested are also resistant to penicillin G, methicillin, oxacillin, gentamicin, and streptomycin.

[p] Positive reactions are with the Staph latex agglutination test (Remel) that detects clumping factor and/or protein A.

[q] Positive with the STAPH-ZYM tests but negative with the API STAPH tests (43).

A commercial PYR broth and PYR reagent (Remel) recommended for the identification of streptococci are useful for distinguishing certain staphylococcal species. A loopful of a 24-h agar slant culture or several well-isolated colonies are dispersed in the PYR broth (containing 0.01% PYR) to a turbidity of a 2 McFarland standard. The suspension is incubated at 35°C for 2 h. After incubation, 2 drops of PYR reagent are added to each tube without mixing. The development of red within 2 min is indicative of positive activity. Yellow, orange, or pink is considered a negative result. The basic features of the test have been incorporated into several of the commercial biochemical test panels for the identification of staphylococcal species. *S. haemolyticus, S. lugdunensis, S. schleiferi,* and *S. intermedius* are usually pyrrolidonase positive.

Ornithine Decarboxylase Activity

Positive ornithine decarboxylase activity can identify the species *S. lugdunensis* with considerable accuracy. Ornithine decarboxylase activity can be determined as follows. Decarboxylase basal medium (BD) is prepared according to the instructions of the manufacturer, 1% (wt/vol) L-ornithine dihydrochloride is added, and the final medium is adjusted to pH 6 with 1 N sodium hydroxide before sterilization. The medium is dispensed in 3- to 4-ml amounts into small (13 by 100 mm) screw-cap tubes and autoclaved at 121°C for 10 min. A loopful of an overnight agar slant culture or several well-isolated colonies are dispersed in the test broth, followed by overlaying of each tube with 4 to 5 mm of sterile mineral oil. Inoculated tubes should be incubated at 35 to 37°C for up to 24 h. They can be read initially at as early as 8 h for the positive identification of most strains of *S. lugdunensis;* at this time, *S. epidermidis* will produce negative results. A positive reaction is indicated by alkalinization of the medium, with a change in the initial grayish color or slight yellowing (caused by the initial fermentation of glucose) to violet (caused by decarboxylation of L-ornithine). Yellow at 24 h indicates a negative result.

Urease Activity

Conventional urea broth or agar (BD and Oxoid) can be used to detect urease activity in staphylococcal species. Miniaturization of the broth urease test has been incorporated into several of the commercial biochemical test systems for species-level identification of staphylococci. *S. epidermidis, S. intermedius,* and most strains of *S. saprophyticus* are usually urease positive.

ß-Galactosidase Activity

Detection of high levels of ß-galactosidase activity for the differentiation of certain staphylococcal species can be accomplished by commercial biochemical test systems that use 2-naphthol-ß-D-galactopyranoside as a substrate. Fast blue BB salt in 2-methoxyethanol is added to the test well after an appropriate incubation period to detect free ß-naphthol released by ß-galactosidase. Positive activity is indicated by plum purple. By this assay, *S. intermedius* and most strains of *S. saprophyticus* are ß-galactosidase positive; *S. schleiferi* is delayed or weakly positive.

Acetoin Production

Acetoin production from glucose or pyruvate is a useful alternative characteristic to distinguish *S. aureus* (positive) from another coagulase-positive species, *S. intermedius* (negative), and coagulase-positive strains of *S. hyicus*

TABLE 3 Key tests for identification of the most clinically significant *Staphylococcus* species

Species	Result of test for[a]:								
	Colony pigment-ation[b]	Staphylo-coagulase	Clumping factor[b]	Heat-stable nuclease	Alkaline phosphatase	Pyrrolidonyl arylamidase[b]	Ornithine decarboxylase	Urease[b]	β-Galactosidase[b]
S. aureus subsp. *aureus*	+	+	+	+	+	−	−	*d*	−
S. epidermidis	−	−	−	−	+	−	(*d*)	+	−
S. haemolyticus	*d*	−	−	−	−	+	−	−	−
S. hyicus (veterinary)	−	*d*	−	+	+	−	−	*d*	−
S. intermedius (veterinary)	−	+	*d*	+	+	+	−	+	+
S. lugdunensis	*d*	−	(+)	−	−	+	+	*d*	−
S. schleiferi subsp. *schleiferi*	−	−	+	+	+	+	−	−	(+)
S. saprophyticus subsp. *saprophyticus*	*d*	−	−	−	−	−	−	+	+

[a] Symbols: +, 90% or more species or strains positive; ±, 90% or more species or strains weakly positive; −, 90% or more species or strains negative; *d*, 11 to 89% of species or strains positive. Parentheses indicate a delayed reaction.
[b] Descriptions are the same as those in Table 2.

(negative). The conventional Voges-Proskauer test tube method with an incubation of 72 h may be used. For speed and convenience, acetoin production can be determined by a miniaturized Voges-Proskauer test incorporated into several of the commercial biochemical test systems for staphylococcal species identification.

Novobiocin Resistance

A disk diffusion test for estimating novobiocin susceptibility and distinguishing *S. saprophyticus* from other clinically important species can be performed using a 5-μg novobiocin disk on Mueller-Hinton agar or tryptic soy sheep blood agar. With an inoculum suspension equivalent in turbidity to a 0.5 McFarland opacity standard and incubation at 35 to 37°C for overnight to 24 h, novobiocin resistance is indicated by an inhibition zone diameter of ≤16 mm with any of these media. Rapid disk elution procedures with either manual or automated instrument interpretation have also been reported to predict reliably novobiocin resistance after only 4 to 5 h of incubation (71). Novobiocin resistance is intrinsic to *S. saprophyticus* and several other species (Table 2) but is uncommon in the other clinically important species.

Polymyxin B Resistance

A disk diffusion test to estimate polymyxin B susceptibility using a 300-U polymyxin B disk can be performed on any of the media mentioned above for estimation of novobiocin resistance, although the largest database has been obtained for tryptic soy sheep blood agar. Test conditions are as described above for novobiocin resistance. The 5-μg novobiocin disk and the 300-U polymyxin B disk can be tested on the same inoculated plate. Polymyxin B resistance is indicated by an inhibition zone diameter of <10 mm. *S. aureus, S. epidermidis, S. hyicus*, and *S. chromogenes* are usually resistant. Some strains of *S. lugdunensis* are also resistant.

Acid Production from Carbohydrates

Acid production from carbohydrates can be detected by the agar plate method of Kloos and Schleifer (92). A wide range of individual diagnostic tests can be performed using Diatabs, which are available from Rosco, Taastrup, Denmark. Carbohydrate reactions are also incorporated into several of the commercial biochemical test systems for staphylococcal species identification. These systems use a more acid-sensitive indicator than the bromcresol purple (pH ≤5.2) in the agar plate method. For this and other reasons, results with conventional carbohydrate tests (Tables 2 and 3) may be slightly different from those obtained with rapid commercial biochemical test systems. The production of acid from maltose and sucrose and the absence of acid production from trehalose and mannitol can distinguish *S. epidermidis* from other novobiocin-susceptible species. Some uncommon strains of this species may produce acid from trehalose. These isolates can be distinguished from other species on the basis of phosphatase activity, anaerobic growth in thioglycolate, polymyxin B resistance, colony morphology, and the absence of ornithine decarboxylase and pyrrolidonase activities. Production of acid from trehalose, mannose, maltose, and sucrose and the absence of acid production from mannitol can identify *S. lugdunensis*. *S. schleiferi* produces acid from mannose and sometimes from trehalose but does not produce acid from mannitol, maltose, or sucrose. The production of acid from sucrose and turanose and the absence of acid production from mannose, xylose, cellobiose, arabinose, and raffinose can distinguish *S. saprophyticus* from other novobiocin-resistant species.

Identification of Species by Commercial Biochemical or Nucleic Acid Test Systems

Commercial kit identification systems and automated instruments (see chapter 15) can identify a number of the *Staphylococcus* species with an accuracy of 70 to >90% with relative speed and simplicity. Since their introduction, systems have been improved and expanded to include more species. *S. aureus, S. epidermidis, S. capitis, S. haemolyticus, S. saprophyticus, S. simulans*, and *S. intermedius* are identified reliably by most of the commercial systems now available. For some systems, reliability depends on additional testing as

Result of test for[a]:											
Acetoin production	Novobiocin resistance[b]	Polymyxin B resistance[b]	Acid production (aerobically) from:								
			D-Trehalose	D-Mannitol	D-Mannose	D-Turanose	D-Xylose	D-Cellobiose	Maltose	Sucrose
+	−	+	+	+	+	+	−	−	+	+
+	−	+	−	−	(+)	(d)	−	−	+	+
+	−	−	+	d	−	(d)	−	−	+	+
−	−	+	+	−	+	−	−	−	−	+
−	−	−	+	(d)	+	d	−	−	(±)	+
+	−	d	+	−	+	(d)	−	−	+	+
+	−	−	d	−	+	−	−	−	−	−
+	+	−	+	d	−	+	−	−	+	+

suggested by the manufacturer. This might include determining coagulase, clumping factor, or ornithine decarboxylase activity, anaerobic growth in thioglycolate, or novobiocin resistance. Identification systems now available include the following: RAPIDEC Staph (identification of *S. aureus*, *S. epidermidis*, and *S. saprophyticus*), and API STAPH, VITEK, a fully automated microbiology system that uses a gram-positive identification card, and the more recent Vitek 2 (all from bioMérieux); the MicroScan Pos ID panel (read manually or automatically on MicroScan instrumentation) and the MicroScan Rapid Pos ID panel (read by the WalkAway systems; in addition, the ID panels are available with antimicrobial agents for susceptibility testing [Dade MicroScan, Inc., West Sacramento, Calif.]); the Crystal gram-positive identification system, Crystal rapid gram-positive identification system, Pasco MIC/ID gram-positive panel, and BD Phoenix, an automated identification system (BD); the GP MicroPlate test panel (read manually with the Biolog MicroLog system or automatically with the Biolog MicroStation system; Biolog, Hayward, Calif.); the MIDI Sherlock identification system; microbial identification system that automates microbial identification by combining cellular fatty acid analysis with computerized high-resolution gas chromatography (MIDI, Newark, Del.); and the RiboPrinter microbial characterization system (Qualicon, Inc., Wilmington, Del.), based on ribotype pattern analysis. Rapid identification of the species *S. aureus* can be made using the AccuProbe culture identification test for *S. aureus* (Gen-Probe, Inc., San Diego, Calif.). This test is a DNA probe assay directed against rRNA and is reported to be very accurate (≥95% specificity) (2, 172). Coagulase-negative and slide agglutination test-negative strains of *S. aureus* should be identified correctly by the AccuProbe test. Real-time PCR and melt curve analysis based on amplification of a portion of the 16S rRNA gene are reported to give accurate results for nine common staphylococcal species (including *S. aureus* and *S. epidermidis*) (171).

Micrococcus and Related Species, *Alloiococcus*, and *R. mucilaginosa*

Pigment production and colony morphology may be used as simple tests in the presumptive identification of *Micrococcus* species and other related gram-positive cocci. *Micrococcus lylae* can be distinguished from *Micrococcus luteus* by its cream-white or unpigmented colonies, lack of growth on organic nitrogen agar, and lysozyme resistance. However, a small percentage of *Micrococus luteus* strains produce cream-white colonies. *Micrococcus* species can be distinguished from species of the genus *Kocuria* on the basis of their inability to produce acid, aerobically, from D-glucose and β-D-fructose. Furthermore, the species *Kocuria varians* and *Kocuria rosea* can be distinguished from micrococci by the former species' nitrate reduction and negative or only weak oxidase activity, and *Kocuria kristinae* can be distinguished from micrococci by the former's production of acid, aerobically, from glycerol and D-mannose, production of acetoin, and hydrolysis of esculin. The orange-pigmented species *Dermacoccus nishinomiyaensis* can be distinguished from micrococci by the former's small, pale orange colonies, nitrate reduction, and lack of growth on 7.5% NaCl agar. *Kytococcus sedentarius* differs from other micrococci by being resistant to penicillin and methicillin and exhibiting arginine dihydrolase activity. Colonies of this species may produce a brownish water-soluble pigment and grow more slowly than those of micrococci. *Nesterenkonia halobia* can easily be separated from micrococci because it requires at least 5% NaCl for growth.

Alloiococci form small, alpha-hemolytic colonies on blood agar after 48 h of incubation. Isolates can be distinguished from other similar organisms by their inability to utilize carbohydrates, obligate aerobic nature, and negative oxidase activity. On routine blood agar, colonies of *R. mucilaginosa* are mucoid or sticky, transparent to white, and nonhemolytic and often adhere to the agar. This organism is distinguished from other similar organisms by its inability to grow in the presence of 5% NaCl and its ability to hydrolyze gelatin and esculin.

TYPING SYSTEMS

Typing is used in the clinical setting to investigate the relationship between strains of the same bacterial species associated with a cluster of infections (such as during a suspected outbreak of MRSA infections) or to track the spread of strains such as MRSA strains between units or hospitals. This information is central to the effective functioning of infection control. Typing may also be used for patients with recurrent staphylococcal infections to indicate whether a second episode is due to relapse or recurrence. Identification of the same bacterial species with identical genotype during independent episodes of infection in a given patient has a high probability of representing relapse, although the possibility that a single colonizing strain has caused both infections cannot be excluded.

A wide range of typing techniques have been described, but the most common technique used worldwide is pulsed-field gel electrophoresis (PFGE). This is particularly suitable for the investigation of local outbreaks. It may also be used to compare banding patterns of *S. aureus* between centers, although this has been hampered by a lack of reproducibility both within and between laboratories. Considerable efforts have been made to standardize PFGE methodology for the typing of MRSA (130, 131). Multilocus sequence typing (MLST) is a sequence-based approach that has the advantage of being highly reproducible (48), but it depends on the availability of sequencing facilities, is expensive, and requires highly experienced personnel. Comparison of MLST and PFGE in a microepidemiological setting has demonstrated similar discriminatory abilities (142). Although the use of MLST may become more widespread, it is predominantly a research tool at the present time.

Other typing techniques include ribotyping (186), which can be performed using an automated system such as the RiboPrinter microbial characterization system (Qualicon) (40, 124), and random amplified polymorphic DNA (122, 137, 188). PCR amplification methodology includes analysis of the 16S to 23S rRNA intergenic spacer region (69, 98), restriction digestion or sequencing of *coa* (encoding coagulase) (35, 63, 167), and sequencing of *spa* (encoding protein A) (96, 136). The PCR-based technique termed variable-number tandem repeat analysis has been used to study *S. aureus*. A scheme using five variable-number tandem repeat loci (*sdr, clfA, clfB, ssp,* and *spa*) has been reported to be equivalent to PFGE in terms of discriminatory power and reproducibility (121, 159). GeneChip technology (Affymetrix Inc.) (47) and matrix-assisted laser desorption ionization–time of flight mass spectrometry (10) have been described for the study of *S. aureus* but are currently research tools.

ANTIMICROBIAL SUSCEPTIBILITIES

Staphylococci may be susceptible to a wide range of antimicrobial agents, and testing of a panel of drugs is common. However, the major emphasis in contemporary laboratories is the isolation and identification of MRSA. Methicillin-resistant strains emerged soon after the introduction of methicillin into clinical practice. This was followed from the mid-1970s by outbreaks of MRSA infection in many countries, mostly caused by a single epidemic strain that was transferred between hospitals. The picture of MRSA within the hospital setting is now one of both epidemic and sporadic infection caused by a broader range of strains. In addition to being a nosocomial pathogen, MRSA has become a community pathogen. High-risk groups including intravenous drug users, individuals with a serious underlying disease, those on antimicrobial therapy, and those recently discharged from the hospital accounted for the first reports of MRSA infection in the community (106). Skin and soft tissue infections are the most commonly reported diseases involving community-associated MRSA, particularly in correctional facilities (30), among competitive sports participants (29) and military recruits (207), and in hospital nursery and maternity units (17, 160). Community-associated isolates typically possess the Panton-Valentine leukocidin locus, share a type IV staphylococcal cassette chromosome *mec* (SCC*mec*), and may be categorized into two to three PFGE clonal groups (39, 133, 135, 190). Although the community-associated MRSA isolates typically are susceptible to various antimicrobial classes, sole empiric therapy to treat these infections may prove unsuccessful as resistance to clindamycin and induced resistance to macrolide-lincosamide-streptogramin have been observed (19, 84, 133).

MRSA strains are often heteroresistant to beta-lactam antibiotics in that two subpopulations (one susceptible and the other resistant) coexist within a culture (32). Each cell in the population may carry the genetic information for resistance, but only a small fraction (10^{-8} to 10^{-4}) express the resistant phenotype under in vitro test conditions. The resistant subpopulation usually grows much more slowly than the susceptible subpopulation and may be missed during laboratory testing. The successful detection of heteroresistant strains depends largely on promoting the growth of the resistant subpopulations, which is favored by neutral pH, cooler temperatures (30 to 35°C), the presence of NaCl (2 to 4%), and possibly prolonged incubation (up to 48 h) (18). Cefoxitin disk (30 μg) diffusion is a better indicator of the presence of *mecA*-mediated resistance than the oxacillin disk (149, 192). Detection of oxacillin resistance in staphylococci can be done by the methods recommended by the Clinical and Laboratory Standards Institute (CLSI; formerly the National Committee for Clinical Laboratory Standards [NCCLS]) guidelines (36) and those described in chapters 73 and 74 of this Manual. To increase the accuracy of methicillin susceptibility testing, recent changes in the CLSI guidelines have given *S. lugdunensis* the same MIC breakpoints as *S. aureus* but susceptibility breakpoints separate from those of other CoNS isolates. Difficulties in the differentiation of MRSA isolates from borderline oxacillin-resistant strains of *S. aureus,* which are resistant due to the hyperproduction of beta-lactamase rather than the presence of the *mecA* determinant, may be problematic to many clinical laboratories not routinely utilizing PCR as their standard method of detecting MRSA. However, to date, there have been no reports of treatment failure with penicillinase-resistant penicillins in cases of infection with these organisms.

New chromogenic media, MRSA ID (bioMérieux) and CHROMagar MRSA (BD), have the ability to identify *S. aureus* isolates and differentiate MRSA isolates (44, 72, 145). The application of a cefoxitin disk to CHROMagar Staph aureus and *S. aureus* ID media may be an alternative means to detect MRSA and has the added benefit of preventing growth inhibition of MRSA on the whole agar surface (72).

A signal-amplified, sandwich hybridization kit, EVIGENE MRSA (AdvanDX) (107), is available for the rapid identification of *mecA* from either positive blood cultures or clinical isolates, although it is for research-only use in the United States. Rapid detection of the *mecA* gene product in *S. aureus* is also possible by using a commercial slide latex agglutination test (23, 134, 155). Accurate differentiation of MRSA from borderline oxacillin-resistant *S. aureus* by using a slide latex agglutination test has also been reported (114). Genotypic testing for detecting the presence of *mecA* may be performed using PCR (51, 67, 82, 155, 168, 181). Some investigators include PCR detection of a second gene such as *femA, femB, orfX,* or *sa442* (80, 155, 168) or the *S. aureus*-specific marker gene *nuc* (thereby providing simultaneous identification) (38), and multiplex PCR may be performed to detect several genes associated with resistance to different antibiotic groups (143). A quadriplex PCR targeting the 16S RNA gene (*Staphylococcus* genus specific), *nuc* (*S. aureus* species specific), *mecA*, and *mupA* (a determinant of mupirocin resistance) (205) demonstrates the potential scope of this rapidly developing technology. The use of real-time PCR is increasing and provides the potential for rapid results. The GenoType MRSA test kit (Hain Lifescience, Nehren, Germany) detects *mecA* plus an *S. aureus*-specific sequence by using PCR and reverse hybridization (138). The probe-based Velogene rapid MRSA identification assay (ID Biomedical Corp., Vancouver, Canada) is based on a chimeric probe to detect the *mecA* gene (115). This test is reported to be accurate and has the advantage that it does not rely on PCR technology.

Antimicrobial susceptibility testing of SCVs of *S. aureus* presents a challenge for the clinical microbiology laboratory. Since SCVs have minimal amounts of ATP available and cannot effectively transport aminoglycosides into the cell, resistance to gentamicin and other aminoglycosides can be expected (152). Resistance to trimethoprim-sulfamethoxazole is observed in thymidine auxotrophs (151). The slow growth of SCVs limits the usefulness of antimicrobials directed against the cell wall. No approved method has been developed to determine the susceptibility profiles of SCVs. Susceptibililty profiles have been determined by using the broth or agar dilution MIC method with low levels of auxotroph supplements, disk diffusion under NCCLS guidelines with MH agar supplemented with blood, and the E test (AB Biodisk, Skolna, Sweden) with Mueller-Hinton (MH) agar supplemented with blood (83, 151).

With the increase in methicillin resistance in *Staphylococcus* species, other antibiotics have been used in the treatment of serious infections caused by this group of bacteria. The glycopeptide vancomycin has been regarded as the drug of choice for the treatment of infections due to methicillin-resistant staphylococci. The appearance of vancomycin-intermediate (MICs, 8 to 16 μg/ml) *S. aureus* (VISA), VRSA (MICs, ≥32 μg/ml), and resistant CoNS requires the prudent use of vancomycin (12, 28, 31, 184). The Centers for Disease Control and Prevention have developed a recommended algorithm for testing *S. aureus* with vancomycin (see http://www.cdc.gov/ncidod/hip/vanco/vanco.htm). Automated susceptibility systems and disk diffusion are not reliable means to detect VISA or VRSA. A vancomycin-intermediate or -resistant result for a staphylococcal isolate should be verified by repeating a validated MIC method (broth microdilution reference MIC, agar dilution reference MIC, or the E test), and the organism should be identified (36). Detecting vancomycin-heteroresistant populations of staphylococci appears to be a challenge similar to that of detecting methicillin-heteroresistant populations. Heterogeneous VISA poulations include two populations of cells, the majority of which are susceptible to vancomycin (175). The heteroresistant populations are associated with clinical failure of glycopeptide therapy, and the use of other antimicrobials such as linezolid along with surgical intervention may be necessary to effectively treat the infection (78, 109, 156). An evaluation of methods used to detect staphylococcal isolates with reduced susceptibility to glycopeptides suggests that the E test with an inoculum with a 2.0 McFarland standard on brain heart infusion yields the highest sensitivity and specificity, with values of 88 and 88%, respectively (198). Interim guidelines have been established to prevent and control staphylococcal infections associated with reduced susceptibility to vancomycin (27).

Reviews have summarized the antimicrobial susceptibilities of staphylococcal species to various drugs (105, 141). Multidrug resistance is more frequent in *S. haemolyticus, S. epidermidis, S. hominis,* and *S. aureus* than in other staphylococcal species isolated in the clinical laboratory. Increased levels of resistance to antimicrobial agents used for therapy, including aminoglycosides, glycopeptides, quinolones, tetracyclines, macrolides, lincosamides, and trimethoprim-sulfamethoxazole, make the treatment of multidrug-resistant-staphylococcus infections difficult. Recent reviews provide a summary of a variety of new compounds being investigated or utilized for the therapy of MRSA infections, including daptomycin and linezolid (4, 166). Several studies comparing vancomycin and linezolid therapy indicate that linezolid may give a better outcome for patients with complicated skin and soft tissue infections (108, 199), pneumonia (202), and surgical site infections (200) caused by MRSA. It is important to note that clinical failures have occurred with linezolid (148, 157).

Micrococci appear to be susceptible to most antibiotics. Successful treatment has been accomplished using vancomycin, penicillin, gentamicin, clindamycin, or a combination of these antibiotics (120). Strains of alloiococci show resistance to both erythromycin and trimethoprim-sulfamethoxazole and relative resistance to beta-lactams (15). *R. mucilaginosa* appears to be variable in its antimicrobial susceptiblity (194, 195). The observation that *R. mucilaginosa* exhibits poor to no growth on MH agar and MH agar with sheep blood may make susceptibility testing a challenge for clinical microbiology laboratories.

INTERPRETATION AND REPORTING OF RESULTS

The first critical step when interpreting a culture that is positive for staphylococci is to distinguish between *S. aureus* and other species. The laboratory tests required to reach this point are essential in all cases. It is also important to have an appreciation of the quality of the specimen under consideration. A positive culture taken from a sterile site is relatively straightforward to interpret, but one from a contaminated site cannot be interpreted accurately away from the bedside. Clinical features and the results of other investigations should be taken into account during the interpretative process. There is no replacement for good communication between laboratory staff and primary physicians.

Identification of the causative pathogen represents the "gold standard" for the diagnosis of staphylococcal disease; serological testing lacks specificity and predictive accuracy. Isolation of *S. aureus* from a sterile-site culture (such as aspirated pus, blood, or cerebrospinal fluid) should be considered clinically significant unless there is strong evidence to the contrary. Contamination of high-quality samples by *S. aureus* is rare, and further samples should be taken if there is clinical doubt. Interpreting the isolation of *S. aureus* from specimens contaminated with normal flora requires consideration of setting, clinical features, and recent interventions. For example, interpretation of the significance of *S. aureus* in bronchoalveolar lavage fluid from a ventilated patient will require an evaluation of the features of pneumonia such as fever, raised peripheral white blood count, new pulmonary infiltrates upon chest radiography, increasing oxygen requirements, and increased production of respiratory secretions. Quantitative culture may be helpful, for example, when interpreting a bronchoalveolar lavage or urine sample. Isolation of *S. aureus* from surgical wounds and other sites such as ulcers may represent infection or colonization, and clinical response to the culture should be strongly guided by the presence of features of infection. Colonization alone is an insufficient reason to treat, unless the patient is colonized by MRSA and decolonization is undertaken as part of a specific infection control policy. Susceptibility testing, and in particular the detection of methicillin resistance, should always be carried out following the identification of *S. aureus*.

Interpreting the significance of cultures that are positive for other staphylococcal species is more challenging. It is almost inevitable that samples taken from colonized sites will contain CoNS, and blood samples taken without careful skin cleaning will become contaminated with skin flora. Interpretation of blood cultures positive for CoNS requires knowledge of the presence of prosthetic material in the intravascular compartment, risk factors for true CoNS sepsis such as prematurity or the presence of an immunocompromised immune system, and clinical features of sepsis (the nature of which will vary depending on the clinical scenario). A review of CoNS infections has summarized factors that are helpful in distinguishing between true positive and contaminated cultures taken from a patient with clinical features of infection (89). These include (i) isolation of a strain in pure culture from the infected site or body fluid (most contaminated clinical specimens produce mixed cultures of different strains and/or species; however, some infections may be the consequence of more than one strain or species) and (ii) the repeated isolation of the same strain or combination of strains over the course of the infection. Thus, repeated acquisition of high-quality samples may prove extremely helpful, where clinically possible. If a patient with suspected bacteremia is due to start antibiotics, then independent blood samples may be taken from different sites over a relatively short period of time. The presence of the same CoNS on an intravenous catheter tip and in a blood culture is supportive evidence for intravenous catheter-associated bacteremia. Isolation of CoNS from peritoneal dialysis fluid or cerebrospinal fluid taken from ventricular shunts in a patient suspected of having infection is usually significant. Again, culture of more than one sample may provide helpful confirmation. Cultures of explanted prosthetic material such as pacemakers and joint replacements are often positive for CoNS and may contain mixed flora. When infection is considered likely and treatment is required, each species should be identified and all species should be tested for antimicrobial susceptibilities, after which the choice of therapy may be based on the combined antibiogram. If mixed colony morphology is observed in a potentially significant culture, one or more aged (≥72 h) colonies of a particular morphotype should be isolated from the primary isolation plate for each culture to be identified. The practice of pooling two or more young (24- to 48-h) colonies in the preparation of an inoculum or culture carries the risk of producing a mixed culture, resulting in an erroneous identification and accompanying antibiogram. Selecting only one young colony from a primary isolation plate carries the risk of missing the actual etiologic agent.

Interpretation of other samples will be influenced by sample type. For example, it is recognized that *S. saprophyticus* is a common cause of urinary tract infection, and laboratory tests that distinguish this species are often performed on urine specimens. Colony counts of ≥100,000 CFU/ml in two or more cultures of midstream urine are taken to indicate significant bacteriuria (180), but staphylococci grow relatively slow in urine and lower counts may be significant in the symptomatic patient. Isolation of CoNS from other samples taken from colonized sites rarely represents a clinically significant result. If doubt remains, repeated sampling (if possible, a higher-quality sample) can be performed.

Given the problems of interpreting cultures containing CoNS, it is worthwhile to develop a sampling strategy for complicated patients who probably have a true CoNS infection. This is particularly pertinent when dealing with patients with low-grade infection associated with implanted prosthetic material such as a joint replacement or vascular graft. These patients may require prolonged courses of antibiotics, and optimizing culture techniques may prove crucial to accurate diagnosis, therapy, and cure. As an example, deep-site samples taken by direct visualization from an area of suspected osteomyelitis during an operative procedure, particularly when the lesion communicates with the exterior, should include samples from each anatomical layer or region, and fresh instruments should be used to gather deep-site samples (5).

All CoNS associated with true infection require susceptibility testing. The decision about when to undertake species-level identification of CoNS associated with infection is a matter for debate. It is often helpful to identify to the species level when there are mixed populations (based on colony morphologies) in a clinically significant sample or when samples from different sites or serial samples are positive. The antibiogram is often used as a surrogate marker for the presence of the same or different strains or species, but this is not 100% reliable. It is also prudent to identify organisms from deep-tissue infections and from the bloodstreams of patients with suspected endocarditis, since the identification of *S. lugdunensis* raises the index of suspicion for aggressive disease. However, species-level identification of CoNS rarely leads to an intervention or to changes in therapy, and there is no compelling clinical reason to identify to the species level in many cases. Species-level identification of pathogenic CoNS contributes epidemiological information, but this is probably not sufficient justification to identify all CoNS to the species level in routine diagnostic laboratories. Contaminants do not require susceptibility testing or identification.

REFERENCES

1. **Aguirre, M., and M. D. Collins.** 1992. Phylogenetic analysis of *Alloiococcus otitis* gen. nov., sp. nov., an organism from human middle ear fluid. *Int. J. Syst. Bacteriol.* **42:**79–83.
2. **Allaouchiche, B., H. Meugnier, J. Freney, J. Fleurette, and J. Motin.** 1996. Rapid identification of *Staphylococcus aureus* in bronchoalveolar lavage fluid using a DNA probe (Accuprobe). *Intensive Care Med.* **22:**683–687.
3. **Altuntas, F., O. Yildiz, B. Eser, K. Gundogan, B. Sumerkan, and M. Cetin.** 2004. Catheter-related bacteremia due to *Kocuria rosea* in a patient undergoing peripheral blood stem cell transplantation. *BMC Infect. Dis.* **4:**62.
4. **Anstead, G. M., and A. D. Owens.** 2004. Recent advances in the treatment of infections due to resistant *Staphylococcus aureus*. *Curr. Opin. Infect. Dis.* **17:**549–555.
5. **Atkins, B. L., N. Athanasou, J. J. Deeks, D. W. Crook, H. Simpson, T. E. Peto, P. McLardy-Smith, A. R. Berendt, and the Osiris Collaborative Study Group.** 1998. Prospective evaluation of criteria for microbiological

diagnosis of prosthetic-joint infection at revision arthroplasty. *J. Clin. Microbiol.* **36:**2932–2939.

6. **Baba, T., F. Takeuchi, M. Kuroda, H. Yuzawa, K. Aoki, A. Oguchi, Y Nagai, N. Iwama, K. Asano, T. Naimi, H. Kuroda, L. Cui, K. Yamamoto, and K. Hiramatsu.** 2002. Genome and virulence determinants of high virulence community-acquired MRSA. *Lancet* **359:**1819–1827.
7. **Becker, K., R. Roth, and G. Peters.** 1998. Rapid and specific detection of toxigenic *Staphylococcus aureus:* use of two multiplex PCR enzyme immunoassays for amplification and hybridization of staphylococcal enterotoxin genes, exfoliative toxin genes, and toxic shock syndrome toxin 1 gene. *J. Clin. Microbiol.* **36:**2548–2553.
8. **Bergan, T., and M. Kocur.** 1982. *Stomatococcus mucilaginosus* gen. nov., sp. nov., ep. rev., a member of the family *Micrococcaceae. Int. J. Syst. Bacteriol.* **32:**374–377.
9. **Bernardini, J., B. Piraino, J. Holley, J. R. Johnston, and R. Lutes.** 1996. A randomized trial of *Staphylococcus aureus* prophylaxis in peritoneal dialysis patients: mupirocin calcium ointment 2% applied to the exit site versus cyclic oral rifampin. *Am. J. Kidney Dis.* **27:**695–700.
10. **Bernardo, K., N. Pakulat, M. Macht, O. Krut, H. Seifert, S. Fleer, F. Hunger, and M. Kronke.** 2002. Identification and discrimination of *Staphylococcus aureus* strains using matrix-assisted laser desorption/ionization-time of flight mass spectrometry. *Proteomics* **2:**747–753.
11. **Beswick, A. J., B. Lawley, A. P. Fraise, A. L. Pahor, and N. L. Brown.** 1999. Detection of *Alloiococcus otitis* in mixed bacterial populations from middle-ear effusions of patients with otitis media. *Lancet* **354:**386–389.
12. **Biavasco, F., C. Vignaroli, and P. E. Varaldo.** 2000. Glycopeptide resistance in coagulase-negative staphylococci. *Eur. J. Clin. Microbiol. Infect. Dis.* **19:**403–417.
13. **Blake, J. E., and M. A. Metcalfe.** 2001. A shared noncapsular antigen is responsible for false-positive reactions by *Staphylococcus epidermidis* in commercial agglutination tests for *Staphylococcus aureus*. *J. Clin. Microbiol.* **39:**544–550.
14. **Boelaert, J. R., H. W. Van Landuyt, C. A. Godard, R. F. Daneels, M. L. Schurgers, E. G. Matthys, Y. A. De Baere, D. W. Gheyle, B. Z. Gordts, and L. A. Herwaldt.** 1993. Nasal mupirocin ointment decreases the incidence of *Staphylococcus aureus* bacteraemias in haemodialysis patients. *Nephrol. Dial. Transplant.* **8:**235–239.
15. **Bosley, G. S., A. M. Whitney, J. M. Pruckler, C. W. Moss, M. Daneshvar, T. Sih, and D. F. Talkington.** 1995. Characterization of ear fluid isolates of *Alloiococcus otitidis* from patients with recurrent otitis media. *J. Clin. Microbiol.* **33:**2876–2880.
16. **Bradley, S. F., M. A. Ramsey, T. M. Morton, and C. A. Kauffman.** 1995. Mupirocin resistance: clinical and molecular epidemiology. *Infect. Control Hosp. Epidemiol.* **16:**354–358.
17. **Bratu, S.** 2005. Community-associated methicillin-resistant *Staphylococcus aureus* in hospital nursery and maternity units. *Emerg. Infect. Dis.* **11:**808–813.
18. **Brown, D. F. J.** 2001. Detection of methicillin/oxacillin resistance in staphylococci. *J. Antimicrob. Chemother.* **48** (Suppl. S1)**:**65–70.
19. **Buescher, E. S.** 2005. Community-acquired methicillin-resistant *Staphylococcus aureus* in pediatrics. *Curr. Opin. Pediatr.* **17:**67–70.
20. **Calvo, J., J. L. Hernandez, M. C. Farinas, D. Garcia-Palomo, and J. Aguero.** 2000. Osteomyelitis caused by *Staphylococcus schleiferi* and evidence of misidentification of this *Staphylococcus* species by an automated bacterial identification system. *J. Clin. Microbiol.* **38:**3887–3889.
21. **Carretto, E., D. Barbarini, I. Couto, D. De Vitis, P. Marone, J. Verhoef, H. De Lencastre, and S. Brisse.** 2005. Identification of coagulase-negative staphylococci other than *Staphylococcus epidermidis* by automated ribotyping. *Clin. Microbiol. Infect.* **11:**177–184.
22. **Cato, E. P., and E. Stackebrandt.** 1989. Taxonomy and phylogeny, p. 1–26. *In* N. P. Minton and D. J. Clarke (ed.), *Clostridia*. Plenum Press, New York, N.Y.
23. **Cavassini, M., A. Wenger, K. Jaton, D. S. Blanc, and J. Bille.** 1999. Evaluation of MRSA-Screen, a simple anti-PBP 2a slide latex agglutination kit, for rapid detection of methicillin resistance in *Staphylococcus aureus*. *J. Clin. Microbiol.* **37:**1591–1594.
24. **Cavdar, C., T. Atay, M. Zeybel, A. Celik, A. Ozder, S. Yildiz, Z. Gulay, and T. Camsari.** 2004. Emergence of resistance in staphylococci after long-term mupirocin application in patients on continuous ambulatory peritoneal dialysis. *Adv. Perit. Dial.* **20:**67–70.
25. **Celard, M., F. Vandenesch, H. Darbas, J. Grando, H. Jean-Pierre, G. Kirkorian, and J. Etienne.** 1997. Pacemaker infection caused by *Staphylococcus schleiferi,* a member of the human preaxillary flora: four case reports. *Clin. Infect. Dis.* **24:**1014–1015.
26. **Centers for Disease Control and Prevention.** 1997. Case definitions for infectious conditions under public health surveillance. *Morb. Mortal. Wkly. Rep.* **46:**1–55.
27. **Centers for Disease Control and Prevention.** 1997. Interim guidelines for the prevention and control of staphylococcal infections associated with reduced susceptibility to vancomycin. *Morb. Mortal. Wkly. Rep.* **46:**626–628, 635–636.
28. **Centers for Disease Control and Prevention.** 2002. Vancomycin-resistant *Staphylococcus aureus*—Pennsylvania, 2002. *Morb. Mortal. Wkly. Rep.* **51:**902.
29. **Centers for Disease Control and Prevention.** 2003. Methicillin-resistant *Staphylococcus aureus* infections among competitive sports participants—Colorado, Indiana, Pennsylvania, and Los Angeles County, 2000–2003. *Morb. Mortal. Wkly. Rep.* **52:**793–795.
30. **Centers for Disease Control and Prevention.** 2003. Methicillin-resistant *Staphylococcus aureus* infections in correctional facilities—Georgia, California, and Texas, 2001–2003. *Morb. Mortal. Wkly. Rep.* **52:**992–996.
31. **Centers for Disease Control and Prevention.** 2004. Vancomycin-resistant *Staphylococcus aureus*—New York, 2004. *Morb. Mortal. Wkly. Rep.* **53:**322–323.
32. **Chambers, H. F.** 1988. Methicillin-resistant staphylococci. *Clin. Microbiol. Rev.* **1:**173–186.
33. **Chapin, K., and M. Musgnug.** 2003. Evaluation of three rapid methods for the direct identification of *Staphylococcus aureus* from positive blood cultures. *J. Clin. Microbiol.* **41:**4324–4327.
34. **Chesneau, O., A. Morvan, F. Grimont, H. Labischinski, and N. El Solh.** 1993. *Staphylococcus pasteuri* sp. nov., isolated from human, animal, and food specimens. *Int. J. Syst. Bacteriol.* **43:**237–244.
35. **Chiou, C. S., H. L. Wei, and L. C. Yang.** 2000. Comparison of pulsed–field gel electrophoresis and coagulase gene restriction profile analysis techniques in the molecular typing of *Staphylococcus aureus*. *J. Clin. Microbiol.* **38:**2186–2190.
36. **Clinical and Laboratory Standards Institute.** 2005. *Performance Standards for Antimicrobial Susceptibility Testing.* Document M100-S15. NCCLS, Wayne, Pa.
37. **Collins, M. D., R. A. Hutson, V. Båverud, and E. Falsen.** 2000. Characterization of a *Rothia*-like organism from a mouse: description of *Rothia nasimurium* sp. nov. and reclassification of *Stomatococcus mucilaginosus* as *Rothia mucilaginosa* comb. nov. *Int. J. Syst. Evol. Microbiol.* **50:**1247–1251.
38. **Costa, A. M., I. Kay, and S. Palladino.** 2005. Rapid detection of *mecA* and *nuc* genes in staphylococci by real-time multiplex polymerase chain reaction. *Diagn. Microbiol. Infect. Dis.* **51:**13–17.
39. **Daum, R. S., T. Ito, K. Hiramatsu, F. Hussain, K. Mongkolrattanothai, M. Jamklang, and S. Boyle-Vavra.** 2002. A novel methicillin-resistance cassette in community-acquired methicillin-resistant *Staphylococcus aureus* isolates of diverse genetic backgrounds. *J. Infect. Dis.* **186:**1344–1347.

40. **Deshpande, L. M., T. R. Fritsche, and R. N. Jones.** 2004. Molecular epidemiology of selected multidrug-resistant bacteria: a global report from the SENTRY Antimicrobial Surveillance Program. *Diagn. Microbiol. Infect. Dis.* **49:** 231–236.
41. **Devriese, L. A.** 1984. A simplified scheme for biotyping *Staphylococcus aureus* strains isolated from different animal species. *J. Appl. Bacteriol.* **56:**215–220.
42. **Devriese, L. A.** 1986. Coagulase-negative staphylococci in animals, p. 51–57. *In* P.-A. Mårdh and K. H. Schleifer (ed.), *Coagulase-Negative Staphylococci.* Almqvist & Wiksell International, Stockholm, Sweden.
43. **Devriese, L. A., M. Vancanneyt, M. Baele, M. Vaneechoutte, E. De Graef, C. Snauwaert, I. Cleenwerck, P. Dawyndt, J. Swings, A. Decostere, and F. Haesebrouck.** 2005. *Staphylococcus pseudintermedius* sp. nov., a coagulase-positive species from animals. *Int. J. Syst. Evol. Microbiol.* **55:**1569–1573.
44. **Diederen, B., I. van Duijn, A. van Belkum, P. Willemse, P. van Keulen, and J. Kluytmans.** 2005. Performance of CHROMagar MRSA medium for detection of methicillin-resistant *Staphylococcus aureus. J. Clin. Microbiol.* **43:** 1925–1927.
45. **Dinges, M. M., P. M. Orwin, and P. M. Schlievert.** 2000. Exotoxins of *Staphylococcus aureus. Clin. Microbiol. Rev.* **13:**16–34.
46. **D'Souza, H. A., and E. J. Baron.** 2005. BBL CHROMagar Staph aureus is superior to mannitol salt for detection of *Staphylococcus aureus* in complex mixed infections. *Am. J. Clin. Pathol.* **123:**806–808.
47. **Dunman, P. M., W. Mounts, F. McAleese, F. Immermann, D. Macapagal, E. Marsilio, L. McDougal, F. C. Tenover, P. A. Bradford, P. J. Petersen, S. J. Projan, and E. Murphy.** 2004. Uses of *Staphylococcus aureus* GeneChips in genotyping and genetic composition analysis. *J. Clin. Microbiol.* **42:**4275–4283.
48. **Enright, M. C., N. P. Day, C. E. Davies, S. J. Peacock, and B. G. Spratt.** 2000. Multilocus sequence typing for the characterization of methicillin-resistant and methicillin-susceptible clones of *Staphylococcus aureus. J. Clin. Microbiol.* **38:**1008–1015.
49. **Faden, H., and D. Dryja.** 1989. Recovery of a unique bacterial organism in human middle ear fluid and its possible role in chronic otitis media. *J. Clin. Microbiol.* **27:**2488–2491.
50. **Faller, A., and K. H. Schleifer.** 1981. Modified oxidase and benzidine tests for separation of staphylococci from micrococci. *J. Clin. Microbiol.* **13:**1031–1035.
51. **Fang, H., and G. Hedin.** 2003. Rapid screening and identification of methicillin-resistant *Staphylococcus aureus* from clinical samples by selective-broth and real-time PCR assay. *J. Clin. Microbiol.* **41:**2894–2899.
52. **Flayhart, D., C. Lema, A. Borek, and K. C. Carroll.** 2004. Comparison of the BBL CHROMagar Staph aureus agar medium to conventional media for detection of *Staphylococcus aureus* in respiratory samples. *J. Clin. Microbiol.* **42:**3566–3569.
53. **Foster, G., H. M. Ross, R. A. Hutson, and M. D. Collins.** 1997. *Staphylococcus lutrae* sp. nov., a new coagulase-positive species isolated from otters. *Int. J. Syst. Bacteriol.* **47:**724–726.
54. **Fournier, J.-M., A. Bouvet, D. Mathieu, F. Nato, A. Boutonnier, R. Gerbal, P. Brunengo, C. Saulnier, N. Sagot, B. Slizewicz, and J.-C. Mazie.** 1993. New latex reagent using monoclonal antibodies to capsular polysaccharide for reliable identification of both oxacillin-susceptible and oxacillin-resistant *Staphylococcus aureus. J. Clin. Microbiol.* **31:**1342–1344.
55. **Fowler, V. G., Jr, J. M. Miro, B. Hoen, C. H. Cabell, E. Abrutyn, E. Rubinstein, G. R. Corey, D. Spelman, S. F. Bradley, B. Barsic, P. A. Pappas, K. J. Anstrom, D. Wray, C. Q. Forters, I. Anguera, E. Athan, P. Jones, J. T. van der Meer, T. S. Elliot, D. P. Levine, A. S. Bayer, et al.** 2003. Clinical identifiers of complicated *Staphylococcus aureus* bacteremia. *Arch. Intern. Med.* **163:**2066–2072.
56. **Francois, P., D. Pittet, M. Bento, B. Pepey, P. Vaudaux, D. Lew, and J. Schrenzel.** 2003. Rapid detection of methicillin-resistant *Staphylococcus aureus* directly from sterile or nonsterile clinical samples by a new molecular assay. *J. Clin. Microbiol.* **41:**254–260.
57. **Frank, D. N., G. B. Spiegelman, W. Davis, E. Wagner, E. Lyons, and N. R. Pace.** 2003. Culture-independent molecular analysis of microbial constituents of the healthy human outer ear. *J. Clin. Microbiol.* **41:**295–303.
58. **Gaillot, O., M. Wetsch, N. Fortineau, and P. Berche.** 2000. Evaluation of CHROMagar Staph aureus, a new chromogenic medium, for isolation and presumptive identification of *Staphylococcus aureus* from human clinical specimens. *J. Clin. Microbiol.* **38:**1587–1591.
59. **Gill, S. R., D. E. Fouts, G. L. Archer, E. F. Mongodin, R. T. Deboy, J. Ravel, I. T. Paulsen, J. F. Kolonay, L. Brinkac, M. Beanan, R. J. Dodson, S. C. Daugherty, R. Madupu, S. V. Angiuoli, A. S. Durkin, D. H. Haft, J. Vamathevan, H. Khouri, T. Utterback, C. Lee, G. Dimitrov, L. Jiang, H. Qin, J. Weidman, K. Tran, K. Kang, I. R. Hance, K. E. Nelson, and C. M. Fraser.** 2005. Insights on evolution of virulence and resistance from the complete genome analysis of an early methicillin-resistant *Staphylococcus aureus* strain and a biofilm-producing methicillin-resistant *Staphylococcus epidermidis* strain. *J. Bacteriol.* **87:**2426–2438.
60. **Gillet, Y., B. Issartel, P. Vanhems, J. C. Fournet, G. Lina, M. Bes, F. Vandenesch, Y. Piemont, N. Brousse, D. Floret, and J. Etienne.** 2002. Association between *Staphylococcus aureus* strains carrying gene for Panton-Valentine leukocidin and highly lethal necrotising pneumonia in young immunocompetent patients. *Lancet* **359:**753–759.
61. **Girard, C., and R. Higgins.** 1999. *Staphylococcus intermedius* cellulitis and toxic shock in a dog. *Can. Vet. J.* **40:**501–502.
62. **Goh, S. H., Z. Santucci, W. E. Kloos, M. Faltyn, C. G. George, D. Driedger, and S. M. Hemmingsen.** 1997. Identification of *Staphylococcus* species and subspecies by the chaperonin 60 gene identification method and reverse checkerboard hybridization. *J. Clin. Microbiol.* **35:**3116–3121.
63. **Goh, S. H., S. K. Byrne, J. L. Zhang, and A. W. Chow.** 1992. Molecular typing of *Staphylococcus aureus* on the basis of coagulase gene polymorphisms. *J. Clin. Microbiol.* **30:**1642–1645.
64. **Goldman, M., U. B. Chaudhary, A. Greist, and C. A. Fausel.** 1998. Central nervous system infections due to *Stomatococcus mucilaginosus* in immunocompromised hosts. *Clin. Infect. Dis.* **27:**1241–1246.
65. **Gomez-Hernando, C., C. Toro, M. Gutierrez, A. Enriquez, and M. Baquero.** 1999. Isolation of *Alloiococcus otitidis* from the external ear in children. *Eur. J. Clin. Microbiol. Infect. Dis.* **18:**69–70.
66. **Granlund, M., M. Linderholm, M. Norgren, C. Olofsson, A. Wahlin, and S. E. Holm.** 1996. *Stomatococcus mucilaginosus* septicemia in leukemic patients. *Clin. Microbiol. Infect.* **2:**179–185.
67. **Grisold, A. J., E. Leitner, G. Muhlbauer, E. Marth, and H. H. Kessler.** 2002. Detection of methicillin-resistant *Staphylococcus aureus* and simultaneous confirmation by automated nucleic acid extraction and real-time PCR. *J. Clin. Microbiol.* **40:**2392–2397.
68. **Gupta, H., N. McKinnon, L. Louie, M. Louie, and A. E. Simor.** 1998. Comparison of six rapid agglutination tests for the identification of *Staphylococcus aureus*, including methicillin-resistant strains. *Diagn. Microbiol. Infect. Dis.* **31:**333–336.
69. **Gurtler, V., and H. D. Barrie.** 1995. Typing of *Staphylococcus aureus* strains by PCR-amplification of variable length

16S–23S rDNA spacer regions: characterization of spacer sequences. *Microbiology* **141:**1255–1265.

70. **Hagen, R. M., I. Seegmuller, J. Navai, I. Kappstein, N. Lehn, and T. Miethke.** 2005. Development of a real-time PCR assay for rapid identification of methicillin-resistant *Staphylococcus aureus* from clinical samples. *Int. J. Med. Microbiol.* **295:**77–86.
71. **Harrington, B. J., and J. M. Gaydos.** 1984. Five-hour novobiocin test for differentiation of coagulase-negative staphylococci. *J. Clin. Microbiol.* **19:**279–280.
72. **Hedin, G., and H. Fang.** 2005. Evaluation of two new chromogenic media, CHROMagar MRSA and S. aureus IS, for identifying *Staphylococcus aureus* and screening methicillin-resistant *S. aureus*. *J. Clin. Microbiol.* **43:**4242–4244.
73. **Heikens, E., A. Fleer, A. Paauw, A. Florijn, and A. C. Fluit.** 2005. Comparison of genotypic and phenotypic methods for species-level identification of clinical isolates of coagulase-negative staphylococci. *J. Clin. Microbiol.* **43:**2286–2290.
74. **Hendolin, P. H., U. Karkkainen, T. Himi, A. Markkanen, and J. Ylikoski.** 1999. High incidence of *Alloiococcus otitis* in otitis media with effusion. *Pediatr. Infect. Dis. J.* **18:**860–865.
75. **Hernández, J. L., J. Calvo, R. Sota, J. Agüero, J. D. García-Palomo, and M. C. Fariñas.** 2001. Clinical and microbiological characteristics of 28 patients with *Staphylococcus schleiferi* infection. *Eur. J. Clin. Microbiol. Infect. Dis.* **20:**153–158.
76. **Holden, M. T., E. J. Feil, J. A. Lindsay, S. J. Peacock, N. P. Day, M. C. Enright, T. J. Foster, C. E. Moore, L. Hurst, R. Atkin, A. Barron, N. Bason, S. D. Bentley, C. Chillingworth, T. Chillingworth, C. Churcher, L. Clark, C. Corton, A. Cronin, J. Doggett, L. Dowd, T. Feltwell, Z. Hance, B. Harris, H. Hauser, S. Holroyd, K. Jagels, K. D. James, N. Lennard, A. Line, R. Mayes, S. Moule, K. Mungall, D. Ormond, M. A. Quail, E. Rabbinowitsch, K. Rutherford, M. Sanders, S. Sharp, M. Simmonds, K. Stevens, S. Whitehead, B. G. Barrell, B. G. Spratt, and J. Parkhill.** 2004. Complete genomes of two clinical *Staphylococcus aureus* strains: evidence for the rapid evolution of virulence and drug resistance. *Proc. Natl. Acad. Sci. USA* **101:**9786–9791.
77. **Holton, D. L., L. E. Nicolle, D. Diley, and K. Bernstein.** 1991. Efficacy of mupirocin nasal ointment in eradicating *Staphylococcus aureus* nasal carriage in chronic haemodialysis patients. *J. Hosp. Infect.* **17:**133–137.
78. **Howden, B. P., P. B. Ward, P. G. Charles, T. M. Korman, A. Fuller, P. du Cros, E. E. Grabsch, S. A. Roberts, J. Robson, K. Read, N. Bak, J. Hurley, P. D. Johnson, A. J. Morris, B. C Mayall, and M. L. Grayson.** 2004. Treatment outcomes for serious infections caused by methicillin-resistant *Staphylococcus aureus* with reduced vancomycin susceptibility. *Clin. Infect. Dis.* **38:**521–528.
79. **Huang, C.-R., C.-H. Lu, J.-J. Wu, H.-W. Chang, C.-C. Chien, C.-B. Lei, and W.-N. Chang.** 2005. Coagulase-negative staphylococcal meningitis in adults: clinical characteristics and therapeutic outcomes. *Infection* **33:**56–60.
80. **Huletsky, A., R. Giroux, V. Rossbach, M. Gagnon, M. Vaillancourt, M. Bernier, F. Gagnon, K. Truchon, M. Bastien, F. J. Picard, A. van Belkum, M. Ouellette, P. H. Roy, and M. G. Bergeron.** 2004. New real-time PCR assay for rapid detection of methicillin-resistant *Staphylococcus aureus* directly from specimens containing a mixture of staphylococci. *J. Clin. Microbiol.* **42:**1875–1884.
81. **Igimi, S., E. Takahashi, and T. Mitsuoka.** 1990. *Staphylococcus schleiferi* subsp. *coagulans* subsp. nov., isolated from the external auditory meatus of dogs with external ear otitis. *Int. J. Syst. Bacteriol.* **40:**409–411.
82. **Jonas, D., M. Speck, F. D. Daschner, and H. Grundmann.** 2002. Rapid PCR-based identification of methicillin-resistant *Staphylococcus aureus* from screening swabs. *J. Clin. Microbiol.* **40:**1821–1823.
83. **Kahl, B., H. Herrmann, A. S. Everding, H. G. Koch, K. Becker, E. Harms, R. A. Proctor, and G. Peters.** 1998. Persistent infection with small colony variant strains of *Staphylococcus aureus* in patients with cystic fibrosis. *J. Infect. Dis.* **177:**1023–1029.
84. **Kaplan, S. L., K. G. Hulten, B. E. Gonzalez, W. A. Hammerman, L. Lamberth, J. Versalovic, and E. O. Mason, Jr.** 2005. Three-year surveillance of community-acquired *Staphylococcus aureus* infections in children. *Clin. Infect. Dis.* **40:**1785–1797.
85. **Khambaty, F. M., R. W. Bennet, and D. B. Shah.** 1994. Application of pulsed-field gel electrophoresis to epidemiological characterization of *Staphylococcus intermedius* implicated in a food-related outbreak. *Epidemiol. Infect.* **113:**75–81.
86. **Kilpper, R., U. Buhl, and K. H. Schleifer.** 1980. Nucleic acid homology studies between *Peptococcus saccharolyticus* and various anaerobic and facultative anaerobic Gram-positive cocci. *FEMS Microbiol. Lett.* **8:**205–210.
87. **Kloos, W. E.** 1980. Natural populations of the genus *Staphylococcus*. *Annu. Rev. Microbiol.* **34:**559–592.
88. **Kloos, W. E.** 1986. Ecology of human skin, p. 37–50. *In* P.-A. Mårdh and K. H. Schleifer (ed.), *Coagulase-Negative Staphylococci*. Almqvist & Wiksell International, Stockholm, Sweden.
89. **Kloos, W. E., and T. L. Bannerman.** 1994. Update on clinical significance of coagulase-negative staphylococci. *Clin. Microbiol. Rev.* **7:**117–140.
90. **Kloos, W. E., C. G. George, J. S. Olgiati, L. Van Pelt, M. L. McKinnon, B. L. Zimmer, E. Muller, M. P. Weinstein, and S. Mirrett.** 1998. *Staphylococcus hominis* subsp. *novobiosepticus* subsp. nov., a novel trehalose- and *N*-acetyl-D-glucosamine-negative, novobiocin- and multiple antibiotic-resistant subspecies isolated from human blood cultures. *Int. J. Syst. Bacteriol.* **48:**799–812.
91. **Kloos, W. E., and M. S. Musselwhite.** 1975. Distribution and persistence of *Staphylococcus* and *Micrococcus* species and other aerobic bacteria on human skin. *Appl. Microbiol.* **30:**381–395.
92. **Kloos, W. E., and K. H. Schleifer.** 1975. Isolation and characterization of staphylococci from human skin. II. Descriptions of four new species: *Staphylococcus warneri*, *Staphylococcus capitis*, *Staphylococcus hominis*, and *Staphylococcus simulans*. *Int. J. Syst. Bacteriol.* **25:**62–79.
93. **Klutymans, J., A. van Belkum, and H. Verbrugh.** 1997. Nasal carriage of *Staphylococcus aureus*: epidemiology, underlying mechanisms, and associated risks. *Clin. Microbiol. Rev.* **10:**505–520.
94. **Kluytmans, J. A., M. J. Manders, E. van Bommel, and H. Verbrugh.** 1996. Elimination of nasal carriage of *Staphylococcus aureus* in hemodialysis patients. *Infect. Control Hosp. Epidemiol.* **17:**793–797.
95. **Koch, C., and E. Stackebrandt.** 1995. Reclassification of *Micrococcus agilis* (Ali-Cohen 1889) to *Arthrobacter* as *Arthrobacter agilis* comb. nov. and emendation of the genus *Arthrobacter*. *Int. J. Syst. Bacteriol.* **45:**837–839.
96. **Koreen, L., S. V. Ramaswamy, E. A. Graviss, S. Naidich, J. M. Musser, and B. N. Kreiswirth.** 2004. *spa* typing method for discriminating among *Staphylococcus aureus* isolates: implications for use of a single marker to detect genetic micro- and macrovariation. *J. Clin. Microbiol.* **42:**792–799.
97. **Kotilainen P., P. Huovinen, and E. Eerola.** 1991. Application of gas-liquid chromatographic analysis of cellular fatty acids for species identification and typing of coagulase-negative staphylococci. *J. Clin. Microbiol.* **29:**315–322.
98. **Kumari, D. N., V. Keer, P. M. Hawkey, P. Parnell, N. Joseph, J. F. Richardson, and B. Cookson.** 1997. Comparison and application of ribosome spacer DNA amplicon polymorphisms and pulsed-field gel electrophoresis for differentiation of methicillin-resistant *Staphylococcus aureus* strains. *J. Clin. Microbiol.* **35:**881–885.

99. **Kuroda, M., T. Ohta, I. Uchiyama, T. Baba, H. Yuzawa, I. Kobayashi, L. Cui, A. Oguchi, K. Aoki, Y. Nagai, J. Lian, T. Ito, M. Kanamori, H. Matsumaru, A. Maruyama, H. Murakami, A. Hosoyama, Y. Mizutani-Ui, N. K. Takahashi, T. Sawano, T. Inoue, C. Kaito, K. Sekimizu, H. Hirakawa, S. Kuhara, S. Goto, J. Yabuzaki, M. Kanehisa, A. Yamashita, K. Oshima, K. Furuya, C. Yoshino, T. Shiba, M. Hattori, N. Ogasawara, H. Hayashi, and K. Hiramatsu.** 2001. Whole genome sequencing of methicillin-resistant *Staphylococcus aureus*. *Lancet* **357:**1225–1240.
100. **Kwok, A. Y., and A. W. Chow.** 2003. Phylogenetic study of *Staphylococcus* and *Macrococcus* species based on partial hsp60 gene sequences. *Int. J. Syst. Evol. Microbiol.* **53:**87–92.
101. **Kwok, A. Y. C., S.-C. Su, R. P. Reynolds, S. J. Bay, Y. Av-Gay, N. J. Dovichi, and A. W. Chow.** 1999. Species identification and phylogenetic relationships based on partial HSP60 gene sequences within the genus *Staphylococcus*. *Int. J. Syst. Bacteriol.* **49:**1181–1192.
102. **Ladhani, S., C. L. Joannou, D. P. Lochrie, R. W. Evans, and S. M. Poston.** 1999. Clinical, microbial and biochemical aspects of the exfoliative toxins causing scalded-skin syndrome. *Clin. Microbiol. Rev.* **12:**224–242.
103. **Lambotte, O., T. Debord, C. Soler, and R. Roue.** 1999. Pneumonia due to *Stomatococcus mucilaginosus* in an AIDS patient: case report and literature review. *Clin. Microbiol. Infect.* **5:**112–114.
104. **Laupland, K. B., and J. M. Conly.** 2003. Treatment of *Staphylococcus aureus* colonization and prophylaxis for infection with topical intranasal mupirocin: an evidence-based review. *Clin. Infect. Dis.* **37:**933–938.
105. **Laverdiere, M., K. Weiss, R. Rivest, and J. Delorme.** 1998. Trends in antibiotic resistance of staphylococci over an eight-year period: differences in the emergence of resistance between coagulase-positive and coagulase-negative staphylococci. *Microb. Drug Resist.* **4:**119–122.
106. **Layton, M. C., W. J. Hierholzer, and J. E. Patterson.** 1995. The evolving epidemiology of methicillin-resistant *Staphylococcus aureus* at a university hospital. *Infect. Control Hosp. Epidemiol.* **16:**12–17.
107. **Levi, K., and K. J. Towner.** 2003. Detection of methicillin-resistant *Staphylococcus aureus* (MRSA) in blood with the EVIGENE MRSA detection kit. *J. Clin. Microbiol.* **41:**3890–3892.
108. **Li, J. Z., R. J. Willke, B. E. Rittenhouse, and M. J. Rybak.** 2003. Effect of linezolid versus vancomycin on length of hospital stay in patients with complicated skin and soft tissue infections caused by known or suspected methicillin-resistant staphylococci: results from a randomized clinical trial. *Surg. Infect.* **4:**57–70.
109. **Liu, C., and H. F. Chambers.** 2003. *Staphylococcus aureus* with heterogeneous resistance to vancomycin: epidemiology, clinical significance, and critical assessment of methods. *Antimicrob. Agents Chemother.* **47:**3040–3045.
110. **Liu, H., Y. Xu, Y. Ma, and P. Zhou.** 2000. Characterization of *Micrococcus antarcticus* sp. nov., a psychrophilic bacterium from Antarctica. *Int. J. Syst. Evol. Microbiol.* **50:**715–719.
111. **Lobbedez, T., M. Gardam, H. Dedier, D. Burdzy, M. Chu, S. Izatt, J. M. Bargman, S. V. Jassal, S. Vas, J. Brunton, and D. G. Orepoulos.** 2004. Routine use of mupirocin at the peritoneal catheter exit site and mupirocin resistance: still low after 7 years. *Nephrol. Dial. Transplant.* **19:**3140–3143.
112. **Loeb, M., C. Main, C. Walker-Dilks, and A. Eady.** 2003. Antimicrobial drugs for treating methicillin-resistant *Staphylococcus aureus* colonization. *Cochrane Database Syst. Rev.* [Online.] DOI:10.1002/14651858.CD00340.
113. **Looney, W. J.** 2000. Small-colony variants of *Staphylococcus aureus*. *Br. J. Biomed. Sci.* **57:**317–322.
114. **Louie, L., J. Goodfellow, P. Mathieu, A. Glatt, M. Louie, and A. E. Simor.** 2002. Rapid detection of methicillin-resistant staphylococci from blood culture bottles by using a multiplex PCR assay. *J. Clin. Microbiol.* **40:** 2786–2790.
115. **Louie, L., S. O. Matsumura, E. Choi, M. Louie, and A. E. Simor.** 2000. Evaluation of three rapid methods for detection of methicillin resistance in *Staphylococcus aureus*. *J. Clin. Microbiol.* **38:**2170–2173.
116. **Lowry, T. R., and J. A. Brennan.** 2005. *Stomatococcus mucilaginosis* infection leading to early cervical necrotizing fasciitis. *Otolaryngol. Head Neck Surg.* **132:**658–660.
117. **Ludwig, W., K. H. Schleifer, G. E. Fox, E. Seewaldt, and E. Stackebrandt.** 1981. A phylogenetic analysis of staphylococci, *Peptococcus saccharolyticus* and *Micrococcus mucilaginosus*. *J. Gen. Microbiol.* **125:**357–366.
118. **Ludwig, W., E. Seewaldt, R. Kilpper-Bälz, K. H. Schleifer, L. Magrum, C. R. Woese, G. F. Fox, and E. Stackebrandt.** 1985. The phylogenetic position of *Streptococcus* and *Enterococcus*. *J. Gen. Microbiol.* **131:**543–551.
119. **Maes, N., Y. de Gheldre, R. de Ryck, M. Vaneechoutte, H. Meugnier, J. Etienne, and M. J. Struelens.** 1997. Rapid and accurate identification of *Staphylococcus* species by tRNA intergenic spacer length polymorphism analysis. *J. Clin. Microbiol.* **35:**2477–2481.
120. **Magee, J. T., I. A. Burnett, J. M. Hindmarch, and R. C. Spencer.** 1990. *Micrococcus* and *Stomatococcus* spp. from human infections. *J. Infect.* **16:**67–73.
121. **Malachowa, N., A. Sabat, M. Gniadkowski, J. Krzyszton-Russjan, J. Empel, J. Miedzobrodzki, K. Kosowska-Shick, P. C. Appelbaum, and W. Hryniewicz.** 2005. Comparison of multiple-locus variable-number tandem-repeat analysis with pulsed-field gel electrophoresis, *spa* typing, and multilocus sequence typing for clonal characterization of *Staphylococcus aureus* isolates. *J. Clin. Microbiol.* **43:**3095–3100.
122. **Marquet-Van Der Mee, N., S. Mallet, J. Loulergue, and A. Audurier.** 1995. Typing of *Staphylococcus epidermidis* strains by random amplification of polymorphic DNA. *FEMS Microbiol. Lett.* **128:**39–44.
123. **Marsou, R., M. Bes, M. Boudouma, Y. Brun, H. Meugnier, J. Freney, F. Vandenesch, and J. Etienne.** 1999. Distribution of *Staphylococcus sciuri* subspecies among human clinical specimens, and profile of antibiotic resistance. *Res. Microbiol.* **150:**531–541.
124. **McAleese, F., E. Murphy, T. Babinchak, G. Singh, B. Said-Salim, B. Kreiswirth, P. Dunman, J. O'Connell, S. J. Projan, and P. A. Bradford.** 2005. Use of ribotyping to retrospectively identify methicillin-resistant *Staphylococcus aureus* isolates from phase 3 clinical trials for tigecycline that are genotypically related to community-associated isolates. *Antimicrob. Agents Chemother.* **49:**4521–4529.
125. **Mehrotra, M., G. Wang, and W. M. Johnson.** 2000. Multiplex PCR for detection of genes for *Staphylococcus aureus* enterotoxins, exfoliative toxins, toxic shock syndrome toxin 1, and methicillin resistance. *J. Clin. Microbiol.* **38:**1032–1035.
126. **Mendoza, M., H. Meugnier, M. Bes, J. Etienne, and J. Freney.** 1998. Identification of *Staphylococcus* species by 16S–23S rDNA intergenic spacer PCR analysis. *Int. J. Syst. Bacteriol.* **48:**1049–1055.
127. **Merlino, J., M. Leroi, R. Bradbury, D. Veal, and C. Harbour.** 2000. New chromogenic identification and detection of *Staphylococcus aureus* and methicillin-resistant *S. aureus*. *J. Clin. Microbiol.* **38:**2378–2380.
128. **Miwa, K., M. Fukuyama, R. Sakai, S. Shimizu, N. Ida, M. Endo, and H. Igarashi.** 2000. Sensitive enzyme-linked immunosorbent assays for the detection of bacterial

superantigens and antibodies against them in human plasma. *Microbiol. Immunol.* **44**:519–523.

129. **Monday, S. R., and G. A. Bohach.** 1999. Use of multiplex PCR to detect classical and newly described pyrogenic toxin genes in staphylococcal isolates. *J. Clin. Microbiol.* **37**:3411–3414.
130. **Mulvey, M. R., L. Chui, J. Ismail, L. Louie, C. Murphy, N. Chang, M. Alfa, and the Canadian Committee for the Standardization of Molecular Methods.** 2001. Development of a Canadian standardized protocol for subtyping methicillin-resistant *Staphylococus aureus* by using pulsed-field gel electrophoresis. *J. Clin. Microbiol.* **39**:3481–3489.
131. **Murchan, S., M. E. Kaufmann, A. Deplano, R. de Ryck, M. Struelens, C. E. Zinn, V. Fussing, S. Salmenlinna, J. Vuopio-Varkila, N. El Solh, C. Cuny, W. Witte, P. T. Tassios, N. Legakis, W. van Leeuwen, A. van Belkum, A. Vindel, I. Laconcha, J. Garaizar, S. Haeggman, B. Olsson-Liljequist, U. Ransjo, G. Coombes, and B. Cookson.** 2003. Harmonization of pulsed-field gel electrophoresis protocols for epidemiological typing of strains of methicillin-resistant *Staphylococcus aureus*: a single approach developed by consensus in 10 European laboratories and its application for tracing the spread of related strains. *J. Clin. Microbiol.* **41**:1574–1585.
132. **Muto, C. A., J. A. Jernigan, B. E. Ostrowsky, H. M. Pichet, W. R. Jarvis, J. M. Boyce, and B. M. Farr.** 2003. SHEA guideline for preventing nosocomial transmission of multidrug-resistant strains of *Staphylococcus aureus* and *Enterococcus*. *Infect. Control Hosp. Epidemiol.* **24**:362–386.
133. **Naimi, T. S., K. H. LeDell, K. Como-Sabetti, S. M. Borchardt, D. J. Boxrud, J. Etienne, S. K. Johnson, F. Vandenesch, S. Fridkin, C. O'Boyle, R. N. Danila, and R. Lynfield.** 2003. Comparison of community- and health care-associated methicillin-resistant *Staphylococcus aureus* infection. *JAMA* **290**:2976–2984.
134. **Nakatomi, Y., and J. Sugiyama.** 1998. A rapid latex agglutination assay for the detection of penicillin-binding protein 2′. *Microbiol. Immunol.* **42**:739–743.
135. **Okuma, K., K. Iwakawa, J. D. Turnidge, W. B. Grubb, J. M. Bell, F. G. O'Brien, G. W. Coombs, J. W. Pearman, F. C. Tenover, M. Kapi, C. Tiensasitorn, T. Ito, and K. Hiramatsu.** 2002. Dissemination of new methicillin-resistant *Staphylococcus aureus* clones in the community. *J. Clin. Microbiol.* **40**:4289–4294.
136. **Oliveira, D. C., I. Crisóstomo, I. Santos-Sanches, P. Major, C. R. Alves, M. Aires-de-Sousa, M. K. Thege, and H. de Lencastre.** 2001. Comparison of DNA sequencing of the protein A gene polymorphic region with other molecular typing techniques for typing epidemiologically diverse collections of methicillin-resistant *Staphylococcus aureus*. *J. Clin. Microbiol.* **39**:574–580.
137. **Olmos, A., J. J. Camarena, J. M. Nogueira, J. C. Navarro, J. Risen, and R. Sánchez.** 1998. Application of an optimized and highly discriminatory method based on arbitrarily primed PCR for epidemiologic analysis of methicillin-resistant *Staphylococcus aureus* nosocomial infections. *J. Clin. Microbiol.* **36**:1128–1134.
138. **Otte, K. M., S. Jenners, and H. V. Wulffen.** 2005. Identification of methicillin-resistant *Staphylococcus aureus* (MRSA): comparison of a new molecular genetic test kit (GenoType MRSA) with standard diagnostic methods. *Clin. Lab.* **51**:389–393.
139. **Oudiz, R. J., A. Widlitz, X. J. Beckmann, D. Camanga, J. Alfie, B. H. Brundage, and R. J. Barst.** 2004. *Micrococcus*-associated central venous catheter infection in patients with pulmonary arterial hypertension. *Chest* **126**:90–94.
140. **Palomares, C., M. J. Torres, A. Torres, J. Aznar, and J. C. Palomares.** 2003. Rapid detection and identification of *Staphylococcus aureus* from blood culture specimens using real-time fluorescence PCR. *Diagn. Microbiol. Infect. Dis.* **45**:183–189.
141. **Peacock, S. J.** 2005. *Staphylococcus*, p. 771–832. *In* S. P. Borriello, P. R. Murray, and G. Funke (ed.), *Topley & Wilson's Microbiology and Microbial Infections*, 10th ed. Hodder Arnold, London, United Kingdom.
142. **Peacock, S. J, G. D. I. de Silva, A. Justice, A. Cowland, C. E. Moore, C. G. Winearls, and N. P. Day.** 2002. Comparison of multilocus sequence typing and pulsed-field gel electrophoresis as typing tools for *S. aureus* in a micro-epidemiological setting. *J. Clin. Microbiol.* **40**:3764–3770.
143. **Perez-Roth, E., F. Claverie-Martin, J. Villar, and S. Mendez-Alvarez.** 2001. Multiplex PCR for simultaneous identification of *Staphylococcus aureus* and detection of methicillin and mupirocin resistance. *J. Clin. Microbiol.* **39**:4037–4041.
144. **Perl, T. M., J. J. Cullen, R. P. Wenzel, M. B. Zimmerman, M. A. Pfaller, D. Sheppard, J. Twombley, P. P. French, L. A. Herwaldt, and the Mupirocin and the Risk of *Staphylococcus aureus* Study Team.** 2002. Intranasal mupirocin to prevent postoperative *Staphylococcus aureus* infections. *N. Engl. J. Med.* **346**:1871–1877.
145. **Perry, J. D., A. Davies, L. A. Butterworth, A. L. Hopley, A. Nicholson, and F. K. Gould.** 2004. Development and evaluation of a chromogenic agar medium for methicillin-resistant *Staphylococcus aureus*. *J. Clin. Microbiol.* **42**:4519–4523.
146. **Perry, J. D., C. Rennison, L. A. Butterworth, A. L. Hopley, and F. K. Gould.** 2003. Evaluation of S. aureus ID, a new chromogenic agar medium for detection of *Staphylococcus aureus*. *J. Clin. Microbiol.* **41**:5695–5698.
147. **Pfaller, M. A., and L. A. Herwaldt.** 1988. Laboratory, clinical, and epidemiological aspects of coagulase-negative staphylococci. *Clin. Microbiol. Rev.* **1**:281–299.
148. **Potoski, B. A., J. E. Mangino, and D. A. Goff.** 2002. Clinical failures of linezolid and implications for the clinical microbiology laboratory. *Emerg. Infect. Dis.* **8**:1519–1520.
149. **Pottumarthy, S., T. R. Fritsche, and R. N. Jones.** 2005. Evaluation of alternative disk diffusion methods for detecting *mec*A-mediated oxacillin resistance in an international collection of staphylococci: validation report from SENTRY Antimicrobial Surveillance Program. *Diagn. Microbiol. Infect. Dis.* **51**:57–62.
150. **Probst, A. J., C. Hertel, L. Richter, L. Wassill, W. Ludwig, and W. P. Hammes.** 1998. *Staphylococcus condimenti* sp. nov., from soy sauce mash, and *Staphylococcus carnosus* (Schleifer and Fischer 1982) subsp. *utilis* subsp. nov. *Int. J. Syst. Bacteriol.* **48**:651–658.
151. **Proctor, R. A., B. Kahl, C. von Eiff, P. E. Vandaux, D. P. Lew, and G. Peters.** 1998. Staphylococcal small-colony variants have novel mechanisms for antibiotic resistance. *Clin. Infect. Dis.* **27**(Suppl. 1):S68–S74.
152. **Proctor, R. A., and G. Peters.** 1998. Small colony variants in staphylococcal infections: diagnostic and therapeutic implications. *Clin. Infect. Dis.* **27**:419–423.
153. **Proctor, R. A., P. van Langevelde, M. Kristjansson, J. M. Maslow, and R. D. Arbeit.** 1995. Persistent and relapsing infections associated with small-colony variants of *Staphylococcus aureus*. *Clin. Infect. Dis.* **20**:95–102.
154. **Reuther, J. W. A., and W. C. Noble.** 1993. An ecological niche for *Staphylococcus saprophyticus*. *Microbial Ecol. Health Dis.* **6**:209–212.
155. **Rohrer, M., M. Tschierske, R. Zbinden, and B. Berger-Bächi.** 2001. Improved methods for detection of methicillin-resistant *Staphylococcus aureus*. *Eur. J. Clin. Microbiol. Infect. Dis.* **20**:267–270.

155a. **Rosypal, S., A. Rosypalora, and J. Horejs.** 1966. The classification of micrococci and staphylococci based on their DNA base composition and adansonian analysis. *J. Gen. Microbiol.* **44:**281–292.

156. **Ruef, C.** 2004. Epidemiology and clinical impact of glycopeptide resistance in *Staphylococcus aureus*. *Infection* **32:**315–327.

157. **Ruiz, M. E., I. C. Guerrero, and C. U. Tuazon.** 2002. Endocarditis caused by methicillin-resistant *Staphylococcus aureus:* treatment failure with linezolid. *Clin. Infect. Dis.* **35:**1018–1020.

158. **Rupp, M. E., and G. L. Archer.** 1994. Coagulase-negative staphylococci: pathogens associated with medical progress. *Clin. Infect. Dis.* **19:**231–245.

159. **Sabat, A., J. Krzyszton-Russjan, W. Strzalka, R. Filipek, K. Kosowska, W. Hryniewicz, J. Travis, and J. Potempa.** 2003. New method for typing *Staphylococcus aureus* strains: multiple-locus variable-number tandem repeat analysis of polymorphism and genetic relationships of clinical isolates. *J. Clin. Microbiol.* **41:**1801–1804.

160. **Saiman, L., M. O'Keefe, P. L. Graham, F. Wu, B. Said-Salim, B. Kreiswirth, A. LaSala, P. M. Schlievert, and P. Della-Latta.** 2003. Hospital transmission of community-acquired methicillin-resistant *Staphylooccus aureus* among postpartum women. *Clin. Infect. Dis.* **37:**1313–1319.

161. **Samra, Z., O. Ofir, and J. Bahar.** 2004. Optimal detection of *Staphylococcus aureus* from clinical specimens using a new chromogenic medium. *Diagn. Microbiol. Infect. Dis.* **49:**243–247.

162. **Schleifer, K. H.** 1986. Gram-positive cocci, p. 999–1002. *In* J. G. Holt, P. H. A. Sneath, N. S. Mair, and M. S. Sharpe (ed.), *Bergey's Manual of Systematic Bacteriology*, vol. 2. The Williams & Wilkins Co., Baltimore, Md.

163. **Schleifer, K. H.** 1986. Taxonomy of coagulase-negative staphylococci, p. 11–26. *In* P.-A. Mårdh and K. H. Schleifer (ed.), *Coagulase-Negative Staphylococci*. Almqvist & Wiksell International, Stockholm, Sweden.

164. **Schmitz, F. J., M. Steiert, B. Hofmann, J. Verhoef, U. Hadding, H. P. Heinz, and K. Kohrer.** 1998. Development of a multiplex-PCR for direct detection of the genes for enterotoxin B and C, and toxic shock syndrome toxin-1 in *Staphylococcus aureus* isolates. *J. Med. Microbiol.* **47:**335–340.

165. **Seifert, H., M. Kaltheuner, and F. Perdreau-Remington.** 1995. *Micrococcus luteus* endocarditis: case report and review of literature. *Zentbl. Bakteriol.* **282:**431–435.

166. **Shah, P. M.** 2005. The need for new therapeutic agents: what is in the pipeline? *Clin. Microbiol. Infect.* **3**(Suppl.)**:** 36–42.

167. **Shopsin, B., M. Gomez, M. Waddington, M. Riehman, and B. N. Kreiswirth.** 2000. Use of coagulase gene *(coa)* repeat region nucleotide sequences for typing of methicillin-resistant *Staphylococcus aureus* strains. *J. Clin. Microbiol.* **38:**3453–3456.

168. **Shrestha, N. K., M. J. Tuohy, G. S. Hall, C. M. Isada, and G. W. Procop.** 2002. Rapid identification of *Staphylococcus aureus* and the *mecA* gene from BacT/ALERT blood culture bottles by using the Lightcycler systems. *J. Clin. Microbiol.* **40:**2659–2661.

169. Reference deleted.

170. **Sivadon, V., M. Rottman, J. C. Quincampoix, V. Avettand, S. Chaverot, P. de Mazancourt, P. Trieu-Cuot, and J. L. Gaillard.** 2004. Use of *sodA* sequencing for the identification of clinical isolates of coagulase-negative staphylococci. *Clin. Microbiol. Infect.* **10:**939–942.

171. **Skow, A., K. A. Mangold, M. Tajuddin, A. Huntington, B. Fritz, R. B. Thomson, Jr., and K. L. Kaul.** 2005. Species-level identification of staphylococcal isolates by real-time PCR and melt curve analysis. *J. Clin. Microbiol.* **43:**2876–2880.

172. **Skulnick, M., A. E. Simor, M. P. Patel, H. E. Simpson, K. J. O'Quinn, D. E. Low, and A. M. Phillips.** 1994. Evaluation of three methods for the rapid identification of *Staphylococcus aureus* in blood cultures. *Diagn. Microbiol. Infect. Dis.* **19:**5–8.

173. **Spergser, J., M. Wieser, M. Taubel, R. A. Rossello-Mora, R. Rosengarten, and H. J. Busse.** 2003. *Staphylococcus nepalensis* sp. nov., isolated from goats of the Himalayan region. *Int. J. Syst. Evol. Microbiol.* **53:**2007–2011.

174. **Squier, C., J. D. Rihs, A. Sagnimeni, M. M. Wagener, J. Stout, R. R. Muder, and N. Singh.** 2002. *Staphylococcus aureus* rectal carriage and its association with infections in patients in a surgical intensive care unit and a liver transplant unit. *Infect. Control Hosp. Epidemiol.* **23:**495–501.

175. **Srinivasan, A., J. D. Dick, and T. M. Perl.** 2002. Vancomycin resistance in staphylococci. *Clin. Microbiol. Rev.* **15:**430–438.

176. **Stackebrandt, E., C. Koch, O. Gvozdiak, and P. Schumann.** 1995. Taxonomic dissection of the genus *Micrococcus*: *Kocuria*, gen. nov., *Nesterenkonia* gen. nov., *Kytococcus* gen. nov., *Dermacoccus* gen. nov., and *Micrococcus* Cohn 1872 gen. emend. *Int. J. Syst. Bacteriol.* **45:**682–692.

177. **Stackebrandt, E., B. J. Lewis, and C. R. Woese.** 1980. The phylogenetic structure of the coryneform group of bacteria. *Zentbl. Bakteriol. Parasitenkd. Infektkrankh. Hyg. Abt. 1 Orig. Reihe C* **2:**137–149.

178. **Stackebrandt, E., and M. Teuber.** 1988. Molecular taxonomy and phylogenetic position of lactic acid bacteria. *Biochimie* **70:**317–324.

179. **Stackebrandt, E., and C. R. Woese.** 1979. A phylogenetic dissection of the family *Micrococcaceae*. *Curr. Microbiol.* **2:**317–322.

180. **Stamm, W. E.** 1988. Protocol for diagnosis of urinary tract infection: reconsidering the criterion for significant bacteriuria. *Urology* **32**(Suppl.)**:**6–10.

181. **Swenson, J. M., P. P. Williams, G. Killgore, C. M. O'Hara, and F. C. Tenover.** 2001. Performance of eight methods, including two new rapid methods, for detection of oxacillin resistance in a challenge set of *Staphylococcus aureus* organisms. *J. Clin. Microbiol.* **39:**3785–3788.

182. **Tacconelli, E., Y. Carmeli, A. Aizer, G. Ferreira, M. G. Foreman, and E. M. D'Agata.** 2003. Mupirocin prophylaxis to prevent *Staphylococcus aureus* infection in patients undergoing dialysis: a meta-analysis. *Clin. Infect. Dis.* **37:**1629–1638.

183. **Tanasupawat, S., Y. Hasimoto, T. Ezaki, M. Kozaki, and K. Komagata.** 1992. *Staphylococcus piscifermentans* sp. nov., from fermented fish in Thailand. *Int. J. Syst. Bacteriol.* **42:**577–581.

184. **Tenover, F. C., J. W. Biddle, and M. V. Lancaster.** 2001. Increasing resistance to vancomycin and other glycopeptides in *Staphylococcus aureus*. *Emerg. Infect. Dis.* **7:**327–332.

185. **Thodis, E., S. Bhaskaran, P. Pasadakis, J. M. Bargman, S. I. Vas, and D. G. Oreopoulos.** 1998. Decrease in *Staphylococcus aureus* exit-site infections and peritonitis in CAPD patients by local application of mupirocin ointment at the catheter exit site. *Perit. Dial. Int.* **18:**261–270.

186. **Thomson-Carter, F. M., P. E. Carter, and T. H. Pennington.** 1989. Differentiation of staphylococcal species and strains by ribosomal RNA gene restriction patterns. *J. Gen. Microbiol.* **135:**2093–2097.

187. **Uttley, L., A. Vardhan, S. Mahajan, A. Hutchison, and R. Gokal.** 2004. Decrease in infection with the introduction of mupirocin cream at the peritoneal dialysis catheter exit site. *J. Nephrol.* **17:**242–245.

188. **Van Belkum, A., J. Kluytmans, W. van Leeuwen, R. Bax, W. Quint, E. Peters, A. Fluit, C. Vandenbroucke-Grauls, A. van den Brule, H. Koeleman, W. Melchers, J. Meis, A. Elaichouni, M. Vaneechoutte, F. Moonens,

N. Maes, M. Struelens, F. Tenover, and H. Verbrugh. 1995. Multicenter evaluation of arbitrarily primed PCR for typing of *Staphylococcus aureus* strains. *J. Clin. Microbiol.* **33:**1537–1547.

189. **Vandenesch, F., J. Etienne, M. E. Reverdy, and S. J. Eykyn.** 1993. Endocarditis due to *Staphylococcus lugdunensis:* report of 11 cases and review. *Clin. Infect. Dis.* **17:**871–876.
190. **Vandenesch, F., T. Naimi, M. C. Enright, G. Lina, G. R. Nimmo, H. Heffernan, N. Liassine, M. Bes, T. Greenland, M. E. Reverdy, and J. Etienne.** 2003. Community-acquired methicillin-resistant *Staphylococcus aureus* carrying Panton-Valentine leukocidin genes: worldwide emergence. *Emerg. Infect. Dis.* **9:**978–984.
191. **Van Griethuysen, A., M. Bes, J. Etienne, R. Zbinden, and J. Kluytmans.** 2001. International multicenter evaluation of latex agglutination tests for identification of *Staphylococcus aureus*. *J. Clin. Microbiol.* **39:**86–89.
192. **Velasco, D., M. del Mar Tomas, M. Cartelle, A. Becerio, A. Perez, F. Molina, R. Moure, R. Villanueva, and G. Bou.** 2005. Evaluation of different methods for detecting methicillin (oxacillin) resistance in *Staphylococcus aureus*. *J. Antimicrob. Chemother.* **55:**379–382.
193. **Vernozy-Rozand, C., C. Mazuy, H. Meugnier, M. Bes, Y. Lasne, F. Fiedler, J. Etienne, and J. Freney.** 2000. *Staphylococcus fleurettii* sp. nov., isolated from goat's milk cheese. *Int. J. Syst. Evol. Microbiol.* **50:**1521–1527.
194. **von Eiff, C., M. Herrman, and G. Peters.** 1995. Antimicrobial susceptibilities of *Stomatococcus mucilaginosus* and of *Micrococcus* spp. *Antimicrob. Agents Chemother.* **39:**268–270.
195. **von Eiff, C., and G. Peters.** 1998. In vitro activity of ciprofloxacin, ofloxacin, and levofloxacin against *Micrococcus* species and *Stomatococcus mucilaginosus* isolated from healthy subjects and neutropenic patients. *Eur. J. Clin. Microbiol. Infect. Dis.* **17:**890–892.
196. **von Eiff, C., K. Becker, K. Machka, H. Stammer, G. Peters, et al.** 2001. Nasal carriage as a source of *Staphylococcus aureus* bacteremia. *N. Engl. J. Med.* **344:**11–16.
197. **von Eiff, C., G. Peters, and C. Heilmann.** 2002. Pathogenesis of infections due to coagulase-negative staphylococci. *Lancet Infect. Dis.* **2:**677–685.
198. **Walsh, T. R., A. Bolmström, A. Qwärnström, P. Ho, M. Wootton, R. A. Howe, A. P. MacGowen, and D. Diekema.** 2001. Evaluation of current methods for detection of staphylococci with reduced susceptibility to glycopeptides. *J. Clin. Microbiol.* **39:**2439–2444.
199. **Weigelt, J., K. Itani, D. Stevens, W. Lau, M. Dryden, C. Knirsch, and the Linezolid CSSTI Study Group.** 2005. Linezolid versus vancomycin in treatment of complicated skin and soft tissue infections. *Antimicrob. Agents Chemother.* **49:**2260–2266.
200. **Weigelt, J., H. M. Kaafarani, K. M. Itani, and R. N. Swanson.** 2004. Linezolid eradicates MRSA better than vancomycin from surgical-site infections. *Am. J. Surg.* **188:**760–766.
201. **Wellinghausen, N., B. Wirths, A. Essig, and L. Wassill.** 2004. Evaluation of the Hyplex BloodScreen multiplex PCR-enzyme-linked immunosorbent assay system for direct identification of gram-positive cocci and gram-negative bacilli from positive blood cultures. *J. Clin. Microbiol.* **42:**3147–3152.
202. **Wunderink, R. G., J. Rello, S. K. Cammarata, R. V. Croos-Dabrera, and M. H. Kollef.** 2003. Linezolid vs. vancomycin: analysis of two double-blind studies of patients with methicillin-resistant *Staphylococcus aureus* nosocomial pneumonia. *Chest* **124:**1789–1797.
203. **Yugueros, J., A. Temprano, B. Berzal, M. Sánchez, C. Hernanz, J. M. Luengo, and G. Naharro.** 2000. Glyceraldehyde-3-phosphate dehydrogenase-encoding gene as a useful taxonomic tool for *Staphylococcus* spp. *J. Clin. Microbiol.* **38:**4351–4355.
204. **Zakrzewska-Bode, A., H. L. Muytjens, and K. D. Liem.** 1995. Mupirocin resistance in coagulase-negative staphylococci, after topical prophylaxis for the reduction of colonization of central venous catheters. *J. Hosp. Infect.* **31:**189–193.
205. **Zhang, K., J. Sparling, B. L. Chow, S. Elsayed, Z. Hussain, D. L. Church, D. B. Gregson, T. Louie, and J. M. Conly.** 2004. New quadriplex PCR assay for detection of methicillin and mupirocin resistance and simultaneous discrimination of *Staphylcoccus aureus* from coagulase-negative staphylococci. *J. Clin. Microbiol.* **42:**4947–4955.
206. **Zhang, Y. Q., S. X. Ren, H. L. Li, Y. X. Wang, G. Fu, J. Yang, Z. Q. Qin, Y. G. Miao, W. Y. Wang, R. S. Chen, Y. Shen, Z. Chen, Z. H. Yuan, G. P. Zhao, D. Qu, A. Danchin, and Y. M. Wen.** 2003. Genome-based analysis of virulence genes in a non-biofilm-forming *Staphylococcus epidermidis* strain (ATCC 12228). *Mol. Microbiol.* **49:**1577–1593.
207. **Zinderman, C. E., B. Conner, M. A. Malakooti, J. E. LaMar, A. Armstrong, and B. K. Bohnker.** 2004. Community-acquired methicillin-resistant *Staphylococcus aureus* among military recruits. *Emerg. Infect. Dis.* **10:**941–944.

*Streptococcus**

BARBARA SPELLERBERG AND CLAUDIA BRANDT

29

TAXONOMY

The taxonomy of streptococci has experienced a number of changes during the last 20 years mostly due to the application of molecular biology techniques such as DNA-DNA reassociation experiments and 16S rRNA gene sequencing. Among the currently established 17 different genera of catalase-negative gram-positive cocci are several genera that were split off from the genus *Streptococcus* some time ago such as *Enterococcus* and *Lactococcus*, or more recently *Abiotrophia, Granulicatella, Facklamia,* and *Globicatella*. For an excellent review on the topic reflecting many of the recent changes, see reference 34. Molecular 16S rRNA analysis of streptococci has shown that species designation based solely on the hemolysis reaction, colony size, and the presence of Lancefield antigens does not correspond well with the molecular analysis in all cases. Taxonomic changes will certainly continue in the future. However, the traditional streptococcal classification system is well established and still of value to the clinical microbiologist. The phenotypic classification system correlates with clinical syndromes caused by different species and enables a first distinction of broad categories of streptococci that is useful for the choice of further tests and guidance of empirical treatments. The information and the identification schemes presented in this chapter therefore adhere in many aspects to this well-known phenotypic classification system.

The classical phenotypic differentation of streptococci separates the group of beta-hemolytic streptococci, which are discussed first in this chapter, from the group of non-beta-hemolytic streptococcal species. Beta-hemolytic streptococci, also referred to as pyogenic streptococci, include the species *S. pyogenes, S. agalactiae, S. dysgalactiae, S. equi,* and *S. canis*. The designation pyogenic streptococci is more precise, since the group includes species that are non-beta-hemolytic like *S. dysgalactiae* subsp. *dysgalactiae,* which is closely related to several beta-hemolytic species, and the term excludes beta-hemolytic strains of the *S. anginosus* group, which are more appropriately placed into the viridans streptococcal group. The small colony size of streptococci from the anginosus group (<0.5 mm) helps to distinguish them from the large-colony-forming (>0.5 mm) streptococci of the pyogenic group. Species from the pyogenic or beta-hemolytic group are further characterized by the presence of Lancefield antigens, which correlates in the case of group A streptococci fairly well but not precisely with the species designation *S. pyogenes*. While the B antigen appears to be limited to *S. agalactiae*, the Lancefield group A antigen has been detected not only in *S. pyogenes* but also in *S. dysgalactiae* subsp. *equisimilis* isolates (16) and in species from the *S. anginosus* group, (Table 1). Correlation with the other Lancefield antigens is even more complicated, which led to the need for novel species designations, presented below and in Table 1.

The group of nonpyogenic streptococci includes mostly α-hemolytic as well as nonhemolytic and even beta-hemolytic streptococcal species from the large category of viridans streptococci. In a study of the genus *Streptococcus* based on sequence comparisons of small-subunit (16S) rRNA genes, five species groups of viridans streptococci were demonstrated (57) in addition to the pyogenic group (beta-hemolytic, large-colony formers). These nonpyogenic groups were designated the *S. mitis* group, the *S. anginosus* group, the *S. mutans* group, the *S. salivarius* group, and the *S. bovis* group. A few streptococcal species were not unequivocally assigned and remain ungrouped. Descriptions of the species in the nonpyogenic groups follow the discussion on *S. pneumoniae*. Among α-hemolytic streptococci, *S. pneumoniae* can be separated from other streptococci of the viridans group through bile solubility and optochin susceptibility. However, phenotypic characterization and taxonomic considerations place *S. pneumoniae* into the *S. mitis* group (57). The relationship of *S. pneumoniae* to other species of the *S. mitis* group is so close that 16S rRNA gene analysis reveals greater than 99% identity to the nucleotide sequences of *S. mitis* and *S. oralis*. A novel, closely related species, *S. pseudopneumoniae,* has recently been split off from *S. pneumoniae,* following DNA-DNA hybridization studies and phenotypic characterization (1). Strains are nonencapsulated and insoluble in bile, and their clinical significance is currently uncertain.

S. mitis, S. sanguinis, S. parasanguinis, S. gordonii, S. cristatus, S. oralis, S. infantis, S. peroris (58), and *S. pneumoniae* are members of the *S. mitis* group. These species form a group whose classification and nomenclature have been a source of considerable confusion in the past. Among the changes that were made is the reclassification of the original *S. mitis* type strain as an *S. gordonii* strain and the subsequent replacement by a new *S. mitis* type strain (NCTC12261^{T}) (61). Further

* This chapter contains information presented in chapter 29 by Kathryn L. Ruoff, R. A. Whiley, and D. Beighton in the eighth edition of this Manual.

TABLE 1 Phenotypic characteristics of beta-hemolytic streptococci[a]

Species	Lancefield group	Colony size[e]	Hosts	Bacitracin	PYR[f]	CAMP[g]	VP[i]	Hippurate hydrolysis	Trehalose	Sorbitol
S. pyogenes	A	Large	Humans	+	+	–[h]	–	–	+	–
S. agalactiae	B	Large	Humans, cows	–	–	+	–	+	v	–
S. dysgalactiae subsp. *dysgalactiae*[b]	C	Large	Animals	–	–	–	–	–	+	v
S. dysgalactiae subsp. *equisimilis*	A, C, G, L	Large	Humans	–	–	–	–	–	+	–
S. equi subsp. *equi*	C	Large	Animals	–	–	–	–	–	–	–
S. equi subsp. *zooepidemicus*	C	Large	Animals, humans[c]	–	–	–	–	–	–	+
S. canis	G	Large	Dogs, humans[c]	–	–	+	–	–	v	–
S. anginosus group[d]	A, C, G, F, none	Small	Humans	–	–	–	+	–	+	–
S. porcinus	E, P, U, V, none	Large	Swine, humans[c]	–	+	+	+	v	+	+

[a] Symbols and abbreviations: +, positive; –, negative; v, variable.
[b] *S. dysgalactiae* subsp. *dysgalactiae* is α-hemolytic on sheep blood agar plates.
[c] *S. equi* subsp. *zooepidemicus*, *S. canis*, and *S. porcinus* are primarily animal pathogens that are only rarely isolated from humans.
[d] Species included in the *S. anginosus* group can be beta-hemolytic, alpha-hemolytic, or nonhemolytic on sheep blood agar plates.
[e] Large colony size refers to colonies >0.5 mm after 24 h of incubation, whereas small colony size is <0.5 mm.
[f] Presence of the enzyme pyrrolidonyl aminopeptidase.
[g] CAMP factor reaction (synergistic hemolysis in the presence of *S. aureus* β-hemolysin).
[h] *S. pyogenes* may occasionally yield a false-positive CAMP factor reaction.
[i] Voges-Proskauer test (formation of acetoin from glucose fermentation).

confusion is caused by the use of the term "biotype," especially for the species *S. sanguinis*. While the biotypes differ in phenotypic reactions, biotypes are not included in the approved lists of bacterial names and appear to vary between different studies (7, 61), and in most cases, no type strains are available. Based on phenotypic reactions (especially arginine hydrolysis and esculin tests), the *S. mitis* group can be further subdivided into the *S. sanguinis* and the *S. mitis* groups (34), but based on 16S rRNA analysis, these two groups appear to belong together (57). Since correlation of the renamed streptococcal species with human infections is still difficult, we chose to present these species as part of the *S. mitis* group until further information becomes available.

The small-colony-forming *S. anginosus* group consists of the three distinct species *S. anginosus*, *S. constellatus*, and *S. intermedius* (118). It includes streptococcal species previously referred to as Lancefield group F streptococci, "*S. milleri*" group or "*S. milleri*." The species "*S. milleri*" has no standing taxonomically. The *S. mutans* group comprises the species *S. mutans*, *S. sobrinus*, *S. criceti*, and *S. ratti* and numerous species that have been identified only from animals thus far (*S. downei*, *S. ferus*, *S. macacae*, and *S. hyovaginalis*).

The human species *S. salivarius*, *S. vestibularis*, and *S. thermophilus*, which is found in dairy products, belong to the *S. salivarius* group. Whether *S. thermophilus* was a subspecies of *S. salivarius* was controversial, although DNA-DNA reassociation experiments determined that they are two separate species (96). The whole *S. salivarius* group is closely related to the *S. bovis* group. Some streptococcal species that are currently part of the *S. bovis* group (*S. infantarius* and *S. alactolyticus*) (94) were formerly part of the *S. salivarius* group (34).

The *S. bovis* group has experienced extensive taxonomic changes (28, 80, 88, 94, 95). Four DNA clusters are currently recognized. DNA cluster I consists of the species formerly known as animal strains of *S. bovis* and *S. equinus*. Molecular analyses of these strains showed that they belong to a single species (41), and the earlier species name *S. equinus* has been formally adopted. DNA cluster II consists of one species, *S. gallolyticus*, with three subspecies: subspecies *gallolyticus* (formerly *S. bovis* biotype I), subspecies *pasteurianus* (formerly *S. bovis* biotype II.2), and subspecies *macedonicus*. DNA cluster III consists of one species, *S. infantarius* (formerly *S. bovis* biotype II.1), with two subspecies: subspecies *infantarius* and subspecies *coli* (formerly called *S. lutetiensis*). DNA cluster IV consists of one species, *S. alactolyticus*. These changes were made because DNA-DNA reassociation studies revealed considerable heterogeneity among the human isolates described as *S. bovis* biotypes.

DESCRIPTION OF THE GENUS

Bacterial species belonging to the genus *Streptococcus* are catalase-negative, gram-positive cocci of less than 2 μm that tend to grow in chains in liquid media. The cell wall composition is typical for gram-positive bacteria and consists mainly of peptidoglycan with glucosamine and muramic acid as amino sugars and galactosamine as a variable component. A variety of carbohydrates, surface protein antigens, and teichoic acid are attached to the cell wall and are, among other characteristics, responsible for species differences and clonal differences among streptococci. Most species of the genus *Streptococcus* have a low G+C content of DNA that lies in the range of 34 to 46%. Streptococci are facultative anaerobic bacteria. Due to a lack of heme compounds, streptococci are incapable of respiratory metabolism. Some species of the viridans streptococcal group and *S. pneumoniae* require 5% CO_2 levels for adequate growth, and the growth of many streptococcal species is enhanced in the presence of 5% CO_2. The temperature optimum for most streptococci is around 37°C, while some species like *S. uberis* also grow at temperatures as low as 10°C. The complex nutritional requirements of streptococci are usually provided by the addition of blood or serum to the growth medium. Glucose and other carbohydrates are metabolized fermentatively, with lactic acid as the major metabolic end product. The addition of glucose or other carbohydrates to liquid medium enhances growth but lowers the pH, resulting in growth inhibition unless the medium is highly buffered (e.g., Todd-Hewitt broth [THB]). Leucine aminopeptidase (LAP) is produced by all streptococci and enterococci but can also be found in lactococci, pediococci, and other catalase-negative gram-positive cocci. It helps to distinguish these species from the LAP-negative *Aerococcus* species and *Leuconostoc*. All streptococci are catalase negative upon exposure to 3% hydrogen peroxide. False-positive reactions may occur if bacteria are grown on blood-containing media.

EPIDEMIOLOGY AND TRANSMISSION

Streptococci can cause infections in humans and in many different animal species including mammals and fish. Different species of streptococci are frequently found as commensal bacteria on mucous membranes. Occasionally streptococci are present as transient skin microbiota. Several streptococcal species exhibit high virulence potential, but even the highly virulent streptococcal species are frequently found as colonizing strains without any apparent effect on the host. *S. pneumoniae* was responsible for approximately 40,000 invasive infections in the United States in 2003, leading to an estimated 5,500 deaths (http://www.cdc.gov/abcs), and was found as a colonizing bacterial species in many asymptomatic carriers. The asymptomatic carriage rate for *S. pneumoniae* differs considerably between children and adults. Detection rates of 30 to 70% have been reported for young children, depending on the sampling method, while carriage rates among healthy adults are often reported to be below 5% (47, 51, 90). Evidence for household transmission between parents and their children has been found, demonstrating colonization rates for adults living in a household with young children that are significantly higher than in adults with no contact with preschool children (51).

Due to active bacterial surveillance in the emerging infections program network (99), reliable epidemiologic data on invasive infections due to *S. pneumoniae* (described above), *S. pyogenes* (group A), and *S. agalactiae* (group B) have been obtained for a population of 17 to 30 million people in the United States during 2003. *S. pyogenes* caused an estimated 11,300 cases of invasive disease and 1,800 deaths, with the peak of infections in people older than 65 years. Invasive infections due to *S. agalactiae* were second to those due to *S. pneumoniae,* with an estimated 20,400 cases and 2,200 deaths in 2003. Reflecting the ongoing changes in the epidemiology of group B streptococcal disease, the highest attack rates were observed for patients less than 1 year and adults greater than 65 years of age. Apart from causing invasive infections, both of these streptococcal species are frequently encountered as colonizing strains. While asymptomatic colonization of the nasopharynx with *S. pyogenes* occurs in less than 5% of the adult population in most studies, *S. agalactiae* colonization rates of the urogenital and gastrointestinal tracts can be demonstrated in 10 to 30% of the female as well as the male population. No significant differences are observed in the colonization rates of pregnant and nonpregnant women.

Transmission of streptococcal infections can occur by different routes. Pathogenic species like *S. pyogenes* and *S. pneumoniae* are primarily transmitted through droplets or direct contact. Transmission can first lead to colonization with the potential for the development of a subsequent infection. The tooth decay-causing species *S. mutans* is transmitted from mother to child during early infancy, most probably through oral secretions. Transmission from mother to child is also the typical transmission mode for neonatal invasive *S. agalactiae* infections. Newborns acquire the bacteria usually during delivery, although transmissions, shortly after birth, from the mother or health care personnel to infants have been documented, especially in late-onset neonatal infections. Endogenous infections most often occur by viridans streptococci as part of the oral microbiota.

Streptococcal infections do not represent classical zoonoses, although most species have a preferred host. While occasional animal-to-human transmissions do occur, as in the case of *Streptococcus suis* (67), genotypic and phenotypic analyses of animal and human strains demonstrated that the strains causing human infections were distinct from the strains causing animal infections. For beta-hemolytic group C and G streptococci, such an analysis led to an important change in species designations (111). Human group C and group G streptococcal strains were demonstrated to belong to a separate subspecies, designated *S. dysgalactiae* subsp. *equisimilis,* while animal group C, G, and L streptococci are classified as *S. dysgalactiae* subsp. *dysgalactiae, S. canis, S. equi* subsp. *equi,* and *S. equi* subsp. *zooepidemicus* (27, 40). The reservoir for *S. dysgalactiae* subsp. *equisimilis* strains is the human host, and transmission usually occurs among humans.

CLINICAL SIGNIFICANCE

Streptococcus pyogenes (Group A Streptococci)

S. pyogenes colonizes the human throat and skin and has developed complex virulence mechanisms to avoid host defenses (20, 31). The upper respiratory tract and skin lesions serve as primary focal sites of infections and principal reservoirs of transmission. *S. pyogenes* can cause superficial or deep infections due to toxin- and immunologically mediated mechanisms of disease. *S. pyogenes* is the most common cause of bacterial pharyngitis and impetigo. In the past, *S. pyogenes* was a common cause of childbed fever or puerperal sepsis. *S. pyogenes* is responsible for deep or invasive infections, especially bacteremia; sepsis; deep soft tissue infections, such as erysipelas; cellulitis; and necrotizing fasciitis. Less common presentations include myositis, osteomyelitis, septic arthritis, pneumonia, meningitis, endocarditis, pericarditis, and severe neonatal infections following intrapartum transmission. One or more erythrogenic exotoxins produced by *S. pyogenes* may cause a confluent erythematous sandpaper-like rash characteristic of scarlet fever. While systemic toxic effects occur rarely with scarlet fever, severe clinical manifestations in streptococcal toxic shock syndrome (STSS) may result from massive superantigen-induced cytokine and lymphokine production. Nonsuppurative complications include poststreptococcal glomerulonephritis and acute rheumatic fever. While either of these conditions may follow pharyngitis, only glomerulonephritis is linked with skin infections due to *S. pyogenes*. *S. pyogenes* has also been associated with pediatric autoimmune neuropsychiatric disorders (106).

Causes of the emergence of STSS, frequently accompanied by necrotizing fasciitis, and the resurgence of invasive *S. pyogenes* infections since the mid-1980s are mostly unexplained (105). *S. pyogenes* remains exquisitely sensitive to penicillin. Despite the continuous exposure and subsequent type-specific immunity, the most prevalent

M types associated with STSS continue to be M1 and M3, together accounting for approximately 50% of invasive infections. Since identical strains have accounted for less serious infections (78), host factors and comorbid conditions account for different diseases. The incidence of STSS seems highest among young children, particularly those with varicella, and the elderly. Other persons at risk include those with diabetes mellitus, chronic cardiac or pulmonary diseases, human immunodeficiency virus infection, intravenous drug abuse, and alcohol use. The risk for severe invasive infection in contacts has been estimated to be 200 times greater than for the general population, but most contacts are asymptomatically colonized (23).

Streptococcus agalactiae (Group B Streptococci [GBS])

S. agalactiae was first identified as the cause of bovine mastitis at the end of the 19th century. Since the 1970s it has been increasingly reported as the cause of invasive neonatal infections. Neonatal infections present as two different clinical entities: early-onset neonatal disease, characterized by sepsis and pneumonia within the first 7 days of life; and late-onset disease with meningitis and sepsis between 7 days and 3 months of age. The most important risk factor for the development of invasive neonatal disease is the colonization of the maternal urogenital or gastrointestinal tract by *S. agalactiae,* which is found in 10 to 30% of pregnant women. Prevention of early-onset neonatal infections can be achieved in the majority of cases by administration of intrapartum antibiotic prophylaxis starting at least 4 h before delivery. Official CDC recommendations for the prevention of neonatal *S. agalactiae* infections were first issued in 1996 (100), were revised in 2002 (97), and resulted in a substantial decline of early-onset neonatal GBS disease (98). Invasive *S. agalactiae* infections of adult patients may be observed as postpartum infections or in immunocompromised adult patients with alcoholism, diabetes mellitus, cancer, or human immunodeficiency virus infection (39). The spectrum of infections in adult patients includes pneumonia, bacteremia, endocarditis, urinary tract infections, skin and soft tissue infections, and osteomyelitis.

Streptococcus dysgalactiae subsp. *equisimilis* (Human Group C and G Streptococci)

Human isolates of large-colony-forming beta-hemolytic streptococci harboring the Lancefield group C or group G antigens belong to *Streptococcus dysgalactiae* subsp. *equisimilis,* a novel species described in 1996 (111). While most isolates of this species possess either the Lancefield group C or the G antigen, strains harboring the Lancefield group L as well as the group A antigen (16) have been described. The clinical spectrum of disease caused by *S. dysgalactiae* subsp. *equisimilis* resembles infections caused by *S. pyogenes,* consistent with strains harboring genes similar to virulence factor genes of *S. pyogenes,* such as *emm*-like genes. These organisms are associated with upper respiratory tract infections, skin infections, soft tissue infections, and invasive infections such as necrotizing fasciitis, STSS, bacteremia, and endocarditis. Similar to *S. pyogenes* infections, cases of glomerulonephritis and acute rheumatic fever have been reported (5, 49) following *S. equi* subsp. *zooepidemicus* and *S. dysgalactiae* subsp. *equisimilis* infections.

Streptococcus anginosus Group

Species from the *Streptococcus anginosus* group (*S. anginosus, S. constellatus,* and *S. intermedius*) are regarded generally as harmless commensals of the oropharyngeal, urogenital, and gastrointestinal microbiota. However, these organisms are strongly associated with abscess formation in the brain, the oropharynx, or the peritoneal cavity. A subspecies of *S. constellatus, S. constellatus* subsp. *pharyngis,* has also been described and associated with pharyngitis (119). All species of this group are small-colony-forming bacteria (colony size, <0.5 mm) that can display variable patterns of hemolysis (alpha, beta, or gamma). Since they can also harbor the Lancefield group antigens A, C, F, or G (or none at all), it is especially important to reliably distinguish them from large-colony-forming (>0.5 mm) beta-hemolytic streptococci of the pyogenic group. Association of certain species with specific isolation sites has been reported. Whereas *S. anginosus* is frequently found in specimens from the urogenital or gastrointestinal tracts, *S. constellatus* is commonly isolated from the respiratory tract and *S. intermedius* is most often identified in abscesses of the brain or liver.

Streptococcus pneumoniae

S. pneumoniae is described separately in this section due to its clinical features that distinguish it from other species of the *S. mitis* group. *S. pneumoniae* is the most frequently isolated respiratory pathogen in community-acquired pneumonia. In as many as 30% of community-acquired pneumonia cases, *S. pneumoniae* can be found in peripheral blood cultures of patients. *S. pneumoniae* is also a major cause of meningitis, leading to high morbidity and mortality in pediatric and adult patients. The most frequently observed infection due to *S. pneumoniae* is otitis media, with an estimate of one infection for every child up to the age of 6 in the United States. Other infections due to *S. pneumoniae* include sinusitis, endocarditis, and rare cases of peritonitis. *S. pneumoniae* colonizes the upper respiratory tract commonly in individuals, especially children, without evidence of infection. Prevention of pneumococcal infections can be achieved by immunization with a 23-valent capsular polysaccharide vaccine in adults or the 7-valent conjugate vaccine in children. Widespread use of these vaccines has resulted in a reduction of invasive pneumococcal infections during the past several years.

Streptococcus mitis Group

S. mitis, S. sanguinis, S. parasanguinis, S. gordonii, S. cristatus, S. oralis, S. infantis, S. peroris (58), and *S. pneumoniae* are members of the *Streptococcus mitis* group. The *S. mitis* group members are regular commensals of the oral cavity, the gastrointestinal tract, and the female genital tract. Isolation of these species from blood cultures in asymptomatic patients often does not require antibiotic treatment, if it is due to a transient bacteremia. The *S. mitis* group members can also be found as transient microbiota of the normal skin and often represent contaminants when isolated from blood cultures. At the same time these species are the most frequently isolated bacteria in bacterial endocarditis in native valve and, less frequently, in prosthetic valve infections. Careful evaluation of the clinical situation is therefore crucial to correctly interpret the clinical significance of blood culture isolates from the *S. mitis* group. In neutropenic patients, streptococcal species from the *S. mitis* group are often responsible for life-threatening sepsis and pneumonia cases following immunosuppression by chemotherapy (14).

Streptococcus salivarius Group

Streptococcal species that belong to the *Streptococcus salivarius* group and have been isolated from human sources include *S. salivarius* and *S. vestibularis*. Another species of this group, *S. thermophilus,* has been identified only from dairy products. *S. salivarius* has been repeatedly reported as a cause of bacteremia, endocarditis, and meningitis (sometimes iatrogenic), whereas *S. vestibularis* has not been clearly associated with human infection. Isolation of *S. salivarius* from blood cultures does correlate to some extent with intestinal neoplasia (93).

Streptococcus mutans Group

S. mutans and *S. sobrinus* belong to the *Streptococcus mutans* group. They are the most commonly isolated species of the group that originate from human clinical specimens, usually obtained from the oral cavity. *S. criceti* and *S. ratti* have occasionally been identified from human sources, while the other streptococcal species of the *S. mutans* group (*S. downei, S. ferus, S. macacae,* and *S. hyovaginalis*) have been identified only in animals. *S. mutans* is the primary etiologic agent of dental caries, and infection is transmissible. By 18 years of age, 85% of the population have at least one caries lesion (103). Permanent colonization with *S. mutans* occurs under normal living conditions in the Western world between the second year and the end of the third year of life (103). Molecular analysis of mother and infant isolates reveals that strains are usually acquired from the mother and that the colonization rate of infants depends on the bacterial load of the mother (17). Analyses of streptococcal blood culture isolates show that *S. mutans* is the most frequently isolated species of this group in cases of bacteremia.

Streptococcus bovis Group

The *Streptococcus bovis* group includes *S. equinus, S. gallolyticus, S. infantarius,* and *S. alactolyticus*. Species from this group are frequently encountered in blood cultures of patients with bacteremia, sepsis, and endocarditis. The clinical significance of blood cultures growing streptococci from the *S. bovis* group lies in the association of *S. gallolyticus* subsp. *gallolyticus* with gastrointestinal cancer and of *S. gallolyticus* subsp. *pasteurianus* with meningitis (4, 43, 63, 82). Extensive taxonomic changes have occurred in this group, and strains formerly known as human *S. bovis* isolates are now designated as different species (see "Taxonomy" above).

Other Streptococci Infrequently Isolated from Human Specimens

Streptococcal species that are primarily animal pathogens are sometimes isolated from human hosts, in most cases from humans that are in close contact with animals. *S. suis, S. porcinus,* and *S. iniae* belong to this category. *S. suis* is a swine pathogen that has occasionally been isolated from cases of human meningitis and bacteremia (67). *S. suis* is encapsulated and appears alpha-hemolytic on sheep blood agar plates, although some strains are beta-hemolytic on horse blood agar. *S. suis* strains are positive for the Lancefield group antigens R, S, or T. These antigens help to distinguish them from the phenotypically similar species *S. gordonii, S. sanguinis,* and *S. parasanguinis*. Similar to *S. suis, S. porcinus* (Lancefield groups E, P, U, and V) is primarily a swine pathogen. Beta-hemolytic *S. porcinus* strains have rarely been isolated from human sources such as peripheral blood, wounds, and the female genital tract (35). *S. porcinus* can be misidentified as *S. agalactiae* due to its isolation from the female genital tract, false-positive reactions with commercially available group B antisera, and a positive CAMP test reaction. *S. porcinus* is PYR (pyrrolidonyl aminopeptidase) positive, in contrast to *S. agalactiae*. *S. iniae* is a fish pathogen that is beta-hemolytic but does not possess any Lancefield group antigens. It has been isolated from soft tissue infections, bacteremia, endocarditis, and meningitis in people handling fish (36, 115). *S. iniae* isolates resemble *S. pyogenes* strains due to the fact that they are PYR positive. Beta-hemolysis of the species can be observed only around agar stabs or under anaerobic culture conditions. Commercial identification systems do not correctly identify the species; the failure to react with Lancefield group antisera is important to notice, since it is rare among beta-hemolytic streptococci.

COLLECTION, TRANSPORT, AND STORAGE OF SPECIMENS

Specimens suspected of harboring streptococci should be collected by methods outlined elsewhere in this Manual (chapters 5 and 20). Since many streptococcal species lose viability fairly quickly, it is best to place swabs in an appropriate moist transport medium and process specimens rapidly. If transport time is below 1 to 2 h, a special transport system is not absolutely necessary. *S. pyogenes* can safely be transported on dry swabs; desiccation enhances recovery from mixed cultures by suppression of accompanying microbiota (70). Detailed recommendations for collection and storage of swabs from pregnant women to detect *S. agalactiae* colonization have been issued by the U.S. Centers for Disease Control and Prevention. These recommendations are summarized below under "Special Procedures for *S. agalactiae* (GBS)."

DIRECT EXAMINATION

Microscopy

Microscopic examination shows streptococci as gram-positive bacteria growing in chains of varying length. *S. pneumoniae* organisms most often present as gram-positive diplococci with an elongated appearance. In blood culture specimens, *S. pneumoniae* tends to form chains of varying length, similar to other streptococci. Direct identification of streptococci by microscopic methods is most helpful in the case of clinical specimens from sterile body sites, such as cerebrospinal fluid (CSF). Tiny, irregular cocci in clumps of chains seen in abscess- or peritonitis-associated aspirates are suggestive of the *S. anginosus* group. Interpretation of Gram stain results from nonsterile body sites is difficult, due to the residential microbiota of mucous membranes that frequently include streptococci. Thus, for example, throat swabs should not be examined by Gram stain for diagnosis of "strep" throat. Identification of *S. pneumoniae* by direct microscopic evaluation can be aided by the Neufeld Quellung reaction, which can be performed directly on clinical specimens (for instructions, see below). This procedure is not established in most clinical microbiological laboratories today.

Direct Antigen Detection of *S. pyogenes* from Throat Specimens

S. pyogenes is the most common cause of acute pharyngitis and accounts for 15 to 30% of cases of acute pharyngitis in children and 5 to 10% of cases in adults. If diagnosis can be provided rapidly, antibiotic therapy can be initiated promptly to relieve symptoms, to avoid sequelae, and to reduce transmission. Numerous assays for direct detection of the group A-specific carbohydrate antigen in throat swabs by agglutination methods or immunoassays (enzyme, liposome, or optical), also referred to as "rapid antigen assays," have become commercially available during the past 2 decades.

A list of FDA-cleared tests is accessible via the Internet (http://www.accessdata.fda.gov/scripts/cdrh/cfdocs/cfRL/LSTSimpleSearch.cfdm). Although these tests provide rapid results and allow early treatment decisions, sensitivities and specificities have never equaled those of culture, ranging from 58 to 96% and 63 to 100%, respectively (38, 110). The throat culture remains the "gold standard," and national advisory committees recommend confirmation of negative rapid test results with a conventional throat culture. Currently, the low positive predictive value of rapid group A antigen tests in the adult population frequently results in prescribing unnecessary antimicrobial therapy (83).

Antigen Detection of *S. pneumoniae* in Urine Samples

An immunochromatographic membrane test relying on the detection of the cell wall-associated polysaccharide that is common to all *S. pneumoniae* serotypes (C-polysaccharide antigen) (Binax NOW; Binax Inc., Portland, Maine) has proven helpful for the identification of *S. pneumoniae* infections in adult patients, especially in patients that already received antibiotic treatment. Compared to conventional diagnostic methods, reported sensitivities of antigen detection in urine samples range between 50 and 80% and specificities are approximately 90% (48, 75). Due to the fact that the test is also positive in *S. pneumoniae* carriage without infection, as is often observed among infants (30), it is of limited value for pediatric patients. The test should not be used for children below the age of 6 (30), and comprehensive studies on schoolchildren with lower colonization rates have not been performed. It can currently be recommended only for adults as an addition to conventional diagnostic culture techniques for *S. pneumoniae* (69) and is probably most helpful for patients who received antimicrobial treatment before cultures were obtained.

Antigen Detection of *S. agalactiae* in Urogenital Tract Samples

Several different commercially available antigen detection tests have been developed for the identification of *S. agalactiae* in samples from the urogenital tract. Independent from the technique involved (latex agglutination, enzyme immunoassay, or optical immunoassay), all of the currently available tests lack sufficient sensitivities to detect bacterial colonization with *S. agalactiae* (107). They are not recommended for screening of pregnant women by the CDC. Even though modified protocols with an incubation of the samples in selective broth prior to antigen testing appear to increase assay sensitivities, the current CDC recommendations rely on selective broth culture performed at 35 to 37 weeks of gestation for this purpose (see "Special Procedures for *S. agalactiae* (GBS)."

Streptococcal Antigen Detection in CSF

Commercially available antigen detection tests for the detection of pathogenic microorganisms in CSF samples include reagents for the detection of *S. agalactiae* and *S. pneumoniae*. These tests have also been used on positive blood culture specimens. The tests are not recommended for routine use, as the results should not be used to change decisions about empiric therapy based on clinical and laboratory criteria (108). It has also been shown that the sensitivity of direct antigen detection in CSF is low (<30%) and offers no advantage over a conventional Gram stain (72).

Nucleic Acid Detection Techniques

S. pyogenes

A rapid method for the detection of *S. pyogenes* in pharyngeal specimens is based on a single-stranded chemiluminescent nucleic acid probe assay to identify specific rRNA sequences (Group A Streptococcus Direct Test; Gen-Probe, Inc., San Diego, Calif.). This test has a reported sensitivity and specificity of 89 and 93.5%, respectively, compared with the results of culture (50, 85). Moreover, a real-time PCR assay (LightCycler Strep A assay; Roche Diagnostics, Indianapolis, Ind.) has been recently developed for the detection of *S. pyogenes* in throat swabs (110). Real-time PCR proved to be more sensitive than the standard culture method in one study, and it appears to be unnecessary to perform cultures when results of the real-time PCR are negative. Real-time PCR allows the detection of beta-hemolytic species *S. pyogenes* and *S. dysgalactiae* subsp. *equisimilis*.

S. agalactiae

A rapid method for the detection of *S. agalactiae* colonization in pregnant women at the time of delivery has recently been developed and evaluated (11). The test is based on the detection of the *S. agalactiae cfb* gene (84) by a fluorogenic real-time PCR assay (IDI-Strep B; Becton Dickinson, Sparks, Md.), and results can be obtained in a few hours with a reported sensitivity of 94% and specificity of 95.9% (24). The test has been evaluated and approved by the FDA for combined rectal and vaginal swabs. The IDI-Strep B test is commercially available and performed well in a multicenter evaluation study (24). If real-time PCR is used at the time of delivery, only a vaginal swab (minus the rectal sample) should be tested. A major advantage is that results are available within a short time frame, and the vaginal colonization status can be assessed at the time of delivery. In comparison with the gold standard of selective broth culture, as recommended by the CDC, the test may offer an alternative for the future.

S. pneumoniae

Several different PCR assays have been developed for the identification of *S. pneumoniae* from culture isolates. Tests are based on the detection of the genes for autolysin *lytA*, the pneumococcal surface antigen *psaA*, and the pneumolysin gene *ply*. Comparison of the ability to distinguish difficult-to-identify *S. pneumoniae* strains and closely related atypical streptococci revealed that the *lytA*-based PCR was the most specific method (73). While results based on the detection of *psaA* are also acceptable, the different pneumolysin-targeted methods appear to be relatively nonspecific. Nucleic acid probes for the detection of cultured isolates of *S. pyogenes*, *S. agalactiae*, and *S. pneumoniae* are commercially available (AccuProbe; GenProbe) (21, 25). Detection relies on hybridization of a specific probe to 16S rRNA sequences. These tests are not routinely performed for standard identification procedures but can aid in the identification of atypical streptococcal isolates. Atypical organisms include *S. pneumoniae* isolates with unusual patterns of bile solubility and optochin susceptibility, nonhemolytic *S. agalactiae* strains, or beta-hemolytic streptococci harboring the Lancefield group A antigen with questionable species identification.

ISOLATION PROCEDURES

General Procedures

Streptococci are usually grown on agar media supplemented with blood because the assessment of the hemolytic reaction is important for identification. Growth of streptococci is often enhanced in the presence of an exogenous catalase source. Streptococcal species with low or absent hydrogen peroxide production, such as *S. agalactiae,* can be grown on other commonly used nonselective media without blood.

Agar media selective for gram-positive bacteria (e.g., phenylethyl alcohol-containing agar or Columbia agar with colistin and nalidixic acid) support the growth of streptococci. The optimal incubation temperature range for most streptococcal species lies between 35 and 37°C. Supplemental carbon dioxide (5% CO_2) and anaerobic conditions enhance the growth of many streptococcal species, since streptococci are facultative anaerobes. Although some streptococci grow well in ambient air, incubation in 5% CO_2 is recommended for the culture of *S. pneumoniae* and other streptococcal species of the viridans group.

Special Procedures for *Streptococcus pyogenes* Throat Cultures

A properly performed and interpreted throat culture remains the gold standard for the diagnosis of *S. pyogenes* acute pharyngitis. The recovery of *S. pyogenes* from throat swabs on 5% sheep blood agar with Trypticase soy base and incubated in air is a reliable and well-accepted method (77). Lack of hemolysis, overgrowth and production of toxic bacterial metabolites by normal upper respiratory tract microbiota, or depletion of substrates often leads to false-negative results or delays caused by labor-intensive reisolation steps. More rigorous standards for the isolation of *S. pyogenes* include an additional blood agar plate containing sulfamethoxazole-trimethoprim, which inhibits the normal respiratory microbiota (65). *Streptococcus* selective medium is highly sensitive for isolation of *S. pyogenes,* suppressing the growth of commensal respiratory microbiota including other beta-hemolytic streptococci (116). Incubation in anaerobic or CO_2-enriched atmosphere more frequently leads to the isolation of non-*S. pyogenes* beta-hemolytic streptococci (77). Important details have been summarized (13, 59). The isolation of a few colonies of *S. pyogenes* does not differentiate a carrier from an acutely infected individual and may reflect inadequate specimen collection (12).

After 18 to 24 h of incubation, culture plates should be examined for growth of beta-hemolytic colonies. Negative cultures should be reexamined after an additional 24-h incubation period. Presumptive identification of *S. pyogenes* can be achieved by susceptibility to bacitracin or testing for PYR activity. Other beta-hemolytic streptococci are occasionally positive in one of these tests, but not in both. Definitive diagnosis includes the demonstration of the Lancefield group A antigen by immunoassay. Although other species may rarely possess the group A antigen (Table 1), they lack PYR activity (34).

Special Procedures for *S. agalactiae* (GBS)

Early-onset neonatal group B streptococcal (*S. agalactiae*) (GBS) infections can be prevented by administration of antibiotic prophylaxis during delivery (97). An essential requirement for efficient prophylaxis is the reliable detection of colonization with *S. agalactiae* in pregnant women before delivery. Screening should be performed between weeks 35 and 37 of pregnancy. A lower vaginal swab and a rectal swab (i.e., insert swab through the anal sphincter) should be obtained with either one or two different swabs and placed in an appropriate transport medium (Amies or Stuart's without charcoal; see chapter 20). While culture counts decline to some extent, viability of *S. agalactiae* is preserved in transport medium kept at room temperature or 4°C for up to 4 days. To reduce costs, vaginal and rectal swabs can be placed in a single transport medium tube and cultured together. Swabs should be cultured in selective broth medium for 18 to 24 h at 35 to 37°C in ambient air or 5% CO_2 and subsequently plated on Trypticase soy blood agar plates. Selective broth medium is commercially available (Trans-Vag broth supplemented with 5% sheep blood [Remel Inc., Lenexa, Kans.] or LIM broth [BBL Microbiology Systems, Cockeysville, Md.]). Selective broth can also be prepared by supplementation of Todd-Hewitt broth (THB) with nalidixic acid (15 μg/ml) and colistin (10 μg/ml) or supplementation of THB with nalidixic acid (15 μg/ml) and gentamicin (8 μg/ml). Trypticase soy blood agar plates should be checked for typical colonies (narrow zone of beta-hemolysis) of *S. agalactiae* after 24 and 48 h of incubation at 35 to 37°C. Identification of *S. agalactiae* is then achieved by standard techniques as described below. Selective media relying on the detection of the *S. agalactiae* pigment (StrepB Carrot broth [Hardy Diagnostics, Santa Maria, Calif.] or GBS broth [Northeast Laboratory Services, Waterville, Maine]) are highly specific and sensitive (91, 113). Subculture is needed to detect nonhemolytic strains with pigment-dependent selective media. Methods to detect *S. agalactiae* by nucleic acid probes (AccuProbe; GenProbe) following overnight enrichment have also been published (15, 121). Commercially available antigen detection tests cannot be recommended for the detection of *S. agalactiae* colonization, due to poor sensitivities in comparison to selective broth isolation procedures (107).

IDENTIFICATION

Description of Colonies

Colonies of streptococci usually appear gray or almost white with moist or glistening features. Dry colonies are rarely encountered. Colony size varies between the different beta-hemolytic species and helps to distinguish groups of streptococci. Beta-hemolytic streptococci of the pyogenic group (*S. pyogenes, S. agalactiae,* and *S. dysgalactiae* subsp. *equisimilis*) form colonies of >0.5 mm after 24 h of incubation, in contrast to beta-hemolytic strains of the *S. anginosus* group (formerly called "*S. milleri*" group), which present with pinpoint colonies of <0.5 mm after the same incubation time (Fig. 1). Members of the *S. anginosus* group emit a distinct odor resembling butterscotch or caramel, presumably due to the production of diacetyl (18) by the species belonging to this group. Among the beta-hemolytic species of the pyogenic group, *S. agalactiae* produces the largest colonies with a relatively small zone of hemolysis. Nonhemolytic *S. agalactiae* strains do occur and look like enterococci.

Within the group of alpha-hemolytic streptococci, *S. pneumoniae* has a distinct colony morphology that helps to distinguish pneumococcal isolates from other streptococci of the viridans group. Due to the production of capsular polysaccharide, colonies glisten and appear moist. Colonies may be large and mucoid if large amounts of capsular

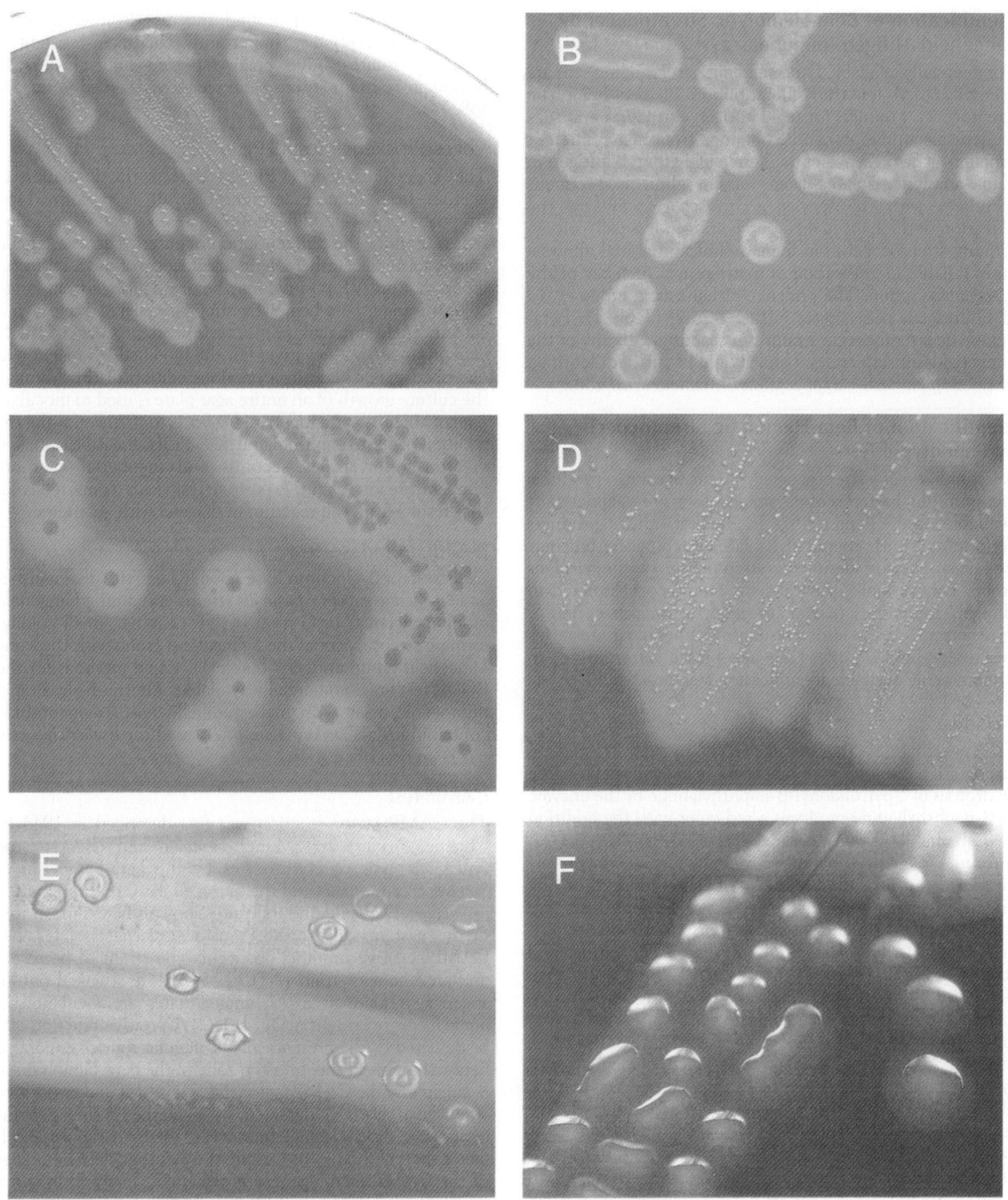

FIGURE 1 Colony morphology of clinical isolates of selected streptococci. (A) *S. pyogenes*; (B) *S. agalactiae*; (C) *S. dysgalactiae* subsp. *equisimilis* (Lancefield group G); (D) *S. anginosus* (note the pinpoint size colonies); (E) *S. pneumoniae* (note the central depression of the colonies); (F) *S. pneumoniae* (note the mucoid appearance of the colonies). (Courtesy of Tim Pietzcker, University of Ulm, Germany.)

polysaccharide are made, a feature often encountered in serotype 3 strains. The mucoid appearance is usually very typical for *S. pneumoniae* but can also occasionally be observed in *S. pyogenes*. Another feature characterizing *S. pneumoniae* isolates is the central navel-like depression of the colonies that is caused by the pneumococcal autolysin. Colonies of other viridans streptococci lack this feature and have a dome-like appearance. Nonhemolytic gray colonies are typical for species of the *S. bovis* and *S. salivarius* groups. Typical streptococcal colony morphologies are presented in Fig. 1.

Identification of Beta-Hemolytic Streptococci by Lancefield Antigen Immunoassays

Commercially available Lancefield antigen grouping sera are primarily used for the differentiation of beta-hemolytic streptococci. Products for rapid antigen extraction and subsequent agglutination can be obtained from many different suppliers. The presence of the Lancefield group B antigen in beta-hemolytic isolates from human clinical specimens correlates with the species *S. agalactiae*. Similarly, the detection of the Lancefield group F antigen in small-colony-forming streptococci from human clinical material allows a fairly reliable identification of a strain as a member of the *S. anginosus* group. The presence of Lancefield group A, C, or G antigens necessitates further testing (Table 1). Beta-hemolytic streptococcal strains not reacting with any of the Lancefield antisera are rare and should be further identified by phenotypic tests or application of nucleic acid probes.

Identification of Beta-Hemolytic Streptococci by Phenotypic Tests

A number of streptococcal identification products incorporating batteries of physiologic tests are commercially available (see chapter 15). In general, these products perform well with commonly isolated streptococci but may lack accuracy for identifying streptococci of the viridans group. For the bulk of pathogenic streptococci isolated in clinical laboratories (e.g., *S. pyogenes*, *S. agalactiae*, and *S. pneumoniae*), serologic or presumptive physiologic tests (as described below) offer an acceptable alternative to commercially available identification systems.

PYR Test

The presence of the enzyme PYR is often tested to distinguish *S. pyogenes* from other beta-hemolytic streptococci. Hydrolysis of L-pyrrolidonyl-β-naphthylamide by the enzyme to β-naphthylamine produces a red color with the addition of cinnamaldehyde reagent (chapter 21). *S. iniae* and *S. porcinus*, which are also positive with this test, are only rarely identified in human clinical specimens since they are primarily animal-associated species. PYR spot tests are commercially available. It is important to distinguish *Streptococcus* from *Enterococcus* prior to PYR testing, and strains of other related genera may be PYR positive (including the genera *Abiotrophia*, *Aerococcus*, *Enterococcus*, *Gemella*, and *Lactococcus*). However, PYR-positive beta-hemolytic enterococcal isolates typically present with a different colonial morphology, and when combined with other phenotypic characteristics (see chapter 30), may be distinguished from streptococci. To avoid false-positive reactions caused by other PYR-positive bacterial species (for example, staphylococci), the test should be performed only on pure cultures.

Bacitracin Susceptibility

S. pyogenes displays bacitracin susceptibility, in contrast to other beta-hemolytic streptococci found in humans. Together with Lancefield antigen determination, it can be used for the identification of *S. pyogenes* since beta-hemolytic strains of other streptococcal species that may contain the group A antigen are bacitracin-resistant. The test can also be used to distinguish *S. pyogenes* from other PYR-positive beta-hemolytic streptococci (*S. iniae* and *S. porcinus*). A bacitracin disk (0.04 U) is applied to a sheep blood agar plate that has been heavily inoculated with 3 or 4 colonies of a pure culture of the strain to be tested. After overnight incubation at 35°C in 5% CO_2, any zone of inhibition around the disk is interpreted as indicating susceptibility. Importantly, bacitracin-resistant *S. pyogenes* isolates have been reported and clusters of bacitracin-resistant strains were recently observed in Europe (68, 74).

Voges-Proskauer Test (VP)

The Voges-Proskauer (VP) test detects the formation of acetoin from glucose fermentation. It is performed on streptococci as a modification of the classical VP reaction that is used for the differentiation of enteric bacteria. Small-colony-forming beta-hemolytic streptococci of the *S. anginosus* group that are VP positive may be distinguished from large-colony-forming beta-hemolytic streptococci harboring identical Lancefield antigens (A, C, or G). Streptococci of the *S. mitis* group are VP negative. For the modified VP reaction as described by Facklam in a previous edition of this Manual, the culture growth of an entire agar plate is used to inoculate 2 ml of VP broth and incubated at 35°C for 6 h. Following the addition of 5% α-naphthol and 40% KOH, the tube is shaken vigorously for a few seconds and incubated at room temperature for 30 min. A positive test yields a pink-red color that results from the reaction of diacetyl with guanidine.

β-Glucuronidase Test

Detection of β-glucuronidase (BGUR) activity distinguishes *S. dysgalactiae* subsp. *equisimilis* strains containing Lancefield group antigens C or G from BGUR-negative, small-colony-forming streptococci of the *S. anginosus* group with the same Lancefield group antigens (Table 1). Rapid methods for the BGUR test are commercially available. Alternatively, a rapid fluorogenic assay with methylumbelliferyl-β-D-glucuronide containing MacConkey agar, often used for *Escherichia coli*, has been described (62).

CAMP Test

The CAMP factor reaction was first described in 1944 by Christie, Atkins, and Munch-Petersen and refers to the synergistic lysis of erythrocytes by the beta-hemolysin of *Staphylococcus aureus* and the extracellular CFB protein of *S. agalactiae*. The gene and its expression can be demonstrated in the vast majority (>98%) of *S. agalactiae* isolates, but CAMP-negative mutants do occur. The strain to be tested and an *S. aureus* strain (ATCC 25923) are streaked onto a sheep agar plate at a 90° angle. Plates are incubated in ambient air overnight at 36 ± 1°C. A positive reaction can be detected by the presence of a triangular zone of enhanced beta-hemolysis in the diffusion zone of the beta-hemolysin of *S. aureus* and the CAMP factor (Fig. 2). CAMP factor-positive strains can also be detected by a method using β-lysin-containing disks (Remel Inc.) (120) or by a rapid CAMP factor spot method (89). Despite the fact that close homologs of the CAMP factor gene are present in many *S. pyogenes* strains, beta-hemolytic streptococci other than *S. agalactiae* are usually negative in the above-described CAMP factor test. Several gram-positive rods including corynebacteria and *Listeria monocytogenes* strains may be CAMP factor positive.

Hippurate Hydrolysis Test

The ability to hydrolyze hippurate is an alternative test for the presumptive identification of *S. agalactiae*. A rapid version of the test, as it is used for campylobacters, can be performed by incubating a turbid suspension of bacterial cells in 0.5 ml of 1% aqueous sodium hippurate for 2 h at 35°C. Glycine formed as an end product of hippurate hydrolysis is detected by adding ninhydrin reagent and

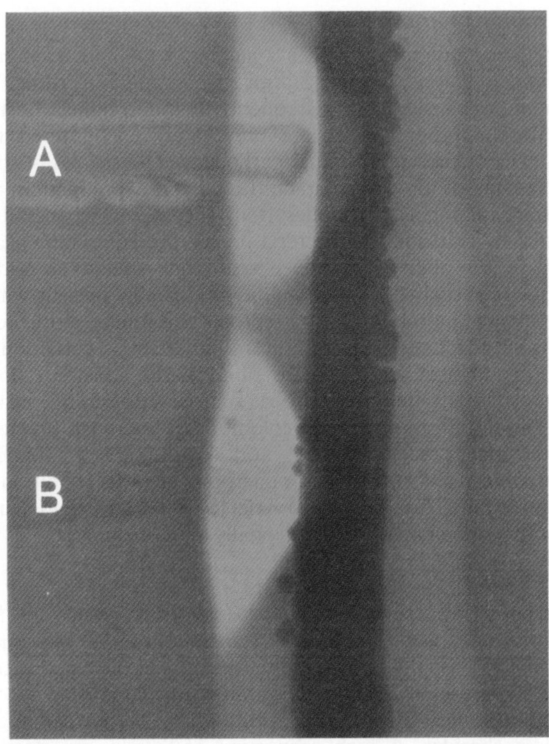

FIGURE 2 CAMP factor test. Arrowhead-shaped zone of hemolysis in the zone of *S. aureus* β-hemolysin. (A) Beta-hemolytic *S. agalactiae* strain O90R; (B) nonhemolytic *S. agalactiae* strain R268.

observing the development of a deep purple color, signifying a positive test (chapter 21) (53). Streptococci other than *S. agalactiae* may also be hippurate hydrolysis positive (114), especially viridans streptococci.

Identification of *S. pneumoniae* and Viridans Group Streptococci

The correct species identification of viridans group streptococci other than *S. pneumoniae* is challenging. Recent taxonomic changes and identification of novel streptococcal species have further complicated matters. The number of recognized species in this group is now greater than 30. The viridans group includes alpha-hemolytic, nonhemolytic (*S. salivarius* group and *S. bovis* group), and beta-hemolytic (*S. anginosus* group) streptococcal strains. All of the viridans streptococci are LAP positive and PYR negative. Conventional microbiologic tests are limited with respect to species identification but are helpful in placing isolates into the correct streptococcal groups (Table 2). Beighton et al. described an identification scheme based on phenotypic tests that allowed the differentiation and correct species identification of the majority of viridans group species (7). The scheme requires the evaluation of enzymatic reactions performed by in-house fluorogenic tests that are not commercially available. Importantly, most clinical laboratories must strive for group, instead of species, classifications with current phenotypic test panels.

The API tests (bioMerieux, Marcy l'Etoile, France) offer species identification of viridans group streptococci. While many species from this group are identified with acceptable accuracy, several species have not been included in the database. Comparisons of molecular species identification by DNA reassociation studies with the results of the API Rapid ID 32 Strep system showed that more than 85% of 156 strains from streptococcal species included in the database were correctly identified (60). However, in the same study, more than 50% of six species not included in the database were incorrectly identified by the test (60). Evaluation studies performed under routine clinical conditions appear to yield less favorable results (46). In conclusion, reliable phenotypic identification of viridans group streptococci can currently be achieved only to the group level.

Molecular methods may offer alternative approaches to conventional phenotypic identification schemes. The most common molecular identification method, 16S rRNA gene sequencing, does not yield reliable species identification for several species including *S. mitis*, *S. oralis*, and *S. pneumoniae*. The 16S rRNA gene sequences are more than 99% identical (57). Whole-cell protein analyses were unable to yield good correlation with species identification by other methods. Sequence determination of the manganese-dependent superoxide dismutase gene *sodA* appears promising (87, 88). In contrast to 16S rRNA gene sequencing, it allows the differentiation of *S. mitis*, *S. oralis*, and *S. pneumoniae* and the correct identification of almost 30 different streptococcal species including 16 species from the viridans group.

Descriptions of the species belonging to the nonpyogenic groups are given below, and physiological traits of the groups are shown in Table 2.

TABLE 2 Phenotypic characteristics of viridans streptococcal groups[a]

Streptococcal group	Arginine hydrolysis	Esculin	Mannitol	Sorbitol	Urea hydrolysis	VP
S. mitis	v[b]	v	–	v	–	–
S. anginosus	+	+	–	–	–	+
S. mutans	–	+	+	+	–	+
S. salivarius	–	v	–	–	v[d]	+
S. bovis	–	+	v[c]	–	–	+

[a] Symbols and abbreviations: +, positive; –, negative; v, variable.

[b] The species *S. cristatus*, *S. gordonii*, *S. parasanguinis*, and *S. sanguinis* are arginine hydrolysis positive; other species of the *S. mitis* group are arginine hydrolysis negative.

[c] *S. gallolyticus* subsp. *gallolyticus* is positive for the acidification of mannitol, and the other species of the *S. bovis* group are negative for mannitol acidification.

[d] *S. salivarius* is variable for urea hydrolysis, and *S. vestibularis* is positive for urea hydrolysis. All other species of the *S. salivarius* group are negative for urea hydrolysis.

S. mitis Group

Streptococcal species belonging to the *S. mitis* group include *S. mitis*, *S. sanguinis*, *S. parasanguinis*, *S. gordonii*, *S. cristatus*, *S. oralis*, *S. infantis* (58), *S. peroris* (58), and *S. pneumoniae*, which is discussed separately. This group of predominantly alpha-hemolytic streptococci includes several species of known clinical significance together with others for which few or no clinical data have been collected. Among the phenotypic characteristics of the species in this group, extracellular polysaccharide production is negative for *S. mitis* strains but a variable characteristic of *S. oralis* isolates. This feature correlates with the smooth colony surface of many *S. oralis* strains and the rough and dry appearance of *S. mitis* colonies.

S. anginosus Group

The small-colony-forming species *S. anginosus*, *S. constellatus*, and *S. intermedius* belong to the *S. anginosus* group, which is sometimes referred to as the "*S. milleri*" group. Strains of the *S. anginosus* group may be non-, alpha-, or beta-hemolytic on blood agar plates, with some variations between the species. While *S. constellatus* is frequently beta-hemolytic, most isolates of *S. intermedius* are nonhemolytic. For many strains, growth is enhanced in the presence of CO_2, with some strains requiring anaerobic conditions. *S. anginosus* and *S. constellatus* strains may possess Lancefield group antigens A, C, F, or G. Most *S. constellatus* or *S. intermedius* strains react with antisera against Lancefield group F antigen or are nongroupable.

The species *S. constellatus* has been further subdivided into two subspecies, *S. constellatus* subsp. *constellatus* and *S. constellatus* subsp. *pharyngis* (119). *S. constellatus* subsp. *constellatus* is phenotypically different from *S. constellatus* subsp. *pharyngis*, which usually possesses the Lancefield group antigen C, is beta-hemolytic, and has been associated with pharyngitis. Detailed phenotypic characteristics of the *S. anginosus* group are shown in Table 3.

TABLE 3 Phenotypic characteristics of streptococcal species of the *S. anginosus* group[a]

Test	*S. anginosus*	*S. constellatus*	*S. intermedius*
β-D-Fucosidase	–	–/+[c]	+
β-D-Acetylglucosaminidase	v	–/+[c]	+
β-D-Acetylgalactosaminidase	–	–/+[c]	+
Neuraminidase	–	–	+
α-D-Glucosidase	v	+	+
β-D-Glucosidase	+	–/+[c]	v
α-D-Galactosidase	v	–	–
β-D-Galactosidase	v	v	+
Amygdalin (acidification)	+	v	v
Mannitol (acidification)	v	–	–
Sorbitol (acidification)	–	–	–
Lactose (acidification)	+	v	+
Melibiose (acidification)	v	v	v
Arginine hydrolysis	+	+	+
Esculin hydrolysis	+	v	+
VP[b]	+	+	+
Urease	–	–	–
Hyaluronidase	–	+	+

[a] Symbols and abbreviations: +, positive; –, negative; v, variable.
[b] Voges-Proskauer test (formation of acetoin from glucose fermentation).
[c] The species *S. constellatus* subsp. *pharyngis* is positive for β-D-fucosidase, β-D-acetylglucosaminidase, β-D-acetylgalactosaminidase, and β-D-glucosidase activities. In contrast, *S. constellatus* subsp. *constellatus* is negative for these enzymatic activities.

S. mutans Group

The *S. mutans* group includes *S. mutans*, *S. sobrinus*, *S. criceti*, *S. ratti*, *S. downei*, *S. ferus*, *S. hyovaginalis*, and *S. macacae*. *S. mutans* and *S. sobrinus* are frequently found in human hosts, while the other species are only rarely encountered in humans or represent animal pathogens. The species of the *S. mutans* group are characterized by the production of extracellular polysaccharides from sucrose, which can be tested by culturing the bacteria on sucrose-containing agar and by the ability to produce acid from a relatively wide range of carbohydrates. *S. mutans* strains may present with an atypical morphology for streptococci, forming short rods on solid media or in broth culture under acidic conditions. On blood agar, colonies are often hard, adherent, and usually alpha-hemolytic. On sucrose-containing agar, species from this group form colonies that are rough (frosted glass appearance), heaped, and surrounded by liquid-containing glucan. Under anaerobic growth conditions, some strains are beta-hemolytic. *S. sobrinus* strains are mostly nonhemolytic or occasionally alpha-hemolytic.

S. salivarius Group

Streptococcal species in the *S. salivarius* group are *S. salivarius*, *S. vestibularis*, and *S. thermophilus*. *S. salivarius* strains are usually non- or alpha-hemolytic on blood agar. On sucrose-containing agar, strains form large mucoid or hard colonies due to the production of extracellular polysaccharides. A high proportion of *S. salivarius* strains react with the Lancefield group K antiserum. Species in this group may also react with the streptococcal group D antiserum. It is unclear if these strains truly possess the group D antigen or yield a nonspecific cross-reaction. *S. vestibularis* is alpha-hemolytic, and the failure of this species to produce extracellular polysaccharides on sucrose-containing agar is helpful in distinguishing *S. vestibularis* from *S. salivarius* strains. *S. thermophilus* is found in dairy products but has not been isolated from clinical specimens.

S. bovis Group

The species belonging to the *S. bovis* group (*S. equinus*, *S. gallolyticus*, *S. infantarius*, and *S. alactolyticus*) are non-enterococcal group D streptococci, grow on bile esculin agar, and are unable to grow in 6.5% NaCl. On blood agar, strains are either nonhemolytic or alpha-hemolytic. Strains of the *S. bovis* group share phenotypic characteristics with *S. mutans* strains, such as production of glucan, fermentation of mannitol, and growth on bile esculin agar. However, the *S. bovis* group does not ferment sorbitol, is able to ferment starch or glycogen, and gives a Lancefield group D reaction. Species of the *S. bovis* group may resemble *S. salivarius* strains. Differentiation of these two groups on the basis of the Lancefield group D reaction, ability to grow on bile esculin agar, fermentation of mannitol, and production of inulin, starch, and urease has been suggested (92). Strains from the *S. bovis* group are usually β-galactosidase negative and α-galactosidase positive, in contrast to *S. salivarius*. As described, strains formerly known as *S. bovis* currently belong to several species of the *S. bovis* group.

Physiologic Tests

Optochin Test

Most *S. pneumoniae* isolates are optochin susceptible. Before application of the optochin disk, several colonies of a pure culture are streaked on a sheep blood agar plate. Optochin testing should be performed on plates that are incubated at 35 to 36°C overnight in 5% CO_2 because up to 8% of strains do not grow under ambient conditions. *S. pneumoniae* isolates show inhibition zones of ≥14 mm with a 6-mm disk (containing 5 μg of optochin) and inhibition zones of ≥16 mm with a 10-mm disk. Incubation in 5% CO_2 yielded increased specificity (1). Optochin-resistant *S. pneumoniae* strains have been reported as well as optochin-susceptible *S. mitis* isolates (especially when tested in ambient conditions). Since optochin testing may miss up to 4% of bile-soluble *S. pneumoniae* isolates (1), strains displaying a smaller zone of inhibition (9 to 13 mm for the 6-mm disk) should be subjected to additional testing for bile solubility to confirm species identification.

Application of an optochin disk onto the primary culture medium may facilitate a rapid presumptive identification but may miss pneumococcal isolates in a mixed culture. The optochin susceptibility test should be repeated with a pure culture in cases of mixed cultures, or additional tests should be performed (e.g., bile solubility).

Bile Solubility Test

Bile solubility can be performed either in a test tube or by direct application of the reagent to an agar plate. For the test tube method, a saline suspension of a pure culture is adjusted to a McFarland standard of 0.5 to 1.0, and 0.5 ml of the suspension is added to a small tube. The bacterial suspension is mixed with 0.5 ml of 10% sodium deoxycholate (bile) and incubated at 35°C. A control containing 0.5 ml of bacterial suspension with 0.5 ml of saline should be prepared for each strain tested. A positive result is characterized by clearing of the bile suspension within 5 to 15 min and allows the identification of a strain as *S. pneumoniae*. For the plate method, one drop of 10% sodium deoxycholate is placed directly on a colony of the strain in question and incubated at 35°C for 15 min in ambient air. It is important to keep the plates in a horizontal position in order to prevent the reagent from washing away the colony. Colonies of *S. pneumoniae* will disappear or demonstrate a flattened colony morphology, while other viridans streptococci will appear unchanged.

Bile Esculin Test

Bile esculin medium (available from commercial sources) in either plates or slants should be inoculated with one to three colonies of the organism to be tested and incubated at 35°C in ambient air for up to 48 h. Optimal results can be achieved by using media supplemented with 4% oxgall (equivalent of 40% bile) (Remel) and a standardized inoculum of 10^6 CFU (19). A definitive blackening of plated media or blackening of at least one-half of an agar slant is considered a positive test, indicative of species belonging to the *S. bovis* group or enterococci. Occasional other viridans streptococci are positive with this test or display weakly positive reactions that are difficult to interpret (92). Isolates from patients with serious infections (e.g., endocarditis) should be more completely characterized.

Arginine Hydrolysis

Arginine hydrolysis is a key reaction for the identification of viridans streptococci. Discrepancies can occur among test methods (117). Two commonly used methods are detailed here. Moeller's decarboxylase broth containing arginine (Becton Dickinson and other sources) should be inoculated with the test organism, overlaid with mineral oil, and incubated at 35 to 37°C for up to 7 days. Degradation of arginine results in elevated pH, indicated by development of a purple color. Negative results are indicated by a yellow color, which is due to acid accumulation from metabolism of glucose only. For the microtiter plate method (8), 3 drops of the arginine-containing reagent are inoculated with 1 drop of an overnight THB culture and incubated for 24 h at 37°C anaerobically. Production of ammonia is detected by the appearance of an orange color following the addition of 1 drop of Nessler's reagent.

Urea Hydrolysis

Christensen urea agar (Becton Dickinson and other sources) is inoculated and incubated aerobically at 35°C for up to 7 days. Development of a pink color indicates a positive reaction. An alternative format is to dispense Christensen's medium without agar into a microtiter tray well and, after inoculation, overlay it with mineral oil prior to incubation.

Voges-Proskauer (VP) Test

The VP test can be performed as described for the identification of beta-hemolytic streptococci. A standard method for performing the VP test, requiring extended incubation, is described in chapter 21.

Esculin Hydrolysis

Esculin agar slants (Becton Dickinson and other sources) are inoculated and incubated for up to 1 week. A positive reaction appears as a blackening of the medium; no change in color indicates a negative esculin hydrolysis test.

Hyaluronidase Production

Hyaluronidase activity can be detected on brain heart infusion agar plates supplemented with 2 mg of sodium hyaluronate per liter (Sigma-Aldrich, St. Louis, Mo.) (104). The strains to be tested are inoculated by stabbing into the agar, and plates are incubated anaerobically at 37°C overnight. After the plate is flooded with 2 M acetic acid, hyaluronidase activity is indicated by the appearance of a clear zone around the stab. A quantitative method for determining hyaluronidase activity can be performed in microtiter trays (52).

Production of Extracellular Polysaccharide

Strains may be isolated as single colonies on sucrose-containing agar. The two most commonly used media are (i) mitis-salivarius agar containing 0.001% (wt/vol) potassium tellurite (Becton Dickinson) and (ii) tryptone-yeast-cystine agar (Lab M, Bury, United Kingdom). Incubation may require up to 5 days at 37°C.

TYPING SYSTEMS

In the majority of cases, typing of streptococci has no immediate clinical or therapeutic consequences. It is most often performed by reference laboratories for the purposes of epidemiologic studies and the evaluation of vaccine efficacy. Although classical antibody-dependent typing systems for capsular serotypes and surface proteins have been used for years, molecular methods have become attractive, since they do not require special techniques or the maintenance of rarely used reagents such as a large antibody panel. Another advantage lies in the fact that the interrogation of DNA sequences is independent of culture conditions and gene expression. For the differentiation of distinct clones, pulsed-field gel electrophoresis (PFGE) and multilocus sequence typing (MLST) systems have been established for many streptococcal species (32).

S. pneumoniae comprises 90 antigenically distinct capsular serotypes that can be detected by the Neufeld test (Quellung reaction), which is still regarded as the gold standard for epidemiologic studies. Pure cultures of pneumococci are grown on a freshly prepared 5% sheep blood agar plate or a 10% horse blood agar plate at 35 to 37°C and 5% CO_2 for 18 to 24 h. A small amount of bacterial growth (less than a 10-μl loop) is resuspended in a droplet of phosphate-buffered or physiological saline (McFarland standard of approximately 0.5). A few microliters of the saline suspension are mixed with an equal amount of specific pneumococcal rabbit antisera on a glass slide. The specimen is subsequently evaluated for capsular swelling (a clear area surrounding the bacterial cells) by phase-contrast microscopy (×1,000 magnification; oil immersion) (2). The reaction is stable for approximately 30 min. The best results are achieved when 10 to 50 bacterial cells are visible per high-power (×1,000) microscopic field. To increase the visibility of the result, it is possible to add 0.3% aqueous methylene blue in the same amount as the antiserum to the mixture. Following the same principle, commercially available kits (Pneumotest; Statens Serum Institut, Copenhagen, Denmark) allow rapid testing of *S. pneumoniae* serotypes with pooled antisera by a checkerboard method. A rapid antigen detection test using pooled antisera coupled to latex beads (Statens Serum Institut) has been developed (102). Due to strain discrepancies, confirmation by the Neufeld Quellung reaction is recommended. For the distinction of single clones, PFGE (66, 71) or MLST typing schemes (32) have been used in pneumococcal investigations.

Nine different antibody-defined capsular polysaccharides have been described for *S. agalactiae* (Ia, Ib, and II through VIII). The percentage of nontypeable strains can be minimized by optimization of capsular expression (10). In addition to antibody detection of capsular serotypes, recently developed PCR- and DNA sequencing-based techniques allow the detection of capsular serotypes (64). Individual clones of *S. agalactiae* have been detected either by MLST (55) or PFGE (9, 45).

Conventional typing of *S. pyogenes* is based upon the antigenic specificity of the surface-expressed T and M proteins (54). The function of the trypsin-resistant T protein is unknown. The T type can be identified by agglutination with commercially available serologic assays utilizing approximately 20 accepted anti-T sera. M proteins are major antiphagocytic virulence factors of *S. pyogenes* (42). N-terminal sequence variation in genes encoding these highly protective antigens is the basis of the *S. pyogenes* precipitation typing system. At present, 83 M serotypes are unequivocally validated and internationally recognized to be serologically unique and are designated M1 to M93 in the Lancefield classification (37). M serotypes that are not included are from non-*S. pyogenes* organisms or correspond to an existing M serotype.

A molecular serotyping system has been established on the basis of nucleotide sequences encoding the amino termini of M proteins. The *emm* gene sequences encode M proteins and have been correlated with Lancefield M serotypes. This methodology allows assignment to a validated M protein gene sequence (*emm1* through *emm124*) and identification of new *emm*-sequence types and subtypes. Molecular serotyping has evolved into the gold standard molecular methodology of *S. pyogenes* typing (37). A large database of approximately 350 *emm* gene sequences from strains originally used for Lancefield serotyping and including *emm* sequences from beta-hemolytic groups C, G, and L streptococci has been developed by the CDC (http://www.cdc.gov/ncidod/biotech/infotech_hp.html). Recently, MLST has been developed for *S. pyogenes*. Population genetic studies demonstrated stable associations between *emm* type and MLST among isolates obtained decades apart and/or from different continents (33).

In outbreak situations that include *S. pyogenes*, restriction enzyme-mediated digestion of *emm* amplicons is a valuable tool for rapid identification of isolates containing similar *emm* genes (6). For clusters of isolates sharing the same *emm* type, PFGE profiles may be helpful for distinguishing similar strains (79).

SEROLOGIC TESTS

Determination of streptococcal antibodies is indicated for the diagnosis of poststreptococcal disease, such as acute rheumatic fever or glomerulonephritis (101). A fourfold rise in antibody titer is regarded as definitive proof of an antecedent streptococcal infection. Multiple variables, including site of infection, time since the onset of infection, age, the background prevalence of streptococcal infections (3), antimicrobial therapy, and other comorbidities, influence antibody levels. The most widely used antibodies are anti-streptolysin O and anti-DNase B.

Antibodies against streptolysin O (ASO) reach a maximum at 3 to 6 weeks after infection. While ASO responses following streptococcal upper respiratory tract infections are usually elevated, pyoderma caused by *S. pyogenes* does not elicit a strong ASO response. *Streptococcus dysgalactiae* subsp. *equisimilis* can also produce streptolysin O, and thus elevated ASO titers are not specific for *S. pyogenes* infections.

Among the four streptococcal DNases produced, the host response is most consistent against DNase B. Anti-DNase B titers may not reach maximum titers for 6 to 8 weeks, but they remain elevated longer than ASO titers and are more reliable than ASO for the confirmation of a preceding streptococcal skin infection. Moreover, since only 80 to 85% of patients with rheumatic fever have elevated ASO titers, additional anti-DNase B titers may be helpful.

Due to frequent exposure to *S. pyogenes*, ASO and anti-DNase B titers are higher in children in the United States from 2 to 12 years of age. Geometric mean values of 89 Todd U (ASO) and 112 U (anti-DNase B) and 240 Todd U and 640 U, respectively, represent the upper limits of normal values (56). Prompt antibiotic therapy of streptococcal infections can reduce the titer but does not abolish antibody production. Streptococcal carriers do not experience a rise in streptococcal antibody titers.

The hemagglutination-based streptozyme test (Streptozyme; Carter-Wallace, Inc., Cranbury, N.J.) was developed to detect antibodies against multiple extracellular streptococcal products. However, variabilities in test standardization and inconsistent specificities have been reported (44).

ANTIMICROBIAL SUSCEPTIBILITIES

Beta-Hemolytic Streptococci

Penicillin remains the drug of choice for the treatment of streptococcal infections due to beta-hemolytic streptococci, because in contrast to *S. pneumoniae* and other alpha-hemolytic streptococci, beta-hemolytic streptococci remain uniformly susceptible to penicillin. Reports of penicillin-resistant strains of beta-hemolytic streptococci have not been confirmed by reference laboratories. Due to suspected or confirmed penicillin allergies in more than 10% of patients, macrolides are often given as an alternative treatment. Macrolide resistance rates among isolates of *S. pyogenes* and *S. agalactiae* have been increasing in North America as well as in Europe (26). Resistance rates correlate with the use of macrolides in clinical practice, and geographic differences in resistance rates are often due to differences in macrolide use. In the United States, macrolide resistance among *S. agalactiae* isolates rose from 12 to 20% from 1990 to 2000 (76). Two major mechanisms are responsible for macrolide resistance in streptococci. Resistance encoded by the *mefA* gene results in low-level erythromycin but not clindamycin resistance due to increased drug efflux from the bacterial cell. Methylation of the macrolide binding site within 23S rRNA by methylases encoded by *erm* genes mediates resistance to macrolides, lincosamides, and streptogramin group B (MLS_B) agents. The methylation causes high-level macrolide resistance and is either inducible or constitutively expressed. Strains with inducible MLS_B resistance are resistant to erythromycin and susceptible to clindamycin in vitro. In contrast, strains with constitutive MLS_B resistance demonstrate resistance to both erythromycin and clindamycin. The majority of macrolide-resistant *S. pyogenes* isolates from North America harbor the *mefA* gene, and macrolide resistance due to the presence of *erm* genes is less common in *S. pyogenes*. Among *S. agalactiae* isolates from North America, the predominant macrolide resistance mechanism is methylation of 23S rRNA due to the *erm* methylase genes (*ermTR* and *ermB*), and only a few strains harbor the efflux gene *mefA* (26). Beta-hemolytic streptococcal isolates with a reduced susceptibility to vancomycin have not been reported.

S. pneumoniae and Viridans Streptococci

In view of the development of penicillin resistance in *S. pneumoniae* and other alpha-hemolytic streptococci, penicillin can no longer be recommended as the initial treatment of choice in many countries. Penicillin is considered a preferred antimicrobial agent only for *S. pneumoniae* and other alpha-hemolytic streptococci with demonstrated susceptibilities to penicillin. Penicillin resistance in *S. pneumoniae* is caused by altered penicillin-binding proteins.

Approximately 20% or more of *S. pneumoniae* isolates are not fully susceptible to penicillin in many geographic regions (http://www.cdc.gov/abcs). *S. pneumoniae* infections should be treated according to current guidelines (69). Depending on the clinical situation, treatment options include extended-spectrum cephalosporins, macrolides, fluoroquinolones, and vancomycin. In addition, more than one-third of blood culture isolates of the viridans group collected in the late 1990s in the United States were not susceptible to penicillin (29). Especially *S. mitis* and *S. salivarius* isolates show high percentages of penicillin-resistant strains.

S. pneumoniae was uniformly susceptible to macrolides until the late 1980s in the United States, but macrolide resistance is now evident in 25% of *S. pneumoniae* strains (109). Macrolide resistance in *S. pneumoniae* is caused by ErmB-mediated methylation of 23S rRNA, causing a high-level resistance phenotype, or MefA-mediated efflux of macrolides resulting in a low-level resistance phenotype. In contrast to the United States, where two-thirds of macrolide resistance is mediated by MefA, a higher overall prevalence of macrolide resistance is found in some parts of Europe and most European macrolide-resistant *S. pneumoniae* isolates contain the *ermB* gene (81).

The increased use of fluoroquinolones to treat *S. pneumoniae* infections has been accompanied by a rise in fluoroquinolone-resistant *S. pneumoniae* strains. Resistance occurs in a stepwise fashion and is due to mutations in DNA topoisomerase IV or a subunit of DNA gyrase. While the overall prevalence of fluoroquinolone resistance is below 1% according to ABC surveillance data (http://www.cdc.gov/abcs), the increase in resistant strains during recent years emphasizes the need for close monitoring. Clinical failures of levofloxacin therapy due to resistance have been reported (22). Vancomycin-resistant *S. pneumoniae* isolates have not been described. However, the isolation of a vancomycin-resistant *S. bovis* isolate has been reported (86).

EVALUATION, INTERPRETATION, AND REPORTING OF RESULTS

Streptococci from the pyogenic group and *S. pneumoniae* are important human pathogens. Timely identification of these species in clinical specimens is therefore crucial to treat infections adequately and to reduce transmission. Detection of *S. pyogenes* strains in throat specimens allows adequate therapy and reduces nonsuppurative sequelae. Because *S. dysgalactiae* subsp. *equisimilis* (human group C and G streptococci) has been documented as an agent of pharyngitis including cases complicated by nonsuppurative sequelae, the presence of *S. dysgalactiae* subsp. *equisimilis* in throat cultures should be reported. To avoid unnecessary antibiotic treatment, it is important to correctly differentiate these pathogens from the small-colony-forming beta-hemolytic species of the *S. anginosus* group that constitute part of the oropharyngeal microbiota. However, *S. anginosus* group species isolated from wound specimens or abscesses are likely to represent true pathogens. While invasive neonatal *S. agalactiae* infections are declining due to improved prenatal screening and peripartal antibiotic prophylaxis, increased detection of *S. agalactiae* from adult patients has been reported. Thorough identification and reporting of this organism should therefore not be confined to screening swabs during pregnancy or in newborns.

The correct identification of viridans streptococci to the species or group level is often difficult and should be reserved for strains isolated from serious infections, such as endocarditis, abscesses, and infections in neutropenic patients. While in the normal host, transient bacteremia with viridans streptococci is generally cleared without adverse sequelae, prolonged bacteremia, particularly that caused by *S. mitis* in neutropenic patients, has become recognized as a distinct clinical entity that can be complicated by adult respiratory distress syndrome. Severe bacteremic infections with viridans streptococci have also been reported from low-birth-weight term and preterm neonates. Many *S. mitis* isolates are no longer penicillin-susceptible, and special attention should be paid to susceptibility testing. For *S. pneumoniae*, the elevated prevalence of resistance to penicillins, macrolides, ketolides, and fluoroquinolones varies worldwide. Careful identification of, and interpretation of susceptibility testing for, invasive and noninvasive *S. pneumoniae* isolates is required to guide appropriate antimicrobial therapy and to monitor the further spread of resistant pathogens. Due to the association of *S. gallolyticus* subsp. *gallolyticus* with malignancies of the gastrointestinal tract, and in view of the recent taxonomic changes within the *S. bovis* group, reports of novel species designations should include information about former species names (112).

REFERENCES

1. **Arbique, J. C., C. Poyart, P. Trieu-Cuot, G. Quesne, G. Carvalho Mda, A. G. Steigerwalt, R. E. Morey, D. Jackson, R. J. Davidson, and R. R. Facklam.** 2004. Accuracy of phenotypic and genotypic testing for identification of *Streptococcus pneumoniae* and description of *Streptococcus pseudopneumoniae* sp. nov. *J. Clin. Microbiol.* **42:**4686–4696.
2. **Austrian, R.** 1976. The quellung reaction, a neglected microbiologic technique. *Mt. Sinai J. Med.* **43:**699–709.
3. **Ayoub, E. M., B. Nelson, S. T. Shulman, D. J. Barrett, J. D. Campbell, G. Armstrong, J. Lovejoy, G. H. Angoff, and S. Rockenmacher.** 2003. Group A streptococcal antibodies in subjects with or without rheumatic fever in areas with high or low incidences of rheumatic fever. *Clin. Diagn. Lab. Immunol.* **10:**886–890.
4. **Ballet, M., G. Gevigney, J. P. Gare, F. Delahaye, J. Etienne, and J. P. Delahaye.** 1995. Infective endocarditis due to *Streptococcus bovis*. A report of 53 cases. *Eur. Heart J.* **16:**1975–1980.
5. **Barnham, M., T. J. Thornton, and K. Lange.** 1983. Nephritis caused by *Streptococcus zooepidemicus* (Lancefield group C). *Lancet* **i:**945–948.
6. **Beall, B., R. R. Facklam, J. A. Elliott, A. R. Franklin, T. Hoenes, D. Jackson, L. Laclaire, T. Thompson, and R. Viswanathan.** 1998. Streptococcal *emm* types associated with T-agglutination types and the use of conserved *emm* gene restriction fragment patterns for subtyping group A streptococci. *J. Med. Microbiol.* **47:**893–898.
7. **Beighton, D., J. M. Hardie, and R. A. Whiley.** 1991. A scheme for the identification of viridans streptococci. *J. Med. Microbiol.* **35:**367–372.
8. **Beighton, D., R. R. Russell, and H. Hayday.** 1981. The isolation of characterization of *Streptococcus mutans* serotype *h* from dental plaque of monkeys *(Macaca fascicularis)*. *J. Gen. Microbiol.* **124:**271–279.
9. **Benson, J. A., and P. Ferrieri.** 2001. Rapid pulsed-field gel electrophoresis method for group B streptococcus isolates. *J. Clin. Microbiol.* **39:**3006–3008.
10. **Benson, J. A., A. E. Flores, C. J. Baker, S. L. Hillier, and P. Ferrieri.** 2002. Improved methods for typing nontypeable isolates of group B streptococci. *Int. J. Med. Microbiol.* **292:**37–42.
11. **Bergeron, M. G., D. Ke, C. Menard, F. J. Picard, M. Gagnon, M. Bernier, M. Ouellette, P. H. Roy, S. Marcoux, and W. D. Fraser.** 2000. Rapid detection of group B streptococci in pregnant women at delivery. *N. Engl. J. Med.* **343:**175–179.
12. **Bisno, A. L.** 2001. Acute pharyngitis. *N. Engl. J. Med.* **344:**205–211.
13. **Bisno, A. L., M. A. Gerber, J. M. Gwaltney, Jr., E. L. Kaplan, R. H. Schwartz, and the Infectious Diseases Society of America.** 1997. Diagnosis and management of group A streptococcal pharyngitis: a practice guideline. *Clin. Infect. Dis.* **25:**574–583.
14. **Bochud, P. Y., T. Calandra, and P. Francioli.** 1994. Bacteremia due to viridans streptococci in neutropenic patients: a review. *Am. J. Med.* **97:**256–264.
15. **Bourbeau, P. P., B. J. Heiter, and M. Figdore.** 1997. Use of Gen-Probe AccuProbe Group B streptococcus test to detect group B streptococci in broth cultures of vaginal-anorectal specimens from pregnant women: comparison with traditional culture method. *J. Clin. Microbiol.* **35:**144–147.
16. **Brandt, C. M., G. Haase, N. Schnitzler, R. Zbinden, and R. Lutticken.** 1999. Characterization of blood culture isolates of *Streptococcus dysgalactiae* subsp. *equisimilis* possessing Lancefield's group A antigen. *J. Clin. Microbiol.* **37:** 4194–4197.
17. **Caufield, P. W., G. R. Cutter, and A. P. Dasanayake.** 1993. Initial acquisition of mutans streptococci by infants: evidence for a discrete window of infectivity. *J. Dent. Res.* **72:**37–45.
18. **Chew, T. A., and J. M. Smith.** 1992. Detection of diacetyl (caramel odor) in presumptive identification of the "*Streptococcus milleri*" group. *J. Clin. Microbiol.* **30:**3028–3029.
19. **Chuard, C., and L. B. Reller.** 1998. Bile-esculin test for presumptive identification of enterococci and streptococci: effects of bile concentration, inoculation technique, and incubation time. *J. Clin. Microbiol.* **36:**1135–1136.
20. **Cunningham, M. W.** 2000. Pathogenesis of group A streptococcal infections. *Clin. Microbiol. Rev.* **13:**470–511.
21. **Daly, J. A., N. L. Clifton, K. C. Seskin, and W. M. Gooch III.** 1991. Use of rapid, nonradioactive DNA probes in culture confirmation tests to detect *Streptococcus agalactiae, Haemophilus influenzae, and Enterococcus* spp. from pediatric patients with significant infections. *J. Clin. Microbiol.* **29:**80–82.
22. **Davidson, R., R. Cavalcanti, J. L. Brunton, D. J. Bast, J. C. de Azavedo, P. Kibsey, C. Fleming, and D. E. Low.** 2002. Resistance to levofloxacin and failure of treatment of pneumococcal pneumonia. *N. Engl. J. Med.* **346:** 747–750.
23. **Davies, H. D., A. McGeer, B. Schwartz, K. Green, D. Cann, A. E. Simor, D. E. Low, and the Ontario Group A Streptococcal Study Group.** 1996. Invasive group A streptococcal infections in Ontario, Canada. *N. Engl. J. Med.* **335:**547–554.
24. **Davies, H. D., M. A. Miller, S. Faro, D. Gregson, S. C. Kehl, and J. A. Jordan.** 2004. Multicenter study of a rapid molecular-based assay for the diagnosis of group B Streptococcus colonization in pregnant women. *Clin. Infect. Dis.* **39:**1129–1135.
25. **Denys, G. A., and R. B. Carey.** 1992. Identification of *Streptococcus pneumoniae* with a DNA probe. *J. Clin. Microbiol.* **30:**2725–2727.
26. **Desjardins, M., K. L. Delgaty, K. Ramotar, C. Seetaram, and B. Toye.** 2004. Prevalence and mechanisms of erythromycin resistance in group A and group B *Streptococcus:* implications for reporting susceptibility results. *J. Clin. Microbiol.* **42:**5620–5623.
27. **Devriese, L. A., J. Hommez, R. Kilpper-Balz, and K. H. Schleifer.** 1986. *Streptococcus canis* sp. nov.: a species of group G streptococci from animals. *Int. J. Syst. Bacteriol.* **36:**422–425.
28. **Devriese, L. A., P. Vandamme, B. Pot, M. Vanrobaeys, K. Kersters, and F. Haesebrouck.** 1998. Differentiation between *Streptococcus gallolyticus* strains of human clinical and veterinary origins and *Streptococcus bovis* strains from the intestinal tracts of ruminants. *J. Clin. Microbiol.* **36:**3520–3523.
29. **Doern, G. V., M. J. Ferraro, A. B. Brueggemann, and K. L. Ruoff.** 1996. Emergence of high rates of antimicrobial resistance among viridans group streptococci in the United States. *Antimicrob. Agents Chemother.* **40:**891–894.
30. **Dowell, S. F., R. L. Garman, G. Liu, O. S. Levine, and Y. H. Yang.** 2001. Evaluation of Binax NOW, an assay for the detection of pneumococcal antigen in urine samples, performed among pediatric patients. *Clin. Infect. Dis.* **32:**824–825.
31. **Efstratiou, A.** 2000. Group A streptococci in the 1990s. *J. Antimicrob. Chemother.* **45**(Suppl.):3–12.
32. **Enright, M. C., and B. G. Spratt.** 1999. Multilocus sequence typing. *Trends Microbiol.* **7:**482-487.
33. **Enright, M. C., B. G. Spratt, A. Kalia, J. H. Cross, and D. E. Bessen.** 2001. Multilocus sequence typing of *Streptococcus pyogenes* and the relationships between *emm* type and clone. *Infect. Immun.* **69:**2416–2427.

34. **Facklam, R.** 2002. What happened to the streptococci: overview of taxonomic and nomenclature changes. *Clin. Microbiol. Rev.* **15:**613–630.
35. **Facklam, R., J. Elliott, N. Pigott, and A. R. Franklin.** 1995. Identification of *Streptococcus porcinus* from human sources. *J. Clin. Microbiol.* **33:**385–388.
36. **Facklam, R., J. Elliott, L. Shewmaker, and A. Reingold.** 2005. Identification and characterization of sporadic isolates of *Streptococcus iniae* isolated from humans. *J. Clin. Microbiol.* **43:**933–937.
37. **Facklam, R. F., D. R. Martin, M. Lovgren, D. R. Johnson, A. Efstratiou, T. A. Thompson, S. Gowan, P. Kriz, G. J. Tyrrell, E. Kaplan, and B. Beall.** 2002. Extension of the Lancefield classification for group A streptococci by addition of 22 new M protein gene sequence types from clinical isolates: *emm103* to *emm124*. *Clin. Infect. Dis.* **34:**28–38.
38. **Facklam, R. R.** 1987. Specificity study of kits for detection of group A streptococci directly from throat swabs. *J. Clin. Microbiol.* **25:**504–508.
39. **Farley, M.** 1995. Group B streptococcal infection in older patients. Spectrum of disease and management strategies. *Drugs Aging* **6:**293–300.
40. **Farrow, J., and M. D. Collins.** 1984. Taxonomic studies on streptococci of serological groups C, G and L and possibly related taxa. *Syst. Appl. Microbiol.* **5:**483–493.
41. **Farrow, J., J. Kruze, B. Phillips, A. Bramley, and M. D. Collins.** 1984. Taxonomic studies on *Streptococcus bovis* and *Streptococcus equinus:* description of *Streptococcus alactolyticus* sp. nov. and *Streptococcus saccharolyticus* sp. nov. *Syst. Appl. Microbiol.* **5:**467–482.
42. **Fischetti, V. A.** 1989. Streptococcal M protein: molecular design and biological behavior. *Clin. Microbiol. Rev.* **2:**285–314.
43. **Gavin, P. J., R. B. Thomson, Jr., S. J. Horng, and R. Yogev.** 2003. Neonatal sepsis caused by *Streptococcus bovis* variant (biotype II/2): report of a case and review. *J. Clin. Microbiol.* **41:**3433–3435.
44. **Gerber, M. A., L. L. Wright, and M. F. Randolph.** 1987. Streptozyme test for antibodies to group A streptococcal antigens. *Pediatr. Infect. Dis. J.* **6:**36–40.
45. **Gordillo, M. E., K. V. Singh, C. J. Baker, and B. E. Murray.** 1993. Typing of group B streptococci: comparison of pulsed-field gel electrophoresis and conventional electrophoresis. *J. Clin. Microbiol.* **31:**1430–1434.
46. **Gorm Jensen, T., H. Bossen Konradsen, and B. Bruun.** 1999. Evaluation of the Rapid ID 32 Strep system. *Clin. Microbiol. Infect.* **5:**417–423.
47. **Greenberg, D., A. Broides, I. Blancovich, N. Peled, N. Givon-Lavi, and R. Dagan.** 2004. Relative importance of nasopharyngeal versus oropharyngeal sampling for isolation of *Streptococcus pneumoniae* and *Haemophilus influenzae* from healthy and sick individuals varies with age. *J. Clin. Microbiol.* **42:**4604–4609.
48. **Gutierrez, F., M. Masia, J. C. Rodriguez, A. Ayelo, B. Soldan, L. Cebrian, C. Mirete, G. Royo, and A. M. Hidalgo.** 2003. Evaluation of the immunochromatographic Binax NOW assay for detection of *Streptococcus pneumoniae* urinary antigen in a prospective study of community-acquired pneumonia in Spain. *Clin. Infect. Dis.* **36:**286–292.
49. **Haidan, A., S. R. Talay, M. Rohde, K. S. Sriprakash, B. J. Currie, and G. S. Chhatwal.** 2000. Pharyngeal carriage of group C and group G streptococci and acute rheumatic fever in an Aboriginal population. *Lancet* **356:**1167–1169.
50. **Heiter, B. J., and P. P. Bourbeau.** 1993. Comparison of the Gen-Probe Group A Streptococcus Direct Test with culture and a rapid streptococcal antigen detection assay for diagnosis of streptococcal pharyngitis. *J. Clin. Microbiol.* **31:**2070–2073.
51. **Hendley, J. O., M. A. Sande, P. M. Stewart, and J. M. Gwaltney, Jr.** 1975. Spread of *Streptococcus pneumoniae* in families. I. Carriage rates and distribution of types. *J. Infect. Dis.* **132:**55–61.
52. **Homer, K. A., L. Denbow, R. A. Whiley, and D. Beighton.** 1993. Chondroitin sulfate depolymerase and hyaluronidase activities of viridans streptococci determined by a sensitive spectrophotometric assay. *J. Clin. Microbiol.* **31:**1648–1651.
53. **Hwang, M. N., and G. M. Ederer.** 1975. Rapid hippurate hydrolysis method for presumptive identification of group B streptococci. *J. Clin. Microbiol.* **1:**114–115.
54. **Johnson, D. R., and E. L. Kaplan.** 1993. A review of the correlation of T-agglutination patterns and M-protein typing and opacity factor production in the identification of group A streptococci. *J. Med. Microbiol.* **38:**311–315.
55. **Jones, N., J. F. Bohnsack, S. Takahashi, K. A. Oliver, M. S. Chan, F. Kunst, P. Glaser, C. Rusniok, D. W. Crook, R. M. Harding, N. Bisharat, and B. G. Spratt.** 2003. Multilocus sequence typing system for group B streptococcus. *J. Clin. Microbiol.* **41:**2530–2536.
56. **Kaplan, E. L., C. D. Rothermel, and D. R. Johnson.** 1998. Antistreptolysin O and anti-deoxyribonuclease B titers: normal values for children ages 2 to 12 in the United States. *Pediatrics* **101:**86–88.
57. **Kawamura, Y., X. G. Hou, F. Sultana, H. Miura, and T. Ezaki.** 1995. Determination of 16S rRNA sequences of *Streptococcus mitis* and *Streptococcus gordonii* and phylogenetic relationships among members of the genus *Streptococcus*. *Int. J. Syst. Bacteriol.* **45:**406–408.
58. **Kawamura, Y., X. G. Hou, Y. Todome, F. Sultana, K. Hirose, S. E. Shu, T. Ezaki, and H. Ohkuni.** 1998. *Streptococcus peroris* sp. nov. and *Streptococcus infantis* sp. nov., new members of the *Streptococcus mitis* group, isolated from human clinical specimens. *Int. J. Syst. Bacteriol.* **48**(Pt. 3)**:**921–927.
59. **Kellogg, J. A.** 1990. Suitability of throat culture procedures for detection of group A streptococci and as reference standards for evaluation of streptococcal antigen detection kits. *J. Clin. Microbiol.* **28:**165–169.
60. **Kikuchi, K., T. Enari, K. Totsuka, and K. Shimizu.** 1995. Comparison of phenotypic characteristics, DNA-DNA hybridization results, and results with a commercial rapid biochemical and enzymatic reaction system for identification of viridans group streptococci. *J. Clin. Microbiol.* **33:**1215–1222.
61. **Kilian, M., L. Mikkelsen, and J. Henrichsen.** 1989. Taxonomic study of viridans streptococci: description of *Streptococcus gordonii* sp. nov. and emended descriptions of *Streptococcus sanguis* (White and Niven 1946), *Streptococcus oralis* (Bridge and Sneath 1982), and *Streptococcus mitis* (Andrews and Horder 1906). *Int. J. Syst. Bacteriol.* **39:**471–484.
62. **Kirby, R., and K. L. Ruoff.** 1995. Cost-effective, clinically relevant method for rapid identification of beta-hemolytic streptococci and enterococci. *J. Clin. Microbiol.* **33:** 1154–1157.
63. **Klein, R. S., R. A. Recco, M. T. Catalano, S. C. Edberg, J. I. Casey, and N. H. Steigbigel.** 1977. Association of *Streptococcus bovis* with carcinoma of the colon. *N. Engl. J. Med.* **297:**800–802.
64. **Kong, F., S. Gowan, D. Martin, G. James, and G. L. Gilbert.** 2002. Serotype identification of group B streptococci by PCR and sequencing. *J. Clin. Microbiol.* **40:** 216–226.
65. **Kurzynski, T. A., and C. K. Meise.** 1979. Evaluation of sulfamethoxazole-trimethoprim blood agar plates for recovery of group A streptococci from throat cultures. *J. Clin. Microbiol.* **9:**189–193.
66. **Lefevre, J. C., G. Faucon, A. M. Sicard, and A. M. Gasc.** 1993. DNA fingerprinting of *Streptococcus pneumoniae* strains by pulsed-field gel electrophoresis. *J. Clin. Microbiol.* **31:**2724–2728.

67. **Lutticken, R., N. Temme, G. Hahn, and E. W. Bartelheimer.** 1986. Meningitis caused by *Streptococcus suis:* case report and review of the literature. *Infection* **14:** 181–185.
68. **Malhotra-Kumar, S., S. Wang, C. Lammens, S. Chapelle, and H. Goossens.** 2003. Bacitracin-resistant clone of *Streptococcus pyogenes* isolated from pharyngitis patients in Belgium. *J. Clin. Microbiol.* **41:**5282–5284.
69. **Mandell, L. A., J. G. Bartlett, S. F. Dowell, T. M. File, Jr., D. M. Musher, and C. Whitney.** 2003. Update of practice guidelines for the management of community-acquired pneumonia in immunocompetent adults. *Clin. Infect. Dis.* **37:**1405–1433.
70. **Martin, D. R., J. M. Stanhope, and L. A. Finch.** 1977. Delayed culture of group-A streptococci: an evaluation of variables in methods of examining throat swabs. *J. Med. Microbiol.* **10:**249–253.
71. **McDougal, L. K., J. K. Rasheed, J. W. Biddle, and F. C. Tenover.** 1995. Identification of multiple clones of extended-spectrum cephalosporin-resistant *Streptococcus pneumoniae* isolates in the United States. *Antimicrob. Agents Chemother.* **39:**2282–2288.
72. **Mein, J., and G. Lum.** 1999. CSF bacterial antigen detection tests offer no advantage over Gram's stain in the diagnosis of bacterial meningitis. *Pathology* **31:**67–69.
73. **Messmer, T. O., J. S. Sampson, A. Stinson, B. Wong, G. M. Carlone, and R. R. Facklam.** 2004. Comparison of four polymerase chain reaction assays for specificity in the identification of *Streptococcus pneumoniae*. *Diagn. Microbiol. Infect. Dis.* **49:**249–254.
74. **Mihaila-Amrouche, L., A. Bouvet, and J. Loubinoux.** 2004. Clonal spread of *emm* type 28 isolates of *Streptococcus pyogenes* that are multiresistant to antibiotics. *J. Clin. Microbiol.* **42:**3844–3846.
75. **Murdoch, D. R., R. T. Laing, G. D. Mills, N. C. Karalus, G. I. Town, S. Mirrett, and L. B. Reller.** 2001. Evaluation of a rapid immunochromatographic test for detection of *Streptococcus pneumoniae* antigen in urine samples from adults with community-acquired pneumonia. *J. Clin. Microbiol.* **39:**3495–3498.
76. **Murdoch, D. R., and L. B. Reller.** 2001. Antimicrobial susceptibilities of group B streptococci isolated from patients with invasive disease: 10-year perspective. *Antimicrob. Agents Chemother.* **45:**3623–3624.
77. **Murray, P. R., A. D. Wold, C. A. Schreck, and J. A. Washington II.** 1976. Effects of selective media and atmosphere of incubation on the isolation of group A streptococci. *J. Clin. Microbiol.* **4:**54–56.
78. **Musser, J. M., B. M. Gray, P. M. Schlievert, and M. E. Pichichero.** 1992. *Streptococcus pyogenes* pharyngitis: characterization of strains by multilocus enzyme genotype, M and T protein serotype, and pyrogenic exotoxin gene probing. *J. Clin. Microbiol.* **30:**600–603.
79. **Musser, J. M., V. Kapur, J. Szeto, X. Pan, D. S. Swanson, and D. R. Martin.** 1995. Genetic diversity and relationships among *Streptococcus pyogenes* strains expressing serotype M1 protein: recent intercontinental spread of a subclone causing episodes of invasive disease. *Infect. Immun.* **63:**994–1003.
80. **Nelms, L. F., D. A. Odelson, T. R. Whitehead, and R. B. Hespell.** 1995. Differentiation of ruminal and human *Streptococcus bovis* strains by DNA homology and 16S rRNA probes. *Curr. Microbiol.* **31:**294–300.
81. **Perez-Trallero, E., C. Fernandez-Mazarrasa, C. Garcia-Rey, E. Bouza, L. Aguilar, J. Garcia-de-Lomas, and F. Baquero.** 2001. Antimicrobial susceptibilities of 1,684 *Streptococcus pneumoniae* and 2,039 *Streptococcus pyogenes* isolates and their ecological relationships: results of a 1-year (1998-1999) multicenter surveillance study in Spain. *Antimicrob. Agents Chemother.* **45:**3334–3340.
82. **Pergola, V., G. Di Salvo, G. Habib, J. F. Avierinos, E. Philip, J. M. Vailloud, F. Thuny, J. P. Casalta, P. Ambrosi, M. Lambert, A. Riberi, A. Ferracci, T. Mesana, D. Metras, J. R. Harle, P. J. Weiller, D. Raoult, and R. Luccioni.** 2001. Comparison of clinical and echocardiographic characteristics of *Streptococcus bovis* endocarditis with that caused by other pathogens. *Am. J. Cardiol.* **88:**871–875.
83. **Peterson, L. R., and R. B. Thomson, Jr.** 1999. Use of the clinical microbiology laboratory for the diagnosis and management of infectious diseases related to the oral cavity. *Infect. Dis. Clin. N. Am.* **13:**775–795.
84. **Podbielski, A., O. Blankenstein, and R. Lutticken.** 1994. Molecular characterization of the *cfb* gene encoding group B streptococcal CAMP-factor. *Med. Microbiol. Immunol.* (Berlin) **183:**239–256.
85. **Pokorski, S. J., E. A. Vetter, P. C. Wollan, and F. R. Cockerill III.** 1994. Comparison of Gen-Probe Group A streptococcus Direct Test with culture for diagnosing streptococcal pharyngitis. *J. Clin. Microbiol.* **32:**1440–1443.
86. **Poyart, C., C. Pierre, G. Quesne, B. Pron, P. Berche, and P. Trieu-Cuot.** 1997. Emergence of vancomycin resistance in the genus *Streptococcus:* characterization of a *vanB* transferable determinant in *Streptococcus bovis*. *Antimicrob. Agents Chemother.* **41:**24–29.
87. **Poyart, C., G. Quesne, S. Coulon, P. Berche, and P. Trieu-Cuot.** 1998. Identification of streptococci to species level by sequencing the gene encoding the manganese-dependent superoxide dismutase. *J. Clin. Microbiol.* **36:**41–47.
88. **Poyart, C., G. Quesne, and P. Trieu-Cuot.** 2002. Taxonomic dissection of the *Streptococcus bovis* group by analysis of manganese-dependent superoxide dismutase gene *(sodA)* sequences: reclassification of '*Streptococcus infantarius* subsp. *coli*' as *Streptococcus lutetiensis* sp. nov. and of *Streptococcus bovis* biotype 11.2 as *Streptococcus pasteurianus* sp. nov. *Int. J. Syst. Evol. Microbiol.* **52:**1247–1255.
89. **Ratner, H. B., L. S. Weeks, and C. W. Stratton.** 1986. Evaluation of spot CAMP test for identification of group B streptococci. *J. Clin. Microbiol.* **24:**296–297.
90. **Regev-Yochay, G., M. Raz, R. Dagan, N. Porat, B. Shainberg, E. Pinco, N. Keller, and E. Rubinstein.** 2004. Nasopharyngeal carriage of *Streptococcus pneumoniae* by adults and children in community and family settings. *Clin. Infect. Dis.* **38:**632–639.
91. **Rosa-Fraile, M., J. Rodriguez-Granger, M. Cueto-Lopez, A. Sampedro, E. B. Gaye, J. M. Haro, and A. Andreu.** 1999. Use of Granada medium to detect group B streptococcal colonization in pregnant women. *J. Clin. Microbiol.* **37:**2674–2677.
92. **Ruoff, K. L., M. J. Ferraro, J. Holden, and L. J. Kunz.** 1984. Identification of *Streptococcus bovis* and *Streptococcus salivarius* in clinical laboratories. *J. Clin. Microbiol.* **20:** 223–226.
93. **Ruoff, K. L., S. I. Miller, C. V. Garner, M. J. Ferraro, and S. B. Calderwood.** 1989. Bacteremia with *Streptococcus bovis* and *Streptococcus salivarius:* clinical correlates of more accurate identification of isolates. *J. Clin. Microbiol.* **27:** 305–308.
94. **Schlegel, L., F. Grimont, E. Ageron, P. A. Grimont, and A. Bouvet.** 2003. Reappraisal of the taxonomy of the *Streptococcus bovis/Streptococcus equinus* complex and related species: description of *Streptococcus gallolyticus* subsp. *gallolyticus* subsp. nov., *S. gallolyticus* subsp. *macedonicus* subsp. nov. and *S. gallolyticus* subsp. *pasteurianus* subsp. nov. *Int. J. Syst. Evol. Microbiol.* **53:**631–645.
95. **Schlegel, L., F. Grimont, M. D. Collins, B. Regnault, P. A. Grimont, and A. Bouvet.** 2000. *Streptococcus infantarius* sp. nov., *Streptococcus infantarius* subsp. *infantarius* subsp. nov. and *Streptococcus infantarius* subsp. *coli* subsp. nov., isolated from humans and food. *Int. J. Syst. Evol. Microbiol.* **50**(Pt. 4)**:**1425–1434.

96. **Schleifer, K. H., M. Ehrmann, U. Krusch, and H. Neve.** 1991. Revival of the species *Streptococcus thermophilus* (ex Orla-Jensen, 1919) nom. rev. *Syst. Appl. Microbiol.* **14:**386–388.
97. **Schrag, S., R. Gorwitz, K. Fultz-Butts, and A. Schuchat.** 2002. Prevention of perinatal group B streptococcal disease. Revised guidelines from CDC. *Morb. Mortal. Wkly. Rep. Recomm. Rep.* **51:**1–22.
98. **Schrag, S. J., S. Zywicki, M. M. Farley, A. L. Reingold, L. H. Harrison, L. B. Lefkowitz, J. L. Hadler, R. Danila, P. R. Cieslak, and A. Schuchat.** 2000. Group B streptococcal disease in the era of intrapartum antibiotic prophylaxis. *N. Engl. J. Med.* **342:**15–20.
99. **Schuchat, A., T. Hilger, E. Zell, M. M. Farley, A. Reingold, L. Harrison, L. Lefkowitz, R. Danila, K. Stefonek, N. Barrett, D. Morse, and R. Pinner.** 2001. Active bacterial core surveillance of the emerging infections program network. *Emerg. Infect. Dis.* **7:**92–99.
100. **Schuchat, A., C. Whitney, and K. Zangwill.** 1996. Prevention of perinatal group B streptococcal disease: a public health perspective. *Morb. Mortal. Wkly. Rep.* **45**(No. RR-7)**:**1–24.
101. **Shet, A., and E. L. Kaplan.** 2002. Clinical use and interpretation of group A streptococcal antibody tests: a practical approach for the pediatrician or primary care physician. *Pediatr. Infect. Dis. J.* **21:**420–426; quiz 427–430.
102. **Slotved, H. C., M. Kaltoft, I. C. Skovsted, M. B. Kerrn, and F. Espersen.** 2004. Simple, rapid latex agglutination test for serotyping of pneumococci (Pneumotest-Latex). *J. Clin. Microbiol.* **42:**2518–2522.
103. **Smith, D. J.** 2002. Dental caries vaccines: prospects and concerns. *Crit. Rev. Oral Biol. Med.* **13:**335–349.
104. **Smith, R. F., and N. P. Willett.** 1968. Rapid plate method for screening hyaluronidase and chondroitin sulfatase-producing microorganisms. *Appl. Microbiol.* **16:** 1434–1436.
105. **Stevens, D. L.** 2001. Invasive streptococcal infections. *J. Infect. Chemother.* **7:**69–80.
106. **Swedo, S. E., H. L. Leonard, B. B. Mittleman, A. J. Allen, J. L. Rapoport, S. P. Dow, M. E. Kanter, F. Chapman, and J. Zabriskie.** 1997. Identification of children with pediatric autoimmune neuropsychiatric disorders associated with streptococcal infections by a marker associated with rheumatic fever. *Am. J. Psychiatry* **154:**110–112.
107. **Thinkhamrop, J., S. Limpongsanurak, M. R. Festin, S. Daly, A. Schuchat, P. Lumbiganon, E. Zell, T. Chipato, A. A. Win, M. J. Perilla, J. E. Tolosa, and C. G. Whitney.** 2003. Infections in international pregnancy study: performance of the optical immunoassay test for detection of group B streptococcus. *J. Clin. Microbiol.* **41:**5288–5290.
108. **Thomas, J. G.** 1994. Routine CSF antigen detection for agents associated with bacterial meningitis: another point of view. *Clin. Microbiol. Newsl.* **16:**89–95.
109. **Thornsberry, C., D. F. Sahm, L. J. Kelly, I. A. Critchley, M. E. Jones, A. T. Evangelista, and J. A. Karlowsky.** 2002. Regional trends in antimicrobial resistance among clinical isolates of *Streptococcus pneumoniae, Haemophilus influenzae,* and *Moraxella catarrhalis* in the United States: results from the TRUST Surveillance Program, 1999-2000. *Clin. Infect. Dis.* **34**(Suppl. 1)**:**S4–S16.
110. **Uhl, J. R., S. C. Adamson, E. A. Vetter, C. D. Schleck, W. S. Harmsen, L. K. Iverson, P. J. Santrach, N. K. Henry, and F. R. Cockerill.** 2003. Comparison of LightCycler PCR, rapid antigen immunoassay, and culture for detection of group A streptococci from throat swabs. *J. Clin. Microbiol.* **41:**242–249.
111. **Vandamme, P., B. Pot, E. Falsen, K. Kersters, and L. A. Devriese.** 1996. Taxonomic study of Lancefield streptococcal groups C, G, and L *(Streptococcus dysgalactiae)* and proposal of *S. dysgalactiae* subsp. *equisimilis* subsp. nov. *Int. J. Syst. Bacteriol.* **46:**774–781.
112. **van't Wout, J. W., and H. A. Bijlmer.** 2005. Bacteremia due to *Streptococcus gallolyticus,* or the perils of revised nomenclature in bacteriology. *Clin. Infect. Dis.* **40:**1070–1071.
113. **Votava, M., M. Tejkalova, M. Drabkova, V. Unzeitig, and I. Braveny.** 2001. Use of GBS media for rapid detection of group B streptococci in vaginal and rectal swabs from women in labor. *Eur. J. Clin. Microbiol. Infect. Dis.* **20:**120–122.
114. **Waitkins, S. A.** 1980. Evaluation of rapid methods of identifying group B streptococci. *J. Clin. Pathol.* **33:**302–305.
115. **Weinstein, M. R., M. Litt, D. A. Kertesz, P. Wyper, D. Rose, M. Coulter, A. McGeer, R. Facklam, C. Ostach, B. M. Willey, A. Borczyk, D. E. Low, and the *S. iniae* Study Group.** 1997. Invasive infections due to a fish pathogen, *Streptococcus iniae*. *N. Engl. J. Med.* **337:**589–594.
116. **Welch, D. F., D. Hensel, D. Pickett, and S. Johnson.** 1991. Comparative evaluation of selective and nonselective culture techniques for isolation of group A beta-hemolytic streptococci. *Am. J. Clin. Pathol.* **95:**587–590.
117. **West, P. W., H. A. Foster, Q. Electricwala, and A. Alex.** 1996. Comparison of five methods for the determination of arginine hydrolysis by viridans streptococci. *J. Med. Microbiol.* **45:**501–504.
118. **Whiley, R. A., and D. Beighton.** 1991. Emended descriptions and recognition of *Streptococcus constellatus, Streptococcus intermedius,* and *Streptococcus anginosus* as distinct species. *Int. J. Syst. Bacteriol.* **41:**1–5.
119. **Whiley, R. A., L. M. Hall, J. M. Hardie, and D. Beighton.** 1999. A study of small-colony, beta-haemolytic, Lancefield group C streptococci within the anginosus group: description of *Streptococcus constellatus* subsp. *pharyngis* subsp. nov., associated with the human throat and pharyngitis. *Int. J. Syst. Bacteriol.* **49**(Pt. 4)**:**1443–1449.
120. **Wilkinson, H. W.** 1977. CAMP-disk test for presumptive identification of group B streptococci. *J. Clin. Microbiol.* **6:**42–45.
121. **Williams-Bouyer, N., B. S. Reisner, and G. L. Woods.** 2000. Comparison of gen-probe AccuProbe group B streptococcus culture identification test with conventional culture for the detection of group B streptococci in broth cultures of vaginal-anorectal specimens from pregnant women. *Diagn. Microbiol. Infect. Dis.* **36:**159–162.

Enterococcus

LÚCIA MARTINS TEIXEIRA, MARIA DA GLÓRIA SIQUEIRA CARVALHO, AND RICHARD R. FACKLAM

30

TAXONOMY

Microorganisms that are now included in the genus *Enterococcus* were related mainly to the "streptococci of fecal origin" or "enterococci" (26). These microorganisms were considered for a long time to be a major division of the genus *Streptococcus,* differentiated by their higher resistance to chemical and physical agents and accommodating most of the serological group D streptococci. In the last decades, however, the enterococci have undergone considerable changes in taxonomy, which started with the splitting of the genus *Streptococcus,* and the recognition of *Enterococcus* as a separate genus (89). Definite evidence that *Streptococcus faecalis* and *Streptococcus faecium* were sufficiently different from the other members of the genus to merit allocation into a separate genus was provided by studies using molecular approaches (89). The other enterococcal species were then transferred to the new genus, and several new species have been described and proposed for inclusion in the genus *Enterococcus* (25, 26). Some of the proposed new enterococcal species were not validated because they were shown to belong to previously described enterococcal species or did not belong to the genus *Enterococcus* at all (24, 26, 75, 104).

The phylogenetic analysis of genera of catalase-negative gram-positive cocci based on the comparison of the 16S rRNA gene sequences has revealed that *Enterococcus* organisms are more closely related to *Vagococcus, Tetragenococcus,* and *Carnobacterium* than they are to *Streptococcus* and *Lactococcus,* genera to which they have been phenotypically associated (17, 26).

Current criteria for inclusion in the genus *Enterococcus* and for the description of new enterococcal species encompass a polyphasic approach resulting from a combination of different molecular techniques (frequently involving DNA-DNA reassociation experiments, 16S rRNA gene sequencing, and whole-cell protein profiling analysis) and phenotypic tests. Partial or nearly entire sequencing of the 16S rRNA genes is now considered a practical and powerful tool in aiding the identification of enterococccal species, and it has been performed for all recognized species of *Enterococcus*. Figure 1 shows the phylogenetic relationships, based on the analysis of 16S rRNA gene sequences, among the species of *Enterococcus* that have their sequences already available at the GenBank database (as of December 2005). More recently, a variety of other nucleic acid-based methods have been used as additional tools to assess the phylogenetic relationships among enterococcal species and to formulate the descriptions of new species (26, 30, 74, 97, 98), but their use is still limited. The long-chain fatty acid composition of enterococcal cells, as revealed by gas-liquid chromatography analysis, is also of taxonomic value and has been used to discriminate species (30, 42, 89, 109).

DESCRIPTION OF THE GENUS

The members of the genus *Enterococcus* are catalase-negative gram-positive cocci that occur singly or arranged in pairs or as short chains. Cells are sometimes coccobacillary when Gram stains are prepared from growth on solid medium but tend to be ovoid and in chains when grown in thioglycolate broth. After growth on blood agar media for 24 h, colonies are usually between 1 and 2 mm in diameter although some variants may appear smaller. Some (about one-third) cultures of *Enterococcus faecalis* may be β-hemolytic on agar containing rabbit, horse, or human blood but nonhemolytic on agar containing sheep blood. Some cultures of *Enterococcus durans* are β-hemolytic regardless of the type of blood used. All other species are usually α-hemolytic or nonhemolytic. Enterococci are facultative anaerobes with a homofermentative metabolism that follows the Embden-Meyerhof-Parnas pathway resulting in the production of lactic acid as the end product of glucose fermentation. Because of their ability to ferment carbohydrates to lactic acid, the enterococci are referred to as typical lactic acid bacteria. Gas is not produced. These microorganisms are usually able to grow in temperatures ranging from 10 to 45°C, with optimum growth at 35°C. The majority of the species grow in broth containing 6.5% NaCl, and they hydrolyze esculin in the presence of bile salts (bile-esculin [BE] test). They also hydrolyze leucine-β-naphthylamide (LAP) by producing leucine aminopeptidase (LAPase). Most enterococci, apart from *Enterococcus cecorum, Enterococcus columbae* (16), *Enterococcus pallens, Enterococcus saccharolyticus,* and some strains of the recently described species *Enterococcus canintestini, Enterococcus devriesei,* and *Enterococcus moraviensis,* hydrolyze L-pyrrolidonyl-β-naphthylamide (PYR) by producing pyrrolidonyl arylamidase (pyrrolidonase [PYRase]). A few species are motile (*Enterococcus casseliflavus* and *Enterococcus gallinarum*), and some are pigmented (*E. casseliflavus, Enterococcus gilvus, Enterococcus mundtii, E. pallens,* and *Enterococcus sulfureus*) (17, 26, 43). Methods used for

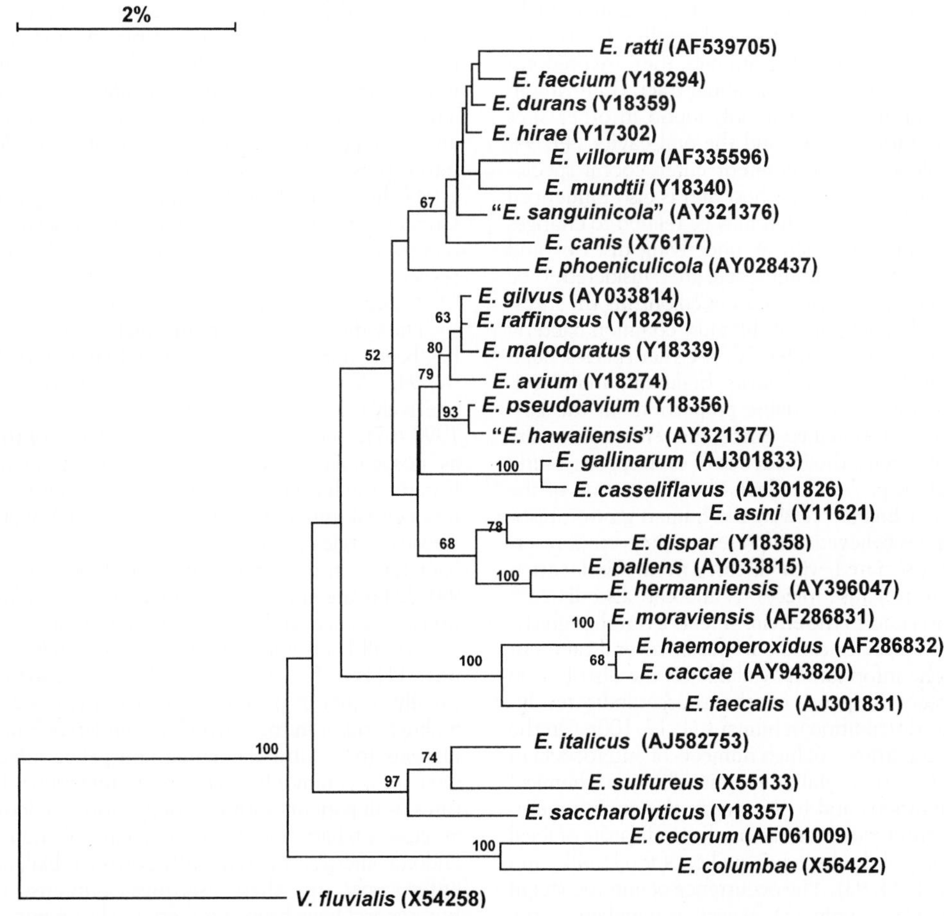

FIGURE 1 Phylogenetic tree based on comparative analysis of 16S rRNA gene sequences, showing the relationships among type strains of species of *Enterococcus*. *Vagococcus fluvialis* was used as an out-group, and bootstrap values at the nodes were displayed as percentages.

detection of enterococcal motility have to be selected carefully, as differences in motility due to the composition of the medium have been demonstrated (111). Enterococci are not able to synthesize porphyrins and, therefore, do not produce cytochrome enzymes (17, 43). However, cytochrome activity is sometimes expressed when strains of *E. faecalis* are grown on blood-containing media, and a weak effervescence is observed in the catalase test. Positive catalase testing has been reported for strains of *Enterococcus haemoperoxidus*, when cultivated on blood-agar media (96). Most enterococcal strains produce a cell wall-associated glycerol teichoic acid that is identified as Lancefield's serological group D antigen. The G+C content of the DNA ranges from 32 to 44 mol%. The genome size is in the range of approximately 2,000 to 3,500 kb (58, 91).

The other genera of catalase-negative gram-positive cocci and the characteristics that distinguish them from the enterococci are discussed in chapters 29 and 31. No phenotypic criteria are available for clearly distinguishing the genus *Enterococcus* unequivocally from other genera, since there are no particular characteristics that are common to all enterococci. However, there are certain characteristics that are usually found in most strains of all the enterococcal species. Accurate presumptive identification of a catalase-negative gram-positive coccus as an *Enterococcus* can be accomplished by demonstrating that the unknown strain is positive for BE, PYR, and LAP tests and grows in the presence of 6.5% NaCl and at 45°C. Because strains of *Lactococcus, Leuconostoc, Pediococcus,* and *Vagococcus* with phenotypic similarities have been isolated from human infections (28, 102), the presumptive identification of enterococci based only on BE reaction and growth in 6.5% NaCl broth can be erroneous. Demonstrating the presence of group D antigen by serological reaction may be helpful in the identification, although antigen is detected in only about 80% of the enterococcal strains. On the other hand, pediococci and leuconostocs (28), as well as some vagococcal strains (102), can also react with anti-group D serum. Reactivity with the AccuProbe *Enterococcus* Culture Identification Test (a genetic probe manufactured by Gen-Probe, Inc., San Diego, Calif.) can also be used to confirm an unknown strain as an *Enterococcus*. Except for the type strains of *Enterococcus asini, Enterococcus canis, E. cecorum, E. columbae, E. haemoperoxidus, E. moraviensis, E. pallens,* and *E. saccharolyticus*, strains of most known species of *Enterococcus* react with this probe. However, *Vagococcus* strains also react with the *Enterococcus* genetic probe (90, 102).

EPIDEMIOLOGY AND TRANSMISSION

Several intrinsic characteristics of the enterococci allow them to grow and survive in harsh environments and to persist almost everywhere. Enterococci are widespread in nature and can be found in soil, plants, water, food, and in animals, including mammals, birds, insects, and reptiles (1, 16, 17, 100, 101). In humans, as in other animals, they are predominantly inhabitants of the gastrointestinal tract, occurring in high numbers, and are less commonly found in other sites such as the genitourinary tract and the oral cavity (44, 94, 100). The prevalence of the different enterococcal species appears to vary according to the host and is also influenced by age, diet, and other factors that may be related to changes in physiologic conditions, such as underlying diseases and prior antimicrobial therapy. Enterococci are considered to be the most abundant gram-positive coccus colonizing the intestine, with *E. faecalis* being one of the most common bacteria isolated from this site (17, 23, 94, 100). Other species, such as *E. faecium* as well as *E. casseliflavus*, *E. durans*, and *E. gallinarum*, are also found in variable proportions in the gastrointestinal tract of humans. Since the enterococci are opportunistic pathogens, the incidence of each species found in human infections probably reflects the distribution of the different species of *Enterococcus* in the human gastrointestinal tract. This site is believed to represent an important reservoir for strains associated with disease; from this location they may migrate to cause infections and can also disseminate to other hosts and to the environment. Even though the same enterococcal species can be found in several different animal species, the information available on the distribution of distinct enterococcal species in other sources indicates differences from the distribution in humans (1, 17, 100). On the other hand, the occurrence of high numbers of enterococci in the feces, as well as their ability to resist different chemical and physical conditions and to survive in the environment, implies that the enterococci can be used as indicators of fecal contamination and of the hygienic quality of food, milk, and drinking water (31, 33, 93). The occurrence of enterococci in natural nonhuman reservoirs (1), as well as members of the intestinal microbiota of humans (100), and the relationship between the presence of enterococci in foods and human safety (31, 33) have been extensively reviewed recently. Overall, several aspects of the ecology of the enterococci and the real incidence of the different species as members of the microbiota in body sites or in environmental sources merit further evaluation, especially in the light of the changing classification and taxonomic approaches to the genus and of the increasing resistance to antimicrobial agents.

CLINICAL SIGNIFICANCE

The enterococci are commensal microorganisms that act as opportunistic agents of infections, particularly in elderly patients with serious underlying diseases and other immunocompromised patients who have been hospitalized for prolonged periods, have been treated with invasive devices, and/or have received broad-spectrum antimicrobial therapy. From the site of colonization, the microorganism must evade host clearance and produce pathologic changes in the host, either by direct toxic activity or indirectly by inducing an inflammatory response. Several potential virulence factors have been identified in enterococci (13, 22, 39, 44, 47, 66, 84, 94), but none has been established as having a major contribution to virulence in humans. On the other hand, the resistance traits of enterococci may be crucial to allow members of this genus to survive for extended periods of time in the host or environment (44), leading to their persistence and role as prominent nosocomial pathogens. Although the enterococci can cause human infections in the community and in the hospital, these microorganisms began to be recognized with increasing frequency as common causes of hospital-acquired infections in the late 1970s, paralleling the increasing resistance to most currently used antimicrobial agents. As a result, enterococci have emerged as one of the leading therapeutic challenges when associated with serious or life-threatening infections. This trend is likely to continue as the overall population ages and more people become at risk for infection (59). The ubiquitous presence of enterococci, however, requires caution in establishing the clinical significance of a particular isolate. Unnecessary work and potentially misleading laboratory reports should be avoided whenever possible, especially with respect to in vitro susceptibility testing decisions (see "Antimicrobial Susceptibilities" below).

The variety of infections in which enterococci are involved has been thoroughly reviewed and summarized (39, 55, 63, 67, 94). Although the spectrum of infections has remained relatively unchanged since the extensive review by Murray in 1990 (67), trends to increasing prevalence of these organisms as nosocomial pathogens have been frequently observed. Enterococci have become the second or third leading cause of nosocomial urinary tract infections (UTIs), wound infections (mostly surgical, decubitus ulcers, and burn wounds), and bacteremia in the United States (39, 50, 55, 63, 67, 76, 88, 94). UTIs are the most common of the enterococcal infections: enterococci have been implicated in approximately 10% of all UTIs and in up to approximately 16% of nosocomial UTIs (55, 63, 76, 88, 94). Enterococcal bacteruria usually occurs in patients with underlying structural abnormalities and/or in those who have undergone urologic manipulations (63). Intra-abdominal and pelvic infections are the next most commonly encountered infections. However, cultures from patients with peritonitis, intra-abdominal or pelvic abscesses, biliary tract infections, surgical site infections, and endomyometritis are frequently polymicrobial, and the role of enterococci in these settings remains controversial. Enterococci have been considered to be an important cause of endocarditis since early descriptions and are estimated to account for about 20% of cases of native valve bacterial endocarditis and for about 6 to 7% of prosthetic valve endocarditis (59). Whereas endocarditis is a serious enterococcal infection, it is less common than bacteremia. Enterococcal infections of the respiratory tract or the central nervous system, as well as otitis, sinusitis, septic arthritis, and endophthalmitis, may occur but are rare (39, 67, 94). There is evidence for a role of enterococci in dental infections (95). The significance of isolates from some of these sites should be carefully evaluated before any clinical decisions are made.

E. faecalis is the most frequent enterococcal species isolated from human clinical specimens, representing 80 to 90% of the isolates, followed by *E. faecium*, which is found in 5 to 10% of enterococcal infections (6, 27, 35, 64). However, the ratios of isolation of the different enterococcal species can vary according to each setting and can be affected by a number of aspects, including the increasing dissemination of outbreak-related strains such as vancomycin-resistant *E. faecium*. For example, in one recent report, the ratio of *E. faecalis* to *E. faecium* isolates recovered from blood cultures was about 2.5:1.0 (50). Other enterococcal species are identified less frequently, even though clusters of infections associated with *E. casseliflavus* (77) and *E. raffinosus* (113) have been reported. Although less frequently or even rarely, several other enterococcal species, including *E. avium*, *E. caccae*, *E. cecorum*, *E. dispar*, *E. durans*, *E. gallinarum*, *E. gilvus*, "*E. hawaiiensis*," *E. hirae*, *E. italicus*, *E. malodoratus*, *E. mundtii*, *E. pallens*, *E. pseudoavium*, "*E. sanguinicola*," and *E. faecalis* variant strains, have also been isolated from human sources (12, 27, 35, 42, 62, 64, 109). Isolation of the other species of enterococci has not yet been documented from human sources.

COLLECTION, TRANSPORT, AND STORAGE OF SPECIMENS

The standard methods of collecting blood, urine, wound samples, and other secretions or swab specimens are adequate (see chapters 5 and 20). No special methods or procedures are usually necessary for transporting clinical specimens containing enterococci because these microorganisms are easily recovered and are relatively resistant to environmental changes. Transport can be performed on almost any transport media or on swabs that are kept dry. Like most clinical samples, the material should be cultured as soon as possible, preferably within 1 h.

Enterococcal strains can be stored indefinitely when lyophilized. In our experience, cultures frozen at –70°C or less can be stored for several years as heavy cell suspensions made directly in defibrinated sheep or rabbit blood or in a skim milk (10%) solution containing glycerol (10%). Most strains of enterococci survive several months at 4°C on agar slants prepared with ordinary agar bases, such as brain heart infusion and Trypticase soy agar.

DIRECT EXAMINATION

The direct microscopic examination of Gram-stained smears of normally sterile clinical specimens, such as blood, may be useful for the diagnosis of enterococcal infections. Direct examination of certain nonsterile specimens may also be informative, but should not be overemphasized. In any case only a presumptive report of the "presence of gram-positive cocci" should be made, as microscopy by itself cannot differentiate the enterococci from most of the other gram-positive cocci. Culture and appropriate identification techniques should be performed for confirmation.

As the occurrence of vancomycin-resistant enterococci (VRE) represents an important problem worldwide, hospitals should consider the implementation of surveillance programs for VRE detection. In an attempt to overcome the inherent limitations of culture-based methods of detection (discussed in "Isolation Procedures"), conventional PCR and real-time PCR-based methods have been evaluated for direct detection of these microorganisms in clinical and surveillance specimens (80, 86, 92). The LightCycler *vanA/vanB* detection assay (commercially available from Roche Diagnostics, Indianapolis, Ind.) has shown promise for screening of VRE in rectal or perianal swabs and has been evaluated for identification of VRE in blood cultures (92). Relatively few methods for direct detection of enterococci from blood samples or blood cultures have been reported. Results of a recent report indicate the potential usefulness of the commercially available DNA probe (AccuProbe, Gen-Probe, Inc.) for the direct detection of enterococci in blood cultures (54).

ISOLATION PROCEDURES

Trypticase soy–5% sheep blood agar, brain heart infusion–5% sheep blood agar, or any blood agar base containing 5% animal blood supports the growth of enterococci. Enterococci grow well at 35 to 37°C and do not require an atmosphere containing increased levels of CO_2, although some strains grow better in this atmosphere. If the sample to be cultured is likely to contain gram-negative bacteria, commercially prepared media containing bile, esculin, and azide are excellent options for primary isolation. These media have traditionally been used and are supplied under different designations by the various manufacturers. More recently, media containing chromogenic substrates have been proposed for the isolation and presumptive identification of enterococci and their use in clinical laboratories is gaining acceptance (18, 60). The use of selective media for the isolation of enterococci has been previously reviewed (17). An extensive review of the diversity of media used for the isolation of enterococci from fecal and clinical specimens, as well as water, food, feeds, and environmental sources, was recently presented by Domig et al. (18).

The increasing incidence of vancomycin resistance among the enterococci has raised the importance of selective isolation of VRE. Early identification of infection or colonization by VRE is recommended to prevent the spread of these microorganisms (41, 70). Current recommendations for hospital infection control include VRE fecal surveillance cultures, but the optimal methods for these cultures are still unclear. Several different selective agar and/or broth media and procedures have been employed for the isolation of VRE from sources containing commensal microbiota, such as stool samples and rectal or perianal swab specimens (18, 78, 80, 85, 86). Most of them are variations of selective media differing with regard to the antimicrobial agents or the antimicrobial concentrations used. Depending on the specific purposes, direct plating techniques give some indication of the number of VRE present in the sample, but enrichment procedures are mainly applied to detect VRE present in low numbers. Although there is not a single generally accepted screening method for isolation at this point, the use of a selective-enrichment broth to enhance the recovery of VRE seems to be the most effective procedure. Enterococcosel broth (a bile-esculin azide medium supplied by Becton Dickinson Microbiology Systems, Sparks, Md.) has been used in a number of studies as the base medium supplemented with different concentrations of vancomycin, with 6 μg/ml being the most common concentration. In some of the protocols proposed, vancomycin and other antimicrobial agents, such as aztreonam and clindamycin, have been used in the enrichment broth as well as in the subculture medium. It would be prudent, however, to use a nonselective agar as well for subculturing from a selective-enrichment broth, as some strains may be inhibited to the point of very poor or no growth. In some circumstances, it may be necessary to recover VRE from environmental surfaces for epidemiologic studies. Isolation of the organisms from these surfaces can be accomplished by swabbing the surfaces with premoistened swabs and placing them either into a selective-enrichment broth or onto agar plates. Alternatively, the Rodac imprint method may be employed by applying the agar surface directly to the environmental surface to be cultured (37). Overall, culture-based screening methods for VRE may be especially demanding and can take several days to complete, besides having variable degrees of sensitivity, which affects the timely implementation of infection control procedures. Therefore, some microbiology laboratories have recently considered the introduction of molecular techniques to facilitate the rapid and accurate identification of VRE and to improve the ability for detecting this pathogen. However, most of the approaches described in the literature still require bacterial growth in culture prior to detection, requiring 24 h or more to complete. More rapid detection of VRE directly from patient samples is still an area for which there is an important clinical need and relatively little published literature, as already mentioned (see "Direct Examination" above). Because a laboratory report that indicates the presence of VRE may initiate a cascade of infection control events that are time-consuming and costly (10, 41, 70), laboratories should be confident in the epidemiologic importance of any suspected VRE isolate. Transferable and high-level vancomycin resistance, encoded by the *vanA* or the *vanB* genes and most frequently associated with *E. faecalis* and *E. faecium* isolates, is the major focus of infection control efforts. In contrast, the intrinsically low-level VanC resistance, which is not transferable and is not associated with dissemination of resistant strains, is less likely to be important to infection control surveillance efforts (10, 44, 85, 86). While the isolation of VRE from clinical and surveillance specimens is important, the need for protocols to rapidly determine the likely underlying mechanism of resistance associated with different genetic determinants (see "Antimicrobial Susceptibilities" below; see also chapters 71 and 78) is equally important (15, 85, 86).

IDENTIFICATION

Identification by Conventional Physiologic Testing

Once it is established that an unknown catalase-negative, gram-positive coccus is an *Enterococcus* or closely related genus (see "Description of the Genus"), the conventional tests (see reference 28 and chapters 14, 15, 29, and 31 for methods) listed in Table 1 can be used to identify the species. Most of the information presented here is related to phenotypic characteristics of strains isolated from humans.

TABLE 1 Phenotypic characteristics used for the identification of *Enterococcus* species and some physiologically related species of other gram-positive cocci

Species	Phenotypic characteristic[a]											
	MAN	SOR	ARG	ARA	SBL	RAF	TEL	MOT	PIG	SUC	PYU	MGP
Group I												
E. avium	+	+	–	+	+	–	–	–	–	+	+	V
E. raffinosus	+	+	–	+	+	+	–	–	–	+	+	V
E. gilvus	+	+	–	–	+	+	–	–	+	+	+	–
E. pallens	+	+	–	–	+	+	–	–	+	+	–	+
E. saccharolyticus[b]	+	+	–	–	+	+	–	–	–	+	–	+
E. malodoratus	+	+	–	–	+	+	–	–	–	+	+	V
E. pseudoavium	+	+	–	–	+	–	–	–	–	+	+	+
"*E. hawaiiensis*"	+	+	–	–	+	–	–	–	–	–	+	–
Group II												
E. faecium	+[c]	–	+	+	V	V	–	–	–	+[c]	–	–
E. casseliflavus	+	–	+[c]	+	V	+	–[c]	+[c]	+[c]	+	V	+
E. gallinarum	+	–	+[c]	+	–	+	–	+[c]	–	+	–	+
E. mundtii	+	–	+	+	V	+	–	–	+	+	–	–
E. faecalis	+[c]	–	+[c]	–	+	–	+	–	–	+[c]	+	–
E. haemoperoxidus[b]	+[d]	–	+[d]	–	–	–	–	–	–	+	–	+
"*E. sanguinicola*"	+	–	+	–	–	–	+[e]	–	–	+	–	–
Lactococcus sp.	+	–	+	–	–	–	–	–	–	V	–	–
Group III												
E. dispar	–	–	+	–	–	+	–	–	–	+	+	+
E. hirae	–	–	+	–	–	+	–	–	–	+	–	–
E. durans	–	–	+	–	–	–	–	–	–	–	–	–
E. ratti	–	–	+	–	–	–	–	–	–	–	–	–
E. villorum	–	–	+	–	–	–	–	–	–	–	–	–
Group IV												
E. cecorum[b]	–	–	–	–	–	+	–	–	–	+	+	–
E. phoeniculicola[b]	–	–	–	+	–	+	–	–	–	+	–	+
E. sulfureus	–	–	–	–	–	+	–	–	+	+	–	+
E. asini[b]	–	–	–	–	–	–	–	–	–	+	–	–
E. caccae	–	–	–	–	–	–	–	–	–	+	+	+[d]
Group V												
E. canis[b]	+	–	–	+	–	–	–	–	–	+	+	+
E. columbae[b]	+	–	–	+	+	+	–	–	–	+	+	–
E. moraviensis[b]	+	–	–	+	–	–	–	–	–	+	+	+
E. hermanniensis	+	–	–	–	–	–	–	–	–	–	–	–
E. italicus	V	–	–	–	V	–	–	–	–	+	+	+
Vagococcus fluvialis	+	–	–	–	+	–	–	+	–	+	–	+

[a] Abbreviations and symbols: MAN, mannitol; SOR, sorbose; ARG, arginine; ARA, arabinose; SBL, sorbitol; RAF, raffinose; TEL, 0.04% tellurite; MOT, motility; PIG, pigment; SUC, sucrose; PYU, pyruvate; MGP, methyl-α-D-glucopyranoside; +, 90% or more of the strains are positive; –, 90% or more of the strains are negative; V, variable (11 to 89% of the strains are positive).

[b] Phenotypic characteristics based on data from type strains.

[c] Occasional exceptions occur (<3% of strains show aberrant reactions).

[d] Late positive (3 days of incubation or longer).

[e] Weak reaction.

Enterococcal species can be separated into five physiologic groups of species based on acid formation from mannitol and sorbose, and hydrolysis of arginine (Table 1). Identification of enterococcal species by conventional tests is not rapid and may require up to 10 days of incubation. However, most identifications can be made after 2 days of incubation.

Group I consists of *E. avium*, *E. gilvus*, "*E. hawaiiensis*," *E. malodoratus*, *E. pallens*, *E. pseudoavium*, *E. raffinosus*, and *E. saccharolyticus* (Table 1). "*E. hawaiiensis*" is a denomination that has been recently proposed (L. M. Teixeira, M. G. S. Carvalho, A. G. Steigerwalt, R. E. Morey, P. L. Shewmaker, E. Falsen, and R. R Facklam, *Abstr. 2nd Int. ASM-FEMS Conf. Enterococci*, abstr. A15, 2005) for the new species previously designated *Enterococcus* sp. nov. CDC PNS-E3 (7). If the results of conventional tests compare to the results originally reported (98), *E. devriesei*, a recently described species, will be grouped with the enterococcal species in group I.

Group II comprises *E. faecalis*, *E. faecium*, *E. casseliflavus*, *E. gallinarum*, *E. haemoperoxidus*, *E. mundtii*, and "*E. sanguinicola*." These species form acid from mannitol and hydrolyze arginine but fail to form acid from sorbose. The majority of the isolates from human sources belong to species included in this group. Atypical strains that fail to hydrolyze arginine or form acid from mannitol have been documented. *Lactococcus* sp. is also listed in this group because the phenotypic characteristics of some strains can lead to the misidentification as an *Enterococcus*. If nonmotile variants of *E. casseliflavus* and *E. gallinarum* are encountered, production of acid from methyl-α-D-glucopyranoside (MGP) can be used to help in the identification of these species. "*E. sanguinicola*" is the denomination recently proposed (Teixeira et al., *Abstr. 2nd Int. ASM-FEMS Conf. Enterococci*) for the new species previously designated *Enterococcus* sp. nov. CDC PNS-E2 (7).

Group III consists of *E. dispar*, *E. durans*, *E. hirae*, *E. ratti* (101), and *E. villorum*. Three of these species (*E. durans*, *E. ratti*, and *E. villorum*) have very similar phenotypic profiles in the tests listed in Table 1. They can be differentiated by clotting reactions in litmus milk, hydrolysis of hippurate, and acid formation from trehalose and xylose. *E. durans* forms acid and clot, *E. villorum* forms acid but no clot, and *E. ratti* does not form acid or clot in litmus milk. *E. durans* hydrolyzes hippurate, while *E. villorum* does not. *E. ratti* is variable in the hippurate hydrolysis test. *E. durans* forms acid from trehalose but not from xylose, *E. villorum* forms acid from both trehalose and xylose, and *E. ratti* does not form acid from either trehalose or xylose. The other members of this group are easily identified by the reactions shown in Table 1. Uncommon mannitol-negative variant strains of *E. faecalis* and *E. faecium* resemble species in this group. However, *E. faecalis* strains are positive in the pyruvate test but not for acid formation from arabinose, raffinose, or sucrose, and E. *faecium* variant strains form acid from arabinose. In all likelihood *E. canintestini*, a recently described species (74), will also fall into enterococcal group III.

Group IV is composed by *E. asini*, *E. caccae*, *E. cecorum*, *E. phoeniculicola*, and *E. sulfureus* (Table 1). *E. caccae* is a recently proposed new species (8). If the results of conventional tests compare to the results originally reported (97), *E. aquimarinus*, a recently described species, will be grouped with the enterococcal species in group IV. Group V consists of *E. canis*, *E. columbae*, *E. hermanniensis*, *E. italicus*, and *E. moraviensis*. Variant strains of *E. casseliflavus*, *E. gallinarum*, and *E. faecalis* that fail to hydrolyze arginine resemble the microorganisms included in this group. However, these variant strains have characteristics similar to those of the strains that hydrolyze arginine and can be differentiated by the same phenotypic tests. *Vagococcus fluvialis* is listed here because the phenotypic characteristics of this species are very similar to those of the genus *Enterococcus* and some strains may be identified as enterococci (102). *E. italicus* corresponds to the new species previously designated *Enterococcus* sp. nov. CDC PNS-E1 (7, 30; Teixeira et al., *Abstr. 2nd Int. ASM-FEMS Conf. Enterococci*).

Identification by Commercial Systems or Molecular Methods

There are several commercially available miniaturized, manual, semiautomated, and automated identification systems for the identification of *Enterococcus* species. Since their introduction, these systems have been updated to improve their performance characteristics and expand their identification capabilities, as investigators have become more aware of inaccuracies (14, 32, 38, 46, 113). In general, these systems are reliable for the identification of *E. faecalis*, and, to a lesser extent, *E. faecium*. Accurate identification of other species, by most systems, depends on additional testing, although improvements have been observed with updated formats and databases. Commercial systems available for the identification of enterococcal species include the API 20S and the API Rapid ID 32 Strep systems (bioMérieux Vitek, Inc., Hazelwood, Mo.), the Crystal Gram-Positive and the Crystal Rapid Gram-Positive identification systems (Becton Dickinson Microbiology Systems), the Gram Positive Identification Card of the Vitek system (bioMérieux), and the Gram-Positive Identification panel of the MicroScan Walkaway system (Dade MicroScan, West Sacramento, Calif.). The accuracy of identification by some of these systems in comparison to identification by molecular techniques has been evaluated (3, 46). In general, a large proportion of enterococcal isolates are accurately identified by any one of these systems; however, the accuracy is dependent on the distribution of species found in each specific setting. Identification of unusual species by a commercial system should be confirmed by a reference method before being reported.

Molecular methods based on the analyses of different target molecules, such as DNA-DNA hybridization and sequencing of the 16S rRNA genes, have been used primarily for taxonomic purposes in special laboratories. In the past 15 years, however, the application of molecular techniques for the identification of *Enterococcus* species has expanded dramatically in an attempt to develop more rapid and accurate identification methods potentially adaptable for use in clinical microbiology laboratories. A variety of molecular procedures have been proposed for the identification of enterococcal species as recently reviewed and summarized (19, 26). These alternate methods include sodium dodecyl sulfate-polyacrylamide gel electrophoresis (SDS-PAGE) analysis of whole-cell protein (WCP) profiles, vibrational spectroscopic analysis, proton magnetic resonance spectroscopic analysis, randomly amplified polymorphic DNA analysis, sequencing analysis of the 16S rRNA gene, restriction fragment-length polymorphism analysis of the PCR-amplified 16S rRNA gene, broad-range amplification of the 16S rRNA gene or of the *groESL* gene, sequencing of the domain V of the 23S rRNA gene, amplification of the tRNA or the rRNA intergenic spacers, amplification of the D-ala:D-ala ligases *(ddl)* and the vancomycin resistance *(van)* genes, sequencing of the *ddl* genes, amplification and probing of the *Enterococcus* protein A *(efaA)* genes or of the *E. faecalis* adhesin for collagen *(ace)* gene, amplification of the elongation factor EF-Tu *(tuf)* or the pEM1225 genes, sequencing of the manganese-dependent superoxide dismutase *(sodA)* gene, sequencing of the chaperonin 60 *(cpn60)* gene, sequencing of the RNA polymerase β subunit *(rpoB)* gene (21), sequencing of the RNA polymerase α subunit (*rpoA*) and the phenylalanyl-tRNA synthase (*pheS*) genes (72), and sequencing of the α subunit of the ATP synthase (*atpA*) gene (73). Many of these molecular procedures have been performed in only one or a few laboratories and have not been evaluated for the majority of the species of *Enterococcus*. Most of them are potentially applicable to all enterococcal species, and others are species specific.

Among the molecular techniques proposed to identify the different enterococcal species, SDS-PAGE analysis of WCP profiles and sequencing of the 16S rRNA genes have been evaluated in reference laboratories. SDS-PAGE analysis of WCP profiles appears to be a reliable tool for the differentiation and identification of *Enterococcus* strains, since WCP profiles are species specific (7, 26, 61, 101). Apart from minor differences among strains, each of the known enterococcal species corresponds to a unique WCP profile. WCP profiles of related species of *Lactococcus* and *Vagococcus* are also unique and different from those of the enterococci (90, 102-104). Table 1 depicts the phenotypic characteristics of *Enterococcus* species discussed in this chapter, is based on correlations between the WCP profiles and the phenotypic tests, and may include findings of DNA-DNA reassociation experiments and 16S rRNA gene sequencing. Sequencing of the 16S rRNA gene is a frequently used nucleic acid-based method for identification of enterococcal species (81). The 16S rRNA gene sequences are available for comparison purposes via public databanks of nucleotide sequences such as GenBank. Comparisons can be made by using one of the several sequence-comparing software packages, many of which are available for public access. Figure 1 shows a dendrogram generated by comparison of 16S rRNA gene sequences of the type strains of the species included in the genus *Enterococcus*. Accession numbers of the reference sequences used for comparative analyses are indicated in the figure. Clear-cut identification is not obtained for all enterococcal species, since several species differ by only 1 to 3 bases in the entire 16S rRNA gene (approximately 1,500 bp). Together with phenotypic characterization and other alternative molecular methods such as analyses of WCP profiles, DNA sequencing can be an important tool to establish species identity.

TYPING METHODS

The increasing documentation of *Enterococcus* as a leading nosocomial pathogen frequently exhibiting resistance to several antimicrobial agents and the evidence supporting the concept of exogenous acquisition of enterococcal infections have generated demand for strain typing and epidemiologic studies. Besides outbreak analysis, the methods used for epidemiologic investigation of enterococcal isolates must be able to track enterococcal dissemination in different environments and hosts and the evolution of multidrug-resistant strains. Classic phenotypic methods used to investigate the diversity among isolates of a given enterococcal species have frequently failed to adequately discriminate among strains, and they have limited value in epidemiologic studies. However, phenotypic information in association with molecular data can contribute valuable information (19, 26, 115). Discriminatory molecular typing methods demonstrated that strains can be exogenously acquired by direct and indirect contact among patients. Intrahospital transmission and interhospital spread have also been documented for antimicrobial-resistant enterococci (4, 19, 26, 55, 94, 115, 116).

Improved discrimination among enterococcal strains involved analyses of chromosomal DNA restriction endonuclease profiles by pulsed-field gel electrophoresis (PFGE) (4, 19, 26, 34, 36, 69, 83). Multilocus enzyme electrophoresis (9, 107), ribotyping (23, 35, 52, 116), and PCR-based typing methods, such as randomly amplified polymorphic DNA PCR assay and repetitive element sequence-based PCR, have also been used to investigate genetic relationships among enterococcal strains (45, 56). Sequencing of PCR products and restriction fragment length polymorphism analyses of PCR products have been used to trace and determine differences among antibiotic resistance genes in enterococci (20, 51, 82, 114).

Results from a number of investigations indicate that analysis of SmaI restriction digests of genomic DNA by PFGE is widely useful for studying enterococcal species (26), showing definite advantages in strain discrimination. PFGE is considered to be the "gold standard" for the epidemiologic analyses of enterococcal infections. Several protocols for performing PFGE analyses of enterococcal strains have been published. However, the development of standardized protocols as a result of collaborative studies is needed in order to allow for interlaboratory comparisons. Most of the information accumulated during the past several years is related to *E. faecium* and *E. faecalis*. Although PFGE is quite discriminatory, epidemiologic interpretation of PFGE profiles is not always clear-cut. The occurrence of genetic events can be associated with substantial changes in the PFGE profiles, leading to problems in clonality assessment (51, 65, 87). There is not a single definitive typing technique for enterococci. A strong match among the results of several typing techniques, particularly those based on different genomic polymorphisms, can be used to indicate a high degree of relatedness. The use of PFGE in conjunction with at least one additional typing technique or independent PFGE analyses using different restriction enzymes is highly recommended to help in clarifying epidemiologic interpretations. General principles proposed for the interpretation of molecular typing data based on fragment differences are usually applied to interpret PFGE profiles obtained for enterococcal strains (26, 105). Well-characterized control strains should be evaluated along with unknown isolates. For that purpose, two reference strains, *E. faecalis* OG1RF (ATCC 47077) and *E. faecium* GE1 (ATCC 51558), have been proposed (105).

Two additional powerful molecular techniques, multilocus sequence typing (MLST) and multiple-locus variable-number tandem repeat analysis (MLVA), were developed more recently and have already been used to identify clonal complexes within enterococcal populations and for investigating genetic relatedness between strains. MLST typing schemes have been applied to explore the population structure of *E. faecalis* and *E. faecium* (5, 40, 71). Application of MLST typing has revealed the occurrence of host-specific genogroups of *E. faecium* and a specific genetic lineage that seems to have emerged recently worldwide, associated with nosocomial outbreaks. Two simultaneously published studies described the development of MLVA typing schemes for *E. faecalis* (106) and *E. faecium* (108). The data indicate that this technique can achieve a high degree of discrimination and is suitable for easy interlaboratory data exchange. However, neither MLVA nor MLST is currently feasible for most laboratories.

ANTIMICROBIAL SUSCEPTIBILITIES

Resistance to several commonly used antimicrobial agents is a remarkable characteristic of most enterococcal species. Moreover, most of this information is based on studies with *E. faecalis* and *E. faecium*, the two species most frequently associated with human infections. Antimicrobial resistance can be classified as either intrinsic or acquired. Intrinsic resistance is related to inherent or natural chromosomally encoded characteristics present in all or most of the enterococci. Furthermore, certain specific mechanisms of intrinsic resistance to some antimicrobial agents are typically associated with a particular enterococcal species or groups of species. In contrast, the occurrence of acquired resistance is more variable, resulting from either mutations in existing DNA or acquisition of new genetic determinants found in plasmids or transposons (44, 48, 67, 68, 94). Intrinsic resistance among enterococci involves two major groups of antimicrobial agents, the aminoglycosides and the β-lactams. Because of the poor activity of several antimicrobial agents against enterococci due to intrinsic resistance, the recommended therapy for serious infections (i.e., endocarditis, meningitis, and other systemic infections, especially in immunocompromised patients) includes a combination of a cell wall-active agent, such as a β-lactam (usually penicillin) or vancomycin, combined with an aminoglycoside (usually gentamicin or streptomycin). These combinations overcome the intrinsic resistance exhibited by enterococci, and a synergistic bactericidal effect is generally achieved since the intracellular penetration of the aminoglycoside is facilitated by the cell wall-active agent.

In addition to the intrinsic resistance traits, enterococci have acquired different genetic determinants that confer resistance to several classes of antimicrobial agents, including chloramphenicol, tetracyclines, macrolides, lincosamides and streptogramins, aminoglycosides, β-lactams, glycopeptides, and, more recently, quinolones. During the past several decades, the occurrence of acquired antimicrobial resistance among enterococci, especially high-level resistance (HLR) to aminoglycosides, β-lactams, and resistance to glycopeptides (especially vancomycin), has been increasingly reported. Isolates that are resistant to the cell wall-active agent or have HLR to aminoglycosides are resistant to the synergistic effects of combination therapy and constitute an even more serious problem. Therefore, the detection of resistance to these groups of antimicrobial agents is important in order to predict the likelihood of synergy by using antimicrobial combinations as a therapeutic strategy. Enterococcal isolates exhibiting HLR to one or more aminoglycosides have been described with increasing frequencies (35, 44, 48, 64, 67, 68, 94) and are now present in large proportions in several geographic areas. Strains expressing acquired HLR to aminoglycosides frequently have MICs of >2,000 μg/ml and cannot be detected by diffusion tests with conventional disks. Special tests using high-content gentamicin and streptomycin disks, as well as a single-dilution method, were developed to screen for this type of resistance (see chapters 73 and 74). Strains exhibiting high-level resistance to penicillin and ampicillin due to altered penicillin-binding proteins have also disseminated widely (44, 48, 67, 68, 94), while strains producing β-lactamase have been rarely identified (35, 67).

The emergence of vancomycin resistance as a therapeutic problem in enterococcal strains was first documented in western Europe and in the United States (49, 53, 110). Thereafter, the isolation of VRE has been continuously reported in diverse geographic locations (10, 44, 48, 66, 94). VRE strains have been classified according to phenotypic and genotypic features. Six types of glycopeptide resistance have already been described among enterococci, including three common phenotypes. The VanA phenotype, with inducible high-level resistance to vancomycin as well as to teicoplanin, encoded by the *vanA* gene; the VanB phenotype, with variable (moderate to high) levels of inducible resistance to vancomycin only, encoded by the *vanB* (*vanB*1 and *vanB2*) genes; and the VanC phenotype, encoded by the *vanC* genes, conferring noninducible low-level resistance to vancomycin. VanA and VanB are considered the most clinically relevant phenotypes and are usually associated with *E. faecium* and *E. faecalis* isolates, while VanC resistance is an intrinsic characteristic of *E. gallinarum* (*vanC1* genotype) and *E. casseliflavus* (*vanC2* and *vanC3* genotypes) strains (10, 11, 44, 68, 82). Three additional types of glycopeptide resistance, encoded by the *vanD* (79), *vanE* (29), and *vanG* (57) genes, seem to occur rarely among enterococci. Furthermore, the isolation of vancomycin-dependent (99) and vancomycin-heteroresistant (2) enterococcal strains from clinically significant infections, although still sporadically reported, may represent additional serious threats for the treatment and control of enterococcal infections.

Although β-lactams other than penicillin or ampicillin (e.g., mezlocillin, piperacillin, azlocillin, amoxicillin-clavulanate, ampicillin-sulbactam, and imipenem) do not offer any significant advantages over ampicillin when they are used against enterococci, they may be useful against polymicrobial infections involving enterococci and gram-negative bacilli. Ampicillin testing, along with a test for β-lactamase production, can be used to predict resistance to other β-lactam antibiotics. Susceptibility testing for the other β-lactams is rarely necessary. A positive test for β-lactamase production (see chapter 74) indicates resistance to ampicillin and the acylureidopenicillins (i.e., azlocillin, mezlocillin, or piperacillin). Resistance to ampicillin revealed by disk diffusion or dilution methods indicates the presence of penicillin-binding protein-mediated resistance to these agents, as well as to β-lactam-β-lactamase inhibitor combinations and imipenem (67, 94, 112).

While in vitro methods for detecting vancomycin resistance are discussed in detail in chapters 73 and 74, some aspects regarding VanC-containing species (i.e., *E. gallinarum* and *E. casseliflavus*) need to be emphasized. Resistance usually associated with *vanC* genotypes is not detected by disk diffusion, but VanC strains usually grow on vancomycin agar screen tests. Because the clinical significance of VanC is still uncertain, the implications of susceptibility testing for patient management may be unclear. However, the need to differentiate VanA or VanB strains from VanC strains is quite evident for therapeutic, infection control, and surveillance reasons. Because growth on the vancomycin agar screen fails to help with this important distinction, species identification is necessary. VanC resistance in *E. faecalis* or *E. faecium* is yet to be described, so growth on the vancomycin agar by either of these species is likely due to VanA or VanB resistance. Although rare, the occurrence of the other kinds of vancomycin resistance may also be considered. Additionally, VanA resistance together with VanC resistance has been described for *E. gallinarum* so that identification of a species that usually harbors only VanC resistance does not completely rule out moderate to high levels of vancomycin resistance. In this regard, determining vancomycin MICs is useful as VanC resistance frequently results in MICs of <16 μg/ml, whereas VanA and VanB usually result in MICs of >32 μg/ml. Resistance to other agents such as ampicillin and aminoglycosides also is uncommon among VanC isolates. Because of limited alternatives, VRE isolates may be tested for susceptibilities to chloramphenicol, erythromycin, tetracycline (or doxycycline or minocycline), and rifampin. Testing of quinupristin-dalfopristin, daptomycin, or linezolid is recommended for reporting of vancomycin-resistant *E. faecium*.

Since enterococci are often discussed in terms of their multidrug resistance phenotypes, two of the most problematic resistance profiles, ampicillin and vancomycin resistance, are most commonly associated with *E. faecium* (44, 48). This is important in terms of resistance surveillance. Because both ampicillin resistance and vancomycin resistance are less commonly seen in *E. faecalis* than in *E. faecium*, widespread emergence and dissemination of these resistance traits in *E. faecalis* would significantly add to the current problem of multiply resistant enterococci. Therefore, enterococcal species identification is important for the purposes of therapy and meaningful surveillance.

Molecular methods (see reference 26 and chapter 78) have been used to detect specific antimicrobial resistance genes and have substantially contributed to the understanding of the spread of acquired resistance among enterococci, especially resistance to vancomycin. However, because of their high specificity, molecular methods do not detect antimicrobial resistance due to mechanisms, including emerging resistance mechanisms, not targeted by testing.

EVALUATION, INTERPRETATION, AND REPORTING OF RESULTS

The diversity and, in some cases, species specificity of emerging antimicrobial resistance traits among enterococcal isolates created an additional need for accurate identification at the species level and for in vitro evaluation of susceptibility to antimicrobial agents. The significance of a particular enterococcal isolate is a major factor in determining when antimicrobial testing should be done. Once the need to test a particular isolate has been established, selection of the appropriate antimicrobial agents for testing must be considered on the basis of the site of infection. Testing of antimicrobial agents to which enterococci are intrinsically resistant is contraindicated. The drugs that should not be tested include aminoglycosides at standard concentrations, aztreonam, cephalosporins, clindamycin, methicillin (or oxacillin), and trimethoprim-sulfamethoxazole. These drugs may appear active for enterococci in vitro but are not effective clinically, and isolates should not be reported as susceptible to these agents. Due to difficulties with some phenotypic methods for detection of HLR to aminoglycosides and resistance to vancomycin, updated guidelines for the selection of antimicrobial agents should be followed for routine testing and reporting. The in vitro methods for detecting antimicrobial resistance in enterococcal isolates were reviewed and summarized by Facklam et al. (26) and are also discussed in detail in chapters 73 and 74.

As already mentioned, synergy testing should be done with any enterococcal isolate implicated in infections for which combination therapy is indicated (e.g., for systemic infections). Enterococci are also frequently encountered in polymicrobial infections associated with the gastrointestinal tract or superficial wounds of hospitalized patients. Their pathogenic significance in such settings is uncertain, but susceptibility testing is warranted when predominant or heavy growth is observed (63). Testing of enterococcal isolates from lower UTIs is optional, as these infections usually respond to therapy with ampicillin. However, many hospital infection control programs require routine testing as a means of surveillance for VRE. For those instances when testing a urinary tract isolate is appropriate, ciprofloxacin, levofloxacin, nitrofurantoin, norfloxacin, or tetracycline could be selected, in addition to ampicillin (44, 55, 94). In cases of treatment failure, testing is always warranted.

REFERENCES

1. **Aarestrup, F. M., P. Butaye, and W. Witte.** 2002. Nonhuman reservoirs of enterococci, p. 55–99. *In* M. S. Gilmore, D. B. Clewell, P. Courvalin, G. M. Dunny, B. E. Murray, and L. B. Rice (ed.), *The Enterococci: Pathogenesis, Molecular Biology, and Antibiotic Resistance*. ASM Press, Washington, D.C.
2. **Alam, M. R., S. Donabedian, W. Brown, J. Gordon, J. W. Chow, M. J. Zervos, and E. Hershberger.** 2001. Heteroresistance to vancomycin in *Enterococcus faecium*. *J. Clin. Microbiol.* **39:**3379–3381.
3. **Angeletti, S., G. Lorino, G. Gherardi, F. Battistoni, M. D. Cesaris, and G. Dicuonzo.** 2001. Routine molecular identification of enterococci by gene-specific PCR and 16S ribosomal DNA sequencing. *J. Clin. Microbiol.* **39:**794–797.
4. **Bischoff, W. E., T. M. Reynolds, G. O. Hall, R. P. Wenzel, and M. B. Edmond.** 1999. Molecular epidemiology of vancomycin-resistant *Enterococcus faecium* in a large urban hospital over a 5-year period. *J. Clin. Microbiol.* **37:**3912–3916.
5. **Bonora, M. G., M. Ligozzi, M. De Fatima, L. Bragagnolo, A. Goglio, G. C. Guazzotti, and R. Fontana.** 2004. Vancomycin-resistant *Enterococcus faecium* isolates causing hospital outbreaks in northern Italy belong to the multilocus sequence typing C1 lineage. *Microb. Drug Resist.* **10:** 114–123.
6. **Buschelman, B. J., B. J. Bale, and R. N. Jones.** 1993. Species identification and determination of high-level aminoglycoside resistance among enterococci. Comparison study of sterile body fluid isolates, 1985–1991. *Diagn. Microbiol. Infect. Dis.* **16:**119–122.
7. **Carvalho, M. G. S., A. G. Steigerwalt, R. E. Morey, P. L. Shewmaker, L. M. Teixeira, and R. R. Facklam.** 2004. Characterization of three new enterococcal species, *Enterococcus* sp. nov. CDC PNS-E1, *Enterococcus* sp. nov. CDC PNS-E2, and *Enterococcus* sp. nov. CDC PNS-E3, isolated from human clinical specimens. *J. Clin. Microbiol.* **42:**1192–1198.
8. **Carvalho, M. G. S., P. L. Shewmaker, A. G. Steigerwalt, R. E. Morey, A. J. Sampson, K. Joyce, T. J. Barrett, L. M. Teixeira, and R. R. Facklam.** 2006. *Enterococcus caccae* sp. nov., isolated from human stools. *Int. J. Syst. Evol. Microbiol.* **56:**1505–1508.
9. **Carvalho, M. G. S., M. C. E. Vianni, J. A. Elliott, M. Reeves, R. R. Facklam, and L. M. Teixeira.** 1997. Molecular analysis of *Lactococcus garvieae* and *Enterococcus gallinarum* isolated from water buffalos with subclinical mastitis. *Adv. Exp. Med. Biol.* **418:**401–404.
10. **Cetinkaya, Y., P. Falk, and C. G. Mayhall.** 2000. Vancomycin-resistant enterococci. *Clin. Microbiol. Rev.* **13:**686–707.
11. **Clark, N. C., L. M. Teixeira, R. R. Facklam, and F. C. Tenover.** 1998. Detection and differentiation of the *vanC-1*, *vanC-2*, and *vanC-3* glycopeptide resistance genes in enterococci. *J. Clin. Microbiol.* **36:**2294–2297.
12. **Collins, M. D., U. M. Rodrigues, N. E. Pigott, and R. R. Facklam.** 1991. *Enterococcus dispar* sp. nov., a new *Enterococcus* species from human sources. *Lett. Appl. Microbiol.* **12:**95–98.
13. **Creti, R., M. Imperi, L. Bertuccini, F. Fabretti, G. Orefici, R. Di Rosa, and L. Baldassarri.** 2004. Survey for virulence determinants among *Enterococcus faecalis* isolated from different sources. *J. Med. Microbiol.* **53:**13–20.
14. **d'Azevedo, P. A., C. A. G. Dias, A. L. S. Goncalves, F. Rowe, and L. M. Teixeira.** 2001. Evaluation of an automated system for the identification and antimicrobial susceptibility testing of enterococci. *Diagn. Microbiol. Infect. Dis.* **42:**157–161.
15. **Depardieu, F., B. Perichon, and P. Courvalin.** 2004. Detection of the *van* alphabet and identification of enterococci and staphylococci at the species level by multiplex PCR. *J. Clin. Microbiol.* **42:**5857–5860.
16. **Devriese, L. A., K. Ceyssens, U. M. Rodrigues, and M. D. Collins.** 1990. *Enterococcus columbae*, a species from pigeon intestines. *FEMS Microbiol. Lett.* **71:**247–252.

17. **Devriese, L. A., M. D. Collins, and R. Wirth.** 1992. The genus *Enterococcus*, p. 1465–1481. *In* A. Balows, H. G. Truper, M. Dworkin, W. Harder, and K. H. Schleifer (ed.), *The Prokaryotes. A Handbook on the Biology of Bacteria: Ecophysiology, Isolation, Identification, Applications,* 2nd ed. Springer-Verlag, New York, N.Y.
18. **Domig, K. J., H. K. Mayer, and W. Kneifel.** 2003. Methods used for the isolation, enumeration, characterisation and identification of *Enterococcus* spp. 1. Media for isolation and enumeration. *Int. J. Food Microbiol.* **88:**147–164.
19. **Domig, K. J., H. K. Mayer, and W. Kneifel.** 2003. Methods used for the isolation, enumeration, characterisation and identification of *Enterococcus* spp. 2. Pheno- and genotypic criteria. *Int. J. Food Microbiol.* **88:**165–188.
20. **Donabedian, S., E. Hershberger, L. A. Thal, J. W. Chow, D. B. Clewell, B. Robinson-Dunn, and M. J. Zervos.** 2000. PCR fragment length polymorphism analysis of vancomycin-resistant *Enterococcus faecium*. *J. Clin. Microbiol.* **38:**2885–2888.
21. **Drancourt, M., V. Roux, P. E. Fournier, and D. Raoult.** 2004. *rpoB* gene sequence-based identification of aerobic gram-positive cocci of the genera *Streptococcus, Enterococcus, Gemella, Abiotrophia,* and *Granulicatella*. *J. Clin. Microbiol.* **42:**497–504.
22. **Eaton, T. J., and M. J. Gasson.** 2001. Molecular screening of *Enterococcus* virulence determinants and potential for genetic exchange between food and medical isolates. *Appl. Env. Microbiol.* **67:**1628–1635.
23. **Endtz, H. P., N. van den Braak, A. van Belkum, J. A. J. W. Kluytmans, J. G. M. Koeleman, L. Spanjaard, A. Voss, A. J. L. Weersink, C. J. E. Vanderbroucke-Grauls, A. G. M. Buiting, A. van Duin, and H. A. Verbrugh.** 1997. Fecal carriage of vancomycin-resistant enterococci in hospitalized patients and those living in the community in The Netherlands. *J. Clin. Microbiol.* **35:**3026–3031.
24. **Ennahar, S., and Y. Cai.** 2005. Biochemical and genetic evidence for the transfer of *Enterococcus solitarius* Collins *et al.* 1989 to the genus *Tetragenococcus* as *Tetragenococcus solitarius* comb. nov. *Int. J. Syst. Evol. Microbiol.* **55:**589–592.
25. **Euzéby, J. P.** 1997. List of bacterial names with standing in nomenclature: a folder available on the internet. *Int. J. Syst. Bacteriol.* **47:**590–592. *(List of Prokaryotic Names with Standing in Nomenclature.* [Online.] http://www.bacterio.net. Last full update January 10, 2006.)
26. **Facklam, R. R., M. G. S. Carvalho, and L. M. Teixeira.** 2002. History, taxonomy, biochemical characteristics, and antibiotic susceptibility testing of enterococci, p. 1–54. *In* M. S. Gilmore, D. B. Clewell, P. Courvalin, G. M. Dunny, B. E. Murray, and L. B. Rice (ed.), *The Enterococci: Pathogenesis, Molecular Biology, and Antibiotic Resistance*. ASM Press, Washington, D.C.
27. **Facklam, R. R., and M. D. Collins.** 1989. Identification of *Enterococcus* species isolated from human infections by a conventional test scheme. *J. Clin. Microbiol.* **27:**731–734.
28. **Facklam, R. R., and J. A. Elliott.** 1995. Identification, classification, and clinical relevance of catalase-negative, gram-positive cocci, excluding the streptococci and enterococci. *Clin. Microbiol. Rev.* **8:**479–495.
29. **Fines, M., B. Perichon, P. Reynolds, D. F. Sahm, and P. Courvalin.** 1999. VanE, a new type of acquired glycopeptide resistance in *Enterococcus faecalis* BM4405. *Antimicrob. Agents Chemother.* **43:**2161–2164.
30. **Fortina, M. G., G. Ricci, D. Mora, and P. L. Manachini.** 2004. Molecular analysis of artisanal Italian cheeses reveals *Enterococcus italicus* sp. nov. *Int. J. Syst. Evol. Microbiol.* **54:**1717–1721.
31. **Franz, C. M., M. E. Stiles, K. H. Schleifer, and W. H. Holzapfel.** 2003. Enterococci in foods—a conundrum for food safety. *Int. J. Food Microbiol.* **88:**105–122.
32. **Garcia-Garrote, F., E. Cercenado, and E. Bouza.** 2000. Evaluation of a new system, VITEK 2, for identification and antimicrobial susceptibility testing of enterococci. *J. Clin. Microbiol.* **38:**2108–2111.
33. **Giraffa, G.** 2002. Enterococci from foods. *FEMS Microbiol. Rev.* **26:**163–171.
34. **Gordillo, M. E., K. V. Singh, and B. E. Murray.** 1993. Comparison of ribotyping and pulsed-field gel electrophoresis for subspecies differentiation of strains of *Enterococcus faecalis*. *J. Clin. Microbiol.* **31:**1570–1574.
35. **Gordon, S., J. S. Swenson, B. C. Hill, N. E. Pigott, R. R. Facklam, R. C. Cooksey, C. Thornsberry, the Enterococcal Study Group, W. R. Jarvis, and F. C. Tenover.** 1992. Antimicrobial susceptibility patterns of common and unusual species of enterococci causing infections in the United States. *J. Clin. Microbiol.* **30:**2373–2378.
36. **Green, M., K. Barbadora, S. Donabedian, and M. J. Zervos.** 1995. Comparison of field inversion gel electrophoresis with contour-clamped homogeneous electric field electrophoresis as a typing method for *Enterococcus faecium*. *J. Clin. Microbiol.* **33:**1554–1557.
37. **Hacek, D. M., W. E. Trick, S. M. Collins, G. A. Noskin, and L. R. Peterson.** 2000. Comparison of the Rodac imprint method to selective enrichment broth for recovery of vancomycin-resistant enterococci and drug-resistant *Enterobacteriaceae* from environmental surfaces. *J. Clin. Microbiol.* **38:**4646–4648.
38. **Hamilton-Miller, J. M. T., and S. Shah.** 1999. Identification of clinically isolated vancomycin-resistant enterococci: comparison of API and BBL Crystal systems. *J. Med. Microbiol.* **48:**695–696.
39. **Hancock, L. E., and M. S. Gilmore.** 2000. Pathogenicity of enterococci, p. 251–258. *In* V. A. Fischetti, R. P. Novick, J. J. Ferretti, D. A. Portnoy, and J. I. Rood (ed.), *Gram-Positive Pathogens*. ASM Press, Washington, D.C.
40. **Homan, W. L., D. Tribe, S. Poznanski, M. Li, G. Hogg, E. Spalburg, J. D. Van Embden, and R. J. Willems.** 2002. Multilocus sequence typing scheme for *Enterococcus faecium*. *J. Clin. Microbiol.* **40:**1963–1971.
41. **Hospital Infection Control Practices Advisory Committee.** 1995. Recommendations for preventing the spread of vancomycin resistance. *Infect. Control Hosp. Epidemiol.* **16:**105–113.
42. **Hsueh, P. R., L. J. Teng, Y. C. Chen, P. C. Yang, S. W. Ho, and K. T. Luh.** 2000. Recurrent bacteremic peritonitis caused by *Enterococcus cecorum* in patients with liver cirrhosis. *J. Clin. Microbiol.* **38:**2450–2452.
43. **Huycke, M. M.** 2002. Physiology of enterococci, p. 133–175. *In* M. S. Gilmore, D. B. Clewell, P. Courvalin, G. M. Dunny, B. E. Murray, and L. B. Rice (ed.), *The Enterococci: Pathogenesis, Molecular Biology, and Antibiotic Resistance*. ASM Press, Washington, D.C.
44. **Huycke, M. M., D. F. Sahm, and M. S. Gilmore.** 1998. Multiple-drug resistant enterococci: the nature of the problem and an agenda for the future. *Emerg. Infect. Dis.* **4:** 239–249.
45. **Issack, M. J., E. G. M. Power, and G. L. French.**1996. Investigation of an outbreak of vancomycin-resistant *Enterococcus faecium* by random amplified polymorphic DNA (RAPD) assay. *J. Hosp. Infect.* **33:**191–200.
46. **Jackson, C. R., P. J. Fedorka-Cray, and J. B. Barrett.** 2004. Use of a genus- and species-specific multiplex PCR for identification of enterococci. *J. Clin. Microbiol.* **42:** 3558–3565.
47. **Jett, B. D., M. M. Huycke, and M. S. Gilmore.** 1994. Virulence of enterococci. *Clin. Microbiol. Rev.* **7:**462–478.
48. **Kak, V., and J. W. Chow.** 2002. Acquired antibiotic resistances in enterococci, p. 355–383. *In* M. S. Gilmore, D. B. Clewell, P. Courvalin, G. M. Dunny, B. E. Murray, and L. B.

Rice (ed.), *The Enterococci: Pathogenesis, Molecular Biology, and Antibiotic Resistance*. ASM Press, Washington, D.C.

49. **Kaplan, A. H., P. H. Gilligan, and R. R. Facklam.** 1988. Recovery of resistant enterococci during vancomycin prophylaxis. *J. Clin. Microbiol.* **26:**1216–1218.
50. **Karlowsky, J. A., M. E. Jones, D. C. Draghi, C. Thornsberry, D. F. Sahm, and G. A. Volturo.** 2004. Prevalence and antimicrobial susceptibilities of bacteria isolated from blood cultures of hospitalized patients in the United States in 2002. *Ann. Clin. Microbiol. Antimicrob.* **10:**3–7.
51. **Kawalec, M., M. Gniadkowski, and W. Hryniewicz.** 2000. Outbreak of vancomycin-resistant enterococci in a hospital in Gdansk, Poland, due to horizontal transfer of different Tn*1546*-like transposon variants and clonal spread of several strains. *J. Clin. Microbiol.* **38:**3317–3322.
52. **Kühn, I., L. G. Burman, S. Haeggman, K. Tullus, and B. E. Murray.** 1995. Biochemical fingerprinting compared with ribotyping and pulsed-field gel electrophoresis of DNA for epidemiological typing of enterococci. *J. Clin. Microbiol.* **33:**2812–2817.
53. **Leclercq, R., E. Derlot, J. Duval, and P. Courvalin.** 1988. Plasmid-mediated resistance to vancomycin and teicoplanin in *Enterococcus faecium*. *N. Engl. J. Med.* **319:**157–161.
54. **Lindholm, L., and H. Sarkkinen.** 2004. Direct identification of Gram-positive cocci from routine blood cultures by using AccuProbe tests. *J. Clin. Microbiol.* **42:**5609–5613.
55. **Malani, P. N., C. A. Kauffman, and M. J. Zervos.** 2002. Enterococcal disease, epidemiology, and treatment, p. 385–408. *In* M. S. Gilmore, D. B. Clewell, P. Courvalin, G. M. Dunny, B. E. Murray, and L. B. Rice (ed.), *The Enterococci: Pathogenesis, Molecular Biology, and Antibiotic Resistance*. ASM Press, Washington, D.C.
56. **Malathum, K., K. V. Singh, G. M. Weinstock, and B. E. Murray.** 1998. Repetitive sequence-based PCR versus pulsed-field gel electrophoresis for typing of *Enterococcus faecalis* at the subspecies level. *J. Clin. Microbiol.* **36:**211–215.
57. **McKessar, S. J., A. M. Berry, J. M. Bell, J. D. Turnidge, and J. C. Paton.** 2000. Genetic characterization of *vanG*, a novel vancomycin resistance locus of *Enterococcus faecalis*. *Antimicrob. Agents Chemother.* **44:**3224–3228.
58. **McShan, W. M., and N. Shankar.** 2002. The genome of *Enterocccus faecalis* V583: a tool for discovery, p. 409–415. *In* M. S. Gilmore, D. B. Clewell, P. Courvalin, G. M. Dunny, B. E. Murray, and L. B. Rice (ed.), *The Enterococci: Pathogenesis, Molecular Biology, and Antibiotic Resistance*. ASM Press, Washington, D.C.
59. **Megran, D. W.** 1992. Enterococcal endocarditis. *Clin. Infect. Dis.* **15:**63–71.
60. **Merlino, J., S. Siarakas, G. J. Robertson, G. R. Funnel, T. Gottlieb, and R. Bradbury.** 1996. Evaluation of CHROMagar Orientation for differentiation and presumptive identification of gram-negative bacilli and *Enterococcus* species. *J. Clin. Microbiol.* **34:**1788–1793.
61. **Merquior, V. L. C., J. M. Peralta, R. R. Facklam, and L. M. Teixeira.** 1994. Analysis of electrophoretic whole-cell protein profiles as a tool for characterization of *Enterococcus* species. *Curr. Microbiol.* **28:**149–153.
62. **Miranda, G., L. Lee, C. Kelly, F. Solorzano, B. Leanos, O. Munoz, and J. E. Patterson.** 2001. Antimicrobial resistance from enterococci in a pediatric hospital. Plasmids in *Enterococcus faecalis* isolates with high-level gentamicin and streptomycin resistance. *Arch. Med. Res.* **32:**159–163.
63. **Moellering, R. C., Jr.** 1992. Emergence of *Enterococcus* as a significant pathogen. *Clin. Infect. Dis.* **14:**1173–1178.
64. **Mondino, S. S. B., A. C. D. Castro, P. J. J. Mondino, M. G. S. Carvalho, K. M. F. Silva, and L. M. Teixeira.** 2003. Phenotypic and genotypic characterization of clinical and intestinal enterococci isolated from inpatients and outpatients in two Brazilian hospitals. *Microb. Drug Resist.* **9:**167–174.
65. **Morrison, D., N. Woodford, S. P. Barrett, P. Sisson, and B. D. Cookson.** 1999. DNA banding pattern polymorphism in vancomycin-resistant *Enterococcus faecium* and criteria for defining strains. *J. Clin. Microbiol.* **37:**1084–1091.
66. **Mundy, L. M., D. F. Sahm, and M. Gilmore.** 2000. Relationships between enterococcal virulence and antimicrobial resistance. *Clin. Microbiol. Rev.* **13:**513–522.
67. **Murray, B. E.** 1990. The life and times of the *Enterococcus*. *Clin. Microbiol. Rev.* **3:**46–65.
68. **Murray, B. E.** 1998. Diversity among multidrug-resistant enterococci. *Emerg. Infect. Dis.* **4:**37–47.
69. **Murray, B. E., K. V. Singh, J. D. Heath, B. R. Sharma, and G. M. Weinstock.** 1990. Comparison of genomic DNAs of different enterococcal isolates using restriction endonucleases with infrequent recognition sites. *J. Clin. Microbiol.* **28:**2059–2063.
70. **Muto, C. A., J. A. Jernigan, B. E. Ostrowsky, H. M. Richet, W. R. Jarvis, J. M. Boyce, and B. M. Farr.** 2003. SHEA guideline for preventing nosocomial transmission of multidrug-resistant strains of *Staphylococcus aureus* and *Enterococcus*. *Infect. Control Hosp. Epidemiol.* **24:**362–386.
71. **Nallapareddy, S. R., R. W. Duh, K. V. Singh, and B. E. Murray.** 2002. Molecular typing of selected *Enterococcus faecalis* isolates: pilot study using multilocus sequence typing and pulsed-field gel electrophoresis. *J. Clin. Microbiol.* **40:**868–876.
72. **Naser, S. M., F. L. Thompson, B. Hoste, D. Gevers, P. Dawyndt, M. Vancanneyt, and J. Swings.** 2005. Application of multilocus sequence analysis (MLSA) for rapid identification of *Enterococcus* species based on *rpoA* and *pheS* genes. *Microbiology* **151:**2141–2150.
73. **Naser, S., F. L. Thompson, B. Hoste, D. Gevers, K. Vandemeulebroecke, I. Cleenwerck, C. C. Thompson, M. Vancanneyt, and J. Swings.** 2005. Phylogeny and identification of enterococci by *atpA* gene sequence analysis. *J. Clin. Microbiol.* **43:**2224–2230.
74. **Naser, S. M., M. Vancanneyt, E. De Graef, L. A. Devriese, C. Snauwaert, K. Lefebvre, B. Hoste, P. Švec, A. Decostere, F. Haesebrouck, and J. Swings.** 2005. *Enterococcus canintestini* sp. nov., from faecal samples of healthy dogs. *Int. J. Syst. Evol. Microbiol.* **55:** 2177–2182.
75. **Naser, S. M., M. Vancanneyt, B. Hoste, C. Snauwaert, K. Vandemeulebroecke, and J. Swings.** 2006. Reclassification of *Enterococcus flavescens* Pompei *et al.* 1992 as a later synonym of *Enterococcus casseliflavus* (*ex* Vaughan *et al.* 1979) Collins *et al.* 1984 and *Enterococcus saccharominimus* Vancanneyt *et al.* 2004 as a later synonym of *Enterococcus italicus* Fortina *et al.* 2004. *Int. J. Syst. Evol. Microbiol.* **56:**413–416.
76. **National Nosocomial Infections Surveillance System.** 2004. National Nosocomial Infections Surveillance (NNIS) System Report, data summary from January 1992 through June 2004, issued October 2004. *Am. J. Infect. Control* **32:**470–485.
77. **Nauschuetz, W. F., S. B. Trevino, L. S. Harrison, R. N. Longfield, L. Fletcher, and W. G. Wortham.** 1993. *Enterococcus casseliflavus* as an agent of nosocomial bloodstream infections. *Med. Microbiol. Lett.* **2:**102–108.
78. **Novicki, T. J., J. M. Schapiro, B. K. Ulness, A. Sebeste, L. Busse-Johnston, K. M. Swanson, S. R. Swanzy, W. Leisenring, and A. P. Limaye.** 2004. Convenient selective differential broth for isolation of vancomycin-resistant *Enterococcus* from fecal material. *J. Clin. Microbiol.* **42:**1637–1640.
79. **Ostrowsky, B. E., N. C. Clark, C. Thauvin-Eliopoulos, L. Venkataraman, M. H. Samore, F. C. Tenover, G. M. Eliopoulos, R. C. Moellering, Jr., and H. S. Gold.** 1999. A cluster of VanD vancomycin-resistant *Enterococcus faecium*: molecular characterization and clinical epidemiology. *J. Infect. Dis.* **180:**1177–1185.

80. **Palladino, S., I. D. Kay, J. P. Flexman, I. Boehm, A. M. G. Costa, E. J. Lambert, and K. J. Christiansen.** 2003. Rapid detection of *vanA* and *vanB* genes directly from clinical specimens and enrichment broths by real-time multiplex PCR assay. *J. Clin. Microbiol.* **41:**2483–2486.
81. **Patel, R., K. E. Piper, M. S. Rouse, J. M. Steckelberg, J. R. Uhl, P. Kohner, M. K. Hopkins, F. R. Cockerill, and B. C. Kline.** 1998. Determination of 16S rRNA sequences of enterococci and application to species identification of nonmotile *Enterococcus gallinarum* isolates. *J. Clin. Microbiol.* **36:**3399–3407.
82. **Patel, R., J. R. Uhl, P. Kohner, K. K. Hopkins, and F. R. Cockerill III.** 1997. Multiplex PCR detection of *vanA*, *vanB*, *vanC-1*, and *vanC-2/3* genes in enterococci. *J. Clin. Microbiol.* **35:**703–707.
83. **Pegues, D. A., C. F. Pegues, P. L. Hibberd, D. S. Ford, and D. C. Hooper.** 1997. Emergence and dissemination of a highly vancomycin-resistant *vanA* strain of *Enterococcus faecium* at a large teaching hospital. *J. Clin. Microbiol.* **35:**1565–1570.
84. **Pillar, C. M., and M. S. Gilmore.** 2004. Enterococcal virulence-pathogenicity island of *E. faecalis*. *Front. Biosci.* **9:**2335–2346.
85. **Sahm, D. F., L. Free, C. Smith, M. Eveland, and L. M. Mundy.** 1997. Rapid characterization schemes for surveillance isolates of vancomycin-resistant enterococci. *J. Clin. Microbiol.* **35:**2026–2030.
86. **Satake, S., N. Clark, D. Rimland, F. S. Nolte, and F. C. Tenover.** 1997. Detection of vancomycin-resistant enterococci in fecal samples by PCR. *J. Clin. Microbiol.* **35:** 2325–2330.
87. **Savor, C., M. A. Pfaller, J. A. Kruszynski, R. J. Hollis, G. A. Noskin, and L. R. Peterson.** 1998. Comparison of genomic methods for differentiating strains of *Enterococcus faecium:* assessment using clinical epidemiologic data. *J. Clin. Microbiol.* **36:**3327–3331.
88. **Schaberg, D. R., D. H. Culver, and R. P. Gaynes.** 1991. Major trends in the microbial etiology of nosocomial infection. *Am. J. Med.* **91:**79S–82S.
89. **Schleifer, K. H., and R. Kilpper-Balz.** 1984. Transfer of *Streptococcus faecalis* and *Streptococcus faecium* to the genus *Enterococcus* nom. rev. as *Enterococcus faecalis* comb. nov. and *Enterococcus faecium* comb. nov. *Int. J. Syst. Bacteriol.* **34:**31–34.
90. **Shewmaker, P. L., A. G. Steigerwalt, R. E. Morey, M. G. S. Carvalho, J. A. Elliott, K. Joyce, T. J. Barrett, L. M. Teixeira, and R. R. Facklam.** 2004. *Vagococcus carniphilus* sp. nov., isolated from ground beef. *Int. J. Syst. Evol. Microbiol.* **54:**1505–1510.
91. **Singh, K. V., and B. E. Murray.** 1994. Revised estimates of enterococcal chromosomal sizes. *DNA Cell Biol.* **13:** 1145–1146.
92. **Sloan, L. M., J. R. Uhl, E. A. Vetter, C. D. Schleck, W. S. Harmsen, J. Manahan, R. L. Thompson, J. E. Rosenblatt, and F. R. Cockerill III.** 2004. Comparison of the Roche LightCycler *vanA/vanB* detection assay and culture for detection of vancomycin-resistant enterococci from perianal swabs. *J. Clin. Microbiol.* **42:**2636–2643.
93. **Stiles, M. E., and W. H. Holzapfel.** 1997. Lactic acid bacteria of foods and their current taxonomy. *Int. J. Food Microbiol.* **36:**1–29.
94. **Strausbaugh, L. J., and M. S. Gilmore.** 2000. Enterococcal infections, p. 280–301. *In* D. L. Stevens and E. L. Kaplan (ed.), *Streptococcal Infections: Clinical Aspects, Microbiology, and Molecular Pathogenesis*. Oxford University Press, Inc., New York, N.Y.
95. **Sundqvist, G., D. Figdor, S. Persson, and U. Sjogren.** 1998. Microbiologic analysis of teeth with failed endodontic treatment and the outcome of conservative re-treatment. *Oral Surg. Oral Med. Oral Pathol.* **85:**86–93.
96. **Švec, P., L. A. Devriese, I. Sedlacek, M. Baele, M. Vancanneyt, F. Haesbrouck, J. Swings, and J. Doskar.** 2001. *Enterococcus haemoperoxidus* sp. nov. and *Enterococcus moraviensis* sp. nov., isolated from water. *Int. J. Syst. Evol. Microbiol.* **51:**1567–1574.
97. **Švec, P., M. Vancanneyt, L. A. Devriese, S. M. Naser, C. Snauwaert, K. Lefebvre, B. Hoste, and J. Swings.** 2005. *Enterococcus aquimarinus* sp. nov., isolated from sea water. *Int. J. Syst. Evol. Microbiol.* **55:**2183–2187.
98. **Švec, P., M. Vancanneyt, J. Koort, S. M. Naser, B. Hoste, E. Vihavainen, P. Vandamme, J. Swings, and J. Björkroth.** 2005. *Enterococcus devriesei* sp. nov., associated with animal sources. *Int. J. Syst. Evol. Microbiol.* **55:**2479–2484.
99. **Tambyah, P. A., J. A. Marx, and D. G. Maki.** 2004. Nosocomial infection with vancomycin-dependent enterococci. *Emerg. Infect. Dis.* **10:**1277–1281.
100. **Tannock, G. W., and G. Cook.** 2002. Enterococci as members of the intestinal microflora of humans, p. 101–132. *In* M. S. Gilmore, D. B. Clewell, P. Courvalin, G. M. Dunny, B. E. Murray, and L. B. Rice (ed.), *The Enterococci: Pathogenesis, Molecular Biology, and Antibiotic Resistance*. ASM Press, Washington, D.C.
101. **Teixeira, L. M., M. G. S. Carvalho, M. M. B. Espinola, A. G. Steigerwalt, M. P. Douglas, D. J. Brenner, and R. R. Facklam.** 2001. *Enterococcus porcinus* sp. nov. and *Enterococcus ratti* sp. nov. associated with enteric disorders in animals. *Int. J. Syst. Evol. Microbiol.* **51:**1737–1743.
102. **Teixeira, L. M., M. G. S. Carvalho, V. L. Merquior, A. G. Steigerwalt, D. J. Brenner, and R. R. Facklam.** 1997. Phenotypic and genotypic characterization of *Vagococcus fluvialis*, including strains isolated from human sources. *J. Clin. Microbiol.* **35:**2778–2781.
103. **Teixeira, L. M., R. R. Facklam, A. G. Steigerwalt, N. E. Pigott, V. L. C. Merquior, and D. J. Brenner.** 1995. Correlation between phenotypic characteristics and DNA relatedness with *Enterococcus faecium* strains. *J. Clin. Microbiol.* **33:**1520–1523.
104. **Teixeira, L. M., V. L. C. Merquior, M. C. E. Vianni, M. G. S. Carvalho, S. E. L. Fracalanzza, A. G. Steigerwalt, D. J. Brenner, and R. R. Facklam.** 1996. Phenotypic and genotypic characterization of atypical *Lactococcus garvieae* strains isolated from water buffalos with subclinical mastitis and confirmation of *L. garvieae* as a senior subjective synonym of *Enterococcus seriolicida*. *Int. J. Syst. Bacteriol.* **46:**664–668.
105. **Tenover, F. C., R. D. Arbeit, R. V. Goering. P. A. Mickelsen, B. E. Murray, D. H. Persing, and B. Swaminathan.** 1995. Interpreting chromosomal DNA restriction patterns produced by pulsed-field gel electrophoresis: criteria for bacterial strain typing. *J. Clin. Microbiol.* **33:**2233–2239.
106. **Titze-de-Almeida, R., R. J. Willems, J. Top, I. P. Rodrigues, R. F. Ferreira II, H. Boelens, M. C. Brandileone, R. C. Zanella, M. S. S. Felipe, and A. van Belkum.** 2004. Multilocus variable-number tandem-repeat polymorphism among Brazilian *Enterococcus faecalis* strains. *J. Clin. Microbiol.* **42:**4879–4881.
107. **Tomayko, J. F., and B. E. Murray.** 1995. Analysis of *Enterococcus faecalis* isolates from intercontinental sources by multilocus enzyme electrophoresis and pulsed-field gel electrophoresis. *J. Clin. Microbiol.* **33:**2903–2907.
108. **Top, J., L. M. Schouls, M. J. Bonten, and R. J. Willems.** 2004. Multiple-locus variable-number tandem repeat analysis, a novel typing scheme to study the genetic relatedness and epidemiology of *Enterococcus faecium* isolates. *J. Clin. Microbiol.* **42:**4503–4511.
109. **Tyrrell, G. J., L. Turnbull, L. Teixeira, M. G. S. Carvalho, J. Lefebvre, R. R. Facklam, and M. Lovgren.** 2002. Description of *Enterococcus gilvus* sp. nov. and

Enterococcus pallens sp. nov. isolated from human clinical specimens. *J. Clin. Microbiol.* **40:**1140–1145.

110. **Uttley, A. H. C., C. H. Collins, J. Naidoo, and R. C. George.** 1988. Vancomycin-resistant enterococci. *Lancet* **i:**57–58.
111. **Van Horn, K., C. Tóth, R. Kariyama, R. Mitsuhata, and H. Kumon.** 2002. Evaluation of 15 motility media and a direct microscopic method for detection of motility in enterococci. *J. Clin. Microbiol.* **40:**2476–2479.
112. **Weinstein, M. P.** 2001. Comparative evaluation of penicillin, ampicillin, and imipenem MICs and susceptibility breakpoints for vancomycin-susceptible and vancomycin-resistant *Enterococcus faecalis* and *Enterococcus faecium*. *J. Clin. Microbiol.* **39:**2729–2731.
113. **Wilke, W. W., S. A. Marshall, S. L. Coffman, M. A. Pfaller, M. B. Edmund, R. P. Wenzel, and R. N. Jones.** 1997. Vancomycin-resistant *Enterococcus raffinosus*: molecular epidemiology, species identification error, and frequency of occurrence in a national resistance surveillance program. *Diagn. Microbiol. Infect. Dis.* **28:**43–49.
114. **Willems, R. J. L., J. Top, N. van den Braak, A. van Belkum, A. van den Bogaard, and J. D. A. van Embden.** 2000. Host specificity of vancomycin-resistant *Enterococcus faecium*. *J. Infect. Dis.* **182:**816–823.
115. **Willey, B. M., A. J. McGree, M. A. Ostrowski, B. N. Kreiswirth, and D. E. Low.** 1994. The use of molecular typing techniques in the epidemiologic investigation of resistant enterococci. *Infect. Control Hosp. Epidemiol.* **15:**548–556.
116. **Woodford, N., D. Morrison, A. P. Johnson, V. Briant, R. C. George, and B. Cookson.** 1993. Application of DNA probes for rRNA and *vanA* genes to investigation of a nosocomial cluster of vancomycin-resistant enterococci. *J. Clin. Microbiol.* **31:**653–658.

Aerococcus, Abiotrophia, and Other Aerobic Catalase-Negative, Gram-Positive Cocci

KATHRYN L. RUOFF

31

TAXONOMY

The bacteria included in this chapter are taxonomically diverse catalase-negative, gram-positive cocci. All, however, share the characteristic of being infrequent clinical isolates found as opportunistic agents of infection in hosts who are usually compromised. Most of these organisms resemble other, more well known clinical isolates (e.g., streptococci and enterococci) and consequently may be mistaken for members of those genera. These bacteria may have been misidentified or overlooked in clinical cultures in the past or may represent emerging pathogens in compromised patient populations. Table 1 lists the organisms included here along with some of their basic characteristics.

Most organisms discussed in this chapter exhibit fairly low G+C contents (30 to 45 mol%) and are not currently affiliated with taxa above the genus level. Two additional infrequently isolated gram-positive cocci (*Rothia mucilaginosa* and *Alloiococcus* sp.) can display positive catalase reactions. The catalase-variable *R. mucilaginosa* (29), formerly called *Stomatococcus mucilaginosus* (G+C content, 50 to 60 mol%), was historically included with staphylococci in the family *Micrococcaceae* (101). The sole species of the catalase-positive genus *Alloiococcus* is *Alloiococcus otitis* (1) (see chapter 28).

The genus *Lactococcus* is composed of organisms formerly classified as Lancefield group N streptococci (102). Motile *Lactococcus*-like organisms with the Lancefield group N antigen (a teichoic acid antigen) have been classified in the genus *Vagococcus* (25, 116). The vagococci also resemble the enterococci, and Facklam and Elliott (51) reported that *Vagococcus* isolates examined at the Centers for Disease Control and Prevention, Atlanta, Ga., gave positive reactions in a commercially available nucleic acid probe test (Gen-Probe, San Diego, Calif.) for enterococci.

The genera *Abiotrophia* and *Granulicatella* have been proposed to accommodate organisms previously known as nutritionally variant or satelliting streptococci (34, 72). These bacteria were initially considered to be nutritional mutants of viridans group streptococcal strains, most notably of the species *Streptococcus mitis*. The work of Bouvet and colleagues (15) suggested that these organisms were really members of two novel streptococcal species given the names *Streptococcus defectivus* and *Streptococcus adjacens*. A comparative analysis of 16S rRNA sequences led Kawamura and coworkers to propose the creation of a new genus, *Abiotrophia*, containing two species, *Abiotrophia defectiva* and *Abiotrophia adiacens,* to accommodate these bacteria (72). A third species from human sources, *Abiotrophia elegans,* was described in 1998 (97). Kanamoto et al. noted the heterogeneity among *Abiotrophia* strains and proposed a fourth species, *Abiotrophia para-adiacens* (71). Most recently, Collins and Lawson proposed a new genus, *Granulicatella*, with *Granulicatella adiacens* and *Granulicatella elegans* encompassing strains formerly called *A. adiacens* and *A. elegans*. *A. defectiva* remains as the sole *Abiotrophia* species (34).

Taxonomic changes among the intrinsically vancomycin-resistant, catalase-negative, gram-positive cocci include the formation of the genus *Weissella* to accommodate the species formerly known as *Leuconostoc paramesenteroides* and related species (38). The vancomycin-susceptible species *Pediococcus halophilus*, formerly included in the otherwise intrinsically vancomycin-resistant *Pediococcus* genus, was reclassified in the genus *Tetragenococcus* (39). The organism formerly called *Enterococcus solitarius* has also been transferred to the *Tetragenococcus* genus as *Tetragenococcus solitarius* (48). Little is known about the role of the tetragenococci in human infection.

The organism we now know as *Gemella morbillorum* was noted in 1917 by Tunicliff (111), who was searching for the etiologic agent of measles. The organism she isolated from blood cultures from numerous measles patients was originally named *Diplococcus rubeolae*. This bacterium was also known as *Diplococcus morbillorum, Peptostreptococcus morbillorum,* and *Streptococcus morbillorum* until a proposal to include it in the genus *Gemella* was made in 1988 (74). *Gemella haemolysans* was originally classified as a *Neisseria* species due to its gram-variable or even gram-negative nature and its cellular morphology (diplococci with flattened adjacent sides). Collins and coworkers described two additional *Gemella* species isolated from human sources, *Gemella bergeri* (originally named *Gemella bergeriae*) (31) and *Gemella sanguinis* (32). The genus *Dolosigranulum* shows phenotypic similarities to *Gemella,* although it is not phylogenetically closely related to *Gemella* strains (3, 79).

Aerococcus urinae, described in 1992, is negative for pyrrolidonyl arylamidase production (PYR) and positive for leucine aminopeptidase production (LAP), showing reactions opposite those of *Aerococcus viridans* in these important identification tests (2). In spite of these phenotypic differences, molecular taxonomic studies suggest that *A. urinae*

TABLE 1 Basic phenotypic characteristics of catalase-negative, gram-positive cocci[a]

Organism (reference[s])	PYR	LAP	NaCl	BE	ESC	MOT	HIP	SAT	ARG	BGUR	MORPH	VAN
Abiotrophia defectiva (21, 34, 72)	+	+	−	−		−	−	+	−	−	Chains	S
Aerococcus christensenii (33, 52)	−	+	+	−	−	−	+	−	−	−	Clusters	S
Aerococcus sanguinicola (52, 82)	+	+	+	+	+	ND	+	−	−	+	Clusters	ND
Aerococcus urinae (22, 23, 52)	−	+	+	−	V	−	+	−	−	+	Clusters	S
Aerococcus urinaehominis (52, 81)	−	−	+	−	+	ND	+	−	−	+	Clusters	ND
Aerococcus viridans[b] (51, 52)	+	−	+	V	+	−	V	−	−	ND	Clusters	S
Dolosicoccus (37)	+	−	−	ND	ND	−	ND	−	ND	ND	Chains	S
Dolosigranulum (3, 52, 79)	+	+	+	−	+[c]	−	−	−	−	−	Clusters	S
Enterococcus[d,e] (51)	+	+	+	+	+	V	ND	−	ND	ND	Chains	S/R
Facklamia languida[f] (79, 80)	+	+	+	ND	−	−	−	−	−	−	Clusters	S
Facklamia spp.[f] (28, 30, 35, 79)	+	+	+	ND	−	−	+	−	V	ND	Chains	S
Gemella haemolysans[g] (51)	+	+	−	−	−	−	ND	−	ND	ND	Clusters	S
Gemella spp.[g] (31, 32, 51)	+	+	−	−	ND	−	ND	−	−	ND	Chains	S
Globicatella (24, 50, 51, 104)	V	−	+	+	+	−	+	−	−	ND	Chains	S
Granulicatella adiacens[h] (21, 34, 72)	+	+	−	−	ND	−	−	+	−	+	Chains	S
Granulicatella elegans[h] (21, 34, 72)	+	+	−	−	ND	−	+	+	+	−	Chains	S
Helcococcus kunzii[b] (26, 51)	+	−	+	−	+	−	−	−	−	−	Clusters	S
Ignavigranum (36, 50, 79)	+	+	+	−	−	−	−	V	−	ND	Chains	S
Lactococcus[e,i] (51)	V	+	V	+	+	−	ND	−	ND	ND	Chains	S
Leuconostoc (51)	−	−	+	V	ND	−	ND	−	ND	ND	Chains	R
Pediococcus (51)	−	+	V	+	ND	−	ND	−	ND	ND	Clusters	R
Streptococcus[i,j] (51)	V	+	V	V	V	−	ND	−	ND	ND	Chains	S
Tetragenococcus (51)	−	+	+	+	ND	−	ND	ND	ND	ND	Clusters	S
Vagococcus[d] (51)	+	+	V	+	+	+	ND	−	ND	ND	Chains	S
Weissella (57, 89)	V	ND	ND	+	+	−	ND	ND	+	ND	Short rods or coccobacilli in pairs and chains	R

[a] Abbreviations and symbols: PYR, production of pyrrolidonyl arylamidase; LAP, production of leucine aminopeptidase; NaCl, growth in 6.5% NaCl; BE, hydrolysis of esculin in the presence of 40% bile; ESC, hydrolysis of esculin; MOT, motility; HIP, hydrolysis of hippurate; SAT, satelliting behavior; ARG, hydrolysis of arginine; BGUR, production of β-glucuronidase; MORPH, cellular arrangement; VAN, susceptibility to vancomycin; +, ≥90% of strains positive; −, ≤10% of strains positive; V, variable (60 to 90% of strains positive); ND, no data; chains, cells arranged primarily in pairs and chains; clusters, cells arranged primarily in clusters, tetrads, or irregular groups; S, susceptible; R, resistant.

[b] Although *H. kunzii* shares some phenotypic traits with *A. viridans*, *H. kunzii* is facultative and usually nonhemolytic, in contrast to *A. viridans*, which favors an aerobic growth atmosphere and is alpha-hemolytic. Two additional species of *Helcococcus* (*H. sueciensis* and "*H. pyogenes*") have been proposed (27, 91), both based on the isolation of single strains. These new species display negative reactions in the PYR test, in contrast to *H. kunzii*.

[c] LaClaire and Facklam (79) note that strains of *Dolosigranulum* are esculin hydrolysis positive when tested on conventional media, but the original description of this organism notes a lack of esculin hydrolysis activity (3).

[d] Most enterococcal strains are capable of growth at 45°C, which differentiates them from vagococci, which may be phenotypically similar. Strains of vagococci have been reported as testing positive with a commercially available nucleic acid probe for members of the genus *Enterococcus*.

[e] Phenotypically similar strains of enterococci and lactococci can be differentiated with a commercially available nucleic acid probe for members of the genus *Enterococcus*.

[f] *F. languida* cells are characteristically arranged in clusters, and cells of other *Facklamia* species are arranged in pairs and chains.

[g] *G. haemolysans* cells are arranged in pairs and clusters, and the cells of other *Gemella* species are arranged in pairs and chains.

[h] Formerly classified as a member of the genus *Abiotrophia*.

[i] Most lactococcal strains are capable of growth at 10°C, which differentiates them from streptococci, which may be phenotypically similar.

[j] *Streptococcus pyogenes* and some strains of *S. pneumoniae* are PYR positive.

should remain in the *Aerococcus* genus. Organisms currently included in the *A. urinae* species are fairly heterogeneous and can probably be subdivided into at least two subspecies (23). *Aerococcus christensenii*, isolated from the human genitourinary tract, was described by Collins and coworkers in 1999 (33) and was joined by the species *Aerococcus sanguinicola* (originally named *Aerococcus sanguicola*) (52, 82) and *Aerococcus urinaehominis* (81) in 2001.

The genera *Facklamia*, *Ignavigranum*, and *Dolosicoccus* are related to, but distinct from, *Globicatella sanguinus*, an organism initially named *Globicatella sanguis*, which was described in 1992 (24). The genus *Facklamia* currently contains four species isolated from human sources: *Facklamia hominis* (28), *Facklamia sourekii* (30), *Facklamia ignava* (35), and *Facklamia languida* (80). The genus *Ignavigranum*, currently consisting of a single species, *Ignavigranum ruoffiae*, was described by Collins and coworkers (36), along with the genus *Dolosicoccus* and its single species, *Dolosicoccus paucivorans* (37).

The genus *Helcococcus* was originally composed of the single species *Helcococcus kunzii* (26), which was joined by a new species isolated from humans, *Helcococcus sueciensis*, in 2004 (27). A third human species, "*Helcococcus pyogenes*," has been proposed but to date has not received official taxonomic standing (91).

The examination of gram-positive cocci with molecular taxonomic methods has encouraged the delineation of new groups of organisms and the refinement of a genetically based taxonomy for the catalase-negative, gram-positive cocci.

DESCRIPTION OF THE GENERA

The organisms included in this chapter form gram-positive coccoid cells, but *G. haemolysans* may appear to be gram variable or gram negative due to the ease with which its cells are decolorized. Cell shape and arrangement can aid in dividing these organisms into two broad groups: those with a streptococcal-like Gram stain morphology (coccobacilli in pairs and chains) and those with a staphylococcal-like Gram stain morphology (more spherical cocci in pairs, tetrads, clusters, or irregular groups). Members of the genera *Abiotrophia* and *Granulicatella* (formerly the nutritionally variant streptococci) form coccobacilli arranged in pairs and chains, but these organisms may also appear pleomorphic, especially when grown under less than optimal nutritional conditions (21). *Weissella* strains form coccobacilli or short rods arranged in pairs and chains (89). Dividing these diverse bacteria into two groups based on cellular shape and arrangement serves only as an aid in identification; no relatedness of organisms is implied by this grouping. With the exception of the infrequently isolated vagococci, these organisms are nonmotile.

Members of most of the genera are catalase-negative facultative anaerobes, but *A. viridans* is classified as a microaerophile that grows poorly if at all under anaerobic conditions. Some strains of *Aerococcus* may exhibit weakly positive catalase reactions due to nonheme catalase activity. None of the members of the genera are beta-hemolytic on routinely employed blood agars, but *G. haemolysans* is described as producing beta-hemolysis on agars supplemented with rabbit or horse blood (95), and some strains of *G. bergeri* and *G. sanguinis* may exhibit hemolytic reactions on horse blood agar (31, 32).

NATURAL HABITATS

Some of the genera discussed here are members of normal flora of the oral cavity or upper respiratory tract *(Gemella, Abiotrophia,* and *Granulicatella)* or colonize the skin (*Helcococcus*). Foods and vegetation are normal habitats for lactococci, pediococci, and leuconostocs (59, 60); members of the genera *Lactococcus, Pediococcus,* and *Leuconostoc* may also be found as normal flora of the alimentary tract, but thorough data supporting this contention are lacking. Aerococci are environmental isolates that can also be found on human skin. Although the organisms have been isolated from human sources, the natural habitats of many of the organisms mentioned here are not well characterized.

CLINICAL SIGNIFICANCE

Although the organisms included in this chapter may be present as contaminants in clinical cultures, they are also isolated infrequently as opportunistic pathogens. These bacteria appear to be of low virulence and are usually pathogenic only in compromised hosts. Infection often occurs in previously damaged tissues (e.g., heart valves) or may be nosocomial and associated with prolonged hospitalization, antibiotic treatment, invasive procedures, and the presence of foreign bodies. Specimens likely to yield significant numbers of isolates of these bacteria are blood, cerebrospinal fluid, urine, and wound specimens.

Lactococcus

Difficulties in distinguishing lactococci from either streptococci or enterococci have probably led to the misidentification of clinical *Lactococcus* isolates in the past and may have contributed to the paucity of reports concerning the clinical role of these bacteria. Elliott and coworkers (45) studied the phenotypic characteristics of a number of lactococcal strains isolated from blood, specimens from patients with urinary tract infections, and an eye wound specimen culture. The authors observed that three blood culture isolates were obtained from patients diagnosed with prosthetic valve endocarditis. Other reports have noted cases of lactococcal native valve endocarditis (56, 84, 94), septicemia in an immunosuppressed patient (86), osteomyelitis (69), and liver abscess (4).

Vagococcus

To date, only a handful of *Vagococcus* isolates from human sources have been reported in the literature. Teixeira and coworkers (110) described strains isolated from blood, peritoneal fluid, and a wound specimen. Vagococci are motile organisms that, like lactococci, express the Lancefield group N antigen (51). Difficulties encountered in identifying vagococci may partially account for their infrequent recognition in clinical cultures.

Abiotrophia and *Granulicatella*

Organisms formally known as nutritionally variant streptococci are normal residents of the oral cavity but have been identified as agents of endocarditis involving both native and prosthetic valves (68). These organisms have also been isolated in cases of ophthalmic infections (87, 90), a brain abscess following neurosurgery (14), and iatrogenic meningitis following myelography (100).

Leuconostoc, Pediococcus, and *Weissella*

The vancomycin-resistant genera *Leuconostoc* and *Pediococcus* have been recognized in clinical specimens since the mid-1980s. Handwerger and colleagues (66) noted host defense impairment, invasive procedures breaching the integument, gastrointestinal symptoms, and prior antibiotic treatment as common features among adult patients infected with *Leuconostoc*. They also observed a predisposition to *Leuconostoc* bacteremia among neonates, suggesting that infants may become colonized during delivery by leuconostocs inhabiting the maternal genital tract. In addition to causing bacteremia, leuconostocs have been isolated from cerebrospinal fluid, peritoneal dialysate fluid, and wound specimens. Case reports have implicated leuconostocs as agents of infection in osteomyelitis (119), ventriculitis (43), and postsurgical endophthalmitis (76).

Pediococcus strains have been isolated in cases of bacteremia, sepsis, and hepatic abscess in compromised patients (9, 62, 85, 105). Barros and coworkers (9) noted that *Pediococcus acidilactici* was isolated from clinical specimens more frequently than *Pediococcus pentosaceus* and was also more commonly isolated in cases of bacteremia. Barton and coworkers noted the role of *Pediococcus* in bacteremia in infants with gastrointestinal malformations requiring surgical correction (10).

Weissella confusa, formerly classified as *Lactobacillus confusus*, has been reported infrequently as an agent of bacteremia and endocarditis (57, 89).

Gemella

G. haemolysans has been isolated as a pathogen in cases of endocarditis (20), meningitis (58), brain abscess (83), and total knee arthroplasty (44). *G. morbillorum* has been isolated (when still classified as a streptococcus; see "Taxonomy") from blood cultures and cultures of respiratory, genitourinary, wound, and abscess specimens (53). This *Gemella* species has been implicated in cases of empyema and lung abscess (41), septic shock (115), endocarditis (55, 61, 118), brain abscess (108), osteomyelitis (114), peritonitis (6), and infection in an arteriovenous shunt (7). The clinical significance of *G. bergeri* and *G. sanguinis* is not well described, but strains of these species have been isolated from blood cultures, and they may also function as agents of endocarditis (31, 32).

Dolosigranulum

Little is known about the clinical significance of *Dolosigranulum*, a genus that is phenotypically similar, but not closely related to, *Gemella* (3). Strains of *Dolosigranulum pigrum*, the sole species in the genus, have been isolated from blood and eye and respiratory specimens (77), and this organism has been cited as a probable agent in a case of synovitis (65).

Aerococcus

Although aerococci appear as contaminants in clinical cultures, occasional reports have noted a clinically significant role for these organisms in cases of endocarditis and bacteremia (40, 73, 92). Until the early 1990s, *A. viridans* was the only species reported from human specimens, but four additional species isolated from humans have been described to date. *A. urinae* (2, 63) has been implicated as a urinary tract pathogen in patients predisposed to infection (22) and also as an agent of endocarditis (75, 107), lymphadenitis (99), and spondylodiscitis (5). Little is currently known about the clinical significance of *A. christensenii* (isolated from vaginal specimens) (33), *A. urinaehominis* (isolated from urine) (81), and *A. sanguinicola* (isolated from blood and urine) (52, 82).

Globicatella

G. sanguinis, the sole *Globicatella* species isolated from humans, has been implicated in cases of bacteremia, urinary tract infection, and meningitis (24). A second species in the genus, *Globicatella sulfidifaciens*, has been isolated in cases of purulent infections in domestic mammals (113).

Facklamia

Members of the *Facklamia* genus are closely related to, but phenotypically and phylogenetically distinct from, members of the *Globicatella* genus (28). Strains of the four *Facklamia* species isolated from humans have been recovered from blood, wound, and genitourinary sites (28, 30, 35, 80), and a patient with chorioamnionitis (67).

Ignavigranum

Only a few strains of *I. ruoffiae*, the sole species of the genus *Ignavigranum*, have been described to date. Sites of isolation include a wound and an ear abscess (36).

Dolosicoccus

Strains of *D. paucivorans*, the only species currently included in the genus *Dolosicoccus*, have been recovered from blood cultures (37, 50).

Helcococcus

H. kunzii has been recovered from intact skin of the lower extremities (64), as well as from wound specimen cultures (notably those from foot ulcers) containing mixtures of bacteria (26). Consequently, the clinical significance of this organism is difficult to interpret, since it may be present merely as a colonizer of the wound site. The ability of this species to function as an opportunist was, however, suggested by its isolation in pure culture from an infected sebaceous cyst (93) and a breast abscess (19). Classification of two additional species isolated from humans, *H. sueciensis* and "*H. pyogenes*," is based on single isolates from a wound and a prosthetic joint infection specimen, respectively (27, 91).

COLLECTION, TRANSPORT, AND STORAGE OF SPECIMENS

The organisms described in this chapter have all been isolated from routine cultures of clinical specimens, and special requirements for collection and processing of specimens have not been described. Since these bacteria are facultative anaerobes or microaerophiles, aerobic collection, transport, and storage methods as described in chapter 5 of this Manual should allow for their isolation.

ISOLATION PROCEDURES

Generally, there are no special requirements for isolation of the group of bacteria discussed here; general recommendations for the culture of blood, body fluids, and other specimens should be followed (see chapters 5, 6, and 20). These organisms are likely to be isolated on rich, nonselective media (e.g., blood and chocolate agars and thioglycolate broth) since they are nutritionally fastidious. If selective isolation of members of the vancomycin-resistant genera *Leuconostoc* and *Pediococcus* is desired, Thayer-Martin medium may be used to inhibit normal flora or other contaminating microorganisms (98). Members of some of the genera (e.g., *Helcococcus*) grow slowly, forming tiny colonies that may not be visible unless extended incubation (48 to 72 h) is employed. The recovery of members of many of the genera included in this chapter may be enhanced by CO_2 enrichment of the incubation atmosphere.

Members of the genera *Abiotrophia* and *Granulicatella* usually grow on chocolate agar, on brucella agar with 5% horse blood, and in thioglycolate broth but not on Trypticase soy agar with 5% sheep blood. These organisms can be cultured on nonsupportive media that have been appropriately supplemented (see "*Abiotrophia* and *Granulicatella*" under "Additional Procedures for Characterization of Selected Genera with Negative Catalase Reactions" below).

IDENTIFICATION

The phenotypic characteristics detailed here may not always be sufficient for accurate identification of the aerobic catalase-negative, gram-positive cocci encountered infrequently in clinical laboratories. Although Gram stain morphology is prone to subjective interpretation, it has been employed as a major decision point in the identification protocols, with two general categories: Gram stain morphology resembling that of streptococci, meaning cocci or coccobacilli in pairs and chains, and staphylococcal morphology, meaning coccoid cells arranged in pairs, clusters, tetrads, or irregular groups. Broth-grown cells (thioglycolate broth is suitable) should be used for making morphological determinations. The flowcharts in this chapter (Fig. 1 and 2) should not be used for definitive identification. In most cases, additional procedures (Table 1) are recommended before identification to the genus level is made. Identifications of unfamiliar organisms from important specimens should be confirmed by a reference laboratory. Molecular methods such as 16S rRNA

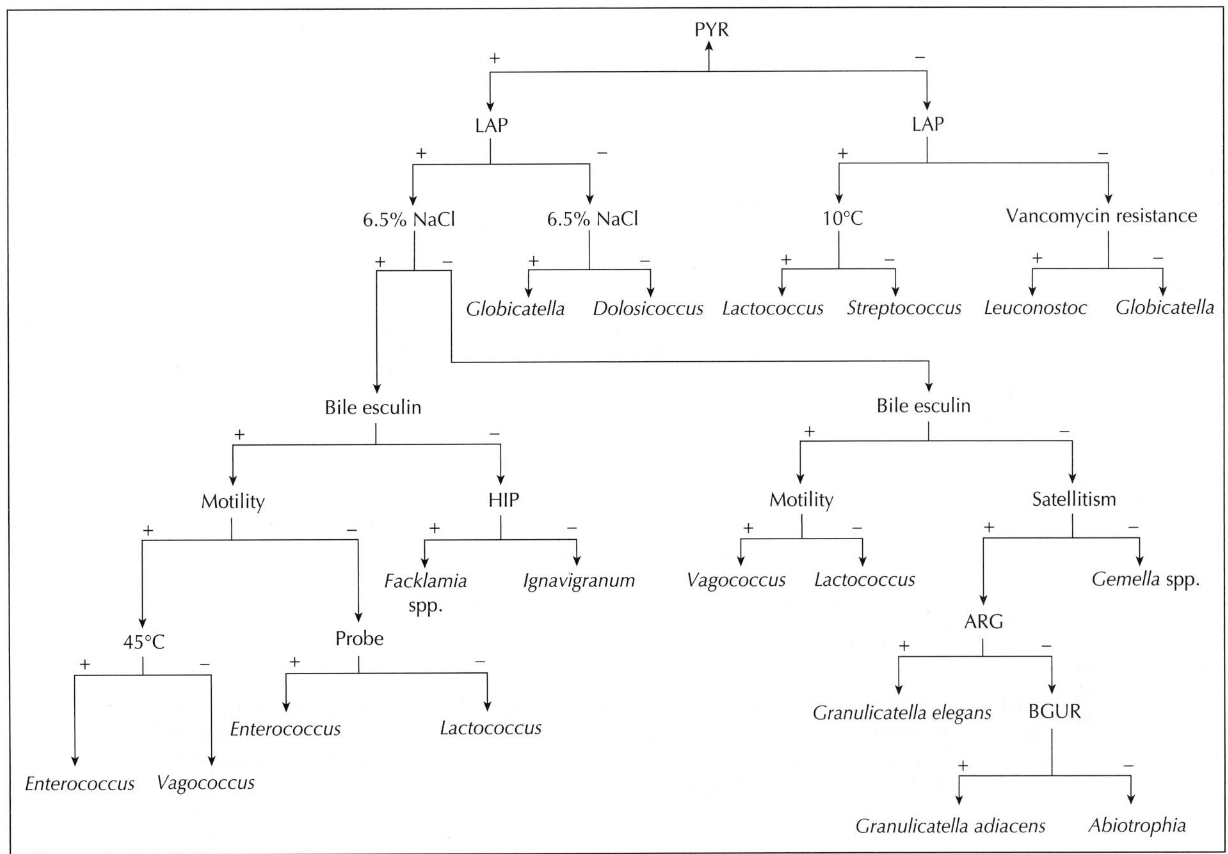

FIGURE 1 Identification of catalase-negative, gram-positive cocci that grow aerobically with cells arranged in pairs or chains. Abbreviations: PYR, pyrrolidonyl arylamidase activity; LAP, leucine aminopeptidase activity; 6.5% NaCl, growth in broth containing 6.5% NaCl; bile esculin, hydrolysis of esculin in the presence of 40% bile; motility, motility in motility test medium; 45°C, growth at 45°C; 10°C, growth at 10°C; probe, reaction with commercially available nucleic acid probe for the genus *Enterococcus;* HIP, hydrolysis of hippurate; satellitism, satelliting growth behavior; ARG, arginine hydrolysis activity; BGUR, β-glucuronidase activity.

gene-based DNA sequencing or the use of alternative genetic targets may be useful for genus- and species-level identification (117).

Procedures for Initial Differentiation of Genera with Negative Catalase Reactions

Initial testing procedures for catalase-negative isolates with streptococcal (Fig. 1) or staphylococcal (Fig. 2) Gram stain morphology are represented in the flowcharts. Note that *Gemella* and *Facklamia* strains may display either type of cellular morphology, depending on the species (see "Additional Procedures for Characterization of Genera with Negative Catalase Reactions" below). Descriptions of tests for these organisms follow.

Catalase Test

If a positive or weakly positive catalase reaction is observed with growth from blood-containing media, growth from a medium devoid of blood (e.g., brain heart infusion agar) should be used to repeat the catalase test. A loopful of growth is transferred onto a microscope slide or empty petri dish and observed for the evolution of bubbles after the addition of a drop of 3% H_2O_2. It may be necessary to use a hand lens to detect weakly positive reactions.

PYR Test

See chapter 21 and reference 51 for a description of the PYR test. Rapid disk tests are commercially available, and an assay for PYR is contained in some commercially available identification kits (e.g., API 20 Strep; bioMerieux, Durham, N.C.).

LAP Test

The LAP test determines the presence of the enzyme leucine aminopeptidase, also called leucine arylamidase. See chapter 21 for a description of this test. An assay for this enzyme is contained in some commercially available identification kits (e.g., API 20 Strep; bioMerieux), and a rapid disk test for LAP is also available commercially (BD Diagnostic Systems, Sparks, Md.; Remel, Lenexa, Kans.). The manufacturer's instructions should be followed when the test is performed (51, 54).

Growth in 6.5% NaCl

Heart infusion broth supplemented with 6.0% NaCl, with or without the acid-base indicator bromcresol purple, may be

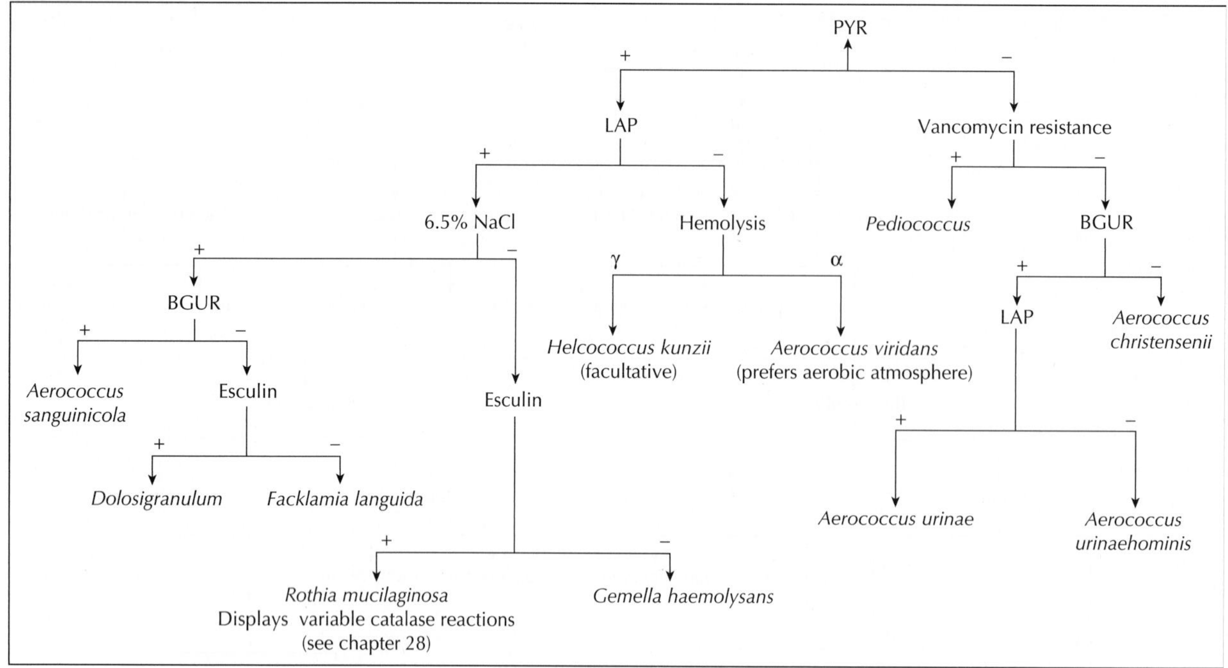

FIGURE 2 Identification of catalase-negative, gram-positive cocci that grow aerobically with cells arranged in pairs, tetrads and clusters, or irregular groups. Abbreviations: PYR, pyrrolidonyl arylamidase activity; LAP, leucine aminopeptidase activity; 6.5% NaCl, growth in broth containing 6.5% NaCl; esculin, hydrolysis of esculin; BGUR, β-glucuronidase activity.

used to test for growth in 6.5% NaCl. The broth is inoculated with two to three colonies of the organism to be tested and incubated at 35°C for up to 72 h. Turbidity with or without a color change from purple to yellow (due to production of acid) indicates growth (51, 54).

Bile Esculin Test

The ability to hydrolyze esculin in the presence of 40% bile is tested by culturing the test organism on bile esculin agar in an ambient-atmosphere incubator at 35°C for up to 48 h. Blackening of the agar indicates a positive reaction (54).

Motility Test

The motility test is performed by stab inoculating modified motility test medium and incubating at 30°C (instead of 35°C) for up to 48 h, according to the method of Facklam and Elliott (51).

Hippurate Hydrolysis Test

Facklam and Elliott recommend a conventional broth medium for determining hippurate hydrolysis (51). This test may also be contained in commercially available identification kits.

Satellitism Test

In a test for satelliting behavior, the strain to be examined is streaked for confluent growth on a medium that fails to support growth or supports only weak growth (e.g., sheep blood agar or brain heart infusion agar). A single cross streak of *Staphylococcus aureus* (ATCC 25923 or another suitable strain) is applied to the inoculated area. After incubation at 35°C in an atmosphere containing an elevated CO_2 level, strains of *Abiotrophia* or *Granulicatella* will grow only in the vicinity of the staphylococcal growth. Alternatively, media can be supplemented with pyridoxal in the form of an aqueous stock solution of filter-sterilized 0.01% pyridoxal hydrochloride. This solution, which can be stored frozen, should be added to media to achieve a final concentration of 0.001%. Disks containing pyridoxal may also be used in the satelliting test and are commercially available (Remel). Some strains of *Ignavigranum* may show satelliting behavior (36).

Arginine Hydrolysis Test

The arginine hydrolysis test can be performed with Moeller's decarboxylase broth containing arginine (51).

β-Glucuronidase Test

A test for β-glucuronidase is included in a number of commercially available identification products or may be performed using commercially prepared disks.

Vancomycin Susceptibility Test

Several colonies are streaked over half of a plate containing Trypticase soy agar with 5% sheep blood. After placing of a 30-μg vancomycin disk in the center of the inoculated area, the plate is incubated overnight in a CO_2-enriched atmosphere at 35°C. Any zone of inhibition indicates susceptibility, and resistant strains exhibit no inhibition zone (51, 54).

Esculin Hydrolysis Test

Esculin agar slants (heart infusion agar containing 0.1% esculin and 0.5% ferric citrate) are employed for the esculin hydrolysis test. After inoculation, slants are incubated at 35°C for up to 7 days. Partial or complete blackening of the agar indicates a positive reaction (51).

Additional Procedures for Characterization of Selected Genera with Negative Catalase Reactions

Lactococcus

Facklam and colleagues (51, 54) recommend growth temperature tests for distinguishing lactococci from streptococci and enterococci. Consult Fig. 1 for growth temperature characteristics of each of the genera. Broths (heart infusion broth containing 1% glucose and bromcresol purple indicator) are inoculated with a single colony or a drop of broth culture of the test strain and incubated at 35°C for up to 7 days. A water bath is recommended for incubation of cultures at 45°C. Turbidity with or without a change in the broth's indicator to yellow indicates a positive test.

If it is important to rule out enterococci, suspicious isolates can be tested with a commercially available nucleic acid probe test for the genus *Enterococcus*. *Lactococcus lactis* and *Lactococcus garvieae* are the *Lactococcus* species most commonly isolated from clinical specimens. Further information on the differentiation of *Lactococcus* isolates to the species level may be found in references 45, 47, and 102.

Abiotrophia and *Granulicatella*

Lists of additional phenotypic traits for *Abiotrophia* and *Granulicatella* species can be found in references 11, 16, 21, and 34. Davis and Peel (42) reported that the API 20 Strep system (bioMerieux) is superior to the Rapid ID 32 Strep system (bioMerieux) for identification of these organisms. They found that accurate results were obtained when a dense inoculum (confluent growth from two blood agar plates) was employed.

Leuconostoc and *Pediococcus*

Members of the genera *Leuconostoc* and *Pediococcus* produce small, alpha- or nonhemolytic colonies on blood agar that can appear similar to those of viridans streptococci. In addition to having differing cellular morphologies (Table 1), members of these vancomycin-resistant genera, along with vancomycin-resistant strains of lactobacilli that form short coccoid cells, may be separated by tests for gas production from glucose and arginine hydrolysis. Leuconostocs produce gas and are always arginine negative. Lactobacilli are variable in both tests, but a positive arginine test for a gas-producing strain would rule out the identification of the organism as a leuconostoc. Pediococci are gas production negative and show variable reactions in the arginine test, although *P. acidilactici* and *P. pentosaceus*, the two species commonly found in clinical material, are arginine positive.

Gas production is measured by inoculating MRS (deMan, Rogosa, Sharpe) broth (BD Diagnostic Systems; Hardy Diagnostics, Santa Maria, Calif.) with the test organism, sealing the culture with melted petrolatum, and incubating for up to 7 days at 35°C. Gas production is evidenced by displacement of the petrolatum plug (51, 54). The arginine hydrolysis test can be performed with Moeller's decarboxylase broth containing arginine (51). The Lancefield group D antigen can be detected in pediococci (54). References 8, 9, 46, 51, 54, and 96 should be consulted for further information on the identification of *Leuconostoc* and *Pediococcus* to the species level.

Tetragenococcus

The organisms formerly known as *P. halophilus* and *E. solitarius* were reclassified in the *Tetragenococcus* genus as *Tetragenococcus halophilus* and *T. solitarius* (39, 48). Although these organisms share some phenotypic characteristics with pediococci, they are vancomycin susceptible. Although little is know about the participation of these organisms in human infection, they should be suspected if vancomycin-susceptible, *Pediococcus*-like strains are encountered.

Weissella

Weissella strains may be misidentified as leuconostocs or lactobacilli. These organisms produce gas from glucose. The few clinical isolates reported in the literature have been described as vancomycin resistant and positive for hydrolysis of arginine. Characteristics useful for the identification of strains of the infrequently isolated *Weissella* genus are found in Table 1 and references 57 and 89.

Gemella

Facklam and Washington (54) state that all *Gemella* species are PYR positive but that *G. morbillorum* displays a weakly positive reaction. Findings of earlier studies (12, 13) generally support these observations, but the previous studies describe some isolates of both *G. haemolysans* and *G. morbillorum* as being negative in the PYR test. Facklam and Washington note that a large inoculum must be used when these bacteria are tested for the pyrrolidonyl arylamidase enzyme. Leucine aminopeptidase is usually absent in isolates of *G. haemolysans* but present in strains of *G. morbillorum* (12, 13). On sheep blood agar media, gemellas form small colonies that are similar in appearance to those of viridans group streptococci. Slow growth of some *Gemella* strains may lead to confusion of these organisms with *Abiotrophia* or *Granulicatella* organisms (formerly called nutritionally variant streptococci). A test for satelliting behavior will separate these two groups of bacteria (54).

Cells of *G. haemolysans* are easily decolorized and resemble those of neisserias, since they occur in pairs with the adjacent sides flattened. *G. haemolysans* favors an aerobic growth atmosphere. *G. morbillorum* cells are gram positive and are arranged in pairs and short chains; individual cells in a given pair may be of unequal sizes. *G. morbillorum* is described as favoring anaerobic growth conditions. Only a small number of strains of *G. bergeri* and *G. sanguinis* have been reported on to date. Information on phenotypic characteristics of these *Gemella* species can be found in references 31 and 32.

Aerococcus

In addition to the traits listed in Table 1, *A. viridans* is characterized by displaying weak or no growth when incubated in an anaerobic atmosphere (49). This trait can be tested by incubating duplicate blood agar plate cultures of the organism in question in an anaerobic and an aerobic atmosphere and comparing growth after 24 to 48 h. When grown aerobically, *A. viridans* forms alpha-hemolytic colonies that may be confused with those of either viridans group streptococci or enterococci. *A. urinae* forms small (0.5 mm in diameter after 24 h of incubation), alpha-hemolytic, convex, shiny, transparent colonies on blood agar media. *A. urinae* is PYR negative and LAP positive, in contrast to *A. viridans* (2). Additional information on the identifying characteristics of *A. urinae* can be found in reference 22, and a second biotype (esculin hydrolysis positive) of this species is described in reference 23. Information on phenotypic traits of the recently described species *A. christensenii*, *A. sanguinicola*, and *A. urinaehominis* can be found in Table 1 and references 33, 52, 81, and 82.

Helcococcus

In addition to the characteristics shown in Table 1, most isolates of *H. kunzii* produce an API 20 Strep (bioMerieux) profile of 4100413. Colonial morphology (tiny, gray, usually slightly alpha-hemolytic colonies), good growth under anaerobic conditions, and stimulation of growth by the addition of 1% horse serum or 0.1% Tween 80 to the medium differentiate *H. kunzii* from aerococci (26).

ANTIBIOTIC SUSCEPTIBILITIES

The lack of standardized methods and interpretation criteria for antibiotic susceptibility testing results, along with relatively small collections of clinical isolates for some of the genera discussed in this chapter, makes it difficult to accurately assess antimicrobial susceptibility patterns. With the exception of *Leuconostoc*, *Pediococcus,* and *Weissella*, members of all of the genera display susceptibility to vancomycin. Since many of the bacteria presented in this chapter are fairly fastidious, investigators have often employed blood-supplemented Mueller-Hinton medium and, if necessary for good growth, incubation in a CO_2-enriched atmosphere. Pyridoxal hydrochloride (0.001%) should also be added to blood-supplemented media for testing strains of *Abiotrophia* and *Granulicatella*. Most studies have employed streptococcal (other than *Streptococcus pneumoniae*) interpretative criteria for determining susceptibility. Details of susceptibility testing methodology and interpretive criteria can be found in reference 88.

Limited information on the in vitro antimicrobial susceptibilities of *L. lactis* and *L. garvieae* strains isolated from humans suggests that *L. garvieae* isolates are less susceptible to penicillin and cephalothin than are strains of *L. lactis*. The uniform resistance of *L. garvieae* to clindamycin contrasts with the uniform susceptibility of the *L. lactis* strains examined by Elliott and Facklam (47) and led them to propose a test for clindamycin susceptibility as an aid in differentiation of these two species. In clinical practice, patients with lactococcal endocarditis have been successfully treated either with penicillin alone or with penicillin and gentamicin (84, 94).

Teixeira and colleagues examined a small collection of *Vagococcus* isolates and observed that all strains tested were susceptible to ampicillin, cefotaxime, and trimethoprim-sulfamethoxazole. All strains were resistant to clindamycin, lomefloxacin, and ofloxacin. Variable results were observed with other antimicrobial agents (110).

Members of the vancomycin-resistant genera *Leuconostoc* and *Pediococcus* are also resistant to teicoplanin. Although they are usually susceptible to imipenem, minocycline, chloramphenicol, and gentamicin, MICs of penicillin for these strains correspond to the moderately susceptible category (109).

There is a range of MICs of penicillin for *Abiotrophia* and *Granulicatella* isolates, with the majority of strains classified as either susceptible or relatively resistant. There is also variability in susceptibilities to aminoglycosides, but no cases of high-level resistance have been reported. A synergistic effect between beta-lactam agents and aminoglycosides has been demonstrated for isolates of *Abiotrophia* (70). Tuohy and colleagues examined a collection of 27 *G. adiacens* and 12 *A. defectiva* strains, noting susceptibilities of all isolates to clindamycin, rifampin, levofloxacin, ofloxacin, and quinupristin-dalfopristin. These authors noted that the percentage of isolates of *G. adiacens* and *A. defectiva* examined that were susceptible to other agents tested was as follows: penicillin, 55 and 8%; amoxicillin, 81 and 92%; ceftriaxone, 63 and 83%; and meropenem, 96 and 100%, respectively (112). Zheng and coworkers reported high rates of beta-lactam and macrolide resistance in a collection of pediatric *Abiotrophia* and *Granulicatella* isolates (120).

A. viridans and *G. haemolysans* appear to be susceptible to penicillin and display a low level of resistance to aminoglycosides (17, 18). Buu-Hoi and colleagues (17) noted that although *A. viridans* seems to be naturally susceptible to macrolides, tetracyclines, and chloramphenicol, resistance to these agents has been observed. *A. urinae* has been described as susceptible to penicillin, amoxicillin, piperacillin, cefipime, rifampin, and nitrofurantoin but resistant to sulfonamides and netilmicin. Isolates display variable susceptibilities to trimethoprim and cotrimoxazole (22, 103, 106). *A. sanguinicola* isolates display susceptibilities to penicillin, amoxicillin, cefotaxime, cefuroxime, erythromycin, chloramphenicol, quinupristin-dalfopristin, rifampin, linezolid, and tetracycline (52). Buu-Hoi and coworkers (18) demonstrated a synergistic effect of penicillin and gentamicin against *G. haemolysans*.

A collection of 27 clinical isolates of *D. pigrum* studied by LaClaire and Facklam (77) all exhibited susceptibilities to penicillin, amoxicillin, cefotaxime, cefuroxime, clindamycin, levofloxacin, meropenem, quinupristin-dalfopristin, rifampin, and tetracycline. Various susceptibilities to erythromycin were noted, and one of the 27 strains was resistant to trimethoprim-sulfamethoxazole. A small number of *Helcococcus* isolates displayed susceptibilities to penicillin and clindamycin, and most strains were resistant to erythromycin (19, 93). MICs of a variety of antibiotics for strains of *Facklamia* varied (78). A study of 27 strains of *G. sanguinis* reported susceptibilities of all isolates to amoxicillin but various levels of resistance to other antimicrobials tested (104).

EVALUATION, INTERPRETATION, AND REPORTING OF RESULTS

Since the gram-positive cocci included in this chapter may appear in clinical cultures as contaminants or part of normal microbiota, efforts to identify them should be made only when isolates are considered to be clinically significant (e.g., when isolated repeatedly, when grown in pure culture, or when recovered from normally sterile sites). It should be remembered that these bacteria are opportunists: isolation from an immunocompetent patient may not have the same significance as isolation from a compromised host. Communication with clinicians should guide the microbiology laboratory in evaluating the significance of these infrequently isolated organisms.

Vancomycin susceptibility testing should be performed routinely on significant isolates. Documenting resistance to this antibiotic will not only guide therapy but also aid in identification of the isolates. The method mentioned in this chapter, using a nonstandardized inoculum, seems to be fairly reliable for determining susceptibility to this drug for identification purposes. Since standardized susceptibility testing methods do not exist for these infrequently isolated gram-positive cocci, caution should be observed in interpretation of in vitro susceptibility test results. A reference laboratory should be consulted for identification or confirmation of the identity of unfamiliar organisms.

REFERENCES

1. **Aguirre, M., and M. D. Collins.** 1992. Phylogenetic analysis of *Alloiococcus otitis* gen. nov., sp. nov., an organism from human middle ear fluid. *Int. J. Syst. Bacteriol.* **42:**79–83.
2. **Aguirre, M., and M. D. Collins.** 1992. Phylogenetic analysis of some *Aerococcus*-like organisms from urinary tract infections: description of *Aerococcus urinae* sp. nov. *J. Gen. Microbiol.* **138:**401–405.
3. **Aguirre, M., D. Morrison, B. D. Cookson, F. W. Gay, and M. D. Collins.** 1993. Phenotypic and phylogenetic

characterization of some *Gemella*-like organisms from human infections: description of *Dolosigranulum pigrum* gen. nov., sp. nov. *J. Appl. Bacteriol.* **75:**608–612.

4. **Antolin, J., R. Ciguenza, I. Saluena, E. Vazquez, J. Hernandez, and D. Espinos.** 2004. Liver abscess caused by *Lactococcus lactis cremoris:* a new pathogen. *Scand. J. Infect. Dis.* **36:**490–491.
5. **Astudillo, L., L. Sailler, L. Porte, J. C. Lefevre, P. Massip, and E. Arlet-Suau.** 2003. Spondylodiscitis due to *Aerococcus urinae:* a first report. *Scand. J. Infect. Dis.* **35:**890–891.
6. **Azap, O. K., G. Yapar, F. Timurkaynak, S. Sezer, and N. Ozdemir.** 2005. *Gemella morbillorum* peritonitis in a patient being treated with continuous ambulatory peritoneal dialysis. *Nephrol. Dial. Transplant.* **20:**853–854.
7. **Bannatyne, R. M., and I. W. Fong.** 1992. *Gemella morbillorum* infection in an arteriovenous shunt. *Clin. Microbiol. News.* **14:**7–8.
8. **Barreau, C., and G. Wagener.** 1990. Characterization of *Leuconostoc lactis* strains from human sources. *J. Clin. Microbiol.* **28:**1728–1733.
9. **Barros, R. R., M. D. Carvalho, J. M. Peralta, R. R. Facklam, and L. M. Teixeira.** 2001. Phenotypic and genotypic characterization of *Pediococcus* strains isolated from human clinical sources. *J. Clin. Microbiol.* **39:**1241–1246.
10. **Barton, L. L., E. D. Rider, and R. W. Coen.** 2001. Bacteremic infection with *Pediococcus:* vancomycin-resistant opportunist. *Pediatrics* **107:**775–776.
11. **Beighton, D., K. A. Homer, A. Bouvet, and A. R. Storey.** 1995. Analysis of enzymatic activities for differentiation of two species of nutritionally variant streptococci, *Streptococcus defectivus* and *Streptococcus adjacens*. *J. Clin. Microbiol.* **33:**1584–1587.
12. **Berger, U.** 1985. Prevalence of *Gemella haemolysans* on the pharyngeal mucosa of man. *Med. Microbiol. Immunol.* **174:**267–274.
13. **Berger, U., and A. Pervanidis.** 1986. Differentiation of *Gemella haemolysans* (Thjotta and Boe 1938) Berger 1960, from *Streptococcus morbillorum* (Prevot 1933) Holdeman and Moore 1974. *Zentbl. Bakteriol. Mikrobiol. Hyg.* **A 261:** 311–321.
14. **Biermann, C., G. Fries, P. Jehnichen, S. Bhakdi, and M. Husmann.** 1999. Isolation of *Abiotrophia adiacens* from a brain abscess which developed in a patient after neurosurgery. *J. Clin. Microbiol.* **37:**769–771.
15. **Bouvet, A., F. Grimont, and P. A. D. Grimont.** 1989. *Streptococcus defectivus* sp. nov. and *Streptococcus adjacens* sp. nov., nutritionally variant streptococci from human clinical specimens. *Int. J. Syst. Bacteriol.* **39:**290–294.
16. **Bouvet, A., F. Villeroy, F. Cheng, C. Lamesch, R. Williamson, and L. Gutmann.** 1985. Characterization of nutritionally variant streptococci by biochemical tests and penicillin-binding proteins. *J. Clin. Microbiol.* **22:**1030–1034.
17. **Buu-Hoi, A., C. LeBouguenec, and T. Horaud.** 1989. Genetic basis of antibiotic resistance in *Aerococcus viridans*. *Antimicrob. Agents Chemother.* **33:**529–534.
18. **Buu-Hoi, A., A. Sapoetra, C. Branger, and J. F. Acar.** 1982. Antimicrobial susceptibility of *Gemella haemolysans* isolated from patients with subacute endocarditis. *Eur. J. Clin. Microbiol.* **1:**102–106.
19. **Chagla, A. H., A. A. Borczyk, R. R. Facklam, and M. Lovgren.** 1998. Breast abscess associated with *Helcococcus kunzii*. *J. Clin. Microbiol.* **36:**2377–2379.
20. **Chatelain, R., J. Croize, P. Rouge, C. Massot, H. Dabernat, J. C. Auvergnat, A. Buu-Hoi, J. P. Stahl, and F. Bimet.** 1982. Isolment de *Gemella haemolysans* dans trois cas d'endocardites bacteriennes. *Med. Mal. Infect.* **12:**25–30.
21. **Christensen, J. J., and R. R. Facklam.** 2001. *Granulicatella* and *Abiotrophia* species from human clinical specimens. *J. Clin. Microbiol.* **39:**3520–3523.
22. **Christensen, J. J., H. Vibits, J. Ursing, and B. Korner.** 1991. *Aerococcus*-like organism, a newly recognized potential urinary tract pathogen. *J. Clin. Microbiol.* **29:**1049–1053.
23. **Christensen, J. J., A. M. Whitney, L. M. Teixeira, A. G. Steigerwalt, R. R. Facklam, B. Korner, and D. J. Brenner.** 1997. *Aerococcus urinae:* intraspecies genetic and phenotypic relatedness. *Int. J. Syst. Bacteriol.* **47:**28–32.
24. **Collins, M. D., M. Aguirre, R. R. Facklam, J. Shallcross, and A. M. Williams.** 1992. *Globicatella sanguis* gen. nov., sp. nov., a new Gram-positive catalase negative bacterium from human sources. *J. Appl. Bacteriol.* **73:**433–437.
25. **Collins, M. D., C. Ash, J. A. E. Farrow, S. Wallbanks, and A. M. Williams.** 1989. 16S ribosomal ribonucleic acid sequence analyses of lactococci and related taxa. Description of *Vagococcus fluvialis* gen. nov., sp. nov. *J. Appl. Bacteriol.* **67:**453–460.
26. **Collins, M. D., R. R. Facklam, U. M. Rodrigues, and K. L. Ruoff.** 1993. Phylogenetic analysis of some *Aerococcus*-like organisms from clinical sources: description of *Helcococcus kunzii* gen. nov., sp. nov. *Int. J. Syst. Bacteriol.* **43:**425–429.
27. **Collins, M. D., E. Falsen, K. Brownlee, and P. A. Lawson.** 2004. *Helcococcus sueciensis* sp. nov., isolated from a human wound. *Int. J. Syst. Evol. Microbiol.* **54:**1557–1560.
28. **Collins, M. D., E. Falsen, J. Lemozy, E. Åkervall, B. Sjödén, and P. A. Lawson.** 1997. Phenotypic and phylogenetic characterization of some *Globicatella*-like organisms from human sources: description of *Facklamia hominis* gen. nov., sp. nov. *Int. J. Syst. Bacteriol.* **47:**880–882.
29. **Collins, M. D., R. A. Hutson, V. Baverud, and E. Falsen.** 2000. Characterization of a *Rothia*-like organism from a mouse: description of *Rothia nasimurium* sp. nov. and reclassification of *Stomatococcus mucilaginosus* as *Rothia mucilaginosa* comb. nov. *Int. J. Syst. Evol. Microbiol.* **50:**1247–1251.
30. **Collins, M. D., R. A. Hutson, E. Falsen, and B. Sjoden.** 1999. *Facklamia sourekii* sp. nov., isolated from human sources. *Int. J. Syst. Bacteriol.* **49:**635–638.
31. **Collins, M. D., R. A. Hutson, E. Falsen, B. Sjoden, and R. R. Facklam.** 1998. *Gemella bergeriae* sp. nov., isolated from human clinical specimens. *J. Clin. Microbiol.* **36:**1290–1293.
32. **Collins, M. D., R. A. Hutson, E. Falsen, B. Sjoden, and R. R. Facklam.** 1998. Description of *Gemella sanguinis* sp. nov., isolated from human clinical specimens. *J. Clin. Microbiol.* **36:**3090–3093.
33. **Collins, M. D., M. R. Jovita, R. A. Hutson, M. Ohlen, and E. Falsen.** 1999. *Aerococcus christensenii* sp. nov., from the human vagina. *Int. J. Syst. Bacteriol.* **49:**1125–1128.
34. **Collins, M. D., and P. A. Lawson.** 2000. The genus *Abiotrophia* (Kawamura et al.) is not monophyletic: proposal of *Granulicatella* gen. nov., *Granulicatella adiacens* comb. nov., *Granulicatella elegans* comb. nov. and *Granulicatella balaenopterae* comb. nov. *Int. J. Syst. Evol. Microbiol.* **50:**365–369.
35. **Collins, M. D., P. A. Lawson, R. Monasterio, E. Falsen, B. Sjoden, and R. R. Facklam.** 1998. *Facklamia ignava* sp. nov., isolated from human clinical specimens. *J. Clin. Microbiol.* **36:**2146–2148.
36. **Collins, M. D., P. A. Lawson, R. Monasterio, E. Falsen, B. Sjoden, and R. R. Facklam.** 1999. *Ignavigranum ruoffiae* sp. nov., isolated from human clinical specimens. *Int. J. Syst. Bacteriol.* **49:**97–101.
37. **Collins, M. D., M. Rodriguez Jovita, R. A. Hutson, E. Falsen, B. Sjoden, and R. R. Facklam.** 1999. *Dolosicoccus paucivorans* gen. nov., sp. nov., isolated from human blood. *Int. J. Syst. Bacteriol.* **49:**1439–1442.
38. **Collins, M. D., J. Samelis, J. Metaxopoulos, and S. Wallbanks.** 1993. Taxonomic studies on some leuconostoc-like organisms from fermented sausages: description of a new genus *Weissella* for the *Leuconostoc paramesenteroides* group of species. *J. Appl. Bacteriol.* **75:**595–603.

39. **Collins, M. D., A. M. Williams, and S. Wallbanks.** 1990. The phylogeny of *Aerococcus* and *Pediococcus* as determined by 16S rRNA sequence analysis: description of *Tetragenococcus* gen. nov. *FEMS Microbiol. Lett.* **70:**255–262.
40. **Colman, G.** 1967. *Aerococcus*-like organisms isolated from human infections. *J. Clin. Pathol.* **20:**294–297.
41. **da Costa, C. T., C. Porter, K. Parry, A. Morris, and A. H. Quoraishi.** 1996. Empyema thoracis and lung abscess due to *Gemella morbillorum*. *Eur. J. Clin. Microbiol. Infect. Dis.* **15:**75–77.
42. **Davis, J. M., and M. M. Peel.** 1994. Identification of ten clinical isolates of nutritionally variant streptococci by commercial streptococcal identification systems. *Aust. J. Med. Sci.* **15:**52–55.
43. **Dye, G., J. Lewis, J. Patterson, and J. Jorgensen.** 2003. A case of *Leuconostoc* ventriculitis with resistance to carbapenem antibiotics. *Clin. Infect. Dis.* **37:**869.
44. **Eggelmeijer, F., P. Petit, and B. A. C. Dijkmans.** 1992. Total knee arthroplasty infection due to *Gemella haemolysans*. *Br. J. Rheumatol.* **31:**67–69.
45. **Elliott, J. A., M. D. Collins, N. E. Pigott, and R. R. Facklam.** 1991. Differentiation of *Lactococcus lactis* and *Lactococcus garvieae* from humans by comparison of whole-cell protein patterns. *J. Clin. Microbiol.* **29:**2731–2734.
46. **Elliott, J. A., and R. R. Facklam.** 1993. Identification of *Leuconostoc* spp. by analysis of soluble whole-cell protein patterns. *J. Clin. Microbiol.* **31:**1030–1033.
47. **Elliott, J. A., and R. R. Facklam.** 1996. Antimicrobial susceptibilities of *Lactococcus lactis* and *Lactococcus garvieae* and a proposed method to discriminate between them. *J. Clin. Microbiol.* **34:**1296–1298.
48. **Ennahar, S., and Y. Cai.** 2005. Biochemical and genetic evidence for the transfer of *Enterococcus solitarius* Collins et al. 1989 to the genus *Tetragenococcus* as *Tetragenococcus solitarius* comb. nov. *Int. J. Syst. Evol. Microbiol.* **55:**589–592.
49. **Evans, J. B.** 1986. Genus *Aerococcus* Williams, Hirch and Cowan 1953, 475[AL], p. 1080. *In* P. H. A. Sneath, N. S. Mair, M. E. Sharpe, and J. G. Holt (ed.), *Bergey's Manual of Systematic Bacteriology*, vol. 2. Williams and Wilkins, Baltimore, Md.
50. **Facklam, R.** 2002. What happened to the streptococci: overview of taxonomic and nomenclature changes. *Clin. Microbiol. Rev.* **15:**613–630.
51. **Facklam, R., and J. A. Elliott.** 1995. Identification, classification, and clinical relevance of catalase-negative, gram-positive cocci, excluding the streptococci and enterococci. *Clin. Microbiol. Rev.* **8:**479–495.
52. **Facklam, R., M. Lovgren, P. L. Shewmaker, and G. Tyrrell.** 2003. Phenotypic description and antimicrobial susceptibilities of *Aerococcus sanguinicola* isolates from human clinical samples. *J. Clin. Microbiol.* **41:**2587–2592.
53. **Facklam, R. R.** 1977. Physiological differentiation of viridans streptococci. *J. Clin. Microbiol.* **5:**184–201.
54. **Facklam, R. R., and J. A. Washington II.** 1991. *Streptococcus* and related catalase-negative gram-positive cocci, p. 238–257. *In* A. Balows, W. J. Hausler, Jr., K. L. Herrmann, H. D. Isenberg, and H. J. Shadomy (ed.), *Manual of Clinical Microbiology*, 5th ed. American Society for Microbiology, Washington, D.C.
55. **Farmaki, E., E. Roilides, E. Darilis, M. Tsivitanidou, C. Panteliadis, and D. Sofianou.** 2000. *Gemella morbillorum* endocarditis in a child. *Pediatr. Infect. Dis. J.* **19:**751–753.
56. **Fefer, J. J., K. R. Ratzan, S. E. Sharp, and E. Saiz.** 1998. *Lactococcus garvieae* endocarditis: report of a case and review of the literature. *Diagn. Microbiol. Infect. Dis.* **32:** 127–130.
57. **Flaherty, J. D., P. N. Levett, F. E. Dewhirst, T. E. Troe, J. R. Warren, and S. Johnson.** 2003. Fatal case of endocarditis due to *Weissella confusa*. *J. Clin. Microbiol.* **41:**2237–2239.
58. **Garcia-Marcos, J. A., M. Meseguer, and F. Baquero.** 1992. Meningitis due to *Gemella haemolysans*. *Clin. Microbiol. News.* **14:**142–143.
59. **Garvie, E. I.** 1986. Genus *Leuconostoc* van Tieghem 1878, 198[AL] emend mut. char. Hucker and Pederson 1930, 66[AL], p. 1071–1075. *In* P. H. A. Sneath, N. S. Mair, M. E. Sharpe, and J. G. Holt (ed.), *Bergey's Manual of Systematic Bacteriology*, vol. 2. Williams and Wilkins, Baltimore, Md.
60. **Garvie, E. I.** 1986. Genus *Pediococcus* Claussen 1903, 68[AL], p. 1075–1079. *In* P. H. A. Sneath, N. S. Mair, M. E. Sharpe, and J. G. Holt (ed.), *Bergey's Manual of Systematic Bacteriology*, vol. 2. Williams and Wilkins, Baltimore, Md.
61. **Gimigliano, F., M. Carletti, G. Carducci, F. Iodice, and L. Ballerini.** 2005. *Gemella morbillorum* endocarditis in a child. *Pediatr. Infect. Dis. J.* **24:**190.
62. **Golledge, C. L., N. Stingemore, M. Aravena, and K. Joske.** 1990. Septicemia caused by vancomycin-resistant *Pediococcus acidilactici*. *J. Clin. Microbiol.* **28:**1678–1679.
63. **Grude, N., A. Jenkins, Y. Tveten, and B.-E. Kristiansen.** 2003. Identification of *Aerococcus urinae* in urine samples. *Clin. Microbiol. Infect.* **9:**976–979.
64. **Haas, J., S. L. Jernick, R. J. Scardina, J. Teruya, A. M. Caliendo, and K. L. Ruoff.** 1997. Colonization of skin by *Helcococcus kunzii*. *J. Clin. Microbiol.* **35:**2759–2761.
65. **Hall, G. S., S. Gordon, S. Schroeder, K. Smith, K. Anthony, and G. W. Procop.** 2001. Case of synovitis potentially caused by *Dolosigranulum pigrum*. *J. Clin. Microbiol.* **39:**1202–1203.
66. **Handwerger, S., H. Horowitz, K. Coburn, A. Kolokathis, and G. P. Wormser.** 1990. Infection due to *Leuconostoc* species: six cases and review. *Rev. Infect. Dis.* **12:**602–610.
67. **Healy, B., R. W. Beukenholt, D. Tuthill, and C. D. Ribeiro.** 2005. *Facklamia hominis* causing chorioamnionitis and puerperal bacteraemia. *J. Infect.* **50:**353–355.
68. **Houpikian, P., and D. Raoult.** 2005. Blood culture-negative endocarditis in a reference center: etiologic diagnosis of 348 cases. *Medicine* **84:**162–173.
69. **James, P. R., S. M. Hardman, and D. L. Patterson.** 2000. Osteomyelitis and possible endocarditis secondary to *Lactococcus garvieae*: a first case report. *Postgrad. Med. J.* **76:**301–303.
70. **Johnson, C. C., and A. R. Tunkel.** 1995. Viridans streptococci and groups C and G streptococci, p. 1845–1861. *In* G. L. Mandell, J. E. Bennett, and R. Dolin (ed.), *Mandell, Douglas and Bennett's Principles and Practice of Infectious Diseases*, 4th ed. Churchill Livingstone, New York, N.Y.
71. **Kanamoto, T., S. Sato, and M. Inoue.** 2000. Genetic heterogeneities and phenotypic characteristics of strains of the genus *Abiotrophia* and proposal of *Abiotrophia paraadiacens* sp. nov. *J. Clin. Microbiol.* **38:**492–498.
72. **Kawamura, Y., X. Hou, F. Sultana, S. Liu, H. Yamamoto, and T. Ezaki.** 1995. Transfer of *Streptococcus adjacens* and *Streptococcus defectivus* to *Abiotrophia* gen. nov. as *Abiotrophia adiacens* comb. nov. and *Abiotrophia defectiva* comb. nov., respectively. *Int. J. Syst. Bacteriol.* **45:**798–803.
73. **Kern, W., and E. Vanek.** 1987. *Aerococcus* bacteremia associated with granulocytopenia. *Eur. J. Clin. Microbiol.* **6:**670–673.
74. **Kilpper-Balz, R., and K. H. Schleifer.** 1988. Transfer of *Streptococcus morbillorum* to the genus *Gemella* as *Gemella morbillorum* comb. nov. *Int. J. Syst. Bacteriol.* **38:**442–443.
75. **Kristensen, B., and G. Nielsen.** 1995. Endocarditis caused by *Aerococcus urinae*, a newly recognized pathogen. *Eur. J. Clin. Microbiol. Infect. Dis.* **14:**49–51.
76. **Kumudhan, D., and S. Mars.** 2004. *Leuconostoc mesenteroides* as a cause of postoperative endophthalmitis—a case report. *Eye* **18:**1023–1024.
77. **LaClaire, L., and R. Facklam.** 2000. Antimicrobial susceptibility and clinical sources of *Dolosigranulum pigrum* cultures. *Antimicrob. Agents. Chemother.* **44:**2001–2003.

78. **LaClaire, L., and R. Facklam.** 2000. Antimicrobial susceptibilities and clinical sources of *Facklamia* species. *Antimicrob. Agents Chemother.* **44:**2130–2132.
79. **LaClaire, L. L., and R. R. Facklam.** 2000. Comparison of three commercial rapid identification systems for the unusual gram-positive cocci *Dolosigranulum pigrum*, *Ignavigranum ruoffiae*, and *Facklamia* species. *J. Clin. Microbiol.* **38:**2037–2042.
80. **Lawson, P. A., M. D. Collins, E. Falsen, B. Sjoden, and R. R. Facklam.** 1999. *Facklamia languida* sp. nov., isolated from human clinical specimens. *J. Clin. Microbiol.* **37:**1161–1164.
81. **Lawson, P. A., E. Falsen, M. Ohlen, and M. D. Collins.** 2001. *Aerococcus urinaehominis* sp. nov., isolated from human urine. *Int. J. Syst. Evol. Microbiol.* **51:**683–686.
82. **Lawson, P. A., E. Falsen, K. Truberg-Jensen, and M. D. Collins.** 2001. *Aerococcus sanguicola* sp. nov., isolated from a human clinical source. *Int. J. Syst. Evol. Microbiol.* **51:**475–479.
83. **Lee, M. R., S.-O. Lee, S.-Y. Kim, S. M. Yang, Y.-H. Seo, and Y. K. Cho.** 2004. Brain abscess due to *Gemella haemolysans*. *J. Clin. Microbiol.* **42:**2338–2340.
84. **Mannion, P. T., and M. M. Rothburn.** 1990. Diagnosis of bacterial endocarditis caused by *Streptococcus lactis*. *J. Infect.* **21:**317–318.
85. **Mastro, T. D., J. S. Spika, P. Lozano, J. Appel, and R. R. Facklam.** 1990. Vancomycin-resistant *Pediococcus acidilactici*: nine cases of bacteremia. *J. Infect. Dis.* **161:**956–960.
86. **Mofredj, A., D. Baraka, G. Kloeti, and J. L. Dumont.** 2000. *Lactococcus garvieae* septicemia with liver abscess in an immunosuppressed patient. *Am. J. Med.* **109:**513–514.
87. **Namdari, H., K. Kintner, B. A. Jackson, S. Namdari, J. L. Hughes, R. R. Peairs, and D. J. Savage.** 1999. *Abiotrophia* species as a cause of endophthalmitis following cataract extraction. *J. Clin. Microbiol.* **37:**1564–1566.
88. **National Committee for Clinical Laboratory Standards.** 2003. *Methods for Dilution Antimicrobial Susceptibility Tests for Bacteria that Grow Aerobically*, 6th ed. Approved standard M7-A6. National Committee for Clinical Laboratory Standards, Wayne, Pa.
89. **Olano, A., J. Chua, S. Schroeder, A. Minari, M. La Salvia, and G. Hall.** 2001. *Weissella confusa* (basonym: *Lactobacillus confusus*) bacteremia: a case report. *J. Clin. Microbiol.* **39:**1604–1607.
90. **Ormerod, L. D., K. L. Ruoff, D. M. Meisler, P. J. Wasson, J. C. Kinter, S. P. Dunn, J. H. Lass, and I. Van de Rijn.** 1991. Infectious crystalline keratopathy. Role of nutritionally variant streptococci and other bacterial factors. *Ophthalmology* **98:**159–169.
91. **Panackal, A. A., Y. B. Houze, J. Prentice, S. S. Leopold, B. T. Cookson, W. C. Liles, and A. P. Limaye.** 2004. Prosthetic joint infection due to "*Helcococcus pyogenica*." *J. Clin. Microbiol.* **42:**2872–2874. (Author's correction, **42:**5966.)
92. **Parker, M. T., and L. C. Ball.** 1976. Streptococci and aerococci associated with systemic infection in man. *J. Med. Microbiol.* **9:**275–302.
93. **Peel, M. M., J. M. Davis, K. J. Griffin, and D. L. Freedman.** 1997. *Helcococcus kunzii* as sole isolate from an infected sebaceous cyst. *J. Clin. Microbiol.* **35:**328–329.
94. **Pellizzer, G., P. Benedetti, F. Biavasco, V. Manfrin, M. Franzetti, M. Scagnelli, C. Scarparo, and F. de Lalla.** 1996. Bacterial endocarditis due to *Lactococcus lactis* subsp. *cremoris*: case report. *Clin. Microbiol. Infect.* **2:**230–232.
95. **Reyn, A.** 1986. Genus *Gemella* Berger 1960, 253[AL], p. 1081–1082. *In* P. H. A. Sneath, N. S. Mair, M. E. Sharpe, and J. G. Holt (ed.), *Bergey's Manual of Systematic Bacteriology*, vol. 2. Williams and Wilkins, Baltimore, Md.
96. **Riebel, W. J., and J. A. Washington.** 1990. Clinical and microbiologic characteristics of pediococci. *J. Clin. Microbiol.* **28:**1348–1355.
97. **Roggenkamp, A., M. Abele-Horn, K.-H. Trebesius, U. Tretter, I. B. Autenreith, and J. Heesemann.** 1998. *Abiotrophia elegans* sp. nov., a possible pathogen in patients with culture-negative endocarditis. *J. Clin. Microbiol.* **36:**100–104.
98. **Ruoff, K. L., D. R. Kuritzkes, J. S. Wolfson, and M. J. Ferraro.** 1988. Vancomycin-resistant gram-positive bacteria isolated from human sources. *J. Clin. Microbiol.* **26:**2064–2068.
99. **Santos, R., E. Santos, S. Goncalves, A. Marques, J. Sequeira, P. Abecasis, and M. Cadete.** 2003. Lymphadenitis caused by *Aerococcus urinae* infection. *Scand. J. Infect. Dis.* **35:**353–354.
100. **Schlegel, I., C. Merlet, J. M. Laroche, A. Fremaux, and P. Geslin.** 1999. Iatrogenic meningitis due to *Abiotrophia defectiva* after myelography. *Clin. Infect. Dis.* **28:**155–156.
101. **Schleifer, K. H.** 1986. Family I. *Micrococcaceae* Prevot 1961, 31[AL], p. 1003–1035. *In* P. H. A. Sneath, N. S. Mair, M. E. Sharpe, and J. G. Holt (ed.), *Bergey's Manual of Systematic Bacteriology*, vol. 2. Williams and Wilkins, Baltimore, Md.
102. **Schleifer, K. H., J. Kraus, C. Dvorak, R. Kilpper-Balz, M. D. Collins, and W. Fischer.** 1985. Transfer of *Streptococcus lactis* and related streptococci to the genus *Lactococcus* gen. nov. *Sys. Appl. Microbiol.* **6:**183–195.
103. **Schurr, P. M. H., M. E. E. V. Kasteren, L. Sabbe, M. C. Vos, M. M. P. C. Janssens, and A. G. M. Buiting.** 1997. Urinary tract infections with *Aerococcus urinae* in the south of the Netherlands. *Eur. J. Clin. Microbiol. Infect. Dis.* **16:**871–875.
104. **Shewmaker, P. L., A. G. Steigerwalt, L. Shealey, R. Weyant, and R. R. Facklam.** 2001. DNA relatedness, phenotypic characteristics, and antimicrobial susceptibilities of *Globicatella sanguinis* strains. *J. Clin. Microbiol.* **39:**4052–4057.
105. **Sire, J. M., P. Y. Donnio, R. Mensard, P. Pouedras, and J. L. Avril.** 1992. Septicemia and hepatic abscess caused by *Pediococcus acidilactici*. *Eur. J. Clin. Microbiol. Infect. Dis.* **11:**623–625.
106. **Skov, R., J. J. Christensen, B. Korner, N. Frimodt-Moeller, and F. Espersen.** 2001. *In vitro* antimicrobial susceptibility of *Aerococcus urinae* to 14 antibiotics, and time-kill curves for penicillin, gentamicin and vancomycin. *J. Antimicrob. Chemother.* **48:**653–658.
107. **Skov, R. L., M. Klarlund, and S. Thorsen.** 1995. Fatal endocarditis due to *Aerococcus urinae*. *Diagn. Microbiol. Infect. Dis.* **21:**219–221.
108. **Spagnoli, D., L. Innocenti, M. L. Ranzi, G. Tomei, and R. M. Villani.** 2003. Cerebral abscess due to *Gemella morbillorum*. *Eur. J. Clin. Microbiol. Infect. Dis.* **22:**515–517.
109. **Swenson, J. M., R. R. Facklam, and C. Thornsberry.** 1990. Antimicrobial susceptibility of vancomycin-resistant *Leuconostoc*, *Pediococcus*, and *Lactobacillus* species. *Antimicrob. Agents Chemother.* **34:**543–549.
110. **Teixeira, L. M., M. G. Carvalho, V. L. Merquior, A. G. Steigerwalt, D. J. Brenner, and R. R. Facklam.** 1997. Phenotypic and genotypic characterization of *Vagococcus fluvialis*, including strains isolated from human sources. *J. Clin. Microbiol.* **35:**2778–2781.
111. **Tunicliff, R.** 1917. The cultivation of a micrococcus from blood in pre-eruptive and eruptive stages of measles. *JAMA* **68:**1028–1030.
112. **Tuohy, M. J., G. W. Procop, and J. A. Washington.** 2000. Antimicrobial susceptibility of *Abiotrophia adiacens* and *Abiotrophia defectiva*. *Diagn. Microbiol. Infect. Dis.* **38:**189–191.
113. **Vandamme, P.** 2001. *Globicatella sulfidifaciens* sp. nov., isolated from purulent infections in domestic animals. *Int. J. Syst. Evol. Microbiol.* **51:**1745–1749.

114. **van Dijk, M., B. J. van Royen, P. I. Wuisman, T. A. Hekker, and C. van Guldener.** 1999. Trochanter osteomyelitis and ipsilateral arthritis due to *Gemella morbillorum*. *Eur. J. Clin. Microbiol. Infect. Dis.* **18:**600–602.
115. **Vasishtha, S., H. D. Isenberg, and S. K. Sood.** 1996. *Gemella morbillorum* as a cause of septic shock. *Clin. Infect. Dis.* **22:**1084–1086.
116. **Wallbanks, S., A. J. Martinez-Murcia, J. L. Fryer, B. A. Phillips, and M. D. Collins.** 1990. 16S rRNA sequence determination for members of the genus *Carnobacterium* and related lactic acid bacteria and description of *Vagococcus salmoninarum* sp. nov. *Int. J. Syst. Bacteriol.* **40:**224–230.
117. **Woo, P. C. Y., K. H. L. Ng, S. K. P. Lau, K. Yip, A. M. Y. Fung, K. Leung, D. M. W. Tam, T. Que, and K. Yuen.** 2003. Usefulness of the MicroSeq 500 16S ribosomal DNA-based bacterial identification system for identification of clinically significant bacterial isolates with ambiguous biochemical profiles. *J. Clin. Microbiol.* **41:**1996–2001.
118. **Zakir, R. M., A. Al-Dehneh, L. Dabu, R. Kapila, and M. Saric.** 2004. Mitral bioprosthetic valve endocarditis caused by an unusual microorganism, *Gemella morbillorum*, in an intravenous drug user. *J. Clin. Microbiol.* **42:**4893–4896.
119. **Zaoui, A., C. Brousse, O. Bletry, L.W. Augouard, and B. Boisaubert.** 2005. *Leuconostoc* osteomyelitis. *Joint Bone Spine* **72:**79–81.
120. **Zheng, X., A. F. Freeman, J. Villafranca, D. Shortridge, J. Beyer, W. Kabat, K. Dembkowski, and S. T. Shulman.** 2004. Antimicrobial susceptibilities of invasive pediatric *Abiotrophia* and *Granulicatella* isolates. *J. Clin. Microbiol.* **42:**4323–4326.

Bacillus and Other Aerobic Endospore-Forming Bacteria*

NIALL A. LOGAN, TANJA POPOVIC, AND ALEX HOFFMASTER

32

TAXONOMY

Molecular taxonomic methods have had a huge impact on the classification of aerobic endospore-forming bacteria. The 1986 edition of *Bergey's Manual of Systematic Bacteriology* listed 40 valid *Bacillus* species, and since then 218 further species have been newly described or revived among *Bacillus* and the genera derived from it: *Alicyclobacillus* (112), *Paenibacillus* (5), *Brevibacillus* (93), *Aneurinibacillus* (93), *Virgibacillus* (50), *Gracilibacillus* (107), *Salibacillus* (107; subsequently merged with *Virgibacillus* [51]), *Geobacillus* (75), *Marinibacillus* (114), and *Ureibacillus* (37). Three species formerly classified within *Bacillus*, *B. pasteurii*, *B. globisporus*, and *B. psychrophilus*, have been transferred (113) to the long-established genus of aerobic endospore-forming cocci, *Sporosarcina*, which now contains six species. Furthermore, 15 new genera containing 33 new species have been proposed to accommodate novel aerobic endospore formers not previously assigned to *Bacillus* (over one-half of these genera have only one species, and over one-half of the species were proposed on the basis of single isolates); they are, in order of validation, *Sulfobacillus*, *Amphibacillus*, *Halobacillus*, *Ammoniphilus*, *Anoxybacillus*, *Thermobacillus*, *Filobacillus*, *Jeotgalibacillus*, *Lentibacillus*, *Oceanobacillus*, *Paraliobacillus*, *Cerasibacillus*, *Pontibacillus*, *Tenuibacillus*, and *Salinibacillus*. Overall, therefore, there have been proposals for 25 new genera containing 234 new or revived species or new combinations, and yet only six proposals for merging species were made in that time. Unfortunately, taxonomic progress has not always revealed readily determinable features characteristic of each genus. They show wide ranges of sporangial morphologies and phenotypic test patterns. Many novel species represent genomic groups disclosed by DNA-DNA pairing experiments or single isolates whose distinction from existing species rests chiefly upon 16S rRNA gene sequence analysis, and routine phenotypic characters for distinguishing some of them are very few and of unproven value.

Bacillus continues to accommodate the best-known species such as *B. subtilis* (the type species), *B. anthracis*, *B. cereus*, *B. licheniformis*, *B. megaterium*, *B. pumilus*, *B. sphaericus*, and *B. thuringiensis*. It still remains a large genus, with over 100 species, as losses to other genera have been balanced by new species proposals. Members of the *B. cereus* group, *B. anthracis*, *B. cereus*, and *B. thuringiensis*, are considered to be pathovars of a single species (104).

DESCRIPTIONS OF THE GENERA

Although the production of resistant endospores in the presence of oxygen remains the defining feature for *Bacillus* and the new genera derived from it, the definition was undermined by the discovery of *Bacillus infernus* and *B. arseniciselenatis*, which are strictly anaerobic, and spores have not been detected in *B. infernus* and *B. subterraneus*.

However, those members likely to be isolated in a clinical laboratory are gram-positive (in young cultures) but sometimes gram-variable or clearly gram-negative, rod-shaped, endospore-forming organisms which may be aerobic or facultatively anaerobic. They are mostly catalase positive and may be motile by means of peritrichous flagella. Most species are mesophilic, but *Bacillus* contains some thermophiles and psychrophiles, and *Paenibacillus* contains one psychrophilic species. *Alicyclobacillus*, *Gracilibacillus*, *Marinibacillus*, and *Ureibacillus* strains and members of the 15 new genera not derived from *Bacillus* are unlikely to be encountered in a clinical laboratory, and clinical isolates of *Geobacillus* and *Sporosarcina* have not been reported, so these genera will not be considered further.

NATURAL HABITATS

Most aerobic endospore formers are saprophytes widely distributed in the natural environment, but some species are opportunistic or obligate pathogens of animals, including humans, other mammals, and insects. The main habitats are soils of all kinds, ranging from acid to alkaline, hot to cold, and fertile to desert, and the water columns and bottom deposits of fresh and marine waters. Their spores readily survive distribution in soils, dusts, and aerosols from these natural environments to a wide variety of other habitats; for example, strains of *B. fumarioli* showing similar phenotypic behavior and substantial genotypic similarity have been isolated from volcanic soils in continental Antarctica and from Candlemas Island, which is some 5,600 km distant in the South Sandwich archipelago, and from gelatin production plants in Belgium, France, and the United States (28). Dried foods such as spices, milk powders, and farinaceous products

*This chapter contains information presented in chapter 32 by Niall A. Logan and Peter C. B. Turnbull in the eighth edition of this Manual.

are often quite heavily contaminated with spores. *B. anthracis* is, to all intents and purposes, an obligate pathogen of animals and humans. Its close relative, *B. cereus*, is now well established as an opportunistic pathogen, and other aerobic endospore formers can also be opportunistic pathogens occasionally. Six organisms are important as insect pathogens: *B. thuringiensis* (another close relative of *B. anthracis*), *B. popilliae, B. lentimorbus, B. sphaericus, P. larvae* subsp. *larvae*, and *P. larvae* subsp. *pulvifaciens*.

CLINICAL SIGNIFICANCE AND INTERPRETATION OF RESULTS

The majority of aerobic endospore-forming species apparently have little or no pathogenic potential and are rarely associated with disease. The principal exceptions to this are *B. anthracis*, the agent of anthrax, and *B. cereus*, but a number of other species, particularly *B. licheniformis*, have been implicated in food poisoning and other human and animal infections. The resistance of the spores to heat, radiation, disinfectants, and desiccation also results in aerobic endospore formers being troublesome contaminants in the operating room, on surgical dressings, in pharmaceutical products, and in foods.

Apart from *B. anthracis*, the majority of species are common environmental contaminants, and isolation from a single clinical specimen is generally not a sufficient basis for incriminating one of these organisms as the etiological agent. Moderate or heavy growth of aerobic endospore formers from wounds is usually significant, however, and *B. cereus* infections of the eye are emergencies which should always be taken seriously and reported to the physician immediately.

In the clinical laboratory, the most important questions to ask about an aerobic spore-forming isolate are as follows. Was it isolated in pure culture or at least apparently dominating the flora? Was it isolated in large numbers? Was it isolated more than once? Low-level contamination of foodstuffs by aerobic endospore formers is common, as is asymptomatic transient fecal carriage. Therefore, in foodborne-illness investigations, qualitative isolation tests are insufficient. The ideal criteria for establishing that an aerobic endospore former is the etiological agent are (i) isolation of significant numbers ($>10^5$ CFU/g) of the organism from the epidemiologically incriminated food (and, in the case of suspected *B. cereus* food poisoning, detection of emetic toxin and/or enterotoxin) and (ii) recovery of the same strain (biovar, serovar, phage type, plasmid type, etc.) in significant numbers from acute phase specimens (feces or vomitus) from the patients, but not from healthy controls.

B. anthracis continues to be generally regarded as an obligate pathogen; its continued existence in the ecosystem appears to depend on a periodic multiplication phase within an animal host, and its environmental presence reflects contamination from an animal source at some time rather than self-maintenance within the environment. In human and animal specimens, it is usually sought only when the case history suggests that it is reasonable to suspect anthrax. Demonstration of capsulating *B. anthracis*, even in low numbers, confirms the clinical suspicion of anthrax, because the bacterium is rapidly destroyed by putrefactive processes after the host's death.

Bacillus anthracis

Anthrax remains the most widely recognized clinical condition caused by a *Bacillus* species. It is primarily a disease of domestic or wild animals, and prior to the availability of an effective veterinary vaccine in the late 1930s, anthrax was one of the foremost causes worldwide of mortality in cattle, sheep, goats, and horses. Humans almost invariably contract anthrax directly or indirectly from animals. The use of veterinary and human vaccines together with improvements in factory hygiene and sterilization procedures for imported animal products and the increased use of man-made alternatives to animal hides or hair have resulted over the past half-century in a marked decline in the incidence of anthrax in both animals and humans. Nevertheless, the disease continues to be endemic in many countries, particularly those that lack efficient vaccination policies (77). Because anthrax spores remain viable in soil for many years and their persistence does not depend on animal reservoirs, *B. anthracis* is exceedingly difficult to eradicate from an area where it is endemic; regions of nonendemicity must be constantly on the alert for the arrival of *B. anthracis* in imported animal products. Anthrax is not contagious, and transmission to humans is usually restricted to direct contact with infected animals or contaminated fomites, including such oddities as communal loofahs and contaminated syringes (84). Direct animal-to-animal transmission within a species (i.e., excluding scavengers feeding on anthrax carcasses) is also very rare.

Circumstantial evidence shows that humans are moderately resistant to anthrax compared with obligate herbivores. Human anthrax has traditionally been classified as either (i) nonindustrial, resulting from close contact with infected animals or their carcasses after death from the disease, or (ii) industrial, i.e., acquired by those employed in processing wool, hair, hides, bones, or other animal products. Dependent on the route of infection, there are three major clinical forms of anthrax: cutaneous, inhalation, and gastrointestinal. Anthrax meningitis can develop as a complication of any of these forms (92). Only a few reports of laboratory-acquired infections exist (18). A major outbreak of anthrax occurred in April 1979 in the city of Sverdlovsk, former USSR (now Yekaterinburg, Russia), in the Urals as a result of the accidental release of spores from a military production facility.

B. anthracis has been subjected to military research, development, and occasional deployment in several countries over many years, following attacks on livestock during the First World War, and it has remained high on the list of agents that could be used in biological warfare or bioterrorism. The natural disease is readily controllable, but the 2001 bioterrorism-related anthrax outbreak in the United States increased public concern about this disease (see chapter 9).

Cutaneous anthrax accounts for about 99% of naturally acquired human anthrax worldwide—an estimated 2,000 cases are reported annually. Infection occurs through a break in the skin. Following the incubation period of usually 2 to 3 days, a small papule appears, progressing over the next 24 h to a ring of vesicles, with subsequent ulceration and formation of a characteristic blackened eschar. Subsequent eschar formation may become thick and surrounded by extensive edema. Fever and pus and pain at the site are normally absent; their presence probably indicates a secondary bacterial infection. Before the availability of antimicrobial agents and vaccines, 10 to 20% of untreated cases of cutaneous anthrax were fatal. Less than 1% of cases are fatal today, and they are due mainly to obstruction of the airways by the edema that accompanies lesions on the face or neck or to the progression of the cutaneous disease into systemic infection.

Gastrointestinal anthrax is not uncommon in regions of endemicity worldwide, where socioeconomic conditions are poor and people eat raw or undercooked meat of animals that have died suddenly (77, 96); asymptomatic infections and symptomatic infections with recovery may not be uncommon. The symptoms of gastrointestinal anthrax are the result of ulcerations developing primarily in the cecal and terminal ileal mucosae: vomiting, nausea, and abdominal pain, accompanied by fever. This can rapidly progress to bloody diarrhea and systemic infection. Mortality ranges from 4 to 50% (96), greatly due to the nonspecific nature of the early symptoms and late initiation of antimicrobial therapy.

Prior to the bioterrorist attack of 2001, 18 cases of naturally acquired inhalation anthrax had been recorded in the United States since 1900, with 16 (88.9%) of them being fatal (12); figures in the United Kingdom show a similar picture. Among the 22 cases of the bioterrorism-related outbreak in the United States in late 2001, in which spores were delivered in mailed letters and packages, early recognition and treatment of the 11 patients with confirmed inhalation anthrax resulted in 60% survival (9, 58). In inhalation anthrax the inhaled spores are ingested by macrophages and carried from the lungs to the lymphatic system, where the infection progresses. During transit to lymph nodes, spores germinate into vegetative cells, begin to replicate, and produce the capsule and toxins that lead to bacteremia and associated hemorrhage and necrosis. The replacement of the older name for this form of the disease, "pulmonary anthrax," with the newer name, "inhalation anthrax," is a reflection of the fact that active infection occurs in the lymph nodes rather than the lung itself. Analysis of 10 of the cases associated with the bioterrorist events of 2001 (58) revealed a median incubation period of 4 days (range, 4 to 6 days). All 11 patients with inhalation anthrax had severe illness and were hospitalized (6). Their clinical presentation included fever or chills ($n = 11$), fatigue or malaise ($n = 11$), minimal or nonproductive cough ($n = 10$), dyspnea ($n = 9$), nausea or vomiting ($n = 9$), chest pain ($n = 7$), and sweats ($n = 7$). All patients had abnormal chest X-ray images with pleural effusion ($n = 8$), infiltrates ($n = 7$), and mediastinal widening ($n = 7$).

Regardless of the form of the diseases, the generalized symptoms that are usually mild (fatigue, malaise, fever, and/or gastrointestinal symptoms) can rapidly develop into the fulminant state, characterized by dyspnea, cyanosis, severe pyrexia, and disorientation followed by circulatory failure, shock, coma, and death (57, 58). Depending on the host, there is a rapid buildup of the bacteria in the blood over the last few hours to terminal levels of 10^7 to 10^9 organisms/ml in the most susceptible species. Enhancing clinical and laboratory expertise and conducting prospective surveillance are critical components of rapid anthrax diagnosis and of preparedness for bioterrorism (40).

Opportunistic Pathogens

Opportunistic infections with *Bacillus* species other than *B. anthracis* have been reported since the late 19th century. It is important to assess isolates of *Bacillus* in the light of any other species cultured and the clinical context and to be wary of dismissing them as mere contaminants.

Bacillus cereus Group

Bacillus cereus is next in importance to *B. anthracis* as a pathogen of humans (and other animals), causing foodborne illness and opportunistic infections, and its ubiquity ensures that cases are not uncommon.

In relation to foodborne illness, *B. cereus* is the etiological agent of two distinct food poisoning syndromes (31, 62): (i) the diarrheal type, characterized by abdominal pain with diarrhea 8 to 16 h after ingestion of the contaminated food and associated with a diversity of foods from meats and vegetable dishes to pastas, desserts, cakes, sauces, and milk; and (ii) the emetic type, characterized by nausea and vomiting 1 to 5 h after eating the offending food, predominantly oriental rice dishes, although occasionally other foods such as pasteurized cream, milk pudding, pastas, and reconstituted formulas have been implicated. One outbreak followed the mere handling of contaminated rice in a children's craft activity, and fulminant liver failure associated with the emetic toxin has been reported. Both syndromes arise as a direct result of the fact that *B. cereus* spores can survive normal cooking procedures; under conditions of improper storage after cooking, the spores germinate and the vegetative cells multiply. Strains of *B. thuringiensis*, which are close relatives of *B. cereus*, may also produce the diarrheal toxin (24).

The toxigenic basis of *B. cereus* food poisoning and other *B. cereus* infections has begun to be elucidated, and a complex picture is emerging (14). A toxin that is possibly associated with *B. licheniformis* food poisoning has been identified (70), but in general, for species outside the *B. cereus* group, toxins or virulence factors associated with foodborne illness have not been identified.

B. cereus is also a destructive ocular pathogen. Endophthalmitis may follow penetrating trauma of the eye or hematogenous spread and evolve very rapidly. Loss of both vision and the eye is likely if appropriate treatment is instituted too late (26). *B. cereus* keratitis associated with contact lens wear has also been reported (80). Other *B. cereus* infections occur mainly, though not exclusively, in persons predisposed by neoplastic disease, immunosuppression, alcoholism and other drug abuse (including a case associated with contaminated heroin), the presence of catheters (49) or implants such as fluid shunts, or some other underlying condition, and fatalities occasionally result. Reported conditions include bacteremia, septicemia, fulminant sepsis with hemolysis, meningitis, brain hemorrhage, ventricular shunt infections, endocarditis (23), pneumonia, exacerbation of bronchiectasis, empyema, pleurisy, lung abscess, brain abscess (23), liver abscess, osteomyelitis, salpingitis, urinary tract infection, and primary cutaneous infections. Wound infections, mostly in otherwise healthy persons, have been reported following surgery (associated, in one report, with contaminated incontinence pads), road traffic and other accidents, scalds, burns, plaster fixation, drug injection, and close-range gunshot and nail bomb injuries; some became necrotic and gangrenous (25, 66). A fatal inflammation was caused by a blank firearm injury; blank cartridge propellants are commonly contaminated with the organism. Neonates also appear to be particularly susceptible to *B. cereus* (100), especially with umbilical stump infections; respiratory tract infections associated with contaminated ventilation systems have also occurred (105). Recently, a near-fatal *B. cereus* pneumonia in an otherwise normal patient was reported (54). Such severe infection in healthy individuals is more typical of *B. anthracis*. Interestingly, the isolate from this case was found to harbor a plasmid (pBCXO1) that was 99.6% similar to the pXO1 virulence plasmid of *B. anthracis* (54); its role, if any, in the virulence of this isolate is not known. A hospital pseudo-outbreak of *B. cereus* infection was associated with contaminated ethanol used as a skin disinfectant.

There have been reports of wound, burn, and ocular infections with *B. thuringiensis* (24), but there is as yet no evidence of infections associated with the use of this organism as an insecticide. The safety of using *B. thuringiensis* as a biopesticide on crop plants has been reviewed (11). Strains of this species commonly carry genes for *B. cereus* enterotoxins, but it was found that the main pesticide strains assayed produced low titers of enterotoxin. Occupational exposure to the organism has been connected with the presence of the organism in feces but without gastrointestinal symptoms. Cases of illness caused by *B. thuringiensis* may have been diagnosed as caused by *B. cereus*, as the former may not produce its characteristic insecticidal toxin crystals when incubated at 37°C, owing to the loss of the plasmids carrying the toxin genes (44). Strains of *B. cereus* and *B. thuringiensis* have been isolated in association with periodontitis (47). *B. cereus* also causes infections in domestic animals. It is a well-recognized agent of mastitis and abortion in cattle and can cause these conditions in other livestock.

Other Species

Reports of infections with non-*B. cereus* group species are comparatively rare but very diverse (see reference 66 for the earlier literature), and there have been several hospital pseudoepidemics associated with contaminated blood culture systems. *B. licheniformis* has been reported from ventriculitis following the removal of a meningioma, cerebral abscess after penetrating orbital injury, septicemia following arteriography, bacteremia associated with indwelling central venous catheters, bacteremia during pregnancy with eclampsia and acute fibrinolysis, peritonitis in a chronic ambulatory peritoneal dialysis patient and in a patient with volvulus and small-bowel perforation, ophthalmitis, and corneal ulcer after trauma. Most bizarre, perhaps, are two reports of bacteremia in cases of Munchausen's syndrome: one case followed self-inoculation with organic drain cleaner (46), and in another *B. pumilus* and *Paenibacillus polymyxa* were also isolated (39). There have also been reports of L-form organisms, phenotypically similar to *B. licheniformis*, occurring in human blood and other body fluids (66). *B. licheniformis* can cause foodborne diarrheal illness and has been associated with an infant fatality (70). This organism is frequently associated with bovine abortion and has been shown to have a tropism for the bovine placenta; it has also been associated with abortion in water buffalo and occasionally with bovine mastitis. These types of *B. licheniformis* and *B. cereus* infections are associated with wet and dirty conditions during winter housing, particularly when the animals lie in spilled silage, and in one outbreak a water tank contaminated with *B. licheniformis* was implicated.

The name *B. subtilis* was often used in the past to mean any aerobic, endospore-forming organism, but since 1970 there have been reports of infection in which the identification of this species appears to have been made accurately. They include cases of pneumonia, bacteremia, and septicemia associated with neoplastic disease; breast prosthesis and ventriculoatrial shunt infections; isolations from surgical wound drainage sites; endocarditis in a drug abuser; meningitis following a head injury; bacteremia associated with trauma; cholangitis associated with kidney and liver disease; and isolation from dermatolymphangioadenitis associated with filarial lymphedema. The administration of a probiotic preparation marketed for the treatment or prevention of intestinal disorders and allegedly containing *B. subtilis* led to a fatal septicemia in an immunocompromised patient (76). Subsequently, the organism concerned was identified as *B. clausii* (97). The authors of the latter report reported another *B. clausii* infection, cholangitis in polycystic kidney disease in a 15-year-old French boy who had undergone renal transplant, but the source of the organism was unclear. *B. subtilis* has also been associated with cases of bovine mastitis and ovine abortion (66). *B. subtilis* has been implicated in foodborne illness: vomiting has been the commonest symptom, but with accompanying diarrhea frequently reported; the onset periods have been short (ranging from 10 min to 14 h; median; 2.5 h), the bacterial loads of the organism were high (10^5 to 10^9 CFU/g), and the implicated foods were often prepared dishes in which meat or fish was served with cereal-based components such as bread, pastry, rice, or stuffing (63). *B. amyloliquefaciens*, a close relative of *B. subtilis*, is widely used industrially for enzyme and amino acid production, but human consumption of L-tryptophan manufactured in an organism genetically engineered from a strain of this species was associated with a large epidemic of eosinophilia-myalgia syndrome with 37 deaths (71); the causative agent has not been identified with certainty (71). Environmental strains of this species producing a heat-stable, nonprotein toxin have been isolated in association with building-related health problems (71).

Organisms identified as *B. circulans* have been isolated from cases of meningitis, a cerebrospinal fluid shunt infection, endocarditis, a wound infection in a cancer patient, a bite wound, endophthalmitis, and epidemic endophthalmitis associated with a contaminated product used during cataract surgery (89). It must be noted, however, that many isolates previously identified as *B. circulans* might have been misallocated (see comments on *B. circulans* below). *B. coagulans* has been isolated from corneal infection, bacteremia, and bovine abortion. *B. pumilus* has been found in cases of pustule and rectal fistula infection, bacteremia in an immunosuppressed patient, bacteremia in a patient with Munchausen's syndrome (39) and in association with bovine mastitis. Toxigenic strains of *B. pumilus* have been isolated in association with foodborne illness and from clinical and environmental specimens (98). *B. sphaericus* has been implicated in a fatal lung pseudotumor and in meningitis (66). Among 18 cancer patients with 24 bacteremic episodes, Banerjee et al. (7) isolated *B. cereus* (eight cases), *B. circulans* (three cases), *B. subtilis* (two cases), *B. coagulans* (one case), *B. licheniformis* (one case), *B. pumilus* (one case), *B. sphaericus* (one case), and six unidentified aerobic endospore formers. *B. megaterium* (eight isolates), *B. pumilus* (six isolates), *Brevibacillus brevis* (five isolates), *B. licheniformis* (two isolates), and *B. subtilis* (one isolate), all from chewing tobacco, were found to produce potent exogenous virulence factors that caused plasma exudation and tissue dysfunction in an animal model (90).

Bacillus brevis has been isolated from corneal infection and implicated in several incidents of food poisoning; since the time of these reports, the species has been split (see "Taxonomy" above) and transferred to the new genus *Brevibacillus*. Strains of the new species, *Brevibacillus agri*, have been isolated in association with an outbreak of waterborne illness in Sweden; *Brevibacillus centrosporus* was isolated from bronchoalveolar lavage fluid, *Brevibacillus parabrevis* was found in a breast abscess, and both species have been isolated from human blood (68). *Brevibacillus laterosporus* has been reported in association with a severe case of endophthalmitis (66).

Paenibacillus alvei has been isolated from cases of meningitis and endophthalmitis, from a prosthetic hip infection in a patient with sickle cell anemia, from a wound infection, and, in association with *Clostridium perfringens*, from a case of gas gangrene. *P. macerans* has been isolated from a wound infection following removal of a malignant melanoma, from a brain abscess following penetrating periorbital injury, from a catheter-associated infection in a leukemic patient, and from bovine abortion, and *P. polymyxa* has been isolated from ovine abortion (66) and a bacteremic case of Munchausen's syndrome (39). *P. popilliae* has been reported from endocarditis, and a new *Paenibacillus* species, *P. hongkongensis*, was discovered in a child with neutropenic fever and pseudobacteremia (99), a case in which the organism was found in only one of four blood cultures and was considered to be an environmental contaminant.

COLLECTION, TRANSPORT, AND STORAGE OF SPECIMENS

Clinical specimens for isolation of *Bacillus* species other than *B. anthracis* can be handled without special precautions. *Bacillus* species will normally survive transport in freshly collected specimens or in a standard transport medium. Local transport of specimens (over a few hours) can be done at room temperature or at 2 to 8°C for most specimens, including serum. Generally, if specimens such as swabs, stool, sputum, pleural fluid, and blood are to be shipped overnight or longer, they should be sent at 2 to 8°C. Fresh tissue and serum samples should be shipped frozen, whereas formalin-fixed tissues can be sent at room temperature primarily for detection using immunohistochemistry and (much less suitable) for PCR. For blood specimens in which PCR will be used to detect *B. anthracis* DNA, collection tubes containing EDTA or citrate as anticoagulants are preferable to those containing heparin.

Safety Aspects in Relation to Anthrax

The infectious doses in human anthrax are considered to be high, with the 50% lethal dose as high as 2,500 to 55,000 (34, 57) but as low as 1 to 3 spores (79) or 2 to 9 spores (34). In general, precautions need to be sensible, not extreme. When collecting specimens for suspected anthrax, personnel should wear disposable gloves, disposable apron or overalls, and boots which can be disinfected after use; for dusty samples that might contain many spores, the use of personal protective equipment such as a face shield and/or a respirator should be considered. It should be noted that although hand washing with soap and water or with chlorhexidine gluconate and the use of hypochlorite-releasing towels may all reduce endospore contamination of the skin, waterless rubs containing ethanol are ineffective at removing spores; the model organism in this study was *B. atrophaeus*, a close relative of *B. subtilis* (110). Disposable items should be discarded into suitable containers for autoclaving. Nonautoclavable items should be immersed overnight in 10% formalin (5% formaldehyde solution), glutaraldehyde (5%), a pH 7-adjusted 1:10 dilution of household bleach, or an aqueous solution of chlorine dioxide (500 mg/liter). Items that cannot be immersed should be bagged and sent for formaldehyde fumigation. Ethylene oxide and hydrogen peroxide vapor are also effective fumigants, but the latter is inappropriate if organic matter is being treated. The best disinfectant for specimen spills is formalin. In cases where this is considered impractical, a 1:10 dilution of household bleach (6,000-mg/liter hypochlorite solution) (http://www.epa.gov/pesticides/factsheets/chemicals/bleachfactsheet.htm) can be used, although its limitations should be appreciated; it is rapidly neutralized by organic matter, and it corrodes metals. Other strong oxidizing agents, such as hydrogen peroxide (5%) and peracetic acid (1%), are also effective but likewise inactivated by organic matter.

When working with pure cultures of *B. anthracis*, direct and indirect contact of broken skin with cultures and contaminated laboratory surfaces, accidental parenteral inoculation, and rarely, exposure to infectious aerosols are the primary hazards to laboratory personnel. Isolation and presumptive identification of *B. anthracis* can be performed safely in the routine clinical microbiology laboratory, provided that the usual good laboratory practice is observed; vaccination is not required for minimal handling of the organism (20).

All of the other species of aerobic endospore-forming bacteria that may be isolated from clinical specimens can be handled safely on the open bench. Efforts should be made to avoid methods that produce aerosols. Any procedures that have the potential to generate aerosols should be done in a biological safety cabinet. In addition, all centrifuging should be done using an aerosol-tight rotor and rotors should be opened within the biological safety cabinet. Centrifuges are the most frequently contaminated pieces of laboratory equipment. Laboratories that frequently centrifuge *B. anthracis* suspensions should use an aerosol-tight rotor that can be repeatedly autoclaved; the rotor and rotor lid should be swabbed regularly to monitor for contamination, and contaminated rotors can be autoclaved before reuse. Biosafety level 2 practices, containment equipment, and facilities are recommended for activities using clinical materials and diagnostic quantities of infectious cultures. Biosafety level 3 practices, containment equipment, and facilities are recommended for work involving production quantities or concentrations of cultures and for activities likely to produce aerosols (20).

Specimens from Suspected Anthrax Patients

In all cases, specimens from possible sources of infection (carcass, hides, hair, bones, etc.) should be sought in addition to patient specimens.

Cutaneous Anthrax

For cutaneous anthrax, collect sufficient vesicular fluid with swabs to allow both culture and a smear for visualizing the capsule. For immunohistochemical analysis of cutaneous lesions, a full-thickness punch biopsy fixed in 10% buffered formalin from a papule or vesicle lesion and including adjacent skin should be taken. Biopsy specimens should also be taken from both vesicle and eschar if present (94).

Intestinal Anthrax

Intestinal anthrax will be suspected only if an adequate history of the patient is known. If the patient is not severely ill, a fecal specimen may be collected, but isolation may not be successful. If the patient is severely ill, blood should also be cultured, although isolation may not be possible after antimicrobial treatment; treatment should not await laboratory results. A blood smear may reveal the capsulated rods or, if treatment has started, capsule "ghosts."

Postmortem blood collected by venipuncture (a characteristic of anthrax is nonclotting blood at death [103]) should be examined by smear (for capsule) and culture. Any hemorrhagic fluid from the nose, mouth, or anus should be cultured. If these are positive, no further specimens are needed. If they are negative, specimens of peritoneal fluid, spleen, and/or mesenteric lymph nodes, aspirated by techniques avoiding spillage of fluids, may be collected for smear and culture.

Inhalation (Pulmonary) Anthrax

As with the intestinal form, inhalational anthrax will be suspected only if the patient's history suggests it. If the patient is severely ill, blood smear and culture should be done. Following the bioterrorist attacks of 2001 in the United States, PCR on pleural fluid specimens was very useful, even when the specimens were collected after antimicrobial therapy had begun;

specimens from three patients were negative by culture but still had positive PCR results even when taken ≥24 h after treatment had begun (53), but results depend somewhat on previous treatment. Serology is also useful for the diagnosis of cases when culture fails due to previous treatment. Sera should be taken <7 days after symptoms appear (or after exposure, if known) and again at >14 days. Postmortem, the approach given above for intestinal anthrax should be followed. If the patient is not severely ill, immediate specimen collection is likely to be unfruitful and the person should be treated and simply observed; paired sera (when first seen and >10 days later) may be useful for confirmation of diagnosis.

Specimens from Animals with Suspected Anthrax

Anthrax should be considered as the possible cause of death in herbivorous animals which have died suddenly and unexpectedly, particularly if hemorrhage from the nose, mouth, or anus has occurred and if death has taken place at a site with a history of anthrax (even several decades previously).

Carcasses 1 to 2 Days Old

Due to the nonclotting nature of blood in anthrax victims, in the case of 1- or 2-day-old carcasses it is usually possible to aspirate a few drops of blood from a vein for (i) M'Fadyean-stained smear and (ii) direct plate culture on blood agar.

Pigs frequently do not develop the enormous terminal bacteremia seen in herbivores, and the capsulated rods may not be visible in blood smears. When cervical edema is present, smears and cultures should be made of fluid aspirated from the enlarged mandibular and suprapharyngeal lymph nodes. In porcine intestinal anthrax, possibly obvious only at necropsy, rods are usually visible in stained smears made from mesenteric lymph nodes.

Older Putrefying Carcasses

B. anthracis competes poorly with putrefactive organisms and may not be seen in smears after 2 to 3 days, so culture is necessary for diagnostic confirmation for older putrefying carcasses. Sections of tissue or any blood-stained material should be collected. If the animal has been opened, spleen or lymph node specimens should be taken. With putrefied and very old carcasses, swabs of the nostrils and eye sockets are likely to yield *B. anthracis*, but the best specimens may be samples of contaminated soil beneath the nose and anus.

Other Specimens

Tests for the presence of *B. anthracis* may be requested on a variety of other specimens, such as animal products (e.g., wool, hides, hair, or bonemeal) from regions of endemicity, soil or other materials from old burial sites or tannery or laboratory sites due for redevelopment, or other environmental materials associated with outbreaks (e.g., sewage sludge). At present, culture by the selective agar techniques described below is the only approach. Suitably equipped laboratories are beginning to use PCR techniques for rapid detection of *B. anthracis* in such samples, but at present it is advisable to confirm positives by conventional methods.

Potential Bioterrorism-Related Specimens

In 1999, a Laboratory Response Network (LRN) was established in the United States by the Centers for Disease Control and Prevention (CDC) in partnership with the Association of Public Health Laboratories, the Federal Bureau of Investigation, and the United States Army Medical Research Institute of Infectious Diseases (USAMRIID) to provide the public health laboratory response to acts of bioterrorism (74). This network links local laboratories (sentinel) to laboratories with more specialized testing and increased biosafety level at the state (reference) and federal (national) level. There are reference level laboratories in all 50 states able to detect agents, including *B. anthracis*, rapidly. State public health laboratories are part of the LRN and will be able to provide guidance, or the LRN can be accessed using the Internet (http://www.bt.cdc.gov/lrn/). State and territorial public health laboratory contact information and sentinel laboratory guidelines are also available on the American Society for Microbiology website at http://www.asm.org. Emergency response guidelines for state, local, and tribal public health personnel can be found at http://www.bt.cdc.gov/ under "Additional Topics and Resources" and a 24-h hotline number for urgent advice is 770-488-7100. Although initially limited to the United States, there are now 152 national and international laboratories within the LRN, including Canada, Great Britain, Australia, Germany (U.S. military base), and South Korea (U.S. military base), which are capable of providing a rapid response to acts of biological terrorism, emerging infectious diseases, and other public health threats and emergencies.

ISOLATION PROCEDURES

Specimens with Mixed Microbiota

In specimens submitted for food-poisoning investigations or for isolation of *B. anthracis* from old carcasses, animal products, or environmental specimens, the organisms will be present mostly as spores. Heating (62.5 to 80°C for 10 to 30 min) will both heat shock the spores and effectively destroy non-spore-forming contaminants. A variety of approaches are used to process solid samples prior to heat treatment. Direct plate cultures are made on blood, nutrient, or, selective agars, as appropriate, by spreading up to 100-μl volumes from undiluted and 10- and 100-fold dilutions of the treated sample.

Enrichment procedures are generally inappropriate for isolations from clinical specimens, but when searching for *B. cereus* in stools ≥3 days after a food-poisoning episode, nutrient or tryptic soy broth with polymyxin (100,000 U/liter) may be added to the heat-treated specimen. There is no effective enrichment method for *B. anthracis* in old animal specimens or environmental samples; isolation from these is best done with polymyxin-lysozyme EDTA-thallous acetate (PLET) agar (61; see also chapter 21). A differential/selective chromogenic medium has recently been introduced by R&F Laboratories, Downers Grove, Il. (R&F Anthracis Chromogenic Medium), but it has yet to be thoroughly evaluated. Aliquots (100 μl) of the undiluted and 1:10 and 1:100 dilutions of heat-treated suspension of the specimen are spread across PLET plates, which are read after incubation for 36 to 40 h at 37°C. Roughly circular, creamy white colonies, 1 to 3 mm in diameter, with a ground-glass texture are subcultured on (i) blood agar plates to test for gamma phage and for hemolysis and (ii) directly or subsequently in blood to look for capsule production by using M'Fadyean's stain or, less reliably, India ink negative stain (the ink coagulates the blood and makes interpretation difficult); 2.5 ml of blood (defibrinated horse blood seems best; horse or fetal calf serum is quite good) is inoculated with a pinhead quantity of growth from the suspect colony, incubated statically for 6 to 18 h at 37°C, and then stained. PCR-based methods are being used increasingly for the direct detection of *B. anthracis* in clinical specimens and environmental samples (53).

Several media have been designed for isolation, identification, and enumeration of *B. cereus*. They exploit the organism's egg yolk reaction positivity and acid-from-mannitol negativity;

pyruvate and polymyxin may be included for selectivity. Three satisfactory formulations are MEYP or MYP (mannitol, egg yolk, polymyxin B agar [MEYP]; Oxoid, Basingstoke, United Kingdom; MYP; Difco, BD, Franklin Lakes, N.J.), PEMBA (polymyxin B, egg yolk, mannitol, bromthymol blue agar; Oxoid), and BCM (*Bacillus cereus* Medium; LabM, Bury, United Kingdom) (106) (see chapter 21). There are no selective media for other *Bacillus* species, but spores can be selected for by heat treating part of the specimen, as described above; the vegetative cells of both spore formers and non-spore-formers will be killed, but the heat-resistant spores not only will survive but also may be heat shocked into subsequent germination. The other part of the specimen is cultivated without heat treatment in case spores are very heat sensitive or absent. Heat treatment is not appropriate for fresh clinical specimens, in which spores are usually sparse or absent.

IDENTIFICATION OF *B. ANTHRACIS*

Gram Stain

Inevitably the first examination of smears and cultures will be with the Gram stain. In the past, it has been regarded as being of limited value in anthrax diagnosis because it does not reveal the capsule. In recent bioterrorism cases such preparations were clearly considered to be of great value (Fig. 1a), but caution is still necessary. In a well-developed country, it is unlikely that large numbers of gram-positive bacteria in the blood at death are going to be anything but *B. anthracis*, particularly when supported by the recent events. In other circumstances, and in animals in particular, the blood or other specimen may not be collected soon after death and before putrefactive organisms appear; *B. anthracis* may then be indistinguishable without the use of the proper capsule stain.

The M'Fadyean polychrome methylene blue staining test dates from 1903 and has proved to be a remarkably successful rapid diagnostic test over the decades. However, reliable stain and adequate quality control of its performance are becoming hard to guarantee. A rapid immunochromatographic on-site test has been developed (13) but is not commercially available.

It is generally easy to distinguish virulent *B. anthracis* from other members of the *B. cereus* group. *B. anthracis* isolates are characterized by a typical microscopic appearance (Fig. 1c and 2a) and colonial morphology (Fig. 3a): colonies are white or gray, nonhemolytic or only weakly hemolytic, susceptible to the diagnostic "gamma phage" (inquiries

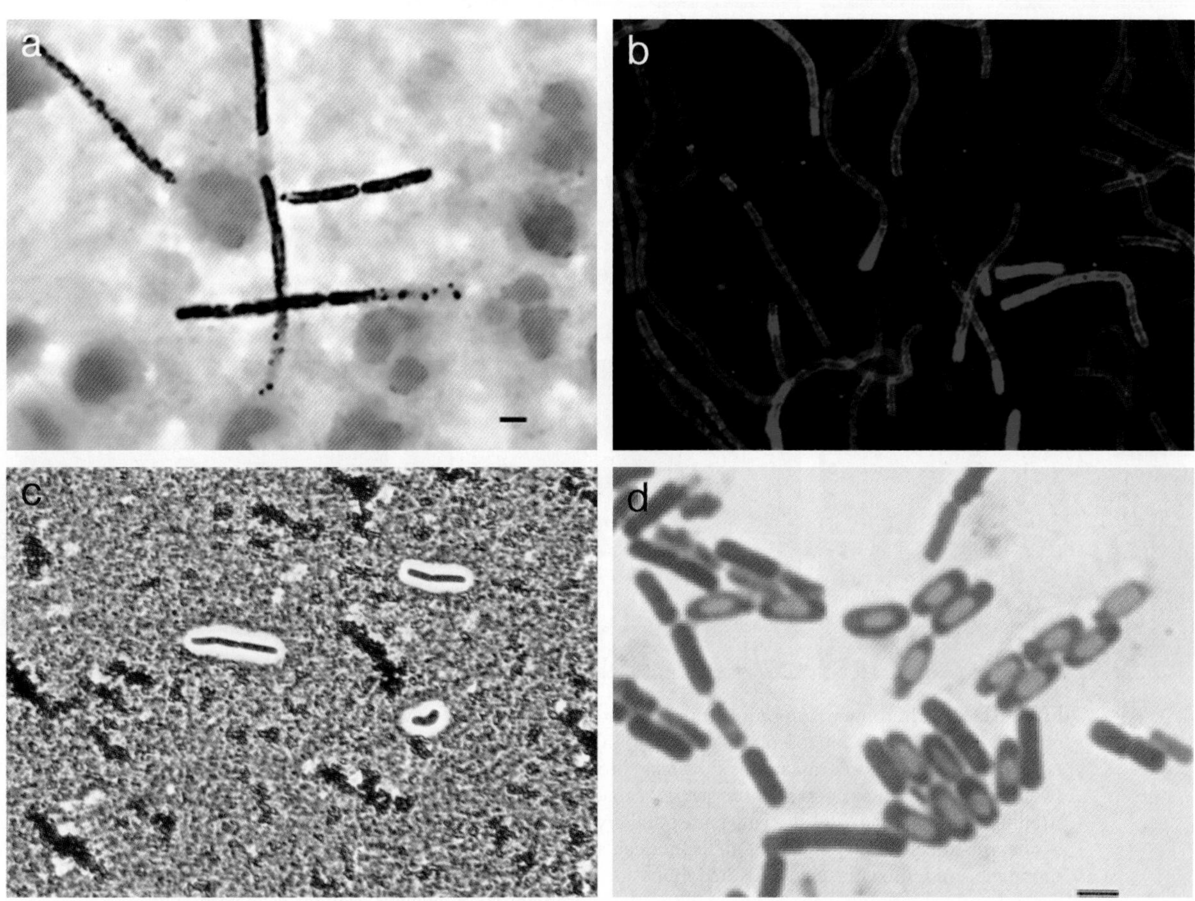

FIGURE 1 (a) Gram stain of *B. anthracis*, associated with a bioterrorism attack, showing gram-positive rods in peripheral blood buffy coat following admission of patient; bar, 3 μm. Courtesy of H. Masur. (b) DFA-stained preparation of *B. anthracis* using an antibody specific for the poly-γ-D-glutamic acid capsule. (c) India ink stain of *B. anthracis* incubated in horse blood. Clear zones surrounding the rods are due to the exclusion of the India ink by the capsule. (d) Spore-stained preparation of *B. cereus* sporangia, viewed by bright-field microscopy. Spores are stained green and vegetative cells are counterstained red. Bar, 2 μm. (Photograph kindly provided by M. Rodriguez-Diaz.)

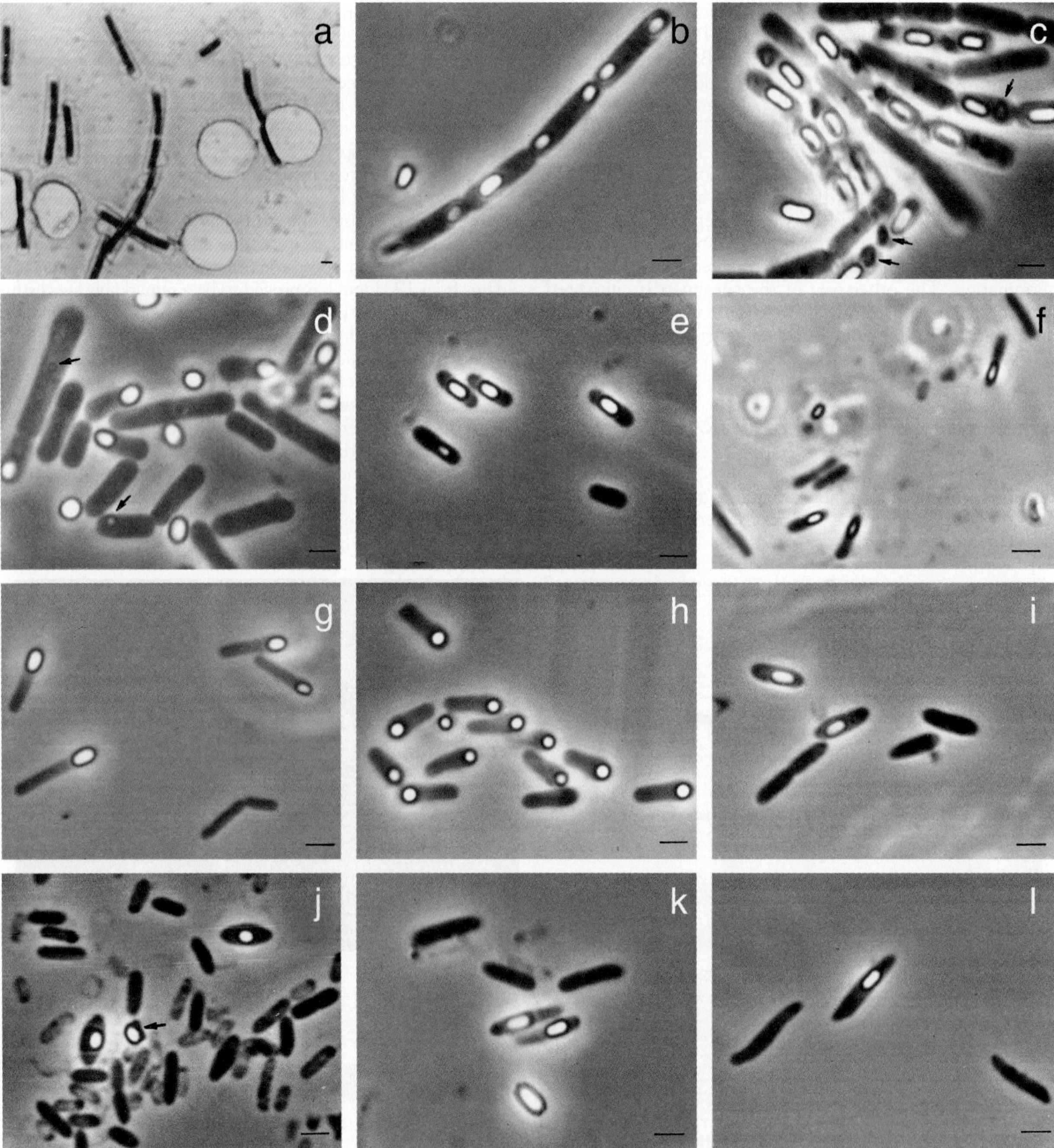

FIGURE 2 Photomicrographs of endospore-forming bacteria viewed by bright-field (a) and phase-contrast (b to l) microscopy. Bars, 2 μm. (a) *B. anthracis,* M'Fadyean stain showing capsulate rods in guinea pig blood smear; (b) *B. cereus,* broad cells with ellipsoidal, subterminal spores, not swelling the sporangia; (c) *B. thuringiensis,* broad cells with ellipsoidal, subterminal spores, not swelling the sporangia, and showing parasporal crystals of insecticidal toxin (arrowed); (d) *B. megaterium,* broad cells with ellipsoidal and spherical, subterminal and terminal spores, not swelling the sporangia, and showing poly-β-hydroxybutyrate inclusions (arrowed); (e) *B. subtilis,* ellipsoidal, central and subterminal spores, not swelling the sporangia; (f) *B. pumilus,* slender cells with cylindrical, subterminal spores, not swelling the sporangia; (g) *B. circulans,* ellipsoidal, subterminal spores, swelling the sporangia; (h) *B. sphaericus,* spherical, terminal spores, swelling the sporangia; (i) *Brevibacillus brevis,* ellipsoidal, subterminal spores, one swelling its sporangium slightly; (j) *Brevibacillus laterosporus,* ellipsoidal, central spores with thickened rims on one side (arrowed), swelling the sporangia; (k) *Paenibacillus polymyxa,* ellipsoidal, paracentral to subterminal spores, swelling the sporangia slightly; (l) *Paenibacillus alvei,* cells with tapered ends, ellipsoidal, paracentral to subterminal spores, not swelling the sporangium.

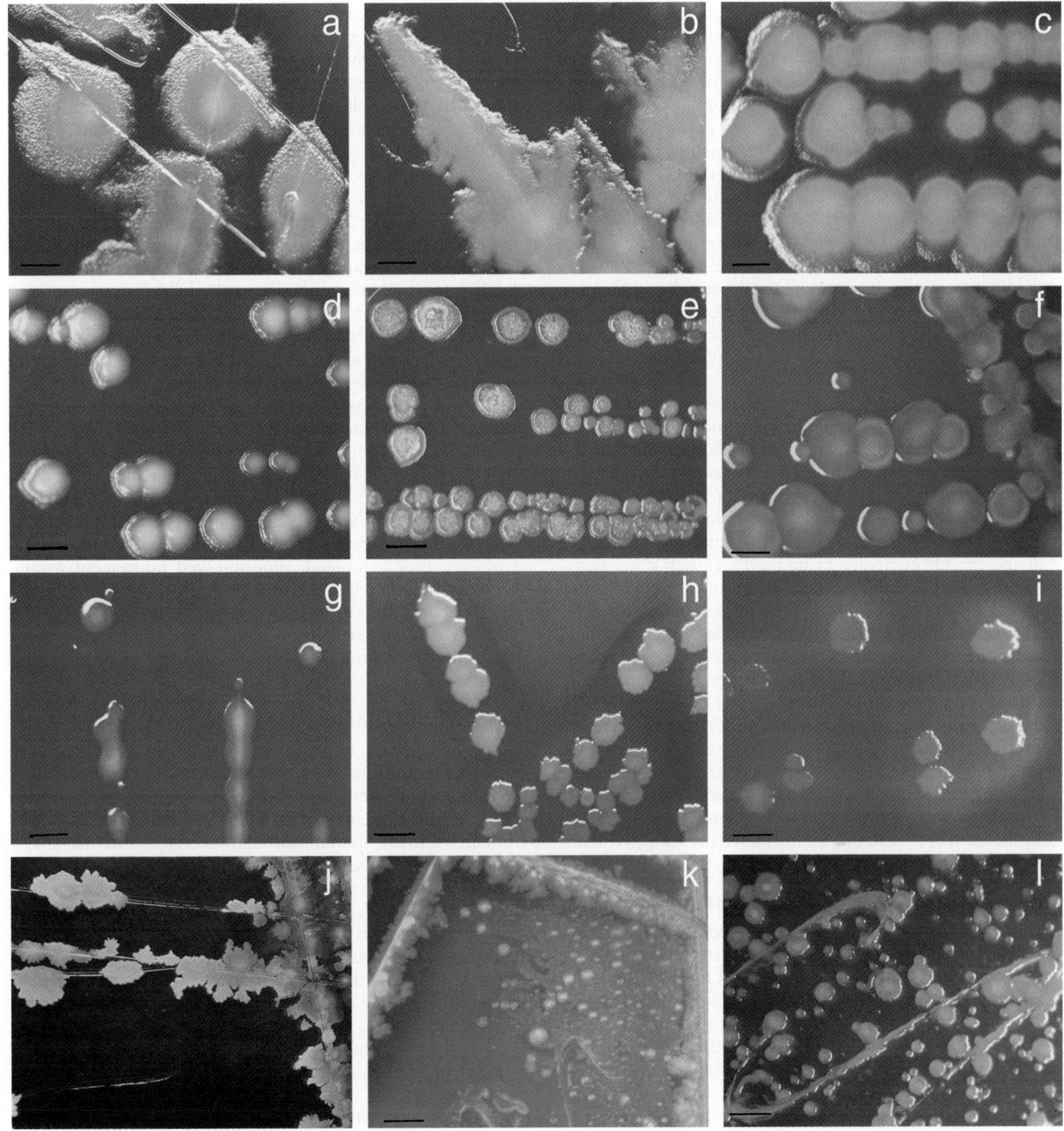

FIGURE 3 Colonies of endospore-forming bacteria on blood agar (a to i) and nutrient agar (j to l) after 24 to 36 h at 37°C. Bars, 2 mm. (a) *B. anthracis;* (b) *B. cereus;* (c) *B. thuringiensis;* (d) *B. megaterium;* (e) *B. pumilus;* (f) *B. sphaericus;* (g) *Brevibacillus brevis;* (h) *Brevibacillus laterosporus;* (i) *Paenibacillus polymyxa;* (j) *B. subtilis;* (k) *Paenibacillus* strain formerly assigned to *B. circulans;* (l) *Paenibacillus alvei.*

about gamma phage should be addressed to the Diagnostics Systems Division, USAMRIID, Fort Detrick, Frederick, MD 21702-5011), generally susceptible to penicillin, nonmotile, and able to produce the characteristic capsule, as shown by M'Fadyean staining (Fig. 2a) or India ink staining (103) (Fig. 1c). As an alternative to culture in blood, the capsule of virulent *B. anthracis* can be demonstrated on nutrient agar containing 0.7% sodium bicarbonate, incubated overnight under 5 to 7% CO_2 (candle jars perform well). Colonies of the capsulated organism appear mucoid, and the capsule can be visualized by M'Fadyean or India ink staining of smears or by direct fluorescent antibody (DFA) staining (Fig. 1b; see below) or indirect antibody staining (inquiries about indirect fluorescent antibody capsule staining should be addressed as above to the Diagnostics Systems Division, USAMRIID).

In addition to phenotypic analysis, molecular and antigenic detection assays are available for the rapid identification of *B. anthracis*. The LRN PCR (restricted to LRN laboratories; see "Potential Bioterrorism-Related Specimens" above) targets three distinct loci on the *B. anthracis* chromosome, pXO1 virulence plasmid, and pXO2 virulence plasmid (54). Using several loci increases specificity and allows for the detection of avirulent strains (lacking pXO1 or pXO2). The anthrax toxin genes (*pagA*, *lef*, and *cya*) are located on pXO1, whereas the genes required for capsule biosynthesis (*capBCA*) are located on pXO2. Isolates lacking pXO2 or both plasmids are found mostly in the environment and are frequently mistaken for *B. cereus*, due to the lack of a capsule, and discarded (102). A commercial kit is also available for the detection of the *B. anthracis* toxin gene, *pagA*, and the capsule gene, *capB* (Roche, Mannheim, Germany) (8). These genes have been widely used as *B. anthracis* specific gene targets; however, there have been recent reports of these genes being found in species other than *B. anthracis* (41, 54). Recently, several laboratories have developed specific PCR assays for *B. anthracis* that target chromosomal genes such as *rpoB*, *gyrA*, and *plcR* (30, 56, 82).

A two-component DFA assay has been used to identify encapsulated vegetative cells of *B. anthracis* (27, 33). This assay uses two different monoclonal antibodies specific for a *B. anthracis* cell wall antigen and the *B. anthracis* capsule (Fig. 1b). Neither antigen is 100% specific for *B. anthracis;* however, only *B. anthracis* has been found to be positive for both antigens, and thus the assay is 100% specific when both cell wall and capsule components are used together; it was heavily used at the CDC during the 2001 bioterrorism-associated outbreak for the rapid (<4-h) identification of isolates (27).

Tetracore, Inc. (Gaithersburg, Md.) has produced a rapid (within 15 min) immunochromatographic test (RedLine Alert) utilizing an antibody specific for one of the *B. anthracis* S-layer proteins. This assay has been approved by the Food and Drug Administration (FDA) for use on nonhemolytic *Bacillus* species colonies cultured on sheep blood agar plates. Manufacturer's data suggest that the test was 98.6% sensitive when tested on 145 *B. anthracis* isolates and 45 nonhemolytic, non-*B. anthracis* isolates; however, such identification of *B. anthracis* is considered presumptive and it should not be used as a stand-alone test.

Molecular Characterization of *B. anthracis*

Although *B. anthracis* is a genetically monomorphic species, the development of a multiple-locus variable-number tandem repeat analysis (MLVA) has allowed for effective strain differentiation (59). This method was relied on during the 2001 bioterrorism-associated outbreak in the United States, and MLVA of the attack strain implicated the Ames laboratory strain (52). Recently, Keim et al. proposed adding canonical single nucleotide polymorphisms, expanding MLVA from 8 to 15 loci, and analyzing four single nucleotide repeats to increase genotyping accuracy and resolution (60). In addition, although not in widespread use, the availability of genome data has led to the use of microarray technology to detect differences between strains of *B. anthracis* and other *Bacillus* species (86, 116) (see also "Molecular Typing" below).

Direct Detection of *B. anthracis* in Clinical Specimens

In addition to culturing *B. anthracis*, there are molecular and antigen-based detection methods available for direct detection in clinical and environmental samples. These are essential when cultures fail, as they particularly do after the initiation of antimicrobial therapy. Several methods, including a *B. anthracis*-specific LRN PCR assay, immunohistochemical (IHC) assays, and serology, were useful for confirmation of cases during the 2001 bioterrorism-associated outbreak, particularly when culture failed (45, 53, 83, 85, 94). At least two such tests need to be positive for a case to be considered laboratory confirmed.

The most widely used and available detection method in the U.S. public health system is the LRN PCR as previously described (53). Following the 2001 anthrax attacks in the United States, this assay was negative on all specimens (n = 142) from patients in whom anthrax was excluded (100% specific). In addition, testing of specimens from inhalation anthrax patients produced a positive result in 33% (29/87) of the specimens which were culture negative, with pleural fluid appearing to be the best specimen even after the initiation of antimicrobial therapy. The IHC assay, as performed at the CDC, uses the same antibodies as the DFA assay (specific to cell wall antigen or the capsule) to detect *B. anthracis* in formalin-fixed, paraffin-embedded tissues. This method was particularly useful in the diagnosis of cutaneous cases during the 2001 bioterrorism-associated outbreak. Skin biopsy specimens from cutaneous lesions from 8 of 10 patients were positive for both the capsule and cell wall antigens (94).

The many reports on the use of different PCR assays to detect or identify *B. anthracis* cannot be summarized here. Although PCR is currently the most widely used detection technology (29), there are increasing reports on novel technologies or improvements to existing ones such as mass spectrometry, flow cytometry, time-resolved fluorescent assays, high-performance liquid chromatography, and even the use of engineered B-cells to detect *B. anthracis* (2, 55, 87, 111, 115). With further improvements and validations, these assays may increasingly be used to detect *B. anthracis* in the future.

Serological Detection of Anthrax

Serological assays for the detection of antibody response against the anthrax toxin protein, protective antigen (PA), were used in combination with PCR or IHC assay results to confirm anthrax cases when culture failed. A quantitative human anti-PA immunoglobulin G (IgG) enzyme-linked immunosorbent assay was performed at the CDC during the 2001 outbreak and was positive only on sera from individuals with anthrax or vaccinated with Anthrax Vaccine Adsorbed (BioThrax; BioPort, Lansing, Mich.) (85). More recently, a commercially available, FDA-approved, qualitative kit (QuickELISA Anthrax-PA Kit) from Immunetics (Boston, Mass.) has become available for the detection of anti-PA IgG and IgM antibodies in human serum. Serological assays aided in the effort to confirm cases in the 2001 attack, particularly cutaneous ones; however, the time to seroconversion after infection limits its usefulness in terms of the rapid diagnosis necessary for treatment and a public health response.

IDENTIFICATION OF SPECIES OTHER THAN *B. ANTHRACIS*

Remember that these organisms do not always stain gram positive. Before attempting to identify to the species level, it is important to establish that the isolate really is an aerobic endospore former and that other inclusions are not being mistaken for spores. A Gram-stained smear showing cells with unstained areas suggestive of spores can be stripped of oil with acetone or alcohol, washed, and then stained for spores. Spores are stained in heat-fixed smears by flooding with 10% aqueous malachite green for up to 45 min (without heating), followed by washing and counterstaining with 0.5% aqueous safranin for 30 s; spores are green within pink/red cells at a magnification of ×1,000 (Fig. 1d). Phase-contrast microscopy (at a magnification of ×1,000) should be used if available, as it is superior to spore staining and more convenient. Spores are larger, more phase bright, and more regular in shape, size, and position than other kinds of inclusion such as polyhydroxybutyrate (PHB) granules (Fig. 2d), and sporangial appearance is valuable in identification (Fig. 2).

Members of the *B. cereus* group and *B. megaterium* produce large amounts of storage material when grown on carbohydrate media, but on routine media this vacuolate or foamy appearance is rarely sufficiently pronounced to cause confusion. Isolates of other organisms have often been submitted to reference laboratories as *Bacillus* species because they were large, aerobic gram-positive rods, even though sporulation had not been observed, or because PHB granules or other storage inclusions had been mistaken for spores.

Bacillus contains facultative anaerobes as well as strict aerobes, which can be a valuable characteristic in identification. For example, *B. licheniformis* and *B. subtilis,* which have very similar colonial (Fig. 3j) and microscopic morphologies (Fig. 2e), are facultatively anaerobic and strictly aerobic, respectively; likewise, the two large-celled species *B. cereus* and *B. megaterium* (Fig. 2b and d) are facultatively anaerobic and strictly aerobic, respectively.

The most widely used diagnostic schemes use traditional phenotypic tests (42) or miniaturized tests of the API 20E and 50CHB kits used together (67) (bioMérieux, Marcy l'Etoile, France). The API 20E and 50CHB kits can be used for the presumptive distinction of *B. anthracis* from other members of the *B. cereus* group within 48 h. bioMérieux also offers identification cards for *Bacillus* and related genera for the Vitek and Vitek Compact automated identification systems. As many new species have been proposed since these schemes were established, updated API and Vitek databases have been prepared. Biolog Inc. (Hayward, Calif.) also offers a *Bacillus* database. The effectiveness of such kits can vary with the genera and species of aerobic endospore formers concerned, but they are improving with continuing development and enlarged databases (67). The many proposals for new species, often on the basis of single isolates, make the satisfactory expansion of such databases problematic; for a database to be effective in identifying a particular species, its entry for that species needs to reflect the characterization of at least 10 authentic strains from a range of sources, but these requirements can be very difficult or impossible to fulfill. It is stressed that the use of these kits should always be preceded by the basic characterization tests described below.

Other approaches include chemotaxonomic fingerprinting by fatty acid methyl ester profiling, polyacrylamide gel electrophoresis analysis, pyrolysis mass spectrometry, and Fourier-transform infrared spectroscopy. All these approaches have been successfully applied either across the genera or to small groups. As with genotypic profiling methods, large databases of authentic strains are necessary; some of these are commercially available, such as the Microbial Identification System software (Microbial ID Inc., Newark, Del.) database for fatty acid methyl ester analysis.

For diagnostic purposes, the aerobic endospore formers comprise two groups: the reactive ones, which give positive results in various routine biochemical tests and which are therefore easier to identify, and the nonreactive ones, which give few if any positive results in such tests. Nonreactive isolates tend to dominate the identification requests sent to reference laboratories. Table 1 shows reactions for some species belonging to the former group, and the phenotypic test scheme outlined above may be used in conjunction with it. Guidance on identifying members of the nonreactive group is found in reference 68.

Identification of *B. cereus* and *B. thuringiensis*

Colonies of *B. cereus* and relatives are very variable but readily recognized (Fig. 3a, b, and c): they are characteristically large (2 to 7 mm in diameter) and vary in shape from circular to irregular, with entire to undulate, crenate, or fimbriate edges; they have matte or granular textures. Smooth and moist colonies are not uncommon, however. The optimum growth temperature is about 37°C with minima and maxima of 15 to 20°C and 40 to 45°C, respectively. Although colonies of *B. anthracis* and *B. cereus* can be similar in appearance, those of the former are generally smaller and nonhemolytic, may show more spiking or tailing along the lines of inoculation streaks, and are very tenacious compared with the usually more butyrous consistency of *B. cereus* and *B. thuringiensis* colonies, so that they may be pulled into standing peaks with a loop. *Bacillus mycoides* produces characteristic rhizoid or hairy-looking, adherent colonies which readily cover the whole agar surface.

There are key characteristics for recognizing and distinguishing the *B. cereus* group organisms. They display a typical colonial morphology (Fig. 3a, b, and c); large cells are observed, often in chains, producing ellipsoidal spores not swelling the sporangia (Fig. 2b and c), usually within 48 h and often apparent after 24 h; they are facultative anaerobes and positive for the egg yolk reaction (i.e., lecithinase positive). Negative or very weak hemolysis and lack of motility distinguish *B. anthracis* and *B. mycoides* from *B. cereus* and *B. thuringiensis*. *B. cereus, B. mycoides, B. thuringiensis,* and, to a lesser extent, *B. anthracis* synthesize lecithinases, forming opaque zones of precipitation around colonies on egg yolk agar as the colonies grow (i.e., usually after overnight or perhaps 24 h of incubation). Recognition of *B. thuringiensis* is largely dependent on observation of its cuboid or diamond-shaped parasporal crystals in sporulated cultures (after 2 to 5 days) by phase-contrast microscopy (Fig. 2c) or by staining with malachite green counterstained with carbol fuchsin or safranin.

Other Species

Other species show a very wide range of colonial morphologies, both within and between species after 24 to 48 h (Fig. 3). They vary from moist and glossy (Fig. 3f to i) through granular to wrinkled (Fig. 3e); shapes vary from round to irregular (Fig. 3d to i), sometimes spreading (Fig. 3k and l), with entire through undulate or crenate to fimbriate edges (Fig. 3d to j); sizes range from 1 to 5 mm; color commonly ranges from buff or creamy gray to off-white, but some strains may produce an orange pigment; hemolysis may be absent, slight or marked, partial or complete (Fig. 3h); elevations range from effuse through raised to convex; the consistency is usually butyrous, but mucoid and dry, adherent colonies are not uncommon. Despite this diversity, *Bacillus* colonies are not generally difficult to recognize, and some species have characteristic yet seemingly infinitely variable colonial morphologies, as does the *B. cereus* group (Fig. 3a to c).

B. subtilis and *B. licheniformis* produce similar colonies, which are exceptionally variable in appearance and often appear to be mixed cultures (Fig. 3j); colonies are irregular in shape and of moderate diameter (2 to 4 mm), and they range from moist and butyrous or mucoid, with margins varying from undulate to fimbriate through membranous with an underlying mucoid matrix, with or without mucoid beading at the surface, to rough and crusty as they dry. The "licheniform" colonies of *B. licheniformis* tend to be quite adherent.

Rotating and migrating microcolonies, which may show spreading growth (Fig. 3k), have been observed macroscopically

TABLE 1 Characters for differentiating some species of *Bacillus, Geobacillus, Paenibacillus*, and *Virgibacillus*[a]

Character[b]	*Bacillus*								
	B. subtilis group				*B. cereus* group				
	B. subtilis	*B. amyloliquefaciens*	*B. licheniformis*	*B. pumilus*	*B. cereus*[c]	*B. anthracis*	*B. thuringiensis*	*B. mycoides*	*B. megaterium*
Rod mean diameter (μm)	0.8	0.8	0.8	0.7	1.4	1.3	1.4	1.3	1.5
Chains of cells	(−)	(+)	(+)	−	+	+	+	+	+
Motility	+	+	+	+	+	−	+	−	+
Sporangia[d]									
Spore shape	E	E	E (C)	C, E	E (C) [E]	E	E (C)	E	E, S
Spore position	S, C	S, T	S, C	S, C	S, C	S	S	S (C)	S, C
Sporangium swollen	−	−	−	−	−	−	−	−	−
Parasporal crystals	−	−	−	−	−	−	+	−	−
Parasporal bodies	−	−	−	−	−	−	−	−	−
Anaerobic growth	−	−	+	−	+	+	+	+	−
Growth at:									
50°C	v	v	+	v	−	−	−	−	−
65°C	−	−	−	−	−	−	−	−	−
Egg yolk reaction	−	−	−	−	+	+	+	+	−
Casein hydrolysis	+	+	+	+	+	+	+	+	+
Starch hydrolysis	+	+	+	−	+	+	+	+	+
Arginine dihydrolase	−	−	+	−	v[(−)]	−	+	v	−
Indole production	−	−	−	−	−	−	−	−	−
Gelatin hydrolysis	+	+	+	+	+	(+)	+	+	+
Nitrate reduction	+	+	+	−	(+)[+]	+	+	(+)	−
Gas from carbohydrates	−	−	−	−	−	−	−	−	−
Acid from:									
D-Arabinose	−	−	−	−	−	−	−	−	−
Glycerol	+	+	+	+	+[v]	−	+	+	+
Glycogen	+	+	+	−	+[−]	+	+	+	+
Inulin	(+)	−	v	−	−	−	−	−	+
Mannitol	+	+	+	+	−	−	−	−	+
Salicin	+	+	+	+	+[−]	−	(+)	(+)	+
D-Trehalose	+	+	+	+	+	+	+	+	+

[a]Symbols and abbreviations: +, ≥85% positive; (+), 75 to 84% positive; v, variable (26 to 74% positive); (−), 16 to 25% positive; −, 0 to 15% positive.
[b]Arginine dihydrolase, indole production, gelatin hydrolysis, and nitrate reduction reactions were determined using tests in the API 20E strip (bioMérieux). Acid from carbohydrate reactions was determined using the API 50CHB System (bioMérieux).

in about 13% of strains received as *B. circulans*, but this very heterogeneous species continues to undergo radical taxonomic revision, and such spreading strains are now assigned to *Paenibacillus* species (Fig. 3l).

Other species that have been encountered in the clinical laboratory include *B. coagulans, B. megaterium, B. pumilus*, and *B. sphaericus; B. brevis* and *B. laterosporus* (now both in *Brevibacillus*); and *B. macerans* and *B. polymyxa* (now both in *Paenibacillus*), and they do not produce a particularly distinctive growth (Fig. 3d to i).

Microscopic morphologies, particularly of sporangia (Fig. 2), are much more helpful for distinguishing between species. Vegetative cells are usually round-ended, but those of *P. alvei* may be tapered (Fig. 2l). The large cells of *B. megaterium* may accumulate PHB (Fig. 2d) and appear vacuolate or foamy when grown on glucose nutrient agar. Overall, cell widths vary from about 0.5 to 1.5 μm, and cell lengths vary from 1.5 to 8 μm. Most strains of these species are motile. Spore shapes vary from cylindrical (Fig. 2f) through ellipsoidal (Fig. 2b, c to e, g, and i to l) to spherical (Fig. 2d and h); bean- or kidney-shaped, curved-cylindrical, and pear-shaped spores are also seen occasionally. Spores may be terminally (Fig. 2h), subterminally (Fig. 2b, c, f, g, and i), or centrally (Fig. 2e and j) positioned within sporangia and may distend them (Fig. 2g to k). Despite within-species and within-strain variation, sporangial morphologies tend to be characteristic of species and may allow tentative identification by the experienced worker. One species, *Brevibacillus laterosporus*, produces very distinctive ellipsoidal spores that have thickened rims on one side, so that they appear to be laterally displaced in the sporangia (Fig. 2j).

All these species are mesophilic and grow well between 30 and 37°C. Minimum growth temperatures lie mostly between 5 and 20°C, and maxima are mostly between 35 and 50°C. Strains of *B. coagulans* may show slight thermophily and grow up to 55 to 60°C.

GENE SEQUENCING AND SPECIES IDENTIFICATION

Although the sequencing of several genes, such as *rpoB* and *gyrA*, has been used to aid in the identification of bacterial species, the16S rRNA gene remains the one most commonly used, and it provides an abundance of data for comparison

Bacillus				*Geobacillus*		*Paenibacillus*				*Virgibacillus pantothenticus*
B. circulans group										
B. circulans	*B. firmus*	*B. lentus*	*B. coagulans*	*G. stearothermophilus*	*G. thermodenitrificans*	*P. polymyxa*	*P. alvei*	*P. macerans*	*P. validus*	
0.8	0.8	0.8	0.8	0.9	0.8	0.9	0.8	0.7	0.8	0.6
−	−	(+)	v	−	v	−	(−)	−	−	+
+	+	+	+	+	−	+	+	+	+	+
E	E	E	E	E	E	E	E (C)	E	E	E, S
S, T	S (C)	S, C	S, T	S, T	S	S, C	S, C	S, T	S, T	S, T
+	v	v	+	+	−	+	+	+	+	+
−	−	−	−	−	−	−	−	−	−	−
−	−	−	−	−	−	−	−	−	−	−
+	−	−	+	−	−	+	+	+	−	+
−	−	−	+	+	+	−	−	v	v	v
−	−	−	−	+	+	−	−	−	−	−
−	−	−	−	−	−	−	−	−	−	−
−	+	v	v	(+)	(−)	+	+	−	−	+
+	+	+	+	+	+	+	+	+	+	+
(−)	−	−	v	−	−	−	−	−	−	(−)
−	−	−	−	−	−	−	+	−	−	−
−	v	v	−	+	+	+	+	v	−	+
v	(+)	(+)	(−)	v	(+)	v	−	−	v	v
−	−	−	−	−	−	+	−	+	−	−
−	−	−	−	−	−	−	−	+	−	+
v	−	v	+	(+)	v	+	+	+	+	+
+	−	v	−	+	−	+	v	+	v	−
(+)	−	(−)	−	−	−	+	−	+	v	−
+	v	(+)	v	−	v	+	−	+	+	−
+	−	+	+	(−)	v	+	v	+	−	+
+	v	(+)	+	+	+	+	v	+	+	+

[c] Reactions shown in brackets are for the biotype isolated particularly in connection with outbreaks of emetic-type food poisoning and for strains of serovars 1, 3, 5, and 8, which are commonly associated with such outbreaks.

[d] Spore shape: C, cylindrical; E, ellipsoidal; S, spherical. Spore position: C, central or paracentral; S, subterminal; T, terminal. The commonest shapes and positions are listed first, and those shown in parentheses are infrequently observed.

(4, 73, 108). Many species, however, including species within the *B. cereus* group, can be extremely difficult to differentiate on the basis of a single gene sequence. Sacchi et al. reported that while *B. anthracis* and *B. cereus* could be differentiated by 16S rRNA gene sequencing, some strains of *B. cereus* and *B. anthracis* differed at only a single nucleotide position; furthermore, a more recent report identified a *B. anthracis* strain with a sequence identical to that of some *B. cereus* strains (3, 91). With differences so small, the quality of the sequence and its analysis are becoming more critically important. Nonetheless, even if sequencing of a gene, such as the 16S rRNA gene, does not always provide identification to the species level with 100% confidence, it is a very helpful component of the identification process and of phylogenetic analyses.

TYPING AND STRAIN DIFFERENTIATION OF SPECIES OTHER THAN *B. ANTHRACIS*

A strain differentiation system for *B. cereus* based on flagellar (H) antigens is available at the Food Safety Microbiology Laboratory, Health Protection Agency Centre for Infections, Colindale, London, United Kingdom, for investigations of food-poisoning outbreaks or other *B. cereus*-associated clinical problems. *B. thuringiensis* strains are classified on the basis of their flagellar antigens; 82 serovars have been recognized. This classification is done at the Institut Pasteur, Paris, France.

Toxin and Antitoxin Detection

The three protein components of anthrax toxin (protective antigen [PA], lethal factor, and edema factor) and antibodies to them can be used in enzyme immunoassay systems. For routine confirmation of anthrax infection, or for monitoring response to anthrax vaccines, antibodies against PA alone appear to be satisfactory; they have proved useful for epidemiological investigations in humans and animals. In human anthrax, however, early treatment sometimes prevents antibody development. PA is available commercially from List Biological Laboratories, Inc., Campbell, Calif. (http://www.listlabs.com). The current human vaccine in the United States is an aluminum hydroxide-adsorbed vaccine strain culture filtrate containing a relatively high proportion of PA and relatively low amounts of lethal factor and edema factor (101).

In countries of the former USSR, a skin test utilizing Anthraxin (trade mark), a heat-stable extract from a non-capsulate strain of *B. anthracis,* which has been licensed for human and animal use since 1962, is widely acclaimed for the retrospective diagnosis of anthrax (95). The delayed-type hypersensitivity is interpreted as indicating cell-mediated immunity to anthrax and can be used to diagnose anthrax retrospectively or to evaluate the vaccine-induced immune status after periods of several years. Anthraxin does not contain highly specific anthrax antigens and depends on the nature of anthrax rather than the specificity of the antigens involved. This is also true of the Ascoli test, which, dating from 1911, must be one of the oldest antigen detection tests in microbiology. It is a precipitin test using hyperimmune serum raised to *B. anthracis* whole-cell antigen to provide rapid retrospective evidence of anthrax infection in an animal from which the material being tested was derived. The test is still in use in Eastern Europe and Central Asia.

The enterotoxin complex responsible for the diarrheal type of *B. cereus* food poisoning has been increasingly well characterized. Two commercial kits are available for its detection in foods and feces, the Oxoid BCET-RPLA (Oxoid Ltd.) and the TECRA VIA (TECRA Diagnostics, Roseville, NSW, Australia). However, these kits detect different antigens, and there is some controversy about their reliabilities. Other assays, based on tissue culture, have also been developed (36). The emetic toxin of *B. cereus* has been identified as a dodecadepsipeptide, and it may be assayed in food extracts or culture filtrates using HEp-2 cells (35) or boar semen (1).

Molecular Typing

Pulsed-field gel electrophoresis has been applied to differentiate between strains of *Bacillus sphaericus* and between very closely related species such as *Bacillus anthracis, Bacillus cereus, Bacillus mycoides,* and *Bacillus thuringiensis,* and two studies dealt with infrequently reported clinical infections by *B. cereus* (47, 65).

Amplified fragment length polymorphism is based upon a specific combination of PCR and restriction methodologies, and although it is much more complex than random amplified polymorphic DNA and repetitive extragenic palindromic-PCR methods, it is also much more reproducible. It has been used in epidemiological studies of *B. cereus* (88) and for the genetic comparison of *B. anthracis* and its closest relatives (104). For other members of the *B. cereus* group, which are not as monomorphic as *B. anthracis,* several multilocus sequence typing (MLST) schemes have recently been reported (48, 81), and a *B. cereus* MLST website that allows for viewing of data and submission of new data is available at http://pubmlst.org/bcereus/. These methods include the partial sequencing and comparison of seven housekeeping genes to differentiate strains.

MAINTENANCE OF STRAINS

All the clinically significant isolates reported to date are of species that grow, and often sporulate, on routine laboratory media at 37°C. It seems unlikely that many clinically important, but more fastidious, strains are being missed for the want of special media or growth conditions. Maintenance is simple if spores can be obtained, but it is a mistake to assume that a primary culture or subculture on blood agar will automatically yield spores if stored on the bench or in the incubator. It is best to grow the organism on nutrient agar containing 5 mg of manganese sulfate per liter for a few days and refrigerate the culture when microscopy shows that most cells have sporulated. For most species, sporulated cultures on slants of this medium, sealed after incubation, can survive in a refrigerator for years. Alternatively, cultures (preferably sporulated) can be frozen or lyophilized.

B. anthracis is defined as a select agent and an "overlap" agent on the HHS/CDC and USDA/APHIS select agent lists. Thus, possession of the agent in the United States requires registration of the laboratory with either CDC or APHIS. When *B. anthracis* is identified in an unregistered clinical or diagnostic laboratory, the identification of this agent must be reported to CDC or APHIS within 7 days and to other authorities as required by federal, state, or local laws. When *B. anthracis* is isolated in an unregistered laboratory, the organism must either be destroyed on-site by a recognized sterilization or inactivation process or be transferred to a registered laboratory within 7 days. Shipping of this agent requires completion of the APHIS/CDC Form 2 and prior approval from either CDC or APHIS.

ANTIMICROBIAL SUSCEPTIBILITIES

B. anthracis

Most strains of *B. anthracis* remain susceptible to penicillin (22, 72). Of 25 genetically diverse isolates from around the world, 3 strains were resistant to penicillin but were negative for β-lactamase production. Most strains give variable susceptibility results for cephalosporins; in vitro results, even if susceptible, may not predict clinical efficacy, particularly for expanded- and broad-spectrum cephalosporins (22). In a study of 50 historical isolates from humans and animals and 15 clinical isolates from the 2001 bioterrorist attack in the United States, the majority of strains could be regarded as not susceptible to the broad-spectrum cephalosporin ceftriaxone, and three strains were resistant to penicillin (72). Tetracyclines, fluoroquinolones, and chloramphenicol are suitable for the treatment of patients allergic to penicillin (but these are not good choices clinically, regardless of in vitro results); most strains in the previously mentioned study showed only intermediate susceptibility to erythromycin (72). Ciprofloxacin and the newer quinolone gatifloxacin had good in vitro activities against 40 Turkish isolates, but for another new quinolone, levofloxacin, it was observed that MICs were high for 10 strains (32). Other in vitro studies have shown novel fluoroquinolones and a ketolide to be of potential therapeutic value (38). Standards for antimicrobial susceptibility testing of *B. anthracis* have been recently adopted (21).

Postexposure prophylaxis is needed for the prevention of inhalation anthrax following a bioterrorist attack; the recommended regimen is 60 days of antibiotic therapy and three doses of anthrax vaccine (19), and recommended antimicrobial agents include ciprofloxacin, doxycycline, and levofloxacin. Amoxicillin is recommended as an option in cases where the *B. anthracis* strain has been demonstrated to be susceptible to penicillins and when other antimicrobial agents are not considered safe, as in the treatment of children and pregnant or lactating women (16, 17). The use of penicillins for postexposure prophylaxis or for treatment of inhalation anthrax following the use of *B. anthracis* as a bioweapon gives cause for concern, owing to the presence of β-lactamases in *B. anthracis* isolates, and the poor penetration of β-lactams into macrophages, the site of spore germination (9). Combination intravenous antibiotic therapy with two or more antibiotics, begun early, such as with ciprofloxacin and one or more other antibiotics to which the organism is sensitive, appeared to improve survival during the treatment of cases during the 2001 outbreak in the United States (58). Following that outbreak, the recommendation for initial treatment of inhalation anthrax is ciprofloxacin or doxycycline along with one or more agents to which the organism is normally susceptible (15).

B. cereus

There have been rather few studies of the antibiotic sensitivity of *B. cereus*, and most information has to be gleaned from the reports of individual cases or outbreaks. *B. cereus* and *B. thuringiensis* produce a broad-spectrum β-lactamase and are thus resistant to penicillin, ampicillin, and cephalosporins; they are also resistant to trimethoprim. An in vitro study of 54 isolates from blood cultures by disk diffusion assay found that all strains were susceptible to imipenem and vancomycin and that most were sensitive to chloramphenicol, ciprofloxacin, erythromycin, and gentamicin (but a small number of strains showed moderate or intermediate sensitivity), while 22 and 37% of strains showed only moderate or intermediate susceptibilities to clindamycin and tetracycline, respectively (109). Although strains are almost always susceptible to clindamycin, erythromycin, chloramphenicol, vancomycin, and the aminoglycosides and are usually sensitive to tetracycline and sulfonamides, there have been several reports of treatment failures with some of these drugs: a fulminant meningitis which did not respond to chloramphenicol (69); a fulminant infection in a neonate which was refractory to treatment that included vancomycin, gentamicin, imipenem, clindamycin, and ciprofloxacin (100); failure of vancomycin to eliminate the organism from cerebrospinal fluid in association with a fluid shunt infection (10); and persistent bacteremias with strains showing resistance to vancomycin in two hemodialysis patients (A. von Gottberg and W. van Nierop, personal communication). Oral ciprofloxacin has been used successfully in the treatment of *B. cereus* wound infections, bacteremia, and pulmonary infection. Clindamycin with gentamicin, given early, appears to be the best treatment for ophthalmic infections caused by *B. cereus*, and experiments with rabbits suggest that intravitreal corticosteroids and antibiotics may be effective in such cases.

Other Species

Information on treatment of infections with other species is sparse. Gentamicin was effective in treating a case of *B. licheniformis* ophthalmitis, and cephalosporin was effective against *B. licheniformis* bacteremia/septicemia. Resistance to macrolides appears to occur naturally in *B. licheniformis*. *B. subtilis* endocarditis in a drug abuser was successfully treated with cephalosporin, and gentamicin was successful against a *B. subtilis* septicemia. Penicillin, or its derivatives, or cephalosporins probably form the best first choices for treatment of infections attributed to other *Bacillus* species. In the study by Weber et al. (109), over 95% of isolates of *B. megaterium*, *B. pumilus*, *B. subtilis*, *B. circulans*, *B. amyloliquefaciens*, and *B. licheniformis*, along with strains of *B.* (now *Paenibacillus*) *polymyxa* and three unidentified strains from blood cultures, were susceptible to imipenem, ciprofloxacin, and vancomycin; between 75 and 90% were susceptible to penicillins, cephalosporins, and chloramphenicol. Isolates of "*B. polymyxa*" and *B. circulans* were more likely to be resistant to the penicillins and cephalosporins than strains of the other species—it is probable that some or all of the strains identified as *B. circulans* might now be accommodated in *Paenibacillus*, along with "*B. polymyxa*." An infection of a human bite wound with an organism identified as *B. circulans* did not respond to treatment with amoxicillin and flucloxacillin but was resolved with clindamycin (43).

A strain of *B. circulans* showing vancomycin resistance has been isolated from an Italian clinical specimen (64). Vancomycin resistance has been reported for *Paenibacillus popilliae*, a biopesticide, and isolates of this species have been shown to carry genes resembling those responsible for high-level vancomycin resistance in enterococci (78). Of two South African vancomycin-resistant clinical isolates, one was identified as *P. thiaminolyticus* and the other was unidentified but considered to be related to *B. lentus*; the latter was isolated from a case of neonatal sepsis and has been shown to have inducible resistance to vancomycin and teicoplanin; this is in contrast to the *B. circulans* and *P. thiaminolyticus* isolates mentioned above, in which expression of resistance was found to be constitutive (von Gottberg and van Nierop, personal communication).

REFERENCES

1. **Andersson, M. A., R. Mikkola, J. Helin, M. C. Andersson, and M. Salkinoja-Salonen.** 1998. A novel sensitive bioassay for detection of *Bacillus cereus* emetic toxin and related depsipeptide ionophores. *Appl. Environ. Microbiol.* **64:**1338–1343.
2. **Andreotti, P. E., G. V. Ludwig, A. H. Peruski, J. J. Tuite, S. S. Morse, and L. F. Peruski.** 2003. Immunoassay of infectious agents. *BioTechniques* **35:**850–859.
3. **Apetroaie, C., M. A. Andersson, C. Sproer, I. Tsitko, R. Shaheen, E. L. Jaaskelainen, L. M. Wijnands, R. Heikkila, and M. S. Salkinoja-Salonen.** 2005. Cereulide-producing strains of *Bacillus cereus* show diversity. *Arch. Microbiol.* **184:**141–151.
4. **Ash, C., J. A. Farrow, M. Dorsch, E. Stackebrandt, and M. D. Collins.** 1991. Comparative analysis of *Bacillus anthracis*, *Bacillus cereus*, and related species on the basis of reverse transcriptase sequencing of 16S rRNA. *Int. J. Syst. Bacteriol.* **41:**343–346.
5. **Ash, C., F. G. Priest, and M. D. Collins.** 1993. Molecular identification of rRNA group 3 bacilli (Ash, Farrow, Wallbanks and Collins) using a PCR probe test. *Antonie Leeuwenhoek* **64:**253–260.
6. **Baggett, H. C., J. C. Rhodes, S. K. Fridkin, C. P. Quinn, J. C. Hageman, C. R. Friedman, C. A. Dykewicz, V. A. Semenova, S. Romero-Steiner, C. M. Elie, and J. A. Jernigan.** 2001. No evidence of a mild form of inhalational *Bacillus anthracis* infection during a bioterrorism-related inhalational anthrax outbreak in Washington, D.C. *Clin. Infect. Dis.* **41:**991–997.
7. **Banerjee, C., C. I. Bustamante, R. Wharton, E. Talley, and J. C. Wade.** 1988. *Bacillus* infections in patients with cancer. *Arch. Intern. Med.* **148:**1769–1774.
8. **Bell, C. A., J. R. Uhl, T. L. Hadfield, J. C. David, R. F. Meyer, T. F. Smith, and F. R. Cockerill.** 2002. Detection of *Bacillus anthracis* DNA by LightCycler PCR. *J. Clin. Microbiol.* **40:**2897–2902.
9. **Bell, D. M., S. Blank, P. E. Kozarsky, and D. S. Stephens.** 2002. Clinical issues in the prophylaxis, diagnosis, and treatment of anthrax. *Emerg. Infect. Dis.* **8:**222–225.
10. **Berne, R., F. Heinen, K. Pelz, V. van Velthoven, M. Sauer, and R. Korinthenberg.** 1997. Ventricular shunt infection and meningitis due to *Bacillus cereus*. *Neuropediatrics* **28:**333–334.
11. **Bishop, A. H.** 2002. *Bacillus thuringiensis* insecticides, p. 160–175. *In* R. C. W. Berkeley, M. Heyndrickx, N. A. Logan, and P. De Vos (ed.), *Applications and Systematics of* Bacillus *and Relatives*. Blackwell Science, Oxford, United Kingdom.
12. **Brachman, P., and A. Kaufmann.** 1998. Anthrax, p. 95–107. *In* A. Evans and P. Brachman (ed.), *Bacterial Infections of Humans*. Plenum Medical Book Company, New York, N.Y.
13. **Burans, J., A. Keleher, T. O'Brien, J. Hager, A. Plummer, and C. Morgan.** 1996. Rapid method for the diagnosis of

Bacillus anthracis infection in clinical samples using a handheld assay. *Salisbury Med. Bull.* **87**(Spec. Suppl.):36–37.

14. **Callegan, M. C., D. C. Cochran, S. T. Kane, M. S. Gilmore, M. Gominet, and D. Lereclus.** 2002. Contribution of membrane-damaging toxins to *Bacillus* endophthalmitis pathogenesis. *Infect. Immun.* **70:**5381–5389.
15. **Centers for Disease Control and Prevention.** 2001. Update: investigation of bioterrorism-related anthrax and interim guidelines for exposure management and antimicrobial therapy. *Morb. Mortal. Wkly. Rep.* **50:**909.
16. **Centers for Disease Control and Prevention.** 2001. Interim recommendations for antimicrobial prophylaxis for children and breastfeeding mothers and treatment of children with anthrax. *Morb. Mortal. Wkly. Rep.* **50:**1014–1016.
17. **Centers for Disease Control and Prevention.** 2001. Updated recommendations for antimicrobial prophylaxis among asymptomatic pregnant women after exposure to *Bacillus anthracis*. *Morb. Mortal. Wkly. Rep.* **50:**960.
18. **Centers for Disease Control and Prevention.** 2002. Suspected cutaneous anthrax in a laboratory worker-Texas (2002). *Morb. Mortal. Wkly. Rep.* **51:**279–281.
19. **Centers for Disease Control and Prevention.** 2004. Responding to detection of aerosolized *Bacillus anthracis* by autonomous detection systems in the workplace. *Morb. Mortal. Wkly. Rep.* **53**(RR07):1–12.
20. **Centers for Disease Control and Prevention and National Institutes of Health.** 1999. *Biosafety in Microbiological Laboratories*, 4th ed. U.S. Government Printing Office, Washington, D.C.
21. **Clinical and Laboratory Standards Institute.** 2005. *Performance Standards for Antimicrobial Susceptibility Testing: 15th Informational Supplement.* CLSI document M100-S15. CLSI, Wayne, Pa.
22. **Coker, P. R., K. L. Smith, and M. Hugh-Jones.** 2002. Antimicrobial susceptibilities of diverse *Bacillus anthracis* isolates. *Antimicrob. Agents Chemother.* **46:**3843–3845.
23. **Cone, L. A., L. Dreisbach, B. E. Potts, B. E. Comess, and W. A. Burleigh.** 2005. Fatal *Bacillus cereus* endocarditis masquerading as an anthrax-like infection in a patient with acute lymphoblastic leukemia: case report. *J. Heart Valve Dis.* **14:** 37–39.
24. **Damgaard, P. H., P. E. Granum, J. Bresciani, M. V. Torregrossa, J. Eilenberg, and L. Valentino.** 1997. Characterization of *Bacillus thuringiensis* isolated from infections in burn wounds. *FEMS Immunol. Med. Microbiol.* **18:**47–53.
25. **Darbar, A., I. A. Harris, and I. B. Gosbell.** 2005. Necrotizing infection due to *Bacillus cereus* mimicking gas gangrene following penetrating trauma. *J. Orthop. Trauma* **19:**353–355.
26. **Das, T., K. Choudhury, S. Sharma, S. Jalali, and R. Nuthethi.** 2001. Clinical profile and outcome in *Bacillus* endophthalmitis. *Ophthalmology* **108:**1819–1825.
27. **De, B. K., S. L. Bragg, G. N. Sanden, K. E. Wilson, L. A. Diem, C. K. Marston, A. R. Hoffmaster, G. A. Barnett, R. S. Weyant, T. G. Abshire, J. W. Ezzell, and T. Popovic.** 2002. Two-component direct fluorescent-antibody assay for rapid identification of *Bacillus anthracis*. *Emerg. Infect. Dis.* **8:**1060–1065.
28. **De Clerck, E., D. Gevers, K. Sergeant, M. Rodríguez-Díaz, L. Herman, N. A. Logan, J. Van Beeumen, and P. De Vos.** 2004. Genotypic and phenotypic comparison of *Bacillus fumarioli* isolates from geothermal Antarctic soil and gelatine. *Res. Microbiol.* **155:**483–490.
29. **Drago, L., A. Lombardi, E. De Vecchi, and M. R. Gismondo.** 2002. Real-time PCR assay for rapid detection of *Bacillus anthracis* spores in clinical samples. *J. Clin. Microbiol.* **40:**4399.
30. **Easterday, W. R., M. N. Van Ert, S. Zanecki, and P. Keim.** 2005. Specific detection of *Bacillus anthracis* using a TaqMan mismatch amplification mutation assay. *BioTechniques* **38:** 731–735.
31. **Ehling-Schulz, M., M. Fricker, and S. Scherer.** 2004. *Bacillus cereus*, the causative agent of an emetic type of food-borne illness. *Mol. Nutr. Food Res.* **48:**479–487.
32. **Esel, D., M. Doganay, and B. Sumerkan.** 2003. Antimicrobial susceptibilities of 40 isolates of *Bacillus anthracis* isolated in Turkey. *Int. J. Antimicrob. Agents* **22:**70–72.
33. **Ezzell, J. W., Jr., T. G. Abshire, S. F. Little, B. C. Lidgerding, and C. Brown.** 1990. Identification of *Bacillus anthracis* by using monoclonal antibody to cell wall galactose-*N*-acetylglucosamine polysaccharide. *J. Clin. Microbiol.* **28:**223–231.
34. **Fennelly, K. P., A. L. Davidow, S. L. Miller, N. Connell, and J. J. Ellner.** 2004. Airborne infection with *Bacillus anthracis*—from mills to mail. *Emerg. Infect. Dis.* **10:**996–1001.
35. **Finlay, W. J. J., N. A. Logan, and A. D. Sutherland.** 1999. Semiautomated metabolic staining assay for *Bacillus cereus* emetic toxin. *Appl. Environ. Microbiol.* **65:**1811–1812.
36. **Fletcher, P., and N. A. Logan.** 1999. Improved cytotoxicity assay for *Bacillus cereus* diarrhoeal enterotoxin. *Lett. Appl. Microbiol.* **28:**394–400.
37. **Fortina, M. G., R. Pukall, P. Schumann, D. Mora, C. Parini, P. L. Manachini, and E. Stackebrandt.** 2001. *Ureibacillus* gen. nov., a new genus to accommodate *Bacillus thermosphaericus* (Andersson *et al.* 1995), emendation of *Ureibacillus thermosphaericus* and description of *Ureibacillus terrenus* sp. nov. *Int. J. Syst. Evol. Microbiol.* **51:** 447–455.
38. **Frean, J., K. P. Klugman, L. Arntzen, and S. Bukofzer.** 2003. Susceptibility of *Bacillus anthracis* to eleven antimicrobial agents including novel fluoroquinolones and a ketolide. *J. Antimicrob. Chemother.* **52:**297–299.
39. **Galanos, J., S. Perera, H. Smith, D. O'Neal, H. Sheorey, and M. J. Waters.** 2003. Bacteremia due to three *Bacillus* species in a case of Munchausen's syndrome. *J. Clin. Microbiol.* **41:**2247–2248.
40. **Gerberding, J. L., J. M. Hughes, and J. P. Koplan.** 2005. Bioterrorism preparedness and response: clinicians and public health agencies as essential partners. *JAMA* **287:**989–900.
41. **Gill, S. R., D. E. Fouts, G. L. Archer, E. F. Mongodin, R. T. Deboy, J. Ravel, I. T. Paulsen, J. F. Kolonay, L. Brinkac, M. Beanan, R. J. Dodson, S. C. Daugherty, R. Madupu, S. V. Angiuoli, A. S. Durkin, D. H. Haft, J. Vamathevan, H. Khouri, T. Utterback, C. Lee, G. Dimitrov, L. Jiang, H. Qin, J. Weidman, K. Tran, K. Kang, I. R. Hance, K. E. Nelson, and C. M. Fraser.** 2005. Insights on evolution of virulence and resistance from the complete genome analysis of an early methicillin-resistant *Staphylococcus aureus* strain and a biofilm-producing methicillin-resistant *Staphylococcus epidermidis* strain. *J. Bacteriol.* **187:**2426–2438.
42. **Gordon, R. E., W. C. Haynes, and C. H.-N. Pang.** 1973. *The Genus* Bacillus. Agriculture Handbook 427. U.S. Department of Agriculture, Washington, D.C.
43. **Goudswaard, W. B., M. H. Dammer, and C. Hol.** 1995. *Bacillus circulans* infection of a proximal interphalangeal joint after a clenched-fist injury caused by human teeth. *Eur. J. Clin. Microbiol. Infect. Dis.* **14:**1015–1016.
44. **Granum, P. E.** 2002. *Bacillus cereus* and food poisoning, p. 35–46. *In* R. C. W. Berkeley, M. Heyndrickx, N. A. Logan, and P. de Vos (ed.), *Applications and Systematics of* Bacillus *and Relatives*. Blackwell Science, Oxford, United Kingdom.
45. **Guarner, J., J. A. Jernigan, W. J. Sheh, K. Tatti, L. M. Flannagan, D. S. Stephens, T. Popovic, D. A. Ashford, B. A. Perkins, S. R. Zaki, and the Inhalational Anthrax Pathology Working Group.** 2003. Pathology and pathogenesis of bioterrorism-related inhalational anthrax. *Am. J. Pathol.* **163:**701–709.

46. **Hannah, W., and P. T. Ender.** 1999. Persistent *Bacillus licheniformis* bacteraemia associated with an intentional injection of organic drain cleaner. *Clin. Infect. Dis.* **29:**659–661.
47. **Helgason, E., D. A. Caugant, I. Olsen, and A.-B. Kolstø.** 2000. Genetic structure of population of *Bacillus cereus* and *B. thuringiensis* isolates associated with periodontitis and other human infections. *J. Clin. Microbiol.* **38:**1615–1622.
48. **Helgason, E., N. J. Tourasse, R. Meisal, D. A. Caugant, and A. B. Kolstø.** 2004. Multilocus sequence typing scheme for bacteria of the *Bacillus cereus* group. *Appl. Environ. Microbiol.* **70:**191–201.
49. **Hernaiz, C., A. Picardo, J. I. Alos, and J. L. Gomez-Garces.** 2003. Nosocomial bacteremia and catheter infection by *Bacillus cereus* in an immunocompetent patient. *Clin. Microbiol. Infect.* **9:**973–975.
50. **Heyndrickx, M., L. Lebbe, M. Vancanneyt, K. Kersters, P. De Vos, G. Forsyth, and N. A. Logan.** 1998. *Virgibacillus:* a new genus to accommodate *Bacillus pantothenticus* (Proom and Knight 1950). Emended description of *Virgibacillus pantothenticus. Int. J. Syst. Bacteriol.* **48:**99–106.
51. **Heyrman, J., A. Balcaen, L. Lebbe, M. Rodriguez-Diaz, N. A. Logan, J. Swings, and P. De Vos.** 2003. *Virgibacillus carmonensis* sp. nov., *Virgibacillus necropolis* sp. nov. and *Virgibacillus picturae* sp. nov., three new species isolated from deteriorated mural paintings, transfer of the species of the genus *Salibacillus* to *Virgibacillus*, as *Virgibacillus marismortui* comb. nov. and *Virgibacillus salexigens* comb. nov., and emended description of the genus *Virgibacillus. Int. J. Syst. Evol. Microbiol.* **53:**501–511.
52. **Hoffmaster, A. R., C. C. Fitzgerald, E. Ribot, L. W. Mayer, and T. Popovic.** 2002. Molecular subtyping of *B. anthracis* and the 2001 bioterrorism-associated anthrax outbreak, United States. *Emerg. Infect. Dis.* **8:**1111–1116.
53. **Hoffmaster, A. R., R. F. Meyer, M. P. Bowen, C. K. Marston, R. S. Weyant, G. A. Barnet, J. J. Sejvar, J. A. Jernigan, B. A. Perkins, and T. Popovic.** 2002. Evaluation and validation of a real-time polymerase chain reaction assay for rapid identification of *Bacillus anthracis. Emerg. Infect. Dis.* **8:**1178–1181.
54. **Hoffmaster, A. R., J. Ravel, D. A. Rasko, G. D. Chapman, M. D. Chute, C. K. Marston, B. K. De, C. T. Sacchi, C. Fitzgerald, L. W. Mayer, M. C. Maiden, F. G. Priest, M. Barker, L. Jiang, R. Z. Cer, J. Rilstone, S. N. Peterson, R. S. Weyant, D. R. Galloway, T. D. Read, T. Popovic, and C. M. Fraser.** 2004. Identification of anthrax toxin genes in a *Bacillus cereus* associated with an illness resembling inhalation anthrax. *Proc. Natl. Acad. Sci. USA* **101:**8449–8454.
55. **Hurtle, W., E. Bode, R. S. Kaplan, J. Garrison, B. Kearney, D. Shoemaker, E. Henchal and D. Norwood.** 2003. Use of denaturing high-performance liquid chromatography to identify *Bacillus anthracis* by analysis of the 16S-23S rRNA interspacer region and *gyrA* gene. *J. Clin. Microbiol.* **41:** 4758–4766.
56. **Hurtle, W., E. Bode, D. A. Kulesh, R. S. Kaplan, J. Garrison, D. Bridge, M. House, M. S. Frye, B. Loveless, and D. Norwood.** 2004. Detection of the *Bacillus anthracis gyrA* gene by using a minor groove binder probe. *J. Clin. Microbiol.* **42:**179–185.
57. **Inglesby, T. V., T. O'Toole, D. A . Henderson, J. G. Bartlett, M. S. Ascher, E. Eitzen, A. M. Friedlander, J. Gerberding, J. Hauer, J. Hughes, J. McDade, M. T. Osterholm, G. Parker, T. M. Perl, P. K. Russell, and K. Tonat.** 2002. Anthrax as a biological weapon, 2002. Updated recommendations for management. *JAMA* **287:**2236–2252.
58. **Jernigan, J. A., D. S. Stephens, D. A. Ashford, C. Omenaca, M. S. Topiel, M. Galbraith, M. Tapper, T. L. Fisk, S. Zaki, T. Popovic, R. F. Meyer, C. P. Quinn, S. A. Harper, S. K. Fridkin, J. J. Sejvar, C. W. Shepard, M. McConnell, J. Guarner, W.-J. Shieh, J. M. Malecki, J. L. Gerberding, J. M. Hughes, and B. A. Perkins.** 2002. Anthrax bioterrorism investigation. Bioterrorism-related inhalational anthrax: the first 10 cases reported in the United States. *Emerg. Infect. Dis.* **7:**933–944.
59. **Keim, P., L. B. Price, A. M. Klevytska, K. L. Smith, J. M. Schupp, R. Okinaka, P. J. Jackson, and M. E. Hugh-Jones.** 2000. Multiple-locus variable-number tandem repeat analysis reveals genetic relationships within *Bacillus anthracis. J. Bacteriol.* **182:**2928–2936.
60. **Keim, P., M. N. Van Ert, T. Pearson, A. J. Vogler, L. Y. Huynh, and D. M. Wagner.** 2004. Anthrax molecular epidemiology and forensics: using the appropriate marker for different evolutionary scales. *Infect. Genet. Evol.* **4:**205–213.
61. **Knisely, R. F.** 1966. Selective medium for *Bacillus anthracis. J. Bacteriol.* **92:**784–786.
62. **Kotiranta, A., K. Lunatmaa, and M. Haapasalo.** 2000. Epidemiology and pathogenesis of *Bacillus cereus* infections. *Microbes Infect.* **2:**189–198.
63. **Kramer, J. M., and R. J. Gilbert.** 1989. *Bacillus cereus* and other *Bacillus* species, p. 21–70. *In* M. Doyle (ed.), *Foodborne Bacterial Pathogens.* Marcel Dekker, New York, N.Y.
64. **Ligozzi, M., G. L. Cascio, and R. Fontana.** 1998. *vanA* gene cluster in a vancomycin-resistant clinical isolate of *Bacillus circulans. Antimicrob. Agents Chemother.* **42:**2055–2059.
65. **Liu, P. Y. F., S. C. Ke, and S. L. Chen.** 1997. Use of pulsed field electrophoresis to investigate a pseudo-outbreak of *Bacillus cereus* in a pediatric unit. *J. Clin. Microbiol.* **35:**1533–1535.
66. **Logan, N. A.** 1988. *Bacillus* species of medical and veterinary importance. *J. Med. Microbiol.* **25:**157–165.
67. **Logan, N. A.** 2002. Modern identification methods, p. 123–140. *In* R. C. W. Berkeley, M. Heyndrickx, N. A. Logan, and P. de Vos (ed.), *Applications and Systematics of* Bacillus *and Relatives.* Blackwell Science, Oxford, United Kingdom.
68. **Logan, N. A., G. Forsyth, L. Lebbe, J. Goris, M. Heyndrickx, A. Balcaen, A. Verhelst, E. Falsen, Å. Ljungh, H. B. Hansson, and P. De Vos.** 2002. Polyphasic identification of *Bacillus* and *Brevibacillus* strains from clinical, dairy, and industrial specimens and proposal of *Brevibacillus invocatus* sp. nov. *Int. J. Syst. Evol. Microbiol.* **52:**953–966.
69. **Marshman, L. A. G., C. Hardwidge, and P. M. W. Donaldson.** 2000. *Bacillus cereus* meningitis complicating cerebrospinal fluid fistula repair and spinal drainage. *Brit. J. Neurosurg.* **14:**580–582.
70. **Mikkola, R., M. Kolari, M. A. Andersson, J. Helin, and M. S. Salkinoja-Salonen.** 2000. Toxic lactonic lipopeptide from food poisoning isolates of *Bacillus licheniformis. Eur. J. Biochem.* **267:**4068–4074.
71. **Mikkola, R., M. A. Andersson, P. Grigoriev, V. V. Teplova, N.-E. L. Saris, F. A. Rainey, and M. S. Salkinoja-Salonen.** 2004. Toxic lactonic lipopeptide from food poisoning isolates of *Bacillus amyloliquefaciens* strains isolated from moisture-damaged buildings produced surfactin and a substance toxic to mammalian cells. *Arch. Microbiol.* **181:**314–323.
72. **Mohammed, M. J., C. H. Marston, T. Popovic, R. S. Weyant, and F. C. Tenover.** 2002. Antimicrobial susceptibility testing of *Bacillus anthracis*: comparison of results obtained by using the National Committee for Clinical Laboratory Standards broth microdilution reference and Etest agar gradient diffusion methods. *J. Clin. Microbiol.* **40:**1902–1907.
73. **Mollet, C., M. Drancourt, and D. Raoult.** 1997. *rpoB* sequence analysis as a novel basis for bacterial identification. *Mol. Microbiol.* **26:**1005–1011.
74. **Morse, S. A., R. B. Kellogg, S. Perry, R. F. Meyer, D. Bray, D. Nichelson, and J. M. Miller.** 2003. Detecting biothreat agents: the laboratory response network. *ASM News* **69:**433–437.

75. **Nazina, T. N., T. P., Tourova, A. B. Poltaraus, E. V. Novikova, A. A. Grigoryan, A. E. Ivanova, A. M. Lysenko, V. V. Petrunyaka, G. A. Osipov, S. S. Belyaev, and M. V. Ivanov.** 2001. Taxonomic study of aerobic thermophilic bacilli: descriptions of *Geobacillus subterraneus* gen nov, sp. nov. and *Geobacillus uzenensis* sp. nov. from petroleum reservoirs and transfer of *Bacillus stearothermophilus, Bacillus thermocatenulatus, Bacillus thermoleovorans, Bacillus kaustophilus, Bacillus thermoglucosidasius, Bacillus thermodenitrificans* to *Geobacillus* as *Geobacillus stearothermophilus, Geobacillus thermocatenulatus, Geobacillus thermoleovorans, Geobacillus kaustophilus, Geobacillus thermoglucosidasius, Geobacillus thermodenitrificans. Int. J. Syst. Evol. Microbiol.* **51:**433–446.

76. **Oggioni, M., G. Pozzi, P. E. Valensis, P. Galieni, and C. Bigazzi.** 1998. Recurrent septicemia in an immunocompromised patient due to probiotic strains of *Bacillus subtilis. J. Clin. Microbiol.* **36:**325–326.

77. **Oncu, S., S. Oncu, and S. Sakarya.** 2003. Anthrax—an overview. *Med. Sci. Monit.* **9:**RA276–283.

78. **Patel, R., K. Piper, F. R. Cockerill, J. M. Steckelberg, and A. A. Yousten.** 2000. The biopesticide *Paenibacillus popilliae* has a vancomycin resistance gene cluster homologous to the enterococcal VanA vancomycin gene custer. *Antimicrob. Agents Chemother.* **44:**705–709.

79. **Peters, C. J., and D. M. Hartley.** 2002. Anthrax inhalation and lethal human infection. *Lancet* **359:**710–711.

80. **Pinna, A., L. A. Sechi, S. Zanetti, D. Esai, G. Delogu, P. Cappuccinelli, and F. Carta.** 2001. *Bacillus cereus* keratitis associated with contact lens wear. *Ophthalmology* **108:**1830–1834.

81. **Priest, F. G., M. Barker, L. W. Baillie, E. C. Holmes, and M. C. Maiden.** 2004. Population structure and evolution of the *Bacillus cereus* group. *J. Bacteriol.* **186:**7959–7970.

82. **Qi, Y., G. Patra, X. Liang, L. E. Williams, S. Rose, R. J. Redkar, and V. G. DelVecchio.** 2001. Utilization of the *rpoB* gene as a specific chromosomal marker for real-time PCR detection of *Bacillus anthracis. Appl. Environ. Microbiol.* **67:**3720–3727.

83. **Quinn, C. P., P. M. Dull, V. Semenova, H. Li, S. Crotty, T. H. Taylor, E. Steward-Clark, K. L. Stamey, D. S. Schmidt, K. W. Stinson, A. E. Freeman, C. M. Elie, S. K. Martin, C. Greene, R. D. Aubert, J. Glidewell, B. A. Perkins, R. Ahmed, and D. S . Stephens.** 2004. Immune responses to *Bacillus anthracis* protective antigen in patients with bioterrorism-related cutaneous or inhalation anthrax. *J. Infect. Dis.* **190:**1228–1236.

84. **Quinn, C. P., and P. C. B. Turnbull.** 1998. Anthrax, p. 799–818. *In* W. J. Hausler and M. Sussman, *Topley and Wilson's Microbiology and Microbial Infection,* 9th ed. Edward Arnold, London, United Kingdom.

85. **Quinn, C. P., V. A. Semenova, C. M. Elie, S. Romero-Steiner, C. Greene, H. Li, K. Stamey, E. Steward-Clark, D. S. Schmidt, E. Mothershed, J. Pruckler, S. Schwartz, R. F. Benson, L. O. Helsel, P. F. Holder, S. E. Johnson, M. Kellum, T. Messmer, W. L. Thacker, L. Besser, B. D. Plikaytis, T. H. Taylor, Jr., A. E. Freeman, K. J. Wallace, P. Dull, J. Sejvar, E. Bruce, R. Moreno, A. Schuchat, J. R. Lingappa, S. K. Martin, J. Walls, M. Bronsdon, G. M. Carlone, M. Bajani-Ari, D. A. Ashford, D. S. Stephens, and B. A. Perkins.** 2002. Specific, sensitive, and quantitative enzyme-linked immunosorbent assay for human immunoglobulin G antibodies to anthrax toxin protective antigen. *Emerg. Infect. Dis.* **8:**1103–1110.

86. **Read, T. D., S. N. Peterson, N. Tourasse, L. W. Baillie, I. T. Paulsen, K. E. Nelson, H. Tettelin, D. E. Fouts, J. A. Eisen, S. R. Gill, E. K. Holtzapple, O. K. Okstad, E. Helgason, J. Rilstone, M. Wu, J. F. Kolonay, M. J. Beanan, R. J. Dodson, L. M. Brinkac, M. Gwinn, R. T. DeBoy, R. Madpu, S. C. Daugherty, A. S. Durkin, D. H. Haft, W. C. Nelson, J. D. Peterson, M. Pop, H. M. Khouri, D. Radune, J. L. Benton, Y. Mahamoud, L. Jiang, I. R. Hance, J. F. Weidman, K. J. Berry, R. D. Plaut, A. M. Wolf, K. L. Watkins, W. C. Nierman, A. Hazen, R. Cline, C. Redmond, J. E. Thwaite, O. White, S. L. Salzberg, B. Thomason, A. M. Friedlander, T. M. Koehler, P. C. Hanna, A. B. Kolsto, and C. M. Fraser.** 2003. The genome sequence of *Bacillus anthracis* Ames and comparison to closely related bacteria. *Nature* **423:**81–86.

87. **Rider, T. H., M. S. Petrovick, F. E. Nargi, J. D. Harper, E. D. Schwoebel, R. H. Mathews, D. J. Blanchard, L. T. Bortolin, A. M. Young, J. Chen, and M. A. Hollis.** 2003. A B cell-based sensor for rapid identification of pathogens. *Science* **301:**213–215.

88. **Ripabelli, G., J. McLauchlin, V. Mithani, and E. J. Threlfall.** 2000. Epidemiological typing of *Bacillus cereus* by amplified fragment length polymorphism. *Lett. Appl. Microbiol.* **30:**358–363.

89. **Roy, M., J. C. Chen, M. Miller, D. Boyaner, O. Kasner, and E. Edelstein.** 1997. Epidemic *Bacillus* endophthalmitis after cataract surgery. *Ophthalmology* **104:**1768–1772.

90. **Rubinstein, I., and G. W. Pedersen.** 2002. *Bacillus* species are present in chewing tobacco sold in the United States and evoke plasma exudation from the oral mucosa. *Clin. Diagn. Lab. Immunol.* **9:**1057–1060.

91. **Sacchi, C. T., A. M. Whitney, L. W. Mayer, R. Morey, A. Steigerwalt, A. Boras, R. S. Weyant, and T. Popovic.** 2002. Sequencing of 16S rRNA gene: a rapid tool for identification of *Bacillus anthracis. Emerg. Infect. Dis.* **8:** 1117–1123.

92. **Sejvar, J. J., F. C. Tenover, and D. S. Stephens.** 2005. Management of anthrax meningitis. *Lancet Infect. Dis.* **5:**287–295.

93. **Shida, O., H. Takagi, K. Kadowaki, and K. Komagata.** 1996. Proposal for two new genera, *Brevibacillus* gen. nov. and *Aneurinibacillus* gen. nov. *Int. J. Syst. Bacteriol.* **46:** 939–946.

94. **Shieh, W. J., J. Guarner, C. Paddock, P. Greer, K. Tatti, M. Fischer, M. Layton, M. Philips, E. Bresnitz, C. P. Quinn, T. Popovic, B. A. Perkins, S. R. Zaki, and the Anthrax Bioterrorism Investigation Team.** 2003. The critical role of pathology in the investigation of bioterrorism-related cutaneous anthrax. *Am. J. Pathol.* **163:**1901–1910.

95. **Shlyakhov, E., and E. Rubinstein.** 1994. Human live anthrax vaccine in the former USSR. *Vaccine* **12:**727–730.

96. **Sirisanthana, T., and A. E. Brown.** 2002. Anthrax of the gastrointestinal tract. *Emerg. Infect. Dis.* **8:**649–651.

97. **Spinosa, M. R., F. Wallet, R. J. Courcol, and M. R. Oggioni.** 2000. The trouble in tracing opportunistic pathogens: cholangitis due to *Bacillus* in a French hospital caused by a strain related to an Italian product? *Microb. Ecol. Health Dis.* **12:**99–101.

98. **Suominen, I., M. A. Andersson, M. C. Andersson, A. M. Hallaksella, P. Kämpfer, F. A. Rainey, and M. Salkinoja-Salonen.** 2001. Toxic *Bacillus pumilus* from indoor air, recycled paper pulp, Norway spruce, food poisoning outbreaks and clinical samples. *Syst. Appl. Microbiol.* **24:**267–276.

99. **Teng, J. L. L., P. C. Y. Woo, K. W. Leung, S. K. P. Lau, M. K. M. Wong, and K. Y. Yuen.** 2003. Pseudobacteraemia in a patient with neutropenic fever caused by a novel paenibacillus species: *Paenibacillus hongkongensis* sp. nov. *J. Clin. Pathol. Mol. Pathol.* **56:** 29–35.

100. **Tuladhar, R., S. K. Patole, T. H. Koh, R. Norton, and J. S. Whitehall.** 2000. Refractory *Bacillus cereus* infection in a neonate. *Int. J. Clin. Pract.* **54:**345–347.

101. **Turnbull, P. C. B.** 2000. Current status of immunization against anthrax: old vaccines may be here to stay for a while. *Curr. Opin. Infect. Dis.* **13:**113–120.
102. **Turnbull, P. C. B., R. A. Hutson, M. J. Ward, M. N. Jones, C. P. Quinn, N. J . Finnie, C. J. Duggleby, J. M. Kramer, and J. Melling.** 1992. *Bacillus anthracis* but not always anthrax. *J. Appl. Bacteriol.* **72:**21–28.
103. **Turnbull, P. C. B., R. Böhm, O. Cosivi, M. Doganay, M. E. Hugh-Jones, D. D. Joshi, M. K. Lalitha, and V. de Vos.** 1998. *Guidelines for the Surveillance and Control of Anthrax in Humans and Animals;* 3rd ed. WHO/EMC/ZDI/98.6. World Health Organization, Geneva, Switzerland.
104. **Turnbull, P. C. B., P. J. Jackson, K. K. Hill, A.-B. Kolstø, P. Keim, and D. J. Beecher.** 2002. Longstanding taxonomic enigmas with the '*Bacillus cereus* group' are on the verge of being resolved by far-reaching molecular developments. Forecasts on the possible outcome by an *ad hoc* team, p. 23–36. *In* R. C. W. Berkeley, M. Heyndrickx, N. A. Logan, and P. de Vos (ed.), *Applications and Systematics of* Bacillus *and Relatives*. Blackwell Science, Oxford, United Kingdom.
105. **Van der Zwet, W. C., G. A. Parlevliet, P. H. Savelkoul, J. Stoof, A. M. Kaiser, A. M. Van Furth, and C. M. Vandenbroucke-Grauls.** 2000. Outbreak of *Bacillus cereus* infections in a neonatal intensive care unit traced to balloons used in manual ventilation. *J. Clin. Microbiol.* **38:**4131–4136.
106. **van Netten, P., and J. M. Kramer.** 1992. Media for the detection and enumeration of *Bacillus cereus* in foods: a review. *Int. J. Food Microbiol.* **17:**85–99.
107. **Wainø, M., B. J. Tindall, P. Schumann, and K. Ingvorsen.** 1999. *Gracilibacillus* gen. nov., with description of *Gracilibacillus halotolerans* gen. nov., sp. nov. : transfer of *Bacillus dipsosauri* to *Gracilibacillus dipsosauri* comb. nov., and *Bacillus salexigens* to the genus *Salibacillus* gen. nov., as *Salibacillus salexigens* comb. nov. *Int. J. Syst. Bacteriol.* **49:**821–831.
108. **Wang, J. C.** 1996. DNA topoisomerases. *Annu. Rev. Biochem.* **65:**635–692.
109. **Weber, D. J., S. M. Saviteer, W. A. Rutala, and C. A. Thomann.** 1988. In vitro susceptibility of *Bacillus* spp. to selected antimicrobial agents. *Antimicrob. Agents Chemother.* **32:**642–645.
110. **Weber, D. J., E. Sickbert-Bennett, M. F. Gergen, and W. A. Rutala.** 2003. Efficacy of selected hand hygiene agents used to remove *Bacillus atrophaeus* (a surrogate of *Bacillus anthracis*) from contaminated hands. *JAMA* **289:**1274–1277.
111. **Whiteaker, J., J. Karns, C. Fenselau, and M. L. Perdue.** 2004. Analysis of *Bacillus anthracis* spores in milk using mass spectrometry. *Foodborne Pathog. Dis.* **1:**185–194.
112. **Wisotzkey, J. D., P. Jurtshuk, Jr., G. E. Fox, G. Deinhard, and K. Poralla.** 1992. Comparative sequence analyses on the 16S rRNA (rDNA) of *Bacillus acidocaldarius, Bacillus acidoterrestris,* and *Bacillus cycloheptanicus* and proposal for creation of a new genus, *Alicyclobacillus* gen. nov. *Int. J. Syst. Bacteriol.* **42:**263–269.
113. **Yoon, J.-H., K.-C. Lee, N. Weiss, Y. H. Kho, K. H. Kang, and Y.-H. Park.** 2001. *Sporosarcina aquimarina* sp. nov., a bacterium isolated from seawater in Korea, and transfer of *Bacillus globisporus* (Larkin and Stokes 1967), *Bacillus psychrophilus* (Nakamura 1984), and *Bacillus pasteurii* (Chester 1898) to the genus *Sporosarcina* as *Sporosarcina globispora* comb. nov., *Sporosarcina psychrophila* comb. nov. and *Sporosarcina pasteurii* comb. nov., and emended description of the genus *Sporosarcina. Int. J. Syst. Evol. Microbiol.* **51:**1079–1086.
114. **Yoon, J.-H., N. Weiss, K.-C. Lee, I.-S. Kho, K. H. Kang, and Y.-H. Park.** 2001. *Jeotgalibacillus alimentarius* gen. nov., sp. nov., a novel bacterium isolated from jeotgal with L-lysine in the cell wall, and reclassification of *Bacillus marinus* Rüger 1983 as *Marinibacillus marinus* gen. nov., comb. nov. *Int. J. Syst. Evol. Microbiol.* **51:** 2087–2093.
115. **Zahavy, E., M. Fisher, A. Bromberg, and U. Olshevsky.** 2003. Detection of frequency resonance energy transfer pair on double-labeled microsphere and *Bacillus anthracis* spores by flow cytometry. *Appl. Env. Microbiol.* **69:** 2330–2339.
116. **Zwick, M. E., F. McAfee, D. J. Cutler, T. D. Read, J. Ravel, G. R. Bowman, D. R. Galloway, and A. Mateczun.** 2005. Microarray-based resequencing of multiple *Bacillus anthracis* isolates. *Genome Biol.* **6:**R10.

Listeria and *Erysipelothrix**

JACQUES BILLE

33

LISTERIA

Taxonomy

Listeria and *Brochothrix* form one of several sublines within the *Clostridium* subdivision. The *Listeria-Brochothrix* subline is approximately equidistant from the *Bacillus* and *Enterococcus-Carnobacterium* sublines. On the basis of 23S rRNA gene sequences, *Listeria* is most similar to *Bacillus* and *Staphylococcus*. Phylogenetically, *Listeria* is sufficiently remote from *Lactobacillus* to justify its exclusion from the family *Lactobacillaceae* and formation of a separate *Listeria-Brochothrix* family (20). The phylogenetic position of *Listeria* is consistent with the low G+C content of its DNA (36 to 42 mol%) (20, 49, 82).

Listeria monocytogenes is the type species and one of six species in the genus *Listeria*. The other species are *L. ivanovii*, *L. innocua*, *L. seeligeri*, *L. welshimeri*, and *L. grayi* (73). Two subspecies of *L. ivanovii* have been described: *L. ivanovii* subsp. *ivanovii* and *L. ivanovii* subsp. *londoniensis*. Based on the results of DNA-DNA hybridization, multilocus enzyme analysis, and 16S rRNA gene sequencing, the six species in the genus *Listeria* are divided into two lines of descent: (i) *L. monocytogenes* and its closely related species, namely, *L. innocua*, *L. ivanovii* (subspecies *ivanovii* and *londoniensis*), *L. welshimeri*, and *L. seeligeri*, and (ii) *L. grayi* (12, 13, 20, 71, 73, 74). Within the genus *Listeria*, only *L. monocytogenes* and *L. ivanovii* are considered to be pathogenic, as evidenced by their 50% lethal doses in mice and their ability to grow in mouse spleen and liver. *L. monocytogenes* is a human pathogen of high public health concern; *L. ivanovii* is primarily an animal pathogen.

Description of the Genus

Members of the genus *Listeria* are asporogenous, nonbranching, regular, short (0.5 to 2 by 0.4 to 0.5 μm), gram-positive rods that occur singly or in short chains. Filaments of 6 to 20 μm long may occur in older or rough cultures. The organisms are motile at 28°C by means of one to five peritrichous flagella but are much less motile at 37°C. Colonies are small (1 to 2 mm in diameter after 1 or 2 days of incubation at 37°C), smooth, and blue-gray on nutrient agar when examined with obliquely transmitted light. The optimum growth temperature is between 30 and 37°C, but growth occurs at 4°C within a few days. *Listeria* spp. are facultatively anaerobic. Catalase is produced except in a few strains (24), and the oxidase test is negative. Acid is produced from D-glucose and other sugars. The Voges-Proskauer and methyl red tests are positive. Esculin is hydrolyzed in a few hours. Urea and gelatin are not hydrolyzed. Neither indole nor H_2S is produced. The cell wall contains a directly cross-linked peptidoglycan based on *meso*-diaminopimelic acid, as well as lipoteichoic acid, but no mycolic acid; the major menaquinone contains seven isoprene units (MK-7). The two predominant cellular fatty acids are $C_{ai15:0}$ and $C_{ai17:0}$ (branched-chain type) (5).

Natural Habitats

Listeria species are widely distributed in the environment. They have been isolated from soil, decaying vegetable matter, silage, sewage, water, animal feed, fresh and frozen poultry, fresh and processed meats, raw milk, cheese, slaughterhouse waste, and asymptomatic human and animal carriers (26). *L. monocytogenes* has been isolated from numerous species of mammals, birds, fish, crustaceans, and insects (25). Nevertheless, the primary habitats of *L. monocytogenes* are considered to be the soil and decaying vegetable matter, in which it survives and grows saprophytically. Because of its widespread occurrence, *L. monocytogenes* has many opportunities to enter food production and processing environments and, because of its ability to grow at 4°C, to cause human disease in persons ingesting colonized food (25, 74).

Clinical Significance

In nonpregnant human adults, *L. monocytogenes* causes primarily meningitis, encephalitis, and/or septicemia (55, 80). Elderly patients or persons with predisposing conditions that lower cell-mediated immunity, such as transplants, lymphomas, and human immunodeficiency virus infection, are especially susceptible. On rare occasions, patients have no known predisposing conditions. The tropism of *L. monocytogenes* for the central nervous system leads to severe disease, often with high mortality (20 to 50%) or with neurologic sequelae among survivors (17). In pregnant women, *L. monocytogenes* often causes an influenza-like bacteremic illness that, if untreated, may lead to placentitis and/or amnionitis and infection of the fetus, resulting in abortion, stillbirth, or premature birth, because the pathogen is able to cross the placenta (46) Early diagnosis can be made in some

*This chapter contains information presented in chapter 33 by Jacques Bille, Jocelyne Rocourt, and Bala Swaminathan in the eighth edition of this Manual.

cases by detecting *L. monocytogenes* in maternal blood cultures; at birth, the diagnosis is made by detecting the organism in cerebrospinal fluid (CSF), blood, amniotic fluid, respiratory secretions, placental or cutaneous swabs, gastric aspirate, or meconium of the neonate. Direct microscopic visualization of gram-positive rods in these specimens may be invaluable in early diagnosis of the disease.

Focal infections rarely occur after an episode of bacteremia. However, primary cutaneous listeriosis with or without bacteremia has been reported among veterinarians and abattoir workers, who acquire the illness through contact with infected animal tissues (53). Endocarditis, arthritis, osteomyelitis, intra-abdominal abscesses, endophthalmitis, and pleuropulmonary infections have been described infrequently (48).

The incubation period and infective dose have not been firmly established. Reported incubation times vary from a few days to 2 to 3 months. Gastrointestinal symptoms such as diarrhea have been observed in some individuals with systemic listeriosis. A transient healthy carrier state exists in 2 to 20% of animals and humans (25, 35). In the past decade, several outbreaks of febrile gastroenteritis caused by *L. monocytogenes* have been documented (38). Implicated foods were chocolate milk, rice salad, corn-and-tuna salad, cold smoked trout, corned beef and ham, delicatessen meat, and cheese. These gastroenteritis outbreaks differ from the invasive outbreaks in several respects. They affect persons with no known predisposing risk factors for listeriosis. Illness typically occurs 24 h after ingestion of a large inoculum of bacteria (1.9×10^5 to 1×10^9 CFU/g or ml) and usually lasts 2 days. Common symptoms include fever, watery diarrhea, nausea, headache, and pain in joints and muscles (63). Therefore, the possibility of infection with *L. monocytogenes* should be considered in investigations of gastroenteritis in which routine enteric pathogens have been ruled out. Cervicovaginal carriage in women (including pregnant ones) seems to be nonexistent.

Listeriosis is observed mainly in industrialized countries. It can occur sporadically or epidemically; in both cases, contaminated foods are the primary mode of transmission. A few limited, non-food-related nosocomial outbreaks, mainly in nurseries, have been described (51) due to cross-infection and on one occasion caused by contaminated mineral oil for bathing (79). The number of sporadic cases of listeriosis in countries that report the illness is typically in the range of 0.5 to 0.8 cases per 100,000 persons (75); during foodborne-disease outbreaks, the incidence may rise to 5 cases per 100,000 persons (8). Foods implicated as vehicles of infection are ready-to-eat food stored at refrigeration temperatures and able to sustain *Listeria* growth, including coleslaw (cabbage), soft cheeses, paté, poultry, turkey frankfurters, mushrooms, milk, pork tongue in jelly, and smoked fish. Large numbers of organisms ($>10^3$ CFU/g) were detected in foods quantitatively assayed for the organism (25).

Major progress has been made recently in the understanding of *Listeria* pathogenesis. After contaminated food has been ingested, the development of an invasive infection in some individuals depends on several factors: host susceptibility, gastric acidity, inoculum size, virulence factors of the organism, and the type of food. After penetrating the epithelial barrier of the intestinal tract, *L. monocytogenes* can grow within hepatic and splenic macrophages, due to a number of virulence factors (21), and then spread to the central nervous system or pregnant uterus, due to the interaction between internalin, a major *Listeria* virulence factor, and E-cadherin, a placental receptor (46). Immunity to listeriosis relies mainly on T-cell-mediated activation of macrophages by lymphokines; the role of humoral defenses is not fully understood (74).

Determination of Pathogenicity

Methods using laboratory animals for evaluation of the virulence potential of *Listeria* isolates are available but are not used routinely. Such tests include intraperitoneal inoculation of mice, inoculation of the chorioallantoic membranes of embryonated eggs, and inoculation of the conjunctivas of rabbits (Anton test). Also, cell culture cytotoxicity assays using the human intestinal epithelial cell line Caco-2 have been developed to determine the virulence potential of *Listeria* isolates in vitro (74). Although the results generally agree with those of animal tests, cytotoxicity assays do not provide as quantitative a measure of virulence (50% lethal dose) as the animal tests do. Also, some outbreak-associated *L. monocytogenes* isolates show very little cytotoxicity in the Caco-2 cell assays (66, 83).

Collection, Transportation, and Storage of Specimens

Laboratory Safety

The infectious dose for listeriosis has not been determined, and it may depend, in part, on the susceptibility of the host. Therefore, laboratorians working with *L. monocytogenes* should be made aware of this potential risk and advised to be particularly cautious when working with this organism. Because *L. monocytogenes* takes advantage of the localized immunosuppression at the maternal-fetal interface and attacks the fetus with devastating consequences (stillbirths and abortions) while causing only mild, flu-like symptoms in the mother, pregnant women should be particularly careful working in a laboratory where *L. monocytogenes* is propagated or handled (18).

Specimens

Clinical

L. monocytogenes is readily isolated from clinical specimens obtained from normally sterile sites (blood, CSF, amniotic fluid, placenta, or fetal tissue). These specimens should be immediately cultured at 35°C or stored at 4°C for up to 48 h. Stool specimens are more productive than rectal swabs when epidemiologic studies of carriage rates are undertaken. One gram of stool can be inoculated into 100 ml of a selective University of Vermont (UVM) enrichment broth or polymyxin-acriflavin-lithium chloride-ceftazidime esculin-mannitol (PALCAM) (87) (see chapter 21) and then shipped at room temperature by overnight mail. If this is not possible, stools should be shipped frozen on dry ice by overnight mail. Other nonsterile-site specimens may be stored at 4°C for 24 to 48 h. To avoid overgrowth of *L. monocytogenes* by contaminating microflora during longer periods of storage, freezing of specimens at −20°C is recommended. Routine stool cultures performed in clinical laboratories should not include *Listeria* detection.

Foods

Food samples must be collected aseptically in sterile containers. Whenever possible, foods packaged in original containers must be collected. Attempts should be made to collect at least 100 g of a sample. Samples may be placed in sterile bags and shipped on ice by overnight mail. Ice cream and other frozen products are best transported in the frozen state in the original container and must be thawed immediately before analysis. Although *L. monocytogenes* is relatively resistant to freezing, repeated freezing and thawing may adversely affect the viability of the bacteria.

Isolates

Cultures of *Listeria* spp. may be shipped to a distant laboratory on a non-glucose-containing agar slant (such as heart infusion agar or tryptic soy agar) packaged to conform with the requirements for interstate shipment of etiologic agents (e.g., U.S. Code of Federal Regulations, 42CFR, part 72).

Isolation Procedures

Culture

Clinical specimens from normally sterile sites can be plated directly onto tryptic soy agar containing 5% sheep, horse, or rabbit blood. Samples for blood culture can be inoculated into conventional blood culture broth. Clinical specimens obtained from nonsterile sites and foods and environmental specimens should be selectively enriched for *Listeria* spp. before being plated.

The U.S. Department of Agriculture method and The Netherlands Government Food Inspection Service method are used together at the Centers for Disease Control and Prevention to isolate *L. monocytogenes* from nonsterile-site clinical specimens and foods (37). Individually, the two methods are approximately 75% sensitive; in conjunction with each other, they are 90% sensitive. The U.S. Department of Agriculture method involves enrichment of the specimen in UVM primary selective enrichment broth (1 part sample plus 9 parts of broth) at 30°C. After 24 h, 0.1 ml of the enrichment culture is plated onto lithium chloride-phenylethanol-moxalactam (LPM) (47) agar and Oxford or modified Oxford agar (see chapter 21). Another 0.1 ml of the enrichment culture is added to 10 ml of UVM secondary selective enrichment broth, which is then incubated for an additional 24 h. The secondary enrichment culture is plated as described above. The plates are incubated at 35°C and examined after 24 and 48 h. All of the media named above are described in the compendium by Atlas and Parks (2) and in chapter 21 of this Manual.

The Netherlands Government Food Inspection Service method involves enrichment of the specimen in liquid PALCAM-egg yolk broth (see chapter 21) (87) at 30°C and plating of the enrichment culture onto PALCAM agar at 24 and 48 h. PALCAM agar is incubated at 30°C for 48 h under microaerobic conditions (5% oxygen, 7.5% carbon dioxide, 7.5% hydrogen, and 80% nitrogen).

LPM agar (47) was developed as a highly selective but nondifferential medium for the isolation of *Listeria* species. Colonies on LPM agar are examined under a stereozoom microscope (magnification, ×15 to ×25), with oblique lighting directed to the microscope stage by a concave mirror positioned at a 45° angle to the incident light (Henry illumination). *Listeria* colonies appear blue, and colonies of other bacteria appear yellowish or orange.

Oxford and PALCAM agars contain selective differential chemicals that eliminate the need for examination under oblique lighting (87). On Oxford and modified Oxford agars, *Listeria* colonies appear black, are 1 to 3 mm in diameter, and are surrounded by a black halo after 24 to 48 h of incubation at 37°C. Color formation is due to the hydrolysis of esculin by *Listeria* spp. and the formation of black iron-phenol compounds in the medium. On PALCAM agar, *Listeria* colonies appear gray-green, are approximately 2 mm in diameter, and have black sunken centers; esculin, ferric iron, D-mannitol, and phenol red contribute to this color formation. New chromogenic media improve the isolation of *L. monocytogenes* (6, 68). They rely on the production by *L. monocytogenes* —but not by other species of *Listeria*—of a phosphatidylinositol-specific phospholipase C which produces an opaque halo around the colonies. Several formulations are available: ALOAgar (Biolife, Milano, Italy) (89), BCM *L. monocytogenes* (Biosynth, Staad, Switzerland) (69), and CHROMagar (BD, Sparks, Md.) (28). To rule out *Listeria* gastroenteritis in an outbreak situation, at least one selective agar plate medium specific for *Listeria* spp. (Oxford or PALCAM) and/or for *L. monocytogenes* (ALOAgar or CHROMagar) should be added to conventional media used for bacterial stool culture.

Rapid Detection

Many rapid and/or automated methods have been developed to speed up the recovery and identification of *L. monocytogenes* from food. They rely on genus- or species-specific immunoassays, as well as on DNA or RNA (indicating cell viability) amplification methods (6). These kits are for use with food products only; they are not designed for the analysis of clinical specimens or for diagnosis and/or treatment.

L. monocytogenes DNA in CSF and tissue (fresh or in paraffin blocks) can be specifically detected by PCR-based tests (42, 79). The PCR assay is highly sensitive and specific and may be particularly useful when prior administration of antimicrobial agents compromises culture.

Identification

Genus Identification

A simplified identification is based on the following tests: Gram staining, observation of tumbling motility in a wet mount, and tests for a positive catalase reaction and esculin hydrolysis. Acid production from D-glucose and positive Voges-Proskauer and methyl red reactions are confirmatory test results.

Differentiation of the Genus *Listeria* from Other Genera

Because they share some characteristics, *Listeria* spp. and some other gram-positive bacteria may be confused. *Streptococcus* and *Enterococcus* spp. may be differentiated from *Listeria* spp. on the basis of Gram stain morphology, motility, and catalase activity. *Erysipelothrix* spp. differ from *Listeria* spp. in motility, catalase reaction, and ability to grow at 4°C (*Erysipelothrix* spp. do not grow at that temperature). Among background microflora of foods, *Lactobacillus* spp. are usually nonmotile and catalase negative, *Brochothrix* spp. are unable to grow at 37°C, and *Kurthia* spp. are strictly aerobic and esculin negative.

Species Identification

The scheme for identification of *Listeria* species is shown in Table 1. Identification of *Listeria* isolates to the species level is crucial, because all species can contaminate foods but only *L. monocytogenes* is of public health concern. Identification is based on a limited number of biochemical markers, among which hemolysis is essential to differentiating between *L. monocytogenes* and the most frequently isolated nonpathogenic *Listeria* species, *L. innocua*.

Hemolysis

Only three species, *L. monocytogenes*, *L. seeligeri*, and *L. ivanovii*, are hemolytic on sheep blood agar plates. Recent studies indicated hemolysin to be the major virulence factor of *L. monocytogenes;* however, hemolysis alone cannot be used as an indicator of the presence of a virulent species because *L. seeligeri* is hemolytic but nonpathogenic. *L. monocytogenes*

TABLE 1 Biochemical differentiation of species in the genus *Listeria*[a]

Characteristic	*L. grayi*	*L. innocua*	*L. ivanovii* subsp. *ivanovii*	*L. ivanovii* subsp. *londoniensis*	*L. monocytogenes*	*L. seeligeri*	*L. welshimeri*
Beta-hemolysis	−	−	++[b]	++	+	+	−
CAMP[c] test reaction							
S. aureus	−	−	−	−	+	+	−
R. equi	−	−	+	+	V	−	−
Acid production from:							
Mannitol	+	−	−	−	−	−	−
α-Methyl-D-mannoside	+	+	−	−	+	−	+
L-Rhamnose	V	V	−	−	+	−	V
Soluble starch	+	−	−	−	−	ND	ND
D-Xylose	−	−	+	+	−	+	+
Ribose	V	−	+	−	−	−	−
N-Acetyl-β-D-mannosamine	ND	ND	V	+	ND	ND	ND
Hippurate hydrolysis	−	+	+	+	+	ND	ND
Reduction of nitrate	V	−	−	−	−	ND	ND
Associated serovar(s)	S	4ab, US, 6a, 6b	5	5	1/2a, 1/2b, 1/2c, 3a, 3b, 3c, 4ab, 4b, 4c, 4d, 4e, 7	1/2a, 1/2b, 1/2c, 4a, US, 4b, 4d, 6b	1/2b, 4c, 6a, 6b, US

[a] See references 13 and 82. Symbols and abbreviations: +, ≥90% of strains are positive; −, ≥90% of strains are negative; ND, not determined; V, variable; US, undesignated serotype; S, specific.
[b] ++, usually a wide zone or multiple zones.
[c] See text and Fig. 2.

and *L. seeligeri* produce narrow zones of hemolysis that frequently do not extend much beyond the edges of the colonies, whereas *L. ivanovii* exhibits a wide zone of hemolysis (Fig. 1).

The CAMP (Christie, Atkins, Munch-Peterson) test uses a β-lysin-producing *Staphylococcus aureus* or *Rhodococcus equi* strain streaked in one direction on a sheep blood agar plate and test cultures of *Listeria* spp. streaked at right angles to (but not touching) the *S. aureus* and *R. equi* lines. According to *Bergey's Manual of Systematic Bacteriology* (82), hemolysis of *L. monocytogenes* and *L. seeligeri* is enhanced in the vicinity of the *S. aureus* streak, and *L. ivanovii* hemolysis is enhanced in the vicinity of *R. equi* (resulting in a shovel shape) (Fig. 2). However, because many investigators have reported observing a synergistic hemolysis reaction between *L. monocytogenes* and *R. equi*, this CAMP reaction must be interpreted with caution. A β-lysin disk (Remel, Lenexa,

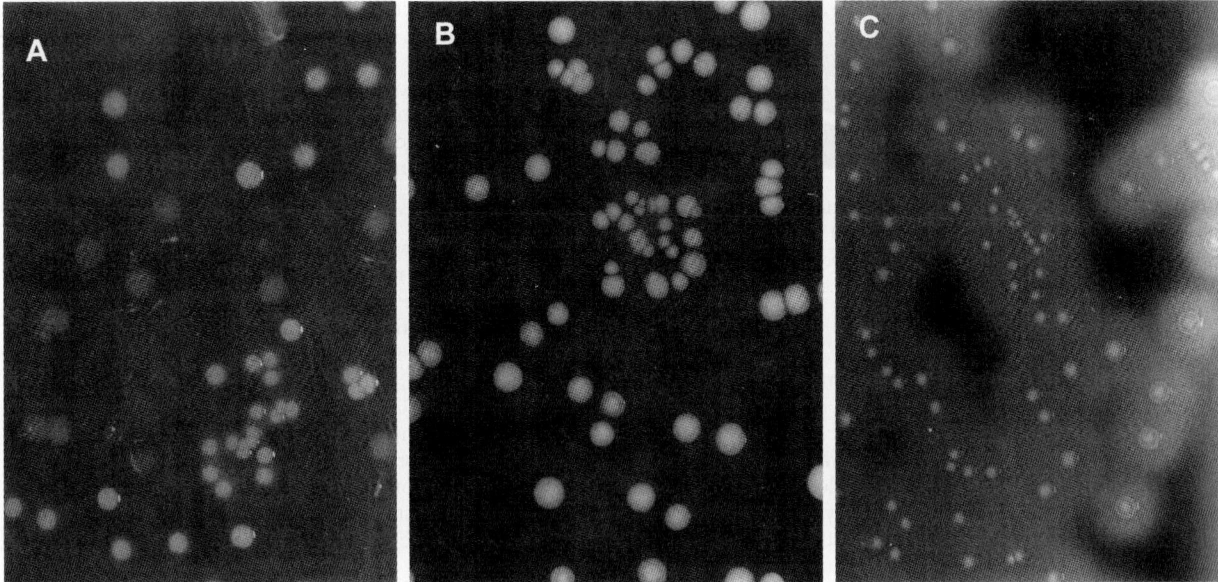

FIGURE 1 Macroscopic view of colonies on 5% human blood agar plates after 24 h of incubation. (A) *L. monocytogenes*: discrete zone of beta-hemolysis under the removed colonies. (B) *L. innocua*: no hemolysis. (C) *L. ivanovii*: wide zone of beta-hemolysis around the colonies.

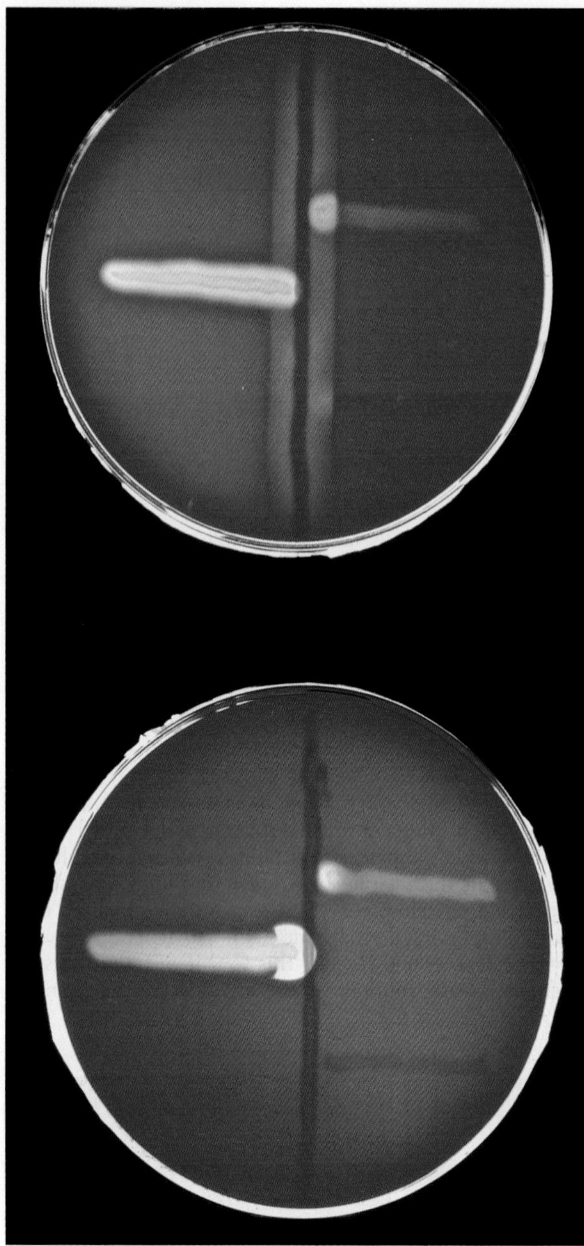

FIGURE 2 CAMP test done with *S. aureus* CIP 5710 (top plate) and *R. equi* CIP 5869 (bottom plate) after 24 h of incubation. Upper right, *L. monocytogenes*; lower right, *L. innocua*; middle left, *L. ivanovii*.

Kans.) may be used to observe enhancement of *L. monocytogenes* with β-lysin from *S. aureus*.

Acid Production from Carbohydrates

L. monocytogenes is always D-xylose negative and α-methyl-D-mannoside positive. Rare atypical strains may be L-rhamnose negative. Test tubes are incubated for 7 days at 37°C in an aerobic incubator.

Miniaturized Biochemical Tests

The API-Listeria test (bioMérieux Vitek, Inc., Hazelwood, Mo.) was specifically designed for *Listeria* and includes 10 biochemical differentiation tests in a microtube format. It includes a patented DIM test, based on the absence or presence of arylamidase, which distinguishes between *L. monocytogenes* (negative) and *L. innocua* (positive) without further tests for hemolytic activity (9). The API Coryne System (bioMérieux) correctly identifies *Listeria* isolates to the genus level (29).

Automated Identification Systems

Both Vitek 2 (bioMérieux) and Phoenix (BD) automated systems have *Listeria* spp. on the list of organisms for their gram-positive identification cards; Vitek 2 (with the new colorimetric gram-positive card) but not Phoenix is able to differentiate *Listeria* colonies to the species level. No independent evaluation is currently available on their performance in identifying *Listeria* spp. at the species or genus level.

DNA Probe Assay for Colony Confirmation

A 30-min chemiluminescence DNA probe assay is available (Gen-Probe, San Diego, Calif.) for the rapid confirmation of *L. monocytogenes* from colonies on primary isolation plates. This assay was highly specific for *L. monocytogenes* in two independent evaluations (56, 62).

Typing Systems

Serotyping

Strains of *Listeria* species are divided into serotypes on the basis of somatic ("O") and flagellar (H) antigens (81). Thirteen serotypes (1/2a, 1/2b, 1/2c, 3a, 3b, 3c, 4a, 4ab, 4b, 4c, 4d, 4e, and 7) of *L. monocytogenes* are known; 4bX, a variant of serotype 4b, was implicated in a listeriosis outbreak traced to contaminated paté in England (52). Serotyping antigens are shared among *L. monocytogenes*, *L. innocua*, *L. seeligeri*, and *L. welshimeri*. Most human disease is caused by serotypes 1/2a, 1/2b, and 4b; therefore, serotyping alone is not sufficiently discriminating for subtyping purposes. Nevertheless, serotyping is useful as a first-level discriminator. Also, unlike those of other subtyping methods, serotype designations are universal. Determination of the serotype also facilitates selection of appropriate controls for molecular subtyping methods. A commercial kit (Denka Seiken, Tokyo, Japan) which relies on the slide agglutination method (78) has been adapted to an enzyme-linked immunosorbent assay format (64). Recently, a multiplex PCR assay has been designed to separate the four major *L. monocytogenes* serovars (1/2a, 1/2b, 1/2c, and 4b) into distinct groups (23).

Phage Typing

Because of the poor discriminating ability of serotyping, phage typing was the only means of distinguishing strains of the same serotype before the introduction of molecular methods (72) which have largely replaced it today. In addition, phage typing is hampered by the nontypeability of some strains.

MLEE

Multilocus enzyme electrophoresis (MLEE) has been extremely useful for taxonomic studies and for characterization of the evolution of strains within the species (7, 11, 12, 65, 79); however, it does not have adequate discriminatory power for use as the sole subtyping method for epidemiologic investigations.

DNA Microrestriction Pattern Analysis

Characterization of chromosomal DNA by restriction endonuclease analysis or ribosomal DNA gene restriction patterns (ribotyping) has been used to differentiate *L. monocytogenes* strains of different serotypes and those within a given serotype, in particular serotype 4b, which is most frequently involved in outbreaks. Microrestriction patterns generated by high-frequency-cutting restriction enzymes (e.g., EcoR1) have proved useful in epidemiologic investigations (3, 57), although the complexity of patterns makes it difficult to compare the patterns of several strains. Ribotyping simplifies the microrestriction patterns by rendering visible only the DNA fragments containing part or all of the ribosomal genes, but its discriminating ability, particularly for serotype 4b, may not be adequate (3, 33, 40, 41, 58). A completely automated RiboPrinter system (Qualicon, Wilmington, Del.) facilitates rapid and easy subtyping of *L. monocytogenes* within 8 h. Although ribotyping alone does not have adequate discriminating power for epidemiologic investigations of outbreaks, the automated RiboPrinter is invaluable for preliminary recognition of disease clusters and for identification of transient and long-term-resident strains of *L. monocytogenes* in food processing plants and their environments (22, 59).

DNA Macrorestriction PFGE Pattern Analysis

Brosch et al. (16) evaluated the pulsed-field gel eletrophoresis (PFGE) method for the World Health Organization multicenter international typing study of *L. monocytogenes*. Four laboratories participated in using PFGE to analyze 80 coded strains. Two restriction endonucleases (ApaI and SmaI) were used by all laboratories; one laboratory used an additional restriction endonuclease (AscI). Agreement of typing data among the four laboratories ranged from 79 to 90%. Sixty-nine percent of the strains were placed in exactly the same genomic groups by all four laboratories; most of the epidemiologically related strains were correctly identified by all four laboratories. This study validated the previous claims that PFGE is a highly discriminating and reproducible method for subtyping *L. monocytogenes* and is particularly useful for subtyping serotype 4b isolates, which are not typed satisfactorily by most other typing methods.

In the United States, the Centers for Disease Control and Prevention has established a network (PulseNet) of public health and food regulatory laboratories that routinely subtype foodborne pathogenic bacteria to rapidly detect foodborne disease clusters that may have a common source. PulseNet laboratories use highly standardized protocols for subtyping of bacteria by PFGE and are able to quickly compare PFGE patterns of foodborne pathogens from different locations within the country via the Internet (84) (PFGE@cdc.gov). A 1-day standardized protocol for PFGE subtyping of *L. monocytogenes* was added to PulseNet in 1998 (34). Routine and timely subtyping of *L. monocytogenes* by participating PulseNet laboratories has significantly enhanced the ability to recognize and investigate outbreaks. For several years now, PFGE has been the standard subtyping method to detect listeriosis outbreaks.

RAPD

Random amplification of polymorphic DNA (RAPD) analysis is a rapid and relatively simple technique for epidemiological typing of *L. monocytogenes* isolates by using several short (10-mer) primers (14, 91). Despite its simplicity and high discriminating ability, RAPD suffers from inconsistent reproducibility of patterns.

MLST

Multilocus sequence typing (MLST) is currently being established for *L. monocytogenes* typing. It is based on the comparative sequencing of housekeeping genes or genes coding for virulence factors. The discriminatory power of MLST is very high, and sequence data comparisons are easily done (70, 76, 93).

Present Status of Subtyping

The vast majority of *L. monocytogenes* strains causing sporadic infections or outbreaks belong to serotypes 1/2a, 1/2b, and 4b. Strains of serotype 1/2a are highly heterogeneous and thus are easily differentiated by any of the molecular methods. In contrast, strains of serotype 4b are more closely related and probably necessitate the combined use of several methods to be optimally differentiated (10). PFGE is considered to be the most effective typing method; it is time and cost efficient and highly discriminative (30).

Serodiagnosis

Serologic responses to whole-cell antigens cannot be used for diagnosis because of antigenic cross-reactivity between *L. monocytogenes* and other gram-positive bacteria such as staphylococci, enterococci, and *Bacillus* species. Furthermore, patients with culture-confirmed listeriosis have had undetectable antibody levels (79). Determination of levels of antibody to listeriolysin O may be of value both for invasive listeriosis and for febrile gastroenteritis (4). Although a serologic method based on the detection of antibodies against recombinant truncated forms of listeriolysin O may be more specific (31), serological tests are not recommended at the present time.

Antimicrobial Susceptibilities

The pattern of antimicrobial susceptibility and resistance of *L. monocytogenes* has been relatively stable for many years (86). In vitro, the organism is susceptible to penicillin, ampicillin, gentamicin, erythromycin, tetracycline, rifampin, and chloramphenicol (77, 92) but only moderately susceptible to quinolones (39). However, many of these antimicrobial agents are only bacteriostatic. Penicillin or ampicillin with or without an aminoglycoside is usually recommended for the treatment of listeriosis. Studies in vitro and in animal models have shown that an aminoglycoside enhances the activity of penicillin against *L. monocytogenes* (54). Trimethoprim-sulfamethoxazole and aminoglycosides are among the few anti-infective agents that are bactericidal to *L. monocytogenes;* only trimethoprim-sulfamethoxazole has been used occasionally with success. Resistance plasmids conferring resistance to chloramphenicol, macrolides, and tetracyclines have been found in several clinical isolates of *L. monocytogenes* and have raised concern for the future (36). *L. monocytogenes* appears to be susceptible in vitro to newly released antibiotics such as linezolid, daptomycin, and tigecyclin, but few strains have been tested. Cephalosporins are ineffective in vivo, although in vitro tests may indicate susceptibility, and should never be administered when listeriosis is suspected.

Evalutation, Interpretation, and Reporting of Results

Colonies from blood, CSF, or other normally sterile-site specimens that show subdued beta-hemolysis on blood agar should be subjected to motility tests, Gram staining, catalase testing, and esculin hydrolysis to confirm identification. They may resemble group B streptococcal colonies on blood agar plates. The CAMP test is not necessary on a routine basis, and the β-lysin test may be substituted for it. Use of the API-Listeria test may eliminate the need for enhanced hemolysis testing altogether. If *L. monocytogenes* is present in low numbers in

CSF, the direct examination of Gram-stained clinical specimens may be of little or no value. Also, Gram-stained *Listeria* cells closely resemble other gram-positive bacteria, such as streptococci, enterococci, and corynebacteria. If antimicrobial therapy was initiated before a CSF specimen was obtained, culture results may be negative. In these instances, Gram staining may be useful, as well as molecular detection of DNA by PCR. Although numerous PCR-based detection methods have been developed and tested with food products, a very limited number of applications to clinical samples have been described, using either a single PCR or multiplex PCR (30).

ERYSIPELOTHRIX

Taxonomy

Included at one time in the coryneform group, *Erysipelothrix* is now classified with the regular non-spore-forming gram-positive rods, a group that comprises the genera *Listeria* and *Lactobacillus*. The genus *Erysipelothrix* has two validated species, *E. rhusiopathiae* and *E. tonsillarum* (85). A third species, *E. inopinata*, has been recently proposed (88). *E. rhusiopathiae*, which is widely distributed in nature and can be carried by a variety of animals, has been recognized for more than 100 years as the agent of swine erysipelas and occasionally causes erysipeloid, a human cutaneous infection usually localized to the hands and fingers (67).

Description of the Genus

Erysipelothrix organisms are mesophilic, facultatively anaerobic, non-spore-forming, non-acid-fast, gram-positive bacteria that appear microscopically as short rods (0.2 to 0.5 μm by 0.8 to 2.5 μm) with rounded ends and occur singly, in short chains, or in long, nonbranching filaments (60 μm or more in length). They are nonmotile and grow in complex media at a wide range of temperatures (5 to 42°C; optimum, 30 to 37°C) and at alkaline pHs (pH 6.7 to 9.2; optimum, pH 7.2 to 7.6). Like *Listeria* organisms, they can grow in the presence of high concentrations of sodium chloride (up to 8.5%). Metabolically, *Erysipelothrix* organisms are catalase negative and oxidase negative, do not hydrolyze esculin, and weakly ferment glucose without the production of gas. They are methyl red and Voges-Proskauer negative and do not produce indole or hydrolyze urea but distinctively produce H_2S in triple sugar iron agar. Key fatty acids are $C_{16:0}$ and $C_{18:cis9}$ (5).

Natural Habitats

E. rhusiopathiae is widespread in nature and is remarkably persistent under environmental conditions such as low temperature and alkaline pH and within organic matter favoring survival. The organism is parasitic on mammals, birds, and fish but is most frequently associated with pigs. Contamination of water and soil from the feces and urine of sick and asymptomatic animals often occurs.

E. tonsillarum has been recovered from water and from the tonsils of healthy swine.

Clinical Significance

Infection with *E. rhusiopathiae* is a zoonosis. Many animal species, especially turkeys and swine, carry the organism in their digestive tracts or tonsils. *E. rhusiopathiae* causes chronic or acute swine erysipelas. Erysipelas can present in several clinical manifestations: skin infection, arthritis, septicemia, and endocarditis. Other domestic and wild animals and birds also can be affected, in particular sheep, rabbits, cattle, and turkeys. Infection is most likely acquired by ingestion of contaminated matter (67).

In humans, *E. rhusiopathiae* causes mostly erysipeloid, a localized cellulitis developing within 2 to 7 days around the inoculation site. The disease is contracted through skin abrasion, injury, or a bite on the hands or arms of individuals handling animals or animal products. Erysipeloid is an occupational disease, occurring most frequently among veterinarians, butchers, and particularly fish handlers. The lesion usually is violaceous and painful, indurated with edema and inflammation but without suppuration, and clearly delineated at the border. Regional lymphangitis may be present, as well as an adjacent arthritis. Dissemination and endocarditis can occur, especially in immunocompromised patients; their prognosis is generally poor (32). Healing of erysipeloids usually takes 2 to 4 weeks, sometimes months, and relapses are common. No apparent immunity develops after an episode of erysipeloid.

E. tonsillarum has not yet been recovered from humans.

Collection, Transport, and Storage of Specimens

Biopsy specimens from erysipeloid lesions are the best source of *E. rhusiopathiae*. Care should be taken to cleanse and disinfect the skin before sampling. The organisms typically are located deep in the subcutaneous layer of the leading edge of the lesion; hence, a biopsy of the entire thickness of the dermis at the periphery of the lesion should be taken for Gram staining and culture. Swabs from the surface of the skin are not useful. In disseminated disease, the organism can be cultured from blood without special procedures.

Isolation Procedures

Microscopic Examination

Generally, direct examination of Gram-stained biopsy specimens is of little value. However, the presence of long, slender, gram-positive rods in tissue from an individual with a consonant history is suggestive of erysipeloid.

Culture

Biopsy specimens should be plated onto blood agar or chocolate blood agar, placed in tryptic soy or Schaedler broth, and incubated at 35°C aerobically or in 5% CO_2 for 7 days. Blood from patients with septicemia or endocarditis can be plated directly onto blood agar plates for primary isolation or inoculated into commercial blood culture systems. *E. rhusiopathiae* colonies generally develop in 1 to 3 days, appearing as pinpoints (<0.1 to 0.5 mm in diameter) on blood agar plates after 24 h of incubation; at 48 h, two distinct colony types can be observed. The smaller, smooth colonies are 0.3 to 1.5 mm in diameter, transparent, convex, and circular with entire edges. Larger, rough colonies are flatter and more opaque and have a matte surface and an irregular, fimbriated edge. A zone of greenish discoloration frequently develops underneath the colonies on blood agar plates after 2 days of incubation (43).

Rapid Detection

PCR initially developed for rapid diagnosis in swine (50) has been used with human samples (15). The target is the 16S rRNA or the 23S rRNA gene.

Identification

Gram Staining of Colonies from a 24-h Blood Agar Plate

Cells stain gram positive but can decolorize and appear gram negative, with gram-positive granules giving a beaded effect. Cells from smooth colonies appear as rods or coccobacilli, sometimes in short chains. Cells from rough colonies appear as long filaments, often more than 60 μm.

Biochemical Identification of *E. rhusiopathiae*

E. rhusiopathiae is catalase negative; glucose, lactose, and H_2S positive; and nitrate, urease, esculin, gelatin, xylose, mannose, maltose, and sucrose negative. *E. tonsillarum* differs biochemically from *E. rhusiopathiae* by being sucrose positive. Vitek automated systems, as well as API Coryne, usually identify *E. rhusiopathiae* correctly.

Differentiation of *Erysipelothix* from Related Genera

Genera that have morphological and physiological characteristics in common with *Erysipelothrix* include *Lactobacillus*, *Listeria*, *Brochothrix*, and *Kurthia*. All are regular nonpigmented, non-spore-forming, gram-positive rods (44). A major discriminatory characteristic is that *E. rhusiopathiae* produces H_2S in triple sugar iron whereas species of the other genera do not. Furthermore, *Listeria*, *Brochothrix*, and *Kurthia* species are catalase positive. In addition, *Listeria* isolates are motile, are esculin positive, and are not alpha-hemolytic. *Brochothrix* isolates strongly ferment carbohydrates, are Voges-Proskauer positive, and do not grow at above 30°C. *Kurthia* species are strict aerobes and are motile and nonhemolytic (45). Corynebacteria and streptococci also can be confused with *E. rhusiopathiae*, but careful examination of cell morphology should facilitate the distinction. The production of H_2S in triple sugar iron by a gram-positive bacterium is usually indicative of *E. rhusiopathiae* because very few gram-positive bacteria of clinical origin produce H_2S. Exceptions include some *Bacillus* strains, but they are easily differentiated from *E. rhusiopathiae* by cellular morphology, spore formation, and catalase reaction. An additional trait highly characteristic of *E. rhusiopathiae* is its "pipe cleaner" pattern of growth in gelatin stab cultures incubated at 22°C (43, 90).

Typing Systems

Twenty-two serovars of *E. rhusiopathiae* have been identified on the basis of heat-stable somatic antigens. Although most isolates are serovar 1 or 2, no serotyping schemes are available for routine use in clinical laboratories. Both MLEE and ribotyping methods have been applied to *Erysipelothrix* strains and have shown an enormous genetic diversity (1, 19, 61). PFGE with SmaI seems to be the best method for epidemiological studies of *E. rhusiopathiae* isolates (60). In these studies, serotyping was unreliable for use as an epidemiologic tool.

Pathogenicity Testing

Most strains of *E. rhusiopathiae* are virulent for mice in a mouse protection test (43).

Serological Tests

Since humans apparently do not develop immunity after an episode of erysipeloid, there are no serological tests for routine use to demonstrate antibodies to *E. rhusiopathiae*. Active immunization of animals with a live attenuated vaccine protects against erysipelas (67); however, a natural erysipeloid infection in humans does not prevent relapses or reinfection from occurring.

Antibiotic Susceptibility

E. rhusiopathiae isolates are generally susceptible to penicillin, cephalosporins, clindamycin, imipenem, tetracycline, chloramphenicol, erythromycin, and the fluoroquinolones; they are usually resistant to aminoglycosides, sulfonamides, and vancomycin (27). Penicillin is the treatment of choice for both localized and systemic infections (32).

REFERENCES

1. **Ahrné, S., I.-M. Stenström, N. E. Jensen, B. Pettersson, M. Uhlén, and G. Molin.** 1995. Classification of *Erysipelothrix* strains on the basis of restriction fragment length polymorphisms. *Int. J. Syst. Bacteriol.* **45:**382–385.
2. **Atlas, R. M., and L. C. Parks (ed.).** 1993. *Handbook of Microbiological Media*. CRC Press, Inc., Boca Raton, Fla.
3. **Baloga, A. O.,** and **S. K. Harlander.** 1991. Comparison of methods for discrimination between strains of *Listeria monocytogenes* from epidemiological surveys. *Appl. Environ. Microbiol.* **57:**2324–2331.
4. **Berche, P., K. A. Reich, M. Bonnichon, J.-L. Beretti, C. Geoffroy, J. Raveneau, P. Cossart, J.-L. Gaillard, P. Geslin, H. Kreis, and M. Véron.** 1990. Detection of anti-listeriolysin O for serodiagnosis of human listeriosis. *Lancet* **335:**624–627.
5. **Bernard, K. A., M. Bellefeuille, and E. P. Ewan.** 1991. Cellular fatty acid composition as an adjunct to the identification of asporogenous, aerobic gram-positive rods. *J. Clin. Microbiol.* **29:**83–89.
6. **Beumer, R. R., and W. C. Hazeleger.** 2003. *Listeria monocytogenes*: diagnostic problems. *FEMS Immunol. Med. Microbiol.* **35:**191–197.
7. **Bibb, W. F., B. G. Gellin, R. Weaver, B. Schwartz, B. D. Plikaytis, M. W. Reeves, R. W. Pinner, and C. V. Broome.** 1990. Analysis of clinical and food-borne isolates of *Listeria monocytogenes* in the United States by multilocus enzyme electrophoresis and application of the method to epidemiologic investigations. *Appl. Environ. Microbiol.* **56:**2133–2141.
8. **Bille, J.** 1990. Epidemiology of human listeriosis in Europe, with special reference to the Swiss outbreak, p. 71–74. *In* A. J. Miller, J. L. Smith, and G. A. Somkuti (ed.), *Food-Borne Listeriosis*. Elsevier, Amsterdam, The Netherlands.
9. **Bille, J., B. Catimel, E. Bannerman, C. Jacquet, M.-N. Yersin, I. Caniaux, D. Monget, and J. Rocourt.** 1992. API-Listeria, a new and promising one-day system to identify *Listeria* isolates. *Appl. Environ. Microbiol.* **58:**1857–1860.
10. **Bille, J., and J. Rocourt.** 1996. WHO international multicenter *Listeria monocytogenes* subtyping study—rationale and set-up of the study. *Int. J. Food Microbiol.* **32:**251–262.
11. **Boerlin, P., and J.-C. Piffaretti.** 1991. Typing of human, animal, food, and environmental isolates of *Listeria monocytogenes* by multilocus enzyme electrophoresis. *Appl. Environ. Microbiol.* **57:**1624–1629.
12. **Boerlin, P., J. Rocourt, and J.-C. Piffaretti.** 1991. Taxonomy of the genus *Listeria* by using multilocus enzyme electrophoresis. *Int. J. Syst. Bacteriol.* **41:**59–64.
13. **Boerlin, P., J. Rocourt, F. Grimont, P. A. D. Grimont, C. Jacquet, and J.-C. Piffaretti.** 1992. *Listeria ivanovii* subsp. *londoniensis* subsp. nov. *Int. J. Syst. Bacteriol.* **42:**69–73.
14. **Boerlin, P., E. Bannerman, F. Ischer, J. Rocourt, and J. Bille.** 1995. Typing of *Listeria monocytogenes*: a comparison of random amplification of polymorphic DNA with 5 other methods. *Res. Microbiol.* **146:**35–49.
15. **Brooke, C. J., and T. V. Riley.** 1999. *Erysipelothrix rhusiopathiae:* bacteriology, epidemiology and clinical manifestations of an occupational pathogen. *J. Med. Microbiol.* **48:**789–799.
16. **Brosch, R., M. Brett, B. Catimel, J. B. Luchansky, B. Ojeniyi, and J. Rocourt.** 1996. Genomic fingerprinting of 80 strains from the WHO multicenter international typing study of *Listeria monocytogenes* via pulsed-field gel electrophoresis (PFGE). *Int. J. Food Microbiol.* **32:**343–355.

17. **Büla, C. J., J. Bille, and M. P. Glauser.** 1995. An epidemic of food-borne listeriosis in Western Switzerland: description of 57 cases involving adults. *Clin. Infect. Dis.* **20:**66–72.
18. **Centers for Disease Control and Prevention and National Institutes of Health.** 1999. *Biosafety in Microbiological and Biomedical Laboratories (BMBL)*, 4th ed. U.S. Government Printing Office, Washington, D.C.
19. **Chooromoney, K. N., D. J. Hampson, G. J. Eamens, and M. J. Turner.** 1994. Analysis of *Erysipelothrix rhusiopathiae* and *Erysipelothrix tonsillarum* by multilocus enzyme electrophoresis. *J. Clin. Microbiol.* **32:**371–376.
20. **Collins, M. D., S. Wallbanks, D. J. Lane, J. Shah, R. Nietupski, J. Smida, M. Dorsch, and E. Stackebrandt.** 1991. Phylogenetic analysis of the genus *Listeria* based on reverse transcriptase sequencing of 16S rRNA. *Int. J. Syst. Bacteriol.* **41:**240–246.
21. **Cossart, P., and P. J. Sansonetti.** 2004. Bacterial invasion: the paradigms of enteroinvasive pathogens. *Science* **304:**242–248.
22. **De Cesare, A., J. L. Bruce, T. R. Dambaugh, M. E. Guerzoni, and M. Wiedmann.** 2001. Automated ribotyping using different enzymes to improve discrimination of *Listeria monocytogenes* isolates, with a particular focus on serotype 4b strains. *J. Clin. Microbiol.* **39:**3002–3005.
23. **Doumith, M., C. Buchrieser, P. Glaser, C. Jacquet, and P. Martin.** 2004. Differentiation of the major *Listeria monocytogenes* serovars by multiplex PCR. *J. Clin. Microbiol.* **42:**3819–3822.
24. **Elsner, H.-A., I. Sobottka, A. Bubert, H. Albrecht, R. Laufs, and D. Mack.** 1996. Catalase-negative *Listeria monocytogenes* causing lethal sepsis and meningitis in an adult hematologic patient. *Eur. J. Clin. Microbiol. Infect. Dis.* **15:**965–967.
25. **Farber, J. M., and P. I. Peterkin.** 1991. *Listeria monocytogenes*, a food-borne pathogen. *Microbiol. Rev.* **55:**476–511.
26. **Fenlon, D. R.** 1999. *Listeria monocytogenes* in the natural environment, p. 30–40. *In* E. T. Ryser and E. H. Marth (ed.), *Listeria, Listeriosis, and Food Safety*, 2nd ed. Marcel Dekker, Inc., New York, N.Y.
27. **Fidalgo, S. G., C. J. Longbottom, and T. V. Riley.** 2002. Susceptibility of *Erysipelothrix rhusiopathiae* to antimicrobial agents and home disinfectants. *Pathology* **34:**462–465.
28. **Foret, J., and F. Dorey.** 1997. Evaluation d'un nouveau milieu de culture pour la recherche de *Listeria monocytogenes* dans le lait cru. *Sci. Aliments* **17:**219–225.
29. **Funke, G., F. N. R. Renaud, J. Freney, and P. Riegel.** 1997. Multicenter evaluation of the updated and extended API (RAPID) Coryne Database 2.0. *J. Clin. Microbiol.* **35:**3122–3126.
30. **Gasanov, U., D. Hughes, and P. M. Hansbro.** 2005. Methods for the isolation and identification of *Listeria* spp. and *Listeria monocytogenes:* a review. *FEMS Microbiol. Rev.* **29:**851–875.
31. **Gholizadeh, Y., C. Poyart, M. Juvin, J.-L. Beretti, J. Croizé, P. Berche, and J.-L. Gaillard.** 1996. Serodiagnosis of listeriosis based upon detection of antibodies against recombinant truncated forms of listeriolysin O. *J. Clin. Microbiol.* **34:**1391–1395.
32. **Gorby, G. L., and J. E. Peacock, Jr.** 1988. *Erysipelothrix rhusiopathiae* endocarditis: microbiologic, epidemiologic, and clinical features of an occupational disease. *Rev. Infect. Dis.* **10:**317–325.
33. **Graves, L. M., B. Swaminathan, M. W. Reeves, and J. Wenger.** 1991. Ribosomal DNA fingerprinting of *Listeria monocytogenes* using a digoxigenin-labeled DNA probe. *Eur. J. Epidemiol.* **7:**77–82.
34. **Graves, L. M., and B. Swaminathan.** 2001. PulseNet standardized protocol for subtyping *Listeria monocytogenes* by macrorestriction and pulsed-field gel electrophoresis. *Int. J. Food Microbiol.* **65:**55–62.
35. **Grif, K., G. Patscheider, M. P. Dierich, and F. Allerberger.** 2003. Incidence of fecal carriage of *Listeria monocytogenes* in three healthy volunteers: a one-year prospective stool survey. *Eur. J. Clin. Microbiol. Infect. Dis.* **22:**16–20.
36. **Hadorn, K., H. Hächler, A. Schaffner, and F. H. Kayser.** 1993. Genetic characterization of plasmid-encoded multiple antibiotic resistance in a strain of *Listeria monocytogenes* causing endocarditis. *Eur. J. Clin. Microbiol. Infect. Dis.* **12:** 928–937.
37. **Hayes, P. S., L. M. Graves, B. Swaminathan, G. W. Ajello, G. B. Malcolm, R. E. Weaver, R. Ransom, K. Deaver, B. D. Plikaytis, A. Schuchat, J. D. Wenger, R. W. Pinner, C. V. Broome, and the Listeria Study Group.** 1992. Comparison of three selective enrichment methods for the isolation of *Listeria monocytogenes* from naturally contaminated foods. *J. Food Prot.* **55:**952–959.
38. **Hof, H.** 2001. *Listeria monocytogenes:* a causative agent of gastroenteritis? *Eur. J. Clin. Microbiol. Infect. Dis.* **20:**369–373.
39. **Hof, H., T. Nichterlein, and M. Kretschmar.** 1997. Management of listeriosis. *Clin. Microbiol. Rev.* **10:**345–357.
40. **Jacquet, C., S. Aubert, N. El Sohl, and J. Rocourt.** 1992. Use of rRNA gene restriction patterns for the identification of *Listeria* species. *Syst. Appl. Microbiol.* **15:**42–46.
41. **Jacquet, C., J. Bille, and J. Rocourt.** 1992. Typing of *Listeria monocytogenes* by restriction fragment length polymorphism of the ribosomal ribonucleic acid gene region. *Zentbl. Bakteriol.* **276:**356–365.
42. **Jaton, K., R. Sahli, and J. Bille.** 1992. Development of polymerase chain reaction assays for detection of *Listeria monocytogenes* in clinical cerebrospinal fluid samples. *J. Clin. Microbiol.* **30:**1931–1936.
43. **Jones, D.** 1986. Genus *Erysipelothrix* Rosenbach 1909, 367^{AL}, p. 1245–1249. *In* P. H. A. Sneath, N. S. Mair, M. E. Sharpe, and J. G. Holt (ed.), *Bergey's Manual of Systematic Bacteriology*, vol. 2. Williams & Wilkins, Baltimore, Md.
44. **Kandler, O., and N. Weiss.** 1986. Regular, nonsporing Gram-positive rods, p. 1208–1209. *In* P. H. A. Sneath, N. S. Mair, M. E. Sharpe, and J. G. Holt (ed.), *Bergey's Manual of Systematic Bacteriology*, vol. 2. Williams & Wilkins., Baltimore, Md.
45. **Keddie, R. M., and S. Shaw.** 1986. Genus *Kurthia Trevisan* 1885, 92^{AL}, p. 1255–1257. *In* P. H. A. Sneath, N. S. Mair, M. E. Sharpe, and J. G. Holt (ed.), *Bergey's Manual of Systematic Bacteriology*, vol. 2. Williams & Wilkins, Baltimore, Md.
46. **Lecuit, M., D. M. Nelson, S. D. Smith, H. Kuhn, M. Huerre, M.-C. Vacher-Lavenu, J. I. Gordon, and P. Cossart.** 2004. Targeting and crossing of the human maternofetal barrier by *Listeria monocytogenes:* role of internalin interaction with trophoblast E-cadherin. *Proc. Natl. Acad. Sci. USA* **101:**6152–6157.
47. **Lee, W. H., and D. McClain.** 1986. Improved *Listeria monocytogenes* selective agar. *Appl. Environ. Microbiol.* **52:**1215–1217.
48. **Lorber, B.** 2005. *Listeria monocytogenes*, p. 2478–2484. *In* G. L. Mandell, J. E. Bennett, and R. Dolin (ed.), *Principles and Practice of Infectious Diseases*, 6th ed. Elsevier Churchill Livingstone, Philadelphia, Pa.
49. **Ludwig, W., K.-H. Schleifer, and E. Stackebrandt.** 1984. 16S rRNA analysis of *Listeria monocytogenes* and *Brochothrix thermosphacta*. *FEMS Microbiol. Lett.* **25:**199–204.
50. **Makino, S.-I., Y. Okada, T. Maruyama, K. Ishikawa, T. Takahashi, M. Nakamura, T. Ezaki, and H. Morita.** 1994. Direct and rapid detection of *Erysipelothrix rhusiopathiae* DNA in animals by PCR. *J. Clin. Microbiol.* **32:**1526–1531.
51. **McLauchlin, J., and P. N. Hoffman.** 1989. Neonatal cross-infection from *Listeria monocytogenes*. *Communicable Dis. Rep.* **16:**3–4.
52. **McLauchlin, J., S. M. Hall, S. K. Velani, and R. J. Gilbert.** 1991. Human listeriosis and paté: a possible association. *Br. Med. J.* **303:**773–775.

53. **McLauchlin, J., and J. C. Low.** 1994. Primary cutaneous listeriosis in adults: an occupational disease of veterinarians and farmers. *Vet. Rec.* **135:**615–617.
54. **Moellering, R. C., G. Medoff, I. Leech, C. Wennersten, and L. J. Kunz.** 1972. Antibiotic synergism against *Listeria monocytogenes*. *Antimicrob. Agents Chemother.* **1:**30–34.
55. **Nieman, R. E., and B. Lorber.** 1980. Listeriosis in adults, a changing pattern: report of eight cases and a review of the literature, 1968–1978. *Rev. Infect. Dis.* **2:**207–227.
56. **Ninet, B., E. Bannerman, and J. Bille.** 1992. Assessment of the Accuprobe *Listeria monocytogenes* culture identification reagent kit for rapid colony confirmation and its application in various enrichment broths. *Appl. Environ. Microbiol.* **58:**4055–4059.
57. **Nocera, D., E. Bannerman, J. Rocourt, K. Jaton Ogay, and J. Bille.** 1990. Characterization by DNA restriction endonuclease analysis of *Listeria monocytogenes* strains related to the Swiss epidemic of listeriosis. *J. Clin. Microbiol.* **28:**2259–2263.
58. **Nocera, D., M. Altwegg, G. Martinetti Lucchini, E. Bannerman, F. Ischer, J. Rocourt, and J. Bille.** 1993. Characterization of *Listeria* strains from a foodborne listeriosis outbreak by rDNA gene restriction patterns compared to four other typing methods. *Eur. J. Clin. Microbiol. Infect. Dis.* **12:**162–169.
59. **Norton, D. M., M. A. McCamey, K. L. Gall, J. M. Scarlett, K. J. Boor, and M. Wiedmann.** 2001. Molecular studies on the ecology of *Listeria monocytogenes* in the smoked fish processing industry. *Appl. Environ. Microbiol.* **67:**198–205.
60. **Okatani,T. A., T. Uto, T. Taniguchi, T. Horisaka, T. Horikita, K. Kaneko, and H. Hayashidani.** 2001. Pulsed-field gel electrophoresis in differentiation of erysipelothrix species strains. *J. Clin. Microbiol.* **39:**4032–4036.
61. **Okatani, T. A., M. Ishikawa, S. Yoshida, M. Sekiguchi, K. Tanno, M. Ogawa, T. Horikita, T. Horisaka, T. Taniguchi, Y. Kato, and H. Hayashidani.** 2004. Automated ribotyping, a rapid typing method for analysis of *Erysipelothrix* spp. strains. *J. Vet. Med. Sci.* **66:**729–733.
62. **Okwumabua, O., B. Swaminathan, P. Edmonds, J. Wenger, J. Hogan, and M. Alden.** 1992. Evaluation of a chemiluminescent DNA probe assay for the rapid confirmation of *Listeria monocytogenes*. *Res. Microbiol.* **143:**183–189.
63. **Ooi, S. T., and B. Lorber.** 2005. Gastroenteritis due to *Listeria monocytogenes*. *Clin. Infect. Dis.* **40:**1327–1332.
64. **Palumbo, J. D., M. K. Borucki, R. E. Mandrell, and L. Gorski.** 2003. Serotyping of *Listeria monocytogenes* by enzyme-linked immunosorbent assay and identification of mixed-serotype cultures by colony immunoblotting. *J. Clin. Microbiol.* **41:**564–571.
65. **Piffaretti, J.-C., H. Kressebuch, M. Aeschbacher, J. Bille, E. Bannerman, J. M. Musser, R. K. Selander, and J. Rocourt.** 1989. Genetic characterization of clones of the bacterium *Listeria monocytogenes* causing epidemic disease. *Proc. Natl. Acad. Sci. USA* **86:**3818–3822.
66. **Pine, L., S. Kathariou, F. Quinn, V. George, J. D. Wenger, and R. E. Weaver.** 1991. Cytopathogenic effects in enterocytelike Caco-2 cells differentiate virulent from avirulent *Listeria* strains. *J. Clin. Microbiol.* **29:**990–996.
67. **Reboli, A. C., and W. E. Farrar.** 1989. *Erysipelothrix rhusiopathiae*: an occupational pathogen. *Clin. Microbiol. Rev.* **2:**354–359.
68. **Reissbrodt, R.** 2004. New chromogenic plating media for detection and enumeration of pathogenic *Listeria* spp.—an overview. *Int. J. Food Microbiol.* **95:**1–9.
69. **Restaino, L., E. W. Frampton, R. M. Irbe, G. Schabert, and H. Spitz.** 1999. Isolation and detection of *Listeria monocytogenes* using fluorogenic and chromogenic substrates for phosphatidylinositol-specific phospholipase C. *J. Food Prot.* **62:**244–251.
70. **Revazishvili, T., M. Kotetishvili, O. C. Stine, A. S. Kreger, J. G. Morris, Jr., and A. Sulakvelidze.** 2004. Comparative analysis of multilocus sequence typing and pulsed-field gel electrophoresis for characterizing *Listeria monocytogenes* strains isolates from environmental and clinical sources. *J. Clin. Microbiol.* **42:**276–285.
71. **Rocourt, J.** 1999. The genus *Listeria* and *Listeria monocytogenes*: phylogenetic position, taxonomy, and identification, p. 1–20. *In* E. T. Ryser and E. H. Marth (ed.), *Listeria, Listeriosis, and Food Safety,* 2nd ed. Marcel Dekker, New York, N.Y.
72. **Rocourt, J., A. Audurier, A. L. Courtieu, J. Durst, S. Ortel, A. Schrettenbrunner, and A. G. Taylor.** 1985. A multicenter study on the phage typing of *Listeria monocytogenes*. *Zentbl. Bakteriol.* **259:**489–497.
73. **Rocourt, J., P. Boerlin, F. Grimont, C. Jacquet, and J.-C. Piffaretti.** 1992. Assignment of *Listeria grayi* and *Listeria murrayi* to a single species, *Listeria grayi*, with a revised description of *Listeria grayi*. *Int. J. Syst. Bacteriol.* **42:**171–174.
74. **Rocourt, J., and P. Cossart.** 1997. *Listeria monocytogenes,* p. 337–352. *In* M. P. Doyle, L. R. Beuchat, and T. J. Montville (ed.), *Food Microbiology: Fundamentals and Frontiers*. ASM Press, Washington, D.C.
75. **Rocourt, J., C. Jacquet, and J. Bille.** 1997. *Human Listeriosis, 1991–1992.* WHOFNU/FOS/97.1.1997. Food Safety Unit Division of Food and Nutrition, WHO, Geneva, Switzerland.
76. **Salcedo, C., L. Arreaza, B. Alcala, L. de la Fuente, and J. A. Vazquez.** 2003. Development of a multilocus sequence typing method for analysis of *Listeria monocytogenes* clones. *J. Clin. Microbiol.* **41:**757–762.
77. **Scheld, W. M.** 1983. Evaluation of rifampin and other antibiotics against *Listeria monocytogenes* in vitro and in vivo. *Rev. Infect. Dis.* **5**(Suppl. 3):S593–S599.
78. **Schonberg, A., E. Bannerman, A. L. Courtieu, R. Kiss, J. McLauchlin, S. Shah, and D. Wilhelms.** 1996. Serotyping of 80 strains from the W. H. O. multicenter international typing study of *Listeria monocytogenes*. *Int. J. Food Microbiol.* **32:**279–287.
79. **Schuchat, A., C. Lizano, C. V. Broome, B. Swaminathan, C. Kim, and K. Winn.** 1991. Outbreak of neonatal listeriosis associated with mineral oil. *Pediatr. Infect. Dis.* **10:**183–189.
80. **Schuchat, A., B. Swaminathan, and C. V. Broome.** 1991. Epidemiology of human listeriosis. *Clin. Microbiol. Rev.* **4:**169–183.
81. **Seeliger, H. P. R., and K. Hohne.** 1979. Serotyping of *Listeria monocytogenes* and related species. *Methods Microbiol.* **13:**31–49.
82. **Seeliger, H. P. R., and D. Jones.** 1986. Genus *Listeria* Pirie, 1940, 383[AL], p. 1235–1245. *In* P. H. A. Sneath, N. S. Mair, M. E. Sharpe, and J. G. Holt (ed.), *Bergey's Manual of Systematic Bacteriology*, vol. 2. Williams & Wilkins, Baltimore, Md.
83. **Sheenan, B., C. Kocks, S. Dramsi, A. D. Klarsfeld, J. Mengaud, and P. Cossart.** 1994. Molecular and genetic determinants of the *Listeria monocytogenes* infectious process. *Curr. Top. Microbiol. Immunol.* **192:**187–216.
84. **Swaminathan, B., T. J. Barrett, S. B. Hunter, and R. V. Tauxe.** 2001. PulseNet: the molecular subtyping network for foodborne bacterial disease surveillance, United States. *Emerg. Infect. Dis.* **7:**382–389.
85. **Takahashi, T., T. Fujisawa, Y. Tamura, S. Suzuki, M. Muramatsu, T. Sawada, Y. Benno, and T. Mitsuoka.** 1992. DNA relatedness among *Erysipelothrix rhusiopathiae* strains representing all twenty-three serovars and *Erysipelothrix tonsillarum*. *Int. J. Syst. Bacteriol.* **42:** 469–473.
86. **Troxler, R., A. von Graevenitz, G. Funke, B. Wiedemann, and I. Stock.** 2000. Natural antibiotic susceptibility of *Listeria* species: *L. grayi, L. innocua, L. ivanovii,*

L. monocytogenes, L. seeligeri, and L. welshimeri strains. *Clin. Microbiol. Infect.* **6:**525–535.

87. **van Netten, P., I. Perales, A. van de Moosdijk, G. D. W. Curtis, and D. A. A. Mossel.** 1989. Liquid and solid differential media for the detection and enumeration of *Listeria monocytogenes* and other *Listeria* spp. *Int. J. Food Microbiol.* **8:**299–316.
88. **Verbarg, S., H. Rheims, S. Emus, A. Fruhling, R. M. Kroppenstedt, E. Stackebrandt, and P. Schumann.** 2004. *Erysipelothrix inopinata* sp. nov., isolated in the course of sterile filtration of vegetable peptone broth, and description of *Erysipelothrichaceae* fam. nov. *Int. J. Syst. Evol. Microbiol.* **54:**221–225.
89. **Vlaemynck, G., V. Lafarge, and S. Scotter.** 2000. Improvement of the detection of *Listeria monocytogenes* by the application of ALOA, a diagnostic, chromogenic isolation medium. *J. Appl. Microbiol.* **88:**430–441.
90. **Weaver, R. E.** 1985. *Erysipelothrix*, p. 209–210. *In* E. H. Lennette, A. Balows, W. J. Hausler, Jr., and H. J. Shadomy (ed.), *Manual of Clinical Microbiology*, 4th ed. American Society for Microbiology, Washington, D.C.
91. **Wernars, K., P. Boerlin, A. Audurier, E. G. Russell, G. D. W. Curtis, L. Herman, and V. van der Mee-Marquet.** 1996. The WHO multicenter study on *Listeria monocytogenes* subtyping: random amplification of polymorphic DNA (RAPD). *Int. J. Food Microbiol.* **32:**325–341.
92. **Wiggins, G. L., W. L. Albritton, and J. C. Feeley.** 1978. Antibiotic susceptibility of clinical isolates of *Listeria monocytogenes*. *Antimicrob. Agents Chemother.* **12:**854–860.
93. **Zhang, W., and S. J. Knabel.** 2005. Multiplex PCR assay simplifies serotyping and sequence typing of *Listeria monocytogenes* associated with human outbreaks. *J. Food Prot.* **68:**1907–1910.

Coryneform Gram-Positive Rods

GUIDO FUNKE AND KATHRYN A. BERNARD

34

This chapter deals with aerobically growing, asporogenous, irregularly shaped, non-partially acid-fast, gram-positive rods generally called "coryneforms." The term "coryneform" is actually somewhat misleading, since only true *Corynebacterium* spp. exhibit a typical club-shaped ("*coryne*," meaning "club" in ancient Greek) morphology, whereas all the other bacteria discussed in this chapter show an irregular morphology. However, in our experience, the term "coryneforms" is a common and convenient expression used by many clinical microbiologists, and therefore, the term will be used in this chapter.

The coryneform bacteria which were, for didactical reasons, not included in this chapter comprise *Actinomyces* spp. (in particular, the most frequently encountered species on aerobic plates, *A. europaeus, A. neuii, A. radingae,* and *A. turicensis*), *Actinobaculum* spp., *Propionibacterium* spp., and *Propioniferax innocua* (see chapter 56), whereas *Arcanobacterium* spp. are included. *Gardnerella vaginalis* is included in this chapter but is discussed separately. Regularly shaped aerobically growing gram-positive rods (*Bacillus, Listeria* and *Erysipelothrix, Lactobacillus,* and *Clostridium tertium*) are covered in chapters 32, 33, 56, and 57, respectively. Taxa which might be initially misidentified as coryneform bacteria also include partially acid-fast bacteria and other actinomycetes (see chapter 35) as well as rapidly growing mycobacteria (see chapter 38).

GENERAL TAXONOMY

The bacteria discussed in this chapter all belong to the class *Actinobacteria*, the genera of which are characterized by specific 16S rRNA gene signature nucleotides (134). All the genera described in this chapter except *Exiguobacterium* and *Gardnerella* belong to the lineage of the gram-positive bacteria with high guanine-plus-cytosine (G+C) content. The coryneform bacteria are most diverse and are differentiated by chemotaxonomic features (Table 1). Phylogenetic investigations, in particular 16S rRNA gene sequencing, have, in general, confirmed the framework set by chemotaxonomic investigations. The 16S rRNA gene sequencing data demonstrate that the genera *Corynebacterium* and *Turicella* are more closely related to the partially acid-fast bacteria and to the genus *Mycobacterium* than to the other coryneform organisms covered in this chapter (62, 104, 123). The genus *Arthrobacter*, which contains rods, is phylogenetically intermixed with the genus *Micrococcus* (and genera formerly called *Micrococcus*), which contains cocci (44, 79). The genus *Rothia* contains both rod-forming organisms, represented by *Rothia dentocariosa*, and a coccus-forming species, *Rothia mucilaginosa,* the former *Stomatococcus mucilaginosus* (19). Other genera which are phylogenetically closely related include *Oerskovia, Cellulosimicrobium,* and *Cellulomonas* (8, 55, 125, 133), as well as *Arcanobacterium* and *Actinomyces* (105).

DESCRIPTIONS OF THE GENERA

Genus *Corynebacterium*

The genus *Corynebacterium* is presently composed of 67 species (and two taxon groups), 40 (and the two taxon groups) of which are medically relevant. Five of the *Corynebacterium* species have been defined since the last edition of this Manual (Table 2).

The cell wall of corynebacteria contains *meso*-diaminopimelic acid (*m*-DAP) as the diamino acid as well as short-chain mycolic acids with 22 to 36 carbon atoms (17). *C. amycolatum, C. atypicum,* and *C. kroppenstedtii* are the only genuine *Corynebacterium* species which do not possess mycolic acids (16, 18, 69). The corynebacterial cell wall also contains arabinose and galactose (17). Palmitic ($C_{16:0}$), oleic ($C_{18:1\omega9c}$), and stearic ($C_{18:0}$) acids are the main cellular fatty acids (CFAs) in all corynebacteria, and tuberculostearic acid (TBSA) can also be found in some species like *C. urealyticum, C. confusum,* and *C. appendicis* (3, 52, 151). The G+C content of *Corynebacterium* spp. varies from 46 to 74 mol%, indicating the enormous diversity within this genus. The phylogenetic relationships within the genus *Corynebacterium* have been outlined (104, 123), creating an extensive and reliable database for future comparative 16S rRNA gene studies, e.g., for the delineation of new species.

Gram staining of corynebacteria shows slightly curved, gram-positive rods with sides not parallel and sometimes slightly wider ends, giving some of the bacteria a typical club shape (Fig. 1a). Corynebacteria whose morphologies differ from this morphology include *C. durum, C. matruchotii,* and *C. sundsvallense* (see below under each species). Cells infrequently stain unevenly. If *Corynebacterium* cells are taken from fluid media, they are arranged as single cells, in pairs, in V forms, in palisades, or in clusters with a so-called Chinese letter appearance. It is again emphasized that the club-shaped form of the rods is observed only for true

TABLE 1 Some chemotaxonomic features of the bacteria covered in this chapter

Genus	Major CFAs	Mycolic acids	Peptidoglycan diamino acid[a]	Acyl type
Corynebacterium	18:1ω9c, 16:0, 18:0	+[b]	*m*-DAP	Acetyl
Turicella	18:1ω9c, 16:0, 18:0	–	*m*-DAP	Glycolyl
Arthrobacter	15:0*ai*, 17:0*ai*, 15:0*i*	–	LYS	Acetyl
Brevibacterium	15:0*ai*, 17:0*ai*, 15:0*i*	–	*m*-DAP	Acetyl
Dermabacter	17:0*ai*, 15:0*ai*, 16:0*i*	–	*m*-DAP	ND[c]
Rothia	15:0*ai*, 17:0*ai*, 16:0*i*	–	LYS	ND
Exiguobacterium	17:0*ai*, 15:0*ai*, 16:0, 13:0*i*	–	LYS	ND
Oerskovia	15:0*ai*, 15:0*i*, 17:0*ai*	–	LYS	Acetyl
Cellulomonas	15:0*ai*, 16:0, 17:0*ai*	–	ORN	Acetyl
Cellulosimicrobium	15:0*ai*, 15:0*i*, 17:0*ai*	–	LYS	Acetyl
Microbacterium	15:0*ai*, 17:0*ai*, 16:0*i*	–	LYS, ORN	Glycolyl
Curtobacterium	15:0*ai*, 17:0*ai*, 16:0*i*	–	ORN	Acetyl
Leifsonia	17:0*ai*, 15:0*ai*, 16:0*i*	–	DAB	ND
Janibacter	17:1, 16:0*i*, 17:0	–	*m*-DAP	Acetyl
Pseudoclavibacter	15:0*ai*, 17:0*ai*, 16:0*i*, 16:0	–	DAB	Acetyl
Brachybacterium	15:0*ai*, 16:0*i*, 17:0*ai*	–	*m*-DAP	Acetyl
Knoellia	17:1*i*, 15:0*i*, 16:0*i*, 17:0*i*	–	*m*-DAP	Acetyl
Arcanobacterium	18:1ω9c, 16:0, 18:0	–	LYS	ND
Gardnerella	16:0, 18:1ω9c, 14:0	–	LYS	ND

[a] *m*-DAP, *meso*-diaminopimelic acid; LYS, lysine; ORN, ornithine; DAB, diaminobutyric acid.
[b] Exceptions: *C. amycolatum*, *C. atypicum*, and *C. kroppenstedtii*.
[c] ND, no data.

Corynebacterium spp. Corynebacteria are always catalase positive, and the medically relevant species are all nonmotile. The genus *Corynebacterium* includes both fermenting and nonfermenting species.

Genus *Turicella*

The genus *Turicella* is phylogenetically closely related to *Corynebacterium* but contains *T. otitidis* as the only species. The cell wall contains *m*-DAP, but mycolic acids are not present (62). The main CFAs for *T. otitidis* are the same as those for *Corynebacterium* spp., but all *T. otitidis* strains also contain significant amounts of TBSA (2 to 10% of all CFAs) (62). *T. otitidis* is the only coryneform bacterium that has a polar lipid profile without glycolipids. The G+C content varies between 65 and 72 mol% (62).

Gram staining shows relatively long gram-positive rods (Fig. 1b). *T. otitidis* is catalase positive, nonmotile, and an oxidizer.

Genus *Arthrobacter*

The genera *Arthrobacter* and *Micrococcus* are so closely related phylogenetically that it has been stated that micrococci are, in fact, arthrobacters which are unable to express rod forms (79). Presently, the genus *Arthrobacter* contains over 50 species, of which only a few have been recovered from human clinical specimens. Lysine is the diamino acid of the cell wall, and $C_{15:0ai}$ is the overall dominating CFA, which represents more than 50% of all CFAs in most *Arthrobacter* species. The G+C content varies between 59 and 70 mol%, indicating the diversity within this genus.

Gram staining may demonstrate a rod-coccus cycle (i.e., rod forms in younger cultures and cocci in older colonies) when cells are grown on rich media (e.g., Columbia base agar). Jointed rods (i.e., rods in a rectangular form, which contributed to the designation of this genus, as "*arthros*" means "joint" in ancient Greek) may also be observed in younger cultures (i.e., after 24 h) but may not be demonstrable for every species. Arthrobacters are catalase positive, motility is variable, and they are always oxidizers.

Genus *Brevibacterium*

The genus *Brevibacterium* presently comprises 17 species, of which 7 species are medically relevant. *m*-DAP is the

TABLE 2 Chronology of recently proposed or reclassified medically relevant coryneform bacteria since publication of the previous edition of this Manual

Yr of definition	Taxon (reference[s])
2002	*Corynebacterium appendicis* (151)
2003	*Brevibacterium luteolum*[a] (146), *Corynebacterium atypicum* (69), *Microbacterium paraoxydans* (82)
2004	*Pseudoclavibacter*/*Zimmermannella* (87, 90), black-pigmented CDC fermentative group 4 bacteria as *Corynebacterium aurimucosum* and *Rothia dentocariosa* (21), *Corynebacterium tuberculostearicum* (35), *Brevibacterium sanguinis* (147)
2005	*Curtobacterium* spp. (38), *Arthrobacter scleromae* (75), *Janibacter* spp. (31, 88), *Brachybacterium* spp. (K. A. Bernard, unpublished observation), *Knoellia* sp. (K. A. Bernard, unpublished observation), *Corynebacterium resistens* (103), *Cellulomonas denverensis* (7)
2006	*Corynebacterium tuscaniae* (114), *Cellulosimicrobium funkei* (8)

[a] This species had originally been designated *Brevibacterium lutescens*.

diamino acid of the cell wall. $C_{15:0ai}$ and $C_{17:0ai}$ usually represent more than 75% of all CFAs (40). The G+C content varies between 60 and 70 mol%.

Gram staining demonstrates relatively short rods which may develop into cocci when cultures are getting older (after 3 days). Brevibacteria are catalase positive, nonmotile, and oxidizers.

Genus *Dermabacter*

The genus *Dermabacter* presently comprises only one species, *D. hominis*. *m*-DAP is the diamino acid of the cell wall, and $C_{15:0ai}$ and $C_{17:0ai}$ usually account for 40 to 60% of all CFAs. The G+C content range is between 60 and 62 mol% (76).

Gram staining shows very short rods (Fig. 1c), which are often initially misinterpreted as cocci. *D. hominis* strains are catalase positive, nonmotile, and glucose fermenters.

Genus *Rothia*

For didactical reasons, the genus *Rothia* is also included in this chapter because some species are rod-like. The genus *Rothia* belongs to the family *Micrococcaceae*. Collins and colleagues reclassified *Stomatococcus mucilaginosus* as *Rothia mucilaginosa* (19). Since *Rothia mucilaginosa* exhibits coccoid forms in the Gram stain, the genus *Rothia* is also covered in chapter 31 (on the catalase-positive, gram-positive cocci). However, the species *R. dentocariosa* clearly exhibits mainly rod forms and is therefore covered in this chapter on coryneform bacteria.

Lysine is the diamino acid of the cell wall, and $C_{15:0ai}$ and $C_{17:0ai}$ usually represent 40 to 60% of all CFAs. The G+C content ranges between 47 and 56 mol%. *Rothia* strains can be quite pleomorphic by Gram staining, but filamentous forms are normally not observed. They have a variable catalase reaction, are nonmotile, and exhibit a fermentative metabolism.

Genus *Exiguobacterium*

The genus *Exiguobacterium* is phylogenetically related to the so-called group 2 bacilli. Seven species are included in this genus, of which only *E. acetylicum* has been mentioned in any publication as being isolated from human clinical material. Lysine is the diamino acid of the cell wall, and $C_{15:0ai}$ and $C_{17:0ai}$ represent only about 30 to 40% of the total CFAs. *E. acetylicum* contains significant amounts of $C_{13:0}$ and $C_{13:0ai}$, which are not found in any other coryneform taxon (3). The G+C content is about 47 mol%.

Exiguobacteria present as relatively short rods in young cultures. Strains are catalase positive and motile and have a fermentative metabolism.

Genus *Oerskovia*

In older textbooks, oerskoviae were assigned to the nocardioform group of organisms due to their morphological features. This includes branching vegetative substrate hyphae and penetration into agar, but they have no aerial hyphae. However, there is now phylogenetic evidence that *Oerskovia*, including the reclassified *Promicromonospora* (133), is more closely related to genera like *Cellulomonas* than to the mycolic acid-containing genera like *Nocardia*. Representatives of the type species, *O. turbata*, were recovered from soil, but human pathogens originally identified as *O. turbata* have now been placed in *Cellulosimicrobium funkei* (8). Lysine is the diamino acid of the cell wall, and $C_{15:0ai}$ is the main CFA in oerskoviae. The G+C content is 70 to 75 mol%.

Gram staining shows coccoid to rod-shaped bacteria which originate from the breaking up of mycelia. Oerskoviae strains are catalase positive, motility is variable, and they are fermentative.

Genus *Cellulomonas*

The genus *Cellulomonas* presently comprises 13 species, of which only *C. hominis* and *C. denverensis* have been described as being isolated from humans (7, 55). Ornithine is the diamino acid of the cell wall, and $C_{15:0ai}$ and $C_{16:0}$ are the main CFAs. The G+C content is 71 to 76 mol%.

Gram staining shows small, thin rods. All *Cellulomonas* spp., except *C. fermentans* and *C. humilata*, are catalase positive, their motility is variable, the environmental *Cellulomonas* strains are cellulolytic (whereas *C. hominis* did not hydrolyze cellulose in the test system used [55]), and they have a fermentative metabolism.

Genus *Cellulosimicrobium*

The genus *Cellulosimicrobium* presently comprises three species. The medically relevant species are *C. funkei* and *C. cellulans*, which had been designated *Cellulomonas cellulans* or *Oerskovia xanthineolytica* in the past (125). The reason for removing *C. cellulans* from the genus *Cellulomonas* was that the topology of the 16S rRNA gene dendrogram indicated that the branching point of this taxon was outside *Cellulomonas* proper. In addition, the chemotaxonomic characteristic of lysine as diamino acid supported the reclassification. Predominant CFAs include $C_{15:0ai}$, $C_{15:0i}$, $C_{16:0i}$, and $C_{16:0}$. The major menaquinone (MK) is MK-9(H_4), and the G+C content is 74 mol%. It should be noted that the genus *Cellulosimicrobium* is related to the genus *Oerskovia* but nevertheless distinct.

In young cultures, a mycelium is produced that fragments later into irregular, curved, and club-shaped rods. Catalase activity is detected, and strains are nonmotile. All strains have a fermentative metabolism.

Genus *Microbacterium*

It had been known since the mid-1990s that the genera *Microbacterium* and *Aureobacterium* are phylogenetically intermixed (109). The diamino acid in the third position of the tetrapeptide of the peptidoglycan was considered one of the most important chemotaxonomical markers. L-Lysine is present in microbacteria, and D-ornithine is present in the former aureobacteria. Because in some genera (e.g., *Propionibacterium* and *Bifidobacterium*) there is not a good correlation between the type of the diamino acid in their peptidoglycan and their phylogenetic trees and because a set of signature nucleotides within the 16S rRNA gene of both microbacteria and aureobacteria was demonstrated, it has been proposed to unify the two genera in a redefined genus, *Microbacterium* (135).

To date, over 35 *Microbacterium* species have been validated, but only a minority of them have been demonstrated to be of clinical importance. Microbacteria are frequently encountered in environmental specimens (e.g., soil). $C_{15:0ai}$ and $C_{17:0ai}$ are the two main CFAs, often representing up to 75% of the total CFAs (42, 65, 135). The G+C content of *Microbacterium* spp. is 65 to 76 mol%, indicating the diversity within the genus.

Gram staining often shows thin or short rods with no branching. Catalase activity and motility are variable. Microbacteria can be either fermenters or oxidizers.

Genus *Curtobacterium*

Curtobacterium spp., like microbacteria, belong to the peptidoglycan type B actinomycetes (i.e., cross-linkage between positions 2 and 4 of the two peptide subunits). Ornithine is the diamino acid and the only amino acid composing the interpeptide bridge. Curtobacteria have an acetyl peptidoglycan acyl-type and menaquinone MK-9 as major MK, whereas

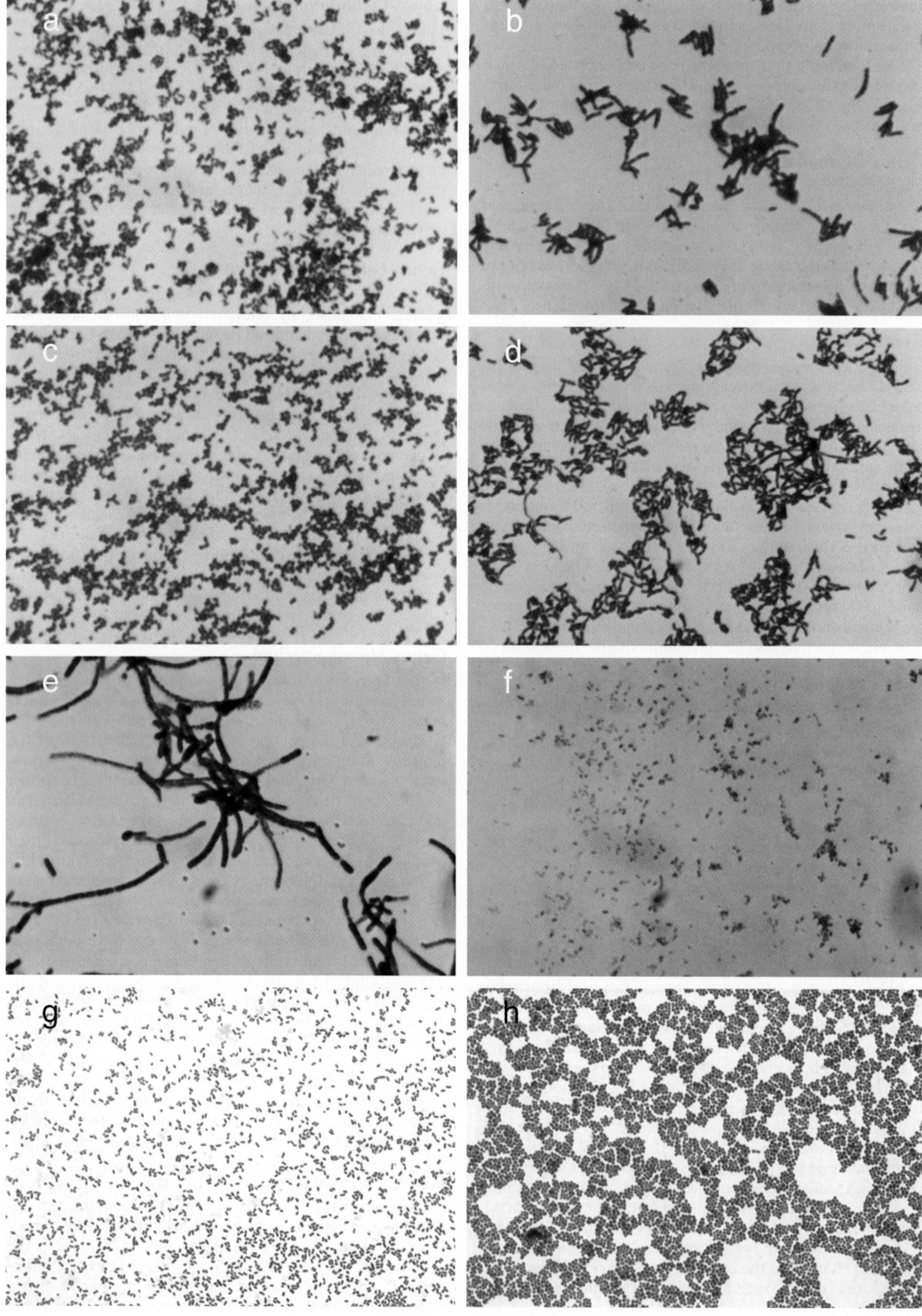
a
b
c
d
e
f
g
h

microbacteria possess a glycolyl type and MK-11,12 (Table 1). For most curtobacteria, $C_{15:0ai}$ and $C_{17:0ai}$ represent more than 75% of all CFAs (38). The G+C contents range from 68 to 75 mol%. Six *Curtobacterium* species are validly described.

Gram staining shows small and short rods with no branching. Catalase activity is positive, motility is observed in most strains, and all strains show a respiratory metabolism which proceeds slowly in oxidizing carbohydrates.

Genus *Leifsonia*

The former "*Corynebacterium aquaticum*" has been transferred into the new genus *Leifsonia* as *L. aquatica* (34). This species is the only medically relevant species in this genus. *L. aquatica* strains belong to the peptidoglycan B type actinomycetes and therefore cannot be true corynebacteria, which actually possess an A type of peptidoglycan (i.e., cross-linkage between positions 3 and 4 of the two peptide subunits). Diaminobutyric acid is the diamino acid of the cell wall peptidoglycan, and $C_{15:0ai}$ and $C_{17:0ai}$, as in microbacteria, are the main CFAs but represent <75% of all CFAs (65). The G+C content is about 70 mol%.

Gram staining shows thin rods. The strains are catalase and oxidase positive (the latter is an untypical feature for coryneform bacteria), always motile, and oxidizers.

Genus *Janibacter* and Other Unusual Coryneforms

Recent examinations of coryneform bacteria by using primarily sequence-based identification approaches have shown that additional genera could be recovered from human clinical materials.

Genus *Janibacter*

Strains of the genus *Janibacter* (91) were found to be associated with bacteremia and recovered from blood cultures (31, 88; Bernard, unpublished) and are the first medically relevant coryneforms reported from the family *Intrasporangiaceae*. *Janibacter* strains can have gram-variable or gram-positive coccoidal to rod forms in singles, pairs, or irregular clumps. The DNA base composition is 69 to 73 mol% G+C, with an unusual CFA profile consisting of significant volumes of CFAs $C_{16:0i}$, $C_{17:1}$, and $C_{17:0}$. These bacteria are described as oxidizers, with white, creamy, or yellowish pigments. They are nonmotile, and optimal growth may occur at 25 to 30°C.

Genus *Pseudoclavibacter*

The genus *Pseudoclavibacter* was described in 2004 for a previous "*Brevibacterium helvolum*" strain (90). The novel genus *Zimmermannella*, described shortly afterwards, is a later synonym of *Pseudoclavibacter* (87). *Z. alba* strains were recovered from urine, and *Z. bifida* strains were recovered from blood cultures and wounds. By Gram staining, these species were found to be short or medium gram-positive rods, with *Z. bifida* demonstrating some rudimentary branching. The DNA base composition is 62 to 68 mol% G+C. Major CFAs are $C_{15:0ai}$, $C_{16:0}$, $C_{16:0i}$, and $C_{17:0ai}$. These strains are oxidizers, with white or yellowish colonies. Optimal growth occurs at 30°C.

Genera *Brachybacterium* and *Knoellia*

Two isolates from the genus *Brachybacterium* and one strain from the genus *Knoellia*, all recovered from blood cultures, have been characterized (K. A. Bernard, unpublished observations). *Brachybacterium* spp. (15) are members of the familiy *Dermabacteraceae* and so are most closely related to the genus *Dermabacter*. Members of this genus grow at 37°C, exhibit gram-positive coccoidal and rodlike forms, and have a G+C content of 68 to 73 mol%. The *Brachybacterium* blood culture isolates were metabolically fermentative and had branched-chained-type CFAs. The genus *Knoellia* (68), like the genus *Janibacter*, is a member of the family *Intrasporangiaceae*. Cells are irregular gram-positive rods or cocci, with major CFAs of the branched-chain type, and the G+C content is 68 to 69 mol%. The single *Knoellia* blood culture isolate was capnophilic, growing best in 5% CO_2 at 37°C.

Genus *Arcanobacterium*

The genus *Arcanobacterium* presently contains six species, of which *A. haemolyticum*, *A. bernardiae*, and *A. pyogenes* have been recovered from human clinical specimens. Lysine is the diamino acid of the cell wall, whereas in the phylogenetically closely related *Actinomyces* spp. lysine or ornithine is found. Arcanobacteria contain menaquinones of the MK-9(H_4) type, whereas the *Actinomyces* spp. examined so far have MK-10(H_4). The main CFAs of arcanobacteria are $C_{16:0}$, $C_{18:1\omega9c}$, and $C_{18:0}$ (as in *Corynebacterium* spp. and *T. otitidis*), but in contrast to corynebacteria significant amounts of $C_{10:0}$, $C_{12:0}$, and $C_{14:0}$ may also be detected (3). The G+C content is 48 to 52 mol%.

Gram staining of arcanobacteria shows irregular gram-positive rods. All clinically relevant arcanobacteria are catalase negative, nonmotile, and fermenters.

NATURAL HABITAT

Many species of the corynebacteria are part of the normal flora of the skin and mucous membranes in humans and mammals. The habitat for some medically irrelevant corynebacteria (e.g., *C. terpenotabidum* and *C. halotolerans*) is the environment. It is noteworthy that not all corynebacteria are equally distributed over skin and mucous membranes but many of them occupy a specific niche. *C. diphtheriae* can be isolated from the nasopharynx as well as from skin lesions, which actually represent a reservoir for the spread of diphtheria. Important opportunistic pathogens like *C. amycolatum*, *C. striatum*, and *D. hominis* are part of the normal human skin flora but have thus far not been recovered from throat swabs from healthy individuals (144). Coryneform bacteria prominent in the oropharynx include *C. durum* and *R. dentocariosa* (144). *C. auris* and *T. otitidis* seem to have an almost exclusive preference for the external auditory canal (73). In nearly every instance that *C. macginleyi* has been isolated, it has been recovered from eye specimens (53). Another *Corynebacterium* species with a distinctive niche is *C. glucuronolyticum*, which is almost exclusively isolated from genitourinary specimens from humans (39) and also from animals (24). *C. urealyticum*, another genitourinary pathogen, has, like *C. jeikeium*, also been cultured from the inanimate hospital environment.

The natural habitat of arcanobacteria is not fully understood, but *A. haemolyticum* is recovered from throat as well as from wound swabs, whereas *A. bernardiae* has been found mainly in abscesses adjacent to skin (G. Funke, unpublished

FIGURE 1 Gram stain morphologies of *Corynebacterium diphtheriae* ATCC 14779 after 48 h of incubation (a), *Turicella otitidis* DSM 8821 (48 h) (b), *Dermabacter hominis* ATCC 51325 (48 h) (c), *Corynebacterium durum* DMMZ 2544 (72 h) (d), *Corynebacterium matruchotii* ATCC 14266 (24 h) (e), *Gardnerella vaginalis* ATCC 14018 (48 h) (f), *Corynebacterium aurimucosum* HC-NML 91-0032 (24 h) (g), and a black-pigmented *Rothia dentocariosa* HC-NML 77-0298 (24 h) (h).

observation). It is unclear whether the two species are part of the normal skin and/or the gastrointestinal flora. *A. pyogenes* is found on mucous membranes of cattle, sheep, and swine. Brevibacteria can be found on dairy products (e.g., cheese) but are also inhabitants of the human skin (40). Arthrobacters are some of the most frequently isolated bacteria when soil samples are cultured, but at least *Arthrobacter cumminsii* also seems to be present on human skin (54). Members of the genera *Exiguobacterium, Oerskovia, Cellulomonas, Cellulosimicrobium,* and *Microbacterium* have their habitats in the inanimate environment (e.g., soil and activated sludge). *Microbacterium* spp. have also been recovered from hospital environments (42). Curtobacteria are primarily plant pathogens (38).

CLINICAL SIGNIFICANCE

Estimating the clinical significance of coryneform bacteria isolated from clinical specimens is often confusing for clinical microbiologists. This is in part due to the natural habitat of coryneform bacteria, which may lead to their recovery if specimens were not taken correctly. The reader is referred to the guidelines on minimal microbiological requirements in publications on disease associations of coryneform bacteria (64).

Coryneform bacteria should be identified to the species level if they are isolated (i) from normally sterile body sites, e.g., blood (except if only one of multiple specimens became positive); (ii) from adequately collected clinical material if they are the predominant organisms; and (iii) from urine specimens if they are the only bacteria encountered and the bacterial count is $>10^4$/ml or if they are the predominant organisms and the total bacterial count is $>10^5$/ml.

The clinical significance of coryneform bacteria is strengthened by the following findings: (i) multiple specimens are positive for the same coryneform bacteria; (ii) coryneform bacteria are seen in the direct Gram stain, and a strong leukocyte reaction is also observed; and (iii) other organisms recovered from the same material are of low pathogenicity.

For a comprehensive summary of case reports on individual coryneform bacteria, the reader is referred to review articles (2, 64). The most frequently reported coryneforms, as well as their established disease associations, are listed in Table 3.

Historically, diphtheria caused by *C. diphtheriae* (or *C. ulcerans*) is the most prominent infectious disease for which coryneform bacteria are responsible. Therefore, special attention is given to that disease in this chapter. Due to immunization programs, the disease has nearly disappeared in countries with high socioeconomic standards. However, the disease is still endemic in some subtropical and tropical countries as well as among individuals of certain ethnic groups (e.g., indigenous peoples in the Americas and Australia). In the 1990s, diphtheria reemerged in the states of the former Soviet Union. However, despite increased global travel activities, only a few imported cases have been reported by countries with well-developed health care systems.

TABLE 3 Most frequently reported disease associations of coryneform bacteria in humans

Taxon	Disease or disease association	Reference(s)[a]
C. amycolatum	Wound infections, foreign body infections, bacteremia, sepsis, urinary tract infections, respiratory tract infections	46, 83
C. aurimucosum	Genitourinary tract infections (mainly females)	126, 127
CDC group F-1	Urinary tract infections	
CDC group G/ *C. tuberculostearicum*	Catheter infections, bacteremia, endocarditis, wound infections, eye infections	
C. diphtheriae (toxigenic)	Throat diphtheria, cutaneous diphtheria	30
C. diphtheriae (nontoxigenic)	Endocarditis, foreign body infections, pharyngitis	25, 37, 111
C. glucuronolyticum	Genitourinary tract infections (mainly males)	39
C. jeikeium	Endocarditis, bacteremia, foreign body infections, wound infections	115
C. kroppenstedtii	Granulomatous lobular mastitis	106
C. macginleyi	Eye infections	53
C. minutissimum	Wound infections, urinary tract infections, respiratory tract infections	154
C. pseudodiphtheriticum	Respiratory tract infections, endocarditis	
C. pseudotuberculosis	Lymphadenitis (occupational)	
C. resistens	Bacteremia	103
C. riegelii	Urinary tract infections (females)	49
C. striatum	Wound infections, respiratory tract infections, foreign body infections	
C. ulcerans (toxigenic)	Respiratory diphtheria	
C. urealyticum	Urinary tract infections, bacteremia, wound infections	130
Arthrobacter spp.	Bacteremia, foreign body infections, urinary tract infections	44, 54
Brevibacterium spp.	Bacteremia, foreign body infections, malodorous feet	40
D. hominis	Wound infections, bacteremia	61
Rothia spp.	Endocarditis, bacteremia, respiratory tract infections	
Cellulomonas spp.	Bacteremia, wound infections	7, 55
Cellulosimicrobium sp.	Foreign body infections, bacteremia	8, 93
Microbacterium spp.	Bacteremia, foreign body infections, wound infections	42, 82, 85
A. bernardiae	Abscess formation (together with mixed anaerobic flora)	57
A. haemolyticum	Pharyngitis in older children, wound and tissue infections	89
A. pyogenes	Abscess formation, wound and soft tissue infections	
G. vaginalis	Bacterial vaginosis, endometritis, postpartum sepsis	10

[a] References for taxa without references are our observations. For further information, see references 2 and 64.

The main manifestation of diphtheria is an upper respiratory tract illness with a sore throat, dysphagia, lymphadenitis, low-grade fever, malaise, and headache. A nasopharyngeal adherent membrane which may occasionally lead to obstruction is characteristic. The severe systemic effects of diphtheria include myocarditis, neuritis, and kidney damage caused by the *C. diphtheriae* exotoxin, which is encoded by a bacteriophage carrying the *tox* gene. *C. diphtheriae* may also cause cutaneous diphtheria or endocarditis (with either toxin-positive or toxin-negative strains). Some people with poor hygienic standards (e.g., drug and alcohol abusers) are prone to colonization (on the skin more often than in the pharynx) by *C. diphtheriae* strains, which are often nontoxigenic.

COLLECTION, TRANSPORT, AND STORAGE OF SPECIMENS

In general, coryneform bacteria do not need special handling when samples are collected.

C. diphtheriae

The diagnosis of diphtheria is primarily a clinical one. The physician should notify the receiving laboratory immediately of suspected diphtheria. In case of respiratory diphtheria, material for culture should be obtained on a swab (either a cotton- or a polyester-tipped swab) from the inflamed areas in the nasopharynx. Multisite sampling (nasopharynx) is thought to increase sensitivity. If membranes are present and can be removed (swabs from beneath the membrane are most valuable), they should also be sent to the microbiology laboratory (although *C. diphtheriae* might not be culturable from those in every instance). Nasopharyngeal swabs should be obtained from suspected carriers. It is preferable that the swabs be immediately transferred to the microbiology laboratory for culturing. If the swabs must be sent to the laboratory, semisolid transport media (e.g., Amies) ensure the maintenance of the bacteria. All coryneform bacteria are relatively resistant to drying and moderate temperature changes. Material from patients with suspected cases of wound diphtheria can be obtained by swab or aspiration.

After the appropriate isolation media have been inoculated (see "Isolation Procedures and Incubation" below), the swabs taken from diphtheritic membranes may be subjected to Neisser or Loeffler methylene blue staining (positive if metachromatic granules [polar bodies] are seen). However, it is noteworthy that the sensitivity of the microscopic examination is limited.

A PCR-based direct detection system for diphtheria toxin has been described by the Centers for Disease Control and Prevention (CDC) (98). Their system had the highest sensitivity when Dacron polyester-tipped swabs were used and when silica gel packages were stored at 4°C rather than at room temperature. The approach of a PCR-based direct detection system was successfully used in a retrospective study for which only formalin-fixed clinical specimens were available (80). However, direct detection for diphtheria toxin as the sole, primary test for clinical specimens has not been recommended, and microbiological culture is essential for confirming diphtheria (29).

Long-term preservation in skim milk at −70°C is applicable to all coryneform bacteria. The same skim milk tube except for those containing lipophilic corynebacteria can be thawed and put into the freezer again, and this can be done several times (Funke, unpublished). For nonlipophilic coryneforms, good results were also observed with Microbank tubes (Pro Lab Diagnostics, Austin, Tex.) (Funke, unpublished). The advantage of using these tubes is that individual beads can be taken out of the tube. Coryneform bacteria can also be stored for decades when they are kept lyophilized in an appropriate medium (e.g., 0.9% NaCl containing 2% bovine serum albumin).

ISOLATION PROCEDURES AND INCUBATION

Coryneform bacteria including *C. diphtheriae* can be readily isolated from a 5% sheep blood agar (SBA)-based selective medium containing 100 μg of fosfomycin per ml (plus 12.5 μg of glucose-6-phosphate per ml), since nearly all coryneforms (except *Actinomyces* spp. and *D. hominis*) are highly resistant to this compound (139, 144). It is also possible to put disks containing 50 μg of fosfomycin (plus 50 μg of glucose-6-phosphate [already incorporated in the disk]) (BD Diagnostics, Sparks, Md.) on a SBA plate and then examine the colonies which grow around the disk. Selective media for coryneform bacteria containing 50 to 100 μg of furazolidone/ml (Sigma, St. Louis, Mo.) have also been described. If lipophilic corynebacteria like *C. jeikeium* or *C. urealyticum* are sought, then 0.1 to 1.0% Tween 80 (Merck, Darmstadt, Germany) should be added to a SBA plate (add Tween 80 before pouring the medium). It is also possible to streak sterile filtered Tween 80 with a cotton swab onto SBA plates. Coryneform bacteria do not grow on MacConkey agar. However, if "coryneform" bacteria are recovered from this medium, they should be examined carefully to rule out rapidly growing mycobacteria.

With very few exceptions (some arthrobacters, microbacteria, and curtobacteria, which have optimal growth temperatures of between 30 and 35°C), the medically relevant coryneform bacteria all grow at 37°C. It is desirable to culture specimens for coryneform bacteria in a CO_2-enriched atmosphere, since some taxa, e.g., *Rothia* and *Arcanobacterium* spp., grow much better under those conditions. Nearly all medically relevant coryneform bacteria grow within 48 h, so that primary culture plates should not be incubated longer than that. However, if liquid media are used (e.g., for specimens from normally sterile body sites), these should be checked after 5 days by Gram staining for the presence of coryneform bacteria (only if growth is observed with the naked eye) before they are discarded.

It is recommended that urine specimens be incubated for longer than 24 h to check for the presence of *C. urealyticum* but only when patients are symptomatic or have alkaline urine or struvite crystals in their urine sediment.

C. diphtheriae

The primary plating media for the cultivation of *C. diphtheriae* should be SBA plus one selective medium (e.g., Cystine-Tellurite blood agar [CTBA] or freshly prepared Tinsdale medium) (29, 30). If silica gel is used as a transport medium, the desiccated swabs need to be additionally incubated overnight in broth (supplemented with either plasma or blood), which should then be streaked onto the primary plating medium. The plates are read after 18 to 24 h of incubation at 37°C, preferably in a 5% CO_2-enriched atmosphere. Tellurite inhibits the growth of many noncoryneform bacteria, but even a few *C. diphtheriae* strains are sensitive to potassium tellurite and will therefore not grow on CTBA but may grow on SBA. It is noteworthy that growth on CTBA and tellurite reduction are not specific for *C. diphtheriae,* since many other coryneforms may also produce black (albeit smaller) colonies. The best medium for direct culturing of *C. diphtheriae* is probably Tinsdale medium (30).

However, the limitations of Tinsdale medium are its relatively short shelf life (<4 weeks) and the necessity to add horse serum to it. On Tinsdale plates, both tellurite reductase activity (as shown by black colonies) and cystinase activity (as shown by a brown halo around the colonies) can be observed (see Fig. 3i). If neither CTBA nor Tinsdale medium is available, colistin-nalidixic acid blood agar plates are recommended for the isolation of *C. diphtheriae* or any other coryneform bacterium. It is necessary to pick multiple colonies from CNA plates to rule out *C. diphtheriae* (first Gram staining, then subculturing, and then subsequent biochemical testing). Nonselective Loeffler serum slants are no longer recommended for the primary isolation of *C. diphtheriae* because of overgrowth by other bacteria (but *C. diphtheriae* cells with polar bodies are produced on Loeffler or Pai slants only).

IDENTIFICATION AND TYPING SYSTEMS

Basic tests available in every microbiology laboratory are of great value for the identification of coryneform bacteria. The Gram staining morphology of the cells can exclude the assignment to many genera and may even lead to the assignment to the correct genus (e.g., to the genus *Corynebacterium*, *Turicella*, or *Dermabacter*) (Fig. 1). Morphology, size, pigment, odor, and hemolysis of colonies are also valuable criteria in the differential diagnosis of coryneform bacteria.

von Graevenitz and Funke (143) had outlined a biochemical identification system for coryneform bacteria which was based on previous results from the CDC Special Bacteriology Reference Laboratory (71). This system includes the following reactions: catalase, test for fermentation or oxidation (in our experience, this is best observed in semisolid cystine Trypticase agar medium [rather than on triple sugar iron or oxidation-fermentation media], with fermentation indicated by acid or alkali production in the entire tube and oxidation found at the surface of the tube); motility; nitrate reduction (24-h incubation); urea hydrolysis (24-h incubation); esculin hydrolysis (up to 48 h of incubation); acid production from glucose, maltose, sucrose, mannitol, and xylose (48-h incubation); CAMP reaction (24-h incubation) with a β-hemolysin-producing strain of *Staphylococcus aureus* (e.g., strain ATCC 25923), i.e., positive reaction indicated by an augmentation of the effect of *S. aureus* β-hemolysin on erythrocytes, resulting in a complete hemolysis in an arrowhead configuration (Fig. 2); and a test for lipophilia (24-h incubation), which is performed only for catalase-positive colonies <0.5 mm in diameter. For the test for lipophilia, colonies are subcultured onto ordinary SBA and onto a 0.1 to 1% Tween 80-containing SBA plate. Lipophilic corynebacteria develop colonies up to 2 mm in diameter after 24 h on Tween-supplemented agar. It has also been suggested that growth in brain heart infusion broth with and without supplementation of 1% Tween 80 be compared and strains which grow only in the supplemented broth can be called lipophilic. The identification protocols given in this chapter are, in principle, based on the identification system of von Graevenitz and Funke (143) mentioned above (Tables 4 and 5).

The currently recommended identification systems include the API (RAPID) Coryne system (bioMérieux, Marcy l'Etoile, France) and the RapID CB Plus system (Remel, Lenexa, Kans.). The API Coryne system contains 49 taxa in its present database (version 2.0). In a comprehensive multicenter study, it was found that 90.5% of the strains belonging to the taxa included were correctly identified, with additional tests needed for correct identification for 55.1% of all strains tested (60). The results were highly reproducible if the manufacturer's recommendations for use were rigorously followed. It was concluded that the system is a useful tool for the identification of the diverse group of coryneform bacteria encountered in the routine clinical laboratory. The RapID CB Plus system correctly identified 80.9% of the strains to the genus and the species levels, and an additional 12.2% strains were correctly identified to the genus level but with less accurate species designations; it was also concluded that this system may perform well under the conditions of a routine clinical laboratory (58). However, it is always important to question critically the identifications provided by any commercial identification system and to correlate the results with simple basic characteristics such as macroscopic morphology and Gram staining results. Furthermore, it is important to note that for both commercially available identification systems the databases have not been updated since 1997 and therefore the recently described taxa are not covered.

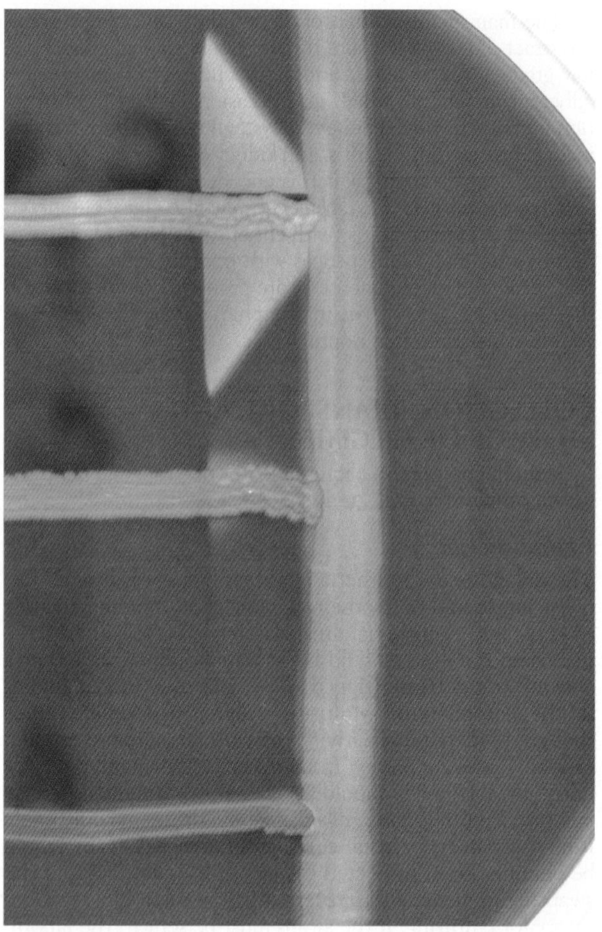

FIGURE 2 CAMP reactions of different coryneform bacteria after 24 h. (Top) *C. glucuronolyticum* DMMZ 891 (positive reaction). (Middle) *C. diphtheriae* ATCC 14779 (negative reaction). (Bottom) *A. haemolyticum* ATCC 9345 (CAMP inhibition reaction). The vertical streak is *S. aureus* ATCC 25923.

For some identifications, the commercial API 50CH system (bioMérieux) has been found to be useful. For example, when applying the AUX medium (usually attached to the kit

TABLE 4 Identification of medically relevant *Corynebacterium* spp.[a]

Species	Fermentation/ oxidation	Lipophilism	Nitrate reduction	Urease	Esculin hydrolysis	Pyrazinamidase	Alkaline phosphatase	Acid production from: Glucose	Maltose	Sucrose	Mannitol	Xylose	CAMP reaction	Other traits
C. accolens	F	+	+	–	–	V	–	+	–	V	V	–	–	
C. afermentans subsp. *afermentans*	O	–	–	–	–	+	+	–	–	–	–	–	V	
C. afermentans subsp. *lipophilum*	O	+	–	–	–	+	+	–	–	–	–	–	V	
C. amycolatum	F	–	V	V	–	+	+	+	V	V	–	–	–	Most O/129 resistant, propionic detected
C. appendicis	F	+	–	+	–	+	+	+	+	–	–	–	ND	Huge amounts of TBSA present
C. argentoratense	F	–	–	–	–	+	V	+	–	–	–	–	–	Chymotrypsin may be positive; propionic detected[b]
C. atypicum	F	–	–	–	–	–	–	+	+	+	–	–	ND	Pinpoint colonies, β-glucuronidase positive
C. aurimucosum	F	–	–	–	V	+	+	+	+	+	–	–	ND	Most strains exhibit grayish black pigment, some pitting agar
C. auris	O	–	–	–	–	+	+	–	–	–	–	–	+	Slight adherence to agar, cleaved mycolics
C. bovis[c]	F	+	–	–	–	–	+	+	–	–	–	–	–	TBSA positive; fructose positive
C. confusum	F	–	+	–	–	+	+	(+)	–	–	–	–	–	Tyrosine negative, propionic detected
C. coyleae	F	–	–	–	–	+	+	(+)	–	–	–	–	+	
CDC group F-1	F	+	V	+	–	+	–	+	+	+	–	–	–	
CDC group G	F	+	V	–	–	+	+	+	V	V	–	–	–	Fructose positive, anaerobic growth positive
C. diphtheriae biotype *gravis*	F	–	+	–	–	–	–	+	+	–	–	–	–	Glycogen positive, propionic detected
C. diphtheriae biotype *intermedius*	F	+	+	–	–	–	–	+	+	–	–	–	–	Propionic detected

(*Continued on next page*)

TABLE 4 Identification of medically relevant *Corynebacterium* spp.[a] *(Continued)*

Species	Fermentation/ oxidation	Lipophilism	Nitrate reduction	Urease	Esculin hydrolysis	Pyrazin-amidase	Alkaline phos-phatase	Acid production from: Glucose	Maltose	Sucrose	Mannitol	Xylose	CAMP reaction	Other traits
C. diphtheriae biotype *mitis* and *belfanti*	F	–	+/–[d]	–	–	–	–	+	+	–	–	–	–	Glycogen negative, propionic detected
C. durum	F	–	+	(V)	(V)	+	–	+	+	+	V	–	–	Adherent to agar, propionic detected
C. falsenii	F	–	–	(+)	–	(+)	+	(+)	V	–	–	–	–	Yellowish
C. freneyi	F	–	V	–	–	+	+	+	+	+	–	–	ND	α-Glucosidase positive, grows at 20 and 42°C
C. glucuronolyticum	F	–	V	V	V	+	V	+	V	+	–	V	+	β-Glucuronidase positive, propionic detected
C. imitans	F	–	–	–	–	(+)	+	+	+	(+)	–	–	+	Tyrosine negative, O/129 resistant
C. jeikeium	O	+	–	–	–	+	+	+	V	–	–	–	–	Fructose negative, anaerobic growth negative
C. kroppenstedtii	F	+	–	–	+	+	–	+	V	+	–	–	–	Lacking mycolic acids, propionic detected
C. lipophiloflavum	O	+	–	–	–	+	+	–	–	–	–	–	–	Yellow
C. macginleyi	F	+	+	–	–	–	+	+	–	+	V	–	–	
C. matruchotii	F	–	+	–	V	+	–	+	+	+	–	–	–	"Whip handle" (upon Gram staining); propionic detected
C. minutissimum	F	–	–	–	–	+	+	+	+	V	V	–	–	Tyrosine positive
C. mucifaciens	O	–	–	–	–	+	+	+	–	V	–	–	–	Very mucoid yellowish colonies
C. propinquum	O	–	+	–	–	V	V	–	–	–	–	–	–	Tyrosine positive
C. pseudodiphtheriticum	O	–	+	+	–	+	V	–	–	–	–	–	–	
C. pseudotuberculosis	F	–	V	+	–	–	V	+	+	V	–	–	REV	Propionic detected
C. resistens	F	+	–	–	–	–	+	+	–	–	–	–	–	Slow growth in anaerobic atmosphere
C. riegelii	F	–	–	+	–	V	V	–	(+)	–	–	–	–	
C. singulare	F	–	–	+	–	+	+	+	+	+	–	–	–	Tyrosine positive
C. simulans[e]	F	–	+	–	–	V	+	+	–	+	–	–	–	Reduces nitrite
C. striatum	F	–	+	–	–	+	+	+	–	V	–	–	V	Tyrosine positive
C. sundsvallense	F	–	–	+	–	V	V	+	+	+	–	–	–	Sticky colonies
C. thomssenii	F	–	–	+	–	+	+	+	+	+	–	–	–	N-Acetyl-β-glucosaminidase positive, sticky colonies

C. tuberculostearicum	F	+	V	−	−	+	V	+	V	V	−	−	ND	
C. tuscaniae	O	−	−	−	−	+	+	+	+	−	−	−	−	Hippurate positive, tyrosine negative
C. ulcerans	F	−	−	+	−	−	+	+	+	−	−	−	REV	Glycogen positive, propionic detected
C. urealyticum	O	+	−	+	−	+	V	−	−	−	−	−	−	
C. xerosis	F	−	V	−	−	+	+	+	+	+	−	−	−	O/129 susceptible, propionic not detected

[a] Abbreviations and symbols: F, fermentation; O, oxidation; +, positive; −, negative; V, variable; ( ), delayed or weak reaction; ND, no data; REV, CAMP inhibition reaction.

[b] Propionic acid as a glucose fermentation product.

[c] Blood culture isolate (4) was also ONPG positive, oxidase positive, weakly maltose positive but negative by API Coryne, propionic acid was not detected; β-galactosidase was not observed using two methods (API Coryne, API Zym); API Coryne code obtained, 0101104.

[d] *C. diphtheriae* biotype *mitis* is nitrate reductase positive, and *C. diphtheriae* biotype *belfanti* is nitrate reductase negative.

[e] *C. simulans* (145) is a strong nitrite reducer at low and high concentrations; nitrate reduction may appear to be negative unless further tested using zinc dust; one strain was catalase negative (4).

for gram-negative nonfermenters [bioMérieux]) to the API 50CH system, utilization reactions which allow the differentiation of *Brevibacterium* spp. or some *Arthrobacter* spp. can be observed (40, 44).

A reference laboratory would also use chromatographic techniques for further characterization of coryneform bacteria. The presence of mycolic acids and their chain lengths can be detected by thin-layer chromatography (TLC), gas chromatography and mass spectrometry, or high-performance liquid chromatography (22). These methods can be useful for the differentiation of *Corynebacterium* spp. (mycolic acids of 22 to 36 carbon atoms) from the partially acid-fast bacteria (mycolic acids of 30 to 78 carbon atoms) but may also provide evidence that a coryneform bacterium is not a *Corynebacterium* (exceptions are *C. amycolatum*, *C. atypicum*, and *C. kroppenstedtii*) if mycolic acids are not detected. The detection of the diamino acid of the peptidoglycan by one-dimensional TLC is of certain value for determining the genus to which a particular strain belongs (Table 1). In some cases, partial hydrolysates of the peptidoglycan are separated by two-dimensional TLC to reveal the interpeptide bridge of the peptidoglycan in order to distinguish between genera having the same diamino acid in the peptide moiety. For example, some of the yellow-pigmented microbacteria and all curtobacteria have ornithine as their diamino acids, but microbacteria have (glycine)-ornithine as the interpeptide bridge, whereas curtobacteria possess ornithine only.

The analysis of CFAs by means of gas-liquid chromatography with the Sherlock system (MIDI Inc., Newark, Del.) is an extremely useful method for the identification of coryneform bacteria. This system is, in general, able to identify coryneform bacteria to the genus level, but identification to the species level is in most cases impossible, although the commercial database suggests that it is possible. This is because of the very closely related CFA profiles of coryneform bacteria belonging to the same genus (3) and because the quantitative profiles observed depend strongly on the incubation conditions. When a laboratory creates its individual database based on its own entries, species identification becomes possible in some cases (Bernard, unpublished). The mycolic acids of some corynebacteria (e.g., *C. auris*) are cleaved at the temperature (300°C) produced in the injection port of the system, resulting in fatty acids which were identified as, e.g., $C_{17:1\omega6c}$ to $C_{\omega9c}$, by the Sherlock system (47).

Molecular genetic-based identification systems for coryneform bacteria have been outlined in recent years. Restriction fragment length polymorphism analysis of the partly amplified and digested 16S rRNA gene has been demonstrated to be of use for the identification of species within the genera *Corynebacterium* and *Brevibacterium* (9, 140). Some corynebacteria may also be identified to the species level by examination of the length of the 16S-23S rRNA intergenic spacer region (1). rRNA gene restriction fragment polymorphism analysis (ribotyping) has been demonstrated to allow the identification of corynebacteria if three different restriction enzymes (BstEII, SmaI, and SphII) are used (5). Another interesting approach for the identification of true corynebacteria is the sequencing of a 434- to 452-bp fragment of the *rpoB* gene (using primers designated C2700F and C3130R), since this particular region of the gene displays a high degree of polymorphism within the genus *Corynebacterium* (77, 78). This approach for molecular identification needs to be evaluated with other genera. For pure taxononomic investigations of coryneform bacteria and in cases of growth of coryneform bacteria from difficult to obtain clinical material (122), full-length 16S rRNA gene

TABLE 5 Identification of medically relevant coryneform bacteria other than *Corynebacterium* spp.[a]

Taxon	Catalase	Fermentation/ oxidation	Motility	Nitrate reduction	Urease	Esculin hydrolysis	Acid production from: Glucose	Maltose	Sucrose	Mannitol	Xylose	Other traits
Turicella otitidis	+	O	−	−	−	−	−	−	−	−	−	CAMP reaction positive, long rods
Arthrobacter spp.	+	O	V	V	V	V	V	V	V	−	−	
Brevibacterium spp.	+	O	−	V	−	−	V	V	V	−	−	Odor cheese-like
Dermabacter hominis	+	F	−	−	−	+	+	+	+	−	V	Small rods
Rothia dentocariosa	V	F	−	+	−	+	+	+	+	−	−	Some strains adherent, grayish-black-pigmented strains exist
Exiguobacterium acetylicum	+	F	+	V	−	+	+	+	+	+	−	Golden yellow pigment
Oerskovia turbata	+	F	V	+	−	+	+	+	+	−	+	Xanthine not hydrolyzed
Cellulomonas spp.	+	F	V	+	−	+	+	+	+	V	+	
Cellulosimicrobium spp.	+	F	V	V	V	+	+	+	+	−	+	Hydrolysis of xanthine
Microbacterium spp.	V	F/O	V	V	V	V	+	+	V	V	V	
Curtobacterium spp.	+	O	V	−	−	+	+	V	V	V	+	
Leifsonia aquatica	+	O	+	V	−	V	+	V	V	+	+	
Arcanobacterium haemolyticum	−	F	−	−	−	−	+	+	V	−	−	CAMP inhibition reaction
Arcanobacterium pyogenes	−	F	−	−	−	V	+	V	V	V	+	
Arcanobacterium bernardiae	−	F	−	−	−	−	+	+	−	−	−	Glycogen positive
Gardnerella vaginalis	−	F	−	−	−	−	+	+	V	−	−	Decolorized cells in Gram stain

[a] Abbreviations and symbols: +, positive reaction; −, negative reaction; V, variable reaction; O, oxidation; F, fermentation.

sequencing might be indicated. Determination of the complete 16S rRNA gene sequence is a rational approach for identifying corynebacteria, since nearly all established species exhibit 3% or greater divergence except for *C. afermentans*, *C. coyleae*, and *C. mucifaciens* (<2%), *C. aurimucosum*, *C. minutissimum*, and *C. singulare* (<2%), *C. sundsvallense* and *C. thomssenii* (<1.5%), and *C. ulcerans* and *C. pseudotuberculosis* (<2%) (2). In very few selected cases, quantitative DNA-DNA hybridizations might be necessary but will be clearly restricted to the reference laboratory. Because of the ever-growing number of coryneform taxa encountered in clinical specimens, it becomes more difficult to readily differentiate all taxa biochemically, so it appears that sequencing studies are most likely to replace some of the biochemical testing in the near future.

The commercial MicroSeq 500 16S bacterial sequencing kit (Perkin-Elmer, Foster City, Calif.) has been applied to the identification of coryneform bacteria, but discordant results (with extensive phenotyping as the "gold standard") were observed for >30% of the *Corynebacterium* isolates, mainly because of the present database of the commercial system (136). However, due to the short running time of approximately 15 to 19 h, this and other similar systems will further spread to the routine clinical laboratory, in which case direct costs should drop and databases will be improved.

It is emphasized that unidentifiable, clinically significant coryneform bacteria should be sent to an established reference laboratory experienced in corynebacterial identification.

DESCRIPTIONS OF GENERA AND SPECIES

Genus *Corynebacterium*

C. accolens

C. accolens (101) is found in specimens from eyes, ears, the nose, and the oropharynx. Endocarditis of native aortic and mitral valves due to this agent has been described. Colonies are, as for all other lipophilic corynebacteria, convex, smooth, and <0.5 mm in diameter on SBA. *C. accolens* strains had initially been described to exhibit satellitism in the vicinity of *S. aureus* strains, attributable to its lipophilism (for the recommended method to demonstrate lipophilism, see "Identification and Typing Systems" above). *C. accolens* has a variable pyrazinamidase reaction but is negative for alkaline phosphatase, thus differentiating it from the morphologically and biochemically closely related CDC group G bacteria (Table 4). The API Coryne and RapID CB Plus systems correctly identify *C. accolens* (58, 60). *C. accolens* strains are susceptible to a broad spectrum of antibiotics.

C. afermentans subsp. *afermentans*

C. afermentans subsp. *afermentans* (116) is part of the normal human skin flora and has so far been isolated mainly from blood cultures. Colonies are whitish, convex with regular edges, creamy, and about 1 to 1.5 mm in diameter after 24 h of incubation. *C. afermentans* subsp. *afermentans* has an oxidative metabolism. The API Coryne system provides the numerical code of 2100004 for this species. About 60% of all strains of this taxon are CAMP reaction positive. *C. afermentans* subsp. *afermentans* can be differentiated from *C. auris* and *T. otitidis* (both of which give the same API numerical code) by the consistency of its colonies (*C. auris* is slightly adherent to agar) and morphology on Gram staining (*T. otitidis* has longer cells). Further differential reactions include the carbohydrate utilization reactions tested with either the Biolog GP plate (Biolog, Hayward, Calif.) or the bioMérieux biotype 100 gallery (47). By chemotaxonomic means, both *C. afermentans* subspecies and *C. auris* contain mycolates, whereas *T. otitidis* lacks them, but these techniques are not applicable in a routine clinical laboratory. *C. afermentans* subsp. *afermentans* is generally susceptible to β-lactam antibiotics.

C. afermentans subsp. *lipophilum*

Strains belonging to the species *C. afermentans* subsp. *lipophilum* (116) have been isolated mainly from blood cultures as well as from superficial wounds. Colonies are, typically for lipophilic corynebacteria, convex, smooth, and <0.5 mm in diameter after 24 h. *C. afermentans* subsp. *lipophilum* has an oxidative metabolism and does not produce acid from any of the carbohydrates usually tested (Table 4). It is the only species of lipophilic corynebacteria which may exhibit a positive CAMP reaction. *C. afermentans* subsp. *lipophilum* is not included in the API Coryne database. The numerical profile observed for the species is 2100004, and so by that method it cannot be discerned from more robustly growing *C. afermentans* subsp. *afermentans*, *C. auris*, or *T. otitidis*. Strains are usually susceptible to β-lactam antibiotics.

C. amycolatum

C. amycolatum is part of the normal human skin flora but was not recovered from throat swabs from healthy persons (144). *C. amycolatum* is the most frequently encountered *Corynebacterium* species in human clinical material (64). It is also the most frequently isolated nonlipophilic *Corynebacterium* in dairy cows with mastitis (74). *C. amycolatum* strains are often multidrug resistant (59). Colonies are very typically dry, waxy, and grayish white with irregular edges and are 1 to 2 mm in diameter after 24 h of incubation. *C. amycolatum* actually has a fermentative metabolism, but when CTA media are used for the observation of acid production from carbohydrates, *C. amycolatum* appears to resemble an oxidizer (i.e., main acid production at the surface of the medium). Strains of *C. amycolatum* are remarkable for their variability in basic biochemical reactions (Table 4) and had been often misidentified in the past as the biochemically similar species *C. xerosis*, *C. striatum*, or *C. minutissimum* (46, 148, 154). These four species can be differentiated by the following reactions: *C. amycolatum* and *C. minutissimum* do not grow at 20°C, but *C. xerosis* and *C. striatum* do; in addition, *C. xerosis* does not ferment glucose at 42°C whereas the other three species do, and *C. minutissimum* and *C. striatum* produce alkali from formate but *C. amycolatum* and *C. xerosis* do not (148). When tested on Mueller-Hinton agar supplemented with 5% sheep blood, nearly all *C. amycolatum* strains were resistant to the vibriocidal compound O/129 (150-μg disks) (Oxoid, Basingstoke, United Kingdom), as indicated by no zone of inhibition around the disk (46). In contrast, only 4% of all *C. amycolatum* strains were resistant to O/129 when tested on Mueller-Hinton agar with 5% horse blood (83). The API Coryne system identifies this species very well, but in every case additional reactions must be carried out in order to confirm the identification of *C. amycolatum* (60). All *C. amycolatum* strains produce propionic acid as the major end product of glucose metabolism. In contrast to many other corynebacteria, *C. amycolatum* exhibits only weak or no leucine arylamidase activity. The identification may also be suggested by the absence of mycolic acids. In addition, it may be shown that acyl phosphatidylglycerol is a major phospholipid in *C. amycolatum*, in contrast to other *Corynebacterium* spp., in which other phospholipids are predominant.

C. appendicis

The one strain of *C. appendicis* described in the literature was isolated from a patient with appendicitis accompanied with abscess formation (151). This lipophilic species contains huge amounts of TBSA (up to 50% of all CFAs) not seen in any other *Corynebacterium* species. It is differentiated from CDC coryneform group F-1 bacteria by a positive alkaline phosphatase reaction but negative reactions for nitrate reduction and sucrose fermentation.

C. argentoratense

C. argentoratense (118) has been isolated from the human throat as well as, in one instance, from a blood culture (4). Colonies are cream colored, nonhemolytic, slightly rough, and 2 mm in diameter after 48 h of incubation. Phenotypically, *C. argentoratense* may appear to be very similar to (rare) ribose negative strains of *C. coyleae*. However, glucose fermentation by *C. argentoratense* is quite rapid compared to the slowly fermenting species *C. coyleae*. As well, CAMP-negative *C. argentoratense* produces propionic acid as a fermentation product, but CAMP-positive *C. coyleae* does not (4, 56). *C. argentoratense* is the only medically relevant *Corynebacterium* species expressing α-chymotrypsin activity, which can be observed in the API ZYM (bioMérieux) system; however, the blood culture isolate was not observed to produce that enzyme (4). Although *C. argentoratense* is phylogenetically closely related to *C. diphtheriae*, it does not harbor the *tox* gene coding for the diphtheria toxin.

C. atypicum

Although this species clearly belongs to the genus *Corynebacterium*, corynomycolic acids, like in *C. amycolatum* and *C. kroppenstedtii*, are not detected (69). *C. atypicum* is not lipophilic but shows only pinpoint colonies after 48 h of incubation. It is the only medically relevant *Corynebacterium* not expressing pyrazinamidase but β-glucuronidase activity.

C. aurimucosum

The initial description of *C. aurimucosum* was based on a single strain which exhibited slightly yellow and sticky colonies on 5% SBA plates but on Trypticase soy agar without blood had colorless and slimy colonies (150). The basic biochemical profile of this particular *C. aurimucosum* strain was similar to that of *C. minutissimum*. The number of *C. aurimucosum* strains was significantly enhanced when it was demonstrated that some former CDC coryneform group 4 bacteria actually belong to *C. aurimucosum* (21). It is important to note that many strains of *C. aurimucosum* exhibit a grayish black pigment that is not seen in any other true *Corynebacterium*. Strains that were originally designated "*C. nigricans*" (126) were shown to be a later synonym of *C. aurimucosum* (21). Some strains of *R. dentocariosa* can also exhibit a charcoal black pigment (21); these strains are differentiated from *C. aurimucosum* by being constantly nitrate reductase positive, a possible negative catalase reaction, and having branched-chain CFAs as opposed to straight-chain-type CFAs for *C. aurimucosum*. API Coryne codes for pigmented *C. aurimucosum* strains include 0000125, 2000125, and 2100327 (126).

C. auris

C. auris (47) has been isolated almost exclusively from the ear region. Colonies are dryish, are slightly adherent to but do not penetrate agar, become slightly yellowish with time, and have diameters ranging from 1 to 2 mm after 48 h of incubation. *C. auris* does not produce acid from any carbohydrates usually tested. However, utilization reactions applying either the Biolog GP plate or the bioMérieux biotype 100 system may help in distinguishing *C. auris* from *C. afermentans* subsp. *afermentans* and *T. otitidis*, but in the clinical routine laboratory this can also be achieved by morphologic differentiation (see "*C. afermentans* subsp. *afermentans*"). All *C. auris* strains are strongly CAMP test positive. The API Coryne system provides the numerical code 2100004 for this species. Abundant degradation products of mycolic acids are indirectly observed when CFA patterns are determined with the Sherlock system (47). It is noteworthy that the MICs of β-lactam antibiotics for *C. auris* strains are elevated, but the molecular mechanism for this is not known at present (59).

C. bovis

Occasionally, but not in the recent era, human infections had been attributed to the lipophilic bovine species, *C. bovis*. Characterization of lipophilic-like corynebacteria based solely on the use of phenotypic tests was probably incorrect in the absence of modern polyphasic methods or identification schemes such as those found in Table 4. This species had not been definitively recovered for many years from human clinical material, as previously reviewed (64). Recently, however, a human blood culture isolate of *C. bovis* was identified based on a polyphasic approach, including phenotypic, chemotaxonomic, and genotypic characteristics, with an API Coryne code of 0101104 (4).

C. confusum

C. confusum has been isolated from patients with foot infections, a blood culture (52), and a breast abscess (4). Colonies are whitish, glistening, convex, creamy, and up to 1.5 mm in diameter after 48 h. Acid from glucose is produced only very weakly, becoming visible in the API Coryne or the API 50CH gallery only after 48 to 72 h. Weak growth under anaerobic conditions corresponds to slow fermentative acid production. It is advisable to incubate the API Coryne system after 24 h for another day in those cases in which the results for acid production are ambiguous (i.e., only a slight change in the color of the indicator). After 48 h of incubation, the API Coryne system provides the numerical code 3100304 for this species; the breast abscess strain had a code of 3100104. Interestingly, the breast abscess strain was also CAMP positive, making it potentially more difficult to discern from *C. coyleae* isolates (4). *C. confusum* is correctly identified by the RapID CB Plus system (58). If glucose fermentation is judged to be negative, *C. confusum* strains can be misidentified as *C. propinquum*. However, in contrast to that species, *C. confusum* does not hydrolyze tyrosine and contains small amounts of TBSA (1 to 3%), whereas *C. propinquum* hydrolyzes tyrosine but does not contain TBSA. *C. confusum* is differentiated from *C. coyleae* and *C. argentoratense* by its ability to reduce nitrate.

C. coyleae

C. coyleae (56) has been isolated mainly from cultures of blood and other normally sterile body fluids, but it may also be recovered from genitourinary specimens (4; Funke, unpublished). Colonies are whitish and slightly glistening with entire edges and are about 1 mm in diameter after 24 h. The consistency of the colonies is either creamy or sticky. A slow fermentative acid production from glucose and a strongly positive CAMP reaction are the most significant phenotypic characteristics. *C. coyleae* is positive for cystine arylamidase, which is not observed for many other corynebacteria. Various API Coryne numerical codes have been observed, especially 2100304 and 6100304. *C. coyleae* is always positive for ribose fermentation, whereas the biochemically similar species *C. argentoratense* is variable for this reaction. The API Coryne database lists only 6% glucose-fermenting *C. coyleae* strains, and therefore, when applying this commercial identification system, the clinical microbiologist may not receive a correct identification (60). However, the two numerical profiles given above combined with a positive CAMP reaction are highly indicative of *C. coyleae*. This species is correctly identified by the RapID CB Plus system (58).

CDC Group F-1 Bacteria

CDC group F-1 bacteria (119) have not been given a species name. Although genetically distinct, no distinguishing phenotypic markers that clearly allow their separation from other defined *Corynebacterium* spp. have been found. The characteristics of the CDC group F-1 bacteria are consistent with the definition of the genus *Corynebacterium* in all respects. The strains are lipophilic and are the only lipophilic fermentative *Corynebacterium* species able to hydrolyze urea. Of note is the negative alkaline phosphatase reaction (Table 4). CDC group F-1 strains are usually susceptible to penicillin but are often resistant to macrolides.

CDC Group G Bacteria

CDC group G bacteria possess all chemotaxonomic features of true corynebacteria but cannot be given a species name since it has so far been impossible to find phenotypic traits allowing for a unanimous definition (119). At least some strains of CDC group G have been found to be consistent with *C. tuberculostearicum* (Bernard, unpublished). These lipophilic strains can be separated from *C. jeikeium* by anaerobic growth and fermentative acid production from fructose (115). Further biochemical features of CDC group G bacteria are given in Table 4. The API Coryne system correctly identifies CDC group G bacteria. They might be multidrug resistant, but the most frequently observed resistance is to macrolides and lincosamides.

C. diphtheriae

In 2003, the complete genome sequence of a *Corynebacterium diphtheriae* strain representative for the diphtheria outbreak in the former Soviet Union states in the 1990s was determined (11). The genome consists of a single circular chromosome of 2,488,635 bp with no plasmids. A complete set of enzymes for the glycolysis, gluconeogenesis, and pentose-phosphate pathways are present, as well as all the de novo amino acid biosynthesis pathways. Fimbrial and fimbria-related genes and sialidase (neuraminidae) genes, as well as iron uptake systems, have been detected as pathogenicity factors.

C. diphtheriae is commonly divided into four biotypes, *gravis*, *mitis*, *belfanti*, and *intermedius*; biotype differentiation is recommended by WHO (29, 30), although biotypes cannot be assigned separate subspecies status (120), nor is biotyping satisfactory for epidemiologic tracking. Initially, these biotypes were defined by differences in colony morphology and biochemical reactions (Table 4). However, only *C. diphtheriae* biotype *intermedius* can be identified on the basis of colonial morphology (small, gray, or translucent lipophilic colonies) (20) as well as positive dextrin fermentation. Other *C. diphtheriae* biotypes produce larger (up to 2 mm after 24 h) white or opaque colonies (Fig. 3b), which are indistinguishable from one another. The lipophilic *C. diphtheriae* biotype *intermedius* occurs only rarely in clinical infections, and *C. diphtheriae* biotype *belfanti* strains almost never harbor the diphtheria toxin gene.

Presumptive identification of C. *diphtheriae* (as well as of C. *pseudotuberculosis* and C. *ulcerans*) may be made by testing suspicious gram-positive rods for the presence of cystinase (as detected by using Tinsdale medium or diagnostic tablets [Rosco, Taastrup, Denmark]) and the absence of pyrazinamidase (diagnostic tablets are available from Key Scientific Products, Round Rock, Tex.). The API Coryne system identifies C. *diphtheriae* strains, with additional tests needed for the differentiation of C. *diphtheriae* biotype *mitis*, C. *diphtheriae* biotype *belfanti*, and C. *diphtheriae* biotype *intermedius* (60). Usually, C. *diphtheriae* strains do not ferment sucrose, but in Brazil sucrose-positive strains have been described (23). Large amounts of propionic acid are produced as the end product of glucose metabolism (36). C. *diphtheriae* strains are distinct from all other coryneform bacteria (except C. *pseudotuberculosis* and C. *ulcerans*) in their CFA patterns by the presence of a large volume of $C_{16:1\omega7c}$ (3).

Diphtheria Toxin Testing

It is recommended that at least 10 colonies of C. *diphtheriae* and related species be tested for diphtheria toxin by the Elek method, modified as described by Engler (32), in a laboratory with personnel skilled in performing the test and in interpreting the test results. The modified Elek method described by the WHO Diphtheria Reference Unit was initially used to characterize strains from the 1990s epidemic in Russia and Ukraine and was found to be faster and less technically problematic than the original version. Antitoxins from various suppliers (e.g., Swiss Serum and Vaccine Institute, Bern, Switzerland; Pasteur Mérieux, Lyon, France; CDC Biological Products Division, Atlanta, Ga.), applied to blank filter disks at 10 IU/disk, have been successfully used with the modified Elek test (32), and precipitin lines can be read as early as 24 h (Fig. 4). A similar modification of the Elek test, which can test up to 24 isolates on the same plate, has been described (112). A 3-h enzyme-linked immunosorbent assay for the detection of diphtheria toxin from clinical isolates of *Corynebacterium* spp. has been developed by the WHO Diphtheria Reference Unit (33).

PCR-based methods for the detection of the diphtheria toxin gene (*tox*) in isolated bacteria have been developed and validated (29, 70). Recently, a real-time fluorescence PCR assay for detecting the A and B subunits of the *tox* gene has been described and evaluated directly with clinical specimens (96). *tox* PCR assays applied directly to clinical specimens are acceptable, particularly because isolation is not always possible for patients already receiving antibiotics. However, a PCR-positive patient from whom bacteria are not isolated or without a histopathologic diagnosis and without an epidemiologic linkage to a patient with a laboratory-confirmed case of diphtheria should be classified as having a "probable case" of diphtheria, since to date there are insufficient data to conclude that a PCR-positive result always implies diphtheria. Also, detection of the toxin gene in samples by PCR cannot automatically be attributed to one species, because C. *diphtheriae* as well as C. *ulcerans* and C. *pseudotuberculosis* may harbor the bacteriophage which carries the diphtheria toxin gene. Furthermore, *tox*-containing, nontoxigenic isolates have been described and characterized further (12). A comprehensive review on the biology and molecular epidemiology of the diphtheria toxin has been given by Holmes (72). Nontoxigenic strains of C. *diphtheriae*, i.e., those which do not express toxin in the Elek test or those which lack a detectable diphtheria toxin gene by PCR, have caused serious disease such as cases or outbreaks of skin disease and endocarditis and occasional mortality among homeless people, alcoholics, and intravenous drug abusers (37, 64, 111). For nontoxigenic C. *diphtheriae* strains circulating in the United Kingdom, it has been shown that the diphtheria toxin repressor (*dtxR*) genes are functional, so that if these strains are lysogenized by a bacteriophage, they could represent a reservoir for toxigenic C. *diphtheriae* (28).

Typing Methods

Outbreaks of C. *diphtheriae* in the states of the former Soviet Union and other locations have been studied by whole-cell peptide analysis, whole-genome restriction fragment length polymorphism analysis, ribotyping, pulsed-field gel electrophoresis, PCR-single-strand conformation polymorphism analysis of *tox* and *dtxR* (i.e., the regulatory element of the diphtheria toxin) as well as of the 16S-23S rRNA spacer region, amplified fragment length polymorphisms, random amplification of polymorphic DNA (RAPD), and multilocus enzyme electrophoresis (26, 27, 99, 108). An international database for C. *diphtheriae* ribotypes using endonuclease BstEII has been established (67). Recently, a spoligotyping system (similar to the spacer oligonucleotide typing for *Mycobacterium tuberculosis*) checking for the presence or absence of 21 different spacers has been described for C. *diphtheriae* (95). Sequencing studies with C. *diphtheriae* strains from the epidemic in the former Soviet Union have shown that point mutations within the *tox* gene were silent mutations, whereas multiple point mutations (which even led to amino acid substitutions) were observed for the *dtxR* gene, corresponding to the heterogeneity of outbreak strains as revealed by PCR-single-strand conformation polymorphism analysis (97). Molecular epidemiologic studies using RAPD have been used to rapidly screen a large number of C. *diphtheriae* strains to identify the epidemic clonal group associated with the outbreak in the former Soviet Union. Isolates derived from specific populations in the United States and Canada and characterized using multilocus enzyme electrophoresis, ribotyping, and RAPD were found to be members of persistent endemic strains, rather than being imported from other countries where diphtheria is endemic.

Antibiotic treatment is required to eliminate C. *diphtheriae* and prevent its spread; however, it is not a substitute for antitoxin prevention, with antibiotics of choice being penicillins or macrolides. Sporadic isolates of C. *diphtheriae* resistant to erythromycin or rifampin have been reported. Penicillin and some of the newer ketolides were tested against a large collection of geographically diverse strains and were found to generally demonstrate significant efficacy against C. *diphtheriae* but reduced ketolide activity against some Southeast Asian strains. It is believed that between 20 and 60% of adults in the United States lack protective antibodies to diphtheria toxin because of declining antibody titers in immunized persons and because many individuals were never immunized, which could pose a potentially significant public health risk and could result in the reemergence of this disease.

C. *durum*

C. *durum* (117) was originally described as being exclusively isolated from respiratory tract specimens. Well-characterized isolates have now been recovered from additional sites, including the gingiva, blood cultures, or abscesses (110). C. *durum* strains were originally isolated after 2 or 3 days from nonselective charcoal-buffered yeast extract plates inoculated with sputa or bronchial washings. C. *durum* is the

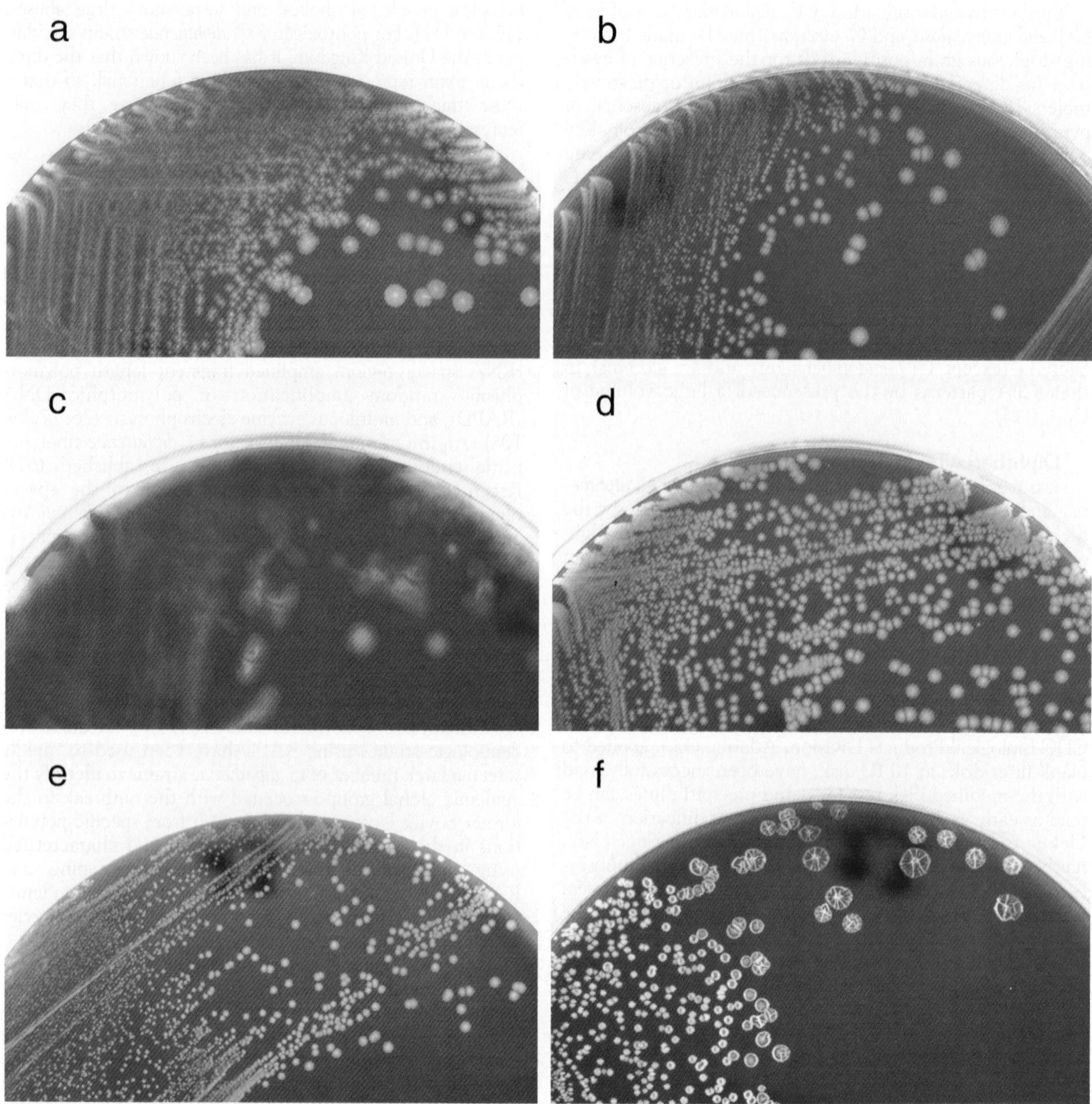

FIGURE 3 Colony morphologies of different coryneform bacteria after 48 h of incubation on SBA. (a) *C. amycolatum* LCDC 91-0077; (b) *C. diphtheriae* ATCC 14779; (c) *C. mucifaciens* LCDC 97-0202; (d) *C. striatum* ATCC 6940; (e) *D. hominis* ATCC 51325; (f) *R. dentocariosa* LCDC 95-0154; (g) *C. aurimucosum* HC-NML 91-0032 (after 96 h); (h) black-pigmented *Rothia dentocariosa* HC-NML 77-0298 (after 96 h); (i) *C. diphtheriae* biotype *gravis* colonies on a Tinsdale agar plate. Panel i was kindly provided by C. Hinnebusch and M. Cohen, UCLA School of Medicine, Los Angeles, Calif.

most frequent *Corynebacterium* isolated from throat swabs from healthy persons (144). Its pathogenic potential is unclear at present. *C. durum* is a peculiar nonlipophilic organism that forms colonies of only 0.5 to 1 mm in diameter after aerobic incubation for 72 h. The original description of this bacterium cited beige and rough colonies with convolutions, with an irregular margin, and strongly adhering to agar if grown under aerobic conditions (117). However, strains described in a later publication were found to be sometimes smoother and not necessarily adherent to agar (110). Gram staining of aerobic cultures shows long and filamentous rods, with occasional "bulges," but true *C. durum* isolates do not have *C. matruchotii*-like "whip handles" (Fig. 1d and e). Long forms are not otherwise found among other *Corynebacterium* species, nor are they observed for *C. durum* when cells are grown in a 10% CO_2-enriched

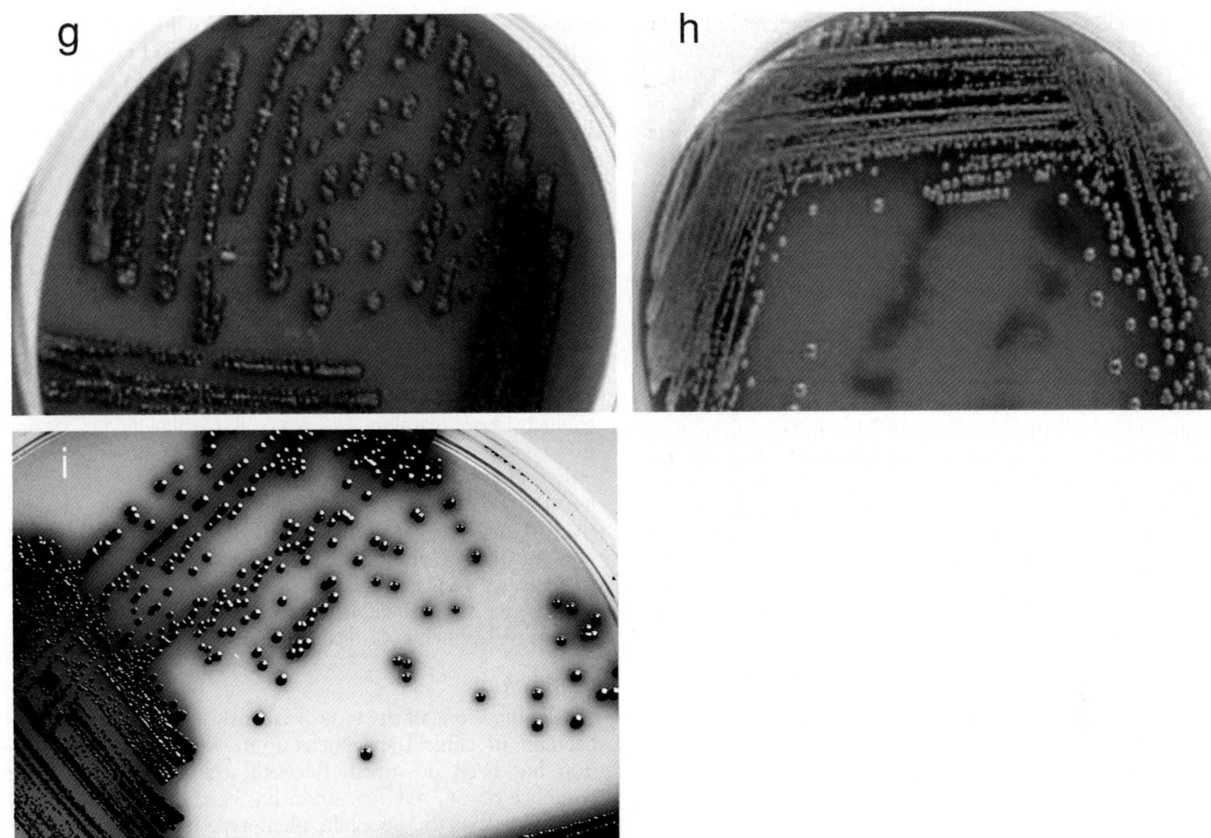

FIGURE 3 *(Continued)*

atmosphere (117). Strains grow only weakly under anaerobic conditions. They always reduce nitrate, and some may exhibit weak and delayed urease and esculinase activities. The majority (but not all [144]) of *C. durum* strains ferment mannitol, which is another very unusual feature for true corynebacteria (Table 4). API Coryne codes observed for *C. durum* include 3000135, 3001135, 3040135, 3400115, 3400135, 3400305, 3400325, and 3400335 (117), as well as 3040325, 3040335, 3440335, and 3441335 (110). This suggests that most strains are negative for alkaline phosphatase and all appear to be negative for pyrrolidonyl arylamidase. Only a small number of *C. durum* strains have been tested with the RapID system, and all were correctly identified (58). It is most likely that some strains identified as *C. matruchotii* in the past may actually have been *C. durum* strains and that differentiation can be difficult if phenotypic methods alone are used. Both species produce propionic acid as a fermentation product (4). *C. durum* usually ferments galactose and very often mannitol, whereas *C. matruchotii* is usually negative for those sugars. The *C. matruchotii* type strain exhibits α-glucosidase activity, which is not observed in *C. durum* (117). It has been shown that some *C. durum* strains also express β-galactosidase activity and ferment ribose (144).

C. falsenii

C. falsenii strains (129) have so far been isolated only from sterile body fluids. Colonies are whitish, glistening, and smooth with entire edges and are 1 to 2 mm in diameter after 24 h. After 72 h, most strains described to date

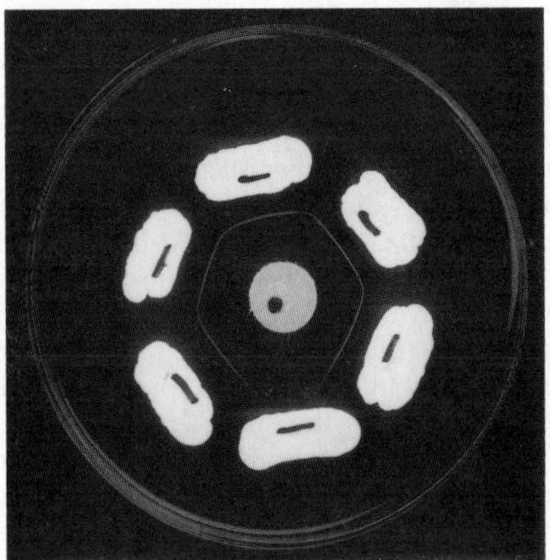

FIGURE 4 Modified Elek test (see the text) with antitoxin disk in the center. Strains are (clockwise starting at noon) NCTC 3984 (weakly toxin-positive *C. diphtheriae* biotype *gravis*), NCTC 10648 (strongly toxin-positive *C. diphtheriae* biotype *gravis*), a test strain (which was found to be a toxin producer), NCTC 10356 (nontoxigenic *C. diphtheriae* biotype *belfanti*), another test strain (also a toxin producer), and (again) NCTC 10648. The photo was kindly supplied by K.-H. Engler (WHO Diphtheria Reference Unit, Central Public Health Laboratory, London, United Kingdom).

exhibit a yellowish pigment that becomes even more intense after 120 h. This pigment is not observed in any other nonlipophilic *Corynebacterium* encountered in clinical specimens, except in the rarely found species *C. xerosis* (the colonies of the latter are dry, in contrast to *C. falsenii* colonies). The most characteristic biochemical features of *C. falsenii* are a slow but fermentative acid production from glucose, a weak pyrazinamidase reaction, and a weak urease activity which becomes visible in either Christensen's urea broth or the API Coryne system after overnight incubation only. API Coryne codes observed for *C. falsenii* are 2101104 and 2101304 (4, 129).

C. freneyi

This species has been outlined based on the study of three strains (113). All these strains had been isolated from skin-related material. There is now evidence that *C. freneyi* is also isolated from genitourinary specimens (43). *C. freneyi* is phylogenetically closely related to *C. xerosis*. Colonies of *C. freneyi* are whitish, dry, and rough, have irregular edges, and are 0.5 to 1 mm in diameter after 48 h of incubation, but *C. freneyi* strains are nonlipophilic. The basic biochemical profile (Table 4) is also similar to that of *C. xerosis*. All *C. freneyi* strains studied so far exhibit α-glucosidase activity, which is not frequently observed in other *Corynebacterium* species (very few *C. amycolatum* and all *C. xerosis* strains express this enzyme). *C. freneyi* can be differentiated from *C. xerosis* by glucose fermentation at 42°C and growth at 20°C, whereas *C. xerosis* is negative for these two reactions.

C. glucuronolyticum

C. seminale is a junior synonym of *C. glucuronolyticum* (24, 39). This species is probably part of the normal genitourinary flora of males, while its presence in females is uncertain. Colonies are whitish-yellowish, convex, and creamy, and they measure 1 to 1.5 mm in diameter after 24 h. The fermentative species *C. glucuronolyticum* is remarkable for its variability in basic biochemical reactions (Table 4). It is the only medically relevant, large-colony *Corynebacterium* species exhibiting β-glucuronidase activity. When urease activity is present, it is abundant in Christensen's urea broth, becoming positive after only 5 min of incubation at room temperature (39). *C. glucuronolyticum* is also one of the very few corynebacteria which are able to hydrolyze esculin. All *C. glucuronolyticum* strains are CAMP reaction positive (Fig. 2). With the exception of strains which are alkaline phosphatase positive, the API Coryne strip identifies *C. glucuronolyticum* well (60), although the profiles obtained from human strains may differ from those of animal isolates (24). Propionic acid is one of the major end products of glucose metabolism. *C. glucuronolyticum* strains are often tetracycline resistant and may also exhibit resistance to macrolides and lincosamides (59). 16S rRNA gene sequences derived from fluids of patients with prostatitis have been found to be homologous with sequences derived for this species, indicating that *C. glucuronolyticum* might be involved in selected cases of prostatitis (137).

C. imitans

C. imitans was originally isolated from a nasopharyngeal specimen of a child suspected of having throat diphtheria, as well as from three adult contacts (41). This was the first well-documented case of person-to-person transmission of a *Corynebacterium* other than *C. diphtheriae* in a nonhospital setting. Additional strains of *C. imitans* have been recovered from blood cultures (4). Colonies are whitish-grayish and glistening, with entire edges; are creamy; and measure 1 to 2 mm in diameter. The strain did not produce a brown halo on Tinsdale medium but was tellurite reductase positive. Interestingly, Neisser staining was positive for polar bodies. Pyrazinamidase activity was weak only, as was fermentation of sucrose, which may lead to the initial misidentification as an atypical *C. diphtheriae* strain. It is not unlikely that *C. imitans* may also have been misidentified as *C. minutissimum* in the past, since the basic biochemical reactions of the two taxa are quite similar (Table 4). However, *C. imitans* is CAMP reaction positive and does not hydrolyze tyrosine, whereas the opposite reactions are observed for *C. minutissimum*. The API Coryne system provided the numerical codes 1100325, 2100324, and 3100325 for *C. imitans*, indicating a negative α-glucosidase reaction, whereas all *C. diphtheriae* strains express this enzyme. *C. imitans* strains do not produce propionic acid as a fermentation product, unlike *C. diphtheriae* (4), and the CFA composition profiles for each species qualitatively differ, as *C. diphtheriae* and closely related species have a unique pattern among the *Corynebacterium* spp. Diphtheria toxin assays using the Elek test or a PCR for the *tox* gene were all negative for *C. imitans* strains (4, 41). *C. imitans* is resistant to O/129, while *C. diphtheriae* is not.

C. jeikeium

C. jeikeium is one of the most frequently encountered coryne-bacteria in clinical specimens (64). Nosocomial transmission has been described. Recently, the complete genome sequence of a *C. jeikeium* strain has been determined (138), indicating that the lipophilic phenotype of *C. jeikeium* originates from the absence of fatty acid synthase. *C. jeikeium* is often resistant to multiple antibiotics (including penicillin and gentamicin), but this cannot be used as a taxonomic characteristic because the phenotypically closely related CDC group G bacteria may also demonstrate multidrug resistance. Quantitative DNA-DNA hydridization experiments had shown that *C. jeikeium* includes two genomospecies for which penicillin and gentamicin MICs are low, but as they could otherwise not be differentiated phenotypically from the resistant *C. jeikeium* strains, they were not proposed as independent species (115). Colonies of *C. jeikeium* are tiny, low, entire, and grayish white. *C. jeikeium* is a strict aerobe which may oxidatively produce acid from glucose and sometimes from maltose but not from fructose (CDC group G bacteria are positive for acid production from fructose). The RapID CB Plus system correctly identifies *C. jeikeium*, as does the API Coryne system if ancillary tests are used (58, 60). As for all other lipophilic corynebacteria, imperfectly cleaved mycolic acids coeluting with CFAs at or near equivalent chain lengths of 14.966 to 15.000 or of 16.7 to 16.8 have never been observed among *C. jeikeium* strains (3; Bernard, unpublished).

C. kroppenstedtii

C. kroppenstedtii (18) is a rarely recovered species originally isolated from the sputum of a patient with pulmonary disease. Additional strains have been isolated from a lung biopsy specimen, sputum, a breast abscess, and patients with granulomatous lobular mastitis (4, 106). Apart from *C. amycolatum* and *C. atypicum*, it is the only *Corynebacterium* species lacking mycolic acids. Colonies are grayish, translucent, slightly dry, and less than 0.5 mm in diameter after 24 h of incubation at 37°C. *C. kroppenstedtii* is lipophilic and is one of the few medically relevant *Corynebacterium* species exhibiting esculinase activity. Other biochemical characteristics are given in Table 4. API Codes of *C. kroppenstedtii* are 0101104,

2040104, and 2040105 (4). It can be differentiated from C. *durum*, C. *matruchotii*, and C. *glucuronolyticum* by its colony morphology and from C. *glucuronolyticum* also by its negative CAMP reaction.

C. *lipophiloflavum*

C. *lipophiloflavum* (45) is represented by only a single strain, which has been isolated from vaginal discharge from a patient with bacterial vaginosis. It has the same biochemical screening pattern as C. *urealyticum*, except that it exhibits a strong yellow pigment and weaker urease activity (Table 4). In contrast to most C. *urealyticum* strains, the C. *lipophiloflavum* strain observed was not multidrug resistant.

C. *macginleyi*

C. *macginleyi* (119) has been isolated almost exclusively from eye specimens, whether from diseased (53) or healthy conjunctiva. Colonies are typical for lipophilic corynebacteria (see above). When grown on Tween 80-SBA plates (better growth is usually found on plates supplemented with 0.1% Tween 80 than on those supplemented with 1.0% Tween 80), some C. *macginleyi* strains exhibit a rose pigment which is not seen for any other lipophilic *Corynebacterium* species. C. *macginleyi* is one of the very few *Corynebacterium* species not expressing pyrazinamidase activity (Table 4). Most strains ferment mannitol, while the majority of other corynebacteria are unable to do so. The API Coryne system correctly identifies C. *macginleyi* (60). Strains belonging to this species are susceptible to a broad spectrum of antibiotics (53).

C. *matruchotii*

C. *matruchotii* is thought to be a natural inhabitant of the oral cavity, particularly on calculus and plaque deposits, and so has been much studied by oral microbiologists (110). Otherwise, it is a very rare human pathogen. Microcolonies appear flat, filamentous, and spider-like, but macrocolonies have a variable appearance. C. *matruchotii* demonstrates a very unusual appearance by Gram staining in that so-called whip handles (i.e., filamentous bacteria with a single short bacillus adjacent to the end of the filament, creating the illusion of a whip) are observed (Fig.1e). This microscopic presentation is consistent even when isolates that had been preserved for many years in a culture collection are stained. It has recently been demonstrated that heterogeneity existed among C. *matruchotii* strains obtained from international culture collections and that some strains represented were misidentified C. *durum* isolates (110). C. *matruchotii* strains are consistently negative for galactose, whereas C. *durum* strains can be positive. The API Coryne system database does not contain C. *matruchotii*; the numerical codes observed for C. *matruchotii* include 7000325, 7010325, and 7050325.

C. *matruchotii*-Like Strain

This species is represented by a single strain, ATCC 43833 (110). It had been deposited in ATCC as C. *matruchotii*, but it is a distinct species as revealed by dot-blot hybridization and 16S rRNA gene sequencing data. Colonies are pinpoint to 0.1 mm in diameter, grayish white, with a smooth, nonadherent texture. Biochemical screening reactions are similar to those of C. *minutissimum*, except that strain ATCC 43833 exhibits esculinase activity in the API Coryne system. The numerical API Coryne profile for this unvalidated taxon is 2140325.

C. *minutissimum*

C. *minutissimum* is part of the normal human skin flora. Its association with erythrasma is highly questionable (154). Colonies of C. *minutissimum* are whitish-grayish, shiny, moist, convex, and circular; have entire edges; and are about 1 to 1.5 mm in diameter after 24 h. Most of the colonies are creamy, but some may also have a sticky consistency. C. *minutissimum* strains have a fermentative metabolism and produce acid from sucrose variably. Very few C. *minutissimum* strains are also able to produce acid from mannitol (154). The API Coryne system identifies C. *minutissimum*, with additional tests being necessary for most of the strains (60). Many C. *minutissimum* strains are pyrrolidonyl arylamidase positive. C. *minutissimum* strains exhibit DNase activity (154), and nearly all strains hydrolyze tyrosine, whereas only a very few strains exhibit a positive CAMP reaction. Lactic and succinic acids are the major end products of glucose metabolism (36, 154). Some isolates possess TBSA in their cell membranes. Nearly all C. *minutissimum* strains are susceptible to O/129 (150-μg disk); i.e., they exhibit an inhibition zone around the disk (usually between 20 and 35 mm in diameter).

C. *mucifaciens*

C. *mucifaciens* (48) has been isolated mainly from blood cultures and other sterile body fluids, but it has also been recovered from abscesses, soft tissue, and dialysate (4). Colonies are very distinct because they are slightly to overtly yellow and very mucoid (Fig. 3c) (with very few strains not being mucoid [Funke, unpublished]). C. *mucifaciens* is the only presently known *Corynebacterium* species exhibiting such mucoid colonies; this characteristic strongly reminds the bacteriologist of *Rhodococcus equi* colonies. An extracellular substance (probably polysaccharides) causing connective filaments between the cells has been demonstrated as the ultrastructural correlate of the mucoid colonies. Colonies are about 1 to 1.5 mm after 24 h of incubation and have entire edges. They appear less mucoid after extended incubation for 96 h. C. *mucifaciens* has an oxidative metabolism. It consistently produces acid from glucose, but acid production from sucrose is variable. The API Coryne numerical codes 2000004, 2000104, 2000105, 2100104, 2100105, 6000004, 6100104, and 6100105 have been observed for C. *mucifaciens*, suggesting that occasionally glucose oxidation may be too slow to be observed by that method. C. *mucifaciens* is enzymatically less active than *R. equi*, which exhibits α- and β-glucosidase activities not observed for C. *mucifaciens*. In addition, C. *mucifaciens* produces acid from fructose and may produce acid from glycerol and mannose, but acid production from these sugars is not seen in *R. equi* strains. Tuberculostearic acid can be detected in amounts of 1 to 2% of the total CFAs. β-Lactam antibiotics and aminoglycosides show very good activities against C. *mucifaciens*.

C. *propinquum*

C. *propinquum* is the closest phylogenetic relative of C. *pseudodiphtheriticum* (104, 123) and has the same niche (i.e., the oropharynx) as C. *pseudodiphtheriticum*. Colonies are whitish and somewhat dryish, have entire edges, and measure 1 to 2 mm in diameter after 24 h of incubation. This species reduces nitrate and hydrolyzes tyrosine but does not hydrolyze urea (Table 4). The API Coryne system and the RapID CB Plus system correctly identify C. *propinquum* strains (58, 60).

C. *pseudodiphtheriticum*

C. *pseudodiphtheriticum* is part of the normal oropharyngeal flora. As described in Table 3, this species has been well documented to cause pneumonia in various patient populations. Colonies are whitish and slightly dry, have entire edges, and measure 1 to 2 mm in diameter after 48 h of incubation. This nonfermenting species reduces nitrate and hydrolyzes urea but does not produce acid from any of the commonly tested carbohydrates (Table 4). Some strains hydrolyze tyrosine. The API Coryne system and the RapID CB Plus system correctly identify *C. pseudodiphtheriticum* strains (58, 60). For this species, imperfectly cleaved mycolic acids coeluting with CFAs have been demonstrated (3). *C. pseudodiphtheriticum* strains are susceptible to β-lactam antibiotics, but resistance to macrolides and lincosamides has been observed.

C. pseudotuberculosis

C. pseudotuberculosis is phylogenetically closely related to *C. diphtheriae* (104, 123), may harbor the diphtheria toxin gene, produces propionic acid as a fermentation product, and contains large amounts of the CFA $C_{16:1\omega7c}$ (3). Colonies are yellowish white, opaque, convex, and about 1 mm in diameter after 24 h. Like *C. ulcerans*, *C. pseudotuberculosis* is positive for urease and the CAMP inhibition test (complete inhibition of the effect of *S. aureus* β-hemolysin on sheep erythrocytes is achieved by streaking the presumed *C. pseudotuberculosis* strain in a right angle toward *S. aureus* and overnight incubation; a β-hemolysin inhibition zone in the form of a triangle is observed, as is the case for *A. haemolyticum* [Fig. 2]). *C. pseudotuberculosis* is not susceptible to O/129, whereas *C. ulcerans* strains are (74). *C. pseudotuberculosis* is variable for both nitrate reduction and sucrose fermentation. The API Coryne system and the RapID CB Plus panel correctly identify this species (58, 60).

C. resistens

This recently defined species (103) has entire, grayish-whitish, and glistening colonies and is lipophilic. It is unusual in having a negative pyrazinamidase reaction, which differentiates it from the phenotypically related *C. jeikeium* or CDC coryneform group G strains. In addition, *C. resistens* grows slowly under anaerobic conditions, whereas *C. jeikeium* is unable to do so. The *C. resistens* strains reported in the literature were resistant to penicillin, cephalosporins, aminoglycosides, clindamycin, and ciprofloxacin but remained susceptible to glycopeptides. It is presently unknown whether true *C. resistens* strains are often misidentified as *C. jeikeium* in the routine laboratory.

C. riegelii

C. riegelii strains were originally described as being isolated from females with urinary tract infections (49), but additional strains have been recovered from blood cultures, including cord blood (4). Colonies are whitish, glistening, and convex; have entire margins; and measure up to 1.5 mm in diameter after 48 h of incubation. Some colonies are of a creamy consistency, whereas others are sticky. *C. riegelii* strains exhibit a very strong urease activity with Christensen's urea broth, becoming positive within 5 min after inoculation at room temperature. A very peculiar characteristic of *C. riegelii* is the slow fermentation of maltose but not glucose. No other defined *Corynebacterium* exhibits this feature (Table 4). The weak anaerobic growth of *C. riegelii* corresponds to the weak fermentative metabolism. The API Coryne system codes observed for *C. riegelii* include 0101224, 2001224, and 2101224.

C. simulans

This species has been delineated from some *C. striatum*-like strains (145). The three strains described in the original publication came from skin-related specimens (foot abscess, lymph node biopsy specimen, and boil). Two additional strains have been characterized, one from bile and one from a blood culture (4). Colonies of *C. simulans* (grayish white, glistening, creamy, and 1 to 2 mm in diameter) are very similar to those of *C. minutissimum*, *C. singulare*, and *C. striatum*, all of which are the closest phylogenetic neighbors. *C. simulans* is the only valid *Corynebacterium* species described to date that reduces nitrite. Further characteristics which differentiate *C. simulans* from the closely related nonlipophilic, fermentative corynebacteria are the inability to acidify ethylene glycol and the inability to grow at 20°C (in contrast to *C. striatum*). API Coryne profiles include 0100305, 2100105, 2100301, 2100305, and 3000125 (including the falsely negative nitrate reduction reaction because of the strong nitrite reduction).

C. singulare

C. singulare colonies are circular and slightly convex with entire margins and are of a creamy consistency, as observed for *C. minutissimum* and *C. striatum* (121). Key biochemical reactions are like those for *C. minutissimum*, except that urease activity is observed (Table 4). The numerical API Coryne system profile is 6101125, indicative that pyrrolidonyl arylamidase activity is observed. Like *C. minutissimum* and *C. striatum*, *C. singulare* also hydrolyzes tyrosine. *C. singulare* can be differentiated from the much more frequently isolated *C. minutissimum* with use of the bioMérieux biotype 100 gallery, but this is not a usual clinical microbiology laboratory test. *C. singulare* does not produce propionic acid as a fermentation product, differentiating it from *C. amycolatum*.

C. striatum

C. striatum is part of the normal human skin flora. Nosocomial transmission of *C. striatum* has been documented (86). Colonies are convex, circular, shiny, moist, and creamy with entire edges and are about 1 to 1.5 mm in diameter after 24 h of incubation. Some investigators have described *C. striatum* colonies as somewhat like those of small coagulase-negative staphylococci. *C. striatum* has a fermentative metabolism, and acid production from sucrose is variable. The API Coryne system identifies *C. striatum*, but additional tests are needed in most of the cases (60). All *C. striatum* strains hydrolyze tyrosine, and some strains are CAMP reaction positive; however, the CAMP reaction of *C. striatum* strains is usually not as strong as that of other CAMP test-positive species (e.g., *C. auris* or *C. glucuronolyticum*). Lactic and succinic acids are the major end products of glucose metabolism (36). All *C. striatum* strains are susceptible to O/129. Resistance to macrolides and lincosamides due to the presence of an rRNA methylase has been described. *C. striatum* may also be resistant to quinolones and tetracyclines.

C. sundsvallense

C. sundsvallense (4, 14) is a newly described species that has been isolated from blood cultures, a vaginal swab, and a sinus drainage from an infected groin. Colonies of this nonlipophilic species are buff or slightly yellowish and adherent to agar and have a sticky consistency. Gram staining shows bulges or knobs at the ends of some rods, and these are not seen in any other corynebacteria. Fermentation of glucose, lactose, and sucrose is slow (Table 4). *C. sundsvallense* can be differentiated from *C. durum* by its positive α-glucosidase reaction and its inability to ferment galactose. It is further differentiated from *C. matruchotii* by expressing urease but not nitrate reductase activity and by not producing propionic acid as an end product of glucose metabolism (4, 14).

C. thomssenii

C. thomssenii (153) is a rarely found species, originally repeatedly isolated from a patient with pleural effusion; a second strain was recovered from the environment in Canada (4). This species is fastidious and slowly growing, resulting in colonies <0.5 mm after 48 h, but it is not lipophilic. After 96 h, colonies are molar tooth-like, very sticky, and slightly adherent to agar. The clinical strain of *C. thomssenii* is the only *Corynebacterium* species expressing *N*-acetyl-β-glucosaminidase activity, which can be observed in either the API Coryne or the API ZYM system. Acid is slowly and fermentatively produced from glucose, maltose, and sucrose, and the resulting API Coryne code for *C. thomssenii* is 2121125.

C. tuberculostearicum

C. tuberculostearicum was recently revived for a never validly published taxon and also included a strain of the unvalidated species "*C. pseudogenitalium*" (35). This lipophilic species has some variable biochemical key reactions (Table 4) and can be differentiated from CDC group G and *C. accolens* only through the presence of TBSA. However, as CFA analysis cannot be routinely performed in every clinical laboratory, it is unknown how many tentatively identified CDC group G strains are in fact *C. tuberculostearicum* strains. Unfortunately, the published report on *C. tuberculostearicum* did not provide any further features to differentiate this species from the phenotypically closely related CDC group G bacteria.

C. tuscaniae

C. tuscaniae, a recently described species, has been isolated from blood cultures of a patient suffering from endocarditis (114). *C. tuscaniae* does not grow under anaerobic conditions, which distinguishes this species from the phenotypically closely related *C. minutissimum*. In addition, *C. tuscaniae* hydrolyzes hippurate but not tyrosine, whereas *C. minutissimum* has opposite reactions (Table 4). *C. tuscaniae* colonies are rounded and regular, in contrast to the biochemically closely related *C. amycolatum* colonies, which exhibit irregular edges.

C. ulcerans

Phylogenetically, *C. ulcerans* (120) is, together with *C. pseudotuberculosis*, the closest relative of *C. diphtheriae* (104, 123) and contains significant amounts of $C_{16:1\omega7c}$. *C. ulcerans* can harbor the diphtheria toxin gene, but differences in the receptor-binding and translocation domains have been described, and a *C. ulcerans* diphtheria toxin-specific PCR has been developed (128). Disease associated with this bacterium is rare, but if the organism is recovered from pseudomembranous material, the disease must be treated like a case of diphtheria (29, 30). Recent reports have described the transmission of *C. ulcerans* from domestic dogs and cats to humans (84). Colonies are somewhat dry, waxy, and gray-white with light hemolysis, being 1 to 2 mm in diameter after 24 h. *C. ulcerans* may be differentiated from *C. diphtheriae* by urease activity and a CAMP inhibition reaction (Table 4). Strains of *C. ulcerans* are positive for glycogen, starch, and trehalose fermentation. The API Coryne system and the RapID CB Plus identification strip correctly identify *C. ulcerans* (58, 60).

C. urealyticum

C. urealyticum is one of the more frequently isolated, clinically significant corynebacteria in clinical specimens (64). *C. urealyticum* is strongly associated with urinary tract infections. Recovery of this bacterium is often associated with urine with an alkaline pH, resulting in struvite crystals. As for all other lipophilic corynebacteria, colonies are pinpoint, convex, smooth, and whitish-grayish on regular SBA. *C. urealyticum* is a strict aerobe and has very strong urease activity (Table 4). Commercial identification systems correctly identify *C. urealyticum*. *C. urealyticum* is almost always multidrug resistant (64, 130), but rare penicillin-susceptible strains have also been described.

C. xerosis

Colonies are dry, granular, and yellowish, have irregular edges, and are 1 to 1.5 mm in diameter after 24 h. It must be emphasized that nearly all "*C. xerosis*" strains that appeared in the literature before 1996 may have been misidentified *C. amycolatum* strains (46). *C. striatum* strains were also misidentified as *C. xerosis* in the past. *C. xerosis* has a fermentative metabolism, is variable for the presence of nitrate reductase, but always expresses α-glucosidase as well as leucine arylamidase activities. Because *C. xerosis* was thought to be rarely encountered in clinical specimens, it was not included in the API Coryne system version 2.0 database. The numerical profiles observed for *C. xerosis* strains include 2110325 and 3110325. The RapID CB Plus system correctly identifies *C. xerosis* (58). Lactic acid is the major end product of glucose metabolism, and strains are susceptible to O/129.

Biochemical Reactions for Other Genera

The key biochemical reactions for the genera other than *Corynebacterium* are given in Table 5.

Genus *Turicella*

T. otitidis is almost exclusively isolated from clinical specimens from the ear region, but it does not cause otitis media with effusion in children (73). Colonies are whitish, convex, and creamy, have entire edges, and measure 1 to 1.5 mm in diameter after 48 h of incubation. Some young colonies show a greenish appearance when taken away from the plates with a swab. The distinctive Gram stain morphology of *T. otitidis* is shown in Fig. 1b. Differentiation from *C. auris* and *C. afermentans* subsp. *afermentans* is readily achieved by morphologic features, but utilization reactions may also assist in the differentiation of these taxa (47). All *T. otitidis* strains are strongly CAMP reaction positive and give the numerical code 2100004 in the API Coryne system. The MICs of β-lactam antibiotics for many strains are very low; some strains might be resistant to macrolides and clindamycin (59).

Genus *Arthrobacter*

Arthrobacter spp. might be part of the indigenous normal human flora, but their main habitat is soil. *A. cumminsii* seems to be a normal commensal in humans and appears to be the most frequently isolated *Arthrobacter* species in human clinical specimens (54). *Arthrobacter* colonies are usually whitish-grayish, slightly glistening, and creamy and are 2 mm or greater in diameter after 24 h. *A. cumminsii* is slightly smaller than the other arthrobacters and may also exhibit a sticky consistency (54). *Arthrobacter* spp. usually do not oxidize any of the carbohydrates routinely tested and do not express a cheese-like smell, as is often found for the phenotypically closely related brevibacteria. Some arthrobacters are motile, whereas brevibacteria are always nonmotile. Like brevibacteria, *Arthrobacter* spp. express DNase and have gelatinase activity (44). The identification of arthrobacters to the species level might be achieved by carbohydrate utilization tests, but this is recommended for the reference laboratory only. The recently described *A. albus* is phylogenetically closely related to *A. cumminsii* but might be differentiated phenotypically by being resistant to desferrioxamine, whereas *A. cumminsii* is susceptible. *A. cumminsii* has a distinctive CFA pattern, with $C_{14:0i}$ and $C_{14:0}$ each representing 2 to 4% of all CFAs (54). The penicillin MICs for most *Arthrobacter* strains are low (44). Aminoglycosides and quinolones show only very weak activities against *A. cumminsii* strains (54).

Genus *Brevibacterium*

Some *Brevibacterium* spp. are part of the normal human skin flora. Colonies are whitish-grayish (or yellowish like *B. luteolum* [146]), convex, and mostly creamy, and are 2 mm or greater in diameter after 24 h. *B. mcbrellneri* colonies have a more granular appearance and are dryer than those of other brevibacteria. Some brevibacteria may develop a yellowish or greenish pigment after prolonged incubation. Many *Brevibacterium* strains isolated from human clinical material give off a distinctive cheese-like odor. Brevibacteria are nonmotile, are halotolerant (6.5% NaCl), and form methanethiol from methionine, but this test is specific for brevibacteria only when it is read within 2 h (40). Brevibacteria can be identified to the species level by carbohydrate utilization tests. More than 90% of all clinical *Brevibacterium* isolates are *B. casei* (40). *B. sanguinis* is very similar to *B. casei* and can be differentiated from this species by susceptibility to thallium acetate (147). The MICs of β-lactam antibiotics for brevibacteria are often elevated (59, 139).

Genus *Dermabacter*

D. hominis strains are part of the normal skin flora. Colonies are whitish, convex, of a creamy or sticky consistency, and 1 to 1.5 mm in diameter after 48 h (Fig. 3e). *D. hominis* strains are sometimes mistaken for small-colony coagulase-negative staphylococci. The Gram stain result is distinctive, with coccobacillary or coccoidal forms (Fig. 1c). The key biochemical reactions are given in Table 5. *D. hominis* is one of the few coryneform bacteria with a variable reaction for xylose fermentation. It is the only catalase-positive coryneform bacterium (except *Actinomyces neuii* [36]) that is able to decarboxylate lysine and ornithine (61). The API Coryne system and the RapID CB Plus panel correctly identify this species (58, 60). *D. hominis* strains may be resistant to aminoglycosides (61, 139).

Genus *Rothia*

This genus presently comprises five validated species, of which only two are clinically relevant: *R. mucilaginosa* (formerly designated *Stomatococcus mucilaginosus*), *R. dentocariosa* (the type species), as well as *R. dentocariosa* genomovar II (19, 81). The last organism has not been formally named because it has not been possible to biochemically distinguish it from authentic *R. dentocariosa* sensu stricto (genomovar I) (81). Some of the former CDC coryneform group 4 bacteria (Fig. 3h) were also shown to be representatives of *R. dentocariosa* (21). These grayish strains were isolated primarily from respiratory materials, pus, or blood cultures, in contrast to *C. aurimucosum* strains, which were derived from the female urogenital tract.

Colonies of *R. dentocariosa* are whitish (or more rarely grayish black), raised, and smooth or rough or have a "spoke wheel" form (Fig. 3f), and they are up to 2 mm in diameter after 48 h. *Rothia* strains usually grow slightly better in a CO_2-enriched atmosphere. The biochemical features of *R. dentocariosa* are given in Table 5. The API Coryne system correctly identifies *R. dentocariosa* (60). Its CFA composition is of the branched-chain type (3), which allows differentiation from the biochemically similar species *C. durum*, *C. matruchotii*, and *Actinomyces viscosus* (see chapter 56), all of which also occupy the oropharynx. *R. dentocariosa* may also be confused with *D. hominis* and *Propionibacterium avidum* (see chapter 55) (142), both of which, in contrast, always exhibit smooth colonies. As shown in a study on the pharyngeal bacterial flora of healthy adults, one-third of all *R. dentocariosa* strains isolated were negative for the key biochemical reaction catalase (144). The MICs of aminoglycosides for some *R. dentocariosa* strains are elevated, whereas penicillins usually show good in vitro activities against *Rothia* strains.

Genus *Exiguobacterium*

It is not known whether exiguobacteria are part of the indigenous bacterial flora of humans. Colonies of *E. acetylicum* are smooth, golden-yellow to orange, and up to 2 mm in diameter after 24 h of incubation. Acid from carbohydrates is rapidly produced by fermentative metabolism. Exiguobacteria are motile and often oxidase positive. They might be confused with microbacteria, but CFA analysis provides a clear-cut distinction between the two genera (Table 1). The pathogenic potential of *E. acetylicum* seems to be rather low, since it has been isolated from different sources (e.g., skin, wounds, and cerebrospinal fluid [71]), but case reports on infectious diseases due to *E. acetylicum* are not extant. Cases of pseudobacteremia due to *E. acetylicum* have been observed.

Genus *Oerskovia*

O. turbata is usually acquired from the environment (e.g., soil). Colonies are pale yellow to phosphorous yellow, convex, and creamy; they penetrate agar; and they are approximately 1 to 2 mm in diameter after 24 h. *O. turbata* rapidly produces acid from sugars by fermentation; it also exhibits a very strong esculin reaction. The genus is well identified by the API Coryne system (60). *O. turbata* does not hydrolyze xanthine or hypoxanthine, whereas the related *C. cellulans* is able to do so.

Genus *Cellulomonas*

Cellulomonas strains are usually acquired from the environment. Colonies are first whitish or pale or bright yellow, but after 7 days nearly all *Cellulomonas* strains are somewhat yellow. Colonies vary between 0.5 and 1.5 mm in diameter after 24 h, are convex and creamy, and have entire edges. *Cellulomonas* spp. are variable for the fermentation of mannitol. Other key biochemical reactions of *Cellulomonas* spp. are given in Table 5. The majority of *Cellulomonas* strains express cellulase activity, demonstrated by incubating a heavy bacterial suspension (McFarland no. 6 standard) with a piece of sterile copy paper in a 0.9% NaCl solution for 10 days, resulting in dissolution of the paper (55). The recently described *C. denverensis* can be differentiated from *C. hominis* by its positive reaction for D-sorbitol fermentation (7).

Genus *Cellulosimicrobium*

Colonies of *C. cellulans* are similar to those of *O. turbata* (see above) and also pit the agar. In addition, *C. cellulans* exhibits a biochemical screening profile which is very similar to that of *O. turbata* (Table 5). However, *C. cellulans* hydrolyzes either xanthine or hypoxanthine whereas *O. turbata* does not, and *O. turbata* strains might be motile whereas *C. cellulans* strains are not (71, 125). The recently described *C. funkei* strains can be differentiated from *C. cellulans* (former *O. xanthinolytica*) by their negative inulin and raffinose fermentation reactions (8); in addition, *C. funkei* strains are motile but *C. cellulans* strains are not.

Genus *Microbacterium*

Microbacteria account for the majority of yellow-pigmented coryneform bacteria isolated from clinical specimens. All shades of yellow pigment are observed, ranging from pale to bright yellow and orange. Most of the strains are catalase positive, but catalase-negative strains might be observed. Some microbacteria grow under anaerobic conditions but only weakly. Some microbacteria are nitrate reductase negative, which distinguishes them from the phenotypically closely related genus *Cellulomonas*, all presently defined species of which are nitrate reductase positive (Table 5). Microbacteria may ferment mannitol but not xylose, whereas the lack of xylose fermentation has not been observed for *Cellulomonas* strains described so far.

Species identification is almost impossible since for many defined *Microbacterium* species the type strain is the only representative, preventing the creation of a comprehensive database. Final identification to the species level is best achieved by chemotaxonomic (interpeptide bridges) and molecular genetic (e.g., 16S rRNA gene sequencing) investigations. The most frequently isolated, validated microbacteria in clinical specimens include *M. oxydans, M. paraoxydans, M. aurum,* and *M. lacticum* (66, 82).

Microbacteria are usually susceptible to vancomycin (except *M. resistens* [50]), but susceptibility to other antimicrobial agents is unpredictable (in particular, resistance to aminoglycosides has been observed [42]), and therefore every individual clinically significant strain must be tested.

Genus *Curtobacterium*

Curtobacteria are very infrequently isolated yellow- or yellow-orange-pigmented oxidative coryneform bacteria. In contrast to most microbacteria, they produce acid from carbohydrates very slowly (within 4 to 7 days) (38). Curtobacteria are usually nitrate reductase negative but strongly hydrolyze esculin (Table 5). *C. pusillum* and related strains have a most unusual CFA composition that is not observed in any other coryneform bacteria, with a ω-cyclohexyl fatty acid identified as feature 7 ($C_{18:1\omega7c/\omega9c/\omega12t}$) representing more than 50% of all CFAs (38). Again, the differentiation of curtobacteria is very difficult and should be performed in a reference laboratory. The MICs of macrolides and rifampin for curtobacteria are very low.

Genus *Leifsonia*

Leifsonia aquatica is very rarely encountered in clinical specimens. It is always motile, does not hydrolyze either gelatin or casein, and has a stronger DNase activity than most microbacteria (65). *L. aquatica* is the only species within the genus *Leifsonia* which is able to grow in broth enriched with 5% NaCl (34). Its yellow pigment develops relatively slowly within 3 to 4 days. The MICs of vancomycin for some *L. aquatica* strains were shown to be elevated (8 μg/ml) (65), but the precise mechanism of this resistance is not known.

Genera *Janibacter, Pseudoclavibacter/Zimmermannella,* and *Knoellia*

Strains belonging to genera *Janibacter, Pseudoclavibacter/Zimmermannella,* and *Knoellia* have been derived from the environment, foods, or animals but have also been recovered recently from clinical materials and characterized using 16S rRNA gene sequencing. These taxa were described as having white, creamy, or yellowish pigment, and all were nonmotile. *Janibacter, Pseudoclavibacter/Zimmermannella,* and *Knoellia* were oxidative, and *Brachybacterium* strains were fermentative. All strains tested so far were susceptible to vancomycin. Since no comprehensive biochemical data based on a large number of strains are available at present, these genera were not included in Table 5.

Genus *Arcanobacterium*

The genus *Arcanobacterium* comprises six species, all of which except *A. pluranimalium* exhibit beta-hemolysis on SBA. The three medically relevant species, *A. haemolyticum, A. pyogenes,* and *A. bernardiae,* are all catalase negative. All species show a fermentative glucose metabolism, with succinic and lactic acids as their major end products. All arcanobacteria grow and express hemolysis best in a CO_2-enriched atmosphere.

The colonies of the type species, *A. haemolyticum,* are 0.5 mm in diameter after 48 h of incubation at 37°C, and two morphotypes have been described: one rough type isolated mainly from the respiratory tract and one smooth type isolated mainly from wounds. The biochemical reactions of *A. haemolyticum* are given in Table 5. Of major value for the identification of *A. haemolyticum* is the so-called CAMP inhibition test (see the description of the CAMP inhibition test in the section on *C. pseudotuberculosis*) (Fig. 2). The protein responsible for this phenomenon is a phospholipase D excreted by *A. haemolyticum,* and this protein is genetically and functionally similar to the ones expressed by *C. ulcerans* and *C. pseudotuberculosis*. *A. haemolyticum* and the two other medically relevant arcanobacteria are correctly identified by the API Coryne system (60).

A. pyogenes colonies are the largest of all arcanobacterium colonies, with diameters of up to 1 mm after 48 h of incubation. Of all the arcanobacteria, this species also shows the sharpest zone of beta-hemolysis on SBA. The protein responsible for hemolysis, named pyolysin, is also an important virulence factor in vivo. Gram stains may show some branching rods. *A. pyogenes* is the only *Arcanobacterium* species of medical relevance that expresses β-glucuronidase activity and that is capable of fermenting xylose.

A. bernardiae (57, 105) shows glassy, whitish colonies of <0.5 mm in diameter after 48 h. Some colonies have a creamy consistency, whereas others are sticky. Gram staining shows relatively short rods without branching. Most *A. bernardiae* strains belong to the very few coryneform bacteria that are able to ferment glycogen. Another peculiar feature of *A. bernardiae* strains is their ability to produce acid faster from maltose than from glucose.

The MICs of all β-lactams, rifampin, and tetracycline for arcanobacteria are very low, whereas aminoglycosides and quinolones have reduced activities against arcanobacteria (Funke, unpublished). Macrolides also exhibit excellent activities against arcanobacteria and are an alternative to β-lactam antibiotics for the treatment of infections, since treatment failures due to β-lactam antibiotics because of the inability of β-lactam antibiotics to act intracellularly have been reported.

ANTIMICROBIAL SUSCEPTIBILITIES

The susceptibility patterns for each taxon were given with the descriptions of each taxon (see above). Since the antimicrobial susceptibility of coryneform bacteria is not predictable in every case, susceptibility testing should always be performed with clinically significant isolates (see "Clinical Significance"). Due to the emergence of vancomycin-resistant gram-positive organisms, it has become inappropriate to recommend glycopeptides as first-line drugs for the treatment of infections caused by coryneform bacteria. It is also noteworthy that some coryneform bacteria (e.g., *Microbacterium resistens*) are intrinsically vancomycin resistant.

The Clinical and Laboratory Standards Institute has recently published testing conditions and interpretive criteria for susceptibility testing of coryneform bacteria by use of a broth microdilution method (13). Direct colony suspensions equivalent to a 0.5 McFarland standard are prepared, and strains are incubated in cation-adjusted Mueller-Hinton broth with 2 to 5% (vol/vol) lysed horse blood at 35°C in ambient air for up to 48 h. Interpretive categories for the MICs obtained are presently available for 16 antimicrobial agents including newer drugs like quinupristin-dalfopristin (63) or linezolid (51). Very few studies comparing broth microdilution and disk diffusion results for susceptibility testing of coryneform bacteria (149) have been performed.

In the past, MICs have been determined by either the E test (AB Biodisk, Solna, Sweden) or the agar dilution or broth microdilution method. The results of the E test have been shown to correlate well with those of both the broth microdilution and the agar dilution methods for *Corynebacterium* spp. (92, 152). The E test should be carried out on Mueller-Hinton agar supplemented with 5% sheep blood. The same medium is used for the agar dilution method (59), but this method is not applicable in the routine laboratory; rather, it should be used in studies with individual antimicrobial agents.

EVALUATION, INTERPRETATION, AND REPORTING OF RESULTS

The guidelines related to when coryneform bacteria should be identified to the species level (see "Clinical Significance") are also applicable for evaluating and interpreting culture results; i.e., whenever coryneform bacteria are identified to the species level, the results should be reported.

In the rare case of microscopically suspected *C. diphtheriae* (i.e., a positive Neisser staining result), the physician in charge of the patient should be notified immediately, although culture results and toxin testing results become available only later.

It is evident that repeated isolation of a predominant strain of a coryneform bacterium or a coryneform bacterium growing in pure culture suggests an etiological relationship to the patient's disease. If coryneform bacteria are present in blood cultures, the physician in charge should be notified immediately, and it should be emphasized when reporting this result that the clinical significance of the coryneform bacteria must be carefully examined by cooperation between the microbiology laboratory and the physician. In our experience, one positive blood culture out of two or three aerobically and anaerobically incubated pairs of blood cultures is hardly ever clinically significant (except in cases of treated endocarditis). Care must be taken in the interpretation of the results for those patients for whom half or more of the blood specimens taken for culture become positive for coryneform bacteria, in particular when lipophilic corynebacteria are cultured, since not all blood samples taken from patients with endocarditis due to lipophilic corynebacteria may eventually become positive.

On the other hand, coryneform bacteria should be reported as "normal flora" when they are grown in equal or smaller numbers from nonsterile sites together with other resident flora. It is suggested that the primary isolation plates be retained for at least 72 h before they are discarded in order to have the opportunity to assess the bacterial population retrospectively.

APPENDIX 1

Genus *Gardnerella*

The genus *Gardnerella* does not have a particular phylogenetic relationship to any of the established genera described in this chapter. It is remotely related to the genus *Bifidobacterium* (94), and these genera share some important features, such as production of acetic and lactic acids as fermentation products. A 16S rRNA gene PCR product selected for detection of a *G. vaginalis*-specific sequence was found to have some less-than-specific homology with several *Bifidobacterium* species (100). *G. vaginalis* is the only species belonging to the genus *Gardnerella*. Studies on the ultrastructure of the cell wall of *G. vaginalis* have demonstrated that it has a cell wall similar to but much thinner than the cell walls of other gram-positive bacteria (i.e., there is a smaller peptidoglycan layer) (124). Lysine is the diamino acid of the cell wall, and CFAs are similar to those detected in *Actinomyces* spp., *Arcanobacterium* spp., and *Corynebacterium* spp., with $C_{16:0}$ and $C_{18:1\omega9c}$ predominating. The G+C content of 42 to 44 mol% is lower than that of every other genus described in this chapter.

Gram stains show thin gram-variable rods or coccobacilli (Fig. 1f). Catalase is not produced, and cells are nonmotile and have a slow fermentative metabolism.

Natural habitat

G. vaginalis can be found in the anorectal flora of healthy adults of both sexes as well as in that of children (10). It is also part of the endogenous vaginal flora in women of reproductive age. The optimal pH for the growth of *G. vaginalis* is between 6 and 7. The organism can also be recovered from the urethras of the male partners of women with bacterial vaginosis (BV) (10).

Clinical significance

G. vaginalis is associated with BV; its causative role in the syndrome is controversial (131, 132). Recurrent BV is due to reinfection rather than to relapse (i.e., overgrowth of the previously colonizing biotype). In pregnant women, BV may lead to preterm birth, premature rupture of membranes, and chorioamnionitis (10). *G. vaginalis* may also be recovered from cultures of blood from patients with postpartum or postabortal fevers and may also cause infections in newborns. Although it might be recovered from the urethras of males, its association with disease in males is questionable. Serious infections in sites other than those associated with the genital tract or obstetrics are rare but have been reported.

Collection, transport, and storage of specimens

Vaginal and extravaginal specimens can be collected with cotton-tipped swabs. It is best to take one swab for direct examination and to take another swab for culture if necessary, such as for epidemiologic studies. If culture media cannot be directly inoculated, then the swab should be placed in a transport medium (e.g., Amies) and culture should be done within 24 h. It is noteworthy that *G. vaginalis* is susceptible to sodium polyanethol sulfonate (SPS), so an SPS-free medium (or an SPS medium supplemented with gelatin) should be used in order to achieve optimal recovery of *G. vaginalis* from blood culture systems whenever *G. vaginalis* is suspected.

Isolation and identification

The gold standard for the diagnosis of BV is direct examination of vaginal secretions and not the culture of *G. vaginalis*, since *G. vaginalis* can also be recovered from healthy women. A bedside test for BV is examination of the vaginal discharge to detect the typical "fishy" trimethylamine odor, which is enhanced after alkalinization with 10% KOH. The typical smear of vaginal discharge from BV patients shows "clue cells" (bacteria covering epithelial cell margins) together with mixed flora consisting of large numbers of small gram-negative (predominantly *Prevotella* and *Porphyromonas* spp.) and gram-variable (*G. vaginalis*) rods and coccobacilli, whereas lactobacilli are almost always absent. It is recommended that a standardized Gram staining interpretative scheme be used in order to improve the reproducibility of this method (102, 132). Detection of *G. vaginalis* in vaginal specimens processed using a DNA probe-based system, Affirm VPIII (Becton Dickinson), has been reported to be useful as a surrogate for wet mount cell examination (6). Although not recommended for routine laboratory procedures, the isolation of *G. vaginalis* can support the diagnosis of BV. Vaginal swabs are cultured on Vaginalis agar (see chapter 20 for the preparation) and should be semiquantitatively streaked out with a loop. Incubation is at 35 to 37°C in a 5% CO_2-enriched atmosphere or in a candle jar. Beta-hemolysis is observed on human or rabbit blood-containing media but not on SBA. Plates may be checked for the growth of diffuse beta-hemolytic colonies of <0.5 mm in diameter after 24 h, but very often *G. vaginalis* is best observed after 48 h. Gram staining of the suspected colonies confirms the diagnosis of *G. vaginalis*.

Eight *G. vaginalis* biotypes had been proposed on the basis of the reactions for lipase, β-galactosidase, and hippurate hydrolysis (107), with biotypes 1, 5, and 6 being most common. The diagnostic value of these biotypes is questionable since they have not been demonstrated to be associated with certain diseases or certain forms of disease. They may have some value for longitudinal studies, but molecular genetic typing methods are likely to be superior to biotyping. *G. vaginalis* strains are consistently α-glucosidase and starch hydrolysis positive, but only 90% of all *G. vaginalis* strains hydrolyze hippurate. The API Coryne system identifies *G. vaginalis* well (60). Confirmation of the identification of *G. vaginalis* can also be achieved by antimicrobial agent disk inhibition tests with 50 μg of metronidazole (inhibition present), 5 μg of trimethoprim (inhibition present), and 1 mg of sulfonamide (inhibition absent).

"*G. vaginalis*-like" organisms recovered from patients with BV have been demonstrated to represent *Actinomyces turicensis* strains (141). *G. vaginalis* can be differentiated from these organisms in that it has acetic acid as the main end product of glucose fermentation and is unable to produce acid from xylose, whereas *A. turicensis* strains have succinic acid as the end product and produce acid from xylose.

Antimicrobial susceptibilities

Metronidazole is the drug of choice both for local therapy of BV and for systemic therapy of extravaginal infections caused by BV-associated flora. Systemic infections due to *G. vaginalis* alone can be treated with ampicillin or amoxicillin, since β-lactamase-producing *G. vaginalis* strains have not been observed so far. Susceptibility testing for *G. vaginalis* is not recommended.

REFERENCES

1. **Aubel, D., F. N. R. Renaud, and J. Freney.** 1997. Genomic diversity of several *Corynebacterium* species identified by amplification of the 16S-23S rRNA gene spacer regions. *Int. J. Syst. Bacteriol.* **47:**767–772.
2. **Bernard, K. A.** 2005. *Corynebacterium* species and coryneforms: an update on taxonomy and diseases attributed to these taxa. *Clin. Microbiol. Newsl.* **27:**9–18.
3. **Bernard, K. A., M. Bellefeuille, and E. P. Ewan.** 1991. Cellular fatty acid composition as an adjunct to the identification of asporogenous, aerobic gram-positive rods. *J. Clin. Microbiol.* **29:**83–89.
4. **Bernard, K. A., C. Munro, D. Wiebe, and E. Ongsansoy.** 2002. Characteristics of rare or recently described *Corynebacterium* species recovered from human clinical material in Canada. *J. Clin. Microbiol.* **40:**4375–4381.
5. **Björkroth, J., H. Korkeala, and G. Funke.** 1999. rRNA gene RFLP as an identification tool for *Corynebacterium* species. *Int. J. Syst. Bacteriol.* **49:**983–989.
6. **Briselden, A. M., and S. L. Hillier.** 1994. Evaluation of Affirm VP Microbial Identification test for *Gardnerella vaginalis* and *Trichomonas vaginalis*. *J. Clin. Microbiol.* **32:** 148–152.
7. **Brown, J. M., R. P. Frazier, R. E. Morey, A. G. Steigerwalt, G. J. Pellegrini, M. I. Daneshvar, D. G. Hollis, and M. McNeil.** 2005. Phenotypic and genetic characterization of clinical isolates of CDC coryneform group A-3: proposal of a new species of *Cellulomonas*, *Cellulomonas denverensis* sp. nov. *J. Clin. Microbiol.* **43:**1732–1737.
8. **Brown, J. M., A. G. Steigerwalt, R. E. Morey, M. I. Daneshvar, L.-J. Romero, and M. M. McNeil.** 2006. Characterization of clinical isolates previously identified as *Oerskovia turbata*: proposal of *Cellulosimicrobium funkei* sp. nov. and emended description of the genus *Cellulosimicrobium*. *Int. J. Syst. Evol. Microbiol.* **56:**801–804.
9. **Carlotti, A., and G. Funke.** 1994. Rapid distinction of *Brevibacterium* species by restriction analysis of rDNA generated by polymerase chain reaction. *Syst. Appl. Microbiol.* **17:**380–386.
10. **Catlin, B. W.** 1992. *Gardnerella vaginalis*: characteristics, clinical considerations, and controversies. *Clin. Microbiol. Rev.* **5:**213–237.
11. **Cerdeño-Tárraga, A. M., A. Efstratiou, L. G. Dover, M. T. G. Holden, M. Pallen, S. D. Bentley, G. S. Besra, C. Churcher, K. D. James, A. De Zoysa, T. Chillingworth, A. Cronin, L. Dowd, T. Feltwell, N. Hamlin, S. Holroyd, K. Jagels, S. Moule, M. A. Quail, E. Rabbinowitsch, K. M. Rutherford, N. R. Thomson, L. Unwin, S. Whitehead, B. G. Barrell, and J. Parkhill.** 2003. The complete genome sequence and analysis of *Corynebacterium diphtheriae* NCTC13129. *Nucleic Acids Res.* **31:** 6516–6523.
12. **Cianciotto, N. P., and N. B. Groman.** 1997. Characterization of bacteriophages from *tox*-containing, nontoxigenic isolates of *Corynebacterium diphtheriae*. *Microb. Pathog.* **22:**343–351.
13. **Clinical and Laboratory Standards Institute.** 2006. *Methods for Antimicrobial Dilution and Disk Susceptibility Testing of Infrequently Isolated or Fastidious Bacteria. Document* M45. CLSI, Wayne, Pa.
14. **Collins, M. D., K. A. Bernard, R. A. Hutson, B. Sjöden, A. Nyberg, and E. Falsen.** 1999. *Corynebacterium sundsvallense* sp. nov., from human clinical specimens. *Int. J. Syst. Bacteriol.* **49:**361–366.
15. **Collins, M. D., J. Brown, and D. Jones.** 1988. *Brachybacterium faecium* gen. nov., sp. nov., a coryneform bacterium from poultry deep litter. *Int. J. Syst. Bacteriol.* **38:**45–48.
16. **Collins, M. D., R. A. Burton, and D. Jones.** 1988. *Corynebacterium amycolatum* sp. nov. a new mycolic acid-less *Corynebacterium* species from human skin. *FEMS Microbiol. Lett.* **49:**349–352.
17. **Collins, M. D., and C. S. Cummins.** 1986. Genus *Corynebacterium*, p. 1266–1276. *In* P. H. A. Sneath, N. S. Mair, M. E. Sharpe, and J. G. Holt (ed.), *Bergey's Manual of Systematic Bacteriology*, vol. 2. The Williams & Wilkins Co., Baltimore, Md.
18. **Collins, M. D., E. Falsen, E. Akervall, B. Sjöden, and A. Alvarez.** 1998. *Corynebacterium kroppenstedtii* sp. nov., a

novel corynebacterium that does not contain mycolic acids. *Int. J. Syst. Bacteriol.* **48:**1449–1454.

19. **Collins, M. D., R. A. Hutson, V. Baverud, and E. Falsen.** 2000. Characterization of a *Rothia*-like organism from a mouse: description of *Rothia nasimurium* sp. nov. and reclassification of *Stomatococcus mucilaginosus* as *Rothia mucilaginosa* comb. nov. *Int. J. Syst. Evol. Bacteriol.* **50:**1247–1251.
20. **Coyle, M. B., D. J. Nowowiejski, J. Q. Russell, and N. B. Groman.** 1993. Laboratory review of reference strains of *Corynebacterium diphtheriae* indicates mistyped *intermedius* strains. *J. Clin. Microbiol.* **31:**3060–3062.
21. **Daneshvar, M. I., D. G. Hollis, R. S. Weyant, J. G. Jordan, J. P. MacGregor, R. E. Morey, A. M. Whitney, D. J. Brenner, A. G. Steigerwalt, L. O. Helsel, P. M. Raney, J. B. Patel, P. N. Levett, and J. M. Brown.** 2004. Identification of some charcoal-black-pigmented CDC fermentative coryneform group 4 isolates as *Rothia dentocariosa* and some as *Corynebacterium aurimucosum*: proposal of *Rothia dentocariosa* emend. Georg and Brown 1967, *Corynebacterium aurimucosum* emend. Yassin et al. 2002, and *Corynebacterium nigricans* Shukla et al. 2003 pro synon. *Corynebacterium aurimucosum*. *J. Clin. Microbiol.* **42:**4189–4198.
22. **de Briel, D., F. Couderc, P. Riegel, F. Jehl, and R. Minck.** 1992. High-performance liquid chromatography of corynomycolic acids as a tool in identification of *Corynebacterium* species and related organisms. *J. Clin. Microbiol.* **30:** 1407–1417.
23. **de Mattos-Guaraldi, A. L., and L. C. Formiga.** 1998. Bacteriological properties of a sucrose-fermenting *Corynebacterium diphtheriae* strain isolated from a case of endocarditis. *Curr. Microbiol.* **37:**156–158.
24. **Devriese, L. A., P. Riegel, J. Hommez, M. Vaneechoutte, T. de Baere, and F. Haesebrouck.** 2000. Identification of *Corynebacterium glucuronolyticum* strains from the urogenital tract of humans and pigs. *J. Clin. Microbiol.* **38:**4657–4659.
25. **DeWinter, L. M., K. A. Bernard, and M. G. Romney.** 2005. Human clinical isolates of *Corynebacterium diphtheriae* and *Corynebacterium ulcerans* collected in Canada from 1999 to 2003 but not fitting reporting criteria for cases of diphtheria. *J. Clin. Microbiol.* **43:**3447–3449.
26. **De Zoysa, A., and A. Efstratiou.** 2000. Use of amplified fragment length polymorphisms for typing *Corynebacterium diphtheriae*. *J. Clin. Microbiol.* **38:**3843–3845.
27. **De Zoysa, A. S., and A. Efstratiou.** 1999. PCR typing of *Corynebacterium diphtheriae* by random amplification of polymorphic DNA. *J. Med. Microbiol.* **48:**335–340.
28. **De Zoysa, A., A. Efstratiou, and P. M. Hawkey.** 2005. Molecular characterization of diphtheria toxin repressor (*dtxR*) genes present in nontoxigenic *Corynebacterium diphtheriae* strains isolated in the United Kingdom. *J. Clin. Microbiol.* **43:**223–228.
29. **Efstratiou, A., K. H. Engler, I. K. Mazurova, T. Glushkevich, J. Vuopio-Varkila, and T. Popovic.** 2000. Current approaches to the laboratory diagnosis of diphtheria. *J. Infect. Dis.* **181**(Suppl. 1):S138–S145.
30. **Efstratiou, A., and R. C. George.** 1999. Laboratory guidelines for the diagnosis of infections caused by *Corynebacterium diphtheriae* and *C. ulcerans*. World Health Organization. *Commun. Dis. Public Health* **2:**250–257.
31. **Elsayed, S., and K. Zhang.** 2005. Bacteremia caused by *Janibacter melonis*. *J. Clin. Microbiol.* **43:**3537–3539.
32. **Engler, K. H., T. Glushkevich, I. K. Mazurova, R. C. George, and A. Efstratiou.** 1997. A modified Elek test for detection of toxigenic corynebacteria in the diagnostic laboratory. *J. Clin. Microbiol.* **35:**495–498.
33. **Engler, K. H., and A. Efstratiou.** 2000. Rapid enzyme immunoassay for determination of toxigenicity among clinical isolates of corynebacteria. *J. Clin. Microbiol.* **38:** 1385–1389.
34. **Evtushenko, L. I., L. V. Dorofeeva, S. A. Subbotin, J. R. Cole, and J. M. Tiedje.** 2000. *Leifsonia poae* gen. nov., sp. nov., isolated from nematode gall on *Poa annua*, and reclassification of '*Corynebacterium aquaticum*' Leifson 1962 as *Leifsonia aquatica* (ex Leifson 1962) gen. nov., nom. rev., comb. nov. and *Clavibacter xyli* Davis et al. 1984 with two subspecies as *Leifsonia xyli* (Davis et al. 1984) gen. nov., comb. nov. *Int. J. Syst. Evol. Microbiol.* **50:**371–380.
35. **Feurer, C., D. Clermont, F. Bimet, A. Candrea, M. Jackson, P. Glaser, C. Bizet, and C. Dauda.** 2004. Taxonomic characterization of nine strains isolated from clinical and environmental specimens, and proposal of *Corynebacterium tuberculostearicum* sp. nov. *Int. J. Syst. Evol. Microbiol.* **54:**1055–1061.
36. **Früh, M., A. von Graevenitz, and G. Funke.** 1998. Use of second-line biochemical and susceptibility tests for the differential diagnosis of coryneform bacteria. *Clin. Microbiol. Infect.* **4:**332–338.
37. **Funke, G., M. Altwegg, L. Frommelt, and A. von Graevenitz.** 1999. Emergence of related nontoxigenic *C. diphtheriae* biotype *mitis* strains in Western Europe. *Emerg. Infect. Dis.* **5:**477–480.
38. **Funke, G., M. Aravena-Roman, and R. Frodl.** 2005. First description of *Curtobacterium* spp. isolated from human clinical specimens. *J. Clin. Microbiol.* **43:**1032–1036.
39. **Funke, G., K. A. Bernard, C. Bucher, G. E. Pfyffer, and M. D. Collins.** 1995. *Corynebacterium glucuronolyticum* sp. nov. isolated from male patients with genitourinary infections. *Med. Microbiol. Lett.* **4:**204–215.
40. **Funke, G., and A. Carlotti.** 1994. Differentiation of *Brevibacterium* spp. encountered in clinical specimens. *J. Clin. Microbiol.* **32:**1729–1732.
41. **Funke, G., A. Efstratiou, D. Kuklinska, R. A. Hutson, A. de Zoysa, K. H. Engler, and M. D. Collins.** 1997. *Corynebacterium imitans* sp. nov. isolated from patients with suspected diphtheria. *J. Clin. Microbiol.* **35:**1978–1983.
42. **Funke, G., E. Falsen, and C. Barreau.** 1995. Primary identification of *Microbacterium* spp. encountered in clinical specimens as CDC coryneform group A-4 and A-5 bacteria. *J. Clin. Microbiol.* **33:**188–192.
43. **Funke, G., R. Frei, and R. Frodl.** Comprehensive study of *Corynebacterium freneyi* and emended description of *Corynebacterium freneyi* Renaud, Aubel, Riegel, Meugnier, and Bollet (2001). Submitted for publication.
44. **Funke, G., R. A. Hutson, K. A. Bernard, G. E. Pfyffer, G. Wauters, and M. D. Collins.** 1996. Isolation of *Arthrobacter* spp. from clinical specimen and description of *Arthrobacter cumminsii* sp. nov. and *Arthrobacter woluwensis* sp. nov. *J. Clin. Microbiol.* **34:**2356–2363.
45. **Funke, G., R. A. Hutson, M. Hilleringmann, W. R. Heizmann, and M. D. Collins.** 1997. *Corynebacterium lipophiloflavum* sp. nov. isolated from a patient with bacterial vaginosis. *FEMS Microbiol. Lett.* **150:**219–224.
46. **Funke, G., P. A. Lawson, K. A. Bernard, and M. D. Collins.** 1996. Most *Corynebacterium xerosis* strains identified in the routine clinical laboratory correspond to *Corynebacterium amycolatum*. *J. Clin. Microbiol.* **34:**1124–1128.
47. **Funke, G., P. A. Lawson, and M. D. Collins.** 1995. Heterogeneity within Centers for Disease Control and Prevention coryneform group ANF-1-like bacteria and description of *Corynebacterium auris* sp. nov. *Int. J. Syst. Bacteriol.* **45:**735–739.
48. **Funke, G., P. A. Lawson, and M. D. Collins.** 1997. *Corynebacterium mucifaciens* sp. nov., an unusual species from human clinical material. *Int. J. Syst. Bacteriol.* **47:**952–957.
49. **Funke, G., P. A. Lawson, and M. D. Collins.** 1998. *Corynebacterium riegelii* sp. nov., an unusual species isolated from female patients with urinary tract infections. *J. Clin. Microbiol.* **36:**624–627.

50. **Funke, G., P. A. Lawson, F. S. Nolte, N. Weiss, and M. D. Collins.** 1998. *Aureobacterium resistens* sp. nov. exhibiting vancomycin resistance and teicoplanin susceptibility. *FEMS Microbiol. Lett.* **158:**89–93.
51. **Funke, G., and C. Nietznik.** 2005. Minimal inhibitory concentrations of linezolid against clinical isolates of coryneform bacteria. *Eur. J. Clin. Microbiol. Infect. Dis.* **24:**612–614.
52. **Funke, G., C. R. Osorio, R. Frei, P. Riegel, and M. D. Collins.** 1998. *Corynebacterium confusum* sp. nov., isolated from human clinical specimens. *Int. J. Syst. Bacteriol.* **48:**1291–1296.
53. **Funke, G., M. Pagano-Niederer, and W. Bernauer.** 1998. *Corynebacterium macginleyi* has to date been isolated exclusively from conjunctival swabs. *J. Clin. Microbiol.* **36:**3670–3673.
54. **Funke, G., M. Pagano-Niederer, B. Sjöden, and E. Falsen.** 1998. Characteristics of *Arthrobacter cumminsii*, the most frequently encountered *Arthrobacter* species in human clinical specimens. *J. Clin. Microbiol.* **36:**1539–1543.
55. **Funke, G., C. Pascual Ramos, and M. D. Collins.** 1995. Identification of some clinical strains of CDC coryneform group A-3 and group A-4 bacteria as *Cellulomonas* species and proposal of *Cellulomonas hominis* sp. nov. for some group A-3 strains. *J. Clin. Microbiol.* **33:**2091–2097.
56. **Funke, G., C. Pascual Ramos, and M. D. Collins.** 1997. *Corynebacterium coyleae* sp. nov., isolated from human clinical specimens. *Int. J. Syst. Bacteriol.* **47:**92–96.
57. **Funke, G., C. Pascual Ramos, J. Fernandez-Garayzabal, N. Weiss, and M. D. Collins.** 1995. Description of human-derived Centers for Disease Control coryneform group 2 bacteria as *Actinomyces bernardiae* sp. nov. *Int. J. Syst. Bacteriol.* **45:**57–60.
58. **Funke, G., K. Peters, and M. Aravena-Roman.** 1998. Evaluation of the RapID CB Plus system for identification of coryneform bacteria and *Listeria* spp. *J. Clin. Microbiol.* **36:**2439–2442.
59. **Funke, G., V. Pünter, and A. von Graevenitz.** 1996. Antimicrobial susceptibility patterns of some recently established coryneform bacteria. *Antimicrob. Agents Chemother.* **40:**2874–2878.
60. **Funke, G., F. N. R. Renaud, J. Freney, and P. Riegel.** 1997. Multicenter evaluation of the updated and extended API (RAPID) Coryne database 2.0. *J. Clin. Microbiol.* **35:**3122–3126.
61. **Funke, G., S. Stubbs, G. E. Pfyffer, M. Marchiani, and M. D. Collins.** 1994. Characteristics of CDC group 3 and group 5 coryneform bacteria isolated from clinical specimens and assignment to the genus *Dermabacter*. *J. Clin. Microbiol.* **32:**1223–1228.
62. **Funke, G., S. Stubbs, G. E. Pfyffer, M. Marchiani, and M. D. Collins.** 1994. *Turicella otitidis* gen. nov., sp. nov., a coryneform bacterium isolated from patients with otitis media. *Int. J. Syst. Bacteriol.* **44:**270–273.
63. **Funke, G., and R. Troxler.** 2005. In vitro activity of quinupristin and dalfopristin in combination and alone against coryneform bacteria. *Eur. J. Clin. Microbiol. Infect. Dis.* **24:**769–771.
64. **Funke, G., A. von Graevenitz, J. E. Clarridge III, and K. A. Bernard.** 1997. Clinical microbiology of coryneform bacteria. *Clin. Microbiol. Rev.* **10:**125–159.
65. **Funke, G., A. von Graevenitz, and N. Weiss.** 1994. Primary identification of *Aureobacterium* spp. isolated from clinical specimens as "*Corynebacterium aquaticum*." *J. Clin. Microbiol.* **32:**2686–2691.
66. **Gneiding, K., R. Frodl, and G. Funke.** Distribution of *Microbacterium* species encountered in clinical specimens. Submitted for publication.
67. **Grimont, P. A. D., F. Grimont, A. Efstratiou, A. De Zoysa, I. Mazurova, C. Ruckly, M. Lejay-Collin, S. Martin-Delautre, B. Regnault, and the European Laboratory Working Group on Diphtheria.** 2004. International nomenclature for *Corynebacterium diphtheriae* ribotypes. *Res. Microbiol.* **155:**162–166.
68. **Groth, I., P. Schumann, B. Schütze, K. Augsten, and E. Stackebrandt.** 2002. *Knoellia sinensis* gen. nov., sp. nov. and *Knoellia subterranea* sp. nov., two novel actinobacteria isolated from a cave. *Int. J. Syst. Evol. Microbiol.* **52:**77–84.
69. **Hall, V., M. D. Collins, R. A. Hutson, P. A. Lawson, E. Falsen, and B. I. Duerden.** 2003. *Corynebacterium atypicum* sp. nov., from a human clinical source, does not contain corynomycolic acids. *Int. J. Syst. Evol. Microbiol.* **53:**1065–1068.
70. **Hauser, D., M. R. Popoff, M. Kiredjian, P. Boquet, and F. Bimet.** 1993. Polymerase chain assay for diagnosis of potentially toxigenic *Corynebacterium diphtheriae* strains: correlation with ADP-ribosylation activity assay. *J. Clin. Microbiol.* **31:**2720–2723.
71. **Hollis, D. G., and R. E. Weaver.** 1981. *Gram-Positive Organisms: a Guide to Identification*. Special Bacteriology Section, Centers for Disease Control, Atlanta, Ga.
72. **Holmes, R. K.** 2000. Biology and molecular epidemiology of diphtheria toxin and the *tox* gene. *J. Infect. Dis.* **181**(Suppl. 1)**:**S156–S167.
73. **Holzmann, D., G. Funke, T. Linder, and D. Nadal.** 2002. *Turicella otitidis* and *Corynebacterium auris* do not cause otitis media with effusion in children. *Pediatr. Infect. Dis.* **21:**1124–1126.
74. **Hommez, J., L. A. Devriese, M. Vaneechoutte, P. Riegel, P. Butaye, and F. Haesebrouck.** 1999. Identification of nonlipophilic corynebacteria isolated from dairy cows with mastitis. *J. Clin. Microbiol.* **37:**954–957.
75. **Huang, Y., N. Zhao, L. He, L. Wang, Z. Liu, M. You, and F. Guan.** 2005. *Arthrobacter scleromae* sp. nov. isolated from human clinical specimens. *J. Clin. Microbiol.* **43:**1451–1455.
76. **Jones, D., and M. D. Collins.** 1988. Taxonomic studies on some human cutaneous coryneform bacteria: description of *Dermabacter hominis* gen. nov. sp. nov. *FEMS Microbiol. Lett.* **123:**167–172.
77. **Khamis, A., D. Raoult, and B. La Scola.** 2004. *rpoB* gene sequencing for identification of *Corynebacterium* species. *J. Clin. Microbiol.* **42:**3925–3931.
78. **Khamis, A., D. Raoult, and B. La Scola.** 2005. Comparison between *rpoB* and 16S rRNA gene sequencing for molecular identification of 168 clinical isolates of *Corynebacterium*. *J. Clin. Microbiol.* **43:**1934–1936.
79. **Koch, C., F. A. Rainey, and E. Stackebrandt.** 1994. 16S rDNA studies on members of *Arthrobacter* and *Micrococcus*: an aid for their future taxonomic restructuring. *FEMS Microbiol. Lett.* **123:**167–172.
80. **Komiya, T., N. Shibata, M. Ito, M. Takahashi, and Y. Arakawa.** 2000. Retrospective diagnosis of diphtheria by detection of *Corynebacterium diphtheriae tox* gene in a formaldehyde-fixed throat swab using PCR and sequencing analysis. *J. Clin. Microbiol.* **38:**2400–2402.
81. **Kronvall, G., M. Lanner-Sjöberg, L. V. von Stedingk, H.-S. Hanson, B. Pettersson, and E. Falsen.** 1998. Whole cell protein and partial 16S rRNA gene sequence analysis suggest the existence of a second *Rothia* species. *Clin. Microbiol. Infect.* **4:**255–263.
82. **Laffineur, K., V. Avesani, G. Cornu, J. Charlier, M. Janssens, G. Wauters, and M. Delmée.** 2003. Bacteremia due to a novel *Microbacterium* species in a patient with leukemia and description of *Microbacterium paraoxydans* sp. nov. *J. Clin. Microbiol.* **41:**2242–2246.
83. **Lagrou, K., J. Verhaegen, M. Janssens, G. Wauters, and L. Verbist.** 1998. Prospective study of catalase-positive coryneform organisms in clinical specimens: identification,

clinical relevance, and antibiotic susceptibility. *Diagn. Microbiol. Infect. Dis.* **30:**7–15.

84. **Lartigue, M.-F., X. Monnet, A. Le Fléche, P. A. D. Grimont, J.-J. Benet, A. Durrbach, M. Fabre, and P. Nordmann.** 2005. *Corynebacterium ulcerans* in an immunocompromised patient with diphtheria and her dog. *J. Clin. Microbiol.* **43:**999–1001.

85. **Lau, S. K. P., P. C. Y. Woo, G. K. S. Woo, and K.-Y. Yuen.** 2002. Catheter-related *Microbacterium* bacteremia identified by 16S rRNA gene sequencing. *J. Clin. Microbiol.* **40:**2681–2685.

86. **Leonard, R. B., D. J. Nowowiejski, J. J. Warren, D. J. Finn, and M. B. Coyle.** 1994. Molecular evidence of person-to-person transmission of a pigmented strain of *Corynebacterium striatum* in intensive care units. *J. Clin. Microbiol.* **32:**164–169.

87. **Lin, Y. C., K. Uemori, D. A. de Briel, V. Arunpairojana, and A. Yokota.** 2004. *Zimmermannella helvola* gen. nov., sp. nov., *Zimmermannella alba* sp. nov., *Zimmermannella bifida* sp. nov., *Zimmermannella faecalis* sp. nov. and *Leucobacter albus* sp. nov., novel members of the family *Microbacteriaceae*. *Int. J. Syst. Evol. Microbiol.* **54:**1669–1676.

88. **Loubinoux, J., B. Rio, L. Mihaila, E. Foïs, A. Le Fleche, P. A. D. Grimont, J.-P. Marie, and A. Bouvet.** 2005. Bacteremia caused by an undescribed species of *Janibacter*. *J. Clin. Microbiol.* **43:**3564–3566.

89. **Mackenzie, A., L. A. Fuite, F. T. H. Chan, J. King, U. Allen, N. MacDonald, and F. Diaz-Mitoma.** 1995. Incidence and pathogenicity of *Arcanobacterium haemolyticum* during a 2-year study in Ottawa. *Clin. Infect. Dis.* **21:**177–181.

90. **Manaia, C. M., B. Nogales, N. Weiss, and O. C. Nunes.** 2004. *Gulosibacter molinativorax* gen. nov., sp. nov., a molinate-degrading bacterium, and classification of '*Brevibacterium helvolum*' DSM 20419 as *Pseudoclavibacter helvolus* gen. nov., sp. nov. *Int. J. Syst. Evol. Microbiol.* **54:**783–789.

91. **Martin, K., P. Schumann, F. A. Rainey, B. Schuetze, and I. Groth.** 1997. *Janibacter limosus* gen. nov., sp. nov., a new actinomycete with *meso*-diaminopimelic acid in the cell wall. *Int. J. Syst. Bacteriol.* **47:**529–534.

92. **Martinez-Martinez, L., M. C. Ortega, and A. I. Suarez.** 1995. Comparison of E-test with broth microdilution and disk diffusion for susceptibility testing of coryneform bacteria. *J. Clin. Microbiol.* **33:**1318–1321.

93. **McNeil, M. M., J. M. Brown, M. E. Carvalho, D. G. Hollis, R. E. Morey, and L. B. Reller.** 2004. Molecular epidemiologic evaluation of endocarditis due to *Oerskovia turbata* and CDC group A-3 associated with contaminated homograft valves. *J. Clin. Microbiol.* **42:**2495–2500.

94. **Miyake, T., K. Watanabe, T. Watanabe, and H. Oyaizu.** 1998. Phylogenetic analysis of the genus *Bifidobacterium* and related genera based on 16S rDNA sequences. *Microbiol. Immunol.* **42:**661–667.

95. **Mokrousov, I., O. Narvskaya, E. Limeschenko, and A. Vyazovaya.** 2005. Efficient discrimination within a *Corynebacterium diphtheriae* epidemic clonal group by a novel macroarray-based method. *J. Clin. Microbiol.* **43:** 1662–1668.

96. **Mothershed, E. A., P. K. Cassiday, K. Pierson, L. W. Mayer, and T. Popovic.** 2002. Development of a real-time fluorescence PCR assay for rapid detection of the diphtheria toxin gene. *J. Clin. Microbiol.* **40:**4713–4719.

97. **Nakao, H., I. K. Mazurova, T. Glushkevich, and T. Popovic.** 1997. Analysis of heterogeneity of *Corynebacterium diphtheriae* toxin gene, *tox*, and its regulatory element, *dtxR*, by direct sequencing. *Res. Microbiol.* **148:**45–54.

98. **Nakao, H., and T. Popovic.** 1997. Development of a direct PCR assay for detection of the diphtheria toxin gene. *J. Clin. Microbiol.* **35:**1651–1655.

99. **Nakao, H., and T. Popovic.** 1998. Development of a rapid ribotyping method for *Corynebacterium diphtheriae* by using PCR single-strand conformation polymorphism: comparison with standard ribotyping. *J. Microbiol. Methods* **31:**127–134.

100. **Nath, K., J. W. Sarosy, and S. P. Stylianou.** 2000. Suitability of a unique 16S rRNA gene PCR product as an indicator of *Gardnerella vaginalis*. *BioTechniques* **28:** 222–226.

101. **Neubauer, M., J. Sourek, M. Ryc, J. Bohacek, M. Mara, and J. Mnukova.** 1991. *Corynebacterium accolens* sp. nov., a gram-positive rod exhibiting satellitism, from clinical material. *Syst. Appl. Microbiol.* **14:**46–51.

102. **Nugent, R. P., M. A. Krohn, and S. L. Hillier.** 1991. Reliability of diagnosing bacterial vaginosis is improved by a standardized method of Gram stain interpretation. *J. Clin. Microbiol.* **29:**297–301.

103. **Otsuka, Y., Y. Kawamura, T. Koyama, H. Iihara, K. Ohkusu, and T. Ezaki.** 2005. *Corynebacterium resistens* sp. nov., a new multidrug-resistant coryneform bacterium isolated from human infection. *J. Clin. Microbiol.* **43:** 3713–3717.

104. **Pascual, C., P. A. Lawson, J. A. E. Farrow, M. Navarro Gimenez, and M. D. Collins.** 1995. Phylogenetic analysis of the genus *Corynebacterium* based on 16S rRNA gene sequences. *Int. J. Syst. Bacteriol.* **45:**724–728.

105. **Pascual Ramos, C., G. Foster, and M. D. Collins.** 1997. Phylogenetic analysis of the genus *Actinomyces* based on 16S rRNA gene sequences: description of *Arcanobacterium phocae* sp. nov., *Arcanobacterium bernardiae* comb. nov., and *Arcanobacterium pyogenes* comb. nov. *Int. J. Syst. Bacteriol.* **47:**46–53.

106. **Paviour, S., S. Musaad, S. Roberts, G. Taylor, S. Taylor, K. Shore, S. Lang, and D. Holland.** 2002. *Corynebacterium* species isolated from patients with mastitis. *Clin. Infect. Dis.* **35:**1434–1440.

107. **Piot, P., E. van Dyck, M. Peeters, J. Hale, P. A. Totten, and K. K. Holmes.** 1984. Biotypes of *Gardnerella vaginalis*. *J. Clin. Microbiol.* **20:**677–679.

108. **Popovic, T., I. K. Mazurova, A. Efstratiou, J. Vuopio-Varkila, M. W. Reeves, A. de Zoysa, T. Glushkevich, and P. Grimont.** 2000. Molecular epidemiology of diphtheria. *J. Infect. Dis.* **181**(Suppl. 1)**:**S168–S177.

109. **Rainey, F., N. Weiss, H. Prauser, and E. Stackebrandt.** 1994. Further evidence for the phylogenetic coherence of actinomycetes with group B-peptidoglycan and evidence for the phylogenetic intermixing of the genera *Microbacterium* and *Aureobacterium* as determined by 16S rDNA analysis. *FEMS Microbiol. Lett.* **118:** 135–140.

110. **Rassoulian Barrett, S. L., B. T. Cookson, L. C. Carlson, K. A. Bernard, and M. B. Coyle.** 2001. Diversity within reference strains of *Corynebacterium matruchotii* includes *Corynebacterium durum* and a novel organism. *J. Clin. Microbiol.* **39:**943–948.

111. **Reacher, M., M. Ramsay, J. White, A. De Zoysa, A. Efstratiou, G. Mann, A. Mackay, and R. C. George.** 2000. Nontoxigenic *Corynebacterium diphtheriae:* an emerging pathogen in England and Wales? *Emerg. Infect. Dis.* **6:**640–645.

112. **Reinhardt, D. J., A. Lee, and T. Popovic.** 1998. Antitoxin-in-membrane and antitoxin-in-well assays for detection of toxigenic *Corynebacterium diphtheriae*. *J. Clin. Microbiol.* **36:**207–210.

113. **Renaud, F. N. R., D. Aubel, P. Riegel, H. Meugnier, and C. Bollet.** 2001. *Corynebacterium freneyi* sp. nov., alpha-glucosidase-positive strains related to *Corynebacterium xerosis*. *Int. J. Syst. Evol. Microbiol.* **51:**1723–1728.

114. **Riegel, P., R. Creti, R. Mattei, A. Nieri, and C. von Hunolstein.** 2006. Isolation of *Corynebacterium tuscaniae*

sp. nov. from blood cultures of a patient with endocarditis. *J. Clin. Microbiol.* **44:**307–312.

115. **Riegel, P., D. de Briel, G. Prevost, F. Jehl, and H. Monteil.** 1994. Genomic diversity among *Corynebacterium jeikeium* strains and comparison with biochemical characteristics. *J. Clin. Microbiol.* **32:**1860–1865.
116. **Riegel, P., D. de Briel, G. Prevost, F. Jehl, H. Monteil, and R. Minck.** 1993. Taxonomic study of *Corynebacterium* group ANF-1 strains: proposal of *Corynebacterium afermentans* sp. nov. containing the subspecies *C. afermentans* subsp. *afermentans* subsp. nov. and *C. afermentans* subsp. *lipophilum* subsp. nov. *Int. J. Syst. Bacteriol.* **43:**287–292.
117. **Riegel, P., R. Heller, G. Prevost, F. Jehl, and H. Monteil.** 1997. *Corynebacterium durum* sp. nov., from human clinical specimens. *Int. J. Syst. Bacteriol.* **47:**1107–1111.
118. **Riegel, P., R. Ruimy, D. de Briel, G. Prevost, F. Jehl, F. Bimet, R. Christen, and H. Monteil.** 1995. *Corynebacterium argentoratense* sp. nov., from human throat. *Int. J. Syst. Bacteriol.* **45:**533–537.
119. **Riegel, P., R. Ruimy, D. de Briel, G. Prevost, F. Jehl, R. Christen, and H. Monteil.** 1995. Genomic diversity and phylogenetic relationships among lipid-requiring diphtheroids from humans and characterization of *Corynebacterium macginleyi* sp. nov. *Int. J. Syst. Bacteriol.* **45:** 128–133.
120. **Riegel, P., R. Ruimy, D. de Briel, G. Prevost, F. Jehl, R. Christen, and H. Monteil.** 1995. Taxonomy of *Corynebacterium diphtheriae* and related taxa, with recognition of *Corynebacterium ulcerans* sp. nov., nom. rev. *FEMS Microbiol. Lett.* **126:**271–276.
121. **Riegel, P., R. Ruimy, F. N. R. Renaud, J. Freney, G. Prevost, F. Jehl, R. Christen, and H. Monteil.** 1997. *Corynebacterium singulare* sp. nov., a new species for urease-positive strains related to *Corynebacterium minutissimum*. *Int. J. Syst. Bacteriol.* **47:**1092–1096.
122. **Roux, V., M. Drancourt, A. Stein, P. Riegel, D. Raoult, and B. La Scola.** 2004. *Corynebacterium* species isolated from bone and joint infections identified by 16S rRNA gene sequence analysis. *J. Clin. Microbiol.* **42:** 2231–2233.
123. **Ruimy, R., P. Riegel, P. Boiron, H. Monteil, and R. Christen.** 1995. Phylogeny of the genus *Corynebacterium* deduced from analyses of small-subunit ribosomal DNA sequences. *Int. J. Syst. Bacteriol.* **45:**740–746.
124. **Sadhu, K., P. A. G. Domingue, A. W. Chow, J. Nelligan, N. Cheng, and J. W. Costerton.** 1989. *Gardnerella vaginalis* has a gram-positive cell-wall ultrastructure and lacks classical cell-wall lipopolysaccharide. *J. Med. Microbiol.* **29:**229–235.
125. **Schumann, P., N. Weiss, and E. Stackebrandt.** 2001. Reclassification of *Cellulomonas cellulans* (Stackebrandt and Keddie 1986) as *Cellulosimicrobium cellulans* gen. nov., comb. nov. *Int. J. Syst. Evol. Microbiol.* **51:**1007–1010.
126. **Shukla, S. K., K. A. Bernard, M. Harney, D. A. Frank, and K. D. Reed.** 2003. *Corynebacterium nigricans* sp. nov.: proposed name for a black-pigmented *Corynebacterium* species recovered from the human female urogenital tract. *J. Clin. Microbiol.* **31:**4353–4358.
127. **Shukla, S. K., M. Harney, B. Jhaveri, K. Andrews, and K. D. Reed.** 2003. Is a black-pigmented *Corynebacterium* species an opportunistic pathogen during pregnancy? Literature review and report of 3 new cases. *Clin. Infect. Dis.* **37:**834–837.
128. **Sing, A., M. Hogardt, S. Bierschenk, and J. Heesemann.** 2003. Detection of differences in the nucleotide and amino acid sequences of diphtheria toxin from *Corynebacterium diphtheriae* and *Corynebacterium ulcerans* causing extrapharyngeal infections. *J. Clin. Microbiol.* **41:** 4848–4851.
129. **Sjöden, B., G. Funke, A. Izquierdo, E. Akervall, and M. D. Collins.** 1998. Description of some coryneform bacteria isolated from human clinical specimens as *Corynebacterium falsenii* sp. nov. *Int. J. Syst. Bacteriol.* **48:**69–74.
130. **Soriano, F., J. M. Aguado, C. Ponte, R. Fernandez-Roblas, and J. L. Rodriguez-Tudela.** 1990. Urinary tract infection caused by *Corynebacterium* group D2: report of 82 cases and review. *Rev. Infect. Dis.* **12:**1019–1034.
131. **Spiegel, C. A.** 1991. Bacterial vaginosis. *Clin. Microbiol. Rev.* **4:**485–502.
132. **Spiegel, C. A.** 1999. Bacterial vaginosis: changes in laboratory practice. *Clin. Microbiol. Newsl.* **21:**33–37.
133. **Stackebrandt, E., S. Breymann, U. Steiner, H. Prauser, N. Weiß, and P. Schumann.** 2002. Re-evaluation of the status of the genus *Oerskovia*, reclassification of *Promicromonospora enterophila* (Jager et al. 1983) as *Oerskovia enterophila* comb. nov. and description of *Oerskovia jenensis* sp. nov. and *Oerskovia paurometabola* sp. nov. *Int. J. Syst. Evol. Microbiol.* **52:**1105–1111.
134. **Stackebrandt, E., F. Rainey, and N. L. Ward-Rainey.** 1997. Proposal for a new hierarchic classification system, *Actinobacteria* classis nov. *Int. J. Syst. Bacteriol.* **47:**479–491.
135. **Takeuchi, M., and K. Hatano.** 1998. Union of the genera *Microbacterium* Orla-Jensen and *Aureobacterium* Collins et al. in a redefined genus *Microbacterium*. *Int. J. Syst. Bacteriol.* **48:**739–747.
136. **Tang, Y.-W., A. von Graevenitz, M. G. Waddington, M. K. Hopkins, D. H. Smith, H. Li, C. P. Kolbert, S. O. Montgomery, and D. H. Persing.** 2000. Identification of coryneform bacterial isolates by ribosomal DNA sequence analysis. *J. Clin. Microbiol.* **38:**1676–1678.
137. **Tanner, M. A., D. Shoskes, A. Shahed, and N. R. Pace.** 1999. Prevalence of corynebacterial 16S rRNA sequences in patients with bacterial and "nonbacterial" prostatitis. *J. Clin. Microbiol.* **37:**1863–1870.
138. **Tauch, A., O. Kaiser, T. Hain, A. Goesmann, B. Weisshaar, A. Albersmeier, T. Bekel, N. Bischoff, I. Brune, T. Chakraborty, J. Kalinowski, F. Meyer, O. Rupp, S. Schneiker, P. Viehoever, and A. Pühler.** 2005. Complete genome sequence and analysis of the multiresistant nosocomial pathogen *Corynebacterium jeikeium* K411, a lipid-requiring bacterium of the human skin flora. *J. Bacteriol.* **187:**4671–4682.
139. **Troxler, R., G. Funke, A. von Graevenitz, and I. Stock.** 2001. Natural antibiotic susceptibility of recently established coryneform bacteria. *Eur. J. Clin. Microbiol. Infect. Dis.* **20:**315–323.
140. **Vaneechoutte, M., P. Riegel, D. de Briel, H. Monteil, G. Verschraegen, A. De Rouck, and G. Claeys.** 1995. Evaluation of the applicability of amplified rDNA-restriction analysis (ARDRA) to identification of species of the genus *Corynebacterium*. *Res. Microbiol.* **146:**633–641.
141. **van Esbroeck, M., P. Vandamme, E. Falsen, M. Vancanneyt, E. Moore, B. Pot, F. Gavini, K. Kersters, and H. Goossens.** 1996. Polyphasic approach to the classification and identification of *Gardnerella vaginalis* and unidentified *Gardnerella vaginalis*-like coryneforms present in bacterial vaginosis. *Int. J. Syst. Bacteriol.* **46:**675–682.
142. **von Graevenitz, A.** 2004. *Rothia dentocariosa:* taxonomy and differential diagnosis. *Clin. Microbiol. Infect.* **10:** 399–402.
143. **von Graevenitz, A., and G. Funke.** 1996. An identification scheme for rapidly and aerobically growing gram-positive rods. *Zentbl. Bakteriol. Parasitenkd. Infektkrankh. Hyg. Abt. 1 Orig.* **284:**246–254.
144. **von Graevenitz, A., V. Pünter-Streit, P. Riegel, and G. Funke.** 1998. Coryneform bacteria in throat cultures of healthy individuals. *J. Clin. Microbiol.* **36:**2087–2088.
145. **Wattiau, P., M. Janssens, and G. Wauters.** 2000. *Corynebacterium simulans* sp. nov., a non-lipophilic,

fermentative *Corynebacterium*. *Int. J. Syst. Evol. Microbiol.* **50:**347–353.

146. **Wauters, G., V. Avesani, K. Laffineur, J. Charlier, M. Janssens, B. Van Bosterhaut, and M. Delmée.** 2003. *Brevibacterium lutescens* sp. nov., from human and environmental samples. *Int. J. Syst. Evol. Microbiol.* **53:**1321–1325.
147. **Wauters, G., G. Haase, V. Avesani, J. Charlier, M. Janssens, J. Van Broeck, and M. Delmée.** 2004. Identification of a novel *Brevibacterium* species isolated from humans and description of *Brevibacterium sanguinis* sp. nov. *J. Clin. Microbiol.* **42:**2829–2832.
148. **Wauters, G., B. van Bosterhaut, M. Janssens, and J. Verhaegen.** 1998. Identification of *Corynebacterium amycolatum* and other nonlipophilic fermentative corynebacteria of human origin. *J. Clin. Microbiol.* **36:**1430–1432.
149. **Weiss, K., M. Laverdiere, and R. Rivest.** 1996. Comparison of antimicrobial susceptibilities of *Corynebacterium* species by broth microdilution and disk diffusion methods. *Antimicrob. Agents Chemother.* **40:** 930–933.
150. **Yassin, A. F., U. Steiner, and W. Ludwig.** 2002. *Corynebacterium aurimucosum* sp. nov. and emended description of *Corynebacterium minutissimum* Collins and Jones (1983). *Int. J. Syst. Evol. Microbiol.* **52:**1001–1005.
151. **Yassin, A. F., U. Steiner, and W. Ludwig.** 2002. *Corynebacterium appendicis* sp. nov. *Int. J. Syst. Evol. Microbiol.* **52:**1165–1169.
152. **Zapardiel, J., E. Nieto, M. I. Gegundez, I. Gadea, and F. Soriano.** 1994. Problems in minimum inhibitory concentration determinations in coryneform organisms—comparison of an agar dilution and the Etest. *Diagn. Microbiol. Infect. Dis.* **19:**171–173.
153. **Zimmermann, O., C. Spröer, R. M. Kroppenstedt, E. Fuchs, H. G. Köchel, and G. Funke.** 1998. *Corynebacterium thomssenii* sp. nov., a *Corynebacterium* with *N*-acetyl-β-glucosaminidase activity from human-clinical specimens. *Int. J. Syst. Bacteriol.* **48:**489–494.
154. **Zinkernagel, A. S., A. von Graevenitz, and G. Funke.** 1996. Heterogeneity within *Corynebacterium minutissimum* strains is explained by misidentified *Corynebacterium amycolatum* strains. *Am. J. Clin. Pathol.* **106:**378–383.

Nocardia, Rhodococcus, Gordonia, Actinomadura, Streptomyces, and Other Aerobic Actinomycetes*

PATRICIA S. CONVILLE AND FRANK G. WITEBSKY

35

TAXONOMY

The word "actinomycete" is derived from two Greek roots (actino- and -mycete) meaning "ray" (and hence also "rod") and "fungus," respectively. The anaerobic organisms now in the genus *Actinomyces* and the aerobic organisms grouped together as the "aerobic actinomycetes" were previously presumed to be related to one another on the basis of shared features of organismal and colonial morphology. The aerobic actinomycetes, a group for which no agreed-upon operational definition currently exists, are now known to be an evolutionarily heterogeneous assemblage of genera. At some stage they all form gram-positive rods, and most of the more commonly isolated species exhibit at least rudimentary branching under certain growth conditions; all grow better under aerobic than anaerobic conditions, a feature distinguishing them from organisms in the genus *Actinomyces*. The organisms containing mycolic acids in their cell walls (included in the genera *Dietzia, Gordonia, Nocardia, Rhodococcus,* and *Tsukamurella*) are rather closely related on the basis of molecular genetic studies (51, 221); these mycolic-acid-containing genera appear phylogenetically more closely related to the genera *Corynebacterium* and *Mycobacterium* (both of which are sometimes considered to be aerobic actinomycetes) than to the other non-mycolic-acid-containing genera usually also included with the aerobic actinomycetes. According to a recent classification scheme, the various genera are placed in several different suborders, emphasizing the lack of close evolutionary relationships among some of them (221). Regardless of their actual evolutionary relationships, several genera (such as *Gordonia* and *Rhodococcus*) exhibit similar colonial and microscopic morphologic features.

The number of recognized pathogenic species of aerobic actinomycetes has been rising rapidly. Only genera containing species of clinical significance are dealt with in this chapter; the genus *Tropheryma* is discussed in a separate chapter. Ultimately the increasingly fine discrimination of species may result in delineation of important species-specific differences in geographic distribution, pathogenic and other biological mechanisms, disease associations, and antimicrobial susceptibility patterns. However, the enormous proliferation of distinct species for which association with human disease has been claimed presents several problems for the clinical microbiologist. First, phenotypic testing has been rendered virtually useless for accurate discrimination among species. Particularly for the aerobic actinomycetes, the number of phenotypic tests available in the clinical laboratory (and in most research laboratories) is far too small for differentiation among so many species, and often information on the percent positivity for a specific reaction in a given species is not known. Furthermore, precisely the same biochemical testing format has generally not been employed with isolates of all the species being compared, making the usefulness of multistudy comparisons uncertain. Second, some types of testing, such as analysis of cell wall constituents and of whole-cell sugars, are available in only a few research settings and are rarely of use for species level identification. Some general information regarding these features is provided herein, but the references should be consulted for performance procedures and additional details. Third, only nucleic acid-based techniques are currently adequately discriminatory, reproducible, and sufficiently widely available to be useful for precise species identifications in clinical laboratories. Fourth, because of the growing problems with accurate species determinations, the clinical literature is rife with erroneous identifications; nowhere is this problem more apparent than with organisms in the genus *Nocardia*. Additionally, as some species have been described on the basis of only a single isolate, and for others only a handful of reports exist, little if any meaningful clinical information can be associated with many species names. Particularly when molecular methods are not available, precise identification of isolates may be impossible—and is also frequently not of immediate clinical utility.

There are a few terminological issues that, while they pertain to all bacteria, seem to cause confusion particularly frequently with regard to the aerobic actinomycetes. First, for every bacterial species, there is only one "type strain," the strain on which the original description of the species was based. Other strains that are thought to belong to the same species as a given type strain could be referred to as "reference strains," but they are not type strains. Second, the term "sensu stricto" means "in the strict sense." The term, when used with a species name, should be restricted to mean organisms belonging to that particular species, as determined by the best available methods. So, to refer to isolates

*This chapter contains information presented in chapter 35 by June M. Brown and Michael M. McNeil in the eighth edition of this Manual.

that are "*Nocardia asteroides* sensu stricto" should mean isolates that by molecular methods are identical to the type strain of *N. asteroides* (ATCC 19247^T).

DESCRIPTION OF THE GENERA

Actinomadura

The microscopic and colonial morphology of organisms in the genus *Actinomadura,* which contains approximately 57 validly named species, is very similar to those in the genus *Streptomyces*. Microscopically, they are thin, short, branching gram-positive rods (175) (see Fig. 2A) that are modified acid-fast stain negative. Colonies are wrinkled, some aerial mycelium may be present, and the color of the colonies may vary considerably among different isolates (Fig. 1A). Cell walls contain the sugar madurose, a feature shared only with organisms in the genus *Dermatophilus*.

Amycolata and *Amycolatopsis*

The genera *Amycolata* and *Amycolatopsis* were proposed by Lechevalier et al. for nocardia-like organisms that were gram positive (Fig. 2B) and modified acid-fast negative (152). Aerial hyphae are frequently produced (Fig. 1F). Among the species transferred to the genus *Amycolatopsis* was *Nocardia orientalis,* two isolates of which were reported from clinical specimens (99). A study based on 16S rRNA sequences recommended combining the genera *Amycolata* and *Pseudonocardia* into an emended genus, *Pseudonocardia* (252). Currently there are 4 validly named species in the genus *Amycolata* and 26 validly named species in the genus *Amycolatopsis*.

Dermatophilus

The two species currently making up the genus *Dermatophilus* are probably not closely related to most of the other organisms considered in this chapter; by molecular methods this genus was placed in the suborder *Micrococcineae*, whereas the majority of the aerobic actinomycete human pathogens were placed in the suborder *Corynebacterineae* (221). *Dermatophilus congolensis* colonies are somewhat heaped, are opaque, show β-hemolysis on blood agar, and may develop a yellow to orange color with age (275). Aerial mycelium may be produced if the organism is grown in an atmosphere of increased CO_2; the organisms are facultatively anaerobic (95). The microscopic morphology is unusual and striking; this branching organism, with hyphae 0.6 to 1.0 μm in diameter, develops both longitudinal and transverse septa (Fig. 2D). The resulting chains of coccoid cells may occur in as many as eight parallel rows (275). The organisms are gram positive but modified acid-fast negative. The coccoid cells may develop into motile zoospores under favorable environmental conditions.

Dietzia

The species *Dietzia maris* was removed from the genus *Rhodococcus* because of chemotaxonomic and 16S rRNA sequence differences from *Rhodococcus* species (203). Two additional species have since been included in the genus. These organisms apparently rarely, if ever, branch, but like organisms in the genus *Rhodococcus*, they may show coccal and rod forms and are modified acid-fast positive (89).

Gordonia

The biology of the genus *Gordonia* has been recently reviewed (7). Colonies are typically orange and usually wrinkled (Fig. 1I). On Gram stain, *Gordonia* species appear coryneform and show no significant branching; these organisms could easily be mistaken for a component of normal oral flora in sputum specimens (154) (Fig. 2C). The genus "*Gordona*" (now *Gordonia*), originally described by Tsukamura, was revived in 1988 by Stackebrandt et al. (222) to contain species with mycolic acids of approximately 46 to 66 carbon atoms in length (90) and a predominant menaquinone of nine isoprene units. *Gordonia* and *Rhodococcus* were also found to be separable on the basis of their 16S rRNA sequences. There are approximately 19 validly named species in the genus.

Nocardia

The most commonly isolated aerobic actinomycete human pathogens belong to the genus *Nocardia*. In direct Gram smears, organisms generally appear as very long, obviously branching, thin (0.5 to 1.0 μm in diameter), and finely beaded gram-positive rods (Fig. 2E, F, and N). Unlike the individual cells composing a streptococcal chain, the beads generally do not abut one another. Occasionally, chains, or what appear to be clumps, of beads are the only clue to the presence of a *Nocardia*-like organism (Fig. 2F). Organisms may not be detectable with a Gram stain, and a modified acid-fast stain should be done on direct patient material when a nocardial infection is suspected. While nearly all isolates of *Nocardia* are modified acid-fast positive, not all organisms, or even the entirety of a given organism, will necessarily retain the acid-fast stain (Fig. 2H and O) (see "Microscopic Morphology" below). Particularly when prepared from cultures, smears may show streptococcus-like chains or small branching filaments, probably as a result of the fragile nocardial mycelium breaking during smear preparation (189, 190).

Colonial morphology varies from species to species and frequently varies from isolate to isolate within a species. Colonies can be white, gray, buff, salmon, or orange (Fig. 1D, E, G, and L). Colony color may best be seen on the reverse when colonies are grown on translucent media, as color may become obscured on the surface by powdery aerial hyphae typically produced. Such aerial hyphae are formed to at least some extent by nearly all nocardial isolates, but they are also found with isolates in other aerobic actinomycete genera.

Of the nearly 70 species of *Nocardia* currently recognized, over 25 have been reported as human isolates, and several others have been reported as pathogens of other animals. Importantly, isolates in many reports of infection, even in the recent literature, are incorrectly identified because of failure to use optimal identification methods.

A brief account of the nomenclatural history of the designation "*Nocardia asteroides*" is necessary to clarify a confusing and widely unappreciated taxonomic issue. In 1888 Edmond Nocard obtained an isolate of an organism thought to be the causative agent of bovine farcy; this organism was given the name *Nocardia farcinica* by Trevisan in 1889, and thereupon it became the type strain for both the genus and species. Gordon and Mihm (98) found, using their battery of phenotypic tests, that *N. farcinica* could not be distinguished from isolates to which the name *Nocardia asteroides* had been applied. Because of some uncertainty relating to the isolate obtained by Nocard and what was presumed to be the conspecificity of the organisms then known as *N. farcinica* and *N. asteroides*, an appeal was made to the Judicial Commission to have the type species of the genus changed to *N. asteroides,* with strain ATCC 19247^T selected as the type strain of the species. The appeal was accepted, but the isolate

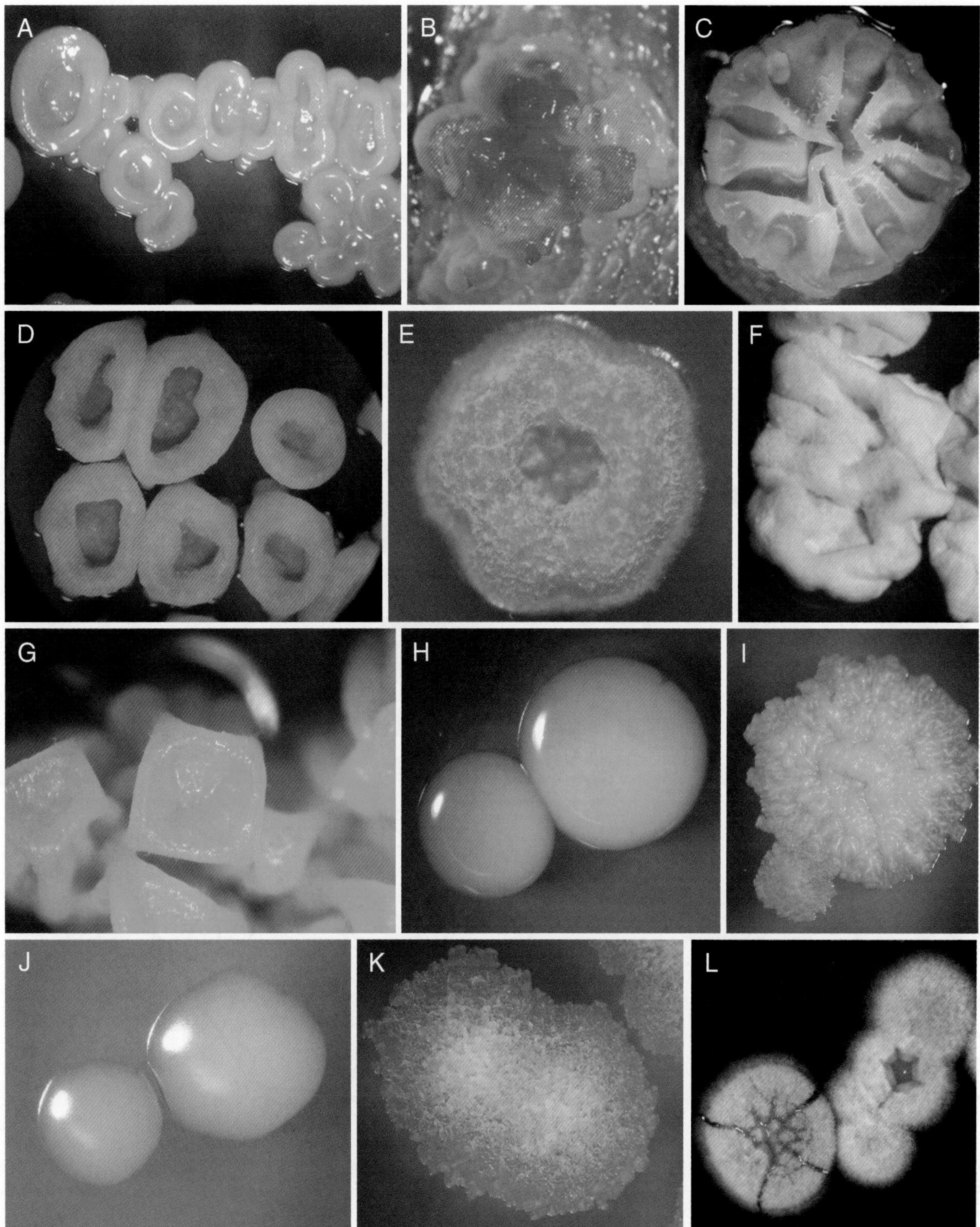

FIGURE 1 Colonial morphology of type strains of various aerobic actinomycetes grown on Sabouraud dextrose agar (Emmons modification). While appearances are typical for the species illustrated, the extent of possible colonial variation within a given species is not known. (A) *Actinomadura latina* at 21 days; smooth umbilicate colonies with no aerial hyphae; (B) *Actinomadura pelletieri* at 10 days; ropy but smooth-surfaced colony with no aerial hyphae; (C) *Streptomyces griseus* at 10 days; rugose colony with some aerial hyphae; (D) *Nocardia brasiliensis* at 10 days; umbilicate colonies; sparse aerial hyphae present, but visible only on microscopic inspection of colonies; (E) *Nocardia carnea* at 25 days; aerial hyphae present; (F) *Amycolatopsis orientalis* at 21 days; aerial hyphae present; (G) *Nocardia otitidiscaviarum* at 7 days; rugose colony; sparse aerial hyphae present, visible only on careful microscopic inspection; (H) *Rhodococcus equi* at 10 days; smooth colonies with no aerial hyphae; (I) *Gordonia bronchialis* at 10 days; irregular but smooth surface with no aerial hyphae; (J) *Tsukamurella pulmonis* at 10 days; smooth colonies with no aerial hyphae; (K) *Tsukamurella strandjordii* at 10 days; rough colonies with no aerial hyphae; (L) *Nocardia cyriacigeorgica* at 10 days; dense powdery aerial hyphae cover most or all the surface of the colonies.

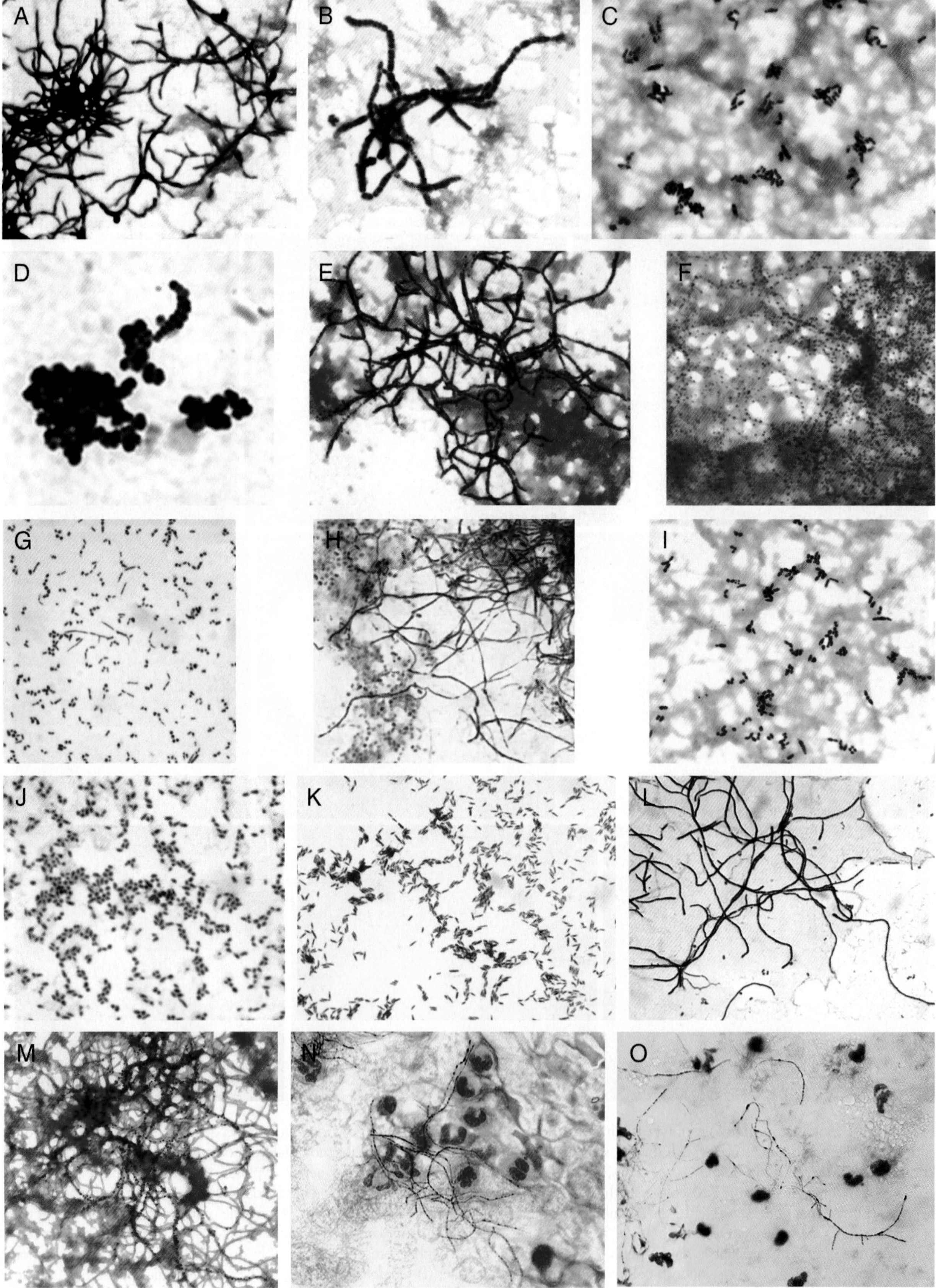
A
B
C
D
E
F
G
H
I
J
K
L
M
N
O

of *N. farcinica* was retained as the type strain for that particular species, as not all were convinced that the two species were truly identical.

Nocardiopsis

The genus *Nocardiopsis* was originally described by Meyer to accommodate an organism that at the time was called *Actinomadura dassonvillei* but differed chemotaxonomically and in certain colonial morphologic features from other organisms in the genus *Actinomadura*. The cell wall of this organism does not contain madurose. The substrate mycelium fragments into coccal forms, and the aerial hyphae fragment into variable-sized spores. Colonies are described as wrinkled or folded; the aerial mycelium varies from sparse to abundant (178). Currently, there are approximately 27 validly named species in the genus, and PCR primers specific for the genus *Nocardiopsis* have been described (209).

Pseudonocardia

Currently, there are approximately 24 validly published species names in the genus *Pseudonocardia*. See "*Amycolata*" above.

Rhodococcus

Species in the genus *Rhodococcus* tend to form smooth to mucoid colonies that may become increasingly pigmented and appear rougher with age. Colony color may vary from essentially colorless through yellow to red (Fig. 1H). At 37°C colonies may be only about 1 mm in diameter after 24 h of incubation. An aerial mycelium is generally not macroscopically visible but may occasionally be seen microscopically (89). The microscopic morphology of rhodococci can range from coccoid to bacillary depending on species and specimen type and on the stage of growth of the organism; cells may be observed intracellularly in macrophages (64). The organisms exhibit a rod-coccus growth cycle; rod forms are best visualized by growing isolates in a liquid medium, and under such conditions some branching of individual cells may be found. Generally, however, the organisms appear as gram-positive, beaded to solidly staining coccobacilli (Fig. 2I). Rhodococci are aerobic, catalase positive, and nonmotile; they are modified acid-fast positive, but the modified acid-fast stain needs to be performed and interpreted with particular care when dealing with isolates that may belong to this genus, as only a tiny fraction of the cells may retain the stain (Fig. 2J). Acid-fast smears prepared from isolates growing on trypticase soy agar with 5% sheep blood or chocolate agar may appear to be acid-fast negative (78). An important caveat regarding *Rhodococcus* species and *Gordonia* species is that they can easily be dismissed as "diphtheroids" because of their Gram stain morphology (Fig. 2C and I) and their frequent failure to develop obvious pigmentation during the first few days of growth. There are chemotaxonomic and 16S rRNA sequence differences between the two genera (see Table 5) (90). The genus and the species often included within it have been the subject of several recent reviews (19, 92, 103). Some data suggest that it may be justifiable to separate the species into several additional genera (103). There are approximately 34 validly named species in the genus.

Streptomyces

Species in the genus *Streptomyces* form branching, gram-positive rods (from 0.5 to 2.0 μm in diameter) that may appear more solidly gram positive than is typical for *Nocardia* species. Filaments may be fragmented (166), and beading may be seen (Fig. 2L and M). Members of the genus are modified acid-fast negative. The colonial morphology of these organisms may be similar to that of *Nocardia* species; an aerial mycelium is generally formed (Fig. 1C). The genus and species level taxonomy of this huge group, which contains approximately 517 validly named species, remains problematic (5, 172). Many of these species have been patented because of the commercially useful products they synthesize (5).

Tsukamurella

The genus *Tsukamurella* (named to honor the microbiologist Michio Tsukamura) was created to accommodate organisms with mycolic acids with chains of 62 to 78 carbon atoms in length (90); menaquinones of the MK-9 type are predominant (90). *Tsukamurella* species generally appear as long, straight to slightly curved, thin rods with no apparent branching; they are gram positive and modified acid-fast positive (Fig. 2K). Colonies tend to be small and can be smooth to rough but do not produce an aerial mycelium; the color varies from whitish to orange (Fig. 1J and K). The type species of the genus, *T. paurometabola* (corrected from *T. paurometabolum*), was previously known as *Corynebacterium paurometabolum*. There are approximately eight validly named species in the genus.

FIGURE 2 Microscopic morphology of various aerobic actinomycetes. (A) *Actinomadura latina;* Gram stain from Tween-albumin broth (TAB) at 4 days; long, branching, relatively solidly staining rods. (B) *Amycolata autotrophica;* Gram stain from TAB at 4 days; long, beaded rods with some branching. (C) *Gordonia bronchialis;* Gram stain from TAB at 4 days; coryneform rods with no obvious branching. (D) *Dermatophilus congolensis;* Gram stain from SAB at 14 days in CO_2; dense aggregates of cells of varying sizes; note chains of longitudinally and transversely dividing cells. (E) *Nocardia abscessus;* Gram stain from TAB at 4 days; long, branching rods; this is a rather solidly staining example, but some beading can be seen. (F) *Nocardia abscessus;* Gram stain from TAB at 10 days; long, beaded, branching rods; note that the beads generally do not abut one another. (G) *Nocardia farcinica;* modified acid-fast stain from horse blood agar at 2 to 3 days; many coccal forms are present; it is mostly these that are staining modified acid-fast positive. (H) *Nocardia veterana;* modified acid-fast stain from TAB at 25 days; some long, branching forms are staining modified acid-fast positive. (I) *Rhodococcus equi;* Gram stain from TAB at 4 days; coccobacilli and short coryneform rods without obvious branching. (J) *Rhodococcus equi;* modifed acid-fast stain from charcoal yeast extract agar at 10 days; only a small percentage of the cells stain positive. (K) *Tsukamurella pulmonis;* modified acid-fast stain from Lowenstein-Jensen medium at 4 days; thin rods, many of which stain positive. (L) *Streptomyces griseus;* Gram stain from SAB at 4 days; long, branching, fairly uniformly staining rods with little beading evident. (M) *Streptomyces candidus;* Gram stain from TAB at 10 days; long, thin, branching rods not distinguishable from *Nocardia* species. (N) Direct Gram stain of sputum which grew a *Nocardia* species; note lacey network of long, thin, branching, beaded rods. (Courtesy Daniel P. Fedorko.) (O) Direct modified acid-fast stain of *Nocardia* sp. in the same specimen as in panel N; the beads are purplish, but the intervening areas of the organism stain positive. (Courtesy Daniel P. Fedorko.)

NATURAL HABITATS

While the aerobic actinomycetes are widely distributed in the environment, the extent to which particular species are geographically restricted is not well known. Their primary ecological niche is probably the decomposition of plant material (172).

Epidemiology and Transmission

The majority of infections caused by aerobic actinomycetes stem from environmental sources, and even most nosocomial infections appear attributable to an environmental source such as dust from construction work (23). There has not yet been a documented case of direct patient-to-patient spread of an aerobic actinomycete infection without the intermediation of another human agent or of environmental contamination.

Most of the reports of outbreaks and pseudo-outbreaks of infection caused by aerobic actinomycetes have been attributed to *Nocardia* species. A 1979 outbreak in a renal intensive care unit involved at least seven patients. A patient on the unit was found to have been excreting, for 7 months from a nephrostomy, what was eventually identified as *N. asteroides*. An investigation resulted in the isolation of the organism from air and dust in the unit. The environmental contamination probably arose more from aerosols produced during disposal of the nephrostomy urine (115, 160, 227). Reports from other institutions involving *Nocardia* species also suggested nosocomial transmission and involved renal transplant recipients (12, 109), heart transplant patients (79), and patients with postoperative wound infections (23, 259).

A seven-patient outbreak of *Gordonia bronchialis* sternal wound infections was traced to a nurse from whose hands and other body sites the organism was isolated; it was also isolated from two of the nurse's dogs (204).

Two pseudo-outbreaks of infection with *N. asteroides* associated with the use of the BACTEC 460 TB system and inadequate needle sterilization have been reported (159, 193).

An outbreak of pseudoinfection attributed to *T. paurometabola*, involving specimens from 10 different patients and attributed to a common source somewhere in the laboratory, has also been reported (10).

CLINICAL SIGNIFICANCE

Table 1 lists the majority of species of aerobic actinomycetes, other than those in the genus *Nocardia*, that have been isolated from human specimens to date. Table 2 contains a listing of species of *Nocardia* that have been reported as human isolates to date. More commonly isolated species of aerobic actinomycetes of particular significance are dealt with in the sections below. For many of the newly described species there is a paucity of data to establish that the organisms were indeed agents of disease or to establish any clinically significant differences, such as in geographic distribution or susceptibility pattern, among the species. The source of bacterial names used is J. P. Euzéby (*List of Bacterial Names with Standing in Nomenclature;* http://www.bacterio.net). Representative examples of colonial and microscopic morphologies are shown in Fig. 1 and 2.

Actinomadura

A useful clue to the identification of organisms in the genus *Actinomadura* is the nature of the lesion from which an isolate originates. Most commonly this organism causes a mycetoma, a chronic, invasive, slowly progressive infection usually occurring in the foot ("Madura foot") and nearby anatomic structures, and nearly always resulting from traumatic implantation of the organism. Draining sinuses are typically present in a mycetoma; macroscopically visible grains (organism aggregates or microcolonies) may be visible in the discharge from the lesions. There are not adequate data available to allow using grain color for species or even genus level discrimination of the etiologic agent. The infection occurs most frequently in tropical regions, where people are more likely to walk barefoot. The word "mycetoma" is used only to describe the clinical nature of the infection, not the etiologic agent. Actinomycotic mycetomas are caused by aerobic actinomycetes; eumycotic mycetomas are caused by true fungi. Organisms in this genus have very rarely been implicated in other types of infection. Only three species have been reported as pathogens: *Actinomadura latina*, *A. madurae*, and *A. pelletieri*, with *A. madurae* being most commonly isolated. A set of 21 phenotypic tests was found useful for species level identification of isolates causing mycetoma (234). The same study also suggested that additional species other than the few commonly said to be etiologically involved remained to be described. In many reports mentioning the species causing mycetomas, identification has been made solely on the basis of the histological appearance of the grains, on the basis of a small number of phenotypic tests, or in ways not specified in any detail (45, 137, 163, 164). As with virtually all the aerobic actinomycetes, molecular methods are the only practical procedures for clinical or even reference laboratories to use for definitive species level identification of organisms in this genus.

Amycolata and *Amycolatopsis*

There are no recent reports documenting human infection caused by species in either of the genera *Amycolata* and *Amycolatopsis*. A newly described species, *Amycolatopsis palatopharyngis*, was isolated from what was described as "the infected palatopharyngeal mucosa" of an elderly male, but no further clinical information was provided (116). Three recently described species and several other aerobic actinomycete species may be causative agents of equine placental infection and abortion (145).

Dermatophilus

D. congolensis causes dermatitis in a wide variety of animals worldwide, including cattle, horses, goats, and sheep, but has only rarely been noted as a cause of human infection (233). In humans, the organism has been reported to cause a variety of cutaneous manifestations, including scaling and exudative lesions, pustules, pitted keratolysis (86), and "hairy" leukoplakia of the tongue (37). Filamentous and coccoid forms of the organism may be visualized directly in tissue specimens. Optimal therapy has not been defined, but infections may be self-limiting. *Dermatophilus chelonae* has been reported to cause disease in several species of animals (168, 257).

Dietzia

Only *Dietzia maris* has been associated with human infection. In one reported case the organism was isolated from blood and from an intravascular catheter; biochemical and chemotaxonomic studies of the isolate were performed (20), but the isolate was noted to be modified Kinyoun-stain negative, although *D. maris* would be expected to be modified acid-fast positive. The other reported case involved infection of a hip prosthesis; a variety of identification techniques were employed, including 16S rRNA

TABLE 1 Species of aerobic actinomycetes in genera other than *Nocardia* reported as human isolates[a]

Genus and species	Site(s) of isolation	Approximate no. of patients	Reference(s)
Actinomadura latina	Mycetoma	3	Euzéby[b]
A. madurae	Mycetoma	Many	158, 235
	Peritonitis	1	263
	Pneumonia and bacteremia	1	175
	Sputum	24	174
	Various sites	Few	172, 174
A. pelletieri	Mycetoma	Many	158, 235
Amycolatopsis orientalis	Cerebrospinal fluid	1	99
(reported as *Nocardia orientalis*)	Unspecified	1	99
A. palatopharyngis	Pharynx	1	Euzéby
Dermatophilus congolensis	Skin lesions	Few	86, 106, 233
	Tongue leukoplakia	1	37
Dietzia maris	Catheter-related bacteremia	1	20
	Hip bone	1	197
Gordonia bronchialis	Sternal wound infection	7	204
	Bacteremia	1	217
G. polyisoprenivorans	Catheter-related bacteremia	1	135
G. otitidis	Ear drainage	1	Euzéby
	Pleural fluid	1	Euzéby
G. rubripertincta	Pulmonary infection	1	107
G. sputi	Mediastinitis	1	144
G. terrae	CNS infection	2	72, 73
	Catheter-related bacteremia	5	196
	Hand mycetoma after trauma	1	13
	Mastitis after nipple piercing	1	274
Gordonia species	Bacteremia	1	205
	Catheter-related bacteremia	2	36
	Catheter-related bacteremia and endocarditis	1	154
Nocardiopsis dassonvillei	Mycetoma	1	2
	Bacteremia	1	17
	Pulmonary infection	2	References in reference 17
	Conjunctivitis	1	References in reference 17
	Cutaneous infection	Few	References in reference 17
N. synnemataformans	Sputum	1	270
Rhodococcus aurantiacus	Abscesses	1	237
(see text—probable *T. inchonensis*)	Peritonitis	1	43
	Pulmonary	1	238
	Meningitis	1	202
R. equi	Pulmonary infection, bacteremia, many other body sites	Many	8, 48, 64, 134, 185, 201, 256
R. erythropolis	Disseminated skin infection	1	243
	Endophthalmitis	1	245
R. fascians (reported as *R. luteus*)	Endophthalmitis	1	245
R. globerulus	Keratitis	1	66
R. gordoniae	Bacteremia	1	124
R. rhodochrous	Corneal ulcer	1	94
Rhodococcus species	Peritonitis	1	31
	Skin lesion	1	167
	Meningitis	1	69
	Pneumonia and bacteremia	1	219
	Various sites	Few	172, 219
Streptomyces albus	Mycetoma	1	5
S. bikiniensis	Bacteremia	1	180
S. griseus	Blood, brain, wound, other	Few	172, 174
S. thermovulgaris	Bacteremia	1	77
S. somaliensis	Mycetoma	Many	14, 172

(Continued on next page)

TABLE 1 Species of aerobic actinomycetes in genera other than *Nocardia* reported as human isolates[a] *(Continued)*

Genus and species	Site(s) of isolation	Approximate no. of patients	Reference(s)
Streptomyces species[c]	Pneumonia, various sites	Few	40, 74, 172
Tsukamurella inchonensis	Bacteremia	1	Euzéby
	Lung	1	46, 268; Euzéby
T. paurometabola	Catheter-related bacteremia	4	125, 214; Euzéby
(see text—probable *T. inchonensis*)	Skin infection	1	101
T. pulmonis	Sputum	1	Euzéby
	Catheter-related bacteremia	4	162, 211
	Conjunctivitis	1	261
T. strandjordii	Catheter-related bacteremia	1	133, 211; Euzéby
T. tyrosinosolvans	Bacteremia	2	Euzéby
	Pneumonia	2	Euzéby
	Catheter-related bacteremia	2	211, 215
	Conjunctivitis	2	261
Tsukamurella species	Knee prosthesis	1	148
	Pneumonia	1	3
	Peritonitis	1	212
	Implanted cardioverter-defibrillator	1	4

[a] Data in this table are based largely on the English-language literature accessible through web-based search engines; the species listing provided should not be regarded as complete. Several of the review articles refer to reports that we have not reviewed ourselves. In some cases, insufficient data are presented to determine whether or not the organism isolated was in fact a cause of disease. Many of the isolates were identified only phenotypically; the application of modern molecular identification techniques might have resulted in a different identification from that reported.

[b] The reference for the isolation of this species is the publication initially describing the organism as listed in J. P. Euzéby, *List of Bacterial Names with Standing in Nomenclature*; http://www.bacterio.net.

[c] The review articles mention several additional *Streptomyces* species that have been reported as human isolates.

sequencing, which showed 98% similarity with the *D. maris* type strain (197). The patient responded to treatment with teicoplanin.

Gordonia

There have been relatively few reports of infections attributed to species in the genus *Gordonia* (Table 1). One of the very few clusters of infection attributable to any aerobic actinomycete involved seven patients who developed sternal wound infections following coronary artery bypass surgery (204). The organism involved, *Gordonia bronchialis* (then called *Rhodococcus bronchialis*), was identified by biochemical testing and cell wall mycolic acid analysis. There have also been case reports of bacteremia, central nervous system (CNS) infections, pulmonary disease, and soft tissue infection caused by various *Gordonia* species. An immunocompromised state and the presence of foreign bodies appear to have been contributing factors for some of the patients. The techniques and interpretive criteria used to identify the organisms involved differ significantly among the various reports. For Table 1, when an isolate was not assigned to a particular species, or when such identification details as were presented made the identification problematic, cases were attributed to *Gordonia* species (Table 1).

Nocardia

Nocardia infections generally result either from trauma-related introduction of the organism or, particularly in immunocompromised patients, from inhalation and the resulting establishment of a pulmonary focus. It should be noted that the brain is one of the most common secondary sites of infection (190). A great advance in the clinically useful categorization of pathogenic nocardial isolates was provided by Wallace and his coworkers (249). They divided organisms phenotypically resembling *N. asteroides* into six different drug pattern types and one additional miscellaneous group. With more recent work, numerous different species have been described within this set of organisms, which came to be known as the *Nocardia asteroides* complex, and included *N. farcinica* (drug pattern type V), *Nocardia nova* (drug pattern type III), and isolates of drug pattern types I, II, IV, and VI. Subsequent work has resulted in the description of at least one separate species in almost all these drug pattern types. Undoubtedly, by using current species definition criteria, numerous species of *Nocardia* remain to be described. Roth et al., in their examination of the nearly complete 16S rRNA gene sequence of 74 *Nocardia* strains representing 25 established species, noted 10 taxa that appeared to be substantially different from each one's most closely related species. These 10 taxa probably represent undescribed species (207).

Given the current state of the literature, it is possible to make only the most tentative statements regarding geographic distribution and disease correlates of different species. Fortunately, with the use of a few selected phenotypic tests (see below), it is possible to assign some isolates in this genus to certain species or species groups with moderate confidence and thus to make some predictions regarding their likely antimicrobial susceptibility patterns. Nonetheless, susceptibility testing of all clinically significant isolates is recommended.

Nocardia abscessus

Nocardia abscessus was formally named in 2000 by Yassin et al. (271). ATCC strain 23824, the reference strain of *N. asteroides* drug pattern type I (207, 226), was one of the

TABLE 2 *Nocardia* species reported as human pathogens

Species[a]	Role as pathogen[b]	Site(s) of isolation	Approximate no. of patients
N. abscessus	Definite	See text	See text
N. africana	Unclear	Sputum	8
N. anaemiae	Unclear	Unknown	1
N. aobensis	Unclear	Unknown	5
N. araoensis	Possible	Pulmonary	1
N. arthritidis	Unclear	Sputum	1
N. asiatica	Unclear	Pulmonary, granuloma	6
N. asteroides	See text	See text	See text
N. beijingensis	Probable	Mostly pulmonary	19
N. brasiliensis	Definite	See text	See text
N. brevicatena complex	Definite	See text	See text
N. carnea[c]	Unclear	Eye, pleural fluid	3
N. concava	Probable	Skin	2
N. cyriacigeorgica	Definite	See text	See text
N. elegans	Possible	Sputum	1
N. farcinica	Definite	See text	See text
N. higoensis[d]	Unclear	Pulmonary	1
N. inohanensis	Unclear	Unknown	1
N. kruczakiae	Definite	Pulmonary	2
N. mexicana	Probable	Mycetoma	3
N. niigatensis	Probable	Skin abscesses	4
N. nova	Definite	See text	See text
N. orientalis	See under *Amycolatopsis*		
N. otitidiscaviarum	Definite	See text	See text
N. paucivorans	Definite	See text	See text
N. pneumoniae	Unclear	Sputum	1
N. pseudobrasiliensis	Definite	See text	See text
N. senatus	Unclear	Sputum	1
N. testacea	Unclear	Sputum	1
N. transvalensis	Definite	See text	See text
N. veterana	Definite	See text	See text
N. vinaceae[e]	Unclear	Unknown	1
N. yamanashiensis	Unclear	Skin abscess	1

[a] Unless otherwise noted, the reference for the isolation of each of these species is the publication initially describing the organism as listed in J. P. Euzéby, *List of Bacterial Names with Standing in Nomenclature.* http://www.bacterio.net.

[b] The role of an organism was considered unclear if the site of isolation was unknown, if it was isolated from only one patient without substantial corroborating information that the isolate was a pathogen, or if it was obtained only once from respiratory specimens or other unspecified sites from more than one patient, without information establishing the pathogenicity for any isolate. The role was considered possible if it was isolated more than once from one patient, but without other significant information provided. The role was considered probable if it was isolated from more than one patient from a mycetoma or skin abscess. The role was considered definite if a substantial amount of corroborating data was provided.

[c] See reference 99.

[d] See reference 129.

[e] See reference 130.

isolates found to be *N. abscessus* on the basis of 16S rRNA sequencing and DNA-DNA hybridization. Several of the strains in the report naming the species were from abscesses; in a subsequent report from Japan, several isolates from pulmonary sources and one from a brain abscess were reported (128). Two isolates have been reported from Germany, one from pericardial fluid (258) and the other from a posttraumatic wound (114). In their description in 1988 of the antimicrobial susceptibility patterns of 78 clinical isolates of *Nocardia* from various sources, Wallace et al. noted that 20% of the isolates had this drug pattern type. By the testing procedures and interpretive criteria employed, the organisms were susceptible to amikacin, ampicillin, carbenicillin, broad-spectrum cephalosporins, minocycline, and sulfamethoxazole; half of the isolates had high MICs to imipenem (249).

Nocardia asteroides and the "*N. asteroides* Complex"

There are innumerable reports of human infection attributed to *N. asteroides;* at least until recently, it has probably been considered to be the most commonly isolated human pathogenic *Nocardia* species. Notably, molecular analyses of the pathogenic isolates attributed to this species that have been conducted thus far have indicated that all belong to some other named or as-yet-unnamed species.

Infection has been reported to occur in patients immunocompromised as a result of human immunodeficiency virus (HIV) infection (198); systemic lupus erythematosis (100); chronic granulomatous disease (71); malignancies of various types (230); and organ transplantation including bone marrow (47), heart (194), kidney (160), liver (81), and lung (119). Trauma (218) and the presence of intravenous catheters (161) also predispose patients to infection. In immunocompromised patients the lung appears to be the most common initial site of infection, presumably acquired by inhalation from an environmental source. Infection may become disseminated, and the organism has been isolated from almost every conceivable body site, including blood (141), natural and prosthetic cardiac valves (68, 253), testes (156), thyroid (41), and peritonsillar abscess (1). Ocular involvement can occur either as a metastatic lesion (138) or as a result of ocular trauma (117). The brain is a relatively frequent site of metastatic infection (218). In a report on 21 patients with nocardial meningitis, 43% were noted to have a concomitant brain abscess (29).

The term "*N. asteroides* complex" has been used for organisms phenotypically resembling the *N. asteroides* type strain. However, several distinct species have now been described within that complex, and precisely what the complex is intended to designate is often no longer clear. The designation should be used, if at all, only if the species intended to be included are clearly stated.

Nocardia brasiliensis

N. brasiliensis appears to be the most common cause of actinomycotic mycetoma (see "*Actinomadura*" above) in the Western Hemisphere, especially in Mexico (44, 45). The organism probably occurs worldwide; there are reports of infection from Australia (85), West Bengal (164), and Europe (165) and many from North America (216). A variety of cutaneous manifestations in addition to mycetoma have been reported, including cellulites, abscesses, and lymphocutaneous infection. Nearly all cases are a result of trauma, including that caused by thorns (165), cat scratch (27), and insect bite (191). Most of the trauma-related infections have occurred in immunocompetent individuals. Disseminated infection, usually originating from a pulmonary focus, has also been reported (216); such infections are more likely to occur in immunocompromised patients (140). Some cases, such as one of a brain abscess resulting from dissemination from a pulmonary focus (184), do occur in patients who appear to be immunocompetent. However, most of the cases of invasive disease, as well as some of the cases of cutaneous infection, attributed to *N. brasiliensis* prior to 1995 may have been due to *N. pseudobrasiliensis*. In that year Wallace et al. (247) reported that a subset of organisms that had been identified as *N. brasiliensis* but were predominantly associated with noncutaneous invasive disease appeared to belong to another taxon, formally named *N. pseudobrasiliensis* the following year (208). Unlike true *N. brasiliensis* isolates, most *N. pseudobrasiliensis* isolates hydrolyze adenine, are susceptible to ciprofloxacin and clarithromycin, and are resistant to minocycline. The two species also differed in their mycolic acid patterns, 16S rRNA gene sequences, and restriction fragment length polymorphism (RFLP) patterns for both the 16S rRNA and 65-kDa heat shock protein genes.

Nocardia brevicatena Complex

Brown et al. suggested in 1997 that *Nocardia* isolates sharing both an unusual drug susceptibility pattern and one or another of three different RFLP patterns of an amplified portion of the 65-kDa heat shock protein gene should be considered to form the *Nocardia brevicatena* complex (B. A. Brown, R. W. Wilson, V. A. Steingrube, Z. Blacklock, and R. J. Wallace, Jr., *Abstr. 97th Gen. Meet. Am. Soc. Microbiol.* 1997, abstr. C-65, p. 131, 1997). These organisms included 19 clinical isolates from the United States, 10 clinical isolates from Australia, and three ATCC reference strains of *N. brevicatena*. The 19 U.S. clinical isolates had the type II *N. asteroides* drug pattern (249), being sensitive to ampicillin, carbenicillin, broad-spectrum cephalosporins, minocycline, sulfamethoxazole, and kanamycin. All 32 isolates studied were also susceptible to amikacin and tobramycin but resistant to gentamicin. There have been no subsequent reports of clinical isolates or taxonomic studies of these organisms. Given the different RFLP patterns involved, several different species may be included in the complex. Some workers include *N. paucivorans* in this complex. The 16S rRNA sequences of the type strains of the two species are 99.5% similar, but DNA-DNA hybridization results indicate that *N. brevicatena* and *N. paucivorans* are separate species (269).

Nocardia cyriacigeorgica

N. cyriacigeorgica (spelling corrected from the original *N. cyriacigeorgici*) was described on the basis of an isolate obtained from the sputum of a patient with chronic bronchitis (272). Subsequent isolates were obtained from brain abscesses in an immunocompromised patient (84) and from a patient with pneumonia following a near-drowning incident, from whom *N. farcinica* and several other pathogens were also isolated (240). Isolates of this species were reported to constitute 13 of 96 (14%) clinical isolates of *Nocardia* from Thailand (199) and 13 of 86 (15%) of such isolates from Belgium (254). It should be noted that the 16S rRNA sequence of the type strain of this species (1,400 bp) is identical to that of the reference strain of "*N. asteroides* drug pattern type VI" (ATCC 14759) (207, 226). As there are no published results of DNA-DNA hybridization studies of these two strains, it is remotely possible that they may in fact belong to different species. In the original work describing the different *N. asteroides* drug pattern types, type VI was the most commonly isolated variety (35%) (249), so should DNA-DNA hybridization prove them to be the same, *N. cyriacigeorgica* may be the most frequent human nocardial pathogen, at least in areas where actinomycotic mycetomas are relatively rare. Note that if one speaks of "*N. asteroides* drug pattern type VI sensu stricto," this should mean isolates corresponding (using the best available methods) to the isolate deposited as the "reference" strain of this drug pattern type. However, the designation "*N. asteroides* drug pattern type VI" is not a valid species name. This drug pattern type was initially characterized by resistance to penicillin and susceptibility to broad-spectrum cephalosporins (249).

Nocardia farcinica

The organisms initially described by Wallace et al. as belonging to the group "*N. asteroides* drug pattern type V" (249) were subsequently found to belong to *N. farcinica* (250). Isolates of this species are perhaps the most resistant of all *Nocardia* isolates; they are typically resistant to cefotaxime, cefamandole, ampicillin, gentamicin, and tobramycin and susceptible to amikacin, sulfamethoxazole, and usually also to ciprofloxacin and imipenem (249). Isolates that showed in vitro resistance to trimethoprim-sulfamethoxazole have been reported to respond to meropenem alone (112) and to the combination of linezolid and minocycline (155). This species may have a particular propensity for causing disseminated disease; Wallace et al. reported that among 30 patients for which disease extent was known, 57% had disseminated disease and one-third had CNS involvement (250). Most patients infected by this species, especially those with disseminated disease, have some type of immunocompromise (231, 250), but cutaneous and other infections have been reported to occur in the apparently immunocompetent as well (210). The lung is a common site of involvement, affecting 43% of patients in one review, while 30% had brain or meningeal involvement (231). The organism has been isolated from blood from a number of patients (50) and from many other sites in addition to the lungs and the CNS; more unusual sites have included the eye of a patient who washed her contact lenses in basin-stored water (75), the site of a cochlear implant (147), and the larynx of an immunocompromised patient for whom no other site of involvement was detected (56). Isolates of this species were also reported to make up 34 of 96 (35%) clinical isolates of *Nocardia* from Thailand (199) and 38 of 86 (44%) of such isolates from Belgium (254). The complete genomic sequence of a clinical isolate (*N. farcinica* IFM 10152) has been determined (121). The genome was found to consist of a single circular chromosome; two circular plasmids were also present. Among the notable findings were the presence of three copies of the rRNA operon and a number of genes that were thought to contribute to the virulence and drug resistance of the organism.

Nocardia nova

N. nova was described by Tsukamura in 1982 and was distinguished from *N. asteroides* by several phenotypic tests (236) and confirmed to be a separate and distinct species by DNA-DNA hybridization (266). Wallace et al. found that 18% of 78 clinical isolates fell into their type III pattern, characterized by susceptibility to ampicillin and erythromycin and resistance to carbenicillin (249). In a subsequent study of 223 clinical isolates, employing both biochemical and susceptibility testing procedures, 17% of the isolates, as well as the type strain of *N. nova*, had similar characteristics, including the type III drug pattern; these isolates were all then considered members of *N. nova* (248). Of the patients for whom clinical information was available, 35% were thought to have disseminated disease; organisms were obtained from many sites, including blood, lung, CNS, skin and soft tissue, joints, and cornea. An upper extremity sporotrichoid form of nocardiosis attributed to *N. nova* in an HIV-positive patient who sustained a thumb injury while working in a field has been reported (120). More recent investigations have revealed that the organisms identified as *N. nova* by phenotypic testing, as well as by the RFLP patterns obtainable from the *hsp65* gene, actually may belong to other species in addition to *N. nova,* including *N. africana*, *N. kruczakiae*, and *N. veterana* (59). These species can be distinguished from one another and from *N. nova* sensu stricto only by detailed molecular analysis. Isolates identified only by phenotypic testing as belonging to one or another of these species are probably best reported as members of the "*N. nova* complex."

Nocardia otitidiscaviarum

The initial isolate of the species *N. otitidiscaviarum*, described by Snijders in 1924, was obtained from the infected middle ear of a guinea pig; for a time this species was known as *N. caviae* (97). This species is a relatively infrequent cause of human infection. Clark et al. reviewed 28 cases of cutaneous infection, including several of mycetoma, attributed to this species; many of those for which information was available were considered trauma related (52). There are a few reports of infection at other sites, including brain abscess (110), pyothorax (273), catheter-related infection (153), and disseminated infection (195). This species is relatively reliably identified on the basis of its decomposition reactions; it decomposes xanthine and hypoxanthine but not casein or tyrosine. In a recent molecular study of numerous clinical isolates, several different sequences were obtained from nine different strains that had been phenotypically identified as *N. otitidiscaviarum* (192). These results were interpreted as suggesting the presence of several different species within this group, but some of the results also suggested that individual isolates might contain two or more differing copies of the 16S rRNA gene.

Nocardia paucivorans

The species *N. paucivorans* was described by Yassin et al. in 2000 on the basis of a respiratory tract isolate from a patient with chronic lung disease (269). A subsequent isolate was reported from a patient with cerebral nocardiosis; by the susceptibility testing procedure used, the isolate was susceptible to nearly every drug tested (76). Another isolate from a brain abscess attributed to this species that showed 98.4% 16S rRNA gene similarity to a "reference" strain has also been reported; this organism was susceptible by the procedure employed to all drugs tested (258). An isolate from a mitral valve has been reported (28), and 2 of 86 (2.3%) clinical isolates from Belgium were identified as belonging to this species (254). The sensitivity pattern of two of the reported isolates is similar to that of drug pattern type II (see "*Nocardia brevicatena*" above), but both appeared susceptible to gentamicin.

Nocardia pseudobrasiliensis

N. pseudobrasiliensis is more often a cause of noncutaneous invasive infection, although it can cause cutaneous infection as well. Most infections have occurred in immunocompromised patients; cases have been reported from North and South America, Japan, and Australia (30, 127, 247) (see "*Nocardia brasiliensis*" above).

Nocardia transvalensis

N. transvalensis was originally described in 1927 on the basis of an isolate from an African patient with a mycetoma. In 1992 McNeil et al. reported on 16 patients from whom isolates attributed to this species had been obtained (173). The isolates from 10 of the patients were considered clinically significant; the other isolates were considered colonizers or of uncertain significance. A variety of sites of infection were involved; some of the infections were disseminated, and several patients were known to be immunocompromised. Wilson et al. subsequently distinguished four taxa that they proposed be grouped together as the "*N. transvalensis* complex" (260); included among these was the type strain of *N. transvalensis*. All isolates were considered resistant to at least one of the aminoglycosides tested, and the majority were resistant to amikacin, suggesting that they might all be grouped with organisms exhibiting drug pattern type IV, originally defined as resistance to all aminoglycosides and susceptibility to ciprofloxacin (249). There are a few other case reports of disseminated infection attributed to this species, including one in a liver transplant patient (255) and one in a heart transplant patient (157). The isolate from the heart transplant patient developed sulfonamide resistance during the course of treatment (157). A total of 11 clinical isolates assigned to this species have been reported from Japan and Thailand (131, 199).

Nocardia veterana

N. veterana was first described on the basis of an isolate obtained from the bronchial lavage fluid of a patient with pulmonary lesions, but that isolate was thought not to be clinically significant (104). Subsequently, there appeared several case reports that indicated that this species could cause human disease; these included reports of a patient with a mycetoma (132), three patients with pulmonary disease (200), and ascitic fluid infection in an HIV patient

(87). In a subsequent report of three additional clinical isolates, two of which were shown to have been causative agents of pulmonary disease, it was noted that the isolates had an antimicrobial susceptibility pattern essentially identical to the patterns of *N. africana* and *N. nova* (60), demonstrating that species identification could not be definitively established by susceptibility testing alone. It was also noted that the isolates of this species that were studied showed 16S rRNA gene similarities to the type strains of *N. africana* and *N. nova* of 99.0 and 97.7%, respectively. In a collection of 101 isolates initially identified as *N. nova*, further analysis using molecular procedures indicated that at least 15 were most probably isolates of *N. veterana* (R. W. Wilson, P. S. Conville, L. Mann, B. A. Brown-Elliott, C. Crist, F. G. Witebsky, and R. J. Wallace, Jr. *Abstr. 104th Gen. Meet. Am. Soc. Microbiol.* 2004, abstr. U-075, p. 636).

Nocardiopsis

Nearly all the very few infections attributed to organisms in the genus *Nocardiopsis* have been attributed to *N. dassonvillei*. In a letter to the editor regarding a case of actinomycetoma attributed to this species, it was stated that *N. dassonvillei* was "regularly encountered" at the Centers for Disease Control and Prevention, with 21 isolates having been identified from 1981 through 1986; no clinical details were provided (2). There are also a few case reports attributing other types of infection to this species (Table 1). One other species in the genus has been reported as isolated from a human specimen (Table 1).

Rhodococcus

The most commonly isolated pathogen in the genus *Rhodococcus* is *Rhodococcus equi*. While other species have occasionally been reported to cause disease (Table 1), it is impossible to obtain reliable species level identifications without resorting to molecular methods (19, 92). *R. equi* itself may be split into several different species (170). Infections caused by *R. equi* have been the subject of several reviews (8, 63, 134, 232). The organism has long been known as a significant pulmonary pathogen in horses (hence the species name) (201). The initial report of human disease caused by the organism (reported as *Corynebacterium equi*) involved a patient on high-dose steroids with a pulmonary abscess; he had worked briefly in stockyards contaminated with animal feces shortly before the onset of his illness (88). Herbivore manure provides an ideal growth medium for the organism, and inhalation of the organism is presumed to be the major mode of infection in horses (201) and is probably also the principal mechanism for human infections. Direct inoculation and oral ingestion are other possible routes of infection (256). Most patients who develop *R. equi* infection are immunocompromised, and at least until recently approximately two-thirds of infected patients were also HIV infected (256). Essentially any body site can be involved, but the lung is a site of involvement in approximately 80% of immunocompromised patients and at least 40% of immunocompetent patients infected with this species. Bacteremia has been reported in >80% of immunocompromised patients and approximately 30% of immunocompetent patients (256). Pulmonary cavitation is a frequent finding. Malacoplakia, an aggregation of histiocytes containing concentrically layered basophilic structures known as Michaelis-Gutmann bodies, has been noted as a histopathologic finding in several studies (102, 232). Two virulence-associated antigens (VapA and VapB) encoded by plasmids have been identified; isolates producing the VapA antigen are the predominant, possibly the sole, cause of disease in horses, but isolates producing the VapA antigen, the VapB antigen, or neither antigen have been isolated from human cases of infection (194). A combination of antimicrobials is generally used for the treatment of infections. Agents used include aminoglycosides, erythromycin, imipenem, quinolones, rifampin, and vancomycin; linezolid may also be efficacious (256). Some rifampin-resistant strains with *rpoB* gene mutations have been reported (9).

Streptomyces

The most common type of infection attributed to species in the genus *Streptomyces* is mycetoma (see "*Actinomadura*" above), and the most commonly mentioned etiologic agent is *Streptomyces somaliensis*, although in many reports the identification procedures employed could not have ensured that other species were not involved. There are a few reports implicating other species in the genus as occasional pathogens. In case reports of bacteremias attributed to *Streptomyces bikiniensis* (180) and *Streptomyces thermovulgaris* (77), molecular methods were used in identifying the isolates, and such methods were described in detail in a case report of a mycetoma attributed to *Streptomyces albus* (166). While the majority of isolates from nonmycetomatous lesions probably represent either contamination or colonization, these organisms are capable of occasionally causing disease.

Tsukamurella

There are case reports attributing a variety of infections to different species in the genus *Tsukamurella* (Table 1). In the older literature there are a few reports of infection attributed to *Rhodococcus aurantiacus*, such as pulmonary infection, meningitis, peritonitis, and subcutaneous abscesses (43, 237). Recently, *R. aurantiacus* ATCC 25938 (the initial type strain of the species), which has had a convoluted taxonomic history (58), has been placed in *T. inchonensis* (133, 268). Organisms isolated from clinical material and thought to belong to this genus have generally been found to resemble strain ATCC 25938. The organisms reported to cause an outbreak of pseudoinfection (10) (and quite possibly most or all of the organisms involved in clinical infections and identified as *T. paurometabola*) were in fact almost certainly what is now called *Tsukamurella inchonensis*.

Other Genera

Some other genera of aerobic actinomycetes do have roles in human diseases but are unlikely to be encountered in the clinical laboratory. Organisms in three genera of thermophilic aerobic actinomycetes, *Saccharomonospora*, *Saccharopolyspora*, and *Thermoactinomyces*, have been implicated in the etiology of hypersensitivity pneumonitis. Spores of these organisms may be encountered when performing air sampling; molecular methods are helpful for species level identification when needed (108, 264). There are currently approximately 7, 10, and 8 validly published species names in the genera *Saccharomonospora*, *Saccharopolyspora*, and *Thermoactinomyces*, respectively. *Crossiella equi* is an aerobic actinomycete that can cause equine placentitis (70), but there are no reports of human infection attributed to this organism.

COLLECTION, TRANSPORT, AND STORAGE

In temperate climates the respiratory tract is the most frequent portal of entry for the aerobic actinomycetes and therefore the primary site of nocardial infections in the immunocompromised host. Sputum is the most easily obtained pulmonary specimen, and examination of several fresh early-morning samples collected on separate days (90, 251) may maximize the chances of organism recovery; recovery of an aerobic actinomycete from multiple samples may help to establish the clinical significance of the isolated organism (90, 142). *Nocardia* species may, however, be difficult to recover from sputum even in documented cases of pulmonary infection (190), either because of low numbers of organisms present in the sample or because contaminating bacteria in the sample may overgrow the more slowly growing aerobic actinomycetes. More invasive procedures, such as bronchoalveolar lavage or fine needle or open lung biopsy, may be required to obtain a definitive diagnosis (190). These more invasive procedures may be necessary for diagnosis of as many as 44% of primary pulmonary infections (85); macrophage-rich samples may be necessary to maximize recovery of organisms such as rhodococci, which tend to localize within these cells (64).

Exudates from abscesses or mycetomas should be delivered to the laboratory in a sterile container for examination for characteristic granules and for smear and culture. In the case of disseminated cutaneous lesions or small lesions secondary to trauma, a skin biopsy can be useful. The use of swabs is not recommended, as fibers can make smear interpretation difficult (251). To optimize isolation of *Dermatophilus*, scabs or crusty lesions should be removed and soaked in sterile distilled water, and the fluid should be inoculated onto blood agar plates (275).

In immunocompromised patients the aerobic actinomycetes, especially *Nocardia*, can disseminate to almost any organ. A biopsy sample or aspirate, when obtainable, may be the best specimen to evaluate for the presence of such organisms. Normally sterile body fluids should be collected in a sterile container and sent immediately to the laboratory. *Nocardia* isolates are infrequently recovered from cerebrospinal fluid, even if numerous brain lesions are present, because the organisms may be confined to the brain abscess itself. Blood should be inoculated directly into blood culture media; many commercially available blood culture or lysis centrifugation systems have been shown to support the growth of *Nocardia* species. Various aerobic actinomycetes have been implicated as the cause of catheter-related bacteremia; potentially infected catheter tips should be transported to the laboratory in a sterile container and cultured by appropriate methods.

In all cases where infection with an aerobic actinomycete is suspected, it is of utmost importance that the laboratory be notified of the suspected diagnosis. This will ensure that samples will receive appropriate handling, that the correct direct smears will be prepared, and that the sample will be inoculated onto the appropriate media and incubated for an extended period of time at the appropriate temperature.

All samples should be transported promptly to the laboratory following the specimen collection and handling procedures outlined in chapters 5 and 20.

DIRECT EXAMINATION

Careful microscopic examination of clinical specimens suspected of containing aerobic actinomycetes is extremely important. The observation of organisms characteristic of *Nocardia* and other aerobic actinomycetes should alert laboratory personnel to inoculate appropriate media and to extend incubation at the appropriate temperature. In addition, the detection of organisms directly in the patient specimen may assist in the interpretation of culture results.

Smears can be made directly from sputum, drainages, and aspirates; however, liquid specimens such as bronchoalveolar lavage or normally sterile body fluids that are not excessively cellular should be concentrated before smear preparation and media inoculation. For tissue samples, smears can be made from ground material and from touch preps. Two important stains that should be used in the clinical laboratory for direct samples are the Gram stain and the modified acid-fast stain. Histopathologic examination of fixed tissue by use of special stains may also reveal the presence of organisms (262).

The modified acid-fast stain used on direct specimens may more accurately reflect the true partially acid-fast nature of the organisms than do modified acid-fast stains prepared from colonial growth (Fig. 2O). The modified acid-fast stain uses a weaker decolorizer (1% H_2SO_4) than does the mycobacterial stain (3% HCl) (see chapters 21 and 36 for details on reagent preparation and staining methodology). Because of the difficulty of standardizing this technique, it is imperative that positive and negative controls be run simultaneously with patient smears. The control slides can be made from growing suspensions of *Streptomyces* species (negative control) and *Nocardia* species (positive control). Smears should be evaluated by experienced laboratory personnel, and the quality of the stain itself should be evaluated before results are reported. *Gordonia, Nocardia, Rhodococcus,* and *Tsukamurella* (and possibly *Dietzia*) are known to be partially acid fast with this stain.

Careful attention should be paid to the cellular material present in the sample. Phagocytized gram-positive or acid-fast organisms can sometimes be seen within macrophages and mononuclear cells; in the modified acid-fast smear these may appear as beaded cells with strongly acid-fast granules within non-acid-fast or weakly acid-fast rods (189).

In cases of suspected actinomycetoma, aspirated material should be examined grossly for the presence of granules by spreading the sample in a sterile petri dish. Granules found should be washed and crushed. Smears should be prepared from the crushed material and appropriate media should be inoculated.

Recently, Couble et al. reported on a method for direct detection of *Nocardia* isolates from clinical samples by using PCR along with DNA probes directed to a portion of the 16S rRNA gene. Analysis of 18 patient samples that were culture positive for various *Nocardia* species gave positive results for all samples; specimens containing *Mycobacterium tuberculosis* gave negative results (65). Further assessment of this technique will be needed to assess its clinical utility.

ISOLATION

Blood agar, chocolate agar, brain heart infusion agar, Sabouraud dextrose agar, and Lowenstein-Jensen medium will support the growth of aerobic actinomycetes. *Dermatophilus congolensis* may not grow on Sabouraud dextrose agar or Lowenstein-Jensen medium (275). Buffered charcoal yeast extract agar (BCYE) is particularly useful for the recovery of *Nocardia* species. Specimens from sterile sites or concentrated sterile body fluids can be inoculated directly onto these media. Specimens from respiratory sites, skin, and other potentially contaminated sites, such as mycetomas, should additionally be inoculated onto selective media, such as modified Thayer Martin agar (183) and selective BCYE (containing polymyxin B, anisomycin, and either vancomycin or cefamandole) (244). Sabouraud agar with added chloramphenicol may not be useful, as it may also suppress the growth of some *Nocardia* species (105). A specialized medium for the recovery of *R. equi,* using a Mueller-Hinton agar-based medium with added ceftazidime and novobiocin, has been described (246).

Cultures for aerobic actinomycetes should be handled as fungal cultures, thus ensuring that the cultures will be held and regularly examined over an extended period. Two BCYE plates (for samples from sterile sites) or selective BCYE plates (for respiratory or other potentially contaminated sites) should be inoculated. One BCYE or selective BCYE should be incubated at 30°C and the other at 35°C, both in ambient air. It should be noted, however, that *Streptomyces* species may show best growth at 25°C and that *D. congolensis* grows better and shows enhanced production of aerial hyphae in increased CO_2 (275). For all cultures, plates should be held for a minimum of 2 weeks, preferably for up to 3 weeks, and should be sealed to prevent dehydration.

A low-pH decontamination procedure has been successfully used for pretreatment of heavily contaminated specimens suspected of harboring *Nocardia* species. The sample is diluted 1:10 in 0.2 M HCl–0.2 M KCl at pH 2.2, mixed, and allowed to stand for 3 to 5 min, after which it is inoculated onto selective and nonselective media (26, 244). Murray et al. report a drop in viability of *Nocardia* species after 30-min exposures to *N*-acetyl-L-cysteine (NALC), NaOH-NALC, or Zephiran-TSP (182). The key to improved recovery of *Nocardia* from NaOH-NALC-treated specimens may be a shorter exposure to the decontaminating reagents (15 min), as is in fact also recommended for the recovery of mycobacteria (136).

Aerobic actinomycetes have been recovered from blood by using a variety of commercially available blood culture systems, including conventional two-bottle systems, biphasic bottles, systems using radiometric and nonradiometric detection, and lysis-centrifugation systems. By use of various blood culture systems, aerobic actinomycetes have been recovered after 3 to 19 days of incubation, which in some cases included the incubation times of terminal subcultures (180, 242). Studies employing newer blood culture systems have resulted in a recommendation that extended incubation is no longer necessary (15); however, such studies have not established that such shorter incubation would generally be adequate for the isolation of aerobic actinomycetes. If the possibility of bacteremia with a member of one of these genera is anticipated, it would be advisable to request fungal blood cultures or to perform terminal subcultures if the incubation period of routine blood cultures cannot be extended.

Cultures from all sources should be examined daily for the first week of incubation and then weekly thereafter, preferably using a dissecting microscope, which will allow detection of tiny colonies. Such microscopic examination is particularly important for specimens that contain contaminating flora, as an aerobic actinomycete can be quickly overgrown by more rapidly growing organisms. Care should also be exercised when examining Lowenstein-Jensen or Middlebrook media for mycobacteria or when examining BCYE plates for *Legionella* species, as *Nocardia* and other aerobic actinomycetes will grow on these media.

IDENTIFICATION

Microscopic Morphology

Gram-stained and modified acid-fast-stained smears should be prepared as the initial step in organism identification. Numerous fields should be reviewed to determine the most prevalent morphology and to detect the sometimes rare branching forms. Care should be taken not to confuse perpendicular aligning of the organisms with true branching (Fig. 2).

A properly prepared and carefully interpreted modified acid-fast smear can assist in the preliminary identification of the organism (Fig. 2G, H, J, and K). Quality control slides should be stained along with stains of colonies from cultures. With the modified acid-fast stain, the background should be blue; slides that have a pink background may be inadequately decolorized and should be repeated. The smear should be scanned for areas where individual cells can be seen or areas where single layers of cells allow clear differentiation of cell borders. The acid-fast reaction of tightly packed clumps of organisms may not represent the true partially acid-fast nature of the cells; be wary of large clumps of cells which all appear to be acid-fast positive. Acid-fast cells will be clearly red; cells that stain purple or light pink may or may not be truly acid fast. A stain that shows an unambiguous acid-fast positive reaction may frequently show only a few clearly red cells, with a majority of blue cells. Frequently, only the "beads" will appear acid-fast positive. If modified acid-fast stain results are ambiguous, transfer of the organism to a lipid-rich medium, such as Lowenstein-Jensen medium or Middlebrook 7H11 agar, and repeat staining may give a more clear-cut stain result. Similar enhancements of the acid-fast reaction have been noted after growth in glycerol nutrient broth, litmus milk, or media containing certain amino acids (142, 239). Acid fastness may become more evident as colonies age; the acid-fast reaction has been reported to be most reliable when performed from colonies after 1 to 4 weeks of growth (239). Occasionally, coccoid forms of *Streptomyces* may appear partially acid fast; hyphae, however, are acid-fast negative. Because of the difficulties of interpretation of the modified acid-fast smear, results of this stain should be considered preliminary and must be used only in conjunction with results from other tests.

Slide Cultures

Slide cultures may be used to evaluate the microscopic morphology of actively growing cultures. Small blocks of a minimal agar (such as tap water agar) are inoculated on the side with the organism of interest, and a coverslip is placed on the top of the block. The slide culture is incubated in a humid environment at 25°C for 2 to 3 weeks and examined regularly for the characteristic features of the various genera. Vegetative mycelia (also called substrate hyphae) grow beneath the surface of the agar and show various degrees of branching. *Gordonia* and *Tsukamurella* show rudimentary to no branching, while the branching of *Actinomadura*, *Nocardia*, and *Streptomyces* is generally extensive. Vegetative hyphae of *Amycolata*, *Amycolatopsis*, and *Nocardia* fragment into bacillary, coccal, or square forms; the vegetative hyphae of *Actinomadura* and *Streptomyces* show little to no fragmentation. The substrate growth of *Rhodococcus* initially appears as short rods, which either remain unchanged in shape or evolve into filaments with side projections or into filaments with elementary to extensively branched hyphae. These forms all rapidly fragment to a coccal or short rod form (113). The rhodococcal colony itself is a mass of these coccoid or coccobacillary forms. The vegetative hyphae of *D. congolensis* are characteristic for the genus and show long, tapering filaments which branch laterally at right angles, with septa forming in transverse and longitudinal planes (113).

Colonial Morphology

The colonial appearance of members of the aerobic actinomycetes is extremely variable among genera and even between isolates of the same species (Fig. 1). Environmental factors such as growth medium, incubation temperature, air circulation, presence of CO_2, and age of culture can affect the size and consistency of the colonies and the production of aerial hyphae (21, 142). Some species produce a diffusible pigment that can vary from strain to strain (142) (see genus and species descriptions above for information on specific colonial morphologies).

Aerial Hyphae

Aerial hyphae project away from the surface of the colony into the air but may not be apparent until 7 to 14 days for most species that form such hyphae. *Nocardia* and *Streptomyces* usually produce abundant aerial hyphae that give the colonies their characteristic powdery or velvety appearance (Fig. 1E and L); rare strains of *Nocardia* produce sparse or no aerial hyphae (Fig. 1D and G). *Actinomadura, Amycolata,* and *Amycolatopsis* show variable production of aerial hyphae. *Rhodococcus* may rarely form rudimentary aerial hyphae (113). Of the genera that are partially acid fast, only *Nocardia* regularly produces aerial hyphae. The presence of spores and their relative number and arrangement on the aerial hyphae can also give some clue to the genus identification (113).

Phenotypic Identification

Limitations

Given the increasing number of species of aerobic actinomycetes, the use of only a limited number of phenotypic tests to obtain exact species or even genus level identification has become impossible. When a precise identification is required for a significant patient isolate, referral to a reference laboratory for molecular testing is strongly recommended.

Genus Assignment

To determine the genus of an unknown isolate, observation of colonial morphology, specifically the presence of aerial hyphae, is especially important. *Nocardia* and *Streptomyces* generally produce aerial hyphae, with other less commonly isolated genera also showing this morphologic trait (see Table 5). Results of a carefully prepared and carefully interpreted modified acid-fast smear will help to distinguish *Nocardia* from the other genera.

Nocardia and *Tsukamurella* (both modified acid-fast positive organisms) are resistant to lysozyme and show good growth in lysozyme broth; of these, only *Nocardia* species show aerial hyphae. *Gordonia* shows variable growth in lysozyme broth but does not show aerial hyphae. Lysozyme catalyzes the hydrolysis of certain polysaccharides in the cell wall, resulting in a weakening of the cell wall. Berd (21) recommends the use of a very small inoculum into glycerol broth with 0.005% lysozyme and a second similarly inoculated glycerol broth without lysozyme as a control. After 4 weeks of incubation, results are interpreted by comparing organism growth in the broths with and without lysozyme. All *Nocardia* isolates tested in one study (Brown et al., *Abstr. 97th Gen. Meet. Am. Soc. Microbiol.* 1997) were resistant to lysozyme, except for 10 lysozyme-susceptible isolates that belonged to the *N. brevicatena* complex. Lysozyme broth is commercially available from Remel (Lenexa, Kans.) and BD Diagnostics (Sparks, Md.).

Species Assignment

Biochemicals

Some useful phenotypic tests are not commercially available. Tables 3 and 4 present antibiotic susceptibility patterns and basic biochemical results that may provide preliminary identifications of frequently isolated *Nocardia* species or complexes obtained from clinical specimens. Most (but not all) of the isolates of a given species show the results listed in Table 4. When performing biochemical tests, it is extremely important to include appropriate positive and negative controls to ensure that tests are inoculated, incubated, and interpreted correctly. See "Evaluation, Interpretation, and Reporting" below for recommendations on reporting preliminary identifications obtained using these methods.

TABLE 3 Typical in vitro antimicrobial susceptibility patterns of various *Nocardia* species[a,b,c]

Drug	*N. abscessus*	*N. brasiliensis*	*N. cyriacigeorgica*	*N. farcinica*	*N. nova* complex[d]	*N. otitidiscaviarum*	*N. pseudobrasiliensis*	*N. transvalensis* complex[e]
AMC[f]	S	S	R	—	R	R	R	—
Amikacin	S	—	—	S	—	S	—	R
Ampicillin	S	R	R	R	S	R	R	—
Carbenicillin	S	S	—	—	R	R	S	—
Cefamandole	—	R	—	R	—	—	R	—
Ceftriaxone	S	—	S	R	—	R	—	—
Ciprofloxacin	R	R	R	S	—	S	S	S
Clarithromycin	R	R	R	R	S	—	S	R
Erythromycin	R	—	—	R	S	—	—	R
Gentamicin	—	—	—	R	—	S	—	R
Imipenem	R	—	—	S	—	R	—	S
Kanamycin	—	R	—	—	—	S	R	R
Linezolid	S	S	S	S	S	S	S	S
Minocycline	—	S	—	—	—	—	R	—
Sulfamethoxazole	S	S	—	S	—	S	S	—

[a] Abbreviations: S, susceptible; R, resistant; —, no result.
[b] From references 35 and 249.
[c] Based on interpretation of MICs, using CLSI breakpoints.
[d] Includes *N. nova* sensu stricto, *N. africana, N. kruczakiae,* and *N. veterana.*
[e] Includes *N. transvalensis* sensu stricto and *N. asteroides* drug pattern type IV.
[f] AMC, amoxicillin-clavulanic acid.

TABLE 4 Phenotypic characteristics of selected *Nocardia* spp. known to cause human disease[a,b]

Species	Growth at 45°C	Production of:			Hydrolysis of:						Utilization of:			
		Arylsulfatase (14 days)	Nitrate reductase	Urease	Adenine	Casein	Esculin	Hypoxanthine	Tyrosine	Xanthine	Acetamide[c]	Citrate[d]	L-Rhamnose[d]	D-Sorbitol[d]
N. abscessus	−	−	+	+	−	−	−	−	−	−	−	+	−	−
N. africana	+	+	−	−	−	+	−	−	−	−	NA	−	−	−
N. aobensis	−	NA	NA	+	−	−	NA	−	−	−	NA	−	−	−
N. asiatica	−	−	+	V	−	−	−	−	−	−	NA	+	+	−
N. beijingensis	−	NA	NA	+	−	−	−	−	−	+	NA	+	+	+
N. brasiliensis	−	−	+	+	−	+	+	+	+	−	−	+	−	−
N. brevicatena	−	−	−	−	−	−	+	−	−	−	−	−	−	−
N. carnea	−	NA	+	−	−	−	+	−	−	−	NA	−	−	+
N. cyriacigeorgica	+	NA	+	−	−	−	−	−	−	−	+	−	−	−
N. farcinica	+	−	−	+	−	−	+	−	−	−	+	−	+	−
N. kruczakiae	+[e]	+	NA	NA	−	−	+	−	−	−	−	+	−	−
N. mexicana	−	−	NA	+	+	−	NA	+	−/W	−	NA	NA	+	+
N. niigatensis	−	NA	NA	V	−	−	NA	W	−	−	NA	−	−	−
N. nova	−	+	+	+	−	−	−	−	−	−	−	−	−	−
N. otitidiscaviarum	V	NA	+	+	−	−	+	+	−	+	−	−	−	−
N. paucivorans	+	NA	−	+	−	−	+	−	−	−	−	−	−	−
N. pseudobrasiliensis	−	−	−	+	+	+	+	+	+	−	NA	+	−	−
N. transvalensis complex	V	−	+	+	−	−	+	+	−	−	−	+	−	V
N. veterana	+	−	−	+	−	−	−	−	−	−	−	−	—[f]	−

[a] Symbols and abbreviations: −, negative; +, positive; NA, not available; V, variable; W, weak.
[b] From reference 34.
[c] Utilization as sole source of carbon and nitrogen.
[d] Utilization as sole source of carbon.
[e] Optimal growth.
[f] Results differ in separate publications (60, 103).

Acetamide Hydrolysis

The enzyme acylamidase hydrolyzes acetamide with the production of ammonia after incubation for 7 days at 35°C. The appropriate color change in the medium must be seen, as acetamide may be assimilated but not hydrolyzed (Remel Technical Information TI #60012-A). A positive result is a distinguishing characteristic for *N. farcinica* (250).

Antibiotic Susceptibility Testing

While various species of *Nocardia* are known to have typical antibiotic susceptibility patterns (Table 3), the use of these patterns alone for species identification should be avoided. Species belonging to "complexes" (for example, the members of the *N. nova* complex) may have identical antibiograms (59).

Arylsulfatase

The enzyme arylsulfatase hydrolyzes the bond between the sulfate group and the aromatic ring of potassium phenolphthalein disulfate incorporated in the medium. With the addition of an alkali (sodium carbonate), free phenolphthalein is released, resulting in a change of color to red in the medium (136). The CDC Actinomycete Laboratory uses a modified methodology of the Kubica method, increasing the phenolphthalein concentration from 0.001 M to 0.008 M. The test can be read at 3 days and again at 2 weeks, with most strains of *N. nova* showing positive results by 14 days. Arylsulfatase medium is available commercially, but the concentration of phenolphthalein in the product being used must be considered when comparing results obtained with results reported in the literature.

Acid Production with Carbohydrates

The "Gordon" method utilizes basal medium with individual carbohydrates; the pH indicator bromcresol purple is used (96). Oxidation of carbohydrates results in a change in medium color from purple to yellow (acid) after 3 weeks of incubation at 25 or 35°C (21). The media are not available from commercial sources.

Utilization of Carbohydrates as a Sole Carbon Source

The "Goodfellow" method tests the ability of organisms to utilize various carbohydrates as a sole source of carbon. Basal medium with a single carbon source added is inoculated with an organism suspension; positive results are noted as heavier growth on medium containing the carbohydrate than is observed on basal medium without carbohydrates, after 3 weeks of incubation at 25 or 35°C (91). The media are not available commercially.

When preparing media for both the Gordon and Goodfellow tests, some substrates must be filter sterilized rather than autoclaved.

Other Compounds as a Sole Source of Carbon

The ability of organisms to utilize compounds such as sodium citrate and gluconate as a sole carbon source is also frequently used in identification schemes.

Esculin Hydrolysis

The esculin hydrolysis test determines the ability of an organism to hydrolyze the glycoside esculin through the action of the enzyme esculinase. This test is commercially available in broth or agar form.

Gelatin Hydrolysis

The ability of an organism to produce the proteolytic gelatinases (which liquefy or hydrolyze gelatin) helps to differentiate *N. brasiliensis* and *N. pseudobrasiliensis* from the other *Nocardia* species (139). This medium is commercially available from several sources. After inoculation the test is incubated at 35°C for up to 7 days; tubes must be placed at 4°C for 15 min prior to checking for hydrolysis (139).

Middlebrook Opacification

Flores and Desmond (80) describe the ability of isolates of *N. farcinica* to opacify Middlebrook 7H10 or 7H11 agar within 2 to 10 days of incubation at 28 or 35°C. Opacification was not seen with isolates of *N. asteroides*, although in a study of a limited number of organisms, rare isolates of *N. otitidiscaviarum* and *Rhodococcus terrae* were positive for this characteristic (42).

Nitrate Reduction

This procedure tests the ability of an organism to reduce nitrate to nitrites or free nitrogen gas through the action of nitrate reductase (169). The medium is available from commercial sources.

Substrate Decomposition

The differential abilities of organisms to degrade or hydrolyze the amino acid tyrosine, the purine adenine, the purine derivatives xanthine and hypoxanthine, and the milk protein casein have been shown to be useful for differentiation of some members of *Nocardia*, *Rhodococcus*, and *Tsukamurella* (139). Typically, heavy inocula of the test organisms are placed on each of the substrate-containing agars; positive reactions are seen as clearing of the medium surrounding the colonial growth. All tests should be evaluated weekly; casein results should be recorded after 14 days' total incubation, xanthine after 3 weeks of incubation, and adenine, hypoxanthine, and tyrosine after 4 weeks' total incubation. Not all of these substrates are commercially available.

Temperature Studies

Growth at various temperatures can help differentiate among *Tsukamurella* species and among the thermophilic actinomycetes. Replicates of the same medium (usually sheep blood agar or Sabouraud dextrose agar) are inoculated with a standardized inoculum and incubated at 35 and 45°C; after 3 days of incubation (139) the amounts of growth on the two tubes or plates are compared to determine temperature tolerances. If the presence of a thermotolerant species is suspected, additional media should be incubated at 50°C.

Urease

Urease hydrolyzes urea with the production of ammonia. Wauters et al. recommend the use of a 1% urea broth with cresol red as an indicator (254). Commercially prepared urease test media are also available.

Test Systems

Several studies investigating the use of commercial panels for the identification of *Nocardia* and other aerobic actinomycetes have been published. Test systems studied include the API Zym panels (bioMérieux, Durham, N.C.) (25), Rapid Anaerobe ID and Haemophilus/Neisseria ID panels (Dade Behring, Deerfield, Ill.) (22), the API 32C Yeast panel (bioMérieux) (181), the API (Rapid) Coryne panel (with an extended database) (bioMérieux), and the RapID CB Plus System (Remel, Lenexa, Kans.) (82, 83). To date, there is insufficient evidence to establish the utility of any of these tests for the identification of the increasing number of described species.

Identification schemes proposed by Kiska et al. (139) and Wauters et al. (254) utilize phenotypic and/or enzymatic tests and have been shown to be useful for the identification of several of the commonly isolated *Nocardia* species. Neither of these algorithms has been extensively evaluated by other investigators, nor have studies been done with recently described species.

Cell Wall and Cell Membrane

Some characteristics of the cell wall and cell membranes of genera of the aerobic actinomycetes are given in Table 5. Analysis of whole-cell hydrolysates using paper and thin-layer chromatography has been used to identify various forms of diaminopimelic acid and sugars present in the peptidoglycan layer of the cell walls; the type of sugars present, combined with the type of diaminopimelic acid, allowed classification of the various genera into cell wall types (67, 224).

Since members of the aerobic actinomycetes and related genera are known to contain elevated levels of cell wall lipids, analysis of the variations in chain length, differences in the degree of saturation, and the presence of various functional groups on cell wall lipids has been evaluated for identification to the genus or species level (241). McNabb et al. used high-performance liquid chromatography and the Microbial Identification System (MIDI, Inc., Newark, Del.) to analyze the fatty acids of aerobic actinomycetes. Their results showed distinct clustering of genera into two groups based on the presence or absence of branching of the cell wall fatty acids. Results also showed significant heterogeneity among species subsequently found to be heterogeneous by molecular methods (171).

Mycolic acids, high-molecular-weight fatty acids with an α-branched, β-hydroxy structure, are thought to contribute to the staining characteristics and pathogenicity of these organisms (16). The corynebacteria and mycobacteria (which also contain mycolic acids) and those aerobic actinomycetes containing mycolic acids can be differentiated based on the number of carbon atoms of their constituent mycolic acids (Table 5). It should be noted that the number of carbon atoms making up the mycolic acids of some genera varies from one report to another.

A variety of methods have been used to evaluate the cell wall lipids and mycolic acids of the aerobic actinomycetes, including thin-layer chromatography (179), gas chromatography with mass spectrometry (11), and high-performance liquid chromatography (38). By using these methods, differences have been noted among nocardiae belonging to the *N. asteroides* complex, among *Rhodococcus* species, and among the genera *Dietzia*, *Gordonia*, and *Rhodococcus* (39, 187, 188).

Isoprenoid quinones are present in the cell membranes of most bacteria; they function in electron transport, oxidative phosphorylation, and perhaps active transport (241). Menaquinones, the type of isoprenoid quinone present in the cell membranes of the aerobic actinomycetes, vary in the number of isoprene units and in the degree of unsaturation of the C_3 isoprenyl side chain. These variations have been

TABLE 5 Morphologic and chemotaxonomic characteristics of genera of aerobic actinomycetes[a]

Genus	Aerial hyphae	Acid fast	Cell wall type[b]	Mycolic acids	No. of carbon atoms in mycolic acid	Growth in lysozyme	Menaquinone
Actinomadura	V	Neg	III	Neg	NA	NF	MK-9(H4H6H8)
Amycolatopsis	V	Neg	IV	Neg	NA	Neg	MK-9(H_2H_4)
Corynebacterium[c]	Neg	Neg	IV	Pos	22–38	NT	MK-8(H_2) or MK-9(H_2)
Dermatophilus	Pos	Neg	III	Neg	NA	NF	NF
Dietzia	Neg	Neg[d]	IV	Pos	34–38	NT	MK-8(H_2)
Gordonia	Neg	W	IV	Pos	46–66	V	MK-9(H_2)
Mycobacterium[c]	V	Pos	IV	Pos	60–90	Pos	MK-9(H_2)
Nocardia	Pos[e]	W	IV	Pos	44–64	Pos	MK-8(H_4) or MK-9(H_2)
Nocardiopsis	Pos	Neg	III	Neg	NA	NF	MK-10($H_2H_4H_6$)
Pseudonocardia	V	Neg	IV	Neg	NA	NF	MK-9(H_4)
Rhodococcus	Neg[f]	W	IV	Pos	34–52	Neg	MK-8(H_2) or MK-9(H_2)
Saccharomonospora	Pos	Neg	IV	Neg	NA	Neg	MK-9(H_4)
Saccharopolyspora	Pos	Neg	IV	Neg	NA	Neg	MK-9(H_4)
Streptomyces	Pos	Neg	I	Neg	NA	V	MK-9(H_6H_8)
Thermoactinomyces	V	NF	III	NF	NF	Pos	NF
Tsukamurella	Neg	W	IV	Pos	62–78	Pos	MK-9

[a] From references 5, 34, 57, 90, 93, 95, 111, 143, and 152. Abbreviations: V, variable; Neg, negative; NA, not applicable; Pos; positive; NT, not tested; NF, test result not found; W, weak positive.
[b] Cell wall types: I, L-DAP, no sugars; III, meso-DAP, madurose, or no sugars; IV, *meso*-DAP, arabinose, and galactose.
[c] Included for completeness; some consider *Corynebacterium* and *Mycobacterium* to be aerobic actinomycetes.
[d] Original description was Pos.
[e] Occasionally no aerial hyphae produced.
[f] Occasional rudimentary aerial hyphae seen.

found to be helpful in the differentiation of members of the aerobic actinomycetes to the genus level (57, 267). Menaquinone analysis has been particularly useful for distinguishing *Nocardia* species from other mycolic acid-containing aerobic actinomycetes (Table 5).

The equipment required for modern chromatographic procedures is generally available only in research or reference laboratories. In addition, these techniques are not applicable for identification to the species level.

Molecular Identification

Molecular techniques are currently the only methods that can provide definitive identification of most isolates of aerobic actinomycetes. These methods have the added benefit of providing identifications in a fraction of the time needed for biochemical tests.

PCR and REA

The use of PCR enables the identification of aerobic actinomycetes that have unique gene regions (chapter 16). This method has been applied to various genes such as the 16S rRNA gene (for genus level identification of *Nocardia* and *Nocardiopsis* species and species level identification of *R. equi*), the *choE* gene (*R. equi*), and a putative nonribosomal peptide synthetase gene (*N. farcinica*) (18, 32, 146, 151, 209).

PCR paired with restriction endonuclease analysis (REA) is useful for the identification of commonly isolated *Nocardia* species. The procedure takes advantage of the presence of sites within the variable regions of an organism's gene sequence (chapter 16). With REA of a portion of the heat shock protein gene (HSP), Steingrube et al. were able to differentiate among eight species of *Nocardia* and the six drug pattern types of *N. asteroides* described by Wallace (225, 229, 249). Refinement of this technique with a different restriction endonuclease set eliminated the intraspecies variability seen with the initial method and allowed recognition of *A. madurae*, *R. equi*, and *T. paurometabola* (226). In 2000, an REA technique utilizing a portion of the 16S rRNA gene which allowed differentiation of 10 species of *Nocardia* was described. Comparison of identifications obtained by REA of the 16S rRNA gene and by REA of the HSP gene showed good correlation between the two methods for most *Nocardia* isolates. Some isolates, however, gave discrepant or unknown RFLP patterns with either or both of the two genes. Subsequent 16S rRNA gene sequencing showed these isolates to be different from species already described (61). By using REA of the two gene regions, reliable identifications can be obtained for the species listed in Table 6. Species not listed are not identifiable by using the 16S rRNA gene and the listed combinations of restriction endonucleases. Two or more species, including numerous newly described species, may give identical RFLP patterns with REA of the 16S rRNA gene as determined experimentally or deduced from the 16S rRNA sequences of the organisms as listed in GenBank. RFLP patterns from REA of the HSP gene for some recently described species are not determinable, due to the lack of HSP gene sequence data. As the number of recognized species increases, the applicability of the REA method will be diminished.

In addition to its use for the identification of *Nocardia* species, REA has been used for differentiation among numerous genera of aerobic actinomycetes and for identification of some species of thermophilic actinomycetes (63, 108).

Other Molecular Methods

Ribotyping (chapter 16) has been used to identify isolates of *N. farcinica* (176) and to discriminate among four members of the *N. asteroides* complex (150). Ribotyping of *Rhodococcus* species has shown specific patterns for all rhodococcal type

TABLE 6 RFLP patterns of the type strains of selected *Nocardia* species; results of PCR-REA of the 16S rRNA gene (999 bp) and of the 65-kDA HSP gene (441 bp)[a]

Species[b]	16S rRNA RFLP					HSP RFLP		
	Expected sizes of fragments (bp)[c] after digestion with:					Expected sizes of fragments (bp)[c,d] after digestion with:		
	HinPI 1	DpnII	BstEII	SphI	HindI	MspI	HinfI	BsaHI
N. abscessus	420-350-225	700-200-95	Uncut	Uncut	—[g]	180-130-120[e]	Uncut	—
N. cyriacigeorgica	420-350-225	455-250-200-95	—	—	565-435	180-(145-130)-(120-115)	Uncut	(320-270)-75-65
N. brasiliensis	420-350-225	700-200-95	730-270	835-165	—	180-(145-130)-(120-115)	315-125	185-80-70-65
N. nova	420-350-225	640-200-95-60	—	—	—	130-110-75	Uncut	—
N. otitidiscaviarum	420-350-150-75	455-250-200-95	—	—	—	180-(145-130)-(120-115) or 305-145	315-125	(270-188)-100-80
N. pseudobrasiliensis	420-350-225	525-200-175-95	—	—	—	180-130	225-190	—
N. transvalensis complex[f]	645-350	705-200-95	—	—	—	265-180 or 265-110-70	260-190	—

[a] From references 61 and 226.
[b] Only the species listed can be discriminated by these methods; see the text.
[c] Rounded to the nearest 5 bp.
[d] Fragment sizes in parentheses indicate the range of possible fragment sizes.
[e] The HSP gene RFLP pattern for *N. abscessus* was derived from the HSP gene sequence for that organism.
[f] Includes *N. transvalensis* sensu stricto and *N. asteroides* drug pattern type IV; the 16S rRNA gene RFLP pattern for *N. asteroides* drug pattern type IV was determined experimentally.
[g] —, not needed for identification.

strains and heterogeneous patterns for members of *R. equi* and *R. rhodochrous* (126, 149).

The use of the PCR-randomly amplified polymorphic DNA (RAPD) technique (chapter 16) has shown species-specific patterns for some species of *Nocardia;* Isik et al. report that *N. nova, N. pseudobrasiliensis, N. transvalensis,* and isolates identified as *N. asteroides* show a variety of patterns (122); it is not clear if the variations reported by these authors represent the presence of additional unrecognized species, within-species variation, or both.

The use of DNA probes has been evaluated for *Streptomyces* species (223), and Brownell reported that six different probes were needed to hybridize with isolates identified as "*N. asteroides*" (33).

Gene Sequencing

Gene sequencing has become a powerful tool for the identification of this complex group of organisms. Sequence analysis of the 16S rRNA gene has been used for the species level identification of members of nearly all genera of the aerobic actinomycetes (7, 17, 116, 133, 166, 185, 203, 207, 264).

The presence of a variable region, located near the 5′ terminus of the gene (61), has made partial 16S rRNA sequencing of a 500-bp region of the gene a useful method for the presumptive identification of many *Nocardia* species. Cloud et al. (54) compared identifications obtained with the MicroSeq 500 System (Applied BioSystems, Foster City, Calif.) with results obtained using phenotypic identifications and with sequencing results from a 999-bp region of the same gene. The 500-bp-based identification of 94 clinical isolates representing 10 species showed 72% agreement with identification obtained by phenotypic methods and 90% agreement with those obtained by sequencing a larger portion of the gene. Sequencing a larger region of the gene is necessary for the separation of members of some species pairs which have identical or nearly identical sequences within the 500-bp region (for example, *N. abscessus* and *N. asiatica,* which differ by 1 bp, and *N. elegans* and *N. veterana,* which have no base pair differences in this region). Patel et al. used the MicroSeq 500 system to determine the 16S rRNA gene sequences of 28 reference strains and 71 clinical isolates and found significant sequence heterogeneity among isolates identified as *N. asteroides* drug pattern type II, *N. nova, N. otitidiscaviarum,* and *N. transvalensis*. This method was also shown to be useful for the identification of *Gordonia, Rhodococcus, Streptomyces,* and *Tsukamurella* species to the genus level (192). At present, the MicroSeq 500 System is capable of distinguishing among the more commonly isolated *Nocardia* species. However, as the number of described species increases, the number of species that can be unambiguously identified using 500-bp sequences will probably decrease.

Sequence analysis of a 441-bp fragment of the 65-kDa heat shock protein gene has been shown to have sufficient variation to allow identification of 42 type or reference strains of *Nocardia* (206) and may be more discriminatory than sequence analysis of the 16S rRNA gene.

The use of an alternative gene, the *secA1* gene, has been reported (P. S. Conville, A. M. Zelazny, and F. G. Witebsky. *Abstr. 105th Gen. Meet. Am. Soc. Microbiol.* 2005, abstr. C-152, p. 134). Analysis of the *secA1* gene sequences of 31 species of *Nocardia* has shown this gene to be more variable than the 16S rRNA gene; it therefore provides greater discrimination among *Nocardia* species. In addition, in the case of genes that code for essential proteins, translation of the gene sequence into an amino acid sequence may be useful to eliminate some within-species microheterogeneities.

For some genera, such as *Nocardia*, sequence analysis of more than one gene may be useful for the recognition of new species.

There is no consensus on how similar sequences must be to consider isolates to belong to the same species. This is a very real problem with isolates of *Nocardia*, as some species possess 16S rRNA gene sequences that are between 99.5 and 99.8% similar to those of another species, yet are distinct species by DNA-DNA hybridization (59, 269). In addition, users of gene sequence data must be careful to consider gene similarity data in relation to the size of the region sequenced; some sequence differences may not be significant if a larger portion of the gene is analyzed (53).

The presence of multiple 16S rRNA genes in *N. nova* isolates has recently been reported (62). It is unclear how the presence of multiple genes with significant sequence differences will affect the ability to identify these isolates.

Species described based on characteristics of a single isolate present problems for laboratories attempting to make identification decisions; the phenotypic characteristics described may not reflect the typical reactions of the species that would be determined if more isolates were analyzed (123). In addition, for single isolates there is no information available concerning sequence variability (49) (see also chapter 19).

Users of any sequence database used for species identification should be aware of the limitations inherent in that database. The GenBank database includes the most extensive collection of sequences, and an informed user can utilize it to make identification decisions. The proprietary database used with the MicroSeq System (Applied BioSystems) for the identification of *Nocardia* species is limited in the species represented and in the number of sequences of each species it contains. Cloud et al. expanded this database with additional entries to obtain better matches for query organisms (54). The Ribosomal Differentiation of Medical Microorganisms (RIDOM) is a quality-controlled database (177), but the portion pertaining to *Nocardia* is not available for public use. Ideally, the isolate from which the top-choice sequence was obtained should be the type strain of the species, and because of method improvements, it should have been submitted after 1995. Any top choice that appears to be out of place with other closely related sequences should be further examined to ensure that it has not appeared as a result of errors in its sequence or its identification.

DNA-DNA Hybridization

Despite the lack of a single standardized DNA-DNA hybridization procedure (220), the use of the procedure may be required for definitive species level discrimination of some isolates which have a high degree of sequence similarity (59).

TYPING SYSTEMS

In a study of *N. farcinica* isolates recovered from heart transplant recipients, Exmelin et al. compared the use of RAPD and ribotyping techniques for strain typing. They found RAPD better able than ribotyping to differentiate outbreak strains from unrelated strains (79). For strain typing with RAPD, isolates initially must be proven to belong to the same species; in this case chemotaxonomic and phenotypic methods identified the outbreak strains as *N. farcinica* (79). Blümel et al. used pulsed-field gel electrophoresis to demonstrate the relatedness of 18 isolates of *N. farcinica* from postoperative wound infections in a surgical ward over an 11-year period; these isolates were unrelated to isolates recovered from other environmental locations (23).

Recently, Yamamura used repetitive sequence-based PCR (rep-PCR) to distinguish strains identified as *N. asteroides* from unrelated clinical isolates and from different ecologic sources (265). This study showed each isolate to have a distinct banding pattern.

SEROLOGIC METHODS

Serologic methods for the detection of antibody response to nocardial infections have been shown to be lacking in sensitivity and specificity. A variety of methodologies and antigens have been evaluated, including immunodiffusion, complement fixation, enzyme-linked immunosorbent assay, and immunoblot techniques. Cell-free culture filtrates, cell homogenates, and specific high-molecular-weight proteins have been studied as sources of antigens. Most methods show considerable cross-reactivity with antibodies produced against *M. tuberculosis*. Such cross-reactivity is problematic, as tuberculosis usually is included in the differential diagnosis of patients with suspected pulmonary or CNS nocardiosis. In addition, serologic assays may not be sensitive enough to detect antibodies in patients who have diminished immunologic responses, and these are the very ones who are most prone to nocardial infections (6, 24, 118, 213, 227, 228).

SUSCEPTIBILITY TESTING

The Clinical Laboratory Standards Institute (CLSI, formerly NCCLS) has published an approved standard for susceptibility testing of both mycobacteria and aerobic actinomycetes (186). The recommended procedure for the aerobic actinomycetes is broth microdilution (55). The applicability of the procedure to the genera other than *Nocardia*, such as *Rhodococcus*, is currently under discussion. Incubation of plates is at 37°C in ambient air for 3 to 5 days, the length of time depending on the particular species being tested. Both an MIC value and an interpretation of the MIC result should be provided. Currently the interpretive breakpoints for three drugs, amikacin, minocycline, and sulfamethoxazole, differ from the breakpoints recommended for rapidly growing aerobic bacteria (55).

Susceptibility testing should be performed on all isolates of aerobic actinomycetes thought to be of possible clinical significance and especially for isolates from patients for whom a sulfonamide cannot be used. It is recommended that laboratories not performing such testing on a regular basis send isolates to an experienced reference laboratory. Antimicrobial agents recommended for primary susceptibility testing are amikacin, amoxicillin-clavulanic acid, ceftriaxone, ciprofloxacin, clarithromycin, imipenem, linezolid, minocycline, sulfamethoxazole or trimethoprim-sulfamethoxazole, and tobramycin. Agents to be considered for secondary testing include cefepime, cefotaxime, doxycycline, or moxifloxacin, and gentamicin. A few drugs with trailing endpoints, such as the sulfonamides and linezolid, may present interpretive problems. Most isolates of *Nocardia* species are susceptible to trimethoprim-sulfamethoxazole; one should be careful not to assume too readily that an isolate is resistant to this combination of drugs. Additionally, most, if not all, isolates of *Nocardia* species are susceptible in vitro to linezolid (35).

Table 3 shows the typical susceptibility patterns for the different *Nocardia* species for which adequate data are available.

EVALUATION, INTERPRETATION, AND REPORTING

The aerobic actinomycetes are widespread in the environment. Therefore, particularly when an aerobic actinomycete is isolated in culture without having been visualized in the direct patient specimen, it may be impossible for the laboratory to know if the isolate is the result of specimen or laboratory contamination, patient colonization, or actual infection. Some indication of the quantity of organism present should be given for any isolate of an aerobic actinomycete. Discussion between the clinical and laboratory staff is extremely useful for selection of additional patient specimens and laboratory procedures for determination of the clinical significance of an isolate from a given patient. Identification of an organism to the genus level may help determine its significance. However, even for accurate genus assignment, molecular methods may need to be employed.

When an isolate is reported to the species level, the laboratory should be certain that clinicians are aware of the reliability of the identification method used. It is possible to identify the more commonly encountered aerobic actinomycetes, particularly *Nocardia* species, with moderate accuracy to the species level by using phenotypic methods (Table 4) (254), but some will inevitably be misidentified by such procedures. Precise identification can be achieved only by molecular methods. For accurate determination of both identification and susceptibility pattern, referral to a laboratory with expertise in working with these organisms may be necessary.

We gratefully acknowledge the assistance of Yvonne R. Shea in the preparation of the colony photographs.

REFERENCES

1. **Adair, J. C., I. J. Amber, and J. M. Johnston.** 1987. Peritonsillar abscess caused by *Nocardia asteroides*. *J. Clin. Microbiol.* **25:**2214–2215.
2. **Ajello, L., and J. Brown.** 1987. Actinomycetoma caused by *Nocardiopsis dassonvillei*. *Arch. Dermatol.* **123:**426.
3. **Alcaide, M. L., L. Espinoza, and L. Abbo.** 2004. Cavitary pneumonia secondary to *Tsukamurella* in an AIDS patient. First case and a review of the literature. *J. Infect.* **49:**17–19.
4. **Almehmi, A., A. K. Pfister, R. McCowan, and S. Matulis.** 2004. Implantable cardioverter-defibrillator infection caused by *Tsukamurella*. *W. V. Med. J.* **100:**185–186.
5. **Anderson, A. S., and E. M. H. Wellington.** 2001. The taxonomy of *Streptomyces* and related genera. *Int. J. Syst. Evol. Microbiol.* **51:**797–814.
6. **Angeles, A. M., and A. M. Sugar.** 1987. Rapid diagnosis of nocardiosis with an enzyme immunoassay. *J. Infect. Dis.* **155:**292–296.
7. **Arenskötter, M., D. Bröker, and A. Steinbücher.** 2004. Biology of the metabolically diverse genus *Gordonia*. *Appl. Environ. Microbiol.* **70:**3195–3204.
8. **Arya, B., S. Hussian, and S. Hariharan.** 2004. *Rhodococcus equi* pneumonia in a renal transplant patient: a case report and review of literature. *Clin. Transplant.* **18:**748–752.
9. **Asoh, N., H. Watanabe, M. Fines-Guyon, K. Watanabe, K. Oishi, W. Kositsakulchai, T. Sanchai, K. Kunsuikmengrai, S. Kahintapong, B. Khantawa, P. Tharavichitkul, T. Sirisanthana, and T. Nagatake.** 2003. Emergence of rifampin-resistant *Rhodococcus equi* with several types of mutations in the *rpoB* gene among AIDS patients in northern Thailand. *J. Clin. Microbiol.* **41:**2337–2340.
10. **Auerbach, S. B., M. M. McNeil, J. M. Brown, B. A. Lasker, and W. R. Jarvis.** 1992. Outbreak of pseudoinfection with *Tsukamurella paurometabolum* traced to laboratory contamination: efficacy of joint epidemiological and laboratory investigation. *Clin. Infect. Dis.* **14:**1015–1022.
11. **Baba, T., Y. Nishiuchi, and I. Yano.** 1997. Composition of mycolic acid molecular species as a criterion in nocardial classification. *Int. J. Syst. Bacteriol.* **47:**795–801.
12. **Baddour, L. M., V. S. Baselski, M. J. Herr, G. D. Christensen, and A. L. Bisno.** 1986. Nocardiosis in recipients of renal transplants: evidence for nosocomial acquisition. *Am. J. Infect. Control* **14:**214–219.
13. **Bakker, X. R., P. H. M. Spauwen, and W. M. V. Dolmans.** 2004. Mycetoma of the hand caused by *Gordona terrae*: a case report. *J. Hand Surg.* **29B:**188–190.
14. **Baril, L., P. Boiron, V. Manceron, S. O. O. Ely, P. Jamet, E. Favre, E. Caumes, and F. Bricaire.** 1999. Refractory craniofacial actinomycetoma due to *Streptomyces somaliensis* that required salvage therapy with amikacin and imipenem. *Clin. Infect. Dis.* **29:**460–461.
15. **Baron, E. J., J. D. Scott, and L. S. Tompkins.** 2005. Prolonged incubation and extensive subculturing do not increase recovery of clinically significant microorganisms from standard automated blood cultures. *Clin. Infect. Dis.* **41:**1677–1680.
16. **Beaman, B. L., and L. Beaman.** 1994. *Nocardia* species: host-parasite relationships. *Clin. Microbiol. Rev.* **7:**213–264.
17. **Beau, F., C. Bollet, T. Coton, E. Garnotel, and M. Drancourt.** 1999. Molecular identification of a *Nocardiopsis dassonvillei* blood isolate. *J. Clin. Microbiol.* **37:**3366–3368.
18. **Bell, K. S., J. C. Philip, N. Christofi, and D. W. J. Aw.** 1996. Identification of *Rhodococcus equi* using the polymerase chain reaction. *Lett. Appl. Microbiol.* **23:**72–74.
19. **Bell, K. S., J. C. Philp, D. W. J. Aw, and N. Christofi.** 1998. The genus *Rhodococcus*. *J. Appl. Microbiol.* **85:**195–210.
20. **Bemer-Melchior, P., A. Haloun, P. Riegel, and H. B. Drugeon.** 1999. Bacteremia due to *Dietzia maris* in an immunocompromised patient. *Clin. Infect. Dis.* **29:**1338–1340.
21. **Berd, D.** 1973. Laboratory identification of clinically important aerobic actinomycetes. *Appl. Microbiol.* **25:**665–681.
22. **Biehle, J. R., S. J. Cavalieri, T. Felland, and B. L. Zimmer.** 1996. Novel method for rapid identification of *Nocardia* species by detection of preformed enzymes. *J. Clin. Microbiol.* **34:**103–107.
23. **Blümel, J., E. Blümel, A. F. Yassin, H. Schmidt-Rotte, and K. P. Schaal.** 1998. Typing of *Nocardia farcinica* by pulsed-field gel electrophoresis reveals an endemic strain as source of hospital infections. *J. Clin. Microbiol.* **36:**118–122.
24. **Blumer, S. O., and L. Kaufman.** 1979. Microimmunodiffusion test for nocardiosis. *J. Clin. Microbiol.* **10:**308–312.
25. **Boiron, P., and F. Provost.** 1990. Enzymatic characterization of *Nocardia* spp. and related bacteria by API ZYM profile. *Mycopathologia* **110:**51–56.
26. **Bopp, C. A., J. W. Sumner, G. K. Morris, and J. G. Wells.** 1981. Isolation of *Legionella* spp. from environmental water samples by low-pH treatment and use of a selective medium. *J. Clin. Microbiol.* **13:**714–719.
27. **Bottei, E., J. P. Flaherty, L. J. Kaplan, and L. Duffee-Kerr.** 1994. Lymphocutaneous *Nocardia brasiliensis* infection transmitted via a cat scratch: a second case. *Clin. Infect. Dis.* **18:**649–650.
28. **Breitkopf, C., D. Hammel, H. H. Scheld, G. Peters, and K. Becker.** 2005. Impact of a molecular approach to improve the microbiological diagnosis of infective heart valve endocarditis. *Circulation* **111:**1415–1421.
29. **Bross, J. E., and G. Gordon.** 1991. Nocardial meningitis: case reports and review. *Rev. Infect. Dis.* **13:**160–165.
30. **Brown, B. A., J. O. Lopes, R. W. Wilson, J. M. Costa, A. C. deVargas, S. H. Alves, C. Klock, G. O. Onyi, and R. J. Wallace, Jr.** 1999. Disseminated *Nocardia pseudobrasiliensis* infection in a patient with AIDS in Brasil. *Clin. Infect. Dis.* **28:**144–145.

31. **Brown, E., and E. Hendler.** 1989. *Rhodococcus* peritonitis in a patient treated with peritoneal dialysis. *Am. J. Kidney Dis.* **14:**417–418.
32. **Brown, J. M., K. N. Pham, M. M. McNeil, and B. A. Lasker.** 2004. Rapid identification of *Nocardia farcinica* clinical isolates by a PCR assay targeting a 314-base-pair species-specific DNA fragment. *J. Clin. Microbiol.* **42:**3655–3660.
33. **Brownell, G. H., and K. E. Belcher.** 1990. DNA probes for the identification of *Nocardia asteroides*. *J. Clin. Microbiol.* **28:**2082–2086.
34. **Brown-Elliott, B. A., J. M. Brown, P. S. Conville, and R. J. Wallace, Jr.** 2006. Clinical and laboratory features of the *Nocardia* spp. based on current molecular taxonomy. *Clin. Microbiol. Rev.* **19:**259–282.
35. **Brown-Elliott, B. A., S. C. Ward, C. J. Crist, L. B. Mann, R. W. Wilson, and R. J. Wallace, Jr.** 2001. In vitro activities of linezolid against multiple *Nocardia* species. *Antimicrob. Agents Chemother.* **45:**1295–1297.
36. **Buchman, A. L., M. M. McNeil, J. M. Brown, B. A. Lasker, and M. E. Ament.** 1992. Central venous catheter sepsis caused by unusual *Gordona (Rhodococcus)* species: identification with a digoxigenin-labeled rDNA probe. *Clin. Infect. Dis.* **15:**694–697.
37. **Bunker, M. L., L. Chewning, S. E. Wang, and M. A. Gordon.** 1988. *Dermatophilus congolensis* and "hairy" leukoplakia. *Am. J. Clin. Pathol.* **89:**683–687.
38. **Butler, W. R., D. G. Ahearn, and J. O. Kilburn.** 1986. High-performance liquid chromatography of mycolic acids as a tool in the identification of *Corynebacterium*, *Nocardia*, *Rhodococcus*, and *Mycobacterium* species. *J. Clin. Microbiol.* **23:**182–185.
39. **Butler, W. R., J. O. Kilburn, and G. P. Kubica.** 1987. High performance liquid chromatography analysis of mycolic acids as an aid in laboratory identification of *Rhodococcus* and *Nocardia* species. *J. Clin. Microbiol.* **25:**2126–2131.
40. **Carey, J., M. Motyl, and D. C. Perlman.** 2001. Catheter-related bacteremia due to *Streptomyces* in a patient receiving holistic infusions. *Emerg. Infect. Dis.* **7:**1043–1045.
41. **Carriere, C., H. Marchandin, J. M. Andrieu, A. Vandome, and C. Perez.** 1999. *Nocardia* thyroiditis: unusual location of infection. *J. Clin. Microbiol.* **37:**2323–2325.
42. **Carson, M., and A. Hellyar.** 1994. Opacification of Middlebrook agar as an aid in distinguishing *Nocardia farcinica* within the *Nocardia asteroides* complex. *J. Clin. Microbiol.* **32:**2270–2271.
43. **Casella, P., A. Tommasi, and A. M. Tortotano.** 1987. Peritonite da *Gordona aurantiaca (Rhodococcus aurantiacus)* in dialisi peritoneale ambulatoria continua. *Microbiologia Medica* **2:**47–48.
44. **Castro, L. G. M., W. Belda, Jr., A. Salebian, and L. C. Cucé.** 1993. Mycetoma: a retrospective study of 41 cases seen in São Paulo, Brazil, from 1978 to 1989. *Mycoses* **36:**89–95.
45. **Chávez, G., R. Estrada, and A. Bonifaz.** 2002. Perianal actinomycetoma experience of 20 cases. *Int. J. Dermatol.* **41:**491–493.
46. **Chong, Y., K. Lee, C. Y. Chon, M. J. Kim, O. H. Kwon, and H. J. Lee.** 1997. *Tsukamurella inchonensis* bacteremia in a patient who ingested hydrochloric acid. *Clin. Infect. Dis.* **24:**1267–1268.
47. **Chouciño, C., S. A. Goodman, J. P. Greer, R. S. Stein, S. N. Wolff, and J. S. Dummer.** 1996. Nocardial infections in bone marrow transplant recipients. *Clin. Infect. Dis.* **23:**1012–1019.
48. **Chow, K. M., C. C. Szeto, V. C.-Y. Chow, T. Y. -H. Wong, and P. K.-T. Li.** 2003. *Rhodococcus equi* peritonitis in continuous ambulatory peritoneal dialysis. *J. Nephrol.* **16:**736–739.
49. **Christensen, H., M. Bisgaard, W. Frederiksen, R. Mutters, P. Kuhnert, and J. E. Olsen.** 2001. Is characterization of a single isolate sufficient for valid publication of a new genus or species? Proposal to modify Recommendation 30b of the *Bacteriological Code* (1990 Revision). *Int. J. Syst. Evol. Microbiol.* **51:**2221–2225.
50. **Christidou, A., S. Maraki, E. Scoulica, E. Mantadakis, S. Agelaki, and G. Samonis.** 2004. Fatal *Nocardia farcinica* bacteremia in a patient with lung cancer. *Diagn. Microbiol. Infect. Dis.* **50:**135–139.
51. **Chun, J., S.-O. Kang, Y. C. Hah, and M. Goodfellow.** 1996. Phylogeny of mycolic acid-containing actinomycetes. *J. Ind. Microbiol.* **17:**205–213.
52. **Clark, N. M., D. K. Braun, A. Pasternak, and C. E. Chenoweth.** 1995. Primary cutaneous *Nocardia otitidiscaviarum* infection: case report and review. *Clin. Infect. Dis.* **20:**1266–1270.
53. **Clarridge, J. E.** 2004. Impact of 16S rRNA gene sequence analysis for identification of bacteria on clinical microbiology and infectious diseases. *Clin. Microbiol. Rev.* **17:**840–862.
54. **Cloud, J. L., P. S. Conville, A. Croft, D. Harmsen, F. G. Witebsky, and K. C. Carroll.** 2004. Evaluation of partial 16S ribosomal DNA sequencing for identification of *Nocardia* species by using the MicroSeq 500 system with an expanded database. *J. Clin. Microbiol.* **42:**578–584.
55. **CLSI.** 2005. *Performance Standards for Antimicrobial Susceptibility Testing: Fifteenth Informational Supplement.* CLSI document M100-S15. Clinical and Laboratory Standards Institute, Wayne, Pa.
56. **Cohen, E., D. Blickstein, E. Inbar, Z. Samra, and M. Weinberger.** 2000. Unilateral vocal cord paralysis as a result of a *Nocardia farcinica* laryngeal abscess. *Eur. J. Clin. Microbiol. Infect. Dis.* **19:**224–227.
57. **Collins, M. D., M. Goodfellow, D. E. Minnikin, and G. Alderson.** 1985. Menaquinone composition of mycolic acid-containing actinomycetes and some sporoactinomycetes. *J. Appl. Bacteriol.* **58:**77–86.
58. **Collins, M. D., J. Smida, M. Dorsch, and E. Stackebrandt.** 1988. *Tsukamurella* gen. nov. harboring *Corynebacterium paurometabolum* and *Rhodococcus aurantiacus*. *Int. J. Syst. Bacteriol.* **38:**385–391.
59. **Conville, P. S., J. M. Brown, A. G. Steigerwalt, J. W. Lee, V. L. Anderson, J. T. Fishbain, S. M. Holland, and F. G. Witebsky.** 2004. *Nocardia kruczakiae* sp. nov., a pathogen in immunocompromised patients and a member of the "*N. nova* complex." *J. Clin. Microbiol.* **42:**5139–5145.
60. **Conville, P. S., J. M. Brown, A. G. Steigerwalt, J. W. Lee, D. E. Byrer, V. L. Anderson, S. E. Dorman, S. M. Holland, B. Cahill, K. C. Carroll, and F. G. Witebsky.** 2003. *Nocardia veterana* as a pathogen in North American patients. *J. Clin. Microbiol.* **41:**2560–2568.
61. **Conville, P. S., S. H. Fischer, C. P. Cartwright, and F. G. Witebsky.** 2000. Identification of *Nocardia* species by restriction endonuclease analysis of an amplified portion of the 16S rRNA gene. *J. Clin. Microbiol.* **38:**158–164.
62. **Conville, P. S., and F. G. Witebsky.** 2005. Multiple copies of the 16S rRNA gene in *Nocardia nova* isolates and implications for sequence-based identification procedures. *J. Clin. Microbiol.* **43:**2881–2885.
63. **Cook, A. E., and P. R. Meyers.** 2003. Rapid identification of filamentous actinomycetes to the genus level using genus-specific 16S rRNA gene restriction fragment patterns. *Int. J. Syst. Evol. Microbiol.* **53:**1907–1915.
64. **Cornish, N., and J. A. Washington.** 1999. *Rhodococcus equi* infections: clinical features and laboratory diagnosis. *Curr. Clin. Top. Infect. Dis.* **19:**198–215.
65. **Couble, A., V. Rodríguez-Nava, M. P. de Montclos, P. Boiron, and F. Laurent.** 2005. Direct detection of *Nocardia*

spp. in clinical samples by a rapid molecular method. *J. Clin. Microbiol.* **43:**1921–1924.

66. **Cuello, O. H., M. J. Caorlin, V. E. Reviglio, L. Carvajal, C. P. Juarez, E. P. deGuerra, and J. D. Luna.** 2002. *Rhodococcus globerulus* keratitis after laser in situ keratomileusis. *J. Cataract Refract. Surg.* **28:**2235–2237.
67. **Cummins, C. S.** 1962. Chemical composition and antigenic structure of cell walls of *Corynebacterium, Mycobacterium, Nocardia, Actinomyces* and *Arthrobacter*. *J. Gen. Microbiol.* **28:**35–50.
68. **Daikos, G. L., V. Syriopoulou, M. Horianopoulou, M. Kanellopoulou, M. Martsoukou, and E. Papafrangas.** 2003. Successful antimicrobial chemotherapy for *Nocardia asteroides* prosthetic valve endocarditis. *Am. J. Med.* **115:**330–332.
69. **DeMarais, P. L., and F. E. Kocka.** 1995. *Rhodococcus* meningitis in an immunocompetent host. *Clin. Infect. Dis.* **20:**167–169.
70. **Donahue, J. M., N. M. Williams, and D. P. Labeda.** 2002. *Crossiella equi* sp. nov., isolated from equine placentas. *Int. J. Syst. Evol. Microbiol.* **52:**2169–2173.
71. **Dorman, S. E., S. V. Guide, P. S. Conville, E. S. DeCarlo, H. L. Malech, J. I. Gallin, F. G. Witebsky, and S. M. Holland.** 2002. *Nocardia* infection in chronic granulomatous disease. *Clin. Infect. Dis.* **35:**390–394.
72. **Drancourt, M., M. M. McNeil, J. M. Brown, B. A. Lasker, M. Maurin, M. Choux, and D. Raoult.** 1994. Brain abscess due to *Gordona terrae* in an immunocompromised child: case report and review of infections caused by *G. terrae*. *Clin. Infect. Dis.* **19:**258–262.
73. **Drancourt, M., J. Pelletier, A. Ali Cherif, and D. Raoult.** 1997. *Gordona terrae* central nervous system infection in an immunocompetent patient. *J. Clin. Microbiol.* **35:**379–382.
74. **Dunne, E. F., W. J. Burman, and M. L. Wilson.** 1998. *Streptomyces* pneumonia in a patient with human immunodeficiency virus infection: case report and review of the literature on invasive *Streptomyces* infections. *Clin. Infect. Dis.* **27:**93–96.
75. **Eggink, C. A., P. Wesseling, P. Boiron, and J. F. G. M. Meis.** 1997. Severe keratitis due to *Nocardia farcinica*. *J. Clin. Microbiol.* **35:**999–1001.
76. **Eisenblätter, M., U. Disko, G. Stoltenburg-Didinger, H. Scherübl, K. P. Schaal, A. Roth, R. Ignatius, M. Zeitz, H. Hahn, and J. Wagner.** 2002. Isolation of *Nocardia paucivorans* from the cerebrospinal fluid of a patient with relapse of cerebral nocardiosis. *J. Clin. Microbiol.* **40:**3532–3534.
77. **Ekkelenkamp, M. B., W. de Jong, W. Hustinx, and S. Thijsen.** 2004. *Streptomyces thermovulgaris* bacteremia in Crohn's disease patient. *Emerg. Infect. Dis.* **10:**1883–1885.
78. **Emmons, W., B. Reichwein, and D. L. Winslow.** 1991. *Rhodococcus equi* infection in the patient with AIDS: literature review and report of an unusual case. *Rev. Infect. Dis.* **13:**91–96.
79. **Exmelin, L., B. Malbruny, M. Vergnaud, F. Provost, P. Boiron, and C. Morel.** 1996. Molecular study of nosocomial nocardiosis outbreak involving heart transplant recipients. *J. Clin. Microbiol.* **34:**1014–1016.
80. **Flores, M., and E. P. Desmond.** 1993. Opacification of Middlebrook agar as an aid in identification of *Nocardia farcinica*. *J. Clin. Microbiol.* **31:**3040–3041.
81. **Forbes, G. M., F. A. H. Harvey, J. N. Philpott-Howard, J. G. O'Grady, R. D. Jensen, M. Sahathevan, M. W. Casewell, and R. Williams.** 1990. Nocardiosis in liver transplantation: variation in presentation, diagnosis and therapy. *J. Infect.* **20:**11–19.
82. **Funke, G., K. Peters, and M. Aravena-Roman.** 1998. Evaluation of the RapID CB Plus system for identification of coryneform bacteria and *Listeria* spp. *J. Clin. Microbiol.* **36:**2439–2442.
83. **Funke, G., F. N. R. Renaud, J. Freney, and P. Riegel.** 1997. Multicenter evaluation of the updated and extended API (RAPID) Coryne Database 2. 0. *J. Clin. Microbiol.* **35:** 3122–3126.
84. **Fux, C., T. Bodmer, H. R. Ziswiler, and S. L. Leib.** 2003. *Nocardia cyriacigeorgici*. First report of invasive human infection. *Dtsch. Med. Wochenschr.* **128:**1038–1041.
85. **Georghiou, P. R., and Z. M. Blacklock.** 1992. Infection with *Nocardia* species in Queensland. *Med. J. Aust.* **156:**692–697.
86. **Gillum, R. L., S. M. H. Qadri, M. N. Al-Ahdal, D. H. Connor, and A. J. Strano.** 1988. Pitted keratolysis: a manifestation of human dermatophilosis. *Dermatologica* **177:**305–308.
87. **Godreuil, S., M.-N. Didelot, C. Perez, A. Leflèche, P. Boiron, J. Reynes, F. Laurent, H. Jean-Pierre, and H. Marchandin.** 2003. *Nocardia veterana* isolated from ascitic fluid of a patient with human immunodeficiency virus infection. *J. Clin. Microbiol.* **41:**2768–2773.
88. **Golub, B., G. Falk, and W. Spink.** 1967. Lung abscess due to *Corynebacterium equi*. *Ann. Intern. Med.* **66:** 1174–1177.
89. **Goodfellow, M.** 1989. Genus *Rhodococcus* Zopf 1891, p. 2362–2371. *In* S. T. Williams, M. E. Sharpe, and J. G. Holt (ed.), *Bergey's Manual of Systematic Bacteriology,* vol. 4. Williams and Wilkins, Baltimore, Md.
90. **Goodfellow, M.** 1998. *Nocardia* and related genera, p. 463–489. *In* L. Collier, A. Balows, and M. Sussman (ed.), *Topley and Wilson's Microbiology and Microbial Infections,* vol. 2. Arnold, London, United Kingdom.
91. **Goodfellow, M.** 1971. Numerical taxonomy of some nocardioform bacteria. *J. Gen. Microbiol.* **69:**33–80.
92. **Goodfellow, M., G. Alderson, and J. Chun.** 1998. Rhodococcal systematics: problems and developments. *Antonie Leeuwenhoek* **74:**3–20.
93. **Goodfellow, M., and M. P. Lechevalier.** 1989. Genus *Nocardia* Trevisan 1889, p. 2350–2361. *In* S. T. Williams, M. E. Sharpe, and J. G. Holt (ed.), *Bergey's Manual of Systematic Bacteriology,* vol. 4. Williams and Wilkins, Baltimore, Md.
94. **Gopaul, D., C. Ellis, A. Maki, Jr., and M. G. Joseph.** 1988. Isolation of *Rhodococcus rhodochrous* from a chronic corneal ulcer. *Diagn. Microbiol. Infect. Dis.* **10:**185–190.
95. **Gordon, M. A.** 1989. Genus *Dermatophilus*, p. 2409–2410. *In* S. T. Williams, M. E. Sharpe, and J. G. Holt (ed.), *Bergey's Manual of Systematic Bacteriology,* vol. 4. Williams and Wilkins, Baltimore, Md.
96. **Gordon, R. E., D. A. Barnett, J. E. Handerhan, and C. H.-N. Pang.** 1974. *Nocardia coeliaca, Nocardia autotrophica*, and the nocardin strain. *Int. J. Syst. Bacteriol.* **24:**54–63.
97. **Gordon, R. E., and J. M. Mihm.** 1962. Identification of *Nocardia caviae* (Erikson) nov. comb. *Ann. N. Y. Acad. Sci.* **98:**628–636.
98. **Gordon, R. E., and J. M. Mihm.** 1962. The type species of the genus *Nocardia*. *J. Gen. Microbiol.* **27:**1–10.
99. **Gordon, R. E., S. K. Mishra, and D. A. Barnett.** 1978. Some bits and pieces of the genus *Nocardia: N. carnea, N. vaccinii, N. transvalensis, N. orientalis* and *N. aerocolonigenes*. *J. Gen. Microbiol.* **109:**69–78.
100. **Gorevic, P. D., E. I. Katler, and B. Agus.** 1980. Pulmonary nocardiosis occurrence in men with systemic lupus erythematosus. *Arch. Intern. Med.* **140:**361–363.
101. **Granel, F., A. Lozniewski, A. Barbaud, C. Lion, M. Dailloux, M. Weber, and J.-L. Schmutz.** 1996. Cutaneous infection caused by *Tsukamurella paurometabolum*. *Clin. Infect. Dis.* **23:**839–840.
102. **Guerrero, M. F., J. M. Ramos, G. Renedo, I. Gadea, and A. Alix.** 1999. Pulmonary malacoplakia associated with

Rhodococcus equi infection in patients with AIDS: case report and review. *Clin. Infect. Dis.* **28:**1334–1336.

103. **Gürtler, V., B. C. Mayall, and R. Seviour.** 2004. Can whole genome analysis refine the taxonomy of the genus *Rhodococcus*? *FEMS Microbiol. Rev.* **28:**377–403.
104. **Gürtler, V., R. Smith, B. C. Mayall, G. Pötter-Reinemann, E. Stackebrandt, and R. M. Kroppenstedt.** 2001. *Nocardia veterana* sp. nov., isolated from human bronchial lavage. *Int. J. Syst. Evol. Microbiol.* **51:**933–936.
105. **Gutmann, L., F. W. Goldstein, M. D. Kitzis, B. Hautefort, C. Darmon, and J. F. Acar.** 1983. Susceptibility of *Nocardia asteroides* to 46 antibiotics, including 22 β-lactams. *Antimicrob. Agents Chemother.* **23:**248–251.
106. **Harman, M., S. Sekin, and S. Akdeniz.** 2001. Human dermatophilosis mimicking ringworm. *Br. J. Dermatol.* **145:**170–171.
107. **Hart, D. H. L., M. M. Peel, J. H. Andrew, and J. G. W. Burdon.** 1988. Lung infection caused by *Rhodococcus*. *Aust. N. Z. J. Med.* **18:**790–791.
108. **Harvey, I., Y. Cormier, C. Beaulieu, V. N. Akimov, A. Mériaux, and C. Duchaine.** 2001. Random amplified ribosomal DNA restriction analysis for rapid identification of thermophilic actinomycete-like bacteria involved in hypersensitivity pneumonitis. *Syst. Appl. Microbiol.* **24:**277–284.
109. **Hellyar, A. G.** 1988. Experience with *Nocardia asteroides* in renal transplant recipients. *J. Hosp. Infect.* **12:**13–18.
110. **Hemmersbach-Miller, M., A. C. Martel, A. Bordes Benítez, and A. O. Sosa.** 2004. Brain abscess due to *Nocardia otitidiscaviarum*: report of a case and review. *Scand. J. Infect. Dis.* **36:**381–383.
111. **Henssen, A.** 1989. Genus *Pseudonocardia*, p. 2376–2378. *In* S. T. Williams, M. E. Sharpe, and J. G. Holt (ed.), *Bergey's Maunual of Systematic Bacteriology*, vol. 4. Williams and Wilkins, Baltimore, Md.
112. **Hitti, W., and M. Wolff.** 2005. Two cases of multidrug resistant *Nocardia farcinica* infection in immunosuppressed patients and implications for empiric therapy. *Eur. J. Clin. Microbiol. Infect. Dis.* **24:**142–144.
113. **Holt, J. G., N. R. Kreig, P. H. A. Sneath, J. T. Staley, and S. T. Williams.** 1994. *Bergey's Manual of Determinative Bacteriology*, 9th ed. Williams and Wilkins, Baltimore, Md.
114. **Horré, R., G. Schumacher, G. Marklein, H. Stratmann, E. Wardelmann, S. Gilges, G. S. de Hoog, and K. P. Schaal.** 2002. Mycetoma due to *Pseudallescheria boydii* and co-isolation of *Nocardia abscessus* in a patient injured in road accident. Med. Mycol. **40:**525–527.
115. **Houang, E. T., I. S. Lovett, F. D. Thompson, A. R. Harrison, A. M. Joekes, and M. Goodfellow.** 1980. *Nocardia asteroides* infection—a transmissible disease. *J. Hosp. Infect.* **1:**31–40.
116. **Huang, Y., M. Pasciak, Z. Liu, Q. Xie, and A. Gamian.** 2004. *Amycolatopsis palatopharyngis* sp. nov., a potentially pathogenic actinomycete isolated from a human clinical source. *Int. J. Syst. Evol. Microbiol.* **54:**359–363.
117. **Hudson, J. D., R. P. Danis, U. Chaluvadi, and S. D. Allen.** 2003. Posttraumatic exogenous *Nocardia* endophthalmitis. *Am. J. Ophthalmol.* **135:**915–917.
118. **Humphreys, D. W., J. G. Crowder, and A. White.** 1975. Serological reactions to *Nocardia* antigens. *Am. J. Med. Sci.* **269:**323–326.
119. **Husain, S., K. McCurry, J. Dauber, N. Singh, and S. Kusne.** 2002. *Nocardia* infection in lung transplant recipients. *J. Heart Lung Transplant.* **21:**354–359.
120. **Inamadar, A. C., A. Palit, B. V. Peerapur, and S. D. Rao.** 2004. Sporotrichoid nocardiosis caused by *Nocardia nova* in a patient infected with human immunodeficiency virus. *Int. J. Dermatol.* **43:**824–826.
121. **Ishikawa, J., A. Yamashita, Y. Mikami, Y. Hoshino, H. Kurita, K. Hotta, T. Shiba, and M. Hattori.** 2004. The complete genomic sequence of *Nocardia farcinica* IFM 10152. *Proc. Natl. Acad. Sci. USA* **101:**14925–14930.
122. **Isik, K., and M. Goodfellow.** 2002. Differentiation of *Nocardia* species by PCR-randomly amplified polymorphic DNA fingerprinting. *Syst. Appl. Microbiol.* **25:**60–67.
123. **Janda, J. M., and S. L. Abbott.** 2002. Bacterial identification for publication: when is enough enough? *J. Clin. Microbiol.* **40:**1887–1891.
124. **Jones, A. L., J. M. Brown, V. Mishra, J. D. Perry, A. G. Steigerwalt, and M. Goodfellow.** 2004. *Rhodococcus gordoniae* sp. nov., an actinomycete isolated from clinical material and phenol-contaminated soil. *Int. J. Syst. Evol. Microbiol.* **54:**407–411.
125. **Jones, R. S., T. Fekete, A. L. Truant, and V. Satishchandran.** 1994. Persistent bacteremia due to *Tsukamurella paurometabolum* in a patient undergoing hemodialysis: case report and review. *Clin. Infect. Dis.* **18:**830–832.
126. **Jorks, S.** 1996. Differentiation of *Rhodococcus* species by ribotyping. *J. Basic Microbiol.* **36:**399–406.
127. **Kageyama, A., H. Sato, M. Nagata, K. Yazawa, M. Katsu, Y. Mikami, K. Kamei, and K. Nishimura.** 2002. First human case of nocardiosis caused by *Nocardia pseudobrasiliensis* in Japan. *Mycopathologia* **156:**187–192.
128. **Kageyama, A., K. Yazawa, T. Kudo, H. Taniguchi, K. Nishimura, and Y. Mikami.** 2004. First isolates of *Nocardia abscessus* from humans and soil in Japan. *Jpn. J. Med. Mycol.* **45:**17–21.
129. **Kageyama, A., K. Yazawa, A. Mukai, M. Kinoshita, N. Takata, K. Nishimura, R. M. Kroppenstedt, and Y. Mikami.** 2004. *Nocardia shimofusensis* sp. nov., isolated from soil, and *Nocardia higoensis* sp. nov., isolated from a patient with lung nocardiosis in Japan. *Int. J. Syst. Evol. Microbiol.* **54:**1927–1931.
130. **Kageyama, A., K. Yazawa, K. Nishimura, and Y. Mikami.** 2005. *Nocardia anaemiae* sp. nov. isolated from an immunocompromised patient and the first isolation report of *Nocardia vinacea* from humans. *Jpn. J. Med. Mycol.* **46:**21–26.
131. **Kageyama, A., K. Yazawa, J. Ishikawa, K. Hotta, K. Nishimura, and Y. Mikami.** 2004. Nocardial infections in Japan from 1992 to 2001, including the first report of infection by *Nocardia transvalensis*. *Eur. J. Epidemiol.* **19:**383–389.
132. **Kashima, M., R. Kano, H. Takahama, M. Ito, A. Hasegawa, and M. Mizoguchi.** 2005. A successfully treated case of mycetoma due to *Nocardia veterana*. *Br. J. Dermatol.* **152:**1349–1352.
133. **Kattar, M. M., B. T. Cookson, L. C. Carlson, S. K. Stiglich, M. A. Schwartz, T. T. Nguyen, R. Daza, C. K. Wallis, S. L. Yarfitz, and M. B. Coyle.** 2001. *Tsukamurella strandjordae* sp. nov., a proposed new species causing sepsis. *J. Clin. Microbiol.* **39:**1467–1476.
134. **Kedlaya, I., M. B. Ing, and S. S. Wong.** 2001. *Rhodococcus equi* infections in immunocompetent hosts: case report and review. *Clin. Infect. Dis.* **32:**e39–e47.
135. **Kempf, V. A. J., M. Schmalzing, A. F. Yassin, K. P. Schaal, D. Baumeister, M. Arenskötter, A. Steinbüchel, and I. B. Autenrieth.** 2004. *Gordonia polyisoprenivorans* septicemia in a bone marrow transplant patient. *Eur. J. Clin. Microbiol. Infect. Dis.* **23:**226–228.
136. **Kent, P. T., and G. P. Kubica.** 1985. *Public Health Mycobacteriology. A Guide for the Level III Laboratory.* U. S. Department of Health and Human Services, Centers for Disease Control, Atlanta, Ga.
137. **Khatri, M. L., H. M. Al-Halali, M. F. Khalid, S. A. Saif, and M. C. R. Vyas.** 2002. Mycetoma in Yemen: clinicoepidemiologic and histopathologic study. *Int. J. Dermatol.* **41:**586–593.

138. **Kim, J. E., R. E. Landon, T. B. Connor, Jr., and J. D. Kivlin.** 2004. Endogenous ocular nocardiosis. *J. AAPOS* **8:**194–195.
139. **Kiska, D. L., K. Hicks, and D. J. Pettit.** 2002. Identification of medically relevant *Nocardia* species with an abbreviated battery of tests. *J. Clin. Microbiol.* **40:**1346–1351.
140. **Koll, B. S., A. E. Brown, T. E. Kiehn, and D. Armstrong.** 1992. Disseminated *Nocardia brasiliensis* infection with septic arthritis. *Clin. Infect. Dis.* **15:**469–472.
141. **Kontoyiannis, D. P., K. Ruoff, and D. C. Hooper.** 1998. *Nocardia* bacteremia, report of 4 cases and review of the literature. *Medicine* (Baltimore) **77:**255–267.
142. **Kurup, P. V., H. S. Randhawa, and N. P. Gupta.** 1970. Nocardiosis: a review. *Mycopathol. Mycol. Appl.* **40:**193–219.
143. **Kurup, V. P., and J. N. Fink.** 1975. A scheme for the identification of thermophilic actinomycetes associated with hypersensitivity pneumonitis. *J. Clin. Microbiol.* **2:**55–61.
144. **Kuwabara, M., T. Onitsuka, K. Nakamura, M. Shimada, S. Ohtaki, and Y. Mikami.** 1999. Mediastinitis due to *Gordona sputi* after CABG. *J. Cardiovasc. Surg.* (Torino) **40:**675–677.
145. **Labeda, D. P., J. M. Donahue, N. M. Williams, S. F. Sells, and M. M. Henton.** 2003. *Amycolatopsis kentuckyensis* sp. nov., *Amycolatopsis lexingtonensis* sp. nov. and *Amycolatopsis pretoriensis* sp. nov., isolated from equine placentas. *Int. J. Syst. Evol. Microbiol.* **53:**1601–1605.
146. **Ladrón, N., M. Fernández, J. Agüero, B. G. Zörn, J. A. Vásques-Boland, and J. Navas.** 2003. Rapid identification of *Rhodococcus equi* by a PCR assay targeting the *choE* gene. *J. Clin. Microbiol.* **41:**3241–3245.
147. **Lanotte, P., S. Watt, R. Ruimy, P. Boiron, A. Robier, and R. Quentin.** 2001. *Nocardia farcinica* infection of a cochlear implant in an immunocompetent boy. *Eur. J. Clin. Microbiol. Infect. Dis.* **20:**880–882.
148. **Larkin, J. A., L. Lit, J. Sinnott, T. Wills, and A. Szentivanyi.** 1999. Infection of a knee prosthesis with *Tsukamurella* species. *South. Med. J.* **92:**831–832.
149. **Lasker, B. A., J. M. Brown, and M. M. McNeil.** 1992. Identification and epidemiological typing of clinical and environmental isolates of the genus *Rhodococcus* with use of a digoxigenin-labeled rDNA gene probe. *Clin. Infect. Dis.* **15:**223–233.
150. **Laurent, F., A. Carlotti, P. Boiron, J. Villard, and J. Freney.** 1996. Ribotyping: a tool for taxonomy and identification of the *Nocardia asteroides* complex species. *J. Clin. Microbiol.* **34:**1079–1082.
151. **Laurent, F. J., F. Provost, and P. Boiron.** 1999. Rapid identification of clinically relevant *Nocardia* species to genus level by 16S rRNA gene PCR. *J. Clin. Microbiol.* **37:**99–102.
152. **Lechevalier, M. P., H. Prauser, D. P. Labeda, and J.-S. Ruan.** 1986. Two new genera of nocardioform actinomycetes: *Amycolata* gen. nov. and *Amycolatopsis* gen. nov. *Int. J. Syst. Bacteriol.* **36:**29–37.
153. **Lee, A. C. W., K. Y. Yuen, and Y. L. Lau.** 1994. Catheter-associated nocardiosis. *Pediatr. Infect. Dis. J.* **13:**1023–1024.
154. **Lesens, O., Y. Hansmann, P. Riegel, R. Heller, M. Benaissa-Djelloulo, M. Martinot, H. Petit, and D. Christmann.** 2000. Bacteremia and endocarditis caused by a *Gordonia* species in a patient with a central venous catheter. *Emerg. Infect. Dis.* **6:**382–385.
155. **Lewis, K. E., P. Ebden, S. L. Wooster, J. Rees, and G. A. J. Harrison.** 2003. Multi-system infection with *Nocardia farcinica*—therapy with linezolid and minocycline. *J. Infect.* **46:**199–202.
156. **López, E., M. Ferrero, C. Lumbreras, C. Gimeno, I. Gonzáles-Pinto, and E. Palengue.** 1994. A case of testicular nocardiosis and literature review. *Eur. J. Clin. Microbiol. Infect. Dis.* **13:**310–313.
157. **Lopez, F. A., F. Johnson, D. M. Novosad, B. L. Beaman, and M. Holodniy.** 2003. Successful management of disseminated *Nocardia transvalensis* infection in a heart transplant recipient after development of sulfonamide resistance: case report and review. *J. Heart Lung Transplant.* **22:**492–497.
158. **Lopez Martinez, R., L. J. Mendez Tovar, P. Lavelle, O. Welsh, and E. Macotela Ruiz.** 1992. Epidemiologia del micetoma en México: estudio de 2105 casos. *Gac. Med. Mex.* **128:**477–481.
159. **Louie, L., M. Louie, and A. E. Simor.** 1997. Investigation of a pseudo-outbreak of *Nocardia asteroides* infection by pulsed-field gel electrophoresis and randomly amplified polymorphic DNA PCR. *J. Clin. Microbiol.* **35:**1582–1584.
160. **Lovett, I. S., E. T. Houang, S. Burge, M. Turner-Warwick, F. D. Thompson, A. R. Harrison, A. M. Joekes, and M. C. Parkinson.** 1981. An outbreak of *Nocardia asteroides* infection in a renal transplant unit. *Q. J. Med.* **50:**123–135.
161. **Lui, W. Y. S., A. C. W. Lee, and T. L. Que.** 2001. Central venous catheter-associated *Nocardia* bacteremia. *Clin. Infect. Dis.* **33:**1613–1614.
162. **Maertens, J., P. Wattiau, J. Verhaegen, M. Boogaerts, L. Verbist, and G. Wauters.** 1998. Catheter-related bacteremia due to *Tsukamurella pulmonis*. *Clin. Microbiol. Inf.* **4:**51–53.
163. **Mahe, A., M. Develoux, C. Lienhardt, S. Keita, and P. Bobin.** 1996. Mycetomas in Mali: causative agents and geographic distribution. *Am. J. Trop. Med. Hyg.* **54:**77–79.
164. **Maiti, P. K., A. Ray, and S. Bandyopadhyay.** 2002. Epidemiological aspects of mycetoma from a retrospective study of 264 cases in West Bengal. *Trop. Med. Int. Health* **7:**788–792.
165. **Maraki, S., E. Scoulica, K. Alpantaki, M. Dialynas, and Y. Tselentis.** 2003. Lymphocutaneous nocardiosis due to *Nocardia brasiliensis*. *Diagn. Microbiol. Infect. Dis.* **47:**341–344.
166. **Martín, M. C., A. Manteca, M. Castillo, F. Vázquez, and F. J. Méndez.** 2004. *Streptomyces albus* isolated from a human actinomycetoma and characterized by molecular techniques. *J. Clin. Microbiol.* **42:**5957–5960.
167. **Martin, T., D. J. Hogan, F. Murphy, I. Natyshak, and E. P. Ewan.** 1991. *Rhodococcus* infection of the skin with lymphadenitis in a nonimmunocompromised girl. *J. Am. Acad. Dermatol.* **24:**328–332.
168. **Masters, A. M., T. M. Ellis, J. M. Carson, S. S. Sutherland, and A. R. Gregory.** 1995. *Dermatophilus chelonae* sp. nov., isolated from chelonids in Australia. *Int. J. Syst. Bacteriol.* **45:**50–56.
169. **McFaddin, J. F.** 2000. *Biochemical Tests for Identification of Medical Bacteria*, 3rd ed. Lippincott Williams and Wilkins, Philadelphia, Pa.
170. **McMinn, E. J., G. Alderson, H. I. Dodson, M. Goodfellow, and A. C. Ward.** 2000. Genomic and phenomic differentiation of *Rhodococcus equi* and related strains. *Antonie Leeuwenhoek* **78:**331–340.
171. **McNabb, A., R. Shuttleworth, R. Behme, and W. D. Colby.** 1997. Fatty acid characterization of rapidly growing pathogenic aerobic actinomycetes as a means of identification. *J. Clin. Microbiol.* **35:**1361–1368.
172. **McNeil, M. M., and J. M. Brown.** 1994. The medically important aerobic actinomycetes: epidemiology and microbiology. *Clin. Microbiol. Rev.* **7:**357–417.
173. **McNeil, M. M., J. M. Brown, P. R. Georghiou, A. M. Allworth, and Z. M. Blacklock.** 1992. Infections due to *Nocardia transvalensis:* clinical spectrum and antimicrobial therapy. *Clin. Infect. Dis.* **15:**453–463.
174. **McNeil, M. M., J. M. Brown, W. R. Jarvis, and L. Ajello.** 1990. Comparison of species distribution and

antimicrobial susceptibility of aerobic actinomycetes from clinical specimens. *Rev. Infect. Dis.* **12:**778–783.

175. **McNeil, M. M., J. M. Brown, G. Scalise, and C. Piersimoni.** 1992. Nonmycetomic *Actinomadura madurae* infection in a patient with AIDS. *J. Clin. Microbiol.* **30:** 1008–1010.

176. **McNeil, M. M., S. Ray, P. E. Kozarsky, and J. M. Brown.** 1997. *Nocardia farcinica* pneumonia in a previously healthy woman: species characterization with use of a digoxigenin-labeled cDNA probe. *Clin. Infect. Dis.* **25:**933–934.

177. **Mellmann, A., J. L. Cloud, S. Andrees, K. Blackwood, K. C. Carroll, A. Kabani, A. Roth, and D. Harmsen.** 2003. Evaluation of RIDOM, MicroSeq, and GenBank services in the molecular identification of *Nocardia* species. *Int. J. Med. Microbiol.* **293:**359–370.

178. **Meyer, J.** 1976. *Nocardiopsis*, a new genus of the order *Actinomycetales*. *Int. J. Syst. Bacteriol.* **26:**487–493.

179. **Mordarska, H.** 1968. A trial of using lipids for the classification of actinomycetes. *Arch. Immunol. Ther. Exp.* (Warsz.) **16:**45–50.

180. **Moss, W. J., J. A. Sager, J. D. Dick, and A. Ruff.** 2003. *Streptomyces bikiniensis* bacteremia. *Emerg. Infect. Dis.* **9:**273–274.

181. **Muir, D. B., and R. C. Pritchard.** 1997. Use of the BioMerieux ID 32C Yeast Identification System for identification of aerobic actinomycetes of medical importance. *J. Clin. Microbiol.* **35:**3240–3243.

182. **Murray, P. R., R. L. Heeren, and A. C. Niles.** 1987. Effect of decontamination procedures on recovery of *Nocardia* spp. *J. Clin. Microbiol.* **25:**2010–2011.

183. **Murray, P. R., A. C. Niles, and R. L. Heeren.** 1988. Modified Thayer-Martin medium for recovery of *Nocardia* species from contaminated specimens. *J. Clin. Microbiol.* **26:**1219–1220.

184. **Naguib, M. T., and D. P. Fine.** 1995. Brain abscess due to *Nocardia brasiliensis* hematogenously spread from a pulmonary infection. *Clin. Infect. Dis.* **21:**459–460.

185. **Napoleão, F., P. V. Damasco, T. C. F. Camello, M. D. do Vale, A. F. B. de Andrade, R. Hirata, Jr., and A. L. de Mattos-Guaraldi.** 2005. Pyogenic liver abscess due to *Rhodococcus equi* in an immunocompetent host. *J. Clin. Microbiol.* **43:**1002–1004.

186. **NCCLS.** 2003. *Susceptibility Testing of Mycobacteria, Nocardiae and Other Aerobic Actinomycetes; Approved Standard, NCCLS Document M24-A.* NCCLS, Wayne, Pa.

187. **Nishiuchi, Y., T. Baba, H. H. Hotta, and I. Yano.** 1999. Mycolic acid analysis in *Nocardia* species. The mycolic acid compositions of *Nocardia asteroides, N. farcinica,* and *N. nova*. *J. Microbiol. Methods* **37:**111–122.

188. **Nishiuchi, Y., T. Baba, and I. Yano.** 2000. Mycolic acids from *Rhodococcus, Gordonia,* and *Dietzia*. *J. Microbiol. Methods* **40:**1–9.

189. **Osoagbaka, O. U., and A. N. U. Njoku-Obi.** 1987. Presumptive diagnosis of pulmonary nocardiosis: value of sputum microscopy. *J. Appl. Bacteriol.* **63:**27–38.

190. **Palmer, D. L., R. L. Harvey, and J. K. Wheeler.** 1974. Diagnostic and therapeutic considerations in *Nocardia asteroides* infection. *Medicine* (Baltimore) **53:**391–401.

191. **Paredes, B. E., R. E. Hunger, L. R. Braathen, and C. U. Brand.** 1999. Cutaneous nocardiosis caused by *Nocardia brasiliensis* after an insect bite. *Dermatology* **198:**159–161.

192. **Patel, J. B., R. J. Wallace, Jr., B. A. Brown-Elliott, T. Taylor, C. Imperatrice, D. G. B. Leonard, R. W. Wilson, L. Mann, K. C. Jost, and I. Nachamkin.** 2004. Sequence-based identification of aerobic actinomycetes. *J. Clin. Microbiol.* **42:**2530–2540.

193. **Patterson, J. E., K. Chapin-Robertson, S. Waycott, P. Farrel, A. McGeer, M. M. McNeil, and S. Edberg.** 1992. Pseudoepidemic of *Nocardia asteroides* associated with a mycobacterial culture system. *J. Clin. Microbiol.* **30:** 1357–1360.

194. **Peraira, J. R., J. Segovia, R. Fuentes, J. Jiménez-Mazuecos, R. Arroyo, B. Fuertes, P. Mendaza, and L. A. Pulpon.** 2003. Pulmonary nocardiosis in heart transplant recipients: treatment and outcome. *Transplant. Proc.* **35:**2006–2008.

195. **Peterson, D. L., L. D. Hudson, and K. Sullivan.** 1978. Disseminated *Nocardia caviae* with positive blood cultures. *Arch. Intern. Med.* **138:**1164–1165.

196. **Pham, A. S., I. Dé, K. V. Rolston, J. J. Tarrand, and X. Y. Han.** 2003. Catheter-related bacteremia caused by the nocardioform actinomycete *Gordonia terrae*. *Clin. Infect. Dis.* **36:**524–527.

197. **Pidoux, O., J.-N. Argenson, V. Jacomo, and M. Drancourt.** 2001. Molecular identification of a *Dietzia maris* hip prosthesis infection isolate. *J. Clin. Microbiol.* **39:**2634–2636.

198. **Pintado, V., E. Gómez-Mampaso, J. Cobo, C. Quereda, M. A. Meseguer, J. Fortún, E. Navas, and S. Moreno.** 2003. Nocardial infection in patients infected with the human immunodeficiency virus. *Clin. Microbiol. Inf.* **9:**716–720.

199. **Poonwan, N., N. Mekha, K. Yazawa, S. Thunyaharn, A. Yamanaka, and Y. Mikami.** 2005. Characterization of clinical isolates of pathogenic *Nocardia* strains and related actinomycetes in Thailand from 1996 to 2003. *Mycopathologia* **159:**361–368.

200. **Pottumarthy, S., A. P. Limaye, J. L. Prentice, Y. B. Houze, S. R. Swanzy, and B. T. Cookson.** 2003. *Nocardia veterana*, a new emerging pathogen. *J. Clin. Microbiol.* **41:**1705–1709.

201. **Prescott, J. F.** 1991. *Rhodococcus equi:* an animal and human pathogen. *Clin. Microbiol. Rev.* **4:**20–34.

202. **Prinz, G., É. Bán, S. Fekete, and Z. Szabó.** 1985. Meningitis caused by *Gordona aurantiaca (Rhodococcus aurantiacus)*. *J. Clin. Microbiol.* **22:**472–474.

203. **Rainey, F. A., S. Klatte, R. M. Kroppenstedt, and E. Stackebrandt.** 1995. *Dietzia*, a new genus including *Dietzia maris* comb. nov., formerly *Rhodococcus maris*. *Int. J. Syst. Bacteriol.* **45:**32–36.

204. **Richet, H. M., P. C. Craven, J. M. Brown, B. A. Lasker, C. D. Cox, M. M. McNeil, A. D. Tice, W. R. Jarvis, and O. C. Tablan.** 1991. A cluster of *Rhodococcus (Gordona) bronchialis* sternal-wound infections after coronary-artery bypass surgery. *N. Engl. J. Med.* **324:**104–109.

205. **Riegel, P., R. Ruimy, D. De Briel, F. Eichler, J.-P. Bergerat, R. Christen, and H. Montiel.** 1996. Bacteremia due to *Gordona sputi* in an immunocompromised patient. *J. Clin. Microbiol.* **34:**2045–2047.

206. **Rodríguez-Nava, V., A. Couble, G. Devulder, J.-P. Flandrois, P. Boiron, and F. Laurent.** 2006. Use of PCR-restriction enzyme pattern analysis and sequencing database for *hsp65* gene-based identification of *Nocardia* sp. *J. Clin. Microbiol.* **44:**536–546.

207. **Roth, A., S. Andrees, R. M. Kroppenstedt, D. Harmsen, and H. Mauch.** 2003. Phylogeny of the genus *Nocardia* based on reassessed 16S rRNA gene sequences reveals underspeciation and division of strains classified as *Nocardia asteroides* into three established species and two unnamed taxons. *J. Clin. Microbiol.* **41:**851–856.

208. **Ruimy, R., P. Riegel, A. Carlotti, P. Boiron, G. Bernardin, H. Monteil, R. J. Wallace, Jr., and R. Christen.** 1996. *Nocardia pseudobrasiliensis* sp. nov., a new species of *Nocardia* which groups bacterial strains previously identified as *Nocardia brasiliensis* and associated with invasive diseases. *Int. J. Syst. Bacteriol.* **46:**259–264.

209. **Salazar, O., I. González, and O. Genilloud.** 2002. New genus-specific primers for the PCR identification of novel isolates of the genera *Nocardiopsis* and *Saccharothrix*. *Int. J. Syst. Evol. Microbiol.* **52:**1411–1421.

210. **Schiff, T. A., M. M. McNeil, and J. M. Brown.** 1993. Cutaneous *Nocardia farcinica* infection in a nonimmunocompromised patient: case report and review. *Clin. Infect. Dis.* **16:**756–760.
211. **Schwartz, M. A., S. R. Tabet, A. C. Collier, C. K. Wallis, L. C. Carlson, T. T. Nguyen, M. M. Kattar, and M. B. Coyle.** 2002. Central venous catheter-related bacteremia due to *Tsukamurella* species in the immunocompromised host: a case series and review of the literature. *Clin. Infect. Dis.* **35:**e72-e77.
212. **Shaer, A. J., and C. A. Gadegbeku.** 2001. *Tsukamurella* peritonitis associated with continuous ambulatory peritoneal dialysis. *Clin. Nephrol.* **56:**241–246.
213. **Shainhouse, J. Z., A. C. Pier, and D. A. Stevens.** 1978. Complement fixation antibody test for human nocardiosis. *J. Clin. Microbiol.* **8:**516–519.
214. **Shapiro, C. L., R. F. Haft, N. M. Gantz, G. V. Doern, J. C. Christenson, R. O'Brien, J. C. Overall, B. A. Brown, and R. J. Wallace, Jr.** 1992. *Tsukamurella paurometabolum:* a novel pathogen causing catheter-related bacteremia in patients with cancer. *Clin. Infect. Dis.* **14:**200–203.
215. **Sheridan, E. A. S., S. Warwick, A. Chan, M. Dall'Antonia, M. Koliou, and A. Sefton.** 2003. *Tsukamurella tyrosinosolvens* intravascular catheter infection identified using 16S ribosomal DNA sequencing. *Clin. Infect. Dis.* **36:**e69–e70.
216. **Smego, R. A., and H. A. Gallis.** 1984. The clinical spectrum of *Nocardia brasiliensis* infection in the United States. *Rev. Infect. Dis.* **6:**164–180.
217. **Sng, L.-H., T. H. Koh, S. R. Toney, M. Floyd, W. R. Butler, and B. H. Tan.** 2004. Bacteremia caused by *Gordonia bronchialis* in a patient with sequestrated lung. *J. Clin. Microbiol.* **42:**2870–2871.
218. **Sorrell, T. C., D. H. Mitchell, and J. R. Iredell.** 2005. *Nocardia* species, p. 2916–2924. *In* G. L. Mandell, J. E. Bennett, and R. Dolin (ed.), *Mandel, Douglas and Bennett's Principles and Practice of Infectious Diseases*, 6th ed., vol. 2. Elsevier, Churchill Livingstone, Philadelphia, Pa.
219. **Spark, R. P., M. M. McNeil, J. M. Brown, B. A. Lasker, M. A. Montano, and M. D. Garfield.** 1993. *Rhodococcus* species fatal infection in an immunocompetent host. *Arch. Pathol. Lab. Med.* **117:**515–520.
220. **Stackebrandt, E.** 2003. The richness of prokaryotic diversity: there must be a species somewhere. *Food Technol. Biotechnol.* **41:**17–22.
221. **Stackebrandt, E., F. A. Rainey, and N. L. Ward-Rainey.** 1997. Proposal for a new hierarchic classification system, *Actinobacteria* classis nov. *Int. J. Syst. Bacteriol.* **47:**479–491.
222. **Stackebrandt, E., J. Smida, and M. D. Collins.** 1988. Evidence of phylogenetic heterogeneity within the genus *Rhodococcus:* revival of the genus *Gordona* (Tsukamura). *J. Gen. Appl. Microbiol.* **34:**341–348.
223. **Stackebrandt, E., D. Witt, C. Kemmerling, R. Kroppenstedt, and W. Liesack.** 1991. Designation of streptomycete 16S and 23S rRNA-based target regions for oligonucleotide probes. *Appl. Environ. Microbiol.* **57:**1468–1477.
224. **Staneck, J. L., and G. D. Roberts.** 1974. Simplified approach to identification of aerobic actinomycetes by thin-layer chromatography. *Appl. Microbiol.* **28:**226–231.
225. **Steingrube, V. A., B. A. Brown, J. L. Gibson, R. W. Wilson, J. Brown, Z. Blacklock, K. Jost, S. Locke, R. F. Ulrich, and R. J. Wallace, Jr.** 1995. DNA amplification and restriction endonuclease analysis for differentiation of 12 species and taxa of *Nocardia*, including recognition of four new taxa within the *Nocardia asteroides* complex. *J. Clin. Microbiol.* **33:**3096–3101.
226. **Steingrube, V. A., R. W. Wilson, B. A. Brown, K. C. Jost, Jr., Z. Blacklock, J. L. Gibson, and R. J. Wallace, Jr.** 1997. Rapid identification of clinically significant species and taxa of aerobic actinomycetes, including *Actinomadura*, *Gordona*, *Nocardia*, *Rhodococcus*, *Streptomyces*, and *Tsukamurella* isolates, by DNA amplification and restriction endonuclease analysis. *J. Clin. Microbiol.* **35:**817–822.
227. **Stevens, D. A., A. C. Pier, B. L. Beaman, P. A. Morozumi, I. S. Lovett, and E. T. Houang.** 1981. Laboratory evaluation of an outbreak of nocardiosis in immunocompromised hosts. *Am. J. Med.* **71:**928–934.
228. **Sugar, A. M., G. K. Schoolnik, and D. A. Stevens.** 1985. Antibody response in human nocardiosis: identification of two immunodominant culture-filtrate antigens derived from *Nocardia asteroides*. *J. Infect. Dis.* **151:**895–901.
229. **Telenti, A., F. Marchesi, M. Balz, F. Bally, E. C. Böttger, and T. Bodmer.** 1993. Rapid identification of mycobacteria to the species level by polymerase chain reaction and restriction enzyme analysis. *J. Clin. Microbiol.* **31:**175–178.
230. **Torres, H. A., B. T. Reddy, I. I. Raad, J. Tarrand, G. P. Bodey, H. A. Hanna, K. V. I. Rolston, and D. P. Kontoyiannis.** 2002. Nocardiosis in cancer patients. *Medicine* (Baltimore) **81:**388–397.
231. **Torres, O. H., P. Domingo, R. Pericas, P. Boiron, J. A. Montiel, and G. Vázquez.** 2000. Infection caused by *Nocardia farcinica:* case report and review. *Eur. J. Clin. Microbiol. Infect. Dis.* **19:**205–212.
232. **Torres-Tortosa, M., J. Arrizabalaga, J. L. Villanueva, J. Gálvez, M. Leyes, M. E. Valencia, J. Flores, J. M. Peña, E. Pérez-Cecilia, and C. Quereda.** 2003. Prognosis and clinical evaluation of infection caused by *Rhodococcus equi* in HIV-infected patients. *Chest* **123:**1970–1976.
233. **Towersey, L., E. S. Martins, A. T. Londero, R. J. Hay, P. J. S. Filho, C. M. Takiya, C. C. Martins, and O. F. Gompertz.** 1993. *Dermatophilus congolensis* human infection. *J. Am. Acad. Dermatol.* **29:**351–354.
234. **Trujillo, M. E., and M. Goodfellow.** 2003. Numerical phenetic classification of clinically significant aerobic sporoactinomycetes and related organisms. *Antonie Leeuwenhoek* **84:**39–68.
235. **Trujillo, M. E., and M. Goodfellow.** 1997. Polyphasic taxonomic study of clinically significant *Actinomadurae* including the description of *Actinomadura latina* sp. nov. *Zentbl. Bakteriol.* **285:**212–233.
236. **Tsukamura, M.** 1982. Numerical analysis of the taxonomy of nocardiae and rhodococci. *Microbiol. Immunol.* **26:**1101–1119.
237. **Tsukamura, M., K. Hikosaka, K. Nishimura, and S. Hara.** 1988. Severe progressive subcutaneous abscesses and necrotizing tenosynovitis caused by *Rhodococcus aurantiacus*. *J. Clin. Microbiol.* **26:**201–205.
238. **Tsukamura, M., and K. Kawakami.** 1982. Lung infection caused by *Gordona aurantiaca (Rhodococcus aurantiacus)*. *J. Clin. Microbiol.* **16:**604–607.
239. **Uesaka, I., and N. M. McClung.** 1961. On the morphology of *Nocardia*, especially on its acid-fastness. *Jpn. J. Tuberc.* **8:**116–117.
240. **van Dam, A. P., M. T. C. Pruijm, B. I. J. Harinck, L. B. S. Gelinck, and E. J. Kuijper.** 2005. Pneumonia involving *Aspergillus* and *Rhizopus* spp. after a near-drowning incident with subsequent *Nocardia cyriacigeorgici* and *N. farcinica* coinfection as a late complication. *Eur. J. Clin. Microbiol. Infect. Dis.* **24:**61–64.
241. **Vandamme, P., B. Pot, M. Gillis, K. De Vos, K. Kersters, and J. Swings.** 1996. Polyphasic taxonomy, a consensus approach to bacterial systematics. *Microbiol. Rev.* **60:**407–438.
242. **Vannier, A. M., B. H. Ackerman, and L. F. Hutchins.** 1992. Disseminated *Nocardia asteroides* diagnosed by

blood culture in a patient with disseminated histoplasmosis. *Arch. Pathol. Lab. Med.* **116:**537–539.

243. **Vernazza, P. L., T. Bodmer, and R. L. Galeazzi.** 1991. *Rhodococcus-erythropolis*-Infektion bei HIV-assoziierter Immunschwäche. *Schweiz. Med. Wschr.* **121:**1095–1098.
244. **Vickers, R. M., J. D. Rihs, and V. L. Yu.** 1992. Clinical demonstration of isolation of *Nocardia asteroides* on buffered charcoal-yeast extract media. *J. Clin. Microbiol.* **30:**227–228.
245. **von Below, H., C. M. Wilk, K. P. Schaal, and G. O. H. Naumann.** 1991. *Rhodococcus luteus* and *Rhodococcus erythropolis* chronic endophthalmitis after lens implantation. *Am. J. Ophthalmol.* **112:**596–597.
246. **von Graevenitz, A., and V. Pünter-Streit.** 1995. Development of a new selective plating medium for *Rhodococcus equi*. *Microbiol. Immunol.* **39:**283–284.
247. **Wallace, R. J., Jr., B. A. Brown, Z. Blacklock, R. Ulrich, K. Jost, J. M. Brown, M. M. McNeil, G. Onyi, V. A. Steingrube, and J. Gibson.** 1995. New *Nocardia* taxon among isolates of *Nocardia brasiliensis* associated with invasive disease. *J. Clin. Microbiol.* **33:**1528–1533.
248. **Wallace, R. J., Jr., B. A. Brown, M. Tsukamura, J. M. Brown, and G. O. Onyi.** 1991. Clinical and laboratory features of *Nocardia nova*. *J. Clin. Microbiol.* **29:**2407–2411.
249. **Wallace, R. J., Jr., L. C. Steele, G. Sumter, and J. M. Smith.** 1988. Antimicrobial susceptibility patterns of *Nocardia asteroides*. *Antimicrob. Agents Chemother.* **32:**1776–1779.
250. **Wallace, R. J., Jr., M. Tsukamura, B. A. Brown, J. Brown, V. A. Steingrube, Y. Zhang, and D. R. Nash.** 1990. Cefotaxime-resistant *Nocardia asteroides* strains are isolates of the controversial species *Nocardia farcinica*. *J. Clin. Microbiol.* **28:**2726–2732.
251. **Warren, N. G.** 1996. Actinomycosis, nocardiosis, and actinomycetoma. *Dermatol. Clin.* **14:**85–95.
252. **Warwick, S., T. Bowen, H. McVeigh, and T. M. Embley.** 1994. A phylogenetic analysis of the family *Pseudonocardiaceae* and the genera *Actinokineospora* and *Saccharothrix* with 16S rRNA sequences and a proposal to combine the genera *Amycolata* and *Pseudonocardia* in an emended genus *Pseudonocardia*. *Int. J. Syst. Bacteriol.* **44:**293–299.
253. **Watson, A., P. French, and M. Wilson.** 2001. *Nocardia asteroides* native valve endocarditis. *Clin. Infect. Dis.* **32:**660–661.
254. **Wauters, G., V. Avesani, J. Charlier, M. Janssens, M. Vaneechoutte, and M. Delmée.** 2005. Distribution of *Nocardia* species in clinical samples and their routine rapid identification in the laboratory. *J. Clin. Microbiol.* **43:**2624–2628.
255. **Weinberger, M., A. Eid, L. Schreiber, M. Shapiro, Y. Ilan, E. Libson, T. Sacks, and R. Tur-Kaspa.** 1995. Disseminated *Nocardia transvalensis* infection resembling pulmonary infarction in a liver transplant recipient. *Eur. J. Clin. Microbiol. Infect. Dis.* **14:**337–341.
256. **Weinstock, D. M., and A. E. Brown.** 2002. *Rhodococcus equi*: an emerging pathogen. *Clin. Infect. Dis.* **34:**1379–1385.
257. **Wellehan, J. F. X., C. Turenne, D. J. Heard, C. J. Detrisac, and J. J. O'Kelley.** 2004. *Dermatophilus chelonae* in a king cobra *(Ophiophagus hannah)*. *J. Zoo Wildl. Med.* **35:**553–556.
258. **Wellinghausen, N., T. Pietzcker, W. Kern, A. Essig, and R. Marre.** 2002. Expanded spectrum of *Nocardia* species causing clinical nocardiosis detected by molecular methods. *Int. J. Med. Microbiol.* **292:**277–282.
259. **Wenger, P. N., J. M. Brown, M. M. McNeil, and W. R. Jarvis.** 1998. *Nocardia farcinica* sternotomy site infections in patients following open heart surgery. *J. Infect. Dis.* **178:**1539–1543.
260. **Wilson, R. W., V. A. Steingrube, B. A. Brown, Z. Blacklock, K. C. Jost, Jr., A. McNabb, W. D. Colby, J. R. Biehle, J. L. Gibson, and R. J. Wallace, Jr.** 1997. Recognition of a *Nocardia transvalensis* complex by resistance to aminoglycosides, including amikacin, and PCR-restriction fragment length polymorphism analysis. *J. Clin. Microbiol.* **35:**2235–2242.
261. **Woo, P. C. Y., A. H. Y. Ngan, S. K. P. Lau, and K.-Y. Yuen.** 2003. *Tsukamurella* conjunctivitis: a novel clinical syndrome. *J. Clin. Microbiol.* **41:**3368–3371.
262. **Woods, G. L., and D. H. Walker.** 1996. Detection of infection or infectious agents by use of cytologic and histologic stains. *Clin. Microbiol. Rev.* **9:**382–404.
263. **Wüst, J., H. Lanzendörfer, A. von Graevenitz, H. J. Gloor, and B. Schmid.** 1990. Peritonitis caused by *Actinomadura madurae* in a patient on CAPD. *Eur. J. Clin. Microbiol. Infect. Dis.* **9:**700–701.
264. **Xu, J., J. R. Rao, B. C. Millar, J. S. Elborn, J. Evans, J. G. Barr, and J. E. Moore.** 2002. Improved molecular identification of *Thermoactinomyces* spp. associated with mushroom worker's lung by 16S rDNA sequence typing. *J. Med. Microbiol.* **51:**1117–1127.
265. **Yamamura, H., M. Hayakawa, Y. Nakagawa, and Y. Iimura.** 2004. Characterization of *Nocardia asteroides* isolates from different ecological habitats on the basis of repetitive extragenic palindromic-PCR fingerprinting. *Appl. Environ. Microbiol.* **70:**3149–3151.
266. **Yano, I., T. Imaeda, and M. Tsukamura.** 1990. Characterization of *Nocardia nova*. *Int. J. Syst. Bacteriol.* **40:**170–174.
267. **Yassin, A. F., H. Brzezinka, K. P. Schaal, H. G. Trüper, and G. Pulverer.** 1988. Menaquinone composition in the classification and identification of aerobic actinomycetes. *Zentbl. Bakteriol. Mikrobiol. Hyg. [A]* **267:**339–356.
268. **Yassin, A. F., F. A. Rainey, H. Brzezinka, J. Burghardt, H. J. Lee, and K. P. Schaal.** 1995. *Tsukamurella inchonensis* sp. nov. *Int. J. Syst. Bacteriol.* **45:**522–527.
269. **Yassin, A. F., F. A. Rainey, J. Burghardt, H. Brzezinka, M. Mauch, and K. P. Schaal.** 2000. *Nocardia paucivorans* sp. nov. *Int. J. Syst. Evol. Microbiol.* **50:**803–809.
270. **Yassin, A. F., F. A. Rainey, J. Burghardt, D. Gierth, J. Ungerechts, I. Lux, P. Seifert, C. Bal, and K. P. Schaal.** 1997. Description of *Nocardiopsis synnemataformans* sp. nov., elevation of *Nocardiopsis alba* subsp. *prasina* to *Nocardiopsis prasina* comb. nov., and designation of *Nocardiopsis antarctica* and *Nocardiopsis alborubida* as later subjective synonyms of *Nocardiopsis dassonvillei*. *Int. J. Syst. Bacteriol.* **47:**983–988.
271. **Yassin, A. F., F. A. Rainey, U. Mendrock, H. Brzezinka, and K. P. Schaal.** 2000. *Nocardia abscessus* sp. nov. *Int. J. Syst. Evol. Microbiol.* **50:**1487–1493.
272. **Yassin, A. F., F. A. Rainey, and U. Steiner.** 2001. *Nocardia cyriacigeorgici* sp. nov. *Int. J. Syst. Evol. Microbiol.* **51:**1419–1423.
273. **Yoshida, K., S. Bandoh, J. Fujita, M. Tokuda, K. Negayama, and T. Ishida.** 2004. Pyothorax caused by *Nocardia otitidiscaviarum* in a patient with rheumatoid vasculitis. *Intern. Med.* **43:**615–619.
274. **Zardawi, I. M., F. Jones, D. A. Clark, and J. Holland.** 2004. *Gordonia terrae*-induced suppurative granulomatous mastitis following nipple piercing. *Pathology* (Philadelphia) **36:**275–278.
275. **Zaria, L. T.** 1993. *Dermatophilus congolensis* infection (dermatophilosis) in animals and man! An update. *Comp. Immunol. Microbiol. Infect. Dis.* **16:**179–222.

Mycobacterium: General Characteristics, Laboratory Detection, and Staining Procedures*

GABY E. PFYFFER

36

Many species within the genus *Mycobacterium* are prominent pathogens, e.g., the members of the *Mycobacterium tuberculosis* complex as well as *M. leprae* and *M. ulcerans.* In addition, numerous species of environmental mycobacteria called nontuberculous mycobacteria (NTM) (formerly "atypical mycobacteria" or "mycobacteria other than tubercle bacilli") are responsible for various kinds of mycobacterioses.

Tuberculosis remains a major global public health problem (35). The actual global prevalence of *M. tuberculosis* infection is 32%, corresponding to approximately 1.9 billion people (51). According to the World Health Organization (229), there were 8.8 million estimated new cases (case rate, 140/100,000) of pulmonary tuberculosis, including 3.9 million smear-positive (and hence highly infectious) cases, in 2003. An estimated 1.9 million people died of tuberculosis, including patients coinfected with human immunodeficiency virus (HIV; 229,000). Analysis of epidemiological trends suggests that numbers of new cases are rising globally, but more people are being cured and death rates are falling (229). Reducing the burden of tuberculosis depends largely on how rapidly DOTS (directly observed therapy, short course) programs can be implemented. Among the prime obstacles for DOTS program expansion are shortages of trained staff, lack of political commitment, weak laboratory services, and the global impact of multidrug resistance (54), together with often inadequate management of multidrug resistance cases as well as people infected with HIV. In the Western Hemisphere, the number of reported cases is steadily decreasing (approximate case rate, 6.8/100,000), reflecting the effectiveness of prevention strategies and control measures implemented by the health authorities, among them the use of more rapid and efficient laboratory algorithms to detect *M. tuberculosis* and susceptibility testing with antituberculosis drugs. In this context, the clinical mycobacteriology laboratory plays an important role (55, 71).

With the advent of new laboratory techniques, new NTM species are being discovered, some of which are sources of diseases in humans (153). Rapid and reliable identification of NTM is thus mandatory but is becoming increasingly complex. The level of service and the choice of methods should, finally, be determined by the patient population served by the laboratory and by the resources available.

TAXONOMY AND DESCRIPTION OF THE GENUS

The genus *Mycobacterium* is the only genus in the family *Mycobacteriaceae* (216) and is related to other mycolic acid-containing genera. The high G+C contents of the DNA of *Mycobacterium* species (61 to 71 mol%, except that of *M. leprae* [55 mol%]) (144) are within the range of those of members of the other mycolic acid-containing genera, *Gordonia* (63 to 69 mol%), *Tsukamurella* (68 to 74 mol%), *Nocardia* (64 to 72 mol%), and *Rhodococcus* (63 to 73 mol%) (38).

Mycobacteria are aerobic (though some species are able to grow under a reduced-O_2 atmosphere), non-spore-forming, nonmotile, slightly curved or straight rods, 0.2 to 0.6 μm by 1.0 to 10 μm, which may branch. Colony morphology varies among the species, ranging from smooth to rough and from nonpigmented (nonphotochromogens) to pigmented. Colonies of the latter type are regularly or variably yellow, orange, or, rarely, pink, usually due to carotenoid pigments. Some species require light to form pigment (photochromogens); other species form pigment in either the light or the dark (scotochromogens). Aerial filaments are very rarely formed and never visible without magnification. Filamentous or mycelium-like growth may sometimes occur but, on slight disturbance, easily fragments into rods or coccoid elements (144).

The cell wall peptidoglycolipid contains *meso*-diaminopimelic acid, alanine, glutamic acid, glucosamine, muramic acid, arabinose, and galactose. Mycolic acids (number of carbon atoms ranging from 70 to 90), together with free lipids (e.g., trehalose-6,6′-dimycolate), provide for a hydrophobic permeability barrier (106, 112). Other important fatty acids are waxes, phospholipids, and mycoserosic and phthienoic acids. Various patterns of cellular fatty acids (number of carbon atoms ranging from 10 to 20) are found as well, among which is tuberculostearic (10-*R*-methyloctadecanoic) acid, a unique cell component for a number of members of the *Actinomycetales* (106).

The high content of complex lipids of the cell wall prevents access of common aniline dyes. Although not readily stained by Gram's method, mycobacteria are usually considered gram-positive. Once stained with special procedures, however, mycobacteria are not easily decolorized, even with

*This chapter contains information presented in chapter 36 by Gaby E. Pfyffer, Barbara A. Brown-Elliott, and Richard J. Wallace, Jr., and in chapter 37 by Véronique Vincent, Barbara A. Brown-Elliott, Kenneth C. Jost, Jr., and Richard J. Wallace, Jr., in the eighth edition of this Manual.

acid-alcohol; i.e., they are acid fast. However, acid fastness can be partly or completely lost at some stage of growth by a proportion of the cells of some species, particularly the rapidly growing ones.

A natural division exists between slowly and rapidly growing species of mycobacteria. Slow growers require more than 7 days to produce colonies on solid media from a dilute inoculum under ideal culture conditions. Rapid growers, by definition, require less than 7 days when subcultured on Löwenstein-Jensen (L-J) medium but may take several weeks to appear upon primary culture from clinical specimens.

NUTRITIONAL REQUIREMENTS AND GROWTH

Most species adapt readily to growth on relatively simple substrates, using ammonia or amino acids as nitrogen sources and glycerol as a carbon source in the presence of mineral salts. A few species (e.g., *M. haemophilum* and *M. genavense*) are fastidious and require supplements such as mycobactin, hemin, or other iron compounds. To date, *M. leprae* has not been cultured outside living cells. Growth of mycobacteria is stimulated by carbon dioxide and by fatty acids which may be provided in the form of egg yolk or oleic acid, even though the latter is toxic in higher concentrations (≥1%) and has to be neutralized by albumin.

With the genome of *M. tuberculosis* deciphered some years ago, functional genomics have provided new insights into its physiological and metabolic regulation and relation to virulence. For instance, genes involved in pathways of carbon metabolism (e.g., *fadD28*) and in electron transport (*nhA* and *cydA*) and genes encoding glycan biosynthesis (e.g., *Fbp*) have been described previously (219).

Optimum temperatures for growth vary widely among species (from <30 to 45°C). Compared to that of other bacteria, the growth of most mycobacterial species is slow, with generation times of up to approximately 20 h on commonly used media. Depending upon the species, visible colonies may appear after a few days to 6 weeks of incubation under optimum conditions.

SUSCEPTIBILITY TO PHYSICAL AND CHEMICAL AGENTS

Mycobacteria are able to survive for weeks to months on inanimate objects if protected from sunlight. Members of the *M. tuberculosis* complex, for instance, survive for several months on surfaces or in soil or cow dung, from which other animals may be infected (123). Mycobacteria are easily killed by heat (>65°C for at least 30 min) and by UV (sun) light but not by freezing or desiccation. They are more resistant to acids, alkalies, and some chemical disinfectants than most other non-spore-forming bacteria. Quaternary ammonium compounds, hexachlorophene, and chlorhexidine are bacteriostatic at best. The concentration of malachite green in egg-based media (e.g., L-J medium) was selected to maximize the growth of mycobacteria while inhibiting that of other microorganisms. Other commonly used sterilants, such as ethylene oxide and formaldehyde vapor, as well as disinfectants such as chlorine compounds, 70% ethanol, 2% alkaline glutaraldehyde, peracetic acid, and stabilized hydrogen peroxide, are effective in killing *M. tuberculosis*. However, agents that are inactivated in the presence of organic matter (e.g., alcohols) cannot be relied upon to disinfect sputum and other protein-containing materials. With iodophors, the bactericidal effect depends on the content of available iodine as well as on the presence of organic matter (14).

HABITATS

The genus *Mycobacterium* includes obligate pathogens, opportunistic pathogens, and saprophytes. The major ecological niche for the *M. tuberculosis* complex and *M. leprae*, incapable of replication in the inanimate environment, is tissues of humans and warm-blooded animals. In contrast, the NTM are free-living mycobacteria and are usually found in association with watery habitats such as lakes, rivers, and wet soil, etc. Some human pathogenic NTM species, however, have yet to be recovered from soil or water, e.g., *M. ulcerans, M. haemophilum, M. asiaticum, M. shimoidei*, and *M. szulgai* (5). Some other NTM species have rarely been recovered from natural waters or soils but are readily recovered from tap water in settings where disease caused by NTM is frequent or cultures from clinical specimens are often positive. Examples are *M. kansasii, M. xenopi, M. malmoense*, and *M. simiae* (5). The *M. avium* complex (MAC), *M. gordonae*, and rapidly growing mycobacteria have been recovered from tap water as well and also occur in association with nosocomial disease and pseudo-outbreaks (5, 83, 208). Although not components of the normal bacterial flora of humans or animals, NTM may be isolated from the skin, upper respiratory tract, and intestinal and genital tracts of asymptomatic individuals (57). Due to their ubiquitous nature, the question of their clinical significance is important but not always easy to answer (5).

A well-known source for positive cultures is bronchoscopes and related devices. Organisms isolated were *M. tuberculosis* (170), *M. xenopi* (12), and *M. chelonae* (66), as well as other NTM.

CLINICAL SIGNIFICANCE AND DESCRIPTION OF SPECIES

With the advent of molecular techniques for appropriate identification, close to 200 mycobacterial species have now been described. This chapter will focus on the slowly growing mycobacteria; rapidly growing mycobacteria are described in chapter 38.

M. tuberculosis Complex

The *M. tuberculosis* complex taxon includes *M. tuberculosis, M. bovis* (*M. bovis* subsp. *bovis, M. bovis* subsp. *caprae*, and *M. bovis* BCG), *M. africanum, M. microti, M. canettii*, and *M. pinnipedii*, which form a tight, discrete group of organisms and display >95% DNA-DNA homology. Recent comparative genomics using the complete DNA sequence of *M. tuberculosis* have provided information on regions of the genome that are deleted in other members of the complex (4, 67). Identification to the species level is justified for epidemiologic, public health, and therapeutic reasons.

M. tuberculosis

M. tuberculosis has an extremely low level of genetic variation, suggesting that the entire population of *M. tuberculosis* organisms resulted from clonal expansion after an evolutionary bottleneck some 35,000 years ago (C. Gutierrez, S. Brisse, R. Brosch, M. Fabre, B. Omais, M. Marmiesse, P. Supply, and V. Vincent, *Abstr. 26th Annu. Congr. Eur. Soc. Mycobacteriol.*, abstr. L-3, 2005).

In today's industrialized world, a higher prevalence of tuberculosis occurs among the medically underserved ethnic minorities, the urban poor, homeless persons, prison inmates, alcoholics, intravenous drug users, the elderly in general, foreign-born persons from areas of high prevalence, and contacts of persons with active tuberculosis. Today, HIV infection is the greatest known risk factor for progression of latent infection to active tuberculosis. Combined HIV and tuberculosis infections, especially in combination with drug resistance, have caused outbreaks with extremely high mortality rates (30, 31). Groups with a higher likelihood of progression also include individuals with underlying medical conditions, persons who have been infected within the past 2 years, children ≤4 years old, and persons with fibrotic and cancerous lesions detected on chest radiographs.

M. tuberculosis is carried in airborne particles (droplet nuclei) generated when patients with pulmonary tuberculosis cough. These particles, 1 to 5 μm in diameter, are kept suspended by normal air currents. Infection occurs when a susceptible person inhales the droplet nuclei. Once in the alveoli, the organisms are engulfed by alveolar macrophages. Usually, the host cell-mediated immune response limits the multiplication and spread of *M. tuberculosis*. However, some bacilli can remain viable but dormant for many years after the initial infection. Patients latently infected with *M. tuberculosis* usually have a positive purified protein derivative (PPD) skin test but are asymptomatic and not infectious. In general, persons with a latent infection have a 10% risk during their lifetime for development of active tuberculosis. By contrast, patients with HIV infection have a 10 to 15% risk per year for progression to manifest disease (2).

Tuberculosis in adults is a slowly progressive process characterized by chronic inflammation and caseation and formation of cavities. These foci may rupture into the bronchi, allowing very large numbers of organisms to spread to other areas of the lungs and to be aerosolized by coughing, hence infecting other persons. The clinical features of pulmonary tuberculosis are cough, weight loss, night sweats, low-grade fever, dyspnea, and chest pain. Extrapulmonary manifestations of *M. tuberculosis* infection include cervical lymphadenitis, pleuritis, pericarditis, synovitis, meningitis, and infections of the skin, joints, bones, and internal organs (85). Relative to the ordinary clinical picture of tuberculosis, pulmonary disease in AIDS patients often differs in radiologic findings, is usually rapidly progressive, and disseminates more frequently, sometimes even without the formation of granulomas.

In culture, colonies of *M. tuberculosis* are off-white and rough on solid media (Fig. 1), although on moist media they may tend to be smoother. In addition to the classical

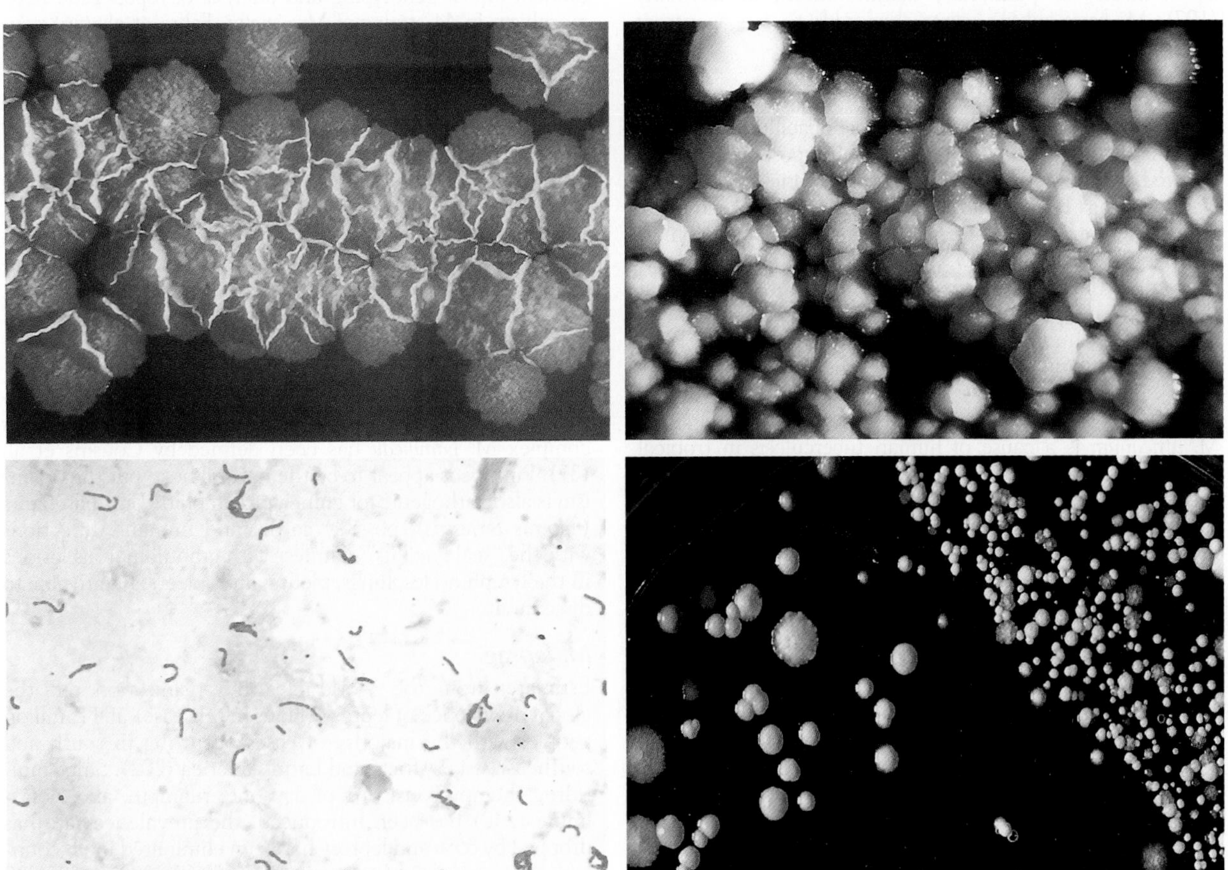

FIGURE 1 (top left) *Mycobacterium tuberculosis* on Middlebrook 7H10 agar. Note the dry and rough colonies, sometimes with a nodular or wrinkled surface.

FIGURE 2 (top right) *Mycobacterium bovis* BCG on Middlebrook 7H10 agar. Colonies may be flat as well as round with irregular edges.

FIGURE 3 (bottom left) Acid-fast staining (Ziehl-Neelsen) of *Mycobacterium microti*. Note the characteristic curved ("croissant-like") microscopic morphology. (Photograph kindly provided by D. van Soolingen, RIVM, Bilthoven, The Netherlands.)

FIGURE 4 (bottom right) *Mycobacterium canettii* on Middlebrook 7H10 agar. Note the heterogeneous colony morphology consisting of some flat and smooth but predominantly domed and glossy colonies. (Photograph kindly provided by D. van Soolingen.)

M. *tuberculosis*, there exists an Asian variant which is susceptible to thiophene-2-carboxylic acid hydrazide. In contrast to M. *tuberculosis*, Asian variant strains often contain few to no IS*6110* elements in their genomes (see chapter 37).

M. *bovis*

M. *bovis* causes tuberculosis in warm-blooded animals such as cattle, dogs, cats, pigs, parrots, badgers, and some birds of prey but also in primates and humans. Human disease is very similar to that caused by M. *tuberculosis* and is treated accordingly, except that pyrazinamide is inefficient due to the inherent resistance of most M. *bovis* strains. The organism grows poorly on L-J medium, but growth is stimulated if glycerol is replaced by pyruvate. In contrast to most members of the M. *tuberculosis* complex, M. *bovis* is able to grow in a reduced-O_2 atmosphere. Colonies on egg-based media are small and rounded, with irregular edges and a granular surface, and on agar media colonies are small and flat (216).

M. *bovis* subsp. *caprae* (6, 53), easily recognized by its susceptibility to pyrazinamide, is not only seen in cattle but accounts for 31% of human M. *bovis*-associated tuberculosis cases, mostly as pulmonary manifestations, in Germany (107). M. *bovis* subsp. *caprae* thus adds to the agents of human tuberculosis contracted from animals.

M. *bovis* BCG

In many parts of the world, M. *bovis* bacillus Calmette-Guérin (BCG) is still used for vaccine purposes. It was distributed by Calmette in 1924 to laboratories around the world and has been maintained in vitro by serial passages. Today, there exists a genetically heterogeneous conglomerate of BCG strains (Fig. 2) (11, 183) which predominantly conform to the properties described for M. *bovis* except that they are more attenuated in virulence. In rare instances, BCG may disseminate as a complication of intravesical BCG immunostimulation against bladder cancer (1).

M. *africanum*

M. *africanum* is a cause of human tuberculosis in tropical Africa. Colonies of M. *africanum* resemble those of M. *tuberculosis*, and physiological and biochemical properties position the organism between M. *tuberculosis* and M. *bovis*. Prior to molecular genetics methods, the definition of M. *africanum* was difficult and its validity was questioned by some authors. Recent genotypic analyses based on variable-number tandem repeats and other molecular characteristics have set M. *africanum* clearly apart from other members of the complex (64, 206). Likewise, Mostowy et al. (126) and Niemann et al. (133) consider M. *africanum* a unique species within the M. *tuberculosis* complex. The distribution of deleted sequences suggests that M. *africanum* subtype II isolates are situated among strains of "modern" M. *tuberculosis* while subtype I isolates are heterogenous and constitute two distinct evolutionary branches within the M. *tuberculosis* complex.

M. *microti*

Originally isolated from rodents such as voles and shrews, M. *microti* causes naturally acquired tuberculosis in guinea pigs, rabbits, llamas, cats, and other warm-blooded animals. It has been identified as a causative agent of tuberculosis in both immunocompetent and immunosuppressed humans (204). Usually revealing a characteristic, "croissant"-like morphology in stained smears (Fig. 3), the organism normally fails to grow in culture. At least the vole type of M. *microti* can easily be recognized upon spacer oligotyping (see chapter 37) since it contains an exceptionally short genomic direct repeat region resulting in identical two-spacer sequence reactions (204).

M. *canettii*

M. *canettii* was first collected by Georges Canetti back in 1969. van Soolingen et al. (205) and Pfyffer et al. (147) reported M. *canettii* causing lymphadenitis in a child and generalized tuberculosis in an HIV-positive patient, respectively. Its natural reservoir was unknown. The facts that both patients were exposed in Africa and that more cases of cervical lymphadenitis have been reported from Djibouti (56) support the hypothesis that M. *canettii* may be more abundant on the African continent. In 2002, pulmonary manifestation of M. *canettii* infection was reported (122).

With its smooth, round, and glossy colonies (Fig. 4), it differs considerably from all other members of the M. *tuberculosis* complex and can even be mistaken for an NTM. Studies by Brosch et al. (20) and Marmiesse et al. (113) of 20 regions where insertion-deletion events took place in the genome of M. *tuberculosis* suggest that M. *canettii* diverged first from the rest of the M. *tuberculosis* complex. Based on variable-number tandem repeat genotyping and analysis of *hsp65* gene polymorphism in 44 strains of M. *canettii*, Fabre et al. (56) confirmed that M. *canettii* is the most probable source species of the M. *tuberculosis* complex rather than just another branch of the taxon. In fact, it is assumed that M. *canettii* appeared some 2.8 million years ago and may, therefore, be the ancestor of all members of the M. *tuberculosis* complex. Moreover, the amount of synonymous nucleotide variation in housekeeping genes suggests that early tubercle bacilli were contemporaneous with the early hominids in East Africa and have thus been coevolving with their human hosts much longer than previously thought (Gutierrez et al., *Abstr. 26th Annu. Congr. Eur. Soc. Mycobacteriol.*).

M. *pinnipedii* sp. nov.

On the basis of host preference and phenotypic and genotypic characteristics, the new member of the M. *tuberculosis* complex M. *pinnipedii* has been defined by Cousins et al. (37). Pinnipeds appear to be the natural host, but the organism is also pathogenic for guinea pigs, rabbits, Brazilian tapirs (*Tapirus terrestris*), possibly cattle, and humans. Infections with the "seal bacillus" manifest with granulomatous lesions in the lymph nodes, lungs, pleura, and spleen and are able to disseminate.

M. leprae

Estimates from the World Health Organization put the global prevalence of leprosy (Hansen's disease) at 11 million people, with the majority of cases occurring in south and southeast Asia, Africa, and Latin America (202). Since multidrug therapy consisting of dapsone, rifampin, and clofazimine (230) has been introduced, the prevalence rate has dropped by 85% and leprosy has been eliminated in 98 countries. The number of new cases (about 600,000 to 700,000 per year) has, however, shown no substantial decline despite multidrug therapy (228). In the past centuries, leprosy occurred on a large scale also in Europe, in particular in Norway. Even though the disease has remained endemic in small pockets in the United States (Texas, California, Louisiana, Hawaii, and Puerto Rico) (114), the majority of infections now seen in North America have been acquired abroad. These imported cases appear to present a negligible risk for transmission within the United States.

Leprosy is a chronic, granulomatous, and debilitating disease (77). Its principal manifestations include anesthetic skin lesions and peripheral neuropathy with nerve thickening. The term leprosy encompasses a continuous spectrum of disease, from a form with very few demonstrable bacilli (tuberculoid leprosy) to a progressive, widespread form with massive numbers of organisms due to the absence of cell-mediated immunity (lepromatous leprosy). The majority of leprosy patients show manifestations between these two polar forms and are clinically unstable. Medical complications arise from nerve damage and immune reactions (77).

Shedding from the nose, rather than from skin lesions, is important for transmission, which results most likely from prolonged and intimate contact with a person with multibacillary disease. The natural reservoir for M. *leprae* is not well established, but naturally occurring infections in the nine-banded armadillo (*Dasypus novemcinctus*) have been documented in Texas and Louisiana.

M. *leprae* differs from all other mycobacteria in that it cannot be cultured in vitro. There is, to date, one single report in which M. *leprae* was claimed to show sparse growth in a special medium at 32°C (135). By tradition, the diagnosis of leprosy is essentially a clinical one, based on finding one or more signs of disease which are supported by the presence of acid-fast bacilli (AFB) on slit skin smears or in skin biopsy specimens. In the case of lepromatous disease, nodules and plaques are the preferred sites for biopsies, which will reveal numerous AFB. Conversely, in patients with tuberculoid leprosy, the rims of lesions should be biopsied and usually only a few or no AFB are found. A number of PCR assays have been established to conclusively identify the organism (140, 142).

Nontuberculous Mycobacteria Frequently Involved in Human Disease

Slowly Growing Species

M. *avium* Complex

MAC organisms have been isolated from water, soil, plants, and other environmental sources. They are important pathogens of poultry and swine but were not recognized as a cause of human disease until the 1940s. Generally, these organisms are of low pathogenicity. Single positive specimens with low numbers of AFB as colonizers are not infrequently observed in individuals without apparent disease. This complicates the interpretation of culture results, particularly from specimens of the respiratory tract (5, 57). However, as a result of the AIDS pandemic, the MAC has become the most common environmental NTM causing disease in humans.

Before the advent of AIDS, the most common presentation of MAC infection was pulmonary disease showing several different clinical patterns, i.e., tuberculosis-like infiltrates, nodular bronchiectasis, solitary nodules, and diffuse infiltrates in immunocompromised patients (209). Tuberculosis-like upper lobe fibrocavitary disease due to the MAC occurs typically in white men 45 to 60 years of age who are heavy smokers, many of whom abuse alcohol, and some of whom have preexisting lung disease. The clinical presentation is similar to that of tuberculosis. Nodular bronchiectasis occurs usually in elderly, nonsmoking women with no predisposing disorders of the lungs or immune system other than associated bronchiectasis ("Lady Windermere syndrome") (46). These patients usually present with persistent cough only. The MAC is also isolated from up to 20% of young adults with cystic fibrosis, particularly in the southeastern United States, but its contribution to the disease process has not been established (100). Further, it is also the leading cause of localized mycobacterial lymphadenitis in children, especially in those 1 to 5 years of age (223). The lymphadenitis is usually unilateral and involves lymph nodes in the submandibular, submaxillary, or periauricular area. Less frequent are thoracic infections in otherwise healthy children (59).

Although disseminated MAC infections in non-AIDS patients are extremely rare (87), patients with AIDS may present with disseminated or focal infections (86). Disseminated infection occurs mostly when the CD4 count is below 100 cells/mm^3. Bacteremia occurs in almost all such patients, its magnitude ranging from <1 to 10^2 CFU/ml. The organism is found almost exclusively in circulating monocytes. Almost any organ (e.g., lungs and intestines) may be involved, with levels of mycobacteria as high as 10^{10} CFU/g of tissue. Focal infections commonly involve the lungs or the gastrointestinal tract and occasionally also peripheral lymph nodes (89).

MAC organisms are well-known for their heterogeneous colony morphology. Glossy, whitish colonies may often occur together with smaller, translucent colonies. A third, less frequent morphology resembles the dry and flat colonies of M. *tuberculosis*. Some MAC strains may develop a yellowish pigment with age. The MAC comprises a heterogeneous group of AFB that are divided into the two species M. *avium* and M. *intracellulare*. Serovars 1 to 6, 8 to 11, and 21 are M. *avium*, and serovars 7, 12 to 20, and 22 to 28 are M. *intracellulare*. Inclusion of M. *scrofulaceum* (serovars 41 to 43) in the group as the M. *avium*-M. *intracellulare*-M. *scrofulaceum* complex is no longer appropriate, given the advances in mycobacterial systematics (214, 215). M. *avium* and M. *intracellulare* are easily distinguishable by genetic methods, such as the use of DNA probes, 16S rRNA gene sequencing, and analysis of the restriction enzyme patterns of the 65-kDa heat shock protein gene (*hsp*) (185). There is evidence for a third species within the MAC which is generally referred to as the MAC-X (215). Those strains are recognized by the commercial DNA MAC AccuProbe (Gen-Probe, San Diego, Calif.) but not by the M. *avium* and M. *intracellulare* probes (Gen-Probe). More than 90% of MAC organisms isolated from AIDS patients are M. *avium* (as are most of the pathogenic isolates from pigs and cattle). In these patients, distinct serovars of M. *avium* have been found to account for the majority of infections (serovars 4, 6, 8, 9, and 11 [95] and serovars 1, 4, and 8 [165]).

Based on phenotypic and genetic characteristics, three subspecies of M. *avium* have been proposed: M. *avium* subsp. *avium*, M. *avium* subsp. *paratuberculosis* (187), and M. *avium* subsp. *silvaticum*. The latter is an obligate pathogen of ruminants (Johne's disease). In humans M. *avium* subsp. *paratuberculosis* is suspected to be involved in Crohn's disease. With the many new genetic tools available, taxonomy of this group becomes more difficult. Results of comparative DNA sequencing (49) are consistent with the hypothesis that M. *avium* subsp. *paratuberculosis* type I strains are an evolutionary intermediate between M. *avium* subsp. *avium* and M. *avium* subsp. *paratuberculosis* type II isolates or share a subset of M. *avium* subsp. *avium* type-specific loci through horizontal transfer. Recently, a new subspecies of M. *avium*, M. *avium* subsp. *hominissuis*, has been proposed by Mijs et al. (121).

M. *genavense*

M. *genavense* is a slowly growing NTM that was isolated in 1991 from the blood of an AIDS patient in Geneva,

Switzerland (19), and subsequently in the United States and in several European countries (39, 57, 195). It has been associated with enteritis, genital and soft tissue infections, and lymphadenitis in HIV-positive and in HIV-negative immunocompromised individuals. Clinically, disseminated disease in HIV-positive patients is similar to that caused by the MAC. However, stool specimens are more often smear-positive in *M. genavense* infections (136). *M. genavense* is also the most common cause of mycobacterial disease in a variety of pet birds, including parrots and parakeets (84, 152).

Analysis of the 16S rRNA gene sequences indicates that this species is most closely related to *M. simiae*. The organism was first isolated in BACTEC 13A medium, but only after extended incubation (6 to 8 weeks). It fails to grow on L-J medium, 7H11 agar, or other media commonly used for the isolation of mycobacteria. Middlebrook 7H11 agar supplemented with mycobactin J (Allied Monitor, Fayette, Mo.), however, supports the growth of *M. genavense* (39), as do microaerophilic conditions (156), the radiometric BACTEC 7H12 PZA test medium (197), and the addition of blood and charcoal to acidified Middlebrook agar (155).

M. haemophilum

M. haemophilum was first isolated in 1978 from a subcutaneous lesion in a patient with Hodgkin's disease (169). Approximately 50% of infections have been in patients with AIDS, with a relatively large number reported from New York City (25). The other cases have been in other immunosuppressed individuals (169, 210) but also in immunocompetent pediatric patients with localized cervical lymphadenopathy (168) or with a pulmonary nodule (220). The classical clinical presentation is that of multiple skin nodules appearing in clusters or without a definite pattern, commonly involving the extremities, and occasionally associated with abscesses, draining fistulas, cellulitis, and osteomyelitis (57).

M. haemophilum infections may be underrecognized because of the organism's predilection for a low incubation temperature (30°C) and its unique requirement for ferric ammonium citrate or hemin for growth. If *M. haemophilum* is suspected in a clinical specimen but culture remains negative, the organism may be recovered by using a chocolate agar plate.

M. kansasii

In the United States and many other countries, *M. kansasii* is second only to the MAC as a cause of NTM lung disease (5, 57). The organism has been cultured from tap water in municipalities around the world where clinical disease occurs. *M. kansasii* lung disease is common in mine workers in both the United Kingdom and South Africa (35) and differs from that due to the MAC in that the response to chemotherapy is much better (5).

Chronic pulmonary disease resembling classical tuberculosis is the most common manifestation of *M. kansasii* infection; it often involves the upper lobes. Extrapulmonary infections are uncommon and include cervical lymphadenitis in children (232), cutaneous and soft tissue infections, and musculoskeletal disease (13). *M. kansasii* infection rarely disseminates, except in patients with severely impaired cellular immunity (e.g., due to organ transplants) or in patients with AIDS (5).

M. kansasii is a photochromogenic species. Studies of the base sequences of the 16S rRNA gene suggest that phylogenetically it is closely related to the slowly growing, nonpigmented species *M. gastri*. Molecular studies have defined five genotypes of *M. kansasii*, all of which are able to cause human disease (148).

M. malmoense

The species name *M. malmoense* is derived from the city of Malmö in Sweden, where the first strains were isolated from patients in 1977. Disease due to this organism was later found in other European countries (5, 81, 194). It remains rare in the United States (21), Canada (3), and other areas of the world. However, in these countries, *M. malmoense* infection may be more common than suspected, because it may require 8 to 12 weeks to isolate some strains, which is longer than many laboratories in North America hold mycobacterial cultures.

Patients with *M. malmoense* infection are usually young children with cervical lymphadenitis or adults with chronic pulmonary disease (5, 57), mostly middle-aged men with previously documented pneumoconiosis. Extrapulmonary and disseminated infections have rarely been reported. The species has been recovered from soil and water (5).

M. marinum

M. marinum causes cutaneous infections as a result of trauma to the skin and subsequent exposure to contaminated freshwater fish tanks ("fish tank granuloma") or salt water (109). The disease occurs worldwide. In the United States, it is most common in southern coastal states (92). The most typical presentation is a single papulonodular lesion confined to one extremity, usually the elbow, knee, foot, toe, or finger. It appears 2 to 3 weeks after inoculation and, with time, may become verrucous or ulcerated (57). A second type resembles cutaneous sporotrichosis, in which the primary inoculation is followed by spread along the lymphatics. More severe complications include tenosynovitis, arthritis, bursitis, and osteomyelitis. Disseminated infections, including infections in patients with AIDS or persons undergoing systemic steroid therapy, have been rare.

M. marinum is photochromogenic and requires incubation at 28 to 30°C upon primary isolation. Recently, Israeli *M. marinum* isolates from humans and fish were compared by direct sequencing of the 16S rRNA and *hsp65* genes, restriction mapping, and amplified fragment length polymorphism analysis. Surprisingly, significant molecular differences separated all clinical isolates from the piscine isolates (201).

M. simiae

M. simiae was first isolated in 1965 from monkeys. Clinical isolates have come from a few geographic areas, including the southwestern United States (5, 164), Israel (88), and the Caribbean (5). The organism has been recovered from tap water in some of these areas, and most positive cultures from humans have come from single positive specimens with low colony counts, suggesting that most positive cultures represent environmental contamination. Clinical manifestations such as osteomyelitis and chronic pulmonary and disseminated disease are rare (for references, see reference 57). Cases of *M. simiae* infection mimicking MAC infection in AIDS patients have been reported (88). *M. simiae* is one of the very few NTM synthesizing niacin. Unless tested for pigment production under the influence of light, it may be misidentified as *M. tuberculosis* by inexperienced observers.

M. szulgai

M. szulgai was first described as a distinct species in 1972. Its distribution appears to be worldwide, but the natural reservoir is unknown. Patients are almost exclusively middle-aged men presenting with chronic pulmonary disease indistinguishable from tuberculosis (196). The remaining presentations include rare cases of bursitis, cervical adenitis, tenosynovitis, cutaneous infections, and osteomyelitis (5, 57). Cases of M. *szulgai* infection in AIDS patients and disseminated disease in an immunocompetent patient have been reported as well.

Although M. *szulgai* is closely related to M. *malmoense* based on the 16S rRNA gene sequences, phenotypic distinction between the two species is easy. M. *szulgai* is scotochromogenic at 37°C and photochromogenic at 25°C (97).

M. *ulcerans*

The frequency of M. *ulcerans* infection has long been underestimated due to difficulties in isolating the pathogen. Today, M. *ulcerans* infection is the third most frequent mycobacterial disease in humans after tuberculosis and leprosy. In Africa the disease is known as Buruli ulcer, and in Australia it is known as Bairnsdale ulcer (5, 57, 68). Closely associated with tropical wetlands, M. *ulcerans* most likely proliferates in mud beneath stagnant waters. Disease likely occurs via direct contact with a contaminated environment or via water-dwelling fauna such as insects. It typically begins as a painless lump under the skin at the site of previous trauma on the lower extremities. After a few weeks, a shallow ulcer develops at the site of the lump. M. *ulcerans* produces a toxin that causes necrosis (203). The type of disease ranges from a localized nodule or ulcer to widespread ulcerative or nonulcerative disease including osteomyelitis. If untreated, severe limb deformities with contractures and scarring are common. There is growing evidence that M. *ulcerans* also produces disease in wild animals such as lizards, opossums, koala bears, armadillos, rats, mice, and cattle (151).

Failure to cultivate this organism in the past was due to its fastidious, heat-sensitive nature (optimum temperature, 30°C) as well as to a long generation time relative to that of other environmental mycobacteria. Many conventional decontamination protocols used in mycobacteriology interfere with the viability of M. *ulcerans*. Treatment with mild hydrochloric acid (final concentration, 0.03 N) (138) or oxalic acid (233) as a decontamination agent provides the best results. A mixture of polymyxin B, amphotericin B, nalidixic acid, trimethoprim, and azlocillin (PANTA) may control secondary contamination. Good recovery of M. *ulcerans* is obtained on L-J medium with glycerol (137, 233). Reduced oxygen tension enhances the rate of recovery in the BACTEC 460TB system (137). Molecular techniques have been developed which may help to lead to more rapid diagnosis (162).

M. *xenopi*

M. *xenopi* was first isolated in 1957 from skin lesions on an African toad *(Xenopus laevis)*, but it was not recognized as a human pathogen until 1965. By 1979, 50 cases of M. *xenopi* infections in humans had been reported, primarily from the United Kingdom, France, Denmark, Australia, and the United States (5, 57). In some areas such as Canada and southeast England, it is second only to the MAC as an NTM clinical isolate (5). A recent case report of M. *xenopi* spondylodiscitis in an AIDS patient not only highlights its potential pathogenic role but also points to the uncertainties in therapeutic management (119). Increased isolation of M. *xenopi* from clinical specimens may also be due to improved laboratory techniques (50). The optimum growth temperature for the species is 45°C, and it seems to occur frequently in hot-water systems. Nosocomial infection and pseudo-infection via water storage tanks in hospitals have been described previously (176).

Pulmonary disease is the most common manifestation of infection (5, 93), usually occurring in male adult patients with underlying lung disease such as chronic obstructive pulmonary disease or bronchiectasis. Extrapulmonary infections such as septic arthritis (96), spondylitis (42), and dissemination (98) in immunocompromised individuals have also been described.

Nontuberculous Slowly Growing Mycobacteria Rarely Recovered or Rarely Causing Human Disease

Several species of slowly growing mycobacteria including M. *gordonae*, M. *scrofulaceum*, and the M. *terrae* complex are not infrequently recovered but are rarely associated with human disease. Some of the case reports of infections attributable to these mycobacteria, especially from the era before the introduction of molecular laboratory techniques, lack sufficient documentation of identification or disease association. Other species (such as M. *asiaticum* and M. *shimoidei*) are so rarely recovered that most laboratories will never see them.

M. asiaticum

M. *asiaticum* was not recognized as a distinct species until 1971, although it had previously been isolated from monkeys. The first published report of human disease described five patients in Australia with pulmonary disease (17). The organism has since infrequently been isolated from patients with respiratory disease in the United States and elsewhere (184). Cases of bursitis and tenosynovitis have been described. M. *asiaticum* is similar to M. *gordonae*, differing primarily in that M. *gordonae* is scotochromogenic whereas M. *asiaticum* is photochromogenic (214).

M. celatum

First described in 1993 (23), M. *celatum* has been isolated from diverse geographic areas, e.g., throughout the United States, Finland, and Somalia, and mostly from respiratory tract specimens but also from stool and blood. In one study, 32% of the patients from whom it was isolated were infected with HIV (23). M. *celatum* has also been isolated from immunocompetent patients, e.g., from a child suffering from lymphadenitis and from an elderly female patient with a fatal pulmonary infection.

M. *celatum* shares morphological and biochemical characteristics with the MAC, M. *malmoense*, and M. *shimoidei* and can, thus, not be identified with conventional tests. Within the bacterial chromosome, M. *celatum* has two copies of the 16S rRNA gene (157). Several subtypes (1 to 3) have been identified (23), with the use of 16S rRNA gene sequencing or restriction fragment length polymorphism analysis of the gene encoding the 65-kDa heat shock protein (149). Due to high similarities in the 16S rRNA gene sequence with that of M. *tuberculosis*, a few strains have been misidentified as members of the M. *tuberculosis* complex by using a commercially available DNA probe (189) or as M. *xenopi* on account of similar biochemical and cultural features. Unlike M. *xenopi*, M. *celatum* usually shows resistance to even high concentrations of rifampin (23).

M. gordonae

M. *gordonae* is the most commonly encountered nonpathogenic species in clinical mycobacteriology laboratories. This scotochromogenic species is widely distributed in soil and water. A pseudo-outbreak associated with drinking water in a French hospital underlined the necessity for proper maintenance of water supply equipment (108). In only 1 of 38 published reports of M. *gordonae* infection was there convincing evidence that the organism played a role in disease (214). There are also reports of peritonitis in patients undergoing continuous ambulatory peritoneal dialysis (75). Eckburg et al. (52) have reviewed clinical and chest radiographic findings among persons with sputum cultures positive for M. *gordonae* and concluded that it is a nonpathogenic colonizing organism, even among persons with local or general immune suppression and abnormal chest X-ray findings.

M. *scrofulaceum*

The name M. *scrofulaceum* was derived from scrofula, a historical term used to describe mycobacterial infections of the cervical lymph glands. Until the 1980s, M. *scrofulaceum* was the most common cause of mycobacterial cervical lymphadenitis in children. Since then it has been replaced primarily by the MAC (223). Other types of clinical disease are rare. They include pulmonary disease, conjunctivitis, osteomyelitis, meningitis, granulomatous hepatitis, and disseminated disease (for references, see reference 57). M. *scrofulaceum* accounted for 14% of the isolates tested in respiratory specimens collected from South African miners (34).

M. *shimoidei*

M. *shimoidei* was first described in 1988 in a Japanese patient with chronic cavitary lung disease. Only a few clinical cases have been reported since (115). It is a thermophilic organism growing well at 45°C. Biochemically, the organism is similar to the M. *terrae* complex but can be separated by catalase and β-galactosidase tests. The unique sequences of the 16S rRNA gene and the 16S-23S rRNA gene spacer region allow unambiguous identification of the organism (104).

M. *terrae* Complex

The M. *terrae* complex consists of three species, M. *terrae*, M. *nonchromogenicum*, and M. *triviale*. Clinical disease due to M. *terrae* is generally limited to pulmonary disease and tenosynovitis of the hand following local trauma (173). M. *nonchromogenicum*, ubiquitous in the aquatic environment, was the cause of bacteremia in an AIDS patient (116). Separation of the members of the complex, especially M. *terrae* from M. *nonchromogenicum*, requires molecular methods.

New Species of Nontuberculous Mycobacteria

Most new NTM species have been described within the last 5 to 10 years (192). Much less is known about these species than about those mentioned previously, and clinical cases of infection are limited to a very few.

M. *bohemicum*

M. *bohemicum* is a bright yellow-pigmented species originally described in 1998 after being isolated from a patient with Down's syndrome and tuberculosis (158). Rare cases of cervical lymphadenitis in children (193) have been reported, as well as a fatal case of an elderly female with generalized eczema, lesions, and scattered nodules that spread from her hands (191). Isolates have been recovered from veterinary (goat) and environmental (freshwater) sources (191). For identification, analysis of the 16S rRNA gene sequence is required (158, 193).

M. *branderi*

M. *branderi* was first described in 1992 after characterization of 14 respiratory isolates collected in Finland. Since then, M. *branderi* has also been isolated from an infected hand wound (222). Identification of the organism requires 16S rRNA gene sequence analysis (103, 222), which shows that the species is most closely related to M. *celatum*, M. *cookii*, and M. *xenopi*.

M. *conspicuum*

M. *conspicuum* was first isolated in 1995 from two AIDS patients with disseminated disease (180). The organism grew at 22 to 31°C and produced pale yellow colonies on solid media. Unusually, the strains do not grow at 37°C except in BACTEC 12B medium. Based on its 16S rRNA gene sequence, it is most closely related to M. *asiaticum* and M. *gordonae*. To date, only two strains have been isolated. Since the organism prefers a rather low temperature for growth, it may, however, be missed in the laboratory.

M. *heckeshornense*

M. *heckeshornense* was described in 2000 as a scotochromogenic species (159, 163) recovered in multiple cultures from the lung of an immunocompetent patient with severe bilateral cavitary disease. On the basis of its unique 16S rRNA and 16S-23S spacer gene sequences, it appears to be a new species (159, 163). M. *heckeshornense* is reported to grow poorly on Middlebrook agar and egg-based media. Colonies resemble those of M. *xenopi*.

M. *heidelbergense*

The nonphotochromogenic organism M. *heidelbergense* was described in 1997 as an isolate from a child with recurrent cervical lymphadenitis (70). An M. *heidelbergense* infection was also found to mimic a lung tumor in a previously healthy woman. Biochemically, M. *heidelbergense* is indistinguishable from M. *malmoense* but unable to grow under microaerophilic conditions. Sequencing of the 16S rRNA gene, however, positions the organism on a branch separate from M. *malmoense* but within a group of slowly growing mycobacteria with a high degree of similarity to M. *simiae* (70).

M. *interjectum*

M. *interjectum* was recovered from children with chronic lymphadenitis (45) and from an AIDS patient with diarrhea (69). Colonies are smooth and scotochromogenic. Visible growth is produced within 21 to 28 days. Fatty acid patterns revealed by gas-liquid chromatography are similar to those of M. *scrofulaceum*. By 16S rRNA gene sequencing, the organism is shown to be most closely related to M. *simiae*.

M. *intermedium*

The photochromogenic species M. *intermedium* was repeatedly isolated from a patient with chronic pulmonary disease and can be easily confused with M. *asiaticum*, although differences exist in colony morphologies (118).

M. *kubicae*

Described in 2000 (63), most strains of the scotochromogenic organism M. *kubicae* have been isolated from respiratory sources. Its pathogenic potential remains, however, unknown. Based on sequence analysis of the 16S rRNA gene, it clusters with the group of M. *simiae*-related slow growers.

M. *lacus*

The new species M. *lacus* was cultured from the synovia of a 68-year-old female presenting with bursitis of the elbow following a local trauma. Granulomas were detected in the bursa upon its excision (200).

M. lentiflavum

M. lentiflavum was first described in 1996 as a cluster of slowly growing pigmented organisms. The majority of the isolates were from respiratory specimens. The organism has been reported as an etiological agent of cervical lymphadenitis and of disseminated infection in an HIV-positive patient. It does not grow at 45°C (181). The organism has a bright yellow pigment and distinct patterns of mycolic acids and cellular fatty acids.

M. palustre

The only strain of *M. palustre* isolated so far originated from a 4-year-old girl with lymphadenitis. Gene sequencing indicates a close relationship with *M. kubicae* and *M. simiae*-like organisms (190).

M. parmense

Closely related to *M. lentiflavum* and *M. simiae*, *M. parmense* has been isolated from a cervical lymph node of a 3-year-old child (58).

M. sherrisii

Five strains (some of which were of clinical origin), previously considered to be *M. simiae* serotype 2, have recently been characterized as a novel group of mycobacteria. Qualitative whole-genomic DNA hybridization analysis confirmed that this group is genetically distinct from *M. simiae* and *M. triplex* (171).

M. triplex

M. triplex was characterized in 1996 as an unusual cluster of slowly growing mycobacteria that strongly resembled the MAC (62) but were DNA MAC probe negative. The majority of organisms were from either lymph nodes or respiratory samples. *M. triplex* has caused disseminated mycobacteriosis in an HIV-positive patient during antiretroviral therapy and in a liver transplant patient. According to 16S rRNA gene sequencing, the organism is most closely related to *M. genavense* and *M. simiae*. It differs from *M. simiae* in not producing any pigment and from *M. genavense* in growing easily on solid media (62).

M. tusciae

The yellow pigmented organism *M. tusciae*, first described in 1999, has been found in tap water but also in a few clinical specimens, i.e., in a lymph node of an immunocompromised child and in a respiratory specimen from a patient with cystic fibrosis (198).

SAFETY AND TRANSPORT ISSUES

Laboratory Safety Procedures

Nosocomial transmission of *M. tuberculosis* from patients or specimens is of major concern to health care workers (24). Because of the low infective dose of *M. tuberculosis* for humans (50% infective dose, <10 bacilli), specimens from suspected or known cases of tuberculosis must be considered potentially infectious and handled with appropriate precautions (32). Control of aerosols and other forms of mycobacterial contamination is achieved in the laboratory by the use of properly functioning biological safety cabinets (BSC), centrifuges with safety carriers, and meticulous processing techniques (see also chapter 8).

Classification of mycobacteriology laboratory practices should be based on risk assessment (i.e., volume of tests, types of testing, prevalence of tuberculosis, and frequency of multidrug-resistant *M. tuberculosis*). Biosafety level 2 practices and facilities are required for laboratory work assessed as low risk. Aerosol-generating manipulations should be conducted in a class I or II BSC. More rigorous biosafety level 3 practices and level 3 facilities are required for laboratories associated with higher risk. These laboratories process specimens for mycobacterial culture and propagate and manipulate cultures of *M. tuberculosis* (e.g., perform identification and susceptibility testing). Such practices require that laboratory access be restricted, that directional airflow be used to maintain the laboratory under negative pressure, and that workers wear special laboratory clothing and gloves. Biosafety level 3 practices and facilities are required for those laboratories growing *M. tuberculosis* to high volumes, working with large numbers of resistant isolates, or performing tests with unknown risk. For a detailed description of safety requirements in the mycobacteriology laboratory, refer to the Centers for Disease Control and Prevention and National Institutes of Health biosafety guide for laboratories (32).

All respiratory protective devices (respirators) used in the workplace should be certified by the National Institute for Occupational Safety and Health (NIOSH) (130). Respirators that contain a NIOSH-certified N-series filter with a 95% efficiency (N-95) rating are appropriate for use. They meet the recommendations from the Centers for Disease Control and Prevention for selection of respirators for protection against *M. tuberculosis*, i.e., (i) the unloaded filter must filter particles 0.3 μm in diameter with an efficiency of 95% at flow rates of up to 50 liters/min; (ii) the respirator must be qualitatively or quantitatively fit tested to obtain a face seal leakage rate of no more than 10%; (iii) it must fit different facial sizes and characteristics, which is accomplished by making the respirators available in at least three sizes; and (iv) it must be checked for face piece fit by the person wearing the respirator each time it is worn in accordance with Occupational Safety and Health Administration (OSHA) standards. Surgical masks are not NIOSH-certified respirators and must not be worn to provide respiratory protection.

The determination of when and if to use respiratory protective devices in the laboratory should be based on risk assessment. A respirator program should be implemented by the laboratory and should include a written protocol describing situations when respirator use is necessary and procedures addressing (i) selection of the appropriate respirator, (ii) conducting of fit testing, and (iii) training of personnel in the use, fit checking, and storage of the respirator.

All work involving specimens or cultures, such as making smears, inoculating media, adding reagents to biochemical tests, opening centrifuge cups, and performing sonication, must be carried out in a BSC. The handling of all specimens suspected of containing mycobacteria (including specimens processed for other microorganisms), with the exception of centrifugation for concentration purposes, must be done within the BSC. Specimens that are to be taken out of the BSC should be covered before transport. All work surfaces, including bench tops and the inside of the BSC, should be cleaned with an appropriate disinfectant before and after work. Effective disinfectants include Amphyl (Reckitt Benckiser North America, Wayne, N.J.) and other phenol-soap mixtures and 0.05 to 0.5% sodium hypochlorite (concentration varies according to the nature of the contaminated surface). Five-percent phenol is no longer recommended as a surface disinfectant due to the documented toxicity of this compound to personnel. UV light is a useful adjunct for surface decontamination and may be used to radiate the work area when it is not in use. Centrifuges should be used with aerosol-free safety carriers to contain debris in the event that tubes break. Use of electric incinerators rather than open flames is recommended. The excess inoculum from inoculating loops, wire, or spades may be removed by dipping the tool into a container of 95% ethanol in washed sand prior to insertion into an incinerator. Disposable inoculating loops are recommended, as are syringes with permanently attached needles if needles are required. An autoclave should be available in an easily accessible area and used to decontaminate infectious waste before removal to disposal areas.

Personnel should be regularly monitored with the Mantoux PPD skin test (annually and more often if a conversion in the laboratory or the institution has been documented) to demonstrate conversions. Those with positive skin tests should be evaluated for active tuberculosis with a chest X ray and clinical evaluation. Physical examinations should be performed when necessary. New converters should be referred to the employee health and infection control departments for epidemiological evaluation. Laboratories should have written protocols describing procedures for handling laboratory accidents. In case of a laboratory accident with possible formation of aerosols, personnel should hold their breath as much as possible, make sure that BSC are on and centrifuges are turned off, and then leave the room with the door closed for at least 30 min (the amount of time depends on the type of accident and the amount of risk). Using appropriate respiratory protection devices, personnel can return to the accident area to clean the spill. PPD-negative personnel should be skin tested at 3 and 6 months after the accident. The QuantiFERON-TB Gold (Cellestis, Valencia, Calif.) cellular immune response assay may have a role in such testing in the near future (116a). Persons who are immunocompromised should be discouraged from working in the mycobacteriology laboratory (32).

Transportation and Transfer of Biological Agents

Mycobacteria are on the list of infectious agents being regulated for shipping and transfer. Recent, more stringent regulations for the transportation of biological agents have been enacted in the United States to ensure that the public and workers in the transportation chain are protected from exposure to any infectious agents (for other countries, please consult the specific regulations). Protection is achieved through (i) the requirements for rigorous packaging that will withstand rough handling and contain all liquid material within the package without leakage to the outside, (ii) appropriate labeling of the package with the biohazard symbol and other labels to alert the workers in the transportation chain to the hazardous contents of the package, (iii) documentation of hazardous contents of the package should such information be necessary in an emergency situation, and (iv) training of workers in the transportation chain to familiarize them with the hazardous contents in order to be able to respond to emergency situations.

The reader is referred to the following regulatory documents for further information.

Public Health Service. 42 CFR Part 72. *Interstate Transportation of Etiologic Agents.* This regulation is in revision to harmonize it with the other U.S. and international regulations. A copy of the current regulation may be obtained from the Internet at http://www.cdc.gov/od/ohs/biosfty/shipregs.htm.

Department of Transportation. 49 CFR Parts 171–178. *Hazardous Materials Regulations.* Applies to the shipment of both biological agents and clinical specimens. Information may be obtained from the Internet at http://www.access.gpo.gov/cgi-bin/cfrassemble.cgi?title=199849.

U.S. Postal Service. 39 CFR Part 111. *Mailability of Etiologic Agents.* Codified in the *Domestic Mail Manual 124:38: Etiologic Agents Preparations.* A copy of the *Domestic Mail Manual* may be obtained from the Government Printing Office by calling 1-202-512-1800 or from the Internet at http://www.access.gpo.gov/cgi.bin/cfrassemble.cgi?title=199839.

OSHA. 29 CFR Part 1910.1030. *Occupational Exposure to Bloodborne Pathogens.* Provides minimal packaging and labeling requirements for transport of blood and body fluids. Information may be obtained from the local OSHA office or from the Internet at http://www.osha.gov/pls/oshaweb/owadisp.show_document?p_table=STANDARDS&p_id=10051.

International Air Transport Association. *Dangerous Goods Regulations.* These regulations provide packaging and labeling requirements for infectious substances and materials, as well as for clinical specimens that have a low probability of containing an infectious substance. A copy of the *Dangerous Goods Regulations* may be obtained by calling 1-800-716-6326 or through the Internet at http://www.iata.org/ps/publications/9065.htm.

There is also a Saf-T-Pak CD including updates available at http://www.saftpak.com/cdupdatedetails.htm.

Permits *must* be obtained for importation and exportation of biological and infectious agents. These are obtained by contacting the Centers for Disease Control and Prevention, Atlanta, Ga. (http://www.cdc.gov).

COLLECTION AND STORAGE OF SPECIMENS

General Rules

Many different types of clinical specimens may be collected for mycobacteriological analyses (90). The majority originate from the respiratory tract (sputum, tracheal and bronchial aspirates, and bronchoalveolar lavage specimens), but urine, gastric aspirates, tissues, biopsy specimens, normally sterile body fluids such as cerebrospinal fluid, and pleural and pericardial aspirates are other commonly submitted specimens. Blood and fecal specimens are usually submitted from immunocompromised patients only.

Specimens should always be collected and submitted in sterile, leak-proof, disposable, appropriately labeled laboratory-approved containers without any fixatives. Waxed containers must not be used because they may yield false-positive AFB smear results (97). Generally, transport media or preservatives are not necessary owing to the robust nature of mycobacteria. Minute biopsy material (e.g., fine-needle aspirates) may be immersed in a small amount of sterile physiological saline. Collection should bypass areas of possible contamination as much as possible, e.g., tap water, since the presence of environmental mycobacteria may result in false-positive smear and/or culture results (208). In general, swabs are not optimal for the recovery of AFB since they provide limited material and the hydrophobicity of the mycobacterial cell envelope often compromises a transfer from swabs onto solid or into broth media. If transport to the laboratory is delayed more than 1 h, specimens (except blood) should be refrigerated at 4°C. Likewise, upon arrival in the laboratory, specimens should be refrigerated until processed (see chapters 5 and 20 for additional information on specimen collection).

Sputum

Sputum, expectorated or induced, is the principal specimen obtained for the diagnosis of pulmonary tuberculosis. An early-morning specimen should be collected on three consecutive days. Pooled sputum specimens are unacceptable for mycobacterial processing because of increased contamination (97). Since the yield of culture from smear-positive specimens is high, two AFB smear-positive specimens are considered enough for the initial evaluation of pulmonary tuberculosis (182). Nelson et al. (131) demonstrated that the majority of culture-proven pulmonary tuberculosis cases are diagnosed from the first or second sputum specimen and that only rarely is a third specimen of diagnostic value. Another study, however, still concluded that three respiratory specimens are needed despite highly sensitive culture techniques (76). Follow-up cultures should be considered because it is culture (and not smears) that yields a definite answer of whether chemotherapy has been effective (120). Children may have difficulties producing sputum. In this age group, a gastric aspirate is usually the specimen of choice for the diagnosis of pulmonary tuberculosis.

Bronchial Aspirates, Bronchoalveolar Lavage Specimens, Fine-Needle Aspirates, and Lung Biopsy Specimens

In some patients unable to produce sputum, invasive collection techniques such as bronchoscopy may be necessary to diagnose pulmonary tuberculosis or mycobacteriosis. Special care is imperative for cleansing the bronchoscope to avoid cross-contamination with AFB from a preceding patient who underwent bronchoscopy (12, 66, 170). Also, the bronchoscope should not be in contact with tap water, which may contain environmental mycobacteria. Specimens collected by other invasive techniques such as fine-needle aspiration and open-lung biopsy may be submitted in difficult-to-diagnose cases.

Gastric Lavage Fluids

Aspiration of swallowed sputum from the stomach by gastric lavage may be necessary for infants, young children, and the obtunded. Early-morning specimens from fasting patients are recommended in order to obtain sputum swallowed during sleep. Samples of 5 to 10 ml, adjusted to neutral pH, should be collected on three consecutive days. If they cannot be processed within 4 h, the laboratory should provide sterile disposable containers with 100 mg of sodium carbonate for collection. Nonneutralized specimens are not acceptable because long-term exposure to acid is detrimental to mycobacteria.

Urine

The first morning urine specimen should be collected on three consecutive days at midstream (by clean catch) into a sterile container. The first morning specimen provides the best results because organisms accumulate in the bladder overnight. A minimum of 40 ml of urine is usually required for culture. Twenty-four-hour pooled specimens and small-volume specimens (unless a larger volume is not obtainable) are unacceptable. Catheterization should be used only if a midstream sample cannot be obtained.

Body Fluids

As much body fluid as possible (e.g., cerebrospinal, pleural, peritoneal, pericardial, or synovial fluid) is aseptically collected by aspiration or during surgical procedures. Bloody specimens may be anticoagulated with sodium polyanethol sulfonate. Because certain body fluids (such as cerebrospinal fluid and peritoneal dialysis effluent) may contain very small numbers of mycobacteria, it is advisable to submit larger specimen volumes (e.g., >5 ml for cerebrospinal fluid) than are required for other specimen types to increase culture yields and the chance to detect mycobacterial organisms.

Tissues (Lymph Node, Skin, and Other Biopsy Material)

At least 1 g of tissue, if possible, should be aseptically collected into a sterile container. It must not be immersed in saline or other liquid or wrapped in gauze. For cutaneous ulcers, biopsy material should be collected from the periphery of the lesion and incubated at both 30 and 37°C. Specimens submitted in formalin are unacceptable for smear and culture. Minute biopsy material may be moistened with a small amount of sterile saline.

Abscess Contents, Aspirated Pus, and Wound Specimens

As much material as possible should be aspirated aseptically. In cutaneous lesions, material is aspirated from beneath the margin of the lesion. Also, for this type of specimen, a second set of cultures has to be incubated at 30°C since one of the organisms with a lower optimum temperature (e.g., *M. haemophilum*, *M. marinum*, or *M. ulcerans*) may be the infectious agent.

Blood

The majority of disseminated mycobacterial infections are due to the MAC; therefore, if this organism is isolated from blood, it is always associated with clinical disease (78). If blood has to be transported before inoculation of the medium, sodium polyanethylene sulfate, heparin, or citrate may be used as an anticoagulant; blood collected in EDTA and coagulated blood are not acceptable. Direct inoculation of blood onto a solid medium is not recommended. The MAC survives for prolonged periods in Isolator lysis-centrifugation tubes (Wampole Laboratories, Cranbury, N.J.). Therefore, processing of Isolator tubes can be delayed for 24 h if absolutely necessary (79). If blood cannot be immediately processed by the laboratory, it should be stored at room temperature. The use of Isolator blood sediments to inoculate BACTEC 12B medium is contraindicated because one of the components, polypropylene glycol, is inhibitory to mycobacteria in the BACTEC 12B system (213). An identical effect on the growth of mycobacteria has also been reported for the Septi-Chek AFB liquid medium and the Mycobacteria Growth Indicator Tube (MGIT) broth (65), but this is controversial (73).

For many years, the Isolator system and the radiometric BACTEC 13A blood culture bottle (BD Diagnostics, Sparks, Md.) were the only reliable and, therefore, recommended systems for mycobacterial blood cultures (7). Very recently, the BACTEC 13A medium was, however, discontinued. Therefore, cultures from blood and bone marrow specimens have to be obtained by using alternative media, e.g., the MYCO/F LYTIC bottles (BD) (7, 207) or the MB/BacT ALERT blood medium (bioMérieux, Marcy-L'Etoile, France) (74). A recent study demonstrated that the continuously monitored systems (BACTEC MYCO/F LYTIC and MB/BacT ALERT) were as sensitive as and faster for the detection of MAC bacteremia than the heretofore standard manual Isolator system and the radiometric BACTEC 13A medium (41).

Stool Specimens

Stool specimens (>1 g) have been used for detection of the MAC from the gastrointestinal tracts of patients with AIDS, in conjunction with specimens from other sites. Past recommendations have been that stool be cultured for mycobacteria only if the direct smear of unprocessed stool is positive for AFB. The sensitivity of the stool smear, however, is only 32 to 34% (124), suggesting that its results should not determine whether a culture for mycobacteria be performed. Screening with smears is, therefore, not an effective way to identify patients at risk for developing disseminated MAC infection (78, 79).

Inadequate Specimens

Processing of inappropriate clinical specimens for mycobacteria is a waste of both financial and personnel resources. There are quite a few reasons why a specimen should not be accepted (and the clinician should be notified), e.g., (i) too small an amount is submitted (ii) specimens consist of saliva, (iii) dried swabs are submitted (biopsy specimens are preferable), (iv) pooled sputum or urine is submitted, (v) sample containers are broken, and (vi) the interval between specimen collection and processing was too long (>7 days) (139). Clinical staff must be properly trained to prevent submission of unacceptable specimens.

ISOLATION PROCEDURES

Because mycobacteria are usually growing slowly and require long incubation times, a variety of microorganisms other than mycobacteria can overgrow cultures of specimens obtained from nonsterile sites. Appropriate pretreatment and processing procedures (homogenization, decontamination, and concentration [90, 97]), culture media, and conditions of incubation must be selected to facilitate optimum recovery of mycobacteria (see also chapter 37). In particular, pretreatment of specimens has to be done carefully, i.e., by eliminating contaminants as much as possible while not seriously affecting the viability of mycobacteria.

Processing of Specimens

Decontamination of a specimen should be attempted only if it is thought to be contaminated. Tissues or body fluids collected aseptically usually do not require pretreatment. If the need to decontaminate a specimen is not clear, the specimen may be refrigerated until routine bacteriologic cultures are checked the next day. It may, however, be easier to initially inoculate a chocolate agar plate to check for sterility before a sample is processed for mycobacteria.

Normally Sterile Specimens

Normally sterile tissue samples may be ground in sterile 0.85% saline or 0.2% bovine albumin and then inoculated directly to the media. Because body fluids commonly contain only small numbers of mycobacteria, they should be concentrated to maximize the yield of mycobacteria before inoculation of media, i.e., centrifuged at ≥3,000 × g for 15 min prior to inoculation of the sediment. If the volume of fluid submitted for culture is small and fluid cannot be obtained again, it may be added directly to liquid media.

Contaminated Specimens

The majority of specimens submitted for mycobacterial culture consist of a complex organic matrix contaminated with a variety of organisms. Mucin may trap mycobacterial cells and protect contaminating bacteria from the action of decontaminating agents. Thus, mycobacteria are recovered optimally from clinical specimens through the use of procedures which reduce or eliminate contaminating bacteria while releasing mycobacteria trapped in mucin and cells. Liquefaction of certain specimens, particularly sputum, is often necessary. Mycobacteria are then concentrated to enhance detection in stained smears and culture.

Digestion and Decontamination Methods

Sodium hydroxide, the most commonly used decontaminant, also serves as a mucolytic agent but must be used cautiously because it is only somewhat less harmful to tubercle bacilli than to the contaminating organisms. The stronger the alkali, the higher its temperature during the time it acts on the specimen, and the longer it is allowed to act, the greater will be the killing action on both contaminants and mycobacteria (105). Harsh decontamination can kill 20 to 90% of the mycobacteria in a clinical specimen (97). Homogenization should occur by centrifugal swirling, and this swirling should not be vigorous enough to allow material to rise to the cap. After agitation, there should be at least a 15-min delay before opening the tube to allow any fine aerosol droplets formed during the mixing to settle. All such procedures should be carried out in a class II BSC.

Most commonly, a combination liquefaction-decontamination mixture is used. *N*-acetyl-L-cysteine (NALC), dithiothreitol, and several enzymes effectively liquefy sputum. These agents have no direct inhibitory effect on bacterial cells; however, their use permits treatment with lower concentrations of sodium hydroxide, thereby indirectly improving the recovery of mycobacteria. Addition of cetylpyridinium chloride (CPC; see Appendix 1) to specimens mailed from remote collection stations to a central processing station has yielded good recovery of *M. tuberculosis* without overgrowth by contaminating bacteria (175), but based on our experience, this agent seriously compromises culture in the BACTEC 460TB system.

For rural areas, the use of sodium carbonate, CPC, and sodium borate has been recommended to allow *M. tuberculosis* to remain viable for 5 to 18 days (18). Under field conditions, liquefaction and concentration of sputum for acid-fast staining may be conducted by treating the specimens with equal volumes of 5% sodium hypochlorite solution (undiluted household bleach) and waiting 15 min before centrifugation (97, 166). Such a treated specimen can, however, not be cultured because the chemical seriously affects the viability of AFB. The major limitation is, therefore, that a second specimen must be collected for culture. The method is very useful, however, for rapid smear preparation and interpretation in laboratories that do not process specimens for culture or that do not have a BSC.

No one method of digestion and decontamination is ideal for all clinical specimens, for all laboratories, and for all circumstances. The laboratorian must be aware of the inherent limitations of the various methods used. Even under the best of conditions, all currently available procedures are toxic for mycobacteria to some extent. Thus, the best yield of mycobacteria may be expected to result from the use of the mildest decontamination procedure that sufficiently controls contaminants. Strict adherence to specimen processing protocols is mandatory to ensure survival of the maximal number of mycobacteria. Most laboratories process specimens in batches; current recommendations suggest that specimen batches should be processed daily (186). The most widely used digestion-decontamination method is the

NALC-2% NaOH method (97) (see Appendix 1), which is compatible with the radiometric BACTEC 460TB system and other commercially available newer broth culture systems. Pretreatment of clinical specimens with sodium dodecyl (lauryl) sulfate (SDS)-NaOH is, by contrast, not suitable for the MGIT cultivation method (145) since it results in poor recovery of mycobacteria and a delayed mean time to detection of AFB. Sodium hydroxide, oxalic acid, and to a lesser extent, mild HCl have a detrimental impact on the viability of *M. ulcerans* (138). A novel procedure for processing respiratory specimens utilizing C_{18}-carboxypropylbetaine has also been described previously (188). Although culture and smear sensitivity significantly improved compared to that with the NALC-NaOH procedure, the contamination rate was extremely high (20.8%).

Commonly used digestion-decontamination methods are described with step-by-step instructions in the guide by Kent and Kubica (97), the *Clinical Microbiology Procedures Handbook* (90), and Appendix 1 of this chapter. In general, the specimen is diluted with an equal volume of digestant and allowed to incubate for some time. A neutralizing buffer is added, and the specimen is centrifuged in order to sediment any AFB present. Centrifugation should be carried out at $\geq$3,000 $\times$ *g* for 15 min to get maximum recovery. The sediment is then inoculated to the appropriate liquid and solid media.

Whatever method is used, care must be taken to prevent laboratory cross-contamination of patient specimens during processing due to aerosols (8, 22, 172). A single false-positive culture for *M. tuberculosis* could easily be the basis of a diagnosis of tuberculosis, with profound consequences for clinical management, epidemiologic investigations, and public health control measures (see chapter 2).

Optimization of Decontamination Procedures

While no contamination or very low rates of contamination indicate that the pretreatment conditions were too harsh and eliminated not only bacteria and fungi but also mycobacteria, a rate exceeding 5% of all digested and decontaminated specimens cultured is generally defined as excessive contamination. A high contamination rate suggests either too weak decontamination or incomplete digestion. One or a combination of several of the following measures may be used to help decrease the contamination rate.

1. Cautiously and slightly increase the strength of the alkali treatment. Be aware that 4% NaOH will in time probably kill most tubercle bacilli.
2. Use a selective medium (one containing antibiotics) in addition to a nonselective primary culture medium to inhibit the growth of bacterial and fungal contaminants. Selective 7H11 agar (Mitchison medium), Mycobactosel agar (BD), or the Gruft modification of L-J medium should be considered. The most useful media for recovering the MAC from stool specimens have been Mitchison's selective 7H11 agar and Mycobactosel L-J medium (231).
3. Make sure specimens are completely digested; partially digested specimens may not be completely decontaminated. Increase the NALC concentration to digest thick, mucoid specimens.
4. Use an alternative digestion-decontamination procedure for problem specimen types. Respiratory secretions from patients with cystic fibrosis, often overgrown with pseudomonads, can successfully be decontaminated with NALC-NaOH followed by the addition of 5% oxalic acid to the concentrated sediment.

To determine the decontaminating capabilities of each new batch of reagents, the laboratory may wish to inoculate blood agar plates with four to six decontaminated sputum specimens in addition to inoculating mycobacterial media. Numbers of contaminants that grow after 48 h of incubation at 35°C should be minimal to none (97).

Acid-Fast Staining Procedures

Smear microscopy is still one of the most rapid and most inexpensive ways to diagnose tuberculosis. In parallel, it is a rapid means to identify the most contagious patients. Normally, its predictive value for M. *tuberculosis* in expectorated sputum is >90% (111).

The common Gram stain is not suitable for mycobacteria. They may be Gram stain invisible, may appear as clear zones or "ghosts," or may appear as beaded gram-positive rods, particularly rapidly growing mycobacteria (199). Special acid-fast staining procedures are necessary to promote the uptake of dyes. Although the exact nature of the acid-fast staining reaction is not completely understood, phenol allows penetration of the stain, which is facilitated by higher temperatures as applied, for instance, with Ziehl-Neelsen staining. Mycobacteria are able to form stable complexes with certain arylmethane dyes such as fuchsin and auramine O. The cell wall mycolic acid residues retain the primary stain even after exposure to acid-alcohol or strong mineral acids. This resistance to decolorization is required for an organism to be termed acid fast. Certain staining protocols include a counterstain to highlight the stained organisms for easier microscopic recognition. Information about specific staining procedures (those for carbol fuchsin and fluorochrome) is given in chapter 21.

Because acid-fast artifacts may be present in a smear, it is necessary to view the cell morphology carefully. AFB are approximately 1 to 10 μm long and typically are slender rods, 0.2 to 0.6 μm wide, that may appear curved or bent. Individual bacilli may display heavily stained areas and areas of alternating stain, producing a beaded appearance. Assessing AFB morphology for presumptive identification of mycobacterial species has to be done with caution and requires ample training and experience of the laboratory personnel. In liquid medium, M. *tuberculosis* often exhibits serpentine cording, but cords are also seen with some NTM species (125). NTM may appear pleomorphic, showing as long filaments or coccoid forms, with uniform staining properties. M. *kansasii* organisms can often be suspected in stained sputum smears because of their large size and cross-banding appearance (9). Cells of rapidly growing mycobacteria may be <10% acid fast and may not stain with the fluorochrome stain (94). If the presence of a rapid grower is suspected and acid-fast stains, in particular fluorochrome stains, are negative, it may be worthwhile to stain the smear with carbol fuchsin and use a weaker decolorizing process. Organisms that are truly acid fast are difficult to overdecolorize. The laboratory must be aware that there are nonmycobacterial organisms with various degrees of acid fastness such as *Rhodococcus* species, *Nocardia* species, and *Legionella micdadei*, as well as the cysts of *Cryptosporidium, Isospora, Cyclospora*, and *Microsporidium* spores. Based on a recent study, Kinyoun's cold carbol fuchsin method is inferior to both the Ziehl-Neelsen and fluorochrome methods (179).

Each slide made from a clinical specimen should be thoroughly examined for the presence of AFB. When a carbol fuchsin-stained smear is read, a minimum of 300 fields should be examined (magnification of $\times$1,000) before the smear is reported as negative (90, 97). A fluorochrome stained smear is read at a lower power (×250) than a carbol fuchsin stained smear; therefore, more material can be examined in a given period. At the lower magnification, a minimum of 30 fields of view should be examined. This requires as little as 90 s. This ease of detection of AFB with the fluorochrome stain makes it the preferred staining method for clinical specimens, although an inexperienced observer may misinterpret fluorescent debris as bacilli.

All smears in which no AFB have been seen should be reported as negative. Conversely, when acid-fast organisms are detected on a smear, the smear should be reported as AFB positive and the staining method should be specified. It is best to confirm positive smears by having them reviewed by another experienced reader. Ideally, all positive fluorochrome-stained smears should be confirmed by a carbol fuchsin-based staining method, e.g., Ziehl-Neelsen, and slides should be stored for future reference (97). The widely accepted practice of confirming positive fluorochrome stains may be challenged in the future. In a recent study, Murray et al. (127) demonstrated that applying a stain to a liquefied (dithiothreitol), concentrated sample and examining the sample before the decontamination process (NaOH) is the most effective method for the detection of AFB.

Information about the quantity of AFB observed on the smear should be provided. The recommended interpretations and reporting of smear results are given in Table 1. If only one or two organisms are seen on an entire smear, this result should be noted but not reported. Confirmation of this finding should be attempted by preparation of additional smears from the same specimen or, if possible, smears from a new specimen. Observations made with the fluorochrome smears should be converted into a format that equates these observations with those made with a 100× oil immersion objective.

However, the reliability of smear microscopy is highly dependent not only on the experience of the laboratory technician but also on the number of AFB present in the specimen. While 10^6 AFB/ml of specimen usually result in a positive smear, only 60% of the smears are positive if 10^4 AFB/ml are present (55).The overall sensitivity of the smear has been reported to range from 22 to 80% (111). An important factor influencing sensitivity is the minimum amount of sputum submitted to the laboratory. In a long-term study, the sensitivity of a concentrated smear from >5 ml of sputum was significantly greater than the sensitivity of a smear processed regardless of volume (211). Other factors influencing smear sensitivity include the type of specimens examined, staining techniques, the experience of the reader, the patient population being evaluated, and pretreatment or lack of pretreatment of the specimens (indirect versus direct smears). Respiratory specimens yield the highest smear positivity rate (111). In practice, the fluorochrome stain is more sensitive than the carbol fuchsin stain, even when smears are read at lower magnification, probably because the fluorochrome-stained smears are easier to read.

The specificity of the smear for the detection of mycobacteria is very high. Prolonged or very harsh specimen decontamination and short incubation of cultures may account for smear-positive, but culture-negative, results. Patients with pulmonary tuberculosis may have positive smears with negative cultures (for 2 to 10 weeks on average) during a course of appropriate treatment (101).

Cytocentrifugation of sputum has resulted in controversial results concerning the sensitivity of smear microscopy (166, 224). Concentration of sputum by centrifugation after liquefaction with 5% sodium hypochlorite is a possible means of increasing smear sensitivity, particularly in developing countries.

The diagnostic yield of acid-fast staining of body fluids is less than that of respiratory specimens because the number of mycobacteria is usually lower. A variety of techniques have been used to concentrate mycobacteria from cerebrospinal fluid and other body fluids, but comparative data are lacking. Centrifugation is not an effective way to concentrate mycobacteria in body fluids since mycobacteria have a buoyant density of approximately 1 and, therefore, many organisms remain in the supernatant (102). Sequential layering of several drops of uncentrifuged fluid onto a slide or polycarbonate membrane filtration is probably the most effective means of concentrating mycobacteria for microscopy (174).

With each new batch of staining reagents, good laboratory practice includes the preparation of a positive and a negative smear for internal quality assessment. Smears containing *M. tuberculosis* or an NTM (positive control) and a gram-positive organism, preferentially a *Nocardia* sp. strain which is not totally acid fast (negative control), may be prepared in advance. Cross-contamination of slides during the staining process and the use of water contaminated with NTM during staining procedures are potential sources of false-positive results (48, 208). Staining jars or dishes should not be used. Transfer of AFB in the oil used for microscopy may also occur. Troubleshooting protocols to prevent false-positive and false-negative smear results have been

TABLE 1 Acid-fast smear evaluation and reporting[a]

Report	No. of AFB seen by staining method and magnification		
	Fuchsin stain	Fluorochrome stain	
	×1,000	×250	×450
No AFB seen	0	0	0
Doubtful; repeat	1–2/300 F[b] (3 sweeps)[c]	1–2/30 F (1 sweep)	1–2/70 F (1.5 sweeps)
1+	1–9/100 F (1 sweep)	1–9/10 F	2–18/50 F (1 sweep)
2+	1–9/10 F	1–9/F	4–36/10 F
3+	1–9/F	10–90/F	4–36/F
4+	>9/F	>90/F	>36/F

[a] Adapted from reference 97.
[b] F, microscope fields.
[c] In all cases, one full sweep refers to scanning the full length (2 cm) of a smear 1 cm wide by 2 cm long.

established by the Association of State and Territorial Public Health Laboratory Directors and the Centers for Disease Control and Prevention (8).

Culture

In detecting as few as 10^1 to 10^2 viable organisms/ml of specimen, culture is more effective than smears. Media available for the recovery of mycobacteria (97) include nonselective and selective ones, the latter containing one or more antibiotics to prevent overgrowth by contaminating bacteria or fungi. Broth media are preferred for rapid initial isolation of mycobacteria.

Solid Media

Egg-Based Media

Egg-based media contain whole eggs or egg yolk, potato flour, salts, and glycerol and are solidified by inspissation. These media have a good buffer capacity and a long shelf life (several months when refrigerated) and support good growth of most mycobacteria. Also, materials in the inoculum or medium toxic to mycobacteria are neutralized. Disadvantages of these media include variations from batch to batch depending on the quality of the eggs used, difficulties in distinguishing colonies from debris, and the inability to achieve accurate and consistent drug concentrations for susceptibility testing. When egg-based media become contaminated, they may liquefy.

Of the egg-based media, L-J medium is most commonly used in clinical laboratories. In general, it recovers *M. tuberculosis* well but is not as reliable for the recovery of other species. Petragnani medium contains about twice as much malachite green as does L-J medium and is most commonly used for recovery of mycobacteria from heavily contaminated specimens. American Trudeau Society medium contains a lower concentration of malachite green than L-J medium and is, therefore, more easily overgrown by contaminants, but the growth of mycobacteria is less inhibited, resulting in earlier growth of larger colonies.

Agar-Based Media

Agar-based media are chemically better defined than egg-containing media. Agar-based media are transparent and provide a ready means for detecting early growth of microscopic colonies easily distinguished from inoculum debris. Colonies may be observed in 10 to 12 days, in contrast to 18 to 24 days with egg-based media. Microscopic examination can be performed by simply turning over the plate and examining it by focusing on the agar surface through the bottom of the plate at a magnification of ×10 to ×100. This type of examination may provide both earlier detection of growth than unaided visual examination and presumptive identification of the species of mycobacteria present. The use of plates with thinly poured 7H11 agar (10 by 90 mm; Remel, Lenexa, Kans.) facilitates this process as microcolonies are visible after 11 days (217). This method is an alternative to broth cultures for some laboratories. Agar-based media can be used for susceptibility testing. They do not readily support the growth of contaminants (97); however, the plates are expensive to prepare, and their shelf life is relatively short (1 month in the refrigerator). Care should be exercised in preparation, incubation, and storage of the media, because excessive heat or light exposure may result in deterioration and in the release of formaldehyde, which is toxic to mycobacteria.

Middlebrook medium contains 2% glycerol, which enhances the growth of the MAC. Nonantibiotic supplements may be helpful for recovery of other mycobacteria and for use in special situations. The addition of 0.2% pyruvic acid is recommended if the presence of *M. bovis* is suspected (47), and 0.25% L-asparagine or 0.1% potassium aspartate added to 7H10 agar maximizes production of niacin (99). The addition of 0.1% enzymatic hydrolysate of casein to the Middlebrook 7H11 formulation (the only difference from 7H10) improves the recovery of isoniazid-resistant strains of *M. tuberculosis*.

Selective Media

The addition of antimicrobial agents may be helpful in eliminating the growth of contaminating organisms. If a selective medium is used for a particular specimen, it should not be used alone but in conjunction with a nonselective agar- or egg-based medium. Egg-based selective media include L-J Gruft with penicillin and nalidixic acid and Mycobactosel L-J medium with cycloheximide, lincomycin, and nalidixic acid. Mitchison selective 7H11 (7H11S) medium and its modifications contain carbenicillin (especially useful for inhibiting pseudomonads), polymyxin B, trimethoprim lactate, and amphotericin B.

Heme-Containing Medium for the Growth of *M. haemophilum*

M. haemophilum will grow on egg- or agar-based media only if they are supplemented with hemin, hemoglobin, or ferric ammonium citrate (169). Thus, specimens from skin lesions, joints, or bone should be inoculated not only onto chocolate agar but also onto Middlebrook 7H10 agar with hemolyzed sheep erythrocytes, hemin, or a factor X disk or onto L-J medium containing 1% ferric ammonium citrate to enhance recovery of this organism. Broth media should be similarly supplemented. *M. haemophilum* can also be isolated from radiometric BACTEC 12B medium as well as from MB Redox broth (168).

Biphasic Media

The Septi-Chek system (BD) is a mycobacterial culture system consisting of a capped bottle containing 20 ml of modified 7H9 broth in an enhanced (20%) CO_2 atmosphere and a paddle containing three types of solid media, i.e., modified L-J medium, Middlebrook 7H11 agar, and chocolate agar, encased in a plastic tube. Bacterial contamination is detected on the chocolate agar. Cultures are inoculated by removing the bottle cap, adding the processed specimen, and then attaching the paddle to the bottle. Solid media are inoculated after 24 h of incubation in an upright position by inverting the bottles. A supplement containing glucose, glycerol, oleic acid, pyridoxal HCl, catalase, albumin, and antibiotics (PANTA) is added to the culture bottle before inoculation. During the incubation period, the bottles are periodically tipped to reinoculate the solid media as cultures are being read. The sensitivity of this system is comparable to that of the BACTEC 460TB system (91). Although the average time to detection of growth is longer than that with the radiometric BACTEC, it is shorter than that with conventional media.

Liquid Media

Broth media may be used for both primary isolation and subculturing of mycobacteria. Cultures based on liquid media yield significantly more rapid results than solid medium-based cultures. Also, isolation rates for mycobacteria are higher. Middlebrook 7H9 and Dubos Tween albumin broths are commonly used for subculturing stock strains of mycobacteria and preparing the inoculum for drug susceptibility tests and other in vitro tests. 7H9 broth is used as the basal medium for several biochemical tests. Tween 80 can be added to liquid media and acts as a surfactant which allows the dispersal of clumps of mycobacteria, resulting in more homogeneous growth.

At present, a number of elaborate commercially available culture systems marketed for the isolation of mycobacteria range from simple bottles and tubes such as the MGIT (BD) and MB Redox (Heipha Diagnostica Biotest, Heidelberg, Germany) to semiautomated systems (the BACTEC 460TB system; BD) and fully automated systems (e.g., the BACTEC 9000 MB and BACTEC MGIT 960 [BD]; the ESP Culture System II [Trek Diagnostic Systems, Westlake, Ohio]; and the MB/BacT ALERT 3D system [bioMérieux]).

MB Redox

MB Redox (Heipha Diagnostica Biotest) is a nonradiometric medium based on a modified Kirchner medium enriched with growth-promoting additives, antibiotic compounds, and a colorless tetrazolium salt as a redox indicator which is reduced to colored formazan by actively growing mycobacteria. With the naked eye, AFB are detected in the medium as pink to purple pinhead-sized particles. Recovery rates are similar to those observed with other liquid systems (178). Overall, it is a cost-efficient alternative with the disadvantage that it requires much handling during visual reading.

MGIT

The MGIT (BD) contains a modified Middlebrook 7H9 broth in conjunction with a fluorescence quenching-based oxygen sensor (silicon rubber impregnated with a ruthenium pentahydrate) to detect the growth of mycobacteria. The large amount of oxygen initially present in the medium quenches the fluorescence of the sensor. The growth of mycobacteria or other microorganisms in the broth depletes the oxygen, and the indicator fluoresces brightly when the tubes are illuminated with UV light at 365 nm. For the manual version, a Wood's lamp or a transilluminator can be used as the UV light source, and in the automated BACTEC MGIT 960 system (see below), tubes are continuously monitored by the instrument. Prior to use, the 7H9 broth is supplemented with oleic acid-albumin-dextrose to promote the growth of mycobacteria and with PANTA to suppress the growth of contaminants.

Overall, the sensitivity and time to growth detection of the MGIT system are similar to those of the BACTEC 460TB system and have been superior to those of solid media in clinical evaluations (36, 146). However, contamination rates for the MGIT system are currently higher than those for the BACTEC 460TB system, probably owing to the enrichments added to the MGIT broth, which enhance the growth of both mycobacteria and nonmycobacterial organisms.

The principal advantages of the manual MGIT system over the BACTEC 460TB system include reduced opportunity for cross-contamination of cultures, no need for needle inoculation, no radioisotopes, and no need for special instrumentation other than the UV light source. Its limitations include higher contamination rates, masking of fluorescence by blood or grossly bloody specimens, and possible lack of compatibility with some methods of digestion and decontamination of specimens (145). For susceptibility testing of primary drugs, the MGIT is an equivalent replacement for the BACTEC 460TB system, in both the manual and automated versions (see chapter 77).

BACTEC 460TB System

^{14}C-labeled palmitic acid as a carbon source in the medium is metabolized by microorganisms into $^{14}CO_2$, which is monitored by the instrument. The amount of $^{14}CO_2$ and the rate at which the gas is produced are directly proportional to the growth rate of the organism in the medium.

An antimicrobial mixture serving as a growth-promoting supplement (PANTA; see above) is added to BACTEC 12B medium inoculated with decontaminated specimens in order to suppress residual contaminants. To potentially sterile specimens, polyoxyethylene stearate is added to enhance mycobacterial growth. For pretreatment of nonsterile specimens, the NALC-NaOH protocol is the method of choice, although some other procedures such as the SDS-NaOH method are compatible with the BACTEC 460TB system as well (167). Specimens processed by the Zephiran-trisodium phosphate, benzalkonium chloride, or CPC method can, however, not be used with the BACTEC 460TB system because residual quantities of these substances in the inoculum inhibit mycobacterial growth.

The use of the BACTEC 460TB method has significantly improved recovery rates and times of mycobacterial isolation from respiratory secretions and other specimens (161). Organisms in smear-positive specimens usually grow within a few days. The average detection time is 9 to 14 days for *M. tuberculosis* and <7 days for NTM. This short detection time is also obvious with smear-negative specimens and specimens from treated patients. BACTEC 13A medium, traditionally used for blood and bone marrow aspirate specimens, was recently discontinued. Other limitations of the BACTEC 460TB system include the inability to observe colony morphology, difficulty in recognizing mixed cultures, overgrowth by contaminants, cost, radioisotope disposal, and extensive use of syringes with its potential for needle punctures among laboratory technicians. Since it is only semiautomated, vials have to be transferred to the incubator once the growth index (GI) has been read by the instrument.

The BACTEC 460TB system allows efficient antimicrobial susceptibility testing as well (see chapter 77). Generally, the initial positive vial can be used directly for identification and drug susceptibility testing. It is good laboratory practice to confirm acid fastness and to subculture positive BACTEC vials to a chocolate agar to check for potential contaminants or, if suspected, for mixed cultures.

Automated, Continuously Monitoring Systems

Several automated, continuously monitoring systems have recently been developed for the growth and detection of mycobacteria, i.e., the BACTEC 9000 MB (BD), the BACTEC MGIT 960 (BD), the ESP Culture System II (Trek Diagnostic Systems), and the MB/BacT ALERT 3D (bioMérieux). All have in common that they are no longer based on the use of radioisotopes. The BACTEC 9000 MB system uses the same fluorescence quenching-based oxygen sensor as the MGIT system to detect growth. The technology used in the ESP Culture System II is based on the detection of pressure changes in the headspace above the broth medium in a sealed bottle resulting from gas production or consumption due to the growth of microorganisms. The MB/BacT ALERT 3D system, finally, employs a colorimetric carbon dioxide sensor in each bottle to detect the growth of mycobacteria. Each of the systems includes a broth similar to 7H9 supplemented with a variety of growth factors and antimicrobial agents.

These systems have similar performance and operational characteristics. In clinical evaluations, recovery rates were similar to those of the BACTEC 460TB system and superior to those of conventional solid media (BACTEC 9000 MB [143], BACTEC MGIT 960 [72, 221], ESP Culture System II [225]; and MB/BacT ALERT 3D [150, 221]). Time to detection of mycobacteria is almost the same as in the radiometric BACTEC 460TB technique. Throughout, contamination rates reported have been higher with these new systems than with the BACTEC 460TB system. All share the advantages over the radiometric broth system of having no potential for cross-contamination by the instrument, being less labor-intensive, having continuous monitoring, using no radioisotopes, addressing safety more appropriately, and offering electronic data management. Since these systems are monitoring continuously, bottles are incubated in the instruments for their entire life in the laboratory. As a consequence, these systems are both instrument and space intensive. Some automated systems also lack the versatility of the BACTEC 460TB system in that direct inoculation of blood is, so far, not possible. The same holds for the incubation of cultures harboring mycobacteria with a lower optimum temperature such as *M. haemophilum*, *M. marinum*, and *M. ulcerans*. Except in the case of the BACTEC 9000 MB system, susceptibility testing applications for the primary antituberculosis drugs, including pyrazinamide (in some systems), are available (see chapter 77).

Medium Selection

Medium selection for the isolation of mycobacteria and culture reading schedules are usually based on personal preferences and/or laboratory tradition. Both should be optimized for the most rapid detection of positive cultures and identification of mycobacterial isolates. The variety of media and methods available today is sufficient to permit laboratories to develop an algorithm that is optimal for their patient population and administrative needs. Workload, financial resources, and in particular, the limited amounts of processed sediments are, however, restraining factors in working with too many different types of media. Thus, cultivation of mycobacteria always involves a compromise.

Today, it is generally accepted that the use of a liquid medium in combination with at least one solid medium is essential for good laboratory practice in the isolation of mycobacteria. The addition of a solid medium is advantageous for those strains which occasionally do not grow in liquid medium, aids in the detection of mixed mycobacterial infections, and can serve as a backup for broth with its higher contamination rate. All positive cultures, even if identified directly from the broth, must be subcultured to solid media to detect mixed cultures and to correlate direct identification results with colony morphology. The Septi-Chek system can be used as a stand-alone system. In contrast, the radiometric BACTEC 460TB system and the new, nonradiometric growth systems such as the BACTEC 9000, BACTEC MGIT 960, ESP Culture System II, and MB/BacT ALERT 3D cannot serve as stand-alone culture systems for mycobacteria for reasons stated above. In a recent meta-analysis of 10 published studies encompassing 1,381 strains from 14,745 clinical specimens, the BACTEC MGIT 960 and BACTEC 460TB systems revealed sensitivities and specificities in detecting mycobacteria of 81.5 and 99.6% and 85.8 and 99.9%, respectively. Combined with solid media, the sensitivities of the two systems increased to 87.7 and 89.7%, respectively (40).

Detection of colonies on solid medium certainly offers several advantages over detection of growth in broth, because colonial morphology can provide clues for identification and facilitate the selection of confirmatory tests, including DNA probe tests. However, smears from broth-based systems can sometimes provide microscopic clues such as cord formation (see above), and it is possible to use the sediment from such cultures for confirmation by gene probes before growth is detected on solid media. The criterion of cord formation for presumptive identification of *M. tuberculosis* should be applied with caution since the phenomenon is also being observed with some NTM species (9, 125).

Incubation

Temperature

The optimum incubation temperature for most cultures is 35 to 37°C. Exceptions to this rule include cultures obtained from skin and soft tissue suspected to contain *M. marinum*, *M. ulcerans*, *M. chelonae*, or *M. haemophilum*, which has a lower optimum temperature. For such specimens, a second set of media should be inoculated and incubated at 25 to 33°C. BACTEC 460TB vials should be incubated at 36 to 38°C because optimum metabolism of the radiolabeled substrate occurs at 37 to 37.5°C for most species. Lower temperatures increase detection time. The newer liquid medium-based culture automated systems do not offer the possibility to incubate at temperatures lower than 36 ± 1°C.

Atmosphere

Five to 10% CO_2 in air stimulates the growth of mycobacteria in primary isolation cultures using conventional media (10). Middlebrook agar requires a CO_2 atmosphere to ensure growth, while it is necessary to incubate egg media under CO_2 for only the first 7 to 10 days after inoculation, i.e., the log phase of growth. Subsequently, L-J cultures can be removed to ambient-air incubators if space is limited. In the absence of CO_2 incubators, plates may be incubated in commercially available bags with CO_2-generating tablets. Candle extinction jars are unacceptable for use in the mycobacteriology laboratory because the oxygen tension is less than that required for the growth of mycobacteria. Broth systems usually do not require incubation at increased CO_2 concentrations.

Time

Mycobacterial cultures on solid and in liquid media are generally held for 6 to 8 weeks before being discarded as negative. Specimens with positive smears that are culture negative should be held for an additional 4 weeks. The same is true for culture-negative specimens which were positive for mycobacteria by one of the nucleic acid-based amplification assays or for cases with a persisting suspicion of tuberculosis. Plates should be incubated with the medium side down until the entire inoculum has been absorbed. Once this has happened, media should be incubated inverted in CO_2-permeable polyethylene bags or sealed with CO_2-permeable shrink-seal or cellulose bands to prevent them from drying up during the incubation period. Tubed media should be incubated in a slanted position with the screw caps loose for at least a week until the inoculum has been absorbed; they can then be incubated upright if space is at a premium. Caps on the tubes should be tightened at 2 to 3 weeks to prevent desiccation of the media. Specimens from skin lesions should be incubated for 8 to 12 weeks if the presence of *M. ulcerans* is suspected.

Reading Schedule

Mycobacteria are relatively slowly growing organisms, and thus cultures can be examined less frequently than routine bacteriologic cultures. All solid media should be examined within 3 to 5 days after inoculation to permit early detection of rapidly growing mycobacteria and to enable prompt removal of contaminated cultures. Young cultures (up to 4 weeks of age) should be examined twice a week, whereas older cultures may be examined at weekly intervals. Use of a hand lens for opaque media and a microscope for agar media will facilitate early detection of microcolonies.

Septi-Chek and the manual MGIT may be inspected for growth several times per week or daily for the first 1 to 2 weeks; Septi-Chek bottles should be inverted for reinoculation of the agar medium if growth is not observed. Afterwards, these systems are inspected twice weekly or weekly for growth.

For BACTEC 460TB vials, the reading schedule varies according to the laboratory workload. Low-volume laboratories may read cultures three times a week for the first 2 or 3 weeks and weekly thereafter for a total of 6 weeks, and high-volume laboratories may read cultures twice a week for the first 2 weeks and weekly thereafter. Some laboratories prioritize smear-positive specimens by separating them from smear-negative specimens and test the former more frequently. In addition, separation of "probable positive" cultures from negative ones will decrease the possibility of vial cross-contamination by the instrument. With more frequent testing of all specimens, however, earlier detection of positive cultures is expected. Readings of negative cultures in 12B medium usually remain below a GI of 10; a GI of 10 or more is considered presumptively positive. At this point, the vials should be separated and tested daily. Acid-fast staining is performed when the GI is >50 to determine whether the culture contains mycobacteria. The morphology of mycobacteria seen in smears from 12B medium may be used by experienced laboratory personnel to presumptively identify the *M. tuberculosis* complex and to decide how to proceed with identification methods (9). In addition, a smear of the broth from the vial may be Gram stained and/or the broth may be subcultured onto a sheep blood agar or chocolate agar plate to determine whether contamination is present. When the GI is 500 or more, BACTEC 460TB antimicrobial susceptibility testing can be performed (see below).

When using one of the new continuously monitoring systems (BACTEC 9000, BACTEC MGIT 960, ESP Culture System II, and MB/BacT ALERT 3D), technicians are automatically alerted by the instrument if a specimen turns positive. Irrespective of the system used, the acid fastness of the organism has to be confirmed by smear staining. Also, it is highly advisable to subculture the broth on a sheep blood or chocolate agar plate to rule out contaminants. Once the growth of AFB is detected, susceptibility testing can be performed, always following the instructions specified by the manufacturers.

IMMUNODIAGNOSTIC TESTS FOR TUBERCULOSIS

A variety of immunodiagnostic tests for tuberculosis based on the recognition of specific host responses to the infecting organism have been described previously. Historically, the first immunodiagnostic test was the tuberculin skin test. The shortcomings of this test include the inability to distinguish active disease from past sensitization and unknown predictive values (177).

Much effort has been devoted to the development of serological tests for tuberculosis, but no test has found widespread clinical use (43). The specificity of serological tests with crude antigen preparations is too low for clinical application. Specificity can be increased by using purified antigens, but since not all patients respond to the same antigens, the increased specificity often results in decreased sensitivity (33, 43). Sensitivity and specificity increase if enzyme-linked immunosorbent assay (44) results obtained with a set of purified antigens are combined. Antigens tested in serological assays are, for instance, the 38-kDa antigen, lipoarabinomannan, antigen 60, the antigen 85 complex, and glycolipids including phenolic glycolipid Tb1, 2,3-diacyltrehalose, and lipooligosaccharide. Weldingh et al. (218) have recently assessed the serodiagnostic potential of 35 *M. tuberculosis* proteins and identified four novel serological antigens.

A number of antigen capture assays based on enzyme-linked immunosorbent assays or radioimmunoassays or agglutination of antibody-coated latex particles have been described previously. The sensitivities of immunoassays for the detection of mycobacterial antigens in cerebrospinal fluid ranged from 65.8 to 100% and the specificities ranged from 95 to 100% in six major studies (43). Experience with sputum and other specimens is limited. The use of antigen tests cannot be recommended at this time.

Although broad experience is not yet available, the recently developed, commercially available whole-blood gamma interferon assays are promising candidates to improve the current level of diagnostic accuracy for tuberculosis infection, in particular if skin tests are equivocal. Guidelines for using the QuantiFERON-TB test (Cellestis Ltd.) (132) for diagnosing latent *M. tuberculosis* infection are available (117). Ferrara et al. (60) have demonstrated that the QuantiFERON-TB Gold test (Cellestis Ltd.) has higher specificity than the tuberculin skin test when used for selected populations. The QuantiFERON-TB Gold test is (i) less affected by BCG for vaccination than the common skin tests, (ii) able to discriminate responses due to NTM, and (iii) less prone to variability and subjectivity associated with placing and reading of the tuberculin skin test. Another approach is based on the overlapping *M. tuberculosis* antigens ESAT-6 and CFP-10 and similarly offers increased specificity over the PPD skin test when used in an ex vivo enzyme-linked immunospot (CTL Laboratory, Cleveland, Ohio) assay for gamma interferon detection for the diagnosis of *M. tuberculosis* infection from recent exposure (82, 110).

CROSS-CONTAMINATION

With the advent of molecular techniques designed for molecular epidemiology, cross-contamination linked either to laboratory procedures or, more rarely, to contaminated bronchoscopes can easily be proven (12, 66, 170). False-positive results may be generated at any step from specimen collection to reading of cultures (8, 61). Laboratory personnel should be alerted for a possible laboratory error if (i) the culture result is not compatible with the clinical picture, (ii) there is a late-appearing cluster of cultures which have scanty growth (<10 colonies on solid medium) or a significant delay in recovering mycobacteria from a liquid system, (iii) there is a large number of isolates of a particular species that is usually rare in the laboratory or of an organism that is normally considered an environmental contaminant, or (iv) there is only one positive culture from multiple specimens submitted from a single patient. Practices which can lead to false-positive culture results are numerous and include inadequate sterilization of instruments or equipment (such as bronchoscopes), use of contaminated water for specimen collection or for laboratory procedures, transfer of organisms from one specimen to another through direct contact or via common reagents or equipment, mix-up of testing samples or lids of specimen containers, and failure to take precautions which minimize the production of aerosols, etc. Laboratory aspects of cross-contamination are addressed in more detail in the following section.

QUALITY ASSURANCE

General Aspects

Much of the information in this section was obtained from recent publications (5, 8, 90, 97, 128, 129). In addition to the specific recommendations listed here, standard components of laboratory quality assurance, such as personnel competency, procedure manuals, proficiency testing, and quality control (QC) of media, tests, and reagents, should be in place.

The Public Health Service introduced the levels of service concept for mycobacteriology laboratories in 1967. In this scheme, laboratories define the level of service which best fits the needs of the patient population they serve, the experience of their personnel, their laboratory facilities, and the number of specimens they receive. The concept of levels of service is supported by the Centers for Disease Control and Prevention and the American Thoracic Society (80). The College of American Pathologists proposed extents of service for participation in mycobacterial interlaboratory comparison surveys. American Thoracic Society levels I, II, and III correlate with College of American Pathologists extents 2, 3, and 4, respectively. Five types of mycobacteriology laboratories have been defined by the Clinical Laboratory Improvement Amendments (CLIA). These are modified from the extents described by the College of American Pathologists, but the definitions are awaiting consensus and thus may be modified in the future (226). All specimens submitted for mycobacterial examination should have cultures as well as smears performed. The American Thoracic Society and Centers for Disease Control and Prevention recommend that laboratories examine a minimum of 10 to 15 smears per week to maintain proficiency in performance and interpretation and that they process and culture 20 specimens per week to maintain proficiency in the culture and identification of *M. tuberculosis*. The Association of State and Territorial Public Health Laboratory Directors proposed that only two levels of service be designated: (i) specimen collection, specimen transport, and (optional) microscopy of at least 20 smears per week and (ii) complete mycobacteriology service from microscopy to complete species identification and drug susceptibility testing (212).

Personnel working in the clinical mycobacteriology laboratory must have proper training and certification in the specific functions that they perform. All laboratories performing mycobacteriology testing must be enrolled in a proficiency program which monitors a laboratory's performance by using external samples which are sent for testing. These programs must follow the specifications outlined by the CLIA.

Multiple test parameters are monitored by adherence to the quality assurance guidelines described in the recent NCCLS (now the Clinical and Laboratory Standards Institute) standard document (128). Acceptable results derived from testing QC reference strains do not guarantee accurate results with all clinical isolates. If inconsistent results are seen with clinical isolates, the test should be repeated in an attempt to ensure accuracy. Each laboratory should put its own policies into effect regarding the verification of atypical test results.

QC is vital for monitoring a laboratory's effectiveness in detecting and isolating mycobacteria. The CLIA and accreditation programs represent the minimum acceptable standards of practice (226), and laboratories performing mycobacterial testing should follow QC recommendations in the scientific literature and in ad hoc publications (8, 90, 128).

The laboratory must maintain a collection of well-characterized mycobacterial strains that are used for QC of test systems. These controls may be obtained from the American Type Culture Collection and proficiency testing programs. Frequently used stock cultures can be maintained on L-J slants or in 7H9 broth at 37°C or at room temperature if subcultured monthly. Cultures on L-J slants may be held for up to 1 year if stored at 4°C. Such maintenance is not recommended for strains with drug resistance. Freezing of organisms suspended in skim milk or broth medium and storage at −20 to −70°C is the best option for long-term maintenance of stock cultures.

Routine QC tests are recommended with new lots of media used with commercial systems (90). Laboratories that prepare their own media must also document the performance characteristics of each new lot.

QC of Smear, Culture, and Molecular Tests

Ideally, positive control slides should be prepared from a concentrated sputum sample obtained from a patient with active tuberculosis. In practice, many laboratories use suspensions of stock cultures or seeded negative sputa as positive controls for acid-fast staining procedures. The *Clinical Microbiology Procedures Handbook* (90) describes a method for preparing control slides. Control slides are also commercially available. An increase in the percentage of smear-positive but culture-negative specimens of >2% that cannot be attributed to a response to mycobacterial therapy or the presence of AFB in the negative controls suggests that water or reagents used in the pretreatment or staining procedures were contaminated with NTM (97). *M. gordonae* or the *M. terrae* complex is most often involved. A procedure for detection of AFB in working solutions and reagents is described in the Association of State and Territorial Public Health Laboratory Directors and Centers for Disease Control and Prevention document (8). AFB may also be carried over from one slide to another if slides are not set properly apart from each other during the staining process. AFB may also be found in the oil used with the immersion lens after a positive slide is examined. The sensitivity of the AFB smear is directly related to the relative centrifugal force (RCF, or *g* force) attained during centrifugation. Thus, laboratories should calculate the RCF of their centrifuge and periodically monitor and document that they are reaching sufficient RCF by checking the revolutions per minute with a tachometer (97).

Laboratories should also monitor contamination rates (percentages of specimens producing contaminating growth on culture media) for decontaminated specimens. Contamination rates of 3 to 5% are generally considered acceptable. Lower rates usually indicate that the decontamination procedure is too harsh and the procedure needs to be modified to minimize the lethal effect on mycobacteria. Contamination rates above 5% often indicate a too-weak decontamination which could compromise mycobacterial cultures due to overgrowth of contaminants. It should be emphasized that the widespread use of liquid media increases the generation of aerosols; as a consequence, the risk of contamination between samples also increases. Laboratories that handle large numbers of isolates of the MAC, *M. abscessus*, or specimens from patients with cystic fibrosis will probably have much higher contamination rates due to the high incidence of colonization of the sputum with gram-negative bacteria, especially *Pseudomonas aeruginosa*.

Culturing of mycobacteria is naturally prone to errors because of the multiple steps involved in processing of cultures, the viability of mycobacteria for long periods in the laboratory environment, and the large number of mycobacteria present in some specimens (22). False-positive cultures may result from mislabeling, specimen switching during handling, specimen carryover (including proficiency testing specimens), contaminated reagents, or cross-contamination between culture tubes or vials (22, 29). Inclusion of a positive control (e.g., a suspension of *M. tuberculosis*) in the processing of patient specimens is discouraged due to the risk of cross-contamination. Cross-contamination of culture vials in the BACTEC 460 TB system due to inadequately sterilized sample needles has been documented (15). Standardized laboratory procedures that minimize the potential for errors leading to false-positive cultures should be followed, and mechanisms should be in place to rapidly recognize the occurrence of false-positive cultures. Transfers or inoculation of cultures must be accomplished by using individual transfer pipettes, single-delivery diluent tubes, or disposable labware. The order in which specimens are processed and media are inoculated should be recorded. Processing of a negative control specimen following processing of patient specimens with the same digestion or decontamination solution can be used for detecting possible specimen contamination of the solutions (8). Alternatively, processing solutions may be planted directly. Laboratories should prospectively track positivity rates and establish a threshold which, when exceeded, will prompt an investigation (172). The significance of an isolate may be determined by reviewing the order in which specimens were handled for all manipulations (e.g., initial processing, liquid medium readings, and subculturing), the direct-smear results, the time to positivity, and the clinical history. Cross-contamination in the BACTEC 460TB system or other automated systems is probably rare if the manufacturer's recommendations for operation and maintenance are closely followed.

Since the introduction of molecular fingerprinting of *M. tuberculosis* strains, false-positive cultures have been demonstrated to occur more frequently than previously assumed, accounting for from 1 to more than 10% of positive cultures (154, 172). The deleterious impact of these undesirable events may be minimized if the evidence of false positivity is established in a timely manner and a rapid molecular method of fingerprinting is available. It has been suggested that single positive cultures of *M. tuberculosis* strains grown from AFB smear-negative specimens should be analyzed by a PCR-derived typing technique to rule out laboratory contamination (154). Cultures of strains with identical fingerprints isolated within a 1-week period from different patients should be considered probably falsely positive (172).

The Centers for Disease Control and Prevention and others have recommended that AFB smear results be available and that positive results be reported within 24 h of specimen receipt (8, 186). The time required for identification and susceptibility testing of *M. tuberculosis* should average 14 to 21 days and 15 to 30 days from the time of specimen receipt, respectively (8, 26, 227). Recently, Pascopella et al. (141) have evaluated laboratory reporting of tuberculosis test results and patient treatment initiation in California.

Nucleic acid amplification (NAA)-based assays require several levels of controls (e.g., to detect amplification inhibition as well as contamination between specimens) in addition to positive or negative controls (129). When used as approved by the Food and Drug Administration, NAA tests for *M. tuberculosis* infection diagnosis do not replace any previously recommended tests (28). Laboratories that test patient specimens by using research or home brew methods or commercially available NAA assays for nonapproved or off-label indications and report their results must validate the assays and establish their performance characteristics prior to diagnostic use. Available information is often insufficient to guide test interpretation. Approved guidelines for molecular diagnostic methods in clinical microbiology are available from the Clinical and Laboratory Standards Institute; in these documents, the development, validation, quality assurance, and routine use of NAA assays are addressed in detail (129). However, basing the identification of *M. tuberculosis* on a sole positive home brew PCR result is not recommended because the results of such assays vary considerably (8, 27).

Potential probes and/or primers must be selected for sensitivity by using multiple clinical and reference strains of the target organism. Additionally, specificity must be evaluated by testing for cross-hybridization with other organisms which may be present in patient samples (129).

Several types of validation tests are used to evaluate the presence of target nucleic acid in the sample and to determine that it was isolated in a manner in which the target has not been introduced. Testing to assess amplification should include positive and negative controls and controls for detection of the presence of inhibitors, such as endogenous nucleic acid. Other QC measures include those referring to assays of restriction enzymes and reagents, inspection of equipment, and laboratory design (i.e., separate areas for processing, amplification, and detection steps) (129). Excellent proficiency testing schemes to assess laboratory performance of NAA tests are currently available both in the United States (160) and in Europe (134).

EVALUATION, INTERPRETATION, AND REPORTING OF RESULTS

Adequate funding and focused training are critical in maintaining state-of-the-art mycobacteriology laboratories (16, 128, 129, 226). Laboratories play a pivotal role in the diagnosis and control of tuberculosis, and every effort should be made to implement sensitive and rapid methods for the detection, identification, and susceptibility testing of the *M. tuberculosis* complex as well as other mycobacterial species. Specifically, these include (i) the use of fluorochrome staining for mycobacteria in smears, (ii) the use of a broth-based or microcolony method for culture, (iii) the use of rapid identification methods (e.g., gene probes and line probe assays), and (iv) direct susceptibility testing of smear-positive specimen concentrates.

The 24-h turnaround time for AFB smear results presents a challenge for most laboratories. The daily processing of specimens required to meet this goal adds considerable expense to the laboratory budget. Turnaround time goals for AFB smear results should be established for each institution after consultation with infection control practitioners and infectious-disease specialists.

NAA assays offer the promise of same-day detection and identification of *M. tuberculosis*. Implementation of these new technologies presents several new challenges. Although the performance characteristics of many of these assays are quite good for smear-positive respiratory specimens, limited information exists on the use of these tests for the diagnosis of paucibacillary pulmonary or extrapulmonary disease. The new technology will supplement rather than replace culture. Culture will still be required to obtain organisms for susceptibility testing and detect mycobacteria other than *M. tuberculosis*.

The significance of the isolation of NTM may be difficult to assess since many species are opportunistic pathogens, and the reader is referred to the criteria suggested by the American Thoracic Society for the evaluation (5). In addition to these criteria, accurate identification of NTM will prevent rarely encountered pathogens from being mistaken for nonpathogenic species.

Thus, accurate and timely reporting of the results of AFB microscopy, culture, identification, and drug susceptibility testing is essential to the effective management of individual patients and to the appropriate implementation of public health and infection control measures.

APPENDIX 1
Commonly Used Digestion-Decontamination Methods

Refer to references 90 and 97 for details.

NALC-NaOH method

Reagents

Digestant: For each 100 ml, combine 50 ml of sterile 0.1 M (2.94%) trisodium citrate with 50 ml of 4% NaOH. The NaOH and citrate mixtures can be mixed, sterilized, and stored for future use. To this solution, add 0.5 g of powdered NALC just before use. Use within 24 h of addition of the NALC because the mucolytic action of NALC is inactivated on exposure to air.

Phosphate buffer: The buffer is 0.067 M and pH 6.8. Mix 50 ml of solution A (0.067 M Na_2HPO_4; 9.47 g of anhydrous Na_2HPO_4 in 1 liter of distilled water) and 50 ml of solution B (0.067 M KH_2PO_4; 9.07 g of KH_2PO_4 in 1 liter of distilled water). If the final buffer requires pH adjustment, add solution A to raise the pH or solution B to lower it.

BSA (optional): Use sterile 0.2% bovine serum albumin (BSA) fraction V (pH 6.8).

Procedure

1. Transfer up to 10 ml of specimen to a sterile, graduated, 50-ml plastic centrifuge tube labeled with appropriate identification. The tube should have a leakproof, aerosol-free screw cap. Add an equal volume of the NALC-NaOH solution. The final concentration of NaOH in the tube is 1%.

2. Tighten the cap completely. Invert the tube so that the NALC-NaOH solution contacts all the inside surfaces of the tube and cap, and then mix the contents for approximately 20 s on a Vortex mixer. If liquefaction is not complete during this time, agitate the solution at intervals during the following decontamination period.

3. Allow the mixture to stand for 15 min at room temperature with occasional gentle shaking by hand. Avoid movement that causes aeration of the specimen. A small pinch of crystalline NALC may be added to viscous specimens for better liquefaction. Specimens should remain in contact with the decontaminating agent for only 15 min, since overprocessing results in reduced recovery of mycobacteria. If more active decontamination is needed, slightly increase the concentration of NaOH.

4. Add phosphate buffer (pH 6.8) up to the 50-ml mark on the tube.

5. Centrifuge the solution for at least 15 min at $\geq$3,000 × *g*.

6. Decant the supernatant fluid into a splashproof discard container containing a suitable disinfectant. Do not touch the lip of the tube to the discard container. Wipe the lip of each tube with disinfectant-soaked gauze (separate piece for each tube) to absorb drips, and recap.

7. Using a separate sterile pipette for each tube, add to the sediment 1 to 2 ml of sterile, 0.2% BSA fraction V (pH 6.8) or 1 to 2 ml of phosphate buffer (pH 6.8), and resuspend the sediment with the pipette or by shaking the tube gently by hand. BSA may have a buffering and detoxifying effect on the sediment and increases the adhesion of the specimen to solid media. However, BSA may lengthen detection times (for instance, in the BACTEC 460TB system).

8. Inoculate the specimens onto appropriate solid culture media and into broth media. Use a separate disposable capillary pipette for each specimen to deliver 3 drops to solid medium.

9. Prepare a smear for acid-fast staining. Use a sterile disposable pipette to place 1 drop of the sediment onto a clean, properly labeled microscope slide, covering an area approximately 1 by 2 cm. Place the smears on an electric slide warmer at 65 to 75°C for 2 h to dry and fix them. Alternatively, air dry the smears and fix them by passing the slide three or four times through the blue cone of a flame (heat fixing does not always kill mycobacteria, and the slides are potentially infectious).

10. Refrigerate the remaining sediment for later use if needed (direct susceptibility testing, further treatment if the specimen is contaminated, etc.).

The NALC-NaOH method can be used to process gastric lavage specimens, tissues, stool, urine, and other body fluids. For neutralized gastric lavage specimens and other body fluids ($\geq$10 ml), centrifuge at $\geq$3,000 × *g* for 30 min in sterile screw-cap 50-ml centrifuge tubes, decant the supernatants, resuspend the sediments in 2 to 5 ml of sterile distilled water, and proceed as for sputum. If a gastric lavage specimen is mucopurulent, add 50 mg of NALC powder per 50 ml of lavage fluid and vortex before centrifugation. Tissue that is not collected aseptically can be ground, placed in a tube, homogenized by vortexing, and processed as for sputum. For stool specimens, place approximately 1 g of a formed specimen or 1 to 5 ml of a liquid specimen in a total volume of 10 ml of 7H9 broth, sterile water, or sterile saline; vortex vigorously for 30 s; and then allow large particles to settle to the bottom of the tube for 15 min. Remove 7 to 8 ml of supernatant, place into a 50-ml centrifuge tube, and process as for sputum.

Sodium hydroxide method

Reagents

Digestant: NaOH solution (2 to 4%). Sterilize by autoclaving.

2 N HCl: Dilute 33 ml of concentrated HCl to 200 ml with water. Sterilize by autoclaving.

Phenol red indicator: Combine 20 ml of phenol red solution (0.4% in 4% NaOH) and 85 ml of concentrated HCl with distilled water to make 1,000 ml.

Phosphate buffer: The buffer is 0.067 M and pH 6.8. See the NALC-NaOH procedure for buffer preparation.

Procedure

Follow the steps described for the NALC-NaOH method, substituting 2% NaOH for the NALC-alkali digestant.

1. Transfer a maximum volume of 10 ml of specimen to a sterile 50-ml screw-cap plastic centrifuge tube. Add an equal volume of NaOH.

2. With the cap tightened, invert the tube and then agitate the mixture vigorously for 15 min on a mechanical mixer, or vortex

vigorously and let stand for exactly 15 min. If it is necessary to reduce excessive contamination, the NaOH concentration can be increased to 3 or 4%.

3. Add phosphate buffer (pH 6.8) up to the 50-ml mark on the tube. Recap the tube, and swirl by hand to mix well.

4. Centrifuge the specimen at ≥3,000 × *g* for 15 min, decant the supernatant, and add a few drops of phenol red indicator to the sediment. Neutralize the sediment with HCl. Thoroughly mix the contents of the tube. Stop acid addition when the solution is persistently yellow.

5. Resuspend the sediment in 1 to 2 ml of phosphate buffer or sterile 0.1% BSA fraction V.

6. Inoculate the resuspended sediment to appropriate culture media, and prepare a smear.

Zephiran-trisodium phosphate method

Principle

This system can be used when the laboratory cannot monitor the amount of time of exposure to the decontaminating agent, since the timing of this digestion-decontamination process is not critical. Benzalkonium chloride (Zephiran), a quaternary ammonium compound, together with trisodium phosphate selectively destroys many contaminants while having little activity on tubercle bacilli. Zephiran is bacteriostatic to mycobacteria, and so the digested, centrifuged sediment must be neutralized with buffer before being inoculated onto agar medium. The phospholipids of egg medium neutralize this compound. It is incompatible with the BACTEC 460TB system.

Reagents

Zephiran-trisodium phosphate digestant: Dissolve 1 kg of trisodium phosphate ($Na_3PO_4 \cdot 12H_2O$) in 4 liters of hot distilled water. Add 7.5 ml of Zephiran concentrate (17% benzalkonium chloride [Winthrop Laboratories, New York, N.Y.]), and mix. Store at room temperature.

Neutralizing buffer: Neutralizing buffer has a pH of 6.6. Add 37.5 ml of 0.067 M disodium phosphate solution to 62.5 ml of 0.067 M monopotassium phosphate solution (for preparation of buffer solutions, see the NALC-NaOH procedure).

Procedure

1. Transfer a maximum volume of 10 ml of specimen to a sterile, 50-ml screw-cap plastic centrifuge tube. Add an equal volume of the Zephiran-trisodium phosphate digestant.

2. Tighten the cap, invert the tube, and then agitate the mixture vigorously for 30 min on a mechanical shaker. Permit the material to stand, without shaking, for an additional 20 to 30 min at room temperature.

3. Centrifuge the specimen at ≥3,000 × *g* for 15 min, decant the supernatant, and add 20 ml of neutralizing buffer. Vortex for 30 s to thoroughly suspend the sediment in the buffer (the neutralizing buffer serves to inactivate traces of Zephiran in the sediment, which is critical if inoculation of an agar-based medium is intended).

4. Centrifuge the specimen again for 15 min.

5. Decant the supernatant, retaining some fluid to resuspend the sediment.

6. Inoculate egg-based medium, and make a smear. The phospholipids of egg medium provide neutralization for this quaternary compound.

Oxalic acid method

Principle

The oxalic acid method is superior to alkali methods for processing specimens consistently contaminated with *Pseudomonas* species and certain other contaminants. Specimens processed by this method may be used with the BACTEC 460TB system. This method can also be used to decontaminate a previously processed sediment when cultures are contaminated with *Pseudomonas*.

Reagents

5% oxalic acid
Physiological saline (0.85%)
4% NaOH
Phenol red indicator or pH paper

Procedure

1. Add an equal volume of 5% oxalic acid to 10 ml or less of specimen in a 50-ml centrifuge tube (1:1, vol/vol).

2. Vortex the solution, and then allow it to stand at room temperature for 30 min with occasional shaking.

3. Add sterile saline up to the 50-ml mark on the centrifuge tube. Recap the tube, and invert it several times to mix the contents.

4. Centrifuge for 15 min at ≥ 3,000 × *g*, decant the supernatant fluid, and add a few drops of phenol red indicator to the sediment. Alternatively, use pH paper.

5. Neutralize with 4% NaOH.

6. Resuspend the sediment, inoculate it to media, and make a smear.

CPC method

Principle

CPC, a quaternary ammonium compound, is used to decontaminate specimens, while sodium chloride effects liquefaction. CPC is bacteriostatic for mycobacteria inoculated onto agar-based media. This effect is not neutralized in the digestion process, and thus sediments from specimens treated with CPC should be inoculated only on egg-based media. This method is incompatible with the BACTEC 460TB system.

This method is a means of digesting and decontaminating specimens in transit (>24 h). Mycobacteria remain viable for 8 days in the solution.

Reagents

CPC digestant-decontaminant: Dissolve 10 g of CPC and 20 g of NaCl in 1,000 ml of distilled water. The solution is self-sterilizing and remains stable if protected from light, extreme heat, and evaporation. Dissolve with gentle heat any crystals that might form in the working solution. Other reagents used in processing include sterile water and sterile saline or 0.2% sterile BSA fraction V.

Procedure

1. Collect 10 ml or less of sputum in a 50-ml screw-cap centrifuge tube.

2. Inside a BSC, add an equal volume of CPC-NaCl, cap securely, and shake by hand until the specimen liquefies.

3. Package the specimen appropriately as specified by current postal regulations, and send it to a processing laboratory.

4. Upon receipt in the processing laboratory (allow at least 24 h for digestion-decontamination to be completed), dilute the digested-decontaminated specimen to the 50-ml mark with sterile distilled water and recap securely. Invert the tube several times to mix the contents.

5. Centrifuge at ≥3,000 × *g* for 15 min, decant the supernatant fluid, and suspend the sediment in 1 to 2 ml of sterile water, saline, or 0.2% BSA fraction V.

6. Inoculate the resuspended sediment onto egg medium, and make a smear.

Sulfuric acid method

Principle

The sulfuric acid method may be useful for urine and other body fluids that yield contaminated cultures when processed by one of the alkaline digestants.

Reagents

4% sulfuric acid
4% sodium hydroxide
Sterile distilled water
Phenol red indicator

Procedure

1. Centrifuge the entire specimen for 30 min at ≥3,000 × *g*. This may require several tubes.

2. Decant the supernatant fluids; pool the sediments if several tubes were used for a single specimen.

3. Add an equal volume of 4% sulfuric acid to the sediment.

4. Vortex, and let stand for 15 min at room temperature.

5. Fill the tube to the 50-ml mark with sterile water.

6. Centrifuge at ≥3,000 × *g* for 15 min, and decant the supernatant.

7. Add 1 drop of phenol red indicator, and neutralize with 4% NaOH until a persistent pale pink color forms.

8. Inoculate the media, and make a smear.

REFERENCES

1. **Abramowsky, C., B. Gonzalez, and R. U. Sorensen.** 1993. Disseminated Bacillus Calmette-Guérin infections in patients with primary immunodeficiencies. *Am. J. Clin. Pathol.* **100:**52–56.
2. **Allen, S., J. Batungwanayo, K. Kerlikowske, A. R. Lifson, W. Wolf, R. Granich, H. Taelman, P. van de Perre, A. Serufilira, J. Bogaerts, et al.** 1993. Two-year incidence of tuberculosis in cohorts of HIV-infected and uninfected urban Rwandan women. *Am. Respir. Dis.* **146:**1439–1444.
3. **Al-Moamary, M. A., W. Black, and K. Elwood.** 1998. Pulmonary disease due to *Mycobacterium malmoense* in British Columbia. *Can. Respir. J.* **5:**135–138.
4. **Amadio, A., M. I. Romano, F. Bigi, I. Etchechoury, T. Kubica, S. Niemann, A. Castaldi, and K. Caimi.** 2005. Identification and characterization of genomic variations between *Mycobacterium bovis* and *M. tuberculosis* H37Rv. *J. Clin. Microbiol.* **43:**2481–2484.
5. **American Thoracic Society.** 1997. Diagnosis and treatment of disease caused by nontuberculous mycobacteria. *Am. J. Respir. Crit. Care Med. Suppl.* **156:**S1–S25.
6. **Aranaz, A., E. Liebana, E. Gomez-Mampaso, J. C. Galan, D. Cousins, A. Ortega, J. Blazquez, F. Baquero, A. Mateos, G. Suarez, and L. Dominguez.** 1999. *Mycobacterium tuberculosis* subsp. *caprae* subsp. nov.: a taxonomic study of the *Mycobacterium tuberculosis* complex isolated from goats in Spain. *Int. J. Syst. Bacteriol.* **49:**1263–1273.
7. **Archibald, L. K., L. C. McDonald, R. M. Addison, C. McKnight, T. Byrne, H. Dobbie, O. Nwanyanwu, P. Kezembe, L. B. Reller, and W. R. Jarvis.** 2000. Comparison of BACTEC MYCO/F LYTIC and WAMPOLE ISOLATOR 10 (lysis-centrifugation) systems for detection of bacteremia, mycobacteremia, and fungemia in a developing country. *J. Clin. Microbiol.* **38:**2994–2997.
8. **Association of State and Territorial Public Health Laboratory Directors and Centers for Disease Control and Prevention.** 1997. *Recognition and Prevention of False-Positive Test Results in Mycobacteriology. A Laboratory Training Program.* Centers for Disease Control and Prevention, Atlanta, Ga.
9. **Attorri, S., S. Dunbar, and J. E. Clarridge III.** 2000. Assessment of morphology for rapid presumptive identification of *Mycobacterium tuberculosis* and *Mycobacterium kansasii. J. Clin. Microbiol.* **38:**1426–1429.
10. **Beam, E. R., and G. P. Kubica.** 1968. Stimulatory effects of carbon dioxide on the primary isolation of tubercle bacilli on agar containing medium. *Am. J. Clin. Pathol.* **50:**395–397.
11. **Behr, M. A., and P. M. Small.** 1999. A historical and molecular phylogeny of BCG strains. *Vaccine* **17:**915–922.
12. **Bennett, S. N., D. E. Peterson, D. R. Johnson, W. N. Hall, B. Robinson-Dunn, and S. Dietrich.** 1994. Bronchoscopy-associated *Mycobacterium xenopi* pseudoinfections. *Am. J. Respir. Crit. Care Med.* **150:**245–250.
13. **Bernard, L., V. Vincent, O. Lortholary, L. Raskine, C. Vettier, D. Colaitis, D. Mechali, F. Bricaire, E. Bouvet, F. B. Sadr, V. Lalande, and C. Perronne.** 1999. *Mycobacterium kansasii* septic arthritis: French retrospective study of 5 years and review. *Clin. Infect. Dis.* **29:**1455–1460.
14. **Best, M., S. A. Sattar, V. S. Springthorpe, and M. E. Kennedy.** 1990. Efficacies of selected disinfectants against *Mycobacterium tuberculosis. J. Clin. Microbiol.* **28:**2234–2239.
15. **Bignardi, G. E., S. P. Barrett, R. Hinkins, P. A. Jenkins, and M. P. Rebec.** 1994. False-positive *Mycobacterium avium-intracellulare* cultures with the BACTEC 460 TB system. *J. Hosp. Infect.* **26:**203–210.
16. **Bird, B. R., M. M. Denniston, R. E. Huebner, and R. C. Good.** 1996. Changing practices in mycobacteriology: a follow-up survey of state and territorial public health laboratories. *J. Clin. Microbiol.* **34:**554–559.
17. **Blacklock, Z., D. Dawson, D. Kane, and D. McEvoy.** 1983. *Mycobacterium asiaticum* as a potential pulmonary pathogen for humans. A clinical and bacteriologic review of five cases. *Am. Rev. Respir. Dis.* **127:**241–244.
18. **Bobadilla-del-Valle, M., A. Ponce-de-Leon, M. Kato-Maeda, A. Hernandez-Cruz, J. J. Calva-Mercado, B. Chavez-Mazari, B. A. Caballero-Rivera, J. C. Nolasco-Garcia, and J. Sifuentes-Osornio.** 2003. Comparison of sodium bicarbonate, cetyl-pyridinium chloride, and sodium borate for preservation of sputa for culture of *Mycobacterium tuberculosis. J. Clin. Microbiol.* **41:**4487–4488.
19. **Böttger, E. C., A. Teske, P. Kirschner, S. Bost, H. R. Chang, V. Beer, and B. Hirschel.** 1991. Disseminated "*Mycobacterium genavense*" infection in patients with AIDS. *Lancet* **340:**76–80.
20. **Brosch, R., S. V. Gordon, M. Marmiesse, P. Brodin, C. Buchrieser, K. Eiglmeier, T. Garnier, C. Gutierrez, G. Hewinson, K. Kremer, L. M. Parsons, A. S. Pym, S. Samper, D. van Soolingen, and S. T. Cole. 2002.** A new evolutionary scenario for the *Mycobacterium tuberculosis* complex. *Proc. Natl. Acad. Sci. USA* **99:**3684–3689.
21. **Buchholz, U. T., M. M. McNeil, L. E. Keyes, and R. C. Good.** 1998. *Mycobacterium malmoense* infections in the United States, January 1993 through June 1995. *Clin. Infect. Dis.* **27:**551–558.
22. **Burman, W. J., and R. R. Reves.** 2000. Review of false-positive cultures for *Mycobacterium tuberculosis* and recommendations for avoiding unnecessary treatment. *Clin. Infect. Dis.* **31:**1390–1395.
23. **Butler, W. R., S. P. O'Connor, M. A. Yakrus, R. W. Smithwick, B. B. Plikaytis, C. W. Moss, M. M. Floyd, C. L. Woodley, J. O. Kilburn, F. S. Vadney, and W. M. Gross.** 1993. *Mycobacterium celatum. Int. J. Syst. Bacteriol.* **43:**539–548.
24. **Castro, K. G., and S. W. Dooley.** 1993. *Mycobacterium tuberculosis* transmission in healthcare settings: is it influenced by coinfection with human immunodeficiency virus? *Infect. Control Hosp. Epidemiol.* **14:**65–66.
25. **Centers for Disease Control.** 1991. *Mycobacterium haemophilum* infections, New York City Metropolitan Area, 1990–1991. *Morb. Mortal. Wkly. Rep.* **40:**636–643.
26. **Centers for Disease Control.** 1992. National MDR-TB Task Force, National Action Plan to combat multi-drug resistant tuberculosis. *Morb. Mortal. Wkly. Rep.* **41:**1–71.
27. **Centers for Disease Control and Prevention.** 1993. Diagnosis of tuberculosis by nucleic acid amplification methods applied to clinical specimens. *Morb. Mortal. Wkly. Rep.* **42:**686.
28. **Centers for Disease Control and Prevention.** 1996. Nucleic acid amplification tests for tuberculosis. *Morb. Mortal. Wkly. Rep.* **45:**950–952.
29. **Centers for Disease Control and Prevention.** 1997. Multiple misdiagnoses of tuberculosis resulting from laboratory error—Wisconsin 1996. *Morb. Mortal. Wkly. Rep.* **46:**797–801.
30. **Centers for Disease Control and Prevention.** 1997. USPHS/IDSA guidelines for the prevention of opportunistic infections in persons infected with human immunodeficiency virus. *Morb. Mortal. Wkly. Rep.* **46**(RR-12)**:**1–46.

31. **Centers for Disease Control and Prevention.** 1998. Tuberculosis morbidity—United States, 1997. *Morb. Mortal. Wkly. Rep.* **47:**253–257.
32. **Centers for Disease Control and Prevention and National Institutes of Health.** 1999. *Biosafety in Microbiological and Biomedical Laboratories*, 4th ed. U.S. Government Printing Office, Washington, D.C.
33. **Chan, S. L., Z. Reggiardo, T. M. Daniel, D. J. Girling, and D. A. Mitchison.** 1990. Serodiagnosis of tuberculosis using an ELISA with antigen 5 and a hemagglutination assay with glycolipid antigens. Results in patients with newly diagnosed pulmonary tuberculosis ranging in extent of disease from minimal to extensive. *Am. Rev. Respir. Dis.* **142:**385–389.
34. **Corbett, E. L., M. Hay, G. J. Churchyard, T. Clayton, B. G. Williams, D. Hayes, D. Mulder, and K. M. de Cock.** 1999. *Mycobacterium kansasii* and *M. scrofulaceum* isolates from HIV-negative South African gold miners: incidence, clinical significance and radiology. *Int. J. Tuberc. Lung Dis.* **3:**501–507.
35. **Corbett, L., and M. Raviglione.** 2005. Global burden of tuberculosis: past, present, and future, p. 3–12. *In* S. T. Cole, K. D. Eisenach, D. N. McMurray, and W. R. Jacobs, Jr. (ed.), *Tuberculosis and the Tubercle Bacillus.* ASM Press, Washington, D.C.
36. **Cornfield, D. B., K. G. Beavis, J. A. Greene, M. Bojac, and J. Bondi.** 1997. Mycobacterial growth and bacterial contamination in the Mycobacteria Growth Indicator Tube and BACTEC 460 culture systems. *J. Clin. Microbiol.* **35:**2068–2071.
37. **Cousins, D. V., R. Bastida, A. Cataldi, V. Quse, S. Redrobe, S. Dow, P. Duignan, A. Murray, C. Dupont, N. Ahmed, D. M. Collins, W. R. Butler, D. Dawson, D. Rodriguez, J. Loureiro, M. I. Romano, A. Alito, M. Zumarraga, and A. Bernardelli.** 2003. Tuberculosis in seals caused by a novel member of the *Mycobacterium tuberculosis* complex: *Mycobacterium pinnipedii* sp. nov. *Int. J. Syst. Evol. Microbiol.* **53:**1305–1314.
38. **Coville, P. S., and F. G. Witebsky.** 2005. *Nocardia* and other aerobic actinomycetes, p. 1137–1180. *In* S. P. Boriello, P. R. Murray, and G. Funke (ed.), *Topley & Wilson's Microbiology and Microbial Infections, Bacteriology*, 10th ed. Hodder Arnold, London, United Kingdom.
39. **Coyle, M. B., L. Carlson, C. Wallis, R. Leonard, V. Raisys, J. Kilburn, M. Samadpour, and E. Böttger.** 1992. Laboratory aspects of *Mycobacterium genavense*, a proposed species isolated from AIDS patients. *J. Clin. Microbiol.* **30:**3206–3212.
40. **Cruciani, M., C. Scarpaio, M. Malena, O. Bosco, G. Serpelloni, and C. Mengoli.** 2004. Meta-analysis of BACTEC MGIT 960 and BACTEC 460 TB, with or without solid media, for detection of mycobacteria. *J. Clin. Microbiol.* **42:**2321–2325.
41. **Crump, J. A., D. C. Tanner, S. Mirrett, C. M. McKnight, and L. B. Reller.** 2003. Controlled comparison of BACTEC 13A, MYCO/F LYTIC, BacT/ALERT MB, and ISOLATOR 10 systems for detection of mycobacteremia. *J. Clin. Microbiol.* **41:**1987–1990.
42. **Danesh-Clough, T., J. C. Theis, and A. van der Linden.** 2000. *Mycobacterium xenopi* infection of the spine: a case report and literature review. *Spine* **25:**626–628.
43. **Daniel, T. M.** 1989. Rapid diagnosis of tuberculosis: laboratory techniques applicable in developing countries. *Rev. Infect. Dis.* **11**(Suppl.)**:**S471–S478.
44. **Daniel, T. M., and S. M. Debanne.** 1987. The serodiagnosis of tuberculosis and other mycobacterial diseases by enzyme-linked immunosorbent assay. *Am. Rev. Respir. Dis.* **135:**1137–1151.
45. **De Baere, T., M. Moerman, L. Rigouts, C. Dhooge, H. Vermeersch, G. Verschraegen, and M. Vaneechoutte.** 2001. *Mycobacterium interjectum* as causative agent of cervical lymphadenitis. *J. Clin. Microbiol.* **39:**725–727.
46. **Dhillon, S. S., and C. Watanakunakorn.** 2000. Lady Windermere syndrome: middle lobe bronchiectasis and *Mycobacterium avium* complex infection due to voluntary cough suppression. *Clin. Infect. Dis.* **30:**572–575.
47. **Dixon, J. M. S., and E. H. Cuthbert.** 1967. Isolation of tubercle bacilli from uncentrifuged sputum on pyruvic acid medium. *Am. Rev. Respir. Dis.* **96:**119–122.
48. **Dizon, D., C. Mihailescu, and H. C. Bae.** 1976. Simple procedure for detection of *Mycobacterium gordonae* in water causing false-positive acid-fast smears. *J. Clin. Microbiol.* **3:**211.
49. **Dohmann, K., B. Strommenger, K. Stevenson, L. de Juan, J. Stratmann, V. Kapur, T. J. Bull, and G.-F. Gerlach.** 2003. Characterzation of genetic differences between *Mycobacterium avium* subsp. *paratuberculosis* type I and type II isolates. *J. Clin. Microbiol.* **41:**5212–5223.
50. **Donnabella, V., J. Salazar-Schicchi, S. Bonk, B. Hanna, and W. N. Rom.** 2000. Increasing incidence of *Mycobacterium xenopi* at Bellevue Hospital: an emerging pathogen or a product of improved laboratory methods? *Chest* **118:**1365–1370.
51. **Dye, C., S. Scheele, P. Dolin, V. Pathania, and M. C. Raviglione.** 1999. Global burden of tuberculosis. Estimated incidence, prevalence, and mortality by country. *JAMA* **282:**677–686.
52. **Eckburg, P. B., E. O. Buadu, P. Stark, P. S. A. Sarinas, R. K. Chitkara, and W. G. Kuschner.** 2000. Clinical and chest radiographic findings among persons with sputum culture positive for *Mycobacterium gordonae*. *Chest* **117:**96–102.
53. **Erler, W., G. Martin, K. Sachse, L. Naumann, D. Kahlau, J. Beer, M. Bartos, G. Nagy, Z. Cvetnic, M. Zolnir-Dovc, and I. Pavlik.** 2004. Molecular fingerprinting of *Mycobacterium bovis* subsp. *caprae* isolates from Central Europe. *J. Clin. Microbiol.* **42:**2234–2238.
54. **Espinal, M. A., and M. Salfinger.** 2005. Global impact of multidrug resistance, p. 101–114. *In* S. T. Cole, K. D. Eisenach, D. N. McMurray, and W. R. Jacobs, Jr. (ed.), *Tuberculosis and the Tubercle Bacillus*, ASM Press, Washington, D.C.
55. **European Society of Mycobacteriology.** 1991. *Manual of Diagnostic and Public Health Mycobacteriology*, p. 57–64. Bureau of Hygiene and Tropical Disease, London, United Kingdom.
56. **Fabre, M., J.-L. Koeck, P. Le Flèche, F. Simon, V. Hervé, G. Vergnaud, and C. Pourcel.** 2004. High genetic diversity revealed by variable-number tandem repeat genotyping and analysis of *hsp65* gene polymorphism in a large collection of "*Mycobacterium canettii*" strains indicates that the *M. tuberculosis* complex is a recently emerged clone of "*M. canettii*." *J. Clin. Microbiol.* **42:**3248–3255.
57. **Falkinham, J. O.** 1996. Epidemiology of infection by nontuberculous mycobacteria. *Clin. Microbiol. Rev.* **9:**178–215.
58. **Fanti, F., E. Tortoli, L. Hall, G. D. Roberts, R. M. Kroppenstedt, I. Dodi, S. Conti, L. Polonelli, and C. Chezzi.** 2004. *Mycobacterium parmense* sp. nov. *Int. J. Syst. Evol. Microbiol.* **54:**1123–1127.
59. **Fergie J. E., T. W. Milligan, B. M. Henderson, and W. W. Stafford.** 1997. Intrathoracic *Mycobacterium avium* complex infection in immunocompetent children: case report and review. *J. Infect. Dis.* **24:**250–253.
60. **Ferrara, G., M. Losi, M. Meacci, B. Meccugni, R. Piro, P. Roversi, B. M. Bergamini, R. D'Amico, P. Marchegiano, F. Rumpianesi, L. M. Fabbri, and L. Richeldi.** 2005. Routine hospital use of a new commercial whole blood interferon-gamma assay for the diagnosis of tuberculosis infection. *Am. J. Respir. Crit. Care Med.* **172:**519–521.
61. **Fitzpatrick, L., C. Braden, W. Cronin, J. English, E. Campbell, S. Valway, and I. Onorato.** 2004. Investigation of laboratory cross-contamination of *Mycobacterium tuberculosis* cultures. *Clin. Infect. Dis.* **15:**52–54.

62. **Floyd, M. M., L. S. Guthertz, V. A. Silcox, P. S. Duffey, Y. Jang, E. P. Desmond, J. T. Crawford, and W. R. Butler.** 1996. Characterization of an SAV organism and proposal of *Mycobacterium triplex* sp. nov. *J. Clin. Microbiol.* **34:** 2963–2967.
63. **Floyd, M. M., W. M. Gross, A. Bonato, V. A. Silcox, R. W. Smithwick, B. Metchock, J. T. Crawford, and W. R. Butler.** 2000. *Mycobacterium kubicae* sp. nov., a slowly growing, scotochromogenic mycobacterium. *Int. J. Syst. Evol. Microbiol.* **50:**1811–1816.
64. **Frothingham, R., P. L. Strickland, G. Bretzel, S. Ramaswamy, J. M. Musser, and D. L. Williams.** 1999. Phenotypic and genotypic characterization of *Mycobacterium africanum* isolates from West Africa. *J. Clin. Microbiol.* **37:**1921–1926.
65. **Gamboa, F., Z. de la Rosa, J. Bustillo, M. P. Mora, I. Hernandez, and F. Mirque.** 2000. Negative effect of the components of the lysis-centrifugation system in the growth of mycobacteria in MGIT and Septi-Chek AFB liquid media. *Enferm. Infect. Microbiol. Clin.* **18:**439–444.
66. **Gillespie, T. G., L. Hogg, E. Budge, A. Duncan, and J. E. Coia.** 2000. *Mycobacterium chelonae* isolated from rinse water within an endoscope washer-disinfectant. *J. Hosp. Infect.* **45:**332–334.
67. **Gordon, S. V., R. Brosch, A. Billault, T. Garnier, K. Eigelmeier, and S. Cole.** 1999. Identification of variable regions in the genomes of tubercle bacilli using bacterial artificial chromosome arrays. *Mol. Microbiol.* **32:**643–655.
68. **Goutzamanis, J. J., and G. L. Gilbert.** 1995. *Mycobacterium ulcerans* infection in Australian children: report of eight cases and review. *Clin. Infect. Dis.* **21:** 1186–1192.
69. **Green, B. A., and B. Afessa.** 2000. Isolation of *Mycobacterium interjectum* in an AIDS patient with diarrhea. *AIDS* **16:**1282–1284.
70. **Haas, W. H., W. R. Butler, P. Kirschner, B. B. Plikaytis, M. B. Coyle, B. Amthor, A. G. Steigerwalt, D. J. Brenner, M. Salfinger, J. T. Crawford, E. C. Böttger, and H. J. Bremer.** 1997. A new agent of mycobacterial lymphadenitis in children: *Mycobacterium heidelbergense* sp. nov. *J. Clin. Microbiol.* **35:**3203–3209.
71. **Hale, Y. M., G. E. Pfyffer, and M. Salfinger.** 2001. Laboratory diagnosis of mycobacterial infections: new tools and lessons learned. *Clin. Infect. Dis.* **33:**834–846.
72. **Hanna, B. A., A. Ebrahimzadeh, L. B. Elliott, M. A. Morgan, S. M. Novak, S. Rüsch-Gerdes, M. Acio, D. F. Dunbar, T. M. Holmes, C. H. Rexer, C. Savthyakumar, and A. M. Vannier.** 1999. Multicenter evaluation of the BACTEC MGIT 960 System for recovery of mycobacteria. *J. Clin. Microbiol.* **37:**748–752.
73. **Hanna, B. A., S. B. Walters, S. J. Bonk, and L. J. Tick.** 1995. Recovery of mycobacteria from blood in Mycobacteria Growth Indicator Tube and Löwenstein-Jensen slant after lysis-centrifugation. *J. Clin. Microbiol.* **33:**3315–3316.
74. **Hanscheid, T., C. Monteiro, J. Melo Cristino, L. Marques Lito, and M. J. Salgano.** 2005. Growth of *Mycobacterium tuberculosis* in conventional BacT/ALERT FA blood culture bottles allows reliable diagnosis of mycobacteremia. *J. Clin. Microbiol.* **43:**890–891.
75. **Harro, C., G. L. Braden, A. B. Morris, G. S. Lipkowitz, and R. L. Madden.** 1997. Failure to cure *Mycobacterium gordonae* peritonitis associated with continuous ambulatory peritoneal dialysis. *Clin. Infect. Dis.* **24:**955–957.
76. **Harvell, J. D., W. K. Hadley, and V. L. Ng.** 2000. Increased sensitivity of the BACTEC 460 mycobacterial radiometric broth culture system does not decrease the number of respiratory specimens required for a definite diagnosis of pulmonary tuberculosis. *J. Clin. Microbiol.* **38:**3608–3611.
77. **Hastings, R. C., T. P. Gillis, J. L. Krahenbuhl, and S. G. Franzblau.** 1988. Leprosy. *Clin. Microbiol. Rev.* **1:**330–348.
78. **Havlik, J., C. Horsburgh, B. Metchock, P. William, S. Fan, and S. Thompson.** 1992. Disseminated *Mycobacterium avium* complex infection: clinical identification and epidemiologic trends. *J. Infect. Dis.* **165:**577–580.
79. **Havlik, J. A., B. Metchock, S. E. Thompson III, K. Barrett, D. Rimland, and C. R. Horsburgh, Jr.** 1993. A prospective evaluation of *Mycobacterium avium* complex colonization of the respiratory and gastrointestinal tracts of persons with human immunodeficiency virus infection. *J. Infect. Dis.* **168:**1045–1048.
80. **Hawkins, J. E., R. C. Good, G. P. Kubica, P. R. J. Gangadharam, H. M. Gruft, K. D. Stottmeier, H. M. Sommers, and L. G. Wayne.** 1983. Levels of laboratory services for mycobacterial diseases: official statement of the American Thoracic Society. *Am. Rev. Respir. Dis.* **128:**213.
81. **Henriques, B., S. E. Hoffner, B. Petrini, I. Juhlin, P. Wahlen, and G. Kallenius.** 1994. Infection with *Mycobacterium malmoense* in Sweden: report of 221 cases. *Clin. Infect. Dis.* **18:**596–600.
82. **Hill, P. C., D. Jackson-Sillah, A. Fox, K. L. Franken, M. D. Lugos, D. J. Jeffries, S. A. Donkor, A. S. Hammond, R. A. Adegbola, T. H. Ottenhoff, M. R. Klein, and R. H. Brookes.** 2005. ESAT-6/CFP-10 fusion protein and peptides for optimal diagnosis of *Mycobacterium tuberculosis* infection by ex vivo enzyme-linked immunospot assay in the Gambia. *J. Clin. Microbiol.* **43:**2070–2074.
83. **Hillebrand-Haverkort, M. E., A. H. Kolk, L. F. Kox, J. J. ten Velden, and J. H. ten Veen.** 1999. Generalized *Mycobacterium genavense* infection in HIV-infected patients: detection of the mycobacterium in hospital tap water. *Scand. J. Infect. Dis.* **31:**63–68.
84. **Hoop, R. K., E. C. Böttger, and G. E. Pfyffer.** 1996. Etiological agents of mycobacterioses in pet birds between 1986 and 1995. *J. Clin. Microbiol.* **34:**991–992.
85. **Hopewell, P. C., and R. M. Jasmer.** 2005. Overview of clinical tuberculosis, p. 15–31. *In* S. T. Cole, K. D. Eisenach, D. N. McMurray, and W. R. Jacobs, Jr. (ed.), *Tuberculosis and the Tubercle Bacillus.* ASM Press, Washington, D.C.
86. **Horsburgh, C., B. Metchock, J. McGowan, Jr., and S. Thompson.** 1992. Clinical implications of recovery of *Mycobacterium avium* complex from the stool or respiratory tract of HIV-infected individuals. *AIDS* **6:**512–514.
87. **Horsburgh, C. R., Jr., U. G. Mason III, D. C. Farhi, and M. D. Iseman.** 1985. Disseminated infection with *Mycobacterium avium intracellulare.* A report of 13 cases and review of the literature. *Medicine* **64:**36–48.
88. **Huminer, D., S. Dux, Z. Samra, L. Kaufman, A. Lavy, C. S. Block, and S. D. Pitlik.** 1993. *Mycobacterium simiae* infection in Israeli patients with AIDS. *Clin. Infect. Dis.* **17:**508–509.
89. **Inderlied, C., C. Kempler, and L. Bermudez.** 1993. The *Mycobacterium avium* complex. *Clin. Microbiol. Rev.* **6:**266–310.
90. **Isenberg, H. D.** 2004. *Clinical Microbiology Procedures Handbook,* 2nd ed. ASM Press, Washington, D.C.
91. **Isenberg, H. D., R. F. D'Amato, L. Heifets, P. R. Murray, M. Scardamaglia, M. C. Jacobs, P. Alperstein, and A. Niles.** 1991. Collaborative feasibility study of a biphasic system (Roche Septi-Chek AFB) for rapid detection and isolation of mycobacteria. *J. Clin. Microbiol.* **29:**1719–1722.
92. **Jernigan, J. A., and B. M. Farr.** 2000. Incubation period and sources for cutaneous *Mycobacterium marinum* infection: case report and review of the literature. *Clin. Infect. Dis.* **31:**439–443.
93. **Jiva, T. M., H. M. Jacoby, L. A. Weymouth, D. A. Kaminski, and A. C. Portmore.** 1997. *Mycobacterium xenopi*: innocent bystander or emerging pathogen? *Clin. Infect. Dis.* **24:**226–232.

94. **Joseph, S., E. Vaichulis, and V. Houk.** 1967. Lack of auramine rhodamine fluorescence of Runyon group IV mycobacteria. *Am. Rev. Respir. Dis.* **95:**114–115.
95. **Julander, I., S. Hoffner, B. Petrini, and L. Ostlund.** 1996. Multiple serovars of *Mycobacterium avium* complex in patients with AIDS. *APMIS* **104:**318–320.
96. **Kelly, M., L. Thibert, and C. Sinave.** 1999. Septic arthritis in the knee due to *Mycobacterium xenopi* in a patient undergoing hemodialysis. *Clin. Infect. Dis.* **29:**1342–1343.
97. **Kent, P. T., and G. P. Kubica.** 1985. *Public Health Mycobacteriology: a Guide for the Level III Laboratory.* U.S. Department of Health and Human Services, Centers for Disease Control, Atlanta, Ga.
98. **Kesten, S., and C. Chaparro.** 1999. Mycobacterial infections in lung transplant recipients. *Chest* **115:**741–745.
99. **Kilburn, J. O., K. D. Stottmeier, and G. P. Kubica.** 1968. Aspartic acid as a precursor for niacin synthesis by tubercle bacilli grown on 7H10 agar medium. *Am. J. Clin. Pathol.* **50:**582–586.
100. **Kilby, J., P. Gilligan, J. Yankaskas, W. Highsmith, Jr., L. Edwards, and M. Knowles.** 1992. Nontuberculous mycobacteria in adult patients with cystic fibrosis. *Chest* **102:**70–75.
101. **Kim, T. C., R. S. Blackman, K. M. Heatwole, T. Kim, and D. F. Rochester.** 1984. Acid-fast bacilli in sputum smears of patients with pulmonary tuberculosis. Prevalence and significance of negative smears pretreatment and positive smears post treatment. *Am. Rev. Respir. Dis.* **129:**264–268.
102. **Klein, G. C., M. M. Cummings, and C. H. Fish.** 1952. Efficiency of centrifugation as a method of concentrating tubercle bacilli. *Am. J. Clin. Pathol.* **22:**581–585.
103. **Koukila-Kähkölä, P., B. Springer, E. C. Böttger, L. Paulin, E. Jantzen, and M. L. Katila.** 1995. *Mycobacterium branderi* sp. nov., a new potential human pathogen. *Int. J. Syst. Bacteriol.* **45:**549–553.
104. **Koukila-Kähkölä, P., L. Paulin, E. Brander, E. Jantzen, M. Eho-Remes, and M. L. Katila.** 2000. Characterization of a new isolate of *Mycobacterium shimoidei* from Finland. *J. Med. Microbiol.* **49:**937–940.
105. **Krasnow, I., and L. G. Wayne.** 1969. Comparison of methods for tuberculosis bacteriology. *Appl. Microbiol.* **18:**915–917.
106. **Kremer, L., and G. S. Besra.** 2005. A waxy tale, by *Mycobacterium tuberculosis*, p. 287–305. *In* S. T. Cole, K. D. Eisenach, D. N. McMurray, and W. R. Jacobs, Jr. (ed.), *Tuberculosis and the Tubercle Bacillus*, ASM Press, Washington, D.C.
107. **Kubica, T., S. Rüsch-Gerdes, and S. Niemann.** 2003. *Mycobacterium bovis* subsp. *caprae* caused one-third of human *M. bovis*-associated tuberculosis cases reported in Germany between 1999 and 2001. *J. Clin. Microbiol.* **41:**3070–3077.
108. **Lalande, V., F. Barbut, A. Vernerot, M. Febvre, D. Nesa, S. Wadel, V. Vincent, and J. C. Petit.** 2001. Pseudo-outbreak of *Mycobacterium gordonae* associated with water from refrigerated fountains. *J. Hosp. Infect.* **48:**76–79.
109. **Lewis, M. T., B. J. Marsh, and C. Fordham von Reyn.** 2003. Fish tank exposure and cutaneous infections due to *Mycobacterium marinum:* tuberculin skin testing, treatment, and prevention. *Clin. Infect. Dis.* **37:**390–397.
110. **Liebeschütz, S., S. Bamber, K. Ewer, J. Deeks, A. A. Pathan, and A. Lalvani.** 2004. Diagnosis of tuberculosis in South African children with a T cell-based assay: a prospective cohort study. *Lancet* **364:**2196–2203.
111. **Lipsky, B. A., J. Gates, F. C. Tenover, and J. J. Plorde.** 1984. Factors affecting the clinical value of microscopy for acid-fast bacilli. *Rev. Infect. Dis.* **6:**214–222.
112. **Mahapatra, S., J. Basu, P. J. Brennan, and D. C. Crick.** 2005. Structure, biosynthesis, and genetics of the mycolic acid-arabinogalactan-peptidoglycan complex, p. 275–285. *In* S. T. Cole, K. D. Eisenach, D. N. McMurray, and W. R. Jacobs, Jr. (ed.), *Tuberculosis and the Tubercle Bacillus*, ASM Press, Washington, D.C.
113. **Marmiesse, M., P. Brodin, C. Buchrieser, C. Gutierrez, N. Simoes, V. Vincent, P. Glaser, S. T. Cole, and R. Brosch.** 2004. Macro-array and bioinformatics analyses reveal mycobacterial 'core' genes, variation in the ESAT-6 gene family and new phylogenetic markers for the *Mycobacterium tuberculosis* complex. *Microbiology* **150:**483–496.
114. **Mastro, T. D., S. C. Redd, and R. F. Breiman.** 1992. Imported leprosy in the United States, 1978 through 1988: an epidemic without secondary transmission. *Am. J. Public Health* **82:**1127–1130.
115. **Mayall, B., V. Gurtler, L. Irving, A. Marzec, and D. Leslie.** 1999. Identification of *Mycobacterium shimoidei* by molecular techniques: case report and summary of the literature. *Int. J. Tuberc. Lung Dis.* **3:**169–173.
116. **Mayo, J., J. Collazos, and E. Martinez.** 1998. *Mycobacterium nonchromogenicum* bacteremia in an AIDS patient. *Emerg. Infect. Dis.* **4:**124–125.
116a. **Mazurek, G. H., J. Jereb, P. Lobue, M. F. Iademarco, B. Metchock, and A. Vernon.** 2005. Guidelines for using the QuantiFERON-TB Gold test for detecting *Mycobacterium tuberculosis* infection, United States. *MMWR Recomm. Rep.* **54**(RR-15):49–55.
117. **Mazurek, G. H., and M. E. Villarino.** 2003. Guidelines for using the QuantiFERON-TB test for diagnosing latent *Mycobacterium tuberculosis* infection. Centers for Disease Control and Prevention. *MMWR Recomm. Rep.* **52**(RR-2):15–18.
118. **Meier, A., P. Kirschner, K.-H. Schröder, J. Wolters, R. M. Kroppenstedt, and E. C. Böttger.** 1993. *Mycobacterium intermedium* sp. nov. *Int. J. Syst. Bacteriol.* **43:**204–209.
119. **Meybeck, A., C. Fortin, S. Abgrall, H. Adle-Biassette, G. Hayem, R. Ruimy, and P. Yeni.** 2005. Spondylitis due to *Mycobacterium xenopi* in a human immunodeficiency virus type 1-infected patient: case report and review of the literature. *J. Clin. Microbiol.* **43:**1465–1466.
120. **Migliori, G. B., M. C. Raviglione, T. Schaberg, P. D. Davies, J. P. Zellweger, M. Grzemska, T. Mihaescu, L. Clancy, L. Casali, et al.** 1999. Tuberculosis management in Europe. *Eur. Respir. J.* **14:**978–992.
121. **Mijs, W., P. de Haas, R. Rossau, T. van der Laan, L. Rigouts, F. Portaels, and D. van Soolingen.** 2002. Molecular evidence to support a proposal to reserve the designation *Mycobacterium avium* subsp. *avium* for the bird-type isolates and *M. avium* subsp. *hominissuis* for the human/porcine type of *M. avium*. *Int. J. Syst. Evol. Microbiol.* **52:**1505–1518.
122. **Miltgen, J., M. Morillon, J. L. Koeck, A. Varnerot, J. F. Briant, G. Nguyen, D. Verrot, D. Bonnet, and V. Vincent.** 2002. Two cases of pulmonary tuberculosis caused by *Mycobacterium tuberculosis* subsp. *canettii*. *Emerg. Infect. Dis.* **8:**1350–1352.
123. **Mitscherlich, E., and E. H. Marth.** 1984. *Microbial Survival in the Environment*, p. 232–266. Springer Verlag, New York, N.Y.
124. **Morris, A., L. B. Reller, M. Salfinger, K. Jackson, A. Sievers, and B. Dwyer.** 1993. Mycobacteria in stool specimens: the nonvalue of smears for predicting culture results. *J. Clin. Microbiol.* **31:**1385–1387.
125. **Morris, A. J., and L. B. Reller.** 1993. Reliability of cord formation in BACTEC media for presumptive identification of mycobacteria. *J. Clin. Microbiol.* **31:**2533–2534.
126. **Mostowy, S., A. Onipede, S. Gagneux, S. Niemann, K. Kremer, E. P. Desmond, M. Kato-Maeda, and M. Behr.** 2004. Genomic analysis distinguishes *Mycobacterium africanum*. *J. Clin. Microbiol.* **42:**3594–3599.

127. **Murray, S. J., A. Barrett, J. G. Magee, and R. Freeman.** 2003. Optimisation of acid-fast smears for the direct detection of mycobacteria in clinical samples. *J. Clin. Pathol.* **56:**613–615.
128. **National Committee for Clinical Laboratory Standards.** 2000. *Susceptibility Testing of Mycobacteria, Nocardia and Other Aerobic Actinomycetes.* Approved standard M24-A. NCCLS, Wayne, Pa.
129. **National Committee for Clinical Laboratory Standards.** 2005. *Molecular Diagnostic Methods for Infectious Diseases.* Proposed guideline, 2nd ed. MM3-P2. NCCLS, Wayne, Pa.
130. **National Institute for Occupational Safety and Health.** 1995. Respiratory protective devices: final rules and notice. 42 CFR part 84. *Fed. Regist.* **60:**30335–30398.
131. **Nelson, S. M., M. A. Deike, and C. P. Cartwright.** 1998. Value of examining multiple sputum specimens in the diagnosis of pulmonary tuberculosis. *J. Clin. Microbiol.* **36:**467–469.
132. **Nguyen, M., S. Perry, and J. Parsonnet.** 2005. QuantiFERON-TB predicts tuberculin skin test boosting in U.S. foreign-born. *Int. J. Tuberc. Lung Dis.* **9:**985–991.
133. **Niemann, S., T. Kubica, F. C. Bange, O. Adjei, E. N. Browne, M. A. Chinbuah, R. Diel, J. Gyapong, R. D. Horstmann, M. L. Joloba, C. G. Meyer, R. D. Mugerwa, A. Okwera, I. Osei, E. Owusu-Darbo, S. K. Schwander, and S. Rüsch-Gerdes.** 2004. The species *Mycobacterium africanum* in the light of new molecular markers. *J. Clin. Microbiol.* **42:**3958–3962.
134. **Noordhoek, G. T., S. Mulder, P. Wallace, and A. M. van Loon.** 2004. Multicentre quality control study for detection of *Mycobacterium tuberculosis* in clinical samples by nucleic amplification methods. *Clin. Microbiol. Infect.* **10:**295–301.
135. **Osawa, N.** 1997. Growth of *Mycobacterium leprae* in vitro. *Proc. Jpn. Acad. Ser. B* **73:**144–149.
136. **Ostergaard Thompson, V., U. B. Dragsted, J. Bauer, K. Fuursted, and J. Lundgren.** 1999. Disseminated infection with *Mycobacterium genavense:* a challenge to physicians and mycobacteriologists. *J. Clin. Microbiol.* **37:**3901–3905.
137. **Palomino, J. C., A. M. Obiang, L. Realini, W. M. Meyers, and F. Portaels.** 1998. Effect of oxygen on growth of *Mycobacterium ulcerans* in the BACTEC system. *J. Clin. Microbiol.* **36:**3420–3422.
138. **Palomino, J. C., and F. Portaels.** 1998. Effects of decontamination methods and culture conditions on viability of *Mycobacterium ulcerans* in the BACTEC system. *J. Clin. Microbiol.* **36:**402–408.
139. **Paramasivan, C. N., A. S. L. Narayana, R. Prabhakar, M. S. Rajagopal, P. R. Somasundaram, and S. P. Tripathy.** 1983. Effect of storage of sputum specimens at room temperature on smear and culture results. *Tubercle* **64:**119–124.
140. **Park, H., H. Jang, E. Song, C. L. Chang, M. Lee, S. Jeong, J. Park, B. Kang, and C. Kim.** 2005. Detection and genotyping of *Mycobacterium* species from clinical isolates and specimens by oligonucleotide array. *J. Clin. Microbiol.* **43:**1782–1788.
141. **Pascopella, L., S. Kellam, J. Ridderhof, D. P. Chin, A. Reingold, E. Desmond, J. Flood, and S. Royce.** 2004. Laboratory reporting of tuberculosis test results and patient treatment initiation in California. *J. Clin. Microbiol.* **42:**4209–4213.
142. **Patrocinio, L. G., I. M. Goulart, J. A. Patrocinio, F. R. Ferriera, and R. N. Fleury.** 2005. Detection of *Mycobacterium leprae* in nasal mucosa biopsies by the polymerase chain reaction. *FEMS Immunol. Med. Microbiol.* **44:**311–316.
143. **Pfyffer, G. E., C. Cieslak, H. M. Welscher, P. Kissling, and S. Rüsch-Gerdes.** 1997. Rapid detection of mycobacteria in clinical specimen by using the automated BACTEC 9000 MB System and comparison with radiometric and solid culture systems. *J. Clin. Microbiol.* **35:**2229–2234.
144. **Pfyffer, G. E., and V. Vincent.** 2005. *Mycobacterium tuberculosis* complex, *Mycobacterium leprae,* and other slowly growing mycobacteria, p. 1181–1235. *In* S. P. Boriello, P. R. Murray, and G. Funke (ed.), *Topley & Wilson's Microbiology and Microbial Infections: Bacteriology,* 10th ed. Hodder Arnold, London, United Kingdom.
145. **Pfyffer, G. E., H. M. Welscher, and P. Kissling.** 1997. Pretreatment of clinical specimens with sodium dodecyl (lauryl) sulfate is not suitable for the Mycobacteria Growth Indicator Tube cultivation method. *J. Clin. Microbiol.* **35:**2142–2144.
146. **Pfyffer, G. E., H. M. Welscher, P. Kissling, C. Cieslak, M. J. Casal, J. Gutierrez, and S. Rüsch Gerdes.** 1997. Comparison of the Mycobacteria Growth Indicator Tube (MGIT) with radiometric and solid culture for recovery of acid fast bacilli. *J. Clin. Microbiol.* **35:**364–368.
147. **Pfyffer, G. E., R. Auckenthaler, J. D. A. van Embden, and D. van Soolingen.** 1998. *Mycobacterium canettii,* the smooth variant of *M. tuberculosis,* isolated from a Swiss patient exposed in Africa. *Emerg. Infect. Dis.* **4:**631–634.
148. **Picardeau, M., G. Prod'hom, L. Raskine, M. P. LePennec, and V. Vincent.** 1997. Genotypic characterization of five subspecies of *Mycobacterium kansasii. J. Clin. Microbiol.* **35:**25–32.
149. **Picardeau, M., T. J. Bull, G. Prod'hom, A. L. Pozniak, D. C. Shanson, and V. Vincent.** 1997. Comparison of a new insertion element, IS*1407*, with established molecular markers for the characterization of *Mycobacterium celatum. Int. J. Syst. Bacteriol.* **47:**640–644.
150. **Piersimoni, C., C. Scarparo, A. Callegaro, C. Passerini Tosi, D. Nista, S. Bornigia, M. Scagnelli, A. Rigon, G. Ruggiero, and A. Goglio.** 2001. Comparison of MB/BacT ALERT 3D system with radiometric BACTEC System and Löwenstein-Jensen medium for recovery and identification of mycobacteria from clinical specimen: a multicenter study. *J. Clin. Microbiol.* **39:**651–657.
151. **Portaels, F., K. Chemlal, P. Elsen, P. D. R. Johnson, J. A. Hayman, J. Hibble, R. Kirkwood, and W. M. Meyers.** 2001. *Mycobacterium ulcerans* in wild animals. *Rev. Sci. Tech. Off. Int. Epizoot.* **20:**252–264.
152. **Portaels, F., L. Realini, L. Bauwens, H. Hirschel, W. M. Meyers, and W. De Meurichy.** 1996. Mycobacteriosis caused by *Mycobacterium genavense* in birds kept in a zoo: 11 year survey. *J. Clin. Microbiol.* **34:**319–323.
153. **Primm, T. P., C. A. Lucero, and J. O. Falkinham III.** 2004. Health impacts of environmental mycobacteria. *Clin. Microbiol. Rev.* **17:**98–106.
154. **Ramos, M., H. Soini, G. C. Roscanni, M. Jaques, M. C. Villares, and J. M. Musser.** 1999. Extensive cross-contamination of specimens with *Mycobacterium tuberculosis* in a reference laboratory. *J. Clin. Microbiol.* **37:**916–919.
155. **Realini, L., K. de Ridder, B. Hirschel, and F. Portaels.** 1999. Blood and charcoal added to acidified agar media promote growth of *Mycobacterium genavense. Diagn. Microbiol. Infect. Dis.* **34:**45–50.
156. **Realini, L., K. de Ridder, J. Palomino, B. Hirschel, and F. Portaels.** 1998. Microaerophilic conditions promote growth of *Mycobacterium genavense. J. Clin. Microbiol.* **36:**2565–2570.
157. **Reischl, U., K. Feldmann, L. Naumann, B. J. Gaugler, B. Ninet, B. Hirschel, and S. Emler.** 1998. 16S rRNA sequence diversity in *Mycobacterium celatum* strains caused by the presence of two different copies of 16S rRNA gene. *J. Clin Microbiol.* **36:**1761–1764.
158. **Reischl, U., S. Emler, Z. Horak, J. Kaustova, R. M. Kroppenstedt, N. Lehn, and L. Naumann.** 1998. *Mycobacterium bohemicum* sp. nov., a new slowly-growing

scotochromogenic mycobacterium. *Int. J. Syst. Bacteriol.* **48:**1349–1355.

159. **Richter, E., S. Niemann, S. Rüsch-Gerdes, and D. Harmsen.** 2001. Description of *Mycobacterium heckeshornense* sp. nov. *J. Clin. Microbiol.* **39:**3023–3024.
160. **Ridderhof, J. C., L. O. Williams, S. Legois, P. A. Shult, B. Metchock, L. N. Kubista, J. H. Handsfield, R. J. Fehd, and P. H. Robinson.** 2003. Assessment of laboratory performance of nucleic acid amplification tests for detection of *Mycobacterium tuberculosis*. *J. Clin. Microbiol.* **41:**5258–5261.
161. **Roberts, G. D., N. L. Goodman, L. Heifets, H. W. Larsh, T. H. Lindner, J. K. McClatchy, M. R. McGinnis, S. H. Siddiqi, and P. Wright.** 1983. Evaluation of the BACTEC radiometric method for recovery of myobacteria and drug susceptibility testing of *Mycobacterium tuberculosis* from acid-fast smear-positive specimens. *J. Clin. Micobiol.* **18:**689–696.
162. **Rondini, S., C. Horsfield, E. Mensah-Quainoo, T. Junghanss, S. Lucas, and G. Pluschke.** 2006. Contiguous spread of *Mycobacterium ulcerans* in Buruli ulcer lesions analysed by histopathology and real-time PCR quantification of mycobacterial DNA. *J. Pathol.* **208:**119–128.
163. **Roth, A., U. Reischl, N. Schönfeld, L. Naumann, S. Emler, M. Fischer, H. Mauch, R. Loddenkemper, and R. Kroppenstedt.** 2000. *Mycobacterium heckeshornense* sp. nov., a new pathogenic slowly growing *Mycobacterium* sp. causing cavitary lung disease in an immunocompetent patient. *J. Clin. Microbiol.* **38:**4102–4107.
164. **Rynkiewicz, D. L., G. D. Cage, W. R. Butler, and N. M. Ampel.** 1998. Clinical and microbiological assessment of *Mycobacterium simiae* isolates from a single laboratory in southern Arizona. *Clin. Infect. Dis.* **26:**625–630.
165. **Saad, M. H., V. Vincent, D. J. Dawson, M. Palaci, L. Ferrazoli, and S. Fonseca Lde.** 1997. Analysis of *Mycobacterium avium* complex serovars isolated from AIDS patients from southeast Brazil. *Mem. Inst. Oswaldo Cruz* **92:**471–475.
166. **Saceanu, C., N. Pfeiffer, and T. McLean.** 1993. Evaluation of sputum smears concentrated by cytocentrifugution for detection of acid fast bacilli. *J. Clin. Microbiol.* **31:**2371–2374.
167. **Salfinger, M., and F. Kafader.** 1987. Comparison of two pretreatment methods for the detection of mycobacteria of BACTEC and Löwenstein-Jensen slants. *J. Microbiol. Methods* **6:**315–321.
168. **Samra, Z., L. Kaufman, A. Zeharia, S. Ashkenazi, J. Amir, J. Bahar, U. Reischl, and L. Naumann.** 1999. Optimal detection and identification of *Mycobacterium haemophilum* in specimens from pediatric patients with cervical lymphadenopathy. *J. Clin. Microbiol.* **37:**832–834.
169. **Saubolle, M. A., T. E. Kiehn, M. H. White, M. F. Rudinsky, and D. Armstrong.** 1996. *Mycobacterium haemophilum:* microbiology and expanding clinical and geographic spectra of diseases in humans. *Clin. Microbiol. Rev.* **9:**435–447.
170. **Schoch, O. D., G. E. Pfyffer, D. Buhl, and A. Paky.** 2003. False-positive *Mycobacterium tuberculosis* culture revealed by restriction fragment length polymorphism analysis. *Infection* **31:**189–191.
171. **Selvarangan R., W.-K. Wu, T. T. Nguyen, L. D. C. Carlson, C. K. Wallis, S. K. Stiglich, Y.-C. Chen, K. C. Jost, Jr., J. L. Prentice, R. J. Wallace, Jr., S. L. Rassoulian Barrett, B. T. Cookson, and M. B. Coyle.** 2004. Characterization of a novel group of mycobacteria and proposal of *Mycobacterium sherrisii* sp. nov. *J. Clin. Microbiol.* **42:**52–59.
172. **Small, P., N. McClenny, S. Sigh, G. Schoolnik, L. Tompkins, and P. Mickelsen.** 1993. Molecular strain typing of *Mycobacterium tuberculosis* to confirm cross contamination in the mycobacteriology laboratory and modification of procedures to minimize occurrence of false positive cultures. *J. Clin. Microbiol.* **31:**1677–1682.
173. **Smith, D. S., P. Lindholm-Levy, G. A. Huitt, L. B. Heifets, and J. L. Cook.** 2000. *Mycobacterium terrae:* case reports, literature review, and in vitro antibiotic susceptibility testing. *Clin. Infect. Dis.* **30:**444–453.
174. **Smithwick, R. W., and C. B. Stratigos.** 1981. Acid-fast microscopy on polycarbonate membrane filter sputum sediments. *J. Clin. Microbiol.* **13:**1109–1113.
175. **Smithwick, R. W., C. B. Stratigos, and H. L. David.** 1975. Use of cetylpyridinium chloride and sodium chloride for the decontamination of sputum specimens that are transported to the laboratory for the isolation of *Mycobacterium tuberculosis*. *J. Clin. Microbiol.* **1:**411–413.
176. **Sniadack, D. H., S. M. Ostroff, M. A. Karlix, R. W. Smithwick, B. Schwartz, M. A. Sprauer, V. A. Silcox, and R. C. Good.** 1993. A nosocomial pseudo outbreak of *Mycobacterium xenopi* due to a contaminated potable water supply: lessons in prevention. *Infect. Control Hosp. Epidemiol.* **14:**636–641.
177. **Snider, D. E., Jr.** 1982. The tuberculin skin test. *Am. Rev. Respir. Dis.* **125:**108–118.
178. **Somoskövi, A., and P. Magyar.** 1999. Comparison of the Mycobacteria Growth Indicator Tube with MB Redox, Löwenstein-Jensen, and Middlebrook 7H11 media for recovery of mycobacteria in clinical specimens. *J. Clin. Microbiol.* **37:**1366–1369.
179. **Somoskövi, A., J. E. Hotaling, M. Fitzgerald, D. O'Donnell, L. M. Parsons, and M. Salfinger.** 2001. Lessons from a proficiency testing event for acid-fast microscopy. *Chest* **120:**250–257.
180. **Springer, B., E. Tortoli, I. Richter, R. Grünewald, S. Rüsch-Gerdes, K. Uschmann, F. Suter, M. D. Collins, R. M. Kroppenstedt, and E. C. Böttger.** 1995. *Mycobacterium conspicuum* sp. nov., a new species isolated from patients with disseminated infections. *J. Clin. Microbiol.* **33:**2805–2811.
181. **Springer, B., W.-K. Wu, T. Bodmer, G. Haase, G. E. Pfyffer, R. M. Kroppenstedt, K.-H. Schröder, S. Emler, J. O. Kilburn, P. Kirschner, A. Telenti, M. B. Coyle, and E. C. Böttger.** 1996. Isolation and characterization of a unique group of slowly growing mycobacteria: description of *Mycobacterium lentiflavum* sp. nov. *J. Clin. Microbiol.* **34:**1100–1107.
182. **Stone, B. L., W. J. Burman, M. V. Hildred, E. A. Jarboe, R. R. Reves, and M. L. Wilson.** 1997. The diagnostic yield of acid-fast bacillus smear-positive specimens. *J. Clin. Microbiol.* **35:**1030–1031.
183. **Supply, P., E. Mazars, S. Lesjean, V. Vincent, B. Gicquel, and C. Locht.** 2000. Variable human minisatellite-like regions in the *Mycobacterium tuberculosis* genome. *Mol. Microbiol.* **36:**762–771.
184. **Taylor, L. Q., A. J. Williams, and S. Santiago.** 1990. Pulmonary disease caused by *Mycobacterium asiaticum*. *Tubercle* **71:**303–305.
185. **Telenti, A., F. Marchesi, M. Balz, F. Bally, E. C. Böttger, and T. Bodmer.** 1993. Rapid identification of mycobacteria to the species level by polymerase chain reaction and restriction enzyme analysis. *J. Clin. Microbiol.* **31:**175–178.
186. **Tenover, F., J. Crawford, R. Huebner, L. Getter, C. R. Horsburgh, Jr., and R. C. Good.** 1993. The resurgence of tuberculosis: is your laboratory ready? *J. Clin. Microbiol.* **32:**767–770.
187. **Thorel, M.-F., M. Krichevsky, and V. Levy-Frébault.** 1990. Numerical taxonomy of mycobactin dependent mycobacteria, emended description of *Mycobacterium avium*, and description of *Mycobacterium avium* subsp. *avium* subsp. nov., *Mycobacterium avium* subsp. *paratuberculosis* subsp. nov., and *Mycobacterium avium* subsp. *silvaticum* subsp. nov. *Int. J. Syst. Bacteriol.* **40:**254–260.

188. **Thornton, C. G., K. M. McLellan, T. L. Brink, Jr., D. E. Lockwood, M. Romagnoli, J. Turner, W. G. Merz, R. S. Schwalbe, M. Moody, Y. Lue, and S. Passen.** 1998. Novel method for processing respiratory specimens for detection of mycobacteria by using C_{18}-carboxypropylbetaine: blinded study. *J. Clin. Microbiol.* **36:**1996–2003.
189. **Tjhie, J. H. T., A. F. van Belle, M. Dessenkroon, and D. van Soolingen.** 2001. Misidentification and diagnostic delay caused by a false-positive amplified *Mycobacterium tuberculosis* direct test in an immunocompetent patient with a *Mycobacterium celatum* infection. *J. Clin. Microbiol.* **39:**2311–2312.
190. **Torkko, P., S. Suomalainen, E. Iivanainen, E. Tortoli, M. Suutari, J. Seppänen, L. Paulin, and M. L. Katila.** 2002. *Mycobacterium palustre* sp. nov, a potentially pathogenic slow-growing mycobacterium isolated from veterinary and clinical specimens, and Finnish stream water. *Int. J. Syst. Evol. Microbiol.* **52:**1519–1525.
191. **Torkko, P., S. Suomalainen, E. Iivanainen, M. Suutari, L. Paulin, E. Rudback, E. Tortoli, V. Vincent, R. Mattila, and M. L. Katila.** 2001. Characterization of *Mycobacterium bohemicum* isolated from human, veterinary, and environmental sources. *J. Clin. Microbiol.* **39:** 207–211.
192. **Tortoli, E.** 2003. Impact of genotypic studies in mycobacterial taxonomy: the new mycobacteria of the 1990s. *Clin. Microbiol. Rev.* **16:**319–354.
193. **Tortoli, E., A. Bartoloni, V. Manfrin, A. Mantella, C. Scarparo, and E. C. Böttger.** 2000. Cervical lymphadenitis due to *Mycobacterium bohemicum. Clin. Infect. Dis.* **30:**210–211.
194. **Tortoli, E., C. Piersimoni, A. Bartoloni, C. Burrini, A. P. Callegaro, G. Caroli, D. Colombri, A. Goglio, A. Mantella, C. P. Tosi, and M. T. Simonetti.** 1997. *Mycobacterium malmoense* in Italy: the modern Norman invasion? *Eur. J. Epidemiol.* **13:**314–316.
195. **Tortoli, E., F. Brunello, A. E. Cagni, D. Colombrita, D. Dionisio, L. Grisendi, V. Manfrin, M. Moroni, C. Passerini Tosi, G. Pinsi, C. Scarparo, and M. Tullia Simonetti.** 1998. *Mycobacterium genavense* in AIDS patients: report of 24 cases in Italy and review of the literature. *Eur. J. Epidemiol.* **14:**219–224.
196. **Tortoli, E., G. Besozzi, C. Lacchini, V. Penati, M. T. Simonetti, and S. Emler.** 1998. Pulmonary infection due to *Mycobacterium szulgai:* case report and review of the literature. *Eur. Respir. J.* **11:**975–977.
197. **Tortoli, E., M. Tullia Simonetti, D. Dionisio, and M. Meli.** 1994. Cultural studies on two isolates of *Mycobacterium genavense* from patients with acquired immunodeficiency syndrome. *Diagn. Microbiol. Infect. Dis.* **18:**7–12.
198. **Tortoli, E., R. M. Kroppenstedt, A. Bartoloni, G. Caroli, I. Jan, J. Pawlowski, and S. Emler.** 1999. *Mycobacterium tusciae* sp. nov. *Int. J. Syst. Bacteriol.* **49:**1839–1844.
199. **Trifiro, S., A.-M. Bourgault, F. Lebel, and P. René.** 1990. Ghost mycobacteria on Gram stain. *J. Clin. Microbiol.* **28:**146.
200. **Turenne, C., P. Chedore, J. Wolfe, F. Jamieson, G. Broukhanski, K. May, and A. Kabani.** 2002. *Mycobacterium lacus* sp. nov., a novel slowly growing, nonchromogenic clinical isolate. *Int. J. Syst. Evol. Microbiol.* **52:**2135–2140.
201. **Ucko, M., and A. Colorni.** 2005. *Mycobacterium marinum* infections in fish and humans in Israel. *J. Clin. Microbiol.* **43:**892–895.
202. **van Baers, S. M., M. Y. L. de Witt, and P. R. Klatser.** 1996. The epidemiology of *Mycobacterium leprae:* recent insight. *FEMS Microbiol. Lett.* **136:**221–230.
203. **van der Werf, T. S., W. T. A. van der Graaf, J. W. Tappero, and K. Asiedu.** 1999. *Mycobacterium ulcerans* infection. *Lancet* **354:**1013–1018.
204. **van Soolingen, D., A. G. M. van der Zanden, P. E. W. de Haas, G. T. Noordhoek, A. Kiers, N. A. Foudraine, F. Portaels, A. H. J. Kolk, K. Kremer, and J. D. A. van Embden.** 1998. Diagnosis of *Mycobacterium microti* infections among humans by using novel genetic markers. *J. Clin. Microbiol.* **36:**1840–1845.
205. **van Soolingen, D., T. Hoogenboezem, P. E. W. de Haas, P. W. M. Hermans, M. A. Koedam, K. S. Teppema, P. J. Brennan, G. S. Besra, F. Portaels, J. Top, L. M. Schouls, and J. D. van Embden.** 1997. A novel pathogenic taxon of the *Mycobacterium tuberculosis* complex, Canettii: characterization of an exceptional isolate from Africa. *Int. J. Syst. Bacteriol.* **47:**1236–1245.
206. **Viana-Niero, C., C. Gutierrez, C. Sola, I. Filliol, F. Boulahbal, V. Vincent, and N. Rastogi.** 2001. Genetic diversity of *Mycobacterium africanum* clinical isolates based on IS*6110*-restriction fragment length polymorphism analysis, spoligotyping, and variable number of tandem DNA repeats. *J. Clin. Microbiol.* **39:**57–65.
207. **Waite, R. T., and G. L. Woods.** 1998. Evaluation of BACTEC MYCO/F lytic medium for recovery of mycobacteria and fungi from blood. *J. Clin. Microbiol.* **36:**1176–1179.
208. **Wallace, R.** 1987. Nontuberculous mycobacteria and water: a love affair with increasing clinical importance. *Infect. Dis. Clin. N. Am.* **1:**677–686.
209. **Wallace, R. J., Jr., Y. Zhang, B. A. Brown, D. Dawson, D. T. Murphy, R. Wilson, and D. Griffith.** 1998. Polyclonal *Mycobacterium avium* complex infections in patients with nodular bronchiectasis. *Am. J. Respir. Crit. Care Med.* **158:**1235–1244.
210. **Wang, S. X., L. H. Sng, H. N. Leong, and B. H. Tan.** 2004. Direct identification of *Mycobacterium haemophilum* in skin lesions of immunocompromised patients by PCR-restriction endonuclease assay. *J. Clin. Microbiol.* **42:**3336–3338.
211. **Warren, J. R., M. Bhattacharya, K. N. De Almeida, K. Trakas, and L. R. Peterson.** 2000. A minimum 5.0 ml of sputum improves the sensitivity of acid-fast smear for *Mycobacterium tuberculosis. Am. J. Respir. Crit. Care Med.* **161:**1559–1562.
212. **Warren, N. G., and J. R. Cordts.** 1996. Clinical mycobacteriology. Activities and recommendations by the Association of State and Territorial Public Health Laboratory Directors. *Clin. Lab. Med.* **16:**731–743.
213. **Wasilauskas, B. L., and R. M. Morrell, Jr.** 1997. Isolator component responsible for inhibition of *Mycobacterium avium-M. intracellulare* in BACTEC 12B medium. *J. Clin. Microbiol.* **35:**588–590.
214. **Wayne, L., and H. Sramek.** 1992. Agents of newly recognized or infrequently encountered mycobacterial diseases. *Clin. Microbiol. Rev.* **5:**1–25.
215. **Wayne, L., R. Good, M. Krichevsky, Z. Blacklock, H. David, D. Dawson, W. Gross, J. Hawkins, V. Levy Frebault, C. McManus, F. Portaels, S. Rüsch-Gerdes, K. Schröder, V. Silcox, M. Tsukamura, L. Van den Breen, and M. Yakrus.** 1991. Fourth report of the cooperative open ended study of slowly growing mycobacteria of the International Working Group on Mycobacterial Taxonomy. *Int. J. Syst. Bacteriol.* **41:**463–472.
216. **Wayne, L. G., and G. P. Kubica.** 1986. *Mycobacterium,* p. 1435–1457. *In* P. H. A. Sneath, N. S. Mair, M. E. Sharpe, and J. G. Holt (ed.), *Bergey's Manual of Systematic Bacteriology,* vol. 2. Williams & Wilkins, Baltimore, Md.
217. **Welch, D., A. Guruswamy, S. Sides, C. Shaw, and M. Gilchrist.** 1993. Timely culture of mycobacteria which utilizes a microcolony method. *J. Clin. Microbiol.* **31:** 2178–2184.
218. **Weldingh, K., I. Rosenkrands, L. M. Okkels, T. M. Doherty, and P. Andersen.** 2005. Assessing the serodiagnostic potential of 35 *Mycobacterium tuberculosis* proteins

and identification of four novel serological antigens. *J. Clin. Microbiol.* **43:**57–65.

219. **Wheeler, P. R., and J. S. Blanchard.** 2005. General metabolism and biochemical pathways of tubercle bacilli, p. 309–339. *In* S. T. Cole, K. D. Eisenach, D. N. McMurray, and W. R. Jacobs, Jr. (ed.), *Tuberculosis and the Tubercle Bacillus*, ASM Press, Washington, D.C.
220. **White, D. A., T. E. Kiehn, A. Y. Bondoc, and S. A. Massarella.** 1999. Pulmonary nodule due to *Mycobacterium haemophilum* in an immunocompetent host. *Am. J. Respir. Crit. Care Med.* **160:**1366–1368.
221. **Whyte, T., B. Hanahoe, T. Collins, G. Corbett-Feeney, and M. Cormican.** 2000. Evaluation of the BACTEC MGIT 960 and MB/BacT systems for routine detection of *Mycobacterium tuberculosis*. *J. Clin. Microbiol.* **38:**3131–3132.
222. **Wolfe, J., C. Turenne, M. Alfa, G. Harding, L. Thibert, and A. Kabani.** 1999. *Mycobacterium branderi* from both a hand infection and a case of pulmonary disease. *J. Clin. Microbiol.* **38:**3896–3899.
223. **Wolinsky, E.** 1995. Mycobacterial lymphadenitis in children: a prospective study of 105 nontuberculous cases with long-term follow-up. *Clin. Infect. Dis.* **20:**954–963.
224. **Woods, G. L., E. Pentony, M. J. Boxley, and A. M. Gatson.** 1995. Concentration of sputum by cytocentrifugation for preparation of smears for detection of acid-fast bacilli does not increase sensitivity of the fluorochrome stain. *J. Clin. Microbiol.* **33:**1915–1916.
225. **Woods, G. L., G. Fish, M. Plaunt, and T. Murphy.** 1997. Clinical evaluation of Difco ESP Culture System II for growth and detection of mycobacteria. *J. Clin. Microbiol.* **35:**121–124.
226. **Woods, G. L., T. A. Long, and F. G. Witebsky.** 1996. Mycobacterial testing in clinical laboratories that participate in the College of American Pathologists Mycobacteriology Surveys. Changes in practices based on responses to 1992, 1993, and 1995 questionnaires. *Arch. Pathol. Lab. Med.* **120:**429–435.
227. **Woods, G. L., and J. C. Ridderhof.** 1996. Quality assurance in the mycobacteriology laboratory. *Clin. Lab. Med.* **16:**657–675.
228. **World Health Organization.** 2002. Leprosy global situation. *Wkly. Epidemiol. Rec.* **77:**1–8.
229. **World Health Organization.** 2005. *World Health Organization Report 2005. Global Tuberculosis Control: Surveillance, Planning, and Financing.* World Health Organization, Geneva, Switzerland.
230. **World Health Organization Study Group**. 1982. *World Health Organization Technical Report Series,* no. 847. Report of the Study Group on Chemotherapy of Leprosy for Control Programs. World Health Organization, Geneva, Switzerland.
231. **Yajko, D. M., P. S. Nassos, C. A. Sanders, P. C. Gonzalez, A. L. Reingold, C. R. Horsburgh, P. Hopewell, D. P. Chin, and W. K. Hadley.** 1993. Comparison of four decontamination methods for recovery of *Mycobacterium avium* complex from stools. *J. Clin. Microbiol.* **31:**302–306.
232. **Yamauchi, T., P. Ferrieri, and B. F. Anthony.** 1980. The etiology of acute cervical adenitis in children: serological and bacteriological studies. *J. Med. Microbiol.* **13:**37–43.
233. **Yeboah-Manu, D., T. Bodmer, E. Mensah-Quainoo, S. Owusu, D. Ofori-Adjei, and G. Pluschke.** 2004. Evaluation of decontamination methods and growth media for primary isolation of *Mycobacterium ulcerans* from surgical specimens. *J. Clin. Microbiol.* **42:** 5875–5876.

Mycobacterium: Laboratory Characteristics of Slowly Growing Mycobacteria*

VÉRONIQUE VINCENT AND M. CRISTINA GUTIÉRREZ

37

IDENTIFICATION OF MYCOBACTERIA

Mycobacteria should always be identified to the species level if possible. They are usually preliminarily identified by traits such as growth rate and pigmentation which will direct the selection of key biochemical tests to further characterize them. Unfortunately, different species may present convergent biochemical profiles and morphological features (Table 1). Similarly, variation occurs among strains, and the strains' properties may not match those of the type strain. Traditional methods are well established, standardized, reproducible, and relatively inexpensive but limited in scope to the species of which large numbers of strains have been studied. Thus, identification errors may result, especially because no characteristic phenotype has been identified for several recently described species recognized on the basis of new 16S rRNA gene sequences.

Alternative laboratory methods for mycobacterial identification include analysis of mycolic acids by chromatography, genetic investigations using nucleic acid probes, and nucleic acid sequencing. It is now recommended to undertake mycobacterial identification with a strategy combining phenotypic and genotypic tests. For obvious reasons, laboratories should perform identification of the *Mycobacterium tuberculosis* complex (MTBC) by using a rapid method (103) to facilitate prompt identification and reporting of results to physicians.

Phenotypic Tests

Table 1 shows characteristic test results for the most commonly encountered species. Detailed descriptions of methods, procedures, and controls can be found elsewhere (40, 48, 115; see also chapter 36).

Growth Rate and Preferred Growth Temperature

Growth rate refers to the length of time required to form mature, isolated colonies visible without magnification on solid media. Mycobacteria forming colonies within 7 days are termed rapid growers, while those requiring longer periods are termed slow growers. Genome analyses support this separation, since slowly growing mycobacteria have been shown to have only one copy of the genes encoding rRNA whereas rapidly growing mycobacteria, except for *M. chelonae* and *M. abscessus,* have two sets of those genes (6). Moreover, comparative 16S rRNA gene sequencing data clearly separate the rapidly growing mycobacteria from the slowly growing species (95).

Isolated colonies are observed after media are inoculated with 0.1 ml of a 10^{-4} dilution of a standard culture suspension (SCS) prepared at an optical density at 580 nm of 0.25 by using a tube with a 2-cm diameter; this roughly corresponds to a suspension of 1 mg (wet weight) of bacilli per ml (115). The cultures are incubated at 35 to 37°C. Some species have special nutrient or temperature requirements for growth (see the previous chapter for details). Cultures are observed at 5 to 7 days and weekly thereafter for visible colonies. Growth in relation to temperature can usually be adequately determined by observing cultures at 37 and 30°C. When more definitive identification is needed, isolates should be incubated at 28, 30, 35 to 37, and 42 or 45°C.

Pigmentation and Photoreactivity

Mycobacteria are classified into three groups based on the production of pigments. Photochromogens produce nonpigmented colonies when grown in the dark and pigmented colonies only after exposure to light. Scotochromogens produce deep-yellow- to orange-pigmented colonies when grown in either light or darkness (some strains show increased pigment production upon continuous exposure to light). Nonchromogens are nonpigmented in both the light and the dark or have only a pale yellow, buff, or tan pigment that does not intensify after light exposure. These responses to light exposure were originally delineated to aid in the identification of nontuberculous mycobacteria (NTM). Members of the MTBC, however, are considered nonchromogens, and pigmented mycobacteria may be preliminarily reported as NTM.

Testing for pigment production should be done on isolated colonies from young cultures. Three tubes of media are inoculated with an SCS diluted to yield isolated colonies as described above. Two tubes are wrapped to be shielded from light, and the third is left uncovered. When growth is detected in the unshielded tube, one of the wrapped tubes should be examined. If colonies are not pigmented, the newly unshielded tube with its cap loosened is exposed to light (100-W tungsten bulb or fluorescent equivalent, placed

*This chapter contains information presented in chapter 37 by Véronique Vincent, Barbara A. Brown-Elliott, Kenneth C. Jost, Jr., and Richard J. Wallace, Jr., in the eigth edition of this Manual.

TABLE 1 Distinctive properties of cultivable, slowly growing mycobacterial species encountered in clinical specimens[a]

Descriptive term	Species	Optimal temp (°C)	Usual colony morpho-logy[b]	Pigmen-tation[c]	Niacin	Growth on T2H (10 μg/ml)	Nitrate reduction	Semi-quantitative catalase (mm of bubbles)	68°C catalase	Tween hydrolysis	Tellurite reduc-tion	Tolerance to 5% NaCl	Arylsul-fatase, 3 days	Urease	Pyrazin-amidase, 4 days	16S rRNA gene ref. no.	Nucleic acid probes available
TB complex	*M. tuberculosis*	37	R	N (100)	+ (95)	+	+ (97)	<45 (89)	− (1)	± (68)	−/+ (36)	− (0)	− (0)	± (64)	+	X58890	+[d]
	M. bovis	37	Rt	N (100)	−	−	− (9)	<45 (69)	− (2)	− (21)	ND	− (0)	− (0)	± (50)	−	IDEM	+[d]
	M. bovis BCG	37	R	N (100)	−	−	−	<45	−	+/−	ND	−	−	+	−	IDEM	+[d]
	M. africanum	37	R	N (100)	V	V	V	<45	−	−	−	−	−	+	+	IDEM	+[d]
	M. canettii	37	Sm	N (100)	−	+	+	<45	−	−	ND	ND	−	ND	+	IDEM	+[d]
	M. microti	37	Sm	N (100)	+	−	V	<45	−	ND	ND	ND	ND	+	+	IDEM	+[d]
	M. caprae	37	Sm	N (100)	−	−	−	<45	−	+/−	ND	−	−	ND	ND	IDEM	+[d]
	M. pinnipedii	37	R	N (100)	V	ND	−	<45	−	−	ND	ND	ND	ND	ND	IDEM	+[d]
Nonchro-mogens	*M. avium*	35–37	Smt/R	N	−	+	−	<45	±	−	+	−	−	−	+	X52198	+[i]
	M. intracellulare	35–37	Smt/R	N	−	+	−	<45	±	−	+	−	−	−	+	X52927	+[i]
	M. haemophilum[e]	30	R	N	ND	+	−	<45	−	−	−	−	−	−	+	X88923	−
	M. malmoense	30	Sm	N (88)	− (0)	+	− (1)	<45 (99)	−/+	+ (99)	+ (74)	− (0)	− (0)	− (9)	+	X52930	−
	M. shimoidei	37	R	N	−	+	−	<45	−	+	ND	−	−	−	+	AJ005005	−
	M. genavense	37	Smt	N	−	+	−	>45	+	−	ND	ND	−	+	+	X60070	−
	M. celatum	35	Sm/Smt	N (100)	−	+	− (0)	<45 (100)	+ (100)	− (0)	+ (100)	− (0)	+ (100)	− (0)	+ (100)	L08170, L08169	−
	M. ulcerans	30	R	N	−	+	−	<45	+	−	ND	−	−	V	−	X58954	−
	M. terrae complex	35	Sm/R	N (93)	− (1)	+	± (67)	>45 (93)	+ (92)	+ (99)	−/+ (46)	− (2)	− (2)	− (13)	V	X52925 (*M. terrae*)	−
	M. triviale	37	R	N (100)	− (0)	+	+ (89)	>45 (100)	+ (100)	+ (100)	− (25)	+ (100)	± (56)	−/+ (33)	V	X88924	−
	M. gastri	35	Sm/SR/R	N (100)	− (0)	+	− (0)	<45 (100)	− (11)	+ (100)	± (50)	− (0)	− (0)	−/+ (44)	−	X52919	−
	M. branderi	35	Sm	N (100)	−	ND	−	−	−	−	ND	ND	−[f]	−	+	X82234	−
	M. heidelbergense	35	Sm	N (100)	−	ND	−	−	+	+	−	−	−	+	+	X70960	−
	M. triplex	35	Sm	N (100)	− (0)	+ (100)	+ (100)	>45 (100)	+ (100)	− (0)	ND	− (0)	− (0), + (50)[f]	+ (100)	+	U57632	−
	M. sherrisii	37	Sm	N	+/− (60)	ND	− (0)	−/+ (40)	+ (100)	− (100)	ND	ND	− (100)	+ (100)	−/+ (40)	AY353699	−
	M. lacus	37–42	SR	N	−	ND	+	<45	−	Weak	+	−	Weak	+	+	AF406783	−
Chromogens	*M. kansasii*	35	Sm/SR/R	P (96)	− (4)	+	+ (99)	>45 (93)	+ (91)	+ (99)	−/+ (31)	− (0)	− (0)	−/+ (49)	−	X15916	+
	M. marinum	30	Sm/SR/R	P (100)	−/+ (21)	+	− (0)	<45	− (30)	+ (97)	−/+ (39)	− (0)	−/+ (41)[f]	+ (83)	+	X52920	−
	M. avium	35–37	Sm/R	S	−	+	−	<45	±	−	+	−	−	−	+	X52198	+
	M. intracellulare	35–37	Sm/R	S	−	+	−	<45	±	−	+	−	−	−	+	X52927	+
	M. simiae	37	Sm	P (90)	± (63)	+	− (28)	>45 (93)	+ (95)	− (9)	+ (82)	− (0)	− (0)	+	+	X52931	−
	M. asiaticum	37	Sm	P (86)	− (0)	+	− (5)	>45 (95)	+ (95)	+ (95)	− (20)	− (0)	− (0)	− (10)	−	X55604	−
	M. xenopi	42	Sm	N/S[g]	−	+	−	<45	+/−	−	ND	− (0)	+	−	ND	X52929	−
	M. gordonae	37	Sm	S (99)	− (0)	+	− (1)	>45 (90)	+ (96)	+ (100)	− (29)	− (0)	V	V (31)	−/+	X52923	+

M. scrofulaceum	37	Sm	S (97)	− (0)	+	− (5)	>45 (84)	+ (94)	− (2)	± (64)	− (0)	V	+	±	X52924	−
M. szulgai	37	Sm or R	S/P (93)	− (0)	+	+ (100)	>45 (98)	+ (93)	−/+ (49)	± (53)	− (0)	−	+ (72)	+	X52926	−
M. flavescens	37	Sm	S (100)	− (0)	+	+ (92)	>45 (94)	+ (100)	+ (100)	−/+ (44)	± (62)	− (0)	+ (72)	+	X52932	−
M. parmense	37	Sm	S	−	+	−	<45	+	+	−	−	−	+	ND	AF466821	−
M. kubicae	37	Sm	S	ND	ND	−	>45	ND	−	ND	ND	− (20)	−	ND	AF133902	−
M. palustre	37–42	Sm	S/P	ND	ND	V (54)	<45	ND	+ (100)	ND	ND	V (46)	+ (100)	+ (100)	AJ308603	−
M. intermedium	35	Sm	P	−	ND	−	ND	+	+	ND	ND	+[h]	+/− (V)	−	X67847	−
M. lentiflavum	35	Sm	S	−	ND	−	± (V)	± (V)	−	ND	ND	−	−	± (V)	AF317658	−
M. interjectum	35	Sm	S	−	ND	−	V	+	−	ND	ND	V	+	+	X70961	−
M. bohemicum	37–40	Sm	S	−	ND	−	<45	+	−	ND	−	−	Weak	−	U84502	−
M. conspicuum	30	Sm	S		+	−	<45	− (100)	+	−	−	+[h]	−	−	X88922	−
M. tusciae	30	R	S	−	+	+	−		+ (10 days)	ND	−	−[f]	+	ND	AF058299	−
M. heckeshornense	35	Sm	S	−	ND	−	−	+	−	ND	−	−	−	−	AF174290	−

[a] Modified from references 27, 29, 40, 48, 87, 105, 106, 109, 120, and 121. Plus and minus signs indicate the presence and absence, respectively, of the feature: V, variable; ±, usually present; −/+, usually absent; ND, not determined; ref. no., reference number. The percentage of strains positive in each test is given in parentheses, and the test result is based on these percentages.

[b] R, rough; Sm, smooth; SR, intermediate in roughness; Smt, smooth and transparent; Rt, rough and thin or transparent.

[c] P, photochromogenic; S, scotochromogenic; N, nonchromogenic (*M. szulgai* is scotochromogenic at 37°C and photochromogenic at 24°C; *M. palustre* is scotochromogenic at 37°C, and 85% of isolates are photochromogenic at 42°C).

[d] Probe identifies the MTBC.

[e] Requires hemin as growth factor.

[f] Arylsulfatase reaction at 14 days is positive.

[g] Young cultures may be nonchromogenic or possess only pale pigment that may intensify with age.

[h] Results for 3-day arylsulfatase reaction not available; 10-day arylsulfatase reaction positive.

[i] A MAC nucleic acid probe that recognizes *M. avium*, *M. intracellulare*, and the "X" strains is commercially available.

20 cm from the culture) for 1 to 5 h. Maximal oxygenation of the culture (loose cap, isolated colonies) is necessary for induction of the pigment, which is controlled by an oxygen-dependent, photoinducible enzyme. The tube is then reshielded and reincubated, and the colonies in the light-exposed tube are compared with those in the shielded tube after 24 h. Variations within species occur.

Colony Morphology

Colony morphology of mycobacteria can be evaluated, according to the scheme developed by Runyon (84a), by microscopically observing young (5- to 14-day-old), isolated colonies on plates inverted under the 10× power objective of a stereomicroscope with transmitted light. The best medium is a clear solid one like Middlebrook 7H10 or 7H11 agar. The large numbers of NTM species have made it increasingly difficult to provide a tentative identification of an NTM species by this method, and so the information gained by this technique is often used to direct the diagnostic procedure to other, more specific tests. The morphology of *M. tuberculosis* usually allows for a tentative identification of this species. Examination of the morphologies of colonies is also important for the detection of mixed cultures. Figure 1 shows the colony types of some frequently isolated species.

Arylsulfatase

Arylsulfatase hydrolyzes the bond between the sulfate group and the aromatic ring of tripotassium phenolphthalein disulfate to form free phenolphthalein, which is easily detected by a red appearance when alkali is added. Arylsulfatase activity can be detected in all mycobacteria after prolonged incubation. Performing the test after only 3 days helps in identifying several slowly growing mycobacteria such as *M. xenopi* and *M. celatum*.

Cultures in Dubos liquid medium (2 ml) containing 0.08 M phenolphthalein disulfate (tripotassium salt) are tested after 3 days of incubation by adding 0.3 ml of 1 M Na_2CO_3. The development of pink indicates a positive reaction. *M. xenopi* and *M. avium* can be used as positive and negative controls, respectively.

Catalase

Catalase is an intracellular, soluble enzyme capable of degrading hydrogen peroxide into water and oxygen. Two tests are used to detect catalase activity, a semiquantitative test that reflects differences in enzyme kinetics and a heat tolerance test. The enzyme is detected by adding H_2O_2 to a culture and observing for the formation of bubbles in the reaction mixture.

The semiquantitative test divides the mycobacteria into two groups, those producing low catalase activity and those producing high catalase activity, based on the sizes of the columns of bubbles produced (less or more than 45 mm). A butt (not a slant) of a Löwenstein-Jensen (L-J) medium tube (16 by 150 mm) is inoculated with 0.2 ml of an SCS prepared as described above for growth rate determination. Tubes are incubated for 2 weeks at 35°C with the caps loosened. Then 1 ml of a reagent consisting of a 1:1 mixture of 10% Tween 80 and 30% H_2O_2 is added. Be sure to loosen the caps and place the tubes on an adsorbent surface in case bubbles overflow. The column of bubbles yielded is measured (in millimeters) after the tube has stood upright for 5 min at room temperature. *M. tuberculosis* H37Ra and *M. kansasii* can be used as controls for low and high catalase activity, respectively.

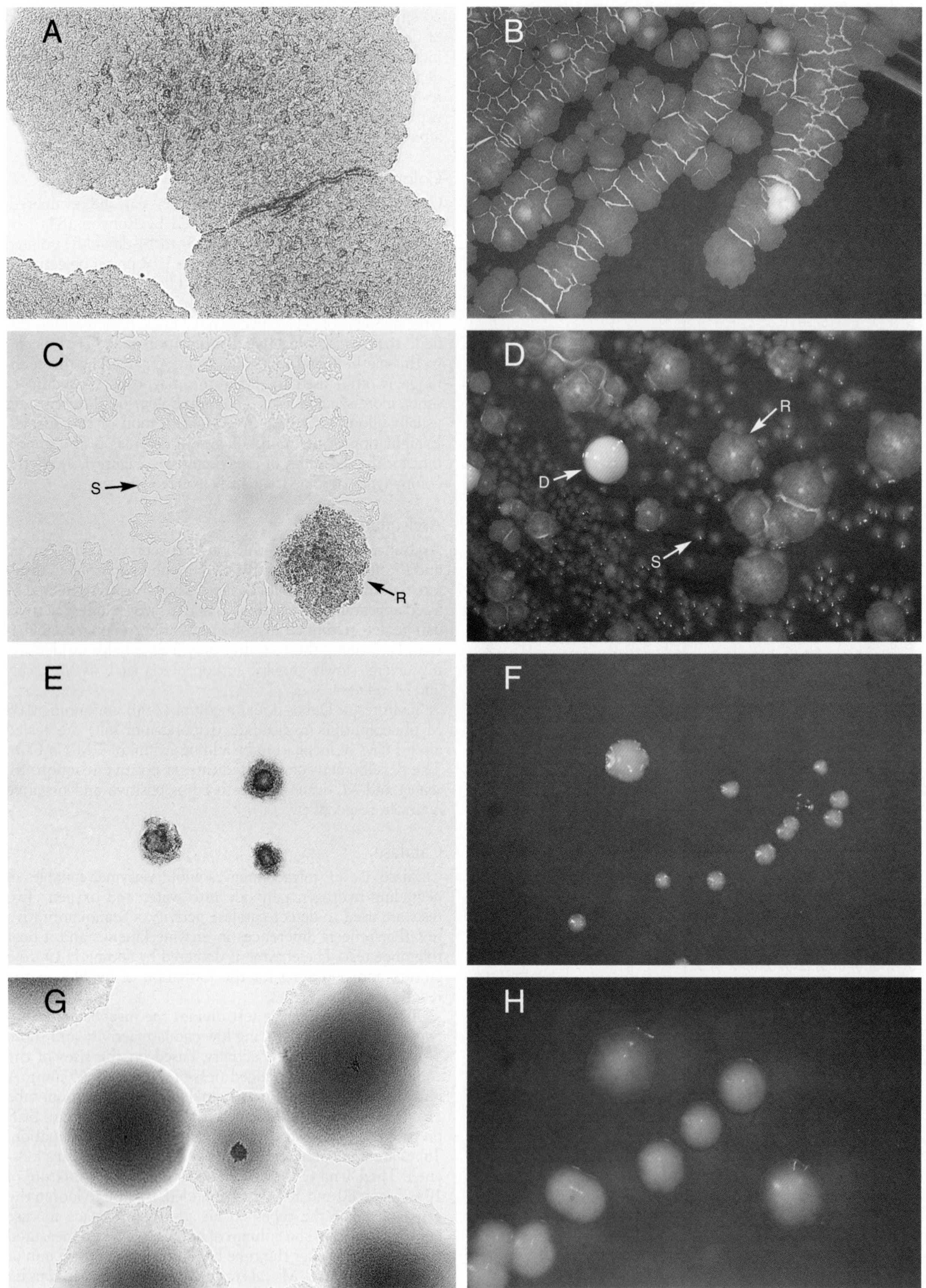

(Continued on next page)

(Continued)

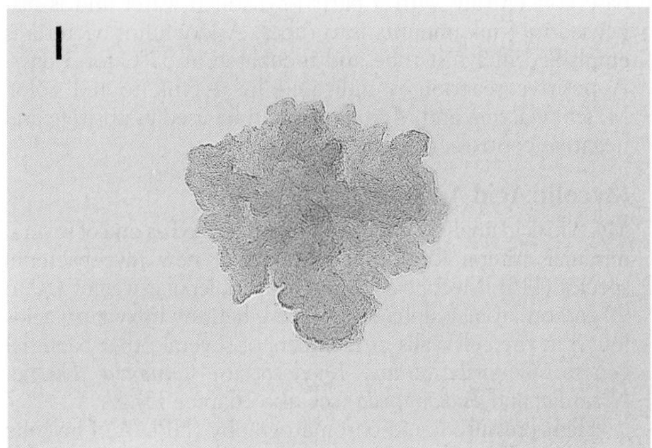

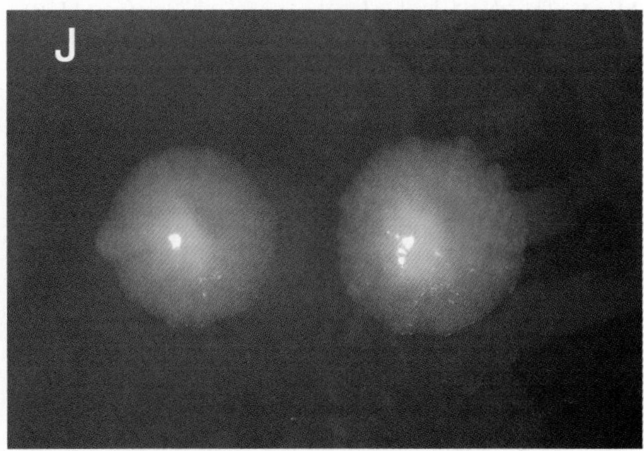

FIGURE 1 (A) M. *tuberculosis* growth after 15 days. Thin, nonpigmented, rough colonies are seen on 7H11 agar; cording is apparent. (B) M. *tuberculosis* growth after 10 days. Dry, buff, wrinkled colonies are visible on 7H11 agar. (C) M. *avium* growth after 10 days. A flat, nonpigmented, smooth (S) colony with an irregular edge and a compact, nonpigmented, rough (R) colony are seen on 7H11 agar. (D) M. *avium* growth after 10 days. Nonpigmented colony variants are visible on 7H11 agar; smooth-flat (S), dome (D), and rough (R) variants are indicated. (E) M. *xenopi* growth after 15 days. Nonpigmented, compact, rough colonies with irregular peripheries are seen on 7H11 agar; the colonies resemble a bird's nest. (F) M. *xenopi* growth after 15 days. Smooth, dome-shaped, and slightly yellow colonies are visible on 7H11 agar. (G) M. *gordonae* growth after 10 days. Orange, smooth, opaque entire colonies and orange, smooth, opaque colonies with irregular edge tints are seen on 7H11 agar. (H) M. *gordonae* growth after 10 days. Smooth, orange, hemispheric colonies are seen on 7H11 agar. (I) M. *kansasii* growth after 10 days in the dark. Nonpigmented, rough colonies are seen on 7H11 agar; stranding of bacilli is seen (similar to cording). (J) M. *kansasii* growth after 15 days. A smooth colony with the center elevated and thickened and with a thin, rough periphery is seen on 7H11 agar; it is orange after light exposure. (Photographs courtesy of Daniel Fedorko and Yvonne Shea, Department of Laboratory Medicine, Microbiology Service, National Institutes of Health, 2002.)

Niacin Accumulation Test

Niacin (nicotinic acid) functions as a precursor in the biosynthesis of coenzymes NAD and NADP. Although all mycobacteria produce nicotinic acid, some have a block in the NAD scavenging pathway and excrete niacin. The niacin accumulated in the culture medium is then detected by its reaction with a cyanogen halide in the presence of a primary amine. Niacin-negative M. *tuberculosis* isolates are extremely rare. A positive niacin test result should not be used alone to identify M. *tuberculosis*, however, because some strains of M. *simiae* and other mycobacteria, although infrequently encountered, also accumulate niacin. Performance of the supportive tests for nitrate reduction and 68°C catalase are necessary for confirming the identification of M. *tuberculosis*.

A niacin paper strip version is available commercially (BD, Sparks, Md., and Remel Inc., Lenexa, Kans.). A heavily grown L-J culture medium is covered with 1 ml of distilled water, and the tube is placed horizontally to allow extraction for 20 min. Then 0.5 ml of the liquid is transferred to a tube. The strip is inserted, and the tube is sealed immediately. After 15 min at room temperature, yellow coloration of the liquid (not the strip) indicates a positive test result. M. *tuberculosis* H37Ra and M. *avium* can be used as positive and negative controls, respectively.

Nitrate Reduction

Mycobacteria differ quantitatively in their abilities to reduce nitrate to nitrite. The nitrate reduction test is performed by adding 2 ml of $NaNO_3$ substrate to a bacterial heavy suspension prepared with two loopfuls of bacteria emulsified in 0.2 ml of distilled water. The tube is shaken manually and incubated upright for 2 h in a 37°C water bath. After the tube is removed from the bath, 1 drop of reagent 1 (50 ml of HCl in 50 ml of H_2O), 2 drops of reagent 2 (0.2 g of sulfanilamide in 100 ml of H_2O), and 2 drops of reagent 3 (0.1 g of *N*-napthylthylenediamine dihydrochloride in 100 ml of H_2O) are added to the SCS. Immediate development of a pink tone is considered to indicate positivity. M. *tuberculosis* H37Ra and M. *avium* can be used as positive and negative controls, respectively.

Pyrazinamidase

The enzyme pyrazinamidase hydrolyzes pyrazinamide (PZA) into ammonia and pyrazinoic acid, which can be detected by the addition of ferric ammonium sulfate. This test is most useful in separating M. *marinum* from M. *kansasii* and M. *bovis* from M. *tuberculosis*. In addition, one mechanism of PZA resistance of M. *tuberculosis* appears to be the inability of the organism to produce pyrazinoic acid, which is assumed to be the active component of the drug PZA. A pyrazinamidase-negative M. *tuberculosis* isolate is assumed to be PZA resistant as well.

The test medium consists of Dubos broth base containing 0.1 g of PZA, 2.0 g of pyruvic acid, and 15.0 g of agar per liter. The medium is dispensed in 5-ml amounts, autoclaved, and solidified in a tube in an upright position. The agar medium is heavily inoculated with growth from the culture so that the inoculum should be visible. After incubation at 37°C for 4 days, 1 ml of 1% ferrous ammonium sulfate is added. The preparation is observed for up to 4 h for a pink band in the agar, which indicates a positive test result. M. *avium* and uninoculated medium are used as positive and negative controls, respectively.

Sodium Chloride Tolerance

M. triviale is the only slowly growing mycobacterium able to grow in the presence of, or tolerate, 5% sodium chloride.

L-J medium containing 5% NaCl or lacking salt is inoculated with 0.2 ml of an SCS and incubated at 30 or 35°C. Growth or no growth is scored at 4 weeks. *M. triviale* and *M. tuberculosis* H37Ra can be used as positive and negative controls, respectively.

Inhibition by Thiophene-2-Carboxylic Acid Hydrazide

Inhibition by thiophene-2-carboxylic acid hydrazide (T2H) is used to distinguish niacin-positive *M. bovis* from *M. tuberculosis* and other nonchromogenic slowly growing mycobacteria. Most *M. bovis* isolates are susceptible to T2H, whereas *M. tuberculosis* and most other slowly growing mycobacteria are resistant.

Middlebrook 7H11 medium containing 10 μg of T2H (Aldrich Chemical Co., Milwaukee, Wis.) per ml is dispensed in 5-ml amounts onto slants. Tubes with and without T2H are inoculated with 0.2 ml of the 10^{-2} and 10^{-4} SCS dilutions. When growth is visible on the control tubes, the colonies are counted. The organism is recorded as resistant if growth on the T2H medium is >1% of the growth on the control. *M. tuberculosis* H37Ra and *M. bovis* can be used as positive and negative controls, respectively.

Tellurite Reduction

Tellurite reductase reduces colorless potassium tellurite into a black metallic tellurium precipitate. The tellurite reduction test is used to separate *M. avium* and *M. intracellulare* from most other nonchromogens. Some rapid growers can similarly produce a positive tellurite test result.

Two drops of a 0.2% aqueous solution of potassium tellurite are added to 5-ml cultures (7 days old) in Middlebrook 7H9. Cultures are incubated and examined daily for 4 days or more. A positive test result is shown by a jet black precipitate. *M. avium* and *M. kansasii* can be used as positive and negative controls, respectively.

Tween 80 Hydrolysis

Lipases produced by some mycobacterial species hydrolyze the detergent polyoxyethylene sorbitan monooleate (Tween 80) into oleic acid and polyoxyethylene sorbitol. Neutral red in the pH 7 test medium is bound by Tween 80 and has an amber color at a neutral pH. If Tween 80 is hydrolyzed, however, neutral red is no longer bound and reverts to its usual red color at pH 7. The Tween 80 hydrolysis test allows for differentiation among the slowly growing NTM species.

The substrate solution consists of 0.5 ml of Tween 80 in 100 ml of 0.067 M phosphate buffer (pH 7.0) to which 2 ml of a 1% aqueous solution of neutral red is added. The solution is dispensed in screw-cap tubes in 4-ml amounts and autoclaved. A loopful of bacteria is suspended in a tube and incubated at 37°C. A change in color from amber to pink or red is recorded after 24 h and 5 and 10 days of incubation as a positive reaction. *M. kansasii* and *M. avium* can be used as positive and negative controls, respectively.

Urease

The ability of an isolate to hydrolyze urea into ammonia and CO_2 is useful in identifying both scotochromogens and nonchromogens. *M. scrofulaceum* is urease positive, whereas *M. avium* and *M. intracellulare* organisms are urease negative. The urease test is particularly helpful in the recognition of pigmented strains of *M. avium*.

The test medium is prepared by mixing 1 part of urea agar base concentrate with 9 parts of distilled water and is dispensed in 4-ml amounts into tubes. A loopful of bacteria is emulsified in a test tube and incubated at 37°C for 3 days. A positive reaction is indicated by a pink to red color. *M. scrofulaceum* and *M. gordonae* can be used as positive and negative controls, respectively.

Mycolic Acid Analysis

Mycolic acid analysis has been recommended as one of several minimal criteria for the description of new mycobacterial species (115). Mycolic acids are high-molecular-weight (20 to 90 carbon atoms) alpha-substituted, beta-hydroxy fatty acids found in the cell walls of members of several other bacterial genera: *Corynebacterium*, *Rhodococcus*, *Gordonia*, *Dietzia*, *Nocardia*, and *Tsukamurella* (see also chapter 35).

High-pressure liquid chromatography (HPLC) of mycolic acid esters has been demonstrated to be a rapid and reliable method for identification of many *Mycobacterium* species. A standardized method that includes sample preparation and chromatographic analysis has been described previously (14). One to two loopfuls of cells grown on solid medium are suspended in a methanolic potassium hydroxide solution and saponified by heating. After acidification and extraction with chloroform, free mycolic acids are derivatized to para-bromophenacyl esters. Internal-standard molecular weight markers are added, and the sample is injected. The mycolic acid esters are separated on a reversed-phase C_{18} column by a methanol-methylene chloride gradient elution and detected by UV spectrophotometry (UV-HPLC). An extract prepared from *M. intracelluare* ATCC 13950 is used as a positive control and provides an external standard peak naming reference. The high biomass requirement of UV-HPLC can be reduced at least 200-fold by derivatizing mycolic acids to 6,7-dimethoxy-4-coumarinyl-methyl esters, which are measured by fluorescence detection HPLC (FL-HPLC). The increased analytical sensitivity of FL-HPLC allows the identification of acid-fast bacilli from smear-positive clinical specimens, liquid medium cultures, and minute amounts of biomass from solid medium (42). MTBC identification by FL-HPLC has been reported to achieve a sensitivity of 99% with BACTEC 12B medium with a growth index of ≥50 (42).

HPLC patterns can be identified to the species or group level by visual or mathematical means. A pattern atlas derived from a multicenter study of more than 350 strains, representing 23 species, that illustrates species patterns is available on the Centers for Disease Control and Prevention website at http://www.cdc.gov/ncidod/dastlr/TB/TB_HPLC.htm. Additionally, pattern overlays of closely related species have been presented along with pattern variations produced by strains of a single species. However, *M. tuberculosis* and *M. bovis* produce indistinguishable patterns. The standardized method (14) recommends a visual comparison of a sample HPLC pattern to an atlas of reference strain patterns in combination with the use of peak height ratios. This approach was reported to achieve an accuracy of 96.1% (104). Libraries that report both an identification and the quality of a match are commercially available (Pirouette and INSTEP software [Infometrix Inc., Woodinville, Wash.] and the Sherlock mycobacterium identification system [MIDI, Inc., Newark, Del.]).

Although HPLC initial equipment costs are high (approximately $50,000) and considerable expertise is required to operate nonautomated systems, material costs per test are economical compared with those for commercial molecular probes. Sample preparation is simple, and many mycobacterial species or groups can be identified in a single analysis. However, mycolic acid analysis does not provide the specificity or the sensitivity of molecular approaches as described below.

Mycobacterial Genomes

The complete genome sequence of M. *tuberculosis* H37Rv comprises 4,411,529 bp and contains approximately 4,000 genes (20). M. *tuberculosis* has an extremely clonal population structure, with genomic variation caused largely by insertion sequence movement rather than point mutation (10, 46, 94). A recent study showed that, similar to *Yersinia pestis* (2) and *Salmonella enterica* serotype Typhi (49), the MTBC consists of a successful clonal population that recently emerged from a much more ancient and larger bacterial species group encompassing M. *canettii* and additional genetic groups of smooth strains (36).

Additional genome sequences are available or are being determined for several mycobacteria. More information can be found at the websites http://genolist.pasteur.fr/TubercuList/index.html for M. *tuberculosis* H37Rv, http://www.tigr.org./tigr-scripts/CMR2/GenomePage3.spl?database = gmt for M. *tuberculosis* CDC1551, http://www.sanger.ac.uk/Projects/M_bovis for M. *bovis*, and http://genolist.pasteur.fr/Leproma/index.html for M. *leprae*.

Genotypic Identification of Mycobacterial Strains

PCR-REA

In 1993, Telenti and colleagues proposed a method for rapid identification of mycobacteria to the species level based on PCR amplification of a 439-bp fragment of the gene encoding the 65-kDa heat shock protein (*hsp65*) followed by restriction enzyme digestion using BstEII and HaeIII (102). The method has been extensively used for the identification of slowly growing mycobacteria (77). M. *tuberculosis* is easily differentiated from the NTM by a characteristic band with HaeIII restriction endonuclease digestion. However, members of the MTBC are not discriminated by PCR-restriction enzyme analysis (PCR-REA). By contrast, most NTM can be recognized by their PCR-REA patterns. Several alleles have been identified in M. *gordonae* and M. *kansasii* yielding several distinct PCR-REA patterns for a single species (77). Some other gene sequences (including those of *rpoB*, *dnaJ*, and the 16S-23S rRNA gene spacer) have been tentatively used for PCR-REA, but none have been studied as extensively as that of *hsp65*.

The advantages of PCR-REA are that equipment is not very expensive and the method is relatively rapid and identifies most mycobacterial species, including some not identified by phenotypic methods and/or HPLC. The disadvantages are that it is a relatively complex procedure and, due to the increase of newly described species, it may not allow unambiguous species identification but may assign to groups of mycobacterial species. A multicenter evaluation of the method showed that differences in gel running conditions and lack of training in interpretation of patterns contributed to low accuracy (58). Furthermore, it is not commercialized or Food and Drug Administration (FDA) approved and it requires a significant amount of in-house validation.

Commercially Available Identification Probes

AccuProbe

Acridinium ester-labeled DNA probes based on the detection of rRNA (Gen-Probe Inc., San Diego, Calif.) specific for the MTBC, the M. *avium* complex (MAC), M. *kansasii*, and M. *gordonae* (as well as separate probes for M. *avium* and M. *intracellulare*) are FDA approved and commercially available. The current total test time for the AccuProbe assay is less than 2 h (17, 59). Briefly, target 16S rRNA is released from the organism by sonication. The labeled DNA probe combines with the organism's rRNA to form a DNA-rRNA hybrid. The labeled product is detected in a luminometer.

Tests with DNA probes can be performed using isolates from solid media or from broth cultures. Combining the probes with a broth culture system has the advantage of optimizing rapid detection and identification of mycobacteria present in clinical samples (17, 43). Procedural modifications are necessary for testing isolates recovered from liquid medium. An aliquot of the broth culture is concentrated by centrifugation, and the pellet is resuspended in culture identification reagent. Testing then follows the procedure for testing colonies from solid media (as described in the AccuProbe technical insert). To eliminate high nonspecific chemiluminescence, BACTEC (BD) 13A broth medium containing blood is pretreated with 100 μl of 10% sodium dodecyl sulfate–50 mM EDTA (pH 7.2) before microcentrifugation to allow lysis of the erythrocytes and sorbitolization of the membranes. Appropriate positive and negative control organisms should be included in each assay run.

It has been shown that specificity is 100% for testing of mycobacterial colonies. Sensitivity, however, varies with the species or species complexes: 95.2 to 97.2% for the MAC, 100% for the MTBC, 100% for M. *gordonae*, and 97.4 to 100% for M. *kansasii* (33, 59, 80, 108). Later studies using AccuProbe on more than 11,000 positive BACTEC cultures also showed 100% specificity and >85 to 100% sensitivity for all species tested (17, 79).

Advantages of this test include the simplicity and rapidity (within 2 h) with which mycobacteria can be identified. The use of a nonradioactive procedure and the extended shelf life of the chemiluminescent probes offer the potential for widespread application in most clinical laboratory settings (33, 59).

A few limitations of using AccuProbe have been described. These include misidentification of M. *celatum* as MTBC due to the similarity of the 16S rRNA genes of these two species in the probe region (92). The specificity of the MTBC probe has been increased by extending the length of the selection reagent incubation step to 10 min, and a temperature of 60 to 61°C is recommended to eliminate cross-reactivity with other species, including M. *terrae* and M. *celatum* (92). Greater biomass in the test suspensions may also result in decreased specificity of the test (92). It has been shown that the use of a higher cutoff (at 80,000 relative light units instead of 30,000 relative light units) may prevent false-positive results when the MAC probe is tested with broth cultures (19). As with all laboratory tests, the user is reminded that the probe should be repeated or the results should be confirmed by an alternate method if results do not correlate with clinical or cultural observations. The MTBC probe does not differentiate among members of the MTBC.

Strip Tests

Two line probe assays have been developed, one targeting the 16S-23S rRNA internal transcribed spacer region (INNO-LiPA Mycobacteria version 2; Innogenetics, Ghent, Belgium) and the other one targeting the 23S rRNA gene (GenoType Mycobacteria; Hain Lifescience, Nehren, Germany).

Strip assays are based on the reverse hybridization of biotinylated PCR products to their complementary probes immobilized as parallel lines on a membrane strip. Kits may be applied to strains subcultured on solid or in liquid media. Lines on the strips include probes for the identification of the

Mycobacterium genus and probes for the identification of various frequently encountered or clinically relevant mycobacterial species, 16 species in the INNO-LiPA Mycobacteria version 2 and 13 species in the GenoType Mycobacteria. The overall concordance with other identification methods (AccuProbe and PCR-REA of *hsp65* or 16S sequences) has been good when tested with reference strains and mycobacterial cultures from clinical specimens (60, 81, 86, 107).

The main advantage of the kits is that a range of several species can be identified by a single PCR assay, and unlike the AccuProbe, they do not require a tentative selection of the adequate probe. The kits are commercially available in Europe at the present time and available only for research in the United States. Tests are performed in 6 h, including the preliminary PCR amplification. They require several time-consuming washes. An automated machine, Auto-LiPA (Innogenetics), which runs the washes and ensures the gentle shaking necessary for several steps of the procedure, greatly contributes to time saving and ease of application in clinical laboratories. However, the cost of this apparatus may hamper its introduction into many laboratories.

DNA Sequencing

The availability of DNA sequencing technologies constitutes a great benefit for mycobacterial identification, owing to the peculiar slow growth of mycobacterial organisms. Recent improvements in automation of target amplification and sequence analysis have led to practical implementation of DNA sequencing in the clinical laboratory. Moreover, the cost has decreased dramatically (106). Sequencing of the entire 16S rRNA gene (*rrs* gene, approximately 1,500 bp) or the *hsp65* gene (approximately 4,400 bp) cannot be done in a routine clinical laboratory. However, identification of species-specific signatures within variable regions of these highly conserved genes allows the design of simple PCR protocols followed by the direct sequencing of the PCR-amplified products. Catalogues of sequences of mycobacterial species may be retrieved from databases (GenBank/EMBL website at http://www.ncbi.nlm.nih.gov) and conveniently imported and stored in a file in the laboratory. Liquid cultures or colonies from solid medium may be used for DNA extraction by boiling the sample without any further purification. The polymorphism of several conserved genes has been investigated for identifying mycobacterial species, such as the gene encoding the 32-kDa protein (91), the *dnaJ* gene (101), the *sod* gene encoding the superoxide dismutase (126), the *gyrB* gene coding for the gyrase subunit B (45), the *rpoB* gene coding for the RNA polymerase (51), the internal transcribed spacer 16S-23S sequence (67, 84), and the *secA1* gene coding for a key component of the major pathway of protein secretion across the cytoplasmic membrane (124). The most widely used targets are 16S rRNA (*rrs* gene) and the *hsp65* gene.

The strategy for sequencing and identification of the signature sequences of the 16S rRNA gene has been extensively described (52). Specific primers for mycobacteria (Table 2) have been designed for the amplification of the 16S rRNA gene to avoid contamination and enhance specificity. Amplification of a 1,030-bp region encompassing the 16S rRNA gene sequence is performed with primers 285 and 264. The sequencing reaction is performed with primer 244 by using sequencing kits for automated DNA sequencers to characterize the hypervariable region A, located on the 5′ side of the *rrs* gene, corresponding to *Escherichia coli* 16S rRNA gene positions 129 to 267. 16S rRNA genes reflect a limited conserved region of the entire genome, and the molecular clock of the marker is rather slow. Species of recent divergence thus may contain 16S rRNA gene

TABLE 2 Oligonucleotides used for mycobacterial identification by DNA sequencing

Target	Primer[a]	Sequence	Position[b]
rrs	285	5′ GAGAGTTTGATCCTGGCTCAG 3′	9–29
rrs	264	5′ TGCACACAGGCCACAAGGGA 3′	1046–1027
rrs	244	5′ CCCACTGCTGCCTCCCGTAG 3′	361–342
hsp65	Tb11	5′ ACCAACGATGGTGTGTCCAT 3′	396–415
hsp65	Tb12	5′ CTTGTCGAACCGCATACCCT 3′	836–817

[a] Primers are described in references 44 and 52.
[b] "Position" refers to the *E. coli* 16S rRNA gene numbering for the *rrs* gene and to the *M. tuberculosis* numbering for the *hsp65* gene.

sequences that are highly similar. Moreover, no single 16S rRNA gene interstrain nucleotide sequence difference value that unequivocally defines species boundaries has been established for the genus *Mycobacterium* (119). For instance, *M. szulgai* and *M. malmoense* present a 2-nucleotide difference only in the 1,384-nucleotide segment examined whereas some *M. intracellulare* serotypes reveal microheterogeneity with 1 to 7 different nucleotides in a 782-nucleotide segment (119). For routine identification, strains should be identified according to a 16S rRNA hypervariable region A matching the type strain sequence. Additional investigation using another molecular marker (e.g., *hsp65*) may be required for accurate identification since hypervariable region A cannot be used to discriminate between some species encountered in clinical specimens, i.e., *M. kansasii* and *M. gastri*, *M. ulcerans* and *M. marinum*, and *M. shimoidei* and *M. triviale* (52). In addition, no polymorphisms are present among the different species in the MTBC.

Partial sequencing of the *hsp65* gene is performed using primers Tb11 and Tb12 (44) for the amplification of a 441-bp region (nucleotides 396 to 836 according to the numbering of the *M. tuberculosis hsp65* gene) (88). As indicated above for the PCR-REA method, several *hsp65* alleles may be identified within a species. The polymorphism in the *hsp65* gene allows unambiguous identification of species with close 16S rRNA gene sequences such as *M. gastri* and *M. kansasii*. As with the 16S rRNA gene, all MTBC members have the same *hsp65* allele except *M. africanum* and *M. canettii*, which show a single nucleotide polymorphism within the gene (30, 36).

Genotypic Markers for Species Identification within the MTBC

Although *M. tuberculosis* is the most prevalent tubercle bacillus isolated in clinical laboratories, identification of other members of the MTBC is of the utmost epidemiological importance and may govern the management of contact-tracing investigations and/or treatment. Incomplete identification of tubercle bacilli can lead to misdiagnosis of *M. bovis* BCG infections in patients treated for bladder cancer or misdiagnosis of nosocomial BCG infections in cancer patients (97, 116, 117). Moreover, the identification of *M. bovis* allows public health investigation and tracing of epidemics possibly due to cattle-to-human transmission (37). A retrospective study (1980 to 1997) of active pediatric tuberculosis in a United States-Mexico cross-border region showed that *M. bovis* accounted for 10.8% of all tuberculosis cases and for 33.9% of cases with positive cultures (23). The main risk factor was exposure to a zoonotic source, namely, ingestion of unpasteurized dairy products (7, 23). Similarly, rare agents of tuberculosis (*M. microti*, *M. canettii*, *M. caprae*, and *M. pinnipedii*) have to be properly identified for documentation of their epidemiology at the national level (37).

The MTBC members cannot be differentiated by the AccuProbe test. Similarly, the *hsp65* gene and the PCR-REA patterns are identical for *M. tuberculosis* and *M. bovis*. However, strains may be differentiated according to conventional identification tests (Table 1) as well as host range and virulence. The sequence polymorphism of the *oxyR* and *pncA* genes led to the development of allele-specific PCR tests which allow differentiation of *M. bovis* from all other MTBC members (25). The distribution of deletions (RD sequences) among the tubercle bacilli contributes to the identification of the different members of the MTBC: this approach is based on PCR tests only (Table 3). Since many laboratories use amplification procedures, it has been proposed that this PCR-based approach be incorporated into the laboratory routine by clinical mycobacteriology laboratories (68). A commercialized strip assay relying on *gyrB* probes has been recently developed for the differentiation of the MTBC members (Hain Lifescience). An evaluation study showed that the species were unequivocally identified but *M. tuberculosis* and *M. canettii* shared a common pattern (81). Moreover, as mentioned below, spoligotyping confirms the specific identification.

Molecular tests should be carried out on *M. tuberculosis* strains with phenotypes which do not fully match that of the type strain, e.g., strains which hybridize with the MTBC probe and do not yield rough, cream, cauliflower-like colonies or do not produce niacin or nitrate reductase. Monoresistance to PZA has been shown to be of poor predictive value as an initial screening tool for *M. bovis* (24, 38). If molecular analysis is not available in the laboratory, strains should be sent to a reference laboratory.

Direct NAA Tests

Three nucleic acid amplification (NAA) kits designed to detect MTBC bacilli directly from patient specimens are commercially available. The amplified *M. tuberculosis* direct test (AMTD; Gen-Probe) consists of transcription-mediated amplification of a specific 16S rRNA target performed at constant temperature for the detection of MTBC rRNA in smear-positive and -negative respiratory samples. The Amplicor *M. tuberculosis* PCR assay (Roche Molecular Systems, Branchburg, N.J.) consists of PCR amplication of a 584-bp region of the 16S rRNA gene sequence. Incorporation of dUTP instead of dTTP prevents carrier contamination in the amplification reaction, and the use of uracil-*N*-glycosylase enzymatically cleaves any contaminating amplicons from previous reactions.

Both of these tests are FDA approved for respiratory samples, the AMTD for both smear-positive and smear-negative specimens and the Amplicor for smear-positive specimens only. Moreover, investigators have shown that, with specific modifications, the tests may also detect *M. tuberculosis* in nonrespiratory specimens (76). The overall AMTD specificity ranged from 92.1 to 100%. For respiratory specimens, the sensitivity was between 91.7 and 100% for smear-positive specimens and decreased to between 65.5 and 92.9% for smear-negative specimens. For nonrespiratory specimens, the sensitivity was between 88 and 100% for smear-positive specimens and between 63.6 and 100% for smear-negative specimens (76). Regarding the Amplicor assay, specificity was similar to the AMTD value for smear-positive specimens and ranged from 90 to 100% for respiratory specimens and from 87.5 to 100% for extrapulmonary specimens. However, sensitivity was lower for smear-negative samples, from 50 to 95.9% for respiratory specimens and from 17.2 to 70.8% for extrapulmonary specimens. Inhibition has been detected in less than 1 to 5% of clinical specimens with the AMTD and up to 20% with the Amplicor assay. The Amplicor assay showed a significantly higher inhibition rate for nonrespiratory specimens and false-positive results were related to cross-reactions with mycobacteria other than tubercle bacilli (76).

The BDProbeTec strand displacement amplification (BD) is an isothermal enzymatic process that coamplifies sequences of IS*6110* (specific to the MTBC) and the 16S rRNA gene (common to most mycobacterial species). The process is based on the nicking of the recognition sequence in double-stranded DNA by a restriction endonuclease and further extension of that site with DNA polymerase that synthesizes a new strand of DNA while displacing the existing one. The sensitivity of the test has been shown to be between 98.5 and 100% for smear-positive specimens and between 33.3 and 85.7% for smear-negative and extrapulmonary specimens, with inhibition rates between 0.3 and 14% (76).

Since tuberculosis of the central nervous system is one of the most malignant forms of human tuberculosis, the rapid and accurate laboratory diagnosis of tuberculous meningitis is of prime importance. Conventional bacteriology methods are usually inefficient (negative microscopy and late positive culture if any). Recently, a systematic review and meta-analysis documented the diagnostic accuracy of NAA tests for tuberculous meningitis. The summary estimates were as follows: sensitivity, 0.56 (95% confidence interval [CI], 0.46 to 0.66); specificity, 0.98 (95% CI, 0.97 to 0.99); positive likelihood ratio, 35.1 (95% CI, 19.0 to 64.6); and negative likelihood ratio, 0.44 (95% CI, 0.33 to 0.60). Consequently, commercial NAA tests show a potential role in confirming tuberculous meningitis diagnosis, although their overall low sensitivity precludes the use of these tests to rule out tuberculous meningitis with certainty (66).

NAA tests can be performed in as few as 6 to 8 h on processed specimens and, therefore, offer the promise of same-day reporting of results for detection and identification of *M. tuberculosis*. Used as approved by the FDA, NAA tests for *M. tuberculosis* detection do not replace any previously recommended tests and supplement rather than replace culture (16). A recent multicenter study stressed the need for external quality control (64).

TABLE 3 Genotypic characteristics of the MTBC members[a]

Strain	*oxyR*/285	*pncA*/169	RD4	RD9	RD12	RD[b] specific
M. tuberculosis	G	C	+	+	+	TbD1[c]
M. bovis	A	G	−	−	−	
M. bovis BCG	A	G	−	−	−	RD1
M. africanum	G	C	+	−	+	
M. canettii	G	C	+	+	+	RDcan[d]
M. microti	G	C	+	−	+	RDmic[e]
M. caprae	A	C	+	−	−	
M. pinnipedii	G	C	+	−	+	RDpin[f]

[a] Data from references 5, 11, 25, 31, 113, and 114. +, present; −, absent.
[b] RD locus numbering according to reference 31.
[c] TbD1 region is absent from "modern" *M. tuberculosis* only and present in all members of the MTBC (11).
[d] RDcan corresponds to a region specifically absent from *M. canettii* only that partially overlaps RD12 (11).
[e] RDmic corresponds to a region specifically absent from *M. microti* only that partially overlaps RD1 (11).
[f] RDpin corresponds to a region specifically absent from *M. pinnipedii* only that partially overlaps RD2 (11).

MYCOBACTERIAL STRAIN TYPING

Molecular Typing Methods for MTBC Strains

Historically, unusual drug susceptibility patterns and phage typing have been used for epidemiological studies of tuberculosis, but they have significant limitations. The description of the repetitive insertion sequence IS*6110* marked a major advance in the molecular epidemiology of tuberculosis (110). Since then, additional sequences of interest for *M. tuberculosis* fingerprinting have been described (32, 111). *M. tuberculosis* DNA fingerprinting has proven to be a powerful epidemiological tool for tracing of transmission groups and determination of their risk factors, for differentiation of exogenous reinfection and relapse, and for detection of laboratory cross-contamination, among other applications (15, 22, 111).

IS*6110* RFLP

The restriction fragment length polymorphism (RFLP) technique using the IS*6110* repetitive sequence as a probe was the first extensively used method for typing MTBC strains. IS*6110* is an insertion sequence present in variable copy numbers, from 0 to 26 in MTBC strains (15). A standardized protocol, based on the use of the restriction enzyme PvuII, has been proposed for IS*6110* RFLP comparison. Standardization of the procedure facilitates interlaboratory comparability of patterns (110).

The IS*6110* RFLP technique is widely applicable to *M. tuberculosis* since fewer than 0.1% of strains tested have no copies of the element (61). However, several sites of IS*6110* insertion are preferential loci for integration into the genome, contributing to reducing the potential diversity of fingerprint patterns (15). The RFLP technique requires approximatively 2 μg of high-quality DNA and hence has to be performed with large quantities of cells. A subculture of the isolate or heavy growth on the original slant and a long turnaround time are required. The technical steps are both labor-intensive and lengthy. Moreover, sophisticated computer image analysis software is required for image analysis, and the availability of well-trained users is sparse. Owing to these difficulties, the IS*6110* RFLP technique cannot be carried out in clinical laboratories and is limited to reference laboratories. PCR-based methods targeting IS*6110* have been developed to reduce the time lag for obtaining IS*6110* RFLP patterns. Although their differentiation levels are close to that of the IS*6110* RFLP technique, the methods suffer from similar drawbacks (lack of accuracy for strains with few IS*6110* copies and lack of expertise for the interpretation of the image patterns) and have not been widely applied (53, 55, 78).

Spoligotyping

The spoligotyping (which stands for "spacer oligotyping") method (Table 4) is based on the polymorphism of the direct repeat (DR) locus. This region, present in all MTBC strains in a unique locus, contains multiple, well-conserved 36-bp repeats interspersed with nonrepetitive short spacer sequences of 34 to 41 bp. Strains are tested by hybridizing their PCR-amplified DR regions to a membrane which consists of an array of 43 covalently bound oligonucleotides representing the polymorphic spacers identified in the *M. tuberculosis* H37Rv DR sequence and in the sequence of *M. bovis* BCG. The method has the clear advantage of being able to simultaneously discriminate among the members of the MTBC and differentiate the clinical isolates in one assay. Spoligotypes appear highly stable, suggesting that isolates with different spoligotypes are rarely related (111). Moreover, spoligotyping allows the identification of prevalent genotypes, especially the Beijing genotype, frequently encountered in China, in other regions of Asia, in the former USSR, and in other geographical areas (54). In the United States, the largest known epidemic associated with drug-resistant strains was due to the so-called "W" strain, an evolutionary branch of the Beijing family (8).

The discriminative power of spoligotyping is less than that of the IS*6110* RFLP technique, and the method tends to group strains in large clusters (111). Spoligotyping, however, is more discriminating for strains with no or few copies of IS*6110* and has been recommended for *M. bovis* since most *M. bovis* strains have few IS*6110* copies (111). Used for the detection of *M. tuberculosis* directly in clinical specimens, spoligotyping failed to yield reproducible patterns. Spoligotyping use in routine clinical laboratories may be difficult to implement due to the multistep hybridization procedures required by the method.

PCR Strategies Targeting Tandem Repeats

Genetic loci containing variable-number tandem repeats (VNTR) have been identified in the *M. tuberculosis* genome (32). VNTR are a source of allelic polymorphism which can be analyzed by amplification of each locus by using primers specific for flanking regions and estimation of the sizes of the PCR products, which reflect the number of VNTR copies. Results can be conveniently coded in a simple numerical format, corresponding to the number of repeated units in each locus. Initial VNTR typing based on limited sets of loci lacked discriminatory ability (55). However, a VNTR method based on 12 loci of a type of VNTR sequences called mycobacterial interspersed repetitive units (MIRUs) has been developed (89, 100). The 12 MIRU-VNTR loci present two to eight alleles which correspond to a potential of over 16 million different combinations. The method yields a discriminatory power close to that of IS*6110* RFLP typing (better for low-copy-number IS*6110* strains) and accurately clusters epidemiologically related strains (39, 56, 93, 99). The MIRU-VNTR method can be performed either in a manual format or on a fluorescence-based DNA analyzer with automation by using multiplex PCRs (99). A microfluidic labchip instrument has been used for rapid typing based on MIRU-VNTR (21). Thanks to its feasibility, portability, high reproducibility, and discriminatory power, the MIRU-VNTR technique is progressively replacing the IS*6110* RFLP method (9, 22, 53).

Whole-Genome Fingerprinting Methods

Promising results have been obtained with DNA arrays. The Affymetrix-GeneChip system has been applied to identify genomic deletions in *M. tuberculosis* isolates (46). It relies on the use of a high-density oligonucleotide microarray harboring 20 probe pairs targeted to every open reading frame and intergenic region of *M. tuberculosis* H37Rv, thus totaling 111,488 probe pairs after exclusion of noninformative probes. Hybridized DNA is detected with a confocal laser scanner. In a small-scale evaluation, the patterns of deletions detected were identical for epidemiologically related clones but differed between different clones, suggesting that the system is suitable for epidemiological studies (46). However, the system is not practical for analyzing large numbers of strains. High-density oligonucleotide microarrays will become commercially available to be used for clinical laboratory purposes in the future.

Single-nucleotide polymorphisms based on the synonymous mutations have been detected in *M. tuberculosis*. Since *M. tuberculosis* displays restricted allelic variation (94), the

TABLE 4 Characteristic spoligotypes of some MTBC members

Strain	Spoligotype[a] (1 … 9 … 19 … 29 … 39 … 43)
M. tuberculosis H37Rv	■■■■■■■■■■■■■■■■■■■□□■■■■■■■■■■■□□□□■■■■■■■
M. tuberculosis Beijing or W	□□□□□□□□□□□□□□□□□□□□□□□□□□□□□□□□□□■■■■■■■■■
M. bovis BCG Pasteur	■■□■■■■■□■■■■■■□■■■■■■■■■■■■■■■■■■■■■■□□□□□
M. africanum ATCC 25420	■■■■■■□□□■■■■□■■■■■□■■■■■■■■■■■■■■■■■■□■■■■
M. canettii	□□□□□□□□□□□□□□□□□□□□□□□□□□□□□■□□□□□■□□□□□□□
M. microti	□□□□□□□□□□□□□□□□□□□□□□□□□□□□□□□□□□□□■■□□□□□
M. caprae	□■□□□□□□□□□□□□□□■■■■■■■■■■■□■□□□□■■■■■□□□□□
M. pinnipedii	□□□■■■■□□□□□□□□□□□□□□□■■■■■■■■■■■■■■■■□□□□□

[a] ■, positive hybridization; □, negative hybridization.

sequencing of several entire genomes allowed the identification of approximately only 400 single-nucleotide polymorphisms based on the synonymous mutations (28). The technique may represent a useful typing method for M. *tuberculosis* isolates for epidemiologic studies provided that high throughput technology becomes available and affordable for clinical laboratories.

Molecular Typing Methods for Slowly Growing NTM

Typing methods have to be applied to isolates belonging to the same species. The precise species identification of such isolates is thus a prerequisite for molecular typing. Assignment of the isolates to the complex level (especially the MAC) cannot be considered an accurate characterization. For mycobacteria, relevant typing methods use specific molecular markers (RFLP methods), apply to the whole genome (e.g., pulsed-field gel electrophoresis [PFGE]), or rely on the polymorphism provided by VNTR.

PFGE can be applied in the absence of knowledge of the specific content of a species genome. However, PFGE is a fastidious technique which requires an actively growing culture and several days for completion. Standardization may be hampered by cell clumping and difficulties in controlling cell lysis, resulting in different DNA yields from strain to strain, even from batch to batch of the same strain. These difficulties may result in uneven patterns (light and overloaded lanes) since agarose cubes may release various DNA amounts. Moreover, because of DNA degradation, some strains or species are untypeable by PFGE (71, 118).

RFLP analysis is easier to perform and does not require living cells, although a consistent amount of DNA is needed. With both RFLP analysis and PFGE, the degree of strain discrimination varies from species to species and may vary within a species from type to type. A comprehensive review of the various methods used for molecular epidemiology studies of the slowly growing mycobacterial species has been published (26).

M. avium Typing Methods

The first strain-typing method for M. *avium* was serotyping, based on a tedious seroagglutination procedure. Combined use of serotyping and species-specific DNA probes has shown that serovars 1 through 6 and 8 through 11 are M. *avium* and that serovars 7, 12 through 17, 19, 20, and 25 are M. *intracellulare* (85). Multilocus enzyme electrophoresis has been shown to provide a wider range of polymorphisms than serotyping (122).

These methods are of limited epidemiological value and have been replaced by discriminant genomic methods utilizing PFGE or RFLP analysis with the repetitive element IS*1245* or IS*1311*. With the use of a standardized IS*1245* RFLP typing method (112), M. *avium* isolates from humans show highly polymorphic patterns with a median number of 16 to 20 bands (35, 72). A PCR method based on amplification of sequences located between the homologous sequences IS*1245* and IS*1311* has been developed for rapid strain typing of M. *avium*, with a level of discrimination similar to that of IS*1245* RFLP analysis (74). The wide genetic variability of clinical strains demonstrated by using IS*1245* is similarly shown by PFGE, with highly discriminant patterns. Pattern polymorphism is comparable in the PFGE and IS*1245* RFLP techniques. Isolates recovered from single patients exhibit stable IS*1245* RFLP or PFGE patterns over months or even years (62, 72, 82).

Strains from birds share a characteristic IS*1245* three-band pattern, whereas human or porcine isolates display polymorphic, multiband IS*1245* patterns (63, 82). It has been recently shown that the three-band bird pattern consists of one copy of IS*1245* and two copies of IS*1311* (41). The designations M. *avium* subsp. *avium* and M. *avium* subsp. *hominissuis* have been proposed. These designations indicate that birds represent an unusual source of M. *avium* infection in human immunodeficiency virus-infected or -uninfected patients (63, 82).

MIRUs identified in M. *avium* subsp. *paratuberculosis* allow the differentiation from M. *avium* subsp. *avium* (13) and differentiate six subtypes, providing a limited molecular typing tool (65). The identification of multilocus short-sequence repeat sequences consisting of mono-, di-, and trinucleotide repeat sequences dispersed throughout the M. *avium* subsp. *paratuberculosis* genome allows high-resolution subtyping of the strains. Twenty distinct subtypes were identified among 33 strains from various sources (human, ovine, bovine, caprine, rabbit, soil, deer, and murine) and from various geographic origins (4). These results are of specific interest since the concern of possible regular exposure of humans to these bacteria has been demonstrated due to the remarkable thermostability of the bacteria during pasteurization and their presence in milk for consumers (34). Although the role of M. *avium* subsp. *paratuberculosis* as an etiologic agent of Crohn's disease is still under debate, a significant correlation between the presence of M. *avium* subsp. *paratuberculosis* in intestinal biopsy specimens and Crohn's disease has been recently shown (12). Moreover, detection of M. *avium* subsp. *paratuberculosis* in river water in an area where paratuberculosis is endemic among the livestock and where a significant increase in Crohn's disease has been reported stresses the potential exposure to aerosols carrying M. *avium* subsp. *paratuberculosis* and generated from the river (75).

M. kansasii Typing Methods

In Europe, the use of various molecular markers showed five subspecies within M. *kansasii* (3, 71). However, strains from the United States were shown to belong exclusively to subspecies I. These results demonstrate that subspecies I is predominant in the United States as it is in Europe and that this genotype I is highly clonal, with the same major genotype responsible for human infection worldwide (125).

Typing Methods for Other Slowly Growing NTM Species

For the other slowly growing species, information on the degree of polymorphism displayed by the different techniques is limited.

Molecular epidemiology of M. *intracellulare* can rely only on PFGE since the M. *avium* insertion sequences IS*1245* and IS*1311* are absent from all strains of M. *intracellulare* (35). Polymorphic PFGE patterns have been obtained for epidemiologically unrelated strains (62, 90).

IS*1395*, a specific insertion sequence, has been detected in M. *xenopi*. All M. *xenopi* strains have the element in 3 to 18 copies. Despite this high copy number, the element provides limited polymorphism, and unrelated strains were shown to share several bands in IS*1395* RFLP patterns. Comparable results were obtained with PFGE, suggesting high homogeneity of the M. *xenopi* genome (73).

Although rarely clinically significant, M. *gordonae* is a common laboratory contaminant and is frequently the cause of pseudo-outbreaks related to endoscopy, tap water, ice machines, or refrigerated fountains (118). Several molecular markers have been detected in M. *gordonae*, including the polymorphic GC-rich sequence (PGRS) and MPTR repetitive elements, also present in the MTBC and in M. *kansasii*, and two insertion sequences, IS*1511* and IS*1512*, which display high polymorphism (70). PFGE has also been successfully applied to M. *gordonae* (57).

The molecular epidemiology of M. *celatum* clearly differentiates M. *celatum* type 1 from M. *celatum* type 2 (69). A specific insertion sequence, IS*1407*, is present in M. *celatum* type 1 only. M. *celatum* type 2 displays polymorphic PFGE patterns, whereas M. *celatum* type 1 presents a single pattern.

A limited polymorphism was demonstrated within M. *haemophilum* with either a repetitive element in an RFLP study (50) or PFGE (123). Random amplification of polymorphic DNA typing also showed some polymorphism in M. *malmoense* (47). Two distinct repeated sequences, IS*2404* (83, 96) and IS*2406* (96), both present in high copy numbers (>50 copies), were identified in M. *ulcerans*. Interestingly, although comparative genetic analysis of M. *ulcerans* and M. *marinum* showed a very close phylogenetic relationship, both elements are absent from M. *marinum*. These data led to the hypothesis that M. *ulcerans* recently diverged from M. *marinum* by the acquisition of IS*2404* and IS*2606*, the species diversity being driven mainly by the genetic activity of the insertion sequences (96). Due to their high copy numbers, the two repeated elements are of poor value for typing M. *ulcerans* strains. Amplified fragment length polymorphism and IS*2404* RFLP analysis showed six types within M. *ulcerans* which correlated with the geographic origins of the strains (18). A novel-category VNTR allows the identification of eight genotypes within M. *ulcerans* and five genotypes within M. *marinum* (1, 98).

REFERENCES

1. **Ablordey, A., J. Swings, C. Hubans, K. Chemlal, C. Locht, F. Portaels, and P. Supply.** 2005. Multilocus variable-number tandem repeat typing of *Mycobacterium ulcerans*. *J. Clin. Microbiol.* **43:**1546–1551.
2. **Achtman, M., K. Zurth, G. Morelli, G. Torrea, A. Guiyoule, and E. Carniel.** 1999. *Yersinia pestis*, the cause of plague, is a recently emerged clone of *Yersinia pseudotuberculosis*. *Proc. Natl. Acad. Sci. USA* **96:**14043–14048.
3. **Alcaide, F., I. Richter, C. Bernasconi, B. Springer, C. Hagenau, R. Schulze-Röbbecke, E. Tortoli, R. Martin, E. C. Böttger, and A. Telenti.** 1997. Heterogeneity and clonality among isolates of *Mycobacterium kansasii:* implications for epidemiological and pathogenicity studies. *J. Clin. Microbiol.* **35:**1959–1964.
4. **Amonsin, A., L. L. Li, Q. Zhang, J. P. Bannantine, A. S. Motiwala, S. Sreevatsan, and V. Kapur.** 2004. Multilocus short sequence repeat sequencing approach for differentiating among *Mycobacterium avium* subsp. *paratuberculosis* strains. *J. Clin. Microbiol.* **42:**1694–1702.
5. **Aranaz, A., E. Liebana, E. Gomez-Mampaso, J. C. Galan, D. Cousins, A. Ortega, J. Blazquez, F. Baquero, A. Mateos, G. Suarez, and L. Dominguez.** 1999. *Mycobacterium tuberculosis* subsp. *caprae* subsp. nov.: a taxonomic study of a new member of the *Mycobacterium tuberculosis* complex isolated from goats in Spain. *Int. J. Syst. Bacteriol.* **49:**1263–1273.
6. **Bercovier, H., O. Kafri, and S. Sela.** 1986. Mycobacteria possess a surprisingly small number of ribosomal RNA genes in relation to the size of their genome. *Biochem. Biophys. Res. Commun.* **136:**1136–1141.
7. **Besser, R. E., B. Pakiz, J. M. Schulte, S. Alvarado, E. R. Zell, T. A. Kenyon, and I. M. Onorato.** 2001. Risk factors for positive mantoux tuberculin skin tests in children in San Diego, California: evidence for boosting and possible foodborne transmission. *Pediatrics* **108:**305–310.
8. **Bifani, P. J., B. Mathema, N. E. Kurepina, and B. N. Kreiswirth.** 2002. Global dissemination of the *Mycobacterium tuberculosis* W-Beijing family strains. *Trends Microbiol.* **10:**45–52.
9. **Blackwood, K. S., J. N. Wolfe, and A. M. Kabani.** 2004. Application of mycobacterial interspersed repetitive unit typing to Manitoba tuberculosis cases: can restriction fragment length polymorphism be forgotten? *J. Clin. Microbiol.* **42:**5001–5006.
10. **Brosch, R., S. V. Gordon, K. Eiglmeier, T. Garnier, F. Tekaia, E. Yeramian, and S. T. Cole.** 2000. Genomics, biology, and evolution of the *Mycobacterium tuberculosis* complex, p. 19–36. *In* G. F. Hatfull and W. R. Jacobs (ed.), *Molecular Genetics of Mycobacteria.* ASM Press, Washington, D.C.
11. **Brosch, R., S. V. Gordon, M. Marmiesse, P. Brodin, C. Buchrieser, K. Eiglmeier, T. Garnier, C. Gutiérrez, G. Hewinson, K. Kremer, L. M. Parsons, A. S. Pym, S. Samper, D. van Soolingen, and S. T. Cole.** 2002. A new evolutionary scenario for the *Mycobacterium tuberculosis* complex. *Proc. Natl. Acad. Sci. USA* **99:**3684–3689.
12. **Bull, T. J., E. J. McMinn, K. Sidi-Boumedine, A. Skull, D. Durkin, P. Neild, G. Rhodes, R. Pickup, and J. Hermon-Taylor.** 2003. Detection and verification of *Mycobacterium avium* subsp. *paratuberculosis* in fresh ileocolonic mucosal biopsy specimens from individuals with and without Crohn's disease. *J. Clin. Microbiol.* **41:**2915–2923.
13. **Bull, T. J., K. Sidi-Boumedine, E. J. McMinn, K. Stevenson, R. Pickup, and J. Hermon-Taylor.** 2003. Mycobacterial interspersed repetitive units (MIRU) differentiate *Mycobacterium avium* subspecies *paratuberculosis* from other species of the *Mycobacterium avium* complex. *Mol. Cell. Probes* **17:**157–164.
14. **Butler, W. R., M. M. Floyd, V. A. Silcox, G. Cage, E. Desmond, P. S. Duffey, L. S. Guthertz, W. M. Gross, K. C. Jost, L. S. Ramos, L. Thibert, and N. G. Warren.** 1999.

Mycolic Acid Standards for HPLC Identification of Mycobacteria. Centers for Disease Control and Prevention, U.S. Department of Health and Human Services, Atlanta, Ga.

15. **Cave, M. D., M. Murray, and E. Nardell.** 2005. Molecular epidemiology of *Mycobacterium tuberculosis*, p. 33–48. *In* S. T. Cole, K. Eisenach, D. McMurray, and W. R. Jacobs, Jr. (ed.), *Tuberculosis and the Tubercle Bacillus.* ASM Press, Washington, D.C.
16. **Centers for Disease Control and Prevention.** 1996. Nucleic acid amplification tests for tuberculosis. *Morb. Mortal. Wkly. Rep.* **45:**950–952.
17. **Chapin-Robertson, K., S. Dahlberg, S. Waycott, J. Corrales, C. Kontnick, and S. C. Edberg.** 1993. Detection and identification of *Mycobacterium* directly from BACTEC bottles by using a DNA-rRNA probe. *Diagn. Microbiol. Infect. Dis.* **17:**203–207.
18. **Chemlal, K., G. Huys, P. A. Fonteyne, V. Vincent, A. G. Lopez, L. Rigouts, J. Swings, W. M. Meyers, and F. Portaels.** 2001. Evaluation of PCR-restriction profile analysis, and IS*2404* restriction fragment length polymorphism and amplified fragment length polymorphism fingerprinting for identification and typing of *Mycobacterium ulcerans* and *M. marinum. J. Clin. Microbiol.* **39:**3272–3278.
19. **Cloud, J. L., K. C. Carroll, S. Cohen, C. M. Anderson, and G. L. Woods.** 2005. Interpretive criteria for use of AccuProbe for identification of *Mycobacterium avium* complex directly from 7H9 broth cultures. *J. Clin. Microbiol.* **43:**3474–3478.
20. **Cole, S. T., R. Brosch, J. Parkhill, T. Garnier, C. Churcher, D. Harris, S. V. Gordon, K. Eiglmeier, S. Gas, C. E. Barry III, F. Tekaia, K. Badcock, D. Basham, D. Brown, T. Chillingworth, R. Connor, R. Davies, K. Devlin, T. Feltwell, S. Gentles, N. Hamlin, S. Holroyd, T. Hornsby, K. Jagels, B. G. Barrell, et al.** 1998. Deciphering the biology of *Mycobacterium tuberculosis* from the complete genome sequence. *Nature* **393:**537–544.
21. **Cooksey, R. C., J. Limor, G. P. Morlock, and J. T. Crawford.** 2003. Identifying *Mycobacterium* species and strain typing using a microfluidic labchip instrument. *BioTechniques* **35:**786–794.
22. **Crawford, J. T.** 2003. Genotyping in contact investigations: a CDC perspective. *Int. J. Tuberc. Lung Dis.* **7:**S453–S457.
23. **Dankner, W. M., and C. E. Davis.** 2000. *Mycobacterium bovis* as a significant cause of tuberculosis in children residing along the United States-Mexico border in the Baja California region. *Pediatrics* **105:**E79.
24. **de Jong, B. C., A. Onipede, A. S. Pym, S. Gagneux, R. S. Aga, K. DeRiemer, and P. M. Small.** 2005. Does resistance to pyrazinamide accurately indicate the presence of *Mycobacterium bovis? J. Clin. Microbiol.* **43:**3530–3532.
25. **Espinosa de los Monteros, L. E., J. C. Galan, M. Gutierrez, S. Samper, J. F. Garcia Marin, C. Martin, L. Dominguez, L. de Rafael, F. Baquero, E. Gomez-Mampaso, and J. Blazquez.** 1998. Allele-specific PCR method based on *pncA* and *oxyR* sequences for distinguishing *Mycobacterium bovis* from *Mycobacterium tuberculosis*: intraspecific *M. bovis pncA* sequence polymorphism. *J. Clin. Microbiol.* **36:**239–242.
26. **Falkinham, J. O. I.** 1999. Molecular epidemiology: other mycobacteria, p. 136–160. *In* C. Ratledge and J. Dale (ed.), *Mycobacteria: Molecular Biology and Virulence.* Blackwell Science, Oxford, England.
27. **Fanti, F., E. Tortoli, L. Hall, G. D. Roberts, R. M. Kroppenstedt, I. Dodi, S. Conti, L. Polonelli, and C. Chezzi.** 2004. *Mycobacterium parmense* sp. nov. *Int. J. Syst. Evol. Microbiol.* **54:**1123–1127.
28. **Fleischmann, R. D., D. Alland, J. A. Eisen, L. Carpenter, O. White, J. Peterson, R. DeBoy, R. Dodson, M. Gwinn, D. Haft, E. Hickey, J. F. Kolonay, W. C. Nelson, L. A. Umayam, M. Ermolaeva, S. L. Salzberg, A. Delcher, T. Utterback, J. Weidman, H. Khouri, J. Gill, A. Mikula, W. Bishai, W. R. Jacobs, Jr., J. C. Venter, and C. M. Fraser.** 2002. Whole-genome comparison of *Mycobacterium tuberculosis* clinical and laboratory strains. *J. Bacteriol.* **184:**5479–5490.
29. **Floyd, M. M., W. M. Gross, D. A. Bonato, V. A. Silcox, R. W. Smithwick, B. Metchock, J. T. Crawford, and W. R. Butler.** 2000. *Mycobacterium kubicae* sp. nov., a slowly growing, scotochromogenic *Mycobacterium. Int. J. Syst. Evol. Microbiol.* **50:**1811–1816.
30. **Goh, K. S., E. Legrand, C. Sola, and N. Rastogi.** 2001. Rapid differentiation of "*Mycobacterium canettii*" from other *Mycobacterium tuberculosis* complex organisms by PCR-restriction analysis of the *hsp65* gene. *J. Clin. Microbiol.* **39:**3705–3708.
31. **Gordon, S. V., R. Brosch, A. Billault, T. Garnier, K. Eiglmeier, and S. T. Cole.** 1999. Identification of variable regions in the genomes of tubercle bacilli using bacterial artificial chromosome arrays. *Mol. Microbiol.* **32:**643–655.
32. **Gordon, S. V., and P. Supply.** 2005. Repetitive DNA in the *Mycobacterium tuberculosis* complex, p. 191–202. *In* S. T. Cole, K. Eisenach, D. McMurray, and W. R. Jacobs, Jr. (ed.), *Tuberculosis and the Tubercle Bacillus.* ASM Press, Washington, D.C.
33. **Goto, M., S. Oka, K. Okuzumi, S. Kimura, and K. Shimada.** 1991. Evaluation of acridinium-ester-labeled DNA probes for identification of *Mycobacterium tuberculosis* and *Mycobacterium avium-Mycobacterium intracellulare* complex in culture. *J. Clin. Microbiol.* **29:**2473–2476.
34. **Grant, I. R., H. J. Ball, and M. T. Rowe.** 2002. Incidence of *Mycobacterium paratuberculosis* in bulk raw and commercially pasteurized cows' milk from approved dairy processing establishments in the United Kingdom. *Appl. Environ. Microbiol.* **68:**2428–2435.
35. **Guerrero, C., C. Bernasconi, D. Burki, T. Bodmer, and A. Telenti.** 1994. IS*1245*: a novel insertion element from *Mycobacterium avium* is a specific marker for analysis of strain relatedness. *J. Clin. Microbiol.* **33:**304–307.
36. **Gutiérrez, M. C., S. Brisse, R. Brosch, M. Fabre, B. Omaïs, M. Marmiesse, P. Supply, and V. Vincent.** 2005. Ancient origin and gene mosaicism of the progenitor of *Mycobacterium tuberculosis. PLOS Pathog.* **1:**e5.
37. **Hale, Y. M., G. E. Pfyffer, and M. Salfinger.** 2001. Laboratory diagnosis of mycobacterial infections: new tools and lessons learned. *Clin. Infect. Dis.* **33:**834–846.
38. **Hannan, M. M., E. P. Desmond, G. P. Morlock, G. H. Mazurek, and J. T. Crawford.** 2001. Pyrazinamide-monoresistant *Mycobacterium tuberculosis* in the United States. *J. Clin. Microbiol.* **39:**647–650.
39. **Hawkey, P. M., E. G. Smith, J. T. Evans, P. Monk, G. Bryan, H. H. Mohamed, M. Bardhan, and R. N. Pugh.** 2003. Mycobacterial interspersed repetitive unit typing of *Mycobacterium tuberculosis* compared to IS*6110*-based restriction fragment length polymorphism analysis for investigation of apparently clustered cases of tuberculosis. *J. Clin. Microbiol.* **41:**3514–3520.
40. **Isenberg, H. D.** 2004. *Clinical Microbiology Procedures Handbook*, 2nd ed. ASM Press, Washington, D.C.
41. **Johansen, T. B., B. Djonne, M. R. Jensen, and I. Olsen.** 2005. Distribution of IS*1311* and IS*1245* in *Mycobacterium avium* subspecies revisited. *J. Clin. Microbiol.* **43:**2500–2502.
42. **Jost, K. C., Jr., D. F. Dunbar, S. S. Barth, V. L. Headley, and L. B. Elliott.** 1995. Identification of *Mycobacterium tuberculosis* and *M. avium* complex directly from smear-positive sputum specimens and BACTEC 12B cultures by high-performance liquid chromatography with fluorescence detection and computer-driven pattern recognition models. *J. Clin. Microbiol.* **33:**1270–1277.
43. **Kaminski, D. A., and D. J. Hardy.** 1995. Selective utilization of DNA probes for identification of *Mycobacterium* species on the basis of cord formation in primary BACTEC 12B cultures. *J. Clin. Microbiol.* **33:**1548–1550.

44. **Kapur, V., L. L. Li, M. R. Hamrick, B. B. Plikaytis, T. M. Shinnick, A. Telenti, W. R. Jacobs, A. Banerjee, S. T. Cole, K. Y. Yuen, J. E. Clarridge, B. N. Kreiswirth, and J. M. Musser.** 1995. Rapid species assignment and unambiguous identification of mutations associated with antimicrobial resistance in *Mycobacterium tuberculosis* by automated DNA sequencing. *Arch. Pathol. Lab. Med.* **119:**131–138.
45. **Kasai, H., T. Ezaki, and S. Harayama.** 2000. Differentiation of phylogenetically related slowly growing mycobacteria by their *gyrB* sequences. *J. Clin. Microbiol.* **38:**301–308.
46. **Kato-Maeda, M., J. T. Rhee, T. R. Gingeras, H. Salamon, J. Drenkow, N. Smittipat, and P. M. Small.** 2001. Comparing genomes within the species *Mycobacterium tuberculosis. Genome Res.* **11:**547–554.
47. **Kauppinen, J., R. Mäntyjärvi, and M.-L. Katila.** 1994. Random amplified polymorphic DNA genotyping of *Mycobacterium malmoense. J. Clin. Microbiol.* **32:**1827–1829.
48. **Kent, P. T., and G. P. Kubica.** 1985. *Public Health Mycobacteriology: a Guide for the Level III Laboratory.* Centers for Disease Control, U.S. Department of Health and Human Services, Atlanta, Ga.
49. **Kidgell, C., U. Reichard, J. Wain, B. Linz, M. Torpdahl, G. Dougan, and M. Achtman.** 2002. *Salmonella typhi*, the causative agent of typhoid fever, is approximately 50,000 years old. *Infect. Genet. Evol.* **2:**39–45.
50. **Kikuchi, K., E. M. Bernard, T. E. Kiehn, D. Armstrong, and L. W. Riley.** 1994. Restriction fragment length polymorphism analysis of clinical isolates of *Mycobacterium haemophilum. J. Clin. Microbiol.* **32:**1763–1767.
51. **Kim, B. J., S. H. Lee, M. A. Lyu, S. J. Kim, G. H. Bai, G. T. Chae, E. C. Kim, C. Y. Cha, and Y. H. Kook.** 1999. Identification of mycobacterial species by comparative sequence analysis of the RNA polymerase gene *(rpoB)*. *J. Clin. Microbiol.* **37:**1714–1720.
52. **Kirschner, R. A., B. Springer, U. Vogel, A. Meier, A. Wrede, M. Kieckenbeck, F. C. Bange, and E. C. Böttger.** 1993. Genotypic identification of mycobacteria by nucleic acid sequence determination: report of a 2-year experience in a clinical laboratory. *J. Clin. Microbiol.* **31:**2882–2889.
53. **Kremer, K., C. Arnold, A. Cataldi, M. C. Gutiérrez, W. H. Haas, S. Panaiotov, R. A. Skuce, P. Supply, A. G. van der Zanden, and D. van Soolingen.** 2005. Discriminatory power and reproducibility of novel DNA typing methods for *Mycobacterium tuberculosis* complex strains. *J. Clin. Microbiol.* **43:**5628–5638.
54. **Kremer, K., J. R. Glynn, T. Lillebaek, S. Niemann, N. E. Kurepina, B. N. Kreiswirth, P. J. Bifani, and D. van Soolingen.** 2004. Definition of the Beijing/W lineage of *Mycobacterium tuberculosis* on the basis of genetic markers. *J. Clin. Microbiol.* **42:**4040–4049.
55. **Kremer, K., D. van Soolingen, R. Frothingham, W. H. Haas, P. W. Hermans, C. Martin, P. Palittapongarnpim, B. B. Plikaytis, L. W. Riley, M. A. Yakrus, J. M. Musser, and J. D. van Embden.** 1999. Comparison of methods based on different molecular epidemiological markers for typing of *Mycobacterium tuberculosis* complex strains: interlaboratory study of discriminatory power and reproducibility. *J. Clin. Microbiol.* **37:**2607–2618.
56. **Kwara, A., R. Schiro, L. S. Cowan, N. E. Hyslop, M. F. Wiser, S. Roahen Harrison, P. Kissinger, L. Diem, and J. T. Crawford.** 2003. Evaluation of the epidemiologic utility of secondary typing methods for differentiation of *Mycobacterium tuberculosis* isolates. *J. Clin. Microbiol.* **41:**2683–2685.
57. **Lalande, V., F. Barbut, A. Varnerot, M. Febvre, D. Nesa, S. Wadel, V. Vincent, and J. C. Petit.** 2001. Pseudo-outbreak of *Mycobacterium gordonae* associated with water from refrigerated fountains. *J. Hosp. Infect.* **48:**76–79.
58. **Leao, S. C., J. L. Mello Sampaio, A. Martin, J. C. Palomino, and F. Portaels.** 2005. Profiling *Mycobacterium ulcerans* with *hsp65*. *Emerg. Infect. Dis.* **11:**1795–1796.
59. **Lebrun, L., F. Espinasse, J. D. Poveda, and V. Vincent-Lévy-Frébault.** 1992. Evaluation of nonradioactive DNA probes for identification of mycobacteria. *J. Clin. Microbiol.* **30:**2476–2478.
60. **Lebrun, L., F. X. Weill, L. Lafendi, F. Houriez, F. Casanova, M. C. Gutiérrez, D. Ingrand, P. Lagrange, V. Vincent, and J. L. Herrmann.** 2005. Use of the INNO-LiPA-MYCOBACTERIA assay (Version 2) for identification of *Mycobacterium avium-Mycobacterium intracellulare-Mycobacterium scrofulaceum* complex isolates. *J. Clin. Microbiol.* **43:**2567–2574.
61. **Lok, K. H., W. H. Benjamin, Jr., M. E. Kimerling, V. Pruitt, M. Lathan, J. Razeq, N. Hooper, W. Cronin, and N. E. Dunlap.** 2002. Molecular differentiation of *Mycobacterium tuberculosis* strains without IS*6110* insertions. *Emerg. Infect. Dis.* **8:**1310–1313.
62. **Mazurek, G. H., S. Hartman, Y. Zhang, B. A. Brown, J. S. R. Hector, D. T. Murphy, and R. J. Wallace, Jr.** 1993. Large DNA selection fragment polymorphisms in the *Mycobacterium avium-M. intracellulare* complex: a potential epidemiological tool. *J. Clin. Microbiol.* **31:**390–394.
63. **Mijs, W., P. de Haas, R. Rossau, T. Van der Laan, L. Rigouts, F. Portaels, and D. van Soolingen.** 2002. Molecular evidence to support a proposal to reserve the designation *Mycobacterium avium* subsp. *avium* for bird-type isolates and '*M. avium* subsp. *hominissuis*' for the human/porcine type of *M. avium. Int. J. Syst. Evol. Microbiol.* **52:**1505–1518.
64. **Noordhoek, G. T., S. Mulder, P. Wallace, and A. M. van Loon.** 2004. Multicentre quality control study for detection of *Mycobacterium tuberculosis* in clinical samples by nucleic amplification methods. *Clin. Microbiol. Infect.* **10:**295–301.
65. **Overduin, P., L. Schouls, P. Roholl, A. van der Zanden, N. Mahmmod, A. Herrewegh, and D. van Soolingen.** 2004. Use of multilocus variable-number tandem-repeat analysis for typing *Mycobacterium avium* subsp. *paratuberculosis. J. Clin. Microbiol.* **42:**5022–5028.
66. **Pai, M., L. L. Flores, N. Pai, A. Hubbard, L. W. Riley, and J. M. Colford, Jr.** 2003. Diagnostic accuracy of nucleic acid amplification tests for tuberculous meningitis: a systematic review and meta-analysis. *Lancet Infect. Dis.* **3:**633–643.
67. **Park, H., H. Jang, C. Kim, B. Chung, C. L. Chang, S. K. Park, and S. Song.** 2000. Detection and identification of mycobacteria by amplification of the internal transcribed spacer regions with genus- and species-specific PCR primers. *J. Clin. Microbiol.* **38:**4080–4085.
68. **Parsons, L. M., R. Brosch, S. T. Cole, A. Somoskovi, A. Loder, G. Bretzel, D. Van Soolingen, Y. M. Hale, and M. Salfinger.** 2002. Rapid and simple approach for identification of *Mycobacterium tuberculosis* complex isolates by PCR-based genomic deletion analysis. *J. Clin. Microbiol.* **40:**2339–2345.
69. **Picardeau, M., T. J. Bull, G. Prod'hom, A. L. Pozniak, D. C. Shanson, and V. Vincent.** 1997. Comparison of a new insertion element, IS*1407*, with established molecular markers for the characterization of *Mycobacterium celatum. Int. J. Syst. Bacteriol.* **47:**640–644.
70. **Picardeau, M., T. J. Bull, and V. Vincent.** 1997. Identification and characterization of IS-like elements in *Mycobacterium gordonae. FEMS Microbiol. Lett.* **154:**95–102.
71. **Picardeau, M., G. Prod'hom, L. Raskine, M. P. LePennec, and V. Vincent.** 1997. Genotypic characterization of five subspecies of *Mycobacterium kansasii. J. Clin. Microbiol.* **35:**25–32.
72. **Picardeau, M., A. Varnerot, T. Lecompte, F. Brel, T. May, and V. Vincent.** 1997. Use of different molecular typing techniques for bacteriological follow-up in a clinical trial with AIDS patients with *Mycobacterium avium* bacteremia. *J. Clin. Microbiol.* **35:**2503–2510.
73. **Picardeau, M., and V. Vincent.** 1995. Development of a species-specific probe for *Mycobacterium xenopi. Res. Microbiol.* **146:**237–243.

74. **Picardeau, M., and V. Vincent.** 1996. Typing of *Mycobacterium avium* isolates by PCR. *J. Clin. Microbiol.* **34:**389–392.
75. **Pickup, R. W., G. Rhodes, S. Arnott, K. Sidi-Boumedine, T. J. Bull, A. Weightman, M. Hurley, and J. Hermon-Taylor.** 2005. *Mycobacterium avium* subsp. *paratuberculosis* in the catchment area and water of the River Taff in South Wales, United Kingdom, and its potential relationship to clustering of Crohn's disease cases in the city of Cardiff. *Appl. Environ. Microbiol.* **71:**2130–2139.
76. **Piersimoni, C., and C. Scarparo.** 2003. Relevance of commercial amplification methods for direct detection of *Mycobacterium tuberculosis* complex in clinical samples. *J. Clin. Microbiol.* **41:**5355–5365.
77. **Rastogi, N., E. Legrand, and C. Sola.** 2001. The mycobacteria: an introduction to nomenclature and pathogenesis. *Rev. Sci. Tech.* **20:**21–54.
78. **Reisig, F., K. Kremer, B. Amthor, D. van Soolingen, and W. H. Haas.** 2005. Fast ligation-mediated PCR, a fast and reliable method for IS*6110*-based typing of *Mycobacterium tuberculosis* complex. *J. Clin. Microbiol.* **43:**5622–5627.
79. **Reisner, B. S., A. M. Gatson, and G. L. Woods.** 1994. Use of Gen-Probe AccuProbes to identify *Mycobacterium avium* complex, *Mycobacterium tuberculosis* complex, *Mycobacterium kansasii*, and *Mycobacterium gordonae* directly from BACTEC TB broth cultures. *J. Clin. Microbiol.* **32:**2995–2998.
80. **Richter, E., S. Niemann, S. Rüsch-Gerdes, and S. Hoffner.** 1999. Identification of *Mycobacterium kansasii* by using a DNA probe (AccuProbe) and molecular techniques. *J. Clin. Microbiol.* **37:**964–970.
81. **Richter, E., M. Weizenegger, A. M. Fahr, and S. Rüsch-Gerdes.** 2004. Usefulness of the GenoType MTBC assay for differentiating species of the *Mycobacterium tuberculosis* complex in cultures obtained from clinical specimens. *J. Clin. Microbiol.* **42:**4303–4306.
82. **Ritacco, V., K. Kremer, T. van der Laan, J. E. M. Pijnenburg, P. E. W. de Haas, and D. van Soolingen.** 1998. Use of IS*901* and IS*1245* in RFLP typing of *Mycobacterium avium* complex: relatedness among serovar reference strains, human and animal isolates. *Int. J. Tuberc. Lung Dis.* **2:**242–251.
83. **Ross, B. C., L. Marino, F. Oppedisano, R. Edwards, R. M. Robins-Browne, and P. D. Johnson.** 1997. Development of a PCR assay for rapid diagnosis of *Mycobacterium ulcerans* infection. *J. Clin. Microbiol.* **35:**1696–1700.
84. **Roth, A., M. Fischer, M. E. Hamid, S. Michalke, W. Ludwig, and H. Mauch.** 1998. Differentiation of phylogenetically related slowly growing mycobacteria based on 16S-23S rRNA gene internal transcribed spacer sequences. *J. Clin. Microbiol.* **36:**139–147.
84a. **Runyon, E. H. 1970.** Identification of mycobacterial pathogens using colony characteristics. *Am. J. Clin. Pathol.* **54:**578–586.
85. **Saito, H., H. Tomioka, K. Sato, H. Tasaka, and D. J. Dawson.** 1990. Identification of various serovar strains of *Mycobacterium avium* complex by using DNA probes specific for *Mycobacterium avium* and *Mycobacterium intracellulare*. *J. Clin. Microbiol.* **28:**1694–1697.
86. **Sarkola, A., J. Makinen, M. Marjamaki, H. J. Marttila, M. K. Viljanen, and H. Soini.** 2004. Prospective evaluation of the GenoType Assay for routine identification of mycobacteria. *Eur. J. Clin. Microbiol. Infect. Dis.* **23:**642–645.
87. **Selvarangan, R., W. K. Wu, T. T. Nguyen, L. D. Carlson, C. K. Wallis, S. K. Stiglich, Y. C. Chen, K. C. Jost, Jr., J. L. Prentice, R. J. Wallace, Jr., S. L. Barrett, B. T. Cookson, and M. B. Coyle.** 2004. Characterization of a novel group of mycobacteria and proposal of *Mycobacterium sherrisii* sp. nov. *J. Clin. Microbiol.* **42:**52–59.
88. **Shinnick, T. M.** 1987. The 65-kilodalton antigen of *Mycobacterium tuberculosis*. *J. Bacteriol.* **169:**1080–1088.
89. **Skuce, R. A., T. P. McCorry, J. F. McCarroll, S. M. Roring, A. N. Scott, D. Brittain, S. L. Hughes, R. G. Hewinson, and S. D. Neill.** 2002. Discrimination of *Mycobacterium tuberculosis* complex bacteria using novel VNTR-PCR targets. *Microbiology* **148:**519–528.
90. **Slutsky, A. M., R. D. Arbeit, T. W. Barber, J. Rich, C. F. von Reyn, W. Pieciak, M. A. Barlow, and J. N. Maslow.** 1994. Polyclonal infections due to *Mycobacterium avium* complex in patients with AIDS detected by pulsed-field gel electrophoresis of sequential clinical isolates. *J. Clin. Microbiol.* **32:**1773–1778.
91. **Soini, H., E. C. Böttger, and M. K. Viljanen.** 1994. Identification of mycobacteria by PCR-based sequence determination of the 32-kilodalton protein gene. *J. Clin. Microbiol.* **32:**2944–2947.
92. **Somoskovi, A., J. E. Hotaling, M. Fitzgerald, V. Jonas, D. Stasik, L. M. Parsons, and M. Salfinger.** 2000. False-positive results for *Mycobacterium celatum* with the AccuProbe *Mycobacterium tuberculosis* complex assay. *J. Clin. Microbiol.* **38:**2743–2745.
93. **Spurgiesz, R. S., T. N. Quitugua, K. L. Smith, J. Schupp, E. G. Palmer, R. A. Cox, and P. Keim.** 2003. Molecular typing of *Mycobacterium tuberculosis* by using nine novel variable-number tandem repeats across the Beijing family and low-copy-number IS*6110* isolates. *J. Clin. Microbiol.* **41:**4224–4230.
94. **Sreevatsan, S., X. Pan, K. E. Stockbauer, N. D. Connell, B. N. Kreiswirth, T. S. Whittam, and J. M. Musser.** 1997. Restricted structural gene polymorphism in the *Mycobacterium tuberculosis* complex indicates evolutionarily recent global dissemination. *Proc. Natl. Acad. Sci. USA* **94:**9869–9874.
95. **Stahl, D. A., and J. W. Urbance.** 1990. The division between fast- and slow-growing species corresponds to natural relationships among the mycobacteria. *J. Bacteriol.* **172:**116–124.
96. **Stinear, T. P., G. A. Jenkin, P. D. Johnson, and J. K. Davies.** 2000. Comparative genetic analysis of *Mycobacterium ulcerans* and *Mycobacterium marinum* reveals evidence of recent divergence. *J. Bacteriol.* **182:**6322–6330.
97. **Stone, M. M., A. M. Vannier, S. K. Storch, C. Peterson, A. T. Nitta, and Y. Zhang** 1995. Meningitis due to iatrogenic BCG infection in two immunocompromised children. *N. Engl. J. Med.* **333:**561–563.
98. **Stragier, P., A. Ablordey, W. M. Meyers, and F. Portaels.** 2005. Genotyping *Mycobacterium ulcerans* and *Mycobacterium marinum* by using mycobacterial interspersed repetitive units. *J. Bacteriol.* **187:**1639–1647.
99. **Supply, P., S. Lesjean, E. Savine, K. Kremer, D. van Soolingen, and C. Locht.** 2001. Automated high-throughput genotyping for study of global epidemiology of *Mycobacterium tuberculosis* based on mycobacterial interspersed repetitive units. *J. Clin. Microbiol.* **39:**3563–3571.
100. **Supply, P., E. Mazars, S. Lesjean, V. Vincent, B. Gicquel, and C. Locht.** 2000. Variable human minisatellite-like regions in the *Mycobacterium tuberculosis* genome. *Mol. Microbiol.* **36:**762–771.
101. **Takewaki, S. I., K. Okuzumi, I. Manabe, M. Tanimura, K. Miyamura, K. I. Nakahara, Y. Yazaki, A. Ohkubo, and R. Nagai.** 1994. Nucleotide sequence comparison of the mycobacterial *dnaJ* gene and PCR-restriction fragment length polymorphism analysis for identification of mycobacterial species. *Int. J. Syst. Bacteriol.* **44:**159–166.
102. **Telenti, A., F. Marchesi, M. Balz, F. Bally, E. C. Bottger, and T. Bodmer.** 1993. Rapid identification of mycobacteria to the species level by polymerase chain reaction and restriction enzyme analysis. *J. Clin. Microbiol.* **31:**175–178.
103. **Tenover, F. C., J. T. Crawford, R. E. Huebner, L. J. Geiter, C. R. Horsburgh, Jr., and R. C. Good.** 1993. The

resurgence of tuberculosis: is your laboratory ready? *J. Clin. Microbiol.* **31:**767–770.

104. **Thibert, L., and S. Lapierre.** 1993. Routine application of high-performance liquid chromatography for identification of mycobacteria. *J. Clin. Microbiol.* **31:**1759–1763.

105. **Torkko, P., S. Suomalainen, E. Iivanainen, E. Tortoli, M. Suutari, J. Seppanen, L. Paulin, and M. L. Katila.** 2002. *Mycobacterium palustre* sp. nov., a potentially pathogenic, slowly growing mycobacterium isolated from clinical and veterinary specimens and from Finnish stream waters. *Int. J. Syst. Evol. Microbiol.* **52:**1519–1525.

106. **Tortoli, E.** 2003. Impact of genotypic studies on mycobacterial taxonomy: the new mycobacteria of the 1990s. *Clin. Microbiol. Rev.* **16:**319–354.

107. **Tortoli, E., A. Mariottini, and G. Mazzarelli.** 2003. Evaluation of INNO-LiPA MYCOBACTERIA v2: improved reverse hybridization multiple DNA probe assay for mycobacterial identification. *J. Clin. Microbiol.* **41:** 4418–4420.

108. **Tortoli, E., M. T. Simonetti, and F. Lavinia.** 1996. Evaluation of reformulated chemiluminescent DNA probe (AccuProbe) for culture identification of *Mycobacterium kansasii*. *J. Clin. Microbiol.* **34:**2838–2840.

109. **Turenne, C., P. Chedore, J. Wolfe, F. Jamieson, G. Broukhanski, K. May, and A. Kabani.** 2002. *Mycobacterium lacus* sp. nov., a novel slowly growing, nonchromogenic clinical isolate. *Int. J. Syst. Evol. Microbiol.* **52:** 2135–2140.

110. **van Embden, J. D., M. D. Cave, J. T. Crawford, J. W. Dale, K. D. Eisenach, B. Gicquel, P. Hermans, C. Martin, R. McAdam, T. M. Shinnick, and P. M. Small.** 1993. Strain identification of *Mycobacterium tuberculosis* by DNA fingerprinting: recommendations for a standardized methodology. *J. Clin. Microbiol.* **31:** 406–409.

111. **van Soolingen, D.** 2001. Molecular epidemiology of tuberculosis and other mycobacterial infections: main methodologies and achievements. *J. Intern. Med.* **249:** 1–26.

112. **van Soolingen, D., J. Bauer, V. Ritacco, S. C. Leao, I. Pavlik, V. Vincent, N. Rastogi, A. Gori, T. Bodmer, C. Garzelli, and M. J. Garcia.** 1998. IS*1245* restriction fragment length polymorphism typing of *Mycobacterium avium* isolates: proposal for standardization. *J. Clin. Microbiol.* **36:**3051–3054.

113. **van Soolingen, D., T. Hoogenboezem, P. E. de Haas, P. W. Hermans, M. A. Koedam, K. S. Teppema, P. J. Brennan, G. S. Besra, F. Portaels, J. Top, L. M. Schouls, and J. D. van Embden.** 1997. A novel pathogenic taxon of the *Mycobacterium tuberculosis* complex, Canetti: characterization of an exceptional isolate from Africa. *Int. J. Syst. Bacteriol.* **47:**1236–1245.

114. **van Soolingen, D., A. G. van der Zanden, P. E. de Haas, G. T. Noordhoek, A. Kiers, N. A. Foudraine, F. Portaels, A. H. Kolk, K. Kremer, and J. D. van Embden.** 1998. Diagnosis of *Mycobacterium microti* infections among humans by using novel genetic markers. *J. Clin. Microbiol.* **36:**1840–1845.

115. **Vincent Lévy-Frébault, V., and F. Portaels.** 1992. Proposed minimal standards for the genus *Mycobacterium* and for description of new slowly growing *Mycobacterium* species. *Int. J. Syst. Bacteriol.* **42:**315–323.

116. **Vos, M. C., P. E. de Haas, H. A. Verbrugh, N. H. Renders, N. G. Hartwig, P. de Man, A. H. Kolk, H. van Deutekom, J. L. Yntema, A. G. Vulto, M. Messemaker, and D. van Soolingen.** 2003. Nosocomial *Mycobacterium bovis*-bacille Calmette-Guerin infections due to contamination of chemotherapeutics: case finding and route of transmission. *J. Infect. Dis.* **188:**1332–1335.

117. **Waecker, N. J., Jr., R. Stefanova, M. D. Cave, C. E. Davis, and W. M. Dankner.** 2000. Nosocomial transmission of *Mycobacterium bovis* bacille Calmette-Guerin to children receiving cancer therapy and to their health care providers. *Clin. Infect. Dis.* **30:**356–362.

118. **Wallace, R. J., Jr., B. A. Brown, and D. E. Griffith.** 1998. Nosocomial outbreaks/pseudo-outbreaks caused by nontuberculous mycobacteria. *Annu. Rev. Microbiol.* **52:**453–490.

119. **Wayne, L. G., R. C. Good, E. C. Böttger, R. Butler, M. Dorsch, T. Ezaki, W. Gross, V. Jonas, J. Kilburn, P. Kirschner, M. I. Krichevsky, M. Ridell, T. M. Shinnick, B. Springer, E. Stackebrandt, I. Tarnok, Z. Tarnok, H. Tasaka, V. Vincent, N. G. Warren, C. A. Knott, and R. Johnson.** 1996. Semantide- and chemotaxonomy-based analyses of some problematic phenotypic clusters of slowly growing mycobacteria, a cooperative study of the International Working Group on Mycobacterial Taxonomy. *Int. J. Syst. Bacteriol.* **46:**280–297.

120. **Wayne, L. G., and G. P. Kubica.** 1986. Genus *Mycobacterium*, p. 1436–1457. *In* P. H. A. Sneath, N. S. Mair, M. E. Sharpe, and J. G. Holt (ed.), *Bergey's Manual of Systematic Bacteriology*, vol. 2. Williams and Wilkins, Baltimore, Md.

121. **Wayne, L. G., and H. A. Sramek.** 1992. Agents of newly recognized or infrequently encountered mycobacterial diseases. *Clin. Microbiol. Rev.* **5:**1–25.

122. **Yakrus, M. A., M. W. Reeves, and S. B. Hunter.** 1992. Characterization of isolates of *Mycobacterium avium* serotypes 4 and 8 from patients with AIDS by multilocus enzyme electrophoresis. *J. Clin. Microbiol.* **30:**1474–1478.

123. **Yakrus, M. A., and W. L. Straus.** 1994. DNA polymorphisms detected in *Mycobacterium haemophilum* by pulsed-field gel electrophoresis. *J. Clin. Microbiol.* **32:**1083–1084.

124. **Zelazny, A. M., L. B. Calhoun, L. Li, Y. R. Shea, and S. H. Fischer.** 2005. Identification of *Mycobacterium* species by *secA1* sequences. *J. Clin. Microbiol.* **43:**1051–1058.

125. **Zhang, Y., L. B. Mann, R. W. Wilson, B. A. Brown-Elliott, V. Vincent, Y. Iinuma, and R. J. Wallace, Jr.** 2004. Molecular analysis of *Mycobacterium kansasii* isolates from the United States. *J. Clin. Microbiol.* **42:**119–125.

126. **Zolg, J. W., and S. Philippi-Schulz.** 1994. The superoxide dismutase gene, a target for detection and identification of mycobacteria by PCR. *J. Clin. Microbiol.* **32:**2801–2812.

Mycobacterium: Clinical and Laboratory Characteristics of Rapidly Growing Mycobacteria*

BARBARA A. BROWN-ELLIOTT AND RICHARD J. WALLACE, JR.

38

TAXONOMY AND DESCRIPTION OF ORGANISMS

During the past 2 decades, there has been an increasing awareness of nontuberculous mycobacteria (NTM), including the rapidly growing mycobacteria (RGM), of which numerous species and phylogenetic groups are clearly established human pathogens. These include primarily the *Mycobacterium fortuitum* group; the *M. chelonae-M. abscessus* group, previously known collectively as the *M. fortuitum* complex; and to a lesser extent the *M. smegmatis* group. Three rare pathogens each belong to separate groups and have been associated with clinical disease: *M. mucogenicum*, *M. mageritense,* and *M. wolinskyi* (1, 4, 5, 47, 49, 64, 68).

The RGM are generally defined as nontuberculous species that grow within 7 days on laboratory media. Most clinically significant (pathogenic) species or groups are not pigmented. Only one pathogenic group (the *M. smegmatis* group) is pigmented, developing a slowly apparent or late pigment (4, 5, 68). All RGM contain long-chain fatty acids known as mycolic acids that can be quantitated using chromatographic techniques such as high-performance liquid chromatography (HPLC).

For many years, the *M. fortuitum* group comprised *M. fortuitum* (formerly *M. fortuitum* biovariant *fortuitum*), *M. peregrinum* (formerly *M. fortuitum* biovariant *peregrinum*), and the *M. fortuitum* third biovariant complex. Recent studies have shown that each of the latter two species comprise multiple additional species or "taxa" (47). *M. peregrinum* was found to contain two taxa originally designated *M. peregrinum* type I and type II (3). Taxonomic studies have now shown that isolates of *M. peregrinum* type II are human isolates of *M. senegalense* (60). In 1991, the third biovariant complex was described as containing two major subgroups (sorbitol positive and sorbitol negative) (63). In the last 7 years, seven new species have been identified from this "unnamed" complex. The sorbitol-positive subgroup currently consists of *M. houstonense, M. brisbanense,* and *M. mageritense*, and the sorbitol-negative subgroup consists of *M. porcinum, M. boenickei, M. neworleansense,* and *M. septicum* (28, 46, 47, 64, 65).

The *M. chelonae-M. abscessus* group is composed of at least three species, including *M. chelonae* (formerly *M. chelonae* subsp. *chelonae*), *M. abscessus* (formerly *M. chelonae* subsp. *abscessus*), and the newly described species *M. immunogenum* (5, 74).

The *M. smegmatis* group was initially described as composed of three species: *M. smegmatis* sensu stricto and two new species, *M. goodii* (4) and *M. wolinskyi* (4). Previously, these species were known as *M. smegmatis* types I, II, and III, respectively (68). This grouping was based on the absence of 3-day arylsulfatase activity in all three species. Current studies based on DNA sequence analysis suggest that *M. wolinskyi* is phylogenetically distinct from the other two species and likely belongs in a separate group (1).

M. mucogenicum, originally known as the *M. chelonae*-like organism, or MCLO, also constitutes a separate phylogenetic group distinct from all others, as does *M. mageritense* (1).

Unfortunately, many clinical laboratories do not take advantage of the new techniques for identifying isolates as identification of the RGM to the species level has traditionally been given low priority. This reluctance to provide identification to the species level partially reflects the lack of available simple, inexpensive, and accurate methods. Although combination analysis of results of biochemical tests, including those for carbohydrate utilization and susceptibility patterns, allows satisfactory identification of the majority of clinically significant isolates of RGM, these tests may be technically difficult to interpret and time-consuming for an inexperienced laboratory. Since no DNA probes are available in the United States for identification of the RGM and since HPLC alone cannot adequately identify most species of RGM, molecular testing by a reference laboratory is now necessary to accurately identify most of the 22 currently known pathogenic RGM to the species level.

CLINICAL SIGNIFICANCE

The RGM are opportunistic pathogens that produce disease in a variety of clinical settings. The three major clinically important species of RGM responsible for disease in humans include *M. fortuitum*, *M. chelonae,* and *M. abscessus*. Names of other potentially pathogenic and clinically significant RGM species have been included in Table 1 (4, 5, 47, 60, 64,

*This chapter contains information presented in chapter 36 by Gaby E. Pfyffer, Barbara A. Brown-Elliott, and Richard J. Wallace, Jr., and in chapter 37 by Véronique Vincent, Barbara A. Brown-Elliott, Kenneth C. Jost, Jr., and Richard J. Wallace, Jr., in the eighth edition of this Manual.

TABLE 1 Currently recognized species of RGM

Species	Characteristic				
	Established clinical significance	Pigmentation	Unique phenotype	Unique *hsp*65 REA pattern	Unique (complete) 16*S* sequence
Common human pathogens					
M. abscessus	Yes	No	No	Yes	Yes
M. chelonae	Yes	No	Yes	Yes	Yes
M. fortuitum	Yes	No	Yes	Yes	Yes
Less common human pathogens (>10 clinical isolates or cases)					
M. boenickei	Yes	No	No	Yes	Yes
M. goodii	Yes	Yes	No	Yes	Yes
M. houstonense	Yes	No	No	No	No[a]
M. immunogenum	Yes	No	No	Yes	Yes
M. mucogenicum	Yes	No	Yes	Yes	Yes
M. peregrinum	Yes	No	No	Yes	No[a]
M. porcinum	Yes	No	No	Yes	Yes
M. senegalense	Yes	No	No	Yes	Yes
M. smegmatis	Yes	Yes	No	Yes	Yes
Rare human pathogens (<10 cases or isolates)					
M. brisbanense	Yes	No	No	Yes	Yes
M. brumae	Yes	No	No	ND[b]	Yes
M. canariasense	Yes	No	No	Yes	Yes
M. elephantis	Yes	Yes	No	Yes	Yes
M. lacticola	Yes	Yes	Unknown	Yes	Yes
M. mageritense	Yes	No	Yes	Yes	Yes
M. neworleansense	Yes	No	No	No	Yes
M. novocastrense	Yes	Yes	No	ND	No
M. septicum	Yes	No	No	Yes	No[a]
M. wolinskyi	Yes	No	No	Yes	Yes
Unproven human pathogens					
M. agri	No	Yes	No	ND	Yes
M. aichiense	No	No	No	ND	Yes
M. alvei	No	No	No	ND	No
M. aurum	No	Yes	No	ND	Yes
M. austroafricanum	No	Yes	No	ND	Yes
M. chitae	No	No	No	ND	Yes
M. chlorophenolicum	No	Yes	No	ND	Yes
M. chubuense	No	Yes	No	ND	Yes
M. confluentis	No	No	No	ND	Yes
M. diernhoferi	No	Yes	No	ND	ND
M. duvalii	No	Yes	No	ND	Yes
M. fallax[c]	No	No	No	ND	Yes
M. flavescens	No	Yes	No	ND	Yes
M. frederiksbergense	No	Yes	No	ND	No
M. gadium	No	Yes	No	ND	Yes
M. gilvum	No	Yes	No	ND	Yes
M. hassiacum	No	Yes	No[d]	ND	Yes
M. hodleri	No	Yes	No[e]	ND	No
M. holsaticum	No	Yes	No	Yes	Yes
M. komossense	No	Yes	No	ND	Yes
M. madagascariense	No	Yes	No	ND	Yes
M. moriokaense	No	No	No	ND	Yes
M. murale	No	Yes	No	ND	Yes
M. obuense	No	Yes	No	ND	Yes
M. parafortuitum	No	Yes	No	ND	Yes
M. phlei	No	Yes	No	ND	Yes
M. psychrotolerans	No	Yes	No	ND	Yes

(Continued on next page)

TABLE 1 *(Continued)*

Species	Characteristic				
	Established clinical significance	Pigmentation	Unique phenotype	Unique *hsp*65 REA pattern	Unique (complete) 16S sequence
M. rhodesiae	No	Yes	No	ND	Yes
M. sphagni	No	Yes	No	ND	Yes
M. thermoresistibile	No	Yes	No	ND	Yes
M. tokaiense	No	Yes	No	ND	Yes
M. vaccae	No	Yes	No	ND	Yes
M. vanbaalenii	No	Yes	No	ND	Yes

[a] *M. houstonense* is 100% identical to *M. farcinogenes*, and *M. peregrinum* (type I) is 100% identical to *M. septicum*.
[b] ND, not determined.
[c] RGM at 30°C, slowly growing at 35°C.
[d] Grows at 65°C.
[e] Grows on or degrades a variety of organic substrates.

65, 73, 74). RGM are presumed to be common in the environment but have been most often identified in tap water when associated with wound infections (15). The specific reservoir for *M. abscessus* chronic lung infections has yet to be identified.

Wound Infections

The most common infection seen with the RGM is posttraumatic wound infection. Aside from the injury, the patients are generally healthy, and drug-induced immune suppression is associated with minimal increase in risk for this type of infection. The *M. fortuitum* group accounts for approximately 60% of cases of localized cutaneous infections, but any of the 22 pathogenic RGM species listed in Table 1 can cause disease (4, 5, 60, 64, 65, 68, 73).

Traumatic wound infections, especially open fractures, often involve species within the *M. fortuitum* third biovariant complex (47, 63, 65). More than 75% of the infections reported in connection with a series of 85 isolates of the *M. fortuitum* third biovariant complex from the United States and the Queensland, Australia, state laboratory were associated with skin, soft tissue, or bone infections (63). The majority of infections occurred 4 to 6 weeks following puncture wounds or open fractures. Metal puncture wounds (48%) and motor vehicle accidents (26%) were the most common antecedent injuries, and approximately 40% of the injury sites involved the foot or leg. Stepping on a nail was the most frequently related scenario. None of the isolates in this series were studied by molecular techniques that would identify them as one of the newly described species within the *M. fortuitum* third biovariant complex (i.e., *M. houstonense, M. boenickei, M. porcinum,* or *M. mageritense*).

In a 1989 report (67), approximately 80% of RGM wound isolates related to cardiac surgery were from seven southern coastal states, including Texas, Louisiana, Georgia, Maryland, Alabama, Florida, and South Carolina. A second report published in the same year showed that 92% of 37 identified cases of surgical wound infection following augmentation mammaplasty were also in patients in southern coastal states, with the majority in Texas, Florida, and North Carolina (61).

Sporadic cases of localized wound infections following medical or surgical procedures, including needle injections, can occur with *M. chelonae* but are less common than those with *M. fortuitum*. The clinical picture of posttraumatic wound infection ranges from localized cellulitis or abscesses to osteomyelitis (70). Localized or disseminated infections with *M. chelonae* most frequently occur in patients receiving long-term corticosteroid treatment and/or chemotherapy, organ transplant recipients, and patients with rheumatoid arthritis or other autoimmune disorders or those receiving immunosuppressive therapy (62). However, immune suppression in diseases such as AIDS has not been a significant risk factor for development of localized or disseminated *M. chelonae* infections.

Less frequently, *M. wolinskyi* and the *M. smegmatis* group, including *M. goodii* and *M. smegmatis* sensu stricto, have been reported in cases of infection following traumatic injury and surgical or medical procedures such as cardiac surgery, breast reduction surgery, and face lift plastic surgery. Cellulitis and localized abscesses are the most common manifestations (4).

Starting in 2000, an outbreak of furunculosis caused by *M. fortuitum* on the lower extremities occurred in 32 otherwise healthy patients who were patrons of a nail salon in California. The organism was also cultured from contaminated foot baths, and shaving the legs prior to the foot bath and pedicure was identified as a risk factor (48, 75, 76). Other species, including *M. abscessus* and *M. mageritense*, have subsequently been recovered in other cases of furunculosis.

Pulmonary Infections

Chronic lung infections can occur with RGM, most often in nonsmoking older women with bronchiectasis (sometimes associated with the *M. avium* complex [MAC] as well). The causative agent in more than 80% of cases of pulmonary disease due to RGM is *M. abscessus* (24).

Similarities exist between patients infected with the MAC and those infected with *M. abscessus* such that a common pathogenicity or host susceptibility factor may be involved (24). Multiple cultures of *M. abscessus* from respiratory samples are usually associated with significant pulmonary disease.

Patients with cystic fibrosis (CF) may also become infected with *M. abscessus* (16, 37). Recovery of *M. abscessus* in this setting is being reported more frequently than previously. *M. abscessus* is the second most common species of NTM recovered from CF patients (after the MAC) and may be the most common species associated with clinical disease in this setting (37). Patients with CF also have bronchiectasis in addition to chronic, recurrent airway and parenchymal infections that may be the primary risk factors for susceptibility to NTM disease.

Rarely, other RGM, including *M. chelonae*, the *M. smegmatis* group, and *M. fortuitum*, can be involved in pulmonary disease. *M. fortuitum* has been reported as a pathogen in half of the cases of chronic aspiration disease secondary to underlying gastroesophageal disorders such as achalasia (24). Pulmonary disease with *M. chelonae* and *M. smegmatis* has been described in only a few cases, including one case of lipoid pneumonia (4, 5, 58, 68, 70).

Hypersensitivity pneumonitis among metal grinders working in industrial plants with contaminated metalworking fluids has been associated with a newly described species of RGM, *M. immunogenum*. This species is able to grow and remain viable in degraded metalworking fluid (74). This species has not been reported to be recovered from open lung biopsy specimens from these patients.

Disseminated Cutaneous Disease

Disseminated cutaneous disease due to members of the *M. fortuitum* group (including *M. fortuitum*) is rare even in immunocompromised patients, including those with AIDS (5, 7, 70). In the modern taxonomic era, we have seen fewer than five well-documented cases of disseminated cutaneous disease due to *M. fortuitum*.

Disseminated cutaneous disease due to *M. chelonae* is much more common. It typically presents as multiple, chronic, painful red nodules, usually involving the lower extremities. These lesions then drain spontaneously, with the drainage usually acid-fast bacillus smear positive. Almost all patients are immunosuppressed, usually from low-dose corticosteroid therapy for diseases such as rheumatoid arthritis and other autoimmune diseases or organ transplantation. Although the disease is presumably a consequence of hematogenous spread, bacteremia is rarely identified. A portal of entry for the pathogen is rarely evident (5, 62, 71). For a series of 100 clinical isolates from skin and soft tissue, it was reported that 53% were from patients with disseminated cutaneous infections (62). Approximately 75% of cases of disseminated cutaneous infection are due to *M. chelonae*, and about 20% are due to *M. abscessus* (5, 70). Disseminated disease involves other sites (blood and internal organs) only in severely immunosuppressed individuals, although immune suppression such as that occurring with AIDS has not been a significant risk factor for the development of disseminated cutaneous or extracutaneous disease.

Disseminated cutaneous disease due to *M. abscessus* occurs rarely but is serious (70). Like those of disseminated *M. chelonae* disease, most cases occur in chronically immunosuppressed patients receiving corticosteroids, and the pathogen has no apparent portal of entry. Also like those of *M. chelonae* infection, cases of *M. abscessus* disseminated cutaneous infection rarely involve detectable bacteremia and/or endocarditis, but patients usually present with multiple draining cutaneous nodules, usually in the lower extremities.

Health Care-Associated Infections

Health care-associated disease with the RGM has been reported most commonly with *M. fortuitum*, *M. chelonae*, *M. abscessus*, and *M. mucogenicum*, although any species may be involved. Most infections follow contamination with tap water harboring the infecting RGM. Types of infections include postsurgical wound infections, catheter sepsis, infections following hemodialysis (27, 61, 70, 72), postinjection abscesses, vaccine-related outbreaks (5, 11, 22, 55, 57, 61), and otitis media following tympanostomy tube replacement (21). These have been seen as both sporadic cases and localized outbreaks. Recent outbreaks have involved cosmetic procedures such as liposuction (35) and infections following nail salon procedures (23, 48, 75, 76).

Central catheter-associated infections are the most common health care-associated infections due to the RGM (5, 43, 46, 70). They are the most common cause of RGM bacteremia, but the disease may also present as local wound drainage as part of an exit site or tunnel infection (5, 28, 43). Other types of catheters, including peritoneal catheters, ventriculoperitoneal shunts, and shunts for hemodialysis, can also become infected (5).

Surgical wound infections due to RGM are a well-recognized clinical entity. In the 1970s and 1980s, these were most commonly associated with augmentation mammaplasty and coronary artery bypass surgery, and multiple disease outbreaks occurred (57). Infections following these types of surgery are now less common, and mastectomies for breast carcinoma, liposuction, and knee replacements have replaced these procedures as the most common causes of disease.

Infections following the insertion of prosthetic devices, including prosthetic heart valves, artificial knees and hips, lens implants, and metal rods inserted into the vertebrae to stabilize bones following fractures, have also been described (4, 5, 70). Again, *M. fortuitum* is the most common pathogen, but any of the pathogenic RGM, including the *M. smegmatis* group, can be associated with this type of infection (4, 5). The infection usually presents with watery drainage, wound breakdown, and low-grade fever.

In addition to true outbreaks of infection, numerous health care-associated pseudo-outbreaks have been described. Contaminated or malfunctioning bronchoscopes (5, 25, 57), automated endoscope cleaning machines (33, 57, 61, 74), and contaminated laboratory reagents and ice (27, 31) have been implicated (61).

Bone and Joint Infection

Infection with the RGM may also result in bone and joint infection. Like bacterial disease, osteomyelitis may follow open bone fractures, puncture wounds, and hematogenous spread from another source. The most common scenario is an open fracture of the femur, often followed by orthopedic surgical procedures. The most frequent pathogen recovered in this setting is the *M. fortuitum* group, including two newly described species, *M. houstonense* and *M. boenickei* (5, 47).

Vertebral osteomyelitis has also been described (40, 45). Sarria and colleagues identified 15 cases, and clinical information was available for six of the cases. Four of the six cases of RGM vertebral osteomyelitis involved *M. fortuitum*, and all of the patients had some type of underlying condition (45).

Bone involvement secondary to a puncture wound is likely the second major cause of osteomyelitis. Infections most commonly involve the *M. fortuitum* group (5, 58, 59). *M. fortuitum* infections associated with prosthetic knees and joints have also been reported.

The two newly described species, *M. goodii* and *M. wolinskyi*, have also been associated with osteomyelitis. In a recent report, 13 (36%) of 36 patients with infection caused by these two species were diagnosed with osteomyelitis (4).

Generally, osteomyelitis due to RGM is treated with surgical debridement and antimicrobial therapy for a minimum of 6 months (5, 66).

MISCELLANEOUS DISEASES

Other diseases associated with the RGM are summarized in the following paragraphs.

CNS Disease

Central nervous system (CNS) disease involving the RGM is rare, but morbidity and mortality are high. Most of the reported cases have been associated with *M. fortuitum* (5, 12). In a review by Flor et al., 52 isolates of NTM were reported that were associated with meningitis, of which 12% were identified as *M. fortuitum* (19).

Treatment of CNS infections due to RGM is difficult and often requires extended multiple-antimicrobial treatment (6 to 12 months) in addition to surgical intervention (5).

Corneal Infections (Keratitis)

The number of RGM recovered from ocular infections has been increasing over the last 20 years. A retrospective review of cases of NTM keratitis from 1982 to1997 at an eye institute in Florida showed that 19 of 24 cases were due to RGM (20).

A review of the literature involving keratitis due to the NTM from 1965 to 1992 found that 21 (55%) of 38 isolates were identified as *M. fortuitum*, 16 (42%) of 38 belonged to the *M. chelonae*-*M. abscessus* group, and 1 (2%) was identified only as "group IV mycobacteria." However, prior to 1978, isolates from all of the cases reported were incompletely identified as "*M. fortuitum*," so it is not possible to ascertain modern species classifications (6).

Since the early 1990s, other descriptions of eye infections associated with the RGM have been published, including cases occurring after keratoplasty and laser in situ keratomileusis (LASIK) surgery (5).

Corneal infections have an indolent course, and often scraping or biopsy following debridement of the epithelial layer is necessary to obtain appropriate specimens for culture. Treatment of patients with keratitis due to RGM is difficult. The most widely used antimicrobial treatment involves the use of topical aminoglycosides and/or systemic amikacin, gentamicin, kanamycin, or neomycin. Other topical therapies have also included clarithromycin drops for infections due to *M. abscessus* or *M. chelonae*, tobramycin for infections due to *M. chelonae*, and ciprofloxacin for infections due to the *M. fortuitum* group. However, most of these antimicrobials have been shown to penetrate poorly through intact corneal epithelium (5, 6).

For patients who do not respond to topical treatments, surgical intervention including penetrating keratoplasty, corneal graft, lamellar keractectomy, and/or superficial debridement is recommended and was required in the majority of the previously reviewed cases (20).

Cervical Lymphadenitis

Although the most common mycobacterial cause of lymphadenitis is *M. tuberculosis* in adults and the MAC in children, RGM have also been implicated. At least 19 cases of cervical lymphadenitis due to *M. fortuitum* have been reported in the literature. Details were not available for all of the cases reviewed (10, 70). The majority of the patients responded to therapy with either complete resolution or significant decrease in the sizes of the affected lymph nodes (10).

Treatment for RGM lymphadenitis usually involves incision and drainage, followed by a combination of antimicrobials that includes an initial course of intravenous amikacin and concludes with one or more oral antibiotics. The recommended duration of therapy is at least 6 months (5, 10, 66).

Otitis Media

The most common NTM species associated with chronic otitis media is *M. abscessus*. In a 1988 outbreak of 17 cases of otitis media in two ear-nose-throat clinics, patients presented with chronic ear drainage, with a perforated tympanic membrane and prior insertion of a tympanostomy tube (32). In another series of infections, 20 of 21 cases of sporadic chronic otitis media (some with associated mastoiditis) were due to *M. abscessus* following ear tube placement. Therapy included removal of the ear tubes, surgical debridement, and antibiotic therapy including initial amikacin for susceptible isolates and either cefoxitin or imipenem for 3 to 6 weeks, followed by long-term oral therapy with erythromycin (preclarithromycin era) or clarithromycin. Approximately one-half of the isolates from these cases were also aminoglycoside resistant, resulting from the long-term use of aminoglycoside ear drops (21).

Otitis media or mastoiditis due to RGM other than *M. abscessus* has been infrequently reported (70).

IDENTIFICATION OF RGM

Collection, Transport, and Storage of Specimens

Details of standard methods for collection, transport, and storage of specimens are included in chapter 20.

Direct Examination and Isolation Procedures

Direct examination and isolation procedures are generally detailed in chapter 36. Primary isolation of RGM requires culture at 28 to 30°C rather than 35°C for wound cultures, especially for recovery of *M. chelonae*.

Biochemical Testing

As previously stated, the RGM are defined as NTM that grow within 7 days (most species within 3 to 4 days) (41, 56). Until the advent of molecular techniques, conventional laboratory identification of the RGM was based primarily upon growth rate, pigmentation, colonial morphology, and results of selected biochemical tests. These standard tests include those for arylsulfatase production, tolerance to 5% NaCl, nitrate reductase activity, and iron uptake. All members of the *M. fortuitum* group and the *M. chelonae*-*M. abscessus* group exhibit a strongly positive arylsulfatase reaction at 3 days (5, 41, 56). The *M. smegmatis* group (*M. smegmatis* and *M. goodii*) and *M. wolinskyi* are similar in growth rates but do not exhibit arylsulfatase activity at 3 days (4, 68). Approximately 95% of the isolates of *M. smegmatis* (sensu stricto) and 80% of *M. goodii* isolates develop a late (7 to 10 days) yellow-orange pigmentation. *M. wolinskyi* differs from the other two species in that it remains nonpigmented (4, 68).

Previously, a study by the former International Working Group on Mycobacterial Taxonomy (30) showed that growth in 5% NaCl was discriminatory for *M. abscessus* and *M. chelonae*. In this study, 100% of the isolates of *M. abscessus* grew in the presence of 5% NaCl but only 17% of the isolates of *M. chelonae* were viable in the same medium. The same study also reported that *M. abscessus* isolates were citrate negative and that 100% of *M. chelonae* isolates grew in the presence of citrate as a sole carbon source (30). These data have subsequently been corroborated by other investigators (4, 77).

Routine conventional testing has generally proven inadequate for recognition of other established species of RGM, such as *M. peregrinum*, and is definitely lacking for identification of most of the newly described species of RGM (4, 5, 47, 74).

Supplemented Biochemical Testing: Carbohydrate Utilization

The supplementation of the standard biochemical tests with a test for the utilization of carbohydrates (mannitol, inositol, sorbitol, rhamnose, and citrate) (Table 2) has allowed more complete and accurate laboratory identification of established species and discrimination of some (but not all) newly described species (5, 56, 59). It is no longer acceptable to fail to identify RGM isolates to the species level, especially isolates considered to be clinically significant. This differentiation is most critical for *M. chelonae* and *M. abscessus* (5).

One point that should be emphasized is that many of the studies involving carbohydrate utilization by the RGM have been performed with media prepared in-house. There have been few studies of currently available commercial media to ascertain if these will provide equivalent results. With this in mind, the use of commercial products will require careful in-house validation. One example of this problem was noted by Conville and Witebsky in the identification of strains of *M. mucogenicum* by using commercially manufactured carbohydrates (14).

Antimicrobial Susceptibility Tests

As discussed above, other adjunctive nonmolecular tests, including antimicrobial susceptibility tests, have also been utilized for the identification of the RGM. The polymyxin B disk diffusion method is used to distinguish between the *M. fortuitum* group and the *M. chelonae-M. abscessus* group. Generally, isolates of the *M. fortuitum* group exhibit a partial or clear zone of inhibition of ≥10 mm around the polymyxin disk whereas isolates of the *M. chelonae-M. abscessus* group show no zone of inhibition (69). Isolates of the *M. fortuitum* group are usually susceptible to a broader range of antimicrobials, including amikacin, quinolones, sulfonamides, linezolid, and imipenem. Most of the isolates of this group appear to be intrinsically resistant to the macrolides through the presence of an inducible *erm* gene (36).

Although originally considered to be two subspecies within one species, *M. chelonae* and *M. abscessus* are in fact two separate species, and infections with these species have distinctly different clinical manifestations. *M. chelonae* is most often associated with skin and soft tissue infections, especially in patients receiving chronic steroid therapy (62), and is rarely a cause of chronic lung disease (24, 70). *M. abscessus* may also cause skin and soft tissue infections but is primarily a lung pathogen, being responsible for more than 80% of the chronic lung disease cases caused by RGM (5, 24, 70). Thus, it is extremely important to differentiate these RGM to the species level and perform susceptibility testing so that appropriate antibiotic therapy can be initiated (5, 66).

M. chelonae and *M. abscessus* also have different antimicrobial susceptibility patterns. One of the major differences between the two species is in resistance to cefoxitin. In agar disk diffusion tests, *M. chelonae* shows complete resistance to cefoxitin, with no partial or complete zones of inhibition, in contrast to the partial or complete zones of inhibition seen with *M. abscessus*. MICs of cefotoxin for isolates of *M. chelonae* are ≥ 256 μg/ml. *M. abscessus* is intermediately susceptible; modal MICs for *M. abscessus* isolates are 32 μg/ml. MICs of amikacin for isolates of *M. abscessus* are also lower, and *M. abscessus* is resistant to tobramycin, whereas tobramycin is more active than amikacin against *M. chelonae*. Additionally, isolates of *M. chelonae* are more susceptible in vitro to some of the newer antibiotics, including linezolid and gatifloxacin, than are isolates of *M. abscessus* (5).

With these differences in susceptibility patterns of the rapidly growing species in mind, tentative identification of the most commonly encountered species of RGM is possible and optimal therapeutic regimens can be designed. However, as with other phenotypic tests, susceptibility testing does not provide definitive species identification, which currently requires molecular testing for almost all RGM species (5).

HPLC Identification

HPLC analysis of mycobacterial cell wall mycolic acid content is routinely used in large reference or state health department laboratories to identify isolates of NTM (9, 53) but has been problematic with species of RGM (9).

HPLC can be helpful for placing RGM into groups but is not specific enough to identify them to the species level with a high degree of accuracy, even with the adoption of standardized growth conditions. Thus, laboratory identification based on HPLC analysis of mycolic acid profiles alone is not adequate for the identification of the pathogenic species of RGM.

MOLECULAR IDENTIFICATION METHODS

Nucleic Acid Probes

The INNO LiPA multiplex probe assay (Innogenetics, Ghent, Belgium) is a molecular biology-based product available outside the United States and utilizes the principle of reverse hybridization (54, 56). Biotinylated DNA obtained by PCR amplification of the 16S-23S internal transcribed spacer region is hybridized with specific oligonucleotide probes immobilized as parallel lines on membrane strips. The addition of streptavidin labeled with alkaline phosphatase and a chromogenic substrate results in a purple-brown precipitate on the hybridized lines. This system was evaluated with multiple species of mycobacteria, including some RGM. The main advantage of this system is that a large variety of species may be identified by a single assay without the need to select an appropriate probe. One limitation of the assay is the cross-reactivity that may be detected with strains of *M. fortuitum* (54, 56). Additionally, it failed to differentiate isolates of *M. chelonae* from those of *M. abscessus*.

Sequence Analysis Identification of RGM

16S rRNA Gene Sequence Analysis

Slowly growing mycobacterial species, with some exceptions such as *M. terrae*, contain one copy of the 16S rRNA operon, whereas the RGM, except for *M. chelonae* and *M. abscessus*, have two copies (2, 18). Routine sequencing of the entire 1,500-nucleotide sequence of the 16S rRNA gene is not feasible for most clinical laboratories. Two main hypervariable domains known as region A and region B are located on the 5′ end of the 16S rRNA gene. These regions correspond to the *Escherichia coli* positions 129 to 267 and 430 to 500, respectively. Hypervariable region A, especially, contains most of the species-specific sequence variations (so-called "signature sequences") in mycobacterial species, and sequencing of this region allows taxonomic identification of most mycobacteria, including most species of RGM (26, 29).

The MicroSeq 500 system (Applied Biosystems, Foster City, Calif.) analyzes approximately 500 bp of the 16S rRNA gene at the 5′ end, including hypervariable region A. Previous studies showed that the MicroSeq assay was able to identify

TABLE 2 Laboratory phenotypic features of the 15 most clinically important species of nonpigmented RGM[a]

Species or complex	Former designation(s)	Pigment	3-Day arylsulfatase	Nitrate reduction	Iron uptake	Carbohydrate utilization				Growth in 5% NaCl
						Mannitol	Inositol	Citrate	Sorbitol	
M. chelonae-M. abscessus group										
M. abscessus	*M. chelonae* subsp. *abscessus*	−	+	−	−	−	−	−	−	+
M. chelonae	*M. borstelense*, *M. chelonei*, *M. chelonae* subsp. *chelonae*	−	+	−	−	−	−	+	−	−
M. immunogenum	*M. immunogen*	−	+	−	−	−	−	−	−	−
M. fortuitum group										
M. fortuitum	*M. ranae*, *M. fortuitum* bv. *fortuitum*	−	+	+	+	−	−	−	−	+
M. peregrinum[b]	*M. fortuitum* bv. *peregrinum* (pipemidic acid susceptible), *M. peregrinum* (type 1)	−	+	+	+	+	−	−	−	+
M. senegalense	*M. fortuitum* bv. *peregrinum* (pipemidic acid resistant), *M. peregrinum* (type 2)	−	+	+	+	+	−	−	−	+
M. fortuitum third biovariant complex										
M. houstonense	*M. fortuitum* third biovar (sorbitol positive)	−	+	+	+	+	+	−	+	+
M. brisbanense	*M. fortuitum* third biovar (sorbitol positive)	−	+	+	+	+	+	−	+	+
M. porcinum	*M. fortuitum* third biovar (sorbitol negative)	−	+	+	+	+	+	−	−	+
M. neworleansense	*M. fortuitum* third biovar (sorbitol negative)	−	+	+	+	+	+	−	−	+
M. boenickei	*M. fortuitum* third biovar (sorbitol negative)	−	+	+	+	+	+	−	−	+
M. mucogenicum	*M. chelonae*-like organism, or MCLO	−	+	±	−[c]	+	−	+	−	−
M. smegmatis group										
M. smegmatis sensu stricto	*M. smegmatis* (group 1)	±	−	+	+	+	+	±	+	+
M. wolinskyi	*M. smegmatis* (group 2)	−	−	+	+	+	+	±	+	+
M. goodii	*M. smegmatis* (group 3)	±	−	+	+	+	+	±	+	+

[a] +, ≥90%; −, <10%; ±, 11 to 89% or late.
[b] *M. peregrinum* (type 1) has the same REA pattern as the *M. fortuitum* third biovariant (sorbitol negative), whereas *M. peregrinum* (type 2) has the same REA pattern as *M. houstonense* (*M. fortuitum* third biovariant [sorbitol positive]). Biochemical testing is necessary for differentiation of these species.
[c] Tan appearance.

most isolates of RGM to the species level (13, 26, 39). Of the discordant isolates, 61% were unusual isolates that were difficult to identify by phenotypic methods and 56% could not be identified using molecular methods. MicroSeq is limited by the fact that analysis of the first 500-bp sequence cannot discriminate between several closely related RGM species, including *M. chelonae* and *M. abscessus*, *M. houstonense* and *M. senegalense*, *M. peregrinum* and *M. septicum*, and *M. houstonense* and *M. farcinogenes* (26, 60). Another major limitation of the MicroSeq system is that the database contains only one entry per species (the type strain). This is especially problematic with isolates that do not have an exact match in the database. Newly reported species are often not in the database. Therefore, the MicroSeq 500 system requires the use of additional sequence databases (13).

A reporting criterion such as (i) distinct species, (ii) related to a species, or (iii) most closely related to a species, depending upon the amount of sequence difference between the unknown isolate and the 16S rRNA gene database entries (39), has been recommended but not validated. This is important as currently there is no standard recommendation for a cutoff value used to interpret sequencing data (13, 26, 39).

Finally, the expense of the MicroSeq assay prevents its application in many clinical laboratories (26).

Sequencing of the *hsp65* Gene

Although the gene for the 65-kDa heat shock protein (*hsp65*) is highly conserved among species of mycobacteria, it exhibits greater interspecies and intraspecies polymorphism than the 16S rRNA gene sequence. This variability can be advantageous in the development of other strategies for the identification of genetically related species of the RGM (44, 54). Like most genes, it has both highly conserved and highly variable nucleotide regions (42). Most sequencing or restriction fragment length polymorphism analysis has utilized a 441-bp sequence identified by Telenti et al. (51) and often referred to as the Telenti fragment.

Studies based on DNA sequencing have demonstrated interspecies allelic diversity within the RGM (38). Detailed studies of several RGM species including *M. peregrinum*, *M. porcinum*, *M. senegalense*, *M. chelonae*, and *M. abscessus* have shown four to six sequence variants (sequevars) per species that differ by 2 to 6 nucleotides within the 441-bp Telenti fragment (44, 60, 65).

Additionally, unlike 16S rRNA gene sequence analysis, the *hsp65* sequencing method was easily able to differentiate isolates of *M. abscessus* from those of *M. chelonae* (they differ by almost 30 bp in the 441-bp *hsp65* sequence compared to only 4 bp in the entire 1,500-bp 16S rRNA gene sequence). In contrast to 16S rRNA gene sequences, sequences of the *hsp65* gene allow even RGM species with a high degree of 16S rRNA gene similarity, such as *M. fortuitum*, *M. septicum*, *M. peregrinum*, *M. houstonense*, and *M. senegalense*, to be distinguished as distinct species (60).

A limitation of sequencing of the *hsp65* gene is that few or no sequences from more recently described RGM species are available in databases and detailed sequencing of older species (i.e., multiple strains) has not been done so only one sequence per species is generally available. This means that in-house validation is essential (34).

PCR-REA of the *hsp65* Gene

PCR-restriction enzyme analysis (PCR-REA) of the gene for the 65-kDA heat shock protein (*hsp*) has become a valuable tool used in the identification of the RGM.

The advantage of REA nonsequencing of the *hsp65* gene is that minor differences (sequevars) within the species rarely involve a restriction site, so most species have only one REA pattern. REA requires less equipment expenditure than sequencing. However, as in sequencing, the system is only as good as its database. Also, there is no commercial system for *hsp65* REA. Ten taxonomic groups of RGM were initially evaluated (a total of 129 reference and clinical isolates of RGM) with 24 restriction endonucleases, and BstEII, HaeIII, CfoI, and AciI were found to give the best species separation (50). A number of additional RGM species were described after this study, and most have shown unique or identifying restriction fragment length polymorphism patterns by this method. These species include *M. immunogenum* (74), *M. mageritense* (64), *M. porcinum* (47, 65), *M. boenickei* (47), *M. goodii* (4), *M. wolinskyi* (4), *M. septicum* (47), and *M. senegalense* (60). Species that could still not be separated include *M. houstonense* and *M. neworleansense* (47). Algorithms for identification of mycobacterial species including RGM by using PCR-restriction fragment length polymorphism analysis of the *hsp65* gene have been proposed (17).

Thus, currently the 441-bp Telenti fragment of the *hsp65* gene remains the most useful sequence for REA identification of the RGM, although it has not been evaluated extensively in the pigmented RGM (4, 50, 51). The advantages of REA are that the method of identification does not rely upon growth rate and nutritional requirements, the equipment is relatively inexpensive, and the results for a large number of mycobacterial species can be generated rapidly. The disadvantages are that it requires knowledge of PCR and is a relatively complex procedure that requires extensive in-house validation since the method is not approved by the Food and Drug Administration.

Sequencing of Other Secondary Gene Targets

Other molecular targets for taxonomic identification, including the gene encoding the 32-kDA protein, the superoxide dismutase gene (*sod*), the *dnaJ* gene, the *rpoB* gene, the 16S-23S rRNA internal transcribed spacer, the *secA1* gene, and the *recA* gene, have been suggested for mycobacterial identification utilizing either REA or direct sequencing (1, 60, 65). However, preliminary data suggest that the sequences of these genes are more variable than that of the *hsp65* gene and to date these sequences have been less commonly utilized in the laboratory identification of the species of RGM (1, 56, 60, 65).

Molecular Typing Methods

PFGE

Pulsed-field gel electrophoresis (PFGE) is the most widely used method for molecular strain typing of the RGM. Although PFGE has never been standardized for RGM, most investigators concur that small (2- to 3-band) differences between isolates indicate that the isolates are closely related; differences of 4 to 6 bands indicate that the strains are possibly related, and ≥7-band differences indicate that the isolates are genetically different (52). Because unrelated strains of most RGM contain highly diverse PFGE patterns, this technique has been useful in epidemiological investigations. With recent modifications of the original method, it is now possible to perform PFGE on all species of RGM (79).

Clinical usage of PFGE for genetic comparison of *M. fortuitum* strains was detailed in a report of an outbreak of respiratory tract colonization with this species in an alcoholism rehabilitation ward in Washington, D.C. (8). Since that report, several other epidemiological investigations of RGM by using PFGE have been performed (27, 33, 35, 72, 79).

RAPD-PCR

In the random amplified polymorphic DNA PCR (RAPD-PCR) using one arbitrary primer and low-stringency conditions, the primer hybridizes to both strands of template DNA, where it is matched or partially matched, resulting in strain-specific heterogeneous DNA products. Zhang and colleagues (78) applied the RAPD-PCR or arbitrarily primed PCR analysis method to comparing strains of *M. abscessus*. They were able to confirm several previous observations about prior outbreaks of nosocomial RGM infection, including a 1988 epidemic of otitis media due to aminoglycoside-resistant *M. abscessus* in children who had previously received tympanostomy tubes (32) and an outbreak associated with cardiac surgery (67).

The need for RAPD-PCR for strain typing of *M. abscessus* is now reduced as recent studies have shown the use of thiourea to prevent the DNA lysis that related to the Tris-borate-EDTA in the PFGE running buffer (79). Whether RAPD-PCR is less or more discriminatory as a typing method than PFGE for RGM has not been established.

EVALUATION, INTERPRETATION, AND REPORTING OF RESULTS

The major species of RGM each have different virulence levels in different clinical settings, and they have different drug susceptibilities as well. *M. mucogenicum*, e.g., is a recognized cause of catheter sepsis but, when recovered from sputum, is usually a contaminant. Thus, all clinically significant RGM should be identified to the species level. The recommended species identification methods are evolving, with declining interest in and accuracy of phenotypic testing, including HPLC, and increasing availability and accuracy of molecular methods. Currently, molecular methods are preferred and generally are the only way to identify more recently described species such as *M. goodii*, *M. mucogenicum*, and *M. senegalense*. Phenotypic tests are still useful (e.g., citrate utilization to separate *M. chelonae* from *M. abscessus*) but work best when combined with molecular methods. Smaller labs should consider referring RGM isolates to a large reference laboratory.

REFERENCES

1. **Adékambi, T., and M. Drancourt.** 2004. Dissection of phylogenetic relationships among 19 rapidly growing *Mycobacterium* species by 16S rRNA, *hsp65*, *sodA*, *recA* and *rpoB* gene sequencing. *Int. J. Syst. Evol. Microbiol.* **54:**2095–2105.
2. **Bercovier, H., O. Kafri, and S. Sela.** 1986. Mycobacteria possess a surprisingly small number of ribosomal RNA genes in relation to the size of their genome. *Biochem. Biophys. Res. Commun.* **136:**1136–1141.
3. **Blom-Potar, M.-C., H. L. David, and N. Rastogi.** 1989. Isoenzymes as tools to discriminate various subdivisions in the *Mycobacterium fortuitum* complex. *Acta Leprol.* **7**(Suppl. 1):39–43.
4. **Brown, B. A., B. Springer, V. A. Steingrube, R. W. Wilson, G. E. Pfyffer, M. J. Garcia, M. C. Menendez, B. Rodriguez-Salgado, K. C. Jost, S. H. Chiu, G. O. Onyi, E. C. Böttger, and R. J. Wallace, Jr.** 1999. *Mycobacterium wolinskyi* sp. nov. and *Mycobacterium goodii* sp. nov., two new rapidly growing species related to *Mycobacterium smegmatis* and associated with human wound infections: a cooperative study from the International Working Group on Mycobacterial Taxonomy. *Int. J. Syst. Bacteriol.* **49:** 1493–1511.
5. **Brown-Elliott, B. A., and R. J. Wallace, Jr.** 2002. Clinical and taxonomic status of pathogenic nonpigmented or late-pigmenting rapidly growing mycobacteria. *Clin. Microbiol. Rev.* **15:**716–746.
6. **Bullington, R. H., J. D. Lanier, and R. L. Font.** 1992. Nontuberculous mycobacterial keratitis. *Arch. Ophthalmol.* **110:**519–524.
7. **Burns, D. N., P. K. Rohatgi, R. Rosenthal, M. Seiler, and F. M. Gordin.** 1990. Disseminated *Mycobacterium fortuitum* successfully treated with combination therapy including ciprofloxacin. *Am. Rev. Respir. Dis.* **142:**468–470.
8. **Burns, D. N., R. J. Wallace, Jr., M. E. Schultz, Y. Zhang, S. Q. Zubairi, Y. Pang, C. L. Gibert, B. A. Brown, E. S. Noel, and F. M. Gordin.** 1991. Nosocomial outbreak of respiratory tract colonization with *Mycobacterium fortuitum:* demonstration of the usefulness of pulsed-field gel electrophoresis in an epidemiologic investigation. *Am. Rev. Respir. Dis.* **144:**1153–1159.
9. **Butler, W. R., and L. S. Guthertz.** 2001. Mycolic acid analysis by high-performance liquid chromatography for identification of *Mycobacterium* species. *Clin. Microbiol. Rev.* **14:**704–726.
10. **Butt, A. A.** 1998. Cervical adenitis due to *Mycobacterium fortuitum* in patients with acquired immunodeficiency syndrome. *Am. J. Med. Sci.* **315:**50–55.
11. **Carmago, D., C. Saad, F. Ruiz, M. E. Ramirez, M. Lineros, G. Rodriguez, E. Navarro, B. Pulido, and L. C. I. Orozco.** 1996. Iatrogenic outbreak of *M. chelonae* skin abscesses. *Epidemiol. Infect.* **117:**113–119.
12. **Cegielski, J. P., and R. J. Wallace, Jr.** 1997. Infections due to nontuberculous mycobacteria, p. 445–461. *In* W. M. Scheld, R. J. Whitley, and D. T. Durack (ed.), *Infections of the Central Nervous System,* 2nd ed. Lippincott-Raven Publishers, Philadelphia, Pa.
13. **Cloud, J. L., H. Neal, R. Rosenberry, C. Y. Turenne, M. Jama, D. R. Hillyard, and K. C. Carroll.** 2002. Identification of *Mycobacterium* spp. by using a commercial 16S ribosomal DNA sequencing kit and additional sequencing libraries. *J. Clin. Microbiol.* **40:**400–406.
14. **Conville, P. S., and F. G. Witebsky.** 2001. Lack of usefulness of carbon utilization tests for identification of *Mycobacterium mucogenicum*. *J. Clin. Microbiol.* **39:**2725–2728.
15. **Covert, T. C., M. R. Rodgers, A. L. Reyes, and G. N. Stelma, Jr.** 1999. Occurrence of nontuberculous mycobacteria in environmental samples. *Appl. Environ. Microbiol.* **65:**2492–2496.
16. **Cullen, A. R., C. L. Cannon, E. J. Mark, and A. A. Colin.** 2000. *Mycobacterium abscessus* infection in cystic fibrosis. *Am. J. Respir. Crit. Care Med.* **161:**641–645.
17. **Devallois, A., K. S. Goh, and N. Rastogi.** 1997. Rapid identification of mycobacteria to species level by PCR-restriction fragment length polymorphism analysis of the *hsp65* gene and proposition of an algorithm to differentiate 34 mycobacterial species. *J. Clin. Microbiol.* **35:**2969–2973.
18. **Domenech, P., M. C. Menendez, and M. J. Garcia.** 1994. Restriction fragment length polymorphisms of 16S rRNA genes in the differentiation of fast-growing mycobacterial species. *FEMS Microbiol. Lett.* **116:**19–24.
19. **Flor, A., J. A. Capdevila, N. Martin, J. Gavaldà, and A. Pahissa.** 1996. Nontuberculous mycobacterial meningitis: report of two cases and review. *Clin. Infect. Dis.* **23:** 1266–1273.

20. **Ford, J. G., A. J. W. Huang, S. C. Pfugfelder, E. C. Alfonso, R. K. Forster, and D. Miller.** 1998. Nontuberculous mycobacterial keratitis in south Florida. *Ophthalmology* **105:**1652–1658.
21. **Franklin, D. J., J. R. Starke, M. T. Brady, B. A. Brown, and R. J. Wallace, Jr.** 1994. Chronic otitis media after tympanostomy tube placement caused by *Mycobacterium abscessus:* a new clinical entity? *Am. J. Otol.* **15:**313–320.
22. **Galil, K., L. A. Miller, M. A. Yakrus, R. J. Wallace, Jr., D. G. Mosley, B. England, G. Huitt, M. M. McNeill, and B. A. Perkins.** 1999. Abscesses due to *Mycobacterium abscessus* linked to injection of unapproved alternative medication. *Emerg. Infect. Dis.* **5:**681–687.
23. **Gira, A. K., H. Reisenauer, L. Hammock, U. Nadiminti, J. T. Macy, A. Reeves, C. Burnett, M. A. Yakrus, S. Toney, B. J. Jensen, H. M. Blumberg, S. W. Caughman, and F. S. Nolte.** 2004. Furunculosis due to *Mycobacterium mageritense* associated with footbaths at a nail salon. *J. Clin. Microbiol.* **42:**1813–1817.
24. **Griffith, D. E., W. M. Girard, and R. J. Wallace, Jr.** 1993. Clinical features of pulmonary disease caused by rapidly growing mycobacteria: an analysis of 154 patients. *Am. Rev. Respir. Dis.* **147:**1271–1278.
25. **Gubler, J. G. H., M. Salfinger, and A. von Graevenitz.** 1992. Pseudoepidemic of nontuberculous mycobacteria due to a contaminated bronchoscope cleaning machine: report of an outbreak and review of the literature. *Chest* **101:**1245–1249.
26. **Hall, L., K. A. Doerr, S. L. Wohlfiel, and G. D. Roberts.** 2003. Evaluation of the MicroSeq system for identification of mycobacteria by 16S ribosomal DNA sequencing and its integration into a routine clinical mycobacteriology laboratory. *J. Clin. Microbiol.* **41:**1447–1453.
27. **Hector, J. S. R., Y. Pang, G. H. Mazurek, Y. Zhang, B. A. Brown, and R. J. Wallace, Jr.** 1992. Large restriction fragment patterns of genomic *Mycobacterium fortuitum* DNA as strain-specific markers and their use in epidemiologic investigation of four nosocomial outbreaks. *J. Clin. Microbiol.* **30:**1250–1255.
28. **Hogg, G. G., M. F. Schinsky, M. M. McNeil, B. A. Lasker, V. A. Silcox, and J. M. Brown.** 1994. Central line sepsis in a child due to a previously unidentified mycobacterium. *J. Clin. Microbiol.* **37:**1193–1196.
29. **Kirschner, P., B. Springer, U. Vogel, A. Meier, A. Wrede, M. Kiekenbeck, F. C. Bange, and E. C. Böttger.** 1993. Genotypic identification of mycobacteria by nucleic acid sequence determination: report of a 2-year experience in a clinical laboratory. *J. Clin. Microbiol.* **31:**2882–2889.
30. **Kubica, G. P., I. Baess, R. E. Gordon, P. A. Jenkins, J. B. G. Kwapinski, C. McDurmont, S. R. Pattyn, H. Saito, V. Silcox, J. L. Stanford, K. Takeya, and M. Tsukamura.** 1972. A co-operative numerical analysis of rapidly growing mycobacteria. *J. Gen. Microbiol.* **73:**55–70.
31. **Lai, K. K., B. A. Brown, J. A. Westerling, S. A. Fontecchio, Y. Zhang, and R. J. Wallace, Jr.** 1998. Long-term laboratory contamination by *Mycobacterium abscessus* resulting in two pseudo-outbreaks: recognition with use of random amplified polymorphic DNA (RAPD) polymerase chain reaction. *Clin. Infect. Dis.* **27:**169–175.
32. **Lowry, P. W., W. R. Jarvis, A. D. Oberle, L. A. Bland, R. Silberman, J. A. Bocchini, Jr., H. D. Dean, J. M. Swenson, and R. J. Wallace, Jr.** 1988. *Mycobacterium chelonae* causing otitis media in an ear-nose-and-throat practice. *N. Engl. J. Med.* **319:**978–982.
33. **Maloney, S., S. Welbel, B. Daves, K. Adams, S. Becker, L. Bland, M. Arduino, R. J. Wallace, Jr., Y. Zhang, G. Buck, P. Risch, and W. Jarvis.** 1994. *Mycobacterium abscessus* pseudoinfection traced to an automated endoscope washer: utility of epidemiologic and laboratory investigation. *J. Infect. Dis.* **169:**1166–1169.
34. **McNabb, A., D. Eisler, K. Adie, M. Amos, M. Rodrigues, G. Stephens, W. A. Black, and J. Isaac-Renton.** 2004. Assessment of partial sequencing of the 65-kilodalton heat shock protein gene *(hsp65)* for routine identification of *Mycobacterium* species isolated from clinical sources. *J. Clin. Microbiol.* **42:**3000–3011.
35. **Meyers, H., B. A. Brown-Elliott, D. Moore, J. Curry, C. Truong, Y. Zhang, and R. J. Wallace, Jr.** 2002. An outbreak of *Mycobacterium chelonae* following liposuction. *Clin. Infect. Dis.* **34:**1500–1507.
36. **Nash, K. A., Y. Zhang, B. A. Brown-Elliott, and R. J. Wallace, Jr.** 2005. Molecular basis of intrinsic macrolide resistance in clinical isolates of *Mycobacterium fortuitum. J. Antimicrob. Chemother.* **55:**170–177.
37. **Olivier, K. N., D. J. Weber, R. J. Wallace, Jr., A. R. Faiz, J.-H. Lee, Y. Zhang, B. A. Brown-Elliott, A. Handler, R. W. Wilson, M. S. Schechter, L. J. Edwards, S. Chakraborti, and M. R. Knowles for the Nontuberculous Mycobacteria in Cystic Fibrosis Study Group.** 2003. Nontuberculous mycobacteria. I. Multicenter prevalence study in cystic fibrosis. *Am. J. Respir. Crit. Care Med.* **167:** 828–834.
38. **Pai, S., N. Esen, X. Pan, and J. M. Musser.** 1997. Routine rapid *Mycobacterium* species assignment based on species-specific allelic variation in the 65-kilodalton heat shock protein gene *(hsp65)*. *Pathol. Lab. Med.* **121:**859–864.
39. **Patel, J. B., D. G. B. Leonard, X. Pan, J. M. Musser, R. E. Berman, and I. Nachamkin.** 2000. Sequence-based identification of *Mycobacterium* species using the MicroSeq 500 16S rDNA bacterial identification system. *J. Clin. Microbiol.* **38:**246–251.
40. **Pettijean, G., U. Fluckiger, S. Schären, and G. Laifer.** 2004. Vertebral osteomyelitis caused by non-tuberculous mycobacteria. *Clin. Microbiol. Infect.* **10:**951–953.
41. **Pfyffer, G. E., B. A. Brown-Elliott, and R. J. Wallace, Jr.** 2003. *Mycobacterium:* general characteristics, isolation, and staining procedures, p. 532–559. *In* P. R. Murray, E. J. Baron, J. H. Jorgensen, M. A. Pfaller, and R. H. Yolken (ed.), *Manual of Clinical Microbiology,* 8th ed. ASM Press, Washington, D.C.
42. **Plikaytis, B. B., B. D. Plikaytis, M. A. Yakrus, W. R. Butler, C. L. Woodley, V. A. Silcox, and T. M. Shinnick.** 1992. Differentiation of slowly growing *Mycobacterium* species, including *Mycobacterium tuberculosis,* by gene amplification and restriction fragment length polymorphism analysis. *J. Clin. Microbiol.* **30:**1815–1822.
43. **Raad, I. I., S. Vartivarian, A. Khan, and G. P. Bodey.** 1991. Catheter-related infections caused by the *Mycobacterium fortuitum* complex: 15 cases and review. *Rev. Infect. Dis.* **13:**1120–1125.
44. **Ringuet, H., C. Akoua-Koffi, S. Honore, A. Varnerot, V. Vincent, P. Berche, J. L. Gaillard, and C. Pierre-Audigier.** 1999. *hsp65* sequencing for identification of rapidly growing mycobacteria. *J. Clin. Microbiol.* **37:**852–857.
45. **Sarria, J. C., N. B. Chutkan, J. E. Figueroa, and A. Hull.** 1998. Atypical mycobacterial vertebral osteomyelitis: case report and review. *Clin. Infect. Dis.* **26:**503–505.
46. **Schinsky, M. F., M. M. McNeil, A. M. Whitney, A. G. Steigerwalt, B. A. Lasker, M. M. Floyd, G. C. Hogg, D. J. Brenner, and J. M. Brown.** 2000. *Mycobacterium septicum* sp. nov., a new rapidly growing species associated with catheter-related bacteraemia. *Int. J. Syst. Evol. Microbiol.* **50:**575–581.
47. **Schinsky, M. F., R. E. Morey, A. G. Steigerwalt, M. P. Douglas, R. W. Wilson, M. M. Floyd, W. R. Butler, M. I. Daneshvar, B. A. Brown-Elliott, R. J. Wallace, Jr., M. M. McNeil, D. J. Brenner, and J. M. Brown.** 2004. Taxonomic variation in the *Mycobacterium fortuitum* third biovariant complex: description of *Mycobacterium boenickei* sp. nov., *Mycobacterium houstonense* sp. nov., *Mycobacterium*

neworleansense sp. nov., and *Mycobacterium brisbanense* sp. nov., and recognition of *Mycobacterium porcinum* from human clinical isolates. *Int. J. Syst. Evol. Microbiol.* **54:**1653–1667.

48. **Sniezek, P. J., B. S. Graham, H. Byers Busch, E. R. Lederman, M. L. Lim, K. Poggemyer, A. Kao, M. Mizrahi, G. Washabaugh, M. Yakrus, and K. L. Winthrop.** 2003. Rapidly growing mycobacterial infections after pedicures. *Arch. Dermatol.* **139:**629–634.
49. **Springer, B., E. C. Böttger, P. Kirschner, and R. J. Wallace, Jr.** 1995. Phylogeny of the *Mycobacterium chelonae*-like organism based on partial sequencing of the 16S rRNA gene and proposal of *Mycobacterium mucogenicum* sp. nov. *Int. J. Syst. Bacteriol.* **45:**262–267.
50. **Steingrube, V. A., J. L. Gibson, B. A. Brown, Y. Zhang, R. W. Wilson, M. Rajagopalan, and R. J. Wallace, Jr.** 1995. PCR amplification and restriction endonuclease analysis of a 65-kilodalton heat shock protein gene sequence for taxonomic separation of rapidly growing mycobacteria. *J. Clin. Microbiol.* **33:**149–153. (Erratum, **33:** 1686.)
51. **Telenti, A., F. Marchesi, M. Balz, F. Bally, E. C. Böttger, and T. Bodmer.** 1993. Rapid identification of mycobacteria to the species level by polymerase chain reaction and restriction enzyme analysis. *J. Clin. Microbiol.* **31:**175–178.
52. **Tenover, F. C., R. D. Arbeit, R. V. Goering, P. A. Mickelsen, B. E. Murray, D. H. Persing, and B. Swaminathan.** 1995. Interpreting chromosomal DNA restriction patterns produced by pulsed-field gel electrophoresis: criteria for bacterial strain typing. *J. Clin. Microbiol.* **33:**2233–2239.
53. **Thibert, L., and S. LaPierre.** 1993. Routine application of high-performance liquid chromatography for identification of mycobacteria. *J. Clin. Microbiol.* **31:**1759–1763.
54. **Tortoli, E.** 2003. Impact of genotypic studies on mycobacterial taxonomy: the new mycobacteria of the 1990s. *Clin. Microbiol. Rev.* **16:**319–354.
55. **Villaneuva, A., R. V. Calderon, B. A. Vargas, F. Ruiz, S. Aguero, Y. Zhang, B. A. Brown, and R. J. Wallace, Jr.** 1997. Report on an outbreak of post-injection abscesses due to *Mycobacterium abscessus*, including management with surgery and clarithromycin therapy and comparison of strains by random amplified polymorphic DNA polymerase chain reaction. *Clin. Infect. Dis.* **24:**1147–1153.
56. **Vincent, V., B. A. Brown-Elliott, K. C. Jost, Jr., and R. J. Wallace, Jr.** 2003. *Mycobacterium:* phenotypic and genotypic identification, p. 560–584. *In* P. R. Murray, E. J. Baron, J. H. Jorgensen, M. A. Pfaller, and R. H. Yolken (ed.), *Manual of Clinical Microbiology,* 8th ed. ASM Press, Washington, D.C.
57. **Wallace, R. J., Jr., and V. R. Koppaka.** 2004. Nontuberculous mycobacteria, p. 667–683. *In* C. G. Mayhall (ed.), *Hospital Epidemiology and Infection Control,* 3rd ed. Lippincott Williams & Wilkins, Philadelphia, Pa.
58. **Wallace, R. J., Jr.** 1989. The clinical presentation, diagnosis, and therapy of cutaneous and pulmonary infections due to the rapidly growing mycobacteria, M. *fortuitum* and M. *chelonae*. *Clin. Chest Med.* **10:**419–429.
59. **Wallace, R. J., Jr., and B. A. Brown.** 1999. *Mycobacterium fortuitum, chelonae, abscessus*, p. 372–379. *In* D. Schlossberg (ed.), *Tuberculosis and Nontuberculous Mycobacterial Infections.* W. B. Saunders Co., Philadelphia, Pa.
60. **Wallace, R. J., Jr., B. A. Brown, J. Brown, A. G. Steigerwalt, L. Hall, G. Woods, J. Cloud, L. Mann, R. Wilson, C. Crist, K. C. Jost, Jr., D. E. Byrer, J. Tang, E. Stamenova, B. Campbell, J. Wolfe, and C. Turenne.** 2005. Polyphasic characterization of *Mycobacterium peregrinum* type II: demonstration as a human pathogen and recognition as human isolates of *Mycobacterium senegalense*. *J. Clin. Microbiol.* **12:**5925–5935.
61. **Wallace, R. J., Jr., B. A. Brown, and D. E. Griffith.** 1998. Nosocomial outbreaks/pseudo-outbreaks caused by nontuberculous mycobacteria. *Annu. Rev. Microbiol.* **2:**453–490.
62. **Wallace, R. J., Jr., B. A. Brown, and G. Onyi.** 1992. Skin, soft tissue, and bone infections due to *Mycobacterium chelonae* subspecies *chelonae*—importance of prior corticosteroid therapy, frequency of disseminated infections, and resistance to oral antimicrobials other than clarithromycin. *J. Infect. Dis.* **166:**405–412.
63. **Wallace, R. J., Jr., B. A. Brown, V. A. Silcox, M. Tsukamura, D. R. Nash, L. C. Steele, V. A. Steingrube, J. Smith, G. Sumter, Y. Zhang, and Z. Blacklock.** 1991. Clinical disease, drug susceptibility, and biochemical patterns of the unnamed third biovariant complex of *Mycobacterium fortuitum*. *J. Infect. Dis.* **163:**598–603.
64. **Wallace, R. J., Jr., B. A. Brown-Elliott, L. Hall, G. Roberts, R. W. Wilson, L. B. Mann, C. J. Crist, S. H. Chiu, R. Dunlap, M. J. Garcia, J. T. Bagwell, and K. C. Jost, Jr.** 2002. Clinical and laboratory features of *Mycobacterium mageritense*. *J. Clin. Microbiol.* **40:**2930–2935.
65. **Wallace, R. J., Jr., B. A. Brown-Elliott, R. W. Wilson, L. Mann, L. Hall, Y. Zhang, K. C. Jost, Jr., J. M. Brown, A. Kabani, M. F. Schinsky, A. G. Steigerwalt, C. J. Crist, G. D. Roberts, Z. Blacklock, M. Tsukamura, V. Silcox, and C. Turenne.** 2004. Clinical and laboratory features of *Mycobacterium porcinum*. *J. Clin. Microbiol.* **42:**5689–5697.
66. **Wallace, R. J., Jr., J. L. Cook, J. Glassroth, D. E. Griffith, K. N. Olivier, and F. Gordin.** 1997. American Thoracic Society statement: diagnosis and treatment of disease caused by nontuberculous mycobacteria. *Am. Respir. Crit. Care Med.* **156:**S1–S25.
67. **Wallace, R. J., Jr., J. M. Musser, S. I. Hull, V. A. Silcox, L. C. Steele, G. D. Forrester, A. Labidi, and R. K. Selander.** 1989. Diversity and sources of rapidly growing mycobacteria associated with infections following cardiac bypass surgery. *J. Infect. Dis.* **159:**708–716.
68. **Wallace, R. J., Jr., D. R. Nash, M. Tsukamura, Z. M. Blacklock, and V. A. Silcox.** 1988. Human disease due to *Mycobacterium smegmatis*. *J. Infect. Dis.* **158:**52–59.
69. **Wallace, R. J., Jr., J. M. Swenson, V. A. Silcox, and R. C. Good.** 1982. Disk diffusion testing with polymyxin and amikacin for differentiation of *Mycobacterium fortuitum* and *Mycobacterium chelonei*. *J. Clin. Microbiol.* **16:** 1003–1006.
70. **Wallace, R. J., Jr., J. M. Swenson, V. A. Silcox, R. C. Good, J. A. Tschen, and M. S. Stone.** 1983. Spectrum of disease due to rapidly growing mycobacteria. *Rev. Infect. Dis.* **5:**657–679.
71. **Wallace, R. J., Jr., D. Tanner, P. J. Brennan, and B. A. Brown.** 1993. Clinical trial of clarithromycin for cutaneous (disseminated) infection due to *Mycobacterium chelonae*. *Ann. Intern. Med.* **119:**482–486.
72. **Wallace, R. J., Jr., Y. Zhang, B. A. Brown, V. Fraser, G. H. Mazurek, and S. Maloney.** 1993. DNA large restriction fragment patterns of sporadic and epidemic nosocomial strains of *Mycobacterium chelonae* and *Mycobacterium abscessus*. *J. Clin. Microbiol.* **31:**2697–2701.
73. **Wayne, L. G., and H. A. Sramek.** 1992. Agents of newly recognized or infrequently encountered mycobacterial diseases. *Clin. Microbiol. Rev.* **5:**1–25.
74. **Wilson, R. W., V. A. Steingrube, E. C. Böttger, B. Springer, B. A. Brown-Elliott, V. Vincent, K. C. Jost, Jr., Y. Zhang, M. J. Garcia, S. H. Chiu, G. O. Onyi, H. Rossmoore, D. R. Nash, and R. J. Wallace, Jr.** 2001. *Mycobacterium immunogenum* sp. nov., a novel species related to *Mycobacterium abscessus* and associated with clinical disease, pseudo-outbreaks, and contaminated metalworking fluids: an international cooperative study on mycobacterial taxonomy. *Int. J. Syst. Evol. Microbiol.* **51:**1751–1764.

75. **Winthrop, K. L., M. Abrams, M. Yakrus, I. Swartz, J. Ely, D. Gillies, and D. J. Vugia.** 2002. An outbreak of mycobacterial furunculosis associated with footbaths at a nail salon. *N. Engl. J. Med.* **346:**1366–1371.
76. **Winthrop, K. L., K. Albridge, D. South, P. Albrecht, M. Abrams, M. C. Samuel, W. Leonard, J. Wagner, and D. J. Vugia.** 2004. The clinical management and outcome of nail salon-acquired *Mycobacterium fortuitum* skin infection. *Clin. Infect. Dis.* **38:**38–44.
77. **Yakrus, M. A., S. M. Hernandez, M. M. Floyd, D. Sikes, W. R. Butler, and B. Metchock.** 2001. Comparison of methods for identification of *Mycobacterium abscessus* and *M. chelonae* isolates. *J. Clin. Microbiol.* **39:**4103–4110.
78. **Zhang, Y., M. Rajagopalan, B. A. Brown, and R. J. Wallace, Jr.** 1997. Randomly amplified polymorphic DNA PCR for comparison of *Mycobacterium abscessus* strains from nosocomial outbreaks. *J. Clin. Microbiol.* **35:**3132–3139.
79. **Zhang, Y., M. A. Yakrus, E. A. Graviss, N. Williams-Bouyer, C. Turenne, A. Kabani, and R. J. Wallace, Jr.** 2004. Pulsed-field gel electrophoresis study of *Mycobacterium abscessus* isolates previously affected by DNA degradation. *J. Clin. Microbiol.* **42:**5582–5587.

*Neisseria**

WILLIAM M. JANDA AND CHARLOTTE A. GAYDOS

39

TAXONOMY OF THE GENUS *NEISSERIA*

At this time, members of the genus *Neisseria* are classified in the family *Neisseriaceae* along with the genera *Kingella*, *Eikenella*, *Simonsiella*, and *Alysiella*. This family is now placed in the β-subgroup of the Phylum *Proteobacteria*.

DESCRIPTION OF THE GENUS *NEISSERIA*

Members of the genus *Neisseria* are coccal or rod-shaped gram-negative organisms that occur in pairs or short chains. Diplococcal species have adjacent sides that are flattened, giving them a "coffee bean" appearance. Currently, *Neisseria* species (except the three *N. elongata* subspecies and *N. weaveri*) are the only true coccal members of the family *Neisseriaceae*. *N. elongata* subspecies and *N. weaveri* are medium to large, plump rods that appear in gram-stained smears as pairs or short chains (5, 51). All species in the genus *Neisseria* inhabit the mucous membrane surfaces of warm-blooded hosts. These organisms are aerobic and non-motile and do not form spores; most species grow optimally at 35 to 37°C. Growth of *Neisseria* species is stimulated by CO_2 and humidity; some gonococcal isolates have an obligate requirement for CO_2 for initial isolation and growth of subsequent subcultures. Those *Neisseria* species that produce acid from carbohydrates do so by an oxidative pathway. All members of the genus are oxidase positive and, except for *N. elongata* subspecies *elongata* and subspecies *nitroreducens*, are catalase positive.

While most *Neisseria* species are not exacting in their nutritional requirements for growth, the pathogenic species, and *N. gonorrhoeae* in particular, are more nutritionally demanding. *N. gonorrhoeae* does not grow in the absence of cysteine and a usable energy source (i.e., glucose, pyruvate, or lactate). Some gonococcal strains display requirements for specific amino acids, pyrimidines, and purines as a result of defective or altered biosynthetic pathways. Demonstration of these growth requirements forms the basis for a typing method for gonococci called auxotyping (see below). The neisseriae can grow under anaerobic conditions if an alternative electron acceptor (e.g., nitrites) is present.

*This chapter contains information presented in chapter 38 by William M. Janda and Joan S. Knapp in the eighth edition of this Manual.

EPIDEMIOLOGY AND TRANSMISSION

N. gonorrhoeae is the causative agent of gonorrhea. In the United States, the incidence of gonorrhea increased during the 1960s and early 1970s, with the highest incidence—over 460 cases per 100,000 population—occurring in 1975. From the mid-1980s and into the 1990s, the incidence of gonorrhea steadily declined. In 1994, reported cases of *Chlamydia trachomatis* infection exceeded reported cases of gonococcal infection for the first time. The decline in the incidence of gonorrhea ceased toward the mid-1990s; from 1998 to 2002, the incidence of gonococcal infections plateaued at 128 to 130 cases per 100,000. In the United States, the incidence of gonorrhea remains high among sexually active teenagers and young adults, with the highest attack rates found among 15- to 19-year-old women (34). In regions where collected statistics include sexual orientation, rates of gonococcal infection more than tripled from 1995 to 2003 among men who have sex with other men (MSM) (30). Maintenance and transmission of gonorrhea are related to a social subset of "core transmitters" who have unprotected intercourse with multiple new partners and either are asymptomatic or choose to ignore symptoms (91). Both social risk factors (i.e., low socioeconomic status, urban residence, lack of education, poor access to health care, unmarried status, race/ethnicity, male homosexuality, prostitution, and histories of other sexually transmitted diseases) and behavioral risk factors (i.e., unprotected intercourse, multiple partners, other high-risk partners, and drug use) have been identified for targeting by outreach/intervention and sexually transmitted disease control programs.

The risk of acquiring gonorrhea is multifactorial and is related to the number and sites of exposure. For heterosexual males, the risk of acquiring urethral infection from an infected female is about 20% for a single exposure and up to 80% for four exposures. Due to anatomical considerations, the risk of infection for females from a single exposure to an infected male is about 50 to 70% (69). Anogenital sexual contact resulting in rectal infection is also efficient, and studies among MSM have demonstrated that urethral infection following fellatio with an infected partner may account for up to 26% of urethral infections diagnosed in this population (68).

N. meningitidis causes a disease spectrum ranging from occult sepsis with rapid recovery to fulminant fatal disease. The major virulence factor of disease-associated meningococci is the polysaccharide capsule. Thirteen meningococcal capsular polysaccharide serogroups (A, B, C, D, H, I, K, L, X, Y, Z, W135, and 29E) have been described, and most infections are caused by organisms belonging to serogroups A, B, C, Y, and W135. Meningococci cause epidemic and endemic meningitis, and serogroups A, B, and C are responsible for 90% of cases globally. Humans are the only natural host for *N. meningitidis*, and the organism is spread from person to person via the respiratory route. Meningococci also may be carried asymptomatically in the oropharynx and nasopharynx. Carriage rates range from about 8 up to 20%, with older children and young adults having higher rates than young children. Carriage may be transient, intermittent, or persistent (105). Carriage strains may be encapsulated (groupable) or nonencapsulated (nongroupable) and result in the formation of serogroup-specific antibodies and broadly cross-reactive antibodies against several other outer membrane antigens. Individuals colonized with nongroupable strains also develop antibody titers against groupable strains, probably due to shared antigenic determinants. This immune response does not eliminate carriage, but it may protect the host from overt disease.

Worldwide, pathogenic clones of *N. meningitidis* composed of different serogroups, serotypes, serosubtypes, and immunotypes are responsible for both endemic and epidemic disease (95). Endemic meningococcal disease occurs at rates of 1 to 3 cases per 100,000 persons in the United States, and in 10 to 25 cases per 100,000 persons in developing countries (95, 100). In the United States, the annual incidence of meningococcal disease has been 0.8 to 1/100,000 population, with infants, the elderly, and the immunocompromised being at greatest risk. Attack rates are highest among children aged 3 months to 1 year and among older teenagers and young adults. Changes in meningococcal epidemiology in the United States during the 1990s have included increases in the incidence of community-acquired serogroup C infections and an increased incidence of disease among teenagers and young adults of high school and college age (54). Outbreaks on college campuses have been associated with bar patronage, drinking, cigarette smoking, and dormitory residence (57). Substantial amounts of meningococcal disease have also been reported among non-first-year students and students living in off-campus housing. With the licensure of the new tetravalent (serogroups A, C, Y, and W135) meningococcal conjugate vaccine (Menactra; Sanofi Pasteur, Inc., Swiftwater, Pa.) in January 2005, the Advisory Committee on Immunization Practices now recommends routine vaccination of adolescents aged 11 to 12 years, and for those past this age, routine immunization before entry into high school or college (29). With this approach, all adolescents will receive either the tetravalent polysaccharide or tetravalent conjugate meningococcal vaccine beginning at age 11 years by the year 2008.

CLINICAL SIGNIFICANCE

Members of the genus *Neisseria* that are found in humans include *N. gonorrhoeae*, *N. meningitidis*, *N. lactamica*, *N. sicca*, *N. subflava* (biovars subflava, flava, and perflava), *N. mucosa*, *N. flavescens*, *N. cinerea*, *N. polysaccharea*, and *N. elongata* subspecies *elongata*, *glycolytica*, and *nitroreducens*. *N. gonorrhoeae* subspecies *kochii*, an extremely rare isolate, has no official taxonomic standing. *N. canis* and *N. weaveri* are found as part of the normal respiratory tract flora of dogs, *N. denitrificans* is present in the respiratory tract of guinea pigs, and *N. macacae*, *N. dentiae*, and *N. iguanae* constitute part of the oral flora in rhesus monkeys, cows, and iguanid lizards, respectively. Most human *Neisseria* species are normal inhabitants of the upper respiratory tract and are not considered pathogens; occasionally these organisms may be isolated from infections, particularly in settings of underlying disease and/or immunosuppression. *N. gonorrhoeae* is always considered a pathogen, regardless of the site of isolation. *N. meningitidis* causes significant and often life-threatening disease but may colonize the nasopharynx without causing disease.

In males, *N. gonorrhoeae* causes an acute urethritis with dysuria and urethral discharge. The incubation period averages 2 to 7 days. After this time, 95 to 99% of infected males experience a purulent urethral discharge. About 2.5% of men presenting to sexually transmitted disease clinics are asymptomatic; the prevalence of asymptomatic urogenital gonorrhea in males in the general population may be as high as 5%. If left untreated, most cases of gonorrhea in men resolve spontaneously. Complications of ascending infection are uncommon and include epididymitis, penile lymphangitis, acute prostatitis, periurethral abscess, seminal vesiculitis, infections of the Tyson's and Cowper's glands, and urethral stricture.

In females, the primary gonococcal infection is present in the endocervix, with concomitant urethral infection occurring in 70 to 90% of cases. After an incubation period of 8 to 10 days, women may present with cervicovaginal discharge, abnormal or intermenstrual bleeding, and abdominal/pelvic pain. Gonococcal infection of the vaginal squamous epithelium of postpubertal women is uncommon, and in women with hysterectomies, the urethra is the most common site of infection. Symptoms of uncomplicated endocervical gonorrhea may resemble other conditions, such as cystitis or vaginal infections. Infection of Bartholin's and Skene's glands may occur in about one-third of women with genital infections, and careful manipulation of these glands can sometimes provide purulent material for direct examination and culture. Endocervical gonorrhea may complicate pregnancy and is a cofactor for spontaneous abortion, chorioamnionitis, premature rupture of membranes, premature delivery, and infant morbidity. Infants born to women with gonorrhea are at risk for developing conjunctival ("ophthalmia neonatorum") or pharyngeal gonococcal infection. Ascending infection may occur in 10 to 20% of infected women and can result in acute pelvic inflammatory disease (PID) manifested as salpingitis (infection of the fallopian tubes), endometritis, and/or tubo-ovarian abscess, all of which can result in scarring, ectopic pregnancies, sterility, and chronic pelvic pain (15). Symptoms of gonococcal PID include lower abdominal pain, abnormal cervical discharge and bleeding, pain on motion, fever, and peripheral leukocytosis. PID caused by *N. gonorrhoeae* generally occurs early in infection and often during or shortly after the onset of menstruation.

N. gonorrhoeae may also cause pharyngeal and anorectal infections. Oropharyngeal infections occur in MSM and heterosexual women who engage in orogenital sexual contact with an infected partner. Oropharyngeal gonococcal infections are usually asymptomatic and are diagnosed by culture of the organism from the throat (12). Rarely, oropharyngeal gonococcal infection may cause acute, exudative pharyngitis or tonsillitis with cervical lymphadenopathy (9). Anorectal gonococcal infection is seen in MSM as a result of unprotected anal intercourse. Women may also acquire rectal infections by this route, but most are due to perianal contamination with cervicovaginal secretions. Rectal infections are often asymptomatic, but some individuals may develop acute proctitis with anorectal pain, a mucopurulent discharge, bleeding, tenesmus, and constipation 5 to 7 days following infection (82). Anoscopic examination of the anal canal reveals an edematous and erythematous rectal mucosa and a purulent discharge associated with the anal crypts.

In 0.5 to 3% of infected individuals, gonococci may invade the bloodstream, resulting in disseminated gonococcal infection (DGI) (71). Disseminated disease may develop following infection at genital or extragenital sites, and repeated bouts of DGI may occur in individuals with certain complement component deficiencies (i.e., C7, C8, or C9) (40). DGI is characterized by low-grade fever, chills, hemorrhagic skin lesions, tenosynovitis, migratory polyarthralgias, and frank arthritis. Skin lesions are usually painful and appear as papules that evolve into necrotic pustules on an erythematous base. Very few lesions may be present, and most are found on the extremities. In 30 to 40% of cases, organisms from the bloodstream may localize in one or more joints to cause a purulent, destructive gonococcal arthritis (11). Joint involvement is usually asymmetric and commonly involves knee, elbow, wrist, fingers, or ankle joints. Rare complications of DGI include endocarditis and meningitis. Gonococcal endocarditis usually involves the aortic valve and follows a rapid and destructive course (90). Gonococcal meningitis has features typical of meningitides caused by other organisms. Pericarditis, pericardial effusions, and adult respiratory distress syndrome may also complicate gonococcal bacteremia. DGI may also present atypically in those with underlying diseases, including human immunodeficiency virus infection and systemic lupus erythematosus (59).

In addition to gonococcal ophthalmia neonatorum, ocular infections have been reported in adults who become infected via genital secretions (55). Laboratory personnel working with cultures may also become accidentally infected if care is not taken to protect the eyes. Eye infection results in painful periorbital cellulitis, profuse purulent discharge, conjunctival injection, eyelid edema and erythema, and epithelial and stromal keratitis. *N. cinerea* has also been reported to cause conjunctival infections, so it is important to perform confirmatory identification tests on gram-negative, oxidase-positive diplococci recovered from ocular sites (37).

Gonococcal infections in children during the newborn period are the result of ocular contamination during vaginal delivery. However, gonococcal infections beyond the immediate neonatal period are indicators of sexual abuse (3). In female children, *N. gonorrhoeae* causes vaginitis with a discharge, rather than cervicitis, because the epithelium of the prepubertal vagina is composed of columnar epithelial cells, which are the cell types that *N. gonorrhoeae* preferentially infects. With the onset of puberty, these vaginal cells are replaced by stratified squamous epithelium that is not susceptible to gonococcal infection. Urethral infection in male children resembles that seen in adults, and pharyngeal and rectal gonococcal infections, as in adults, are usually asymptomatic in children.

The clinical manifestations of infection with *N. meningitidis* can be highly variable, ranging from transient bacteremia with low-grade fever to fulminant, rapidly fatal disease. In all cases, the meningococcal strain becomes established in the upper respiratory tract and enters the bloodstream to initiate systemic disease. Invasive disease occurs in those who are newly infected with a strain against which bactericidal meningococcal serogroup-specific antibodies are lacking. Concurrent viral or mycoplasmal respiratory tract infections facilitate systemic invasion by the organism. The risk of meningococcal disease is also higher among those with complement component deficiencies (e.g., C5, C6, C7, C8, and C9) (41). Other underlying conditions, such as hepatic failure, systemic lupus erythematosus, multiple myeloma, and asplenia, may also predispose to serious meningococcal disease.

The clinical spectrum of meningococcal disease includes meningoencephalitis, meningitis with or without meningococcemia, meningococcemia without meningitis, and bacteremia without septic complications. These presentations may occur discretely or can blend into one another during clinical disease progression. Classic signs of meningitis (e.g., confusion, headache, fever, and nuchal rigidity) may be seen only in about one-half of the patients, and vomiting may be part of the presentation, particularly in children. Meningococcemia and organism dissemination are heralded by the development of a pink, maculopapular eruption that becomes petechial. Rapidly progressive disease may result in purpuric or ecchymotic skin lesions that are hemorrhagic and necrotic. Fulminant shock may dominate the clinical picture of meningococcal meningitis and acute meningococcal sepsis (100). Gangrenous changes in the extremities may occur due to peripheral vasoconstriction, and death may supervene as a result of disseminated intravascular coagulation. The classic finding of acute hemorrhagic necrosis of the adrenal glands represents the hallmark of the Waterhouse-Friderichsen syndrome (1). Meningococcal meningitis with sepsis may have a mortality rate of up to 30%.

N. meningitidis may also cause acute or chronic meningococcemia without meningitis. Patients present with fever, headache, malaise, and leukocytosis, and meningococci are recovered from blood cultures. By that time, the patient is usually clinically well and no therapy or a short course of therapy is administered. Patients with chronic meningococcemia are usually symptomatic, with a presentation clinically similar to the gonococcal arthritis-dermatitis syndrome. Individuals with deficiencies in late complement components, other hypocomplementeric states (e.g., systemic lupus erythematosus), and human immunodeficiency virus infection are also at risk for serious meningococcal disease (41).

Meningococcal pneumonia occurs infrequently and presents as a community-acquired infection that is indistinguishable clinically from other acute bacterial pneumonias. Pneumonia occurs primarily in older individuals with preexisting pulmonary compromise (102). Diagnosis is complicated by the presence of the organisms in the nasopharynx, resulting in contamination of expectorated sputum specimens. Bacteremic epiglottitis and supraglottitis have also been reported in association with serogroup B, C, and Y meningococcal infections (89). Other infections associated with *N. meningitidis* that result from hematogenous dissemination include osteomyelitis, arthritis, cellulitis, endophthalmitis, and spontaneous bacterial peritonitis.

Meningococcal conjunctivitis has been described in adults, children, and neonates and may develop as a complication of systemic meningococcal disease or as a primary infection (6). Complications limited to the eye include corneal ulcers, keratitis, subconjunctival hemorrhage, endophthalmitis, and iritis. *N. meningitidis* may also be isolated from the male urethra, the female genital tract, and the anal canal. In these sites, meningococci may cause infections that are clinically indistinguishable from gonococcal infections, including acute purulent urethritis, cervicitis, salpingitis, and proctitis (74). Orogenital, anogenital, and oroanal sexual practices are believed to be responsible for the presence of meningococci in these anatomic sites (97).

NEISSERIA GONORRHOEAE

Collection, Transport, and Storage of Specimens

Details of specimen collection are given in chapters 5 and 20.

The collection of specimens for diagnosis of gonococcal infection depends on the sex and sexual practices of the patient and on the clinical presentation. In all cases, specimens from genital sites should be collected. If the patient has a history of orogenital or anogenital sexual contacts, collection of oropharyngeal or anal canal specimens is also appropriate. In cases of suspected DGI, blood cultures and specimens from genital and extragenital sites should be obtained. Appropriate sites for culture are summarized in Table 1.

Specimens should be collected with Dacron or rayon swabs. Calcium alginate may be toxic to gonococci, and some brands of cotton swabs may contain fatty acids that may be inhibitory for gonococci. These swab types should be used only if specimens are inoculated directly onto culture growth media or are transported in nonnutritive swab transport media. Some transport media contain charcoal to inactivate toxic materials present in the swab material or in the specimen itself. Instruments used to facilitate specimen collection (e.g., vaginal specula) should be lubricated with warm water or saline because water- and oil-based lubricants may also inhibit organism growth.

The role of the clinical microbiology laboratory in diagnosing gonococcal infections in children involves the proper handling of appropriately collected specimens and the accurate identification of isolated organisms. For prepubertal females, specimens should be obtained from the vagina or urethra, the oropharynx, and the rectum and inoculated onto media as described below. Vaginal specimens are collected by swabbing the vaginal wall for 10 to 15 s to absorb any secretions, or, if the hymen is intact, the specimen is collected from the vaginal orifice. Specimens for diagnosis of rectal, urethral, and oropharyngeal gonococcal infections in children are collected as for adults.

Maximal recovery of gonococci is obtained when specimens are plated directly onto growth medium after collection. However, this technique might not always be possible or practical and various transport systems are available, as described below.

Nonnutritive Swab Transport Systems

Stuart's or Amies buffered semisolid transport media are used for transport of swab specimens for *N. gonorrhoeae*. Some swab transport systems use sponges soaked with transport medium, while others use a semisolid medium with or without activated charcoal. Studies with newer swab collection devices (Copan Transystems; Copan Diagnostics, Inc., Corona, Calif., now marketed as BBL CultureSwab Plus, BD Biosciences, Sparks, Md.) suggest that semisolid Amies transport medium with or without charcoal may preserve the viability of gonococci for as long as 48 h, although the viability of many gonococcal isolates may decrease noticeably after 24 h. Semisolid transport media are superior to devices that use medium-soaked sponges. Sponge materials in some swab transport systems may contain substances (e.g., sulfur or quaternary ammonium compounds) that may inhibit or injure fastidious organisms such as gonococci. While some recent studies have shown that gonococci may survive refrigeration in some swab transport systems up to 48 h (7), other studies have demonstrated that refrigeration beyond 6 h may result in significant reductions in viable organisms, regardless of the transport system used (39, 56). In order to prevent loss of organism viability, swab specimens submitted in transport medium should not be refrigerated and should be inoculated onto growth medium within 6 h after collection.

Culture Medium Transport Systems

Transport of specimens already inoculated onto culture media presents several advantages over swab transport systems. Commercially available systems include JEMBEC plates containing various selective media (Remel, Inc., Lenexa, Kans.), the Gono-Pak (BD Biosciences), and the InTray GC system (BioMed Diagnostics, Inc., San Jose, Calif.) (16). While the Gono-Pak and JEMBEC products require refrigerated storage, the sealed InTray system permits storage of the medium at room temperature for up to 1 year. Media are inoculated with the specimen from a swab and placed in an impermeable plastic bag with a bicarbonate-citric acid pellet. Contact of the pellet with moisture via evaporation from the medium during incubation or by crushing an ampoule of water adjacent to the pellet generates a CO_2-enriched environment within the bag. Organisms remain viable in the CO_2-enriched environment

TABLE 1 Body sites or specimens and culture media for the isolation of *N. gonorrhoeae* and *N. meningitidis*

Species	Syndrome	Gender	Site(s) or specimen(s)	Media
N. gonorrhoeae	Uncomplicated	Female	Endocervix (Bartholin's glands), rectum,[a] urethra, pharynx[a]	Selective
		Male, heterosexual	Urethra	Selective
		Male, homosexual, bisexual	Urethra, rectum,[a] pharynx[a]	Selective
	PID	Female	Endocervix endometrium,[b] fallopian tubes	Selective, nonselective
	DGI	Female/male	Endocervix, (urethra), urethra (male), skin lesions	Selective, nonselective
			Joint fluid	Nonselective, selective
			Blood	Blood culture medium
	Ophthalmia	Female/male	Conjunctivae	Nonselective
N. meningitidis	Meningitis	Female/male	CSF, skin lesions	Nonselective
			Blood	Blood culture medium
			Nasopharynx	Selective, nonselective

[a] If there is a history of oral-genital or anal-genital exposure.
[b] If a laparoscopic examination is performed.

during transport to a reference laboratory, but incubation for 18 to 24 h at 35°C prior to transport allows some initial outgrowth of the organisms and enhances survival.

Direct Examination of Clinical Specimens

Microscopy

The diagnosis of gonococcal urethritis in men can be made by observing gram-negative diplococci within or closely associated with polymorphonuclear leukocytes (PMNs) on a smear prepared from the urethral discharge (Fig. 1). When properly performed, the Gram stain has a sensitivity of 90 to 95% and a specificity of 95 to 100% for diagnosing genital gonorrhea in symptomatic men. For females, Gram stains of endocervical specimens collected under direct visualization of the cervix may also be helpful in diagnosis (see "Collection, Transport, and Storage of Specimens" above). Gram-stained smears of such specimens have a sensitivity of 50 to 70%, depending on the adequacy of the specimen and the patient population. An endocervical smear showing gram-negative intracellular diplococci, particularly from a woman with other signs and symptoms of gonococcal infection, is highly predictive. For patients with symptomatic proctitis, smears collected under direct visualization through an anoscope may provide a diagnosis for 70 to 80% of such patients, as opposed to blind collection, where Gram-stained smears have a sensitivity of only 40 to 60% (Fig. 2). Because of the presence of other gram-negative coccobacilli and bipolar staining bacilli in rectal and endocervical specimens contaminated with vaginal secretions, care must be taken not to overinterpret smears obtained from these sites. Gram-stained smears have no value in the diagnosis of pharyngeal gonococcal infection. Gram-stained smears should not be relied upon for diagnosis of gonorrhea and should be used adjunctively along with more specific tests.

Smears for Gram stain should be prepared from urethral and endocervical sites and should be collected with a swab other than that used for the collection of specimen for culture. The swab is rolled gently over the surface of a glass slide in one direction only to minimize distortion of PMNs and preserve the characteristic appearance of the microorganisms. Gram-stained smears from males with urethral discharge usually show moderate amounts to many PMNs with two or more gram-negative intracellular diplococci (Fig. 1). Smears prepared from specimens submitted in transport media may be difficult to interpret due to distortion of the PMNs or to interfering substances (e.g., charcoal). Smears from normally sterile or minimally contaminated sites (e.g., joint fluid) should also be prepared.

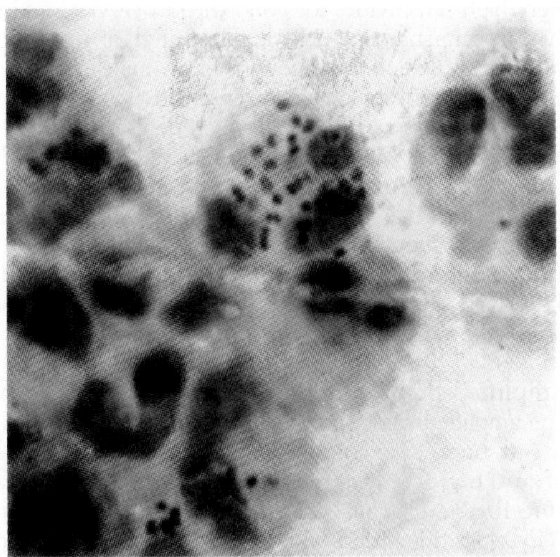

FIGURE 1 Gram stain of male urethral exudate. Some PMNs contain many diplococci; others contain none. Magnification, ×1,500.

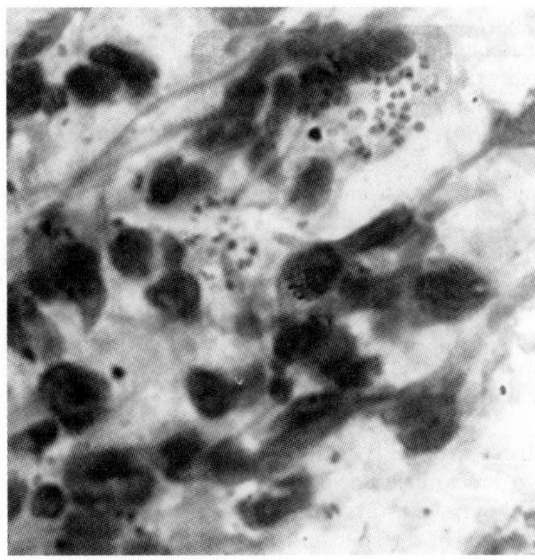

FIGURE 2 Gram stain of mucopurulent rectal exudate showing many diplococci inside PMNs. Magnification, ×1,500.

Antigen Detection

The only commercially available antigen detection test available for diagnosis of gonorrhea is the Binax NOW Gonorrhea Test (Binax, Inc., Portland, Maine). This immunochromatographic strip-based assay can be performed with male urine specimens and both vaginal and endocervical specimens. The test requires no additional materials and takes about 30 min to perform. In a comparative evaluation of the Binax NOW test performed on voided urine with conventional culture of urethral swab specimens from males, the NOW test had a sensitivity of 94.1% and a specificity of 95.8%, with corresponding positive and negative predictive values of 96.9% and 92.0%, respectively (92). The NOW test was shown to have a lower limit of detection of about 1×10^4 CFU of gonococci per ml of urine.

Nucleic Acid Detection Techniques

Nucleic acid detection techniques allow direct detection of *N. gonorrhoeae* in clinical samples and do not require viable organisms. Assays often allow the concurrent detection of *Chlamydia trachomatis*. For *N. gonorrhoeae*, these assays may be divided into three types: (i) direct probe hybridization to the target nucleic acid with direct detection of the hybrid; (ii) nucleic acid amplification tests (NAATs); and (iii) amplified-signal probe tests, which hybridize with nucleic acid and then amplify the signal of the probe. The direct probe tests only slightly increase the sensitivity of culture with a proficient specimen transport system, but the NAATs can appreciably increase sensitivity. The advantages of the tests are that specimens may be transported from geographically distant areas and stored for several days prior to testing in the laboratory. These samples can be maintained frozen prior to testing. The NAATs also allow use of noninvasive specimen types such as urine and vaginal swabs. The disadvantages of using nonculture nucleic acid probe or amplification tests include unavailability of a viable isolate for antimicrobial susceptibility testing and the possibility of a positive test after treatment, since nucleic acids from organisms may persist for a period of time after successful therapy. One report noted that gonococcal DNA for the ligase chain reaction test remained for a mean of 1.7 days in male urine and 2.8 days in female urine, but 2.8 days in vaginal specimens (8). In contrast, chlamydia DNA may remain detectable for about 2 weeks and the recommended time for retesting is 3 weeks (43). Thus, amplification tests should not be used immediately to assess the success of therapy. Results of probe tests and NAATs may be used only to make a presumptive diagnosis of gonococcal infection and are inadmissible evidence in medicolegal cases in the United States at this time.

Direct Probe Hybridization

Two direct nucleic acid probe assays, the Gen-Probe PACE 2 and PACE 2C assays (Gen-Probe Inc., San Diego, Calif.), are approved by the Food and Drug Administration (FDA) for detecting *N. gonorrhoeae*. In the Gen-Probe tests, an acridinium ester-labeled DNA probe for a specific sequence of *N. gonorrhoeae* rRNA is allowed to hybridize with any complementary rRNA in the specimen (65). An acridinium ester hybridization protection assay detects any hybrids, and chemiluminescence generated by the acridinium ester in the hybrids is detected with a luminometer, resulting in a numerical readout. The PACE 2C test detects both *N. gonorrhoeae* and *C. trachomatis* in a single test. A probe competition assay may also be used to augment the specificity of the test. Compared to culture as the "gold standard," reported sensitivity ranged from 90.8 to 96.3% for women and 99.1 to 99.6% for men in the manufacturer's package insert, while specificity ranged from 97.5 to 100% for men and women. Evaluations of the assay in public health settings have supported the high sensitivity and specificity of the test (52).

NAATs

NAATs are designed to amplify *N. gonorrhoeae*-specific nucleic acid sequences from a particular gene target with up to a billion-fold amplification of as little as theoretically a single copy of the target nucleic acid, either DNA or RNA, depending on the specific assay. Currently, there are four commercially available NAATs for the detection of *N. gonorrhoeae:* one based on PCR, Roche AMPLICOR (Roche Molecular Diagnostics, Indianapolis, Ind.); one based on strand displacement amplification (BDProbeTec; Becton Dickinson); and two based on transcription-mediated amplification: APTIMA Combo2, which is for dual detection of gonorrhea and chlamydia, and APTIMA AGC, which is available for detection of only gonorrhea (both from GenProbe) (44, 70, 99). The AGC assay is presently available as an analyte-specific reagent.

The ligase chain reaction-based assay Abbott LCx (Abbott Laboratories Inc., Abbott Park, Ill.), which was commercially available and used by many laboratories, is no longer available due to manufacturing problems.

PCR for *N. gonorrhoeae* detects a 201-bp sequence in the cytosine methyltransferase gene. Although this assay has been used with sensitivity well above 90% for the detection of gonorrhea agents in cervical specimens, the clinical trial did not achieve a high enough sensitivity (64.8%) for the detection of gonorrhea in urine samples from women for FDA clearance, although it is highly accurate with male urine (Table 2) (70). PCR has been shown to detect gonorrhea in male urine with great accuracy with a sensitivity of 94.1% and a specificity of 99.9% in 1,291 symptomatic men, having a sensitivity which is somewhat lower (73.1%) in 721 asymptomatic men (70). It has also been used quite successfully in research settings with self-administered vaginal swabs from women, although it is not FDA cleared for use with vaginal swabs (101). Recently, this assay has been reported to have false-positive results caused by nonpathogenic *Neisseria* spp., such as *N. subflava*, *N. flavescens*, *N. lactamica*, and *N. cinerea* (77). These false-positive assays have been thought to be due to the interspecies genetic recombination potential that occurs among *Neisseria* spp., thus indicating the need for confirmation of positive PCR assays in extragenital specimens and those from low prevalence populations (77).

TABLE 2 Nucleic acid amplification tests for *Neisseria gonorrhoeae*[a]

Assay and specimen	Sensitivity (%)	Specificity (%)
PCR(COBAS)		
Cervical	92.4	99.5
Female urine	64.8	99.8
Male urine	94.1	99.9
Strand displacement amplification		
Cervical	96.6	98.9–99.8
Female urine	84.9	98.8–99.8
Male urine	98.1	96.8–98.7
Male urethral	98.1	96.8–98.7
Transcription-mediated amplification		
Cervical	99.2	98.7
Female urine	91.3	99.3
Male urine	97.1	99.2
Male urethral	98.8	98.2

[a] Percentages indicate comparisons with infected patient status; data from package inserts and clinical trials.

The strand displacement amplification assay (ProbeTec) is approved for detection of gonorrhea in cervical, male urethral, and female and male urine samples and has achieved widespread use in clinical laboratories throughout the United States and Europe (Table 2) (99). The BD ProbeTec ET system has very high sensitivities for gonorrhea in cervical and male urethral specimens and has demonstrated a sensitivity of 97.9% for the detection of gonorrhea in male urine in 680 patients, but it has a somewhat lower sensitivity in female urine (84.9%) (99). This assay has also been demonstrated to produce false positives with nonpathogenic *Neisseria* spp. (77).

TMA (APTIMA Combo2) has been shown to be perhaps the most sensitive assay for gonorrhea (44). It has sensitivities uniformly above 97% for cervical and male urine and urethral samples and well above 91% for female urine (Table 2). This assay has not been shown to produce false-positive results with nonpathogenic neisseriae (49).

Amplified-Signal Probe Test

The amplified-signal probe test employs hybridization of a probe with nucleic acid of the organism and then amplifies the signal of the probe. It is represented by the Digene Hybrid Capture II test (Digene, Silver Spring, Md.), which employs RNA hybridization probes which are specific for both genomic DNA and cryptic plasmid DNA sequences of *N. gonorrhoeae* and *C. trachomatis* (72). The RNA-DNA hybrids are captured in microtiter plate wells by specific antibodies, which are detected by alkaline phosphatase-labeled anti-RNA-DNA hybrid antibodies. The signal is amplified using a chemiluminescent substrate detected by a luminometer. The test is positive if either chlamydia or gonorrhea is present, and then an organism-specific test is performed. It is approved only for cervical samples.

One study reported that the Digene assay was 92.2% sensitive and that the specificity was greater than 99% compared to culture adjudicated by direct fluorescent-antibody (DFA) staining and PCR (32). In another evaluation, compared to *N. gonorrhoeae* culture, it had a sensitivity of 93% (87/94) and a specificity of 98.5% (1,244/1,263) (87).

Additional Considerations for NAATs

Confirmation Tests for NAATs

Because of the potential for false-positive tests in low-prevalence populations, the Centers for Disease Control and Prevention (CDC) has suggested that confirmatory tests should be performed for patients testing positive from populations with a positive predictive value of <90% (26). Suggestions for confirmation include testing a second specimen with a different test using a different target; testing the original specimen with a different test that uses a different target or format; repeating the original test on the original specimen with a blocking antibody or competitive probe; or repeating the original test on the original specimen (26). The requirement for confirmatory testing for positive NAAT results is controversial, and analysis of the particular population under study will influence the decision by a laboratory as to whether to confirm these assays (86). The particular assay in use also plays a role in this decision (49, 86). At present, the only commercial assay with the capability to confirm a positive test with another gene target using the same platform is the Gen-Probe APTIMA assay, with the ACT and AGC stand-alone assays, which can be used to confirm either chlamydia or gonorrhea tests, respectively. These assays are also the only NAATs that are FDA cleared for use with vaginal swabs at present.

Noninvasive Sample Collection and Inhibitors

The ability to detect *N. gonorrhoeae* in noninvasive urine and vaginal samples, avoiding the necessity to obtain an endocervical specimen from women or a urethral swab from men, is an important advantage of NAATs over tests which require invasive specimen collection procedures. However, some specimens contain inherent inhibitors which may result in false-negative results by NAATs. The use of amplification controls in commercial NAATs can indicate when a specimen contains inhibitors by failure of the nonspecific amplification control to be amplified. When inhibition occurs, steps such as heating or dilution can be performed and the test can then be repeated. A discussion of inhibitors in amplification assays can be found on the Association of Public Health Laboratories website (http://www.aphl.org/chlamydia_lab.cfm).

Choice of NAAT and Cost Considerations

Amplified assays are more costly than culture and other detection methods. They have become widely used in clinical microbiology laboratories because of the ability to also test the sample for chlamydia and the ability to test "noninvasive" samples such as urine, as well as the convenience of transport of the sample. Factors that influence whether to choose to perform amplified testing for *N. gonorrhoeae,* as well as which test to choose, include the level of expertise in the laboratory, consideration of costs, training and equipment issues, the population being served, and whether transportation of specimens for culture is a problem. Also a consideration is whether isolates are required for susceptibility testing. The choice of which NAAT to use will also be based on sensitivity and specificity estimates, specimen types being tested (i.e., vaginal, urethral, cervical, or urine), testing that also includes chlamydia, and whether the laboratory wishes to confirm positive NAAT samples (45, 86).

Isolation Procedures

Various selective media allow recovery of *N. gonorrhoeae* from body sites harboring an endogenous bacterial flora. Enriched selective media include modified Thayer-Martin (MTM) medium, Martin-Lewis (ML) medium, GC-Lect medium (BD Biosciences), and New York City (NYC) medium. MTM, ML, and GC-Lect are chocolate agar-based media that are supplemented with additional growth factors, whereas NYC medium is a clear peptone-corn starch agar-based medium containing yeast dialysate, citrated horse plasma, and lysed horse erythrocytes. These media contain antimicrobial agents that inhibit other microorganisms and allow the selective recovery of *N. gonorrhoeae*, *N. meningitidis*, and *N. lactamica*. Vancomycin and colistin, antimicrobials present in all four formulations, inhibit gram-positive and gram-negative bacteria (including saprophytic *Neisseria* species), respectively. Trimethoprim is added to inhibit the swarming of *Proteus* spp. present in rectal and, occasionally, in cervicovaginal specimens. Nystatin (MTM medium), amphotericin B (NYC and GC-Lect media), or anisomycin (ML medium) is added to inhibit yeasts and molds. NYC medium also supports the growth of rapidly growing genital mycoplasmas and ureaplasmas. Media are available in either petri dishes or JEMBEC plates.

Media for the pathogenic *Neisseria* should be at room temperature before inoculation and should not be excessively dry or moist. Swab specimens are rolled in a "Z" pattern on selective medium and cross-streaked with a bacteriologic loop. If nonselective chocolate agar is also inoculated, these plates are streaked for isolation. Plates are incubated in a CO_2 incubator or a candle extinction jar at 35 to 37°C. The CO_2 level of the incubator should be 3 to 7%; higher CO_2 concentrations may inhibit growth of some strains. The atmosphere should be moist; with candle jars, moisture evaporating from the medium during incubation is usually sufficient for organism growth. If candle jars are used, candles should be made of white wax or beeswax; scented or colored candles release volatile products that may inhibit organism growth. CO_2 incubators that are not equipped with humidifiers can be kept moist by placing a pan of water on the lower shelf. Plates are inspected at 24, 48, and 72 h before a final report of "no growth" is issued. Suspect colonies are subcultured to chocolate agar, incubated, and used as inocula for identification procedures.

Presumptive Identification

Colony Morphology

Gonococci produce several colony types that are related to piliation of organisms in the colony. Typical colonies tend to be small (about 0.5 mm in diameter), glistening, and raised. With subculture of individual piliated colonies, the culture can be maintained in this colonial type. With nonselective subculture (i.e., a "sweep" of growth), the other colony types become evident, with all colonies eventually becoming the nonpiliated varieties. These colonies are larger (about 1 mm in diameter) and flatter and do not have the high profile and glistening highlights of piliated colony types. The presence of multiple colony types on a subculture from a primary plate may give the appearance of a mixed culture. Careful scrutiny and subculture with the use of a dissecting microscope (10×)

enable one to become familiar with these colony types. Some *N. gonorrhoeae* strains grow on commercially available sheep blood agar, although growth takes longer and is not as luxuriant as on chocolate agar. However, other strains do not grow on sheep blood agar at all.

Gram Stain and Oxidase Test

Smears prepared from suspicious colonies should be examined with the Gram stain. The Gram stain of organisms from colonial growth should show uniform, characteristic gram-negative diplococci. Some of the organisms may appear as tetrads, particularly on smears prepared from young colonies. Organisms on smears prepared from older cultures may appear swollen and variable in counterstaining intensity, while smears prepared from partially autolyzed colonies may be uninterpretable. Examination by Gram stain is essential for presumptive identification because other organisms may occasionally grow on selective media, particularly when oropharyngeal specimens are cultured (discussed below).

Oxidase test results are obtained with the tetramethyl derivative of the oxidase reagent (*N,N,N,N*-tetramethyl-1,4-phenylenediamine, 1% aqueous solution). A drop of this reagent is placed on a piece of filter paper and a portion of colonial growth is rubbed onto the reagent with a platinum loop, a cotton swab, or a wooden applicator stick. With fresh cultures, a dark purple color will appear on the filter paper within 10 s. Excellent results are obtained with the oxidase reagents that are packaged in crushable glass ampoules (e.g., BACTIDROP Oxidase; Remel, Inc.).

Superoxol Test

Superoxol (30% hydrogen peroxide) is another helpful test for rapid presumptive identification of *N. gonorrhoeae* (84). *N. gonorrhoeae* strains produce immediate, brisk bubbling when the colony material is emulsified with the reagent on a glass slide. Both *N. meningitidis* and *N. lactamica*, the other species that grow on selective media, generally produce weak, delayed bubbling, although some isolates of *N. meningitidis* may also produce immediate, brisk bubbling similar to the gonococcus in this test. Isolates of oxidase-positive, gram-negative diplococci that are recovered from urogenital sites and that grow on selective media may be presumptively identified as *N. gonorrhoeae*. The superoxol test provides an additional presumptive test for identifying these isolates. Confirmatory identification tests are recommended for all isolates and are required for identification of isolates from extragenital sites (i.e., throat, rectum, blood, joint fluid, and cerebrospinal fluid [CSF]).

Differentiation of Other Organisms on Selective Media

Presumptive and confirmatory identification of *N. gonorrhoeae* depends on the ability to differentiate this organism from others that may also grow on selective media. These organisms include *Kingella denitrificans*, *Moraxella catarrhalis*, other *Moraxella* species, *Acinetobacter* species, and *Capnocytophaga* species. *K. denitrificans* grows on MTM medium and produces colony types resembling those of *N. gonorrhoeae*. Whereas gonococci produce vigorous bubbling when colonial growth is immersed in 3% H_2O_2 or in superoxol, *K. denitrificans* produces a negative catalase reaction. *Moraxella* species are both oxidase positive and catalase positive; these organisms can be differentiated from *Neisseria* by the penicillin disk test (21). The organism is subcultured to a Trypticase-soy blood agar plate and streaked to obtain confluent growth. A penicillin susceptibility disk (10 U) is placed on the inoculum, and after overnight incubation in CO_2, a Gram stain is prepared from growth at the edge of the zone of inhibition. *Neisseria* species and *M. catarrhalis* retain their diplococcal morphology, although the cells may appear to be swollen (Fig. 3). Coccobacillary *Moraxella* species and *K. denitrificans* form filaments or spindle-shaped cells under the influence of subinhibitory concentrations of penicillin. *Acinetobacter* spp. can exhibit diplococcal morphology, but these organisms are oxidase negative. *Capnocytophaga* species appear as gram-negative, slightly curved, fusiform bacteria and are oxidase negative and catalase negative. *Capnocytophaga* spp. tend to spread over the agar surface due to gliding motility and may impede recovery of gonococci from oropharyngeal specimens incubated longer than 48 h.

Confirmatory Identification Tests for *Neisseria* Species

Confirmatory tests for *N. gonorrhoeae*, *N. meningitidis*, and other *Neisseria* species include carbohydrate acidification

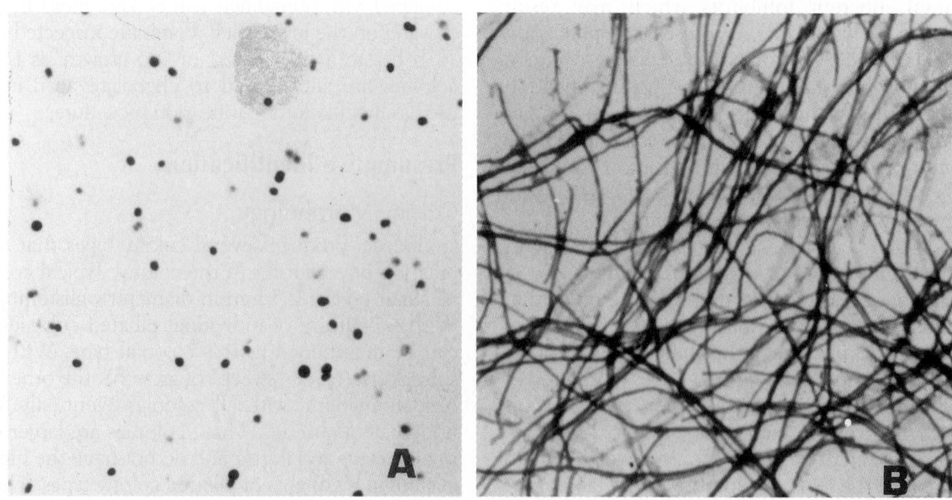

FIGURE 3 Cocci (A) and bacilli (B) exposed to subinhibitory concentrations of penicillin. Some cocci are swollen but still coccoid; bacilli form long strings. Magnification, ×1,000.

tests, chromogenic enzyme substrate tests, immunologic tests (e.g., fluorescent antibody or staphylococcal coagglutination), multitest identification systems, and DNA probe tests. Carbohydrate acidification tests and the multitest identification systems can be used to identify *N. gonorrhoeae*, *N. meningitidis*, and other *Neisseria* species (Table 3). Chromogenic substrate identification procedures are limited to those isolates that grow on selective media (i.e., *N. gonorrhoeae*, *N. meningitidis*, *N. lactamica*, and some strains of *M. catarrhalis*). Fluorescent-antibody, coagglutination, and other immunologic tests and the DNA probe culture confirmation test are available for identification of *N. gonorrhoeae* only. Most nucleic acid hybridization and NAAT procedures are approved for direct detection of *N. gonorrhoeae* in genital tract and urine specimens only.

Acid Production from Carbohydrates

Conventional CTA Carbohydrates

The traditional technique for identification of *Neisseria* species employs cystine-tryptic digest semisolid agar-base (CTA) medium containing 1% carbohydrate and a phenol red pH indicator (2). The usual test battery includes CTA-glucose, -maltose, -sucrose, and -lactose, plus a carbohydrate-free CTA control. The lactose structural analogue, *o*-nitrophenyl-β-D-galactopyranoside (ONPG), may be substituted for the lactose tube, and the addition of CTA-fructose is helpful for identifying the *N. subflava* biovars. Some CTA formulations may be supplemented with ascitic fluid to support growth of more fastidious strains. CTA media are inoculated with a dense suspension of the organism from a pure 18- to 24-h culture on chocolate agar. Either the inoculum is prepared in 0.5 ml of saline and divided among the tubes, or each tube is individually inoculated with a loopful of the organism. The inoculum is restricted to the top 0.5 in. of the agar-deep tubes. The tubes are incubated in a non-CO_2 incubator at 35°C with the caps tightened firmly. With a heavy inoculum, many isolates produce changes in the color of the phenol red indicator within 24 h. Some strains may change the indicator within 4 h, while other gonococcal strains may require 24 to 72 h to produce sufficient acid to change the indicator. Because CTA media containing 1% carbohydrate are used primarily for detection of acid by fermentative organisms, the small amounts of acid produced oxidatively by some strains of *Neisseria* species may not be detected. This method may be problematic for differentiating *N. gonorrhoeae* and *N. cinerea*. Consequently, it is no longer favored for the detection of acid production from carbohydrates. Table 3 shows the carbohydrate acidification profiles and other useful tests for the identification of *Neisseria* spp. recovered from humans.

Rapid Carbohydrate Tests

The rapid carbohydrate test is a non-growth-dependent method for detection of acid production from carbohydrates by *Neisseria* species. Small volumes (0.10 ml) of a balanced salts solution (0.04 g of K_2HPO_4 per liter, 0.01 g of KH_2PO_4 per liter, and 0.80 g of KCl per liter, pH 7.0) with phenol red indicator (0.5 ml of a 1% aqueous solution/liter) are dispensed in nonsterile tubes to which single drops of 20% filter-sterilized aqueous carbohydrates are added. A dense suspension of the organism is prepared in balanced salts solution, and 1 drop of this suspension is added to each of the carbohydrate-containing tubes. Tubes are incubated for 4 h at 35°C in a non-CO_2 incubator or a water bath. This method is economical, the reagents are easy to prepare and inoculate, and the results are clear-cut. The key to this technique is the use of reagent grade carbohydrates. Maltose from some bacteriologic media companies may produce positive or equivocal results for *N. gonorrhoeae* in this procedure, presumably due to the presence of contaminant glucose. Inocula may be obtained from the primary culture if sufficient colonies are present and if the growth is less than 24 h old. Since growth does not occur in the test medium, small numbers of contaminants do not interfere with the 4-h result. However, incubation cannot be continued overnight. The RIM-*Neisseria* Test (Rapid Identification Method-Neisseria; Remel, Inc.), the Gonobio-Test (I.A.F. Production, Inc., Laval, Quebec, Canada), and the Neisseria-Kwik test (MicroBio Logics, St. Cloud, Minn.) are commercial modifications of the rapid carbohydrate utilization test, and evaluations have reported good agreement with conventional methods, although these tests may not provide adequate differentiation between *N. gonorrhoeae* and *N. cinerea* (35, 36).

Chromogenic Enzyme Substrate Tests

Enzymatic identification systems use specific substrates that, after hydrolysis by bacterial enzymes, yield a colored end product that is detected directly or after the addition of a diazo dye-coupling reagent. These tests are used to identify species that are able to grow on selective media—*N. gonorrhoeae*, *N. meningitidis*, and *N. lactamica*. Because some *M. catarrhalis* strains grow on selective media, these systems also provide a presumptive identification of this organism as well. Chromogenic substrate identification tests should not be used to identify organisms recovered on blood and/or chocolate agar without prior subculture of the isolate to selective media. Enzymatic activities that are detected in these systems include β-galactosidase, γ-glutamylaminopeptidase, and prolyl-hydroxyprolyl aminopeptidase. β-Galactosidase and γ-glutamylaminopeptidase are specific for *N. lactamica* and *N. meningitidis*, respectively. The absence of these activities and the presence of prolyl-hydroxyprolyl aminopeptidase identify an organism as *N. gonorrhoeae*. Some *N. meningitidis* strains produce both γ-glutamyl aminopeptidase and prolyl-hydroxyprolyl aminopeptidase. *M. catarrhalis* lacks all three of these enzymatic activities. The Gonochek II (EY Labs, San Mateo, Calif.) is a commercial system that detects all three enzyme activities in a single tube (35). The BactiCard *Neisseria* (Remel, Inc.) uses filter paper pads that are impregnated with substrates for the three enzymes, plus an indoxyl butyrate substrate for identification of *M. catarrhalis* (62). The interpretive guidelines for these tests do not allow for the fact that some nongonococcal neisseria isolates (e.g., *N. subflava* bv. perflava) may be isolated on gonococcal selective media. These species are also prolyl-hydroxyprolyl aminopeptidase positive and may be misidentified as *N. gonorrhoeae* if additional tests are not performed. Recently, gonococcal strains lacking prolyl-hydroxyprolyl aminopeptidase have been isolated in Denmark and the United Kingdom (2, 42).

Immunologic Methods for Culture Confirmation

Direct Fluorescent Monoclonal Antibody Test

The DFA culture confirmation procedure uses monoclonal antibodies that recognize epitopes on the PorI (Protein I) outer membrane protein (OMP) of *N. gonorrhoeae*. The DFA test (*Neisseria gonorrhoeae* Culture Confirmation Test; Trinity Biotech, Wicklow, Ireland) is performed by preparing a smear on a DFA slide, overlaying the smear with DFA reagent, and incubating the smear for 15 min. After rinsing and mounting, the slide is examined with a fluorescence microscope. Gonococci appear as apple-green fluorescent

TABLE 3 Characteristics of *Neisseria* species of human origin[a]

Species	Colony morphology on chocolate agar	Growth on:			Acid from:					Reduction of NO_3	Polysaccharide from SUC
		MTM, ML, and NYC media (35°C)	Chocolate or blood agar (22°C)	Nutrient agar (35°C)	GLU	MAL	LAC	SUC	FRU		
N. gonorrhoeae[b]	Beige to gray-brown, translucent, smooth, 0.5–1 mm in diameter	+	0	0	+	0	0	0	0	0	0
N. meningitidis	Beige to gray-brown, translucent, smooth, 1–3 mm in diameter	+	0	V	+	+	0	0	0	0	0
N. lactamica	Beige to gray-brown, translucent, smooth, 1–2 mm in diameter	+	V	+	+	+	+	0	0	0	0
N. cinerea[c]	Beige to gray-brown to yellowish, translucent, smooth, 1–2 mm in diameter	V	0	+	0	0	0	0	0	0	0
N. polysaccharea	Beige to gray-brown to yellow, translucent, smooth, 1–2 mm in diameter	V	+	+	+	+	0	V	0	0	+
N. subflava[d]	Greenish, yellow, opaque, 1–3 mm in diameter, smooth to rough, sometimes adherent	V	+	+	+	+	0	V	V	0	V
N. sicca	White, opaque, 1–3 mm in diameter, adherent, wrinkled with age	0	+	+	+	+	0	+	+	0	+
N. mucosa	Greenish yellow, opaque, 1–3 mm in diameter	0	+	+	+	+	0	+	+	+	+
N. flavescens	Yellow, opaque, 1–2 mm in diameter	0	+	+	0	0	0	0	0	0	+
N. elongata[e]	Gray-brown, translucent, smooth, 1–2 mm in diameter, glistening, dry, claylike consistency	0	+	+	0	0	0	0	0	0	0

[a] Symbols and abbreviations: +, strains typically positive but genetic mutants may be negative; V, strain dependent; 0, negative; GLU, glucose; MAL, maltose; LAC, lactose; SUC, sucrose; FRU, fructose.

[b] *N. kochii* is considered to be a subspecies of *N. gonorrhoeae;* isolates of *N. kochii* exhibit characteristics of both *N. gonorrhoeae* and *N. meningitidis*, but are identified as *N. gonorrhoeae* by tests routinely used for identification of *Neisseria* spp.

[c] Some strains grow on selective media.

[d] Includes biovars subflava, flava, and perflava. *N. subflava* bv. perflava strains produce acid from sucrose and fructose and produce polysaccharide from sucrose; *N. subflava* bv. flava strains produce acid from fructose; *N. subflava* bv. subflava strains do not produce polysaccharide from sucrose.

[e] Rod-shaped organism. The catalase test is weakly positive or negative compared with those of other *Neisseria* spp. (catalase positive). Results in the table are for *N. elongata* subsp. *elongata*. Strains of *N. elongata* subsp. *glycolytica* may produce a weak acid reaction from D-glucose, are catalase positive, and do not reduce nitrate but do reduce nitrite. Strains of *N. elongata* subsp. *nitroreducens* (formerly CDC group M-6) may produce a weak acid reaction from D-glucose, are catalase negative, and reduce both nitrate and nitrite.

diplococci. The currently available kit is the same product that was developed and marketed by Syva in 1986. At that time, the DFA reagent was highly sensitive and specific; however, at present, many strains of *N. gonorrhoeae* fail to stain with this reagent (63). Serotyping and pulsed-field gel electrophoresis (PFGE) data indicate that gonococcal strains that are negative with the DFA reagent belong to a variety of serovars (17, 63). Since the monoclonal antibody cocktail used in this product has not been modified since 1986, package insert claims of 99.6% sensitivity and 100% specificity are no longer valid. Therefore, isolates that do not stain with the DFA reagent must be identified by another method. This limits the advantages of the DFA procedure, which included its rapidity, ability to test colonies directly from primary cultures, and the small amount of growth required for test performance. The DFA test is not intended for direct identification of organisms in smears from patient specimens.

Coagglutination Tests

Two coagglutination tests for the identification of *N. gonorrhoeae* are currently available: the Phadebact Monoclonal GC test (Boule Diagnostics AB, Huddinge, Sweden) and the GonoGen I (New Horizons Diagnostics, Columbia, Md.). The Phadebact Monoclonal GC test uses anti-PorI monoclonal antibodies bound to staphylococcal cells. Unlike the GC OMNI test previously marketed by Boule Diagnostics, this monoclonal GC test contains one reagent that reacts with serogroup WI *N. gonorrhoeae* strains and a second reagent that reacts with serogroup WII/WIII strains. Since a negative control reagent is not included, gonococcal isolates react with either the WI or the WII/WIII reagent, depending on the PorI epitopes expressed by an individual isolate. A suspension (0.5 McFarland standard) prepared in buffered saline (pH 7.2 to 7.4) is boiled and mixed with the two test reagents on a cardboard slide. Agglutination within 1 min is a positive test. Freshly subcultured serogroup WI (ATCC 19424) and serogroup WII/III (ATCC 23051) strains are recommended for quality control but are not provided with the kit. The GonoGen I coagglutination test also uses staphylococcal cells coated with anti-PorI monoclonal antibodies. This test kit contains test and control coagglutination reagents, and positive and negative test control suspensions are also included. GonoGen I also uses a boiled organism suspension (McFarland standard of 3) for testing, and agglutination with the test but not the control reagent constitutes a positive test. Attention to procedural details is necessary to prevent false-positive and false-negative results with these coagglutination tests. Some gonococci may not react with these reagents, and cross-reactions with other *Neisseria* species (i.e., *N. meningitidis*, *N. lactamica*, and *N. cinerea*) and *K. denitrificans* have been reported (2, 35, 63).

GonoGen II

GonoGen II (New Horizons Diagnostics) uses anti-PorI monoclonal antibodies conjugated to red-colored metal sol particles as the detection reagent. Colonies from agar medium are suspended in a solubilizing buffer that releases PorI-antigen-containing complexes from the cell wall. A drop of the antibody-sol particles is added, and the PorI antigen binds to the antibody-sol particles. After 5 min, 2 drops of this mixture are passed through a membrane filter that retains antigen-antibody complexes. Concentration of these complexes on the filter turns the filter red, identifying the organism as *N. gonorrhoeae*. Nongonococcal isolates do not produce these, so the entire suspension passes through the filter, resulting in the filter remaining white or pale pink. *N. gonorrhoeae* strains that do not react with the conjugate are not identified, and false-positive reactions have been noted with some *N. meningitidis* and *N. lactamica* strains (3, 63).

Multitest Identification Systems

Kit systems that identify *Neisseria* spp., *Haemophilus* spp., and other fastidious gram-negative organisms are available. These systems are the RapID NH *(Neisseria-Haemophilus)* (Remel, Inc.), the Vitek NHI (*Neisseria-Haemophilus* Identification) card (bioMerieux, Inc., Hazelwood, Mo.), the *Haemophilus-Neisseria* identification (HNID) panel (Dade Behring, Sacramento, Calif.), and the API NH (bioMerieux, Inc., La Balme-les-Grottes, France) (2, 10, 60, 61). These kits use modified conventional tests and chromogenic substrates to provide identifications within 2 to 4 h. The NHI card identifies the pathogenic *Neisseria* spp., *N. lactamica*, and *N. cinerea* (61). At present, a new NHI card is being developed for use with the Vitek-2 instrument. *N. cinerea* is not included in the database of the MicroScan HNID panel, resulting in misidentifications as *N. gonorrhoeae* or *M. catarrhalis*, and some *N. meningitidis* strains do not produce clear-cut reactions with key tests (60). RapID NH includes tests that enable identification of the pathogenic *Neisseria* and *N. cinerea* (2). The API NH system identifies gonococci, meningococci, and *N. lactamica* within 2 h; other *Neisseria* species required additional tests for correct species identification (2, 10).

DNA Probe Test for Culture Confirmation

The Accuprobe *Neisseria gonorrhoeae* Culture Confirmation Test (Gen Probe) identifies *N. gonorrhoeae* by the detection of species-specific rRNA sequences. Organisms from agar medium are lysed and mixed with a chemiluminescent acridinium ester-labeled single-stranded DNA probe that is complementary to gonococcal rRNA. DNA probe/rRNA hybrids are selected by a chemical process, and the presence of the probe is detected by hydrolysis of the acridinium ester and the consequent release of light energy. This energy is detected by a chemiluminometer and reported in relative light units. The Accuprobe test is more sensitive and specific than biochemical or immunologic culture confirmation tests and is particularly useful for confirming problem isolates (63).

NAATs

Theoretically, any of the FDA-cleared NAATs could be used to confirm the identification of an isolate from a culture. However, this particular use of the tests is not cleared by the FDA.

Typing Systems

Phenotypic and genotypic typing methods are used to differentiate between strains of *N. gonorrhoeae*. The specific characteristics chosen depend on the question(s) being asked. Antimicrobial resistance is frequently the subject of investigation or surveillance. Using the CLSI-approved method, susceptibilities to several agents are determined (i.e., penicillin, tetracycline, spectinomycin, an extended-spectrum cephalosporin [ceftriaxone or cefixime], a fluoroquinolone [ciprofloxacin or ofloxacin], and a macrolide [erythromycin or azithromycin]), and results are interpreted according to CLSI breakpoints (31, 73). Gonococcal strains are usually described by their pattern of penicillin-tetracycline susceptibilities (penicillin-tetracycline resistance phenotype) (79). Penicillin-tetracycline resistance phenotypes include penicillin resistant (PenR), tetracycline resistant (TetR), chromosomally mediated resistance to penicillin and tetracycline (CMRNG), β-lactamase-positive (PPNG), plasmid-mediated resistance to tetracycline (TRNG), strains with plasmid-mediated resistance to both penicillin and tetracycline (PP/TR), and isolates susceptible to both penicillin and tetracycline (Susc.) (104). PPNG and TRNG isolates may exhibit chromosomally mediated resistance to tetracycline (PPNG, TetR) and penicillin (TRNG, PenR), respectively. Intermediate resistance or resistance to other antimicrobial agents is appended to the penicillin-tetracycline resistance phenotype. For example, a PPNG isolate exhibiting resistance to ciprofloxacin (CipR) would be designated PPNG, CipR.

Phenotypic characterization also includes the determination of requirements for growth using a chemically defined medium (auxotyping) and serotyping with a panel of 12 monoclonal antibodies in coagglutination tests to define serovars (85). Strains have been classified with a dual auxotype-serovar system to provide greater discrimination among strains than is possible with either typing system alone. Auxotyping involves determining growth requirements of individual strains for discrete metabolites on a chemically defined medium. For example, if a strain does not grow on a medium from which arginine has been omitted, the strain is recorded as requiring arginine. Strains with single or multiple growth requirements may be identified. Serotyping is performed with a panel of monoclonal antibody coagglutination reagents directed against epitopes on the PorI (protein I) molecule in the gonococcal outer membrane (85). Strains are divided into two major serogroups, serogroups IA and IB, based on the protein I species expressed by the strain; subdivision into serovars is then made according to the reactions observed with a panel of six protein IA- and six protein IB-specific antibody reagents. These typing methods are used to compare isolates in epidemiologic investigations, including studies on the dynamics of gonococcal strains in communities and the geographic spread of resistant strains, and for comparisons between strains for medicolegal investigations (85).

Gonococcal isolates may also be characterized by additional characteristics related to antimicrobial resistance. At least six different β-lactamase plasmids have been described in the gonococcus; these as well as two conjugative plasmids (one possessing a *tet*M determinant) have also been used to study the distribution of gonococcal strains (85). Strains possessing the *tet*M determinant may, with PCR-based tests, be assigned to one of two types: American or Dutch (58). Mutations in the *gyrA* and *parC* genes in strains exhibiting decreased susceptibilities to fluoroquinolones may also be characterized (33).

Molecular typing methods that characterize either specific genes or the entire chromosome have been used more recently to differentiate gonococcal isolates. With older methods, such as PFGE and restriction endonuclease analysis, the chromosome is digested into fragments with restriction enzymes that are resolved in polyacrylamide gels. Restriction endonuclease typing permitted differentiation among isolates belonging to the same serovar; however, restriction patterns are complex and are sometimes difficult to interpret. PFGE is tedious to perform and results in large fragments of DNA that are difficult to separate on conventional gels.

Recently developed typing methods involve amplification and restriction typing of individual genes or gene clusters. The Lip typing system permits the grouping of gonococcal isolates based on the number and sequence of pentamer amino acid repeats within the *lip* gene (94). Opa typing is based on identifying the restriction patterns of a family of 11 distinct and highly variable *opa* genes to give an *opa*-type (75). One disadvantage of the Opa typing system is that new types may evolve very rapidly, resulting in every isolate having a different type unless it is from a sexual partner or a short chain of sexual partners (75). A system for typing the variable regions of the *porB* gene using oligonucleotide probes has also been developed (93). This system can detect differences in *porB* among isolates belonging to the same serovar; however, this method requires the use of different hybridization conditions for individual probes. Real-time PCR amplification of the *porB* gene followed by pyrosequence analysis of highly polymorphic segments of the *porB1a* or *porB1b* alleles has been reported to provide a rapid, highly discriminatory approach to typing gonococcal isolates (96). *PorB* genotyping using probes or sequencing has been used along with amplification and sequence analysis of other genes (e.g., *gyrA* and *parC*) to characterize isolates with acquired resistance to antimicrobial agents used for the treatment of gonococcal infections (47). Use of molecular methods for detection of antimicrobial resistance may provide a molecular approach to surveillance whereby strain variation and dissemination of antimicrobial resistance can be monitored.

In addition, two typing methods that characterize the entire chromosome are based on amplification fragment length polymorphism analysis. These methods use different restriction enzymes to digest the DNA (76, 91). The fluorescent amplification fragment length polymorphism approach has the same discriminatory power as the Opa typing system but is more stable than the latter system (76).

Antimicrobial Susceptibilities

Resistance of *N. gonorrhoeae* to antimicrobial agents is a major problem in the control of gonorrhea. Resistance occurs both as chromosomally mediated resistance to a variety of antibiotics and plasmid-mediated resistance to penicillins (penicillinase [β-lactamase]-producing) and to tetracycline (tetracycline-resistant *N. gonorrhoeae*). The Centers for Disease Control and Prevention (CDC) recommended the use of fluoroquinolones or broad-spectrum cephalosporins for the treatment of gonorrhea (28). Now, however, because of the emergence of resistance to fluoroquinolones (primarily ciprofloxacin and ofloxacin) (66), the CDC now recommends that if symptoms persist after treatment with one of the recommended therapies, patients should be reevaluated for *N. gonorrhoeae* infection by culture and the susceptibilities of any resulting gonococcal isolate should be determined (27). Strains with clinically significant resistance to fluoroquinolones, failure to respond to 500 mg of ciprofloxacin or 400 mg of ofloxacin, or MIC of ciprofloxacin $\geq$1.0 μg/ml or MIC of ofloxacin $\geq$2.0 μg/ml are now widespread in the Far East and have been isolated from a number of cities in the United States, the United Kingdom, Australia, and Canada (23, 24, 66).

The Gonococcal Isolate Surveillance Project (GISP) in 24 to 26 sentinel sites in the United States was implemented by the CDC to monitor changes in antimicrobial susceptibilities in *N. gonorrhoeae* on a monthly basis, but this project monitors only males and only approximately 3% of gonococcal isolates (24). A similar program was established by the World Health Organization and is called GASP (Gonococcal Antimicrobial Surveillance Program) (104). The GISP tests susceptibility to penicillin, tetracycline, spectinomycin, ceftriaxone, cefixime, ciprofloxacin, and azithromycin, and the results are published annually (24). Antimicrobial resistance patterns for *N. gonorrhoeae* vary geographically within the United States, and conducting local antimicrobial susceptibility studies can provide a more accurate assessment with which to judge appropriate treatment recommendations.

Susceptibilities of gonococcal isolates can be determined by an agar dilution method, either on antibiotic-containing media, the E test, or by a disk diffusion method recommended by the Clinical Laboratory Standards Institute (CLSI), formerly NCCLS (73). Susceptibilities to penicillin, tetracycline, spectinomycin, an extended-spectrum cephalosporin, a fluoroquinolone, and azithromycin should be determined for surveillance purposes.

Azithromycin is not presently recommended for the routine treatment of uncomplicated gonococcal infections, although it may be used for the treatment of gonorrhea in geographic areas where fluoroquinolone-resistant isolates are prevalent and if spectinomycin is not available. The 2-g dose as cleared by the FDA should be used and not the 1-g dose recommended for the primary treatment of chlamydial infections (53). However, one recent report that studied the efficacy of a 1-g dose found only one failure of the 1-g therapy among 226 gonorrhea-infected patients in the United Kingdom (50).

With increasing testing for gonorrhea being performed by NAATs, monitoring of resistance has become more difficult. However, as understanding of molecular mechanisms of resistance increases, it may be possible in the future to determine antimicrobial resistance by using molecular techniques on specimens submitted for NAATs (47, 98, 106). Since worldwide resistance to fluoroquinolones (QRNG) has increased dramatically, there is an increased need to monitor susceptibility trends in different geographical areas and for different population types; and there is a great need for additional single-dose antibiotic regimes in order to control gonorrhea (46). Resistance in *N. gonorrhoeae* and QRNG has been reviewed (46, 106). Data from California indicated that as of 2003, the rate of QRNG had risen from <1% in 1999 to 20.2% in the last half of 2003 (14). The emergence and spread of QRNG seemingly has evolved from sporadic cases to endemic transmission among heterosexuals and particularly among MSM (14).

Culture remains the only test that can be used to identify *N. gonorrhoeae* for legal purposes and for the performance of susceptibility tests. As such, maintaining the ability to perform culture in local areas is an essential component of gonorrhea control programs.

Evaluation, Interpretation, and Reporting of Results

The level of testing and the format for reporting of results should be directed by the sociodemographic characteristics (e.g., age and gender) of the patient clientele served and a knowledge of the incidence and prevalence of clinically significant disease caused by *Neisseria* species, e.g., gonorrhea, in that population. When specimens are collected from patients at high risk for gonorrhea and there are no sociologic or medicolegal implications of a diagnosis of gonorrhea, a presumptive identification of *N. gonorrhoeae* may be sufficient if the diagnosis is intended to facilitate prompt and effective treatment. However, when specimens are collected to confirm a clinical diagnosis for patients such as women and children at low risk for gonorrhea, special concerns apply to laboratory processing and retention of specimens because of the medicolegal consequences that may ensue if an organism is identified as *N. gonorrhoeae*.

Special protocols should be developed for processing specimens from alleged victims of sexual abuse and assault. Suspect gonococci isolated from children must be confirmed by at least two different methods that involve different principles (3). Tests may include carbohydrate utilization, immunologic methods, enzymatic procedures, or the DNA probe culture confirmation test (see below). Of these, tests which detect acid production from glucose and the probe confirmation test provide the least equivocal results. Nongonococcal isolates may cross-react in coagglutination tests, and gonococcal isolates may not react in the monoclonal immunofluorescence test (63). Nongonococcal isolates may produce positive prolyl-hydroxyprolyl aminopeptidase reactions in enzyme substrate tests, as do gonococcal isolates. Therefore, communication between the clinician and the laboratory is essential to ensure that specimens of medicolegal importance are processed according to these criteria.

In general, with the exception of high-risk patients for whom presumptive identifications may suffice, similar principles apply to the identification of all gram-negative, oxidase-positive diplococci. Although many tests for identification of *Neisseria* and related species are marketed as confirmatory tests, most do not provide sufficient data to accurately identify an isolate to the species level without additional tests. Some different isolates may produce identical reactions with some tests, e.g., maltose-negative *N. meningitidis* and *K. denitrificans* may give reactions identical to those of *N. gonorrhoeae* in acid production tests. In addition, problems have been identified with most tests for the identification of *N. gonorrhoeae* and related species, e.g., false-negative acid production reactions from glucose with *N. gonorrhoeae* or false-positive reactions for glucose acidification with *N. cinerea*.

Culture confirmation tests are preferred for the identification of *Neisseria* and related species because they require the isolation of an organism which can be examined by multiple tests if the results of the primary tests are equivocal. Multitest identification systems provide the most information about biochemical characteristics that may, in some cases, allow the identification of an isolate. Rapid identification tests, including serologic and nucleic acid probe or amplification tests, that provide a "yes-no" answer, i.e., an isolate either is or is not *N. gonorrhoeae*, may be adequate if it is necessary only to eliminate *N. gonorrhoeae* as the causative agent; these tests are of limited usefulness when identification to the species level is required.

Because of the consequences of misdiagnosing gonorrhea or misidentifying strains of *N. gonorrhoeae*, three levels are recommended for reporting diagnoses of gonorrhea. These levels are "suggestive," which is defined on the basis of clinical findings, "presumptive," and "definitive," with the last two levels including the results of laboratory tests. A suggestive diagnosis is defined by (i) the presence of a mucopurulent endocervical or urethral exudate on physical examination and (ii) sexual exposure to a person infected with *N. gonorrhoeae*. A presumptive diagnosis of gonorrhea is made on the basis of two of the following three criteria: (i) typical gram-negative intracellular diplococci on microscopic examination of a smear of urethral exudate (men) or endocervical secretions (women); (ii) growth of *N. gonorrhoeae* from the urethra (men) or endocervix (women) on culture media and demonstration of typical colonial morphology, positive oxidase reaction, and typical gram-negative morphology; and/or (iii) detection of *N. gonorrhoeae* by nonculture tests (e.g., antigen detection, nucleic acid probe tests, or NAATs). Definitive diagnosis requires (i) isolation of *N. gonorrhoeae* from sites of exposure (e.g., urethra, endocervix, throat, or rectum) by culture (usually on a selective medium) and demonstration of typical colonial morphology, positive oxidase reaction, and typical gram-negative morphology; and (ii) confirmation by biochemical, enzymatic, serologic, or nucleic acid tests, e.g., carbohydrate utilization, rapid enzyme substrate tests, serologic methods, or the DNA probe culture confirmation test.

For reporting purposes, the laboratory should perform species level identification and confirmation with appropriate tests in order to report a definitive result of "*N. gonorrhoeae* confirmed" for the clinician unless otherwise requested. If an organism suspected to be *N. gonorrhoeae* is tested by rapid tests but not by additional confirmatory tests that compensate for problems associated with the primary test and is reported as "presumptive *N. gonorrhoeae*," it is important that the clinician understands that additional tests may be required to confirm this identification. Ideally, to avoid confusion, an organism should be reported only as "gram-negative, oxidase-positive diplococcus isolated" unless it has been identified to the species level with sufficient tests to ensure the accuracy of the identification.

NEISSERIA MENINGITIDIS

Collection, Transport, and Storage of Specimens

Specimens helpful in the diagnosis of meningococcal disease include CSF, blood, aspirates, biopsy specimens, and nasopharyngeal and oropharyngeal swabs (Table 1). Occasionally, meningococci may be sought in sputum and bronchoalveolar lavage specimens. Genital, rectal, and oropharyngeal isolates of *N. meningitidis* may be recovered using the collection and inoculation procedures described for *N. gonorrhoeae*. Incubation conditions for inoculated media are the same as those described for *N. gonorrhoeae*. Meningococci grow well on all selective media for the pathogenic neisseriae, and vancomycin-susceptible strains have not been described. Recovery of both gonococci and meningococci from blood cultures may be adversely affected by the anticoagulant sodium polyanethol sulfonate that is present in blood culture media. This effect may be neutralized by addition of sterile gelatin (1% final concentration) to the media or by processing the blood specimen by lysis-centrifugation (i.e., Isolator, Wampole Laboratories, Cranbury, N.J.).

Laboratory Safety

N. meningitidis is classified as a biosafety level 2 organism, which means that a biological safety cabinet should be used for the manipulation of specimens that have a substantial risk for the generation of aerosols (e.g., centrifuging, grinding, and blending). Reports of laboratory-acquired meningococcal infections suggest, however, that manipulation of cultures, rather than patient specimens, increases the risk of infection for microbiology laboratory technologists (22, 25). Such manipulations may include the preparation of heavy organism suspensions for inoculation of identification systems and for serogrouping of isolates. Use of a biological safety cabinet when manipulating cultures for these purposes helps to provide protection of the laboratorian from aerosolized organisms. Alternative measures for protection from droplet aerosols, such as the use of splash guards and masks, are currently being assessed. Education and adherence to established laboratory safety precautions should minimize the risk of meningococcal infection for workers in the clinical microbiology laboratory. Laboratory policies should also be developed for situations that may require administration of chemoprophylaxis to employees who are exposed to meningococci. Laboratories may also consider offering the quadrivalent meningococcal vaccine (which includes serogroups A, C, Y, and W135) to microbiology laboratory staff. Vaccination would decrease, but not eliminate, the potential risk of laboratory-acquired infections.

Direct Examination

Microscopy

A presumptive diagnosis of meningococcal meningitis can be made by direct examination of CSF, using the Gram stain. If sufficient (i.e., more than 1 to 2 ml) CSF is received, the specimen should be centrifuged to obtain a pellet of material for examination and culture. Cytocentrifugation of CSF specimens enhances detection of small numbers of organisms and increases the sensitivity of the Gram stain in comparison with conventionally centrifuged or uncentrifuged specimens. On Gram-stained smears prepared from clinical specimens, meningococci appear as Gram-negative diplococci both inside and outside PMNs. Organisms may display considerable size variation and tend to resist decolorization. Heavily encapsulated strains may have a distinct pink halo around the cells. Because the presence of inflammatory cells has prognostic value (e.g., with fulminant, rapidly fatal disease, many organisms and few inflammatory cells are present), the Gram stain report to the physician should include quantitation of both organisms and PMNs.

Antigen Detection

Direct tests for detection of meningococcal capsular polysaccharides in CSF, serum, and urine are also available. Direct antigen tests use antibody-sensitized latex agglutination or coagglutination to detect capsular antigens of meningococcal serogroups A, B, C, Y, and W135. The serogroup B reagent also detects the cross-reacting *Escherichia coli* K1 antigen. These reagents are available from several vendors (BD Biosciences for latex tests; Boule Diagnostics AB for coagglutination tests). A negative test does not rule out meningitis, and false-positive latex agglutination tests may occur, particularly with urine specimens. Due to the enhanced sensitivity of the Gram stain provided by specimen cytocentrifugation and the problems with the specificity of the antigen detection assays, most laboratories in the United States no longer perform these tests routinely and they are not recommended.

Nucleic Acid Detection Techniques

Molecular methods for direct detection of *N. meningitidis* in clinical specimens are not currently available.

Isolation Procedures

For recovery of *N. meningitidis*, CSF specimens should be inoculated onto nonselective chocolate agar and sheep blood agar. Specimens that may harbor other organisms (e.g., oropharyngeal and nasopharyngeal swab specimens) should be inoculated onto both selective and nonselective media. Plates are incubated in 5 to 7% CO_2 at 35°C (CO_2 incubator or candle extinction jar) and inspected after 24, 48, and 72 h before a final report of "no growth" is issued. Suspicious colonies are subcultured to blood and chocolate agar for further identification.

Identification

Colony Morphology

Colonies of *N. meningitidis* are larger than gonococcal colonies, usually attaining a diameter of about 1 mm or more after 18 to 24 h of incubation. Colonies are low and convex, with a smooth, moist entire edge and a glistening surface. On sheep blood agar, colonies are usually gray; heavily encapsulated strains may be mucoid. The medium beneath and adjacent to the colonies may exhibit a gray-green cast, particularly in areas of confluent growth. Young cultures have a smooth consistency, while older cultures become gummy due to autolysis.

Identification Procedures

N. meningitidis is identified by acid production tests or by chromogenic enzyme substrate tests. Identification procedures for meningococci produce the best results when inoculated from fresh 18- to 24-h subcultures on chocolate or blood agar. *N. meningitidis* acidifies glucose and maltose, but not sucrose, fructose, or lactose (Table 3). Isolates recovered on selective media can be identified with chromogenic enzyme substrate tests. *N. meningitidis* strains produce γ-glutamyl aminopeptidase; some strains also produce prolyl-hydroxyprolyl aminopeptidase. Glucose-negative, maltose-negative, and asaccharolytic *N. meningitidis* strains may also be isolated occasionally. For these isolates, chromogenic substrate confirmatory tests or serogrouping should be performed.

Serogrouping and Typing

Slide agglutination is commonly used for serogrouping meningococci. A dense suspension of the organism is prepared in 0.5 to 1.0 ml of phosphate-buffered saline (pH 7.2) from a 12- to 18-h subculture on Trypticase-soy blood agar. One drop of this suspension is mixed with 1 drop of meningococcal antisera on a sectored slide, and the slide is rotated for 2 to 4 min. Groupable strains agglutinate strongly within this time. Although isolates from systemic infections usually agglutinate rapidly, those from carriers may fail to agglutinate (nongroupable strains) or may autoagglutinate in saline. Use of younger cultures from blood agar (6 to 8 h) or use of a serum-enriched medium, such as Trypticase-soy agar containing 10% decomplemented horse serum, may resolve these problems. Antisera for the major meningococcal serogroups are available from BD Biosciences. Some nongroupable strains may actually be *N. polysaccharea;* testing for production of polysaccharide from sucrose helps identify this species (see below) (18).

N. meningitidis isolates may be serotyped and subserotyped based on OMP and lipooligosaccharide antigens (95). Meningococcal isolates can be subdivided into 20 serotypes based on class 2 and 3 OMP or PorB antigens, 10 serosubtypes based on class 1 OMP (PorA) antigens, and 13 immunotypes based on lipooligosaccharide antigens. Multilocus isoenzyme electrophoresis typing and multilocus sequence typing have been used to identify genetically defined clonal groups responsible for both epidemic and sporadic, endemic disease. Meningococcal serogroup antigen gene sequencing by sialytransferase gene PCR can be used to confirm serologic grouping results and to determine the genetic grouping of serologically "nongroupable" strains (19). Other molecular methods, including DNA fingerprinting, restriction fragment length polymorphisms, PFGE, ribotyping, repetitive element-based PCR, random-amplified PCR, *porA* gene sequencing, and PCR-amplicon endonuclease analysis, have also been developed for monitoring the epidemiology of pathogenic *N. meningitidis* locally and globally (13, 80, 103).

Antimicrobial Susceptibilities

Despite the occasional recovery of *N. meningitidis* strains with decreased susceptibility to penicillin, penicillin G remains the drug of choice for treatment of meningococcal meningitis. Several broad-spectrum cephalosporins reach therapeutic levels in CSF and are also recommended treatment options. Patients may also require intensive supportive care and monitoring for detection of complications and disease progression (100). Other biological agents (e.g., antiendotoxin and anticytokine monoclonal antibodies) may also play important roles as adjunctive therapies in the management of meningococcal septic shock.

As in the gonococcus, the antimicrobial susceptibility of *N. meningitidis* strains is also evolving (83). Historically, penicillin-susceptible strains of *N. meningitidis* have penicillin MICs of ≤0.06 μg/ml. Rare β-lactamase-producing meningococcal isolates have been encountered sporadically since 1983 in Canada, South Africa, and Spain; these isolates have penicillin MICs of >256 μg/ml. Since 1987, β-lactamase-negative *N. meningitidis* strains with penicillin MICs of >0.06 μ/ml have been isolated in the United Kingdom, Europe, Greece, South America, South Africa, Asia, and the United States (83). These strains are referred to as being relatively resistant to penicillin, being moderately susceptible to penicillin, and having diminished susceptibility to penicillin. Strains with decreased susceptibility to penicillin have MICs ranging from 0.10 to 1.0 μg/ml, and resistant strains are defined as having penicillin MICs of ≥2 μg/ml. Diminished penicillin susceptibility is due to decreased binding of penicillin by altered meningococcal cell wall penicillin-binding proteins (PBP 2 and PBP 3). In the case of the PBP 2 proteins, decreased binding of penicillin to the altered binding protein results from a mutation in the nucleotide sequence of the PBP 2 gene, *penA*. Similar low-affinity forms of PBP 2 are found in penicillin-resistant strains of *N. lactamica*, *N. flavescens*, *N. polysaccharea*, and *N. gonorrhoeae* (20). The altered PBP 2 found in these *N. meningitidis* strains apparently arose from recombinational events that resulted in replacement of nucleotide sequences in the native meningococcal *penA* gene with corresponding genetic material from the commensal *Neisseria* species.

The clinical significance of diminished penicillin susceptibility in *N. meningitidis* is unclear at present. Although both treatment failures and higher rates of complications have been observed in patients infected with relatively resistant strains, the administration of higher doses of penicillin has been clinically effective. Broad-spectrum cephalosporins, such as ceftriaxone and cefotaxime, are active against both susceptible and moderately susceptible *N. meningitidis* strains, but MICs for some agents (e.g., cefuroxime, aztreonam, and imipenem) may be significantly higher than those of susceptible strains (78).

N. meningitidis strains may also demonstrate resistance to other antimicrobial agents (64). High-level chloramphenicol resistance due to production of chloramphenicol acetyltransferase has been reported in isolates from France and Vietnam. High-level resistance to sulfonamides, including trimethoprim-sulfamethoxazole, is widespread. Rifampin resistance has also emerged, even during the administration of rifampin prophylaxis, and is due to alterations in cell membrane permeability or to mutations in the *rpoB* gene coding for the β-subunit of the meningococcal RNA polymerase. In 2000, an *N. meningitidis* strain with decreased susceptibility to ciprofloxacin (MIC of 0.25 μg/ml) was isolated from a patient with invasive meningococcal disease in Australia (88). Susceptible strains have ciprofloxacin MICs of ≤0.03 μg/ml. Finally, some *N. meningitidis* strains have acquired the *tetM* tetracycline resistance determinant. Resistance to the extended-spectrum cephalosporins that may be used for treatment in developed countries has not been described.

For antimicrobial susceptibility testing of *N. meningitidis* isolates, MIC determinations are the methods of choice. Disk diffusion tests with penicillin, ampicillin, and rifampin for *N. meningitidis* are unreliable. The CLSI recommends either broth microdilution or agar dilution MIC testing of *N. meningitidis* using cation-adjusted Mueller-Hinton broth supplemented with 2 to 5% lysed horse blood or Mueller-Hinton agar with 5% (vol/vol) defibrinated sheep blood, respectively (31). For optimal growth of some *N. meningitidis* strains, this medium may require supplementation with IsoVitalex (1%) (BD Biosciences) or GCHI enrichment (Remel, Inc.). The E test may also be valuable for determining the antimicrobial susceptibility of individual meningococcal isolates. Since most clinical microbiology laboratories are not equipped to perform agar dilution tests, isolates from patients who are not responding to appropriate antimicrobial chemotherapy and any presumptively penicillin-resistant isolates should be tested for β-lactamase production with the chromogenic cephalosporin test (Cefinase nitrocefin disks; BD Biosciences) and forwarded to a reference laboratory for agar or broth dilution susceptibility testing.

Evaluation, Interpretation, and Reporting

Meningococci are isolated most frequently from the oro- or nasopharynges of asymptomatic carriers along with other normal flora. *N. meningitidis* isolated from throat cultures should not be reported, since reporting implies that the organism is behaving as a pathogen and requires treatment. Meningococci from oropharyngeal cultures represent carriage strains. Meningococcal carriage may be transient, intermittent, or chronic, and carriage alone is not predictive of the development of life-threatening disease (105). While chemoprophylaxis with rifampin, ciprofloxacin, or ceftriaxone is recommended for close contacts of individuals with severe disease, treatment of meningococcal carriers is not recommended. Unless selective media are employed, colonies of *N. meningitidis* may not be noticed among the other members of the resident flora. *N. meningitidis* recovered from CSF, blood, and other normally sterile sites should be identified and reported. Isolates from sputum cultures must be interpreted with regard to clinical presentation and in consultation with clinicians caring for the patient. Because meningococci may be isolated from anogenital sites infected by gonococci, it is necessary to identify neisserial isolates from these sites to the species level by using confirmatory tests.

OTHER *NEISSERIA* SPECIES

Neisseria lactamica

N. lactamica resembles *N. meningitidis* in colony morphology and was initially thought to be a lactose-positive variant of *N. meningitidis*. This species is found in the throat and is isolated more frequently from children than from adults (48). *N. lactamica* grows on all types of selective media and produces acid from glucose, maltose, and lactose (Table 3). ONPG is also hydrolyzed and can be used as a substitute for lactose. Some strains may cause false-positive reactions with commercial coagglutination tests.

N. cinerea

N. cinerea is part of the commensal flora of the upper respiratory tract and has been isolated from other sites, including the cervix, rectum, conjunctivae, blood, and CSF (37, 38, 67). *N. cinerea* grows on both blood and chocolate agar. On chocolate agar after 24 h of incubation, colonies of *N. cinerea* resemble the large-colony types of *N. gonorrhoeae*, are about 1 mm in diameter, and are smooth with entire edges. The organism does not produce acid from carbohydrates in either CTA-based media or the rapid acid production test (Table 3). Weak positive reactions with glucose after overnight incubation have been reported with some identification systems, and its positive prolyl-hydroxyprolyl aminopeptidase reaction may also result in misidentifications of *N. cinerea* as *N. gonorrhoeae* (45, 79). Most *N. cinerea* isolates, however, do not grow well on MTM or other selective media, which precludes testing using chromogenic substrate tests such as the BactiCard-*Neisseria* (Remel, Inc.). *N. cinerea* can be differentiated from the asaccharolytic species *N. flavescens* by its inability to produce polysaccharide from sucrose (see below) and the lack of a discernible yellow pigment. This species is differentiated from the asaccharolytic diplococcal species *M. catarrhalis* by its negative nitrate reduction, DNase, and tributyrin hydrolysis reactions.

The colistin susceptibility test is helpful for differentiating *N. cinerea* from *N. gonorrhoeae*. A suspension of the organism (0.5 McFarland turbidity standard) is prepared in broth and is swabbed onto a chocolate or blood agar plate as for a disk diffusion susceptibility test. A 10-μg colistin disk is placed on the inoculum, and the plate is incubated in CO_2 for 18 to 24 h. *N. cinerea* is colistin susceptible and has a zone that is larger than or equal to 10 mm around the disk. Generally, *N. gonorrhoeae* grows up to the edge of the disk.

Neisseria flavescens

N. flavescens is found in the upper respiratory tract and is rarely associated with infectious processes. This organism forms smooth, yellowish colonies on blood, chocolate, and nutrient agar at 35°C. Most strains also grow at room temperature on chocolate or blood agar. This organism synthesizes iodine-positive polysaccharide from sucrose (see discussion below) and can be differentiated from *M. catarrhalis* by its yellow pigmentation, inability to reduce nitrate, and negative DNase and tributyrin hydrolysis reactions.

Neisseria subflava Biovars, *Neisseria mucosa*, and *Neisseria sicca*

N. subflava, *N. mucosa*, and *N. sicca* make up part of the normal human upper respiratory tract flora and are occasional isolates from infectious processes, including endocarditis, bacteremia, meningitis, empyema, pericarditis, and pneumonia. Identification of the "nonpathogenic" *Neisseria* species is not generally necessary unless the organism is determined to be clinically significant or is isolated from a systemic site (e.g., blood or CSF) or in pure culture. Identification is based on colony morphology, growth on simple nutrient media, inability to grow on selective media, acid production from carbohydrates, reduction of nitrate and nitrite, and synthesis of a starch-like, iodine-staining polysaccharide from sucrose. Nitrate reduction and nitrite reduction are determined in tryptic-soy or heart infusion broth containing 0.1% (wt/vol) KNO_3 or 0.01% (wt/vol) KNO_2, respectively. Polysaccharide synthesis is determined by inoculating the organism onto brain heart infusion agar containing 1% sucrose. Medium lacking sucrose is inoculated as a negative control. After incubation at 35°C for 48 h, the plates are flooded with Gram's or Lugol's iodine (1:4 dilution). A positive test is indicated by the development of a deep blue color in and around the colonies synthesizing the polysaccharide.

N. subflava strains can be subdivided into three biovars (biovars subflava, flava, and perflava) based on acid production from fructose and sucrose, synthesis of iodine-positive polysaccharide from sucrose, and reduction of nitrate and nitrite (Table 3). All three biovars reduce nitrite but not nitrate. *N. mucosa* has a carbohydrate utilization pattern similar to that of *N. subflava* bv. perflava and also produces the iodine-positive polysaccharide, but *N. mucosa* is able to reduce both nitrate and nitrite to nitrogen gas. All of these organisms display varying degrees of yellow pigmentation. *N. sicca* strains are biochemically identical to *N. subflava* bv. perflava, but they grow as dry, adherent, leathery colonies on agar media.

Neisseria polysaccharea

N. polysaccharea is found in the human oropharynx. This organism is an oxidase-positive, catalase-positive, gram-negative diplococcus that forms smooth yellow colonies (81). Growth on selective media for the pathogenic *Neisseria* is a variable characteristic of *N. polysaccharea* due to the colistin susceptibility of some strains (4). The organisms are resistant to vancomycin. After 24 h of growth, *N. polysaccharea* forms colonies of about 2 mm in diameter on chocolate or blood agar. Acid is produced from glucose and maltose but not from fructose or lactose. Acid production from sucrose is variable and appears to depend on the types of media used to determine this characteristic. *N. polysaccharea* produces an amylosucrase enzyme that synthesizes amylopectin, an extracellular polysaccharide from sucrose. Nitrate is not reduced, whereas nitrite frequently is reduced. *N. polysaccharea* can be differentiated from *N. meningitidis* by polysaccharide synthesis and the γ-glutamylaminopeptidase test. *N. polysaccharea* produces iodine-positive polysaccharide from sucrose and is γ-glutamyl aminopeptidase negative, whereas *N. meningitidis* does not produce iodine-positive polysaccharide from sucrose and is γ-glutamyl aminopeptidase positive. Like *N. gonorrhoeae*, *N. lactamica*, and some *N. meningitidis* strains, *N. polysaccharea* is L-hydroxyprolyl aminopeptidase positive (4). The organism requires cysteine for growth and does not grow on nutrient agar or on chocolate agar at 22°C.

Neisseria elongata Subspecies

N. elongata subspecies *elongata*, *glycolytica*, and *nitroreducens* are rod-shaped members of the genus *Neisseria*. All subspecies are members of the human upper respiratory tract flora, and all have been isolated from infectious processes, including endocarditis (51). These subspecies can be differentiated on the basis of catalase reactivity, acid production from glucose, and reduction of nitrate (Table 3).

REFERENCES

1. **Agraharkar, M., M. Fahlen, M. Siddiqui, and S. Rajaraman.** 2000. Waterhouse-Friderichsen syndrome and bilateral cortical necrosis in meningococcal sepsis. *Am. J. Kidney Dis.* **36:**396–400.
2. **Alexander, S., and C. Ison.** 2005. Evaluation of commercial kits for the identification of *Neisseria gonorrhoeae*. *J. Med. Microbiol.* **54:**827–831.
3. **American Academy of Pediatrics Committee on Child Abuse and Neglect.** 1998. Gonorrhea in prepubertal children. *Pediatrics* **101:**134–135.
4. **Anand, C. M., F. Ashton, H. Shaw, and R. Gordon.** 1991. Variability in growth of *Neisseria polysaccharea* on colistin-containing selective media for *Neisseria* spp. *J. Clin. Microbiol.* **29:**2434–2437.
5. **Andersen, B. M., A. G. Steigerwalt, S. P. O'Connor, D. G. Hollis, R. S. Weyant, R. E. Weaver, and D. J. Brenner.** 1993. *Neisseria weaveri* sp. nov., formerly CDC group M-5, a gram-negative bacterium associated with dog bite wounds. *J. Clin. Microbiol.* **31:**2456–2466.
6. **Andreoli, C. M., H. E. Wiley, M. L. Durand, and L. M. Watkins.** 2004. Primary meningococcal conjunctivitis in an adult. *Cornea* **23:**738–739.
7. **Arbique, J. C., K. R. Forward, and J. LeBlanc.** 2000. Evaluation of four commercial transport media for the survival of *Neisseria gonorrhoeae*. *Diagn. Microbiol. Infect. Dis.* **36:**163–168.
8. **Bachmann, L. H., R. A. Desmond, J. Stephens, A. Hughes, and E. W. Hook III.** 2002. Duration of persistence of gonococcal DNA detected by ligase chain reaction in men and women following recommended therapy for uncomplicated gonorrhea. *J. Clin. Microbiol.* **40:**3596–3601.
9. **Balmelli, C., and H. F. Guntard.** 2003. Gonococcal tonsillar infection—a case report and literature review. *Infection* **31:**L362–L365.
10. **Barbe, G., M. Babolet, J. M. Boeufgras, D. Monget, and J. Freney.** 1994. Evaluation of API NH, a new 2-hour system for identification of *Neisseria* and *Haemophilus* species and *Moraxella catarrhalis* in a routine clinical laboratory. *J. Clin. Microbiol.* **32:**187–189.
11. **Bardin, T.** 2003. Gonococcal arthritis. *Best Pract. Res. Clin. Rheumatol.* **17:**201–208.
12. **Barlow, D.** 1997. The diagnosis of oropharyngeal gonorrhea. *Genitourin. Med.* **73:**16–17.
13. **Bart, A., I. G. Schuurman, M. Achtman, D. A. Caugant, J. Dankert, and A. van der Ende.** 1998. Randomly amplified polymorphic DNA genotyping of serogroup A meningococci yields results similar to those obtained by multilocus enzyme electrophoresis and reveals new genotypes. *J. Clin. Microbiol.* **36:**1746–1749.
14. **Bauer, H. M., K. E. Mark, M. Samuel, S. A. Wang, P. Weismuller, D. Moore, R. A. Gunn, C. Peter, A. Vannier, N. DeAugustine, J. D. Klausner, and J. S. Knapp.** 2005. Prevalence of and associated risk factors for fluoroquinolone-resistant *Neisseria gonorrhoeae* in California, 2000–2003. *Clin. Infect. Dis.* **41:**795–803.
15. **Beigi, R. H., and H. C. Wiesenfeld.** 2003. Pelvic inflammatory disease: new diagnostic criteria and treatment. *Obstet. Gynecol. Clin. N. Am.* **30:**777–793.
16. **Beverly, A., J. R. Bailey-Griffin, and J. R. Schwebke.** 2000. InTray GC medium versus modified Thayer-Martin agar plates for diagnosis of gonorrhea from endocervical specimens. *J. Clin. Microbiol.* **38:**3825–3826.
17. **Billings, S. D., D. Fuller, A. M. LeMonte, T. E. Davis, and A. L. Hartstein.** 1997. Characterization of DFA-negative, probe-positive *Neisseria gonorrhoeae* by pulsed field electrophoresis. *Diagn. Microbiol. Infect. Dis.* **29:**281–283.
18. **Boquete, M. T., C. Marcos, and J. A. Saez-Nieto.** 1986. Characterization of *Neisseria polysaccharea* sp. nov. (Riou, 1983) in previously identified noncapsulated strains of *Neisseria meningitidis*. *J. Clin. Microbiol.* **23:**973–975.
19. **Borrow, R., H. Claus, U. Chaudhry, M. Guiver, E. B. Kaczmarski, M. Frosch, and A. J. Fox.** 1998. *siaD* PCR ELISA for confirmation and identification of serogroup Y and W135 meningococcal infections. *FEMS Microbiol. Lett.* **159:**209–214.
20. **Bowler, L. D., Q.-Y. Zhang, J.-Y. Riou, and B. G. Spratt.** 1994. Interspecies recombination between the *penA* genes of *Neisseria meningitidis* and commensal *Neisseria* species during the emergence of penicillin resistance in *N. meningitidis:* natural events and laboratory simulation. *J. Bacteriol.* **176:**333–337.
21. **Catlin, B. W.** 1975. Cellular elongation under the influence of antibacterial agents: way to differentiate coccobacilli from cocci. *J. Clin. Microbiol.* **1:**102–105.
22. **Centers for Disease Control and Prevention.** 1999. *Biosafety in Microbiological and Biomedical Laboratories,* 4th ed. U.S. Department of Health and Human Services, Atlanta, Ga.
23. **Centers for Disease Control and Prevention.** 2000. Fluoroquinolone-resistance in *Neisseria gonorrhoeae,* Hawaii, 1999, and decreased susceptibility to azithromycin in *N. gonorrhoeae,* Missouri, 1999. *Morb. Mortal. Wkly. Rep.* **49:**833.
24. **Centers for Disease Control and Prevention.** 2000. *2000 Sexually Transmitted Disease Surveillance. Gonococcal Isolate Surveillance Project (GISP) Supplement.* [Online.] http://www.cdc.gov/nchstp/dstd/Stats_Trends/Stats_and_Trends.htm. Centers for Disease Control and Prevention, Atlanta, Ga.
25. **Centers for Disease Control and Prevention.** 2002. Laboratory-acquired meningococcal disease—United States, 2000. *Morb. Mortal. Wkly. Rep.* **71:**141–144.
26. **Centers for Disease Control and Prevention.** 2002. Screening tests to detect *Chlamydia trachomatis* and *Neisseria gonorrhoeae* infections—2002. *Morb. Mortal. Wkly. Rep.* **51**(RR-15)**:**1–38.

27. **Centers for Disease Control and Prevention.** 2002. Sexually transmitted disease treatment guidelines 2002. *Morb. Mortal. Wkly. Rep.* **51**(RR-6)**:**1–78.
28. **Centers for Disease Control and Prevention.** 2003. *Sexually Transmitted Disease Surveillance, 2002.* U.S. Department of Health and Human Services, Atlanta, Ga.
29. **Centers for Disease Control and Prevention.** 2005. Prevention and control of meningococcal disease. Recommendations of the Advisory Committee on Immunization Practices. *Morb. Mortal. Wkly. Rep.* **55**(RR07)**:**1–21.
30. **Chen, S. Y., S. Gibson, M. H. Katz, J. D. Klausner, J. W. Dilley, S. K. Schwarcz, T. A. Kellogg, and W. McFarland.** 2002. Continuing increases in sexual risk behavior and sexually transmitted diseases among men who have sex with men: San Francisco, California, 1999–2001, U.S.A. *Am. J. Public Health* **92:**1387–1388.
31. **Clinical and Laboratory Standards Institute.** 2005. *Performance Standards for Antimicrobial Susceptibility Testing; Fifteenth Informational Supplement.* CLSI document M100-S15. Clinical and Laboratory Standards Institute, Wayne, Pa.
32. **Darwin, L. D., A. P. Cullen, P. M. Arthur, C. D. Long, K. R. Smith, J. L. Girdner, E. W. Hook III, J. C. Quinn, and A. T. Lorincz.** 2002. Comparison of Digene hybrid capture 2 and conventional culture for detection of *Chlamydia trachomatis* and *Neisseria gonorrhoeae* in cervical specimens. *J. Clin. Microbiol.* **40:**641–644.
33. **Deguchi, T., M. Yasuda, M. Nakano, S. Ozeki, T. Ezaki, I. Saito, and Y. Kawada.** 1996. Quinolone-resistant *Neisseria gonorrhoeae:* correlations of alterations in the GyrA subunit of DNA gyrase and the ParC subunit of topoisomerase IV with antimicrobial susceptibility profiles. *Antimicrob. Agents Chemother.* **40:**1020–1023.
34. **Dicker, L. W., D. J. Mosure, S. M. Berman, and W. C. Levine.** 2003. Gonorrhea prevalence and coinfection with *Chlamydia trachomatis* in women in the United States, 2000. *Sex. Transm. Dis.* **30:**472–476.
35. **Dillon, J. R., M. Carballo, and M. Pauze.** 1988. Evaluation of eight methods for identification of pathogenic *Neisseria* species: *Neisseria*-Kwik, RIM-N, Gonobio Test, Gonochek II, GonoGen, Phadebact GC OMNI test, and Syva MicroTrak test. *J. Clin. Microbiol.* **26:**493–497.
36. **Dolter, J., L. Bryant, and J. M. Janda.** 1990. Evaluation of five rapid systems for the identification of *Neisseria gonorrhoeae*. *Diagn. Microbiol. Infect. Dis.* **13:**265–267.
37. **Dolter, J., J. Wong, and J. M. Janda.** 1998. Association of *Neisseria cinerea* with ocular infections in paediatric patients. *J. Infect.* **36:**49–52.
38. **Dossett, J. H., P. C. Applebaum, J. S. Knapp, and P. S. Totten.** 1985. Proctitis associated with *Neisseria cinerea* misidentified as *Neisseria gonorrhoeae* in a child. *J. Clin. Microbiol.* **21:**575–577.
39. **Drake, C., J. Barenfanger, J. Lawhorn, and S. Verhulst.** 2005. Comparison of easy-flow Copan liquid Stuart's and Starplex swab transport systems for recovery of fastidious aerobic bacteria. *J. Clin. Microbiol.* **43:**1301–1303.
40. **Ellison, R. T., III, J. G. Curd, P. F. Kohler, L. B. Reller, and F. N. Judson.** 1987. Underlying complement deficiency in patients with disseminated gonococcal infection. *Sex. Transm. Dis.* **14:**201–204.
41. **Fijen, C. A. P., E. J. Kuijper, M. T. te Bulte, M. R. Daha, and J. Dankert.** 1999. Assessment of complement deficiency in patients with meningococcal disease in the Netherlands. *Clin. Infect. Dis.* **28:**98–105.
42. **Fjeldsoe-Nielsen, H., M. Unemo, H. Fredlund, S. V. Hjorth, L. M. Berthelsen, H. M. Palmer, and A. Friis-Moller.** 2005. Phenotypic and genotypic characterization of prolyliminopeptidase-negative *Neisseria gonorrhoeae* isolates in Denmark. *Eur. J. Clin. Microbiol. Infect. Dis.* **24:**280–283.
43. **Gaydos, C. A., K. A. Crotchfelt, M. R. Howell, S. Kralian, P. Hauptman, and T. C. Quinn.** 1998. Molecular amplification assays to detect *Chlamydia trachomatis* infections in urine specimens from high school female students and to monitor the persistence of chlamydial DNA after therapy. *J. Infect. Dis.* **177:**417–424.
44. **Gaydos, C. A., T. C. Quinn, D. Willis, A. Weissfeld, E. W. Hook, D. H. Martin, D. V. Ferrero, and J. Schachter.** 2003. Performance of the APTIMA Combo 2 assay for the multiplex detection of *Chlamydia trachomatis* and *Neisseria gonorrheae* in female urine and endocervical swab specimens. *J. Clin. Microbiol.* **41:**304–309.
45. **Gaydos, C. A., M. Theodore, N. Dalesio, B. J. Wood, and T. C. Quinn.** 2004. Comparison of three nucleic acid amplification tests for detection of *Chlamydia trachomatis* in urine specimens. *J. Clin. Microbiol.* **42:**3041–3045.
46. **Ghanem, K. G., I. G. Giles, and J. M. Zenilman.** 2005. Fluoroquinolone-resistant *Neisseria gonorrhoeae:* the inevitable epidemic. *Infect. Dis. Clin. N. Am.* **19:**351–365.
47. **Giles, J. A., J. Falconio, J. D. Yuenger, J. M. Zenilman, M. Dan, and M. C. Bash.** 2004. Quinolone resistance-determining region mutations and *por* type of *Neisseria gonorrhoeae* isolates: resistance surveillance and typing by molecular methodologies. *J. Infect. Dis.* **189:**2085–2093.
48. **Gold, R., I. Goldschneider, M. L. Lepow, T. F. Draper, and M. Randolph.** 1978. Carriage of *Neisseria meningitidis* and *Neisseria lactamica* in infants and children. *J. Infect. Dis.* **137:**112–121.
49. **Golden, M. R., J. P. Hughes, L. E. Cles, K. Crouse, K. Gudgel, J. Hu, P. D. Swenson, W. E. Stamm, and H. H. Handsfield.** 2004. Positive predictive value of Gen-Probe APTIMA Combo 2 testing for *Neisseria gonorrhoeae* in a population of women with low prevalence of *N. gonorrhoeae* infection. *Clin. Infect. Dis.* **39:**1387–1390.
50. **Habib, A., and R. Fernando.** 2004. Efficacy of azithromyin 1 g single dose in the management of uncomplicated gonorrhoea. *Int. J. STD AIDS* **15:**240–242.
51. **Haddow, L. J., C. Mulgrew, A. Ansari, J. Miell, G. Jackson, H. Malnick, and G. G. Rao.** 2003. *Neisseria elongata* endocarditis: case report and literature review. *Clin. Microbiol. Infect.* **9:**426–430.
52. **Hale, Y. M., M. E. Melton, J. S. Lewis, and D. E. Willis.** 1993. Evaluation of the PACE 2 *Neisseria gonorrhoeae* assay by three public health laboratories. *J. Clin. Microbiol.* **31:** 451–453.
53. **Handsfield, H. H., Z. A. Dalu, D. H. Martin, J. M. Douglas, J. M. McCarty, D. Schlossberg, and the Azithromycin Gonorrhea Study Group.** 1994. Multicenter trial of single-dose azithromycin vs. ceftriaxone in the treatment of uncomplicated gonorrhea. *Sex. Transm. Dis.* **21:**107–111.
54. **Harrison, L. H., D. M. Dwyer, C. T. Maples, and L. Billiman.** 1999. The risk of meningococcal infection in college students. *JAMA* **281:**1906–1910.
55. **Hegde, V., G. Smith, J. Choi, and S. Pagliarini.** 2005. A case of gonococcal keratoconjunctivitis mimicking orbital cellulitis. *Acta Ophthalmol. Scand.* **83:**511–512.
56. **Human, R. P., and G. A. Jones.** 2006. Evaluation of swab transport systems against a published standard. *J. Clin. Pathol.* **57:**762–763.
57. **Imrey, P. B., L. A. Jackson, P. H. Ludwinski, A. C. England III, G. A. Fella, B. C. Fox, L. B. Isdale, M. W. Reeves, and J. D. Wenger.** 1996. Outbreak of serogroup C meningococcal disease associated with campus bar patronage. *Am. J. Epidemiol.* **143:**624–630.
58. **Ison, C. A., N. Tekki, and M. J. Gill.** 1993. Detection of the *tet*M determinant in *Neisseria gonorrhoeae*. *Sex. Transm. Dis.* **20:**329–333.
59. **Jacoby, H. M., and B. J. Mady.** 1995. Acute gonococcal sepsis in an HIV-infected woman. *Sex. Transm. Dis.* **22:**380–382.
60. **Janda, W. M., J. J. Bradna, and P. Ruther.** 1989. Identification of *Neisseria* spp., *Haemophilus* spp., and other fastidious gram-negative bacteria with the MicroScan

Haemophilus-Neisseria identification panel. *J. Clin. Microbiol.* **27:**869–873.

61. **Janda, W. M., P. J. Malloy, and P. C. Schreckenberger.** 1987. Clinical evaluation of the Vitek *Neisseria-Haemophilus* identification card. *J. Clin. Microbiol.* **25:**37–41.
62. **Janda, W. M., M. Montero, and L. M. Wilcoski.** 2002. Evaluation of the BactiCard *Neisseria* for identification of pathogenic *Neisseria* species and *Moraxella catarrhalis*. *Eur. J. Clin. Microbiol. Infect. Dis.* **21:**875–879.
63. **Janda, W. M., L. M. Wilcoski, K. L. Mandel, P. Ruther, and J. M. Stevens.** 1993. Comparison of monoclonal antibody-based methods and a ribosomal ribonucleic acid probe test for *Neisseria gonorrhoeae* culture confirmation. *Eur. J. Clin. Microbiol. Infect. Dis.* **12:**177–184.
64. **Jorgensen, J. H., S. A. Crawford, and K. R. Fiebelkorn.** 2005. Susceptibility of *Neisseria meningitidis* to 16 antimicrobial agents and characterization of resistance mechanisms affecting some agents. *J. Clin. Microbiol.* **43:**3162–3171.
65. **Kluytmans, J. A., W. H. Goessens, J. H. Van Rijsoort-Vos, H. G. M. Niesters, and E. Stolz.** 1994. Improved performance of PACE 2 with modified collection system in combination with probe competition assay for detection of *Chlamydia trachomatis* in urethral specimens from males. *J. Clin. Microbiol.* **32:**568–570.
66. **Knapp, J. S., K. K. Fox, D. L. Trees, and W. L. Whittington.** 1997. Fluoroquinolone resistance in *Neisseria gonorrhoeae*. *Emerg. Infect. Dis.* **3:**33–39.
67. **Knapp, J. S., P. A. Totten, M. H. Mulks, and B. H. Minshew.** 1984. Characterization of *Neisseria cinerea*, a nonpathogenic species isolated on Martin-Lewis medium selective for pathogenic *Neisseria* spp. *J. Clin. Microbiol.* **19:**63–67.
68. **Lafferty, W., J. P. Hughes, and H. H. Handsfield.** 1997. Sexually transmitted diseases among men who have sex with men: acquisition of gonorrhea and non-gonococcal urethritis by fellatio and implications for STD/HIV prevention. *Sex. Transm. Dis.* **24:**272–278.
69. **Lin, J.-S., S. P. Donegan, T. C. Heeren, M. Greenberg, E. E. Flaherty, R. Haivanis, X. H. Su, D. Dean, W. J. Newhall, J. S. Knapp, S. K. Sarafian, R. J. Rice, S. A. Morse, and P. A. Rice.** 1998. Transmission of *Chlamydia trachomatis* and *Neisseria gonorrhoeae* among men with urethritis and their female sex partners. *J. Infect. Dis.* **178:**1707–1712.
70. **Martin, D. H., C. Cammarata, B. Van Der Pol, R. B. Jones, T. C. Quinn, C. A. Gaydos, K. Crotchfelt, J. Schachter, J. Moncada, D. Jungkind, B. Turner, and C. Peyton.** 2000. Multicenter evaluation of the AMPLICOR and automated COBAS AMPLICOR CT/NG tests for *N. gonorrhoeae*. *J. Clin. Microbiol.* **38:**3544–3549.
71. **Mehrany, K., J. M. Kist, W. J. O'Connor, and D. J. DiGaudio.** 2003. Disseminated gonococcemia. *Int. J. Dermatol.* **42:**208–209.
72. **Modarress, K. J., A. P. Cullen, W. J. S. Jaffurs, G. L. Troutman, N. Mousavi, R. A. Hubbard, S. Henderson, and A. T. Lorincz.** 1999. Detection of *Chlamydia trachomatis* and *Neisseria gonorrhoeae* in swab specimens by the Hybrid Capture II and PACE 2 nucleic acid probe tests. *Sex. Transm. Dis.* **26:**303–308.
73. **National Committee for Clinical Laboratory Standards.** 2001. *Methods for Dilution Antimicrobial Susceptibility Tests for Bacteria That Grow Aerobically*. Approved standard M7-A5. National Committee for Clinical Laboratory Standards, Wayne, Pa.
74. **Orden, B., R. Martinez-Ruiz, C. Gonzalez-Manjavacas, T. Mombiela, and R. Millan.** 2004. Meningococcal urethritis in a heterosexual man. *Eur. J. Clin. Microbiol. Infect. Dis.* **23:**646–647.
75. **O'Rourke, M., C. A. Ison, A. M. Renton, and B. G. Spratt.** 1995. Opa-typing: a high-resolution tool for studying the epidemiology of gonorrhoea. *Mol. Microbiol.* **17:**865–875.
76. **Palmer, H. M., and C. Arnold.** 2001 Genotyping *Neisseria gonorrhoeae* using fluorescent amplified fragment length polymorphism analysis. *J. Clin. Microbiol.* **39:**2325–2329.
77. **Palmer, H. M., H. Mallinson, R. L. Wood, and A. J. Herring.** 2003. Evaluation of the specificities of five DNA amplification methods for the detection of *Neisseria gonorrhoeae*. *J. Clin. Microbiol.* **41:**835–837.
78. **Perez-Trallero, E., J. M. Garcia-Arenzana, I. Ayestaran, and J. Munoz-Baroja.** 1989. Comparative activity in vitro of 16 antimicrobial agents against penicillin-susceptible meningococci and meningococci with diminished susceptibility to penicillin. *Antimicrob. Agents Chemother.* **33:**1622–1623.
79. **Rice, R. J., and J. S. Knapp.** 1994. Comparative in vitro activities of penicillin G, amoxicillin-clavulanic acid, selected cephalosporins and quinolone antimicrobial agents against representative resistance phenotypes of *Neisseria gonorrhoeae*. *Antimicrob. Agents Chemother.* **38:**155–158.
80. **Riesbeck, K., P. Orvelid-Molling, H. Fredlund, and P. Olcen.** 2000. Long-term persistence of a discotheque-associated invasive *Neisseria meningitidis* group C strain as proven by pulsed-field gel electrophoresis and *porA* gene sequencing. *J. Clin. Microbiol.* **38:**1638–1640.
81. **Riou, J. -Y., and M. Guibourdenche.** 1987. *Neisseria polysaccharea* sp. nov. *Int. J. Syst. Bacteriol.* **37:**163–165.
82. **Rompalo, A. M.** 1999. Diagnosis and treatment of sexually acquired proctitis and proctocolitis: an update. *Clin. Infect. Dis.* **28**(Suppl.):S84–S90.
83. **Rosenstein, N. E., S. A. Stocker, T. Popovic, F. C. Tenover, and B. A. Perkins.** 2000. Antimicrobial resistance of *Neisseria meningitidis* in the U.S., 1997. *Clin. Infect. Dis.* **30:**212–213.
84. **Saginur, R., B. Clecner, J. Portnoy, and J. Mendelson.** 1982. Superoxol (catalase) test for identification of *Neisseria gonorrhoeae*. *J. Clin. Microbiol.* **15:**475–477.
85. **Sarafian, S. K., and J. S. Knapp.** 1989. Molecular epidemiology of gonorrhea. *Clin. Microbiol. Rev.* **2:**S49–S55.
86. **Schachter, J., E. W. Hook, D. H. Martin, D. Willis, P. Fine, D. Fuller, J. Jordan, W. M. Janda, and M. Chernesky.** 2005. Confirming positive results of nucleic acid amplification tests (NAATs) for *Chlamydia trachomatis*: all NAATs are not created equal. *J. Clin. Microbiol.* **43:**1372–1373.
87. **Schachter, J., E. W. Hook III, W. M. McCormack, J. C. Quinn, M. Chernesky, S. Chong, J. L. Girdner, P. B. Dixon, L. DeMeo, E. Williams, A. Cullen, and A. Lorincz.** 1999. Ability of the digene hybrid capture II test to identify *Chlamydia trachomatis* and *Neisseria gonorrhoeae* in cervical specimens. *J. Clin. Microbiol.* **37:**3668–3671.
88. **Schultz, T. R., J. W. Tapsall, P. A. White, and P. J. Newton.** 2000. An invasive isolate of *Neisseria meningitidis* showing decreased susceptibility to quinolones. *Antimicrob. Agents Chemother.* **45:**909–911.
89. **Schwam, E., and J. Cox.** 1999. Fulminant meningococcal supraglottitis: an emerging infectious syndrome. *Emerg. Infect. Dis.* **5:**464–467.
90. **Shetty, A., D. Ribeiro, A. Evans, and S. Linnane.** 2004. Gonococcal endocarditis: a rare complication of a common disease. *J. Clin. Pathol.* **57:**780–781.
91. **Spaargaren, J., J. Stoof, H. Fennema, R. Coutinho, and P. Savelkoul.** 2001. Amplified fragment length polymorphism fingerprinting for identification of a core group of *Neisseria gonorrhoeae* transmitters in the population attending a clinic for treatment of sexually transmitted diseases in Amsterdam, The Netherlands. *J. Clin. Microbiol.* **39:**2335–2337.
92. **Suzuki, K., T. Matsumoto, H. Murakami, K. Tateda, N. Ishii, and K. Yamaguchi.** 2004. Evaluation of a rapid antigen detection test for *Neisseria gonorrhoeae* in urine sediment for diagnosis of gonococcal urethritis in males. *J. Infect. Chemother.* **10:**208–211.

93. **Thompson, D. K., C. D. Deal, C. A. Ison, J. M. Zenilman, and M. C. Bash.** 2000. A typing system for *Neisseria gonorrhoeae* based on biotinylated oligonucleotide probes to PIB gene variable regions. *J. Infect. Dis.* **181:**1652–1660.
94. **Trees, D. L., A. J. Schultz, and J. S. Knapp.** 2000. Use of the neisserial lipoprotein (Lip) for subtyping *Neisseria gonorrhoeae*. *J. Clin. Microbiol.* **38:**2914–2916.
95. **Tzeng, Y.-L., and D. S. Stephens.** 2000. Epidemiology and pathogenesis of *Neisseria meningitidis*. *Microbes Infect.* **2:**687–700.
96. **Unemo, M., P. Olcen, J. Jonasson, and H. Fredlund.** 2004. Molecular typing of *Neisseria gonorrhoeae* isolates by pyrosequencing of highly polymorphic segments of the *porB* gene. *J. Clin. Microbiol.* **42:**2926–2934.
97. **Urra, E., M. Alkorta, M. Sota, B. Alcala, I. Martinez, J. Barron, and R. Cisterna.** 2005. Orogenital transmission of *Neisseria meningitidis* serogroup C confirmed by genotyping techniques. *Eur. J. Clin. Microbiol. Infect. Dis.* **24:**51–53.
98. **Uthman, A., C. Heller-Vitouch, A. Stary, A. Bilina, A. Kuchinka-Koch, J. Soltz-Szots, and E. Tschachler.** 2004. High-frequency of quinolone-resistant *Neisseria gonorrhoeae* in Austria with a common pattern of triple mutations in GyrA and ParC genes. *Sex. Transm. Dis.* **31:**616–628.
99. **Van Der Pol, B., D. Ferrero, L. Buck-Barrington, E. W. Hook III, C. Lenderman, T. C. Quinn, C. A. Gaydos, J. Moncada, G. Hall, M. J. Tuohy, and B. R. Jones.** 2001. Multicenter evaluation of the BD ProbeTec ET system for the detection of *Chlamydia trachomatis* and *Neisseria gonorrhoeae* in urine specimens, female endocervical swabs, and male urethral swabs. *J. Clin. Microbiol.* **39:**1008–1016.
100. **Van Deuren, M., P. Brandtzaeg, and J. W. M. van der Mer.** 2000. Update on meningococcal disease with emphasis on pathogenesis and clinical management. *Clin. Microbiol. Rev.* **13:**144–166.
101. **Wiesenfeld, H. C., D. L. B. Lowry, R. P. Heine, M. A. Krohn, H. Bittner, K. Kellinger, M. Schultz, and R. L. Sweet.** 2001. Self-collection of vaginal swabs for the detection of chlamydia, gonorrhea, and trichomonas. *Sex. Transm. Dis.* **28:**321–325.
102. **Winstead, J. M., D. S. McKinsey, S. Tasker, M. A. DeGroote, and L. M. Baddour.** 2000. Meningococcal pneumonia: characterization and review of cases seen over the past 25 years. *Clin. Infect. Dis.* **30:**87–94.
103. **Woods, C. R., T. Koeuth, M. M. Estabrook, and J. R. Lupski.** 1996. Rapid determination of outbreak-related strains of *Neisseria meningitidis* by repetitive element-based polymerase chain reaction. *J. Infect. Dis.* **174:**760–767.
104. **World Health Organization Western Pacific Gonococcal Antimicrobial Surveillance Programme.** 2003. Surveillance of antibiotic resistance in *Neisseria gonorrhoeae* in the WHO Western Pacific Region, 2002. *Commun. Dis. Intell.* **27:**487–490.
105. **Yazdankhah, S. P., and D. A. Caugant.** 2004. *Neisseria meningitidis:* an overview of the carriage state. *J. Med. Microbiol.* **53:**821–832.
106. **Zhou, W., W. Du, H. Cao, J. Zhao, S. Yang, W. Li, Y. Shen, S. Zhang, W. Du, and X. Zhang.** 2004. Detection of *gyrA* and *parC* mutations associated with ciprofloxacin resistance in *Neisseria gonorrhoeae* by use of oligonucleotide biochip technology. *J. Clin. Microbiol.* **42:**5819–5824.

Actinobacillus, Capnocytophaga, Eikenella, Kingella, Pasteurella, and Other Fastidious or Rarely Encountered Gram-Negative Rods

ALEXANDER von GRAEVENITZ, REINHARD ZBINDEN, AND REINIER MUTTERS

40

The bacterial genera covered in this chapter are taxonomically diverse, but common traits justify their discussion as a group. They are facultatively anaerobic gram-negative rods that belong neither to the families *Enterobacteriaceae, Vibrionaceae,* and *Aeromonadaceae* nor to the *Rickettsiales;* they are rather part of the families *Pasteurellaceae, Neisseriaceae, Cardiobacteriaceae, Flavobacteriaceae, Porphyromonadaceae,* and *Fusobacteriaceae* (51).

These bacteria grow aerobically but require, with the exception of *Chromobactrium* and some *Pasteurella* species, supplemented media for growth, grow slowly, often requiring 48 h at 37°C, and do not grow on enteric media such as MacConkey or desoxycholate agar. A 5 to 10% CO_2 atmosphere may be necessary for initial growth and improves growth on subcultures. Some isolates may be gram-variable; many species show limited viability. With the exception of *Chromobacterium,* they do not possess flagella but may show gliding or twitching motility, resulting in limited spreading of colonies and pitting of the agar (66).

Most species may be part of the flora of the nasopharynx and/or the oral cavity of animals and/or humans and, thus, are parasitic, in contrast to the environmental *Chromobacterium.* Only those isolated from humans are covered in this chapter. Transmission from animals to humans occurs by contact (e.g., bites or licking of wounds for *Pasteurella*), and from human to human by droplets (e.g., directly for *Kingella* or via paraphernalia or human bites for *Eikenella*); only *Chromobacterium* is transmitted by soil. Endogenous infections may occur as well (e.g., endocarditis).

The collection of specimens should follow the guidelines described in chapters 5 and 20. The low viability of many species makes use of transport media mandatory. Serological tests have not been tried on large numbers of cases.

The use of blood or chocolate agar and, wherever no normal flora is present, of enriched liquid media is mandatory. Selective media are mentioned below for each organism.

Phenotypic identification may present numerous difficulties. Identification to the species level often requires the use of multiple substrates not altogether available in many automated systems (17, 36, 60); databases of the latter also may not contain all relevant species. Similar biochemical characteristics, e.g., in *Actinobacillus* spp., may call for species confirmation by molecular methods (44, 52, 90). Triple-sugar iron or Kligler's agar may not support growth, e.g., of *Eikenella.* Gas formation, if present, is generally scant and may not be seen in these media. Media used to check acid formation from carbohydrates should be rich in peptones (e.g., cystine-trypticase agar), but serum should not be used, if at all possible, because it may split maltose. An alternative would be the use of Trypticase agar with 1% carbohydrate and a large inoculum (cell paste or agar block). Indole formation may take 2 days and may require extraction with xylene. The indole spot test is reliable only for *Pasteurella multocida* (103). Oxidase must be tested from colonies on blood-containing media with tetramethyl-*p*-phenylenediamine dihydrochloride (57). Catalase should preferably be checked in a liquid medium in order to avoid false-positive reactions on slides due to transfer of blood and false negatives due to weak reactions.

Except for a very recent report on *Pasteurella* spp. (30), there are no Clinical and Laboratory Standards Institute (CLSI) (formerly NCCLS) data for disk susceptibility testing of members of the group. MIC determinations require either dilution systems or E tests (55–56, 74, 80, 94). Most species are susceptible to many antimicrobials. There may even be small zones around 5-μg vancomycin disks (42).

Members of the group may cause infections anywhere in the human body. Those present in the oropharynx of animals often cause bite infections which may develop into systemic disease, particularly in immunosuppressed individuals. A disease particular to members of the group is HACEK endocarditis, named after the bacteria involved (*Haemophilus parainfluenzae, Haemophilus aphrophilus, Actinobacillus actinomycetemcomitans, Cardiobacterium, Eikenella,* and *Kingella* spp.) (19). It is characterized by a long interval between first symptoms and diagnosis (2 weeks to 6 months), frequent embolization, and large vegetations on left-side valves. Native and prosthetic valves may be affected. Prognosis is good with appropriate antibiotic treatment. In modern automated blood culture systems, HACEK organisms grow within 5 days (35, 62). In a few instances, blood cultures were negative but microscopy of the resected valve and/or broad-range PCR of valve or emboli led to the diagnosis (98, 101). *Cardiobacterium, Capnocytophaga,* and *Eikenella* may also participate in noma lesions (108), whereas the latter two genera and *Actinobacillus actinomycetemcomitans* (as the predominant agent) participate in periodontal lesions (102).

PASTEURELLA

The genus *Pasteurella* belongs, together with the genera *Haemophilus* and *Actinobacillus* and several nonhuman ones, to the family *Pasteurellaceae* (51). These genera have identical cellular fatty acid composition, with C16:1ω7c, C16:0, and C14:0 as the principal components. There is no single phenotypic feature that distinguishes the genera *Pasteurella* and *Actinobacillus*. The guanine-plus-cytosine (G+C) content of the DNA for *Pasteurella* is between 37.7 and 45.9 mol%. Members of one group of pasteurellae, however, are by DNA-DNA hybridization more closely related to the other two genera and have been marked *[P.]* (5), whereas the other group are called *Pasteurella* sensu stricto.

Pasteurellae are coccoid to small, nonmotile, facultatively anaerobic gram-negative rods that occur singly, in pairs, or in short chains. Bipolar staining is frequent. The "related" species generally have a more pronounced rod-like morphology and may even grow on MacConkey agar. All pasteurellae are hemin and CO_2 independent, but a few strains require factor V (nicotine adenine dinucleotide) (80). Colonies are 1 to 2 mm in diameter after 24 h of growth on blood agar at 37°C and opaque-grayish. Encapsulated strains tend to be mucoid. A slight greening underneath them may be observed. The indole-positive species exhibit a mouse-like odor.

Pasteurellae are widespread in healthy and diseased wild and domestic animals. Their habitats are the nasopharynx and the gingiva. Those occurring in animals only (particularly in birds and mammals) (25) are not covered here. *P. multocida*, the species most frequently isolated from humans, also occurs in many animals including dogs and cats. In spite of the genotypical homogeneity of *P. multocida*, phenotypically diverse lineages have been observed, e.g., infections of wounds from bites by large cats may be due to sucrose-negative variants (27). Virulence factors (capsule serotypes A to F, a cytotoxin, filamentous hemagglutinins, and iron acquisition proteins) have been identified in animal models (63), but their role in human pathology remains to be elucidated. Most human cases are due to serotypes A, D, and F (37).

Human infections are predominantly those of wounds or soft tissues following bites, scratches, or licking of skin lesions by carnivores. Of 159 human isolates of *Pasteurella* sensu stricto, 60% were *P. multocida* subsp. *multocida*, 18% were *P. canis*, 13% were *P. multocida* subsp. *septica*, 5% were *P. stomatis*, and 3% were *P. dagmatis* (all except *P. canis* are associated with both dogs and cats) (68). Infected cat bite wounds contain pasteurellae (mostly subsp. *multocida* and *septica*) significantly more often than infected dog bite wounds, reflecting a higher oropharyngeal colonization rate in cats (50 to 90% versus 55 to 60%) (24). Two species may even be encountered in one sample (142). The second most common site not only of infection but also of colonization is the respiratory tract, where pasteurellae sensu stricto may also cause sinusitis and bronchitis as well as pneumonia and empyema (with a poor prognosis), mostly in patients with underlying disease (24, 141). Finally, systemic diseases (meningitis, peritonitis, septicemia, arthritis, endocarditis, and osteomyelitis) have also been reported, with underlying medical conditions, particularly liver cirrhosis, present in many individuals affected (8, 143). An association exists between subspecies and clinical presentation: subsp. *septica* is more often associated with wounds than with respiratory and systemic infections, whereas subsp. *multocida* predominates in respiratory infections and bacteremias (24, 37). Cases of human infection with *P. gallinarum* (3, 6) (now *Avibacterium gallinarum*) (13) have to be regarded with circumspection (45); nevertheless, a case of neonatal meningitis (1) seems to be beyond reproach.

Of the "related" species, *[P.] caballi* has primarily been isolated from horses (120) and also from horse bite wounds in humans (41). *[P.] bettyae* (formerly HB-5), of uncertain habitat, has been isolated from infections of the male and female genital tracts and of newborns (15, 33). *[P.] aerogenes* has been detected primarily in pigs and hamsters and was isolated from bite wounds from those animals (39, 46). *[P.] pneumotropica* corresponds in habitat and transmission to *P. multocida*, but human infections (bites, systemic disease) are rare (44). The former *[P.] haemolytica*, also of animal origin, has now been subdivided into trehalose-positive strains, named *[P.] trehalosi*, and trehalose-negative strains, named *Mannheimia haemolytica* (5). Cases of human infection are somewhat doubtful (89, 111, 141); one case of endocarditis (132) seems to conform to the former description of the *[P.] haemolytica* complex.

Media containing vancomycin, clindamycin, and/or amikacin have been used to select pasteurellae (9). Biochemical reactions of species isolated from humans are listed in Table 1. In view of the phenotypic similarity of some species and the presence of some unclassified taxa (12, 25), species identification requires tests that may not be included in automated diagnostic systems (61). Beta-hemolysis is observed only in the former *[P.] haemolytica* complex. PCR (71), repetitive extragenic palindromic PCR (24), and 16S rRNA gene sequencing (44) have been used for diagnostic confirmation. Typing of pasteurellae has employed multilocus enzyme electrophoresis, PCR profiling, restriction endonuclease analysis, pulsed-field gel electrophoresis, and ribotyping (27, 71).

Pasteurellae are generally susceptible to β-lactam antibiotics including penicillin, cephalosporins (except oral narrow-spectrum agents), tetracyclines, quinolones, and trimethoprim-sulfamethoxazole and are generally resistant to macrolides and amikacin; other aminoglycosides are only moderately active (54, 55, 56, 57, 143). A few β-lactamase-positive strains of *P. multocida* (100) and *[P.] bettyae* (15) have been reported; they were susceptible to a combination of penicillin and clavulanic acid.

ACTINOBACILLUS

The genus *Actinobacillus*, in the family *Pasteurellaceae* (51), resembles *Pasteurella* in the composition of cellular fatty acids but has a narrower G+C content of the DNA (between 40 and 43%).

Actinobacilli are nonmotile, facultatively anaerobic coccoid to small gram-negative rods on solid media but are longer in liquid media or in those containing glucose or maltose and show a tendency to bipolar staining. Arrangement is single, in pairs, and (rarely) in short chains. Growth requires enriched media but not necessarily hemin and is improved by a 5 to 10% CO_2 atmosphere.

Many species have been isolated only from animals and are not discussed here. Species isolated from humans belong either to *Actinobacillus* sensu stricto (26) or to *A. actinomycetemcomitans*. The former include *A. lignieresii* (primary habitat in the oral cavity of sheep and cattle), *A. equuli* subsp. *equuli* (oral cavity of horses and pigs), *A. equuli* subsp. *haemolyticus* and *A. suis* (oral cavity of pigs), and the exclusively human species *A. ureae* (formerly *Pasteurella ureae*) and *A. hominis*. The species *A. actinomycetemcomitans* is of uncertain taxonomic status because 16S rRNA gene sequencing and DNA-DNA hybridization place it more

TABLE 1 Biochemical reactions of *Pasteurella* spp. and related species [a,b,c]

Reaction	*P. multocida*[d]	*P. canis*	*P. dagmatis*	*P. stomatis*	*Avibacterium gallinarum*	*[P.] aerogenes*	*[P.] bettyae*	*[P.] caballi*	*[P.] pneumotropica*	*[P.] trehalosi*[e]	*M. haemolytica*[e]
Catalase	+	+	+	+	+	+	−	−	+	v	+
Oxidase	+	+	+	+	+	+	v	+	+	+	+
Indole	+	+	+	+	−	−	+[w]	−	+	−	−
Urease	−	−	+	−	−	+	−	−	+	−	−
Ornithine decarboxylase	+	+	−	−	v	v	−	+	+	−	−
Growth on MacConkey agar	−	−	−	−	v	+	v	−	v	+	+
Gas from glucose	−	−	v	−	−	+	+[w]	+	−	−	−
Acid from:											
Lactose	−	−	−	−	−	v	−	+	−	−	ND
Sucrose	+	+	+	+	+	+	−	+	+	+	+
Xylose	v	−	−	−	v	v	−	+	+	−	+
Maltose	−	−	+	−	+	+	−	+	+	+	+
Mannitol	+	−	−	−	−	−	−	+	−	+	+

[a] Data from references 12, 25, 120, and 135.
[b] +, ≥90% of strains positive; −, ≥90% of strains negative; v, variable; w, weak; ND, no data available.
[c] All species reduce nitrate to nitrite and are negative for arginine dihydrolase and esculin hydrolysis.
[d] The three subspecies *multocida, septica*, and *gallicida* can be separated on the basis of sorbitol and dulcitol fermentation (+/− in subsp. *multocida*, −/− in subsp. *septica*, and −/+ in the mostly avian subsp. *gallicida*); weakly sorbitol-positive strains of subsp. *multocida* can be recognized by a negative α-glucosidase test and a specific PCR profile (52).
[e] Beta-hemolytic; *[P.] trehalosi* is trehalose positive; *Mannheimia haemolytica* is trehalose negative.

closely to the genus *Haemophilus* than to *Actinobacillus* (105). Its transfer to the genus *Haemophilus* (110), however, was not favored by the International Committee on Systematic Bacteriology Subcommittee on *Pasteurellaceae* and Related Organisms (72). Its habitat is the oral cavity of humans and of some primates (65).

Colonies of actinobacilli sensu stricto are approximately 2 mm in diameter after 24 h of growth at 37°C, are smooth or rough, are viscous, and often adhere to the agar surface. Smooth colonies are dome-shaped and have a bluish hue when viewed by transmitted light. *A. actinomycetemcomitans* colonies initially show a central dot and a slightly irregular edge, which, on further incubation, develops into a star-like configuration resembling "crossed cigars," and pit the agar (Fig. 1). After several subcultures, this rough morphology may give way to smooth and opaque, nonpitting colonies, reflecting loss of fimbriae. In liquid media, the bacterium forms granules which adhere to the sides and to the bottom of the tube.

A. lignieresii causes actinobacillosis, a granulomatous disease in cattle and sheep in which, in a fashion similar to actinomycosis, sulfur granules are formed in tissues (116). A few human soft tissue infections, originating from cattle or sheep bite wounds or contact, have been reported (109). The *A. equuli* subspecies and *A. suis* cause a variety of diseases in horses and pigs (25); human infections are mostly due to horse or pig bites or contact (7, 40). Both species have also been isolated from the human upper respiratory tract (117, 135). *A. ureae* has been isolated most often as a commensal from the human respiratory tract but also from meningitis patients following trauma or surgery (137) and other infections in immunocompromised patients (77). *A. hominis* was also encountered in such patients, as well as a commensal, albeit rarely (48).

A. actinomycetemcomitans is one of the major agents of adult and juvenile periodontitis (102). Furthermore, it has caused endocarditis (HACEK) (19) and soft tissue and other infections (75, 107). In sulfur granules, it may occur in combination with *Actinomyces* spp. (75).

Virulence factors of actinobacilli belong to the RTX (repeats-in-toxin) family, i.e., poreforming (hemolytic or cohemolytic) and cytolytic proteins (47). *A. actinomycetemcomitans* forms an RTX toxin termed leukotoxin, an epithelial distending toxin, some less well characterized immunomodulatory toxins, and fimbriae responsible for adherence (65).

Selective media have been devised for isolation of *A. actinomycetemcomitans* from dental samples. The clear Tryptic soy-serum-bacitracin-vancomycin medium allows observation of colonial morphology and catalase activity (127). It was recently modified (4). PCR has been used for detection, targeting the leukotoxin gene or specific 16S rRNA sequences (50).

Biochemical reactions are listed in Table 2. Species of *Actinobacillus* sensu stricto are easily separated from *A. actinomycetemcomitans* by urease production and sucrose fermentation. The latter and catalase and ONPG (*o*-nitrophenyl-β-D-galactopyranoside) reactions separate *A. actinomycetemcomitans* from *Haemophilus aphrophilus*, an important differentiation in the clinical laboratory which cannot always be accomplished if commercial systems are employed (17, 36). Separation of *A. equuli* subsp. *equuli* and *A. suis* may be impossible by phenotypic tests; the organisms share the same 16S rRNA gene sequence (26) but have different RTX toxin profiles (83).

On the basis of surface polysaccharides determined by tube agglutination or multiplex PCR (131), six serotypes of

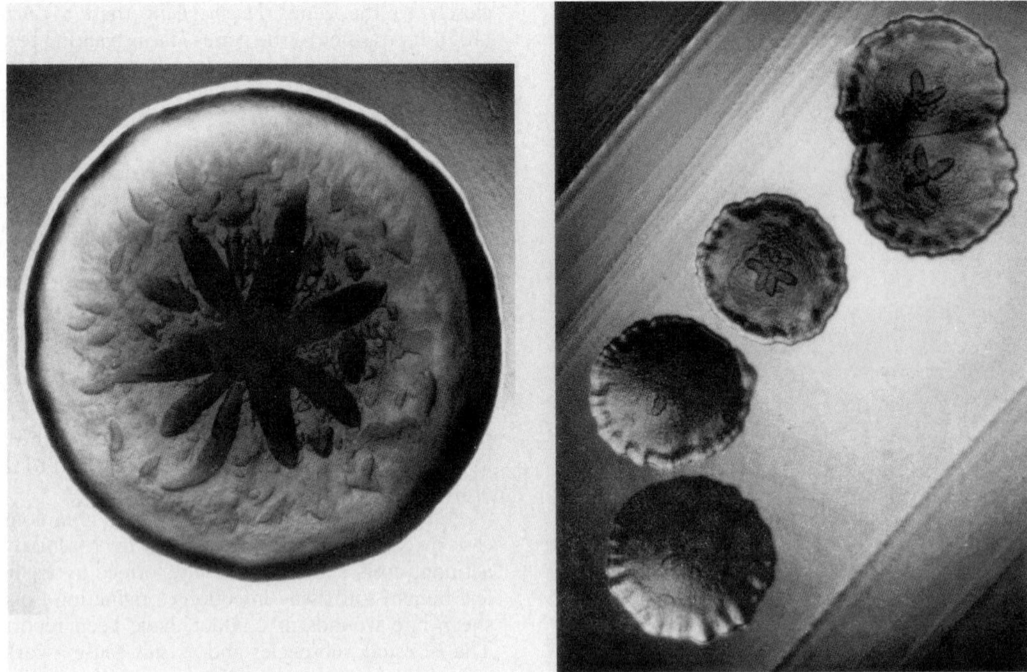

FIGURE 1 Star-shaped colonies of *Actinobacillus actinomycetemcomitans.*

A. actinomycetemcomitans can be distinguished, of which a, b, and c are most common. Serotype b is associated with periodontitis, penicillin resistance, and endocarditis, whereas serotype c is associated with other extraoral infections but also with periodontal health (106). Other typing systems (65, 107), also used on strains of *A. suis* and *A. equuli* (26), have been of less clinical relevance.

Susceptibility studies are extant for a few isolates of *A. ureae* and *A. hominis* that are susceptible to many antimicrobials including penicillin (48, 77). *A. actinomycetemcomitans* is usually susceptible to cephalosporins, ampicillin, doxycycline, and aminoglycosides; resistance to penicillin and macrolides is not uncommon (75, 80, 94, 107, 128). Penicillinase, however, has not been detected (94, 128).

CHROMOBACTERIUM

The genus *Chromobacterium*, in the *Neisseriaceae* family, contains one species, *C. violaceum* (51). It is a facultatively anaerobic, straight gram-negative rod which differs from all

TABLE 2 Biochemical reactions of *Actinobacillus* spp. and *Haemophilus aphrophilus*[a,b,c]

Reaction	*A. lignieresii*	*A. equuli* subsp. *equuli*	*A. equuli* subsp. *haemolyticus*	*A. suis*	*A. ureae*	*A. hominis*	*A. actinomycetemcomitans*	*H. aphrophilus*
Beta-hemolysis	−	−	+	+	−	−	−	−
Catalase	v	v	$+^w$	$+/+^w$	v	+	+	−
Oxidase	+	+	+	+	+	+	v	v
Esculin hydrolysis	−	−	−	+	−	−	−	−
Urease	+	+	+	+	+	+	−	−
ONPG	+	+	+	+	−	+	−	+
Growth on MacConkey agar	v	+	+	v	−	+	−	v
Gas from glucose	−	−	−	−	−	−	v	+
Acid from:								
Lactose	v	+	+	+	−	+	−	$+^D$
Sucrose	+	+	+	+	+	+	−	+
Xylose	+	+	+	+	−	+	v	−
Maltose	+	+	+	+	+	+	v	+
Mannitol	+	+	v	−	+	+	v	−
Trehalose	−	+	+	+	−	+	−	$+^D$
Melibiose	−	+	+	+	−	+	−	−

[a]Data from references 26, 48, 109, 117, and 135.
[b]+, ≥90% of strains positive; −, ≥90% of strains negative; D, delayed reaction; ONPG, *o*-nitrophenyl-β-D-galactosidase; v, variable; w, weak.
[c]All species are indole and ornithine decarboxylase negative and reduce nitrate to nitrite.

other species covered in this chapter by being motile by one polar and one to four lateral flagella, by growth on most enteric media, by an optimal growth temperature below 37°C, and an environmental origin. Colonies are 1 to 2 mm in diameter after 24 h of growth at 30 to 35°C, are round and smooth, have an almond-like smell, and may be beta-hemolytic. Most colonies produce a violet pigment called violacein, which is soluble in ethanol but not in water. Nonpigmented strains are known, however. The G+C value of the DNA is between 65 and 68 mol%.

C. violaceum inhabits soil and water in tropical and subtropical climates between latitudes of 35°N and 35°S (South Africa, Southeast Asia, Australia, southeastern United States). Human infections are rare. The portal of entry is usually the skin, but oral intake has also been reported. Wound infections, abscesses, and septicemia may develop. Infections are significantly associated with neutrophil dysfunction (glucose-6-phosphate dehydrogenase deficiency, chronic granulomatous disease [CGD]). Children without CGD and children with bacteremia show a high fatality rate (88, 123). A number of virulence factors other than endotoxin (adhesions, invasins, and cytolytic proteins) have been described (18).

Biochemical reactions are listed in Table 3. Identification of *C. violaceum* is easy if violacein is produced, although in those cases the oxidase reaction may be difficult to detect. Nonpigmented strains may be confused with *Aeromonas* spp. but are lysine, maltose, and mannitol negative. The principal cellular fatty acids do not differentiate between these genera.

C. violaceum is usually resistant to many antimicrobials but is often susceptible to imipenem, fluoroquinolones, gentamicin, tetracycline, and trimethoprim-sulfamethoxazole (2, 88).

EIKENELLA

The genus *Eikenella* belongs to the family *Neisseriaceae* (51). Thus far, only one species, *E. corrodens*, has been recognized, but DNA-DNA hybridization, composition of cellular carbohydrates, and the occurrence of biochemically aberrant (among them, catalase-positive) isolates suggest that there may be more than one genomospecies (76). The G+C content is between 56 and 58 mol%.

Eikenellae are slender, straight, small, nonmotile, facultatively anaerobic gram-negative rods (Fig. 2A). With a few exceptions, they require hemin for growth unless 5 to 10% CO_2 is present (53) and, therefore, grow poorly or not at all on triple-sugar iron or Kligler's agar. Colonies are 1 to 2 mm in diameter after 48 h of growth and show clear centers that are often surrounded by spreading growth, and they may pit the agar. They smell of hypochlorite and assume a slightly yellow hue after several days. In liquid media, granules are formed.

The habitat of *E. corrodens* is the oral cavity and perhaps the gastrointestinal tract of humans and some mammals from whom it can be transmitted via saliva (bites, syringes) to other individuals. The organism is associated with adult and juvenile periodontitis (102) and is also an agent of oral, pleuropulmonary, abdominal, joint, bone, and wound (e.g., human bite) infections (108, 122). These are often indolent and mixed with other members of the oropharyngeal flora. Risk factors are dental manipulations and intravenous drug abuse. Endocarditis is of the HACEK type if monomicrobial; polymicrobial cases, however, are known (19).

Detection is improved by use of a selective medium containing clindamycin (124) and by PCR (50). Biochemical reactions are recorded in Table 3. A typical isolate fails to form acid from carbohydrates and is ornithine decarboxylase and nitratase positive. Typing has been done by arbitrarily primed PCR (49) and restriction endonuclease analysis (23), demonstrating unstable polyclonality in the oral cavity.

E. corrodens is susceptible to many antimicrobials including penicillin, expanded- and broad-spectrum cephalosporins, carbapenems, doxycycline, and fluoroquinolones and is often resistant to macrolides (54, 55, 56). β-Lactamase-positive strains have become more frequent, but their resistance can be overcome by β-lactamase inhibitors (85).

KINGELLA

The genus *Kingella*, consisting of the species *K. kingae*, *K. denitrificans*, *K. oralis*, and *K. potus*, also belongs to the family *Neisseriaceae* (51). The G+C content of the DNA is between 47 and 58 mol%.

Its members are short, nonmotile, facultatively anaerobic gram-negative rods with square ends which lie together in pairs or clusters (Fig. 2B) and tend to decolorize unevenly on Gram stain. Colonies develop to 1- to 2-mm diameter in 48 h of growth, one type being smooth with a central papilla, the other showing spreading edges and pitting of the medium. *K. kingae*, as the only species, shows a small but distinct zone of hemolysis on blood agar. CO_2 (5 to 10%) enhances growth. Viability is limited.

K. kingae colonizes the throat but not the nasopharynx of many children aged 6 months to 4 years (139). The natural habitats of *K. denitrificans* and *K. potus* are unknown. *K. oralis* has been isolated from the healthy human mouth (22).

Infections with *K. kingae* show a predilection for bones and joints of previously healthy children under 4 years of age (139). Septic arthritis, diskitis, and osteomyelitis of the lower extremities but also occult bacteremia are conspicuous. Stomatitis and/or upper respiratory tract infections may precede systemic disease, which suggests possible interaction with viral disease(s) (139). Infections in adults occur more commonly in immunocompromised individuals (139) or may present as endocarditis (HACEK) (19). Ribotyping and pulsed-field gel electrophoresis have shown that person-to-person transmission via respiratory droplets may occur (125). *K. denitrificans* has been reported mostly as an agent of endocarditis (96). *K. oralis* has been isolated from patients with periodontitis, but its relationship to the disease is unclear (22). *K. potus* has caused a wound infection following a bite of a kinkajou (87).

Recovery of *K. kingae* from body fluids and pus can be difficult because these specimens seem to be inhibitory to the bacteria. The use of various blood culture media has significantly improved the detection rate (139). In a study using blood culture media for simulated synovial fluids, BacT/Alert (BioMérieux, Inc., Durham, N.C.) proved to be superior to BACTEC (Becton Dickinson, Cockeysville, Md.) blood cultures with regard to sensitivity and detection time (70), but comparative studies with clinical samples are not extant. Broad-range PCR has even detected *K. kingae*-specific sequences in synovial fluids that did not show growth in blood culture media (97). For isolation from areas with normal flora, solid media containing clindamycin (34) or vancomycin (140) as well as Thayer-Martin agar (140) have been recommended.

Biochemical test results are listed in Table 3. In addition to microscopic and colonial morphology, they serve to differentiate kingellae from rod-shaped members of the genus *Neisseria* (Table 4).

TABLE 3 Biochemical reactions of rod-shaped species of the *Neisseriaceae* and of the *Cardiobacteriaceae* [a,b,c]

Reaction	*Chromobacterium violaceum*	*Eikenella corrodens*	*Kingella kingae*	*Kingella denitrificans*	*Kingella oralis*	*Kingella potus*	*Simonsiella muelleri*	Group EF-4a	*Cardiobacterium hominis*	*Cardiobacterium valvarum*	*Suttonella indologenes*
Catalase	+	–	–	–	–	–	–	–	–	–	v
Oxidase	v	+	+	+	+	+	+	+	+	+	+
Indole	v	–	–	–	–	–	–	–	+[w]	v	+
Arginine dihydrolase	+	–	–	–	–	–	–	v	–	ND	–
Nitrate to nitrite	+	+	–	+/G	–	–	v	+/G	–	–[d]	–
Esculin hydrolysis	–	–	–	–	–	–	–	–	–	–	–
Ornithine decarboxylase	–	+	–	–	–	–	–	–	–	ND	–
Growth on MacConkey agar	+	–	–	–	–	–	–	v	–	ND	–
Alkaline phosphatase[e]	+	–	+	–	+	–	–	–	–	ND	+
Acid from:											
Glucose	+[f]	–[g]	+	+	+[w]	–	+	+	+	v	+
Lactose	–	–	–	–	–	–	–	–	–	–	–
Sucrose	v	–	–	–	–	–	–	–	+	v	+
Xylose	–	–	–	–	–	–	–	–	–	–	–
Maltose	–	–	+	–	–	–	+	–	+	v	+
Mannitol	–	–	–	–	–	–	–	–	+	–	–
Special features	Violacein v	LD v	Beta-hemolytic			DNase +, yellow pigment	Microscopic morphology	Yellowish or no pigment			
Main cellular fatty acids	18:1ω7c, 16:0, 14:0	16:0, 18:1ω7c, 16:1ω7c	14:0, 16:1ω7c, 16:0	16:0, 14:0, 18:2, 18:1ω9c	ND	16:0, 18:1ω7c	16:1ω7c, 12:0, 14:0	16:0, 16:1ω7c, 18:1ω7c	18:1ω7c, 16:0, 14:0	18:1ω7c, 16:0, 14:0	16:0, 18:1ω7c, 16:1ω7c, 14:0

[a]Data from references 34, 61, 76, 81, 87, and 135.
[b]+, ≥90% of strains positive; –, ≥90% of strains negative; G, gas; LD, lysine decarboxylase; ND, no data; v, variable; w, weak.
[c]All species are negative for urease.
[d]One possible isolate (69; see text) was nitratase positive.
[e]APIZYM system (76).
[f]Some strains form small amounts of gas.
[g]Weakly positive reactions may be observed in O/F media (76).

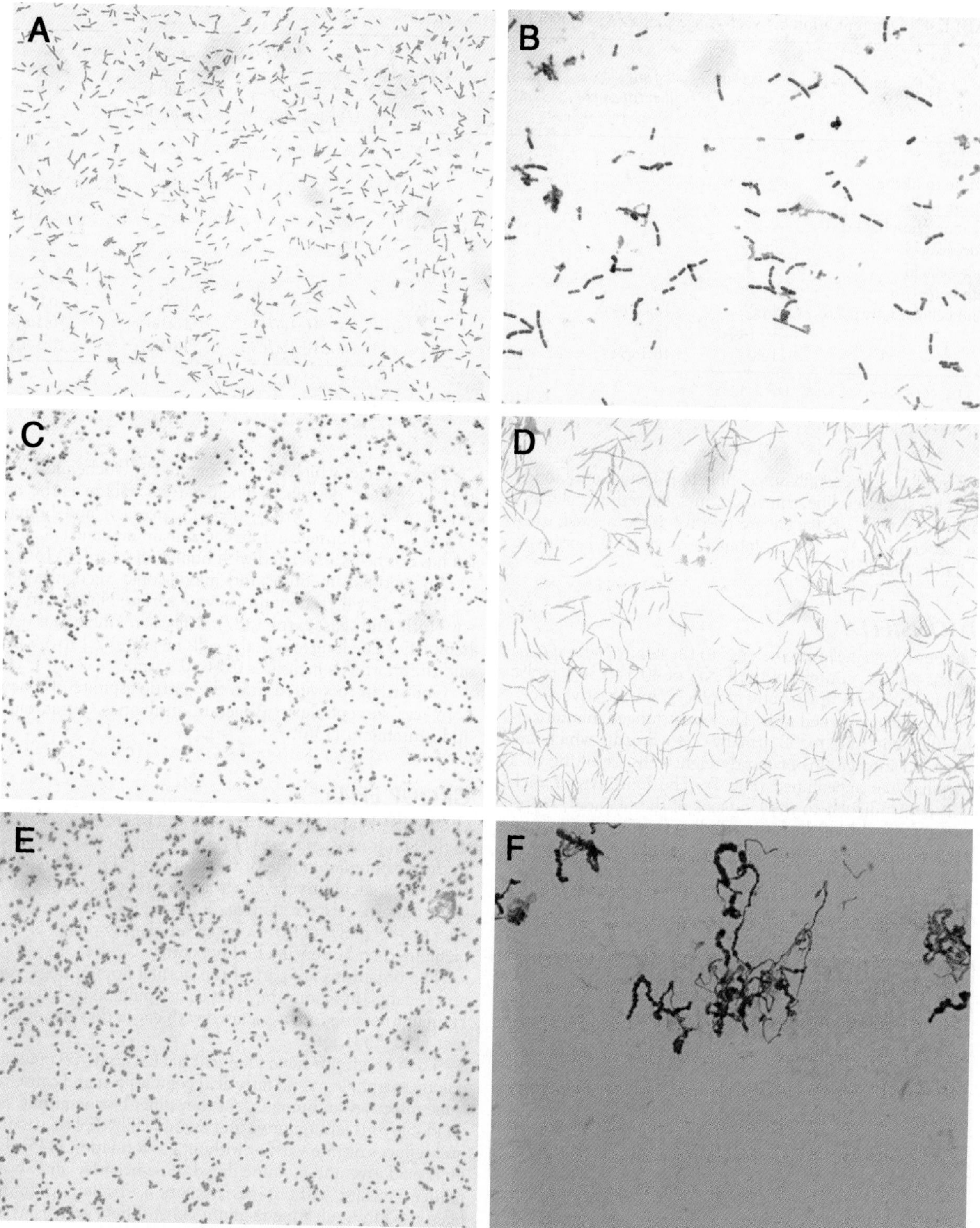

FIGURE 2 (A) *Eikenella corrodens* (Gram stain); (B) *Kingella kingae* (Gram stain); (C) Group EF-4a (Gram stain); (D) *Capnocytophaga ochracea* (Gram stain); (E) *Dysgonomonas capnocytophagoides* (Gram stain); (F) *Streptobacillus moniliformis* (Gram stain of a 48-h culture grown on sheep blood agar). (Courtesy of D. Fedorko, Bethesda, Md.)

TABLE 4 Differentiation between *Kingella* and rod-shaped *Neisseria* species[a,b]

Feature	*Kingella kingae*	*Kingella denitrificans*	*Kingella oralis*	*Kingella potus*	*Neisseria elongata* subsp. *glycolytica*	*Neisseria elongata* subsp. *nitroreducens*	*Neisseria weaveri*
Catalase	−	−	−	−	+	−	+
Nitrate to nitrite	−	+	−	−	−	+	−
Nitrate to gas	−	+	−	−	−	−	−
Alkaline phosphatase[c]	+	−	+	ND	−	−	ND
Glucose acid	+	+	$+^w$	−	$+^w$	v	−
Maltose acid	+	−	−	−	−	−	−
Beta-hemolysis	+	−	−	−	−	−	−
Main cellular fatty acids	14:0, 16:1ω7c, 16:0	16:0, 14:0, 18:2, 18:1ω9c	ND	16:0, 18:1ω7c	16:0, 16:1ω7c, 18:1ω7c	16:0, 16:1ω7c, 18:1ω7c	16:0, 16:1ω7c, 18:1ω7c

[a]Data from references 22, 87, 114, and 135.
[b]+, ≥90% of strains positive; −, ≥90% of strains negative; ND, no data available; v, variable; w, weak.
[c]APIZYM system (76).

Kingellae are generally susceptible to β-lactam antibiotics, macrolides, doxycycline, trimethoprim-sulfamethoxazole, and quinolones (139). β-Lactamase-positive isolates exist; they are susceptible to the combination with β-lactamase inhibitors (96, 129).

SIMONSIELLA

The genus *Simonsiella* also belongs to the family *Neisseriaceae* and has a G+C content of the DNA of 40.3 to 50.1 mol% (51). Its members are strictly aerobic gram-negative, nonmotile, crescent-shaped rods. They are arranged in multicellular filaments, 10 to 50 μm by 2 to 8 μm, which are segmented into groups of mostly eight cells, resulting in a caterpillar-like appearance (Fig. 3). The long axis of each cell is perpendicular to the long axis of the filament, representing the width of the latter. Gliding motility and incomplete decolorization with Gram stain are usually observed. Simonsiellae grow well on blood agar but not on enteric media. Colonies are 1 to 2 mm in diameter after 24 h at 37°C and produce a pale yellow pigment.

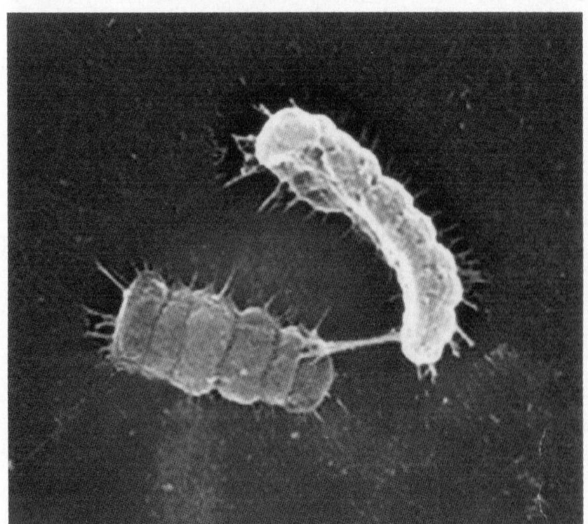

FIGURE 3 Scanning electron micrograph of *Simonsiella* sp. with two multicellular filaments giving the appearance of caterpillars. (Courtesy of L. Corboz, Zürich, Switzerland.)

Three species which can be separated by biochemical tests (81) have been described. Their natural habitat is the oral cavity of sheep (*S. crassa*), dogs (*S. steedae*), and humans (*S. muelleri*); simonsiellae from cats remain unnamed. *S. muelleri* has not been associated with human disease (20, 136).

An optimal medium for microscopic recognition is BSTSY agar, which contains bovine serum, glucose, tryptic soy broth, and yeast extract (82). *S. muelleri* (Table 3) is beta-hemolytic. The long axis of the cells measures 2.1 to 3.5 μm, and the short axis measures 0.5 to 0.9 μm.

One strain recovered from the gastric aspirate of a newborn was susceptible to β-lactam antibiotics, tetracycline, and gentamicin (136).

GROUP EF-4a

Groups EF-4a and EF-4b (EF, eugonic fermenter) also belong to the family *Neisseriaceae* (114), although they are not listed in the taxonomic outline of the bacteria (51). Group EF-4a consists of facultatively anaerobic, nonmotile, coccoid to short gram-negative rods (Fig. 2C) with a G+C content of 49.3 to 50.9 mol% (114). Colonies are slightly yellow or nonpigmented and often smell of popcorn.

The organisms are part of the normal flora of dogs, cats, and rodents, in whom they may cause pulmonary infection. Human infections are associated with cat or dog bite or contact (112, 133).

The two groups have identical habitats, microscopic and colony morphology, and fatty acid composition and cause the same infections in humans, but they differ biochemically. EF-4a (Table 3) is fermentative and arginine dihydrolase variable and reduces nitrate with or without gas formation (135). EF-4b is oxidative and arginine dihydrolase negative and always reduces nitrate without gas formation. Trimethoprim has been used in a selective medium (112). EF-4a organisms are susceptible to aminopenicillins, expanded- and broad-spectrum cephalosporins, fluoroquinolones, and trimethoprim-sulfamethoxazole and variably susceptible to penicillin, aminoglycosides, and macrolides (55, 92). β-Lactamases have not been found in any strain (92).

CARDIOBACTERIUM

The genus *Cardiobacterium*, which belongs to the family *Cardiobacteriaceae* (51), consists of *C. hominis* and a newly described species, provisionally named *C. valvarum*, until now represented by five (61) and possibly another (69) isolate from which it differs in nitrate reduction but with whom it shares similar cellular fatty acids and a 99.4% 16S rRNA sequence similarity. The G+C content of the DNA is 59 to 60 mol%.

C. hominis occurs in short chains, pairs, or rosettes, showing bulbous ends and staining irregularly. Addition of yeast extract to the medium (e.g., in chocolate agar) seems to abolish this pleomorphism. Initial growth requires 5 to 10% CO_2. Colonies on blood agar attain a diameter of approximately 1 mm after 48 h at 37°C, are circular, smooth, and opaque, and may pit the agar. Colonies of *C. valvarum* are of the same or a smaller size (0.2-mm diameter), barely grow on chocolate agar, and show pleomorphism and sometimes pitting on that medium.

The normal habitat of *C. hominis* is the human upper respiratory tract and possibly also the gastrointestinal and genitourinary tracts (126). Human disease is mainly endocarditis (HACEK) (19, 31); on rare occasions, *C. hominis* has been isolated from other body sites (84, 108). In blood culture-negative cases, the diagnosis has been made by broad-range PCR and stains from heart valve or embolic tissue (98, 101).

Biochemical tests are recorded in Table 3. The indole test is weakly positive for *C. hominis* and was strongly positive for only one *C. valvarum* isolate (61). A positive indole reaction may initially suggest *Pasteurella* or *Suttonella;* identification must, therefore, include tests for catalase and mannitol fermentation.

C. hominis and *C. valvarum* are susceptible to many antimicrobials (30) including penicillin. β-Lactamase production is very rare and can be inhibited by clavulanic acid (93).

SUTTONELLA

The genus *Suttonella* is the second one in the family *Cardiobacteriaceae* (51). It contains one species, *S. indologenes* (formerly *Kingella indologenes*), a plump, irregularly staining, nonmotile, facultatively anaerobic gram-negative rod whose colonies may show spreading and/or pitting (135). The G+C value is 49 mol%. Characteristics differentiating *Suttonella* from morphologically and biochemically similar species are listed in Table 3. The organism, whose natural habitat is unknown, has only rarely been isolated from human sources, e.g., from diseased eyes (130, 135) and from blood cultures of patients with endocarditis (73, 135). Its susceptibility resembles that of *C. hominis*.

CAPNOCYTOPHAGA

The genus *Capnocytophaga,* in the family *Flavobacteriaceae* (51), consists of seven species. The G+C content of the DNA is 34 to 40 mol%.

Cells are mainly fusiform, medium to long, with tapered ends (Fig. 2D). Primary isolation requires 5 to 10% CO_2 and enriched media. Growth may differ depending on the composition of the blood agar base (38). Colonies are very small after 24 h at 37°C, reach 2 to 4 mm in diameter after 2 to 4 days, are convex or flat and often slightly yellow when scraped off the agar, show regular or spreading edges, and adhere to the agar surface.

The oxidase- and catalase-negative species *C. ochracea*, *C. gingivalis*, *C. sputigena*, *C. haemolytica*, and *C. granulosa* are normal inhabitants of the human mouth. The first three are also associated with juvenile and adult periodontitis (66, 102), whereas the latter two have been isolated from supragingival plaque of healthy adults as well as from subgingival plaque in adult periodontitis (28). All five species may cause septicemia and other infections (endocarditis, endometritis, osteomyelitis, abscesses, peritonitis, and keratitis) in immunocompetent and immunosuppressed (mainly neutropenic) patients (16, 108). They produce an immunosuppressive factor (104).

The oxidase- and catalase-positive species *C. canimorsus* and *C. cynodegmi* reside in the oral cavity of healthy dogs and cats (*C. canimorsus* is found in approximately 25% of dogs and 15% of cats) (14). Infections are associated mainly with dog and cat bites or contact. Patients infected with *C. canimorsus* most often present with septicemia and have been splenectomized or are alcoholics. In fulminant cases with a poor prognosis, disseminated intravascular coagulation, acute renal failure, respiratory distress syndrome, and shock may develop (91). Hemolytic-uremic syndrome and thrombotic thrombocytopenic purpura are other possible sequelae (78, 99). Meningitis, arthritis, eye infections (91), and endocarditis (118) have been reported as well. *C. cynodegmi* has rarely been isolated from localized and systemic infections (119). Both organisms are able to multiply intracellularly in mouse macrophages; *C. canimorsus* also produces a cytotoxin (43).

For detection of *Capnocytophaga* spp. in mixed cultures, various selective media containing bacitracin, polymyxin B, vancomycin, and trimethoprim (29) have been used, as has PCR (64). The organisms also grow on Thayer-Martin and Martin-Lewis agar. Inhibition by sodium polyanethol sulfonate has been reported (121).

Biochemical test results are listed in Table 5. Phenotypic species differentiation in the oxidase-negative group may be inconclusive (28), which has frequently resulted in the identification of the organism as "*Capnocytophaga* sp." 16S rRNA PCR-restriction fragment length polymorphism backed up by 16S rRNA gene sequencing has proven to be a reliable method for identification (28). Typing by restriction fragment length polymorphism has been undertaken (16).

Capnocytophaga spp. are usually susceptible to broad-spectrum β-lactams, macrolides, doxycycline, and fluoroquinolones but are resistant to aminoglycosides and to colistin (115). β-Lactamase-positive isolates have occasionally been found; they were susceptible to combinations with β-lactam inhibitors (74).

DYSGONOMONAS AND RELATED BACTERIA

In the genus *Dysgonomonas* of the family *Porphyromonadaceae*, three species have been recognized: *D. capnocytophagoides* (formerly CDC group DF-3), *D. gadei* (so far represented by one strain only) (68), and *D. mossii* (three strains) (86). The G+C content of the DNA has been approximately 38 mol%. The related DF-3-like bacteria have not been investigated further since their first description (32).

All resemble *Capnocytophaga* spp. in their growth characteristics; *D. mossii* has been reported to be dependent on heme (86). They are coccoid to small, nonmotile gram-negative rods (Fig. 2E). Colonies are entire, measure 1 to 2 mm in diameter after 24 h of growth, have a strawberry-like odor, and are neither adherent nor spreading.

Most *D. capnocytophagoides* strains have been isolated from stools of immunocompromised patients, and a few strains were from other sources (95). Diarrhea was reported to occur for one-half of 20 patients with fecal isolates, whereas routine stool cultures yielded the organism for 1.1 to 2.3% of individuals (95). One blood isolate was found by

TABLE 5 Biochemical reactions of *Capnocytophaga* spp., *Dysgonomonas* and related species, and *Streptobacillus*[a,b,c]

Reaction	*C. ochracea*	*C. sputigena*	*C. gingivalis*	*C. granulosa*	*C. haemolytica*	*C. canimorsus*	*C. cynodegmi*	*D. capnocytophagoides*[d]	*D. mossii*	DF-3-like	*S. moniliformis*
Catalase	−	−	−	−	−	+	+	−	−	−	−
Oxidase	−	−	−	−	−	+	+	−	−	−	−
Indole	−	−	−	−	−	−	−	−	+	+	−
Arginine dihydrolase	−	−	−	ND	ND	+	+	−	−	−	+
Nitrate to nitrite	−	v	−	−	+	−	v	−	−	−	−
Esculin hydrolysis	+	+	−	−	+	v	+	v	+	+	v
Gelatinase	−	v	−	ND	ND	−	−	−	−	v	−
Starch hydrolysis	+	−	−	ND	ND	ND	ND	ND	+	ND	ND
ONPG	+	+	−	+	+	+	+	+	+	+	−
Acid from:											
Lactose	v	v	−	+	+	+	+	+	+	+	−
Sucrose	+	+	+	+	+	−	+	+	+	−	−
Xylose	−	−	−	−	−	−	−	+	+	−	−
Main cellular fatty acids	i-15:0, 3OH-17:0	i-15:0, 3OH-17:0	i-15:0, 3OH-17:0	i-15:0, 3OH-17:0	i-15:0, 3OH-17:0	i-15:0, 3OH-17:0	i-15:0, 3OH-17:0	ai-15:0, i14:0, 15:0, i-3-OH-16:0	ND	ai-15:0, i-15:0, 16:0, 18:2, i-3-OH-17:0	16:0, 18:1, 18:2, 18:0

[a]Data from references 11, 32, 67, and 135.
[b]+, ≥90% of strains positive; −, ≥90% of strains negative; ND, no data available; v, variable.
[c]All species are negative for urease and ornithine decarboxylase and form acid from glucose.
[d]The isolate of *D. gadei* was catalase and indole positive (67).

ribotyping to be identical to one in the stool of the same patient (58). The natural habital of the other species is unknown.

A selective medium containing cefoperazone, vancomycin, and amphotericin B has been used for stool cultures (58). The species show few biochemical differences (Table 5). Aerobically growing isolates of *Leptotrichia buccalis* may be confused with *Dysgonomonas;* however, the former have a different cellular fatty acid profile (mainly C16:0 and C11/t9/t6C18:1) and produce lactic acid from glucose whereas *Dysgonomonas* produces propionic and succinic acid (11).

Only *D. capnocytophagoides* strains have been checked for antimicrobial susceptibility, and they were found to be mostly susceptible to doxycycline, clindamycin, erythromycin, and trimethoprim-sulfamethoxazole, resistant to cephalosporins, aminoglycosides, and fluoroquinolones, and variably susceptible to other β-lactam antibiotics and imipenem (58, 95).

STREPTOBACILLUS

The genus *Streptobacillus,* in the family *Fusobacteriaceae,* consists of one species, *S. moniliformis,* with a G+C content of the DNA of 24 to 26 mol%.

The species is a facultatively anaerobic, nonmotile gram-negative rod with a pleomorphic appearance. For culture, media enriched with sheep or rabbit blood (15% seems to be optimal), serum, or ascitic fluid and a 5 to 10% CO_2 atmosphere are required. As a culture consisting of small- to medium-size rods ages, some organisms develop into 100- to 150-μm-long filaments which contain granules, bulbs (often in series), and bands (Fig. 2F). Coccal forms and Gram variability may also be observed. Eubacterial and L-phase colonies may be present in the same culture. The former are 1 to 3 mm in diameter after 48 h of growth on blood agar, are round and smooth, and develop optimally after approximately 72 h in 10% CO_2 at 37°C. L-phase colonies develop better on clear, serum-supplemented media and yield the characteristic "fried egg" appearance with irregular outlines and coarse granular lipid globules. In liquid media, growth occurs mainly in the form of "puff balls" at the bottom of the tube. The organism dies quickly unless subcultured.

S. moniliformis occurs naturally in the nasopharynx of wild and laboratory rats and other rodents (mice, squirrels, ferrets, weasels, and gerbils) and occasionally of dogs and cats that prey on rodents. Human infections result either from bites of those animals or from consumption of contaminated food or water. The former infection is called rat-bite fever, and the latter is called Haverhill fever. The characteristic picture of irregular fever, chills, myalgias, and arthralgias is followed in a few days by a maculopapular rash on the extremities and, sometimes, polyarthritis. Complications such as endocarditis (113), myocarditis, pericarditis, meningitis, pneumonia, amnionitis, and abscesses may develop (59).

The organism is best isolated from blood, joint fluid, or abscess material, which has to be collected and transported in the usual way (see chapters 5 and 20). It is inhibited by sodium polyanethol sulfonate present in blood culture media (138). Nalidixic acid has been used in selective media (138). In culture-negative cases, broad-range PCR of fluids has been employed (10, 134). Serological tests are unreliable (21).

S. moniliformis is biochemically inert (Table 5). Glucose is acidified weakly and in a delayed fashion (135). Identification may be confirmed by 16S rRNA gene sequencing (10) or by fatty acid analysis.

S. moniliformis is susceptible to many antimicrobials, particularly to penicillin and doxycycline, the mainstays of treatment (59). It is resistant to trimethoprim-sulfamethoxazole, nalidixic acid, and colistin. The MICs of aminoglycosides and ciprofloxacin are near breakpoint levels (138).

REFERENCES

1. **Ahmed, K., P. P. Sein, M. Shahnawaz, and A. A. Hoosen.** 2002. *Pasteurella gallinarum* neonatal meningitis. *Clin. Microbiol. Infect.* **8:**55–57.
2. **Aldridge, K. E., G. T. Valainis, and C. V. Sanders.** 1988. Comparison of the *in vitro* activity of ciprofloxacin and 24 other antimicrobial agents against clinical strains of *Chromobacterium violaceum. Diagn. Microbiol. Infect. Dis.* **10:**31–39.
3. **Al Fadel Saleh, M., M. S. Al-Madan, H. H. Erwa, I. Defonseka, S. Z. Sohel, and S. K. Sanyal.** 1995. First case of human infection caused by *Pasteurella gallinarum* causing infective endocarditis in an adolescent 10 years after surgical correction for truncus arteriosus. *Pediatrics* **95:**944–948.
4. **Alsina, M., E. Olle, and J. Frias.** 2001. Improved, low-cost selective culture medium for *Actinobacillus actinomycetemcomitans. J. Clin. Microbiol.* **39:**509–513.
5. **Angen, O., R. Mutters, D. A. Caugant, J. E. Olsen, and M. Bisgaard.** 1999. Taxonomic relationships of the *[Pasteurella] haemolytica* complex as evaluated by DNA-DNA hybridizations and 16S rRNA sequencing with proposal of *Mannheimia haemolytica* gen. nov., comb. nov., *Mannheimia granulomatis* comb. nov., *Mannheimia glucosida* sp. nov., *Mannheimia ruminalis* sp. nov. and *Mannheimia varigena* sp. nov. *Int. J. Syst. Bacteriol.* **49:**67–86.
6. **Arashima, Y., K. Kato, R. Kakuta, T. Fukui, K. Kumasaka, T. Tsuchiya, and K. Kawano.** 1999. First case of *Pasteurella gallinarum* isolation from blood of a patient with symptoms of acute gastroenteritis in Japan. *Clin. Infect. Dis.* **29:**698–699.
7. **Ashhurst-Smith, C., R. Norton, W. Thoreau, and M. M. Peel.** 1998. *Actinobacillus equuli* septicemia: an unusual zoonotic infection. *J. Clin. Microbiol.* **36:**2789–2790.
8. **Ashley, B. D., M. Nonne, A. D. Dwarakanath, and H. Malnick.** 2004. Fatal *Pasteurella dagmatis* peritonitis and septicaemia in a patient with cirrhosis: a case report and review of the literature. *J. Clin. Pathol.* **57:**210–212.
9. **Avril, J.-L., P.-Y. Donnio, and P. Pouedras.** 1990. Selective medium for *Pasteurella multocida* and its use to detect oropharyngeal carriage in pig breeders. *J. Clin. Microbiol.* **28:**1438–1440.
10. **Berger, C., M. Altwegg, A. Meyer, and D. Nadal.** 2001. Broad range polymerase chain reaction for diagnosis of rat-bite fever caused by *Streptobacillus moniliformis. Pediatr. Infect. Dis. J.* **20:**1181–1182.
11. **Bernard, K., C. Cooper, S. Tessier, and E. P. Ewan.** 1991. Use of chemotaxonomy as an aid to differentiate among *Capnocytophaga* species, CDC group DF-3, and aerotolerant strains of *Leptotrichia buccalis. J. Clin. Microbiol.* **29:**2263–2265.
12. **Bisgaard, M., and R. Mutters.** 1986. Characterization of some previously unclassified "*Pasteurella*" spp. obtained from the oral cavity of dogs and cats and description of a new species tentatively classified with the family *Pasteurellaceae* Pohl 1981 and provisionally called taxon 16. *Acta Pathol. Microbiol. Immunol. Scand. Sect. B* **94:**177–184.
13. **Blackall, P. J., H. Christensen, T. Beckenham, L. L. Blackall, and M. Bisgaard.** 2005. Reclassification of *Pasteurella gallinarum, [Haemophilus] paragallinarum, Pasteurella avium* and *Pasteurella volantium* as *Avibacterium gallinarum* gen. nov., comb. nov., *Avibacterium paragallinarum* comb. nov., *Avibacterium avium* comb. nov., *Avibacterium avium* comb. nov. and *Avibacterium volantium* comb. nov. *Int. J. Syst. Evol. Microbiol.* **55:**353–362.

14. **Blanche, P., E. Bloch, and D. Sicard.** 1998. *Capnocytophaga canimorsus* in the oral flora of dogs and cats. *J. Infect.* **36:**134.
15. **Bogaerts, J., J. Verhaegen, W. M. Tello, S. Allen, L. Verbist, E. Van Dyck, and P. Piot.** 1990. Characterization, in vitro susceptibility, and clinical significance of CDC group HB-5 from Rwanda. *J. Clin. Microbiol.* **28:**2196–2199.
16. **Bonatti, H., D. W. Rossboth, D. Nachbaur, M. Fille, C. Aspöck, I. Hend, K. Hourmont, L. White, H. Malnick, and F. J. Allerberger.** 2003. A series of infections due to *Capnocytophaga* spp. in immunosuppressed and immunocompetent patients. *Clin. Microbiol. Infect.* **9:**380–387.
17. **Brands, U., and W. Mannheim.** 1996. Use of two commercial rapid test kits for the identification of *Haemophilus* and related organisms—reactions of authentic strains. *Med. Microbiol. Lett.* **5:**133–144.
18. **Brito, C. F., C. B. Carvalho, F. Santos, R. T. Gazzinelli, S. C. Oliveira, V. Azevedo, and S. M. Teixeira.** 2004. *Chromobacterium violaceum* genome: molecular mechanisms associated with pathogenicity. *Genet. Mol. Res.* **3:**148–161.
19. **Brouqui, P., and D. Raoult.** 2001. Endocarditis due to rare and fastidious bacteria. *Clin. Microbiol. Rev.* **14:**177–207.
20. **Carandina, G., M. Bacchelli, A. Virgili, and R. Strumia.** 1984. *Simonsiella* filaments isolated from erosive lesions of the human oral cavity. *J. Clin. Microbiol.* **19:**931–933.
21. **Centers for Disease Control and Prevention.** 1998. Rat-bite fever, New Mexico, 1996. *JAMA* **279:**740–741.
22. **Chen, C.** 1996. Distribution of a newly described species, *Kingella oralis*, in the human oral cavity. *Oral Microbiol. Immunol.* **11:**425–427.
23. **Chen, C.-K. C., G. J. Sunday, J. J. Zambon, and M. E. Wilson.** 1990. Restriction endonuclease analysis of *Eikenella corrodens*. *J. Clin. Microbiol.* **28:**1265–1270.
24. **Chen, H. I., K. Hulten, and J. E. Clarridge III.** 2002. Taxonomic subgroups of *Pasteurella multocida* correlate with clinical presentation. *J. Clin. Microbiol.* **40:**3438–3441.
25. **Christensen, H., and M. Bisgaard.** 2006. The genus *Pasteurella*, p. 1062–1090. *In* M. Dworkin, S. Falkow, E. Rosenberg, K.-H. Schleifer, and E. Stackebrandt (ed.), *The Prokaryotes*, 3rd ed., vol. 6. *Proteobacteria: Gamma Subclass.* Springer, New York, N.Y.
26. **Christensen, H., and M. Bisgaard.** 2004. Revised definition of *Actinobacillus sensu stricto* isolated from animals. A review with special emphasis on diagnosis. *Vet. Microbiol.* **99:**13–30.
27. **Christensen, H., M. Bisgaard, Ø. Angen, W. Frederiksen, and J. E. Olsen.** 2005. Characterization of sucrose-negative *Pasteurella multocida* variants, including isolates from large-cat bite wounds. *J. Clin. Microbiol.* **43:**259–270.
28. **Ciantar, M., H. N. Newman, M. Wilson, and D. A. Spratt.** 2005. Molecular identification of *Capnocytophaga* spp. via 16S rRNA PCR-restriction fragment length polymorphism analysis. *J. Clin. Microbiol.* **43:**1894–1901.
29. **Ciantar, M., D. A. Spratt, H. N. Newman, and M. Wilson.** 2000. Assessment of five culture media for the growth and isolation of *Capnocytophaga* spp. *Clin. Microbiol. Infect.* **7:**158–160.
30. **Citron, D. M., Y. A. Warren, H. T. Fernandez, M. A. Goldstein, K. L. Tyrrell, and E. J. C. Goldstein.** 2005. Broth microdilution and disk diffusion tests for susceptibility testing of *Pasteurella* species isolated from human clinical specimens. *J. Clin. Microbiol.* **43:**2485–2488.
31. **Currie, P. F., M. Codispoti, P. S. Mankad, and M. J. Goodman.** 2000. Late aortic homograft valve endocarditis caused by *Cardiobacterium hominis*: a case report and review of the literature. *Heart* **83:**579–581.
32. **Daneshvar, M. I., D. G. Hollis, and C. W. Moss.** 1991. Chemical characterization of clinical isolates which are similar to CDC group DF-3 bacteria. *J. Clin. Microbiol.* **29:**2351–2353.
33. **De Leon, J. P., R. F. Sandfort, and J. D. Wong.** 2000. *Pasteurella bettyae*: report of nine cases and evidence of an emerging neonatal pathogen. *Clin. Microbiol. Newsl.* **22:**190–192.
34. **Dewhirst, F. E., C.-K. C. Chen, B. J. Paster, and J. J. Zambon.** 1993. Phylogeny of species in the family *Neisseriaceae* isolated from human dental plaque and description of *Kingella oralis* sp. nov. *Int. J. Syst. Bacteriol.* **43:**490–499. (Erratum, **44:**376, 1994.)
35. **Doern, G. V., R. Davaro, M. George, and P. Campognone.** 1996. Lack of requirement for prolonged incubation of Septi-Chek blood culture bottles in patients with bacteremia due to fastidious bacteria. *Diagn. Microbiol. Infect. Dis.* **24:**141–143.
36. **Dogan, B., S. Asikainen, and H. Jousimies-Somer.** 1999. Evaluation of two commercial kits and arbitrarily primed PCR for identification and differentiation of *Actinobacillus actinomycetemcomitans*, *Haemophilus aphrophilus*, and *Haemophilus paraphrophilus*. *J. Clin. Microbiol.* **37:**742–747.
37. **Donnio, P.-Y., A.-L. Lerestif-Gautier, and J.-L. Avril.** 2004. Characterization of *Pasteurella* spp. strains isolated from human infections. *J. Comp. Pathol.* **130:**137–142.
38. **Dusch, H., R. Zbinden, and A. von Graevenitz.** 1995. Growth differences of *Capnocytophaga canimorsus* strains and some other fastidious organisms on various Columbia-based blood agar media. *Zentbl. Bakteriol.* **282:**362–366.
39. **Ejlertsen, T., B. Gahrn-Hansen, P. Sogaard, O. Heltberg, and W. Frederiksen.** 1996. *Pasteurella aerogenes* isolated from ulcers or wounds in humans with occupational exposure to pigs: a report of 7 Danish cases. *Scand. J. Infect. Dis.* **28:**567–570.
40. **Escande, F., A. Bailly, S. Bone, and J. Lemozy.** 1996. *Actinobacillus suis* infection after a pig bite. *Lancet* **348:**888.
41. **Escande, F., E. Vallée, and F. Aubart.** 1997. *Pasteurella caballi* infection following a horse bite. *Zentbl. Bakteriol.* **285:**440–444.
42. **Fenollar, F., and D. Raoult.** 2000. Comparison of a commercial disk test with vancomycin and colimycin susceptibility testing for identification of bacteria with abnormal Gram staining reactions. *Eur. J. Clin. Microbiol. Infect. Dis.* **19:**33–38.
43. **Fischer, L. J., R. S. Weyant, E. H. White, and F. D. Quinn.** 1995. Intracellular multiplication and toxic destruction of cultured macrophages by *Capnocytophaga canimorsus*. *Infect. Immun.* **63:**3484–3490.
44. **Frebourg, N. B., G. Berthelot, R. Hocq, A. Chibani, and J.-F. Lemeland.** 2002. Septicemia due to *Pasteurella pneumotropica*: 16S rRNA sequencing for diagnosis confirmation. *J. Clin. Microbiol.* **40:**687–689.
45. **Frederiksen, W., and B. Tonning.** 2001. Possible misidentification of *Haemophilus aphrophilus* as *Pasteurella gallinarum*. *Clin. Infect. Dis.* **32:**987–989.
46. **Freeman, A. F., X. T. Zheng, J. C. Lane, and S. T. Shulman.** 2004. *Pasteurella aerogenes* hamster bite peritonitis. *Pediatr. Infect. Dis. J.* **23:**368–370.
47. **Frey, J., and P. Kuhnert.** 2002. RTX toxins in *Pasteurellaceae*. *Int. J. Med. Microbiol.* **292:**149–158.
48. **Friis-Moller, A., J. J. Christensen, V. Fussing, A. Hesselbjerg, J. Christiansen, and B. Bruun.** 2001. Clinical significance and taxonomy of *Actinobacillus hominis*. *J. Clin. Microbiol.* **39:**930–935.
49. **Fujise, O., W. Chen, S. Rich, and C. Chen.** 2004. Clonal diversity and stability of subgingival *Eikenella corrodens*. *J. Clin. Microbiol.* **42:**2036–2042.
50. **Furcht, C., K. Eschrich, and K. Merte.** 1996. Detection of *Eikenella corrodens* and *Actinobacillus actinomycetemcomitans* by use of the polymerase chain reaction (PCR) in vitro and in subgingival plaque. *J. Clin. Periodontol.* **23:**891–897.
51. **Garrity, G. M., J. A. Bell, and T. G. Lilburn.** 2005. Taxonomic outline of the Archaea and Bacteria, p. 207–220.

In G. M. Garrity (ed.-in-chief), *Bergey's Manual of Systematic Bacteriology*, 2nd ed., vol. 2. Springer, New York, N.Y.

52. **Gerardo, S. H., D. M. Citron, M. C. Claros, H. T. Fernandez, and E. J. C. Goldstein.** 2001. *Pasteurella multocida* subsp. *multocida* and *P. multocida* subsp. *septica* differentiation by PCR fingerprinting and α-glucosidase activity. *J. Clin. Microbiol.* **39:**2558–2564.
53. **Goldstein, E. J. C., E. O. Agyare, and R. Silletti.** 1981. Comparative growth of *Eikenella corrodens* on 15 media in three atmospheres of incubation. *J. Clin. Microbiol.* **13:**951–953.
54. **Goldstein, E. J. C., D. M. Citron, C. V. Merriam, Y. A. Warren, K. Tyrrell, and H. Fernandez.** 2001. Comparative *in vitro* activity of ertapenem and 11 other antimicrobial agents against aerobic and anaerobic pathogens isolated from skin and soft tissue animal and human bite wound infections. *J. Antimicrob. Chemother.* **48:**641–651.
55. **Goldstein, E. J. C., D. M. Citron, C. V. Merriam, Y. A. Warren, K. L. Tyrrel, and H. T. Fernandez.** 2002. Comparative *in vitro* activity of faropenem and 11 other antimicrobial agents against 405 aerobic and anaerobic pathogens isolated from skin and soft tissue infections from animal and human bites. *J. Antimicrob. Chemother.* **50:**411–420.
56. **Goldstein, E. J. C., D. M. Citron, and G. A. Richwald.** 1988. Lack of *in vitro* efficacy of oral forms of certain cephalosporins, erythromycin, and oxacillin against *Pasteurella multocida*. *Antimicrob. Agents Chemother.* **32:**213–215.
57. **Grehn, M., and F. Müller.** 1989. The oxidase reaction of *Pasteurella multocida* strains cultured on Mueller-Hinton medium. *J. Microbiol. Methods* **9:**333–336.
58. **Grob, R., R. Zbinden, C. Ruef, M. Hackenthal, I. Diesterweg, M. Altwegg, and A. von Graevenitz.** 1999. Septicemia caused by dysgonic fermenter 3 in a severely immunocompromised patient and isolation of the same microorganism from a stool specimen. *J. Clin. Microbiol.* **37:**1617–1618.
59. **Hagelskjaer, L., I. Sorensen, and E. Randers.** 1998. *Streptobacillus moniliformis* infection: 2 cases and a literature review. *Scand. J. Infect. Dis.* **30:**309–311.
60. **Hamilton-Miller, J. M. T.** 2002. Distinguishing *Pasteurella* spp. from *Haemophilus* spp.: the problem revisited. *Clin. Microbiol. Infect.* **8:**245.
61. **Han, X. Y., and E. Falsen.** 2005. Characterization of oral strains of *Cardiobacterium valvarum* and emended description of the organism. *J. Clin. Microbiol.* **43:**2370–2374.
62. **Hardy, D. J., B. B. Hulbert, and P. C. Migneault.** 1992. Time to detection of positive BacT/Alert blood cultures and lack of need for routine subculture of 5- to 7-day negative cultures. *J. Clin. Microbiol.* **30:**2743–2745.
63. **Harper, M., J. D. Boyce, I. W. Wilkie, and B. Adler.** 2003. Signature-tagged mutagenesis of *Pasteurella multocida* identifies mutants displaying differential virulence characteristics in mice and chickens. *Infect. Immun.* **71:**5440–5446.
64. **Hayashi, F., M. Okada, X. Zhong, and K. Miura.** 2001. PCR detection of *Capnocytophaga* species in dental plaque samples from children aged 2 to 12 years. *Microbiol. Immunol.* **45:**17–22.
65. **Henderson, B., S. P. Nair, J. M. Ward, and M. Wilson.** 2003. Molecular pathogenicity of the oral opportunistic pathogen *Actinobacillus actinomycetemcomitans*. *Ann. Rev. Microbiol.* **57:**29–55.
66. **Henrichsen, J.** 1983. Twitching motility. *Ann. Rev. Microbiol.* **37:**81–93.
67. **Hofstad, T., I. Olsen, E. R. Eribe, E. Falsen, M. D. Collins, and P. A. Lawson.** 2000. *Dysgonomonas* gen. nov. to accommodate *Dysgonomonas gadei* sp. nov., an organism isolated from a human gall bladder, and *Dysgonomonas capnocytophagoides* (formerly CDC group DF-3). *Int. J. Syst. Evol. Microbiol.* **50:**2189–2195.
68. **Holst, E., J. Rollof, L. Larsson, and J. P. Nielsen.** 1992. Characterization and distribution of *Pasteurella* species recovered from infected humans. *J. Clin. Microbiol.* **30:**2984–2987.
69. **Hoover, S. E., S. H. Fischer, R. Shaffer, B. M. Steinberg, and D. R. Lucey.** 2005. Endocarditis due to a novel *Cardiobacterium* species. *Ann. Intern. Med.* **142:**229–230.
70. **Host, B., H. Schumacher, J. Prag, and M. Arpi.** 2000. Isolation of *Kingella kingae* from synovial fluids using four commercial blood culture bottles. *Eur. J. Clin. Microbiol. Infect. Dis.* **19:**608–611.
71. **Hunt, M. L., B. Adler, and K. M. Townsend.** 2000. The molecular biology of *Pasteurella multocida*. *Vet. Microbiol.* **72:**3–25.
72. **ICSB Subcommittee on *Pasteurellaceae* and Related Organisms.** 1987. Minutes of the meetings, 6 and 10 September 1986, Manchester, England. *Int. J. Syst. Bacteriol.* **37:**474.
73. **Jenny, D. B., P. W. Letendre, and G. Iverson.** 1987. Endocarditis caused by *Kingella indologenes*. *Rev. Infect. Dis.* **9:**787–789.
74. **Jolivet-Gougeon, A., Z. Tamanai-Shacoori, L. Desbordes, N. Burggraeve, M. Cormier, and M. Bonnaure-Mallet.** 2004. Genetic analysis of an Ambler class A extended-spectrum beta-lactamase from *Capnocytophaga ochracea*. *J. Clin. Microbiol.* **42:**888–890.
75. **Kaplan, A. H., D. J. Weber, E. Z. Oddone, and J. R. Perfect.** 1989. Infection due to *Actinobacillus actinomycetemcomitans*: 15 cases and review. *Rev. Infect. Dis.* **11:**46–63.
76. **Kasten, R., R. Mutters, and W. Mannheim.** 1998. Catalase-positive *Eikenella corrodens* and *Eikenella*-like isolates of human and canine origin. *Zentbl. Bakteriol.* **288:**319–329.
77. **Kaur, P. P., C. T. Derk, M. Chatterji, and R. J. Dehoratius.** 2004. Septic arthritis caused by *Actinobacillus ureae* in a patient with rheumatoid arthritis receiving anti-tumor necrosis factor-alpha therapy. *J. Rheumatol.* **31:**1663–1666.
78. **Kok, R. H., M. J. Wolfhagen, B. M. Mooi, and J. J. Offerman.** 1999. A patient with thrombotic thrombocytopenic purpura caused by *Capnocytophaga canimorsus* septicemia. *Clin. Microbiol. Infect.* **5:**297–298.
79. **Krause, T., H. U. Bertschinger, L. Corboz, and R. Mutters.** 1987. V-factor dependent strains of *Pasteurella multocida* subsp. *multocida*. *Zentbl. Bakteriol.* **266:**255–260.
80. **Kugler, K. C., D. J. Biedenbach, and R. N. Jones.** 1999. Determination of the antimicrobial activity of 29 clinically important compounds tested against fastidious HACEK group organisms. *Diagn. Microbiol. Infect. Dis.* **34:**73–76.
81. **Kuhn, D. A., and D. A. Gregory.** 1978. Emendation of *Simonsiella muelleri* Schmid and description of *Simonsiella steedae* sp. nov., with designations of the respective proposed neotype and holotype strains. *Curr. Microbiol.* **1:**11–14.
82. **Kuhn, D. A., D. A. Gregory, G. E. Buchanan, Jr., M. D. Nyby, and K. R. Daly.** 1978. Isolation, characterization, and numerical taxonomy of *Simonsiella* strains from the oral cavities of cats, dogs, sheep and humans. *Arch. Microbiol.* **118:**235–241.
83. **Kuhnert, P., H. Berthoud, R. Straub, and J. Frey.** 2003. Host cell specific activity of RTX toxins from haemolytic *Actinobacillus equuli* and *Actinobacillus suis*. *Vet. Microbiol.* **92:**161–167.
84. **Kuzucu, C., G. Yetkin, G. Kocak, and V. Nisanoglu.** 2005. An unusual case of pericarditis caused by *Cardiobacterium hominis*. *J. Infect.* **50:**346–347.
85. **Lacroix, J. M., and C. Walker.** 1991. Characterization of a beta-lactamase found in *Eikenella corrodens*. *Antimicrob. Agents Chemother.* **35:**886–891.

86. **Lawson, P. A., E. Falsen, E. Inganäs, R. S. Weyant, and M. D. Collins.** 2002. *Dysgonomonas mossii* sp. nov., from human sources. *Syst. Appl. Microbiol.* **25:**194–197.
87. **Lawson, P. A., H. Malnick, M. D. Collins, J. J. Shah, M. A. Chattaway, R. Bendall, and J. W. Hartley.** 2005. Description of *Kingella potus* sp. nov., an organism isolated from a wound caused by an animal bite. *J. Clin. Microbiol.* **43:**3526–3529.
88. **Lee, J., J. S. Kim, C. H. Nahm, J. W. Choi, J. Kim, S. H. Pai, K. H. Moon, K. Lee, and Y. Chong.** 1999. Two cases of *Chromobacterium violaceum* infection after injury in a subtropical region. *J. Clin. Microbiol.* **37:**2068–2070.
89. **Lejbkowicz, F., V. Davidkin, and S. Gorenshtein.** 2003. *Pasteurella haemolytica* in human urine. *Scand. J. Infect. Dis.* **35:**512–514.
90. **Lindberg, J., W. Frederiksen, B. Gahrn-Hansen, and B. Bruun.** 1998. Problems of identification in clinical microbiology exemplified by pig bite wound infections. *Zentbl. Bakteriol.* **288:**491–499.
91. **Lion, C., F. Escande, and J. C. Burdin.** 1996. *Capnocytophaga canimorsus* infections in human: review of the literature and cases report. *Eur. J. Epidemiol.* **12:**521–533.
92. **Lion, C., P. de Monchy, M. Weber, M. C. Conroy, F. Mory, and J. C. Burdin.** 1992. Sensibilité aux antibiotiques de quarante-quatre souches de bactéries du groupe EF4: étude des concentrations minimales inhibitrices par dilution en gélose. *Pathol. Biol.* **40:**471–478.
93. **Lu, P.-L., P.-R. Hsueh, C.-C. Hung, L.-J. Teng, T.-N. Jang, and K.-T. Luh.** 2000. Infective endocarditis complicated with progressive heart failure due to β-lactamase-producing *Cardiobacterium hominis*. *J. Clin. Microbiol.* **38:**2015–2017.
94. **Madinier, I. M., T. B. Fosse, C. Hitzig, Y. Charbit, and L. R. Hannoun.** 1999. Resistance profile survey of 50 periodontal strains of *Actinobacillus actinomycetemcomitans*. *J. Periodontol.* **70:**888–892.
95. **Martinez-Sanchez, L., F. J. Vasallo, F. Garcia-Garrote, L. Alcala, M. Rodriguez-Créixems, and E. Bouza.** 1998. Clinical isolation of a DF-3 microorganism and review of the literature. *Clin. Microbiol. Infect.* **4:**344–346.
96. **Minamoto, G. Y., and E. M. Sordillo.** 1992. *Kingella denitrificans* as a cause of granulomatous disease in a patient with AIDS. *Clin. Infect. Dis.* **15:**1052–1053.
97. **Moumile, K., J. Merckx, C. Glorion, P. Berche, and A. Ferroni.** 2003. Osteoarticular infections caused by *Kingella kingae* in children: contribution of polymerase chain reaction to the microbiologic diagnosis. *Pediatr. Infect. Dis. J.* **22:**837–839.
98. **Mueller, N. J., V. Kaplan, R. Zbinden, and M. Altwegg.** 1999. Diagnosis of *Cardiobacterium hominis* endocarditis by broad-range PCR from arterio-embolic tissue. *Infection* **27:**278–279.
99. **Mulder, A. H., P. G. G. Gerlag, L. H. M. Verhoef, and A. W. L. van den Wall Bake.** 2001. Hemolytic uremic syndrome after *Capnocytophaga canimorsus* (DF-2) septicemia. *Clin. Nephrol.* **55:**167–170.
100. **Naas, T., F. Benaoudia, L. Lebrun, and P. Nordmann.** 2001. Molecular identification of TEM-1 beta-lactamase in a *Pasteurella multocida* isolate of human origin. *Eur. J. Clin. Microbiol. Infect. Dis.* **20:**210–213.
101. **Nikkari, S., R. Gotoff, P. P. Bourbeau, R. E. Brown, N. R. Kamal, and D. A. Relman.** 2002. Identification of *Cardiobacterium hominis* by broad-range bacterial polymerase chain reaction analysis in a case of culture-negative endocarditis. *Arch. Intern. Med.* **162:**477–479.
102. **Nonnemacher, C., R. Mutters, and L. Flores de Jacoby.** 2001. Microbiological characteristics of subgingival microbiota in adult periodontitis, localized juvenile periodontis and rapidly progressive periodontitis subjects. *Clin. Microbiol. Infect.* **7:**213–217.
103. **Oberhofer, T. R.** 1981. Characteristics and biotypes of *Pasteurella multocida* isolated from humans. *J. Clin. Microbiol.* **13:**566–571.
104. **Ochiai, K., H. Senpuku, and T. Kurita-Ochiai.** 1998. Purification of immunosuppressive factor from *Capnocytophaga ochracea*. *J. Med. Microbiol.* **47:**1087–1095.
105. **Olsen, J., H. N. Shah, and S. E. Gharbia.** 1999. Taxonomy and biochemical characteristics of *Actinobacillus actinomycetemcomitans* and *Porphyromonas gingivalis*. *Periodontology* **20:**14–52.
106. **Paju, S., P. Carlson, H. Jousimies-Somer, and S. Asikainen.** 2000. Heterogeneity of *Actinobacillus actinomycetemcomitans* strains in various human infections and relationships between serotype, genotype, and antimicrobial susceptibility. *J. Clin. Microbiol.* **38:**79–84.
107. **Paju, S., P. Carlson, H. Jousimies-Somer, and S. Asikainen.** 2003. *Actinobacillus actinomycetemcomitans* and *Haemophilus aphrophilus* in systemic and nonoral infections in Finland. *APMIS* **111:**653–657.
108. **Paster, B. J., W. A. Falkler, Jr., C. O. Enwonwu, E. O. Idigbe, K. O. Savage, V. A. Levanos, M. A. Tamer, R. L. Ericson, C. N. Lau, and F. E. Dewhirst.** 2002. Prevalent bacterial species and novel phylotypes in advanced noma lesions. *J. Clin. Microbiol.* **40:**2187–2191.
109. **Peel, M. M., K. A. Hornidge, M. Luppino, A. M. Stacpoole, and R. E. Weaver.** 1991. *Actinobacillus* spp. and related bacteria in infected wounds of humans bitten by horses and sheep. *J. Clin. Microbiol.* **29:**2535–2538.
110. **Potts, T. V., J. J. Zambon, and R. J. Genco.** 1985. Reassignment of *Actinobacillus actinomycetemcomitans* to the genus *Haemophilus* as *Haemophilus actinomycetemcomitans* comb. nov. *Int. J. Syst. Bacteriol.* **33:**337–341.
111. **Rivera, M., G. C. Hunter, J. Brooker, C. W. O'Berg, S. H. Smythe, and V. M. Bernhard.** 1994. Aortic graft infection due to *Pasteurella haemolytica* and group C β-hemolytic streptococcus. *Clin. Infect. Dis.* **19:**941–943.
112. **Roebuck, J. D., and J. T. Morris.** 1999. Chronic otitis media due to EF-4 bacteria. *Clin. Infect. Dis.* **29:**1343–1344.
113. **Rordorf, T., C. Züger, R. Zbinden, A. von Graevenitz, and M. Pirovino.** 2000. *Streptobacillus moniliformis* endocarditis in an HIV-positive patient. *Infection* **28:**393–394.
114. **Rossau, R., G. Vandenbussche, S. Thielemans, P. Segers, H. Grosch, E. Göthe, W. Mannheim, and J. de Ley.** 1989. Ribosomal ribonucleic acid cistron similarities and deoxyribonucleic acid homologies of *Neisseria*, *Kingella*, *Eikenella*, *Simonsiella*, *Alysiella*, and Centers for Disease Control groups EF-4 and M-5 in the emended family *Neisseriaceae*. *Int. J. Syst. Bacteriol.* **39:**185–198.
115. **Rummens, J.-L., B. Gordts, and H. W. van Landuyt.** 1986. In vitro susceptibility of *Capnocytophaga* species to 29 antimicrobial agents. *Antimicrob. Agents Chemother.* **30:**739–742.
116. **Rycroft, A. N., and L. H. Garside.** 2000. *Actinobacillus* species and their role in animal disease. *Vet. J.* **159:**18–36.
117. **Sakazaki, R., E. Yoshizaki, K. Tamura, and S. Kuramochi.** 1984. Increased frequency of isolation of *Pasteurella* and *Actinobacillus* species and related organisms. *Eur. J. Clin. Microbiol. Infect. Dis.* **3:**244–248.
118. **Sandoe, J. A. T.** 2004. *Capnocytophaga canimorsus* endocarditis. *J. Med. Microbiol.* **53:**245–248.
119. **Sarma, P. S., and S. Mohanty.** 2001. *Capnocytophaga cynodegmi* cellulitis, bacteremia, and pneumonitis in a diabetic man. *J. Clin. Microbiol.* **39:**2028–2029.
120. **Schlater, L. K., D. J. Brenner, A. G. Steigerwalt, C. W. Moss, M. A. Lambert, and R. A. Packer.** 1989. *Pasteurella caballi*, a new species from equine clinical specimens. *J. Clin. Microbiol.* **27:**2169–2174.
121. **Shawar, R., J. Sepulveda, and J. E. Clarridge.** 1990. Use of the RapID-ANA system and sodium polyanetholesulfonate

disk susceptibility testing in identifying *Haemophilus ducreyi*. *J. Clin. Microbiol.* **28:**108–111.

122. **Sheng, W.-S., P.-R. Hsueh, C.-C. Hung, L.-J. Teng, Y.-C. Chen, and K.-T. Luh.** 2001. Clinical features of patients with invasive *Eikenella corrodens* infections and microbiological characteristics of the causative isolates. *Eur. J. Clin. Microbiol. Infect. Dis.* **20:**213–236.
123. **Sirinavin, S., C. Techasaensiri, S. Benjaponpitak, R. Pornkul, and M. Vorachit.** 2005. Invasive *Chromobacterium violaceum* infection in children: case report and review. *Pediatr. Infect. Dis. J.* **24:**559–561.
124. **Slee, A. M., and J. M. Tanzer.** 1978. Selective medium for isolation of *Eikenella corrodens* from periodontal lesions. *J. Clin. Microbiol.* **8:**459–462.
125. **Slonim, A., E. S. Walker, E. Mishori, N. Porat, R. Dagan, and P. Yagupsky.** 1998. Person-to-person transmission of *Kingella kingae* among day care center attendees. *J. Infect. Dis.* **178:**1843–1846.
126. **Slotnick, I. J.** 1968. *Cardiobacterium hominis* in genitourinary specimens. *J. Bacteriol.* **95:**1175.
127. **Slots, J.** 1982. Selective medium for isolation of *Actinobacillus actinomycetemcomitans*. *J. Clin. Microbiol.* **15:**606–609.
128. **Slots, J., R. T. Evans, P. M. Lobbins, and R. J. Genco.** 1980. In vitro anti-microbial susceptibility of *Actinobacillus actinomycetemcomitans*. *Antimicrob. Agents Chemother.* **18:**9–12.
129. **Sordillo, E. M., M. Rendel, R. Sood, J. Belinfanti, O. Murray, and D. Brook.** 1993. Septicemia due to β-lactamase-positive *Kingella kingae*. *Clin. Infect. Dis.* **17:**818–819.
130. **Sutton, R. G. A., M. F. O'Keeffe, M. A. Bundock, J. Jeboult, and M. P. Tester.** 1972. Isolation of a new *Moraxella* from corneal abscess. *J. Med. Microbiol.* **5:**148–150.
131. **Suzuki, N., Y. Nakano, Y. Yoshida, D. Ikeda, and T. Koga.** 2001. Identification of *Actinobacillus actinomycetemcomitans* serotypes by multiplex PCR. *J. Clin. Microbiol.* **39:**2002–2005.
132. **Takeda, S., Y. Arashima, K. Kato, M. Ogawa, K. Kono, K. Watanabe, and T. Saito.** 2003. A case of *Pasteurella haemolytica* sepsis in a patient with mitral disease who developed a splenic abscess. *Scand. J. Infect. Dis.* **35:**764–765.
133. **Talan, D. A., D. M. Citron, F. M. Abrahamian, G. J. Moran, and E. J. C. Goldstein.** 1999. Bacteriologic analysis of infected dog and cat bites. *N. Engl. J. Med.* **340:**85–92.
134. **Wallet, F., C. Savage, C. Loïez, E. Renaux, P. Tischedda, and R. J. Courcol.** 2003. Molecular diagnosis of arthritis due to *Streptobacillus moniliformis*. *Diagn. Microbiol. Infect. Dis.* **47:**623–624.
135. **Weyant, R. S., C. W. Moss, R. E. Weaver, D. G. Hollis, J. G. Jordan, E. C. Cook, and M. I. Daneshvar.** 1996. *Identification of Unusual Pathogenic Gram-Negative Aerobic and Facultatively Anaerobic Bacteria*, 2nd ed. Williams & Wilkins, Baltimore, Md.
136. **Whitehouse, R. L. S., H. Jackson, M. C. Jackson, and M. M. Ramji.** 1987. Isolation of *Simonsiella* sp. from a neonate. *J. Clin. Microbiol.* **25:**522–525.
137. **Whitelaw, A. C., I. M. Shankland, and B. G. Elisha.** 2002. Use of 16S rRNA sequencing for identification of *Actinobacillus ureae* isolated from a cerebrospinal fluid sample. *J. Clin. Microbiol.* **40:**666–668.
138. **Wullenweber, M.** 1994. *Streptobacillus moniliformis*—a zoonotic pathogen. Taxonomic considerations, host species, diagnosis, therapy, geographical distribution. *Lab. Anim.* **29:**1–15.
139. **Yagupsky, P.** 2004. *Kingella kingae:* from medical rarity to an emerging paediatric pathogen. *Lancet Infect. Dis.* **4:**358–367.
140. **Yagupsky, P., M. Merires, J. Bahar, and R. Dagan.** 1995. Evaluation of novel vancomycin-containing medium for primary isolation of *Kingella kingae* from upper respiratory tract specimens. *J. Clin. Microbiol.* **33:**1426–1427.
141. **Yaneza, A. L., H. Jivan, P. Kumari, and M. S. Togoo.** 1991. *Pasteurella haemolytica* endocarditis. *J. Infect.* **23:**65–67.
142. **Zbinden, R., P. Sommerhalder, and U. von Wartburg.** 1988. Co-isolation of *Pasteurella dagmatis* and *Pasteurella multocida* from cat-bite wounds. *Eur. J. Clin. Microbiol. Infect. Dis.* **7:**203–204.
143. **Zurlo, J. J.** 2005. *Pasteurella* species, p. 2687–2691. *In* G. L. Mandell, J. E. Bennett, and R. Dolin (ed.), *Principles and Practice of Infectious Diseases*, 6th ed. Elsevier-Churchill Livingstone, Philadelphia, Pa.

Haemophilus

MOGENS KILIAN

41

TAXONOMY AND DESCRIPTION OF THE GENUS

Members of the genus *Haemophilus* are gram-negative, non-acid-fast, nonmotile, and non-spore-forming rods that may range from small coccobacilli to filamentous rods. They are obligate parasites that, with a few misclassified exceptions (e.g., *Haemophilus ducreyi*), are exclusively adapted to human mucosal membranes in the respiratory tract. Most species of animal origin originally included in the genus *Haemophilus* have been transferred to the genus *Pasteurella* or the genus *Actinobacillus*, which together with the genus *Haemophilus* and several newly described genera of bacteria from animals constitute the family *Pasteurellaceae* (62).

The currently recognized *Haemophilus* species associated with humans are *H. influenzae, H. aegyptius, H. haemolyticus, H. parainfluenzae, H. parahaemolyticus, H. ducreyi, H. aphrophilus, H. paraphrophilus, H. segnis, H. pittmaniae*, and the poorly defined species *H. paraphrohaemolyticus* (36, 60).

All *Haemophilus* species are facultatively anaerobic. The genus name refers to the fact that in vitro growth requires accessory growth factors contained in blood: X factor (hemin; "X" for unknown) and V factor (NAD; "V" for vitamin). *H. influenzae* requires both of these compounds, whereas most other species require only one of them (Table 1). Strains of a few species grow better in a humid atmosphere with added 5 to 10% CO_2. The optimal temperature is about 33 to 37°C (see below).

Haemophilus species ferment a characteristic range of carbohydrates; end products from the fermentation of glucose are succinic, lactic, and acetic acids. Strains of some species (e.g., *H. aphrophilus*) produce gas in fermentation media. All *Haemophilus* strains reduce nitrate and produce alkaline phosphatase (35). The G+C content of DNA of *Haemophilus* species ranges from 37 to 44 mol% (35). Predominant cell wall fatty acids are *n*-tetradecanoate (14:0), 3-hydroxytetradecanoate (3-OH-14:0), hexadecanoate (16:1), and *n*-hexadecanoate (16:0) (36).

Separate subpopulations of *H. influenzae* express polysaccharide capsules, of which six different serotypes, termed serotypes a through f, have been described.

By traditional taxonomic criteria, it is unjustified to maintain the recognition of *H. influenzae* and *H. aegyptius* as separate species (10). However, one formal obstacle to combining the two is that the name *H. aegyptius* has priority over *H. influenzae*. Moreover, population genetic analyses reveal that they do constitute distinct populations of bacteria, and clinical experience indicates that they have distinct pathogenic potentials. This is even truer for the so-called *H. influenzae* biogroup aegyptius, which is the closest relative of *H. aegyptius* (7, 37). Likewise, several studies have questioned the validity of *H. paraphrophilus* as a species separate from *H. aphrophilus* (37).

According to nucleic acid hybridization studies and 16S rRNA sequence homologies, the species *H. ducreyi* does not belong in the genus *Haemophilus*, although it is a valid member of the family *Pasteurellaceae* (37, 62). *Actinobacillus actinomycetemcomitans* is closely related to *H. aphrophilus, H. paraphrophilus*, and *H. segnis* (62, 71). However, as *A. actinomycetemcomitans* lacks significant homology to the type species *H. influenzae*, the proposal to transfer *A. actinomycetemcomitans* to the genus *Haemophilus* has gained limited support (71). Rather, *A. actinomycetemcomitans* and its close relatives among the *Haemophilus* species warrant recognition as a separate genus in the family *Pasteurellaceae*.

EPIDEMIOLOGY AND TRANSMISSION

Haemophilus bacteria constitute approximately 10% of the normal bacterial flora of the healthy upper respiratory tract. The predominant species is *H. parainfluenzae*, which accounts for three-fourths of the *Haemophilus* flora both in the oral cavity and in the pharynx but is absent in the nasal cavity. Noncapsulate *H. influenzae* strains, predominantly of biotypes II or III, are present in the pharynx of most healthy children but normally constitute less than 2% of the total bacterial flora (19, 37).

Nasopharyngeal colonization by *H. influenzae* is a dynamic phenomenon characterized by constant turnover of a mixture of clones, with a mean duration of carriage of 1.4 to 2 months (19, 74, 80). During local infection a single clone of *H. influenzae* usually dominates the bacterial flora in the pharynx and nasal cavity. With increasing age of the individual, carriage of *H. influenzae* in the upper respiratory tract becomes less frequent (37). In contrast to the situation in the upper respiratory tract, patients with chronic obstructive pulmonary disease are often persistently colonized by a single or multiple clones of noncapsulate *H. influenzae* (54). In most populations without vaccination, *H. influenzae* serotype b carriage by

TABLE 1 Principal differential characteristics of *Haemophilus* species

Species	Growth factor requirement		Hemolysis	Fermentation of:					Presence of catalase	β-Galactosidase (ONPG[b] test)	CO_2 enhances growth
	X[a]	V		Glucose	Sucrose	Lactose	Mannose	Xylose			
H. influenzae[c]	+	+	−	+	−	−	−	+[d]	+	−	−
H. aegyptius[c]	+	+	−	+	−	−	−	−	+	−	−
H. haemolyticus	+	+[e]	+/−	+	−	−	−	+[d]	+	−	−
H. ducreyi	+	−	−[f]	−	−	−	−	−	−	−	−
H. parainfluenzae	−	+	−	+	+	−	+	−	D[g]	D	−
H. parahaemolyticus	−	+[e]	+	+	+	−	−	−	+	−	−
H. segnis	−	+	−	w[h]	w	−	−	−	D	−	−
H. paraphrophilus[i]	−	+	−	+	+	+	+	D	−	+	+
H. aphrophilus[i]	−	−	−	+	+	+	+	−	−	+	+
H. pittmaniae	−	+[e]	+	+	+	−	+	−	−/w	+	−

[a] As determined by the porphyrin test.
[b] ONPG, *o*-nitrophenyl-β-D-galactopyranoside.
[c] For further characteristics, see Table 2.
[d] More than 90% of isolates are positive.
[e] Due to V factor being released from blood cells in blood agar (bovine, horse, and rabbit blood) by the bacterial hemolysin, symbiosis can be demonstrated only on blood-free media.
[f] Detection requires special media; see text.
[g] D, differences encountered.
[h] w, weak reaction.
[i] For further characteristics, see Table 3.

healthy individuals is below 1% during the first 6 months of life but averages 3 to 5% throughout the rest of childhood, although it may be considerably higher in selected populations (74, 86). Crowding seems to be a factor contributing to a higher carriage rate (33, 74). In most populations, vaccination of children resulted in a significantly reduced carriage of *H. influenzae* serotype b as a result of antibodies induced by the conjugate vaccine (81), but there are unexplained exceptions to this pattern (3, 33).

The association between pharyngeal colonization with *H. influenzae* type b and the occurrence and transmission of disease remains poorly understood. Factors that seem to contribute to the lack of direct association are differences in virulence of individual clones of *H. influenzae* type b (56, 57) and in the disease susceptibility of individuals (33, 66). Carriage in healthy individuals of *H. aegyptius* and *H. influenzae* biogroup aegyptius has not been demonstrated.

The species *H. parainfluenzae, H. pittmaniae, H. aphrophilus, H. paraphrophilus,* and *H. segnis,* but not *H. influenzae,* are part of the normal microflora of the oral cavity in front of the palatinal arches. The species *H. aphrophilus, H. paraphrophilus,* and *H. segnis* occur predominantly on tooth surfaces in the biofilm known as dental plaque. Carriage of *H. parahaemolyticus* and *H. haemolyticus* in healthy individuals appears to be rare. Human saliva contains a mean number of more than 10^7 haemophili per ml (36). Symptomless cervical carriage of the venereal pathogen *H. ducreyi* may occur (29, 85). Spread of the *Haemophilus* species that colonize the upper respiratory tract typically occurs by respiratory droplets, and spread of *H. ducreyi* is by sexual intercourse.

CLINICAL SIGNIFICANCE

H. influenzae

Until the implementation of vaccination in many countries, *H. influenzae* was one of the three leading causes of bacterial meningitis worldwide. Most of these cases were in young children between the ages of 3 months and 3 years, with a peak incidence of infection at 6 to 7 months of age. Virtually all were caused by serotype b, and the majority belonged to biotype I. Both characteristics make them distinct from commensal strains. Strains with the same characteristics were also a major etiological agent of acute epiglottitis (obstructive laryngitis) associated with septicemia. The annual number of invasive *H. influenzae* serotype b infections in the United States is now below 100, most of which occur in unvaccinated or incompletely vaccinated children (1, 11). However, disease still occurs in selected vaccinated populations (27, 28, 43) and *H. influenzae* type b remains a leading cause of meningitis among unvaccinated children in many Asian and developing countries. It is estimated that at least 3 million cases of serious disease and 400,000 to 700,000 deaths occur in young children per year worldwide (66). Occasional cases of invasive infection caused by noncapsulate strains or strains possessing a capsule, primarily of serotype f, occur, mostly in patients with significant underlying disease, such as malignancy, chronic obstructive pulmonary disease, alcoholism, and human immunodeficiency virus infection (22). In children, underlying diseases are less common (26% of cases), and pneumonia and meningitis are equally represented (88). Strains that carry a capsule of serotype a, c, d, or e are occasionally isolated from patients with infections as well as from the healthy respiratory tract (38, 51, 86, 92). Among Navajo and White Mountain Apache children a relatively high incidence (20.2 cases per 100,000 population aged <5 years) of invasive disease with serotype a strains is observed, but with no absolute increase in numbers in the period after vaccination against *H. influenzae* type b (51).

Invasion of the bloodstream by encapsulated strains of *H. influenzae* may also result in septic arthritis, osteomyelitis, cellulitis, and pericarditis (66, 86). Primary *H. influenzae* pneumonia is being recognized with increasing frequency in both children and adults and is sometimes complicated by bacteremia (44, 53, 58). A recent literature review revealed that *H. influenzae* accounted for 7% of identified etiologic agents of childhood community-acquired pneumonia in North America and Europe and for 21% of such agents in Africa and South America (58). Most isolates from patients with pneumonia are non-type b strains. Pneumonia was the predominant clinical syndrome in patients with *H. influenzae* serotype f disease (88).

Noncapsulate *H. influenzae* strains (often collectively referred to by the misnomer "nontypeable"), indistinguishable from strains found in the healthy respiratory tract (predominantly biotypes II and III), are frequent causes of infections in children. Infections with noncapsulate *H. influenzae* usually occur at sites contiguous with the upper respiratory tract (21, 53) and typically do not include bacteremia, although occasional cases are reported (21, 63). Noncapsulate *H. influenzae* is, after *Streptococcus pneumoniae*, the second most frequent cause of otitis media, the most common cause of purulent bacterial conjunctivitis, and an important cause of sinusitis and chronic or acute exacerbations of lower respiratory tract infections in patients with and without cystic fibrosis (21, 24, 53, 86). *H. influenzae* otitis media is usually associated with significantly increased proportions (>50% of total bacterial flora) of the same clone in the nasopharynx (18, 42). *H. influenzae* occasionally causes obstetric and neonatal infections, and in some countries these are predominantly due to biotype IV strains that are genetically distinct from other *H. influenzae* (73, 93). Both *H. influenzae* and *H. parainfluenzae* have been implicated in urinary tract infections and peritonitis (2, 73, 86, 93). Occasional cases of meningitis caused by noncapsulate *H. influenzae* are often associated with underlying medical problems including ventriculoperitoneal shunts (21, 63).

H. aegyptius

H. aegyptius (Koch-Weeks bacillus) is associated with an acute purulent and contagious form of conjunctivitis ("pink eye") that occurs in seasonal endemics, especially in hot climates (69, 86). In the mid-1980s and early 1990s bacteria that share many of the properties of *H. aegyptius* caused small epidemics of a fulminant pediatric disease known as Brazilian purpuric fever (BPF), manifested by high fever, hemorrhagic skin lesions, septicemia, vascular collapse, hypotensive shock, and death, usually within 48 h of onset (7). The disease is characteristically preceded by purulent conjunctivitis that has resolved before the onset of fever. Although invasive, these bacteria are noncapsulate and have been designated *H. influenzae* biogroup aegyptius (7), a term sometimes erroneously also applied to strains of *H. aegyptius*. Cases clinically similar to BPF were observed in Australia and in the United States, but these were caused by strains genetically related to but distinct from Brazilian BPF isolates (7, 37).

H. ducreyi

H. ducreyi causes the venereal disease soft chancre or chancroid. The genital lesion begins as a tender papule that becomes pustular and then ulcerated over the course of 2 days. Lesions may merge to form larger ulcers that may be accompanied by unilateral inguinal lymphadenitis (bubo formation). *H. ducreyi* infection is an important cause of genital ulcers in Asia, Africa, and Latin America, but is a less important cause of such infections in North America and most parts of Europe. However, PCR detection of *H. ducreyi* suggests that the prevalence of chancroid is underreported (64, 88). The disease has received renewed attention because it facilitates the transmission of human immunodeficiency virus in populations in which it is endemic. Extragenital lesions may occur but are rare (39, 70, 88).

Other Species

In my experience *H. parahaemolyticus* is often isolated from patients with pharyngitis in whom no other bacterial pathogen is detected, from patients with lower respiratory tract infections, and from patients with local abscesses in the oral cavity. Some *Haemophilus* isolates from lower respiratory tract samples from patients with chronic obstructive pulmonary disease are *H. haemolyticus*, some of which, disturbingly, are nonhemolytic and impossible to distinguish from *H. influenzae* by phenotypic analysis (55). Further studies on the clinical significance of these species in causing respiratory tract infections are needed.

Some of the oral *Haemophilus* species (*H. parainfluenzae, H. pittmaniae, H. aphrophilus, H. paraphrophilus,* and *H. segnis*) are occasionally implicated in subacute endocarditis, brain abscesses, sinusitis, arthritis, and osteomyelitis (2, 15, 76), which may follow a temporary bacteremic condition in association with dental treatments that cause a break of the oral mucosal barrier. Reported cases of meningitis ascribed to *H. parainfluenzae* can probably be explained by misidentification of *H. influenzae* isolates as described below.

COLLECTION, TRANSPORT, AND STORAGE

Specimens of patient blood and cerebrospinal fluid (CSF) are obtained and processed as described in chapters 5 and 20. Prompt transport of these samples to the laboratory is mandatory to ensure the fastest possible diagnosis and survival of microorganisms in the sample. Additional specimens from which *Haemophilus* organisms may be isolated include aspirated synovial fluid, pericardial fluid, pleural fluid, pus, nasopharyngeal or throat swabs, sputum, purulent discharge from infected eyes, urine, and occasionally vaginal swabs. It is important that samples taken from the respiratory tract remain representative of the infecting flora by avoidance of contamination with commensals as far as possible. Thus, throat swabs must be collected from the pharynx and not surfaces in front of the palatinal arches. Because most children carry *H. influenzae* in the upper respiratory tract, its mere detection is of no value for establishment of the etiology of otitis media (18).

Samples must be transported to the laboratory in a suitable transport medium or should be spread directly onto appropriate agar media whenever possible (especially conjunctival specimens). The viability of most *Haemophilus* organisms is readily lost as a result of drying out, and they do not survive more than a few days in clinical samples. This is particularly true for the more fastidious species such as *H. aegyptius*.

Genital specimens for *H. ducreyi* culture should be collected from the base and the undermined margins of the chancroid lesion with a saline- or broth-moistened swab. Cultivation may be supplemented by aspiration of pus from infected bubonic lymph nodes, but isolation of *H. ducreyi* from pus is usually less successful than isolation from ulcer material (17, 85). Direct plating on selective media is preferable as it results in the highest recovery. The use of transport media is a viable alternative only if a reliable source of refrigeration is available, as the viability of *H. ducreyi* in various transport media is completely lost within 1 day at room temperature. Best results were obtained by using thioglycolate-hemin-based transport media containing various combinations of selenium dioxide, albumin, and glutamine (14). After storage at 4°C for up to 4 days, 71% of samples from patients clinically diagnosed with chancroid yielded growth of *H. ducreyi.*

Haemophilus isolates may be stored for many years at room temperature after lyophilization in skim milk or at −135°C on dry cotton swabs heavily inoculated with bacteria from an agar culture transferred to a sterile empty vial. An alternative method of storage is freezing below −60°C of 24-h broth cultures or suspensions of freshly grown cells in broth medium containing 10% glycerol. Biweekly transfers on agar media can also maintain most strains. However, strains of *H. aegyptius* and *H. ducreyi* will rapidly die out.

DIRECT EXAMINATION

Microscopic Examination

CSF

A smear of CSF previously concentrated by centrifugation at 10,000 × *g* or by filtration is stained by Gram's method or with methylene blue. Cytocentrifugation of CSF significantly increases the sensitivity of the Gram stain (79). Care should be exercised in destaining because the coccobacillary form of *H. influenzae* may morphologically resemble pneumococci. However, in CSF the organism may be relatively pleomorphic, with coccoid, coccobacillary, short-rod, long-rod, and filamentous forms. The bacteria may be few in number but are usually detected along with granulocytes by careful examination.

Capsules present on bacteria in CSF can be demonstrated by several techniques, provided that a sufficient number of bacteria are present. The simplest method is by demonstration of the capsular swelling reaction (Quellung reaction). A drop of CSF is mixed on a slide with a drop of an antiserum against each of the capsular serotypes (Becton Dickinson Diagnostic Systems, Sparks, Md.). When mixed with the relevant antiserum, the capsule will appear swollen and sharply delineated by phase-contrast microscopy when it is compared with a control smear without added antiserum. Immunofluorescence staining achieved by addition of a secondary layer of fluorescein-conjugated anti-rabbit immunoglobulins (DAKO, Carpinteria, Calif.) provides another excellent means of identifying and serotyping encapsulated strains of *H. influenzae* in clinical samples. It is important to include controls that rule out direct binding of the fluorescent-labeled secondary antibodies to the bacteria.

Respiratory Tract Specimens

The presence of small, pleomorphic gram-negative rods in sputum samples in areas of the sample that contain polymorphonuclear leukocytes and no squamous epithelial cells strongly suggests that a *Haemophilus* species is etiologically involved, but the final diagnosis must be established by cultivation. Due to their small size and staining reaction, *Haemophilus* bacteria may easily be missed in Gram-stained smears of sputa. Direct microscopy is also an important tool in cases in which fluid is collected by bronchoalveolar lavage or transthoracic needle aspiration.

Other Specimens

Due to the fastidious nature of *H. aegyptius,* microscopic examination of Gram-stained smears of conjunctival scrapings, particularly from patients with seasonal conjunctivitis, is a useful supplement to cultivation. *H. aegyptius* organisms appear as long, slender gram-negative rods (Fig. 1).

There is some doubt about the value of direct examination of Gram-stained smears or dark-field microscopy as an aid in the diagnosis of chancroid. Most genital ulcers have a polymicrobial flora, and the arrangements of *H. ducreyi* cells as long chains or "schools of fish," previously considered typical, appear to be more characteristic of smears prepared from cells grown in vitro (85). The sensitivity of Gram staining does not exceed 50% (85). The development of assays for the direct detection of *H. ducreyi* in smears by immunofluorescence has been hindered, in part, by the poor specificities of polyclonal antisera. Monoclonal antibodies against various surface epitopes on *H. ducreyi* have been developed and used in field studies. Many show satisfactory specificities and sensitivities compared with the results of culture techniques (85), but none appear to be commercially available.

Antigen Detection

Various immunochemical techniques for detection of capsular antigen of serotype b in CSF and other body fluids have been developed, but with the rarity of this serotype in many countries and the limited sensitivity that these tests offer over microscopy of Gram-stained smears, they are now of limited clinical value (49).

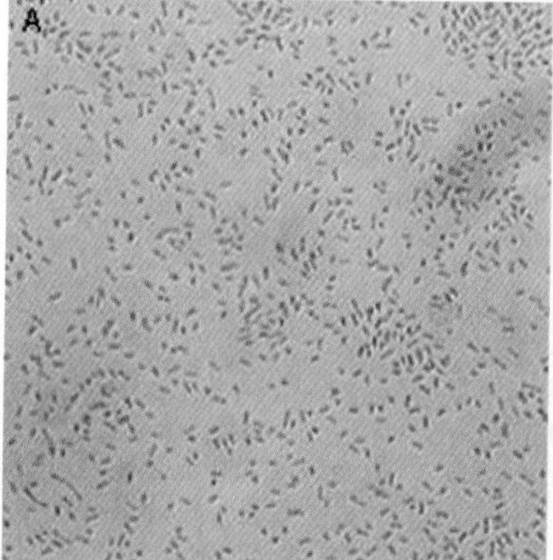

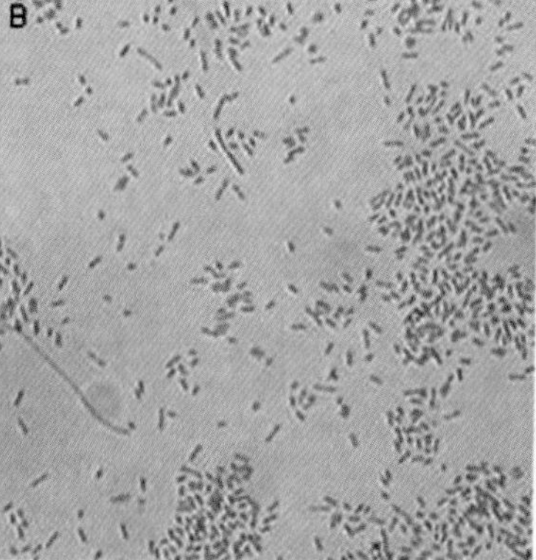

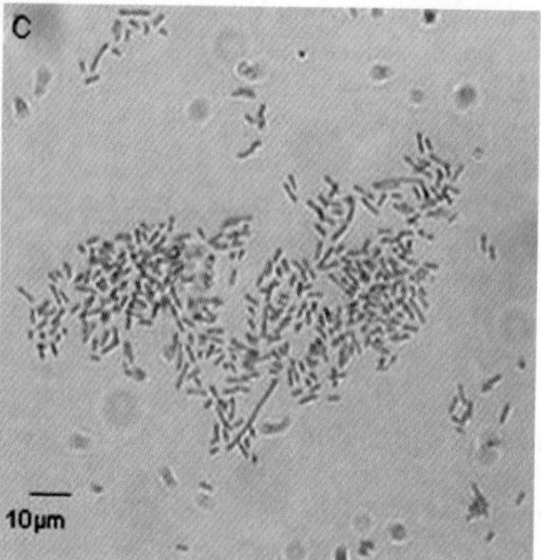

FIGURE 1 Gram-stained smears of *H. influenzae* (A), *H. aegyptius* (B), and *H. influenzae* biogroup aegyptius (C) showing the elongated slender rod morphology of the last two.

Nucleic Acid Detection Techniques

Real-time PCR-based technology for simultaneous detection of *H. influenzae* (serotypes b and c), *Neisseria meningitidis* (multiple serogroups), and *S. pneumoniae* (multiple serotypes) or for specific detection of *H. influenzae* type b in clinical samples of CSF, plasma, serum, and whole blood has been described (12, 47). Multiplex PCR may also be used for simultaneous detection of the four principal middle-ear pathogens *H. influenzae, S. pneumoniae, Moraxella catarrhalis*, and *Alloiococcus otitis* and of the major etiologic agents of genital ulcer disease, *H. ducreyi, Treponema pallidum*, and herpes simplex virus types 1 and 2. The sensitivity of these methods exceeds that of standard culture techniques, and their specificity is generally high (6, 12, 30, 47, 50, 64, 82). None of the methods are commercially available.

ISOLATION TECHNIQUES

Media

Attempts to isolate *Haemophilus* species must take into account the particular growth requirements of this group of bacteria (Table 1). The two growth factors hemin (X factor) and NAD (V factor) are contained in blood cells, but only X factor is directly available in conventional blood agar. To release V factor, the blood cells must be broken up by brief heating as in chocolate agar and in Levinthal's medium. In addition to liberating V factor, heat treatment inactivates V factor-destroying enzymes (NADase) present in blood. The heat treatment is obtained by adding the blood (5% sheep, bovine, or horse blood) to the medium base when its temperature is reduced to approximately 80°C immediately after autoclaving. A comparison of six medium bases showed that a medium consisting of GC agar base plus 5% chocolatized sheep blood and 1% yeast autolysate promoted the best growth of *H. influenzae, H. parainfluenzae,* and most other species that may be isolated from humans, excluding *H. ducreyi* (75).

For *H. aegyptius*, which is particularly fastidious, chocolate agar supplemented with 1% growth factor supplements (IsoVitaleX [Becton Dickinson Diagnostic Systems]; Vitox [Oxoid, Basingstoke, United Kingdom]; or cofactors-vitamin-amino acids [CVA; Gibco Diagnostics, Grand Island, N.Y.]) provides a good medium for isolation, although primary growth from clinical samples is never luxuriant (13, 91).

Growth on conventional blood agar may be achieved by adding a source of V factor, traditionally done by cross-streaking the inoculated plate with a staphylococcus or enterococcus strain. These bacteria excrete V factor and allow detection of *Haemophilus* species that grow as satellite colonies (Fig. 2). Alternatively, V factor may be supplied by applying a filter paper disk or a strip saturated with V factor (BD Diagnostic Systems, Franklin Lakes, N.J.; or Rosco A/S, Taastrup, Denmark) to the surface of the medium.

Due to the relatively slow growth and small size of *Haemophilus* colonies, their presence in cultures from sites with a mixed flora may easily be overlooked. When necessary, this problem may be solved by including selective agents or by a special incubation procedure. This is particularly important for attempts to detect *H. ducreyi*. GC-HgS agar, which consists of GC agar (GIBCO Laboratories) supplemented with 3 mg of vancomycin per liter, 1% hemoglobin, 5% fetal bovine serum, 1% IsoVitaleX (Becton Dickinson Diagnostics), or some other comparable enrichment, has a high sensitivity for isolation of *H. ducreyi* from clinical specimens, as does Mueller-Hinton agar (BBL) supplemented with 5% chocolatized horse blood, 1% IsoVitaleX, and 3 mg of vancomycin per liter (MH-HB agar) (14). Strains of *H. ducreyi* that are inhibited by 3 mg of vancomycin per liter have been reported (32). However, this observation needs to be confirmed in other laboratories. It is generally accepted that the combined use of two media, e.g., GC-HgS and MH-HB, is optimal for the detection and isolation of *H. ducreyi*, possibly because of differences in nutritional requirements between strains (85), but the sensitivity of culture techniques for *H. ducreyi* is never 100% (14, 17, 85). Some lots of fetal calf serum inhibit growth of *H. ducreyi*. Fetal calf serum can be replaced by either activated charcoal or bovine albumin, but not by newborn calf serum (84).

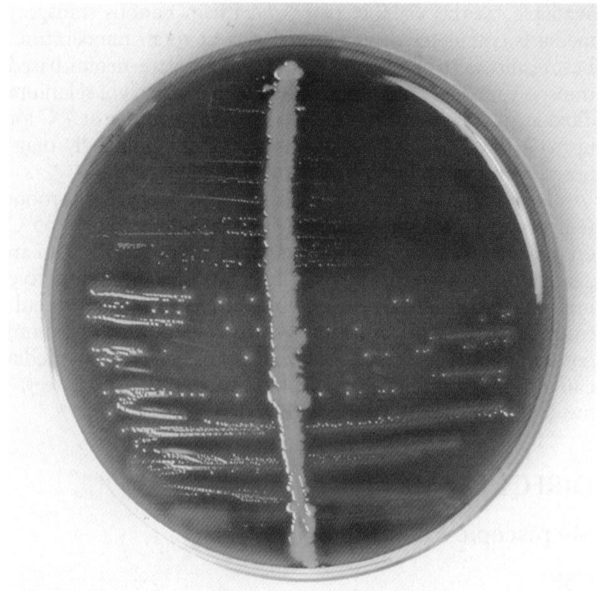

FIGURE 2 Growth of *Haemophilus* isolates on horse blood agar around a streak of *Staphylococcus aureus*. The upper half shows typical satellite growth characteristic of most *Haemophilus* species. The lower part shows characteristic lack of satellite growth of a strain of *H. parahaemolyticus* in spite of its requirement for V factor. Note that the colonies of *H. parahaemolyticus* resemble those of pyogenic streptococci on blood agar.

The problem of overgrowth of *H. influenzae* by *Pseudomonas aeruginosa* in cultures of sputa from patients with cystic fibrosis has been solved with some success by anaerobic incubation of inoculated chocolate agar plates containing 300 mg of bacitracin per liter. Detection of *Haemophilus* bacteria in cultures from the upper respiratory tract is also considerably improved by use of the latter medium (36). However, to be able to evaluate the relative proportion of haemophili in the microflora, a nonselective medium must be included.

Lower respiratory tract secretions and aspirates or swabs of pus from localized infections should be inoculated both on 5% blood agar cross-inoculated with a feeder strain and on chocolate agar.

Cultures of all *Haemophilus* organisms except *H. ducreyi* should be incubated at 35 to 37°C. *H. ducreyi* grows significantly better at 33°C. A moist atmosphere supplemented with 5 to 10% CO_2 is preferred by most strains and is mandatory for the isolation of *H. ducreyi* and many strains of *H. aphrophilus* and *H. paraphrophilus*. Given optimal conditions, most *Haemophilus* species grow to colonies of at least 1 to 2 mm in diameter after incubation for 18 to 24 h. Fresh isolates of *H. aegyptius* and *H. ducreyi* require incubation for 3 to 4 days.

Modern commercial blood culture systems show excellent recovery of *Haemophilus* species from blood samples. However, the same systems fail to recover *Haemophilus* species from normally sterile body fluids like pleural fluids, joint fluids, ascitic fluid, or dialysates unless blood (e.g., human blood, 1:8, vol/vol) or X- and V-factor enrichments are added (26, 67). Cultivation of spinal fluid or subcultivation from blood cultures should be performed on both chocolate agar and blood agar.

Appearance of Growth

With the exception of *H. aphrophilus* and *H. ducreyi*, all *Haemophilus* species that may be isolated from humans require V factor. Therefore, on blood agar these species will grow as satellite colonies around the staphylococcus streak. Colonies of *H. parahaemolyticus* and some strains of *H. haemolyticus* are surrounded by strong beta-hemolytic zones on horse, bovine, and rabbit blood agar. In contrast, *Haemophilus* species are nonhemolytic on sheep blood agar. Colonies of the three hemolytic species *H. parahaemolyticus*, *H. haemolyticus*, and *H. pittmaniae* usually do not show satellite growth on agar media with blood that they are capable of lysing and may be mistaken for pyogenic streptococci (Fig. 2).

H. influenzae colonies on chocolate agar are grayish, semiopaque, smooth, and flat convex and reach a diameter of 1 to 2 mm after incubation for 24 h. In dense areas of the plate, encapsulated strains tend to grow confluently, in contrast to colonies of noncapsulate strains, which remain separate. On clear agar media such as Levinthal's agar, colonies of encapsulated strains show a bright iridescence (red, blue, green, and yellow) when light is obliquely transmitted from behind. The phenomenon is most clearly detected in young (10- to 18-h) cultures and gradually disappears during prolonged incubation. In some strains with capsules of serotypes other than type b, iridescence is not always clear-cut. Noncapsulate strains examined in the same way show a more uniform bluish green color. Strains from cases of meningitis and epiglottitis virtually always produce indole, and so do many noncapsulate isolates (e.g., biovar II). Release of indole gives the growth on agar media a characteristic pungent smell similar to that of *Escherichia coli*. Otherwise, *Haemophilus* strains emit a "mouse-nest" smell.

Colonies of *H. parainfluenzae* may be up to 2 mm in diameter after incubation for 24 h and appear either smooth or rough and wrinkled. Most colonies are flat, grayish, and semiopaque. *H. aphrophilus* and *H. paraphrophilus* grow as rough, raised colonies that rarely attain a diameter exceeding 1 mm. When incubated in air without extra CO_2, these species grow, if at all, in colonies of varying sizes; the growth mimics that of a mixed culture. Fresh isolates of *H. aegyptius* and *H. segnis* grow as small (<1 mm), smooth colonies. Colonies of *H. ducreyi* are smooth and semitranslucently gray and attain a diameter of 0.1 to 0.5 mm on enriched chocolate agar after incubation for 3 days. They are characteristically cohesive and can be pushed intact across the surface of the agar.

Microscopy of Cultures

Gram-stained smears of *Haemophilus* isolates show small gram-negative rods with varying degrees of polymorphism (Fig. 1). The most extensive polymorphism, which may include long filamentous forms, is observed with the X-factor-independent species. *H. ducreyi* often appears as parallel rows of small rods in chains with a "school of fish," "railroad track," or "fingerprint" appearance.

IDENTIFICATION

X- and V-Factor Requirement

The satellite phenomenon, which may be detected in primary blood agar plate cultures, provides a convenient means for a tentative genus identification of all of the V-factor-requiring species that are regularly isolated from humans. However, other bacteria, such as occasional strains of *Pasteurella multocida*, some animal-pathogenic *Actinobacillus* and *Pasteurella* species (59, 62), and some streptococci may also show satellite growth, although it is not always due to V-factor requirement.

A small 5.25-kb plasmid that is normally present in *H. ducreyi* has been found to confer independence of V factor in occasional isolates of *H. parainfluenzae* (46, 94). How widespread such V-factor-independent strains of *H. parainfluenzae* are is not known.

A prerequisite for detection of the satellite phenomenon is an agar medium that lacks V factor. Since ordinary blood agar contains various amounts of free V factor, depending on the method of preparation and length of storage, it is sometimes difficult to achieve convincing satellite growth on this medium. The special problem associated with hemolytic strains has already been mentioned. In case of doubtful reactions, far better results are obtained on a blood agar medium to which the blood (5 to 10%) is added before autoclaving. Since NAD is heat labile, this medium is completely devoid of V factor but otherwise satisfies all growth requirements of *Haemophilus* species, including X factor.

Determination of a requirement for X factor is done in some laboratories by demonstrating growth around an X-factor-containing paper disk (Becton Dickinson Diagnostic Systems) on an agar medium or by comparing growth on medium with blood to growth on medium without blood. However, even when particular care is being exercised to avoid carrying over X factor with the inoculum, this method results in erroneous results in up to 20% of cases (M. Kilian, unpublished observations). If the identity is not confirmed by biochemical tests, *H. influenzae* strains are often misidentified as *H. parainfluenzae* and occasionally vice versa. This undoubtedly explains some of the reported cases of meningitis ascribed to *H. parainfluenzae*. The porphyrin test (34) provides a more accurate and rapid means of determining the X-factor requirement.

Porphyrin Test

The porphyrin test is based on the observation that hemin-independent *Haemophilus* strains excrete porphobilinogen and porphyrins, both of which are intermediates in the hemin biosynthetic pathway (Fig. 3), when supplied with δ-aminolevulinic acid. X-factor-requiring strains do not excrete these compounds because of a lack of enzymes involved in the biosynthesis of heme (36).

The substrate consists of 2 mM δ-aminolevulinic acid hydrochloride (Sigma Chemical Co., St. Louis, Mo.) and 0.8 mM $MgSO_4$ in 0.1 M phosphate buffer at pH 6.9. It is distributed in 0.5-ml quantities in small glass tubes and may be stored for several months in a refrigerator. Sterility is not required. The substrate is inoculated by suspending a heavy loopful of bacteria from an agar plate culture. After incubation for 4 h at 37°C, the mixture is exposed to UV light (wavelength, approximately 360 nm), preferably in a dark room. A red fluorescence from the bacterial cells or from the fluid indicates the presence of porphyrins; i.e., growth of the strain is not dependent on X factor. In cases of doubtful

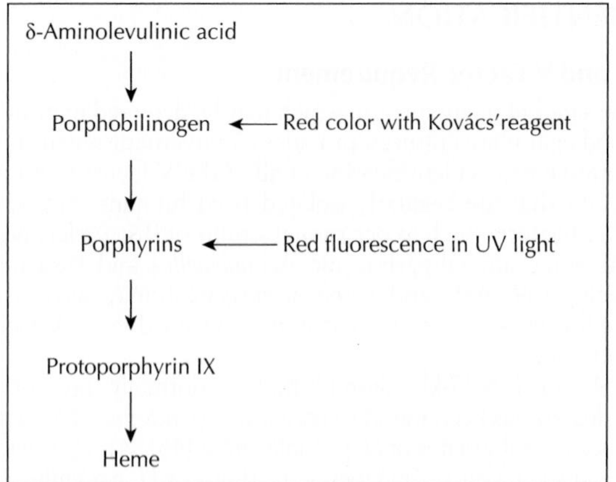

FIGURE 3 Principal steps of the heme biosynthetic pathway and methods for detection of intermediate compounds.

reactions, tubes may be reincubated for up to 24 h. An alternative way is to add 0.5 ml of Kovács' reagent (p-dimethylaminobenzaldehyde, 5 g; amyl alcohol, 75 ml; concentrated HCl, 25 ml), shake the mixture vigorously, and allow the phases to separate. A red color in the lower water phase is indicative of porphobilinogen. When this method of reading is used, it is advisable to include an inoculated tube without δ-aminolevulinic acid as a negative control. Kovács' reagent also gives a red color reaction with indole, which, however, will be present in the upper alcohol phase. Still, indole-positive strains of *H. influenzae* may erroneously be identified as X-factor independent in the absence of an appropriate control. Another disadvantage of this method of reading is that further incubation of samples with doubtful reactions is not possible.

Hemolysis

Hemolysis induced by isolates of *H. haemolyticus, H. parahaemolyticus,* and *H. pittmaniae* may be detected on agar plates with horse, bovine, or rabbit (quad plates) blood but not on sheep blood agar. Demonstration of the hemolytic activity of *H. ducreyi* requires specialized media. Reproducible results have been obtained with bilayer horse blood agar plates consisting of GC agar base, 1% X factor-V factor supplement, and 5% horse blood. All strains examined were less hemolytic on sheep blood agar (83).

Biochemical Tests, General

Table 1 shows key reactions for further differentiation of the *Haemophilus* species. Tests for fermentation of glucose, sucrose, and lactose are important for species identification. They are performed in 1% solutions of the respective carbohydrates in phenol red broth base (Becton Dickson Diagnostic Systems) supplemented with X and V factors (10 mg/liter each; Sigma Chemical Co.) after autoclaving (35). Reactions are usually clear-cut after 24 h of incubation, but some species such as *H. segnis* and *H. aegyptius* show weak reactions.

The ability to reduce nitrate, which is a characteristic of all *Haemophilus* species, can be demonstrated after 5 days of growth in Levinthal's broth with 0.1% (wt/vol) of potassium nitrate. Strains of *H. aphrophilus* and *H. paraphrophilus* may, however, reduce nitrate beyond nitrite, which may result in a negative reaction for nitrite (35).

Direct Enzyme Tests

Three biochemical reactions are important tools in the differentiation of some of the *Haemophilus* species and for differentiation from species of other *Pasteurellaceae* genera: indole production, urease, and ornithine decarboxylase activities (Table 2). The three biochemical reactions used in identification and in biotyping (see below) of *H. influenzae* and *H. parainfluenzae* may preferably be performed as rapid tests that bypass the problems of special growth requirements (35). All three test media (0.3- to 0.5-ml quantities) are inoculated with a heavy loopful of bacteria from an agar culture, and the results are read after incubation for 4 h. (The test for ornithine decarboxylase may in some cases require additional incubation for 18 to 20 h.)

Indole Test

The substrate for the indole test is 1% L-tryptophan in 0.05 M phosphate buffer at pH 6.8. After inoculation and incubation for 4 h, 1 volume of Kovács' reagent is added and the mixture is shaken. A red color in the upper alcohol phase indicates the presence of indole.

Urease Test

The substrate for the urease test is 0.1 g of KH_2PO_4, 0.1 g of K_2HPO_4, 0.5 g of NaCl, and 0.5 ml of 1:500 phenol red in 100 ml of distilled water. The pH is adjusted to 7.0 with NaOH, and 10.4 ml of a 20% (wt/vol) aqueous solution of urea is added (for 1:500 phenol red, dissolve 0.2 g of phenol red in NaOH and add distilled water to 100 ml). The development of a red color within 4 h after inoculation indicates urease activity.

TABLE 2 Differential tests for *H. influenzae, H. parainfluenzae, H. aegyptius, H. parahaemolyticus,* and *H. segnis* and for biotyping of *H. influenzae* and *H. parainfluenzae*

Species and biotype	Indole	Urease	Ornithine decarboxylase
H. influenzae			
Biotype I	+	+	+
Biotype II	+	+	–
Biotype III	–	+	–
Biotype IV	–	+	+
Biotype V	+	–	+
Biotype VI	–	–	+
Biotype VII	+	–	–
Biotype VIII	–	–	–
H. aegyptius[a]	–	+	–
H. influenzae biogroup aegyptius[a]	–	+	–
H. parainfluenzae			
Biotype I	–	–	+
Biotype II	–	+	+
Biotype III	–	+	–
Biotype IV	+	+	+
Biotype V	–	–	–
Biotype VI	+	–	+
Biotype VII	+	+	–
Biotype VIII	+	–	–
H. parahaemolyticus	–	+	–
H. segnis	–	–	–

[a] For differentiation of *H. aegyptius, H. influenzae* biotype III, and *H. influenzae* biogroup aegyptius, see text for further information.

Ornithine Decarboxylase Test

The substrate for ornithine decarboxylase is the medium used regularly for other bacteria (see chapter 21). For *Haemophilus* organisms it is to be inoculated with a heavy loopful of bacteria from an agar plate culture. A purple color developing within 4 to 24 h indicates ornithine decarboxylase activity.

Alternative Methods

Several commercial kits are available for identification of *Haemophilus* species once the V-factor requirement has been determined; e.g., API NH (bioMérieux Inc., Hazelwood, Mo.), Vitek NHI Card V1308 (bioMérieux), the Haemophilus ID Test kit (Remel, Lenexa, Kans.), the RIM-H system (Austin Biological Laboratories, Austin, Tex.), and RapidID NF (Innovative Diagnostics, Norcross, Ga.) (65, 72). However, most of these kits do not provide sufficient information to accurately identify an isolate to the species level without additional tests. Therefore, it is advisable that more unusual findings be confirmed with traditional tests.

DNA-Based Identification

If the technology is available, isolates of most *Haemophilus* species and related genera may easily be identified by determining a partial 16S rRNA gene sequence and comparing it with sequences of type strains available in databases accessible on the Internet (e.g., http://www.ncbi.nlm.nih.gov/BLAST/ or http://rdp.cme.msu.edu/index.jsp, which allows a BLAST search against only type strains). Because of their close similarities, the technique does not differentiate between *H. influenzae*, *H. aegyptius*, and *H. influenzae* biogroup aegyptius and between *H. aphrophilus* and *H. paraphrophilus*.

A review of various published methods for identification of virulence-associated properties and identification probes and a comprehensive compilation of primer and probe sequences have been prepared by Van Belkum and van Alphen (89).

Particular Identification Problems

The differentiation of *H. influenzae, H. aegyptius,* and *H. influenzae* biogroup aegyptius by standard laboratory techniques is impossible at present. The three taxa form distinct clusters by phylogenetic analysis based on multiple genetic and phenotypic traits including electrophoretic mobility of selected housekeeping enzymes (as determined by multilocus enzyme electrophoresis) (37). Both *H. aegyptius* and *H. influenzae* biogroup aegyptius have the same key biochemical characteristics as *H. influenzae* biotype III (Table 2). Since the latter does not possess the invasive potential of BPF strains or the ability to cause serious endemic conjunctivitis, as *H. aegyptius* strains do, it is important to develop means for exact identification. *H. aegyptius* and *H. influenzae* biogroup aegyptius lack the ability to ferment xylose, in contrast to the vast majority of *H. influenzae* strains (7, 35). Additional characteristics that may be of use in the separation of *H. aegyptius* from *H. influenzae* are its poorer in vitro growth, its more slender and rod-like shape (Fig. 1), and its ability to agglutinate human erythrocytes as a result of more stable pilus expression (36). It has been reported that the distinct outer membrane protein profiles of *H. aegyptius* and *H. influenzae* biotype III may be used as an adjunct to differentiate the two species (9).

Recently it has become clear that identification of *H. haemolyticus* poses special problems. Some strains of *H. haemolyticus* are clearly nonhemolytic and cannot be distinguished from *H. influenzae* by phenotypic analysis (55). The prevalence and clinical significance of *H. haemolyticus* are therefore not clear.

Isolates of *H. ducreyi* may be presumptively identified by their adherent colony characteristics, by their appearance in Gram-stained smears, and by a positive oxidase and negative catalase reaction. Confirmation can be achieved by demonstrating a negative porphyrin test result, the inability to ferment carbohydrates, and a positive reaction for nitrate reduction. However, commercial identification systems fail to reveal the ability to reduce nitrate, and a positive oxidase reaction is obtained only with tetramethyl-*p*-phenylenediamine (36, 52).

H. aphrophilus and *A. actinomycetemcomitans* are not easily distinguished from certain *Pasteurella* species, which potentially may explain two reports of the isolation of *Pasteurella gallinarum* from human cases of endocarditis and bacteremia (25). Criteria for the identification of such bacteria may be found elsewhere (62; see also chapter 40).

Biochemical reactions that are valuable in separating *H. aphrophilus* and *H. paraphrophilus* from the closely related *A. actinomycetemcomitans* and other resembling species are provided in Table 3.

TYPING SYSTEMS

Capsular Serotyping

Due to significant differences in pathogenic potentials of noncapsulate and individual serotypes of encapsulated strains of *H. influenzae,* capsule detection and serotyping have been important in the analysis of clinical isolates. The separation of the six serotypes of *H. influenzae* is based on structurally distinct capsular polysaccharides. Until vaccination against *H. influenzae* type b was introduced, identification of serotype b strains was of particular practical significance, as invasive pathogenicity was almost exclusively associated with that serotype. There is no doubt that the exclusive focus on serotype b in many laboratories has resulted in an underestimation of infections caused by other serotypes.

The evaluation of cases of apparent vaccine failure necessitates definitive serotyping. Furthermore, the decline of *H. influenzae* serotype b carriage raised concerns about an increase of *H. influenzae* carriage and disease caused by other serotypes and by noncapsulate strains. A study of Alaskan residents aged 10 years and older suggests such an increase (from 0.5 to 1.1 per 100.000 per year) (68).

Capsular serotyping may be carried out by slide agglutination, by coagglutination with staphylococci or latex particles coated with type-specific antibodies, by a capsular swelling test, and by immunofluorescence microscopy. A recent multicenter comparison of the outcome of slide agglutination serotyping with PCR-based detection of capsule biosynthesis genes in 141 invasive H. influenzae isolates showed discrepancies in 40% of the isolates characterized. Discrepancies were due mainly to false-positive reactions obtained with isolates that were noncapsulate. An overall 94% agreement was achieved when the slide agglutination method was performed correctly (38). It is therefore advisable that laboratories that are unable to perform appropriate serotyping of isolates refer these to reference laboratories.

Bacterial suspensions used for serological typing of isolates must be prepared from a young (12- to 18-h) agar culture, since the capsular structure tends to deteriorate in older cultures. A smooth suspension of bacteria is made in normal saline containing formalin (0.5%, vol/vol) and must be of sufficient density to permit the antigen-antibody reaction to proceed to completion within 1 min. In a strong positive slide

TABLE 3 Differential tests for *H. aphrophilus*, *H. paraphrophilus*, and some related species

Species	X factor required	V factor required	Indole	Urease	Ornithine decarboxylase	Lysine decarboxylase	Fermentation of: Glucose	Sucrose	Lactose	Mannitol	Nitrate reduction	Presence of catalase
H. aphrophilus	−	−	−	−	−	−	+	+	+	−	+	−
H. paraphrophilus	−	+	−	−	−	−	+	+	+	−	+	−
A. actinomycetemcomitans	−	−	−	−	−	−	+	−	−	D[a]	+	+
Eikenella corrodens	−	−	−	−	+	+	−	−	−	−	+	−
Cardiobacterium hominis	−	−	+	−	−	−	+	+	−	+	−	−
Suttonella indologenes	−	−	+	−	−	−	+	+	−	−	−	−
H. haemoglobinophilus	+	−	+	−	−	−	+	+	−	+	+	+

[a]D, differences encountered.

agglutination reaction, all bacteria are agglutinated, and the fluid between the clusters is clear.

As polyclonal antisera contain various proportions of antibodies to somatic antigens, agglutination may occur as a result of reaction with somatic antigens. This problem may result in simultaneous agglutination in antisera against several serotypes. Only strong reactions occurring within 1 min should be taken as a positive reaction. Antisera for serotyping of encapsulated *H. influenzae* isolates are available from Becton Dickinson Diagnostic Systems and from some state laboratories. A coagglutination test for detection of serotype b is available under the product name Phadebact (Boule Diagnostics AB, Huddinge, Sweden).

PCR-Based Capsule Typing

While traditional serotyping in inexperienced hands is liable to frequent misinterpretations, the capsule serotype of an isolate may be unequivocally determined by detection of serotype-specific gene sequences. The most attractive method is PCR capsular genotyping, which is easier to perform than probe analysis as there is no need for lengthy DNA extractions, Southern blotting, and hybridization. This PCR methodology may also be used to detect deletion mutants and the amplification pattern of the *capB* locus (21, 90), which differentiates two distinct evolutionary divisions (divisions I and II) of *H. influenzae* type b with different pathogenic potentials (56). Primers specific for the *bexA* gene, which is required for capsule transport and present in strains of all six serotypes, can be used to differentiate between noncapsulate and capsulate isolates (90). Primers for the *bexA* gene (Primers HI-1 and HI-2) and three-primer sets for amplification of each of the six serotype-specific gene sequences are shown in Table 4.

TABLE 4 Capsule transport gene *(bexA)* and serotype-specific three-primer sets for demonstration of capsule production and capsular serotype-specific genes in *H. influenzae*[a]

Primer name	Primer sequences[b]
HI-1 (*bexA*)	CGT TTG TAT GAT GTT GAT CCA GAC
HI-2 (*bexA*)	TGT CCA TGT CTT CAA AAT GAT G
a_1	CTA CTC ATT GCA GCA TTT GC
a_2	GAA TAT GAC CTG ATC TTC TG
a_3	AGT GGA CTA TTC CTG TTA CAC
b_1	GCG AAA GTG AAC TCT TAT CTC TC
b_2	GCT TAC GCT TCT ATC TCG GTG AA
b_3	ACC ATG AGA AAG TGT TAG CG
c_1	TCT GTG TAG ATG ATG GTT CA
c_2	CAG AGG CAA GCT ATT AGT GA
c_3	TGG CAG CGT AAA TAT CCT AA
d_1	TGA TGA CCG ATA CAA CCT GT
d_2	TCC ACT CTT CAA ACC ATT CT
d_3	CTC TTC TTA GTG CTG AAT TA
e_1	GGT AAC GAA TGT AGT GGT AG
e_2	GCT TTA CTG TAT AAG TCT AG
e_3	CAG CTA TGA ACA AGA TAA CG
f_1	GCT ACT ATC AAG TCC AAA TC
f_2	CGC AAT TAT GGA AGA AAG CT
f_3	AAT GCT GGA GTA TCT GGT TC

[a]The data are from references 20 and 31.

[b]Primers labeled "3" represent sequences between primers labeled "1" and "2" and may, in combination with one of the primary primers, be used for confirmation in second rounds of PCR using the first-round PCR product as a template.

Occasional strains that have lost the ability to produce a serotype b capsule (b⁻mutants) are identified by a positive result in the type-b-specific PCR and a negative result with the *bexA* gene primers (21).

Other Typing Methods

H. influenzae and *H. parainfluenzae* may be subdivided into eight biotypes or biovars each (35, 36) on the basis of indole production, urease, and ornithine decarboxylase activities (Table 2). Biotypes of *H. influenzae* show a relationship to source of isolation (35, 61) and to capsular serotype (35) in agreement with the fact that the serotypes constitute separate evolutionary lineages, in contrast to serotypes of *S. pneumoniae* (48, 56, 57). The vast majority of serotype a, b, and f strains belong to biotype I, serotype c strains are usually biotype II, and strains with serotype d or e capsules are biotype IV (35). Subtyping on the basis of outer membrane proteins, lipopolysaccharides, or isoenzymes has also been done. However, for epidemiological purposes, typing by DNA-based techniques (DNA fingerprinting, ribotyping, pulsed-field gel electrophoresis, and multilocus sequence typing [MLST]) is preferred because of their superior discriminatory power (41, 48, 77). The optimal typing method is MLST, which is based on sequencing of parts of seven selected housekeeping genes (*adk, atpG, frdB, fucK, mdh, pgi,* and *recA*) (48). The method has the advantage that results are electronically portable and easily comparable between laboratories. In addition, by taking advantage of the MLST database (http://haemophilus.mlst.net/) it is possible to see one's own observations in a global context.

ANTIBIOTIC SUSCEPTIBILITY

Wild-type strains of the *Haemophilus* species are susceptible to ampicillin, cephalosporins, chloramphenicol, sulfonamides, tetracycline, and the macrolide-azalide-ketolide group of antimicrobials. However, mainly because of the spread of conjugative plasmids, a large proportion of clinical isolates are resistant to ampicillin and most other β-lactam antibiotics, to chloramphenicol, and to the tetracyclines (5, 8, 23, 45). The likelihood that an *H. influenzae* isolate will be resistant to ampicillin varies from 5 to 60% in different countries. This development has effectively removed the aminopenicillins (without the addition of a β-lactamase inhibitor) and certain cephalosporins as options for empirical treatment of infections in which *H. influenzae* is a suspected pathogen. Resistance to β-lactams is in most cases a result of a TEM-1 and, to a lesser extent, ROB-1-type β-lactamase production. There are also β-lactamase-negative strains for which ampicillin MICs are increased due to mutations in the penicillin-binding proteins (4, 5, 78, 87). Those strains are referred to as β-lactamase-negative, ampicillin resistant (BLNAR). The prevalence of BLNAR *H. influenzae* in the United States is still below 1%, but recent surveys from several European countries show prevalences from 2 to 20% among *H. influenzae* isolates (33). In contrast to other cephalosporins tested, cefixime is still fully active against *H. influenzae* with the BLNAR phenotype (31).

The rate of macrolide nonsusceptibility is about 1% for azithromycin and 10% for clarithromycin and is in most cases categorized as intermediate resistance. Resistance to fluoroquinolones is still rare (the reported rate in Spain is 0.1%) (16, 45).

Considerable geographical and temporal differences in the antimicrobial susceptibilities of *H. ducreyi* isolates have been recorded. There is very little information concerning chromosomally mediated resistance in *H. ducreyi*. However, most clinical isolates contain plasmids, which may encode resistance, either separately or in combination, to sulfonamides, aminoglycosides, tetracyclines, chloramphenicol, and β-lactam antibiotics. It is not unusual for a single isolate to contain multiple resistance plasmids. Both TEM-1 and ROB-1 β-lactamases have been identified in isolates from Thailand (85). Recommended drugs are azithromycin, ceftriaxone, ciprofloxacin, or erythromycin (95). Strains for which the erythromycin MIC is 4 mg/liter have been isolated in Thailand and Singapore (85). In general, the prevalence and spectrum of antimicrobial resistance make it important that clinical isolates of *H. ducreyi* be routinely monitored for resistance.

Comprehensive and up-to-date in vitro susceptibility data for other *Haemophilus* species are not available. However, there are indications that the prevalence of resistance in these species is higher than in *H. influenzae*. Both β-lactamase-mediated resistance and non-β-lactamase-mediated resistance to ampicillin have been observed in *H. parainfluenzae*. A PCR-based screening of nasopharyngeal haemophili of a group of individuals in the United Kingdom revealed that 59% carried plasmids encoding β-lactamase. Of these, 83% were in *H. parainfluenzae* and 17% were in *H. influenzae* (40). Transmissible resistance to chloramphenicol and aminoglycosides in *H. parainfluenzae, H. parahaemolyticus,* and *H. paraphrophilus* has been described (36).

EVALUATION, INTERPRETATION, AND REPORTING

Detection of *Haemophilus* species by culture is uncomplicated and reliable provided that correct media and incubation procedures are being applied. Only for *H. ducreyi* do isolation procedures show suboptimal sensitivity. Once they become commercially available, PCR methods will become important in the diagnosis of *H. ducreyi* infections.

Interpretation of laboratory findings is also, in most cases, uncomplicated. Isolation of *Haemophilus* species from sites other than the upper respiratory tract and from normally sterile sites is almost always clinically significant. The mere detection of *H. influenzae* in a sample from the nasopharynx is of no clinical significance. However, strong predominance in the flora suggests an impaired balance that may be associated with sinusitis, otitis media, or other local infection in the area. It is therefore important that findings be interpreted on this basis and that they be reported in semiquantitative terms. It is also unavoidable that sputum samples are contaminated with haemophili during passage through the pharynx and oral cavity. The sample must be evaluated by microscopy prior to culture to make sure that small gram-negative rods in the sample are associated with inflammatory cells and not with squamous epithelial cells from the upper respiratory tract. Even in samples that bypass the upper respiratory tract, a mixture of bacteria often renders the interpretation difficult.

Detection of *H. ducreyi* in samples from genital ulcers or in inguinal lymph node aspirates is always clinically relevant and should be followed by proper antibacterial therapy.

With the virtual elimination of *H. influenzae* serotype b disease in many countries, the demands on the clinical microbiology laboratory in this area have changed dramatically. Methods specifically designed to detect antigens of *H. influenzae* type b are of less importance, and more emphasis should be placed on other serotypes. In this context, it is important to realize that observations made for one human population do not necessarily apply to other populations. Population genetic analyses of *H. influenzae* suggest that individual clones of *H. influenzae* may be strictly adapted to humans with a particular genetic background and do not spread freely among human populations (57). As there is significant coupling of gene loci (linkage disequilibrium) in the *H. influenzae* population, such differences may include antibiotic resistance markers as well as virulence traits.

REFERENCES

1. **Adams, W. G, K. A. Deaver, S. L. Cochi, B. D. Plikaytis, E. R. Zell, C. V. Broome, and J. D. Wenger.** 1996. Decline in childhood *Haemophilus influenzae* type b (Hib) disease in the vaccine era. *JAMA* **269:**221–226.
2. **Albritton, W. L.** 1982. Infections due to *Haemophilus* species other than *H. influenzae*. *Annu. Rev. Microbiol.* **36:**199–216.
3. **Barbour, M. L.** 1996. Conjugate vaccines and the carriage of *Haemophilus influenzae* type b. *Emerg. Infect. Dis.* **2:**176–182.
4. **Barry, A. L., P. C. Fuchs, and S. D. Brown.** 2001. Identification of β-lactamase-negative, ampicillin-resistant strains of *Haemophilus influenzae* with four methods and eight media. *Antimicrob. Agents Chemother.* **45:**1585–1588.
5. **Barry, A. L., P. C. Fuchs, and M. A. Pfaller.** 1993. Susceptibilities of beta-lactamase-producing and -nonproducing ampicillin-resistant strains of *Haemophilus influenzae* to ceftibuten, cefaclor, cefuroxime, cefixime, cefotaxime, and amoxicillin-clavulanic acid. *Antimicrob. Agents Chemother.* **37:**14–18.
6. **Black, C. M., and S. A. Morse.** 2000. The use of molecular techniques for the diagnosis and epidemiologic study of sexually transmitted infections. *Curr. Infect. Dis.* **2:**31–43.
7. **Brenner, D. J., L. W. Mayer, G. M. Carlone, L. H. Harrison, W. F. Bibb, M. C. C. Brandileone, F. O. Sottnek, K. Irino, M. W. Reeves, J. M. Swenson, K. A. Birkness, R. S. Weyant, S. F. Berkley, T. C. Woods, A. G. Steigerwalt, P. A. D. Grimont, R. M. McKinney, D. W. Fleming, L. L. Gheesling, R. C. Cooksey, R. J. Akko, C. V. Broome, and The Brazilian Purpuric Fever Study Group.** 1988. Biochemical, genetic, and epidemiologic characterization of *Haemophilus influenzae* biogroup aegyptius (*Haemophilus aegyptius*) strains associated with Brazilian purpuric fever. *J. Clin. Microbiol.* **26:**1524–1534.
8. **Campos, J., S. Garcia-Tornel, J. M. Gairi, and I. Fabregues.** 1986. Multiply resistant *Haemophilus influenzae* type b causing meningitis: comparative clinical and laboratory study. *J. Pediatr.* **108:**897–902.
9. **Carlone, G. M., F. O. Sottnek, and B. D. Plikaytis.** 1985. Comparison of outer membrane protein and biochemical profiles of *Haemophilus aegyptius* and *Haemophilus influenzae* biotype III. *J. Clin. Microbiol.* **22:**708–713.
10. **Casin, I., F. Grimont, and P. A. Grimont.** 1986. Deoxyribonucleic acid relatedness between *Haemophilus aegyptius* and *Haemophilus influenzae*. *Ann. Inst. Pasteur Microbiol.* **137B:** 155–163.
11. **Centers for Disease Control and Prevention.** 1999. Impact of vaccines universally recommended for children—United States, 1900–1998. *Morb. Mortal. Wkly. Rep.* **48:**243–248.
12. **Corless, C. E., M. Guiver, R. Borrow, V. Edwards-Jones, A. J. Fox, and E. B. Kaczmarski.** 2001. Simultaneous detection of *Neisseria meningitidis*, *Haemophilus influenzae*, and *Streptococcus pneumoniae* in suspected cases of meningitis and septicemia using real-time PCR. *J. Clin. Microbiol.* **39:**1553–1558.
13. **Dangor, Y., S. D. Miller, H. J. Koornhof, and R. C. Ballard.** 1992. A simple medium for the primary isolation of *Haemophilus ducreyi*. *Eur. J. Microbiol. Infect. Dis.* **11:**930–934.
14. **Dangor, Y., F. Radebe, and R. C. Ballard.** 1993. Transport media for *Haemophilus ducreyi*. *Sex. Transm. Dis.* **20:**5–9.
15. **Darras-Joly, C., O. Lortholary, J.-L. Mainardi, J. Etienne, L. Guillevin, J. Acar, and the *Haemophilus* Endocarditis Study Group.** 1997. *Haemophilus* endocarditis: report of 42 cases in adults and review. *Clin. Infect. Dis.* **24:**1087–1094.
16. **Doern, G. V., R. N. Jones, M. A. Phaller, K. Kugler, and the SENTRY Participants Group.** 1999. *Haemophilus influenzae* and *Moraxella catarrhalis* from patients with community-acquired respiratory tract infections: antimicrobial susceptibility patterns from the SENTRY Antimicrobial Surveillance Program (United States and Canada, 1997). *Antimicrob. Agents Chemother.* **43:**385–389.
17. **Dylewski, J., H. Nisanze, G. Maitha, and A. Ronald.** 1986. Laboratory diagnosis of *Haemophilus ducreyi*: sensitivity of culture media. *Diagn. Microbiol. Infect. Dis.* **4:**241–245.
18. **Faden, H., J. Stanievich, L. Brodsky, J. Bernstein, and P. L. Ogra.** 1990. Changes in nasopharyngeal flora during otitis media of childhood. *Pediatr. Infect. Dis. J.* **9:**623–626.
19. **Faden, H., L. Duffy, A. Williams, D. A. Krystofik, and J. Wolf.** 1995. Epidemiology of nasopharyngeal colonization with nontypeable *Haemophilus influenzae* in the first 2 years of life. *J. Infect. Dis.* **172:**132–135.
20. **Falla, T. J., D. W. Crook, L. N. Brophy, D. Maskell, J. S. Kroll, and E. R. Moxon.** 1994. PCR for capsular typing of *Haemophilus influenzae*. *J. Clin. Microbiol.* **32:**2382–2386.
21. **Falla, T. J., S. R. Dobson, D. W. Crook, W. A. Kraak, W. W. Nichols, E. C. Anderson, J. Z. Jordens, M. P. Slack, D. Mayon-White, and E. R. Moxon.** 1993. Population-based study of non-typeable *Haemophilus influenzae* invasive disease in children and neonates. *Lancet* **341:**851–854.
22. **Farley, M. M. D. S. Stephens, P. S. Brachman, Jr., R. C. Harvey, J. D. Smith, J. D. Wenger, and The CDC Meningitis Surveillance Group.** 1992. Invasive *Haemophilus influenzae* disease in adults. A prospective, population-based surveillance. *Ann. Intern. Med.* **116:**806–812.
23. **Fluit, A. C., A. Florijn, J. Verhoef, and D. Milatovic.** 2005. Susceptibility of European β-lactamase-positive and -negative *Haemophilus influenzae* isolates from the periods 1997/1998 and 2002/2003. *J. Antimicrob. Chemother.* **56:**133–138.
24. **Foxwell, A. R., J. M. Kyd, and A. W. Cripps.** 1998. Nontypeable *Haemophilus influenzae*: pathogenesis and prevention. *Microbiol. Mol. Biol. Rev.* **62:**294–308.
25. **Frederiksen, W., and B. Tønning.** 2001. Possible misidentification of *Haemophilus aphrophilus* as *Pasteurella gallinarum*. *Clin. Infect. Dis.* **32:**987–988.
26. **Fuller, D. D., T. E. Davis, P. C. Kibsey, L. Rosmus, L. W. Ayers, M. Ott, M. A. Saubolle, and D. L. Sewell.** 1994. Comparison of BACTEC Plus 26 and 27 media with and without fastidious organism supplement with conventional methods for culture of sterile body fluids. *J. Clin. Microbiol.* **32:**1488–1491.
27. **Galil, K., R. Singleton, O. S. Levine, M. A. Fitzgerald, L. Bulkow, M. Getty, B. A. Perkins, and A. Parkinson.** 1999. Reemergence of invasive *Haemophilus influenzae* type b disease in a well-vaccinated population in remote Alaska. *J. Infect. Dis.* **179:**101–106.
28. **Garner, D., and V. Weston.** 2003. Effectiveness of vaccination for *Haemophilus influenzae* type b. *Lancet* **361:**395–396.
29. **Hawkes, S., B. West, S. Wilson, H. Whittle, and D. Mabey.** 1995. Asymptomatic carriage of *Haemophilus ducreyi* confirmed by the polymerase chain reaction. *Genitourin. Med.* **71:**224–227.
30. **Hendolin, P. H., L. Paulin, and J. Ylikoski.** 2000. Clinically applicable multiplex PCR for four middle ear pathogens. *J. Clin. Microbiol.* **38:**125–132.
31. **Jacobs, M. R., S. Bajaksouzian, A. Zilles, G. Lin, G. A. Pankuch, and P. C. Appelbaum.** 1999. Susceptibilities of *Streptococcus pneumoniae* and *Haemophilus influenzae* to 10 oral antimicrobial agents based on pharmacodynamic parameters: 1997 U.S. surveillance study. *Antimicrob. Agents Chemother.* **43:**1901–1908.
32. **Jones, C., T. Rosen, J. Clarridge, and S. Collins.** 1990. Chancroid: results from an outbreak in Houston, Texas. *South. Med. J.* **83:**1384–1389.

33. **Karlowsky, J. A., I. A. Critchley, R. S. Blosser-Middleton, E. A. Karginova, M. E. Jones, C. Thorsberry, and D. F. Sahm.** 2002. Antimicrobial surveillance of *Haemophilus influenzae* in the United States during 2000–2001 leads to detection of clonal dissemination of a β-lactamase-negative and ampicillin-resistant strain. *J. Clin. Microbiol.* **40:**1063–1066.
34. **Kilian, M.** 1974. A rapid method for the differentiation of *Haemophilus* strains. The porphyrin test. *Acta Pathol. Microbiol. Scand. Sect. B* **82:**835–842.
35. **Kilian, M.** 1976. A taxonomic study of the genus *Haemophilus* with the proposal of a new species. *J. Gen. Microbiol.* **93:**9–62.
36. **Kilian, M.** 2005. *Haemophilus* Winslow, Broadhurst, Buchanan, Krumwiede, Rogers and Smith 1917, 561, p. 883–904. *In* D. J. Brenner, N. R. Krieg, J. T. Staley, and G. M. Garrity (ed.), *Bergey's Manual of Systematic Bacteriology*, 2nd ed., vol. 2: *The Proteobacteria*. Springer-Verlag, New York, N.Y.
37. **Kilian, M., K. Poulsen, and H. Lomholt.** 2002. Evolution of the paralogous *hap* and *iga* genes in *Haemophilus influenzae:* evidence for a conserved *hap* pseudogene associated with microcolony formation in the recently diverged *Haemophilus aegyptius* and *H. influenzae* biogroup aegyptius. *Mol. Microbiol.* **46:**1367–1380.
38. **LaClaire, L. L., M. L. C. Tondella, D. S. Beall, C. A. Noble, P. L. Raghunathan, N. E. Rosenstein, T. Popovic, and the Active Bacterial Core Surveillance Team Members.** 2003. Identification of *Haemophilus influenzae* serotyping and PCR-based capsule typing. *J. Clin. Microbiol.* **41:**393–396.
39. **Lagergård, T.** 1995. *Haemophilus ducreyi*: pathogenesis and protective immunity. *Trends Microbiol.* **3:**87–91.
40. **Leaves, N. I., I. Dimopoulou, I. Hayes, S. Kerridge, T. Falla, O. Secka, R. A. Adegbola, M. P. Slack, T. E. Peto, and D. W. Crook.** 2000. Epidemiological studies of large resistance plasmids in *Haemophilus*. *J. Antimicrob. Chemother.* **45:**599–604.
41. **Leaves, N. I., and J. Z. Jordens.** 1994. Development of a ribotyping scheme for *Haemophilus influenzae* type b. *Eur. J. Clin. Microbiol. Infect. Dis.* **13:**1038–1045.
42. **Long, S. S., F. M. Henretig, M. J. Teter, and K. L. McGowan.** 1983. Nasopharyngeal flora and acute otitis media. *Infect. Immun.* **41:**987–991.
43. **Lucher, L. A., M. Reeves, T. Hennessy, O. S. Levine, T. Popovic, N. Rosenstein, and A. J. Parkinson.** 2002. Reemergence, in Southwestern Alaska, of invasive *Haemophilus influenzae* type b disease due to strains indistinguishable from those isolated from vaccinated children. *J. Infect. Dis.* **186:**958–965.
44. **Macfarlane, J., W. Holmes, P. Gard, R. Macfarlane, D. Rose, V. Weston, M. Leinonen, P. Saikku, and S. Myint.** 2001. Prospective study of the incidence, aetiology and outcome of adult lower respiratory tract illness in the community. *Thorax* **56:**109–114.
45. **Marco, F., J. García-de-Lomas, C. García-Rey, E. Bouza, L. Aguilar, C. Fernández-Mazarrasa, and The Spanish Surveillance Group for Respiratory Pathogens.** 2001. Antimicrobial susceptibilities of 1,730 *Haemophilus influenzae* respiratory tract isolates in Spain in 1998–1999. *Antimicrob. Agents Chemother.* **45:**3226–3228.
46. **Martin, P. R., R. J. Shea, and M. H. Mulks.** 2001. Identification of a plasmid-encoded gene from *Haemophilus ducreyi* which confers NAD independence. *J. Bacteriol.* **183:**1168–1174.
47. **Marty, A., O. Greiner, P. J. R. Day, S. Gunziger, K. Mühlemann, and D. Nadal.** 2004. Detection of *Haemophilus influenzae* type b by real-time PCR. *J. Clin. Microbiol.* **42:**3813–3815.
48. **Meats, M., E. J. Feil, S. Stringer, A. J. Cody, R. Goldstein, J. S. Kroll, T. Popovic, and B. G. Spratt.** 2003. Characterization of encapsulated and noncapsulated *Haemophilus influenzae* and determination of phylogenetic relationships by multilocus sequence typing. *J. Clin. Microbiol.* **41:**1623–1636.
49. **Mein, J., and G. Lum.** 1999. CSF bacterial antigen detection tests offer no advantage over Gram's stain in the diagnosis of bacterial meningitis. *Pathology* **31:**67–69.
50. **Mertz, K. J., J. B. Weiss, R. M. Webb, W. C. Levine, J. S. Lewis, K. A. Orle, P. A. Totten, J. Overbaugh, S. A. Morse, M. M. Currier, M. Fishbein, and M. E. St. Louis.** 1998. An investigation of genital ulcers in Jackson, Mississippi, with use of a multiplex polymerase chain reaction assay: high prevalence of chancroid and human immunodeficiency virus infection. *J. Infect. Dis.* **178:**1060–1066.
51. **Millar, E. V., K. L. O'Brien, J. P. Watt, J. Lingappa, R. Pallipamu, N. Rosenstein, D. Hu, R. Reid, and M. Santosham.** 2005. Epidemiology of invasive *Haemophilus influenzae* type a disease among Navajo and White Mountain Apache children, 1988–2003. *Clin. Infect. Dis.* **40:**823–830.
52. **Morse, S. A., D. L. Trees, Y. Htun, F. Radebe, K. A. Orle, Y. Dangor, C. M. Beck-Sague, S. Schmid, G. Fehler, J. B. Weiss, and R. C. Ballard.** 1997. Comparison of clinical diagnosis and standard laboratory and molecular methods for the diagnosis of genital ulcer disease in Lesotho: association with human immunodeficiency virus infection. *J. Infect. Dis.* **175:**583–589.
53. **Murphy, T. F.** 2003. Respiratory infections caused by non-typeable *Haemophilus influenzae*. *Curr. Opin. Infect. Dis.* **16:**129–134.
54. **Murphy, T. F., A. L. Brauer, A. T. Schiffmacher, and S. Sethi.** 2004. Persistent colonization by *Haemophilus influenzae* in chronic obstructive pulmonary disease. *Am. J. Respir. Crit. Care Med.* **170:**266–272.
55. **Murphy, T. F., A. L. Brauer, S. Sethi, M. Kilian, and A. J. Lesse.** 2005. *Haemophilus haemolyticus* in the human respiratory tract, abstr. B90. Abstr. *ASM Conf.* Pasteurellaceae, October 23–26, 2005, Kohala Coast, Big Island, Hawaii. American Society for Microbiology, Washington, D.C.
56. **Musser, J. M., D. M. Granoff, P. E. Pattison, and R. K. Selander.** 1985. A population genetic framework for the study of invasive diseases caused by serotype b strains of *Haemophilus influenzae*. *Proc. Natl. Acad. Sci. USA* **82:**5078–5082.
57. **Musser, J. M., J. S. Kroll, D. M. Granoff, E. R. Moxon, B. R. Brodeur, J. Campos, H. Dabernat, W. Frederiksen, J. Hamel, G. Hammond, E. A. Høiby, K. E. Jonsdottir, M. Kabeer, I. Kallings, W. N. Khan, M. Kilian, K. Knowles, H. J. Koornhof, B. Law, K. I. Li, J. Montgomery, P. E. Pattison, J.-C. Piffaretti, A. K. Takala, M. L. Thong, R. A. Wall, J. I. Ward, and R. K. Selander.** 1990. Global genetic structure and molecular epidemiology of encapsulated *Haemophilus influenzae*. *Rev. Infect. Dis.* **12:**75–111.
58. **Nascimento-Carvalho, C. M.** 2001. Etiology of childhood community acquired pneumonia and its implications for vaccination. *Braz. J. Infect. Dis.* **5:**87–97.
59. **Niven, D. F., and T. O'Reilly.** 1990. Significance of V-factor dependency in the taxonomy of *Haemophilus* species and related organisms. *Int. J. Syst. Bacteriol.* **40:**1–4.
60. **Nørskov-Lauritsen, N., B. Bruun, and M. Kilian.** 2005. Multilocus sequence phylogenetic study of the genus *Haemophilus* with description of *Haemophilus pittmaniae* sp. nov. *Int. J. Syst. Evol. Microbiol.* **55:**449–456.
61. **Oberhofer, T. R., and A. E. Back.** 1979. Biotypes of *Haemophilus* encountered in clinical laboratories. *J. Clin. Microbiol.* **10:**168–174.
62. **Olsen, I., F. E. Dewhirst, B. J. Paster, and H.-J. Busse.** 2005. Family *Pasteurellaceae* Pohl 1981, 382; p. 851–856. *In* D. J. Brenner, N. R. Krieg, J. T. Staley, and G. M. Garrity (ed.), *Bergey's Manual of Systematic Bacteriology,* 2nd ed., vol. 2. *The Proteobacteria*, Springer-Verlag, New York, N.Y.
63. **O'Neill, J. M., J. W. St. Geme III, D. Cutter, E. E. Adderson, J. Anyanwu, R. F. Jacobs, and G. E. Schutze.** 2003. Invasive disease due to nontypeable *Haemophilus*

influenzae among children in Arkansas. *J. Clin. Microbiol.* **41**:3064–3069.

64. **Orle, K. A., C. A. Gates, D. H. Martin, B. A. Body, and J. B. Weiss.** 1996. Simultaneous PCR detection of *Haemophilus ducreyi, Treponema pallidum,* and herpes simplex virus types 1 and 2 from genital ulcers. *J. Clin. Microbiol.* **34**:49–54.
65. **Palladino, S., B. J. Leahy, and T. L. Newall.** 1990. Comparison of the RIM-H rapid identification kit with conventional tests for the identification of *Haemophilus* spp. *J. Clin. Microbiol.* **28**:1862–1863.
66. **Peltola, H.** 2000. Worldwide *Haemophilus influenzae* type b disease at the beginning of the 21st century: global analysis of the disease burden 25 years after the use of the polysaccharide vaccine and a decade after the advent of conjugates. *Clin. Microbiol. Rev.* **13**:302–317.
67. **Pennekamp, A., R. Zbinden, and A. von Graevenitz.** 1996. Detection of *Haemophilus influenzae* and *Haemophilus parainfluenzae* from body fluids in blood culture bottles. *J. Microbiol. Methods* **25**:303–307.
68. **Perdue, D. G., L. R. Bulkow, B. G. Gellin, M. Davidson, K. M. Petersen, R. J. Singleton, and A. J. Parkinson.** 2000. Invasive *Haemophilus influenzae* disease in Alaskan residents aged 10 years and older before and after infant vaccination programs. *JAMA* **283**:3089–3094.
69. **Pittman, M., and D. J. Davis.** 1950. Identification of the Koch-Weeks bacillus *(Hemophilus aegyptius)*. *J. Bacteriol.* **59**:413–426.
70. **Plummer, F. A., L. J. D'Costa, H. Nisanze, J. Dylewski, P. Karasira, and A. R. Ronald.** 1983. Epidemiology of *Haemophilus ducreyi* in Nairobi, Kenya. *Lancet* **ii**:1293–1295.
71. **Potts, T. V., J. J. Zambon, and R. J. Genco.** 1985. Reassignment of *Actinobacillus actinomycetemcomitans* to the genus *Haemophilus* as *Haemophilus actinomycetemcomitans* comb. nov. *Int. J. Syst. Bacteriol.* **35**:337–341.
72. **Quentin, R., I. Dubarry, C. Martin, B. Catteier, and A. Goudeau.** 1992. Evaluation of four commercial methods for identification and biotyping of genital and neonatal strains of *Haemophilus* species. *Eur. J. Clin Microbiol. Infect. Dis.* **11**:546–549.
73. **Quentin, R., R. Ruimy, A. Rosenau, J. M. Musser, and R. Christen.** 1996. Genetic identification of cryptic genospecies of *Haemophilus* causing urogenital and neonatal infections by PCR using specific primers targeting genes coding for 16S rRNA. *J. Clin. Microbiol.* **34**:1380–1385.
74. **Raymond, J., L. Armand-Lefevre, F. Moulin, H. Dabernat, A. Commeau, D. Gendrel, and P. Berche.** 2001. Nasopharyngeal colonization by *Haemophilus influenzae* in children living in an orphanage. *Pediatr. Infect. Dis. J.* **20**:779–784.
75. **Rennie, R., T. Gordon, Y. Yaschuk, P. Tomlin, P. Kibsey, and W. Albritton.** 1992. Laboratory and clinical evaluations of media for the primary isolation of *Haemophilus* species. *J. Clin. Microbiol.* **30**:1917–1921.
76. **Saez-Llorens, X., J. Velarde, and C. Canton.** 1994. Pediatric osteomyelitis in Panama. *Clin. Infect. Dis.* **19**:323–324.
77. **Saito, M., A. Umeda, and S.-I. Yoshida.** 1999. Subtyping of *Haemophilus influenzae* strains by pulsed-field gel electrophoresis. *J. Clin. Microbiol.* **37**:2142–2147.
78. **Scriver, S. R., S. L. Walmsley, C. L. Kau, D. J. Hoban, J. Brunton, A. McGeer, T. C. Moore, and E. Witwicki.** 1994. Determination of antimicrobial susceptibilities of Canadian isolates of *Haemophilus influenzae* and characterization of their beta-lactamases. Canadian *Haemophilus* study group. *Antimicrob. Agents Chemother.* **38**:1678–1680.
79. **Shanholtzer, C. J., P. J. Schaper, and L. R. Peterson.** 1982. Concentrated Gram-stained smears prepared with a cytospin centrifuge. *J. Clin. Microbiol.* **16**:1052–1056.
80. **Smith-Vaughan, H. C., A. J. Leach, T. M. Shelby-James, K. Kemp, D. J. Kemp, and J. D. Mathews.** 1996. Carriage of multiple ribotypes of non-encapsulated *Haemophilus influenzae* in aboriginal infants with otitis media. *Epidemiol. Infect.* **116**:177–183.
81. **Takala, A. K., J. Eskola, M. Leinonen, H. Käyhty, A. Nissinen, E. Pekkanen, and P. H. Mäkelä.** 1991. Reduction of oropharyngeal carriage of *Haemophilus influenzae* type b (Hib) in children immunized with an Hib conjugate vaccine. *J. Infect. Dis.* **164**:982–986.
82. **Totten, P. A., J. M. Kuypers, C.-Y. Chen, M. J. Alfa, L. M. Parsons, S. M. Dutro, S. A. Morse, and N. B. Kiviat.** 2000. Etiology of genital ulcer disease in Dakar, Senegal, and comparison of PCR and serologic assays for detection of *Haemophilus ducreyi*. *J. Clin. Microbiol.* **38**:268–273.
83. **Totten, P. A., D. V. Norn, and W. E. Stamm.** 1995. Characterization of the hemolytic activity of *Haemophilus ducreyi*. *Infect. Immun.* **63**:4409–4416.
84. **Totten, P. A., and W. E. Stamm.** 1994. Clear broth and plate media for culture of *Haemophilus ducreyi*. *J. Clin. Microbiol.* **32**:2019–2023.
85. **Trees, D. L., and S. A. Morse.** 1995. Chancroid and *Haemophilus ducreyi*: an update. *Clin. Microbiol. Rev.* **8**:357–375.
86. **Turk, D. C.** 1984. The pathogenicity of *Haemophilus influenzae*. *J. Med. Microbiol.* **18**:1–16.
87. **Ubukata, K., Y. Shibasaki, K. Yamamoto, N. Chiba, K. Hasegawa, Y. Takeuchi, K. Sunakawa, M. Inoue, and M. Konno.** 2001. Association of amino acid substitutions in penicillin-binding protein 3 with β-lactam resistance in β-lactamase-negative ampicillin-resistant *Haemophilus influenzae*. *Antimicrob. Agents Chemother.* **45**:1693–1699.
88. **Urwin, G., J. A. Krohn, K. Deaver-Robinson, J. D. Wenger, M. M. Farley, and the *Haemophilus influenzae* Study Group.** 1996. Invasive disease due to *Haemophilus influenzae* serotype f: clinical and epidemiological characteristics in the *H. influenzae* serotype b vaccine era. *Clin. Infect. Dis.* **22**:1077–1078.
89. **Van Belkum, A., and L. van Alphen.** 1998. Diagnosis of infection, p. 71–92. *In* M. A. Herbert, D. Crook, and E. R. Moxon (ed.), *Molecular Methods for* Haemophilus influenzae. Humana Press Inc., Totowa, N.J.
90. **Van Ketel, R. J., B. de Weber, and L. van Alphen.** 1990. Detection of *Haemophilus influenzae* in cerebrospinal fluid by polymerase chain reaction DNA amplification. *J. Med. Microbiol.* **33**:271–276.
91. **Vastine, D. W., C. R. Dawson, I. Hoshiwara, C. Yoneda, T. Daghfous, and M. Messadi.** 1974. Comparison of media for the isolation of *Haemophilus* species from cases of seasonal conjunctivitis associated with severe endemic trachoma. *Appl. Microbiol.* **28**:688–690.
92. **Waggoner-Fountain, L. A., J. O. Hendley, E. J. Cody, A. A. Perriello, and L. G. Donowitz.** 1995. The emergence of *Haemophilus influenzae* types e and f as significant pathogens. *Clin. Infect. Dis.* **21**:1322–1324.
93. **Wallace, R. J., C. J. Baker, F. J. Quinones, D. G. Hollis, R. E. Weaver, and K. Wiss.** 1983. Nontypeable *Haemophilus influenzae* (biotype 4) as a neonatal, maternal and genital pathogen. *Rev. Infect. Dis.* **5**:123–135.
94. **Windsor, H. M., R. C. Gromkova, and H. J. Koornhof.** 1991. Plasmid-mediated NAD independence in *Haemophilus parainfluenzae*. *J. Gen. Microbiol.* **137**:2415–2421.
95. **Workowski, K. A., and W. C. Levine.** 2002. Sexually transmitted diseases guidelines—2002. *Morb. Mortal. Wkly. Rep.* **51**(RR06):1–80.

Enterobacteriaceae: Introduction and Identification

J. J. FARMER III, K. D. BOATWRIGHT, AND J. MICHAEL JANDA

42

In the fifth edition of this Manual in 1991, Farmer and Kelly commented that it was becoming more difficult to cover the family *Enterobacteriaceae* in a single chapter. The family includes many important organisms (see Tables 1 to 7) such as the plague bacillus *Yersinia pestis,* the typhoid bacillus *Salmonella enterica* serotype Typhi *(Salmonella typhi),* four genera with species that often cause diarrhea and other intestinal infections, seven species that frequently cause nosocomial infections, many other organisms that occasionally cause human or animal infections, dozens of species that occasionally occur in human clinical specimens, and many other species that do not occur in human clinical specimens but can be confused with those that do. In the sixth edition, the material on *Enterobacteriaceae* was divided among three chapters: an introduction to the family that described the overall plan for isolation and identification; a chapter that covered *Salmonella, Shigella, Escherichia coli,* and *Yersinia,* the enteric pathogens; and a chapter that covered the remaining genera and species in the family. In the seventh edition, a fourth chapter was added that covered *Klebsiella, Enterobacter, Citrobacter,* and *Serratia.* In the eighth edition, there were also four chapters. However, *Yersinia* was assigned to its own chapter, and *Klebsiella, Enterobacter, Citrobacter, Serratia,* and *Plesiomonas* (see this chapter) and the remaining *Enterobacteriaceae* were grouped together. This organization has been maintained for the ninth edition.

Because of space limitations, many topics in the present chapter are discussed briefly and only a few primary literature citations are given. Several books, reviews, and chapters are recommended for more detailed information (5, 12–14, 16, 24, 32, 37, 38, 43, 45, 49, 55, 63, 68, 69, 82, 90, 92).

NOMENCLATURE AND CLASSIFICATION

The nomenclature and classification of the genera, species, subspecies, biogroups, and serotypes of *Enterobacteriaceae* have always been topics for heated debate and differing opinions (12–14, 24, 31–34, 37, 38, 55, 63). Until recently, genera and species were defined by biochemical and antigenic analysis. Today, newer techniques such as nucleic acid hybridization and nucleic acid sequencing, which measure evolutionary distance (see chapters 16 and 19 in this Manual), have made it possible to determine the evolutionary relationships among organisms in the family (12–16, 21, 37, 38, 55). The use of these molecular techniques has led to the discovery of many new species and has resulted in the proposed reclassification of others (12–14, 37).

This chapter includes the different names and classifications that clinical microbiologists are likely to encounter in the scientific literature and in material accompanying commercial products. The nomenclature and classification given in Tables 1 to 5 are a compromise based on all available evidence. They include most of the genera, species, subspecies, biogroups, and unnamed Enteric Groups included in the family. If two names are widely used for the same organism, both are mentioned in this chapter with one in parentheses. Many of the "nonclinical" organisms in the family are also included, because there is a possibility that they will be isolated from a human clinical specimen in the future (12–14, 16, 37, 55).

Most of the newly described organisms are very rarely found in clinical specimens (26, 32, 37). This is illustrated by the published listings of organisms that most often cause bacteremia, nosocomial infections, and infections of the gastrointestinal tract (see Tables 6 and 7). The National Library of Medicine's Internet taxonomy database has a useful list of organisms in the family *Enterobacteriaceae* and its relatives (http://www.ncbi.nlm.nih.gov/Taxonomy/Browser/wwwtax.cgi?id=543). This list may also be accessed through http://www.ncbi.nlm.nih.gov/entrez/query.fcgi?db=Taxonomy by selecting "Taxonomy" in the "Search" field and typing "Enterobacteriaceae" in the adjacent "for" field. The Internet site of J. P. Euzéby (http://www.bacterio.cict.fr) gives nomenclature, classifications, original literature citations, and other information for all of the genera and species in the family *Enterobacteriaceae* and its relatives. Unfortunately, the Euzéby site has no alphabetical list of the genera included in the family.

New Species That Occur in Human Clinical Specimens

Names of several new organisms and several "proposed alternative classifications" have been published since the previous edition of this Manual (Table 2), and several of the new organisms occur in human clinical specimens. It is becoming more and more difficult to update the biochemical reaction table (Table 3) of clinically important *Enterobacteriaceae.* For example, *Klebsiella granulomatis (Calymmatobacterium granulomatis)* does not grow on most bacteriological media and lacks a type strain that can be grown and described based on

TABLE 1 Genera and species of *Enterobacteriaceae* that cause,[a] or are associated with, specific or unusual human diseases, syndromes, or conditions[b]

Disease, syndrome, or condition	Organism(s)	Comment
Brain abscesses	*Citrobacter diversus, Enterobacter sakazakii*	Severe, often fatal disease in neonates, survivors have severe mental impairment; cause outbreaks in hospital nurseries.
Dysentery[c]	*Shigella*	One the most important human diarrheal diseases ("invasive" strains of *Escherichia coli* cause a similar but often milder disease)
Granuloma inguinale	*Klebsiella granulomatis (Calymmatobacterium granulomatis)*	Chronic genital ulcerative disease; organism is difficult to demonstrate microbiologically because it does not grow on laboratory media (see text).
Hemorrhagic colitis[c]	*Escherichia coli* O157:H7	Other Shiga toxin-producing strains can also causes a similar, but often milder disease.[b]
Histamine poisoning (scombroid poisoning)	*Proteus morganii, Klebsiella=Raoultella,* others	Caused by bacteria that produce large amounts of histamine and histamine-like substances (scombrotoxin) when they multiply and spoil fish tissues (via bacterial histidine decarboxylase)
Intestinal infection preceded by *Entamoeba histolytica* infection	*Edwardsiella tarda*	Several interesting studies suggest that the protozoan infection must precede *Edwardsiella tarda* in order for it to cause infection.
Meningitis and sepsis in neonates caused by ingesting contaminated infant formula	*Enterobacter sakazakii*	Nursery outbreaks in which infants acquire the strain from dried infant formula that is contaminated with the bacterium; other coliform organisms have also been isolated from formula samples.
Neutropenic patients—initial fever and fever after empirical antibiotic treatment	*Escherichia coli, Klebsiella, Enterobacter*	
Ozena	*Klebsiella ozaenae*	Chronic atrophic rhinitis (ozena), foul smelling discharge from the nose: causative role is uncertain; it may be just colonization.
Paratyphoid fever	*Salmonella* serotypes Paratyphi A, B, C, and others	Causation: paratyphoid fever is an enteric fever that is similar to typhoid fever[b].
Plague (pneumonic and bubonic plague)	*Yersinia pestis*	One of the most important human diseases—the "Black Death" of the Middle Ages
Pneumonia associated with alcoholism—"Friedländer's pneumonia"	*Klebsiella pneumoniae*	Capsular types K1–K6 are most frequently isolated.
Pseudoappendicitis	*Yersinia enterocolitica*	The appendix is normal after surgical removal.
Rhinoscleroma	*Klebsiella rhinoscleromatis*	Chronic granulomatous infection of the nasal passages and respiratory tract; usually seen in the tropics
Reiters syndrome (reactive arthritis)	*Salmonella, Shigella,* enteropathogenic strains of *Yersinia enterocolitica*	Sometimes occurs after gastrointestinal infection; more common in patients with the HLA-B27 histocompatibility antigen
Salmonellosis[c]	*Salmonella*—any of the named or numbered serotypes	One of the most important human diarrheal diseases
Shigellosis[c]	*Shigella*—any of the named and provisional serotypes	One of the most important human diarrheal diseases
Tropical sprue/enteropathy	*Klebsiella, Enterobacter, Hafnia,* others	"Syndrome of enigmatic origin" characterized by prolonged diarrhea and malabsorption by certain residents of the tropics (68); strong presumption for causation (68)
Typhoid fever[c]	*Salmonella* serotype Typhi	One of the most important human diseases

[a] See reference 68 for more details and the evidence for causation versus association in each.

[b] "Adherent-invasive *Escherichia coli*–strains" have been isolated from some patients with Crohn's disease (10), and this organism is being investigated for a causal role (along with many other unrelated organisms).

[c] See reference 68 and chapter 43 for discussions.

TABLE 2 Newly proposed genera, species, and subspecies of *Enterobacteriaceae*,[a] including several "proposed alternative classifications" for previously described organisms

Organism	Occurrence in human clinical specimens	Proposed as: comments	Reference
Averyella dalhousiensis (formerly classified as Enteric Group 58)	Yes	New genus and new species that colonize or infect traumatic injuries; septicemia in a patient receiving total parenteral nutrition (TPN) through a subcutaneous port	56
Citrobacter Group 139	Yes	Proposed alternative classification[b] for Enteric Group 139, which caused a small hospital outbreak	94[b]
Enterobacter cloacae subsp. *dissolvens*	Yes	Proposed alternative classification for *Enterobacter dissolvens;* isolated from plants, blood, skin abscess, abdomen	51
Enterobacter ludwigii	Yes	New species, 16 clinical isolates from blood, urine, etc.; formerly included in *Enterobacter cloacae;* now part of this species complex	52
Enterobacter radicincitans	No	New species isolated from phyllosphere of winter wheat; fixes nitrogen, promotes plant growth	59
Escherichia albertii	Yes	New species; originally misidentified as "Shiga toxin-producing *Hafnia alvei*"	53
Klebsiella singaporensis	No	New species represented by a single isolate from soil	67
Klebsiella variicola	Yes	New species that is phenotypically almost identical to *Klebsiella pneumoniae;* isolated from plants but also from human blood	81
Kluyvera intermedia	No	Proposed alternative classification for *Enterobacter intermedius*	74
Photorhabdus asymbiotica subsp. *australis*	Yes	New subspecies isolated from blood and wounds of patients in Australia	2
Photorhabdus luminescens subsp. *kayaii* and subsp. *thracensis*	No	Two new subspecies isolated from nematodes in Turkey	48
Salmonella enterica	Yes	An old species, but newly made legitimate (see text)	58
Samsonia erythrinae	No	New species isolated from diseased erythrina trees (*Erythrina* sp.)	89
Serratia marcescens subsp. *sakuensis*	No	New subspecies; reported to produce endospores; isolated from wastewater	1
Serratia quinivorans	No	Proposed alternative classification of *Serratia proteamaculans* subsp. *quinivora;* isolated from plants and insects	3
Yersinia aleksiciae	Yes (feces only)	New species represented by only five strains, formerly included in *Yersinia kristensenii* serogroup O:16; isolated from human feces, pork products, and rats/moles	87
Yersinia enterocolitica subspecies *palearctica*	Yes	New subspecies that was proposed to include one of the three evolutionary groups in the species	72
Xenorhabdus budapestensis, *X. ehlersii*, *X. inexii*, *X. szentirmaii*	No	Four new species that are symbiotic in nematodes of the genus *Steinernema* (family *Steinernematidae*) and that are insect pathogens	65

[a] This table includes organisms that were not included in this chapter in the 8th edition of the Manual.
[b] This chapter should be cited as the reference for *Citrobacter* Group 139 as a proposed alternative classification for Enteric Group 139.

simple phenotypic methods. Another problem has been the unavailability of certain strains (62). Other new organisms are almost identical to older organisms in their phenotypic properties. For example, *Klebsiella variicola* will be very difficult to differentiate from *K. pneumoniae* and other *Klebsiella* species. All the newly described species of *Enterobacteriaceae* need to be characterized and added to Table 3.

Organisms That Do Not Occur in Human Clinical Specimens

New or unusual *Enterobacteriaceae* that do not occur in human clinical specimens are listed in Tables 1 to 5, and more information and literature citations can be found at the Internet sites previously cited and in the new edition of *Bergey's Manual of Systematic Bacteriology* (16). These new organisms should be characterized and added to Table 3.

The Expanding Number of *Enterobacteriaceae* Species

How many species of *Enterobacteriaceae* are there? There are probably many hundreds, if not thousands. This is becoming more apparent as methods such as DNA-DNA hybridization and 16S rRNA sequencing (14, 16) are being used to study strains isolated from human clinical specimens, plants, animals,

TABLE 3 Biochemical reactions[a] of the named species, subspecies, biogroups, and Enteric Groups of the family *Enterobacteriaceae*

Organism	Indole production	Methyl red	Voges-Proskauer	Citrate (Simmons)	Hydrogen sulfide (TSI)	Urea hydrolysis	Phenylalanine deaminase	Lysine decarboxylase	Arginine dihydrolase	Ornithine decarboxylase	Motility	Gelatin hydrolysis (22°C)	Growth in KCN	Malonate utilization	D-Glucose, acid	D-Glucose, gas	Lactose fermentation	Sucrose fermentation	D-Mannitol fermentation	Dulcitol fermentation	Salicin fermentation	Adonitol fermentation	*myo*-Inositol fermentation	D-Sorbitol fermentation	L-Arabinose fermentation	Raffinose fermentation	L-Rhamnose fermentation	Maltose fermentation	D-Xylose fermentation	Trehalose fermentation	Cellobiose fermentation	α-Methyl-D-glucoside fermentation	Erythritol fermentation	Esculin hydrolysis	Melibiose fermentation	D-Arabitol fermentation	Glycerol fermentation	Mucate fermentation	Tartrate, Jordan's	Acetate utilization	Lipase (corn oil)	DNase (25°C)	Nitrate → nitrite	Oxidase, Kovacs	ONPG test	Yellow pigment (25°C)	D-Mannose fermentation	Tyrosine hydrolysis
Genus *Averyella*																																																
*A. dalhousiensis**[b]	0	100	0	85	0	70	0	100	0	85	100	0	100	85	100	85	30	0	100	85	100	0	0	100	100	0	100	100	100	100	100	55	0	0	0	0	30	0	60	45	0	0	100	0	100	0	100	0
Genus *Budvicia*																																																
*B. aquatica**	0	93	0	0	80	33	0	0	0	0	27	0	0	0	100	53	87	0	60	0	0	0	0	0	80	0	100	0	93	0	0	0	0	0	0	27	0	20	27	0	0	0	100	0	93	0	0	0
Genus *Buttiauxella*																																																
B. agrestis	0	100	0	100	0	0	0	0	0	100	100	0	80	60	100	100	100	0	100	0	100	0	0	0	100	100	100	100	100	100	100	0	0	100	100	0	60	100	60	0	0	0	100	0	100	0	100	0
B. brennerae	0	100	0	0	0	0	0	0	0	33	100	0	100	100	100	100	0	0	100	0	100	67	0	0	100	100	33	100	100	100	100	0	0	100	100	67	67	67	0	0	0	0	100	0	100	0	100	0
B. ferragutiae	0	100	0	0	0	0	0	100	0	80	60	0	40	0	100	100	0	0	100	0	100	0	0	100	100	0	100	100	100	100	100	40	0	100	0	0	0	60	0	0	0	0	100	0	100	0	100	0
B. gaviniae	0	100	0	20	0	0	0	0	20	0	80	0	60	100	100	40	60	0	100	0	100	100	0	0	100	0	100	60	100	100	100	0	0	100	0	80	0	80	40	0	0	0	100	0	100	0	100	0
B. izardii	0	100	0	0	0	0	0	0	0	100	100	0	67	100	100	100	100	0	100	0	100	0	0	0	100	33	100	100	100	100	100	0	0	100	67	0	33	100	67	0	0	0	100	0	100	0	100	0
*B. noackiae**	33	100	0	33	0	0	100	0	67	0	100	0	100	100	100	100	0	0	100	0	100	0	0	0	100	0	100	100	100	100	100	33	0	100	0	0	0	100	100	0	0	0	100	0	100	0	100	0
B. warmboldiae	0	100	0	33	0	0	100	0	0	0	100	0	33	100	100	100	0	0	100	0	100	0	67	0	100	0	100	100	100	100	100	0	0	100	0	0	0	0	0	0	0	0	100	0	100	0	100	0
Genus *Cedecea*																																																
*C. davisae**	0	100	50	95	0	0	0	0	50	95	95	0	86	91	100	70	19	100	100	0	99	0	0	0	0	10	0	100	100	100	100	5	0	45	0	100	0	0	0	0	91	0	100	0	90	0	100	0
*C. lapagei**	0	40	80	99	0	0	0	0	80	0	80	0	100	99	100	100	60	0	100	0	100	0	0	0	0	0	0	100	0	100	100	0	0	100	0	100	0	0	0	60	100	0	100	0	99	0	100	0
*C. neteri**	0	100	50	100	0	0	0	0	100	0	100	0	65	100	100	100	35	100	100	0	100	0	0	100	0	0	0	100	100	100	100	0	0	100	0	100	0	0	0	0	100	0	100	0	100	0	100	0
C. species 3*	0	100	50	100	0	0	0	0	100	0	100	0	100	0	100	100	0	50	100	0	100	0	0	0	0	100	0	100	100	100	100	50	0	100	100	100	0	0	0	50	100	0	100	0	100	0	100	0
C. species 5*	0	100	50	100	0	0	0	0	50	50	100	0	100	0	100	100	0	100	100	0	100	0	0	100	0	100	0	100	100	100	100	0	0	100	100	100	0	0	0	50	50	0	100	0	100	0	100	0
Genus *Citrobacter*																																																
*C. freundii** (A)[c]	33	100	0	78	78	44	0	0	67	0	89	0	89	11	100	89	78	89	100	11	0	0	0	100	100	44	100	100	89	100	44	11	0	0	100	0	100	100	100	44	0	0	100	0	89	0	100	0
*C. youngae** (A)	15	100	0	75	65	80	0	0	50	5	95	0	95	5	100	75	25	20	100	85	10	0	5	100	100	10	100	95	100	100	45	0	0	5	10	5	90	100	100	65	0	0	85	0	90	0	100	0
*C. braakii** (A)	33	100	0	87	60	47	0	0	67	93	87	0	100	0	100	93	80	7	100	33	0	0	0	100	100	7	100	100	100	100	73	33	0	0	80	0	87	100	93	53	0	0	100	0	80	0	100	0
*C. murliniae** (A)	100	100	0	100	67	67	0	0	67	0	100	0	100	0	100	100	67	33	100	100	33	0	0	100	100	33	100	100	100	100	100	0	0	0	33	0	100	100	100	33	0	0	100	0	100	0	100	0
*C. werkmanii** (A)	0	100	0	100	100	100	0	0	100	0	100	0	100	100	100	100	17	0	100	0	0	0	0	100	100	0	100	100	100	100	0	0	0	0	0	0	100	100	100	100	0	0	100	0	100	0	100	0
*C. gillenii** (A)	0	100	0	33	67	0	0	0	33	0	67	0	100	100	100	100	67	33	100	0	0	0	0	100	100	0	100	100	100	100	67	0	0	0	67	0	67	67	100	0	0	0	100	0	67	0	100	0
*C. amalonaticus** (B)	100	100	0	95	5	85	0	0	85	95	95	0	99	1	100	97	35	9	100	1	30	0	0	99	99	5	100	99	99	100	100	2	0	5	0	0	60	96	96	86	0	0	99	0	97	0	100	0
*C. farmeri** (B)	100	100	0	10	0	59	0	0	85	100	97	0	93	0	100	96	15	100	100	2	9	0	0	98	100	100	100	100	100	100	100	75	0	0	100	0	65	100	93	80	0	0	100	0	100	0	100	0
C. Group 137* (B)	100	100	0	0	0	70	0	0	20	100	100	0	100	0	100	0	100	100	100	0	100	0	0	100	100	100	100	100	100	100	100	80	0	100	100	0	100	100	50	100	0	0	100	0	100	0	100	0
*C. rodentium** (B)	0	100	0	0	0	100	0	0	0	100	0	0	0	100	100	100	100	0	100	0	0	0	0	100	100	0	100	100	100	100	100	0	0	0	0	0	0	100	100	0	0	0	100	0	100	0	100	0
*C. sedlakii** (B)	100	100	0	95	5	85	0	0	85	95	95	0	99	1	100	97	35	9	100	1	30	0	0	99	99	5	100	99	99	100	100	2	0	5	0	0	60	96	96	86	0	0	99	0	97	0	100	0
C. diversus (*C. koseri*)* (C)	100	100	0	10	0	59	0	0	85	100	97	0	93	0	100	96	15	100	100	2	9	0	0	98	100	100	100	100	100	100	100	75	0	0	100	0	65	100	93	80	0	0	100	0	100	0	100	0
Genus *Edwardsiella*																																																
*E. tarda**	99	100	0	1	100	0	0	100	0	100	98	0	0	0	100	100	0	0	0	0	0	0	0	0	9	0	0	100	0	0	0	0	0	0	0	0	30	0	25	0	0	0	100	0	0	0	100	0
E. tarda biogroup 1*	100	100	0	0	0	0	0	100	0	100	100	0	0	0	100	50	0	100	100	0	0	0	0	0	100	0	0	100	0	0	0	0	0	0	0	0	0	0	0	0	0	0	100	0	0	0	100	0
*E. hoshinae**	50	100	0	0	0	0	0	100	0	95	100	0	0	100	100	35	0	100	100	0	50	0	0	0	13	0	0	100	0	100	0	0	0	0	0	0	65	0	0	0	0	0	100	0	0	0	100	0
E. ictaluri	0	0	0	0	0	0	0	100	0	65	0	0	0	0	100	50	0	0	0	0	0	0	0	0	0	0	0	100	0	0	0	0	0	0	0	0	0	0	0	0	0	0	100	0	0	0	100	0
Genus *Enterobacter*																																																
*E. aerogenes**	0	5	98	95	0	2	0	98	0	98	97	0	98	95	100	100	95	100	100	5	100	98	95	100	100	96	99	99	100	100	100	95	0	98	99	100	98	90	95	50	0	0	100	0	100	0	95	0
*E. cloacae**	0	5	100	100	0	65	0	0	97	96	95	0	98	75	100	100	93	97	100	15	75	25	15	95	100	97	92	100	99	100	99	85	0	30	90	15	40	75	30	75	0	0	99	0	99	0	100	0
"*E. agglomerans* complex"*	20	50	70	50	0	20	20	0	0	0	85	2	35	65	100	20	40	75	100	15	65	7	15	30	95	30	85	89	93	97	55	7	0	60	50	50	30	40	25	30	0	0	85	0	90	75	98	0
*E. gergoviae**	0	5	100	99	0	93	0	90	0	100	90	0	0	96	100	98	55	98	99	0	99	0	0	0	99	97	99	100	99	100	99	2	0	97	97	97	100	2	97	93	0	0	99	0	97	0	100	0
*E. sakazakii**	11	5	100	99	0	1	50	0	99	91	96	0	99	18	100	98	99	100	100	5	99	0	75	0	100	99	100	100	100	100	100	96	0	100	100	0	15	1	1	96	0	0	99	0	100	98	100	0
E. taylorae (*E. cancerogenus*)*	0	5	100	100	0	1	0	0	94	99	99	0	98	100	100	100	10	0	100	0	92	0	0	1	100	0	100	99	100	100	100	1	0	90	0	0	1	75	0	35	0	0	100	0	100	0	100	
E. amnigenus biogroup 1*	0	7	100	70	0	0	0	0	9	55	92	0	100	91	100	100	70	100	100	0	91	0	0	9	100	100	100	100	100	100	100	55	0	91	100	0	0	35	9	0	0	0	100	0	91	0	100	0
E. amnigenus biogroup 2*	0	65	100	100	0	0	0	0	35	100	100	0	100	100	100	100	35	0	100	0	100	0	0	100	100	0	100	100	100	100	100	100	0	100	100	0	0	100	0	0	0	0	100	0	100	0	100	0
*E. asburiae**	0	100	2	100	0	60	0	0	21	95	0	0	97	3	100	95	75	100	100	0	100	0	0	100	100	70	5	100	97	100	100	95	0	95	0	0	11	21	30	87	0	0	100	0	100	0	100	0

TABLE 3 *(Continued)*

Organism	Indole production	Methyl red	Voges-Proskauer	Citrate (Simmons)	Hydrogen sulfide (TSI)	Urea hydrolysis	Phenylalanine deaminase	Lysine decarboxylase	Arginine dihydrolase	Ornithine decarboxylase	Motility	Gelatin hydrolysis (22°C)	Growth in KCN	Malonate utilization	D-Glucose, acid	D-Glucose, gas	Lactose fermentation	Sucrose fermentation	D-Mannitol fermentation	Dulcitol fermentation	Salicin fermentation	Adonitol fermentation	*myo*-Inositol fermentation	D-Sorbitol fermentation
*E. hormaechei**	0	57	100	96	0	87	4	0	78	91	52	0	100	100	100	83	9	100	100	87	44	0	0	0
E. cancerogenus	0	0	100	100	0	0	0	0	100	100	100	0	100	100	100	100	0	0	100	0	100	0	0	0
E. dissolvens	0	0	100	100	0	100	0	0	100	100	0	0	100	100	100	100	0	100	100	0	100	0	0	100
E. nimipressuralis	0	100	100	0	0	0	0	0	0	100	0	0	100	100	100	100	0	0	100	0	100	0	0	100
E. pyrinus	0	29	86	0	0	86	0	100	0	100	43	0	0	86	100	100	14	100	100	0	100	0	100	0
Genera *Escherichia* and *Shigella*																								
*E. coli**	98	99	0	1	1	1	0	90	17	65	95	0	3	0	100	95	95	50	98	60	40	5	1	94
E. coli, inactive*	80	95	0	1	1	1	0	40	3	20	5	0	1	0	100	5	25	15	93	40	10	3	1	75
*S. dysenteriae** (Serogroup A)	45	99	0	0	0	0	0	0	2	0	0	0	0	0	100	0	0	0	0	5	0	0	0	30
*S. flexneri** (Serogroup B)	50	100	0	0	0	0	0	0	5	0	0	0	0	0	100	3	1	1	95	1	0	0	0	29
*S. boydii** (Serogroup C)	25	100	0	0	0	0	0	0	18	2	0	0	0	0	100	0	1	0	97	5	0	0	0	43
*S. sonnei** (Serogroup D)	0	100	0	0	0	0	0	0	2	98	0	0	0	0	100	0	2	1	99	0	0	0	0	2
*E. fergusonii**	98	100	0	17	0	0	0	95	5	100	93	0	0	35	100	95	0	0	98	60	65	98	0	0
*E. hermannii**	99	100	0	1	0	0	0	6	0	100	99	0	94	0	100	97	45	45	100	19	40	0	0	0
*E. vulneris**	0	100	0	0	0	0	0	85	30	0	100	0	15	85	100	97	15	8	100	0	30	0	0	1
E. blattae	0	100	0	50	0	0	0	100	0	100	0	0	0	100	100	100	0	0	0	0	0	0	0	0
Genus *Ewingella*																								
*E. americana**	0	84	95	95	0	0	0	0	0	0	60	0	5	0	100	0	70	0	100	0	80	0	0	0
Genus *Hafnia*																								
*H. alvei**	0	40	85	10	0	4	0	100	6	98	85	0	95	50	100	98	5	10	99	0	13	0	0	0
H. alvei biogroup 1	0	85	70	0	0	0	0	100	0	45	0	0	0	45	100	0	0	0	55	0	55	0	0	0
Genus *Klebsiella*																								
*K. pneumoniae** (A)	0	10	98	98	0	95	0	98	0	0	0	0	98	93	100	97	98	99	99	30	99	90	95	99
*K. ozaenae** (A)	0	98	0	30	0	10	0	40	6	3	0	0	88	3	100	50	30	20	100	2	97	97	55	65
*K. rhinoscleromatis** (A)	0	100	0	0	0	0	0	0	0	0	0	0	80	95	100	0	0	75	100	0	98	100	95	100
*K. oxytoca** (B)	99	20	95	95	0	90	1	99	0	0	0	0	97	98	100	97	100	100	99	55	100	99	98	99
*K. ornithinolytica** (C)	100	96	70	100	0	100	0	100	0	100	0	0	100	100	100	100	100	100	100	10	100	100	95	100
*K. planticola** (C)	20	100	98	100	0	98	0	100	0	0	0	0	100	100	100	100	100	100	100	15	100	100	100	92
K. terrigena (C)	0	60	100	40	0	0	0	100	0	20	0	0	100	100	100	80	100	100	100	20	100	100	80	100
Genus *Kluyvera*																								
*K. ascorbata**	92	100	0	96	0	0	0	97	0	100	98	0	92	96	100	93	98	98	100	25	100	0	0	40
*K. cryocrescens**	90	100	0	80	0	0	0	23	0	100	90	0	86	86	100	95	95	81	95	0	100	0	0	45
*K. georgiana**	100	100	0	100	0	0	0	100	0	100	100	0	83	50	100	17	83	100	100	33	100	0	0	0
*K. intermedia**	0	100	100	65	0	0	0	0	0	89	89	0	65	100	100	100	100	65	100	100	100	0	0	100
Genus *Leclercia*																								
*L. adecarboxylata**	100	100	0	0	0	48	0	0	0	0	79	0	97	93	100	97	93	66	100	86	100	93	0	0
Genus *Leminorella*																								
*L. grimontii**	0	100	0	100	100	0	0	0	0	0	0	0	0	0	100	33	0	0	0	83	0	0	0	0
*L. richardii**	0	0	0	0	100	0	0	0	0	0	0	0	0	0	100	0	0	0	0	0	0	0	0	0
Genus *Moellerella*																								
*M. wisconsensis**	0	100	0	80	0	0	0	0	0	0	0	0	70	0	100	0	100	100	60	0	0	100	0	0

Organism	L-Arabinose fermentation	Raffinose fermentation	L-Rhamnose fermentation	Maltose fermentation	D-Xylose fermentation	Trehalose fermentation	Cellobiose fermentation	α-Methyl-D-glucoside fermentation	Erythritol fermentation	Esculin hydrolysis	Melibiose fermentation	D-Arabitol fermentation	Glycerol fermentation	Mucate fermentation	Tartrate, Jordan's	Acetate utilization	Lipase (corn oil)	DNase (25°C)	Nitrate → nitrite	Oxidase, Kovacs	ONPG test	Yellow pigment (25°C)	D-Mannose fermentation	Tyrosine hydrolysis
*E. hormaechei**	100	0	100	100	96	100	100	83	0	0	0	0	4	96	13	74	0	0	100	0	95	0	100	0
E. cancerogenus	100	0	100	100	100	100	100	0	0	100	0	0	0	100	0	33	0	0	100	0	100	0	100	0
E. dissolvens	100	100	100	100	100	100	100	100	0	100	100	0	0	100	0	100	0	0	100	0	100	0	100	0
E. nimipressuralis	100	0	100	100	100	100	100	100	0	100	100	0	0	100	0	0	0	0	100	0	100	0	100	0
E. pyrinus	100	0	100	100	0	100	100	0	0	100	0	0	0	0	0	0	0	0	100	0	100	0	100	0
Genera *Escherichia* and *Shigella*																								
*E. coli**	99	50	80	95	95	98	2	0	0	35	75	5	75	95	95	90	0	0	100	0	95	0	98	0
E. coli, inactive*	85	15	65	80	70	90	2	0	0	5	40	5	65	30	85	40	0	0	98	0	45	0	97	0
*S. dysenteriae** (Serogroup A)	45	0	30	15	4	90	0	0	0	0	0	0	10	0	75	0	0	0	99	0	30	0	100	0
*S. flexneri** (Serogroup B)	60	40	5	30	2	65	0	0	0	0	55	1	10	0	30	8	0	0	99	0	1	0	100	0
*S. boydii** (Serogroup C)	94	0	1	20	11	85	0	0	0	0	15	0	50	0	50	0	0	0	100	0	10	0	100	0
*S. sonnei** (Serogroup D)	95	3	75	90	2	100	5	0	0	0	25	0	15	10	90	0	0	0	100	0	90	0	100	0
*E. fergusonii**	98	0	92	96	96	96	96	0	0	46	0	100	20	0	96	96	0	0	100	0	83	0	100	0
*E. hermannii**	100	40	97	100	100	100	97	0	0	40	0	8	3	97	35	78	0	0	100	0	98	98	100	0
*E. vulneris**	100	99	93	100	100	100	100	25	0	20	100	0	25	78	2	30	0	0	100	0	100	50	100	0
E. blattae	100	0	100	100	100	75	0	0	0	0	0	0	100	50	50	0	0	0	100	0	0	0	100	0
Genus *Ewingella*																								
*E. americana**	0	0	23	16	13	99	10	0	0	50	0	99	24	0	35	10	0	0	97	0	85	0	99	0
Genus *Hafnia*																								
*H. alvei**	95	2	97	100	98	95	15	0	0	7	0	0	95	0	70	15	0	0	100	0	90	0	100	0
H. alvei biogroup 1	0	0	0	0	0	70	0	0	0	0	0	0	0	0	30	0	0	0	100	0	30	0	100	0
Genus *Klebsiella*																								
*K. pneumoniae** (A)	99	99	99	98	99	99	98	90	0	99	99	98	97	90	95	75	0	0	99	0	99	0	99	0
*K. ozaenae** (A)	98	90	55	95	95	98	92	70	0	80	97	95	65	25	50	2	0	0	80	0	80	0	100	0
*K. rhinoscleromatis** (A)	100	90	96	100	100	100	100	0	0	30	100	100	50	0	50	0	0	0	100	0	0	0	100	0
*K. oxytoca** (B)	98	100	100	100	100	100	100	98	2	100	99	98	99	93	98	90	0	0	100	0	100	1	100	0
*K. ornithinolytica** (C)	100	100	100	100	100	100	100	100	0	100	100	100	100	96	100	95	0	0	100	0	100	0	100	0
*K. planticola** (C)	100	100	100	100	100	100	100	100	0	100	100	100	100	100	100	62	0	0	100	0	100	1	100	0
K. terrigena (C)	100	100	100	100	100	100	100	100	0	100	100	100	100	100	100	20	0	0	100	0	100	0	100	0
Genus *Kluyvera*																								
*K. ascorbata**	100	98	100	100	99	100	100	98	0	99	99	0	40	90	35	50	0	0	100	0	100	0	100	0
*K. cryocrescens**	100	100	100	100	91	100	100	95	0	100	100	0	5	81	19	86	0	0	100	0	100	0	100	0
*K. georgiana**	100	100	83	100	100	100	100	100	0	100	100	0	33	83	50	83	0	0	100	0	100	0	100	0
*K. intermedia**	100	100	100	100	100	100	100	100	0	100	100	0	100	100	100	0	0	0	100	0	100	0	100	0
Genus *Leclercia*																								
*L. adecarboxylata**	100	66	100	100	100	100	100	0	0	100	100	96	3	93	83	28	0	0	100	0	100	37	100	0
Genus *Leminorella*																								
*L. grimontii**	100	0	0	0	83	0	0	0	0	0	0	0	17	100	100	0	0	0	100	0	0	0	0	0
*L. richardii**	100	0	0	0	100	0	0	0	0	0	0	0	0	50	100	0	0	0	100	0	0	0	0	0
Genus *Moellerella*																								
*M. wisconsensis**	0	100	0	30	0	0	0	0	0	0	100	75	10	0	30	10	0	0	90	0	90	0	100	0

(Continued)

TABLE 3 Biochemical reactions[a] of the named species, subspecies, biogroups, and Enteric Groups of the family *Enterobacteriaceae* (*Continued*)

Organism	Indole production	Methyl red	Voges-Proskauer	Citrate (Simmons)	Hydrogen sulfide (TSI)	Urea hydrolysis	Phenylalanine deaminase	Lysine decarboxylase	Arginine dihydrolase	Ornithine decarboxylase	Motility	Gelatin hydrolysis (22°C)	Growth in KCN	Malonate utilization	D-Glucose, acid	D-Glucose, gas	Lactose fermentation	Sucrose fermentation	D-Mannitol fermentation	Dulcitol fermentation	Salicin fermentation	Adonitol fermentation	*myo*-Inositol fermentation	D-Sorbitol fermentation
Genus *Morganella*																								
M.morganii subsp. *morganii**	95	95	0	0	20	95	95	1	0	95	95	0	98	1	99	90	1	0	0	0	0	0	0	0
M. morganii biogroup 1*	100	95	0	0	15	100	100	100	0	80	0	0	90	5	100	93	0	0	0	0	0	0	0	0
M. morganii subsp. *sibonii**	50	86	0	0	7	100	93	29	0	64	79	0	79	0	100	86	0	7	0	0	0	0	0	0
Genus *Obesumbacterium*																								
O. proteus biogroup 2	0	15	0	0	0	0	0	100	0	100	0	0	0	0	100	0	0	0	0	0	0	0	0	0
Genus *Pantoea*																								
P. dispersa	0	82	64	100	0	0	9	0	0	0	100	0	82	9	100	0	0	1	100	0	0	0	0	0
Genus *Photorhabdus*																								
P. luminescens (25°C)	50	0	0	50	0	25	0	0	0	0	100	50	0	0	75	0	0	0	0	0	0	0	0	0
*P. asymbiotica**	0	0	0	20	0	60	0	0	0	0	100	80	20	0	100	0	0	0	0	0	0	0	0	0
Genus *Plesiomonas*																								
*P. shigelloides**	100	90	0	0	0	0	3	100	98	99	95	0	1	0	100	0	80	0	0	0	0	0	95	0
Genus *Pragia*																								
P. fontium	0	100	0	89	89	0	22	0	0	0	100	0	0	0	100	0	0	0	0	0	78	0	0	0
Genus *Proteus*																								
*P. mirabilis**	2	97	50	65	98	98	98	0	0	99	95	90	98	2	100	96	2	15	0	0	0	0	0	0
*P. vulgaris**	98	95	0	15	95	95	99	0	0	0	95	91	99	0	100	85	2	97	0	0	50	0	0	0
*P. penneri**	0	100	0	0	30	100	99	0	0	0	85	50	99	0	100	45	1	100	0	0	0	0	0	0
P. myxofaciens	0	100	100	50	0	100	100	0	0	0	100	100	100	0	100	100	0	100	0	0	0	0	0	0
Genus *Providencia*																								
*P. rettgeri**	99	93	0	95	0	98	98	0	0	0	94	0	97	0	100	10	5	15	100	0	50	100	90	1
*P. stuartii**	98	100	0	93	0	30	95	0	0	0	85	0	100	0	100	0	2	50	10	0	2	5	95	1
*P. alcalifaciens**	99	99	0	98	0	0	98	0	0	1	96	0	100	0	100	85	0	15	2	0	1	98	1	1
*P. rustigianii**	98	65	0	15	0	0	100	0	0	0	30	0	100	0	100	35	0	35	0	0	0	0	0	0
P. heimbachae	0	85	0	0	0	0	100	0	0	0	46	0	8	0	100	0	0	0	0	0	0	92	46	0
Genus *Rahnella*																								
*R. aquatilis**	0	88	100	94	0	0	95	0	0	0	6	0	0	100	100	98	100	100	100	88	100	0	0	94
Genus *Salmonella*																								
*S. enterica** (Group I[d])	1	100	0	95	95	1	0	98	70	97	95	0	0	0	100	96	1	1	100	96	0	0	35	95
Serotype Typhi*	0	100	0	0	97	0	0	98	3	0	97	0	0	0	100	0	1	0	100	0	0	0	0	99
Serotype Choleraesuis*	0	100	0	25	50	0	0	95	55	100	95	0	0	0	100	95	0	0	98	5	0	0	0	90
Serotype Paratyphi A*	0	100	0	0	10	0	0	0	15	95	95	0	0	0	100	99	0	0	100	90	0	0	0	95
Serotype Gallinarum*	0	100	0	0	100	0	0	90	10	1	0	0	0	0	100	0	0	0	100	90	0	0	0	1
Serotype Pullorum*	0	90	0	0	90	0	0	100	10	95	0	0	0	0	100	90	0	0	100	0	0	0	0	10
Group II strains*	2	100	0	100	100	0	0	100	90	100	98	2	0	95	100	100	1	1	100	90	5	0	5	100
Group IIIa strains*	1	100	0	99	99	0	0	99	70	99	99	0	1	95	100	99	15	1	100	0	0	0	0	99
Group IIIb strains*	2	100	0	98	99	0	0	99	70	99	99	0	1	95	100	99	85	5	100	1	0	0	0	99
Group IV strains*	0	100	0	98	100	2	0	100	70	100	98	0	95	0	100	100	0	0	98	0	60	5	0	100
S. bongori (Group V)*	0	100	0	94	100	0	0	100	94	100	100	0	100	0	100	94	0	0	100	94	0	0	0	100
Group VI strains*	0	100	0	89	100	0	0	100	67	100	100	0	0	0	100	100	22	0	100	67	0	0	0	0
Genus *Serratia*																								
*S. marcescens**	1	20	98	98	0	15	0	99	0	99	97	90	95	3	100	55	2	99	99	0	95	40	75	99
S. marcescens biogroup 1*	0	100	60	30	0	0	0	55	4	65	17	30	70	0	100	0	4	100	96	0	92	30	30	92

Organism	L-Arabinose fermentation	Raffinose fermentation	L-Rhamnose fermentation	Maltose fermentation	D-Xylose fermentation	Trehalose fermentation	Cellobiose fermentation	α-Methyl-D-glucoside fermentation	Erythritol fermentation	Esculin hydrolysis	Melibiose fermentation	D-Arabitol fermentation	Glycerol fermentation	Mucate fermentation	Tartrate, Jordan's	Acetate utilization	Lipase (corn oil)	DNase (25°C)	Nitrate → nitrite	Oxidase, Kovacs	ONPG test	Yellow pigment (25°C)	D-Mannose fermentation	Tyrosine hydrolysis
Genus *Morganella*																								
M.morganii subsp. *morganii**	0	0	0	0	0	0	0	0	0	0	0	0	5	0	95	0	0	0	90	0	10	0	98	99+
M. morganii biogroup 1*	0	0	0	0	0	0	0	0	0	0	0	0	100	0	100	0	0	0	90	0	20	0	100	99+
M. morganii subsp. *sibonii**	0	0	0	0	0	100	0	0	0	0	0	0	7	7	100	0	0	0	100	0	0	0	100	99+
Genus *Obesumbacterium*																								
O. proteus biogroup 2	0	0	15	50	15	85	0	0	0	0	0	0	0	0	15	0	0	0	100	0	0	0	85	0
Genus *Pantoea*																								
P. dispersa	100	0	91	82	100	100	55	0	0	0	0	100	27	0	9	100	0	0	91	0	91	27	100	0
Genus *Photorhabdus*																								
P. luminescens (25°C)	0	0	0	25	0	0	0	0	0	0	0	0	0	0	50	0	0	0	0	0	0	50	100	0
*P. asymbiotica**	0	0	0	0	0	0	0	0	0	0	0	0	0	0	60	20	0	0	0	0	0	60	100	0
Genus *Plesiomonas*																								
*P. shigelloides**	0	0	0	95	0	100	0	0	0	0	70	0	35	0	50	8	0	0	100	99	90	0	10	0
Genus *Pragia*																								
P. fontium	0	0	0	0	0	0	0	0	0	78	0	0	0	0	0	0	0	0	100	0	0	0	0	0
Genus *Proteus*																								
*P. mirabilis**	0	1	1	0	98	98	1	0	0	0	0	0	70	0	87	20	92	50	95	0	0	0	0	99+
*P. vulgaris**	0	1	5	97	95	30	0	60	1	50	0	0	60	0	80	25	80	80	98	0	1	0	0	99+
*P. penneri**	0	1	0	100	100	55	0	80	0	0	0	0	55	0	85	5	45	40	90	0	1	0	0	99+
P. myxofaciens	0	0	0	100	0	100	0	100	0	0	0	0	100	0	100	0	100	50	100	0	0	0	0	99+
Genus *Providencia*																								
*P. rettgeri**	0	5	70	2	10	0	3	2	75	35	5	100	60	0	95	60	0	0	100	0	5	0	100	99+
*P. stuartii**	1	7	0	1	7	98	5	0	0	0	0	0	50	0	90	75	0	10	100	0	10	0	100	99+
*P. alcalifaciens**	1	1	0	1	1	2	0	0	0	0	0	0	15	0	90	40	0	0	100	0	1	0	100	99+
*P. rustigianii**	0	0	0	0	0	0	0	0	0	0	0	0	5	0	50	25	0	0	100	0	0	0	100	99+
P. heimbachae	0	0	100	54	8	0	0	0	0	0	0	92	0	0	69	0	0	0	100	0	0	0	100	99+
Genus *Rahnella*																								
*R. aquatilis**	100	94	94	94	94	100	100	0	0	100	100	0	13	30	6	6	0	0	100	0	100	0	100	0
Genus *Salmonella*																								
*S. enterica** (Group I[d])	99	2	95	97	97	99	5	2	0	5	95	0	5	90	90	90	0	2	100	0	2	0	100	0
Serotype Typhi*	2	0	0	97	82	100	0	0	0	0	100	0	20	0	100	0	0	0	100	0	0	0	100	0
Serotype Choleraesuis*	0	1	100	95	98	0	0	0	1	0	45	1	0	0	85	1	0	0	98	0	0	0	95	0
Serotype Paratyphi A*	100	0	100	95	0	100	5	0	0	0	95	0	10	0	0	0	0	0	100	0	0	0	100	0
Serotype Gallinarum*	80	10	10	90	70	50	10	0	1	0	0	0	0	50	100	0	0	10	100	0	0	0	100	0
Serotype Pullorum*	100	1	100	5	90	90	5	0	0	0	0	0	0	0	0	0	0	0	100	0	0	0	100	0
Group II strains*	100	0	100	100	100	100	0	8	0	15	8	0	25	96	50	95	0	0	100	0	15	0	95	0
Group IIIa strains*	99	1	99	98	100	99	1	1	0	1	95	1	10	90	5	90	0	2	100	0	100	0	100	0
Group IIIb strains*	99	1	99	98	100	99	1	1	0	1	95	1	10	30	20	75	0	2	100	0	92	0	100	0
Group IV strains*	100	0	98	100	100	100	50	0	0	0	100	5	0	0	65	70	0	0	100	0	0	0	100	0
S. bongori (Group V)*	94	0	88	100	100	100	0	0	0	0	94	0	0	88	0	100	0	0	100	0	94	0	100	0
Group VI strains*	100	0	100	100	100	100	0	0	0	0	89	0	33	89	100	89	0	0	100	0	44	0	100	0
Genus *Serratia*																								
*S. marcescens**	0	2	0	96	7	99	5	0	1	95	0	0	95	0	75	50	98	98	98	0	95	0	99	0
S. marcescens biogroup 1*	0	0	0	70	0	100	4	0	0	96	0	0	92	0	50	4	75	82	83	0	75	0	100	0

TABLE 3 *(Continued)*

Organism	Indole production	Methyl red	Voges-Proskauer	Citrate (Simmons)	Hydrogen sulfide (TSI)	Urea hydrolysis	Phenylalanine deaminase	Lysine decarboxylase	Arginine dihydrolase	Ornithine decarboxylase	Motility	Gelatin hydrolysis (22°C)	Growth in KCN	Malonate utilization	D-Glucose, acid	D-Glucose, gas	Lactose fermentation	Sucrose fermentation	D-Mannitol fermentation	Dulcitol fermentation	Salicin fermentation	Adonitol fermentation	*myo*-Inositol fermentation	D-Sorbitol fermentation	L-Arabinose fermentation	Raffinose fermentation	L-Rhamnose fermentation	Maltose fermentation	D-Xylose fermentation	Trehalose fermentation	Cellobiose fermentation	α-Methyl-D-glucoside fermentation	Erythritol fermentation	Esculin hydrolysis	Melibiose fermentation	D-Arabitol fermentation	Glycerol fermentation	Mucate fermentation	Tartrate, Jordan's	Acetate utilization	Lipase (corn oil)	DNase (25°C)	Nitrate → nitrite	Oxidase, Kovacs	ONPG test	Yellow pigment (25°C)	D-Mannose fermentation	Tyrosine hydrolysis
S. liquefaciens complex*	1	93	93	90	0	3	0	95	0	95	95	90	90	2	100	75	10	98	100	0	97	5	60	95	98	85	15	98	100	100	5	5	0	97	75	0	95	0	75	40	85	85	100	0	93	0	100	0
*S. rubidaea**	0	20	100	95	0	2	0	55	0	0	85	90	25	94	100	30	100	99	100	0	99	99	20	1	100	99	1	99	99	100	94	1	0	94	99	85	20	0	70	80	99	99	100	0	100	0	100	0
S. odorifera biogroup 1*	60	100	50	100	0	5	0	100	0	100	100	95	60	0	100	0	70	100	100	0	98	50	100	100	100	100	95	100	100	100	100	0	0	95	100	0	40	5	100	60	35	100	100	0	100	0	100	0
S. odorifera biogroup 2*	50	60	100	97	0	0	0	94	0	0	100	94	19	0	100	13	97	0	97	0	45	55	100	100	100	7	94	100	100	100	100	0	7	40	96	0	50	0	100	65	65	100	100	0	100	0	100	0
*S. plymuthica**	0	94	80	75	0	0	0	0	0	0	50	60	30	0	100	40	80	100	100	0	94	0	50	65	100	94	0	94	94	100	88	70	0	81	93	0	50	0	100	55	70	100	100	0	70	0	100	0
*S. ficaria**	0	75	75	100	0	0	0	0	0	0	100	100	55	0	100	0	15	100	100	0	100	0	55	100	100	70	35	100	100	100	100	8	0	100	40	100	0	0	17	40	77	100	92	8	100	0	100	0
S. entomophila	0	20	100	100	0	0	0	0	0	0	100	100	100	0	100	0	0	100	100	0	100	0	0	0	0	0	0	100	40	100	0	0	0	100	0	60	0	0	100	80	20	100	100	0	100	0	100	0
"*Serratia*" *fonticola**	0	100	9	91	0	13	0	100	0	97	91	0	70	88	100	79	97	21	100	91	100	100	30	100	100	100	76	97	85	100	6	91	0	100	98	100	88	0	58	15	0	0	100	0	100	0	100	0
Genus *Tatumella*																																																
*T. ptyseos**	0	0	5	2	0	0	90	0	0	0	0	0	0	0	100	0	0	98	0	0	55	0	0	0	0	11	0	0	9	93	0	0	0	0	25	0	7	0	0	0	0	0	98	0	0	0	100	0
Genus *Trabulsiella*																																																
*T. guamensis**	40	100	0	88	100	0	0	100	50	100	100	0	100	0	100	100	0	0	100	0	13	0	0	100	100	0	100	100	100	100	100	0	0	40	0	0	0	100	50	88	0	0	100	0	100	0	100	0
Genus *Xenorhabdus*																																																
X. nematophilus	40	0	0	0	0	0	0	0	0	0	100	80	0	0	80	0	0	0	0	0	0	0	0	0	0	0	0	0	0	0	0	0	0	0	0	0	0	0	60	0	0	20	20	0	0	60	80	0
Genus *Yersinia*																																																
*Y. pestis** (A)	0	80	0	0	0	5	0	0	0	0	0	0	0	0	100	0	0	0	97	0	70	0	0	50	100	0	1	80	90	100	0	0	0	50	20	0	50	0	0	0	0	0	85	0	50	0	100	0
*Y. pseudotuberculosis** (A)	0	100	0	0	0	95	0	0	0	0	0	0	0	0	100	0	0	0	100	0	25	0	0	0	50	15	70	95	100	100	0	0	0	95	70	0	50	0	50	0	0	0	95	0	70	0	100	0
*Y. enterocolitica** (B)	50	97	2	0	0	75	0	0	0	95	2	0	2	0	100	5	5	95	98	0	20	0	30	99	98	5	1	75	70	98	75	0	0	25	1	40	90	0	85	15	55	5	98	0	95	0	100	0
*Y. frederiksenii** (B)	100	100	0	15	0	70	0	0	0	95	5	0	0	0	100	40	40	100	100	0	92	0	20	100	100	30	99	100	100	100	100	0	0	85	0	100	85	5	55	15	55	0	100	0	100	0	100	0
*Y. intermedia** (B)	100	100	5	5	0	80	0	0	0	100	5	0	10	5	100	18	35	100	100	0	100	0	15	100	100	45	100	100	100	100	96	77	0	100	80	45	60	6	88	18	12	0	94	0	90	0	100	0
*Y. kristensenii** (B)	30	92	0	0	0	77	0	0	0	92	5	0	0	0	100	23	8	0	100	0	15	0	15	100	77	0	0	100	85	100	100	0	0	0	0	45	70	0	40	8	0	0	100	0	70	0	100	0
*Y. rohdei** (B)	0	62	0	0	0	62	0	0	0	25	0	0	0	0	100	0	0	100	100	0	0	0	0	100	100	62	0	0	38	100	25	0	0	0	50	0	38	0	100	0	0	0	88	0	50	0	100	0
Y. aldovae (B)	0	80	0	0	0	60	0	0	0	40	0	0	0	0	100	0	0	20	80	0	0	0	0	60	60	0	0	0	40	80	0	0	0	0	0	0	0	0	100	0	0	0	100	0	0	0	100	0
*Y. bercovieri** (B)	0	100	0	0	0	60	0	0	0	80	0	0	0	0	100	0	20	100	100	0	20	0	0	100	100	0	0	100	100	100	100	0	0	20	0	0	0	0	100	0	0	0	100	0	80	0	100	0
*Y. mollaretii** (B)	0	100	0	0	0	20	0	0	0	80	0	0	0	0	100	0	40	100	100	0	20	0	0	100	100	0	0	60	60	100	100	0	0	0	0	0	20	0	100	0	0	0	100	0	20	0	100	0
"*Yersinia*" *ruckeri** (C)	0	97	10	0	0	0	0	50	5	100	0	30	15	0	100	5	0	0	100	0	0	0	0	50	5	5	0	95	0	95	5	0	0	0	0	0	30	0	30	0	30	0	75	0	50	0	100	0
Genus *Yokenella*																																																
*Y. regensburgei** (*K. trabulsii*)	0	100	0	92	0	0	0	100	8	100	100	0	92	0	100	100	0	0	100	0	8	0	0	0	100	25	100	100	100	100	100	0	0	67	92	0	0	0	0	25	0	0	100	0	100	0	100	0
CDC Enteric Groups																																																
Enteric Group 59*	10	100	0	100	0	0	30	0	60	0	100	0	80	90	100	100	80	0	100	0	100	0	0	0	100	0	100	100	100	100	100	10	0	100	0	10	10	60	50	50	0	0	100	0	100	25	100	0
Enteric Group 60*	0	100	0	0	0	50	0	0	0	100	75	0	0	100	100	100	0	0	50	0	0	0	0	0	25	0	75	0	0	100	0	0	0	0	0	0	75	0	75	0	0	0	100	0	100	0	100	0
Enteric Group 63	0	100	0	0	0	0	0	100	0	100	65	0	0	0	100	100	0	0	100	0	100	0	0	100	100	0	100	100	100	100	100	65	0	100	0	0	0	65	0	0	0	0	100	0	100	0	100	0
Enteric Group 64	0	100	0	50	0	0	0	0	50	0	100	0	100	100	100	50	100	0	100	0	100	100	0	0	100	0	100	100	100	100	100	0	0	100	0	100	0	100	50	0	0	0	100	0	100	0	100	0
Enteric Group 68*	0	100	50	0	0	0	0	0	0	0	0	0	100	0	100	0	0	100	100	0	50	0	0	0	0	0	0	50	0	100	0	0	0	0	0	0	50	0	0	0	0	100	100	0	0	0	100	0
Enteric Group 69	0	0	100	100	0	0	0	0	100	100	100	0	100	100	100	100	100	25	100	100	100	0	0	100	100	100	100	100	100	100	100	100	0	100	100	0	0	100	0	25	0	0	100	0	100	0	100	0

Matrix 1, Version 11, February 2006

[a] Each number is the percentage of positive reactions after 2 days of incubation at 36°C (unless a different temperature is indicated). The vast majority of these positive reactions occur within 24 h. Reactions that become positive after 2 days are not considered. Abbreviations: TSI, triple sugar iron agar; ONPG, *o*-nitrophenyl-β-D-galactopyranoside. Several "species" in the table are composed of two or more DNA-DNA hybridization groups, so the term "complex" should be understood to follow the species name (see text).

[b] An asterisk by the name of an organism indicates that it occurs in human clinical specimens.

[c] Species in the same genus are grouped with their closest phenotypic and evolutionary relatives (14, 16, 38) rather than being listed alphabetically. For example, the three "subgroups" of the genus *Citrobacter* are defined as "A," "B," and "C" and are listed together.

[d] The Roman numerals refer to the seven *Salmonella* groups that are also biochemically and genetically distinct (see text).

TABLE 4 New, unusual, fastidious, or unculturable genera and species that have been classified[a] (14) in the family *Enterobacteriaceae*

Human pathogen
Klebsiella granulomatis (Calymmatobacterium granulomatis)—causes donovanosis (granuloma inguinale) (see text)

Associated with plants, but some species may occasionally cause or be associated with human clinical infections (see text)
Pantoea, 7 species, 2 subspecies

Pathogenic for or associated with plants; not isolated from human clinical specimens
Brenneria, 6 species; causes a variety of diseases of deciduous trees and walnut trees
Dickeya, 6 species (4 new species plus 2 additional species from other genera) (83)
Erwinia, 9 to 28 species, several named subspecies; major plant pathogen, also exists as a saprophyte and epiphyte
Pectobacterium, 4 to 6 species, several named subspecies; causes soft rot and a variety of other plant diseases, including blights, cankers, die back, leaf spot, and wilts
Phlomobacter fragariae—unculturable species that occurs in the sieve tubes of phloem tissue of plants.

Pathogenic for or associated with insects; not isolated from human clinical specimens
Arsenophonus—2 species, *A. nasoniae,* which is culturable and was originally described as causing the "son-killer" trait in a parasitic wasp, and *A. tiatominarum,* which has not been cultured
Buchnera aphidicola—Cannot be cultivated outside of the aphid host; it is essential for the survival of the aphid.
Photorhabdus—3 species, 3 subspecies. Two species are found only in nematodes and insects that are infected by the nematode. One species, *P. asymbiotica,* causes bacteremia and wound infections in humans (see text).
Wigglesworthia glossinidia—Obligate intracellular endosymbiont of tsetse flies
Xenorhabdus—several species; found only in nematodes and the insects that the nematodes infect; insect pathogens

Associated with extreme environments, not isolated from human clinical specimens
Alterococcus agarolyticus—habitat is coastal hot springs

[a] The unculturable and extremely fastidious organisms have been classified in the family *Enterobacteriaceae* based mainly on 16S rRNA sequencing data. This table includes some organisms whose eventual classification may be as "relatives" of *Enterobacteriaceae*. For more information about each organism, see the Internet site of J. P. Euzéby at http://www.bacterio.cict.fr.

and the environment. One example is the study by Müller et al. (71), who found six new species of *Buttiauxella* and two new species of *Kluyvera* in a large collection of strains isolated from snails. Similarly, additional DNA-DNA hybridization subgroups, which are probably new species (sometimes called genomospecies), have been found in systematic studies of *Enterobacter cloacae* (12), *Proteus vulgaris* (73), *Rahnella aquatilis* (17), *Klebsiella* (67, 81), *Enterobacter* (48, 52, 54, 59), *Yersinia* (7, 8), and *Citrobacter* (15, 18, 94). Most of the *Enterobacteriaceae* that clinical microbiologists encounter every day belong to just a few of the many species described (32). However, the expanding number of *Enterobacteriaceae* species is becoming a serious problem for reference laboratories and for commercial identification systems, whose identification methods are becoming inadequate for complete and accurate identification. When a commercial identification system gives an unusual organism for a final identification, there are several possibilities to consider (56): the identification is correct, just unusual; the identification is incorrect because another aerobic or anaerobic organism is present (42) and the biochemical profile is the result of the metabolic activities of the mixture; or a handling or coding error was made somewhere along the way. Before a final report of an unusual organism is issued, it is advisable to do as much checking as possible. This checking could include repeating the biochemical tests with the same commercial system after confirming the absence of a contaminating aerobic or anaerobic organism (42), testing the isolate with another commercial identification system (56) or with tube tests, and comparing the strain's antibiogram with known patterns reported for this organism. If these steps do not resolve the problem, the state health department or a reference laboratory can be contacted for advice, and the culture will often be accepted for further study. Different commercial systems often give different identifications for the same strain. The "gold standard" for identification is DNA-DNA hybridization; however, it is unavailable except in a few research laboratories. A different standard is evolving that is based on 16S rRNA sequencing. Although less accurate, it is a readily available alternative, and unusual strains can be submitted to a commercial laboratory (Accugenix, Newark, Del. [http://www.accugenix.com] or Midi, Newark, Del. [http://www.midi-inc.com]) for a "fee-for-service" identification. Clinical isolates reported with results obtained with these commercial tests should be reported with a disclaimer to indicate their research ("non-Clinical Laboratory Improvement Amendment [CLIA]") status. We suspect that a reference laboratory's identification based on phenotypic characteristics will be the final result for most difficult strains and will be done at state or national health departments or commercial reference laboratories.

Changes in Classification: "Proposed Alternative Classifications"

Contrary to popular opinion, there is no designated international body that considers every proposed change in classification and then issues an official classification. For almost 75 years, the Subcommittee on *Enterobacteriaceae* (http://www.the-icsp.org/subcoms/Enterobacteriaceae.htm) of the International Committee on Prokaryotes (http://www.the-icsp.org/default.htm) has studied and discussed the nomenclature and classification of the family. When the *Enterobacteriaceae* Subcommittee studies a specific "proposed reclassification," it can only make a recommendation, which can then be accepted or rejected by individuals in the scientific community. It should be emphasized that changes in classification are decided by usage, not by a judicial decision or action (see chapter 19 for further discussion). Sometimes two classifications are widely used, and both can be "correct." Classifications are correct if they conform to all the

TABLE 5 *Enterobacteriaceae* that are difficult to differentiate and identify completely; use of the term "complex"[a] as a solution for reporting cultures[b]

Vernacular name	Organisms included, definition, and comment
Citrobacter freundii complex	In addition to *C. freundii,* this term includes *C. braakii, C. gillenii, C. murliniae, C. rodentium, C. sedlakii, C. werkmanii,* and *C. youngae,* which are difficult to differentiate (15, 18).
Enterobacter agglomerans complex	This term includes over 60 named organisms: over a dozen "*Enterobacter agglomerans* DNA-DNA hybridization groups,"[c] the species of *Brenneria, Dickeya, Erwinia, Pectobacterium, Pantoea,* and perhaps also *Enterobacter cowanii,* all of which are difficult or impossible to differentiate.
Enterobacter cloacae complex	*E. cloacae* is made up of at least five DNA-DNA hybridization groups (12). The definition of the complex would include *Enterobacter ludwigii* plus these unnamed groups. For practical identification schemes, the term includes *Enterobacter amnigenus* and *Enterobacter kobei,* which are difficult to differentiate.
Klebsiella pneumoniae complex	In addition to *K. pneumoniae,* the term includes the closely related species (subspecies) *K. ozaenae* and *K. rhinoscleromatis* and the new species *K. ludwigii.* For practical identification schemes, the term includes *Klebsiella (Raoultella) planticola* and *K. terrigena,* which are very difficult to differentiate. *Klebsiella (Raoultella) ornithinolytica* is ornithine$^+$ and thus phenotypically distinct.
Kluyvera-Buttiauxella complex	This complex includes two genera with almost a dozen species (Table 3) and now includes *Kluyvera intermedia,* formerly classified as *Enterobacter intermedium.*
Proteus vulgaris complex	*P. vulgaris* is made up of at least four DNA-DNA hybridization groups. The definition of the complex could be expanded to include the closely related species *P. penneri* and *P. hauseri,* which can often be differentiated.
Rahnella aquatilis complex	*R. aquatilis* is made up of at least three DNA-DNA hybridization groups.
Serratia liquefaciens complex	The term includes *S. liquefaciens* and three closely related species *S. grimesii, S. proteamaculans,* and *S. quinovorans,* which are difficult to differentiate.
Yersinia enterocolitica complex	In addition to *Y. enterocolitica,* the term includes the closely related species *Y. aldovae, Y. bercovieri, Y. frederiksenii, Y. intermedia, Y. kristensenii,* and *Y. mollaretii,* which are difficult to differentiate.

[a] The word "group" is an alternative term for complex; e.g., the *Enterobacter agglomerans* group, which is also a vernacular name.
[b] An alternative approach would be to report only the genus name (i.e., *Citrobacter* species, *Kluyvera* species, or *Kluyvera-Buttiauxella* species). However, the terms in this table have a narrower definition.
[c] Some of the *Enterobacter agglomerans* DNA-DNA hybridization groups can rarely occur in human clinical specimens.

rules in the *Bacteriological Code (International Code of Nomenclature of Bacteria)*. However, classifications can be useful or not useful and can be frequently used in the literature or rarely used (14, 16, 38).

Proposed Changes in Classification and Other Changes in Table 3

Several "alternative classifications" have been proposed in the literature. Some of these appear to be totally justified and have been incorporated into Table 3. However, others have not been fully discussed or widely accepted by the scientific community (28). Table 3 gives the nomenclature and classification that one of us (J.J.F.) has incorporated into tables, data matrices, and computer programs used to identify clinical and nonclinical isolates of *Enterobacteriaceae*. It will differ from other nomenclatures and classifications.

In the seventh edition, the genus *Plesiomonas* was classified in the family *Vibrionaceae* along with *Aeromonas*. Because *Plesiomonas* is closer to *Enterobacteriaceae* than to *Vibrionaceae* based on 16S rRNA sequencing and because it contains the enterobacterial common antigen, it was included in the family *Enterobacteriaceae* in the eighth edition, and this classification has been maintained in the ninth edition. However, *Plesiomonas* is oxidase positive, a characteristic not shared with other species of *Enterobacteriaceae,* and is a distant relative of *E. coli,* the type species of the type genus of *Enterobacteriaceae* (14). Thus, the classification of *Plesiomonas* in the family *Enterobacteriaceae* might best be viewed as tentative.

In Table 3, the organism originally classified (9, 40) as *Xenorhabdus luminescens* DNA hybridization group 5 is now classified as *Photorhabdus asymbiotica* (44). It has caused rare cases of bacteremia and wound infection in the United States (40) and Australia (75). These Australian strains are distinct in some ways and have been proposed (Table 2) as *Photorhabdus asymbiotica* subspecies *australis* (2).

The names *Citrobacter diversus* and *Citrobacter koseri* have both been used in the literature for some time, but the name *Citrobacter diversus* has been used much more frequently. Many workers recognized the phenotypic similarity of these two organisms and thought that they might be the same. The species have different type strains, and so considering them to be the same will always be a subjective matter. They can be considered subjective synonyms but not objective synonyms (which must have the same type strain). The name *Citrobacter diversus* became the correct name for this organism on 1 January 1980, when the *Approved Lists of Bacterial Names* was issued, because under the laws of priority it was the older name. However, in 1993 the Judicial Commission of the International Committee on Systematic Bacteriology issued an Opinion (57) that the name *Citrobacter koseri* should be conserved over the name *Citrobacter diversus,* even though the name *Citrobacter diversus* was the older name, was on the

TABLE 6 *Salmonella* isolates in the United States for 1993 to 2003[a]

Rank for 2003	Serotype name (or formula[b])	No. of isolates:	
		1993–2002	2003
1	Typhimurium	83,873	6,631
2	Enteritidis	74,241	4,863
3	Newport	24,637	3,847
4	Heidelberg	19,837	1,810
5	Javiana	9,186	1,659
6	Montevideo	7,918	849
7	Saintpaul	4,838	823
8	Munchen	6,904	781
9	Oranienburg	6,093	554
10	Infantis	5,477	539
11	Branderup	4,824	530
12	Agona	6,068	510
13	1, 4, [5], 12:i:–[b]	628	498
14	Thompson	5,766	494
15	Mississippi	2,389	438
16	Typhi	3,979	359
17	Paratyphi B (L-tartrate$^+$)	3,014	331
18	Hadar	6,197	280
19	Bareilly	1,419	234
20	Stanley	2,157	224
	Paratyphi A	822	108
	Paratyphi C	9	0
	Choleraesuis	675	19
	Choleraesuis variety Kunzendorf		13
	Other serotypes		5,239
	Incomplete or no typing		2,105
	Total	354,093	33,589

[a] Surveillance data are from the Centers for Disease Control and Prevention. A free copy of the annual *Salmonella* surveillance reports can be obtained from the Centers for Disease Control and Prevention, Foodborne and Diarrheal Diseases Branch, Mail Stop A38, 1600 Clifton Rd., Atlanta, GA 30333. Recent surveillance reports can also be viewed on the Internet at http://www.cdc.gov/ncidod/dbmd/phlisdata/salmonella.htm. Note: the entire document for a given year can be very large, so it may be necessary to download individual tables to avoid time and computer data storage problems. A paper copy (619 pages in color) of CDC's very useful *Salmonella* atlas (22) is also available without charge (contact Richard Bishop at rqb7@cdc.gov).

[b] This serotype is referred to by its antigenic formula because it does not have a formal serotype name, unlike the other 19 serotypes. Its O antigens are 1, 4, [5], 12 ([5] indicates that serofactor 5 may or may not be present); its H antigen for phase one is "i," and it does not have a phase two H antigen.

Approved Lists of Bacterial Names, was the correct name under the rules of the *Bacteriological Code,* and was the name used most frequently in the literature. This opinion needs much more discussion by the scientific community, which is beyond the scope of this chapter; therefore, both names are included in Table 3.

Phenotypic and 16S rRNA sequencing data indicate that *Kluyvera cochleae* is almost identical to *Enterobacter intermedium,* and the proposed reclassification of this organism as *Kluyvera intermedia* (74) appears to solve several problems (Tables 2 and 3).

Another change in Table 3 is that species in the same genus are now grouped with their closest phenotypic and evolutionary relatives (14, 16, 38) rather than listed alphabetically. For example, three subgroups of the genus *Citrobacter* are defined as A, B, and C and listed together. In addition, we propose that Enteric Group 139 be reclassified as *Citrobacter* Group 139. A similar notation is used in Table 3 for other genera; Tables 2 and 4 and the text give explanations.

Other Proposed Changes in Nomenclature and Classification

Proposed Classification of Three *Klebsiella* Species in *Raoultella*

In 2001, Drancourt et al. (28) proposed that *Klebsiella planticola, K. ornithinolytica,* and *K. terrigena* be classified in a new genus, *Raoultella,* as *R. planticola, R. ornithinolytica,* and *R. terrigena.* These three species are extremely similar to *Klebsiella pneumoniae* in their phenotypic properties (37), making differentiation very difficult (Table 3). This proposed alternative classification needs further evaluation; however, we agree that these three species should be grouped together and have done this in Table 3.

Enterobacter agglomerans Group–*Pantoea*

The *Enterobacter agglomerans–Pantoea* complex is a confusing subject, and writers continue to make errors in the definition

TABLE 7 *Shigella* isolates in the United States for 2003[a]

Rank	Serotype	Isolates
1	*Shigella sonnei* (serogroup D)	9,263
2	*Shigella flexneri* (serogroup B)	1,660
3	*Shigella boydii* (serogroup C)	125
4	*Shigella dysenteriae* (serogroup A)	41
	Not (completely) serotyped	463
	Total *Shigella* isolates	11,552

[a] Data are from the Centers for Disease Control and Prevention at http://www.cdc.gov/ncidod/dbmd/phlisdata/shigella.htm. Surveillance reports for previous years are also at this Internet address. Note: the entire document for a given year is typically very large so it may be prudent to download individual tables to avoid time and computer data storage problems.

and circumscription (boundaries) of *Pantoea agglomerans.* In 1972, Ewing and Fife redefined the name *Enterobacter agglomerans* to include a wide variety of organisms known under many different names (32). These investigators also defined 11 different biogroups to recognize the phenotypic diversity of the many strains included in *Enterobacter agglomerans.* This name has become useful for clinical microbiologists, and it has been used extensively in the literature. Systematic analysis by Brenner and coworkers using DNA-DNA hybridization indicated that *Enterobacter agglomerans* is very heterogeneous, with at least 14 DNA hybridization groups (12). For this reason, the names "*Enterobacter agglomerans* complex" and "*Enterobacter agglomerans* group" (37) have been used to better indicate the heterogeneity of this "species" (Tables 3 and 5). However, it has been very difficult to find simple tests to differentiate and identify all of the DNA hybridization groups (37). For this reason, workers have been reluctant to subdivide the *Enterobacter agglomerans* group until a definitive classification could be proposed (37). Gavini et al. (46) took the first step toward more logical classification for this complex group by proposing that the group of six strains defined by Brenner et al. as "DNA hybridization group 13 of *Enterobacter agglomerans*" be classified in a new genus, *Pantoea,* as *P. agglomerans.* They also defined a new species in the genus, *Pantoea dispersa* (46), previously classified as *Enterobacter agglomerans* DNA hybridization group 3 by Brenner (12).

However, this new classification has caused communication problems. Some authors have broadened the original definition of Gavini et al. for *Pantoea agglomerans* to include organisms that are not phylogenetically related. Since DNA-DNA hybridization is not routinely done and since simple tests are not available to definitively identify strains to the level of DNA hybridization group, it seems prudent to retain the vernacular name "*Enterobacter agglomerans* complex" as a convenient name for clinical microbiologists to use in reporting clinical isolates (Tables 3 and 5). This term is defined biochemically in Table 3, and it should be emphasized that it is used merely for convenience because the name *Enterobacter agglomerans* is well understood and widely used in the literature. Eventually, this term will be replaced with a better classification. When definitive testing in a reference laboratory (usually including DNA hybridization) is done, more precise names can be used in reporting. Examples could include *Pantoea agglomerans* (limited to strains that fall into DNA hybridization group 13), *Pantoea dispersa* (limited to strains that fall into DNA hybridization group 3), and *Enterobacter agglomerans* DNA hybridization group 1, etc. Tables 3 and 5 use and define the vernacular name *Enterobacter agglomerans* complex, a term that may prove useful for reporting isolates in most microbiology laboratories because almost none can do DNA-DNA hybridization. A less desirable vernacular name for this group of organisms is the "*Pantoea agglomerans* complex."

Enterobacter taylorae–Enterobacter cancerogenus

Enterobacter taylorae and *Enterobacter cancerogenus* may be two names for the same organism (47). However, they have different type strains; therefore, they are not objective synonyms under the rules of the *Bacteriological Code.* Until the identity of these two organisms is universally accepted, both names will be used (Table 3).

Nomenclature, Classification, and Reporting of the Genus *Salmonella*

After much study and a lengthy judicial process (58), there is now good agreement on many issues in the nomenclature and classification of the genus *Salmonella* (32, 41, 58, 70, 76, 78, 79). The recent decision of the Judicial Commission on the International Committee on Systematics of Prokaryotes (58) to replace *Salmonella choleraesuis* with *Salmonella enterica* stabilizes this issue which has caused confusion and the use of illegitimate names in the literature for many years. In 2005 (58), *Salmonella enterica* finally became the legitimate species name to include most of the most important serotype names. Three 2005 references (58, 78, 91) and the Internet site of J. P. Euzéby (http://www.bacterio.cict.fr) provide additional historical insights and alternative perspectives on the issues.

Until the 1970s, the species concept in the genus *Salmonella* was based on epidemiology, host range, biochemical reactions, and antigenic structure (the O antigen, phases 1 and 2 of the H antigen, and the Vi antigen, if present), and strains that differed in one or all of these properties were given distinct names. Names such as *Salmonella typhi, Salmonella cholerae-suis* (originally some names such as this one were written with a hyphen, which was eventually dropped because of changes in the *Bacteriological Code*), *Salmonella paratyphi* A, *Salmonella paratyphi* A var. *durazzo, Salmonella typhimurium, Salmonella typhimurium* var. *copenhagen, Salmonella enteritidis,* and *Salmonella newport* began to appear, and the list rapidly expanded to include hundreds of names. Some workers believed that these names really represented biological species, but others thought that they were antigenic and biochemical varieties with an uncertain evolutionary relationship. However, there was universal agreement that the names were an extremely useful way to communicate about the particular serotypes and the diseases they caused. Most authors wrote the serotype names in italics as a species in the genus *Salmonella,* for example, *Salmonella typhimurium* (32, 41). Several proposals to the Judicial Commission of the International Committee on Systematic Bacteriology have requested that important serotype names be preserved (31, 33, 34) to preserve stability in nomenclature, but it is not clear whether this is a matter that will be decided by judicial action or by usage.

In 1973, Crosa et al. (25) used DNA-DNA hybridization to show that *Salmonella* strains could be grouped into five main evolutionary groups. Two (possibly three) additional groups are now known (11, 78, 79). The vast majority of strains that cause human infections occur in DNA hybridization group 1 (*Salmonella* group I). Strains isolated from animals and the environment clustered into the four other groups, designated DNA groups 2 (II), 3a (IIIa), 3b (IIIb), and 4 (IV). Over the years, different authors have used different terms to refer to these evolutionary groups: DNA-DNA hybridization groups (25, 41), multilocus enzyme electrophoresis clusters (11, 79), subgenera, species (see the *Approved Lists of Bacterial Names* and http://www.bacterio.cict.fr), and subspecies (70, 76, 77). Crosa et al. (25) showed that all five groups of *Salmonella* were very highly related genetically. With the operational species definition usually used in DNA hybridization, these five groups were considered to belong to the same species. Under the rules of the *Bacteriological Code,* the name of this species had to be *Salmonella choleraesuis.* However, this species name is a cause of confusion, since *Salmonella choleraesuis* would have two totally different meanings, a broad one as a species and a narrow one as a serotype. There was support for making an exception to the rules of the *Bacteriological Code* and using a name that has never been used as a serotype name to avoid confusion. There was a formal proposal in 1999 to coin a new name, *Salmonella enterica* (31), which would replace the name *Salmonella choleraesuis* as the species name to represent most of the serotypes of *Salmonella.* However, the proposal to replace the name *Salmonella choleraesuis* with *Salmonella enterica* was denied by the Judicial Commission of the International Committee on Systematic Bacteriology. Thus, *Salmonella choleraesuis* remained the correct name until a variation of the original proposal to the Judicial Commission was approved in 2005 (58). Even though it was an illegitimate name, the name *Salmonella enterica* had already been used by the World Health Organization's International Center for *Salmonella* (76) and by many of the World Health Organization's national centers for *Salmonella.* The name had also been used widely in the literature. Fortunately, the 2005 decision of the Judicial Commission has made *Salmonella enterica* the correct name, which is gaining universal acceptance.

Another point of confusion concerns the method of writing serotype names. For almost 100 years, serotype names have been written as species (the serotype-as-species nomenclature), for example, *Salmonella enteritidis.* The World Health Organization's International Center for *Salmonella* at the Institut Pasteur, Paris, France, introduced a different nomenclature in which the serotype name is capitalized and not written in italics. In this nomenclature, the name *Salmonella enteritidis* would be written in one of the following ways: "*Salmonella enterica* serovar Enteritidis," "*Salmonella* serovar Enteritidis," "*Salmonella* ser. Enteritidis," or "*Salmonella* Enteritidis." The nomenclature described by McWhorter-Murlin and Hickman-Brenner (70) is similar, but these authors use the term "serotype" instead of "serovar." The main advantage of these nomenclatures is that they do not artificially treat the serotypes as species. The main disadvantage is that they create a new nomenclature that differs from one that has been widely accepted and used for more than 70 years. There have been literally hundreds of thousands of uses of the serotype-as-species nomenclature in the literature. The International Center for *Salmonella*'s nomenclature appears in the second edition of *Bergey's Manual* (78) and is being used (sometimes with modifications) by the national centers for *Salmonella* (19, 70). However, many published articles and books continue to use the nomenclature. Since *Salmonella* names are being written differently by different authors and different national centers for *Salmonella,* it is not surprising that the literature is beginning to reflect this confusion. Recent examples of the way "serotype Typhimurium" is being written include *Salmonella* serotype Typhimurium, *Salmonella* ser. Typhimurium, *Salmonella typhimurium, Salmonella* Typhimurium, *Salmonella* typhimurium, *Salmonella* serovar Typhimurium, and *Salmonella* serovar *Typhimurium* or simply Typhimurium (omitting the genus name *Salmonella* entirely) (88). When the variations are combined with the four species and subspecies possibilities, i.e., *Salmonella choleraesuis, Salmonella choleraesuis* subspecies *choleraesuis, Salmonella enterica,* and *Salmonella enterica* subspecies *enterica,* the number of possible variations is multiplied considerably. One example of the almost endless possibilities is *Salmonella enterica* subspecies *enterica* serovar Typhimurium.

The current disagreements in *Salmonella* nomenclature and classification include the use of the term "serotype" (19, 70) versus "serovar" (76, 77) (both terms are often abbreviated as "ser."); the best way to write the names of the serotypes; the use of names versus antigenic formulas for some of the serotypes; the argument over whether some well-known serotype names should be eliminated and combined with other serotypes (19, 70, 76, 77); and the question of how to name the distinct DNA hybridization groups.

Most clinical microbiology laboratories identify *Salmonella* isolates with a commercial identification system and then with commercial *Salmonella* "polyvalent grouping antisera," which will agglutinate only those strains with the O antigen groups contained in the polyvalent serum (often only groups A through E). These two methods usually give definitive results, and a simple report can be issued such as "*Salmonella* serogroup B," avoiding the problems described above. Abbreviating "serotype" and "serovar" as "ser." would be a further simplification and would avoid the disagreement over these two terms. Reference laboratories that do complete serotyping and biochemical testing can issue a definitive report such as "*Salmonella* serotype Typhimurium" or "*Salmonella enterica* serotype Typhimurium."

Nomenclature for Shiga Toxins/Verotoxins Produced by *E. coli* and *Shigella*

Several different names are being used in the literature for the cytotoxins produced by *E. coli* and *Shigella.* This topic is critical because of the importance of *E. coli* O157 and other strains that produce these toxins (see chapter 43 of this Manual). Several different commercial assays for these toxins are being marketed; therefore, it is essential to read the package insert carefully to determine exactly which toxin(s) the kit is detecting and to word laboratory reports accordingly.

For almost 100 years, it has been known that *Shigella dysenteriae* serogroup O1 produces a potent cytotoxin known as Shiga toxin. More recently, it has been shown that certain strains of *E. coli* that cause intestinal infections produce a similar toxin, which was first detected because it was cytotoxic for Vero cells in tissue culture. A number of recent studies have defined these proteins from *S. dysenteriae* O1 and *E. coli,* and there is agreement that they constitute a family of toxins. They are being referred to in the literature as Shiga toxin (ST), Shiga-like toxins (SLT), verocytotoxin(s), and verotoxin(s) (VT), and at least five different toxins are involved (20, 86). This complex subject was recently reviewed by Scheutz and Strockbine (86). The *E. coli* strains that produce these toxins are often referred to as STEC and VTEC. Calderwood et al. (20) summarized the data available and proposed that strains of *E. coli* that produce these toxins be called "Shiga toxin-producing" *E. coli,* which would replace the previous term, "Shiga-like toxin producing." They also recommended that the new toxin name be cross-referenced with the corresponding verotoxin name. With this nomenclature, a laboratory report for a stool culture might be worded, "Positive for *E. coli* O157:H7, which produces Shiga toxins Stx1 (VT1) and Stx2 (VT2)." Hopefully, the differences between those using the two different nomenclatures will be resolved, resulting in a single nomenclature.

Proposed Reclassification of *Calymmatobacterium granulomatis* as *Klebsiella granulomatis*

Calymmatobacterium granulomatis has received little attention in industrialized countries. In the seventh edition of this Manual, *Calymmatobacterium* was mentioned only twice (pages 25 and 50). It was listed as an aerobic bacterium that can be found in the genital area, and under the topic "Specimen Management" it was mentioned under the disease granuloma inguinale, or ulcerative donovanosis, with the notes "mostly a tropical disease" and "culture is nonproductive." *Calymmatobacterium granulomatis* has been described as a highly pleomorphic gram-negative rod that does not grow on laboratory media. Diagnosis of granuloma inguinale has been based on showing the presence of "Donovan bodies" in Giemsa-stained smears of mononuclear cells or histiocytes from the patient's genital ulcers.

It had been assumed for almost a century that *Calymmatobacterium granulomatis* has no relationship to the "easy-to-culture" organisms of the family *Enterobacteriaceae.* However, Carter et al. (21) proposed that *Calymmatobacterium granulomatis* be reclassified in the genus *Klebsiella* as *Klebsiella granulomatis.* This proposal was based both on nucleotide sequence relatedness and on disease similarity. Granuloma inguinale is a disease similar to rhinoscleroma, also a tropical disease (nasal infection) caused by (or associated with) *Klebsiella rhinoscleromatis.* While this alternative classification is being evaluated and tested, it would be helpful to write both scientific names, with the writer's preference listed first: "*Klebsiella granulomatis (Calymmatobacterium granulomatis)*" (which we prefer) or "*Calymmatobacterium granulomatis (Klebsiella granulomatis).*" Other diseases of unknown etiology may be caused by unculturable *Enterobacteriaceae.*

DESCRIPTION OF THE FAMILY *ENTEROBACTERIACEAE*

Most genera and species in the family *Enterobacteriaceae* share the following properties: they are gram negative and rod shaped; do not form spores; are motile with peritrichous flagella or are nonmotile; grow on peptone or meat extract media without the addition of other supplements or sodium chloride; grow well on MacConkey agar; grow both aerobically and anaerobically; are often active biochemically; ferment (rather than oxidize) D-glucose and other sugars, often with gas production; are catalase positive and oxidase negative; reduce nitrate into nitrite; contain the enterobacterial common antigen; and have 39 to 59% guanine-plus-cytosine (G+C) contents in DNA (5, 12–14, 38, 55). Host-adapted species that are unculturable, difficult to culture, or slow growing appear to have evolved in some genera (14) (Table 4).

When techniques that measure evolutionary distance are used, genera and species in the family should also be more closely related to *E. coli,* the type species of the type genus of the family, than they are to organisms in other families (14, 38). Tables 1 to 5 expand on this definition and give most of the exceptions.

NATURAL HABITATS

Enterobacteriaceae are widely distributed on plants and in soil, water, and the intestines of humans and animals (5, 14, 43, 55). Some species occupy very limited ecological niches. *Salmonella* serotype Typhi causes typhoid fever and is found only in humans (50, 68). In contrast, strains of *Klebsiella pneumoniae* are distributed widely in the environment and contribute to biochemical and geochemical processes (63). However, strains of *K. pneumoniae* also cause human infections, ranging from asymptomatic colonization of the intestinal, urinary, and respiratory tracts to fatal pneumonia, septicemia, and meningitis.

CLINICAL SIGNIFICANCE

Some *Enterobacteriaceae* are associated with or cause specific humans diseases (Table 1) (14, 55, 68, 69, 82). Many cause, or are isolated from, abscesses, pneumonia, meningitis, septicemia, and infections of wounds, the urinary tract, and the intestine (68, 69). They are a major component of the normal intestinal flora of humans but are relatively uncommon as normal flora of other body sites. Several species of *Enterobacteriaceae* are very important causes of nosocomial infections (69). *Enterobacteriaceae* may account for 80% of clinically significant isolates of gram-negative bacilli and 50% of clinically significant bacteria in clinical microbiology laboratories (30). They account for nearly 50% of septicemia cases, more than 70% of urinary tract infections, and a significant percentage of intestinal infections (68, 69).

Human Extraintestinal Infections

Except for the species of *Shigella,* which rarely cause infections outside the gastrointestinal tract, many species of *Enterobacteriaceae* commonly cause extraintestinal infections. However, a small number of species, i.e., *E. coli, Klebsiella pneumoniae, Klebsiella oxytoca, Proteus mirabilis, Enterobacter aerogenes,* the *Enterobacter cloacae* complex, and *Serratia marcescens,* account for most of these infections. Urinary tract infections, primarily cystitis, are the most common (85), followed by respiratory, wound, bloodstream (27), and central nervous system infections. Many of these infections, especially sepsis and meningitis, are life threatening and are often hospital acquired. Because of the severity of these infections, prompt isolation, identification, and susceptibility testing of *Enterobacteriaceae* isolates are essential.

Human Intestinal Infections

Several organisms in the family *Enterobacteriaceae* are also important causes (Tables 6 and 7) of intestinal infections of humans and animals worldwide. Although other species in the family have been associated with diarrhea (93) or even implicated as causes of diarrhea, only organisms in four genera, *Escherichia* (29, 36, 55, 61), *Salmonella* (25, 41, 50, 78), *Shigella* (32, 68), and *Yersinia* (7, 60, 68, 80), have been clearly documented as enteric pathogens. These four genera are discussed in chapters 43 and 44 of this Manual. Other *Enterobacteriaceae* such as *Citrobacter, Edwardsiella, Hafnia, Morganella, Proteus, Klebsiella, Enterobacter,* and *Serratia* may have an association with diarrhea in certain studies (39, 93), and some authors have gone as far as to implicate them as actually causing diarrhea (5, 93). Strains of these *Enterobacteriaceae* that produce "biologically active" compounds (often vastly overstated as being "enterotoxin-producing strains") have been isolated from people with diarrhea (93), but the causal role of these strains in diarrhea is uncertain. One possible way to emphasize the drastic change in the stool flora would be to issue a report such as "*Klebsiella pneumoniae* isolated in essentially pure culture

(10 of 10 colonies tested); please consult the laboratory to discuss possible significance." The patient's antibody response, or lack of one, would be a helpful way to assess the particular organism's causative role. There is no evidence that strains of these other genera are important causes of diarrhea.

In contrast to the arguable role of the organisms listed above, the evidence for the causal role of *Plesiomonas shigelloides* (see chapter 45 in this Manual) in diarrhea is somewhat stronger. A safe generalization would be that "certain strains of *P. shigelloides* may cause diarrhea in certain people under certain conditions, but it is probably not an intrinsic pathogen." For an intrinsic pathogen, most strains would cause diarrhea in most people, under most conditions (39).

Surveillance at the National and International Levels

Many countries provide surveillance data on the Internet for plague, typhoid fever, salmonellosis, shigellosis, diarrheagenic *E. coli*, institutional infections, bacteremia, meningitis, antibiotic resistance, and other enteric and nonenteric infections. Often the word "infection" or a similar word is used when the term "clinical microbiology isolate" would be more appropriate. Care must be used in interpreting these data because "association" and "clinical microbiology isolate" do not equate with "causation" and "infection" in each instance (39). For example, few would argue with the use of the term "infection" for a clinical isolate of *Salmonella* serotype Typhi from the stool of a patient with typhoid fever. In contrast, the word "infection" would be an overstatement if used to describe a stool isolate of a nonenteropathogenic *Yersinia enterocolitica* serotype (such as O10) or one of the other six species of the *Y. enterocolitica* group (Table 3). Check to see if surveillance data make these important distinctions.

SPECIMEN COLLECTION, TRANSPORT, AND PROCESSING

Extraintestinal Specimens

Enterobacteriaceae are recovered from infections at many different body sites, and normal practices (see chapters 5 and 20 of this Manual) for collecting blood, respiratory, wound, urine, and other specimens should be followed.

Intestinal Specimens

Stool cultures are usually submitted to the laboratory with a request to isolate and identify the cause of a possible intestinal infection, usually manifested as diarrhea (see chapter 20). The groups of *Enterobacteriaceae* usually associated with diarrhea in the United States are *Salmonella* (22), *Shigella* (23), and certain pathogenic strains of *E. coli* and *Yersinia enterocolitica.*

Stool specimens require special attention to both collection and transportation and should be obtained early in the course of illness, when the causative agent is likely to be present in the largest numbers in feces. At this stage, the use of enrichment broths should be unnecessary. If rapid processing (within 2 h of collection) is not possible, a small portion of feces or a swab coated with feces should be placed in transport medium, such as Stuart, Amies, Cary-Blair, or buffered glycerol saline. Cary-Blair is probably the best overall transport medium for diarrheal stools. In cases of diarrhea that do not yield a causative agent, a tube of frozen stool can be invaluable for looking for new causative agents or for testing against the patient's convalescent serum. More information about the isolation, identification, typing, and virulence testing of isolates of *Salmonella, Shigella, E. coli,* and *Y. enterocolitica* is given in chapters 43 and 44.

Macroscopic and Microscopic Examination

Stool specimens should be examined visually for the presence of blood or mucus, but microscopic examination is less helpful because of its lack of specificity (84). Although identification by fluorescent-antibody staining is theoretically possible for all enteric pathogens, it has been of limited success because the method is difficult and there are many serological cross-reactions among the species of *Enterobacteriaceae* (32). This technique was most often used to detect *Salmonella* strains (primarily in the food industry) and certain serogroups of *E. coli* and to aid in outbreak investigations.

ISOLATION

Extraintestinal Specimens

Most strains of *Enterobacteriaceae* grow readily on the plating media commonly used in clinical microbiology laboratories (see chapter 20). MacConkey agar, generally interchangeable with eosin methylene blue agar, is usually used, because it allows a preliminary grouping of enteric and other gram-negative bacteria. The most common isolates of *Enterobacteriaceae* have a characteristic appearance on blood agar and MacConkey agar that is useful for preliminary identification (Table 8). Broth enrichment can increase the isolation rate if small numbers of *Enterobacteriaceae* are present, but this step is not normally required.

Intestinal Specimens

Media that can be used routinely for intestinal specimens include a nonselective medium such as blood agar, a differential medium of low to moderate selectivity such as MacConkey agar, and a more selective differential medium such as xylose-lysine-deoxycholate (XLD) agar or Hektoen enteric agar (HE). A broth enrichment substance such as selenite (or GN [gram-negative broth] or tetrathionate) can be included, particularly if the specimen is not optimal. A highly selective medium such as brilliant green agar, bismuth sulfite, Rambach, or CHROM agar *Salmonella* (BD Diagnostics, Sparks, Md.) can also be included for isolating strains of *Salmonella.* A special plate, such as sorbitol-MacConkey agar (or one of its modifications), can be added to enhance the isolation of Shiga toxin-producing strains of *E. coli* O157:H7. This medium should be used if the stool is frankly bloody or if the patient has a diagnosis of hemolytic-uremic syndrome, and it can be used for all fecal specimens if resources permit (see chapter 42). When the presence of *Yersinia enterocolitica* is suspected, a selective-differential medium, such as CIN (cefsulodin-Irgasan-novobiocin) agar (also called *Yersinia* selective agar), can be added (see chapter 44). A complete stool culture procedure should also include media for isolation of *Campylobacter* and possibly *Vibrio* strains in areas where cholera and other *Vibrio* infections are common. Several new plating media appear to be more sensitive or specific and are gaining in popularity (see chapters 43 and 44).

IDENTIFICATION

There are many different approaches to identifying strains of *Enterobacteriaceae* (14, 37, 38).

TABLE 8 Colonial appearance of the most common *Enterobacteriaceae* on MacConkey agar and sheep blood agar[a]

Genus or species	Appearance and typical colony diameter on:	
	MacConkey agar	Sheep blood agar[b]
Salmonella and *Shigella*	Colorless, flat, 2–3 mm	Smooth, 2–3 mm
Escherichia coli (lactose positive)	Red, usually surrounded by precipitated bile, 2–3 mm	Smooth, 2–3 mm
Escherichia coli (lactose negative)	Colorless, 2–3 mm	Smooth, 2–3 mm
Yersinia enterocolitica	Colorless, less than 1 mm	Smooth, less than 1 mm
Klebsiella pneumoniae	Pink, mucoid, 3–4 mm	Mucoid, 3–4 mm
Enterobacter	Pink, not as mucoid as *Klebsiella*, 2–4 mm	Smooth, 3–4 mm
Proteus vulgaris and *Proteus mirabilis*	Colorless, flat, often swarm slightly, 2–3 mm	Swarm in waves to cover plate
Other *Proteus*, *Providencia*, and *Morganella* species	Colorless, flat, no swarming, 2–3 mm	Flat, 2–3 mm, no swarming

[a] Most strains appear this way, but there are exceptions.

[b] Most strains of *Enterobacteriaceae* are nonhemolytic, which is in contrast to many strains of *Aeromonas* and *Vibrio*, which are hemolytic. A few strains of *E. coli* are strongly hemolytic, as are occasional strains of other *Enterobacteriaceae*.

Conventional Biochemical Tests in Tubes

Tube testing was once used by all clinical microbiology laboratories, and it is still widely used in reference and public health laboratories (32, 37). Although some laboratories prepare their own media from commercial dehydrated powders, most of the common media are also available commercially in glass tubes that are ready to use. Growth from a single colony is inoculated into each tube, and the tests are read at 24 h and usually also at 48 h. In many reference laboratories, most tests are often kept for 7 days to detect delayed reactions. Unfortunately, the media and tests are not completely standardized, and few laboratories use exactly the same formulations or procedures. Even with these variables, this approach usually results in correct identifications of the common species of *Enterobacteriaceae.* Table 3 gives the results for *Enterobacteriaceae* in 48 tests (for the media and methods used to generate the data in this table, see references 32, 35, and 37).

Computer Analysis To Assist in Identification

Two microcomputer programs were developed in the 1980s at the Centers for Disease Control and Prevention (CDC)'s Enteric Reference Laboratories to assist with the identification of *Enterobacteriaceae* cultures. "George" and "Strain Matcher" were described in the 1985 review of the family (37). One of us (J.J.F.) plans to revise and update these programs to run on current operating systems and make them more available. These plans include modifying the *Enterobacteriaceae* data matrix in Table 3 and other data matrices to be compatible with the probabilistic identification program *PIBWin* that is free and can be downloaded from the Internet (http://www.som.soton.ac.uk/staff/tnb/pib.htm).

Screening Tests, Using All Information Available

Over the years, the Enteric Reference Laboratories at CDC have found that many genera, species, and serotypes can be tentatively identified with a number of screening tests (Table 9). More precise identification can be made by using a complete set of tests or commercial identification systems. Because of the limited availability of certain reagents (bacteriophage O1 and *Yersinia* typing sera, etc.), these screening tests may be more useful in a reference or research laboratory.

Example 1. A urine isolate has the following properties: colonies on MacConkey agar are 2 to 3 mm in diameter, are bright red and nonmucoid, and have precipitated bile around them; it is indole positive and 4-methylumbelliferyl-β-D-glucuronidase (MUG) positive; it grows at 44.5°C; and it is antibiotic resistant. These results are completely compatible with *E. coli.*

Example 2. An isolate from the feces of a diarrhea patient has the following properties: colonies on MacConkey agar are 2 to 3 mm in diameter and colorless; colonies on XLD agar are 2 to 3 mm and black; the isolate agglutinates in *Salmonella* polyvalent O serum and in O-group B serum; the MUCAP test (hydrolysis of 4-methylumbelliferyl caprylate; Biolife, Milan, Italy) and lysis by bacteriophage O1 are positive; and it is antibiotic resistant. All these results are compatible with *Salmonella* serogroup B.

Commercial "Kits" for Identification

A commercial kit is defined as a panel of miniaturized or standardized tests that are available commercially. The tests incorporated in the kits are often a subset of those given in Table 3. The approach for using kits is similar to the conventional tube method, with the main differences being in the miniaturization, the number of tests available, the suspending medium, and the method of reading and interpreting results (sometimes by machine). Kits are now used by most American laboratories and are discussed in chapter 15. Kits often give the correct identification for the most common species of *Enterobacteriaceae,* but they may not be as accurate for some of the new species. It is important to check the instruction manual to determine which organisms have been included in the database and the number of strains that were used to define each organism. The main problem with kit-based identification is that the tests used (usually about 20 tests) are becoming inadequate to differentiate all of the current species of *Enterobacteriaceae* given in Tables 1 to 5. This is also becoming a problem with conventional tube tests, even when the 48 tests listed in Table 3 are used. Unusual identifications or "no identification" obtained with a kit could be verified by other methods or approaches (56), but referral to a reference laboratory may be the best alternative. Other methods might

TABLE 9 Screening test for the enteric pathogens *Salmonella, Shigella, Escherichia coli, Yersinia,* and for the other important *Enterobacteriaceae* and those most frequently isolated from human clinical specimens[a]

Organism (genus, species, or serotype)	Test or property[b]
Salmonella	Lactose⁻, sucrose⁻, H_2S^+, O1 phage[+c], MUCAP[+d], agglutinates in polyvalent serum,[b] typical colonies on media selective/differential for *Salmonella* (brilliant green agar, SS agar, Rambach agar, CHROM agar, etc.), lysed by the *Salmonella*-specific "bacteriophage O1"[c], often antibiotic resistant
Salmonella typhi	Ornithine$^-$, H_2S^+ (trace amount only), L-rhamnose$^-$, no gas produced during fermentation, agglutinates in group D serum, Vi serum, and flagella "d" serum
Shigella	Nonmotile, lysine$^-$, gas$^-$, agglutinates in polyvalent serum, biochemically inactive, often antibiotic resistant, PhoE$^+$ (molecular test)[d]
Shigella dysenteriae	Agglutinates in group A serum, D-mannitol$^-$
Shigella dysenteriae O1	Catalase$^-$, agglutinates in O1 serum, Shiga toxin$^+$
Shigella flexneri	Agglutinates in group B serum, D-mannitol$^+$
Shigella boydii	Agglutinates in group C serum, D-mannitol$^+$
Shigella sonnei	Agglutinates in group D serum, D-mannitol$^+$, ornithine decarboxylase$^+$, lactose$^+$ (delayed), characteristic colony variation from smooth to rough
Escherichia coli	Extremely variable biochemically, indole$^+$, MUG$^+$, grows at 44.5°C, sometimes antibiotic resistant, PhoE$^+$ (molecular test)[d]
Escherichia coli O157:H7	Colorless colonies on sorbitol-MacConkey agar (SMAC), red colonies on MacConkey agar, MUG$^-$, D-sorbitol$^-$ (or delayed), agglutinates in O157 serum and H7 serum; many commercial media and tests are available (95)
Escherichia coli—invasive strains	Many strains resemble *Shigella* because they are "inactive" biochemically: lactose$^-$, nonmotile, lysine$^-$; O antigen groups O28, O29, O112, O124, O136, O143, O144, O152, O164, O167, and others; no commercial assay or simple way to isolate and identify
Yersinia	Grows on CIN agar, often more active biochemically at 25 than 36°C ; motile at 25°C, nonmotile at 36°C, urea$^+$
Yersinia enterocolitica, pathogenic serotypes	Smaller colonies (often less than 1 mm) than other *Enterobacteriaceae* species on enteric plating media, CR-MOX$^+$, pyrazinamidase$^-$, salicin$^-$, esculin$^-$, agglutinate in O-typing sera for "enteric pathogenic" serotypes: 3; 4,32; 5,27; 8; 9; 13a,13b; 18; 20; or 21
Yersinia enterocolitica O3 (a pathogenic serotype)	D-Xylose$^-$, agglutinates in O3 serum, tiny colonies at 24 h on plating media; in most countries it is the most frequently isolated pathogenic serotype
Yersinia enterocolitica, nonpathogenic serotypes	CR-MOX$^-$, pyrazinamidase$^+$, salicin$^+$, esculin$^+$, do not agglutinate in O-typing sera for "enteric pathogenic" serotypes: 3; 4,32; 5,27; 8; 9; 13a,13b; 18; 20; or 21
Citrobacter	Citrate$^+$, lysine decarboxylase$^-$, often grows on CIN agar, strong characteristic odor
Enterobacter	Variable biochemically, citrate$^+$, VP$^+$, resistant to cephalothin
Enterobacter sakazakii	Yellow colonies (more pigmented at 25 than 36°C), often "tough as leather"; grows on several selective media designed for its isolation; D-sorbitol negative, delayed positive DNase at 36°C
Hafnia	Lysed by *Hafnia*-specific bacteriophage 1672,[c] often more active biochemically at 25 than 36°C
Klebsiella	Mucoid colonies, encapsulated cells, nonmotile, lysine$^+$, very active biochemically, ferment most sugars, VP$^+$, malonate$^+$, resistant to carbenicillin and ampicillin
Proteus-Providencia-Morganella	Phenylalanine$^+$, tyrosine hydrolysis$^+$, often urea$^+$, resistant to colistin
Proteus	Swarms on blood agar, pungent odor, H_2S^+, gelatin$^+$, lipase$^+$
Proteus mirabilis	Urea$^+$, indole$^-$, ornithine$^+$, maltose$^-$
Proteus vulgaris	Urea$^+$, indole$^+$, ornithine$^-$, maltose$^+$
Providencia	No swarming, H_2S^-, ornithine$^-$, gelatin$^-$, lipase$^-$
Morganella	Very inactive biochemically, no swarming, citrate$^-$, H_2S^-, ornithine$^+$, gelatin$^-$, lipase$^-$, urea$^+$
Plesiomonas shigelloides	Oxidase$^+$, lysine$^+$, arginine$^+$, ornithine$^+$, *myo*-inositol$^+$
Serratia	DNase$^+$, gelatinase$^+$, lipase$^+$, resistant to colistin and cephalothin
Serratia marcescens	L-Arabinose$^-$
Serratia, other species	L-Arabinose$^+$

[a] This table gives only the general properties of the genera, species, and serogroups, so there will be exceptions. See Table 3 in this chapter and following chapters for more details and more precise data. The properties listed for a genus or group of genera generally apply to each of its species, and the properties listed for a species generally apply to each of its serotypes.

[b] See Table 3 for biochemical test results given as percentages. The serological tests refer to slide agglutination in group or individual antisera (O1, O3, etc.) for *Salmonella, Shigella, Escherichia coli,* or *Yersinia,* respectively.

[c] These are two bacteriophage tests useful for identification. The *Hafnia*-specific bacteriophage 1672 (HER 272) is available from the American Type Culture Collection (ATCC 51873-B1).

[d] Abbreviations: CIN, cefsulodin-Irgasan-novobiocin agar (a plating medium selective for *Yersinia*); CR-MOX, Congo red, magnesium oxalate agar (a differential medium useful for distinguishing pathogenic from nonpathogenic strains of *Yersinia*); MUCAP, 4-methylumbelliferyl caprylate (a genus-specific test for *Salmonella*); MUG, 4-methylumbelliferyl-β-D-glucuronidase; ONPG, *o*-nitrophenyl-β-D-galactopyranoside; PhoE, a research test done by PCR that is sensitive and specific for *E. coli/Shigella* (57); VP, Voges Proskauer.

include a different kit (which will have similar limitations), a kit that contains more tests (such as those in 96-well plastic plates), or more expensive research techniques such as molecular tests or 16S rRNA sequencing (56).

Molecular Methods of Identification

Molecular methods have proved extremely useful for identification to the level of family, genus, species, serotype, clone, and strain and for differentiating pathogenic from nonpathogenic strains (see chapter 16 of this Manual). For example, a PCR test for the *phoE* gene appears to be a sensitive and specific test for determining if a strain belongs to the *Escherichia-Shigella* group (88). However, few if any of these molecular methods are commercially available. In the United States, commercial diagnostic tests must often be approved by the Food and Drug Administration if they are used on human clinical specimens. Regulatory and cost limitations have greatly restricted the use of molecular methods in clinical microbiology laboratories. However, they have proved extremely useful in a research setting. In the United States, to conform to the CLIA regulations of 1988, also called CLIA '88, it is necessary to report these research results with a disclaimer unless all the CLIA requirements have been met.

Problem Strains

Most strains of *Enterobacteriaceae* grow rapidly on plating media and on media used for biochemical identification, but occasionally a slow-growing or fastidious strain is encountered. Some strains grow poorly on blood agar but much better on chocolate agar incubated in a candle jar. This characteristic suggests a possible nutritional requirement or a mutation involving respiration. There are slow-growing strains of *E. coli, Klebsiella pneumoniae,* and *Serratia marcescens,* and typical biochemical reactions of these strains usually require extended incubation. Another type of problem organism is sometimes isolated from patients being treated with antimicrobial agents. Li et al. described such "pleiotropic" (having multiple phenotypic expression) mutants of *S. marcescens* (66) and *Salmonella* after exposure to gentamicin. These strains react atypically in many of the standard biochemical tests and are difficult to identify. A different type of pleiotropic mutant induced by chemical exposure was reported by Lannigan and Hussian (64). A *Salmonella* strain lost the ability to produce hydrogen sulfide, reduce nitrate to nitrite, and produce gas from glucose because of chlorate resistance acquired after exposure to Dakin's solution (a solution that contains chlorate and is found in hospitals). Similarly, "dwarf" colony forms of *Salmonella* serotype Typhi have been known for many years. They are only 0.2 to 0.3 mm in diameter after 24 h of incubation but are normal size if the medium is supplemented with sulfite or thiosulfate. Some atypical and slowly growing strains become more typical and grow better after they have been transferred several times. Laboratories occasionally isolate strains that grow rapidly but have a biochemical reaction profile that does not fit (Table 3) any of the described species, biogroups, or Enteric Groups of *Enterobacteriaceae* (56). At present, this type of culture can be reported only as "unidentified." It may be an atypical strain of one of the organisms listed in Tables 1 to 5, or it may belong to a new species that has not been described (37, 56, 94). Additional testing at a state, national, or international reference laboratory can often answer the question about the culture's identity and has led to the discovery of new causes of human infections (12–18, 37, 55, 56, 71, 94).

Commercial Products and Services

A wide variety of commercial products and diagnostic services are available for *Enterobacteriaceae,* but availability is constantly changing. The best approach is to go to a suppliers' Internet site to check availability, technical information, and price. Products include routine and reference identification products and kits (with or without antimicrobial susceptibility tests), combination isolation-identification products, dehydrated media, ready-to-use media in tubes and plates, antisera, reagents, antibiotic products, cultures, and bacteriophages. Services include serodiagnosis, isolation, identification, antimicrobial susceptibility testing, molecular testing, serotyping, and subtyping. For more information, see chapters 15 and 16 of this Manual, the U. S. Food and Drug Administration's *BAM Manual Online* (http://www.cfsan.fda.gov/~ebam/bam-toc.html), and references 55 and 92.

ANTIBIOTIC SUSCEPTIBILITY

Several methods are available for testing the antibiotic susceptibility of *Enterobacteriaceae,* but the most popular are disk diffusion (6) and broth dilution (see chapters 17 and 70 to 78). Several textbook and infectious disease reviews describe antibiotic usage in clinical practice (4, 68, 69, 82).

When antibiotics were first introduced, there was only slight resistance among the species of *Enterobacteriaceae.* Today, antibiotic resistance is much more common among strains isolated from humans and animals. Resistance patterns vary depending on the organism and its origin (4, 68, 69, 82).

Intrinsic Resistance

Intrinsic resistance is a genetic property of most strains of a species and evolved long before the clinical use of antibiotics. For example, essentially all strains of *Serratia marcescens* have intrinsic resistance to penicillin G, colistin, and cephalothin. This evolution of resistance can best be shown by studying strains isolated and stored before the antibiotic era or by studying a large collection of strains from a wide variety of sources including strains that have had little or no exposure to antibiotics. Table 10 lists some common *Enterobacteriaceae* and their intrinsic resistance patterns.

The Antibiogram as a Marker in Epidemiological Studies

Antibiotic susceptibility testing is usually done on isolates that are clinically significant and provides an antibiogram that is useful for comparing isolates in epidemiologic studies. When the selective ecological pressure of antibiotics is changed, the resistance patterns of epidemic (or endemic) strains may also change (4, 68, 69, 82). These changes have been documented in outbreaks that have lasted for several months or longer. Even with these limitations in stability, the antibiogram is probably the most useful and practical laboratory marker for comparing strains and can be extremely helpful in recognizing and analyzing infection problems.

Use of Antibiograms for Identification

The antibiogram of a culture can be compared with those of known isolates (Table 10) to provide a different approach to identification. When the antibiogram and identification are incompatible (for example, a strain of *Klebsiella* that is susceptible to ampicillin and carbenicillin or a culture of *Enterobacter* that is susceptible to cephalothin), the culture should be streaked and checked for purity. In addition, both the identification and the antibiogram may have to be repeated.

TABLE 10 Intrinsic antimicrobial resistance in some common *Enterobacteriaceae* species

Genus/species	Most strains are resistant to:
Buttiauxella species	Cephalothin
Cedecea species	Polymyxins, ampicillin, cephalothin
Citrobacter amalonaticus	Ampicillin
Citrobacter freundii	Cephalothin
Citrobacter diversus (*C. koseri*)	Cephalothin, carbenicillin
Edwardsiella tarda	Colistin
Enterobacter cloacae	Cephalothin
Enterobacter aerogenes	Cephalothin
Many other *Enterobacter* species	Cephalothin
Escherichia hermannii	Ampicillin, carbenicillin
Ewingella americana	Cephalothin
Hafnia alvei	Cephalothin
Klebsiella pneumoniae	Ampicillin, carbenicillin
Kluyvera ascorbata	Ampicillin
Kluyvera cryocrescens	Ampicillin
Proteus mirabilis	Polymyxins, tetracycline, nitrofurantoin
Proteus vulgaris	Polymyxins, ampicillin, nitrofurantoin, tetracycline
Morganella morganii	Polymyxins, ampicillin, cephalothin
Providencia rettgeri	Polymyxins, cephalothin, nitrofurantoin, tetracycline
Other *Providencia*[a] species	Polymyxins, nitrofurantoin
Serratia marcescens[b]	Polymyxins, cephalothin, nitrofurantoin
Serratia fonticola	Ampicillin, carbenicillin, cephalothin
Other *Serratia* species	Polymyxins,[c] cephalothin

[a] Most strains of *Providencia stuartii* are also resistant to cephalothin and tetracycline.

[b] *Serratia marcescens* can also be resistant to ampicillin, carbenicillin, streptomycin, and tetracycline.

[c] Most *Serratia* species are resistant to polymyxins, but some strains have unusual zones of inhibition from 10 to 12 mm or larger, even though they are resistant when tested by other methods.

Some of the material in this chapter was taken from or adapted from chapters and reviews of the family Enterobacteriaceae *that J.J.F. wrote while an employee or "guest researcher" of the U.S. Government. Under U.S. copyright law, these publications are defined to be "works of the U.S. Government" and thus are not subject to copyright under the U.S. Code.*

Special thanks are expressed to the many people who did biochemical testing at CDC of over 10,000 cultures whose results are tabulated in Table 3.

REFERENCES

1. **Ajithkumar, B., V. P. Ajithkumar, R. Iriye, Y. Doi, and T. Sakai.** 2003. Spore-forming *Serratia marcescens* subsp. *sakuensis* subsp. nov., isolated from a domestic wastewater treatment tank. *Int. J. Syst. Evol. Microbiol.* **53:**253–258.
2. **Akhurst, R. J., N. E. Boemare, P. H. Janssen, M. M. Peel, D. A. Alfredson, and C. E. Beard.** 2004. Taxonomy of Australian clinical isolates of the genus *Photorhabdus* and proposal of *Photorhabdus asymbiotica* subsp. *asymbiotica* subsp. nov. and *P. asymbiotica* subsp. *australis* subsp. nov. *Int. J. Syst. Evol. Microbiol.* **54:**1301–1310.
3. **Ashelford, K. E., J. C. Fry, M. J. Bailey, and M. J. Day.** 2002. Characterization of *Serratia* isolates from soil, ecological implications and transfer of *Serratia proteamaculans* subsp. *quinovora* Grimont et al. 1983 to *Serratia quinivorans* corrig., sp. nov. *Int. J. Syst. Evol. Microbiol.* **52:**2281–2289.
4. **Baddour, L. M., and S. L. Gorbach (ed.).** 2003. *Therapy of Infectious Diseases.* Saunders, Phildelphia, Pa.
5. **Balows, A., H. G. Trüper, M. Dworkin, W. Harder, and K.-H. Schleifer (ed.).** 1992. *The Prokaryotes,* 2nd ed., vol. 3, p. 2673–2937. Springer-Verlag KG, Berlin, Germany.
6. **Bauer, A. W., W. M. M. Kirby, J. C. Sherris, and M. Turck.** 1966. Antibiotic susceptibility testing by a standardized single disk method. *Am. J. Clin. Pathol.* **45:**493–496.
7. **Bercovier, H., D. J. Brenner, J. Ursing, A. G. Steigerwalt, G. R. Fanning, J. M. Alonso, G. A. Carter, and H. H. Mollaret.** 1980. Characterization of *Yersinia enterocolitica sensu stricto. Curr. Microbiol.* **4:**201–206.
8. **Bercovier, H., J. Ursing, D. J. Brenner, A. G. Steigerwalt, G. R. Fanning, G. P. Carter, and H. H. Mollaret.** 1980. *Yersinia kristensenii:* a new species of *Enterobacteriaceae* composed of sucrose-negative strains (formerly called *Yersinia enterocolitica* or *Yersinia enterocolitica*-like). *Curr. Microbiol.* **4:**219–224.
9. **Boemare, N. E., R. J. Akhurst, and R. G. Mourant.** 1993. DNA relatedness between *Xenorhabdus* spp. *(Enterobacteriaceae),* symbiotic bacteria of entomopathogenic nematodes, and a proposal to transfer *Xenorhabdus luminescens* to a new genus, *Photorhabdus* gen. nov. *Int. J. Syst. Bacteriol.* **43:**249–255.

9a. **Borriello, S. P., P. R. Murray, and G. Funke (ed.).** 2005. *Bacteriology,* vol. 1 and 2. *Topley and Wilson's Microbiology & Microbial Infections,* 10th ed. Arnold Health Sciences Publishing, London, England.

10. **Boudeau J., A. L. Glasser, E. Masseret, B. Joly, and A. Darfeuille-Michaud.** 1999. Invasive ability of an *Escherichia coli* strain isolated from the ileal mucosa of a patient with Crohn's disease. *Infect. Immun.* **67:**4499–4509.
11. **Boyd, E. F., F.-S. Wang, T. S. Whittam, and R. K. Selander.** 1996. Molecular genetic relationships of the salmonellae. *Appl. Environ. Microbiol.* **62:**804–808.
12. **Brenner, D. J.** 1992. Additional genera of *Enterobacteriaceae,* p. 2922–2937. *In* A. Balows, H. G. Trüper, M. Dworkin, W. Harder, and K.-H. Schleifer (ed.), *The Prokaryotes,* 2nd ed. Springer-Verlag KG, Berlin, Germany.
13. **Brenner, D. J.** 1992. Introduction to the family *Enterobacteriaceae,* p. 2673–2695. *In* A. Balows, H. G. Trüper, M. Dworkin, W. Harder, and K.-H. Schleifer (ed.), *The Prokaryotes,* 2nd ed. Springer-Verlag KG, Berlin, Germany.

14. **Brenner, D. J., and J. J. Farmer III.** 2005. Introduction to the family *Enterobacteriaceae*, p. 587–607. *In* D. J. Brenner, N. R. Krieg, J. T. Staley, and G. M. Garrity (ed.), *Bergey's Manual of Systematic Bacteriology*, 2nd ed., vol. 2. *The Proteobacteria,* part B, *The Gammaproteobacteria.* Springer, New York, N.Y.
15. **Brenner, D. J., P. A. D. Grimont, A. G. Steigerwalt, G. R. Fanning, E. Ageron, and C. F. Riddle.** 1993. Classification of citrobacteria by DNA hybridization: designation of *Citrobacter farmeri* sp. nov., *Citrobacter youngae* sp. nov., *Citrobacter braakii* sp. nov., *Citrobacter werkmanii* sp. nov., *Citrobacter sedlakii* sp. nov., and three unnamed *Citrobacter* genomospecies. *Int. J. Syst. Bacteriol.* **43:**645–658.
16. **Brenner, D. J., N. R. Krieg, J. T. Staley, and G. M. Garrity (ed.).** 2005. *Bergey's Manual of Systematic Bacteriology*, 2nd ed., vol. 2. *The Proteobacteria*, part B. *The Gammaproteobacteria,* p. 587–850. Springer, New York, N.Y.
17. **Brenner, D. J., H. E. Müller, A. G. Steigerwalt, A. M. Whitney, C. M. O'Hara, and P. Kämpfer.** 1998. Two new *Rahnella* genomospecies that cannot be phenotypically differentiated from *Rahnella aquatilis. Int. J. Syst. Bacteriol.* **48:**141–149.
18. **Brenner, D. J., C. M. O'Hara, P. A. D. Grimont, J. M. Janda, E. Falsen, E. Aldova, E. Ageron, J. Schindler, S. L. Abbott, and A. G. Steigerwalt.** 1999. Biochemical identification of *Citrobacter* species defined by DNA hybridization and description of *Citrobacter gillenii* sp. nov. (formerly *Citrobacter* genomospecies 10) and *Citrobacter murliniae* sp. nov. (formerly *Citrobacter* genomospecies 11). *J. Clin. Microbiol.* **37:**2619–2624.
19. **Brenner, F. W., R. G. Villar, F. J. Angulo, R. Tauxe, and B. Swaminathan.** 2000. *Salmonella* nomenclature. *J. Clin. Microbiol.* **38:**2465–2467.
20. **Calderwood, S. B., D. W. K. Acheson, G. T. Keusch, T. J. Barrett, P. M. Griffin, N. A. Strockbine, B. Swaminathan, J. B. Kaper, M. M. Levine, B. S. Kaplan, H. Karch, A. D. O'Brien, T. G. Obrig, Y. Takeda, P. I. Tarr, and I. K. Wachsmuth.** 1996. Proposed new nomenclature for SLT (VT) family. *ASM News* **62:**118–119.
21. **Carter, J. S., F. J. Bowden, I. Bastian, G. M. Myers, K. S. Sriprakash, and D. J. Kemp.** 1999. Phylogenetic evidence for reclassification of *Calymmatobacterium granulomatis* as *Klebsiella granulomatis* comb. nov. *Int. J. Syst. Bacteriol.* **49:**1695–1700.
22. **Centers for Disease Control and Prevention.** 2001. *An Atlas of* Salmonella *in the United States.* Centers for Disease Control and Prevention, Atlanta, Ga.
23. **Centers for Disease Control and Prevention.** 2001. Shigella *Surveillance: Annual Summary, 2000.* Centers for Disease Control and Prevention, Atlanta, Ga.
24. **Collier, L., A. Balows, and M. Sussman (ed).** 1998. *Topley and Wilson's Microbiology and Microbial Infections,* 9th ed., vol. 2 and 3. Edward Arnold, London, England.
25. **Crosa, J. H., D. J. Brenner, W. H. Ewing, and S. Falkow.** 1973. Molecular relationships among the salmonelleae. *J. Bacteriol.* **115:**307–315.
26. **Dickey, R. S., and C. H. Zumoff.** 1988. Emended description of *Enterobacter cancerogenus* comb. nov. (formerly *Erwinia cancerogena*). *Int. J. Syst. Bacteriol.* **38:**371–374.
27. **Diekema, D. J., M. A. Pfaller, R. N. Jones, G. V. Doern, P. L. Winokur, A. C. Gales, H. S. Sader, K. Kugler, and M. Beach.** 1999. Survey of bloodstream infections due to gram-negative bacilli: frequency of occurrence and antimicrobial susceptibility of isolates collected in the United States, Canada, and Latin America for the SENTRY antimicrobial surveillance program, 1997. *Clin. Infect. Dis.* **29:**595–607.
28. **Drancourt, M., C. Bollet, A. Carta, and P. Rousselier.** 2001. Phylogenetic analysis of *Klebsiella* species delineate *Klebsiella* and *Raoultella* gen. nov. with description of *Raoultella ornithinolytica* comb. nov., *Raoultella terrigena* comb. nov. and *Raoultella planticola* comb. nov. *Int. J. Syst. Evol. Microbiol.* **51:**925–932.
29. **DuPont, H. L., S. B. Formal, R. B. Hornick, M. J. Snyder, J. P. Libonati, D. G. Sheahan, E. H. LaBrec, and J. P. Kalas.** 1971. Pathogenesis of *Escherichia coli* diarrhea. *N. Engl. J. Med.* **285:**1–9.
30. **Edmond, M. B., S. E. Wallace, D. K. McClish, M. A. Pfaller, R. N. Jones, and R. P. Wenzel.** 1999. Nosocomial bloodstream infections in United States hospitals: a three-year analysis. *Clin. Infect. Dis.* **29:**239–244.
31. **Euzeby, J. P.** 1999. Revised *Salmonella* nomenclature: designation of *Salmonella enterica* (ex Kauffmann and Edwards) Le Minor and Popoff 1987 sp. nov., nom. rev. as the neotype species of the genus *Salmonella* Lignieres 1900 (Approved Lists 1980), rejection of the name *Salmonella choleraesuis* (Smith 1894) Weldin 1927 (Approved Lists 1980), and conservation of the name *Salmonella typhi* (Schroeter 1886) Warren and Scott 1930 (Approved Lists 1980). Request for an opinion. *J. Syst. Bacteriol.* **49:**927–930.
32. **Ewing, W. H.** 1986. *Edwards and Ewing's Identification of Enterobacteriaceae,* 4th ed. Elsevier Science Publishing Co., New York, N.Y.
33. **Ezaki, T., M. Amano, Y. Kawamura, and E. Yabuuchi.** 2000. Proposal of *Salmonella paratyphi* sp. nov., nom. rev. and request for an opinion to conserve the epithet *paratyphi* in the binary combination *Salmonella paratyphi* as *nomen epitheton conservandum. Int. J. Syst. Evol. Microbiol.* **50:**941–944.
34. **Ezaki, T., Y. Kawamura, and E. Yabuuchi.** 2000. Recognition of the nomenclatural standing of *Salmonella typhi* (Approved Lists 1980), *Salmonella enteritidis* (Approved Lists 1980) and *Salmonella typhimurium* (Approved Lists 1980), and conservation of the specific epithets *enteritidis* and *typhimurium.* Request for an opinion. *Int. J. Syst. Evol. Microbiol.* **50:**945–947.
35. **Farmer, J. J., III, M. A. Asbury, F. W. Hickman, D. J. Brenner, and The *Enterobacteriaceae* Study Group.** 1980. *Enterobacter sakazakii:* a new species of "*Enterobacteriaceae*" isolated from clinical specimens. *Int. J. Syst. Bacteriol.* **30:**569–584.
36. **Farmer, J. J., III, and B. R. Davis.** 1985. H7 antiserum-sorbitol fermentation medium: a single tube screening medium for detecting *Escherichia coli* O157:H7 associated with hemorrhagic colitis. *J. Clin. Microbiol.* **22:**620–625. (*Note:* This paper has a misprint in the formula for MacConkey sorbitol agar. The paper says to use 22.2 g of MacConkey agar base; the correct amount is 40 g, which is given in the instructions on the bottle.)
37. **Farmer, J. J., III, B. R. Davis, F. W. Hickman-Brenner, A. McWhorter, G. P. Huntley-Carter, M. A. Asbury, C. Riddle, H. G. Wathen, C. Elias, G. R. Fanning, A. G. Steigerwalt, C. M. O'Hara, G. K. Morris, P. B. Smith, and D. J. Brenner.** 1985. Biochemical identification of new species and biogroups of *Enterobacteriaceae* isolated from clinical specimens. *J. Clin. Microbiol.* **21:**46–76.
38. **Farmer, J. J., III, M. K. Farmer, and B. Holmes.** 2005. *Enterobacteriaceae*: general characteristics, p. 1317–1359. *In* S. P. Boriello, P. R. Murray, and G. Funke, *Bacteriology,* vol. 2, *Topley and Wilson's Microbiology & Microbial Infections,* 10th ed. Arnold Health Sciences Publishing, London, England.
39. **Farmer, J. J., III, R. E. Gangarosa, and E. J. Gangarosa.** 2004. Commentary. Does *Laribacter hongkongensis* cause diarrhoea, or does diarrhoea "cause" *L. hongkongensis. Lancet* **363:** 1923–1924.
40. **Farmer, J. J., III, J. H. Jorgensen, P. A. D. Grimont, R. J. Akhurst, G. O. Poinar, Jr., E. Ageron, G. V. Pierce, J. A. Smith, G. P. Carter, K. L. Wilson, and F. W. Hickman-Brenner.** 1989. *Xenorhabdus luminescens* (DNA hybridization group 5) from human clinical specimens. *J. Clin. Microbiol.* **27:**1594–1600.
41. **Farmer, J. J., III, A. C. McWhorter, D. J. Brenner, and G. K. Morris.** 1984. The *Salmonella-Arizona* group of

Enterobacteriaceae: nomenclature, classification and reporting. *Clin. Microbiol. Newsl.* **6:**63–66.

42. **Farmer, J. J., III, C. F. Riddle, M. D. Stargel, H. Iida, T. Aikawa, D. Achanzar, and W. I. Taylor.** 1976. Unusual *Enterobacteriaceae:* H_2S^+ *Shigella sonnei*, one authentic and one false positive due to contamination with the obligate anaerobe *Eubacterium lentum*. *J. Clin. Microbiol.* **3:**206–208.
43. **Farmer, J. J., III, J. G. Wells, P. M. Griffin, and I. K. Wachsmuth.** 1987. *Enterobacteriaceae* infections, p. 233–296. *In* B. B. Wentworth (ed.), *Diagnostic Procedures for Bacterial Infections*, 7th ed. American Public Health Association, Washington, D.C.
44. **Fischer-Le Saux, M., V. Viallard, B. Brunel, P. Normand, and N. Boemare.** 1999. Polyphasic classification of the genus *Photorhabdus* and proposal of new taxa: *P. luminescens* subsp. *luminescens* subsp. nov., *P. luminescens* subsp. *akhurstii* subsp. nov., *P. luminescens* subsp. *laumondii* subsp. nov., *P. temperata* sp. nov., and *P. asymbiotica* sp. nov. *Int. J. Syst. Bacteriol.* **49:**1645–1656.
45. **Fratamico, P. M., A. K. Bhunia, and J. L. Smith.** 2005. *Foodborne Pathogens: Microbiology and Molecular Biology.* Caister Academic Press, Norwich, United Kingdom.
46. **Gavini, F., J. Mergaert, A. Beji, C. Mielcarek, D. Izard, K. Kersters, and J. De Ley.** 1989. Transfer of *Enterobacter agglomerans* (Beijerinck 1888) Ewing and Fife 1972 to *Pantoea* gen. nov. as *Pantoea agglomerans* comb. nov. and description of *Pantoea dispersa* sp. nov. *Int. J. Syst. Bacteriol.* **39:**337–345.
47. **Grimont, P. A. D., and E. Ageron.** 1989. *Enterobacter cancerogenus* (Urosevic, 1966) Dickey and Zumoff 1988, a senior subjective synonym of *Enterobacter taylorae* Farmer et al. (1985). *Res. Microbiol.* **140:**459–465.
48. **Hazir, S., E. Stackebrandt, E. Lang, P. Schumann, R. U. Ehlers, and N. Keskin.** 2004. Two new subspecies of *Photorhabdus luminescens*, isolated from *Heterorhabditis bacteriophora* (Nematoda: *Heterorhabditidae*): *Photorhabdus luminescens* subsp. *kayaii* subsp. nov. and *Photorhabdus luminescens* subsp. *thracensis* subsp. nov. *Syst. Appl. Microbiol.* **27:**36–42.
49. **Heymann, D. L. (ed.).** 2004. *Control of Communicable Diseases Manual*, 18th ed. American Public Health Association, Washington, D.C.
50. **Hickman, F. W., and J. J. Farmer III.** 1978. *Salmonella typhi:* identification, antibiograms, serology, and bacteriophage typing. *Am. J. Med. Technol.* **44:**1149–1159.
51. **Hoffmann, H., S. Stindl, W. Ludwig, A. Stumpf, A. Mehlen, J. Heesemann, D. Monget, K. H. Schleifer, and A. Roggenkamp.** 2005. Reassignment of *Enterobacter dissolvens* to *Enterobacter cloacae* as *E. cloacae* subspecies *dissolvens* comb. nov. and emended description of *Enterobacter asburiae* and *Enterobacter kobei*. *Syst. Appl. Microbiol.* **28:**196–205.
52. **Hoffmann, H., S. Stindl, A. Stumpf, A. Mehlen, D. Monget, J. Heesemann, K. H. Schleifer, and A. Roggenkamp.** 2005. Description of *Enterobacter ludwigii* sp. nov., a novel *Enterobacter* species of clinical relevance. *Syst. Appl. Microbiol.* **28:**206–212.
53. **Huys, G., M. Cnockaert, J. M. Janda, and J. Swings.** 2003. *Escherichia albertii* sp. nov., a diarrhoeagenic species isolated from stool specimens of Bangladeshi children. *Int. J. Syst. Evol. Microbiol.* **53:**807–810.
54. **Inoue, K., K. Sugiyama, Y. Kosako, R. Sakazaki, and S. Yamai.** 2000. *Enterobacter cowanii* sp. nov., a new species of the family *Enterobacteriaceae*. *Curr. Microbiol.* **41:**417–420.
55. **Janda, J. M., and S. L. Abbott.** 2006. *The Enterobacteria*, 2nd ed. ASM Press, Washington, D.C.
56. **Johnson, A. S., C. Tarr, B. H. Brown, Jr., K. M. Birkhead, and J. J. Farmer III.** 2005. First case of septicemia due to Enteric Group 58 (Enterobacteriaceae): and its designation as *Averyella dalhousiensis* gen. nov., sp. nov. based on strains from 20 additional cases. *J. Clin. Microbiol.* **43:**5195–5201.
57. **Judicial Commission of the International Committee on Systematic Bacteriology.** 1993. Rejection of the name *Citrobacter diversus* Werkman and Gillen. *Int. J. Syst. Bacteriol.* **43:**392.
58. **Judicial Commission of the International Committee on Systematics of Prokaryotes.** 2005. The type species of the genus *Salmonella* Lignieres 1900 is *Salmonella enterica* (ex Kauffmann and Edwards 1952) Le Minor and Popoff 1987, with the type strain LT2T, and conservation of the epithet *enterica* in *Salmonella enterica* over all earlier epithets that may be applied to this species. Opinion 80. *Int. J. Syst. Evol. Microbiol.* **55:**519–520.
59. **Kampfer, P., S. Ruppel, and R. Remus.** 2005. *Enterobacter radicincitans* sp. nov., a plant growth promoting species of the family *Enterobacteriaceae*. *Syst. Appl. Microbiol.* **28:**213–221.
60. **Kandolo, K., and G. Wauters.** 1985. Pyrazinamidase activity in *Yersinia enterocolitica* and related organisms. *J. Clin. Microbiol.* **21:**980–982.
61. **Karmali, M. A.** 1989. Infection by verocytotoxin-producing *Escherichia coli*. *Clin. Microbiol. Rev.* **2:**15–38.
62. **Kosako, Y., K. Tamura, R. Sakazaki, and K. Miki.** 1996. *Enterobacter kobei* sp. nov., a new species of *Enterobacteriaceae* resembling *Enterobacter cloacae*. *Curr. Microbiol.* **33:**261–265.
63. **Krieg, N. R., and J. G. Holt (ed.).** 1984. *Bergey's Manual of Systematic Bacteriology*, vol. 1, p. 408–516. The Williams & Wilkins Co., Baltimore, Md.
64. **Lannigan, R., and Z. Hussian.** 1993. Wound isolate of *Salmonella typhimurium* that became chlorate resistant after exposure to Dakin's solution: concomitant loss of hydrogen sulfide production, gas production, and nitrate reduction. *J. Clin. Microbiol.* **31:**2497–2498.
65. **Lengyel, K., E. Lang, A. Fodor, E. Szallas, P. Schumann, and E. Stackebrandt.** 2005. Description of four novel species of *Xenorhabdus*, family *Enterobacteriaceae: Xenorhabdus budapestensis* sp. nov., *Xenorhabdus ehlersii* sp. nov., *Xenorhabdus innexi* sp. nov., and *Xenorhabdus szentirmaii* sp. nov. *Syst. Appl. Microbiol.* **28:**115–122.
66. **Li, K., J. J. Farmer III, and A. Coppola.** 1974. A novel type of resistant bacteria induced by gentamicin. *Trans. N. Y. Acad. Sci.* **36:**369–396.
67. **Li, X., D. Zhang, F. Chen, J. Ma, Y. Dong, and L. Zhang.** 2004. *Klebsiella singaporensis* sp. nov., a novel isomaltulose-producing bacterium. *Int. J. Syst. Evol. Microbiol.* **54:**2131–2136.
68. **Mandell, G. L., J. E. Bennett, and R. Dolin (ed.).** 2005. *Mandell, Douglas, and Bennett's Principles and Practice of Infectious Diseases*, 6th ed. Elsevier, Philadelphia, Pa.
69. **Mayhall, C. G.** 2000. *Hospital Epidemiology and Infection Control*, 2nd ed. Lippincott Williams and Wilkins, Philadelphia, Pa.
70. **McWhorter-Murlin, A. C., and F. W. Hickman-Brenner.** 1994. *Identification and Serotyping of* Salmonella *and an Update of the Kauffmann-White Scheme; Appendix A, Kauffmann-White Scheme, Alphabetical List of* Salmonella *Serotypes (Updated 1994); Appendix B, Kauffmann-White Scheme, List of* Salmonella *Serotypes by O Group (Updated 1994)*. Foodborne and Diarrheal Diseases Laboratory Section, Centers for Disease Control and Prevention, Atlanta, Ga.
71. **Müller, H. E., D. J. Brenner, G. R. Fanning, P. A. D. Grimont, and P. Kämpfer.** 1996. Emended description of *Buttiauxella agrestis* with recognition of six new species of *Buttiauxella* and two new species of *Kluyvera: Buttiauxella ferragutiae* sp. nov., *Buttiauxella gaginiae* sp. nov., *Buttiauxella brennerae* sp. nov., *Buttiauxella izardii* sp. nov., *Buttiauxella noackiae* sp. nov., *Buttiauxella warmboldiae* sp. nov., *Kluyvera cochleae* sp. nov., and *Kluyvera georgiana* sp. nov. *Int. J. Syst. Bacteriol.* **46:**50–63.

72. **Neubauer, H., S. Aleksic, A. Hensel, E.-J Finke, and H. Meyer.** 2000. *Yersinia enterocolitica* 16S rRNA gene types belong to the same genospecies but form three homology groups. *Int. J. Med. Microbiol.* **290:**61–64.
73. **O'Hara, C. M., F. W. Brenner, A. G. Steigerwalt, B. C. Hill, B. Holmes, P. A. D. Grimont, P. M. Hawkey, J. L. Penner, J. M. Miller, and D. J. Brenner.** 2000. Classification of *Proteus vulgaris* biogroup 3 with recognition of *Proteus hauseri* sp. non., nom. rev. and unnamed *Proteus* genomospecies 4, 5 and 6. *Int. J. Syst. Evol. Microbiol.* **50:**1869–1875.
74. **Pavan, M. E., R. J. Franco, J. M. Rodriguez, P. Gadaleta, S. L. Abbott, J. M. Janda, and J. Zorzopulos.** 2005. Phylogenetic relationships of the genus *Kluyvera:* transfer of *Enterobacter intermedius* Izard et al. 1980 to the genus *Kluyvera* as *Kluyvera intermedia* comb. nov. and reclassification of *Kluyvera cochleae* as a later synonym of *K. intermedia. Int. J. Syst. Evol. Microbiol.* **55:**437–442.
75. **Peel, M. M., D. A. Alfredson, J. G. Gerrard, J. M. Davis, J. M. Robson, R. J. McDougall, B. L. Scullie, and R. J. Akhurst.** 1999. Isolation, identification, and molecular characterization of strains of *Photorhabdus luminescens* from infected humans in Australia. *J. Clin. Microbiol.* **37:**3647–3653.
76. **Popoff, M. Y.** 2001. *Antigenic Formulas of the* Salmonella *Serovars,* 8th ed. WHO Collaborating Centre for Reference and Research on *Salmonella,* Institut Pasteur, Paris, France.
77. **Popoff, M. Y.** 2001. *Guidelines for the Preparation of* Salmonella *Antisera.* WHO Collaborating Centre for Reference and Research on *Salmonella,* Institut Pasteur, Paris, France.
78. **Popoff, M. Y., and L. E. LeMinor.** 2005. Genus XXXIII. *Salmonella* Ligières 1900, 389^{AL}, p. 764–799. *In* D. J. Brenner, N. R. Krieg, J. T. Staley, and G. M. Garrity (ed.), *Bergey's Manual of Systematic Bacteriology,* 2nd ed., vol. 2. *The Proteobacteria,* part B. *The Gammaproteobacteria.* Springer, New York, N.Y.
79. **Reeves, M. W., G. M. Evins, A. A. Heiba, B. D. Plikaytis, and J. J. Farmer III.** 1989. Clonal nature of *Salmonella typhi* and its genetic relatedness to other salmonellae as shown by multilocus enzyme electrophoresis, and proposal of *Salmonella bongori* comb. nov. *J. Clin. Microbiol.* **27:**313–320.
80. **Riley, G., and S. Toma.** 1989. Detection of pathogenic *Yersinia enterocolitica* by using Congo red-magnesium oxalate agar medium. *J. Clin. Microbiol.* **27:**213–214.
81. **Rosenblueth, M., L. Martinez, J. Silva, and E. Martinez-Romero.** 2004. *Klebsiella variicola,* a novel species with clinical and plant-associated isolates. *Syst. Appl. Microbiol.* **27:**27–35.
82. **Ryan, K. J., and C. G. Ray (ed.).** 2004. *Sherris Medical Microbiology: an Introduction to Infectious Diseases,* 4th ed. McGraw-Hill, New York, N.Y.
83. **Samson, R., J. B. Legendre, R. Christen, M. Fischer-Le Saux, W. Achouak, and L. Gardan.** 2005. Transfer of Pectobacterium chrysanthemi (Burkholder et al. 1953) Brenner et al. 1973 and Brenneria paradisiaca to the genus Dickeya gen. nov. as Dickeya chrysanthemi comb. nov. and Dickeya paradisiaca comb. nov. and delineation of four novel species, Dickeya dadantii sp. nov., Dickeya dianthicola sp. nov., Dickeya dieffenbachiae sp. nov. and Dickeya zeae sp. nov. *Int. J. Syst. Evol. Microbiol.* **55:**1415–1427.
84. **Savola, K. L., E. J. Baron, L. S. Tompkins, and D. J. Passaro.** 2001. Fecal leukocyte stain has diagnostic value for outpatients but not inpatients. *J. Clin. Microbiol.* **39:**266–269.
85. **Schaberg, D. R.** 1991. Major trends in the microbial etiology of nosocomial infections. *Ann. Intern. Med.* **91**(Suppl. 3B):72S–75S.
86. **Scheutz, F., and N. A. Strockbine.** 2005. Genus I. *Escherichia* Castellani and Chalmers 1919, 941T^{AL}, p. 607–624. *In* D. J. Brenner, N. R. Krieg, J. T. Staley, and G. M. Garrity (ed.), *Bergey's Manual of Systematic Bacteriology,* 2nd ed., vol. 2. *The Proteobacteria,* part B. *The Gammaproteobacteria.* Springer, New York, N.Y.
87. **Sprague, L. D., and H. Neubauer.** 2005. *Yersinia aleksiciae* sp. nov. *Int. J. Syst. Evol. Microbiol.* **55:**831–835.
88. **Sprierings, G., C. Ockhuijsen, H. Hofstra, and J. Tommassen.** 1993. Polymerase chain reaction for the specific detection of *Escherichia coli/Shigella. Res. Microbiol.* **144:**557–564.
89. **Sutra, L., R. Christen, C. Bollet, P. Simoneau, and L. Gardan.** 2001. *Samsonia erythrinae* gen. nov., sp. nov., isolated from bark necrotic lesions of *Erythrina* sp., and discrimination of plant-pathogenic *Enterobacteriaceae* by phenotypic features. *Int. J. Syst. Evol. Microbiol.* **51:**1291–1304.
90. **Threlfall, E. J.** 2005. *Salmonella,* p. 1398–1434. *In* S. P. Boriello, P. R. Murray, and G. Funke, *Bacteriology,* vol. 2. *Topley and Wilson's Microbiology & Microbial Infections,* 10th ed. Arnold Health Sciences Publishing, London, England.
91. **Tindall, B. J., P. A. Grimont, G. M. Garrity, and J. P. Euzeby.** 2005. Nomenclature and taxonomy of the genus *Salmonella. Int. J. Syst. Evol. Microbiol.* **55:**521–524.
92. **Truant, A. L. (ed.).** 2002. *Manual of Commercial Methods in Clinical Microbiology.* ASM Press, Washington, D.C.
93. **Wadstrom, T., A. Aust-Kettis, D. Habte, J. Holmgren, G. Meeuwisse, R. Mollby, and O. Soderlind.** 1976. Enterotoxin-producing bacteria and parasites in stool of Ethiopian children with diarrhoeal disease. *Arch. Dis. Child.* **51:**865–870.
94. **Warren, J. R., J. J. Farmer III, F. E. Dewhirst, K. Birkhead, T. Zembower, L. R. Peterson, L. Sims, and M. Bhattacharya.** 2000. Outbreak of nosocomial infections due to extended-spectrum β-lactamase-producing strains of Enteric Group 137, a new member of the family *Enterobacteriaceae* closely related to *Citrobacter farmeri* and *Citrobacter amalonaticus. J. Clin. Microbiol.* **38:**3946–3952.
95. **Wells, J. G., B. R. Davis, I. K. Wachsmuth, L. W. Riley, R. S. Remis, R. Sokolow, and G. K. Morris.** 1983. Laboratory investigation of hemorrhagic colitis outbreaks associated with a rare *Escherichia coli* serotype. *J. Clin. Microbiol.* **18:**512–520.

Escherichia, Shigella, and *Salmonella**

JAMES P. NATARO, CHERYL A. BOPP, PATRICIA I. FIELDS, JAMES B. KAPER, AND NANCY A. STROCKBINE

43

TAXONOMY

Escherichia, Shigella, and *Salmonella* are classified in the family *Enterobacteriaceae,* which is addressed in chapter 42 of this Manual (35). Species in these three genera are gram-negative rods that grow well on MacConkey agar (MAC). When these organisms are motile, it is by peritrichous flagella; however, all strains of *Shigella* spp. and some strains of *Escherichia* and *Salmonella* are nonmotile. All ferment D-glucose; *Escherichia* and *Salmonella* strains usually produce gas. *Shigella* is phenotypically similar to *Escherichia coli* and, with the exception of *Shigella boydii* serotype 13, would be considered the same species by DNA-DNA hybridization analysis (16). Findings from recent phylogenetic studies with nucleotide sequences of internal fragments from 14 housekeeping genes show that *S. boydii* 13 strains cluster in a neighbor-joining tree with *Escherichia albertii,* a newly described species of *Escherichia* associated with diarrheal disease in Bangladeshi children (48, 49).

NATURAL HABITATS

Escherichia, Shigella, and *Salmonella* are most frequently isolated from the intestines of humans and animals. Because *E. coli* is ubiquitous in human and animal feces, the presence of this species in water is considered to be an indicator of fecal contamination. Some species or serotypes are isolated primarily from humans (e.g., all species of *Shigella* and *Salmonella* serotype Typhi), while others (e.g., *Salmonella* serotype Gallinarum and *Salmonella* serotype Marina) are strongly associated with certain animal hosts. These genera can be isolated from fecally contaminated foods or water but probably do not occur as free-living organisms in the environment. *Salmonella* strains can, however, survive for long periods of time, perhaps years, in the environment (58).

COLLECTION, TRANSPORT, AND STORAGE OF FECAL SPECIMENS

Information on the collection, transport, and storage of specimens from extraintestinal sites is provided in chapters 5 and 20 of this Manual. Fecal specimens can include whole stools, swabs prepared from whole stools, or rectal swabs with visible fecal staining. Transport of fecal specimens to the laboratory in a timely fashion is critical, particularly for more delicate organisms such as *Shigella* (119). Ideally, fecal specimens should be examined as soon as they are received in the laboratory, but if not processed immediately, they should be either refrigerated or frozen at −70°C. Fecal specimens that will not be examined within 1 to 2 h after collection and all rectal swabs should be immediately placed in chilled transport medium and stored refrigerated. If specimens in transport medium are not to be examined within 3 days, they should be frozen immediately at −70°C.

Many of the commercially available transport media (e.g., Cary-Blair, Stuart's, and Amies transport media) are satisfactory for these organisms. Although acceptable for the transport of *E. coli, Salmonella,* and *Shigella,* buffered glycerol saline should not be used for specimens that must also be tested for *Campylobacter* and *Vibrio.*

ESCHERICHIA

Description of the Genus

The genus *Escherichia* is composed of motile or nonmotile bacteria that conform to the definitions of the family *Enterobacteriaceae* (35). There are six species in this genus: *Escherichia albertii, E. blattae, E. coli, E. fergusonii, E. hermannii,* and *E. vulneris.* The type species is *E. coli.* Typical biochemical reactions are listed in Table 1.

Clinical Significance

Of the six *Escherichia* species, *E. coli* is the species usually isolated from human specimens. It is a nearly ubiquitous constituent of the bowel flora of healthy individuals; however, certain strains may cause extraintestinal and intestinal infections in healthy as well as immunocompromised individuals. Urinary tract infections, bacteremia, meningitis, and diarrheal disease are the most frequent clinical syndromes, caused primarily by a limited number of pathogenic clones of *E. coli* (53). In particular, *E. coli* organisms bearing the K1 capsule are isolated with high frequency from cases of neonatal sepsis and meningitis. Uropathogenic *E. coli* strains are not easily identified by conventional microbiologic methods. *E. hermannii* and *E. vulneris* are most often obtained from

*This chapter contains information presented in chapter 42 by Cheryl A. Bopp, Frances W. Brenner, Patricia I. Fields, Joy G. Wells, and Nancy A. Strockbine in the eighth edition of this Manual.

TABLE 1 Biochemical reactions of the six species of *Escherichia* and selected members of the family *Enterobacteriaceae*[a]

Species/biogroup	Indole production	Voges-Proskauer	Motility (35°C)	Yellow pigment	Lysine decarboxylase	Ornithine decarboxylase	Growth in KCN	Acetate utilization	Mucate utilization	D-Glucose, gas	Adonitol, acid	L-Arabinose, acid	D-Arabitol, acid	Cellobiose, acid	Dulcitol, acid	Lactose, acid	Sucrose, acid	D-Mannitol, acid	Raffinose, acid	L-Rhamnose, acid	D-Sorbitol, acid	D-Xylose
Escherichia albertii/ biogroup 1 [*n* = 5] (e.g., Albert 19982)	0	0	0	0	100	100	0	40	0	100	0	100	0	0	0	0	0	100	0	0	100	0
Escherichia albertii/ biogroup 2 [*n* = 10] (e.g., former *S. boydii* 13)	100	0	0	0	0	100	0	0	0	40	0	100	0	0	0	0	0	100	0	0	0	0
Escherichia blattae	0	0	0	0	100	100	0	0	50	100	0	100	0	0	0	0	0	0	0	100	0	100
Escherichia coli	98	0	95	0	90	65	0	90	95	95	5	99	5	2	60	95	50	98	50	80	94	95
Escherichia coli (inactive biotypes)	80	0	5	0	40	20	1	40	30	5	3	85	5	2	40	25	15	93	15	65	75	70
Escherichia fergusonii	98	0	93	0	95	100	0	96	0	95	98	98	100	96	60	0	0	98	0	92	0	96
Escherichia hermannii	99	0	99	98	6	100	94	78	97	97	0	100	8	97	19	45	45	100	40	97	0	100
Escherichia vulneris	0	0	100	50	85	0	15	30	78	97	0	100	0	100	0	15	8	100	99	93	1	100
Shigella boydii[b]	23	0	0	0	0	0	0	0	0	0	0	94	0	0	12	1	0	7	0	1	34	16
Shigella dysenteriae	40	0	0	0	0	0	0	0	0	0	0	45	0	0	4	0	0	0	0	30	29	3
Shigella flexneri	42	0	0	0	0	0	0	8	0	3	0	60	1	0	2	0	1	91	33	5	30	3
Shigella sonnei	0	0	0	0	0	98	0	0	10	0	0	95	15	5	0	2	1	99	3	77	1	1
Hafnia alvei	0	85	85	0	100	98	95	15	0	98	0	95	0	15	0	5	10	99	2	97	0	98
Hafnia alvei/biogroup 1	0	70	0	0	100	45	0	0	0	0	0	0	0	0	0	0	0	55	0	0	0	0
Salmonella serotype Paratyphi A	0	0	95	0	0	95	0	0	0	99	0	100	0	5	90	0	0	100	0	100	95	0
Salmonella serotype Choleraesuis	0	0	95	0	95	100	0	1	0	95	0	0	1	0	5	0	0	98	1	100	90	98
Yersinia ruckeri	0	10	0	0	50	100	15	0	0	5	0	5	0	5	0	0	0	100	5	0	50	0

[a] Values are percentages of isolates tested with positive test results within 1 or 2 days of incubation at 35 to 37°C. Reactions for isolates that become positive after 2 days are not considered. Data were compiled from findings published by Ewing (34), Wathen-Grady et al. (117, 118), Ansaruzzaman et al. (5), Pryamukhina and Khomenko (88), and Farmer (37) and from unpublished findings from the reference laboratory at the CDC, 1972 to 2005.

[b] Excludes strains previously identified as *S. boydii* 13.

wound infections but have also been isolated from infections at other body sites, while *E. fergusonii* is most frequently identified from human feces (9). *E. albertii* has recently been implicated as a possible diarrheal pathogen in humans (see below) (104). *E. blattae,* which is a commensal organism of cockroaches, is not recovered from human specimens.

Diarrheagenic *E. coli*

There are at least five categories of recognized diarrheagenic *E. coli:* Shiga toxin (ST)-producing *E. coli* (STEC) (also referred to as enterohemorrhagic *E. coli* [EHEC]), enterotoxigenic *E. coli* (ETEC), enteropathogenic *E. coli* (EPEC), enteroaggregative *E. coli* (EAEC), and enteroinvasive *E. coli* (EIEC) (53, 72). The clinical significance of several other groups of putative diarrheagenic *E. coli*, particularly diffusely adherent *E. coli* (DAEC), is unclear.

STEC: O157 and Other STEC Serogroups

We refer to the STEC category of diarrheagenic *E. coli* according to the toxins that these organisms produce, e.g., STEC rather than EHEC, because the essential genetic features that define organisms capable of causing hemorrhagic colitis and hemolytic-uremic syndrome (HUS) are not clear. *E. coli* serotypes O157:H7 and O157:nonmotile (NM) (O157 STEC) produce one or more Shiga toxins, also called verocytotoxins, and are the most frequently identified diarrheagenic *E. coli* serotypes in North America and Europe. Each year an estimated 73,000 cases of illness and 60 deaths are caused by O157 STEC in the United States (69).

E. coli O157:H7 and other STEC serotypes cause illness that can present as mild nonbloody diarrhea, severe bloody diarrhea (hemorrhagic colitis), and HUS (reviewed in reference 42). Additional symptoms of *E. coli* O157:H7 infection include abdominal cramps and lack of a high fever. Of patients with O157 STEC diarrhea, 4% or more develop HUS (90), a condition characterized by microangiopathic hemolytic anemia, thrombocytopenia, and acute renal failure. The fatality rate of HUS has declined in recent years due to improvements in case management.

O157 STEC is thought to cause at least 80% of cases of HUS in North America and is recognized as a common cause of bloody diarrhea in developed countries (90). In the United States, the rate of isolation of O157 STEC from fecal specimens is highest in the Northern tier states, where it may approach the rates of common diarrheal pathogens. Many U.S. clinical laboratories do not routinely culture stools for O157 STEC; as a result, many illnesses are not detected (24).

O157 STEC colonizes dairy and beef cattle and, therefore, ground beef has caused more O157 STEC outbreaks than any other vehicle of transmission (101). Other known vehicles of transmission include raw milk, sausage, roast beef, unchlorinated municipal water, apple cider, raw vegetables, and sprouts; these vehicles are typically exposed to water contaminated by bovine manure. O157 STEC spreads easily from person to person because the infectious dose is low (<200 CFU); outbreaks associated with person-to-person spread have occurred in schools, long-term-care institutions, families, and day-care facilities.

More than 150 non-O157 STEC serotypes have been isolated from persons with diarrhea or HUS (http://www.microbionet.com.au/frames/feature/vtec/brief01.html). In some countries, non-O157 STEC strains, particularly *E. coli* serotypes O111:NM and O26:H11, are more commonly isolated than O157 STEC, although most outbreaks and cases of HUS are attributed to the latter (serotypes characteristic of diarrheagenic *E. coli* pathotypes are presented in Table 2). In the United States, *E. coli* O157:H7 is the most frequently isolated STEC but increasingly non-O157 STEC are identified as causes of outbreaks and sporadic illness (23). At the CDC's *E. coli* Reference Laboratory, 72% of all non-O157 STEC isolates received between 1983 and 2000 belonged to eight serogroups (O26, O111, O103, O121, O45, O145, O165, and O113) (N. A. Strockbine, unpublished data). Because most laboratory methods for the detection of O157 STEC do not detect non-O157 STEC, the numbers of infections with serotypes other than O157:H7 or O157:NM are probably underestimated.

ETEC

ETEC, which produces heat-labile *E. coli* enterotoxin (LT) and/or heat-stable *E. coli* enterotoxin (ST), is an important cause of diarrhea in developing countries, particularly among young children (72). ETEC also is a frequent cause of traveler's diarrhea. Ten U.S. outbreaks were reported to the CDC from 1995 to 2001, whereas only 15 outbreaks occurred during the preceding 25 years (C. A. Bopp, unpublished data) (30). ETEC is infrequently identified in the United States, but this may be attributable in part to the fact that few laboratories are capable of identifying this pathogen. ETEC strains, particularly those associated with outbreaks, tend to cluster in a few serotypes (Table 2).

The most prominent symptoms of ETEC illness are diarrhea and abdominal cramps, sometimes accompanied by nausea and headache, but usually with little vomiting or fever (30). Although ETEC is usually associated with relatively mild watery diarrhea, illness in some recent ETEC outbreaks has been notable for its prolonged duration.

EPEC

In the past, EPEC strains were defined as certain *E. coli* serotypes that were epidemiologically associated with infantile diarrhea but did not produce enterotoxins or Shiga toxins and were not invasive. The traditional EPEC serotypes are listed in Table 2; typically these serotypes show a distinct pattern of localized adherence to HeLa and HEp-2 cells (115). These serotypes usually also demonstrate actin aggregation in the fluorescent actin stain test, which correlates with the attaching-and-effacing lesion in vivo (72). Because of the lack of simple diagnostic methods for EPEC, few laboratories attempt to identify these organisms. Full EPEC pathogenicity requires two genetic elements: the EPEC adherence factor (EAF) plasmid, which encodes most importantly the bundle-forming pilus, and the chromosomal locus of enterocyte effacement (LEE), which mediates the attaching-and-effacing phenotype. The term "typical EPEC" has been suggested for those organisms harboring both the EAF plasmid and the LEE pathogenicity island (see below). Typical

TABLE 2 Frequently encountered serotypes of diarrheagenic *E. coli*[a]

ETEC	EPEC	EIEC	STEC		EAEC
O6:NM	**O55:NM**	O28:NM	O22:H5	O118:H16	O3:H2
O6:H16	**O55:H6**	O29:NM	O22:H8	O119:NM	O15:H18
O8:H9	O55:H7	O112:NM	**O26:NM**	O119:H4	**O44:H18**
O15:H11	O86:NM	O124:NM	**O26:H11**	O119:H25	O51:H11
O20:NM	O86:H34	O124:H7	O28:H25	**O121:H19**	O77:H18
O25:NM	**O111:NM**	**O124:H30**	O45:H2	O128:NM	O86:H2
O25:H42	**O111:H2**	O136:NM	O55:H7	O128:H2	O111ab:H21
O27:NM	O111:H12	**O143:NM**	O84:NM	O128:H45	O126:H27
O27:H7	O111:H21	O144:NM	O88:H25	**O145:NM**	O141:H49
O27:H20	**O114:NM**	O152:NM	O91:NM	O146:H21	ONT:H21
O49:NM	**O114:H2**	**O164:NM**	O91:H14	O153:H2	ONT:H33
O63:H12	**O119:H6**	O167:NM	O91:H21	O153:H25	
O78:H11	**O125:H21**	**ONT:NM**	**O103:H2**	**O157:NM**	
O78:H12	O126:NM		**O104:H21**	**O157:H7**	
O128:H7	O126:H27		**O111:NM**	O165:NM	
O148:H28	**O127:NM**		**O111:H2**	O165:H25	
O153:H45	**O127:H6**		**O111:H8**	O172:NM	
O159:NM	O127:H9		**O113:H21**	O174:H21	
O159:H4	O127:H21		**O118:H2**	O174:H28	
O159:H20	**O128:H2**		O118:H12		
O167:H5	O128:H7				
O169:NM	O128:H12				
O169:H41	**O142:H6**				
	O157:H45				

[a] Outbreak-related serotypes are shown in bold type. NM, nonmotile; NT, not typeable.

EPEC correspond to EPEC of the classical serotypes and are important causes of diarrhea in developing countries (32, 72); these organisms were implicated in highly lethal nursery outbreaks in the United States and the United Kingdom before 1970. The infection is currently rare in the industrialized world. More recently, atypical EPEC have been implicated as enteric pathogens in the United States, including in several outbreaks of diarrheal disease (113). These strains possess a functional LEE apparatus but do not carry the EAF plasmid. The full role of these pathogens has yet to be elucidated, but they may be considered as potential causes of diarrheal outbreaks when no other pathogens are identified.

The symptoms of often severe, prolonged, and nonbloody diarrhea, vomiting, and fever in infants or young toddlers are characteristic of EPEC illness (72). Infection with EPEC has been associated with chronic diarrhea; sequelae may include malabsorption, malnutrition, weight loss, and growth retardation.

EIEC

EIEC strains invade cells of the colon and produce a generally watery, but occasionally bloody, diarrhea by a pathogenic mechanism similar to that of *Shigella*. EIEC is rare in the United States and is less common than ETEC or EPEC in the developing world (72). EIEC strains, like ETEC and EPEC, are associated with a few characteristic serotypes (Table 2). Three large outbreaks of diarrhea caused by EIEC have been reported in the United States (72).

EAEC

EAEC, as originally defined by its specific pattern of aggregative adherence to HEp-2 cells in culture, has been associated with diarrhea in a variety of clinical settings, including endemic diarrhea in children of both impoverished and industrialized countries, epidemic diarrhea, diarrhea of travelers to developing countries, and persistent diarrhea among patients with human immunodeficiency virus/AIDS infection (47). The pathogenicity of EAEC has been confirmed in volunteer studies (73) and by implication of EAEC in diarrhea outbreaks (28). Early studies frequently failed to find an association of EAEC with pediatric diarrhea, but this association has been strengthened by the use of molecular techniques, which discriminate the true pathogens exhibiting the aggregative pattern (29, 95). The term "typical EAEC" describes organisms harboring virulence genes under the control of the global EAEC regulator AggR (95). Typical EAEC may be a common cause of pediatric diarrhea in U.S. infants (29) and should be considered as a potential cause of foodborne outbreaks and diarrhea in human immunodeficiency virus/AIDS patients (47). EAEC diarrhea is accompanied by signs and symptoms of mild inflammation (abdominal pain and fever), but stools usually do not contain blood or fecal leukocytes (47).

Putative Diarrheagenic *E. coli*

Several putative pathotypes have been described. For none of these types has virulence clearly been demonstrated in volunteer strudies or outbreak investigations. DAEC strains, which exhibit a characteristic diffuse pattern of adherence to HEp-2 cells, have been implicated as causes of diarrhea in some epidemiologic studies but not others (72), and a prototype DAEC strain did not elicit diarrhea in adult volunteers (109). In several studies, DAEC infections have been significantly associated with watery diarrhea among children 1 to 5 years of age but were not associated with illness among infants (59). DAEC may occur in industrialized countries (72). A complex signal transduction cascade has been suggested as the mechanism of DAEC pathogenesis (99).

Cytotoxic necrotizing factor (CNF)-producing *E. coli* strains produce a toxin that induces morphological alterations (multinucleation) and death in tissue cultures (20). Two forms have been described: CNF1 and CNF2. CNF1-producing strains were originally detected in infants with enteritis and later from humans with extraintestinal infections (13, 20). Most CNF1-producing strains are also hemolytic, although the toxin is distinct from hemolysin. CNF2-producing strains have been isolated from animals with diarrhea (31, 80, 102). The role of these strains in human diarrheal disease has not been definitively determined (72).

Cytolethal distending toxin-producing *E. coli* strains produce a heat-labile factor that induces cytotonic and cytotoxic changes in Chinese hamster ovary cells similar to those caused by LT (51). This factor does not affect Y-1 cells. The results of one study in Bangladesh suggested that cytolethal distending toxin-producing *E. coli* strains are associated with diarrhea (3), but other studies are needed to establish their status as etiologic agents.

Several diarrheal outbreaks have been linked to *E. coli* strains that do not belong to any of the established pathotypes. Some of these strains carry the gene encoding the enteroaggregative ST-like toxin (EAST1), which is related to the ETEC ST enterotoxin. Further studies are needed to prove the pathogenicity of these strains, but the EAST1 gene can be identified using molecular techniques (68).

Isolation Procedures

Isolation procedures for extraintestinal infections are covered in chapter 20.

Isolation Procedures for STEC

All fecal specimens submitted for culture of bacterial enteric pathogens in areas of high endemicity or from patients with bloody diarrhea should be examined for O157 STEC (106). Culture for non-O157 STEC is indicated for patients with HUS and/or bloody diarrhea and should be considered for other patients with diarrhea based on severity of illness, age, and epidemiologic or exposure information.

Because there is no selective isolation medium for non-O157 STEC, testing for the presence of Shiga toxin in fecal specimens is the best approach for detecting these organisms. Commercial enzyme-linked immunoassays are a sensitive means of detecting Shiga toxin (33, 63). Isolation and serotyping of STEC from fecal specimens that are positive by nonculture assays should always be attempted because serotype information is important for public health purposes and may also help in clinical decisions.

Enrichment

Although broth enrichment is widely used for the recovery of O157 STEC from foods, there is little evidence that it enhances isolation from human fecal specimens. However, immunomagnetic separation (IMS), a technique shown to increase the rate of isolation of O157 STEC from food specimens, has been adapted to culture of fecal specimens (54). IMS enhances the detection of O157 STEC from patients with HUS, patients presenting an extended period of time after the onset of illness, asymptomatic carriers, or specimens that have been stored or transported improperly. IMS beads for O157, O111, and O26 are available commercially (Table 3), or laboratories may produce beads with other O-specific antibodies (81).

TABLE 3 Partial listing of commercial suppliers of reagents for detection of STEC[a]

Antisera for tube agglutination
- Difco Laboratories (Division of Becton Dickinson and Co., Sparks, Md.)
  - O157 and H7 antisera
- SA Scientific, San Antonio, Tex.
  - O157 and H7 antisera
- Denka Seiken Co., Ltd., Tokyo, Japan
  - O157, H7, O145, O128, O111, O103, O91, O26, and other *E. coli* O antisera

Latex slide agglutination reagents
- Denka Seiken Co., Ltd., Tokyo, Japan
  - O157, O111, and O26 reagents
- Oxoid Inc., Ogdensburg, N.Y.
  - O157, O145, O128, O111, O103, O91, and O26 reagents
- ProLab Diagnostics, Inc., Ontario, Canada
  - O157 and H7 reagents
- Remel, Inc., Lenexa, Kans.
  - O157 and H7 reagents

Immunomagnetic beads
- Dynal Biotech Inc., Lake Success, N.Y.
  - Anti-O157 labeled beads
- Denka Seiken Co., Ltd., Tokyo, Japan
  - Anti-O157, anti-O111, and anti-O26 labeled beads

O157 immunoassays
- Meridian Diagnostics Inc., Cincinnati, Ohio
  - For testing stool specimens or enrichment broths for O157 antigen
- Denka Seiken Co., Ltd., Tokyo, Japan
  - For testing colony sweeps or individual colonies for O157, O111, or O26 antigens

Shiga toxin immunoassays
- Meridian Diagnostics Inc., Cincinnati, Ohio
  - For testing stool specimens, enrichment broths, colony sweeps, or individual colonies for Shiga toxin
- Remel, Inc., Lenexa, Kans.
  - For testing stool specimens or enrichment broths for Shiga toxin
- Denka Seiken Co., Ltd., Tokyo, Japan
  - For testing colony sweeps or individual colonies for Shiga toxin
- Oxoid Inc., Ogdensburg, N.Y.
  - For testing individual colonies for Shiga toxin

Chromogenic agars (for visual detection of O157:H7 colonies upon direct inoculation of agar plates)
- Merck KGaA, Darmstadt, Germany
- Biomerieux Inc., Hazelwood, Mo.
- Biosynth International, Inc., Naperville, Il.
- Biolog, Inc., Hayward, Calif.
- CHROMagar; available under license to Becton Dickinson and Co., Franklin Lakes, N.J.

[a] Not intended to be a comprehensive listing. The U.S. Food and Drug Administration has not approved all of these reagents for use with clinical specimens. This table does not include reagents or tests specifically intended for examination of food, water, or environmental specimens. The online version of the *Bacteriological Analytical Manual* lists many tests for food specimens (http://www.fda.gov). Inclusion does not constitute endorsement by the CDC or ASM.

Plating Media

Because O157 STEC strains ferment lactose, they are impossible to differentiate from other lactose-fermenting organisms on lactose-containing media. Most O157 STEC strains do not ferment the carbohydrate D-sorbitol overnight, in contrast to the approximately 80% of other *E. coli* strains that ferment sorbitol rapidly. Thus, sorbitol-containing MacConkey agar (SMAC) is used for isolation of O157 STEC. Sorbitol-nonfermenting colonies are suspected (but not definitively) to be O157:H7 (67). In some areas of central Europe, sorbitol-fermenting O157 STEC strains are commonly isolated from patients with HUS (12); these organisms are very rare in North America (Strockbine, unpublished).

Specific culture media have been developed to exploit biochemical and antibiotic resistance traits that are characteristic of STEC strains. Several chromogenic agar media are available commercially to assist in rapid identification (Table 3); these media generally perform well for O157:H7 and for some non-O157 STEC (10, 65, 77) Cefixime-tellurite SMAC (CT-SMAC) has also proved to be a useful selective medium for O157:H7. It has been used mainly for culture of animal and food specimens because of its selectivity, but it has also been applied to culture of human fecal specimens (25, 124). It has been reported that some O157:NM strains fail to grow on CT-SMAC (54).

As noted above, *E. coli* strains with particular virulence in the urinary tract cannot be easily distinguished from organisms of lower virulence, and any *E. coli* isolated in high numbers (particularly $>10^5$ CFU/ml of urine) should be considered a potential pathogen. *E. coli* with increased virulence in the urinary tract is commonly hemolytic on sheep blood agar and expresses one or more of several urinary tract adhesins. Several chromogenic media have been proposed for use in detecting uropathogenic *E. coli;* these have been compared in published studies (6, 26).

Commercial Rapid Diagnostic Methods

A number of commercial immunoassays (Table 3) are now available for detecting Shiga toxin or O157 antigen in fecal specimens, enrichment broth cultures, colony sweeps, or individual colonies. Isolation of STEC from fecal specimens that are positive by one of these rapid diagnostic methods is important for public health purposes. Determination of the subtype of O157 STEC and the serotype of a non-O157 STEC isolate is valuable for outbreak investigations and surveillance purposes (see "Subtyping" and "Identification" below).

Screening Procedures for STEC Strains

For the isolation of O157 STEC from SMAC, colorless (nonfermenting) colonies are tested with O157 antiserum or latex reagent (103) (Table 3). If the O157 latex reagent is used, it is important to test positive colonies with the latex control reagent to rule out nonspecific reactions. The manufacturers of these kits recommend that strains reacting with both the antigen-specific and control latex reagents be heated and retested. However, in a study that followed this procedure, none of the nonspecifically reacting strains were subsequently identified as O157 STEC (14).

Unlike most other *E. coli* strains, O157 STEC do not express beta-glucuronidase; therefore, the MUG reaction (4-methylumbelliferyl-beta-D-glucuronide for detection of beta-glucuronidase activity) is helpful for screening for

O157 STEC (98). MUG-positive, urease-positive O157 STEC strains have been isolated in the United States but are still rare (45) (Strockbine, unpublished).

For the recovery of STEC from stool specimens which test positive for Shiga toxin, either SMAC or MacConkey agar should be inoculated. It is advantageous to use SMAC because O157 STEC can be quickly and easily identified. If sorbitol-nonfermenting colonies are negative with O157 latex, then sorbitol-fermenting colonies (because most non-O157 STEC ferment sorbitol) and a representative sample of sorbitol-nonfermenting colonies may be selected for Shiga toxin testing. Latex reagents and antisera (Table 3) for detecting certain non-O157 STEC serotypes are now available and could also be used to test colonies from Shiga toxin-positive specimens or to serogroup Shiga toxin-positive isolates.

Virtually all O157 STEC and 60 to 80% of non-O157 STEC produce a characteristic *E. coli* hemolysin, referred to as enterohemolysin (Ehly), which is distinct from the α-hemolysin, produced by other *E. coli* strains (11). A special medium, washed sheep blood agar supplemented with calcium (WSBA-Ca), is used as a differential medium for the detection of enterohemolytic activity (11). Ehly-producing colonies can be differentiated from α-hemolysin-producing colonies on WSBA-Ca because the latter are visible after 3 to 4 h of incubation. After 3 to 4 h, colonies are marked for the appearance of α-hemolysin, and the plates are examined again after 18 to 24 h. Incorporation of mitomycin C into the WSBA-Ca enhances the appearance of the Ehly hemolysis and increases the proportion of non-O157 STEC that exhibit this activity (107). Because many non-O157 STEC strains do not demonstrate the enterohemolytic phenotype and because enterohemolytic nontoxigenic strains have been reported, additional screening methods should be used in conjunction with WSBA-Ca medium (96).

Presumptive STEC isolates should be sent to a reference laboratory or a public health laboratory for further characterization.

Isolation Methods for Diarrheagenic *E. coli*

Methods for the identification of ETEC, EPEC, EIEC, EAEC, and the putative diarrheagenic *E. coli* are generally available only in reference or research settings. Public health and reference laboratories usually examine specimens for these pathogens only when an outbreak has occurred and specimens are negative for routine bacterial pathogens. EAEC should be considered as a possible etiologic agent of watery diarrhea for which no other pathogen has been identified (29), and ETEC should be considered for travelers. EPEC should be considered as a possible pathogen in outbreaks of severe nonbloody diarrhea occurring in infants or young toddlers, particularly in nursery or day care settings. EIEC and EAEC should be considered as possible etiologic agents in outbreaks of diarrhea, bloody or nonbloody.

To capture *E. coli* for further testing, fecal specimens should be plated on a differential medium of low selectivity (e.g., MAC). Five to 20 colonies, mostly lactose fermenting but with a representative sample of nonfermenting colonies, should be selected and inoculated to nonselective agar slants (such as L agar or nutrient agar). These colonies are then sent to a reference laboratory for testing or are screened for virulence-associated characteristics if assays are available. Strains can be kept frozen for long periods in L broth with 15 to 50% glycerol at −80°C. Arrangements for sending *E. coli* isolates from well-characterized outbreaks to the CDC for testing can be made through local and state health departments.

Screening Procedures for ETEC, EPEC, EAEC, and EIEC Strains

E. coli pathotypes other than STEC cannot be distinguished from other *E. coli* strains by biochemical screening techniques. Many EIEC strains are nonmotile and fail to decarboxylate lysine; however, some EIEC strains are motile or lysine positive. Use of commercial antisera to the classical EPEC somatic (O) and capsular (K) antigens is no longer recommended.

Identification

Biochemical Identification

Biochemical identification of presumptive O157 STEC isolates is necessary because other species may cross-react with O157 antiserum or latex reagents, including *Salmonella* O group N, *Yersinia enterocolitica* serotype O9, *Citrobacter freundii*, and *E. hermannii*. Special biochemical tests (cellobiose fermentation and growth in the presence of KCN) may be necessary to differentiate *E. hermannii* from *E. coli*, but because *E. hermannii* is rarely detected in stool specimens, use of these tests is not cost-effective for most laboratories.

Identification of *E. albertii* with commercial identification systems is problematic at present because representative strains of this species are not yet included in commercial databases (1). Abbott and colleagues, who extensively characterized five strains of *E. albertii* by conventional biochemical methods and by commercial identification panels, reported that *E. albertii* is an indole-negative species that ferments D-mannitol but not D-xylose (1). In their study, *E. albertii* strains were identified by commercial systems as *Hafnia alvei*; *Salmonella* or *S. enterica* serotype Cholerasuis; *E. coli*, inactive or serotype O157:H7; or *Yersinia ruckeri*. Although some strains would have been clearly misidentified, the majority of the strains generated probability scores for the final identification that were unacceptable or the identification was inconsistent with the source of the specimen (e.g., the fish pathogen *Y. ruckeri* from a human specimen), which should have triggered additional biochemical tests to establish a more reliable identification. The authors found that the most reliable clue to the possible presence of *E. albertii* was an unacceptable first-choice identification of *H. alvei* for an isolate that is both L-rhamnose and D-xylose negative.

Biochemical tests that can help discriminate *E. albertii* strains from selected members of the *Enterobacteriaceae* family with similar biochemical phenotypes are shown in Table 1. Two biogroups of *E. albertii* are listed in Table 1. These correlate with two of the distinct clusters of strains identified in the *E. albertii* lineage by phylogenetic studies (49). Biogroup 1 is comprised of the five strains isolated from Bangladeshi children with diarrhea, while biogroup 2 is comprised of strains formerly identified as *S. boydii* 13. The strains in the two biogroups differ from each other in their abilities to produce indole from tryptophane, decarboxylate lysine, and ferment D-sorbitol. Antigenic relationships between members of the *E. albertii* lineage and other members of the *Enterobacteriaceae* family have been observed (e.g., *S. boydii* 7 and *E. coli* O28). A diagnostic PCR assay using three housekeeping genes was described by Hyma et al. (49) for *E. albertii*; this assay is independent of biochemical or antigenic phenotypes and should facilitate studies to learn about the diversity within the lineage, their natural habitat, and their role in enteric disease.

Serotyping

The serologic classification of *E. coli* is generally based on the O antigen (somatic) and the H antigen (flagellar) (9).

The O and H antigens of *E. coli* are stable and reliable strain characteristics, and although 181 O antigens and 56 H antigens have been described (a few of which are no longer recognized), the actual number of serotype combinations associated with diarrheal disease is limited (Table 2). Determination of the O and H serotypes of *E. coli* strains implicated in diarrheal disease is particularly useful in epidemiologic investigations (Table 2). Even though antisera for the tube agglutination test are available from several manufacturers, most laboratories do not attempt to complete E. coli serotyping because it is costly. For well-characterized outbreaks with no identified etiologic agent, arrangements may be made through state health departments to send *E. coli* isolates to the CDC for virulence testing and serotyping.

Serologic Confirmation of O157 STEC

Confirmation of *E. coli* O157:H7 requires identification of the H7 flagellar antigen. H7-specific antisera and latex reagents are commercially available (Table 3), but detection of the H7 flagellar antigen often requires multiple passages (103). Isolates that are nonmotile or negative for the H7 antigen should be tested for the production of Shiga toxins or the presence of Shiga toxin gene sequences.

Approximately 85% of O157 isolates from humans received by the CDC are serotype O157:H7, 12% are nonmotile, and 3% are H types other than H7 (Strockbine, unpublished). *E. coli* O157:NM strains frequently produce Shiga toxin and are otherwise very similar to O157:H7, but no O157 strain from human illness with an H type other than H7 has been found to produce Shiga toxin (Strockbine, unpublished) (38).

Virulence Testing

Detection of diarrheagenic pathotypes is typically performed on *E. coli* colonies selected from selective or nonselective media. If PCR techniques are used, a sweep of confluent growth from a MAC plate may be screened; if the PCR assay is positive, isolated colonies may then be picked and screened individually. Multiplex PCR assays are capable of simultaneously detecting multiple *E. coli* pathotypes (75).

STEC

Two distinct Shiga toxins, Stx1 and Stx2, also referred to as verocytotoxins, have been described. In addition, there are several variant forms of Stx2, including Stx2c, Stx2d, Stx2e, and Stx2f, which in one study were more frequently identified from asymptomatic carriers than HUS (40). All of these toxins are similar to the Shiga toxin expressed by *Shigella dysenteriae* serotype 1, and the Stx1 toxins produced by O157 STEC and other STEC serotypes are virtually identical. STEC may produce either Stx1 or Stx2 or both toxins. The production of Stx or the genes encoding Stx can be detected by a variety of biologic, immunologic, or nucleic acid-based assays (72). Protocols for several of these tests (e.g., cell culture, DNA probing, and PCR) are available (79). Stx has also been directly detected in the blood of HUS patients by using flow cytometry even in the absence of serologic or microbiologic evidence of STEC infection (111).

STEC strains represent a spectrum of virulence potential ranging from the highly virulent O157:H7 serotype that has been responsible for the majority of outbreak cases to avirulent serotypes that have been isolated only from nonhuman sources. The presence of additional virulence factors other than Stx correlates with disease potential. The most important of these virulence factors are the intimin adhesin and the type III secretion system encoded on the LEE pathogenicity island (53). The *eae* gene probe for intimin and the *hlyA (ehxA)* gene probe for a plasmid-encoded hemolysin have been the most frequently employed methods to determine virulence potential, but probes for at least 25 different virulence-associated genes have been employed to characterize STEC strains (86). STEC have been classified into five "seropathotypes" (A through E) based on the occurrence of serotypes in human disease, in outbreaks, and in severe disease (HUS or hemorrhagic colitis) and on possession of specific virulence genes (55).

ETEC

The ST and LT enterotoxins produced by ETEC may be detected by a variety of biologic, immunologic, and nucleic acid-based assays (72). Two distinct ST variants (STh and STp) have been identified in human strains. Strains that produce ST only or ST in combination with LT have caused most ETEC outbreaks in the United States (30).

Immunoassays for the identification of ST or LT from culture supernatants of ETEC strains are available from at least two commercial sources (Table 3). The ST EIA assay (Denka Seiken Co., Ltd., and Oxoid Ltd.) is a competitive enzyme immunoassay for the detection of ST only (97). A reversed passive latex agglutination assay (VET-RPLA; Oxoid; a similar kit is available from Denka Seiken) detects both cholera toxin and LT, which are highly related antigenically. The effectiveness of the VET-RPLA may be optimized by use of a culture medium designed for LT production such as Biken's medium rather than the medium recommended by the manufacturer (122).

EPEC

EPEC, EAEC, and DAEC can be detected by the characteristic patterns of adherence to HEp-2 or HeLa cells in culture (115). These patterns are also observed on formalin or glutaraldehyde-fixed cells, obviating the need to prepare cells expressly for the assay (70).

EPEC are defined on the basis of the attaching/effacing (A/E) histopathology produced on epithelial cells and the lack of Stx (reviewed in references 32 and 53). The A/E phenotype can be detected by tissue culture cell assays or by DNA probe or PCR tests for the *eae* gene encoding intimin or the LEE pathogenicity island. The EAF plasmid of typical EPEC (see above) is detected by fragment or oligonucleotide probes or PCR primers (72). Atypical EPEC possess only the A/E phenotype/LEE pathogenicity island but do not possess the EAF plasmid.

EAEC

Several simple assays have been described as surrogates to the cell adherence test for identification of EAEC. These include a simple biofilm formation assay on polystyrene (123) and screening for the presence of a pellicle at the surface of broth media (4). EAEC can be more definitively identified by a specific DNA probe (the AA or CVD432 probe) (7), which is superior to tissue culture adherence assays in identifying pathogenic strains of EAEC (29). More recent data suggest that the AA probe corresponds to a putative virulence gene called *aatA* (76), which is under the control of a regulator termed AggR. AggR in turn controls several other virulence factors (95). Thus, the *aggR* gene (which defines typical EAEC) may represent a superior diagnostic target.

EIEC

EIEC can be identified by various in vivo assays, immunoassays, and nucleic acid-based assays for invasiveness, but no commercial kits or reagents are available. Cell culture invasion assays or DNA-based assays for the *ipaC* or *ipaH* invasion-related factors are, for the most part, practical only in research settings (72). Plasmid DNA electrophoresis may be used to detect the large 120- to 140-MDa plasmid associated with invasiveness, but this plasmid is easily lost when the isolate is subcultured. Because of shared invasiveness-related characteristics, these assays also detect *Shigella* strains.

DAEC

DAEC were initially defined on the basis of a diffuse adherence pattern to cultured epithelial cells, but this phenotype is not specific for enteric strains (99). Various DNA probes and PCR assays have been proposed for DAEC identification as reviewed (72).

Extraintestinal *E. coli*

The presence of any *E. coli* in urine specimens at 10^5 CFU/ml (or lower in some situations) or in cerebrospinal fluid or blood specimens in any amount is indicative of infection and the need for treatment. Numerous virulence factors have been identified for extraintestinal *E. coli* (53), particularly the K1 antigen, but these are usually identified only in epidemiological studies.

Subtyping

Several methods of subtyping have been used for *E. coli* O157:H7 isolates. In particular, pulsed-field gel electrophoresis (PFGE) methods are useful (72). A national molecular subtyping network, PulseNet, was established in 1996 by the CDC to facilitate subtyping of bacterial foodborne pathogens, including *E. coli* O157:H7, *Shigella,* nontyphoidal *Salmonella* serotypes, and *Listeria monocytogenes* (108). Successful detection of outbreaks by this network of state and local public health laboratories is dependent upon submission of isolates by clinical laboratories for confirmation and subtyping.

Determination of the serotype and the antimicrobial susceptibility pattern is usually adequate for defining outbreak strains of ETEC, EPEC, and EIEC. Plasmid typing or PFGE methods may also be helpful for distinguishing between sporadic isolates and outbreak strains, but neither method has been widely used for these groups of *E. coli.*

Serodiagnostic Tests

At the present time, serodiagnostic tests for diarrheagenic *E. coli* are valuable only for seroepidemiology surveys and are not useful for the diagnosis of sporadic infections. Assays that measure serum antibody response to lipopolysaccharide (LPS) have been used to detect STEC infection in culture-negative HUS patients (72). Enzyme-linked immunosorbent assays have been described to detect saliva antibodies to LPS (62) and serum antibodies to the secreted EspB protein in HUS patients (100).

Antimicrobial Susceptibilities

STEC

Antimicrobial therapy for O157 STEC diarrhea or HUS is controversial: some publications have suggested that antibiotics increase the risk of HUS (42, 121), while a meta-analysis of published reports found no significantly increased risk (94). Until recently, *E. coli* O157:H7 isolates were almost uniformly sensitive to antimicrobial agents. However, since the early 1990s, O157 and other STEC strains have demonstrated slowly increasing levels of resistance to certain antibiotics, particularly streptomycin, sulfonamides, and tetracycline (see http://www.cdc.gov/narms/).

ETEC, EPEC, EIEC, EAEC, and Other Diarrheagenic *E. coli* Strains

Treatment with an appropriate antibiotic can reduce the severity and duration of symptoms of ETEC infection (72). Antimicrobial resistance, particularly to tetracycline, is common among ETEC strains isolated from outbreaks in the United States (30). Antibiotic treatment may be helpful for diarrhea caused by EPEC (72). Most EPEC strains associated with outbreaks are resistant to multiple antimicrobial agents (32). EAEC are commonly resistant to most antibiotics, though these strains are typically sensitive to fluoroquinolones. Clinical studies have demonstrated the effectiveness of ciprofloxacin for travelers with diarrhea caused by EAEC (41). Little information about the efficacy of antimicrobial treatment or the prevalence of resistance is available for EIEC or other putative diarrheagenic *E. coli* strains, but determination of the antimicrobial susceptibility pattern may be helpful in establishing whether the isolates are associated with an outbreak.

Interpretation and Reporting of Results

STEC

A presumptive diagnosis of an O157 STEC (isolate positive for O157 antigen) or a non-O157 STEC (isolate positive for Shiga toxin) infection should be reported to the clinician as soon as the laboratory obtains this result. It is advisable to indicate on negative reports that non-O157 STEC strains can cause diarrhea and HUS. Clusters and outbreaks of STEC should be reported to public health authorities. Presumptive STEC isolates should be confirmed by demonstration of the O157 and H7 antigens or assay for Shiga toxin and should be identified biochemically as *E. coli.* STEC isolates should be forwarded to a local or state public health laboratory for serotyping and/or molecular subtyping.

ETEC, EPEC, EAEC, and EIEC

Generally, the ETEC, EPEC, EAEC, and EIEC classes of diarrheagenic *E. coli* are identified only during outbreak investigations. A laboratorian reporting these results, which usually will be a retrospective diagnosis obtained by a reference laboratory, should provide an explanation of the clinical significance of these organisms and may refer the clinician to the reference laboratory for further information. All suspected outbreaks should be reported to public health authorities.

SHIGELLA

Description of the Genus and Taxonomy

The genus *Shigella* is composed of nonmotile bacteria that conform to the definition of the family *Enterobacteriaceae* (35). There are four subgroups of *Shigella* that historically have been treated as species: subgroup A as *S. dysenteriae,* subgroup B as *Shigella flexneri,* subgroup C as *Shigella boydii,* and subgroup D as *Shigella sonnei.* From a genetic standpoint, the four species of *Shigella* and *E. coli* represent a single genomospecies (56). Using a genetic definition for species, the four species of *Shigella* would be regarded as serologically defined anaerogenic biotypes of *E. coli.* The current nomenclature of *Shigella* is maintained largely for medical purposes because of the useful association of the genus epithet with

TABLE 4 Differentiation of *E. coli* and *Shigella*

Test	Result[a] of test with:		
	Shigella	Inactive *E. coli*[b]	*E. coli*
Lysine decarboxylase	–	d	+
Motility	–	–	+
Gas from glucose	–	–	+
Acetate utilization	–	d	+
Mucate	–	d	+
Lactose	–	d	+

[a] Abbreviations: +, 90% or more positive within 1 or 2 days;–, no reaction (90% or more) in 7 days; d, different reactions [+, (+), –]. Adapted from Ewing (35).

[b] Nonmotile, anaerogenic biotypes sometimes referred to as Alkalescens-Dispar bioserotypes.

the distinctive disease (shigellosis) caused by these organisms. The type species is *S. dysenteriae*. *Shigella* does not form gas from fermentable carbohydrates, with the exception of certain strains of *S. flexneri* serotype 6 and *S. boydii* serotype 14. Compared with *Escherichia*, *Shigella* strains are less active in their use of carbohydrates (Table 4). *S. sonnei* strains ferment lactose on extended incubation, but other species generally do not use this substrate in conventional medium.

Recent findings from phylogenetic studies show that *S. boydii* 13 strains, some of which can produce gas from glucose, are more appropriately regarded as *E. albertii* (49). *S. boydii* 13 strains were first described in 1952 and then added to the *Shigella* scheme in 1958 (36).

Epidemiology and Transmission

Humans and other large primates are the only natural reservoirs of *Shigella* bacteria. Most transmission is by person-to-person spread, but infection is also caused by ingestion of contaminated food or water. Shigellosis is most common in situations in which hygiene is compromised (e.g., child care centers and other institutional settings). In developing populations without running water and indoor plumbing, shigellosis can become endemic. Sexual transmission of *Shigella* among men who have sex with men also occurs.

In the United States, an estimated 450,000 cases of shigellosis occur each year, with 70 deaths (69). Up to 20% of all U.S. cases of shigellosis are related to international travel. Most infections in the United States and other developed countries are caused by *S. sonnei; S. flexneri* is the second most common serogroup (44). In the developing world, the most prevalent *Shigella* species are *S. flexneri* and *S. dysenteriae* 1, with the latter being the most frequent cause of epidemic dysentery. Infection with *S. dysenteriae* 1 is associated with high rates of morbidity and mortality in developing countries, particularly when antimicrobial resistance or its misdiagnosis delays appropriate treatment.

Clinical Significance

Members of the genus *Shigella* have been recognized since the late 19th century as causative agents of bacillary dysentery. *Shigella* causes bloody diarrhea (dysentery) and nonbloody diarrhea. Shigellosis often begins with watery diarrhea accompanied by fever and abdominal cramps but may progress to classic dysentery with scant stools containing blood, mucus, and pus. Ulcerations, which are restricted to the large intestine and rectum, typically do not penetrate beyond the lamina propria. Bloodstream infections can occur but are rare. All four subgroups of *Shigella* are capable of causing dysentery, but *S. dysenteriae* serotype 1 has been associated with a particularly severe form of illness thought to be related in part to its production of Shiga toxin. Infection can occasionally be asymptomatic, particularly infection with *S. sonnei* strains. Complications of shigellosis include HUS, which is associated with *S. dysenteriae* 1 infection, and Reiter chronic arthritis syndrome, which is associated with *S. flexneri* infection (2). The identification of *Shigella* species is important for both clinical and epidemiologic purposes.

Isolation Procedures

Enrichment and Plating Media

There is no reliable enrichment medium for all *Shigella* isolates, but gram-negative broth and Selenite broth are frequently used. For the optimal isolation of *Shigella*, two different selective media should be used: a general-purpose plating medium of low selectivity (e.g., MAC) and a more selective agar medium (e.g., xylose lysine desoxycholate agar [XLD]). Desoxycholate citrate agar (DCA) and Hektoen Enteric agar (HE) are suitable alternatives to XLD as media with moderate to high selectivities. Salmonella-Shigella agar (SS) should be used with caution because it inhibits the growth of some strains of *S. dysenteriae* 1.

Screening Procedures

Shigella strains appear as lactose- or xylose-nonfermenting colonies on the isolation media described above. *S. dysenteriae* 1 colonies may be smaller on all of these media, and these strains generally grow best on media with low selectivities (e.g., MAC). *S. dysenteriae* 1 colonies on XLD agar are frequently very tiny, unlike other *Shigella* species. *S. sonnei* colonies often appear flattened and spread out on blood agar plates.

Suspect colonies may be screened biochemically or serologically on Kligler iron agar [KIA] or triple sugar iron agar [TSI]. *Shigella* species characteristically produce an alkaline slant and an acid butt (K/A) but do not produce gas or H_2S. A few strains of *S. flexneri* 6 and a very few strains of *S. boydii* produce gas in KIA or TSI. The motility and the lysine decarboxylase tests are characteristically negative for *Shigella* and can be used to further screen isolates before serologic testing (Table 4). Isolates that react appropriately with the screening biochemicals should then be identified with a complete set of biochemical tests, with automated systems or self-contained commercial kits being satisfactory, and should be tested with grouping antisera. Confirmation requires both biochemical and serologic identification, and laboratories that do not perform both types of tests should send *Shigella* isolates to a reference laboratory for confirmation.

Identification

Biochemical

Because the somatic antigens of most serotypes of *Shigella* are either identical or related to those of *E. coli*, suspicious cultures that are serologically negative should be tested further biochemically (35). *Shigella* and inactive *E. coli* (anaerogenic or lactose nonfermenting) are frequently difficult to distinguish by routine biochemical tests. See Table 4 for the biochemical reactions characteristic of *Shigella* spp. Although *S. dysenteriae* and *S. sonnei* are biochemically distinct, *S. flexneri* and *S. boydii* are often biochemically indistinguishable, so that serologic grouping is essential.

Serotyping

Serologic testing is essential for the identification of *Shigella*. Three of the four subgroups, A *(S. dysenteriae)*, B *(S. flexneri)*, and C *(S. boydii)*, are made up of a number of serotypes. Subgroup A has 15 serotypes; subgroup B has 8 serotypes (with serotypes 1 to 5 subdivided into 11 subserotypes); and subgroup C has 19 serotypes numbered 1 through 20, with *S. boydii* 13 reclassified as *E. albertii*. Subgroup D *(S. sonnei)* is made up of a single serotype. Subgroups A and C are rare. Several provisional *Shigella* serotypes have also been described, which are held sub judice until findings from the characterization of representative isolates show them to be unique. Antisera for the identification of provisional serotypes are typically available only at reference laboratories.

Serologic identification is typically performed by slide agglutination with polyvalent somatic (O) antigen grouping sera, followed, in some cases, by testing with monovalent antisera for specific serotype identification. Monovalent antiserum to *S. dysenteriae* 1 is required to identify this serotype and is not widely available. Because of the potentially serious nature of illness associated with this serotype, isolates that agglutinate in subgroup A reagent should be sent to a reference laboratory immediately for further serotyping.

Biochemically typical *Shigella* isolates that agglutinate poorly or that do not agglutinate at all should be suspended in saline and heated in a water bath at 100°C for 15 to 30 min. After cooling, the antigen suspension is tested in normal saline to determine if it is rough (agglutinates spontaneously). If the heated and cooled suspension is not rough, it may then be retested for agglutination in antisera.

Subtyping

A variety of methods have been used to subtype *Shigella*, including colicin typing (particularly for *S. sonnei*), plasmid profiling, restriction fragment length polymorphism analysis, PFGE, and ribotyping (105). For an overview of the epidemiologic use of typing methods, refer to chapter 12 in this Manual.

Serodiagnostic Tests

Several serodiagnostic assays based on different antigens possessed by *Shigella* have been described (61, 114). These assays are practical only in research settings for seroepidemiology surveys and are not currently used for the diagnosis of infection in individual patients.

Antimicrobial Susceptibilities

Shigella infections are often treated with antimicrobial agents. Because of the widespread antimicrobial resistance among *Shigella* strains, all isolates should undergo susceptibility testing (http://www.cdc.gov/narms/). Reporting of susceptibility results to the clinician is particularly important for *S. dysenteriae* 1 isolates. Infections caused by these strains are often acquired during international travel to areas where most strains are multidrug resistant (110). In many areas of Africa and Asia, *S. dysenteriae* 1 strains are resistant to all locally available antimicrobial agents, including nalidixic acid, but are still susceptible to the fluoroquinolones (93); however, fluoroquinolone-resistant strains have been reported in south Asia.

Interpretation and Reporting of Results

A preliminary report of suspected *Shigella* infection may be issued if biochemical or serologic screening tests are positive. If serotyping results are available, these should also be reported, particularly if the isolate is *S. dysenteriae* 1. All *Shigella* isolates should be tested for antimicrobial susceptibility. Before issuing a final report, isolates should be confirmed by both serologic and biochemical methods. Isolates, particularly those from individuals with dysentery-like illness, that are biochemically identified as *Shigella* but that are serologically negative may be new serotypes of *Shigella* and should be sent to a reference laboratory for further characterization. Isolates from sites other than the gastrointestinal tract and which resemble *Shigella* should be carefully scrutinized for gas production and other differentiating characteristics. These isolates should be sent to a reference laboratory for confirmation because they are more likely to be anaerogenic *E. coli*, certain strains of which may cross-react with *Shigella* antiserum.

SALMONELLA

Description of the Genus

The genus *Salmonella* is composed of motile bacteria that conform to the definition of the family *Enterobacteriaceae* (35). The nomenclature employed to describe the genus *Salmonella* had been problematic for many years, due to the use of multiple schemes in the literature and the historical practice of considering different serotypes of *Salmonella* to be different species. The publication of Judicial Opinion 80 in 2005 (112) will hopefully serve to clarify nomenclatural issues regarding the genus *Salmonella*, and the conventions set forth in that opinion are used here. *Salmonella* history and nomenclature are reviewed at the following website: http://www.bacterio.cict.fr/s/salmonella.html.

The genus *Salmonella* is composed of two species, *Salmonella enterica* and *Salmonella bongori* (formerly subspecies V) (91). *Salmonella enterica* has been subdivided into six subspecies: *S. enterica* subsp. *enterica*, designated subspecies I; *S. enterica* subsp. *salamae*, subspecies II; *S. enterica* subsp. *arizonae*, subspecies IIIa; *S. enterica* subsp. *diarizonae*, subspecies IIIb; *S. enterica* subsp. *houtenae*, subspecies IV; and *S. enterica* subsp. *indica*, subspecies VI. The type species is *S. enterica* subsp. *enterica*. Subspecies IIIa and IIIb represent organisms originally described in the genus *"Arizona"*; subspecies IIIa contains the monophasic strains and subspecies IIIb contains the diphasic strains of "*Arizona*" (92). Despite their common history, subspecies IIIa and IIIb are more closely related to some of the other subspecies of *Salmonella enterica* than they are to each other and thus should be considered separate entities (120).

Subspecies I strains are commonly isolated from humans and warm-blooded animals. Subspecies II, IIIa, IIIb, IV, and VI strains and *S. bongori* are usually isolated from cold-blooded animals and the environment. Non-subspecies I strains are typically considered rare human pathogens; they make up about 1 to 2% of *Salmonella* isolates reported to the U.S. National *Salmonella* surveillance system (22). The biochemical tests useful for identification of *Salmonella* and for subspecies differentiation are given in Table 5.

Salmonella Serotypes

Salmonella serotyping is a subtyping method based on the immunologic characterization of three surface structures: O antigen, which is the outermost portion of the LPS layer that covers the bacterial cell; H antigen, which is the filament portion of the bacterial flagella; and Vi antigen, which is a capsular polysaccharide present in specific serotypes. Serotyping of *Salmonella* is commonly performed to facilitate public health

TABLE 5 Biochemical reactions useful for differentiating *Salmonella* species and subspecies[a]

Test	Species or subspecies (no. of strains tested)						
	S. enterica						*S. bongori* (16)
	I (650)	II (146)	IIIa (120)	IIIb (155)	IV (120)	VI (9)	
Dulcitol	+	+	–	–	–	d[b]	+
Lactose	–	–	–[c]	+[d]	–	d[e]	–
ONPG (*o*-nitrophenyl-β-D-galactopyranoside)	–	–[f]	+	+	–	d[g]	+
Salicin	–	–	–	–	+[h]	–	–
Sorbitol	+	+	+	+	+	–	+
Galacturonate	–	+	–	+	+	+	+
Malonate	–	+	+	+	–	–	–
Mucate	+	+	+	–[i]	–	+	+
Growth in KCN	–	–	–	–	+	–	+
Gelatin (strip)	–	+	+	+	+	+	–
L(+)-Tartrate (*d*-tartrate[j])	+	–	–	–	–	–	–

[a] Reactions after incubation at 37°C. +, 90% or more positive within 1 or 2 days; (+), positive reaction after 3 or more days; –, no reaction (90% or more) in 7 days; d, different reactions [+, (+), –]; KCN, potassium cyanide. Adapted from Ewing (35).

[b] A total of 67% were positive.

[c] A total of 15% were positive.

[d] A total of 85% were positive.

[e] A total of 22% were positive.

[f] A total of 15% were positive.

[g] A total of 44% were positive.

[h] A total of 60% were positive.

[i] A total of 30% were positive.

[j] Sodium potassium tartrate (35).

surveillance for *Salmonella* infection and to aid in the recognition of outbreaks. The serotype of an isolate often correlates with a particular disease syndrome or food vehicle, making serotype data particularly useful in identifying cases and defining outbreaks. For example, *Salmonella* serotype Typhi causes typhoid fever, a more severe disease syndrome than those caused by most other *Salmonella* serotypes. *Salmonella* serotype Enteritidis is associated with infections acquired from chicken or egg products (82). Further, *Salmonella* serotyping is performed worldwide and has aided in the recognition of international outbreaks (64). *Salmonella* serotypes Enteritidis and Typhimurium are the two most common serotypes in the United States, making up approximately 35 to 40% of all culture-confirmed infections (22).

Clinical Significance

Strains of *Salmonella* are categorized as typhoidal and nontyphoidal, corresponding to the disease syndrome with which they are associated. Strains of nontyphoidal *Salmonella* usually cause an intestinal infection (accompanied by diarrhea, fever, and abdominal cramps) that often lasts 1 week or longer (46). Less commonly, nontyphoidal *Salmonella* can cause extraintestinal infections (e.g., bacteremia, urinary tract infection, or osteomyelitis), especially in immunocompromised persons. Persons of all ages are affected; the incidence is highest in infants and young children. *Salmonella* is ubiquitous in animal populations, and human illness is usually linked to foods of animal origin. Salmonellosis also is transmitted by direct contact with animals, by nonanimal foods, by water, and occasionally, by human contact. Each year, an estimated 1.4 million cases of illness and 600 deaths are caused by nontyphoidal salmonellosis in the United States (69).

Typhoid fever, caused by *Salmonella* serotype Typhi, is a serious bloodstream infection common in the developing world. However, it is rare in the United States, where an estimated 800 cases, with fewer than 5 deaths, occur each year; >70% of U.S. cases are related to foreign travel (69). Typhoid fever typically presents with a sustained debilitating high fever and headache. Adults characteristically present without diarrhea. Illness is milder in young children, where it may manifest as nonspecific fever. Humans are the only reservoir for *Salmonella* serotype Typhi, indicating that this serotype is adapted to the human host; healthy carriers have been noted. Typhoid fever typically has a low infectious dose (<10^3) and a long, highly variable incubation period (1 to 6 weeks). It is transmitted through person-to-person contact or fecally contaminated food and water. Fatal complications of typhoid most commonly occur in the second or third week of illness.

A syndrome similar to typhoid fever is caused by "paratyphoidal" strains of *Salmonella*, *Salmonella* serotypes Paratyphi A, Paratyphi B, and Paratyphi C. Serotypes Paratyphi A and Paratyphi C are rare in the United States (22). Serotype Paratyphi B is a diverse serotype that is associated with both paratyphoid fever and gastroenteritis (87). The two pathovars are typically differentiated on the basis of the ability to ferment tartrate; isolates causing paratyphoid fever, the systemic pathovar, are tartrate negative. Isolates associated with gastroenteritis, the enteric pathovar, are typically tartrate positive and are referred to as *Salmonella* Paratyphi B var. L(+)-tartrate + or *Salmonella* Paratyphi B var. Java. The systemic pathovar of *Salmonella* Paratyphi B is considered to be rare in the United States; however, the tartrate reaction is often not reported, making it impossible to distinguish between the two pathovars (22).

Salmonella serotypes Choleraesuis and Dublin are host adapted to cattle and pigs, respectively, causing serious disease in these two animal species. They rarely cause human infection, but such infections are typically severe, with spread to extraintestinal sites (66, 116). *Salmonella* serotype

Dublin has been shown to share virulence traits with *Salmonella* serotype Typhi, which may contribute to its invasiveness in humans (71, 83).

Isolation Procedures

Enrichment

Maximal recovery of *Salmonella* from fecal specimens is obtained by using an enrichment broth, although isolation from acutely ill persons is usually possible by direct plating of specimens. Enrichment broths for *Salmonella* are usually highly selective and inhibit certain serotypes of *Salmonella,* particularly *Salmonella* serotype Typhi. The three selective enrichment media most widely used to isolate *Salmonella* from fecal specimens are tetrathionate broth, tetrathionate broth with brilliant green, and Selenite broth (SEL). SEL may also be used for the recovery of *Salmonella* serotype Typhi and *Shigella,* although its value as enrichment for the latter has not been clearly established. Specimens that might contain organisms inhibited by selective enrichment broths should be plated directly or cultured in a nonselective enrichment broth (e.g., gram-negative broth).

A number of commercial rapid diagnostic tests are available for the testing of foods, but to our knowledge, none has been evaluated in the literature for use with fecal specimens.

Plating Media

Many differential plating media, varying from slightly selective to highly selective, are available for isolation of *Salmonella* from fecal specimens. Media of low selectivity include MAC and eosin methylene blue. Media of intermediate selectivity include XLD, desoxycholate citrate agar, Salmonella-Shigella agar, and HE. Highly selective media include bismuth sulfite agar, the preferred medium for the isolation of *Salmonella* serotype Typhi, and brilliant green agar. Bismuth sulfite agar, XLD, and HE all have H_2S indicator systems, which are helpful for the detection of lactose-positive *Salmonella*. Most laboratories today use HE or XLD because these media may also be used for the isolation of *Shigella*.

In the developing world, typhoid fever is frequently diagnosed solely on clinical grounds, but isolation of the causative organism is necessary for a definitive diagnosis. *Salmonella* serotype Typhi is more frequently isolated from blood cultures than from fecal specimens. Blood cultures are positive for 80% of typhoid patients during the first week of fever but show decreasing positive results thereafter.

Screening Procedures

A latex agglutination kit has been described for screening for *Salmonella* from SEL enrichment broth (Wellcolex Color *Salmonella;* Remel Inc., Lenexa, Kans.) (15). This kit can also be used to screen individual colonies from primary plates. In using this kit, it should be kept in mind that it identifies only those *Salmonella* isolates belonging to the more common O serogroups and it does not differentiate between O groups C_1 and C_2.

Suspect colonies may be inoculated onto a screening medium such as KIA or TSI. On KIA or TSI, most *Salmonella* strains produce a K/AG + reaction, indicating that glucose is fermented with gas, and H_2S is produced. On these media, *Salmonella* serotype Typhi isolates are characteristically K/A but do not produce gas and only a small amount of H_2S is visible at the site of the stab and in the stab line. Lysine iron agar is also a useful screening medium because most *Salmonella* isolates, even those that ferment lactose, decarboxylate lysine and produce H_2S. Alternately, isolates may be identified by a battery of biochemical tests or by slide agglutination with antisera for *Salmonella* O groups. Isolates suspected of being *Salmonella* serotype Typhi should be tested serologically with *Salmonella* Vi and O group D antisera (see below).

If the biochemical reactions for a particular isolate are not characteristic but *Salmonella* antigens are found, the cultures should be plated on MAC or eosin methylene blue to obtain a pure culture, tested with a complete set of biochemical tests, or forwarded to a reference laboratory.

Identification

Clinical laboratories may issue a preliminary report of *Salmonella* when an isolate is positive either with *Salmonella* O group antisera or by biochemical identification methods. An isolate is confirmed as *Salmonella* when the specific O serogroup has been determined and biochemical identification has been completed.

Biochemical Identification

Suspect colonies from one of the differential plating media mentioned above can be identified biochemically as *Salmonella* spp. with traditional media in tubes or commercial biochemical systems. Methods of biochemical identification and specific commercial manual and automated identification systems are covered in chapter 15. The species and subspecies of *Salmonella* can be identified biochemically, as indicated in Table 5.

Serotyping

O serogroup determination is adequate for confirmation of isolates as *Salmonella.* Full serotype determination is useful for public health surveillance but is beyond the scope of most routine clinical laboratories. The methods described below for serotyping are intended primarily for reference laboratories. *Salmonella* isolates are serotyped based on the antigenic properties of their O (somatic) antigens, H (flagellar) antigens, and Vi (capsular) antigen (17). O antigen is a carbohydrate antigen and is the outermost component of LPS. It is a polymer of O subunits; each O subunit is typically composed of four to six sugars depending on the O antigen. O antigens are designated by numbers and are divided into O serogroups based on antigenic factors associated with the O subunit. Many of the common O groups were originally designated by letter and are still commonly referred to by letter (e.g., serotype Typhimurium belongs to group O:4 or group B, serotype Enteritidis belongs to group O:9 or group D1). Additional O antigenic factors have been identified for specific O groups. They are typically associated with a side sugar that is added to the basic O subunit structure, and they are often variably present or variably expressed within O groups or within serotypes.

H antigen is a protein antigen called flagellin; multiple flagellin subunits make up the flagellar filament. The ends of flagellin are conserved and give the flagellum its characteristic filament structure; the antigenically variable portion of flagellin is the middle region, which is surface exposed. Salmonellae are unique among the enteric bacteria in that they commonly express two different flagellin antigens, although specific serotypes such as Typhi and Enteritidis possess only one flagellar antigen. The two flagellar antigens are referred to as phase 1 and phase 2; monophasic and diphasic strains express one or two flagellar antigens, respectively. Individual flagellar antigens can be composed of multiple antigenic factors. For example, the phase 2 flagellar antigen of serotype Typhimurium is antigen 1,2, which is composed of two antigenic factors, 1 and 2.

Many of the O and H antigenic types are found in multiple subspecies, and isolates from different subspecies can have the same antigenic profile. Thus, subspecies determination is an integral component of serotype determination for *Salmonella*. The serotype for all *Salmonella* strains can be designated by an antigenic formula; additionally, serotypes belonging to subspecies I are given a name which is typically related to the geographical place where the serotype was first isolated (84). The antigenic formulae of *Salmonella* serotypes are listed in the Kauffmann-White scheme and are expressed as follows: O antigen(s), Vi (when present): phase 1 H antigen(s): phase 2 H antigen(s) (when present). For example, the antigenic formula for *Salmonella* serotype Typhimurium is 4,5,12:i:1,2. Serotype names for subspecies I serotypes are written in roman (not italicized) letters, and the first letter is a capital letter (for example, *Salmonella* serotype [ser.] Typhimurium or *Salmonella* Typhimurium [19]). Serotypes belonging to other subspecies are designated by their antigenic formulae following the subspecies name (for example, *S. enterica* subsp. *salamae* ser. 50:z:e,n,x or *Salmonella* serotype II 50:z:e,n,x).

The WHO Collaborating Centre for Reference and Research on *Salmonella,* which is located at the Pasteur Institute in Paris, France, maintains the Kauffmann-White Scheme for the designation of *Salmonella* serotypes (84). The Kauffmann-White scheme is updated annually with a listing of new serotypes (85). Currently, there are 2,541 recognized *Salmonella* serotypes; the majority belong to subspecies I (1,504 serotypes [85]). Most common serotypes belong to O groups A, B, C_1, C_2, D_1, and E_1 (also known as groups O:2, O:4, O:7; O:8; O:9, and O:3,10, respectively). Serotypes belonging to subspecies II (502 serotypes), IIIa (95 serotypes), IIIb (333 serotypes), IV (72 serotypes), VI (13 serotypes), and *S. bongori* (22 serotypes) are primarily found in O groups O:11 (F) through O:67 (commonly referred to as the higher O groups).

Determination of O Antigens

O (heat-stable, somatic) antigens are identified by first testing the isolate in antisera that detects one or multiple antigenic factors corresponding to the O groups (O grouping antisera). Once the O group is determined, antisera that recognize single antigenic factors are used to confirm the O group and identify any additional antigenic factors that are associated with that O group (O single-factor antisera) (18). The approach most commonly used for determining O antigens is to initially test the isolates by slide agglutination in antisera against O groups A to E_1 because approximately 95% of *Salmonella* isolates belong to one of these O groups. If no agglutination occurs in antisera for these O groups, the isolate is tested in pools containing the remaining *Salmonella* O antisera, O:11 through O:67.

Determination of H Antigens

H (flagellar) antigens are typically determined by tube agglutination tests using broth cultures. Isolates are initially tested with H typing antisera, which recognize individual or multiple antigenic factors, and then with H single-factor antisera, which recognize individual antigenic factors. Typically, the flagellar antigens in a diphasic strain are coordinately regulated so that only one is expressed at time in a single bacterial cell; however, both phases may be detected in the whole culture, particular with a fresh clinical isolate. When only one phase is detected (either phase 1 or phase 2), the strain should be inoculated into a semisolid medium to which sterile antiserum to the detected flagellar antigen has aseptically been added. Growth of the strain in this semisolid agar immobilizes cells expressing the detected antigen and allows the growth of bacteria expressing the antigen in the other phase. After phase reversal, the strain is tested in appropriate H typing and single-factor antisera to complete the serotyping. A strain must be actively motile to ensure the good expression of H antigens; sometimes it must be passed through one or more tall tubes of semisolid agar to enhance motility before H antigens can be detected.

Detection of the Vi Antigen and Identification of *Salmonella* Serotype Typhi (9,12,[Vi]:d:-)

The Vi antigen, a heat-labile capsular polysaccharide, is useful for the identification of *Salmonella* serotype Typhi. It is also occasionally detected in *Salmonella* serotype Dublin, *Salmonella* serotype Paratyphi C, and some *Citrobacter* strains, so its detection does not constitute definitive evidence of *Salmonella* serotype Typhi. Vi antigen is identified by slide agglutination with specific antiserum.

If *Salmonella* serotype Typhi is suspected, the culture is first tested live (unheated) in O group D antiserum (which contains antibodies to O antigens 9 and 12) and Vi antiserum on a slide. The Vi capsular polysaccharide can mask the O antigens, blocking their reactivity with the O grouping antiserum. If only the Vi antiserum is positive, the bacterial suspension is heated in boiling water for 15 min to remove the capsule, cooled, and tested again in the same antisera. After heating, *Salmonella* serotype Typhi isolates will be negative in the Vi antiserum but positive in the O group D antiserum. Expression of the Vi antigen by *Salmonella* serotype Typhi is variable but tends to occur more frequently in freshly isolated cultures than in cultures that have been subcultured. If the strain is typical for *Salmonella* serotype Typhi on TSI or KIA (see "Screening Procedures" above), is urease negative, and reacts in O group D or Vi antiserum, a presumptive report is made. The identity of the isolate is confirmed by biochemical testing (Table 5) and determination of the H (flagellar) antigen (see below) before a final report is issued. *Salmonella* serotype Typhi strains typically express only one flagellar antigen, Hd.

Identification Problems

Several potential problems may prevent accurate serotype determination. The strain may express the Vi capsular antigen, which can block the binding of antibodies against the O antigens. The strain may be rough, i.e., fails to make complete O antigens. Rough strains have a tendency to weakly agglutinate in multiple O grouping antisera. The strain may be mucoid and not agglutinate in any O antisera, or isolates can be nonmotile and not express any flagellar antigens. Among isolates submitted to the National *Salmonella* Reference Laboratory at the CDC, isolates from urine are frequently rough, mucoid, and/or nonmotile. When O antigen and/or H antigens are not detected, a strain is confirmed as a *Salmonella* species by characterization of any antigens that are expressed and by biochemical testing (Table 5).

Many laboratories are likely to overlook *Salmonella* serotype Paratyphi A because they do not screen with O group A antiserum or because it is H_2S negative, lysine negative, and citrate negative. *Salmonella* serotypes Paratyphi B and Paratyphi B var. L(+)-tartrate + (var. Java) can be confused because they have an identical antigenic formula (4,5,12:b:1,2), but they are distinguished biochemically by their tartrate reaction. Similarly, *Salmonella* serotype Choleraesuis and *Salmonella* serotype Paratyphi C have the same antigenic formula (6,7:c:1,5) but are differentiated biochemically. *Salmonella* serotype Paratyphi C may express the

Vi antigen. *Citrobacter* and *E. coli* strains may possess O, H, or Vi antigens that are related to those of *Salmonella;* biochemical identification may be necessary to confirm that an isolate is *Salmonella* (see Table 5 in this chapter and Table 1 in chapter 42).

Subtyping

For rarer serotypes, serotype identification may be all that is necessary to identify clusters of temporally related isolates. However, additional subtyping methods are typically required for more common serotypes (e.g., Typhimurium, Enteritidis, and Newport). A variety of phenotypic (e.g., phage typing, antimicrobial susceptibility pattern determination, and biotyping) and genotyping methods (e.g., plasmid fingerprinting, PFGE, IS*200* profiling, and random amplified polymorphic DNA analysis) have been developed for subtyping within serotypes of *Salmonella* (74, 108). PFGE is the current method of choice for the subtyping of most *Salmonella* serotypes since it is universally applicable and provides good strain discrimination for most serotypes. PulseNet, an international subtyping network that tracks *Salmonella,* is based on PFGE (108). *Salmonella* serotype Enteritidis has limited diversity in PFGE analysis; as a result, phage typing is still commonly used to characterize strains, particularly in an outbreak setting (39, 82).

Serodiagnostic Tests

The Widal test, which measures agglutinating antibodies to the O and H antigens of *Salmonella* serotype Typhi, produces false-negative and false-positive reactions and does not provide a definitive diagnosis of individual cases of infection. Two other rapid serodiagnostic tests have proved more useful than the Widal test for the serodiagnosis of typhoid fever (78) (Tubex; IDL Biotech, Sollentuna, Sweden; and TyphiDot; Malaysian Biodiagnostic Research SDN BHD, Kuala Lumpur, Malaysia).

Antimicrobial Susceptibilities

Antimicrobial therapy is not recommended for uncomplicated *Salmonella* gastroenteritis, and routine susceptibility testing of fecal isolates is not warranted for treatment purposes. However, determination of antimicrobial resistance patterns is often valuable for surveillance purposes and may be performed periodically to monitor the development and spread of antimicrobial resistance among *Salmonella* isolates.

In contrast to uncomplicated salmonellosis, treatment with the appropriate antimicrobial agent can be crucial for patients with invasive *Salmonella* and typhoidal infections, and the susceptibilities of these isolates should be reported as soon as possible (57). Testing methods are detailed in chapter 73. The untreated case mortality rate for typhoid fever is >10%; when patients with typhoid fever are treated with appropriate antibiotics, the rate should be <1%. However, increasing levels of resistance to one or more antimicrobial agents in *Salmonella* isolates, particularly in *Salmonella* serotype Typhi, make selection of an appropriate antibiotic problematic. In particular, reduced susceptibility to ciprofloxacin among *Salmonella* serotype Typhi isolates and increasing numbers of treatment failures are of concern (52, 89).

Antimicrobial resistance, particularly multiple drug resistance, has been noted in several nontyphoidal serotypes of *Salmonella.* A strain of *Salmonella* serotype Typhimurium phage type DT104 resistant to five antimicrobials (ampicillin, chloramphenicol, streptomycin, sulfonamides, and tetracycline, or ACSSuT) emerged in the late 1990s and is now recognized worldwide. In 2002, 21% of *Salmonella* serotype Typhimurium isolates in the United States had the ACSSuT resistance profile (21). The ACSSuT resistance determinant has been found in *Salmonella* serotype Agona strains (27). The genomic element that carries this ACSSuT determinant has been found to harbor these and other resistance determinants in a variety of serotypes, indicating that the element may spread horizontally to other serotypes and acquire additional resistance determinants (60).

The emergence of a clone of *Salmonella* serotype Newport resistant to at least nine antimicrobials, including expanded-spectrum cephalosporins, was first noted in 2000 in the northeastern United States (43) and has now been found in many regions of the United States (8). In 2002, this strain made up 22% of all serotype Newport strains in the United States. Similarly resistant strains of *Salmonella* serotype Newport were recently reported in Japan, documenting the potential for worldwide spread of multiply resistant strains (50). Additional information regarding these and other antimicrobial resistant strains can be found at the CDC's NARMS website (http://www.cdc.gov/narms/).

Interpretation and Reporting of Results

A preliminary report can be issued as soon as a presumptive identification of *Salmonella* is obtained. In most situations, a presumptive identification would be based on biochemical findings obtained either by traditional or commercial systems or by a serologic reaction in *Salmonella* O grouping antisera. A confirmed identification requires both biochemical and serologic identification methods. Because the National *Salmonella* Surveillance System depends on the receipt of serotype information for *Salmonella* strains isolated in the United States for the tracking of outbreaks of infection, laboratories should follow the procedures recommended by their state health departments for submitting isolates for further characterization, including complete serotyping. The antimicrobial susceptibility of typhoidal *Salmonella* strains and strains from normally sterile sites should be determined, and the strains should be forwarded to a reference or public health laboratory for complete biochemical and serologic characterization.

REFERENCES

1. **Abbott, S. L., J. O'Connor, T. Robin, B. L. Zimmer, and J. M. Janda.** 2003. Biochemical properties of a newly described *Escherichia* species, *Escherichia albertii. J. Clin. Microbiol.* **41:**4852–4854.
2. **Acheson, D. W. K., and G. T. Keusch.** 1995. *Shigella* and enteroinvasive *Escherichia coli*, p. 763–784. *In* M. J. Blaser, J. I. Ravdin, H. B. Greenberg, and R. L. Guerrant (ed.), *Infections of the Gastrointestinal Tract.* Raven Press, New York, N.Y.
3. **Albert, M. J., S. M. Faruque, A. S. Faruque, K. A. Bettelheim, P. K. Neogi, N. A. Bhuiyan, and J. B. Kaper.** 1996. Controlled study of cytolethal distending toxin-producing *Escherichia coli* infections in Bangladeshi children. *J. Clin. Microbiol.* **34:**717–719.
4. **Albert, M. J., F. Qadri, A. Haque, and N. A. Bhuiyan.** 1993. Bacterial clump formation at the surface of liquid culture as a rapid test for identification of enteroaggregative *Escherichia coli. J. Clin. Microbiol.* **31:**1397–1399.
5. **Ansaruzzaman, M., A. K. M. G. Kibriya, A. Rahman, P. K. B. Neogi, A. S. G. Faruque, B. Rowe, and M. J. Albert.** 1995. Detection of provisional serovars of *Shigella dysenteriae* and designation as *S. dysenteriae* serotypes 14 and 15. *J. Clin. Microbiol.* **33:**1423–1425.
6. **Aspevall, O., B. Osterman, R. Dittmer, L. Sten, E. Lindback, and U. Forsum.** 2002. Performance of four chromogenic urine culture media after one or two days of

incubation compared with reference media. *J. Clin. Microbiol.* **40:**1500–1503.

7. **Baudry, B., S. J. Savarino, P. Vial, J. B. Kaper, and M. M. Levine.** 1990. A sensitive and specific DNA probe to identify enteroaggregative *Escherichia coli*, a recently discovered diarrheal pathogen. *J. Infect. Dis.* **161:**1249–1251.
8. **Berge, A. C., J. M. Adaska, and W. M. Sischo.** 2004. Use of antibiotic susceptibility patterns and pulsed-field gel electrophoresis to compare historic and contemporary isolates of multi-drug-resistant *Salmonella enterica* subsp. *enterica* serovar Newport. *Appl. Environ. Microbiol.* **70:**318–323.
9. **Bettelheim, K. A.** 1992. The genus *Escherichia*, p. 2696–2736. *In* A. Balows, H. G. Truper, M. Dworkin, W. Harder, and K.-H. Schleifer (ed.), *The Prokaryotes*, 2nd ed. Springer-Verlag KG, Berlin, Germany.
10. **Bettelheim, K. A.** 2005. Reliability of O157:H7 ID agar (O157 H7 ID-F) for the detection and isolation of verocytotoxigenic strains of *Escherichia coli* belonging to serogroup O157. *J. Appl. Microbiol.* **99:**408–410.
11. **Beutin, L., M. A. Montenegro, I. Orskov, F. Orskov, J. Proada, S. Zimmerman, and R. Stephan.** 1989. Close association of verocytotoxin (Shiga-like toxin) production with enterohemolysin production in strains of *Escherichia coli*. *J. Clin. Microbiol.* **27:**2559–2564.
12. **Bitzan, M., K. Ludwig, M. Klemt, H. Konig, J. Buren, and D. E. Muller-Wiefel.** 1993. The role of *Escherichia coli* O157 infections in the classical (enteropathic) haemolytic uraemic syndrome: results of a Central European multicentre study. *Epidemiol. Infect.* **110:**183–196.
13. **Blanco, J. E., J. Blanco, M. Blanco, M. P. Alonso, and W. H. Jansen.** 1994. Serotypes of CNF1-producing *Escherichia coli* strains that cause extraintestinal infections in humans. *Eur. J. Epidemiol.* **10:**707–711.
14. **Borczyk, A. A., N. Harnett, M. Lombos, and H. Lior.** 1990. False-positive identification of *Escherichia coli* O157 by commercial latex agglutination tests. *Lancet* **336:** 946–947.
15. **Bouvet, P. J., and S. Jeanjean.** 1992. Evaluation of two colored latex kits, the Wellcolex Colour Salmonella Test and the Wellcolex Colour Shigella Test, for serological grouping of *Salmonella* and *Shigella* species. *J. Clin. Microbiol.* **30:** 2184–2186.
16. **Brenner, D. J.** 1992. Introduction to the family *Enterobacteriaceae*, p. 2673–2695. *In* A. Balows, H. G. Truper, M. Dworkin, W. Harder, and K.-H. Schleifer (ed.), *The Prokaryotes*, 2nd ed. Springer-Verlag KG, Berlin, Germany.
17. **Brenner, F. W.** 1998. *Modified Kauffmann-White Scheme.* Centers for Disease Control and Prevention, Atlanta, Ga.
18. **Brenner, F. W., and A. C. McWhorter-Murlin.** 1998. *Identification and Serotyping of* Salmonella. Centers for Disease Control and Prevention, Atlanta, Ga.
19. **Brenner, F. W., R. G. Villar, F. J. Angulo, R. Tauxe, and B. Swaminathan.** 2000. *Salmonella* nomenclature. *J. Clin. Microbiol.* **38:**2465–2467.
20. **Caprioli, A., V. Falbo, L. G. Roda, F. M. Ruggeri, and C. Zona.** 1983. Partial purification and characterization of an *Escherichia coli* toxic factor that induces morphological cell alterations. *Infect. Immun.* **39:**1300–1306.
21. **Centers for Disease Control and Prevention.** 2004. *National Antimicrobial Resistance Monitoring System for Enteric Bacteria (NARMS): 2002 Human Isolates Final Report.* U.S. Department of Health and Human Services, CDC, Atlanta, Ga.
22. **Centers for Disease Control and Prevention.** 2004. Salmonella *Surveillance: Annual Summary, 2003.* U.S. Department of Health and Human Services, CDC, Atlanta, Ga.
23. **Centers for Disease Control and Prevention.** 2000. *Escherichia coli* O111:H8 outbreak among teenage campers—Texas, 1999. *Morb. Mortal. Wkly. Rep.* **49:**321–324.
24. **Centers for Disease Control and Prevention.** 2001. Preliminary FoodNet data on the incidence of foodborne illnesses—selected sites, United States, 2000. *Morb. Mortal. Wkly. Rep.* **50:**241–246.
25. **Chapman, P. A., and C. A. Siddons.** 1996. A comparison of immunomagnetic separation and direct culture for the isolation of verocytotoxin-producing *Escherichia coli* O157 from cases of bloody diarrhoea, non-bloody diarrhoea and asymptomatic contacts. *J. Med. Microbiol.* **44:**267–271.
26. **Chaux, C., M. Crepy, S. Xueref, C. Roure, Y. Gille, and A. M. Freydiere.** 2002. Comparison of three chromogenic agar plates for isolation and identification of urinary tract pathogens. *J. Clin. Microbiol.* **8:**641–645.
27. **Cloeckaert, A., K. Sidi Boumedine, G. Flaujac, H. Imberechts, I. D'Hooghe, and E. Chaslus-Dancla.** 2000. Occurrence of a *Salmonella enterica* serovar Typhimurium DT104-like antibiotic resistance gene cluster including the *floR* gene in *S. enterica* serovar Agona. *Antimicrob. Agents Chemother.* **44:**1359–1361.
28. **Cobeljic, M., B. Miljkovic-Selimovic, D. Paunovic-Todosijevic, Z. Velickovic, Z. Lepsanovic, N. Zec, D. Savic, R. Ilic, S. Konstantinovic, B. Jovanovic, and V. Kostic.** 1996. Enteroaggregative *Escherichia coli* associated with an outbreak of diarrhoea in a neonatal nursery ward. *Epidemiol. Infect.* **117:**11–16.
29. **Cohen, M. B., J. P. Nataro, D. I. Bernstein, J. Hawkins, N. Roberts, and M. A. Staat.** 2005. Prevalence of diarrheagenic *Escherichia coli* in acute childhood enteritis: a prospective controlled study. *J. Pediatr.* **146:**54–61.
30. **Dalton, C. B., E. D. Mintz, J. G. Wells, C. A. Bopp, and R. V. Tauxe.** 1999. Outbreaks of enterotoxigenic *Escherichia coli* infection in American adults: a clinical and epidemiologic profile. *Epidemiol. Infect.* **123:**9–16.
31. **De Rycke, J., J. F. Guillot, and R. Boivin.** 1997. Cytotoxins in nonenterotoxigenic strains of *Escherichia coli* isolated from feces of diarrheic calves. *Vet. Microbiol.* **15:**137–150.
32. **Donnenberg, M. S.** 2002. Enteropathogenic *Escherichia coli*, p. 595–612. *In* M. J. Blaser, P. D. Smith, J. I. Ravdin, H. B. Greenberg, and R. L. Guerrant (ed.), *Infections of the Gastrointestinal Tract*, 2nd ed. Lippincott Williams and Wilkins, Philadelphia, Pa.
33. **Dylla, B. L., E. A. Vetter, J. G. Hughes, and F. R. Cockerill III.** 1995. Evaluation of an immunoassay for direct detection of *Escherichia coli* O157 in stool specimens. *J. Clin. Microbiol.* **33:**222–224.
34. **Ewing, W. H.** 1971. *Biochemical Reactions of* Shigella. Center for Disease Control, Atlanta, Ga.
35. **Ewing, W. H.** 1986. *Edwards and Ewing's Identification of* Enterobacteriaceae, 4th ed. Elsevier Science Publishing Co. Inc., New York, N.Y.
36. **Ewing, W. H., R. W. Reavis, and B. R. Davis.** 1958. Provisional *Shigella* serotypes. *Can. J. Microbiol.* **4:**89–107.
37. **Farmer, J. J., III.** 2003. *Enterobacteriaceae:* introduction and identification, p. 636–653. *In* P. R. Murray, E. J. Baron, J. H. Jorgensen, M. A. Pfaller, and R. H. Yolken (ed.), *Manual of Clinical Microbiology*, 8th ed., vol. 1. ASM Press, Washington, D.C.
38. **Fields, P. I., K. Blom, H. J. Hughes, L. O. Helsel, P. Feng, and B. Swaminathan.** 1997. Molecular characterization of the gene encoding H antigen in *Escherichia coli* and development of a PCR-restriction fragment length polymorphism test for identification of *E. coli* O157:H7 and O157:NM. *J. Clin. Microbiol.* **35:**1066–1070.
39. **Fisher, I. S.** 2004. Dramatic shift in the epidemiology of *Salmonella enterica* serotype Enteritidis phage types in western Europe, 1998–2003—results from the Enter-net international salmonella database. *Euro Surveill.* **9:**45–47.
40. **Friedrich, A. W., M. Bielaszewska, W. L. Zhang, M. Pulz, T. Kuczius, A. Ammon, and H. Karch.** 2002. *Escherichia coli* harboring Shiga toxin 2 gene variants: frequency and

association with clinical symptoms. *J. Infect. Dis.* **185:** 74–84.

41. **Glandt, M., J. A. Adachi, J. J. Mathewson, Z. D. Jiang, D. DiCesare, D. Ashley, C. D. Ericsson, and H. L. DuPont.** 1999. Enteroaggregative *Escherichia coli* as a cause of traveler's diarrhea: clinical response to ciprofloxacin. *Clin. Infect. Dis.* **29:**335–338.
42. **Griffin, P. M., P. S. Mead, and S. Sivapalasingam.** 2002. *Escherichia coli* O157:H7 and other enterohemorrhagic *Escherichia coli,* p. 627–642. *In* M. J. Blaser, J. I. Ravdin, H. B. Greenberg, and R. L. Guerrant (ed.), *Infections of the Gastrointestinal Tract,* 2nd ed. Lippincott Williams & Wilkins, New York, N.Y.
43. **Gupta, A., J. Fontana, C. Crowe, B. Bolstorff, A. Stout, S. Van Duyne, M. P. Hoekstra, J. M. Whichard, T. J. Barrett, and F. J. Angulo.** 2003. Emergence of multidrug-resistant *Salmonella enterica* serotype Newport infections resistant to expanded-spectrum cephalosporins in the United States. *J. Infect. Dis.* **188:**1707–1716.
44. **Gupta, A., C. S. Polyak, R. D. Bishop, J. Sobel, and E. D. Mintz.** 2004. Laboratory-confirmed shigellosis in the United States, 1989–2002: epidemiologic trends and patterns. *Clin. Infect. Dis.* **38:**1372–1377.
45. **Hayes, P. S., K. Blom, P. Feng, J. Lewis, N. A. Strockbine, and B. Swaminathan.** 1995. Isolation and characterization of a β-glucuronidase-producing strain of *Escherichia coli* O157:H7 in the United States. *J. Clin. Microbiol.* **33:** 3347–3348.
46. **Hohmann, E. L.** 2001. Nontyphoidal salmonellosis. *Clin. Infect. Dis.* **32:**263–269.
47. **Huang, D. B., H. Koo, and H. L. DuPont.** 2004. Enteroaggregative *Escherichia coli:* an emerging pathogen. *Curr. Infect. Dis. Rep.* **6:**83–86.
48. **Huys, G., M. Cnockaert, J. M. Janda, and J. Swings.** 2003. *Escherichia albertii* sp. nov., a diarrhoeagenic species isolated from stool specimens of Bangladeshi children. *Int. J. Syst. Evol. Microbiol.* **53:**807–810.
49. **Hyma, K. E., D. W. Lacher, A. M. Nelson, A. C. Bumbaugh, J. M. Janda, N. A. Strockbine, V. B. Young, and T. S. Whittam.** 2005. Evolutionary genetics of a new pathogenic *Escherichia* species: *Escherichia albertii* and related *Shigella boydii* strains. *J. Bacteriol.* **187:**619–628.
50. **Ishiguro, F., Y. Kyota, M. Mochizuki, T. Fuseda, S. Omoya, H. Izumiya, and H. Watanabe.** 2005. Comparison of multidrug-resistant *Salmonella enterica* serovar Newport isolates from a patient and sewages in Fukui Prefecture. *Kansen-shogaku Zasshi* **79:**270–275.
51. **Johnson, W. M., and H. Lior.** 1988. A new heat-labile cytolethal distending toxin (CLDT) produced by *Escherichia coli* isolates from clinical material. *Microb. Pathog.* **4:**103–113.
52. **Kadhiravan, T., N. Wig, A. Kapil, S. K. Kabra, K. Renuka, and A. Misra.** 2005. Clinical outcomes in typhoid fever: adverse impact of infection with nalidixic acid-resistant *Salmonella typhi. BMC Infect. Dis.* **5:**37.
53. **Kaper, J. B., J. P. Nataro, and H. L. Mobley.** 2004. Pathogenic *Escherichia coli. Nat. Rev. Microbiol.* **2:**123–140.
54. **Karch, H., C. Janetzki-Mittman, S. Aleksic, and M. Datz.** 1996. Isolation of enterohemorrhagic *Escherichia coli* O157 strains from patients with hemolytic-uremic syndrome by using immunomagnetic separation, DNA-based methods, and direct culture. *J. Clin. Microbiol.* **34:**516–519.
55. **Karmali, M. A., M. Mascarenhas, S. Shen, K. Ziebell, S. Johnson, R. Reid-Smith, J. Isaac-Renton, C. Clark, K. Rahn, and J. B. Kaper.** 2003. Association of genomic O island 122 of *Escherichia coli* EDL 933 with verocytotoxin-producing *Escherichia coli* seropathotypes that are linked to epidemic and/or serious disease. *J. Clin. Microbiol.* **41:** 4930–4940.
56. **Lan, R., M. C. Alles, K. Donohoe, M. B. Martinez, and P. R. Reeves.** 2004. Molecular evolutionary relationships of enteroinvasive *Escherichia coli* and *Shigella* spp. *Infect. Immun.* **72:**5080–5088.
57. **Lee, L. A., N. D. Puhr, E. K. Mahoney, N. H. Bean, and R. V. Tauxe.** 1994. Increase in antimicrobial-resistant *Salmonella* infections in the United States, 1989–1990. *J. Infect. Dis.* **170:**128–134.
58. **Le Minor, L.** 1992. The genus *Salmonella,* p. 2760–2774. *In* A. Balows, H. G. Truper, M. Dworkin, W. Harder, and K.-H. Schleifer (ed.), *The Prokaryotes,* 2nd ed. Springer-Verlag KG, Berlin, Germany.
59. **Levine, M. M., C. Ferreccio, V. Prado, M. Cayazzo, P. Abrego, J. Martinez, L. Maggi, M. M. Baldini, W. Martin, D. Maneval, B. Kay, L. Guers, H. Lior, S. S. Wasserman, and J. P. Nataro.** 1993. Epidemiologic studies of *Escherichia coli* diarrheal infections in a low socioeconomic level peri-urban community in Santiago, Chile. *Am. J. Epidemiol.* **138:**849–869.
60. **Levings, R. S., D. Lightfoot, S. R. Partridge, R. M. Hall, and S. P. Djordjevic.** 2005. The genomic island SGI1, containing the multiple antibiotic resistance region of *Salmonella enterica* serovar Typhimurium DT104 or variants of it, is widely distributed in other *S. enterica* serovars. *J. Bacteriol.* **187:**4401–4409.
61. **Lindberg, A. A., P. D. Cam, N. Chan, L. K. Phu, D. D. Trach, G. Lindberg, K. Karlsson, A. Karnell, and E. Ekwall.** 1991. Shigellosis in Vietnam: seroepidemiologic studies with use of lipopolysaccharide antigens in enzyme immunoassays. *Rev. Infect. Dis.* **13:**S213–S237.
62. **Ludwig, K., E. Grabhorn, M. Bitzan, C. Bobrowski, M. J. Kemper, I. Sobottka, R. Laufs, H. Karch, and D. E. Muller-Wiefel.** 2002. Saliva IgM and IgA are a sensitive indicator of the humoral immune response to *Escherichia coli* O157 lipopolysaccharide in children with enteropathic hemolytic uremic syndrome. *Pediatr. Res.* **52:**307–313.
63. **Mackenzie, A. M., P. Lebel, E. Orrbine, P. C. Rowe, L. Hyde, F. Chan, W. Johnson, P. N. McLaine, and The SYNSORB Pk Study Investigators.** 1998. Sensitivities and specificities of Premier *E. coli* O157 and Premier EHEC enzyme immunoassays for diagnosis of infection with verotoxin (Shiga-like toxin)-producing *Escherichia coli. J. Clin. Microbiol.* **36:**1608–1611.
64. **Mahon, B. E., A. Ponka, W. N. Hall, K. Komatsu, S. E. Dietrich, A. Siitonen, G. Cage, P. S. Hayes, M. A. Lambert-Fair, N. H. Bean, P. M. Griffin, and L. Slutsker.** 1997. An international outbreak of *Salmonella* infections caused by alfalfa sprouts grown from contaminated seeds. *J. Infect. Dis.* **175:**876–882.
65. **Manafi, M., and B. Kremsmaier.** 2001. Comparative evaluation of different chromogenic/fluorogenic media for detecting *Escherichia coli* O157:H7 in food. *Int. J. Food Microbiol.* **71:**257–262.
66. **Mandal, B. K., and J. Brennand.** 1988. Bacteraemia in salmonellosis: a 15 year retrospective study from a regional infectious diseases unit. *Brit. Med. J.* **297:**1242–1243.
67. **March, S. B., and S. Ratnam.** 1986. Sorbitol-MacConkey medium for detection of *Escherichia coli* O157:H7 associated with hemorrhagic colitis. *J. Clin. Microbiol.* **23:**869–872.
68. **McVeigh, A., A. Fasano, D. A. Scott, S. Jelacic, S. L. Moseley, D. C. Robertson, and S. J. Savarino.** 2000. IS1414, an *Escherichia coli* insertion sequence with a heat-stable enterotoxin gene embedded in a transposase-like gene. *Infect. Immun.* **68:**5710–5715.
69. **Mead, P. S., L. Slutsker, V. Dietz, L. F. McCaig, J. S. Bresee, C. Shapiro, P. M. Griffin, and R. V. Tauxe.** 1999. Food-related illness and death in the United States. *Emerg. Infect. Dis.* **5:**607–625.
70. **Miqdady, M. S., Z. D. Jiang, J. P. Nataro, and H. L. DuPont.** 2002. Detection of enteroaggregative *Escherichia coli* with formalin-preserved HEp-2 cells. *J. Clin. Microbiol.* **40:**3066–3067.

71. **Morris, C., C. K. Tam, T. S. Wallis, P. W. Jones, and J. Hackett.** 2003. *Salmonella enterica* serovar Dublin strains which are Vi antigen-positive use type IVB pili for bacterial self-association and human intestinal cell entry. *Microb. Pathog.* **35:**279–284.
72. **Nataro, J. P., and J. B. Kaper.** 1998. Diarrheagenic *Escherichia coli*. *Clin. Microbiol. Rev.* **11:**142–201.
73. **Nataro, J. P., D. Yikang, S. Cookson, A. Cravioto, S. J. Savarino, L. D. Guers, M. M. Levine, and C. O. Tacket.** 1995. Heterogeneity of enteroaggregative *Escherichia coli* virulence demonstrated in volunteers. *J. Infect. Dis.* **171:** 465–468.
74. **Navaro, F., T. Llovett, M. A. Echeita, P. Coll, A. Aladueña, M. A. Usera, and G. Prats.** 1996. Molecular typing of *Salmonella enterica* serovar Typhi. *J. Clin. Microbiol.* **34:**2831–2834.
75. **Nguyen, T. V., P. Le Van, C. Le Huy, K. N. Gia, and A. Weintraub.** 2005. Detection and characterization of diarrheagenic *Escherichia coli* from young children in Hanoi, Vietnam. *J. Clin. Microbiol.* **43:**755–760.
76. **Nishi, J., J. Sheikh, K. Mizuguchi, B. Luisi, V. Burland, A. Boutin, D. J. Rose, F. R. Blattner, and J. P. Nataro.** 2003. The export of coat protein from enteroaggregative *Escherichia coli* by a specific ATP-binding cassette transporter system. *J. Biol. Chem.* **278:**45680–45689.
77. **Novicki, T. J., J. A. Daly, S. L. Mottice, and K. C. Carroll.** 2000. Comparison of sorbitol MacConkey agar and a two-step method which utilizes enzyme-linked immunosorbent assay toxin testing and a chromogenic agar to detect and isolate enterohemorrhagic *Escherichia coli*. *J. Clin. Microbiol.* **38:**547–551.
78. **Olsen, S. J., J. Pruckler, W. Bibb, T. M. Nguyen, M. T. Tran, S. Sivapalasingam, A. Gupta, T. P. Phan, T. C. Nguyen, V. C. Nguyen, D. C. Phung, and E. D. Mintz.** 2004. Evaluation of rapid diagnostic tests for typhoid fever. *J. Clin. Microbiol.* **42:**1885–1889.
79. **Olsvik, O., and N. A. Strockbine.** 1993. PCR detection of heat-stable, heat-labile, and Shiga-like toxin genes in *Escherichia coli*, p. 271–276. *In* D. H. Persing, T. F. Smith, F. C. Tenover, and T. J. White (ed.), *Diagnostic Molecular Microbiology: Principles and Applications*. American Society for Microbiology, Washington, D.C.
80. **Oswald, E., J. DeRycke, J. F. Guillot, and R. Boivin.** 1989. Cytotoxic effect of multinucleation in HeLa cell cultures associated with the presence of Vir plasmid in *Escherichia coli* strains. *FEMS Microbiol. Lett.* **58:**95–100.
81. **Paton, A. W., R. M. Ratcliff, R. M. Doyles, J. Seymour-Murray, D. Davos, J. A. Lanser, and J. C. Paton.** 1996. Molecular microbiological investigation of an outbreak of hemolytic-uremic syndrome caused by dry fermented sausage contaminated with Shiga-like toxin-producing *Escherichia coli*. *J. Clin. Microbiol.* **34:**1622–1627.
82. **Patrick, M. E., P. M. Adcock, T. M. Gomez, S. F. Altekruse, B. H. Holland, R. V. Tauxe, and D. L. Swerdlow.** 2004. *Salmonella enteritidis* infections, United States, 1985–1999. *Emerg. Infect. Dis.* **10:**1–7.
83. **Pickard, D., J. Wain, S. Baker, A. Line, S. Chohan, M. Fookes, A. Barron, P. O. Gaora, J. A. Chabalgoity, N. Thanky, C. Scholes, N. Thomson, M. Quail, J. Parkhill, and G. Dougan.** 2003. Composition, acquisition, and distribution of the Vi exopolysaccharide-encoding *Salmonella enterica* pathogenicity island SPI-7. *J. Bacteriol.* **185:** 5055–5065.
84. **Popoff, M. Y.** 2001. *Antigenic Formulas of the* Salmonella *Serovars*, 8th rendition. WHO Collaborating Centre for Reference and Research on Salmonella, Pasteur Institute, Paris, France.
85. **Popoff, M. Y., J. Bockemuhl, and L. L. Gheesling.** 2004. Supplement 2002 (no. 46) to the Kauffmann-White scheme. *Res. Microbiol.* **155:**568–570.
86. **Prager, R., S. Annemuller, and H. Tschape.** 2005. Diversity of virulence patterns among shiga toxin-producing *Escherichia coli* from human clinical cases—need for more detailed diagnostics. *Int. J. Med. Microbiol.* **295:** 29–38.
87. **Prager, R., W. Rabsch, W. Streckel, W. Voigt, E. Tietze, and H. Tschape.** 2003. Molecular properties of *Salmonella enterica* serotype Paratyphi B distinguish between its systemic and its enteric pathovars. *J. Clin. Microbiol.* **41:** 4270–4278.
88. **Pryamukhina, N. S., and N. A. Khomenko.** 1988. Suggestion to supplement *Shigella flexneri* classification scheme with the subserovar *Shigella flexneri* 4c: phenotypic characteristics of strains. *J. Clin. Microbiol.* **26:**1147–1149.
89. **Rahman, M. M., J. A. Haq, M. A. Morshed, and M. A. Rahman.** 2005. *Salmonella enterica* serovar Typhi with decreased susceptibility to ciprofloxacin—an emerging problem in Bangladesh. *Int. J. Antimicrob. Agents.* **25:** 345–346.
90. **Rangel, J. M., P. H. Sparling, C. Crowe, P. M. Griffin, and D. L. Swerdlow.** 2005. Epidemiology of *Escherichia coli* O157:H7 outbreaks, United States, 1982–2002. *Emerg. Infect. Dis.* **11:**603–609.
91. **Reeves, M. W., G. M. Evins, A. A. Heiba, B. D. Plikaytis, and J. J. Farmer III.** 1989. Clonal nature of *Salmonella typhi* and its genetic relatedness to other salmonellae as shown by multilocus enzyme electrophoresis and proposal of *Salmonella bongori* comb. nov. *J. Clin. Microbiol.* **27:**313–320.
92. **Rohde, R.** 1979. Serological integration of all known *Arizona* species into the Kauffmann-White schema. *Zentbl. Bakteriol. Parasitenkd. Infektkrankh. Hyg. I Abt. Orig. Reihe A* **243:**148–176.
93. **Sack, R. B., M. Rahman, M. Yunus, and E. H. Khan.** 1997. Antimicrobial resistance in organisms causing diarrheal disease. *Clin. Infect. Dis.* **24:**S102–S105.
94. **Safdar, N., A. Said, R. E. Gangnon, and D. G. Maki.** 2002. Risk of hemolytic uremic syndrome after antibiotic treatment of *Escherichia coli* O157:H7 enteritis: a meta-analysis. *JAMA* **288:**996–1001.
95. **Sarantuya, J., J. Nishi, N. Wakimoto, S. Erdene, J. P. Nataro, J. Sheikh, M. Iwashita, K. Manago, K. Tokuda, M. Yoshinaga, K. Miyata, and Y. Kawano.** 2004. Typical enteroaggregative *Escherichia coli* is the most prevalent pathotype among *E. coli* strains causing diarrhea in Mongolian children. *J. Clin. Microbiol.* **42:**133–139.
96. **Schmidt, H., and H. Karch.** 1996. Enterohemolytic phenotypes and genotypes of Shiga toxin-producing *Escherichia coli* O111 strains from patients with diarrhea and hemolytic-uremic syndrome. *J. Clin. Microbiol.* **34:**2364–2367.
97. **Scotland, S. M., G. A. Willshaw, B. Said, H. R. Smith, and B. Rowe.** 1989. Identification of *Escherichia coli* that produce heat-stable enterotoxin STA by a commercially available enzyme-linked immunoassay and comparison of the assay with infant mouse and DNA probe tests. *J. Clin. Microbiol.* **27:**1697–1699.
98. **Scotland, S. M., T. Cheasty, A. Thomas, and B. Rowe.** 1991. Beta-glucuronidase activity of Vero cytotoxin-producing strains of *Escherichia coli*, including serogroup O157, isolated in the United Kingdom. *Lett. Appl. Microbiol.* **13:**42–44.
99. **Servin, A. L.** 2005. Pathogenesis of Afa/Dr diffusely adhering *Escherichia coli*. *Clin. Microbiol. Rev.* **18:**264–292.
100. **Sjogren, A. C., J. B. Kaper, A. Caprioli, and D. Karpman.** 2004. Enzyme-linked immunosorbent assay for detection of Shiga toxin-producing *Escherichia coli* infection by antibodies to *Escherichia coli* secreted protein B in children with hemolytic uremic syndrome. *Eur. J. Clin. Microbiol. Infect. Dis.* **23:**208–211.

101. **Slutsker, L., A. A. Ries, K. D. Greene, J. G. Wells, L. Hutwagner, and P. M. Griffin.** 1997. *Escherichia coli* O157:H7 diarrhea in the United States: clinical and epidemiologic features. *Ann. Intern. Med.* **126:**505–513.
102. **Smith, H. W.** 1974. A search for transmissible pathogenic characters in invasive strains of *Escherichia coli:* the discovery of a plasmid-controlled toxin and a plasmid-controlled lethal character closely associated, or identical, with colicine V. *J. Gen. Microbiol.* **83:**95–111.
103. **Sowers, E. G., J. G. Wells, and N. A. Strockbine.** 1996. Evaluation of commercial latex reagents for identification of O157 and H7 antigens of *Escherichia coli. J. Clin. Microbiol.* **34:**1286–1289.
104. **Stock, I., M. A. Rahman, K. J. Sherwood, and B. Wiedemann.** 2005. Natural antimicrobial susceptibility patterns and biochemical identification of *Escherichia albertii* and *Hafnia alvei* strains. *Diagn. Microbiol. Infect. Dis.* **51:**151–163.
105. **Strockbine, N. A., J. Parsonnet, K. Greene, J. A. Kiehlbauch, and I. K Wachsmuth.** 1991. Molecular epidemiologic techniques in analysis of epidemic and endemic *Shigella dysenteriae* type 1 strains. *J. Infect. Dis.* **163:**406–409.
106. **Subcommittee of the PHLS Advisory Committee on Gastrointestinal Infections.** 2000. Guidelines for the control of infection with Vero cytotoxin producing *Escherichia coli* (VTEC). *Commun. Dis. Pub. Health* **3:**14–23.
107. **Sugiyama, K., K. Inoue, and R. Sakazaki.** 2001. Mitomycin-supplemented washed blood agar for the isolation of Shiga toxin-producing *Escherichia coli* other than O157:H7. *Lett. Appl. Microbiol.* **33:**193–195.
108. **Swaminathan, B., T. J. Barrett, S. B. Hunter, and R. V. Tauxe.** 2001. PulseNet: the molecular subtyping network for foodborne bacterial disease surveillance, United States. *Emerg. Infect. Dis.* **7:**382–389.
109. **Tacket, C. O., S. L. Moseley, B. Kay, G. Losonsky, and M. M. Levine.** 1990. Challenge studies in volunteers using *Escherichia coli* strains with diffuse adherence to HEp-2 cells. *J. Infect. Dis.* **162:**550–552.
110. **Tauxe, R. V., N. D. Puhr, J. G. Wells, N. Hargrett-Bean, and P. A. Blake.** 1990. Antimicrobial resistance of *Shigella* isolates in the USA: the importance of international travelers. *J. Infect. Dis.* **162:**1107–1111.
111. **Tazzari, P. L., F. Ricci, D. Carnicelli, A. Caprioli, A. E. Tozzi, G. Rizzoni, R. Conte, and M. Brigotti.** 2004. Flow cytometry detection of Shiga toxins in the blood from children with hemolytic uremic syndrome. *Cytometry B Clin. Cytom.* **61:**40–44.
112. **Tindall, B. J., P. A. Grimont, G. M. Garrity, and J. P. Euzeby.** 2005. Nomenclature and taxonomy of the genus *Salmonella. Int. J. Syst. Evol. Microbiol.* **55:**521–524.
113. **Trabulsi, L. R., R. Keller, and T. A. Tardelli Gomes.** 2002. Typical and atypical enteropathogenic *Escherichia coli. Emerg. Infect. Dis.* **8:**508–513.
114. **Verbrugh, H. A., D. R. Mekkes, R. P. Verkoyen, and J. E. Landbeer.** 1987. Widal type serology using live antigen for diagnosis of *Shigella flexneri* dysentery. *Eur. J. Clin. Microbiol. Infect. Dis.* **5:**540–542.
115. **Vial, P. A., J. J. Mathewson, H. L. DuPont, L. Guers, and M. M. Levine.** 1990. Comparison of two assay methods for patterns of adherence to HEp-2 cells of *Escherichia coli* from patients with diarrhea. *J. Clin. Microbiol.* **28:**882–885.
116. **Vugia, D. J., M. Samuel, M. M. Farley, R. Marcus, B. Shiferaw, S. Shallow, K. Smith, and F. J. Angulo.** 2004. Invasive *Salmonella* infections in the United States, FoodNet, 1996–1999: incidence, serotype distribution, and outcome. *Clin. Infect. Dis.* **38** (Suppl. 3)**:**S149–S156.
117. **Wathen-Grady, H. G., B. R. Davis, and G. K. Morris.** 1985. Addition of three new serotypes of *Shigella boydii* to the *Shigella* schema. *J. Clin. Microbiol.* **21:**129–132.
118. **Wathen-Grady, H. G., L. E. Britt, N. A. Strockbine, and I. K. Wachsmuth.** 1990. Characterization of *Shigella dysenteriae* serotypes 11, 12, and 13. *J. Clin. Microbiol.* **28:**2580–2584.
119. **Wells, J. G., and G. K. Morris.** 1981. Evaluation of transport methods for isolating *Shigella* spp. *J. Clin. Microbiol.* **13:**789–790.
120. **Whittam, T. S., and A. C. Bumbaugh.** 2002. Inferences from whole-genome sequences of bacterial pathogens. *Curr. Opin. Genet. Dev.* **12:**719–725.
121. **Wong, C. S., S. Jelacic, R. L. Habeeb, S. L. Watkins, and P. I. Tarr.** 2000. The risk of hemolytic uremic syndrome after antibiotic treatment of *Escherichia coli* O157:H7 infections. *N. Engl. J. Med.* **342:**1930–1936.
122. **Yam, W. C., M. L. Lung, and M. H. Ng.** 1992. Evaluation and optimization of a latex agglutination assay for detection of cholera toxin and *Escherichia coli* heat-labile toxin. *J. Clin. Microbiol.* **30:**2518–2520.
123. **Yamamoto, T., Y. Koyama, M. Matsumoto, E. Sonoda, S. Nakayama, M. Uchimura, W. Paveenkittiporn, K. Tamura, T. Yokota, and P. Echeverria.** 1992. Localized, aggregative, and diffuse adherence to HeLa cells, plastic, and human small intestines by *Escherichia coli* isolated from patients with diarrhea. *J. Infect. Dis.* **166:**1295–1310.
124. **Zadik, P. M., P. A. Chapman, and C. A. Siddons.** 1993. Use of tellurite for the selection of verocytotoxigenic *Escherichia coli* O157. *J. Med. Microbiol.* **39:**155–158.

*Yersinia**

AUDREY WANGER

44

TAXONOMY AND HISTORY OF THE GENUS

Yersinia pseudotuberculosis and *Y. pestis* were included in the genus *Pasteurella* until 1944, when van Loghem suggested that a new genus be formed due to the significant phenotypic and genotypic differences among the organisms. It was not until 1964 that *Y. enterocolitica* was renamed by Frederiksen from the previous name of *Bacterium enterocolitica* assigned in 1939 following a report of several cases of gastrointestinal disease. This diverse group of organisms was further divided into a subgroup initially designated *Y. enterocolitica*-like organisms and later into an additional four species (*Y. intermedia*, *Y. frederiksenii*, *Y. kristensenii*, and *Y. aldovae*) based on sugar fermentation and DNA relatedness. Subsequent species designations included *Y. ruckeri*, *Y. rohdei*, *Y. mollaretii*, and *Y. bercovieri*. The newest member of the genus is *Y. aleksiciae*, named after the German scientist Stojanca Aleksic (54) and previously included in the species *Y. kristensenii*. Although phenotypically identical, the two species were differentiated by multilocus enzyme electrophoresis (MLEE) typing and 16S rRNA analysis. A further breakdown of *Y. enterocolitica* into subspecies (*enterocolitica* and *palearctica*) differentiable based only on 16S rRNA gene sequencing has been proposed (37).

Although most species of the genus have been isolated from humans, with the exception of *Y. aldovae*, the only species that are considered human pathogens are *Y. pestis*, *Y. pseudotuberculosis*, and *Y. enterocolitica*. These species, in addition to *Y. ruckeri* serogroup 01, which is the cause of enteric red mouth disease in rainbow trout, are the only members of the genus that are pathogenic for animals. All of the other species are considered to be nonpathogenic, environmental isolates.

As a group, members of the genus *Yersinia* have a G+C content of 46 to 50% and are related to the rest of the members of the family *Enterobacteriaceae* by 10 to 32%. Intraspecies relatedness is very variable, ranging from 55 to 74% with the exception of that of *Y. pestis* and *Y. pseudotuberculosis*, which demonstrate more than 90% relatedness. Based on multilocus sequence typing (MLST) of the housekeeping genes, the two species are very closely related. *Y. pestis* is believed to have evolved from *Y. pseudotuberculosis* prior to the first plague pandemic (1, 12, 64). Detailed analysis of genetic differences between the species was later described by Hinchliffe et al. using DNA microarrays (22). The entire genome of *Y. pestis* has recently been sequenced, and work is in progress to sequence the genome of *Y. pseudotuberculosis*. Data collected from these studies will likely provide definitive information regarding the ancestry of these organisms (42). However, despite the high degree of relatedness between the two species, they have not been combined due to the significant epidemiologic and clinical differences that exist between them.

DESCRIPTION OF THE AGENTS

As are all members of the family *Enterobacteriaceae*, *Yersinia* is a gram-negative, non-spore-forming bacillus that exhibits bipolar staining particularly when seen in primary specimens stained with Giemsa or Wayson's dye, although Wayson's dye is not readily available in most routine clinical laboratories. The bacilli are smaller than other members of their family (0.5 to 0.8 μm in diameter and 1 to 3 μm in length) and tend to grow more slowly as well. With the exception of *Y. pestis*, which is nonmotile, all of the members of the genus are motile at room temperature and nonmotile at 37°C due to the presence of peritrichous or paripolar flagella.

Yersinia species are facultative anaerobes that grow at a wide range of temperatures (4 to 43°C), but optimal growth conditions are 25 to 28°C. *Yersinia* ferments glucose with the production of acid and no gas. Most strains will grow on MacConkey agar as well as various selective media; however, most exhibit poor growth in liquid media and do not form a turbid suspension (62). *Yersinia* is catalase positive and oxidase negative.

The cell walls and antigenic structures of *Yersinia* species are also very similar to those of other members of the *Enterobacteriaceae* family, with an O-specific side chain and only minor variations in the lipopolysaccharides of various serogroups. *Y. enterocolitica* has more than 70 serotypes, *Y. pseudotuberculosis* has 15 (7), and *Y. pestis* lacks the O antigen.

Although all three pathogenic *Yersinia* species, *Y. pestis*, *Y. enterocolitica*, and *Y. pseudotuberculosis*, are associated with different clinical entities, they all have in common the possession of a 70- to 75-kb virulence plasmid that contains the major virulence factors, including the *Yersinia* outer membrane proteins (Yops) and the processing and regulatory proteins for the Yops: Ysc (*Yersinia* secretion) and Lcr (low-calcium response) (6).

The gene for enterotoxin production in *Y. enterocolitica* and *Y. pseudotuberculosis* as well as those for other invasion factors such as invasin is located on the chromosome. *Y. pestis* has two

*This chapter contains information presented in chapter 43 by Jochen Bockemühl and Jane D. Wong in the eigth edition of this Manual.

plasmids that carry the genes for plasminogen activator (Pla), the bacteriocin pesticin (Pst), murine toxin (Ymr), and fraction 1 protein capsule (F1). *Y. pestis*, *Y. pseudotuberculosis*, and some strains of *Y. enterocolitica* also have a chromosomally located high-pathogenicity island that carries the genes for yersiniabactin, a siderophore that provides the organisms with iron. Additionally, *Y. pestis* contains the gene *hsm*, responsible for a hemin storage system. A comprehensive review of the virulence mechanisms and pathogenesis of *Yersinia* species has been recently published (61).

EPIDEMIOLOGY AND TRANSMISSION

The natural reservoir for *Y. pestis* is rodents, which have an inapparent infection and are not a common source of infection for humans. Although many different species of fleas infect more than 100 rodent species that can be specific to geographic locations, transmission of plague is classically associated with the rat flea *(Xenopsylla cheopis)* (18). Approximately 3,000 human cases of plague are identified every year in the world, and about 12 to 15 are identified in the United States (35), where 90% of cases occur in New Mexico, Arizona, Colorado, and California. Transmission to humans is usually through the bite of an infected rodent flea and regurgitation by the flea during a blood meal. *Yersinia* can survive in the stomach and proventriculus of the flea and actually multiply there and block the proventriculus, causing the flea to bite its host mammal repeatedly, thereby increasing chances for disease transmission (43). Interestingly, when the environmental temperature is above 80°F, *Y. pestis* does not produce coagulase, so blockage of the proventriculus is unlikely to occur in the flea, which makes transmission to humans less likely to occur (51). The most common reservoir in the United States for plague transmission is the squirrel. A secondary mode of transmission of disease to humans is through contact with infected cats, either by scratches, bites, or inhalation of aerosolized organisms. Cats become infected by ingestion of contaminated rodents. Human-to-human transmission is very rare and occurs only with the pneumonic form by inhalation of aerosolized particles, which might occur in a bioterrorism attack (see chapter 9). Death can occur within 2 to 4 days. Pneumonic plague is a very rare sequela in patients appropriately treated with antibiotics (<5%) (29). Rare cases of person-to-person transmission from patients with pneumonic plague have been documented. Several of the virulence factors of *Y. pestis* aid in dissemination, including plasminogen activator (Pla), the Yops, and pH 6 antigen. These virulence factors are involved in cell lysis, suppression of the immune system, and survival of the organisms within macrophages. Once *Y. pestis* enters the human host, other virulence factors such as F1 capsular antigen and the yersiniabactin iron scavenging system aid the organism in survival within phagocytes. Endotoxin produced by the organism is associated with the subsequent septic shock and systemic response. *Y. pestis* has been known to survive for days to weeks outside of the vector or mammalian host (in flea feces, dead rodents, or soil), which allows for further transmission.

Plague Pandemics

There have been three plague pandemics, each in different parts of the world and all believed to have been due to one of three biovars of *Y. pestis* differentiated by their abilities to ferment glycerol and to reduce nitrate (see "Identification"). The earliest pandemic, called the Justinian plague, in the fifth through seventh centuries in Africa was associated with biovar Antiqua. Biovar Medievalis, which was identified in Central Asia, was associated with the pandemic known as the Black Death during the 13th to 15th centuries. Modern plague, which originally was identified in southern China and is now worldwide, is associated with biovar Orientalis (29). Using microarray analysis, Zhou et al. (63) proposed a new, fourth biovar, Microtus, which includes strains previously part of the biovar Medievalis but separated based on biochemical, molecular, and pathogenicity differences. Biovar Microtus is pathogenic to the rodent genus *Microtus* (voles), mice, and other small rodents but not to large mammals, including humans (65).

There are more than 70 serotypes of *Y. enterocolitica,* and only a few are associated with disease in animals or humans, five of which are associated with human disease. Serotypes seem to be location specific. *Y. enterocolitica* organisms are widely distributed in nature and are found in the gastrointestinal tracts of many animal species, most commonly swine, rodents, and dogs. Due to their enhanced growth in cold temperatures, geographic distribution is mostly in the northern portions of the United States and in colder portions of Europe. Food products, particularly raw and poorly cooked meats, are frequently found to contain these organisms, although the majority of them are of nonpathogenic serotypes.

Y. pseudotuberculosis is also found in the environment (soil and water) and in a diverse group of wild and domesticated animal species. The main reservoirs for the organism are rodents, rabbits, and wild birds. The mode of transmission of *Y. pseudotuberculosis* is unknown, although due to its similarity to *Y. enterocolitica* (both are found in the environment), it has been speculated that transmission is via contaminated food or water.

CLINICAL SIGNIFICANCE

There are three forms of plague: pneumonic, septicemic, and bubonic. Bubonic plague is the most common clinical presentation. Following the bite of an infected flea, *Y. pestis* migrates through the blood and proliferates in the regional lymph nodes. Following a 2- to 8-day incubation period, the patient develops a fever and a painful swelling (bubo) in the area of the affected node.

Pneumonic plague can be a rare complication of bubonic plague or can be the primary infection following inhalation of aerosolized organisms either from contact with infected animals or from a bioterrorism event. After an incubation period of 1 to 6 days, symptoms include high fever and cough with hemoptysis and chest pain (24). An even higher mortality rate is associated with this form of plague than with bubonic plague.

Septicemic plague can occur when the organisms inoculated by the infected flea spread to the bloodstream without localizing in regional lymph nodes. This form of the disease is more common in children and is rapidly fatal. Septicemic plague can also occur following bubonic plague that is not adequately treated.

The most common form of disease due to *Y. enterocolitica* is gastroenteritis associated with consumption of contaminated food or water. It is not unusual to isolate *Y. enterocolitica* from raw meats including beef, lamb, pork, and chicken. The organism has also been found as a contaminant of cooked, prepackaged deli meat. The majority of strains isolated from human food sources are of the nonpathogenic serotypes. Carriage of the pathogenic serotypes of *Y. enterocolitica* is more common in swine; therefore, consumption of raw or poorly cooked pork, such as chitterlings, is the main risk factor for gastroenteritis (11, 26). Severity of disease is related to the serotype and can range from self-limited gastroenteritis to terminal ileitis and mesenteric lymphadenitis, often misdiagnosed as appendicitis. Young children most commonly develop gastroenteritis and present with fever, diarrhea, and abdominal pain following consumption of food contaminated by *Yersinia*. Although symptoms typically resolve within approximately 7 days, patients can carry the organism in their gastrointestinal tracts for as long as several months. Organisms can migrate out of the gut via the lymphatics into local lymph nodes. An uncommon complication of gastroenteritis is septicemia, which is associated with the patient's HLA type. Persons at high risk for septicemia include the elderly and immunocompromised patients, particularly those with underlying metabolic diseases that are associated with iron overload (hemochromatosis), cancer, liver disease, and steroid therapy.

The production of urease allows the organism to survive in the stomach and colonize the small intestine of the human host. Pathogenic strains contain YoPs which allow them to resist the normal phagocytic and complement killing process that takes place in the Peyer's patches (58).

Y. enterocolitica is the most common cause of transfusion-related infections due to contaminated red blood cells. Since the organism is able to survive and multiply at refrigeration temperatures, donated blood contaminated with small numbers of organisms from an asymptomatic person can transmit infection to the transfused patient (31).

Reactive arthritis is an uncommon sequela of diarrhea due to *Y. enterocolitica*. Patients at increased risk include those who are carriers of the HLA-B27 allele and those with other immunologic disorders. Reactive arthritis is differentiated from rheumatoid arthritis by the asymmetrical involvement of multiple joints, most commonly the sacroiliac and the spine. Symptoms appear several days to months after the onset of diarrhea and may persist for months. Other, less common diseases associated with *Y. enterocolitica* infection include inflammatory bowel disease, most commonly associated with serotype O:3 (48), and autoimmune thyroid disorders such as Graves' disease and Hashimoto's thyroiditis (14). Both *Y. enterocolitica* and *Y. pseudotuberculosis* have been isolated from patients with Crohn's disease, although a causal relationship has not been proven (23).

Y. pseudotuberculosis usually produces a self-limiting disease, particularly in children and young adults. Rarely, *Y. pseudotuberculosis* can cause mesenteric lymphadenitis that clinically mimics appendicitis and septicemia and that occurs usually in immunocompromised patients (diabetics and those with liver cirrhosis or iron overload) (15). Long-term sequlae of *Y. pseudotuberculosis* infection include erythema nodosum, Reiter's syndrome, and nephritis. *Y. pseudotuberculosis* has also recently been implicated as a cause of foodborne illness following an outbreak of gastroenteritis-pseudoappendicitis associated with consumption of contaminated lettuce (40).

The other *Yersinia* species are not known to be human pathogens. Some of the other *Yersinia* species have also been shown to produce an enterotoxin and therefore may be associated with enteric disease in some patients (58). Elderly patients, more commonly women and those being treated with acid blockers, are more likely to develop gastroenteritis due to *Yersinia* species other than *Y. enterocolitica* and to have a prolonged course of disease related to these organisms (33).

COLLECTION, TRANSPORT, AND STORAGE OF SPECIMENS

Y. pestis is on the list of agents of bioterrorism (see chapter 9), and therefore all routine procedures performed with this organism should be done in a facility with a biosafety level of at least 2. Processes which are high risk for creating an aerosol should be performed under biosafety level 3 conditions. Routine clinical laboratories or sentinel laboratories should notify their local public health departments in the case of a presumptive diagnosis of plague. Clinical laboratories should be aware of the protocols as outlined by the American Society for Microbiology (http://www.asm.org/Policy/index.asp?bid=520).

Diagnosis of plague can be made by detection of *Y. pestis* in a bubo aspirate or by growth of *Y. pestis* from the blood. Patients with bubonic plague may shed organisms into the blood intermittently, so obtaining multiple sets of blood cultures over a 24-h period increases the sensitivity of detection. Blood cultures should be incubated at both 28 and 35°C to increase chances of recovery of the organism (3, 24). Other sources appropriate for culture include respiratory samples such as sputum, throat swabs, and throat washing specimens; however, due to contamination of these specimens with normal flora, a bronchial alveolar washing or lavage specimen would be preferable (3). Tissue samples should be collected in a sterile container with a small amount of sterile nonbactericidal saline to avoid drying of tiny pieces. Swab specimens are not recommended due to the poor recovery of the organisms. Blood or tissue specimens can also be collected from animals suspected to have died from *Y. pestis* infection for culture or direct fluorescent-antibody testing for the presence of the F1 antigen. Sera can also be collected from dead infected animals to test for antibody to *Y. pestis*. Material from fleas can be inoculated into mice for culture or direct fluorescent-antibody testing. If clinical suspicions are high and cultures of animal material fail to yield *Y. pestis*, PCR can be attempted. Specimens should be sent to the laboratory immediately, and if a delay in transit of more than 2 h is expected, the sample should be transported at 2 to 8°C, with the exception of blood, which should be transported under ambient conditions.

The appropriate specimen for culture of *Y. enterocolitica* and *Y. pseudotuberculosis* as well as other *Yersinia* species is stool, blood, or lymph nodes, depending on the disease form suspected. If food is suspected as the source of an outbreak, the local health department should be involved in processing of such specimens (see chapter 12). Maintain food at 4°C, and transport it as soon as possible. Swabs should be transported to the laboratory at 4°C in Cary-Blair, Amies, or Stuart's medium. Stool specimens can also be placed in transport media and should be maintained at 4°C if transport is expected to take longer than 2 to 4 h.

MICROSCOPY

Yersinia species are small (1 to 2 μm by 0.5 μm) gram-negative bacilli that appear either as single cells or as pairs or short chains, particularly when stains are prepared from liquid medium. Direct microscopy of a tissue specimen by using either Wright, Giemsa, Wayson's, or methylene blue stain may be helpful in presumptive identification of *Y. pestis* since the organisms appear to be safety pin shaped due to bipolar staining (Fig. 1). This morphology is not always evident following Gram staining or staining of colonies from culture media. Other, more specific direct staining methods include the use of fluorescently labeled antibody to the capsular F1 antigen, which is confirmatory for *Y. pestis*. However, rare strains of *Y. pestis* may lack the F1 antigen, and therefore the LcrV antigen, a key virulence factor that is secreted by the organism, has been used to develop a more sensitive diagnostic tool.

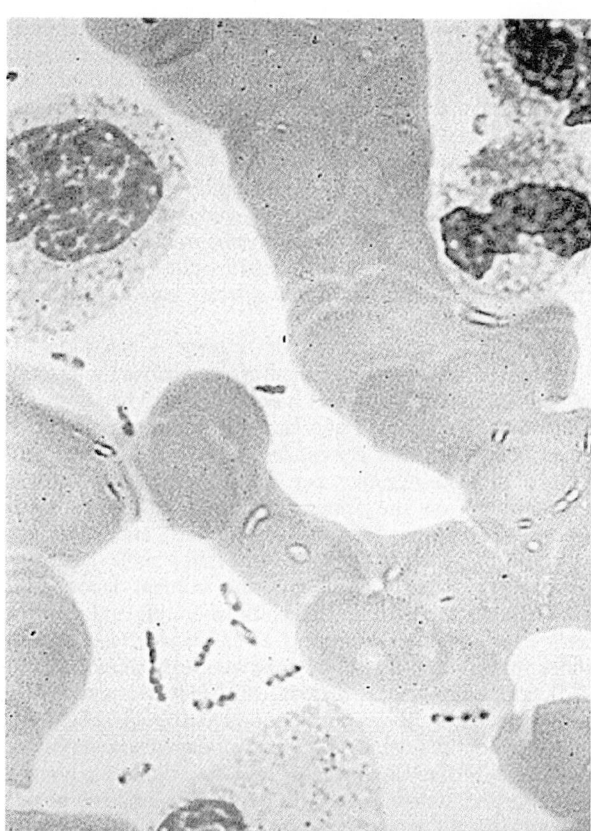

FIGURE 1 Giemsa stain of a blood smear from a patient with *Y. pestis* infection. Note the bipolar-staining "closed safety pin"-shaped cells. (Courtesy of the Centers for Disease Control and Prevention.)

DIRECT DETECTION

An antigen capture enzyme-linked immunosorbent assay (ELISA) using monoclonal antibody to the LcrV antigen detects as little as 0.5 ng of purified *Y. pestis* LcrV in blood or sputum (20). The only disadvantage is that the assay cannot distinguish *Y. pestis* from the other *Yersinia* species, although it would be less likely to find other species in respiratory specimens or blood cultures. A capture ELISA for detection of *Y. pestis* in bubo aspirates can also be applied to serum. This assay was tested on patients in Madagascar and was found to have a high sensitivity (100% with bubos and 90% with sera; limit of detection, 4 ng/ml) and specificity (approximately 99%) (52). Chanteau et al. modified the ELISA to use two different monoclonal antibodies, both directed at the F1 capsular antigen and designed in a dipstick format, to be used in the field for rapid diagnosis of plague in humans or animals (13). The only disadvantage of this assay is the inability to detect strains that lack the F1 capsule; however, this is a rare occurrence (53). Unfortunately, commercial sources for this antigen are not currently available.

Tissue biopsy specimens fixed in formalin can also be stained with an immunohistochemical stain that is based on a monoclonal antibody to the F1 capsular antigen of *Y. pestis*. This is a rapid method for diagnosis of plague that does not rely on having fresh tissue or live organisms (21).

Assays for the direct detection of nucleic acid in patient specimens have been developed to increase the sensitivity of detection of *Y. pestis*, especially in cases of suspected bioterrorism. Initial assays designed to detect the 16S rRNA gene were not found to be useful due to cross-reactivity with *Y. pseudotuberculosis* (45). The most sensitive assay at this time uses primers directed at the plasminogen activator gene (*pla*) that is located in a high copy number on a *Y. pestis*-specific plasmid. Development of a real-time PCR assay to detect the *pla* gene in sputum samples spiked with *Y. pestis* decreased the time to detection to 2 h and increased the sensitivity to 1.5 bacteria per ml (34). This assay also has the advantage of being useful for real-time diagnosis in the field in regions of the world where plague is endemic and culture methods are impractical (45). Following the sequencing of the entire genome of *Y. pestis* (42), so-called signature genes could be identified on the chromosome of *Y. pestis* that allow for its distinction from *Y. pseudotuberculosis* (63).

PCR has also been used as a sensitive method to detect small numbers of *Y. enterocolitica* in foodstuff (59), as well as in stored red blood cells to prevent transfusion reactions (49). Use of a multiplex PCR assay containing primer sets directed at four different virulence genes to test food samples allows for the distinction between pathogenic and nonpathogenic serotypes and specifically identifies the presence of *Y. enterocolitica* serotype O:3 (59).

ISOLATION PROCEDURES

Yersinia species grow on most routine media including blood, chocolate, and MacConkey agars incubated at 35°C in ambient air. Eosin-methylene blue, xylose-lysine-deoxycholate agar, and Hektoen enteric agars do not provide any advantage in the isolation of *Y. enterocolitica* and the differentiation of *Yersinia* species from other normal stool flora. Due to their ability to ferment sucrose and the fact that *Yersinia* species grow more slowly than most *Enterobacteriaceae*, a selective medium is recommended for specifically culturing for *Yersinia* from nonsterile sites. There are various selective media for the recovery of *Y. enterocolitica*, including cefsulodin-Irgasan-novobiocin (CIN) agar, which inhibits the growth of many other organisms from the family *Enterobacteriaceae*. Another selective medium is salmonella-shigella deoxycholate calcium chloride agar (17). CIN agar has been found to provide better recovery rates for *Yersinia* than either MacConkey or salmonella-shigella agar incubated at room temperature. Growth of many strains of *Y. pseudotuberculosis* can be inhibited on CIN agar, and therefore MacConkey agar is preferred for isolation.

Recovery of *Y. enterocolitica* from food is more difficult than recovery from human clinical specimens, and samples are usually referred to a public health laboratory (see chapter 12). Food must be enriched with saline (or a selective broth such as modified Rappaport broth containing magnesium chloride, malachite green, and carbenicillin [MRB]) at cold temperatures for approximately 21 days (2 to 4 days in MRB) (17).

Selective media are not commonly used for the isolation of *Y. pestis*, since when isolated from sterile sites organisms will grow on MacConkey agar and seem to be inhibited to some extent on CIN agar selective for *Y. enterocolitica*. Ber et al. developed a new medium, BIN (brain heart infusion supplemented with Irgasan, cholate salt, crystal violet, and nystatin), for the isolation of *Y. pestis* from specimens likely to be contaminated with normal flora, such as respiratory specimens (4), bubo aspirates, and stool specimens. Plates should be incubated at room temperature in 5% CO_2 for fastest growth. Cultures from suspected plague patients should be incubated for 5 days and up to 7 days if the patient has been treated for more than a few days with an appropriate antimicrobial.

Acute and convalescent serum samples should be collected for serologic testing from pretreated patients for whom cultures do not grow after this period of time.

Y. pestis colonies are slow growing and are only 1 to 2 mm in diameter after 48 h of incubation, with an irregular, "hammered copper" appearance. No hemolysis is seen on blood agar media. Viewed with a dissecting microscope, the colonies are raised with irregular edges, appearing as a "fried egg" (Fig. 2). Organisms growing in broth appear in clumps along the side of the tube in flocculant or stalactite-like formations if the tube is not shaken. After 24 h of incubation, the clumps settle to the bottom of the tube. Colonies of *Y. pestis* growing on BIN agar have a bluish color in the center and a transparent precipitate around the colony.

Colonies of *Y. enterocolitica* have a bull's eye appearance with a red center on CIN agar. Other members of the *Enterobacteriaceae* family, which grow on CIN agar, such as *Serratia*, *Morganella*, and *Citrobacter* spp., produce colonies similar in appearance to those of *Yersinia*, but larger. The use of pectin agar has also been described for isolation of *Y. enterocolitica* from stool and differentiation from other *Enterobacteriaceae*. Although the medium was more sensitive than other currently used selective media and the only other member of the family able to grow and demonstrate a similar colony morphology was *Klebsiella oxytoca*, the medium is not currently commercially available (9).

IDENTIFICATION

Yersinia are catalase positive and oxidase negative and ferment glucose, as do all other members of the family *Enterobacteriaceae*. *Y. enterocolitica* and *Y. pseudotuberculosis* can be presumptively identified by reactions on triple sugar iron (TSI) and lysine iron agar slants. *Y. enterocolitica* produces a yellow color in the entire TSI tube without gas production, and *Y. pseudotuberculosis* produces an alkaline slant and an acid butt, similar to *Shigella*. Both species are lysine decarboxylase negative and therefore produce a yellow butt in lysine iron agar slants. *Yersinia* species are included in the databases of some automated systems; however, most species have not been thoroughly evaluated due to the small number of *Yersinia* isolates tested. Although *Y. pestis* is included in the databases of many of the manual and automated systems (41), commercial systems may not adequately identify *Yersinia* species (particularly *Y. pestis*) due in part to their slow growth and biochemical inactivity. In addition, *Y. pestis* has been misidentified as *Y. pseudotuberculosis* and as *Shigella*, *Salmonella*, and *Acinetobacter* species. API 20E was shown to have the highest sensitivity and specificity for the identification of *Y. enterocolitica* and *Y. pseudotuberculosis* (39). A miniaturized, automated system (MICRONAUT; Merlin, Bornheim-Hersel, Germany) available only outside of the United States shows promise in the identification of *Yersinia* species based on enzyme reactivity (38).

Presumptive identification of *Y. pestis* is based on the detection of bipolar-staining, small gram-negative bacilli forming pinpoint colonies after 24 h on blood, with better growth at 28 than at 35°C, and non-lactose-fermenting colonies on MacConkey agar that are catalase positive and indole, oxidase, and urease negative. See "Basic Protocols for Sentinel Laboratories" on the American Society for Microbiology website for specific information, pictures, and flowcharts (http://www.asm.org/Policy/index.asp?bid=520). Following presumptive identification, routine clinical laboratories should notify the local public health laboratory and refer the isolate for confirmatory testing. *Y. pseudotuberculosis* can be differentiated from *Y. pestis* by negative urease activity.

Y. pestis can further be separated into biovars based on phenotypic methods. Biovars Antiqua and Medievalis are glycerol and arabinose positive, and biovar Antiqua is nitrate positive and biovar Medievalis is negative. Biovar Orientalis is glycerol negative and arabinose and nitrate positive, and the newest biovar, Microtus, is glycerol positive and arabinose and nitrate negative (65).

Presumptive identification of *Y. enterocolitica* can be made based on typical morphology on CIN agar, reactivity on TSI agar, and urease positivity. Identification of the other *Yersinia* species can be performed by biochemical analysis (Table 1).

Y. enterocolitica has six biogroups which can be differentiated based on reactivity to esculin, indole, D-xylose, trehalose, pyrazinamidase, β-D-glucosidase, and lipase. Although the issue is controversial, biogroup 1A is thought to be nonpathogenic and biotypes 1B and 2 through 5 are pathogenic. Strains belonging to biotype 1A can be differentiated from the

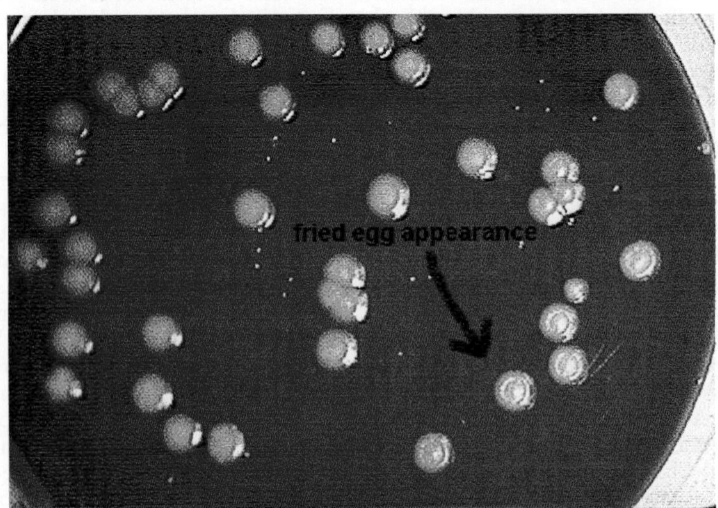

FIGURE 2 Typical fried egg-shaped colonies of *Y. pestis* on sheep blood agar. (Courtesy of the Centers for Disease Control and Prevention.)

TABLE 1 Biochemical reactivity of *Yersinia* species[a]

Yersinia species	Reaction or characteristic[b]													
	Motility (25°C)	Ornithine decarboxylase	Urease	VP (25°C)	Citrate (25°C)	Indole	Rhamnose	Sucrose	Cellobiose	Sorbose	Sorbitol	Melibiose	Raffinose	Fucose
Y. pestis	–	–	–	–	–	–	–	–	–	–	–	V	–	ND
Y. pseudotuberculosis	+	–	+	–	–	–	+	–	–	–	–	+	V	–
Y. enterocolitica	+	+	+	+	–	V	–	+	+	+	+	–	–	V
Y. frederiksenii	+	+	+	+	V	+	+	+	+	+	+	–	–	+
Y. kristensenii	+	+	+	–	–	V	–	–	+	+	+	–	–	V
Y. ruckeri	V	+	–	V	+	–	–	–	–	–	–	–	–	ND
Y. mollaretii	+	+	+	–	–	–	–	+	+	+	+	–	–	–
Y. bercovieri	+	+	+	–	–	–	–	+	+	–	+	–	–	+
Y. rohdei	+	V	V	–	–	–	–	+	+	ND	+	V	V	ND
Y. aldovae	+	+	+	+	+	–	+	–	–	ND	+	–	–	V
Y. intermedia	+	+	+	+	+	+	+	+	+	ND	+	+	+	V

[a]From references 56 and 62.
[b]Incubation is at 35°C except where indicated. VP, Voges-Proskauer; V, variable; ND, not done; –, negative; +, positive.

others by salicin and pyrazinamidase positivity (Table 2) (25). Serotyping could also help determine the pathogenicity of the isolate since only 11 of the 60 known serotypes are pathogenic; however, antisera are not readily available. Other methods that have been evaluated to determine the pathogenicity of *Y. enterocolitica* are based on the presence of the virulence plasmid and include autoagglutination, calcium dependency testing, and Congo red binding. Selective media containing Congo red as well as PCR assays have been evaluated for differentiation of virulent from avirulent strains but are currently being used only in research laboratories (5, 60).

TYPING SYSTEMS

Methods used for the evaluation of the relatedness of *Yersinia* species include serotyping, biotyping, antibiogram analysis, and bacteriophage typing as well as genetic methods. *Y. enterocolitica* can be divided into six biogroups, 1A, 1B, 2, 3, 4, and 5, by using biochemical analysis. These biogroups vary in geographic locations and pathogenic potentials (50). *Y. enterocolitica* also contains more than 70 serotypes, although serotyping is not often performed in routine clinical laboratories since the antisera are not readily available. Pulsed-field gel electrophoresis has long been considered the "gold standard" for typing of *Yersinia* species. Pulsed-field gel electrophoresis was found to be a more useful tool than ribotyping for typing of pathogenic isolates of *Y. enterocolitica* (59). Patterns generated by the restriction enzyme NotI alone or combined with ApaI and XhoI were highly discriminatory (36).

Recently, MLEE has been evaluated for its discriminatory power among *Yersinia* species. Sequencing of a single gene unique to an organism, such as 16S rRNA, has also been used for strain analysis of *Yersinia* species (30). An approach that combines the ease of MLEE testing with the specificity of genome sequencing is MLST. Comparing the sequences of multiple unique genes allows for better discrimination than comparing only 16S rRNA. This technique has recently been applied to *Yersinia* (2). MLST analysis of a large collection of *Yersinia* species was further studied by Kotetishvili et al. (30). With the use of six genes, all of the *Y. pestis* isolates appeared to be homogeneous and also were found to be identical to *Y. pseudotuberculosis*. Most of the other species of *Yersinia* tested also appeared to be homogeneous, with the exception of *Y. enterocolitica*, *Y. frederiksenii*, *Y. kristensenii*, and *Y. mollaretii*, which were more heterogeneous.

SEROLOGIC TESTS

The gold standard for the diagnosis of plague is isolation of the organism from blood or aspirate; however, serology can play a role, particularly for retrospective diagnostic and epidemiologic studies in areas where plague is endemic (46). Most patients with plague seroconvert 1 to 2 weeks following the onset of symptoms (47). Diagnosis can be made based only on a fourfold rise in antibody titers between acute and convalescent serum samples. Assay methods include passive hemagglutination, which is the method recommended by the World Health Organization due to its low cost and ease of performance. However, the assay lacks both sensitivity and specificity due to lack of standardization and lack of commercialization of reagents. The most commonly used antigen in serologic assays for *Y. pestis* is the capsular F1 antigen, which is a highly immunogenic, stable antigen and present in high concentrations in sera and bubo fluids of plague patients even after several days of appropriate antimicrobial therapy.

TABLE 2 Biotypes of *Y. enterocolitica*[a] after incubation at 25°C for 48 h

Test	Reaction[b] for biotype:					
	1A	1B	2	3	4	5
Lipase (Tween esterase)	+	+	−	−	−	−
Esculin	+	−	−	−	−	−
Salicin	+	−	−	−	−	−
Indole	+	+	(+)	−	−	−
Xylose	+	+	+	+	−	d
Trehalose	+	+	+	+	+	−
$NO_3 \rightarrow NO_2$	+	+	+	+	+	−
DNase	−	−	−	−	+	+
Pyrazinamidase[c]	+	−	−	−	−	−

[a]Modified from reference 62a with permission of the publisher, S. Karger AG, Basel, Switzerland.

[b]+, ≥90% of strains positive; d, 11 to 89% of strains positive; −, ≥90% of strains negative; (+), weakly positive reaction.

[c]According to Kandolo and Wauters (27a).

Other assays include ELISA, which is not standardized either and must be confirmed by using a Western blot assay.

Serology can be used as an adjunct in the diagnosis of disease due to *Y. enterocolitica* or *Y. pseudotuberculosis*. Antibody is detectable within the first week of illness and returns to normal levels 3 to 6 months later. The specificity of serologic assays ranges from 82 to 95% due to cross-reactivity between the two species and also with *Brucella*, *Franciscella*, and *Vibrio* species, *Borrelia burgdorferi*, *Chlamydia pneumoniae*, and some *Escherichia coli* serogroups. Another disadvantage of using serology for diagnosis is that antibodies to *Y. enterocolitica* O antigens can be found in many normally healthy patients due to the frequency of exposure to nonpathogenic serotypes. Most human infections with *Y. enterocolitica* involve serotypes O:3, O:5, 27, O:8, and O:9. Serotype O:3 is the most common cause of gastroenteritis. However, as mentioned above, antisera are available only to public health and research laboratories.

Antibody to outer membrane proteins (Yops) that are present only in virulent strains of *Y. enterocolitica* may be more helpful. In a small study of normally healthy blood donors, immunoglobulin M (IgM) antibody to Yops was 97% specific for acute infection (57). Testing of blood donors for anti-Yop IgA in New Zealand, which has a high incidence of *Y. enterocolitica* gastroenteritis, showed promise in preventing transfusion-related infections (28). The presence of IgG and IgA antibodies to *Y. enterocolitica* Yops is also used as an aid in the diagnosis of autoimmune disorders that occur post-infection, such as reactive arthritis, erythema nodosum, Graves' disease, and Hashimoto's thyroiditis (14). Increased sensitivity and specificity are seen with the Western blot assay compared to complement fixation and ELISA; however, cross-reactivity is still seen, particularly with *B. burgdorferi*, which can be associated with arthritis that is clinically indistinguishable from that due to *Y. enterocolitica* (47).

ANTIMICROBIAL SUSCEPTIBILITIES

Pneumonic plague is nearly 100% fatal if not treated within the first 24 h of development of symptoms. The drug of choice for the treatment of plague, pneumonic, septicemic, or bubonic, is streptomycin. However, due to the lack of availability of streptomycin and the threats of *Y. pestis*'s being used as an agent of bioterrorism, other agents have been evaluated in vitro and in animal models. The only other antibiotic currently approved for treatment of plague is doxycycline; however, other alternatives would be gentamicin and a fluoroquinolone (8). Antibiotic resistance among isolates of *Y. pestis* has been described, but only in rare case reports of resistance to tetracycline or streptomycin. Fluoroquinolone resistance has been induced in vitro, but naturally occurring resistance has not been documented (16). Steward et al. documented the efficacy of fluoroquinolones in the mouse model of systemic and pneumonic plague (55). Rapid detection of ciprofloxacin-resistant strains of *Y. pestis* can be accomplished by using real-time PCR and assessing point mutations in the DNA gyrase gene (32). An isolate of *Y. pestis* from a single infected patient in Madagascar was found to be multidrug resistant, with resistance to streptomycin, sulfonamides, tetracycline, and chloramphenicol (19). The treatment of choice for plague meningitis is chloramphenicol.

Most cases of *Y. enterocolitica* gastroenteritis do not require treatment; however, treatment is necessary in cases of systemic disease, especially in immunosuppressed patients. Treatment options include trimethoprim-sulfamethoxazole and a fluoroquinolone. *Y. enterocolitica* produces two different β-lactamases, one of which is a class A constitutive enzyme and the other of which is an inducible class C enzyme that is not inhibited by β-lactamase inhibitors. The presence of one or both of these enzymes varies depending on the biogroup (10). Although the β-lactamase confers resistance to penicillin on *Y. enterocolitica,* the organism remains uniformly susceptible to the extended-spectrum cephalosporins (44). Resistance to fluoroquinolones is due to either a mutation in the *gyrA* gene or efflux mechanisms. In a study conducted in Spain, 23% of *Y. enterocolitica* strains isolated from patients with gastroenteritis were nalidixic acid resistant. All resistant isolates had a mutation in *gyrA,* and some were resistant based on an efflux mechanism as well (10). *Y. enterocolitica* strains are susceptible in vitro to aminoglycosides, chloramphenicol, tetracycline, trimethoprim-sulfamethoxazole, and extended-spectrum cephalosporins.

Y. pseudotuberculosis is susceptible to ampicillin, tetracycline, chloramphenicol, cephalosporins, and aminoglycosides. Although infections due to *Y. pseudotuberculosis* are not usually treated, patients with septicemia should be treated with ampicillin, streptomycin, or tetracycline.

Y. aldovae and *Y. ruckeri* are also susceptible to penicillin. *Y. frederiksenii, Y. intermedia,* and *Y. rhodei* produce a β-lactamase similar to that of *Y. enterocolitica*, which is expressed at different levels in different strains (56).

EVALUATION, INTERPRETATION, AND REPORTING OF RESULTS

Y. pestis, *Y. enterocolitica,* and *Y. pseudotuberculosis* are the primary pathogens in the genus *Yersinia.* Isolation of *Y. pestis* from any body site warrants further investigation. Isolation of *Y. enterocolitica* or *Y. pseudotuberculosis* from stool culture is not sufficient for causal evidence of disease since nonpathogenic serotypes may be normal stool flora. However, no readily available methods except those using routine biochemicals, which are not usually maintained in routine clinical laboratories, are available for differentiation of pathogenic serotypes. Isolation of either species in pure culture from a symptomatic patient with no other diagnosis should be considered suspect. Isolation of either species from blood or other normally sterile sites should also be considered significant.

It has not been shown to be cost-effective to screen all stools for *Y. enterocolitica* by using CIN agar. Isolation rates vary based on geographic locations, with the highest incidence in the colder portions of the country (27), so the decision to routinely rule out these organisms in stool cultures should be evaluated in individual laboratories after consultation with the infectious disease physicians.

Although the other *Yersinia* species besides *Y. pestis*, *Y. enterocolitica*, and *Y. pseudotuberculosis* are not considered human pathogens, they have been isolated from the gastrointestinal tracts of symptomatic patients with no other diagnosis. It has been recommended that the presence of these *Yersinia* species in pure culture be reported and that antibiotic susceptibility testing be performed to assess these organisms' pathogenic potentials. These organisms may be underrecognized pathogens (33).

Due to the lack of accuracy of commercial systems for the identification of *Y. pestis* and the implications related to bioterrorism with its identification, isolates should be sent to a local public health laboratory for confirmation.

REFERENCES

1. **Achtman, M., G. Morelli, and P. Zhu.** 2004. Microevolution and history of the plague bacillus, *Yersinia pestis*. *Proc. Natl. Acad. Sci. USA* **101:**17837–17842.
2. **Achtman, M., K. Zurth, G. Morelli, G. Torrea, A. Guiyoule, and E. Carniel.** 1999. *Yersinia pestis*, the cause of plague, is a recently emerged clone of *Yersinia pseudotuberculosis*. *Proc. Natl. Acad. Sci. USA* **96:**14043–14048.
3. **American Society for Microbiology.** 15 August 2005, posting date. *Sentinel Laboratory Guidelines for Suspected Agents of Bioterrorism:* Yersinia pestis. [Online.] American Society for Microbiology, Washington, D.C. http://www.asm.org/ASM/files/LeftMarginHeaderList/DOWNLOADFILENAME/000000000524/ypestis81505.pdf.
4. **Ber, R., E. Mamroud, M. Aftalion, A. Tidhar, D. Gur, Y. Flashner, and S. Cohen.** 2003. Development of an improved selective agar medium for isolation of *Yersinia pestis*. *Appl. Environ. Microbiol.* **69:**5787–5792.
5. **Bhaduri, S., C. Turner-Jones, and R. V. Lachica.** 1991. Convenient agarose medium for simultaneous determination of the low-calcium response and Congo red binding by virulent strains of *Yersinia enterocolitica*. *J. Clin. Microbiol.* **29:**2341–2344.
6. **Bleves, S., and G. R. Cornelis.** 2000. How to survive in the host: the *Yersinia* lesson. *Microbes Infect.* **2:**1451–1460.
7. **Bogdanovich, T., E. Carniel, H. Fukushima, and M. Skurnik.** 2003. Use of O-antigen gene cluster-specific PCRs for the identification and O-genotyping of *Yersinia pseudotuberculosis* and *Yersinia pestis*. *J. Clin. Microbiol.* **41:**5103–5112.
8. **Boulanger, L. L., P. Ettestad, J. D. Fogarty, D. T. Dennis, D. Romig, and G. Mertz.** 2004. Gentamicin and tetracyclines for the treatment of human plague: review of 75 cases in New Mexico, 1985–1999. *Clin. Infect. Dis.* **38:**663–669.
9. **Bowen, J. H., and S. D. Kominos.** 1979. Evaluation of a pectin agar medium for isolation of *Yersinia enterocolitica* within 48 hours. *Am. J. Clin. Pathol.* **72:**586–590.
10. **Capilla, S., J. Ruiz, P. Goni, J. Castillo, M. C. Rubio, M. T. Jimenez de Anta, R. Gomez-Lus, and J. Vila.** 2004. Characterization of the molecular mechanisms of quinolone resistance in *Yersinia enterocolitica* O:3 clinical isolates. *J. Antimicrob. Chemother.* **53:**1068–1071.
11. **Centers for Disease Control and Prevention.** 2003. *Yersinia enterocolitica* gastroenteritis among infants exposed to chitterlings—Chicago, Illinois, 2002. *Morb. Mortal. Wkly. Rep.* **52:**956–958.
12. **Chain, P. S., E. Carniel, F. W. Larimer, J. Lamerdin, P. O. Stoutland, W. M. Regala, A. M. Georgescu, L. M. Vergez, M. L. Land, V. L. Motin, R. R. Brubaker, J. Fowler, J. Hinnebusch, M. Marceau, C. Medigue, M. Simonet, V. Chenal-Francisque, B. Souza, D. Dacheux, J. M. Elliott, A. Derbise, L. J. Hauser, and E. Garcia.** 2004. Insights into the evolution of *Yersinia pestis* through whole-genome comparison with *Yersinia pseudotuberculosis*. *Proc. Natl. Acad. Sci. USA* **101:**13826–13831.
13. **Chanteau, S., L. Rahalison, L. Ralafiarisoa, J. Foulon, M. Ratsitorahina, L. Ratsifasoamanana, E. Carniel, and F. Nato.** 2003. Development and testing of a rapid diagnostic test for bubonic and pneumonic plague. *Lancet* **361:**211–216.
14. **Chatzipanagiotou, S., J. N. Legakis, F. Boufidou, V. Petroyianni, and C. Nicolaou.** 2001. Prevalence of *Yersinia* plasmid-encoded outer protein (Yop) class-specific antibodies in patients with Hashimoto's thyroiditis. *Clin. Microbiol. Infect.* **7:**138–143.
15. **Deacon, A. G., A. Hay, and J. Duncan.** 2003. Septicemia due to *Yersinia pseudotuberculosis*—a case report. *Clin. Microbiol. Infect.* **9:**1118–1119.
16. **Frean, J., K. P. Klugman, L. Arntzen, and S. Bukofzer.** 2003. Susceptibility of *Yersinia pestis* to novel and conventional antimicrobial agents. *J. Antimicrob. Chemother.* **52:**294–296.
17. **Fredriksson-Ahomaa, M., and H. Korkeala.** 2003. Low occurrence of pathogenic *Yersinia enterocolitica* in clinical, food, and environmental samples: a methodological problem. *Clin. Microbiol. Rev.* **16:**220–229.
18. **Gage, K. L., and M. Y. Kosoy.** 2005. Natural history of plague: perspectives from more than a century of research. *Annu. Rev. Entomol.* **50:**505–528.
19. **Galimand, M., A. Guiyoule, G. Gerbaud, B. Rasoamanana, S. Chanteau, E. Carniel, and P. Courvalin.** 1997. Multidrug resistance in *Yersinia pestis* mediated by a transferable plasmid. *N. Engl. J. Med.* **337:**677–680.
20. **Gomes-Solecki, M. J., A. G. Savitt, R. Rowehl, J. D. Glass, J. B. Bliska, and R. J. Dattwyler.** 2005. LcrV capture enzyme-linked immunosorbent assay for detection of *Yersinia pestis* from human samples. *Clin. Diagn. Lab. Immunol.* **12:**339–346.
21. **Guarner, J., W. J. Shieh, P. W. Greer, J. M. Gabastou, M. Chu, E. Hayes, K. B. Nolte, and S. R. Zaki.** 2002. Immunohistochemical detection of *Yersinia pestis* in formalin-fixed, paraffin-embedded tissue. *Am. J. Clin. Pathol.* **117:**205–209.
22. **Hinchliffe, S. J., K. E. Isherwood, R. A. Stabler, M. B. Prentice, A. Rakin, R. A. Nichols, P. C. Oyston, J. Hinds, R. W. Titball, and B. W. Wren.** 2003. Application of DNA microarrays to study the evolutionary genomics of *Yersinia pestis* and *Yersinia pseudotuberculosis*. *Genome Res.* **13:**2018–2029.
23. **Homewood, R., C. P. Gibbons, D. Richards, A. Lewis, P. D. Duane, and A. P. Griffiths.** 2003. Ileitis due to *Yersinia pseudotuberculosis* in Crohn's disease. *J. Infect.* **47:**328–332.
24. **Inglesby, T. V., D. T. Dennis, D. A. Henderson, J. G. Bartlett, M. S. Ascher, E. Eitzen, A. D. Fine, A. M. Friedlander, J. Hauer, J. F. Koerner, M. Layton, J. McDade, M. T. Osterholm, T. O'Toole, G. Parker, T. M. Perl, P. K. Russell, M. Schoch-Spana, K. Tonat, et al.** 2000. Plague as a biological weapon: medical and public health management. *JAMA* **283:**2281–2290.
25. **Janda, J., and S. Abbott.** 2005. *The Enterobacteria*, 2nd ed. ASM Press, Washington, D.C.
26. **Jones, T. F.** 2003. From pig to pacifier: chitterling-associated yersiniosis outbreak among black infants. *Emerg. Infect. Dis.* **9:**1007–1009.
27. **Kachoris, M., K. L. Ruoff, K. Welch, W. Kallas, and M. J. Ferraro.** 1988. Routine culture of stool specimens for *Yersinia enterocolitica* is not a cost-effective procedure. *J. Clin. Microbiol.* **26:**582–583.

27a. **Kandolo, K., and G. Wauters.** 1985. Pyrazinamidase activity in *Yersinia enterocolitica* and related organisms. *J. Clin. Microbiol.* **21:**980–982.

28. **Kendrick, C. J., B. Baker, A. J. Morris, and P. W. O'Toole.** 2001. Identification of *Yersinia*-infected blood donors by anti-Yop IgA immunoassay. *Transfusion* **41:** 1365–1372.

29. **Kool, J. L.** 2005. Risk of person-to-person transmission of pneumonic plague. *Clin. Infect. Dis.* **40:**1166–1172.

30. **Kotetishvili, M., A. Kreger, G. Wauters, J. G. Morris, Jr., A. Sulakvelidze, and O. C. Stine.** 2005. Multilocus sequence typing for studying genetic relationships among *Yersinia* species. *J. Clin. Microbiol.* **43:**2674–2684.

31. **Leclercq, A., L. Martin, M. L. Vergnes, N. Ounnoughene, J. F. Laran, P. Giraud, and E. Carniel.** 2005. Fatal *Yersinia enterocolitica* biotype 4 serovar O:3 sepsis after red blood cell transfusion. *Transfusion* **45:**814–818.

32. **Lindler, L. E., W. Fan, and N. Jahan.** 2001. Detection of ciprofloxacin-resistant *Yersinia pestis* by fluorogenic PCR using the LightCycler. *J. Clin. Microbiol.* **39:**3649–3655.

33. **Loftus, C. G., G. C. Harewood, F. R. Cockerill III, and J. A. Murray.** 2002. Clinical features of patients with novel *Yersinia* species. *Dig. Dis. Sci.* **47:**2805–2810.

34. **Loiez, C., S. Herwegh, F. Wallet, S. Armand, F. Guinet, and R. J. Courcol.** 2003. Detection of *Yersinia pestis* in sputum by real-time PCR. *J. Clin. Microbiol.* **41:**4873–4875.

35. **Lowell, J. L., D. M. Wagner, B. Atshabar, M. F. Antolin, A. J. Vogler, P. Keim, M. C. Chu, and K. L. Gage.** 2005. Identifying sources of human exposure to plague. *J. Clin. Microbiol.* **43:**650–656.

36. **Lukinmaa, S., U. M. Nakari, M. Eklund, and A. Siitonen.** 2004. Application of molecular genetic methods in diagnostics and epidemiology of food-borne bacterial pathogens. *APMIS* **112:**908–929.

37. **Neubauer, H., S. Aleksic, A. Hensel, E. J. Finke, and H. Meyer.** 2000. *Yersinia enterocolitica* 16S rRNA gene types belong to the same genospecies but from three homology groups. *Int. J. Med. Microbiol.* **290:**61–64.

38. **Neubauer, H., M. Molitor, L. Rahalison, S. Aleksic, H. Backes, S. Chanteau, and H. Meyer.** 2000. A miniaturised semiautomated system for the identification of *Yersinia* species within the genus *Yersinia*. *Clin. Lab.* **46:**561–567.

39. **Neubauer, H., T. Sauer, H. Becker, S. Aleksic, and H. Meyer.** 1998. Comparison of systems for identification and differentiation of species within the genus *Yersinia*. *J. Clin. Microbiol.* **36:**3366–3368.

40. **Nuorti, J. P., T. Niskanen, S. Hallanvuo, J. Mikkola, E. Kela, M. Hatakka, M. Fredriksson-Ahomaa, O. Lyytikainen, A. Siitonen, H. Korkeala, and P. Ruutu.** 2004. A widespread outbreak of *Yersinia pseudotuberculosis* O:3 infection from iceberg lettuce. *J. Infect. Dis.* **189:** 766–774.

41. **O'Hara, C. M.** 2005. Manual and automated instrumentation for identification of *Enterobacteriaceae* and other aerobic gram-negative bacilli. *Clin. Microbiol. Rev.* **18:**147–162.

42. **Parkhill, J., B. W. Wren, N. R. Thomson, R. W. Titball, M. T. Holden, M. B. Prentice, M. Sebaihia, K. D. James, C. Churcher, K. L. Mungall, S. Baker, D. Basham, S. D. Bentley, K. Brooks, A. M. Cerdeno-Tarraga, T. Chillingworth, A. Cronin, R. M. Davies, P. Davis, G. Dougan, T. Feltwell, N. Hamlin, S. Holroyd, K. Jagels, A. V. Karlyshev, S. Leather, S. Moule, P. C. Oyston, M. Quail, K. Rutherford, M. Simmonds, J. Skelton, K. Stevens, S. Whitehead, and B. G. Barrell.** 2001. Genome sequence of *Yersinia pestis*, the causative agent of plague. *Nature* **413:**523–527.

43. **Perry, R. D.** 2003. A plague of fleas—survival and transmission of *Yersinia pestis*. *ASM News* **69:**336–340.

44. **Pham, J. N., S. M. Bell, L. Martin, and E. Carniel.** 2000. The beta-lactamases and beta-lactam antibiotic susceptibility of *Yersinia enterocolitica*. *J. Antimicrob. Chemother.* **46:**951–957.

45. **Rahalison, L., E. Vololonirina, M. Ratsitorahina, and S. Chanteau.** 2000. Diagnosis of bubonic plague by PCR in Madagascar under field conditions. *J. Clin. Microbiol.* **38:** 260–263.

46. **Rasoamanana, B., F. Leroy, P. Boisier, M. Rasolomaharo, P. Buchy, E. Carniel, and S. Chanteau.** 1997. Field evaluation of an immunoglobulin G anti-F1 enzyme-linked immunosorbent assay for serodiagnosis of human plague in Madagascar. *Clin. Diagn. Lab. Immunol.* **4:**587–591.

47. **Rawlins, M. L., C. Gerstner, H. R. Hill, and C. M. Litwin.** 2005. Evaluation of a Western blot method for the detection of *Yersinia* antibodies: evidence of serological cross-reactivity between *Yersinia* outer membrane proteins and *Borrelia burgdorferi*. *Clin. Diagn. Lab. Immunol.* **12:** 1269–1274.

48. **Saebo, A., E. Vik, O. J. Lange, and L. Matuszkiewicz.** 2005. Inflammatory bowel disease associated with *Yersinia enterocolitica* O:3 infection. *Eur. J. Intern. Med.* **16:**176–182.

49. **Sen, K.** 2000. Rapid identification of *Yersinia enterocolitica* in blood by the 5' nuclease PCR assay. *J. Clin. Microbiol.* **38:**1953–1958.

50. **Sharma, S., P. Ramnani, and J. S. Virdi.** 2004. Detection and assay of beta-lactamases in clinical and non-clinical strains of *Yersinia enterocolitica* biovar 1A. *J. Antimicrob. Chemother.* **54:**401–405.

51. **Slack, M. P.** 1999. *Infectious Diseases*, vol. 2. Mosby, Philadelphia, Pa.

52. **Splettstoesser, W. D., R. Grunow, L. Rahalison, T. J. Brooks, S. Chanteau, and H. Neubauer.** 2003. Serodiagnosis of human plague by a combination of immunomagnetic separation and flow cytometry. *Cytometry* A **53:**88–96.

53. **Splettstoesser, W. D., L. Rahalison, R. Grunow, H. Neubauer, and S. Chanteau.** 2004. Evaluation of a standardized F1 capsular antigen capture ELISA test kit for the rapid diagnosis of plague. *FEMS Immunol. Med. Microbiol.* **41:**149–155.

54. **Sprague, L. D., and H. Neubauer.** 2005. *Yersinia aleksiciae* sp. nov. *Int. J. Syst. Evol. Microbiol.* **55:**831–835.

55. **Steward, J., M. S. Lever, P. Russell, R. J. Beedham, A. J. Stagg, R. R. Taylor, and T. J. Brooks.** 2004. Efficacy of the latest fluoroquinolones against experimental *Yersinia pestis*. *Int. J. Antimicrob. Agents* **24:**609–612.

56. **Stock, I., and B. Wiedemann.** 2003. Natural antimicrobial susceptibilities and biochemical profiles of *Yersinia enterocolitica*-like strains: *Y. frederiksenii*, *Y. intermedia*, *Y. kristensenii* and *Y. rohdei*. *FEMS Immunol. Med. Microbiol.* **38:**139–152.

57. **Strobel, E., J. Heesemann, G. Mayer, J. Peters, S. Muller-Weihrich, and P. Emmerling.** 2000. Bacteriological and serological findings in a further case of transfusion-mediated *Yersinia enterocolitica* sepsis. *J. Clin. Microbiol.* **38:** 2788–2790.

58. **Sulakvelidze, A.** 2000. *Yersiniae* other than *Y. enterocolitica*, *Y. pseudotuberculosis*, and *Y. pestis*: the ignored species. *Microbes Infect.* **2:**497–513.

59. **Thisted Lambertz, S., and M.-L. Danielsson-Tham.** 2005. Identification and characterization of pathogenic *Yersinia enterocolitica* isolates by PCR and pulsed-field gel electrophoresis. *Appl. Environ. Microbiol.* **71:**3674–3681.

60. **Thoerner, P., C. I. Bin Kingombe, K. Bogli-Stuber, B. Bissig-Choisat, T. M. Wassenaar, J. Frey, and T. Jemmi.** 2003. PCR detection of virulence genes in *Yersinia enterocolitica* and *Yersinia pseudotuberculosis* and investigation of virulence gene distribution. *Appl. Environ. Microbiol.* **69:** 1810–1816.

61. **Viboud, G. I., and J. B. Bliska.** 2005. *Yersinia* outer proteins: role in modulation of host cell signalling responses and pathogenesis. *Annu. Rev. Microbiol.* **59:**69–89.

62. **Wanger, A.** 1998. *Yersinia*, p. 1051–1063. *In* A. Balows and B. Duerden (ed.), *Topley & Wilson's Microbiology and*

Microbial Infections, vol. 2. Arnold, London, United Kingdom.

62a. **Wauters, G., K. Kandolo, and M. Janssens.** 1987. Revised biogrouping scheme of *Yersinia enterocolitica*. *Contrib. Microbiol. Immunol.* **9:**14–21.

63. **Zhou, D., Y. Han, E. Dai, D. Pei, Y. Song, J. Zhai, Z. Du, J. Wang, Z. Guo, and R. Yang.** 2004. Identification of signature genes for rapid and specific characterization of *Yersinia pestis*. *Microbiol. Immunol.* **48:**263–269.

64. **Zhou, D., Y. Han, Y. Song, P. Huang, and R. Yang.** 2004. Comparative and evolutionary genomics of *Yersinia pestis*. *Microbes Infect.* **6:**1226–1234.

65. **Zhou, D., Z. Tong, Y. Song, Y. Han, D. Pei, X. Pang, J. Zhai, M. Li, B. Cui, Z. Qi, L. Jin, R. Dai, Z. Du, J. Wang, Z. Guo, P. Huang, and R. Yang.** 2004. Genetics of metabolic variations between *Yersinia pestis* biovars and the proposal of a new biovar, microtus. *J. Bacteriol.* **186:**5147–5152.

Klebsiella, Enterobacter, Citrobacter, Serratia, Plesiomonas, and Other *Enterobacteriaceae*

SHARON L. ABBOTT

45

TAXONOMY

Taxonomic changes within the *Enterobacteriaceae* have become commonplace and undoubtedly will continue at a rapid pace for the foreseeable future. Three major taxonomic changes in the *Enterobacteriaceae* included in the eighth edition of this Manual merit mention again. The oxidase-positive organism, *Plesiomonas shigelloides,* which clusters with *Proteus* in phylogenetic studies using 16S and 5S rRNA sequencing is now a member of the family *Enterobacteriaceae* (98, 99, 125). The *Enterobacteriaceae* will be redefined in the next edition of *Bergey's Manual* to accommodate an oxidase-positive organism and other organisms that defy the traditional definition of this family. Inclusion of *Calymmatobacterium granulomatis,* a nonculturable organism causing a sexually transmitted disease, in the genus *Klebsiella* as *K. granulomatis* was another major change (28, 85). This move was based on 16S rRNA and *phoE* gene sequencing. Lastly, it should be remembered that *Enterobacter agglomerans* now resides in the genus *Pantoea; P. agglomerans* remains heterogeneous at the DNA level (46). Members of the *Enterobacteriaceae* covered in this chapter, including new taxa or taxonomic changes, are listed in Tables 1 and 2. When laboratories adopt taxonomic changes, which are dictated by common usage in the literature, the older epithet should be included in parentheses following the new name.

Because of the genetic heterogeneity within the genus, taxonomic changes occur frequently in *Enterobacter*. To start, two new species, *E. radicincitans* and *E. ludwigii,* have been added to the genus (64, 81). *E. radicincitans* is a plant growth-promoting bacterium isolated from the phyllosphere of wheat, and *E. ludwigii,* which is isolated from human clinical specimens, was formerly a genomovar within the *E. cloacae* complex. Two other clusters of organisms previously included in the *E. cloacae* complex are now subspecies of *E. hormaechei*. Strains previously known as *E. hormaechei* are now subsp. *hormaechei,* and there are two newly created subspecies, subsp. *oharae* and subsp. *steigerwaltii;* all three subspecies are isolated from human clinical specimens from multiple sites and from plants (63). *Enterobacter intermedius,* which clustered with the type strain of *Kluyvera cochleae* by 16S rRNA sequencing, has been moved to the genus *Kluyvera* (118). The older legitimate epithet, *intermedius,* has replaced *cochleae* as the species name, resulting in the new designation *Kluyvera intermedia. E. dissolvens,* which was previously suspected to belong in *E. cloacae,* is now *E. cloacae* subsp. *dissolvens;* strains formerly known as *E. cloacae* are now *E. cloacae* subspecies *cloacae* (62). *E. cloacae* remains a heterogeneous species with several DNA groups residing within it, and as with *P. agglomerans* groups, these groups remain unnamed because they are not separable by phenotypic tests (61). *Hafnia alvei* is composed of two distinct DNA hybridization groups, and studies are in progress to name DNA hybrization group 2 (74).

Several additions have been proposed for the genus *Serratia. S. marcescens* subsp. *sakuensis* is a strain isolated from activated sludge from a wastewater treatment plant in Japan and reportedly is a spore former; strains known as *S. marcescens* assume subspecies status as subsp. *marcescens* (2). Of the two new species added to *Serratia,* one is a urea-utilizing organism isolated from water in India, named *S. ureilytica,* of which only a single strain is known, and the other is a nonculturable symbiont found in aphids and provisionally designated "*Candidatus* Serratia symbiotica" (17, 104).

In the genus *Klebsiella,* a group of nitrogen-fixing strains isolated from plants (banana, rice, sugar cane, and maize) and human clinical samples, primarily blood, have been named *K. variicola* (124). A second new species, *K. singaporensis,* has been proposed for a single strain isolated from soil collected from sugar cane roots in Singapore (93).

Two new species have been created within the genus *Photorhabdus, P. temperata* and *P. asymbiotica,* and three subspecies (*luminescens, laumondii,* and *akhurstii*) were described for the existing species, *P. luminescens* (43). *P. temperata,* like *P. luminescens,* is a symbiont of nematodes that causes disease in insects. However, *P. asymbiotica* contains only isolates from human infections and has two subspecies, *asymbiotica* and *australis,* isolated in the United States and Australia, respectively (3). Four new species, all symbionts in entomopathogenic nematodes, have been proposed for the genus *Xenorhabdus* including *X. budapestensis, X. ehlersii, X. innexi,* and *X. szentirmaii* (92).

Two new genera, *Averyella* and *Dickeya,* have been proposed for the *Enterobacteriaceae* (78, 127). *Averyella dalhousiensis* strains, previously known as enteric group 58, are isolated primarily from human wound specimens, although the organism was recently isolated from blood (78). The genus *Dickeya* includes two species transferred from *Pectobacterium* (*chrysanthemi*) and *Brenneria* (*paradisiaca*) as well as four novel species (*dadantii, dianthicola, dieffenbachiae,*

TABLE 1 Nomenclature, isolation source, and significance of selected genera of the family *Enterobacteriaceae*[a]

Current (previous) designation	Clinical data			Environmental data
	Frequency	Source	Significance	
Averyella dalhousiensis (enteric group 58)	Unk	Wound, blood	2	Unk
Citrobacter				
C. amalonaticus	++	**Feces,** blood, wound, UT, RT	2	Unk, one isolate from an animal
C. braakii	++	**Feces,** UT, wound	2	Similar to *C. freundii*
C. farmeri (*C. amalonaticus* biogroup 1)	++	**Feces,** UT, blood, wound, RT	2	Unk
C. freundii	++++	All sites, feces most common	1	Water, soil, fish, animals, food
C. koseri (*C. diversus*)	++	All sites, CSF most common	1	Unk
C. rodentium	–			Pathogenic for mice
C. sedlakii	+	Feces, UT, blood, wound	3	Same as for *C. braakii*
C. werkmanii	+	**Feces,** blood, wound	3	Same as for *C. braakii*
C. youngae	+++	**Feces,** UT, blood, wound	3	Same as for *C. braakii*
C. gillenii (*Citrobacter* DNA group 10)	+	**Feces,** UT, blood	3	Same as for *C. braakii*
C. murlinae (*Citrobacter* DNA group 11)	+	Feces, blood, UT, wound	3	Same as for *C. braakii*
Enterobacter				
E. aerogenes	++++	All sites	1	Water, soil, sewage, animals, dairy products
E. amnigenus biogroup 1	–			Plants
E. amnigenus biogroup 2	–			Water
E. asburiae	++	**UT,** RT, feces, wound, blood	2	Water
E. cancerogenus (*E. taylorae*)	++	**Wound,** RT, feces	2	Animals, water
E. cloacae subsp. *cloacae*	++++	All sites	1	Water, soil, sewage, meat
E. cloacae subsp. *dissolvens* (*Enterobacter dissolvens*)	–			Diseased corn stalks
E. cowanii (*P. agglomerans*/ Japanese NIH group 42)	Unk	UT, RT, blood, wound	3	Unk
E. gergoviae	++	RT, UT, blood	2	Water, cosmetics
E. hormaechei subsp. *hormaechei*	++	RT, wound, blood	1	Unk, one isolate from a frog
E. hormaechei subsp. *oharae*	++	All sites	1	Plants
E. hormaechei subsp. *steigerwaltii*	++	All sites	1	Plants
E. kobei	Unk	Unk	Unk	Food
E. ludwigii (*E. cloacae*)	Unk	UT, RT, blood, stool	2	Food
E. nimipressuralis (*Erwinia*)	–			Diseased elms
E. pyrinus (*Erwinia*)	–			Diseased pear trees
E. radicincitans	–			Phyllosphere of winter wheat
E. sakazakii	++	RT, wound, CSF	1	Unk
Hafnia alvei DNA Group 1 and DNA Group 2	++	**Feces,** blood, RT	2	Ubiquitous
Klebsiella				
K. pneumoniae	++++	All sites, RT and UT most common	1	Ubiquitous, including foods and water
K. granulomatis (*Calymmatobacterium*)	++	Genital tract	1	None
K. pneumoniae subsp. *ozaenae*	++	**Nasal discharge,** RT, UT, blood	1	Unk
K. pneumoniae subsp. *rhinoscleromatis*	++	Nasal discharge	2	Unk
K. oxytoca	++++	All sites	2	Ubiquitous, including foods and water
K. variicola	++	Blood	1	Plants
K. singaporensis	–			Soil

(*Continued on next page*)

TABLE 1 Nomenclature, isolation source, and significance of selected genera of the family *Enterobacteriaceae*[a] *(Continued)*

Current (previous) designation	Clinical data			Environmental data
	Frequency	Source	Significance	
Morganella morganii subsp. *morganii* and subsp. *sibonii*	++	All sites	1	Unk, isolations from mammalian and reptile gastrointestinal tracts
Pantoea agglomerans (*Enterobacter*)	+++	All sites	2	Plants
Photorhabdus	++	Wound	2	Unknown, possibly insects
P. asymbiotica subsp. *asymbiotica* and subsp. *australis*				
P. luminescens	–			Nematodes infecting insects
P. temperata	–			Nematodes infecting insects
Plesiomonas shigelloides	+++	**Feces,** blood	1	Aquatic habitats and animals
Proteus				
P. hauseri (*P. vulgaris* genomospecies 3)	+	Unk	Unk	Unk, probably like *P. mirabilis*
P. mirabilis	++++	**UT,** blood, CSF	1	Animals, birds, fish, foods
P. myxofaciens	–			Gypsy moth
P. penneri	++	**UT,** blood, wound, feces, eye	1	Probably similar to *P. mirabilis*
P. vulgaris	+++	**UT,** wound, stool, RT	1	Probably similar to *P. mirabilis*
Providencia				
P. alcalifaciens	+++	All sites, UT and feces common	1	Mammals, water
P. heimbachae	+	Feces	3	Penguins
P. rettgeri	+++	All sites, UT most common	1	Same as for *P. alcalifaciens*, insects
P. rustigianii	+	Feces	3	Unk
P. stuartii	+++	All sites, UT most common	1	Mammals
Raoultella				
R. ornithinolytica (*Klebsiella*)	+	Wound, UT, blood	2	Food
R. planticola (*Klebsiella*)	Unk	Similar to *K. pneumoniae?*	3	Plants, water
R. terrigena (*Klebsiella*)	Unk	Similar to *K. pneumoniae?*	3	Soil, water
Serratia				
S. entomophila	–			New Zealand grass grub, water
S. ficaria	+	RT, wound	3	Fig wasps, figs, plants
S. fonticola	+	**Wound,** RT	3	Water, birds
S. liquefaciens complex (*S. liquefaciens* sensu stricto, *S. proteamaculans*, *S. grimesii*)	+++	RT, wound	2	Plants, insects, mammals, birds, dairy products
S. marcescens subsp. *marcescens*	++++	All sites, RT most common	1	Water, soil, plants, vegetables, animals, insects
S. marcescens subsp. *marcescens* biogroup 1	+	**UT,** RT	2	Unk
S. marcescens subsp. *sakuensis*	–			Wastewater
S. odorifera biogroup 1 and biogroup 2	+	RT, wound, feces, blood, UT	2	Plants
S. plymuthica	+	RT	3	Water, plants, small mammals
S. rubidaea	+	RT, wound, blood, UT, feces	2	Water, plants
S. ureilytica	–			Water
"*Candidatus* Serratia symbiotica"	–			Aphid symbiont

[a] Abbreviations and symbols: ++++, frequent; +++, occasional; ++, rare; +, very rare; –, not yet isolated from humans; CSF, cerebral spinal fluid; RT, respiratory tract; Unk, unknown; UT, urinary tract; 1, major pathogenic species of humans; 2, proven cause of disease in rare instances; 3, isolated from humans, significance unknown. Bold denotes most common source. Data are from references 2, 3, 17, 21, 23, 37, 42, 46, 50, 51, 52, 68, 71, 74, 78, 89, 97, 104, 106, 111, 112, 113, 118, 130, and 133.

TABLE 2 Other members of the family *Enterobacteriaceae*[a]

Human pathogens or opportunists	Primarily environmental strains[b]	Nonhuman isolates
Edwardsiella tarda	*Budvicia aquatica*[c] (9, 20)	*Alterococcus agarolytica*[c] (131)
Ewingella americana	*Buttiauxella noackiae*[d] (105)	*Arsenophonus nasoniae*[e] (47, 140)
Cedecea davisae	*Edwardsiella hoshinae*[c,d] (55)	*Brenneria* species[f] (57)
Cedecea lapagei	*Trabulsiella guamensis*[c] (101)	*Buchnera aphidicola*[e] (107)
Cedecea neteri	*Pragia fontium*[c] (8)	*Buttiauxella* species[b,c,e] (34, 105)
Cedecea genomospecies 3		"*Candidatus* Hamiltonella defensa"[e] (104)
Cedecea genomospecies 5		"*Candidatus* Regiella insecticola"[e] (104)
Kluyvera ascorbata		"*Candidatus* Phlomobacter fragariae"[f] (147)
Kluyvera cryocrescens		*Dickeya* species[f] (127)
Kluyvera georgiana		*Erwinia* species[b,f] (79, 114, 129)
Leclercia adecarboxylata		*Edwardsiella ictaluri*[d] (58)
Leminorella grimontii		*Kluyvera intermedia*[f] (*Enterobacter intermedius* and *Kluyvera cochleae*) (105, 118)
Leminorella richardii		*Obesumbacterium proteus*[c] (71)
Leminorella genomospecies 3		*Pantoea* species[b,c,f] (33, 57 ,80)
Moellerella wisconsensis		*Pectobacterium* species[f] (57)
Rahnella aquatilis		*Samsonia erythrinae*[f] (134)
Rahnella genomospecies 2 (22)		*Sodalis glossinidius*[e] (32, 100)
Rahnella genomospecies 3		*Wigglesworthia glossinidia*[e] (4)
Tatumella ptyseos		*Xenorhabdus* species[e] (18, 92)

[a] References are given in parentheses. Genomospecies listed cannot be biochemically separated from other species within their genus and/or only a single strain exists.
[b] Rare human isolates of no, or questionable, significance.
[c] Environmental isolates.
[d] Fish, marine, animal, or bird isolates.
[e] Insect isolate or pathogen.
[f] Plant isolate or phytopathogens.

and *zeae*); *Dickeya* species are not isolated from human specimens (127).

Miscellaneous genera within the *Enterobacteriaceae* are given in Table 2. Numbered genomospecies designations within a genus are given when they are comprised of a single strain, if too few organisms exist to be named, or if they cannot be differentiated from other members of their genus with available phenotypic tests. The genera listed in the last two columns of Table 2 are not isolated from human clinical specimens or are isolated but may not be significant, and most of these taxa will be unfamiliar to clinical microbiologists. However, it should be noted that a *Pantoea dispersa*-like organism and a strain of *Pantoea ananatis* have been reported recently from bacteremic patients (33, 129). *Erwinia persicinus* and *Buttiauxella gaviniae* have been isolated from a urinary tract infection (UTI) and a spinal cord patient with urinary bladder pathology, respectively (34, 114). A number of the organisms in the third column cannot be grown on laboratory media, so they are unlikely to be confused with, or necessitate separation from, those genera seen in humans. References have been included for those organisms that are isolated only from nonhuman sources, and they will not be discussed further.

DESCRIPTION OF GENERA

Members belonging to the family *Enterobacteriaceae* are gram-negative, facultative anaerobic rods or coccobacilli ranging in width from 0.3 to 1.0 μm and in length from 0.6 to 6.0 μm. A proposed subspecies of *Serratia*, *S. marcescens* subsp. *sakuensis*, is the only reportedly spore-forming organism in this family (2). Prototrophic strains grow readily on ordinary media. Among these genera, auxotrophic strains from clinical specimens are rare. However, cysteine-requiring urinary isolates of *K. pneumoniae*, which grow as pinpoint colonies on routine media, do occur. If encountered, these strains require supplementation of biochemical media or commercial identification systems with 0.63 mM cysteine for accurate identification. A number of newer genera are not culturable in vitro but have been assigned to the *Enterobacteriaceae* based upon analysis of the genetic sequences of their genome. A proposal to create a "*Candidatus*" status for these types of organisms has been made (108). Other genera, including *K. (C.) granulomatis* and many insect symbionts, are culturable only by cell culture techniques.

Of the organisms in Tables 1 and 2 isolated from human specimens, all *Klebsiella*, *Leminorella*, *Moellerella*, *Tatumella*, and *Enterobacter asburiae* strains are nonmotile, although any strain of any genus may be nonmotile and recent data for *E. asburiae* indicate that some strains may be motile (62). Some strains of *S. plymuthica* may not grow at 37°C, but most other members of the genera discussed in this chapter grow well between 25 and 37°C. Essentially only *Klebsiella* and *Raoultella* (previously *Klebsiella*) spp. are encapsulated, but strains from all genera may grow as mucoid or rough colonies. Five genera produce pigment. Some strains of *S. marcescens* and most *S. rubidaea* and *S. plymuthica* strains produce a red pigment, prodigiosin, which may appear throughout the entire colony or only as a red center or margin. Most strains of *E. sakazakii* and some strains of *P. agglomerans*, *Leclercia adecarboxylata*, and *Photorhabdus asymbiotica* form yellow-pigmented colonies that range from bright to pale yellow. Weak pigment producers may be detected only by observing growth placed on a swab or filter paper. Yellow pigment may be enhanced by incubation at 25°C. *Photorhabdus luminescens* and *P. asymbiotica* cultures are luminescent, giving a visible glow in a darkroom after 5 min. *S. odorifera*, as indicated by its name, and some *Cedecea* spp. strains, produce a pungent (potato-like) odor due to the production of alkyl-methoxypyrazines (50). Species of *Proteus* and *Providencia* oxidatively deaminate α-amino acids, producing pyruvic acids. L-phenylalanine deamination yields a green color when ferric chloride is added; however, deamination of *dl*-tryptophan produces the deep reddish brown pigment often seen in media inoculated with these organisms without the addition of ferric chloride (120). *Proteus* species also produce swarmer cells, which are elongated forms that are created when cells fail to septate or divide. These cells, which are profusely covered with flagella, act in concert to produce swarming motility on solid media (14).

Plesiomonas shigelloides organisms are also gram-negative, facultative anaerobes growing as straight rods similar in size to other *Enterobacteriaceae*. However, unlike other *Enterobacteriaceae, P. shigelloides* strains are oxidase positive, do not produce gas from glucose (*Enterobacteriaceae* are variable), and are susceptible to vibriostatic agent O/129 (2,4-diamino-6,7-diisopropylpteridine). Both *P. shigelloides* and enterobacteria grow at similar salt concentrations (0 to 5%) and pH ranges (4.0 to 8.0).

NATURAL HABITAT AND CLINICAL SIGNIFICANCE

The *Enterobacteriaceae* are widespread throughout the environment (Tables 1 and 2). Many species of the genera in Table 1 are commonly recognized nosocomial pathogens. The *Enterobacteriaceae* comprise 50% of all isolates from hospital-acquired infections and 80% of all gram-negative isolates (83). *Enterobacter* and *Klebsiella* spp. rank between fifth and ninth among common agents of bloodstream infections (35, 82, 143). Although less prevalent than a number of other etiologic agents, *Klebsiella* and *Enterobacter* cause significant infections. In one study, when found intraoperatively, *Klebsiella* and *Enterobacter* species had a 68 and 100% probability, respectively, of causing a wound infection; probability rates for *Escherichia coli* or *Staphylococcus aureus*, which were isolated three times more often during surgery, were only 31 and 55%, respectively (137). While *K. pneumoniae* and *E. cloacae* cause sepsis four to five times less often than gram-positive organisms, they are twice as likely to cause patient mortality (138). Species of both genera were among the most common organisms involved in relapse or reinfection in a study on recurrent bacteremia (139). *S. marcescens* and *Citrobacter* spp. constitute 1 to 2% and <1% of bloodstream infections, respectively (143). *Klebsiella* spp. rank as the second to fourth most common species in hospital-acquired UTIs and are the third to fourth most common agent in community-acquired UTIs (42, 49). In 2000, *Klebsiella* spp. accounted for 20, 23, and 58% of UTIs in Latin America, Europe, and North America, respectively (49). In this survey, *P. mirabilis, Enterobacter* spp., and *Citrobacter* spp. ranked as the fifth, sixth, and seventh most common agents of UTIs in Latin America, Europe, and North America, respectively (49). *Proteus mirabilis* continues to be an important cause of UTIs in Europe and North America, causing 4 to 6% of community-acquired UTIs and 3 to 6% of nosocomial infections including pyelonephritis (42, 49).

Klebsiella is carried in the nasopharynx and the bowel; however, feces are probably the most significant source of patient infections (103). Approximately one-third of patients carry *Klebsiella* in their stool, but rates may increase as much as threefold with hospitalization and antimicrobial usage in adults. Fecal carriage rates for children may be as high as 90 to 100% without antimicrobial therapy. *K. pneumoniae* has emerged as an important cause of community-acquired pyogenic liver abscess (PLA) worldwide (91, 121, 146). Diabetes and underlying biliary disease are major risk factors. The majority of patients with PLA due to *Klebsiella* are Asian males, 50 to 60 years of age, who present primarily with a right-lobe, solitary, monomicrobial abscess. *Klebsiella*-associated PLA mortality rates are lower than rates seen with other bacterial agents. *K. rhinoscleromatis* and *K. ozaenae* cause granulomatous infections termed rhinoscleroma and atrophic rhinitis, respectively. Both are chronic diseases of the upper respiratory tract; although atrophic rhinitis is restricted to the nose, rhinoscleroma may spread to the trachea and larynx (71). Both diseases occur most frequently in tropical areas of the world; transmission is thought to be from person to person, although prolonged contact with persons producing airborne nasal secretions is required. *K. (C.) granulomatis* causes chronic genital ulcers and also occurs predominantly in tropical countries (56). It is believed that *K. (C.) granulomatis* is sexually transmitted and that the only known reservoir is humans. *Raoultella (Klebsiella) planticola* and *Raoultella (Klebsiella) terrigena* are difficult to distinguish from *Klebsiella pneumoniae* without special tests. Studies in Europe have found that 3.5 to 19% of clinical strains initially identified as *Klebsiella* are actually *R. planticola* and that these strains have pathogenicity characteristics similar to those found in *K. pneumoniae* (119). In a survey of 436 *Klebsiella* strains isolated from newborns in the United States, however, only one isolate could be identified as *R. planticola,* indicating that its prevalence may vary geographically (141). Notably, all of the human strains of the new species *K. variicola* were reportedly isolated from blood (124). No further information on the human isolates was presented, but it would appear that this species is, at the very least, an opportunistic pathogen. As with other klebsiellae, plants appear to be the natural habitat of this organism.

Nosocomial *Enterobacter* colonization and infection are frequently associated with contaminated medical devices and instrumentation; however, *Enterobacter* spp. are commonly consumed in food and an endogeneous source should also be considered (71). *E. ludwigii* and the three subspecies of *E. hormaechei* are isolated from a variety of human sources including blood (63, 64). A nonhuman source for *E. ludwigii* has not been reported, but plants appear to be the natural habitat of *E. hormaechei* subspecies. A number of *Enterobacter* spp. were previously members of the genus *Erwinia* and are isolated from plants or trees (Table 1), where they may cause disease. The clinical microbiologist should be aware of these species as potential transients or commensals in clinical specimens.

Although *Serratia* spp. are seldom a cause of primary infections, they are notorious nosocomial pathogens and colonizers. The predominant mode of transmission is from person to person, but various medical apparatuses, intravenous fluids, and other solutions have often been implicated as well (71). Patients with indwelling catheters, particularly those for UTIs, serve as a primary reservoir for transmission via hospital personnel. For children, the gastrointestinal tract is a common source of infections. Outbreaks transmitted by hand are often insidious, occurring over long periods of time, and may subside and peak a number of times before recognition and infection control efforts can contain them. Pigment production in *S. marcescens* appears to be a marker that the strain is environmental in origin and of low virulence (11). Community-acquired infections are rare, except for *S. marcescens* contact lens-induced acute red eye (66). Most of the other species of *Serratia* have also been isolated from humans, where they too are usually transients or cause opportunistic infections.

The citrobacteria are considered inhabitants of the intestinal tract primarily, and their presence in the environment may reflect fecal excretion by humans and animals; however, the natural habitat of some newer *Citrobacter* species is unknown. Sepsis involving *Citrobacter* is often polymicrobic, with reported mortality rates as high as 48 to 50%; death is associated more often with polymicrobic than with monomicrobic infections (71). *Citrobacter* meningitis is almost exclusively associated with *C. koseri* and involves children less than 2 months of age, with the highest onset rates noted in neonates with a mean age of 7 days (71). An exceedingly high number (>75%) of these infants develop brain abscesses, and those who survive are generally afflicted with neurological defects. The most prominent risk factor is prior colonization; during outbreaks, colonization rates of 27% have been noted, in contrast to the normal rate of <1% (94, 142). Person-to-person spread from hospital personnel and, less often, mother-to-offspring infections are the most likely pathways; sampling of inanimate or environmental reservoirs in hospitals usually fails to yield *Citrobacter*. *Citrobacter* species previously belonging to the *Citrobacter freundii* complex, including *C. gillenii* and *C. murlinae*, have been found in human clinical, animal, food, and environmental specimens (21, 23). It is unclear what role many of these species may play in human infections; for some, the numbers of strains available are insufficient to either determine clinical significance in humans or establish a reservoir for infections. *C. rodentium* is the cause of murine colonic hyperplasia (97). This disease is self-limiting in adult mice but causes significant morbidity and mortality in infant mice when outbreaks occur in mouse colonies (97).

Proteus, Providencia, and *Morganella* are widespread in the environment and are normal inhabitants of the gut. While *Proteus* spp., especially *P. mirabilis*, are common causes of uncomplicated UTI, they frequently affect the upper urinary tract as well, causing renal scarring and kidney stone formation (102). Ammonia and CO_2 production from urine caused by the urease of *Proteus* lowers the pH, causing precipitation of soluble ions and the formation of stones, composed of struvite and apatite crystals, within the urinary tract. These crystals, which can be visualized within urine agar (filter-sterilized human urine solidified with agar) that has been inoculated with *Proteus*, are composed of magnesium ammonium phosphate or calcium phosphate (102). Since *P. mirabilis, P. penneri, Morganella,* and *P. alcalifaciens* have been isolated with greater frequency from diarrheal stools than from normal stools, it has been speculated that they may cause diarrhea. However, of these agents, only *P. alcalifaciens* plays a potential role in gastroenteritis. Studies by several groups have shown that *P. alcalifaciens* is invasive in HEp-2 cell assays (6, 77) and elicits diarrhea in the RITARD (reversible intestinal tie-adult rabbit diarrhea) model (6). However, some strains isolated in pure culture or in large numbers from diarrheal stools have failed to invade cell lines. The inability of noninvasive strains to penetrate epithelial cells may be explained by the fact that they appear unable to adhere to cell lines, a prerequisite to invasion (86).

Hafnia alvei has also been linked to gastrointestinal disease. *Hafnia* isolated from the diarrheal stool of a 9-month-old child in pure culture has been found to produce fluid in a rabbit intestinal tie model (5). A 1994 study of tourists returning to Finland found that 5% of patients with diarrhea had *Hafnia* in their stool whereas >300 asymptomatic individuals were negative for *Hafnia* (123). To date, putative virulence characteristics have not been demonstrated in hafniae. Prototypal *Hafnia alvei* isolates from Bangladesh originally identified as diarrheal strains, thought to possess the *eae* gene (attaching-effacing) and thus giving credence to *Hafnia*'s role in diarrhea, were eventually found to be a new species of *Escherichia, E. albertii* (7, 67, 73). Extraintestinal infections caused by *H. alvei* are unusual but can occur in immunocompetent individuals as well as those with underlying diseases, although the latter group is more likely to be affected (122). These infections are often community acquired and are believed to arise from the gastrointestinal tract. *Hafnia* appears to have a predilection for the biliary tree and may produce abscesses at the site of infection (122).

Averyella dalhousiensis is predominantly isolated from human wounds, where it is probably a contaminant since it appears to play no role in these infections (78). However, a recent isolation from blood indicates that it may be an opportunistic pathogen in compromised patients.

In humans, *Plesiomonas shigelloides* is primarily associated with diarrheal disease in infections occurring most frequently in individuals who live in or travel to tropical countries; a history of seafood consumption is common (76, 84). Bacteremia, which is primarily community acquired, is rare, with underlying biliary tract disease and advanced age (>75 years) as major risk factors (145). *Plesiomonas* bacteremias are polymicrobial; the gastrointestinal tract appears to serve as the primary source of infection since concomitantly isolated bacteria are all gastrointestinal agents. A retrospective study of *Plesiomonas* diarrheal infections undertaken in Hong Kong found an infection rate of 5.9% over a four-year period, with increasing numbers of isolations during three of the four years of the study (144). Most infections are self-limiting; however, hospitalization may be required for severe infections and/or for patients with underlying conditions. Symptoms associated with *Plesiomonas* diarrhea vary, and patients may present with either a secretory or a dysenteric type of disease. In the study of Wong et al. (144), 73% of cases had watery diarrhea and 25% had bloody diarrhea. Of 38 Bangladeshi children with monomicrobial *Plesiomonas* diarrhea, 76% were < 2 years of age and 74% were male (84). Vomiting was a significant feature (71%) of infections in these children, but in contrast to other reports, dehydration and fever were less prominent symptoms (23 and 8%, respectively), and the majority of infections were treated with oral rehydration alone. Patients may also report chronic diarrhea for 2 weeks or longer (76, 84). Association of *P. shigelloides* with diarrheal disease has been hampered by the inability to demonstrate putative virulence factors and the lack of an animal model. However, *Plesiomonas* has recently been observed both in membrane-bound vacuoles and free within the cytosol of cultured human colon cells examined by transmission electron microscopy (136). A beta-hemolysin described previously and now shown to be calcium and iron dependent probably plays a role in the infectious process by releasing *P. shigelloides* from intracellular vacuoles (12, 72). The dysenteric form of diarrhea seen with some patients may be explained by the ability to invade and multiply within human gastrointestinal cells. Association of *Plesiomonas* with secretory diarrheal infections is more tenuous, although cholera-like, heat-stable, and heat-labile toxins have been described (70). The lipopolysaccharide of *Plesiomonas* may also play a role in the infectious process in view of the fact that the O17 antigen belonging to the most common serogroup of *Plesiomonas* and the form 1 antigen of *S. sonnei* share almost identical gene regions (29). Although plesiomonads have an aquatic reservoir, wound infections associated with water contact and similar to those found with *Aeromonas* spp. are not encountered. *Plesiomonas* has been isolated from a wide range of mammals (other than humans), birds, fish, and water-dwelling reptiles and amphibians, but with the possible exception of cats, there is no evidence to suggest that it plays a role in diarrheal disease in any of these species (69).

Edwardsiella tarda is typically associated with animals that inhabit water. It is an infrequent cause of gastroenteritis in humans, with most infections occurring after contact with fish or turtles. However, a low carriage rate in humans, except in tropical areas of the world, and the ability to produce a cell-associated hemolysin and invade HEp-2 cells suggest that *E. tarda* is a diarrheal agent (76). Serious wound infections, including myonecrosis, have been reported in immunocompetent individuals who had aquatic exposure (132). Systemic infections usually occur in patients with liver disease or iron overload conditions.

Except for *E. tarda*, the other *Enterobacteriaceae* listed in the left-hand column of Table 2 cause opportunistic infections and are not frequently encountered in clinical laboratories (71). Some, like *Cedecea* spp., *Leminorella* spp., *Moellerella*, and *Tatumella*, are rarely isolated from nonhuman sources, making it difficult to determine reservoirs for these organisms (53, 59, 60, 65, 71). Strains of *Ewingella, Leclercia,* and *Kluyvera* spp. have been found in a variety of foods, water, or animals (snails and slugs) and are probably, like many *Enterobacteriaceae,* ubiquitous in the environment (40, 54, 71, 135). Other genera that have been isolated from human specimens have more specific natural habitats. These include *Rahnella* (71), all of whose initially described isolates were recovered from water, which probably serves as the reservoir for human infections, or *Yokenella* and both subspecies of *Photorhabdus asymbiotica,* which are common in insects and have caused infections following insect bites (3, 41, 88).

ISOLATION

For the most part, none of the clinically relevant strains covered in this chapter present difficulties in isolation from sterile body sites. Cockerill et al. (31) did find, however, that in blood cultures both *E. cloacae* and *S. marcescens* grew significantly better in aerobic culture than in nonvented or anaerobic culture; no difference was noted for other major species of the genera included in this chapter. Isolation from nonsterile body or environmental sites may require specialized media.

A number of chromogenic media have been developed to isolate and differentiate urinary tract pathogens based on the colony color produced by the enzymatic action of the organism on chromogenic substrates in the medium. Of these, CHROMagar Orientation (Becton Dickinson, Sparks, Md.) and CPS ID2 (bioMérieux, Hazelwood, Mo.) perform similarly for the detection of the UTI pathogens covered in this chapter and can reliably replace commonly used media such as MacConkey and blood agars (BA) (26, 128). However, CHROMagar is more sensitive for the isolation of *E. coli* because it detects beta-galactosidase while CPS ID2 detects beta-glucuronidase (26, 128). Although *Proteus, Providencia, Morganella, Klebsiella, Citrobacter,* and *Enterobacter* are all easily identified on both of these media, further biochemical tests are required to identify them to the species level. Both media prevent swarming of *Proteus,* and mucoid colonies allowing for easier detection of multiple pathogens and antimicrobial susceptibility tests can be performed directly without the need for subculturing. Ohkusu (115) expanded the usage of CHROMagar Orientation to cover isolation of pathogenic organisms from wound, stool, and a variety of other specimens in addition to urine. Using colony color on CHROMagar in combination with indole, lysine, and ornithine decarboxylase tests and serology, 466 of 472 (98.7%) isolates were correctly identified.

Both of the diarrheal pathogens covered in this chapter are easily isolated. *E. tarda,* which is a lactose-negative, H_2S-positive organism, is indistinguishable from *Salmonella* on enteric plating media (opaque or opaque with black centers). A positive indole reaction and lack of agglutination in specific *Salmonella* antisera differentiate *E. tarda* strains. *Plesiomonas* grows as 2- to 3-mm, opaque, convex colonies on BA or as non-lactose-, non-sucrose-fermenting colonies on enteric plating media. It does not grow on thiosulfate-citrate-bile salts-sucrose medium but does grow well on, and can be isolated from, cefsulodin-irgasan-novobiocin (CIN) medium. Because *Plesiomonas* does not ferment mannitol, the colonies are opaque without a pink center on CIN medium. It must be distinguished from other oxidase-positive organisms *(Pseudomonas, Aeromonas)* that can also grow on this medium, although *Aeromonas* should have a pink center with an opaque apron. Inositol fermentation and a positive reaction in Moeller's lysine, arginine, and ornithine tests differentiate *Plesiomonas* from other organisms.

Other *Enterobacteriaceae* that are involved in opportunistic infections and that may be isolated from a variety of specimen types generally grow well on commonly used laboratory media (71). Some genera are lactose or sucrose fermenters and give the appearance of normal flora on enteric plating media, while others may produce H_2S and appear *Salmonella*-like. *Rahnella, Ewingella,* and *Tatumella* may require 48 h for growth. *Tatumella* also grows poorly on Mueller-Hinton agar, and a broth dilution method may be required for susceptibility testing. Strains of *Tatumella* do not survive well at room temperature and should be stored at $-70°C$.

K. (C.) granulomatis, as with many of the organisms in the third column of Table 2, does not grow on conventional laboratory media. Since it does not stain well with gram reagents, Giemsa- or Wright-stained Donovan bodies have been the method most commonly used to detect this organism. However, Donovan bodies, which are pleomorphic, bipolar staining bodies shaped like a closed safety pin, are not always present and are not reliable for diagnosis. Recently, growth in HEp-2 monolayers has been achieved (27). Primers to the *phoE* and *scrA* (sucrose regulon) genes have been used to identify and distinguish *K. (C.) granulomatis* (*phoE* positive) from *Klebsiella* species (*phoE* and *scrA* positive) (28).

IDENTIFICATION

The biochemical tests most useful for differentiating species within each genus are given in Tables 3 through 13. Full biochemical profiles for most species can be found in chapter 42. Correct identification to the species level is increasingly important in recognizing strains that are of high risk for carrying extended-spectrum beta-lactamases, cephalosporinases, or carbapenemases (95). Identification problems arising from the use of commercial systems vary with each genus. Of the *Klebsiella, K. ozaenae* and *K. rhinoscleromatis* do the poorest in commercial systems, probably as a result of slow growth. These species can be difficult to distinguish using conventional biochemicals as well. *R. (Klebsiella) planticola* and *R. (Klebsiella) terrigena* cannot be readily separated from other *Klebsiella* without temperature growth or carbon assimilation tests, neither of which are readily available in most clinical laboratories.

TABLE 3 Separation of members of the genus *Citrobacter*[a]

Species	Indole	ODC	Malonate	Acid[b] from:			
				Sucrose	Dulcitol	Melibiose	Adonitol
C. amalonaticus	+	+	−	−	−	−	−
C. braakii	V	+	−	−	V	+	−
C. farmeri	+	+	−	+	−	+	−
C. freundii (sensu stricto)	V	−	V	V	V	+	−
C. koseri	+	+	+	V	V	−	+
C. rodentium	−	+	+	−	−	−	−
C. sedlakii	V	+	+	−	+	+	−
C. werkmanii	−	−	+	−	−	V	−
C. youngae	V	−	−	V	V	+	−
C. gillenii	−	−	+	V	−	V	−
C. murlinae	+	−	−	V	+	V	−

[a] Abbreviations and symbols: ODC, ornithine decarboxylase; +, ≥85%; V, 15 to 85%; −, ≤15%.
[b] Fermentation reactions in commercial systems should be similar to reactions in conventional fermentation broths (1% carbohydrate in broth with indicator).

Growth at 10°C, utilization of histamine, and no gas production from lactose at 44.5°C can be used to separate *Raoultella* spp. from *K. pneumoniae* and *K. oxytoca; R. terrigena* can be distinguished from *R. planticola* by fermentation of β-gentibiose. The new species, *K. variicola*, is not in commercial systems; *K. variicola* strains do not ferment adonitol (some strains are L-rhamnose negative as well), and reportedly only this trait separates it from *K. pneumoniae* (124).

Members of the genus *Enterobacter* appear to confound commercial systems more often than other genera in the *Enterobacteriaceae*, probably because of the heterogeneity of several of the species (71). Most major commercial systems include at least nine *Enterobacter* species, and they all identify the three major *Enterobacter* species *(E. cloacae, E. aerogenes,* and *E. sakazakii)* at an acceptable accuracy rate of ≥90% (71). The percentage of correct identifications with many

TABLE 4 Differentiation of *Pantoea agglomerans* and members of the genus *Enterobacter*[a,b]

Species	LDC	ADH	ODC	VP	Acid[c] from:							Yellow pigment
					Sucrose	Adonitol	D-Sorbitol	L-Rhamnose	α-Methyl-D-glucoside	Esculin	Melibiose	
Human species												
E. aerogenes	+	−	+	+	+	+	+	+	+	+	+	−
P. agglomerans	−	−	−	V	V	−	V	V	−	V	V	V
E. amnigenus biogroup 1	−	−	V	+	+	−	−	+	V	+	+	−
E. asburiae	−	V	+	−	+	−	+	−	+	+	−	−
E. cancerogenus	−	+	+	+	−	−	−	+	−	+	−	−
E. cloacae subsp. *cloacae*	−	+	+	+	+	V	+	+	V	V	+	−
E. cowanii[d]	−	−	−	+	+	−	+	+	−	+	+	V
E. gergoviae	+	−	+	+	+	−	−	+	−	+	+	−
E. hormaechei subsp. *hormaechei*	−	V	+	+	+	−	−	+	V	−	−	−
E. kobei	−	+	+	−	+	−	+	+	+	V	+	−
E. sakazakii	−	+	+	+	+	−	−	+	+	+	+	+
Environmental species												
E. amnigenus biogroup II	−	V	+	+	−	−	+	+	+	+	+	−
E. cloacae subsp. *dissolvens*	−	+	+	+	+	−	+	+	+	+	+	−
E. nimipressuralis	−	−	+	+	−	−	+	+	+	+	+	−
E. pyrinus[e]	NA	NA	NA	+	+	−	−	+	−	+	+	−
E. radicincitans	−	+	−	+	+	−	+	+	−	+	−	−

[a] See the text for *E. ludwigii* and *E. hormaechei* subsp. *steigerwaltii* and *oharae* identification.
[b] Abbreviations and symbols: LDC, lysine decarboxylase; ADH, arginine dihydrolase; ODC, ornithine decarboxylase; VP, Voges-Proskauer; +, ≥90%; V, 11 to 89%; −, ≤10%; NA, not available.
[c] See Table 3, footnote *b*.
[d] Separated from *P. agglomerans* by a negative malonate reaction and fermentation of D-sorbitol (68).
[e] Separated from *E. gergoviae* by positive reactions in potassium cyanide broth and *myo*-inositol.

TABLE 5 Separation of some members of the genera *Klebsiella* and *Raoultella*[a,b]

Species	Indole	ODC	VP	Malonate	ONPG	Growth at:		Acid[c] from D-melezitose
						10°C	44°C	
R. ornithinolytica	+	+	V	+	+	+	NA	NA
K. oxytoca	+	−	+	+	+	−	+	−
K. ozaenae	−	−	−	−	V	NA	NA	NA
K. pneumoniae[d]	−	−	+	+	+	−	+	−
R. planticola	V	−	+	+	+	+	−	−
R. terrigena	−	−	+	+	+	+	−	+
K. rhinoscleromatis	−	−	−	+	−	NA	NA	NA

[a] *K. singaporensis* biochemicals are not available; only a single strain is known.
[b] Abbreviations and symbols: ODC, ornithine decarboxylase; VP, Voges-Proskauer; ONPG, *o*-nitrophenyl-β-D-galactopyranoside; NA, not available; +, ≥90%; V, 11 to 89%; −, ≤10%.
[c] See Table 3, footnote *b*.
[d] *K. variicola* is separated from *K. pneumoniae* by negative adonitol reaction; some strains are also L-rhamnose negative.

commercial systems increases significantly when "low probability" identifications are included as correct identifications or when additional biochemical tests are performed following initial testing results. Neither *E. ludwigii* nor the subspecies of *E. hormaechei* can be separated from other clinically relevant *Enterobacter* spp. by biochemicals readily available in most clinical laboratories. In the Biotype 100 system (bioMerieux, Marcy l'Etoile, France), *E. ludwigii* can be separated from *E. cloacae,* the most common species that it resembles phenotypically, by growth on 3-0-methyl-D-glucopyranose and putrescine (64). Likewise, *E. hormaechei* subspecies can be separated from *E. cloacae* in the Biotype 100 system by growth on L-fucose and 1-0-methyl-α-galactopyranoside for subsp. *hormaechei,* growth on D-arabitol and adonitol for subsp. *steigerwaltii,* and growth on 3-hydroxybutyrate for subsp. *oharae* (63).

Serratia spp. are generally easily identified by commercial systems, except for the *S. liquefaciens* group; differentiation of members within this group requires carbon assimilation tests (71). These tests can be performed using a combination of API 50 CH and API ZYM (carbohydrate and enzymatic panels, respectively) (bioMérieux, Hazelwood, Mo.) strips (50).

Most automated system databases now contain the newer *Citrobacter* spp., at least to subgroups (*C. braakii-C. freundii-C. sedlakii, C. werkmanii-C. youngae,* and *C. koseri-C. amalonaticus*); however, subgroup identification requires further biochemical testing by standard methodologies to identify strains to the species level, and this delays final identification (71). A PYR (L-pyroglutamic acid to detect pyrrolidonyl peptidase [Oxoid PYR Test]) test may be useful for separating biochemically atypical strains of *Citrobacter* (positive) and *Salmonella* (negative) (15).

Two members of the genus *Proteus* can be rapidly identified with minimal testing. Gram-negative and oxidase-negative organisms with colonies that swarm on BA and appear flat with tapered edges on MacConkey agar may be reported as *Proteus*. *Proteus* spp. that are spot indole negative and ampicillin susceptible may be reported as *P. mirabilis* (13).

TABLE 6 Biochemical characterization of members of the genus *Serratia*[a,b]

Species	LDC	ODC	Mal	Acid[c] from:								Red pigment	Odor
				Arabinose	L-Rhamnose	D-Xylose	Sucrose	Adonitol	D-Sorb	Cello	D-Ara		
S. entomophila[d]	−	−	−	−	−	V	+	−	−	−	V	−	−
S. ficaria	−	−	−	+	V	+	+	−	+	+	+	−	V
S. fonticola	+	+	V	+	V	V	V	+	+	−	+	−	−
S. liquefaciens group	+	+	−	+	V	+	+	−	+	−	−	−	−
S. marcescens subsp. *marcescens*	+	+	−	−	−	−	+	V	+	−	−	V	−
S. marcescens biogroup 1	V	+	−	−	−	−	+	V	+	−	−	NA	−
S. odorifera biogroup 1	+	+	−	+	+	+	+	V	+	+	−	−	+
S. odorifera biogroup 2	+	−	−	+	+	+	−	V	+	+	−	−	+
S. plymuthica[e]	−	−	−	+	−	+	+	−	V	V	−	+	−
S. rubidaea	V	−	+	+	−	+	+	+	−	+	V	+	−

[a] *S. marcescens* subsp. *sakuensis* is reportedly a spore-forming organism; *S. ureilytica* is urea positive; only a single strain is known.
[b] Abbreviations and symbols: LDC, lysine decarboxylase; ODC, ornithine decarboxylase; Mal, malonate; D-Ara, D arabitol; D-Sorb, D-sorbitol; Cello, cellobiose; +, ≥90%; V, 11 to 89%; −, ≤10%; NA, information not available.
[c] See Table 3, footnote *b*.
[d] Growth at 37°C but biochemical characterization optimal at 30°C.
[e] May fail to grow at 37°C.

TABLE 7 Separation of members of the genera *Proteus, Providencia,* and *Morganella*[a]

Organism	Indole	H_2S	Urea	ODC	Acid[b] from:				
					Maltose	D-Adonitol	D-Arabitol	Trehalose	*myo*-Inositol
Proteus									
P. hauseri	+	V	+	−	+	−	−	+	−
P. mirabilis	−	+	+	+	−	−	−	+	−
P. penneri	−	V	+	−	+	−	−	V	−
P. vulgaris[c]	+	V	+	−	+	−	−	−	−
Providencia									
P. alcalifaciens	+	−	−	−	−	+	−	−	−
P. heimbachae	−	−	−	−	V	+	+	−	V
P. rettgeri	+	−	+	−	−	+	+	−	+
P. rustigianii	+	−	−	−	−	−	−	−	−
P. stuartii	+	−	V	−	−	−	−	+	+
Morganella									
M. *morganii* subsp. *morganii*	+	−[d]	+	+[e]	−	−	−	−	−
M. *morganii* subsp. *sibonii*	V	−[d]	+	+[e]	−	−	−	+	−

[a] Abbreviations and symbols: H_2S, hydrogen sulfide; ODC, ornithine decarboxylase; +, ≥90%; V, 11 to 89%; −, ≤10%.
[b] See Table 3, footnote *b*.
[c] *P. vulgaris* genomospecies 4, 5, and 6 cannot be differentiated phenotypically.
[d] Some members of some biogroups are H_2S positive.
[e] Some members of some biogroups are ornithine decarboxylase negative.

P. penneri, which is a rare clinical isolate, also fits the above description but can be separated from *P. mirabilis* by its negative reactions in ornithine decarboxylase and maltose. Spot indole-positive, ampicillin-resistant strains are reported as *P. vulgaris* (13). *P. hauseri,* previously a subgroup of *P. vulgaris,* can be differentiated from *P. vulgaris* by a negative salicin or esculin reaction (110). Although it is found in clinical specimens, *P. hauseri* is infrequently seen in the laboratory (75). If an organism does not fit any of the above qualifications, it must be fully identified by commercial or conventional biochemical methods (13). Most commercially available systems satisfactorily identify *Proteus,* with reports varying between 95 and 100% accuracy for different systems. *Providencia* spp., however, are not identified with the same level of accuracy in commercial systems, and the rates vary from 79 to 100% (110). When *Providencia* spp. are misidentified, they are usually called *Morganella* or *Proteus.* Urea-positive *P. stuartii* may be misidentified as *P. rettgeri,* or the system may require additional tests for identification. *P. heimbachae* is not in commercial system databases (110). M. *morganii* subsp. *morganii* is identified 100% of the time in commercial systems according to most studies, although 2-h identification methods misidentify it about 66% of the time.

M. *morganii* subsp. *sibonii* is not included in most databases and may be distinguished from subsp. *morganii* only by a positive reaction in trehalose.

Hafnia alvei, which biochemically most closely resembles members of the genus *Enterobacter,* and *Yokenella regensburgei* (Table 11) are usually correctly identified in commercial systems. Biogroup 2 strains of *H. alvei* can be separated from *H. alvei* sensu stricto by a positive malonate reaction (74).

Averyella dalhousiensis is not included in commercial system databases; it is an indole-, VP-, H_2S-negative, lysine decarboxylase-positive organism that gives variable reactions in citrate, urea, and dulcitol (78). It most closely resembles *Kluyvera ascorbata* but differs from it by negative reactions in indole, melibiose, and mucate. It also may be misidentified as *Salmonella enterica* in commercial systems but can be differentiated from *Salmonella* subgroup 1 strains by a negative reaction in H_2S, a positive reaction for urease at 48 h, and fermentation of cellobiose. *Averyella* strains are *o*-nitrophenyl-β-D-galactopyranoside (ONPG)-, malonate-, and potassium cyanide-positive and ferment dulcitol and salicin, traits shared with *Salmonella* subgroups 2, 3, and 4.

The two agents of gastroenteritis, *Plesiomonas* (Table 13) and *E. tarda* (Table 12), are easily separated both from other

TABLE 8 Separation of *Cedecea* from selected *Enterobacter* species (VP, ADH, and ODC variable or positive)[a]

Organism	Acid[b] from:					
	D-Sorbitol	Raffinose	L-Rhamnose	Melibiose	D-Arabitol	Sucrose
C. *davisae*	−	−	−	−	−	+
C. *lapagei*	−	−	−	+	+	−
E. *cloacae*	+	+	+	+	V	−
E. *sakazakii*	−	+	+	+	−	+
E. *cancerogenus*	−	−	+	−	−	−

[a] Abbreviations and symbols: VP, Voges-Proskauer; ADH, arginine dihyrolase; ODC, ornithine decarboxylase; +, ≥90%; V, 11 to 89%; −, ≤10%.
[b] See Table 3, footnote *b*.

TABLE 9 Differentiation of *Klyuvera* from commonly seen indole-positive, VP-negative organisms[a]

Organism	Citrate	Urea	LDC	KCN
Kluyvera[b]	–	–	+	+
C. koseri	+	V	–	–
Morganella	–	+	–	+
Providencia	V	+	–	+
E. coli	–	–	+	–

[a] Abbreviations and symbols: VP, Voges-Proskauer; LDC, lysine decarboxylase; KCN, potassium cyanide; +, ≥90%; V, 11 to 89%; –, ≤10%. *Leclercia* and *E. tarda* are also indole positive and VP negative and can be found in Tables 10 and 12, respectively.

[b] Includes *K. intermedia* (*K. cochleae* and *Enterobacter intermedius* combined) (118).

enteric pathogens and from normal flora, and their identification presents no difficulty in either conventional or commercial systems. Sequencing data have shown that the somatic antigen that occurs in the most common serogroup of *Plesiomonas* (serogroup O17) and the form 1 antigen of *S. sonnei* share almost identical gene regions (29). Thus, if *Shigella* serotyping is mistakenly performed with strains of *Plesiomonas*, cross-reactions may occur.

Reactions to identify other enterobacteria isolated from clinical specimens can be found in Tables 8 through 12. The organisms are grouped with the genera with which they would most likely be confused and from which they must be differentiated. Many of the agents in these tables are in commercial system databases. Unfortunately, the number of strains available for use in challenge studies is very limited; therefore, the ability of these systems to accurately identify these organisms is really unknown. *Ewingella* and *Tatumella* are biochemically inactive, and the latter organism grows poorly in vitro. *Kluyvera* can be identified only to genus level by these systems; species determination requires an ascorbate test and irgasan susceptibility and/or gas-liquid chromatography profiles (71). *Photorhabdus asymbiotica* is not included in most commercial databases. *Pantoea dispersa*, *P. ananatis*, and *Erwinia persicinus* most closely resemble *P. agglomerans*. *P. dispersa* and *E. persicinus* may be distinguished from *P. agglomerans* by negative reactions for raffinose, salicin, and sucrose and by negative reactions for maltose and D-xylose, respectively. *P. ananatis* is more difficult to differentiate, and all suspected isolates of this organism, as with other rare *Enterobacteriaceae*, should be sent to a reference laboratory for confirmation.

At this time, 16S rRNA sequencing is not used extensively to identify this group of organisms and not all species are included in currently available databases. The use of molecular methods (see chapter 16) to determine the presence and/or identity of bacteria directly from clinical specimens or from isolates is increasingly reported but not universally available. These methods offer a great advantage when bacteria are difficult or impossible to culture, such as *K. (C.) granulomatis*, or in the case of diseases such as keratitis, where cultures are negative 40 to 60% of the time (87). Testing of specimens from sterile sites with universal primers based on conserved regions of the bacterial chromosome (with the exception of *K. granulomatis*) can be used to determine if a patient has a bacterial infection in 1 h (16). Normally sterile clinical specimens found negative by these assays would not then require culturing, saving considerably on laboratory resources. However, numerous problems remain to be worked out with these methods for bacterial identification. For rRNA sequencing these include, but are not limited to, DNA extraction protocols, ambiguous profiles arising from testing mixed cultures, the presence of too few species in the databases, and percent similarity cutoff guidelines for identification to the species or genus level (36).

The ability to trace the spread or involvement of nosocomial pathogens in outbreaks caused by the *Enterobacteriaceae* has become a major responsibility for the laboratory. Biotyping using commercially available identification systems is seldom suitably discriminating, unless an unusual marker or profile is present. Biotyping schemes using carbon assimilation tests have been developed, particularly for *Serratia*, but may be difficult and costly to perform (50). Typing all genera for which traditional typing methods are available (serotyping, bacteriocins, and bacteriophages) would necessitate multiple sets of reagents, which are not readily available and/or are economically prohibitive. Molecular techniques including plasmid analysis, ribotyping, pulsed-field gel electrophoresis (PFGE), and various PCR methodologies all appear satisfactorily discriminatory, some working better for a specific genus or species than others (see chapter 16). The variety of PCR techniques is proliferating at an astonishing pace, especially repetitive-element PCR methods for the *Enterobacteriaceae*. Care in the performance and interpretation of these assays is critical since many PCR techniques have not been standardized (38, 48). For now, since a single method applicable to the most strains is preferable, at least economically, PFGE remains the most universally accepted standardized technique for epidemiological studies.

TABLE 10 Separation of LDC-, ODC-, and ADH-negative unusual *Enterobacteriaceae* found in clinical specimens[a]

Organism	Motility	Gas from glucose	KCN	VP	Acid[b] from:		
					Sucrose	L-Arabitol	Trehalose
Ewingella	V	–	–	+	–	–	+
Leclercia	+	+	+	–	+	+	+
Moellerella	+	+	V	–	–	+	+
Rahnella	–	+	–	+	+	+	+
Tatumella	–	–	–	–	+	–	+
Photorhabdus asymbiotica[c]	+	–	–	–	–	–	–

[a] Abbreviations and symbols: LDC, lysine decarboxylase; ODC, ornithine decarboxylase; ADH, arginine dihydrolase; KCN, potassium cyanide; VP, Voges-Proskauer; +, ≥90%; V, 11 to 89%; –, ≤10%. *Budvicia* is also LDC, ODC, and ADH negative and can be found in Table 12.

[b] See Table 3, footnote *b*.

[c] *Photorhabdus* subsp. *australis* can be separated from subsp. *asymbiotica* by fermentation of maltose and glycerol.

TABLE 11 Separation of *Yokenella* from *Hafnia*[a]

Organism	VP	Malonate	Citrate	Acid[b] from:	
				Melibiose	Glycerol
Yokenella	−	−	+	+	−
Hafnia alvei	+	+	−	−	+
H. alvei biogroup 2	+	−	V	−	+

[a] Abbreviations and symbols: VP, Voges-Proskauer; +, ≥90%; V, 11 to 89%; −, ≤10%. Data from reference 74.
[b] See Table 3, footnote *b*.

The disadvantage of a long turn-around time (usually 4 days) has been partially overcome by a rapid PFGE protocol that is suitable for most enteric bacteria as well as other common clinical strains (45).

ANTIMICROBIAL SUSCEPTIBILITY

The number of strains harboring extended-spectrum β-lactamases (ESBL), cephalosporinases and carbapenemases that mediate resistance to the β-lactam antibiotics (Table 14) (for resistance mechanisms, see chapters 71, 74, and 78), and the increase in resistance to quinolones are major issues with members of the *Enterobacteriaceae* (10, 143). In one study, of >380,000 blood, respiratory, and urine isolates of *Enterobacteriaceae* tested against 14 antimicrobials, susceptibilities of <90% were recorded for eight (46 to 89%) and three (57 to 84%) drugs for intensive care unit (ICU) and non-ICU patients, respectively (83). Ceftazidime, cefotaxime, and ceftriaxone susceptibility rates were up to 10% lower for isolates from ICU patients than from non-ICU patients; however, only three isolates were carbapenem resistant, two of which were *E. aerogenes*. Only fluoroquinolone susceptibility decreased over a 4-year period, and fluoroquinolone-resistant *Enterobacteriaceae* were frequently resistant to extended-spectrum cephalosporins, aminoglycosides, and trimethoprim-sulfamethoxazole (SXT) (83). Ciprofloxacin resistance, influenced by antibiotic usage and clonal spread of strains containing ESBLs among patients, has been found in strains of *K. pneumoniae* and *K. oxytoca*, with rates as high as 7.2 and 3.4%, respectively (24). Imipenem resistance has been noted worldwide among the *Enterobacteriaceae*; it typically emerges during long therapy to treat ceftazidime- and aminoglycoside-resistant strains and appears reversible with cessation of therapy (1, 19). Cefepime resistance in *Enterobacter* spp. and *K. oxytoca* strains has been reported (126).

The spread of ESBL-producing strains can be controlled, without restricting antimicrobial usage, by using barrier precautions and cohorting patients after discharge from ICUs, since transmission occurs primarily on the hands of hospital staff (96, 117). However, Paterson and Yu (117) recommend a three-prong effort to control ESBL-producing organisms, which includes enhancing surveillance and control within the ICU, increasing laboratory capability in the detection of ESBLs, and limiting empirical use of antibiotics. Restriction of specific antimicrobials may reduce resistance in one or several species but select for resistance in others, substituting one problem for another (90). Further, resistance to one drug found in a multi-drug-resistant isolate will be maintained or accelerate in patient populations even if use of the drug is discontinued, as long as the other drugs to which the strain is also resistant are prescribed (83).

The effective infection control of organisms harboring ESBLs necessitates that the laboratory provides testing methods that will detect these strains. The question of whether it is cost-effective for laboratories to test for ESBL-producing organisms because their detection isn't likely to affect patient outcome has not been resolved (39). Studies to determine the outcomes of serious infections caused by organisms considered cephalosporin "susceptible" or "intermediate" in vitro found that 54% of patients who were treated with a cephalosporin experienced therapy failure (116). These patients either succumbed to their infections or required a change in therapy to achieve a cure. UTIs caused by ESBL-producing organisms can be successfully treated with cephalosporins, eliminating the need to test urine isolates for ESBL production for therapeutic consideration; however, testing may be required for infection control efforts to prevent horizontal transfer of these strains. Appropriate broth microdilution and disk diffusion testing procedures for ESBL-producing *Klebsiella* spp. are described in chapter 74.

Strains of *P. mirabilis* are resistant to nitrofurantoin but susceptible to trimethoprim-sulfamethoxazole, ampicillin, amoxicillin, piperacillin, cephalosporins, aminoglycosides, and imipenem. Although most strains are susceptible to ciprofloxacin, resistance occurs with unrestricted use of the drug (110). *P. penneri* and *P. vulgaris* have resistance profiles similar to that of *Morganella*, although *P. penneri* is more resistant to penicillin than *P. vulgaris*. All three organisms are susceptible to broad-spectrum cephalosporins, cefoxitin,

TABLE 12 Separation of *Enterobacteriaceae* that may be H_2S positive[a]

Organism	LDC	ODC	Urea	Acid[b] from L-arabinose	Citrate	KCN	ONPG
Leminorella spp.	−	−	−	+	V[c]	−	−
Edwardsiella tarda	+	+	−	−	−	−	−
Budvicia aquatilis[d]	−	−	+	V	−	−	+
Pragia fontium[d]	−	−	−	−	−	−	−
Trabulsiella guamensis[d]	+	+	−	+	V	+	+
Salmonella subgroup 1	+	+	−	+	+	−	−
Citrobacter	−	V	V	+	V	+	+
Proteus	−	V	+	−	V	+	−

[a] Abbreviations and symbols: LDC, lysine decarboxylase; ODC, ornithine decarboxylase; KCN, potassium cyanide; ONPG, *o*-nitrophenol-β-D-galactopyranoside; +, ≥90%; V, 11 to 89%; −, ≤10%.
[b] See Table 3, footnote *b*.
[c] *L. grimontii* is positive, *L. richardii* is negative.
[d] Found in clinical specimens but of questionable or no significance.

TABLE 13 Differentiation of *P. shigelloides* from other clinically significant members of the *Vibrionaceae* and the *Aeromonadaceae*[a]

Organism	LDC	ODC	ADH	Gas from glucose	Acid[b] from:		Growth in:		O/129 susceptibility
					Sucrose	Inositol	TCBS	0% NaCl	
Plesiomonas	+	+	+	−	−	+	−	+	+
Aeromonas spp.	V	−[c]	+	V	V	−	−	+	−
Vibrio spp.[d]	+	+	−	−	V	−	+	V	+

[a] Abbreviations and symbols: LDC, lysine decarboxylase; ODC, ornithine decarboxylase; ADH, arginine dihydrolase; TCBS, thiosulfate-citrate-bile salts-sucrose agar; O/129, 2,4-diamino-6,7-diisopropylpteridine; +, ≥90%; V, 11 to 89%; −, ≤10%.

[b] See Table 3, footnote *b*.

[c] Only *A. veronii* biotype *veronii* is positive.

[d] *V. hollisae* is LDC, ODC, and ADH negative; only *V. fluvialis* and *V. furnissii* are ADH positive; *V. furnissii* produces gas; *V. cincinnatiensis* ferments *myo*-inositol; *V. cholerae* and *V. mimicus* grow in 0% NaCl.

cefepime, aztreonam, aminoglycosides, and imipenem. They are resistant to piperacillin, amoxicillin, ampicillin, cefoperazone, cefuroxime, and cefazolin. *Providencia rettgeri* and *P. stuartii* are resistant to gentamicin and tobramycin but susceptible to amikacin. Urine isolates are susceptible to broad- and expanded-spectrum cephalosporins, ciprofloxacin, amoxicillin-clavulanic acid, imipenem, and SXT. *Providencia heimbachae,* although infrequently seen in humans, is resistant to tetracycline, most cephalosporins, gentamicin, and amikacin. Human isolates of *E. tarda* are susceptible to cephalosporins, aminoglycosides, imipenem, ciprofloxacin, aztreonam, and antibiotic-β-lactamase inhibitor combination agents (30). Isolates from fish and fish ponds may be more resistant because of the prophylactic use of antibiotics in fish farming. Most strains of *E. tarda* produce β-lactamases, even though they are susceptible to β-lactams. *P. shigelloides* is resistant to ampicillin, carbenicillin, piperacillin, and ticarcillin and is variably resistant to most aminoglycosides and tetracycline (70). Cephalosporins, quinolones, carbapenems, and SXT show good activity against *P. shigelloides*.

Freney et al. (44) performed susceptibility studies with 120 isolates of uncommonly seen species of *Klebsiella, Enterobacter,* and *Serratia* and found their susceptibilities to be similar to those of conventional species within each genus. Because they are infrequently seen in clinical laboratories, resistance profiles of many of the other *Enterobacteriaceae* are found only in individual case reports. Susceptibilities vary from isolate to isolate even within a genus, so that no empirical guidelines are available for therapy prior to susceptibility testing of the suspected strain.

EVALUATION, INTERPRETATION, AND REPORTING OF RESULTS

When any of the species included in this chapter are identified with a high level of accuracy (>90% probability) by a commercial system, the identification is probably reliable. However, if the organism is isolated from a source where it may be considered significant, such as blood or

Table 14 Extended-spectrum β-lactamases, cephalosporinases, and carbapenemases of the *Enterobacteriaceae*[a]

Ambler class	Bush class	Enzyme class	Substrate	Clavulanic acid	Organism	Location
Serine β-lactamase						
A	2b	Restricted-spectrum β-lactamase	Aminopenicillins, carboxypenicillins	S	*K. pneumoniae* Several other genera	Plasmid Chromosome
A	2be	Extended-spectrum β-lactamase	Extended-spectrum β-lactams	S	*Klebsiella* spp., *S. marcescens, Enterobacter* spp., *Proteus* spp., *C. freundii, M. morganii*	Plasmid
A	2f	Carbapenemase	Carbapenems, aztreonam	S	*Enterobacter* spp., *S. marcescens*	Chromosome
A	2e	Cefuroximase	Cephalosporins	S	*Proteus* spp., *C. koseri*	Chromosome
C	1	Cephalosporinase	Extended-spectrum β-lactam, cephamycins, aztreonam	R	*K. pneumoniae,* several other genera	Plasmid
C	1	Cephalosporinase	Extended-spectrum β-lactams, aztreonam	R	*Enterobacter* spp., *C. freundii, S. marcescens, Proteus* spp., *M. morganii*	Chromosome
Metallo-β-lactamase						
B	3	Carbapenemase	Oxyamino-cephalosporins, aztreonam	R	*K. pneumoniae* *S. marcescens*	Plasmid Chromosome

[a] Abbreviations: S, susceptible; R, resistant. Data from references 25 and 109.

cerebrospinal fluid, and the identification has a probability of <90%, the isolate should be identified by conventional methods or sent to a reference laboratory using these techniques. In the interim, the isolate may be reported to the physician with a presumptive identification. For those strains seen more commonly, the antimicrobial susceptibility profile may be a helpful adjunct for deciding if identifications with lower probabilities are reliable. Rare species that are identified with low probabilities should always be sent to a reference laboratory accompanied by a brief history. Colony appearance on MacConkey and blood agar plates, spot oxidase and indole reactions, and ampicillin susceptibility or resistance are sufficient for reporting *P. mirabilis* and *P. vulgaris* (13). At the very least, susceptibility testing of strains of *Klebsiella* that appear to contain ESBLs should be tested by the methods described in chapter 74. Any strain of *Enterobacteriaceae* that has been shown to have an ESBL or AmpC cephalosporinase should be reported as resistant to all penicillins, expanded-spectrum cephalosporins, and aztreonam (117).

REFERENCES

1. **Ahmad, M., C. Urban, N. Mariano, P. A. Bradford, E. Calcagni, S. J. Projan, K. Bush, and J. J. Rahal.** 1999. Clinical characteristics and molecular epidemiology associated with imipenem-resistant *Klebsiella pneumoniae*. *Clin. Infect. Dis.* **29:**352–355.
2. **Ajithkumar, B., V. P. Ajithkumar, R. Iriye, Y. Doi, and T. Sakai.** 2003. Spore-forming *Serratia marcescens* subsp. *sakuensis* subsp. nov. isolated from a domestic wastewater treatment plant. *Int. J. Syst. Evol. Microbiol.* **53:**253–258.
3. **Akhurst, R. J., N. E. Boemare, P. H. Janssen, M. M. Peel, D. A. Alfredson, and C. E. Beard.** 2004. Taxonomy of Australian clinical isolates of the genus *Photorhabdus* and proposal of *Photorhabdus asymbiotica* subsp. *asymbiotica* subsp. nov. and *P. asymbiotica* subsp. *australis* subsp. nov. *Int. J. Syst. Evol. Microbiol.* **54:**1301–1310.
4. **Aksoy, S.** 1995. *Wigglesworthia* gen. nov. and *Wigglesworthia glossinidia* sp. nov., taxa consisting of the mycetocyte-associated, primary endosymbionts of tsetse flies. *Int. J. Syst. Bacteriol.* **45:**848–851.
5. **Albert, M. J., K. Alam, M. M. Islam, J. Montanaro, A. S. Rhaman, K. Haider, M. A. Hossain, A. K. Kibriyan, and S. Tzipori.** 1991. *Hafnia alvei*, a probable cause of diarrhea in humans. *Infect. Immun.* **59:**1507–1513.
6. **Albert, M. J., M. Ansaruzzaman, N. A. Bhuiyan, P. K. B. Neogi, and A. S. G. Faruque.** 1995. Characteristics of invasion of HEp-2 cells by *Providencia alcalifaciens*. *J. Med. Microbiol.* **42:**186–190.
7. **Albert, M. J., S. M. Faruque, M. Ansaruzzaman, M. M. Islam, K. Haider, K. Alam, I. Kabir, and R. Robbins-Browne.** 1992. Sharing of virulence-associated properties at the phenotypic and genetic levels between enteropathogenic *Escherichia coli* and *Hafnia alvei*. *J. Med. Microbiol.* **37:**310–314.
8. **Aldova, E., O. Hausner, D. J. Brenner, D. Kocmoud, J. Schindler, B. Potuznikova, and P. Petras.** 1988. *Pragia fontium* gen. nov., sp. nov. of the family *Enterobacteriaceae*, isolated from water. *Int. J. Syst. Bacteriol.* **38:**183–189.
9. **Aldova, E., O. Hausner, and M. Gabrhelova.** 1984. *Budvicia*–a new genus of *Enterobacteriaceae*. Data on phenotypic characters. *J. Hyg. Epidemiol. Microbiol. Immunol.* **28:**234–237.
10. **ASCP Susceptibility Group.** 1997. United States geographic bacteria susceptibility patterns. *Diagn. Microbiol. Infect. Dis.* **35:**143–151.
11. **Aucken, H. M., and T. L. Pitt.** 1998. Antibiotic resistance and putative virulence factors of *Serratia marcescens* with respect to O and K serotypes. *J. Med. Microbiol.* **47:**1105–1113.
12. **Baratela, K. C., H. O. Saridakis, L. C. J. Gaziri, and J. S. Pelayo.** 2001. Effects of medium composition, calcium, iron and oxygen in haemolysin production by *Plesiomonas shigelloides* isolated from water. *J. Appl. Microbiol.* **90:**482–487.
13. **Baron, E. J.** 2001. Rapid identification of bacteria and yeast: summary of a national committee for clinical laboratory standards proposed guidelines. *Clin. Infect. Dis.* **33:**220–225.
14. **Belas, R.** 1992. The swarming phenomenon of *Proteus mirabilis*. *ASM News* **58:**15–22.
15. **Bennett, A. R., S. MacPhee, R. Betts, and D. Post.** 1999. Use of pyrrolidonyl peptidase to distinguish *Citrobacter* from *Salmonella*. *Lett. Appl. Microbiol.* **28:**175–178.
16. **Bergeron, M. G.** 2000. Genetic tools for the simultaneous identification of bacterial species and their antibiotic resistance genes: impact on clinical practice. *Int. J. Antimicrob. Agents* **16:**1–3.
17. **Bhadra, B., P. Roy, and R. Chakraborty.** 2005. *Serratia ureilytica* sp. nov., a novel urea utilizing species. *Int. J. Syst. Evol. Microbiol.* **55:**2155–2158.
18. **Boemare, N. E., R. J. Akhurst, and R. G. Mourant.** 1993. DNA relatedness between *Xenorhabdus* spp. (*Enterobacteriaceae*), symbiotic bacteria of entomopathogenic nematodes, and a proposal to transfer *Xenorhabdus luminescens* to a new genus, *Photorhabdus* gen. nov. *Int. J. Syst. Microbiol.* **43:**249–255.
19. **Bornet, C., A. Davin-Regli, C. Bosi, J.-M. Pages, and C. Bollet.** 2000. Imipenem resistance of *Enterobacter aerogenes* mediated by outer membrane permeability. *J. Clin. Microbiol.* **38:**1048–1052.
20. **Bouvet, O. M. M., P. A. D. Grimont, C. Richard, E. Aldova, O. Hausner, and M. Gabrhelova.** 1985. *Budvicia aquatica* gen. nov.: a hydrogen sulfide-producing member of the *Enterobacteriaceae*. *Int. J. Syst. Bacteriol.* **35:**60–64.
21. **Brenner, D. J., P. A. D. Grimont, A. G. Steigerwalt, G. R. Fanning, E. Ageron, and C. F. Riddle.** 1993. Classification of citrobacteria by DNA hybridization: designation of *Citrobacter farmeri* sp. nov., *Citrobacter youngae* sp. nov., *Citrobacter braakii* sp. nov., *Citrobacter werkmanii* sp. nov., *Citrobacter sedlakii* sp. nov., and three unnamed *Citrobacter* genomospecies. *Int. J. Syst. Bacteriol.* **43:**645–658.
22. **Brenner, D. J., H. E. Muller, A. G. Steigerwalt, A. M. Whitney, C. M. O'Hara, and P. Kampfer.** 1998. Two new *Rahnella* genomospecies that cannot be phenotypically differentiated from *Rahnella aquatilis*. *Int. J. Syst. Bacteriol.* **48:**141–149.
23. **Brenner, D. J., C. M. O'Hara, P. A. D. Grimont, J. M. Janda, E. Falsen, E. Aldova, E. Ageron, J. Schindler, S. L. Abbott, and A. G. Steigerwalt.** 1999. Biochemical identification of *Citrobacter* species defined by DNA hybridization and description of *Citrobacter gillenii* sp. nov. (formerly *Citrobacter* genomospecies 10) and *Citrobacter murlinae* sp. nov. (formerly *Citrobacter* genomospecies 11). *J. Clin. Microbiol.* **37:**2619–2624.
24. **Brisse, S., D. Milatovic, A. C. Fluit, J. Verhoef, and F.-J. Schmitz.** 2000. Epidemiology of quinolone resistance of *Klebsiella pneumoniae* and *Klebsiella oxytoca* in Europe. *Eur. J. Clin. Microbiol. Infect. Dis.* **19:**64–68.
25. **Bush, K., G. A. Jacoby, and A. A. Medeiros.** 1995. A functional classification scheme for β-lactamases and its correlation with molecular structure. *Antimicrob. Agents Chemother.* **39:**1211–1233.
26. **Carricajo, A., S. Boiste, J. Thore, G. Aubert, Y. Gille, and A. M. Freydiere.** 1999. Comparative evaluation of five chromogenic media for detection, enumeration and identification of urinary tract pathogens. *Eur. J. Clin. Microbiol. Infect. Dis.* **18:**796–803.

27. **Carter, J., S. Hutton, K. S. Sriprakash, D. J. Kemp, G. Lum, J. Savage, and F. J. Bowden.** 1997. Culture of the causative organism of donovanosis *(Calymmatobacterium granulomatis)* in HEp-2 cells. *J. Clin. Microbiol.* **35:**2915–2917.
28. **Carter, J. S., F. J. Bowden, I. Bastain, G. M. Myers, K. S. Sriprakash, and D. J. Kemp.** 1999. Phylogenetic evidence for reclassification of *Calymmatobacterium granulomatis* as *Klebsiella granulomatis* comb. nov. *Int. J. Syst. Bacteriol.* **49:** 1695–1700.
29. **Chida, T., N. Okamura, K. Ohtani, Y. Yoshida, E. Arakawa, and H. Watanabe.** 2000. The complete DNA sequence of the O antigen gene region of *Plesiomonas shigelloides* serotype O17 which is identical to *Shigella sonnei* form I antigen. *Microbiol. Immunol.* **44:**161–172.
30. **Clark, R. B., P. D. Lister, and J. M. Janda.** 1991. In vitro susceptibilities of *Edwardsiella tarda* to 22 antibiotics and antibiotic-β-lactamase-inhibitor agents. *Diagn. Microbiol. Infect. Dis.* **14:**173–175.
31. **Cockerill, F. R., III, J. G. Hughes, E. A. Vetter, R. A. Mueller, A. L. Weaver, D. M. Ilstrup, J. E. Rosenblatt, and W. R. Wilson.** 1997. Analysis of 281,797 consecutive blood cultures performed over an eight-year period: trends in microorganisms isolated and the value of anaerobic culture of blood. *Clin. Infect. Dis.* **24:**403–418.
32. **Dale, C., and I. Maudlin.** 1999. *Sodalis* gen. nov. and *Sodalis glossinidius* sp. nov., a microaerophilic secondary endosymbiont of the tsetse fly *Glossinia morsitans morsitans*. *Int. J. Syst. Bacteriol.* **49:**267–275.
33. **De Baere, T., R. Verhelst, C. Labit, G. Verschraegen, G. Wauters, G. Claeys, and M. Vaneechoutte.** 2004. Bacteremic infection with *Pantoea ananatis*. *J. Clin. Microbiol.* **42:**4393–4395.
34. **De Baere, T., G. Wauters, P. Kampfer, C. Labit, G. Claeys, G. Verschraegen, and M. Vaneechoutte.** 2002. Isolation of *Buttiauxella gaviniae* from a spinal cord patient with urinary bladder pathology. *J. Clin. Microbiol.* **40:**3867–3870.
35. **Diekma, D. J., M. A. Pfaller, R. N. Jones, and the SENTRY Participants Group.** 2002. Age-related trends in pathogen frequency and antimicrobial susceptibility of bloodstream isolates in North America SENTRY Antimicrobial Surveillance Program, 1997-2000. *Int. J. Antimicrob. Agents* **20:**412–418.
36. **Drancourt, M., C. Bollet, A. Carlioz, R. Martelin, J.-P. Gayral, and D. Raoult.** 2000. 16S ribosomal DNA sequence analysis of a large collection of environmental and clinical unidentifiable bacterial isolates. *J. Clin. Microbiol.* **38:**3623–3630.
37. **Drancourt, M., C. Bollet, A. Carta, and P. Rousselier.** 2001. Phylogenetic analyses of *Klebsiella* species delineate *Klebsiella* and *Raoultella* gen. nov., with description of *Raoultella ornithinolytica* comb. nov. *Int. J. Syst. Evol. Microbiol.* **51:**925–932.
38. **Ehrlich, G. D.** 1991. Caveats of PCR. *Clin. Microbiol. Newsl.* **13:**149–151.
39. **Emery, C. L., and L. A. Weymouth.** 1997. Detection and clinical significance of extended-spectrum β-lactamases in a tertiary-care medical center. *J. Clin. Microbiol.* **35:**2061–2067.
40. **Farmer, J. J., III, G. R. Fanning, G. P. Huntley-Carter, B. Holmes, F. W. Hickman, C. Richard, and D. J. Brenner.** 1981. *Kluyvera*, a new (redefined) genus in the family *Enterobacteriaceae:* identification of *Kluyvera ascorbata* sp. nov. and *Kluyvera cryocrescens* sp. nov. in clinical specimens. *J. Clin. Microbiol.* **13:**919–933.
41. **Farmer, J. J., III, J. H. Jorgeson, P. A. D. Grimont, R. J. Akhurst, G. O. Poinar, E. Ageron, G. V. Pierce, and J. A. Smith.** 1989. *Xenorhabdus luminescens* (DNA hybrization group 5) from human clinical specimens. *J. Clin. Microbiol.* **27:**1594–1600.
42. **Farrell, D. J., I. Morrissey, D. De Rubeis, M. Robbins, and D. Felmingham.** 2003. A UK multicentre study of the antimicrobial susceptibility of bacterial pathogens causing urinary tract infection. *J. Infect.* **46:**94–100.
43. **Fischer-LeSaux, M., V. Viallard, B. Brunel, P. Normand, and N. Boemare.** 1999. Polyphasic classification of the genus *Photorhabdus* and proposal of new taxa: *P. luminescens* subsp. *luminescens* subsp. nov., *P. luminescens* subsp. *akhurstii* subsp. nov., *P. luminescens* subsp. *laumondii* subsp. nov., *P. temperata* sp. nov., and *P. asymbiotica* sp. nov. *Int. J. Syst. Bacteriol.* **49:**1645–1656.
44. **Freney, J., M. O. Husson, F. Gavini, S. Madier, A. Martra, D. Izard, H. Leclerc, and J. Fleurette.** 1988. Susceptibilities to antibiotics and antiseptics of new species of the family *Enterobacteriaceae. Antimicrob. Agents Chemother.* **32:**873–876.
45. **Gautom, R. K.** 1997. Rapid pulsed-field gel electrophoresis protocol for typing of *Escherichia coli* O157:H7 and other gram-negative organisms in 1 day. *J. Clin. Microbiol.* **35:** 2977–2980.
46. **Gavini, E., J. Mergaert, A. Beji, C. Mielcarek, D. Izard, K. Kersters, and J. De Ley.** 1989. Transfer of *Enterobacter agglomerans* (Beijerinck 1988) Ewing and Fife 1972 to *Pantoea* gen. nov. as *Pantoea agglomerans* comb. nov. and description of *Pantoea dispersa* sp. nov. *Int. J. Syst. Bacteriol.* **39:**337–345.
47. **Gherna, R. L., J. H. Werren, W. Weisburg, R. Cote, C. R. Woese, L. Mandelco, and D. J. Brenner.** 1991. *Arsenophonas nasoniae* gen. nov., sp. nov., the causative agent of the son-killer trait in the parasitic wasp *Nasonia vitripennis*. *Int. J. Syst. Bacteriol.* **41:**563–565.
48. **Goering, R. V.** 1998. The molecular epidemiology of nosocomial infection. *In* S. Specter, M. Bendinella, and H. Friedman (ed.), *Rapid Detection of Infectious Agents*. Plenum Press, New York, N.Y.
49. **Gordon, K. A., R. N. Jones, and SENTRY Participants Groups (Europe, Latin America, North America).** 2003. Susceptibility patterns of orally administered antimicrobials among urinary tract infection pathogens from hospitalized patients in North America: comparison report to Europe, and Latin America. Results from the SENTRY Antimicrobial Program (2000). *Diagn. Microbiol. Infect. Dis.* **45:**295–301.
50. **Grimont, F., and P. A. D. Grimont.** 1981. The genus *Serratia*, p. 2822–2848. *In* M. P. Starr, H. Stolp, H. G. Truper, and H. G. Schlegel (ed.), *The Prokaryotes: a Handbook on Habitats, Isolation, and Identification of Bacteria*. Springer-Verlag, Berlin, Germany.
51. **Grimont, F., and P. A. D. Grimont.** 1991. The genus *Enterobacter*, p. 2797–2815. *In* A. Balows, H. G. Truper, M. Dworkin, W. Harder, and K.-H. Schleifer (ed.), *The Prokaryotes: a Handbook on the Biology of Bacteria: Ecophysiology, Isolation, Identification, Applications*, 2nd ed. Springer-Verlag, Berlin, Germany.
52. **Grimont, F., P. A. D. Grimont, and C. Richard.** 1991. The genus *Klebsiella*, p. 2775–2796. *In* M. P. Starr, H. Stolp, H. G. Trüper, A. Balows, and H. G. Schlegel (ed.), *The Prokaryotes: a Handbook on the Biology of Bacteria: Ecophysiology, Isolation, Identification, Applications*. Springer-Verlag, Berlin, Germany.
53. **Grimont, P. A. D., F. Grimont, J. J. Farmer III, and M. A. Asbury.** 1981. *Cedecea davisae* gen. nov., sp. nov., new *Enterobacteriaceae* from clinical specimens. *Int. J. Syst. Bacteriol.* **31:**317–326.
54. **Grimont, P. A. D., J. J. Farmer III, F. Grimont, M. A. Asbury, D. J. Brenner, and C. Deval.** 1983. *Ewingella americana* gen. nov., sp. nov., a new *Enterobacteriaceae* isolated from clinical specimens. *Ann. Microbiol.* (Paris) **134A:**39–52.
55. **Grimont, P. A. D., F. Grimont, C. Richard, and R. Sakazaki.** 1980. *Edwardsiella hoshinae*, a new species of Enterobacteriaceae. *Curr. Microbiol.* **4:**347–351.

56. **Hart, C. A., and S. K. Rao.** 1999. Donovanosis. *J. Med. Microbiol.* **48:**707–709.
57. **Hauben, L., E. R. B. Moore, L. Vauterin, M. Steenackers, J. Maegaert, L. Verdonck, and J. Swings.** 1999. Phylogenetic position of phytopathogens within the *Enterobacteriaceae*. *System. Appl. Microbiol.* **21:**384–397.
58. **Hawke, J. P., A. C. McWhorter, A. G. Steigerwalt, and D. J. Brenner.** 1981. *Edwardsiella ictaluri* sp. nov., the causative agent of enteric septicemia of catfish. *Int. J. Syst. Bacteriol.* **31:**396–400.
59. **Hickman-Brenner, F. W., G. P. Huntley-Carter, Y. Saitoh, A. G. Steigerwalt, J. J. Farmer III, and D. J. Brenner.** 1984. *Moellerella wisconsensis*, a new genus and species of *Enterobacteriaceae* found in human stool specimens. *J. Clin. Microbiol.* **19:**460–463.
60. **Hickman-Brenner, F. W., M. P. Vohra, G. P. Huntley-Carter, G. R. Fanning, V. A. Lowery III, D. J. Brenner, and J. J. Farmer III.** 1985. *Leminorella*, a new genus of *Enterobacteriaceae:* identification of *Leminorella grimontii* sp. nov. and *Leminorella richardii* sp. nov. found in clinical specimens. *J. Clin. Microbiol.* **21:**234–239.
61. **Hoffmann, H., and A. Roggenkamp.** 2003. Population genetics of the nomenspecies *Enterobacter cloacae*. *Appl. Environ. Microbiol.* **69:**5306–5318.
62. **Hoffmann, H., S. Stindl, W. Ludwig, A. Stumpf, A. Mehlen, J. Heesemann, D. Monget, K. H. Schleifer, and A. Roggenkamp.** 2005. Reassignment of *Enterobacter dissolvens* to *Enterobacter cloacae* as *E. cloacae* subspecies *dissolvens* comb. nov. and emended description of *Enterobacter asburiae* and *Enterobacter kobei*. *Syst. Appl. Microbiol.* **28:**196–205.
63. **Hoffmann, H., S. Stindl, W. Ludwig, A. Stumpf, A. Mehlen, D. Monget, D. Pierard, S. Ziesing, J. Heesemann, A. Roggenkamp, and K. H. Schleifer.** 2005. *Enterobacter hormaechei* subsp. *oharae* subsp. nov., *E. hormaechei* subsp. *hormaechei* comb. nov., and *E. hormaechei* subsp. *steigerwaltii* subsp. nov., three new subspecies of clinical importance. *J. Clin. Microbiol.* **43:**3297–3303.
64. **Hoffmann, H., S. Stindl, A. Stumpf, A. Mehlen, D. Monget, J. Heesemann, K. H. Schleifer, and A. Roggenkamp.** 2005. Description of *Enterobacter ludwigii* sp. nov., a novel *Enterobacter* species of clinical relevance. *Syst. Appl. Microbiol.* **28:**206–212.
65. **Hollis, D. G., F. W. Hickman, G. R. Fanning, J. J. Farmer III, R. E. Weaver, and D. J. Brenner.** 1981. *Tatumella ptyseos* gen. nov., sp. nov., a member of the family *Enterobacteriaceae* found in clinical specimens. *J. Clin. Microbiol.* **14:**79–88.
66. **Hume, E. B. H., M. D. P. Willcox, D. F. Sweeney, and B. A. Holden.** 1996. An examination of the clonal variants of *Serratia marcescens* that infect the eye during contact lens wear. *J. Med. Microbiol.* **45:**127–132.
67. **Huys, G., M. Cnockaert, J. M. Janda, and J. Swings.** 2003. *Escherichia albertii* sp. nov., a diarrhoeagenic species isolated from stool specimens of Bangladeshi children. *Int. J. Syst. Evol. Microbiol.* **53:**1237–1270.
68. **Inoue, K., K. Sugiyama, Y. Kosako, R. Sakazaki, and S. Yamai.** 2000. *Enterobacter cowanii* sp. nov., a new species of the family *Enterobacteriaceae*. *Curr. Microbiol.* **41:**417–420.
69. **Jagger, T. D.** 2000. *Plesiomonas shigelloides*–a veterinary perspective. *Infect. Dis. Rev.* **2:**199–210.
70. **Janda, J. M.** 2001. *Aeromonas* and *Plesiomonas*, p. 1237–1270. *In* M. Sussman (ed.), *Molecular Medical Microbiology*, vol. 2. Academic Press, Ltd., London, United Kingdom.
71. **Janda, J. M., and S. L. Abbott.** 2005. *The Enterobacteria*, 2nd ed. ASM Press, Washington, D.C.
72. **Janda, J. M., and S. L. Abbott.** 1993. Expression of hemolytic activity in *Plesiomonas shigelloides*. *J. Clin. Microbiol.* **31:**1206–1208.
73. **Janda, J. M., S. L. Abbott, and M. J. Albert.** 1999. Prototypal diarrheagenic strains of *Hafnia alvei* are actually members of the genus *Escherichia*. *J. Clin. Microbiol.* **37:**2399–2401.
74. **Janda, J. M., S. L. Abbott, S. Bystrom, and W. S. Probert.** 2005. Identification of two distinct hybridization groups in the genus *Hafnia* by 16S rRNA gene sequencing and phenotypic methods. *J. Clin. Microbiol.* 43:3320–3323.
75. **Janda, J. M., S. L. Abbott, S. Khashe, and W. Probert.** 2001. Biochemical identification and characterization of DNA groups within the *Proteus vulgaris* complex. *J. Clin. Microbiol.* **39:**1231–1234.
76. **Janda, J. M., S. L. Abbott, J. G. Morris.** 1995. *Aeromonas*, *Plesiomonas* and *Edwardsiella*, p. 905–917. *In* M. J. Blaser, P. D. Smith, J. I. Ravdin, H. B. Greenberg, and R. L. Guerrant (ed.), *Infections of the Gastrointestinal Tract*. Raven Press, Ltd., New York, N.Y.
77. **Janda, J. M., S. L. Abbott, D. Woodward, and S. Khashe.** 1998. Invasion of HEp-2 and other eukaryotic cell lines by *Providenciae:* further evidence supporting the role of *Providencia alcalifaciens* in bacterial gastroenteritis. *Curr. Microbiol.* **37:**159–165.
78. **Johnson, A. S., C. L. Tarr, B. H. Brown, Jr., K. M. Birkhead, and J. J. Farmer III.** 2005. First case of septicemia due to a strain belonging to enteric group 58 *(Enterobacteriaceae)* and its designation as *Averyella dalhousiensis* gen. nov., sp. nov., based on analysis of strains from 20 additional cases. *J. Clin. Microbiol.* **43:**5195–5201.
79. **Kado, C. I.** 2000. *Erwinia* and related genera. *In* M. Dworkin, S. Falkow, E. Rosenberg, K.-H. Schleifer, and E. Stackebrandt (ed.), *The Prokaryotes: an Evolving Electronic Resource for the Microbiological Community*, 3rd ed. [Online.] Springer-Verlag, New York. N.Y. http://141.150.157.117:8080/prokPUB/index.htm. (latest update release 3.2; July 2000).
80. **Kageyama, B., M. Nakae, S. Yagi, and T. Sonoyama.** 1992. *Pantoea punctata* sp. nov., *Pantoea citrea* sp. nov., and *Pantoea terrea* sp. nov. isolated from fruit and soil samples. *Int. J. Syst. Bacteriol.* **42:**203–210.
81. **Kampfer, P., S. Ruppel, and R. Remus.** 2005. *Enterobacter radicincitans* sp. nov., a plant growth promoting species of the family *Enterobacteriaceae*. *Syst. Appl. Microbiol.* **28:**213–221.
82. **Karlowsky, J. A., M. E. Jones, D. C. Draghi, C. Thornsberry, D. F. Sahm, and G. A. Volturo.** 2004. Prevalence and antimicrobial susceptibilities of bacteria isolated from blood cultures of hospitalized patients in the United States in 2002. *Ann. Clin. Microbiol. Antimicrob.* **3:**7–15.
83. **Karlowsky, J. A., M. E. Jones, C. Thornsberry, I. R. Friedland, and D. F. Sahm.** 2003. Trends in antimicrobial susceptibilities among *Enterobacteriaceae* isolated from hospitalized patients in the United States from 1998 to 2001. *Antimicrob. Agents Chemother.* **47:**1672–1680.
84. **Khan, A. M., A. S. G. Faruque, M. S. Hossain, S. Sattar, G. J. Fuchs, and M. A. Salam.** 2004. *Plesiomonas shigelloides*-associated diarrhoea in Bangladeshi children: a hospital-based surveillance study. *J. Trop. Pediatr.* **50:**354–356.
85. **Kharsany, A. B. M., A. A. Hoosens, P. Kiepela, P. Kirby, and A. W. Sturm.** 1999. Phylogenetic analysis of *Calymmatobacterium granulomatis* based on rRNA gene sequences. *J. Med. Microbiol.* **48:**841–847.
86. **Khashe, S., D. J. Scales, S. L. Abbott, and J. M. Janda.** 2001. Non-invasive *Providencia alcalifaciens* strains fail to attach to HEp-2 cells. *Curr. Microbiol.* **43:**414–417.
87. **Knox, C. M., V. Cevellos, and D. Dean.** 1998. 16S ribosomal DNA typing for identification of pathogens in patients with bacterial keratitis. *J. Clin. Microbiol.* **36:**3492–3496.
88. **Kosako, Y., R. Sakazaki, and E. Yoshizaki.** 1984. *Yokenella regensburgei* gen. nov., sp. nov.: a new genus and species in the family *Enterobacteriaceae*. *Jpn. J. Med. Sci. Biol.* **37:**117–124.

89. **Kosako, Y., K. Tamura, R. Sakazaki, and K. Miki.** 1996. *Enterobacter kobei* sp. nov., a new species of the family *Enterobacteriaceae* resembling *Enterobacter cloacae*. *Curr. Microbiol.* **33:**261–265.
90. **Landman, D., M. Chocklingam, and J. M. Quale.** 1999. Reduction in the incidence of methicillin-resistant *Staphylococcus aureus* and ceftazidime-resistant *Klebsiella pneumoniae* following changes in a hospital antibiotic formulary. *Clin. Infect. Dis.* **28:**1062–1066.
91. **Lederman, E. R., and N. F. Crum.** 2005. Pyogenic liver abscess with a focus on *Klebsiella pneumoniae* as a primary pathogen: an emerging disease with unique clinical characteristics. *Am. J. Gastroenterol.* **100:**322–331.
92. **Lengyel, K., E. Lang, A. Fodor, E. Szallas, P. Schumann, and E. Stackebrandt.** 2005. Description of four novel species of *Xenorhabdus*, family *Enterobacteriaceae*: *Xenorhabdus budapestensis* sp. nov., *Xenorhabdus ehlersii* sp. nov., *Xenorhabdus innexi* sp. nov., and *Xenorhabdus szentirmaii* sp. nov. *Syst. Appl. Microbiol.* **28:**115–122.
93. **Li, X., D. Zhang, F. Chen, J. Ma, Y. Dong, and L. Zhang.** 2004. *Klebsiella singaporensis* sp. nov., a novel isomaltulose-producing bacterium. *Int. J. Syst. Evol. Microbiol.* **54:**2131–2136.
94. **Lin, F.-Y. C., W. F. Devoe, C. Morrison, J. Libonati, P. Powers, R. J. Gross, B. Rowe, E. Israel, and J. G. Morris.** 1987. Outbreak of neonatal *Citrobacter diversus* meningitis in a suburban hospital. *Pediatr. Infect. Dis. J.* **6:**50–55.
95. **Livermore, D. M.** 1995. β-Lactamases in laboratory and clinical resistance. *Clin. Microbiol. Rev.* **8:**557–584.
96. **Lucet, J.-C., D. Decre, A. Fichelle, M.-L. Joly-Guillou, M. Pernet, C. Deblangy, M.-J. Kosmann, and B. Regnier.** 1999. Control of a prolonged outbreak of extended-spectrum β-lactamase-producing Enterobacteriaceae in a university hospital. *Clin. Infect. Dis.* **29:**1411–1418.
97. **Luperchio, S. A., J. V. Newman, C. A Dangler, M. D. Schrenzel, D. J. Brenner, A. G. Steigerwalt, and D. B. Schauer.** 2000. *Citrobacter rodentium*, the causative agent of transmissible murine colonic hyperplasia, exhibits clonality: synonymy of *C. rodentium* and mouse-pathogenic *Escherichia coli*. *J. Clin. Microbiol.* **38:**4343–4350.
98. **MacDonell, M. T., and R. R. Colwell.** 1985. Phylogeny of the *Vibrionaceae*, and recommendation for two new genera, *Listonella* and *Shewanella*. *Syst. Appl. Microbiol.* **6:**171–182.
99. **Martinez-Murcia, A. J., S. Beniloch, and M. D. Collins.** 1992. Phylogenetic interrelationships of members of the genera *Aeromonas* and *Plesiomonas* as determined by 16S ribosomal DNA sequencing: lack of congruence with results of DNA-DNA hybridizations. *Int. J. Syst. Bacteriol.* **42:**412–421.
100. **Matthew, C. Z., A. C. Darby, S. A. Young, L. H. Hune, and S. C. Welburn.** 2005. The rapid isolation and growth dynamics of the tsetse symbiont *Sodalis glossinidius*. *FEMS Microbiol. Lett.* **248:**69–74.
101. **McWhorter, A. C., R. L. Haddock, F. A. Nocon, A. G. Steigerwalt, D. J. Brenner, S. Aleksic, J. Bockmuhl, and J. J. Farmer III.** 1991. *Trabulsiella guamensis*, a new genus and species of the family *Enterobacteriaceae* that resembles *Salmonella* subgroups 4 and 5. *J. Clin. Microbiol.* **29:** 1480–1485.
102. **Mobley, H. L.** 2000. Virulence of the two primary uropathogens. *ASM News* **66:**403–410.
103. **Montgomerie, J. Z.** 1979. Epidemiology of *Klebsiella* and hospital-associated infections. *Rev. Infect. Dis.* **1:**736–753.
104. **Moran, N. A., J. A. Russell, R. Koga, and T. Fukatsu.** 2005. Evolutionary relationships of three new species of *Enterobacteriaceae* living as symbionts of aphids and other insects. *Appl. Environ. Microbiol.* **71:**3302–3310.
105. **Muller, H. E., D. J. Brenner, G. R. Fanning, P. A. D. Grimont, and P. Kampfer.** 1996. Emended description of *Buttiauxella agrestis* with recognition of six new species of *Buttiauxella* and two new species of *Kluyvera*: *Buttiauxella ferragutiae* sp. nov., *Buttiauxella gaviniae* sp. nov., *Buttiauxella brennerae* sp. nov., *Buttiauxella izardii* sp. nov., *Buttiauxella noackiae* sp. nov., *Buttiauxella warmboldiae* sp. nov., *Kluyvera cochleae* sp. nov., and *Kluyvera georgiana* sp. nov. *Int J. Syst. Bacteriol.* **46:**50–63.
106. **Muller, H. E., C. M. O'Hara, G. R. Fanning, F. W. Hickman-Brenner, J. M. Swenson, and D. J. Brenner.** 1986. *Providencia heimbachae*, a new species of *Enterobacteriaceae* isolated from animals. *Int. J. Syst. Bacteriol.* **36:**252–256.
107. **Munson, M. A., P. Baumann, and M. G. Kinsey.** 1991. *Buchnera* gen. nov. and *Buchnera aphidicola* sp. nov., a taxon consisting of the mycetocyte-associated, primary endosymbionts of aphids. *Int. J. Syst. Bacteriol.* **41:**566–568.
108. **Murray, R. G. E., and K. H. Schleifer.** 1994. Taxonomic notes: a proposal for recording the properties of putative taxa of procaryotes. *Int. J. Syst. Bacteriol.* **44:**174–176.
109. **Nordmann, P.** 1998. Trends in β-lactam resistance among Enterobacteriaceae. *Clin. Infect. Dis.* **27**(Suppl. 1)**:** S100–S106.
110. **O'Hara, C. M., F. W. Brenner, and J. M. Miller.** 2000. Classification, identification, and clinical significance of *Proteus*, *Providencia*, and *Morganella*. *Clin. Microbiol. Rev.* **13:**534–546.
111. **O'Hara, C. M., F. W. Brenner, A. G. Steigerwalt, B. C. Hill, B. Holmes, P. A. D. Grimont, P. M. Hawkey, J. L. Penner, J. M. Miller, and D. J. Brenner.** 2000. Classification of *Proteus vulgaris* biogroup 3 with recognition of *Proteus hauseri* sp. nov., nom. rev. and unnamed *Proteus* genomospecies 4, 5, and 6. *Int. J. Syst. Evol. Microbiol.* **50:**1869–1875.
112. **O'Hara, C. M., A. G. Steigerwalt, D. Green, M. McDowell, B. C. Hill, D. J. Brenner, and J. M. Miller.** 1999. Isolation of *Providencia heimbachae* from human feces. *J. Clin. Microbiol.* **37:**3048–3050.
113. **O'Hara, C. M., A. G. Steigerwalt, B. C. Hill, J. J. Farmer III, G. R. Fanning, and D. J. Brenner.** 1989. *Enterobacter hormaechei*, a new species of the family *Enterobacteriaceae* formerly known as enteric group 75. *J. Clin. Microbiol.* **27:**2046–2049.
114. **O'Hara, C. M., A. G. Steigerwalt, B. C. Hill, J. M. Miller, and D. J. Brenner.** 1998. First report of a human isolate of *Erwinia persicinus*. *J. Clin. Microbiol.* **36:**248–250.
115. **Ohkusu, K.** 2000. Cost-effective and rapid presumptive identification of gram-negative bacilli in routine urine, pus, and stool cultures: evaluation of the use of CHROMagar orientation medium in conjunction with simple biochemical tests. *J. Clin. Microbiol.* **38:**4586–4592.
116. **Paterson, D. L., W.-C. Ko, A. Von Gottberg, J. M. Casellas, L. Mulazimoglu, K. P. Klugman, R. A. Bonomo, L. B. Rice, J. G. McCormack, and V. L. Yu.** 2001. Outcome of cephalosporin treatment for serious infections due to apparently susceptible organisms producing extended-spectrum β-lactamases: implications for the clinical microbiology laboratory. *J. Clin. Microbiol.* **39:**2206–2212.
117. **Paterson, D. L., and V. L. Yu.** 1999. Editorial response: extended-spectrum β-lactamases: a call for improved detection and control. *Clin. Infect. Dis.* **29:**1419–1422.
118. **Pavan, M. E., R. J. Franco, J. M. Rodriguez, P. Gadaleta, S. L. Abbott, J. M. Janda, and J. Zorzopulos.** 2005. Phylogenetic relationships of the genus *Kluyvera*: transfer of *Enterobacter intermedius* Izard *et al.* 1980 to the genus *Kluyvera* as *Kluyvera intermedia* comb. nov. and reclassification of *Kluyvera cochleae* as a later synonym of *K. intermedia*. *Int. J. Syst. Evol. Microbiol.* **55:**437–442.
119. **Podschun, R., A. Fischer, and U. Ullman.** 2000. Expression of putative virulence factors by clinical isolates of *Klebsiella planticola*. *J. Med. Microbiol.* **49:**115–119.

120. **Polster, M., and M. Svobodova.** 1964. Production of reddish-brown pigment from *dl*-tryptophan by Enterobacteria of the Proteus-Providencia group. *Experimentia* **20:**637–638.
121. **Rahimian, J., T. Wilson, V. Oram, and R. S. Holzman.** 2004. Pyogenic liver abscess: recent trends in etiology and mortality. *Clin. Infect. Dis.* **39:**1654–1659.
122. **Ramos, A., and D. Damaso.** 2000. Extraintestinal infection due to *Hafnia alvei. Eur. J. Microbiol. Infect. Dis.* **19:**708–710.
123. **Ridell, J., A. Siitonen, L. Paulin, L. Mattila, H. Korkeala, and M. J. Albert.** 1994. *Hafnia alvei* in stool specimens from patients with diarrhea and healthy controls. *J. Clin. Microbiol.* **32:**2335–2337.
124. **Rosenblueth, M., L. Martinez, J. Silva, and E. Martinez-Romero.** 2004. *Klebsiella variicola*, a novel species with clinical and plant-associated isolates. *System. Appl. Microbiol.* **27:**27–35.
125. **Ruimy, R., V. Breittmayer, P. Elbaze, B. Lafay, O. Boussemart, M. Gauthier, and R. Christen.** 1994. Phylogenetic analysis and assessment of the genera *Vibrio, Photobacterium, Aeromonas*, and *Plesiomonas* deduced from small-subunit rRNA sequences. *Int. J. Syst. Bacteriol.* **44:**416–426.
126. **Sabella, C., M. Touhy, G. Hall, A. C. Gales, M. E. Erwin, and R. N. Jones.** 2000. Emergence of cefepime-resistance in *Klebsiella oxytoca* clinical isolate due to alteration in the outer membrane permeability. *Clin. Microbiol. Newsl.* **22:**37–39.
127. **Samson, R., J. B. Legendre, R. Christen, W. Achouak, and L. Gardan.** 2004. Transfer of *Pectobacterium chrysanthemi* (Brenner *et al.* 1973) Hauben *et al.* 1998 and *Brenneria paradisiaca* to the genus *Dickeya* gen. nov. as *D. chrysanthemi* comb. nov. and *D. paradisiaca* comb. nov. and delineation of four novel species: *D. dadantii* sp. nov., *D. dianthicola* sp. nov., *D. dieffenbachiae* sp. nov. and *D. zeae* sp. nov. *Int. J. Syst. Evol. Microbiol.* **55:**1415–1427.
128. **Scarparo, C., P. Piccoli, P. Ricordi, and M. Scagnelli.** 2002. Comparative evaluation of two commercial chromogenic media for detection and presumptive identification of urinary tract pathogens. *Eur. J. Clin. Microbiol. Infect. Dis.* **21:**283–289.
129. **Schmid, H., C. Weber, J. R. Bogner, and S. Schubert.** 2003. Isolation of a *Pantoea dispersa*-like strain from a 71-year-old woman with acute myeloid leukemia and multiple myeloma. *Infection* **31:**66–67.
130. **Schonheyder, H. C., K. T. Jensen, and W. Frederiksen.** 1994. Taxonomic notes: synonymy of *Enterobacter cancerogenus* (Urosevic 1966) Dickey and Zumoff 1988 and *Enterobacter taylorae* Farmer et al. 1985 and resolution of an ambiguity in the biochemical profile. *Int. J. Syst. Bacteriol.* **44:**586–587.
131. **Shieh, W. Y., and W. D. Jean.** 1998. *Alterococcus agarolyticus*, gen. nov., sp. nov., a halophilic thermophilic bacterium capable of agar degradation. *Can. J. Microbiol.* **44:**637–645.
132. **Slaven, E. M., F. A. Lopez, S. M. Hart, and C. V. Sanders.** 2001. Myonecrosis caused by *Edwardsiella tarda:* a case report and case series of extraintestinal *E. tarda* infections. *Clin. Infect Dis.* **32:**1430–1433.
133. **Sproer, C., U. Mendrock, J. Swiderski, E. Lang, and E. Stackebrandt.** 1999. The phylogenetic position of *Serratia, Buttiauxella* and some other genera of the family *Enterobacteriaceae*. *Int. J. Syst. Bacteriol.* **49:**1433–1438.
134. **Sutra, L., R. Christen, C. Bollet, P. Simoneau, and L. Gardan.** 2001. *Samsonia erythrinae* gen. nov., sp. nov., isolated from bark necrotic lesions of *Erythrina* sp., and discrimination of plant-pathogenic *Enterobacteriaceae* by phenotypic features. *Int. J. Syst. Evol. Bacteriol.* **51:**1291–1304.
135. **Tamura, K., R. Sakazaki, Y. Kosako, and E. Yoshizaki.** 1986. *Leclercia adecarboxylata* gen. nov., comb. nov., formerly known as *Escherichia adecarboxylata*. *Curr. Microbiol.* **13:**179–184.
136. **Theodoropoulos, T., H. Wong, M. O'Brien, and D. Stenzel.** 2001. *Plesiomonas shigelloides* enters polarized human intestinal Caco-2 cells in an in vitro model system. *Infect. Immun.* **69:**2260–2269.
137. **Twum-Danso, K., C. Grant, S. A. Al-Suleiman, S. Abdel-Khader, M. S. Al-Awami, H. Al-Breiki, S. Taha, A.-A. Ashoor, and L. Wosornu.** 1992. Microbiology of postoperative wound infection: a prospective study of 1770 wounds. *J. Hosp. Infect.* **21:**29–37.
138. **Vallis, J., C. Leon, and F. Alvarez-Lerma.** 1997. Nosocomial bacteremia in critically ill patients: a multicenter study evaluating epidemiology and prognosis. *Clin. Infect. Dis.* **24:**387–395.
139. **Wendt, C., S. A. Messer, R. J. Hollis, M. A. Pfaller, R. P. Wenzel, and L. A. Herwaldt.** 1999. Recurrent gram-negative bacteremia: incidence and clinical patterns. *Clin. Infect. Dis.* **28:**611–617.
140. **Werren, J. H., S. W. Skinner, and A. M. Huger.** 1986. Male-killing bacteria in a parasitic wasp. *Science* **231:** 990–992.
141. **Westbrook, G. L., C. M. O'Hara, S. B. Roman, and J. M. Miller.** 2000. Incidence and identification of *Klebsiella planticola* in clinical isolates with emphasis on newborns. *J. Clin. Microbiol.* **38:**1495–1497.
142. **Williams, W. W., J. Mariano, M. Spurrier, H. D. Donnell, Jr., R. L. Breckenridge, Jr., R. L. Anderson, I. K. Wachsmuth, C. Thornsberry, D. R. Graham, D. W. Thibeault, and J. R. Allen.** 1984. Nosocomial meningitis due to *Citrobacter diversus* in neonates: new aspects of epidemiology. *J. Infect. Dis.* **150:**229–235.
143. **Wisplinghoff, H., T. Bischoff, S. M. Tallent, H. Seifert, R. P. Wenzel, and M. B. Edmond.** 2004. Nosocomial bloodstream infections in US hospitals: analysis of 24,179 cases from a prospective nationwide surveillance study. *Clin. Infect. Dis.* **39:**309–317.
144. **Wong, T. Y., H. Y. Tsui, M. K. So, J. Y. Lai, C. W. S. Tse, and T. K. Ng.** 2000. *Plesiomonas shigelloides* infection in Hong Kong: retrospective study of 167 laboratory-confirmed cases. *Hong Kong Med. J.* **6:**375–380.
145. **Woo, P. C. Y., S. K. P. Lau, and K.-Y. Yuen.** 2005. Biliary tract disease as a risk factor for *Plesiomonas shigelloides* bacteraemia: a nine-year experience in a Hong Kong hospital and review of the literature. *New Microbiol.* **28:**45–55.
146. **Yang, C.-C., C.-H. Yen, M.-W. Ho, and J.-H. Wang.** 2004. Comparison of pyogenic liver abscess caused by non-*Klebsiella pneumoniae* and *Klebsiella pneumoniae*. *J. Microbiol. Immunol. Infect.* **37:**176–184.
147. **Zreik, L., J. M. Bove, and M. Garnier.** 1998. Phylogenetic characterization of the bacterium-like organism associated with marginal chlorosis of strawberry and proposition of a *Candidatus* taxon for the organism, '*Candidatus* Phlomobacter fragariae.' *Int. J. Syst. Bacteriol.* **48:**257–261.

Aeromonas

AMY J. HORNEMAN, AFSAR ALI, AND SHARON L. ABBOTT

46

TAXONOMY

The genus *Aeromonas* resides within the family *Aeromonadaceae* (8) and the newly proposed order *Aeromonadales*, ord. nov., along with the genera *Oceanimonas* and *Tolumonas* (30). *Aeromonas* is the only one of these three genera that is pathogenic for humans. The frequent reclassifications and constant amended or extended descriptions within *Aeromonas* taxonomy can often be initially puzzling to microbiologists not working with these organisms on a daily basis; however, the information in this chapter should clarify the identification and significance of those species most often associated with human disease (Table 1). DNA hybridization group numbers, which no longer serve a meaningful purpose, and synonymous species designations for *Aeromonas veronii* bv. sobria (*A. ichthiosmia*) and *A. trota* (*A. enteropelogenes*) (7) are not included for simplicity. *Aeromonas* group 501, which is made up of *A. schubertii*-like organisms, and *Aeromonas* sp. DNA hybridization group 11 (31), which is made up of *A. eucrenophila*/*A. encheleia*-like organisms, are also not addressed in the table. These groups contain few strains, their taxonomic status has yet to be resolved and is still highly debated, and most importantly, neither group has been shown to be significant in human or animal disease. Newly proposed *Aeromonas* species and subspecies since the publication of the previous edition of this Manual include *A. hydrophila* subspecies *hydrophila*, sensu stricto (19); *A. hydrophila* subsp. *dhakensis*, isolated from pediatric diarrheal cases in Bangladesh (19); *A. hydrophila* subsp. *ranae*, isolated from septic frogs in Thailand (20); *A. culicicola*, isolated from mosquitoes and drinking water (11, 38); *A. simiae*, isolated from monkey feces (16); and *A. molluscorum*, isolated from bivalve mollusks (34). Because of its clinical significance, it should be noted that clinical strains formerly referred to as "*A. sobria*" are, in fact, *A. veronii* bv. sobria (esculin hydrolysis and ornithine decarboxylase negative and arginine dihydrolase positive) and should be reported as such. Nearly all rapid identification databases, excepting API 20E strips (BioMerieux, Hazelwood, Mo.), have converted their *A. sobria* identifications to *A. veronii* bv. sobria. This is especially important because of *A. veronii* bv. sobria's association with more severe, extraintestinal infections, such as septicemia, meningitis following leech therapy, and disseminated intravascular gas production (36, 43). It usually is not necessary to definitively separate members of the *A. hydrophila* complex (*A. hydrophila, A. bestiarum,* and *A. salmonicida*) or the *A. caviae* complex (*A. caviae, A. media,* and *A. eucrenophila*), especially when they are isolated from feces (see "Interpretation and Reporting of Results" below).

The type strain *Aeromonas hydrophila* ATCC 7966^T recently had its 4.7-megabase genome completely sequenced and is undergoing manual annotation at The Institute for Genomic Research (TIGR). Preliminary data can be accessed at the TIGR Homepage at http://www.tigr.org under the link for "Unfinished Genomes," and the entire genome will eventually be available in GenBank at NCBI.

DESCRIPTION OF THE GENUS

Members of the genus *Aeromonas* are gram-negative facultative anaerobes that are straight, coccobacillary to bacillary cells with rounded ends, 0.3 to 1.0 μm in diameter and 1.0 to 3.5 μm in length. They can occur singly, in pairs, or rarely in short chains. Most species are motile by a single, polar flagellum of 1.7-μm wavelength, but peritrichous flagella may be formed on solid media in young cultures and lateral flagella occur in some species. Aeromonads are usually oxidase positive and catalase positive and are generally resistant to 150 μg of the vibriostatic agent 2,4 diamino-6,7-diisopropylpteridine (O/129). They are chemoorganotrophic, displaying oxidative and fermentative metabolism of glucose. Acid and often acid with gas are produced from many carbohydrates, especially glucose, and nitrate is reduced to nitrite. A variety of exoenzymes such as arylamidases, amylase, DNase, esterases, peptidases, proteases, chitinase, chondroitinase, and hemolysins are produced. The main cellular fatty acids produced are hexadecanoic acid (16:0), hexadecenoic acid (16:1), and octadecenoic acid (18:1). Human (mesophilic) strains grow between 10 and 42°C, but occasional isolates may be more active in some biochemical assays at 22 to 25°C. Psychrophilic strains from fish and the environment (*A. popoffii* and *A. salmonicida*) seldom grow above 37°C and preferentially grow at 22 to 25°C. In brain heart infusion broth at 28°C, growth occurs between pH 4.5 and 9.0 and at salt concentrations between 0 and 4%. The mol% G+C of the DNA is 57 to 63%.

NATURAL HABITATS

Aeromonads are inhabitants of aquatic ecosystems worldwide. These include groundwater and drinking water at treatment plants and in distribution systems and reservoirs as well as

TABLE 1 Members of the genus *Aeromonas*[a]

Organism	Human isolation (extraintestinal/fecal)	Human pathogen (extraintestinal/fecal)	Frequency in humans	Pathogenic for animals, fish, reptiles
A. hydrophila complex				
A. hydrophila				
subsp. *hydrophila*	Yes	Yes	Yes	Yes
subsp. *dhakensis*	Yes	Yes	Rare	No
subsp. *ranae*	No	No	—	Yes
A. bestiarum	No/yes	—/no	One case	Yes
A. salmonicida[b]	No/yes	No/no	Rare	
subsp. *salmonicida*				Yes
subsp. *achromogenes*				Yes
subsp. *masoucida*				Yes
subsp. *smithia*				Yes
subsp. *pectinolytica*				No
A. caviae complex				
A. caviae	Yes	Yes	Common	Yes
A. media	No/yes	—/yes	Rare	No
A. eucrenophila	Yes	No/—	Very rare	No
A. veronii complex				
A. veronii bv. sobria	Yes	Yes	Common	Yes
A. veronii bv. veronii	Yes	Yes	Rare	No
A. jandaei	Yes	Yes/unknown	Rare	No
A. trota	Yes	Neither	Rare	No
A. schubertii	Yes/no	Yes/—	Rare	No
A. encheleia	Yes/no	No/—	One case	No
A. allosaccharophila	No/yes	—/no	Rare	Yes
A. sobria	Neither	—	—	No
A. popoffii	Yes	Yes	Rare	No
A. culicicola	No	No	—	No
A. simiae	No	No	—	No
A. molluscorum	No	No	—	No

[a] Abbreviations and symbols: bv., biovar; —, not applicable.
[b] There are motile strains of *A. salmonicida* that grow at 37°C and resemble clinical *A. hydrophila* strains that have been isolated from human feces; these can be distinguished using the tests in Table 3.

clean or polluted lakes and rivers. *Aeromonas* may also be found in marine environments but only in brackish water or water with a low saline content. Most *Aeromonas* species, particularly those associated with human infections, are found in a wide variety of fresh produce, meat (beef, poultry, and pork), and dairy products (raw milk and ice cream) (24). *A. veronii* bv. sobria is a symbiont in the gut of medicinal leeches, where it may grow as a pure culture (15). In fisheries, psychrophilic strains of *Aeromonas* cause severe infections resulting in considerable economic loss. Infections in frogs, pigs, cattle, birds, and marine animals have also been reported (24).

CLINICAL SIGNIFICANCE

Aeromonas gastroenteritis ranges from an acute watery diarrhea (most common form) to dysenteric illness to chronic illness. Stools from acute watery diarrhea are loose (take the shape of their container), and erythrocytes and fecal leukocytes are absent. Accompanying symptoms include abdominal pain (60 to 70%), fever and vomiting (20 to 40%), and nausea (40%) (22). Infections are usually self-limiting, but children may require hospitalization due to dehydration. *A. caviae* is the most common species associated with these infections and can even mimic inflammatory bowel disease in children (48). *A. veronii* bv. sobria strains may be associated with rare cholera-like disease characterized by abdominal pain (60%) and fever and nausea (20%) (22). In dysenteric diarrhea resembling shigellosis, patients suffer from severe abdominal pain and have bloody stools containing mucus and polymorphonuclear leukocytes. About 10 to 15% of patients with either cholera-like or dysenteric diarrhea are coinfected with another enteric pathogen(s).

A comprehensive study done in Bangladesh in 2000 found that the presence of loose stools was associated with *Aeromonas* strains possessing an *alt* gene encoding a heat-labile cytotonic enterotoxin (4). Patients with more severe disease and watery diarrhea had strains that possessed both the *alt* gene and a second gene, *ast,* which encodes a heat-stable cytotonic enterotoxin. A total of seven different *Aeromonas* species were associated with diarrhea in this study. This was followed by a large 2003 study of traveler's diarrhea associated with *Aeromonas* species in Spain, where the predominant species isolated were *A. veronii* bv. veronii and *A. caviae* (49). Finally, a large 2004 study completed in Kolkata, India, found seven different species of *Aeromonas* among hospitalized diarrheal cases, with *A. caviae* predominating, followed by *A. hydrophila* and *A. veronii* bv. sobria. They also found the *alt* and *act* genes in 71.9 and 20.1% of the isolates, respectively, and only 2.4% of the isolates carried the *ast* gene (44).

Complications from *Aeromonas* diarrheal disease include hemolytic uremic syndrome (5) or kidney disease requiring kidney transplantation (12). These more severe infections are usually associated with *A. hydrophila* or *A. veronii* bv. sobria. Also, nonresolvable, intermittent diarrhea can occur months after the initial infection and may persist for months or several years.

Aeromonas can also be isolated from a variety of extraintestinal sites, although blood and wounds are the most common sources. *Aeromonas* septicemia occurs rarely in immunocompetent hosts; most cases involve patients with liver disease and hematological malignancies. The more commonly isolated species from septicemia are *A. hydrophila, A. veronii* bv. sobria, and *A. jandaei,* with a recent third case report (33) of septicemia with an *A. veronii* bv. veronii strain (arginine dihydrolase negative, esculin hydrolysis positive, and ornithine decarboxylase positive). Fatality rates in these infections range from 30 to 50%. Wound infections are usually preceded by traumatic injury that occurs in contact with water, where the predominant species is *A. hydrophila.* These infections range from uncomplicated cases of cellulitis to myonecrotic infections with a poor prognosis. Two such scenarios are the reported outbreak of wound infections with *A. hydrophila* associated with mud football (47) and wound infections among the 2004 Asian tsunami survivors (29). Surveys indicate that only 17 to 52% of *Aeromonas* wound infections are monomicrobic (24). Use of medicinal leeches postoperatively to enhance blood flow to surgical sites has resulted in wound infection rates of 20%, primarily with *A. veronii* bv. sobria (15). Other extraintestinal infections include ocular, respiratory, and urinary tract infections; meningitis; osteomyelitis; cholecystitis; endocarditis; and peritonitis (23). Two recent examples were the isolation of *A. caviae* from keratitis associated with contact lens wear (39) and the isolation of *A. popoffii* from a urinary tract infection (18).

COLLECTION, TRANSPORT, AND STORAGE OF SPECIMENS

Aeromonads survive well in specimens; any of the widely used transport media are acceptable for transport, including buffered glycerol in saline (chapter 20). Feces are always preferable to rectal swabs for isolation of enteric pathogens, and stools should be collected in the acute phase of disease.

ISOLATION PROCEDURES

Aeromonads generally grow well on a variety of enteric differential and selective agars, although sucrose- and/or lactose-fermenting strains usually resemble nonpathogens on these media. Blood agar (BA) with 20 μg of ampicillin per ml (ABA) is useful for isolating all *Aeromonas* species except *A. trota,* which is intrinsically susceptible to ampicillin, and a substantial percentage (15 to 57%) of *A. caviae* isolates (6, 27). Since most clinically relevant species are beta-hemolytic, including an increasing number of *A. caviae* strains, beta-hemolytic colonies on BA should be screened with oxidase and a spot indole test. Any colonies positive for both tests should be characterized further, although occasional indole-negative *A. caviae* isolates and nearly all known *A. schubertii* strains (which are generally associated with severe aquatic wounds) are indole negative (2). Modified cefsulodin-Irgasan-novobiocin (CIN) (which contains 4 μg of cefsulodin per ml versus 15 μg/ml in unmodified CIN) is also an excellent isolation medium for aeromonads. On this medium, *Aeromonas* colonies have a pink center with an uneven, clear apron and are indistinguishable from *Yersinia enterocolitica* morphologically. One can incubate CIN at 25°C to enhance the recovery of *Yersinia* and still be able to recover *Aeromonas* within 24 h at this temperature. For optimal isolation, use of both ABA and modified CIN is recommended (26). A xylose-galactosidase medium (XGM), containing novobiocin, bile salts, xylose, and two galactopyranosides, has been evaluated in Europe for the isolation of *Aeromonas, Salmonella, Shigella,* and *Yersinia* spp. (14). *Aeromonas* species, which form green colonies, were isolated more frequently from XGM agar (36%) than from any other medium except CIN (43%), but XGM had fewer false positives (11% for XGM versus 60% for CIN). Thiosulfate-citrate-bile salts-sucrose (TCBS) medium is usually inhibitory to aeromonads. Enrichment in alkaline peptone water enhances recovery of *Aeromonas* from populations that generally would be expected to shed low numbers of organisms (carriers, convalescent-phase patients, and those with subclinical infections). For patients with acute diarrhea, enrichment is probably unnecessary (40).

IDENTIFICATION

Aeromonas spp. are most easily confused in the laboratory with other oxidase-positive fermenters, i.e., *Vibrio* and *Plesiomonas* spp. *Plesiomonas* is easily differentiated from *Aeromonas* by positive reactions in Moeller's lysine, ornithine, and arginine tests and by fermentation of *m*-inositol. Vibrios may be more difficult to distinguish from aeromonads (1), which is particularly true for *Vibrio fluvialis* and *A. caviae,* and in laboratories where the sole means of identification is a rapid miniaturized system (21, 45). Resistance to the vibriostatic agent O/129 and the inability to grow in salt concentrations of ≥6% usually indicate the genus *Aeromonas. Vibrio cholerae* O139, a cholera toxin-positive, non-salt-requiring, O/129-resistant vibrio, is a major exception to this rule. However, the decarboxylase pattern (positive for lysine and ornithine) and negative reactions for arginine dihydrolase, production of gas from glucose, and fermentation of salicin separate this organism from most aeromonads. Unfortunately, strains of "ornithine decarboxylase-positive" *A. veronii* bv. veronii yield an "excellent to very good ID" for *V. cholerae* with a rapid identification kit, and serotyping and/or additional testing are required to resolve the issue. *A. veronii* bv. veronii would be String test negative, O/129 resistant, and able to produce gas from glucose fermentation, would not require additional salt for growth, and would be inhibited on TCBS agar, whereas *V. cholerae* strains would have the opposite reactions. Once it has been determined that you have a glucose-fermenting, oxidase-positive, motile gram-negative rod that is resistant to O/129, a small number of biochemical tests can be used for separating *Aeromonas* species into the three major species complexes (Table 2). If warranted, even more discriminatory tests for separating members of each complex can be found in boldface type in Table 3 (2), which should replace earlier published tests for species identification (3).

The sequencing of a single housekeeping gene 16S rRNA (32) and the development of an extended method using 16S rRNA restricted fragment length polymorphism analysis that followed (10) were both initially promising as methods to identify aeromonads to the species level. However, very recently published data on the intragenomic heterogeneity within the 16S rRNA gene in *Aeromonas* strains suggest caution in using this gene for anything beyond genus level identification (35). Therefore, the use of other housekeeping genes as multiple molecular markers, such as *gyrB* and *rpoD*

TABLE 2 Biochemical identification of *Aeromonas* to complex level

Test	No. of strains identified as belonging to[a]:		
	A. hydrophila complex (*A. hydrophila, A. bestiarum, A. salmonicida)*	*A. caviae* complex (*A. caviae, A. media, A. eucrenophila)*	*A. veronii* complex (*A. veronii* HG8,[b] *A. jandaei, A. schubertii, A. trota)*
Esculin	87 (92, 81, 85)	71 (76, 55, 78)	0
Voges-Proskauer	75 (88, 63, 62)	0	54 (88, 87, 17, 0)
Glucose (gas)	81 (92, 69, 77)	16 (0, 0, 78)	87 (92, 100, 0, 69)
L-Arabinose	93 (84, 100, 100)	96 (100, 100, 78)	4 (12, 0, 0, 0)

[a] The first number is the overall percent positive for each complex for a given trait; the numbers in parentheses are the percentages of positives for each species listed within that complex. Data are derived and modified from Table 5 in reference 2.

[b] Biovar sobria (DNA hybridization group 8); the separation of *A. veronii* biovar veronii (DNA hybridization group 10) from *A. veronii* biovar sobria is achieved with *A. veronii* bv. veronii having positive reactions for ornithine decarboxylase and esculin hydrolysis and a negative reaction for arginine dihydrolase.

(46), or an even broader approach using multilocus sequence typing seems to be the future avenue for accurate species identification.

Because isolates do not survive well at room or refrigerator temperature in the laboratory for long periods (>1 month), placing aeromonads in media such as Trypticase soy broth with 30% glycerol and deep freezing at −80°C are recommended for their long-term storage.

SEROLOGIC RESPONSE

Most serologic assays that have been used to detect antibodies to *Aeromonas* (tube agglutination, immunoblot, and enzyme-linked immunoassay) have low sensitivity and specificity and are not considered reliable. An immunoglobulin A (IgA fecal antibody) response to *Aeromonas* somatic lipopolysaccharides and exotoxins has been reported (9). Crivelli et al. (9) found secretory IgA to *Aeromonas* in 10 of 13 stools from patients when the stool was extracted with Jacalin, a lectin with high affinity for human IgA.

ANTIBIOTIC SUSCEPTIBILITIES

Two recent articles on *Aeromonas* antimicrobial susceptibilities (25, 37) included only strains well characterized to the species level and expand previously known susceptibility information on aeromonads isolated less frequently from clinical specimens. A general antimicrobial susceptibility profile for *Aeromonas* derived from both of these investigations as well as other studies (22, 28, 50) is given in Table 4. Ciprofloxacin, commonly used to treat gram-negative infections, remains active against all species of *Aeromonas*, with little or no resistance reported in studies in the United States and most of Europe (25, 37). However, a recent Spanish study of 43 strains, identified as *A. hydrophila, A. veronii* bv. sobria, and *A. caviae*, found 26 and 20% of the *A. caviae* and *A. hydrophila* strains, respectively, and 88% of the *A. veronii* bv. sobria strains to be resistant to nalidixic acid and pipemidic acid. This means that these organisms, though still susceptible to ciprofloxacin, are known to already have a mutation in the *gyrA* gene and could easily develop a second mutation resulting in resistance to ciprofloxacin (49). Two to three percent of *A. caviae, A. hydrophila,* and *A. veronii* bv. sobria strains in Asia have been reported to be ciprofloxacin resistant (28). Antimicrobial susceptibility testing of local isolates is necessary for the detection of species-related patterns, such as continued susceptibility to cephalothin in *A. veronii* bv. sobria isolates, and because susceptibilities may differ from one geographic area to another. *Aeromonas* species can express three chromosomal β-lactam-induced β-lactamases, including a group 1 molecular class C cephalosporinase, a group 2d molecular class D penicillinase, and a group 3 molecular class B metallo-β-lactamase (carbapenemase) (42). The presence of these β-lactamases in *Aeromonas*, in particular the carbapenemase, may not be detected by conventional susceptibility methods (42). It may be necessary to test strains of species known to potentially carry carbapenemases (*A. hydrophila, A. veronii* bv. sobria, *A. veronii* bv. veronii, and *A. jandaei)* with a higher-than-standard inoculum if imipenem or meropenem therapy is being considered. CphA, one of several enzymes responsible for resistance to carbapenems, hydrolyzes nitrocefin poorly or not at all, indicating that the nitrocefin test is not reliable for detecting carbapenemases (17, 42). A case of sepsis due to an extended-spectrum β-lactamase (ESBL)-producing *A. hydrophila* in a pediatric patient with diarrhea and pneumonia (41) and a case of *A. hydrophila* necrotizing fasciitis with probable "in vivo" transfer of a TEM-24 plasmid-borne ESBL gene from *Enterobacter aerogenes* have been reported (13).

INTERPRETATION AND REPORTING OF RESULTS

Regardless of the site of isolation (intestinal or extraintestinal), aeromonads should be identified either as belonging to the *A. hydrophila* or *A. caviae* complex or as *A. veronii* bv. sobria and not "*A. sobria.*" For routine isolates recovered from uncomplicated cases of gastroenteritis, this level of identification may be sufficient. Although there is strong evidence that some aeromonads are gastrointestinal pathogens, there is no convincing evidence at present that all fecal isolates of *Aeromonas* are involved in diarrheal disease. Thus, the significance of the recovery of aeromonads from stool specimens should be interpreted cautiously and must rely on both laboratory information and clinical interpretation. Because of this, the relative quantity of *Aeromonas* recovered on enteric media (few colonies, moderate growth, or predominant organism) should be reported in conjunction with the *Aeromonas* complex or species identification. For complicated cases of diarrhea, i.e., prolonged bloody diarrhea in pediatric patients or chronic gastroenteritis of >1-month duration or in cancer patients with positive fecal cultures in whom *Aeromonas* tends to disseminate, a definitive species identification is warranted.

For extraintestinal isolates (from blood or wounds), the same general rules should apply to species identification of aeromonads. Although it is clear that both the in vitro and in vivo pathogenic potentials of *Aeromonas* species and strains vary considerably, for the present, there are no universal markers or indicators available that dictate when

TABLE 3 Tests useful in the separation of members within the *Aeromonas* species complexes

Test	Result[a]									
	A. hydrophila	*A. bestiarum*	*A. salmonicida*	*A. caviae*	*A. media*	*A. eucrenophila*	*A. veronii*[b]	*A. jandaei*	*A. schubertii*	*A. trota*
Utilization of:										
Citrate	**+(92)**	**V(38)**	**+(85)**	**+(88)**	**V(82)**	**−(0)**	V(52)	**+(87)**	**V(58)**	**+(94)**
DL-Lactate	**V(84)**	**−(0)**	**−(0)**	**+(96)**	**V(56)**	**−(0)**	−(0)	−(7)	V (58)	+(88)
Urocanic acid	**V(16)**	**+(94)**	**+(100)**	**+(100)**	**+(100)**	**−(0)**	−(0)	−(7)	−(0)	V(75)
Gluconate oxidation	**V(64)**	**−(13)**	**−(0)**	−(0)	−(0)	−(0)	V(60)	V(60)	−(0)	−(0)
Gas from D-Glucose	+(92)	V(69)	V(77)	**−(0)**	**−(0)**	**V(78)**	**+(92)**	**+(100)**	**−(0)**	**V(69)**
PZA	V(24)	V(50)	V(31)	**+(88)**	**V(18)**	**+(100)**				
Indole	+(96)	+(100)	+(100)	V(84)	+(100)	+(89)	**+(100)**	**+(100)**	**V(17)**	**+(100)**
Voges-Proskauer	+(92)	V(63)	V(62)	−(0)	−(0)	−(0)	**+(92)**	**+(87)**	**V(17)**	**−(0)**
Lipase (corn oil)	+(100)	+(88)	+(92)	V(76)	V(82)	+(89)	**+(92)**	**+(100)**	**+(100)**	**−(0)**
Acid from:										
Cellobiose	**−(4)**	**V(38)**	**V(69)**	+(100)	+(100)	V(56)	**V(20)**	**V(20)**	**−(0)**	**+(100)**
Lactose	**V(64)**	**−(13)**	**+(92)**	V(60)	V(64)	−(11)	−(12)	−(0)	−(0)	−(0)
L-Rhamnose	**V(24)**	**V(69)**	**−(0)**	−(0)	−(0)	V(22)	−(0)	−(0)	−(0)	−(0)
D-Sorbitol	**−(0)**	**−(0)**	**+(85)**	−(4)	−(0)	−(0)	−(0)	−(0)	−(0)	−(0)
Glucose 1-phosphate	ND	ND	ND	**−(4)**	**+(100)**	**+(100)**	ND	ND	ND	ND
Glucose 6-phosphate	ND	ND	ND	**−(4)**	**+(100)**	**+(100)**	ND	ND	ND	ND
Lactulose	ND	ND	ND	**V(68)**	**V(55)**	**−(0)**	ND	ND	ND	ND
D-Mannose	+(100)	+(100)	+(100)	**V(32)**	**+(100)**	**+(100)**		+(100)	+(92)	+(100)
Glycerol	+(96)	+(100)	+(100)	V(68)	V(55)	−(11)	**+(100)**	**+(100)**	**−(0)**	**+(94)**
D-Mannitol	+(96)	+(100)	+(100)	+(100)	+(100)	+(100)	**+(100)**	**+(100)**	**−(0)**	**V(69)**
Sucrose	+(100)	+(94)	+(100)	+(100)	+(100)	V(33)	**+(100)**	**−(0)**	**−(0)**	**V(19)**
Amp^r	+(100)	+(94)	+(85)	+(100)	V(73)	+(100)	**+(100)**	**+(93)**	**+(92)**	**−(6)**

[a] +, ≥85% of the strains positive; −, <15% positive; V, 15 to 85% positive (results at 48 h); numbers in parentheses indicate the percentages of positives for the test at the final day of reading: gluconate, 2 days; DL-lactate and urocanic acid, 3 days; citrate, 4 days; carbohydrates, indole, and lipase, 7 days; PZA (pyrazinamidase), 2 days; Amp^r, resistance to 10 μg of ampicillin, 1 day; Voges-Proskauer, 3 days; ND, not done. For each of the three *Aeromonas* species complexes, the discriminatory reactions between the species within each complex are in boldface type.

[b] Biovar sobria (DNA hybridization group 8); the separation of *A. veronii* biovar veronii (DNA hybridization group 10) from *A. veronii* biovar sobria is achieved with *A. veronii* bv. veronii having positive reactions for ornithine decarboxylase and esculin hydrolysis and a negative reaction for arginine dihydrolase.

TABLE 4 *Aeromonas* species susceptibilities

Susceptibility[a]	Antibiotic agent
Resistant	Ampicillin (except *A. trota* [100% susceptible] and *A. caviae* [35% susceptible][b])
Variable	Ticarcillin or piperacillin (except *A. veronii* bv. veronii [100% resistant] and *A. trota* [100% susceptible])
	Cephalothin
	Cefazolin
	Cefoxitin (except *A. veronii* bv. veronii [100% susceptible])
	Cefuroxime
	Ceftriaxone
	Cefotaxime
Susceptible	Ciprofloxacin[c]
	Gentamicin
	Amikacin
	Tobramycin (*A. veronii* bv. veronii [42% resistant])
	Imipenem (*A. jandaei* [65% resistant], *A. veronii* bv. veronii [67% resistant])
	Trimethoprim-sulfamethoxazole

[a] Resistant or susceptible, ≥90% of all isolates are resistant or susceptible; variable, 10 to 90% of isolates are susceptible (data from reference 2).

[b] Data for *A. caviae* susceptibility are from references 6 and 27.

[c] Data for resistance to nalidixic acid and pipemidic acid in 26 and 20% of *A. caviae* and *A. hydrophila* isolates, respectively, and 88% in *A. veronii* clinical strains suggest possible future resistance to fluoroquinolones (49).

isolates should be definitively identified to the species level. Thus, for extraintestinal isolates, identification of aeromonads beyond complexes should be reserved for strains isolated from sterile body sites (blood or cerebrospinal fluid) and serious wound infections (cellulitis and necrotizing fasciitis); for strains exhibiting unusual resistance patterns, associated with nosocomial outbreaks; or for publications describing traditional species associated with new disease processes or newly described species isolated from new anatomic sites.

REFERENCES

1. **Abbott, S. L., L. S. Seli, M. Catino, Jr., M. A. Hartley, and J. M. Janda.** 1998. Misidentification of unusual *Aeromonas* species as members of the genus *Vibrio*: a continuing problem. *J. Clin. Microbiol.* **36:**1103–1104.
2. **Abbott, S. L., W. K. W. Cheung, and J. M. Janda.** 2003. The genus *Aeromonas*: biochemical characteristics, atypical reactions, and phenotypic schemes. *J. Clin. Microbiol.* **41:**2348–2357.
3. **Abbott, S. L., W. K. W. Cheung, S. Kroske-Bystrom, T. Malekzadeh, and J. M. Janda.** 1992. Identification of *Aeromonas* strains to the genospecies level in the clinical laboratory. *J. Clin. Microbiol.* **30:**1262–1266.
4. **Albert, M. J., M. Ansaruzzaman, K. A. Talukder, A. K. Chopra, I. Kuhn, M. Rahman, A. S. G. Faruque, M. S. Islam, R. B. Sack, and R. Mollby.** 2000. Prevalence of enterotoxin genes in *Aeromonas* spp. isolated from children with diarrhea, healthy controls, and the environment. *J. Clin. Microbiol.* **38:**3785–3790.
5. **Bogdanovic, R., M. Cobeljic, V. Markovic, V. Nikolic, M. Ognjanovic, L. Sarjanovic, and D. Makic.** 1991. Haemolytic-uremic syndrome associated with *Aeromonas hydrophila* enterocolitis. *Pediatr. Nephrol.* **5:**293–295.
6. **Carnahan, A. M., and S. W. Joseph.** 1993. Systematic assessment of geographically and clinically diverse aeromonads. *Syst. Appl. Microbiol.* **16:**72–84.
7. **Collins, M. D., A. J. Martinez-Murcia, and J. Cai.** 1994. *Aeromonas enteropelogenes* and *Aeromonas ichthiosmia* are identical to *Aeromonas trota* and *Aeromonas veronii*, respectively, as revealed by small-subunit rRNA sequence analysis. *Int. J. Syst. Bacteriol.* **43:**855–856.
8. **Colwell, R. R., M. R. MacDonell, and J. DeLey.** 1986. Proposal to recognize the family *Aeromonadaceae* fam. nov. *Int. J. Syst. Bacteriol.* **36:**473–477.
9. **Crivelli, C., A. Demarta, and R. Peduzzi.** 2001. Intestinal secretory immunoglobulin A (sIgA) response to *Aeromonas* exoproteins in patients with naturally acquired *Aeromonas* diarrhea. *FEMS Immunol. Med. Microbiol.* **30:**31–35.
10. **Figueras, M. J., L. Soler, M. R. Chacon, J. Guarro, and A. J. Martinez-Murcia.** 2000. Extended method for discrimination of *Aeromonas* spp. by 16S rDNA RFLP analysis. *Int. J. Syst. Evol. Microbiol.* **6:**2069–2073.
11. **Figueras, M. J., A. Suarez-Franquet, M. R. Chacon, L. Soler, M. Navarro, C. Alejandre, B. Grasa, A. J. Martinez-Murcia, and J. Guarro.** 2005. First record of the rare species *Aeromonas culicicola* from a drinking water supply. *Appl. Environ. Microbiol.* **71:**538–541.
12. **Filler, G., J. H. H. Ehrich, E. Strauch, and L. Beutin.** 2000. Acute renal failure in an infant associated with cytotoxic *Aeromonas sobria* isolated from patient's stool and from aquarium water as suspected source of infection. *J. Clin. Microbiol.* **38:**469–470.
13. **Fosse, T., C. Giraud-Morin, I. Madinier, F. Mantoux, J. P. Lacour, and J. P. Ortonne.** 2004. *Aeromonas hydrophila* with plasmid-borne class A extended-spectrum β-lactamase TEM-24 and three chromosomal class B, C, and D β-lactamases, isolated from a patient with necrotizing fasciitis. *Antimicrob. Agents Chemother.* **48:**2342–2343.
14. **Garcia-Arguayo, J. M., P. Ubedo, and M. Gobernado.** 1999. Evaluation of xylose-galactosidase medium, a new plate for the isolation of *Salmonella, Shigella, Yersinia* and *Aeromonas* species. *Eur. J. Clin. Microbiol. Infect. Dis.* **18:**77–78.
15. **Graf, J.** 1999. Symbiosis of *Aeromonas veronii* biovar sobria and *Hirudo medicinalis*, the medicinal leech: a novel model for digestive tract associations. *Infect. Immun.* **67:**1–7.
16. **Harf-Monteil, C., A. L. Fleche, P. Riegel, G. Prevost, D. Bermond, P. A. Grimont, and H. Monteil.** 2004. *Aeromonas simiae* sp. nov., isolated from monkey faeces. *Int. J. Syst. Evol. Microbiol.* **54:**481–485.
17. **Hayes, M. V., C. J. Thomson, and S. G. B. Amyes.** 1996. The "hidden" carbapenemase of *Aeromonas hydrophila*. *J. Antimicrob. Chemother.* **37:**33–44.
18. **Hua, H. T., C. Bollet, S. Tercian, M. Crancourt, and D. Raoult.** 2004. *Aeromonas popoffii* urinary tract infection. *J. Clin. Microbiol.* **42:**5427–5428.
19. **Huys, G., P. Kampfer, M. J. Albert, I. Kuhn, R. Denys, and J. Swings.** 2002. *Aeromonas hydrophila* subsp. *dhakensis* subsp. nov., isolated from children with diarrhea in Bangladesh, and extended description of *Aeromonas hydrophila* subsp. *hydrophila* (Chester 1901) Stanier 1943 (approved lists 1980). *Int. J. Syst. Evol. Microbiol.* **52:**705–712.
20. **Huys, G., M. Pearson, P. Kampfer, R. Denys, M. Cnockaert, V. Inglis, and J. Swings.** 2003. *Aeromonas hydrophila* subsp. *ranae* subsp. nov., isolated from septicaemic farmed frogs in Thailand. *Int. J. Syst. Evol. Microbiol.* **53:**885–891.
21. **Israil, A. M., M. C. Balotescu, I. Alexandru, and G. Dobre.** 2003. Discordancies between classical and API 20E microtest biochemical identification of *Vibrio* and *Aeromonas* strains. *Bacteriol. Virusol. Parazitol. Epidemiol.* **48:**141–143.

22. **Janda, J. M.** 2001. *Aeromonas* and *Plesiomonas*, p. 1237–1270. *In* M. Sussman (ed.), *Molecular Medical Microbiology*, vol. 2. Academic Press, London, United Kingdom.
23. **Janda, J. M., and S. L. Abbott.** 1998. Evolving concepts regarding the genus *Aeromonas:* an expanding panorama of species, disease presentations, and unanswered questions. *Clin. Infect. Dis.* **27:**332–344.
24. **Janda, J. M., S. L. Abbott, and J. G. Morris.** 1995. *Aeromonas, Plesiomonas* and *Edwardsiella*, p. 905–917. *In* M. J. Blaser, P. D. Smith, J. I. Ravdin, H. B. Greenberg, and R. L. Guerrant (ed.), *Infections of the Gastrointestinal Tract.* Raven Press, Ltd., New York, N.Y.
25. **Kampfer, P., C. Christmann, J. Swings, and G. Huys.** 1999. In vitro susceptibilities of *Aeromonas* genomic species to 69 antimicrobial agents. *Syst. Appl. Microbiol.* **22:**662–669.
26. **Kelly, M. T., E. M. D. Stroh, and J. Jessop.** 1988. Comparison of blood agar, ampicillin blood agar, MacConkey-ampicillin-Tween agar, and modified cefsulodin-irgasan-novobiocin agar for isolation of *Aeromonas* spp. from stool specimens. *J. Clin. Microbiol.* **26:**1738–1740.
27. **Kilpatrick, M. E., J. Escamilla, A. L. Bourgeois, H. J. Adkins, and R. C. Rockhill.** 1987. Overview of four U.S. Navy overseas research studies on *Aeromonas*. *Experientia* **43:**365–367.
28. **Ko, W. C., K. W. Yu, C. Y. Liu, C. T. Huang, H. S. Leu, and Y. C. Chuang.** 1996. Increasing antibiotic resistance in clinical isolates of *Aeromonas* strains in Taiwan. *Antimicrob. Agents Chemother.* **40:**1260–1262.
29. **Maegele, M., S. Gregor, E. Steinhausen, B. Bouillon, M. M. Heiss, W. Perbix, F. Wappler, D. Rixen, J. Geisen, B. Berger-Schreck, and R. Schwarz.** 2005. The long-distance tertiary air transfer and care of tsunami victims: injury pattern and microbiological and psychological aspects. *Crit. Care Med.* **33:**1178–1180.
30. **Martin-Carnahan, A., and S. W. Joseph.** 2005. *Aeromonas*, p. 556–578. *In* D. J. Brenner, N. R. Krieg, J. T. Staley, and G. M. Garrity (ed.), *Bergey's Manual of Systematic Bacteriology*, 2nd ed., vol. 2. Springer-Verlag, New York, N.Y.
31. **Martinez-Murcia, A. J.** 1999. Phylogenetic positions of *Aeromonas encheleia, Aeromonas popoffii, Aeromonas* DNA hybridization group 11 and *Aeromonas* group 501. *Int. J. Syst. Bacteriol.* **49:**1403–1408.
32. **Martinez-Murcia, A. J., S. Benlloch, and M. D. Collins.** 1992. Phylogenetic interrelationships of members of the genera *Aeromonas* and *Plesiomonas* as determined by 16S ribosomal DNA sequencing: lack of congruence with results of DNA-DNA hybridizations. *Int. J. Syst. Bacteriol.* **42:**412–421.
33. **Mencacci, A., E. Cenci, R. Mazzolla, S. Farinelli, F. D'Alo, M. Vitali, and F. Bistoni.** 2003. *Aeromonas veronii* biovar veronii septicaemia and acute suppurative cholangitis in a patient with hepatitis B. *J. Med. Microbiol.* **52:**727–730.
34. **Minana-Galvis, D., F. Maribel, M. Carme Fuste, and J. Gaspar Loren.** 2004. *Aeromonas molluscorum* sp. nov., isolated from bivalve mollusks. *Int. J. Syst. Evol. Microbiol.* **54:**2073–2078.
35. **Morandi, A., O. Zhaxybayeva, J. P. Gogarten, and J. Graf.** 2005. Evolutionary and diagnostic implications of intragenomic heterogeneity in the 16S rRNA gene in *Aeromonas* strains. *J. Bacteriol.* **187:**6561–6564.
36. **Ouderkirk, J. P., D. Bekhor, G. S. Turett, and R. Murali.** 2004. *Aeromonas* meningitis complicating medicinal leech therapy. *Clin. Infect. Dis.* **38:**36–37.
37. **Overman, T. L., and J. M. Janda.** 1999. Antimicrobial susceptibility patterns of *Aeromonas jandaei, A. schubertii, A. trota,* and *A. veronii* biotype veronii. *J. Clin. Microbiol.* **37:**706–708.
38. **Pidiyar, V., A. Kaznowski, N. B. Narayan, M. Patole, and Y. S. Shouche.** 2002. *Aeromonas culicicola* sp. nov., from the midgut of *Culex quinquefasciatus*. *Int. J. Syst. Evol. Microbiol.* **52:**1723–1728.
39. **Pinna, A., L. A. Sechi, S. Zanetti, D. Usai, and F. Carta.** 2004. *Aeromonas caviae* keratitis associated with contact lens wear. *Ophthalmology* **111:**348–351.
40. **Robinson, J., J. Beaman, L. Wagener, and V. Burke.** 1986. Comparison of direct plating with the use of enrichment culture for isolation of *Aeromonas* spp. from faeces. *J. Med. Microbiol.* **22:**315–317.
41. **Rodriguez, C. N., R. Campos, B. Pastran, I. Jimenez, A. Garcia, P. Meijomil, and A. J. Rodriguez-Morales.** 2005. Sepsis due to extended-spectrum β-lactamase producing *Aeromonas hydrophila* in a pediatric patient with diarrhea and pneumonia. *Clin. Infect. Dis.* **41:**421–422.
42. **Rossolini, G. M., T. Walsh, and G. Amicosante.** 1996. The *Aeromonas* metallo-β-lactamases: genetics, enzymology, and contribution to drug resistance. *Microb. Drug Resist.* **2:**245–251.
43. **Shiina, Y., K. Ii, and M. Iwanaga.** 2004. An *Aeromonas veronii* biovar sobria infection with disseminated intravascular gas production. *J. Infect. Chemother.* **10:**37–41.
44. **Sinha, S., T. Shimada, T. Ramamurthy, S. K. Bhattacharya, S. Yamasaki, Y. Takeda, and G. B. Nair.** 2004. Prevalence, serotype distribution, antibiotic susceptibility and genetic profiles of mesophilic *Aeromonas* species isolated from hospitalized diarrhoeal cases in Kolkata, India. *J. Med. Microbiol.* **53:**527–534.
45. **Soler, L., F. Marco, J. Vila, M. R. Chacon, J. Guarro, and M. J. Figueras.** 2003. Evaluation of two miniaturized systems, MicroScan W/A and BBL Crystal E/NF, for identification of clinical isolates of *Aeromonas* sp. *J. Clin. Microbiol.* **41:**5732–5734.
46. **Soler, L., M. A. Yanez, M. R. Chacon, M. G. Aguilera-Arreola, V. Catalan, M. J. Figueras, and A. J. Martinez-Murcia.** 2004. Phylogenetic analysis of the genus *Aeromonas* based on two housekeeping genes. *Int. J. Syst. Evol. Microbiol.* **54:**1511–1519.
47. **Vally, H., A. Whittle, S. Cameron, G. K. Dowse, and T. Watson.** 2004. Outbreak of *Aeromonas hydrophila* wound infections associated with mud football. *Clin. Infect. Dis.* **38:**1084–1089.
48. **van der Gaag, E. J., E. Roelofsen, and R. F. Tummers.** 2005. *Aeromonas caviae* infection mimicking inflammatory bowel disease in a child. *Ned. Tijdschr. Geneeskd.* **149:**712–714.
49. **Vila, J., J. Ruiz, F. Gallardo, M. Vargas, L. Soler, M. J. Figueras, and J. Gascon.** 2003. *Aeromonas* spp. and traveler's diarrhea: clinical features and antimicrobial resistance. *Emerg. Infect. Dis.* **9:**552–555.
50. **Vila, J., F. Marco, L. Soler, M. Chacon, and M. J. Figueras.** 2002. *In vitro* antimicrobial susceptibility of clinical isolates of *Aeromonas caviae, Aeromonas hydrophila,* and *Aeromonas veronii* biotype sobria. *J. Antimicrob. Chemother.* **49:**701–702. (Letter.)

Vibrio and Related Organisms*

SHARON L. ABBOTT, J. MICHAEL JANDA, JUDITH A. JOHNSON, AND J. J. FARMER III

47

TAXONOMY

Vibrio is the type genus of the family *Vibrionaceae*, with *V. cholerae*, the causative agent of pandemic cholera, as the type species (25, 26). The genus is extremely diverse with greater than 75 validly published species to date (http://www.bacterio.cict.fr/). Of these 75 named species, 12 have been associated with or isolated from infections in humans. Phylogenetic investigations indicate that multiple clades (separate or distant groups in a phylogenetic sense) exist within this genus, indicating that many *Vibrio* species may eventually be reclassified to different genera (58). Several formal proposals have already been made over the years (26) including the classification of *V. hollisae* in the genus *Grimontia* as *G. hollisae* (77) and the classification of *V. damsela* in the genus *Photobacterium* as *P. damselae* (73).

Changes in Classification for This Edition

In this chapter we accept the taxon *Grimontia hollisae* and use it rather than *Vibrio hollisae*. Studies based on DNA-DNA hybridization, 16S rRNA and *recA* sequencing, biochemical reactions, and other phenotypic characters (antibiotic susceptibility, poor growth on thiosulfate-citrate-bile salts-sucrose [TCBS], fastidious nature, metabolic inactivity, etc.) all indicate that *Vibrio hollisae* has diverged significantly from *Vibrio cholerae* and *V. mimicus*, the core species of the genus *Vibrio* (26). We suggest that clinical microbiology reports list both names to avoid confusion, with the reporter's choice listed first, i.e., *Grimontia hollisae (Vibrio hollisae)* or *Vibrio hollisae (Grimontia hollisae)*.

DESCRIPTION OF THE GENUS *VIBRIO*

A majority of *Vibrio* species have the following characteristics: gram-negative, facultatively anaerobic straight, curved, or comma-shaped rods, 0.5 to 0.8 μm in width and 1.4 to 2.6 μm in length, that are catalase and oxidase positive (26). Vibrios are motile by means of sheathed monotrichous or multitrichous polar flagella when grown in liquid media. Strains of some species, such as *V. parahaemolyticus* and *V. alginolyticus*, swarm on solid media by production of numerous lateral flagella (26, 51). All *Vibrio* species require Na^+ for growth, and the halophilic species usually require that NaCl be added to media (such as commercial decarboxylase broths) that do not include NaCl in their formulas. Most media formulated with peptone and meat extracts contain enough salt for *V. cholerae* and *V. mimicus* to grow. The minimal concentration for optimum growth varies from 0.029 to 4.1% NaCl (26). Vibrios ferment D-glucose but rarely produce gas, reduce nitrate to nitrite, and grow on TCBS medium. The G+C content of the DNA is 38 to 51 mol% (26). Key properties or characteristics useful in separating members of the genus *Vibrio* from phylogenetically or phenotypically related species are listed in Table 1. The description of the genus *Grimontia* is based on its single species and is given in Tables 2 and 4.

NATURAL HABITATS

Vibrios are primarily aquatic residents, and their relative distributions in such environs are typically dependent upon temperature, Na^+ concentration, available nutrients in the water column, and the presence of various plants and vertebrate and invertebrate animal species that inhabit such ecosystems (78). Vibrios that require small amounts of Na^+ for growth, such as *V. cholerae* and *V. mimicus*, can be found in freshwater rivers and lakes as well as estuarine and marine environments. Some *Vibrio* species, such as *V. fischeri* and *V. harveyi*, have evolved close symbiotic associations over thousands of years with marine inhabitants such as *Eupryema scolopes*, the Hawaiian small bobtail squid (59). In marine and estuarine environments, vibrios are commonly isolated from sediment, the water column, plankton, various bivalves (oysters, clams, and mussels), crabs, shrimp, and prawns (30, 47, 78). In temperate climates, *Vibrio* concentrations peak during the warmer months of the year (7). A "viable but nonculturable" state has been described for several *Vibrio* species including *V. cholerae* and *V. vulnificus* (9). It is unclear if the term "viable but nonculturable" represents a new idea or is just a subpart of the well-documented term "injured bacterial cell" that has been known for many decades, particularly in water microbiology. In either instance its significance is unknown.

CLINICAL SIGNIFICANCE

Vibrios are isolated from and actually cause a wide variety of human illnesses, both intestinal and extraintestinal. These

*This chapter contains information presented in chapter 46 by J. J. Farmer III, J. Michael Janda, and Karen Birkhead in the eighth edition of this Manual.

TABLE 1 Properties of the genus *Vibrio* and differentiation from other phenotypically similar genera

Test or property	Reaction or property of[a]:				
	Vibrio	*Photobacterium*	*Aeromonas*	*Plesiomonas*	*Enterobacteriaceae*
Associated with diarrhea and extraintestinal infections in humans	+	–[d]	+	+	+
Oxidase reaction	+	+	+	+	–
Na^+ is required for growth or stimulates growth	+	+	–	–	–
Sensitive to the vibriostatic compound O/129[b]	+	+	–	+	–
D-Mannitol fermentation	+	–	+	–	+
Growth on TCBS[c]	+	+	+	–	–

[a] Symbols: +, most species and strains are positive; –, most species and strains are negative.
[b] 2,4-diamino-6,7-diisopropylpteridine phosphate (150 μg per disk); resistance to O/129 has become common in *V. cholerae* from parts of India and Bangladesh.
[c] Relative growth of *Aeromonas* on TCBS is dependent on the commercial manufacturer.
[d] *Photobacterium damselae* is an exception if this classification is used.

include diarrhea, localized (cellulitis) and invasive (necrotizing fasciitis) wound infections, eye and ear infections, and septicemia (26). In individual cases of both diarrhea and extraintestinal infection it may be difficult to determine if a positive culture result represents true infection, colonization, or simply the transient presence of the organism because of its occurrence in sea- and estuarine water. Twelve vibrio species occur in human clinical specimens: *V. alginolyticus, V. cholerae, V. cincinnatiensis, V. damsela (P. damselae), V. fluvialis, V. furnissii, V. harveyi (= V. carchariae), Grimontia hollisae (V. hollisae), V. metschnikovii, V. mimicus, V. parahaemolyticus,* and *V. vulnificus* (26, 55). The clinical importance of some of these species in individual cases of infection is sometimes unclear. *V. cholerae* is the only species that causes endemic, epidemic, and pandemic cholera (68), but several other species are important causes of intestinal infections. *V. parahaemolyticus* is the foremost cause of food poisoning in Japan and Southeast Asia and is the leading cause of intestinal infections due to vibrios in the United States (81, 84).

Extraintestinal *Vibrio* infections are frequently associated with injuries or exposure to estuarine or marine waters and may result in severe tissue destruction and/or lead to systemic infection (63). Primary septicemia may occur after ingestion of raw seafood (oysters) or as a secondary bacteremia subsequent to a wound infection. Septicemia due to *V. vulnificus* tends to be fulminant with a fatality rate exceeding 50% (56) and is often accompanied by secondary skin lesions called bullae (63). *Vibrio vulnificus* is the most common cause of vibrio septicemia, but other vibrios may also cause bacteremia including *V. cholerae* non-O1.

V. cholerae

V. cholerae is the most important species in the genus *Vibrio*. It has caused many epidemics of cholera and millions of deaths (21, 68). It is now divided into three major subgroups: *V. cholerae* O1, *V. cholerae* O139, and *V. cholerae* non-O1.

V. cholerae O1

V. cholerae serogroup O1 is the organism responsible for seven pandemics of cholera (1816–1817, 1829, 1852, 1863, 1881, 1889, and 1961–present) (66, 68). While the majority of persons ingesting toxigenic *V. cholerae* O1 have asymptomatic infections or self-limiting diarrhea (≥75%), severe cholera ("cholera gravis") usually results in massive diarrhea and large volumes of "rice water stools" (clear fluid with flecks of mucus) passed painlessly; fluid loss can reach 200 ml/kg of body weight/day. If left untreated, the patient becomes prostrate with symptoms of severe dehydration, electrolyte imbalance, painful muscle cramps, watery eyes, loss of skin elasticity, and anuria. Dehydration subsequently leads to hypovolemic shock, acidosis, circulatory collapse, and death, even in healthy adults (42). Interestingly, there is a correlation between human blood types and susceptibility to *V. cholerae* infection with persons of O blood group presenting with more severe symptoms. In the United States, occasional cases of cholera are seen in travelers returning from regions of endemicity; rarely such illnesses are due to an O1 strain indigenous to the Gulf of Mexico. Treatment consists of fluid replacement by oral rehydration therapy and/or intravenous fluids.

The ability of *V. cholerae* serogroup O1 to uniquely cause this fulminant form of diarrhea is due to the presence of virulence "cassette" regions and pathogenicity islands on the bacterial chromosome. These regions encode a number of key virulence factors including cholera enterotoxin responsible for the large excretion of fluids and electrolytes into the lumen and the toxin coregulated pilus responsible for attachment of *V. cholerae* to the gastrointestinal epithelium (27). Traditional (classic) cholera can be produced by two different biotypes of *V. cholerae* O1, designated Classical and El Tor. These biotypes can be differentiated by a number of phenotypic tests including hemolysis of sheep erythrocytes, production of acetylmethylcarbinol (Voges-Proskauer test), and resistance to polymyxin B, all positive for the El Tor biotype (40). The first six pandemics were thought to be due to the Classical biotype, whereas the ongoing seventh pandemic that began in 1961 is caused by the El Tor biotype, which was first isolated in 1905 (68).

Although extremely rare, O1 strains have been known to cause severe extraintestinal infections. A 2001 report from Malawi describes three cases of *V. cholerae* O1 bacteremia in two adults and one neonate (34). All three patients died as a direct or indirect result of their infections.

V. cholerae O139

Until the last decade, only *V. cholerae* serogroup O1 was believed to cause epidemic cholera. In 1992, cholera cases due to a new serogroup of *V. cholerae*, O139 (synonym, *V. cholerae* O139 Bengal), appeared in India and Bangladesh and spread rapidly throughout Asia (4). This new serogroup probably resulted from the lateral transfer of a novel somatic antigen and capsule from an unknown bacterium to an El Tor strain (4). O139 strains carry cholera enterotoxin and other critical virulence factors that O1 strains harbor including the toxin coregulated pilus (54). The clinical diseases due to O1 and

O139 *V. cholerae* are strikingly similar, except that adults are more frequently affected than children since previous infection with O1 cholerae is not protective (2, 28). *V. cholerae* O139 replaced O1 as the cause of epidemic cholera between 1994 and 1995 in many areas of Southeast Asia, including Bangladesh. However, in this setting O1 reemerged in 1996. In 2002, O139 reemerged in Bangladesh, causing an estimated 30,000 cases of cholera, mostly in older patients than typically observed with O1 infections (28). Some researchers speculate that the emergence of O139 may be the beginning of the eighth cholera pandemic (4).

V. cholerae Non-O1

V. cholerae non-O1 strains do not agglutinate in O1 or O139 antisera but are otherwise phenotypically identical to O1 and O139 *V. cholerae* strains in their biochemical reactions. *V. cholerae* non-O1 strains are the third most commonly isolated vibrios in clinical laboratories in the United States, following *V. parahaemolyticus* and *V. vulnificus* (37). They typically do not produce cholera toxin and are usually isolated from patients with mild watery diarrhea, although the diarrhea is occasionally severe (57). However, unlike O1 strains, non-O1 isolates are commonly associated with extraintestinal infections such as septicemia. Persons at increased risk of developing non-O1 bacteremia include those with liver disease/cirrhosis or hematologic malignancies. The case fatality rate ranges from 47 to 65% (44, 69). Strains have also been isolated from ears, wounds, the respiratory tract, and urine (39, 56).

V. mimicus

V. mimicus is a nonhalophilic vibrio species that is biochemically similar to *V. cholerae* except that it is sucrose negative. It has been recovered from patients with diarrhea, which usually occurred after the consumption of uncooked seafood, particularly raw oysters (23). Rare strains carry the cholera toxin gene and can produce cholera-like symptoms. Human infections are uncommon. Symptoms include abundant watery diarrhea, vomiting, and severe dehydration. There has been one recent report of *V. mimicus* diarrhea in Costa Rica that involved 33 patients over a 3-year period (12).

V. parahaemolyticus

In Asia, *V. parahaemolyticus* is the leading cause of foodborne intestinal infections, almost always associated with the consumption of raw fish or shellfish (84). Fifty to 70% of the cases of foodborne diarrhea in Japan alone are due to *V. parahaemolyticus*. It is also the *Vibrio* species most frequently isolated from clinical specimens in the United States and is primarily associated with diarrhea, but it has occasionally been isolated from extraintestinal sites. *V. parahaemolyticus* causes gastroenteritis with nausea, vomiting, abdominal cramps, low-grade fever, and chills. The diarrhea is usually watery but can on rare occasions be bloody. Fatalities are extremely rare but can occur in cases of severe dehydration. Rehydration is usually the only treatment needed, but in some severe cases the patient requires hospital admission. Antimicrobial therapy may be beneficial.

A pandemic clone of *V. parahaemolyticus* serotype O3:K6 emerged worldwide in 1997 (62). Strains of this serotype caused an unusually high proportion of *V. parahaemolyticus* foodborne disease outbreaks in Taiwan from 1996 to 1999, suggesting something unusual in the organism's ecology, epidemiology, or virulence (17). This pandemic clone has continued to spread throughout Asia, to the United States, Canada, Russia, Chile, and Mozambique (6, 32). Recently, new pandemic serogroups have emerged that have been shown to be genetically closely related to the O3:K6 strain. These include O4:K68, O1:K25, O1:K41, and O1:KUT (UT, untypeable) (17).

V. vulnificus

V. vulnificus causes primary septicemia and wound infection and is responsible for more than 90% of deaths due to vibrios in the United States each year (63). Primary septicemia has a fatality rate that exceeds 50% even with hospitalization (15, 74) and occurs predominantly in men over 50. Cases generally have predisposing conditions such as liver disease, immunosuppression, increased serum iron, or other chronic diseases (74). Data from CDC showed that more than 95% of patients had consumed raw oysters within the last 7 days. Patients typically present with symptoms including a sudden onset of fever and chills, vomiting, diarrhea, and abdominal pain. Secondary skin lesions often appear, progressing to bulla formation and necrosis. Endotoxic shock often occurs and can rapidly lead to death. Blood cultures and biopsy specimens (scrapings) from skin lesions are usually positive.

V. vulnificus also causes severe wound infections usually after trauma and exposure to marine animals or the marine environment (63). Wound infections may progress to cellulitis with extensive necrosis (often requiring surgical debridement), myositis, necrotizing fasciitis that may mimic gas gangrene, and secondary septicemia. The fatality rate for wound infections ranges from 20 to 30%.

Three biogroups have now been defined for *V. vulnificus*. Most infections in the United States are due to biogroup 1 (see Table 5). *V. vulnificus* biogroup 2 was originally isolated from diseased eels, but in 1995 Amaro and Biosca (5) isolated it from a human wound infection from Rhode Island. To date, no other isolations of biogroup 2 from clinical specimens have been reported. *V. vulnificus* biogroup 3 was described in 1999 by Bisharat et al. (10), who isolated it from patients with wound infections and bacteremia. Cases have been limited to Israel and were acquired from exposure to live fish (tilapia) grown in aquaculture. One case report strongly suggests that *V. vulnificus* biogroup 3 can survive on fish skin for at least 24 h (19).

V. alginolyticus

V. alginolyticus is very common in the marine environment and is the fourth most commonly isolated *Vibrio* species in the United States. *V. alginolyticus* has most frequently been isolated from ear infections (otitis externa and otitis media) (29) and wound infections following exposure to seawater. *V. alginolyticus* has also been isolated from ocular infections and from infrequent cases of monomicrobic or polymicrobic bacteremia, mostly in immunocompromised persons (16). It is occasionally isolated from diarrheal stool (79), but there is no strong evidence that it can actually cause diarrhea or intestinal infections.

V. damsela (*Photobacterium damselae*)

V. damsela, originally isolated from wound infections in damselfish, is an important though infrequent cause of serious and aggressive wound infections (necrotizing fasciitis) and bacteremia (31, 33, 83). Risk factors for infection include puncture wounds (from a fish fin or a fish hook) and exposure of open wounds to seawater. Although the case fatality rate is unknown, many reports in the literature describe fatal *V. damsela* infections, suggesting a fairly high case fatality rate. The enhanced virulence of this species is thought to be related to the production of a damselysin (phospholipase-D).

V. fluvialis

V. fluvialis appears to cause sporadic cases of diarrhea worldwide (75). Although in the past it has only rarely been isolated from extraintestinal sites, several recent reports of cellulitis, cerebritis, peritonitis, and bacteremia have been attributed to *V. fluvialis* (38, 45, 67).

V. furnissii

V. furnissii is rarely isolated from human clinical specimens, but when it is recovered it is invariably from fecal specimens of patients with diarrhea (22). There is no convincing evidence that it can actually infect the intestinal tract or cause diarrhea, although this merits further investigation (22).

V. harveyi (originally known as *V. carchariae*)

A single case of a *V. harveyi* (the name *V. carchariae* was used in the report describing this organism [64]) wound infection, resulting from a shark bite, has been published (64). Subsequently, it was shown by DNA-DNA hybridization that the type strains of *V. carchariae* and *V. harveyi* are 88% related (65). The two organisms also have identical or almost identical 16S rRNA sequences. Since the two species appear to be synonyms (subjective), *V. harveyi,* being the older name, has priority.

Grimontia hollisae (Vibrio hollisae)

G. hollisae is a halophilic vibrio species that is primarily associated with moderate to severe cases of diarrhea (1), for which there is evidence for a causative role. It has been rarely isolated from extraintestinal sites such as bacteremia (35).

V. metschnikovii

V. metschnikovii has frequently been isolated from fresh, brackish, and marine waters. In 1981 Jean-Jacques et al. (41) reported that it caused peritonitis and bacteremia in a patient with an inflamed gallbladder. Subsequently, *V. metschnikovii* has been isolated from additional patients with bacteremia and rarely from wound infections (46). It has also been isolated from cases of cholecystitis, diarrhea, and pneumonia (46, 80). There is no convincing evidence that it can actually infect the intestinal tract or cause diarrhea, although this merits further investigation (46).

V. cincinnatiensis

V. cincinnatiensis was first reported by Brayton et al. (11) from a patient with bacteremia and meningitis. Subsequent isolates have been from feces (intestine), the ear, a foot or leg wound, animals, and water.

COLLECTION, TRANSPORT, AND STORAGE OF SPECIMENS

As with all stools, specimens should be collected in the acute stage of disease before initiation of treatment (13). If stool is unavailable, rectal swabs (or vomitus) are reliable from acute cases but should not be used when the numbers of organisms present may be small, as occurs with contacts to known cases or for convalescing patients. Vibrios are particularly susceptible to desiccation; therefore, any specimen that cannot be inoculated onto plating media within 2 to 4 h should be placed in a transport medium. Cary-Blair, which maintains the viability of vibrios up to 4 weeks, or most commercially available transport media are satisfactory; but because some lots of glycerol may be toxic to vibrios, buffered glycerol in saline is unacceptable. Specimens collected in the field may be transported in tellurite-taurocholate-peptone or alkaline peptone water enrichment broths only if they can be plated within 12 to 24 h and are delivered by courier. If necessary, liquid stool may be placed on strips of blotting paper or gauze, inserted in airtight plastic bags with a few drops of saline to maintain moisture, and submitted to the laboratory. Detailed information on the collection and transport of specimens for vibrio isolation is available (13).

Direct microscopic detection of vibrios in stool is not routinely recommended, since it may not be possible to distinguish pathogenic vibrios from other enteric flora. Detection of *V. cholerae* directly from stool using an "O1 (or O139) serum immobilization" method is described in a subsequent section.

Special methods for the collection and processing of extraintestinal specimens (blood and wounds, etc.) for vibrio isolation are not required; vibrios are, as a rule, isolated in pure culture from these sites, and the concentration of salt in primary plating media is usually sufficient for their recovery. Once isolated, however, salt may need to be added to subsequent media to attain growth of salt-requiring vibrios.

ISOLATION PROCEDURES

Since it is not common practice to use special isolation media for vibrios, inclusion of pertinent clinical history (when known) should accompany specimens to alert the laboratory to include vibrio isolation techniques (media or reagents) in their stool workup (49). Such information includes consumption of seafood, any activity associated with marine or brackish water or wounds associated with such exposure, and hobbies associated with aquaria. Examination of blood agar plates for oxidase-positive colonies may also improve recovery of vibrios as well as *Aeromonas* spp. and *Plesiomonas shigelloides*.

Vibrios associated with human disease generally grow on MacConkey agar and when present appear as colorless colonies (with the exception of the lactose-fermenting species, *V. vulnificus*). Sucrose-fermenting vibrios associated with human disease such as *V. cholerae, V. fluvialis,* or *V. alginolyticus* cannot be differentiated from other sucrose-fermenting normal enteric flora on sucrose-containing agars such as Hektoen or xylose-lysine-desoxycholate. Additionally, *Grimontia hollisae* may grow poorly or not at all on any enteric isolation medium, including TCBS, and is most reliably isolated from blood agar. Plating efficiency on TCBS may be less for *V. cincinnatiensis* than that observed for other vibrio species, and it may be reduced for *V. metschnikovii* when the plate is incubated at 36°C. Although there are a number of selective media suitable for the isolation of vibrios, TCBS is generally used for the isolation of vibrios associated with human disease and is readily available from a number of commercial sources (26). Since this medium does not require autoclaving, powdered media may be kept available in the laboratory and readily prepared by boiling whenever needed. The use of TCBS is particularly useful in coastal areas, where vibrios are isolated with greater frequency. It is not cost-effective to use it for every stool specimen. The inclusion of sucrose in TCBS allows for preliminary differentiation of *Vibrio* species, with *V. cholerae, V. fluvialis,* and *V. alginolyticus* producing yellow colonies whereas *V. parahaemolyticus, V. mimicus,* and most strains of *V. vulnificus* produce green colonies, indicating sucrose was not fermented. Yellow colonies on TCBS may convert to green colonies if plates are refrigerated after incubation. It should be noted that oxidase testing is unreliable when performed directly on colonies growing on TCBS and should not be attempted. A chromogenic agar, CHROMagar

Vibrio (CHROMagar Microbiology, Paris, France), has been developed primarily for the recovery of *V. parahaemolyticus* from seafood and supports the growth of other vibrios as well (36). Vibrio colonies on this medium range in color from milk white to pale blue to violet; other enteric flora, with the exception of *Proteus mirabilis* and *Providencia rettgeri,* which also produce milk white colonies, do not grow. Marine agar (BD Biosciences, Sparks, Md.), which does not contain any inhibitory or selective ingredients, may be more appropriate for isolation of vibrios from the environment, especially salt-requiring vibrios. It is common for pure cultures of vibrios to produce multiple colony morphologies on any medium, but this is most readily noticeable on nonselective media such as blood or heart infusion agars. Morphologies can range from smooth, convex to flat, spreading colonies to rough; occasionally, rugose (extremely wrinkled) colonies are encountered.

Alkaline peptone water (1% NaCl, pH 8.5) is the most commonly used enrichment broth for human specimens and is available from a number of commercial sources. Alkaline peptone water is incubated at 36°C and subcultured at 18 h. Occasionally, vibrios are recovered only when subcultured after 6 h of incubation. Longer incubation times of such specimens may fail to yield a vibrio, probably due to overgrowth by other flora.

DIRECT DETECTION OF *V. CHOLERAE* O1 IN FECES

Direct detection of *V. cholerae* from stool requires experience to correctly interpret results and is typically done only in laboratories in areas where cholera is common or in situations where laboratory services are unavailable. One of the oldest assays, the microscopic immobilization test, detects loss of motility of *V. cholerae* O1 organisms in the presence of O1 antibody and can be used to detect *V. cholerae* O139 by using O139 antibody (66). Coagglutination, direct fluorescent-antibody (New Horizons Diagnostics Corp., Columbia, Md.; FDA approval pending), and latex agglutination (Denka Seiken, Tokyo, Japan; not FDA approved for human clinical specimens) assays are all commercially available.

IDENTIFICATION

Biochemical properties that separate members of the *Vibrionaceae* from the *Enterobacteriaceae* (including *Plesiomonas shigelloides*) and the *Aeromonadaceae* are listed in Table 1. Useful tests for separating *Vibrio* species are described in Tables 2 and 3, and comprehensive biochemical profiles of the 12 species that occur in human clinical specimens are given in Table 4. All vibrios are negative to 10% positive for H_2S in triple sugar iron agar, urea (except *V. parahaemolyticus* [15%]), phenylalanine deaminase (except *V. vulnificus* biogroup 1 [35%]), malonate, mucate production, yellow pigment production, and fermentation of D-adonitol, dulcitol, erythritol, melibiose (except *V. vulnificus* biogroup 1 [40%]), raffinose, L-rhamnose (except *V. furnissii* [45%]), D-sorbitol (except *V. metschnikovii* [45%]), and α-methyl-β-D-galactoside and D-xylose (except for 57 and 43% of *V. cincinnatiensis* isolates, respectively). Variable reactions are seen with methyl red, growth in potassium cyanide broth, D-galactose, glycerol, Jordan's tartrate, sodium acetate, DNase at 25°C, lipase, and tyrosine clearing. All vibrio species are 99 to 100% positive for growth in 1% NaCl, and fermentation of maltose (except *V. hollisae* [0%]) and D-mannose (except *V. cholerae* [78%] and *V. harveyi* [50%]). Many commercial standard tube tests have sufficient

TABLE 2 Key differential tests for the six groups of 12 *Vibrio* species that occur in clinical specimens

Test	Reactions of the species in[a]:											
	Group 1		Group 2,	Group 3,	Group 4,	Group 5		Group 6				
	V. cholerae	*V. mimicus*	*V. metschnikovii*	*V. cincinnatiensis*	*G. hollisae*	*V. damsela*	*V. fluvialis*[b]	*V. alginolyticus*	*V. parahaemolyticus*	*V. vulnificus*	*V. harveyi*
Growth in nutrient broth with:											
No NaCl added[c]	+	+	–	–	–	–	–	–	–	–	–
1% NaCl added	+	+	+	+	+	+	+	+	+	+	+
Oxidase production			–	+	+	+	+	+	+	+	+
Nitrate reduced to nitrite			–	+	+	+	+	+	+	+	+
myo-Inositol fermentation			V	+	–	–	–	–	–	–	–
Arginine dihydrolase					–/NG	+	+	–	–	–	–
Lysine decarboxylase					–/NG	V	–	+	+	+	+
Ornithine decarboxylase					–/NG						

[a] All data except those for oxidase production and nitrate reduction are for reactions that occur within 2 days at 35 to 37°C; oxidase production and nitrate reduction reactions are done only at day 1. Symbols: +, 90 to 100% positive; V, variable, 11 to 89% of strains are positive; –, negative, 0 to 10% positive; NG, no growth, possibly because the NaCl concentration is too low, even when 1% NaCl is added. See Table 3 for the exact percentages.

[b] Includes *V. furnissii,* which differs from *V. fluvialis* primarily by production of gas in D-glucose.

[c] Species that require salt should have salt added to each biochemical tested.

TABLE 3 Key differential biochemicals to separate species within Groups 1, 5, and 6

Test	% Positive for[a]:							
	Group 1		Group 5		Group 6			
	V. cholerae	*V. mimicus*	*V. damsela*	*V. fluvialis*[a]	*V. alginolyticus*	*V. parahaemolyticus*	*V. vulnificus*	*V. harveyi*
Voges-Proskauer (1% NaCl)	75	9	95	0	95	0	0	50
Motility	99	98	25	70–89	99	99	99	0
Acid production from:								
Sucrose	100	0	5	100	99	1	15	50
D-Mannitol	99	99	0	97	100	100	45	50
Cellobiose	8	0	0	30	3	5	99	50
Salicin	1	0	0	0	4	1	95	0

[a] The numbers indicate the percentages of strains that are positive after 48 h of incubation at 36°C (unless other conditions are indicated). Most of the positive reactions occur during the first 24 h.

salt to support growth without salt supplementation (0.5 to 1%), but the Microbial Disease Laboratory adds 1% salt to all biochemicals (except for the 0% salt broth) for all NaCl-requiring species. Voges-Proskauer, Moeller's decarboxylases and dihydrolase, and nitrate broth may contain no or insufficient NaCl to support growth of some NaCl-requiring strains, and these biochemicals should always have salt added (to a final concentration of 1%) to them when testing these species. Sensitivity to the vibriostatic compound O/129 (Remel, Lenexa, Kans.) should be used with caution, as many *V. cholerae* isolates from Bangladesh and surrounding areas are now resistant to O/129.

Correct identification of vibrios by commercial identification systems is problematic at best, and published evaluations of these kits are based upon specific lot numbers, software versions, and microbial databases. No commercial automated or manual identification system includes all 12 clinical vibrio species in their databases, and some manual systems do not contain any vibrio species (60, 61). Six commonly used identification systems claim that they are capable of identifying *V. cholerae, V. parahaemolyticus, V. vulnificus, V. alginolyticus,* and *V. damsela* (61). However, even when tested against only those species listed in their databases, the API 20E (bioMerieux Inc., Durham, N.C.), Crystal E/NF (BD Biosciences), MicroScan Neg ID type 2 and type 3 (MicroScan, West Sacramento, Calif.), and Vitek GNI+ and ID-GNB cards (bioMerieux) correctly identified only 63.1 to 80.9% of vibrios to the species level (61). Accurate identification by these systems for the three most commonly isolated species varied. Correct identification of *V. cholerae* ranged from 50.0 to 96.7%, with API 20E and Crystal being the least and most accurate, respectively; for *V. parahaemolyticus* the range was 40.0 to 96.6%, with Rapid Neg ID3 faring the worst and API 20E and GNI+ being the best; and for *V. vulnificus* (biogroup 1 strains) the range was 50.0 to 90%, with GNI+ and Crystal showing the lowest and highest correct identification rates, respectively. Only Crystal was able to correctly identify ≥90% of *V. cholerae* or *V. vulnificus* strains, and only API 20E and the two Vitek cards correctly identified ≥90% of *V. parahaemolyticus* strains. For *V. vulnificus* biotype 3 strains, the MicroScan (98.0%) and Phoenix (90.2%) systems did the best in identifying 51 well-characterized isolates to the correct species, while the identification rate obtained by Vitek (13.7%) was much less satisfactory (20). The manufacturer's instructions should be checked prior to testing salt-requiring vibrios to determine if salt supplementation is required. Identification of vibrios from seafood and environmental sources is problematic. Many newly identified "nonclinical" species are published with poor phenotypic descriptions, and identification is based on 16S rRNA.

In areas of the world where cholera is common, isolates of *V. cholerae* may be presumptively identified simply by agglutination with O1 or O139 antisera. In other areas of the world, complete biochemical testing should be performed, and cultures identified as *V. cholerae* should be sent to public health laboratories for O1 and O139 agglutination and cholera toxin testing. *V. cholerae* O1 isolates should be biotyped (see "*V. cholerae* O1" under "Clinical Significance" above) to determine whether they are El Tor or Classical biotypes. *V. cholerae* O139 strains are phenotypically similar to *V. cholerae* O1 El Tor. Strains of *V. cholerae* that fail to agglutinate in either O1 or O139 antisera are reported as *V. cholerae* non-O1. These strains may also be serotyped; however, this testing is available only in a limited number of reference laboratories. *V. cholerae* is distinguished from other vibrios, except *V. mimicus,* by Na^+ requirement (Table 2), and *V. cholerae* can be differentiated from *V. mimicus* by sucrose and Voges-Proskauer tests (Table 3). Strains of *V. mimicus* may produce cholera toxin.

Strains of *V. parahaemolyticus, V. alginolyticus,* and *V. damsela* may be urea positive. As with most vibrios isolated from humans, these species produce a buff or tan pigment; occasional strains of *V. parahaemolyticus* may produce a dark brown pigment. *G. hollisae* generally grows poorly, especially in Moeller's decarboxylases and dihydrolase broths even after salt supplementation, and produce extremely large zones of inhibition, often necessitating the use of two plates when performing antimicrobial susceptibility testing. Because it is oxidase negative, *V. metschnikovii* is the most difficult vibrio to detect, but it is easily separated from other vibrios by negative reactions for nitrate reduction, indole production (most strains), and ornithine decarboxylase and fermentation of sucrose. *V. fluvialis* and *V. furnissii* are frequently confused with *Aeromonas caviae,* especially as some strains are poorly halophilic and only moderately susceptible to O/129, and some strains of *A. caviae* grow on TCBS. *V. furnissii* is the only vibrio isolated from humans that is positive for gas production from glucose. Rapid, correct identification of *V. vulnificus* strains is critical because of the mortality associated with this organism. Occasionally, strains of *V. vulnificus* are sucrose positive, which may add to the confusion in identifying it; it is unique among human *Vibrio*

TABLE 4 Biochemical test results and other properties of the 12 *Vibrio* species that occur in human clinical specimens

Test[a]	% Positive for[b]:											
	V. cholerae	*V. mimicus*	*V. metschnikovii*	*V. cincinnatiensis*	*G. hollisae*	*V. damsela*	*V. fluvialis*	*V. furnissii*	*V. alginolyticus*	*V. parahaemolyticus*	*V. vulnificus* biogroup 1	*V. harveyi*
Indole production (HIB, 1% NaCl)*	99	98	20	8	97	0	13	11	85	98	97	100
Voges-Proskauer (1% NaCl)*	75	9	96	0	0	95	0	0	95	0	0	50
Citrate (Simmons)	97	99	75	21	0	0	93	100	1	3	75	0
Urea hydrolysis	0	1	0	0	0	0	0	0	0	15	1	0
Arginine (Moeller's; 1% NaCl)*	0	0	60	0	0	95	93	100	0	0	0	0
Lysine (Moeller's; 1% NaCl)*	99	100	35	57	0	50	0	0	99	100	99	100
Ornithine (Moeller's; 1% NaCl)*	99	99	0	0	100	0	0	0	50	95	55	0
Motility (36°C)	99	98	74	86	0	25	70	89	99	99	99	0
Gelatin hydrolysis (1% NaCl, 22°C)	90	65	65	0	0	6	85	86	90	95	75	0
D-Glucose, acid production	100	100	100	100	100	100	100	100	100	100	100	50
D-Glucose, gas production	0	0	0	0	0	10	0	100	0	0	0	0
Acid production from:												
L-Arabinose*	0	1	0	100	97	0	93	100	1	80	0	0
Lactose*	7	21	50	0	0	0	3	0	0	1	85	0
Sucrose*	100	0	100	100	0	5	100	100	99	1	15	50
ONPG test*	94	90	50	86	0	0	40	35	0	5	75	0
Growth in nutrient broth with:												
0% NaCl*	100	100	0	0	0	0	0	0	0	0	0	0
6% NaCl*	53	49	78	100	83	95	96	100	100	99	65	100
8% NaCl*	1	2	44	62	0	0	71	78	94	80	0	2
10% NaCl*	0	0	4	0	0	0	4	0	69	2	0	2
O/129, zone of inhibition[c]	99	95	90	25	40	90	31	0	19	20	98	100

[a] Symbols and abbreviations: *, the test is recommended as part of the routine set for *Vibrio* identification; 1% NaCl, 1% NaCl has been added to the standard media to enhance growth; HIB, heart infusion broth; TSI, triple sugar iron agar; ONPG, *o*-nitrophenyl-β-D-galactopyranoside; a positive string test indicates that cells are lysed when they are suspended in a 0.5% sodium deoxycholate solution.

[b] The numbers indicate the percentages of strains that are positive after 48 h of incubation at 36°C (unless other conditions are indicated). Most of the positive reactions occur during the first 24 h.

[c] The content of the disk was 150 μg.

species because it ferments lactose, salicin, and cellobiose and is ONPG (*o*-nitrophenyl-β-D-galactopyranoside) positive. Table 5 gives biochemicals useful in separating the biogroups of *V. vulnificus* (10).

Although identification of vibrios by conventional methods is challenging, there is limited use of molecular methods for detection and identification of vibrios. Molecular methods are expensive, and vibrios are relatively rare pathogens in areas where cholera is not endemic. 16S sequencing has been used to identify clinically important *Vibrio* spp. The use of 16S sequencing alone is less than ideal for identification of vibrios, as the sequence differences between some species are very small and polymorphism has been shown to be fairly common in 16S rRNA genes of vibrios (53). There are few if any commercial molecular products with FDA approval for human clinical specimens. In-house molecular methods used in the United States for testing human clinical specimens will require extensive efforts to evaluate and implement in order to comply with all the Clinical Laboratory Improvement Amendments (CLIA) regulations. In a research setting, molecular methods for vibrios have proved to be very useful.

COMMERCIAL PRODUCTS FOR DETECTING CHOLERA TOXIN AND THE THERMOSTABLE DIRECT HEMOLYSIN OF *V. PARAHAEMOLYTICUS*

In reference laboratories, cholera toxin may be detected by fluid accumulation in animal assays or detection of a cytopathic effect in Y1 adrenal or Chinese hamster ovary cell cultures (40). However, a reverse passive latex agglutination assay produced by Denka Seiken, Tokyo, Japan, is commercially available (Oxoid, Inc., Ogdensburg, N.Y.).

The majority of human strains of *V. parahaemolyticus* produce a thermostable direct hemolysin (TDH) encoded by two genes, *tdh* and *tdh2x*. These toxins are rarely encountered in environmental strains of *V. parahaemolyticus* but have been detected in *V. cholerae* non-O1, *V. mimicus*, and *G. hollisae* strains. This hemolysin can be detected by observing hemolysis of red blood cells on Watgatsuma agar (Kanagawa test), a specialized agar, difficult to make. Like cholera toxin, TDH can be detected by a commercial latex assay (also available from Oxoid), but there are no commercial products that detect a second hemolysin seen in *V. parahaemolyticus* strains, i.e., thermostable-related hemolysin. PCR assays for TDH and thermostable-related hemolysin have been developed but are not commercially available (24).

TABLE 5 Differentiation of the three biogroups of *V. vulnificus*[a]

Test	Result for biogroup[b]:		
	1	2	3
Ornithine decarboxylase	V	–	+
Indole production	+	–	+
Acid produced by:			
D-Mannitol	V	–	–
D-Sorbitol	–	+	–
Cellobiose	+	+	–
Salicin	+	+	–

[a] Data from reference 10.
[b] V, variable (11 to 89% of strains are positive); +, positive (90 to 100% positive); –, negative (0 to 10% positive).

TYPING SYSTEMS

The usefulness of typing systems for determining strain relatedness among *Vibrio* isolates of the same species has very limited applicability for most clinical laboratories in the United States since, with the exception of very rare *V. parahaemolyticus* outbreaks, virtually all other *Vibrio* illnesses are sporadic in nature. Even then, state or federal reference laboratories will probably perform such extensive typing procedures. These typing schemes can basically be broken down into two groups, conventional (traditional) and molecular.

Among conventional techniques, serotyping is by far the most widely utilized procedure. Typing schemes have been described for a number of vibrio species including *V. cholerae*, *V. parahaemolyticus*, and *V. vulnificus* (40, 71, 72). However, commercial-grade typing sera are available only for *V. cholerae* and *V. parahaemolyticus*. *V. cholerae* O1 (polyclonal, serovars Inaba and Ogawa) and O139 antisera in one of several forms (slide, colorimetric) are available from Difco (Beckton Dickinson), Denka Seiken (Campbell, Calif.), Oxoid (Remel), and New Horizons (Columbia, Md.). *V. parahaemolyticus* antisera (O-group O1-O11 and K-group K1-K32) are available from Denka Seiken. *V. cholerae* isolates can also be typed by determining the sensitivity pattern to lytic bacteriophages (not commercially available), which may be another useful tool for tracking the spread of cholera. Phage (not commercially available) can be used for differentiating Classical from El Tor biotypes of *V. cholerae* O1 and O139 isolates (3, 14). The use of phage typing is limited to a few reference laboratories by the availability of typing phage and a lack of consensus in the typing schemes. Antibiograms, such as resistance to streptomycin, trimethoprim, and furazolidone, have been used to subtype *V. cholerae* O1 and O139 strains on a limited basis (8, 50). Such techniques are more useful in Southeast Asia, where unusual resistance patterns in isolates are observed more frequently than in the United States.

A large number of molecular typing methods have been successfully used in tracking the spread of *V. cholerae* epidemics and the clonal migration of *V. parahaemolyticus* strains and for phylogenetic analysis. However, these are primarily epidemiologic and taxonomic research techniques and not commercially available or easily adapted to clinical laboratories. Pulsed-field gel electrophoresis has been used extensively for both *V. cholerae* and *V. parahaemolyticus* (50, 52). Sequencing of single genes such as *ctxA*, *ctxB*, *hsp60*, and *recA* shows promise as a molecular typing method (42).

SEROLOGIC TESTS

Serodiagnosis of cholera can be established with a high degree of certainty by titration of acute- and convalescent-phase sera in agglutination, vibriocidal, or antitoxin tests (48). The reagents are not commercially available, so this technique will normally be limited to a few reference laboratories.

ANTIMICROBIAL SUSCEPTIBILITY TESTING

Antibiotic resistance is more uncommon in *Vibrio* than in members of the family *Enterobacteriaceae*. However, all clinical *Vibrio* isolates should be tested against a number of therapeutically active compounds, since resistance can be acquired through plasmid transfer or exposure to antimicrobials and spread quickly through global travel. The Clinical and Laboratory Standards Institute (CLSI, formerly NCCLS) has interpretive guidelines only for *V. cholerae* limited to ampicillin, tetracyclines, folate pathway inhibitors, and chloramphenicol (18). Because most vibrios grow rapidly and are similar to enteric bacteria in many ways, a first approximation might be to use interpretive guidelines for the *Enterobacteriaceae* for *Vibrio* species other than *V. cholerae* when testing agents that are not currently covered by the CLSI document.

There have been only limited susceptibility studies involving vibrios in recent times. Most strains of *V. cholerae* (O1, O139, and non-O1) are susceptible (>90%) in vitro to aminoglycosides, azithromycin, fluoroquinolones, extended-spectrum cephalosporins, carbapenems, and monobactams (70, 82). However, O1 El Tor and O139 strains from India and Bangladesh demonstrate moderate to high-level resistance to sulfamethoxazole, trimethoprim, and chloramphenicol (82). The fluoroquinolones alone or the synergistic combination of ciprofloxacin and cefotaxime shows excellent in vitro activity against *V. vulnificus* strains (43, 76). Most vibrios are also susceptible to tetracyclines, gentamicin, chloramphenicol (except *V. damsela*), monobactams, carbapenems, and fluoroquinolones.

INTERPRETATION AND REPORTING OF RESULTS

The isolation of *V. cholerae* O1 or O139 should be reported immediately to the attending physician because of the severe dehydration that cholera can produce. The case should also be reported by telephone to public health authorities, and the isolate should be sent to a public health laboratory for confirmation and toxin testing. Similarly, isolation of a vibrio from a sterile body site or a wound should be reported by telephone to the attending physician immediately so that rapid and appropriate antibiotic therapy can be initiated. *Vibrio* septicemia and/or meningitis have a high mortality rate associated with infection, and wound infections can frequently cause extensive tissue damage.

The clinical significance of *Vibrio* strains in many other specimens is more difficult to determine. Since physicians are not familiar with many *Vibrio* species, it would be helpful to provide a telephone consultation when a *Vibrio* isolate is identified. *Vibrio* isolates should also be submitted to public health laboratories, as they are monitored under the CDC emerging infections program and Vibrio Surveillance System; they may also be needed for confirmation and toxin testing. *Vibrio* species that are known to cause diarrhea should be considered clinically significant, particularly if they are present in large numbers and no other potential pathogens are present. Isolation of vibrios from stool in small numbers may reflect only transitory colonization. *V. cholerae*, *V. mimicus*, and *V. parahaemolyticus* have documented virulence factors that correlate with their ability to cause intestinal infections. Laboratory tests are helpful in determining pathogenic potential but are likely to be done only in reference laboratories. The same warning should be emphasized for *Vibrio* isolates from other specimens such as ears or wounds. The isolation of vibrios could represent infection, transient colonization, or merely the vibrio flora that is always present in seawater or brackish water.

REFERENCES

1. **Abbott, S. L., and J. M. Janda.** 1994. Severe gastroenteritis associated with *Vibrio hollisae* infection: report of two cases and review. *Clin. Infect. Dis.* **18:**310–312.
2. **Albert, M. J.** 1994. *Vibrio cholerae* O139 Bengal. *J. Clin. Microbiol.* **32:**2345–2349.
3. **Albert, M. J., N. A. Bhuiyan, A. Rahman, A. N. Ghosh, K. Hultenby, A. Weintraub, S. Nahar, A. K. Kibriya, M. Ansaruzzaman, and T. Shimada.** 1996. Phage specific for *Vibrio cholerae* O139 Bengal. *J. Clin. Microbiol.* **34:**1843–1845.
4. **Albert, M. J., and G. B. Nair.** 2005. *Vibrio cholerae* O139 – 10 years on. *Rev. Med. Microbiol.* **16:**135–143.
5. **Amaro, C., and E. G. Biosca.** 1996. *Vibrio vulnificus* biotype 2, pathogenic for eels, is also an opportunistic pathogen for humans. *Appl. Environ. Microbiol.* **62:**1454–1457.
6. **Ansaruzzaman, M., M. Lucas, J. L. Deen, N. A. Bhuiyan, X.-Y. Wang, A. Safa, M. Sultana, A. Chowdhury, G. B. Nair, D. A. Sack, L. von Seidlein, M. K. Puri, M. Ali, C.-L. Chaignat, J. D. Clemens, and A. Barreto.** 2005. Pandemic serovars (O3:K6 and O4:K68) of *Vibrio parahaemolyticus* associated with diarrhea in Mozambique: spread of the pandemic into the African continent. *J. Clin. Microbiol.* **43:**2559–2562.
7. **Barbieri, E., L. Falzono, C. Fiorentini, A. Pianetti, W. Baffone, A. Fabbri, P. Matarrese, A. Casiere, M. Katouli, I. Kühn, R. Möllby, F. Bruscolini, and G. Donelli.** 1999. Occurrence, diversity, and pathogenicity of halophilic *Vibrio* spp. and non-O1 *Vibrio cholerae* from estuarine waters along the Italian Adriatic coast. *Appl. Environ. Microbiol.* **65:** 2748–2753.
8. **Basu, A., P. Garg, S. Datta, S. Chakraborty, T. Bhattacharya, A. Khan, T. Ramamurthy, S. K. Bhattacharya, S. Yamasaki, Y. Takeda, and G. B. Nair.** 2000. *Vibrio cholerae* O139 in Calcutta, 1992–1998: incidence, antibiograms, and genotypes. *Emerg. Infect. Dis.* **6:**139–147.
9. **Binsztein, N., M. C. Costagliola, M. Pichel, V. Jurquiza, F. C. Ramírez, R. Akselman, M. Vacchino, A. Huq, and R. R. Colwell.** 2004. Viable but nonculturable *Vibrio cholerae* O1 in the aquatic environment. *Appl. Environ. Microbiol.* **70:**7481–7486.
10. **Bisharat, N., V. Agmon, R. Finkelstein, R. Raz, G. Ben-Dror, L. Lerner, S. Soboh, R. Colodner, D. N. Cameron, D. L. Wykstra, D. L. Swerdlow, J. J. Farmer III, and the Israel *Vibrio* Study Group.** 1999. Clinical, epidemiological, and microbiological features of *Vibrio vulnificus* biogroup 3 causing outbreaks of wound infection and bacteraemia in Israel. *Lancet* **354:**1421–1424.
11. **Brayton, P. R., R. B. Bode, R. R. Colwell, M. T. MacDonell, H. L. Hall, D. J. Grimes, P. A. West, and T. N. Bryant.** 1986. *Vibrio cincinnatiensis* sp. nov., a new human pathogen. *J. Clin. Microbiol.* **23:**104–108.
12. **Campos, E., H. Bolaños, M. T. Acuña, G. Díaz, M. C. Matamoros, H. Raventós, L. M. Sánchez, C. Barquero, and Red Nacional De Laboratorios Para Cólera, Costa Rica.** 1996. *Vibrio mimicus* diarrhea following ingestion of raw turtle eggs. *Appl. Environ. Microbiol.* **62:**1141–1144.
13. **Centers for Disease Control and Prevention.** 1999. *Laboratory Methods for the Diagnosis of Epidemic Dysentery and Cholera.* Centers for Disease Control and Prevention, Atlanta, Ga.
14. **Chattopadhyay, D. J., B. L. Sarkar, M. Q. Ansari, B. K. Chakrabarti, M. K. Roy, A. N. Ghosh, and S. C. Pal.** 1993. New phage typing scheme for *Vibrio cholerae* O1 biotype El Tor strains. *J. Clin. Microbiol.* **31:**1579–1585.
15. **Chiang, S.-R., and Y.-C. Chuang.** 2003. *Vibrio vulnificus* infection: clinical manifestations, pathogenesis, and antimicrobial therapy. *J. Microbiol. Immunol.* **36:**81–88.
16. **Chien, J. Y., J. T. Shih, P. R. Hsueh, P. C. Yang, and K. T. Luh.** 2002. *Vibrio alginolyticus* as the cause of pleural emyema and bacteremia in an immunocompromised patient. *Eur. J. Clin. Microbiol. Infect. Dis.* **21:**401–403.
17. **Chowdhury, N. R., S. Chakraborty, T. Ramamurthy, M. Nishibuchi, S. Yamasaki, Y. Takeda, and G. B. Nair.** 2000. Molecular evidence of clonal *Vibrio parahaemolyticus* pandemic strains. *Emerg. Infect. Dis.* **6:**631–636.

18. **Clinical Laboratory Standards Institute.** 2005. *Performance Standards for Antimicrobial Susceptibility Testing.* Eighth informational supplement. NCCLS document M100-S8. National Committee for Clinical Laboratory Standards, Wayne, Pa.
19. **Colodner, R., B. Chszan, J. Kopelowitz, Y. Keness, and R. Raz.** 2002. Unusual portal of entry of *Vibrio vulnificus:* evidence of its prolonged survival on the skin. *Clin. Infect. Dis.* **34:**714–715.
20. **Colodner, R., R. Raz, I. Meir, T. Lazarovich, L. Lerner, J. Kopelowitz, Y. Keness, W. Sakran, S. Ken-Dror, and N. Bisharat.** 2004. Identification of the emerging pathogen *Vibrio vulnificus* biotype 3 by commercially available phenotypic methods. *J. Clin. Microbiol.* **42:**4137–4140.
21. **Colwell, R. R.** 2004. Infectious disease and environment: cholera as a paradigm for waterborne disease. *Int. Microbiol.* **7:**285–289.
22. **Dalsgaard, A., P. Glerup, L.-L. Høybe, A.-M. Paarup, R. Meza, M. Bernal, T. Shimada, and D. N. Taylor.** 1997. *Vibrio furnissii* isolated from humans in Peru: a possible human pathogen? *Epidemiol. Infect.* **119:**143–149.
23. **Davis, B. R., G. R. Fanning, J. M. Madden, A. G. Steigerwalt, H. B. Bradford, Jr., H. L. Smith, Jr., and D. J. Brenner.** 1981. Characterization of biochemically atypical *Vibrio cholerae* strains and designation of a new pathogenic species, *Vibrio mimicus*. *J. Clin. Microbiol.* **14:**631–639.
24. **DePaola, A., J. Ulaszek, C. A. Kaysner, B. J. Tenge, J. L. Nordstrom, J. Wells, N. Puhr, and S. M. Gendel.** 2003. Molecular, serological, and virulence characteristics of *Vibrio parahaemolyticus* isolated from environmental, food, and clinical resources in North America and Asia. *Appl. Environ. Microbiol.* **69:**3999–4005.
25. **Farmer, J. J., III, and J. M. Janda.** 2005. Family I. Vibrionaceae Veron 1965, 5245[AL], p. 491–494. *In* D. Brenner, N. Krieg, J. T. Staley, and G. Garrity (ed.), *Bergey's Manual of Systematic Bacteriology*, vol. 2. *The Proteobacteria*, part B. The Gammaproteobacteria. Springer, New York, N.Y.
26. **Farmer, J. J., III, J. M. Janda, F. W. Brenner, D. N. Cameron, and K. M. Birkhead.** 2005. Genus I. Vibrio Pacini 1854, 411[AL], p. 494–546. *In* D. Brenner, N. Krieg, J. T. Staley, and G. Garrity (ed.), *Bergey's Manual of Systematic Bacteriology*, vol. 2. *The Proteobacteria*, part B. The Gammaproteobacteria. Springer, New York, N.Y.
27. **Faruque, S. H., M. J. Albert, and J. J. Mekalanos.** 1998. Epidemiology, genetics, and ecology of toxigenic *Vibrio cholerae*. *Microbiol. Mol. Biol. Rev.* **62:**1301–1314.
28. **Faruque, S. M., N. Chowdhury, M. Kamruzzaman, Q. S. Ahmad, A. S. G. Faruque, M. A. Salam, T. Ramamurthy, G. B. Nair, A. Weintraub, and D. A. Sack.** 2003. Reemergence of epidemic *Vibrio cholerae* O139, Bangladesh. *Emerg. Infect. Dis.* **9:**1116–1122.
29. **Feingold, M. H., and M. L. Kumar.** 2004. Otitis media associated with *Vibrio alginolyticus* in a child with pressure-equalizing tubes. *Pediatr. Infect. Dis. J.* **23:**475–476.
30. **Feldhusen, F.** 2000. The role of seafood in bacterial foodborne diseases. *Microbes Infect.* **2:**1651–1660.
31. **Fraser, S. L., B. K. Purcell, B. Delgado, Jr., A. E. Baker, and A. C. Whelen.** 1997. Rapidly fatal infection due to *Photobacterium (Vibrio) damsela*. *Clin. Infect. Dis.* **25:**935–936.
32. **Gonzalez-Escalona, N., V. Cachicas, C. Acevedo, M. L. Rioseco, J. A. Vergara, F. Cabello, J. Romero, and R. T. Espejo.** 2005. *Vibrio parahaemolyticus* diarrhea, Chile, 1998 and 2004. *Emerg. Infect. Dis.* **11:**129–131.
33. **Goodell, K. H., M. R. Jordan, R. Graham, C. Cassidy, and S. A. Nasraway.** 2004. Rapidly advancing necrotizing fasciitis caused by *Photobacterium (Vibrio) damsela:* a hyperaggressive variant. *Crit. Care Med.* **32:**278–281.
34. **Gordon, M. A., A. L. Walsh, S. R. K. Rogerson, K. C. Magomero, C. E. Machili, J. E. Corkill, and C. A. Hart.** 2001. Three cases of bacteremia caused by *Vibrio cholerae* O1 in Balatyre, Malawi. *Emerg. Infect. Dis.* **7:**1059–1061.
35. **Gras-Rouzet, S., P. Y. Donnio, F. Juguet, P. Plessis, J. Minet, and J. L. Avril.** 1996. First European case of gastroenteritis and bacteremia due to *Vibrio hollisae*. *Eur. J. Clin. Microbiol. Infect. Dis.* **15:**864–866.
36. **Hara-Kudo, Y., T. Nishina, H. Nakagawa, H. Konuma, J. Hasegawa, and S. Kumagai.** 2001. Improved method for detection of *Vibrio parahaemolyticus* in seafood. *Appl. Environ. Microbiol.* **67:**5819–5823.
37. **Hlady, W. G., and K. C. Klontz.** 1996. The epidemiology of *Vibrio* infections in Florida, 1981–1993. *J. Infect. Dis.* **173:**1176–1183.
38. **Huang, K.-C., and R. W.-W. Hsu.** 2005. *Vibrio fluvialis* hemorrhagic cellulitis and cerebritis. *Clin. Infect. Dis.* **40:**e75–e77.
39. **Hughes, J. M., D. G. Hollis, E. J. Gangarosa, and R. E. Weaver.** 1978. Non-cholera vibrio infections in the United States. *Ann. Intern. Med.* **88:**602–606.
40. **Janda, J. M., C. Powers, R. G. Bryant, and S. L. Abbott.** 1988. Current perspectives on the epidemiology and pathogenesis of clinically significant *Vibrio* sp. *Clin. Microbiol. Rev.* **1:**245–267.
41. **Jean-Jacques, W., K. R. Rajashekaraiah, J. J. Farmer III, F. W. Hickman, J. G. Morris, and C. A. Kallick.** 1981. *Vibrio metschnikovii* bacteremia in a patient with cholecystitis. *J. Clin. Microbiol.* **14:**711–712.
42. **Kaper, J. B., J. G. Morris, Jr., and M. M. Levine.** 1995. Cholera. *Clin. Microbiol. Rev.* **8:**48–86.
43. **Kim, D.-M., Y. Lym, S. J. Jang, H. Han, Y. G. Kim, C.-H. Chung, and S. P. Hong.** 2005. In vitro efficacy of the combination of ciprofloxacin and cefotaxime against *Vibrio vulnificus*. *Antimicrob. Agents Chemother.* **49:**3489–3491.
44. **Ko, W.-C., Y.-C. Chuang, G.-C. Huang, and S.-Y. Hsu.** 1998. Infections due to non-O1 *Vibrio cholerae* in southern Taiwan: predominance in cirrhotic patients. *Clin. Infect. Dis.* **27:**774–780.
45. **Lai, C. H., C. K. Hwang, C. Chin, H. H. Lin, W. W. Wong, and C. Y. Liu.** 2006. Severe watery diarrhea and bacteraemia caused by *Vibrio fluvialis:* a first case report. *J. Infect.* **52:**e95–e98.
46. **Linde, H.-J., R. Kobuch, S. Jayasinghe, U. Reischl, N. Lehn, S. Kaulfuss, and L. Beutin.** 2004. *Vibrio metschnikovii*, a rare cause of wound infection. *J. Clin. Microbiol.* **42:**4909–4911.
47. **Lipp, E. K., and J. B. Rose.** 1997. The role of seafood in foodborne diseases in the United States of America. *Rev. Sci. Tech.* **16:**620–640.
48. **Losonsky, G. A., and M. M. Levine.** 1997. Immunologic methods for diagnosis of infections caused by diarrheagenic members of the families *Enterobacteriaceae* and *Vibrionaceae*, p. 484–497. *In* N. R. Rose, E. C. de Macario, J. D. Folds, H. C. Lane, and R. M. Nakamura (ed.), *Manual of Clinical Immunology*, 5th ed. ASM Press, Washington, D.C.
49. **Marano, N. N., N. A. Daniels, A. N. Easton, A. Mc Shan, B. Ray, J. G. Wells, P. M. Griffin, and F. J. Angulo.** 2000. A survey of stool culturing practices for *Vibrio* species at clinical laboratories in Gulf Coast states. *J. Clin. Microbiol.* **38:**2267–2270.
50. **Matsumoto, M., M. Suzuki, R. Hiramatsu, M. Yamazaki, H. Matsui, K. Sakae, Y. Suzuki, and Y. Miyazaki.** 2002. Epidemiological investigation of a fatal case of cholera in Japan by phenotypic techniques and pulsed-field gel electrophoresis. *J. Med. Microbiol.* **51:**264–268.
51. **McCarter, L. L.** 2001. Polar flagellar motility of the *Vibrionaceae*. *Microbiol. Mol. Biol. Rev.* **65:**445–462.
52. **McLaughlin, J. B., A. DePaola, C. A. Bopp, K. A. Martinek, N. P. Napolilli, C. G. Allison, S. L. Murray, E. C. Thompson, M. M. Bird, and J. P. Middaugh.** 2005. Outbreak of *Vibrio parahaemolyticus* gastroenteritis associated with Alaskan oysters. *N. Engl. J. Med.* **353:**1463–1470.
53. **Moreno, C. O., J. Romero, and R. T. Espejo.** 2002. Polymorphism in repeated 16S rRNA genes is a common

property of type strains and environmental isolates of the genus. *Microbiology* **148:**1233–1239.

54. **Morris, J. G., Jr.** 1995. *Vibrio cholerae* O139 Bengal: emergence of a new epidemic strain of cholera. *Infect. Agents Dis.* **4:**41–46.
55. **Morris, J. G., Jr.** 2003. Cholera and other types of vibriosis: a story of human pandemics and oysters on the half shell. *Clin. Infect. Dis.* **37:**272–280.
56. **Morris, J. G., and G. B. Nair.** 2001. "Non-cholera" vibrio infections. *In* M. J. Blaser, P. D. Smith, J. I. Ravdin, H. B. Greenberg, and R. L. Guerrant (ed.), *Infections of the Gastrointestinal Tract*, 2nd ed. Lippincott, Williams, and Wilkins, Philadelphia, Pa.
57. **Morris, J. G., Jr., R. Wilson, B. R. Davis, I. K. Wachsmuth, C. F. Riddle, H. G. Wathen, R. A. Pollard, and P. A. Blake.** 1981. Non-O Group 1 *Vibrio cholerae* gastroenteritis in the United States. *Ann. Intern. Med.* **94:**656–658.
58. **Nishiguchi, M. K., and V. S. Nair.** 2003. Evolution of symbiosis in the Vibrionaceae: a combined approach using molecules and physiology. *Int. J. Syst. Evol. Microbiol.* **53:**2019–2026.
59. **Nyholm, S. V., and M. J. McFall-Ngai.** 2004. The winnowing: establishing the squid-Vibrio symbiosis. *Nat. Rev. Microbiol.* **2:**632–642.
60. **O'Hara, C. M.** 2005. Manual and automated instrumentation for identification of *Enterobacteriaceae* and other aerobic gram-negative bacilli. *J. Clin. Microbiol.* **18:**147–162.
61. **O'Hara, C. M., E. G. Sowers, C. A. Bopp, S. B. Duda, and N. A. Strockbine.** 2003. Accuracy of six commercially available systems for identification of members of the family *Vibrionaceae*. *J. Clin. Microbiol.* **41:**5654–5659.
62. **Okuda, J., M. Ishibashi, E. Hayakawa, T. Nishino, Y. Takeda, A. K. Mukhopadhyay, S. Garg, S. K. Bhattacharya, G. B. Nair, and M. Nishibuchi.** 1997. Emergence of a unique O3:K6 clone of *Vibrio parahaemolyticus* in Calcutta, India, and isolation of strains from the same clonal group from Southeast Asian travelers arriving in Japan. *J. Clin. Microbiol.* **35:**3150–3155.
63. **Oliver, J. D.** 2005. Wound infections caused by *Vibrio vulnificus* and other marine bacteria. *Epidemiol. Infect.* **133:**383–391.
64. **Pavia, A. T., J. A. Bryan, K. L. Maher, T. R. Hester, Jr., and J. J. Farmer III.** 1989. *Vibrio carchariae* infection after a shark bite. *Ann. Intern. Med.* **111:**85–86.
65. **Pedersen, K., L. Verdonck, B. Austin, D. A. Austin, A. R. Blanch, P. A. D. Grimont, J. Jofre, S. Koblavi, J. L. Larsen, T. Tiainen, M. Vigneulle, and J. Swings.** 1998. Taxonomic evidence that *Vibrio carchariae* Grimes *et al.* 1985 is a junior synonym of *Vibrio harveyi* (Johnson and Shunk 1936) Baumann *et al.* 1981. *Int. J. Syst. Bacteriol.* **48:**749–758.
66. **Pollitzer, R.** 1959. *Cholera*. World Health Organization, Geneva, Switzerland.
67. **Ratnaraja, N., T. Blackmore, J. Byrne, and S. Shi.** 2005. *Vibrio fluvialis* peritonitis in a patient receiving continuous ambulatory peritoneal dialysis. *J. Clin. Microbiol.* **43:**514–515.
68. **Sack, D. A., R. B. Sack, G. B. Nair, and A. K. Siddique.** 2004. Cholera. *Lancet* **363:**223–233.
69. **Safrin, S., J. G. Morris, Jr., M. Adams, V. Pons, R. Jacobs, and J. E. Conte, Jr.** 1988. Non-O1 *Vibrio cholerae* bacteremia: case report and review. *Rev. Infect. Dis.* **10:**1012–1017.
70. **Sciortino, C. V., J. A. Johnson, and A. Hamad.** 1996. Vitek system antimicrobial susceptibility testing of O1, O139, and non-O1 *Vibrio cholerae*. *J. Clin. Microbiol.* **34:**897–900.
71. **Shimada, T., E. Arakawa, K. Itoh, T. Okitsu, A. Matushima, Y. Asai, S. Yamai, T. Nakazato, G. B. Nair, M. J. Albert, and Y. Takeda.** 1994. Extended serotyping scheme for *Vibrio cholerae*. *Curr. Microbiol.* **28:**175–178.
72. **Shimada, T., and R. Sakazaki.** 1984. On the serology of *Vibrio vulnificus*. *Jpn. J. Med. Sci. Biol.* **37:**241–246.
73. **Smith, S. K., D. C. Sutton, J. A. Fuerst, and J. L. Reichelt.** 1991. Evaluation of the genus *Listonella* and reassignment of *Listonella damsela* (Love et al.) MacDonald and Colwell to the genus *Photobacterium* as *Photobacterium damsela* comb. nov. with an emended description. *Int. J. Syst. Bacteriol.* **41:**529–534.
74. **Strom, M. S., and R. N. Paranjpye.** 2000. Epidemiology and pathogenesis of *Vibrio vulnificus*. *Microbes Infect.* **2:**177–188.
75. **Tacket, C. O., F. Hickman, G. V. Pierce, and L. F. Mendoza.** 1982. Diarrhea associated with *Vibrio fluvialis* in the United States. *J. Clin. Microbiol.* **16:**991–992.
76. **Tang, H.-J., M.-C. Chang, W.-C. Ko, K.-Y. Huang, C.-L. Lee, and Y.-C. Chuang.** 2002. In vitro and in vivo activities of newer fluoroquinolones against *Vibrio vulnificus*. *Antimicrob. Agents Chemother.* **46:**3580–3584.
77. **Thompson, F. L., B. Hoste, K. Vandemeulebroecke, and J. Swings.** 2003. Reclassification of *Vibrio hollisae* as *Grimontia hollisae* gen. nov., comb. nov. *Int. J. Syst. Evol. Microbiol.* **53:**1615–1617.
78. **Thompson, F. L., T. Iida, and J. Swings.** 2004. Biodiversity of vibrios. *Microbiol. Mol. Biol. Rev.* **68:**403–431.
79. **Uh, Y., J.-S. Park, G.-Y. Hwang, I. H. Jang, K.-J. Yoon, H.-C. Park, and S.-O. Hwang.** 2001. *Vibrio alginolyticus* gastroenteritis: report of two cases. *Clin. Microbiol. Infect.* **7:**104–106.
80. **Wallet, F., M. Tachon, S. Nseir, R. J. Courcol, and M. Roussel-Delvallez.** 2005. *Vibrio metschnikovii* pneumonia. *Emerg. Infect. Dis.* **11:**1641–1642.
81. **Wong, H. C., S. H. Liu, L. W. Ku, I. Y. Lee, T. K. Wang, Y. S. Lee, C. L. Lee, L. P. Kuo, and D. Y. Shih.** 2000. Characterization of *Vibrio parahaemolyticus* isolates obtained from foodborne illness outbreaks during 1992 through 1995 in Taiwan. *J. Food Prot.* **63:**900–906.
82. **Yamamoto, T., G. B. Nair, M. J. Albert, C. C. Parodi, and Y. Takeda.** 1995. Survey of in vitro susceptibilities of *Vibrio cholerae* O1 and O139 to antimicrobial agents. *Antimicrob. Agents Chemother.* **39:**241–244.
83. **Yamane, K., J. Asato, N. Kawade, H. Takahashi, B. Kimura, and Y. Arakawa.** 2004. Two cases of fatal necrotizing fasciitis caused by *Photobacterium damsela* in Japan. *J. Clin. Microbiol.* **42:**1370–1372.
84. **Yeung, P. S. M., and K. J. Boor.** 2004. Epidemiology, pathogenesis, and prevention of foodborne *Vibrio parahaemolyticus*. *Foodborne Pathog. Dis.* **1:**74–88.

*Pseudomonas**

EDITH BLONDEL-HILL, DEBORAH A. HENRY, AND DAVID P. SPEERT

48

TAXONOMY

Pseudomonas is a large and complex genus of gram-negative bacteria of importance, as it includes species with both clinical and environmental implications. The genus *Pseudomonas* first proposed by Migula in 1894 (91) has undergone many taxonomic revisions as methodologies of identification to the species level continue to improve. The genus *Pseudomonas* was comprised of five unrelated groups, as determined by ribosomal RNA-DNA hybridization studies in the early 1970s. *Pseudomonas* (sensu stricto) is rRNA homology group I (28), in the gamma subclass of the *Proteobacteria.* The other rRNA homology groups are II, *Burkholderia* species; III, *Comamonas, Acidovorax,* and *Hydrogenophaga* genera; IV, *Brevundimonas* species; and V, *Stenotrophomonas* and *Xanthomonas* genera (69). Currently there are 160 species within the *Pseudomonas* genus, with only 12 (described herein) of clinical interest. The closest phylogenetic neighbors of the *Pseudomonas* genus are the genera of *Azomonas, Azotobacter, Cellvibrio, Chrysomonas,* and *Flavimonas.*

Several of the clinically relevant *Pseudomonas* species demonstrate marked heterogeneity and have been subdivided into biovars or genomovars. Genomovars are genetically distinct groups that warrant species designation but lack phenotypically defining characteristics and that are determined by DNA-DNA reassociation experiments and 16S rRNA gene sequencing in combination with chemotaxonomic total fatty acid analysis and total protein pattern analysis (49).

The highest level of genetic diversity of any species known is found in *Pseudomonas stutzeri,* which has at least 18 genomovars (131), with clinical isolates being found in genomovars 1 and 2. There are no consistent phenotypic differences to justify splitting *P. stutzeri* into unique species (49).

Pseudomonas fluorescens was originally divided into biotypes A, B, C, D, E, F, and G (biotypes A to E are also referred to as biovars I, II, III, IV, and V). Biotype B was reclassified as *Pseudomonas marginalis.* Biotypes D and E (*Pseudomonas chlororaphis* and *Pseudomonas aureofaciens*) have now been combined into the single species *P. chlororaphis,* which is no longer considered a member of the fluorescent pseudomonad group.

Pseudomonas putida consists of biovars A and B. Biovar A should be regarded as the typical *P. putida* (34), while biovar B may have a closer affinity with *P. fluorescens.* More biovars of *P. putida* are warranted (34).

Great heterogeneity is found within the species of *P. stutzeri, P. fluorescens,* and *P. putida,* which are of interest mainly to plant, marine, soil, and biotechnical sciences. They are of limited importance in clinical medicine. As polyphasic taxonomy continues to advance, more changes will doubtlessly arise; the clinical laboratory must keep abreast of such changes in order to differentiate these isolates from the more clinically important *Pseudomonas* species.

GENERAL DESCRIPTION

Pseudomonas spp. are aerobic, non-spore-forming, gram-negative rods which are straight or slightly curved and 0.5 to 1.0 by 1.5 to 5.0 μm in size (63). They are usually motile, with one or several polar flagella. They possess a strictly aerobic respiratory metabolism with oxygen as the terminal electron acceptor; in some cases nitrate can be used as an alternative electron acceptor that allows anaerobic growth. Most species of clinical interest are oxidase positive (except *Pseudomonas luteola* and *Pseudomonas oryzihabitans*). *Pseudomonas* spp. are catalase positive and are chemolithotrophs.

NATURAL HABITATS

Most *Pseudomonas* species can reside in a wide variety of environmental niches. Since their preferred temperature requirements are between 4 and 36°C and they can utilize an extraordinarily varied range of nutrients, they can be found throughout nature, provided that a moist environment is available. For example, *P. putida* is commonly found in soil, water, plants, and hospital sources such as sinks and floors. When isolated from human specimens, they are usually of indeterminate clinical significance. Due to their opportunistic nature, *Pseudomonas* species such as *Pseudomonas veronii,* found in mineral water (32), may account for unusual isolates that may infect immunocompromised patients.

*This chapter contains information presented in chapter 47 by Deanna L. Kiska and Peter H. Gilligan in the eighth edition of this Manual.

EPIDEMIOLOGY AND TRANSMISSION

P. aeruginosa is hydrophilic and can be readily recovered from moist environments, such as sink drains, vegetables, river water, and even antiseptic solutions. The propensity of *P. aeruginosa* to colonize raw vegetables might pose a risk to immunocompromised (particularly neutropenic) patients (118). However, none of these environmental reservoirs poses a great risk to most individuals; ingestion does not appear to induce gastrointestinal colonization unless antibiotic therapy has altered the normal bacterial flora.

Pseudomonas species, and in particular the human pathogen *P. aeruginosa,* rarely colonize healthy humans (136). The throat, intact skin, or stools of healthy individuals are heavily colonized by normal flora, which does not include *Pseudomonas* species. Indeed, if *P. aeruginosa* (and in particular the mucoid variant) is recovered from a throat culture of an otherwise healthy individual, an explanation should usually be sought. The gastrointestinal tracts of healthy humans and mice are heavily colonized with other bacteria that likely provide colonization resistance against *P. aeruginosa*. Healthy mice fed 10^7 CFU of *P. aeruginosa* fail to sustain intestinal colonization unless they have been pretreated with antibiotics (72).

Individuals (such as neutropenic cancer patients) receiving frequent courses of antibiotic therapy are at risk of gastrointestinal colonization with *P. aeruginosa;* it is from this reservoir that they are then at risk for *P. aeruginosa* septicemia. Such autoinfection has been demonstrated by recovering *P. aeruginosa* from the stools of neutropenic hosts prior to a bout of sepsis with the same strain (149). Similar observations have been made for neutropenic mice (72).

P. aeruginosa can be recovered from body sites that remain moist, such as the outer ear of children who swim frequently or the endotracheal tubes of patients receiving mechanical ventilation (93). For reasons which remain poorly understood, *P. aeruginosa* can also colonize the upper respiratory tracts of patients in intensive care units; this may be due in part to the alteration of the buccal epithelial cells with loss of fibronectin and attendant loss of the cells' antiadhesive properties (163). Adults receiving mechanical ventilation or neutropenic patients are at high risk for developing ventilator-associated or other pneumonias caused by *P. aeruginosa* (17), particularly after or during treatment with broad-spectrum antimicrobial agents (121). Patients at greatest risk are adults undergoing cancer chemotherapy or marrow ablation for bone marrow transplantation; children with similar conditions are at lesser risk for *P. aeruginosa* bacteremia. Individuals with congenital neutropenia or cyclic neutropenia do not appear to be at much risk for invasive infection with *P. aeruginosa*. Normal skin does not support *P. aeruginosa* colonization, but burned skin is an attractive site for this bacterium, which is one of the leading causes of burn wound sepsis.

P. aeruginosa is the predominant respiratory tract pathogen in patients with cystic fibrosis (CF) (47), but its mode of acquisition is poorly understood (133). Several studies have each demonstrated a common clone in particular groups of patients who have received their care at the same center (7, 18, 68); this is most likely due to patient-to-patient spread. However, in most patients with CF, it appears that the infecting strain undergoes a switch from the environmental phenotype (lipopolysaccharide [LPS] smooth, nonmucoid, and motile) to the CF phenotype (LPS rough, mucoid, and nonmotile) during the course of infection (135). That patients each tend to carry a unique strain during the course of infection (101, 137) suggests that the infection was acquired from an environmental source. One large study performed in Vancouver, Canada, over more than 20 years failed to demonstrate patient-to-patient spread of *P. aeruginosa* except between siblings (137). Infection control policies applicable to CF patients for transmission prevention should be determined by local epidemiological experience (154).

CLINICAL SIGNIFICANCE

P. aeruginosa

Individuals with intact host defenses are not at risk for serious infection with *P. aeruginosa,* but those whose circulating neutrophil counts are profoundly depressed (such as patients with cancer receiving chemotherapy) are at risk for invasive infection (134). Neutropenic hosts who develop antibodies against specific serotypes of *P. aeruginosa* appear to be protected against infection with those types during periods of neutropenia (109), illustrating the important role for opsonization in protection against blood-borne infection. Individuals with thermal burns are at risk for invasive disease because the dermal barrier can be breached, and patients on mechanical ventilation are at risk for pneumonia because the normal respiratory mucociliary clearance is compromised.

Recovery of *P. aeruginosa* from respiratory tract cultures of patients receiving mechanical ventilation may not indicate a true infection, and the significance of its presence in the culture should be interpreted with caution.

P. aeruginosa has a particular tropism for CF epithelial cells and can resist normal respiratory tract host defenses. Once infection is established, it usually persists, and the bacteria undergo a transition to the CF phenotype consisting of the following: (i) a rough LPS (53), in which the O-polysaccharide is incompletely expressed, rendering the bacteria susceptible to the bactericidal effect of human serum; (ii) mucoid colonial morphology (80) resulting from the exuberant production of a mucoid expolysaccharide composed of O-acetylated guluronic and mannuronic acids; (iii) nonmotility (87), meaning that the bacteria lack normal functional flagellar function; and (iv) hypoexpression of various exotoxins and other exoproducts (11). Some of these changes may be under global regulation, but they can also be expressed individually. Transition of *P. aeruginosa* from nonmucoid to mucoid in the CF patient's lung is usually associated with an accelerated decline in pulmonary function and an adverse prognosis (106), perhaps because of the capacity of the mucoid exopolysaccharide to interfere with normal host phagocytic defenses (47, 136) and to facilitate the formation of biofilms (76). Biofilm formation may also be enhanced by another colonial form, small-colony variants (previously known as dwarf colonies) (56). Furthermore, CF patients receive frequent courses of antipseudomonas antimicrobial therapy, often rendering the bacterium with which they are chronically infected resistant to a wide range of antimicrobial agents (54).

Thermal burns of the skin inhibit an essential component of the body's defense against infection, the physical barrier of the intact dermis (113). The resulting damaged tissue is a rich culture medium and is at great risk for colonization and infection by *P. aeruginosa;* such infections have been one of the leading causes of morbidity and mortality in victims of burns. Topical therapy is designed to prevent *P. aeruginosa* and other pathogens from causing infection. Infections of burn wounds with gram-negative bacteria (in particular *P. aeruginosa*) typically occur about 1 week after the injury. The extent of the burn has a profound influence on the risk of infection and prognosis (113). Prevention of bacterial burn wound infection has become so effective over the past decade that it is now very rare, and in many centers fungal infections predominate.

P. aeruginosa is the most common cause of osteochondritis of the dorsum of the foot following penetrating wounds (20). The typical scenario involves a child who has stepped on a nail which pierces the foot after passing through the sole of a running shoe. The prevalence of *P. aeruginosa* as the etiological agent may be due to its propensity to survive in the rubber of old running shoes (35).

Because *P. aeruginosa* can survive up to 42°C, hot tub users are at risk of *P. aeruginosa* folliculitis (48), a self-limiting condition for normal hosts that resolves rapidly. People who spend extended periods for time swimming are at risk for external ear infections ("swimmer's ear"), another self-limiting condition in immunocompetent people that responds readily to therapy with topical antimicrobial agents (9). The cornea is relatively resistant to infection except when its integrity has been broken. Users of contact lenses are at risk of *P. aeruginosa* conjunctivitis, especially if hygiene is poor or lenses are worn for extended periods of time (142).

P. aeruginosa can cause meningitis (usually following trauma or surgery) (36), malignant otitis externa in diabetics (122), sepsis and meningitis in newborns (145), endocarditis or osteomyelitis in intravenous drug users (126), community-acquired pneumonia in people with underlying lung disease such as bronchiectasis (43), urinary tract infections in patients with complex urinary tract abnormalities (120), and peritonitis (97). Each of these presentations is unusual and is superimposed on some inhibition of normal host defenses.

Other *Pseudomonas* Species

Healthy individuals are resistant to serious infections by all *Pseudomonas* species, including *P. aeruginosa*. However, immunocompromised hosts are occasionally infected with one of the many non-*P. aeruginosa* species (Table 1). Several of these species have been recovered from the respiratory secretions of patients with CF, but their role in pathogenesis of lung disease has not been determined. Some of these species have the capacity, like *P. aeruginosa,* to grow in hostile environments, such as antiseptic solutions; they can therefore be the cause of pseudobacteremia. Because of their low virulence, infections due to these species are often iatrogenic and are associated with the administration of contaminated solutions, medicines, and blood products or with the presence of indwelling catheters. *P. fluorescens* and *P. putida* have the ability to grow at 4°C, and *P. fluorescens* can be isolated from the skin of a small proportion of blood donors (128), resulting in occasional transfusion-associated septicemia in the recipient.

COLLECTION, TRANSPORT, AND STORAGE OF SPECIMENS

Pseudomonas spp. are able to survive in diverse environments. These organisms are easily recovered from clinical specimens by using standard collection, transport, and storage techniques as outlined in chapters 5 and 20.

DIRECT EXAMINATION

Pseudomonas organisms are gram-negative, non-spore-forming, straight or slightly curved bacilli measuring 0.5 to 0.8 μm by

TABLE 1 Non-*P. aeruginosa* isolates of *Pseudomonas* spp. recovered from human clinical specimens

Organism	Source	Reference(s)
P. fluorescens	Respiratory isolates from CF patients, transfusion-associated septicemia, pseudobacteremia	128
P. putida	Nosocomial infections including bacteremia, pneumonia, and urinary tract infections following external instrumentation/catheterization. CF, elderly, and immunocompromised patients are most vulnerable.	74, 165
P. veronii	Associated with an intestinal inflammatory pseudotumor	19
P. monteilii	Recovered from stool, bile, placenta, bronchial aspirates, pleural fluid, and urine, but of uncertain clinical significance	33
P. mosseilii	Various clinical specimens of uncertain clinical significance	26
P. stutzeri	Respiratory isolates of CF patients, alcoholics with pneumonia; immunocompromised patients with bacteremia, meningitis, and pneumonia; and patients with osteomyelitis, iatrogenic endophthalmitis, pseudobacteremia, and bacteremia from contaminated hemodialysis fluid. Also recovered from respiratory tracts of intubated patients, from urine, and from wound specimens in which pathogenic role was uncertain.	15, 45, 67, 70, 99, 112, 117, 119
P. mendocina	Rare cases of endocarditis	6
P. alcaligenes	One reported case of catheter-related endocarditis in a bone marrow transplant recipient	90
P. pseudoalcaligenes	A case of meningitis. Also isolated from sputum and urine. May be coisolated with other pathogens in wounds in which clinical significance is uncertain.	24
P. luteola	Associated with bacteremia, cellulitis, osteomyelitis, peritonitis, endocarditis, and postsurgical meningitis	115, 116
P. oryzihabitans	Bacteremia in immunocompromised patients with central venous access devices, peritonitis in peritoneal dialysis patients, cellulitis, abscesses, wound infections, and postsurgical meningitis	89, 115

1.5 to 3.0 μm. The Gram stain morphology cannot easily distinguish *Pseudomonas* spp. from other nonfermenting bacilli, although they are usually thinner than *Enterobacteriaceae*. Among the pseudomonads, there is some variation in Gram stain morphology. Certain strains of *P. putida* can appear elongated. Organisms from older cultures may appear slightly pleomorphic. Mucoid strains may be distinguished on direct examination by the presence of clusters or long filaments of short gram-negative bacilli surrounded by darker pink staining material (alginate). It is important to note this on direct examination since the organisms may grow very slowly or not at all. The presence of these mucoid forms should be documented on clinical reports. Because *Pseudomonas* spp. may be colonizers, their isolation does not always link them to clinical disease. However, their intracellular presence in polymorphonuclear cells is clinically significant and should be documented and direct further workup. Flagellar stains reveal one or more polar flagella (Table 2). *P. aeruginosa* has a single polar flagellum.

NUCLEIC ACID DETECTION TECHNIQUES

P. aeruginosa and other *Pseudomonas* species are detected ordinarily by culture techniques; these methods are particularly important for determining antimicrobial susceptibility, as these organisms have a high degree of intrinsic and acquired resistance (54, 83). When a more rapid method is desired, such as for screening environmental niches or for rapidly evaluating the sputum of patients with CF (22, 138), methods that can be used include PCR amplification of various genomic regions, such as genes for ribosomal RNA (65), heat shock protein (22), or exotoxin A (71). Conventional and real-time PCR (RT-PCR) (65) are both useful, and the amplification of multiple targets is valuable in the identification of non-*aeruginosa Pseudomonas* species (114). Fluorescence in-situ hybridization (FISH) is very specific, although it lacks sensitivity below 10^4 CFU (62). Both RT-PCR and FISH are rapid, cost-effective methods, and FISH doesn't require costly technical equipment (159). Probes directed at species-specific 16S rRNA (50, 141) may have a role in the identification of clinically relevant, biochemically inactive *Pseudomonas* species including certain strains of *P. aeruginosa* (114). PCR amplification of 16S rRNA followed by restriction fragment length polymorphism (RFLP) analysis has been used to successfully identify and characterize members of the fluorescent pseudomonad group (75). Since RFLP of the 16S gene does not provide sufficient resolution among genomovars of a species, a more discriminatory test may be used, such as sequencing the internally transcribed 16S-23S rRNA spacer internal transcribed spacer 1 regions, believed to have more genetic variability among genomovars (49). It should be noted that commercial probes are not yet available.

CULTURE AND ISOLATION

Pseudomonas species have very simple nutritional requirements and grow well on standard broth and solid laboratory media such as tryptic soy or columbia agar with 5% sheep blood, chocolate agar, and MacConkey agar, which are recommended to isolate *Pseudomonas* spp. from clinical specimens. MacConkey agar is also a differential medium helpful in identifying different strains of *Pseudomonas* spp., including mucoid strains of *P. aeruginosa* from CF patients. Multiple selective media containing inhibitors such as acetamide, nitrofurantoin, phenanthroline, 9-chloro-9-[4-(diethyamino)phenyl]-9,10-dihydro-10-phenylacridine hydrochloride (C-390), and cetrimide (14, 58) have been used for the isolation and presumptive identification of *P. aeruginosa* from clinical and environmental samples. Inhibition of some strains of *P. aeruginosa* from CF sputum specimens has been reported to occur with the use of a selective agar containing cetrimide (200 mg/liter) and nalidixic acid (15 mg/liter) (37), emphasizing the need to use both selective and nonselective media for recovery of bacteria from these patients. Some of the non-*aeruginosa* pseudomonads may grow better at lower temperatures of 28 to 30°C. Good growth is usually achieved after 24 to 48 h of incubation. For cultures from CF patients, it is recommended that solid media plates be held at 35 to 37°C for 5 days.

IDENTIFICATION

Fluorescent Group

Members of the fluorescent pseudomonad group produce pyoverdin (fluorescein), a water-soluble yellow-green or yellow-brown pigment that fluoresces under short-wavelength UV light. Many strains of *P. aeruginosa* can produce the blue pigment pyocyanin. When pyoverdin combines with the blue water-soluble phenazine pigment pyocyanin, the bright green color characteristic of *P. aeruginosa* is created. This organism may also produce other water-soluble pigments such as pyorubrin (red) or pyomelanin (brown/black). Conditions of iron limitation enhance pigment production, as these pigments act as siderophores in iron uptake systems of the bacteria. Non-dye-containing media enhance visualization of pigments.

P. aeruginosa

Most *P. aeruginosa* are easily recognizable on primary isolation media on the basis of characteristic colonial morphology, production of diffusible pigments, and a grape-like odor. Older cultures may exhibit a corn taco-like odor. Colonies are usually flat and spreading and have a serrated edge and a metallic sheen that is often associated with autolysis of the colonies (166). Other morphologies exist, including smooth, mucoid, and dwarf (small-colony variants) (104, 155). Mucoid colonial variants are particularly prevalent in respiratory tract specimens from CF patients.

P. aeruginosa is distinct from the rest of the clinically relevant fluorescent pseudomonads in its ability to grow at 42°C (see Table 2 for other tests). In addition to pigment production, other tests that confirm its identification are positive oxidase and arginine tests and an alkaline over no-change reaction in a triple-sugar iron agar slant.

Microbiologists must be aware of certain variations in the phenotypes of *P. aeruginosa*. Isolates lacking oxidase activity have occasionally been reported, but they exhibit the other characteristic features; prior antibiotic therapy with agents that affect protein synthesis may cause the aberrant phenotype (52). Mucoid isolates of *P. aeruginosa* from CF patients may undergo several phenotypic changes including slow growth, loss of motility, and loss of pigment production. Small colony variants may require prolonged incubation, lack motility, be hyperpiliated, adhere to agar surface, and show autoaggregative properties in liquid medium (155).

P. fluorescens and *P. putida*

P. fluorescens and *P. putida* do not possess distinctive colony morphology or odor. Their inability to reduce nitrates to

TABLE 2 Characteristics of *Pseudomonas* species found in clinical specimens[a]

Test	*P. aeruginosa* (n = 201)	*P. fluorescens* (n = 155)	*P. putida* (n = 16)	*P. veronii* (n = 8)	*P. monteilii* (n = 10)	*P. mosseilii* (n = 12)	*P. stutzeri* (n = 28)	*P. mendocina* (n = 4)	*P. pseudoalcaligenes* (n = 34)	*P. alcaligenes* (n = 26)	*P. luteola* (n = 34)	*P. oryzihabitans* (n = 36)
Oxidase	99	97	100	100	100	100	100	100	100	96	0	0
Growth:												
MacConkey	100	100	100	ND[c]	ND	ND	100	100	100	96	100	100
Cetrimide	94	89	81 (6)	ND	90	100	4	75 (25)	56 (18)	15	0	25 (28)
6% NaCl	65	43	100	ND	0	100[e]	80 (16)	100	62 (6)	41	74	62
42°C	100	0	0	0	0	0	69	100	94	V[f]	94	33
Nitrate reduction	98	19	0	100	0	0	100	100	100	54	62	6
Gas from nitrate	93	3	0	100	0	0	100	100	0	0	0	0
Pyoverdin	65	96	93	100	100	100	0	0	0	0	0	0
Arginine dihydrolase	100	97	100	100	100	100	0[d]	100	78	12	100	14
Lysine decarboxylase	0	0	0	ND	0	0	0	0	0	0	0	7
Ornithine decarboxylase	0	0	0	ND	0	0	0	0	0	0	0	3
Hydrolysis:												
Urea	48 (9)	21 (31)	31 (44)	25	50	ND	33 (22)	50	3 (6)	0	26 (38)	77
Gelatin[g]	82	100	0	13	0	92	0	0	0	0	61	17
Acetamide	100	6 (12)	0	0	0	ND	0	0	ND	ND	ND	ND
Esculin	0	0	0	ND	0	0	0	0	0	0	100	0
Starch	0	0	0	ND	0	8	100	0	0	0	0	0
Acid from[b]:												
Glucose	97	100	100	100	100	100	96 (4)	100	9	0	100	100
Fructose	ND	ND	ND	100	100	100	ND	ND	79 (21)	0	ND	ND
Xylose	90	100	100	100	0	0	93 (7)	75 (25)	18 (12)	0	100	100
Lactose	<1	24	25 (13)	ND	0	0	0	0	0	0	3 (24)	14 (22)
Sucrose	0	48	0	100	0	17	0	0	0	0	12	25
Maltose	<1	2	31	ND	0	17	100	0	0	0	100	97
Mannitol	70	53	25	ND	0	75	89 (4)	0	0	0	76 (18)	100
Simmons citrate	95	93	94 (6)	ND	100	100	82 (14)	100	26 (9)	57 (8)	100	97
No. of flagella	1	>1	>1	1	ND	1	1	1	1	1	>1	1

[a] Results are given as percentages of positive strains; percentages in parentheses represent strains with delayed reactions. Data are from references 26, 32, 33, 63, and 160.
[b] Oxidative-fermentative basal medium with 1% carbohydrate.
[c] ND, no data.
[d] *P. stutzeri*-like organisms (formerly CDC group 3b) are arginine dihydrolase positive.
[e] Growth at 3 to 5% NaCl but not at 7% NaCl.
[f] V, variable, many strains can grow at 41°C; see comment in text under "Identification."
[g] Results are for 7-day incubation.

nitrogen gas and their ability to produce acid from xylose distinguish these two species from the other fluorescent pseudomonads. *P. fluorescens* can be differentiated from *P. putida* by its ability to grow at 4°C and to hydrolyze gelatin. *P. fluorescens* isolates may require 4 to 7 days of incubation for accurate detection of gelatin hydrolysis. The package insert for API 20NE (bioMérieux Vitek, Hazelwood, Mo.) states that only 39% of *P. fluorescens* isolates hydrolyze gelatin in 24 to 48 h in this test system.

P. veronii, P. monteilii, and *P. mosselii*

P. veronii can reduce nitrates to nitrogen gas but is unable to hydrolyze acetamide. The type strain of *P. veronii* (LMG 17761) is negative for acid from lactose and maltose and does not grow at 36°C (D. A. Henry, personal observation). *P. monteilii* can be distinguished from the other members of the fluorescent group by its inability to reduce nitrates to nitrites or nitrogen gas, to hydrolyze gelatin, or to produce acid from xylose. *P. mosselii* can reduce nitrates neither to nitrites nor to nitrogen gas, nor can it produce acid from xylose; but most isolates (92%) can hydrolyze gelatin (Table 2).

Other fluorescent pseudomonads are rarely encountered in clinical specimens. Many of these isolates are negative for arginine dihydrolase activity. Identification as "*Pseudomonas* species not *aeruginosa*" and susceptibility testing of the isolates, when appropriate, are sufficient in most circumstances. When necessary, these isolates can be referred to reference laboratories.

Nonfluorescent Group

P. stutzeri and *P. mendocina*

Most *P. stutzeri* isolates are easily recognized on primary isolation media by their distinctive dry, wrinkled colony morphology, similar to that of *Burkholderia pseudomallei*. *P. stutzeri* can be distinguished from the latter species by its lack of arginine dihydrolase activity and inability to produce acid from lactose. *P. stutzeri* colonies can pit or adhere to the agar and are buff to brown in color. The adherence can make removal of colonies from agar medium difficult. Because of the difficulty in making suspensions of specific turbidity, commercial susceptibility systems may not work well with this organism. Not all isolates of *P. stutzeri* produce wrinkled colonies; such strains can be distinguished from other pseudomonads by their ability to hydrolyze starch, a unique reaction for this species.

P. mendocina colonies are smooth and flat and produce a brownish yellow pigment. Key biochemical characteristics include the ability to reduce nitrates to nitrogen gas, positive arginine dihydrolase activity, and inability to hydrolyze acetamide.

P. alcaligenes and *P. pseudoalcaligenes*

P. alcaligenes and *P. pseudoalcaligenes* have rarely been encountered in clinical samples and do not have a distinctive colony morphology. Compared to other pseudomonads, they are biochemically inactive. Characteristics that distinguish them from other biochemically inactive gram-negative rods are a positive oxidase reaction, motility due to a polar flagellum, and growth on MacConkey agar. *P. alcaligenes* is distinguished from *P. pseudoalcaligenes* by its inability to oxidize fructose. Although growth at 42°C was thought to be a distinguishing feature between them, further studies now indicate that growth at 41°C (and probably 42°C) is also present in most strains of *P. alcaligenes* (N. Palleroni, personal communication). These organisms are difficult to identify by many commercial systems, and for most clinical situations they can simply be referred to as "*Pseudomonas* spp. not *aeruginosa*." If the clinical situation dictates a definitive identification, assistance from reference laboratories should be sought.

P. luteola and *P. oryzihabitans*

P. luteola and *P. oryzihabitans* (formerly CDCVe-1 and CDCVe-2, respectively) can be distinguished from other pseudomonads by their negative oxidase reaction and production of an intracellular, nondiffusible yellow pigment. Both organisms typically exhibit rough, wrinkled, adherent colonies or, more rarely, smooth colonies. *P. luteola* can be differentiated from *P. oryzihabitans* on the basis of its ability to hydrolyze *o*-nitrophenyl-β-D-galactopyranoside (ONPG) and esculin.

Use of Commercial Identification Systems

Commercial identification systems are used increasingly in many laboratories to identify *Pseudomonas* spp. Commercial products can be divided into manual and automated systems. The more frequently used manual systems are the API 20NE (bioMérieux Vitek), Crystal E/NF (Becton Dickinson, Sparks, Md.), and RapID NF Plus (Remel Inc., Lenexa, Kans.). The manual systems usually provide accurate identification of *P. aeruginosa,* including mucoid isolates as well as other *Pseudomonas* species, and are preferred over automated systems for isolates from CF patients.

Automated systems (see chapter 15) are commonly used in many medium-to-large clinical laboratories. As *P. aeruginosa* is easily identified by a few conventional biochemical tests, it is not necessary to use a more expensive commercial system. Several of the automated systems are not very accurate and may require additional testing for non-*P. aeruginosa* species; thus, their labor-, cost-, and time-saving benefits are lost. Automated systems can identify *P. aeruginosa* from non-CF patient sources with 90 to 100% accuracy (40, 103), but some systems such as the Autoscan-W/A (Dade Behring Microscan Inc., West Sacramento, Calif.) may require additional tests to achieve these results (102, 147). Most reviews focus on the evaluation of *P. aeruginosa* with only a few, if any, other *Pseudomonas* species represented in the organisms being tested. When other *Pseudomonas* species were included, the new Vitek 2GN panel performed well (39, 103) while the Autoscan and BD Phoenix (Becton Dickinson) often relied on additional testing to obtain an identification (30, 102, 140, 147). Hence, it is wise to consider carefully the clinical significance, colonial morphology, and other key features before accepting results from automated systems.

Identification of *Pseudomonas* species, especially those isolated from CF patients, is not always optimal with rapid systems. The Autoscan-W/A system (Negative Combo 15) performed poorly for CF isolates when they were incubated for 20 to 24 h according to the manufacturer's method, with only 57% of nonmucoid and 40% of mucoid *P. aeruginosa* isolates correctly identified (125). Extension of incubation to 48 h improved accuracy to 86 and 83%, respectively. Misidentified species were most commonly identified as either *Alcaligenes* spp. or *P. fluorescens/P. putida.* Other automated systems have not been evaluated to date specifically for the identification of CF patient isolates, so caution in interpreting results is advised.

TYPING SYSTEMS

Genotypic methods have generally supplanted conventional schemes based on phenotypic characteristics (reviewed in reference 133) such as LPS serotyping and phage typing. Several different genotypic methods for typing *P. aeruginosa* for epidemiological purposes are useful, even for typing isolates from patients with CF, but they are not available in most clinical diagnostic laboratories, and their use is often dependent upon local availability.

RFLP

This method relies upon the genetic diversity that exists upstream of the gene for exotoxin A (*exoA*) in *P. aeruginosa* (101). In a study of different typing methods, *exoA* RFLP proved superior to all phenotypic methods for typing *P. aeruginosa* (151). Pilin gene RFLP has demonstrated that individual CF patients are durably infected with the same strain despite changes in pilin protein expression (101). The disadvantages of RFLP are its relatively weak discriminatory power compared to that of newer methods, its cumbersome nature, and its predominant use of radioactive probes.

PFGE

P. aeruginosa has substantial genetic plasticity, so there can be more than three band differences among isolates typed by pulsed-field gel electrophoresis (PFGE) (see chapter 11) and considered epidemiologically to be from the same strain, even though Tenover's criteria state that if there are three or fewer banding differences between two isolates, they should be considered to be from the same strain, as such differences are likely to be due to only one genetic event (150). The advantages of PFGE are its universal utility for typing virtually any bacterial species and its high discriminatory power. The major disadvantages are its requirement for specialized equipment and its inability to evaluate a large number of isolates rapidly.

PCR-Based Typing Methods

PCR-based methods used for typing *P. aeruginosa* are directed at known elements within the genome or against random but relatively frequently encoded sequences. The latter method, random amplified polymorphic DNA analysis (RAPD), has proved quite robust for typing *P. aeruginosa* (88), but it must be run consistently on the same equipment to yield reproducible results. Data from RAPD analysis usually are highly consistent with those from PFGE. PCR-amplified products can be digested with restriction enzymes to yield more discriminatory data (127).

Multilocus Sequence Typing

Multilocus sequence typing has only recently been employed for typing *P. aeruginosa*. It is likely to be the most highly discriminatory among the genetic typing tools, but it is extremely time-consuming and expensive to employ. The method entails PCR amplification of specific genes and then sequencing of the gene products. This can be done only in very specialized centers, but it has the power to provide highly reliable data on relatedness among isolates. Standards are currently being developed, and a large study is evaluating the suitability of this method for typing *P. aeruginosa* (25).

ANTIMICROBIAL SUSCEPTIBILITY

P. aeruginosa possesses intrinsic resistance to many antibiotic classes and has the ability to develop resistance by mutations in different chromosomal loci or by horizontal acquisition of resistance genes carried on plasmids, transposons, or integrons. The frequent acquisition of antimicrobial resistance in *P. aeruginosa* limits the utility of antimicrobial susceptibility patterns as a tool in epidemiologic typing.

Mechanisms of Resistance

Intrinsic Resistance

P. aeruginosa has two main mechanisms of intrinsic resistance: an inducible chromosomal AmpC β-lactamase that renders it resistant to ampicillin, amoxicillin, amoxicillin-clavulanate, narrow-spectrum and expanded-spectrum cephalosporins, cefotaxime, and ceftriaxone (81); and several efflux pump systems (83).

Acquired Resistance

Various antibiotics overcome the intrinsic resistance of *P. aeruginosa*. These include extended-spectrum penicillins (piperacillin and ticarcillin), certain expanded-spectrum cephalosporins (ceftazidime and cefipime), carbapenems (imipenem and meropenem), monobactams (aztreonam), fluoroquinolones (ciprofloxacin and levofloxacin), aminoglycosides (gentamicin, tobramycin, and amikacin), and colistin. Unfortunately, mutational resistance to all the antipseudomonal antibiotics can develop.

A mutation at the AmpD locus, selected by therapy with antipseudomonal penicillins or ceftazidime (82), can result in partial or total derepression of the AmpC enzyme, which may account for 30% of β-lactamase resistance in *P. aeruginosa* (16).

Target mutations to topoisomerases II (*gyrA* and *gyrB* subunits) and IV (*parC* and *parE* subunits) confer quinolone resistance more readily in *P. aeruginosa* than in *Enterobacteriaceae*. Selection of mutants occurs after exposure to quinolones, and evidence suggests that levofloxacin has a greater potential to induce these mutations than ciprofloxacin (44).

Although multidrug efflux pump systems play a significant role in the intrinsic resistance of *P. aeruginosa*, they also are critical to the development of multidrug resistance (98). MexAB-OprM is expressed constitutively in all strains of *P. aeruginosa*. Upregulation or a mutation in the *mexR* repressor gene (*nalB* mutant) results in efflux pump overproduction and significant increase in the MICs of multiple antibiotics (111).

Efflux pump mutants may appear under conditions favoring high bacterial density as found in abscesses, empyemas, diabetic foot infections, and chronic lung infections. In one study, efflux pump-overproducing mutants were found in isolates from 80% of CF patients who had received earlier treatment with ciprofloxacin (66). Overexpression of efflux pumps may also be selected by the use of antiseptics and biocides (79). Evidence of multiple resistance determinants including an efflux transport system encoded by a transmissible plasmid in environmental bacteria (148) would be of grave concern if these genetic elements were to be transferred to *Pseudomonas* species.

Impermeability mutations may result in resistance to carbapenem, aminoglycosides, colistin, and quinolones. They are important in carbapenem resistance and result from the loss of the OprD porin, which is associated with low-level (MIC, 8 to 32 μg/ml) imipenem resistance and decreased susceptibility to meropenem (73). Resistance by this mechanism depends on the continued expression of the chromosomal AmpC β-lactamase. Selection of imipenem resistance following imipenem therapy is more frequent than selection of resistance to any other β-lactam agent (152).

Mutational impermeability is also associated with reduced aminoglycoside transport into the cell and lack of susceptibility to all aminoglycosides. Impermeability may be the major mechanism of aminoglycoside resistance, especially in CF patients (85), but it is clear that efflux systems also contribute (3).

Membrane changes most likely account for colistin resistance, which is rare but increasing, especially in CF patients who receive inhalational colistin (78). It appears that regulatory genes for the outer membrane protein OprH, specifically the LPS component of the outer membrane, may be involved in both aminoglycoside and colistin resistance (77, 110). Decreased uptake as a result of porin reduction contributes to quinolone resistance but seems to be synergistically linked to upregulation of efflux pumps (79).

The acquisition of β-lactamases is not as common for *P. aeruginosa* as it is for *Enterobacteriaceae* (81). Nevertheless, β-lactamases are being recognized increasingly and are very diverse in this organism. The most common β-lactamases are PSE-1 and PSE-4, which do not affect ceftazidime, cefipime, aztreonam, or carbapenems (83). Other enzymes have been found in limited geographic locations, suggesting a specific ecological niche. More recently, extended-spectrum β-lactamases (ESBLs) in *P. aeruginosa* have been described. Genes for ESBLs are carried on plasmids, integrons in plasmids, or in the bacterial chromosome (83, 157). This group of enzymes is inhibited by clavulanic acid and only marginally inhibited by tazobactam. With minor variations, substrates for most of these enzymes include antipseudomonal penicillins, ceftazidime, cefipime, and aztreonam (64).

The OXA family of enzymes (Ambler Molecular Class D) (4) are found most commonly in *P. aeruginosa* (96, 146). Genes for these enzymes are located in plasmids, on transposons, or on integrons, making their further dissemination likely. They confer resistance predominantly to antipseudomonal penicillins, ceftazidime, cefipime, and aztreonam but not carbapenems. Their activity is inhibited poorly by clavulanic acid or tazobactam (108).

With the exception of GES-2 (an ESBL that hydrolyzes carbapenems), all carbapenemases in *P. aeruginosa* belong to Ambler Class B, commonly referred to as metalloenzymes. Metalloenzymes are not inhibited by clavulanic acid but are inhibited by divalent ion chelators such as EDTA. They hydrolyze all β-lactam antibiotics, except aztreonam, and are associated with high-level (MIC, >32 μg/ml) carbapenem resistance. Underreporting of carbapenem resistance may occur, as expression of the carbepenemases varies, resulting in a wide range of MIC values (2 to 128 μg/ml) that may go undetected in clinical laboratories that rely only on automated systems. In many cases, carbapenem resistance, especially to meropenem, is derived from a synergistic combination of mechanisms (105), resulting in enhanced resistance. For example, diminished expression of OprD porin or activation of an efflux system enhances the activity of a β-lactamase by increasing extracellular accumulation of the antibiotic.

Although impermeability mutations can result in aminoglycoside resistance, especially in CF and intensive care patients, drug inactivation by plasmid or chromosomally encoded enzymes is the most common mechanism for resistance worldwide to aminoglycosides (110). Aminoglycoside-modifying enzymes have been detected in *P. aeruginosa* for over 30 years, resulting in various combinations of resistance to gentamicin, tobramycin, and/or amikacin. These enzymes are often encoded on transposons and/or integrons that carry resistance determinants for other classes of antibiotics such as sulfonamides, β-lactams, and chloramphenicol. Multiresistance genes for both aminoglycosides and extended-spectrum β-lactamases and metalloenzymes are of particular concern (110). Aminoglycoside-modifying enzymes can occur together with impermeability mutations (92), resulting in broad-spectrum aminoglycoside resistance.

The discovery of a plasmid-borne quinolone resistance determinant (*qnr*) in gram-negative organisms (156) is of significance for several reasons: it has been transferred by conjugation to multiple organisms including *P. aeruginosa;* it is associated with high-level quinolone resistance (up to 250-fold increase in MICs); it appears to be associated with integrons that carry resistance determinants to β-lactams and aminoglycosides; and it expands the spectrum of high-level plasmid-mediated resistance to quinolones.

Antibiotic Tolerance

Biofilm-producing *P. aeruginosa* isolates appear to be protected from killing by antibiotics (144). Although this is widely accepted to indicate antibiotic resistance, a more appropriate term is antibiotic tolerance. Although slower or stationary growth phase has classically been thought to account for relative antibiotic tolerance, many other mechanisms have been proposed. These include quorum sensing (130), decreased diffusion of antibiotics through the matrix polysaccharide alginate (59), synthesis of glucans that specifically bind antibiotics (86), phenotypic variability (31, 38), presence of persister cells (139), and anaerobic growth of biofilm bacteria, which affects the activity of multiple antibiotics (10, 55).

Multidrug Resistance

Worldwide, antimicrobial resistance, including multidrug (three or more antimicrobial classes) resistance among *P. aeruginosa,* is widespread and increasing. In 2003, the European MYSTIC study group reported considerable country-to-country variation in the proportion of multidrug-resistant *P. aeruginosa* isolates within Europe, ranging from 50% to less than 3% (46). The SENTRY Antimicrobial Surveillance Program confirmed geographic variation in Latin America but emphasized the rapid increase in multidrug-resistant strains with rates approaching 35% (123). From 1993 to 2002, in the United States, the rates of multidrug resistance increased from 4 to 14%, with highest rates of increase reported for ciprofloxacin, imipenem, tobramycin, and aztreonam (100). Globally, multidrug resistance was found in 10% of *P. aeruginosa* strains analyzed (41).

Antimicrobial Susceptibility Testing

It may be difficult to estimate the true prevalence of antimicrobial resistance in *P. aeruginosa* because detection of resistance by routine tests agrees poorly with MIC data (5, 60). Susceptibility testing of *P. aeruginosa* is challenging due to multiple mechanisms of resistance, both intrinsic and acquired, which are frequently expressed concurrently, often at low levels.

In clinical laboratories, susceptibility testing for *Pseudomonas* species may be performed by disk diffusion, agar or broth dilution, E test (AB Biodisk, Solna, Sweden), or automated susceptibility systems using broth microdilution. Disk diffusion tests are standardized in North America and perform satisfactorily for most clinical isolates of *P. aeruginosa* (23). Limitations of this method include the lack of a quantitative result (MIC) and the potential to miss low-level resistance. Agar dilution is a well-accepted, reliable MIC method, especially for mucoid isolates, but it is time-consuming and too expensive for most routine clinical laboratories. The E test (see chapter 73) has been shown to correlate well with agar dilution for isolates from CF (13) and non-CF patients (29).

Good correlation with reference methods has been reported for most automated systems (57, 140) when testing *Pseudomonas* isolates from non-CF patients. Results evaluating the performance of various automated systems must be interpreted with caution, as the numbers of isolates tested is often limited, especially for non-*P. aeruginosa* strains. Whereas most *P. aeruginosa* isolates grow well on agar media, growth of some isolates in broth is variable and may pose difficulties for laboratories that rely solely on automated systems. Alternatively, a liquid medium improves the detection of the efflux resistance phenotype, which may not be detected by solid-media-based testing (2, 30). This may account for some of the discrepancies reported when comparing different susceptibility methods.

Several antibiotics pose specific challenges to susceptibility testing. Carbapenem susceptibility testing results are difficult to interpret due to several factors that include rapid imipenem degradation (153), variable levels of efflux pump expression, and unstable impermeability mutations. Carbapenemase detection is especially challenging because it is associated with a wide range of MICs and lacks a simple test for detection. Susceptibility testing of imipenem with and without EDTA (disks or E-test strips) may be used but has been associated with variable results (164). Meropenem or ceftazidime, with or without EDTA, may be better substrates than imipenem, and testing these combinations may increase the sensitivity of the test (107). Reproducibility of carbapenem resistance results by using various susceptibility methods is poor, and it is recommended that initial carbapenem resistance be confirmed by a second antimicrobial susceptibility method (143). Although still restricted to reference laboratories, there are PCR-based methods for detection of carbapenemase production (158).

Colistin is being used more frequently in the treatment of multidrug-resistant *P. aeruginosa*. Disk diffusion testing does not correlate well with MIC results, and underreporting of resistance has been reported (42). Susceptibility testing of colistin should be performed by an MIC method such as agar dilution, E test, or broth microdilution. Prolonged incubation of 48 h is recommended for broth microdilution (61).

Isolates of *P. aeruginosa* from CF patients pose specific difficulties for microbiology laboratories. Isolates from these patients often exhibit mixed morphotypes including mucoid phenotypes, small-colony variants, and bacterial microcolonies in biofilms. Susceptibility testing is complicated by several factors including lack of correlation between susceptibility results and clinical response (132), different susceptibility patterns within a morphotype (38), lack of reproducibility of susceptibility tests, falsely positive susceptibility results, and the presence of hypermutable strains (51, 104). Mucoid and nonmucoid phenotypes of *P. aeruginosa* are often coisolated in specimens from patients with CF. Mucoid isolates tend to be more susceptible and have lower β-lactamase activity than nonmucoid isolates (21). One explanation may be that these isolates are protected from selective antibiotic pressure. Selective antibiotic pressure, notably from inhalational tobramycin or colistin therapy, gives rise to small-colony variants of *P. aeruginosa* with properties of increased antimicrobial resistance, autoaggregative growth behavior, and enhanced ability to form biofilms (155). In turn, bacterial cells in biofilms adapt into symbiotic bacterial communities in which the mucoid alginate-producing bacterial cells provide physical protection to the biofilm, while the highly antibiotic-resistant nonmucoid cells protect against antibiotic killing (21). The increased ability of biofilm bacteria to acquire resistance phenotypes (27) and the selection of hypermutable strains following antimicrobial therapy (51, 104) may explain the lack of eradication of *P. aeruginosa* from chronically infected CF patients. Since for bacteria found in biofilms MICs are 100- to 1,000-fold greater than for free-living, planktonic bacteria (95), routine susceptibility testing may underestimate resistance and may contribute to treatment failures. In a study of 597 CF isolates (13), both disk diffusion and E test were found to be generally acceptable as routine susceptibility testing methods. However, poor correlation was found with disk diffusion testing of mucoid isolates for piperacillin, piperacillin-tazobactam, and meropenem. Underreporting of resistance was more frequent with disk diffusion than with E test, especially when ceftazidime, piperacillin, and piperacillin-tazobactam were tested.

Hypermutable strains may be detected using either disk diffusion or E-test methods by the presence of resistant subpopulations within the inhibition zones of three or more antibiotics (84).

Mucoid isolates pose a specific challenge for automated systems (8, 12, 30). Overestimation of susceptibility may occur, as mucoid isolates often demonstrate insufficient growth at 24 h. Automated systems that allow for longer incubation may be preferable. On the other hand, overcalling resistance may result from the presence of large amounts of exopolysaccharide, resulting in turbidity without adequate bacterial growth. These limitations have led many microbiologists who routinely work with mucoid isolates of *P. aeruginosa* to choose alternative methods for susceptibility testing.

Isolating and individually testing all the morphotypes of *P. aeruginosa* is labor-intensive and time-consuming and may not provide clinically relevant susceptibility results. Mixed-morphotype testing using phenotypically different colonies directly from sputum cultures or from subcultures of isolated colonies has been shown to correlate well with disk diffusion and MIC susceptibility methods (162) and may provide clinically useful susceptibility data with significant time and cost savings. However, the correlation appears to be better for susceptible strains than for resistant strains (94). Direct sputum susceptibility testing using the E-test method has been suggested as an alternative to morphotype testing in assessing the in vivo situation by evaluating bacterial population susceptibility as well as potential interactions with other organisms, including commensal flora (129).

Other methods have been recommended in an attempt to better predict susceptibility results. Biofilm susceptibility assays which confirm that biofilm inhibitory concentrations are much higher than conventionally determined MICs for multiple antibiotics have been developed (95). Synergy testing, using microtiter checkerboard, time-kill test, broth macrodilution breakpoint combination sensitivity test, or E-test methods (129, 161), has been used to assess the activity of antibiotic combinations in vitro in order to predict in vivo synergistic activity. This testing is labor-intensive, time-consuming, and difficult to reproduce and does not result in better clinical and bacteriological outcomes than those obtained with therapy directed by standard culture and sensitivity techniques (1).

Susceptibility testing of *Pseudomonas* species other than *P. aeruginosa* is rarely indicated, and clinical correlation is required before susceptibility testing is performed. These organisms are generally susceptible to most antipseudomonal antibiotics as well as to trimethoprim-sulfamethoxazole (except most *P. fluorescens* or *P. putida* strains), a property that differentiates them from *P. aeruginosa*. *P. fluorescens*, *P. putida*, and *P. oryzihabitans* may be more resistant to aztreonam and ticarcillin-clavulanic acid. *P. stutzeri* is usually very susceptible to all antipseudomonal agents (124).

EVALUATION, INTERPRETATION, AND REPORTING OF RESULTS

Pseudomonas species represent a diverse group of organisms widely distributed in nature. *P. aeruginosa* may be associated with colonization or clinically significant infections. It is a major pathogen in CF patients and represents an important nosocomial and opportunistic pathogen. Interpretation of the Gram stain often directs the further workup of this organism. The presence of small clusters of gram-negative organisms surrounded by amorphous material is indicative of biofilm formation compatible with a chronic infection. This finding should be reported to physicians, and incubation should be prolonged because these strains usually exhibit slower-growth characteristics. The intracellular presence of these organisms in polymorphonuclear cells is clinically significant. Isolation of *P. aeruginosa* from sterile body sites should always be interpreted as indicative of probable infection. Pseudoinfection from contaminated skin disinfectant solutions can occur and should be considered if the patient is not severely ill and especially if there is a cluster of infections with the same strain of *Pseudomonas* spp. Disinfection solutions should be cultured using the same methods as those recommended for *Pseudomonas* species. Isolation in mixed culture requires correlation with the direct smear, other organisms isolated, and clinical history. Identification of this organism requires only a few simple tests, and commercial tests are not usually needed. Isolates from sites of chronic infection often exhibit multiple morphotypes, frequently with altered characteristics, which can make identification more difficult. Molecular methods increasingly are finding a role in the identification of this organism, especially for epidemiological studies. Susceptibility testing of these organisms is difficult, especially for mucoid isolates, due to increasing resistance, lack of reproducibility of results, and lack of clinical correlation. A basic understanding of the multiple mechanisms of resistance, both intrinsic and acquired, is essential to interpret susceptibility testing results and give therapeutic recommendations to physicians. Optimal treatment to eradicate infection and prevent resistance, especially in chronic infections, remains controversial. Judicious use of antibiotics is necessary to eradicate infections and avoid resistance. Combination therapy is prudent in serious infections such as endocarditis, septicemia, nosocomial pneumonia, central nervous system and prosthetic material-related infections, and bacteremia in neutropenic patients. Strict adherence to infection control measures, including handwashing, is essential to prevent the spread of these organisms within hospitals. Other *Pseudomonas* species are infrequently isolated in the laboratory and are usually not clinically significant. Clinical correlation and correlation with the Gram stain are essential before further workup is undertaken.

REFERENCES

1. **Aaron, S. D., W. Ferris, D. A. Henry, D. P. Speert, and N. E. Macdonald.** 2000. Multiple combination bactericidal antibiotic testing for patients with cystic fibrosis infected with *Burkholderia cepacia*. *Am. J. Respir. Crit. Care Med.* **161:**1206–1212.
2. **Aeschlimann, J. R.** 2003. The role of multidrug efflux pumps in the antibiotic resistance of *Pseudomonas aeruginosa* and other gram-negative bacteria. Insights from the Society of Infectious Diseases Pharmacists. *Pharmacotherapy* **23:**916–924.
3. **Aires, J. R., T. Kohler, H. Nikaido, and P. Plesiat.** 1999. Involvement of an active efflux system in the natural resistance of *Pseudomonas aeruginosa* to aminoglycosides. *Antimicrob. Agents Chemother.* **43:**2624–2628.
4. **Ambler, R. P.** 1980. The structure of beta-lactamases. *Philos. Trans. R. Soc. Lond. B Biol. Sci.* **289:**321–331.
5. **Andrews, J., R. Walker, and A. King.** 2002. Evaluation of media available for testing the susceptibility of *Pseudomonas aeruginosa* by BSAC methodology. *J. Antimicrob. Chemother.* **50:**479–486.
6. **Aragone, M. R., D. M. Maurizi, L. O. Clara, J. L. Navarro Estrada, and A. Ascione.** 1992. *Pseudomonas mendocina*, an environmental bacterium isolated from a patient with human infective endocarditis. *J. Clin. Microbiol.* **30:**1583–1584.
7. **Armstrong, D. S., G. M. Nixon, R. Carzino, A. Bigham, J. B. Carlin, R. M. Robins-Browne, and K. Grimwood.** 2002. Detection of a widespread clone of *Pseudomonas aeruginosa* in a pediatric cystic fibrosis clinic. *Am. J. Respir. Crit. Care Med.* **166:**983–987.
8. **Balke, B., L. Hoy, H. Weissbrodt, and S. Haussler.** 2004. Comparison of the Micronaut Merlin automated broth microtiter system with the standard agar dilution method for antimicrobial susceptibility testing of mucoid and nonmucoid *Pseudomonas aeruginosa* isolates from cystic fibrosis patients. *Eur. J. Clin. Microbiol. Infect. Dis.* **23:**765–771.
9. **Beers, S. L., and T. J. Abramo.** 2004. Otitis externa review. *Pediatr. Emerg. Care* **20:**250–256.
10. **Borriello, G., E. Werner, F. Roe, A. M. Kim, G. D. Ehrlich, and P. S. Stewart.** 2004. Oxygen limitation contributes to antibiotic tolerance of *Pseudomonas aeruginosa* in biofilms. *Antimicrob. Agents Chemother.* **48:**2659–2664.
11. **Burke, V., J. O. Robinson, C. J. L. Richardson, and C. S. Bundell.** 1991. Longitudinal studies of virulence factors of *Pseudomonas aeruginosa* in cystic fibrosis. *Pathology* **23:**145–148.
12. **Burns, J. L., L. Saiman, S. Whittier, J. Krzewinski, Z. Liu, D. Larone, S. A. Marshall, and R. N. Jones.** 2001. Comparison of two commercial systems (Vitek and MicroScan-WalkAway) for antimicrobial susceptibility testing of *Pseudomonas aeruginosa* isolates from cystic fibrosis patients. *Diagn. Microbiol. Infect. Dis.* **39:**257–260.
13. **Burns, J. L., L. Saiman, S. Whittier, D. Larone, J. Krzewinski, Z. Liu, S. A. Marshall, and R. N. Jones.** 2000. Comparison of agar diffusion methodologies for antimicrobial susceptibility testing of *Pseudomonas aeruginosa* isolates from cystic fibrosis patients. *J. Clin. Microbiol.* **38:**1818–1822.
14. **Campbell, M. E., S. W. Farmer, and D. P. Speert.** 1988. A new selective medium for *Pseudomonas aeruginosa* with phenanthroline and 9-chloro-9-[4-(diethylamino)phenyl]-9,10-dihydro-10-phenylacridine (C-390). *J. Clin. Microbiol.* **26:**1910–1912.
15. **Carratala, J., A. Salazar, J. Mascaro, and M. Santin.** 1992. Community-acquired pneumonia due to *Pseudomonas stutzeri*. *Clin. Infect. Dis.* **14:**792.
16. **Cavallo, J. D., R. Fabre, F. Leblanc, M. H. Nicolas-Chanoine, and A. Thabaut.** 2000. Antibiotic susceptibility and mechanisms of beta-lactam resistance in 1310 strains of *Pseudomonas aeruginosa*: a French multicentre study (1996). *J. Antimicrob. Chemother.* **46:**133–136.
17. **Chastre, J., and J. Y. Fagon.** 2002. Ventilator-associated pneumonia. *Am. J. Respir. Crit. Care Med.* **165:**867–903.

18. **Cheng, K., R. L. Smyth, J. R. W. Govan, C. Doherty, C. Winstanley, N. Denning, D. P. Heaf, H. van Saene, and C. A. Hart.** 1996. Spread of B-lactam-resistant *Pseudomonas aeruginosa* in a cystic fibrosis clinic. *Lancet* **348:**639–642.
19. **Cheuk, W., P. C. Woo, K. Y. Yuen, P. H. Yu, and J. K. Chan.** 2000. Intestinal inflammatory pseudotumour with regional lymph node involvement: identification of a new bacterium as the aetiological agent. *J. Pathol.* **192:**289–292.
20. **Chusid, M. J., W. M. Jacobs, and J. R. Sty.** 1979. Pseudomonas arthritis following puncture wounds of the foot. *J. Pediatr.* **94:**429–431.
21. **Ciofu, O., V. Fussing, N. Bagge, C. Koch, and N. Hoiby.** 2001. Characterization of paired mucoid/non-mucoid *Pseudomonas aeruginosa* isolates from Danish cystic fibrosis patients: antibiotic resistance, beta-lactamase activity and RiboPrinting. *J. Antimicrob. Chemother.* **48:**391–396.
22. **Clarke, L., J. E. Moore, B. C. Millar, L. Garske, J. Xu, M. W. Heuzenroeder, M. Crowe, and J. S. Elborn.** 2003. Development of a diagnostic PCR assay that targets a heat-shock protein gene (groES) for detection of *Pseudomonas* spp. in cystic fibrosis patients. *J. Med. Microbiol.* **52:**759–763.
23. **Clinical and Laboratory Standards Institute.** 2005. *Performance Standards for Antimicrobial Susceptibility Testing; Fifteenth Informational Supplement* (M100-S15). CLSI, Wayne, Pa.
24. **Cowlishaw, W. A., M. E. Hughes, and H. C. Simpson.** 1976. Meningitis caused by an alkali-producing pseudomonad. *J. Clin. Pathol.* **29:**1088–1090.
25. **Curran, B., D. Jonas, H. Grundmann, T. Pitt, and C. G. Dowson.** 2004. Development of a multilocus sequence typing scheme for the opportunistic pathogen *Pseudomonas aeruginosa*. *J. Clin. Microbiol.* **42:**5644–5649.
26. **Dabboussi, F., M. Hamze, E. Singer, V. Geoffroy, J. M. Meyer, and D. Izard.** 2002. *Pseudomonas mosselii* sp. nov., a novel species isolated from clinical specimens. *Int. J. Syst. Evol. Microbiol.* **52:**363–376.
27. **Delissalde, F., and C. F. Amabile-Cuevas.** 2004. Comparison of antibiotic susceptibility and plasmid content, between biofilm producing and non-producing clinical isolates of *Pseudomonas aeruginosa*. *Int. J. Antimicrob. Agents* **24:**405–408.
28. **De Vos, P., and J. De Ley.** 1983. Intra- and intergeneric similarities of *Pseudomonas* and *Xanthomonas* ribosomal ribonucleic acid cistrons. *Int. J. Syst. Bacteriol.* **33:** 487–509.
29. **Di Bonaventura, G., E. Ricci, N. Della Loggia, G. Catamo, and R. Piccolomini.** 1998. Evaluation of the E test for antimicrobial susceptibility testing of *Pseudomonas aeruginosa* isolates from patients with long-term bladder catheterization. *J. Clin. Microbiol.* **36:**824–826.
30. **Donay, J. L., D. Mathieu, P. Fernandes, C. Pregermain, P. Bruel, A. Wargnier, I. Casin, F. X. Weill, P. H. Lagrange, and J. L. Herrmann.** 2004. Evaluation of the automated Phoenix system for potential routine use in the clinical microbiology laboratory. *J. Clin. Microbiol.* **42:**1542–1546.
31. **Drenkard, E., and F. M. Ausubel.** 2002. *Pseudomonas* biofilm formation and antibiotic resistance are linked to phenotypic variation. *Nature* **416:**740–743.
32. **Elomari, M., L. Coroler, B. Hoste, M. Gillis, D. Izard, and H. Leclerc.** 1996. DNA relatedness among *Pseudomonas* strains isolated from natural mineral waters and proposal of *Pseudomonas veronii* sp. nov. *Int. J. Syst. Bacteriol.* **46:** 1138–1144.
33. **Elomari, M., L. Coroler, S. Verhille, D. Izard, and H. Leclerc.** 1997. *Pseudomonas monteilii* sp. nov., isolated from clinical specimens. *Int. J. Syst. Bacteriol.* **47:**846–852.
34. **Elomari, M., D. Izard, P. Vincent, L. Coroler, and H. Leclerc.** 1994. Comparison of ribotyping analysis and numerical taxonomy studies of *Pseudomonas putida* biovar A. *System. Appl. Microbiol.* **17:**361–369.
35. **Fisher, M. C., J. F. Goldsmith, and P. H. Gilligan.** 1985. Sneakers as a source of *Pseudomonas aeruginosa* in children with osteomyelitis following puncture wounds. *J. Pediatr.* **106:**607–609.
36. **Fong, I. W., and K. B. Tomkins.** 1985. Review of *Pseudomonas aeruginosa* meningitis with special emphasis on treatment with ceftazidime. *Rev. Infect. Dis.* **7:**604–612.
37. **Fonseca, K., J. MacDougall, and T. L. Pitt.** 1986. Inhibition of *Pseudomonas aeruginosa* from cystic fibrosis by selective media. *J. Clin. Pathol.* **39:**220–222.
38. **Foweraker, J. E., C. R. Laughton, D. F. Brown, and D. Bilton.** 2005. Phenotypic variability of *Pseudomonas aeruginosa* in sputa from patients with acute infective exacerbation of cystic fibrosis and its impact on the validity of antimicrobial susceptibility testing. *J. Antimicrob. Chemother.* **55:**921–927.
39. **Funke, G., and P. Funke-Kissling.** 2004. Evaluation of the new VITEK 2 card for identification of clinically relevant gram-negative rods. *J. Clin. Microbiol.* **42:**4067–4071.
40. **Funke, G., and P. Funke-Kissling.** 2004. Use of the BD PHOENIX Automated Microbiology System for direct identification and susceptibility testing of gram-negative rods from positive blood cultures in a three-phase trial. *J. Clin. Microbiol.* **42:**1466–1470.
41. **Gales, A. C., R. N. Jones, J. Turnidge, R. Rennie, and R. Ramphal.** 2001. Characterization of *Pseudomonas aeruginosa* isolates: occurrence rates, antimicrobial susceptibility patterns, and molecular typing in the global SENTRY Antimicrobial Surveillance Program, 1997–1999. *Clin. Infect. Dis.* **32**(Suppl. 2)**:**S146–S155.
42. **Gales, A. C., A. O. Reis, and R. N. Jones.** 2001. Contemporary assessment of antimicrobial susceptibility testing methods for polymyxin B and colistin: review of available interpretative criteria and quality control guidelines. *J. Clin. Microbiol.* **39:**183–190.
43. **Garau, J., and L. Gomez.** 2003. *Pseudomonas aeruginosa* pneumonia. *Curr. Opin. Infect. Dis.* **16:**135–143.
44. **Gilbert, D. N., S. J. Kohlhepp, K. A. Slama, G. Grunkemeier, G. Lewis, R. J. Dworkin, S. E. Slaughter, and J. E. Leggett.** 2001. Phenotypic resistance of *Staphylococcus aureus*, selected *Enterobacteriaceae*, and *Pseudomonas aeruginosa* after single and multiple in vitro exposures to ciprofloxacin, levofloxacin, and trovafloxacin. *Antimicrob. Agents Chemother.* **45:**883–892.
45. **Goetz, A., V. L. Yu, J. E. Hanchett, and J. D. Rihs.** 1983. *Pseudomonas stutzeri* bacteremia associated with hemodialysis. *Arch. Intern. Med.* **143:**1909–1912.
46. **Goossens, H.** 2003. Susceptibility of multi-drug-resistant *Pseudomonas aeruginosa* in intensive care units: results from the European MYSTIC study group. *Clin. Microbiol. Infect.* **9:**980–983.
47. **Govan, J. R., and V. Deretic.** 1996. Microbial pathogenesis in cystic fibrosis: mucoid *Pseudomonas aeruginosa* and *Burkholderia cepacia*. *Microbiol. Rev.* **60:**539–574.
48. **Gregory, D. W., and W. Schaffner.** 1987. Pseudomonas infections associated with hot tubs and other environments. *Infect. Dis. Clin. N. Am.* **1:**635–648.
49. **Guasp, C., E. R. Moore, J. Lalucat, and A. Bennasar.** 2000. Utility of internally transcribed 16S-23S rDNA spacer regions for the definition of *Pseudomonas stutzeri* genomovars and other *Pseudomonas* species. *Int. J. Syst. Evol. Microbiol.* **50**(Pt. 4)**:**1629–1639.
50. **Gunasekera, T. S., M. R. Dorsch, M. B. Slade, and D. A. Veal.** 2003. Specific detection of *Pseudomonas* spp. in milk by fluorescence in situ hybridization using ribosomal RNA directed probes. *J. Appl. Microbiol.* **94:**936–945.
51. **Gustafsson, I., M. Sjolund, E. Torell, M. Johannesson, L. Engstrand, O. Cars, and D. I. Andersson.** 2003. Bacteria

with increased mutation frequency and antibiotic resistance are enriched in the commensal flora of patients with high antibiotic usage. *J. Antimicrob. Chemother.* **52:**645–650.

52. **Hampton, K. D., and B. L. Wasilauskas.** 1979. Isolation of oxidase-negative *Pseudomonas aeruginosa* from sputum culture. *J. Clin. Microbiol.* **9:**632–634.
53. **Hancock, R. E., L. M. Mutharia, L. Chan, R. P. Darveau, D. P. Speert, and G. B. Pier.** 1983. *Pseudomonas aeruginosa* isolates from patients with cystic fibrosis: a class of serum-sensitive, nontypable strains deficient in lipopolysaccharide O side chains. *Infect. Immun.* **42:**170–177.
54. **Hancock, R. E., and D. P. Speert.** 2000. Antibiotic resistance in *Pseudomonas aeruginosa:* mechanisms and impact on treatment. *Drug Resist. Updat.* **3:**247–255.
55. **Hassett, D. J., J. Cuppoletti, B. Trapnell, S. V. Lymar, J. J. Rowe, S. S. Yoon, G. M. Hilliard, K. Parvatiyar, M. C. Kamani, D. J. Wozniak, S. H. Hwang, T. R. McDermott, and U. A. Ochsner.** 2002. Anaerobic metabolism and quorum sensing by *Pseudomonas aeruginosa* biofilms in chronically infected cystic fibrosis airways: rethinking antibiotic treatment strategies and drug targets. *Adv. Drug Deliv. Rev.* **54:**1425–1443.
56. **Haussler, S., I. Ziegler, A. Lottel, F. von Gotz, M. Rohde, D. Wehmhohner, S. Saravanamuthu, B. Tummler, and I. Steinmetz.** 2003. Highly adherent small-colony variants of *Pseudomonas aeruginosa* in cystic fibrosis lung infection. *J. Med. Microbiol.* **52:**295–301.
57. **Haussler, S., S. Ziesing, G. Rademacher, L. Hoy, and H. Weissbrodt.** 2003. Evaluation of the Merlin, Micronaut system for automated antimicrobial susceptibility testing of *Pseudomonas aeruginosa* and *Burkholderia* species isolated from cystic fibrosis patients. *Eur. J. Clin. Microbiol. Infect. Dis.* **22:**496–500.
58. **Hedberg, M.** 1969. Acetamide agar medium selective for *Pseudomonas aeruginosa. Appl. Microbiol.* **17:**481.
59. **Hentzer, M., G. M. Teitzel, G. J. Balzer, A. Heydorn, S. Molin, M. Givskov, and M. R. Parsek.** 2001. Alginate overproduction affects *Pseudomonas aeruginosa* biofilm structure and function. *J. Bacteriol.* **183:**5395–5401.
60. **Henwood, C. J., D. M. Livermore, D. James, and M. Warner.** 2001. Antimicrobial susceptibility of *Pseudomonas aeruginosa:* results of a UK survey and evaluation of the British Society for Antimicrobial Chemotherapy disc susceptibility test. *J. Antimicrob. Chemother.* **47:**789–799.
61. **Hogardt, M., S. Schmoldt, M. Gotzfried, K. Adler, and J. Heesemann.** 2004. Pitfalls of polymyxin antimicrobial susceptibility testing of *Pseudomonas aeruginosa* isolated from cystic fibrosis patients. *J. Antimicrob. Chemother.* **54:**1057–1061.
62. **Hogardt, M., K. Trebesius, A. M. Geiger, M. Hornef, J. Rosenecker, and J. Heesemann.** 2000. Specific and rapid detection by fluorescent in situ hybridization of bacteria in clinical samples obtained from cystic fibrosis patients. *J. Clin. Microbiol.* **38:**818–825.
63. **Holt, J. G., N. R. Kreig, P. H. A. Sneath, J. T. Staley, and S. T. Williams.** 1994. *Bergey's Manual of Systematic Bacteriology,* 9th ed., p. 93–94. The Williams & Wilkins Co., Baltimore, Md.
64. **Jacoby, G. A., and L. S. Munoz-Price.** 2005. The new beta-lactamases. *N. Engl. J. Med.* **352:**380–391.
65. **Jaffe, R. I., J. D. Lane, and C. W. Bates.** 2001. Real-time identification of *Pseudomonas aeruginosa* direct from clinical samples using a rapid extraction method and polymerase chain reaction (PCR). *J. Clin. Lab. Anal.* **15:**131–137.
66. **Jalal, S., O. Ciofu, N. Hoiby, N. Gotoh, and B. Wretlind.** 2000. Molecular mechanisms of fluoroquinolone resistance in *Pseudomonas aeruginosa* isolates from cystic fibrosis patients. *Antimicrob. Agents Chemother.* **44:**710–712.
67. **Jiraskova, N., and P. Rozsival.** 1998. Delayed-onset *Pseudomonas stutzeri* endophthalmitis after uncomplicated cataract surgery. *J. Cataract Refract. Surg.* **24:**866–867.
68. **Jones, A. M., A. K. Webb, J. R. Govan, C. A. Hart, and M. J. Walshaw.** 2002. *Pseudomonas aeruginosa* cross-infection in cystic fibrosis. *Lancet* **359:**527–528.
69. **Kersters, K., M. Ludwig, P. Vancanneyt, P. De Vos, M. Gillis, and K.-H. Schleifer.** 1996. Recent changes in the classification of the Pseudomonads: an overview. *System. Appl. Microbiol.* **19:**465–477.
70. **Keys, T. F., L. J. Melton III, M. D. Maker, and D. M. Ilstrup.** 1983. A suspected hospital outbreak of pseudobacteremia due to *Pseudomonas stutzeri. J. Infect. Dis.* **147:**489–493.
71. **Khan, A. A., and C. E. Cerniglia.** 1994. Detection of *Pseudomonas aeruginosa* from clinical and environmental samples by amplification of the exotoxin A gene using PCR. *Appl. Environ. Microbiol.* **60:**3739–3745.
72. **Koh, A. Y., G. P. Priebe, and G. B. Pier.** 2005. Virulence of *Pseudomonas aeruginosa* in a murine model of gastrointestinal colonization and dissemination in neutropenia. *Infect. Immun.* **73:**2262–2272.
73. **Kohler, T., M. Michea-Hamzehpour, S. F. Epp, and J. C. Pechere.** 1999. Carbapenem activities against *Pseudomonas aeruginosa:* respective contributions of OprD and efflux systems. *Antimicrob. Agents Chemother.* **43:**424–427.
74. **Korcova, J., J. Koprnova, V. Krcmery, and V. Krcmery.** 2005. Bacteraemia due to *Pseudomonas putida* and other Pseudomonas non-aeruginosa in children. *J. Infect.* **51:**81.
75. **Laguerre, G., L. Rigottier-Gois, and P. Lemanceau.** 1994. Fluorescent *Pseudomonas* species categorized by using polymerase chain reaction (PCR)/restriction fragment analysis of 16S rDNA. *Mol. Ecol.* **3:**479–487.
76. **Lam, J., R. Chan, K. Lam, and J. W. Costerton.** 1980. Production of mucoid microcolonies by *Pseudomonas aeruginosa* within infected lungs in cystic fibrosis. *Infect. Immun.* **28:**546–556.
77. **Li, J., R. L. Nation, R. W. Milne, J. D. Turnidge, and K. Coulthard.** 2005. Evaluation of colistin as an agent against multi-resistant Gram-negative bacteria. *Int. J. Antimicrob. Agents* **25:**11–25.
78. **Li, J., J. Turnidge, R. Milne, R. L. Nation, and K. Coulthard.** 2001. In vitro pharmacodynamic properties of colistin and colistin methanesulfonate against *Pseudomonas aeruginosa* isolates from patients with cystic fibrosis. *Antimicrob. Agents Chemother.* **45:**781–785.
79. **Li, X. Z., and H. Nikaido.** 2004. Efflux-mediated drug resistance in bacteria. *Drugs* **64:**159–204.
80. **Linker, A., and R. S. Jones.** 1966. A new polysaccharide resembling alginic acid isolated from pseudomonads. *J. Biol. Chem.* **241:**3845–3851.
81. **Livermore, D. M.** 1995. beta-Lactamases in laboratory and clinical resistance. *Clin. Microbiol. Rev.* **8:**557–584.
82. **Livermore, D. M.** 1987. Clinical significance of beta-lactamase induction and stable derepression in gram-negative rods. *Eur. J. Clin. Microbiol.* **6:**439–445.
83. **Livermore, D. M.** 2002. Multiple mechanisms of antimicrobial resistance in *Pseudomonas aeruginosa:* our worst nightmare? *Clin. Infect. Dis.* **34:**634–640.
84. **Macia, M. D., N. Borrell, J. L. Perez, and A. Oliver.** 2004. Detection and susceptibility testing of hypermutable *Pseudomonas aeruginosa* strains with the Etest and disk diffusion. *Antimicrob. Agents Chemother.* **48:**2665–2672.
85. **MacLeod, D. L., L. E. Nelson, R. M. Shawar, B. B. Lin, L. G. Lockwood, J. E. Dirk, G. H. Miller, J. L. Burns, and R. L. Garber.** 2000. Aminoglycoside-resistance mechanisms for cystic fibrosis *Pseudomonas aeruginosa* isolates are unchanged by long-term, intermittent, inhaled tobramycin treatment. *J. Infect. Dis.* **181:**1180–1184.
86. **Mah, T. F., B. Pitts, B. Pellock, G. C. Walker, P. S. Stewart, and G. A. O'Toole.** 2003. A genetic basis for *Pseudomonas aeruginosa* biofilm antibiotic resistance. *Nature* **426:**306–310.

87. **Mahenthiralingam, E., M. Campbell, and D. P. Speert.** 1994. Nonmotility and phagocytic resistance of *Pseudomonas aeruginosa* isolates from chronically colonized patients with cystic fibrosis. *Infect. Immun.* **62:**596–605.
88. **Mahenthiralingam, E., M. E. Campbell, J. Foster, J. S. Lam, and D. P. Speert.** 1996. Random amplified polymorphic DNA typing of *Pseudomonas aeruginosa* isolates recovered from patients with cystic fibrosis. *J. Clin. Microbiol.* **34:**1129–1135.
89. **Marin, M., D. Garcia de Viedma, P. Martin-Rabadan, M. Rodriguez-Creixems, and E. Bouza.** 2000. Infection of hickman catheter by *Pseudomonas* (formerly flavimonas) *oryzihabitans* traced to a synthetic bath sponge. *J. Clin. Microbiol.* **38:**4577–4579.
90. **Martino, P., A. Micozzi, M. Venditti, G. Gentile, C. Girmenia, R. Raccah, S. Santilli, N. Alessandri, and F. Mandelli.** 1990. Catheter-related right-sided endocarditis in bone marrow transplant recipients. *Rev. Infect. Dis.* **12:**250–257.
91. **Migula, W.** 1894. Uber ein neues System der Bakterien. *Arb. Bakteriol. Inst. Karlsruhe* **1:**235–238.
92. **Miller, G. H., F. J. Sabatelli, R. S. Hare, Y. Glupczynski, P. Mackey, D. Shlaes, K. Shimizu, and K. J. Shaw.** 1997. The most frequent aminoglycoside resistance mechanisms—changes with time and geographic area: a reflection of aminoglycoside usage patterns? Aminoglycoside Resistance Study Groups. *Clin. Infect. Dis.* **24**(Suppl. 1)**:** S46–S62.
93. **Morehead, R. S., and S. J. Pinto.** 2000. Ventilator-associated pneumonia. *Arch. Intern. Med.* **160:**1926–1936.
94. **Morlin, G. L., D. L. Hedges, A. L. Smith, and J. L. Burns.** 1994. Accuracy and cost of antibiotic susceptibility testing of mixed morphotypes of *Pseudomonas aeruginosa. J. Clin. Microbiol.* **32:**1027–1030.
95. **Moskowitz, S. M., J. M. Foster, J. Emerson, and J. L. Burns.** 2004. Clinically feasible biofilm susceptibility assay for isolates of *Pseudomonas aeruginosa* from patients with cystic fibrosis. *J. Clin. Microbiol.* **42:**1915–1922.
96. **Naas, T., and P. Nordmann.** 1999. OXA-type beta-lactamases. *Curr. Pharm. Des.* **5:**865–879.
97. **Nakamoto, H., Y. Hashikita, A. Itabashi, T. Kobayashi, and H. Suzuki.** 2004. Changes in the organisms of resistant peritonitis in patients on continuous ambulatory peritoneal dialysis. *Adv. Perit. Dial.* **20:**52–57.
98. **Nikaido, H.** 1996. Multidrug efflux pumps of gram-negative bacteria. *J. Bacteriol.* **178:**5853–5859.
99. **Noble, R. C., and S. B. Overman.** 1994. *Pseudomonas stutzeri* infection. A review of hospital isolates and a review of the literature. *Diagn. Microbiol. Infect. Dis.* **19:**51–56.
100. **Obritsch, M. D., D. N. Fish, R. MacLaren, and R. Jung.** 2004. National surveillance of antimicrobial resistance in *Pseudomonas aeruginosa* isolates obtained from intensive care unit patients from 1993 to 2002. *Antimicrob. Agents Chemother.* **48:**4606–4610.
101. **Ogle, J. W., J. M. Janda, D. E. Woods, and M. L. Vasil.** 1987. Characterization and use of a DNA probe as an epidemiological marker for *Pseudomonas aeruginosa. J. Infect. Dis.* **155:**119–126.
102. **O'Hara, C. M., and J. M. Miller.** 2002. Ability of the MicroScan rapid gram-negative ID type 3 panel to identify nonenteric glucose-fermenting and nonfermenting gram-negative bacilli. *J. Clin. Microbiol.* **40:**3750–3752.
103. **O'Hara, C. M., and J. M. Miller.** 2003. Evaluation of the Vitek 2 ID-GNB assay for identification of members of the family *Enterobacteriaceae* and other nonenteric gram-negative bacilli and comparison with the Vitek GNI+ card. *J. Clin. Microbiol.* **41:**2096–2101.
104. **Oliver, A., R. Canton, P. Campo, F. Baquero, and J. Blazquez.** 2000. High frequency of hypermutable *Pseudomonas aeruginosa* in cystic fibrosis lung infection. *Science* **288:**1251–1254.
105. **Pai, H., J. Kim, J. H. Lee, K. W. Choe, and N. Gotoh. 2001.** Carbapenem resistance mechanisms in *Pseudomonas aeruginosa* clinical isolates. *Antimicrob. Agents Chemother.* **45:**480–484.
106. **Pedersen, S. S., N. Hoiby, F. Espersen, and C. Koch.** 1992. Role of alginate in infection with mucoid *Pseudomonas aeruginosa* in cystic fibrosis. *Thorax* **47:**6–13.
107. **Pitout, J. D., D. B. Gregson, L. Poirel, J. A. McClure, P. Le, and D. L. Church.** 2005. Detection of *Pseudomonas aeruginosa* producing metallo-beta-lactamases in a large centralized laboratory. *J. Clin. Microbiol.* **43:**3129–3135.
108. **Poirel, L., G. F. Weldhagen, T. Naas, C. De Champs, M. G. Dove, and P. Nordmann.** 2001. GES-2, a class A beta-lactamase from *Pseudomonas aeruginosa* with increased hydrolysis of imipenem. *Antimicrob. Agents Chemother.* **45:**2598–2603.
109. **Pollack, M., and L. S. Young.** 1979. Protective activity of antibodies to exotoxin A and lipopolysaccharide at the onset of *Pseudomonas aeruginosa* septicemia in man. *J. Clin. Investig.* **63:**276–286.
110. **Poole, K.** 2005. Aminoglycoside resistance in *Pseudomonas aeruginosa. Antimicrob. Agents Chemother.* **49:**479–487.
111. **Poole, K., K. Tetro, Q. Zhao, S. Neshat, D. E. Heinrichs, and N. Bianco.** 1996. Expression of the multidrug resistance operon mexA-mexB-oprM in *Pseudomonas aeruginosa:* mexR encodes a regulator of operon expression. *Antimicrob. Agents Chemother.* **40:**2021–2028.
112. **Potvliege, C., J. Jonckheer, C. Lenclud, and W. Hansen.** 1987. *Pseudomonas stutzeri* pneumonia and septicemia in a patient with multiple myeloma. *J. Clin. Microbiol.* **25:**458–459.
113. **Pruitt, B. A., Jr., A. T. McManus, S. H. Kim, and C. W. Goodwin.** 1998. Burn wound infections: current status. *World J. Surg.* **22:**135–145.
114. **Qin, X., J. Emerson, J. Stapp, L. Stapp, P. Abe, and J. L. Burns.** 2003. Use of real-time PCR with multiple targets to identify *Pseudomonas aeruginosa* and other nonfermenting gram-negative bacilli from patients with cystic fibrosis. *J. Clin. Microbiol.* **41:**4312–4317.
115. **Rahav, G., A. Simhon, Y. Mattan, A. E. Moses, and T. Sacks.** 1995. Infections with *Chryseomonas luteola* (CDC group Ve-1) and *Flavimonas oryzihabitans* (CDC group Ve-2). *Medicine* (Baltimore) **74:**83–88.
116. **Rastogi, S., and S. J. Sperber.** 1998. Facial cellulitis and *Pseudomonas luteola* bacteremia in an otherwise healthy patient. *Diagn. Microbiol. Infect. Dis.* **32:**303–305.
117. **Reisler, R. B., and H. Blumberg.** 1999. Community-acquired *Pseudomonas stutzeri* vertebral osteomyelitis in a previously healthy patient: case report and review. *Clin. Infect. Dis.* **29:**667–669.
118. **Remington, J. S., and S. C. Schimpff.** 1981. Please don't eat the salads. *N. Engl. J. Med.* **304:**433–434.
119. **Roig, P., A. Orti, and V. Navarro.** 1996. Meningitis due to *Pseudomonas stutzeri* in a patient infected with human immunodeficiency virus. *Clin. Infect. Dis.* **22:**587–588.
120. **Ronald, A.** 2002. The etiology of urinary tract infection: traditional and emerging pathogens. *Am. J. Med.* **113**(Suppl. 1A)**:**14S–19S.
121. **Rossolini, G. M., and E. Mantengoli.** 2005. Treatment and control of severe infections caused by multiresistant *Pseudomonas aeruginosa. Clin. Microbiol. Infect.* **11**(Suppl. 4)**:** 17–32.
122. **Rubin Grandis, J., B. F. Branstetter IV, and V. L. Yu.** 2004. The changing face of malignant (necrotising) external

otitis: clinical, radiological, and anatomic correlations. *Lancet Infect. Dis.* **4**:34–39.

123. **Sader, H. S., M. Castanheira, R. E. Mendes, M. Toleman, T. R. Walsh, and R. N. Jones.** 2005. Dissemination and diversity of metallo-beta-lactamases in Latin America: report from the SENTRY Antimicrobial Surveillance Program. *Int. J. Antimicrob. Agents* **25**:57–61.
124. **Sader, H. S., and R. N. Jones.** 2005. Antimicrobial susceptibility of uncommonly isolated non-enteric Gram-negative bacilli. *Int. J. Antimicrob. Agents* **25**:95–109.
125. **Saiman, L., J. L. Burns, D. Larone, Y. Chen, E. Garber, and S. Whittier.** 2003. Evaluation of MicroScan Autoscan for identification of *Pseudomonas aeruginosa* isolates from cystic fibrosis patients. *J. Clin. Microbiol.* **41**:492–494.
126. **Sapico, F. L., and J. Z. Montgomerie.** 1980. Vertebral osteomyelitis in intravenous drug abusers: report of three cases and review of the literature. *Rev. Infect. Dis.* **2**:196–206.
127. **Schutze, G. E., C. H. Gilliam, S. Jin, C. K. Cavenaugh, R. W. Hall, R. W. Bradsher, and R. F. Jacobs.** 2004. Use of DNA fingerprinting in decision making for considering closure of neonatal intensive care units because of *Pseudomonas aeruginosa* bloodstream infections. *Pediatr. Infect. Dis. J.* **23**:110–114.
128. **Scott, J., F. E. Boulton, J. R. Govan, R. S. Miles, D. B. McClelland, and C. V. Prowse.** 1988. A fatal transfusion reaction associated with blood contaminated with *Pseudomonas fluorescens*. *Vox Sang.* **54**:201–204.
129. **Serisier, D. J., G. Jones, A. Tuck, G. Connett, and M. P. Carroll.** 2003. Clinical application of direct sputum sensitivity testing in a severe infective exacerbation of cystic fibrosis. *Pediatr. Pulmonol.* **35**:463–466.
130. **Shih, P. C., and C. T. Huang.** 2002. Effects of quorum-sensing deficiency on *Pseudomonas aeruginosa* biofilm formation and antibiotic resistance. *J. Antimicrob. Chemother.* **49**:309–314.
131. **Sikorski, J., J. Lalucat, and W. Wackernagel.** 2005. Genomovars 11 to 18 of Pseudomonas stutzeri, identified among isolates from soil and marine sediment. *Int. J. Syst. Evol. Microbiol.* **55**:1767–1770.
132. **Smith, A. L., S. B. Fiel, N. Mayer-Hamblett, B. Ramsey, and J. L. Burns.** 2003. Susceptibility testing of *Pseudomonas aeruginosa* isolates and clinical response to parenteral antibiotic administration: lack of association in cystic fibrosis. *Chest* **123**:1495–1502.
133. **Speert, D. P.** 2002. Molecular epidemiology of *Pseudomonas aeruginosa*. *Front. Biosci.* **7**:e354–e361. [Online.]
134. **Speert, D. P.** 1993. *Pseudomonas aeruginosa*-phagocytic cell interaction, p. 163–182. *In* M. Campa, M. Bendinelli, and H. Friedman (ed.), Pseudomonas aeruginosa *as an Opportunistic Pathogen*. Plenum Press, New York, N.Y.
135. **Speert, D. P.** 1994. *Pseudomonas aeruginosa* infections in patients with cystic fibrosis, p. 183–236. *In* A. L. Baltch and R. P. Smith (ed.), Pseudomonas aeruginosa *Infections and Treatment*. Marcel Dekker, Inc., New York. N.Y.
136. **Speert, D. P., M. E. Campbell, A. G. Davidson, and L. T. Wong.** 1993. *Pseudomonas aeruginosa* colonization of the gastrointestinal tract in patients with cystic fibrosis. *J. Infect. Dis.* **167**:226–229.
137. **Speert, D. P., M. E. Campbell, D. A. Henry, R. Milner, F. Taha, A. Gravelle, A. G. Davidson, L. T. Wong, and E. Mahenthiralingam.** 2002. Epidemiology of *Pseudomonas aeruginosa* in cystic fibrosis in British Columbia, Canada. *Am. J. Respir. Crit. Care Med.* **166**:988–993.
138. **Spilker, T., T. Coenye, P. Vandamme, and J. J. LiPuma.** 2004. PCR-based assay for differentiation of *Pseudomonas aeruginosa* from other *Pseudomonas* species recovered from cystic fibrosis patients. *J. Clin. Microbiol.* **42**:2074–2079.
139. **Spoering, A. L., and K. Lewis.** 2001. Biofilms and planktonic cells of *Pseudomonas aeruginosa* have similar resistance to killing by antimicrobials. *J. Bacteriol.* **183:** 6746–6751.
140. **Stefaniuk, E., A. Baraniak, M. Gniadkowski, and W. Hryniewicz.** 2003. Evaluation of the BD Phoenix automated identification and susceptibility testing system in clinical microbiology laboratory practice. *Eur. J. Clin. Microbiol. Infect. Dis.* **22**:479–485.
141. **Stender, H., A. Broomer, K. Oliveira, H. Perry-O'Keefe, J. J. Hyldig-Nielsen, A. Sage, B. Young, and J. Coull.** 2000. Rapid detection, identification, and enumeration of *Pseudomonas aeruginosa* in bottled water using peptide nucleic acid probes. *J. Microbiol. Methods* **42**:245–253.
142. **Stern, G. A.** 1990. Pseudomonas keratitis and contact lens wear: the lens/eye is at fault. *Cornea* **9**(Suppl. 1)**:** S36–S40.
143. **Steward, C. D., J. M. Mohammed, J. M. Swenson, S. A. Stocker, P. P. Williams, R. P. Gaynes, J. E. McGowan, Jr., and F. C. Tenover.** 2003. Antimicrobial susceptibility testing of carbapenems: multicenter validity testing and accuracy levels of five antimicrobial test methods for detecting resistance in *Enterobacteriaceae* and *Pseudomonas aeruginosa* isolates. *J. Clin. Microbiol.* **41**:351–358.
144. **Stewart, P. S., and J. W. Costerton.** 2001. Antibiotic resistance of bacteria in biofilms. *Lancet* **358**:135–138.
145. **Stoll, B. J., N. Hansen, A. A. Fanaroff, L. L. Wright, W. A. Carlo, R. A. Ehrenkranz, J. A. Lemons, E. F. Donovan, A. R. Stark, J. E. Tyson, W. Oh, C. R. Bauer, S. B. Korones, S. Shankaran, A. R. Laptook, D. K. Stevenson, L. A. Papile, and W. K. Poole.** 2002. Late-onset sepsis in very low birth weight neonates: the experience of the NICHD Neonatal Research Network. *Pediatrics* **110**:285–291.
146. **Sturenburg, E., and D. Mack.** 2003. Extended-spectrum beta-lactamases: implications for the clinical microbiology laboratory, therapy, and infection control. *J. Infect.* **47**:273–295.
147. **Sung, L. L., D. I. Yang, C. C. Hung, and H. T. Ho.** 2000. Evaluation of autoSCAN-W/A and the Vitek GNI+ AutoMicrobic system for identification of non-glucose-fermenting gram-negative bacilli. *J. Clin. Microbiol.* **38**:1127–1130.
148. **Szczepanowski, R., I. Krahn, B. Linke, A. Goesmann, A. Puhler, and A. Schluter.** 2004. Antibiotic multiresistance plasmid pRSB101 isolated from a wastewater treatment plant is related to plasmids residing in phytopathogenic bacteria and carries eight different resistance determinants including a multidrug transport system. *Microbiology* **150**:3613–3630.
149. **Tancrede, C. H., and A. O. Andremont.** 1985. Bacterial translocation and gram-negative bacteremia in patients with hematological malignancies. *J. Infect. Dis.* **152:** 99–103.
150. **Tenover, F. C., R. D. Arbeit, R. V. Goering, P. A. Mickelsen, B. E. Murray, D. H. Persing, and B. Swaminathan.** 1995. Interpreting chromosomal DNA restriction patterns produced by pulsed-field gel electrophoresis: criteria for bacterial strain typing. *J. Clin. Microbiol.* **33**:2233–2239.
151. **The International *Pseudomonas aeruginosa* Typing Study Group.** 1994. A multicenter comparison of methods for typing strains of *Pseudomonas aeruginosa* predominantly from patients with cystic fibrosis. *J. Infect. Dis.* **169**:134–142.

152. **Troillet, N., M. H. Samore, and Y. Carmeli.** 1997. Imipenem-resistant *Pseudomonas aeruginosa:* risk factors and antibiotic susceptibility patterns. *Clin. Infect. Dis.* **25:**1094–1098.

153. **Valdezate, S., J. Martinez-Beltran, L. de Rafael, F. Baquero, and R. Canton.** 1996. Beta-lactam stability in frozen microdilution PASCO MIC panels using strains with known resistance mechanisms as biosensors. *Diagn. Microbiol. Infect. Dis.* **26:**53–61.

154. **Vonberg, R. P., and P. Gastmeier.** 2005. Isolation of infectious cystic fibrosis patients: results of a systematic review. *Infect. Control Hosp. Epidemiol.* **26:**401–409.

155. **von Gotz, F., S. Haussler, D. Jordan, S. S. Saravanamuthu, D. Wehmhoner, A. Strussmann, J. Lauber, I. Attree, J. Buer, B. Tummler, and I. Steinmetz.** 2004. Expression analysis of a highly adherent and cytotoxic small colony variant of *Pseudomonas aeruginosa* isolated from a lung of a patient with cystic fibrosis. *J. Bacteriol.* **186:**3837–3847.

156. **Wang, M., J. H. Tran, G. A. Jacoby, Y. Zhang, F. Wang, and D. C. Hooper.** 2003. Plasmid-mediated quinolone resistance in clinical isolates of *Escherichia coli* from Shanghai, China. *Antimicrob. Agents Chemother.* **47:**2242–2248.

157. **Weldhagen, G. F., L. Poirel, and P. Nordmann.** 2003. Ambler class A extended-spectrum beta-lactamases in *Pseudomonas aeruginosa:* novel developments and clinical impact. *Antimicrob. Agents Chemother.* **47:**2385–2392.

158. **Weldhagen, G. F., and A. Prinsloo.** 2004. Molecular detection of GES-2 extended spectrum Beta-lactamase producing *Pseudomonas aeruginosa* in Pretoria, South Africa. *Int. J. Antimicrob. Agents* **24:**35–38.

159. **Wellinghausen, N., J. Kothe, B. Wirths, A. Sigge, and S. Poppert.** 2005. Superiority of molecular techniques for identification of gram-negative, oxidase-positive rods, including morphologically nontypical *Pseudomonas aeruginosa,* from patients with cystic fibrosis. *J. Clin. Microbiol.* **43:**4070–4075.

160. **Weyant, R. C. M., R. E. Weaver, D. G. Hollis, J. G. Jordan, E. C. Cook, and M. I. Daneshvar.** 1995. *Identification of Unusual Pathogenic Gram-Negative Aerobic and Facultatively Anaerobic Bacteria,* p. 318–319, 340–341, 470–503. The Williams & Wilkins Co., Baltimore, Md.

161. **White, R. L., D. S. Burgess, M. Manduru, and J. A. Bosso.** 1996. Comparison of three different in vitro methods of detecting synergy: time-kill, checkerboard, and E test. *Antimicrob. Agents Chemother.* **40:**1914–1918.

162. **Wolter, J. M., G. Kotsiou, and J. G. McCormack.** 1995. Mixed morphotype testing of *Pseudomonas aeruginosa* cultures from cystic fibrosis patients. *J. Med. Microbiol.* **42:**220–224.

163. **Woods, D. E., D. C. Straus, W. G. Johanson, and J. A. Bass.** 1981. Role of fibronectin in the prevention of adherence of *Pseudomonas aeruginosa* to buccal cells. *J. Infect. Dis.* **143:**784–790.

164. **Yan, J. J., J. J. Wu, S. H. Tsai, and C. L. Chuang.** 2004. Comparison of the double-disk, combined disk, and E test methods for detecting metallo-beta-lactamases in gram-negative bacilli. *Diagn. Microbiol. Infect. Dis.* **49:**5–11.

165. **Yang, C. H., T. Young, M. Y. Peng, and M. C. Weng.** 1996. Clinical spectrum of *Pseudomonas putida* infection. *J. Formos. Med. Assoc.* **95:**754–761.

166. **Zierdt, C. H.** 1971. Autolytic nature of iridescent lysis in *Pseudomonas aeruginosa. Antonie Leeuwenhoek* **37:**319–337.

Burkholderia, Stenotrophomonas, Ralstonia, Cupriavidus, Pandoraea, Brevundimonas, Comamonas, Delftia, and *Acidovorax**

JOHN J. LiPUMA, BART J. CURRIE, GARY D. LUM, AND PETER A. R. VANDAMME

49

TAXONOMY

In 1973, the taxonomic heterogeneity of the genus *Pseudomonas* was revealed by the work of Palleroni and coworkers, who identified five major species clusters (referred to as rRNA homology groups) among the pseudomonads (169). DNA-rRNA hybridization experiments led to the gradual dissection of the genus during the following decades (131). The name *Pseudomonas* was confined to rRNA homology group I organisms because they constituted the type species, *Pseudomonas aeruginosa* (see chapter 48).

The nomenclatural rearrangements of the genus *Pseudomonas* entailed the creation of several new genera. Some of these encompassed complete rRNA homology groups (e.g., both rRNA homology group IV species were reclassified into the genus *Brevundimonas*), whereas others encompassed only partial groups. rRNA group II pseudomonads belong to the class of the *β-Proteobacteria* and were reclassified into the genera *Burkholderia* and *Ralstonia* (233, 234). The rRNA group II pseudomonads form a remarkable group of primary and opportunistic human, animal, and plant pathogens, as well as environmental species with considerable potential for biological control, remediation, and plant growth promotion. During the past decade, the interest in several peculiar characteristics of these organisms led to the discovery and description of a multitude of novel species. The genus *Burkholderia* now contains more than 35 validly named species, most of which have been isolated from soil and water samples. Some other novel *Burkholderia*-like species were found to represent a distinct phylogenetic lineage with a position intermediate between those of the genera *Burkholderia* and *Ralstonia* and were classified into the novel genus *Pandoraea* (41).

More recently, Vaneechoutte et al. (205) reported that results of comparative 16S rRNA gene sequence analysis, further supported by phenotypic differences, indicated that two distinct sublineages existed within the genus *Ralstonia*. It was proposed that species of the *Ralstonia eutropha* lineage be classified into a novel genus named *Wautersia*. The name *Ralstonia* was preserved for the sublineage comprising *Ralstonia pickettii*, the type species. Shortly thereafter, Vandamme and Coenye (201) reported that *Wautersia eutropha*, the name of the type species of the genus *Wautersia*, was a junior synonym of *Cupriavidus necator*, the name of the type (and only) species of the genus *Cupriavidus*, an environmental organism which was validly named in 1987, i.e., long before 16S rRNA gene sequence studies were performed routinely (152). Thus, to conform to the International Code of Nomenclature of Bacteria (191), the name *Wautersia* was replaced by *Cupriavidus* and all species of the genus *Wautersia* became species of the genus *Cupriavidus*. Although renaming and subsequent further renaming of bacterial species cause confusion and irritation in the wider microbiological community, adhering to the rules of nomenclature is essential for establishing a truly systematic taxonomy.

Several *Burkholderia* species have been isolated from human clinical samples, but only the *Burkholderia cepacia* complex, *B. mallei*, and *B. pseudomallei* are generally recognized as human or animal pathogens. Recent taxonomic studies using 16S rRNA and *recA* sequence analysis, DNA-DNA hybridization experiments, whole-cell protein and fatty acid analyses, and biochemical characterization revealed that *B. cepacia*-like bacteria belong to at least nine distinct genomic species (genomovars), referred to collectively as the *B. cepacia* complex (54, 204). Ongoing surveys of the diversity of *B. cepacia*-like bacteria recovered from specimens from cystic fibrosis (CF) patients and other specimens revealed the presence of several additional groups in the *B. cepacia* complex which cannot be assigned to one of the established species within this complex by using traditional or molecular identification approaches (178). Further polyphasic taxonomic analyses are needed to determine if these groups represent additional novel species within the *B. cepacia* complex or if they represent new variants of established species. All *B. cepacia* complex species have been recovered from human clinical samples, but primarily *B. multivorans* and *B. cenocepacia* are important opportunistic pathogens in CF patients (99, 178).

Apart from the *B. cepacia* complex species, *B. mallei*, and *B. pseudomallei*, the genus *Burkholderia* now comprises an additional 26 validly described species. Most of these organisms are not associated with human disease and are not discussed further here. Organisms associated with human infections include *B. fungorum*, *B. gladioli* (including strains previously classified as *B. cocovenenans*[45]), and *B. thailandensis* (20, 46). A complete overview of validly named species can be obtained through Internet sites such as http://www.bacterio.cict.fr/ and http://www.dsmz.de/bactnom/genera1.htm.

*This chapter contains information presented in chapter 48 by Peter H. Gilligan, Gary Lum, Peter A. R. Vandamme, and Susan Whittier in the eighth edition of this Manual.

There are now five species in the genus *Ralstonia*. The human pathogens include *Ralstonia pickettii*, *R. mannitolilytica* (previously known as *R. pickettii* biovar 3/'*thomasii*') (72), and *R. insidiosa* (43). *R. paucula* (previously known as Centers for Disease Control group IVc-2) (202), *R. gilardii* (42), *R. respiraculi* (56), *R. taiwanensis* (31), and five additional species, which occur primarily in environmental samples, are now all classified as *Cupriavidus* species (201).

Five distinct species of *Pandoraea*, *Pandoraea apista* (the type species), *P. pulmonicola*, *P. pnomenusa*, *P. sputorum*, and *P. norimbergensis*, were distinguished by sodium dodecyl sulfate-polyacrylamide gel electrophoresis of whole-cell proteins, amplified fragment length polymorphism fingerprinting, DNA-DNA hybridization, and 16S rRNA gene sequence analysis. In addition, four strains, each representing a distinct novel *Pandoraea* species, presently remain unnamed (41, 70).

Organisms in the *Pseudomonas* rRNA homology group III also belong to the *β-Proteobacteria* and are now classified in the family *Comamonadaceae*, which includes the genera *Comamonas*, *Delftia*, and *Acidovorax* (216, 223). The genus *Comamonas* was originally created in 1985 and included a single species, *Comamonas terrigena*. Two years later, *Pseudomonas acidovorans* and *Pseudomonas testosteroni* were reclassified as members of the genus *Comamonas*. *Comamonas acidovorans* was subsequently again reclassified as *Delftia acidovorans* (216). *Comamonas terrigena* encompassed three strain clusters on the basis of DNA-rRNA and DNA-DNA hybridization data and data from protein electrophoretic patterns and immunotyping (226). Wauters et al. (214) reported biochemical differences between these three clusters and consequently described them as separate species. They proposed to rename *Comamonas terrigena* DNA groups 2 and 3 as *Comamonas aquatica* and *Comamonas kerstersii*, respectively. *Comamonas terrigena*, *Comamonas aquatica*, and *Comamonas kerstersii* all occur in human clinical samples. Additional novel species have been isolated from environmental samples (27, 83, 102, 196).

Originally, *Acidovorax facilis* was classified as *Hydrogenomonas facilis* based on its ability to oxidize hydrogen. Poly-β-hydroxybutyrate metabolism studies resulted in the transfer of this species to the genus *Pseudomonas*, along with a new species called *Pseudomonas delafieldii*. A new genus, *Acidovorax*, was proposed which included three species, *A. facilis*, *A. delafieldii*, and *A. temperans*, all members of rRNA homology group III (224). An additional five plant-pathogenic pseudomonads and novel environmental species have been classified as *Acidovorax* species (89, 90, 185, 225).

The genus *Brevundimonas*, consisting of the species *Brevundimonas diminuta* and *Brevundimonas vesicularis*, was proposed for bacteria originally classified as members of *Pseudomonas* rRNA homology group IV (186) and is a member of the *α-Proteobacteria*. Phylogenetic studies by Abraham et al. (2) revealed that the taxonomy of the genera *Brevundimonas* and *Caulobacter* was intertwined. Six *Caulobacter* species and two novel environmental species were therefore described as novel *Brevundimonas* species (2, 87, 139).

Finally, *Pseudomonas maltophilia* represented *Pseudomonas* rRNA homology group V (115). Based on genotypic and phenotypic characteristics, including DNA-rRNA hybridizations, cellular fatty acid composition, and growth parameters, its transfer to the genus *Xanthomonas*, a member of the *γ-Proteobacteria*, was proposed (195). However, many differences were also noted, including flagellum number, nitrate reduction characteristics, fimbriation, and plant pathogenicity. Therefore, the organism was once again reclassified into a novel genus, *Stenotrophomonas* (168). More recently, a novel species, *Stenotrophomonas africana*, was proposed (81). However, Coenye et al. (57) demonstrated that *S. maltophilia* and *S. africana* are the same species and nomenclatural priority was given to the former. Three additional environmental *Stenotrophomonas* species were described recently (11, 85, 228).

DESCRIPTION OF THE AGENTS

Burkholderia, *Ralstonia*, *Cupriavidus*, *Pandoraea*, *Brevundimonas*, *Comamonas*, *Delftia*, and *Acidovorax* spp. are aerobic, non-spore-forming, straight or slightly curved gram-negative rods. They are 1 to 5 μm in length and 0.5 to 1.0 μm in width (113). *Stenotrophomonas* spp. are straight rods and tend to be slightly smaller than members of the other genera (0.7 to 1.8 μm in length and 0.4 to 0.7 μm in width) (113). With the exception of *B. mallei*, these organisms are motile due to the presence of one or more polar flagella (167). These bacteria are catalase positive, and most, with the exception of *Stenotrophomonas* and *B. gladioli*, are either weakly or strongly oxidase positive. All grow on MacConkey agar, except for certain strains of *Brevundimonas vesicularis*, and appear as nonfermenters. The majority of species degrade glucose oxidatively, and most degrade nitrate into either nitrite or nitrogen gas. Certain species have distinctive colony morphologies or pigmentation. They are nutritionally quite versatile, with different species being able to utilize a variety of simple and complex carbohydrates, alcohols, and amino acids as carbon sources. Certain species can multiply at 4°C, but most are mesophilic, with optimal growth temperatures of between 30 and 37°C (167). For some genera, growth at higher temperatures (i.e., up to 42°C) can be useful for species identification.

EPIDEMIOLOGY AND TRANSMISSION

Burkholderia, *Ralstonia*, *Cupriavidus*, *Pandoraea*, *Comamonas*, *Delftia*, *Acidovorax*, *Brevundimonas*, and *Stenotrophomonas* spp. are environmental organisms found in water, soil, and the rhizosphere and in and on plants including fruits and vegetables. They have a worldwide distribution. Members of these genera are widely recognized as phytopathogens, and many species were first described in that context. Because of their ability to survive in aqueous environments, these organisms have become particularly problematic as opportunistic nosocomial pathogens in hospitals and health care settings.

The natural distribution of *B. cepacia* complex species is being intensively studied because of interest in their biotechnological properties and their pathogenicity in persons with CF (99, 144). *B. cepacia* complex bacteria often have antifungal, antinematodal, or plant growth-promoting properties, which makes them attractive as biological pesticides and fertilizers (170). Because of their nutritional versatility, *B. cepacia* complex bacteria also have applications for bioremediation of contaminated soils. Unlike *P. aeruginosa*, *B. cepacia* complex bacteria are rarely recovered from environmental sites such as sinks, swimming pools, showers, and salad bars (99, 157). However, they are frequently recovered from soil and environmental water samples (12, 176), provided that appropriate growth conditions are used to inhibit the growth of vast numbers of other environmental bacteria. Studies of a variety of foodstuffs and bottled water have shown that *B. cepacia* complex bacteria have been found in unpasteurized dairy products (17, 156). Due to their intrinsic resistance to antibiotics and disinfectants, *B. cepacia* complex bacteria are also notorious contaminants of pharmaceutical preparations and medical equipment such as nebulizers, which may be sterilized with contaminated anti-infectives (116, 163).

Genotypic and conventional epidemiologic investigations provide compelling evidence for interpatient transmission of common or epidemic *B. cepacia* complex strains among persons with CF (142). One such strain, referred to as the ET12 (for electrophoretic type 12) lineage, is common among CF patients in eastern Canada and the United Kingdom (124, 174). This organism is a *B. cenocepacia* strain that is characterized by the presence of a distinctive cable-like pilus and an associated adhesin that mediates adherence to the respiratory epithelium (181). *B. cenocepacia* strain PHDC dominates among infected CF patients in the mid-Atlantic region of the United States and has recently been identified in agricultural soil as well as in CF patients in several European countries (30, 53, 148).

B. pseudomallei and *B. thailandensis* are found primarily in tropical and subtropical areas. *B. pseudomallei* is endemic in rodents and is found in moist soil, on vegetables, and on fruit. Both species are particularly prevalent in the rice-growing regions of northern Thailand and southern and central Vietnam because of high concentrations of the organisms in rice paddy surface water (171). Reports have suggested that *B. pseudomallei* can also be found with some frequency on the Indian subcontinent but goes unrecognized (69).

Because of the increasing frequency of nosocomial infections due to *S. maltophilia*, its presence in hospital environments is being more closely examined. Like *P. aeruginosa*, *S. maltophilia* is ubiquitous in aqueous environments and can be readily cultured from water sources in homes and hospitals (77).

Unlike that of certain *B. cepacia* complex strains, evidence for person-to-person transmission of *B. gladioli*, *B. pseudomallei*, *B. mallei*, *S. maltophilia*, and the other species discussed in this chapter is lacking.

CLINICAL SIGNIFICANCE

B. cepacia Complex and *B. gladioli*

B. cepacia has long been recognized as an occasional opportunistic human pathogen capable of causing a variety of infections, including bacteremia, urinary tract infection, septic arthritis, peritonitis, and pneumonia in persons with underlying illness (144, 166). Persons with chronic granulomatous disease (CGD), a primary immunodeficiency in which white blood cells are unable to generate the superoxide and reactive oxidants necessary for intracellular microbicidal activity, are particularly susceptible to infection (227). *B. cepacia* also has a history as a nosocomial pathogen, causing infections associated with contaminated hospital equipment, medications, and disinfectants including povidone-iodine and benzalkonium chloride (143). Nosocomial outbreaks of respiratory tract infections in patients on mechanical ventilation in intensive care units have been attributed to contamination of nebulizers or nebulized medications such as albuterol (177). Contamination of blood culture systems or disinfectants resulting in pseudobacteremia has been described following the isolation of *B. cepacia* from the blood of multiple patients over a short period (60).

During the 1980s, *B. cepacia* emerged as a life-threatening pathogen in persons with CF, which is the most common inherited lethal disease in Caucasians in North America and Europe, affecting about 1 in 2,750 live births (144). Early reports of infection in CF described patients with acute pulmonary deterioration and sepsis (referred to as cepacia syndrome) or chronic respiratory tract infections associated with an accelerated decline in lung function (121, 198). Clinical outcome studies consistently identified *B. cepacia* infection as a significant independent risk factor for morbidity and mortality in CF (59, 140).

The recognition that several closely related species can be distinguished from among organisms previously identified as *B. cepacia* has stimulated interest in the clinical significance of each of these species (141). Approximately 3% of CF patients in the United States are infected with *B. cepacia* complex species, although rates of infection vary from 0 to 20% among CF treatment centers (68). Rates of infection increase with increasing patient age; approximately 6 to 7% of adults with CF are infected (68). Most strains are inherently resistant to currently available antimicrobial agents (see below), and pulmonary infection is generally refractory to therapy. Furthermore, due to the poor postoperative prognosis associated with *B. cepacia* complex infection, most CF treatment centers consider infection to be an absolute contraindication for lung transplantation, which at present is the only therapeutic option for successful intermediate-term survival of persons with end-stage pulmonary disease (142). Thus, respiratory tract infection with these species is a cause of great concern to CF patients and their caregivers.

Although all nine species of the *B. cepacia* complex have been recovered from persons with CF, the distribution of species in this patient population is disproportionate. In the United States, *B. multivorans* and *B. cenocepacia* together account for approximately 85% of infections (178). In Canada and some European countries, *B. cenocepacia* alone accounts for as much as 80% of infections (4, 192). Some *B. cepacia* complex species are recovered only rarely. In a recent survey, *B. stabilis*, *B. ambifaria*, *B. anthina*, and *B. pyrrocinia* each accounted for less than 1% of *B. cepacia* complex infections among 1,218 infected CF patients (178).

Emerging data suggest that *B. cepacia* complex species also vary with respect to their virulence levels and clinical impacts in CF. Studies with lung transplant recipients, for example, indicate that rates of postoperative mortality are greater for persons infected preoperatively with *B. cenocepacia* than for patients infected with other *B. cepacia* complex species (8, 80). However, although it is almost certainly true that *B. cenocepacia* is the species most frequently associated with cepacia syndrome, it remains to be shown whether this species, in general, is disproportionately associated with poor outcome; recent reports document fatal infection associated with other *B. cepacia* complex species, including *B. multivorans*, *B. stabilis*, and *B. dolosa* (18, 73, 164). Thus, although a positive correlation between species frequency and poor clinical outcome seems likely, firm conclusions regarding the relative virulence of *B. cepacia* complex species must await more definitive study. Recent studies also suggest that epidemic strains, particularly ET12, are relatively more virulent in CF (125, 136), but again, further comparative outcome studies are needed before firm conclusions about relative virulence can be drawn.

B. gladioli is most notable as a plant pathogen but is also well recognized to be capable of causing infection in persons with CF or CGD and, occasionally, other immunocompromised patients (101, 180). Anecdotal reports describe acute pulmonary deterioration and recurrent soft tissue abscesses, as well as severe post-lung transplantation infections due to *B. gladioli* in CF patients (15, 126, 132). A more complete appreciation of the epidemiology and clinical significance of *B. gladioli* infection in CF has been confounded by difficulty with accurate identification of this species, which typically is capable of growth on selective media used to isolate the *B. cepacia* complex (38) and is frequently misidentified as a member of the *B. cepacia* complex by commercial test systems (40, 189).

B. pseudomallei and *B. mallei*

B. pseudomallei is the causative agent of the human and animal disease melioidosis, which is endemic in Southeast Asia and tropical northern Australia and is being increasingly recognized on the Indian subcontinent and in Central and South America (32). In locations where the disease is endemic, infection is seasonal, with up to 85% of cases occurring during the monsoon wet season. As travel to Southeast Asia and northern Australia has become more frequent, reports of melioidosis in travelers returning to Europe and the United States are becoming more common (69), including those of infections in persons with CF (162, 184, 211). Infection with this organism should be considered in the differential diagnosis of any individual with a fever of unknown origin or a tuberculosis-like illness who has a history of travel to a region where *B. pseudomallei* infection is endemic.

B. pseudomallei is present in soil and surface water and is acquired either by inoculation through cut or abraded skin or by inhalation. Zoonotic disease is described but is exceedingly uncommon, as are person-to-person transmission and laboratory-acquired infection (32). The association of severe weather events with respiratory infection and high mortality rates has been attributed to a shift from percutaneous inoculation to inhalation (65). This idea supports the potential of *B. pseudomallei* as a bioterrorism agent; its isolation from patients who do not give a history of travel to an area where melioidosis is endemic should be immediately reported to local or state public health authorities. For further details, see chapter 9 or http://www.bt.cdc.gov.

The majority of persons infected with *B. pseudomallei* remain asymptomatic, with rates of seropositivity of over 20% in some locations (128). Latent infection with subsequent reactivation is well recognized, with a recent description of disease onset in the United States, where melioidosis is not endemic, 62 years after presumed infection in Thailand (159). Nevertheless, the vast majority of cases of melioidosis are from recent infection, with an incubation period of 1 to 21 days (mean, 9 days) (64). Risk factors for clinical disease following infection with *B. pseudomallei* include diabetes, excessive alcohol consumption, chronic renal disease, and chronic lung disease (66). Around 20% of patients have no identified risk factor, and mortality in this group is usually low. Disease in children is also uncommon, although parotid abscesses are well recognized as an important manifestation of melioidosis in children in Thailand. Overall rates of mortality from melioidosis vary from 15% in centers where state-of-the-art intensive care therapy is available to over 50% in locations with poor resources (32, 222). Fifty percent of cases present with pneumonia, which can be part of a fatal septicemia or a less severe unilateral infection indistinguishable from other community-acquired pneumonias or a chronic illness mimicking tuberculosis (29, 61). Chronic melioidosis, defined as illness present for over 2 months, occurs in only 10% of cases. Overall, 50% of cases are bacteremic; the presence of >100 CFU/ml of blood and a blood culture showing growth in the first 24 h of incubation are markers for high mortality (199). Other common presentations with or without bacteremia are genitourinary infections, septic arthritis, and osteomyelitis (32, 63, 222). Prostatic abscesses are especially common (63). Abscesses can also occur in the spleen, liver, kidneys, and adrenal glands. Parotitis, lymphadenitis, sinusitis, orchitis, myositis (especially psoas abscesses), mycotic aneurysms, and pericardial and mediastinal collections have all been described. Lesions can be frankly purulent and may include microabscesses or granulomas or a combination of these features. Clinical meningitis is rare, but melioidosis encephalomyelitis syndrome (62, 63, 229) and brain abscesses have also been reported (135). The one presentation that has yet to be described is *B. pseudomallei* endocarditis.

B. mallei is the etiologic agent of glanders, a highly communicable disease of livestock, particularly horses, mules, and donkeys. It can be transmitted to humans and is also identified as a potential agent of bioterrorism. Unlike *B. pseudomallei*, *B. mallei* is a host-adapted pathogen that does not persist in the environment outside its host. Glanders has been eradicated from most countries, but enzootic foci persist in the Middle East, Asia, Africa, and South America. The only human case of glanders in the past 50 years in the United States was a recent laboratory-acquired case in a biodefense scientist (26). Like melioidosis, human glanders can be acute or chronic, with the clinical presentation and course depending on the mode of infection, the inoculation dose, and host risk factors. Respiratory inoculation can result in pneumonia with potential for dissemination to internal organs and septicemia. Cutaneous inoculation can result in skin nodules and regional lymphadenitis, also with potential for disseminated disease. Involvement of lymph nodes, both mediastinal and peripheral, is much more common in glanders than in melioidosis, often with suppurative abscesses in untreated cases.

S. maltophilia

S. maltophilia, although typically not pathogenic for healthy persons, is a well-known opportunistic human pathogen. It is among the most common causes of wound infection due to trauma involving agricultural machinery (3). It is also an important nosocomial pathogen associated with substantial morbidity and mortality, particularly in debilitated or immunocompromised patients and patients requiring ventilatory support in intensive care units (5, 88, 107, 158). The incidence of human infection appears to have increased in recent years, and a variety of clinical syndromes have been described, including bacteremia, pneumonia, urinary tract infection, ocular infection, endocarditis, meningitis, soft tissue and wound infection, mastoiditis, epididymitis, cholangitis, osteochondritis, bursitis, and peritonitis (76, 183). Septicemia can be accompanied by ecthyma gangrenosa, a skin lesion more commonly associated with *P. aeruginosa* and *Vibrio* spp. (206).

The incidence of *S. maltophilia* respiratory tract infection in persons with CF also appears to be increasing (74, 197); however, the unreliability of historical data limits firm conclusions. Approximately 11% of CF patients included in the CF Foundation's patient registry were culture-positive for *S. maltophilia* in 2003 (68). In large multicenter clinical trials, however, *S. maltophilia* was found in a larger proportion of CF patients, being second only to *P. aeruginosa* in frequency of isolation from study subjects (25). Infection or colonization was most frequently transient, with 30% of subjects having at least one sputum culture positive for *S. maltophilia* during the course of 6 months (100). Several case control studies have drawn conflicting conclusions regarding the role that *S. maltophilia* plays in contributing to pulmonary decline in CF (74, 98).

Ralstonia and *Cupriavidus* spp.

As described above, the taxonomy of the genus *Ralstonia* has been recently revised, with several species being assigned to the genus *Cupriavidus* (201). Among the species in these two genera, *R. pickettii* is best known with respect to human infection. Older reports describe this species as being recovered from a variety of clinical specimens (179) and as causing various infections including bacteremia, meningitis, endocarditis, and osteomyelitis (217). *R. pickettii* also has been identified in cases of pseudobacteremias and nosocomial outbreaks due to contamination of intravenous medications, sterile water, saline, chlorhexidine solutions, respiratory therapy solutions, and intravenous catheters (19, 36, 84). This species has also been recovered from the respiratory tracts of persons with CF (25). However, *R. pickettii* is easily confused with *Pseudomonas fluorescens* and members of the *B. cepacia* complex (25, 72, 111). Furthermore, several newly recognized *R. pickettii*-like species are also now known to be involved in human infection, particularly in CF (52). Thus, the role of *R. pickettii* as a human pathogen is difficult to assess based on historical data.

R. mannitolilytica (formerly known as *R. pickettii* biovar 3/'*thomasii*') was recently described as causing nosocomial outbreaks and a case of recurrent meningitis (72). This species accounts for the majority of *Ralstonia* infections in CF patients, being found in more than twice as many CF patients as *R. pickettii* (52). *R. insidiosa* and *Cupriavidus respiraculi* are recently described species recovered from persons with CF (43, 56). *Cupriavidus gilardii* has been recovered from cerebrospinal fluid (42), and cases of *Cupriavidus paucula* bacteremia, peritonitis, and tenosynovitis have been reported (202). Both of these species may be found in sputa from patients with CF (52). Although *Cupriavidus metallidurans* and *Cupriavidus basilensis* are not known to cause human infection, they too have been recovered recently from sputum cultures from patients with CF (52). Despite these observations, the roles of *Ralstonia* and *Cupriavidus* species in human infection, particularly in persons with CF, require further elucidation.

Other Genera

In general, *Brevundimonas*, *Comamonas*, *Delftia*, *Acidovorax*, and *Pandoraea* spp. infrequently cause human infection. Interest in these species focuses primarily on their roles as plant pathogens or on studies of microbial biodiversity and biodegradation.

Brevundimonas spp. are occasionally recovered from clinical specimens (37). *Brevundimonas vesicularis* bacteremia in patients with various underlying illnesses has been reported (92), and the organism has been recognized in cervical specimens because of its ability to produce bright orange colonies on Thayer-Martin agar (165). *Brevundimonas diminuta* has been recovered from blood, urine, and pleural fluid from patients with cancer (105).

Among the *Comamonas* species, *Comamonas testosteroni* has been implicated most often in human infection, with recent reports describing endocarditis, meningitis, and catheter-associated bacteremia due to this species (7, 58, 137). *D. acidovorans* has similarly been reported to cause infection, being identified in cases of bacteremia, endocarditis, ocular infection, and suppurative otitis (82). *Acidovorax* spp. have been isolated from a variety of clinical sources (224), including blood from a patient with a hematological malignancy (232). *Acidovorax* spp., *Comamonas testosteroni*, and *D. acidovorans* have also been recovered from sputa of persons with CF (44; J. J. LiPuma, unpublished data); however, the roles of these species in contributing to lung disease in CF have not been established.

In addition to causing infections in CF (123, 127), *Pandoraea* spp. have been recovered from blood and from patients with chronic obstructive pulmonary disease or CGD (70). Although the roles of these species in contributing to poor outcomes in persons with underlying diseases are unclear, a recent report describes sepsis, multiple organ failure, and death in a patient who underwent lung transplantation due to sarcoidosis (194).

COLLECTION, TRANSPORT, AND STORAGE

The genera described in this chapter include organisms that can survive in a variety of hostile environments and at temperatures found in clinical settings. Therefore, standard collection, transport, and storage techniques as outlined in chapters 5, 6, and 20 are sufficient to ensure the recovery of these organisms from clinical specimens.

DIRECT EXAMINATION

Members of these genera have similar morphologies and, with the exception of *B. pseudomallei*, are not easily distinguished from one another on the basis of Gram staining. *B. pseudomallei* often appears as small, gram-negative bacilli with bipolar staining, making the cells resemble safety pins (Fig. 1). It is not uncommon for the presumptive laboratory diagnosis of *B. pseudomallei* infection to be made upon the examination of the initial Gram-stained smear.

Although PCR-based assays have been described for the identification of *B. cepacia* complex species, *B. pseudomallei*, *B. gladioli*, several *Ralstonia* and *Cupriavidus* species, *Pandoraea* species, and *S. maltophilia* following culture and isolation (see "Identification" below), the use of PCR for direct detection of these species in clinical specimens remains a research tool (71, 153, 220). Studies of CF sputum samples have indicated that some specimens may be PCR positive but culture negative for certain *B. cepacia* complex species, raising important questions about the natural history of infection in CF. However, the sensitivities and specificities of such PCR assays for the intended target species are difficult to determine in the absence of reliable "gold standards." The development of assays employing real-time PCR technology may yield reliable approaches to direct detection of these species in clinical specimens in the near future.

Because septicemia with *B. pseudomallei* is frequently fatal, several rapid direct detection methods have been developed in research laboratories, including urinary antigen detection using latex agglutination (LA) and enzyme immunoassay (EIA), direct fluorescent-antibody (DFA) staining, and PCR (78, 103, 190, 212). The EIA for the detection of urinary antigens is more sensitive than LA, with an overall sensitivity of 71% for patients with melioidosis compared with an LA sensitivity of 62% (with concentrated urine) or only 17.5% (with unconcentrated urine). The EIA has higher sensitivity (84%) with samples from septicemic patients. Cross-reactions with other urinary tract pathogens including *Klebsiella pneumoniae* and *Escherichia coli* have been reported with EIA but not LA; therefore, EIA results must be interpreted cautiously (78, 190).

Antibodies raised against heat-killed whole cells of *B. pseudomallei* have been used to prepare a reagent for DFA staining. When this DFA reagent was used to stain clinical specimens from patients with suspected melioidosis, it showed a sensitivity of 73%, similar to those of other bacterial DFA stains. The reagent (not available commercially) apparently does not cross-react with other organisms, although the number of isolates tested for cross-reaction was small (212).

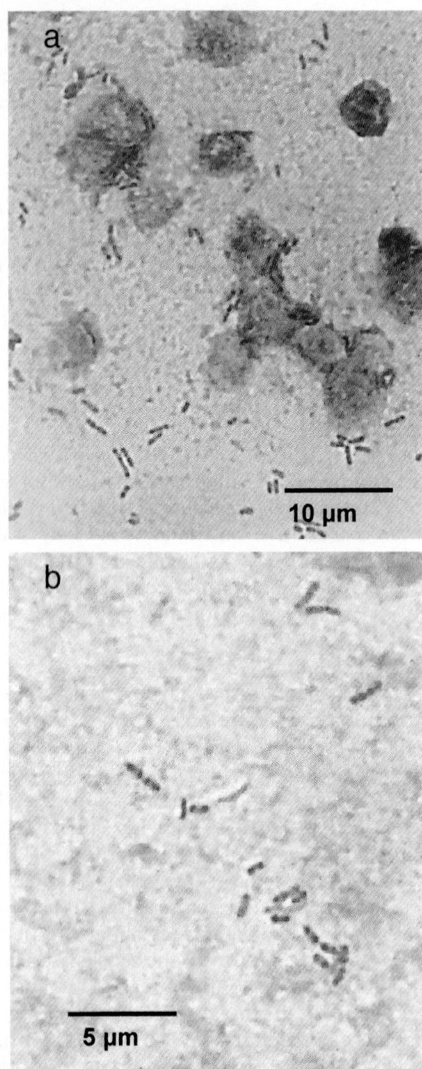

FIGURE 1 (a) Gram stain of *B. pseudomallei* in a blood culture; (b) Gram stain of *B. pseudomallei* from a colony on blood agar.

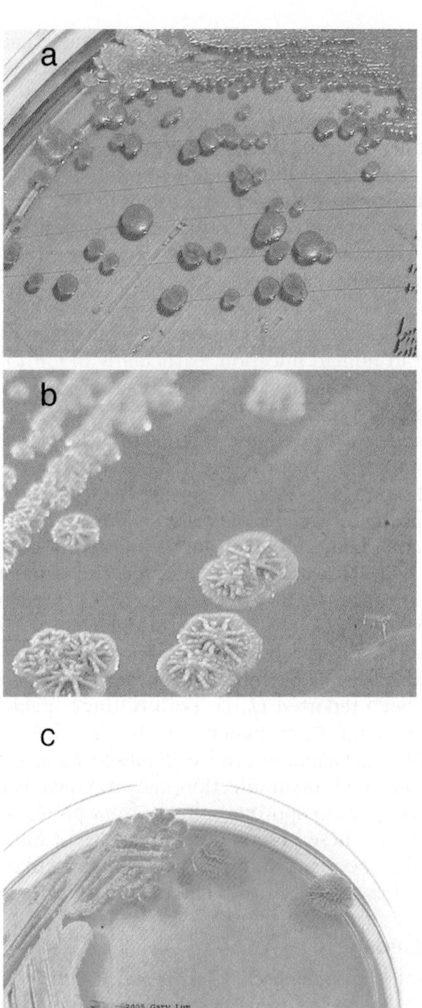

FIGURE 2 (a) *B. pseudomallei* colonies on MacConkey agar; (b) *B. pseudomallei* colonies on blood agar; (c) *B. pseudomallei* colonies on Ashdown medium agar.

Reports on the use of PCR for the direct detection of *B. pseudomallei* in clinical specimens indicate that the currently used primer sets and assay conditions are sensitive but lack specificity, resulting in positive predictive values of only 70% (103).

CULTURE AND ISOLATION

These species grow well on standard laboratory media such as 5% sheep blood and chocolate agars. Such media can be used to recover the organisms from sterile fluid or tissue where a mixed flora is not anticipated (see chapter 20). All species that have been reported to be recovered from blood, including *B. pseudomallei* (199), grow in broth-based blood culture systems within the standard 5-day incubation period, so special blood culture techniques such as lysis-centrifugation and extended incubation periods are not required. The use of selective media facilitates the isolation of these organisms from specimens with mixed microbiota. With the exception of *Brevundimonas vesicularis,* MacConkey agar can be used to isolate most species of these genera.

Burkholderia species grow on MacConkey agar (Fig. 2), but the use of specific selective media with the ability to inhibit *P. aeruginosa* is preferred for the isolation of *B. cepacia* complex species and *B. pseudomallei*. Several selective media have been described, and some are commercially available. A multicenter comparison of three media, PC (for *Pseudomonas cepacia*) agar (BD Diagnostics, Franklin Lakes, N.J.) (94), OFPBL (for oxidation-fermentation base-polymyxin b-bacitracin-lactose) agar (BD Diagnostics) (215), and BCSA (for *B. cepacia* selective agar; Hardy Diagnostics, Santa Maria, Calif.) (109), showed that BCSA was superior, being both more sensitive (more *B. cepacia* isolates were recovered) and more specific (fewer other types of organisms grew) than PC or OFPBL agar (109, 110). More recently, the sensitivities of TB-T (for trypan blue-tetracycline) (104), PC-AT (for *Pseudomonas cepacia* azelaic acid) (23), and BCSA (109, 110) were compared with those of three commercial media, i.e., *B. cepacia* media from MAST Diagnostics (Bootle, Merseyside, United Kingdom), LAB M Ltd. (Bury, United Kingdom), and Oxoid Ltd. (Basingstoke, United Kingdom), through the analysis of 142 clinical and environmental isolates representing all species within the *B. cepacia* complex (209).

BCSA and MAST *B. cepacia* medium supported the growth of *B. cepacia* complex isolates most efficiently. The latter two media were also compared in a study to evaluate the sensitivities and specificities for the isolation of *B. cepacia* complex species from sputum specimens from CF patients (230). BCSA was reported to be equally sensitive as MAST agar but more selective.

Ashdown medium is effective for the isolation of *B. pseudomallei* (Fig. 2); crystal violet and gentamicin act as selective agents. It has been shown to be superior to MacConkey agar or MacConkey agar supplemented with colistin for the recovery of *B. pseudomallei* from clinical specimens containing mixed bacterial microbiota, such as throat, rectal, and sputum specimens (231). An enrichment broth consisting of Ashdown medium supplemented with 50 mg of colistin per liter allowed the recovery of 25% more *B. pseudomallei* isolates than direct plating of clinical specimens on Ashdown agar (213).

For the recovery of *B. pseudomallei* from rectal and throat swabs, selective broth should be inoculated at the bedside and incubated for up to 7 days at 35 to 37°C. The broth can be subcultured to selective media in the laboratory, and solid-phase agar can be kept for an additional 7 days at 35 to 37°C. During the monsoon season, specimens such as sputa, urine (male patients), and wound swabs should be inoculated onto Ashdown agar (213, 229). Subculture from broth should be done earlier if a pellicle at the liquid-air interface is observed or if the broth changes from a deep purple to a deep pink hue due to a change in pH affecting the neutral red indicator.

Recently, a new selective agar, BPSA (for *B. pseudomallei* selective agar), was reported to improve the recovery of *B. pseudomallei* over that with other media (114). BPSA was more inhibitory to *P. aeruginosa* and *B. cepacia* complex species and made recognition of *Burkholderia* species easier due to their distinctive colony morphology. However, in clinical practice this medium may offer only a modest advantage over current commercially available media.

The use of selective media (130) increases the isolation rates for *S. maltophilia* from clinical and environmental samples (75). Denton et al. (75) studied the sensitivity of a selective medium incorporating vancomycin, imipenem, and amphotericin B as selective agents (VIA medium) for isolating *S. maltophilia* from sputum samples collected from children with CF. This study compared the use of VIA medium to an existing in-house method that utilized an imipenem disk placed upon bacitracin-chocolate agar (BC medium) and reported improved detection using VIA medium as a selective medium.

IDENTIFICATION

B. cepacia Complex and *B. gladioli*

Accurate identification of *B. cepacia* complex species presents a challenge (154). Commercial bacterial identification systems are not able to reliably distinguish among the species of the *B. cepacia* complex and often fail to differentiate these species from other closely related species such as *B. gladioli* and *Ralstonia, Cupriavidus,* and *Pandoraea* spp. (21, 111, 133, 189). This failure presents a serious problem for CF patients and their caregivers as detailed in "Clinical Significance" above. The identification of *B. cepacia* complex species from CF sputum culture has a dramatic impact on patient management and is a cause of considerable anxiety for patients with CF (142, 143). Consequently, when *Burkholderia, Ralstonia, Cupriavidus,* or *Pandoraea* species are tentatively identified in a patient with CF by using a commercial system, the identity of the isolate should be confirmed by conventional biochemical testing (111) and, if necessary, molecular techniques. To aid clinical microbiologists in the United States, the CF Foundation has established a *B. cepacia* reference laboratory, which uses a combination of phenotypic and genotypic methods (described below) to confirm the identity of suspected *B. cepacia* complex isolates (146). Further information concerning the *B. cepacia* reference laboratory can be found on the CF Foundation website (http://www.cff.org).

B. cepacia complex species may require 3 days of incubation before colonies are seen on selective media. On MacConkey or Mueller-Hinton agar, these colonies may be punctate and tenacious, and on blood agar or a selective medium such as BCSA, PC agar, or OFPBL agar, the colonies are smooth and slightly raised; occasional isolates are mucoid. On MacConkey agar, colonies of the *B. cepacia* complex frequently become dark pink to red due to oxidation of lactose after extended incubation (4 to 7 days). Most clinical isolates are nonpigmented, but on iron-containing media such as a triple sugar iron slant, many strains produce a bright yellow pigment. *B. cepacia* complex species have a characteristic dirt-like odor.

The species of the *B. cepacia* complex are phenotypically very similar, making their differentiation, even with an extended panel of biochemical tests, rather difficult (Table 1) (111). *B. multivorans, B. stabilis,* and *B. dolosa* rarely oxidize sucrose. *B. stabilis* is ornithine decarboxylase positive, as are most *B. cenocepacia* strains, but is distinctive in that more than two-thirds of strains are *o*-nitrophenyl-β-D-galactopyranoside (ONPG) negative. *B. stabilis* and most *B. ambifaria* strains show poor growth at 42°C. *B. dolosa* is usually lysine decarboxylase negative, whereas only approximately half of *B. multivorans* strains are negative. Other *B. cepacia* complex species are usually lysine decarboxylase positive. *B. vietnamiensis* and most *B. anthina* strains do not oxidize adonitol. *B. anthina* strains show a distinctive creamy morphology on BCSA, which also turns pink (i.e., alkaline) despite the ability of this species to utilize sucrose (203).

Phenotypic differentiation of *B. cepacia* complex species from *B. gladioli* and *Pandoraea* spp. is also difficult (Table 1). Cellular fatty acid analysis is unable to differentiate *B. cepacia* complex species from *B. gladioli* (193). However, in contrast to *B. cepacia* complex species, most *B. gladioli* strains are oxidase negative and whereas most *B. cepacia* complex strains oxidize maltose and lactose, *B. gladioli* typically oxidizes neither. *Pandoraea* spp. do not oxidize maltose, lactose, xylose, sucrose, or adonitol, and most are ONPG negative. *B. cepacia* complex species also may be difficult to differentiate from *Ralstonia* and *Cupriavidus* species. However, several of the latter species show a fast and strong oxidase reaction whereas *B. cepacia* complex species produce a slow, weak-positive oxidase reaction. Further, in contrast to most *B. cepacia* complex species, *Ralstonia* and *Cupriavidus* species are lysine decarboxylase negative and most often ONPG negative.

The difficulty in differentiating *B. cepacia* complex species has prompted the development of molecular genetic diagnostic tests capable of identifying these species individually and distinguishing them (as a group) from biochemically similar species. DNA sequence differences in 16S and 23S rRNA genes have been used to develop species-specific PCR assays for the identification of several *B. cepacia* complex species (16, 146, 207), as well as *B. gladioli* (221). *B. multivorans, B. vietnamiensis,* and *B. dolosa* can be reliably identified with 16S rRNA-targeted assays, but insufficient sequence variation in rRNA genes exists to enable reliable separation of the remaining *B. cepacia* complex species. Fortunately, species-specific

TABLE 1 Characteristics of the *B. cepacia* complex, *B. gladioli*, and *Pandoraea* spp.

Test	% of strains positive										
	B. cepacia complex (genomovar)									*B. gladioli*	*Pandoraea* spp.
	B. cepacia (I)	*B. multivorans* (II)	*B. cenocepacia* (III)	*B. stabilis* (IV)	*B. vietnamiensis* (V)	*B. dolosa* (VI)	*B. ambifaria* (VII)	*B. anthina* (VII)	*B. pyrrocinia* (IX)		
Oxidase[a]	100	98	98	96	99	98	100	100	86	14	57
Growth:											
MacConkey[b]	83	96	84	93	83	100	100	100	100	96	100
BCSA[a]	100	100	100	100	98	100	100	100	100	69	83
42°C[b]	43	100	84	0	100	100	22	60	66	4	89
Yellow pigment[b]	78	2	3	0	0	0	0	0	33	44	0
Brown pigment[b]	4	2	14	0	0	0	6	0	0	33	0
Lysine decarboxylase[a]	98	50	97	100	99	0	98	87	100	1	4
Ornithine decarboxylase[b]	30	0	71	100	0	0	0	0	67	0	0
Acid from[c]:											
Glucose[b]	100	100	96 (95)	100	100	100	100	100	100	100	89 (11)
Maltose[b]	70 (39)	99 (98)	86 (78)	93	100 (97)	100	100	100	100	0	0
Lactose[a]	91	99	92	86	99	98	96	100	100	8	1
Xylose[b]	100 (87)	99 (98)	92 (88)	78 (44)	86 (75)	100	100	100 (94)	100	96	0
Sucrose[a]	84	2	90	6	92	0	94	59	79	1	1
Adonitol[b]	78 (70)	92 (91)	87 (79)	96 (78)	0	100	100	20	100	96 (93)	0
PNPG or ONPG[a,d]	98	99	99	29	99	100	100	83	93	95	11
Nitrate to nitrite reduction[b,e]	4	94	31	4	47	100	67	88	0	33	11
Gelatin liquefaction[b,e]	74	2	55	93	0	0	94	0	66	70	0
Esculin hydrolysis[b,e]	56	2	33	0	0	0	56	6	33	11	0

[a]The number of strains of each species tested was as follows: *B. cepacia*, 122; *B. multivorans*, 715; *B. cenocepacia*, 768; *B. stabilis*, 49; *B. vietnamiensis*, 145; *B. dolosa*, 57; *B. ambifaria*, 51; *B. anthina*, 24; *B. pyrrocinia*, 14; *B. gladioli*, 280; and *Pandoraea* spp., 75. Data are from references 111 and 203 and J. J. LiPuma (unpublished data) and D. A. Henry (unpublished data).

[b]The number of strains of each species tested was as follows: *B. cepacia*, 23; *B. multivorans*, 109; *B. cenocepacia*, 139; *B. stabilis*, 27; *B. vietnamiensis*, 36; *B. dolosa*, 9; *B. ambifaria*, 18; *B. anthina*, 16; *B. pyrrocinia*, 3; *B. gladioli*, 27; and *Pandoraea* spp., 9. Data are from references 111 and 203 and D. A. Henry (unpublished data).

[c]Oxidation test results were recorded after 7 days of incubation (data in parentheses were recorded after 3 days of incubation).

[d]PNPG, *p*-nitrophenyl-β-D-glucoside.

[e]Results presented are from the API 20 NE test strip.

sequence variation does exist in the *recA* gene, and PCR assays targeting this locus enable the reliable identification of *B. multivorans*, *B. cenocepacia*, and *B. ambifaria* (49, 150, 208). Other 16S rRNA- and *recA*-based PCR assays identify all *Burkholderia* spp. (i.e., at the genus level) or all species within the *B. cepacia* complex (i.e., as a group) (146, 150, 172).

Another molecular genetic approach to identifying *B. cepacia* complex species involves restriction fragment length polymorphism (RFLP) analysis of either 16S rRNA or *recA* genes (150, 187). Again, insufficient sequence variation in the 16S rRNA gene limits the use of RFLP analysis of this locus, even when multiple restriction enzymes are used (86, 187, 210). In contrast, *recA* RFLP analysis has proved quite useful in reliably distinguishing all species within the *B. cepacia* complex (150, 172, 208).

Other genomic approaches, including amplified fragment length polymorphism typing, ribotyping, and whole-cell protein profiling, have been proposed for the differentiation of *B. cepacia* complex species (22, 50, 204). However, these methods are time-consuming and expensive and require an extensive validated database before isolates can be reliably identified. These limitations render them impractical for use in a routine diagnostic laboratory. Cellular fatty acid methyl ester analysis is useful for identification of *Burkholderia* strains at the genus level but is not reliable for identification of individual *B. cepacia* complex species and does not differentiate *B. gladioli* (40, 202).

B. pseudomallei and *B. mallei*

If *B. pseudomallei* is suspected, all efforts should be made to confirm or exclude a positive oxidase reaction, production of gas from nitrate, multitrichous polar flagella, and arginine dihydrolase and gelatinase activities (Table 2). The bacterium gives off a distinctive earthy odor such that a clue to its presence can be gleaned upon opening a petri dish (even with a mixed culture). However, active sniffing of cultures is strongly discouraged in order to prevent infection (10). Cellular fatty acid profiles may be useful for differentiating *B. pseudomallei* from other genera, but reports vary on their utility in differentiating *B. thailandensis* and *B. pseudomallei* (117) or other pathogenic *Burkholderia* species including *B. mallei*, *B. cepacia* complex species, and *B. gladioli*.

B. pseudomallei must be differentiated from *Pseudomonas stutzeri* and *B. cepacia* complex species in clinical specimens. *Pseudomonas stutzeri* appears very similar to *B. pseudomallei* after a few days of incubation, and both *B. pseudomallei* and *B. cepacia* complex species may be isolated from persons with CF (162, 184, 211). Whereas *B. pseudomallei* produces gas from nitrate and is arginine dihydrolase positive, most *B. cepacia* complex isolates are negative for both characteristics. *Pseudomonas stutzeri* is negative for arginine dihydrolase, oxidation-fermentation glucose, and gelatin hydrolysis. *Pseudomonas stutzeri* also has only one flagellum, and *B. pseudomallei* has more than one.

There have been reports linking a lack of virulence of *B. pseudomallei* with the ability to assimilate arabinose (6). Environmental strains tend to be arabinose assimilators, and those that do not assimilate arabinose are almost always found as clinical isolates. The name *B. thailandensis* is used to describe arabinose-utilizing strains with low virulence (20).

The Microbact 24E strip (MedVet, Adelaide, Australia) appears to more accurately identify *B. pseudomallei* than does the API 20NE system (bioMérieux, Hazelwood, Mo.) (118). Limited experience with automated systems such as Vitek-1 and Vitek-2 (bioMérieux, Durham, N.C.) and MicroScan WalkAway (Dade International Inc., West Sacramento, Calif.) indicates that they reliably identify *B. pseumomallei*. However, further evaluation of commercially available identification systems is required (96, 119). Because of the difficulty with accurate laboratory identification, referral to a reference laboratory is advised when isolation of *B. pseudomallei* is suspected. This is especially important with the advent of emerging bioterrorism legislation in many countries (see chapter 9).

TABLE 2 Characteristics of *B. mallei*, *B. pseudomallei*, and *B. thailandensis*[a]

Test	*B. mallei*	*B. pseudomallei*	*B. thailandensis*
Oxidase	v	+	+
Growth:			
MacConkey	+	+	+
42°C	−	+	+
Nitrate reduction	+	+	+
Gas from nitrate	−	+	+
Arginine dihydrolase	+	+	+
Lysine decarboxylase	−	−	−
Ornithine decarboxylase	−	−	−
Hydrolysis of:			
Urea	v	v	v
Citrate	−	v	v
Gelatin	−	v	v
Esculin	−	v	v
Acid from:			
Glucose	+	+	+
Xylose	v	+	+
Lactose	v	+	+
Sucrose	−	v	v
Maltose	−	+	+
Mannitol	−	+	+
Arabinose	ND	−	+
Motility	0	100% +	100% +
No. of flagella	0	≥2	≥2

[a]Data from references 20 and 218. +, >90% positive; −, >90% negative; v, variable; ND, not determined.

Ralstonia and *Cupriavidus* spp.

Although *R. pickettii* was considered to be the *Ralstonia* species most frequently isolated from clinical specimens (179), the recent recognition that several other *Ralstonia* and *Cupriavidus* species can be identified from among *R. pickettii*-like isolates limits previous observations. As is the case with *B. cepacia* complex species, *Ralstonia* and *Cupriavidus* species are phenotypically similar, requiring rather extensive biochemical testing to reliably differentiate them; species-level identification with standard biochemical testing is difficult (Table 3). These species may grow slowly on primary isolation media, requiring ≥72 h of incubation before colonies are visible. They are lysine decarboxylase negative and generally catalase positive, although catalase-negative *R. pickettii* strains have been described (42, 202). Most species show a fast and strong oxidase reaction; however, the intensity of the oxidase reaction varies for *R. mannitolilytica*, *R. pickettii*, and *Cupriavidus gilardii*, with some strains showing a weakly positive reaction (42, 202; LiPuma, unpublished). *R. pickettii*, *R. mannitolilytica*, and *R. insidiosa* grow on BCSA; growth of other species is strain dependent. These species do not produce acid from sucrose.

TABLE 3 Characteristics of *Ralstonia* and *Cupriavidus* spp.[a]

Test	*R. pickettii*	*R. mannitolilytica*	*R. insidiosa*	*Cupriavidus respiraculi*	*Cupriavidus gilardii*	*Cupriavidus paucula*
Catalase	v	+	+	+	+	+
Oxidase	+	+	+	+	+	+
Growth:						
BCSA	+	+	+	−	v	v
42°C	v	+	ND	ND	+	v
Colistin resistance	+	+	ND	ND	ND	−
Nitrate reduction	+	−	+	v	−	−
Tween 80 hydrolysis	+	+	ND	ND	−	+
Urease	+	+	v	−	−	+
Lysine decarboxylase	−	−	−	−	−	−
ONPG	−	v	v	−	v	ND
Acid from:						
L-Arabinose	+	+	ND	ND	−	−
D-Arabitol	−	+	ND	ND	ND	−
Glucose	+	+	−	−	−	−
Inositol	−	−	ND	ND	ND	−
Lactose	v	+	−	−	−	−
Maltose	v	+	ND	ND	ND	−
Mannitol	−	+	ND	ND	ND	−
Sucrose	−	−	−	−	−	−
Xylose	+	+	ND	ND	−	−
Motility	+	+	ND	ND	+	+
Flagella	1 polar	1 polar	ND	ND	1 polar	Peritrichous

[a]Data from references 42, 43, 72, and 202, and J. J. LiPuma (unpublished data). +, >90% positive; −, >90% negative; v, variable; ND, not determined.

Most *R. mannitolilytica* strains acidify lactose, whereas most strains from other species do not. *R. insidiosa, Cupriavidus respiraculi, Cupriavidus gilardii,* and *Cupriavidus paucula* are differentiated from *R. pickettii* and *R. mannitolilytica* in failing to acidify glucose. *Cupriavidus gilardii* has a characteristic cellular fatty acid profile different from that of other *Ralstonia* species (42, 72).

Molecular genetic tests have proved quite helpful in differentiating these species. A recently described 16S rRNA-directed PCR assay reliably identifies all *Ralstonia* and *Cupriavidus* species (as a group), allowing their differentiation from the phenotypically similar species in the genera *Burkholderia* and *Pandoraea* (52). Species-specific 16S rRNA-based PCR assays have also been developed recently; these enable the accurate identification of *R. pickettii, R. mannitolilytica, R. insidiosa,* and *Cupriavidus respiraculi* (52, 55, 56).

Pandoraea spp.

Overall, the biochemical profiles of *Pandoraea* strains are similar to those of *Burkholderia* and *Ralstonia* strains isolated from clinical specimens (Table 1) (41, 70, 111). A lack of saccharolytic activity is indicative of *Pandoraea* but is also seen with some *Ralstonia* species. Definitive identification of putative *Pandoraea* isolates requires molecular confirmation. Coenye et al. (48) described 16S rDNA-based PCR assays for the identification of these bacteria. A PCR assay was developed for the identification of *Pandoraea* isolates to the genus level. PCR assays for the identification of *P. apista* and *P. pulmonicola* (as a group), *P. pnomenusa, P. sputorum,* and *P. norimbergensis* were also developed. *Pandoraea* strains can be differentiated from *Burkholderia* and *Ralstonia* strains by their specific 16S rDNA restriction profile (111, 188) and can be identified at the species level through MspI restriction analysis of the *gyrB* gene (47). A quantitative comparison of the whole-cell fatty acid profiles of the members of these three genera allows the differentiation of *Pandoraea* strains from the others (42, 70). However, with the use of the commercially available microbial identification system database (Microbial ID, Inc., Newark, Del.), these organisms are mostly identified with low identification scores as *Burkholderia* or *Ralstonia* species (42, 111) due to a lack of discriminatory fatty acids.

S. maltophilia

Key features for identifying *S. maltophilia* include a negative oxidase reaction, oxidation of glucose and maltose with a more intense reaction with the latter, positive reactions for DNase and lysine decarboxylase, and a tuft of polar flagella (Table 4) (218). Detection of extracellular DNase activity by *S. maltophilia* is a key to differentiating this species from most other glucose-oxidizing, gram-negative bacilli. It can be detected in tube-based or plated DNase medium with a methyl green indicator. DNase-positive organisms produce a zone of clearing around the colonies on this medium. Care must be taken in interpreting the DNase reaction, since one report documented the misidentification of *S. maltophilia* as *B. cepacia* based partially on false-negative DNase reactions that were finalized with 48 h of incubation rather than 72 h (24). Selected isolates of *Flavobacterium* and *Shewanella* spp. may also be DNase positive (see chapters 14 and 21). On sheep blood agar, colonies appear rough and lavender-green and have an ammonia-like odor. *S. maltophilia* has a characteristic cellular fatty acid profile with large amounts (>30%) of 13-methyl tetradecanoic acid ($C_{15:0\ iso}$) and lesser amounts (>10%) of 12-methyl tetradecanoic acid ($C_{15:0\ anteiso}$) and *cis*-9-hexadecanoic acid ($C_{16:1\ cis9}$) (218). To overcome the problems associated with definitive identification of *S. maltophilia*, Whitby et al. (219) developed a species-specific PCR assay targeting the 23S rRNA gene and reported sensitivity and specificity of 100%. This PCR test was recently

TABLE 4 Characteristics of *Acidovorax*, *Brevundimonas*, *Delftia*, *Comamonas*, and *Stenotrophomonas* spp. found in clinical specimens[a]

Test	*A. delafieldii* (*n* = 2)	*A. facilis* (*n* = 2)	*A temperans* (*n* = 2)	*Brevundimonas diminuta* (*n* = 68)	*Brevundimonas vesicularis* (*n* = 94)	*D. acidovorans* (*n* = 69)	*Comamonas* spp. (*n* = 28)	*S. maltophilia* (*n* = 228)
Oxidase	100	100	100	100	98	100	100	0
Growth:								
MacConkey	100	0	100	100	43	100	100	100
Cetrimide	0	0	0	0	0	4	0	2
6.0% NaCl	0	0	0	21	23	6	0	22
42°C	50	0	100	38	19	29	68	48
Nitrate reduction	100	100	100	3	5	99	96	39
Gas from nitrate	0	0	100	0	0	0	0	0
Pigment	Yellow, soluble	None	Yellow, soluble	Brown-tan, soluble	52% yellow-orange, insoluble[d]	26% fluorescent, 44% yellow-tan, soluble	27% yellow-brown, soluble	Brown-tan, soluble
Arginine dihydrolase	100	100	0	0	0	0	0	0
Lysine decarboxylase	0	0	0	0	0	0	0	93
Ornithine decarboxylase	0	0	0	0	0	0	0	0
Indole	0	0	0	0	0	0	0	0
Hemolysis	0	0	0	0	0	0	0	1
Hydrolysis of:								
Urea	100	100	50	13	2	0	7	3
Citrate	100	0	0	1	1	94	47	34
Gelatin	0	100	0	68	25	11	0	93
Esculin	0	0	0	5	88	0	0	39
Acid from:								
Glucose[b]	100	100	100	21	87	0	0	85
Xylose	85	100	0	0	27	0	0	35
Lactose	0	0	0	0	0	0	0	60
Sucrose	0	0	0	0	0	0	0	63
Maltose	0	0	0	0	94	0	0	100
Mannitol	50	100	50	0	0	100	0	0
H_2S[c]	100	100	100	34	49	57	0	95
Motility	100	100	100	100	100	100	100	100
No. of flagella	1–2	1–2	1–2	1–2	1–2	>2	>2	>2

[a]Data are from reference 218. Results are expressed as the percentage of strains positive.
[b]Oxidation-fermentation basal medium with 1% carbohydrate.
[c]Lead acetate paper.
[d]Pigment observed on Thayer-Martin agar.

used as a standard to evaluate the identification of *S. maltophilia* using the API 20NE strip and the Vitek-2 ID-GNB card (95). Both systems showed good reliability compared to PCR. A multiplex PCR assay to identify *P. aeruginosa*, *B. cepacia* complex species, and *S. maltophilia* directly in sputum and oropharyngeal specimens from CF patients has been reported, but only a limited number of *S. maltophilia* isolates were examined (71).

Acidovorax, Brevundimonas, Delftia, and *Comamonas* spp.

Characteristics of *Acidovorax*, *Brevundimonas*, *Delftia*, and *Comamonas* spp. are given in Table 4.

Acidovorax species, rarely encountered in clinical and environmental samples, are straight to slightly curved gram-negative bacilli which occur either singly or in short chains. They are oxidase positive and nonpigmented and have a single polar flagellum. Urease activity varies among strains (218, 224).

Brevundimonas diminuta and *Brevundimonas vesicularis*, infrequently encountered in clinical and environmental samples, have growth requirements for specific vitamins, including pantothenate, biotin, and cyanocobalamin. An additional growth requirement for *Brevundimonas diminuta* is cysteine. Most strains of *Brevundimonas diminuta* grow on MacConkey agar, while only approximately 25% of *Brevundimonas vesicularis* strains do so. On primary isolation media, *Brevundimonas diminuta* colonies are chalk white whereas many strains of *Brevundimonas vesicularis* are characterized by an orange intracellular pigment. These organisms are oxidase positive, have a single polar flagellum, and weakly oxidize glucose (*Brevundimonas vesicularis* more so than *Brevundimonas diminuta*), and the vast majority fail to reduce nitrate to nitrite. The most reliable method for differentiating these two species is the test for esculin hydrolysis. Almost all strains of *Brevundimonas vesicularis* (88%) are reported to hydrolyze this substrate, while *Brevundimonas diminuta* strains rarely do (5%) (Table 4) (218).

Comamonas spp. are straight to slightly curved gram-negative bacilli which occur singly or in pairs. The organisms are catalase and oxidase positive and have a single tuft of polar flagella. All human clinical *Comamonas* species reduce nitrate to nitrite. Phenotypic differentiation of *Comamonas terrigena* from *Comamonas testosteroni* is difficult, and as a result isolates are typically reported as *Comamonas* spp. (Table 4).

D. acidovorans is phenotypically similar to *Comamonas*. Key characteristics of the species include abilities to oxidize fructose and mannitol. One-quarter of the strains produce a fluorescent pigment, and approximately half of the strains may produce a soluble yellow to tan hue (218, 223).

TYPING SYSTEMS

Several molecular genetic methods are available to assess the relatedness of isolates of these genera during nosocomial outbreak investigations. These methods are preferred over phenotypically based systems, which are less discriminatory and reproducible. Analysis of whole-genome macrorestriction profiles with pulsed-field gel electrophoresis (PFGE) has gained acceptance as a preferred genotyping method and has proved useful in numerous studies of *Burkholderia*, *Ralstonia*, and *S. maltophilia* (36, 51, 200). The endonucleases XbaI and SpeI are most frequently used and typically yield a dozen or more DNA fragments for analysis. Care must be taken in interpreting PFGE profiles of *Burkholderia* species, however. These species have unusually large and dynamic multichromosome genomes that are prone to large-scale alterations in content and arrangement (138). Consequently, epidemiologically irrelevant genomic polymorphisms may arise in the short term and confound outbreak investigations (51).

Ribotyping, which relies on polymorphisms in and around rRNA operons, has been used to investigate the epidemiology of the *B. cepacia* complex and *B. pseudomallei* (120, 145, 147). Both PFGE and ribotyping are relatively time-consuming and expensive to perform and are therefore not particularly well suited for routine analysis in clinical microbiology laboratories. A variety of PCR-based methods, including randomly amplified polymorphic DNA typing and repetitive-sequence PCR typing, offer attractive alternatives for genotyping *S. maltophilia* and *Burkholderia*, *Ralstonia*, and *Pandoraea* spp. (30, 44, 134, 151, 188). These methods are inexpensive and can provide rapid, reliable results. Multilocus sequence typing, which assesses DNA sequence variation at several chromosomal loci, has been developed for numerous bacterial species, including the *B. cepacia* complex, *B. pseudomallei*, and *B mallei* (13, 34, 97). This genotyping strategy provides robust, reproducible, and portable results and is quickly becoming the preferred method for investigating bacterial epidemiology, evolution, and population structure. Despite these attributes, however, multilocus sequence typing carries considerable expense and at present is largely a research tool. Typing methods have not been reported for *Brevundimonas*, *Delftia*, *Comamonas*, or *Acidovorax* spp.

SEROLOGIC TESTS

Of the organisms discussed in this chapter, serologic tests have been used clinically to diagnose only infections with *B. pseudomallei*. The indirect hemagglutination assay (IHA), although not available commercially, is the most widely used test in regions where infection is endemic (67). It is performed by using a prepared antigen from strains of *B. pseudomallei* sensitized to sheep cells and includes unsensitized cells as a control. This assay can be adapted to a microtiter plate test system. Because of high antibody background levels in healthy individuals, cross-reactions with other organisms including the *B. cepacia* complex, and the rapid onset of septicemic disease, IHA is of limited clinical value. Interpretation is difficult in areas where infection is endemic, and all results must be viewed in a clinical context. IHA titers may rise to high levels in culture-negative individuals, and a specific titer cutoff that indicates disease has not been established. In regions where infection is endemic, single titers may be reported without interpretation. The need for acute- and convalescent-phase titers along with relevant clinical information to aid in interpretation is paramount in attempting to establish serologically the diagnosis of subacute or chronic *B. pseudomallei* infection (160). Evaluation of recently developed rapid immunochromatographic test kits (Pan-Bio, Windsor, Queensland, Australia) suggests that the immunoglobulin G test may be useful for investigating travelers presenting with possible melioidosis after returning from regions where the disease is endemic but the immunoglobulin M test has low specificity (161).

ANTIMICROBIAL SUSCEPTIBILITY

Specific susceptibility testing interpretative criteria are not available for all of the species discussed in this chapter. For some species, such as the *B. cepacia* complex and *S. maltophilia*, interpretive criteria for disk diffusion testing are available for only a limited number of antibiotics. In general, MIC broth microdilution tests or E tests are preferred for this group of organisms.

B. cepacia complex species are among the most antimicrobial-resistant bacteria encountered in the clinical laboratory. These species are intrinsically resistant to aminoglycoside and polymyxin antibiotics and are often resistant to β-lactam antibiotics due to inducible chromosomal β-lactamases and altered penicillin-binding proteins (106). Antibiotic efflux pumps may mediate resistance to chloramphenicol, fluoroquinolones, and trimethoprim (175). Clinical strains may be susceptible to only a handful of agents, including trimethoprim-sulfamethoxazole (TMP-SMX), ceftazidime, chloramphenicol, minocycline, imipenem, meropenem, and some fluoroquinolones (1, 112, 173). Clinical and Laboratory Standards Institute (formerly NCCLS) interpretative criteria for disk diffusion susceptibility testing are available only for ceftazidime, meropenem, minocycline, and TMP-SMX (39). MIC broth microdilution tests or E tests are preferred methodologies for susceptibility testing of these species. Because isolates that are initially susceptible may become resistant during the course of therapy, susceptibility testing of repeat isolates may be warranted. Furthermore, strains recovered from patients with CF who have received repeated courses of antibiotic therapy are frequently resistant to all currently available antimicrobial agents (1, 93). Combinations of antimicrobial agents may provide synergistic activity against resistant strains; however, antagonism with combinations is also observed in vitro (1). Testing for synergy with both double and triple combinations of agents is available in reference laboratories (http://synergy.columbia.edu) (1). The value of such testing is controversial, however; studies have yet to correlate in vitro synergy testing results with patient response to therapy (1, 155).

B. pseudomallei is resistant to penicillin, aminoglycosides, and macrolides, but several agents have antimicrobial activity in vitro, including ceftazidime, meropenem and imipenem, cefoperazone, amoxicillin-clavulanate, ampicillin-sulbactam, ticarcillin-clavulanate, chloramphenicol, and doxycycline. TMP-SMX is often used clinically; although reported in vitro susceptibility results are variable, most isolates are susceptible by agar dilution testing (122, 129). Resistance to fluoroquinolones is common, and their use has been associated with higher relapse rates (28). E tests have proved satisfactory for determining in vitro resistance or susceptibility, especially for TMP-SMX (158). Disk diffusion techniques have been disappointing, and inaccurate results suggest that they should probably be avoided (149).

Current trends in the management of melioidosis involve an initial 10- to 14-day intensive therapy phase with ceftazidime with or without TMP-SMX, followed by eradication therapy with TMP-SMX with or without doxycycline for at least 3 months (32, 222). Amoxicillin-clavulanate is recommended for eradication therapy in pregnancy and is an alternative to TMP-SMX in children. In critically ill patients requiring intensive care, meropenem or imipenem may be superior to ceftazidime, and granulocyte colony-stimulating factor is being used in some centers (33, 35, 122). According to molecular genotyping studies, relapse following antimicrobial therapy has been observed in as many as 15% of patients (79).

Because of the potential role of *B. mallei* as a bioterrorism agent, studies have been done recently to determine the activities of a variety of agents against this species. *B. mallei* has a susceptibility profile similar to that of *B. pseudomallei*, except that *B. mallei* is susceptible to aminoglycosides and newer macrolides such as clarithromycin and azithromycin whereas *B. pseudomallei* is resistant (108, 129). Current recommended treatment and duration of therapy for glanders are the same as those for melioidosis.

S. maltophilia is intrinsically resistant to many classes of antibiotics. Resistance can also develop rapidly during infection (91). Resistance to β-lactam agents is mediated by at least two β-lactamases, one of which is zinc dependent and resistant to β-lactamase inhibitors and confers resistance to imipenem. Aminoglycoside and quinolone resistance results from mutations in outer membrane proteins. In a recent study of isolates recovered from patients with CF, doxycycline was the most active agent in vitro (182). TMP-SMX is usually active and is often used in combination with ticarcillin-clavulanate, minocycline, or piperacillin-tazobactam (182). Other combinations that may be effective include ciprofloxacin paired with ticarcillin-clavulanate, ciprofloxacin and piperacillin-tazobactam, or doxycycline and ticarcillin-clavulanate. Clinical and Labaratory Standards Institute interpretive criteria for disk diffusion susceptibility testing are available for minocycline, levofloxacin, and TMP-SMX (39). However, broth microdilution, E test, or agar dilution methods are the preferred susceptibility testing methods (9, 235). Many U.S. laboratories comment only on the activity of TMP-SMX but will test additional antibiotics such as minocycline, ceftazidime, ticarcillin-clavulanate, and ciprofloxacin or levofloxacin upon request.

In general, *Comamonas testosteroni* is susceptible to extended- and broad-spectrum cephalosporins, carbapenems, quinolones, and TMP-SMX (14). *D. acidovorans* is frequently resistant to the aminoglycosides.

EVALUATION, INTERPRETATION, AND REPORTING OF RESULTS

These species are found in the natural environment and may occasionally contaminate clinical specimens. Nevertheless, they are increasingly recognized as nosocomial and opportunistic pathogens, especially in certain patient populations, such as persons with CF. They are also frequently misidentified by commercial microbial identification systems. Therefore, their recovery in the clinical laboratory must be given careful consideration. In particular, species of the *B. cepacia* complex are not reliably differentiated by phenotypic analyses and their recovery from persons with CF has serious consequences with respect to patient management and psychosocial well-being (141). Identification of these species should be confirmed by genotypic analyses at a reference laboratory and should promptly be reported to the CF care team. Similarly, identification of *B. pseudomallei*, *B. mallei*, or *B. thailandensis* should be confirmed by a reference laboratory with experience with these species. Care must be given to ensure that culture handling and shipping comply with current biosafety regulations (see chapters 8 and 9). Identification of these species must be reported to public health officials due to the potential of these species as agents of bioterrorism (see chapter 9).

Interpretive criteria for disk diffusion antimicrobial susceptibility testing of most of these species are lacking; MIC broth microdilution and the E test are, therefore, the preferred methodologies for susceptibility testing. For multidrug-resistant strains, consideration should be given to testing for synergy with double or triple combinations of antimicrobial agents in reference laboratories.

REFERENCES

1. **Aaron, S. D., W. Ferris, D. A. Henry, D. P. Speert, and N. E. MacDonald.** 2000. Multiple combination bactericidal antibiotic testing for patients with cystic fibrosis infected with *Burkholderia cepacia*. *Am. J. Respir. Crit. Care Med.* **161:**1206–1212.
2. **Abraham, W. R., C. Strompl, H. Meyer, S. Lindholst, E. R. Moore, R. Christ, M. Vancanneyt, B. J. Tindall, A. Bennasar, J. Smit, and M. Tesar.** 1999. Phylogeny and polyphasic taxonomy of *Caulobacter* species. Proposal of *Maricaulis* gen. nov. with *Maricaulis maris* (Poindexter) comb. nov. as the type species, and emended description of the genera *Brevundimonas* and *Caulobacter*. *Int. J. Syst. Bacteriol.* **49:** 1053–1073.
3. **Agger, W. A., T. H. Cogbill, H. Busch, Jr., J. Landercasper, and S. M. Callister.** 1986. Wounds caused by corn-harvesting machines: an unusual source of infection due to gram-negative bacilli. *Rev. Infect. Dis.* **8:**927–931.
4. **Agodi, A., M. Barchitta, V. Giannino, A. Collura, T. Pensabene, M. L. Garlaschi, C. Pasquarella, F. Luzzaro, F. Sinatra, E. Mahenthiralingam, and S. Stefani.** 2002. *Burkholderia cepacia* complex in cystic fibrosis and non-cystic fibrosis patients: identification of a cluster of epidemic lineages. *J. Hosp. Infect.* **50:**188–195.
5. **Alfieri, N., K. Ramotar, P. Armstrong, M. E. Spornitz, G. Ross, J. Winnick, and D. R. Cook.** 1999. Two consecutive outbreaks of *Stenotrophomonas maltophilia (Xanthomonas maltophilia)* in an intensive-care unit defined by restriction fragment-length polymorphism typing. *Infect. Control Hosp. Epidemiol.* **20:**553–556.
6. **Anuntagool, N., P. Intachote, V. Wuthiekanun, N. J. White, and S. Sirisinha.** 1998. Lipopolysaccharide from nonvirulent Ara^+ *Burkholderia pseudomallei* isolates is immunologically indistinguishable from lipopolysaccharide from virulent Ara^- clinical isolates. *Clin. Diagn. Lab. Immunol.* **5:**225–229.
7. **Arda, B., S. Aydemir, T. Yamazhan, A. Hassan, A. Tunger, and D. Serter.** 2003. *Comamonas testosteroni* meningitis in a patient with recurrent cholesteatoma. *APMIS* **111:**474–476.
8. **Aris, R. M., J. C. Routh, J. J. LiPuma, D. G. Heath, and P. H. Gilligan.** 2001. Lung transplantation for cystic fibrosis patients with *Burkholderia cepacia* complex. Survival linked to genomovar type. *Am. J. Respir. Crit. Care Med.* **164:**2102–2106.
9. **Arpi, M., M. A. Victor, I. Mortensen, A. Gottschau, and B. Bruun.** 1996. In vitro susceptibility of 124 *Xanthomonas maltophilia (Stenotrophomonas maltophilia)* isolates: comparison of the agar dilution method with the E-test and two agar diffusion methods. *APMIS* **104:**108–114.
10. **Ashdown, L. R.** 1992. Melioidosis and safety in the clinical laboratory. *J. Hosp. Infect.* **21:**301–306.
11. **Assih, E. A., A. S. Ouattara, S. Thierry, J. L. Cayol, M. Labat, and H. Macarie.** 2002. *Stenotrophomonas acidaminiphila* sp. nov., a strictly aerobic bacterium isolated from an upflow anaerobic sludge blanket (UASB) reactor. *Int. J. Syst. Evol. Microbiol.* **52:**559–568.
12. **Balandreau, J., V. Viallard, B. Cournoyer, T. Coenye, S. Laevens, and P. Vandamme.** 2001. *Burkholderia cepacia* genomovar III is a common plant-associated bacterium. *Appl. Environ. Microbiol.* **67:**982–985.
13. **Baldwin, A., E. Mahenthiralingam, K. M. Thickett, D. Honeybourne, M. C. J. Maiden, J. Govan, D. Speert, J. J. LiPuma, P. Vandamme, and C. G. Dowson.** 2005. Multilocus sequence typing scheme for the *Burkholderia cepacia* complex. *J. Clin. Microbiol.* **43:**4665–4673.
14. **Barbaro, D. J., P. A. Mackowiak, S. S. Barth, and P. M. Southern, Jr.** 1987. *Pseudomonas testosteroni* infections: eighteen recent cases and a review of the literature. *Rev. Infect. Dis.* **9:**124–129.
15. **Barker, P. M., R. E. Wood, and P. H. Gilligan.** 1997. Lung infection with *Burkholderia gladioli* in a child with cystic fibrosis: acute clinical and spirometric deterioration. *Pediatr. Pulmonol.* **23:**123–125.
16. **Bauernfeind, A., I. Schneider, R. Jungwirth, and C. Roller.** 1999. Discrimination of *Burkholderia multivorans* and *Burkholderia vietnamiensis* from *Burkholderia cepacia* genomovars I, III, and IV by PCR. *J. Clin. Microbiol.* **37:**1335–1339.
17. **Berriatura, E., I. Ziluaga, C. Miguel-Virto, P. Uribarren, R. Juste, S. Laevens, P. Vandamme, and J. R. W. Govan.** 2001. Outbreak of subclinical mastitis in a flock of dairy sheep associated with *Burkholderia cepacia* complex infection. *J. Clin. Microbiol.* **39:**990–994.
18. **Blackburn, L., K. Brownlee, S. Conway, and M. Denton.** 2004. '*Cepacia* syndrome' with *Burkholderia multivorans*, 9 years after initial colonization. *J. Cyst. Fibros.* **3:**133–134.
19. **Boutros, N., N. Gonullu, A. Casetta, M. Guibert, D. Ingrand, and L. Lebrun.** 2002. *Ralstonia pickettii* traced in blood culture bottles. *J. Clin. Microbiol.* **40:**2666–2667.
20. **Brett, P. J., D. DeShazer, and D. E. Woods.** 1998. *Burkholderia thailandensis* sp. nov., a *Burkholderia pseudomallei*-like species. *Int. J. Syst. Bacteriol.* **48:**317–320.
21. **Brisse, S., S. Stefani, J. Verhoef, A. Van Belkum, P. Vandamme, and W. Goessens.** 2002. Comparative evaluation of the BD Phoenix and VITEK 2 automated instruments for identification of isolates of the *Burkholderia cepacia* complex. *J. Clin. Microbiol.* **40:**1743–1748.
22. **Brisse, S., C. M. Verduin, D. Milatovic, A. Fluit, J. Verhoef, S. Laevens, P. Vandamme, B. Tummler, H. A. Verbrugh, and A. van Belkum.** 2000. Distinguishing species of the *Burkholderia cepacia* complex and *Burkholderia gladioli* by automated ribotyping. *J. Clin. Microbiol.* **38:**1876–1884.
23. **Burbage, D. A., and M. Sasser.** 1982. A medium selective for *Pseudomonas cepacia*. *Phytopathology* **76:**706.
24. **Burdge, D. R., M. A. Noble, M. E. Campbell, V. L. Krell, and D. P. Speert.** 1995. *Xanthomonas maltophilia* misidentified as *Pseudomonas cepacia* in cultures of sputum from patients with cystic fibrosis: a diagnostic pitfall with major clinical implications. *Clin. Infect. Dis.* **20:**445–448.
25. **Burns, J. L., J. Emerson, J. R. Stapp, D. L. Yim, J. Krzewinski, L. Louden, B. W. Ramsey, and C. R. Clausen.** 1998. Microbiology of sputum from patients at cystic fibrosis centers in the United States. *Clin. Infect. Dis.* **27:**158–163.
26. **Centers for Disease Control and Prevention.** 2000. Laboratory-acquired human glanders—Maryland, May 2000. *Morb. Mortal. Wkly. Rep.* **49:**532–535.
27. **Chang, Y. H., J. I. Han, J. Chun, K. C. Lee, M. S. Rhee, Y. B. Kim, and K. S. Bae.** 2002. *Comamonas koreensis* sp. nov., a non-motile species from wetland in Woopo, Korea. *Int. J. Syst. Evol. Microbiol.* **52:**377–381.
28. **Chaowagul, W., Y. Suputtamongkul, M. D. Smith, and N. J. White.** 1997. Oral fluoroquinolones for maintenance treatment of melioidosis. *Trans. R. Soc. Trop. Med. Hyg.* **91:**599–601.
29. **Chaowagul, W., N. J. White, D. A. Dance, Y. Wattanagoon, P. Naigowit, T. M. Davis, S. Looareesuwan, and N. Pitakwatchara.** 1989. Melioidosis: a major cause of community-acquired septicemia in northeastern Thailand. *J. Infect. Dis.* **159:**890–899.
30. **Chen, J. S., K. A. Witzmann, T. Spilker, R. J. Fink, and J. J. LiPuma.** 2001. Endemicity and inter-city spread of *Burkholderia cepacia* genomovar III in cystic fibrosis. *J. Pediatr.* **139:**643–649.
31. **Chen, W. M., S. Laevens, T. M. Lee, T. Coenye, P. De Vos, M. Mergeay, and P. Vandamme.** 2001. *Ralstonia taiwanensis* sp. nov., isolated from root nodules of Mimosa species and sputum of a cystic fibrosis patient. *Int. J. Syst. Evol. Microbiol.* **51:**1729–1735.

32. **Cheng, A. C., and B. J. Currie.** 2005. Melioidosis: epidemiology, pathophysiology, and management. *Clin. Microbiol. Rev.* **18:**383–416.
33. **Cheng, A. C., D. A. Fisher, N. M. Anstey, D. P. Stephens, S. P. Jacups, and B. J. Currie.** 2004. Outcomes of patients with melioidosis treated with meropenem. *Antimicrob. Agents Chemother.* **48:**1763–1765.
34. **Cheng, A. C., D. Godoy, M. Mayo, D. Gal, B. G. Spratt, and B. J. Currie.** 2004. Isolates of *Burkholderia pseudomallei* from Northern Australia are distinct by multilocus sequence typing, but strain types do not correlate with clinical presentation. *J. Clin. Microbiol.* **42:**5477–5483.
35. **Cheng, A. C., D. P. Stephens, and B. J. Currie.** 19 July 2004, posting date. Granulocyte-colony stimulating factor (G-CSF) as an adjunct to antibiotics in the treatment of pneumonia in adults. *Cochrane Database Syst. Rev.* **2004:**CD004400. [Online.] doi:10.1002/146S1858.CD004400.pub2.
36. **Chetoui, H., P. Melin, M. J. Struelens, E. Delhalle, M. M. Nigo, R. De Ryck, and P. De Mol.** 1997. Comparison of biotyping, ribotyping, and pulsed-field gel electrophoresis for investigation of a common-source outbreak of *Burkholderia pickettii* bacteremia. *J. Clin. Microbiol.* **35:**1398–1403.
37. **Chi, C. Y., C. P. Fung, W. W. Wong, and C. Y. Liu.** 2004. *Brevundimonas bacteremia:* two case reports and literature review. *Scand. J. Infect. Dis.* **36:**59–61.
38. **Christenson, J. C., D. F. Welch, G. Mukwaya, M. J. Muszynski, R. E. Weaver, and D. J. Brenner.** 1989. Recovery of *Pseudomonas gladioli* from respiratory tract specimens of patients with cystic fibrosis. *J. Clin. Microbiol.* **27:**270–273.
39. **Clinical and Laboratory Standards Institute.** 2005. *Performance Standards for Antimicrobial Susceptibility Testing; Fifteenth Informational Supplement. M100-S15.* Clinical and Laboratory Standards Institute, Wayne, Pa.
40. **Clode, F. E., L. A. Metherell, and T. L. Pitt.** 1999. Nosocomial acquisition of *Burkholderia gladioli* in patients with cystic fibrosis. *Am. J. Respir. Crit. Care Med.* **160:**374–375.
41. **Coenye, T., E. Falsen, B. Hoste, M. Ohlen, J. Goris, J. R. Govan, M. Gillis, and P. Vandamme.** 2000. Description of *Pandoraea* gen. nov. with *Pandoraea apista* sp. nov., *Pandoraea pulmonicola* sp. nov., *Pandoraea pnomenusa* sp. nov., *Pandoraea sputorum* sp. nov. and *Pandoraea norimbergensis* comb. nov. *Int. J. Syst. Evol. Microbiol.* **50:**887–899.
42. **Coenye, T., E. Falsen, M. Vancanneyt, B. Hoste, J. R. Govan, K. Kersters, and P. Vandamme.** 1999. Classification of *Alcaligenes faecalis*-like isolates from the environment and human clinical samples as *Ralstonia gilardii* sp. nov. *Int. J. Syst. Bacteriol.* **49:**405–413.
43. **Coenye, T., J. Goris, P. De Vos, P. Vandamme, and J. J. LiPuma.** 2003. Classification of *Ralstonia pickettii*-like isolates from the environment and clinical samples as *Ralstonia insidiosa* sp. nov. *Int. J. Syst. Evol. Microbiol.* **53:**1075–1080.
44. **Coenye, T., J. Goris, T. Spilker, P. Vandamme, and J. J. LiPuma.** 2002. Characterization of unusual bacteria isolated from respiratory secretions of cystic fibrosis patients and description of *Inquilinus limosus* gen. nov., sp. nov. *J. Clin. Microbiol.* **40:**2062–2069.
45. **Coenye, T., B. Holmes, K. Kersters, J. R. Govan, and P. Vandamme.** 1999. *Burkholderia cocovenenans* (van Damme et al. 1960) Gillis et al. 1995 and *Burkholderia vandii* Urakami et al. 1994 are junior synonyms of *Burkholderia gladioli* (Severini 1913) Yabuuchi et al. 1993 and *Burkholderia plantarii* (Azegami et al. 1987) Urakami et al. 1994, respectively. *Int. J. Syst. Bacteriol.* **49:**37–42.
46. **Coenye, T., S. Laevens, A. Willems, M. Ohlen, W. Hannant, J. R. Govan, M. Gillis, E. Falsen, and P. Vandamme.** 2001. *Burkholderia fungorum* sp. nov. and *Burkholderia caledonica* sp. nov., two new species isolated from the environment, animals and human clinical samples. *Int. J. Syst. Evol. Microbiol.* **51:**1099–1107.
47. **Coenye, T., and J. J. LiPuma.** 2002. Use of the *gyrB* gene for the identification of *Pandoraea* species. *FEMS Microbiol. Lett.* **208:**15–19.
48. **Coenye, T., L. Liu, P. Vandamme, and J. J. LiPuma.** 2001. Identification of *Pandoraea* species by 16S ribosomal DNA-based PCR assays. *J. Clin. Microbiol.* **39:**4452–4455.
49. **Coenye, T., E. Mahenthiralingam, D. Henry, J. J. LiPuma, S. Laevens, M. Gillis, D. P. Speert, and P. Vandamme.** 2001. *Burkholderia ambifaria* sp. nov., a novel member of the *Burkholderia cepacia* complex including biocontrol and cystic fibrosis-related isolates. *Int. J. Syst. Evol. Microbiol.* **51:**1481–1490.
50. **Coenye, T., L. M. Schouls, J. R. Govan, K. Kersters, and P. Vandamme.** 1999. Identification of *Burkholderia* species and genomovars from cystic fibrosis patients by AFLP fingerprinting. *Int. J. Syst. Bacteriol.* **49:**1657–1666.
51. **Coenye, T., T. Spilker, A. Martin, and J. J. LiPuma.** 2002. Comparative assessment of genotyping methods for epidemiologic study of *Burkholderia cepacia* genomovar III. *J. Clin. Microbiol.* **40:**3300–3307.
52. **Coenye, T., T. Spilker, R. Reik, P. Vandamme, and J. J. LiPuma.** 2005. Use of PCR analyses to define the distribution of *Ralstonia* species recovered from patients with cystic fibrosis. *J. Clin. Microbiol.* **43:**3463–3466.
53. **Coenye, T., T. Spilker, A. Van Schoor, J. J. LiPuma, and P. Vandamme.** 2004. Recovery of *Burkholderia cenocepacia* strain PHDC from cystic fibrosis patients in Europe. *Thorax* **59:**952–954.
54. **Coenye, T., P. Vandamme, J. R. Govan, and J. J. LiPuma.** 2001. Taxonomy and identification of the *Burkholderia cepacia* complex. *J. Clin. Microbiol.* **39:**3427–3436.
55. **Coenye, T., P. Vandamme, and J. J. LiPuma.** 2002. Infection by *Ralstonia* species in cystic fibrosis patients: identification of *R. pickettii* and *R. mannitolilytica* by polymerase chain reaction. *Emerg. Infect. Dis.* **8:**692–696.
56. **Coenye, T., P. Vandamme, and J. J. LiPuma.** 2003. *Ralstonia respiraculi* sp. nov., isolated from the respiratory tract of cystic fibrosis patients. *Int. J. Syst. Evol. Microbiol.* **53:**1339–1342.
57. **Coenye, T., E. Vanlaere, E. Falsen, and P. Vandamme.** 2004. *Stenotrophomonas africana* Drancourt et al. 1997 is a later synonym of *Stenotrophomonas maltophilia* (Hugh 1981) Palleroni and Bradbury 1993. *Int. J. Syst. Evol. Microbiol.* **54:**1235–1237.
58. **Cooper, G. R., E. D. Staples, K. A. Iczkowski, and C. J. Clancy.** 2005. *Comamonas (Pseudomonas) testosteroni* endocarditis. *Cardiovasc. Pathol.* **14:**145–149.
59. **Corey, M., and V. Farewell.** 1996. Determinants of mortality from cystic fibrosis in Canada, 1970–1989. *Am. J. Epidemiol.* **143:**1007–1017.
60. **Craven, D. E., B. Moody, M. G. Connolly, N. R. Kollisch, K. D. Stottmeier, and W. R. McCabe.** 1981. Pseudobacteremia caused by povidone-iodine solution contaminated with *Pseudomonas cepacia*. *N. Engl. J. Med.* **305:**621–623.
61. **Currie, B. J.** 2003. Melioidosis: an important cause of pneumonia in residents of and travellers returned from endemic regions. *Eur. Respir. J.* **22:**542–550.
62. **Currie, B. J., D. A. Fisher, D. M. Howard, and J. N. Burrow.** 2000. Neurological melioidosis. *Acta Trop.* **74:**145–151.
63. **Currie, B. J., D. A. Fisher, D. M. Howard, J. N. Burrow, D. Lo, S. Selva-Nayagam, N. M. Anstey, S. E. Huffam, P. L. Snelling, P. J. Marks, D. P. Stephens, G. D. Lum, S. P. Jacups, and V. L. Krause.** 2000. Endemic melioidosis in tropical northern Australia: a 10-year prospective study and review of the literature. *Clin. Infect. Dis.* **31:**981–986.
64. **Currie, B. J., D. A. Fisher, D. M. Howard, J. N. Burrow, S. Selvanayagam, P. L. Snelling, N. M. Anstey, and M. J. Mayo.** 2000. The epidemiology of melioidosis in Australia and Papua New Guinea. *Acta Trop.* **74:**121–127.

65. **Currie, B. J., and S. P. Jacups.** 2003. Intensity of rainfall and severity of melioidosis, Australia. *Emerg. Infect. Dis.* **9:**1538–1542.

66. **Currie, B. J., S. P. Jacups, A. C. Cheng, D. A. Fisher, N. M. Anstey, S. E. Huffam, and V. L. Krause.** 2004. Melioidosis epidemiology and risk factors from a prospective whole-population study in northern Australia. *Trop. Med. Int. Health* **9:**1167–1174.

67. **Cuzzubbo, A. J., V. Chenthamarakshan, J. Vadivelu, S. D. Puthucheary, D. Rowland, and P. L. Devine.** 2000. Evaluation of a new commercially available immunoglobulin M and immunoglobulin G immunochromatographic test for diagnosis of melioidosis infection. *J. Clin. Microbiol.* **38:**1670–1671.

68. **Cystic Fibrosis Foundation.** 2004. *Patient Registry 2003 Annual Data Report to the Center Directors*. Cystic Fibrosis Foundation, Bethesda, Md.

69. **Dance, D. A., M. D. Smith, H. M. Aucken, and T. L. Pitt.** 1999. Imported melioidosis in England and Wales. *Lancet* **353:**208.

70. **Daneshvar, M. I., D. G. Hollis, A. G. Steigerwalt, A. M. Whitney, L. Spangler, M. P. Douglas, J. G. Jordan, J. P. MacGregor, B. C. Hill, F. C. Tenover, D. J. Brenner, and R. S. Weyant.** 2001. Assignment of CDC weak oxidizer group 2 (WO-2) to the genus *Pandoraea* and characterization of three new *Pandoraea* genomospecies. *J. Clin. Microbiol.* **39:**1819–1826.

71. **Da Silva Filho, L. V., A. F. Tateno, F. Velloso Lde, J. E. Levi, S. Fernandes, C. N. Bento, J. C. Rodrigues, and S. R. Ramos.** 2004. Identification of *Pseudomonas aeruginosa*, *Burkholderia cepacia* complex, and *Stenotrophomonas maltophilia* in respiratory samples from cystic fibrosis patients using multiplex PCR. *Pediatr. Pulmonol.* **37:**537–547.

72. **De Baere, T., S. Steyaert, G. Wauters, P. De Vos, J. Goris, T. Coenye, T. Suyama, G. Verschraegen, and M. Vaneechoutte.** 2001. Classification of *Ralstonia pickettii* biovar 3/'thomasii' strains (Pickett 1994) and of new isolates related to nosocomial recurrent meningitis as *Ralstonia mannitolilytica* sp. nov. *Int. J. Syst. Evol. Microbiol.* **51:**547–558.

73. **De Boeck, K., A. Malfroot, L. Van Schil, P. Lebecque, C. Knoop, J. R. Govan, C. Doherty, S. Laevens, and P. Vandamme.** 2004. Epidemiology of *Burkholderia cepacia* complex colonisation in cystic fibrosis patients. *Eur. Respir. J.* **23:**851–856.

74. **Demko, C. A., R. C. Stern, and C. F. Doershuk.** 1998. *Stenotrophomonas maltophilia* in cystic fibrosis: incidence and prevalence. *Pediatr. Pulmonol.* **25:**304–308.

75. **Denton, M., M. J. Hall, N. J. Todd, K. G. Kerr, and J. M. Littlewood.** 2000. Improved isolation of *Stenotrophomonas maltophilia* from the sputa of patients with cystic fibrosis using a selective medium. *Clin. Microbiol. Infect.* **6:**397–398.

76. **Denton, M., and K. G. Kerr.** 1998. Microbiological and clinical aspects of infection associated with *Stenotrophomonas maltophilia*. *Clin. Microbiol. Rev.* **11:**57–80.

77. **Denton, M., N. J. Todd, K. G. Kerr, P. M. Hawkey, and J. M. Littlewood.** 1998. Molecular epidemiology of *Stenotrophomonas maltophilia* isolated from clinical specimens from patients with cystic fibrosis and associated environmental samples. *J. Clin. Microbiol.* **36:**1953–1958.

78. **Desakorn, V., M. D. Smith, V. Wuthiekanun, D. A. Dance, H. Aucken, P. Suntharasamai, A. Rajchanuwong, and N. J. White.** 1994. Detection of *Pseudomonas pseudomallei* antigen in urine for the diagnosis of melioidosis. *Am. J. Trop. Med. Hyg.* **51:**627–633.

79. **Desmarchelier, P. M., D. A. Dance, W. Chaowagul, Y. Suputtamongkol, N. J. White, and T. L. Pitt.** 1993. Relationships among *Pseudomonas pseudomallei* isolates from patients with recurrent melioidosis. *J. Clin. Microbiol.* **31:**1592–1596.

80. **De Soyza, A., A. McDowell, L. Archer, J. H. Dark, S. J. Elborn, E. Mahenthiralingam, K. Gould, and P. A. Corris.** 2001. *Burkholderia cepacia* complex genomovars and pulmonary transplantation outcomes in patients with cystic fibrosis. *Lancet* **358:**1780–1781.

81. **Drancourt, M., C. Bollet, and D. Raoult.** 1997. *Stenotrophomonas africana* sp. nov., an opportunistic human pathogen in Africa. *Int. J. Syst. Bacteriol.* **47:**160–163.

82. **Ender, P. T., D. P. Dooley, and R. H. Moore.** 1996. Vascular catheter-related *Comamonas acidovorans* bacteremia managed with preservation of the catheter. *Pediatr. Infect. Dis. J.* **15:**918–920.

83. **Etchebehere, C., M. I. Errazquin, P. Dabert, R. Moletta, and L. Muxi.** 2001. *Comamonas nitrativorans* sp. nov., a novel denitrifier isolated from a denitrifying reactor treating landfill leachate. *Int. J. Syst. Evol. Microbiol.* **51:**977–983.

84. **Fernandez, C., I. Wilhelmi, E. Andradas, C. Gaspar, J. Gomez, J. Romero, J. A. Mariano, O. Corral, M. Rubio, J. Elviro, and J. Fereres.** 1996. Nosocomial outbreak of *Burkholderia pickettii* infection due to a manufactured intravenous product used in three hospitals. *Clin. Infect. Dis.* **22:**1092–1095.

85. **Finkmann, W., K. Altendorf, E. Stackebrandt, and A. Lipski.** 2000. Characterization of N_2O-producing *Xanthomonas*-like isolates from biofilters as *Stenotrophomonas nitritireducens* sp. nov., *Luteimonas mephitis* gen. nov., sp. nov. and *Pseudoxanthomonas broegbernensis* gen. nov., sp. nov. *Int. J. Syst. Evol. Microbiol.* **50:**273–282.

86. **Fiore, A., S. Laevens, A. Bevivino, C. Dalmastri, S. Tabacchioni, P. Vandamme, and L. Chiarini.** 2001. *Burkholderia cepacia* complex: distribution of genomovars among isolates from the maize rhizosphere in Italy. *Environ. Microbiol.* **3:**137–143.

87. **Fritz, I., C. Strompl, D. I. Nikitin, A. M. Lysenko, and W. R. Abraham.** 2005. *Brevundimonas mediterranea* sp. nov., a non-stalked species from the Mediterranean Sea. *Int. J. Syst. Evol. Microbiol.* **55:**479–486.

88. **Fujita, J., I. Yamadori, G. Xu, S. Hojo, K. Negayama, H. Miyawaki, Y. Yamaji, and J. Takahara.** 1996. Clinical features of *Stenotrophomonas maltophilia* pneumonia in immunocompromised patients. *Respir. Med.* **90:**35–38.

89. **Gardan, L., C. Dauga, P. Prior, M. Gillis, and G. S. Saddler.** 2000. *Acidovorax anthurii* sp. nov., a new phytopathogenic bacterium which causes bacterial leaf-spot of anthurium. *Int. J. Syst. Evol. Microbiol.* **50:**235–246.

90. **Gardan, L., D. E. Stead, C. Dauga, and M. Gillis.** 2003. *Acidovorax valerianellae* sp. nov., a novel pathogen of lamb's lettuce [*Valerianella locusta* (L.) Laterr.]. *Int. J. Syst. Evol. Microbiol.* **53:**795–800.

91. **Garrison, M. W., D. E. Anderson, D. M. Campbell, K. C. Carroll, C. L. Malone, J. D. Anderson, R. J. Hollis, and M. A. Pfaller.** 1996. *Stenotrophomonas maltophilia*: emergence of multidrug-resistant strains during therapy and in an in vitro pharmacodynamic chamber model. *Antimicrob. Agents Chemother.* **40:**2859–2864.

92. **Gilad, J., A. Borer, N. Peled, K. Riesenberg, S. Tager, A. Appelbaum, and F. Schlaeffer.** 2000. Hospital-acquired *Brevundimonas vesicularis* septicaemia following open-heart surgery: case report and literature review. *Scand. J. Infect. Dis.* **32:**90–91.

93. **Gilligan, P. H.** 1991. Microbiology of airway disease in patients with cystic fibrosis. *Clin. Microbiol. Rev.* **4:**35–51.

94. **Gilligan, P. H., P. A. Gage, L. M. Bradshaw, D. V. Schidlow, and B. T. DeCicco.** 1985. Isolation medium for the recovery of *Pseudomonas cepacia* from respiratory secretions of patients with cystic fibrosis. *J. Clin. Microbiol.* **22:**5–8.

95. **Giordano, A., A. Magni, M. Trancassini, P. Varesi, R. Turner, and C. Mancini.** 2006. Identification of respiratory isolates of *Stenotrophomonas maltophilia* by commercial

biochemical systems and species-specific PCR. *J. Microbiol. Methods* **64:**135–138.

96. **Glass, M. B., and T. Popovic.** 2005. Preliminary evaluation of the API 20NE and RapID NF plus systems for rapid identification of *Burkholderia pseudomallei* and *B. mallei*. *J. Clin. Microbiol.* **43:**479–483.
97. **Godoy, D., G. Randle, A. J. Simpson, D. M. Aanensen, T. L. Pitt, R. Kinoshita, and B. G. Spratt.** 2003. Multilocus sequence typing and evolutionary relationships among the causative agents of melioidosis and glanders, *Burkholderia pseudomallei* and *Burkholderia mallei*. *J. Clin. Microbiol.* **41:**2068–2079.
98. **Goss, C. H., K. Otto, M. L. Aitken, and G. D. Rubenfeld.** 2002. Detecting *Stenotrophomonas maltophilia* does not reduce survival of patients with cystic fibrosis. *Am. J. Respir. Crit. Care Med.* **166:**356–361.
99. **Govan, J. R., J. E. Hughes, and P. Vandamme.** 1996. *Burkholderia cepacia*: medical, taxonomic and ecological issues. *J. Med. Microbiol.* **45:**395–407.
100. **Graff, G. R., and J. L. Burns.** 2002. Factors affecting the incidence of *Stenotrophomonas maltophilia* isolation in cystic fibrosis. *Chest* **121:**1754–1760.
101. **Graves, M., T. Robin, A. M. Chipman, J. Wong, S. Khashe, and J. M. Janda.** 1997. Four additional cases of *Burkholderia gladioli* infection with microbiological correlates and review. *Clin. Infect. Dis.* **25:**838–842.
102. **Gumaelius, L., G. Magnusson, B. Pettersson, and G. Dalhammar.** 2001. *Comamonas denitrificans* sp. nov., an efficient denitrifying bacterium isolated from activated sludge. *Int. J. Syst. Evol. Microbiol.* **51:**999–1006.
103. **Haase, A., M. Brennan, S. Barrett, Y. Wood, S. Huffam, D. O'Brien, and B. Currie.** 1998. Evaluation of PCR for diagnosis of melioidosis. *J. Clin. Microbiol.* **36:**1039–1041.
104. **Hagedorn, C., W. D. Gould, T. R. Bardinelli, and D. R. Gustavson.** 1987. A selective medium for enumeration and recovery of *Pseudomonas cepacia* biotypes from soil. *Appl. Environ. Microbiol.* **53:**2265–2268.
105. **Han, X. Y., and R. A. Andrade.** 2005. *Brevundimonas diminuta* infections and its resistance to fluoroquinolones. *J. Antimicrob. Chemother.* **55:**853–859.
106. **Hancock, R. E.** 1998. Resistance mechanisms in *Pseudomonas aeruginosa* and other nonfermentative gram-negative bacteria. *Clin. Infect. Dis.* **27**(Suppl. 1)**:**S93–S99.
107. **Hanes, S. D., K. Demirkan, E. Tolley, B. A. Boucher, M. A. Croce, G. C. Wood, and T. C. Fabian.** 2002. Risk factors for late-onset nosocomial pneumonia caused by *Stenotrophomonas maltophilia* in critically ill trauma patients. *Clin. Infect. Dis.* **35:**228–235.
108. **Heine, H. S., M. J. England, D. M. Waag, and W. R. Byrne.** 2001. In vitro antibiotic susceptibilities of *Burkholderia mallei* (causative agent of glanders) determined by broth microdilution and E-test. *Antimicrob. Agents Chemother.* **45:**2119–2121.
109. **Henry, D., M. Campbell, C. McGimpsey, A. Clarke, L. Louden, J. L. Burns, M. H. Roe, P. Vandamme, and D. Speert.** 1999. Comparison of isolation media for recovery of *Burkholderia cepacia* complex from respiratory secretions of patients with cystic fibrosis. *J. Clin. Microbiol.* **37:**1004–1007.
110. **Henry, D. A., M. E. Campbell, J. J. LiPuma, and D. P. Speert.** 1997. Identification of *Burkholderia cepacia* isolates from patients with cystic fibrosis and use of a simple new selective medium. *J. Clin. Microbiol.* **35:**614–619.
111. **Henry, D. A., E. Mahenthiralingam, P. Vandamme, T. Coenye, and D. P. Speert.** 2001. Phenotypic methods for determining genomovar status of the *Burkholderia cepacia* complex. *J. Clin. Microbiol.* **39:**1073–1078.
112. **Hoban, D. J., S. K. Bouchillon, J. L. Johnson, G. G. Zhanel, D. L. Butler, L. A. Miller, and J. A. Poupard.** 2001. Comparative in vitro activity of gemifloxacin, ciprofloxacin, levofloxacin and ofloxacin in a North American surveillance study. *Diagn. Microbiol. Infect. Dis.* **40:**51–57.
113. **Holt, J., N. R. Krieg, P. H. A. Sneath, J. T. Staley, and S. T. Williams.** 1994. *Bergey's Determinative Bacteriology*, 9th ed., vol. 1. The Williams and Wilkins Co., Philadelphia, Pa.
114. **Howard, K., and T. J. Inglis.** 2003. Novel selective medium for isolation of *Burkholderia pseudomallei*. *J. Clin. Microbiol.* **41:**3312–3316.
115. **Hugh, R., and E. Ryschenkow.** 1961. *Pseudomonas maltophilia*, an *Alcaligenes*-like species. *J. Gen. Microbiol.* **26:**123–132.
116. **Hutchinson, G. R., S. Parker, J. A. Pryor, F. Duncan-Skingle, P. N. Hoffman, M. E. Hodson, M. E. Kaufmann, and T. L. Pitt.** 1996. Home-use nebulizers: a potential primary source of *Burkholderia cepacia* and other colistin-resistant, gram-negative bacteria in patients with cystic fibrosis. *J. Clin. Microbiol.* **34:**584–587.
117. **Inglis, T. J., M. Aravena-Roman, S. Ching, K. Croft, V. Wuthiekanun, and B. J. Mee.** 2003. Cellular fatty acid profile distinguishes *Burkholderia pseudomallei* from avirulent *Burkholderia thailandensis*. *J. Clin. Microbiol.* **41:**4812–4814.
118. **Inglis, T. J., D. Chiang, G. S. Lee, and L. Chor-Kiang.** 1998. Potential misidentification of *Burkholderia pseudomallei* by API 20NE. *Pathology* **30:**62–64.
119. **Inglis, T. J., A. Merritt, G. Chidlow, M. Aravena-Roman, and G. Harnett.** 2005. Comparison of diagnostic laboratory methods for identification of *Burkholderia pseudomallei*. *J. Clin. Microbiol.* **43:**2201–2206.
120. **Inglis, T. J., L. O'Reilly, N. Foster, A. Clair, and J. Sampson.** 2002. Comparison of rapid, automated ribotyping and DNA macrorestriction analysis of *Burkholderia pseudomallei*. *J. Clin. Microbiol.* **40:**3198–3203.
121. **Isles, A., I. Maclusky, M. Corey, R. Gold, C. Prober, P. Fleming, and H. Levison.** 1984. *Pseudomonas cepacia* infection in cystic fibrosis: an emerging problem. *J. Pediatr.* **104:**206–210.
122. **Jenney, A. W., G. Lum, D. A. Fisher, and B. J. Currie.** 2001. Antibiotic susceptibility of *Burkholderia pseudomallei* from tropical northern Australia and implications for therapy of melioidosis. *Int. J. Antimicrob. Agents* **17:**109–113.
123. **Johnson, L. N., J. Y. Han, S. M. Moskowitz, J. L. Burns, X. Qin, and J. A. Englund.** 2004. *Pandoraea bacteremia* in a cystic fibrosis patient with associated systemic illness. *Pediatr. Infect. Dis. J.* **23:**881–882.
124. **Johnson, W. M., S. D. Tyler, and K. R. Rozee.** 1994. Linkage analysis of geographic and clinical clusters in *Pseudomonas cepacia* infections by multilocus enzyme electrophoresis and ribotyping. *J. Clin. Microbiol.* **32:**924–930.
125. **Jones, A. M., M. E. Dodd, J. R. Govan, V. Barcus, C. J. Doherty, J. Morris, and A. K. Webb.** 2004. *Burkholderia cenocepacia* and *Burkholderia multivorans*: influence on survival in cystic fibrosis. *Thorax* **59:**948–951.
126. **Jones, A. M., T. N. Stanbridge, B. J. Isalska, M. E. Dodd, and A. K. Webb.** 2001. *Burkholderia gladioli*: recurrent abscesses in a patient with cystic fibrosis. *J. Infect.* **42:**69–71.
127. **Jorgensen, I. M., H. K. Johansen, B. Frederiksen, T. Pressler, A. Hansen, P. Vandamme, N. Hoiby, and C. Koch.** 2003. Epidemic spread of *Pandoraea apista*, a new pathogen causing severe lung disease in cystic fibrosis patients. *Pediatr. Pulmonol.* **36:**439–446.
128. **Kanaphun, P., N. Thirawattanasuk, Y. Suputtamongkol, P. Naigowit, D. A. Dance, M. D. Smith, and N. J. White.** 1993. Serology and carriage of *Pseudomonas pseudomallei*: a prospective study in 1000 hospitalized children in northeast Thailand. *J. Infect. Dis.* **167:**230–233.
129. **Kenny, D. J., P. Russell, D. Rogers, S. M. Eley, and R. W. Titball.** 1999. In vitro susceptibilities of *Burkholderia mallei* in comparison to those of other pathogenic *Burkholderia* spp. *Antimicrob. Agents Chemother.* **43:**2773–2775.

130. **Kerr, K. G., M. Denton, N. Todd, C. M. Corps, P. Kumari, and P. M. Hawkey.** 1996. A new selective differential medium for isolation of *Stenotrophomonas maltophilia. Eur. J. Clin. Microbiol. Infect. Dis.* **15:**607–610.
131. **Kersters, K., W. Ludwig, M. Vancanneyt, P. De Vos, M. Gillis, and K. H. Schleifer.** 1996. Recent changes in the classification of the pseudomonads: an overview. *Syst. Appl. Microbiol.* **19:**465–477.
132. **Khan, S. U., S. M. Gordon, P. C. Stillwell, T. J. Kirby, and A. C. Arroliga.** 1996. Empyema and bloodstream infection caused by *Burkholderia gladioli* in a patient with cystic fibrosis after lung transplantation. *Pediatr. Infect. Dis. J.* **15:**637–639.
133. **Kiska, D. L., A. Kerr, M. C. Jones, J. A. Caracciolo, B. Eskridge, M. Jordan, S. Miller, D. Hughes, N. King, and P. H. Gilligan.** 1996. Accuracy of four commercial systems for identification of *Burkholderia cepacia* and other gram-negative nonfermenting bacilli recovered from patients with cystic fibrosis. *J. Clin. Microbiol.* **34:**886–891.
134. **Krzewinski, J. W., C. D. Nguyen, J. M. Foster, and J. L. Burns.** 2001. Use of random amplified polymorphic DNA PCR to examine epidemiology of *Stenotrophomonas maltophilia* and *Achromobacter (Alcaligenes) xylosoxidans* from patients with cystic fibrosis. *J. Clin. Microbiol.* **39:**3597–3602.
135. **Lath, R., V. Rajshekhar, and V. George.** 1998. Brain abscess as the presenting feature of melioidosis. *Br. J. Neurosurg.* **12:**170–172.
136. **Ledson, M. J., M. J. Gallagher, M. Jackson, C. A. Hart, and M. J. Walshaw.** 2002. Outcome of *Burkholderia cepacia* colonisation in an adult cystic fibrosis centre. *Thorax* **57:**142–145.
137. **Le Moal, G., M. Paccalin, J. P. Breux, F. Roblot, P. Roblot, and B. Becq-Giraudon.** 2001. Central venous catheter-related infection due to *Comamonas testosteroni* in a woman with breast cancer. *Scand. J. Infect. Dis.* **33:**627–628.
138. **Lessie, T. G., W. Hendrickson, B. D. Manning, and R. Devereux.** 1996. Genomic complexity and plasticity of *Burkholderia cepacia. FEMS Microbiol. Lett.* **144:**117–128.
139. **Li, Y., Y. Kawamura, N. Fujiwara, T. Naka, H. Liu, X. Huang, K. Kobayashi, and T. Ezaki.** 2004. *Sphingomonas yabuuchiae* sp. nov. and *Brevundimonas nasdae* sp. nov., isolated from the Russian space laboratory Mir. *Int. J. Syst. Evol. Microbiol.* **54:**819–825.
140. **Liou, T. G., F. R. Adler, S. C. Fitzsimmons, B. C. Cahill, J. R. Hibbs, and B. C. Marshall.** 2001. Predictive 5-year survivorship model of cystic fibrosis. *Am. J. Epidemiol.* **153:**345–352.
141. **LiPuma, J. J.** 2003. *Burkholderia* and emerging pathogens in cystic fibrosis. *Semin. Respir. Crit. Care Med.* **24:**681–692.
142. **LiPuma, J. J.** 2001. *Burkholderia cepacia* complex: a contraindication to lung transplantation in cystic fibrosis? *Transplant Infect. Dis.* **3:**149–160.
143. **LiPuma, J. J.** 1998. *Burkholderia cepacia* epidemiology and pathogenesis: implications for infection control. *Curr. Opin. Pulm. Med.* **4:**337–341.
144. **LiPuma, J. J.** 1998. *Burkholderia cepacia.* Management issues and new insights. *Clin. Chest Med.* **19:**473–486.
145. **LiPuma, J. J., S. E. Dasen, D. W. Nielson, R. C. Stern, and T. L. Stull.** 1990. Person-to-person transmission of *Pseudomonas cepacia* between patients with cystic fibrosis. *Lancet* **336:**1094–1096.
146. **LiPuma, J. J., B. J. Dulaney, J. D. McMenamin, P. W. Whitby, T. L. Stull, T. Coenye, and P. Vandamme.** 1999. Development of rRNA-based PCR assays for identification of *Burkholderia cepacia* complex isolates recovered from cystic fibrosis patients. *J. Clin. Microbiol.* **37:**3167–3170.
147. **LiPuma, J. J., J. E. Mortensen, S. E. Dasen, T. D. Edlind, D. V. Schidlow, J. L. Burns, and T. L. Stull.** 1988. Ribotype analysis of *Pseudomonas cepacia* from cystic fibrosis treatment centers. *J. Pediatr.* **113:**859–862.
148. **LiPuma, J. J., T. Spilker, T. Coenye, and C. F. Gonzalez.** 2002. An epidemic *Burkholderia cepacia* complex strain identified in soil. *Lancet* **359:**2002–2003.
149. **Lumbiganon, P., U. Tattawasatra, P. Chetchotisakd, S. Wongratanacheewin, and B. Thinkhamrop.** 2000. Comparison between the antimicrobial susceptibility of *Burkholderia pseudomallei* to trimethoprim-sulfamethoxazole by standard disk diffusion method and by minimal inhibitory concentration determination. *J. Med. Assoc. Thai.* **83:**856–860.
150. **Mahenthiralingam, E., J. Bischof, S. K. Byrne, C. Radomski, J. E. Davies, Y. Av-Gay, and P. Vandamme.** 2000. DNA-based diagnostic approaches for identification of *Burkholderia cepacia* complex, *Burkholderia vietnamiensis, Burkholderia multivorans, Burkholderia stabilis,* and *Burkholderia cepacia* genomovars I and III. *J. Clin. Microbiol.* **38:**3165–3173.
151. **Mahenthiralingam, E., M. E. Campbell, D. A. Henry, and D. P. Speert.** 1996. Epidemiology of *Burkholderia cepacia* infection in patients with cystic fibrosis: analysis by randomly amplified polymorphic DNA fingerprinting. *J. Clin. Microbiol.* **34:**2914–2920.
152. **Makkar, N. S., and L. E. Casida.** 1987. *Cupriavidus necator* gen. nov., sp. nov.: a nonobligate bacterial predator of bacteria in soil. *Int. J. Syst. Bacteriol.* **37:**323–326.
153. **McDowell, A., E. Mahenthiralingam, J. E. Moore, K. E. Dunbar, A. K. Webb, M. E. Dodd, S. L. Martin, B. C. Millar, C. J. Scott, M. Crowe, and J. S. Elborn.** 2001. PCR-based detection and identification of *Burkholderia cepacia* complex pathogens in sputum from cystic fibrosis patients. *J. Clin. Microbiol.* **39:**4247–4255.
154. **McMenamin, J. D., T. M. Zaccone, T. Coenye, P. Vandamme, and J. J. LiPuma.** 2000. Misidentification of *Burkholderia cepacia* in US cystic fibrosis treatment centers: an analysis of 1,051 recent sputum isolates. *Chest* **117:**1661–1665.
155. **Moore, J. E., M. Crowe, A. Shaw, J. McCaughan, A. O. Redmond, and J. S. Elborn.** 2001. Antibiotic resistance in *Burkholderia cepacia* at two regional cystic fibrosis centres in Northern Ireland: is there a need for synergy testing? *J. Antimicrob. Chemother.* **48:**319–321.
156. **Moore, J. E., B. McIlhatton, A. Shaw, P. G. Murphy, and J. S. Elborn.** 2001. Occurrence of *Burkholderia cepacia* in foods and waters: clinical implications for patients with cystic fibrosis. *J. Food Prot.* **64:**1076–1078.
157. **Moore, J. E., J. Xu, B. C. Millar, M. Crowe, and J. S. Elborn.** 2002. Improved molecular detection of *Burkholderia cepacia* genomovar III and *Burkholderia multivorans* directly from sputum of patients with cystic fibrosis. *J. Microbiol. Methods* **49:**183–191.
158. **Muder, R. R., A. P. Harris, S. Muller, M. Edmond, J. W. Chow, K. Papadakis, M. W. Wagener, G. P. Bodey, and J. M. Steckelberg.** 1996. Bacteremia due to *Stenotrophomonas (Xanthomonas) maltophilia:* a prospective, multicenter study of 91 episodes. *Clin. Infect. Dis.* **22:**508–512.
159. **Ngauy, V., Y. Lemeshev, L. Sadkowski, and G. Crawford.** 2005. Cutaneous melioidosis in a man who was taken as a prisoner of war by the Japanese during World War II. *J. Clin. Microbiol.* **43:**970–972.
160. **Norzah, A., M. Y. Rohani, P. T. Chang, and G. M. Kamel.** 1996. Indirect hemagglutination antibodies against *Burkholderia pseudomallei* in normal blood donors and suspected cases of melioidosis in Malaysia. *Southeast Asian J. Trop. Med. Public Health* **27:**263–266.
161. **O'Brien, M., K. Freeman, G. Lum, A. C. Cheng, S. P. Jacups, and B. J. Currie.** 2004. Further evaluation of a rapid diagnostic test for melioidosis in an area of endemicity. *J. Clin. Microbiol.* **42:**2239–2240.

162. **O'Carroll, M. R., T. J. Kidd, C. Coulter, H. V. Smith, B. R. Rose, C. Harbour, and S. C. Bell.** 2003. *Burkholderia pseudomallei*: another emerging pathogen in cystic fibrosis. *Thorax* **58:**1087–1091.
163. **Oie, S., and A. Kamiya.** 1996. Microbial contamination of antiseptics and disinfectants. *Am. J. Infect. Control* **24:**389–395.
164. **Otag, F., G. Ersoz, M. Salcioglu, C. Bal, I. Schneider, and A. Bauernfeind.** 2005. Nosocomial bloodstream infections with *Burkholderia stabilis*. *J. Hosp. Infect.* **59:**46–52.
165. **Otto, L. A., B. S. Deboo, E. L. Capers, and M. J. Pickett.** 1978. *Pseudomonas vesicularis* from cervical specimens. *J. Clin. Microbiol.* **7:**341–345.
166. **Pallent, L. J., W. B. Hugo, D. J. Grant, and A. Davies.** 1983. *Pseudomonas cepacia* as contaminant and infective agent. *J. Hosp. Infect.* **4:**9–13.
167. **Palleroni, N. J.** 1984. Genus I. *Pseudomonas* Migula 1984, 237[AL], p. 141–199. *In* J. Holt and N. R. Krieg (ed.), *Bergey's Manual of Systematic Bacteriology,* vol. 1. The Williams and Wilkins Co., Baltimore, Md.
168. **Palleroni, N. J., and J. F. Bradbury.** 1993. *Stenotrophomonas*, a new bacterial genus for *Xanthomonas maltophilia* (Hugh 1980) Swings et al. 1983. *Int. J. Syst. Bacteriol.* **43:**606–609.
169. **Palleroni, N. J., R. Kunisawa, R. Contopoulo, and M. Doudoroff.** 1973. Nucleic acid homologies in the genus *Pseudomonas*. *Int. J. Syst. Bacteriol.* **23:**333–339.
170. **Parke, J. L., and D. Gurian-Sherman.** 2001. Diversity of the *Burkholderia cepacia* complex and implications for risk assessment of biological control strains. *Annu. Rev. Phytopathol.* **39:**225–258.
171. **Parry, C. M., V. Wuthiekanun, N. T. Hoa, T. S. Diep, L. T. Thao, P. V. Loc, B. A. Wills, J. Wain, T. T. Hien, N. J. White, and J. J. Farrar.** 1999. Melioidosis in southern Vietnam: clinical surveillance and environmental sampling. *Clin. Infect. Dis.* **29:**1323–1326.
172. **Payne, G. W., P. Vandamme, S. H. Morgan, J. J. Lipuma, T. Coenye, A. J. Weightman, T. H. Jones, and E. Mahenthiralingam.** 2005. Development of a *recA* gene-based identification approach for the entire *Burkholderia* genus. *Appl. Environ. Microbiol.* **71:**3917–3927.
173. **Pitkin, D. H., W. Sheikh, and H. L. Nadler.** 1997. Comparative in vitro activity of meropenem versus other extended-spectrum antimicrobials against randomly chosen and selected resistant clinical isolates tested in 26 North American centers. *Clin. Infect. Dis.* **24**(Suppl. 2)**:** S238–S248.
174. **Pitt, T. L., M. E. Kaufmann, P. S. Patel, L. C. Benge, S. Gaskin, and D. M. Livermore.** 1996. Type characterisation and antibiotic susceptibility of *Burkholderia (Pseudomonas) cepacia* isolates from patients with cystic fibrosis in the United Kingdom and the Republic of Ireland. *J. Med. Microbiol.* **44:**203–210.
175. **Poole, K., and R. Srikumar.** 2001. Multidrug efflux in *Pseudomonas aeruginosa*: components, mechanisms and clinical significance. *Curr. Top. Med. Chem.* **1:**59–71.
176. **Ramette, A., J. J. LiPuma, and J. M. Tiedje.** 2005. Species abundance and diversity of *Burkholderia cepacia* complex in the environment. *Appl. Environ. Microbiol.* **71:**1193–1201.
177. **Reboli, A. C., R. Koshinski, K. Arias, K. Marks-Austin, D. Stieritz, and T. L. Stull.** 1996. An outbreak of *Burkholderia cepacia* lower respiratory tract infection associated with contaminated albuterol nebulization solution. *Infect. Control Hosp. Epidemiol.* **17:**741–743.
178. **Reik, R., T. Spilker, and J. J. Lipuma.** 2005. Distribution of *Burkholderia cepacia* complex species among isolates recovered from persons with or without cystic fibrosis. *J. Clin. Microbiol.* **43:**2926–2928.
179. **Riley, P. S., and R. E. Weaver.** 1975. Recognition of *Pseudomonas pickettii* in the clinical laboratory: biochemical characterization of 62 strains. *J. Clin. Microbiol.* **1:**61–64.
180. **Ross, J. P., S. M. Holland, V. J. Gill, E. S. DeCarlo, and J. I. Gallin.** 1995. Severe *Burkholderia (Pseudomonas) gladioli* infection in chronic granulomatous disease: report of two successfully treated cases. *Clin. Infect. Dis.* **21:**1291–1293.
181. **Sajjan, U. S., L. Sun, R. Goldstein, and J. F. Forstner.** 1995. Cable (cbl) type II pili of cystic fibrosis-associated *Burkholderia (Pseudomonas) cepacia:* nucleotide sequence of the *cblA* major subunit pilin gene and novel morphology of the assembled appendage fibers. *J. Bacteriol.* **177:**1030–1038.
182. **San Gabriel, P., J. Zhou, S. Tabibi, Y. Chen, M. Trauzzi, and L. Saiman.** 2004. Antimicrobial susceptibility and synergy studies of *Stenotrophomonas maltophilia* isolates from patients with cystic fibrosis. *Antimicrob. Agents Chemother.* **48:**168–171.
183. **Sattler, C. A., E. O. Mason, Jr., and S. L. Kaplan.** 2000. Nonrespiratory *Stenotrophomonas maltophilia* infection at a children's hospital. *Clin. Infect. Dis.* **31:**1321–1330.
184. **Schülin, T., and I. Steinmetz.** 2001. Chronic melioidosis in a patient with cystic fibrosis. *J. Clin. Microbiol.* **39:** 1676–1677.
185. **Schulze, R., S. Spring, R. Amann, I. Huber, W. Ludwig, K. H. Schleifer, and P. Kampfer.** 1999. Genotypic diversity of *Acidovorax* strains isolated from activated sludge and description of *Acidovorax defluvii* sp. nov. *Syst. Appl. Microbiol.* **22:**205–214.
186. **Segers, P., M. Vancanneyt, B. Pot, U. Torck, B. Hoste, D. Dewettinck, E. Falsen, K. Kersters, and P. De Vos.** 1994. Classification of *Pseudomonas diminuta* Leifson and Hugh 1954 and *Pseudomonas vesicularis* Busing, Doll, and Freytag 1953 in *Brevundimonas* gen. nov. as *Brevundimonas diminuta* comb. nov. and *Brevundimonas vesicularis* comb. nov., respectively. *Int. J. Syst. Bacteriol.* **44:**499–510.
187. **Segonds, C., T. Heulin, N. Marty, and G. Chabanon.** 1999. Differentiation of *Burkholderia* species by PCR-restriction fragment length polymorphism analysis of the 16S rRNA gene and application to cystic fibrosis isolates. *J. Clin. Microbiol.* **37:**2201–2208.
188. **Segonds, C., S. Paute, and G. Chabanon.** 2003. Use of amplified ribosomal DNA restriction analysis for identification of *Ralstonia* and *Pandoraea* species: interest in determination of the respiratory bacterial flora in patients with cystic fibrosis. *J. Clin. Microbiol.* **41:**3415–3418.
189. **Shelly, D. B., T. Spilker, E. J. Gracely, T. Coenye, P. Vandamme, and J. J. LiPuma.** 2000. Utility of commercial systems for identification of *Burkholderia cepacia* complex from cystic fibrosis sputum culture. *J. Clin. Microbiol.* **38:**3112–3115.
190. **Smith, M. D., V. Wuthiekanun, A. L. Walsh, N. Teerawattanasook, V. Desakorn, Y. Suputtamongkol, T. L. Pitt, and N. J. White.** 1995. Latex agglutination for rapid detection of *Pseudomonas pseudomallei* antigen in urine of patients with melioidosis. *J. Clin. Pathol.* **48:**174–176.
191. **Sneath, P. H. A. (ed.).** 1992. *International Code of Nomenclature of Bacteria. Bacteriological Code. 1990 Revision.* American Society for Microbiology, Washington, D.C.
192. **Speert, D. P., D. Henry, P. Vandamme, M. Corey, and E. Mahenthiralingam.** 2002. Epidemiology of *Burkholderia cepacia* complex in patients with cystic fibrosis, Canada. *Emerg. Infect. Dis.* **8:**181–187.
193. **Stead, D. E.** 1992. Grouping of plant-pathogenic and some other *Pseudomonas* spp. by using cellular fatty acid profiles. *Int. J. Syst. Bacteriol.* **42:**281–285.
194. **Stryjewski, M. E., J. J. LiPuma, R. H. Messier, Jr., L. B. Reller, and B. D. Alexander.** 2003. Sepsis, multiple organ failure, and death due to *Pandoraea pnomenusa* infection after lung transplantation. *J. Clin. Microbiol.* **41:**2255–2257.
195. **Swing, J., P. de Vos, M. van den Mooter, and J. de Ley.** 1983. Transfer of *Pseudomonas maltophilia* Hugh 1981 to

the genus *Xanthomonas* as *Xanthomonas maltophilia* (Hugh 1981) comb. nov. *Int. J. Syst. Bacteriol.* **33:**409–413.

196. **Tago, Y., and A. Yokota.** 2004. *Comamonas badia* sp. nov., a floc-forming bacterium isolated from activated sludge. *J. Gen. Appl. Microbiol.* **50:**243–248.
197. **Talmaciu, I., L. Varlotta, J. Mortensen, and D. V. Schidlow.** 2000. Risk factors for emergence of *Stenotrophomonas maltophilia* in cystic fibrosis. *Pediatr. Pulmonol.* **30:**10–15.
198. **Thomassen, M. J., C. A. Demko, J. D. Klinger, and R. C. Stern.** 1985. *Pseudomonas cepacia* colonization among patients with cystic fibrosis. A new opportunist. *Am. Rev. Respir. Dis.* **131:**791–796.
199. **Tiangitayakorn, C., S. Songsivilai, N. Piyasangthong, and T. Dharakul.** 1997. Speed of detection of *Burkholderia pseudomallei* in blood cultures and its correlation with clinical outcome. *Am. J. Trop. Med.* **57:**96–99.
200. **Van Couwenberghe, C., and S. Cohen.** 1994. Analysis of epidemic and endemic isolates of *Xanthomonas maltophilia* by contour clamped homogeneous electric field gel electrophoresis. *Infect. Control Hosp. Epidemiol.* **15:**691–696. 119G.
201. **Vandamme, P., and T. Coenye.** 2004. Taxonomy of the genus *Cupriavidus:* a tale of lost and found. *Int. J. Syst. Evol. Microbiol.* **54:**2285–2289.
202. **Vandamme, P., J. Goris, T. Coenye, B. Hoste, D. Janssens, K. Kersters, P. De Vos, and E. Falsen.** 1999. Assignment of Centers for Disease Control group IVc-2 to the genus *Ralstonia* as *Ralstonia paucula* sp. nov. *Int. J. Syst. Bacteriol.* **49:**663–669.
203. **Vandamme, P., D. Henry, T. Coenye, S. Nzula, M. Vancanneyt, J. J. LiPuma, D. P. Speert, J. R. Govan, and E. Mahenthiralingam.** 2002. *Burkholderia anthina* sp. nov. and *Burkholderia pyrrocinia*, two additional *Burkholderia cepacia* complex bacteria, may confound results of new molecular diagnostic tools. *FEMS Immunol. Med. Microbiol.* **33:**143–149.
204. **Vandamme, P., B. Holmes, M. Vancanneyt, T. Coenye, B. Hoste, R. Coopman, H. Revets, S. Lauwers, M. Gillis, K. Kersters, and J. R. Govan.** 1997. Occurrence of multiple genomovars of *Burkholderia cepacia* in cystic fibrosis patients and proposal of *Burkholderia multivorans* sp. nov. *Int. J. Syst. Bacteriol.* **47:**1188–1200.
205. **Vaneechoutte, M., P. Kampfer, T. De Baere, E. Falsen, and G. Verschraegen.** 2004. *Wautersia* gen. nov., a novel genus accommodating the phylogenetic lineage including *Ralstonia eutropha* and related species, and proposal of *Ralstonia [Pseudomonas] syzygii* (Roberts et al. 1990) comb. nov. *Int. J. Syst. Evol. Microbiol.* **54:**317–327.
206. **Vartivarian, S. E., K. A. Papadakis, J. A. Palacios, J. T. Manning, Jr., and E. J. Anaissie.** 1994. Mucocutaneous and soft tissue infections caused by *Xanthomonas maltophilia*. A new spectrum. *Ann. Intern. Med.* **121:**969–973.
207. **Vermis, K., T. Coenye, J. J. LiPuma, E. Mahenthiralingam, H. J. Nelis, and P. Vandamme.** 2004. Proposal to accommodate *Burkholderia cepacia* genomovar VI as *Burkholderia dolosa* sp. nov. *Int. J. Syst. Evol. Microbiol.* **54:**689–691.
208. **Vermis, K., T. Coenye, E. Mahenthiralingam, H. J. Nelis, and P. Vandamme.** 2002. Evaluation of species-specific recA-based PCR tests for genomovar level identification within the *Burkholderia cepacia* complex. *J. Med. Microbiol.* **51:**937–940.
209. **Vermis, K., P. A. Vandamme, and H. J. Nelis.** 2003. *Burkholderia cepacia* complex genomovars: utilization of carbon sources, susceptibility to antimicrobial agents and growth on selective media. *J. Appl. Microbiol.* **95:**1191–1199.
210. **Vermis, K., C. Vandekerckhove, H. J. Nelis, and P. A. Vandamme.** 2002. Evaluation of restriction fragment length polymorphism analysis of 16S rDNA as a tool for genomovar characterisation within the *Burkholderia cepacia* complex. *FEMS Microbiol. Lett.* **214:**1–5.
211. **Visca, P., G. Cazzola, A. Petrucca, and C. Braggion.** 2001. Travel-associated *Burkholderia pseudomallei* infection (melioidosis) in a patient with cystic fibrosis: a case report. *Clin. Infect. Dis.* **32:**E15-E16.
212. **Walsh, A. L., M. D. Smith, V. Wuthiekanun, Y. Suputtamongkol, V. Desakorn, W. Chaowagul, and N. J. White.** 1994. Immunofluorescence microscopy for the rapid diagnosis of melioidosis. *J. Clin. Pathol.* **47:**377–379.
213. **Walsh, A. L., V. Wuthiekanun, M. D. Smith, Y. Suputtamongkol, and N. J. White.** 1995. Selective broths for the isolation of *Pseudomonas pseudomallei* from clinical samples. *Trans. R. Soc. Trop. Med. Hyg.* **89:**124.
214. **Wauters, G., T. De Baere, A. Willems, E. Falsen, and M. Vaneechoutte.** 2003. Description of *Comamonas aquatica* comb. nov. and *Comamonas kerstersii* sp. nov. for two subgroups of *Comamonas terrigena* and emended description of *Comamonas terrigena*. *Int. J. Syst. Evol. Microbiol.* **53:**859–862.
215. **Welch, D. F., M. J. Muszynski, C. H. Pai, M. J. Marcon, M. M. Hribar, P. H. Gilligan, J. M. Matsen, P. A. Ahlin, B. C. Hilman, and S. A. Chartrand.** 1987. Selective and differential medium for recovery of *Pseudomonas cepacia* from the respiratory tracts of patients with cystic fibrosis. *J. Clin. Microbiol.* **25:**1730–1734.
216. **Wen, A., M. Fegan, C. Hayward, S. Chakraborty, and L. I. Sly.** 1999. Phylogenetic relationships among members of the *Comamonadaceae*, and description of *Delftia acidovorans* (den Dooren de Jong 1926 and Tamaoka et al. 1987) gen. nov., comb. nov. *Int. J. Syst. Bacteriol.* **49:**567–576.
217. **Wertheim, W. A., and D. M. Markovitz.** 1992. Osteomyelitis and intervertebral discitis caused by *Pseudomonas pickettii*. *J. Clin. Microbiol.* **30:**2506–2508.
218. **Weyant, R. S., C. W. Moss, R. E. Weaver, D. G. Hollis, J. G. Jordan, E. C. Cook, and M. I. Daneshvar.** 1996. *Identification of Unusual Pathogenic Gram-Negative Aerobic and Facultatively Anaerobic Bacteria*, 2nd ed., vol. 1. The Williams and Wilkins Co., Baltimore, Md.
219. **Whitby, P. W., K. B. Carter, J. L. Burns, J. A. Royall, J. J. LiPuma, and T. L. Stull.** 2000. Identification and detection of *Stenotrophomonas maltophilia* by rRNA-directed PCR. *J. Clin. Microbiol.* **38:**4305–4309.
220. **Whitby, P. W., H. L. Dick, P. W. Campbell III, D. E. Tullis, A. Matlow, and T. L. Stull.** 1998. Comparison of culture and PCR for detection of *Burkholderia cepacia* in sputum samples of patients with cystic fibrosis. *J. Clin. Microbiol.* **36:**1642–1645.
221. **Whitby, P. W., L. C. Pope, K. B. Carter, J. J. LiPuma, and T. L. Stull.** 2000. Species-specific PCR as a tool for the identification of *Burkholderia gladioli*. *J. Clin. Microbiol.* **38:**282–285.
222. **White, N. J.** 2003. Melioidosis. *Lancet* **361:**1715–1722.
223. **Willems, A., J. DeLay, M. Gillis, and K. Kersters.** 1991. *Comamonadaceae*, a new family encompassing the *acidovorans* rRNA complex, including *Variovorax paradoxus* gen. nov., comb nov., for *Alcaligenes paradoxus* (Davis 1969). *Int. J. Syst. Bacteriol.* **41:**445–450.
224. **Willems, A., E. Falsen, B. Pot, E. Jantzen, B. Hoste, P. Vandamme, M. Gillis, K. Kersters, and J. De Ley.** 1990. *Acidovorax*, a new genus for *Pseudomonas facilis*, *Pseudomonas delafieldii*, E. Falsen (EF) group 13, EF group 16, and several clinical isolates, with the species *Acidovorax facilis* comb. nov., *Acidovorax delafieldii* comb. nov., and *Acidovorax temperans* sp. nov. *Int. J. Syst. Bacteriol.* **40:**384–398.
225. **Willems, A., M. Goor, S. Thielemans, M. Gillis, K. Kersters, and J. De Ley.** 1992. Transfer of several phytopathogenic *Pseudomonas* species to *Acidovorax* as *Acidovorax avenae* subsp. *avenae* subsp. nov., comb. nov., *Acidovorax avenae* subsp. *citrulli*, *Acidovorax avenae* subsp. *cattleyae*, and *Acidovorax konjaci*. *Int. J. Syst. Bacteriol.* **42:**107–119.

226. **Willems, A., B. Pot, E. Falsen, P. Vandamme, M. Gillis, K. Kersters, and J. De Ley.** 1991. Polyphasic taxonomic study of the emended genus *Comamonas:* relationship to *Aquaspirillum aquaticum*, E. Falsen group 10, and other clinical isolates. *Int. J. Syst. Bacteriol.* **41:**427–444.
227. **Winkelstein, J. A., M. C. Marino, R. B. Johnston, Jr., J. Boyle, J. Curnutte, J. I. Gallin, H. L. Malech, S. M. Holland, H. Ochs, P. Quie, R. H. Buckley, C. B. Foster, S. J. Chanock, and H. Dickler.** 2000. Chronic granulomatous disease. Report on a national registry of 368 patients. *Medicine* **79:**155–169.
228. **Wolf, A., A. Fritze, M. Hagemann, and G. Berg.** 2002. *Stenotrophomonas rhizophilia* sp. nov., a novel plant-associated bacterium with antifungal properties. *Int. J. Syst. Evol. Microbiol.* **52:**1937–1944.
229. **Woods, M. L., II, B. J. Currie, D. M. Howard, A. Tierney, A. Watson, N. M. Anstey, J. Philpott, V. Asche, and K. Withnall.** 1992. Neurological melioidosis: seven cases from the Northern Territory of Australia. *Clin. Infect. Dis.* **15:**163–169.
230. **Wright, R. M., J. E. Moore, A. Shaw, K. Dunbar, M. Dodd, K. Webb, A. O. Redmond, M. Crowe, P. G. Murphy, S. Peacock, and J. S. Elborn.** 2001. Improved cultural detection of *Burkholderia cepacia* from sputum in patients with cystic fibrosis. *J. Clin. Pathol.* **54:**803–805.
231. **Wuthiekanun, V., D. A. Dance, Y. Wattanagoon, Y. Supputtamongkol, W. Chaowagul, and N. J. White.** 1990. The use of selective media for the isolation of *Pseudomonas pseudomallei* in clinical practice. *J. Med. Microbiol.* **33:**121–126.
232. **Xu, J., J. E. Moore, B. C. Millar, H. D. Alexander, R. McClurg, T. C. Morris, and P. J. Rooney.** 2004. Improved laboratory diagnosis of bacterial and fungal infections in patients with hematological malignancies using PCR and ribosomal RNA sequence analysis. *Leuk. Lymphoma* **45:**1637–1641.
233. **Yabuuchi, E., Y. Kosako, H. Oyaizu, I. Yano, H. Hotta, Y. Hashimoto, T. Ezaki, and M. Arakawa.** 1992. Proposal of *Burkholderia* gen. nov. and transfer of seven species of the genus *Pseudomonas* homology group II to the new genus, with the type species *Burkholderia cepacia* (Palleroni and Holmes 1981) comb. nov. *Microbiol. Immunol.* **36:**1251–1275.
234. **Yabuuchi, E., Y. Kosako, I. Yano, H. Hotta, and Y. Nishiuchi.** 1995. Transfer of two *Burkholderia* and an *Alcaligenes* species to *Ralstonia* gen. nov.: proposal of *Ralstonia pickettii* (Ralston, Palleroni and Doudoroff 1973) comb. nov., *Ralstonia solanacearum* (Smith 1896) comb. nov. and *Ralstonia eutropha* (Davis 1969) comb. nov. *Microbiol. Immunol.* **39:**897–904.
235. **Yao, J. D., M. Louie, L. Louie, J. Goodfellow, and A. E. Simor.** 1995. Comparison of E test and agar dilution for antimicrobial susceptibility testing of *Stenotrophomonas (Xanthomonas) maltophilia*. *J. Clin. Microbiol.* **33:**1428–1430.

Acinetobacter, Achromobacter, Chryseobacterium, Moraxella, and Other Nonfermentative Gram-Negative Rods*

PAUL C. SCHRECKENBERGER, MARYAM I. DANESHVAR, AND DANNIE G. HOLLIS

50

DESCRIPTION OF GENERA

The organisms covered in this chapter belong to a group of taxonomically diverse, nonfermentative gram-negative rods. They all share the common phenotypic features of failing to acidify the butt of Kligler iron agar (KIA) or triple sugar iron (TSI) agar or of oxidative-fermentative (OF) media and grow significantly better under aerobic than under anaerobic conditions; many strains fail to grow anaerobically. Most of the organisms covered in this chapter, with the exception of *Neisseria elongata* subspecies *elongata* and *nitroreducens*, are catalase positive. Oxidase and growth on MacConkey agar are variable. They either are nonmotile or, if motile, often have peritrichous flagella.

The methods used for growth and identification of these organisms are those used for *Pseudomonas* spp. (see chapter 48). Initial incubation should be at 35 to 37°C, although many pink-pigmented strains grow better at ≤30°C and may be detected only on plates left at room temperature after the initial readings. In such cases, all identification tests should be carried out at that temperature. In fact, some of the commercial kits, such as the API 20 NE, are designed to be incubated at 30°C. Growth on certain selective primary media (e.g., MacConkey or Salmonella-Shigella [SS] agar) is variable; and there can be significant lot-to-lot variations in the media. Nonfermenters that grow on MacConkey agar generally form colorless colonies, although some form lavender or purple colonies due to uptake of crystal violet contained in the agar medium.

When laboratory identification of this group of organisms is deemed necessary, a simplified approach is recommended whereby unknown isolates are initially characterized and placed into one of seven groups based on microscopic morphology, oxidase reaction, motility, acidification of carbohydrates, indole production, and production of pink-pigmented colonies (Fig. 1). Further characterization is made on the basis of the biochemical reactions (see Tables 1 through 7) that are examined after 1, 2, and 7 days of incubation. Additional differential tests can be found in other publications (96, 207, 256, 257). Carbohydrate utilization and mode of utilization are based on the King formulation of OF medium (256). In the authors' experience, indole production is best demonstrated by inoculation of heart infusion broth and incubation at 35 to 37°C for 48 h followed by extraction with xylene and addition of Ehrlich's reagent. The oxidase test is performed after overnight incubation using *N, N, N, N*-tetramethyl-*p*-phenylenediamine dihydrochloride (0.5%). Motility is easily determined by performing a wet mount preparation of a young colony from a blood agar plate. For some strains, motility can best be demonstrated after incubation of cultures at room temperature.

Traditional diagnostic systems, e.g., those based on OF media, aerobic low-peptone media, or buffered single substrates, have now been replaced in many laboratories by commercial kits. The ability of commercial kits to identify this group of nonfermenters is variable and often results in identification to the genus or group level only, necessitating the use of supplemental biochemical testing for species identification (10, 123, 135, 147, 175, 223). If such kits are used, the laboratory must be familiar with the extent of the database; organisms not included will be unidentified or identified incorrectly. Because assimilation test results often depend on the basal medium used, most of those results are not included in the tables presented here. Identification of nonfermenters by automated fatty acid analysis has also been attempted (243). In view of the difficulties inherent in this approach (176), it is recommended that fatty acid profiles be used only in conjunction with traditional or commercial diagnostic systems. The fatty acid profiles for the most common species of nonfermenting bacilli have been published by Weyant and colleagues (256) and are included in the tables presented here. Furthermore, rRNA gene sequencing is likely to become the standard for identification of many organisms that are difficult to identify using conventional methods, such as those described in this chapter, and laboratories are encouraged to develop such capabilities. The impact of this technology has already been noted in several publications (38, 63, 180); this method was used to confirm the identification of several new nonfermenting species included in this chapter.

TAXONOMY, NATURAL HABITATS, AND CLINICAL SIGNIFICANCE

Since a large and diverse group of organisms are covered in this chapter, the taxonomy, natural habitats, and clinical significance of the individual species are covered under the individual organism headings.

*This chapter contains information presented in chapter 49 by Paul C. Schreckenberger, Maryam I. Daneshvar, Robbin S. Weyant, and Dannie G. Hollis in the eighth edition of this Manual.

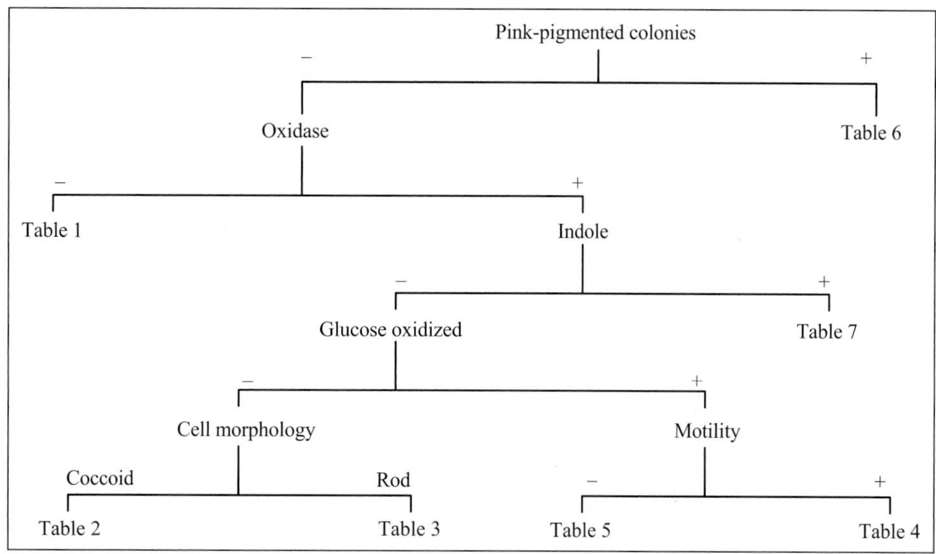

FIGURE 1 Identification of miscellaneous gram-negative nonfermenters.

COLLECTION, TRANSPORT, AND STORAGE OF SPECIMENS

Standard methods for collection, transport, and storage of specimens as detailed in chapters 5 and 20 are satisfactory for this group of organisms.

OXIDASE-NEGATIVE GROUP

See Table 1.

Acinetobacter spp.

General Description

The genus *Acinetobacter* consists of strictly aerobic, gram-negative coccobacillary rods that are oxidase negative, nonmotile, usually nitrate negative, and nonfermentative. Individual cells are 1 to 1.5 by 1.5 to 2.5 μm in size, sometimes difficult to decolorize, and frequently arranged in pairs. Clinical microbiologists should be alert to the fact that *Acinetobacter* species may initially appear as gram-positive cocci in direct smears prepared from positive blood culture bottles (83). In the stationary growth phase and on nonselective agars, coccobacillary forms predominate, whereas early growth in fluid media and growth on plates containing cell wall-active antimicrobial agents yield mostly rods. Colonies are smooth, opaque, and slightly smaller than those of members of the family *Enterobacteriaceae*. Many strains grow on MacConkey agar as either colorless or slightly pinkish colonies. Some strains are fastidious, showing punctate colonies on blood agar, and fail to grow in nutrient broth (256). Certain glucose-oxidizing acinetobacters may also cause a unique brown discoloration of heart infusion agar with tyrosine or blood agar into which glucose is incorporated (213, 256). We have also observed this phenomenon on MacConkey and Mueller-Hinton agars with a clinical isolate of *A. baumannii*. Differential and selective media have been described for isolation of *Acinetobacter* spp. from contaminated specimens. (103, 118).

Taxonomy

The genus was originally placed within the family *Neisseriaceae* but more recently moved to the family *Moraxellaceae* (203). Studies based on DNA-DNA hybridization have resulted in the description of 25 DNA homology groups (also called genomospecies) within the genus *Acinetobacter* (18, 20, 75, 115, 169, 171, 229). While only 11 species have been named (18, 169, 170, 171), differential biochemical and growth tests have been published for at least 19 species (18, 20, 76, 169, 170, 171). Genomospecies 1, 2, 3, and 13 of Tjernberg and Ursing (229) may be difficult to separate in the clinical laboratory and have been referred to as the *Acinetobacter calcoaceticus-Acinetobacter baumannii* complex (76). Because of problems in the clinical laboratory separating the DNA groups by phenotypic tests, we have chosen to separate the *Acinetobacter* species in Table 1 into two groups, saccharolytic and asaccharolytic. Most glucose-oxidizing nonhemolytic clinical strains are *A. baumannii*, most glucose-negative nonhemolytic ones are *Acinetobacter lwoffii*, and most hemolytic ones are *Acinetobacter haemolyticus*.

Natural Habitat and Clinical Significance

Acinetobacter species are widely distributed in nature and in the hospital environment, are the second most commonly isolated nonfermenters in human specimens (*Pseudomonas aeruginosa* being the first), are able to survive on moist and dry surfaces (77), and may be present in foodstuffs (105) and on healthy human skin (208). *Acinetobacter* spp. are generally considered to be nonpathogenic to healthy individuals but may cause infections in debilitated individuals. The species most frequently isolated from humans is *A. baumannii* (with 19 biotypes identified by assimilation tests [19] and 34 serovars [230]).

A. baumannii is the species most often responsible for hospital-acquired infections (152, 244). A biotyping system for differentiating 17 biotypes of *A. baumannii* based on the utilization of six substrates has been established and may be useful for epidemiologic studies (19). Turton and colleagues have reported that integrons are useful markers for epidemic strains of *A. baumannii* and that integron typing provides valuable information for epidemiological studies (232). The ability of this microorganism to acquire antimicrobial multiresistance and its high capacity for survival on most environmental surfaces has led to an increased concern

TABLE 1 Oxidase-negative group[a]

Test	*Acinetobacter* species[b] Asaccharolytic (270)	*Acinetobacter* species[b] Saccharolytic (77)	CDC group EO-5 (*Acetobacter*-like)[c] (10)	CDC group NO-1 (22)	*Bordetella ansorpii*[d] (1)	*Bordetella holmesii* (13)	*Bordetella parapertussis* (12)	*Bordetella trematum* (1)	*Kerstersia gyiorum*[e] (2)	*Pseudomonas oryzihabitans*[f] (36)	*Pseudomonas luteola*[f] (34)
Motility; flagella	0	0	0	0	100; ND	0	0	100; pe	50; pe	100; p, 1–2	100; p, >2
Acid from[g]:											
D-Glucose	0	95(5)	100	0[h]	0	0	0	0	0	100	100
D-Xylose	<1	98	100	0	0	0	0	0	0	100	100
D-Mannitol	0	0	0	0	0	0	0	0	0	100	76(18)
Lactose	0	62(13)	0	0	0	0	0	0	0	14(22)	3(24)
Sucrose	0	0	0	0	0	0	0	0	0	25	12
Maltose	0	17(37)	0	0	0	0	0	0	0	97(3)	100
Catalase	>99	100	100	100	ND	38	100	100	100	94	100
Growth on:											
MacConkey	74(4)	96	10w	5(15)	100	77(23)	100	100	100	100	100
SS	9(2)	10(2)	0	0	ND	0	0	100	100	22	68
Cetrimide	<1	2	0	0	ND	0	0	0	ND	25(28)	0
Simmons citrate	30(3)	63(3)	0	0	100	0	67(8)	100w	100	97	100
Urea, Christensen's	8(18)	22(24)	(10w)	5w	0	0	100	0	0	77	26(38)
Nitrate reduction	6	8	0	100	0	0	0	0[i]	0	6	62
H_2S (lead acetate paper)	51	38	50	5, 45w	ND	62	17	100	ND	97	12
Gelatin hydrolysis[j]	2	6	0	0	100	0	0	0	0	17	61
Pigment:											
Insoluble	0	0	0	0	ND	0	0	0	0	100 yel	97 yel
Soluble	12 yel/tan	22 br-yel-tan	20 yel	0	ND	100 br	100 br	0	ND	0	0
Growth at:											
25°C	98	100	90	20	ND	67	60	100	ND	100	100
35°C	98	100	90	100	100	100	100	100	100	100	100
42°C	48	72	0	15	ND	0	18	0	100	33	94
Esculin hydrolysis	0	0	0	0	0	0	0	0	0	0	100
Lysine decarboxylase	0	10	0	0	ND	0	ND	0	0	7	0
Arginine dihydrolase	9, 6w	19	0	0	0	0	ND	0	0	14	100
Ornithine decarboxylase	0	5	0	0	ND	0	ND	0	0	3	0

Nutrient broth, 0% NaCl	86(1)	99	90	10(5)	ND	46(15)	92	100	100	100	100
Nutrient broth, 6% NaCl	19	13	0	0	ND	0	0	100	50	62	74(3)
Major CFAs[k]	16:0,[l] 16:1ω7c, 18:1ω9c	16:0,[l] 16:1ω7c, 18:1ω9c	16:0, 18:1ω7c	16:0, 16:1ω7c, 18:1ω7c	16:0, 16:1ω7c, 17:0cyc, 18:1ω7c	16:0, 17:0cyc	16:0, 17:0cyc	16:0, 17:0cyc	16:0, 17:0cyc, 18:1ω7c	16:0, 16:1ω7c, 18:1ω7c	16:0, 16:1ω7c, 18:1ω7c

[a]Unless otherwise indicated, data are from the CDC Special Bacteriology Reference Laboratory (256). All taxa were negative (<10% positive) for gas from nitrate, nitrite reduction, indole production, acid in TSI butt, and H_2S in TSI. Numbers indicate the percentage positive at 2 days of incubation; parentheses indicate a delayed reaction (3 to 7 days of incubation); w, weak reaction; pe, peritrichous; p, polar; br, brown; yel, yellow; ND, not determined or not available. Numbers in parentheses after organisms indicate the number of strains.

[b]A total of 25 *Acinetobacter* genomospecies have been described. See the text.

[c]Probable *Acetobacter* species based on three phenotypically similar strains that were identified by 16S rRNA gene sequencing.

[d]Data from reference 138.

[e]Data from reference 41.

[f]Included in table only; see description in chapter 48.

[g]Oxidative-fermentative basal medium with 1% carbohydrate.

[h]Usually does not grow in oxidative-fermentative medium.

[i]Nitrate reduction reported variable by other authors (see chapter 51).

[j]14 days of incubation.

[k]CFA, cellular fatty acid. The number before the colon indicates the number of carbons; the number after the colon is the number of double bonds; ω, the position of the double bond counting from the hydrocarbon end of the carbon chain; c, *cis* isomer; cyc, a cyclopropane ring structure.

[l]Cannot distinguish most *Acinetobacter* species by CFA.

regarding hospital-acquired infections. Corbella et al. have shown that the digestive tract of intensive care unit patients is an important epidemiologic reservoir for multiresistant *A. baumannii* infections in hospital outbreaks, and they suggest that a fecal surveillance program might be considered for early implementation of patient isolation precautions in an outbreak setting (48). Hospital-acquired infections are most likely to involve the respiratory tract (most often related to endotracheal tubes or tracheostomies), urinary tract, and wounds (including catheter sites) and may progress to septicemia (9, 37, 258). Sporadic cases of continuous ambulatory peritoneal dialysis peritonitis, endocarditis, meningitis, osteomyelitis, arthritis, and corneal perforation have also been reported (9). There are an increasing number of reports of *Acinetobacter* species as agents of nosocomial pneumonia, particularly ventilator-associated pneumonia in patients confined to hospital intensive care units (9). Risk factors are antibiotic treatment and/or surgery, instrumentation, mechanical ventilation, and stay in intensive care units; clinical isolates, however, are more often colonizers than infecting agents (9, 37, 258). Hospital outbreaks have been investigated by various typing methods (139, 150, 232). Community-acquired *Acinetobacter* pneumonias in which a fatal outcome was strongly associated with inappropriate initial antibiotic therapy have also been reported (2). Most recently, American troops wounded in Iraq and Afghanistan have suffered severe wound infections and osteomyelitis from multidrug-resistant *A. baumannii* (30, 56).

Other species, such as *Acinetobacter johnsonii, A. lwoffii,* and *Acinetobacter radioresistens,* seem to be natural inhabitants of the human skin and may also be commensals in the oropharynx and vagina (21). *A. lwoffii* has been more commonly associated with meningitis than other *Acinetobacter* species (214). *Acinetobacter ursingii* has been shown to cause bloodstream infections in hospitalized patients (153, 169). *Acinetobacter junii* is a rare cause of ocular infection (190) and bacteremia, particularly in pediatric patients (126, 146). A case of community-acquired *A. radioresistens* bacteremia in a human immunodeficiency virus-positive patient has also been reported (245). *Acinetobacter schindleri* has been recovered from a variety of human specimens (vaginal, cervical, throat, nasal, ear, conjunctiva, and urine) but is mostly regarded as clinically nonsignificant (169).

Antibiotic Susceptibility

Cephalothin is ineffective against *Acinetobacter* spp., but trimethoprim-sulfamethoxazole, imipenem, imipenem-cilastatin, ampicillin-sulbactam, ticarcillin-clavulanate, piperacillin-tazobactam, amoxicillin-clavulanate, doxycycline, and quinolones are effective against most strains (9, 37, 119), but susceptibility testing is required for each clinically significant strain. Multiply resistant strains including carbapenem-resistant *Acinetobacter* species have been reported in nosocomial outbreaks (17, 108, 157, 158). Although the carbapenems are still the most active antimicrobials against *Acinetobacter* species, carbapenem resistance is now becoming common (47, 50, 158, 269).

Antimicrobial susceptibility testing for *Acinetobacter* species is problem prone. Swenson and colleagues at the CDC have shown that results obtained using standardized broth microdilution do not agree with results obtained with the standardized disk diffusion method for certain antibiotics. Very major errors were frequent with the β-lactam and β-lactam inhibitor combination antibiotics, with the broth microdilution method typically showing greater resistance (225). At present, there are no data to indicate which method provides more clinically relevant information.

Treatment

Combined treatment with an aminoglycoside and ticarcillin or piperacillin is synergistic and may be effective in serious infections. For multiply resistant *Acinetobacter* infections, several studies have demonstrated clinical efficacy of sulbactam in combination with ampicillin or cefoperazone (46, 85, 119, 143). The only other antibacterial agent that has been shown to be active against multiply resistant *Acinetobacter* is colistin (78, 121, 144). For a review of the clinical features, molecular epidemiology, and antimicrobial susceptibility of nosocomial *Acinetobacter* infections, consult the reviews by Bergogne-Berezin and Towner (9) and Wisplinghoff et al. (258).

CDC Group EO-5

CDC Eugonic Oxidizer (EO) Group 5 organisms (M. I. Daneshvar, D. G. Hollis, C. W. Moss, J. G. Jordan, J. P. MacGregor, and R. S. Weyant, *Abstr. 98th Gen. Meet. Am. Soc. Microbiol.*, abstr. C-204, 1998) are glucose-oxidizing gram-negative rods that have a biochemical profile similar to that of *A. baumannii*. Based on 16S rRNA sequencing, these are probably *Acetobacter* species (M. I. Daneshvar, unpublished data). They are nonmotile and oxidase negative and fail to grow on MacConkey agar. Some strains produce a yellow soluble pigment. Cellular fatty acid (CFA) analysis is also useful in differentiating EO-5 strains from *A. baumannii*. Other characteristics are given in Table 1. Isolates have been recovered from blood, peritoneal fluid, transtracheal aspirate, gall bladder, and an arm wound. Antibiotic susceptibility data are not available.

CDC Group NO-1

Group NO (nonoxidizer)-1 bacteria (87) are oxidase negative, asaccharolytic, nonmotile, coccoid to medium-sized gram-negative rods forming small colonies on sheep blood agar (SBA). Other differential features are shown in Table 1. Nitrate, but not nitrite, is reduced; however, since approximately 6% of asaccharolytic *Acinetobacter* spp. reduce nitrate, CFA profiles and 16S rRNA gene sequencing are useful for making a definitive identification. Most strains have been isolated from human wounds resulting from dog or cat bites, suggesting that these animals are a reservoir for NO-1 infections (87, 125). They are susceptible to antibiotics used for infections caused by gram-negative organisms, including aminoglycosides, β-lactam antibiotics, tetracyclines, quinolones, and sulfonamides (87).

Bordetella spp.

The *Bordetella* species are discussed in detail in chapter 51 of this Manual. There are eight *Bordetella* spp. that are nonfastidious and will grow on ordinary culture media (i.e., sheep blood and MacConkey agars) and biochemically resemble either *Acinetobacter* spp. or *Alcaligenes/Achromobacter* spp. Four species (*B. ansorpii, B. holmesii, B. parapertussis,* and *B. trematum*) are oxidase negative and are included in Table 1, and four species are oxidase positive (*B. avium, B. bronchiseptica, B. hinzii,* and *B. petrii*) and are included in Table 3. *B. holmesii* (formerly CDC group NO-2) is nitrate negative (differentiating it from NO-1 strains) and produces a brown soluble pigment on heart infusion-tyrosine agar. Other differential tests are given in Table 1. *B. bronchiseptica* is rapid urease positive and must be differentiated from *Cupriavidus pauculus* (Table 3) and *Oligella ureolytica* (Table 2).

Genus *Kerstersia*

Kerstersia is a newly described novel genus that consists of a single species, *K. gyiorum* (Greek *gyion,* meaning "limb," referring to the fact that the majority of strains were isolated from human leg wounds) (41). They appear as gram-negative, small (1 to 2 μm long), coccoid cells that occur singly, in pairs, or in short chains. On nutrient agar, colonies are flat or slightly convex, with smooth margins and color ranging from white to light brown. Growth occurs at 28 and 42°C, motility is strain dependent, and all strains are asaccharolytic. All strains are catalase positive but are negative for oxidase, arginine, lysine and ornithine decarboxylase, β-galactosidase, gelatinase, amylase, urease, DNase, reduction of nitrate and nitrite, and hydrolysis of esculin (Table 1). Strains have been isolated from various human specimens, including feces, sputum, and leg and ankle wounds. Pathogenicity is unknown (41).

OXIDASE-POSITIVE, INDOLE-NEGATIVE, ASACCHAROLYTIC COCCOID NONFERMENTERS

See Table 2.

Psychrobacter phenylpyruvicus, Moraxella catarrhalis, and Other *Moraxella* spp.

Members of the genus *Moraxella* are oxidase-positive, nonmotile, asaccharolytic coccobacilli that are often plump, occur predominantly in pairs and sometimes in short chains, and have a tendency to resist decolorization (54).

Moraxellae are parasitic on human skin and mucous membranes. *M. catarrhalis, M. osloensis, M. nonliquefaciens,* and *M. lincolnii* are part of the normal flora of the human respiratory tract, while most *M. canis* strains have been found in the upper respiratory tracts of dogs and cats. These and other moraxellae are rare agents of infections (conjunctivitis, keratitis, meningitis, septicemia, endocarditis, arthritis, and otolaryngologic infections) (122, 127, 209, 241).

M. catarrhalis has been reported to cause sinusitis and otitis media by contiguous spread of the organisms from a colonizing focus in the respiratory tract (127). However, isolation of *M. catarrhalis* from the upper respiratory tract (i.e., a throat culture) of children with otitis media or sinusitis does not provide evidence that the isolate is the cause of these infections. Rates of upper respiratory tract colonization by *M. catarrhalis* in children vary widely and are influenced by many factors (both environmental and genetic). The presence of the organism in the oropharynx or nasopharynx is not necessarily predictive of infection in contiguous anatomic sites. Isolates from sinus aspirates and middle ear specimens obtained by tympanocentesis should be identified and reported. Similarily, little is known about the pathogenesis of lower respiratory tract infection in adults with chronic lung diseases. Examination of Gram-stained smears of sputum specimens from patients with exacerbations of bronchitis and pneumonia due to *M. catarrhalis* usually reveals an abundance of leukocytes, the presence of many gram-negative diplococci as the exclusive or predominant bacterial morphotype, and the presence of intracellular gram-negative diplococci. Such specimens may yield *M. catarrhalis* in virtually pure culture, and the organism should be identified and reported.

Colonies of *M. catarrhalis* grow well on both blood and chocolate agars, and some strains also grow well on Modified Thayer-Martin and other selective media. Colonies are generally gray to white, opaque, and smooth and measure about

1 to 3 mm after 24 h of incubation. Characteristically, the colonies may be nudged across the plate intact with a bacteriological loop like a "hockey puck." *M. catarrhalis* is strongly oxidase positive and catalase positive. It does not produce acid from glucose or other carbohydrates. Most strains reduce nitrate and nitrite and produce DNase. *M. catarrhalis* may be easily distinguished from *Neisseria* species by its ability to hydrolyze ester-linked butyrate groups (butyrate esterase) (179, 219). A very rapid (2.5-min) and reliable indoxyl-butyrate hydrolysis spot test has been described and is commercially available (Remel, Inc., Lenexa, Kans.) (58).

M. nonliquefaciens is the second most frequently isolated species after *M. catarrhalis*. It forms smooth, translucent to semiopaque colonies 0.1 to 0.5 mm in diameter after 24 h and 1 mm in diameter after 48 h of growth on SBA plates. Occasionally, these colonies spread and pit the agar. The colonial morphologies of *M. lincolnii* (237), *M. osloensis*, and *Psychrobacter phenylpyruvicus* (formerly *M. phenylpyruvica*) are similar, but pitting is rare. On the other hand, pitting is common with *M. lacunata*, whose colonies are smaller and form dark haloes on chocolate agar. Colonies of *M. atlantae* are small (usually 0.5 mm in diameter) and show pitting and spreading (22). Most *M. canis* colonies resemble those of the *Enterobacteriaceae* (large, smooth colonies) and may produce a brown pigment when grown on starch-containing Mueller-Hinton agar (117). Some strains may also produce very slimy colonies resembling colonies of *Klebsiella pneumoniae* (117). Microscopically, *M. canis* resembles *M. catarrhalis*, both appearing as gram-negative diplococci measuring 0.5 to 1.5 μm in diameter. Animal species include *M. bovis*, isolated from healthy cattle and other animals, including horses, *M. boevrei* and *M. caprae* (goats), *M. caviae* (guinea pigs), *M. cuniculi* (rabbits), and *M. ovis* and *M. oblonga* (sheep).

Biochemical reactions for the human isolates are listed in Table 2. Most laboratories do not determine the species of moraxellae, other than *M. catarrhalis*, because of the similarity in pathogenic significance of the species and because many strains are somewhat fastidious and biochemical reactions are often negative or equivocal. *M. atlantae, M. lacunata*, and *M. nonliquefaciens* are similar in many of their features. Growth of *M. atlantae* is stimulated by bile salts and sodium desoxycholate, while *M. lacunata* and *M. nonliquefaciens* are not. Only *M. lacunata* liquefies gelatin, whereas both *M. lacunata* and *M. nonliquefaciens* reduce nitrate to nitrite (22, 182) Separation of *M. lacunata* and nonspreading *M. nonliquefaciens* may prove difficult, because gelatin hydrolysis (with any method) and liquefaction of Loeffler slants may take more than 1 week. In some instances, fatty acid analysis may help determine the species (256); in other cases, quantitative transformation of a high-level streptomycin resistance marker can be used (124). The differential diagnosis of *P. phenylpyruvicus* and *Brucella* spp. is of great practical importance (see the discussion of agents of bioterrorism in chapter 9) and requires microscopy (*Brucella* organisms are tiny coccobacilli) and tests for acidification of xylose and glucose (183, 184). *P. phenylpyruvicus* is asaccharolytic, whereas *Brucella* spp. utilize xylose and usually glucose when a sufficiently sensitive method for detecting acidification of glucose is employed (183). Microbiologists should be aware that *Brucella* species that are unwittingly inoculated into certain commercial identification systems may be misidentified as *P. phenylpyruvicus* or *Haemophilus influenzae* (5, 6, 178). The tributyrin test may be positive for several *Moraxella* spp. and therefore cannot be used to separate them from *M. catarrhalis* (179). Likewise, gamma-glutamyl aminopeptidase occurs not only in *M. canis* but also in some strains of other moraxellae (117).

Most *Moraxella* strains are susceptible to penicillin and its derivatives, cephalosporins, tetracyclines, quinolones, and aminoglycosides (70, 201, 218). Production of beta-lactamase has been only rarely reported in *Moraxella* species other than *M. catarrhalis*, which commonly produces an inducible, cell-associated beta-lactamase (122, 201). Isolates of *M. catarrhalis* are generally susceptible to amoxicillin-clavulanate, expanded-spectrum and broad-spectrum cephalosporins (i.e., cefuroxime, cefotaxime, ceftriaxone, cefpodoxime, ceftibuten, and the oral agents cefixime and cefaclor), macrolides (e.g., azithromycin, clarithromycin, erythromycin), tetracyclines, and rifampin. While most isolates are susceptible to the fluoroquinolones, resistance to these agents has emerged in isolates recovered from patients who were receiving long-term therapy with such agents.

Oligella spp.

The genus *Oligella* consists of two species: *O. urethralis* (formerly *Moraxella urethralis* and CDC group M-4) and *O. ureolytica* (formerly CDC group IVe) (202). *O. urethralis* is nonmotile, while most strains of *O. ureolytica* are motile by peritrichous flagella. Biochemical features that help differentiate *Oligella* spp. from *Moraxella* spp. are shown in Table 2. *O. urethralis* is similar to *Moraxella* spp. in that isolates are coccobacillary, oxidase positive, and nonmotile. Colonies are smaller than those of *M. osloensis* and are opaque to whitish. *O. urethralis* and *M. osloensis* share additional biochemical similarities, e.g., accumulation of poly-β-hydroxybutyric acid and failure to hydrolyze urea, but can be differentiated on the basis of nitrite reduction and alkalinization of formate, itaconate, proline, and threonine (all positive for *O. urethralis* and negative for *M. osloensis*) (185). CFA analysis can also be used to differentiate these two species (256).

Colonies of *O. ureolytica* are slow growing on blood agar, appearing as pinpoint colonies after 24 h but large colonies after 3 days of incubation. Colonies are white, opaque, entire, and nonhemolytic. *O. ureolytica* strains are both phenylalanine deaminase and rapid urease positive, with the urease reaction often turning positive within minutes after inoculation. In this regard, *O. ureolytica* is similar to *Bordetella bronchiseptica* and *Cupriavidus pauculus* from which it must be differentiated. CFA analysis is useful since the CFA profiles are different for each of these species (256).

Both *Oligella* spp. have been isolated chiefly from the human urinary tract, and both have been reported to cause urosepsis (191, 200). A case of septic arthritis due to *O. urethralis* has also been reported (160). *O. urethralis* is generally susceptible to most antibiotics, including penicillin, while *O. ureolytica* exhibits variable susceptibility patterns (70).

Haematobacter spp. (Proposed)

Haematobacter is a proposed new genus of aerobic gram-negative rods that phenotypically most closely resembles *Psychrobacter phenylpyruvicus* (L. O. Helsel, D. Hollis, A. G. Steigerwalt, R. E. Morey, J. Jordan, T. Aye, J. Radosevic, D. Jannat-Kahah, D. R. Lonsway, J. B. Patel, M. I. Daneshvar, and P. N. Levett, *Abstr. 105th Gen. Meet. Am. Soc. Microbiol.*, abstr. C-404, 2005). The genus consists of two named (*H. cherryi* and *H. missouriensis*) and one unnamed genomospecies. All strains are nonmotile and asaccharolytic. They produce catalase, oxidase, urease, and H_2S (lead acetate paper) but do not produce indole, reduce nitrate or nitrite, or hydolyze gelatin or esculin. Colonies of *Haematobacter* are nonpigmented, and most strains grow on MacConkey agar. Additional phenotypic properties are given in Table 2. Strains received at the CDC have been mainly from patients

TABLE 2 Oxidase-positive, indole-negative, asaccharolytic, coccoid nonfermenters[a]

Test	*Moraxella atlantae*[b] (73)	*Moraxella canis* (1)	*Moraxella catarrhalis* (74)	*Moraxella lacunata*[b] (66)	*Moraxella lincolnii* (1)	*Moraxella nonliquefaciens*[b] (243)	*Moraxella osloensis* (163)	*Oligella ureolytica* (37)	*Oligella urethralis* (22)	*Psychrobacter phenylpyruvicus* (50)	*Psychrobacter immobilis* (5)	*Haematobacter* species (proposed) (12)
Motility; flagella	0	0	0	0	0	0	0	100[c]; pe	0	0	0	0
Growth on MacConkey	80 (20)	100	5	2	0	8 (2)	70	62 (27)	96	80 (6)	40	58
Simmons citrate	0	0	0	0	0	0	0	14 (16)	46	0	20	0
Urea, Christensen's	0	0	68	0	0	0	0	97	0	100	(20)	100
Nitrate reduction	0	100	92	98	0	95	24	100	0	68	40 (20)	0
Gas from nitrate	0	0	0	0	0	0	0	60	0	0	0	0
Nitrite reduction	3	ND	86	0	0[d]	0	0	100	100	0	ND	0
H_2S (lead acetate paper)	61	100	73	34	0	83	74	38	9	47	20 (20)	92
Gelatin hydrolysis[e]	0	0	0	42	0	0	0	0	0	0	0	0
Growth at:												
25°C	51	100	85	33	100	93	96	67	50	85	100	100
35°C	99	100	97	73	100	88	98	88	100	100	40	100
42°C	46	100	23	0	0	15	51	18	59	29	20	0
Phenylalanine deaminase	0	100w	ND	17	ND	ND	14	100[f]	100	97	ND	ND
Penicillin sensitivity[g]	100	ND	ND	95	ND	99	92	ND	100	73	ND	ND
Loeffler slant digestion	ND	ND	ND	100	ND	0	0	ND	ND	ND	ND	ND
Sodium acetate alkalinization	ND	ND	ND	0	0	0	100	ND	84	43	ND	ND
Nutrient broth, 0% NaCl	0	100	47	5	0	22	98	19 (3)	96	53	100	67
Nutrient broth, 6% NaCl	0	100w	ND	2	0	0	12	15 (5)	59	19	60	42
DNase[h]	0	100	100	0	0	0	0	0	0	0	ND	ND

Major CFAs[i]	16:0, 18:0, 18:1ω9c, 18:2	18:1ω9c	16:1ω7c, 17:1ω8c, 18:1ω9c	16:0, 16:1ω7c, 16:0alc, 17:1ω8c, 18:0, 18:1ω9c, 18:2, 18:0alc[j]	16:0, 16:1ω7c, 18:1ω9c	16:0, 16:1ω7c, 18:1ω9c	16:1ω7c, 18:1ω9c	16:0, 18:1ω7c	16:0, 18:1ω7c	16:0, 16:1ω7c, 18:1ω9c, 18:2	16:1ω7c, 17:1ω8c, 18:1ω9c	16:0, 18:1ω7c, 19:0 cyc

[a] Unless otherwise indicated, data are from the CDC Special Bacteriology Reference Laboratory (256). All taxa were positive (≥90%) for catalase. All were negative (<10% positive) for acid from D-glucose, D-xylose, D-mannitol, lactose, sucrose, and maltose; growth on SS and cetrimide agars, esculin hydrolysis, acid production in TSI agar, and H_2S production in TSI agar. Numbers indicate the percentage positive at 2 days of incubation; numbers in parentheses indicate a delayed reaction (3 to 7 days of incubation); w, weak reaction; pe, peritrichous; ND, not determined or not available. Numbers in parentheses after the organism indicate the number of strains.

[b] Usually does not grow in OF medium.

[c] Motility may be delayed or difficult to demonstrate.

[d] Nitrite-positive strains have been described (237).

[e] 14 days of incubation.

[f] Data from P. Schreckenberger.

[g] Based on results obtained by streaking a blood agar plate with growth from an 18- to 36-h culture and then placing a 10-U penicillin disk on the streaked area. A positive reaction is indicated by the appearance of a zone of inhibition.

[h] Data from reference 117.

[i] The number before the colon indicates the number of carbons; the number after the colon is the number of double bonds; ω, the position of the double bond counting from the hydrocarbon end of the carbon chain; c, *cis* isomer; alc, alcohol.

[j] Two profiles exist. Most strains of M. *lacunata* II differ from M. *lacunata* I by lower amounts of 17:1ω8c, 16:1ω7c, and 18:1ω9c, higher amounts of 18:0 (16 versus 3%), and higher amounts of 16:0 alc and 18:0 alc. However, there is some overlap in relative amounts of these acids in some strains of both groups which prohibit their differentiation solely on the basis of CFA data (256).

with septicemia. *Haematobacter* strains have low MIC values for amoxicillin, fluoroquinolones, aminoglycosides, and carbapenems but variable MICs for cephalosporins, monobactams, and piperacillin.

OXIDASE-POSITIVE, INDOLE-NEGATIVE, ASACCHAROLYTIC, ROD-SHAPED NONFERMENTERS

See Table 3.

Alcaligenes faecalis and Asaccharolytic *Achromobacter* spp.

Based on taxonomic studies, Yabuuchi et al. transferred the species *Alcaligenes ruhlandii* and *Alcaligenes piechaudii* to the genus *Achromobacter* and proposed the transfer of *Alcaligenes denitrificans* to the genus *Achromobacter* as *Achromobacter xylosoxidans* subsp. *denitrificans* (263), thus automatically creating a second subspecies, *Achromobacter xylosoxidans* subsp. *xylosoxidans*. However, the reclassification of *Alcaligenes denitrificans* as a subspecies of *Achromobacter xylosoxidans* contradicted previous work that showed that the two taxa are distinct species (239). Accordingly, Coenye and colleagues have proposed that *Alcaligenes denitrificans* be reclassified as *Achromobacter denitrificans* (41). In this text we treat these organisms as separate species, referring to them as *Achromobacter xylosoxidans* and *Achromobacter denitrificans*, respectively. *Alcaligenes faecalis* remains the only *Alcaligenes* species of clinical importance.

Members of these genera are rods (0.5 by 1 to 0.5 by 2.6 μm) with peritrichous flagella. Both phylogenetically and biochemically, they are closely related to members of the genus *Bordetella*. They occur mainly in the environment and show limited action on carbohydrates. Colonies are nonpigmented and similar in size to those of *Acinetobacter* spp. Medically important species are divided into the asaccharolytic species (Table 3) including *Alcaligenes faecalis*, *Achromobacter piechaudii* (263), and *Achromobacter denitrificans* (41, 263) and the saccharolytic species (see Table 4) *Achromobacter xylosoxidans* (41, 263) as well as the unnamed Achromobacter groups B, E, and F (89, 90). The asaccharolytic species are rarely observed as human pathogens (14, 134, 248). *A. faecalis* is the most frequently isolated species and characteristically produces colonies with a thin, spreading, irregular edge. Some strains (previously named "*A. odorans*") produce a characteristic fruity odor (sometimes described as the odor of green apples) and cause a greenish discoloration of blood agar medium. A key biochemical feature of this species is its ability to reduce nitrite but not nitrate. It is often found in mixed cultures, particularly in diabetic ulcers of the feet and lower extremities, and its clinical significance is difficult to determine. *Achromobacter piechaudii* has been recovered from blood, recurrent ear discharge, nose, pharynx, and soil (129, 134, 177). In one instance the blood isolate was associated with an infected Hickman catheter in a patient with hematological malignancy (129). *A. faecalis* and *A. piechaudii* have been reported to be resistant to ampicillin, aztreonam, and gentamicin and of variable susceptibility to other antimicrobials (13, 129). The clinical significance of *Achromobacter denitrificans* remains to be elucidated; however, an organism that is biochemically similar, known as *Alcaligenes*-like group 1, has been recovered from blood, urine, knee joint, brain abscess, and bronchial washings, suggesting that it may have greater potential to cause human infection. It can be differentiated from *A. denitrificans* by CFA composition, failure to grow on

TABLE 3 Oxidase-positive, indole-negative, asaccharolytic, rod-shaped nonfermenters[a]

Test	*Achromobacter denitrificans* (4)	*Achromobacter piechaudii* (5)	*Advenella incenata*[b] (6)	*Alcaligenes faecalis* (49)	*Alishewanella fetalis*[c] (1)	CDC *Alcaligenes*-like group 1 (8)	*Aquaspirillum* species (5)
Motility; flagella	100; pe	100; pe	v; ND	100; pe	0	100; pe	60; m; p, 1–2
Acid from D-glucose	0	0	v	0	0	0	0
Catalase	100	100	100	98	ND	100	100
Growth on:							
MacConkey	100	100	ND	100	100	100	0
SS	100	100	ND	100	100	13	0
Cetrimide	25 (25)	80 (20)	0	59	ND	0	0
Simmons citrate	100	100	100	100	0	100	0
Urea, Christensen's	0	0	v	2	0	75	0
Nitrate reduction	100	100	0	0	100	100	20
Gas from nitrate	100	0	0	0	ND	100	0
Nitrite reduction	ND	0	ND	100	100	100	0
H_2S (lead acetate paper)	25w	100[l]	ND	8	ND	13	100
Gelatin hydrolysis[m]	0	0	0	22	100	0	0
Pigment:							
Insoluble	0	0	Lt br	0	ND	0	0
Soluble	25 yel	0	ND	22 yel	ND	0	0
Growth at:							
25°C	100	100	ND	100	ND	100	40
35°C	100	100	100	100	ND	100	100
42°C	25w	60	v	18	100	50	0
Alkalinization of:							
Acetamide	33 (33)	0	0	83	ND	0	ND
Serine	33 (33)	40 (40)	ND	39	ND	(75)	ND
Tartrate	75 (25)	80 (20)	ND	6	ND	0	ND
Arginine dihydrolase	0	0	0	0	0	(33)	ND
Nutrient broth, 0% NaCl	100	100	100	100	ND	100	60
Nutrient broth, 6% NaCl	25	100[o]	v	98 (2)	100	13	0
Major CFAs[p]	16:0, 16:1ω7c, 17:0cyc	16:0, 16:1ω7c, 17:0cyc	ND	3–OH–14:0, 16:0, 16:1ω7c, 17:0cyc	16:1ω7c, 17:1ω8c	16:0, 16:1ω7c, 17:0cyc, 18:1ω7c	ND

[a] Unless otherwise indicated, data are from the CDC Special Bacteriology Reference Laboratory (256). All taxa were negative (<10% positive) for acid production from D-xylose, D-mannitol, lactose, sucrose, and maltose; acid in TSI agar, H_2S production in TSI agar, esculin hydrolysis, lysine decarboxylase and ornithine decarboxylase activity. Numbers indicate the percentage positive at 2 days of incubation; numbers in parentheses indicate a delayed reaction (3 to 7 days of incubation); w, weak reaction; pe, peritrichous; p, polar; ND, not determined or not available; yel, yellow; amb, amber; Lt br, light brown; v, strain dependent. Numbers in parentheses after the organisms indicate the number of strains.

[b] Data from reference 43.

[c] Data from reference 247. Carbohydrate results are from assimilation tests.

[d] Data from references 73 and 252.

[e] *Myroides* genus consists of two phenotypically similar species: *M. odoratus* and *M. odoratimimus*. The type strain of *M. odoratus* did not grow on MacConkey agar; in contrast, the type strain of *M. odoratimimus* grew heavily.

[f] Data from reference 268.

SS agar, failure to alkalinize tartrate and acetamide, and a positive urease reaction (Table 3) (256).

Advenella incenata

Advenella incenata is a gram-negative, small (1- to 2-μm), rod-shaped or coccoid bacterium that occurs singly, in pairs, or in short chains (43). On nutrient agar, colonies are flat or slightly convex with smooth margins and appear light brown in color (43). They are oxidase and catalase positive. Motility and oxidation of OF glucose are strain dependent. Additional characteristics are given in Table 3. Isolates have been recovered from human blood, sputum, and wound specimens (43).

Alishewanella fetalis

Alishewanella fetalis is a halophilic gram-negative rod that grows at temperatures between 25 and 42°C with optimum growth at 37°C. NaCl is required for growth. It can withstand NaCl concentrations of up to 8% but does not grow at 10% NaCl, which helps differentiate this species from *Shewanella algae*, which can grow in 10% NaCl (247). Also, unlike *S. algae*, it is esculin hydrolysis positive. It is oxidase and catalase positive and asaccharolytic. It does not produce H_2S in the butt of TSI and KIA. Other reactions are given in Table 3. It has been isolated from a human fetus at autopsy; however, its association with clinical infection is unknown (247).

Bordetella avium (3[j])	*Bordetella bronchiseptica* (85)	*Bordetella hinzii* (2)	*Bordetella petrii*[d] (2)	*Myroides* species[e] (74)	*Laribacter hongkongensis*[f] (1)	*Neisseria weaveri* (132)	*Neisseria elongata* subsp. *elongata* (15)
100; pe	100; pe	100; pe	0	0	0	0	0
0	0	0	0	0	0	0	0
100	100	100	100	100	100	100	0
100	100	100	100	91 (5)	100	27 (18)	13 (53)
100	99	100	ND	30 (11)	ND	0	0
0	0	0	ND	0	100	0	0
33w	98 (1)	100	100	0	0	0	0
0	99	0	0	100	100	0	0
0	92	0	0	0	100	0	0
0	0	0	0	0	0	0	0
0	ND	0	100	83	ND	100	92
67	74	50	ND	16	ND	86	67
0	0	0	0	96	0	0	0
0	0	0	0[n]	85 yel	0	0	0
33 yel	0	0	ND	0	0	24 yel	13 yel
100	99	100	ND	100	100	94	67
100	100	100	100	100	100	100	100
100	78	100	ND	31	100	41	27
0	0	0	ND	(2w)	0	2	0
(50w)	30 (61)	50	ND	5, 2w	ND	0	0
0	5	0	ND	(2w)	ND	0	0
0	0	50 (50)	ND	(9)	100	0	ND
100	100	100	ND	100	100	85	100
67	82 (5)	100	ND	20 (5)	0	18	0
16:0, 17:0cyc	16:0, 16:1ω7c, 17:0cyc	16:0, 17:0cyc	ND	i15:0	ND	16:0, 16:1ω7c, 18:1ω7c	16:0, 16:1ω7c, 18:1ω7c

[g] Data from reference 39.
[h] Data from reference 42.
[i] Data from reference 32.
[j] All from avian sources.
[k] Acid production may be detected in rapid sugar test base.
[l] H_2S (TSI butt), the line of the stab became dark in 3 to 7 days with three strains.
[m] 14 days of incubation.
[n] Slightly red when grown anaerobically on selenate-containing media (252).
[o] Light growth at 48 h, heavier at 7 days.
[p] The number before the colon indicates the number of carbons; the number after the colon is the number of double bonds; ω, the position of the double bond counting from the hydrocarbon end of the carbon chain; c, *cis* isomer; i, *iso;* 3–OH, a hydroxyl group at the 3 (β) position from the carboxyl end; cyc, a cyclopropane ring structure.

Aquaspirillum Species

The genus *Aquaspirillum* is a heterogeneous group that at present includes 13 species and two subspecies. All species are aerobic and helical and do not grow in the presence of 3% NaCl (60, 188). Colonies on nutrient agar are generally pinpoint in size at 48 h but become larger (up to 2.0 mm in diameter) at 7 days. They are usually convex or umbonate, glistening, opaque, pale yellow, and butyrous (188). They are oxidase and catalase positive and asaccharolytic. Additional reactions are given in Table 3. Aquaspirillae are found in a wide variety of freshwater sources, especially stagnant water sources such as ditch water, canal water, and ponds. They have also been isolated from storage tanks of distilled water in laboratories (188). Three of the isolates characterized at the CDC have been from human blood cultures, one from a patient with diabetes, one from a patient with pneumonia, and one from an individual whose clinical condition is unknown. All three were shown by 16S rRNA sequencing to be *Aquaspirillum* species.

Laribacter hongkongensis

Laribacter hongkongensis belongs to the family *Neisseriaceae* and is a facultatively anaerobic, nonsporulating bacillus. On Gram stain the organisms appear as gram-negative gull-shaped or spiral rods. It grows on sheep blood agar as non-hemolytic, gray colonies 1 mm in diameter after 24 h of

TABLE 3 Oxidase-positive, indole-negative, asaccharolytic, rod-shaped nonfermenters[a] *(Continued)*

Test	*Neisseria elongata* subsp. *glycolytica* (2)	*Neisseria elongata* subsp. *nitroreducens* (26)	*Shewanella algae* (26)	*Cupriavidus pauculus* (36)	*Cupriavidus gilardii*[g] (8)	*Cupriavidus respiraculi*[h] (5)	*Cupriavidus taiwanensis*[i] (9)	Gilardi rod group 1 (15)
Motility; flagella	0	0	100; p, 1–2	100; pe	100; p, 1–2	pe	pe	0
Acid from D-glucose	0[k]	23	0	0	0	0	0	0
Catalase	100	0	ND	100	100	100	100	100
Growth on:								
MacConkey	50 (50)	19 (35)	100	94 (6)	ND	ND	ND	93
SS	0	0	92 (4)	3 (6)	ND	ND	ND	80
Cetrimide	0	0	8	0 (3)	0	ND	0	0
Simmons citrate	0	0	8	100	0	0	100	0
Urea, Christensen's	0	0	42	100	0	0	0	0
Nitrate reduction	0	100	100	11	0	v	100	0
Gas from nitrate	ND	0	ND	0	0	ND	ND	0
Nitrite reduction	50	100	0	ND	0	ND	ND	0
H_2S (lead acetate paper)	100	100	100	51	ND	ND	ND	87
Gelatin hydrolysis[m]	0	0	100	0	0	0	ND	0
Pigment:								
Insoluble	0	0	0	0	0	0	0	60 amb
Soluble	50 yel	15 yel	0	22 yel	0	ND	ND	0
Growth at:								
25°C	100	62	ND	94	ND	100	100	100
35°C	100	100	ND	100	100	100	100	100
42°C	0	23	23	86	100	0	0	80
Alkalinization of:								
Acetamide	0	0	ND	ND	0	ND	ND	0
Serine	0	0	ND	ND	100	ND	ND	0
Tartrate	0	0	ND	100	0	ND	ND	0
Arginine dihydrolase	ND	0	100	ND	0	0	0	0
Nutrient broth, 0% NaCl	100	88	0	100	100	100	100	100
Nutrient broth, 6% NaCl	0	4	100	11	0	0	0	7 (13)
Major CFAs[p]	16:0, 16:1ω7c, 18:1ω7c	16:0, 16:1ω7c, 18:1ω7c	i-15:0, 16:1ω7c, 17:1ω8c	16:0, 16:1ω7c, 17:0cyc, 18:1ω7c	16:0, 16:1ω7c, summed feature 7	14:0, 3–OH 14:0, 16:1ω7c, 16:0, 17:0cyc, 18:1ω7c	ND	14:0, 16:0, 18:1ω7c, 19:0cyc

incubation at 37°C in ambient air. Growth also occurs on MacConkey agar and at 25 and 42°C. No enhancement of growth is observed with 5% CO_2. Most strains are motile with bipolar flagella. All strains are oxidase, catalase, urease, and arginine dihydrolase positive and reduce nitrate but do not ferment, oxidize, or assimilate any carbohydrates (Table 3) (259, 268). *L. hongkongensis* has been isolated from the blood and pleural fluid of a 54-year-old cirrhotic patient (268) and from the stools of patients with community-acquired diarrhea (141, 259, 260, 261). Woo and colleagues have reported an association between *L. hongkongensis* and community-acquired diarrhea, eating fish, and travel (260); however, a causative role has not been shown (69). *L. hongkongensis* has been reported from countries in Asia (China and Japan), Europe (Switzerland), Africa (Tunisia), and Central America (Cuba), suggesting that the bacterium is found worldwide (260). However, as of this writing, no isolates have been reported from North America.

Myroides spp.

Vancanneyt et al. (235) determined that the organism formerly classified as *Flavobacterium odoratum* consisted of a heterogenous group that comprised two distinct species for which they proposed the names *Myroides odoratus* and *Myroides odoratimimus*. Cells of both species are gram-negative rods 0.5 μm in diameter and 1 to 2 μm long. Various colony types may occur, but most colonies are yellow pigmented and form effuse, spreading colonies that may be confused with the colony morphology of a *Bacillus* species. A characteristic fruity odor (similar to the odor of *A. faecalis*) is produced by most strains. *Myroides* grows on most media including MacConkey agar. Growth occurs at 18 to 37°C but not at 42°C. They are asaccharolytic but are oxidase, catalase, urease, and gelatinase positive. Indole is not produced, and nitrite (but not nitrate) is reduced (Table 3). There are no routine phenotypic tests for differentiating the two *Myroides* species, their differences being confined to assimilation tests and CFA profiles (235).

Organisms identified as *M. odoratus* have been reported mostly from urine but have also been found in wound, sputum, blood, and ear specimens (98, 265). Clinical infection with *Myroides* spp. is exceedingly rare; however, cases of rapidly progressive necrotizing fasciitis and bacteremia (112) and recurrent cellulitis with bacteremia (3) have been reported. Most strains are resistant to penicillins, cephalosporins, aminoglycosides, aztreonam, and carbapenems (98).

Neisseria weaveri and *Neisseria elongata*

Although assigned to the genus *Neisseria*, the rod-shaped *Neisseria weaveri* and *Neisseria elongata* morphologically resemble nonfermenting gram-negative bacilli and therefore are placed in Table 3 to help in the differentiation of these phenotypically similar bacteria. The *Neisseria* species are covered in detail in chapter 39.

Shewanella Species

The organism formerly called *Pseudomonas putrefaciens*, *Alteromonas putrefaciens*, *Achromobacter putrefaciens*, and CDC group Ib has now been placed in the genus *Shewanella* (154). Colonies on SBA are convex, circular, smooth, and occasionally mucoid; produce a brown to tan soluble pigment; and cause green discoloration of the medium. Cells are long, short, or filamentous. Motility is due to a single polar flagellum. Ornithine decarboxylase, nitrate reductase, and DNase are always produced, and with few exceptions, hydrogen sulfide (H_2S) is produced in KIA and TSI agar (shewanellae are the only nonfermenters that produce H_2S in these media). The CDC recognizes two biotypes based upon the requirement of NaCl for growth, oxidation of sucrose and maltose, and the ability to grow on SS agar (256). CDC biotype 2 was subsequently assigned to a new species, *S. alga* (173), later corrected to *S. algae* (231). Khashe and Janda (132) have reported that *S. algae* is the predominant human clinical isolate (77%), while *S. putrefaciens* (CDC biotype 1) represents the majority of nonhuman isolates (89%). *S. algae* is halophilic (requires NaCl for growth) and asaccharolytic (Table 3), whereas *S. putrefaciens* is nonhalophilic and saccharolytic (see Table 4). Although infrequently isolated in the clinical laboratory, *S. putrefaciens* and *S. algae* have been recovered from a wide variety of clinical specimens and are associated with a broad range of human infections including skin and soft tissue infection (33), otitis media (102), ocular infection (27), osteomyelitis (16), peritonitis (51) and septicemia (24, 116). Many of these infections were probably caused by *S. algae*. The habitat for *S. algae* is saline habitats, whereas *S. putrefaciens* has been isolated mostly from fish, poultry, and meats as well as fresh water and marine samples. *Shewanella* species are generally susceptible to most antimicrobial agents effective against gram-negative rods except penicillin and cephalothin (70, 248). The mean MICs of *S. algae* to penicillin, ampicillin, and tetracycline are higher than the corresponding MICs of *S. putrefaciens* (132, 246).

Cupriavidus Species

Cupriavidus pauculus was formerly designated CDC Group IVc-2 and *Ralstonia paucula* (236, 238). It is a short to medium-sized gram-negative rod that is asaccharolytic and motile by peritrichous flagella. Cells may stain irregularly. It is rapid urease positive and can be differentiated from the phenotypically similar organisms *B. bronchiseptica* and *O. ureolytica* by a usually negative nitrate reduction test and its CFA composition (Table 3).

Cupriavidus gilardii (formerly *Ralstonia gilardii*) is the new designation for an *Alcaligenes faecalis*-like organism that has been isolated from human clinical sources and the environment (39, 236). *C. gilardii* can be differentiated from *A. faecalis* by the absence of nitrite reduction, failure to utilize acetamide, the presence of polar rather than peritrichous flagella, and CFA composition (Table 3).

Cupriavidus respiraculi (formerly *Ralstonia respiraculi*) has been recovered from the respiratory tract of cystic fibrosis (CF) patients, although the isolates do not grow on *B. cepacia*-selective agar (42, 236). Characteristics that differentiate *C. respiraculi* from other *Cupriavidus* species are given in Table 3.

C. taiwanensis (formerly *Ralstonia taiwanensis*) has also been isolated from the sputum of a CF patient (32, 236). It is a nonsaccharolytic gram-negative rod that is oxidase, catalase, nitrate, and esculin positive. Additional biochemical characteristics are given in Table 3. The *Cupriavidus* species are discussed in more detail in chapter 49.

Gilardi Rod Group 1

Gilardi rod group 1 consists of oval to medium-length asaccharolytic gram-negative rods that resemble *N. weaveri* in many respects except that Gilardi rod group 1 isolates do not reduce nitrite and are strongly phenylalanine deaminase positive, producing a dark green slant after addition of $FeCl_3$ (10%), whereas *N. weaveri*, when positive, produces a weak to moderate reaction. Additional reactions are given in Table 3. There is >98.7% 16S rRNA gene similarity between Gilardi rod group 1 and *Schineria larvae* (K. Bernard, personal communication); however, no formal proposal to name Gilardi rod group 1 has been made as of this writing. Isolates of Gilardi rod group 1 have been recovered from a variety of human sources including leg, arm, and foot wounds, an oral lesion, urine, and blood; however, their pathogenic potential has yet to be determined (166). They are susceptible to many antimicrobial agents including various penicillins, cephalothin, and chloramphenicol (166).

OXIDASE-POSITIVE, INDOLE-NEGATIVE, SACCHAROLYTIC, MOTILE, ROD-SHAPED NONFERMENTERS

See Table 4.

Achromobacter xylosoxidans

Achromobacter xylosoxidans is a relatively frequent agent of infection in immunocompromised patients, causing both local and systemic infections in nosocomial settings (34, 64, 254). *A. xylosoxidans* colonizes the respiratory tract of intubated children and patients with CF, leading to exacerbation of pulmonary symptoms (65). Epidemiologic typing of *A. xylosoxidans* by restriction fragment length polymorphism and PCR has been described (34, 145). Susceptibilities are unpredictable, which requires testing of individual isolates. Strains are frequently resistant to aminoglycosides, ampicillin, narrow- and expanded-spectrum cephalosporins, chloramphenicol, and fluoroquinolones but are usually susceptible to antipseudomonal broad-spectrum cephalosporins, piperacillin, ticarcillin-clavulanic acid, imipenem, and trimethoprim-sulfamethoxazole (13, 218, 248). Panresistance has been reported in at least one clinically significant infection (254).

TABLE 4 Oxidase-positive, indole-negative, saccharolytic, motile, rod-shaped nonfermenters[a]

Test	"*Achromobacter*" group B[b] (3)	"*Achromobacter*" group E[b] (2)	"*Achromobacter*" group F[b] (2)	*Achromobacter xylosoxidans* (135)	*Agrobacterium* yellow group (3)	CDC group Ic (34)	CDC group O-1 (62)	CDC group O-2 (66)	CDC group O-3 (13)
Motility; flagella	100; p, L	100; p, L	100	100; pe	100; p, 1–2[g]	100; p, 1–2	100; p, 1–2[g]	100; p, 1–2 or p, L[g]	100; p, 1–2[g]
Acid from:									
D-Glucose	100	100	100	78	33 (67)	97	69 (31)	73 (11)	100
D-Xylose	100	100	100	99	67 (33)	0	0	2	100
D-Mannitol	(67)	0	100	0	0	0	0	2	0
Lactose	(33)	(100)[h]	ND	0	(100)	0	0	2	0
Sucrose	(100)	(100)	100	0	(100)	0	0	64 (36)	100
Maltose	33 (67)	100	100	0	100	100	0	71 (27)	100
Catalase	100	100	ND	98	100	97	98	91	23, 62w
Growth on:									
MacConkey	100	100	0	100	(33)	100	6 (40)	5 (5)	(38)
SS	100	100	ND	98	0	100	0	0	0
Cetrimide	0	50 (50)	ND	95 (1)	0	94	0	0	0
Simmons citrate	100	100	0	95	0	41 (15)	0	0	0
Urea, Christensen's	100	100	100	0	(33)	18 (15)	2	12	0
Nitrate reduction	100	(100)[i]	100	100	0	100	0	15	8
Gas from nitrate	100	100	0	60	0	0	0	0	0
Nitrite reduction	100[k]	100[k]	0	ND	0	0	0	ND	0
TSI slant, acid	0	0	0	0	0	0	0	18	0
TSI butt, acid	0	0	0	0	0	0	0	20	0
H_2S (TSI butt)	0	(50)	ND	0	0	3	0	0	0
H_2S (lead acetate paper)	(100)	100	ND	0	100	100	93	91	15
Gelatin hydrolysis[j]	0	0	ND	0	0	0	25	38	0
Pigment:									
Insoluble	0	0	ND	0	100 yel	9w pk	100 yel	100 yel	0
Soluble	67 yel	50 tan	ND	5 br	0	32 tan-br	0	0	0
Growth at:									
25°C	100	100	ND	98	100	100	90	89	92
35°C	100	100	ND	100	100	100	100	100	100
42°C	100	100	ND	84	0	97	24	31	40
Esculin hydrolysis	100	100	100	0	67 (33)	0	93 (2)	64	92 (8)
Lysine decarboxylase	0	0	ND	0	0	0	0	0	0
Arginine dihydrolase	100	100	0	13	0	100	0	22	0
Ornithine decarboxylase	0	0	ND	0	0	0	0	6	0
Nutrient broth, 0% NaCl	100	100	ND	100	67 (33)	100	34	92	100
Nutrient broth, 6% NaCl	100	100	ND	69	0	91	0	22	0
3-Ketolactonate	0	0	ND	ND	100	ND	ND	ND	ND
ONPG	100[l]	100[l]	0[l]	0[m]	ND	ND	ND	ND	ND
Major CFAs[n]	18:1ω7c	18:1ω7c	ND	16:0, 16:1ω7c, 17:0cyc	16:0, 18:1ω7c	ND	16:0, 18:1ω7c	ND[o]	16:0, 16:1ω7c, 18:1ω7c

[a] Unless otherwise indicated, data are from CDC Special Bacteriology Reference Laboratory (256). Numbers indicate percentage positive at 2 days of incubation; parentheses, delayed reaction (3 to 7 days of incubation); w, weak reaction; ND, not determined or not available; pe, peritrichous; p, polar; L, lateral; br, brown; yel, yellow; pk, pink. Numbers in parentheses after organisms indicate numbers of strains.

[b] The following tests are useful in identifying to the species level "*Achromobacter*" group B, E, and F: L-rhamnose, D-sorbitol, and cellobiose: B (+, +, +); E (+, −, +), and F (−, ND, +) (89).

[c] Data from reference 249. Carbohydrate results are from assimilation tests.

[d] Data from reference 148.

[e] Colistin resistance has been suggested to differentiate *O. intermedium* (colistin resistant) from *O. anthropi* and *O. tritici* (colistin sensitive), whereas acid production from melibiose is useful in identifying *O. grignonense* (142).

[f] Glycerol and rhamnose oxidation are absent in *S. paucimobilis* and present in *S. parapaucimobilis*.

[g] Motility may be difficult to demonstrate.

Halomonas venusta[c] (15)	*Herbaspirillum* species 3 (1)	*Inquilinus limosus* (3)	*Massilia timonae*[d] (4)	*Ochrobactrum* species[e] (14)	OFBA-1 (6)	*Pseudomonas*-like group 2 (11)	*Rhizobium radiobacter* (66)	*Shewanella putrefaciens* (24)	*Sphingomonas paucimobilis*[f] (1)	*Sphingomonas parapaucimobilis*[f] (2)
100; pe	100; >2p	67; p, 1–2	100; 1p, L	100; pe	100; p, 1–2	100; p, >2	100; pe	100; p, 1–2	100; p, 1–2	100; p, 1–2
100	100	33 (67)	(100w)	93 (7)	100	100	94 (6)	17 (33)	100w	(100)
0	100	33 (67)	100	100	100	100	97 (3)	0	100	100
80	100	33 (67)	0	43 (14)	67 (33)	100	94 (6)	0	0	0
0	100w	33 (67)	0	0	67 (33)	100	79 (21)	0	100	50 (50)
80	0	(100)	0	50	67 (33)	0	95 (5)	96 (4)	100	100
100	0	(100)	100	64	67 (33)	0	97 (3)	92 (8)	100	50 (50)
100	100	67	100	100	100	100	98	100	100	100
ND	100	67 (33)	100	100	100	100	100	100	0	0
ND	0	0	0	100	100	0	20 (5)	(8)	0	0
100	0	67	ND	100	100	0	0	4	0	0
100	100	67	75 (25)	64	33 (33)	100	97 (3)	4 (4)	0	0[i]
100	100	33 (33)	0	100	33 (17)	91 (9)	88 (9)	4 (8)	0	0
ND	67	33	25	86	100	18	83	100	0	0
ND	0	0	0	43	100	0	5	0	0	0
ND	0	0	0	ND	ND	ND	38	ND	ND	ND
ND	0	0	0	0	100	0	0	0	0	100w
0	0	0	0	0	33 (67)	0	0	0	0	0
ND	0	0	0	43	0	0	11 (3)	96	0	0
ND	100	100	ND	100	50	89	100	100	0	100
0	0	0	100	0	50	0	2	65	0	0
ND	0	0	100 straw	0	0	0	0	0	100 yel	100 yel
ND	0	0	0	21 yel	0	0	21 yel	71 br	0	0
ND	100	33	100	100	100	80	100	100	100	100
ND	100	100	100	100	100	100	100	96	100	100
ND	100	33	0	64	100	20	32	38	100w	0
100	0	100	100	29 (7)	0	0	100	0	100	100
0	ND	0	0	0	0	0	0	0	ND	ND
0	ND	0	0	71	100	30	8	0	ND	ND
0	ND	0	0	0	0	0	0	100	ND	ND
ND	100	100	100	100	100	100	100	100	100	100
100	0	0	0	60	75	0	18	43	0	50
ND	ND	ND	ND	0	ND	ND	100	ND	0	0
ND	ND	ND	ND	0[m]	ND	ND	100[m]	ND	100[m]	ND
16:0, 18:1ω9c	16:0, 16:1ω7c, 18:1ω7c	18:1ω7c, 18:1-2OH, 18:0-3OH, 19:0cyloω8c	3–OH–10:0, 16:1ω7c, 16:0, 18:1ω7c	18:0, 18:1ω7c, 19:0cyc	16:0, 19:0cyc	16:0, 16:1ω7c, 18:1ω7c	16:0, 18:1ω7c, 19:0cyc	i-15:0, 16:1ω7c, 17:1ω8c	16:0, 18:1ω7c	16:0, 17:1ω6c, 18:1ω7c

[h] Acid production was detected only after 21 days of incubation.
[i] Reported to be positive (264).
[j] 14 days of incubation.
[k] When tested at 48 h of incubation, nitrite reduction may be observed only in media containing <0.01% nitrite.
[l] Data from reference 96.
[m] Data from P. Schreckenberger.
[n] The number before the colon indicates the number of carbons; the number after the colon is the number of double bonds; ω, the position of the double bond counting from the hydrocarbon end of the carbon chain; c, *cis* isomer; cyc, a cyclopropane ring structure; i, *iso;* ND, not determined.
[o] Fatty acid profile analysis, performed on six strains in our laboratory, indicates that this group is heterogeneous.

Ochrobactrum Species and *Achromobacter* Groups B, E, and F

Ochrobactrum anthropi (97) comprises the urease-positive *Achromobacter* species formerly designated CDC group Vd (biotypes 1 and 2) and *Achromobacter* groups A, C, and D described by Holmes et al. (96). Subsequent studies showed, however, that biogroup C and some strains belonging to biogroup A constitute a homogeneous DNA-DNA hybridization group separate from *O. anthropi*, named *Ochrobactrum intermedium* (242). Both *Ochrobactrum* species are closely related to *Brucella* spp., with *Ochrobactrum intermedium* occupying a phylogenetic position that is intermediate between *O. anthropi* and *Brucella* (242). The two species share identical phenotypic properties. They appear as medium-length rods with peritrichous flagella, but individual cells may have a single flagellum only. Colonies on SBA resemble those of *Enterobacteriaceae*, except that those of *Ochrobactrum* are smaller. Colonies measure about 1 mm in diameter and appear circular, low convex, smooth, shining, and entire.

O. anthropi has been isolated from various environmental and human sources, predominantly from patients with catheter-related bacteremias (97, 131, 204) and rarely with other infections (155) including one case of meningitis (29). Pulsed-field gel electrophoresis and PCR genome fingerprinting based on repetitive chromosomal sequences have both been used successfully for epidemiologic typing of outbreak strains (240). *O. anthropi* strains are usually resistant to β-lactams, such as broad-spectrum penicillins, broad-spectrum cephalosporins, aztreonam, and amoxicillin-clavulanate, but are usually susceptible to aminoglycosides, fluoroquinolones, imipenem, tetracycline, and trimethoprim-sulfamethoxazole (12, 131, 204).

There are no biochemical tests currently available that separate *O. intermedium* from *O. anthropi;* however, it has been suggested that colistin (polymyxin E) and polymyxin B resistance can be used to separate *O. intermedium* (resistant) from *O. anthropi* (susceptible) (242). One case of pyogenic liver infection due to *O. intermedium* has been reported (162), but because of the close phenotypic similarity of *O. anthropi* and *O. intermedium*, it is possible that certain infections thought to be caused by *O. anthropi* were actually caused by *O. intermedium.*

Achromobacter groups B and E constitute biotypes of a single new species that has yet to be named (89, 90, 92). *Achromobacter* group F is genetically distinct from groups B and E (89, 90). *Achromobacter* group B strains susceptible to chloramphenicol, ciprofloxacin, gentamicin, imipenem, tobramycin, and trimethoprim-sulfamethoxazole have been isolated from patients with septicemia (91, 120). Isolates of *Achromobacter* groups E and F have also been recovered from blood (89, 90).

Rhizobium radiobacter

The former genus *Agrobacterium* contained several species of plant pathogens occurring worldwide in soils. Four distinct species of *Agrobacterium* were recognized: *A. radiobacter* (formerly *A. tumefaciens* and CDC group Vd-3), *A. rhizogenes* (subsequently transferred to the genus *Sphingomonas* as *S. rosa*), *A. vitis*, and *A. rubi* (206). More recently, Young and colleagues (267) proposed an emended description of the genus *Rhizobium* to include all species of *Agrobacterium*. Following this proposal the new combinations are *Rhizobium radiobacter, R. rhizogenes, R. rubi,* and *R. vitis* (267). Cells measure 0.6 to 1.0 by 1.5 to 3.0 μm and occur singly and in pairs. Colonies of *R. radiobacter* grow optimally at 25 to 28°C but grow at 35°C as well. They appear circular, convex, smooth, and nonpigmented to light beige on SBA with a diameter of 2 mm at 48 h. Colonies may appear wet looking and become extremely mucoid and pink on MacConkey agar with prolonged incubation (Fig. 2).

R. radiobacter has been most frequently isolated from blood, followed by peritoneal dialysate, urine, and ascitic fluid (66, 114). The majority of cases have occurred in patients with transcutaneous catheters or implanted biomedical prostheses, and effective treatment often requires removal of the device (67). *R. radiobacter* septicemia has also been reported in hospitalized patients with advanced human immunodeficiency virus disease (156). One case of endophthalmitis caused by a *Rhizobium radiobacter*-like (3-ketolactonate-negative) organism has also been reported (161). Most strains are susceptible to broad-spectrum cephalosporins, carbapenems, tetracyclines, and gentamicin but not to tobramycin (66, 248). Testing of individual isolates is recommended for clinically significant cases.

Agrobacterium Yellow Group

Organisms in the *Agrobacterium* yellow group are represented by slender, medium to long gram-negative rods that produce a yellow insoluble growth pigment and most closely resemble *Sphingomonas paucimobilis* and CDC group O-1 and O-2 organisms. Growth on MacConkey agar is variable, motility occurs via a single polar flagellum, oxidase and catalase are positive, and glucose, xylose, lactose, sucrose, and maltose are oxidized, but not mannitol. Only a positive 3-ketolactonate reaction differentiates this organism from *S. paucimobilis* (Table 4). Isolates have been recovered from blood and peritoneal fluid (224, 256).

CDC Group Ic

Members of CDC group Ic are gram-negative, slender, short to long, motile rods with one or two polar flagella. The organisms grow well on MacConkey, SS, and usually cetrimide agars; oxidize glucose and maltose; reduce nitrate to nitrite without gas; produce H_2S on lead acetate paper (usually strong); they are arginine dihydrolase positive, urease and citrate variable, and esculin and gelatin hydrolysis negative; and they grow well at 25, 35, and usually 42°C. Other characteristics are listed in Table 4. Most isolates have come from human sources including urine, sputum, blood, and other sites (256). Antibiotic susceptibility data are not available.

CDC Groups O-1, O-2, and O-3

CDC groups O-1, O-2, and O-3 are phenotypically similar, motile, and usually oxidase-positive, gram-negative rods. Groups O-1 and O-2 are yellow pigmented and most closely resemble *Agrobacterium* yellow group and *Sphingomonas* species. These organisms grow poorly or not at all on MacConkey agar and usually hydrolyze esculin but are otherwise inactive. All are motile, although motility may be difficult to demonstrate. O-1 organisms appear as uniformly short gram-negative rods, O-2 organisms appear as slightly pleomorphic rods with some cells appearing thin in the central portion with thickened ends, and O-3 cells appear as thin, medium to slightly long curved rods with tapered ends (sickle-like) (52, 256). O-3 is the only group in which yellow growth pigment is not produced. Most isolates of O-3 grow well on CAMPY CVA (Campylobacter agar with cefoperazone, vancomycin, and amphotericin B) plates under microaerophilic conditions, thus creating the potential for misidentification of

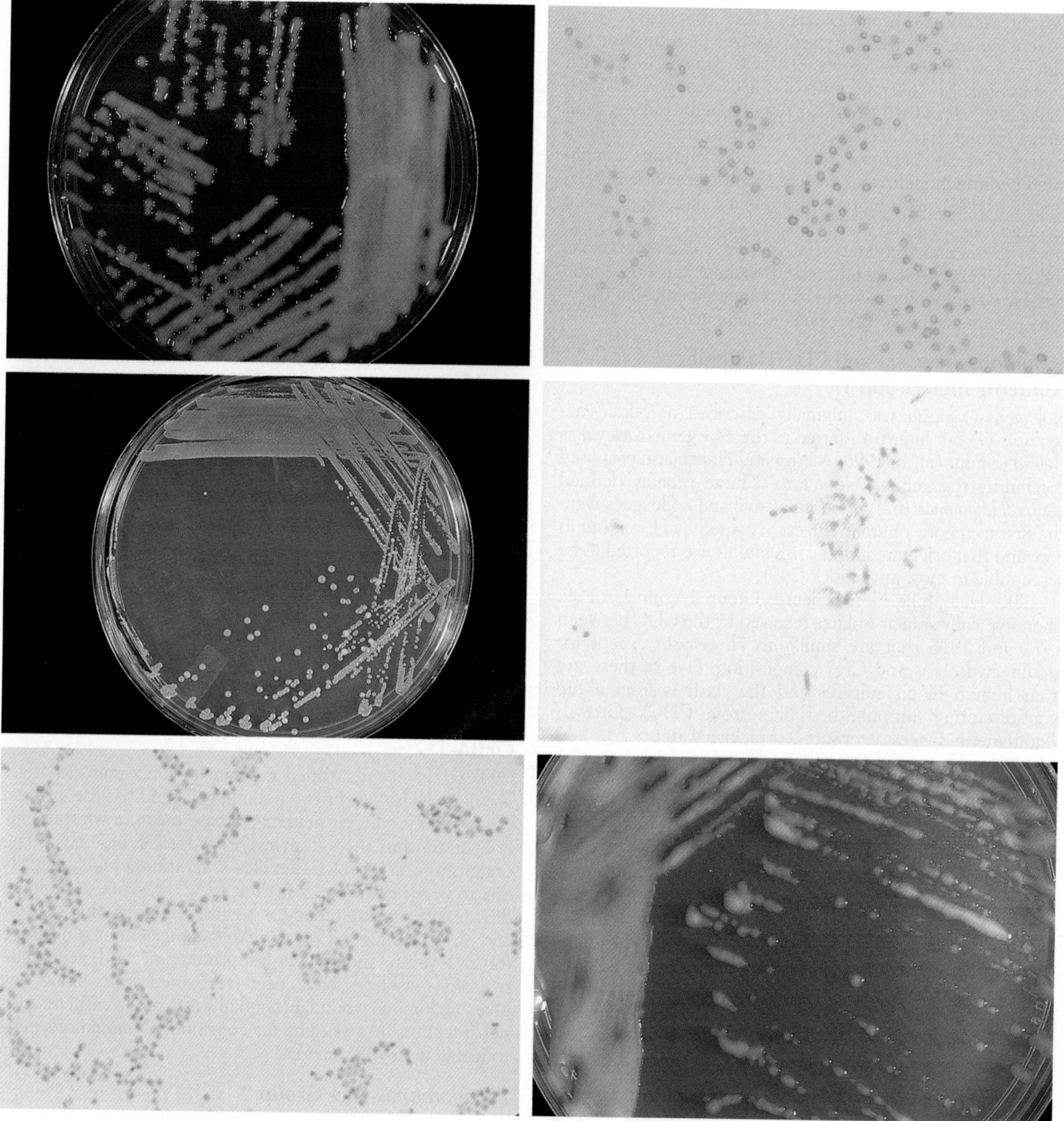

FIGURE 2 (top left) *Rhizobium radiobacter* on MacConkey agar after 48 h of incubation.

FIGURE 3 (top right) Gram stain of *Paracoccus yeei* (EO-2) showing characteristic donut-shaped morphology.

FIGURE 4 (middle left) *Methylobacterium* on Sabouraud's dextrose agar showing coral-pigmented colonies.

FIGURE 5 (middle right) Gram stain of *Methylobacterium* showing pleomorphic gram-negative rods with vacuoles.

FIGURE 6 (bottom left) Gram stain of *Roseomonas* showing gram-negative coccoid rods.

FIGURE 7 (bottom right) *Roseomonas* on Sabouraud's dextrose agar showing pink mucoid colonies.

O-3 organisms as *Campylobacter* (52). 16S rRNA gene sequencing and cell wall fatty acid analysis performed at the CDC show a close match of CDC group O-1 with *Hydrogenophaga palleroni* and of CDC group O-2 with *Caulobacter vibrioides* (Daneshvar, unpublished). Isolates of all three O groups have been recovered from a variety of clinical sources. One case of group O1-associated pneumonia complicated by bronchopulmonary fistula and bacteremia has been reported (192). Antibiotic susceptibility data have been reported only for group O-3. All isolates tested were susceptible to the aminoglycosides, trimethoprim-sulfamethozaxole, and imipenem. Resistance to most β-lactams was noted, and variable susceptibility was noted for chloramphenicol, tetracycline, ciprofloxacin, and amoxicillin-clavulanate (52).

Halomonas venusta and CDC Halophilic Nonfermenter Group 1

Halomonas venusta was originally described as *Alcaligenes venustus* (7) but later transferred to the new genus *Deleya*, as *Deleya venusta* (8). In 1996 Dobson and Franzmann proposed combining the genus *Deleya* into a more broadly defined genus, *Halomonas* (62). von Graevenitz and colleagues were the first to report a human infection caused by *H. venusta* in a wound that originated from a fish bite. It was reported to be susceptible to most antibiotics (249).

CDC Halophilic Nonfermenter Group 1 consists of six phenotypically similar isolates received by the CDC between 1971 and 1998 that are similar to *H. venusta* except for esculin hydrolysis and CFA composition. Five of these are from human blood cultures and the sixth is from a hip wound culture (unpublished data from CDC). Growth requirements suggest exposure to brackish water.

Herbaspirillum Species 3

Herbaspirillum is a gram-negative, generally curved, and sometimes helical bacillus. Individual cells are 0.6 to 0.7 μm wide and 1.5 to 5.0 μm long and have one to three or more flagella on one or both poles (4). A group of clinical isolates, previously described as EF-1, was shown by molecular hybridization to belong to the genus *Herbaspirillum* and was designated as a new unnamed species, *Herbaspirillum* species 3 (4). The organism is oxidase and urease positive; catalase is weak or variable. Other reactions are given in Table 4. Isolates have been recovered from the respiratory tract, feces, urine, ear, eye, and wound sites (4). Antibiotic susceptibility data are not available.

Inquilinus limosus

Inquilinus limosus is a rod-shaped gram-negative bacterium that measures 1.5 to 2 μm in width by 3.5 μm in length, grows at 35 and 42°C but poorly at 25°C, and is either nonmotile or motile with one or two polar flagella. It forms very slimy, nonpigmented colonies on nonselective media. Growth on MacConkey agar is very slight after 3 days. It is polymyxin B resistant and lipase positive, making it appear phenotypically similar to the *B. cepacia* complex (40, 186). The original description of *Inquilinus* stated that there is no utilization of glucose, mannitol, inositol, sorbitol, rhamnose, sucrose, melibiose, amygdalin, or arabinose (40); however, all three isolates tested at CDC showed oxidative utilization of glucose, xylose, mannitol, lactose, sucrose, and maltose either within 2 days or between 3 and 7 days of incubation (Table 4). All strains are positive for catalase, beta-glucosidase, phosphatase, proline aminopeptidase, pyrollidonyl aminopeptidase, and acetoin production and negative for lysine, arginine, ornithine, denitrification, and indole (40). Additional reactions are given in Table 4. All strains have been recovered from respiratory secretions of CF patients and are very mucoid. Identifying the species is difficult because it is not contained in the databases of commercial identification kits and its mucoid appearance may lead to confusion with mucoid *P. aeruginosa* strains (186, 255). Isolates can be recovered on colistin containing *B. cepacia* selective media, but are inhibited on *Burkholderia cepacia* selective agar, which also contains gentamicin (35). The natural habitat of *Inquilinus* is unknown to date, and the clinical impact of chronic colonization with *Inquilinus* sp. remains unclear. Chiron and colleagues reported that for one patient, *Inquilinus* sp. was the only potential pathogen recovered from the sputum and *Inquilinus* acquisition was followed by a worsening of his lung function (35). All isolates are reported to be resistant to penicillins and cephalosporins, kanamycin, tobramycin, colistin, doxycycline, and trimethoprim-sulfamethoxazole and susceptible to imipenem and ciprofloxacin (35, 255).

Massilia timonae

M. timonae is an actively motile (with lateral flagella as well as a single polar flagellum), strictly aerobic gram-negative rod that is oxidase positive, catalase positive, and weakly saccharolytic. Additional phenotypic characteristics are given in Table 4. Colonies appear pale yellow and are distinctively tenacious on agar media and have a tendency to form flocs and films in liquid medium (140). Isolates have been recovered from a surgical wound, cerebrospinal fluid (CSF), the femur of a patient with osteomyelitis, and the blood of several patients (140, 148, 216). *M. timonae* is susceptible to most antibiotics active against gram-negative bacteria with resistance only to ampicillin, cephalothin, and aztreonam (140, 216).

OFBA-1

OFBA-1 is an unclassified medium to long gram-negative, motile rod with one or two polar flagella and has the unusual property of producing acid in OF base medium without carbohydrate, thus the acronym OFBA for OF base acid. The organism most closely resembles *P. aeruginosa* biochemically due to beta-hemolysis, growth at 42°C, presence of arginine dihydrolase, nitrate reduction to gas, and utilization of most carbohydrates (251, 256). Unlike *P. aeruginosa*, it is negative for pyocyanin and pyoverdin production and acetamide hydrolysis. Isolates have been recovered from blood, leg ulcer, abdominal wound, bronchial wash, and a catheter tunnel infection in a patient on continuous ambulatory peritoneal dialysis (251, 256).

Pseudomonas-Like Group 2

The organisms in *Pseudomonas*-like group 2 were previously included in a heterogeneous group of organisms designated CDC group IVd (59). 16S rRNA gene sequencing and cell wall fatty acid analysis performed at the CDC show a close match between *Pseudomonas*-like group 2 and *Herbaspirillum rubrisubalbicans* (Daneshvar, unpublished). Strains are oxidase positive and motile with polar tufts of flagella and are urea, ONPG (*o*-nitrophenyl-β-D-galactopyranoside), and phenylalanine deaminase positive (59). Isolates are similar to *Burkholderia gladioli* but do not oxidize dulcitol or inositol. Other characteristics are given in Table 4. Colonies tend to stick to the agar. Human clinical isolates have come from the respiratory tract, blood, spinal fluid, feces, urine, and dialysate (136).

Sphingomonas spp.

On the basis of its 16S rRNA sequence and the presence of unique sphingoglycolipid and ubiquinone types, the genus

Sphingomonas was created for the organism formerly known as *Pseudomonas paucimobilis* and CDC group IIk-1 (93, 264). Since the original proposal, numerous novel species originating from various environments have been added to the genus *Sphingomonas*.

Members of this genus are known to be decomposers of aromatic compounds and are being developed for use in bioremediation. The genus *Sphingomonas* can be divided into four phylogenetic groups, each representing a different genus. Consequently, three new genera, *Sphingobium, Novosphingobium,* and *Sphingopyxis,* in addition to the genus *Sphingomonas* have been created to accommodate the four phylogenetic groups (226). The emended genus *Sphingomonas* contains at least 12 species, of which only *S. paucimobilis,* designated the type species, and *S. parapaucimobilis* are thought to be important clinically.

S. paucimobilis is characterized by medium to long motile rods with a polar flagellum. However, few cells are actively motile in broth culture, thus making motility a difficult characteristic to demonstrate. Motility occurs at 18 to 22°C but not at 37°C. The oxidase reaction is weakly positive, although occasional strains may be oxidase negative. Colonies are slow growing on blood agar medium, with only small colonies appearing after 24 h of incubation. Older colonies demonstrate a deep yellow (mustard color) pigment. Growth occurs at 37°C but not at 42°C, with optimum growth occurring at 30°C. Isolates are strongly esculin hydrolysis positive and produce a zone of growth inhibition around a vancomycin disk (30 μg) placed on a blood agar plate inoculated with a pure culture isolate (P. Schreckenberger, personal observation). *S. paucimobilis* is widely distributed in the environment, including water, and has been isolated from a variety of clinical specimens, including blood, CSF, peritoneal fluid, urine, wounds, the vagina, the cervix, and from the hospital environment (110, 165, 194). Most strains are susceptible to tetracycline, chloramphenicol, trimethoprim-sulfamethoxazole, and aminoglycosides; susceptibility to other antimicrobial agents including fluoroquinolones varies (70, 110, 194).

The cellular and colonial characteristics of *S. parapaucimobilis* are similar to those of *S. paucimobilis*. It is differentiated from *S. paucimobilis* by blackening of lead acetate paper suspended over KIA, ability to grow and alkalinize Simmons' citrate medium, and a negative extracellular deoxyribonuclease reaction (264). Clinical isolates have been obtained from sputum, urine, and the vagina (264). Antibiotic susceptibility data are not available.

Thermophilic Bacteria

Rabkin and colleagues studied 31 bacterial isolates from clinical specimens received by the CDC that were described as "thermophilic," because they had the unusual feature of growing better when incubated at 42 or 50°C than at 35°C and none grew at 25°C in 18 to 24 h. All were slow growers even at optimum temperatures with colonies appearing circular, usually 0.5 mm or less in diameter after 48 to 72 h at 35°C, and smooth, convex, semitranslucent, and slightly glossy (193). Biochemically, they are oxidase positive, fail to grow on MacConkey agar, and do not ferment glucose. Most strains are oxidative in OF glucose and OF maltose. Isolates have been recovered from blood, CSF, urine, nasopharynx, abscess, wound, and liver biopsy specimens. Two cases of meningitis occurred in previously healthy children. In four other cases, infections occurred in compromised hosts (193). The thermophiles were uniformly susceptible to penicillins and cephalosporins and, with few exceptions, to the aminoglycosides (193).

Ko and colleagues recovered a novel asaccharolytic thermophilic gram-negative bacillus from the bone marrow of a patient who developed febrile neutropenia after induction chemotherapy for treatment of myelogenous leukemia. The isolate grew poorly at 37°C but grew optimally at 50°C. Based on 16S rRNA gene sequencing and fatty acid composition, the isolate was classified as a new species, *Tepidimonas arfidensis* (137).

OXIDASE-POSITIVE, INDOLE-NEGATIVE, SACCHAROLYTIC, NONMOTILE, COCCOID OR ROD-SHAPED NONFERMENTERS

See Table 5.

Sphingobacterium and *Pedobacter*

Sphingobacterium spp. are oxidase-positive, indole-negative gram-negative rods that form yellow-pigmented colonies. They have no flagella but may exhibit sliding motility. They are nonproteolytic and produce acid from carbohydrates. The currently described species of *Sphingobacterium* are *S. multivorum* (formerly *Flavobacterium multivorum* and CDC group IIk-2), *S. spiritivorum* (includes species formerly designated *Flavobacterium spiritivorum, F. yabuuchiae,* and CDC group IIk-3), *S. antarcticum, S. faecium, S. thalpophilum,* and unnamed species *Sphingobacterium* genomospecies 1 and 2 (101, 211, 227, 262). The former *Sphingobacterium* species *S. heparinum* and *S. piscium* have been placed in a new genus, *Pedobacter,* as *P. heparinus* and *P. piscium* (220). The genus *Pedobacter* contains several species of heparinase-producing bacteria found in soil, activated sludge, or fish, but not from human sources. Steyn and colleagues have shown that all these organisms constitute a separate rRNA branch in the rRNA superfamily V for which they have proposed a new family called the *Sphingobacteriaceae* (220).

S. multivorum and *S. spiritivorum* have been most frequently recovered from human clinical specimens. They can be distinguished from the similar organism *Sphingomonas paucimobilis* (formerly IIk-1) by lack of motility, urease production, and resistance to polymyxin B (*S. paucimobilis* is usually motile, urease negative, and usually susceptible to polymyxin B). *S. multivorum* has been isolated from various clinical specimens but has only rarely been associated with serious infections (peritonitis and sepsis) (72, 95, 189). Blood and urine have been the most common sources for the isolation of *S. spiritivorum* (94). *S. mizutaii* has been isolated from blood, CSF, and wound specimens and can be differentiated from *S. multivorum* by its failure to grow on MacConkey agar and usual lack of urease (256). *S. thalpophilum* has been recovered from wounds, blood, eye, abscess, and abdominal incision (256). A positive nitrate test and growth at 42°C differentiate *S. thalpophilum* from other *Sphingobacterium* species.

The organism formerly known as *Sphingobacterium mizutaii* has been transferred to the genus *Flavobacterium* (101) but is included with the sphingobacteria in Table 5 because it is indole negative and phenotypically resembles the *Sphingobacterium* species. *F. mizutaii* has been isolated from blood, CSF, and wound specimens and can be differentiated from *Sphingobacterium* species by its failure to grow on MacConkey agar and usual lack of urease activity (256).

Sphingobacterium species are generally resistant to aminoglycosides and polymyxin B while susceptible in vitro to the quinolones and trimethoprim-sulfamethoxazole. Susceptibility to β-lactam antibiotics is variable, requiring testing of individual isolates (218).

TABLE 5 Oxidase-positive, indole-negative, saccharolytic, nonmotile, coccoid or rod-shaped nonfermenters[a]

Test	*Flavobacterium mizutaii* (6)	*Sphingobacterium multivorum* (22)	*Sphingobacterium spiritivorum* (13)	*Sphingobacterium thalpophilum* (10)	CDC group EF-4b (34)	*Paracoccus yeei* (formerly CDC group EO-2) (11)	CDC group EO-3 (7)	CDC group EO-4[b] (8)	*Pedobacter* spp.[c] (14)	*Psychrobacter immobilis* (saccharolytic strains) (7)
Acid from:										
D-Glucose	67 (33)	100	100	100	70 (26)	91 (9)	100	100	43	57 (43)
D-Xylose	(100)	100	92 (8)	100	0	91 (9)	100	100	ND	57 (43)
D-Mannitol	0	0	100	0	0	0	57 (43)	0	7	0
Lactose	100	100	92 (8)	100	0	45 (55)	71 (29)	0	21	57 (43)
Sucrose	50 (50)	100	100	100	0	0	0	0	21	0
Maltose	50 (50)	100	92 (8)	100	0	(9)	14 (14)	0	ND	0
Catalase	100	100	100	100	100	82	100	100	100	100
Growth on MacConkey	0	100	(46)	100	65 (6)	64 (18)	100	87 (13)	0	40
Simmons citrate	0	0	0	0	14 (6)	64 (36)	29 (71)	87	0	20
Urea, Christensen's	0	95	62 (38)	90 (10)	0	36 (55)	14 (86)	62 (38)	0	(43)
Nitrate reduction	0	0	0	100	97	100	0	0	0	86
Gas from nitrate	0	0	0	0	0	18	0	0	0	0
Nitrite reduction	100[d]	0	0	0	71	0[e]	0[e]	0	ND	0[e]
TSI slant, acid	17	55 (5)	0	100	0	0	0	0	0	0
TSI butt, acid	17	5 (76)	0	10 (70)	6	0	0	0	0	0
H_2S (lead acetate paper)	100	86 (5)	56	100	88	64 (9)	100	100	ND	43 (14)
Gelatin hydrolysis[f]	0	0	15	40	9	0	0	0	0	0
Pigment:										
Insoluble	33 yel[g]	57 light yel	54 pale yel	50 pale yel	50 yel	0	100 yel	75 yel	93 yel	0
Soluble	0	0	0	0	0	55 yel	0	0	0	0
Growth at:										
25°C	100	100	100	100	88	73	100	100	100	100
35°C	100	100	100	100	100	100	100	100	36	57
42°C	0	0	9	100	69	36	14	0	ND	0
Esculin hydrolysis	100	100	100	100	0	0	0	0	100	0
Arginine dihydrolase	25	0	25	0	0	ND	ND	14	0	29
Nutrient broth, 0% NaCl	100	100	100	100	89 (7)	64	71	87	100	43 (57)
Nutrient broth, 6% NaCl	0	25	0	10	0	36	43	13	ND	100
Major CFAs[h]	i-15:0, i-2-OH-15:0, 16:1ω7c	i-15:0, i-2-OH-15:0, 16:1ω7c	i-15:0, i-2-OH-15:0	i-15:0, i-2-OH-15:0, 16:1ω7c	16:0, 16:1ω7c, 18:1ω7c	16:0, 18:1ω7c	18:1ω7c	18:1ω7c	i-15:0, i-2-OH-15:0, 16:1ω7c, 16:0, i-3-OH-17:0	16:1ω7c, 18:1ω9c

[a] Most data are from the CDC Special Bacteriology Reference Laboratory (256). All taxa were negative (≤10% positive) for motility, growth on SS and cetrimide agars, production of H_2S in TSI, lysine decarboxylase, and ornithine decarboxylase activity. Numbers indicate percentage positive at 2 days of incubation; parentheses, delayed reaction (3 to 7 days of incubation); w, weak reaction; ND, not determined or not available; yel, yellow. Numbers in parentheses following organisms indicate number of strains.

[b] Data from Weyant et al., *Abstr. 99th Gen. Meet. Am. Soc. Microbiol.*

[c] Data from reference 220.

[d] A partial reduction may be observed with 0.1% nitrite. A full reduction is observed with 0.01% nitrite.

[e] Fewer than five strains tested.

[f] 14 days of incubation.

[g] Pigment production may be enhanced by room temperature incubation.

[h] The number before the colon indicates the number of carbons; the number after the colon is the number of double bonds; ω, the position of the double bond counting from the hydrocarbon end of the carbon chain; c, *cis* isomer; i, *iso*; 2-OH, a hydroxyl group at the 2 (β) position from the carboxyl end; 3-OH, a hydroxyl group at the 3 (β) position from the carboxyl end.

CDC Group EF4b

EF-4b and EF-4a were originally designated Eugonic Fermenter group 4 (EF-4); however, EF-4b does not ferment glucose, hydrolyze arginine, or produce gas from nitrate, which separates it from the glucose-fermenting strains now designated CDC group EF-4a (see chapter 40). 16S rRNA studies indicate that EF-4b is closely related to *Neisseria canis* (Daneshvar, unpublished). EF-4b strains are coccoid to short rods that are nonmotile and oxidase and catalase positive. Colonies on culture plates are nonpigmented and reported to smell like popcorn. Most isolates have been recovered from human infections following dog and cat bites (256). Antibiotic susceptibility resembles that of EF-4a.

Paracoccus yeei (EO-2), CDC Groups EO-3, EO-4, and *Psychrobacter immobilis*

The classification of the eugenic oxidizers (EO) and the saccharolytic strains of *Psychrobacter immobilis* is incomplete. All are strongly oxidase-positive, nonmotile, saccharolytic coccobacilli and grow, sometimes poorly, on MacConkey agar. In contrast to the EO groups, *P. immobilis* grows best at 20°C and only occasionally at 37°C. EO-3 and many EO-4 strains have a yellow, nondiffusible pigment that is not observed with either *P. yeei* or *P. immobilis*. Daneshvar et al. (53) proposed the name *Paracoccus yeeii*, the epithet being later changed to *yeei* (68), for the former CDC group EO-2. CDC group EO-3 has been shown by 16S rRNA sequencing to closely match *Fulvimarina pelagi* (Daneshvar, unpublished), and CDC EO-4 remains unnamed.

Microscopically, *P. yeei* is characterized by distinctive "O-shaped" cells (Fig. 3) upon Gram stain examination due to the presence of vacuolated or peripherally stained cells, and *P. immobilis* is characterized by paired, coccoid organisms. *P. immobilis* is divided into saccharolytic and asaccharolytic strains. Saccharolytic *P. immobilis* strains (Table 5) share all of the characteristics of the asaccharolytic strains (Table 2) except that glucose, xylose, and lactose, but not sucrose and maltose, are oxidized. Asaccharolytic strains are phenotypically similar to *P. phenylpyruvicus*. The diagnosis of *P. immobilis* can be confirmed by transformation studies, CFA profile, and optimal growth at temperatures of <35°C (167, 256). Many strains of *P. immobilis* have an odor resembling phenylethyl alcohol agar (roses) and are resistant to penicillin but susceptible to most other antibiotics (79, 151). All four groups have been recovered from clinical specimens. *P. yeei* has been isolated from various human wound infections (53). EO-3 has been reported to cause peritonitis in a patient on continuous peritoneal dialysis (49). EO-4 has been recovered from blood, urine, and a nasal sinus, but the clinical significance of these isolates is unknown (R. S. Weyant, M. I. Daneshvar, J. G. Jordan, J. P. MacGregor, and D. G. Hollis, *Abstr. 99th Gen. Meet. Am. Soc. Microbiol.*, abstr. C-196, 1999). One case of ocular infection and one case of infant meningitis have been reported to be caused by *P. immobilis* (79, 151).

PINK-PIGMENTED NONFERMENTERS

See Table 6.

Asaia spp.

Asaia is a recently described genus consisting of two members, *A. bogorensis* (266) and *A. siamensis* (128). The natural habitats of *Asaia* spp. are reported to be in the flowers of the orchid tree, plumbago, and fermented glutinous rice, all originating in hot tropical climates, particularly in Indonesia and Thailand. *Asaia bogorensis* has been reported as a cause of peritonitis in a patient on automated peritoneal dialysis (217). Daneshvar and colleagues identified 14 isolates of a novel *Asaia* species, of which 3 were from a dialysis-associated outbreak (M. I. Daneshvar, L. W. Mayer, A. G. Steigerwalt, A. M. Whitney, R. E. Morey, L. O. Helsel, P. N. Levett, B. J. Paster, F. E. Dewhirst, R. S. Weyant, and D. J. Brenner, Int. Conf. Emerg. Infect. Dis., Atlanta, 2004). *Asaia* species have also been isolated from a batch of fruit-flavored bottled water, which had spoiled as a result of bacterial overgrowth (164). Isolates characterized at the CDC are pink-pigmented, oxidase-negative, motile rods that are oxidative in OF glucose, xylose, and mannitol. Additional characteristics are given in Table 6. Moore reported that *Asaia* spp. were resistant to ceftazidime, meropenem, imipenem, trimethoprim, amikacin, vancomycin, aztreonam, penicillin, and ampicillin by disk diffusion (164). The *A. bogorensis* strain reported by Snyder et al. was susceptible to aminoglycosides (amikacin, tobramycin, and gentamicin) and resistant to ceftazidime and meropenem by disk diffusion (217).

Methylobacterium spp.

Members of the genus *Methylobacterium* are pink-pigmented bacteria able to utilize methanol as a sole source of carbon and energy, although this characteristic may be lost on subculture. They occur mostly on vegetation but may also be found in the hospital environment. The genus currently consists of 20 named species plus additional unassigned biovars recognized on the basis of carbon assimilation type, electrophoretic type, and DNA-DNA homology grouping (74, 80, 81, 233). *Methylobacterium mesophilicum* (formerly *Pseudomonas mesophilica, Pseudomonas extorquens, and Vibrio extorquens*) and *Methylobacterium zatmanii* have been the two most commonly reported species isolated in clinical samples. Methylobacteria are oxidase positive and motile by one polar or lateral flagellum, although motility is often difficult to demonstrate. Isolates are slow growing on ordinary media, producing 1-mm-diameter colonies in 4 to 5 days on SBA, modified Thayer-Martin, Sabouraud, buffered charcoal-yeast extract, and Middlebrook 7H11 agars, with best growth occurring on Sabouraud agar, and usually no growth on MacConkey agar. Optimum growth occurs from 25 to 30°C. Colonies are dry and appear pink or coral in incandescent light (Fig. 4). Under UV light, *Methylobacterium* species appear dark due to absorption of UV light (199). On Gram stain the cells appear as large, vacuolated, pleomorphic rods that stain poorly and may resist decolorization (Fig. 5). Oxidation of sugars (xylose and sometimes glucose) is weak; urea and starch are hydrolyzed.

Methylobacterium species have been reported to cause septicemia, continuous ambulatory peritoneal dialysis-related peritonitis, skin ulcers, synovitis, and other infections often in immunocompromised patients, as well as pseudoinfections (104, 130, 149, 205). Tap water has been implicated as a possible agent of transmission in hospital environments, and methods for monitoring water systems for methylobacteria have been described (197). Active drugs include aminoglycosides and trimethoprim-sulfamethoxazole, whereas β-lactam drugs show variable patterns (26). They are best tested for susceptibility by agar or broth dilution at 30°C for 48 h (26).

Roseomonas and *Azospirillum* spp.

Members of the genus *Roseomonas* (199) are also pink pigmented but differ in morphologic and biochemical characteristics from *Methylobacterium* spp. (Table 6). They are

TABLE 6 Pink-pigmented nonfermenters[a]

Test	*Asaia* spp.[b] (8)	*Methylobacterium* species[c] (90)	*Roseomonas cervicalis* (7)	*Roseomonas gilardii*[d] (21)	*Roseomonas mucosa* (22)	*Roseomonas* genomospecies 4 (3)	*Roseomonas* genomospecies 5 (3)	*Azospirillum* sp. (*Roseomonas* genomospecies 6) (1)	*Azospirillum* sp. (*Roseomonas fauriae*) (5)
Motility; flagella	87; p, 1–2, L	100; p, 1	100; p, 1–2	33; p, 1–2[e]	100; p, 1	67; p, 1–2[f]	0	100; p, 1–2	100; p, 1–2
Acid from:									
D-Glucose	100	40	0	(43)	0	0	0	0	20
D-Xylose	100	94	43	19 (57)	0	100	67	0	80 (20)
D-Mannitol	100	2	0	14 (38)	0 (27)	0	0	0	0
Oxidase	0	96	100	52	27	100	100	100	100
Growth on:									
MacConkey	13 (37)	15	100	43 (52)	50 (50)	100	67(33)	100w	60 (40)
SS	0	0	0	0	0	0	0	0	20
Simmons citrate	0	2 (3)	86 (14)	100	91 (5)	0	33	(100)	60 (20)
Urea, Christensen's	0	29 (26)	86 (14)	71 (29)	95 (5)	67(33)	100	100	100
Nitrate reduction	0	25	0	5	5	100	0	100	100
Gas from nitrate	0	0	0	0	0	0	0	0	20
H_2S (lead acetate paper)	0	47	100	100	100	100	100	100	100
Growth at 42°C	0	12	100	67	100w	100	67	100	100
Esculin hydrolysis	13	0	0	0	0	0	0	100	100
Nutrient broth, 0% NaCl	87	93	100	100	100	100	100	100	100
Nutrient broth, 6% NaCl	13	0	0	24	0	33	0	0	20
Major CFAs[g]	ND	18:1ω7c	16:0, 18:1ω7c	16:0, 18:1ω7c, 19:0cyc, 2–OH–19:0cyc	16:0, 18:1ω7c, 19:0cyc	16:0, 18:1ω7c	16:0, 3–OH–16:0, 18:1ω7c	3–OH–14:0, 16:1ω7c, 18:1ω7c	16:1ω7c, 18:1ω7c

[a] Unless otherwise indicated, data are from the CDC Special Bacteriology Reference Laboratory (256). Numbers indicate the percentage positive at 2 days of incubation; parentheses, delayed reaction (3 to 7 days of incubation); w, weak reaction; ND, not determined or not available; L, lateral; p, polar. All taxa were positive (≥90%) for catalase, growth at 25 and 35°C. All were negative for growth on cetrimide agar, indole production, acid in TSI agar, and H_2S production in TSI agar.

[b] Data from Daneshvar et al. Int. Conf. Emerg. Infect. Dis. Atlanta, 2004.

[c] At least 20 species and additional biovars have been described (see the text).

[d] Two subspecies are proposed: *R. gilardii* subsp. *gilardii* and *R. gilardii* subsp. *rosea* (82).

[e] Motility was more easily demonstrated in OF medium than in motility medium. Motile strains demonstrated either 1 or 2 polar flagella or detached flagella.

[f] Motile strains demonstrated 1 or 2 flagella.

[g] The number before the colon indicates the number of carbons; the number after the colon is the number of double bonds; ω, the position of the double bond counting from the hydrocarbon end of the carbon chain; c, *cis* isomer; OH, a hydroxyl group at the 2(α) or 3(β) position from the carboxyl end; cyc, a cyclopropane ring structure.

nonvacuolated and rather plump and coccoid and form mostly pairs and short chains (Fig. 6). They grow on SBA, modified Thayer-Martin, and usually on MacConkey agars at 37°C, but best growth is observed on Sabouraud's agar. Colonies are mucoid and runny (Fig. 7). They are separated from *Methylobacterium* by their inability to oxidize methanol and assimilate acetamide and by lack of absorption of long-wave UV light (199). All strains are weakly oxidase positive (often after 30 s) or oxidase negative, catalase positive, and urease positive. The original description of the genus *Roseomonas* included three named species, *Roseomonas gilardii* (genomospecies 1), *Roseomonas cervicalis* (genomospecies 2), *Roseomonas fauriae* (genomospecies 3), and three unnamed species, *Roseomonas* genomospecies 4, 5, and 6 (199). More recently, Han et al. proposed a new species, *Roseomonas mucosa*, and a new subspecies, *R. gilardii* subspecies *rosea* (to differentiate from *R. gilardii* subspecies *gilardii*) (82). 16S rRNA gene sequencing of all six *Roseomonas* genomospecies suggests that *Roseomonas* genomospecies 1, 2, 4, and 5 are valid taxa while genomospecies 3 and 6 are not. The invalid *Roseomonas* genomospecies 3 and 6 belong to the genus *Azospirillum*, a nitrogen-fixing plant symbiont that is in a different order of bacteria (44, 82, 228).

Clinical isolates have been recovered from blood, wounds, exudates, abscesses, genitourinary sites, continuous ambulatory peritoneal dialysis fluid, and bone (11, 57, 159, 168, 198, 212, 221, 222). In a review of the laboratory, clinical, and epidemiologic data on 35 patients from whom *Roseomonas* was isolated, Struthers and colleagues reported that *Roseomonas* spp. appear to have a low pathogenic potential for humans but that some species, particularly *R. gilardii*, may be significant pathogens in persons with underlying medical complications (221). In multiple-case reports about 60% of the isolates recovered have been from blood, with about 20% from wounds, exudates, and abscesses and about 10% from genitourinary sites (57, 221).

De et al. summarized susceptibility data from three published reports on a combined 80 strains of *Roseomonas*. All strains were susceptible to amikacin (100%); frequently susceptible to imipenem (99%), ciprofloxacin (90%), and ticarcillin (83%); less susceptible to ceftriaxone (38%), trimethoprim-sulfamethoxazole (30%), and ampicillin (13%); and rarely susceptible to ceftazidime (5%). All strains were resistant to cefepime (57). In catheter-related infections, eradication of the organism has proven difficult unless the infected catheter is removed (198).

OXIDASE-POSITIVE, INDOLE-POSITIVE, NONMOTILE OR MOTILE, YELLOW-PIGMENTED NONFERMENTERS

See Table 7.

Chryseobacterium, Elizabethkingia, Empedobacter, and Unnamed CDC Groups IIc, IIe, IIg, IIh, and IIi

The natural habitats of *Chryseobacterium, Elizabethkingia, Empedobacter,* and the unnamed CDC groups are soil, plants, foodstuffs, and water sources, including those in hospitals. Species in these genera are oxidase positive, indole positive, and nonmotile. The indole reaction is often weak and difficult to demonstrate; therefore, the more sensitive Ehrlich method should be used. Pigment formation with these organisms is variable. Colonies of *Elizabethkingia meningoseptica,* formerly *Chryseobacterium meningosepticum* (133), are smooth and fairly large (1 to 2 mm in diameter after 24 h) but show only weak (if any) production of yellow pigment. In contrast, colonies of *Chryseobacterium indologenes* are deep yellow due to the production of the water-insoluble pigment flexirubin (181). Colonies of *Empedobacter brevis* are pale yellow. Microscopically, cells of *E. meningoseptica, C. indologenes,* and groups IIe, IIh, and IIi are thinner in their central than in their peripheral portions and include filamentous forms; IIh cells are significantly smaller than those of other species. It should be emphasized that test results (e.g., DNase, indole, urea, and starch hydrolysis) in this group are dependent on the choice of medium, reagents, and length of incubation (181). *Chryseobacterium indologenes, C. gleum,* and CDC group IIb are tabulated individually in Table 7. Group IIb is genetically heterogeneous and includes strains of *C. indologenes, C. gleum,* and probably additional genomospecies. Phenotypic separation between *C. indologenes* and *C. gleum* has been difficult; however, acid production from xylose and growth at 41°C are consistently positive in DNA groups clustering around the type strain of *C. gleum* (234).

Chryseobacterium indologenes is the most frequent human isolate, although it rarely has clinical significance (248). It causes bacteremia in hospitalized patients with severe underlying disease, although the mortality is relatively low even among patients who were administered antibiotics without activity against *C. indologenes* (107, 215). Nosocomial infections due to *C. indologenes* have been linked to the use of indwelling devices during hospital stay (109, 111, 174).

Elizabethkingia meningoseptica (133) is most often associated with significant disease in humans, causing neonatal meningitis and nosocomial miniepidemics (15, 36, 215) verifiable by ribotyping (45) and random amplified polymorphic DNA fingerprinting (36), and rarely, adult pneumonia and septicemia (15, 210, 248). A case of respiratory colonization and infection following aerosolized polymyxin B treatment has also been described (25).

Empedobacter brevis and the unnamed CDC groups IIc, IIe, IIg, IIh, and IIi are rarely recovered from clinical material, and little is known about their involvement in clinical disease. One case of meningitis caused by CDC group IIe has been reported (253), and the phenotypic characteristics of several clinical isolates of CDC groups IIc and IIg have been described (86, 88).

The appropriate choice of effective antimicrobial agents for treatment of chryseobacterial infections is difficult. *Chryseobacterium* spp. and *E. meningoseptica* are inherently resistant to many antimicrobial agents commonly used to treated infections caused by gram-negative bacteria (aminoglycosides, β-lactam antibiotics, tetracyclines, and chloramphenicol) but are often susceptible to agents generally used for treating infections caused by gram-positive bacteria (rifampin, clindamycin, erythromycin, sparfloxacin, trimethoprim-sulfamethoxazole, and vancomycin) (70, 218, 248). Although early investigators recommended vancomycin for treating serious infection with *E. meningoseptica* (84, 187), subsequent studies showed greater in vitro activity of minocycline, rifampin, trimethoprim-sulfamethoxazole, and quinolones (15, 71, 218). Among the quinolones, sparfloxacin and levofloxacin are more active than ciprofloxacin and ofloxacin (218). Di Pentima et al. (61) suggested that the combination of intravenous vancomycin and rifampin is an appropriate regimen for initial empirical therapy of *E. meningoseptica* meningitis in newborns. *C. indologenes* is reported to be uniformly resistant to cephalothin, cefotaxime, ceftriaxone, aztreonam,

TABLE 7 Oxidase-positive, indole-positive, nonmotile or motile, nonpigmented or yellow-pigmented nonfermenters[a]

Test	*Elizabethkingia meningoseptica* (149)	*Chryseo-bacterium gleum* (type strain)	*Chryseo-bacterium indologenes* (type strain)	*Empedobacter brevis* (7)	*Weeksella virosa* (87)	*Bergeyella zoohelcum* (41)	*Balneatrix alpica* (1)	CDC group IIb[b] (155)	CDC group IIc (20)	CDC group IIe (30)	CDC group IIg (12)	CDC group IIh (21)	CDC group IIi (23)
Motility; flagella	0	–	–	0	0	0	100; p, 1–2	0	0	0	0	0	0
Acid from:													
D-Glucose	95 (4)	(+)	(+)	85 (15)	0	0	100	92 (6)	100	83 (17)	0	85 (15)	91 (9)
D-Xylose	2 (1)	(+)	–	0	0	0	0	30 (1)	0	0	0	5	87 (13)
D-Mannitol	91 (8)	–	–[b]	0	0	0	(100)	10	0	0	0	0	0
Lactose	42 (15)	–	–	0	0	0	0	0	0	0	0	0	91 (9)
Sucrose	0	–	–	0	0	0	0	13 (1)	100	0	0	0	91 (9)
Maltose	93 (7)	(+)	(+)	85 (15)	0	0	100	92 (6)	100	97 (3)	0	95	91 (9)
Starch	0	–	(+)	75	ND	ND	(100)	100	ND	ND	ND	ND	ND
Trehalose	100	(+)	(+)	0	ND	ND	0	100	ND	ND	ND	ND	ND
ONPG	100	ND	–	0	ND	ND	ND	57	ND	ND	ND	ND	ND
Catalase	100	+	+	100	98	100	100	99	100	100	92	100	100
Oxidase	99	+	+	100	100	100	100	96	100	100	100	100	100
Growth on MacConkey	89 (3)	+	(+)[b]	100	(10)	2	0	54 (9)	0	3	100	0	0
Citrate	9 (3)	+[b]	+	0	0	0	100	2 (1)	0	0	0	0	0
Urea, Christensen's	3 (5)	(+)	–	0	0	100	0	14 (28)	0	0	0	0	14 (18)
Nitrate reduction	0	+	–[b]	0	0	0	100	22	90	0	0	0	0
Nitrite reduction	50[c]	+	–	0[c]	0	0	0	20	90	ND	100	ND	ND
TSI slant, acid	0	–	–	0	0	0	0	1	60 (20)	0	0	0	0
TSI butt, acid	(3)	–	–	0	0	0	0	5 (5)	10 (70)	0	0	5	0
H_2S (lead acetate paper)	98	+	+	100	95	59	100	99	100	87	50	100	70
Gelatin hydrolysis[d]	91	+	+	100	100	98	0	78	20	3	0	7	0
Yellow insoluble pigment	0	+	+	85w	0	0	0	99	0	7w	0	0	22
Growth at:													
25°C	100	+	+	100	58	30	100	100	100	90	100	100	100
35°C	100	+	+	100	100	95	100	100	100	100	100	100	100
42°C	45	+	–	0	70	10	100	42	5	0	90	5	36
Esculin hydrolysis	99	+	+	0	0	0	0	70	100	0	0	100	96

Lysine decarboxylase	0[c]	ND	ND	0	0	0	0	12	0	0	ND	0	0
Arginine dihydrolase	33[c]	ND	ND	0	0	100	0	24	(20)	0	ND	0	0
Nutrient broth, 0% NaCl	100	+	+	100	99	15	100	100	100	97	100	86	100
Nutrient broth, 6% NaCl	7	−	−	0	7	0	0	0	10	3	0	5	9
CFAs[e]	i-15:0, i-2-OH-15:0, i-3-OH-17:0	i-15:0, i-2-OH-15:0, i-17:1ω8c	i-15:0, i-2-OH-15:0, i-17:1ω8c	i-15:0, 16:1ω7c	i-15:0, i-2-OH-15:0	i-15:0	16:0, 16:1ω7c, 18:1ω7c	i-15:0, i-2-OH-15:0, i-17:1ω8c	i-15:0, i-2-OH-15:0, i-3-OH-17:0, i-17:1ω8c	i-15:0, a-15:0, i-2-OH-15:0, i-17:1ω8c	3-OH-14:0, 16:0, 16:1ω7c, 18:1ω7c	i-15:0, a-15:0	i-15:0, i-2-OH-15:0, i-3-OH-17:0

[a] Unless otherwise indicated, data are from the CDC Special Bacteriology Reference Laboratory (256). All taxa were negative (<10% positive) for growth on SS agar, H_2S production in TSI, and ornithine decarboxylase activity. Numbers indicate the percentage positive at 2 days of incubation; parentheses, delayed reaction (3 to 7 days of incubation); w, weak reaction; +, positive; −, negative; ND, not determined or not available; p, polar.

[b] The original description of *C. gleum* lists the type strain as citrate negative. In the original description of *C. indologenes*, 30% of strains (4/13) oxidized mannitol, 46% of strains (6/13) grew on MacConkey agar, and 38% of strains (5/13) reduced nitrate to gas. CDC group IIb includes *C. indologenes* and *C. gleum* (262).

[c] Fewer than five strains tested.

[d] 7 to 14 days of incubation.

[e] The number before the colon indicates the number of carbons; the number after the colon is the number of double bonds; ω, the position of the double bond counting from the hydrocarbon end of the carbon chain; c, *cis* isomer; i, *iso*; a, anteiso; OH, a hydroxyl group at the 2(α) or 3(β) position from the carboxyl end; cyc, a cyclopropane ring structure.

aminoglycosides, erythromycin, clindamycin, vancomycin, and teicoplanin, while susceptibility to piperacillin, cefoperazone, ceftazidime, imipenem, quinolones, minocycline, and trimethoprim-sulfamethoxazole is variable, requiring testing of individual isolates (107, 111, 218, 250). Further complicating the choice of appropriate antimicrobial therapy is the fact that MIC breakpoints for resistance and susceptibility of chryseobacteria have not been established by the Clinical and Laboratory Standards Institute (CLSI) and the results of disk diffusion testing are unreliable in predicting antimicrobial susceptibility to *Chryseobacterium* species (1, 31, 71, 250). The E test is a possible alternative to the standard agar dilution method for testing cefotaxime, ceftazidime, amikacin, minocycline, ofloxacin, and ciprofloxacin but not piperacillin (106). Definitive therapy for clinically significant isolates should be guided by individual susceptibility patterns determined by an MIC method.

Weeksella and *Bergeyella*

Weeksella virosa and *Bergeyella zoohelcum* are morphologically similar organisms measuring 0.6 by 2 to 3 μm, with parallel sides and rounded ends. Both species are oxidase positive and indole positive, fail to grow on MacConkey agar, are nonpigmented, and are nonsaccharolytic. Both species have the unusual feature of being susceptible to penicillin, a feature that allows them to be easily differentiated from the related genera of *Chryseobacterium* and *Sphingobacterium*. *W. virosa* colonies are mucoid and adherent to the agar and develop tan to brown pigmentation; *B. zoohelcum* colonies are sticky and tan to yellow. *W. virosa* is urease negative and polymyxin B susceptible; *B. zoohelcum* is rapid urease positive and polymyxin B resistant. *W. virosa* occurs mainly in urine and vaginal samples (99, 196), whereas *B. zoohelcum* is isolated mainly from wounds caused by animal (mostly dog) bites (100, 195). Meningitis or septicemia due to *B. zoohelcum* has occurred in patients either bitten by a dog (23, 163) or with continuous contact with cats (172). Both organisms are susceptible to most antibiotics; however, at present no specific antibiotic treatment is recommended; therefore, antibiotic susceptibility testing should be performed on significant clinical isolates.

Balneatrix

The genus *Balneatrix* contains a single species, *B. alpica* (55), that was first isolated in 1987 during an outbreak of pneumonia and meningitis among persons who attended a hot (37°C) spring spa in southern France (28, 55, 113). Isolates from eight patients were recovered from blood, CSF, and sputum, and one was recovered from water. The bacterium is described as a gram-negative, straight or curved rod, motile by a single polar flagellum, and strictly aerobic. Growth occurs at 20 to 46°C, producing colonies that are 2 to 3 mm in diameter, convex, and smooth. The center of the colonies is pale yellow after 2 to 3 days and pale brown after 4 days. Growth occurs on chocolate and tryptic soy agars but not on MacConkey agar. It is oxidase positive and nonfermentative but oxidizes glucose, mannose, fructose, maltose, sorbitol, mannitol, glycerol, and inositol. Indole is produced and nitrate is reduced to nitrite (Table 7). Gelatin is weakly hydrolyzed and lecithinase is positive. It is similar to *E. meningoseptica* but can be differentiated by positive motility and nitrate and negative ONPG reactions. *B. alpica* is reported to be susceptible to penicillin G and all other β-lactam antibiotics and to all aminoglycosides, chloramphenicol, tetracycline, erythromycin, sulfonamides, trimethoprim, ofloxacin, and nalidixic acid. It is resistant to clindamycin and vancomycin (28).

EVALUATION, INTERPRETATION, AND REPORTING OF RESULTS

Although certain nonfermenting bacilli (NFBs) can on occasion be frank pathogens, e.g., *Pseudomonas aeruginosa*, *Burkholderia pseudomallei*, and *Elizabethkingia meningoseptica*, NFBs are generally considered to be of low virulence and often occur in mixed cultures, making it difficult to determine when to work up cultures and when to perform susceptibility studies. Decisions regarding the significance of NFBs in a clinical specimen must take into account the clinical condition of the patient and the source of the specimen submitted for culture. In general, the recovery of an NFB in pure culture from a normally sterile site warrants identification and susceptibility testing, whereas predominant growth of an NFB from a nonsterile specimen, such as an endotracheal culture of a patient with no clinical signs or symptoms of pneumonia, would not be worked up further. Because many NFBs exhibit multiple antibiotic resistance, patients who are on antibiotics often become colonized with NFBs. NFB species isolated in mixed cultures can usually be reported by descriptive identification, e.g., "growth of *P. aeruginosa* and two varieties of nonfermenting gram-negative bacilli not further identified." The Gram stain made from the clinical material should be used to guide the laboratory decision on how far to work up the specimen.

Decisions about performing susceptibility testing are complicated by the fact that the CLSI interpretive guidelines for disk diffusion testing of the nonfermenting gram-negative bacilli are limited to *Pseudomonas* spp., *Burkholderia cepacia*, *Stenotrophomonas maltophilia*, and *Acinetobacter* spp. and therefore, except for *Acinetobacter* species, do not include the organisms covered in this chapter. Furthermore, results obtained with certain organisms (e.g., *Acinetobacter* species) by using disk diffusion do not correlate with results obtained by conventional MIC methods (see discussion elsewhere in this chapter). In general, laboratories should try to avoid performing susceptibility testing on the organisms included in this chapter. When clinical necessity dictates that susceptibility testing be performed, an overnight MIC method is recommended.

REFERENCES

1. **Aber, R. C., C. Wennersten, and R. C. Moellering, Jr.** 1978. Antimicrobial susceptibility of flavobacteria. *Antimicrob. Agents Chemother.* **14:**483–487.
2. **Anstey, N. M., B. J. Currie, and K. M. Withnall.** 1992. Community-acquired *Acinetobacter* pneumonia in the northern territory of Australia. *Clin. Infect. Dis.* **14:**83–91.
3. **Bachman, K. H., D. L. Sewell, and L. J. Strausbaugh.** 1996. Recurrent cellulitis and bacteremia caused by *Flavobacterium odoratum. J. Clin. Microbiol.* **22:**1112–1113.
4. **Baldani, J. I., B. Pot, G. Kirchhof, E. Falsen, V. L. D. Baldani, F. L. Olivares, B. Hoste, K. Kersters, A. Hartmann, M. Gillis, and J. Dobereiner.** 1996. Emended description of *Herbaspirillum;* inclusion of *[Pseudomonas] rubrisubalbicans*, a mild plant pathogen, as *Herbaspirillum rubrisubalbicans* comb. nov.; and classification of a group of clinical isolates (EF Group 1) as *Herbaspirillum* species 3. *Int. J. Syst. Bacteriol.* **46:**802–810.
5. **Barham, W. B., P. Church, J. E. Brown, and S. Paparello.** 1993. Misidentification of *Brucella* species with use of rapid bacterial identification systems. *Clin. Infect. Dis.* **17:** 1068–1069.
6. **Batchelor, B. I., R. J. Brindle, G. F. Gilks, and J. B. Selkon.** 1992. Biochemical misidentification of *Brucella melitensis* and subsequent laboratory-acquired infections. *J. Hosp. Infect.* **22:**159–162.
7. **Baumann, L., P. Baumann, M. Mandel, and R. D. Allen.** 1972. Taxonomy of aerobic marine eubacteria. *J. Bacteriol.* **110:**402–429.
8. **Baumann, L., R. D. Bowditch, and P. Baumann.** 1983. Description of *Deleya* gen. nov. created to accommodate the marine species *Alcaligenes aestus, A. pacificus, A. cupidus, A. venustus,* and *Pseudomonas marina. Int. J. Syst. Bacteriol.* **33:**793–802.
9. **Bergogne-Berezin, E., and K. J. Towner.** 1996. *Acinetobacter* spp. as nosocomial pathogens: microbiological, clinical, and epidemiological features. *Clin. Microbiol. Rev.* **9:**148–165.
10. **Bernards, A. T., J. van der Toorn, C. P. A. van Boven, and L. Dijkshoorn.** 1996. Evaluation of the ability of a commercial system to identify *Acinetobacter* genomic species. *Eur. J. Clin. Microbiol. Infect. Dis.* **15:**303–308.
11. **Bibashi, E., D. Sofianou, K. Kontopoulou, E. Mitsopoulos, and E. Kokolina.** 2000. Peritonitis due to *Roseomonas fauriae* in a patient undergoing continuous ambulatory peritoneal dialysis. *J. Clin. Microbiol.* **38:**456–457.
12. **Bizet, C., and J. Bizet.** 1995. Sensibilité comparée de *Ochrobactrum anthropi, Agrobacterium tumefaciens, Alcaligenes faecalis, Alcaligenes denitrificans* subsp. *denitrificans, Alcaligenes denitrificans subsp. xylosidans* et *Bordetella bronchiseptica* vis-à-vis de 35 antibiotiques dont 17 β-lactamines. *Pathol. Biol.* **43:**258–263.
13. **Bizet, C., F. Tekaia, and A. Philippon.** 1993. In-vitro susceptibility of *Alcaligenes faecalis* compared with those of other *Alcaligenes* spp. to antimicrobial agents including seven β-lactams. *J. Antimicrob. Chemother.* **32:**907–910.
14. **Bizet, J., and C. Bizet.** 1997. Strains of *Alcaligenes faecalis* from clinical material. *J. Infect.* **35:**167–169.
15. **Bloch, K. C., R. Nadarajah, and R. Jacobs.** 1997. *Chryseobacterium meningosepticum:* an emerging pathogen among immunocompromised adults. *Medicine* **76:**30–40.
16. **Botelho-Nevers, E., F. Gouriet, C. Rovery, P. Paris, V. Roux, D. Raoult, and P. Brouqui.** 2005. First case of osteomyelitis due to *Shewanella algae. J. Clin. Microbiol.* **43:**5388–5390.
17. **Bou, G., G. Cervero, M. A. Dominguez, C. Quereda, and J. Martinez-Beltran.** 2000. PCR-based DNA fingerprinting (REP-PCR, AP-PCR) and pulsed-field gel electrophoresis characterization of a nosocomial outbreak caused by imipenem- and meropenem-resistant *Acinetobacter baumannii. Clin. Microbiol. Infect.* **6:**635–643.
18. **Bouvet, P. J. M., and P. A. D. Grimont.** 1986. Taxonomy of the genus *Acinetobacter* with the recognition of *Acinetobacter baumannii* sp. nov., *Acinetobacter haemolyticus* sp. nov., *Acinetobacter johnsonii* sp. nov., and *Acinetobacter junii* sp. nov. and emended descriptions of *Acinetobacter calcoaceticus* and *Acinetobacter lwoffii. Int. J. Syst. Bacteriol.* **36:**228–240.
19. **Bouvet, P. J. M., and P. A. D. Grimont.** 1987. Identification and biotyping of clinical isolates of *Acinetobacter. Ann. Inst. Pasteur Microbiol.* **138:**569–578.
20. **Bouvet, P. J. M., and S. Jeanjean.** 1989. Delineation of new proteolytic genomic species in the genus *Acinetobacter. Res. Microbiol.* **140:**291–299.
21. **Bouvet, P. J. M., S. Jeanjean, J. F. Vieu, and L. Dijkshoorn.** 1990. Species, biotype, and bacteriophage type determinations compared with cell envelope protein profiles for typing *Acinetobacter* strains. *J. Clin. Microbiol.* **28:**170–176.
22. **Bovre, K., J. E. Fuglesang, N. Hagen, E. Jantzen, and L. O. Froholm.** 1976. *Moraxella atlantae* sp. nov. and its distinction from *Moraxella phenylpyrouvica. Int. J. Syst. Bacteriol.* **26:**511–521.
23. **Bracis, R., K. Seibers, and R. M. Julien.** 1979. Meningitis caused by Group IIj following a dog bite. *West. J. Med.* **131:**438–440.

24. **Brink, A. J., A. van Straten, and A. J. van Rensburg.** 1995. *Shewanella (Pseudomonas) putrefaciens* bacteremia. *Clin. Infect. Dis.* **20:**1327–1332.
25. **Brown, R. B., D. Phillips, M. J. Barker, R. Pieczarka, M. Sands, and D. Teres.** 1989. Outbreak of nosocomial *Flavobacterium meningosepticum* respiratory infections associated with use of aerosolized polymyxin B. *Am. J. Infect. Control* **17:**121–125.
26. **Brown, W. J., R. L. Sautter, and A. E. Crist, Jr.** 1992. Susceptibility testing of clinical isolates of *Methylobacterium* species. *Antimicrob. Agents Chemother.* **36:**1635–1638.
27. **Butt, A. A., J. Figueroa, and D. H. Martin.** 1997. Ocular infection caused by three unusual marine organisms. *Clin. Infect. Dis.* **24:**740.
28. **Casalta, J. P., Y. Peloux, D. Raoult, P. Brunet, and H. Gallais.** 1989. Pneumonia and meningitis caused by a new nonfermentative unknown gram-negative bacterium. *J. Clin. Microbiol.* **27:**1446–1448.
29. **Centers for Disease Control and Prevention.** 1996. *Ochrobactrum anthropi* meningitis associated with cadaveric pericardial tissue processed with a contaminated solution—Utah, 1994. *Morb. Mortal. Wkly. Rep.* **45:**671–673.
30. **Centers for Disease Control and Prevention.** 2004. *Acinetobacter baumannii* infections among patients at military medical facilities treating injured U.S. service members, 2002–2004. *Morb. Mortal. Wkly. Rep.* **53:**1063–1066.
31. **Chang, J.-C., P.-R. Hsueh, J.-J. Wu, S.-W. Ho, W.-C. Hsieh, and K.-T. Luh.** 1997. Antimicrobial susceptibility of flavobacteria as determined by agar dilution and disk diffusion methods. *Antimicrob. Agents Chemother.* **41:**1301–1306.
32. **Chen, W.-M., S. Laevens, T.-M. Lee, et al.** 2001. *Ralstonia taiwanensis* sp. nov., isolated from root nodules of *Mimosa* species and sputum of a cystic fibrosis patient. *Int. J. Syst. Evol. Microbiol.* **51:**1729–1735.
33. **Chen, Y.-S., Y.-C. Liu, M.-Y. Yen, J.-H. Wang, J.-H. Wang, S.-R. Wann, and D.-L. Cheng.** 1997. Skin and soft-tissue manifestations of *Shewanella putrefaciens* infection. *Clin. Infect. Dis.* **25:**225–229.
34. **Cheron, M., E. Abachin, E. Guerot, M. El-Bez, and M. Simonet.** 1994. Investigation of hospital-acquired infections due to *Alcaligenes denitrificans* subsp. *xylosoxidans* by DNA restriction fragment length polymorphism. *J. Clin. Microbiol.* **32:**1023–1026.
35. **Chiron, R., H. Marchandin, F. Counil, E. Jumas-Bilak, A. M. Freydiere, G. Bellon, M. O. Husson, D. Turck, F. Bremont, G. Chabanon, and C. Segonds.** 2005. Clinical and microbiological features of *Inquilinus* sp. isolates from five patients with cystic fibrosis. *J. Clin. Microbiol.* **43:**3938–3943.
36. **Chiu, C.-H., M. Waddingdon, W.-S. Hsieh, D. Greenberg, P. C. Schreckenberger, and A. M. Carnahan.** 2000. Atypical *Chryseobacterium meningosepticum* and meningitis and sepsis in newborns and the immunocompromised, Taiwan. *Emerg. Infect. Dis.* **6:**481–486.
37. **Cisneros, J. M., M. J. Reyes, J. Pachon, B. Becerril, F. J. Caballero, J. L. Garcia-Garmendia, C. Ortiz, and A. R. Cobacho.** 1996. Bacteremia due to *Acinetobacter baumannii:* epidemiology, clinical findings, and prognostic features. *Clin. Infect. Dis.* **22:**1026–1032.
38. **Clarridge, J. E., III.** 2004. Impact of 16S rRNA gene sequence analysis for identification of bacteria on clinical microbiology and infectious diseases. *Clin. Microbiol. Rev.* **17:**840–862.
39. **Coenye, T., E. Falsen, M. Vancanneyt, B. Hoste, J. R. W. Govan, K. Kersters, and P. Vandamme.** 1999. Classification of *Alcaligenes faecalis*-like isolates from the environment and human clinical samples as *Ralstonia gilardii* sp. nov. *Int. J. Syst. Bacteriol.* **49:**405–413.
40. **Coenye, T., J. Goris, T. Spilker, P. Vandamme, and J. J. LiPuma.** 2002. Characterization of unusual bacteria isolated from respiratory secretions of cystic fibrosis patients and description of *Inquilinus limosus* gen. nov., sp. nov. *J. Clin. Microbiol.* **40:**2062–2069.
41. **Coenye, T., M. Vancanneyt, M. C. Cnockaert, E. Falsen, J. Swings, and P. Vandamme.** 2003. *Kerstersia gyiorum* gen. nov., sp. nov., a novel *Alcaligenes faecalis*-like organism isolated from human clinical samples, and reclassification of *Alcaligenes denitrificans* Rüger and Tan 1983 as *Achromobacter denitrificans* comb. nov. *Int. J. Syst. Evol. Microbiol.* **53:**1825–1831.
42. **Coenye, T., P. Vandamme, and J. J. LiPuma.** 2003. *Ralstonia respiraculi* sp. nov., isolated from the respiratory tract of cystic fibrosis patients. *Int. J. Syst. Evol. Microbiol.* **53:**1339–1342.
43. **Coenye, T., E. Vanlaere, E. Samyn, E. Falsen, P. Larsson, and P. Vandamme.** 2005. *Advenella incenata* gen. nov., sp. nov., a novel member of the *Alcaligenaceae*, isolated from various clinical specimens. *Int. J. Syst. Evol. Microbiol.* **55:**251–256.
44. **Cohen, M. F., X. Y. Han, and M. Mazzola.** 2004. Molecular and physiological comparison of *Azospirillum* spp. isolated from *Rhizoctonia solani* mycelia, wheat rhizosphere, and human skin wounds. *Can. J. Microbiol.* **50:**291–297.
45. **Colding, H., J. Bangsborg, N.-E. Fiehn, T. Bennekov, and B. Bruun.** 1994. Ribotyping for differentiating *Flavobacterium meningosepticum* isolates from clinical and environmental sources. *J. Clin. Microbiol.* **32:**501–505.
46. **Corbella, X., J. Ariza, C. Ardanuy, M. Vuelta, F. Tubau, M. Sora, M. Pujol, and F. Gudiol.** 1998. Efficacy of sulbactam alone and in combination with ampicillin in nosocomial infections caused by multiresistant *Acinetobacter baumannii*. *J. Antimicrob. Chemother.* **42:**793–802.
47. **Corbella, X., A. Montero, M. Pujol, M. A. Dominguez, J. Ayats, M. J. Argerich, F. Garrigosa, J. Ariza, and F. Gudiol.** 2000. Emergence and rapid spread of carbapenem resistance during a large and sustained hospital outbreak of multiresistant *Acinetobacter baumannii*. *J. Clin. Microbiol.* **38:**4086–4095.
48. **Corbella, X., M. Pujol, J. Ayats, M. Sendra, C. Ardanuy, M. A. Dominguez, J. Linares, J. Ariza, and F. Gudiol.** 1996. Relevance of digestive tract colonization in the epidemiology of nosocomial infections due to multiresistant *Acinetobacter baumannii*. *Clin. Infect. Dis.* **23:**329–334.
49. **Daley, D., S. Neville, and K. Kociuba.** 1997. Peritonitis associated with a CDC Group EO-3 organism. *J. Clin. Microbiol.* **35:**3338–3339.
50. **Dalla-Costa, L. M., J. M. Coelho, H. A. P. H. M. Souza, M. E. Castro, C. J. Stier, K. L. Bragagnolo, A. Rea-Neto, S. R. Penteado-Filho, D. M. Livermore, and N. Woodford.** 2003. Outbreak of carbapenem-resistant *Acinetobacter baumannii* producing OXA-23 enzyme in Curitiba, Brazil. *J. Clin. Microbiol.* **41:**3403–3406.
51. **Dan, M., R. Gutman, and A. Biro.** 1992. Peritonitis caused by *Pseudomonas putrefaciens* in patients undergoing continuous ambulatory peritoneal dialysis. *Clin. Infect. Dis.* **14:**359–360.
52. **Daneshvar, M. I., B. Hill, D. G. Hollis, C. W. Moss, J. G. Jordan, J. P. MacGregor, F. Tenover, and R. S. Weyant.** 1998. CDC group O-3: phenotypic characteristics, fatty acid composition, isoprenoid quinone content, and in vitro antimicrobic susceptibilities of an unusual gram-negative bacterium isolated from clinical specimens. *J. Clin. Microbiol.* **36:**1674–1678.
53. **Daneshvar, M. I., D. G. Hollis, R. S. Weyant, A. G. Steigerwalt, A. M. Whitney, M. P. Douglas, J. P. Macgregor, J. G. Jordan, L. W. Mayer, S. M. Rassouli, W. Barchet, C. Munro, L. Shuttleworth, and K. Bernard.** 2003. *Paracoccus yeeii* sp. nov. (formerly CDC group EO-2),

a novel bacterial species associated with human infection. *J. Clin. Microbiol.* **41:**1289–1294.

54. **Das, K., S. Shah, and M. H. Levi.** 1997. Misleading Gram stain from a patient with *Moraxella (Branhamella) catarrhalis* bacteremia. *Clin. Microbiol. Newslett.* **19:**85–88.

55. **Dauga, C., M. Gillis, P. Vandamme, E. Ageron, F. Grimont, K. Kersters, C. de Mahenge, Y. Peloux, and P. A. D. Grimont.** 1993. *Balneatrix alpica* gen. nov., sp. nov., a bacterium associated with pneumonia and meningitis in a spa therapy centre. *Res. Microbiol.* **144:**35–46.

56. **Davis, K. A., K. A. Moran, C. K. McAllister, and P. G. Gray.** 2005. Multidrug-resistant *Acinetobacter* extremity infections in soldiers. *Emerg. Infect. Dis.* **11:**1218–1224.

57. **De, I., K. V. I. Rolston, and X. Y. Han.** 2004. Clinical significance of *Roseomonas* species isolated from catheter and blood samples: analysis of 36 cases in patients with cancer. *Clin. Infect. Dis.* **38:**1579–1584.

58. **Dealler, S. F., M. Abbott, M. J. Croughan, and P. M. Hawkey.** 1989. Identification of *Branhamella catarrhalis* in 2.5 min with an indoxyl butyrate strip test. *J. Clin. Microbiol.* **27:**1390–1391.

59. **Dees, S. B., D. G. Hollis, R. E. Weaver, and C. W. Moss.** 1983. Cellular fatty acid composition of *Pseudomonas marginata* and closely associated bacteria. *J. Clin. Microbiol.* **18:**1073–1078.

60. **Ding, L., and A. Yokota. 2002.** Phylogenetic analysis of the genus *Aquaspirillum* based on 16S rRNA gene sequences. *FEMS Microbiol. Lett.* **212:**165–169.

61. **Di Pentima, M. C., E. O. Mason, Jr., and S. L. Kaplan.** 1998. In vitro antibiotic synergy against *Flavobacterium meningosepticum:* implications for therapeutic options. *Clin. Infect. Dis.* **26:**1169–1176.

62. **Dobson, S. J., and P. D. Franzmann.** 1996. Unification of the genera *Deleya* (Baumann et al. 1983), *Halomonas* (Vreeland et al. 1980), and *Halovibrio* (Fendrich 1988) and the species *Paracoccus halodenitrificans* (Robinson and Gibbons 1952) into a single genus, *Halomonas,* and placement of the genus *Zymobacter* in the family *Halomonadaceae*. *Int. J. Syst. Bacteriol.* **46:**550–558.

63. **Drancourt, M., and D. Raoult.** 2005. Sequence-based identification of new bacteria: a proposition for creation of an orphan bacterium repository. *J. Clin. Microbiol.* **43:**4311–4315.

64. **Duggan, J. M., S. J. Goldstein, C. E. Chenoweth, C. A. Kauffman, and S. F. Bradley.** 1996. *Achromobacter xylosoxidans* bacteremia: report of four cases and review of the literature. *Clin. Infect. Dis.* **23:**569–576.

65. **Dunne, W. M., Jr., and S. Maisch.** 1995. Epidemiological investigation of infections due to *Alcaligenes* species in children and patients with cystic fibrosis: use of repetitive-element-sequence polymerase chain reaction. *Clin. Infect. Dis.* **20:**836–841.

66. **Dunne, W. M., Jr., J. Tillman, and J. C. Murray.** 1993. Recovery of a strain of *Agrobacterium radiobacter* with a mucoid phenotype from an immunocompromised child with bacteremia. *J. Clin. Microbiol.* **31:**2541–2543.

67. **Edmond, M. B., S. A. Riddler, C. M. Baxter, B. M. Wicklund, and A. W. Pasculle.** 1993. *Agrobacterium radiobacter:* a recently recognized opportunistic pathogen. *Clin. Infect. Dis.* **16:**388–391.

68. **Euzeby, J.** 2003. Validation of publication of new names and new combinations previously effectively published outside the IJSEM. *Int. J. Syst. Evol. Microbiol.* **53:**935–937.

69. **Farmer, J. J., III, R. E. Gangarosa, and E. J. Gangarosa.** 2004. Does *Laribacter hongkongensis* cause diarrhoea, or does diarrhoea "cause" *L hongkongensis? Lancet* **363:**1923–1924.

70. **Fass, R. J., and J. Barnishan.** 1980. In vitro susceptibility of nonfermentative gram-negative bacilli other than *Pseudomonas aeruginosa* to 32 antimicrobial agents. *Rev. Infect. Dis.* **2:**841–853.

71. **Fraser, S. L., and J. H. Jorgensen.** 1997. Reappraisal of the antimicrobial susceptibilities of *Chryseobacterium* and *Flavobacterium* species and methods for reliable susceptibility testing. *Antimicrob. Agents Chemother.* **41:**2738–2741.

72. **Freney, J., W. Hansen, C. Ploton, H. Meugnier, S. Madier, N. Bornstein, and J. Fleurette.** 1987. Septicemia caused by *Sphingobacterium multivorum*. *J. Clin. Microbiol.* **25:**1126–1128.

73. **Fry, N. K., J. Duncan, H. Malnick, M. Warner, A. J. Smith, M. S. Jackson, and A. Ayoub.** 2005. *Bordetella petrii* clinical isolate. *Emerg. Infect. Dis.* **11:**1131–1133.

74. **Gallego, V., M. T. Garcia, and A. Ventosa.** 2005. *Methylobacterium isbiliense* sp. nov., isolated from the drinking water system of Sevilla, Spain. *Int. J. Syst. Evol. Microbiol.* **55:**2333–2337.

75. **Gerner-Smidt, P., and I. Tjernberg.** 1993. *Acinetobacter* in Denmark. II. Molecular studies of the *Acinetobacter calcoaceticus-Acinetobacter baumannii* complex. *APMIS* **101:**826–832.

76. **Gerner-Smidt, P., I. Tjernberg, and J. Ursing.** 1991. Reliability of phenotypic tests for identification of *Acinetobacter* species. *J. Clin. Microbiol.* **29:**277–282.

77. **Getchell-White, S. I., L. G. Donowitz, and D. H. M. Gröschel.** 1989. The inanimate environment of an intensive care unit as a potential source of nosocomial bacteria: evidence for long survival of *Acinetobacter calcoaceticus*. *Infect. Control Hosp. Epidemiol.* **10:**402–407.

78. **Giamarellos-Bourboulis, E. J., E. Xirouchaki, and H. Giamarellou.** 2001. Interactions of colistin and rifampin on multidrug-resistant *Acinetobacter baumannii*. *Diagn. Microbiol. Infect. Dis.* **40:**117–120.

79. **Gini, G. A.** 1990. Ocular infection caused by *Psychrobacter immobilis* acquired in the hospital. *J. Clin. Microbiol.* **28:**400–401.

80. **Green, P. N., and I. J. Bousfield.** 1983. Emendation of *Methylobacterium* Patt, Cole, and Hanson 1976; *Methylobacterium rhodinum* (Heumann 1962) comb. nov. corrig.; *Methylobacterium radiotolerans* (Ito and Iizuka 1971) comb. nov. corrig.; and *Methylobacterium mesophilicum* (Austin and Goodfellow 1979) comb. nov. *Int. J. Syst. Bacteriol.* **33:**875–877.

81. **Green, P. N., I. J. Bousfield, and D. Hood.** 1988. Three new *Methylobacterium* species: *M. rhodesianum* sp. nov., *M. zatmanii* sp. nov., and *M. fujisawaense* sp. nov. *Int. J. Syst. Bacteriol.* **38:**124–127.

82. **Han, X. Y., A. S. Pham, J. J. Tarrand, K. V. Rolston, L. O. Helsel, and P. N. Levett.** 2003. Bacteriologic characterization of 36 strains of *Roseomonas* species and proposal of *Roseomonas mucosa* sp. nov. and *Roseomonas gilardii* subsp. *rosea* subsp. nov. *Am. J. Clin. Pathol.* **120:**256–264.

83. **Harrington, B. J.** 1997. Letter. *Clin. Microbiol. Newslett.* **19:**191.

84. **Hawley, H. B., and D. W. Gump.** 1973. Vancomycin therapy of bacterial meningitis. *Am. J. Dis. Child.* **126:**261–264.

85. **Higgins, P. G., H. Wisplinghoff, D. Stefanik, and H. Seifert.** 2004. In vitro activities of the β-lactamase inhibitors clavulanic acid, sulbactam, and tazobactam alone or in combination with β-lactams against epidemiologically characterized multidrug-resistant *Acinetobacter baumannii* strains. *Antimicrob. Agents Chemother.* **48:**1586–1592.

86. **Hollis, D. G., M. I. Daneshvar, C. W. Moss, and C. N. Baker.** 1995. Phenotypic characteristics, fatty acid composition, and isoprenoid quinone content of CDC group IIg bacteria. *J. Clin. Microbiol.* **33:**762–764.

87. **Hollis, D. G., C. W. Moss, M. I. Daneshvar, L. Meadows, J. Jordan, and B. Hill.** 1993. Characterization of Centers for Disease Control group NO-1, a fastidious, nonoxidative, gram-negative organism associated with dog and cat bites. *J. Clin. Microbiol.* **31:**746–748.

88. **Hollis, D. G., C. W. Moss, M. I. Daneshvar, and P. L. Wallace-Shewmaker.** 1996. CDC group IIc: phenotypic characteristics, fatty acid composition, and isoprenoid quinone content. *J. Clin. Microbiol.* **34:**2322–2324.
89. **Holmes, B., M. Costas, A. C. Wood, and K. Kersters.** 1990. Numerical analysis of electrophoretic protein patterns of "*Achromobacter*" group B, E and F strains from human blood. *J. Appl. Bacteriol.* **68:**495–504.
90. **Holmes, B., M. Costas, A. C. Wood, R. J. Owen, and D. D. Morgan.** 1990. Differentiation of *Achromobacter*-like strains from human blood by DNA restriction endonuclease digest and ribosomal RNA gene probe patterns. *Epidemiol. Infect.* **105:**541–551.
91. **Holmes, B., R. Lewis, and A. Trevett.** 1992. Septicaemia due to *Achromobacter* group B: a report of two cases. *Med. Microbiol. Lett.* **1:**177–184.
92. **Holmes, B., C. W. Moss, and M. I. Daneshvar.** 1993. Cellular fatty acid compositions of "*Achromobacter* Groups B and E." *J. Clin. Microbiol.* **31:**1007–1008.
93. **Holmes, B., R. J. Owen, A. Evans, H. Malnick, and W. R. Willcox.** 1977. *Pseudomonas paucimobilis,* a new species isolated from human clinical specimens, the hospital environment, and other sources. *Int. J. Syst. Bacteriol.* **27:**133–146.
94. **Holmes, B., R. J. Owen, and D. G. Hollis.** 1982. *Flavobacterium spiritivorum,* a new species isolated from human clinical specimens. *Int. J. Syst. Bacteriol.* **32:**157–165.
95. **Holmes, B., R. J. Owen, and R. E. Weaver.** 1981. *Flavobacterium multivorum,* a new species isolated from human clinical specimens and previously known as group IIK, biotype 2. *Int. J. Syst. Bacteriol.* **31:**21–34.
96. **Holmes, B., C. A. Pinning, and C. A. Dawson.** 1986. A probability matrix for the identification of Gram-negative, aerobic, non-fermentative bacteria that grow on nutrient agar. *J. Gen. Microbiol.* **132:**1827–1842.
97. **Holmes, B., M. Popoff, M. Kiredjian, and K. Kersters.** 1988. *Ochrobactrum anthropi* gen. nov., sp. nov. from human clinical specimens and previously known as Group Vd. *Int. J. Syst. Bacteriol.* **38:**406–416.
98. **Holmes, B., J. J. S. Snell, and S. P. Lapage.** 1979. *Flavobacterium odoratum:* a species resistant to a wide range of antimicrobial agents. *J. Clin. Pathol.* **32:**73–77.
99. **Holmes, B., A. G. Steigerwalt, R. E. Weaver, and D. J. Brenner.** 1986. *Weeksella virosa* gen. nov., sp. nov. (formerly Group IIf), found in human clinical specimens. *Syst. Appl. Microbiol.* **8:**185–190.
100. **Holmes, B., A. G. Steigerwalt, R. E. Weaver, and D. J. Brenner.** 1986. *Weeksella zoohelcum* sp. nov. (formerly Group IIj), from human clinical specimens. *Syst. Appl. Microbiol.* **8:**191–196.
101. **Holmes, B., R. E. Weaver, A. G. Steigerwalt, and D. J. Brenner.** 1988. A taxonomic study of *Flavobacterium spiritivorum* and *Sphingobacterium mizutae:* proposal of *Flavobacterium yabuuchiae* sp. nov. and *Flavobacterium mizutaii* comb. nov. *Int. J. Syst. Bacteriol.* **38:**348–353.
102. **Holt, H. M., P. Sogaard, and B. Gahrn-Hansen.** 1997. Ear infections with *Shewanella alga:* a bacteriologic, clinical and epidemiologic study of 67 cases. *Clin. Microbiol. Infect.* **3:**329–334.
103. **Holton, J.** 1983. A note on the preparation and use of a selective and differential medium for the isolation of the *Acinetobacter* spp. from clinical sources. *J. Appl. Bacteriol.* **66:**24–26.
104. **Hornei, B., E. Luneberg, H. Schmidt-Rotte, M. Maab, K. Weber. F. Heits, M. Frosch, and W. Solbach.** 1999. Systemic infection of an immunocompromised patient with *Methylobacterium zatmanii. J. Clin. Microbiol.* **37:**248–250.
105. **Houang, E. T. S., Y. W. Chu, C. M. Leung, K. Y. Chu, J. Berlau, K. C. Ng, and A. F. B. Cheng.** 2001. Epidemiology and infection control implications of *Acinetobacter* spp. in Hong Kong. *J. Clin. Microbiol.* **39:**228–234.
106. **Hsueh, P.-R., J.-C. Chang, L.-J. Teng, P.-C. Yang, S.-W. Ho, W.-C. Hsieh, and K.-T. Luh.** 1997. Comparison of Etest and agar dilution method for antimicrobial susceptibility testing of *Flavobacterium* isolates. *J. Clin. Microbiol.* **35:**1021–1023.
107. **Hsueh, P.-R., T.-R. Hsiue, J.-J. Wu, L.-J. Teng, S.-W. Ho, W.-C. Hsieh, and K.-T. Luh.** 1996. *Flavobacterium indologenes* bacteremia: clinical and microbiological characteristics. *Clin. Infect. Dis.* **23:**550–555.
108. **Hsueh, P.-R., L.-J. Teng, C.-Y. Chen, W.-H. Chen, C.-J. Yu, S.-W. Ho, and K.-T. Luh.** 2002. Pandrug-resistant *Acinetobacter baumannii* causing nosocomial infections in a university hospital, Taiwan. *Emerg. Infect. Dis.* **8:**827–832.
109. **Hsueh, P.-R., L.-J. Teng, S.-W. Ho, W.-C. Hsieh, and K.-T. Luh.** 1996. Clinical and microbiological characteristics of *Flavobacterium indologenes* infections associated with indwelling devices. *J. Clin. Microbiol.* **34:**1908–1913.
110. **Hsueh, P.-R., L.-J. Teng, P.-C. Yang, Y.-C. Chen, H.-J. Pan, S.-W. Ho, and K.-T. Luh.** 1998. Nosocomial infections caused by *Sphingomonas paucimobilis:* clinical features and microbiological characteristics. *Clin. Infect. Dis.* **26:**676–681.
111. **Hsueh, P.-R., L.-J. Teng, P.-C. Yang, S.-W. Ho, W.-C. Hsieh, and K.-T. Luh.** 1997. Increasing incidence of nosocomial *Chryseobacterium indologenes* infections in Taiwan. *Eur. J. Clin. Microbiol. Infect. Dis.* **16:**568–574.
112. **Hsueh, P.-R., J.-J. Wu, T.-R. Hsiue, and W.-C. Hsieh.** 1995. Bacteremic necrotizing fasciitis due to *Flavobacterium odoratum. Clin. Infect. Dis.* **21:**1337–1338.
113. **Hubert, B., A. de Mahenge, F. Grimont, C. Richard, Y. Peloux, C. de Mahenge, J. Fleurette, and P. A. D. Grimont.** 1991. An outbreak of pneumonia and meningitis caused by a previously undescribed gram-negative bacterium in a hot spring spa. *Epidemiol. Infect.* **107:**373–381.
114. **Hulse, M., S. Johnson, and P. Ferrieri.** 1993. *Agrobacterium* infections in humans: experience at one hospital and review. *Clin. Infect. Dis.* **16:**112–117.
115. **Ibrahim, A., P. Gerner-Smidt, and W. Liesack.** 1997. Phylogenetic relationship of the twenty-one DNA groups of the genus *Acinetobacter* as revealed by 16S ribosomal DNA sequence analysis. *Int. J. Syst. Bacteriol.* **47:**837–841.
116. **Iwata, M., K. Tateda, T. Matsumoto, N. Furuya, S. Mizuiri, and K. Yamaguchi.** 1999. Primary *Shewanella alga* septicemia in a patient on hemodialysis. *J. Clin. Microbiol.* **37:**2104–2105.
117. **Jannes, G., M. Vaneechoutte, M. Lannoo, M. Gillis, M. Vancanneyt, P. Vandamme, G. Verschraegen, H. van Heuverswyn, and R. Rossau.** 1993. Polyphasic taxonomy leading to the proposal of *Moraxella canis* sp. nov. for *Moraxella catarrhalis*-like strains. *Int. J. Syst. Bacteriol.* **43:**438–449.
118. **Jawad, A., P. M. Hawkey, J. Heritage, and A. M. Snelling.** 1994. Description of Leeds *Acinetobacter* Medium, a new selective and differential medium for isolation of clinically important *Acinetobacter* spp., and comparison with Herellea agar and Holton's agar. *J. Clin. Microbiol.* **32:**2353–2358.
119. **Jellison, T. K., P. S. McKinnon, and M. J. Rybak.** 2001. Epidemiology, resistance, and outcomes of *Acinetobacter baumannii* bacteremia treated with imipenem-cilastatin or ampicillin-sulbactam. *Pharmacotherapy* **21:**142–148.
120. **Jenks, P. J., and E. J. Shaw.** 1997. Recurrent septicaemia due to "*Achromobacter* Group B." *J. Infect.* **34:**143–145.
121. **Jiménez-Mejías, M. E., C. Pichardo-Guerrero, F. J. Márquez-Rivas, D. Martin-Lozano, T. Prados, and J. Pachon.** 2002. Cerebrospinal fluid penetration and pharmacokinetic/pharmacodynamic parameters of intravenously administered colistin in a case of multidrug-resistant

Acinetobacter baumannii meningitis. *Eur. J. Clin. Microbiol. Infect. Dis.* **21:**212–214.

122. **Johnson, D. W., G. Lum, G. Nimmo, and C. M. Hawley.** 1995. *Moraxella nonliquefaciens* septic arthritis in a patient undergoing hemodialysis. *Clin. Infect. Dis.* **21:**1039–1040.
123. **Joyanes, P., M. Del Carmen Conejo, L. Martínez-Martínez, and E. J. Perea.** 2001. Evaluation of the Vitek 2 system for the identification and susceptibility testing of three species of nonfermenting gram-negative rods frequently isolated from clinical specimens. *J. Clin. Microbiol.* **39:**3247–3253.
124. **Juni, E., G. A. Heym, M. J. Maurer, and M. L. Miller.** 1987. Combined genetic transformation and nutritional assay for identification of *Moraxella nonliquefaciens*. *J. Clin. Microbiol.* **25:**1691–1694.
125. **Kaiser, R. M., R. L. Garman, M. G. Bruce, R. S. Weyant, and D. A. Ashford.** 2002. Clinical significance and epidemiology of NO-1, an unusual bacterium associated with dog and cat bites. *Emerg. Infect. Dis.* **8:**171–174.
126. **Kappstein, I., H. Grundmann, T. Hauer, and C. Niemeyer.** 2000. Aerators as a reservoir of *Acinetobacter junii*: an outbreak of bacteraemia in paediatric oncology patients. *J. Hosp. Infect.* **44:**27–30.
127. **Karalus, R., and A. Campagnari.** 2000. *Moraxella catarrhalis*: a review of an important human mucosal pathogen. *Microbes Infect.* **2:**547–559.
128. **Katsura, K., H. Kawasaki, W. Potacharoen, S. Saono, T. Seki, Y. Yamada, T. Uchimura, and K. Komagata.** 2001. *Asaia siamensis* sp. nov., an acetic acid bacterium in the alpha-proteobacteria. *Int. J. Syst. Evol. Microbiol.* **51:**559–563.
129. **Kay, S. E., R. A. Clark, K. L. White, and M. M. Peel.** 2001. Recurrent *Achromobacter piechaudii* bacteremia in a patient with hematological malignancy. *J. Clin. Microbiol.* **39:**808–810.
130. **Kaye, K. M., A. Macone, and P. H. Kazanjian.** 1992. Catheter infection caused by *Methylobacterium* in immunocompromised hosts: report of three cases and review of the literature. *Clin. Infect. Dis.* **14:**1010–1014.
131. **Kern, W. V., M. Oethinger, A. Kaufhold, E. Rozdzinski, and R. Marre.** 1993. *Ochrobactrum anthropi* bacteremia: report of four cases and short review. *Infection* **21:** 306–310.
132. **Khashe, S., and J. M. Janda.** 1998. Biochemical and pathogenic properties of *Shewanella alga* and *Shewanella putrefaciens*. *J. Clin. Microbiol.* **36:**783–787.
133. **Kim, K. K., M. K. Kim, J. H. Lim, H. Y. Park, and S.-T. Lee.** 2005. Transfer of *Chryseobacterium meningosepticum* and *Chryseobacterium miricola* to *Elizabethkingia* gen. nov. as *Elizabethkingia meningoseptica* comb. nov. and *Elizabethkingia miricola* comb. nov. *Int. J. Syst. Evol. Microbiol.* **55:**1287–1293.
134. **Kiredjian, M., B. Holmes, K. Kersters, I. Guilvout, and J. de Ley.** 1986. *Alcaligenes piechaudii*, a new species from human clinical specimens and the environment. *Int. J. Syst. Bacteriol.* **36:**282–287.
135. **Kiska, D. L., A. Kerr, M. C. Jones, J. A. Caracciolo, B. Eskridge, M. Jordan, S. Miller, D. Hughes, N. King, and P. H. Gilligan.** 1996. Accuracy of four commercial systems for identification of *Burkholderia cepacia* and other gram-negative nonfermenting bacilli recovered from patients with cystic fibrosis. *J. Clin. Microbiol.* **34:**886–891.
136. **Knuth, B. D., M. R. Owen, and R. Latorraca.** 1969. Occurrence of an unclassified organism group IVd. *Am. J. Med. Technol.* **35:**227–232.
137. **Ko, K. S., N. Y. Lee, W. S. Oh, J. H. Lee, H. K. Ki, K. R. Peck, and J.-H. Song.** 2005. *Tepidimonas arfidensis* sp. nov., a novel gram-negative and thermophilic bacterium isolated from the bone marrow of a patient with leukemia in Korea. *Microbiol. Immunol.* **49:**785–788.
138. **Ko, K. S., K. R. Peck, W. S. Oh, N. Y. Lee, J. H. Lee, and J.-H. Song.** 2005. New species of *Bordetella, Bordetella ansorpii* sp. nov., isolated from the purulent exudates of an epidermal cyst. *J. Clin. Microbiol.* **43:**2516–2519.
139. **Koeleman, J. G. M., J. Stoof, D. J. Biesmans, P. H. M. Savelkoul, and C. M. J. E. Vandenbroucke-Grauls.** 1998. Comparison of amplified ribosomal DNA restriction analysis, random amplified polymorphic DNA analysis, and amplified fragment length polymorphism fingerprinting for identification of *Acinetobacter* genomic species and typing of *Acinetobacter baumannii*. *J. Clin. Microbiol.* **36:**2522–2529.
140. **La Scola, B., R. J. Birtles, M.-N. Mallet, and D. Raoult.** 1998. *Massilia timonae* gen. nov., sp. nov., isolated from blood of an immunocompromised patient with cerebellar lesions. *J. Clin. Microbiol.* **36:**2847–2852.
141. **Lau, S. K. P., P. C. Y. Woo, W.-T. Hui, M. W. S. Li, J. L. L. Teng, T.-L. Que, W.-K. Luk, R. W. M. Lai, R. W. H. Yung, and K.-Y. Yuen.** 2003. Use of cefoperazone MacConkey agar for selective isolation of *Laribacter hongkongensis*. *J. Clin. Microbiol.* **41:**4839–4841.
142. **Lebuhn, M., W. Achouak, M. Schloter, O. Berge, H. Meier, M. Barakat, A. Hartmann, and T. Heulin.** 2000. Taxonomic characterization of *Ochrobactrum* sp. isolates from soil samples and wheat roots, and description of *Ochrobactrum tritici* sp. nov. and *Ochrobactrum grignonense* sp. nov. *Int. J. Syst. Evol. Microbiol.* **50:**2207–2223.
143. **Levin, A. S.** 2002. Multiresistant *Acinetobacter* infections: a role for sulbactam combinations in overcoming an emerging worldwide problem. *Clin. Microbiol. Infect.* **8:**144–153.
144. **Levin, A. S., A. A. Barone, J. Penco, M. V. Santos, I. S. Marinho, E. A. Arruda, E. I. Manrique, and S. F. Costa.** 1999. Intravenous colistin as therapy for nosocomial infections caused by multidrug-resistant *Pseudomonas aeruginosa* and *Acinetobacter baumannii*. *Clin. Infect. Dis.* **28:** 1008–1011.
145. **Lin, Y.-H., P. Y.-F. Liu, Z.-Y. Shi, Y.-J. Lau, and B.-S. Hu.** 1997. Comparison of polymerase chain reaction and pulsed-field gel electrophoresis for the epidemiological typing of *Alcaligenes xylosoxidans* subsp. *xylosoxidans* in a burn unit. *Diagn. Microbiol. Infect. Dis.* **28:**173–178.
146. **Linde, H.-J., J. Hahn, E. Holler, U. Reischl, and N. Lehn.** 2002. Septicemia due to *Acinetobacter junii*. *J. Clin. Microbiol.* **40:**2696–2697.
147. **Ling, T. K. W., P. C. Tam, Z. K. Liu, and A. F. B. Cheng.** 2001. Evaluation of Vitek 2 rapid identification and susceptibility testing system against gram-negative clinical isolates. *J. Clin. Microbiol.* **39:**2964–2966.
148. **Linquist, D., D. Murrill, W. P. Burran, G. Winans, J. M. Janda, and W. Probert.** 2003. Characteristics of *Massilia timonae* and *Massilia timonae*-like isolates from human patients, with an emended description of the species. *J. Clin. Microbiol.* **41:**192–196.
149. **Liu, J.-W., J.-J. Wu, H.-M. Chen, A.-H. Huang, W.-C. Ko, and Y.-C. Chuang.** 1997. *Methylobacterium mesophilicum* synovitis in an alcoholic. *Clin. Infect. Dis.* **24:**1008–1009.
150. **Liu, P. Y.-F., and W.-L. Wu.** 1997. Use of different PCR-based DNA fingerprinting techniques and pulsed-field gel electrophoresis to investigate the epidemiology of *Acinetobacter calcoaceticus-Acinetobacter baumannii* complex. *Diagn. Microbiol. Infect. Dis.* **28:**19–28.
151. **Lloyd-Puryear, M., D. Wallace, T. Baldwin, and D. G. Hollis.** 1991. Meningitis caused by *Psychrobacter immobilis* in an infant. *J. Clin. Microbiol.* **29:**2041–2042.
152. **Lortholary, O., J.-Y. Fagon, A. B. Hoi, M. A. Slama, J. Pierre, P. Giral, R. Rosenzweig, L. Gutmann, M. Safar, and J. Acar.** 1995. Nosocomial acquisition of multiresistant *Acinetobacter baumannii*: risk factors and prognosis. *Clin. Infect. Dis.* **20:**790–796.

153. **Loubinoux, J., L. Mihaila-Amrouche, A. Le Fleche, E. Pigne, G. Huchon, P. A. Grimont, and A. Bouvet.** 2003. Bacteremia caused by *Acinetobacter ursingii*. *J. Clin. Microbiol.* **41:**1337–1338.

154. **MacDonell, M. T., and R. R. Colwell.** 1985. Phylogeny of the *Vibrionaceae*, and recommendation for two new genera, *Listonella* and *Shewanella*. *Syst. Appl. Microbiol.* **6:**171–182.

155. **Mahmood, M. S., A. R. Sarwari, M. A. Khan, Z. Sophie, E. Khan, and S. Sami.** 2000. Infective endocarditis and septic embolization with *Ochrobactrum anthropi:* case report and review of literature. *J. Infect.* **40:**287–290.

156. **Manfredi, R., A. Nanetti, M. Ferri, A. Mastroianni, O. V. Coronado, and F. Chiodo.** 1999. Emerging gram-negative pathogens in the immunocompromised host: *Agrobacterium radiobacter* septicemia during HIV disease. *Microbiologica* **22:**375–382.

157. **Manikal, V. M., D. Landman, G. Saurina, E. Oydna, H. Lal, and J. Quale.** 2000. Endemic carbapenem-resistant *Acinetobacter* species in Brooklyn, New York: citywide prevalence, interinstitutional spread, and relation to antibiotic usage. *Clin. Infect. Dis.* **31:**101–106.

158. **Manuel, R. J., G. Y. Shin, N. Farrag, and R. Holliman.** 2003. Endemic carbapenem-resistant *Acinetobacter baumannii* in a London hospital. *J. Antimicrob. Chemother.* **52:**141–142.

159. **Marin, M. E., J. Marco Del Pont, E. Dibar, L. Fernandez Caniggia, G. Greco, Y. Flores, and A. Ascione.** 2001. Catheter-related bacteremia caused by *Roseomonas gilardii* in an immunocompromised patient. *Int. J. Infect. Dis.* **5:**170–171.

160. **Mesnard, R., J. M. Sire, P. Y. Donnio, J. Y. Riou, and J. L. Avril.** 1992. Septic arthritis due to *Oligella urethralis*. *Eur. J. Clin. Microbiol. Infect. Dis.* **11:**195–196.

161. **Miller, J. M., C. Novy, and M. Hiott.** 1996. Case of bacterial endophthalmitis caused by an *Agrobacterium radiobacter*-like organism. *J. Clin. Microbiol.* **34:**3212–3213.

162. **Moller, L. V. M., J. P. Arends, H. J. M. Harmsen, A. Talens, P. Terpstra, and M. J. H. Slooff.** 1999. *Ochrobactrum intermedium* infection after liver transplantation. *J. Clin. Microbiol.* **37:**241–244.

163. **Montejo, M., K. Aguirrebengoa, J. Ugalde, L. Lopez, J. A. S. Nieto, and J. L. Hernández.** 2001. *Bergeyella zoohelcum* bacteremia after a dog bite. *Clin. Infect. Dis.* **33:**1608–1609.

164. **Moore, J. E., M. McCalmont, J. Xu, B. C. Millar, and N. Heaney.** 2002. *Asaia* sp., an unusual spoilage organism of fruit-flavored bottled water. *Appl. Environ. Microbiol.* **68:**4130–4131.

165. **Morrison, A. J., and J. A. Shulman.** 1986. Community-acquired bloodstream infection caused by *Pseudomonas paucimobilis:* case report and review of literature. *J. Clin. Microbiol.* **24:**853–855.

166. **Moss, C. W., M. I. Daneshvar, and D. G. Hollis.** 1993. Biochemical characteristics and fatty acid composition of Gilardi Rod Group 1 bacteria. *J. Clin. Microbiol.* **31:**689–691.

167. **Moss, C. W., P. L. Wallace, D. G. Hollis, and R. E. Weaver.** 1988. Cultural and chemical characterization of CDC Groups EO-2, M-5, and M-6, *Moraxella (Moraxella)* species, *Oligella urethralis*, *Acinetobacter* species, and *Psychrobacter immobilis*. *J. Clin. Microbiol.* **26:**484–492.

168. **Nahass, R. G., R. Wisneski, D. J. Herman, E. Hirsh, and K. Goldblatt.** 1995. Vertebral osteomyelitis due to *Roseomonas* species: case report and review of the evaluation of vertebral osteomyelitis. *Clin. Infect. Dis.* **21:**1474–1476.

169. **Nemec, A., T. De Baere, I. Tjernberg, M. Vaneechoutte, T. J. K. van der Reijden, and L. Dijkshoorn.** 2001. *Acinetobacter ursingii* sp. nov. and *Acinetobacter schindleri* sp. nov., isolated from human clinical specimens. *Int. J. Syst. Evol. Microbiol.* **51:**1891–1899.

170. **Nemec, A., L. Dijkshoorn, I. Cleenwerck, T. De Baere, D. Janssens, T. J. K. van der Reijden, P. Jezek, and M. Vaneechoutte.** 2003. *Acinetobacter parvus* sp. nov., a small-colony-forming species isolated from human clinical specimens. *Int. J. Syst. Evol. Microbiol.* **53:**1563–1567.

171. **Nishimura, Y., T. Ino, and H. Hzuka.** 1988. *Acinetobacter radioresistens* sp. nov. isolated from cotton and soil. *Int. J. Syst. Bacteriol.* **38:**209–211.

172. **Noell, F., M. F. Gorce, C. Garde, and C. Bizet.** 1989. Isolation of *Weeksella zoohelcum* in septicaemia. *Lancet* **ii:**332. (Letter.)

173. **Nozue, H., T. Hayashi, Y. Hashimoto, T. Ezaki, K. Hamasaki, K. Ohwada, and Y. Terawaki.** 1992. Isolation and characterization of *Shewanella alga* from human clinical specimens and emendation of the description of *S. alga* Simidu et al., 1990, 335. *Int. J. Syst. Bacteriol.* **42:**628–634.

174. **Nulens, E., B. Bussels, A. Bols, B. Gordts, and H. W. Van Landuyt.** 2001. Recurrent bacteremia by *Chryseobacterium indologenes* in an oncology patient with a totally implanted intravascular device. *Clin. Microbiol. Infect.* **7:**391–393.

175. **O'Hara, C. M., G. L. Westbrook, and J. M. Miller.** 1997. Evaluation of Vitek GNI+ and Becton Dickinson Microbiology Systems Crystal E/NF identification systems for identification of members of the family *Enterobacteriaceae* and other gram-negative, glucose-fermenting and non-glucose-fermenting bacilli. *J. Clin. Microbiol.* **35:**3269–3273.

176. **Osterhout, G. J., V. H. Shull, and J. D. Dick.** 1991. Identification of clinical isolates of gram-negative nonfermentative bacteria by an automated cellular fatty acid identification system. *J. Clin. Microbiol.* **29:**1822–1830.

177. **Peel, M. M., A. J. Hibberd, B. M. King, and H. G. Williamson.** 1988. *Alcaligenes piechaudii* from chronic ear discharge. *J. Clin. Microbiol.* **26:**1580–1581.

178. **Peiris, V., S. Fraser, M. Fairhurst, D. Weston, and E. Kaczmarski.** 1992. Laboratory diagnosis of brucella infection: some pitfalls. *Lancet* **339:**1415–1416.

179. **Perez, J. L., A. Pulido, F. Pantozzi, and R. Martin.** 1990. Butyrate esterase (tributyrin) spot test, a simple method for immediate identification of *Moraxella (Branhamella) catarrhalis*. *J. Clin. Microbiol.* **28:**2347–2348.

180. **Petti, C. A., C. R. Polage, and P. Schreckenberger.** 2005. Is misidentification of microorganisms by conventional methods a laboratory error? Preventing laboratory errors with 16S rRNA gene sequencing. *J. Clin. Microbiol.* **43:**6123–6125.

181. **Pickett, M. J.** 1989. Methods for identification of flavobacteria. *J. Clin. Microbiol.* **27:**2309–2315.

182. **Pickett, M. J.** 1994. Moraxellae: differential features for identification of *Moraxella atlantae*, *M. lacunata*, and *M. nonliquefaciens*. *Med. Microbiol. Lett.* **3:**397–400.

183. **Pickett, M. J.** 1994. Identification of *Brucella* species with a procedure for detecting acidification of glucose. *Clin. Infect. Dis.* **19:**976.

184. **Pickett, M. J., and E. L. Nelson.** 1955. Speciation within the genus *Brucella* IV. Fermentation of carbohydrates. *J. Bacteriol.* **69:**333–336.

185. **Pickett, M. J., A. von Graevenitz, G. E. Pfyffer, V. Pünter, and M. Altwegg.** 1996. Phenotypic features distinguishing *Oligella urethralis* from *Moraxella osloensis*. *Med. Microbiol. Lett.* **5:**265–270.

186. **Pitulle, C., D. M. Citron, B. Bochner, R. Barbers, and M. D. Appleman.** 1999. Novel bacterium isolated from a lung transplant patient with cystic fibrosis. *J. Clin. Microbiol.* **37:**3851–3855.

187. **Plotkin, S. A., and J. C. McKitrick.** 1966. Nosocomial meningitis of the newborn caused by a flavobacterium. *JAMA* **198:**194–196.

188. **Pot, B., and M. Gillis.** 2005. Genus III. *Aquaspirillum* Hylemon, Wells, Krieg and Jannasch 1973b, 361[AL], p. 801–823. *In* G. M. Garrity, D. J. Brenner, N. R. Krieg, and J. T. Staley (ed.), *Bergey's Manual of Systematic Bacteriology*, 2nd ed., vol. 2, part C. Springer, New York, N.Y.
189. **Potvliege, C., C. Dejaegher-Bauduin, W. Hansen, M. Dratwa, F. Collart, C. Tielemans, and E. Yourassowsky.** 1984. *Flavobacterium multivorum* septicemia in a hemodialyzed patient. *J. Clin. Microbiol.* **19:**568–569.
190. **Prashanth, K., M. P. M. Ranga, V. A. Rao, and R. Kanungo.** 2000. Corneal perforation due to *Acinetobacter junii:* a case report. *Diagn. Microbiol. Infect. Dis.* **37:**215–217.
191. **Pugliese, A., B. Pacris, P. E. Schoch, and B. A. Cunha.** 1993. *Oligella urethralis* urosepsis. *Clin. Infect. Dis.* **17:**1069–1070.
192. **Purcell, B. K., and D. P. Dooley.** 1999. Centers for Disease Control and Prevention Group O1 bacterium-associated pneumonia complicated by bronchopulmonary fistula and bacteremia. *Clin. Infect. Dis.* **29:**945–946.
193. **Rabkin, C. S., E. I. Galaid, D. G. Hollis, R. E. Weaver, S. B. Dees, A. Kai, C. W. Moss, K. K. Sandhu, and C. V. Broome.** 1985. Thermophilic bacteria: a new cause of human disease. *J. Clin. Microbiol.* **21:**553–557.
194. **Reina, J., A. Bassa, I. Llompart, D. Portela, and N. Borrell.** 1991. Infections with *Pseudomonas paucimobilis:* report of four cases and review. *Rev. Infect. Dis.* **13:**1072–1076.
195. **Reina, J., and N. Borrell.** 1992. Leg abscess caused by *Weeksella zoohelcum* following a dog bite. *Clin. Infect. Dis.* **14:**1162–1163. (Letter.)
196. **Reina, J., J. Gil, F. Salva, J. Gomez, and P. Alomar.** 1990. Microbiological characteristics of *Weeksella virosa* (formerly CDC Group IIf) isolated from the human genitourinary tract. *J. Clin. Microbiol.* **28:**2357–2359.
197. **Rice, E. W., D. J. Reasoner, C. H. Johnson, and L. A. DeMaria.** 2000. Monitoring for methylobacteria in water systems. *J. Clin. Microbiol.* **38:**4296–4297.
198. **Richardson, J. D.** 1997. Failure to clear a *Roseomonas* line infection with antibiotic therapy. *Clin. Infect. Dis.* **25:**155.
199. **Rihs, J. D., D. J. Brenner, R. E. Weaver, A. G. Steigerwalt, D. G. Hollis, and V. L. Yu.** 1993. *Roseomonas,* a new genus associated with bacteremia and other human infections. *J. Clin. Microbiol.* **31:**3275–3283.
200. **Rockhill, R. C., and L. I. Lutwick.** 1978. Group IVe-like gram-negative bacillemia in a patient with obstructive uropathy. *J. Clin. Microbiol.* **8:**108–109.
201. **Rosenthal, S. L., L. F. Freundlich, G. L. Gilardi, and F. Y. Clodomar.** 1978. In vitro antibiotic sensitivity of *Moraxella* species. *Chemotherapy* **24:**360–363.
202. **Rossau, R., K. Kersters, E. Falsen, E. Jantzen, P. Segers, A. Union, L. Nehls, and J. de Ley.** 1987. *Oligella,* a new genus including *Oligella urethralis* comb. nov. (formerly *Moraxella urethralis*) and *Oligella ureolytica* sp. nov. (formerly CDC Group IVe): relationship to *Taylorella equigenitalis* and related taxa. *Int. J. Syst. Bacteriol.* **37:**198–210.
203. **Rossau, R., A. Van Landschoot, M. Gillis, and J. de Ley.** 1991. Taxonomy of *Moraxellaceae* fam. nov., a new bacterial family to accommodate the genera *Moraxella, Acinetobacter,* and *Psychrobacter* and related organisms. *Int. J. Syst. Bacteriol.* **41:**310–319.
204. **Saavedra, J., C. Garrido, D. Folgueira, M. J. Torres, and J. T. Ramos.** 1999. *Ochrobactrum anthropi* bacteremia associated with a catheter in an immunocompromised child and review of the pediatric literature. *Pediatr. Infect. Dis. J.* **18:**658–660.
205. **Sanders, J. W., J. W. Martin, M. Hooke, and J. Hooke.** 2000. *Methylobacterium mesophilicum* infection: case report and literature review of an unusual opportunistic pathogen. *Clin. Infect. Dis.* **30:**936–938.
206. **Sawada, H., H. Ieki, H. Oyaizu, and S. Matsumoto.** 1993. Proposal for rejection of *Agrobacterium tumefaciens* and revised descriptions for the genus *Agrobacterium* and for *Agrobacterium radiobacter* and *Agrobacterium rhizogenes. Int. J. Syst. Bacteriol.* **43:**694–702.
207. **Schreckenberger, P. C.** 2005. *Practical Approach to the Identification of Glucose Non-Fermenting Gram-Negative Bacilli,* 3rd ed. Loyola University Chicago, Maywood, Ill.
208. **Seifert, H., L. Dijkshoorn, P. Gerner-Smidt, N. Pelzer, I. Tjernberg, and M. Vaneechoutte.** 1997. Distribution of *Acinetobacter* species on human skin: comparison of phenotypic and genotypic identification methods. *J. Clin. Microbiol.* **35:**2819–2825.
209. **Shah, S. S., A. Ruth, and S. E. Coffin.** 2000. Infection due to *Moraxella osloensis:* case report and review of the literature. *Clin. Infect. Dis.* **30:**179–181.
210. **Sheridan, R. L., C. M. Ryan, M. S. Pasternack, J. M. Weber, and R. G. Tompkins.** 1993. Flavobacterial sepsis in massively burned pediatric patients. *Clin. Infect. Dis.* **17:**185–187.
211. **Shivaji, S., M. K. Ray, N. S. Rao, L. Saisree, M. V. Jagannadham, G. S. Kumar, G. S. N. Reddy, and P. M. Bhargava.** 1992. *Sphingobacterium antarcticus* sp. nov., a psychrotrophic bacterium from the soils of Schirmacher Oasis, Antarctica. *Int. J. Syst. Bacteriol.* **42:**102–106.
212. **Shokar, N. K., G. S. Shokar, J. Islam, and A. R. Cass.** 2002. *Roseomonas gilardii* infection: case report and review. *J. Clin. Microbiol.* **40:**4789–4791.
213. **Siau, H., K.-Y. Yuen, P.-L. Ho, W. K. Luk, S. S. Y. Wong, P. C. Y. Woo, R. A. Lee, and W.-T. Hui.** 1998. Identification of acinetobacters on blood agar in presence of D-glucose by unique browning effect. *J. Clin. Microbiol.* **36:**1404–1407.
214. **Siegman-Igra, Y., S. Bar-Yosef, A. Gorea, and J. Avram.** 1993. Nosocomial *Acinetobacter* meningitis secondary to invasive procedures: report of 25 cases and review. *Clin. Infect. Dis.* **17:**843–849.
215. **Siegman-Igra, Y., D. Schwartz, G. Soferman, and N. Konforti.** 1987. *Flavobacterium* group IIb bacteremia: report of a case and review of *Flavobacterium* infections. *Med. Microbiol. Immunol.* **176:**103–111.
216. **Sintchenko, V., P. Jelfs, A. Sharma, L. Hicks, and G. L. Gilbert.** 2000. *Massilia timonae:* an unusual bacterium causing wound infection following surgery. *Clin. Microbiol. Newsl.* **22:**149–151.
217. **Snyder, R. W., J. Ruhe, S. Kobrin, A. Wasserstein, C. Doline, I. Nachamkin, and J. H. Lipschutz.** 2004. *Asaia bogorensis* peritonitis identified by 16S ribosomal RNA sequence analysis in a patient receiving peritoneal dialysis. *Am. J. Kidney Dis.* **44:**E15–E17.
218. **Spangler, S. K., M. A. Visalli, M. R. Jacobs, and P. C. Appelbaum.** 1996. Susceptibilities of non-*Pseudomonas aeruginosa* gram-negative nonfermentative rods to ciprofloxacin, ofloxacin, levofloxacin, D-ofloxacin, sparfloxacin, ceftazidime, piperacillin, piperacillin-tazobactam, trimethoprim-sulfamethoxazole, and imipenem. *Antimicrob. Agents Chemother.* **40:**772–775.
219. **Speeleveld, E., J.-M. Fosspre, B. Gordts, and H. W. Landuyt.** 1994. Comparison of three rapid methods, tributyrine, 4-methylumbelliferyl butyrate, and indoxyl acetate, for rapid identification of *Moraxella catarrhalis. J. Clin. Microbiol.* **32:**1362–1363.
220. **Steyn, P. L., P. Segers, M. Vancanneyt, P. Sandra, K. Kersters, and J. J. Joubert.** 1998. Classification of heparinolytic bacteria into a new genus, *Pedobacter,* comprising four species: *Pedobacter heparinus* comb. nov., *Pedobacter piscium* comb. nov., *Pedobacter africanus* sp. nov. and *Pedobacter saltans* sp. nov. Proposal of the family *Sphingobacteriaceae* fam. nov. *Int. J. Syst. Bacteriol.* **48:**165–177.

221. **Struthers, M., J. Wong, and J. M. Janda.** 1996. An initial appraisal of the clinical significance of *Roseomonas* species associated with human infections. *Clin. Infect. Dis.* **23:**729–733.
222. **Subudhi, C. P. K., A. Adedeji, M. E. Kaufmann, G. S. Lucas, and J. R. Kerr.** 2001. Fatal *Roseomonas gilardii* bacteremia in a patient with refractory blast crisis of chronic myeloid leukemia. *Clin. Microbiol. Infect.* **7:**573–575.
223. **Sung, L. L., D. I. Yang, C. C. Hung, and H. T. Ho.** 2000. Evaluation of autoSCAN-W/A and the Vitek GNI+ AutoMicrobic System for identification of non-glucose-fermenting gram-negative bacilli. *J. Clin. Microbiol.* **38:**1127–1130.
224. **Swann, R. A., S. J. Foulkes, B. Holmes, J. B. Young, R. G. Mitchell, and S. T. Reeders.** 1985. "*Agrobacterium* yellow group" and *Pseudomonas paucimobilis* causing peritonitis in patients receiving continuous ambulatory peritoneal dialysis. *J. Clin. Pathol.* **38:**1293–1299.
225. **Swenson, J. M., G. E. Killgore, and F. C. Tenover.** 2004. Antimicrobial susceptibility testing of *Acinetobacter* spp. by NCCLS broth microdilution and disk diffusion methods. *J. Clin. Microbiol.* **42:**5102–5108.
226. **Takeuchi, M., K. Hamana, and A. Hiraishi.** 2001. Proposal of the genus *Sphingomonas sensu stricto* and three new genera, *Sphingobium, Novosphingobium* and *Sphingopyxis,* on the basis of phylogenetic and chemotaxonomic analyses. *Int. J. Syst. Evol. Microbiol.* **51:**1405–1417.
227. **Takeuchi, M., and A. Yokota.** 1992. Proposals of *Sphingobacterium faecium* sp. nov., *Sphingobacterium piscium* sp. nov., *Sphingobacterium heparinum* comb. nov., *Sphingobacterium thalpophilum* comb. nov. and two genospecies of the genus *Sphingobacterium,* and synonymy of *Flavobacterium yabuuchiae* and *Sphingobacterium spiritivorum. J. Gen. Appl. Microbiol.* **38:**465–482.
228. **Tarrand, J. J., N. R. Krieg, and J. Dobereiner.** 1978. A taxonomic study of the *Spirillum lipoferum* group, with descriptions of a new genus, *Azospirillum* gen. nov. and two species, *Azospirillum lipoferum* (Beijernck) comb. nov. and *Azospirillum brasilense* sp. nov. *Can. J. Microbiol.* **24:**967–980.
229. **Tjernberg, I., and J. Ursing.** 1989. Clinical strains of *Acinetobacter* classified by DNA-DNA hybridization. *APMIS* **97:**595–605.
230. **Traub, W. H., and B. Leonhard.** 1994. Serotyping of *Acinetobacter baumannii* and genospecies 3: an update. *Med. Microbiol. Lett.* **3:**120–127.
231. **Trüper, H. G., and L. De Clari.** 1997. Taxonomic note: necessary correction of specific epithets formed as substantives (Nouns) "in apposition." *Int. J. Syst. Bacteriol.* **47:**908–909.
232. **Turton, J. F., M. E. Kaufmann, J. Glover, J. M. Coelho, M. Warner, R. Pike, and T. L. Pitt.** 2005. Detection and typing of integrons in epidemic strains of *Acinetobacter baumannii* found in the United Kingdom. *J. Clin. Microbiol.* **43:**3074–3082.
233. **Urakami, T., H. Araki, K.-I. Suzuki, and K. Komagata.** 1993. Further studies of the genus *Methylobacterium* and description of *Methylobacterium aminovorans* sp. nov. *Int. J. Syst. Bacteriol.* **43:**504–513.
234. **Ursing, J., and B. Bruun.** 1991. Genotypic heterogeneity of *Flavobacterium* group IIb and *Flavobacterium breve,* demonstrated by DNA-DNA hybridization. *APMIS* **99:** 780–786.
235. **Vancanneyt, M., P. Segers, U. Torck, B. Hoste, J.-F. Bernardet, P. Vandamme, and K. Kersters.** 1996. Reclassification of *Flavobacterium odoratum* (Stutzer 1929) strains to a new genus, *Myroides,* as *Myroides odoratus* comb. nov. and *Myroides odoratimimus* sp. nov. *Int. J. Syst. Bacteriol.* **46:**926–932.
236. **Vandamme, P., and T. Coenye.** 2004. Taxonomy of the genus *Cupriavidus:* a tale of lost and found. *Int. J. Syst. Evol. Microbiol.* **54:**2285–2289.
237. **Vandamme, P., M. Gillis, M. Vancanneyt, B. Hoste, K. Kerster, and E. Falsen.** 1993. *Moraxella lincolnii* sp. nov., isolated from the human respiratory tract, and reevaluation of the taxonomic position of *Moraxella osloensis. Int. J. Syst. Bacteriol.* **43:**474–481.
238. **Vandamme, P., J. Goris, T. Coenye, B. Hoste, D. Janssens, K. Kersters, P. De Vos, and E. Falsen.** 1999. Assignment of Centers for Disease Control group IV c-2 to the genus *Ralstonia* as *Ralstonia paucula* sp. nov. *Int. J. Syst. Bacteriol.* **49:**663–669.
239. **Vandamme, P., M. Heyndrickx, M. Vancanneyt, B. Hoste, P. De Vos, E. Falsen, K. Kersters, and K.-H. Hinz.** 1996. *Bordetella trematum* sp. nov., isolated from wounds and ear infections in humans, and reassessment of *Alcaligenes denitrificans* Rüger and Tan 1983. *Int. J. Syst. Bacteriol.* **46:**849–858.
240. **van Dijck, P., M. Delmee, H. Ezzedine, A. Deplano, and M. J. Struelens.** 1995. Evaluation of pulsed-field gel electrophoresis and rep-PCR for the epidemiological analysis of *Ochrobactrum anthropi* strains. *Eur. J. Clin. Microbiol. Infect. Dis.* **14:**1099–1102.
241. **Vaneechoutte, M., G. Claeys, S. Steyaert, T. De Baere, R. Peleman, and G. Verschraegen.** 2000. Isolation of *Moraxella canis* from an ulcerated metastatic lymph node. *J. Clin. Microbiol.* **38:**3870–3871.
242. **Velasco, J., C. Romero, I. Lopez-Goni, J. Leiva, R. Diaz, and I. Moriyon.** 1998. Evaluation of the relatedness of *Brucella* spp. and *Ochrobactrum anthropi* and description of *Ochrobactrum intermedium* sp. nov., a new species with a closer relationship to *Brucella* spp. *Int. J. Syst. Bacteriol.* **48:**759–768.
243. **Veys, A., W. Callewaert, E. Waelkens, and K. van den Abbeele.** 1989. Application of gas-liquid chromatography to the routine identification of nonfermenting gram-negative bacteria in clinical specimens. *J. Clin. Microbiol.* **27:** 1538–1542.
244. **Villegas, M. V., and A. I. Hartstein.** 2003. *Acinetobacter* outbreaks, 1977–2000. *Infect. Control Hosp. Epidemiol.* **24:**284–295.
245. **Visca, P., A. Petrucca, P. De Mori, A. Festa, E. Boumis, A. Antinori, and N. Petrosillo.** 2001. Community-acquired *Acinetobacter radioresistens* bacteremia in an HIV-positive patient. *Emerg. Infect. Dis.* **7:**1032–1035.
246. **Vogel, B. F., K. Jørgensen, H. Christensen, J. E. Olsen, and L. Gram.** 1997. Differentiation of *Shewanella putrefaciens* and *Shewanella alga* on the basis of whole-cell protein profiles, ribotyping, phenotypic characterization, and 16S rRNA gene sequence analysis. *Appl. Environ. Microbiol.* **63:**2189–2199.
247. **Vogel, B. F., K. Venkateswaran, H. Christensen, E. Falsen, G. Christiansen, and L. Gram.** 2000. Polyphasic taxonomic approach in the description of *Alishewanella fetalis* gen. nov., sp. nov., isolated from a human foetus. *Int. J. Syst. Evol. Microbiol.* **50:**1133–1142.
248. **von Graevenitz, A.** 1985. Ecology, clinical significance, and antimicrobial susceptibility of infrequently encountered glucose-nonfermenting gram-negative rods, p. 181–232. *In* G. L. Gilardi (ed.), *Nonfermentative Gram-Negative Rods: Laboratory Identification and Clinical Aspects.* Marcel Dekker, Inc., New York, N.Y.
249. **von Graevenitz, A., J. Bowman, C. Del Notaro, and M. Ritzler.** 2000. Human infection with *Halomonas venusta* following fish bite. *J. Clin. Microbiol.* **38:**3123–3124.
250. **von Graevenitz, A., and M. Grehn.** 1977. Susceptibility studies on *Flavobacterium* II-b. *FEMS Microbiol. Lett.* **2:**289–292.

251. **von Graevenitz, A., G. E. Pfyffer, M. J. Pickett, R. E. Weaver, and J. Wüst.** 1993. Isolation of an unclassified non-fermentative gram-negative rod from a patient on continuous ambulatory peritoneal dialysis. *Eur. J. Clin. Microbiol. Infect. Dis.* **12:**568–570.
252. **von Wintzingerode, F., A. Schattke, R. A. Siddiqui, U. Rosick, U. B. Gobel, and R. Gross.** 2001. *Bordetella petrii* sp. nov., isolated from an anaerobic bioreactor, and emended description of the genus *Bordetella*. *Int. J. Syst. Evol. Microbiol.* **51:**1257–1265.
253. **Watson, K. C., and I. Muscat.** 1983. Meningitis caused by a *Flavobacterium*-like organism (CDC IIe strain). *J. Infect.* **7:**278–279.
254. **Weitkamp, J.-H., Y.-W. Tang, D. W. Haas, N. K. Midha, and J. E. Crowe, Jr.** 2000. Recurrent *Achromobacter xylosoxidans* bacteremia associated with persistent lymph node infection in a patient with hyper-immunoglobulin M syndrome. *Clin. Infect. Dis.* **31:**1183–1187.
255. **Wellinghausen, N., A. Essig, and O. Sommerburg.** 2005. *Inquilinus limosus* in patients with cystic fibrosis, Germany. *Emerg. Infect. Dis.***11:**457–459.
256. **Weyant, R. S., C. W. Moss, R. E. Weaver, D. G. Hollis, J. G. Jordan, E. C. Cook, and M. I. Daneshvar.** 1996. *Identification of Unusual Pathogenic Gram-Negative Aerobic and Facultatively Anaerobic Bacteria,* 2nd ed. The Williams & Wilkins Co., Baltimore, Md.
257. **Winn, W. C., Jr., S. D. Allen, W. M. Janda, E. W. Koneman, G. Procop, P. C. Schreckenberger, and G. L. Woods.** 2006. *Koneman's Color Atlas and Textbook of Diagnostic Microbiology,* 6th ed., p. 303–391. Lippincott Williams & Wilkins, Philadelphia, Pa.
258. **Wisplinghoff, H., M. B. Edmond, M. A. Pfaller, R. N. Jones, R. P. Wenzel, and H. Seifert.** 2000. Nosocomial bloodstream infections caused by *Acinetobacter* species in United States hospitals: clinical features, molecular epidemiology, and antimicrobial susceptibility. *Clin. Infect. Dis.* **31:**690–697.
259. **Woo, P. C., P. Kuhnert, A. P. Burnens, J. L. Teng, S. K. Lau, T. L. Oue, H. H. Yau, and K. Y. Yuen.** 2003. *Laribacter hongkongensis:* a potential cause of infectious diarrhea. *Diagn. Microbiol. Infect. Dis.* **47:**551–556.
260. **Woo, P. C., S. K. P. Lau, J. L. L. Teng, T. L. Oue, R. W. Yung, W. K. Luk, R. W. Lai, W. T. Hui, S. S. Wong, H. H. Yau, and K. Y. Yuen.** 2004. Association of *Laribacter hongkongensis* in community-acquired gastroenteritis with travel and eating fish: a multicentre case-control study. *Lancet* **363:**1941–1947.
261. **Woo, P. C. Y., S. K. P. Lau, J. L. L. Teng, and K.-Y. Yuen.** 2005. Current status and future directions for *Laribacter hongkongensis,* a novel bacterium associated with gastroenteritis and traveller's diarrhoeae. Curr. *Opin. Infect. Dis.* **18:**413–419.
262. **Yabuuchi, E., T. Kaneko, I. Yano, C. W. Moss, and N. Miyoshi.** 1983. *Sphingobacterium* gen. nov., *Sphingobacterium spiritivorum* comb. nov., *Sphingobacterium multivorum* com. nov., *Sphingobacterium mizutae* sp. nov., and *Flavobacterium indologenes* sp. nov.: glucose-nonfermenting gram-negative rods in CDC groups IIk-2 and IIb. *Int. J. Syst. Bacteriol.* **33:**580–598.
263. **Yabuuchi, E., Y. Kawamura, Y. Kosako, and T. Ezaki.** 1998. Emendation of genus *Achromobacter* and *Achromobacter xylosoxidans* (Yabuuchi and Yano) and proposal of *Achromobacter ruhlandii* (Packer and Vishniac) comb. nov., *Achromobacter piechaudii* (Kiredjian et al.) comb. nov., and *Achromobacter xylosoxidans* subsp. *denitrificans* (Rüger and Tan) comb. nov. *Microbiol. Immunol.* **42:**429–438.
264. **Yabuuchi, E., I. Yano, H. Oyaizu, Y. Hashimoto, T. Ezaki, and H. Yamamoto.** 1990. Proposals of *Sphingomonas paucimobilis* gen. nov. and comb. nov., *Sphingomonas parapaucimobilis* sp. nov., *Sphingomonas yanoikuyae* sp. nov., *Sphingomonas adhaesiva* sp. nov., *Sphingomonas capsulata* comb. nov., and two genospecies of the genus *Sphingomonas*. *Microbiol. Immunol.* **34:**99–119.
265. **Yağci, A., N. Çerikçioğlu, M. E. Kaufmann, H. Malnick, G. Söyletir, F. Babacan, and T. L. Pitt.** 2000. Molecular typing of *Myroides odoratimimus (Flavobacterium odoratum)* urinary tract infections in a Turkish hospital. *Eur. J. Clin. Microbiol. Infect. Dis.* **19:**731–732.
266. **Yamada, Y., K. Katsura, H. Kawasaki, Y. Widyastuti, S. Saono, T. Seki, T. Uchimura, and K. Komagata.** 2000. *Asaia bogorensis* gen. nov., sp. nov., an unusual acetic acid bacterium in the alpha-Proteobacteria. *Int. J. Syst. Evol. Microbiol.* **50:**823–829.
267. **Young, J. M., L. D. Kuykendall, E. Martinez-Romero, A. Kerr, and H. Sawada.** 2001. A revision of *Rhizobium* Frank 1889, with an emended description of the genus, and the inclusion of all species of *Agrobacterium* Conn 1942 and *Allorhizobium undicola* de Lajundie *et al.* 1998 as new combinations: *Rhizobium radiobacter, R. rhizogenes, R. rubi, R. undicola* and *R. vitis*. *Int. J. Syst. Evol. Microbiol.* **51:**89–103.
268. **Yuen, K.-Y., P. C. Y. Woo, J. L. L. Teng, K. W. Leung, M. K. Wong, and S. K. Lau.** 2001. *Laribacter hongkongensis* gen. nov., sp. nov., a novel gram-negative bacterium isolated from a cirrhotic patient with bacteremia and empyema. *J. Clin. Microbiol.* **39:**4227–4232.
269. **Zarrilli, R., M. Crispino, M. Bagattini, E. Barretta, A. Di Popolo, M. Triassi, and P. Villari.** 2004. Molecular epidemiology of sequential outbreaks of *Acinetobacter baumannii* in an intensive care unit shows the emergence of carbapenem resistance. *J. Clin. Microbiol.* **42:**946–953.

Bordetella

MICHAEL J. LOEFFELHOLZ AND GARY N. SANDEN

51

TAXONOMY

The genus *Bordetella*, in the family *Alcaligenaceae*, is named for J. Bordet, who, with O. Gengou, described the bacterium in 1906 (9). A total of eight *Bordetella* species have been described: *B. pertussis*, *B. bronchiseptica*, *B. parapertussis*, *B. avium*, *B. hinzii*, *B. holmesii*, *B. trematum* (5, 61), and the recently described species *B. petrii* (96). An additional organism, *B. ansorpii* sp. nov. (50), currently has no standing in nomenclature (http://www.bacterio.cict.fr/nonvalid.html). Phylogenetic analysis based on 16S rRNA gene sequencing has demonstrated that *B. pertussis, B. parapertussis, B. bronchiseptica*, and *B. holmesii* are very closely related (48). *B. pertussis* and *B. parapertussis* may be recent derivatives of *B. bronchiseptica*, developing unique host ranges and pathogenicity due to gene loss (72). In spite of considerable genetic relatedness among some *Bordetella* species, current literature still refers to distinct species. Evidence suggests that the genetic diversity of *B. pertussis* is decreasing, due to selective pressure of vaccination (84). This may be partially responsible for the reemergence of pertussis, as described later in this chapter.

DESCRIPTION OF THE GENUS

Bordetella organisms are small gram-negative coccobacilli. Some species are motile. With the exception of the recently described *B. petrii*, they are strictly aerobic, with optimal growth at 35 to 37°C. All species possess catalase activity. All species oxidize amino acids, but none ferment carbohydrates. While all species have relatively simple nutritional requirements, fastidiousness varies depending on the degree of sensitivity to toxic substances and metabolites found in common laboratory media. *B. pertussis* is the most fastidious species and is inhibited by constituents present in many media, including fatty acids, metal ions, sulfides, and peroxides. Isolation of *B. pertussis* requires media containing protective substances such as charcoal, blood, or starch. The other *Bordetella* species are less fastidious and will grow on routine agars containing blood and on MacConkey agar. Growth rates of *Bordetella* species are generally inversely related to fastidiousness; *B. pertussis* grows slowly, while *B. avium* and *B. bronchiseptica* grow rapidly. *B. petrii* is unique among the *Bordetella* in that it is capable of growth under both aerobic and anaerobic conditions. Table 1 lists some of the common characteristics used to differentiate *Bordetella* species.

B. pertussis produces a number of virulence factors that are responsible for pathogenesis (61). These virulence factors include toxins (pertussis toxin, adenylate cyclase toxin, and tracheal cytotoxin) and components that mediate adherence to ciliated epithelial cells of the respiratory tract (pertussis toxin [PT], fimbriae, filamentous hemagglutinin [FHA], and pertactin). Other virulence factors include dermonecrosis (heat-labile) toxin, lipopolysaccharide (endotoxin), and tracheal colonization factor. *Bordetella* species other than *B. pertussis* also express virulence factors. *B. parapertussis* and *B. bronchiseptica* produce pertactin and FHA (61). Promoter and structural genes for PT are present in both *B. parapertussis* and *B. bronchiseptica* but are not expressed.

NATURAL HABITATS

With the exception of *B. petrii*, *Bordetella* species are isolated from humans and warm-blooded animals. *B. petrii*, the sole environmental species, was isolated from an anaerobic culture enriched from river sediment (96). *B. pertussis* produces disease only in humans, who also serve as the sole reservoir. *B. parapertussis*, once thought to be strictly a human pathogen, is also found in sheep (61). Genotypic strain analysis showed that human and ovine *B. parapertussis* strains are distinct (93). *B. pertussis* has historically been considered a strict respiratory pathogen, causing localized infection of the ciliated epithelium of the bronchial tree. However, its isolation from blood indicates the potential for invasive infection (13, 47). *B. bronchiseptica* is a respiratory tract pathogen of a variety of animals, including dogs, swine, cats, and rabbits (61). *B. avium* is found in wild and domesticated birds and causes coryza in turkeys (75). *B. hinzii* colonizes the respiratory tracts of poultry, and recent evidence suggests that it may cause disease (78). An organism isolated from a cancer patient undergoing chemotherapy has been designated *B. ansorpii* sp. nov., based on 16S rRNA gene sequence, cellular fatty acid composition, G+C content, and biochemical testing. Although recovered from the exudate from an epidermal cyst, a pathogenic role for this isolate was not established (50). On rare occasions *B. bronchiseptica* and *B. hinzii* cause disease in humans (19, 102). *B. avium* is strictly a veterinary pathogen. *B. holmesii* and *B. trematum* are infrequently associated with nonrespiratory infections in humans (88, 90). Additionally, *B. holmesii* has been linked to respiratory infections with pertussis-like symptoms (103).

TABLE 1 Differential characteristics of *Bordetella* spp.[a]

Characteristic	*B. pertussis*	*B. parapertussis*	*B. bronchiseptica*	*B. avium*	*B. hinzii*	*B. holmesii*	*B. trematum*	*B. petrii*[b]
Oxidase	+	−	+	+	+	−	−	+
Nitrate reduction	−	−	+	−	−	−	V	−
Urease production	−	+ (24 h)	+ (4 h)	−	V	−	−	−
Motility	−	−	+	+	+	−	+	−
Growth on:								
Blood agar	−	+	+	+	+	+	+	+[c]
MacConkey agar	−	V (delayed)	+	+	+	+ (delayed)	+	+

[a]Modified from references 19, 90, and 96 and earlier editions of this Manual. Responses: +, activity or growth present; −, not present; V, variable.
[b]Data from a single strain.
[c]Ulf Göbel, personal communication.

CLINICAL SIGNIFICANCE

The incubation period of pertussis is usually 7 to 10 days, with a range of approximately 4 to 21 days (12). The symptoms that develop following the incubation period can be classified as either typical (classical) or atypical. Classical pertussis consists of a catarrhal stage lasting 1 to 2 weeks, a paroxysmal stage lasting 1 to 6 weeks (as long as 10 weeks), and a convalescent stage lasting 2 to 4 weeks (as long as several months). Patient symptoms during the catarrhal stage are nonspecific and include rhinorrhea, sneezing, low-grade fever, and occasional mild cough. Pertussis is frequently unsuspected during this period. The paroxysmal stage of pertussis is characterized by the presence of one or more of the pathognomonic signs of pertussis: episodes of paroxysmal cough, whoop, and posttussive vomiting. The severity of respiratory symptoms gradually decreases during the convalescent stage. Atypical symptoms in older children and adults consist of a prolonged, nondescript cough. The differential diagnosis of atypical pertussis includes bronchitis and upper respiratory tract infections caused by adenovirus, parainfluenza virus, respiratory syncytial virus, *Chlamydophila* (formerly *Chlamydia*) *pneumoniae*, and *Mycoplasma pneumoniae* (29, 30). Infants with pertussis may present with choking and apnea, while cough may be absent. Morbidity and mortality rates are higher in infants than in other age groups (61). Adults experience more complications from pertussis than do adolescents (21). *Bordetella* infections have recently been shown to play a major role in acute exacerbation of chronic bronchitis (8).

B. pertussis is responsible for the vast majority of pertussis cases and causes more-severe respiratory symptoms than other *Bordetella* species associated with pertussis syndrome. Worldwide, *B. pertussis* causes an estimated 20 million to 40 million cases of pertussis and 200,000 to 400,000 deaths each year, primarily among children in countries lacking organized vaccination programs (http://www.who.int/vaccines/en/pertussis.shtml#summary). *B. pertussis* is transmitted from person to person via respiratory droplets and is highly contagious, infecting 80 to 90% of susceptible contacts (12). Relatively close contact (within several feet) is required for transmission. Transmission is not uncommon in health care facilities and can be associated with high rates of morbidity in this high-risk setting (14).

A carrier state is not recognized for *B. pertussis*. Sensitive nonculture tests such as PCR can detect organisms in asymptomatic immune persons (35), but this is more likely to represent a transient colonization or infection rather than a prolonged carrier state. The disease is endemic, with epidemics consistently occurring every 3 to 5 years (12). The number of reported pertussis cases in the United States has increased steadily since the 1980s, in spite of continued high levels of vaccination coverage. Explanations offered for the increased incidence include heightened awareness and reporting of disease (particularly the atypical presentation, and disease in older persons), and the use of more sensitive laboratory diagnostic tests.

Immunity to pertussis following natural infection or vaccination wanes after 5 to 12 years. As a result, *B. pertussis* is a significant cause of respiratory disease in older children and adults (15, 61, 87) who, in countries with vaccination programs, have replaced young children as the primary reservoir of *B. pertussis*. Serologic evidence indicates that as much as one-third of chronic cough illness in adults is due to *B. pertussis* (15). However, in some studies in which culture was performed, *B. pertussis* was not isolated from any seropositive subjects (64). Therefore, the public health significance of this high seroprevalence is unclear.

Vaccines have dramatically reduced the public health impact of pertussis. The initial heat-killed, whole-cell vaccines have been largely replaced by multicomponent acellular vaccines, which are associated with fewer side effects (73). The efficacy of whole-cell and acellular vaccines is estimated to be between 60 and 90% (12). Until recently, available pertussis vaccines had been formulated and licensed for children younger than 7 years. However, two aspects of recent pertussis epidemiology have stimulated evaluations of the immunogenicity and safety of acellular vaccines in older persons (10). The first is the recognition of the importance of *B. pertussis* as a cause of respiratory disease in adolescents and adults (61, 87); the second is the accumulating evidence for the predominant role of adolescents and adults in transmission of pertussis to infants (7). Acellular booster doses are licensed in Australia, Austria, Canada, France, and most recently, the United States (http://www.cdc.gov/nip/vaccine/tdap/tdap_acip_recs.pdf) for administration to adolescents or adults. Vaccination (with either acellular or whole-cell vaccine) may be selecting for *B. pertussis* strains distinct from those from the prevaccination era (66, 84). The role of the divergence between vaccine and recently circulating strains in the changing epidemiology of pertussis over the last 20 years is still uncertain. There is no epidemiological evidence to suggest that vaccine efficacy in the United States has been compromised by the divergence of circulating strains. Vaccines directed against *B. pertussis* do not confer protection from infections by other *Bordetella* spp.

Septicemia caused by *B. pertussis* has been reported only rarely, but blood cultures showing gram-negative bacilli that are not recovered on routine subculture media should be subcultured on media supporting *B. pertussis* (13, 47).

B. parapertussis causes a pertussis syndrome similar to but usually less severe than that caused by *B. pertussis* (61). While *B. parapertussis* may be quite prominent in isolated outbreaks (56), overall it accounts for 2 to 20% of *Bordetella* isolates (61). Symptomatic *B. parapertussis* infections more commonly present as a nonspecific cough illness or bronchitis. Mixed infections by *B. pertussis* and *B. parapertussis* have been reported, and this should be considered when examining primary cultures from clinical specimens (56). *B. bronchiseptica* (23, 102) and *B. holmesii* (81, 103) have been implicated as infrequent causes of pertussis syndrome and other respiratory illnesses. *B. holmesii* is also a rare cause of bacteremia in asplenic patients (85). Most reported cases of *B. bronchiseptica* respiratory disease have been associated either with underlying conditions such as immunosuppression or with exposure to animals. *B. bronchiseptica* has been associated with pleural effusion in a patient with AIDS (94) and pneumonia in lung transplant recipients (71). *Bordetella* species isolated from cystic fibrosis patients include *B. bronchiseptica* (99) and *B. hinzii* (18).

COLLECTION, TRANSPORT, AND STORAGE OF SPECIMENS

Excellent summaries of specimen collection and handling for optimal detection of *B. pertussis* are available (70), including several earlier editions of this Manual. Preferred specimens for laboratory diagnosis of pertussis are nasopharyngeal (NP) aspirates and posterior NP swabs. When properly collected, these specimens contain the ciliated respiratory epithelial cells for which *B. pertussis* exhibits tropism. NP aspirates yield more positive culture results than do NP swabs (31). Aspirates offer additional advantages over swabs; there is usually sufficient specimen for multiple analyses (important when verifying new test procedures), and the specimen collection technique may be preferred by clinicians and parents of young patients (31). Throat swabs are inferior specimens for culture; they do not sample the ciliated epithelium, and they contain large numbers of members of the normal flora, which can result in overgrowth of isolation media. In one study, significantly fewer infections were detected by culture using throat swabs than by culture using NP swabs (60). However, throat swabs may be suitable for PCR diagnosis of *B. pertussis* infection (25).

To obtain an NP aspirate, a narrow catheter or infant feeding tube is inserted through the nostril to the posterior nasopharynx. A mucous trap and hand-operated vacuum pump are connected to the other end, and suction is applied while the tube is in place and while slowly withdrawing it back through the nostril. Any secretions remaining in the tube should be flushed into the trap by aspirating *Bordetella* transport medium or phosphate-buffered saline. Additionally, the catheter tip can be cut off and placed into suitable transport medium for shipping. Swab specimens are collected by inserting a small swab on a flexible (usually aluminum wire) shaft through the nostril. The placement of the swab is important. Figure 1 depicts the correct positioning of the patient's head and placement of the swab. The swab should then be rotated for several seconds before being withdrawn. It is generally recommended that two NP swab specimens be collected, one through each nostril. This provides separate swabs if multiple laboratory tests are to be performed. Specimens are then either directly plated or placed in a suitable medium for transport.

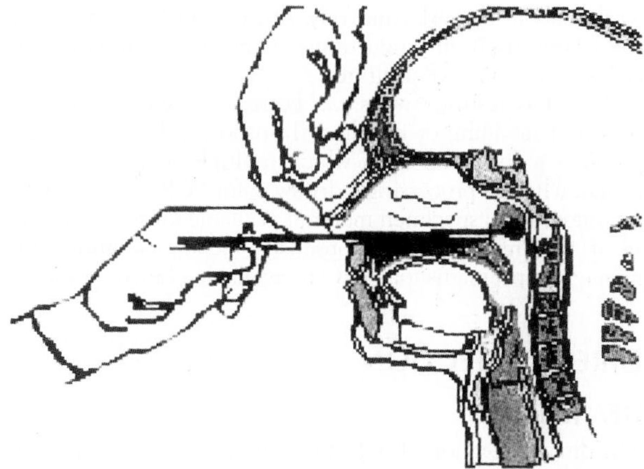

FIGURE 1 Correct positioning of patient's head and placement of the swab for collection of NP specimens (reprinted from reference 12). (Courtesy of Kris Bisgard, Centers for Disease Control and Prevention.)

Several transport media are readily available for NP specimens, including 1% acid-hydrolyzed casein (Casamino Acids; Becton Dickinson, Sparks, Md.) and Amies medium with charcoal. Survival of *B. pertussis* at 4°C in Casamino Acids was substantially greater than in water or phosphate-buffered saline (11). Regan-Lowe (RL) transport medium contains half-strength charcoal agar and horse blood, with cephalexin added to suppress growth of the normal NP flora. Substitution of 2.5 μg of methicillin per ml or 0.625 μg of oxacillin per ml for cephalexin reportedly allows the growth of *B. holmesii* (62). Unlike Casamino Acids and Amies medium, RL transport medium also functions as an enrichment medium for *B. pertussis*. Preincubation of specimens in RL transport medium is controversial. Preincubation at 36°C may enhance the recovery of *B. pertussis* due to multiplication of organisms (76). Some recommend against preincubation because of overgrowth of cephalexin-resistant members of the flora (12). Transport at 4°C provides better recovery of *B. pertussis* than does transport at room temperature (33, 68) but adds additional costs due to packaging and weight.

Swab material should be calcium alginate, Dacron, or rayon if culture isolation is to be performed (17, 44). Cotton contains inhibitors that will decrease isolation rates of *B. pertussis* (44). Dacron or rayon is recommended if PCR testing is performed, since calcium alginate can inhibit PCR (17, 97). The inhibitory effect of calcium alginate on PCR amplification may depend in part on the specimen extraction procedure. Crude proteinase K extracts were completely inhibitory to PCR (97).

Because of the lability of *B. pertussis* outside its normal host environment, proper handling and shipping conditions are critical for optimal culture sensitivity. For culture testing, direct plating of NP specimens onto agar plates provides optimal sensitivity. Kurzynski et al. showed that 14% more NP swab specimens were positive by a plate inoculated bedside than by a plate inoculated after enrichment and transport (54). However, this requires clinician participation and training and is not practical for off-site reference and public health laboratories.

For direct fluorescent-antibody (DFA) testing, the specimen collection kit should contain a glass slide, on which a smear is prepared from an NP swab immediately after collection. The slide is allowed to air dry and is then transported to the laboratory. Alternatively, smears can be prepared at the laboratory from liquid transport medium containing an NP swab or from NP aspirates.

For PCR testing, swabs can be transported dry (57), in transport medium, or in saline. Transport in liquid medium provides a specimen from which multiple aliquots can be tested, whereas processing a dry swab for PCR testing leaves no unextracted specimen material available for repeat analysis if required. Detailed consensus recommendations for managing specimens for PCR are available elsewhere (80).

DIRECT DETECTION

DFA Testing

The direct detection of *B. pertussis* in NP secretions by using fluorochrome-conjugated antibody provides the most rapid and simple diagnosis of pertussis. Commercially available antibodies are polyclonal (Becton Dickinson) or monoclonal, recognizing a lipooligosaccharide epitope (Accu-Mab; Altachem Pharma, Edmonton, Alberta, Canada) (1). The monoclonal antibodies are available as a dual-fluorochrome reagent for the detection of both *B. pertussis* and *B. parapertussis* in a single smear. A head-to-head comparison of the polyclonal and monoclonal reagents showed that they had similar sensitivity (89). Factors to consider when choosing an antibody source include cost and performance in the laboratory's own hands.

Regardless of the antibody used, the direct detection of *B. pertussis* by DFA lacks both sensitivity and specificity. Compared to that of culture, DFA sensitivity in several published studies ranged from 30 to 71% (32, 57). DFA-positive, culture-negative specimens are not unusual. When DFA was compared to an expanded diagnostic standard (e.g., two positive nonculture tests or a clinical diagnosis), its sensitivity ranged from one-half that of culture (32) to threefold greater than that of culture (57). The large range in DFA performance reflects variation in the sensitivities of both the DFA procedure and the culture procedures against which it is compared. The specificity of DFA is highly variable, due to the cross-reactivity of immunological reagents and the subjectivity of fluorescence interpretation. Weak cross-reactivity of the Accu-Mab monoclonal antibody with *B. bronchiseptica* has been reported (63). Polyclonal antibodies cross-react with a number of organisms, including unencapsulated *Haemophilus influenzae* and diphtherioids (61). In a study conducted by Loeffelholz et al., several specimens positive only by DFA were considered to be true positives because of strong clinical or epidemiological evidence of infection (57). Other studies have shown extremely poor DFA specificity (32). Notwithstanding the variable performance, DFA testing can provide valuable information when appropriate quality assurance and quality control measures are implemented to maximize specificity. DFA testing should be performed only as an adjunct to culture or PCR, and the results should be considered presumptive.

Antibody for DFA testing must be appropriately titrated before use. To control for staining specificity, control slides should contain separate smears of *B. pertussis* and *B. parapertussis*. Smears should contain 10 to 100 organisms per oil immersion field. Suspensions of control organisms can be prepared in phosphate-buffered saline with a turbidity equivalent to a McFarland standard of 1. Stained smears are examined under a fluorescent microscope for the presence or absence and degree of fluorescence. Slides are viewed initially at a magnification of ×400. Any fluorescence is examined at a magnification of ×1,000 to confirm morphology. *Bordetella* organisms appear as small coccobacillary rods with pronounced peripheral apple green fluorescence and dark centers. Fluorescence must be intense, and other staining characteristics and morphology must be ignored.

Nucleic Acid Detection

Nucleic acid detection methods such as PCR can provide a test response time similar to that of DFA, while offering enhanced sensitivity and objectivity in results interpretation. These advantages, together with the continuing loss of expertise in interpreting DFA results, have contributed to the ascension of PCR over DFA as the routine nonculture test method in many clinical laboratories. Although the Centers for Disease Control and Prevention recommended in 2000 that PCR be used as a presumptive assay in conjunction with culture (12), this test is rapidly moving from presumptive to diagnostic status and becoming more available.

PCR clinical sensitivity suffers from the same constraints associated with other detection methods, including specimen quality and timing in the disease course and antimicrobic treatment. However, PCR has consistently been reported to be more sensitive than DFA or culture (25, 27, 28, 34, 35, 57, 91, 98). The superiority of PCR performance over that of culture is due in part to variation in the sensitivity of culture. PCR tests themselves vary in sensitivity, depending on the nucleic acid extraction method, the amount of specimen amplified, the amplification conditions and efficiency, the sequence targeted, and the DNA detection format. Presumably because of its greater sensitivity and ability to detect dead organisms, PCR remains positive longer during the course of disease than does culture (91, 98) and is more likely to remain positive following antibiotic therapy (24, 98). Longitudinal analysis of erythromycin-treated infants showed that after 4 days of treatment, 56 and 89% of NP swab specimens were positive by culture and PCR, respectively (24), whereas after 7 days of treatment, no specimens were positive by culture but 56% were still positive by PCR. The higher sensitivity of PCR is also marked among persons with mild or atypical symptoms (83) and among older persons (91, 98).

Despite the increasing use of PCR methods to diagnose pertussis, these assays continue to demonstrate significant shortcomings. There is no standardized or Food and Drug Administration (FDA)-cleared, commercially available PCR test for *B. pertussis* and *B. parapertussis*. In fact, many assays fail to test for *B. parapertussis*, which remains a significant cause of pertussis in some outbreaks (56). Validation criteria vary by regulatory program, but extensive method validation on the part of the laboratory is required before the test can be offered for diagnostic use. Unfortunately, the validation process is easily compromised by insufficient availability of positive specimens and inadequate resolution of discrepant results between the PCR test and the diagnostic standard, especially when the PCR is positive and the comparative standard is negative. The validation criteria specified by the Clinical and Laboratory Standards Institute (http://www.nccls.org) are helpful in designing a validation program and would likely satisfy all state criteria. The laboratory must also develop and implement quality control and an ongoing quality assurance program; these requirements also vary by regulatory program. A widely available and independently certified proficiency testing program is lacking, so it is currently difficult to assess interlaboratory performance.

Because PCR detects nonviable cells and DNA, defining the clinical sensitivity and specificity of PCR tests for pertussis is critical. However, these predictive values for pertussis PCR remain incompletely defined, especially regarding the effect on these values of pertussis prevalence in the host community, host vaccination status and age, and disease severity. Interpretation standards should include relevance of unpredicted results such as multiple consecutive positives. Similarly, results reporting formats also must reflect these limitations and the clinical community must be educated regarding test limitations and reporting criteria. It is strongly recommended that positive test results be confirmed with an additional laboratory test or clinical pertussis ascertainment, until PCR clinical sensitivity and specificity values are more completely defined.

Consensus recommendations for the diagnosis of *B. pertussis* and *B. parapertussis* infections by PCR have been proposed (80). These recommendations focus heavily on quality assurance and control, verification of assay performance (clinical sensitivity and specificity and analytical specificity), and ongoing validation studies and also describe appropriate sample collection, transport, pretreatment, and DNA extraction. Chapter 16 of this Manual describes good laboratory practices to avoid false-positive PCR results due to contamination. Positive and negative controls must be able to monitor the entire PCR assay procedure, including specimen extraction. Internal specimen amplification controls should be included for each specimen; ideally these would be amplified by the same primers as the diagnostic target (36). While there are no established guidelines about the number of negative controls to include in each run, some laboratories routinely include a negative control for approximately every five specimens.

Chromosomal regions targeted by PCR include, but are not limited to, the pertussis toxin promoter region (28, 45), a region upstream of the porin gene (26), repetitive insertion sequences IS*481* of *B. pertussis* (27, 34, 92) and IS*1001* of *B. parapertussis* (92), the adenylate cyclase gene (22), and a region upstream of the flagellin gene (46). A set of primers targeted to the toxin promoter was shown not to detect *B. parapertussis* or *B. bronchiseptica* (28, 45). Primers targeting IS*481* have been shown to detect *B. holmesii* (58) and may cross-react with other *Bordetella* spp. (80). Carriage of IS*481* by strains of several *Bordetella* species makes monitoring the specificity of IS*481* necessary (80). Nested-PCR assays for the detection of *Bordetella* have been described (25, 79). While these assays were reported to be sensitive and specific, nested PCR is inherently more susceptible to contamination than unnested PCR. It is our opinion that when PCR conditions are properly optimized, nesting of PCR is not required for the accurate, sensitive diagnosis of most infectious diseases, including pertussis.

ISOLATION

Culture provides the most specific diagnosis of pertussis and produces isolates for genotypic analysis and antimicrobial susceptibility testing. The sensitivity of culture varies greatly, depending on patient factors (including prior antibiotic therapy, duration of symptoms, age, and vaccination status), specimen transport conditions, the type and quality of media used, and other conditions (38). While PCR testing is also affected by these factors, culture is affected to a greater degree because of its requirement for viable organisms. The highest isolation rates are achieved when specimens are inoculated onto media immediately after collection from the patient. Since this is often not possible, transport media should be used.

Several media for the isolation of *B. pertussis* have been described. Traditional media consist of bases such as potato infusion (Bordet-Gengou [BG] medium) or charcoal (RL medium) supplemented with glycerol, peptones, and horse or sheep blood. An antimicrobial agent is added to reduce the growth of the normal flora. Cephalexin is the agent of choice, yet growth of resistant members of the NP flora is still quite common (70). RL medium provides better isolation of *B. pertussis* than does BG medium (68, 70). The shelf life of media ranges from 5 days for BG medium to 4 to 8 weeks for RL medium (76).

Plates are incubated in ambient air at 35 to 36°C and examined daily for suspicious colonies. In one study, *B. pertussis* colony development was more rapid in ambient air than in air containing 5 to 10% carbon dioxide (43). The humidity must be sufficient to prevent the desiccation of agar plates during the long incubation period. While most *B. pertussis* colonies become visible after 3 to 4 days of incubation (*B. parapertussis* becomes visible after 2 to 3 days), an incubation time of 7 days has historically been recommended. In one study, 12 days of incubation recovered more isolates than did 7 days of incubation (49).

IDENTIFICATION

Phenotypic

On RL agar, young *B. pertussis* colonies are round, domed, mercury-silver colored, and shiny. *B. parapertussis* colonies are similar but are grayer and less domed (Fig. 2). On BG agar, *B. pertussis* and *B. parapertussis* produce zones of hemolysis.

Bordetella organisms appear as gram-negative coccobacilli or short rods. Poly- or monoclonal antibodies are available to confirm identity (Fig. 3). Suspensions of colonies are prepared in phosphate-buffered saline and should be dilute to avoid dulling of fluorescence. Both *B. pertussis* and *B. parapertussis* controls should be included. Fluorescence is interpreted as described earlier in this chapter. For identification by slide agglutination, a heavier suspension is prepared, equivalent to a McFarland standard of 3. Uniform suspensions are best prepared from cultures no more than 3 days old and harvested with a Dacron or rayon swab instead of a bacteriological loop. Cell aggregates can be dispersed by repeatedly forcing the suspension through a pipette and using aerosol precautions. Colonies grown on antibiotic-free RL agar produce more homogeneous suspensions for easier interpretation of agglutination. In addition to identification using specific antisera, *Bordetella* species can be identified by biochemical tests based on differential phenotypic characteristics (Table 1). Oxidase-positive, nonfermentative gram-negative rods, particularly *Oligella ureolytica* and *Ralstonia paucula,* can be misidentified as *B. bronchiseptica. B. bronchiseptica* differs from *R. paucula* by having a positive nitrate reduction test and from *O. ureolytica* by having a negative nitrite reduction test and by showing penicillin susceptibility.

Commercially obtained strains (American Type Culture Collection, Manassas, Va.) or previously characterized clinical isolates can serve as controls for quality control of media and reagents. Clinical isolates should be frozen as soon as possible at −70°C in glycerol. Once plated, cultures lose viability quickly and must be replaced regularly. As per Clinical Laboratory Improvement Amendment regulations, laboratories must maintain thorough documentation of control strains, including strain source/origin and storage conditions. Standard operating procedures must be developed for the maintenance of control strains.

Biosafety level 2 practices are recommended when working with *Bordetella* spp. Routine manipulations of specimens and isolates can be conducted on open bench tops.

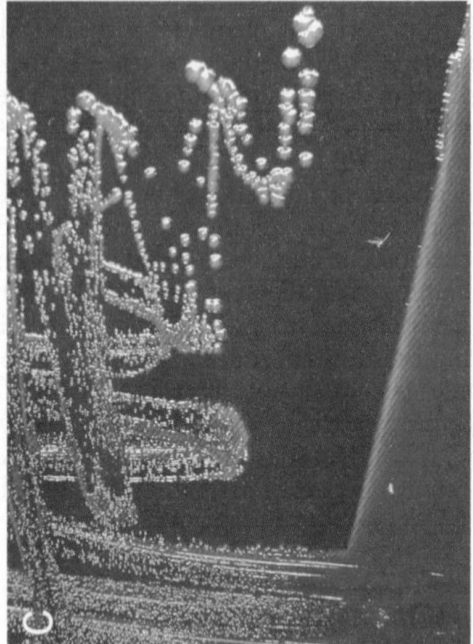

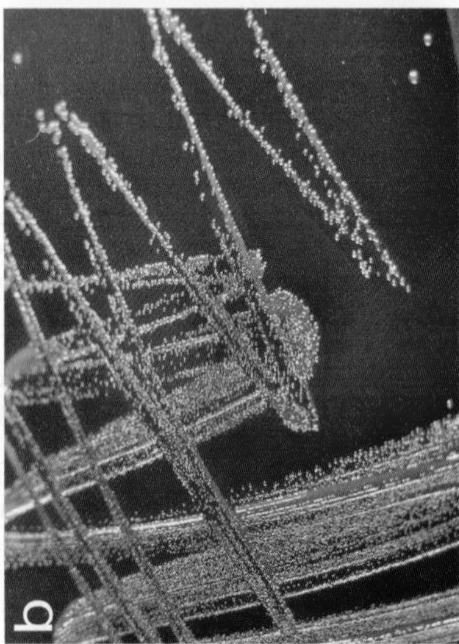

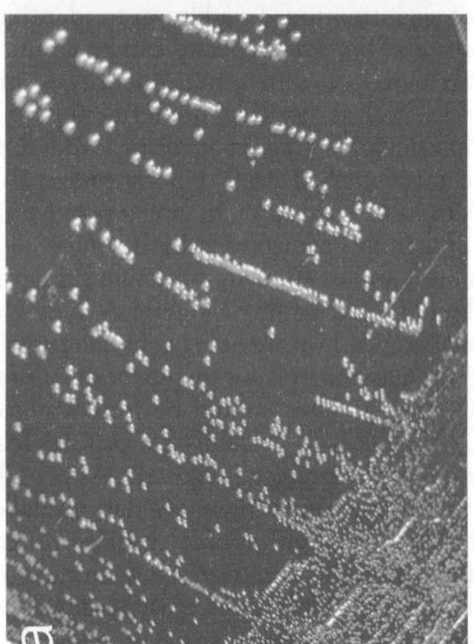

FIGURE 2 Colony morphologies of *Bordetella* after 3 to 5 days of incubation on BG agar. (a) *B. pertussis*; (b) *B. parapertussis*; (c) *B. bronchiseptica*.

Genotypic Strain Typing

Pulsed-field gel electrophoresis (PFGE) methods for the identification of *B. pertussis* strains have been described previously (12, 67). PFGE has been proven to be valuable in tracking outbreak transmission patterns (12, 65). It has also been used to identify *B. parapertussis* (74) and *B. bronchiseptica* isolates (6). The rare-cutting restriction enzyme XbaI is used in most PFGE procedures for typing *B. pertussis, B. parapertussis,* and *B. bronchiseptica* (6, 12, 74). Other genotypic methods used to discriminate *Bordetella* isolates include restriction enzyme analysis (82), arbitrarily primed PCR (randomly amplified polymorphic DNA) (104), PCR targeting a specific repetitive element (65), ribotyping (77), sequence analysis of genes encoding pertactin and the S1 fragment of pertussis toxin (67), and multilocus variable-number repeat analysis (84). Comparative analysis of PFGE and PCR-based typing methods for discrimination of *B. pertussis* isolates showed PFGE to be more discriminatory (65). Standardized approaches to genotypic analysis of *B. pertussis* isolates have focused on PFGE, largely due to the wide availability and demonstrated epidemiological relevance of this approach (12, 67).

SEROLOGIC TESTS

Serologic diagnostic methods are generally limited to the detection of immune responses to *B. pertussis*. In the past, these methods included enzyme-linked immunosorbent assay (ELISA), agglutination, complement fixation, immunoblotting, indirect hemagglutination, and toxin neutralization (70). Assays other than ELISAs, immunoblotting, and toxin neutralization are not common in clinical laboratories. The toxin neutralization assays are generally limited to reference and research institutions to measure functional serum antibodies. Because of ease of use and sensitivity, ELISAs in microwell plate format have become the method of choice.

ELISAs have been used to measure immunoglobulin A (IgA), IgG, and IgM levels to PT, FHA, pertactin, fimbriae, and sonicated *B. pertussis* cells. As measured by ELISAs, at least 90% of infected persons develop IgG to PT and FHA after ≥3 to 4 weeks following onset of symptoms (70). IgG and IgA responses to these antigens are most often used as indicators of *B. pertussis* infection. Responses to PT are specific for *B. pertussis,* since no other *Bordetella* species expresses PT. FHA is expressed by *B. pertussis, B. parapertussis,* and *B. bronchiseptica.* Other bacteria, including *Haemophilus influenzae,* possess epitopes that cross-react with FHA (95). Clinical sensitivity of IgA-specific responses is not as great as for IgG responses, but IgA is rarely detected in uninfected vaccines, and therefore, such responses enhance clinical specificity when present (70, 91). IgM responses do not increase clinical sensitivity and specificity sufficiently over those for IgA and IgG to be widely tested.

The specific strategy used for the serodiagnosis of pertussis is often a function of patient age and vaccination status, and sensitivity and specificity may vary. Currently, the demonstration of seroconversion or a significant rise in the concentration of IgG against PT is widely accepted as the most sensitive and specific serodiagnostic test. Consequently, a suitable strategy for serologic diagnosis in unvaccinated children is the demonstration of increases in the concentrations of IgG or IgA to PT or FHA, although young infants may not produce IgA (91). However, the appropriate collection of acute and convalescent serum specimens is often problematic in pertussis patients of any age (61, 86). True acute-phase specimens are often

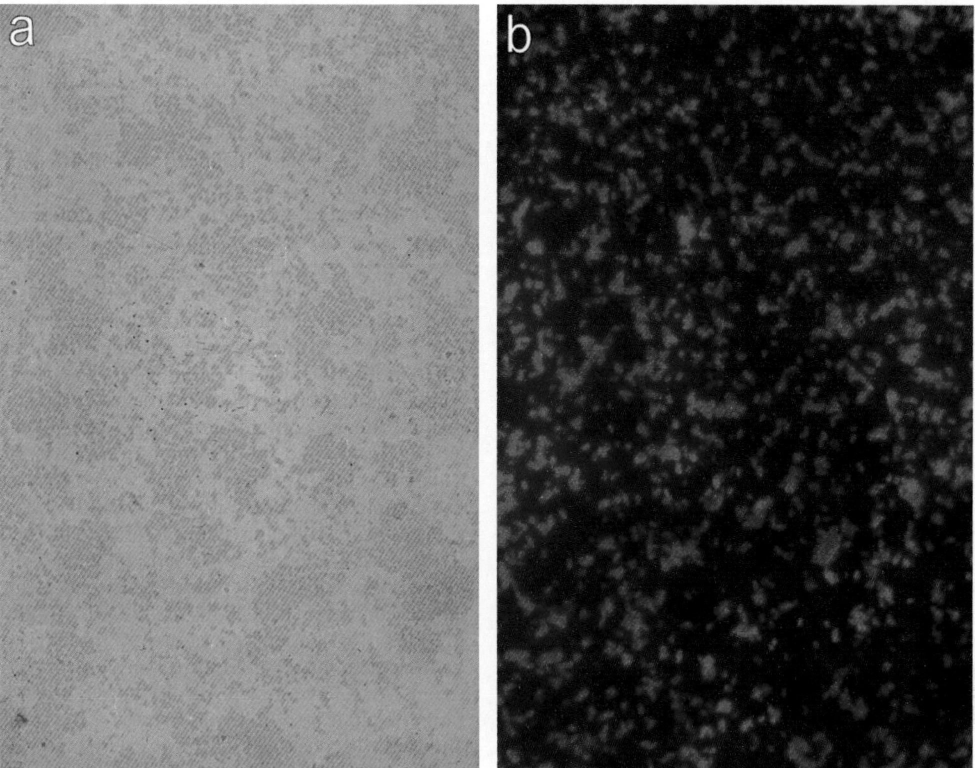

FIGURE 3 (a) Gram stain morphology of *B. pertussis*. (b) Immunofluorescent staining of *B. pertussis*. (Photographs courtesy of Charlotte Parker.)

excluded by the clinical presentation of patients late in the illness due to the nonspecific symptoms early in disease, and convalescent-phase specimens can be compromised by poor patient compliance with recall. Testing of single specimens collected early in the disease (1 to 3 weeks after onset of cough) was reportedly compromised by low sensitivity (101).

Serodiagnosis of pertussis in vaccinated children is even more problematic due to rapid increases in antibody concentration and the consequent difficulty in detecting significant rises in these responses. The tendency to collect "acute"-phase specimens late in this population further contributes to this problem. These conditions among vaccinees suggest that a significant decrease in specific antibodies between late acute- and convalescent-phase specimens may be a valid diagnostic criterion, and one report has demonstrated the feasibility of this approach (86).

Since obtaining acute- and convalescent-phase specimens is problematic, serodiagnosis of pertussis in adolescents and adults based on high antibody concentrations in a single specimen is an attractive strategy (70). The general waning of vaccine-induced serum antibodies in these populations further promotes this approach. Until recently, results from single-serum specimens required interpretation in the context of control values determined for a specific patient population. Epidemiologic studies can stringently identify case-patient controls by age and vaccination status in order to derive serodiagnostic control (cutoff) values related to their study population (16). Although these diagnostic values are limited to specific study populations, potential single-serum IgG anti-PT diagnostic levels with more general diagnostic relevance are emerging from longitudinal studies of the kinetics of IgG anti-PT responses and seroepidemiologic studies of representative samples of populations (4, 20). The specificity of this approach depends on the particular assay and cutoff used. Diagnostic sensitivity has not been widely evaluated for any of the currently proposed diagnostic cutoffs (20).

IgA-, IgG-, and IgM-specific ELISAs are available from a number of manufacturers on several continents, and the immunoblot format is also commercially available (MarBlot; Trinity Biotech, Wicklow, Ireland). Although there is currently no FDA-cleared serodiagnostic test, ELISAs are widely used outside the United States, particularly for testing adolescents and adults. In the United States, the lack of an FDA-cleared test and inadequate supply of standard reference serum specimens severely restrict the use of diagnostic ELISAs. Comparative analyses of serologic testing, culture, DFA, and PCR have generally shown serologic testing to be the most sensitive method for diagnosis of *B. pertussis* infections (28, 32, 91). In one study, PCR was positive for only 21% of patients with positive serology (either high IgG or IgA concentrations in a single specimen or significant increases in antibody concentrations in paired specimens) (91). The authors attributed the low sensitivity of PCR to the collection of specimens relatively late in disease. The same study demonstrated that the sensitivity of both PCR and culture decreases rapidly after the paroxysmal phase. An evaluation of several commercial IgG-based ELISAs showed that individual assay reproducibility was acceptable, but results between tests and between test and reference assays were not concordant (52). Sensitivities with challenge paired serum specimens were 60 to 95%, but none of the assays identified all cases correctly.

ANTIMICROBIAL SUSCEPTIBILITY

Erythromycin, azithromycin, and clarithromycin are the antimicrobial agents of choice for treatment and prophylaxis of pertussis (3, 69). Trimethoprim-sulfamethoxazole (SXT) is an acceptable alternative for patients intolerant of macrolides and for the rare pertussis case caused by macrolide-resistant *B. pertussis* (40). Among the fluoroquinolones, ciprofloxacin, levofloxacin, and gemifloxacin showed the highest activities against *B. pertussis* (42, 69) but are not recommended for treating children because of their potential harmful side effects. The most recent treatment and prophylaxis recommendations can be seen at http://www.cdc.gov/nip/publications/pertussis/guide.htm and http://www.cdc.gov/nip/publications/pertussis/chapter3a_update_macrolides.pdf.

Eleven instances of erythromycin resistance in *B. pertussis* have been reported from Arizona, California, Georgia, Minnesota, New York, and Utah since 1994 (2, 51, 55; K. Bromberg, personal communication), but the true prevalence of resistance in the circulating population is unknown. Susceptibility screening of *B. pertussis* isolates at several enhanced pertussis surveillance sites suggests that the prevalence of resistant strains is too low to justify routine testing of all isolates. However, resistant *B. pertussis* isolates have demonstrated wide geographic distribution and been associated with treatment failure. Consequently, surveillance for resistant organisms is recommended and isolates should be tested if associated with treatment failure (12). Resistance in *B. pertussis* is conferred by a mutation in the macrolide binding domain of the 23S rRNA.

A novel heterogeneous erythromycin resistant/susceptible phenotype has been described (100). This phenotype is distinguished by the appearance of two colony types during the resistance screening test. The first type manifests as susceptible with a zone of inhibition >40 mm after 3 to 4 days of incubation. The second colony type appears up to 8 days later within the zone of inhibition defining the susceptible type. Subculture and susceptibility testing of the resistant colonies yield uniformly resistant cultures, whereas the susceptible phenotype recapitulates the original phenotype with both the resistant and susceptible colonies.

While antibiotics are generally less active against *B. parapertussis* than against *B. pertussis* (53), *B. parapertussis* is susceptible to macrolides, fluoroquinolones, and SXT (39, 69). *B. bronchiseptica* and other *Bordetella* species generally have antimicrobial susceptibility profiles similar to those of other nonfermentative gram-negative bacilli.

Antibiotic susceptibility testing of *B. pertussis* is not standardized. Reported methods include the E test (AB Biodisk, Solna, Sweden), agar dilution, and disk diffusion using a 15-μg erythromycin disk (12, 37, 41, 51). Agar dilution has been performed with Mueller-Hinton agar supplemented with 5% horse blood (41), as well as BG agar containing 20% horse blood (37). RL agar without cephalexin is commonly used for the disk diffusion and E-test methods (37, 55). In most studies, agar dilution has served as the reference method; erythromycin MICs for 47 susceptible isolates were ≤12 μg/ml (37). It is recommended that strains determined to be nonsusceptible by disk diffusion also be tested by agar dilution (12). Studies have demonstrated good agreement among diffusion tests and agar dilution for determining erythromycin resistance in *B. pertussis* (37, 51). Less agreement was observed when testing SXT (37).

EVALUATION AND INTERPRETATION OF RESULTS

The diagnosis of pertussis can be challenging, given the frequent atypical presentation and the shortcomings of laboratory tests. Indeed, no single laboratory test can be considered a perfect diagnostic standard. While culture is virtually 100% specific, its sensitivity is often low due to poorly collected specimens, long specimen transport time, and patient factors such as duration of symptoms and prior antibiotic treatment.

Nucleic acid amplification methods such as PCR generally offer greater sensitivity than does culture. PCR has frequently been shown to provide the specific diagnosis of pertussis when culture is negative. The major shortcomings of nucleic acid amplification methods are the potential for false-positive results due to contamination, the lack of standardization among assays, and the interpretation of a positive result for *B. pertussis* DNA in the absence of a positive culture. While the combination of a positive PCR result and a negative culture result for the same patient can reflect the greater sensitivity of PCR, there are situations when a positive PCR result alone may not have clinical or public health relevance. Therefore, positive PCR results must be interpreted in conjunction with patient symptoms, treatment status, and epidemiological factors. Culture, serology, and, to a greater extent, PCR have shown that asymptomatic *B. pertussis* infections occur (35, 59). In one study, 92% of preschool-aged children with positive PCR results remained free of symptoms during a 6-week follow-up period (35). The authors attributed this to protective immunity. Comparatively, only one-third of older, school-age children remained asymptomatic throughout the follow-up period. During pertussis outbreaks, laboratories may be pressured to test specimens from asymptomatic contacts of patients. In fact, while these individuals may share a day care center or school classroom with a patient, they often do not meet the criteria for exposure to *B. pertussis*. Positive laboratory results (usually by the sensitive PCR test) for these asymptomatic persons confound treatment and outbreak response decisions. Given the general belief that a long-lasting carrier state for pertussis does not exist, PCR-positive asymptomatic persons are unlikely to contribute significantly, if at all, to the spread of pertussis.

Serology has the potential to contribute substantially to the diagnosis of pertussis, when standardized tests and interpretive criteria that reliably diagnose recent infections in vaccinated populations are available. Interpretive criteria for a single serum specimen will have more clinical utility than those that require paired sera. For the optimal use and interpretation of serology and other tests for pertussis, the laboratory must have information on the patient's symptoms, antibiotic treatment, exposure to other ill persons, vaccination status, and age and on the level of disease activity in the community.

REFERENCES

1. **Archambault, D., P. Rondeau, P. Martin, and B. R. Brodeur.** 1991. Characterization and comparative bactericidal activity of monoclonal antibodies to *Bordetella pertussis* lipooligosaccharide A. *J. Gen. Microbiol.* **137:**905–911.
2. **Bartkus, J. M., B. A. Juni, K. Ehresmann, C. A. Miller, G. N. Sanden, P. K. Cassiday, M. Saubolle, B. Lee, J. Long, A. R. Harrison, Jr., and J. M. Besser.** 2003. Identification of a mutation associated with erythromycin resistance in *Bordetella pertussis:* implications for surveillance of antimicrobial resistance. *J. Clin. Microbiol.* **41:**1167–1172.

3. **Bass, J. W.** 1986. Erythromycin for treatment and prevention of pertussis. *Pediatr. Infect. Dis. J.* **5:**154–157.
4. **Baughtman, A. L., K. Bisgard, K. M. Edwards, D. Guris, M. D. Decker, K. Holland, B. D. Meade, and F. Lynn.** 2004. Establishment of diagnostic cutoff points for levels of serum antibodies to pertussis toxin, filamentous hemagglutinin, and fimbrae in adolescents and adults in the United States. *Clin. Diagn. Lab. Immunol.* **11:**1054–1053.
5. **Bergey, D. H., F. C. Harrison, R. S. Breed, B. W. Hammer, and F. M. Huntoon.** 1984. Genus *Bordetella*, p. 388–393. *In* N. R. Krieg and J. G. Holt (ed.), *Bergey's Manual of Determinative Bacteriology*, vol. 1. The Williams and Wilkins Co., Baltimore, Md.
6. **Binns, S. H., A. J. Speakman, S. Dawson, M. Bennett, R. M. Gaskell, and C. A. Hart.** 1998. The use of pulsed-field gel electrophoresis to examine the epidemiology of *Bordetella bronchiseptica* isolated from cats and other species. *Epidemiol. Infect.* **120:**201–208.
7. **Bisgard, K. M., F. B. Pascual, K. R. Ehresmann, C. A. Miller, C. Cianfini, C. E. Jennings, C. A. Rebmann, J. Gabel, S. L. Schauer, and S. M. Lett.** 2004. Infant pertussis: who was the source? *Pediatr. Infect. Dis. J.* **23:**985–989.
8. **Bonhoeffer, J., G. Bar, M. Riffelmann, M. Soler, and U. Heininger.** 2005. The role of *Bordetella* infections in patients with acute exacerbation of chronic bronchitis. *Infection* **33:**13–17.
9. **Bordet, J., and O. Gengou.** 1906. Le microbe de la coqueluche. *Ann. Inst. Pasteur* **20:**731–741.
10. **Campins-Marti, M., H. K. Cheng, K. Forsyth, N. Guiso, S. Halperin, L.-M. Huang, J. Mertsola, G. Oselka, J. Ward, C. H. Wirsing von König, and F. Zepp.** 2002. Recommendations are needed for adolescent and adult pertussis immunization: rationale and strategies for consideration. *Vaccine* **20:**641–646.
11. **Cassiday, P. K., G. N. Sanden, C. Toure Kane, S. M'Boup, and J. M. Barbaree.** 1994. Viability of *Bordetella pertussis* in four suspending solutions at three temperatures. *J. Clin. Microbiol.* **32:**1550–1553.
12. **Centers for Disease Control and Prevention.** 2000. *Guidelines for the Control of Pertussis Outbreaks.* Centers for Disease Control and Prevention, Atlanta, Ga.
13. **Centers for Disease Control and Prevention.** 2004. Fatal case of unsuspected pertussis diagnosed from a blood culture—Minnesota, 2003. *Morb. Mortal. Wkly. Rep.* **53:** 131–132.
14. **Centers for Disease Control and Prevention.** 2005. Outbreaks of pertussis associated with hospitals—Kentucky, Pennsylvania, and Oregon, 2003. *Morb. Mortal. Wkly. Rep.* **54:**67–71.
15. **Cherry, J. D.** 1999. Epidemiological, clinical, and laboratory aspects of pertussis in adults. *Clin. Infect. Dis.* **28:**S112–S117.
16. **Cherry, J. D., E. Grimprel, N. Guiso, U. Heininger, and J. Mertsola.** 2005. Defining pertussis epidemiology. Clinical, microbiologic and serologic perspectives. *Pediatr. Infect. Dis. J.* **24:**S25–S34.
17. **Cloud, J. L., W. Hymas, and K. C. Carroll.** 2002. Impact of nasopharyngeal swab types on detection of *Bordetella pertussis* by PCR and culture. *J. Clin. Microbiol.* **40:**3838–3840.
18. **Coenye, T., J. Goris, T. Spilker, P. Vandamme, and J. J. LiPuma.** 2002. Characterization of unusual bacteria isolated from respiratory secretions of cystic fibrosis patients and description of *Inquilinus limosus* gen. nov., sp. nov. *J. Clin. Microbiol.* **40:**2062–2069.
19. **Cookson, B. T., P. Vandamme, L. C. Carlson, A. M. Larson, J. V. Sheffield, K. Kersters, and D. H. Spach.** 1994. Bacteremia caused by a novel *Bordetella* species, "*B. hinzii.*" *J. Clin. Microbiol.* **32:**2569–2571.
20. **De Melker, H. E., F. G. A. Versteegh, M. A. E. Conyn-van Spaendonck, L. H. Elvers, G. A. M. Berbers, A. van der Zee, and J. F. P. Schellekens.** 2000. Specificity and sensitivity of high levels of immunoglobulin G antibodies against pertussis toxin in a single serum sample for diagnosis of infection with *Bordetella pertussis*. *J. Clin. Microbiol.* **38:**800–806.
21. **De Serres, G., R. Shadmani, B. Duval, N. Boulianne, P. Dery, M. Douville-Fradet, L. Rochette, and S. A. Halperin.** 2000. Morbidity of pertussis in adolescents and adults. *J. Infect. Dis.* **182:**174–179.
22. **Douglas, E., J. G. Coote, R. Parton, and W. McPheat.** 1993. Identification of *Bordetella pertussis* in nasopharyngeal swabs by PCR amplification of a region of the adenylate cyclase gene. *J. Med. Microbiol.* **38:**140–144.
23. **Dworkin, M. S., P. S. Sullivan, S. E. Buskin, R. D. Harrington, J. Olliffe, R. D. MacArthur, and C. E. Lopez.** 1999. *Bordetella bronchiseptica* infection in human immunodeficiency virus-infected patients. *Clin. Infect. Dis.* **28:**1095–1099.
24. **Edelman, K., S. Nikkari, O. Ruuskanen, Q. He, M. Viljanen, and J. Mertsola.** 1996. Detection of *Bordetella pertussis* by polymerase chain reaction and culture in the nasopharynx of erythromycin-treated infants with pertussis. *Pediatr. Infect. Dis. J.* **15:**54–57.
25. **Farrell, D. J., G. Daggard, and T. K. S. Mukkur.** 1999. Nested duplex PCR to detect *Bordetella pertussis* and *Bordetella parapertussis* and its application in diagnosis of pertussis in nonmetropolitan southeast Queensland, Australia. *J. Clin. Microbiol.* **37:**606–610.
26. **Farrell, D. J., M. McKeon, G. Daggard, M. J. Loeffelholz, C. J. Thompson, and T. K. S. Mukkur.** 2000. Rapid-cycle PCR method to detect *Bordetella pertussis* that fulfills all consensus recommendations for use of PCR in diagnosis of pertussis. *J. Clin. Microbiol.* **38:**4499–4502.
27. **Glare, E. M., J. C. Paton, R. R. Premier, A. J. Lawrence, and I. T. Nisbet.** 1990. Analysis of a repetitive DNA sequence from *Bordetella pertussis* and its application to the diagnosis of pertussis using the polymerase chain reaction. *J. Clin. Microbiol.* **28:**1982–1987.
28. **Grimprel, E., P. Begue, I. Anjak, F. Betsou, and N. Guiso.** 1993. Comparison of polymerase chain reaction, culture, and western immunoblot serology for diagnosis of *Bordetella pertussis* infection. *J. Clin. Microbiol.* **31:**2745–2750.
29. **Hagiwara, K., K. Ouchi, N. Tashiro, M. Azuma, and K. Kobayashi.** 1999. An epidemic of a pertussis-like illness caused by *Chlamydia pneumoniae*. *Pediatr. Infect. Dis. J.* **18:**271–275.
30. **Hallander, H. O., J. Gnarpe, H. Gnarpe, and P. Olin.** 1999. *Bordetella pertussis, Bordetella parapertussis, Mycoplasma pneumoniae, Chlamydia pneumoniae* and persistent cough in children. *Scand. J. Infect. Dis.* **31:**281–286.
31. **Hallander, H. O., E. Reizenstein, B. Renemar, G. Rasmuson, L. Mardin, and P. Olin.** 1993. Comparison of nasopharyngeal aspirates with swabs for culture of *Bordetella pertussis*. *J. Clin. Microbiol.* **31:**50–52.
32. **Halperin, S. A., R. Bortolussi, and A. J. Wort.** 1989. Evaluation of culture, immunofluorescence, and serology for the diagnosis of pertussis. *J. Clin. Microbiol.* **27:**752–757.
33. **Halperin, S. A., A. Kasina, and M. Swift.** 1992. Prolonged survival of *Bordetella pertussis* in a simple buffer after nasopharyngeal secretion aspiration. *Can. J. Microbiol.* **38:**1210–1213.
34. **He, Q., J. Mertsola, H. Soini, M. Skurnik, O. Ruuskanen, and M. K. Viljanen.** 1993. Comparison of polymerase chain reaction with culture and enzyme immunoassay for diagnosis of pertussis. *J. Clin. Microbiol.* **31:**642–645.
35. **He, Q., G. Schmidt-Schlapfer, M. Just, H. C. Matter, S. Nikkari, M. K. Viljanen, and J. Mertsola.** 1996. Impact of polymerase chain reaction on clinical pertussis research: Finnish and Swiss experiences. *J. Infect. Dis.* **174:**1288–1295.

36. **Herwegh, S., C. C. Carnoy, F. Wallet, C. Loïez, and R. J. Courcol.** 2005. Development and use of an internal positive control for detection of *Bordetella pertussis* by PCR. *J. Clin. Microbiol.* **48:**2462–2464.
37. **Hill, B. C., C. N. Baker, and F. C. Tenover.** 2000. A simplified method for testing *Bordetella pertussis* for resistance to erythromycin and other antimicrobial agents. *J. Clin. Microbiol.* **38:**1151–1155.
38. **Hoppe, J. E.** 1988. Methods for isolation of *Bordetella pertussis* from patients with whooping cough. *Eur. J. Clin. Microbiol.* **7:**616–620.
39. **Hoppe, J. E., and A. Eichhorn.** 1989. Activity of new macrolides against *Bordetella pertussis* and *Bordetella parapertussis*. *Eur. J. Clin. Microbiol. Infect. Dis.* **8:**653–654.
40. **Hoppe, J. E., U. Halm, H. J. Hagedorn, and A. Kraminer-Hagedorn.** 1989. Comparison of erythromycin ethylsuccinate and co-trimoxazole for treatment of pertussis. *Infection* **17:**227–231.
41. **Hoppe, J. E., and T. Paulus.** 1998. Comparison of three media for agar dilution susceptibility testing of *Bordetella pertussis* using six isolates. *Eur. J. Clin. Microbiol. Infect. Dis.* **17:**391–393.
42. **Hoppe, J. E., E. Rahimi-Galougahi, and G. Seibert.** 1996. In vitro susceptibilities of *Bordetella pertussis* and *Bordetella parapertussis* to four fluoroquinolones (levofloxacin, d-ofloxacin, ofloxacin, and ciprofloxacin), cefpirome, and meropenem. *Antimicrob. Agents Chemother.* **40:**807–808.
43. **Hoppe, J. E., and M. Schlagenhauf.** 1989. Comparison of three kinds of blood and two incubation atmospheres for cultivation of *Bordetella pertussis* on charcoal agar. *J. Clin. Microbiol.* **27:**2115–2117.
44. **Hoppe, J. E., and A. Weiss.** 1987. Recovery of *Bordetella pertussis* from four kinds of swabs. *Eur. J. Clin. Microbiol.* **6:**203–205.
45. **Houard, S., C. Hackel, A. Herzog, and A. Bollen.** 1989. Specific identification of *Bordetella pertussis* by the polymerase chain reaction. *Res. Microbiol.* **140:**477–487.
46. **Hozbor, D., F. Fouque, and N. Guiso.** 1999. Detection of *Bordetella bronchiseptica* by the polymerase chain reaction. *Res. Microbiol.* **150:**333–341.
47. **Janda, W. M., E. Santos, J. Stevens, D. Celig, L. Terrile, and P. C. Schreckenberger.** 1994. Unexpected isolation of *Bordetella pertussis* from a blood culture. *J. Clin. Microbiol.* **32:**2851–2853.
48. **Kattar, M. M., J. F. Chavez, A. P. Limaye, S. L. Rassoulian-Barrett, S. L. Yarfitz, L. C. Carlson, Y. Houze, S. Swanzy, B. L. Wood, and B. T. Cookson.** 2000. Application of 16S rRNA gene sequencing to identify *Bordetella hinzii* as the causative agent of fatal septicemia. *J. Clin. Microbiol.* **38:**789–794.
49. **Katzko, G., M. Hofmeister, and D. Church.** 1996. Extended incubation of culture plates improves recovery of *Bordetella* spp. *J. Clin. Microbiol.* **34:**1563–1564.
50. **Ko, K. S., K. R. Peck, W. S. Oh, N. Y. Lee, J. H. Lee, and J. H. Song.** 2005. New species of *Bordetella*, *Bordetella ansorpii* sp. nov., isolated from the purulent exudate of an epidermal cyst. *J. Clin. Microbiol.* **43:**2516–2519.
51. **Korgenski, E. K., and J. A. Daly.** 1997. Surveillance and detection of erythromycin resistance in *Bordetella pertussis* isolates recovered from a pediatric population in the Intermountain West region of the United States. *J. Clin. Microbiol.* **35:**2989–2991.
52. **Kosters, K., M. Riffelmann, B. Dohrn, and C. H. von Konig.** 2000. Comparison of five commercial enzyme-linked immunosorbent assays for detection of antibodies to *Bordetella pertussis*. *Clin. Diagn. Lab. Immunol.* **7:**422–426.
53. **Kurzynski, T. A., D. M. Boehm, J. A. Rott-Petri, R. F. Schell, and P. E. Allison.** 1988. Antimicrobial susceptibilities of *Bordetella* species isolated in a multicenter pertussis surveillance project. *Antimicrob. Agents Chemother.* **32:**137–140.
54. **Kurzynski, T. A., D. M. Boehm, J. A. Rott-Petri, R. F. Schell, and P. E. Allison.** 1988. Comparison of modified Bordet-Gengou and modified Regan-Lowe media for the isolation of *Bordetella pertussis* and *Bordetella parapertussis*. *J. Clin. Microbiol.* **26:**2661–2663.
55. **Lewis, K., M. A. Saubolle, F. C. Tenover, M. F. Rudinsky, S. D. Barbour, and J. D. Cherry.** 1995. Pertussis caused by an erythromycin-resistant strain of *Bordetella pertussis*. *Pediatr. Infect. Dis. J.* **14:**388–391.
56. **Linnemann, C. C., and E. B. Perry.** 1977. *Bordetella parapertussis*. Recent experience and a review of the literature. *Am. J. Dis. Child.* **131:**560–563.
57. **Loeffelholz, M. J., C. J. Thompson, K. S. Long, and M. J. R. Gilchrist.** 1999. Comparison of PCR, culture, and direct fluorescent-antibody testing for detection of *Bordetella pertussis*. *J. Clin. Microbiol.* **37:**2872–2876.
58. **Loeffelholz, M. J., C. J. Thompson, K. S. Long, and M. J. R. Gilchrist.** 2000. Detection of *Bordetella holmesii* using *Bordetella pertussis* IS*481* PCR assay. *J. Clin. Microbiol.* **38:**467.
59. **Long, S. S., C. J. Welkon, and J. L. Clark.** 1990. Widespread silent transmission of pertussis in families: antibody correlates of infection and symptomatology. *J. Infect. Dis.* **161:**480–486.
60. **Marcon, M. J., A. C. Hamoudi, H. J. Cannon, and M. M. Hribar.** 1987. Comparison of throat and nasopharyngeal swab specimens for culture diagnosis of *Bordetella pertussis* infection. *J. Clin. Microbiol.* **25:**1109–1110.
61. **Mattoo, S., and J. D. Cherry.** 2005. Molecular pathogenesis, epidemiology, and clinical manifestations of respiratory infections due to *Bordetella pertussis* and other *Bordetella* species. *Clin. Microbiol. Rev.* **18:**326–382.
62. **Mazengia, E., E. A. Silva, J. A. Peppe, R. Timperi, and H. George.** 2000. Recovery of *Bordetella holmesii* from patients with pertussis-like symptoms: use of pulsed-field gel electrophoresis to characterize circulating strains. *J. Clin. Microbiol.* **38:**2330–2333.
63. **McNicol, P., S. M Giercke, M. Gray, D. Martin, B. Brodeur, M. S. Peppler, T. Williams, and G. Hammond.** 1995. Evaluation and validation of a monoclonal immunofluorescent reagent for direct detection of *Bordetella pertussis*. *J. Clin. Microbiol.* **33:**2868–2871.
64. **Mink, C. M., J. D. Cherry, P. Christenson, K. Lewis, E. Pineda, D. Shlian, J. A. Dawson, and D. A. Blumber.** 1992. A search for *Bordetella pertussis* infection in university students. *Clin. Infect. Dis.* **14:**464–471.
65. **Moissenet, D., M. Valcin, V. Marchand, E. Grimprel, P. Begue, A. Garbarg-Chenon, and H. Vu-Thien.** 1996. Comparative DNA analysis of *Bordetella pertussis* clinical isolates by pulsed-field gel electrophoresis, randomly amplified polymorphism DNA, and ERIC polymerase chain reaction. *FEMS Microbiol. Lett.* **143:**127–132.
66. **Mooi, F. R., H. van Oirschot, K. Heuvelman, H. G. van der Heide, W. Gaastra, and R. J. Willems.** 1998. Polymorphism in the *Bordetella pertussis* virulence factors P. 69/pertactin and pertussis toxin in The Netherlands: temporal trends and evidence for vaccine-driven evolution. *Infect. Immun.* **66:**670–675.
67. **Mooi, F. R., H. Hallander, C. H. Wirsing von Konig, B. Hoet, and N. Guiso.** 2000. Epidemiological typing of *Bordetella pertussis* isolates: recommendations for a standard methodology. *Eur. J. Clin. Microbiol. Infect. Dis.* **19:**174–181.
68. **Morrill, W. E., J. M. Barbaree, B. S. Fields, G. N. Sanden, and W. T. Martin.** 1988. Effects of transport temperature and medium on recovery of *Bordetella pertussis* from nasopharyngeal swabs. *J. Clin. Microbiol.* **26:**1814–1817.
69. **Mortensen, J. E., and G. L. Rodgers.** 2000. In vitro activity of gemifloxacin and other antimicrobial agents against isolates of *Bordetella pertussis* and *Bordetella parapertussis*. *J. Antimicrob. Chemother.* **45:**47–49.

70. **Müller, F.-M. C., J. E. Hoppe, and C.-H. Wirsing von König.** 1997. Laboratory diagnosis of pertussis: state of the art in 1997. *J. Clin. Microbiol.* **35:**2435–2443.
71. **Ner, Z., L. A. Ross, M. V. Horn, T. G. Keens, E. F. MacLaughlin, V. A. Starnes, and M. S. Woo.** 2003. *Bordetella bronchiseptica* infection in pediatric lung transplant recipients. *Pediatr. Transplant.* **7:**413–417.
72. **Parkhill, J., M. Sebaihia, A. Preston, et al.** 2003. Comparative analysis of the genome sequences of *Bordetella pertussis*, *Bordetella parapertussis* and *Bordetella bronchiseptica*. *Nat. Genet.* **35:**32–40.
73. **Pichichero, M. E., M. A. Deloria, M. B. Rennels, E. L. Anderson, K. M. Edwards, M. D. Decker, J. A. Englund, M. C. Steinhoff, A. Deforest, and B. D. Meade.** 1997. A safety and immunogenicity comparison of 12 acellular pertussis vaccines and one whole-cell pertussis vaccine given as a fourth dose in 15- to 20-month-old children. *Pediatrics* **100:**772–788.
74. **Porter, J. F., K. Connor, and W. Donachie.** 1996. Differentiation between human and ovine isolates of *Bordetella parapertussis* using pulsed-field gel electrophoresis. *FEMS Microbiol. Lett.* **135:**131–135.
75. **Raffel, T. R., K. B. Register, S. A. Marks, and L. Temple.** 2002. Prevalence of *Bordetella avium* infection in selected wild and domesticated birds in the eastern USA. *J. Wildl. Dis.* **38:**40–46.
76. **Regan, J., and F. Lowe.** 1977. Enrichment medium for the isolation of *Bordetella*. *J. Clin. Microbiol.* **6:**303–309.
77. **Register, K. B., A. Boisvert, and M. R. Ackermann.** 1997. Use of ribotyping to distinguish *Bordetella bronchiseptica* isolates. *Int. J. Syst. Bacteriol.* **47:**678–683.
78. **Register, K. B., R. E. Sacco, and G. E. Nordholm.** 2003. Comparison of ribotyping and restriction enzyme analysis for inter- and intraspecies discrimination of *Bordetella avium* and *Bordetella hinzii*. *J. Clin. Microbiol.* **41:**1512–1519.
79. **Reizenstein, E., L. Lindberg, R. Möllby, and H. O. Hallander.** 1996. Validation of nested *Bordetella* PCR in pertussis vaccine trial. *J. Clin. Microbiol.* **34:**810–815.
80. **Riffelmann, M., C. H. Wirsing von König, V. Caro, N. Guiso, and the Pertussis PCR Consensus Group.** 2005. Nucleic acid amplification tests for diagnosis of *Bordetella* infections. *J. Clin. Microbiol.* **43:**4925–4929.
81. **Russel, F. M., J. M. Davis, M. J. Whipp, P. H. Janssen, P. B. Ward, J. R. Vyas, M. Starr, S. M. Sawyer, and N. Curtis.** 2001. Severe *Bordetella holmesii* infection in a previously healthy adolescent confirmed by gene sequence analysis. *Clin. Infect. Dis.* **33:**129–130.
82. **Sacco, R. E., K. B. Register, and G. E. Nordholm.** 2000. Restriction endonuclease analysis discriminates *Bordetella bronchiseptica* isolates. *J. Clin. Microbiol.* **38:**4387–4393.
83. **Schlapfer, G., H. P. Senn, R. Berger, and M. Just.** 1993. Use of the polymerase chain reaction to detect *Bordetella pertussis* in patients with mild or atypical symptoms of infection. *Eur. J. Clin. Microbiol. Infect. Dis.* **12:**459–463.
84. **Schouls, L. M., H. G. van der Heide, L. Vauterin, P. Vauterin, and F. R. Mooi.** 2004. Multiple-locus variable-number tandem repeat analysis of Dutch *Bordetella pertussis* strains reveals rapid genetic changes with clonal expansion during the late 1990s. *J. Bacteriol.* **186:** 5496–5505.
85. **Shepard, C. W., M. I. Daneshvar, R. M. Kaiser, D. A. Ashford, D. Lonsway, J. B. Patel, R. E. Morey, J. G. Jordan, R. S. Weyant, and M. Fischer.** 2004. *Bordetella holmesii* bacteremia: a newly recognized clinical entity among asplenic patients. *Clin. Infect. Dis.* **38:**799–804.
86. **Simondon, F., I. Iteman, M. P. Preziosi, A. Yam, and N. Guiso.** 1998. Evaluation of an immunoglobulin G enzyme-linked immunosorbent assay for pertussis toxin and filamentous hemagglutinin in diagnosis of pertussis in Senegal. *Clin. Diagn. Lab. Immunol.* **5:**130–134.
87. **Strebel, P., J. Nordin, K. Edwards, J. Hunt, J. Besser, S. Burns, G. Amundson, A. Baughman, and W. Wattigney.** 2001. Population-based incidence of pertussis among adolescents and adults, Minnesota, 1995–1996. *J. Infect. Dis.* **183:**1353–1359.
88. **Tang, Y. W., M. K. Hopkins, C. P. Kolbert, P. A. Hartley, P. J. Severance, and D. H. Persing.** 1998. *Bordetella holmesii*-like organisms associated with septicemia, endocarditis, and respiratory failure. *Clin. Infect. Dis.* **26:** 389–392.
89. **Tilley, P. A., M. V. Kanchana, I. Knight, J. Blondeau, N. Antonishyn, and H. Deneer.** 2000. Detection of *Bordetella pertussis* in a clinical laboratory by culture, polymerase chain reaction, and direct fluorescent antibody; accuracy, and cost. *Diagn. Microbiol. Infect. Dis.* **37:**17–23.
90. **Vandamme, P., M. Heyndrickx, M. Vancanneyt, B. Hoste, P. De Vos, E. Falsen, K. Kersters, and K.-H. Hinz.** 1996. *Bordetella trematum* sp. nov., isolated from wounds and ear infections in humans, and reassessment of *Alcaligenes denitrificans* Rüger and Tan 1983. *Int. J. Syst. Bacteriol.* **46:**849–858.
91. **van der Zee, A., C. Agterberg, M. Peeters, F. Mooi, and J. Schellekens.** 1996. A clinical validation of *Bordetella pertussis* and *Bordetella parapertussis* polymerase chain reaction: comparison with culture and serology using samples from patients with suspected whooping cough from a highly immunized population. *J. Infect. Dis.* **174:**89–96.
92. **van der Zee, A., C. Agterberg, M. Peeters, J. Schellekens, and F. R. Mooi.** 1993. Polymerase chain reaction assay for pertussis: simultaneous detection and discrimination of *Bordetella pertussis* and *Bordetella parapertussis*. *J. Clin. Microbiol.* **31:**2134–2140.
93. **van der Zee, A., H. Groenendijk, M. Peeters, and F. R. Mooi.** 1996. The differentiation of *Bordetella parapertussis* and *Bordetella bronchiseptica* from humans and animals as determined by DNA polymorphism mediated by two different insertion sequence elements suggests their phylogenetic relationship. *Int. J. Syst. Bacteriol.* **46:**640–647.
94. **Viejo, G., P. de la Iglesia, L. Otero, M. I. Blanco, B. Gomez, D. De Miquel, A. Del Valle, and B. De la Fuente.** 2002. *Bordetella bronchiseptica* pleural infection in a patient with AIDS. *Scand. J. Infect. Dis.* **34:**628–629.
95. **Vincent, J. M., J. D. Cherry, W. F. Nauschuetz, A. Lipton, C. M. Ono, C. N. Costello, L. K. Sakaguchi, G. Hsue, L. A. Jackson, R. Tachdjian, P. A. Cotter, and J. A. Gornbein.** 2000. Prolonged afebrile nonproductive cough illnesses in American soldiers in Korea: a serological search for causation. *Clin. Infect. Dis.* **30:**534–539.
96. **von Wintzingerode, F., A. Schattke, R. A. Siddiqui, U. Rosick, U. B. Gobel, and R. Gross.** 2001. *Bordetella petrii* sp. nov., isolated from an anaerobic bioreactor, and emended description of the genus *Bordetella*. *Int. J. Syst. Bacteriol.* **51:**1257–1265.
97. **Wadowsky, R. M., S. Laus, T. Libert, S. J. States, and G. D. Ehrlich.** 1994. Inhibition of PCR-based assay for *Bordetella pertussis* by using calcium alginate fiber and aluminum shaft components of a nasopharyngeal swab. *J. Clin. Microbiol.* **32:**1054–1057.
98. **Wadowsky, R. M., R. H. Michaels, T. Libert, L. A. Kingsley, and G. D. Ehrlich.** 1996. Multiplex PCR-based assay for detection of *Bordetella pertussis* in nasopharyngeal swab specimens. *J. Clin. Microbiol.* **34:**2645–2649.
99. **Wallet, F., T. Perez, S. Armand, B. Wallaert, and R. J. Courcol.** 2002. Pneumonia due to *Bordetella bronchiseptica* in a cystic fibrosis patient: 16S rRNA sequencing for diagnosis confirmation. *J. Clin. Microbiol.* **40:**2300–2301.
100. **Wilson, K. E., P. K. Cassiday, T. Popovic, and G. N. Sanden.** 2002. *Bordetella pertussis* isolates with a heterogeneous phenotype for erythromycin resistance. *J. Clin. Microbiol.* **40:**2942–2944.

101. **Wirsing von König, C. H., D. Gounis, S. Laukamp, H. Bogaerts, and H. J. Schmitt.** 1999. Evaluation of a single-sample serological technique for diagnosing pertussis in unvaccinated children. *Eur. J. Clin. Microbiol. Infect. Dis.* **18:**341–345.
102. **Woolfrey, B. F., and J. A. Moody.** 1991. Human infections associated with *Bordetella bronchiseptica*. *Clin. Microbiol. Rev.* **4:**243–255.
103. **Yih, W. K., E. A. Silva, J. Ida, N. Harrington, S. M. Lett, and H. George.** 1999. *Bordetella holmesii*-like organisms isolated from Massachusetts patients with pertussis-like symptoms. *Emerg. Infect. Dis.* **5:**441–443.
104. **Yuk, M. H., U. Heininger, G. Martinez de Tejada, and J. F. Miller.** 1998. Human but not ovine isolates of *Bordetella parapertussis* are highly clonal as determined by PCR-based RAPD fingerprinting. *Infection* **26:**270–273.

Francisella and *Brucella**

DAVID LINDQUIST, MAY C. CHU, AND WILL S. PROBERT

52

Francisella and *Brucella*, while not closely related taxonomically, have been traditionally linked in the mind of the bacteriologist. Both are zoonotic agents capable of producing severe disease in humans. In the laboratory, they are seen as very small to tiny gram-negative coccobacilli that do not seem to grow particularly well and are not particularly active biochemically. The two genera are apt to show cross-reactivity with each other in agglutination-based serologic tests (13, 103, 178). They share a reputation for frequently causing laboratory-acquired infections (50). Finally, *Francisella tularensis*, *Brucella melitensis*, *B. suis*, and *B. abortus* are all considered to be potential bioterrorism agents (68, 138; chapter 9 of this Manual). This circumstance has arguably led to a heightened interest in these agents and has helped prompt development of tests, particularly rapid tests, for their detection, identification, and further characterization.

In the United States, *F. tularensis* and three species of *Brucella*, *B. melitensis*, *B. suis*, and *B. abortus*, are classified as select agents. To transfer, receive, or possess these agents, laboratories must be registered both with the Centers for Disease Control and Prevention (CDC) and with the Animal and Plant Health Inspection Service (APHIS) of the U.S. Department of Agriculture. The registration process includes a U.S. Department of Justice investigation of all personnel having access to select agents. Clinical laboratories are exempt from the registration requirement provided that within 7 calendar days of identifying one of these agents, they transfer it to a registered entity and/or destroy the agent on site. Laboratories identifying an organism as *F. tularensis* or *B. melitensis* are required to report this finding immediately to APHIS or the CDC. The identification of *B. abortus* or *B. suis* is to be reported within 7 calendar days by using the appropriate form. Report forms, contact information, laboratory registration information, and pertinent citations of the U.S. Federal Code may be found at http://www.cdc.gov/od/sap.

FRANCISELLA

Taxonomy

Tularemia, a zoonosis affecting a wide range of animals and humans, is the disease caused by infection with members of the genus *Francisella*. Tularemia was described in detail in the first part of the 20th century (67, 105). The story of its discovery and the elucidation of its pathology and epidemiology are essentially American (159). Several recent publications have reviewed the history and description of the genus *Francisella* (54, 143). The first article describing the etiologic agent of tularemia was published in 1912 by McCoy and Chapin, who isolated the agent from a ground squirrel die-off in Tulare County in California (105). Francis, for whom the genus is named, recognized and confirmed that a number of diverse and epidemiologically distinct clinical entities were really one disease, and he proposed the name "tularemia" to describe the disease in humans (67). In addition to *F. tularensis*, two other species, both first isolated in North America, are included as members of the family *Francisellaceae*. *F. novicida* was recovered in 1951 from water. *F. philomiragia* was isolated in 1969 from muskrats and the surrounding water environment (147). These two species are infrequently isolated and rarely implicated in clinical disease. The genus members have been separated into two pathogenic groups: one that causes serious illness in humans and is often lethal for animals, and one that is considered to be of lesser virulence for humans and animals (84, 89, 147). The pathogenic members of this genus exist as intracellular parasites; therefore, antibiotic therapy may have to be extended in order to eliminate the infection. All genus members are susceptible to aminoglycosides and tetracyclines. It is the widespread epizootic nature of tularemia, its potentially severe and fatal forms in humans, its reputation as a laboratory hazard, and its potential use as a biological warfare agent that have given tularemia its notoriety. *F. tularensis* has been developed as a biological weapon, and projections about its impact, if used as a weapon in an urban setting, depict a scenario devastating to public health and to the economy of health services (49).

The species of *Francisella* share some biochemical activities, a high degree of DNA relatedness (54, 63, 64, 94), and a unique cellular fatty acid (CFA) profile (83, 169). Subspecies designations continue to be in transition as new information about host relationships, geographic origin, virulence, and phenotypic, biochemical, and genetic features is revealed. Four subspecies of *F. tularensis* are listed in the most recent edition of *Bergey's Manual of Systematic Bacteriology* (147): *F. tularensis* subsp. *tularensis* (type A), *F. tularensis* subsp. *holarctica* (type B; formerly known as *F. tularensis* subsp.

*This chapter contains information presented in chapter 51 by May C. Chu and Robbin S. Weyant in the eighth edition of this Manual.

palaearctica), *F. tularensis* subsp. *mediasiatica*, and *F. tularensis* subsp. *novicida*. The last subspecies, a reclassification of *F. novicida*, does not yet have standing in taxonomy. In anticipation of its becoming validated and coming into common usage, *F. tularensis* subsp. *novicida* will be used in this chapter. The members of this genus have been associated with the natural outdoor environment, small mammals, and arthropods. *Wolbachia persica*, a bacterium isolated from *Argas persicus* ticks and two additional tick endosymbionts, from *Dermacentor andersoni* and *Ornithodoros moubata*, have 16S rRNA sequence similarity to *Francisellaceae* (64, 147).

Description of the Genus

The genus *Francisella* comprises tiny gram-negative coccobacilli that can be distinguished from other families by several features (Table 1). Members of the genus take up Gram's counterstain (safranin) poorly; they are strict aerobes, weakly catalase positive, nonmotile, and non-spore forming; and they react with a limited number of carbohydrates (Table 2). Only a few sugars (glucose, maltose, sucrose, and glycerol) are utilized by most of the members of the genus. Acid is produced without gas. Unique fatty acids are associated with the genus (Table 1) (83, 147, 169). For most species, in vitro growth is enhanced by sulfhydryl supplementation. The organisms in this genus show >98% 16S rRNA sequence similarity (147). Rare single plasmids have been associated with individual isolates of *F. tularensis* subsp. *holarctica* and *F. tularensis* subsp. *novicida* and have been found in two strains of *F. philomiragia* (M. Chu, unpublished observation).

Only a few key differences separate the two species of *Francisella* (Table 2). *F. philomiragia* is more biochemically reactive than *F. tularensis*; it differs also by its ability to ferment maltose, and it is oxidase positive using Kovács's modification. Subspecies differentiation is less distinctive; single biochemical differences in glycerol fermentation and glucose utilization are used to define the biovars. *F. tularensis* subsp. *tularensis*, designated type A, is the most virulent of the subspecies, with a 50% lethal dose of <10 cells for laboratory mice and rabbits (84, 89, 119). *F. tularensis* subsp. *tularensis* and *F. tularensis* subsp. *mediasiatica* have the greatest similarity in that they utilize glycerol (2, 54), possess citrulline ureidase activity (141, 147), and along with *F. tularensis* subsp. *novicida*, share the same 16S rRNA signature nucleotide sequence (64, 141). *F. tularensis* subsp. *mediasiatica* differs by its inability to utilize glucose and its comparatively low virulence. Type B organisms (*F. tularensis* subsp. *holarctica*) may be differentiated by their inability to utilize glycerol, an absence of citrulline ureidase activity, and the presence of a unique 16S rRNA signature sequence. *F. tularensis* subsp. *holarctica* is of intermediate virulence, with a 50% lethal dose of <1,000 cells for laboratory animals (84, 89). *F. tularensis* subsp. *novicida* can be distinguished from the other subspecies by its ability to grow independently of cysteine supplementation and by its comparatively large vegetative cell size. *F. tularensis* subsp. *novicida* is considered to be of low virulence, like *F. tularensis* subsp. *mediasiatica* and *F. philomiragia*, but otherwise shares genetic characteristics with *F. tularensis* subsp. *tularensis* (147).

Epidemiology and Transmission

Francisellaceae are distributed widely within the Northern Hemisphere (Holarctic region) in a variety of natural habitats, from the Arctic Circle south to about latitude 20°N (84). Australian and Spanish isolates recovered from patients have been identified as *F. tularensis* subsp. *novicida* by using molecular techniques to augment the standard diagnostic tests (171; Chu, unpublished). *F. philomiragia* has been recovered from a patient with a history of travel to Turkey (69). Turkey has recently reported a waterborne outbreak in its western Black Sea region, an illustration of the continued appearance or reemergence of tularemia in the zone of endemicity (79).

Thus, as techniques and molecular tools are developed, it is likely that we can expect recovery of *F. tularensis*-like organisms from regions beyond the Northern Hemisphere. Tularemia is associated with a wide range of habitats and hosts, with more than 100 species of wild animals, birds, and arthropod vectors being involved (84, 90, 120). Habitats where the *Lagomorpha* (*Sylvilagus* [rabbits], *Lepus* [hares], and *Oryctolagus* [Old World hares]) and the *Rodentia* (water voles, muskrats, lemmings, voles, and beavers) thrive are important in maintaining tularemia enzootic foci (84, 90, 120, 179). Biting arthropod vectors, primarily tabanid flies (*Chrysops* and *Tabanus*), ticks (*Dermacentor*, *Ixodes*, and *Amblyomma*), and mosquitoes (*Culicidae* in Europe and Russia), are implicated in the mechanical transmission of tularemia (53). Amebas also may carry viable *F. tularensis* cells and keep the bacteria viable in water (1). Because of the presence of *Francisella* in the natural environment, infections with *Francisella* are usually acquired in association with outdoor activities via contact with contaminated air, water, soil, vegetation, or sick or dead animals and from infective insect bites.

F. tularensis subsp. *tularensis*, the most virulent member of the genus, has been thought to occur only in North America, where it has been most closely associated with infection in lagomorphs and humans. Though *F. tularensis* subsp. *tularensis* has been recovered from mites and fleas in Europe, no human infection has been found there (159). In contrast, infection with *F. tularensis* subsp. *holarctica* is less virulent; it has a much wider distribution, in both the Old and New Worlds, and is associated with a greater variety of animals, primarily hares and rodents, and with contaminated environmental source outbreaks. *F. tularensis* subsp. *mediasiatica* is found only in circumscribed geographical regions in Kazakhstan and Turkmenistan and has been isolated from hares and ticks but not from humans (147). *F. tularensis* subsp. *novicida* has been found primarily in North America. It has also been found in Australia (171) and in Spain. Of the fewer than 20 known isolates of *F. philomiragia*, most have been from North America, with three single incidences reported from Central and Eastern Europe and Australia.

Since the 1940s, when several thousand cases annually were sometimes reported, the incidence of reported tularemia cases in the United States has steadily declined to 100 to 200 cases each year. All states except Hawaii have reported cases. From 1995 through 1999, tularemia was removed from the nationally notifiable disease list, but it was reinstated in 2000 because of concerns about its potential use as a bioterrorism agent. Despite its absence from the nationally notifiable disease list between 1995 and 1999, the number of cases reported annually to the CDC did not differ substantially from those in previous years. A total of 1,368 human cases were reported to the CDC between 1990 and 2000 (34).

The epidemiology of tularemia in the United States has not changed significantly in the past several decades. Most cases occur in south central and western states. It remains a rural disease. Most patients acquire tularemia from tick or deer fly bites, from contact with infected animals (e.g., by skinning rabbits), or as recently reported, from contact with

TABLE 1 Presumptive differentiation of *Francisella* and *Brucella* from similar gram-negative genera[a]

Test	*F. tularensis*	*Brucella* spp.	*Bartonella* spp.[b]	*Acinetobacter* spp.	*Psychrobacter phenylpyruvicus*[c]	*Oligella ureolytica*	*Bordetella bronchiseptica*	*Haemophilus* spp.[d]	*Ochrobactrum anthropi*
Oxidase	−	+	−	−	+	+	+	v	+
Urease	−	+	−	−	+	+	+	v	+
Gram stain morphology	Very tiny ccb	Tiny ccb	Thin rod	Broad ccb	Broad ccb	Small to tiny ccb	Thin rod	Small ccb	Medium rod
Specimen source	Ulcer, wound, blood, aspirates	Blood, bone marrow	Blood, bone marrow, lymph node	v	v	Urinary tract	v	Blood, cerebrospinal fluid, other	v
X and/or V factor requirement	−	−	−[e]	−	−	−	−	+	−
Cysteine enhancement	+	−	−	−	−	−	−	−	−
Motility	−	−	−	−	−	+[f]	+	−	+
Major CFA[g]	10:0; 14:0; 16:0; 3-OH-16:0; 18:1ω9c; 3-OH-18:0	16:0; 18:1ω7c; 18:0; 19:0cyc[h]	16:0; 17:0; 18:1ω7c	2-OH-12:0; 3-OH-12:0; 16:1ω7c; 16:0; 18:1ω9c	3-OH-12:0; 16:1ω7c; 16:0; 18:2; 18:1ω9c	3-OH-14:0; 16:0; 3-OH-16:0; 18:1ω7c	2-OH-12:0; 3-OH-14:0; 16:1ω7c; 16:0; 17:0cyc	14:0; 3-OH-14:0; 16:1ω7c; 16:0	18:1ω7c; 18:0; 19:0cyc; 2-OH-19:0cyc

[a] +, greater than or equal to 90% positive; −, less than or equal to 10% positive; v, variable (11 to 89% positive); ccb, coccobacilli. Data are from reference 169.

[b] Does not include *Bartonella bacilliformis*, which is the only motile species.

[c] Formerly *Moraxella phenylpyruvica*.

[d] *Haemophilus* spp. requiring X and V factors or V factor only.

[e] While not required, X factor (hemin) enhances growth for many strains.

[f] May be difficult to demonstrate.

[g] The number before the colon indicates the number of carbons; the number after the colon is the number of double bonds; ω indicates the location of the double bond counting from the hydrocarbon end of the carbon chain; OH indicates a hydroxy group at the 2- or 3-position from the carboxyl end; c indicate *cis* isomer; cyc indicates a cyclopropane ring structure. Hydroxy acids listed are at least 2% of the total CFA composition; all others are at least 10%.

[h] *B. canis* lacks 19:0cyc. CFA data for marine mammal strains are not available.

TABLE 2 *Francisella* spp. characteristics

Characteristic	*F. tularensis* subspecies				*F. philomiragia*[c]
	tularensis[a]	*holarctica*[b]	*mediasiatica*	*novicida*[c]	
Gram stain (culture)	Faintly staining, pleomorphic, single, rarely chained, gram-negative coccobacilli	As for subsp. *tularensis*	As for subsp. *tularensis*	As for subsp. *tularensis*	As for subsp. *tularensis*
Cell size (μm)	0.2 by 0.2–0.7	0.2 by 0.2–0.7	0.2 by 0.2–0.7	0.7 by 1.7	0.7 by 1.7
Growth on:					
Standard agar[d]	–	–	–	+	+
CA, 48 h	2–4-mm-diam, raised, gray, smooth, moist, butyrous, entire colonies; usually no agar discoloration	As for subsp. *tularensis*	As for subsp. *tularensis*	As for subsp. *tularensis* but 5 mm in diam	>5-mm-diam, white, smooth, mucoid, entire colonies; no agar discoloration
Cysteine heart blood agar, 48 h	2-mm-diam, pearl-white to ivory colonies with green tint and prominent opalescent sheen; smooth and butyrous; green-yellow discoloration of agar medium	As for subsp. *tularensis*	Not tested	5-mm-diam, colonies with features the same as those of type A and type B	Colonies are >5 mm in diam, creamy white-gray, mucoid, and smooth with purple-tinted opalescent sheen
Requires cystine/cysteine	+	+	+	–	–
Catalase	Weakly +	Weakly +	Weakly +	Weakly +	Weakly +
Oxidase (Kovács)	–	–	–	–	+
Acid from:					
Glucose[e]	+	+	–	+	+
Maltose	+	+	–	V[f]	+
Sucrose	–	–	+	+	V
Glycerol	+	–	+	+	+
Relative virulence (mice)	High	Intermediate	Low	Low	Low
DNA typing					
16S rRNA probe[g]	Type A	Type B	Type A	Type A	Type A
PCR primers[h]	Species specific	Species specific	Species specific	Species specific	Does not react
VNTR and IS probe[i]	Strain specific	Strain specific	Strain specific	Strain specific	Strain specific

[a] Type A, found predominantly in North America and associated with a severe form of disease in humans and rabbits.
[b] Type B, found throughout the Northern Hemisphere and associated with a less severe form of disease in humans; associated with humans and rodents (muskrats, field mice, beaver, voles, and water rats).
[c] Associated with low virulence and infrequently isolated.
[d] Standard bacteriology media: blood, tryptic soy, and brain heart infusion.
[e] Delayed or variable reaction. *F. tularensis* subsp. *mediasiatica* does not ferment glucose.
[f] V, variable or delayed reaction.
[g] Probes that define type A and type B sequences.
[h] PCR primers: Tul-4, T-cell epitope; FopA and p43,000 antigen.
[i] VNTR, variable number of tandem repeats: allelic variation, subspecies and strain specific. IS, insertion element PCR (type B specific) or Southern hybridization pattern (subspecies and strain specific).

pets and zoo animals (6, 36, 82, 87, 106). Cultures recovered in the United States from 1996 to 2001 comprise equal proportions of type A and type B genotypes, and these overwhelmingly predominate. Isolation of *F. tularensis* subsp. *novicida* and *F. philomiragia* is rare.

There is an increasing awareness of unusual occurrences of tularemia in animals and humans. Pet owners, pet owners' family members, and animal care professionals are at risk when handling sick pets. These pets may include both domestic (dogs, cats, and hamsters) and exotic animals (14, 36, 87, 106, 161). Captive prairie dogs caught in the wild have been implicated as well as commercially sold hamsters, monkeys (in monkey colonies), and zoo animals (56, 73, 82, 97, 114, 128, 129, 167). Transport of these animals poses risks to unsuspecting shipping handlers and the public of contracting an unusual and exotic disease, as illustrated by recently reported incidents

(6, 35). Cases of tularemia associated with immunocompromised patients or patients recovering from prosthetic replacement or transplantation surgery have been reported (42, 76, 102, 112, 126, 142). Additional reports on such unusual cases continue, with the recovery of *F. tularensis* subsp. *holarctica* from a patient with metastatic cancer (81) and from a kidney transplant patient (95) and a pneumonic case of *F. tularensis* subsp. *holarctica* in southern Europe. Patients with pneumonic tularemia associated with inhalation of aerosolized infectious particles are at risk of acquiring typhoidal tularemia (61, 157). Though we have gained much knowledge about the epidemiological association of lawn mowing and brush cutting with tularemia in areas like Martha's Vineyard where the disease is endemic, gaps remain in our understanding of the transmission dynamics of tularemia (61, 74, 103, 104).

Clinical Significance

F. tularensis subsp. *tularensis* and *F. tularensis* subsp. *holarctica* are the two members of the genus *Francisella* most commonly encountered in human disease. Tularemia has been known historically by a number of synonyms, such as plague-like disease, rabbit fever, deer fly fever, market men's disease, glandular type of tick fever, conjunctivitis tularensis, Ohara's or Yao-byo disease, and water rat trappers' disease. These synonyms attest to the variety of clinical presentations, the infectious agent's ubiquitous presence in nature, and the means by which humans may acquire the infection.

The clinical spectrum depends on the mode of transmission, the virulence of the infecting strain, the degree of systemic involvement, the immune status of the host, and timely diagnosis and treatment (159). Tularemia can be misdiagnosed early in infection since its symptoms are not unique: sudden onset of chills, fever, headache, and generalized malaise characterize each onset of illness. The differential diagnosis includes a wide range of infectious diseases, such as cat-scratch fever, syphilis, mycobacterial infections, anthrax, brucellosis, legionellosis, and plague. The incubation period averages 3 to 5 days, but onset may occur as early as 2 days to as late as 14 days after infection. Without treatment, nonspecific symptoms—sweats, chills, progressive weakness, and weight loss—usually persist for several weeks to months. Before the advent of antibiotics, the overall mortality from infections with the more severe type A strains was in the range of 5 to 15%; however, fatality rates as high as 30 to 60% have been reported for untreated typhoidal and pneumonic forms of the disease. In the United States, untreated type B strain infections were rarely fatal. The fatality rate for all forms in recent years has been less than 2% (49).

Patients may present with any one or more of the classically described forms of tularemia: ulceroglandular, glandular, oculoglandular, pharyngeal, typhoidal, and pneumonic. The most common form is ulceroglandular disease (45 to 80% of the reported cases), indicating that the portal of entry is via infective insect bite or other inoculation through the skin barrier, usually associated with handling contaminated materials. Pharyngeal lymphadenopathy suggests a portal of entry via ingestion of contaminated water or food, as was the case with the recent food- and waterborne outbreak in Kosovo (134). Typhoidal tularemia is the most difficult form to recognize because there is no identified portal of entry and localization signs are absent. Any of the initial forms of tularemia may be complicated by bacteremic spread, leading to various secondary tularemic symptoms such as pneumonia, sepsis, and meningitis.

Until 1989 *F. tularensis* subsp. *novicida* was defined by a single isolate recovered from water in Utah in 1951. This subspecies was not known to cause human disease. During a subsequent study of 16 unusual human bacterial isolates, 14 were identified as *F. philomiragia* and 2 were identified as *F. tularensis* subsp. *novicida* (83). These two human isolates, two isolates from Texas (37), and the molecular typing of additional isolates from the United States, Australia (171), and more recently Spain all suggest that our knowledge about the prevalence of *F. tularensis* subsp. *novicida* remains incomplete. Fever, chills, cough, shortness of breath, and chest pain are the more common symptoms described in those with airway-acquired disease. In a case from Australia, the organism was isolated from an abscessed toe. Isolates are recovered from blood, granulomatous tissue, and wounds. Patients may also present with skin lesions and cervical lymphadenopathy. Overall, cases are milder than those of disease caused by *F. tularensis* subsp. *tularensis* and *F. tularensis* subsp. *holarctica*, but occasionally some are serious enough to warrant hospitalization.

F. philomiragia is an opportunistic agent infecting patients with a previous underlying condition that renders them more susceptible. More isolates have been recovered and identified since 2000, but overall, fewer than 20 cases have been described since the discovery of this species in 1974 (168). All but one case have involved a host with an impaired physical barrier to infection (near drowning) or impaired immunologic defenses (chronic granulomatous disease or myeloproliferative disease) (146). Most patients reported are from the United States (nine different states) (146). In addition, one case from Switzerland (168), one case from Australia (171), and a fatal water exposure-related case in a patient with a history of travel to Turkey (69) have been reported. In most cases *F. philomiragia* was isolated from normally sterile sites: blood, bone marrow, cerebrospinal fluid, and pericardial fluid. The drowning and water exposure cases were associated with salt water and brackish water, in contrast to *F. tularensis* infections, which are associated with freshwater sources.

Collection, Handling, Storage, and Transport of Specimens

Working with live *F. tularensis* can be hazardous. *F. tularensis* has a long and notorious history of infecting laboratory personnel working with infectious materials. Even though the use of biological safety cabinets and prophylactic antibiotic therapy (as well as vaccination, where available) provides safeguards for laboratory workers, these precautions have not fully eliminated laboratory exposures or modified behavior in the clinical laboratory to minimize risks (95, 140, 145). Clinical specimens should be handled under biosafety level 2 (BSL-2) conditions with universal precautions, with work being done using BSL-3 practices as soon as *F. tularensis* is suspected (50). Hundreds of laboratory-acquired infections have been documented, including infections of the pioneer scientists who first investigated the natural history of tularemia; they acquired infections from handling infected animals, removing arthropods from carcasses, and working with live cultures (17, 121, 140). The greatest risk of laboratory-acquired tularemia is by aerosol inhalation while working with infected materials and cultures. The infectivity of the organisms is high; *F. tularensis* should be handled only by trained and, preferably, vaccinated personnel.

Specimens should be stored chilled in appropriate medium until processed in the laboratory. Freezing of samples, unless they are kept at −80°C, is not recommended because of lysis of live bacteria upon thawing. Though *F. tularensis* may survive for long periods in the environment, successfully culturing it from environmental specimens is difficult. Efforts should be made to maintain the integrity of such specimens and avoid delay in transporting them to the laboratory for testing. Ectoparasites may be stored intact in 2% NaCl and transported to the laboratory for identification and then processed for evidence of *F. tularensis.* Clinical specimens should be placed in Amies agar with charcoal, a commercial transport system designed for anaerobic and aerobic pathogens (BD, Franklin, N.J.). *F. tularensis* should remain viable for 7 days at ambient room temperature when stored in Amies medium (91). Stuart medium, designed for transporting gonococcal specimens, and saline are inadequate for keeping *F. tularensis* viable during transport (91). For PCR, specimens should be collected in guanidine isothiocyanate-containing buffer, which should preserve *F. tularensis* DNA for up to 1 month (91).

Direct Examination of Specimens

The *F. tularensis* subspecies cannot be clearly differentiated from one another by microscopy. Cultures and fresh clinical specimens (ulcer and wound swabs, touch-prep fresh tissues, and aspirates) but not thick blood or environmental samples can be directly examined. Under microscopic examination of Gram-stained specimens or cultures, *Francisella* cells (single and pleomorphic) appear so tiny and stain so faintly that they can be easily missed. Thus, direct Gram staining is usually of no diagnostic value. To improve visualization, direct fluorescent-antibody (DFA) staining using a labeled hyperimmune rabbit polyclonal antibody prepared by immunizations with *F. tularensis* subsp. *tularensis* cells will presumptively identify *F. tularensis* subsp. *tularensis* and *F. tularensis* subsp. *holarctica.* This DFA reagent does not react with *F. tularensis* subsp. *novicida* or *F. philomiragia* or with *Legionella* species. Immunohistochemical (IHC) staining using a monoclonal antibody directed against the lipopolysaccharide (LPS) has been used successfully to visualize *F. tularensis* in formalin-fixed tissues in both intra- and extracellular sites (78). Neither the DFA reagent nor the IHC reagent is commercially available.

The presence of *F. tularensis* in specimens taken from ulcers, wounds, tissues, and the environment (animal feces and urine, water, hay infusion, mud, and ectoparasites) may be determined by detection of the *F. tularensis* LPS antigen by using an antigen capture enzyme-linked immunoassay (cELISA) or a lateral flow assay (127, 143). DNA detection by PCR directed at unique target regions has been widely applied (65, 91, 92, 125, 148, 163). The detection limit is 10^3 bacteria/ml for the cELISA and 10^2 bacteria/ml for PCR. These are specialized tests and are not widely available, although PCR technologies have become more commonly used for screening purposes.

Isolation Procedures

F. tularensis is not readily recovered by culture and is not easily identified even when it is cultured. The pathogenic *F. tularensis* bacteria are fastidious, requiring supplementation with sulfhydryl compounds (cysteine, cystine, thiosulfate, and IsoVitaleX) to grow on artificial medium. *F. tularensis* will grow well on cysteine heart blood agar supplemented with 9% chocolatized sheep blood (CHAB), chocolate agar (CA), buffered charcoal-yeast extract agar, and Thayer-Martin agar. It will grow in thioglycolate broth. When supplemented with 1 to 2% IsoVitaleX, general bacteriological media (tryptic soy broth and Mueller-Hinton broth) will support growth. The organisms grow slowly (60-min generation time); robust growth, therefore, is obtained by prolonged incubation (48 h or longer) or by plating on highly nutritive media such as CHAB. *F. tularensis* cultures should be incubated at 35 to 37°C aerobically and observed daily for 10 to 14 days; CO_2 does not impede growth. Incorporation of antibiotics (penicillin, 100,000 U/ml; polymyxin B sulfate, 100,000 U/ml; and cycloheximide, 0.1 mg/ml) into the medium will help prevent normal flora from overwhelming the *F. tularensis* organisms (125). Freezing of specimens combined with the use of antibiotics in the medium has allowed for a higher recovery rate than ever before (125). Complex protein or nutritionally enriched specimens such as blood or tissue will provide an intrinsic source of sulfhydryl compounds that permit *F. tularensis* growth. Upon subculture, the fastidious nature of *F. tularensis* will become evident as the exogenous compounds are depleted, leading to the loss of the bacterium's viability unless the subculture is propagated on cysteine-supplemented media. If a subculture fails to grow successfully on agar, inoculation of laboratory mice with a suspension of the original specimen or inoculated medium may assist in reviving the culture.

Specimens should be taken on the basis of clinical presentation and before administration of antibiotics. Fresh clinical material that is likely to contain high concentrations of *F. tularensis* organisms such as ulcer and wound specimens and lymphoid tissue (liver, spleen, or affected lymph node tissue) is inoculated directly onto an agar plate by using a sample-laden swab or bacteriological loop. Larger inocula will be necessary for the recovery of *F. tularensis* from specimens that contain a lower concentration of the organisms: blood, aspirates of pharyngeal washes, bronchial wash fluids, pleural fluids, urine, and environmental samples (159). A total of 3 to 10 ml of whole blood should be inoculated into blood culture bottles (147, 159). Environmental specimens, impinged air samples, and collected water are concentrated through a 0.22- or a 0.45-μm-pore-size nitrocellulose filter, and the filter-trapped organisms are released by vigorous agitation of the filter in less than 5 ml of sterile buffer. The inoculum should be spread onto as many agar plates as necessary at a seeding volume of 0.5 ml/agar plate. A portion of the inoculum (0.1 ml) may be injected subcutaneously into mice for enhanced recovery. Other methods for PCR and ameba culture from water have been discussed previously (1, 65). Preserved, formalin-fixed tissues should be examined by IHC staining (78).

Identification

Early recognition that an isolate may be *F. tularensis* is important from the standpoint of laboratory safety as well as helping to establish the cause of the patient's infection. There is also the possibility that a case of tularemia may be due to an act of bioterrorism. Prompt identification of an organism as *F. tularensis* may lead to an earlier recognition of such an event (chapter 9). The isolation of a poorly staining, tiny (indeed, individual cells may be difficult to discern), gram-negative coccobacillus (Fig. 1A) that produces 1- to 2-mm-diameter gray to gray-white colonies on CA after 48 h (and scant to no growth on blood agar) should raise the suspicion of *F. tularensis*. Further work on the isolate should be done in a biological safety cabinet. If further testing according to the algorithms given in chapter 9 does not rule out *F. tularensis* and the laboratory cannot do further confirmatory tests, the isolate needs to be sent to a reference laboratory that can confirm (or rule out) its identification as *F. tularensis*. Proper biohazard shipping procedures must be followed (chapter 9). In the United States, all states have at least one reference laboratory that is part of the Laboratory Response Network (LRN). These CDC- and APHIS-registered LRN laboratories are

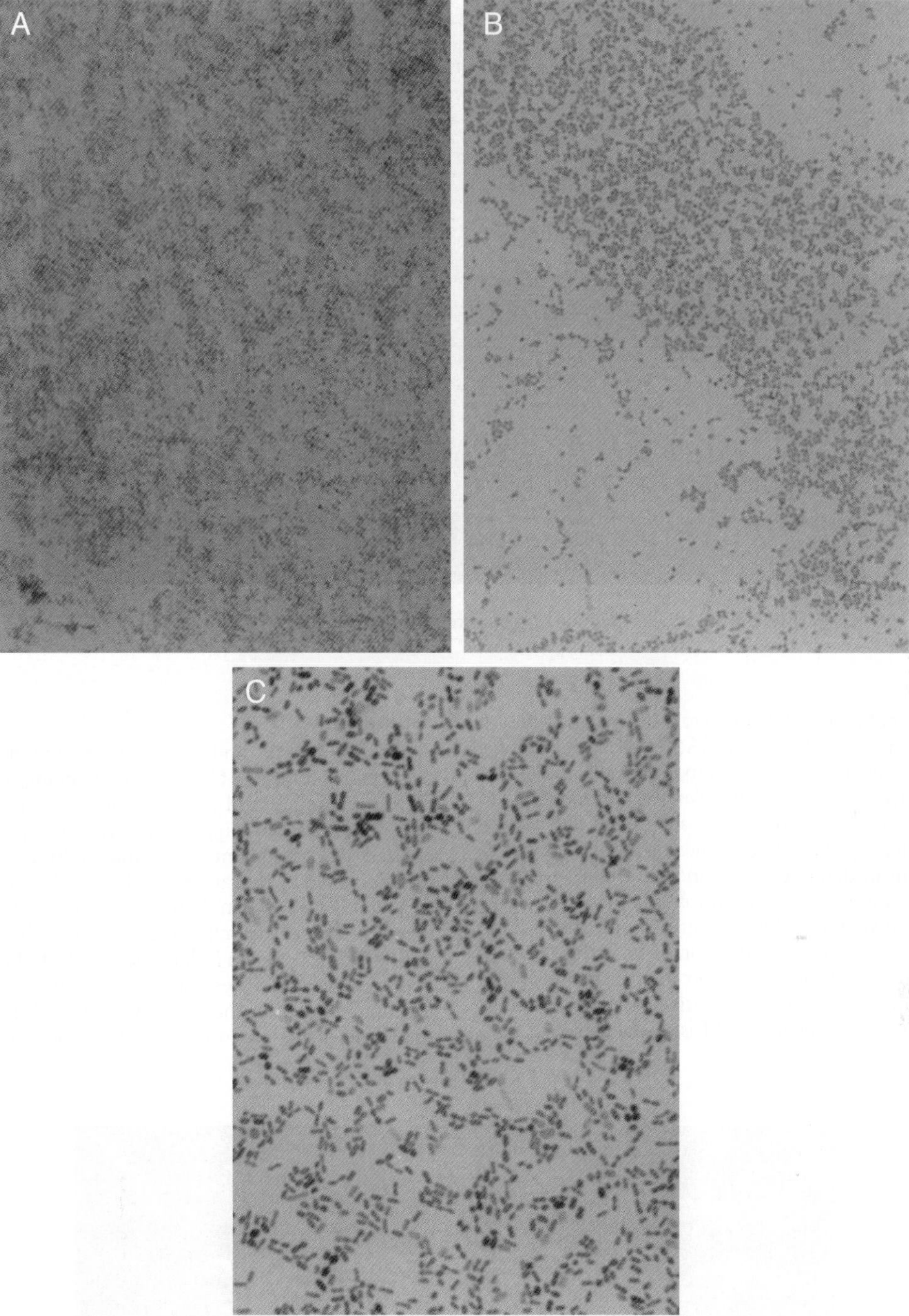

FIGURE 1 Gram stains of *F. tularensis* (A), *B. abortus* (B), and *Acinetobacter* species (C). Magnification, ×1,000.

able to confirm the identification of bacterial select agents, including *F. tularensis*. State public health laboratories can provide additional information, including location, about a state's LRN laboratories. See also http://www.bt.cdc.gov/lrn/.

A positive test result with any one of five methods—DFA staining (Fig. 2), IHC staining, the slide agglutination test, PCR, or a serology test for a single antibody titer—provides a presumptive diagnosis. Confirmation of infection would include identification of a culture as *F. tularensis* and/or a fourfold difference in titers in acute and convalescent serum samples, with one of the paired samples having a positive titer. The slide agglutination test presumptively identifies a suspect culture by mixing polyclonal rabbit anti-*F. tularensis* antibody with safranin-stained cells. Results of biochemical reactions are supportive of identification but are not reliable for confirmation since *Francisella* spp. are not very reactive. Fatty acid profiles may also be used to presumptively identify the organism as belonging to the *Francisella* genus (83, 147, 169). There is no specific bacteriophage lysis test for *F. tularensis*.

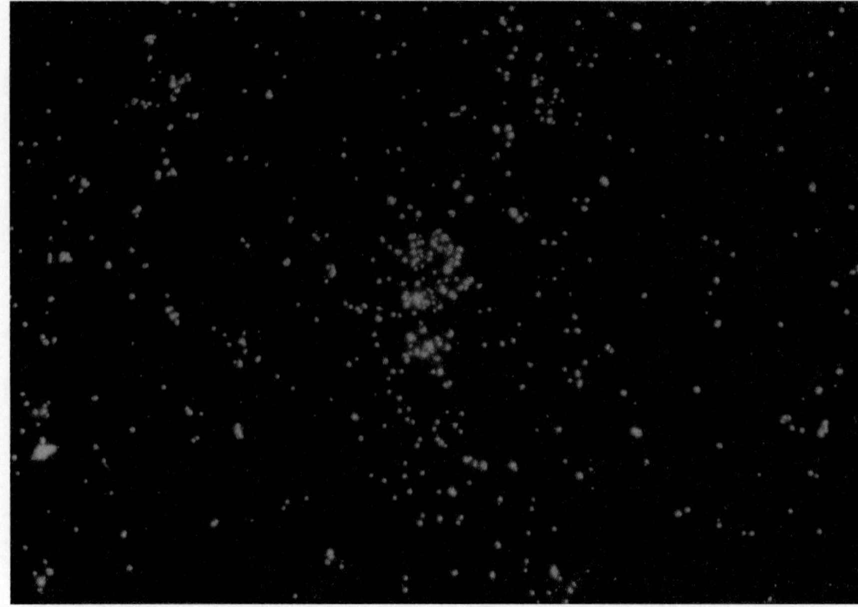

FIGURE 2 DFA staining of a culture of *F. tularensis*. Magnification, ×400.

Colonial morphology of *F. tularensis* is most distinctive when it is grown on CHAB. On CA, *F. tularensis* colonies have an entire edge; they are gray, smooth, raised, and moist, with a butyrous consistency. *F. tularensis* subsp. *novicida* grows more robustly than the other subspecies and is cysteine independent (Table 2). Colonies of *F. philomiragia* on CA are >5 mm in diameter, with an entire edge; they are white, smooth, raised, mucoid, and cysteine independent. On CHAB, *F. tularensis* exhibits a prominent and unique opalescent sheen due to its production of H_2S; this sheen is less prominent in *F. philomiragia* than in *F. tularensis* and is absent in cultures of other gram-negative organisms, such as *Yersinia*, *Brucella*, *Haemophilus*, and *Pasteurella* spp. (Fig. 3).

Typing Systems

F. tularensis biovars and *F. philomiragia* may be differentiated by protein profiling, 16S rRNA sequencing, various types of PCR approaches, and insertion element typing (60, 63, 99, 147) (Table 2). New approaches with the application of specialized PCR fragments targeting multiple-locus, variable-number tandem repeats have identified significant linkages and changes between *F. tularensis* subsp. *tularensis* and *F. tularensis* subsp. *holarctica* (92). Such analysis has revealed relationships between isolates demonstrated by geographical and ecological features and provides an interesting context for understanding the transmission and maintenance of *Francisella* in its environment. With the completion of the

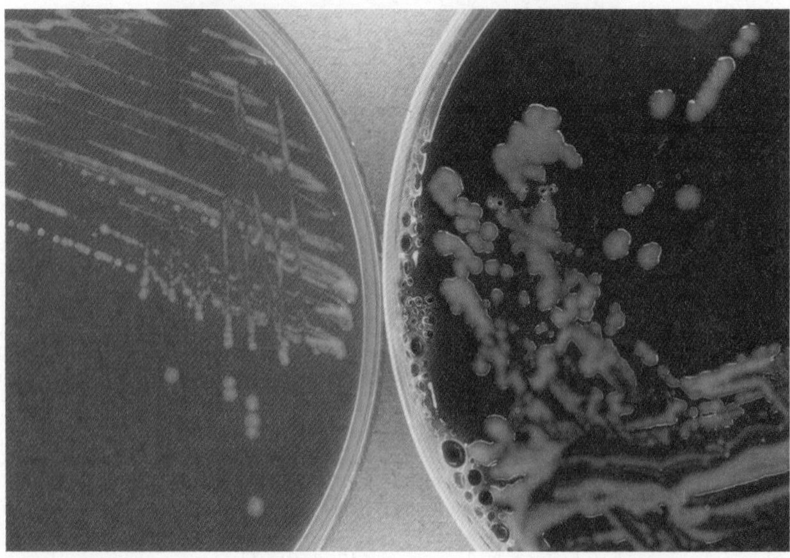

FIGURE 3 *F. tularensis* on CA (right) and cysteine heart blood agar (left) after 3 days of growth.

genomic sequencing of the prototypic type A strain (Schu 4) (98) and its comparison with the prototypic type B strain (live vaccine strain [LVS]), additional target areas may be identified for more precise typing and for study of strain pathogenesis. More recent application of technologies like DNA microarray analysis and surface-enhanced mass spectrometric methods will increase our ability to discriminate among and identify unique genomic regions for finer typing and characterization of the strains (25, 100).

Genus, species, and subspecies strains can be determined using 16S rRNA sequences, a method that has been applied in several instances to identify *Francisella* spp. successfully (69, 81, 145, 171). PCR is more sensitive than recovery by culture (83% compared to 62%) (91). Various PCR methods have been used to type isolates by genus, species, or individual isolates or small groups. Rapid PCR methods using the *Taq*man 5′ nuclease assay have a detection limit of <100 CFU under controlled laboratory conditions. These methods have been refined and applied widely in examining clinical specimens since 2003, with good correlation between culture and PCR results (125, 163).

Serologic Testing

Serology is the most common method by which *F. tularensis* infections are diagnosed (158, 159). Serum, plasma from citrated or heparinized blood, and filter paper-extracted serum proteins (172) can be used in serological assays. Antibodies may be detected as early as 1 week after onset of symptoms (about 2 weeks after infection). By 2 weeks after onset, antibodies may be detected in 89 to 95.4% of samples. Antibodies can persist for more than 10 years (17, 159, 166). Immunoglobulin M (IgM), IgA, and IgG antibodies appear simultaneously (158, 164). IgM antibodies can last for many years; thus, their presence does not indicate early or recent infection (17, 158). Agglutination testing, either by the tube agglutination (TA) or the microagglutination (MA) method, is the standard serology test for determining the presence of antibodies in tularemia (16, 27). A single specimen with a TA titer of ≥1:160 or an MA titer of ≥1:128 can be interpreted to be presumptively positive when compatible symptoms of tularemia are present and there is no history of vaccination or previous exposure. Confirmatory serodiagnosis requires a fourfold difference in titers between acute and convalescent specimens taken at least 14 days apart. One of the pair of serum specimens must show a positive titer by TA or MA. The formalin-killed whole-cell agglutination antigen (BBL Microbiology Systems, Cockeysville, Md.) may have low-level cross-reactivity primarily with *Brucella* antibodies, but the level of reactivity is typically <1:20 and will not interfere with interpretation of a positive result (6, 27, 118).

Enzyme-linked immunoassay (ELISA) formats that identify immunoglobulin class types and antigen detection have been adopted and updated for use in parts of Europe where tularemia is endemic (111, 127, 143). Although recombinant antigens have been used for ELISAs, the LPS extract remains the primary ELISA target to be used in recent test applications. Although ELISAs are more sensitive and specific than agglutination, their limitation of host specificity precludes their wide use in enzootic disease serosurveillance. Antigenic differences between the type A and type B biovars have not been demonstrated, although there is hope that such developments will be forthcoming as a result of the efforts in genomic sequencing and use of various DNA and mass spectrophotometric methods. The serology test materials thus react with anti-type A and anti-type B antibodies and usually do not react with anti-*F. tularensis* subsp. *novicida* and anti-*F. philomiragia* antibodies.

F. tularensis organisms are intracellular bacteria and are capable of eliciting both humoral and cell-mediated immunity (158). The latter response has been known to remain strong 25 years after infection (57). A skin test was previously used to measure specific reactivity by means of an intradermally injected ether extract of *F. tularensis*, but this test is no longer used. Host T cells retain proliferative responses to unique *F. tularensis* membrane proteins, with concomitant increase in interferon and interleukin-2 levels (57, 154, 155, 158). Tests for measuring the cell-mediated immune response are specialized and are not routinely used for diagnosis of tularemia. With the current emphasis on research with biodefense applications, however, new developments in this area for clinical use may be expected.

Antimicrobial Susceptibilities

Antimicrobial susceptibility testing of *F. tularensis* is not usually performed in clinical microbiology laboratories because of safety concerns in working with this organism (30, 121). Mueller-Hinton medium supplemented with 2% IsoVitaleX or CHAB must be used because of the fastidiousness of the pathogenic *F. tularensis*. This medium was recently evaluated as suitable for Clinical and Laboratory Standards Institute (formerly NCCLS) standards (26). Susceptibility of the *F. tularensis* isolate to the antibiotics recommended for treatment and prophylaxis, i.e., chloramphenicol, ciprofloxacin, gentamicin, streptomycin, and tetracycline, should be tested. No known naturally occurring strains resistant to the drugs recommended for treatment exist. Standardized methods have been published for susceptibility testing using broth, agar dilution (7), disk diffusion, and the E test (86, 93; chapter 73). No breakpoint standards have been set since there are no known naturally drug-resistant strains, except for erythromycin-resistant *F. tularensis* subsp. *holarctica* strains in Northern Europe (120).

F. tularensis infections are treatable with narrow-spectrum antibiotics, and drug resistance, with the exception of erythromycin resistance, in wild-type isolates is not known. Appropriate and early treatment, with streptomycin as the drug of choice, is effective. Streptomycin is given intramuscularly to adults in a dosage of 1 g every 12 h for 10 days (49). Gentamicin is an alternative drug that can be given intramuscularly at 3 to 5 mg/kg/day in equally divided doses at 8-h intervals for 10 days. Doxycycline or chloramphenicol may be used in combination with an aminoglycoside or used alone in less severe cases. Treatment with bacteriostatic agents, doxycycline, or chloramphenicol alone may result in treatment failures or relapses. An extended dosage schedule of 14 to 21 days may be necessary to prevent relapses. Ciprofloxacin has been used successfully to treat a limited number of patients; these clinical results, coupled with the low MIC of ciprofloxacin, suggest that this drug may become a useful addition to the armamentarium of drugs recommended for treating tularemia (156, 158). All *Francisella* isolates examined to date are β-lactamase positive, so penicillins and cephalosporins are not effective and should not be used to treat tularemia.

Prevention and Control

F. tularensis is a well-entrenched agent of enzootic disease that is unlikely to be eliminated even from limited natural foci. *F. tularensis* can survive for long periods in a cold, moist environment (15, 90, 120). Recently, extensive emphasis has been placed on understanding the ecology and survival of and the reservoir for *F. tularensis* (1, 65). Avoidance of infective exposure is the principal means of preventing tularemia. The public should be educated about the risks for acquiring the disease in regions where tularemia is endemic and warned especially not to handle dead or sick animals, particularly rabbits, hares, and water rodents. Gloves and protective clothing should be worn when skinning or preparing such animals for food. People should be advised to cook these animals thoroughly before eating them. Repellents should be used to avoid arthropod bites, and ticks should be removed promptly. Chlorinated municipal water is safe from tularemia, but untreated water can be a ready source of infection; outbreaks have followed consumption of water from contaminated wells and streams and even consumption of freshwater crustaceans (4, 134).

Isolation of patients is not necessary, as person-to-person spread does not occur; therefore, treatment of close contacts of tularemia patients is not recommended (49). Universal precautions to avoid direct contact with contaminated secretions is advised. Laboratory personnel are at high risk of acquiring typhoidal or pulmonary tularemia via inhalation. As mentioned above, laboratory personnel should work in a class II biosafety cabinet when handling suspected tularemia specimens. All work should be performed under BSL-3 conditions once an isolate is confirmed (or even suspected) to be *F. tularensis*. People who have a recognized high-risk exposure (e.g., from a spill, aerosal spray, or puncture of skin) to *F. tularensis* should be given oral antibiotic prophylaxis. People subjected to low-risk exposure (e.g., handling a culture in the biosafety cabinet, preparing and making slides) should be placed on fever watch for 10 days and treated if they develop symptoms.

Vaccination may be advised for laboratory personnel who are working with live cultures and for others whose occupational duties put them at risk. A live attenuated vaccine has been used to immunize millions of people living in northern European countries and Russia. A variant of this vaccine, the LVS vaccine, has been used in the United States since 1959 for immunization of personnel who are at risk for laboratory-acquired infection. The vaccine is administered as a single dose of 0.06 ml by scarification. Antibodies develop within 3 weeks and may persist at reduced levels for months or years. Human volunteer studies demonstrated only partial protection against aerosol challenges after vaccination. A review of vaccination records at the U.S. Army microbiological laboratories from 1960 to 1969 revealed that there were 11 cases of laboratory-acquired tularemia (1 case per 1,000 at-risk employee-years) in vaccinated personnel (30). A recent update of this information also illustrates the protective value of vaccination (140). In the United States, vaccination was used for at-risk laboratory workers handling infective *F. tularensis* cultures. Retrospective evaluation of LVS-vaccinated people demonstrated protection against respiratory tularemia and apparent mitigation of the course of ulceroglandular disease (159). Vaccinated people maintain antibody and memory T-cell responses for at least 10 years. However, the LVS vaccine is not licensed and is not currently available in Western countries. With additional biodefense funding, several laboratories are developing vaccines using better-characterized live and killed strains and identifying and assessing the relevance of subcellular fragments for the next generation of vaccines. The challenge is that a yet-undefined mixture of T-cell-reactive bacterial proteins may be required for inducing protection (41, 122).

BRUCELLA

Taxonomy

The genus *Brucella* consists of small gram-negative coccobacilli that are pathogenic for humans and animals. In 1886 and 1887, Sir David Bruce, a British army medical officer working on the island of Malta, made the first isolation of *Brucella*, recovering it from the spleens of patients suffering from Malta fever (28). Bruce called this organism *Micrococcus melitensis*. In 1895, the Danish veterinarian Bernhard Bang isolated an organism, which he called *Bacillus abortus*, from cases of bovine abortion (8). In 1918, the American Alice Evans published her work demonstrating the close similarity of these two organisms (59). Shortly thereafter, Meyer and Shaw proposed the new genus *Brucella*, to include the agents of both Malta fever and Bang's disease as *B. melitensis* and *B. abortus*, respectively (107). In 1929, Huddleston described a third species, *B. suis*, encompassing strains originally isolated by Traum in 1914 from aborted swine (85, 160). Two additional species were identified in the 1950s: *B. ovis*, an agent of reproductive disease in sheep, and *B. neotomae*, isolated from the desert wood rat in Utah (29, 153). In 1968, Carmichael and Bruner described *B. canis*, a cause of canine abortion (31). In addition to host preference, these six species classically have been characterized phenotypically on the basis of their tolerance to dyes, requirement for CO_2, rate of urease reaction, lysis by the *Brucella* Tbilisi phage, H_2S production, agglutination by monospecific antisera, and rough-versus-smooth colony morphology (3).

Since the mid-1990s, several studies have described *Brucella* strains recovered from marine mammals. One of these studies suggested the name "*B. maris*" for these isolates (88). Others have proposed the names "*B. delphini*," "*B. pinnipediae*," and "*B. cetaceae*," based in part on the strains' host specificities (40, 109). None of these names have been validly published. These strains have been found to differ phenotypically from the six nomenspecies by their patterns of substrate-mediated metabolic activity (88).

Brucella, *Ochrobactrum*, and *Mycoplana* form the family *Brucellaceae*. *Mycoplana* species are soil organisms that have not been associated with human disease, and *Ochrobactrum anthropi* is a soil organism and an opportunistic human pathogen. The close phylogenetic relationship among the members of the family *Brucellaceae* suggests that they may have evolved from a common free-living soil organism. The *Brucellaceae* are part of the order *Rhizobiales*, which is in the class *Alphaproteobacteria* of the phylum *Proteobacteria* and the domain *Bacteria* (71). Other members of the *Rhizobiales* associated with human disease include *Bartonella* (family *Bartonellaceae*), *Afipia* (family *Bradyrhyzobiaceae*), and *Methylobacterium* and *Roseomonas* (family *Methylobacteriaceae*).

For most *Brucella* spp., the genome consists of two circular chromosomes of approximately 2.1 and 1.2 Mbp. In contrast to the larger chromosome I, the smaller chromosome II has an origin of replication and a genetic content that suggest that it was derived originally from a megaplasmid. The G+C contents of both chromosomes are 57%. The exception to the two-chromosome genome is that of *B. suis* bv. 3, which possesses a single circular chromosome of 3.1 Mbp with an overall genetic content similar to that of other *Brucella* species. Sequencing of the genomes of *B. suis*, *B. melitensis*, and *B. abortus* recently has been completed, and the sequences have been compared (48, 80, 124). Overall, the genomic content and organization are highly conserved among the sequenced *Brucella* genomes and demonstrate similarities to the plant symbionts *Mesorhizobium loti* and *Sinorhizobium meliloti* and the plant pathogen *Rhizobium radiobacter (Agrobacterium tumefaciens)*. Chromosome I of *Brucella* contains approximately 2,100 to 2,200 open reading frames (ORFs), and chromosome II is predicted to have approximately 1,100 to 1,200 ORFs. Among the three sequenced *Brucella* genomes, the vast majority of the ORFs share greater than 99% sequence identity (80). However, through comparative genomic studies, a limited number of species-specific ORFs and variable ORFs, a significant number of which likely encode surface-exposed proteins, have been identified (80). The recent creation of an *Escherichia coli* library of 3,091 ORFs predicted from the genome of *B. melitensis* and the identification of ORFs encoding unique or highly variable proteins should greatly facilitate investigations into host tropism and *Brucella* pathogenesis, as well as the development of new diagnostic tests that target species-specific genetic sequences or polymorphic regions (52, 80).

The taxonomy of this genus is confounded by a dichotomy between the traditional (phenotypically based) and molecular definitions of its species. DNA relatedness and multilocus enzyme electrophoresis studies indicate that the six validly published nomenspecies, along with the recent marine mammal-derived strains, represent a single species (23, 70, 162). Recent molecular taxonomic studies show that although a high overall level of relatedness exists, the historically recognized species and the marine mammal strains can be differentiated by restriction polymorphisms of major outer membrane genes, insertion sequences, and whole-chromosome preparations (23, 165). This chapter follows the guidelines of the International Committee on Systematic Bacteriology subcommittee on the taxonomy of *Brucella* and retains the historical taxonomy to avoid confusion (43).

Description of the Genus

Brucellae are small, gram-negative coccoid rods, 0.5 to 0.7 μm in diameter and 0.6 to 1.5 μm in length. In Gram stains they are seen predominantly arranged singly (Fig. 1B). They are nonmotile. Their metabolism is aerobic, with oxygen or nitrate acting as the terminal electron acceptor via a cytochrome-based electron transport system. Some carbohydrates and polyhydric alcohols are oxidized; none are fermented. Nitrate is reduced, with some strains of some species producing gas. Strains are positive for catalase and, with the exception of *B. ovis*, *B. neotomae*, and some strains of *B. canis*, positive for oxidase. All species except *B. ovis* hydrolyze urea. Brucellae are negative for indole production, gelatin liquefaction, citrate utilization, and hemolysis. Growth on MacConkey agar is variable. The optimum growth temperature is 35 to 37°C. Chemo-organotrophic, most strains require complex media for growth, especially upon initial isolation. Growth may be improved by serum or blood; hemin (X factor) and NAD (V factor) are not required (3, 46).When grown on blood agar at an optimum temperature and under an optimum atmosphere, colonies are usually 0.5 to 1.0 mm in diameter, raised, and convex, with an entire edge and a smooth, shiny surface. *B. canis* and *B. ovis* characteristically produce rough colonies. Rough variants of the other species also occur (46).

Epidemiology and Transmission

Brucellae are facultative intracellular parasites, taking as their natural habitat a variety of animal species. *B. abortus* is found primarily in cattle but also occurs in camels, buffalo, yaks, and horses. Goats and sheep are the most common hosts for *B. melitensis*. This species is also found in alpacas and camels. In some parts of the world, cattle have emerged as a significant source of *B. melitensis* infections. It has been suggested that when this species occurs in cattle, smaller ruminants have provided the actual reservoir (45, 73, 178). The primary hosts for *B. suis* are swine (biovars 1, 2, and 3) and reindeer and caribou (biovar 4). In some countries, cattle have become a significant source of *B. suis* bv. 1 infection for humans. Maintenance of *B. suis* in cattle may depend on a concomitant pig reservoir (73). *B. canis* is usually isolated from kennel-bred dogs but also has been found in coyotes and foxes. Hosts for the marine mammal brucellae include seals, dolphins, and porpoises (40). Unlike the preceding taxa, *B. ovis* and *B. neotomae* are not known to cause human disease. The former has been isolated from sheep, the latter from the desert wood rat (73). Brucellae localize in their host's reticuloendothelial tissue and reproductive tract. Causing abortion, they are typically transmitted from one host animal to the next via contamination of the environment by the products of abortion (110).

Brucellosis has been described as the world's most widespread zoonosis, taking not only a serious human toll but also a severe economic toll when infecting domestic animals (73). The disease is highly endemic in the Middle East, the Mediterranean basin, Latin America, southeastern Europe, Asia, Africa, and the Caribbean (73). Though *B. abortus* has the broadest geographic distribution, *B. melitensis* causes more cases of human disease. This is attributed to bovine brucellosis's having been controlled more effectively than brucellosis in sheep and goats. In many developing countries, these small ruminants are the most important domestic animals and where they are kept, brucellosis is almost always present (45, 73). In the United States, the epidemiology of brucellosis has changed over the last 30 years. The success of programs to eradicate brucellosis in cattle, swine, sheep, and goats has decreased, though not eliminated, the risk of infection for farmers, veterinarians, and abattoir workers. Brucellosis has become primarily a foodborne disease caused by *B. melitensis* and associated with consumption of unpasteurized goat milk products from countries where caprine brucellosis is endemic (66, 132). Person-to-person transmission does not ordinarily occur but has been reported in connection with tissue transplantation and sexual intercourse (45, 175).

Brucellosis is usually transmitted to humans by direct contact through abraded skin or mucosal surfaces, consumption of contaminated food products, or inhalation. Brucellosis continues to be one of the most common laboratory-acquired infections. Practices associated with transmission in the laboratory include unprotected handling of specimens, sniffing of plates, mouth pipetting, and exposure of the eyes, nose, or mouth to infectious aerosols (50).

Clinical Significance

Of the species causing brucellosis in humans, *B. melitensis* tends to produce the most severe disease, followed by *B. suis* and *B. abortus* (110). While *B. canis* can cause clinical disease similar to that caused by the above-mentioned species, it has reduced virulence for humans (44, 175). Human brucellosis caused by marine mammal strains has been reported more recently (20, 150). The two community-acquired cases in one report presented as neurobrucellosis. The relative risk of infection with and pathogenicity of these strains for humans need further investigation.

The incubation period of brucellosis is usually 1 to 3 weeks but can be much longer. Symptoms are nonspecific.

They include fever (often undulating), malaise, night sweats, backache, muscle aches, and anorexia. The disease may affect a particular organ or organ system, causing osteomyelitis, hepatomegaly, splenomegaly, meningitis and other central nervous system symptoms, epididymo-orchitis, and endocarditis, among other complications. Although endocarditis is rare, when brucellosis is fatal, endocarditis is usually the cause. Chronic brucellosis can be defined as a disease in which compatible signs and symptoms persist for more than a year. Arguably, with brucellosis the definitions of acute and chronic are somewhat arbitrary (175). Though the fatality rate of brucellosis is now less than 2%, principally because of antibiotics, it remains a severe and debilitating disease (110).

Collection, Handling, Storage, and Transport of Specimens

Specimens for the diagnosis of brucellosis in humans include blood and bone marrow for culture and serum for serologic testing. Brucellae may also be cultured from spleen, liver, synovial fluid, or abscess specimens. For best results, multiple blood samples should be drawn during febrile episodes (110). The general collection, handling, storage, and transport guidelines for these specimens given in this Manual are applicable here (see chapters 5 and 20). Specimens for culture should be collected before the initiation of antibiotic therapy. Specimens that cannot be processed within 1 h of collection should be refrigerated. Acute-phase serum specimens should be collected as soon as possible after the onset of symptoms, and convalescent-phase specimens should be collected 14 to 21 days thereafter. Serum specimens should be shipped and stored cold or frozen. If PCR analysis is to be done, the collection method needs to adhere to the requirements of the particular assay method. Specimens from patients with suspected brucellosis should be labeled appropriately so that laboratory exposures to the disease agent can be minimized.

Direct Examination of Specimens

Direct microscopic examination of blood or bone marrow is not sufficiently sensitive to be useful in the diagnosis of brucellosis. There is no laboratory protocol for DFA staining. Direct detection methods using PCR assays have been described. When available for routine use, PCR-based tests will be particularly useful for laboratories serving areas of high endemicity (113, 131, 133). However, most PCR methods are capable of sampling only a small volume of specimen relative to that used to culture *Brucella*.

Isolation Procedures

Isolation of *Brucella* provides proof of the disease. Blood and bone marrow are the usual specimens for culture in cases of human brucellosis. Historically, bone marrow culture has been considered more sensitive, particularly in cases of chronic brucellosis and when the patient has already been treated with antibiotics (75). The greater sensitivity of modern automated blood culture systems may obviate this advantage. For example, in one study Ozturk et al., using the BACTEC 9240 system (Becton Dickinson Diagnostic Instrument Systems, Towson, Md.), cultured both blood and bone marrow specimens from 16 brucellosis patients. For 13 of the patients, *Brucella* was recovered from both specimens. For the remaining three patients, both specimens were culture negative. This study included cases in which antibiotics were given before culture but no chronic cases (123). These findings suggest that the more invasive procedure of bone marrow culture can be reserved for diagnostic problem cases in which blood cultures are negative.

Not all laboratories, particularly those in developing countries, will have an automated blood culture system. The classic biphasic blood culture technique of Casteñeda is one alternative. The culture bottle contains a broth medium with a layer of the same medium solidified with 2 to 3% agar on one side of the bottle (32, 110). Various studies have reported times to detection ranging from less than 6 days to more than 27 days by using this method (75, 137, 144).

Lysis-centrifugation involves osmotic lysis of erythrocytes followed by concentration of bacteria by centrifugation and direct plating of the concentrate onto culture media (19). This technique may be done by using the commercially available Isolator microbial tube (Wampole Laboratories, Cranbury, N.J.) or an in-house method. Lysis-centrifugation has better sensitivity and shorter time to detection than the biphasic bottle method. Since it is also technologically simple, this technique is arguably a better choice than the biphasic (Casteñeda) bottle method for laboratories that do not have an automated blood culture system (58, 101). Lysis-centrifugation also gave improved results compared to those of direct plating when synovial fluid was used for culture of *Brucella* (174). Compared with early versions of automated blood culture systems, such as BACTEC 460 and BACTEC NR, the lysis-centrifugation approach produced reduced times to detection, but in some cases the automated systems produced higher sensitivity rates (96).

Recent studies with the newer continuous-monitoring systems indicate that the BACTEC 9000 series is able to achieve times to detection that are shorter than those of lysis-centrifugation (>95% positive within 7 days of incubation) and has greater sensitivity (173). In general, modern automated blood culture systems can be depended on to detect *Brucella* within the routine incubation period used with these technologies (10, 11).

Because *Brucella* spp. have a slower growth rate than many of the bacteria encountered in the clinical laboratory, they seem more fastidious than they really are. They will grow on most of the media commonly used in this setting, including Trypticase soy agar, heart infusion agar, and brain heart infusion agar. Most strains will grow on Thayer-Martin or Martin-Lewis agar, which may be useful in recovering *Brucella* from contaminated specimens. Some strains will grow better with increased CO_2 (5 to 10%); *B. abortus* may require increased CO_2, particularly upon initial isolation.

Identification

Early recognition that an isolate may be a *Brucella* species is important for reasons of public health and laboratory safety as well as the patient's diagnosis. Brucellosis is a serious infectious disease that is frequently foodborne. Existence of a new case in the community suggests the possibility of additional cases, and *Brucella*, like *F. tularensis*, is considered a possible bioterrorism agent (chapter 9). Because of the hazard of laboratory-acquired infections, possible *Brucella* cultures should be handled using BSL-3 practices, with culture manipulations being done in a biological safety cabinet (50).

Fortunately, *Brucella* has some easily determined salient features that can lead to an early suspicion of the organism's identity. A Gram stain shows tiny, gram-negative coccobacilli. With the exception of *F. tularensis*, *Brucella* is the smallest gram-negative organism likely to be seen in the clinical laboratory. Its reputation for faint staining notwithstanding, *Brucella* may occasionally show a hint of gram positivity, especially with insufficient decolorization, leading to initial misidentification (117). In Fig. 1 the size of *Brucella* (Fig. 1B) may be compared with that of *Acinetobacter* spp. (Fig. 1C). When streaked for isolation, discrete colonies are seldom seen in 1 day. Once evident, colonies are small (1 mm or less in diameter), translucent, soft, and easily emulsified. They are nonhemolytic on blood agar.

Brucella spp. are positive for oxidase and urease. Some of the oxidase- and urease-positive, non-glucose-fermenting, gram-negative taxa that along with *Haemophilus* spp. may be confused with *Brucella* spp. are listed in Table 1. Size difference is helpful in differentiating *Psychrobacter phenylpyruvicus (Moraxella phenylpyruvica)* from *Brucella* spp., the former being about the size of *Acinetobacter* spp. Both morphology and motility are useful in differentiating *Brucella* spp. from *Bordetella bronchiseptica* and *Ochrobactrum anthropi*. Urease-positive biotypes of *Haemophilus* spp., in addition to requiring X and V factor (or only V factor), differ from *Brucella* by not growing on sheep blood agar. *Oligella ureolytica*, also a small organism, may be more difficult to separate from *Brucella* spp. While *O. ureolytica* is described as motile, motility may be delayed or difficult to demonstrate. Most isolations of *O. ureolytica* are made from urine, an unlikely source for *Brucella*. Also, when tested in oxidation-fermentation medium, *Brucella* spp. produce acid from xylose and *O. ureolytica* does not. In all these instances, CFA analysis is another useful differential test. Laboratories using identification kits or automated identification systems need to know if the database includes *Brucella* spp. With most systems, at present, *Brucella* is not included. In the past, some of these test methodologies have been reported to misidentify *Brucella* variously as *Haemophilus influenzae* biotype IV, *Psychrobacter phenylpyruvicus*, and *Ochrobactrum anthropi* (9, 12, 55, 136).

If an identification as *Brucella* sp. cannot be ruled out (also see chapter 9) and the laboratory is unable to do further confirmatory tests, the isolate should be sent to a reference laboratory that can definitively identify and determine the species of brucellae. Use proper biohazard shipping procedures (chapter 9). In the United States, LRN laboratories are able to confirm and identify *Brucella* spp. to the species level. Again, state public health laboratories can provide additional information, including location, about a state's LRN laboratories. See also http://www.bt.cdc.gov/lrn/.

Confirmation of a culture as *Brucella* sp. can be done serologically. A suspension of the isolate equivalent to a 2 McFarland standard is made up in 1% formalin saline. The suspension is allowed to stand for 24 h, which kills the organism. The resulting product is used as an antigen in a TA test using a positive control serum such as Difco/BBL Brucella Positive Control Serum AMS (BD Diagnostics, Sparks, Md.). *B. canis* is not agglutinated by this antiserum, but this procedure will confirm as *Brucella* those species that commonly cause human brucellosis and that cause the most severe human disease, *B. melitensis*, *B. suis*, and *B. abortus*. Serologic cross-reactions have been reported with *Afipia clevelandensis*, *Vibrio cholerae*, *Yersinia enterocolitica* O:9, and *F. tularensis* (51, 178). *A. clevelandensis* is motile and its cells are larger than those of *Brucella*; *V. cholerae* and *Y. enterocolitica* are motile, glucose-fermenting, medium rods; *F. tularensis* is easily differentiated from *Brucella* by the characteristics given in Table 1.

Tests for the species-level identification of *Brucella* include sensitivity to the dyes thionin and basic fuchsin, rapidity of urea hydrolysis, H_2S production, lysis by Tbilisi (Tb) phage at the routine test dilution (RTD) and the RTD $\times 10^4$, and determination of rough versus smooth phase. Dye sensitivities are tested by swabbing a saline suspension of the test organism in a line across a plate of medium such as Trypticase soy agar or heart infusion agar containing the appropriate dye, typically at a concentration of 20 μg/ml. Known cultures of *B. melitensis*, *B. suis*, and *B. abortus* should be included as controls. The rate of urease activity can be tested conveniently by heavily inoculating a Christensen's urea agar slant with fresh growth and leaving it at room temperature for 5 min. A positive reaction will be seen with *B. suis*, *B. canis*, and some strains of *B. melitensis* within this time period. *B. abortus* and most strains of *B. melitensis* will need an additional incubation at 35 to 37°C, up to overnight, to become positive. Production of H_2S is detected using a lead acetate paper strip suspended over an inoculated slant of medium such as heart infusion agar. Read and change the strip daily for up to 6 days or until the strip blackens, indicating a positive result. Tbilisi (Tb) phage, available from the American Type Culture Collection (ATCC 23448-B1), lyses *B. abortus* when used at its RTD. It will also lyse *B. suis* when used at the RTD $\times 10^4$. The RTD is determined by making serial 10-fold dilutions of the phage and applying a 10-μl drop of each dilution to a plate inoculated for confluent growth with a suspension of a known *B. abortus* culture. The highest dilution giving confluent lysis is the RTD. The test organism is similarly inoculated onto a plate for confluent growth, and a 10-μl drop of the RTD and of the RTD $\times$ 10^4 of the phage is applied. *B. canis*, a rough organism, will agglutinate in acriflavine solution; *B. melitensis*, *B. suis*, and *B. abortus*, typically smooth species, will not. For this test, suspend a small amount of growth in a drop of a freshly prepared solution of 1:1,000 neutral acriflavine in distilled water and observe for agglutination (3, 169). For additional details on these tests, see the monograph by Alton et al. (3).

Table 3 summarizes the characteristics of the four validly named species that cause human disease. The dye sensitivity and H_2S reactions noted for *B. suis* are for biovars 1 and 3 and those for *B. abortus* are for biovar 1. These are the biovars of these two species most commonly encountered in human brucellosis (44). For the reactions of the other biovars of these two species, see Alton et al. (3). With *Brucella* identification, as with any bacterial identification, it is necessary to consider the phenotypic picture as a whole before coming to a conclusion. An additional useful test for the identification of *B. canis* is CFA analysis. While *B. melitensis*, *B. suis*, and *B. abortus* all have lactobacillic acid (19:0cyc) as

TABLE 3 Differential characteristics of *Brucella* spp.[a]

Test	*B. melitensis*	*B. suis*	*B. abortus*	*B. canis*
Dye sensitivity				
Thionin	R	R	S	R
Basic fuchsin	R	V[b]	R	S
Time (min) for urea hydrolysis	>5[c]	<5	>5	<5
H_2S production	–	V[d]	+	–
Lysis by Tb[e] phage at RTD	–	–	+	–
Lysis by Tb phage at RTD $\times$ 10^4	–	+	+	–
Agglutination in 1:1,000 acriflavine	–[f]	–[f]	–[f]	+

[a] Data are from references 3 and 169. R, resistant; S, sensitive; V, variable.
[b] Biovar 1, sensitive; biovar 3, resistant.
[c] Some strains are positive in <5 min.
[d] Biovar 1, positive; biovar 3, negative.
[e] Tbilisi, a *Brucella* phage originally isolated in the former USSR.
[f] Occasional strains are rough.

a major component of their CFA profile, *B. canis* lacks this compound (169). Marine mammal strains of *Brucella* are smooth, are resistant to thionin and basic fuchsin, hydrolyze urea (not rapidly), do not produce H_2S, and are variable for lysis by Tb phage (110). Strains not lysed by Tb phage will resemble *B. melitensis*.

The traditional methods of species-level identification of *Brucella* are complex and labor-intensive, involve some hazard, and in part because of the slow growth rate of *Brucella* organisms, take some days to yield a final result. Molecular methods, which involve much less manipulation of viable organisms and yield results much more rapidly, are gaining greater acceptance as a supplement or alternative to the conventional methods of identification. A number of molecular tests are now available for the identification of *Brucella* to the genus and species levels. PCR assays targeting *omp43*, *omp31*, the 16S rRNA gene, 16S to 23S spacer regions, heat shock protein genes, and the perosamine synthetase gene have been developed to detect *Brucella* spp. (18, 47, 113, 116, 130, 131, 135). 16S rRNA gene sequencing of a large panel of isolates has shown perfect sequence conservation among *Brucella* spp., limiting the usefulness of this target for species identification (72). However, resolution to species level is possible through ribotyping, amplified fragment length polymorphism analysis, amplification and DNA sequencing of *omp2* and *omp25*, and PCR assays targeting species-specific insertions of IS*711* elements (22, 38, 39, 62, 77, 115, 130, 133, 170). Several PCR assays have been formatted for use on real-time PCR instrumentation that facilitates rapid detection and reduces the risk of amplicon carryover contamination (18, 115, 130, 131, 133).

Typing Systems

B. melitensis, *B. suis*, and *B. abortus* are further divided into biovars. The three biovars of *B. melitensis* are based on agglutination with monospecific antisera for the *B. abortus* A antigen and the *B. melitensis* M antigen. *B. suis* has five biovars, defined by H_2S production, dye sensitivities, and agglutination patterns with the monospecific antisera. Differentiation among the seven biovars of *B. abortus* uses these same characteristics plus testing for CO_2-dependent growth. See the monograph by Alton et al. for details on these test procedures (3).

Molecular typing methods offer advantages over biovar determination similar to the advantages that molecular biology-based tests have over conventional tests for genus- and species-level identification of *Brucella*. In addition, molecular typing offers much greater discrimination among strains than does biovar determination. Identification beyond the species level has been demonstrated by PCR, RNA mismatch cleavage, and Fourier transform infrared spectroscopy (21, 22, 108). A PCR-based method targeting genetic segments containing variable numbers of tandem repeats has been recently developed for *Brucella* strain typing and promises to provide a useful tool for facilitating epidemiological investigations (24).

Serologic Testing

Serologic testing is a valuable adjunct to culture for the laboratory diagnosis of brucellosis. Demonstration of a specific antibody response can provide useful diagnostic information, and the characterization of the response (predominantly IgM versus IgG) assists in differentiating acute infection from chronic disease (149). The serum agglutination test (SAT) is the most widely used test in the United States (178). This test can be modified to differentiate IgG from IgM titers by pretreatment of specimens with 2-mercaptoethanol. The SAT detects antibodies against *B. abortus*, *B. suis*, and *B. melitensis* but not *B. canis*. A fourfold rise in SAT titer between the acute- and convalescent-phase serum samples is indicative of brucellosis. For single specimens, an SAT titer of ≥1:160 is suggestive of brucellosis. Cross-reactions may be observed with antibodies directed against *F. tularensis*, *Vibrio cholerae*, *Yersinia enterocolitica*, and *Afipia clevelandensis* (51, 178). There are few reports of using the SAT in cases of human brucellosis of marine mammal origin. Of the three reported human cases, two were positive in the SAT and one was negative (20, 150). Other serologic assays that have been described include the Rose Bengal test, the Coombs anti-human globulin test, the complement fixation test, ELISA, and the rapid dipstick test (5, 149, 152). The rapid dipstick assay, a relatively simple screening procedure for *Brucella*-specific IgM, shows promise as a field test in areas without direct access to a reference laboratory.

Antimicrobial Susceptibilities

The development of antibiotic resistance by *Brucella* has not yet been demonstrated. This has been attributed in part to the lack of plasmids (110). Additional reasons for not routinely doing in vitro susceptibility testing with this organism include safety concerns, poor correlation between high levels of in vitro activity and clinical efficacy for many agents including β-lactams and quinolones, and a general lack of well-established interpretive standards (177).

Successful treatment of brucellosis requires long-term combination antibiotic therapy. The regimen that the World Health Organization recommends is doxycycline (200 mg/day) in combination with rifampin (600 to 900 mg/day, orally) for 6 weeks (45). The combination of doxycycline and streptomycin is also effective. In children younger than 8 years, treatment combining trimethoprim-sulfamethoxazole with an aminoglycoside has been successful, without the side effects of tetracyclines in this age group (178).

The question of prophylaxis often arises after potential laboratory exposure to *Brucella*. Universally accepted practices in these cases are lacking. Some have advocated a full 6-week course of antibiotics if there has been significant exposure (151). Use of doxycycline alone for 1 week immediately following exposure (180) as well as a 3-week course of the standard combination of doxycycline and rifampin (136) has been reported.

Evaluation, Interpretation, and Reporting of Results

Isolation of *Brucella* from a patient's blood, bone marrow, or other tissue establishes a diagnosis of brucellosis. Modern blood culture methods can be quite sensitive, especially in acute infections (123, 139). An isolate presumptively identified as *Brucella* should be immediately reported to the physician as a possible *Brucella* sp., and results of confirmatory testing and identification to species level should be reported as soon as these are available. With the SAT, a fourfold or greater rise in titer is considered to indicate positivity (33). A single titer needs to be interpreted in light of epidemiologic and clinical evidence. In many settings a titer of ≥1:160 is considered significant in a patient with compatible symptoms (33, 176).

REFERENCES

1. **Abd, H., T. Johansson, I. Golovliov, G. Sandström, and M. Forsman.** 2003. Survival and growth of *Francisella tularensis* in *Acanthamoeba castellanii*. *Appl. Environ. Microbiol.* **69:**600–606.
2. **Aikimbaev, M. A.** 1996. Taxonomy of genus *Francisella*. *Rep. Acad. Sci. Kaz. SSR Ser. Biol.* **5:**42–44.

3. **Alton, G. G., L. M. Jones, R. D. Angus, and J. M. Verger.** 1988. *Techniques for the Brucellosis Laboratory*. Institut National de la Recherche Agronomique, Paris, France.
4. **Anda, P., J. S. del Pozo, J. M. D. Garcia, R. Escudero, F. J. G. Peña, M. C. L. Velasco, R. E. Sellek, M. R. J. Chillarón, L. P. S. Serrano, and J. F. M. Navarro.** 2001. Waterborne outbreak of tularemia associated with crayfish fishing. *Emerg. Infect. Dis.* **7**:575–582.
5. **Ariza, J., T. Pellicer, R. Pallares, and F. Gudiol.** 1992. Specific antibody profile in human brucellosis. *Clin. Infect. Dis.* **14**:131–140.
6. **Avashia, S. B., J. M. Petersen, C. M. Lindley, M. E. Schriefer, K. L. Gage, M. Cetron, T. A. DeMarcus, D. K. Kim, J. Buck, J. A. Montenieri, J. L. Lowell, M. F. Antolin, M. Y. Kosoy, L. G. Carter, M. C. Chu, K. A. Hendricks, D. T. Dennis, and J. L. Kool.** 2004. First reported prairie dog-to-human tularemia transmission, Texas, 2002. *Emerg. Infect. Dis.* **10**:483–486.
7. **Baker, C. N., D. G. Hollis, and C. Thornsberry.** 1985. Antimicrobial susceptibility testing of *Francisella tularensis* with a modified Mueller-Hinton broth. *J. Clin. Microbiol.* **22**:212–215.
8. **Bang, B.** 1897. The etiology of epizootic abortion. *J. Comp. Pathol. Ther.* **10**:125–149.
9. **Barham, W. B., P. Church, J. E. Brown, and S. Paparello.** 1993. Misidentification of *Brucella* species with the use of rapid bacterial identification systems. *Clin. Infect. Dis.* **17**:1068–1069.
10. **Baron, E. J., M. P. Weinstein, W. M. Dunne, P. Yagupsky, D. F. Welch, and D. M. Wilson.** 2005. *Cumitech 1C, Blood Cultures IV.* Coordinating ed., E. J. Baron. ASM Press, Washington, D.C.
11. **Baron, E. J., J. D. Scott, and L. S. Tompkins.** 2005. Prolonged incubation and extensive subculturing do not increase recovery of clinically significant microorganisms from standard automated blood cultures. *Clin. Infect. Dis.* **41**:1677–1680.
12. **Batchelor, B. I., R. J. Brindle, G. F. Gilks, and J. B. Selkon.** 1992. Biochemical mis-identification of *Brucella melitensis* and subsequent laboratory-acquired infections. *J. Hosp. Infect.* **22**:159–162.
13. **Behan, K. A., and G. C. Klein.** 1982. Reduction of *Brucella* species and *Francisella tularensis* cross-reacting agglutinins by dithiothreitol. *J. Clin. Microbiol.* **16**:756–757.
14. **Behr, M.** 2000. Laboratory-acquired lymphadenopathy in a veterinary pathologist. *Lab. Anim.* **29**:23–25.
15. **Bell, J. F., and S. J. Stewart.** 1975. Chronic shedding tularemia nephritis in rodents: possible relation to occurrence of *Francisella tularensis* in lotic waters. *J. Wildl. Dis.* **11**:421–436.
16. **Bevanger, L., J. A. Maeland, and A. I. Naess.** 1988. Agglutinins and antibodies to *Francisella tularensis* outer membrane antigens in the early diagnosis of disease during an outbreak of tularemia. *J. Clin. Microbiol.* **26**:433–437.
17. **Bevanger, L., J. A. Maeland, and A. I. Kvam.** 1994. Comparative analysis of antibodies to *Francisella tularensis* antigens during the acute phase of tularemia and eight years later. *Clin. Diagn. Lab. Immunol.* **1**:238–240.
18. **Bogdanovich, T., M. Skurnik, P. S. Lübeck, P. Aherns, and J. Hoofar.** 2004. Validated 5′ nuclease PCR assay for rapid identification of the genus *Brucella*. *J. Clin. Microbiol.* **42**:2261–2263.
19. **Braun, W., and J. Kelsh.** 1954. Improved method for cultivation of *Brucella* from the blood. *Proc. Soc. Exp. Biol. Med.* **85**:154–155.
20. **Brew, S. D., L. L. Perrett, J. A. Stack, and A. P. MacMillan.** 1999. Human exposure to *Brucella* recovered from a sea mammal. *Vet. Rec.* **24**:483.
21. **Bricker, B. J.** 1999. Differentiation of hard-to-type bacterial strains by RNA mismatch cleavage. *BioTechniques* **42**:321–326.
22. **Bricker, B. J., and S. M. Halling.** 1994. Differentiation of *Brucella abortus* biovars 1, 2, and 4, *Brucella melitensis*, *Brucella ovis*, and *Brucella suis* biovar 1 by PCR. *J. Clin. Microbiol.* **32**:2660–2666.
23. **Bricker, B. J., D. R. Ewalt, A. P. MacMillan, G. Foster, and S. Brew.** 2000. Molecular characterization of *Brucella* strains isolated from marine mammals. *J. Clin. Microbiol.* **38**:1258–1262.
24. **Bricker, B. J., D. R. Ewalt, and S. M. Halling.** 2003. *Brucella* HOOF-prints: strain typing by multi-locus analysis of variable number tandem repeats (VNTRs). *BMC Microbiol.* **3**:15.
25. **Broekhuijsen, M., P. Larsson, A. Johansson, U. Byström, E. Eriksson, E. Larsson, R. G. Prior, A. Sjöstedt, and R. W. Titball.** 2003. Genome-wide DNA microarray analysis of *Francisella tularensis* strains demonstrates extensive genetic conservation within the species but identifies regions that are unique to the highly virulent *F. tularensis* subsp. *tularensis*. *J. Clin. Microbiol.* **41**:2924–2931.
26. **Brown, S. D., K. Krisher, and M. M. Traczewski.** 2004. Broth microdilution susceptibility testing of *Francisella tularensis:* quality control limits for nine antimicrobial agents and three standard quality control strains. *J. Clin. Microbiol.* **42**:5877–5880.
27. **Brown, S. L., F. T. McKinney, G. C. Klein, and W. L. Jones.** 1980. Evaluation of a safranin-O-stained antigen microagglutination test for *Francisella tularensis* antibodies. *J. Clin. Microbiol.* **11**:146–148.
28. **Bruce, D.** 1887. Note on the discovery of a microorganism in Malta Fever. *Practitioner* **36**:161–170.
29. **Buddle, M. B.** 1956. Studies on *Brucella ovis* (n. sp.), a cause of genital disease of sheep in New Zealand and Australia. *J. Hyg. Camb.* **54**:351–364.
30. **Burke, D. S.** 1977. Immunization against tularemia: analysis of the effectiveness of live *Francisella tularensis* vaccine in prevention of laboratory-acquired tularemia. *J. Infect. Dis.* **135**:55–60.
31. **Carmichael, L. E., and D. W. Bruner.** 1968. Characteristics of a newly recognized species of *Brucella* responsible for infectious canine abortions. *Cornell Vet.* **48**:579–592.
32. **Casteñada, M. R.** 1947. A practical method for routine blood cultures in brucellosis. *Proc. Soc. Exp. Biol. Med.* **64**:114–115.
33. **Centers for Disease Control and Prevention.** 1994. Brucellosis outbreak at a pork processing plant—North Carolina, 1992. *Morb. Mortal. Wkly. Rep.* **43**:113–116.
34. **Centers for Disease Control and Prevention.** 2002. Tularemia—United States, 1990–2000. *Morb. Mortal. Wkly. Rep.* **51**:182–184.
35. **Centers for Disease Control and Prevention.** 2003. Multistate outbreak of monkeypox—Illinois, Indiana, and Wisconsin, 2003. *Morb. Mortal. Wkly. Rep.* **52**:537–540.
36. **Centers for Disease Control and Prevention.** 2005. Tularemia associated with a hamster bite—Colorado, 2004. *Morb. Mortal. Wkly. Rep.* **53**:1202–1203.
37. **Clarridge, J. E., III, T. J. Raich, A. Sjöstedt, G. Sandström, R. O. Darouiche, R. M. Shawar, P. R. Georghiou, C. Osting, and L. Vo.** 1996. Characterization of two unusual clinically significant *Francisella* strains. *J. Clin. Microbiol.* **34**:1995–2000.
38. **Cloeckaert, A., J. Verger, M. Grayon, M. S. Zygmunt, and O. Grepinet.** 1996. Nucleotide sequence and expression of the gene encoding the major 25-kilodalton outer membrane protein of *Brucella ovis:* evidence for antigenic shift, compared with other *Brucella* species, due to a deletion in the gene. *Infect. Immun.* **64**:2047–2055.
39. **Cloeckaert, A., M. Grayon, and O. Grepinet.** 2000. An IS*711* element downstream of the *bp26* gene is a specific marker of *Brucella* spp. isolated from marine mammals. *Clin. Diagn. Lab. Immunol.* **7**:835–839.

40. **Cloeckaert, A., J. Verger, M. Grayon, J. Paquet, B. Garin-Bastuji, G. Foster, and J. Godfroid.** 2001. Classification of *Brucella* spp. isolated from marine mammals by DNA polymorphism at the *omp2* locus. *Microbes Infect.* **3:**729–738.
41. **Conlan, J. W.** 2004. Vaccines against *Francisella tularensis*—past, present and future. *Expert Rev. Vaccines* **3:**307–314.
42. **Cooper, C. L., P. Van Caeseele, J. Canvir, and L. E. Nicoll.** 1999. Chronic prosthetic device infection with *Francisella tularensis*. *Clin. Infect. Dis.* **29:**1589–1591.
43. **Corbel, M. J.** 1988. International committee on systematic bacteriology subcommittee on the taxonomy of *Brucella*. *Int. J. Syst. Bacteriol.* **38:**450–452.
44. **Corbel, M. J.** 1989. Microbiology of the genus *Brucella*, p. 53–72. *In* E. J. Young and M. J. Corbel (ed.), *Brucellosis: Clinical and Laboratory Aspects*. CRC Press, Boca Raton, Fla.
45. **Corbel, M. J.** 1997. Brucellosis: an overview. *Emerg. Infect. Dis.* **3:**213–221.
46. **Corbel, M. J., and W. J. Brinley-Morgan.** 1984. Genus *Brucella*, p. 377–388. *In* N. R. Krieg and J. G. Holt (ed.), *Bergey's Manual of Systematic Bacteriology*, vol. 1. The Williams & Wilkins Co., Baltimore, Md.
47. **Da Costa, M., J. P. Guillou, B. Garin-Bastuji, M. Thiébaud, and G. Dubray.** 1996. Specificity of six gene sequences for the detection of the genus *Brucella* by DNA amplification. *J. Appl. Bacteriol.* **81:**267–275.
48. **DelVecchio, V. G., V. Kapatral, R. J. Redkar, G. Patra, C. Mujer, T. Los, N. Ivanova, I. Anderson, A. Bhattacharyya, A. Lykidis, G. Reznik, L. Jablonski, N. Larsen, M. D'Souza, A. Bernal, M. Mazur, E. Goltsman, E. Selkov, P. H. Elzer, S. Hagius, D. O'Callaghan, J. Letesson, R. Haselkorn, N. Kyrpides, and R. Overbeek.** 2002. The genome sequence of the facultative intracellular pathogen *Brucella melitensis*. *Proc. Natl. Acad. Sci. USA* **99:**443–448.
49. **Dennis, D. T., T. V. Inglesby, D. A. Henderson, J. G. Bartlett, M. S. Ascher, E. Eitzen, A. D. Fine, A. M. Friedlander, J. Hauer, M. Layton, S. R. Lillibridge, J. E. McDade, M. T. Osterholm, T. O'Toole, G. Parker, T. M. Perl, P. K. Russell, and K. Tonat.** 2001. Tularemia as a biological weapon: medical and public health management. *JAMA* **285:**2763–2773.
50. **Department of Health and Human Services, Public Health Service.** 4 June 2002, last reviewed. *Biosafety in Microbiological and Biomedical Laboratories*, 4th ed. HHS publication (CDC) 93-8395. [Online.] Department of Health and Human Services, Washington, D.C. http://www.cdc.gov/od/ohs/biosfty/bmbl4/bmbl4toc.htm.
51. **Drancourt, M., P. Brouqui, and D. Raoult.** 1997. *Afipia clevelandensis* antibodies and cross-reactivity with *Brucella* spp. and *Yersinia enterocolitica* O:9. *Clin. Diagn. Lab. Immunol.* **4:**748–752.
52. **Dricot, A., J. Rual, P. Lamesch, N. Bertin, D. Dupuy, T. Hao, C. Lambert, R. Hallez, J. Delroisse, J. Vandenhaute, I. Lopez-Goñi, I. Moriyon, J. M. Garcia-Lobo, F. J. Sangari, A. P. MacMillan, S. J. Cutler, A. M. Whatmore, S. Bozak, R. Sequerra, L. Doucette-Stamm, M. Vidal, D. E. Hill, J. Letesson, and X. De Bolle.** 2004. Generation of the *Brucella melitensis* ORFeome version 1.1. *Genome Res.* **14:**2201–2206.
53. **Eliasson, H., J. Lindbäck, J. P. Nuorti, M. Arneborn, J. Giesecke, and A. Tegnell.** 2002. The 2000 tularemia outbreak: a case-control study of risk factors in disease-endemic and emergent areas, Sweden. *Emerg. Infect. Dis.* **8:**956–960.
54. **Ellis, J., P. C. Oyston, M. Green, and R. W. Titball.** 2002. Tularemia. *Clin. Microbiol. Rev.* **15:**631–646.
55. **Elsaghir, A., and E. James.** 2003. Misidentification of *Brucella melitensis* as *Ochrobactrum anthropi* by API 20NE. *J. Med. Microbiol.* **52:**441–442.
56. **Emmons, R. W., J. D. Woodie, M. S. Taylor, and G. S. Nygaard.** 1970. Tularemia in a pet squirrel monkey (*Saimiri sciureus*). *Lab. Anim. Care* **30:**1149–1153.
57. **Ericsson, M., G. Sandström, A. Sjöstedt, and A. Tarnvik.** 1994. Persistence of cell-mediated immunity and decline of humoral immunity to the intracellular bacterium *Francisella tularensis*. *J. Infect. Dis.* **170:**110–114.
58. **Etemadi, H., A. Raissadat, M. J. Pickett, Y. Zafari, and P. Vahedifar.** 1984. Isolation of *Brucella* spp. from clinical specimens. *J. Clin. Microbiol.* **20:**586.
59. **Evans, A. C.** 1918. Further studies on *Bacterium abortus* and related bacteria. II. A comparison of *Bacterium abortus* with *Bacterium bronchosepticus* and with the organism which causes Malta fever. *J. Infect. Dis.* **22:**580–593.
60. **Farlow, J., K. L. Smith, J. Wong, M. Abrams, M. Lytle, and P. Keim.** 2001. *Francisella tularensis* strain typing using multilocus variable-number tandem repeat analysis. *J. Clin. Microbiol.* **39:**3186–3192.
61. **Feldman, K. A., R. Enscore, S. Lathrop, B. Matyas, M. McGuill, M. Schriefer, D. Stiles-Enos, D. Dennis, and E. Hayes.** 2001. Outbreak of primary pneumonic tularemia on Martha's Vineyard. *N. Engl. J. Med.* **345:**1601–1606.
62. **Ficht, T. A., H. S. Husseinen, J. Derr, and S. W. Bearden.** 1996. Species-specific sequences at the *omp2* locus of *Brucella* type strains. *Int. J. Syst. Bacteriol.* **46:**329–331.
63. **Forsman, M., G. Sandström, and B. Jaurin.** 1990. Identification of *Francisella* species and discrimination of type A and type B strains of *F. tularensis* by 16S rRNA analysis. *Appl. Environ. Microbiol.* **56:**949–955.
64. **Forsman, M., G. Sandström, and A. Sjöstedt.** 1994. Analysis of 16S ribosomal DNA sequences of *Francisella* strains and utilization for determination of the phylogeny of the genus and for identification of strains by PCR. *Int. J. Syst. Bacteriol.* **44:**38–46.
65. **Forsman, M., A. Nyrén, A. Sjöstedt, L. Sjökvist, and G. Sandström.** 1995. Identification of *Francisella tularensis* in natural water samples by PCR. *FEMS Microbiol. Ecol.* **16:**83–92.
66. **Fosgate, G. T., T. E. Carpenter, B. B. Chomel, J. T. Case, E. E. DeBess, and K. F. Reilly.** 15 July 2002, revision date. Time-space clustering of human brucellosis, California, 1973–1992. *Emerg. Infect. Dis.* **8.** [Online.] http://www.cdc.gov/ncidod/EID/vol8no7/01-0351.htm.
67. **Francis, E.** 1921. The occurrence of tularemia in nature as a disease of man. *Public Health Rep.* **36:**1731–1738.
68. **Franz, E. R., P. B. Jahrling, A. M. Friedlander, D. J. McClain, D. L. Hoover, W. R. Bryne, J. A. Pavlin, G. W. Christopher, and E. M. Eitzen.** 1997. Clinical recognition and management of patients exposed to biological warfare agents. *JAMA* **278:**399–411.
69. **Friis-Møller, A., L. E. Lemming, N. H. Valerius, and B. Bruun.** 2004. Problems in identification of *Francisella philomiragia* associated with fatal bacteremia in a patient with chronic granulomatous disease. *J. Clin. Microbiol.* **42:**1840–1842.
70. **Gandara, B., A. Lopez Merino, M. A. Rogel, and E. Martinez-Romero.** 2001. Limited genetic diversity of *Brucella* spp. *J. Clin. Microbiol.* **39:**235–240.
71. **Garrity, G. M., and J. G. Holt.** 2001. Taxonomic outline of the *Archaea* and *Bacteria*, p. 155–166. *In* D. R. Boone and R. C. Castenholz (ed.), *Bergey's Manual of Systematic Bacteriology*, 2nd ed., vol. 1. Springer-Verlag, New York, N.Y.
72. **Gee, J. E., B. K. De, P. N. Levett, A. M. Whitney, R. T. Novak, and T. Popovic.** 2004. Use of 16S rRNA gene sequencing for rapid confirmatory identification of *Brucella* isolates. *J. Clin. Microbiol.* **42:**3649–3654.
73. **Godfroid, J., A. Cloeckaert, J. Liautard, S. Kohler, D. Fretin, K. Walravens, B. Garin-Bastuji, and J. Letesson.** 2005. From the discovery of the Malta fever's agent to the discovery of a marine mammal reservoir, brucellosis

has continuously been a re-emerging zoonosis. *Vet. Res.* **36:**313–326.

74. **Goethert, H. K., I. Shani, and S. R. Telford.** 2004. Genotypic diversity of *Francisella tularensis* infecting *Dermacentor variabilis* ticks on Martha's Vineyard, Massachusetts. *J. Clin. Microbiol.* **42:**4968–4973.
75. **Gotuzzo, E., C. Carrillo, J. Guerra, and L. Llosa.** 1986. An evaluation of diagnostic methods for brucellosis—the value of bone marrow culture. *J. Infect. Dis.* **153:**122–125.
76. **Greis, D. M., and M. P. Fairchok.** 1996. Typhoidal tularemia in a human immunodeficiency virus-infected adolescent. *Pediatr. Infect. Dis. J.* **15:**838–840.
77. **Grif, K., M. P. Dierich, P. Much, E. Hofer, and F. Allerberger.** 2003. Identifying and subtyping species of dangerous pathogens by automated ribotyping. *Diagn. Microbiol. Infect. Dis.* **47:**313–320.
78. **Guarner, J., P. R. Breer, J. C. Bartlett, M. C. Chu, W. J. Shieh, and S. R. Zaki.** 1999. Immunohistochemical detection of *Francisella tularensis* in formalin-fixed paraffin-embedded tissue. *Appl. Immunohistochem. Mol. Morphol.* **7:**122–126.
79. **Gurcan, S., M. T. Otkun, M. Otkun, O. K. Aridan, and B. Ozer.** 2004. An outbreak of tularemia in Western Black Sea region of Turkey. *Yonsei Med. J.* **45:**17–22.
80. **Halling, S. M., B. D. Peterson-Burch, B. J. Bricker, R. L. Zuerner, Z. Qing, L. Li, V. Kapur, D. P. Alt, and S. C. Olsen.** 2005. Completion of the genome sequence of *Brucella abortus* and comparison to the highly similar genomes of *Brucella melitensis* and *Brucella suis*. *J. Bacteriol.* **187:**2715–2726.
81. **Han, X. Y., L. X. Ho, and A. Safdar.** 2004. *Francisella tularensis* peritonitis in stomach cancer patient. *Emerg. Infect. Dis.* **10:**2238–2240.
82. **Hoelzle, L. E., L. Corboz, P. Ossent, and M. M. Wittenbrink.** 2004. Tularaemia in a captive golden-headed lion tamarin *(Leontopithecus chrysomelas)* in Switzerland. *Vet. Rec.* **155:**60–61.
83. **Hollis, D. G., R. E. Weaver, A. G. Steigerwalt, J. D. Wenger, C. W. Moss, and D. J. Brenner.** 1989. *Francisella philomiragia* comb. nov. (formerly *Yersinia philomiragia*) and *Francisella tularensis* biogroup novicida (formerly *Francisella novicida*) associated with human disease. *J. Clin. Microbiol.* **27:**1601–1608.
84. **Hopla, C. E., and A. K. Hopla.** 1994. Tularemia, p. 113–126. *In* G. W. Beran and J. H. Steele (ed.), *Handbook of Zoonoses*, 2nd ed. CRC Press, Boca Raton, Fla.
85. **Huddleston, I. F.** 1929. Differentiation of the species of the genus *Brucella*. *Am. J. Public Health* **21:**491–498.
86. **Ikäheimo, I., H. Syrjälä, J. Karhukorpi, R. Schildt, and M. Koskela.** 2000. *In vitro* antibiotic susceptibility of *Francisella tularensis* isolated from humans and animals. *J. Antimicrob. Chemother.* **46:**287–290.
87. **Inzana, T. J., G. E. Glindermann, G. Snider, S. Gardner, L. Crofton, B. Bryne, and J. Harper.** 2004. Characterization of a wild-type strain of *Francisella tularensis* isolated from a cat. *J. Vet. Diagn. Investig.* **16:**374–381.
88. **Jahans, K. L., G. Foster, and E. S. Broughton.** 1997. The characterization of *Brucella* strains isolated from marine mammals. *Vet. Microbiol.* **57:**373–382.
89. **Jellison, W. L.** 1974. *Tularemia in North America, 1930–1974*, p. 1–276. University of Montana, Missoula, Mont.
90. **Jellison, W. L., C. R. Owen, J. F. Bell, and G. M. Kohls.** 1961. Tularemia and animal populations: ecology and epizootiology. *Wildl. Dis.* **17:**1–15.
91. **Johansson, A., L. Berglund, U. Eriksson, I. Göransson, R. Wollin, M. Forsman, A. Tärnvik, and A. Sjöstedt.** 2000. Comparative analysis of PCR versus culture for diagnosis of ulceroglandular tularemia. *J. Clin. Microbiol.* **38:**22–26.
92. **Johansson, A., A. Ibrahim, I. Göransson, U. Eriksson, D. Gurycová, J. E. Clarridge III, and A. Sjöstedt.** 2000. Evaluation of PCR-based methods for discrimination of *Francisella* species and subspecies and development of a specific PCR that distinguishes the two major subspecies of *Francisella tularensis*. *J. Clin. Microbiol.* **38:**4180–4185.
93. **Johansson, A., S. K. Urich, M. C. Chu, A. Sjöstedt, and A. Tärnvik.** 2002. In vitro susceptibility to quinolones of *Francisella tularensis* subspecies *tularensis*. *Scand. J. Infect. Dis.* **34:**327–330.
94. **Johansson, A., J. Farlow, P. Larsson, M. Dukerich, E. Chambers, M. Byström, J. Fox, M. Chu, M. Forsman, A. Sjöstedt, and P. Keim.** 2004. Worldwide genetic relationships among *Francisella tularensis* isolates determined by multiple-locus variable-number tandem repeat analysis. *J. Bacteriol.* **186:**5808–5818.
95. **Khoury, J. A., D. L. Bohl, M. J. Hersh, A. C. Argoudelis, and D. C. Brennan.** 2005. Tularemia in a kidney transplant recipient: an unsuspected case and literature review. *Am. J. Kidney Dis.* **45:**926–929.
96. **Kolman, S., M. C. Maayan, G. Gotesman, L. A. Rozenzajn, B. Wolach, and R. Lang.** 1991. Comparison of the BACTEC and lysis concentration methods for recovery of *Brucella* species from clinical specimens. *Eur. J. Clin. Microbiol. Infect. Dis.* **10:**647–648.
97. **La Regina, M. L., J. Longro, and M. Wallace.** 1986. *Francisella tularensis* infection in captive, wild caught prairie dogs. *Lab. Anim. Sci.* **4:**178–180.
98. **Larsson, P., P. C. Oyston, P. Chain, M. C. Chu, M. Dufield, H. H. Fuxelius, E. Garcia, G. Halltorp, D. Johansson, K. E. Isherwood, P. D. Karp, E. Larsson, Y. Liu, S. Michell, J. Prior, R. Prior, S. Malfatti, A. Sjöstedt, K. Svensson, N. Thompson, L. Vergez, J. K. Wagg, B. W. Wren, L. E. Lindler, S. G. Andersson, M. Forsman, and R. W. Titball.** 2005. The complete genome sequence of *Francisella tularensis*, the causative agent of tularemia. *Nat. Genet.* **37:**153–159.
99. **Long, G. W., J. J. Oprandy, R. B. Narayanan, A. H. Fortier, K. R. Porter, and C. A. Nacy.** 1993. Detection of *Francisella tularensis* in blood by polymerase chain reaction. *J. Clin. Microbiol.* **31:**152–154.
100. **Lundquist, M., M. B. Caspersen, P. Wikström, and M. Forsman.** 2005. Discrimination of *Francisella tularensis* subspecies using surface enhanced desorption ionization mass spectrometry and multivariate data analysis. *FEMS Microbiol. Lett.* **243:**303–310.
101. **Mantur, B. G., and S. S. Mangalgi.** 2004. Evaluation of conventional Castaneda and lysis centrifugation blood culture techniques for diagnosis of human brucellosis. *J. Clin. Microbiol.* **42:**4327–4328.
102. **Maranan, M. C., D. Schiff, D. C. Johnson, C. Abrahams, M. Wylam, and S. I. Gerber.** 1997. Pneumonic tularemia in a patient with chronic granulomatous disease. *Clin. Infect. Dis.* **25:**630–633.
103. **Massachusetts Medical Society.** 1985. Case records of the Massachusetts General Hospital (case 27-1985). *N. Engl. J. Med.* **313:**36–42.
104. **Massachusetts Medical Society.** 2000. Case records of the Massachusetts General Hospital (case 14-2000). *N. Engl. J. Med.* **342:**1430–1437.
105. **McCoy, G. W., and C. W. Chapin.** 1912. *Bacterium tularense* the cause of a plague-like disease of rodents. *U.S. Public Health Hosp. Bull.* **53:**17–23.
106. **Meinkoth, K. R., R. J. Morton, and J. H. Meinkoth.** 2004. Naturally occurring tularemia in a dog. *J. Am. Vet. Med. Assoc.* **225:**545–547.
107. **Meyer, K. F., and E. B. Shaw.** 1920. A comparison of the morphologic, culture and biochemical characteristics of *B. abortus* and *B. melitensis:* studies on the genus *Brucella* nov. gen. I. *J. Infect. Dis.* **27:**173–184.

108. **Miguel Gómez, M. A., M. A. Bratos Pérez, F. J. Martín Gil, A. Dueñas Diez, J. F. Martín Rodríguez, P. Gutiérrez Rodríguez, A. Orduña Domingo, and A. Rodríguez Torres.** 2003. Identification of species of *Brucella* using Fourier transform infrared spectroscopy. *J. Microbiol. Methods* **55:**121–131.
109. **Miller, W. G., L. G. Adams, T. A. Ficht, N. F. Cheville, J. P. Payeur, D. R. Harley, C. House, and S. H. Ridgway.** 1999. *Brucella*-induced abortions and infection in bottlenose dolphins *(Tursiops truncatus)*. *J. Zoo Wildl. Med.* **30:**100–110.
110. **Moreno, E., and I. Moriyón.** 2 November 2001, posting date. The genus *Brucella*. *In* M. Dworkin (ed.), *The Prokaryotes: an Evolving Electronic Resource for the Microbiological Community*, 3rd ed., release 3.7. [Online.] Springer-Verlag, New York, N.Y. http://link.springer-ny.com/link/service/books/10125/.
111. **Mörner, T., G. Sandström, and R. Matsson.** 1988. Comparison of serum and lung extracts for surveys of wild animals for antibodies to *Francisella tularensis* biovar *palaearctica*. *J. Wildl. Dis.* **24:**10–14.
112. **Naughton, M., R. Brown, D. Adkins, and J. DiPersio.** 1999. Tularemia—an unusual cause of a solitary pulmonary nodule in the post-transplant setting. *Bone Marrow Transplant.* **24:**197–199.
113. **Navarro, E., M. A. Casao, and J. Solera.** 2004. Diagnosis of human brucellosis using PCR. *Expert Rev. Mol. Diagn.* **4:**115–123.
114. **Nayar, G. P. S., G. J. Crawshaw, and J. L. Neufeld.** 1979. Tularemia in a group of nonhuman primates. *J. Am. Vet. Med. Assoc.* **175:**962–963.
115. **Newby, D. T., T. L. Hadfield, and F. F. Roberto.** 2003. Real-time PCR detection of *Brucella abortus*: a comparative study of SYBR green I, 5′-exonuclease, and hybridization probe assays. *Appl. Environ. Microbiol.* **69:**4753–4759.
116. **Nimri, L. F.** 2003. Diagnosis of recent and relapsed cases of human brucellosis by PCR assay. *BMC Infect. Dis.* **3:**5.
117. **Noviello, S., R. Gallo, M. Kelly, R. Limberger, K. DeAngelis, L. Cain, B. Wallace, and N. Dumas.** 2004. Laboratory-acquired brucellosis. *Emerg. Infect. Dis.* **10:**1848–1850.
118. **Ohara, S., T. Sato, and M. Homma.** 1974. Serological studies on *Francisella tularensis*, *Francisella novicida*, *Yersinia philomiragia*, and *Brucella abortus*. *Int. J. Syst. Bacteriol.* **24:**191–196.
119. **Olsufjev, N. G., and I. S. Meshcheryakova.** 1982. Infraspecific taxonomy of tularemia agent *Francisella tularensis* McCoy et Chapin. *J. Hyg. Epidemiol. Microbiol. Immunol.* **3:**291–299.
120. **Olsufjev, N. G., K. N. Shlygina, and E. V. Ananova.** 1984. Persistence of *Francisella tularensis* McCoy et Chapin tularemia agent in the organism of highly sensitive rodents after oral infection. *J. Hyg. Epidemiol. Microbiol. Immunol.* **28:**441–454.
121. **Overholt, E. I., W. D. Tigertt, P. J. Kadull, M. K. Ward, N. D. Charkes, R. M. Rene, T. E. Salzman, and M. Stephens.** 1961. An analysis of forty-two cases of laboratory-acquired tularemia. *Am. J. Med.* **30:**785–806.
122. **Oyston, P. C., A. Sjöstedt, and R. W. Titball.** 2004. Tularaemia: bioterrorism defence renews interest in *Francisella tularensis*. *Nat. Rev. Microbiol.* **2:**967–978.
123. **Ozturk, R., A. Mert, F. Kocak, R. Ozaras, F. Koksal, F. Tabak, M. Bilir, and Y. Aktuglu.** 2002. The diagnosis of brucellosis by use of BACTEC 9240 blood culture system. *Diagn. Microbiol. Infect. Dis.* **44:**133–135.
124. **Paulsen, I. T., R. Seshadri, K. E. Nelson, J. A. Eisen, J. F. Heidelberg, T. D. Read, R. J. Dodson, L. Umayam, L. M. Brinkac, M. J. Beanan, S. C. Daugherty, R. T. Deboy, A. S. Durkin, J. F. Kolonay, R. Madupu, W. C. Nelson, B. Ayodeji, M. Kraul, J. Shetty, J. Malek, S. E. Van Aken, S. Riedmuller, H. Tettelin, S. R. Gill, O. White, S. L. Salzberg, D. L. Hoover, L. E. Lindler, S. M. Halling, S. M. Boyle, and C. M. Fraser.** 2002. The *Brucella suis* genome reveals fundamental similarities between animal and plant pathogens and symbionts. *Proc. Natl. Acad. Sci. USA* **99:**13148–13153.
125. **Petersen, J. M., E. Schriefer, L. G. Carter, Y. Zhou, T. Sealy, D. Baweic, B. Yockey, S. Urich, N. S. Zeidner, S. Avashia, J. L. Kool, J. Buck, C. Lindley, L. Celeda, J. A. Monterneiri, K. L. Gage, and M. C. Chu.** 2004. Laboratory analysis of tularemia in wild-trapped, commercially traded prairie dogs, Texas, 2002. *Emerg. Infect. Dis.* **10:**419–425.
126. **Pittman, T., D. Williams, and A. D. Friedman.** 1996. A shunt infection caused by *Francisella tularensis*. *Pediatr. Neurosurg.* **24:**50–51.
127. **Porsch-Özcürümez, M., N. Kischel, H. Priebe, W. Splettstösser, E. J. Finke, and R. Grunow.** 2004. Comparison of enzyme-linked immunosorbent assay, Western Blotting, microagglutination, indirect immunofluorescence assay, and flow cytometric serological diagnosis of tularemia. *Clin. Diagn. Lab. Immunol.* **11:**1008–1015.
128. **Posthaus, H., M. Welle, T. Mörner, J. Nicolet, and P. Kuhnert.** 1998. Tularemia in a common marmoset *(Calithrix jacchus)* diagnosed by 16S rRNA sequencing. *Vet. Microbiol.* **61:**145–150.
129. **Preiksaitis, J. K., G. J. Crawshaw, G. S. P. Nayar, and H. G. Stiver.** 1979. Human tularemia at an urban zoo. *Can. Med. Assoc. J.* **121:**1097–1099.
130. **Probert, W. S., K. N. Schrader, N. Y. Khuong, S. L. Bystrom, and M. H. Graves.** 2004. Real-time multiplex PCR assay for detection of *Brucella* spp., *B. abortus*, and *B. melitensis*. *J. Clin. Microbiol.* **42:**1290–1293.
131. **Queipo-Ortuño, M. I., J. D. Colmenero, G. Baeza, and P. Morata.** 2005. Comparison between the LightCycler real-time polymerase chain reaction (PCR) assay with serum and PCR-enzyme-linked immunosorbent assay with whole blood samples for the diagnosis of human brucellosis. *Clin. Infect. Dis.* **40:**260–264.
132. **Radolf, J. D.** 1994. Brucellosis: don't let it get your goat. *Am. J. Med. Sci.* **307:**64–75.
133. **Redklar, R., S. Rose, B. Bricker, and V. delVecchio.** 2001. Real-time detection of *Brucella abortus*, *Brucella melitensis*, and *Brucella suis*. *Mol. Cell. Probes* **15:**43–52.
134. **Reintjes, R., I. Dedushaj, A. Gjini, T. R. Jorgensen, B. Cotter, A. Lieftucht, F. D'Ancona, D. T. Dennis, M. A. Kosoy, G. Mulliqi-Osmani, R. Grunow, A. Kalaveshi, L. Gashi, and I. Humolli.** 2002. Tularemia outbreak investigation in Kosovo: case control and environmental studies. *Emerg. Infect. Dis.* **8:**69–73.
135. **Rijpens, N. P., G. Jannes, M. Van Asbroeck, R. Rossau, and L. M. F. Herman.** 1996. Direct detection of *Brucella* spp. in raw milk by PCR and reverse hybridization with 16S-23S rRNA spacer probes. *Appl. Environ. Microbiol.* **62:**1683–1688.
136. **Robichaud, S., M. Libman, M. Behr, and E. Rubin.** 24 May 2004, posting date. Prevention of laboratory-acquired brucellosis. *Clin. Infect. Dis.* **38:**e119–e122. [Online.] http://www.journals.uchicago.edu/CID/journal/issues/v38n12/33078/33078.html.
137. **Rodriguez-Torrez, A., J. Fermoso, and R. Landinez.** 1983. Brucellosis. *Medicine* **48:**3126–3136. (In Spanish.)
138. **Rotz, L. D., A. S. Kahn, S. R. Lillibridge, S. M. Ostroff, and J. M. Hughes.** 2002. Public health assessment of potential biological terrorism agents. *Emerg. Infect. Dis.* **8:**225–230.
139. **Ruiz, J., I. Lorente, J. Pérez, E. Simmarro, and L. Martínez-Campos.** 1997. Diagnosis of brucellosis by using blood cultures. *J. Clin. Microbiol.* **35:**2417–2418.
140. **Rusnak, J. M., M. G. Kortepeter, R. J. Hawley, A. O. Anderson, E. Boudreau, and E. Eitzen.** 2004. Risk of

occupationally acquired illnesses from biological threat agents in unvaccinated laboratory workers. *Biosecur. Bioterror.* **2:**281–293.

141. **Sandström, G., A. Sjöstedt, M. Forsman, N. V. Pavlovich, and B. N. Mishankin.** 1992. Characterization and classification of strains of *Francisella tularensis* isolated in the Central Asian focus of the Soviet Union, and in Japan. *J. Clin. Microbiol.* **30:**172–175.
142. **Sarria, J. C., A. M. Vidal, R. C. Kimbrough, and J. E. Figueroa.** 2002. Fatal infection caused by *Francisella tularensis* in a neutropenic bone marrow transplant recipient. *Ann. Hematol.* **82:**41–43.
143. **Schmitt, P., W. Splettstosser, M. Porsch-Özcürümez, E. J. Finke, and R. Grunow.** 2005. A novel screening ELISA and a confirmatory Western blot useful for diagnosis and epidemiological studies of tularemia. *Epidemiol. Infect.* **133:**759–766.
144. **Serrano, M. L., J. Llosa, C. Castells, J. Mendoza, J. M. Navarro, and M. de la Rosa.** 1987. Detection radiometrica de bacteriemias por *Brucella. Enferm. Infec. Microbiol. Clin.* **5:**139–142.
145. **Shapiro, D. S., and D. R. Schwartz.** 2002. Exposure of laboratory workers to *Francisella tularensis* despite a bioterrorism procedure. *J. Clin. Microbiol.* **40:**2278–2281.
146. **Sicherer, S. H., E. J. Asturias, J. A. Winkelstein, J. D. Dick, and R. E. Willoughby.** 1997. *Francisella philomiragia* sepsis in chronic granulomatous disease. *Pediatr. Infect. Dis. J.* **16:**420–422.
147. **Sjöstedt, A.** 2004. *Francisella*, p. 200–210. *In* D. J. Brenner, N. R. Kreig, J. T. Staley, and G. M. Garrity (ed.), *Bergey's Manual of Systematic Bacteriology*, 2nd ed., vol. 2, *The Proteobacteria.* Springer-Verlag, New York, N.Y.
148. **Sjöstedt, A., U. Eriksson, L. Berglund, and A. Tärnvik.** 1997. Detection of *Francisella tularensis* in ulcers of patients with tularemia by PCR. *J. Clin. Microbiol.* **35:**1045–1048.
149. **Smits, H. L., M. A. Basahi, R. Diaz, T. Marrodan, J. T. Douglas, A. Rocha, J. Veerman, M. M. Zheludkov, O. W. M. Witte, J. de Jong, G. G. Gussenhoven, M. G. A. Goris, and M. A. W. G. van der Hoorn.** 1999. Development and evaluation of a rapid dipstick assay for serodiagnosis of acute human brucellosis. *J. Clin. Microbiol.* **37:**4179–4182.
150. **Sohn, A. H., W. S. Probert, C. A. Glaser, N. Gupta, A. W. Bollen, J. D. Wong, E. M. Grace, and W. C. McDonald.** 2003. Human neurobrucellosis with intracerebral granuloma caused by a marine mammal *Brucella* spp. *Emerg. Infect. Dis.* **9:**485–488.
151. **Solera, J., E. Martinez-Alfaro, and A. Espinosa.** 1997. Recognition and optimum treatment of Brucellosis. *Drugs* **53:**245–256.
152. **Spink, W. W., N. B. McCullough, L. M. Hutchings, and C. K. Mingle.** 1954. A standardized antigen and agglutination technique for human brucellosis. *Am. J. Clin. Pathol.* **24:**466–468.
153. **Stoenner, H. G., and D. B. Lackman.** 1957. A new species of *Brucella* isolated from the desert woodrat *Neotoma lepida. Am. J. Vet. Res.* **18:**947–951.
154. **Surcel, H. M., J. Ilonen, K. Poikonen, and E. Herva.** 1989. *Francisella tularensis*-specific T-cell clones are human leukocyte antigen class II restricted, secrete interleukin-2 and gamma interferon, and induce immunoglobulin production. *Infect. Immun.* **57:**2906–2908.
155. **Surcel, H. M., M. Sarvas, I. M. Helander, and E. Herva.** 1989. Membrane proteins of *Francisella tularensis* LVS differ in ability to induce proliferation of lymphocytes from tularemia-vaccinated individuals. *Microb. Pathog.* **7:**411–419.
156. **Syrjälä, H., R. Schildt, and S. Räisäinen.** 1991. In vitro susceptibility of *Francisella tularensis* to fluoroquinolones and treatment of tularemia with norfloxacin and ciprofloxacin. *Eur. J. Clin. Microbiol. Infect. Dis.* **10:**68–70.
157. **Syrjälä, H. P., V. Kujala, V. Myllyla, and A. Salminen.** 1985. Airborne transmission of tularemia in farmers. *Scand. J. Infect. Dis.* **17:**371–375.
158. **Tärnvik, A.** 1989. Nature of protective immunity to *Francisella tularensis. Rev. Infect. Dis.* **11:**440–451.
159. **Tärnvik, A., and L. Berglund.** 2003. Tularaemia. *Eur. Respir. J.* **21:**361–373.
160. **Traum, J.** 1914. *Report of the Chief of the Bureau of Animal Industry,* p. 30. U.S. Department of Agriculture, Washington, D.C.
161. **Valentine, B. A., B. M. DeBey, R. J. Sonn, L. R. Stauffer, and L. G. Pielstick.** 2004. Localized cutaneous infection with *Francisella tularensis* resembling ulceroglandular tularemia in a cat. *J. Vet. Diagn. Investig.* **16:**83–85.
162. **Verger, J. M., F. Grimont, P. A. D. Grimont, and M. Grayon.** 1985. *Brucella,* a monospecific genus as shown by deoxyribonucleic acid hybridization. *Int. J. Syst. Bacteriol.* **35:**292–295.
163. **Versage, J. L., D. D. Severin, M. C. Chu, and J. M. Petersen.** 2003. Development of a multitarget real-time Taqman PCR assay for enhanced detection of *Francisella tularensis* in complex specimens. *J. Clin. Microbiol.* **41:**5492–5499.
164. **Viljanen, M. K., T. Nurmi, and A. Salminen.** 1983. Enzyme-linked immunosorbent assay (ELISA) with bacterial sonicate antigen for IgM, IgA, and IgG antibodies to *Francisella tularensis*: comparison with bacterial agglutination test and ELISA with lipopolysaccharide antigen. *J. Infect. Dis.* **148:**715–720.
165. **Vizcaino, N., A. Cloeckaert, J. M. Verger, M. Grayon, and L. Fernandez-Lago.** 2000. DNA polymorphism in the genus *Brucella. Microbes Infect.* **2:**1089–1100.
166. **Waag, D. M., K. T. McKee, Jr., G. Sandström, L. L. K. Pratt, C. R. Bolt, M. J. England, G. O. Nelson, and J. C. Williams.** 1995. Cell-mediated and humoral immune responses after vaccination of human volunteers with the live vaccine strain of *Francisella tularensis. Clin. Diagn. Lab. Immunol.* **2:**143–148.
167. **Waggie, K. S., P. A. Day-Lollini, P. A. Marphy-Hackley, J. R. Blum, and G. W. Morrow.** 1997. Diagnostic exercise: illness, cutaneous hemorrhage, and death in two squirrel monkeys *(Saimiri sciureus). Lab. Anim. Sci.* **47:**647–649.
168. **Wenger, J. D., D. G. Hollis, R. E. Weaver, C. N. Baker, G. R. Brown, D. J. Brenner, and C. V. Broome.** 1989. Infection caused by *Francisella philomiragia* (formerly *Yersinia philomiragia*): a newly recognized human pathogen. *Ann. Intern. Med.* **110:**888–892.
169. **Weyant, R. S., C. W. Moss, R. E. Weaver, D. G. Hollis, J. G. Jordan, E. C. Cook, and M. I. Daneshvar.** 1996. *Identification of Unusual Pathogenic Gram-Negative Aerobic and Facultatively Anaerobic Bacteria,* 2nd ed. The Williams & Wilkins Co., Baltimore, Md.
170. **Whatmore, A. M., T. J. Murphy, S. Shankster, E. Young, S. J. Cutler, and A. P. Macmillan.** 2005. Use of amplified fragment length polymorphism to identify and type *Brucella* isolates of medical and veterinary interest. *J. Clin. Microbiol.* **43:**761–769.
171. **Whipp, M. J., J. M. Davis, G. Lum, J. de Boer, Y. Zhou, S. W. Bearden, J. M. Petersen, M. C. Chu, and G. Hogg.** 2003. Characterization of a novicida-like subspecies of *Francisella tularensis* in Australia. *J. Med. Microbiol.* **52:**839–842.
172. **Wolff, K. L., and B. W. Hudson.** 1974. Paper-strip blood-sampling technique for the detection of antibody to the plague organism *Yersinia pestis. Appl. Microbiol.* **28:**323–325.
173. **Yagupsky, P., N. Peled, J. Press, O. Abramson, and M. Abu-Rashid.** 1997. Comparison of BACTEC 9240 Peds Plus medium and Isolator 1.5 microbial tube for detection

of *Brucella melitensis* from blood cultures. *J. Clin. Microbiol.* **35:**1382–1384.

174. **Yagupsky, P., and N. Peled.** 2002. Use of the Isolator 1.5 microbial tube for detection of *Brucella melitensis* in synovial fluid. *J. Clin. Microbiol.* **40:**3878.

175. **Young, E. J.** 1989. Clinical manifestations of human brucellosis, p. 97–126. *In* E. J. Young and M. J. Corbel (ed.), *Brucellosis: Clinical and Laboratory Aspects*. CRC Press, Boca Raton, Fla.

176. **Young, E. J.** 1995. An overview of human brucellosis. *Clin. Infect. Dis.* **21:**283–290.

177. **Young, E. J.** 1999. *Brucella* species, p. 71–89. *In* V. L. Yu, T. C. Merigan, Jr., and S. L. Barriere (ed.), *Antimicrobial Therapy and Vaccines*. The Williams & Wilkins Co., Baltimore, Md.

178. **Young, E. J.** 2000. *Brucella* species, p. 2386–2393. *In* G. L. Mandell, J. E. Bennett, and R. Dolin (ed.), *Mandell, Douglas, and Bennett's Principles and Practice of Infectious Diseases*, vol. 2. Churchill Livingstone, Inc., Philadelphia, Pa.

179. **Young, L. S., D. S. Bicknell, B. G. Archer, J. M. Clinton, L. J. Leavens, J. C. Feeley, and P. S. Brachman.** 1969. Tularemia epidemic, Vermont, 1968: forty-seven cases linked to contact with muskrats. *N. Engl. J. Med.* **280:**1253–1260.

180. **Zervos, J., and G. Bostic.** 1997. Exposure to *Brucella* in the laboratory. *Lancet* **349:**651.

*Legionella**

PAUL H. EDELSTEIN

53

TAXONOMY

The *Legionellaceae* are composed of a single genus, *Legionella*, and 50 validly named species (http://www.bacterio.cict.fr/l/legionella.html) (Table 1). *Legionella pneumophila, L. micdadei, L. longbeachae,* and *L. dumoffii* are the most important from a clinical standpoint, with *L. pneumophila* causing more than 90% of the cases of Legionnaires' disease (LD). The *Legionellaceae* are most closely related to the *Coxiellaceae,* and these two families constitute the proposed order "*Legionellales,*" within the class *Gammaproteobacteria* and phylum *Proteobacteria* phy. nov. (http://sn2000.taxonomy.nl/Taxonomicon/TaxonTree.aspx?id=111537). *Coxiella burnetii,* the agent of Q fever, shares many characteristics with *L. pneumophila,* including intracellular parasitism and close homologies of several virulence genes (102). Some investigators proposed the use of *Tatlockia* and *Fluoribacter* as additional genera within the *Legionellaceae* (39), but a subsequent study of 16S rRNA demonstrated that the *Legionellaceae* are monophyletic (36); use of these genus names was never widely accepted and is of historical interest only. A number of *Legionella*-like bacteria have been described to grow only within free-living amoebae and have been designated LLAP, for *Legionella*-like amoebal pathogen. One of the LLAPs, *L. lytica,* has been shown to cause human disease, and four have been assigned novel *Legionella* spp.; three of these four have been grown axenically at low temperature (1).

DESCRIPTION OF THE AGENT

The *Legionellaceae* are a diverse group of mesophilic, motile, asaccharolytic, obligately aerobic, nutritionally fastidious gram-negative rods, sharing growth dependence for L-cysteine, growth enhancement by iron, and cellular branched-chain fatty acids and ubiquinones that are unusual for gram-negative bacteria (23). *L. pneumophila* is the most extensively studied of the *Legionella* spp., with relatively little known about most of the other *Legionella* spp. Almost all of the *Legionella* spp. have been isolated from aqueous environmental sources and about one-third of the 50 validly named species have been isolated from both humans and the environment. It is assumed that the natural reservoir of all the *Legionellaceae* is our aqueous environment and that humans are an accidental host of the bacterium. Environmental *L. pneumophila* is a facultative intracellular parasite of several different free-living amoebae, such as *Acanthamoeba* and *Naegleria,* existing in microbial consortia in biofilms and free-flowing water.

L. pneumophila grows optimally at 35 to 37°C and grows less well at temperatures ranging from 20 to 42°C. Growth on solid media is enhanced by increased humidity. Incubation in 2 to 5% CO_2 can enhance the growth of some, but not most, *Legionella* spp. Bacterial phenotype, including immunogenicity, cell size, and virulence, can be altered by growth at different temperatures (23).

Amino acids, rather than carbohydrates, are used as energy sources by the *Legionellaceae* growing in vitro; this is true for intracellular bacteria as well, despite the presence of putative carbohydrate utilization genes in the *L. pneumophila* genome (23). Primary isolation of all known *Legionella* spp. requires medium supplementation with L-cysteine, as does successful propagation of all but a few species. Iron supplementation of growth media is required for optimal growth, although many *Legionella* spp. can grow, albeit poorly, in the absence of the mineral. Growth of *L. pneumophila* is enhanced by the addition of α-ketoglutarate (0.1%) to media, via an unknown, nonnutritive mechanism.

Growth of *L. pneumophila* in artificial media can be inhibited by a number of extraneous factors. These include the presence of high (100 mM, or 0.6%) NaCl concentrations, toxic peroxides, products of other bacteria and fungi, and some lipids (23). In addition, optimal growth occurs over a very narrow pH range, from 6.7 to 6.9. Solid growth media contain activated charcoal to inactivate toxic lipids and peroxides and an organic buffer (MOPS [morpholine propanesulfonic acid] or ACES [*N*-(2-acetamido)-2-aminoethanesulfonic acid]) to reduce sodium content and provide the required pH. Preparation of growth media for *Legionella* spp. can be complex and is usually best left to competent commercial sources or to specialized laboratories.

EPIDEMIOLOGY AND TRANSMISSION

LD was first recognized as a distinct entity when epidemic pneumonia with a 15% fatality rate developed during and after a convention of Pennsylvania State Legionnaires in

*This chapter contains information presented in chapter 52 by Janet E. Stout, John D. Rihs, and Victor L. Yu in the eighth edition of this Manual.

TABLE 1 Selected characteristics of *Legionella* spp.[a]

Legionella sp.[b]	Isolated from humans[c]	No. of recognized serogroups	Color under long-wave UV light	Comments
L. adelaidensis	N	1	NC	
L. anisa	Y	1	BW/YG	
L. beliardensis	N	1	YG	
L. birminghamensis	Y	1	YG	
L. bozemanae	Y	2	BW	AN, *Fluoribacter bozemanae*[d]
L. brunensis	N	1	NC	
L. busanensis	N	1	NC	
L. cherrii	N	1	BW	
L. cincinnatiensis	Y	1	YG	
L. drancourtii	N	NK	NK	Amoebic pathogen; no axenic growth
L. drozanskii	N	1	NC	Grows at 30°C but not at 37°C
L. dumoffii	Y	1	BW	AN, *F. dumoffii*[d]
L. erythra	N	2	R	
L. fairfieldensis	N	1	NC	
L. fallonii	N	1	NC	Grows at 30°C but not at 37°C
L. feeleii	Y	2	NC	
L. geestiana	N	1	NC	
L. gormanii	Y	1	BW	AN, *F. gormanii*[d]
L. gratiana	N	1	NC	
L. gresilensis	N	1	YG	
L. hackeliae	Y	2	YG	
L. israelensis	N	1	NC	
L. jamestowniensis	N	1	YG	
"*L. jeonii*"	N	NK	NK	Amoebic endosymbiont
L. jordanis	Y	1	YG	Partial L-cysteine dependence with serial passage
L. lansingensis	Y	1	NC	
L. londiniensis	N	1	NC	
L. longbeachae	Y	2	YG	
L. lytica	Y	NK	BW	Grows at 30°C but not at 37°C
L. maceachernii	Y	1	YG	AN, *Tatlockia maceachernii*[d]
L. micdadei	Y	1	YG	AN, *T. micdadei*[d]
L. moravica	N	1	NC	
L. nautarum	N	1	NC	
L. oakridgensis	Y	1	YG	Partial L-cysteine dependence with serial passage
L. parisiensis	Y	1	BW	
L. pneumophila	Y	16	YG	Three subspecies recognized
L. quateirensis	N	1	NC	
L. quinlivanii	N	2	YG	
L. rowbothamii	N	1	BW	
L. rubrilucens	N	1	R	
L. sainthelensi	Y	2	YG	
L. santicrucis	N	1	YG	
L. shakespearei	N	1	NC	
L. spiritensis	N	2	YG	Partial L-cysteine dependence with serial passage
L. steigerwaltii	N	1	BW	
L. taurinensis	N	1	R/yg	
L. tucsonensis	Y	1	BW	
L. wadsworthii	Y	1	YG	
L. waltersii	N	1	NC	
L. worsleiensis	N	1	NC	

[a] Abbreviations: Y, yes; N, no; NK, not known; NC, no color; BW, bright blue-white; YG, pale yellow-green; BW/YG, some strains are BW and some are YG; R, dark red; R/yg, majority of strains are red, with remainder YG.

[b] All species listed, except "*L. jeonii*," constitute validly published names. Several other species probably exist.

[c] Severely immunosuppressed patients may acquire infections with *Legionella* spp. not previously isolated from humans.

[d] AN, alternative name; while valid, the genus names *Fluoribacter* and *Tatlockia* are not in widespread usage.

Philadelphia in July 1976 (22, 33). Joseph McDade and colleagues at the CDC determined that a novel gram-negative bacterium was the cause of the outbreak (70). Neither the disease nor the bacterium was found to be novel, with the first known epidemic of LD having occurred in 1957 (78) and isolation of the bacterium having occurred multiple times from the 1940s on.

Environmental studies found that the bacterium was widespread in natural bodies of water and occasionally in high concentration in warm waters found in plumbing systems, water heaters, warm water spas, and cooling towers. Many different *Legionella* spp. exist in nature within free-living amoebae, and as a result these otherwise fastidious bacteria can multiply within the amoebae and be protected from biocides (87). *Legionella*-infected amoebae are often found in complex consortia of microorganisms within biofilms. The bacteria are present in very low concentrations in freely flowing cold water and biocide-treated waters but can multiply in warm, and especially stagnant, water. Devices that aerosolize these contaminated waters serve to disseminate the bacteria.

The usual route of infection is thought to be by aerosol inhalation, although microaspiration of contaminated water may also be a mechanism of acquiring the disease (22). The majority of community epidemics of LD are from *Legionella*-contaminated cooling towers or other aerosol-generating devices. Contaminated potable water systems, such as water heaters and warm water in pipes, can also be a major source of disease, especially in hospitals, although they are not usually the cause of explosive outbreaks of the disease.

The bacterial inoculum required to cause human infection or disease is unknown. Animal studies performed using broth-grown bacteria show the infecting dose to be in the range of 10 to 500 CFU and the fatal dose to be about 10^4 to 10^5 CFU. Since bacterial virulence for cells or animals can be enhanced by growth in amoebae or by infection with the spore-like form, the infective doses may be even lower for naturally grown bacteria (2, 38).

Despite the ubiquity of legionella bacteria in our environment, LD is an unusual cause of pneumonia. It is estimated that 0.5 to 5% of adults requiring hospitalization for pneumonia have LD. Passive reporting indicates that the disease incidence is from 4 to 20 cases per million people per year, and a prospective study estimated that the disease incidence is about 80 cases per million people per year, or between 8,000 to 18,000 LD cases annually in the United States (69). Sporadic community-acquired LD is much more common than epidemic-associated disease, in a ratio of about 4 to 1.

The incubation period of LD is estimated to be between 2 and 14 days, with a median value of about 4 days. A study of a large outbreak extended the incubation period to as long as 19 days, with a median value of 7 days (12).

L. pneumophila causes disease by infecting human mononuclear cells, primarily alveolar macrophages. After the bacterium is inhaled into the lungs, it invades lung macrophages and multiplies in them. Detailed descriptions of pathogenesis can be found elsewhere (22, 23).

CLINICAL SIGNIFICANCE

LD is a type of bacterial pneumonia caused by *L. pneumophila* and other *Legionella* spp. The pneumonia ranges in severity from mild to fatal, with an average fatality rate of 12% (4). Major risk factors for the disease include immunosuppression of the cellular immune system, cigarette smoking, overnight travel outside the home, use of well water, chronic heart or lung disease, and chronic renal failure.

LD cannot be readily distinguished from other forms of community-acquired pneumonia by clinical, roentgenographic, or nonspecific laboratory studies (22). Several attempts at developing a clinical scoring system to distinguish LD from other pneumonias have failed.

The severity of pneumonia at presentation, underlying diseases, and promptness of specific antibiotic therapy are important prognostic factors. Promptly treated, LD can be cured in 95 to 99% of cases occurring in otherwise healthy persons. Less than one-half of patients may respond if there is a delay in therapy, immunosuppression, or respiratory failure (22). Untreated disease causes death in about 15% of previously healthy patients and up to 75% of severely immunocompromised ones.

Prospective, randomized controlled studies of adequate size have not been performed to determine the optimal therapy for LD, so great reliance is placed on experimental tissue culture and animal model studies, as well as results of nonrandomized studies (18, 22). Erythromycin, clarithromycin, azithromycin, a tetracycline, telithromycin, levofloxacin, ciprofloxacin, gatifloxacin, and moxifloxacin all appear to have roughly equivalent efficacy for nonimmunocompromised outpatients with mild LD (22). The quinolone antimicrobials, especially levofloxacin, and azithromycin are the drugs of choice for severe disease and for immunocompromised patients (22, 74).

Pontiac fever is an acute influenza-like illness that has been associated with exposure to *Legionella*-containing environmental aerosols (32, 42). The etiology and pathogenesis of this disease are unknown, but it appears as if the disease is caused by inhalation of bacterial toxins, such as endotoxin, or perhaps an acute allergic reaction to a bacterium. Since multiple microorganisms and endotoxin have been found in aerosols causing Pontiac fever, it is unclear if *Legionella* spp. play any role at all in disease causation. Pontiac fever is self-limited, with no reported deaths, little to no need for hospitalization, and no need for antibiotic therapy.

COLLECTION, STORAGE, AND TRANSPORT

Expectorated sputum and other lower respiratory specimens are the most common sources of *Legionella* spp. Other, less common sources include pleural fluid and blood. Rare sources have included pericardial fluid, kidney, liver, spleen, myocardium, respiratory sinuses, skin and soft tissues, infected wounds, peritoneal fluid, bone marrow, and intestine. Culture of available sputum, bronchoscopy specimens, lung biopsy specimens, and pleural fluid should be routine for laboratory diagnosis of LD. Lung biopsy specimens have the highest yield but may be negative. Culture of expectorated sputum or other lower respiratory tract secretions, second in yield to lung biopsy, should always be performed for optimal detection of legionella infection. Pleural fluid has low yield but should be cultured if it is available. Routine culture of other specimens for *Legionella* spp. is not indicated unless there is a high clinical suspicion of the disease affecting these sites.

Sputum microscopic scoring criteria cannot be used to determine which sputum specimens should be cultured for legionella bacteria because of limited purulence and scanty secretions in patients with LD. Up to 80% of specimens culture positive for *Legionella* spp. may be rejected when using the criterion of the presence of sputum purulence for processing specimens (31, 54).

Urine for antigen detection should be collected in a sterile container (16). Boric acid preserves the antigen, but commercial urine transport systems containing boric acid have not been studied for antigen preservation and freedom from interactions. The urine can be transported to the laboratory at room temperature if no more than a several hour delay is anticipated. Longer transport times require specimen refrigeration; urine specimens should not be frozen, as this may reduce test sensitivity and specificity.

Blood for serum antibody testing is collected in standard tubes and transported at room temperature(19). Test performance is not adversely affected by storage of the clotted unseparated blood at room temperature for several days. Long-term storage is at –20°C in aliquots to allow parallel testing without freeze-thawing, which can lower antibody levels.

Legionella is hardy and generally survives for up to a week in clinical specimens. Sputum and other respiratory tract specimens, including lung biopsy specimens, should be collected in sterile containers and transported to the laboratory promptly at room temperature. Transportation and storage should be at 2 to 5°C if more than a several hour delay is anticipated before the specimen can be plated. Very long-term storage is best at –70°C, although this can reduce bacterial concentration to below the level of detection in cases where the starting concentration is low or the specimen is primarily aqueous. Repeated freeze-thawing is harmful to the bacteria. Some tissues, especially spleen, contain growth-preventing substances and must be plated promptly; even overnight storage at 5°C dramatically reduces culture yield; however, this is not true of lung specimens.

DIRECT SPECIMEN EXAMINATION

Microscopy

L. pneumophila found in lung and sputum is a small coccobacillus to short rod, 3 to 5 μm in length (Fig. 1). This morphology is very different from that observed for the bacterium taken from a culture plate, which is usually a long, filamentous bacillus, 10 to 25 μm in length. *L. pneumophila* is difficult to detect by Gram staining of sputum or lung biopsy specimens. Use of 0.1% basic fuchsin, rather than safranin, greatly enhances the staining of the bacterium from culture plates, but even with use of this stain it is often very difficult to visualize the bacterium in sputum and tissues. Less than 0.1% of *L. pneumophila* present in lung tissue or sputum can be visualized by Gram staining using basic fuchsin. The small

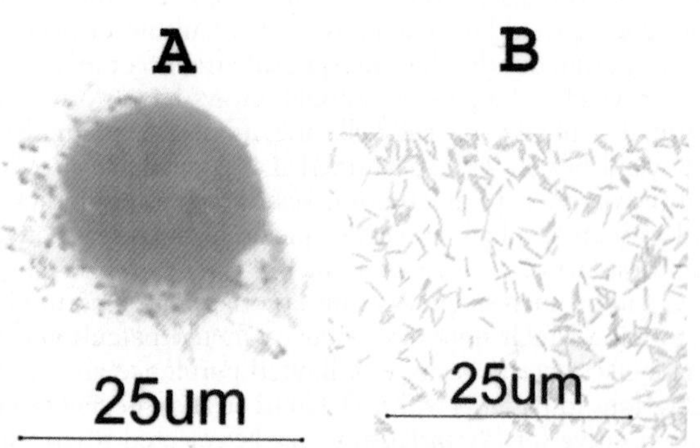

FIGURE 1 Photomicrographs of *L. pneumophila*. (A) Gimenez stain of intracellular bacteria in lung infection. (B) Gram stain using basic fuchsin counterstain of colony taken from BCYEα plate. Note the dramatic size and shape differences between the intracellular and extracellular bacteria.

size of intracellular *L. pneumophila* bacteria, the form present in human tissues, makes visualization difficult with Gram stain, as does stain uptake by the surrounding proteinaceous material found in sputum and tissue.

Use of the Gimenez stain dramatically increases the number of *L. pneumophila* organisms detected in sputum and lung tissue, 100- to 1,000-fold over that visualized with Gram stain using basic fuchsin counterstain. Even so, this stain is very insensitive for the detection of the bacterium in sputum when compared to immunofluorescent microscopy (27). Sensitivity of the Gimenez stain for the detection of *L. pneumophila* in lung tissue has not been studied, but it appears to be high in fulminant cases. Unfortunately, the Gimenez stain is difficult to prepare, is not commercially available, requires filtration before each use, and can be unstable. Finally, the Gimenez stain cannot distinguish between *L. pneumophila* and other bacteria present in sputum and tissues. The stain detects the bacterium in Formalin-fixed, but not embedded, tissues (43).

Enhancement of bacterial staining by silver precipitate stains, such as the Warthin-Starry stain and its modifications and the Dieterle stain (29, 101), was an early approach to the detection of *L. pneumophila* in embedded tissues as well as sputum. These silver stains are useful for detection of the bacterium in embedded tissues but have no present role in the staining of the bacterium in sputum or other nonembedded specimens. Silver stains are not highly sensitive, can produce artifacts, and require expert use and interpretation for optimal sensitivity and specificity.

Immunofluorescent microscopy is the most sensitive and specific microscopic method for the detection of *L. pneumophila* in tissues and sputum (17, 27). Optimal sensitivity and specificity require exacting staining methods and great expertise by the microscopist. Polyclonal antibodies, which are commercially available, can be used to stain the bacterium in fresh, fixed, and embedded tissues and secretions. A commercially available monoclonal antibody (Bio-Rad, Hercules, Calif.) is useful for the highly specific staining of nonfixed tissues and secretions but loses sensitivity when used to stain fixed or embedded tissues (21, 41). Even when performed expertly, immunofluorescent microscopy is insensitive for the detection of *L. pneumophila* in sputum, detecting from 25 to 75% of culture-proven cases. False-positive tests with the polyclonal antibody can result from cross-reactions with non-*Legionella* bacteria, including *Pseudomonas aeruginosa*, *P. fluorescens*, *Bacteroides fragilis*, *Staphylococcus aureus*, *Bordetella pertussis*, *Bacillus* spp., lactobacillus-like bacteria, and candida-like yeasts; the number and variety of these potential cross-reactions make it imperative that the microscopist be skilled in distinguishing the morphology of *L. pneumophila* from those of the cross-reacting bacteria (6). Even so, some false-positive reactions will be recorded by very experienced microscopists. The monoclonal antibody has many fewer cross-reactions but may cross-react with *S. aureus* and *Bacillus* spp. In addition, *Legionella* organisms present in buffers, wash solutions, or Formalin, from specimen containers contaminated during manufacture, and from cross-contaminating, true-positive specimens can all cause false-positive tests. This means that extreme care needs to be taken to keep all slides physically separated from one another, to filter sterilize critical buffers and other aqueous solutions, and to screen specimen containers. Most important is performance of the staining and slide reading by an expert. Performance of these tests by inexperienced technologists can lead to many more false-positive than true-positive results. More details on immunofluorescent microscopy can be found elsewhere (17).

Antigen Detection

LD due to *L. pneumophila* serogroup 1 can often be diagnosed by detection of bacterial antigenuria (16). Several immunoassays are commercially available for this purpose, the most convenient of which is a rapid single-test immunochromatographic card assay (Binax, Scarborough, Maine). Several other assays utilize a microtube-based enzyme immunoassay. Only one kit (Biotest, Denville, N.J.) is designed to detect non-serogroup 1 *L. pneumophila* and appears to be somewhat sensitive for the detection of these infections (52). The strength of all these assays is their ability to detect *L. pneumophila* serogroup 1 infections, and in particular the Pontiac/MAB2/MAB3-1 monoclonal subtype (48–50). The immunochromatographic card assay may be somewhat less sensitive than the microtube-based immunoassays, although its convenience, ease of use, and robustness make up for a slightly lesser sensitivity.

Clinical test performance for all assays is dependent on the pretest probability of *L. pneumophila* serogroup 1 and on the probability of Pontiac monoclonal subtype *L. pneumophila* serogroup 1 infection (48, 50). Infection caused by *L. pneumophila* serogroup 1 Pontiac subtype is most common in epidemic and sporadic community-acquired LD and least common in nosocomial LD, especially that involving immunocompromised patients. About 80 to 90% of community-acquired LD is due to this subtype, whereas up to 60% of nosocomial LD may be caused by other *L. pneumophila* serogroup 1 subtypes, other *L. pneumophila* serogroups, and other *Legionella* species (48, 49). The assays detect about 60 to 70% of *L. pneumophila* serogroup 1 Pontiac monoclonal subtype epidemic infections and up to 90% of sporadic pneumonia caused by this subtype. The differences in test sensitivity for the same bacterial subtype are probably due to differences in disease severity, the other major factor determining test sensitivity. Patients with severe *L. pneumophila* serogroup 1 LD are the most likely to have positive urine antigen tests, for example, those requiring intensive care nursing and ventilator assistance; test sensitivity in this population is probably in the range of 90 to 95% of those infected with the Pontiac monoclonal subtype. On the other hand, urine testing may detect only 50% of outpatients with mild epidemic disease caused by the same monoclonal subtype, perhaps 40% of hospitalized patients with other *L. pneumophila* serogroup 1 subtypes, and fewer than 5 to 40% of those with infections caused by other serogroups and species, with the higher sensitivity value for testing being obtained with the Biotest kit (49, 52). The test may be negative during the first day of illness, but those with severe disease are likely to be positive on presentation to hospital. Repeat testing 2 to 3 days after the onset of illness may detect a small number of infections in patients who had negative tests initially.

Test sensitivity can be enhanced by concentrating the specimen by use of ultrafiltration devices such as Amicon concentrators (Millipore, Billerca, Mass.). In some studies this has increased test sensitivity by about 30%, without affecting specificity (14, 44). Test sensitivity decreases when specimens are frozen for weeks to months before testing.

The urine antigen assays are very specific, in the range of 99 to 99.9%. False-positive results can be due to urine rheumatoid-like factors, freeze-thawing of urine, and excessive urinary sediment. All together, these causes of false-positive results account for no more than a few percent of all positive results. Regardless, all positive results should be confirmed after boiling urine clarified by centrifugation.

Molecular Diagnosis of LD

PCR-based detection of *L. pneumophila* genes in sputum, urine, and blood has been successfully used in reference and research laboratories. The best results show that molecular diagnosis is a more sensitive method of diagnosis than culture, although some studies showed rough equivalence (73). Test sensitivities have been estimated to be 80 to 100%, 30 to 50%, and 50 to 90% for lower respiratory secretions, serum, and urine analytes, respectively; test specificities are estimated to be >90% (73). Both conventional and real-time assays have been utilized (51, 73). Until recently, only home brew assays were available.

One commercial assay, the BD ProbeTec ET *Legionella*, based on the Becton Dickinson ProbeTec methodology, is cleared for marketing by the U.S. FDA (BD Diagnostics, Sparks, Md.). Test sensitivity for 23 culture-proven archived sputum specimens was 91% (95% confidence interval [CI], 72 to 99%), and specificity was 87% (95% CI, 75 to 94%) in one study and 100% (95% CI, 96.8 to 100%) in another study. Several sputum specimens that were apparent false positives were also positive by a second molecular method (U.S. FDA 510K k033861 clearance letter, March 2004; http://www.fda.gov/cdrh/reviews/K033861.doc).

ISOLATION PROCEDURES

Specimen Plating

Optimal yield of *Legionella* spp. from clinical specimens usually requires that specimens be diluted to reduce inhibition by tissue and serum factors as well as antibiotics; that the specimen be pretreated to reduce contaminating flora; and that a variety of selective and nonselective media be used (Table 2). Culture of *Legionella* spp. from normally sterile fluids and tissues, such as pleural fluid, aseptically obtained lung tissue, or blood, is often successful without the use of multiple selective tissues and specimen decontamination.

Dilution (1:10) in tryptic soy broth increases the culture yield of most specimen types including sputum and other liquid respiratory tract specimens, lung tissue, lymph nodes, spleen, and probably other organs such as liver and kidney. Sputum and other respiratory specimens should first be examined in a petri dish for material that appears purulent, and this material should be selected for culture. Tissues (about 1 g) are ground in a tissue grinder with a small amount (1 ml) of broth, which adequately dilutes most tissues except for spleen; this tissue requires an additional 1:10 dilution for the best recovery of bacteria. Liquid specimens are roughly diluted by adding 3 drops of vortex-mixed liquid specimens to 0.9 ml of the dilution broth. Pleural fluid, joint fluid, and blood subcultured from blood culture bottles do not require dilution before plating; in fact, pleural fluid yield may be enhanced by concentration by centrifugation.

Decontamination, by either of two methods, is required to reduce contaminating flora in most sputum specimens and other respiratory tract secretions. The first method consists of diluting (1:10) the specimen in a low pH KCl-HCl buffer (pH 2.2) and incubating the mixture at room temperature (4.0 min) before plating the suspension onto culture media. Timing is critical here, since a low yield may result if the timing is off by as little as 1 min. The culture medium is sufficiently buffered so that the acidified specimen is neutralized upon being plated. The second method, an alternative to specimen acidification, consists of heating the specimen at 50°C for 30 min. Most aseptically collected tissue specimens do not require decontamination, although occasionally lung tissues contain multiple contaminating bacteria and fungi. In this case, heat or acid treatment of tissue ground in sterile distilled water may help; sometimes dilutions of the ground tissues are also required for optimal yield, with or without pretreatment.

TABLE 2 Composition and selectivity of media used to grow *Legionella* spp. from clinical and environmental specimens[a]

Medium	Synonym	Selective agents	Main use	Selectivity[b]
BCYEα	CYE	None	Clinical, culture maintenance	None
BMPA	PAC	Cephamandole, poly B, antifungal	Clinical, environmental	Normal respiratory flora, 3+; enterics, 3+; yeasts, 3+; molds, 1+; *Legionella* spp., 1+ to 4+
PAV	VAP	Vanco, poly B, antifungal	Clinical, environmental	Normal respiratory flora, 2+; enterics, 2+; yeasts, 3+; molds, 1+; *Legionella* spp., 1+
MWY	VGP	Vanco, poly B, antifungal, glycine	Environmental	Normal respiratory flora, 2+; enterics, 2+; yeasts, 3+; molds, 1+; environmental bacteria, 2+; *Legionella* spp., 1+
CCVC		Cephalothin, poly E, vanco, cycloheximide	Environmental	Normal respiratory flora, +; enterics, 3+; yeasts, 2+; molds, 2+; *Legionella* spp., 1+ to 4+
BCYEα-L		None (made without L-cysteine)	Organism identification	*Legionella* spp., 4+ (no growth of *Legionella* spp. on this medium)

[a] Abbreviations: poly B or E, polymyxin B or E; antifungal, either anisomycin or natamycin antifungal compounds; vanco, vancomycin; normal respiratory flora, normal upper respiratory tract bacteria.

[b] Selectivity scale range, 0 to 4+: 0, does not inhibit these organisms; 1+, slight inhibition, allows about 75% growth; 2+, allows about 25 to 50% growth; 3+, allows about 10% growth; 4+, allows less than 1% growth.

Inoculation of Plates

Approximately 0.1 ml is inoculated into each plate, with the bulk of the inoculum applied to the first quadrant. There is a lack of comparative studies showing whether it is better to streak plates for isolation or to uniformly distribute the inoculum over the entire plate. The plates must be thoroughly dry before being inoculated, to aid in absorption of the relatively large volume inoculum and to retard spreading of contaminants throughout the plate.

Culture Media

Buffered charcoal yeast extract medium, usually supplemented with 0.1% α-ketoglutaric acid (BCYEα), is used for isolation and growth of *Legionella* spp. Use of BCYE without α-ketoglutarate supplementation cannot be recommended for clinical use, as this amino acid greatly enhances growth of the bacterium (25).

BCYEα can be made selective by the addition of antimicrobial agents (Table 2). A variety of different antifungal agents are used in the media. Cycloheximide is a poor choice for media used for clinical specimens as it fails to inhibit *Candida albicans*. Both anisomycin and natamycin inhibit more yeasts than does cycloheximide. This dizzying array of media (Table 2) exists because no one selective medium is best for all purposes. Optimal yield of *Legionella* spp. from clinical specimens requires the use of three different media, one nonselective plate medium (BCYEα) and two selective media (BMPA and MWY). BMPA is an excellent selective medium for the vast majority of *L. pneumophila* strains, but the cephamandole present in the medium inhibits the growth of some other *Legionella* spp. and very rare *L. pneumophila* strains. Therefore, use of the less selective medium, MWY, is required for optimal growth of some *Legionella* spp. other than *L. pneumophila*. No selective medium inhibits multiresistant gram-negative bacteria found in hospitals, reducing culture yield in nosocomial disease.

Selective and nonselective media are optimized for the isolation of *L. pneumophila*, and their performance for the isolation of other *Legionella* spp. is not accurately known. One study showed that *L. micdadei* in guinea pig spleen had enhanced recovery on BCYEα medium prepared with 1% bovine serum albumin; the growth was enhanced because of decreased growth inhibition by spleen tissue (71). Whether addition of bovine serum albumin to BCYEα medium enhances *L. micdadei* recovery from human lung or sputum is unknown and probably unlikely. A BCYEα-based selective medium containing natamycin, aztreonam, and vancomycin has been reported to be useful for the isolation of *L. longbeachae* from soil (88).

Medium shelf life is around 1 year for nonselective plates and slants. This long shelf life requires thick plates (25-ml pour), complete drying of plates before storage at 2 to 4°C in sealed plastic bags, and protection from light. Selective media lose selectivity after about 3 months' storage time, but depending on the antibiotic used, they may last considerably longer.

Quality control (QC) testing of media is required before they are put into use. Current Clinical and Laboratory Standards Institute (CLSI) (NCCLS) standards are inadequate for proper QC testing of these media. About 1% of commercial media fail our laboratory QC testing. The CLSI QC testing protocol utilizes a heavy inoculum of medium-adapted *Legionella* strains and a growth/no-growth test. Minor variations in the manufacture of media, such as the addition of excess salt, overlong autoclaving, and degradation of buffers, can all seriously affect the ability of the medium to support wild strain growth, but not necessarily that of medium-adapted strains. The optimal method for medium QC testing is the inoculation of the test media with several hundred non-artificial medium-passed *L. pneumophila* bacteria (obtained from infected guinea pig lung) and quantification of the bacterial colonies after 3 to 4 days of incubation (20). In the absence of the availability of lung-passaged *L. pneumophila* bacteria, low-passage clinical strains should be used, taking care to plate only several hundred bacteria per plate. QC testing of selective media for the ability to suppress non-*Legionella* bacteria can be done by inoculation of the plate with relatively antibiotic-susceptible strains of *Escherichia coli* and *Staphylococcus aureus*, such as ATCC 25922 and 25923; the growth should be markedly suppressed.

Medium Incubation

Inoculated media are incubated at 35 to 37°C in humidified air. Regardless of the humidification method, care must be taken to keep the incubators or jars very clean and to regularly sterilize the containers or incubators. A small amount of CO_2 supplementation (2 to 5%) may enhance the growth of some of the more fastidious *Legionella* spp., such as *L. sainthelensi* and *L. oakridgenensis*. This low level of CO_2 supplementation will not harm the growth of *L. pneumophila*, but CO_2 levels higher than 5% may inhibit growth. Since the more capnophilic species are very rare human isolates, many laboratories do not use CO_2 incubation of media for *Legionella* spp.

Plate Inspection

Legionella colonies begin to appear on culture plates on day 3 of incubation. It is very unusual for the bacterial colonies to appear on plates after five incubation days. Some very rarely isolated *Legionella* spp. may require up to 14 days of incubation before growth appears; this is an extremely rare event. Regardless, it is reasonable to inspect culture plates on days 1 to 5 and then again at day 14.

The late appearance of *Legionella* spp. on culture plates can be used to great advantage if a careful record is kept of the colonies present on days 1 and 2 postincubation. New colonies appearing after day 2 should be suspected of being *Legionella* spp. Very rarely *Legionella* spp. may grow from heavily infected lung (usually from the autopsy of a fatal untreated case) on day 2, so some latitude in growth rate assumptions needs to be applied in the case of autopsy lung cultures. *Legionella* spp. never grow from clinical specimens on day 1 postincubation, a critical point in the distinction of *Pseudomonas aeruginosa* colonies from those of *Legionella* spp., as very early colonies of the latter superficially resemble those of the former.

Proper observation of culture plates requires the use of a dissecting microscope illuminated with direct light aimed at the plate surface at approximately a 30° angle. Failure to use a dissecting microscope or use of improper lighting will result in missed positive cultures, especially when there is mixed bacterial growth on the plates. In addition, very young *Legionella* colonies are very small and difficult to see with the naked eye. Therefore, use of a dissecting microscope can speed up the time to colony detection by as much as 1 day. *Legionella* growth occurs almost exclusively in the first streak quadrant, and sometimes at the edge of the plate.

The size and morphology of *Legionella* colonies change with time. Very young colonies (day 3) are flat, entire, and 0.5 to 1 mm in diameter, and when observed using a dissecting microscope and incident visible light they usually have a speckled blue, blue-green, or red color. Within 6 to 24 h of additional incubation, these colonies become smooth, convex, iridescent, and entire, measure about 1 to 3 mm in diameter, and look opal-like when observed with a dissecting microscope (Fig. 2). A thick string may form when a loop is inserted in the colony and then removed from the colony. In contrast to several mimics, the edges of the colonies are of the same consistency as the central portion and are not watery and clear. In another 1 to 2 days the colonies may increase in size up to 5 to 7 mm, become umbonate, sometimes with tuberculated or inhomogeneous texture, and develop spready edges; their iridescent nature may be lost at this stage. It is these late-stage colonies that are most difficult to distinguish from non-*Legionella* bacteria, making daily plate observation crucial for accurate detection. Very rarely some *Legionella* colonies do not change morphology with prolonged incubation.

Biosafety level 2 precautions should be used for manipulation of *Legionella* spp. cultures. It is safe to inspect culture plates and pick and subculture colonies on the open bench in a properly ventilated laboratory. Making an organism emulsion on microscope slides for the purposes of Gram staining can be safely carried out on the open bench. However, vortexing suspensions, sonication, tissue grinding, primary plating, and manipulations that may result in generation of a high-concentration aerosol should be performed in a biological safety cabinet. No well-documented cases of laboratory-acquired LD have been reported.

Initial Workup of Suspect Colonies and Look-Alike Bacteria

Colonies suspected of being *Legionella* spp. should first be subjected to Gram staining to ascertain that the bacteria are small or sometimes filamentous gram-negative rods. A small amount of the colony should be emulsified in sterile water or saline on a glass slide. It is important to completely suspend

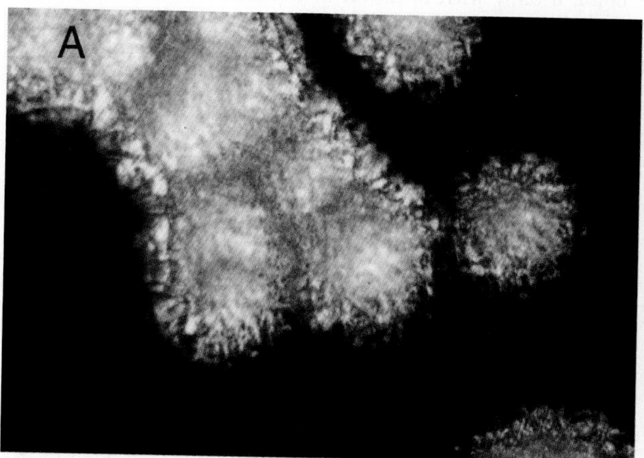

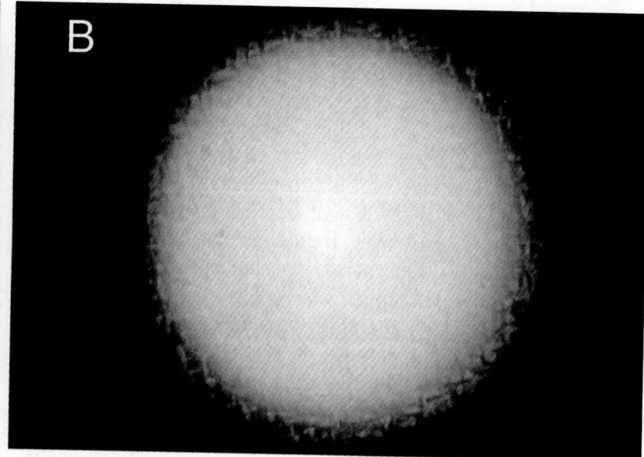

FIGURE 2 Photographs of *L. pneumophila* colonies growing on BCYEα agar. Note the internal speckling and different colors that may be seen, sometimes in the same culture. (Reproduced from Fig. 2, panels A and B, p. 814 of the 8th edition of this Manual.)

the bacteria in the liquid, as nondispersed clumps may stain as gram-positive rods. It is also crucial to use 0.1% basic fuchsin counterstain, because safranin stains these bacteria very poorly. Depending on the colony age and on the strain and species, *Legionella* spp. taken from plates vary in size from short rods measuring 0.5 by 5 μm to very long, filamentous bacteria measuring 1 by 25 μm.

Gram-negative bacteria should then be plated to two different media, BCYEα and either tryptic soy sheep blood agar (BAP) or BCYEα made without L-cysteine (BCYEα-L), in approximately equal amounts in a small (1-cm^2) area; eight or more isolates can be plated to each plate if needed (Fig. 3). Rather large amounts of the picked colony should be inoculated into these media to enable growth after 16 to 18 h of incubation, as the small inocula normally used for other bacteria may otherwise take several days to produce visible colonies on plates. If only a small single colony is available, then it can be emulsified in a small amount (~0.5 ml) of sterile distilled water (not saline) and used for staining, plate inoculation, and seroidentification. *Legionella* spp. should grow in 16 to 36 h on BCYEα medium, but not on BAP or BCYEα-L medium; this takes advantage of the L-cysteine growth dependence of *Legionella* spp. Sometimes *Legionella* spp. will grow poorly on BAP or BCYEα-L media but at most will yield only about 10% of the amount of growth on BCYEα. Nutrient carryover from the primary isolation plate is the explanation for this light growth; this can be proven by making a subculture of growth on BCYEα or BAP on a second plate of the same medium. Rare *Legionella* spp. partially lose growth dependence for L-cysteine on serial passage, but still grow more poorly on BCYEα-L than on BCYEα; these species include *L. spiritensis, L. oakridgensis,* and *L. jordanis,* none of which have been reported to cause more than two cases of LD each. BAP performs almost as well as does BCYEα-L for determining L-cysteine dependence for clinical isolates and may be less expensive, depending on the number of isolates tested per plate. If a blood-containing agar medium is used as the screening plate rather than BCYEα-L for L-cysteine dependence, great care must be taken that the medium base is not too rich. For example, brucella blood agar will support *L. pneumophila* growth almost as well as BCYEα medium, and other blood-containing media have been described to do the same (13). The plates are incubated overnight at 35 to 37°C or until there is visible growth on the BCYEα plate. Compare the relative amounts of growth on each plate to determine if there is L-cysteine dependence. Most *Legionella* spp. produce a very characteristic dank odor when growing in pure growth, which is easily identifiable to the trained nose.

Common mimics of *Legionella* colonies on BCYEα plates include *Eikenella corrodens, P. aeruginosa, Flavobacterium* spp., and some *Bacillus* spp. All of these bacteria grow equally well on BCYEα and BCYEα-L media, but when young they often grow as speckled colonies on BCYEα plates. *Francisella tularensis* can grow well on BCYEα agar but has no resemblance to *Legionella* colonies. However, *F. tularensis* is the only gram-negative bacterium other than *Legionella* spp. that exhibits L-cysteine growth dependence. The colony morphology of *F. tularensis* is not speckled; rather, it is opaque and homogeneous. Adding to the confusion is that some serotyping reagents for *Legionella* spp. may cross-react with *F. tularensis.* There is one case report of the misidentification of *F. tularensis* as *L. pneumophila* (99). Of note, some *Bacillus* sp. mimics can stain as gram-negative rods, have unapparent sporulation, and not grow on BAP (but will grow on BCYEα-L) (91). With prolonged incubation, colonies of both *E. corrodens* and *Flavobacterium* spp. change color and no longer resemble *Legionella* spp.; *E. corrodens* colonies become a light to dark green color, and *Flavobacterium* spp. turn a bright yellow color. Very young *P. aeruginosa* and *Bacillus* spp. colonies resemble the speckled flat to slightly convex young *Legionella* colonies but with prolonged incubation change their morphology, making them easily recognizable as non-*Legionella* colonies. *Bordetella pertussis* colonies may appear late on BCYEα plates, and although this bacterium neither is cysteine dependent nor possesses colony morphology similar to that of *Legionella* spp., *B. pertussis* has been reported to be misidentified as *Legionella* spp., abetted by serological cross-reactivity (76). Because many different bacteria may cross-react with serological reagents used for typing and identifying *Legionella* spp., it is crucial to become familiar with the morphology and growth characteristics of this genus; relying exclusively on serotyping to identify *Legionella* spp. could result in mistaken identification.

Microbiologists should know that some pathogenic fungi and higher bacteria grow well on BCYEα medium, presenting both potential biohazards and the opportunity to diagnose unsuspected infections. *Coccidioides* spp. often grow within a day or two on this medium and can rapidly form arthroconidia, and as such they present a biohazard. *Blastomyces dermatitidis* also grows well and converts to the mold phase within a few days. It is likely that other pathogenic fungi grow equally well on this very rich medium. *Nocardia* spp. and rapidly growing mycobacteria often grow quite well on this medium, making BCYEα medium and its selective variants plating media of choice for the laboratory diagnosis of nocardiosis (57, 98). Nocardia bacteremia can sometimes be diagnosed by subculture of blood culture bottles on BCYEα.

IDENTIFICATION

Basic Identification

Once L-cysteine dependence has been confirmed, further identification of *Legionella* spp. in a clinical laboratory relies almost exclusively on serotyping the bacteria, using either immunofluorescence or agglutination methods (17, 80). Prior to attempting identification by serotyping, the plate should be illuminated with long-wave UV light in a darkroom; some *Legionella* spp. other than *L. pneumophila* fluoresce a brilliant blue-white color, and some a brilliant red; such bacteria are best identified by a reference laboratory and are not *L. pneumophila. L. pneumophila* fluoresces a very pale yellow-green color, usually with diffusion of the fluorescent pigment into the culture medium; this is not specific for this species, and sometimes young cultures are completely nonfluorescent. An excellent and specific FDA-cleared fluorescein isothiocyanate-labeled monoclonal antibody to all serogroups of *L. pneumophila* is available (Monofluo, Bio-Rad). Also, an excellent non-FDA-cleared fluorescein isothiocyanate-labeled *L. pneumophila* serogroup 1 (Philadelphia 1 strain)-specific polyclonal antiserum is available (m-TECH, Atlanta, Ga. [http://www.4m-tech.com/]). Serotyping can also be performed using non-FDA-cleared latex agglutination antisera, available in a variety of formats (Oxoid, Basingstoke, United Kingdom; Denka Seiken, Tokyo, Japan); few data on performance of these reagents are available.

Since more than 90% of *Legionella* isolates are *L. pneumophila* serogroup 1, a reagent- and time-saving technique is to first test with *L. pneumophila* serogroup 1 antibody; strains negative with this antibody can then be tested with the species-specific monoclonal antibody. Extraordinarily rarely, some *L. pneumophila* serogroup 1 strains do not react with Philadelphia 1 strain antibodies, making it possible that a

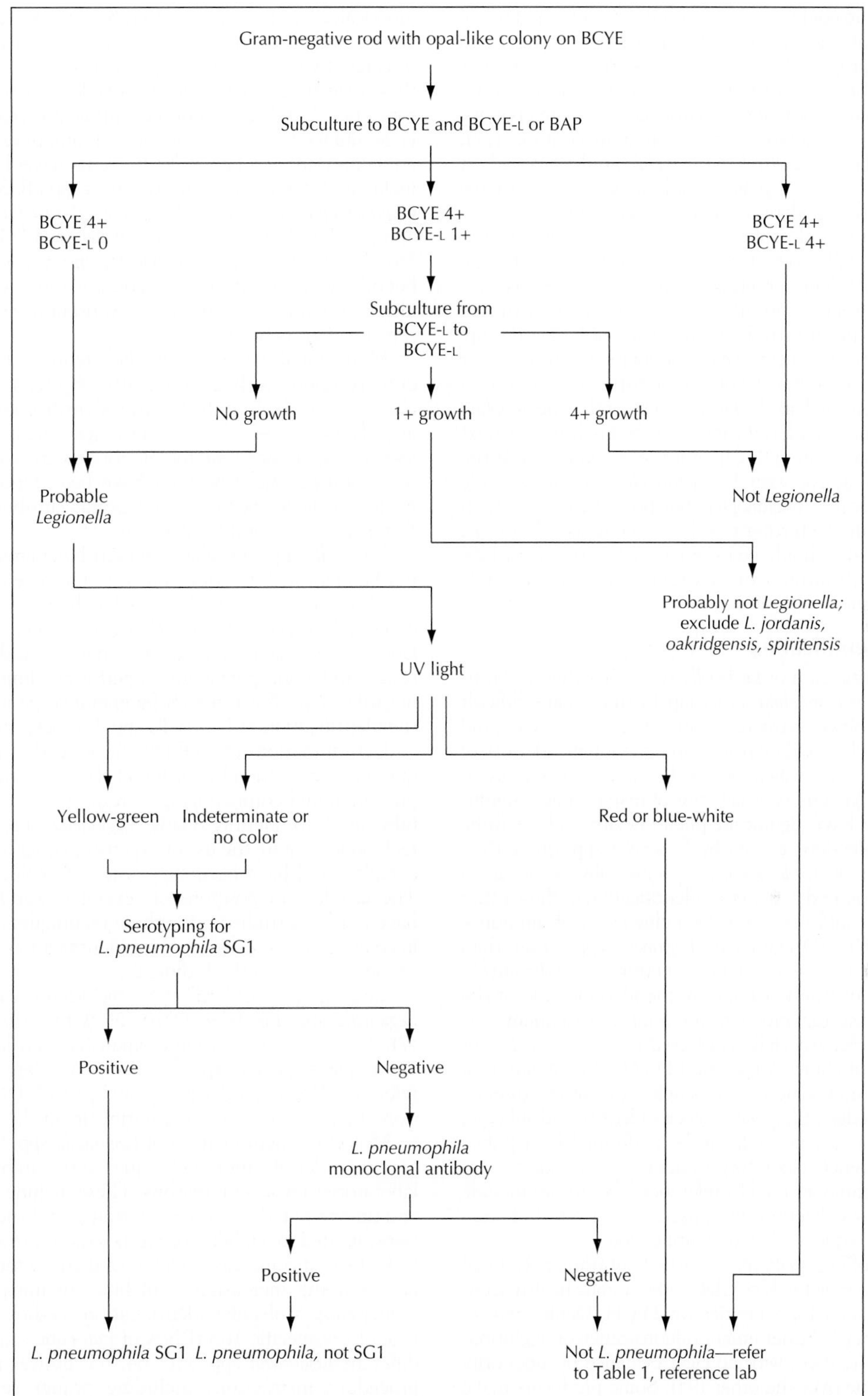

FIGURE 3 Flow scheme for basic identification of *Legionella* spp. grown from a BCYEα plate. Abbreviations: BCYE, BCYEα; BCYE-L, BCYEα made without L-cysteine; BAP, tryptic soy blood agar; UV light, colony fluorescence and color when illuminated with long-wave (360-nm) UV light. Numbers refer to the amount of growth: 4+, good growth; 1+, poor growth; 0, no growth.

serogroup 1 strain could be missed with this reagent; additional serogroup 1 antibodies are available (m-TECH). Testing has to be conducted properly for valid results, with the commonest errors being false-negative results because of a prozone phenomenon and false-positive results from contaminated buffers, wash solutions, or cross-contamination from controls (17). Strains that fail to react with *L. pneumophila* antibodies are best identified by reference or public health laboratories that have other typing sera and identification methods in use.

Gram-negative rods isolated from clinical specimens that are morphologically consistent with *Legionella* spp. and are L-cysteine dependent for growth can be reported as presumptive *Legionella* spp. in the absence of reactivity with typing sera. Gram-negative rods characteristic of *Legionella* spp. that react with *L. pneumophila* monoclonal antibody or *L. pneumophila* serogroup 1 polyvalent antibody can be presumptively identified as *L. pneumophila* or *L. pneumophila* serogroup 1, and the identification can be finalized the next day once L-cysteine growth dependence is confirmed. If the isolate is nonreactive with *L. pneumophila* species-specific antibody, or if it is *L. pneumophila* but not serogroup 1, then the isolate should be further typed by a reference laboratory. All clinical isolates should be frozen at –70°C in TSB in 10% glycerol and subcultured on a BCYEα slant for possible analysis by public health authorities.

Advanced Identification

Accurate identification of *Legionella* spp. other than *L. pneumophila* and *L. pneumophila* serogroup 1 can be quite difficult because of serologic cross-reactivities between species and serogroups, biochemical inertness, and phenotypic identity of different species. Identification to the species or serogroup level for these bacteria is usually not of major clinical significance but may have significant public health and scientific importance. Infections caused by *Legionella* spp. other than *L. pneumophila* or *L. longbeachae* almost always occur in immunocompromised patients, so identification of these other *Legionella* spp. could very rarely be a clue to occult immunosuppression (72). LD caused by *Legionella* spp. other than *L. pneumophila* may respond more poorly to erythromycin therapy (30), but whether knowing the identification of the *Legionella* spp. causing infection would influence patient outcome is debatable, especially since erythromycin is no longer the treatment of choice for severe LD (22). Investigation of LD outbreaks, and sometimes of single cases of the disease, requires knowledge of *Legionella* species identity and subtype; this identification, if needed, can be performed by a public health or reference laboratory as long as the isolates are frozen. The techniques used by reference laboratories include serotyping using collections of antisera, biochemical characterization, and sequence-based identification.

Serotyping of *Legionella* spp. is carried out using polyclonal antisera produced by the U.S. CDC, other public health agencies, and commercial laboratories (m-TECH, Denka Seiken, Oxoid, and others). Either immunofluorescence or agglutination reactions are used, with no clear evidence of superiority of one technique over the other (95). Some producers make polyvalent serum pools that react with a large number of species or serogroups, which can be useful to reduce the number of monovalent antisera used. The specificity of the polyvalent antisera has not been studied in great detail, although at least one product reacted with a number of non-*Legionella* bacteria (24). This makes it important that monovalent typing be carried out and that the bacteria meet minimal phenotypic criteria for *Legionella* spp. Unfortunately, cross-reactions between different species and serogroups occur even when monovalent antisera are used (1, 81, 84, 89, 93, 100). Use of cross-adsorbed polyvalent antisera has been described as a research tool to avoid this problem of cross-reactions, but these reagents are not available outside some research laboratories (5, 92, 94). In addition to intragenus cross-reactions, a large number of cross-reactions of monovalent polyclonal antibodies to non-*Legionella* bacteria have been reported, including *P. aeruginosa*, *Flavobacterium* spp., *Bacteroides fragilis*, *Capnocytophaga ochracea*, *B. pertussis*, *Bordetella bronchiseptica*, and possibly *Burkholderia pseudomallei* (6, 10, 11, 26, 40, 55, 58). Antibody to *L. pneumophila* serogroup 1 is quite specific, but otherwise enough cross-reactions exist to make serological identification only presumptive. Antisera to newer *Legionella* spp. are often unavailable.

Monoclonal typing antibodies reduce the number of cross-reactions with gram-negative bacteria but are commercially available only for the identification of *L. pneumophila* (9, 21, 47, 90). Nevertheless, great care must be used by experienced microbiologists, as cross-reactions with some non-*Legionella* bacteria have been reported with the *L. pneumophila*-specific monoclonal antibody, including *S. aureus*, yeasts, and *Bacillus* spp.

Legionella spp. are relatively inert biochemically and cannot be identified by using conventional tube or commercial panel biochemical tests. The few biochemical characteristics described for *Legionella* spp. that can be determined in most laboratories, such as oxidase, catalase, and β-lactamase tests, can be nonspecific and if performed improperly falsely negative. Use of a research biochemical panel to facilitate the identification of *Legionella* spp. has been described (97).

Determination of cellular fatty acid and isoprenoid quinone composition by gas-liquid chromatography and high-pressure liquid chromatography, respectively, can be successfully used to identify many *Legionella* spp. (61). These techniques require the use of expensive equipment, are highly complex, and have been supplanted by molecular methods. The cellular compositions of several newer *Legionella* spp. have not been studied using these techniques and/or are not in commercial databases, making identification of these newer species by these methods difficult.

The "gold standard" for the identification of new *Legionella* spp. has been DNA-DNA hybridization analysis (7). This method is tedious, expensive, and labor-intensive and requires special expertise as well as a large collection of reference DNA standards. As such, DNA-DNA hybridization analysis is not used to identify already known species.

Molecular identification of *Legionella* spp. is now replacing other identification techniques in research and specialty laboratories for several reasons. These include the labor cost and time required to serotype a strain, serological cross-reactions, limited availability of antibodies to newer strains, the lack of specific and easy biochemical characterization methods, and the increasing availability of inexpensive DNA sequencing. Molecular identification methods take advantage of the specific 16S rRNA or *mip* gene sequences of the different *Legionella* spp. (36, 64, 83, 86). A *mip* database, procedure instructions including primer sequences, *mip* sequence alignment software, and other genomic software tools are all freely available online (http://www.hpa.org.uk/srmd/bioinformatics/ewgli/legionellamips.htm). Sequence analysis of 16S rRNA has been used to identify several new *Legionella* spp. (35, 62, 65, 79). In addition, sequence of the *rpoB* gene has been shown to distinguish between species as well as, or better than, 16S rRNA or *mip* gene sequencing (59). Intergenic 16S-23S ribosomal spacer PCR analysis has been successful for species identification and does not require

DNA sequencing (85). The relative performances of *mip* and 16S rRNA sequencing are not accurately known. In addition, limited numbers of reference strains, especially of some unusual species, have been sequenced using either method, leaving open the possibility of incorrect classifications. A commercial plate DNA hybridization assay has been reported to correctly identify 23 different *Legionella* spp. (28) and is distributed in Japan (Kobayashi Pharmaceutical, Osaka, Japan).

Whether molecular methods can substitute for serologic ones is difficult to know because of several reports of genotypic discordances for identical serogroups and vice versa (8, 45, 66). Sequencing of the *L. pneumophila dnaJ* gene appeared to be able to distinguish between some, but not all, *L. pneumophila* serogroups (64); different serogroups that had very similar genotypes had been shown by other methods to have discordant genotypes and serotypes. More extensive testing of this method needs to be performed before it is put into routine use. Note that several molecular methods are useful for establishing strain clonality in the context of epidemiologic investigations.

TYPING SYSTEMS

Typing of *Legionella* spp. is important for public health investigations to help link culture-positive environmental sites with clinical isolates during an epidemic of the disease. Typing cannot be used by itself to determine the environmental source of an outbreak and must be accompanied by an epidemiologic investigation. Otherwise, incorrect conclusions may be made about epidemic sources (46, 60). This problem is due to clonal distributions of environmental and clinical *Legionella* spp. (3, 53, 63, 82) and to the poor specificity of some typing techniques (15, 82).

L. pneumophila serogroup 1 can be divided into at least 17 or 10 different groups by using cross-absorbed polyclonal or monoclonal antibodies, respectively (56, 96). Neither the cross-absorbed polyclonal typing sera nor all of the original monoclonal antibodies are available. Lück and colleagues made alternative monoclonal antibodies that can be used in a typing scheme (67). Monoclonal antibody typing plays a major role in subtyping *L. pneumophila* serogroup 1 isolates and, when used with molecular methods, can increase typing specificity (34, 37, 82). Used by itself, monoclonal antibody typing may not be specific enough to distinguish between closely related strains.

Sequence-based typing appears to be the most specific and precise molecular subtyping system for both *L. pneumophila* and *L. pneumophila* serogroup 1. Performed according to a standardized protocol, the method provides uniform results between laboratories, with excellent discrimination between strains (37). This method uses determination of portions of sequences of six different *L. pneumophila* genes, *flaA, pilE, asd, mip, mompS,* and *proA*. An online database, an allele subtype assignment tool, and standardized procedures are available on the Internet (http://www.hpa.org.uk/srmd/bioinformatics/ewgli/ewglisbt.htm). Amplified fragment length polymorphism analysis is an alternative molecular typing system with lower between-laboratory precision than sequence-based typing, but with high specificity (34). An amplified fragment length polymorphism analysis online database and allele assignment tool is available (http://www.hpa.org.uk/srmd/bioinformatics/ewgli/ewgliaflp.htm). Pulsed-field gel electrophoresis, plasmid typing, polyacrylamide gel protein electrophoresis, gel analysis of genomic DNA restriction fragments, and several other methods have all been successfully used to subtype *L. pneumophila,* and in some cases *Legionella* spp., but appear to be too nonspecific for epidemiologic investigative purposes.

SEROLOGIC TESTS

LD can be diagnosed by demonstration of an increase in antibodies to killed bacterial cells (19). Enzyme immunoassay, microagglutination, and indirect immunofluorescent assay methods can all be used to detect antibody changes, with indirect immunofluorescent assay considered the gold standard. While most patients develop both immunoglobulin G (IgG) and IgM responses, some develop IgM-only, IgG-only, or IgA-only responses, making it necessary to test for total immunoglobulin response and not just IgG. In addition, IgM antibodies may persist for as long as a year after infection, making IgM presence a poor marker of acute disease (75). About 75% of patients with culture-proven nosocomial *L. pneumophila* serogroup 1 LD develop seroconversion to the bacterium, whereas the test seems to have higher sensitivity in LD epidemics. Test specificity depends on several technical factors, including the method of antigen preparation, the numbers of different bacteria used in antigen preparation, the method of diluting serum, and several other factors. Seroconversion requires weeks to months after infection, with only about a 50% seroconversion rate after 2 weeks; for optimal test sensitivity, acute-phase serum should be frozen while convalescent-phase sera are collected at 2, 4, 6, 9, and 12 weeks postinfection. Sera tested 2 weeks after disease onset have only about a 37% (50% of 75%) chance of detecting seroconversion. Parallel testing of sera is required for the best specificity. Some laboratories test acute-phase sera only for evidence of early antibody production; this approach can be nonspecific and insensitive. The most specific testing is for seroconversion to *L. pneumophila* serogroup 1 only, and the least specific is the use of polyvalent antigen preparations, with approximate test specificities of 99% and 90 to 95%, respectively. Polyvalent antigen preparations are best used for screening purposes only, with follow-up monovalent testing. Almost all commercially available tests use only polyvalent antigen preparations, which can result in nonspecific results. There is also some concern that screening enzyme-linked immunosorbent assays may be insensitive, possibly making such testing both insensitive and nonspecific (68). Serologic diagnosis is best used for epidemiologic studies because of the retrospective nature of serologic diagnosis and limitations on test specificity and sensitivity.

Antimicrobial Susceptibilities and Susceptibility Testing

The antimicrobial susceptibility of *L. pneumophila* grown in broth or on agar can give results having no clinical correlate. This is because of the intracellular location of the bacterium in human infection, to which not all antimicrobial agents gain access and retain activity (18). In addition, the complex broth and agar media used to grow *L. pneumophila* inactivate many drugs. There is no indication for performing antimicrobial susceptibility testing against *Legionella* spp. except in a research setting, when correlative studies of intracellular and experimental animal model infection can be performed. The microbiologist must not assume that a particular drug will be effective for the treatment of LD simply because the drug is active against *L. pneumophila* in vitro, nor should there be an assumption that drugs having low MICs against the bacterium in vitro will be more clinically effective than will drugs with higher MICs for the organism.

Antimicrobial agents having good intracellular activity against *L. pneumophila* include most macrolide, tetracycline, ketolide, and quinolone antimicrobial agents (18, 22). No beta-lactam agent or aminoglycoside has acceptable intracellular activity against the bacterium. It is unknown if the intracellular activity of antimicrobial agents against *L. pneumophila* can be extrapolated to all other *Legionella* spp. and to treatment of infections caused by *Legionella* spp. other than *L. pneumophila*. Some of these other *Legionella* spp. may reside in subcellular compartments different from those where *L. pneumophila* resides and thus may respond differently to antimicrobial agents (77). However, macrolide and quinolone antimicrobials appear to be effective for the treatment of LD caused by *L. micdadei, L. longbeachae, L. bozemanae,* and *L. dumoffii* (72).

EVALUATION, INTERPRETATION, AND REPORTING OF RESULTS

Multiple laboratory methods have to be used for optimal laboratory diagnosis of LD. Culture of *Legionella* bacteria from sputum, lung, or other respiratory sites is the most specific (100%) method for diagnosis of the disease, very sensitive (~80 to 90%) in severe untreated disease and insensitive (~20%) in cases of mild disease. Culture may be the only diagnostic test giving positive results, especially when *Legionella* bacteria other than *L. pneumophila* are causing the infection. In addition, a culture isolate can be used to sort out the source of an epidemic, unlike any of the other diagnostic tests. Because of the technical difficulty of culture diagnosis, its expense, and its low sensitivity for nonsevere disease, several alternative diagnostic methods have been developed. The antigenuria assay is more sensitive than culture for the detection of community-acquired disease, and especially epidemic disease. Nevertheless, the antigenuria test is only about 60% sensitive in the best of circumstances, performs poorly for detection of nosocomial infection, and detects almost exclusively *L. pneumophila* serogroup 1. Antibody detection complements other laboratory diagnostic methods but is retrospective because it requires seroconversion for greater test specificity and sensitivity. In addition, antibody results obtained using only polyvalent antigens must be viewed with circumspection. Commercial molecular amplification tests are just being marketed and have yet to be thoroughly evaluated; prior to adoption, more-extensive studies are required. The performance of all laboratory diagnostic tests for non-*L. pneumophila* serogroup 1 LD is unknown but presumably is not as good as it is for the diagnosis of *L. pneumophila* serogroup 1 disease.

Because of the lack of any one laboratory test that is highly sensitive and specific for the diagnosis of LD caused by *L. pneumophila* serogroup 1, let alone the disease caused by other serogroups and species, multiple test types should be performed if laboratory diagnosis is crucial for clinical or public health reasons. In particular, culture needs to be performed whenever possible to enhance diagnostic yield, for public health reasons, and because it may be the only specific method capable of diagnosing LD caused by *Legionella* species other than *L. pneumophila*.

A major hindrance to the evaluation of all laboratory diagnostic methods is the lack of a good gold standard for LD diagnosis. Culture diagnosis, while very specific, is known to be imperfect and of limited sensitivity, especially for epidemic LD. Relative performance of the diagnostic tests is often compared to culture diagnosis, which tends to overestimate test sensitivity and underestimate specificity.

Positive cultures for all *Legionella* spp. are virtually diagnostic of LD, providing there are supportive clinical findings such as pneumonia. In contrast, single serum specimens showing elevated antibodies to *Legionella* spp. or to *L. pneumophila* are often not the result of LD. Only rises in antibody titers to *L. pneumophila* serogroup 1, evaluated by a test not usually commercially available, are specific enough for diagnosis, but even then use of appropriate techniques is required for optimal specificity. Detection of *L. pneumophila* serogroup 1 antigenuria is almost as specific as a positive culture, once heat-labile factors capable of causing false-positive tests are excluded. Positive test results must be reported promptly to the patient's clinician as well as to public health authorities.

REFERENCES

1. **Adeleke, A. A., B. S. Fields, R. F. Benson, M. I. Daneshvar, J. M. Pruckler, R. M. Ratcliff, T. G. Harrison, R. S. Weyant, R. J. Birtles, D. Raoult, and M. A. Halablab.** 2001. *Legionella drozanskii* sp. nov., *Legionella rowbothamii* sp. nov. and *Legionella fallonii* sp. nov.: three unusual new *Legionella* species. *Int. J. Syst. Evol. Microbiol.* **51:**1151–1160.
2. **Amer, A. O., and M. S. Swanson.** 2002. A phagosome of one's own: a microbial guide to life in the macrophage. *Curr. Opin. Microbiol.* **5:**56–61.
3. **Aurell, H., J. Etienne, F. Forey, M. Reyrolle, P. Girardo, P. Farge, B. Decludt, C. Campese, F. Vandenesch, and S. Jarraud.** 2003. *Legionella pneumophila* serogroup 1 strain Paris: endemic distribution throughout France. *J. Clin. Microbiol.* **41:**3320–3322.
4. **Benin, A. L., R. F. Benson, and R. E. Besser.** 2002. Trends in Legionnaires disease, 1980–1998: declining mortality and new patterns of diagnosis. *Clin. Infect. Dis.* **35:**1039–1046.
5. **Benson, R. F., W. L. Thacker, J. A. Lanser, N. Sangster, W. R. Mayberry, and D. J. Brenner.** 1991. *Legionella adelaidensis*, a new species isolated from cooling tower water. *J. Clin. Microbiol.* **29:**1004–1006.
6. **Benson, R. F., W. L. Thacker, B. B. Plikaytis, and H. W. Wilkinson.** 1987. Cross-reactions in *Legionella* antisera with *Bordetella pertussis* strains. *J. Clin. Microbiol.* **25:**594–596.
7. **Brenner, D. J.** 1987. Classification of the legionellae. *Semin. Resp. Infect.* **2:**190–205.
8. **Brenner, D. J., A. G. Steigerwalt, P. Epple, W. F. Bibb, R. M. McKinney, R. W. Starnes, J. M. Colville, R. K. Selander, P. H. Edelstein, and C. W. Moss.** 1988. *Legionella pneumophila* serogroup Lansing 3 isolated from a patient with fatal pneumonia, and descriptions of *L. pneumophila* subsp. *pneumophila* subsp. nov., *L. pneumophila* subsp. *fraseri* subsp. nov., and *L. pneumophila* subsp. *pascullei* subsp. nov. *J. Clin. Microbiol.* **26:**1695–1703.
9. **Cercenado, E., P. H. Edelstein, L. H. Gosting, and J. C. Sturge.** 1987. *Legionella micdadei* and *Legionella dumoffii* monoclonal antibodies for laboratory diagnosis of *Legionella* infections. *J. Clin. Microbiol.* **25:**2163–2167.
10. **Chen, S., L. Hicks, M. Yuen, D. Mitchell, and G. L. Gilbert.** 1994. Serological cross-reaction between *Legionella* spp. and *Capnocytophaga ochracea* by using latex agglutination test. *J. Clin. Microbiol.* **32:**3054–3055.
11. **Collins, M. T., F. Espersen, N. Høiby, S. N. Cho, A. Friss-Møller, and J. S. Reif.** 1983. Cross-reactions between *Legionella pneumophila* (serogroup 1) and twenty-eight other bacterial species, including other members of the family *Legionellaceae*. *Infect. Immun.* **39:**1441–1456.
12. **den Boer, J. W., E. P. Yzerman, J. Schellekens, K. D. Lettinga, H. C. Boshuizen, J. E. Van Steenbergen, A. Bosman, S. Van den Hof, H. A. Van Vliet, M. F. Peeters, R. J. van Ketel, P. Speelman, J. L. Kool, and M. A. Conyn-van Spaendonck.** 2002. A large outbreak of Legionnaires' disease at a flower show, the Netherlands, 1999. *Emerg. Infect. Dis.* **8:**37–43.

13. **Dennis, P. J., J. A. Taylor, and G. I. Barrow.** 1981. Phosphate buffered, low sodium chloride blood agar medium for *Legionella pneumophila. Lancet* **ii:**636.
14. **Domínguez, J. A., J. M. Manterola, R. Blavia, N. Sopena, F. J. Belda, E. Padilla, M. Gimenez, M. Sabria, J. Morera, and V. Ausina.** 1996. Detection of *Legionella pneumophila* serogroup-1 antigen in nonconcentrated urine and urine concentrated by selective ultrafiltration. *J. Clin. Microbiol.* **34:**2334–2336.
15. **Drenning, S. D., J. E. Stout, J. R. Joly, and V. L. Yu.** 2001. Unexpected similarity of pulsed-field gel electrophoresis patterns of unrelated clinical isolates of *Legionella pneumophila*, serogroup 1. *J. Infect. Dis.* **183:**628–632.
16. **Edelstein, P. H.** 2004. Urinary antigen detection for *Legionella* spp., p. 11.4.1–11.4.6. *In* H. D. Isenberg (ed.), *Clinical Microbiology Procedures Handbook*, 2nd ed. ASM Press, Washington, D.C.
17. **Edelstein, P. H.** 2004. Detection of *Legionella* antigen by direct immunofluorescence, p. 11.3.1–11.3.7. *In* H. D. Isenberg (ed.), *Clinical Microbiology Procedures Handbook*, 2nd ed. ASM Press, Washington, D.C.
18. **Edelstein, P. H.** 1995. Antimicrobial chemotherapy for Legionnaires' disease: a review. *Clin. Infect. Dis.* **21:**S265–S276.
19. **Edelstein, P. H.** 2002. Detection of antibodies to *Legionella* spp., p. 468–476. *In* N. R. Rose, R. G. Hamilton, and B. Detrick (ed.), *Manual of Clinical Laboratory Immunology*, 6th ed. ASM Press, Washington, D.C.
20. **Edelstein, P. H.** 1999. The guinea-pig model of Legionnaires' disease, p. 303–314. *In* O. Zak and M. A. Sande (ed.), *Handbook of Animal Models of Infection.* Academic Press, London, United Kingdom.
21. **Edelstein, P. H., K. B. Beer, J. C. Sturge, A. J. Watson, and L. C. Goldstein.** 1985. Clinical utility of a monoclonal direct fluorescent reagent specific for *Legionella pneumophila:* comparative study with other reagents. *J. Clin. Microbiol.* **22:**419–421.
22. **Edelstein, P. H., and N. P. Cianciotto.** 2005. *Legionella*, p. 2711–2724. *In* G. L. Mandell, J. E. Bennett, and R. Dolin (ed.), *Principles and Practice of Infectious Diseases*. Elsevier Churchill Livingstone, Philadelphia, Pa.
23. **Edelstein, P. H., and N. P. Cianciotto.** 2001. *Legionella* species and Legionnaires' disease. *In* M. Dworkin, S. Falkow, E. Rosenberg, K. H. Schleifer, and E. Stackebrandt (ed.), *The Prokaryotes: An Evolving Electronic Resource for the Microbiological Community*. Springer-Verlag, New York, N.Y.
24. **Edelstein, P. H., and M. A. C. Edelstein.** 1989. Evaluation of the Merifluor-*Legionella* immunofluorescent reagent for identifying and detecting 21 *Legionella* species. *J. Clin. Microbiol.* **27:**2455–2458.
25. **Edelstein, P. H., and S. M. Finegold.** 1979. Use of a semiselective medium to culture *Legionella pneumophila* from contaminated lung specimens. *J. Clin. Microbiol.* **10:**141–143.
26. **Edelstein, P. H., R. M. McKinney, R. D. Meyer, M. A. C. Edelstein, C. J. Krause, and S. M. Finegold.** 1980. Immunologic diagnosis of Legionnaires' disease: cross-reactions with anaerobic and microaerophilic organisms and infections caused by them. *J. Infect. Dis.* **141:**652–655.
27. **Edelstein, P. H., R. D. Meyer, and S. M. Finegold.** 1980. Laboratory diagnosis of Legionnaires' disease. *Am. Rev. Respir. Dis.* **121:**317–327.
28. **Ezaki, T., Y. Hashimoto, H. Yamamoto, M. L. Lucida, S. L. Liu, S. Kusunoki, K. Asano, and E. Yabuuchi.** 1990. Evaluation of the microplate hybridization method for rapid identification of *Legionella* species. *Eur. J. Clin. Microbiol. Infect. Dis.* **9:**213–217.
29. **Faine, S., P. Edelstein, B. D. Kirby, and S. M. Finegold.** 1979. Rapid presumptive bacteriological diagnosis of Legionnaires disease. *J. Clin. Microbiol.* **10:**104–105.
30. **Fang, G.-D., V. L. Yu, and R. M. Vickers.** 1989. Disease due to the *Legionellaceae* (other than *Legionella pneumophila*): historical, microbiological, clinical, and epidemiological review. *Medicine* **68:**116–132.
31. **Ferrer, A., P. Bellver, and P. Royo.** 1995. Screening quality of respiratory samples and *Legionella pneumoniae* (sic). *J. Clin. Microbiol.* **33:**1971.
32. **Fields, B. S., T. Haupt, J. P. Davis, M. J. Arduino, P. H. Miller, and J. C. Butler.** 2001. Pontiac fever due to *Legionella micdadei* from a whirlpool spa: possible role of bacterial endotoxin. *J. Infect. Dis.* **184:**1289–1292.
33. **Fraser, D. W., T. R. Tsai, W. Orenstein, W. E. Parkin, H. J. Beecham, R. G. Sharrar, J. Harris, G. F. Mallison, S. M. Martin, J. E. McDade, C. C. Shepard, and P. S. Brachman.** 1977. Legionnaires' disease: description of an epidemic of pneumonia. *N. Engl. J. Med.* **297:**1189–1197.
34. **Fry, N. K., J. M. Bangsborg, S. Bernander, J. Etienne, B. Forsblom, V. Gaia, P. Hasenberger, D. Lindsay, A. Papoutsi, C. Pelaz, M. Struelens, S. A. Uldum, P. Visca, and T. G. Harrison.** 2000. Assessment of intercentre reproducibility and epidemiological concordance of *Legionella pneumophila* serogroup 1 genotyping by amplified fragment length polymorphism analysis. *Eur. J. Clin. Microbiol. Infect. Dis.* **19:**773–780.
35. **Fry, N. K., T. J. Rowbotham, N. A. Saunders, and T. M. Embley.** 1991. Direct amplification and sequencing of the 16S ribosomal DNA of an intracellular *Legionella* species recovered by amoebal enrichment from the sputum of a patient with pneumonia. *FEMS Microbiol. Lett.* **67:**165–168.
36. **Fry, N. K., S. Warwick, N. A. Saunders, and T. M. Embley.** 1991. The use of 16S ribosomal RNA analyses to investigate the phylogeny of the family *Legionellaceae*. *J. Gen. Microbiol.* **137:**1215–1222.
37. **Gaia, V., N. K. Fry, B. Afshar, P. C. Luck, H. Meugnier, J. Etienne, R. Peduzzi, and T. G. Harrison.** 2005. Consensus sequence-based scheme for epidemiological typing of clinical and environmental isolates of *Legionella pneumophila*. *J. Clin. Microbiol.* **43:**2047–2052.
38. **Garduño, R. A., E. Garduño, M. Hiltz, and P. S. Hoffman.** 2002. Intracellular growth of *Legionella pneumophila* gives rise to a differentiated form dissimilar to stationary-phase forms. *Infect. Immun.* **70:**6273–6283.
39. **Garrity, G. M., A. Brown, and R. M. Vickers.** 1980. *Tatlockia* and *Fluoribacter*: two new genera of organisms resembling *Legionella pneumophila*. *Int. J. Syst. Bacteriol.* **30:**609–614.
40. **Glupczynski, Y., M. Labbe, and E. Yourassowsky.** 1984. Cross-reactivity of environmental bacteria with fluorescent-antibody conjugates for *Legionella pneumophila*. *Eur. J. Clin. Microbiol. Infect. Dis.* **3:**215.
41. **Gosting, L. H., K. Cabrian, J. C. Sturge, and L. C. Goldstein.** 1984. Identification of a species-specific antigen in *Legionella pneumophila* by a monoclonal antibody. *J. Clin. Microbiol.* **20:**1031–1035.
42. **Gotz, H. M., A. Tegnell, J. De, K. A. Broholm, M. Kuusi, I. Kallings, and K. Ekdahl.** 2001. A whirlpool associated outbreak of Pontiac fever at a hotel in Northern Sweden. *Epidemiol. Infect.* **126:**241–247.
43. **Greer, P. W., F. W. Chandler, and M. D. Hicklin.** 1980. Rapid demonstration of *Legionella pneumophila* in unembedded tissue. An adaptation of the Gimenez stain. *Am. J. Clin. Pathol.* **73:**788–790.
44. **Guerrero, C., C. M. Toldos, G. Yague, C. Ramirez, T. Rodriguez, and M. Segovia.** 2004. Comparison of diagnostic sensitivities of three assays (Bartels enzyme immunoassay [EIA], Biotest EIA, and Binax NOW immunochromatographic test) for detection of *Legionella pneumophila* serogroup 1 antigen in urine. *J. Clin. Microbiol.* **42:**467–468.
45. **Harrison, T. G., N. A. Saunders, A. Haththotuwa, N. Doshi, and A. G. Taylor.** 1992. Further evidence that genotypically closely related strains of *Legionella pneumophila* can express different serogroup specific antigens. *J. Med. Microbiol.* **37:**155–161.

46. **Heath, T. C., C. Roberts, B. Jalaludin, I. Goldthrope, and A. G. Capon.** 1998. Environmental investigation of a legionellosis outbreak in western Sydney: the role of molecular profiling. *Aust. N. Z. J. Public Health* **22:**428–431.
47. **Helbig, J. H., P. C. Luck, and W. Witzleb.** 1994. Serogroup-specific and serogroup-cross-reactive epitopes of *Legionella pneumophila*. *Int. J. Med. Microbiol. Virol. Parasitol. Infect. Dis.* **281:**16–23.
48. **Helbig, J. H., S. A. Uldum, S. Bernander, P. C. Luck, G. Wewalka, B. Abraham, V. Gaia, and T. G. Harrison.** 2003. Clinical utility of urinary antigen detection for diagnosis of community-acquired, travel-associated, and nosocomial Legionnaires' disease. *J. Clin. Microbiol.* **41:**838–840.
49. **Helbig, J. H., S. A. Uldum, P. C. Luck, and T. G. Harrison.** 2001. Detection of *Legionella pneumophila* antigen in urine samples by the BinaxNOW immunochromatographic assay and comparison with both Binax Legionella Urinary Enzyme Immunoassay (EIA) and Biotest Legionella Urin Antigen EIA. *J. Med. Microbiol.* **50:**509–516.
50. **Helbig, J. H., S. A. Uldum, P. C. Lück, and T. G. Harrison.** 2003. Detection of *Legionella pneumophila* antigen in urine samples: recognition of serogroups and monoclonal serogroups, p. 204–206. *In* R. Marre, Y. Abu Kwaik, C. Bartlett, N. P. Cianciotto, B. S. Fields, M. Frosch, J. Hacker, and P. C. Lück (ed.), *Legionella*. ASM Press, Washington, D.C.
51. **Herpers, B. L., B. M. de Jongh, K. van der Zwaluw, and E. J. van Hannen.** 2003. Real-time PCR assay targets the 23S-5S spacer for direct detection and differentiation of *Legionella* spp. and *Legionella pneumophila*. *J. Clin. Microbiol.* **41:**4815–4816.
52. **Horn, J.** 2002. Comparison of non-serogroup 1 detection by Biotest and Binax *Legionella* urinary antigen enzyme immunoassays, p. 207–210. *In* R. Marre, Y. Abu Kwaik, C. Bartlett, N. P. Cianciotto, B. S. Fields, M. Frosch, J. Hacker, and P. C. Lück (ed.), *Legionella*. ASM Press, Washington, D.C.
53. **Huang, B., B. A. Heron, B. R. Gray, S. Eglezos, J. R. Bates, and J. Savill.** 2004. A predominant and virulent *Legionella pneumophila* serogroup 1 strain detected in isolates from patients and water in Queensland, Australia, by an amplified fragment length polymorphism protocol and virulence gene-based PCR assays. *J. Clin. Microbiol.* **42:**4164–4168.
54. **Ingram, J. G., and J. F. Plouffe.** 1994. Danger of sputum purulence screens in culture of *Legionella* species. *J. Clin. Microbiol.* **32:**209–210.
55. **Jimenez-Lucho, V., M. Shulman, and J. Johnson.** 1994. *Bordetella bronchiseptica* in an AIDS patient cross-reacts with *Legionella* antisera. *J. Clin. Microbiol.* **32:**3095–3096.
56. **Joly, J. R., R. M. McKinney, J. O. Tobin, W. F. Bibb, I. D. Watkins, and D. Ramsay.** 1986. Development of a standardized subgrouping scheme for *Legionella pneumophila* serogroup 1 using monoclonal antibodies. *J. Clin. Microbiol.* **23:**768–771.
57. **Kerr, E., H. Snell, B. L. Black, M. Storey, and W. D. Colby.** 1992. Isolation of *Nocardia asteroides* from respiratory specimens by using selective buffered charcoal-yeast extract agar. *J. Clin. Microbiol.* **30:**1320–1322.
58. **Klein, G. C.** 1980. Cross-reaction to *Legionella pneumophila* antigen in sera with elevated titers to *Pseudomonas pseudomallei*. *J. Clin. Microbiol.* **11:**27–29.
59. **Ko, K. S., H. K. Lee, M. Y. Park, K. H. Lee, Y. J. Yun, S. Y. Woo, H. Miyamoto, and Y. H. Kook.** 2002. Application of RNA polymerase beta-subunit gene *(rpoB)* sequences for the molecular differentiation of *Legionella* species. *J. Clin. Microbiol.* **40:**2653–2658.
60. **Kool, J. L., U. Buchholz, C. Peterson, E. W. Brown, R. F. Benson, J. M. Pruckler, B. S. Fields, J. Sturgeon, E. Lehnkering, R. Cordova, L. M. Mascola, and J. C. Butler.** 2000. Strengths and limitations of molecular subtyping in a community outbreak of Legionnaires' disease. *Epidemiol. Infect.* **125:**599–608.
61. **Lambert, M. A., and C. W. Moss.** 1989. Cellular fatty acid compositions and isoprenoid quinone contents of 23 *Legionella* species. *J. Clin. Microbiol.* **27:**465–473.
62. **La Scola, B., R. J. Birtles, G. Greub, T. J. Harrison, R. M. Ratcliff, and D. Raoult.** 2004. *Legionella drancourtii* sp. nov., a strictly intracellular amoebal pathogen. *Int. J. Syst. Evol. Microbiol.* **54:**699–703.
63. **Lawrence, C., M. Reyrolle, S. Dubrou, F. Forey, B. Decludt, C. Goulvestre, P. Matsiota-Bernard, J. Etienne, and C. Nauciel.** 1999. Single clonal origin of a high proportion of *Legionella pneumophila* serogroup 1 isolates from patients and the environment in the area of Paris, France, over a 10-year period. *J. Clin. Microbiol.* **37:**2652–2655.
64. **Liu, H., Y. Li, X. Huang, Y. Kawamura, and T. Ezaki.** 2003. Use of the *dnaJ* gene for the detection and identification of all *Legionella pneumophila* serogroups and description of the primers used to detect 16S rDNA gene sequences of major members of the genus *Legionella*. *Microbiol. Immunol.* **47:**859–869.
65. **LoPresti, F., S. Riffard, H. Meugnier, M. Reyrolle, Y. Lasne, P. A. Grimont, F. Grimont, F. Vandenesch, J. Etienne, J. Fleurette, and J. Freney.** 1999. *Legionella taurinensis* sp. nov., a new species antigenically similar to *Legionella spiritensis*. *Int. J. Syst. Bacteriol.* **49**(Pt. 2):397–403.
66. **Luck, P. C., R. J. Birtles, and J. H. Helbig.** 1995. Correlation of MAb subgroups with genotype in closely related *Legionella pneumophila* serogroup 1 strains from a cooling tower. *J. Med. Microbiol.* **43:**50–54.
67. **Lück, P. C., J. H. Helbig, W. Ehret, R. Marre, and W. Witzleb.** 1992. Subtyping of *Legionella pneumophila* serogroup 1 strains isolated in Germany using monoclonal antibodies. *Int. J. Med. Microbiol. Virol. Parasitol. Infect. Dis.* **277:**179–187.
68. **Malan, A. K., T. B. Martins, T. D. Jaskowski, H. R. Hill, and C. M. Litwin.** 2003. Comparison of two commercial enzyme-linked immunosorbent assays with an immunofluorescence assay for detection of *Legionella pneumophila* types 1 to 6. *J. Clin. Microbiol.* **41:**3060–3063.
69. **Marston, B. J., J. F. Plouffe, T. M. File, B. A. Hackman, S. J. Salstrom, H. B. Lipman, M. S. Kolczak, and R. F. Breiman.** 1997. Incidence of community-acquired pneumonia requiring hospitalization—results of a population-based active surveillance study in Ohio. *Arch. Intern. Med.* **157:**1709–1718.
70. **McDade, J. E., C. C. Shepard, D. W. Fraser, T. R. Tsai, M. A. Redus, and W. R. Dowdle.** 1977. Legionnaires' disease: isolation of a bacterium and demonstration of its role in other respiratory disease. *N. Engl. J. Med.* **297:**1197–1203.
71. **Morrill, W. E., J. M. Barbaree, B. S. Fields, G. N. Sanden, and W. T. Martin.** 1990. Increased recovery of *Legionella micdadei* and *Legionella bozemanii* on buffered charcoal yeast extract agar supplemented with albumin. *J. Clin. Microbiol.* **28:**616–618.
72. **Muder, R. R., and V. L. Yu.** 2002. Infection due to *Legionella* species other than *L. pneumophila*. *Clin. Infect. Dis.* **35:**990–998.
73. **Murdoch, D. R.** 2003. Diagnosis of *Legionella* infection. *Clin. Infect. Dis.* **36:**64–69.
74. **Mykietiuk, A., J. Carratalà, N. Fernández-sabé, J. Dorca, R. Verdaguer, F. Manresa, and F. Gudiol.** 2005. Clinical outcomes for hospitalized patients with *Legionella* pneumonia in the antigenuria era: the influence of levofloxacin therapy. *Clin. Infect. Dis.* **40:**794–799.
75. **Nagington, J., T. G. Wreghitt, J. O. Tobin, and A. D. Macrae.** 1979. The antibody response in Legionnaires' disease. *J. Hyg.* **83:**377–381.
76. **Ng, V., L. Weir, M. K. York, and W. K. Hadley.** 1992. *Bordetella pertussis* versus non-*L. pneumophila Legionella* spp.: a continuing diagnostic challenge. *J. Clin. Microbiol.* **30:**3300–3301.

77. **Ogawa, M., A. Takade, H. Miyamoto, H. Taniguchi, and S. Yoshida.** 2001. Morphological variety of intracellular microcolonies of *Legionella* species in Vero cells. *Microbiol. Immunol.* **45:**557–562.
78. **Osterholm, M. T., T. D. Chin, D. O. Osborne, H. B. Dull, A. G. Dean, D. W. Fraser, P. S. Hayes, and W. N. Hall.** 1983. A 1957 outbreak of Legionnaires' disease associated with a meat packing plant. *Am. J. Epidemiol.* **117:**60–67.
79. **Park, M. Y., K. S. Ko, H. K. Lee, M. S. Park, and Y. H. Kook.** 2003. *Legionella busanensis* sp. nov., isolated from cooling tower water in Korea. *Int. J. Syst. Evol. Microbiol.* **53:**77–80.
80. **Pasculle, A. W., and D. McDevitt.** 2004. *Legionella* cultures, p. 3.11.4.1–3.11.4.14. *In* H. D. Isenberg (ed.), *Clinical Microbiology Procedures Handbook*, 2nd ed. ASM Press, Washington, D.C.
81. **Pelaz, C., L. García Albert, and C. M. Bourgon.** 1987. Cross-reactivity among *Legionella* species and serogroups. *Epidemiol. Infect.* **99:**641–646.
82. **Pruckler, J. M., L. A. Mermel, R. F. Benson, C. Giorgio, P. K. Cassiday, R. F. Breiman, C. G. Whitney, and B. S. Fields.** 1995. Comparison of *Legionella pneumophila* isolates by arbitrarily primed PCR and pulsed-field gel electrophoresis: analysis from seven epidemic investigations. *J. Clin. Microbiol.* **33:**2872–2875.
83. **Ratcliff, R. M., J. A. Lanser, P. A. Manning, and M. W. Heuzenroeder.** 1998. Sequence-based classification scheme for the genus *Legionella* targeting the *mip* gene. *J. Clin. Microbiol.* **36:**1560–1567.
84. **Richardson, I. R., and N. F. Lightfoot.** 1992. *Legionella pneumophila* species identification using a commercial latex agglutination kit: a potential cross-reaction problem with serogroup 12. *Med. Lab. Sci.* **49:**144–146.
85. **Riffard, S., F. LoPresti, P. Normand, F. Forey, M. Reyrolle, J. Etienne, and F. Vandenesch.** 1998. Species identification of *Legionella* via intergenic 16S-23S ribosomal spacer PCR analysis. *Int. J. Syst. Bacteriol.* **48**(Pt. 3)**:**723–730.
86. **Riffard, S., F. Vandenesch, M. Reyrolle, and J. Etienne.** 1996. Distribution of *mip*-related sequences in 39 species (48 serogroups) of *Legionellaceae*. *Epidemiol. Infect.* **117:** 501–506.
87. **Rowbotham, T. J.** 1986. Current views on the relationships between amoebae, legionellae and man. *Isr. J. Med. Sci.* **22:**678–689.
88. **Steele, T. W., J. Lanser, and N. Sangster.** 1990. Isolation of *Legionella longbeachae* serogroup 1 from potting mixes. *Appl. Environ. Microbiol.* **56:**49–53.
89. **Tateyama, M.** 1992. Misleading serological identification of *Legionella anisa* as *Legionella bozemanii*. *Kansenshogaku Zasshi* **66:**149–155.
90. **Tenover, F. C., P. H. Edelstein, L. C. Goldstein, J. C. Sturge, and J. J. Plorde.** 1986. Comparison of cross-staining reactions by *Pseudomonas* spp. and fluorescein-labeled polyclonal and monoclonal antibodies directed against *Legionella pneumophila*. *J. Clin. Microbiol.* **23:**647–649.
91. **Thacker, L., R. M. McKinney, C. W. Moss, H. M. Sommers, M. L. Spivack, and T. F. O'Brien.** 1981. Thermophilic sporeforming bacilli that mimic fastidious growth characteristics and colonial morphology of legionella. *J. Clin. Microbiol.* **13:**794–797.
92. **Thacker, W. L., R. F. Benson, R. B. Schifman, E. Pugh, A. G. Steigerwalt, W. R. Mayberry, D. J. Brenner, and H. W. Wilkinson.** 1989. *Legionella tucsonensis* sp. nov. isolated from a renal transplant recipient. *J. Clin. Microbiol.* **27:**1831–1834.
93. **Thacker, W. L., R. F. Benson, H. W. Wilkinson, N. M. Ampel, E. J. Wing, A. G. Steigerwalt, and D. J. Brenner.** 1986. 11th serogroup of *Legionella pneumophila* isolated from a patient with fatal pneumonia. *J. Clin. Microbiol.* **23:**1146–1147.
94. **Thacker, W. L., J. W. Dyke, R. F. Benson, D. H. Havlichek, Jr., B. Robinson-Dunn, H. Stiefel, W. Schneider, C. W. Moss, W. R. Mayberry, and D. J. Brenner.** 1992. *Legionella lansingensis* sp. nov. isolated from a patient with pneumonia and underlying chronic lymphocytic leukemia. *J. Clin. Microbiol.* **30:**2398–2401.
95. **Thacker, W. L., H. W. Wilkinson, and R. F. Benson.** 1983. Comparison of slide agglutination test and direct immunofluorescence assay for identification of *Legionella* isolates. *J. Clin. Microbiol.* **18:**1113–1118.
96. **Thomason, B. M., and W. F. Bibb.** 1984. Use of absorbed antisera for demonstration of antigenic variation among strains of *Legionella pneumophila* serogroup 1. *J. Clin. Microbiol.* **19:**794–797.
97. **Vesey, G., P. J. Dennis, J. V. Lee, and A. A. West.** 1988. Further development of simple tests to differentiate the legionellas. *J. Appl. Bacteriol.* **65:**339–345.
98. **Vickers, R. M., J. D. Rihs, and V. L. Yu.** 1992. Clinical demonstration of isolation of *Nocardia asteroides* on buffered charcoal-yeast extract media. *J. Clin. Microbiol.* **30:**227–228.
99. **Westerman, E. L., and J. McDonald.** 1983. Tularemia pneumonia mimicking Legionnaires' disease: isolation of organism on CYE agar and successful treatment with erythromycin. *South. Med. J.* **76:**1169–1170.
100. **Wilkinson, H. W., W. L. Thacker, A. G. Steigerwalt, D. J. Brenner, N. M. Ampel, and E. J. Wing.** 1985. Second serogroup of *Legionella hackeliae* isolated from a patient with pneumonia. *J. Clin. Microbiol.* **22:**488–489.
101. **Winn, W. C., Jr.** 1985. *Legionella* and Legionnaires' disease: a review with emphasis on environmental studies and laboratory diagnosis. *Crit. Rev. Clin. Lab. Sci.* **21:**323–381.
102. **Zusman, T., G. Yerushalmi, and G. Segal.** 2003. Functional similarities between the *icm/dot* pathogenesis systems of *Coxiella burnetii* and *Legionella pneumophila*. *Infect. Immun.* **71:**3714–3723.

*Bartonella**

BRUNO B. CHOMEL AND JEAN MARC ROLAIN

54

TAXONOMY

The genus *Bartonella* is named for A. L. Barton, who first described the intraerythrocytic bacterium *Bartonella bacilliformis* in 1909. Until recently, this genus consisted of only one species, *B. bacilliformis*. The *Bartonella* genus now combines all the species of the three genera *Bartonella*, *Rochalimaea*, and *Grahamella* and is the only genus of the family *Bartonellaceae*, which has been removed from the order *Rickettsiales* (6, 10). *Bartonella* species are members of the alpha-2 subgroup of the class alpha-proteobacteria within the order *Rhizobiales*. The list of newly recognized species and subspecies has been increasing in the last few years (2, 9). These small gram-negative rods are erythrocyte-adherent bacilli. Based on 16S rRNA gene similarity, *Bartonella* is closely related to *Brucella* and *Agrobacterium*.

DESCRIPTION OF THE GENUS

The present family consists of 19 species and 3 subspecies, of which 10 are human pathogens (Table 1). *B. bacilliformis*, the type species of the genus, is the etiologic agent of Carrion's disease and causes either an acute bacteremic infection called Oroya fever, characterized by sepsis and hemolysis, or a chronic form called verruga peruana, characterized by cutaneous nodular vascular eruptions. *B. quintana*, the agent of trench fever, has also been found to be one of the agents of bacillary angiomatosis (BA), a vascular proliferative lesion observed in immunocompromised individuals, mainly those with AIDS (48). *B. quintana* has also been associated with endocarditis and bacteremia in homeless people (12). BA can also be caused by *B. henselae*. *B. henselae* causes cat scratch disease (CSD) in immunocompetent individuals. Similarly, *B. henselae* has been associated with several cases of endocarditis. The fourth human pathogen, *B. elizabethae*, was isolated from an immunocompetent individual suffering from endocarditis. Since then, *Bartonella vinsonii* subsp. *berkhoffii*, *B. vinsonii* subsp. *arupensis* (24), and *B. koehlerae* have also been associated with human cases of endocarditis (7), and "*B. washoensis*" (proposed species) has been associated with a human case of myocarditis. *B. grahamii* has been associated with a human case of neuroretinitis. *B. vinsonii* subsp. *arupensis* was also isolated from the blood of a rancher with fever and mild neurological symptoms (7). Finally, *B. clarridgeiae* is suspected to be a minor agent of CSD, based on serological evidence only. Most of the *Bartonella* species that are pathogenic to humans (*B. vinsonii* subsp. *berkhoffii*, *B. clarridgeiae*, *B. henselae*, *B. elizabethae*, and "*B. washoensis*") have been associated with various clinical entities, including endocarditis, in domestic dogs (7, 18).

Several other *Bartonella* species, such as *B. vinsonii* subsp. *vinsonii*, *B. doshiae*, *B. taylorii*, *B. peromysci*, *B. birtlesii*, *B. tribocorum*, *B. alsatica*, *B. talpae*, *B. bovis*, *B. chomelii*, *B. schoenbuchensis*, and *B. capreoli*, have only been isolated from the blood of various animal species, including various wild rodents, squirrels, rabbits, felids, canids, and ruminants (cattle, deer, and elk). At present, these species are not known to induce any specific disease in the infected animal.

Bartonella spp. are fastidious, aerobic, short, pleomorphic, gram-negative coccobacillary or bacillary rods (0.2 to 0.6 μm by 0.5 to 1.0 μm). Because of the slow growth of these bacteria, standard biochemical methods for identification may not be applicable. Bartonellae are oxidase and catalase negative and do not produce acid from carbohydrates. All members of the genus take from 5 to 15 days and up to 45 days in the presence of 5% CO_2 on primary culture to form visible colonies on enriched blood-containing media, as they are highly hemin dependent. The optimal growth temperature varies from 25 to 30°C for *B. bacilliformis* to 35 to 37°C for the other *Bartonella* species, such as *B. henselae*, *B. koehlerae*, and *B. elizabethae*. On primary isolation, some *Bartonella* species, such as *B. henselae*, *B. clarridgeiae*, *B. vinsonii*, and *B. elizabethae*, have colonies with a white, rough, dry, raised appearance and pit the medium. They are hard to break up or transfer. Other bartonellae such as *B. quintana* have colonies that are usually smaller, gray, translucent, and somewhat gummy or slightly mucoid. *B. bacilliformis*, *B. clarridgeiae*, *B. capreoli*, and *B. schoenbuchensis* are the only members of the genus that are motile by means of unipolar flagella.

NATURAL HABITATS

Most *Bartonella* species are vector-borne organisms. Some *Bartonella* species are very limited geographically, such as *B. bacilliformis*, which is found only in the Andes mountain region of South America, associated with the limited distribution of its vector, the sand fly *Lutzomyia verrucarum*. Others,

*This chapter contains information presented in chapter 53 by David F. Welch and Leonard N. Slater in the eighth edition of this Manual.

TABLE 1 *Bartonella* species or subspecies presently described, their main reservoirs, and confirmed or possible vectors[a]

Bartonella sp.	Main reservoir	Vector or potential vector
B. bacilliformis	Humans	Pheblotomines (sand flies) (*L. verrucarum*)
B. quintana	Humans	Human body lice (*Pediculus humanus corporis*)
B. henselae	Cats (*Felis catus*)	Fleas (*C. felis*), ticks?
B. clarridgeiae	Cats (*F. catus*)	Fleas (*C. felis*)
B. koehlerae	Cats (*F. catus*)	Fleas (*C. felis*)
B. vinsonii subsp. *vinsonii*	Meadow voles (*Microtus pennsylvanicus*)	Ear mites (*Trombicula microti*)?
B. vinsonii subsp. *arupensis*	White-footed mice (*Peromyscus leucopus*)	Fleas? Ticks?
B. vinsonii subsp. *berkhoffii*	Coyotes (*C. latrans*), dogs (*Canis familiaris*)	Ticks?
B. talpae	Moles (*Talpa europaea*)	?
B. peromysci	Field mice (*Peromyscus* spp.)	Fleas?
B. birtlesii	Wood mice (*Apodemus* spp.)	Fleas?
B. grahamii	Bank voles (*Clethrionomys glareolus*)	Fleas (*Ctenophthalmus nobilis*) (8)
B. taylorii	Wood mice (*Apodemus* spp.)	Fleas (*C. nobilis*)
B. doshiae	Field voles (*Microtus agrestis*)	Fleas?
B. elizabethae	Rats (*Rattus norvegicus*)	Fleas
B. tribocorum	Rats (*R. norvegicus*)	Fleas?
B. alsatica	Rabbits (*Oryctolagus cuniculus*)	Fleas? Ticks?
"*B. washoensis*"	California ground squirrels (*Spermophilus beecheyi*)	Fleas? Ticks?
B. bovis ("*B.weissii*")	Domestic cattle (*Bos taurus*)	Biting flies? Ticks?
B. chomelii	Domestic cattle (*B. taurus*)	Biting flies? Ticks?
B. capreoli	Roe deer (*Capreolus capreolus*)	Biting flies? Ticks?
B. schoenbuchensis	Roe deer (*C. capreolus*)	Biting flies, Ticks?

[a] As reported in reference 81.

such as *B. quintana*, *B. henselae*, and *B. elizabethae*, appear to have a worldwide distribution. *B. quintana* outbreaks had been mainly reported in Europe at the beginning of the 20th century causing hundreds of thousands of human cases of trench fever during World War I (WWI) and WWII. These outbreaks were associated with poor sanitation and personal hygiene and have now reemerged in homeless populations worldwide, associated with infestation by the human body louse, *Pediculus humanus*, possibly by inoculation of arthropod excreta through broken skin (41, 42). Humans are the only known reservoirs and victims of these two *Bartonella* species. In cases of BA caused by *B. quintana*, a history of body louse exposure is usually reported. Most cases of BA caused by *B. henselae* and almost all cases of CSD are associated with cat scratches or exposure.

The domestic cat is a healthy carrier of *B. henselae*, *B. clarridgeiae*, and *B. koehlerae* and constitutes the main reservoir of these organisms. *B. henselae* infection is transmitted from cat to cat mainly by the cat flea, *Ctenocephalides felis* (19), but the role of the cat flea seems limited in human infection. More likely, human infection results from the inoculation of infective flea feces at the time of the scratch (7). Some data have suggested a possible role for ticks in some human *B. henselae* infections (7). Stray cats, cats living outdoors, and young cats are more likely to be bacteremic. The prevalence of infection is usually highest in warm and humid climates where cat fleas are abundant. At least two genotypes of *B. henselae* have been identified, with type I (Houston) more common in cats in the Far East (Japan and the Philippines) and type II (Marseille) predominant in Western Europe, North America, and Australia (7). Coinfection of cats with different *Bartonella* species or genotypes has been reported (30). Additionally, *B. quintana*, *B. koehlerae*, and *B. clarridgeiae* have been detected by molecular methods in cat fleas, suggesting their possible role as vectors for these organisms (83). Domestic and wild canids represent the main reservoir of *B. vinsonii* subsp. *berkhoffii*, with high antibody prevalence in dogs from tropical countries (7), as well as high bacteremia prevalence in coyotes (*Canis latrans*) in California (16). Ticks may be involved in the transmission of *B. vinsonii* subsp. *berkhoffii* to dogs (9). Similarly, *Bartonella* DNA has been identified in questing adult *Ixodes pacificus* ticks from California, including several species pathogenic for humans (15), and *B. henselae* DNA was detected recently in *Ixodes ricinus* ticks collected from humans in Italy (92).

A wide range of rodent species has been reported to be infected with different *Bartonella* species (Table 1). Finally, several *Bartonella* species have been isolated from domestic and wild ruminants (Table 1), and biting flies could be an important vector of infection among these animals (7).

CLINICAL SIGNIFICANCE

Human Pathogens

Oroya Fever and Verruga Peruana (Carrion's Disease): *B. bacilliformis*

The disease caused by *B. bacilliformis*, especially its chronic form known as verruga peruana, has been recognized since pre-Columbian times in populations of the Andes. However, the suspected link between the acute form (Oroya fever) and the chronic form was confirmed in 1885 when Carrion, a medical student, died of Oroya fever after inoculating himself with material from a verruga. The acute form of the disease, usually seen in people who are not natives of the zone of endemicity, is an acute, progressive, severe, and febrile anemia with extravascular hemolysis associated with the presence of *B. bacilliformis* in the erythrocytes. Mortality was reported to be up to 40% of the cases prior to the antibiotic era. Bacteremia is common in the general population in zones of endemicity and nonendemicity (14, 50). The second stage of infection leads in weeks to months to the eruption of nodular angioproliferative cutaneous lesions named verruga peruana; mucosal and internal lesions can occur (80). The lesions can persist for several months, but the prognosis is good at this stage.

Trench Fever, BA, Endocarditis, and Prolonged Fever or Bacteremia Caused by *B. quintana*

Trench or quintan fever is a recurrent fever with three to five, sometimes more, febrile episodes lasting 4 to 5 days each occurring after 15 to 25 days of incubation. Severe headaches and shin pain are common symptoms associated with malaise, anorexia, abdominal pain, restlessness, and insomnia. Mild forms as well as asymptomatic carriage have also been reported (12, 40). Several cases of endocarditis have been associated with *B. quintana* infection (55). In human immunodeficiency virus (HIV)-infected persons, bacteremia caused by *B. quintana* develops insidiously, involving recurrent fever, headaches, and hepatomegaly. *B. quintana* and *B. henselae* are the two *Bartonella* species involved in the etiology of BA. BA, also called epithelioid angiomatosis, is a vascular proliferative disease of the skin characterized by multiple, blood-filled, partially endothelial cell-lined cystic structures (96). It is usually characterized by violaceous or colorless papular and nodular skin lesions that clinically may suggest Kaposi's sarcoma but histologically resemble epithelioid hemangiomas. When visceral parenchymal organs are involved, the condition is referred to as bacillary peliosis hepatis, splenic peliosis, or systemic BA. Fever, weight loss, malaise, and enlargement of affected organs may develop in people with disseminated BA. Subcutaneous and lytic bone lesions are strongly associated with *B. quintana* infection (47).

Zoonotic Bartonellae

CSD

CSD is mainly caused by *B. henselae* (77, 102), even if *B. clarridgeiae* is suspected in some cases based on serological evidence (49, 63). There are now strong arguments against *Afipia felis* being one of the etiologic agents of CSD (54). In CSD, 1 to 3 weeks elapse between the scratch or bite of a cat and the appearance of clinical signs. In 50% of the cases, a small skin lesion, often resembling an insect bite, appears at the inoculation site, usually the hand or forearm, and evolves from a papule to a vesicle and partially healed ulcers. These lesions resolve within a few days to a few weeks. Lymphadenitis develops approximately 3 weeks after exposure and is generally unilateral. It commonly appears in the epitrochlear, axillary, or cervical lymph nodes. Swelling of the lymph node is usually painful and persists for several weeks to several months. In 25% of the cases, suppuration occurs. The large majority of the patients show signs of systemic infection: fever, chills, malaise, anorexia, and headache. In general, the disease is benign and heals spontaneously without sequelae. Atypical manifestations of CSD occur in 5 to 10% of the cases. The most common of these is Parinaud's oculoglandular syndrome (periauricular lymphadenopathy and palpebral conjunctivitis), but also meningitis, encephalitis, osteolytic lesions, and thrombocytopenic purpura may occur. Encephalopathy is one of the most serious complications of CSD and usually occurs 2 to 6 weeks after the onset of lymphadenopathy. However, it usually resolves with complete recovery and few or no sequelae. It is estimated that 22,000 human cases of CSD occur yearly in the United States. From 55 to 80% of CSD patients are <20 years old. There is a seasonal pattern, with most cases seen in autumn and winter.

New clinical presentations associated with *B. henselae* infection have been reported for immunocompetent persons, including neuroretinitis or bacteremia as a cause of chronic fatigue syndrome, and a case of aggressive *B. henselae* endocarditis in a cat owner. *B. henselae* was also determined as a frequent cause of prolonged fever and fever of unknown origin in children. Rheumatic manifestations of *Bartonella* infection have been described for children, including a case of myositis and a case of arthritis and skin nodules. Arthritis has been described in a very limited number of cases. Other rheumatic manifestations related to *Bartonella* infection in humans include erythema nodosum, leukocytoclastic vasculitis, and fever of unknown origin with myalgia and arthralgia (7).

For BA in immunocompromised persons, the symptoms are very different from those of CSD. BA patients with *B. henselae* infection are epidemiologically linked to cat and flea exposure (47). Cutaneous lesions are common with *B. henselae* infection, and peliosis hepatis is associated exclusively with *B. henselae* infection. Fever, weight loss, malaise, and enlargement of affected organs may develop in people with disseminated BA. Endocarditis has also been reported for patients with BA. *B. henselae* and *B. quintana* have been implicated in a few cases of HIV-associated brain lesions, meningoencephalitis and encephalopathy, dementia, and neuropsychological decline (94, 97).

Zoonotic *Bartonella* Species Associated with Endocarditis or Myocarditis

Several zoonotic *Bartonella* spp. have been recognized as causative agents of blood culture-negative endocarditis or myocarditis in humans, including *B. henselae, B. koehlerae, B. elizabethae, B. vinsonii* subsp. *berkhoffii, B. vinsonii* subsp. *arupensis* (24), and "*B. washoensis*" (7). *Bartonella* spp. account for 3 to 4% of all human cases of endocarditis in France, a percentage similar to that of endocarditis cases caused by *Coxiella burnetii*, the agent of Q fever (35, 75).

Zoonotic *Bartonella* Species Associated with Ocular Lesions, Fever, and Neurological Symptoms

Some rodent-borne *Bartonella* species are also associated with cases of neuroretinitis (*B. elizabethae* and *B. grahamii*) or fever with bacteremia and neurological symptoms (*B. vinsonii* subsp. *arupensis*) (46, 98).

Other *Bartonella* Species or Subspecies

The clinical impact on animals or humans of many *Bartonella* species is still unknown. A broad array of manifestations, including endocarditis, has been identified for dogs (9). *B. henselae, B. clarridgeiae,* "*B. washoensis,*" and *B. elizabethae* have been recognized as pathogenic for dogs (18). No specific pathology has been associated yet with *Bartonella* species infecting domestic and wild ruminants or with many rodent-borne *Bartonella* spp.

COLLECTION, TRANSPORT, AND STORAGE OF SPECIMENS

Most specimens used for *Bartonella* isolation are either blood or tissue. Approaches typically used for recovery of other pathogens from such sites are suitable, although the fastidious nature of these organisms requires that precautions be taken to minimize the interval from collection to processing. *Bartonella* spp. are difficult to isolate from blood of immunocompetent individuals, as opposed to the relative ease of isolation from blood of immunocompromised patients. Blood samples can be collected either in Isolator blood lysis tubes (Wampole, Cranbury, N.J.), in sodium citrate tubes, or in plastic EDTA tubes, which is now the most common method used for blood collection in animals. If storage of specimens prior to culture is necessary, samples should be kept frozen (at least −20°C). It was shown that blood collected from *B. henselae*-infected cats into both EDTA and Isolator blood lysis tubes yielded good recovery and no loss of sensitivity for EDTA tubes kept at −65°C for 26 days (11). *Bartonella* spp. are susceptible to a broad spectrum of antimicrobial agents; therefore, specimens should be collected prior to antimicrobial therapy.

Collection of tissue from enlarged lymph nodes, cutaneous lesions, or various organs can be performed and samples cultured after homogenization or processed for DNA extraction and PCR. Fresh tissues are preferred for PCR amplification, but paraffin-embedded tissue may be used (23). Fine-needle aspiration has also been successful for detection of *Bartonella* and is less invasive than biopsy (3).

For animals, bartonellae are isolated from blood collected in plastic EDTA tubes; these tubes prevent breakage during shipment and during storage at low temperature, which facilitates lysis of the red blood cells. Biopsies of visceral or cutaneous lesions can be performed, especially in dogs, as described for humans. Collection of aqueous humor in cat or dog retinitis cases for detection of *Bartonella* bacteria or antibodies has been suggested (51, 70).

DIRECT EXAMINATION

Microscopy

Detection of *Bartonella* in erythrocytes from blood smears is rarely performed, with the exception of stained blood films for patients with Oroya fever, as the number of bacteria present in each erythrocyte is quite low (82), reaching a high of eight bacteria in a *B. birtlesii* model in rats (93). Microscopic detection of *Bartonella* organisms in fixed tissue sections includes Warthin-Starry silver staining, which is not highly specific for *Bartonella* organisms and requires careful attention to the details of the procedure (Fig. 1). Detection of bacilli by Warthin-Starry staining is more likely to occur during the early stage of CSD lymphadenopathy, but not during the granulomatous stage of inflammation. In patients with BA, there is usually a larger number of bacilli that are identifiable by Warthin-Starry silver staining.

Antigen Detection

Immunocytochemical labeling is a specific technique but is not widely available (76). Direct immunofluorescence of blood smears allowed rapid diagnosis of *B. quintana* in a patient with acute trench fever (27) and in bacteremic homeless patients (82). In the United States and Europe, *B. henselae* and *B. quintana* immunofluorescence assay (IFA) slides are available through companies such as Focus Diagnostics, Inc. (Cypress, Calif.).

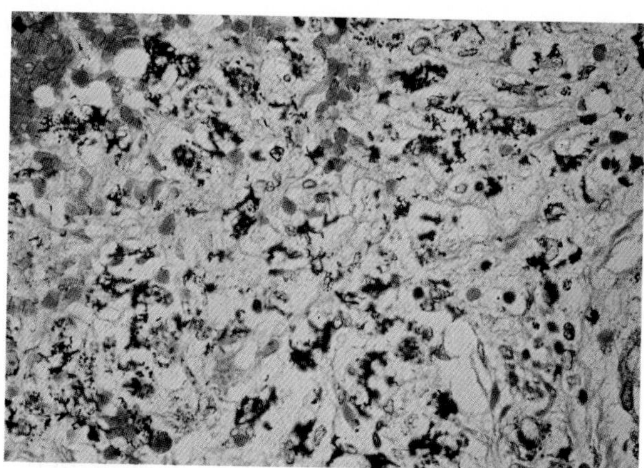

FIGURE 1 Warthin-Starry silver stain of a liver tissue section containing clusters of *B. henselae*. Magnification, ×530.

Nucleic Acid Detection Techniques

Direct detection of *Bartonella* spp. is more often performed by amplification of DNA from tissue, pus, or skin lesions. Molecular genetic methods such as restriction fragment length polymorphism (RFLP) of various genes (see recommended gene targets in Table 2) and, more recently, analysis based on PCR of random, repetitive extragenic palindromic sequences have been used to distinguish strains and species of *Bartonella*. RFLP or sequence analysis of 16S rRNA or citrate synthase genes after PCR amplification, both directly from specimens and from pure cultures, has been largely used for detecting and characterizing *Bartonella*. Identification has also been performed with the amplification of the intergenic spacer region between the 16S and 23S rRNA genes (89) or with protein-coding genes. A new tool has been proposed for the diagnosis of *Bartonella* endocarditis: a real-time nested PCR assay performed on a LightCycler apparatus using serum (23).

ISOLATION PROCEDURES (CULTURE)

Blood

Bartonellae can be recovered from the blood of bacteremic patients, especially persons infected with *B. quintana*, *B. bacilliformis*, and, less frequently, *B. henselae*. In immunocompromised patients, the level of bacteremia is often higher than in immunocompetent people, and most bacteremic patients have fever, chills, and weight loss (48). However, cultures from patients with infective endocarditis caused by *Bartonella* spp. are rarely positive. *Bartonella* species are optimally isolated from blood with the use of Isolator lysis centrifugation tubes or EDTA tubes and plating onto fresh chocolate or heart infusion agar containing 5% fresh rabbit blood in the absence of antibiotics. Commercial sheep or horse blood agar plates have also been used. *B. koehlerae* does not grow well on heart infusion agar and requires fresh chocolate plates (21). Plates inoculated with blood should be incubated at 35°C for at least 4 weeks in 5% CO_2 and at high humidity. Colonies usually appear after 5 to 15 days (48). Considering that the length of time required for detection of *Bartonella* spp. allows other slowly growing pathogens, including *Mycobacterium tuberculosis*, to grow on the same plates, appropriate safety precautions should be taken with positive cultures. Vials used for blood culture (broth-based or biphasic culture systems) can also be used for isolation of *Bartonella*,

TABLE 2 Sequences used as PCR primers or probes to amplify or identify *Bartonella*

Bacterium	Gene[a]	Direction[b]	Primer	Sequence	Reference(s)
B. clarridgeiae	*ribC*	F	PBC5	TACATAACGAGCCAATT	4
	ribC	R	PBC15	TAGCTTTAGAACAATATGGT	4
B. henselae	*ribC*	F	PBH-L1	GATATCGGTTGTGTTGAAGA	4
	ribC	R	PBH-R1	AATAAAAGGTATAAAACGCT	4
B. bacilliformis	*ribC*	F	PBH-L1	GATATCGGTTGTGTTGAAGA	4
	ribC	R	PBB-R1	AAAGGCGCTAACTGTTC	4
B. quintana	*ribC*	F	PBH-L1	GATATCGGTTGTGTTGAAGA	4
	ribC	R	PBQ-R1	AAAGGGCGTGAATTTTG	4
All bartonellae	*ribC*	F	PBH3	CCAAGTGCTACATAACCATC	4
	ribC	R	PBH4	CGGGTTGTTATTGCTCTTAC	4
All bartonellae (except *B. bacilliformis*)	*rrs-rrl* igs	F	16SF	AGAGGCAGGCAACCACGGTA	33, 90
	rrs-rrl igs	R	23S1	GCCAAGGCATCCACC	33, 90
All bartonellae	*rrs-rrl* igs	F	QHVE1	TTCAGATGATGATCCCAA	33, 90
	rrs-rrl igs	R	QHVE2	TTGGGATCATCATCTGAA	33, 90
	rrs-rrl igs	F	QHVE3	GATATATTCAGACATGTT	33, 90
	rrs-rrl igs	R	QHVE4	AACATGTCTGAATATATC	33, 90
B. bacilliformis	*rrs-rrl* igs	F	BABF	CTGGATCACCTCCTTTCTAA	33, 90
	rrs-rrl igs	R	BABR	ATGCCCTTAAGACACTTGAT	33, 90
B. quintana	*rrs-rrl* igs	F	BQF	CTCCACCATTTTAGGTCATC	33, 90
	rrs-rrl igs	R	BQR	GGTTTTGAGAATTCCCTTGC	33, 90
All bartonellae	*rrs-rrl* igs	F	16s1	(C/T)CTTCGTTTCTCTTTCTTCA	43
	rrs-rrl igs	R	16s2	GGATAAACCGGAAAACCTTC	43
	rrs-rrl igs	F	16s3	(C/T)CTTCGTTTCTCTTTCTTCA	43
	rrs-rrl igs	R	16s4	AACCAACTGAGCTACAAGCC	43
	rrs-rrl igs	F	16s5	CTCTTTCTTCAGATGATGATCC	43
	rrs-rrl igs	R	16s6	AACCAACTGAGCTACAAGCCCT	43
	ribC	F	BARTON-1F	TAACCGATATTGGTTGTGTTGAAG	45
	ribC	R	BARTON-2R	TAAAGCTAGAAAGTCTGGCAACATAACG	45
	rrs	S	Probe	ATTTGGTTGGGCACTCTAGGGG	46
	rrs		Rp2a	ACGGCTACCTTGTTAGGACTT	52
	rrs	F	357f	TACGGGAGGCAGCAG	52
	rrs	R	357ra	CTGCTGCCTCCCGTA	52
	rrs	F	536F	CAGCAGCCGCGGTAATAC	52
	rrs	R	536R	GTATTACCGCGGCTGCTG	52
	rrs	F	800F	ATTAGATACCCTGGTAG	52
	rrs	R	800R	CTACCAGGGTATCTAAT	52
	rrs	F	1050F	TGTCGTCAGCTCGTG	52
	rrs	R	1050R	CACGAGCTGACGACA	52
	35-kDa antigen gene	F	35KD1fa	GTCGCTAAAGGCTGATGA	52
	35-kDa antigen gene	R	35KD2ra	GACTGATATCGTGCGTGTG	52
	35-kDa antigen gene	F	35KDs1f	GGTACGACGACAGTAATTGTT	52
	35-kDa antigen gene	R	35KDs2r	GATTTAAGAGATACCAACCA	52
	pap	F	PAP1fa	CTTTAATGACGACTTCTGTT	52
	pap	R	PAP4ra	CCGAAATCTGAGTAACGGTA	52
	pap	R	PAP2r	CCCTAAATGTTTCAAGTTCA	52
	pap	F	PAP3f	GCTGACAGAGAAGACGCAA	52
	groEL	F	BbHs233.p	CGTGAAGTTGCCTCAAAAACC	64
	groEL	R	BbHs1630.n	AATCCATTCCGCCCATTC	64
	rpoB	F	QVE1	TTCAGATGATGATCCCAAGC	79
	rpoB	R	QVE3	AACATGTCTGAATATATCTTC	79
			Bfp1	ATTAATCTGCAYCGGCCAGA	105
			Bfp2	ACVGADACACGAATAACACC	105
			Bfs3	TTACAAAAATCYGTTGATAC	105
			Bfs4	GTATCAACRGATTTTTGTAA	105
	ftsZ	F	BaftsZF	GCTAATCGTATTCGCGAAGAA	105
	ftsZ	R	BaftsZR	GCTGGTATTTCCAAYTGATCT	105
B. henselae, *B. clarridgeiae*	*ftsZ*		Bh ftsZ 1393.n	GCGAACTACGGCTTACTTGC	105
	ftsZ		Bh ftsZ 1247.p	CGGTTGGAGAGCAGTTTCGTC	105

(Continued on next page)

TABLE 2 (*Continued*)

Bacterium	Gene[a]	Direction[b]	Primer	Sequence	Reference(s)
B. quintana	*ftsZ*	F	Bq ftsZseqF	GCACATATTCTTGATGAGAT	105
	ftsZ	R	Bq ftsZseqR	CCCCTATCATCTCATCAAG	105
B. bacilliformis	*ftsZ*	F	Bb ftsZseqF	GCGCATGTTCTTAGTGAAAT	105
	ftsZ	R	Bb ftsZseqR	CCTGTATACGTGATGCATTT	105
All bartonellae	*ftsZ*		FTS1p	GCCTTCTCATCCTCAACTT	105
	ftsZ		FTS2p	CAGCCTCTTCACGATGTG	105
	pap31		PAPn1	TTCTAGGAGTTGAAACCGAT	104
	pap31		PAPn2	GAAACACCACCAGCAACATA	104
	pap31		PAPns2	GCACCAGACCATTTTTCCTT	104
	pap31		PAPns1	CAGAGAAGACGCAAAAACCT	104
	groEL		HSPps1	CAGAAGTTGAAGTGAAAGAAAA	104
	groEL		HSPps2	GCNGCTTCTTCACCNGCATT	104
	groEL		HSPps4	GCTGGNGGTGTTGCNGTTA	104
	groEL		HSPps3	GCTGTNGAAGANGGNATTGT	104
	gltA		BhCS.781p	GGGGACCAGCTCATGGTGG	73
	gltA		BhCS.1137n	AATGCAAAAAGAACAGTAAACA	73
	gltA		CS.877p	GGGGGCCTGCTCACCGCGG	44
	gltA		CS.1258n	ATTGCAAAAAGTACAGTGAACA	44
	gltA		1240F	GATYCTTTCCGCCTTATG	74
	gltA		1497R	GAAATCCTAGAGCTTTTAATG	74
	rrs-rrl igs		321s	AGATGATGATCCCAAGCCTTCTGG	59
	rrs-rrl igs		983As	TGTTCTYACAACAATGATGAT	59
	rpoB		1400F	CGCATTGGCTTACTTCGTATG	79
	rpoB		2300R	GTAGACTGATTAGAACGCTG	79

[a] *rrs-rrl* igs, 16S rRNA-23S rRNA gene intergenic spacer region; *rrs*, 16S rRNA gene.
[b] F, forward; R, reverse.

such as BACTEC Peds Plus vials (Becton Dickinson, Sparks, Md.) (32) inoculated with about ≤5 ml and incubated, with recovery subsequently achieved by subculture onto solid media (42). Acridine orange staining and blind subculture from negative bottles before discarding them at 7 days may increase the likelihood of identifying bartonellae (1). An assay was also developed in which samples of heparinized blood are sedimented and the plasma is collected for inoculation into shell vials (42). Culture is then performed by the centrifugation-shell vial technique using ECV304 human endothelial cell monolayers (48).

In broth, *Bartonella* spp. usually do not produce turbidity or convert enough oxidizable substrate to CO_2 for CO_2 detection-based blood culture systems to indicate growth. A novel, chemically modified, insect-based liquid culture medium has been developed and supports the growth of at least seven *Bartonella* species (60). This medium also supports cocultures consisting of different *Bartonella* species, and it facilitates primary isolation of *B. henselae* from blood and aqueous fluids of naturally infected cats. This liquid growth medium may provide an advantage over conventional direct blood agar plating for the diagnosis of bartonellosis (60).

Tissue

Recovery of *Bartonella* spp. from cutaneous lesions, liver, spleen, or lymph node is not easy but is possible, especially after homogenization in inoculation medium and plating directly onto solid agar. Cocultivation with an endothelial cell line or by the shell vial method is more laborious but can yield bacterial growth on some occasions where nothing else works (48). Such methods have both been applied successfully for isolation of *Bartonella* in endocarditis cases (55). Some liquid media have been developed to allow primary isolation of *B. henselae* from blood and tissue (17, 101) but have not been used widely.

IDENTIFICATION

Bartonella spp.

Colonies of *B. henselae* can be of two morphological types, present in the same culture: (i) irregular, raised, whitish, rough (cauliflower-like), and dry in appearance and (ii) smaller, circular, tan, and moist in appearance, tending to pit and adhere to the agar (Fig. 2) (99). *B. quintana* colonies are usually smooth, flat, and shiny and do not pit the agar (48). *B. clarridgeiae* produces small white, raised, indurated, and cohesive colonies (57). They also can appear to spread on the agar during primary isolation from cats. Most *Bartonella* spp. usually appear as uniformly smooth after repeated subcultures. The bacilli are small (2 by 0.5 μm) and stain best with Gimenez stain (48). With Gram staining, *Bartonella* spp. are only weakly counterstained with safranin O. *Bartonella* spp. appear after Gram staining as small gram-negative slightly curved rods resembling *Campylobacter*, *Helicobacter*, or *Haemophilus* (99). Clumping of cells is quite common. The morphology of the colonies which appear usually after a lengthy incubation (more than 7 days) and negative catalase and oxidase reactions are often sufficient for a presumptive identification of *Bartonella*. After several subcultures, *Bartonella* colonies appear in less than a week. Furthermore, during primary isolation of *B. henselae* from cat blood, colonies appear most often in less than a week, whereas it usually takes 10 to 14 days to observe the first colonies for *B. clarridgeiae* or *B. koehlerae*.

B. bacilliformis, *B. clarridgeiae*, *B. capreoli*, and *B. schoenbuchensis* are the only members of the genus that are motile by means of unipolar flagella. *B. quintana* and *B. henselae* as well as several other *Bartonella* species have a twitching motility associated with fimbriae or pili. These pili are associated with cytoadherence and may mediate specific interaction with host erythrocytes and endothelial cells (62).

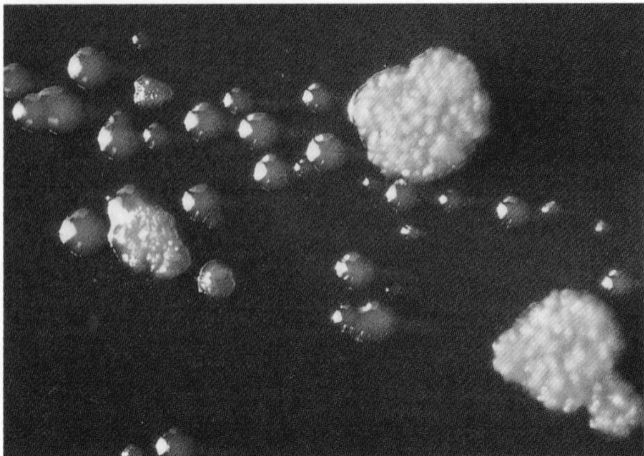

FIGURE 2 *B. henselae* after 7 days of incubation on chocolate agar, showing heterogeneity of colonies. Magnification, ×21.

Measurements of preformed enzymes and standard testing have revealed differences between species. Fatty acid methyl esters are prepared from cells harvested after 7 days of incubation on agar plates under conditions usually used for *Bartonella* isolation (see above). Bartonellae have a unique and characteristic whole-cell fatty acid composition (99). They have gas-liquid chromatography profiles consisting mainly of $C_{18:0}$, $C_{18:1}$, and $C_{16:0}$ acids. *B. elizabethae* contains a greater amount of $C_{17:0}$ than the other species.

Most species are biochemically inert except for the production of peptidases. None of the various commercially available identification systems contain *Bartonella* spp. in their databases. However, the MicroScan Rapid Anaerobe Panel (Baxter Diagnostics, Deerfield, Ill.), the RapID ANA II, and Rapid ID 32 A have been used as aids for identification. The MicroScan Rapid Anaerobe Panel has been reported to provide species identification (code 10077640 for *B. henselae,* code 10073640 for *B. quintana,* and code 10077240 for *B. bacilliformis*) (99). Overall, these identification kits are of limited use for proper diagnosis of *Bartonella* infection.

Identification of *Bartonella* isolates is largely based on molecular techniques, many allowing determination of the species or even some genotypes within a given species. Methods include Southern blotting, gel and capillary electrophoresis, PCR, DNA hybridization, RFLP, and sequence analysis and immunofluorescence detection (1, 84). The most widely targeted genes are those coding for the citrate synthase *(gltA)*, a heat shock protein *(groEL)*, riboflavin synthase *(ribC)*, a cell division protein *(ftsZ)*, and a 17-kDa antigen (23) (Table 2). The 16S rRNA gene *(rrs)* was first used by Relman et al. in 1990 for identification of the microbial etiology in a case of BA (78). However, this gene is not sensitive enough to properly discriminate *Bartonella* at the species level (56). Sequences obtained from the *gltA* and *rpoB* (RNA polymerase beta-subunit) genes are congruent with DNA-DNA hybridization for *Bartonella* species identification (56). The intergenic spacer region between the 16S and 23S rRNA genes has also been useful for *Bartonella* species identification (43, 59, 61). A genomic fingerprinting technique using infrequent restriction site PCR was also proposed to identify pathogenic *Bartonella* species (31). Use of monoclonal antibodies has been proposed for rapid identification of *B. quintana* (58).

Typing Systems

Multilocus sequence typing (MLST) has been used to examine the distribution of polymorphisms within different genes of *B. henselae* isolates (36). MLST distinguished several sequence types that resolved into three distinct lineages, suggesting a clonal population structure for the species. Similarly, multispacer typing was applied for the sequence-based typing of *B. quintana* (25).

SEROLOGICAL TESTS

Serological testing has become the cornerstone of clinical diagnosis, as it is widely used for diagnosis of *Bartonella* infections, especially cases of CSD, because culture and isolation are quite time-consuming and difficult and may yield results only after several weeks. However, cross-reactivity among *Bartonella* species is common, and it may occur with some other pathogenic bacteria such as *C. burnetii* and *Chlamydophila* spp. (53, 65). Antibody response in humans and animals is detected mainly with the IFA or different enzyme immunoassays (EIAs) (68). Western blotting tests have also been developed but are not used as widely (34, 91). In the United States, serological testing for CSD is performed by the Centers for Disease Control and Prevention (CDC) in Atlanta, Ga., by various state public health laboratories, and by commercial laboratories. Commercial slides (such as those from Focus Diagnostics, Inc.) for *B. henselae* and *B. quintana* IFA testing are available and widely used in both the United States and Europe.

B. bacilliformis

IFA and EIAs for the diagnosis of *B. bacilliformis* infection and for use in serological surveys have both been used for many years. A new IFA based on *B. bacilliformis*-infected Vero cells has been developed and shown to be very specific (92% based on 101 healthy controls) and identified 81% (86 of 106) of those with laboratory-diagnosed acute bartonellosis (13). Some other assays have been developed but showed some cross-reactivity with *Brucella* and *Chlamydophila psittaci,* suggesting that test optimization is still required (1).

B. quintana, B. henselae, and *B. clarridgeiae*

Human infection with *B. henselae* or *B. quintana* is evaluated by the presence of immunoglobulin M (IgM) or IgG directed against these bacteria, with cross-reactivity in up to 95% of samples (91). Antigen adsorption can be used to reduce cross-reactivity and to determine to which antigen the antibodies are truly directed (1). For animals, detection of antibodies is usually directed toward IgG. The first serological test for CSD, developed at the CDC, was an IFA based on *B. henselae* bacilli that were cocultivated with Vero cells to inhibit autoagglutination (77). This test was found to have good sensitivity (84 to 95%) and specificity (94 to 98%) (20, 77, 102). Lower sensitivity and specificity were reported from Europe (22, 103). However, commercial slides from at least one specific manufacturer (Focus Diagnostics) have been shown to be more sensitive for detection of cases of CSD, especially in Europe (68, 103). IFA is the most frequently used serological test, and it seems to currently be the most reliable test and the method of choice for the diagnosis of CSD (91). Dilution titers of 256 or higher are usually indicative of ongoing infection; lower titers may indicate an early or late clinical phase of the disease or prior exposure to the bacteria. In cases of endocarditis caused by either *B. henselae* or *B. quintana,* high IgG antibody titers (≥800) are usually detected (28). A titer ≥800 for IgG antibodies to either *B. henselae* or *B. quintana* has a positive predictive value of 0.810 for the detection of chronic *Bartonella* infections in the general population and 0.955 for the detection of *Bartonella* infections among patients with endocarditis.

IFA is time-consuming, requires appropriate equipment and expertise, and is subject to interobserver variation due to the difficulty of reading the test (1). Within the last 10 years, different EIAs have been developed; they are simpler to perform, use readily available equipment, and can be automated (1). However, at present, EIAs have not been widely used and the sensitivity of the tests (17 to 35%) was lower than for one IFA (5). Giladi et al. (29) developed an EIA that used *N*-lauroylsarcosine-insoluble outer membrane antigens from agar-grown *B. henselae* for the detection of anti-*B. henselae* IgG and IgM antibodies in patients with CSD. It was found that when a positive IgG or IgM test result or both are accepted as diagnostic, the sensitivity of the EIA is 85%. Applying stringent criteria, this test is highly specific (98 and 99% for IgG and IgM, respectively), as determined by testing healthy control subjects and patients with lymphadenopathy due to defined non-CSD causes (69). EIA seems more sensitive than IFA for detection of IgM (1).

ANTIMICROBIAL SUSCEPTIBILITY

Antimicrobial susceptibility testing can be performed by incorporation of antibiotics into either blood or chocolate agar or into various media supplemented with blood using a microdilution technique (88, 95). The E test (AB Biodisk, Solna, Sweden) can also be used to determine antibiotic susceptibility (100). Results of susceptibility testing of *Bartonella* spp. are summarized in Table 3. Evaluation of susceptibility to

TABLE 3 MICs for *Bartonella* strains[a]

Antibiotic group and drug name	MIC (μg/ml)				
	B. henselae	*B. quintana*	*B. bacilliformis*	*B. vinsonii*	*B. elizabethae*
Aminoglycosides					
Amikacin	2–4	4–8	2–8	4	1
Gentamicin	0.12–0.25	0.12–2	1–2	0.5	0.12
Streptomycin	ND	ND	4	ND	ND
Tobramycin	0.5–1	0.5–4	2–4	2	0.25
Cephalosporins					
Cefotaxime	0.12–0.25	0.12–0.25	0.03–0.12	0.12	0.06
Cefotetan	0.25–0.5	0.12–0.5	2	1	1
Ceftazidime	0.25–0.5	0.25–0.5	0.12–0.25	0.25	0.5
Ceftriaxone	0.12–0.25	0.06–0.25	0.003–0.006	0.06	0.12
Cephalothin	8–16	8–16	4–8	16	8
Macrolides					
Azithromycin	0.006–0.015	0.006–0.03	0.015	0.015	0.006
Clarithromycin	0.006–0.03	0.006–0.03	0.015–0.03	0.03	0.015
Erythromycin	0.06–0.25	0.06–0.12	0.06	0.25	0.12
Roxithromycin	0.015–0.03	0.015–0.06	0.03	0.12	0.06
Telithromycin	0.003	0.006	0.015	ND	ND
Penicillins					
Amoxicillin	0.6–0.12	0.03–0.06	0.03–0.06	0.06	0.03
Oxacillin	1–2	1–4	0.25–0.5	1	4
Penicillin G	0.03–0.06	0.03	0.015–0.03	0.03	0.015
Ticarcillin	0.25	0.06–0.25	0.06–0.12	0.25	0.12
Quinolones					
Ciprofloxacin	0.25–1	0.5–2	0.25–0.5	1	0.5
Pefloxacin	4–8	2–8	1–2	4	2
Sparfloxacin	0.06	0.06–0.12	0.25	0.06	0.06
Tetracyclines					
Doxycycline	0.12	0.06–0.25	0.03–0.06	0.25	0.06
Miscellaneous					
Clindamycin	2–4	4–16	32–64	8	8
Colistin	4–16	4–16	16	8	4
Fosfomycin	16–32	32–64	8–16	16	16
Imipenem	0.5	0.25–1	0.5–1	2	0.25
Rifampin	0.03–0.06	0.06–0.25	0.003	0.12	0.03
TMP-SXT	1/5	0.25/1.25–1/5	0.4/2–0.8/4	1/5	0.5/2.5
Vancomycin	2–8	8–16	4–8	8	8

[a] Determined by agar dilution with Columbia agar supplemented with 5% horse blood. Table adapted from reference 81. Abbreviations: TMP-SXT, trimethoprim-sulfamethoxazole; ND, not done.

antibiotics has been performed either in cells or without cells, i.e., in axenic media. These various methods of culture could be used for determination of the bacteriostatic activity of antibiotics with similar results. Determination of the antibiotic susceptibility in axenic medium has been carried out either in solid media enriched with 5 to 10% sheep or horse blood or in liquid media (66, 95). It should be noted that the conditions required to grow *Bartonella* during susceptibility testing do not meet standardized criteria established for the Clinical and Laboratory Standards Institute. Bacteria of the genus *Bartonella* are susceptible to many antibiotics when grown axenically, including β-lactams, aminoglycosides, chloramphenicol, tetracyclines, macrolide compounds (including telithromycin), rifampin, fluoroquinolones, and trimethoprim-sulfamethoxazole (66, 67, 72, 86).

In vitro antibiotic susceptibilities also have been examined for *Bartonella* species cocultivated with eukaryotic cells. As with agar-based susceptibilities, these studies demonstrated that *Bartonella* spp. are susceptible to many antibiotics in vitro (37). However, all of these antibiotics (39) had only bacteriostatic activity (38, 39). Only aminoglycosides are bactericidal in vitro against *Bartonella* species grown in liquid medium (88), in endothelial cells (71), or in an erythrocyte coculture model (87).

Choice and Use of Antibiotics In Vivo

CSD typically does not respond to antibiotic therapy. Most investigators have observed no benefit with antibiotic treatment, whereas anecdotal reports have indicated that ciprofloxacin, rifampin, and trimethoprim-sulfamethoxazole may be effective (26, 75, 81).

EVALUATION, INTERPRETATION, AND REPORTING OF RESULTS

Diagnosis of *Bartonella* infection in humans, especially for typical forms of CSD, is mainly based on serological data, which is the most cost-effective approach. As reported by Bergmans et al. (5) and Sander et al. (91), the sensitivities of different IFAs range from 14 to 100%, depending on the antigen used, the cutoff chosen, and the test procedures. For cases of endocarditis, the best approach is serological testing and performing PCR on cardiac valves. A recent procedure using a single-step serological assay against *C. burnetii* and *Bartonella* species found a sensitivity of 100%, and a positive predictive value of 98% for the diagnosis of blood culture-negative endocarditis (85). New methods of culture in liquid media are being developed, as direct isolation from blood or tissues is often negative despite detection of *Bartonella* DNA by PCR tests (60).

REFERENCES

1. **Agan, B. K., and M. J. Dolan.** 2002. Laboratory diagnosis of *Bartonella* infections. *Clin. Lab. Med.* **22:**937–962.
2. **Anderson, B. E., and M. A. Neuman.** 1997. *Bartonella* spp. as emerging human pathogens. *Clin. Microbiol. Rev.* **10:** 203–219.
3. **Avidor, B., M. Varon, S. Marmor, B. Lifschitz-Mercer, Y. Kletter, M. Ephros, and M. Giladi.** 2001. DNA amplification for the diagnosis of cat-scratch disease in small-quantity clinical specimens. *Am. J. Clin. Pathol.* **115:**900–909.
4. **Bereswill, S., S. Hinkelmann, M. Kist, and A. Sander.** 1999. Molecular analysis of riboflavin synthesis genes in *Bartonella henselae* and use of the *ribC* gene for differentiation of *Bartonella* species by PCR. *J. Clin. Microbiol.* **37:**3159–3166.
5. **Bergmans, A. M., M. F. Peeters, J. F. Schellekens, M. C. Vos, L. J. Sabbe, J. M. Ossewaarde, H. Verbakel, H. J. Hooft, and L. M. Schouls.** 1997. Pitfalls and fallacies of cat scratch disease serology: evaluation of *Bartonella henselae*-based indirect fluorescence assay and enzyme-linked immunoassay. *J. Clin. Microbiol.* **35:**1931–1937.
6. **Birtles, R. J., T. G. Harrison, N. A. Saunders, and D. H. Molyneux.** 1995. Proposals to unify the genera *Grahamella* and *Bartonella*, with descriptions of *Bartonella talpae* comb. nov., *Bartonella peromysci* comb. nov., and three new species, *Bartonella grahamii* sp. nov., *Bartonella taylorii* sp. nov., and *Bartonella doshiae* sp. nov. *Int. J. Syst. Bacteriol.* **45:**1–8.
7. **Boulouis, H. J., C. C. Chang, J. B. Henn, R. W. Kasten, and B. B. Chomel.** 2005. Factors associated with the rapid emergence of zoonotic *Bartonella* infections. *Vet. Res.* **36:**383–410.
8. **Bown, K. J., M. Bennet, and M. Begon.** 2004. Flea-borne *Bartonella grahamii* and *Bartonella taylorii* in bank voles. *Emerg. Infect. Dis.* **10:**684–687.
9. **Breitschwerdt, E. B., and D. L. Kordick.** 2000. *Bartonella* infection in animals: carriership, reservoir potential, pathogenicity, and zoonotic potential for human infection. *Clin. Microbiol. Rev.* **13:**428–438.
10. **Brenner, D. J., S. P. O'Connor, H. H. Winkler, and A. G. Steigerwalt.** 1993. Proposals to unify the genera *Bartonella* and *Rochalimaea*, with descriptions of *Bartonella quintana* comb. nov., *Bartonella vinsoni* comb. nov., *Bartonella henselae* comb. nov., and *Bartonella elizabethae* comb. nov., and to remove the family *Bartonellaceae* from the order *Rickettsiales*. *Int. J. Syst. Bacteriol.* **43:**777–786.
11. **Brenner, S. A., J. A. Rooney, P. Manzewitsch, and R. L. Regnery.** 1997. Isolation of *Bartonella (Rochalimaea) henselae*: effects of methods of blood collection and handling. *J. Clin. Microbiol.* **35:**544–547.
12. **Brouqui, P., B. La Scola, V. Roux, and D. Raoult.** 1999. Chronic *Bartonella quintana* bacteremia in homeless patients. *N. Engl. J. Med.* **340:**184–189.
13. **Chamberlin, J., L. Laughlin, S. Gordon, S. Romero, N. Solorzano, and R. L. Regnery.** 2000. Serodiagnosis of *Bartonella bacilliformis* infection by indirect fluorescence antibody assay: test development and application to a population in an area of bartonellosis endemicity. *J. Clin. Microbiol.* **38:**4269–4271.
14. **Chamberlin, J., L. W. Laughlin, S. Romero, N. Solorzano, S. Gordon, R. G. Andre, P. Pachas, H. Friedman, C. Ponce, and D. Watts.** 2002. Epidemiology of endemic *Bartonella bacilliformis:* a prospective cohort study in a Peruvian mountain valley community. *J. Infect. Dis.* **186:**983–990.
15. **Chang, C. C., B. B. Chomel, R. W. Kasten, V. Romano, and N. Tietze.** 2001. Molecular evidence of *Bartonella* spp. in questing adult *Ixodes pacificus* ticks in California. *J. Clin. Microbiol.* **39:**1221–1226.
16. **Chang, C.-C., R. W. Kasten, B. B. Chomel, D. C. Simpson, C. M. Hew, D. L. Kordick, R. Heller, Y. Piemont, and E. B. Breitschwerdt.** 2000. Coyotes *(Canis latrans)* as the reservoir for a human pathogenic *Bartonella* sp.: molecular epidemiology of *Bartonella vinsonii* subsp. *berkhoffii* infection in coyotes from central coastal California. *J. Clin. Microbiol.* **38:**4193–4200.
17. **Chenoweth, M. R., G. A. Somerville, D. C. Krause, K. L. O'Reilly, and F. C. Gherardini.** 2004. Growth characteristics of *Bartonella henselae* in a novel liquid medium: primary isolation, growth-phase-dependent phage induction, and metabolic studies. *Appl. Environ. Microbiol.* **70:**656–663.
18. **Chomel, B. B., H. J. Boulouis, and E. B. Breitschwerdt.** 2004. Cat scratch disease and other zoonotic *Bartonella* infections. *J. Am. Vet. Med. Assoc.* **224:**1270–1279.
19. **Chomel, B. B., R. W. Kasten, K. A. Floyd-Hawkins, B. Chi, K. Yamamoto, J. Roberts-Wilson, A. N. Gurfield, R. C. Abbott, N. C. Pedersen, and J. E. Koehler.** 1996. Experimental transmission of *Bartonella henselae* by the cat flea. *J. Clin. Microbiol.* **34:**1952–1956.

20. **Dalton, M. J., L. E. Robinson, J. Cooper, R. L. Regnery, J. G. Olson, and J. E. Childs.** 1995. Use of *Bartonella* antigens for serologic diagnosis of cat-scratch disease at a national referral center. *Arch. Intern. Med.* **155:**1670–1676.
21. **Droz, S., B. Chi, E. Horn, A. G. Steigerwalt, A. M. Whitney, and D. J. Brenner.** 1999. *Bartonella koehlerae* sp. nov., isolated from cats. *J. Clin. Microbiol.* **37:**1117–1122.
22. **Dupon, M., A. M. Savin de Larclause, P. Brouqui, M. Drancourt, D. Raoult D, A. de Mascarel, and J. Y. Lacut.** 1996. Evaluation of serological response to *Bartonella henselae, Bartonella quintana* and *Afipia felis* antigens in 64 patients with suspected cat-scratch disease. *Scand. J. Infect. Dis.* **28:**361–366.
23. **Fenollar, F., and D. Raoult.** 2004. Molecular genetic methods for the diagnosis of fastidious microorganisms. *APMIS* **112:**785–807.
24. **Fenollar, F., S. Sire, and D. Raoult.** 2005. *Bartonella vinsonii* subsp. *arupensis* as an agent of blood culture-negative endocarditis in a human. *J. Clin. Microbiol.* **43:**945–947.
25. **Foucault, C., B. La Scola, H. Lindroos, S. G. Andersson, and D. Raoult.** 2005. Multispacer typing technique for sequence-based typing of *Bartonella quintana. J. Clin. Microbiol.* **43:**41–48.
26. **Foucault, C., D. Raoult, and P. Brouqui.** 2003. Randomized open trial of gentamicin and doxycycline for eradication of *Bartonella quintana* from blood in patients with chronic bacteremia. *Antimicrob. Agents Chemother.* **47:**2204–2207.
27. **Foucault, C., J. M. Rolain, D. Raoult, and P. Brouqui.** 2004. Detection of *Bartonella quintana* by direct immunofluorescence examination of blood smears of a patient with acute trench fever. *J. Clin. Microbiol.* **42:**4904–4906.
28. **Fournier, P. E., J. L. Mainardi, and D. Raoult.** 2002. Value of microimmunofluorescence for diagnosis and follow-up of *Bartonella* endocarditis. *Clin. Diagn. Lab. Immunol.* **9:**795–801.
29. **Giladi, M., Y. Kletter, B. Avidor, E. Metzkor-Cotter, M. Varon, Y. Golan, M. Weinberg, I. Riklis, M. Ephros, and L. Slater.** 2001. Enzyme immunoassay for the diagnosis of cat-scratch disease defined by polymerase chain reaction. *Clin. Infect. Dis.* **33:**1852–1858.
30. **Gurfield, A. N., H. J. Boulouis, B. B. Chomel, R. Heller, R. W. Kasten, K. Yamamoto, and Y. Piemont.** 1997. Coinfection with *Bartonella clarridgeiae* and *Bartonella henselae* and with different *Bartonella henselae* strains in domestic cats. *J. Clin. Microbiol.* **35:**2120–2123.
31. **Handley, S. A., and R. L. Regnery.** 2000. Differentiation of pathogenic *Bartonella* species by infrequent restriction site PCR. *J. Clin. Microbiol.* **38:**3010–3015.
32. **Heller, R., M. Artois, V. Xemar, D. de Briel, H. Gehin, B. Jaulhac, H. Monteil, and Y. Piemont.** 1997. Prevalence of *Bartonella henselae* and *Bartonella clarridgeiae* in stray cats. *J. Clin. Microbiol.* **35:**1327–1331.
33. **Houpikian, P., and D. Raoult.** 2001. 16S/23S rRNA intergenic spacer regions for phylogenetic analysis, identification, and subtyping of *Bartonella* species. *J. Clin. Microbiol.* **39:**2768–2778.
34. **Houpikian, P., and D. Raoult.** 2003. Western immunoblotting for *Bartonella* endocarditis. *Clin. Diagn. Lab. Immunol.* **10:**95–102.
35. **Houpikian, P., and D. Raoult.** 2005. Blood culture-negative endocarditis in a reference center: etiologic diagnosis of 348 cases. *Medicine* (Baltimore) **84:**162–173.
36. **Iredell, J., D. Blanckenberg, M. Arvand, S. Grauling, E. J. Feil, and R. J. Birtles.** 2003. Characterization of the natural population of *Bartonella henselae* by multilocus sequence typing. *J. Clin. Microbiol.* **41:**5071–5079.
37. **Ives, T. J., P. Manzewitsch, R. L. Regnery, J. D. Butts, and M. Kebede.** 1997. In vitro susceptibilities of *Bartonella henselae, B. quintana, B. elizabethae, Rickettsia rickettsii, R. conorii, R. akari,* and *R. prowazekii* to macrolide antibiotics as determined by immunofluorescent-antibody analysis of infected Vero cell monolayers. *Antimicrob. Agents Chemother.* **41:**578–582.
38. **Ives, T. J., E. L. Marston, R. L. Regnery, and J. D. Butts.** 2001. In vitro susceptibilities of *Bartonella* and *Rickettsia* spp. to fluoroquinolone antibiotics as determined by immunofluorescent antibody analysis of infected Vero cell monolayers. *Int. J. Antimicrob. Agents* **18:**217–222.
39. **Ives, T. J., E. L. Marston, R. L. Regnery, J. D. Butts, and T. C. Majerus.** 2000. *In vitro* susceptibilities of *Rickettsia* and *Bartonella* spp. to 14-hydroxy-clarithromycin as determined by immunofluorescent antibody analysis of infected Vero cell monolayers. *J. Antimicrob. Chemother.* **45:**305–310.
40. **Jackson, L. A., and D. H. Spach.** 1996. Emergence of *Bartonella quintana* infection among homeless persons. *Emerg. Infect. Dis.* **2:**141–144.
41. **Jacomo, V., P. J. Kelly, and D. Raoult.** 2002. Natural history of *Bartonella* infections (an exception to Koch's postulate). *Clin. Diagn. Lab. Immunol.* **9:**8–18.
42. **Jacomo, V., and D. Raoult.** 2000. Human infections caused by *Bartonella* spp. Part 2. *Clin. Microbiol. Newsl.* **22:**9–13.
43. **Jensen, W. A., M. Z. Fall, J. Rooney, D. L. Kordick, and E. B. Breitschwerdt.** 2000. Rapid identification and differentiation of *Bartonella* species using a single-step PCR assay. *J. Clin. Microbiol.* **38:**1717–1722.
44. **Joblet, C., V. Roux, M. Drancourt, J. Gouvernet, and D. Raoult.** 1995. Identification of *Bartonella (Rochalimaea)* species among fastidious gram-negative bacteria on the basis of the partial sequence of the citrate-synthase gene. *J. Clin. Microbiol.* **33:**1879–1883.
45. **Johnson, G., M. Ayers, S. C. C. McClure, S. E. Richardson, and R. Tellier.** 2003. Detection and identification of *Bartonella* species pathogenic for humans by PCR amplification targeting the riboflavin synthase gene *(ribC)*. *J. Clin. Microbiol.* **41:**1069–1072.
46. **Kerkhoff, F. T., A. M. C. Bergmans, A. van der Zee, and A. Rothova.** 1999. Demonstration of *Bartonella grahamii* DNA in ocular fluids of a patient with neuroretinitis. *J. Clin. Microbiol.* **37:**4034–4038.
47. **Koehler, J. E., M. A. Sanchez, C. S. Garrido, M. J. Whitfeld, F. M. Chen, T. G. Berger, M. C. Rodriguez-Barradas, P. E. LeBoit, and J. W. Tappero.** 1997. Molecular epidemiology of *Bartonella* infections in patients with bacillary angiomatosis-peliosis. *N. Engl. J. Med.* **337:**1876–1883.
48. **Koehler, J. E., and J. W. Tappero.** 1993. Bacillary angiomatosis and bacillary peliosis in patients infected with human immunodeficiency virus. *Clin. Infect. Dis.* **17:**612–624.
49. **Kordick, D. L., E. J. Hilyard, T. L. Hadfield, K. H. Wilson, A. G. Steigerwalt, D. J. Brenner, and E. B. Breitschwerdt.** 1997. *Bartonella clarridgeiae,* a newly recognized zoonotic pathogen causing inoculation papules, fever, and lymphadenopathy (cat scratch disease). *J. Clin. Microbiol.* **35:**1813–1818.
50. **Kosek, M., R. Lavarello, R. H. Gilman, J. Delgado, C. Maguina, M. Verastegui, A. G. Lescano, V. Mallqui, J. C. Kosek, S. Recavarren, and L. Cabrera.** 2000. Natural history of infection with *Bartonella bacilliformis* in a non-endemic population. *J. Infect. Dis.* **182:**865–872.
51. **Lappin, M. R., D. L. Kordick, and E. B. Breitschwerdt.** 2000. *Bartonella* spp. antibodies and DNA in aqueous humour of cats. *J. Feline Med. Surg.* **2:**61–68.
52. **La Scola, B., Z. Liang, Z. Zeaiter, P. Houpikian, P. A. D. Grimont, and D. Raoult.** 2002. Genotypic characteristics of two serotypes of *Bartonella henselae. J. Clin. Microbiol.* **40:**2002–2008.
53. **La Scola, B., and D. Raoult.** 1996. Serological cross-reactions between *Bartonella quintana, Bartonella henselae,* and *Coxiella burnetii. J. Clin. Microbiol.* **34:**2270–2274.
54. **La Scola, B., and D. Raoult.** 1999. *Afipia felis* in hospital water supply in association with free-living amoebae. *Lancet* **353:**1330.

55. **La Scola, B., and D. Raoult.** 1999. Culture of *Bartonella quintana* and *Bartonella henselae* from human samples: a 5-year experience (1993 to 1998). *J. Clin. Microbiol.* **37:**1899–1905.
56. **La Scola, B., Z. Zeaiter, A. Khamis, and D. Raoult.** 2003. Gene-sequence-based criteria for species definition in bacteriology: the *Bartonella* paradigm. *Trends Microbiol.* **11:**318–321.
57. **Lawson, P. A., and M. D. Collins.** 1996. Description of *Bartonella clarridgeiae* sp. nov. isolated from the cat of a patient with *Bartonella henselae* septicemia. *Med. Microbiol. Lett.* **5:**64–73.
58. **Liang, Z., and D. Raoult.** 2000. Species-specific monoclonal antibodies for rapid identification of *Bartonella quintana*. *Clin. Diagn. Lab. Immunol.* **7:**21–24.
59. **Maggi, R. G., and E. B. Breitschwerdt.** 2005. Potential limitations of the 16S-23S rRNA intergenic region for molecular detection of *Bartonella* species. *J. Clin. Microbiol.* **43:**1171–1176.
60. **Maggi, R. G., A. W. Duncan, and E. B. Breitschwerdt.** 2005. Novel chemically modified liquid medium that will support the growth of seven *Bartonella* species. *J. Clin. Microbiol.* **43:**2651–2655.
61. **Maillard, R., M. Vayssier-Taussat, C. Bouillin, C. Gandoin, L. Halos, B. Chomel, Y. Piemont, and H. J. Boulouis.** 2004. Identification of *Bartonella* strains isolated from wild and domestic ruminants by a single-step PCR analysis of the 16S-23S intergenic spacer region. *Vet. Microbiol.* **98:**63–69. (Erratum, *Vet. Microbiol.* **100:**139–140.)
62. **Mändle, T., H. Einsele, M. Schaller, D. Neumann, W. Vogel, I. B. Autenrieth, and V. A. Kempf.** 2005. Infection of human CD34+ progenitor cells with *Bartonella henselae* results in intraerythrocytic presence of *B. henselae*. *Blood* **106:**1215–1222.
63. **Margileth, A. M., and D. F. Baehren.** 1998. Chest-wall abscess due to cat-scratch disease (CSD) in an adult with antibodies to *Bartonella clarridgeiae*: case report and review of the thoracopulmonary manifestations of CSD. *Clin. Infect. Dis.* **27:**353–357.
64. **Marston, E. L., J. W. Sumner, and R. L. Regnery.** 1999. Evaluation of intraspecies genetic variation within the 60 kDa heat-shock protein gene (*groEL*) of *Bartonella* species. *Int. J. Syst. Bacteriol.* **49:**1015–1023.
65. **Maurin, M., F. Eb, J. Etienne, and D. Raoult.** 1997. Serological cross-reactions between *Bartonella* and *Chlamydia* species: implications for diagnosis. *J. Clin. Microbiol.* **35:**2283–2287.
66. **Maurin, M., S. Gasquet, C. Ducco, and D. Raoult.** 1995. MICs of 28 antibiotic compounds for 14 *Bartonella* (formerly *Rochalimaea*) isolates. *Antimicrob. Agents Chemother.* **39:**2387–2391.
67. **Maurin, M., and D. Raoult.** 1993. Antimicrobial susceptibility of *Rochalimaea quintana*, *Rochalimaea vinsonii* and the newly recognized *Rochalimaea henselae*. *J. Antimicrob. Chemother.* **32:**587–594.
68. **Maurin, M., J. M. Rolain, and D. Raoult.** 2002. Comparison of in-house and commercial slides for detection by immunofluorescence of immunoglobulins G and M against *Bartonella henselae* and *Bartonella quintana*. *Clin. Diagn. Lab. Immunol.* **9:**1004–1009.
69. **Metzkor-Cotter, E., Y. Kletter, B. Avidor, M. Varon, Y. Golan, M. Ephros, and M. Giladi.** 2003. Long-term serological analysis and clinical follow-up of patients with cat scratch disease. *Clin. Infect. Dis.* **37:**1149–1154.
70. **Michau, T. M., E. B. Breitschwerdt, B. C. Gilger, and M. G. Davidson.** 2003. *Bartonella vinsonii* subspecies *berkhoffii* as a possible cause of anterior uveitis and choroiditis in a dog. *Vet. Ophthalmol.* **6:**299–304.
71. **Musso, D., M. Drancourt, and D. Raoult.** 1995. Lack of bactericidal effect of antibiotics except aminoglycosides on *Bartonella (Rochalimaea) henselae*. *J. Antimicrob. Chemother.* **36:**101–108.
72. **Myers, W. F., D. M. Grossman, and C. L. Wisseman, Jr.** 1984. Antibiotic susceptibility patterns in *Rochalimaea quintana*, the agent of trench fever. *Antimicrob. Agents Chemother.* **25:**690–693.
73. **Norman, A. F., R. Regnery, P. Jameson, C. Greene, and D. C. Krause.** 1995. Differentiation of *Bartonella*-like isolates at the species level by PCR-restriction fragment length polymorphism in the citrate synthase gene. *J. Clin. Microbiol.* **33:**1797–1803.
74. **Patel, R., J. O. Newell, G. W. Procop, and D. H. Persing.** 1999. Use of polymerase chain reaction for citrate synthase gene to diagnose *Bartonella quintana* endocarditis. *Am. J. Clin. Pathol.* **112:**36–40.
75. **Raoult, D., P. E. Fournier, F. Vandenesch, J. L. Mainardi, S. J. Eykyn, J. Nash, E. James, C. Benoit-Lemercier, and T. J. Marrie.** 2003. Outcome and treatment of *Bartonella* endocarditis. *Arch. Intern. Med.* **163:**226–230.
76. **Reed, J. A., D. J. Brigati, S. D. Flynn, N. S. McNutt, K. W. Min, D. F. Welch, and L. N. Slater.** 1992. Immunocytochemical identification of *Rochalimaea henselae* in bacillary (epithelioid) angiomatosis, parenchymal bacillary peliosis, and persistent fever with bacteremia. *Am. J. Surg. Pathol.* **16:**650–657.
77. **Regnery, R. L., J. G. Olson, B. A. Perkins, and W. Bibb.** 1992. Serological response to "*Rochalimaea henselae*" antigen in suspected cat-scratch disease. *Lancet* **339:**1443–1445.
78. **Relman, D. A., J. S. Loutit, T. M. Schmidt, S. Falkow, and L. S. Tompkins.** 1990. The agent of bacillary angiomatosis. An approach to the identification of uncultured pathogens. *N. Engl. J. Med.* **323:**1573–1580.
79. **Renesto, P., J. Gouvernet, M. Drancourt, V. Roux, and D. Raoult.** 2001. Use of rpoB gene analysis for detection and identification of *Bartonella* species. *J. Clin. Microbiol.* **39:**430–437.
80. **Ricketts, W. E.** 1949. Clinical manifestations of Carrion's disease. *Arch. Intern. Med.* **84:**751–781.
81. **Rolain, J. M., P. Brouqui, J. E. Koehler, C. Maguina, M. J. Dolan, and D. Raoult.** 2004. Recommendations for treatment of human infections caused by *Bartonella* species. *Antimicrob. Agents Chemother.* **48:**1921–1933.
82. **Rolain, J. M., C. Foucault, R. Guieu, B. La Scola, P. Brouqui, and D. Raoult.** 2002. *Bartonella quintana* in human erythrocytes. *Lancet* **360:**226–228.
83. **Rolain, J. M., M. Franc, B. Davoust, and D. Raoult.** 2003. Molecular detection of *Bartonella quintana*, *B. koehlerae*, *B. henselae*, *B. clarridgeiae*, *Rickettsia felis*, and *Wolbachia pipientis* in cat fleas, France. *Emerg. Infect. Dis.* **9:**338–342.
84. **Rolain, J. M., F. Gouriet, M. Enea, M. Aboud, and D. Raoult.** 2003. Detection by immunofluorescence assay of *Bartonella henselae* in lymph nodes from patients with cat scratch disease. *Clin. Diagn. Lab. Immunol.* **10:**686–691.
85. **Rolain, J. M., C. Lecam, and D. Raoult.** 2003. Simplified serological diagnosis of endocarditis due to *Coxiella burnetii* and *Bartonella*. *Clin. Diagn. Lab. Immunol.* **10:**1147–1148.
86. **Rolain, J.-M., M. Maurin, A. Bryskier, and D. Raoult.** 2000. In vitro activities of telithromycin (HMR 3647) against *Rickettsia rickettsii*, *Rickettsia conorii*, *Rickettsia africae*, *Rickettsia typhi*, *Rickettsia prowazekii*, *Coxiella burnetii*, *Bartonella henselae*, *Bartonella quintana*, *Bartonella bacilliformis*, and *Ehrlichia chaffeensis*. *Antimicrob. Agents Chemother.* **44:**1391–1393.
87. **Rolain, J. M., M. Maurin, M. N. Mallet, D. Parzy, and D. Raoult.** 2003. Culture and antibiotic susceptibility of *Bartonella quintana* in human erythrocytes. *Antimicrob. Agents Chemother.* **47:**614–619.
88. **Rolain, J. M., M. Maurin, and D. Raoult.** 2000. Bactericidal effect of antibiotics on *Bartonella* and *Brucella* spp.: clinical implications. *J. Antimicrob. Chemother.* **46:**811–814.

89. **Roux, V., and D. Raoult.** 1995. The 16S-23S rRNA intergenic spacer region of *Bartonella (Rochalimaea)* species is longer than usually described in other bacteria. *Gene* **156:**107–111.
90. **Roux, V., and D. Raoult.** 1995. Inter- and intraspecies identification of *Bartonella (Rochalimaea)* species. *J. Clin. Microbiol.* **33:**1573–1579.
91. **Sander, A., R. Berner, and M. Ruess.** 2001. Serodiagnosis of cat scratch disease: response to *Bartonella henselae* in children and a review of diagnostic methods. *Eur. J. Clin. Microbiol. Infect. Dis.* **20:**392–401.
92. **Sanogo, Y. O., Z. Zeaiter, G. Caruso, F. Merola, S. Shpynov, P. Brouqui, and D. Raoult.** 2003. *Bartonella henselae* in *Ixodes ricinus* ticks (Acari: Ixodida) removed from humans, Belluno province, Italy. *Emerg. Infect. Dis.* **9:**329–332.
93. **Schulein, R., A. Seubert, C. Gille, C. Lanz, Y. Hansmann, Y. Piemont, and C. Dehio.** 2001. Invasion and persistent intracellular colonization of erythrocytes. A unique parasitic strategy of the emerging pathogen *Bartonella*. *J. Exp. Med.* **193:**1077–1086.
94. **Schwartzman, W. A., M. Patnaik, F. J. Angulo, B. R. Visscher, E. N. Miller, and J. B. Peter.** 1995. *Bartonella (Rochalimaea)* antibodies, dementia, and cat ownership among men infected with human immunodeficiency virus. *Clin. Infect. Dis.* **21:**954–959.
95. **Sobraquès, M., M. Maurin, R. Birtles, and D. Raoult.** 1999. In vitro susceptibilities of four *Bartonella bacilliformis* strains to 30 antibiotic compounds. *Antimicrob. Agents Chemother.* **43:**2090–2092.
96. **Spach, D. H., and J. E. Koehler.** 1998. *Bartonella*-associated infections. *Infect. Dis. Clin. N. Am.* **12:**137–155.
97. **Spach, D. H., L. A. Panther, D. R. Thorning, J. E. Dunn, J. J. Plorde, and R. A. Miller.** 1992. Intracerebral bacillary angiomatosis in a patient infected with human immunodeficiency virus. *Ann. Intern. Med.* **116:**740–742.
98. **Welch, D. F., K. C. Carroll, E. K. Hofmeister, D. H. Persing, D. A. Robison, A. G. Steigerwalt, and D. J. Brenner.** 1999. Isolation of a new subspecies, *Bartonella vinsonii* subsp. *arupensis*, from a cattle rancher: identity with isolates found in conjunction with *Borrelia burgdorferi* and *Babesia microti* among naturally infected mice. *J. Clin. Microbiol.* **37:**2598–2601.
99. **Welch, D. F., and L. N. Slater.** 2003. *Bartonella* and *Afipia*, p. 824–834. *In* P. R. Murray, E. J. Baron, J. H. Jorgensen, M. A. Pfaller, and R. H. Yolken (ed.), *Manual of Clinical Microbiology*, 8th ed. ASM Press, Washington, D.C.
100. **Wolfson, C., J. Branley, and T. Gottlieb.** 1996. The Etest for antimicrobial susceptibility testing of *Bartonella henselae*. *J. Antimicrob. Chemother.* 38:963–968.
101. **Wong, M. T., D. C. Thornton, R. C. Kennedy, and M. J. Dolan.** 1995. A chemically defined liquid medium that supports primary isolation of *Rochalimaea (Bartonella) henselae* from blood and tissue specimens. *J. Clin. Microbiol.* **33:**742–744.
102. **Zangwill, K. M., D. H. Hamilton, B. A. Perkins, R. L. Regnery, B. D. Plikaytis, J. L. Hadler, M. L. Cartter, and J. D. Wenger.** 1993. Cat scratch disease in Connecticut. Epidemiology, risk factors, and evaluation of a new diagnostic test. *N. Engl. J. Med.* **329:**8–13.
103. **Zbinden, R., N. Michael, M. Sekulovski, A. von Graevenitz, and D. Nadal.** 1997. Evaluation of commercial slides for detection of immunoglobulin G against *Bartonella henselae* by indirect immunofluorescence. *Eur. J. Clin. Microbiol. Infect. Dis.* **16:**648–652.
104. **Zeaiter, Z., P. E. Fournier, and D. Raoult.** 2002. Genomic variation of *Bartonella henselae* strains detected in lymph nodes of patients with cat scratch disease. *J. Clin. Microbiol.* **40:**1023–1030.
105. **Zeaiter, Z., Z. Liang, and D. Raoult.** 2002. Genetic classification and differentiation of *Bartonella* species based on comparison of partial *ftsZ* gene sequences. *J. Clin. Microbiol.* **40:**3641–3647.

Peptostreptococcus, Finegoldia, Anaerococcus, Peptoniphilus, Veillonella, and Other Anaerobic Cocci*

YULI SONG AND SYDNEY M. FINEGOLD

55

TAXONOMY

Gram-positive anaerobic cocci are better known to most bacteriologists as peptococci or peptostreptococci. *Peptococcus* is only remotely related to other species of gram-positive anaerobic cocci and is rarely cultured from human clinical specimens; its main interest lies in its taxonomic significance. *Peptococcus niger* is now the sole remaining representative of this genus. Until recently, most clinical isolates of gram-positive anaerobic cocci were identified to the species level in the genus *Peptostreptococcus*, but this genus is currently under revision. *Peptostreptococcus* was described as a genus in 1936 and was considered the anaerobic equivalent of *Streptococcus*. The genus comprised 16 recognized species, with a G+C range from 27 to 37 mol%, except for *Peptostreptococcus productus* (44 to 45 mol%). Two proposals would restrict the genus *Peptostreptococcus* to *P. anaerobius* (46) and place *Peptostreptococcus magnus* and *Peptostreptococcus micros* in two new genera, *Finegoldia* and *Micromonas*, respectively (45). However, the name *Micromonas* is illegitimate because of the precedence of the microalga *Micromonas*. The name *Peptostreptococcus micros* must continue to be used because it is the single legitimate, validly published name. More recently, Ezaki et al. (19) proposed three new genera: *Anaerococcus*, which includes the saccharolytic, butyrate-producing species (*A. hydrogenalis, A. lactolyticus, A. octavius, A. prevotii, A. tetradius,* and *A. vaginalis*); *Peptoniphilus*, which contains the nonsaccharolytic, butyrate-producing species (*P. asaccharolyticus, P. harei, P. lacrimalis, P. indolicus,* and *P. ivorii*); and *Gallicola* (which contains a single species, *G. barnesae*). Table 1 shows the changes in classification of gram-positive anaerobic coccal species from human clinical specimens.

The taxonomy of the other validly published gram-positive anaerobic cocci from human clinical specimens such as *Streptococcus parvulus, P. productus,* and *Peptostreptococcus saccharolyticus* is also under revision. *S. parvulus* has been transferred to the genus *Atopobium* as *Atopobium parvulum* (13) (see chapter 56). *P. productus* was reclassified in the genus *Ruminococcus* (20); however, it has been recommended that *P. productus* be retained in its present taxonomic position until there is a definitive revision of the classification of ruminococci. *Peptococcus saccharolyticus* has been transferred to the genus *Staphylococcus* based on the analysis of nucleic acid relatedness data and cell wall peptidoglycan structure.

The gram-negative anaerobic cocci have been classified in a single family, the *Veillonellaceae*. *Veillonella, Acidaminococcus,* and *Megasphaera* are genera in this family, and *Anaeroglobus geminatus* gen. nov., sp. nov., was recently described (11). The genus *Veillonella* is currently subdivided into eight species (31). Among them, four have been isolated from human clinical specimens frequently. They include *V. parvula, V. atypica, V. dispar,* and the new species *V. montpellierensis*. The other four species, *V. caviae, V. criceti, V. ratti,* and *V. rodentium*, were found only in animals, except for one *V. ratti* isolate which was recovered from human semen. Phylogenetic analysis showed that the family *Veillonellaceae* did not represent a true clade and could not be considered a relevant taxon. This family has been suppressed from the classification proposed in the latest edition of *Bergey's Manual of Systematic Bacteriology* (24). This classification grouped all genera belonging to the *Sporomusa* subbranch in a single large family named "*Acidaminococcaceae*." The phylogenetic analysis of the *Sporomusa* subbranch is in accordance with the proposed new classification mentioned above.

DESCRIPTION OF THE GROUP

The organisms included in this chapter are obligately anaerobic non-spore-forming, sometimes elongated cocci. The genera *Peptostreptococcus, Anaerococcus, Gallicola, Finegoldia, Peptoniphilus,* and *Peptococcus* are gram-positive, coccobacillary or occasionally coccoid cells. In Gram-stained preparations of pure cultures, cells vary in size from 0.3 to 2.0 μm and can be arranged in pairs, short chains, tetrads, small clusters, or irregular masses; most species are present as either chains or clumps. The ability to utilize carbohydrates varies greatly; some genera are asaccharolytic, but a few are strongly saccharolytic. For most species, the products of protein digestion appear to be the principal energy source. The genus *Staphylococcus* contains two species, *S. saccharolyticus* and *Staphylococcus aureus* subsp. *anaerobius*, that initially grow under anaerobic conditions and become aerotolerant on subcultures (see chapter 28). Strictly anaerobic *Staphylococcus epidermidis* was reported to be occasionally isolated from clinical specimens (53). The genera *Veillonella, Acidaminococcus, Megasphaera,* and *Anaeroglobus*

*This chapter contains information presented in chapter 55 by Bernard J. Moncla and Sharon L. Hillier and chapter 56 by Hannele R. Jousimies-Somer, Paula H. Summanen, Hannah Wexler, Sydney M. Finegold, Saheer E. Gharbia, and Haroun N. Shah in the eighth edition of this Manual.

TABLE 1 Changes in classification of gram-positive anaerobic coccal species from human clinical specimens

Current classification	Previous classification
Peptococcus niger	*Peptococcus niger*
Peptostreptococcus anaerobius	*Peptostreptococcus anaerobius*
Peptostreptococcus micros[a]	*Peptostreptococcus micros*
Peptoniphilus asaccharolyticus	*Peptostreptococcus asaccharolyticus*
Peptoniphilus indolicus	*Peptostreptococcus indolicus*
Peptoniphilus harei	*Peptostreptococcus harei*
Peptoniphilus ivorii	*Peptostreptococcus ivorii*
Peptoniphilus lacrimalis	*Peptostreptococcus lacrimalis*
Anaerococcus prevotii	*Peptostreptococcus prevotii*
Anaerococcus tetradius	*Peptostreptococcus tetradius*
Anaerococcus octavius	*Peptostreptococcus octavius*
Anaerococcus hydrogenalis	*Peptostreptococcus hydrogenalis*
Anaerococcus lactolyticus	*Peptostreptococcus lactolyticus*
Anaerococcus vaginalis	*Peptostreptococcus vaginalis*
Finegoldia magna	*Peptostreptococcus magnus*
Gallicola barnesae	*Peptostreptococcus barnesae*
Slackia heliotrinireducens corrig[b]	*Peptostreptococcus heliotrinreducens*
Atopobium parvulum	*Streptococcus parvulus*
Ruminococcus productus[c]	*Peptostreptococcus productus*
Staphylococcus saccharolyticus	*Peptococcus saccharolyticus*

[a] The name *Micromonas micros* was proposed by Murdoch and Shah (45), but it is illegitimate because it is placed in an illegitimate genus. So, the name *Peptostreptococcus micros* must be used because it is the single legitimate, validly published name.

[b] The specific epithet *heliotrinreducens* [*sic*] has been corrected in the new combination *Slackia heliotrinireducens*. However, the name "*Peptostreptococcus heliotrinireducens*" corrig. was never formally proposed before 14 December 2000. Consequently, in the "List of Prokaryotic Names with Standing in Nomenclature" (http://www.bacterio.cict.fr/index.html), the epithet *heliotrinreducens* [*sic*] has been maintained for *Peptostreptococcus heliotrinreducens*.

[c] *Ruminococcus productus* was proposed recently; however, Willems and Collins have recommended that *P. productus* be retained in its present taxonomic position (67).

are gram-negative cocci. Cells vary in size from 0.3 to 2.5 μm. They characteristically occur in pairs, but single cells, masses, or chains may also occur.

EPIDEMIOLOGY AND TRANSMISSION

Gram-positive anaerobic cocci are part of the normal microbiota of the mouth, upper respiratory and gastrointestinal tracts, female genitourinary system, and skin (42). Gram-positive anaerobic cocci constitute 1 to 15% of the normal oral microbiota (60); *P. micros* is usually considered to be the predominant species of gram-positive anaerobic cocci in the oral microbiota, and *P. anaerobius* and *Finegoldia magna* are also present in the oral cavity. The gastrointestinal tract hosts a wide variety of gram-positive anaerobic cocci, including most recognized species of *Peptostreptococcus*. *P. productus* is one of the most common organisms in the gastrointestinal microbiota; *F. magna* and *A. prevotii* are also common. Several other gram-positive anaerobic cocci are found less often. Large numbers of gram-positive anaerobic cocci can be found in the female genitourinary tract (15). *A. tetradius, A. lactolyticus,* and *A. vaginalis* were first described from vaginal discharges (21, 35); *P. anaerobius, P. asaccharolyticus, P. hydrogenalis, F. magna, P. micros, A. prevotii,* and *Peptococcus niger* have also been isolated from that site (35). The skin microbiota contains gram-positive anaerobic cocci; *F. magna* is the species identified most frequently, followed by *P. asaccharolyticus*.

Gram-negative anaerobic cocci form part of the oral, genitourinary, respiratory, and intestinal flora of humans (30). *Veillonella* species are part of the normal mouth, upper respiratory tract, gastrointestinal tract, and vaginal flora; *Acidaminococcus* and *Megasphaera* are part of the intestinal flora.

CLINICAL SIGNIFICANCE

Estimation of the clinical significance of anaerobic cocci isolated from clinical specimens is often difficult, partly due to their recovery from poorly obtained specimens. Anaerobic gram-positive cocci are opportunistic pathogens, comprising approximately one-quarter of all isolates from anaerobic infections (42). They may be present in a great variety of infections involving all areas of the human body, ranging in severity from mild skin abscesses to more serious and life-threatening infections such as brain abscess, bacteremia, necrotizing pneumonia, and septic abortion. Brain abscess is one of the more serious infections involving anaerobic cocci (10, 33, 36). Anaerobic cocci are involved in as many as 40% of pleuropulmonary infections such as lung abscess, necrotizing pneumonia, aspiration pneumonia, and empyema (37, 64). Anaerobic cocci often are isolated with other organisms in skin and soft tissue infections, including progressive bacterial synergistic gangrene, necrotizing fasciitis, and crepitant cellulitis (4, 44, 58). Other infections in which anaerobic cocci have been recognized as significant pathogens are infections of the female genital tract and intra-abdominal infections (8, 18, 56).

Although most infections involving gram-positive anaerobic cocci are polymicrobial (22), there are many instances of their isolation in pure culture (42); most relate to *F. magna*, but there are also reports of *P. anaerobius*, *P. asaccharolyticus*, *P. indolicus*, *P. micros*, *A. vaginalis*, and *P. harei* in pure culture. *F. magna* is the most pathogenic and one of the most frequently isolated gram-positive anaerobic coccal species found in human clinical specimens. It has been isolated from a wide variety of infections at various body sites in pure culture. These include cases of endocarditis (63), meningitis (10), and pneumonia (47), some of which have been fatal. *F. magna* is most commonly associated with infection of skin and soft tissue and with bone and joint infections, but it has also been isolated from cases of septic arthritis (23), prosthetic implant infections (14), breast abscess (17), diabetic foot infection (29), and upper respiratory tract infection such as sinusitis and otitis media. *P. anaerobius* is involved in polymicrobial infections, including abscesses of the brain, ear, jaw, and pleural cavity; pelvic and urogenital regions; the external genitalia; the abdominal region; and the nasal septum (7, 9, 28). The isolation of *P. anaerobius* from a patient with endocarditis has been reported (39). *P. anaerobius* has been associated with gingivitis (40) and periodontitis (65) and is one of the species found most frequently in the root canals of teeth with periapical abscess (59) and has been isolated from a peritonsillar abscess (12). *P. micros* is increasingly recognized as an important oral pathogen. Although it is considered a natural commensal of the oral cavity, elevated counts of this organism are associated with periodontal destruction (16, 50). It is also commonly isolated from other oral infections such as endodontic lesions and peritonsillar infections (38). *P. micros* is not restricted to the oral cavity; it is often isolated in mixed anaerobic infections from different body sites, including brain abscess, otitis media, sinus infection, human bite wounds, pleural empyema, intra-abdominal infection, anorectal abscess, septicemia, gynecologic infection, vertebral osteomyelitis, and prosthetic joint infection.

Anaerobic gram-negative cocci account for a small percentage of the anaerobic cocci isolated from human specimens (3). *Veillonella* sp. strains are frequently isolated from clinical specimens in aerobic-anaerobic polymicrobial cultures. Rarely, *Veillonella* species have been the only etiologic agents identified in serious infections such as meningitis, osteomyelitis, prosthetic joint infection, pleuropulmonary infection, bacteremia, and endocarditis.

The variety of infections in which anaerobic cocci are involved has been thoroughly reviewed and summarized (42). Although the spectrum of infections has remained relatively unchanged since the extensive review by Murdoch in 1998 (42), the prevalence of these organisms as pathogens is clearly increasing.

COLLECTION, TRANSPORT, AND STORAGE OF CLINICAL SPECIMENS

Most gram-positive anaerobic cocci isolated from human clinical material are not extremely oxygen sensitive. Specimens suspected of harboring anaerobic cocci should be collected, transported, and stored by methods outlined elsewhere (see chapters 5 and 20).

ISOLATION PROCEDURES

Routinely used anaerobic plate media, such as brucella, Columbia, or Schaedler agar base supplemented with 5% sheep blood, vitamin K_1, and hemin, will support the growth of these microorganisms. However, the CDC (Centers for Disease Control and Prevention) agar base gives better recovery of gram-positive anaerobic cocci than brucella agar or other medium formulations. The usual procedures for anaerobes should be followed. Many of these organisms require high moisture content for optimal growth, so fresh medium should be used. Laboratories unable to prepare their own media may wish to consider the use of commercially prepared, prereduced, anaerobically sterilized blood agar (Anaerobe Systems, Morgan Hill, Calif.). These media have an extended shelf life, of up to 6 months, and yield results comparable to or better than those obtained with fresh media.

Gram-positive anaerobic cocci are heterogeneous; a single medium is unlikely to support the growth of all representatives and be reasonably selective. Wren (68) showed that nalidixic acid-Tween blood agar gave better isolation than neomycin blood agar, but recommended that a combination of different media be used to maximize recovery rates. The disadvantage of neomycin blood agar may be the particular inhibitory nature of neomycin to gram-positive anaerobic cocci. Petts et al. (49) reported that oxolinic acid was superior to nalidixic acid for suppression of staphylococci but permitted the growth of non-spore-forming anaerobes, including gram-positive anaerobic cocci. Turng et al. (61) described *P. micros* medium, a selective and differential medium for *P. micros* which contains colistin-nalidixic acid agar (Difco, BD Diagnostics, Sparks, Md.), a selective base for gram-positive cocci that is supplemented with glutathione and lead acetate. Strains of *P. micros* can use the reduced form of glutathione to form hydrogen sulfide, which reacts with lead acetate to form a black precipitate under the colony. Tween 80 supplementation of media may improve growth of some gram-positive anaerobic cocci.

TABLE 2 Differential characteristics of *Peptostreptococcus*, *Peptococcus*, *Peptoniphilus*, *Finegoldia*, and *Anaerococcus*[a]

Species	GLC	Inhibition by SPS	Production of:				Glucose	Production of saccharolytic and proteolytic enzymes									Gram stain and colonial morphology
			Indole	Urease	ALP	ADH		α-Gal	β-Gal	α-Glu	β-Gur	ArgA	ProA	PheA	LeuA	PyrA	
P. asaccharolyticus	A, b	–	d	–	–	–	–	–	–	–	–	+	–	–	d	–	Cells are uniform, in clumps, retaining Gram stain poorly, resembling strains of *Neisseria*. Glistening, low convex, usually whitish to lemon-yellow, musty-odor colonies.
P. indolicus	A, b	–	+	–	+	–	–	–	–	–	–	+	–	+	+	–	Similar to *P. asaccharolyticus*
P. harei	A, b	–	d	–	–	–	–	–	–	–	–	+	–	–	–/w	–	Cells variable in size and shape. Flat, translucent colonies.
P. lacrimalis	A, b	–	–	–	–	–	–	–	–	–	–	+	–	+	+	–	Cells are in short chains or clumps. Pink-white colonies.
"*trisimilis*" group[b]	A, b	–	+	–	d	–	+	–	d	–	–	–	–	–	–	+	Cells are in clumps and tetrads. Gray with white centers, entire and circular colonies.
A. hydrogenalis	B, a	–	+	d	–/w	–	+	–	–	d	–	–	–	–	–	–	Cells variable in size, arranged in clumps, tetrads, and short chains. Gray-white convex colonies, unpleasant odor.

A. prevotii	B, a	−	−	+	−	−	−	+	−	+	+	+	−	d	−	+	Cells variable in size, in clumps or tetrads. Matte gray, low convex colonies.
A. tetradius	B, a	−	−	+	−	−	+	−	−	+	+	+	−	w	+	−/w	Cells variable in size, in clumps and tetrads. Matte gray, low convex colonies.
A. lactolyticus	B, a	−	−	+	+	−	+	−	+	−	−	+	−	−	−	+	Cells are in short chains or clumps. Pink-white colonies.
A. vaginalis	B, a	−	d	−	d	+	+	−	−	−	−	+	−	−	+	−	Cells variable in size, in clumps or tetrads. Gray-white, low convex colonies.
"β-GAL" group[b]	B, a	−	−	−	w	d	+	−	w/+	−/w	−	+	−	−	+	w	Cells variable in size, arranged in clumps. Gray-white, low convex colonies.
A. octavius	B, a, c	−	−	−	−	−	+	−	−	−	−	−	+	−	−	w	Cells are arranged in clumps. Yellowish white, glistening, circular, raised, entire colonies.
P. ivorii	IV	−	−	−	−	−	−	−	−	−	−	−	+	−	−	−	Cells variable in size, arranged in clumps. Yellowish white, low convex colonies.
P. anaerobius	A, IC	+	−	−	−	−	+	−	−	+	−	−	+	−	−	−	Cells are highly pleomorphic, in chains. Colonies are gray with slightly raised off-white centers and a distinctive, sweet odor.
F. magna	A	−	−	−	d	d	−/w	−	−	−	−	+	−	−	+	+	Cells are in pairs, tetrads, or clusters and >0.6 μm in diam. Small colonies, convex and whitish, while others are flatter and translucent.
P. micros	A	−	−	−	+	−	−	−	−	−	−	+	+	+	+	+	Cells in pairs, chains, and clusters. Small colonies; typically white, glistening, and domed and often surrounded by a distinctive yellow-brown halo of discolored agar up to 2 mm wide.
P. productus	A	−	−	−	−	−	+	+	−	+	−	−	−	−	−	−	Cells are ovoid, in pairs or chains; glistening gray colonies.

[a] Data mainly from Murdoch (42) and our unpublished data. Abbreviations and symbols: A, acetate; B, butyrate; IV, isovalerate; IC, isocaproate; C, *n*-caproate; ALP, alkaline phosphatase; ADH, arginine dihydrolase; α-Gal, α-galactosidase; β-Gal, β-galactosidase; α-Glu, α-glucosidase; β-Gur, β-glucuronidase; ArgA, arginine arylamidase; ProA, proline arylamidase; PheA, phenylalanine arylamidase; LeuA, leucine arylamidase; PyrA, pyroglutamyl arylamidase; −, >90% negative; w, weakly positive; +, >90% positive; d, different reactions; w, weakly positive.

[b] Described by Murdoch and Mitchelmore (43).

A recent study (27) tested different media for recovery of *Veillonella* spp. from saliva samples and concluded that a selective medium for *Veillonella* with vancomycin and laked blood gave the greatest recovery of *Veillonella*. This medium can also be used for presumptive identification of *Veillonella* since the colonies produce a red fluorescence.

IDENTIFICATION

Phenotypic Tests

Some gram-positive anaerobic cocci, particularly strains of *P. asaccharolyticus*, decolorize readily by Gram stain and can be confused with gram-negative anaerobes such as *Veillonella*. Gram-positive anaerobic cocci can be distinguished from gram-negative anaerobic cocci by special-potency disks (vancomycin, 5 μg; kanamycin, 1,000 μg; and colistin, 10 μg). The cell morphology of older cultures of gram-positive anaerobic cocci can be very irregular, with many coccobacillary and rod-like forms. It is also important to distinguish gram-positive anaerobic cocci from microaerobic organisms, such as strains of *Streptococcus* species. A simple and reliable test is to apply a 5-μg metronidazole disk to the edge of the inoculum; gram-positive anaerobic cocci show a zone of inhibition of 15 mm or greater, whereas microaerobic strains show no zones of inhibition after incubation for 48 h (43).

P. anaerobius is the only gram-positive anaerobic coccus that gives a zone of inhibition of ≥12 mm around a sodium polyanetholsulfonate (SPS) disk. *P. micros* also exhibits a zone of inhibition with SPS; however, the zone is usually <12 mm. Most *P. anaerobius* strains form distinctive colonies on enriched blood agar; they are 1 mm in diameter after 24 h and gray, with slightly raised off-white centers and a distinctively sweet odor (43). *P. micros* and *F. magna* can be readily distinguished by a combination of colonial morphology and proteolytic enzyme profiles, supported by Gram-stained cell morphology to assess the cell size. An anaerobic coccus with a milky halo around the colonies and small cells (<0.6 μm) can be presumptively identified as *P. micros* (43, 62). *F. magna* cells are larger than those of most peptostreptococci. Published data (42) also indicate that they can be differentiated by enzymatic tests for proteolytic activity such as proline arylamidase, phenylalanine arylamidase, and tyrosine arylamidase.

P. asaccharolyticus is another gram-positive anaerobic coccal species frequently isolated from human clinical specimens, but strains that were identified phenotypically are genetically diverse. To complicate matters further, the type strain of *P. asaccharolyticus* is highly atypical in its whole-cell composition and some biochemical properties. A recent study of ours (unpublished data) indicated that all strains (a total of 33) that were identified as *P. asaccharolyticus* phenotypically shared only a low sequence similarity (<90%) with the corresponding sequence of the type strain of *P. asaccharolyticus*. They all had almost identical 16S rRNA sequences and shared a high sequence similarity (>99%) with another *P. asaccharolyticus* strain, ATCC 29743. The cellular morphology of this group of bacteria is characteristic; the cell size is more uniform than is observed with most species of gram-positive anaerobic cocci, and cells occur in clumps, retaining the Gram stain poorly and often resembling strains of *Neisseria*. The colony morphology is also distinctive; after 5 days of incubation on enriched blood agar, colonies are 2 to 3 mm in diameter, glistening, low convex, and usually whitish to lemon-yellow, and they often have a characteristic musty odor. They produce an enzyme profile very similar to that of *P. harei* strains but can easily be differentiated by their clearly different cell and colonial morphology. Cells of *P. harei* vary considerably in size (diameter, 0.5 to 1.5 μm) and shape (circular, oval, or elliptical). Colonies of 5-day cultures on enriched blood agar are approximately 1 mm in diameter, nonhemolytic, flat, and translucent. *P. indolicus* is phenotypically similar to *P. asaccharolyticus* and can be difficult to identify, but it is rarely isolated from human clinical specimens. *P. indolicus* can be tentatively distinguished from *P. asaccharolyticus* by its ability to produce alkaline phosphatase.

A. prevotii and *A. tetradius* were reported as common species of gram-positive anaerobic cocci in human clinical material in early surveys. However, nucleic acid studies indicate that they are very heterogeneous. Again, our study based on 16S rDNA sequencing indicated that a large percentage of organisms identified as *A. prevotii* or *A. tetradius* are strains of *A. vaginalis*. It is likely that strictly defined strains of *A. prevotii* or *A. tetradius* are only occasionally recovered from most clinical specimens. The activity of pyroglutamic acid arylamidase might be useful for differentiation of *A. prevotii* and *A. tetradius;* however, distinctions cannot be generalized because insufficient numbers of strains of each species have been reliably identified. *A. prevotii* and *A. tetradius* can be distinguished from other recognized species of gram-positive anaerobic cocci by production of α-glucosidase and β-glucuronidase. Strains of other saccharolytic gram-positive anaerobic cocci such as *A. vaginalis* and *A. lactolyticus* can be differentiated by their enzyme profiles.

Table 2 summarizes the differential characteristics of gram-positive anaerobic coccal species. Based on published data and our unpublished data, we developed a flowchart for rapid identification of gram-positive anaerobic cocci (Fig. 1). The identification is based on phenotypic tests that can be performed in many diagnostic laboratories. Most of the information presented here relates to the phenotypic characteristics of strains isolated from humans.

Several systems, such as Rapid ID 32A (bioMérieux, Marcy L'Etoile, France) and RapID ANA II (Remel, Inc., Lenexa, Kans.), are available commercially for the rapid identification of anaerobes. Evaluation of these biochemical kits indicates that they may be valuable for characterizing anaerobic cocci (42). However, these systems are designed to identify a wide range of anaerobes, and they contain many tests of little relevance for identification of anaerobic cocci. Furthermore, databases accompanying the kits are often incomplete or inaccurate, especially for newly described species. Our most recent comparison of the Rapid ID 32A kit with 16S rRNA gene sequencing for identification of gram-positive anaerobic cocci showed that the Rapid ID 32A system is good for accurate identification of *P. micros*, *P. anaerobius*, *F. magna*, and *P. asaccharolyticus*, but not the others.

Gram-positive anaerobic cocci are separated into five groups based on fatty acid end products of metabolism analyzed by gas-liquid chromatography (GLC) (Table 2): (i) an acetate group containing *F. magna*, *P. micros*, and *P. productus* that only produces acetic acid; (ii) a butyrate-acetate group that produces butyric acid as its major terminal volatile fatty acid (VFA) and acetic acid as a second lesser acid (this group contains all of the species in the genus *Anaerococcus*); (iii) an acetate-butyrate group that produces acetic acid as its major terminal VFA and butyric acid as the second acid (this group contains all of the species in the genus *Peptoniphilus* except for *P. ivorii*); (iv) a caproate group whose members produce large quantities of longer-chain VFAs (the most important species in this group is *P. anaerobius*, the only

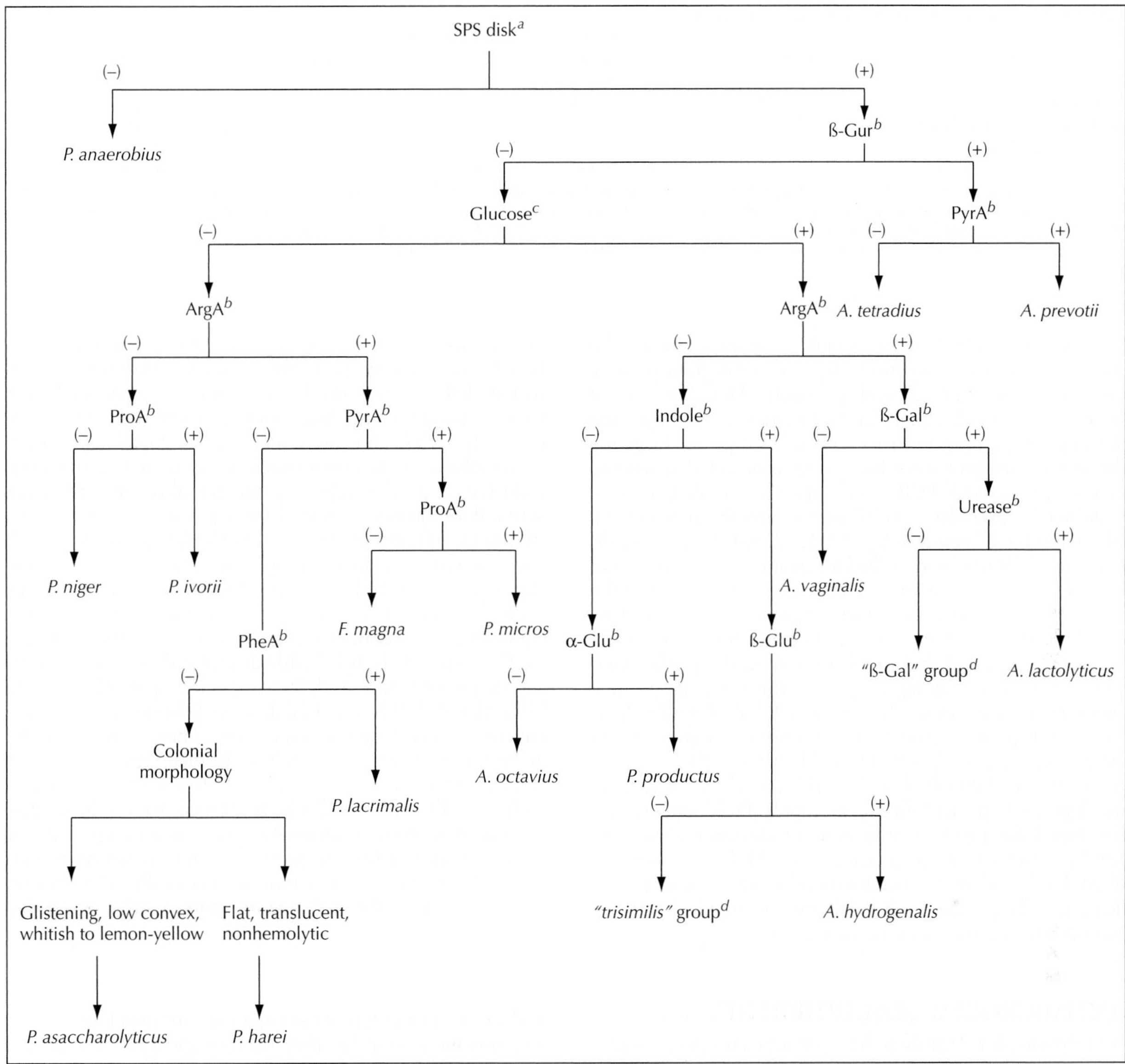

FIGURE 1 Flowchart with key characteristics for identification and differentiation of gram-positive anaerobic cocci. *a*, SPS testing was done using the SPS disk from Anaerobe Systems. All gram-positive anaerobic cocci are resistant to SPS except for *P. anaerobius*, which gives a zone of inhibition of ≥12 mm around an SPS disk. *P. micros* also exhibits a zone of inhibition with SPS; however, the zone is usually <12 mm. +, no zone or the zone of inhibition is <12 mm; −, zone of inhibition is ≥12 mm. *b*, All the enzymatic tests were done using the Rapid ID 32A system (API bioMérieux) according to the manufacturer's instructions. β-Gal, β-galactosidase; α-Glu, α-glucosidase; β-Glu, β-glucosidase; β-Gur, β-glucuronidase; ArgA, arginine arylamidase; ProA, proline arylamidase; PheA, phenylalanine arylamidase; PyrA, pyroglutamyl arylamidase. *c*, Glucose fermentation tests were performed using prereduced, anaerobically sterilized peptone-yeast-glucose (PYG) broth tube (Anaerobe Systems). A pH of ≤5.5 in the PYG tubes was interpreted as a positive result, and a pH of ≥5.9 was interpreted as a negative result. *d*, Described by Murdoch and Mitchelmore (43).

species of gram-positive anaerobic cocci to produce a major terminal peak of isocaproic acid); and (v) an isovaleric acid group that contains *P. ivorii* (this organism is the only species of gram-positive anaerobic cocci that produces a major terminal peak of isovaleric acid). GLC is also useful for identifying the rarely isolated *Peptococcus niger* and *P. octavius*, which produce *n*-caproic acid.

Veillonella, *Acidaminococcus*, and *Megasphaera* comprise the genera of anaerobic gram-negative cocci. Table 3 contains a key for distinguishing these three genera.

Molecular Methods

Molecular methods, such as nucleic acid probe hybridization, PCR amplification, and 16S rRNA gene sequencing,

TABLE 3 Characteristics of gram-negative cocci[a]

Organism(s)	Nitrate reduction	Catalase	Glucose fermentation[b]	Fatty acids from PYG
Veillonella spp.	+	V	−	A, p
Acidaminococcus fermentans	−	−	−	A, B
Megasphaera elsdenii	−	−	+	A, ib, b, iv, v, C

[a] A, acetate; B and b, butyrate; C, *n*-caproate; ib, isobutyrate; iv, isovalerate; v, valeric acid; V, variable; p, propionate; +, positive reaction; −, negative reaction.
[b] Glucose fermentation tests were performed using prereduced, anaerobically sterilized (PRAS) peptone-yeast-glucose (PYG) broth tube (Anaerobe Systems). The PRAS tubes were inoculated from an actively growing broth culture (without carbohydrate). A pH of ≤5.5 in the PRAS tubes was interpreted as a positive result, a pH of 5.6 to 5.8 was interpreted as weakly positive, and a pH of ≥5.9 was interpreted as negative for fermentation.

are not yet standardized or available commercially for the direct demonstration of medically important gram-positive anaerobic cocci from clinical specimens. However, several studies have used molecular techniques to identify and detect gram-positive anaerobic cocci. DNA probes targeting the 16S rRNA gene have been used to detect *P. anaerobius* and *P. micros*, and PCR assays specific for detection of *F. magna*, *P. anaerobius*, and *P. micros* directly from clinical specimens have been developed (51, 52, 55). More recently, real-time PCR has been applied for quantitative detection of *P. micros* in clinical samples (2, 5). Our group evaluated the utility of 16S rRNA gene sequencing as a means of identifying clinically important gram-positive anaerobic cocci (57). Our study indicated that problems exist in the public database. For example, among the 13 type strains of gram-positive anaerobic coccal species that we tested, only 4 gave a "perfect" match with their corresponding sequences in GenBank, whereas the other 9 had lower sequence similarities (<98%) (Table 4). Based on the 16S rRNA sequences we deposited in GenBank, a multiplex PCR scheme was developed for rapid identification of clinically significant gram-positive anaerobic coccal species. Molecular methods undoubtedly will offer a potential option for accurate identification and rapid diagnosis in laboratories supplied with the appropriate equipment and competence.

ANTIMICROBIAL SUSCEPTIBILITIES

New information regarding the antimicrobial susceptibilities of gram-positive anaerobic cocci is sparse compared with the information available for other anaerobic species. Current information is summarized in Table 5. Many reports fail to give results for individual species, opting instead to combine data for the group.

Penicillins are considered to be effective first-line therapy for gram-positive anaerobic cocci. Most evidence suggests that *P. asaccharolyticus*, *F. magna*, and *P. micros* are usually susceptible to penicillins, although Wren (69) reported resistance among isolates of *F. magna* and *P. micros* (16 and 8%, respectively) to penicillin. Cephalosporins are usually, but not always, effective. Carbapenems are extremely active. Several authorities maintain that most gram-positive anaerobic cocci are susceptible to metronidazole, but resistance has frequently been reported. Strains that are microaerobic are much more likely to be resistant to metronidazole. Susceptibilities to clindamycin vary widely, and local geographic variation should be taken into account. A French multicenter study (41) reported clindamycin resistance (28%) among *Peptostreptococcus* spp., and an American study by Sanchez et al. (54) noted >10% resistance of *F. magna* to clindamycin. Wren (69) reported that 9% of *F. magna* isolates were resistant to clindamycin in London, England. Erythromycin, clarithromycin, and azithromycin have similar efficacies and are probably not active enough to be recommended. Several studies (25, 48, 66) indicated that narrow-spectrum quinolones such as ciprofloxacin have only moderate activity, but more recently developed agents such as trovafloxacin and clinafloxacin are extremely active (48). Goldstein et al. (26) reported that gemifloxacin is the most active fluoroquinolone tested for peptostreptococci. In two studies (1, 34), ciprofloxacin and ceftazidime showed much lower activities against gram-positive anaerobic cocci than the other antimicrobial agents tested. In another recent study, Koeth et al. (32) reported that the levofloxacin and clindamycin susceptibility rates of *F. magna* were 72.4 and 84.7%, respectively. It is highly desirable that future investigations present data on different species separately. A study by Brazier et al. (6) presented data on different gram-positive anaerobic coccal species separately. They found that the highest percentage of overall resistance detected among gram-positive anaerobic cocci was 41.6% resistance to tetracycline, followed by 27.4% resistance to erythromycin. Among gram-positive anaerobic cocci as a group, 7.1% of isolates were resistant to penicillin and clindamycin, and 3.5% of isolates were resistant to amoxicillin-clavulanate. There was no resistance among gram-positive anaerobic

TABLE 4 List of type strains and the corresponding accession numbers of 16S rRNA gene sequences in GenBank

Species	Strain	Accession no.
Anaerococcus hydrogenalis	ATCC 49630	D14140
Anaerococcus lactolyticus	ATCC 51172	AF542233
Anaerococcus octavius	CCUG 38493	Y07841
Anaerococcus prevotii	ATCC 9321	AF542232
Anaerococcus tetradius	ATCC 35098	AF542234
Anaerococcus vaginalis	ATCC 51170	AF542229
Finegoldia magna	ATCC 15794	AF542227
Peptoniphilus asaccharolyticus	ATCC 14963	AF542228
Peptoniphilus harei	ATCC BAA-601	Y07839
Peptoniphilus indolicus	ATCC 29427	AY153431
Peptoniphilus ivorii	ATCC BAA-602	Y07840
Peptoniphilus lacrimalis	ATCC 51171	AF542230
Peptostreptococcus anaerobius	ATCC 27337	L04168
Peptostreptococcus micros	ATCC 33270	AF542231
Veillonella atypica	ATCC 17744	AF439641
Veillonella dispar	ATCC 17748	AY995770
Veillonella montpellierensis	ADV 281.99	AF473836
Veillonella parvula	ATCC 10790	AY995767
Acidaminococcus fermentans	ATCC 25085	X65935
Megasphaera elsdenii	ATCC 25940	U95027

TABLE 5 Antimicrobial susceptibilities of gram-positive anaerobic cocci[a]

Species (no. of strains)	Range of MICs (μg/ml)[b]									
	Pen (1)	Amp/Sul[c] (8)	Amox/Clav[c] (8)	Pip/Tazo[c] (64)	Cefox (32)	Imi (8)	Clinda (4)	Metro (16)	Cipro (2)	Trova (4)
A. lactolyticus (2)	≤0.5	≤0.25	0.25		0.5	0.12	≤0.12	1		
A. lactolyticus-I (5)	≤0.5–2[d]	≤0.25–0.5	0.12–0.25	0.5	0.5–2	0.12–0.5	0.25–64[h]	1	0.5–1	
A .*lactolyticus*-II (3)	≤0.5–1	≤0.25			0.5–1	0.12–0.5	≤0.12	4		
A. prevotii (3)	2–16	1–4	2	2	1–4	0.5–1	32–128	1–2	16	
A. tetradius (1)	≤0.5	≤0.25			0.5	≤0.062	0.25	2		
A. vaginalis (16)	≤0.5	0.12–0.25	0.12–0.25	0.062–0.12	≤0.12–0.25	≤0.062–0.12	0.062–0.5	0.25–4	4–8	
F. magna (12)	0.12–1	≤0.25–0.5	0.12–0.25		0.5–2	0.062–0.5	0.062–2	0.25–2	0.12–2	0.062–0.12
P. asaccharolyticus (10)	≤0.5	0.12–0.25	0.12–0.25	0.062	≤0.12	≤0.062	≤0.12	0.5–4		
P. harei (2)	≤0.5–1	≤0.25			0.25	≤0.062	0.5	2		
P. anaerobius (16)	0.12–32[e]	≤0.25–16[g]	0.12–32		0.5–32	≤0.062–2	≤0.062–0.5	0.12–8	1	0.12
P. micros (15)	0.062–64[f]	0.062–0.5	0.062	0.062	0.5–1	0.062–0.12	0.062–1	0.25–1	1–16	0.062

[a] Data were obtained from the Wadsworth Anaerobic Bacteriology Laboratory. Strains were tested by Clinical and Laboratory Standards Institute (NCCLS) agar dilution procedures.

[b] MIC breakpoints are indicated in parentheses next to each antimicrobial agent. Abbreviations: Pen, penicillin; Amp/Sul, ampicillin-sulbactam; Amox/Clav, amoxicillin-clavulanic acid; Pip/Tazo, piperacillin-tazobactam; Cefox, cefoxitin; Imi, imipenem; Clinda, clindamycin; Metro, metronidazole; Cipro, ciprofloxacin; Trova, trovafloxacin.

[c] Results for these three drug combinations given for amoxicillin and piperacillin.

[d] One of 5 strains showed resistance.

[e] Three of 16 strains showed resistance.

[f] Two of 15 strains showed resistance.

[g] Three of 16 strains showed resistance.

[h] One of 5 strains showed resistance.

cocci to piperacillin-tazobactam, chloramphenicol, cefoxitin, imipenem, or metronidazole. Data from our laboratory are presented in Table 5.

EVALUATION, INTERPRETATION, AND REPORTING OF RESULTS

The initial report should provide Gram stain results and bacterial and human cell morphologies. The relative quantities of different organisms seen in the smear give a good overall impression of specimen quality, the nature of the polymicrobial infection, and the relative importance of each organism. In general, bacterial isolates that are predominant, virulent, and resistant to antimicrobial agents should be given the greatest attention. Bacteria present in pure culture or in large numbers are probably of major importance, as are organisms recovered in multiple cultures and isolated from normally sterile sites. Furthermore, Gram stain results can guide the laboratory in choosing media for optimal recovery of the predicted organisms.

The significance of finding anaerobic gram-positive or gram-negative cocci in clinical specimens depends on the specimen and the likelihood that it was contaminated by the microbiota of the skin or mucous membranes. Hence, interpretation of culture results is dependent on the nature and quality of the specimen submitted to the laboratory.

REFERENCES

1. **Aldridge, K. E., D. Ashcraft, K. Cambre, C. L. Pierson, S. G. Jenkins, and J. E. Rosenblatt.** 2001. Multicenter survey of the changing in vitro antimicrobial susceptibilities of clinical isolates of *Bacteroides fragilis* group, *Prevotella, Fusobacterium, Porphyromonas,* and *Peptostreptococcus* species. *Antimicrob. Agents Chemother.* **45:**1238–1243.
2. **Bartz, H., C. Nonnenmacher, C. Bollmann, M. Kuhl, S. Zimmermann, K. Heeg, and R. Mutters.** 2005. *Micromonas (Peptostreptococcus) micros*: unusual case of prosthetic joint infection associated with dental procedures. *Int. J. Med. Microbiol.* **294:**465–470.
3. **Bhatti, M. A., and M. O. Frank.** 2000. *Veillonella* parvula meningitis: case report and review of *Veillonella* infections. *Clin. Infect. Dis.* **31:**839–840.
4. **Bourgault, A.-M., J. E. Rosenblatt, and R. H. Fitzgerald.** 1980. *Peptococcus magnus:* a significant human pathogen. *Ann. Intern. Med.* **93:**244–248.
5. **Boutaga, K., A. J. van Winkelhoff, C. M. Vandenbroucke-Grauls, and P. H. Savelkoul.** 2005. Periodontal pathogens: a quantitative comparison of anaerobic culture and real-time PCR. *FEMS Immunol. Med. Microbiol.* **45:**191–199.
6. **Brazier, J. S., V. Hall, T. E. Morris, M. Gal, and B. I. Duerden.** 2003. Antibiotic susceptibilities of gram-positive anaerobic cocci: results of a sentinel study in England and Wales. *J. Antimicrob. Chemother.* **52:**224–228.
7. **Brook, I.** 1989. Anaerobic bacteria in suppurative genitourinary infections. *J. Urol.* **141:**889–893.
8. **Brook, I.** 2004. Intra-abdominal, retroperitoneal, and visceral abscesses in children. *Eur. J. Pediatr. Surg.* **14:**265–273.
9. **Brook, I., and E. H. Frazier.** 1990. Aerobic and anaerobic bacteriology of wounds and cutaneous abscesses. *Arch. Surg.* **125:**1445–1451.
10. **Brown, M. A., J. N. Greene, R. L. Sandin, and A. L. Vincent.** 1994. Case report: anaerobic meningitis caused by *Peptostreptococcus magnus* after head and neck surgery. *Am. J. Med. Sci.* **308:**184–185.
11. **Carlier, J.-P., H. Marchandin, E. Jumas-Bilak, V. Lorin, C. Henry, C. Carriere, and H. Jean-Pierre.** 2002. *Anaeroglobus*

geminatus gen. nov., sp. nov., a novel member of the family *Veillonellaceae*. *Int. J. Syst. Evol. Microbiol.* **52:**983–986.

12. **Civen, R., M.-L. Väisänen, and S. M. Finegold.** 1993. Peritonsillar abscess, retropharyngeal abscess, mediastinitis, and nonclostridial anaerobic myonecrosis: a case report. *Clin. Infect. Dis.* **16**(Suppl. 4)**:** S299–S303.
13. **Collins, M. D., and S. Wallbanks.** 1992. Comparative sequence analyses of the 16S rRNA genes of *Lactobacillus minutus*, *Lactobacillus rimae* and *Streptococcus parvulus*: proposal for the creation of a new genus *Atopobium*. *FEMS Microbiol. Lett.* **95:**235–240.
14. **Davies, U. M., A. M. Leak, and J. Dave.** 1988. Infection of a prosthetic knee joint with *Peptostreptococcus magnus*. *Ann. Rheum. Dis.* **47:**866–868.
15. **Delaney, M. L., and A. B. Onderdonk.** 2001. Nugent score related to vaginal culture in pregnant women. *Obstet. Gynecol.* **98:**79–84.
16. **Dzink, J. L., A. C. Tanner, A. D. Haffajee, and S. S. Socransky.** 1985. Gram negative species associated with active destructive periodontal lesions. *J. Clin. Periodontol.* **12:**648–659.
17. **Edmiston, C. E., Jr., A. P. Walker, C. J. Krepel, and C. Gohr.** 1990. The nonpuerperal breast infection: aerobic and anaerobic microbial recovery from acute and chronic disease. *J. Infect. Dis.* **162:**695–699.
18. **Egwari, L., V. O. Rotimi, O. O. Abudu, and A. O. Coker.** 1995. A study of the anaerobic bacterial flora of the female genital tract in health and disease. *Cent. Afr. J. Med.* **41:**391–397.
19. **Ezaki, T., Y. Kawamura, N. Li, Z. Y. Li, L. Zhao, and S. Shu.** 2001. Proposal of the genera *Anaerococcus* gen. nov., *Peptoniphilus* gen. nov. and *Gallicola* gen. nov. for members of the genus *Peptostreptococcus*. *Int. J. Syst. Evol. Microbiol.* **51:**1521–1528.
20. **Ezaki, T., N. Li, Y. Hashimoto, H. Miura, and H. Yamamoto.** 1994. 16S ribosomal DNA sequences of anaerobic cocci and proposal of *Ruminococcus hansenii* comb. nov. and *Ruminococcus productus* comb. nov. *Int. J. Syst. Bacteriol.* **44:**130–136.
21. **Ezaki, T., N. Yamamoto, K. Ninomiya, S. Suzuki, and E. Yabuuchi.** 1983. Transfer of *Peptococcus indolicus*, *Peptococcus asaccharolyticus*, *Peptococcus prevotii*, and *Peptococcus magnus* to the genus *Peptostreptococcus* and proposal of *Peptostreptococcus tetradius* sp. nov. *Int. J. Syst. Bacteriol.* **33:**683–698.
22. **Finegold, S. M.** 1995. Anaerobic infections in humans: an overview. *Anaerobe* **1:**3–9.
23. **Fitzgerald, R. H., Jr., J. E. Rosenblatt, J. H. Tenney, and A.-M. Bourgault.** 1982. Anaerobic septic arthritis. *Clin. Orthop. Relat. Res.* **1982**(164)**:**141–148.
24. **Garrity, G. M., and J. G. Holt.** 2001. Taxonomic outlines of the Archaea and Bacteria, p. 155–166. *In* D. R. Boone and R. W. Castenholz (ed.), *Bergey's Manual of Systematic Bacteriology*, 2nd ed. Springer, New York, N.Y.
25. **Goldstein, E. J.** 1993. Patterns of susceptibility to fluoroquinolones among anaerobic bacterial isolates in the United States. *Clin. Infect. Dis.* **16:**S377–S381.
26. **Goldstein, E. J., G. Conrads, D. M. Citron, C. V. Merriam, Y. Warren, and K. Tyrrell.** 2002. *In vitro* activity of gemifloxacin compared to seven other oral antimicrobial agents against aerobic and anaerobic pathogens isolated from antral sinus puncture specimens from patients with sinusitis. *Diagn. Microbiol. Infect. Dis.* **42:**113–118.
27. **Gutierrez de Ferro, M. I., R. E. Ruiz de Valladares, and I. L. Benito de Cardenas.** 2005. Recovery of *Veillonella* from saliva. *Rev. Argent. Microbiol.* **37:**22–25.
28. **Holdeman Moore, L. V., J. L. Johnson, and W. E. C. Moore.** 1986. Genus *Peptostreptococcus*, p. 1083–1092. *In* P. H. A. Sneath, N. S. Mair, M. E. Sharpe, and J. G. Holt (ed.), *Bergey's Manual of Systematic Bacteriology*, vol. 2. The Williams & Wilkins Co., Baltimore, Md.
29. **Johnson, S., F. Lebahn, L. R. Peterson, and D. N. Gerding.** 1995. Use of an anaerobic collection and transport swab device to recover anaerobic bacteria from infected foot ulcers in diabetics. *Clin. Infect. Dis.* **20:**S289–S290.
30. **Jousimies-Somer, H. R., P. Summanen, D. Citron, E. Baron, H. M. Wexler, and S. M. Finegold.** 2002. *Wadsworth-KTL Anaerobic Bacteriology Manual.* Star Publishing, Belmont, Calif.
31. **Jumas-Bilak, E., J. P. Carlier, H. Jean-Pierre, C. Teyssier, B. Gay, J. Campos, and H. Marchandin.** 2004. *Veillonella montpellierensis* sp. nov., a novel, anaerobic, gram-negative coccus isolated from human clinical samples. *Int. J. Syst. Evol. Microbiol.* **54:**1311–1316.
32. **Koeth, L. M., C. E. Good, P. C. Appelbaum, E. J. Goldstein, A. C. Rodloff, M. Claros, and L. J. Dubreuil.** 2004. Surveillance of susceptibility patterns in 1297 European and US anaerobic and capnophilic isolates to co-amoxiclav and five other antimicrobial agents. *J. Antimicrob. Chemother.* **53:**1039–1044.
33. **Korman, T. M., E. Athan, and D. W. Spelman.** 1997. Anaerobic meningitis due to *Peptostreptococcus* species: case report and review. *Clin. Infect. Dis.* **25:**1462–1464.
34. **Kuriyama, T., T. Karasawa, K. Nakagawa, S. Nakamura, and E. Yamamoto.** 2002. Antimicrobial susceptibility of major pathogens of orofacial odontogenic infections to 11 beta-lactam antibiotics. *Oral Microbiol. Immunol.* **17:**285–289.
35. **Li, N., Y. Hashimoto, S. Adnan, H. Miura, H. Yamamoto, and T. Ezaki.** 1992. Three new species of the genus *Peptostreptococcus* isolated from humans: *Peptostreptococcus vaginalis* sp. nov., *Peptostreptococcus lacrimalis* sp. nov., and *Peptostreptococcus lactolyticus* sp. nov. *Int. J. Syst. Bacteriol.* **42:**602–605.
36. **Maniglia, R. J., T. Roth, and E. A. Blumberg.** 1997. Polymicrobial brain abscess in a patient infected with human immunodeficiency virus. *Clin. Infect. Dis.* **24:**449–451.
37. **Marina, M., C. A. Strong, R. Civen, E. Molitoris, and S. M. Finegold.** 1993. Bacteriology of anaerobic pleuropulmonary infections: preliminary report. *Clin. Infect. Dis.* **16:**S256–S262.
38. **Mitchelmore, I. J., A. J. Prior, P. Q. Montgomery, and S. Tabaqchali.** 1995. Microbiological features and pathogenesis of peritonsillar abscesses. *Eur. J. Clin. Microbiol. Infect. Dis.* **14:**870–877.
39. **Montejo, M., G. Ruiz-Irastorza, K. Aguirrebengoa, E. Amutio, J. L. Hernández, and C. Aguirre.** 1995. Prosthetic-valve endocarditis caused by *Peptostreptococcus anaerobius*. *Clin. Infect. Dis.* **20:**1431.
40. **Moore, L. V. H., W. E. C. Moore, and E. P. Cato.** 1987. Bacteriology of human gingivitis. *J. Dent. Res.* **66:**989–995.
41. **Mory, F., A. Lozniewski, S. Bland, A. Sedallian, G. Grollier, F. Girard-Pipau, M. F. Paris, and L. Dubreuil.** 1998. Survey of anaerobic susceptibility patterns: a French multicentre study. *Int. J. Antimicrob. Agents* **10:**229–236.
42. **Murdoch, D. A.** 1998. Gram-positive anaerobic cocci. *Clin. Microbiol. Rev.* **11:**81–120.
43. **Murdoch, D. A., and J. Mitchelmore.** 1991. The laboratory identification of gram-positive anaerobic cocci. *J. Med. Microbiol.* **34:**295–308.
44. **Murdoch, D. A., I. J. Mitchelmore, and S. Tabaqchali.** 1994. The clinical importance of gram-positive anaerobic cocci isolated at St. Bartholomew's Hospital, London, in 1987. *J. Med. Microbiol.* **41:**36–44.
45. **Murdoch, D. A., and H. N. Shah.** 1999. Reclassification of *Peptostreptococcus magnus* (Prevot 1933) Holdeman and Moore 1972 as *Finegoldia magna* comb. nov. and *Peptostreptococcus micros* (Prevot 1933) Smith 1957 as *Micromonas micros* comb. nov. *Anaerobe* **5:**555–559.

46. **Murdoch, D. A., H. N. Shah, S. E. Gharbia, and D. Rajendram.** 2000. Proposal to restrict the genus *Peptostreptococcus* (Kluyver & van Niel 1936) to *Peptostreptococcus anaerobius*. *Anaerobe* **6:**257–260.
47. **Panagou, P., L. Papandreou, and D. Bouros.** 1991. Severe anaerobic necrotizing pneumonia complicated by pyopneumothorax and anaerobic monoarthritis due to *Peptostreptococcus magnus*. *Respiration* **58:**223–225.
48. **Pankuch, G. A., M. R. Jacobs, and P. C. Appelbaum.** 1993. Susceptibilities of 428 gram-positive and -negative anaerobic bacteria to Bay y3118 compared with their susceptibilities to ciproflaxacin, clindamycin, metronidazole, piperacillin, piperacillin-tazobactam, and cefoxitin. *Antimicrob. Agents Chemother.* **37:**1649–1654.
49. **Petts, D. N., W. Champion, and G. Raymond.** 1988. Oxolinic acid as a selective agent for the isolation of nonsporing anaerobes from clinical material. *Lett. Appl. Microbiol.* **6:**65–67.
50. **Rams, T. E., D. Feik, M. A. Listgarten, and J. Slots.** 1992. *Peptostreptococcus micros* in human periodontitis. *Oral Microbiol. Immunol.* **7:**1–6.
51. **Riggio, M. P., and A. Lennon.** 2003. Specific PCR detection of *Peptostreptococcus magnus*. *J. Med. Microbiol.* **52:**309–313.
52. **Riggio, M. P., A. Lennon, and A. Smith.** 2001. Detection of *Peptostreptococcus micros* DNA in clinical samples by PCR. *J. Med. Microbiol.* **50:**249–254.
53. **Rowlinson, M. C., P. LeBourgeois, K. Ward, Y. L. Song, S. M. Finegold, and D. A. Bruckner.** 2006. Isolation of a strictly anaerobic strain of *Staphylococcus epidermidis*. *J. Clin. Microbiol.* **44:**857–860.
54. **Sanchez, M. L., R. N. Jones, and J. L. Croco.** 1992. Use of the Etest to access macrolide-lincosamide resistance patterns among *Peptostreptococcus* species. *Antimicrob. Newsl.* **8:**45–49.
55. **Siqueira, J. F., Jr., I. N. Rocas, A. F. Andrade, and M. de Uzeda.** 2003. *Peptostreptococcus micros* in primary endodontic infections as detected by 16S rDNA-based polymerase chain reaction. *J. Endod.* **29:**111–113.
56. **Smayevsky, J., L. F. Canigia, A. Lanza, and H. Bianchini.** 2001. Vaginal microflora associated with bacterial vaginosis in nonpregnant women: reliability of sialidase detection. *Infect. Dis. Obstet. Gynecol.* **9:**17–22.
57. **Song, Y., C. Liu, M. McTeague, and S. M. Finegold.** 2003. 16S ribosomal DNA sequence-based analysis of clinically significant gram-positive anaerobic cocci. *J. Clin. Microbiol.* **41:**1363–1369.
58. **Summanen, P. H., D. A. Talan, C. Strong, M. McTeague, R. Bennion, J. E. Thompson, Jr., M.-L. Väisänen, G. Moran, M. Winer, and S. M. Finegold.** 1995. Bacteriology of skin and soft-tissue infections: comparison of infections in intravenous drug users and individuals with no history of intravenous drug use. *Clin. Infect. Dis.* **20**(Suppl. 2)**:** S279–S282.
59. **Sundqvist, G.** 1992. Associations between microbial species in dental root canal infections. *Oral Microbiol. Immunol.* **7:**257–262.
60. **Sutter, V. L.** 1984. Anaerobes as normal oral flora. *Rev. Infect. Dis.* **6:**S62–S66.
61. **Turng, B.-F., J. M. Guthmiller, G. E. Minah, and W. A. Falkler, Jr.** 1996. Development and evaluation of a selective and differential medium for the primary isolation of *Peptostreptococcus micros*. *Oral Microbiol. Immunol.* **11:**356–361.
62. **van Dalen, P. J., T. J. van Steenbergen, M. M. Cowan, H. J. Busscher, and J. de Graaff.** 1993. Description of two morphotypes of *Peptostreptococcus micros*. *Int. J. Syst. Bacteriol.* **43:**787–793.
63. **van der Vorm, E. R., A. M. Dondorp, R. J. van Ketel, and J. Dankert.** 2000. Apparent culture-negative prosthetic valve endocarditis caused by *Peptostreptococcus magnus*. *J. Clin. Microbiol.* **38:**4640–4642.
64. **Verma, P.** 2000. Laboratory diagnosis of anaerobic pleuropulmonary infections. *Semin. Respir. Infect.* **15:** 114–118.
65. **Wade, W. G., J. Moran, J. R. Morgan, R. Newcombe, and M. Addy.** 1992. The effects of antimicrobial acrylic strips on the subgingival microflora in chronic periodontitis. *J. Clin. Periodontol.* **19:**127–134.
66. **Watt, B., and F. V. Brown.** 1986. Is ciprofloxacin active against clinically important anaerobes? *J. Antimicrob. Chemother.* **17:**605–613.
67. **Willems, A., and M. D. Collins.** 1995. Phylogenetic analysis of *Ruminococcus flavefaciens*, the type species of the genus *Ruminococcus*, does not support the reclassification of *Streptococcus hansenii* and *Peptostreptococcus productus* as ruminococci. *Int. J. Syst. Bacteriol.* **45:**572–575.
68. **Wren, M. W. D.** 1980. Multiple selective media for the isolation of anaerobic bacteria from clinical specimens. *J. Clin. Pathol.* **33:**61–65.
69. **Wren, M. W. D.** 1996. Anaerobic cocci of clinical importance. *Br. J. Biomed. Sci.* **53:**294–301.

Propionibacterium, Lactobacillus, Actinomyces, and Other Non-Spore-Forming Anaerobic Gram-Positive Rods*

EIJA KÖNÖNEN AND WILLIAM G. WADE

56

TAXONOMY AND DESCRIPTION OF AGENTS

The anaerobic gram-positive non-spore-forming rods are widely distributed among two gram-positive phyla: *Actinobacteria* and *Firmicutes* (Table 1). Several new genera have been described, and numerous taxonomic revisions within the genera covered in this chapter have been performed since the 8th edition of this Manual (Table 2). Although it may be confusing for those in clinical microbiology laboratories, the clarification of taxonomic relationships allows definitive associations between taxa and disease to be uncovered and greater precision in the laboratory identification of pathogens. In addition, molecular ecological analysis of clinical specimens has revealed numerous as-yet-uncultivable bacterial taxa belonging to this group (15, 35, 70, 117, 118, 126).

Phylum *Actinobacteria*

The family *Actinomycetaceae* currently includes five genera: *Actinomyces, Actinobaculum, Arcanobacterium, Varibaculum,* and *Mobiluncus*. It has long been known that species assigned to the genus *Actinomyces* constitute a heterogeneous group. New genera have been proposed to include both newly described species related to, and species formerly included in, *Actinomyces*. For example, *A. bernardiae* and *A. pyogenes* have been moved to the genus *Arcanobacterium* (116) (see chapter 34). *Actinomyces* and related genera contain anaerobic and aerotolerant, non-acid-fast, gram-positive organisms with variable morphology, ranging from characteristic branching rods to coccobacilli. *Actinomyces* contains a rapidly increasing number of species (Table 2) that usually produce succinic acid from glucose. *Actinobaculum* currently includes *A. schaalii* and *A. urinale* from humans and the type species *A. suis* from pigs (63, 97), but the proposal of more new species in the genus is warranted (35, 58). *Varibaculum* (67) is a monophyletic genus related to *Mobiluncus* but distinct on the basis of 16S rRNA gene sequence identity. *Varibaculum cambriensis* is related to *Actinomyces neuii* but would appear to deserve consideration as a separate genus. *Mobiluncus* contains two species, *M. curtisii* and *M. mulieris,* which are strictly anaerobic, curved bacilli with variable Gram reactions and corkscrew motility. They resemble *Actinomyces* in that succinic acid is the major metabolic end product from glucose. It has been shown recently that *Falcivibrio vaginalis* and *Falcivibrio grandis* are later synonyms of *M. curtisii* and *M. mulieris*, respectively (76).

Propionibacterium species are anaerobic and aerotolerant, pleomorphic, gram-positive rods that produce propionic acid from glucose. Four *Propionibacterium* species have been isolated from human clinical infections: *P. acnes, P. avidum, P. granulosum,* and *P. propionicum*. The last species (formerly *Arachnia propionica*) exhibits some characteristics similar to *Actinomyces* species. Two related taxa, formerly members of *Propionibacterium, Propionimicrobium lymphophilum* (146) and *Propioniferax innocua* (172), can also be encountered in clinical material.

Members of the genus *Bifidobacterium* and the closely related genera *Parascardovia* and *Scardovia* are strictly anaerobic or occasionally microaerobic, gram-positive, pleomorphic rods, appearing as uniform to branched or club-shaped. Typically, bifidobacteria produce fructose-6-phosphate phosphoketolase as well as acetic and lactic acids as major metabolic end products. Bifidobacteria are aciduric and are nutritionally fastidious. There are currently 29 *Bifidobacterium* species. Of these, 10 species (*B. bifidum, B. breve, B. gallicum, B. longum, B. adolescentis, B. catenulatum, B. dentium, B. angulatum, B. pseudocatenulatum,* and *B. scardovii*) have been isolated from the human gut and oral cavity. *B. longum* now includes the former species *B. infantis* and *B. suis* (129). Two species isolated from dental plaque, *B. inopinatum* and *B. denticolens* (27), were later shown to represent novel genera on the basis of HSP60 gene sequence relatedness and were transferred to *Scardovia* and *Parascardovia*, respectively (81).

Numerous taxa have been misassigned to *Lactobacillus* in the past, including the so-called "anaerobic lactobacilli," which are now recognized to constitute two new genera, *Atopobium* and *Olsenella*, within the family *Coriobacteriaceae* (26, 30). *Atopobium* species produce lactic acid as the major glucose metabolic end product. *A. minutum* and *A. rimae* were formerly *Lactobacillus* species, and *A. parvulum* and *A. fossor* formerly belonged to the genera *Streptococcus* and *Eubacterium*, respectively (26, 87). *A. vaginae* is a novel species, originally isolated from the healthy vagina (124). The genus *Olsenella* is closely related to *Atopobium* (30) and currently includes two species: *O. uli* (formerly *Lactobacillus uli*) and *O. profusa*, both isolated from the human oral cavity.

Most *Eubacterium* species belong to the *Firmicutes*, but until recently, the genus included a number of species now

* This chapter contains information presented in chapter 55 by Bernard J. Moncla and Sharon L. Hillier in the eighth edition of this Manual.

TABLE 1 Some features of non-spore-forming anaerobic gram-positive genera

Phylum and genus	G+C mol%	Cell characteristics	Aerotolerance[a]	Gram reaction[b]	Major end product(s)[c]	Other features
Actinobacteria						
Actinobaculum	50–57	Straight/slightly curved, branching; singly/in clusters	+/−	(+)	A	Saccharolytic
Actinomyces	55–68	Variable, often branching; singly/in pairs	+/−	+	S, L	Saccharolytic
Atopobium	35–46	Short, elliptical; singly/in pairs/short chains	−/+	+	L	Saccharolytic
Bifidobacterium	57–64	Variable	−/+	+	A, L	Aciduric
Collinsella	60–61	Short; in chains	−	+	A, F, L	Saccharolytic, H_2 production
Cryptobacterium	50–51	Short	−	(+)	None	Asaccharolytic
Eggerthella	62	Coccobacilli/short rods; in pairs/short chains	−	+	(A, L, S)	Asaccharolytic
Mobiluncus	49–52	Curved with tapered ends; singly/in pairs; motile	−	v	S, L, A	Saccharolytic
Olsenella	63–64	Short, elliptical; singly/in pairs/short chains	−	+	L, A	Saccharolytic
Parascardovia	54–56	Small, slender, variable	−	+	A, L	Saccharolytic
Propionibacterium	59–67	Variable	−/+	+	P	Saccharolytic
Propionimicrobium	53–54	Variable; often diphtheroid/club-shaped	−	+	P, A, S	Saccharolytic
Scardovia	44–46	Small, coccoid, variable	−	+	A, L	Saccharolytic
Slackia	60–64	Cocci/coccobacilli/short rods; singly/in clumps	−	(+)	(A)	Asaccharolytic
Varibaculum	52	Short, straight/curved, diphtheroid	−/+	+	L, S	Saccharolytic
Firmicutes						
Anaerofustis	70	Thin rods	−	+	A, B	Saccharolytic
Anaerostipes	46	Thin rods; in short chains	−	(+)	A, B, L	Saccharolytic
Anaerotruncus	54	Thin rods	−	+	A, B	Saccharolytic
Bryantella	50	Short; in pairs/short chains	−	+	A (S, L)	Formate required
Bulleidia	38	Short, straight/slightly curved; singly/in pairs	−	+	A, L	Saccharolytic
Catenibacterium	36–38	Short; in long tangled chains	−	+	A, B, L	Saccharolytic
Dorea	40–46	Short/long; in pairs/in chains	−	+	A, F	Saccharolytic, H_2 production
Eubacterium	30–57	Variable	−	v	B, A, L (F)	Saccharolytic
Faecalibacterium	47–57	Pleomorphic rods	−	−	B, F, L	Saccharolytic
Filifactor	34	Short, regular	−	−	B	Asaccharolytic
Holdemania	38	Short; in pairs/short chains	−	(+)	A, L	Saccharolytic
Lactobacillus	35–53	Short/long, slender; in chains	−/+	+	L	Aciduric
Mogibacterium	41–50	Short; singly/in clumps	−	(+)	PAA	Asaccharolytic
Oribacterium	42	Elongated, ovoid; singly/in pairs; highly motile	−	−	A, L	Saccharolytic
Pseudoramibacter	61	Pleomorphic; in pairs	−	+	A, B, C, F	Saccharolytic
Roseburia	29–42	Thin, pleomorphic rods	−	v	B, L	Saccharolytic, H_2 production
Shuttleworthia	50–51	Short/slightly curved; singly/in pairs/short chains	−	+	B, A (L)	Saccharolytic
Solobacterium	37–39	Short, straight/slightly curved; singly/in pairs	−	+	A, L	Saccharolytic
Turicibacter	37	Irregular, long; in long chains	−	+	L	Saccharolytic

[a] +/− or −/+, variable aerotolerance within the genus; −, the genus contains only strictly anaerobic species.
[b] +, positive; −, negative; v, variable; (+), decolorization in old culture.
[c] A, acetic acid; B, butyric acid; C, caproic acid; F, formic acid; L, lactic acid; P, propionic acid; S, succinic acid; PAA, phenylacetic acid; parentheses, strain variation.

shown to belong to the *Actinobacteria*, such as the former *E. lentum*, now renamed *Eggerthella lenta* (162); *E. aerofaciens*, now *Collinsella aerofaciens* (88); and *E. exiguum*, now *Slackia exigua* (162). *E. lenta* and *C. aerofaciens* are numerically important bacteria in the human intestinal tract (88, 162), whereas *S. exigua* is strongly associated with oral infections (162). Recently, two new *Eggerthella* species, *E. hongkongensis* and *E. sinensis*, have been proposed (96). A novel species found in oral infections, *Cryptobacterium curtum* (108), is related to this group.

Phylum *Firmicutes*

Lactobacillus, a large and heterogeneous genus, contains microaerobic, catalase-negative, non-spore-forming gram-positive rods, which produce lactic acid as their single or major metabolic end product from glucose fermentation. Members of *Lactobacillus* sensu stricto constitute a branch of the *Firmicutes* subdivided into seven groups: *L. buchneri*, *L. casei*, *L. delbrueckii*, *L. plantarum*, *L. reuteri*, *L. sakei*, and *L. salivarius* (69). *Catenibacterium mitsuokai* (84), isolated from human feces, forms a cluster with *L. vitulinus* and *L. catenaformis*, two misclassified *Lactobacillus* species.

Organisms assigned to *Eubacterium* are defined by default; they do not produce propionic acid as a major acid product, lactic acid as the sole major acid product, succinic and lactic acids with small amounts of acetic or formic acids, or acetic and lactic (acetic > lactic) acids, with or without formic acid, as the sole major acid products (103). It has

TABLE 2 Recently classified or reclassified genera and species (from 2002 onwards) of non-spore-forming anaerobic gram-positive rods isolated from humans

Phylum and genus	New genus	Species	Previous nomenclature	Reference
Actinobacteria				
Actinobaculum		*A. massiliae*	New sp.	58
		A. urinale	New sp.	63
Actinomyces		*A. cardiffensis*	New sp.	62
		A. dentalis	New sp.	66
		A. hongkongensis	New sp.	169
		A. nasicola	New sp.	65
		A. oricola	New sp.	64
Bifidobacterium		*B. longum*	*B. infantis, B. longum, B. suis*	129
		B. scardovii	New sp.	77
Eggerthella		*E. hongkongensis*	New sp.	96
		E. sinensis	New sp.	96
Parascardovia	Yes	*P. denticolens*	*Bifidobacterium denticolens*	81
Propionimicrobium	Yes	*P. lymphophilum*	*Propionibacterium lymphophilum*	146
Scardovia	Yes	*S. inopinata*	*Bifidobacterium inopinatum*	81
Varibaculum	Yes	*V. cambriensis*	New sp.	67
Firmicutes				
Anaerofustis	Yes	*A. stercorihominis*	New sp.	48
Anaerostipes	Yes	*A. caccae*	New sp.	140
Anaerotruncus	Yes	*A. colihominis*	New sp.	99
Bryantella	Yes	*B. formatexigens*	New sp.	168
Dorea	Yes	*D. formicigenerans*	*Eubacterium formicigenerans*	152
		D. longicatena	New sp.	152
Faecalibacterium	Yes	*F. prausnitzii*	*Fusobacterium prausnitzii*	37
Lactobacillus		*L. antri*	New sp.	127
		L. gastricus	New sp.	127
		L. kalixensis	New sp.	127
		L. ultunensis	New sp.	127
Mogibacterium		*M. diversum*	New sp.	109
		M. neglectum	New sp.	109
Oribacterium	Yes	*O. sinus*	New sp.	17
Roseburia		*R. intestinalis*	New sp.	36
Shuttleworthia	Yes	*S. satelles*	New sp.	32
Turicibacter	Yes	*T. sanguinis*	New sp.	6

been proposed that *Eubacterium* sensu stricto should be restricted to *E. limosum*, *E. callanderi*, and *E. barkeri* (165). The remaining *Eubacterium* species would therefore require reclassification. Clinically important *Eubacterium* species are widely distributed among the *Firmicutes*. *E. alactolyticum*, a saccharolytic species found in the oral cavity of humans, and a close phylogenetic relative of the strictly defined genus *Eubacterium*, has been moved to a new genus as *Pseudoramibacter alactolyticus* (165). *E. biforme*, *E. cylindroids*, and *E. dolichum* fall within the family *Erysipelotrichaceae* with the recently described saccharolytic species, *Bulleidia extructa*, isolated from the human mouth (34), and *Holdemania filiformis* (166) and *Solobacterium moorei* (86), isolated from human feces. *E. brachy*, *E. infirmum*, *E. minutum*, *E. nodatum*, *E. saphenum*, and *E. sulci* (formerly *Fusobacterium sulci*), together with *Mogibacterium*, a genus of five species indistinguishable by phenotypic tests (109, 110), are a group of asaccharolytic taxa isolated from the human mouth. On the basis of the 16S rRNA phylogeny and their phenotypic characteristics, novel genera should be created for the majority of these species, with the exception of the pairs of species *E. minutum* and *E. nodatum* and *E. sulci* and *E. infirmum*, which are closely related. Many *Eubacterium* species are closely related to clostridia. Spore formation has long been the primary criterion for assignation of gram-positive anaerobic rods to *Clostridium*, but phylogenetic analysis indicates that the taxonomic importance of this characteristic may have been overemphasized. Numerous phylogenetic clusters contain both sporing and nonsporing representatives. *E. budayi*, *E. moniliforme*, and *E. nitritogenes* are found in clostridial Cluster 1 (25), while *E. siraeum* belongs to a clostridial group that includes *Clostridium leptum* and the recently described *Anaerotruncus colihominis* (99). *E. tenue* and *E. yurii* belong to the clostridial Cluster XI described by Collins et al. (25). *E. tenue* is related to *Clostridium ghonii* and *Clostridium sordellii;* further work is required to determine whether these species constitute a novel genus. *E. yurii* is related to the genus *Filifactor*, which includes *F. alocis* (formerly *Fusobacterium alocis*) isolated from oral infections in humans (80). *E. contortum*, *E. eligens*, *E. hadrum*, *E. hallii*, *E. ramulus*, *E. rectale*, *E. saburreum*, and *E. ventriosum* belong to the family *Lachnospiraceae*. *E. rectale* and *E. ramulus* are related to *Roseburia intestinalis* (36). This family also includes the recently described formate-requiring species *Bryantella formatexigens* (168), isolated from human feces without any disease association so far, and *Oribacterium sinus* (17), a highly motile species isolated from pus of a human sinus. *E. eligens* and *Lachnospira pectinoschiza* are close phylogenetic neighbors and are both motile rods whose growth in broth culture is stimulated by the presence of fermentable carbohydrate. *E. eligens* should be transferred to the genus *Lachnospira*. *Anaerostipes caccae* (140) forms a loose group with *E. hallii* and *Coprococcus eutactus*, all common species in human feces.

Turicibacter sanguinis (6) is a recently described gram-positive anaerobic rod from human blood, belonging to the phylum *Firmicutes* but which, on the basis of 16S rRNA sequence comparisons, appears to represent a novel lineage within this phylum. Further work is required to clarify the taxonomic position of this genus. Similarly, *Anaerofustis stercorihominis* (48), isolated from human feces, is another deep-branching gram-positive anaerobic rod within *Firmicutes*.

EPIDEMIOLOGY AND TRANSMISSION

Many of the organisms described in this chapter are integral components of the commensal microbiota associated with the mucocutaneous surfaces of the human and animal digestive tract, being found in the mouth, small and large intestines, urogenital tract, and skin (1, 2, 117, 118, 127, 160). Microbial colonization of an individual occurs in a successive manner during the first weeks and months of life. *Actinomyces* are among the first colonizers in the mouth (134), whereas bifidobacteria and *Collinsella* have been suggested to play a significant role in the development of the gut microbiota (70). *Eubacterium rectale, Faecalibacterium prausnitzii,* and lactobacilli are also among the dominant members of the intestinal microbiota (1, 37, 149). In contrast to previous culture-based reports indicating *L. acidophilus* to be the predominant *Lactobacillus* species in the female genital tract, molecular techniques have revealed significant numbers of *L. crispatus, L. gasseri, L. iners, L. jensenii,* and *L. vaginalis* (2, 145, 160, 161, 164). These species, except for *L. iners,* are responsible for hydrogen peroxide (H_2O_2) production, which may help to control the overgrowth of bacterial vaginosis-associated organisms (2).

CLINICAL SIGNIFICANCE

Non-spore-forming anaerobic gram-positive rods seldom cause infections alone but are typically found in polymicrobial infections associated with mucosal surfaces (Table 3). Many anaerobes involved in infections of the head and neck originate from the oral cavity, and most vaginal and bladder pathogens are of fecal origin. In intra-abdominal infections due to organ perforation, the predominant recoveries reflect the microbiota at the site of the leakage (163). For surgical patients, anaerobes remain a significant cause of morbidity and mortality (39). Anaerobic bacteria can occasionally spread to adjacent tissues and even the bloodstream with serious consequences. In anaerobic bacteremias, the gastrointestinal tract is the most common source, followed by abscesses, gynecologic infections, and wound infections (131). Anaerobic blood culture methods tend to be targeted at *Clostridium* species and *Bacteroides fragilis,* which are aerotolerant and relatively fast growing and do not have complex nutritional requirements.

Actinomyces and Related Bacteria

Actinomyces and related bacteria have been isolated with increased frequency, as contaminants or etiologic agents, from clinical specimens representing a wide range of infections (Table 3). *Actinomyces* and related species occur typically in polymicrobial infections together with anaerobic and/or capnophilic, gram-negative species (23, 102, 128, 136). These include several types of oral infection, such as dental caries, endodontic infections, odontogenic abscesses, and dental implant-associated infections (4, 8, 24, 64, 66, 133, 136, 142). Traditionally, *A. israelii* has been thought to be the etiologic agent of classical actinomycosis but *A. gerencseriae,* which is very similar to *A. israelii, A. graevenitzii,* and *A. meyeri,* has also been isolated from actinomycotic lesions (23, 102, 136, 154). Several recognized *Actinomyces* species, especially *A. israelii* and *A. turicensis* but also *A. naeslundii, A. odontolyticus, A. gerencseriae, A. cardiffensis,* and a novel, closely related species, *V. cambriensis,* have been isolated from intrauterine device-associated infections in the female genital tract (50, 62, 67, 68). In addition, *A. naeslundii* and *A. israelii* have been isolated from infectious hip prostheses (148, 171). *A. turicensis,* in particular, seems to dominate in both female and male genital and urinary tract infections (128). *A. funkei, A. naeslundii, A. odontolyticus,* and *A. turicensis* as well as two *Actinobaculum* species, *A. schaalii* and *A. urinale,* have been isolated from blood (46, 68, 97, 98, 115, 122). Taken together, *A. turicensis, A. radingae, A. israelii,* and *A. naeslundii* seem to be the most frequent *Actinomyces* findings in clinical specimens, present in polymicrobial infections or, occasionally, alone (23, 51, 68, 128).

Propionibacterium

Propionibacteria can be found in various systemic or disseminated opportunistic infections (Table 3), such as endocarditis, central nervous system infections, osteomyelitis, osteitis, and arthritis (11, 29, 43, 51, 79), and in about 20% of infected dog and cat bite wounds (151). When *P. acnes* is isolated from blood, it is mainly seen as a causative agent of clinically insignificant bacteremia (11, 95, 131) or as a contaminant from the skin. Typically, *P. acnes* is isolated from sebaceous follicles and lesions of acne vulgaris (51). However, the pathogenic potential of *P. acnes* should not be underestimated when there are predisposing factors present, such as a foreign body, surgery or trauma, diabetes, or immunosuppression (11, 59, 79, 157). *P. acnes* has been connected with some, often severe, late postsurgical infections after implantation of a foreign body, e.g., intraocular lenses, prosthetic heart valves, ventriculoperitoneal shunts, and posterior implants for scoliosis patients (11, 22, 60, 79, 95, 131, 157). It can be a causal agent in infective endocarditis with a predilection for prosthetic valves and foreign bodies (59, 157). The suggested association of *P. acnes* with SAPHO (synovitis, acne, pustulosis, hyperostosis, and osteomyelitis) syndrome with arthritis is based on its repeated growth in pure cultures from bone specimens (91). *P. acnes* and *P. granulosum* have been recently linked as possible etiologic agents to sarcoidosis (42), in which host factors play an important role. In contrast to *P. acnes* and other propionibacteria, the spectrum of infections with involvement of *P. propionicum* is somewhat similar to that of *Actinomyces;* for example, *P. propionicum* has been isolated from actinomycosis-like eye infections (9) and endodontic infections (18, 142).

Lactobacillus

Despite the reputation of lactobacilli as beneficial organisms, they can be involved in serious infections (Table 3), especially in immunocompromised individuals (10, 12, 16, 45, 89, 111, 130). The most common *Lactobacillus* species isolated from various human infections are *L. rhamnosus, L. casei, L. fermentum, L. gasseri, L. plantarum, L. acidophilus,* and *L. ultunensis* (15, 16, 130). The most frequent infections caused by lactobacilli are bacteremia and endocarditis, which carry a relatively high mortality rate (16). Detection of lactobacilli, alone or with other microorganisms, in blood cultures of patients with underlying diseases may be clinically

TABLE 3 Genera of non-spore-forming anaerobic gram-positive rods detected in human infections

Site/disease association	Genera isolated
Brain and/or central nervous system	*Actinomyces, Eubacterium, Propionibacterium, Pseudoramibacter, Varibaculum*
Eye infections	*Actinomyces, Propionibacterium, Varibaculum*
Mouth	
Abscesses	*Actinomyces, Atopobium, Eubacterium, Filifactor, Mogibacterium, Olsenella, Pseudoramibacter, Slackia, Varibaculum*
Dental caries	*Actinomyces, Bifidobacterium, Lactobacillus, Olsenella, Propionibacterium*
Endodontic infection	*Actinomyces, Atopobium, Bifidobacterium, Eubacterium, Filifactor, Mogibacterium, Lactobacillus, Olsenella, Propionibacterium, Pseudoramibacter, Slackia*
Periodontal diseases	*Cryptobacterium, Eubacterium, Filifactor, Mogibacterium, Olsenella, Pseudoramibacter, Slackia*
Respiratory tract infections	*Actinomyces, Eubacterium, Lactobacillus, Oribacterium*
Abdomen/intestine	
Abscesses	*Actinomyces, Eggerthella, Eubacterium, Lactobacillus*
Appendicitis	*Actinomyces, Eggerthella*
Cholecystitis	*Actinomyces, Lactobacillus*
Peritonitis	*Eggerthella, Lactobacillus*
Genital tract	
Abscesses	*Actinomyces, Atopobium, Eubacterium*
Bacterial vaginosis	*Atopobium, Mobiluncus*
Intrauterine device infections	*Actinomyces, Eubacterium, Varibaculum*
Pelvic inflammatory disease	*Actinomyces, Atopobium, Eubacterium, Lactobacillus*
Preterm labor/delivery	*Mobiluncus*
Urinary tract infections	*Actinobaculum, Actinomyces*
Skin and/or soft tissue	
Abscesses	*Actinobaculum, Actinomyces*
Acne vulgaris	*Propionibacterium*
Cellulitis	*Actinomyces, Pseudoramibacter*
Necrotizing soft tissue infections	*Actinomyces, Eubacterium, Mogibacterium*
Lymphadenitis	*Propionibacterium, Propionimicrobium*
Bone and joint infections	*Actinomyces, Propionibacterium*
Wounds	
Bite wound infections (animal)	*Filifactor, Propionibacterium*
Bite wound infections (human)	*Actinomyces, Collinsella, Eggerthella, Eubacterium, Mogibacterium, Lactobacillus, Propionibacterium*
Postoperative wound infections	*Bifidobacterium, Propionibacterium, Pseudoramibacter*
Diabetic foot infections	*Actinomyces, Propionibacterium*
Cardiovascular sites	
Bacteremia	*Actinobaculum, Actinomyces, Atopobium, Eggerthella, Eubacterium, Lactobacillus, Olsenella, Propionibacterium*
Endocarditis	*Actinomyces, Lactobacillus, Propionibacterium*
Infected atheroma	*Actinomyces*
Foreign body infections	*Actinomyces, Mogibacterium, Propionibacterium*

significant. *L. rhamnosus* was the most frequent species in *Lactobacillus* bacteremia (16, 45, 95, 130). *L. rhamnosus* GG, a common probiotic strain, has been occasionally detected in clinical specimens (93, 101, 120, 130). In two pediatric patients with sepsis, the *Lactobacillus* strain from blood samples was indistinguishable from the probiotic strain ingested (93), suggesting that further work needs to be done. Vancomycin-resistant lactobacilli have been connected to dialysis-related peritonitis after extended use of glycopeptides (89, 111). In contrast to other *Lactobacillus* species, *L. iners* has been associated with an intermediate state of bacterial vaginosis (161). In the oral cavity, lactobacilli form a considerable part of the species present in advanced caries lesions (19), with *L. gasseri* and *L. ultunensis* numerically dominant (15). Interestingly, a dental procedure or condition can be a potential predisposing factor for *Lactobacillus* endocarditis (16).

Eubacterium and Related Bacteria

Low G+C organisms representing the former genus *Eubacterium* are often detected in various oral infections (Table 3). Careful isolation of tiny-colony-forming anaerobes from periodontal pockets in adult patients with advanced periodontitis showed that former *Eubacterium* strains (mostly asaccharolytic) dominated (155), thus suggesting their role in the etiology of chronic periodontitis. Downes et al. (33) characterized *Eubacterium*-like strains from oral infections and found *Mogibacterium timidum* to be among the most frequently detected species. *Mogibacterium vescum, Bulleidia extructa, Filifactor alocis,* and *Pseudoramibacter alactolyticus* were also found among the isolates from severe (some of them requiring treatment in intensive care units) odontogenic infections. Less frequently isolated were *E. sulci*, *E. saburreum*, and *E. yurii* (33). Many species found in odontogenic infections are also common in endodontic infections (71, 107, 109, 141, 143). *F. alocis*, *E. nodatum*, *E. saphenum*, and *M. timidum* have been associated with periodontal diseases (5, 92, 117). Due to their presence in the oral cavity, various *Eubacterium* and related species are among the anaerobic findings in human bite wound infections (150). *Filifactor villosus*, a species of animal origin, has been isolated from infected cat bite wounds in humans (151). *E. nodatum* has been found in infections of the female genital tract (73). *E. tenue* and *E. callanderi*, an environmental anaerobe, have been detected in clinically significant bacteremia (95, 153).

Eggerthella and Related Bacteria

Of the four high G+C content genera previously classified as *Eubacterium*, *Eggerthella* has been shown to possess particular pathogenic potential (Table 3). *E. lenta* has been isolated from a wide range of clinical specimens, mainly from intra-abdominal sites (10, 12, 104, 121). *E. lenta* and two recently described *Eggerthella* species, *E. hongkongensis* and *E. sinensis*, have been found in blood in association with clinically significant infections of relatively high mortality (95, 96). *Cryptobacterium curtum* and *Slackia exigua* have been associated with chronic periodontitis (5, 92), and the latter has also been associated with endodontic infections (71).

Atopobium

The genus *Atopobium* can be isolated from various infections (Table 3) and includes several clinically relevant species. Although *A. vaginae* was first isolated from the healthy vagina (124), it has been increasingly reported to be involved in infections of the genital tract, especially bacterial vaginosis (14, 47, 52, 161). *A. minutum* has been isolated from various infections of the lower part of the body, and *A. parvulum* has been isolated from respiratory specimens (113). In the oral cavity, *A. parvulum* and *A. rimae* have been detected in periodontal pockets (113, 117); however, in another study, these species have been shown to be more prevalent in healthy individuals than in periodontitis patients (92). Among *Eubacterium*-like isolates from severe odontogenic infections, *A. rimae* proved to be the most frequent finding (33). An *Atopobium* species of animal origin, *A. fossor*, has been isolated as one of the most frequent species from horses with pneumonia and lung abscesses (119).

Olsenella

Olsenella species show disease associations similar to those observed for lactobacilli in the oral cavity, *O. profusa* being detected in advanced dental caries lesions (106), and *O. uli*, in particular, in endodontic infections (18, 107, 123). Both species can also be found in subgingival sites of periodontitis patients (30, 113). In addition, *O. uli* has been reported as one of the causative organisms in clinically significant bacteremia (95).

Bifidobacterium and Related Bacteria

Bifidobacteria, one of the dominant bacterial groups in the human intestinal tract (70), are generally considered nonpathogenic but appear in some infectious lesions (Table 3). Dental caries is the most common clinical entity where *Bifidobacterium*, mainly *B. dentium*, and related species *P. denticolens* and *S. inopinata* may have a pathogenic role (4, 19, 27, 81). Some *Bifidobacterium* species, such as *B. adolescentis* and *B. dentium*, are occasionally isolated from other infections, mainly in immunocompromised individuals (10, 12). In addition, a novel *Bifidobacterium* species, *B. scardovii*, has been isolated from human clinical samples, including blood, urine, and the hip (77).

Mobiluncus

The presence of vibrio-like *Mobiluncus* species in smears of vaginal fluid has been widely used as one of the indicators of bacterial vaginosis, the most common infection in the female genital tract (112). Of the two *Mobiluncus* species, *M. curtisii* seldom occurs in the vaginas of healthy women but, instead, is highly associated with bacterial vaginosis and its treatment failure due to the persistence of the organism (138). The disturbed composition of the vaginal microbiota can be a risk for adverse pregnancy outcome when ascending to the upper genital tract (75). In addition to bacterial vaginosis, *M. curtisii* has been occasionally isolated from endometrial smears and pus specimens of the female genital tract (3) and some extragenital infections (40, 57).

COLLECTION, TRANSPORT, AND STORAGE OF SPECIMENS

Careful specimen collection, avoidance of contamination with the commensal microbiota where necessary, and anaerobic transport techniques are essential for the successful recovery of clinically significant anaerobic bacteria (see chapters 5 and 20). Specimens suitable for the isolation of non-spore-forming, gram-positive anaerobic rods present as organisms of etiologic importance include aseptically collected peripheral blood, tissue biopsy specimens, aspirates (e.g., cerebrospinal fluid, joint fluids, and pus), root canal exudates, and subgingival plaque. Mucosal or cutaneous swabs are not recommended (53). A comprehensive description of different specimen collection and transport methods for anaerobic bacteriology can be found elsewhere (83).

DIRECT EXAMINATION

Direct examination is of unequivocal value for the diagnosis of actinomycosis. The presence of "sulfur granules" in pus, which when crushed, Gram stained, and viewed under the microscope reveal a mass of gram-positive branching filaments, is characteristic of this disease. Similarly, in cervical smears of women with an intrauterine contraceptive device, the presence of branching gram-positive organisms suggests an infection with *Actinomyces* (50, 128). Gram stains of vaginal smears have been considered more useful than culture for laboratory confirmation of bacterial vaginosis, and the diagnostic criteria for this common infection have been based on the standardized Nugent scoring system (112). The system relies on Gram stain characteristics of vaginal smears, recognizing individual morphotypes or their combination. Although intercenter reliability for gram-positive cocci was poor, the study documented moderate agreement for large gram-positive rods (lactobacilli) and small gram-variable and/or gram-negative rods (*Gardnerella vaginalis* and *Bacteroides/Prevotella*), and good agreement for curved gram-variable rods (*Mobiluncus*) (112). A simplified assessment of Gram-stained smears, taking lactobacillary and mixed bacterial morphotypes into account, has been proposed (78). It has been noted that the image area observed in microscopes requires standardization, in particular, when interpreting the intermediate state of bacterial vaginosis (94). Subsequently, a strong association between *A. vaginae* and an abnormal vaginal state has been established (47, 161). This gram-positive, variably shaped, often coccoid species may confuse scoring systems relying on the Gram stain.

In cases where there is no typical microbiota associated with a particular infection, it can be difficult to make a preliminary decision regarding appropriate empiric antimicrobial treatment on the basis of the Gram stain. For example, branching/pleomorphic rods can be tentatively identified as facultatively anaerobic *Actinomyces* or strictly anaerobic *E. nodatum* (73), and coccoid cells of *A. radicidentis* may suggest a genus other than *Actinomyces* (24), while easily decolorizing species (e.g., *Eubacterium*-like species) can yield a false gram-negative reaction (33). The misinterpretation can lead to antimicrobial coverage targeted against facultative organisms instead of anaerobes and/or gram-negative bacteria.

CULTURE AND ISOLATION

Specimens should be processed without delay using appropriate culture media, including standard anaerobic blood agar enriched with hemin and vitamin K_1 and a variety of selective media based on the expected microbiota at the collection site, or in the case of bite wounds, on the oral microbiota of the attacker (human or animal). Fresh or prereduced culture media, including phenyl ethyl alcohol blood agar and/or colistin nalidixic acid blood agar, can be useful for enhanced recovery rates of gram-positive organisms (20). Many asaccharolytic species exhibit enhanced growth on solid media augmented with 0.5% arginine (156). In general, members of the aciduric genera *Bifidobacterium* and *Lactobacillus* can be selectively cultured using agar media with an acidic pH, such as Rogosa or deMan Rogosa Sharpe (MRS) agar. However, some nutritionally fastidious *Lactobacillus* strains fail to grow on these agar media. Munson et al. (106) observed that lactobacilli grew as well on nonselective media with neutral pH and suggested that acidic-pH medium is not required for their detection. Notably, *L. iners*, one of the predominant lactobacilli in the vagina, can grow only on blood agar and not on typical solid media used for *Lactobacillus* (44).

Similar species among facultatively anaerobic *Actinomyces*, *A. gerencseriae* and *A. israelii*, can be isolated preferably from aerobically (*A. gerencseriae*) or anaerobically (*A. israelii*) incubated plates (8). On the other hand, to maintain bacterial viability, processing the samples and performing all the steps throughout the protocol in an anaerobic chamber favor the growth of some fastidious anaerobes, e.g., *Eubacterium*-like species (31). An anaerobic atmosphere-generating system has been shown to be superior to an anaerobic chamber in culturing *Eubacterium*-like strains from stock (28). When anaerobic jars are used for incubation, anaerobic growth should not be exposed to oxygen by opening the jar before 48 h of incubation in order to facilitate the detection of fastidious organisms (20). The availability of an anaerobic chamber may enable examination of the culture whenever necessary. For reliable detection of slow-growing organisms, the incubation time should be sufficient; for instance, an extended incubation period may be needed for some clinically relevant *Eubacterium*-like species (33, 73, 108–110, 153). In heart tissue specimens from endocarditis patients, grinding the tissue can improve the detection of anaerobic bacteria (59, 79). A lytic anaerobic medium can increase the recovery rate of anaerobes and facultative bacteria in automated blood culture systems (125).

IDENTIFICATION PROCEDURES

Traditionally, the identification of bacterial isolates in clinical microbiology laboratories is performed by phenotypic tests. For organisms inert in most conventional biochemical tests or with unusual biochemical profiles, as is the case for many *Eubacterium* and related species, or in cases where fastidious organisms require specific nutrients or temperatures, identification strategies based on phenotypic characteristics can be challenging.

Presumptive Identification

The initial differentiation is based on aerotolerance (growth in air or in air plus 5% CO_2), colonial morphology, pigmentation, fluorescence under long-wave UV illumination, and presence of hemolysis. The colonial morphology can provide clues regarding the organism involved; for instance, an easily recognizable "molar tooth" appearance is typical for *A. israelii* but, notably, also for *E. nodatum* (73). Sometimes a species has various colonial morphologies, as is the case for *Shuttleworthia satelles*, with three separate colony types; the last two types (satellite and opaque) appear after incubation for 5 days (32). Other rapidly recognizable features are fluorescence and/or pigment production: *E. lenta* shows orange to red fluorescence under UV light (104), and pigmentation of colonies is typical for *A. odontolyticus*, but *A. graevenitzii* and some other *Actinomyces* species can also produce pigment (68, 135).

Gram stain morphology can be helpful; it can show whether organisms are gram-positive anaerobic rods, which can be very short (e.g., *C. curtum* and *E. lenta*), long (e.g., many *Lactobacillus* species), pleomorphic (e.g., *Bifidobacterium*), branching (e.g., many *Actinomyces* spp.), or curved and motile (e.g., *Mobiluncus* spp.); sometimes a specific cell morphology can be seen, such as "flying birds" (e.g., *P. alactolyticus*). The morphology may vary when cells are grown on different culture media. The two *Mobiluncus* species can be tentatively separated based on the length of the curved, motile cells: in contrast to the short, gram-variable cells of *M. curtisii*, *M. mulieris* reveals clearly longer cells, which often appear as gram negative (139). Although *Actinomyces* organisms have been traditionally described as branching rods, many new species within the genus are nonbranching, and some have very short or even coccoid cells (24, 158). Staining of cells can vary with different culture conditions. Certain gram-positive anaerobes, e.g., *F. alocis* and *M. mulieris*, routinely stain gram negative, whereas older cultures (>3 days) of *Actinobaculum* and some *Eubacterium* species and related genera are gram variable (97, 108, 110). Decolorization of gram-positive organisms may be due to exposure to oxygen or to damage from fixatives and reagents causing a breakdown of the physical integrity of the cell wall; therefore, anaerobic working conditions or, if not available, limited exposure time to oxygen between incubation and staining improves the reliability of the Gram stain for anaerobic bacteria (82). Routine screening of special-potency antibiotic susceptibility disk patterns is valuable to confirm the accuracy of the Gram stain reaction (83): gram-positive species are generally resistant to colistin (10 μg) and susceptible to vancomycin (5 μg) and often to kanamycin (1 mg). However, the intrinsic resistance of some *Lactobacillus* species/strains, e.g., *L. rhamnosus*, to glycopeptides should be considered (16, 45, 89, 111), in addition to intrinsic resistance of *Bifidobacterium* to aminoglycosides (105). *Holdemania filiformis* has been reported to be resistant to vancomycin (34). For rapid confirmation of the Gram reaction, a simple test based on dissolution of gram-negative cell wall and cytoplasmic membrane with a solution of 3% potassium hydroxide

(61) can be used: when suspended in the solution, gram-negative cells display increased viscosity and stringing within 30 s, whereas the absence of stringing, i.e., a negative reaction, suggests that the isolate is gram positive.

Additional rapid tests for initial grouping of non-spore-forming gram-positive anaerobes include testing for production of catalase (H_2O_2 at a concentration of 15%) and indole, nitrate reduction, and motility (20). If presumptive identification to the genus level has been made correctly, this may give valuable information to clinicians in deciding the initial treatment. However, differentiating members of the "normal flora" of human skin and mucous membranes from pathogenic non-spore-forming gram-positive rods can be difficult. Identification of nonsporing gram-positive rods to the species level should be performed whenever they are present in pure cultures in clinical specimens or as the predominant organism from normally sterile sites; otherwise, the potential pathogenicity of these less often suspected species may remain undetected.

Biochemical Testing

For a more advanced phenotypic classification of anaerobic organisms and distinguishing individual species, sugar fermentation reactions, preferably using prereduced, anaerobically sterilized carbohydrates, and enzyme profiles with individual diagnostic tablets, fluorogenic substrate tests, or preformed enzyme kits must be determined. Insufficient growth or poor reproducibility of reactions can cause difficulties in interpretation of results obtained with biochemical tests; therefore, young cultures and heavy inoculum should be used (135). A well-designed selection of key tests provides a tentative identification of various isolates to the species level prior to confirming their identifications by more definitive methods. Table 4 presents some biochemical characteristics of *Actinomyces* and related organisms. Since the description of many novel species, such as *A. dentalis, A. hongkongensis, A. nasicola, A. oricola, A. urinale,* and "*A. massiliae,*" is based on a single strain (58, 63–66, 169), discrepancies in test reactions may appear. Table 5 presents simple enzymatic reactions useful in distinguishing propionibacteria encountered in human infections, and Table 6 shows tests for *Atopobium* and *Olsenella* species. Although the cultivation and identification of *Eubacterium*-like species are very laborious, not only because of their oxygen sensitivity and slow growth but also due to their nonreactivity in conventional biochemical testing, some simple reactions may be helpful for grouping these organisms (Table 7).

In culture-based identification of anaerobic non-spore-forming gram-positive rods, the determination of major volatile fatty acid end products of glucose metabolism, as detected by gas chromatography, is a prerequisite, even for the genus level (Table 1). Typically, *Actinomyces* strains produce succinic and lactic acids as their major metabolic end products but *A. dentalis* seems to lack this characteristic succinic acid (66). An *Actinomyces*-like *Propionibacterium* species, *P. propionicum,* is easily separated from *Actinomyces* based on its production of propionic acid (51). For microaerobic *Lactobacillus* spp., defining characteristics are their ability to grow in acid media and ferment carbohydrates to produce lactic acid as the major end product with or without small amounts of acetate, whereas in the case of *Bifidobacterium* spp. the production of acetic acid dominates that of lactic acid. Downes et al. (33) successfully used the determination of metabolic end products by gas chromatography together with sugar fermentation by prereduced, anaerobically sterilized carbohydrates and enzyme profiles generated by a commercial identification kit (API Rapid ID 32A; bioMérieux, Marcy-l'Etoile, France) for identification of *Eubacterium*-like isolates to the genus and species level; for instance, the lack of enzyme activity and formation of caproic acid or phenylacetic acid distinguish *P. alactolyticus* or *Mogibacterium* spp., respectively, from other related taxa. However, phenotypic criteria are particularly unreliable for identification of many *Actinomyces* species (68) and members of the *L. acidophilus* complex and related species (159). In addition, gas chromatographic analysis of cellular fatty acids and examination of protein patterns by polyacrylamide gel electrophoresis have been used taxonomically to distinguish among strains within a species and among organisms within a genus or family. However, the availability of gas chromatography methods is often restricted to reference laboratories. The precise identification to the species level of heterogeneous groups within non-spore-forming gram-positive bacteria can be difficult, even when using the determination of volatile fatty acids by gas chromatography and biochemical profile analyses because biochemical tests do not accurately reflect genotypic groups (33, 45, 68, 145).

Preformed enzyme and carbohydrate fermentation profiles can be obtained using commercially available identification test kits, such as the API (bioMérieux), RapID (Remel, Lenexa, Kans.), and BBL Crystal (Becton Dickinson Diagnostic Systems, Sparks, Md.) systems, according to manufacturers' instructions. Although this approach is often hindered by similarities in fermentation profiles of separate species within a genus, kits serve as a widely used adjunct to anaerobe diagnostics in most hospital laboratories (53), since they are easy to use and much faster than conventional anaerobic procedures. The main problems with these kits are their incomplete or inaccurate databases (7, 132). The databases of the API Coryne (bioMérieux) and RapID CB Plus (Remel) tests, designed for coryneform bacteria, currently include some aerotolerant *Actinomyces* and *Propionibacterium* species as well. Notably, different test kits and individual tests differ in their substrate specificities so that an indicated reaction can vary depending on the system used (23, 132, 135). For example, one key reaction for *A. naeslundii,* urease production, can remain negative with one test, and thus the strain can be misidentified as *A. israelii,* while another test yields a correctly positive reaction (132, 171). Isolates of a novel *Atopobium* species, *A. vaginae,* have been misidentified as *Gemella morbillorum* by the API Rapid ID 32A (bioMérieux) and RapID ANA II (Remel) test kits (47, 52). In contrast, a clinically relevant *Bifidobacterium* species, *B. scardovii,* was readily separated from other bifidobacteria by using the Rapid ID 32A kit (bioMérieux) (77). The carbohydrate fermentation test kit API 50 CH (bioMérieux), which is specifically designed for lactobacilli, can be valuable in identification to the genus level but fail at the species level (7). Despite the lack of reliability of species level identifications, commercial test kits can be useful for the detection of positive reactions and identification of many organisms from clinical sources to the genus level. Clinical microbiologists should be aware of the possibility of erroneous identification and adjust the interpretation of their results accordingly, in conjunction with cellular and colonial morphology and other information available. Indeed, practical, discriminatory, and cost-effective methods are needed for identification of fastidious gram-positive bacteria. Molecular identification offers an opportunity for the description of new bacterial species encountered in clinical microbiology laboratories, and commercial 16S rRNA gene sequence-based identification kits are coming into the market (170).

TABLE 4 Biochemical characteristics of *Actinomyces* and related bacteria encountered in human infections[a]

Genus and species	Aerotolerance	Pigment	Production of:		Nitrate reduction	Esculin hydrolysis	Production of:			CAMP test	Fermentation of:				
			Catalase	Urease			α-Glu	β-NAG	β-Gal		Mal	Man	Raf	Suc	Tre
Actinobaculum															
A. massiliae	+	–	–	–	–	–	+	–	–	–	+	–	+	ND	+
A. schaalii	+	–	–	–	–	–	+	–	–	Weak	+	–	–	v	v
A. urinale	(+)	–	–	+	–	–	–	–	–	–	v	–	–	v	–
Actinomyces															
A. cardiffensis	(+)	–	–	–	v	–	+	–	–	–	v	–	v	v	–
A. dentalis	–	–	–	–	–	+	+	–	+	–	+	–	+	+	+
A. europaeus	+	–	–	–	v	v	+	–	+	–	+	–	–	v	v
A. funkei	+	–	–	–	+	–	+	v	v	v	v	–	–	+	–
A. georgiae	+	–	–	–	v	+	+	–	+	–	+	–	–	+	+
A. gerencseriae	+	–	–	–	v	+	+	–	+	–	+	v	v	+	v
A. graevenitzii	+	+	–	–	v	–	v	+	+	–	+	–	v	+	v
A. hongkongensis	–	–	–	–	–	–	–	–	–	–	ND	ND	–	ND	–
A. israelii	(+)	–	–	–	+	+	+	–	+	–	+	–	+	+	+
A. meyeri	–	–	–	–	v	–	+	+	+	v	+	–	–	+	–
A. naeslundii	+	–	–	+	+	v	v	–	+	–	+	–	+	+	+
A. nasicola	(+)	–	–	–	–	–	+	+	+	–	–	–	–	–	–
A. neuii															
subsp. *anitratus*	+	–	+	–	–	–	v	–	+	+	+	+	v	+	v
subsp. *neuii*	+	–	+	–	+	–	+	–	+	+	+	+	v	+	v
A. odontolyticus	+	+	–	–	+	v	–	–	+	–	+	–	–	+	–
A. oricola	+	–	–	–	–	+	+	–	v	–	–	–	+	+	+
A. radicidentis	+	+	+	v	v	+	+	–	+	–	+	+	+	+	+
A. radingae	+	–	–	–	v	+	+	+	+	v	+	–	v	+	v
A. turicensis	+	–	–	–	–	–	+	–	–	–	+	–	v	+	v
A. urogenitalis	+	+	–	–	+	+	+	+	+	–	+	–	–	+	+
A. viscosus	+	–	+	v	+	v	v	–	v	–	+	v	+	+	v
Varibaculum															
V. cambriensis	(+)	–	–	–	+	–	+	–	v	–	+	v	–	+	–

[a] Biochemical data from references 51, 58, 62–67, 135, 158, and 169. Symbols and abbreviations: +, positive; –, negative; (+), better growth in anaerobic condition; v, variable; ND, no data; α-Glu, α-glucosidase; β-NAG, β-*N*-acetyl-glucosaminidase; β-Gal, β-galactosidase; Mal, maltose; Man, mannitol; Raf, raffinose; Suc, sucrose; Tre, trehalose.

TABLE 5 Biochemical characteristics of propionibacteria encountered in human infections[a]

Genus and species	Aerotolerance	Catalase	Indole	Nitrate reduction	Esculin hydrolysis
Propionibacterium					
P. acnes	+	+	+	+	−
P. avidum	+	+	−	−	+
P. granulosum	+	+	−	−	−
P. propionicum	−	−	−	+	−
Propionimicrobium					
P. lymphophilum	−	v	−	v	ND

[a] Biochemical data compiled from references 51 and 146. Symbols and abbreviations: +, positive; −, negative; v, variable; ND, no data.

Identification by DNA Sequence Analysis

As mentioned above, the use of conventional and biochemical tests for the identification of this group carries a significant risk of misidentification. Far more precise identifications can be obtained by 16S rRNA gene sequence analysis (90). A major advantage is that methods do not need to be adapted for different groups of organisms; thus, there are no special considerations needed when analyzing gram-positive non-spore-forming anaerobes.

A major impetus to the study of unculturable bacteria has been the development of 16S rRNA/PCR amplification/cloning/sequencing methodology (167). The phylum *Firmicutes*, in particular, has been found to harbor a number of lineages without culturable representatives. For example, branches within the families *Eubacteriaceae* and *Lachnospiraceae* have been found in advanced carious lesions, endodontic infections, and subgingival plaque in periodontitis (19, 107, 117). Similarly, the colonic microbiota includes novel branches within the *Clostridiaceae* and *Erysipelotrichaceae* (149). Culture-independent analysis of the microbiota in bacterial vaginosis identified a novel taxon related to *A. vaginae* (161), and novel taxa belonging to both the *Actinobacteria* and *Firmicutes* were found in a corneal ulcer (137).

SEROLOGICAL TESTS

Serological tests are of little diagnostic value for this group of organisms, which are found almost exclusively in polymicrobial infections. Furthermore, infections are frequently opportunistic in nature, with the causative organism being a member of the commensal microbiota, rendering serological tests difficult to interpret.

ANTIMICROBIAL SUSCEPTIBILITIES

In the clinical setting, empirical information is used for the initial diagnosis of infection and choice of antimicrobial therapy, while awaiting culture and susceptibility test results. Published data regarding antimicrobial susceptibilities of nonsporing gram-positive anaerobes may be difficult to interpret. Changes in the bacterial taxonomy, e.g., among the former *Eubacterium* genus, and more precise classification of tested isolates may result in antimicrobial resistance patterns different from those given in previously published surveys (144). In general, penicillin and other β-lactams exhibit activity against gram-positive bacteria together with parenteral carbapenems, such as imipenem, ertapenem, and meropenem (13, 41, 54, 55, 74, 100, 105, 144). Metronidazole has been considered a drug of choice for treatment of anaerobic infections; however, resistant strains are common among non-spore-forming gram-positive genera with facultative/microaerobic strains, i.e., *Propionibacterium*, *Actinomyces*, *Bifidobacterium*, and *Lactobacillus*, but also among the strictly anaerobic genera *Atopobium* and *Mobiluncus* (3, 47). In addition, some strains of *Eggerthella* and *Eubacterium* resistant to metronidazole have been reported (21, 74, 100). Failures or relapses are common in the treatment of bacterial vaginosis, but whether metronidazole-resistant *A. vaginae* or *M. curtisii* (3, 47, 52) could play a role is not known. Occasional strains among various genera of non-spore-forming gram-positive anaerobic rods show

TABLE 6 Enzyme reactions useful in distinguishing species within the genera *Atopobium* and *Olsenella*[a]

Genus and species	Aerotolerance	Production of:		Nitrate reduction	Hydrolysis of:		Acid phos	β-Gal
		Catalase	Indole		Esculin	Arginine		
Atopobium								
A. minutum	−	−	−	−	ND	+	−	−
A. parvulum	−	−	−	−	v	−	+	+
A. rimae	−	−	−	−	v	v	+	−
A. vaginae	(−)[b]	−	−	−	−	+	+	−
Olsenella								
O. profusa	−	−	−	−	+	−	ND	ND
O. uli	−	−	−	−	+	+	ND	ND

[a] Biochemical data compiled from references 26, 30, 33, 113, and 124. Symbols and abbreviations: +, positive; −, negative; v, variable; ND, no data; Acid phos, acid phosphatase; β-Gal, β-galactosidase.

[b] In the original description, *A. vaginae* is facultatively anaerobic.

TABLE 7 Biochemical characteristics of some human *Eubacterium*-like organisms[a]

Phylum/genus and species	Glucose fermentation	Production of:		Nitrate reduction	Hydrolysis of:		Production of:		
		Catalase	Indole		Esculin	Arginine	β-Gal	β-Glu	β-NAG
Actinobacteria									
Collinsella aerofaciens	+	−	−	−	v	v	v	v	−
Collinsella intestinalis	+	ND	ND	ND	ND	ND	−	−	+
Collinsella stercoris	+	ND	ND	ND	ND	ND	+	Weak	+
Cryptobacterium curtum	−	−	−	−	−	+	ND	ND	ND
Eggerthella hongkongensis	−	+	−	−	ND	+	−	+	−
Eggerthella lenta	−	+	−	+	−	+	−	−	−
Eggerthella sinensis	−	+	−	−	ND	+	−	−	−
Slackia exigua	−	−	−	−	−	+	ND	ND	ND
Firmicutes									
Bulleidia extructa	+	−	−	−	−	+	ND	ND	ND
Catenibacterium mitsuokai	+	−	ND	−	−	ND	ND	ND	ND
Eubacterium brachy	−	−	−	−	−	−	ND	ND	ND
Eubacterium limosum	+	−	−	−	+	v	ND	ND	ND
Eubacterium minutum	−	−	−	−	−	−	ND	ND	ND
Eubacterium nodatum	−	−	−	−	−	+	ND	ND	ND
Eubacterium rectale	+	−	−	−	+	−	ND	ND	ND
Eubacterium saburreum	+	−	+	−	+	+	ND	ND	ND
Eubacterium saphenum	−	−	−	−	−	−	ND	ND	ND
Eubacterium sulci	−	−	−	−	−	−	ND	ND	ND
Eubacterium tenue	Weak	−	+	−	−	ND	ND	ND	ND
Eubacterium yurii	Weak	−	+	−	−	−	ND	ND	ND
Filifactor alocis	−	−	−	−	−	+	ND	ND	ND
Holdemania filiformis	+	−	−	−	+	−	ND	ND	ND
Mogibacterium spp.	−	−	−	−	−	−	ND	ND	ND
Pseudoramibacter alactolyticus	+	−	−	−	−	−	ND	ND	ND
Shuttleworthia satelles	+	−	+	−	+	−	ND	ND	ND
Solobacterium moorei	+	−	−	−	+	+	ND	ND	ND

[a] Biochemical data compiled from references 32, 33, 73, 83–85, 96, 108, 109, 165, and 166. Symbols and abbreviations: +, positive reaction; −, negative reaction; v, variable reaction; ND, no data; β-Gal, β-galactosidase; β-Glu, β-glucosidase; β-NAG, β-*N*-acetyl-glucosaminidase.

resistance to clindamycin (13, 21, 38, 56, 72, 114, 144). For example, of the 304 *P. acnes* isolates collected from various human infections in 13 European countries, 15% of isolates demonstrated resistance to clindamycin (114). Isolates were also resistant to erythromycin (17%) and to tetracycline (3%), whereas all isolates were susceptible to penicillin, vancomycin, and linezolid. Although vancomycin and teicoplanin are considered active against most gram-positive bacteria, species-related resistance to glycopeptides is frequent among species of the genus *Lactobacillus*. Less than one-quarter of the isolates from 80 cases of *Lactobacillus* infections were reported as susceptible to vancomycin (16). Notably, the vancomycin-resistant *L. rhamnosus* is the most common *Lactobacillus* species in clinical specimens (45, 130). In contrast to vancomycin and teicoplanin, ramoplanin, a novel glycolipodepsipeptide, showed good activity against lactobacilli (21, 49). A novel glycopeptide, telavancin, proved to be more active than vancomycin against lactobacilli, except for *L. casei*, and demonstrated very good activity against the tested strains of *Propionibacterium*, *Actinomyces*, *Eggerthella*, and *Eubacterium* (55). Oxazolidinones represent a new class of synthetic antimicrobial agents, having relatively good in vitro activities against gram-positive cocci but also against anaerobes, and ranbezolid may have lower MICs than linezolid (13, 41). Also telithromycin, a novel ketolide, and streptogramin antimicrobial agents, such as pristinamycin and quinupristin-dalfopristin, have considerable activities against non-spore-forming gram-positive rods (13, 56, 105). Fluoroquinolones have a broad spectrum of antibacterial activity and good absorption from the gastrointestinal tract. Novel quinolones, such as garenoxacin, gatifloxacin, and moxifloxacin, exhibit better antianaerobic activity than the older quinolone compounds levofloxacin and ciprofloxacin (13, 38, 72, 100), suggesting their potential in treating mixed organism infections.

The potential presence of anaerobic gram-positive non-spore-forming rods in infections associated with biofilms and increased antimicrobial resistance of biofilms (147) needs to be taken into account. Due to the involvement of biofilms, mechanical intervention (drainage of abscesses, decompression of infected spaces, debridement of necrotic tissue, and removal of foreign bodies) can be critical in the management of these infections. In addition, appropriate coverage for both facultative and anaerobic bacteria is often necessary.

INTERPRETATION AND REPORTING OF RESULTS

Once clinically relevant isolates are recovered, their accurate classification is needed to estimate the seriousness of the infection and to select the appropriate antimicrobial therapy. Conventional identification protocols for anaerobic non-spore-forming gram-positive bacteria to the species level are laborious and time-consuming and involve substantial subjective judgment that can result in inconclusive identification. In reference anaerobic laboratories, the use of gas chromatography and/or sequencing of the 16S rRNA gene provides useful tools for organism identification.

REFERENCES

1. **Ahrné, S., S. Novaek, B. Jeppsson, Y. Adlerberth, A. E. Wold, and G. Molin.** 1998. The normal *Lactobacillus* flora of healthy human rectal and oral mucosa. *J. Appl. Microbiol.* **85:**88–94.
2. **Antonio, M. A., S. E. Hawes, and S. L. Hillier.** 1999. The identification of vaginal *Lactobacillus* species and the demographic and microbiologic characteristics of women colonized by these species. *J. Infect. Dis.* **180:**1950–1956.
3. **Bahar, H., M. M. Torun, F. Ocer, and B. Kocazeybek.** 2005. *Mobiluncus* species in gynaecological and obstetric infections: antimicrobial resistance and prevalence in a Turkish population. *Int. J. Antimicrob. Agents* **25:**268–271.
4. **Becker, M. R., B. J. Paster, E. J. Leys, M. L. Moeschberger, S. G. Kenyon, J. L. Galvin, S. K. Boches, F. E. Dewhirst, and A. L. Griffen.** 2002. Molecular analysis of bacterial species associated with childhood caries. *J. Clin. Microbiol.* **40:**1001–1009.
5. **Booth, V., J. Downes, J. Van den Berg, and W. G. Wade.** 2004. Gram-positive anaerobic bacilli in human periodontal disease. *J. Periodont. Res.* **39:**213–220.
6. **Bosshard, P. P., R. Zbinden, and M. Altwegg.** 2002. *Turicibacter sanguinis* gen. nov., sp. nov., a novel anaerobic, gram-positive bacterium. *Int. J. Syst. Evol. Microbiol.* **52:**1263–1266.
7. **Boyd, M. A., M. A. D. Antonio, and S. L. Hillier.** 2005. Comparison of API 50 CH strips to whole-chromosomal DNA probes for identification of *Lactobacillus* species. *J. Clin. Microbiol.* **43:**5309–5311.
8. **Brailsford, S. R., R. B. Tregaskis, H. S. Leftwich, and D. Beighton.** 1999. The predominant *Actinomyces* spp. isolated from infected dentin of active root caries lesions. *J. Dent. Res.* **78:**1525–1534.
9. **Brazier, J. S., and V. Hall.** 1993. *Propionibacterium propionicum* and infections of the lacrimal apparatus. *Clin. Infect. Dis.* **17:**892–893.
10. **Brook, I.** 1996. Isolation of non-sporing anaerobic rods from infections in children. *J. Med. Microbiol.* **45:**21–26.
11. **Brook, I., and E. H. Frazier.** 1991. Infections caused by *Propionibacterium* species. *Rev. Infect. Dis.* **13:**819–822.
12. **Brook, I., and E. H. Frazier.** 1993. Significant recovery of non-sporulating anaerobic rods from clinical specimens. *Clin. Infect. Dis.* **16:**476–480.
13. **Bryskier, A.** 2001. Anti-anaerobic activity of antibacterial agents. *Expert Opin. Investig. Drugs* **10:**239–267.
14. **Burton, J. P., E. Devillard, P. A. Cadieux, J.-A. Hammond, and G. Reid.** 2004. Detection of *Atopobium vaginae* in postmenopausal women by cultivation-independent methods warrants further investigation. *J. Clin. Microbiol.* **42:**1829–1831.
15. **Byun, R., M. A. Nadkarni, K.-L. Chhour, F. E. Martin, N. A. Jacques, and N. Hunter.** 2004. Quantitative analysis of diverse *Lactobacillus* species present in advanced dental caries. *J. Clin. Microbiol.* **42:**3128–3136.
16. **Cannon, J. P., T. A. Lee, J. T. Bolanos, and L. H. Danziger.** 2005. Pathogenic relevance of *Lactobacillus:* a retrospective review of over 200 cases. *Eur. J. Clin. Microbiol. Infect. Dis.* **24:**31–40.
17. **Carlier, J.-P., G. K'ouas, I. Bonne, A. Lozniewski, and F. Mory.** 2004. *Oribacterium sinus* gen. nov., sp. nov., within the family '*Lachnospiraceae*' (phylum Firmicutes). *Int. J. Syst. Evol. Microbiol.* **54:**1611–1615.
18. **Chavez de Paz, L. E., A. Molander, and G. Dahlén.** 2004. Gram-positive rods prevailing in teeth with apical periodontitis undergoing root canal treatment. *Int. Endod. J.* **37:**579–587.
19. **Chhour, K. L., M. A. Nadkarni, R. Byun, F. E. Martin, N. A. Jacques, and N. Hunter.** 2005. Molecular analysis of microbial diversity in advanced caries. *J. Clin. Microbiol.* **43:**843–849.
20. **Citron, D. M.** 1999. Rapid identification of anaerobes in the clinical laboratory. *Anaerobe* **5:**109–113.
21. **Citron, D. M., C. V. Merriam, K. L. Tyrrell, Y. A. Warren, H. Fernandez, and E. J. Goldstein.** 2003. In vitro activities of ramoplanin, teicoplanin, vancomycin, linezolid, bacitracin, and four other antimicrobials against intestinal anaerobic bacteria. *Antimicrob. Agents Chemother.* **47:**2334–2338.
22. **Clark, W. L., P. K. Kaiser, H. W. Flynn, Jr., A. Belfort, D. Miller, and D. M. Meisler.** 1999. Treatment strategies and visual acuity outcomes in chronic postoperative *Propionibacterium acnes* endophthalmitis. *Ophthalmology* **106:**1665–1670.
23. **Clarridge, J. E., III, and Q. Zhang.** 2002. Genotypic diversity of clinical *Actinomyces* species: phenotype, source, and disease correlation among genospecies. *J. Clin. Microbiol.* **40:**3442–3448.
24. **Collins, M. D., L. Hoyles, S. Kalfas, G. Sundquist, T. Monsen, N. Nikolaitchouk, and E. Falsen.** 2000. Characterization of *Actinomyces* isolates from infected root canals of teeth: description of *Actinomyces radicidentis* sp. nov. *J. Clin. Microbiol.* **38:**3399–3403.
25. **Collins, M. D., P. A. Lawson, A. Willems, J. J. Cordoba, J. Fernandez-Garayzabal, P. Garcia, J. Cai, H. Hippe, and J. A. Farrow.** 1994. The phylogeny of the genus *Clostridium:* proposal of five new genera and eleven new species combinations. *Int. J. Syst. Bacteriol.* **44:**812–826.
26. **Collins, M. D., and S. Wallbanks.** 1992. Comparative sequence analyses of the 16S rRNA genes of *Lactobacillus minutus*, *Lactobacillus rimae* and *Streptococcus parvulus:* proposal for the creation of a new genus *Atopobium*. *FEMS Microbiol. Lett.* **74:**235–240.
27. **Crociani, F., B. Biavati, A. Alessandrini, C. Chiarini, and V. Scardovi.** 1996. *Bifidobacterium inopinatum* sp. nov. and *Bifidobacterium denticolens* sp. nov., two new species isolated from human dental caries. *Int. J. Syst. Bacteriol.* **46:**564–571.
28. **Delaney, M. L., and A. B. Onderdonk.** 1997. Evaluation of the AnaeroPack system for growth of clinically significant anaerobes. *J. Clin. Microbiol.* **35:**558–562.
29. **Delyle, L. G., O. Vittecoq, A. Bourdel, F. Duparc, C. Michot, and X. Le Loet.** 2000. Chronic destructive oligoarthritis associated with *Propionibacterium acnes* in a female patient with acne vulgaris: septic-reactive arthritis? *Arthr. Rheum.* **43:**2843–2847.
30. **Dewhirst, F. E., B. J. Paster, N. Tzellas, B. Coleman, J. Downes, D. A. Spratt, and W. G. Wade.** 2001. Characterization of novel human oral isolates and cloned 16S rDNA sequences that fall in the family *Coriobacteriaceae:* description of *Olsenella* gen. nov., reclassification of *Lactobacillus uli* as *Olsenella uli* comb. nov. and description of *Olsenella profusa* sp. nov. *Int. J. Syst. Evol. Microbiol.* **51:**1797–1804.
31. **Doan, N., A. Contreras, J. Flynn, J. Morrison, and J. Slots.** 1999. Proficiencies of three anaerobic culture systems for recovering periodontal pathogenic bacteria. *J. Clin. Microbiol.* **37:**171–174.
32. **Downes, J., M. A. Munson, D. R. Radford, D. A. Spratt, and W. G. Wade.** 2002. *Shuttleworthia satelles* gen. nov., sp. nov., isolated from the human oral cavity. *Int. J. Syst. Evol. Microbiol.* **52:**1469–1475.
33. **Downes, J., M. A. Munson, D. A. Spratt, E. Kononen, E. Tarkka, H. Jousimies-Somer, and W. G. Wade.** 2001. Characterisation of *Eubacterium*-like strains isolated from oral infections. *J. Med. Microbiol.* **50:**947–951.

34. **Downes, J., B. Olsvik, S. J. Hiom, D. A. Spratt, S. L. Cheeseman, I. Olsen, A. J. Weightman, and W. G. Wade.** 2000. *Bulleidia extructa* gen. nov., sp. nov., isolated from the oral cavity. *Int. J. Syst. Evol. Microbiol.* **50:**979–983.
35. **Drancourt, M., P. Berger, and D. Raoult.** 2004. Systematic 16S rRNA gene sequencing of atypical clinical isolates identified 27 new bacterial species associated with humans. *J. Clin. Microbiol.* **42:**2197–2202.
36. **Duncan, S. H., G. L. Hold, A. Barcenilla, C. S. Stewart, and H. J. Flint.** 2002. *Roseburia intestinalis* sp. nov., a novel saccharolytic, butyrate-producing bacterium from human faeces. *Int. J. Syst. Evol. Microbiol.* **52:**1615–1620.
37. **Duncan, S. H., G. L. Hold, H. J. Harmsen, C. S. Stewart, and H. J. Flint.** 2002. Growth requirements and fermentation products of *Fusobacterium prausnitzii,* and a proposal to reclassify it as *Faecalibacterium prausnitzii* gen. nov., comb. nov. *Int. J. Syst. Evol. Microbiol.* **52:**2141–2146.
38. **Edmiston, C. E., C. J. Krepel, G. R. Seabrook, L. R. Somberg, A. Nakeeb, R. A. Cambria, and J. B. Towne.** 2004. In vitro activities of moxifloxacin against 900 aerobic and anaerobic surgical isolates from patients with intra-abdominal and diabetic foot infections. *Antimicrob. Agents Chemother.* **48:**1012–1016.
39. **Edmiston, C., E., Jr., C. J. Krepel, G. R. Seabrook, and W. G. Jochimsen.** 2002. Anaerobic infections in the surgical patient: microbial etiology and therapy. *Clin. Infect. Dis.* **35**(Suppl. 1):S112–S118.
40. **Edmiston, C. E., Jr., C. J. Krepel, and A. P. Walker.** 1989. Recovery of *Mobiluncus curtisii* subspecies *holmesii* from mixed non-puerperal breast abscess. *Eur. J. Clin. Microbiol. Infect. Dis.* **8:**315–316.
41. **Ednie, L. M., A. Rattan, M. R. Jacobs, and P. C. Appelbaum.** 2003. Antianaerobe activity of RBX 7644 (ranbezolid), a new oxazolidinone, compared with those of eight other agents. *Antimicrob. Agents Chemother.* **47:** 1143–1147.
42. **Eishi, Y., M. Suga, I. Ishige, D. Kobayashi, T. Yamada, T. Takemura, T. Takizawa, M. Koike, S. Kudoh, U. Castabel, J. Guzman, G. Rizzato, M. Gambacorta, R. du Bois, A. G. Nicholson, O. P. Sharma, and M. Ando.** 2002. Quantitative analysis of mycobacterial and propionibacterial DNA in lymph nodes of Japanese and European patients with sarcoidosis. *J. Clin. Microbiol.* **40:**198–204.
43. **Estoppey, O., G. Rivier, C. H. Blanc, F. Widmer, A. Gallusser, and A. K. So.** 1997. *Propionibacterium avidum* sacroiliitis and osteomyelitis. *Rev. Rhum. Engl. Ed.* **64:**54–56.
44. **Falsen, E., C. Pascual, B. Sjödén, M. Ohlén, and M. D. Collins.** 1999. Phenotypic and phylogenetic characterisation of a novel *Lactobacillus* species from human sources: description of *Lactobacillus iners* sp. nov. *Int. J. Syst. Bacteriol.* **49:**217–221.
45. **Felten, A., C. Barreau, C. Bizet, P. H. Lagrange, and A. Philippon.** 1999. *Lactobacillus* species identification, H_2O_2 production, and antibiotic resistance and correlation with human clinical status. *J. Clin. Microbiol.* **37:**729–733.
46. **Fendukly, F., and B. Osterman.** 2005. Isolation of *Actinobaculum schaalii* and *Actinobaculum urinale* from a patient with chronic renal failure. *J. Clin. Microbiol.* **43:**3567–3569.
47. **Ferris, M. J., A. Masztal, K. E. Aldridge, J. D. Fortenberry, P. L. Fidel, Jr., and D. H. Martin.** 2004. Association of *Atopobium vaginae,* a recently described metronidazole resistant anaerobe, with bacterial vaginosis. *BMC Infect. Dis.* **4:**5.
48. **Finegold, S. M., P. A. Lawson, M.-L. Vaisanen, D. R. Molitoris, Y. Song, C. Liu, and M. D. Collins.** 2004. *Anaerofustis stercorihominis* gen. nov., sp. nov., from human feces. *Anaerobe* **10:**41–45.
49. **Finegold, S. M., S. St. John, A. W. Vu, C. M. Li, D. Molitoris, Y. Song, C. Liu, and H. M. Wexler.** 2004. In vitro activity of ramoplanin and comparator drugs against anaerobic intestinal bacteria from the perspective of potential utility in pathology involving bowel flora. *Anaerobe* **10:**205–211.
50. **Fiorino, A. S.** 1996. Intrauterine contraceptive device-associated actinomycotic abscess and *Actinomyces* detection on cervical smear. *Obstet. Gynecol.* **87:**142–149.
51. **Funke, G., A. von Graevenitz, J. E. Clarridge III, and K. E. Bernard.** 1997. Clinical microbiology of coryneform bacteria. *Clin. Microbiol. Rev.* **10:**125–159.
52. **Geissdörfer, W., C. Böhmer, K. Pelz, C. Schoerner, W. Frobenius, and C. Bogdan.** 2003. Tuboovarian abscess caused by *Atopobium vaginae* following transvaginal oocyte recovery. *J. Clin. Microbiol.* **41:**2788–2790.
53. **Goldstein, E. J. C., D. M. Citron, and R. J. Goldman.** 1992. National hospital survey of anaerobic culture and susceptibility testing methods: results and recommendations for improvement. *J. Clin. Microbiol.* **30:**1529–1534.
54. **Goldstein, E. J., D. M. Citron, C. V. Merriam, Y. Warren, K. L. Tyrrell, and H. Fernandez.** 2003. In vitro activities of telithromycin and 10 oral agents against aerobic and anaerobic pathogens isolated from antral puncture specimens from patients with sinusitis. *Antimicrob. Agents Chemother.* **47:**1963–1967.
55. **Goldstein, E. J., D. M. Citron, C. V. Merriam, Y. A. Warren, K. L. Tyrrell, and H. T. Fernandez.** 2004. In vitro activities of the new semisynthetic glycopeptide telavancin (TD-6424), vancomycin, daptomycin, linezolid, and four comparator agents against anaerobic gram-positive species and *Corynebacterium* spp. *Antimicrob. Agents Chemother.* **48:**2149–2152.
56. **Goldstein, E. J., D. M. Citron, C. V. Merriam, Y. A. Warren, K. L. Tyrrell, H. T. Fernandez, and A. Bryskier.** 2005. Comparative in vitro activities of XRP 2868, pristinamycin, quinupristin-dalfopristin, vancomycin, daptomycin, linezolid, clarithromycin, telithromycin, clindamycin, and ampicillin against anaerobic gram-positive species, actinomycetes, and lactobacilli. *Antimicrob. Agents Chemother.* **49:**408–413.
57. **Gomez-Garces, J. L., D. Balas, M. T. Merino, and J. Ignacio Alos.** 1994. *Mobiluncus curtisii* bacteremia following septic abortion. *Clin. Infect. Dis.* **19:**1166–1167.
58. **Greub, G., and D. Raoult.** 2002. "*Actinobaculum massiliae*," a new species causing chronic urinary tract infection. *J. Clin. Microbiol.* **40:**3938–3941.
59. **Günthard, H., A. Hany, M. Turina, and J. Wüst.** 1994. *Propionibacterium acnes* as a cause of aggressive aortic valve endocarditis and importance of tissue grinding: case report and review. *J. Clin. Microbiol.* **32:**3043–3045.
60. **Hahn, F., R. Zbinden, and K. Min.** 2005. Late implant infections caused by *Propionibacterium acnes* in scoliosis surgery. *Eur. Spine J.* **14:**783–788.
61. **Halebian, S., B. Harris, S. M. Finegold, and R. D. Rolfe.** 1981. Rapid method that aids in distinguishing gram-positive from gram-negative anaerobic bacteria. *J. Clin. Microbiol.* **13:**444–448.
62. **Hall, V., M. D. Collins, R. Hutson, E. Falsen, and B. I. Duerden.** 2002. *Actinomyces cardiffensis* sp. nov. from human clinical sources. *J. Clin. Microbiol.* **40:**3427–3431.
63. **Hall, V., M. D. Collins, R. A. Hutson, E. Falsen, E. Inganas, and B. I. Duerden.** 2003. *Actinobaculum urinale* sp. nov., from human urine. *Int. J. Syst. Evol. Microbiol.* **53:** 679–682.
64. **Hall, V., M. D. Collins, R. A. Hutson, E. Inganas, E. Falsen, and B. I. Duerden.** 2003. *Actinomyces oricola* sp. nov., from a human dental abscess. *Int. J. Syst. Evol. Microbiol.* **53:**1515–1518.
65. **Hall, V., M. D. Collins, P. A. Lawson, E. Falsen, and B. I. Duerden.** 2003. *Actinomyces nasicola* sp. nov., isolated from a human nose. *Int. J. Syst. Evol. Microbiol.* **53:**1445–1448.

66. **Hall, V., M. D. Collins, P. A. Lawson, E. Falsen, and B. I. Duerden.** 2005. *Actinomyces dentalis* sp. nov., from a human dental abscess. *Int. J. Syst. Evol. Microbiol.* **55:**427–431.
67. **Hall, V., M. D. Collins, P. A. Lawson, R. A. Hutson, E. Falsen, E. Inganas, and B. Duerden.** 2003. Characterization of some *Actinomyces*-like isolates from human clinical sources: description of *Varibaculum cambriensis* gen. nov., sp. nov. *J. Clin. Microbiol.* **41:**640–644.
68. **Hall, V., P. R. Talbot, S. L. Stubbs, and B. I. Duerden.** 2001. Identification of clinical isolates of *Actinomyces* species by amplified 16S ribosomal DNA restriction analysis (ARDRA). *J. Clin. Microbiol.* **39:**3555–3562.
69. **Hammes, W. P., and C. Hertel.** 2003. The genera *Lactobacillus* and *Carnobacterium*. *In* M. Dworkin (ed.), *The Prokaryotes: an Evolving Electronic Resource for the Microbiological Community,* 3rd ed. [Online.] Springer-Verlag, New York, N.Y. http://link.springer-ny.com/link/service/books/10125/.
70. **Harmsen, H. J., A. C. Wildeboer-Veloo, J. Grijpstra, J. Knol, J. E. Degener, and G. W. Welling.** 2000. Development of 16S rRNA-based probes for the *Coriobacterium* group and the *Atopobium* cluster and their application for enumeration of *Coriobacteriaceae* in human feces from volunteers of different age groups. *Appl. Environ. Microbiol.* **66:**4523–4527.
71. **Hashimura, T., M. Sato, and E. Hoshino.** 2001. Detection of *Slackia exigua, Mogibacterium timidum* and *Eubacterium saphenum* from pulpal and periradicular samples using the polymerase chain reaction (PCR) method. *Int. Endod. J.* **34:**463–470.
72. **Hecht, D. W., and J. R. Osmolski.** 2003. Activities of garenoxacin (BMS-284756) and other agents against anaerobic clinical isolates. *Antimicrob. Agents Chemother.* **47:**910–916.
73. **Hill, G. B., O. M. Ayers, and A. P. Kohan.** 1987. Characteristics and sites of infection of *Eubacterium nodatum, Eubacterium timidum, Eubacterium brachy,* and other asaccharolytic eubacteria. *J. Clin. Microbiol.* **25:**1540–1545.
74. **Hoellman, D. B., L. M. Kelly, K. Credito, L. Anthony, L. M. Ednie, M. R. Jacobs, and P. C. Appelbaum.** 2002. In vitro antianaerobic activity of ertapenem (MK-0826) compared to seven other compounds. *Antimicrob. Agents Chemother.* **46:**220–224.
75. **Holst, E., A. R. Goffeng, and B. Andersch.** 1994. Bacterial vaginosis and vaginal microorganisms in idiopathic premature labor and association with pregnancy outcome. *J. Clin. Microbiol.* **32:**176–186.
76. **Hoyles, L., M. D. Collins, E. Falsen, N. Nikolaitchouk, and A. L. McCartney.** 2004. Transfer of members of the genus *Falcivibrio* to the genus *Mobiluncus,* and emended description of the genus *Mobiluncus*. *Syst. Appl. Microbiol.* **27:**72–83.
77. **Hoyles, L., E. Inganas, E. Falsen, M. Drancourt, N. Weiss, A. L. McCartney, and M. D. Collins.** 2002. *Bifidobacterium scardovii* sp. nov., from human sources. *Int. J. Syst. Bacteriol.* **52:**995–999.
78. **Ison, C. A., and P. E. Hay.** 2002. Validation of a simplified grading of Gram stained vaginal smears for use in genitourinary medicine clinics. *Sex. Transm. Infect.* **78:**413–415.
79. **Jakab, E., R. Zbinden, J. Gubler, C. Ruef, A. von Graevenitz, and M. Krause.** 1996. Severe infections caused by *Propionibacterium acnes:* an underestimated pathogen in late postoperative infections. *Yale J. Biol. Med.* **69:**477–482.
80. **Jalava, J., and E. Eerola.** 1999. Phylogenetic analysis of *Fusobacterium alocis* and *Fusobacterium sulci* based on 16S rRNA gene sequences: proposal of *Filifactor alocis* (Cato, Moore and Moore) comb. nov. and *Eubacterium sulci* (Cato, Moore and Moore) comb. nov. *Int. J. Syst. Bacteriol.* **49:**1375–1379.
81. **Jian, W., and X. Dong.** 2002. Transfer of *Bifidobacterium inopinatum* and *Bifidobacterium denticolens* to *Scardovia inopinata* gen. nov., comb. nov., and *Parascardovia denticolens* gen. nov., comb. nov., respectively. *Int. J. Syst. Evol. Microbiol.* **52:**809–812.
82. **Johnson, M. J., E. Thatcher, and M. E. Cox.** 1995. Techniques for controlling variability in gram staining of obligate anaerobes. *J. Clin. Microbiol.* **33:**755–758.
83. **Jousimies-Somer, H. R., P. Summanen, D. M. Citron, E. J. Baron, H. M. Wexler, and S. M. Finegold.** 2002. *Wadsworth-KTL Anaerobic Bacteriology Manual,* 6th ed. Star Publishing, Belmont, Calif.
84. **Kageyama, A., and Y. Benno.** 2000. *Catenibacterium mitsuokai* gen. nov., sp. nov., a gram-positive anaerobic bacterium isolated from human faeces. *Int. J. Syst. Evol. Microbiol.* **50:**1595–1599.
85. **Kageyama, A., and Y. Benno.** 2000. Emendation of genus *Collinsella* and proposal of *Collinsella stercoris* sp. nov. and *Collinsella intestinalis* sp. nov. *Int. J. Syst. Evol. Microbiol.* **50:**1767–1774.
86. **Kageyama, A., and Y. Benno.** 2000. Phylogenic and phenotypic characterization of some *Eubacterium*-like isolates from human feces: description of *Solobacterium moorei* gen. nov., sp. nov. *Microbiol. Immunol.* **44:**223–227.
87. **Kageyama, A., Y. Benno, and T. Nakase.** 1999. Phylogenic and phenotypic evidence for the transfer of *Eubacterium fossor* to the genus *Atopobium* as *Atopobium fossor* comb. nov. *Microbiol. Immunol.* **43:**389–395.
88. **Kageyama, A., Y. Benno, and T. Nakase.** 1999. Phylogenetic and phenotypic evidence for the transfer of *Eubacterium aerofaciens* to the genus *Collinsella* as *Collinsella aerofaciens* gen. nov., comb. nov. *Int. J. Syst. Bacteriol.* **49:**557–565.
89. **Klein, G., E. Zill, R. Schindler, and J. Louwers.** 1998. Peritonitis associated with vancomycin-resistant *Lactobacillus rhamnosus* in a continuous ambulatory peritoneal dialysis patient: organism identification, antibiotic therapy, and case report. *J. Clin. Microbiol.* **36:**1781–1783.
90. **Kolbert, C. P., and D. H. Persing.** 1999. Ribosomal DNA sequencing as a tool for identification of bacterial pathogens. *Curr. Opin. Microbiol.* **2:**299–305.
91. **Kotilainen, P., R. Merilahti-Palo, O.-P. Lehtonen, I. Manner, I. Helander, T. Möttönen, and E. Rintala.** 1996. *Propionibacterium acnes* isolated from sternal osteitis in a patient with SAPHO syndrome. *J. Rheumatol.* **23:**1302–1304.
92. **Kumar, P. S., A. L. Griffen, J. A. Barton, B. J. Paster, M. L. Moeschberger, and E. J. Leys.** 2003. New bacterial species associated with chronic periodontitis. *J. Dent. Res.* **82:**338–344.
93. **Land, M. H., K. Rouster-Stevens, C. R. Woods, M. L. Cannon, J. Cnota, and A. K. Shetty.** 2005. *Lactobacillus* sepsis associated with probiotic therapy. *Pediatrics* **115:**178–181.
94. **Larsson, P.-G., B. Carlsson, L. Fåhraeus, T. Jakobsson, and U. Forsum.** 2004. Diagnosis of bacterial vaginosis: need for validation of microscopic image area used for scoring bacterial morphotypes. *Sex. Transm. Infect.* **80:**63–67.
95. **Lau, S. K., P. C. Woo, A. M. Fung, K. M. Chan, G. K. Woo, and K. Y. Yuen.** 2004. Anaerobic, non-sporulating, gram-positive bacilli bacteraemia characterized by 16S rRNA gene sequencing. *J. Med. Microbiol.* **53:**1247–1253.
96. **Lau, S. K., P. C. Woo, G. K. Woo A. M. Fung, M. K. Wong, K. M. Chan, D. M. Tam, and K. Y. Yuen.** 2004. *Eggerthella hongkongensis* sp. nov. and *Eggerthella sinensis* sp. nov., two novel *Eggerthella* species, account for half of the cases of *Eggerthella* bacteremia. *Diagn. Microbiol. Infect. Dis.* **49:**255–263.
97. **Lawson, P. A., E. Falsen, E. Akervall, P. Vandamme, and M. D. Collins.** 1997. Characterization of some *Actinomyces*-like isolates from human clinical specimens: reclassification of *Actinomyces suis* (Soltys and Spratling) as *Actinobaculum suis* comb. nov. and description of *Actinobaculum schaalii* sp. nov. *Int. J. Syst. Bacteriol.* **47:**899–903.

98. **Lawson, P. A., N. Nikolaitchouk, E. Falsen, K. Westling, and M. D. Collins.** 2001. *Actinomyces funkei* sp. nov., isolated from human clinical specimens. *Int. J. Syst. Bacteriol.* **51:**853–855.
99. **Lawson, P. A., Y. Song, C. Liu, D. R. Molitoris, M. L. Vaisanen, M. D. Collins, and S. M. Finegold.** 2004. *Anaerotruncus colihominis* gen. nov., sp. nov., from human faeces. *Int. J. Syst. Evol. Microbiol.* **54:**413–417.
100. **Liebetrau, A., A. C. Rodloff, J. Behra-Miellet, and L. Dubreuil.** 2003. In vitro activities of a new des-fluoro(6) quinolone, garenoxacin, against clinical anaerobic bacteria. *Antimicrob. Agents Chemother.* **47:**3667–3671.
101. **Mackay, A. D., M. B. Taylor, C. C. Kibbler, and J. M. Hamilton-Miller.** 1999. *Lactobacillus* endocarditis caused by a probiotic organism. *Clin. Microbiol. Infect.* **5:**290–292.
102. **Miyamoto, M. I., and F. C. Fang.** 1993. Pyogenic liver abscess involving *Actinomyces:* case report and review. *Clin. Infect. Dis.* **16:**303–309.
103. **Moore, W. E. C., and L. V. Holdeman Moore.** 1986. Genus *Eubacterium*, p. 1353–1373. *In* P. H. A. Sneath, N. S. Mair, M. E. Sharpe, and J. G. Holt (ed.), *Bergey's Manual of Systematic Bacteriology*, 1st ed. The Williams and Wilkins Co., Baltimore, Md.
104. **Mosca, A., P. Summanen, S. M. Finegold, G. De Michele, and G. Miragliotta.** 1998. Cellular fatty acid composition, soluble-protein profile, and antimicrobial resistance pattern of *Eubacterium lentum*. *J. Clin. Microbiol.* **36:**752–755.
105. **Moubareck, C., F. Gavini, L. Vaugien, M. J. Butel, and F. Doucet-Populaire.** 2005. Antimicrobial susceptibility of bifidobacteria. *J. Antimicrob. Chemother.* **55:**38–44.
106. **Munson, M. A., A. Banerjee, T. F. Watson, and W. G. Wade.** 2004. Molecular analysis of the microflora associated with dental caries. *J. Clin. Microbiol.* **42:**3023–3029.
107. **Munson, M. A., T. Pitt-Ford, B. Chong, A. Weightman, and W. G. Wade.** 2002. Molecular and cultural analysis of the microflora associated with endodontic infections. *J. Dent. Res.* **81:**761–766.
108. **Nakazawa, F., S. E. Poco, T. Ikeda, M. Sato, S. Kalfas, G. Sundqvist, and E. Hoshino.** 1999. *Cryptobacterium curtum* gen. nov., sp. nov., a new genus of gram-positive anaerobic rod isolated from human oral cavities. *Int. J. Syst. Bacteriol.* **49:**1193–1200.
109. **Nakazawa, F., S. E. Poco, Jr., M. Sato, T. Ikeda, S. Kalfas, G. Sundqvist, and E. Hoshino.** 2002. Taxonomic characterization of *Mogibacterium diversum* sp. nov. and *Mogibacterium neglectum* sp. nov., isolated from human oral cavities. *Int. J. Syst. Evol. Microbiol.* **52:**115–122.
110. **Nakazawa, F., M. Sato, S. E. Poco, T. Hashimura, T. Ikeda, S. Kalfas, G. Sundqvist, and E. Hoshino.** 2000. Description of *Mogibacterium pumilum* gen. nov., sp. nov. and *Mogibacterium vescum* gen. nov., sp. nov., and reclassification of *Eubacterium timidum* (Holdeman et al. 1980) as *Mogibacterium timidum* gen. nov., comb. nov. *Int. J. Syst. Evol. Microbiol.* **50:**679–688.
111. **Neef, P. A., H. Polenakovik, J. E. Clarridge., M. Saklayen, L. Bogard, and J. M. Bernstein.** 2003. *Lactobacillus paracasei* continuous ambulatory peritoneal dialysis-related peritonitis and review of the literature. *J. Clin. Microbiol.* **41:**2783–2784.
112. **Nugent, R. P., M. A. Krohn, and S. L. Hillier.** 1991. Reliability of diagnosing bacterial vaginosis is improved by a standardized method of gram stain interpretation. *J. Clin. Microbiol.* **29:**297–301.
113. **Olsen, I., J. L. Johnson, L. V. Moore, and W. E. Moore.** 1991. *Lactobacillus uli* sp. nov. and *Lactobacillus rimae* sp. nov. from the human gingival crevice and emended descriptions of *Lactobacillus minutus* and *Streptococcus parvulus*. *Int. J. Syst. Bacteriol.* **41:**261–266.
114. **Oprica, C., C. E. Nord, and the ESCMID Study Group on Antimicrobial Resistance in Anaerobic Bacteria.** 2005. European surveillance study on the antibiotic susceptibility of *Propionibacterium acnes*. *Clin. Microbiol. Infect.* **11:**204–213.
115. **Pajkrt, D., A. M. Simoons-Smit, P. H. Savelkoul, J. van den Hoek, W. W. Hack, and A. M. van Furth.** 2003. Pyelonephritis caused by *Actinobaculum schaalii* in a child with pyeloureteral junction obstruction. *Eur. J. Clin. Microbiol. Infect. Dis.* **22:**438–440.
116. **Pascual Ramos, C., G. Foster, and M. D. Collins.** 1997. Phylogenetic analysis of the genus *Actinomyces* based on 16S rRNA gene sequences: description of *Arcanobacterium phocae* sp. nov., *Arcanobacterium bernardiae* comb. nov., and *Arcanobacterium pyogenes* comb. nov. *Int. J. Syst. Bacteriol.* **47:**46–53.
117. **Paster, B. J., S. K. Boches, J. L. Galvin, R. E. Ericson, C. N. Lau, V. A. Levanos, A. Sahasrabudhe, and F. E. Dewhirst.** 2001. Bacterial diversity in subgingival plaque. *J. Bacteriol.* **183:**3770–3783.
118. **Pei, Z., E. J. Bini, L. Yang, M. Zhou, F. Francois, and M. J. Blaser.** 2004. Bacterial biota in the human distal esophagus. *Proc. Natl. Acad. Sci. USA* **101:**4250–4255.
119. **Racklyeft, D. J., and D. N. Love.** 2000. Bacterial infection of the lower respiratory tract in 34 horses. *Aust. Vet. J.* **78:**549–559.
120. **Rautio, M., H. Jousimies-Somer, H. Kauma, I. Pietarinen, M. Saxelin, S. Tynkkynen, and M. Koskela.** 1999. Liver abscess due to a *Lactobacillus rhamnosus* strain indistinguishable from *L. rhamnosus* strain GG. *Clin. Infect. Dis.* **28:**1159–1160.
121. **Rautio, M., H. Saxen, A. Siitonen, R. Nikku, and H. Jousimies-Somer.** 2000. Bacteriology of histopathologically defined appendicitis in children. *Pediatr. Infect. Dis. J.* **19:**1078–1083.
122. **Reinhard, M., J. Prag, M. Kemp, K. Andresen, B. Klemmensen, N. Højlyng, S. H. Sørensen, and J. J. Christensen.** 2005. Ten cases of *Actinobaculum schaalii* infection: clinical relevance, bacterial identification, and antibiotic susceptibility. *J. Clin. Microbiol.* **43:**5305–5308.
123. **Rocas, I. N., and J. F. Siqueira, Jr.** 2005. Species-directed 16S rRNA gene nested PCR detection of *Olsenella* species in association with endodontic diseases. *Lett. Appl. Microbiol.* **41:**12–16.
124. **Rodriguez Jovita, M., M. D. Collins, B. Sjöden, and E. Falsen.** 1999. Characterization of a novel *Atopobium* isolate from the human vagina: description of *Atopobium vaginae* sp. nov. *Int. J. Syst. Bacteriol.* **49:**1573–1576.
125. **Rohner, P., B. Pepey, and R. Auckenthaler.** 1997. Advantage of combining resin with lytic BACTEC blood culture media. *J. Clin. Microbiol.* **35:**2634–2638.
126. **Rolph, H. J., A. Lennon, M. P. Riggio, W. P. Saunders, D. MacKenzie, L. Coldero, and J. Bagg.** 2001. Molecular identification of microorganisms from endodontic infections. *J. Clin. Microbiol.* **39:**3282–3289.
127. **Roos, S., L. Engstrand, and H. Jonsson.** 2005. *Lactobacillus gastricus* sp. nov., *Lactobacillus antri* sp. nov., *Lactobacillus kalixensis* sp. nov. and *Lactobacillus ultunensis* sp. nov., isolated from human stomach mucosa. *Int. J. Syst. Evol. Microbiol.* **55:**77–82.
128. **Sabbe, L. J. M., D. Van de Merwe, L. Schouls, A. Bergmans, M. Vaneechoutte, and P. Vandamme.** 1999. Clinical spectrum of infections due to the newly described *Actinomyces* species *A. turicensis*, *A. radingae*, and *A. europaeus*. *J. Clin. Microbiol.* **37:**8–13.
129. **Sakata, S., M. Kitahara, M. Sakamoto, H. Hayashi, M. Fukuyama, and Y. Benno.** 2002. Unification of *Bifidobacterium infantis* and *Bifidobacterium suis* as *Bifidobacterium longum*. *Int. J. Syst. Evol. Microbiol.* **52:** 1945–1951.

130. **Salminen, M. K., H. Rautelin, S. Tynkkynen, T. Poussa, M. Saxelin, V. Valtonen, and A. Järvinen.** 2004. *Lactobacillus* bacteremia, clinical significance, and patient outcome, with special focus on probiotic *L. rhamnosus* GG. *Clin. Infect. Dis.* **38:**62–69.

131. **Salonen, J. H., E. Eerola, and O. Meurman.** 1998. Clinical significance and outcome of anaerobic bacteremia. *Clin. Infect. Dis.* **26:**1413–1417.

132. **Santala, A.-M., N. Sarkonen, V. Hall, P. Carlson, H. Jousimies-Somer, and E. Könönen.** 2004. Evaluation of four commercial test systems for identification of *Actinomyces* and some closely related species. *J. Clin. Microbiol.* **42:**418–420.

133. **Sarkonen, N., E. Könönen, E. Eerola, M. Könönen, H. Jousimies-Somer, and P. Laine.** 2005. Characterization of *Actinomyces* species isolated from failed dental implant fixtures. *Anaerobe* **11:**231–237.

134. **Sarkonen, N., E. Könönen, P. Summanen, A. Kanervo, A. Takala, and H. Jousimies-Somer.** 2000. Oral colonization with *Actinomyces* species in infants by two years of age. *J. Dent. Res.* **79:**864–867.

135. **Sarkonen, N., E. Könönen, P. Summanen, M. Könönen, and H. Jousimies-Somer.** 2001. Phenotypic identification of *Actinomyces* and related species isolated from human sources. *J. Clin. Microbiol.* **39:**3955–3961.

136. **Schaal, K. P., and H. J. Lee.** 1992. Actinomycete infections in humans—a review. *Gene* **115:**201–211.

137. **Schabereiter-Gurtner, C., S. Maca, S. Kaminsky, S. Rolleke, W. Lubitz, and T. Barisani-Asenbauer.** 2002. Investigation of an anaerobic microbial community associated with a corneal ulcer by denaturing gradient gel electrophoresis and 16S rDNA sequence analysis. *Diagn. Microbiol. Infect. Dis.* **43:**193–199.

138. **Schwebke, J. R., and L. F. Lawing.** 2001. Prevalence of *Mobiluncus* spp. among women with and without bacterial vaginosis as detected by polymerase chain reaction. *Sex. Transm. Dis.* **28:**195–199.

139. **Schwebke, J. R., S. A. Lukehart, M. C. Roberts, and S. L. Hillier.** 1991. Identification of two new antigenic subgroups within the genus *Mobiluncus*. *J. Clin. Microbiol.* **29:**2204–2208.

140. **Schwiertz, A., G. L. Hold, S. H. Duncan, B. Gruhl, M. D. Collins, P. A. Lawson, H. J. Flint, and M. Blaut.** 2002. *Anaerostipes caccae* gen. nov., sp. nov., a new saccharolytic, acetate-utilising, butyrate-producing bacterium from human faeces. *Syst. Appl. Microbiol.* **25:**46–51.

141. **Siqueira, J. F., Jr., and I. N. Rocas.** 2003. Detection of *Filifactor alocis* in endodontic infections associated with different forms of periradicular diseases. *Oral Microbiol. Immunol.* **18:**263–265.

142. **Siqueira, J. F., Jr., and I. N. Rocas.** 2003. Polymerase chain reaction detection of *Propionibacterium propionicus* and *Actinomyces radicidentis* in primary and persistent endodontic infections. *Oral Surg. Oral Med. Oral Pathol. Oral Radiol. Endod.* **96:**215–222.

143. **Siqueira, J. F., Jr., and I. N. Rocas.** 2003. *Pseudoramibacter alactolyticus* in primary endodontic infections. *J. Endod.* **29:**735–738.

144. **Smith, A. J., V. Hall, B. Thakker, and C. G. Gemmell.** 2005. Antimicrobial susceptibility testing of *Actinomyces* species with 12 antimicrobial agents. *J. Antimicrob. Chemother.* **56:**407–409.

145. **Song, Y.-L., N. Kato, Y. Matsumiya, C.-X. Liu, H. Kato, and K. Watanabe.** 1999. Identification of and hydrogen peroxide production by fecal and vaginal lactobacilli isolated from Japanese women and newborn infants. *J. Clin. Microbiol.* **37:**3062–3064.

146. **Stackebrandt, E., P. Schumann, K. P. Schaal, and N. Weiss.** 2002. *Propionimicrobium* gen. nov., a new genus to accommodate *Propionibacterium lymphophilum* (Torrey 1916) Johnson and Cummins 1972, 1057AL as *Propionimicrobium lymphophilum* comb. nov. *Int. J. Syst. Evol. Microbiol.* **52:**1925–1927.

147. **Stewart, P. S., and J. W. Costerton.** 2001. Antibiotic resistance of bacteria in biofilms. *Lancet* **358:**135–138.

148. **Strazzeri, J. C., and S. Anzel.** 1986. Infected total hip arthroplasty due to *Actinomyces israelii* after dental extraction. A case report. *Clin. Orthop. Relat. Res.* **210:**128–131.

149. **Suau, A., R. Bonnet, M. Sutren, J. J. Godon, G. R. Gibson, M. D. Collins, and J. Dore.** 1999. Direct analysis of genes encoding 16S rRNA from complex communities reveals many novel molecular species within the human gut. *Appl. Environ. Microbiol.* **65:**4799–4807.

150. **Talan, D. A., F. M. Abrahamian, G. J. Moran, D. M. Citron, J. O. Tan, and E. J. C. Goldstein for the Emergency Medicine Human Bite Infection Study Group.** 2003. Clinical presentation and bacteriologic analysis of infected human bites in patients presenting to emergency departments. *Clin. Infect. Dis.* **37:**1481–1489.

151. **Talan, D. A., D. M. Citron, F. M. Abrahamian, G. J. Moran, and E. J. C. Goldstein.** 1999. Bacteriologic analysis of infected dog and cat bites. *N. Engl. J. Med.* **340:**85–92.

152. **Taras, D., R. Simmering, M. D. Collins, P. A. Lawson, and M. Blaut.** 2002. Reclassification of *Eubacterium formicigenerans* Holdeman and Moore 1974 as *Dorea formicigenerans* gen. nov., comb. nov., and description of *Dorea longicatena* sp. nov., isolated from human faeces. *Int. J. Syst. Evol. Microbiol.* **52:**423–428.

153. **Thiolas, A., C. Bollet, M. Gasmi, M. Drancourt, and D. Raoult.** 2003. *Eubacterium callanderi* bacteremia: report of the first case. *J. Clin. Microbiol.* **41:**2235–2236.

154. **Tietz, A., K. E. Aldridge, and J. E. Figueroa.** 2005. Disseminated coinfection with *Actinomyces graevenitzii* and *Mycobacterium tuberculosis:* case report and review of the literature. *J. Clin. Microbiol.* **43:**3017–3022.

155. **Uematsu, H., and E. Hoshino.** 1992. Predominant obligate anaerobes in human periodontal pockets. *J. Periodont. Res.* **27:**15–19.

156. **Uematsu, H., N. Sato, M. Z. Hossain, T. Ikeda, and E. Hoshino.** 2003. Degradation of arginine and other amino acids by butyrate-producing asaccharolytic anaerobic gram-positive rods in periodontal pockets. *Arch. Oral Biol.* **48:**423–429.

157. **Vanagt, W. Y., W. J. Daenen, and T. Delhaas.** 2004. *Propionibacterium acnes* endocarditis on an annuloplasty ring in an adolescent boy. *Heart* **90:**e56.

158. **Vandamme, P., E. Falsen, M. Vancanneyt, M. Van Esbroeck, D. Van de Merwe, A. Bergmans, L. Schouls, and L. Sabbe.** 1998. Characterization of *A. turicensis* and *A. radingae* strains from human clinical samples. *Int. J. Syst. Bacteriol.* **48:**503–510.

159. **Vandamme, P., B. Pot, M. Gillis, P. de Vos, K. Kersters, and J. Swings.** 1996. Polyphasic taxonomy, a consensus approach to bacterial systematics. *Microbiol. Rev.* **60:**407–438.

160. **Vasquez, A., T. Jakobsson, S. Ahrné, U. Forsum, and G. Molin.** 2002. Vaginal *Lactobacillus* flora of healthy Swedish women. *J. Clin. Microbiol.* **40:**2746–2749.

161. **Verhelst, R., H. Verstraelen, G. Claeys, G. Verschraegen, J. Delanghe, L. Van Simaey, C. De Ganck, M. Temmerman, and M. Vaneechoutte.** 2004. Cloning of 16S rRNA genes amplified from normal and disturbed vaginal microflora suggests a strong association between *Atopobium vaginae, Gardnerella vaginalis* and bacterial vaginosis. *BMC Microbiol.* **4:**16.

162. **Wade, W. G., J. Downes, D. Dymock, S. J. Hiom, A. J. Weightman, F. E. Dewhirst, B. J. Paster, N. Tzellas, and B. Coleman.** 1999. The family *Coriobacteriaceae:* reclassification of *Eubacterium exiguum* (Poco et al. 1996) and *Peptostreptococcus heliotrinreducens* (Lanigan 1976) as *Slackia exigua* gen. nov., comb. nov. and *Slackia heliotrinireducens*

gen. nov., comb. nov., and *Eubacterium lentum* (Prevot 1938) as *Eggerthella lenta* gen. nov., comb. nov. *Int. J. Syst. Bacteriol.* **49:**595–600.

163. **Walker, A. P., C. J. Krepel, C. M. Gohr, and C. E. Edmiston.** 1994. Microflora of abdominal sepsis by locus of infection. *J. Clin. Microbiol.* **32:**557–558.
164. **Wilks, M., R. Wiggins, A. Whiley, E. Hennessy, S. Warwick, H. Porter, A. Corfield, and M. Millar.** 2004. Identification and H_2O_2 production of vaginal lactobacilli from pregnant women at high risk of preterm birth and relation with outcome. *J. Clin. Microbiol.* **42:**713–717.
165. **Willems, A., and M. D. Collins.** 1996. Phylogenetic relationships of the genera *Acetobacterium* and *Eubacterium* sensu stricto and reclassification of *Eubacterium alactolyticum* as *Pseudoramibacter alactolyticus* gen. nov., comb. nov. *Int. J. Syst. Bacteriol.* **46:**1083–1087.
166. **Willems, A., W. E. Moore, N. Weiss, and M. D. Collins.** 1997. Phenotypic and phylogenetic characterization of some *Eubacterium*-like isolates containing a novel type B wall murein from human feces: description of *Holdemania filiformis* gen. nov., sp. nov. *Int. J. Syst. Bacteriol.* **47:**1201–1204.
167. **Wilson, M. J., A. J. Weightman, and W. G. Wade.** 1997. Applications of molecular ecology in the characterisation of uncultured microorganisms associated with human disease. *Rev. Med. Microbiol.* **8:**91–101.
168. **Wolin, M. J., T. L. Miller, M. D. Collins, and P. A. Lawson.** 2003. Formate-dependent growth and homoacetogenic fermentation by a bacterium from human feces: description of *Bryantella formatexigens* gen. nov., sp. nov. *Appl. Environ. Microbiol.* **69:**6321–6326.
169. **Woo, P. C., A. M. Fung, S. K. Lau, J. L. Teng, B. H. Wong, M. K. Wong, E. Hon, G. W. Tang, and K. Y. Yuen.** 2003. *Actinomyces hongkongensis* sp. nov. a novel *Actinomyces* species isolated from a patient with pelvic actinomycosis. *Syst. Appl. Microbiol.* **26:**518–522.
170. **Woo, P. C. Y., K. H. L. Ng, S. K. P. Lau, K.-T. Yip, A. M. Y. Fung, K.-W. Leung, D. M. W. Tam, T.-L. Que, and K.-Y. Yuen.** 2003. Usefulness of the MicroSeq 500 16S ribosomal DNA-based bacterial identification system for identification of clinically significant bacterial isolates with ambiguous biochemical profiles. *J. Clin. Microbiol.* **41:**1996–2001.
171. **Wüst, J., U. Steiger, H. Vuong, and R. Zbinden.** 2000. Infection of a hip prosthesis by *Actinomyces naeslundii*. *J. Clin. Microbiol.* **38:**929–930.
172. **Yokota, A., T. Tamura, M. Takeuchi, N. Weiss, and E. Stackebrandt.** 1994. Transfer of *Propionibacterium innocuum* Pitcher and Collins 1991 to *Propioniferax* gen. nov. as *Propioniferax innocua* comb. nov. *Int. J. Syst. Bacteriol.* **44:**579–582.

*Clostridium**

ERIC A. JOHNSON, PAULA SUMMANEN, AND SYDNEY M. FINEGOLD

57

TAXONOMY

The genus *Clostridium* comprises obligately anaerobic (or occasionally aerotolerant) rods that usually stain gram positive in young cultures. Clostridia, mainly from our indigenous microbiota, are involved in a variety of infections that are commonly associated with considerable morbidity and mortality (44, 86). Virulence factors (particularly toxins), inoculum size, and other properties play important roles in diseases involving *Clostridium* species. Impaired host defenses also enhance susceptibility to clostridial infections. Currently, 202 clostridial species are validly published (http://www.dsmz.de/bactnom/bactname.htm); however, the number of clinically significant clostridia from human infections is limited (Table 1).

Phylogenetically, the genus *Clostridium* is extremely heterogeneous, with many species intermixed with other spore-forming and non-spore-forming genera (53, 66). Traditionally, the species have been defined based on a few morphological, ultrastructure (72), and physiological features (44, 173). During the past decade, analyses of 16S rRNA gene sequences indicated that the "clostridia" could be divided into 19 clusters and 11 groups (53). Homology group I forms the basis of the genus *Clostridium* and is analogous to group I proposed in 1975 (96, 173). The type species, *Clostridium butyricum* (44), and most of the clinically important *Clostridium* species cluster within homology group I. The heterogeneous non-group I clostridia require reclassification (53, 173), but a difficulty in resolving the heterogeneity within the genus is that 16S rRNA gene sequences may not be adequate alone in distinguishing genera, and it is necessary to find genetic and phenotypic characters that enable rapid discrimination among genera within this group (173; P. Lawson, personal communication).

Since the last edition of this Manual, some new pathogenic species have been designated within the clinically significant *Clostridium* species. Two new species clustering within the *C. coccoides* rRNA group, *C. hathewayi* (174) and *C. bolteae* (169), were described from human feces. Phenotypically, *C. clostridioforme* is a relatively heterogeneous anaerobe. Sequencing analyses of 16S rRNA genes from 107 strains that were previously identified phenotypically as *C. clostridioforme* in various clinical laboratories revealed that "*C. clostridioforme*" in fact represents three distinct species: *C. bolteae*, *C. clostridioforme*, and *C. hathewayi* (67). *C. bartlettii* is another new *Clostridium* species described from human feces (168); the clinical significance of this organism remains unknown. *C. neonatale* was proposed as a novel species recovered from bacteremia in patients with necrotizing enterocolitis (NEC) (9); however, this species is not yet validly published.

Anaerotruncus colihominis is a new genus and species within the *C. leptum* rRNA cluster of organisms originally described from human feces (120), and subsequently found in bacteremia (118). *A. colihominis* was originally described as a non-spore-forming organism; however, further studies have revealed that this organism does produce spores under some conditions (118) and should therefore be considered in *Clostridium* identification schemes.

DESCRIPTION OF THE GENUS

The description of the genus *Clostridium* is outlined in *Bergey's Manual of Systematic Bacteriology* (44) and *The Prokaryotes* (89). Recent analyses of rRNA genes have greatly expanded the clostridia to include 5 new genera and 11 new species combinations (53). The clostridia, as currently named, belong to the phylum *Firmicutes* and comprise a heterogeneous (paraphyletic) group consisting of at least 12 lineages. The clostridia have a wide range of G+C contents, from 22 to 55 mol%, while the toxigenic species have a much narrower range of G+C contents, 24 to 29 mol% (44, 86, 89, 173). Common morphological and phenotypic properties that have traditionally been used to define the genus include (i) the formation of endospores, (ii) an anaerobic energy metabolism, (iii) the inability to reduce sulfate to sulfide, and (iv) a gram-positive cell wall structure (44, 89).

Vegetative cells of *Clostridium* species are rod shaped, commonly pleomorphic, and are often arranged in pairs or short chains; the cells have rounded or sometimes pointed ends (44, 86, 90). Rods may join to form tight coils or spiral configurations in certain species, such as *C. cocleatum* and *C. spiroforme*. Clostridia usually stain gram positive at least in early stages of growth, although some species, such as *C. clostridioforme*, *C. hathewayi*, *C. innocuum*, and *C. ramosum*, almost always appear gram negative. Several species (e.g., *C. tetani*) appear gram negative by the time spores have formed. The cells form oval or spherical endospores (44, 86, 89). The spores are often wider than the vegetative organisms, imparting characteristic

* This chapter contains information presented in chapter 54 by Stephen D. Allen, Christopher L. Emery, and David M. Lyerly in the eighth edition of this Manual.

TABLE 1 Characteristics of *Clostridium* species of clinical significance[a]

Species	Gelatin hydrolysis	Lecithinase	Lipase	Indole	Esculin hydrolysis	Nitrate	Fermentation of:		
							Milk digestion	Glucose	Arabinose
Saccharolytic, proteolytic									
C. bifermentans[b]	+	+	−	+	$+^{-}$	−	+	+	−
C. botulinum[c]									
Types A, B, F	+	−	+	−	+	−	+	$+^{-}$	−
Types B, E, F[d]	+	−	+	−	−	−	−	+	w^{-}
Types C, D	+	$-^{+}$	+	$-^{+}$	−	−	+	+	−
C. cadaveris	+	−	−	+	−	−	+	+	−
C. difficile[e]	+	−	−	−	+	−	−	$+^{w}$	−
C. novyi A	+	+	+	−	−	−	−	+	−
C. perfringens	+	+	−	−	v	v	+	+	−
C. putrificum	+	−	−	−	$-^{+}$	−	+	$+^{w}$	−
C. septicum[f]	+	−	−	−	+	v	+	+	−
C. sordellii[b]	+	+	−	+	$-^{+}$	−	+	+	−
C. sporogenes[f]	+	−	+	−	+	−	+	+	−
Saccharolytic, nonproteolytic									
C. baratii	−	+	−	−	+	$+^{-}$	−	+	−
C. bolteae[g]	−	−	−	−	$-^{+}$	−	−	+	+
C. butyricum	−	−	−	−	+	−	−	+	$+^{-}$
C. carnis[h]	−	−	−	−	+	−	−	+	−
C. clostridioforme[g]	−	−	−	−	+	−	−	+	+
C. glycolicum	−	−	−	−	$-^{+}$	−	−	+	−
C. hathewayi[g]	−	−	−	−	$+^{w}$	−	−	+	v
C. indolis	−	−	−	+	+	$+^{-}$	−	+	w^{-}
C. innocuum[e]	−	−	−	−	+	−	−	+	$-^{+}$
C. paraputrificum	$-^{w}$	−	−	−	+	$-^{+}$	−	+	−
C. ramosum	−	−	−	−	+	−	−	+	−
C. sphenoides	−	−	−	+	+	$+^{-}$	−	+	$-^{w}$
C. symbiosum	$-^{w}$	−	−	−	−	−	−	$+^{w}$	v
C. tertium[h]	−	−	−	−	+	$+^{-}$	−	+	−
Asaccharolytic									
C. argentinense	+	−	−	−	−	−	+	−	−
C. hastiforme	+	−	−	−	−	$-^{+}$	$-^{+}$	−	−
C. histolyticum[h]	+	−	−	−	−	−	+	−	−
C. limosum	+	+	−	−	−	−	+	−	−
C. orbiscindens[i]	$-^{w}$	−	−	v	−	−	−	−	−
C. subterminale	+	$-^{+}$	−	−	$-^{+}$	−	+	−	−
C. tetani[f]	+	−	$-^{w}$	v	−	−	+	−	−

[a] +, positive reaction; −, negative reaction; v, variable reaction; w, weakly positive reaction; ST, subterminal; T, terminal. Superscript indicates rare variability. Capital letters indicate major metabolic products from peptone-yeast-glucose (PYG), lowercase letters indicate minor products, and parentheses indicate a variable reaction for fatty acids as follows: A, acetic; P, propionic; IB, isobutyric; B, butyric; IV, isovaleric; V, valeric; IC, isocaproic; L, lactic; S, succinic; and PA, phenylacetic.

[b] *C. bifermentans* is urease negative, and *C. sordellii* is urease positive. *C. bifermentans* usually forms chalk-white colonies on egg yolk agar.

[c] Toxin neutralization test required for identification. Send suspected isolates or *C. botulinum*-containing material to the appropriate local or state public health agency.

Fermentation of:											Spore location	Metabolic end products from PYG
Cellobiose	Fructose	**Lactose**	Maltose	Mannitol	Mannose	Melibiose	Ribose	Salicin	**Sucrose**	Xylose		
–	$-^{w}$	–	w^{-}	–	$-^{w}$	–	–	–	–	–	ST	A (iv, ic, p, ib, b, l, s)
–	$-^{w}$	–	$-^{w}$	–	–	–	–	–	–	–	ST	A, B, IV, ib (ic, v, p)
–	$+^{w}$	–	$+^{-}$	$-^{w}$	$+^{w}$	$-^{w}$	v	–	$+^{w}$	–	ST	B, A (1)
–	v	–	v	–	v	$-^{w}$	v	–	–	–	T	B, P, A (v, l, s)
–	v	–	–	–	$-^{w}$	–	–	–	–	–	T	B, A
v	$+^{w}$	–	–	w^{+}	v	–	$-^{w}$	$-^{w}$	–	$-^{w}$	ST^{T}	B, A, ic, iv, ib (v, l)
–	$-^{w}$	–	v	–	–	$-^{w}$	v	$-^{w}$	–	–	ST	A, B, P
$-^{+}$	+	+	+	–	+	v	v	$-^{+}$	+	–	ST	A, B, L (p, s)
–	$-^{w}$	–	$-^{w}$	–	–	–	–	–	–	–	T^{ST}	A, B, ib, iv (p, ic, v, l, s)
$+^{w}$	+	+	+	–	+	–	v	v	–	–	ST	B, A (p, l)
–	v	–	w	–	$-^{w}$	–	$-^{w}$	–	–	–	ST	A (IC, p, ib, iv, l)
$-^{w}$	–	–	$-^{w}$	–	–	–	–	–	–	–	ST	A, B, iv, ib (p, ic, v, l, s)
+	+	w^{+}	w^{+}	–	+	$-^{w}$	w^{-}	$+^{-}$	+	–	ST	B, A, L (p, s)
$-^{+}$	+	–	+	–	+		–	$-^{+}$	+	+	ST	A (l)
+	+	+	+	$-^{w}$	+	$+^{w}$	$+^{w}$	$+^{w}$	+	+	ST	B, A (l, s)
w^{+}	v	v	w^{+}	–	w^{+}	–	–	w	w^{+}	–	ST	B, A, L (s)
+	$+^{w}$	+	+	–	+	v	v	+	$+^{w}$	$+^{w}$	ST	A (l)
–	$+^{w}$	–	v	–	–	–	–	–	–	$+^{-}$	ST	A, IV, IB (p, l, s)
+	+	+	+	–	+	+	+	+	+	+	ST	A (l)
$+^{w}$	w^{+}	w^{+}	w^{+}	$-^{w}$	$-^{w}$	$-^{w}$	$-^{w}$	w^{-}	v	v	T	A
+	+	$-^{w}$	–	$+^{w}$	+	–	v	$+^{w}$	$+^{w}$	$-^{w}$	T	B, L, a (s)
+	$+^{w}$	+	+	–	+	–	w^{-}	+	+	–	T^{ST}	B, A, L (s)
+	+	+	+	$+^{-}$	+	$+^{-}$	v	+	+	$-^{w}$	T	A, l (s)
$+^{w}$	$+^{w}$	w^{+}	$+^{w}$	w^{+}	$+^{w}$	v	$-^{w}$	v	w^{-}	v	ST^{T}	A (l, s)
–	+	$-^{+}$	–	–	v	–	–	–	–	–	ST	A, B, L
$+^{w}$	+	+	+	w^{+}	$+^{w}$	$+^{w}$	$+^{w}$	$+^{w}$	+	v	T	A, B, L
–	–	–	–	–	–	–	–	–	–	–	ST	A, b, ib, iv (l)
–	–	–	–	–	–	–	–	–	–	–	T	A, B, iv, ib(p, ic)
–	–	–	–	–	–	–	–	–	–	–	ST	A (l, s)
–	–	–	–	–	–	–	–	–	–	–	ST	A (l, s)
–	–	–	–	–	–	–	$-^{w}$	–	–	–	ST	a, B (l)
–	–	–	–	–	–	–	–	–	–	–	ST	A, B, IV, ib (p, ic, l, s)
–	–	–	–	–	–	–	–	–	–	–	T	A, B, p (l, s)

[d] Nonproteolytic.

[e] L-Proline-aminopeptidase differentiates: C. *difficile* is positive, and C. *innocuum* is negative.

[f] Swarming.

[g] Cigar shaped; C. *bolteae* is lactose and β-NAG negative, C. *clostridioforme* is lactose positive and β-NAG negative, and C. *hathewayi* is lactose and β-NAG positive.

[h] C. *tertium*, C. *carnis*, and most C. *histolyticum* isolates grow aerobically.

[i] Described from a case of bacteremia; frequently isolated from stool specimens.

spindle shapes of clostridia (47, 99). Most strains are motile by means of peritrichous flagella. Nonmotile species from clinical specimens include *C. perfringens, C. ramosum,* and *C. innocuum.*

Clostridium species are metabolically diverse. As currently designated (53, 89), most species are chemoorganotrophic; some species may be chemoautotrophic and chemolithotrophic. They can be saccharolytic, proteolytic, neither, or both; they do not carry out dissimilatory sulfate reduction. They usually produce mixtures of organic acids and alcohols from carbohydrates, proteins and peptides, or purines and pyrimidines (86, 89).

Most species are obligately anaerobic, although the tolerance to oxygen varies widely; some species (e.g., *C. tertium*) will grow but not sporulate in the presence of air, and a few aerotolerant species, such as *C. carnis, C. histolyticum,* and occasional strains of *C. perfringens,* give scant growth on solid media incubated under 5 to 10% CO_2. The distinction between aerotolerant clostridia and certain *Bacillus* species may be made by virtue of the fact that clostridia usually form spores only under anaerobic conditions, they grow better anaerobically than in air, and clostridia usually do not produce catalase. Although *Clostridium* species are usually catalase and superoxide dismutase negative, trace amounts of these enzyme activities may be detected in some strains. In addition, clostridia lack a cytochrome system and are thus oxidase negative. Clostridia often occur in nature and in infections as consortia of mixed species, wherein aerobic and facultative organisms utilize oxygen, provide nutrients or other factors, and create an environment favorable for clostridial growth. Since clostridia often are present as mixed cultures, it is important to carefully ascertain purity by plating for single colonies and by microscopic analysis.

Clostridia produce a diversity of biologically active proteins, including toxins, many of which are important in human disease. The clostridia produce more kinds of protein toxins than any other bacterial genus, and more than 25 toxins lethal to mice have been identified (14, 23, 85). At least 15 species of cluster I *Clostridium* produce protein toxins, and new toxins and virulence proteins have been discovered through traditional isolation techniques and genomic analyses (38, 159). These proteins include neurotoxins, enterotoxins, cytotoxins, collagenases, permeases, necrotizing toxins, lipases, lecithinases, hemolysins, proteinases, hyaluronidases, DNases, ADP-ribosyltransferases, neuraminidases, and some others that are simply known as lethal toxins (85). Certain clostridial toxins have extraordinary potency, and botulinum and tetanus neurotoxins are the most poisonous toxins known, with lethal doses of 0.2 to 10 ng per kg for various animals, including humans (23, 75, 85, 154). The virulence traits of clostridia that cause disease in hosts are incompletely understood. Recently, genomic sequences of pathogenic clostridia have become available (38, 159), which should facilitate a comprehensive approach for understanding virulence factors involved in clostridial pathogenesis.

EPIDEMIOLOGY AND TRANSMISSION

Clostridium species are widespread in the environment partly due to their ability to form resistant endospores. They are commonly found in soil, feces, sewage, and marine sediments (44, 86, 163). The common presence of *C. perfringens* in soil is seldom of clinical significance (165). Infection of war wounds, for example, typically is due to the subject's indigenous microbiota and the lack of sufficient hygiene. On the other hand, the incidences of tetanus and food-borne botulism are commonly related to the incidence of their spores in soil, water, and many foods (86, 164). Outbreaks of hospital-acquired *C. difficile* enteric infections are often traceable to environmental sources and other typical background factors for nosocomial infection (142). Many clostridia are present in large numbers as part of the indigenous microbiota of the intestinal tract of humans and animals (44, 86) and may be found in the female genital tract and oral microbiota as well.

CLINICAL SIGNIFICANCE

Although the exogenous clostridial infections or intoxications such as tetanus, food-borne botulism, and hospital-acquired *C. difficile* colitis are serious, endogenous infections by clostridia that are a part of the host's indigenous microbiota are commonly encountered. Nearly any type of infection in the body may involve clostridia, often in association with non-spore-forming anaerobes and facultative or aerobic organisms. These infections tend to be more severe than comparable infections without clostridia as part of the infecting microbiota. Head and neck infections, brain abscess, sinusitis, otitis, aspiration pneumonia, lung abscess, pleural empyema, cholecystitis, other intra-abdominal infections, gynecologic and obstetric infections, and soft tissue and bone infections all may involve clostridia (79). Common predisposing factors are surgical procedures, trauma, vascular stasis, obstruction, malignancy with or without chemotherapy and immunosuppressive agents, diabetes mellitus, prior aerobic infection, and use of antimicrobial agents with poor activity against clostridia (e.g., trimethoprim-sulfamethoxazole) (64, 83).

Clostridial Bacteremia

C. septicum is isolated only rarely from the feces of healthy individuals but is found in anaerobic blood cultures in bacteremia associated with underlying disease processes, often neoplastic disease, particularly in the ileocecal region. As many as 70 to 85% of patients whose blood cultures are positive for this organism have some underlying malignancy (29, 103). *C. septicum* has been found in the lumen of 10 to 68% of normal appendices (27, 72). Another clinically important association has been observed between *C. septicum* bacteremia, neutropenia of any origin, and neutropenic enterocolitis involving the terminal ileum or cecum (102, 113). Patients with diabetes mellitus, severe atherosclerotic cardiovascular disease, or anaerobic myonecrosis (gas gangrene) may also develop *C. septicum* bacteremia (77, 109). The clinical importance of recognizing *C. septicum* bacteremia and starting appropriate treatment immediately cannot be overemphasized. Patients with this condition are usually gravely ill and may have metastatic spread of myonecrosis to distant anatomic sites. Mortality rates are very high. *C. septicum* has also been recovered from bacteremia in cirrhotic patients, as have *C. perfringens, C. bifermentans,* and other clostridia (49). Some of these patients demonstrated septic shock.

Another clostridial species of importance in patients with serious underlying disease such as malignancy is *C. tertium.* This organism, as well as *C. septicum* and *C. perfringens,* may be seen in bacteremia in such patients, with or without neutropenic enterocolitis (122). *C. tertium* may present special problems in terms of both identification and treatment. This organism may appear gram negative, is aerotolerant, and is resistant to metronidazole, clindamycin, and cephalosporins. *C. tertium* has also been found in bacteremia associated with acute pancreatitis (157).

An important study by Woo et al. (188) involved sequencing of genes encoding 16S rRNA of non-*C. perfringens* clostridia in a study of anaerobic bacteremia. *C. perfringens* accounted for 79% of clinically relevant clostridial bacteremias; 11 other species accounted for 17 other blood cultures positive for clostridia other than *C. perfringens*. There were four bacteremias due to *C. paraputrificum*, three due to *C. ramosum*, two due to *C. tertium*, and one each due to *C. baratii*, *C. difficile*, *C. disporicum*, *C. indolis*, *C. innocuum*, *C. orbiscindens*, *C. septicum*, and *C. sporosphaeroides*. The mortality rate of clinically relevant clostridial bacteremia was 29%. A study of risk factors for mortality in patients with anaerobic bacteremia (187) found, in a multivariate analysis, that the only significant factors were liver disease and patient age. In this study, there were 25 patients with clostridial bacteremia; the crude mortality rate in this group was 35%. The *C. clostridioforme* group (including *C. clostridioforme*, *C. hathewayi*, and *C. bolteae*) has been reported from a number of cases of bacteremia (67, 189).

Enteric Infections

Food Poisoning

C. perfringens is one of the most common bacterial causes of food-borne illness in the United States and Canada (32, 145). Almost all U.S. outbreaks and cases of *C. perfringens* food-borne gastroenteritis appear to be due to type A strains (32, 162). In *C. perfringens* type A food-borne disease, the food vehicle is typically an improperly cooked meat or meat product, such as gravy, that has cooled slowly after cooking or may have been inadequately reheated. Spores surviving the initial cooking germinate, and vegetative cells proliferate during slow cooling or insufficient reheating. Illness results from the ingestion of food containing about 10^8 or more viable vegetative cells, which sporulate in the alkaline environment of the small intestine, producing an enterotoxin (*C. perfringens* enterotoxin [CPE]) in the process. *C. perfringens* type A food-borne illness occurs within 7 to 30 h of ingestion of the suspect food and is generally mild and self-limiting (162). In the very young, the elderly, and the immunocompromised, symptoms are more severe, occasionally resulting in death (33). Enterotoxin-producing *C. perfringens* has been implicated as an etiologic agent of persistent diarrhea in elderly patients in nursing homes and tertiary-care institutions (30) and has been considered to play a role in antibiotic-associated diarrhea (AAD) without pseudomembranous colitis.

C. perfringens strains associated with food poisoning contain the enterotoxin gene *(cpe)* on the chromosome and produce the *C. perfringens* enterotoxin (CPE), which generally acts by forming pores in membranes of host cells (162). *C. perfringens* strains isolated from non-food-borne diseases, such as AAD and sporadic diarrhea, carry *cpe* on a plasmid (41, 68). The plasmid possessing *cpe* may be transmissible, since cases of food-associated diarrhea as well as AAD may be associated with a relatively small number of CPE-positive cells (68, 171, 184). These results indicate that *C. perfringens* strains bear a plasmid-borne enterotoxin gene that should not be disregarded as causative agents of food poisoning.

In addition to CPE, various strains of *C. perfringens* collectively produce about 15 protein toxins, several of which are involved in diseases of animals and livestock (85, 162). Epsilon-toxin is a 33-kDa protein produced by *C. perfringens* types B and D strains and is among the most lethal of clostridial toxins, next to botulinum and tetanus neurotoxins, and epsilon-toxin is considered a potential bioterrorism agent (23, 162). In animals, it causes edema and hemorrhage in the brain, heart, spinal cord, and kidneys (162).

Enteritis Necroticans (Pig-bel and Darmbrand), Necrotizing Enteritis, and NEC

Enteritis necroticans is caused by alpha-toxin- and beta-toxin-producing strains of *C. perfringens* type C, and beta-toxin is probably mainly responsible for the pathogenesis (162, 170). The gene encoding beta-toxin is located on a plasmid in *C. perfringens* (68). Enteritis necroticans is a life-threatening infection with ischemic necrosis of the jejunum (10). It was recognized in Papua New Guinea during the 1960s as the most frequent cause of death in children; it has been associated with pig feasts and occurs both sporadically and in outbreaks (143). Immunization against the beta-toxin resulted in a decreased incidence of the disease in New Guinea (119). Enteritis necroticans has also been recognized in the United States, the United Kingdom, Germany, and other developed nations, especially involving adults who are malnourished or who have chronic illnesses (e.g., diabetes or alcoholic liver disease) (60, 78, 81, 148) and also in a child with neutropenia (124). Enteritis necroticans may be underreported (128). It should be noted that NEC, a disease resembling enteritis necroticans but associated with *C. perfringens* type A, has been found rarely in North America in previously healthy adults (167).

NEC is a serious gastrointestinal disease that affects low-birth-weight (premature) infants who are hospitalized in neonatal intensive care units (110). Kliegman et al. (105) noted that the etiology and pathogenesis of this condition remain speculative in spite of more than 1,000 publications on NEC over the last 4 decades. Pathological similarities between NEC and enteritis necroticans include the patterns of bowel necrosis and inflammation that occur in these conditions (104, 105). Both diseases may manifest intestinal gas cysts (pneumatosis cystoides intestinalis). The sources of the gas, which contains hydrogen, methane, and carbon dioxide, are probably the fermentative activities of intestinal bacteria, including clostridia in particular (104). Epidemiological data support an important role for *C. perfringens* or other gas-producing microorganisms (e.g., *C. neonatale*, certain other clostridia, or *Klebsiella* spp.) in the pathogenesis of NEC (9, 104, 110).

CDAD and Colitis

C. difficile, the major cause of antibiotic-associated pseudomembranous colitis, is also the most frequently identified cause of hospital-acquired diarrhea (97). It has been estimated that *C. difficile* is responsible for more than 250,000 cases of diarrheal disease per year in the United States (186), with a cost exceeding $1 billion (114). *C. difficile* has been isolated from various natural habitats and the feces of domestic animals and humans (129). *C. difficile* is present asymptomatically as part of the bowel microbiota in up to half of all healthy neonates during the first year of life; the carriage rate decreases to the adult rate of 3% or less by the age of 2. Hospitalized patients frequently become colonized with this organism (73). McFarland et al. (136) reported that 21% of 399 patients with negative cultures on admission to a hospital with a high prevalence of *C. difficile*-associated disease (CDAD) acquired *C. difficile* during hospitalization. Of these patients, 63% remained asymptomatic, while 37% developed diarrhea. Antimicrobial agents of all classes and several anticancer chemotherapeutic agents have been implicated in the development of CDAD or pseudomembranous colitis (97). As noted above, certain *C. difficile* strains contain mobilizable transposable elements with antibiotic resistance to chloramphenicol, tetracycline, or erythromycin (4, 172). Metronidazole and vancomycin have been active against all strains tested, but there have been a number of failures with metronidazole therapy recently (20, 146). Higher likelihood of treatment failure was noted in patients who remain on the predisposing antibiotics while undergoing treatment for CDAD (138).

In CDAD, the primary initiating event involves the disruption of the commensal intestinal microbiota during treatment with antibiotics or antineoplastic agents (73, 97, 129). As the levels of antibiotics drop below inhibitory concentrations, nosocomial pathogens such as *C. difficile* are able to grow. Toxigenic as well as nontoxigenic isolates are capable of forming spores and existing in the hospital environment. As a result, either type can infect the colon because of changes in populations of the intestinal microbiota. Only the toxigenic isolates are associated with disease, and nontoxigenic isolates may be protective by competitive exclusion (31). Toxigenic strains produce and release toxins TcdA and/or TcdB. TcdA and TcdB each have a molecular mass of approximately 270 kDa, similar to the TcsH hemorrhagic and TcsL lethal toxins from *C. sordellii* and alpha-toxin from *C. novyi* (179). The cytotoxic actions of these toxins and the associated inflammatory response result in the histopathology of CDAD.

In the early 1990s, an isolate of *C. difficile* that produced only toxin TcdB was described, and detailed studies suggested that the isolate contained a truncated *tcdA* gene (140, 179, 186). Furthermore, bioassays indicated that toxin B from this particular isolate was more toxic than toxin B from typical A^+/B^+ isolates. Multiple reports of atypical $TcdA^-/TcdB^+$ isolates and their association with clinical disease were documented (6, 8, 98, 130). Such isolates may be missed in laboratories that base their diagnosis solely on the use of toxin A-specific tests. In $TcdA^-/TcdB^+$ isolates, a large portion of the *tcdA* gene encoding the repeating region (i.e., the binding portion of the toxin) is deleted (100, 140). In addition to the deletion in TcdA, the active site of the TcdB gene is modified in $TcdA^-/TcdB^+$ isolates, resulting in a TcdB protein that more closely resembles the lethal toxin of *C. sordellii* (129, 140, 179). A limited number of cases of pseudomembranous colitis are caused by $TcdA^-/TcdB^+$ organisms (6, 8, 98, 130). Strains of *C. difficile* may only produce TcdA (97, 130, 179). Recently, *C. difficile* isolates that produce the highly potent iota-toxin, which is related to the iota-toxin of *C. perfringens* and *C. spiroforme*, have been noted (179). Virulent clones of *C. difficile* strains, characterized as toxinotype III, North American PFGE type 1, and PCR ribotype 027 (NAP1/027), have been linked to increased mortality in North America and Europe (135, 147, 181). The severity of CDAD caused by NAP1/027 may be due to hyperproduction of toxins A and B. Dissemination of this strain has led to important changes in the epidemiology of CDAD (181).

C. difficile is responsible for 20% or fewer of cases of AAD (24, 186). Reports suggest that *C. perfringens* is a less frequently identified cause of AAD (30). Enterotoxin-producing *C. perfringens* type A has been isolated from AAD patients who are negative for *C. difficile* and who have no other apparent cause of the disease. Coinfection with *C. difficile* and enterotoxigenic *C. perfringens* type A has been reported for AAD patients (43). The incidence of *C. perfringens*-associated AAD has been estimated at 5 to 20%, but additional epidemiological studies are needed to accurately determine the role of this organism in AAD (43).

C. difficile is an important cause of enteric infection in the elderly and in nursing home residents (160). *C. difficile* may be a problem even when antibiotics are not used, in patients with bowel stasis and those who have had bowel surgery. The clinical picture of *C. difficile* infection ranges from mild diarrhea to pseudomembranous colitis with or without toxic megacolon. In the most severe form, the disease may lead to bowel perforation and death.

Skin and Soft Tissue Infections

Soft tissue infections with clostridia or other organisms are sometimes not regarded as serious. However, it should be appreciated that necrotizing soft tissue infections (such as necrotizing fasciitis and myonecrosis) have a poor prognosis and require early surgical intervention as well as antimicrobial therapy. An interesting study published recently (15) reviewed 166 patients with necrotizing soft tissue infection of various types and with differing etiologies. The overall mortality was 16.9% in this series, and loss of limbs occurred in 26%. Clostridial infection was consistently associated with poor outcome and was an independent predictor for both mortality and limb loss; it was strongly associated with intravenous drug use and high levels of leukocytosis.

Clostridial Myonecrosis

C. perfringens is the clostridial species most commonly isolated from human clinical specimens, excluding feces (78, 79). One of the serious and unique infections in which this organism plays a major role is myonecrosis (gas gangrene) that involves a breakdown of muscle tissue related to the action of potent exotoxins, particularly alpha-toxin (a phospholipase C) and theta-toxin (a thiol-activated cytolysin) (39, 40). Alpha-toxin produces the opaque zone of lecithin hydrolysis products that surrounds colonies of *C. perfringens* growing on egg yolk agar plates. It gives rise to an outer zone of partial hemolysis that surrounds a smaller zone of complete hemolysis produced by theta-toxin (a heat-labile, oxygen-labile hemolysin easily detected around colonies of *C. perfringens* growing on sheep blood agar).

Clostridial myonecrosis is rapidly progressive and has a high mortality rate. Associated systemic manifestations may include shock, renal failure, and sometimes bacteremia with intravascular hemolysis (78, 79). In addition to *C. perfringens*, gas gangrene may involve *C. septicum*, *C. novyi*, *C. histolyticum*, *C. bifermentans*, *C. sordellii*, and other clostridia. Gas gangrene of the uterus, now rare, occurred most frequently as a consequence of illegal or self-induced abortions but has also followed spontaneous abortion, vaginal delivery, and cesarean section (78, 79, 128). Crepitant cellulitis, also called anaerobic cellulitis, is seen principally in diabetic patients and characteristically involves subcutaneous tissues or retroperitoneal tissues and can progress to fulminant systemic disease (78, 79, 128). The muscle and fascia are not involved. When clostridia are involved in this process, the disease may be more severe than when only non-spore-forming anaerobes and other bacteria are responsible.

Other Skin and Soft Tissue Infections

In addition to the well-known exogenous clostridial infections, emerging clostridial diseases have been recognized during the past decade. An emerging infection with a high mortality rate is soft tissue infection and toxic shock among injecting drug users. These individuals manifest hypotension, marked edema, and high leukocyte counts. The principal pathogens have been found to be *C. novyi* type A and *C. perfringens* (21, 36, 144). *C. novyi* types B, C, and D are unlikely to be isolated from human clinical material. Cases of *C. histolyticum* infection with cellulitis, abscess formation, or endocarditis have also been found (21). An outbreak of necrotizing fasciitis due to *C. sordellii* has been reported for black-tar heroin users (101).

C. sordellii is responsible for a rare, rapidly fatal postpartum endometritis in young, previously healthy women with a unique clinical picture of little or no fever or purulent discharge, shock, extensive edema and fluid accumulation in body cavities, and a markedly elevated white blood cell count (137, 151). *C. sordellii* has also been implicated in toxic shock-like syndrome following spontaneous childbirth or abortion; these women had refractory hypotension, multiple effusions, peripheral edema, hemoconcentration, and profound leukocytosis with lack of fever (161, 185). Also, *C. sordellii* was accountable for endophthalmitis after suture removal from a corneal transplant (192).

Botulism

C. botulinum is the cause of the rare but occasionally fatal illness known as botulism. Spores of *C. botulinum* are widely distributed in soil and aquatic habitats (94, 164). *C. botulinum*, along with unique strains of *C. butyricum*, *C. baratii*, and *C. argentinense*, can produce botulinum neurotoxin (BoNT), the most lethal poison known (46, 71, 75, 85, 154). The intravenous lethal dose for BoNT has been estimated as 0.1 to 0.5 ng per kg of body weight, and BoNT is among the most potent protein toxins by oral ingestion, with an estimated oral lethal dose of 0.2 to 1 μg per kg (17, 75, 154). There are seven antigenic serotypes of BoNT (A through G), which serve as useful clinical and epidemiological markers (84, 94, 115). Toxin serotypes A, B, and E of *C. botulinum* are the principal causes of botulism in humans (52, 84, 94). Neurotoxigenic strains of *C. butyricum* (63, 71, 86) and *C. baratii* (86) that produce type E and F neurotoxins, respectively, have been implicated mainly in infant botulism. Type E botulinal toxin-producing *C. butyricum* strains were confirmed by sequencing of the16S rRNA gene (48, 71), leading to the conclusion that neurotoxigenic *C. butyricum* must be regarded as an emergent food-borne pathogen. *C. argentinense*, which produces type G neurotoxin (84), has been isolated from soil in Argentina. Its reported isolation from autopsy materials from five individuals who died suddenly has not been substantiated, and *C. argentinense* has not been clearly implicated in botulism (86). *C. botulinum* types C and D are associated primarily with botulism in birds and mammals (94, 163, 164). Strains of *C. botulinum* that produce more than one serotype of BoNT, generally with one serotype formed in much higher levels, have been isolated from the environment and human and animal botulism cases (71, 84, 93). The BoNTs are coexpressed with nontoxic proteins of toxin gene clusters (34), and evidence suggests that the complexes are much more stable in the gastrointestinal tract (153). The genes for BoNT complex formation are associated with unstable genetic elements in certain serotypes, enabling toxin gene transfer to nonpathogenic clostridia (57, 92, 191).

There are four naturally occurring types of botulism: (i) classical food-borne botulism, an intoxication caused by the ingestion of preformed botulinal toxin in contaminated food; (ii) wound botulism, which results from elaboration of botulinal toxin in vivo after growth of *C. botulinum* in an infected wound; (iii) infant botulism, in which botulinal toxin is elaborated in vivo in the gastrointestinal tract of an infant colonized with *C. botulinum*; and (iv) botulism due to intestinal colonization in children and adults (16, 46, 71, 84, 106, 164). Intestinal colonization in adults has been associated with surgery and administration of antibiotics (80, 84). Recently, *C. botulinum* has been isolated from patients colonized with *C. difficile* (63), with viral infections (62), or with Crohn's disease (80).

Regardless of the category of botulism, the toxin enters the bloodstream at a peripheral site (e.g., gut, wound, or lung) and is transferred to the neuromuscular junctions of motor neurons, where it binds irreversibly to the presynaptic membranes. The site of action of all serotypes of BoNT is the presynaptic terminal of motor neurons (50, 117, 155). Elucidation of the three-dimensional structures of botulinum and tetanus toxins and their constituent domains has provided considerable insights into their mechanisms of action (116, 117, 155, 176). BoNT penetrates the plasma membrane by receptor-mediated endocytosis, and the light chain of 50 kDa (the catalytic domain) is internalized into the nerve cell through a protein channel (117, 155). Once internalized, BoNT specifically cleaves SNARE proteins involved in vesicle trafficking of neurotransmitters to the membrane (155). Exocytosis of acetylcholine is prevented at the nerve terminal to the neuromuscular junction, with consequent blockage of innervation of muscle activity (155). The clinical hallmark of botulism is an acute flaccid paralysis, which begins with bilateral cranial nerve impairment involving muscles of the eyes, face, head, and pharynx and then descends symmetrically to involve muscles of the thorax and extremities. At physiological levels, botulinum toxin, unlike tetanus neurotoxin (TeNT), probably does not enter the central nervous system (CNS). In naturally occurring food-borne botulism, gastrointestinal symptoms (e.g., abdominal cramps, nausea, vomiting, or diarrhea [more often constipation or obstipation]) may precede the neurologic signs of descending flaccid paralysis. Death may result from respiratory failure caused by paralysis of the tongue or muscles of the pharynx leading to occlusion of the upper airway or from paralysis of the diaphragm and intercostal muscles (17, 50). Generally, the patient's hearing remains normal, consciousness is not lost, and the victim is cognizant of the progression of the disease. Certain episodes of botulism have been reported that affect autonomic and sensory functions. A patient's awareness of loss of muscle activity can lead to considerable emotional distress, such as anxiety and depression (50).

Wound Botulism in Intravenous Drug Users

Wound botulism is another exogenous clostridial intoxication that may be found among injecting drug users (37, 133). Although wound botulism is rare in non-drug users, cases occasionally occur, such as a fatal case that occurred in a young girl who had a tooth extracted (182). An association between botulism and subcutaneous injection of Mexican black-tar heroin was reported in the United States and in the United Kingdom (37, 133). A study found 33 clinically diagnosed cases of wound botulism in the United Kingdom and Ireland between 2000 and 2002 (37). All individuals affected had injected black-tar heroin into muscle or by "skin popping." The clinical diagnosis was confirmed by laboratory tests in 20 of these cases; 18 cases were caused by type A toxin and 2 by type B toxin. Users of drugs other than heroin are also at risk of illness caused by clostridia; injection or snorting cocaine has resulted in cases of botulism (112).

Infant Botulism

In the United States, infant botulism is the most frequently recognized form of botulism. Although infant botulism has been documented in at least 15 other countries (16, 70, 71), it is comparatively rare outside the United States, perhaps due to failure of recognition and diagnosis (16). Of the nearly 2,000 cases reported in the United States from the discovery of infant botulism in 1976 (16, 149), approximately 45% of cases were in California, where an intensive epidemiological and microbiological program has been used for recognition and treatment of infant botulism (16).

Across the United States, the geographic distribution of toxin types in infant botulism cases has roughly paralleled the spore distribution of C. *botulinum* toxin types in soil sampled from different locations (16), although certain geographic locations have comparatively high incidences. Type A has been the most frequent BoNT type in cases of infant botulism in states west of the Mississippi River, whereas type B cases have predominated east of the Mississippi River (16, 164). Three known cases have been caused by a strain(s) of C. *botulinum* that produced toxins requiring both type B and F antitoxins for neutralization (84). Type E infant botulism, caused by neurotoxigenic strains of C. *butyricum*, was initially confirmed in two infants from Italy (71, 86), and later in additional patients. Type F infant botulism has been caused by neurotoxigenic C. *baratii* (71, 86).

Although most infants that contract botulism are 3 weeks to 6 months old, the age range is a few hours following birth to 363 days (16). Botulinum spores have not been detected in any food or liquid ingested by these infants other than honey (16). To date, the only clearly defined risk factors have been exposure to soil, dust, and honey (16, 70). It is recommended that honey not be fed to infants less than 1 year of age. Another possible risk factor, although not proven, is that spores could be transmitted in corn syrup, and possibly infant foods within the household environment (95). Whatever the sources, the ingested spores of C. *botulinum* germinate within the intestinal tract, and the vegetative cells multiply and produce the neurotoxin, which is then absorbed into the bloodstream (16, 84). Decreased frequency of bowel movements, a sign of decreased intestinal motility, may be an additional risk factor for infant botulism. The first sign of illness is usually constipation, which is often overlooked. Infants who are ultimately hospitalized develop lethargy and mild weakness, with feeding difficulties, pooled oral secretions, and an altered cry (16). They eventually lose head control and may go on to develop ophthalmoplegia, ptosis, flaccid facial expression, dysphagia, other signs of cranial nerve deficits, and generalized muscular weakness. Respiratory insufficiency and inability to swallow necessitating intubation and intragastric feeding also may occur. There is likely a spectrum of clinical features in infant botulism, ranging from mild illness not requiring hospitalization to severe botulism requiring intensive care. It has been postulated that fulminant, rapid-onset botulism can cause sudden death, which may account for a small percentage of cases of sudden infant death syndrome (17, 25). Human immune globulin that neutralizes BoNT (BabyBIG) is now approved by the FDA for use in therapy of infant botulism; this product has moderate titers of neutralizing antibodies against types A and B toxin, but its efficacy against serotypes E and F is unknown (18, 70).

Aerosolized Botulinum Toxin and Potential Use as a Bioterrorism Agent

Inhalational botulism, which results from aerosolization and inhalation of botulinum toxin, has been considered a fifth category of botulism (17, 150). Botulism could also result from covert contamination of foods (17, 183). These two routes of botulism have been considered most likely to occur in a bioterrorism incident (17, 42) (see chapter 9). Inhalational botulism has been demonstrated experimentally in monkeys (17, 150), accidentally in three veterinary personnel in Germany who were exposed to reaerosolized BoNT from rabbits and guinea pigs with aerosolized BoNT on their fur (17), and three researchers who were exposed to an aerosol during BoNT manipulations (91). Terrorists have attempted to use aerosolized botulinum toxin as a bioweapon in Japan but were not successful. After Operation Desert Storm ended in 1991, Iraq admitted to having produced 19,000 liters of concentrated botulinum toxin and to having loaded more than half of it into specially designed military weapons (e.g., missiles). According to Arnon et al. (17), 19,000 liters of concentrated botulinum toxin is more than enough to kill the entire human population by inhalation. Although inhalational botulism is possible, the toxin is unstable in aerosols and the more likely route of intentional intoxication is by food contamination and oral ingestion.

Tetanus

Tetanus, caused by C. *tetani*, is often associated with puncture wounds that do not appear to be serious. The organism and its spores can be isolated from a variety of sources, including soil and the intestinal contents of numerous animal species. A potent neurotoxin (TeNT), often referred to as tetanospasmin, is elaborated at the site of trauma and rapidly binds to neural tissue, provoking a characteristic paralysis and tonic spasms (28, 65). Tetanus is largely a disease of nonimmunized people, particularly in poor regions of the world and primarily affecting infants, since an effective toxoid for immunization has been used for many years.

Tetanus is an intoxication analogous to botulism except that it occurs solely through wound infection and production of tetanospasmin (TeNT). TeNT is synthesized as a single, inactive polypeptide chain (150 kDa), which is cleaved by an intrinsic protease to produce an active dichain form, consisting of a heavy chain (100 kDa) and a light chain (50 kDa) linked by a disulfide bond (155). The heavy chain is the part of the molecule that binds to neuronal cells, and the three-dimensional structure of this region has been elucidated (155). The light chain, a zinc endopeptidase, enters the cell cytoplasm and traverses from the nerve terminal to the nerve cell body by retrograde axonal transport (28, 155), eventually reaching neurons in the spinal cord and brain stem, where it affects glycinergic and GABA (γ-amino-*n*-butyric acid)-ergic neurotransmission (28, 155). Inhibitory impulses to CNS neurons are blocked, while uninhibited firing of motor nerve transmission continues, resulting in prolonged muscle spasms of both flexor and extensor muscles that can persist for weeks. The mechanism by which exocytosis of neurotransmitter release is inhibited is analogous to that of BoNT; in fact, TeNT cleaves the SNARE protein (VAMP) at the same peptide bond as BoNT B (117). In contrast to the pathophysiology of botulism, TeNT is retrogradely transported in neurons to the CNS and its site of action (28, 155).

In the United States, tetanus is reported most frequently in California, Michigan, Texas, and Florida and areas of the rural South (65). While most cases involve older, nonimmunized persons, injection of drugs (i.e., skin popping) has recently become an important risk factor in younger patients (22). It would be an unusual request for the clinical laboratory to isolate C. *tetani* from a wound, since tetanus usually presents few diagnostic problems for the clinician. The worldwide incidence of tetanus has been estimated to be as many as 500,000 cases per year (28, 65). Neonatal tetanus is endemic in developing countries despite the fact that it could be prevented by immunization of the mother and acquisition of passive antibodies by the fetus.

ADDITIONAL CLOSTRIDIAL SPECIES OF INTEREST

C. *innocuum* is an important organism in infections of immunocompromised hosts. C. *innocuum* has also been recovered from patients with recurrent CDAD (2). It is often resistant to multiple drugs used to treat anaerobic infections (2). *C. ramosum* is the second most common *Clostridium* species (after *C. perfringens*) isolated from clinical specimens, including blood cultures and intra-abdominal and soft tissue infections. This species may be resistant to clindamycin and multiple cephalosporins. As noted earlier, *C. tertium* is often isolated from blood cultures from immunocompromised patients and has been reported as a cause of neutropenic enterocolitis and meningitis (51, 111, 122, 175). *C. hathewayi* and *C. bolteae* have been described from various human infections (67, 189), including fatal sepsis (127). Phenotypically similar *C. clostridioforme* is one of the clostridia most commonly isolated from human infections and appears to be associated with more serious or invasive human infections than *C. hathewayi* or *C. bolteae*.

The emergence of 16S rRNA gene sequencing technology has provided a means for identification of strains that may previously have been misidentified or classified as *Clostridium* without species identification. Examples are bacteremia caused by *C. hathewayi* (189), *C. intestinale* (59), and *C. symbiosum* (58); a fatal sepsis due to *C. fallax* in a previously healthy 16-year-old (87); and abscesses yielding *C. celerecrescens* (76). Microarray analysis of DNA from fecal samples has also been useful in determination of predominant species in the large bowel (180). It is likely that in this era of molecular identification techniques, a more accurate picture of clostridial infections will emerge.

COLLECTION, TRANSPORT, AND STORAGE OF CLINICAL SPECIMENS

As with other anaerobic infections, the proper selection, collection, and transport of clinical specimens are extremely important for the laboratory diagnosis of clostridial infections. For recommended collection and transport procedures in general, refer to chapters 5 and 20. Multiple tissue specimens should be sampled from the active sites of infection when gas gangrene is suspected, because clostridia are often not distributed uniformly in pathologic lesions. In addition to aspirates and tissues, selected clostridial illnesses require special specimens.

Confirmation of *C. perfringens* Food-Borne Illness

A freshly passed fecal specimen is the preferred specimen for *C. perfringens* culture and toxin assay, and appropriate specimens include the suspect food. Swab specimens are inadequate for the toxin assay because the sample volume is insufficient. These specimens should be placed into sterile unbreakable containers. All specimens should be stored at 4°C and shipped on cold packs as soon as possible. For optimal recovery, stool specimens should be processed within 24 h of collection.

Diagnosis of Enteritis Necroticans (*C. perfringens* Type C)

If enteritis necroticans is suspected, the appropriate specimens include three blood cultures from three different venipuncture sites, stool (at least 25 g, or 25 ml if liquid), and bowel luminal contents or tissue from the involved bowel (e.g., surgical specimen or autopsy material). Specimens should be transported in tightly sealed leakproof containers for the following: direct Gram stain, culture, isolation, identification, and typing of *C. perfringens*. PCR assays for genotyping *C. perfringens* are being used in certain research or referral laboratories to aid in diagnosis (170). Accordingly, DNA can be extracted for this purpose from formalin-fixed intestinal tissue or culture and amplified by PCR using primers specific for the *cpa* and *cpb* genes of *C. perfringens* type C.

C. difficile Culture and Toxin Assay

A single, freshly passed fecal specimen (ideally 10 to 20 ml of watery stool; minimum of 5.0 ml or 5 g) is the preferred specimen for *C. difficile* culture and toxin assay. To lessen the chance of obtaining positive culture results from patients merely colonized with the organism, only liquid or unformed stool specimens should be processed. Swab specimens are inadequate for the toxin assay because the sample volume is insufficient. Other appropriate specimens include bowel luminal contents and surgical or autopsy samples of the large bowel. Specimens should be transported in tightly sealed, leakproof plastic or glass containers. For optimal recovery, stool specimens should be cultured within 2 h of collection; although spores will survive in refrigerated stool for several days, there will probably be a large decrease in the number of viable vegetative cells of *C. difficile* in refrigerated specimens. Stools should be placed in an anaerobic environment (anaerobic transport vial or bag) if culture must be performed after storage. Adequate recovery of *C. difficile* may be expected from stools stored at 4°C for up to 2 days. Specimens for toxin assay may be stored at 4°C for up to 3 days and should be frozen at −70°C if performance of the assay is delayed. Freezing at −20°C results in a dramatic loss of cytotoxin activity. *C. difficile* toxin is unstable and will degrade at room temperature within 2 h after collection.

Suspected Neutropenic Enterocolitis Involving *C. septicum*

The specimens of choice for suspected neutropenic enterocolitis involving *C. septicum* are three blood cultures collected from three different venipuncture sites, stool (at least 25 g, or 25 ml if liquid), and luminal contents or tissue from the involved ileocecal area collected at surgery or autopsy and transported in tightly sealed leakproof containers. In addition, a biopsy sample of muscle (or an aspirate of fluid from the involved area, taken with a needle and syringe) should be collected if the patient is also suspected of having myonecrosis or another form of progressive infection.

C. botulinum Culture and Toxin Assay

Most hospital laboratories are not properly equipped to process specimens from patients suspected of having botulism. Before collecting any specimens, the medical care providers who suspect a diagnosis of botulism in a patient should immediately call their state health department's emergency 24-h telephone number or the CDC in Atlanta, Ga. (770-488-7100, 24-h/7-day emergency service), so that appropriate action can be taken to establish the diagnosis, initiate treatment, and investigate the case. Acceptable specimens include feces, enema fluid, gastric aspirates or vomitus, tissue or exudates, and postmortem specimens. These specimens should be placed into sterile unbreakable containers. Serum specimens (preferably >10 ml) should be collected as soon as possible after the onset of symptoms. Clinical swabs should be collected in an anaerobic transport medium; environmental swabs (from which spores may be isolated) may be sent in plastic containers without any medium. Food specimens should be left in their original containers if possible, or placed in sterile unbreakable containers. All specimens should be stored at 4°C and shipped on cold packs as soon as possible. Further information can be found at the CDC botulism website (http://www.bt.cdc.gov/agent/botulism). Laboratories should have all of the pertinent information and contact numbers handy. During investigations of possible bioterrorism, sera, gastric aspirates, feces, and environmental or nasal swabs could be useful for detecting aerosolized botulinum toxin that may have been inhaled (11, 190). All specimens should be refrigerated until they can be transported to the laboratory for testing.

Certain clostridial toxins, particularly BoNT and TeNT and iota-toxin, are extremely toxic molecules and are considered very potent poisons. The CDC recommends biosafety level 3 primary containment and personnel precautions for facilities producing BoNTs for study. Personnel who work in the laboratory may be immunized with a pentavalent (A to E) toxoid available from the CDC. A biosafety manual should be posted in the laboratory and should contain the proper emergency phone numbers and procedures for emergency response. Regulations governing personnel safety for research with select agents are outlined in the *Code of Federal Regulations* and the manual *Biosafety in Microbiological and Biomedical Laboratories* (CDC/NIH; available on the Internet at http://www.cdc.gov/od/ohs/biosfty/ bmbl4/bmbl4toc.htm).

DIRECT EXAMINATION

Gas gangrene and necrotizing fasciitis represent extremely urgent situations requiring rapid clinical diagnoses. The direct examination of a Gram-stained smear of the wound may be useful for supporting the diagnosis of gas gangrene (11). Characteristic findings in *C. perfringens* infections include the absence of leukocytic infiltration and the presence of clostridia in smears prepared from central areas of the lesion. Special note should be made of gram-positive rods, with or without spores, because sporulation in tissue is not common for the two species most frequently encountered in wound and abscess materials, *C. perfringens* and *C. ramosum*. *C. perfringens* usually appears as large, relatively short, fat, gram-positive rods with blunt ends and often in short chains in tissue smears; the cells of *C. ramosum* are more slender and longer (Fig. 4). *C. perfringens* may or may not be encapsulated in smears from wounds; capsules usually are present in smears of endometrial specimens from postabortion *C. perfringens* infections. Spore stains offer no advantage over Gram stains for demonstration of spores, but examination with a phase-contrast or dark-field microscope may be helpful if the spores are close to maturity. If spores are present, shapes (spherical or oval) and positions (terminal, subterminal, or central) in the cells should be noted.

Direct Toxin Detection

Bioassays for BoNT and TeNT are currently the most important laboratory tests for diagnosis of botulism and tetanus (46, 56, 84). The definitive diagnosis of botulism is the detection of BoNT (not the organism) (84). Currently, the only reliable assay for BoNT is the mouse bioassay together with neutralization of mouse toxicity with type-specific antitoxins (84). Detection of neurotoxins is usually performed on fecal specimens, blood (serum), suspect foods in food-borne botulism cases, and culture fluid following enrichment by growth of the organism (46, 84). Enzyme-linked immunosorbent assays (ELISAs) have also been used to detect BoNT (56, 158), and cell culture systems (82) and biosensor platforms (55, 158) are in development for BoNT detection (158). Real-time PCR assays for detection of *C. botulinum* BoNT gene fragments specific to BoNT A, B, and E have been developed as alternatives to the mouse bioassay; this approach was found to demonstrate a sensitivity and specificity similar to those of conventional approaches (5).

Antigen Tests for Diagnosis of *C. difficile* Disease

Controversy exists about which of the multiple methods for the detection of *C. difficile* and its toxins is optimal. Toxin detection and neutralization by a cell culture cytotoxin assay are often considered the "gold standard" when new detection methods are evaluated. A confirmed diagnosis of *C. difficile*-associated enteric disease on the basis of both clinical and laboratory criteria represents the ultimate gold standard. Cytotoxicity assay for toxin B is considered the gold standard due to its high sensitivity (94 to 100%) and high specificity (99%) (35, 54). However, the assay is costly and technically demanding and has a slow turnaround time. Therefore, it is not widely used in clinical laboratories. Cytotoxin B neutralization assays are commercially available (Table 2).

The commercially available enzyme immunoassays (EIAs) (Table 2) generally show lower sensitivities and specificities (45 to 95% and 75 to 100%, respectively) than tissue culture assay (35, 134, 178). In general, the relative sensitivities and specificities for the various tests vary considerably, depending upon the laboratory and the method to which the test is compared. Although the sensitivity is lower, the rapid turnaround time of the EIAs and their ease of use explain the preference of many laboratories for an EIA procedure (186). EIAs that detect both toxins A and B are preferable since some strains of *C. difficile* produce only one toxin or the other (186).

Most of the EIAs for detection of toxin A and/or toxin B in stool are microwell format assays, but several membrane-based EIAs are also available (Table 2). The membrane-based EIAs offer an even faster turnaround time than many of the microwell formats, although that of the microwell EIAs from Meridian Bioscience (Cincinnati, Ohio) and TechLab (Blacksburg, Va.) can be shortened considerably by utilizing a shaking incubation step. The microwell formats offer increased sensitivity and specificity over membrane-based EIAs (61). However, one study found the Triage *C. difficile* Micro Panel (Biosite Diagnostics, San Diego, Calif.) and two new chromatographic immunoassays (Clearview *C. difficile* A [Inverness Medical Professional Diagnostics, Princeton, N.J.] and ColorPac Toxin A [Becton Dickinson, Sparks, Md.]) to be more sensitive than conventional EIAs (178). Similarly, the ImmunoCard Toxins A&B (Meridian Bioscience) was found to provide a high specificity and sensitivity and to be suitable for rapid screening for CDAD (177).

The common antigen glutamate dehydrogenase (GDH) does not differentiate between toxigenic and nontoxigenic strains and cannot establish a diagnosis for CDAD because colonization with *C. difficile* is frequent in hospitalized patients. However, testing for GDH has proven useful as a screening test due to its high negative predictive value. A preferred laboratory approach for the diagnosis of CDAD is to test the stool specimens for GDH and, if positive, to test the specimens by EIA for toxin detection (134, 166). The GDH-positive but toxin-negative specimens should be further tested with a cell culture-based cytotoxin assay. The Triage *C. difficile* Micro Panel provides simultaneous detection of toxin A and GDH. Several studies have found the Triage to provide a suitable, rapid alternative for the diagnosis of CDAD (121, 134, 166, 178). Laboratory results obtained with the commercial kits must be correlated and interpreted within the context of the patient's clinical presentation.

Currently PCR is used mostly as a research tool in laboratories for detecting *C. difficile* toxin genes directly in fecal specimens. Real-time PCR has been successfully used for quantitative detection of C. *difficile* and its toxins in fecal samples (26, 177). Also, a multiplex PCR toxin approach has been designed for simultaneous identification and toxigenic type characterization of C. *difficile* isolates (123).

Tests for Diagnosis of CPE

Testing of food sources of C. *perfringens* illness is a public health function (see chapter 12). Several methods have been described for the detection of CPE in feces, including cell culture assays, ELISA, and reversed-phase latex agglutination (RPLA) (139). The cell culture assay using Vero cells is not as sensitive or reproducible as other methods (19, 69). The RPLA kit (PET-RPLA; Oxoid, Hampshire, United Kingdom, and Remel Inc., Lenexa, Kans.) was reproducible and reasonably sensitive; however, nonspecific interference by fecal matter has been reported (139). Similarly, the background bacterial DNA in stool has been reported to interfere with PCR amplification of the enterotoxin gene (139). While an in-house ELISA system developed by the Food Safety Microbiology Laboratory of the Public Health Laboratory Service has been reported to be the most sensitive assay and considered the gold standard, the TechLab C. *perfringens* enterotoxin ELISA system provided a specific, reliable, and practical tool for detecting CPE in fecal samples (19, 69).

ISOLATION PROCEDURES

A summary of useful procedures for culture and isolation of clostridia is provided below. Clostridia usually produce good growth on commercially available CDC anaerobe blood agar and phenylethyl alcohol blood agar (PEA) after 1 to 2 days of incubation. Brucella agar with 5% sheep blood, Columbia agar, or brain heart infusion agar supplemented with yeast extract, vitamin K, and hemin may also be used as the nonselective blood agar medium. Colony characteristics vary on different media. A few species, such as C. *perfringens,* form colonies after overnight incubation or in as little as 6 h. When clostridia are suspected in wound or abscess specimens (e.g., gas gangrene), egg yolk agar (modified McClung-Toabe formula; see chapter 21) may also be inoculated.

After incubation, the blood agar and PEA cultures should be examined under a dissecting microscope, with attention to the hemolysis pattern, colony structure, and any evidence of swarming or motile colonies. Egg yolk agar should be examined for evidence of lecithinase (Fig. 1) or lipase production. Lecithinase activity is indicated by the development of an insoluble, opaque, whitish precipitate within the agar. An iridescent sheen or oil-on-water appearance (pearly layer) indicates lipase activity. Proteolysis, the third reaction that can be seen on egg yolk agar, is indicated by a zone of translucent clearing in the medium around the colonies. In addition to the modified McClung-Toabe egg yolk agar formulation, the same reactions can be visualized on the hemin-supplemented egg yolk agar formulation recommended by Jousimies-Somer et al. (99) or on Lombard-Dowell egg yolk agar (187a).

Isolation of additional strains in the presence of swarming *Proteus* species or C. *septicum* may require short incubation times (18 to 24 h), subculture onto PEA, or use of anaerobe blood agar with 4% agar ("stiff blood agar"). When isolated colonies can be picked, they should be subcultured to chopped-meat medium, and the culture should be incubated overnight and used for the inoculation of differential media. In addition, prereduced, anaerobically sterilized (PRAS) peptone-yeast-glucose media may be inoculated for gas-liquid chromatography if the laboratory has that capability.

Spore Selection Techniques

Heat (80°C) or ethanol treatment procedures can aid in detecting spores (99, 108). Ethanol may be more effective than heat if the specimen contains relatively heat-sensitive clostridia (e.g., C. *botulinum* type E and some strains of C. *perfringens* involved in food-borne outbreaks). Heat treatment may be more effective than alcohol if homogenization is incomplete and the specimen contains particulate matter that is not penetrated adequately by the alcohol. For any spore selection technique, an untreated control subculture should be prepared.

Alcohol Treatment

To a 1-ml sample of a fecal suspension or homogenate of a wound or exudate, in a sterile screw-cap tube, an equal volume of absolute (or 95%) ethanol is added. The specimen is gently mixed at room temperature (22 to 25°C for 1 h). An Ames aliquot mixer (Miles Laboratories, Inc., Elkhart, Ind.) is a convenient way to provide continuous mixing. The treated material is used to inoculate chopped-meat–glucose or thioglycolate medium, anaerobe blood agar, or egg yolk agar. The culture is incubated and inspected for growth.

Heat Treatment

For heat treatment, a tube of chopped-meat–glucose or thioglycolate medium (5 ml) is preheated in an 80°C water bath for 5 min, and 1 ml of sample suspension is added. The culture is heated for 10 min, and the tube is removed and cooled in cold water. The treated sample suspension is subcultured into an unheated tube of chopped-meat–glucose or thioglycolate medium, anaerobe blood agar, or egg yolk agar. The cultures are incubated anaerobically and examined for growth.

Isolation of *C. difficile*

Culture alone (without subsequent testing of C. *difficile* isolates for toxin production) results in lower specificity and misdiagnosis of CDAD, especially when C. *difficile* carriage is prevalent. Testing isolates with a toxin assay by cell culture or EIA provides the organism for epidemiological studies and for antimicrobial susceptibility testing, if required. To perform a culture for C. *difficile,* a stool specimen should be inoculated directly onto cycloserine-cefoxitin-fructose agar (CCFA) (see chapter 21). The culture should be incubated anaerobically at 35 to 37°C for 18 to 24 h before observation. Following incubation, the plates should be examined by using a dissecting microscope. Colonies of C. *difficile* are yellowish to white, circular to irregular, and flat, with a rhizoid or erose edge and a ground-glass appearance (Fig. 2). The colonies have a distinctive odor like *para*-cresol (or horse manure). In addition, C. *difficile* colonies on CCFA fluoresce chartreuse under UV light (99).

In addition to the use of CCFA medium, C. *difficile* from fecal samples can be isolated by using the alcohol or heat shock spore selection technique. After 18 to 24 h of incubation on blood-containing agar, colonies from treated samples are nonhemolytic, 2 to 4 mm in diameter, creamy yellow to gray-white, and irregular. The colonies have a coarsely mottled to mosaic internal structure and a matte or dull surface, and they are seen to be slightly raised when viewed under a dissecting microscope. The odor is distinctive. Gram staining of C. *difficile* reveals gram-positive to gram-variable rods that are thin, with parallel sides, and 0.5 μm wide by 3 to 5 μm long. If spores are present, they are subterminal. Presumptive

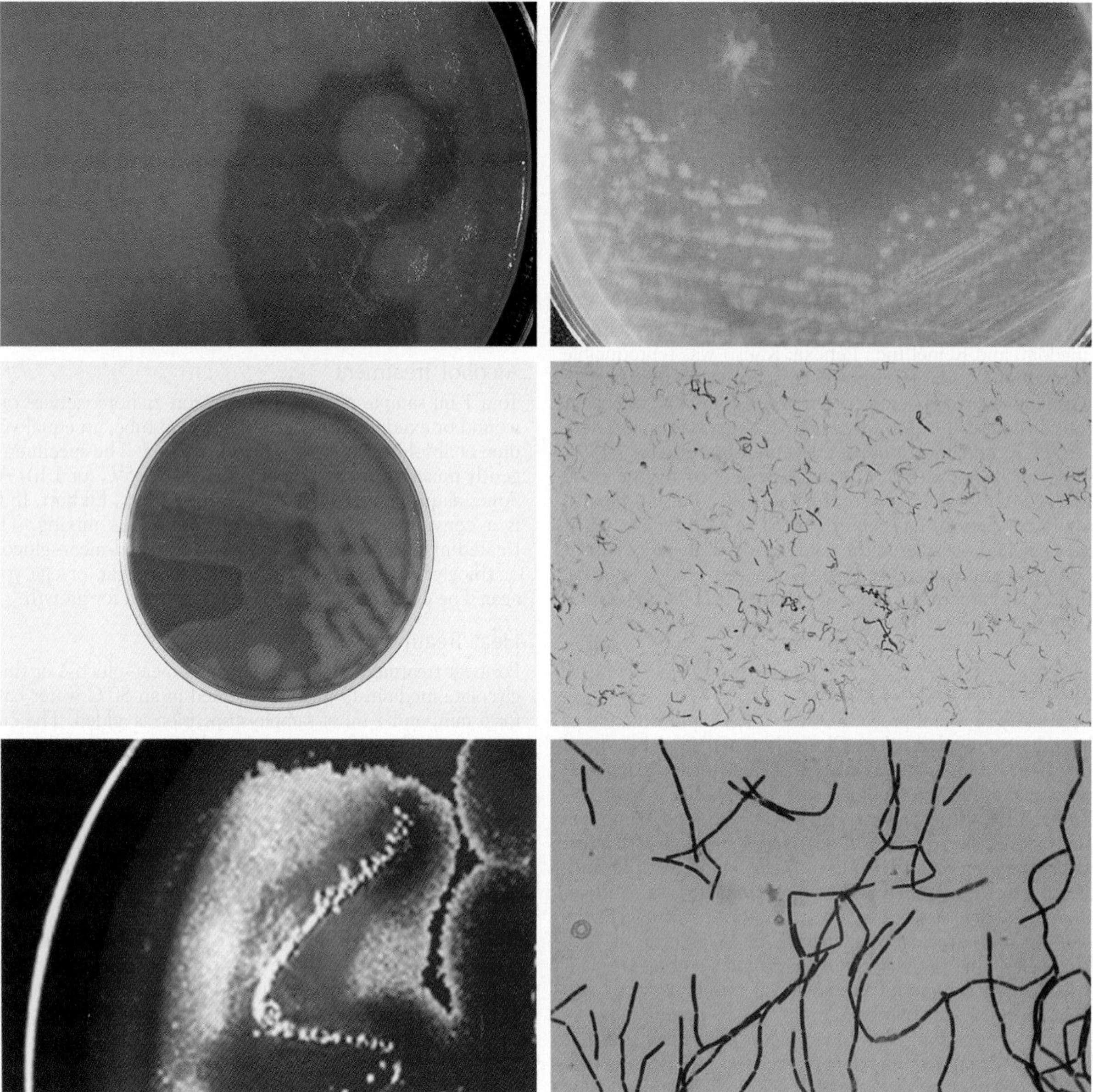

FIGURE 1 (top row, left) Lecithinase reaction on egg yolk agar. Note opacity of agar surrounding colonies due to precipitation of complex fats. (Reprinted with permission from reference 99.)

FIGURE 2 (top row, right) *C. difficile* on CCFA. Note the yellow, ground-glass appearance of colonies. (Reprinted with permission from reference 99.)

FIGURE 3 (middle row, left) *C. perfringens* on blood agar showing double zone of beta-hemolysis. (Reprinted with permission from reference 99.)

FIGURE 4 (middle row, right) Gram stain of *C. ramosum*. Note thin, gram-variable bacilli with distinct spores. (Reprinted with permission from reference 99.)

FIGURE 5 (bottom row, left) *Clostridium septicum* on blood agar after 12 h of incubation. Note spreading colonies. (Courtesy of E. J. Baron.)

FIGURE 6 (bottom row, right) Gram stain of *C. septicum*. Note long, filamentous bacilli with rare spores. (Courtesy of E. J. Baron.)

TABLE 2 Commonly used tests for the diagnosis of C. *difficile* disease

Entity detected	Method	Principal advantages	Principal limitations	Available tests and sources
Organism	Toxigenic culture	Sensitive, specific	Efficiency varies from lab to lab; must add method for toxin detection	CCFA, available from various manufacturers; prereduced media preferred (Anaerobe Systems)
GDH	Latex agglutination	Rapid, simple	Low sensitivity; does not distinguish between toxigenic and nontoxigenic C. *difficile*	CDT (BD) Meritec C. *difficile* (Meridian Bioscience)
	Membrane EIA	Rapid, simple	Higher sensitivity; does not distinguish between toxigenic and nontoxigenic C. *difficile*	Triage Micro C. *difficile* panel (Biosite Diagnostics Inc.) Immunocard C. *difficile* (Meridian Bioscience) C. *diff* Chek (Inverness Medical Professional Diagnostics and TechLab, Inc.)
Toxin B	Tissue culture	Sensitive, specific	Requires 24–48 h to complete; toxin B can be inactivated, resulting in false-negative results	C. *difficile* Toxin/Antitoxin (TechLab) C. *difficile* Tox B Test (Inverness Medical Professional Diagnostics and TechLab)
Toxin A	EIA	Rapid, simple	Sensitivity and specificity vary considerably Does not detect A^-/B^+ isolates	Triage C. *difficile* panel (Biosite Diagnostics) Premier C. *difficile* Toxin A (Meridian Bioscience) ProSpecT-II C. *difficile* Toxin A microplate (Remel Inc.) C. *difficile* Tox-A Test (TechLab) Culturette Toxin CD Test (BD) VIDAS-CDA (bioMerieux)
	Membrane EIA	Rapid, simple	Sensitivity and specificity vary considerably Does not detect A^-/B^+ isolates	Triage C. *difficile* panel (Biosite Diagnostics) ImmunoCard Stat! Toxin A (Meridian Bioscience) C. *difficile* Toxin A (Oxoid and Remel) Clearview C. *difficile* Toxin A (Inverness Medical Professional Diagnostics and Hardy Diagnostics, Santa Maria, Calif.)
	Optical immunoassay	Rapid, simple	Less sensitive than EIA	ColorPAC Toxin A Test Kit (BD) BioStar OIA CdTOX A (Inverness Medical Professional Diagnostics)
Toxins A and B	EIA	Rapid, simple	Sensitivity and specificity vary considerably Detects A^-/B^+ isolates	Premier Toxins A and B (Meridian Bioscience) ProSpecT C. *difficile* Toxin A/B microplate (Remel Inc.) C. *difficile* TOX A/B II (Inverness Medical Professional Diagnostics and TechLab)
	Membrane EIA	Rapid, simple	Sensitivity and specificity vary considerably Detects A^-/B^+ isolates	ImmunoCard Toxins A and B (ICTAB; Meridian) Xpect C. *difficile* Toxin A/B (Remel and Oxoid) Tox A/B Quik Chek (Inverness Medical Professional Diagnostics)

identification of C. *difficile* can be made by demonstrating typical colonies, Gram stain morphology, and characteristic odor. Definitive identification depends on demonstration of the unique pattern of short-chain fatty acid metabolic products by gas-liquid chromatography (GLC) and by biochemical characterization of isolates (12, 74, 90) (see Table 1).

IDENTIFICATION

Preliminary Identification of *Clostridium* Species

Clostridia are typically gram-positive rods by microscopic morphology. Some clostridia appear gram negative, especially *C. ramosum*, *C. innocuum*, and the *C. clostridioforme* group, but the special-potency antibiotic disk pattern will verify the presence of gram-positive organisms. Second, it may be difficult to detect spores, so an ethanol or heat spore treatment may be necessary, and phase-contrast or dark-field microscopy may be helpful. Third, the colonial morphology of pure cultures may be variable, so the culture may appear to be mixed. Subcultures of single, well-isolated colonies yield the same variable morphologies. Examination of colonies by stereomicroscopy is helpful for noting colonial characteristics. Fourth, the aerotolerant clostridia may be confused with *Bacillus* or *Lactobacillus* spp. *Clostridium* species sporulate anaerobically only, grow much better anaerobically (larger colonies), and are almost always catalase negative. *Bacillus* spp. sporulate aerobically only, usually grow better aerobically, and are usually catalase positive. Aerobically grown *C. tertium* shares similar colonial and cellular morphologies with *Lactobacillus* spp. Certain clostridia can be identified with relative ease by Gram stain and colony morphology, indole reaction, hemolysis on blood agar, and tests decribed below (Table 3).

Special-Potency Disks

The isolate should be subcultured on blood agar with special-potency disks containing vancomycin (5 μg), kanamycin (1 mg), or colistin (10 μg). The plates should be incubated anaerobically for 48 to 72 h at 35 to 37°C. Clostridia are colistin resistant and vancomycin susceptible (Table 3), except for occasional *C. innocuum* isolates, which may be only moderately susceptible to vancomycin (7).

Lecithinase and Lipase

The isolate should be subcultured on egg yolk agar and incubated anaerobically for 48 to 72 h at 35 to 37°C. Lecithinase activity is demonstrated by a white, opaque, diffuse zone around the colonies and extending into the medium (Fig. 1). Lipase activity is indicated by an iridescent sheen on the surface of bacterial growth and on the agar surface around the colonies.

Spore Test

Media for the demonstration of spores include chopped-meat agar slant or broth and thioglycolate medium. The culture should be incubated anaerobically at 5 to 7°C below the optimum temperature (30°C) for growth and sporulation of clostridia, except for *C. perfringens* (should be induced at 37°C). Actively growing cultures may stand at room temperature for several days to 1 week, and ethanol or heat spore treatments can be performed as described above.

Definitive Identification of *Clostridium* Species

The traditional method for the phenotypic characterization and identification of clostridia is the use of PRAS media for the determination of fermentation profiles and other characteristics combined with GLC analysis of metabolic end products (99). However, only a few laboratories have PRAS media or GLC available. Table 1 lists characteristics that are useful for definitive identification of clinically relevant clostridia. The key reactions (bold in Table 1) require minimal PRAS media and can be used in conjunction with commercial identification kits or individual preformed-enzyme tests such as Wee Tabs (Key Scientific, Round Rock, Tex.) or Rosco Diagnostic Tablets (Rosco, Taasrup, Denmark). Gelatin and esculin hydrolysis, carbohydrate fermentation reactions, and metabolic end product analysis (Table 1) are based on results obtained with PRAS media (Anaerobe Systems, Morgan Hill, Calif.).

PRAS Biochemical Inoculation

Actively growing broth cultures (without carbohydrate) or cell pastes suspended in broth medium (e.g., peptone-yeast or thioglycolate) may be used to inoculate PRAS media. The cultures are incubated for 48 to 72 h at 35 to 37°C, and overnight incubation may be sufficient for many clostridia.

Gelatin Hydrolysis

A PRAS gelatin tube with an actively growing culture is refrigerated along with an uninoculated tube for at least 1 h. The tubes are removed to room temperature, inverted immediately, and observed for liquefaction every 5 min. In a positive reaction, the gelatin has been hydrolyzed and thus fails to solidify and will drop to the top of the inverted tube immediately. In a negative reaction, the medium fails to liquefy when it reaches room temperature (>30 min).

TABLE 3 Rapid identification of some lecithinase-positive and/or swarming *Clostridium* spp. of clinical significance[a]

Species	Lecithinase	Lipase	Indole	Swarming	Urease	Spore location	Other characteristics
C. bifermentans	+	–	+	–	–	ST	Chalk-white colonies on EYA
C. novyi A	+	+	–	+	–	ST	Robust beta-hemolysis
C. perfringens	+	–	–	–	–	ST	Double zone of beta-hemolysis Reverse CAMP positive
C. sordellii	+	–	+	–	+	ST	Large gram-positive bacilli
C. septicum	–	–	–	+	–	ST	Rare spores Spreading, adherent colonies
C. sporogenes	–	+	–	+	–[+]	ST	Abundant oval spores
C. tetani	–	–[w]	v	+	–	T	Drumstick shaped

[a] EYA, egg yolk agar; for other abbreviations and symbols, see Table 1, footnote *a*.

A weakly positive reaction yields liquid medium at the time it reaches room temperature (<30 min).

Esculin Hydrolysis

Five drops of 1% ferric ammonium citrate are added to a tube of actively growing bacteria in a PRAS esculin tube, and the tube is observed for a color change and fluorescence under UV (366 nm) light. In a positive reaction, a black or dark brown color may develop, and there is no fluorescence under UV light. In a negative reaction no color develops, and the tube fluoresces white-blue under UV light. Since many clostridia produce hydrogen sulfide (H_2S), which also reacts with the reagent to form a black complex, all tubes that darken after the addition of reagent should be confirmed under UV light.

Carbohydrate Fermentation

The pH of actively growing organisms (at least 2+ turbidity) should be measured in a PRAS carbohydrate tube. A positive reaction ("acid") yields a pH below 5.5, and a negative reaction results in a pH exceeding 5.9. "Weak acid" is indicated by a pH of 5.6 to 5.8. Details of GLC procedures used for the analyses of metabolic end products listed in Table 1 are outlined elsewhere (99).

Commercial kits, based on the detection of preformed enzymes with chromogenic or fluorogenic substrates, have been marketed for the rapid identification of anaerobes. These panels include RapID ANA II (Remel), RapID 32A (bioMerieux, Durham, N.C.), Vitek ANI Card (bioMerieux), and BBL Crystal Anaerobe Identification System (BD, Franklin Lakes, N.J.). The overall performance of these panels varies, and the panels are generally not satisfactory as the sole identification method for clostridia. In the RapID ANA II system, 74% of the 130 clostridia tested were correctly identified to the species level (132). Identification was correct for *C. perfringens* and *C. ramosum* but less likely to be correct for other commonly encountered clostridia, such as *C. difficile, C. innocuum,* and *C. clostridioforme* (132). Similarly, in another study, 100% of 20 *C. ramosum* isolates, 24% of 21 *C. innocuum* isolates, 50% of 20 *C. clostridioforme* isolates, and 91% of 11 *C. perfringens* isolates were correctly identified by RapID ANA II (7). In the same study, Rapid ID 32A identified 70% of *C. ramosum* isolates, 0% of *C. innocuum* isolates, 40% of *C. clostridioforme* isolates, and 46% of *C. perfringens* isolates correctly (7). Neither the RapID ANA II nor the Rapid ID 32A test system was found to provide a reliable method for identification of *C. botulinum* (126). The Vitek ANI Card identified only 64% of clostridia correctly; all *C. perfringens* isolates (total of 8) and 64% of *C. difficile* isolates (7 of 11 total isolates) were correctly identified to the species level (156). The BBL Crystal Anaerobe Identification System (BD) correctly identified 79 of 103 (76.7%) *Clostridium* strains, but the system failed to identify any of the 7 *C. innocuum* or 9 *C. tetani* strains tested (45).

In general, Gram reaction, cellular morphologies, colonial characteristics, and aerotolerance of isolates should be determined in conjunction with the use of commercial microsystems. Supplementation of tests in these kits with individual tablets (e.g., Wee Tabs or Rosco Tablets) can be helpful. Other useful supplemental tests for clostridia include the tests outlined above, such as lipase and lecithinase, the reduction of nitrate, gelatin and esculin hydrolysis, carbohydrate fermentation, and metabolic end product analysis using GLC.

Characteristics of Commonly Encountered Clostridia

Key characteristics that aid in the presumptive identification of the most common species are listed below. See Tables 1 and 3.

- *C. bifermentans:* colonies chalk-white on egg yolk agar, irregular, scalloped edge; many free spores, often chaining; urease negative; indole and lecithinase positive. *C. sordellii* is similar but is usually urease positive.
- *C. bolteae:* colonies usually have a slightly irregular edge; greening of agar around colonies; gram negative; tapered ends; spores are rare. Lactose negative and β-*N*-acetylglucosaminidase (β-NAG) negative.
- *C. butyricum:* very large, irregular colonies with mottled to mosaic internal structure; subterminal spores; ferments many carbohydrates.
- *C. cadaveris:* white-gray, entire or slightly irregular, raised to slightly convex; oval terminal spores; spot indole positive.
- *C. clostridioforme:* same as for *C. bolteae* but lactose positive and β-NAG negative.
- *C. difficile:* colonies creamy yellow to gray-white (Fig. 2), irregular, coarse, mottled to mosaic internal structure, matte or dull surface, horse stable odor; subterminal to free spores or spores infrequent; gelatin hydrolysis can be slow. Mannitol and proline positive; colonies fluoresce chartreuse on CCFA.
- *C. glycolicum:* colonies gray-white, entire to scalloped edge, convex; subterminal and free spores.
- *C. hathewayi:* same as for *C. bolteae* but lactose and β-NAG positive.
- *C. innocuum:* gray-white to brilliant greenish colonies, coarsely mottled to mosaic internal structure, entire edge usually; terminal spores may be difficult to find; nonmotile; mannitol positive; lactose, maltose, and proline negative.
- *C. novyi* type A: lecithinase and lipase positive, may swarm, strong beta-hemolysis.
- *C. perfringens:* double zone of beta-hemolysis around colonies (Fig. 3), boxcar-shaped rods, spores rare, lecithinase positive (Fig. 1).
- *C. ramosum:* colonies resemble *Bacteroides fragilis* but usually have a slightly irregular edge; gram-variable, palisading, slender rods; small round or oval terminal spores (Fig. 4); nonmotile; mannitol positive.
- *C. septicum:* swarms (Fig. 5), large, filamentous bacilli (Fig. 6), subterminal spores often "lemon" forms, DNase positive, sucrose negative.
- *C. sporogenes:* medusa-head colonies, possible swarming, colonies adhere firmly to agar; subterminal and many free spores; lipase positive.
- *C. symbiosum:* rods with tapered ends, football shaped, may form chains, often has spores.
- *C. tertium:* aerotolerant, terminal spores when anaerobically incubated.
- *C. tetani:* may form a thin film of growth over entire agar plate, especially on moist media; drumstick spores.

Toxin tests are necessary for the identification of a few species. *C. sporogenes* cannot be differentiated with certainty from the proteolytic group I strains of *C. botulinum* unless toxin tests are used. A few strains of C. *botulinum* produce lecithinase as well as lipase and are difficult to distinguish from C. *novyi* type A except by toxin tests or by the use of a C. *novyi* fluorescent-antibody conjugate (165). An excellent source of diagnostic clostridial antisera is TechLab. As a supplement to the methods described, the various types of C. *botulinum* and other clostridia can be presumptively identified on the basis of differences in their cellular fatty acid profiles (12, 74, 90) and by typing methods such as pulsed-field gel electrophoresis or other molecular analyses. Finegold et al. (67) described a multiplex PCR procedure for the rapid distinction among the three species of the C. *clostridioforme* group.

ANTIMICROBIAL SUSCEPTIBILITIES

Antimicrobial susceptibility studies with strains of a number of clostridial species are summarized in Table 4. Now that more laboratories are identifying anaerobes by 16S rRNA gene sequencing, more accurate species identification will be available and more reliable susceptibility data can be generated. Drugs lacking antimicrobial activity against various clostridia include trimethoprim-sulfamethoxazole (a drug noted for promoting intestinal overgrowth of clostridia [83]), ampicillin, and clindamycin. No resistance of clostridia to ampicillin-sulbactam or piperacillin-tazobactam was noted, and antimicrobial resistance was uncommon among clostridia with respect to imipenem, metronidazole, and vancomycin. Five species (all with small numbers of strains) and C. *perfringens* showed little or no resistance to the antimicrobial agents under consideration (Table 4). Organisms with some resistance to three drugs included C. *ramosum*, C. *innocuum*, and C. *clostridioforme*; two strains of C. *orbiscindens* displayed resistance to ampicillin as well as linezolid.

Multiple studies have described resistance to various antibiotics among clostridia. Resistance to penicillin is especially common in C. *ramosum*, C. *clostridioforme*, and C. *butyricum* (64, 152); these species produce β-lactamases that are induced by β-lactam antibiotics (88). C. *tertium* has resistance features unusual among clostridia, including resistance to β-lactam antibiotics, metronidazole, and clindamycin. Resistance to clindamycin has been documented for strains of C. *perfringens* (as noted above), C. *ramosum*, C. *difficile*, C. *tertium*, C. *subterminale*, C. *butyricum*, C. *sporogenes*, and C. *innocuum* (187a).

Chloramphenicol, piperacillin, metronidazole, imipenem, and combinations of β-lactams with β-lactam inhibitors (e.g., ampicillin-sulbactam) were active against most clostridia (187a). The clostridia are variably resistant to cephalosporins and tetracyclines, and they are usually resistant to the aminoglycosides. Many clostridia other than C. *perfringens* (particularly C. *ramosum*, C. *clostridioforme*, and C. *innocuum*) are resistant to cefoxitin, cefotaxime, ceftazidime, ceftizoxime, cefoperazone, and other broad-spectrum β-lactams (7, 64, 152, 187a). Most strains of C. *innocuum* were only moderately susceptible to vancomycin (7). C. *innocuum* may be intrinsically resistant to this compound (141).

Earlier quinolones, such as ciprofloxacin, levofloxacin, and lomefloxacin, have demonstrated low or intermediate activity against anaerobes, but more recently introduced quinolones, like moxifloxacin, gatifloxacin, trovafloxacin, and garenoxacin, have good activity in vitro against most anaerobes, including clostridia (1, 125). A high frequency of moxifloxacin resistance has been described among C. *difficile*

TABLE 4 Activities of various drugs against *Clostridium* spp. (Wadsworth agar dilution procedure)[a]

Antimicrobial agent	CLSI MIC breakpoint (μg/ml)		% Susceptible[b]																			
	Susceptible	Intermediate	C. *bifermentans*	C. *bolteae*	C. *butyricum*	C. *cadaveris*	C. *clostridioforme*	C. *difficile*	C. *disporicum*	C. *glycolicum*	C. *hathewayi*	C. *innocuum*	C. *orbiscindens*	C. *paraputrificum*	C. *perfringens*	C. *ramosum*	C. *septicum*	C. *sordellii*	C. *sporogenes*	C. *subterminale*	C. *tertium*
Ampicillin[c]	0.5	1	100	67	86	100[d]	67	26	100	100		100	53	94	100	100	100[d]	100	100	100	100
Amoxicillin-clavulanate	4/2	8/4	100	66	100		75	100	100	100	100	100	100	100	100	100		100	100	100[d]	100[d]
Piperacillin-tazobactam	32/4	64/4	100[d]					100				100			100	100		100	100[d]		
Ticarcillin	32	64						100							100	100		100	100[d]		
Clindamycin	2	4	100	100	100	100[d]	90	56	100	92	93	83	100	87	100	82	100[d]	94	8	85	100[d]
Vancomycin	8	16	100	91	100	100[d]	100	100	100	100	100	98	100	100	100	100	100[d]	100	100	100	100
Imipenem	4	8	100[d]	100[d]	100[d]	100[d]		94				100		100[d]	100	100		100	100		
Linezolid	2	4	100	100	85		86	91	100	100	100	94		75	100	12		100	100	83	100[d]
Metronidazole	8	16	100	100	100	100	100	100	100	100	100	98	100	100	97	98	100[d]	95	100	100	100
Trimethoprim-sulfamethoxazole	32	64	0	67	50	0[d]	100	26	78	0		3	12	31	4	57	100[d]	0	0[d]	0	14
Trovafloxacin	2	4		0[d]	100[d]	100[d]	100[d]	86				100	100	100	8	86	100[d]	100	100		

[a] Clinical and Laboratory Standards Institute (CLSI) approved method M11-A6 (50a); data from Wadsworth Anaerobic Bacteriology Laboratory.
[b] According to the CLSI-approved breakpoints (M11-A6) (50a), the intermediate category is susceptible.
[c] Strains producing β-lactamase should be considered resistant.
[d] Five or fewer strains were tested.

isolates (3), and quinolone resistance is a problem among pathogens.

Severe *C. difficile*-associated intestinal disease is usually treated with oral vancomycin or metronidazole, but recently a number of metronidazole failures have been noted. Relapse of disease following antibiotic therapy occurs in about 30% of patients. Surgical therapy is required in the event of bowel perforation and toxic megacolon.

Patients diagnosed with food-borne or wound botulism should immediately receive trivalent (type ABE) antitoxin and intensive respiratory care (17, 46, 84). Early administration of antibodies can decrease the severity of the disease and slow its progression, resulting in a shorter hospital stay and more rapid recovery (16, 18, 84). Convalescence and recovery from botulism are generally prolonged, requiring weeks to months depending on the quantity of toxin exposure and serotype (serotype A has the longest duration, 1 to 6 months), but recovery is usually complete and patients regain normal function (16, 50, 84). Symptoms of fatigue, muscular weakness, and constipation have been reported to persist for months in certain patients (50).

Surgical measures are especially important in the treatment of gas gangrene and a number of *Clostridium* infections. The effect of clindamycin (and metronidazole) on toxin suppression by *C. perfringens* and other gram-positive organisms is an important reason to utilize such an agent in addition to penicillin or other β-lactam agents in the management of serious infections such as anaerobic myonecrosis (gas gangrene).

EVALUATION, INTERPRETATION, AND REPORTING OF RESULTS

The isolation of a *Clostridium* species from a clinical specimen, even a blood culture, may or may not be significant clinically, and culture results should be interpreted in relation to the patient's clinical findings. Clostridia of the patient's own intestinal microbiota may be present on the skin and may contaminate blood samples or other specimens. Bacteremia may be transient or clinically insignificant. In addition, most clostridia currently encountered in wounds, exudates, blood, and other normally sterile body fluids are opportunistic and may not cause serious or progressive disease unless conditions are suitable in the host. As discussed earlier in this chapter, one exception to this generalization is *C. septicum*, which rarely is encountered in blood cultures except from patients who have an underlying malignancy or neutropenic sepsis. *C. septicum* sepsis is an infectious disease emergency that requires prompt and clear communication between the laboratory and the clinician in order to institute early surgical measures and treatment with antimicrobial agents to improve outcomes. *C. tertium*, *C. perfringens*, and other clostridia, to a lesser extent, may be involved in serious infections that require emergency measures. The best approach for preventing tragic consequences that may be avoidable is good communication between microbiologists and clinicians.

The accurate and timely reporting of preliminary results (e.g., findings from direct microscopic examinations of clinical specimens), as well as early culture results (after 24 and 48 h of incubation), can be extremely valuable to the physician. For smaller laboratories without anaerobic chambers, incubation of the appropriate media in anaerobic jars provides acceptable recovery for most clinically significant anaerobes, assuming that optimal collection and transport of specimens are performed. The colony characteristics and microscopic features of some clostridia (e.g., *C. perfringens*, *C. sordellii*, and *C. sporogenes*) may be distinctive, so preliminary or presumptive reports may be released before aerotolerance studies are completed. Accurate, definitive identification is needed to better define the role of clostridia in disease, to aid the clinician in selecting optimal treatment, and for public health purposes (e.g., hospital-acquired *C. difficile* disease).

REFERENCES

1. **Ackermann, G., R. Schaumann, B. Pless, M. C. Claros, E. J. C. Goldstein, and A. C. Rodloff.** 2000. Comparative activity of moxifloxacin *in vitro* against obligately anaerobic bacteria. *Eur. J. Clin. Microbiol. Infect. Dis.* **19:**228–232.
2. **Ackermann, G., Y. J. Tang, S. S. Jang, J. Silva, A. C. Rodloff, and S. H. Cohen.** 2001. Isolation of *Clostridium innocuum* from cases of recurrent diarrhea in patients with prior *Clostridium difficile* associated diarrhea. *Diagn. Microbiol. Infect. Dis.* **40:**103–106.
3. **Ackermann, G., Y. J. Tang, R. Kueper, P. Heisig, A. C. Rodloff, J. Silva, Jr., and S. H. Cohen.** 2001. Resistance to moxifloxacin in toxigenic *Clostridium difficile* isolates is associated with mutations in *gyrA*. *Antimicrob. Agents Chemother.* **45:**2348–2353.
4. **Adams, V., D. Lyras, K. A. Farrow, and J. I. Rood.** 2002. The clostridial mobilisable transposons. *Cell. Mol. Life Sci.* **59:**2033–2043.
5. **Akbulut, D., K. A. Grant, and J. McLauchlin.** 2005. Improvement in laboratory diagnosis of wound botulism and tetanus among injecting illicit-drug users by use of real-time PCR assays for neurotoxin gene fragments. *J. Clin. Microbiol.* **43:**4342–4348.
6. **al-Barrak, A., J. Embil, B. Dyck, K. Olekson, D. Nicoll, M. Alfa, and A. Kabani.** 1999. An outbreak of toxin A negative, toxin B positive *Clostridium difficile*-associated diarrhea in a Canadian tertiary-care hospital. *Can. Commun. Dis. Rep.* **25:**65–69.
7. **Alexander, C. J., D. M. Citron, J. S. Brazier, and E. J. Goldstein.** 1995. Identification and antimicrobial resistance patterns of clinical isolates of *Clostridium clostridioforme*, *Clostridium innocuum*, and *Clostridium ramosum* compared with those of clinical isolates of *Clostridium perfringens*. *J. Clin. Microbiol.* **33:**3209–3215.
8. **Alfa, M. J., A. Kabani, D. Lyerly, S. Moncrief, L. M. Neville, A. Al-Barrak, G. K. Harding, B. Dyck, K. Olekson, and J. M. Embil.** 2000. Characterization of a toxin A-negative, toxin B-positive strain of *Clostridium difficile* responsible for a nosocomial outbreak of *Clostridium difficile*-associated diarrhea. *J. Clin. Microbiol.* **38:**2706–2714.
9. **Alfa, M. J., D. Robson, M. Davi, K. Bernard, P. Van Caeseele, and G. K. M. Harding.** 2002. An outbreak of necrotizing enterocolitis associated with a novel *Clostridium* species in a neonatal intensive care unit. *Clin. Infect. Dis.* **35:**S101–S105.
10. **Allen, S. D.** 1997. Pig-bel and other necrotizing disorders of the gut involving *Clostridium perfringens*, p. 717–724. *In* D. H. Connor, F. W. Chandler, D. A. Schwartz, H. J. Manz, and E. E. Lack (ed.), *Pathology of Infectious Diseases*. Appleton & Lange, Norwalk, Conn.
11. **Allen, S. D., C. L. Emery, and J. A. Siders.** 2002. Anaerobic bacteriology, p. 50–81. *In* A. L. Truant (ed.), *Manual of Commercial Methods in Clinical Microbiology*. ASM Press, Washington, D.C.
12. **Allen, S. D., J. A. Siders, M. J. Riddell, J. A. Fill, and W. S. Wegener.** 1995. Cellular fatty acid analysis in the differentiation of *Clostridium* in the clinical microbiology laboratory. *Clin. Infect. Dis.* **20:**S198–S201.

13. **Alonso, R., C. Munoz, S. Gros, D. Garcia de Viedma, T. Pelaez, and E. Bouza.** 1999. Rapid detection of toxigenic *Clostridium difficile* from stool samples by a nested PCR of toxin B gene. *J. Hosp. Infect.* **41:**145–149.
14. **Alouf, J. E., and M. R. Popoff (ed.).** *The Comprehensive Sourcebook of Bacterial Toxins,* 3rd ed., in press. Elsevier Press, London, United Kingdom.
15. **Anaya, D. A., K. McMahon, A. B. Nathens, S. R. Sullivan, H. Foy, and E. Bulger.** 2005. Predictors of mortality and limb loss in necrotizing soft tissue infections. *Arch. Surg.* **140:**151–157.
16. **Arnon, S. S.** 2004. Infant botulism, p. 1758–1766. *In* R. D. Feigen, J. D. Cherry, G. Demmler, and S. Kaplan (ed.), *Textbook of Pediatric Infectious Diseases,* 5th ed. W. B. Saunders, Philadelphia, Pa.
17. **Arnon, S. S., R. Schechter, T. V. Inglesby, D. A. Henderson, J. G. Bartlett, M. S. Ascher, E. Eitzen, A. D. Fine, J. Hauer, M. Layton, S. Lillibridge, M. T. Osterholm, T. O'Toole, G. Parker, T. M. Perl, P. K. Russell, D. L. Swerdlow, and K. Tonat.** 2001. Botulinum toxin as a biological weapon: medical and public health management. *JAMA* **285:**1059–1070.
18. **Arnon, S. S., R. Schechter, S. E. Maslanka, N. P. Jewell, and C. L. Hatheway.** 2006. Human botulism immune globulin for the treatment of infant botulism. *N. Engl. J. Med.* **354:**462–471.
19. **Asha, N. J., and M. H. Wilcox.** 2002. Laboratory diagnosis of *Clostridium perfringens* antibiotic-associated diarrhoea. *J. Med. Microbiol.* **51:**891–894.
20. **Aslam, S., R. J. Hamill, and D. M. Musher.** 2005. Treatment of *Clostridium difficile*-associated disease: old therapies and new strategies. *Lancet Infect. Dis.* **5:**549–557.
21. **Assadian, O., A. Assadian, C. Senekowitsch, A. Makristathis, and G. Hagmuller.** 2004. Gas gangrene due to *Clostridium perfringens* in two injecting drug users in Vienna, Austria. *Wien. Klin. Wochenschr.* **116:**264–267.
22. **Barsam, A., M. Kerins, and P. Jaye.** 2005. Tetanus and intravenous drug use. *Eur. J. Clin. Microbiol. Infect. Dis.* **24:** 497–498.
23. **Barth, H., K. Aktories, M. R. Popoff, and B. G. Stiles.** 2004. Binary bacterial toxins: biochemistry, biology, and applications of common *Clostridium* and *Bacillus* proteins. *Microbiol. Mol. Biol. Rev.* **68:**373–402.
24. **Bartlett, J. G.** 2002. Clinical practice. Antibiotic-associated diarrhea. *N. Engl. J. Med.* **346:**334–339.
25. **Bartram, U., and D. Singer.** 2004. Infant botulism and sudden infant death syndrome. *Klin. Paediatr.* **216:**26–30.
26. **Belanger, S. D., M. Boissinot, N. Clairoux, F. J. Picard, and M. G. Bergeron.** 2003. Rapid detection of *Clostridium difficile* in feces by real-time PCR. *J. Clin. Microbiol.* **41:**730–734.
27. **Bennion, R. S., E. J. Baron, J. E. Thompson, Jr., J. Downes, P. Summanen, D. A. Talan, and S. M. Finegold.** 1990. The bacteriology of gangrenous and perforated appendicitis—revisited. *Ann. Surg.* **211:**165–171.
28. **Bleck, T. P.** 1991. Tetanus: pathophysiology, management, and prophylaxis. *Dis. Mon.* **37:**545–603.
29. **Bodey, G. P., S. Rodriguez, V. Fainstein, and L. S. Elting.** 1991. Clostridial bacteremia in cancer patients. A 12-year experience. *Cancer* **67:**1928–1942.
30. **Boone, J. H., and R. J. Carman.** 1997. *Clostridium perfringens:* food poisoning and antibiotic-associated diarrhea. *Clin. Microbiol. Newsl.* **19:**65–67.
31. **Borriello, S. P., and F. E. Barclay.** 1986. An in-vitro model of colonisation resistance to *Clostridium difficile* infection. *J. Med. Microbiol.* **21:**299–309.
32. **Borriello, S. P., F. E. Barclay, A. R. Welch, M. F. Stringer, G. N. Watson, R. K. Williams, D. V. Seal, and K. Sullens.** 1985. Epidemiology of diarrhoea caused by enterotoxigenic *Clostridium perfringens*. *J. Med. Microbiol.* **20:**363–372.
33. **Bos, J., L. Smithee, B. McClane, R. F. Distefano, F. Uzal, J. G. Songer, S. Mallonee, and J. M. Crutcher.** 2005. Fatal necrotizing colitis following a foodborne outbreak of enterotoxigenic *Clostridium perfringens* type A infection. *Clin. Infect. Dis.* **40:**E78–E83.
34. **Bradshaw, M., S. S. Dineen, N. D. Maks, and E. A. Johnson.** 2004. Regulation of neurotoxin complex expression in *Clostridium botulinum* strains 62A, Hall A-hyper, and NCTC 2916. *Anaerobe* **10:**321–333.
35. **Brazier, J. S.** 1998. The diagnosis of *Clostridium difficile*-associated disease. *J. Antimicrob. Chemother.* **41**(Suppl. C): 29–40.
36. **Brazier, J. S., T. E. Morris, and B. I. Duerden.** 2003. Heat and acid tolerance of *Clostridium novyi* type A spores and their survival prior to preparation of heroin for injection. *Anaerobe* **9:**141–144.
37. **Brett, M. M., G. Hallas, and O. Mpamugo.** 2004. Wound botulism in the UK and Ireland. *J. Med. Microbiol.* **53:**555–561.
38. **Brüggemann, H., and G. Gottschalk.** 2004. Insights in metabolism and toxin production from the complete genome sequence of *Clostridium tetani*. *Anaerobe* **10:** 53–68.
39. **Bryant, A. E., R. Y. Chen, Y. Nagata, Y. Wang, C. H. Lee, S. Finegold, P. H. Guth, and D. L. Stevens.** 2000. Clostridial gas gangrene. I. Cellular and molecular mechanisms of microvascular dysfunction induced by exotoxins of *Clostridium perfringens*. *J. Infect. Dis.* **182:**799–807.
40. **Bryant, A. E., R. Y. Chen, Y. Nagata, Y. Wang, C. H. Lee, S. Finegold, P. H. Guth, and D. L. Stevens.** 2000. Clostridial gas gangrene. II. Phospholipase C-induced activation of platelet gpIIbIIIa mediates vascular occlusion and myonecrosis in *Clostridium perfringens* gas gangrene. *J. Infect. Dis.* **182:**808–815.
41. **Brynestad, S., M. R. Sarker, B. A. McClane, P. E. Granum, and J. I. Rood.** 2001. Enterotoxin plasmid from *Clostridium perfringens* is conjugative. *Infect. Immun.* **69:**3483–3487.
42. **Burnett, J. C., E. A. Henchal, A. L. Schmaljohn, and S. Bavari.** 2005. The evolving field of biodefence: therapeutic developments and diagnostics. *Nat. Rev. Drug Discov.* **4:**281–297.
43. **Carman, R. J.** 1997. *Clostridium perfringens* in spontaneous and antibiotic-associated diarrhoea of man and other animals. *Rev. Med. Microbiol.* **8:**S43–S45.
44. **Cato, E. P., W. L. George, and S. M. Finegold.** 1986. Genus *Clostridium* Prazmowski 1880, 23 AL, p. 1141–1200. *In* P. H. A. Sneath, N. S. Mair, M. E. Sharpe, and G. H. Holt (ed.), *Bergey's Manual of Systematic Bacteriology,* vol. 2. Williams & Wilkins, Baltimore, Md.
45. **Cavallaro, J. J., L. S. Wiggs, and J. M. Miller.** 1997. Evaluation of the BBL Crystal Anaerobe identification system. *J. Clin. Microbiol.* **35:**3186–3191.
46. **Centers for Disease Control and Prevention.** 1998. *Botulism in the United States 1899–1996: Handbook for Epidemiologists, Clinicians, and Laboratory Workers.* Centers for Disease Control and Prevention, Atlanta, Ga.
47. **Centers for Disease Control and Prevention.** 1998. *Media for Isolation, Characterization, and Identification of Obligately Anaerobic Bacteria.* U.S. Department of Health and Human Services, Public Health Service, Centers for Disease Control and Prevention, Atlanta, Ga.
48. **Chaudry, R., B. Dhawan, and D. Kumar.** 1998. Outbreak of suspected *Clostridium butyricum* botulism in India. *Emerg. Infect. Dis.* **4:**506–507.
49. **Chen, Y. M., H. C. Lee, C. M. Chang, X. C. Chuang, and W. C. Ko.** 2001. *Clostridium* bacteremia: emphasis on the poor prognosis in cirrhotic patients. *J. Microbiol. Immunol. Infect.* **34:**113–118.

50. **Cherington, M.** 2004. Botulism: update and review. *Semin. Neurol.* **24:**155–163.

50a. **Clinical and Laboratory Standards Institute.** 2004. *Methods for Antimicrobial Susceptibility Testing of Anaerobic Bacteria.* Approved method M11-A6. Clinical and Laboratory Standards Institute, Wayne, Pa.

51. **Coleman, N., G. Speirs, J. Kahn, V. Broadbent, D. G. Wight, and R. E. Warren.** 1993. Neutropenic enterocolitis associated with *Clostridium tertium. J. Clin. Pathol.* **46:**180–183.

52. **Collins, M. D., and A. K. East.** 1998. Phylogeny and taxonomy of the food-borne pathogen *Clostridium botulinum* and its neurotoxins. *J. Appl. Microbiol.* **84:**5–17.

53. **Collins, M. D., P. A. Lawson, A. Willems, J. J. Cordoba, J. Fernandez-Garayzabal, P. Garcia, J. Cai, H. Hippe, and J. A. E. Farrow.** 1994. The phylogeny of the genus *Clostridium*—proposal of 5 new genera and 11 new species combinations. *Int. J. Syst. Bacteriol.* **44:**812–826.

54. **Doern, G. V., R. T. Coughlin, and L. Wu.** 1992. Laboratory diagnosis of *Clostridium difficile*-associated gastrointestinal disease: comparison of a monoclonal antibody enzyme immunoassay for toxins A and B with a monoclonal antibody enzyme immunoassay for toxin A only and two cytotoxicity assays. *J. Clin. Microbiol.* **30:**2042–2046.

55. **Dong, M., W. H. Tepp, E. A. Johnson, and E. R. Chapman.** 2004. Using fluorescent sensors to detect botulinum neurotoxin activity *in vitro* and in living cells. *Proc. Natl. Acad. Sci. USA* **101:**14701–14706.

56. **Downes, F. P., and K. Ito (ed.).** 2001. *Compendium of Methods for the Microbiological Examination of Foods,* 4th ed. American Public Health Association, Washington, D.C.

57. **Eklund, M. W., F. T. Poysky, and W. H. Habig.** 1989. Bacteriophages and plasmids in *Clostridium botulinum* and *Clostridium tetani* and their relationship to production of toxins, p. 25–51. *In* L. L. Simpson (ed.), *Botulinum Toxin and Tetanus Toxin.* Academic Press, Inc., San Diego, Calif.

58. **Elsayed, S., and K. Y. Zhang.** 2004. Bacteremia caused by *Clostridium symbiosum. J. Clin. Microbiol.* **42:**4390–4392.

59. **Elsayed, S., and K. Y. Zhang.** 2005. Bacteremia caused by *Clostridium intestinale. J. Clin. Microbiol.* **43:**2018–2020.

60. **Farrant, J. M., Z. Traill, C. Conlon, B. Warren, N. Mortensen, F. V. Gleeson, and D. P. Jewell.** 1996. Pigbel-like syndrome in a vegetarian in Oxford. *Gut* **39:**336–337.

61. **Fedorko, D. P., H. D. Engler, E. M. O'Shaughnessy, E. C. Williams, C. J. Reichelderfer, and W. I. Smith, Jr.** 1999. Evaluation of two rapid assays for detection of *Clostridium difficile* toxin A in stool specimens. *J. Clin. Microbiol.* **37:**3044–3047.

62. **Fenicia, L., F. Anniballi, S. Pulitano, O. Genovese, G. Polidori, and P. Aureli.** 2004. A severe case of infant botulism caused by *Clostridium botulinum* type A with concomitant intestinal viral infections. *Eur. J. Pediatr.* **163:**501–502.

63. **Fenicia, L., L. Da Dalt, F. Anniballi, G. Franciosa, S. Zanconato, and P. Aureli.** 2002. A case of infant botulism due to neurotoxigenic *Clostridium butyricum* type E associated with *Clostridium difficile* colitis. *Eur. J. Clin. Microbiol. Infect. Dis.* **21:**736–738.

64. **Finegold, S. M.** 1989. Therapy of anaerobic infections, p. 793–818. *In* S. M. Finegold and W. L. George (ed.), *Anaerobic Infections in Humans.* Academic Press, Inc., New York, N.Y.

65. **Finegold, S. M.** 1998. Tetanus, p. 693–722. *In* L. Collier, A. Balows, and M. Sussman (ed.), *Topley and Wilson's Microbiology and Microbial Infections,* 9th ed., vol. 3. *Bacterial Infections.* Arnold, London, United Kingdom.

66. **Finegold, S. M., Y. Song, and C. Liu.** 2002. Taxonomy—general comments and update on taxonomy of clostridia and anaerobic cocci. *Anaerobe* **8:**283–285.

67. **Finegold, S. M., Y. Song, C. Liu, D. W. Hecht, P. Summanen, E. Kononen, and S. D. Allen.** 2005. *Clostridium clostridioforme:* a mixture of three clinically important species. *Eur. J. Clin. Microbiol. Infect. Dis.* **24:**319–324.

68. **Fisher, D. J., K. Miyamoto, B. Harrison, S. Akimoto, M. R. Sarker, and B. A. McClane.** 2005. Association of beta2 toxin production with *Clostridium perfringens* type A human gastrointestinal disease isolates carrying a plasmid enterotoxin gene. *Mol. Microbiol.* **56:**747–762.

69. **Forward, L. J., D. S. Tompkins, and M. M. Brett.** 2003. Detection of *Clostridium difficile* cytotoxin and *Clostridium perfringens* enterotoxin in cases of diarrhoea in the community. *J. Med. Microbiol.* **52:**753–757.

70. **Fox, C. K., C. A. Keet, and J. B. Strober.** 2005. Recent advances in infant botulism. *Pediatr. Neurol.* **32:**149–154.

71. **Franciosa, G., P. Aureli, and R. Schechter.** 2003. *Clostridium botulinum,* p. 61–89. *In* M. D. Bier and J. W. Miliotis (ed.), *International Handbook of Foodborne Pathogens.* Marcel Dekker, Inc., New York, N.Y.

72. **George, W. L., and S. M. Finegold.** 1985. Clostridia in the human gastrointestinal flora, p. 1–37. *In* S. P. Borriello (ed.), *Clostridia in Gastrointestinal Disease.* CRC Press, Inc., Boca Raton, Fla.

73. **Gerding, D. N., S. Johnson, L. R. Peterson, M. E. Mulligan, and J. Silva, Jr.** 1995. *Clostridium difficile* associated diarrhea and colitis. *Infect. Control Hosp. Epidemiol.* **16:**459–477.

74. **Ghanem, F. M., A. C. Ridpath, W. E. Moore, and L. V. Moore.** 1991. Identification of *Clostridium botulinum, Clostridium argentinense,* and related organisms by cellular fatty acid analysis. *J. Clin. Microbiol.* **29:**1114–1124.

75. **Gill, D. M.** 1982. Bacterial toxins—a table of lethal amounts. *Microbiol. Rev.* **46:**86–94.

76. **Glazunova, O. O., D. Raoult, and V. Roux.** 2005. First identification of *Clostridium celerecrescens* in liquid drained from an abscess. *J. Clin. Microbiol.* **43:**3007–3008.

77. **Goon, P. K. Y., M. O'Brien, and O. G. Titey.** 2005. Spontaneous *Clostridium septicum* septic arthritis of the shoulder and gas gangrene—a case report. *J. Bone Jt. Surg. Am. Vol.* **87:**874–877.

78. **Gorbach, S. L.** 1998. *Clostridium perfringens* and other clostridia, p. 1925–1933. *In* S. L. Gorbach, J. G. Bartlett, and N. R. Blacklow (ed.), *Infectious Diseases,* 2nd ed. W. B. Saunders Company, Philadelphia, Pa.

79. **Gorbach, S. L.** 1998. Gas gangrene and other clostridial skin and soft tissue infections, p. 915–922. *In* S. L. Gorbach, J. G. Bartlett, and N. R. Blacklow (ed.), *Infectious Diseases,* 2nd ed. W. B. Saunders Company, Philadelphia, Pa.

80. **Griffin, P. M., C. L. Hatheway, R. Rosenbaum, and R. Sokolow.** 1997. Endogenous antibody production to botulinum toxin in an adult with intestinal colonization botulism and underlying Crohn's disease. *J. Infect. Dis.* **175:**633–637.

81. **Gui, L., C. Subramony, J. Fratkin, and M. D. Hughson.** 2002. Fatal enteritis necroticans (pigbel) in a diabetic adult. *Mod. Pathol.* **15:**66–70.

82. **Hall, Y. H. J., J. A. Chaddock, H. J. Moulsdale, E. R. Kirby, F. C. G. Alexander, J. D. Marks, and K. A. Foster.** 2004. Novel application of an *in vitro* technique to the detection and quantification of botulinum neurotoxin antibodies. *J. Immunol. Methods* **288:**55–60.

83. **Haralambie, E., H. K. Mahmoud, G. Linzenmeier, and F. Wendt.** 1983. The clostridial effect of selective decontamination of the human gut with trimethoprim/sulphamethoxazole in neutropenic patients. *Infection* **11:**201–204.

84. **Hatheway, C. L.** 1988. Botulism, p. 111–133. *In* A. Balows, W. J. Hausler, Jr., M. Ohashi, and A. Turano (ed.), *Laboratory Diagnosis of Infectious Diseases: Principles and Practice,* vol. 1. Springer, New York, N.Y.

85. **Hatheway, C. L.** 1990. Toxigenic clostridia. *Clin. Microbiol. Rev.* **3:**66–98.

86. **Hatheway, C. L., and E. A. Johnson.** 1998. *Clostridium:* the spore-bearing anaerobes, p. 731–782. *In* L. Collier, A.

Balows, and B. Duerden (ed.), *Systematic Bacteriology*, 9th ed., vol. 2. Edward Arnold Publisher, New York, N.Y.

87. **Hausmann, R., F. Albert, W. Geissdorfer, and P. Betz.** 2004. *Clostridium fallax* associated with sudden death in a 16-year-old boy. *J. Med. Microbiol.* **53:**581–583.
88. **Hecht, D. W., M. H. Malamy, and F. P. Tally.** 1989. Mechanisms of resistance and resistance transfer in anaerobic bacteria, p. 755–769. *In* S. M. Finegold and W. L. George (ed.), *Anaerobic Infections in Humans*. Academic Press, Inc., New York, N.Y.
89. **Hippe, H., J. R. Andreesen, and G. Gottschalk.** 1992. The genus *Clostridium*—nonmedical, p. 1800–1866. *In* A. Balows, H. G. Trüper, et al. (ed.), *The Prokaryotes*, 2nd ed., vol II. Springer Verlag, New York, N.Y.
90. **Holdeman, L. V., E. P. Cato, and W. E. C. Moore (ed.).** 1977. *Anaerobe Laboratory Manual*, 4th ed. Virginia Polytechnic Institute and State University, Blacksburg.
91. **Holzer, V. E.** 1962. Botulismus dürch inhalation. *Med. Klin.* **41:**1735–1738.
92. **Johnson, E. A.** 2005. Bacteriophages encoding botulinum and diphtheria toxins, p. 280–296. *In* M. Waldor, D. I. Friedman, and S. L. Adhya (ed.), *Phages: Their Role in Bacterial Pathogenesis and Biotechnology*. ASM Press, Washington, D.C.
93. **Johnson, E. A., and M. Bradshaw.** 2001. *Clostridium botulinum* and its neurotoxins: a metabolic and cellular perspective. *Toxicon* **39:**1703–1722.
94. **Johnson, E. A., and M. C. Goodnough.** 1998. Botulism, p. 723–741. *In Topley and Wilson's Current Topics in Microbiology*. Arnold Publishing, London, United Kingdom.
95. **Johnson, E. A., W. H. Tepp, M. Bradshaw, R. J. Gilbert, P. E. Cook, and E. D. G. McIntosh.** 2005. Characterization of *Clostridium botulinum* strains associated with an infant botulism case in the United Kingdom. *J. Clin. Microbiol.* **43:**2602–2607.
96. **Johnson, J. L., and B. S. Francis.** 1975. Taxonomy of the clostridia: ribosomal ribonucleic acid homologies among the species. *J. Gen. Microbiol.* **88:**229–244.
97. **Johnson, S., and D. N. Gerding.** 1998. *Clostridium difficile* associated diarrhea. *Clin. Infect. Dis.* **26:**1027–1034.
98. **Johnson, S., S. A. Kent, K. J. O'Leary, M. M. Merrigan, S. P. Sambol, L. R. Peterson, and D. N. Gerding.** 2001. Fatal pseudomembranous colitis associated with a variant *Clostridium difficile* strain not detected by toxin A immunoassay. *Ann. Intern. Med.* **135:**434–438.
99. **Jousimies-Somer, H. R., P. Summanen, D. M. Citron, E. J. Baron, H. M. Wexler, and S. M. Finegold.** 2002. Wadsworth-KTL. *Anaerobic Bacteriology Manual*. Star Publishing Company, Belmont, Calif.
100. **Kato, H., N. Kato, S. Katow, T. Maegawa, S. Nakamura, and D. M. Lyerly.** 1999. Deletions in the repeating sequences of the toxin A gene of toxin A-negative, toxin B-positive *Clostridium difficile* strains. *FEMS Microbiol. Lett.* **175:**197–203.
101. **Kimura, A. C., J. I. Higa, R. M. Levin, G. Simpson, Y. Vargas, and D. J. Vugia.** 2004. Outbreak of necrotizing fasciitis due to *Clostridium sordellii* among black-tar heroin users. *Clin. Infect. Dis.* **38:**E87–E91.
102. **King, A., A. Rampling, D. G. Wright, and R. E. Warren.** 1984. Neutropenic enterocolitis due to *Clostridium septicum* infection. *J. Clin. Pathol.* **37:**335–343.
103. **Kirchner, J. T.** 1991. *Clostridium septicum* infection. Beware of associated cancer. *Postgrad. Med.* **90:**157–160.
104. **Kliegman, R. M., and A. A. Fanaroff.** 1984. Necrotizing enterocolitis. *N. Engl. J. Med.* **310:**1093–1103.
105. **Kliegman, R. M., W. A. Walker, and R. H. Yolken.** 1993. Necrotizing enterocolitis: research agenda for a disease of unknown etiology and pathogenesis. *Pediatr. Res.* **34:**701–708.
106. **Kobayashi, H., K. Fujisawa, Y. Saito, M. Kamijo, S. Oshima, M. Kubo, Y. Eto, C. Monma, and M. Kitamura.** 2003. A botulism case of a 12-year-old girl caused by intestinal colonization of *Clostridium botulinum* type Ab. *Jpn. J. Infect. Dis.* **56:**73–74.
107. Reference deleted.
108. **Koransky, J. R., S. D. Allen, and V. R. Dowell, Jr.** 1978. Use of ethanol for selective isolation of spore-forming microorganisms. *Appl. Environ. Microbiol.* **35:**762–765.
109. **Koransky, J. R., M. D. Stargel, and V. R. Dowell, Jr.** 1979. *Clostridium septicum* bacteremia. Its clinical significance. *Am. J. Med.* **66:**63–66.
110. **Kosloske, A. M.** 1994. Epidemiology of necrotizing enterocolitis. *Acta Paediatr. Suppl.* **396:**2–7.
111. **Kourtis, A. P., R. Weiner, K. Belson, and F. O. Richards.** 1997. *Clostridium tertium* meningitis as the presenting sign of a meningocele in a twelve-year-old child. *Pediatr. Infect. Dis. J.* **16:**527–529.
112. **Kudrow, D. B., D. A. Henry, D. A. Haake, G. Marshall, and G. E. Mathisen.** 1988. Botulism associated with *Clostridium botulinum* sinusitis after intranasal cocaine abuse. *Ann. Intern. Med.* **109:**984–985.
113. **Kudsk, K. A.** 1992. Occult gastrointestinal malignancies producing metastatic *Clostridium septicum* infections in diabetic patients. *Surgery* **112:**765–770.
114. **Kyne, L., M. B. Hamel, R. Polavaram, and C. N. P. Kelly.** 2002. Health care costs and mortality associated with nosocomial diarrhea due to *Clostridium difficile*. *Clin. Infect. Dis.* **34:**346–353.
115. **Lacy, D. B., and R. C. Stevens.** 1999. Sequence homology and structural analysis of the clostridial neurotoxins. *J. Mol. Biol.* **291:**1091–1104.
116. **Lacy, D. B., W. Tepp, A. C. Cohen, B. R. DasGupta, and R. C. Stevens.** 1998. Crystal structure of botulinum neurotoxin type A and implications for toxicity. *Nat. Struct. Biol.* **5:**898–902.
117. **Lalli, G., S. Bohnert, K. Deinhardt, C. Verastegui, and G. Schiavo.** 2003. The journey of tetanus and botulinum neurotoxins in neurons. *Trends Microbiol.* **11:**431–437.
118. **Lau, S. K., P. C. Woo, G. K. Woo, A. M. Fung, A. H. Ngan, Y. Song, C. Liu, P. Summanen, S. M. Finegold, and K. Y. Yuen.** 2006. Bacteraemia caused by *Anaerotruncus colihominis* and emended description of the species. *J. Clin. Pathol.* **59:**748–752. (First published 7 February 2006; doi:10.1136/jcp.2005.031773.)
119. **Lawrence, G. W., D. Lehmann, G. Anian, C. A. Coakley, G. Saleu, M. J. Barker, and M. W. Davis.** 1990. Impact of active immunisation against enteritis necroticans in Papua New Guinea. *Lancet* **336:**1165–1167.
120. **Lawson, P. A., Y. L. Song, C. X. Liu, D. R. Molitoris, M. L. Vaisanen, M. D. Collins, and S. M. Finegold.** 2004. *Anaerotruncus colihominis* gen. nov., sp. nov., from human faeces. *Int. J. Syst. Evol. Microbiol.* **54:**413–417.
121. **Lee, S. D., D. K. Turgeon, C. W. Ko, T. R. Fritsche, and C. M. Surawicz.** 2003. Clinical correlation of toxin and common antigen enzyme immunoassay testing in patients with *Clostridium difficile* disease. *Am. J. Gastroenterol.* **98:**1569–1572.
122. **Leegaard, T. M., P. Sandven, and P. Gaustad.** 2005. *Clostridium tertium:* 3 case reports. *Scand. J. Infect. Dis.* **37:**230–232.
123. **Lemee, L., A. Dhalluin, S. Testelin, M.-A. Mattrat, K. Maillard, J.-F. Lemeland, and J.-L. Pons.** 2004. Multiplex PCR targeting *tpi* (triose phosphate isomerase), *tcdA* (toxin A), and *tcdB* (toxin B) genes for toxigenic culture of *Clostridium difficile*. *J. Clin. Microbiol.* **42:**5710–5714.
124. **Li, D. Y., A. O. Scheimann, J. G. Songer, R. E. Person, M. Horwitz, T. Resar, and T. B. Schwarz.** 2004. Enteritis

necroticans with recurrent enterocutaneous fistulae caused by *Clostridium perfringens* in a child with cyclic neutropenia. *J. Pediatr. Gastroenterol. Nutr.* **38:**213–215.
125. **Liebetrau, A., A. C. Rodloff, J. Behra-Miellet, and L. Dubreuil.** 2003. In vitro activities of a new des-fluoro(6) quinolone, garenoxacin, against clinical anaerobic bacteria. *Antimicrob. Agents Chemother.* **47:**3667–3671.
126. **Lindstrom, M. K., H. M. Jankola, S. Hielm, E. K. Hyytia, and H. J. Korkeala.** 1999. Identification of Clostridium botulinum with API 20 A, Rapid ID 32 A and RapID ANA II. *FEMS Immunol. Med. Microbiol.* **24:**267–274.
127. **Linscott, A. J., R. B. Flamholtz, D. Shukla, Y. L. Song, C. X. Liu, and S. M. Finegold.** 2005. Fatal septicemia due to *Clostridium hathewayi* and *Campylobacter hominis*. *Anaerobe* **11:**97–98.
128. **Lorber, B.** 2000. Gas gangrene and other *Clostridium* associated diseases, p. 2549–2561. *In* G. L. Mandell, J. E. Bennett, and R. Dolin (ed.), *Mandell, Douglas and Bennett's Principles and Practice of Infectious Diseases,* 4th ed., vol. 2. Churchill Livingstone, Philadelphia, Pa.
129. **Lyerly, D. M., H. C. Krivan, and T. D. Wilkins.** 1988. *Clostridium difficile:* its disease and toxins. *Clin. Microbiol. Rev.* **1:**1–18.
130. **Lyerly, D. M., L. M. Neville, D. T. Evans, J. Fill, S. Allen, W. Greene, R. Sautter, P. Hnatuck, D. J. Torpey, and R. Schwalbe.** 1998. Multicenter evaluation of the *Clostridium difficile* TOX A/B TEST. *J. Clin. Microbiol.* **36:**184–190.
131. **Malizio, C. J., M. C. Goodnough, and E. A. Johnson.** 2000. Purification of *Clostridium botulinum* type A neurotoxin. *Methods Mol. Biol.* **145:**27–39.
132. **Marler, L. M., J. A. Siders, L. C. Wolters, Y. Pettigrew, B. L. Skitt, and S. D. Allen.** 1991. Evaluation of the new Rap-ID-ANA II system for the identification of clinical anaerobic isolates. *J. Clin. Microbiol.* **29:**874–878.
133. **Maselli, R. A., W. Ellis, R. N. Mandler, F. Sheikh, G. Senton, S. Knox, H. Salari-Namin, M. Agius, R. L. Wollman, and D. P. Richman.** 1997. Cluster of wound botulism in California: clinical, electrophysiological, and pathologic study. *Muscle Nerve* **20:**1284–1295.
134. **Massey, V., D. B. Gregson, A. H. Chagla, M. Storey, M. A. John, and Z. Hussain.** 2003. Clinical usefulness of components of the Triage immunoassay, enzyme immunoassay for toxins A and B, and cytotoxin B tissue culture assay for the diagnosis of *Clostridium difficile* diarrhea. *Am. J. Clin. Pathol.* **119:**45–49.
135. **McDonald, L. C., G. E. Killgore, A. Thompson, R. C. Owens, Jr., S. V. Kazakova, S. P. Sambol, S. Johnson, and D. N. Gerding.** 2005. An epidemic, toxin gene-variant strain of *Clostridium difficile*. *N. Engl. J. Med.* **353:** 2433–2441.
136. **McFarland, L. V., M. E. Mulligan, R. Y. Kwok, and W. E. Stamm.** 1989. Nosocomial acquisition of *Clostridium difficile* infection. *N. Engl. J. Med.* **320:**204–210.
137. **McGregor, J. A., D. E. Soper, G. Lovell, and J. K. Todd.** 1989. Maternal deaths associated with *Clostridium sordellii* infection. *Am. J. Obstet. Gynecol.* **161:**987–995.
138. **Modena, S., S. Gollamudi, and F. Friedenberg.** 2006. Continuation of antibiotics is associated with failure of metronidazole for *Clostridium difficile*-associated diarrhea. *J. Clin. Gastroenterol.* **40:**49–54.
139. **Modi, N., and M. H. Wilcox.** 2001. Evidence for antibiotic induced *Clostridium perfringens* diarrhea. *J. Clin. Pathol.* **54:**748–751.
140. **Moncrief, J. S., L. Zheng, L. M. Neville, and D. M. Lyerly.** 2000. Genetic characterization of toxin A-negative, toxin B-positive *Clostridium difficile* isolates by PCR. *J. Clin. Microbiol.* **38:**3072–3075.
141. **Mory, F., A. Lozniewski, V. David, J. P. Carlier, L. Dubreuil, and R. Leclercq.** 1998. Low-level vancomycin resistance in *Clostridium innocuum*. *J. Clin. Microbiol.* **36:**1767–1768.
142. **Mulligan, M. E., L. R. Peterson, R. Y. Kwok, C. R. Clabots, and D. N. Gerding.** 1988. Immunoblots and plasmid fingerprints compared with serotyping and polyacrylamide gel electrophoresis for typing *Clostridium difficile*. *J. Clin. Microbiol.* **26:**41–46.
143. **Murrell, T. G. C.** 1989. Enteritis necroticans, p. 639–659. *In* S. M. Finegold and W. L. George (ed.), *Anaerobic Infections in Humans*. Academic Press, San Diego, Calif.
144. **Noone, M., M. Tabaqchali, and J. B. Spillane.** 2002. *Clostridium novyi* causing necrotising fasciitis in an injecting drug user. *J. Clin. Pathol.* **55:**141–142.
145. **Olsen, S. J., L. C. MacKinnon, J. S. Goulding, N. H. Bean, and L. Slutsker.** 2000. Surveillance for foodborne disease outbreaks—United States, 1993–1997. *Morb. Mortal. Wkly. Rep. CDC Surveill. Summ.* **49:**1–62.
146. **Pepin, J., M. E. Alary, L. Valiquette, E. Raiche, J. Ruel, K. Fulop, D. Godin, and C. Bourassa.** 2005. Increasing risk of relapse after treatment of *Clostridium difficile* colitis in Quebec, Canada. *Clin. Infect. Dis.* **40:**1591–1597.
147. **Pepin, J., L. Valiquette, and B. Cossette.** 2005. Mortality attributable to nosocomial *Clostridium difficile*-associated disease during an epidemic caused by a hypervirulent strain in Quebec. *Can. Med. Assoc. J.* **173:**1037–1042.
148. **Petrillo, T. M., C. M. Beck-Sague, J. G. Songer, C. Abramowsky, J. D. Fortenberry, L. Meacham, A. G. Dean, H. Lee, D. M. Bueschel, and S. R. Nesheim.** 2000. Enteritis necroticans (pigbel) in a diabetic child. *N. Engl. J. Med.* **342:**1250–1253.
149. **Pickett, J., B. Berg, E. Chaplin, and M. A. Brunstetter-Shafer.** 1976. Syndrome of botulism in infancy: clinical and electrophysiologic study. *N. Engl. J. Med.* **295:**770–772.
150. **Pitt, M. L. M., and R. D. LeClaire.** 2005. Pathogenesis by aerosol, p. 65–78. *In* L. E. Lindler, F. J. Lebeda, and G. W. Korch (ed.), *Biological Weapons Defense. Infectious Diseases and Counterbioterrorism.* Humana Press, Inc., Totowa, N.J.
151. **Rorbye, C., I. S. Petersen, and L. Nilas.** 2000. Postpartum *Clostridium sordellii* infection associated with fatal toxic shock syndrome. *Acta Obstet. Gynecol. Scand.* **79:**1134–1135.
152. **Rosenblatt, J. E.** 1989. Susceptibility testing of anaerobic bacteria. *Clin. Lab. Med.* **9:**239–254.
153. **Sakaguchi, G.** 1983. *Clostridium botulinum* toxins. *Pharmacol. Rev.* **19:**165–194.
154. **Schantz, E. J., and E. A. Johnson.** 1992. Properties and use of botulinum toxin and other microbial neurotoxins in medicine. *Microbiol. Rev.* **56:**80–99.
155. **Schiavo, G., M. Matteoli, and C. Montecucco.** 2000. Neurotoxins affecting neuroexocytosis. *Physiol. Rev.* **80:** 717–766.
156. **Schreckenberger, P. C., D. M. Celig, and W. M. Janda.** 1988. Clinical evaluation of the Vitek ANI card for identification of anaerobic bacteria. *J. Clin. Microbiol.* **26:**225–230.
157. **Severin, A., R. Paulet, A. Berth, L. Balgone, J. M. Coudray, and M. Thyrault.** 2005. Acute pancreatitis complicated by *Clostridium tertium* septicaemia. *Presse Med.* **34:**446–447.
158. **Sharma, S. K., and R. C. Whiting.** 2005. Methods for detection of *Clostridium botulinum* toxin in foods. *J. Food Prot.* **68:**1256–1263.
159. **Shimizu, T., K. Ohtani, H. Hirakawa, K. Ohshima, A. Yamashita, T. Shiba, N. Ogasawara, M. Hattori, S. Kuhara, and H. Hayashi.** 2002. Complete genome sequence of *Clostridium perfringens,* an anaerobic flesh-eater. *Proc. Natl. Acad. Sci. USA* **99:**996–1001.
160. **Simor, A. E., S. L. Yake, and K. Tsimidis.** 1993. Infection due to *Clostridium difficile* among elderly residents of a long-term-care facility. *Clin. Infect. Dis.* **17:**672–678.

161. **Sinave, C., G. Le Templier, D. Blouin, F. Leveille, and E. Deland.** 2002. Toxic shock syndrome due to *Clostridium sordellii:* a dramatic postpartum and postabortion disease. *Clin. Infect. Dis.* **35:**1441–1443.
162. **Smedley, J. G., D. J. Fisher, S. Sayeed, G. Chakrabarti, and B. A. McClane.** 2004. The enteric toxins of *Clostridium perfringens. Rev. Physiol. Biochem. Pharmacol.* **152:**183–204.
163. **Smith, G. R.** 1987. Botulism in water birds and its relation to comparative medicine, p. 73–86. *In* M. W. Elklund and V. R. Dowell, Jr. (ed.), *Avian Botulism.* Charles C Thomas, Inc., Springfield, Ill.
164. **Smith, L. D. S., and H. Sugiyama.** 1988. *Botulism. The Organism, Its Toxins, the Diseases.* Charles C Thomas, Springfield, Ill.
165. **Smith, L. D. S., and B. L. Williams.** 1984. *The Pathogenic Anaerobic Bacteria,* 3rd ed. Charles C Thomas, Springfield, Ill.
166. **Snell, H., M. Ramos, S. Longo, M. John, and Z. Hussain.** 2004. Performance of the TechLab *C. DIFF* CHEK-60 enzyme immunoassay (EIA) in combination with the *C. difficile* Tox A/B II EIA kit, the Triage *C. difficile* panel immunoassay, and a cytotoxin assay for diagnosis of *Clostridium difficile*-associated diarrhea. *J. Clin. Microbiol.* **42:**4863–4865.
167. **Sobel, J., C. G. Mixter, P. Kolhe, A. Gupta, J. Guarner, S. Zaki, N. A. Hoffman, J. G. Songer, M. Fremont-Smith, M. Fischer, G. Killgore, P. H. Britz, and C. MacDonald.** 2005. Necrotizing enterocolitis associated with *Clostridium perfringens* type A in previously healthy North American adults. *J. Am. Coll. Surg.* **201:**48–56.
168. **Song, Y. L., C. X. Liu, M. McTeague, P. Summanen, and S. M. Finegold.** 2004. *Clostridium bartlettii* sp. nov., isolated from human faeces. *Anaerobe* **10:**179–184.
169. **Song, Y. L., C. X. Liu, D. R. Molitoris, T. J. Tomzynski, P. A. Lawson, M. D. Collins, and S. M. Finegold.** 2003. *Clostridium bolteae* sp. nov., isolated from human sources. *Syst. Appl. Microbiol.* **26:**84–89.
170. **Songer, J. G.** 1997. Molecular and immunological methods for the diagnosis of clostridial diseases, p. 491–503. *In* J. I. Rood, B. A. McClane, J. G. Songer, and R. W. Titball (ed.), *The Clostridia: Molecular Biology and Pathogenesis.* Academic Press, New York, N.Y.
171. **Sparks, S. G., R. J. Carman, M. R. Sarker, and B. A. McClane.** 2001. Genotyping of enterotoxigenic *Clostridium perfringens* fecal isolates associated with antibiotic-associated diarrhea and food poisoning in North America. *J. Clin. Microbiol.* **39:**883–888.
172. **Spigaglia, P., V. Carucci, F. Barbanti, and P. Mastrantonio.** 2005. ErmB determinants and Tn*916*-like elements in clinical isolates of *Clostridium difficile. Antimicrob. Agents Chemother.* **49:**2550–2553.
173. **Stackebrandt, E., and F. A. Rainey.** 1997. Phylogenetic relationships, p. 3–19. *In* J. I. Rood, B. A. McClane, J. G. Songer, and R. W. Titball (ed.), *The Clostridia: Molecular Biology and Pathogenesis.* Academic Press, New York, N.Y.
174. **Steer, T., M. D. Collins, G. R. Gibson, H. Hippe, and P. A. Lawson.** 2001. *Clostridium hathewayi* sp. nov., from human faeces. *Syst. Appl. Microbiol.* **24:**353–357.
175. **Steyaert, S., R. Peleman, M. Vaneechoutte, T. De Baere, G. Claeys, and G. Verschraegen.** 1999. Septicemia in neutropenic patients infected with *Clostridium tertium* resistant to cefepime and other expanded-spectrum cephalosporins. *J. Clin. Microbiol.* **37:**3778–3779.
176. **Swaminathan, S., and S. Eswaramoorthy.** 2000. Structural analysis of the catalytic and binding sites of *Clostridium botulinum* neurotoxin B. *Nat. Struct. Biol.* **7:**693–699.
177. **van den Berg, R. J., L. S. Bruijnesteijn van Coppenraet, H.-J. Gerritsen, H. P. Endtz, E. R. van der Vorm, and E. J. Kuijper.** 2005. Prospective multicenter evaluation of a new immunoassay and real-time PCR for rapid diagnosis of *Clostridium difficile*-associated diarrhea in hospitalized patients. *J. Clin. Microbiol.* **43:**5338–5340.
178. **Vanpoucke, H., T. De Baere, G. Claeys, M. Vaneechoutte, and G. Verschraegen.** 2001. Evaluation of six commercial assays for the rapid detection of *Clostridium difficile* toxin and/or antigen in stool specimens. *Clin. Microbiol. Infect.* **7:**55–64.
179. **Voth, D. E., and J. E. Ballard.** 2005. *Clostridium difficile* toxins: mechanism of action and role in disease. *Clin. Microbiol. Rev.* **18:**247–263.
180. **Wang, R. F., M. L. Beggs, B. D. Erickson, and C. E. Cerniglia.** 2004. DNA microarray analysis of predominant human intestinal bacteria in fecal samples. *Mol. Cell. Probes* **18:**223–234.
181. **Warny, M., J. Pepin, A. Fang, G. Killgore, A. Thompson, J. Brazier, E. Frost, and L. C. McDonald.** 2005. Toxin production by an emerging strain of *Clostridium difficile* associated with outbreaks of severe disease in North America and Europe. *Lancet* **366:**1079–1084.
182. **Weber, J. T., H. C. Goodpasture, H. Alexander, S. B. Werner, C. L. Hatheway, and R. V. Tauxe.** 1993. Wound botulism in a patient with a tooth abscess—case-report and review. *Clin. Infect. Dis.* **16:**635–639.
183. **Wein, L. M., and Y. F. Liu.** 2005. Analyzing a bioterror attack on the food supply: the case of botulinum toxin in milk. *Proc. Natl. Acad. Sci. USA* **102:**9984–9989.
184. **Wen, Q. Y., and B. A. McClane.** 2004. Detection of enterotoxigenic *Clostridium perfringens* type A isolates in American retail foods. *Appl. Environ. Microbiol.* **70:**2685–2691.
185. **Wiebe, E., E. Guilbert, F. Jacot, C. Shannon, and B. Winikoff.** 2004. A fatal case of *Clostridium sordellii* septic shock syndrome associated with medical abortion. *Obstet. Gynecol.* **104:**1142–1144.
186. **Wilkins, T. D., and D. M. Lyerly.** 2003. *Clostridium difficile* testing: after 20 years, still challenging. *J. Clin. Microbiol.* **41:**531–534.
187. **Wilson, J. R., and A. P. Limaye.** 2004. Risk factors for mortality in patients with anaerobic bacteremia. *Eur. J. Clin. Microbiol. Infect. Dis.* **24:**310–316.

187a. **Winn, W. C., Jr., S. D. Allen, W. M. Janda, E. W. Koneman, G. Procop, P. C. Schreckenberger, and G. Woods.** 2005. *Koneman's Color Atlas and Textbook of Diagnostic Microbiology,* 6th ed. Lippincott Williams & Wilkins, Philadelphia, Pa.

188. **Woo, P. C. Y., S. K. P. Lau, K. M. Chan, A. M. Y. Fung, B. S. F. Tang, and K. Y. Yuen.** 2005. *Clostridium* bacteremia characterized by 16S ribosomal RNA gene sequencing. *J. Clin. Pathol.* **58:**301–307.
189. **Woo, P. C. Y., S. K. P. Lau, G. K. S. Woo, A. M. Y. Fung, V. P. Y. Yiu, and K. Y. Yuen.** 2004. Bacteremia due to *Clostridium hathewayi* in a patient with acute appendicitis. *J. Clin. Microbiol.* **42:**5947–5949.
190. **Woodruff, B. A., P. M. Griffin, L. M. McCroskey, J. F. Smart, R. B. Wainwright, R. G. Bryant, L. C. Hutwagner, and C. L. Hatheway.** 1992. Clinical and laboratory comparison of botulism from toxin types A, B, and E in the United States, 1975–1988. *J. Infect. Dis.* **166:**1281–1286.
191. **Zhou, Y., H. Sugiyama, and E. A. Johnson.** 1993. Transfer of toxigenicity from *Clostridium butyricum* to a nontoxigenic *Clostridium botulinum* type E-like strain. *Appl. Environ. Microbiol.* **59:**3825–3831.
192. **Zink, J. M., R. Singh-Parikshak, A. Sugar, and M. W. Johnson.** 2004. *Clostridium sordellii* endophthalmitis after suture removal from a corneal transplant. *Cornea* **23:**522–523.

Bacteroides, Porphyromonas, Prevotella, Fusobacterium, and Other Anaerobic Gram-Negative Rods*

DIANE M. CITRON, IAN R. POXTON, AND ELLEN JO BARON

58

TAXONOMY

The anaerobic gram-negative bacteria are part of the normal flora of the mouth, upper respiratory tract, intestinal tract, and urogenital tract of humans and animals. Anaerobic spirochetes are covered in chapter 63, and *Campylobacter* spp. other than *Campylobacter rectus, Campylobacter curvus, Campylobacter gracilis*, and *Campylobacter showae* are discussed in chapter 59. The anaerobic gram-negative rods belong to the phyla *Bacteroidetes* and *Fusobacteria* and the families *Bacteroidaceae, Porphyromonadaceae, Prevotellaceae*, and *Fusobacteriaceae*. Species definition is based on biochemical characteristics, nucleic acid base composition, and homology (see chapter 19). *Veillonella* and the other anaerobic gram-negative cocci are covered in chapter 55. In the majority of clinical specimens, organisms of the genera *Bacteroides, Porphyromonas, Prevotella, Fusobacterium, Campylobacter, Sutterella*, and *Bilophila* are most often encountered (65).

The taxonomy of the gram-negative rods has been changing in recent years (14, 25, 64). A number of new genera and species have been named since the last edition of this book (Table 1). The methods used for taxonomic studies have been based mainly on nucleic acid analyses such as DNA-DNA hybridization and 16S rRNA and other gene sequencing (25). The latter classification approach, based on phylogenetic relatedness, does not necessarily correlate with phenotypic characteristics, such as Gram-staining properties, morphology, atmospheric growth requirements, and sporulation, concepts that were earlier considered cornerstones in the classification of anaerobes (68, 102). In fact, several species currently thought of as anaerobic gram-negative rods *(Butyrivibrio* spp., *Catonella morbi, Dialister pneumosintes, Fusobacterium* spp., *Leptotrichia* spp., *Johnsonella ignava, Tissierella* spp., *Mitsuokella multiacida, Selenomonas* spp., *Centipeda periodontii)* cluster within the *Clostridium* subphylum of the gram-positive bacteria (23, 60). Some of them are discussed in chapters 56 and 57.

The genus *Bacteroides* includes bile-resistant species that were formerly described as the "*Bacteroides fragilis*" group (including *Bacteroides eggerthii*) (78, 102, 125). However, the *B. fragilis* group organisms *Bacteroides distasonis, B. goldsteinii*, and *B. merdae* are related to *Tannerella forsythensis* (formerly *Bacteroides forsythus*) and cluster close to *Porphyromonas* on the basis of 16S rRNA sequencing (102, 103). A new genus, *Parabacteroides*, has been proposed to encompass these three species (M. Sakamoto, unpublished data). Similarly, *Bacteroides splanchnicus* falls far outside the group and probably represents a new genus (103). On the other hand, the bile-sensitive *Prevotella heparinolytica* and *Prevotella zoogleoformans* cluster among the *B. fragilis* group (102). Inclusion of these species warrants redefinition of the *B. fragilis* group. The taxonomic positions of other species still included in the genus *Bacteroides* remain uncertain, but all of these will ultimately be transferred to other genera. *Porphyromonas catoniae* is the only nonpigmented taxon in the genus *Porphyromonas* (144). Animal strains similar to *Porphyromonas gingivalis* are called *Porphyromonas gulae* (43). 16S rRNA sequencing results have identified two new closely related gram-negative species named *Alistipes finegoldii*, which is pigmented, bile resistant, and weakly saccharolytic, and *A. putredinis*, which is asaccharolytic and nonpigmented (111). The asaccharolytic, formate- and fumarate-requiring gram-negative rods *Bacteroides ureolyticus, C. gracilis* (formerly *B. gracilis*), *C. curvus, C. rectus* (formerly *Wolinella curva* and *W. recta*), and *Sutterella wadsworthensis* are actually microaerophiles. *Campylobacter hominis* is a truly anaerobic campylobacter from the human gastrointestinal tract (77). *Wolinella succinogenes*, isolated from the bovine rumen, is the only species remaining in the genus *Wolinella*. The taxonomic position of *B. ureolyticus* has remained uncertain; additional studies are required to determine whether these organisms should be transferred to the genus *Campylobacter* or if they represent a new genus (139). Sulfate-reducing *Desulfomonas pigra* was renamed *Desulfovibrio piger*, and the genus *Desulfomonas* is no longer valid (80).

DESCRIPTION OF THE GROUP

The true anaerobic gram-negative bacteria are differentiated from facultatively anaerobic bacteria by their inability to grow in the presence of oxygen and their susceptibility to metronidazole. Metronidazole resistance in these genera is rare and usually due to a laboratory error or an incorrect identification. Some of the species included here are indeed microaerophiles and are often resistant to metronidazole; the appropriate atmospheric requirements should be determined for all isolates. Cell morphology varies from short coccobacilli

*This chapter contains information presented in chapter 56 by Hannele R. Jousimies-Somer, Paula H. Summanen, Hannah Wexler, Sydney M. Finegold, Saheer E. Gharbia, and Haroun N. Shah in the eighth edition of this Manual.

TABLE 1 New anaerobic gram-negative rods named since the last edition of this Manual

New genus or species	Previous designation	Isolated from:	Reference
Alistipes putredinis	*Bacteroides putredinis*	Appendicitis specimens	111
Alistipes finegoldii	New	Appendicitis specimens	111
Bacteroides coprocola	*B. vulgatus-like*	Human feces	69
Bacteroides goldsteinii	*B. distasonis*-like	Human infections (intestinal origin)	126
Bacteroides nordii	*B. uniformis*-like	Human infections (intestinal origin)	127
Bacteroides plebeius	*B. vulgatus*-like	Human feces	69
Bacteroides salyersiae	*B. uniformis*-like	Human infections (intestinal origin)	127
Cetobacterium somerae	New	Children's feces	40
Desulfovibrio piger	*Desulfomonas pigra*	Human infections (intestinal origin)	80
Dialister micraerophilus	New	Human clinical samples	67
Dialister propionicifaciens	New	Human clinical samples	67
Faecalibacterium prausnitzii	*Fusobacterium prausnitzii*	Feces	32
Fusobacterium canifelinum	*F. nucleatum*-like	Oral cavity of cats and dogs; bite infections	24
Fusobacterium equinum	*F. necrophorum*-like	Oral cavity of horses	28
Porphyromonas gulae	*P. gingivalis*—animal strain	Gingival sulcus of animals	43
Porphyromonas somerae	*Porphyromonas levii*-like	Human skin, soft tissue, bone infections	130
Porphyromonas uenonis	*P. endodontalis*-nonoral	Human infections (nonoral)	41
Prevotella baroniae	New	Human oral cavity	30
Prevotella marshii	New	Human oral cavity	30
Prevotella multiformis	*P. denticola*-like	Human subgingival plaque	113
Prevotella multisaccharivorax	New	Human subgingival plaque	117
Prevotella salivae	*P. oris*-like	Human oral cavity	114
Prevotella shahii	*P. loeschii*-like	Human oral cavity	114
Sneathia sanguinegens	*Leptotrichia sanguinegens*	Human blood	22
Tannerella forsythensis	*Bacteroides forsythus*	Human periodontal pockets	115

to long, thin, pointed forms. The age of the culture, nutritional status, and exposure to air strongly affect morphology.

EPIDEMIOLOGY AND TRANSMISSION

Gram-negative anaerobic rods inhabit the mucosa of animals and humans. They are the predominant species in the oral cavity, the gastrointestinal tract, and the vaginal tract (in bacterial vaginosis; otherwise lactobacilli predominate). Most infections are acquired endogenously, when the integrity of the colonized mucosa or lumen is breached by trauma, disease (cancer), or iatrogenically (during surgery). Along the gastrointestinal tract, luminal populations appear to differ from adherent/mucosal strains. *B. vulgatus* and *B. thetaiotaomicron* are luminal and thus more commonly isolated from feces (100, 108). The predilection to adherence among *B. fragilis* may contribute to its predominance among the group as a pathogen, which, along with its relative aerotolerance, allows survival in hostile, oxygenated environments prior to establishment of the infection (112). Aspiration pneumonia, characterized by mixed anaerobes including gram-negative rods from the mouth, occurs during lapses of consciousness or other sedation events. Exceptions to endogenous acquisition of infection include clenched-fist wounds and animal and human bite wounds, which occur when the oral contents of an animal or person are implanted traumatically through the skin into the underlying tissue (131, 132). These infections invariably involve mixed flora, often with aerobic organisms. It is possible that *B. fragilis* is associated with diarrhea in children and that some toxigenic *B. fragilis* group may be transmitted from livestock, but that has not been proven (104).

CLINICAL SIGNIFICANCE

Gram-negative anaerobic rods predominate among anaerobes in clinical infections; they are found in more than one-half of the specimens yielding anaerobes (37, 65). Among the anaerobes encountered in clinical specimens, members of the bile-resistant *B. fragilis* group are the most commonly encountered and are more virulent and resistant to antimicrobial agents than most other anaerobes (91). *B. fragilis* and *Bacteroides thetaiotaomicron* are of the greatest clinical significance (44). Members of the *B. fragilis* group are major constituents of the normal colonic flora but are not common in the genital tract, mouth, or upper respiratory tract (108). These species are often found among the mixed microbiota of abscesses in tissue adjacent to their normal mucosal environments (intra-abdominal abscess or female genital tract abscess, for example). Some *B. fragilis* strains produce a potent zinc-dependent metalloprotease or enterotoxin with a variety of pathological effects on intestinal mucosal cells (119). The enterotoxin induces interleukin-8 production, which probably accounts for the inflammatory damage seen in *B. fragilis* diarrhea (145). *B. fragilis* also possesses lipopolysaccharides (LPS) and capsular polysaccharides of varying structure, antigenicity, and biological activity, which appear to play a role in periodontal disease and abscess formation (137, 141).

The pigmented anaerobic gram-negative rods are composed of saccharolytic and asaccharolytic species of the genera *Prevotella, Porphyromonas,* and *Alistipes finegoldii.* Several species of these genera are found in human clinical specimens. *Prevotella corporis, Prevotella denticola, Prevotella intermedia, Prevotella loescheii, Prevotella melaninogenica, Prevotella nigrescens, Prevotella pallens, Prevotella tannerae, Porphyromonas endodontalis, P. gingivalis,* and the nonpigmented species *P. catoniae* are found in the human oral cavity (116). Some are important pathogens in oral, dental, and bite infections and may produce infections of the head, neck, and lower respiratory tract. *P. gingivalis* and *Tannerella forsythensis* are the putative key pathogens (with *Treponema denticola*) in aggressive forms of adult periodontitis and, together with *P. endodontalis,* are often involved in root canal infections and complications of these infections such as odontogenic sinusitis (56, 115). Some of the above-named pigmented organisms and *Porphyromonas asaccharolytica* and *P. uenonis* are also prevalent in the urogenital or intestinal tracts and are important in infections arising from these sources (25, 41, 111). In addition to *P. uenonis* and the pigmented bile-resistant organisms mentioned above, *P. gingivalis* has also been isolated from extraoral sources, especially from patients with appendicitis (93, 138). *Porphyromonas* spp. of animal origin have been encountered in humans with animal bite infections (19, 45, 57). *Porphyromonas somerae* has been isolated from various types of human clinical infections including pleuropulmonary infections, skin and soft tissue infections, and bacterial vaginosis (130).

The bile-sensitive, nonpigmented, saccharolytic *Prevotella* and related strains recovered from human samples are found in the same settings as the pigmented gram-negative rods (38). *Prevotella bivia* and *Prevotella disiens* are found in female patients with genital tract infections, in patients with soft tissue infections, and less frequently in oral infections (4); these strains are often resistant to the β-lactam antibiotics, including penicillin, aminopenicillins, and cephalosporins (140). *Prevotella oris* and *Prevotella buccae* are found in a variety of oral, pleuropulmonary, and other infections (21, 38, 65). Members of the *P. oralis* group are relatively infrequently encountered in routine human clinical samples but common in oral and dental infections (30, 114).

P. zoogleoformans (indole negative) is rarely isolated from human clinical specimens, whereas *P. heparinolytica* (indole positive) is often found in the oral cavity of humans and animals and in association with oral infections. *Prevotella dentalis* (formerly *Mitsuokella dentalis*) is a common isolate from infected root canals, periodontal pockets, mandibular and gum abscesses, and in sialadenitis (128). *M. multiacida*, a nonmotile gram-negative anaerobic rod, sometimes isolated from rumen and the mammalian intestinal tract, is not related to *P. dentalis* but is most closely related to *Selenomonas* species, which in turn seem to belong to cluster IX of the *Clostridium* subphylum of the gram-positive bacteria (23). The nonpigmented, saccharolytic organism *Megamonas hypermegas* has not been isolated from human clinical specimens.

The nonpigmented, asaccharolytic, or weakly fermentative species *Anaerorhabdus furcosus*, *Bacteroides capillosus*, *Bacteroides coagulans*, *Dialister pneumosintes*, *Alistipes putredinis*, *Desulfovibrio* spp., and *Tissierella praeacuta* inhabit the intestinal tract and have occasionally been recovered from miscellaneous infections (37, 38, 48). *Bacteroides tectus* and the phenotypically similar *Bacteroides pyogenes* are often associated with canine or feline oral flora and are prevalent in infections in humans who have sustained animal bites (1, 38, 132). *Bilophila wadsworthia*, a bile-resistant organism, is present in small numbers in the bowel flora of healthy persons, yet it is the third most common anaerobe recovered from gangrenous or perforated appendixes and is a common constituent of the microbiota in other intra-abdominal infections (5, 7, 11). It has also been isolated from various other clinical specimens including blood, brain abscess, liver abscess, pericardial fluid, joint fluid, and pleural fluid as well as from human feces and vaginal and oral secretions (6, 36). *B. wadsworthia* is easily overlooked in cultures owing to its fastidious growth.

Members of the formate-fumarate-requiring *B. ureolyticus*-*Campylobacter* group, including *B. ureolyticus*, *C. gracilis*, *C. curvus*, *C. rectus*, and *S. wadsworthensis*, have been isolated from various types of infections (122). *B. ureolyticus* has been recovered from pulmonary, head and neck, intra-abdominal, urogenital, bone, and soft tissue infections. *C. gracilis* has been recognized as an important pathogen in serious visceral or head and neck infections and, in general, in infections above the diaphragm, and *S. wadsworthensis* is an important pathogen in infections below the diaphragm, especially abdominal infections (94, 143). *Campylobacter* spp. are primarily oral isolates found in patients with oral infections and periodontitis; they occasionally enter the bloodstream in immunocompromised patients. *C. rectus* has been implicated as a putative pathogen at sites of active periodontal breakdown (58, 110, 122). Many species of oral anaerobes have recently been associated with atherosclerosis, although a causal relationship has not been proved (59, 118, 124).

Among *Fusobacterium* species, *F. nucleatum* is most commonly encountered in clinical infections (13, 65). This organism is found in the mouth and in the genital, gastrointestinal, and upper respiratory tracts. It is often involved in the same types of infections as the pigmented *Prevotella* spp. and *Porphyromonas* spp. *F. nucleatum* may be found as the sole infecting agent in pleuropulmonary infections (21). *Fusobacterium necrophorum* is a very virulent anaerobe that may cause severe infection, usually in children or young adults, originating from pharyngotonsillitis, sometimes in association with infectious mononucleosis (70). It was the most common anaerobe isolated from peritonsillar abscesses in young adults and may in fact be an etiological agent of pharyngitis as often as *Streptococcus pyogenes* (2, 10, 63). Complications include Lemierre's disease, an acute jugular vein septic thrombophlebitis often complicated by sepsis and metastatic abscesses most frequently in the lungs, pleural space, liver, and large joints (63, 70). *F. necrophorum* is now encountered in serious infections less often than in the preantimicrobial agent era, but this makes it more treacherous, because many clinicians may not be familiar with the syndrome (74). There are two subspecies; *F. necrophorum* subsp. *necrophorum* contains lipase-positive, hemagglutinin-producing biovar A, and *F. necrophorum* subsp. *funduliforme* contains lipase-negative, non-hemagglutinin-producing biovar B. *Fusobacterium mortiferum* and *Fusobacterium varium* are encountered mainly in patients with intra-abdominal infections. *Fusobacterium russii* and *F. canifelinum* have been implicated in animal bite infections (24, 38), and *Fusobacterium ulcerans* is found in tropical ulcer. Other fusobacteria are isolated from clinical specimens rarely, usually oropharyngeal or genital sites. The former *F. prausnitzii*, abundant in the human feces, is not a fusobacterium but, rather, is related to the *Clostridium* spp. and has been renamed *Faecalibacterium prausnitzii*. Its pathogenic potential is unknown (26, 32). Other former gram-negative anaerobes closely related to clostridia include *Butyrivibrio fibrisolvens* and *B. hungatei* (from rumen) and *Catonella morbi* and *Johnsonella ignava* (from human gingival crevice). Routine clinical laboratories are unlikely to encounter these organisms.

Capnocytophaga spp. of human origin are often isolated only in anaerobic culture, and they are common in the oral cavity. *Leptotrichia buccalis* is a common mouth organism and may be found in the vagina and intestinal tract. Isolation of *Capnocytophaga* spp. or *Leptotrichia* spp. from blood cultures is often linked to patients (often adolescents) with hematological malignancies and is a direct clue to the presence of oral mucosal lesions in the patient (3, 38, 92). *Sneathia sanguinegens* has been isolated from cultures of blood from pregnant and elderly women and neonates (53).

Selenomonas sputigena, *Selenomonas artemidis*, *Selenomonas dianae*, *Selenomonas flueggei*, *Selenomonas infelix*, and *Selenomonas noxia* are all oral organisms, as is *Centipeda periodontii,* which closely resembles and phylogenetically clusters with *Selenomonas* in the *Clostridium* subphylum of the gram-positive bacteria (23, 133); these organisms are found in subgingival sites in patients with periodontitis (16, 75, 133).

The motile organisms *Succinivibrio dextrinosolvens, Butyrivibrio fibrisolvens,* and *Desulfovibrio* spp. including the nonmotile species *D. piger* are found as members of the normal colonic flora but may occasionally be encountered in patients with clinical infections, such as appendicitis (48). *Desulfovibrio* has been recovered in blood cultures from an immunocompromised patient, an immunocompetent patient, and from a pyogenic liver abscess in another patient (48, 80). The sites of normal carriage of *Anaerobiospirillum succiniciproducens* and *Anaerobiospirillum thomasii* in humans are unknown, but *Anaerobiospirillum* species are common in the fecal flora of cats and dogs (82). Strains of *Anaerobiospirillum* have been isolated from cultures of blood from compromised patients and from fecal specimens of patients with diarrhea (82, 83, 89, 134). In the latter case, a zoonotic role for *Anaerobiospirillum* spp. has been proposed.

COLLECTION, TRANSPORT, AND STORAGE OF SPECIMENS

General guidelines for collection, transport, and storage of specimens are discussed in chapters 5 and 20. Sites normally harboring a rich indigenous flora, such as the intestinal tract or vagina, should not be sampled and cultured for anaerobes except under special circumstances and by using special methods (e.g., quantitative study of upper small bowel flora in patients with the blind loop syndrome). Lower respiratory tract specimens and endometrial samples are especially difficult to obtain without contaminating the sample with indigenous flora. Double-lumen-catheter bronchial brushings and bronchoalveolar lavage fluid transported immediately to the laboratory under anaerobic conditions and cultured quantitatively, as well as pleural fluid, represent good respiratory tract specimens. An endometrial suction curette (Pipelle; Unimar, Wilton, Conn.) biopsy provides a good sample from the endometrium (39). Instructions for collection of specimens from different body sites and by various methods are given in more detail elsewhere (14, 39, 65).

Ulcers should be carefully debrided, and proper tissue samples should be collected from the base or progressive edge, where bacteria actively multiply, rather than from unremoved crust or surface pus, which is often contaminated by other bacteria not reflecting the true infecting flora.

Pus, when present, is best aspirated into a syringe through a needle and injected into an anaerobic transport vial containing an oxidation-reduction indicator. Syringes used for aspiration should not be used as transporters because of the potential danger of needlestick injuries or accidental expulsion and because oxygen diffuses through plastic syringes. Pieces of infected tissue obtained by excision or biopsy are always preferable to pus.

Specimens obtained with a swab are the least desirable and should be discouraged unless special circumstances exist. Swabs are intrinsically aerobic and prone to drying if not in anaerobic transport vials, often carry a volume of sample too small to be cultured on several media or quantitatively, and leave some of the specimen in the transport medium. However, swabs are used in many institutions. One study showed that aerobic and anaerobic organisms in purulent specimens survived for up to 48 h in anaerobic swab transport systems (20). Tissue samples are best transported in anaerobic transport vials or in loosely capped containers sealed in gas-impermeable bags in which an anaerobic atmosphere was generated. For small tissue and biopsy specimens and for subgingival and root canal samples, a semisolid anaerobic transport medium in which the specimen can be submerged may be used (Dental Transport Medium; Anaerobe Systems, Morgan Hill, Calif.). The dental specimens can be collected with a curette or with the use of paper points after careful removal of supragingival plaque (27, 65). The material from curettes or the paper points are transported in a transport medium, such as VMGA III (Viability Medium, Göteborg, anaerobically prepared and sterilized), containing glass beads to facilitate dispersion of aggregates in plaque (27). In the case of failed peri-implants, the whole fixture is placed in VMGA III (27, 65).

The conditions and time of transport should not affect the viability or relative proportions of bacteria present in the specimen if appropriate transport systems are used (8). Rapid transport is important when Gram stain and culture results are needed early for guidance of therapy. Contrary to previous recommendations, specimens in glass may be transported at room temperature or refrigerated (not frozen), as the organisms, especially facultative fastidious species, seem to survive at lower temperatures in newer transport systems (31, 136). More detailed information on transport systems and anaerobic techniques can be found elsewhere (8, 14, 65).

DIRECT EXAMINATION

The gross appearance (purulence, necrotic tissue), fluorescence of the sample under long-wave (366-nm) UV light, and the odor of the specimen can give the laboratory valuable clues to the presence of anaerobes. A fetid or putrid odor due to volatile short-chain fatty acids and amines is always associated with the presence of anaerobes in the sample. Black necrotic tissue and/or red fluorescence of the sample may be indicative of the presence of pigmented gram-negative rods.

Microscopy

The Gram stain is still the fastest, simplest, and the most likely to yield significant information among rapid methods and should be prepared from all specimens accepted for anaerobic culture. The morphotypes and relative quantities of both the host and the bacterial cells present in the preparation should be reported. Furthermore, the Gram stain information also provides quality control for specimen transport and isolation efficiency (39). Thick films from exudates and bloody fluids should be spread thin as for a blood smear. Smears should be fixed in methanol for 30 s to preserve the host and bacterial cell morphologies (87). Standard Gram stain procedures and reagents are used, except that 0.1 to 0.5% basic fuchsin, which enhances the staining of gram-negative anaerobes, is substituted for safranin as the counterstain (65, 87). Dark-field and phase-contrast microscopy may be helpful in the detection of small, poorly staining organisms *(D. pneumosintes),* for the direct observation of motility (*Campylobacter* spp.), for the notation of spores (*Clostridium* spp.), and for the recognition of morphotypes not cultivable on ordinary media (spirochetes). Gram stain using Nugent criteria for interpretation of vaginal discharge is still considered the best method for diagnosis of bacterial vaginosis (76, 120). Chapter 20 outlines this procedure.

Antigen or Product Detection

Although a direct fluorescent antibody for *B. fragilis* has been reported, it is not in routine use (105). Gas-liquid chromatography (GLC) of specimens has been proposed, but it has not gained acceptance. Newer methods for identification of volatile products in specimens, such as the electronic nose, are in developmental stages (54, 106, 135).

Molecular methods, such as nucleic acid probe hybridization, PCR amplification, and direct demonstration of nucleic acid sequences by 16S rRNA gene sequencing, are not used for routine diagnostic studies but are widely used in specialized oral and other research microbiology laboratories (16, 116). Eventually, molecular methods will become more commonplace (see chapter 16) (2).

ISOLATION PROCEDURES

The use of selective media along with nonselective media increases the yield and saves time in terms of recognition and isolation of colonies. Freshly prepared or prereduced and anaerobically sterilized media (Anaerobe Systems) should be used (88, 107). Different basal media differ in their abilities to support the growth of anaerobes; brucella base is superior to Trypticase soy (CDC base agar) and Schaedler base for isolation of gram-negative rods, but CDC base better supports the growth of anaerobic gram-positive cocci. Brain heart infusion base is superior to Trypticase soy in isolation efficiency for *Eubacterium* species but is inferior for pigmented gram-negative rods from subgingival and other samples (65). Fastidious anaerobe agar (Lab M, Bury, England) produces luxuriant growth of fusobacteria and some formate-fumarate-requiring species and can be used as a basal medium with or without selective agents. In academic centers performing large-scale anaerobic bacteriology, it would be ideal to use two different basal media to maximize isolation efficiency (39, 86) (chapter 21).

Isolation methods have been published elsewhere (15, 65, 86) (chapter 20). The minimum medium setup includes (i) a nonselective, enriched, brucella base sheep blood agar plate supplemented with vitamin K_1 and hemin (BAP); (ii) a kanamycin-vancomycin laked sheep blood agar (KVLB) for the selection of *Bacteroides* and *Prevotella* spp. (KVLB allows growth and rapid pigmentation of most *Prevotella* spp., but the concentration of vancomycin [7.5 μg/ml] inhibits most *Porphyromonas* spp.; for the isolation of *Porphyromonas* spp., KVLB medium with a reduced vancomycin concentration [2 μg/ml] may be prepared); and (iii) a *Bacteroides* bile-esculin agar plate (BBE) for specimens from areas below the diaphragm for the selection and presumptive identification of the *B. fragilis* group and *Bilophila* sp. BBE and KVLB are also available as biplates. When indicated, a phenylethyl alcohol-sheep blood agar plate, used to prevent overgrowth by aerobic gram-negative rods and swarming of some clostridia, may be inoculated. When fusobacteria are clinically suspected as the cause of infection, *Fusobacterium* neomycin-vancomycin agar or *Fusobacterium* selective agar may be used for isolation (65). A selective medium for culturing *Anaerobiospirillum* spp. from fecal specimens has been described (83). Use of a metronidazole disk on nonselective agar may help detect strict anaerobes, as resistant colonies would suggest facultative anaerobes or gram-positive anaerobes which are often resistant. After inoculation, the anaerobic plates should immediately be incubated at 36°C in an anaerobic environment, such as an anaerobic bag, jar, or chamber. Alternatively, setup and incubation may all be done in an anaerobic chamber. Plates should not be exposed to air during the first 48 h to avoid death of the more oxygen-sensitive species. In routine clinical microbiology, a total incubation period of at least 5 days for primary plates is recommended. In our experience with shorter incubation times, some anaerobic species, such as *Porphyromonas* and *Bilophila* spp., may not be detected.

Use of anaerobic blood culture media has been controversial, as strict anaerobes now comprise <5% of most clinically relevant blood culture isolates (98, 99). At the least, blood cultures from patients with abdominal or gynecological processes, peritoneal abscess, dirty wound, decubitus ulcers, osteomyelitis, oropharyngeal disease, and elderly patients should be cultured in an anaerobic bottle (9). However, since many facultative organisms may be recovered faster from the anaerobic bottle, both aerobic and anaerobic media are recommended for at least one blood culture set.

IDENTIFICATION

Colonies should be examined with a dissecting microscope to facilitate detection. Use a broken sterile wooden stick point to obtain material from each different colony type. Use this single colony sample to inoculate (i) a brucella BAP to which special-potency antibiotic disks (colistin, 10 μg; kanamycin, 1,000 μg; and vancomycin, 5 μg) are applied (a nitrate disk may also be added) (Fig. 1); (ii) a chocolate agar plate that is incubated in 5 to 10% CO_2 (can be a pie plate) for aerotolerance testing and detection of *Haemophilus* and capnophilic organisms; and finally (iii) an area on a slide for Gram staining. A blood agar pie plate is optional, but it is useful for seeing β-hemolysis of microaerophilic streptococci. A laked rabbit blood agar plate (LRBA) for the rapid demonstration of pigment production (laked rabbit blood agar is the most reliable and effective medium) (57, 65) and an egg yolk agar plate (EYA) for the demonstration of lipase, lecithinase, and proteolytic activities may also be inoculated at this point. The primary plates are reincubated along with the purity and test plates.

Preliminary Examination of Isolates

The characteristics that are noted from BAP include detailed Gram stain and colony morphology, pigment, fluorescence (long-wave UV light) (the results of the last two tests are also recorded from an LRBA), hemolysis, and greening or pitting of the agar. Furthermore, the spot indole reaction (*para*-dimethylaminocinnamaldehyde reagent), the nitrate reduction test, tests for sensitivities to special-potency antibiotic disks (Fig. 1), and catalase (15% H_2O_2) are performed. Most commonly isolated anaerobes are nonmotile, but in case of an unusual strain, motility tests from a broth culture or plate (hanging drop or wet mount) may be performed. Motile isolates are most likely to be *Campylobacter* spp. Instead of spot tests, Lombard-Dowell quadrant plates I, II, and III (Remel, Lenexa, Kans.) developed at the Centers for Disease Control and Prevention can be used to test for kanamycin resistance, indole, esculin, bile, gelatinase, lecithinase, lipase, and several carbohydrate fermentation reactions (35). Good growth is necessary for the proper interpretation of test results on this medium.

The primary plates are reinspected after 4 or more days to detect slow growers, new morphotypes, or late pigmenters. In oral microbiology laboratories, two rapid in situ tests have been used. The rapid differentiation of lactose-fermenting species from lactose-nonfermenting species is determined by applying 4-methylumbelliferyl-D-galactoside reagent (catalog no. M-1633; Sigma Chemical Co., St. Louis, Mo.) to the colonies and screening for fluorescent (lactose-positive) colonies under long-wave UV light. The carboxy-L-arginine-7-amino-4-methylcoumarin amide HCl (CAAM) test demonstrates the trypsin-like activities of suspected colonies of *P. gingivalis;* the colonies are treated with the CAAM reagent (catalog no. C-9396; Sigma) and screened for blue-white fluorescence under long-wave UV light (123).

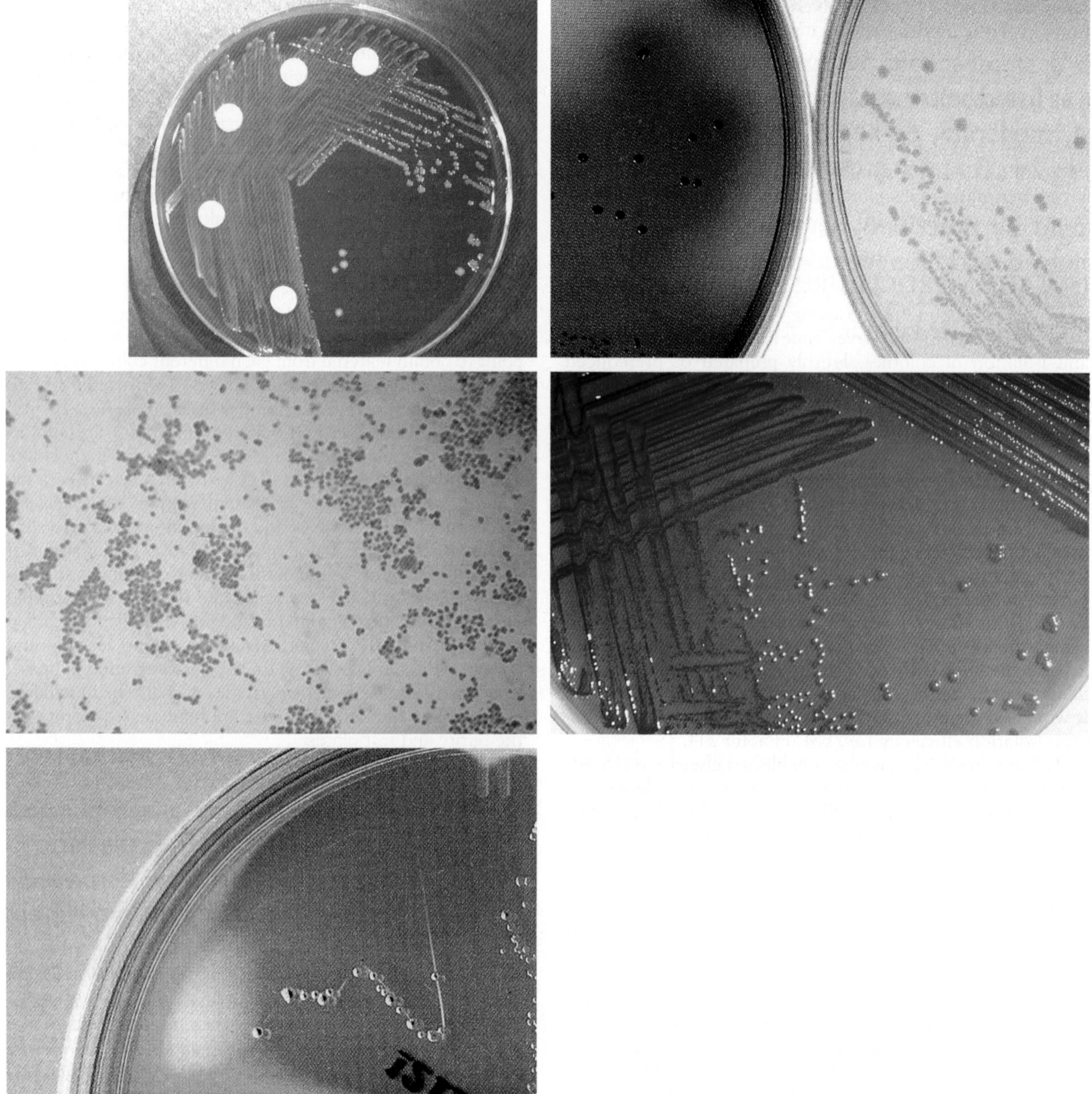

FIGURE 1 (top left) Placement of special-potency antibiotic disks. A blank disk for indole testing may be added (usually after growth has occurred).

FIGURE 2 (top right) Colonies of *Bacteroides fragilis* (left) and *Bacteroides vulgatus* (right) on BBE. Note the blackening of the agar and colonies due to esculin hydrolysis and bile precipitation.

FIGURE 3 (middle left) Coccobacillary cells of *Prevotella melaninogenica*.

FIGURE 4 (middle right) Pigmented colonies of *Porphyromonas* species.

FIGURE 5 (bottom) Colony morphology of *Bilophila wadsworthia* on BBE. Note the black centers due to H_2S production.

Presumptive Identification of Species

Most of the clinically significant gram-negative rods can be placed into broad groups with relatively few tests, and some isolates, including *Bilophila wadsworthia* and *Fusobacterium nucleatum*, can be presumptively identified with ease (Table 2) (101). The special-potency antibiotic disk pattern can be used to separate the gram-negative rods into several groups. A zone size equal to or greater than 10 mm is considered sensitive (65).

Most of the *Bacteroides* and *Prevotella* spp. are resistant to vancomycin and kanamycin and are variable in sensitivity to colistin; *Porphyromonas* spp. are generally sensitive to vancomycin and resistant to colistin. The *B. fragilis* group can be identified presumptively by their resistance to all three special-potency antibiotic disks and by growth equal to or greater than the control growth in 20% bile, as determined by a tube test, by a bile disk test (65), or on BBE (Fig. 2). Coccobacillary organisms that fluoresce red or produce black colonies are in the pigmented *Prevotella* spp.-*Porphyromonas* spp. group (Fig. 3 and 4).

Fusobacterium spp., *B. ureolyticus, Campylobacter* spp., *Bilophila* sp., *Sutterella* sp., and *Leptotrichia* spp. are resistant to vancomycin but sensitive to both colistin and kanamycin. *B. ureolyticus, Campylobacter, Bilophila,* and *Sutterella* colonies are usually much smaller and more translucent than those of fusobacteria and typically reduce nitrate; *Leptotrichia* colonies are large and gray and have a convoluted ("brain surface") texture. Furthermore, the most commonly encountered fusobacteria, *F. nucleatum* and *F. necrophorum,* are indole positive and nitrate negative. On microscopic inspection, fusobacteria are usually larger than the other bacteria with the same identification disk profile, excluding the large tapered cells of *Leptotrichia.* An anaerobic, gram-negative, catalase-negative rod that requires formate and fumarate for growth in broth culture or that pits agar may be presumptively identified as *B. ureolyticus* or a *Campylobacter* sp.; *B. ureolyticus* is urease positive (Table 2, footnote *d*). To document the formate-fumarate requirement, inoculate one tube of peptone yeast (or thioglycolate) broth medium containing the additive (0.3%) and one tube not containing the additive (control) (Table 2, footnote *b*). Compare the two tubes for intensity of growth. A strongly catalase-positive, bile-resistant, often urease-positive gram-negative rod can be presumptively identified as *Bilophila* sp. (Fig. 5). Microaerophilic and catalase- and urease-negative but bile-resistant (by the disk test) organisms growing in *Campylobacter* atmosphere (2 to 6% oxygen) are probably *S. wadsworthensis.*

Desulfovibrio piger (nonmotile), other *Desulfovibrio* spp. (motile), and the capnophilic, often yellow-pigmented *Capnocytophaga* spp. are resistant to vancomycin and colistin but sensitive to kanamycin (142). *Desulfovibrio* cells are curved or spiral; *Capnocytophaga* cells resemble fusobacteria with tapered ends. *Selenomonas* spp. may have the same special-potency disk patterns as *Desulfovibrio* and *Capnocytophaga* spp., but a few strains are sensitive to colistin. *Selenomonas* cells are curved and motile, as are those of *C. periodontii,* a closely related species that forms swarming colonies.

Most organisms not fitting the above-described groupings are *Bacteroides* spp. or *Prevotella* spp. but occasionally are representatives of the other genera listed in Table 1.

Rapid Identification

Whenever possible, simple tests should be used for the rapid and, to the extent that they permit, definitive identification of anaerobes (65, 85, 101). These include tests for colony and microscopic morphologies; the spot indole, catalase, lipase, and lecithinase tests; the nitrate disk test; the bile disk test; growth stimulation tests; and tests for sensitivities to special-potency antibiotic disks. Furthermore, rapid tests based on the presence of preformed enzymes produce clinically meaningful results in a timely fashion (see "Other Approaches to Identification"). See Tables 2 to 7, which incorporate the results of these tests; they can be used for the rapid identification of many commonly encountered anaerobic gram-negative rods.

Identification of the most commonly encountered bile-resistant members of the *B. fragilis* group is based on the special-potency disk profile and the results of a few tests that can be performed rapidly, including the catalase, indole, esculin, and α-fucosidase tests (Table 3, footnote *b*). Based on these reactions, the members of this group can be reported as *B. fragilis* group, most closely related to *B. fragilis,* or other species in this group (Tables 2 and 3). Further tests are performed when indicated. *Porphyromonas* spp. are easily identified even to the species level with the aid of the special-potency disk profile and the results of a few tests including indole, catalase, lipase, and some rapid enzyme tests (see Tables 2 and 6) (57, 66, 85, 138). *Porphyromonas asaccharolytica* may be confused with some *Prevotella* species without the vancomycin special-potency disk results (*Prevotella* spp. are resistant). An indole- and lipase-positive coccobacillus that forms black-pigmented colonies or that fluoresces red may be identified as belonging to *Prevotella intermedia/P. nigrescens* group; *P. pallens* resembles these two species but has lighter pigment and is lipase negative (71, 72). A rapid enzyme test for α-glucosidase (with Rosco Diagnostic Tablets [Rosco Diagnostics, Taastrup, Denmark] or the WEE-Tabs system [Key Scientific Products, Round Rock, Tex.]) is helpful; *P. intermedia/P. nigrescens* and *P. pallens* are positive, and *P. asaccharolytica* is negative (57). Furthermore, *Porphyromonas asaccharolytica* is sensitive to the special-potency vancomycin disk. Any indole-negative strains must be identified further by other biochemical tests. A lipase-positive, indole-negative, pigmented gram-negative rod could be *P. loescheii.*

B. ureolyticus, C. gracilis, other "anaerobic" *Campylobacter* spp., and *Sutterella* sp. are thin gram-negative rods with rounded ends that produce the *Fusobacterium* disk pattern. The colonies are small and translucent or transparent and may produce greening of the agar. Three colony morphotypes exist: smooth and convex, pitting (Fig. 6), and spreading. All colony types can occur in the same culture. These organisms are asaccharolytic and nitrate reducing, and they require supplementation of broth media with formate and fumarate for growth (Table 2, footnote *b*). *C. rectus, C. curvus, C. concisus,* and *C. showae* are motile and oxidase positive; unlike the first three, *C. showae* is catalase positive. *C. gracilis* is nonmotile and urease negative and, thus, is differentiated from urease-positive *B. ureolyticus* (Table 2, footnotes *d* and *e*). *Bilophila* sp., which phenotypically resembles *B. ureolyticus,* is distinguished from the above-mentioned species by its resistance to bile and its strong catalase reaction. *Sutterella* sp. is also resistant to bile but is urease and catalase negative (7, 143).

F. nucleatum is a thin rod with tapering ends (Fig. 7) and is indole positive. The needle-shaped morphology is shared with the microaerophilic, indole-negative *Capnocytophaga* spp. and *Leptotrichia* spp., as discussed above. *F. nucleatum* fluoresces chartreuse under UV light and often produces greening of the agar after exposure to air due to H_2O_2 production. At least three different colony morphotypes of *F. nucleatum* exist (13, 14, 34, 68). Due to considerable phenotypic and genotypic heterogeneity and uncertainty of valid criteria for the separation of the *F. nucleatum* subspecies, it is hard to judge whether the reported colonial morphologies consistently coincide with the subspecies designations. *F. nucleatum* subsp. *nucleatum* colonies may be small, grayish white, and smooth; *F. nucleatum* subsp. *fusiforme* colonies may also be small (<0.5 to 1 mm), granular, and irregular (bread crumb shaped) (Fig. 8); and *F. nucleatum* subsp. *polymorphum* colonies often are large, speckled, smooth, translucent, and butyrous. *F. necrophorum* subsp. *necrophorum* is lipase positive and usually bile sensitive. It is a pleomorphic long rod with round ends and often has bizarre forms, especially in older

TABLE 2 Group identification of anaerobic gram-negative organisms[a]

Group or organism	Vancomycin (5 μg)	Kanamycin (1,000 μg)	Colistin (10 μg)	Growth in 20% bile	Catalase	Indole	Growth stimulated by formate-fumarate[b]
B. fragilis group	R	R	R	+	V	V	
Other *Bacteroides* spp.	R	R	V	$-^{+}$	$-^{+}$	V	
Pigmented species	V	R	V	−	$-^{+}$	V	
Porphyromonas spp.	S	R	R	−	V	$+^{-}$	
Prevotella spp.	R	R^{S}	V	−	−	V	
P. intermedia-P. nigrescens-P. pallens	R	R^{S}	S	−	−	+	
P. loescheii	R	R	V	−	−	−	
Other *Prevotella* spp.	R	R	V	−	$-^{+}$	$-^{+}$	
Campylobacter spp./*B. ureolyticus*	R	S	S	−	$-^{+}$	−	+
B. ureolyticus	R	S	S	−	−	−	+
Campylobacter spp.[g]	R	S	S	−	−	−	+
C. gracilis	R	S	S	−	−	−	+
Sutterella sp.	R	S	S	+	−	−	+
Bilophila sp.[h]	R	S	S	+	+	−	−
Desulfovibrio spp.[i]	R	S	R	V	V	$-^{+}$	−
Fusobacterium spp.	R	S	S	V	−	V	
F. nucleatum	R	S	S	−	−	+	
F. necrophorum	R	S	S	$-^{+}$	−	+	
F. varium/F. mortiferum	R	S	S	+	−	V	
Anaerobiospirillum spp.	R	S	S	−	−	−	
Capnocytophaga spp.	R	S	R	−	−	−	
Centipeda periodontii	R	S	R	−	−	−	
Leptotricihia/Sneathia	R	S	S	$+^{-}$	−	−	
Selenomonas spp.	R	S	R	−	−	−	
Dialister pneumosintes	R	S	R^{S}	−	−	−	
Veillonella spp. (cocci)	R	S	S	−	V	−	

[a] R, resistant; S, susceptible; R^{S}, most strains resistant, some strains susceptible; V, variable; +, positive reaction for majority of strains; −, negative reaction; $+^{-}$, most strains positive but some strains negative; $-^{+}$, most strains negative but some strains positive.

[b] Compare the growth of the organism in an unsupplemented thioglycolate broth with growth in a broth supplemented with formate and fumarate additive: dissolve 3 g of sodium formate, 3 g of fumaric acid, and 20 pellets of sodium hydroxide in 50 ml of distilled water; adjust the pH to 7; and filter sterilize. Add 0.5 ml of additive to 10 ml of culture broth (55, 65).

[c] Use the nitrate disk test (65).

[d] Make a heavy suspension of the organism in 0.5 ml of sterile urea broth (BBL; BD, Franklin Lakes, N.J.) or in sterile water and insert a urea tablet (Rosco Diagnostic Tablets, A/S Rosco, Taastrup, Denmark) or WEE-Tabs (Key Scientific Products; Round Rock, Tex.). Incubate the tubes aerobically for up to 24 h. A bright pink or red is positive; this color usually appears within 15 to 30 min.

TABLE 3 Characteristics of *B. fragilis* group and *B. splanchnicus*[a]

Species	Growth on BBE	Indole	Catalase	Esculin hydrolysis	α-Fucosidase[b]
B. caccae[d]	+	−	$-^{+}$	+	+
B. distasonis[e]	+	−	$+^{-}$	+	−
B. eggerthii	+	+	−	+	−
B. fragilis[d]	+	−	+	+	+
B. goldsteinii	+	−	V	+	−
B. merdae[e]	+	−	$-^{+}$	+	−
B. nordii	+	+		+	−
B. ovatus	+	+	$+^{-}$	+	$+^{-}$
B. salyersiae	+	+	−	+	−
B. stercoris	+	+	$-^{+}$	$+^{-}$	V
B. thetaiotaomicron	+	+	+	+	+
B. uniformis	W^{+}	+	V	+	+
B. vulgatus	+	−	$-^{+}$	$-^{+}$	+
B. splanchnicus	+	+	−	+	+

[a] +, positive reaction for the majority of strains; −, negative reaction; V, variable reaction; W, weak reaction; W^{+}, weak reaction but some strains more strongly positive; $+^{-}$, most strains positive; $-^{+}$, most strains negative, some strains positive; $-^{w}$, most strains negative, some strains weakly positive. For sugars: +, pH < 5.5; W, pH = 5.5 to 5.8; −, pH > 5.8.

[b] Make a heavy suspension (heavier than a McFarland no. 2 standard) of the organism in 0.25 ml of sterile saline. Add a tablet of substrate (Rosco Diagnostic Tablets or WEE-Tabs). Incubate for 4 h (or overnight). Yellow color, positive; colorless, negative.

Nitrate reduction[c]	Lipase	Pigment	Red fluorescence	Urease[d]	Motility[e]	Pitting of agar[f]	Slender cells with pointed ends
–	–		–	–			
–	–			–			
–	V	+	$+^{-}$	–			
–	$-^{+}$	$+^{-}$	$+^{-}$	–			
–	$-^{+}$	+	+	–			
–	$+^{-}$	+	+	–			
–		+	+	–			
–	$-^{+}$	–	–				
+	–			V	V	V	
+	–			+	–	V	
+	–			–	$+^{-}$	V	
+	–			–	–	V	
+	–			–	–	V	
+	–			$+^{-}$	–	–	
V	–			$-^{+}$	$+^{-}$	–	
$-^{+}$	V			–	–		V
–	–			–			+
–	$+^{-}$			–			–
–	–			–			–
–	–			–	+		
–	–			–	–		+
+				–	+		
–	–			–	–		
–	–			–	+		
–	–			–	–		
+	–		V	–	–		

[e] Check motility with a young broth culture supplemented with formate and fumarate or prepare a suspension in broth directly from the blood agar plate.
[f] Formate and fumarate should be added to broth media for this group of organisms.
[g] *C. rectus, C. curvus,* and *C. showae.*
[h] Growth stimulated by 1% pyruvate (final concentration).
[i] Desulfoviridin positive. Swab cell paste from a pure culture on blood agar, add 1 drop of 2N NaOH to the swab, and immediately observe under long-wave (366-nm) UV light. Positive, red fluorescence; negative, no fluorescence.

cultures that have been exposed to air. It produces indole, fluoresces chartreuse, produces greening of the agar, and often demonstrates beta-hemolysis around the grayish to yellow dull, umbonate colonies (Fig. 9). Lipase-negative strains require further biochemical testing. *F. mortiferum* is indole negative and extremely pleomorphic; it has filaments containing swollen areas with large, round bodies and exhibiting irregular staining (Fig. 10). *F. necrophorum* may have a similar

Fermentation of:								Fatty acids from PYG[c]
Arabinose	Cellobiose	Rhamnose	Salicin	Sucrose	Trehalose	Xylose	Xylan	
+	$+^{-}$	$+^{-}$	$-^{+}$	+	+	+	–	A, p, S, (iv)
$-^{+}$	+	V	+	+	+	+	–	A, p, s, (pa, ib, iv, l)
+	$-^{+}$	$+^{-}$	–	–	–	+	+	A, p, S, (ib, iv, l)
–	$+^{-}$	–	–	+	–	+	–	A, p, S, pa, (ib, iv, l)
–	+	+	+	+	+	+	–	A, p, S, (ib, iv)
–	V	+	+	+	+	+	–	A, p, S, (ib, iv)
–	+	+	–	+	–	+	–	
+	+	+	+	+	+	+	+	A, p, S, pa, (ib, iv, l)
+	+	+	–	+	–	+	–	
–	$-^{+}$	+	$-^{+}$	+	–	+	+	A, p, S, (ib, iv)
+	$+^{-}$	+	$-^{+}$	+	+	+	–	A, p, S, pa, (ib, iv, l)
+	+	$-^{+}$	$+^{-}$	+	$-^{w}$	+	–	a, p, l, S, (ib, iv)
+	–	+	–	+	–	+	$-^{+}$	A, p, S
+	–	–	–	–	–	–	–	A, P, S, ib, b, iv, (l)

[c] Capital letters indicate major metabolic products from peptone-yeast-glucose (PYG), lowercase letters indicate minor products, and parentheses indicate a variable reaction for the following fatty acids: A, acetic; P, propionic; IB, isobutyric; B, butyric; IV, isovaleric; V, valeric; L, lactic; S, succinic; PA, phenylacetic. Note that isoacids are primarily from carbohydrate-free media (e.g., peptone-yeast extract) in the case of saccharolytic organisms.
[d] *B. caccae* is L-arabinose positive with Rosco Diagnostic Tablets; *B. fragilis* is negative.
[e] *B. merdae* and *B. goldsteinii* are β-glucuronidase positive with Rosco Diagnostic Tablets; *B. distasonis* is negative. *B. goldsteinii* is α-glucosidase positive; *B. merdae* is negative.

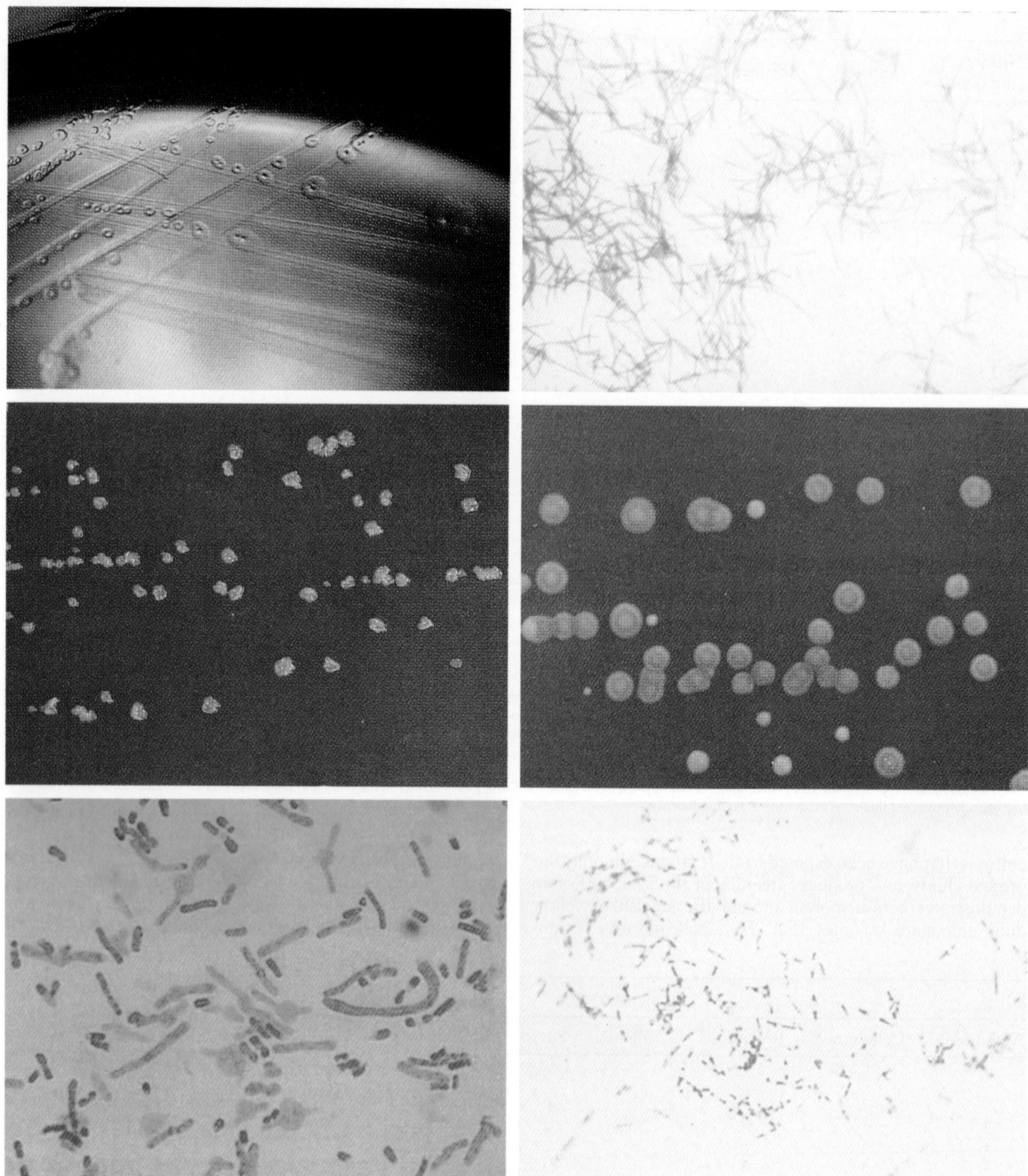

FIGURE 6 (top left) Pitting colonies of *Bacteroides ureolyticus*.

FIGURE 7 (top right) Cells of *Fusobacterium nucleatum*. Note the slender shape with pointed ends.

FIGURE 8 (middle left) Bread crumb-shaped colonies of *Fusobacterium nucleatum*. Note the greening of the agar.

FIGURE 9 (middle right) Umbonate colonies of *Fusobacterium necrophorum*.

FIGURE 10 (bottom left) Microscopic morphology of *Fusobacterium mortiferum*. There is marked pleomorphism and irregularity of staining. Note the filaments with swellings.

FIGURE 11 (bottom right) Pleomorphic, irregularly staining cells of *Bacteroides fragilis*.

morphology but usually has fewer round bodies. A bile-resistant fusobacterium isolated from BBE may be identified as *F. mortiferum* or *F. varium*; *F. mortiferum* is positive for *o*-nitrophenyl-β-D-galactopyranoside (Table 3, footnote *b*), whereas *F. varium* is negative.

Definitive Identification

A definitive identification of an anaerobic isolate should be obtained for all isolates from normally sterile body sites such as blood, spinal fluid, and organs or body cavities; when the patient is gravely ill and not responding to treatment; and when prolonged treatment is necessary. Definitive identification is also indicated in unusual case presentations and in some teaching-hospital settings, particularly if the case is to be published.

The definitive identification of some species requires certain additional biochemical tests, metabolic end product analysis, and/or cell wall fatty acid profiling by GLC (65). Even in good research or reference laboratories, a percentage of strains will not be identified definitively. If such strains are isolated from blood or closed-space infections, molecular methods such as 16S rRNA sequencing may be helpful. Motility may be helpful for characterizing curved rods that are not *Campylobacter*, as shown in Table 2. Organisms with small, translucent, spreading colonies that are not *B. ureolyticus*-like should also be checked for motility. The results in Tables 3 to 7 are based on reactions in prereduced, anaerobically sterilized (PRAS) liquid media (55, 65). A shortened and simplified scheme (spot indole, arabinose, sucrose, trehalose, rhamnose, and xylan tests) for the identification of the *B. fragilis* group with commercial PRAS biochemicals and the addition of bromthymol blue at 24 h postincubation has been described (18, 125). Other systems that depend on color changes of pH-dependent indicators for interpretation of reactions may not yield the same results as reactions in PRAS biochemicals. Gas chromatographic analysis may be performed on peptone-yeast glucose broth that shows good growth of the organism (55, 65). Each lot of uninoculated broth must be assayed in parallel with samples to determine the background amounts of acetic and succinic acids, and if chopped-meat broth is used, an uninoculated broth is assayed for lactic acid. Fermentation end products vary depending on the substrate available to the organism. Use of substrates other than those on which the results in the identification tables are based may lead to misinterpretation of the GLC pattern and misidentification of the organism. For instance, saccharolytic organisms produce larger amounts of isoacids in the absence of a fermentable carbohydrate, and a fermentable carbohydrate is required for the detection of lactic acid.

Colonies of the *B. fragilis* group on brucella BAP are 2 to 3 mm in diameter, circular, entire, convex, and gray to white. The cells may be uniform, bipolarly stained, or pleomorphic (some may contain vacuoles) (Fig. 11); this difference is medium and age dependent. The presence of ovoid cells suggests *B. ovatus*. Good growth in or stimulation by 20% bile (2% oxgall) is characteristic of the *B. fragilis* group; the exception to this rule is the poor growth of *B. uniformis* in bile. Some organisms not belonging to the *B. fragilis* group (non-*B. fragilis* group) are bile resistant. These include *B. splanchnicus*, *B. tectus*, *B. pyogenes*, *M. multiacida*, *Bilophila* sp., *Alistipes* spp., and some fusobacteria (111). Not all of these, however, grow on BBE. Morphologic characteristics, special-potency identification disks, and some biochemical reactions differentiate these species. Most of the *B. fragilis* group organisms blacken the BBE (esculin hydrolyzed), although *B. vulgatus* may not hydrolyze esculin. Table 3 is a key for the differentiation of members of the bile-resistant *B. fragilis* group.

Members of the non-*B. fragilis* group, nonpigmented anaerobic gram-negative rods, form two major subgroups: saccharolytic and asaccharolytic or weakly saccharolytic. Tables 4 and 5 list the more commonly encountered or clinically important species in these groups.

The saccharolytic organisms fall into two categories, i.e., pentose (arabinose and xylose) fermenters and pentose nonfermenters. Pentose fermentation may be difficult to demonstrate owing to suboptimal growth in the test medium; therefore, a screening test for the presence of the preformed enzyme β-xylosidase is recommended (for the procedure, see Table 3, footnote *b*). *P. oris* and *P. buccae* are pentose fermenters (Table 4). They are phenotypically very similar but can be differentiated by the α-fucosidase and *N*-acetyl-β-glucosaminidase tests (Table 3, footnote *b*) (33, 57); furthermore, *P. buccae* is usually sensitive to the special-potency colistin disk, whereas *P. oris* is not. *P. zoogleoformans* and *P. heparinolytica* may also ferment pentoses. Both produce viscous material in broth cultures, and on solid media the colonies often adhere to the agar. The positive indole reaction of *P. heparinolytica* differentiates these two species. The indole production is sometimes very difficult to demonstrate and should be tested from a pure culture on an EYA plate and/or from an old (>5-day-old) culture in chopped-meat broth because in some strains it can be a weak reaction. Other pentose fermenters include bile-resistant *M. multiacida* and *B. splanchnicus* and bile-sensitive *P. dentalis*. Unlike most *Prevotella* and *Bacteroides* species, *M. multiacida* is both nitrate and inositol positive. *P. dentalis* forms characteristic "water-drop," viscous colonies on blood agar. A positive *N*-acetyl-β-glucosaminidase reaction differentiates it from *P. buccae*, and a negative α-fucosidase reaction differentiates it from *P. oris*. The far better growth of *P. dentalis* on CDC blood agar than on brucella blood agar is an additional feature to facilitate the identification of the species.

Salicin, cellobiose, xylan, and sucrose are the key sugars in the differentiation of *P. baroniae*, *P. oralis*, *P. buccalis*, *P. veroralis*, *P. marshii*, *P. oulorum*, and *P. enoeca* (Table 4). In addition, *P. oulorum* produces catalase and is lipase positive (97). Certain strains of the saccharolytic pigmented *Prevotella* spp. require more than 21 days to develop pigment, and these strains (especially *P. loescheii*) closely resemble *P. veroralis*. Darker, more opaque colonies and salicin and cellobiose reactions may aid in differentiation of the strains.

P. bivia and *P. disiens* are both saccharolytic and strongly proteolytic (Table 4). Gelatin and milk are usually digested within 2 to 3 days (milk digestion may take longer). Differentiation is based on lactose fermentation; *P. bivia* is lactose positive, and *P. disiens* is lactose negative. Furthermore, *P. bivia* is both *N*-acetyl-β-glucosaminidase and α-fucosidase positive, but *P. disiens* is negative for both. Under long-wave UV light, *P. bivia* and *P. disiens* colonies may fluoresce light orange to pink (coral), and *P. disiens* also may produce a brown pigment on LRBA that makes differentiation from the phenotypically similar *P. corporis* difficult. *P. bivia* and *P. enoeca* share the same phenotypic characteristics, but *P. enoeca* is gelatin negative; it is usually isolated from oral or oral-associated sources, whereas *P. bivia* is more often found in nonoral samples.

Asaccharolytic, nonpigmented *Bacteroides* spp. and *Tissierella* spp. are infrequently isolated from clinical specimens (Table 5). *Anaerorhabdus furcosus*, another rare species, is currently considered to be within *Bacteroidaceae* but may

TABLE 4 Characteristics of nonpigmented saccharolytic *Prevotella* spp. and other genera[a]

Subgroup and species	Growth in 20% bile	Gelatin	Indole	Esculin hydrolysis	α-Fucosidase[b]	ONPG[b,c]	N-Acetyl-β-glucosaminidase[b]	β-Xylosidase[b]
Pentose fermenters								
M. multiacida	+	−	−	+	+	+	+	+
P. buccae	−	+	−	+	−	+	−	+
P. dentalis	−	−	−	V	−	+	+	V
P. heparinolytica[e]	−	−	+	+	+	+	+	+
P. multisaccharivorax	−	+	−	+	−	V		+
P. oris	−	V	−	+	+	+	+	+
P. zoogleoformans[e]	−	V	−	+	+	+	+	+
Not pentose fermenters								
P. buccalis	−	−	−	+	+	+	+	−
P. baroniae	−	+	−	+	+	+	+	−[f]
P. bivia	−	+	−	−	+	+	+	−
P. disiens	−	+	−	−	−	−	−	−
P. enoeca	−	+	−	V	+	+	+	−
P. marshii	−	+	−	−	+	−	−	−[f]
P. multiformis	−	+	−	−	V	+		−
P. oralis	−	+	−	+	+	+	+	−[f]
P. oulorum[g]	−	−	−	+	−	+	+	−
P. shahii	−	+	−	−	+	W	+	−[f]
P. veroralis	−	V	−	+	+	+	+	−
Other								
Anaerobiospirillum succiniciproducens[h]	−	−	−	−		+		
Capnocytophaga spp.	−		−	$+^{-}$				
Leptotrichia buccalis	$+^{-}$	−	−	+				
Leptotrichia sanguinegens			−	+				
Selenomonas sp.	−		−	V				

[a] See Table 3, footnote *a*.
[b] See Table 3, footnote *b*.
[c] ONPG, *o*-nitrophenyl-β-D-galactopyranoside.
[d] See Table 3, footnote *c*.

TABLE 5 Characteristics of nonpigmented weakly saccharolytic or nonsaccharolytic gram-negative rods[a]

Species	Growth in 20% bile	Glucose	Catalase	Indole	Nitrate	Motility
Alistipes putredinis	$+^{-}$	−	$+^{-}$	+	−	−
Anaerohabdus furcosa	$+^{-}$	W	−	−	−	−
Bilophila wadsworthia[g]	+	−	+	−	+	−
Bacteroides capillosus	$-^{+}$	W^{-h}	−	−	−	−
B. coagulans	+	−	−	−	−	−
B. pyogenes[f]	+	W	−	−	−	−
B. tectus[f]	+	W	−	−	−	−
B. ureolyticus	−	−	$-^{+}$	−	+	−
Campylobacter spp.	−	−	−	−	+	$+^{-}$
C. gracilis	−	−	−	−	+	−
Desulfovibrio piger[g]	+	−	−	−	−	−
D. desulfuricans[g]	−	−	−	−	+	+
D. fairfieldensis[g]	+	−	+	−	+	+
D. vulgaris[g]	+	−	−	+	−	+
Dialister pneumosintes	−	−	−	−	−	−
Sutterella wadsworthensis	+	−	−	−	+	−
Tannerella forsythensis	−	−	−	−	−	−
Tissierella praeacuta	+	−	−	−	V	+

[a] See Table 3, footnote *a*.
[b] F/F, formate-fumarate. See Table 3, footnote *b*.
[c] See Table 2, footnote *i*.
[d] See Table 2, footnote *d*.

Fermentation of:								
Arabinose	Cellobiose	Glucose	Lactose	Salicin	Sucrose	Xylose	Xylan	Fatty acids from PYG[d]
+	+	+	+	+	+	+		A, L, S
+	+	+	+	+	+	+		A, S, (p, ib, iv)
+	+	+	+	−	W	V		A, S
+	+	+	+	+	+	+		A, p, S (iv)
V	+	+	+	V	+	+		A, S, iv
$+^{-}$	+	+	+	+	+	+		A, S, (P, ib, iv)
V	+	+	+	V	+	V		A, P, S, (ib, iv)
−	+	+	+	−	+	−	−	a, iv, S
−	+	+	+	+	+	−		A, S, (l)
−	−	+	+	−	−	−		A, iv, S, (ib)
−	−	+	−	−	−	−		A, S, (p, ib, iv)
−	−	+	+	−	−	−		a, S
−	−	+	−	−	−	−		A, S, (l)
−	+	+	+	−	+	−		A, S, iv
−	+	+	+	+	+	−	−	A, S, (l)
−	−	+	+	−	+	−	−	A, S
−	−	+	+	−	+	−		A, S, (l)
−	+	+	+	−	+	−	+	a, S
−	−	+	+	−	+	−		A, S
−	$-^{+}$	+	V	−	+	−		A, S
$-^{+}$	$+^{-}$	+	$+^{-}$	$+^{-}$	+	−		L, (a, s)
−	+	+	−	+	−	−		L, (a)
−	−	$+^{-}$	V	−	$+^{-}$	−		A, P

[e] Produces viscous sediment in broth and colonies usually adhere to agar.
[f] Positive with 4-methylumbelliferyl substrates (81).
[g] Catalase and lipase positive.
[h] Corkscrew motility.

F/F required[b]	Desulfoviridin[c]	Urease[d]	Esculin hydrolysis	Gelatin hydrolysis	Fatty acids from PYG[e]
−	−	−	−	+	a, P, ib, b, IV, S, (1), pa
−	−	+	+	$-^{w}$	a, l, (s)
−	W	$+^{-}$	−	−	A, (s)
−	−	−	+	$-^{w}$	a, s, (p, l)
−	−	−	−	+	a, (p, 1, s)
−	−	−	+	+	a, P, ib, b, IV, S, (l)
−	−	−	+	+	A, p, iv, S, pa
+	−	+	−	−	A, S
+	−	−	−	−	a, S
+	−	−	−	−	a, S
−	+	−	−	−	A
−	+	+	−	−	A
−	+	+	−	−	A
−	+	−	−	−	A
−	−	−	−	$-^{w}$	a, (l, s)
+	−	−	−	−	a, S
−	−	−	+	+	A, S, pa
−	−	−	−	+	A, p, ib, B, IV, s, (l)

[e] See Table 3, footnote c.
[f] Animal origin; also isolated from bite infections in humans. Quantitative differences between some cellular fatty acids may help in differentiation of these species (42).
[g] *Bilophila* sp. is colistin sensitive; *Desulfovibrio* spp. are colistin resistant.
[h] W^-, most strains weakly positive, some strains negative.

be more related to gram-positive rods. *B. capillosus* coagulates milk and may grow better with Tween 80-supplemented media. *D. pneumosintes* is a very tiny rod best seen by dark-field examination (it almost resembles *Veillonella* spp. by Gram staining) and forms minute colonies that may require magnification to be seen. Other species of *Dialister* from clinical specimens have been described recently (67). *T. forsythensis* is a fusiform rod that exhibits a wide variety of enzyme activities including trypsin-like activity and *N*-acetyl-β-glucosaminidase, α-fucosidase, and β-glucuronidase activities. However, its growth is minimal in broth media, and it requires *N*-acetylmuramic acid; therefore, it is often seen as satellite colonies around colonies of other organisms, especially fusobacteria. *Desulfovibrio* spp. are sulfate-reducing bacteria and can be confirmed by the desulfoviridin test (Table 2, footnote *i*). The species are motile (except for the recently included *D. piger*) and produce copious amounts of H_2S (142).

The pigmented *Prevotella* spp. and *Porphyromonas* spp. (Table 6) vary greatly in the degree and rapidity of pigment production, which ranges from buff to tan to black depending primarily on the type of blood and the composition of the base medium used in the agar. A period of 2 to 21 days may be required even on LRBA to detect pigmentation in some strains. The identities of strains not showing pigmentation must be established by other biochemical tests to avoid confusion with the *P. oralis* group of organisms. The pigmented *Prevotella* and *Porphyromonas* spp. fluoresce pink, orange, or brick red under UV light. Fluorescence is best demonstrated in young cultures; in older cultures, especially on laked blood agar, the fluorescence is more or less masked depending on the intensity of pigment production (66).

The indole-positive species *P. intermedia* and *P. nigrescens* produce dark pigment; the pigment produced by *P. pallens* is lighter. The use of oligonucleotide probes or determination of arbitrarily primed PCR and enzyme electrophoretic mobility profiles are needed for species differentiation (51, 66). The unusual special-potency antibiotic disk pattern (sensitivity to vancomycin), in addition to asaccharolytic properties, separates most *Porphyromonas* spp. from the other pigment producers. *P. asaccharolytica, P. endodontalis, P. uenonis*, and *P. gingivalis* are all asaccharolytic and phenotypically very similar. The key differential tests include tests for phenylacetic acid production, trypsin-like activity, and *N*-acetyl-β-glucosaminidase and α-fucosidase activities (Table 6). Unlike most *Porphyromonas* spp., *P. catoniae, P. levii*, and *P. somerae* (frequently isolated from human clinical specimens) are indole negative and weakly saccharolytic; the latter characteristic is also shared with the animal strains of *Porphyromonas macacae*. Most of the *Porphyromonas* spp. of

TABLE 6 Characteristics of pigmented *Porphyromonas* spp. and *Prevotella* spp.[a]

Species and origin	Indole	Lipase	Catalase	Esculin hydrolysis	α-Fucosidase[b]	α-Galactosidase[b]	β-Galactosidase[b]
Porphyromonas, asaccharolytic or weakly saccharolytic							
Human origin							
P. asaccharolytica	+	−[+]	−	−	+	−	−
P. catoniae[d]	−	−	−	−	+	−[+]	+
P. uenonis	+	−	−	−	−	−	−
P. endodontalis	+	−	−	−	−	−	−
P. gingivalis[e]	+	−	−	−	−	−	−[f]
P. somerae[e]	−	−	−	−	−	−	+
Animal origin[g]							
P. canoris	+	−	+	−	−	−	+
P. cangingivalis	+	−	+	−	−	−	−
P. cansulci	+	−	+[w]	−	−	−	−
P. circumdentaria	+	−	+	−	−	−	−
P. crevioricanis	+		−	−	−		
P. gingivicanis	+		+	−	−		
P. gulae	+	−	+	−	−	−	−[f]
P. levii[e]	−	−	−	−	−	−	+
P. macacae	+	+	+	−	−	+	−[f]
Prevotella, saccharolytic							
P. corporis	−	−	−	−	−	−	−
P. denticola	−	−	−	+[−]	+	+	+
P. intermedia	+	+[−]	−	−	+	−	−
P. loescheii	−	V	−	+[−]	+	+	+
P. melaninogenica	−	−	−	−[+]	+	+	+
P. nigrescens[h]	+	+[−]	−	−	+	−	−
P. pallens	+	−	−	−	+	−	−
P. tannerae	−	−	−	−	+	−	+

[a] See Table 3, footnote *a*. +[w], most strains positive; some strains weakly positive.
[b] Reaction by the API ZYM system or with Rosco Diagnostic Tablets (see Table 3, footnote *b*). Reactivity in these systems is not always identical (see footnote *f*).
[c] See Table 3, footnote c.
[d] Nonpigmented.

animal origin are differentiated from the human strains by a positive catalase reaction; *Porphyromonas crevioricanis*, however, is catalase negative (66).

Table 7 characterizes the more commonly isolated fusobacteria. Bizarre pleomorphic rods with very large, round bodies are suggestive of *F. mortiferum* (Fig. 10). This organism may grow on BBE and turn the agar black due to H_2S production. *F. ulcerans*, isolated from tropical ulcer, closely resembles indole-negative strains of *F. varium* but is nitrate positive. *F. periodonticum*, an oral isolate, is indole positive and bile sensitive. The national anaerobic laboratory of Finland failed to demonstrate glucose, fructose, or galactose fermentation by the type strain; this bacterium is indistinguishable from *F. nucleatum* except by 16S-23S rRNA internal transcribed spacer sequencing (26). *Fusobacterium russii* is indole negative and bile sensitive (26).

Other Approaches to Identification

Several microsystems for the identification of anaerobes are currently available. The API 20A system (bioMérieux Vitek, St. Louis, Mo.) is a microtube biochemical system that uses bromcresol purple as indicator, produces results after 24 to 48 h of incubation, and has a computerized database. The API 20A is best suited for identification of saccharolytic, fast-growing organisms such as members of the *B. fragilis* group and many clostridia. Most asaccharolytic organisms cannot be identified by API 20A, and some fastidious organisms (e.g., some *Prevotella* spp.) fail to grow. Even for many saccharolytic organisms, supplemental tests are often required for definitive identification. The color reactions are not always clear-cut, as shades of brown or no color can make interpretation of the test results difficult.

The rapid (2- to 4-h) identification systems based on detection of preformed (constitutive) enzymes by use of chromogenic or fluorogenic substrates, or a combination of both, include the RapID ANA II system (Remel), Rapid ID 32A, ANI Card, and API ZYM systems (bioMérieux), the MicroScan system (Dade Behring MicroScan, Inc., Sacramento, Calif.), and the BBL Crystal Anaerobe Identification system (Becton Dickinson Diagnostic Systems, Franklin Lakes, N.J.), as mentioned in chapter 15. The overall performance of these systems has varied from moderate to good; 53 to 100% of the isolates are identified to the species level (17, 29, 61, 79, 90, 129). The Crystal Anaerobe (ANR) Identification (ID) system was reported to identify 91% of the *B. fragilis* group and all of the *Prevotella* and *Porphyromonas* strains tested to the species level; 53% of the non-*B. fragilis* group *Bacteroides* spp. were identified correctly (17). The Rapid ID 32A system was found to be 78.4 to 90.6% accurate for the *B. fragilis* group (29, 79); a supplemental test for catalase

N-Acetyl-β glucosaminidase[b]	Chymotrypsin	Trypsin	Fermentation of:				Fatty acids from PYG[c]
			Glucose	Cellobiose	Lactose	Sucrose	
–	–	–	–	–	–	–	
+	$+^{-}$	$-^{+}$	W	–	W	–	A, P, iv, l, S
–	–	–	–	–	–	–	A, p, ib, B, IV, s
–	–	–	–	–	–	–	A, p, ib, B, IV, s
+	+	+	–	–	–	–	A, p, ib, B, IV, s, pa
+	+	–	W	–	W	–	A, p, ib, B, IV, s
+	+	–	–	–	–	–	A, P, ib, b, IV, s
–	–	–	–	–	–	–	A, p, ib, B, IV
–	–	–	–	–	–	–	A, P, ib, B, IV, S, pa
–	–	–	–	–	–	–	A, P, ib, b, IV, s, pa
–	NA	–	–	–	–	–	A, p, ib, B, IV, s
–	NA	–	–	–	–	–	
+	+	+	–	–	–	–	A, p, ib, B, IV, s, pa
+	+	–	W	–	W	–	A, p, ib, B, IV, s
+	+	+	W	–	W	–	A, p, ib, B, IV, s, pa
–	$+^{-}$	–	+	–	–	–	A, ib, iv, S, (b)
+	–	–	+	$-^{+}$	+	+	A, S, (ib, iv, l)
–	–	–	+	–	–	$+^{-}$	A, iv, S, (p, ib)
+	–	–	+	+	+	+	a, S, (1)
+	–	–	+	$-^{+}$	+	+	A, S, (ib, iv, l)
–	–	–	+	–	–	$+^{-}$	A, iv, S, (p, ib)
–	–	–	+	–	–	+	A, S, (p, ib)
+	–	–	+	–	+	V	a, iv, S, (ib)

[e] *P. gingivalis* does not show fluorescence; *P. somerae* and *P. levii*-like may show weak or no fluorescence.
[f] Negative by the API ZYM system; positive by the Rosco *o*-nitrophenyl-β-D-galactopyranoside test.
[g] May be isolated from bite infections.
[h] *P. intermedia* shares the same characteristics. Differentiation based on enzyme electrophoresis, oligonucleotide probe analysis, or arbitrarily primed PCR (93).

TABLE 7 Characteristics of more common *Fusobacterium* species from human clinical samples[a]

Species	Distinctive cellular morphology	Indole	Growth on BBE or 20% bile	Lipase	ONPG[b]	Fermentation of:				Lactate converted to propionate	Threonine converted to propionate	Fatty acids from PYG[c]
						Glucose	Fructose	Lactose	Mannose			
F. nucleatum[d]	Slender, pointed ends	+	–	–	–	$-^{w}$	$-^{w}$	–	–	–	+	A, p, B, (l, s)
F. necrophorum[e]	Large, pleomorphic	+	$-^{+}$	$+^{-}$	–	$-^{w}$	$-^{w}$	–	–	+	+	A, p, B, (l, s)
F. mortiferum	Bizarre; round bodies	–	+	–	+	$+^{w}$	$+^{w}$	+	$+^{w}$	–	+	a, p, B, (v, l, s)
F. varium	Large, rounded ends	$+^{-}$	+	$-^{+}$	–	w^{+}	w^{+}	–	$+^{w}$	–	+	a, p, B, L, (s)
F. gonidiaformans	Gonidial forms	+	–	–	–	–	–	–	–	–	+	A, p, B, (l, s)
F. naviforme	Boat shape	+	–	–	–	w^{-}	–	–	–	–	–	a, B, L, (p, s)
F. russii	Large, rounded ends	–	–	–	–	–	–	–	–	–	–	a, B, L
F. canifelinum	Slender, pointed ends	+	–	–	–	$-^{w}$	$-^{w}$	–	–	–	+	A, p, B, (l, s)
F. ulcerans[f]	Large, rounded ends	–	+	–	–	+	–	–	$+^{-}$	–	+	a, p, B, l, (s)

[a]See Table 3, footnote *a*. $+^{w}$, most strains positive; some strains weakly positive; w^{-}, most strains weakly positive, some strains negative; w^{+}, most strains weakly positive, some strains positive.
[b]ONPG, *o*-nitrophenyl-β-D-galactopyranoside. Reaction by the API ZYM system or with Rosco Diagnostic Tablets (see Table 3, footnote *b*). Reactivity in these systems is not always identical.
[c]See Table 3, footnote *c*.
[d]*F. periodonticum* shares the same characteristics with, and is very similar to, *F. nucleatum*.
[e]Lipase-positive strains, *F. necrophorum* subsp. *necrophorum*; lipase-negative strains, *F. necrophorum* subsp. *funduliforme*.
[f]Nitrate positive.

activity increased the accuracy to 94.6% (61). The Rapid ID 32A system identified 95.5% of the fusobacteria correctly (79); however, poor discrimination between *F. nucleatum* and *F. necrophorum* has been noted (29). Similarly, the Rapid ID 32A system accurately assigned *Prevotella* and *Porphyromonas* species to the genus level, but it less accurately differentiated between the species (29). The RapID ANA II system identified 62% of the gram-negative rods correctly (90). Use of the rapid identification systems is indicated when an identification is not achieved by using the tests described in "Rapid Identification" above but before more time-consuming tests, such as fermentation tests and GLC, are used. These systems are also suited for the identification of slowly growing fastidious gram-negative rods and cocci, since no growth in the test medium is required. When using rapid identification systems, all the information available on the organism should be considered and correspond to the profile number identification. The performance of all these systems is, of course, affected by the source and nature of the isolates and the extent of the system's database; the accuracy can be further increased by certain simple supplemental tests. The API ZYM system, which allows the detection of 19 preformed enzymes in 4 h, does not have a database; only data compiled from different publications are available, but it is a useful supplement for identification of clinically encountered anaerobic bacteria, especially the *Porphyromonas* spp. (Table 6) (33, 138).

Individually available tablets containing single, dual, or triple enzyme substrates (Rosco Diagnostic Tablets [Rosco]; WEE-Tabs [Key Scientific Products]) are much cheaper than commercial kits; they can be applied in a number of situations and allow flexibility in tailoring the set to best suit special needs (33, 57). The use of 4-methylumbelliferone derivatives of many substrates (Sigma) permits rapid and inexpensive spot tests based on fluorescence (84, 85, 95, 109). It should be noted, however, that reactions obtained by fluorogenic and the different chromogenic test applications may not completely agree, owing to divergent substrate concentrations, affinities, and buffering conditions in the different systems. Therefore, it is important to name the system used for identification when reporting enzyme reactions, particularly in publications.

A method for identification of anaerobes based on analysis of whole-cell fatty acids by capillary column GLC has been adopted primarily by some reference laboratories (96). An extensive database (MIDI, Inc., Newark, Del.) for anaerobes has been compiled, largely by the Virginia Polytechnic Institute Anaerobe Laboratory, and it is updated frequently. An option for creating a cumulative database is also available. Nucleic acid probes are not commercially available for the identification of clinically important anaerobes, but they are being used in some dental laboratories (16). Determination of arbitrarily primed PCR profiles may be useful in differentiation of certain species such as *P. intermedia* and *P. nigrescens* (72).

Matrix-assisted laser desorption ionization–time of flight mass spectrometry (MALDI-TOF-MS) may have some utility for rapid identification of anaerobic bacteria (121). Ions from colony paste activated by a pulsed laser beam travel through a tube to a detector, where they are separated by differences in mass-to-ionic charge ratios, which are used to form a pattern. In practice, minimal sample preparation from a single colony is required (121). At the generic level, representative members of *Bacteroides, Prevotella,* and *Porphyromonas* may be readily distinguished. This new tool has not yet been introduced into clinical laboratories.

Identification of isolates by 16S rRNA and other genetic sequencing is gradually being adopted by dental, reference, and clinical laboratories and is also commercially available (see chapter 16) (25, 63, 68, 72, 78, 116, 125).

TYPING SYSTEMS

Due to the endogenous nature of most infections, no generally agreed upon typing systems exist.

SEROLOGICAL TESTS

Serological procedures are not practical for the identification of anaerobic bacteria from colonies. Furthermore, no standardized tests are available for the detection of antibodies or antigens in clinical specimens that would be useful for this group of organisms.

ANTIMICROBIAL SUSCEPTIBILITIES

Susceptibility testing of anaerobes is discussed in chapter 76. The susceptibility patterns for the most commonly encountered gram-negative rods of clinical significance are noted in Table 8. Resistance is increasingly common among anaerobic gram-negative rods. This is particularly true for the members of the *B. fragilis* group, which are not uncommonly resistant to expanded- and broad-spectrum cephalosporins (including β-lactamase-resistant drugs such as cefoxitin) and clindamycin. Strains of the *B. fragilis* group with resistance to imipenem and metronidazole are rarely encountered. The originally reported resistance to several antimicrobial agents in the group containing both *C. gracilis* and *S. wadsworthensis* was found to be partly due to a technical artifact (lack of formate-fumarate additive in susceptibility testing media), highlighting the importance of good growth for these assays. The true resistance seems to be confined to *Sutterella; Sutterella* spp. are more resistant to antimicrobial agents such as metronidazole and some β-lactam drugs than *C. gracilis* (94, 143).

β-Lactamase production (nitrocefin test positivity) and penicillin resistance are present in the species of the *B. fragilis* group; thus, routine testing of known *B. fragilis* group strains is unnecessary. Approximately 50% of *Prevotella* spp. are also β-lactamase producers, and even higher proportions of β-lactamase producers have been reported among certain species when several colonies per plate were tested (62, 73). An increasing number of β-lactamase-positive *F. nucleatum* strains have been encountered. Occasional strains of *C. gracilis, B. coagulans, B. splanchnicus, Desulfovibrio* spp., *F. mortiferum, F. varium, Megamonas hypermegas, M. multiacida,* and *Porphyromonas* spp. may produce β-lactamase (52). Animal-derived *Porphyromonas* spp. are more often β-lactamase producers than those derived from humans (66). *Leptotrichia* spp. as well as *Capnocytophaga* spp. are sometimes β-lactamase producers and are resistant to aminoglycosides and vancomycin; *Leptotrichia* spp. are resistant to erythromycin as well. Erythromycin and all the newer extended-spectrum macrolides except azithromycin, commonly used for the treatment of upper respiratory tract infections, such as tonsillitis, otitis media, and maxillary sinusitis, are not active against fusobacteria.

Piperacillin-tazobactam is active against most strains of anaerobic gram-negative rods, although some members of the *B. fragilis* group are resistant to ampicillin-sulbactam and amoxicillin-clavulanate. Ertapenem, imipenem, and meropenem are also consistently active against most anaerobes (49). A new antimicrobial, tigecycline, (a glycylcycline

TABLE 8 Percent susceptibility of clinically important anaerobic gram negative rods to selected antimicrobial agents[a]

Antimicrobial agent	*B. fragilis*	*B. fragilis* group	*Prevotella*	*Porphyromonas*	*F. nucleatum*	*F. mortiferum/varium*
Carbapenems						
Ertapenem	>95	>95	>95	>95	>95	>95
Imipenem	>95	>95	>95	>95	>95	>95
Meropenem	>95	>95	>95	>95	>95	>95
β-Lactamase inhibitor combinations						
Ampicillin-sulbactam	>95	90	>95	>95	>95	>95
Amoxicillin-clavulanate	>95	90	>95	>95	>95	>95
Piperacillin-tazobactam	>95	>95	>95	>95	>95	>95
Ticarcillin-clavulanate	>95	>95	>95	>95	>95	>95
Penicillins						
Penicillin	0	0	50	95	>95	90
Ampicillin	0	0	50	95	>95	90
Cephalosporins						
Cefoxitin	85	70	90	>95	>95	>95
Ceftizoxime	85	50	90	>95	>95	>95
Chloramphenicol	>95	>95	>95	>95	>95	>95
Tetracyclines						
Tetracycline	20	10	50	90	>95	90
Doxycycline	30	20	80	90	>95	90
Tigecycline	90	90	>95	>95	>95	>95
Lincosamides						
Clindamycin	80	50	90	>95	>95	80
Fluoroquinolones						
Moxifloxacin	90	80	90	>95	>95	90

[a] Data from references 12, 46, 47, and 49 through 52.

derived from minocycline) is also very active against the full spectrum of anaerobic gram-negative rods (12). Resistance to quinolones is increasing, although moxifloxacin remains moderately active against many of these strains (46, 50, 51). Mechanisms of resistance other than β-lactamase (including high-level metalloenzyme production) include changes in penicillin-binding proteins and in outer membrane porin channels. Efflux pumps are present in many *Bacteroides* species and contribute to other mechanisms of quinolone resistance. Plasmids conferring resistance to metronidazole have been reported but have not spread resistance to this antimicrobial agent.

EVALUATION, INTERPRETATION, AND REPORTING OF RESULTS

Because anaerobic bacteriology is time-consuming, several interim reports are desirable. The initial report can give Gram stain results. Bacterial and host cell morphologies and the relative quantities seen in the smear give a good overall impression of the specimen quality, the nature of the polymicrobial infection, and even morphologies suggestive of certain anaerobes. Furthermore, Gram stain results can guide the laboratory in choosing media for the optimal recovery of the predicted organisms. At 24 h, preliminary information on the anaerobic as well as the aerobic and facultatively anaerobic flora is available if the laboratory incubates plates in an anaerobic chamber. At 48 h, more definite information on the nonanaerobes and preliminary but clinically useful information on the anaerobes can be given (39).

Interpretation of results of a mixed culture containing multiple species is difficult. In general, bacterial isolates that are most predominant, empirically most virulent, and most resistant to antimicrobials should be given the most attention. Rough quantitation of the different isolates recovered, together with Gram stain results (provided that the specimen was properly taken and transported), is helpful. The bacteria present in pure culture or in large numbers are probably of major importance, as are organisms recovered on repeat culture and organisms isolated from normally sterile sites. The nature of the bacteria found can also give clues to their importance in the infectious process. Certain taxa, including the *B. fragilis* group, *Fusobacterium* spp., and some *Prevotella* spp., are much more important clinically in terms of the frequency of occurrence, the severity of the infection produced, and antimicrobial resistance.

Microbiologists must be willing to consult with the clinician on interpretation of the relevance of the findings. The laboratory should provide the clinician with a gradual introduction to new taxonomy by reporting both the new and old names in parallel for at least 2 years. Statements of specimen quality and possible limitations of methods used serve as the most important feedback to the clinician. Dialogue between the clinician and the microbiologist should be frequent.

REFERENCES

1. **Alexander, C. J., D. M. Citron, G. S. Hunt, M. C. Claros, D. Talan, and E. J. Goldstein.** 1997. Characterization of saccharolytic *Bacteroides* and *Prevotella* isolates from infected dog and cat bite wounds in humans. *J. Clin. Microbiol.* **35:**406–411.
2. **Aliyu, S. H., R. K. Marriott, M. D. Curran, S. Parmar, N. Bentley, N. M. Brown, J. S. Brazier, and H. Ludlam.** 2004. Real-time PCR investigation into the importance of Fusobacterium necrophorum as a cause of acute pharyngitis in general practice. *J. Med. Microbiol.* **53:**1029–1035.
3. **Baquero, F., J. Fernandez, F. Dronda, A. Erice, O. J. de Perez , J. A. Reguera, and M. Reig.** 1990. Capnophilic and anaerobic bacteremia in neutropenic patients: an oral source. *Rev. Infect. Dis.* **12**(Suppl. 2)**:**S157–S160.
4. **Baron, E., G. H. Cassell, L. B. Duffy, D. A. Eschenbach, J. R. Greenwood, S. M. Harvey, N. E. Madinger, E. M. Peterson, and K. B. Waites.** 1993. *Laboratory Diagnosis of Female Genital Tract Infections*, p. 1–28. American Society for Microbiology, Washington, D.C.
5. **Baron, E. J., R. Bennion, J. Thompson, C. Strong, P. Summanen, M. McTeague, and S. M. Finegold.** 1992. A microbiological comparison between acute and complicated appendicitis. *Clin. Infect. Dis.* **14:**227–231.
6. **Baron, E. J., M. Curren, G. Henderson, H. Jousimies-Somer, K. Lee, K. Lechowitz, C. A. Strong, P. Summanen, K. Tuner, and S. M. Finegold.** 1992. *Bilophila wadsworthia* isolates from clinical specimens. *J. Clin. Microbiol.* **30:**1882–1884.
7. **Baron, E. J., P. Summanen, J. Downes, M. C. Roberts, H. Wexler, and S. M. Finegold.** 1989. Bilophila wadsworthia, gen. nov. and sp. nov., a unique gram-negative anaerobic rod recovered from appendicitis specimens and human faeces. *J. Gen. Microbiol.* **135:**3405–3411.
8. **Baron, E. J., M. L. Vaisanen, M. McTeague, C. A. Strong, D. Norman, and S. M. Finegold.** 1993. Comparison of the Accu-CulShure system and a swab placed in a B-D Port-a-Cul tube for specimen collection and transport. *Clin. Infect. Dis.* **16**(Suppl. 4)**:**S325–S327.
9. **Baron, E. J., M. P. Weinstein, W. M. Dunne, P. Yagupsky, D. F. Welch, and D. M. Wilson.** 2005. *Cumitech 1C: Blood Cultures IV.* ASM Press, Washington, D.C.
10. **Batty, A., and M. W. Wren.** 2005. Prevalence of Fusobacterium necrophorum and other upper respiratory tract pathogens isolated from throat swabs. *Br. J. Biomed. Sci.* **62:**66–70.
11. **Bennion, R. S., E. J. Baron, J. E. Thompson, Jr., J. Downes, P. Summanen, D. A. Talan, and S. M. Finegold.** 1990. The bacteriology of gangrenous and perforated appendicitis—revisited. *Ann. Surg.* **211:**165–171.
12. **Betriu, C., E. Culebras, M. Gomez, I. Rodriguez-Avial, and J. J. Picazo.** 2005. In vitro activity of tigecycline against Bacteroides species. *J. Antimicrob. Chemother.* **56:**349–352.
13. **Bolstad, A. I., H. B. Jensen, and V. Bakken.** 1996. Taxonomy, biology, and periodontal aspects of *Fusobacterium nucleatum*. *Clin. Microbiol. Rev.* **9:**55–71.
14. **Brown, R., J. G. Collee, and I. R. Poxton.** 1996. *Bacteroides, Fusobacterium* and other Gram-negative rods; anaerobic cocci; identification of anaerobes, p. 501–519. *In* J. G. Collee, A. G. Fraser, B. P. Marmion, and A. Simmons (ed.), *Mackie & McCartney's Practical Medical Microbiology*. Churchill Livingston, New York, N.Y.
15. **Byrd, L.** 2004. Examination of primary culture plates for anaerobic bacteria, p. 4.4.1–4.4.6. *In* H. D. Isenberg (ed.), *Clinical Microbiology Procedures Handbook*. ASM Press, Washington, D.C.
16. **Callan, D. P., C. M. Cobb, and K. B. Williams.** 2005. DNA probe identification of bacteria colonizing internal surfaces of the implant-abutment interface: a preliminary study. *J. Periodontol.* **76:**115–120.
17. **Cavallaro, J. J., L. S. Wiggs, and J. M. Miller.** 1997. Evaluation of the BBL Crystal Anaerobe identification system. *J. Clin. Microbiol.* **35:**3186–3191.
18. **Citron, D. M., E. J. Baron, S. M. Finegold, and E. J. Goldstein.** 1990. Short prereduced anaerobically sterilized (PRAS) biochemical scheme for identification of clinical isolates of bile-resistant *Bacteroides* species. *J. Clin. Microbiol.* **28:**2220–2223.
19. **Citron, D. M., G. S. Hunt, M. C. Claros, F. Abrahamian, D. Talan, and E. J. Goldstein.** 1996. Frequency of isolation of Porphyromonas species from infected dog and cat bite

wounds in humans and their characterization by biochemical tests and arbitrarily primed-polymerase chain reaction fingerprinting. *Clin. Infect. Dis.* **23**(Suppl. 1)**:**S78–S82.

20. **Citron, D. M., Y. A. Warren, M. K. Hudspeth, and E. J. Goldstein.** 2000. Survival of aerobic and anaerobic bacteria in purulent clinical specimens maintained in the Copan Venturi Transystem and Becton Dickinson Port-a-Cul transport systems. *J. Clin. Microbiol.* **38:**892–894.
21. **Civen, R., H. Jousimies-Somer, M. Marina, L. Borenstein, H. Shah, and S. M. Finegold.** 1995. A retrospective review of cases of anaerobic empyema and update of bacteriology. *Clin. Infect. Dis.* **20**(Suppl. 2)**:**S224–S229.
22. **Collins, M. D., L. Hoyles, E. Tornqvist, E. R. von Essen, and E. Falsen.** 2001. Characterization of some strains from human clinical sources which resemble "Leptotrichia sanguinegens": description of Sneathia sanguinegens sp. nov., gen. nov. *Syst. Appl. Microbiol.* **24:**358–361.
23. **Collins, M. D., P. A. Lawson, A. Willems, J. J. Cordoba, J. Fernandez-Garayzabal, P. Garcia, J. Cai, H. Hippe, and J. A. Farrow.** 1994. The phylogeny of the genus Clostridium: proposal of five new genera and eleven new species combinations. *Int. J. Syst. Bacteriol.* **44:**812–826.
24. **Conrads, G., D. M. Citron, R. Mutters, S. Jang, and E. J. Goldstein.** 2004. Fusobacterium canifelinum sp. nov., from the oral cavity of cats and dogs. *Syst. Appl. Microbiol.* **27:**407–413.
25. **Conrads, G., D. M. Citron, K. L. Tyrrell, H. P. Horz, and E. J. Goldstein.** 2002. 16S-23S rRNA gene internal transcribed spacer sequences for analysis of the phylogenetic relationships among species of the genus Porphyromonas. *Int. J. Syst. Evol. Microbiol.* **55:**607–613.
26. **Conrads, G., M. C. Claros, D. M. Citron, K. L. Tyrrell, V. Merriam, and E. J. Goldstein.** 2002. 16S-23S rDNA internal transcribed spacer sequences for analysis of the phylogenetic relationships among species of the genus Fusobacterium. *Int. J. Syst. Evol. Microbiol.* **52:**493–499.
27. **Dahlen, G., P. Pipattanagovit, B. Rosling, and A. J. Moller.** 1993. A comparison of two transport media for saliva and subgingival samples. *Oral Microbiol. Immunol.* **8:**375–382.
28. **Dorsch, M., D. N. Love, and G. D. Bailey.** 2001. Fusobacterium equinum sp. nov., from the oral cavity of horses. *Int. J. Syst. Evol. Microbiol.* **51:**1959–1963.
29. **Downes, J., A. King, J. Hardie, and I. Phillips.** 1999. Evaluation of the Rapid ID 32A system for identification of anaerobic Gram-negative bacilli, excluding the Bacteroides fragilis group. *Clin. Microbiol. Infect.* **5:**319–326.
30. **Downes, J., I. Sutcliffe, A. C. Tanner, and W. G. Wade.** 2005. Prevotella marshii sp. nov. and Prevotella baroniae sp. nov., isolated from the human oral cavity. *Int. J. Syst. Evol. Microbiol.* **55:**1551–1555.
31. **Drake, C., J. Barenfanger, J. Lawhorn, and S. Verhulst.** 2005. Comparison of Easy-Flow Copan Liquid Stuart's and Starplex Swab transport systems for recovery of fastidious aerobic bacteria. *J. Clin. Microbiol.* **43:**1301–1303.
32. **Duncan, S. H., G. L. Hold, H. J. Harmsen, C. S. Stewart, and H. J. Flint.** 2002. Growth requirements and fermentation products of Fusobacterium prausnitzii, and a proposal to reclassify it as Faecalibacterium prausnitzii gen. nov., comb. nov. *Int. J. Syst. Evol. Microbiol.* **52:**2141–2146.
33. **Durmaz, B., H. R. Jousimies-Somer, and S. M. Finegold.** 1995. Enzymatic profiles of Prevotella, Porphyromonas, and Bacteroides species obtained with the API ZYM system and Rosco diagnostic tablets. *Clin. Infect. Dis.* **20**(Suppl. 2)**:** S192–S194.
34. **Dzink, J. L., M. T. Sheenan, and S. S. Socransky.** 1990. Proposal of three subspecies of Fusobacterium nucleatum Knorr 1922: Fusobacterium nucleatum subsp. nucleatum subsp. nov., comb. nov.; Fusobacterium nucleatum subsp. polymorphum subsp. nov., nom. rev., comb. nov.; and Fusobacterium nucleatum subsp. vincentii subsp. nov., nom. rev., comb. nov. *Int. J. Syst. Bacteriol.* **40:**74–78.
35. **Engelkirk, P. J., J. Dubin-Engelkirk, and V. R. Dowell, Jr.** 1992. *Principles and Practice of Clinical Anaerobic Bacteriology.* Star Publishing, Belmont, Calif.
36. **Finegold, S., P. Summanen, G. S. Hunt, and E. Baron.** 1992. Clinical importance of Bilophila wadsworthia. *Eur. J. Clin. Microbiol. Infect. Dis.* **11:**1058–1063.
37. **Finegold, S. M.** 1995. Overview of clinically important anaerobes. *Clin. Infect. Dis.* **20**(Suppl. 2)**:**205–207.
38. **Finegold, S. M., and H. Jousimies-Somer.** 1997. Recently described clinically important anaerobic bacteria: medical aspects. *Clin. Infect. Dis.* **25**(Suppl. 2)**:**S88–S93.
39. **Finegold, S. M., H. R. Jousimies-Somer, and H. M. Wexler.** 1993. Current perspectives on anaerobic infections: diagnostic approaches. *Infect. Dis. Clin. N. Am.* **7:**257–275.
40. **Finegold, S. M., M. L. Vaisanen, D. R. Molitoris, T. J. Tomzynski, Y. Song, C. Liu, M. D. Collins, and P. A. Lawson.** 2003. Cetobacterium somerae sp. nov. from human feces and emended description of the genus Cetobacterium. *Syst. Appl. Microbiol.* **26:**177–181.
41. **Finegold, S. M., M. L. Vaisanen, M. Rautio, E. Eerola, P. Summanen, D. Molitoris, Y. Song, C. Liu, and H. Jousimies-Somer.** 2004. *Porphyromonas uenonis* sp. nov., a pathogen for humans distinct from *P. asaccharolytica* and *P. endodontalis*. *J. Clin. Microbiol.* **42:**5298–5301.
42. **Forsblom, B., D. N. Love, E. Sarkiala-Kessel, and H. Jousimies-Somer.** 1997. Characterization of anaerobic, gram-negative, nonpigmented, saccharolytic rods from subgingival sites in dogs. *Clin. Infect. Dis.* **25**(Suppl. 2)**:**S100–S106.
43. **Fournier, D., C. Mouton, P. Lapierre, T. Kato, K. Okuda, and C. Menard.** 2001. Porphyromonas gulae sp. nov., an anaerobic, gram-negative coccobacillus from the gingival sulcus of various animal hosts. *Int. J. Syst. Evol. Microbiol.* **51:**1179–1189.
44. **Goldstein, E. J.** 2002. Intra-abdominal anaerobic infections: bacteriology and therapeutic potential of newer antimicrobial carbapenem, fluoroquinolone, and desfluoroquinolone therapeutic agents. *Clin. Infect. Dis.* **35:**S106–S111.
45. **Goldstein, E. J.** 1998. New horizons in the bacteriology, antimicrobial susceptibility and therapy of animal bite wounds. *J. Med. Microbiol.* **47:**95–97.
46. **Goldstein, E. J., and D. M. Citron.** 1985. Comparative activity of the quinolones against anaerobic bacteria isolated at community hospitals. *Antimicrob. Agents Chemother.* **27:**657–659.
47. **Goldstein, E. J., D. M. Citron, C. V. Merriam, Y. A. Warren, K. Tyrrell, and H. Fernandez.** 2001. Comparative in vitro activity of ertapenem and 11 other antimicrobial agents against aerobic and anaerobic pathogens isolated from skin and soft tissue animal and human bite wound infections. *J. Antimicrob. Chemother.* **48:**641–651.
48. **Goldstein, E. J., D. M. Citron, V. A. Peraino, and S. A. Cross.** 2003. *Desulfovibrio desulfuricans* bacteremia and review of human *Desulfovibrio* infections. *J. Clin. Microbiol.* **41:**2752–2754.
49. **Goldstein, E. J., D. M. Citron, M. C. Vreni, Y. Warren, and K. L. Tyrrell.** 2000. Comparative in vitro activities of ertapenem (MK-0826) against 1,001 anaerobes isolated from human intra-abdominal infections. *Antimicrob. Agents Chemother.* **44:**2389–2394.
50. **Goldstein, E. J., D. M. Citron, Y. A. Warren, K. L. Tyrrell, C. V. Merriam, and H. Fernandez.** 2006. In vitro activity of moxifloxacin against 923 anaerobes isolated from human intra-abdominal infections. *Antimicrob. Agents Chemother.* **50:**148–155.
51. **Goldstein, E. J., G. Conrads, D. M. Citron, C. V. Merriam, Y. Warren, and K. Tyrrell.** 2002. In vitro activity of gemifloxacin compared to seven other oral antimicrobial agents against aerobic and anaerobic pathogens isolated from antral sinus puncture specimens from patients with sinusitis. *Diagn. Microbiol. Infect. Dis.* **42:**113–118.

52. **Goldstein, E. J., P. H. Summanen, D. M. Citron, M. H. Rosove, and S. M. Finegold.** 1995. Fatal sepsis due to a beta-lactamase-producing strain of Fusobacterium nucleatum subspecies polymorphum. *Clin. Infect. Dis.* **20:**797–800.
53. **Hanff, P. A., J. A. Rosol-Donoghue, C. A. Spiegel, K. H. Wilson, and L. H. Moore.** 1995. Leptotrichia sanguinegens sp. nov., a new agent of postpartum and neonatal bacteremia. *Clin. Infect. Dis.* **20**(Suppl. 2)**:**S237–S239.
54. **Hay, P., A. Tummon, M. Ogunfile, A. Adebiyi, and A. Adefowora.** 2003. Evaluation of a novel diagnostic test for bacterial vaginosis: 'the electronic nose'. *Int. J. STD AIDS* **14:**114–118.
55. **Holdeman, L. V., E. P. Cato, and W. E. Moore.** 1977. *Anaerobic Laboratory Manual*. Virginia Polytechnic Institute and State University, Blacksburg, Va.
56. **Holt, S. C., and J. L. Ebersole.** 2005. Porphyromonas gingivalis, Treponema denticola, and Tannerella forsythia: the "red complex," a prototype polybacterial pathogenic consortium in periodontitis. *Periodontol. 2000* **38:**72–122.
57. **Hudspeth, M. K., G. S. Hunt, D. M. Citron, and E. J. Goldstein.** 1997. Growth characteristics and a novel method for identification (the WEE-TAB system) of *Porphyromonas* species isolated from infected dog and cat bite wounds in humans. *J. Clin. Microbiol.* **35:**2450–2453.
58. **Ihara, H., T. Miura, T. Kato, K. Ishihara, T. Nakagawa, S. Yamada, and K. Okuda.** 2003. Detection of Campylobacter rectus in periodontitis sites by monoclonal antibodies. *J. Periodont. Res.* **38:**64–72.
59. **Iwai, T., Y. Inoue, M. Umeda, Y. Huang, N. Kurihara, M. Koike, and I. Ishikawa.** 2005. Oral bacteria in the occluded arteries of patients with Buerger disease. *J. Vasc. Surg.* **42:**107–115.
60. **Jalava, J., and E. Eerola.** 1999. Phylogenetic analysis of Fusobacterium alocis and Fusobacterium sulci based on 16S rRNA gene sequences: proposal of Filifactor alocis (Cato, Moore and Moore) comb. nov. and Eubacterium sulci (Cato, Moore and Moore) comb. nov. *Int. J. Syst. Bacteriol.* **49**(Pt. 4)**:**1375–1379.
61. **Jenkins, S. A., D. B. Drucker, M. G. Keaney, and L. A. Ganguli.** 1991. Evaluation of the RAPID ID 32A system for the identification of Bacteroides fragilis and related organisms. *J. Appl. Bacteriol.* **71:**360–365.
62. **Jousimies-Somer, H.** 1997. Recently described clinically important anaerobic bacteria: taxonomic aspects and update. *Clin. Infect. Dis.* **25**(Suppl. 2)**:**S78–S87.
63. **Jousimies-Somer, H., S. Savolainen, A. Makitie, and J. Ylikoski.** 1993. Bacteriologic findings in peritonsillar abscesses in young adults. *Clin. Infect. Dis.* **16**(Suppl. 4)**:** S292–S298.
64. **Jousimies-Somer, H., and P. Summanen.** 2002. Recent taxonomic changes and terminology update of clinically significant anaerobic gram-negative bacteria (excluding spirochetes). *Clin. Infect. Dis.* **35:**S17–S21.
65. **Jousimies-Somer, H., P. Summanen, D. M. Citron, E. J. Baron, H. M. Wexler, and S. M. Finegold.** 2002. *Wadsworth-KTL Anaerobic Bacteriology Manual*. Star Publishing, Belmont, Calif.
66. **Jousimies-Somer, H. R.** 1995. Update on the taxonomy and the clinical and laboratory characteristics of pigmented anaerobic gram-negative rods. *Clin. Infect. Dis.* **20**(Suppl. 2)**:** S187–S191.
67. **Jumas-Bilak, E., H. Jean-Pierre, J. P. Carlier, C. Teyssier, K. Bernard, B. Gay, J. Campos, F. Morio, and H. Marchandin.** 2005. Dialister micraerophilus sp. nov. and Dialister propionicifaciens sp. nov., isolated from human clinical samples. *Int. J. Syst. Evol. Microbiol.* **55:**2471–2478.
68. **Kapatral, V., N. Ivanova, I. Anderson, G. Reznik, A. Bhattacharyya, W. L. Gardner, N. Mikhailova, A. Lapidus, N. Larsen, M. D'Souza, T. Walunas, R. Haselkorn, R. Overbeek, and N. Kyrpides.** 2003. Genome analysis of F. nucleatum sub spp vincentii and its comparison with the genome of F. nucleatum ATCC 25586. *Genome Res.* **13:**1180–1189.
69. **Kitahara, M., M. Sakamoto, M. Ike, S. Sakata, and Y. Benno.** 2005. Bacteroides plebeius sp. nov. and Bacteroides coprocola sp. nov., isolated from human faeces. *Int. J. Syst. Evol. Microbiol.* **55:**2143–2147.
70. **Koay, C. B., T. Heyworth, and P. Burden.** 1995. Lemierre syndrome—a forgotten complication of acute tonsillitis. *J. Laryngol. Otol.* **109:**657–661.
71. **Kononen, E., E. Eerola, E. V. Frandsen, J. Jalava, J. Matto, S. Salmenlinna, and H. Jousimies-Somer.** 1998. Phylogenetic characterization and proposal of a new pigmented species to the genus Prevotella: Prevotella pallens sp. nov. *Int. J. Syst. Bacteriol.* **48**(Pt. 1)**:**47–51.
72. **Kononen, E., J. Matto, M. L. Vaisanen-Tunkelrott, E. V. Frandsen, I. Helander, S. Asikainen, S. M. Finegold, and H. Jousimies-Somer.** 1998. Biochemical and genetic characterization of a Prevotella intermedia/nigrescens-like organism. *Int. J. Syst. Bacteriol.* **48**(Pt. 1)**:**39–46.
73. **Kononen, E., S. Nyfors, J. Matto, S. Asikainen, and H. Jousimies-Somer.** 1997. beta-lactamase production by oral pigmented Prevotella species isolated from young children. *Clin. Infect. Dis.* **25**(Suppl. 2)**:**S272–S274.
74. **Kuduvalli, P. M., C. M. Jukka, M. Stallwood, C. Battersby, T. Neal, G. Masterson, and G. Marx.** 2005. Fusobacterium necrophorum-induced sepsis: an unusual case of Lemierre's syndrome. *Acta Anaesthesiol. Scand.* **49:**572–575.
75. **Kumar, P. S., A. L. Griffen, M. L. Moeschberger, and E. J. Leys.** 2005. Identification of candidate periodontal pathogens and beneficial species by quantitative 16S clonal analysis. *J. Clin. Microbiol.* **43:**3944–3955.
76. **Larsson, P. G., B. Carlsson, L. Fahraeus, T. Jakobsson, and U. Forsum.** 2004. Diagnosis of bacterial vaginosis: need for validation of microscopic image area used for scoring bacterial morphotypes. *Sex. Transm. Infect.* **80:**63–67.
77. **Lawson, A. J., S. L. On, J. M. Logan, and J. Stanley.** 2001. Campylobacter hominis sp. nov., from the human gastrointestinal tract. *Int. J. Syst. Evol. Microbiol.* **51:**651–660.
78. **Liu, C., Y. Song, M. McTeague, A. W. Vu, H. Wexler, and S. M. Finegold.** 2003. Rapid identification of the species of the Bacteroides fragilis group by multiplex PCR assays using group- and species-specific primers. *FEMS Microbiol. Lett.* **222:**9–16.
79. **Looney, W. J., A. J. Gallusser, and H. K. Modde.** 1990. Evaluation of the ATB 32 A system for identification of anaerobic bacteria isolated from clinical specimens. *J. Clin. Microbiol.* **28:**1519–1524.
80. **Loubinoux, J., F. M. Valente, I. A. Pereira, A. Costa, P. A. Grimont, and A. E. Le Faou.** 2002. Reclassification of the only species of the genus Desulfomonas, Desulfomonas pigra, as Desulfovibrio piger comb. nov. *Int. J. Syst. Evol. Microbiol.* **52:**1305–1308.
81. **Maiden, M. F., A. Tanner, and P. J. Macuch.** 1996. Rapid characterization of periodontal bacterial isolates by using fluorogenic substrate tests. *J. Clin. Microbiol.* **34:**376–384.
82. **Malnick, H.** 1997. Anaerobiospirillum thomasii sp. nov., an anaerobic spiral bacterium isolated from the feces of cats and dogs and from diarrheal feces of humans, and emendation of the genus Anaerobiospirillum. *Int. J. Syst. Bacteriol.* **47:**381–384.
83. **Malnick, H., K. Williams, J. Phil-Ebosie, and A. S. Levy.** 1990. Description of a medium for isolating *Anaerobiospirillum* spp., a possible cause of zoonotic disease, from diarrheal feces and blood of humans and use of the medium in a survey of human, canine, and feline feces. *J. Clin. Microbiol.* **28:**1380–1384.

84. **Mangels, J., I. Edvalson, and M. Cox.** 1993. Rapid presumptive identification of Bacteroides fragilis group organisms with use of 4-methylumbelliferone-derivative substrates. *Clin. Infect. Dis.* **16**(Suppl. 4):S319–S321.
85. **Mangels, J. I.** 2004. Rapid biochemical tests (4 hours or less) for the identification of anaerobes, p. 4.9.1–4. 9.8.2. *In* H. D. Isenberg (ed.), *Clinical Microbiology Procedures Handbook.* ASM Press, Washington, D.C.
86. **Mangels, J. I.** 2004. Culture media for anaerobes, p. 4.4.1–4.4.6. *In* H. D. Isenberg (ed.), *Clinical Microbiology Procedures Handbook.* ASM Press, Washington, D.C.
87. **Mangels, J. I., M. E. Cox, and L. H. Lindberg.** 1984. Methanol fixation. An alternative to heat fixation of smears before staining. *Diagn. Microbiol. Infect. Dis.* **2:** 129–137.
88. **Mangels, J. I., and B. P. Douglas.** 1989. Comparison of four commercial brucella agar media for growth of anaerobic organisms. *J. Clin. Microbiol.* **27:**2268–2271.
89. **Marcus, L., E. W. Gove, M. L. van der Walt, H. J. Koornhof, H. Malnick, and J. G. Kilian.** 1996. First reported African case of Anaerobiospirillum succiniciproducens septicemia. *Eur. J. Clin. Microbiol. Infect. Dis.* **15:** 741–744.
90. **Marler, L. M., J. A. Siders, L. C. Wolters, Y. Pettigrew, B. L. Skitt, and S. D. Allen.** 1991. Evaluation of the new RapID-ANA II system for the identification of clinical anaerobic isolates. *J. Clin. Microbiol.* **29:**874–878.
91. **Marshall, J. C.** 2004. Intra-abdominal infections. *Microbes. Infect.* **6:**1015–1025.
92. **Mathur, P., R. Chaudhry, L. Kumar, A. Kapil, and B. Dhawan.** 2002. A study of bacteremia in febrile neutropenic patients at a tertiary-care hospital with special reference to anaerobes. *Med. Oncol.* **19:**267–272.
93. **Matto, J., S. Asikainen, M. L. Vaisanen, M. Rautio, M. Saarela, P. Summanen, S. Finegold, and H. Jousimies-Somer.** 1997. Role of Porphyromonas gingivalis, Prevotella intermedia, and Prevotella nigrescens in extraoral and some odontogenic infections. *Clin. Infect. Dis.* **25**(Suppl. 2): S194–S198.
94. **Molitoris, E., H. M. Wexler, and S. M. Finegold.** 1997. Sources and antimicrobial susceptibilities of Campylobacter gracilis and Sutterella wadsworthensis. *Clin. Infect. Dis.* **25**(Suppl. 2):S264–S265.
95. **Moncla, B. J., P. Braham, L. K. Rabe, and S. L. Hillier.** 1991. Rapid presumptive identification of black-pigmented gram-negative anaerobic bacteria by using 4-methylumbelliferone derivatives. *J. Clin. Microbiol.* **29:** 1955–1958.
96. **Moore, L. V., D. M. Bourne, and W. E. Moore.** 1994. Comparative distribution and taxonomic value of cellular fatty acids in thirty-three genera of anaerobic gram-negative bacilli. *Int. J. Syst. Bacteriol.* **44:**338–347.
97. **Moore, L. V. H., E. P. Cato, and W. E. Moore.** 1991. *Anaerobic Laboratory Manual Update: a Supplement to the VPI Anaerobe Laboratory Manual.* Virginia Polytechnic Institute and State University, Blacksburg, Va.
98. **Murray, P. R., P. Traynor, and D. Hopson.** 1992. Critical assessment of blood culture techniques: analysis of recovery of obligate and facultative anaerobes, strict aerobic bacteria, and fungi in aerobic and anaerobic blood culture bottles. *J. Clin. Microbiol.* **30:**1462–1468.
99. **Mylotte, J. M., and A. Tayara.** 2000. Blood cultures: clinical aspects and controversies. *Eur. J. Clin. Microbiol. Infect. Dis.* **19:**157–163.
100. **Namavar, F., E. B. Theunissen, A. M. Verweij-Van Vught, P. G. Peerbooms, M. Bal, H. F. Hoitsma, and D. M. MacLaren.** 1989. Epidemiology of the Bacteroides fragilis group in the colonic flora in 10 patients with colonic cancer. *J. Med. Microbiol.* **29:**171–176.
101. **NCCLS.** 2002. *Abbreviated Identification of Bacteria and Yeast; Approved Guideline.* NCCLS, Wayne, Pa.
102. **Olsen, I., and H. N. Shah.** 2001. International Committee on Systematics of Prokaryotes Subcommittee on the taxonomy of Gram-negative anaerobic rods; minutes of the meetings, 9 and 10 July 2000, Manchester, UK. *Int. J. Syst. Evol. Microbiol.* **51:**1943–1944.
103. **Paster, B. J., F. E. Dewhirst, I. Olsen, and G. J. Fraser.** 1994. Phylogeny of *Bacteroides, Prevotella,* and *Porphyromonas* spp. and related bacteria. *J. Bacteriol.* **176:**725–732.
104. **Pathela, P., K. Z. Hasan, E. Roy, K. Alam, F. Huq, A. K. Siddique, and R. B. Sack.** 2005. Enterotoxigenic Bacteroides fragilis-associated diarrhea in children 0–2 years of age in rural Bangladesh. *J. Infect. Dis.* **191:**1245–1252.
105. **Patrick, S., L. D. Stewart, N. Damani, K. G. Wilson, D. A. Lutton, M. J. Larkin, I. Poxton, and R. Brown.** 1995. Immunological detection of Bacteroides fragilis in clinical samples. *J. Med. Microbiol.* **43:**99–109.
106. **Pavlou, A., A. P. Turner, and N. Magan.** 2002. Recognition of anaerobic bacterial isolates in vitro using electronic nose technology. *Lett. Appl. Microbiol.* **35:**366–369.
107. **Peterson, L. R.** 1997. Effect of media on transport and recovery of anaerobic bacteria. *Clin. Infect. Dis.* **25**(Suppl. 2): S134–S136.
108. **Poxton, I. R., R. Brown, A. Sawyerr, and A. Ferguson.** 1997. Mucosa-associated bacterial flora of the human colon. *J. Med. Microbiol.* **46:**85–91.
109. **Rabe, L. K., D. Sheiness, and S. L. Hillier.** 1995. Comparison of the use of oligonucleotide probes, 4-methylumbelliferyl derivatives, and conventional methods for identifying Prevotella bivia. *Clin. Infect. Dis.* **20** (Suppl. 2): S195–S197.
110. **Rams, T. E., D. Feik, and J. Slots.** 1993. Campylobacter rectus in human periodontitis. *Oral Microbiol. Immunol.* **8:**230–235.
111. **Rautio, M., E. Eerola, M. L. Vaisanen-Tunkelrott, D. Molitoris, P. Lawson, M. D. Collins, and H. Jousimies-Somer.** 2003. Reclassification of Bacteroides putredinis (Weinberg et al., 1937) in a new genus Alistipes gen. nov., as Alistipes putredinis comb. nov., and description of Alistipes finegoldii sp. nov., from human sources. *Syst. Appl. Microbiol.* **26:**182–188.
112. **Rocha, E. R., G. Owens, Jr., and C. J. Smith.** 2000. The redox-sensitive transcriptional activator OxyR regulates the peroxide response regulon in the obligate anaerobe *Bacteroides fragilis. J. Bacteriol.* **182:**5059–5069.
113. **Sakamoto, M., Y. Huang, M. Umeda, I. Ishikawa, and Y. Benno.** 2005. Prevotella multiformis sp. nov., isolated from human subgingival plaque. *Int. J. Syst. Evol. Microbiol.* **55:**815–819.
114. **Sakamoto, M., M. Suzuki, Y. Huang, M. Umeda, I. Ishikawa, and Y. Benno.** 2004. Prevotella shahii sp. nov. and Prevotella salivae sp. nov., isolated from the human oral cavity. *Int. J. Syst. Evol. Microbiol.* **54:**877–883.
115. **Sakamoto, M., M. Suzuki, M. Umeda, I. Ishikawa, and Y. Benno.** 2002. Reclassification of Bacteroides forsythus (Tanner et al. 1986) as Tannerella forsythensis corrig., gen. nov., comb. nov. *Int. J. Syst. Evol. Microbiol.* **52:**841–849.
116. **Sakamoto, M., M. Umeda, and Y. Benno.** 2005. Molecular analysis of human oral microbiota. *J. Periodont. Res.* **40:**277–285.
117. **Sakamoto, M., M. Umeda, I. Ishikawa, and Y. Benno.** 2005. Prevotella multisaccharivorax sp. nov., isolated from human subgingival plaque. *Int. J. Syst. Evol. Microbiol.* **55:**1839–1843.
118. **Scannapieco, F. A., R. B. Bush, and S. Paju.** 2003. Associations between periodontal disease and risk for atherosclerosis, cardiovascular disease, and stroke. A systematic review. *Ann. Periodontol.* **8:**38–53.

119. **Sears, C. L.** 2001. The toxins of Bacteroides fragilis. *Toxicon* **39:**1737–1746.

120. **Sha, B. E., H. Y. Chen, Q. J. Wang, M. R. Zariffard, M. H. Cohen, and G. T. Spear.** 2005. Utility of Amsel criteria, Nugent score, and quantitative PCR for *Gardnerella vaginalis, Mycoplasma hominis,* and *Lactobacillus* spp. for diagnosis of bacterial vaginosis in human immunodeficiency virus-infected women. *J. Clin. Microbiol.* **43:** 4607–4612.

121. **Shah, H. N., C. J. Keys, O. Schmid, and S. E. Gharbia.** 2002. Matrix-assisted laser desorption/ionization time-of-flight mass spectrometry and proteomics: a new era in anaerobic microbiology. *Clin. Infect. Dis.* **35:**S58–S64.

122. **Siqueira, J. F., Jr., and I. N. Rocas.** 2003. Campylobacter gracilis and Campylobacter rectus in primary endodontic infections. *Int. Endod. J.* **36:**174–180.

123. **Slots, J.** 1987. Detection of colonies of Bacteroides gingivalis by a rapid fluorescence assay for trypsin-like activity. *Oral Microbiol. Immunol.* **2:**139–141.

124. **Soder, P. O., B. Soder, J. Nowak, and T. Jogestrand.** 2005. Early carotid atherosclerosis in subjects with periodontal diseases. *Stroke* **36:**1195–1200.

125. **Song, Y., C. Liu, M. Bolanos, J. Lee, M. McTeague, and S. M. Finegold.** 2005. Evaluation of 16S rRNA sequencing and reevaluation of a short biochemical scheme for identification of clinically significant *Bacteroides* species. *J. Clin. Microbiol.* **43:**1531–1537.

126. **Song, Y., C. Liu, J. Lee, M. Bolanos, M. L. Vaisanen, and S. M. Finegold.** 2005. "*Bacteroides goldsteinii* sp. nov." isolated from clinical specimens of human intestinal origin. *J. Clin. Microbiol.* **43:**4522–4527.

127. **Song, Y. L., C. X. Liu, M. McTeague, and S. M. Finegold.** 2004. "*Bacteroides nordii*" sp. nov. and "*Bacteroides salyersae*" sp. nov. isolated from clinical specimens of human intestinal origin. *J. Clin. Microbiol.* **42:**5565–5570.

128. **Summanen, P., P. J. Hancher, M. J. Flynn, and J. Slots.** 1996. Obstructive sialadenitis secondary to parotic sialolithiasis: a case report. *Anaerobe* **2:**81–84.

129. **Summanen, P., and H. Jousimies-Somer.** 1988. Comparative evaluation of RapID ANA and API 20 A for identification of anaerobic bacteria. *Eur. J. Clin. Microbiol. Infect. Dis.* **7:**771–775.

130. **Summanen, P. H., B. Durmaz, M. L. Vaisanen, C. Liu, D. Molitoris, E. Eerola, I. M. Helander, and S. M. Finegold.** 2005. *Porphyromonas somerae* sp. nov., a pathogen isolated from humans and distinct from *Porphyromonas levii. J. Clin. Microbiol.* **43:**4455–4459.

131. **Talan, D. A., F. M. Abrahamian, G. J. Moran, D. M. Citron, J. O. Tan, and E. J. Goldstein.** 2003. Clinical presentation and bacteriologic analysis of infected human bites in patients presenting to emergency departments. *Clin. Infect. Dis.* **37:**1481–1489.

132. **Talan, D. A., D. M. Citron, F. M. Abrahamian, G. J. Moran, and E. J. Goldstein for the Emergency Medicine Animal Bite Infection Study Group.** 1999. Bacteriologic analysis of infected dog and cat bites. *N. Engl. J. Med.* **340:** 85–92.

133. **Tanner, A., M. F. Maiden, B. J. Paster, and F. E. Dewhirst.** 1994. The impact of 16S ribosomal RNA-based phylogeny on the taxonomy of oral bacteria. *Periodontol. 2000* **5:**26–51.

134. **Tee, W., T. M. Korman, M. J. Waters, A. Macphee, A. Jenney, L. Joyce, and M. L. Dyall-Smith.** 1998. Three cases of *Anaerobiospirillum succiniciproducens* bacteremia confirmed by 16S rRNA gene sequencing. *J. Clin. Microbiol.* **36:**1209–1213.

135. **Thaler, E. R., and C. W. Hanson.** 2005. Medical applications of electronic nose technology. *Expert. Rev. Med. Devices* **2:**559–566.

136. **Tvede, M., and N. Hoiby.** 1992. Experimental studies of survival of anaerobic bacteria at 4 degrees C and 22 degrees C in two different transport systems. *APMIS* **100:**1048–1052.

137. **Tzianabos, A. O., D. L. Kasper, and A. B. Onderdonk.** 1995. Structure and function of Bacteroides fragilis capsular polysaccharides: relationship to induction and prevention of abscesses. *Clin. Infect. Dis.* **20**(Suppl. 2):S132–S140.

138. **Vaisanen, M. L., M. Kiviranta, P. Summanen, S. M. Finegold, and H. R. Jousimies-Somer.** 1997. Porphyromonas endodontalis-like organisms from extraoral sources. *Clin. Infect. Dis.* **25**(Suppl. 2):S191–S193.

139. **Vandamme, P., M. I. Daneshvar, F. E. Dewhirst, B. J. Paster, K. Kersters, H. Goossens, and C. W. Moss.** 1995. Chemotaxonomic analyses of Bacteroides gracilis and Bacteroides ureolyticus and reclassification of B. gracilis as Campylobacter gracilis comb. nov. *Int. J. Syst. Bacteriol.* **45:**145–152.

140. **Von Gruenigen, V. E., R. L. Coleman, A. J. Li, M. C. Heard, D. S. Miller, and D. L. Hemsell.** 2000. Bacteriology and treatment of malodorous lower reproductive tract in gynecologic cancer patients. *Obstet. Gynecol.* **96:**23–27.

141. **Wang, Y., W. M. Kalka-Moll, M. H. Roehrl, and D. L. Kasper.** 2000. Structural basis of the abscess-modulating polysaccharide A2 from Bacteroides fragilis. *Proc. Natl. Acad. Sci. USA* **97:**13478–13483.

142. **Warren, Y. A., D. M. Citron, C. V. Merriam, and E. J. Goldstein.** 2005. Biochemical differentiation and comparison of *Desulfovibrio* species and other phenotypically similar genera. *J. Clin. Microbiol.* **43:**4041–4045.

143. **Wexler, H. M., D. Reeves, P. H. Summanen, E. Molitoris, M. McTeague, J. Duncan, K. H. Wilson, and S. M. Finegold.** 1996. Sutterella wadsworthensis gen. nov., sp. nov., bile-resistant microaerophilic Campylobacter gracilis-like clinical isolates. *Int. J. Syst. Bacteriol.* **46:**252–258.

144. **Willems, A., and M. D. Collins.** 1995. Reclassification of Oribaculum catoniae (Moore and Moore 1994) as Porphyromonas catoniae comb. nov. and emendation of the genus Porphyromonas. *Int. J. Syst. Bacteriol.* **45:**578–581.

145. **Wu, S., J. Powell, N. Mathioudakis, S. Kane, E. Fernandez, and C. L. Sears.** 2004. *Bacteroides fragilis* enterotoxin induces intestinal epithelial cell secretion of interleukin-8 through mitogen-activated protein kinases and a tyrosine kinase-regulated nuclear factor-kappaB pathway. *Infect. Immun.* **72:**5832–5839.

Campylobacter and *Arcobacter*

COLLETTE FITZGERALD AND IRVING NACHAMKIN

59

TAXONOMY

Three closely related genera, *Campylobacter*, *Arcobacter*, and *Sulfurospirillum*, are included in the family *Campylobacteraceae* (95, 129). The family *Campylobacteraceae* includes 17 species in the genus *Campylobacter*, 6 species in the genus *Arcobacter*, and 6 species in the genus *Sulfurospirillum*. Since the last edition, several new species have been proposed, including *Campylobacter insulaenigrae* (32), isolated from marine mammals. Two new *Arcobacter* species have recently been described: *Arcobacter cibarius*, isolated from chickens (48), and *A. halophilus*, an obligate halophilic species (23). Some isolates previously identified as *C. gracilis* have been renamed as *Sutterella wadsworthensis* and are more closely related to *Alcaligenes* and *Bordetella* species (144).

DESCRIPTION OF AGENTS

Campylobacters are curved, S-shaped, or spiral rods that are 0.2 to 0.9 μm wide and 0.5 to 5 μm long. Certain species, such as *C. hominis*, form straight rods. *Campylobacter* species are gram-negative, non-spore-forming rods that may form spherical or coccoid bodies in old cultures or cultures exposed to air for prolonged periods. Organisms are usually motile by means of a single polar unsheathed flagellum at one or both ends but may lack flagella. Species are generally microaerobic with a respiratory type of metabolism; however, some strains grow aerobically or anaerobically. An atmosphere containing an increased hydrogen concentration is required by some species for microaerobic growth (131).

Arcobacters are gram-negative, slightly curved, curved, S-shaped, or helical non-spore-forming rods that are 0.2 to 0.9 μm wide and 1 to 3 μm long. Organisms are motile with a single polar unsheathed flagellum. Arcobacters grow at 15, 25, and 30°C but have variable growth at 37 and 42°C. Organisms are microaerobic and do not require increased hydrogen for growth. Arcobacters may grow aerobically at 30°C and anaerobically at 35 to 37°C. Most strains are nonhemolytic. *A. skirrowii* may be alpha-hemolytic (133). *A. halophilus* is an obligate halophile and grows poorly on media containing less than 2% NaCl (23).

Originally classified as free-living *Campylobacter* species, *Sulfurospirillum* spp. are slender, curved, gram-negative rods that are 0.1 to 0.5 μm wide and 1 to 3 μm long. All of the species are sulfur reducers and exhibit variable metabolic activities. *Sulfurospirillum deleyianum* is the type species of the genus. These species have no known pathogenicity for humans or animals, are environmental organisms isolated from water sediments, and will not be further discussed in this chapter (129).

EPIDEMIOLOGY AND TRANSMISSION

Campylobacter species are primarily zoonotic, with a variety of animals implicated as reservoirs for human infection (Table 1). In addition to food animals such as poultry, cattle, sheep, and pigs, *Campylobacter* species may be present in domestic pets. Humans appear to be the only recognized reservoirs for the periodontal pathogens, *C. concisus*, *C. rectus*, *C. curvus*, and *C. showae*.

Campylobacter infections are common in both the developed and the developing world. The reported incidences of culture-confirmed infections vary considerably from country to country, and as culturing practices and reporting requirements can vary, direct comparison of the reported incidences can be complex. In the United States, where reporting practices vary from state to state, the food-borne-disease active surveillance program FoodNet (http://www.cdc.gov/foodnet) provides uniform reporting from a panel of sentinel sites, giving an accurate measure of the incidence of diagnosed infections. FoodNet data suggest that numbers of campylobacteriosis cases in the United States reached a peak in the mid-1990s and showed a decline from 1996 to 1999 (110). This decline continued somewhat through 2003 and into 2004, with the incidence of diagnosed *Campylobacter* infections at 12.6 and 12.9 per 100,000 people, respectively, lower than that of salmonellosis (17). A comparison of the data from 1996 to 1998 with the 2004 data shows that the estimated incidence of infection with *Campylobacter* decreased 31%. However, *C. jejuni* subsp. *jejuni*, referred to as *C. jejuni*, continues to be the most common enteric pathogen isolated from patients in some states, according to FoodNet reports, with 1.4 million cases estimated to occur in the United States annually (110). Because of underdiagnosis and underreporting, the actual incidence in any country is substantially greater than the reported incidence. For example, in the United States, it was estimated that the true incidence was 35-fold higher than the reported incidence, or 515 per 100,000 people in 1999 (110).

TABLE 1 Reservoirs for and diseases associated with *Campylobacter* and *Arcobacter* species[a]

Species	Humans	Cattle	Sheep	Pigs	Wild birds	Poultry	Pets	Rodents	Types of infection[b]
C. jejuni subsp. *jejuni*	×	×			×	×	×		GI, B
C. jejuni subsp. *doylei*	×								GI, B
C. coli				×	×	×			GI, B
C. fetus subsp. *fetus*		×	×						GI, B
C. upsaliensis						×	×		GI, B
C. lari					×		×		GI, B
C. hyointestinalis		×		×		×	×	×	GI
C. helveticus							×		NR
C. sputorum	×[c]	×[d,e]	×[e]						GI[c]
C. concisus	×								D
C. curvus	×								D
C. rectus	×								D, GI
C. showae	×								D
C. gracilis	×								D
C. mucosalis				×					NR
A. butzleri		×		×		×			GI, B, T
A. cryaerophilus		×	×	×		×			GI
A. skirrowii		×	×	×		×			GI

[a] The information in this table is from references 66, 83, 112, and 130.
[b] GI, gastrointestinal; B, bloodstream; D, oral or dental; T, soft tissue; NR, not reported to be associated with human infections.
[c] Biovar sputorum.
[d] Biovar paraureolyticus.
[e] Biovar faecalis.

The epidemiology of campylobacteriosis does not appear to have changed over the last 5 years. *Campylobacter* infections are usually sporadic, occurring in the summer months and early fall, and usually follow ingestion of improperly handled or improperly cooked food, primarily poultry products. A large case control study concluded that numerous food sources are associated with *Campylobacter* infections but that a large proportion of infection is attributable to consumption of poultry and other meats in restaurants (33). The incidence of infection follows a bimodal age distribution, with the highest incidence in infants and young children, followed by a second peak in young adults 20 to 40 years old (110). Outbreaks usually occur in the spring and fall months, and in recent years, most outbreaks have been food (poultry and unpasteurized dairy products) or water associated. Milk-borne outbreaks, while common in the 1980s and early 1990s, are less frequently reported now; the most recent milk-borne outbreaks were reported in Wisconsin in 2001 (44) and Michigan in 2003 (http://www.cdc.gov/foodborneoutbreaks/us_outb/fbo2003/summary03.htm).

The incidence of *Campylobacter* infection in developing countries such as Mexico and Thailand is much higher than that in the United States. In developing countries, *Campylobacter* is frequently isolated from individuals who may or may not have diarrheal disease. Most symptomatic infections occur in infancy and early childhood, and incidence decreases with age. Travelers to developing countries are at risk for developing *Campylobacter* infection, with isolation rates from 0 to 39% reported in different studies (91).

CLINICAL SIGNIFICANCE

C. jejuni and *C. coli*

C. jejuni and *C. coli* have been recognized since the early 1970s as agents of gastrointestinal infection. *C. jejuni* is one of the most common causes of bacterial enteritis in the United States. *C. jejuni* and *C. coli* continue to be the most common *Campylobacter* species associated with diarrheal illness and produce clinically indistinguishable infections. Most laboratories do not routinely distinguish between these organisms.

In patients with gastroenteritis caused by *C. jejuni* or *C. coli*, symptoms range from nonexistent to severe and may include fever, abdominal cramping, and diarrhea (with or without blood or fecal white blood cells) that last several days to more than 1 week. Symptomatic infections are usually self-limited, but relapses may occur in 5 to 10% of untreated patients (11). *Campylobacter* infection may mimic acute appendicitis and result in unnecessary surgery. Extraintestinal infections and other complications have been reported following *Campylobacter* enteritis and include bacteremia, hepatitis, cholecystitis, pancreatitis, abortion and neonatal sepsis, nephritis, prostatitis, urinary tract infection, peritonitis, myocarditis, and focal infections including meningitis, septic arthritis, and abscess formation (114). Bacteremia has been reported to occur at a rate of 1.5 per 1,000 intestinal infections, with the highest rate occurring in the elderly (115). Persistent diarrheal illness and bacteremia may occur in immunocompromised hosts, such as patients with human immunodeficiency infection (102), and may be difficult to treat. Deaths attributable to *C. jejuni* infection are uncommon (34). The health burden of campylobacteriosis may be under-recognized (45).

C. jejuni infection is the most often recognized infection preceding the development of Guillain-Barré syndrome (GBS), an acute paralytic disease of the peripheral nervous system (85). Certain heat-stable (HS) serotypes appear to be overrepresented in some GBS cases, such as HS:19 and HS:41; however, other more common serotypes are frequently reported (85). The pathogenesis of *Campylobacter*-induced GBS likely involves host immune responses to ganglioside-like epitopes present in the core region of the lipooligosaccharide (36) which, in the susceptible host, mediate damage to the peripheral nerves, where ganglioside targets are highly enriched (145).

Reactive arthritis sometimes follows *Campylobacter* infection, with the onset of pain and joint swelling occurring an average of 2 weeks after the infection and lasting from a few weeks to nearly a year. Reiter's syndrome may also occur in some patients (114). The pathogenesis of *Campylobacter* infection and joint involvement is unknown, but HLA B27 positivity is strongly associated with reactive arthritis (19).

The pathogenesis of *Campylobacter* enteric infection is still not well understood. The infective dose of *Campylobacter* is not well defined, but as few as 1,000 organisms may be capable of causing illness (9). The signs and symptoms of infection suggest an invasive mechanism of disease. A variety of determinants may be important in the virulence of *C. jejuni* infection, including invasiveness (49), the presence or absence of the large virulence plasmid pVir (64), protein glycosylation (120), and motility (53). *C. jejuni* express a cytolethal distending toxin; however, the role of the toxin in pathogenesis is not understood (63). *Campylobacter* spp. do not produce a classic, cholera-like enterotoxin (142).

Campylobacter Species Other Than *C. jejuni* and *C. coli*

Campylobacter species other than *C. jejuni* and *C. coli* are increasingly isolated from cases of human infection in newer studies using culture methods that are more optimal for the non-*C. jejuni* and non-*C. coli* species.

C. fetus subsp. *fetus* is primarily associated with bacteremia and extraintestinal infections in patients with underlying diseases (11). *C. fetus* is also associated with septic abortions, septic arthritis, abscesses, meningitis, endocarditis, mycotic aneurysm, thrombophlebitis, peritonitis, and salpingitis (11). Although gastroenteritis does occur with this species, the incidence is probably underestimated because the organism may not grow well at 42°C and is usually susceptible to cephalothin, an antimicrobial agent used in some common selective media for stool cultures (135). *C. fetus* subsp. *fetus* produces a surface protein microcapsule composed of a high-molecular-weight surface array protein that is essential for virulence (126). *C. fetus* subsp. *venerealis* causes bovine venereal campylobacteriosis and is a cause of bovine infertility. It has rarely been isolated from cases of human infection (126).

C. upsaliensis is a thermotolerant species that causes diarrhea and bacteremia in humans and is also associated with canine and feline gastroenteritis (39, 135). *C. upsaliensis* is susceptible to many antimicrobial agents present in *C. jejuni*-selective media and, thus, is usually not isolated on routine primary isolation media; it can be recovered using the filtration technique described below.

C. lari is a thermophilic species first isolated from gulls of the genus *Larus* and from other avian species, dogs, cats, and chickens. *C. lari* has been infrequently reported to be isolated from humans with bacteremia and gastrointestinal and urinary tract infections. A waterborne outbreak of infection occurred in 1985 and affected more than 100 individuals (121).

Other *Campylobacter* species have been isolated from clinical specimens from patients with a variety of diseases, but their pathogenic role has not been determined. *C. jejuni* subsp. *doylei* is a nitrate-negative subspecies of *C. jejuni* that is rarely recovered from patients with upper gastrointestinal tract infections and gastroenteritis (39, 118). *C. hyointestinalis* has been occasionally associated with proctitis and diarrhea in human infection (24). *C. concisus* is associated primarily with periodontal disease but has also been isolated from patients with bacteremia, foot ulcers, and upper and lower gastrointestinal tract infections (54, 132). Although *C. concisus* has been isolated from many patients with diarrheal illness, it can also be isolated from the feces of healthy individuals, and there is no convincing evidence to date that it causes diarrhea (28, 137). *C. sputorum* biovars have been associated with lung, axillary, scrotal, and groin abscesses (66). *C. sputorum* bv. paraureolyticus, formerly referred to as catalase-negative, urease-positive campylobacter, has been isolated from patients with diarrhea, but the significance of this finding is unknown (97). *C. mucosalis* was reportedly isolated from two children with enteritis (30), but the isolates were subsequently shown to have been misidentified and were actually *C. concisus* (96). *C. helveticus* (117) has been recovered from domestic cats and dogs and has not been reported to have been isolated from human sources. *C. rectus* is primarily isolated from patients with active periodontal infections but has also been isolated from patients with pulmonary infections (107, 116) and a breast abscess (42). *C. curvus* is also isolated from patients with periodontal infections, but its role in gastrointestinal infections is unknown (28). *C. curvus* was isolated from numerous patients with diarrhea (1) and from patients with a liver abscess and pneumonia (42). *C. showae* has been isolated from the human gingival crevice (29). *C. gracilis* has been isolated from patients with appendicitis and peritonitis, bacteremia, soft-tissue abscesses, and pulmonary infections (81). A more extensive review of the clinical significance of non-*C. jejuni* and non-*C. coli* species was published previously (66).

Arcobacter

Arcobacters are aerotolerant, *Campylobacter*-like organisms frequently isolated from bovine and porcine products of abortion and feces of animals with enteritis (143). Two of the five *Arcobacter* species have been associated with human infection. *A. butzleri* has been isolated from patients with bacteremia, endocarditis, peritonitis, and diarrhea (66, 135). *A. cryaerophilus* strains have been previously classified into two DNA-related groups, 1A and 1B (60). *A. cryaerophilus* group 1B has been isolated from patients with bacteremia and diarrhea (66, 135). Group 1A has been isolated from animal sources (60). *A. butzleri* was reported by Vandenberg et al. to be the fourth most common *Campylobacter*-like organism isolated from patients with diarrhea (135) and may be underrecognized if appropriate culture conditions are not used. *A. nitrofigilis*, a nitrogen-fixing bacterium found on the roots of a small marsh plant in Nova Scotia, is not associated with human disease (77). The recently described *A. cibarius* has been isolated only from poultry carcasses; the clinical significance of this species is unknown (48). *A. halophilus* requires increased salt for growth in culture; however, the medical significance of this species is unknown (23).

COLLECTION, TRANSPORT, AND STORAGE OF SPECIMENS

Fecal Samples

Fecal specimens are preferred for isolating *Campylobacter* species from patients with gastrointestinal infections; however, rectal swabs are acceptable for culture. For hospitalized patients, the 3-day rule (rejection of specimens collected >72 h after admission) should be used as a criterion for acceptability of routine culture requests (40, 47). For routine purposes, testing of a single stool sample has high sensitivity for detection of common enteric pathogens, but testing of two samples may be desirable depending upon clinical circumstances, such as a >2-h delay in transport of the first sample, that could affect recovery (128). A transport medium should be used when a delay of more than 2 h is anticipated and when rectal swabs are transported. Several types of transport media are useful for *Campylobacter*, including alkaline peptone water with thioglycolate and cystine (140), modified Stuart medium (2), and Cary-Blair medium (16). Transport media such as commercial Stuart medium and buffered glycerol saline do not appear to perform well (140). Modified Cary-Blair medium containing reduced agar (1.6 g/liter) appears to be the most suitable single transport medium for *Campylobacter* as well as other enteric pathogens (140). Specimens received in Cary-Blair medium should be stored at 4°C if processing is not performed immediately. Use of Cary-Blair medium supplemented with laked sheep blood may be effective for prolonged storage of stool samples and recovery of *C. jejuni* (141).

Blood

Campylobacter species, primarily *C. fetus*, *C. jejuni*, and *C. upsaliensis*, have been isolated from blood; however, in only a few studies have optimal conditions for isolating *Campylobacter* from blood culture systems been evaluated. Both the BACTEC system (BD, Sparks, Md.; aerobic bottles) and the Septi-Chek system (BD) appear to support the growth of the common *Campylobacter* species (59, 65, 139). Other systems, such as anaerobic broth and lysis-centrifugation, may not be as sensitive (59).

DIRECT EXAMINATION

Microscopy

Clinical microbiologists do not normally consider performing Gram stain analysis of stool samples for diagnosis of bacterial gastroenteritis; however, this is a rapid and sensitive method for presumptive diagnosis of *Campylobacter* enteritis. Campylobacters are not easily visualized with the safranin counterstain commonly used in the Gram stain procedure and are somewhat thinner than other enteric gram-negative bacteria; carbol-fuchsin or 0.1% aqueous basic fuchsin should be used as the counterstain for smears of stools or pure cultures (99, 111, 138). Because of their characteristic microscopic morphology, campylobacters may be detected by direct Gram stain examination of stools obtained from patients with acute enteritis, with sensitivity ranging from 66 to 94% and specificity above 95% (99, 111, 138). Phase-contrast and dark-field microscopy have also been used to directly detect motile campylobacters in fresh stool samples; however, the sensitivities of these approaches have not been studied widely, and in our opinion, these methods require significant microscopic expertise (56, 98).

Fecal white blood cells may be present during *Campylobacter* infection and have been reported in 25 to 80% of culture-proven cases (47). While the likelihood of infection with *Campylobacter* or other enteroinvasive pathogens may be higher in the presence of fecal leukocytes, the absence of fecal leukocytes does not rule out the diagnosis (128). Thus, routine examination of stool samples for fecal leukocytes is not recommended as a test for predicting bacterial infection or for selective culturing for *Campylobacter* or other stool pathogens (40).

Antigen Detection

A commercially available antigen detection system for *Campylobacter* in stool samples is available (ProSpecT *Campylobacter*; Alexon-Trend, Inc. [distributed through Remel, Lenexa, Kans.]). Compared with culture, this immunoassay has been shown to vary in sensitivity from 80 to 96%, and it has good specificity, >97% (21, 46, 127). *C. upsaliensis* was found to cross-react in the enzyme immunoassay (21). Antigen may be detected in stored samples at 4°C for several days (25).

Nucleic Acid Detection Techniques

Amplification techniques have been used to detect *Campylobacter* directly in stool samples (103). Molecular approaches to detecting *Campylobacter* directly may reduce the time to detection and improve abilities to identify isolates to the species level and to identify the less common *Campylobacter* species often missed by conventional culture. A commercially available molecular test for detection of *Campylobacter* spp. in fecal samples is not currently available. Molecular approaches are also more expensive than culture and do not provide an isolate for further characterization.

ISOLATION PROCEDURES

Most *Campylobacter* species require a microaerobic atmosphere containing approximately 5% O_2, 10% CO_2, and 85% N_2 for optimal recovery. Several manufacturers produce microaerobic gas generator packs that are suitable for routine use. A trigas incubator (125) or evacuation and replacement of an anaerobic jar with the approximate gas mixture may also be used for routine cultures (82). The concentration of oxygen generated in candle jars is suboptimal for the isolation of *Campylobacter*, and these jars should not be used for routine laboratory isolation procedures (72).

Some species of *Campylobacter*, such as *C. sputorum*, *C. concisus*, *C. mucosalis*, *C. curvus*, *C. rectus*, and *C. hyointestinalis*, require increased hydrogen for primary isolation and growth. These species will usually not be recovered using the conventional microaerobic conditions since the amount of hydrogen generated in properly used commercial gas packs is <2%. A gas mixture of 10% CO_2 and 6% H_2, with the balance consisting of N_2, in an evacuation-replacement jar is sufficient for isolating hydrogen-requiring species (12). A study by Vandenberg and colleagues reemphasized the requirement for increased hydrogen for isolating certain *Campylobacter* spp. (135).

A number of selective media are recommended for isolating *C. jejuni* and *C. coli*. These include blood-free media, such as charcoal cefoperazone deoxycholate agar (CCDA) (51) and charcoal-based selective medium (CSM) (57), and blood-containing media, such as Campy-CVA medium (L. B. Reller, S. Mirrett, and L. G. Reimer, *Abstr. Annu. Meet. Am. Soc. Microbiol. 1983*, abstr. C-274, p. 357, 1983) and Skirrow medium (113). Charcoal-based medium containing cefoperazone, amphotericin, and teicoplanin (CAT medium) is a selective medium for the primary isolation of *C. upsaliensis* (6). Researchers in two studies, however, did not isolate *C. upsaliensis* from any stool samples by using this medium (28, 46). *C. upsaliensis* may occasionally be recovered on some other selective media. *C. upsaliensis* isolates can also be recovered by using the filtration method, and some strains may grow better in a hydrogen-enriched atmosphere (39, 66).

To achieve the highest yield of *Campylobacter* from stool samples, use of a combination of media including either CCDA or CSM as one of the media appears to be the optimal method (26, 41) and may increase the recovery of *Campylobacter* by as much as 10 to 15% over that with the use of a single medium. If only a single medium can be used because of budgetary constraints, we suggest the Campy-CVA formulation, but a charcoal-based medium such as CCDA works just as well. In a comparative study, CCDA medium was found to be the most sensitive for detecting *C. jejuni* and *C. coli* when compared with Skirrow medium, CAT agar, and the filtration technique (28).

Most of these selective media have one or more antimicrobial agents, mainly cefoperazone, as the primary inhibitors of enteric bacterial flora. Antimicrobial agents such as cephalothin, colistin, and polymyxin B present in some selective medium formulations are inhibitory to some strains of *C. jejuni* and *C. coli* (38, 90), and are inhibitory to *C. fetus* subsp. *fetus*. *C. jejuni* subsp. *doylei*, *C. upsaliensis*, and *A. butzleri* generally will not grow on cephalothin-containing media. We no longer recommend cephalothin-containing formulations for primary isolation of *Campylobacter* and *Arcobacter* from fecal samples.

If *Campylobacter* infection is suspected at the time blood specimens are drawn, broth media should be subcultured after 24 to 48 h to a nonselective blood agar medium and plates should be incubated under microaerobic conditions at 37°C, preferably with increased hydrogen. This will allow for the isolation of thermophilic and nonthermophilic species. Although commonly used blood culture systems should support the growth of *Campylobacter* and give appropriate signals if cultures are positive, it may be prudent to perform a blind subculture. Similarly, blood drawn in Isolator (Wampole Laboratories, Cranbury, N.J.) tubes for bacterial culture should be inoculated onto a nonselective blood agar plate and incubated under microaerobic conditions at 37°C if *Campylobacter* infection is suspected. If a curved, gram-negative rod is observed upon Gram stain examination of a positive blood culture bottle, an aliquot should be cultured on a nonselective blood agar plate and incubated under microaerobic conditions at 37°C. An alternative staining method such as the use of acridine orange may also be effective for detecting campylobacters in blood culture bottles if the Gram stain is negative.

Optimal conditions for recovery of *Arcobacter* from clinical specimens have not been determined. *Arcobacter* spp. were first isolated on semisolid media designed to isolate *Leptospira* spp. (133, 143). *Arcobacter* species are aerotolerant and have been recovered on certain selective media such as Campy-CVA (5) incubated under microaerobic conditions at 37°C and on nonselective media used in the filtration method (135). Several other media have been reported to recover *Arcobacter* species but have not been studied in clinical settings (5, 20, 133).

Enrichment Cultures

Enrichment broths formulated to enhance the recovery of *Campylobacter* from stool include Preston enrichment (13), Campy-thio (109), and *Campylobacter* enrichment broth (76). Enrichment cultures may be beneficial in instances in which low numbers of organisms may be expected due to delayed transport to the laboratory or after the acute stage of disease, when the concentration of organisms may be low, such as in the investigation of GBS following acute *Campylobacter* infection (84). The clinical effectiveness and cost-effectiveness of using enrichment cultures as part of the routine stool culture setup has not been studied adequately.

Filtration

Filtration techniques designed to isolate *C. jejuni* and *C. coli* as well as other *Campylobacter* species (28, 38, 135) and *Arcobacter* spp. (60, 135) that are susceptible to antibiotics present in most selective media (135) should be used to complement direct culture to selective plating media and not as a replacement. The filtration method is based on the principle that campylobacters can pass through membrane filters (pore sizes, 0.45 to 0.65 μm) with relative ease (because organisms are thin and highly motile) while other stool flora are retained during the short processing time. Cellulose acetate membrane filters with a 0.65-μm pore size are recommended for routine use and are available from a number of suppliers (J. G. Wells, N. D. Puhr, C. M. Patton, M. A. Nicholson, M. A. Lambert, and R. Jerris, *Abstr. Annu. Meet. Am. Soc. Microbiol. 1989*, abstr. C231, p. 432, 1989). Filtration is performed by placing a sterile 0.65-μm-pore-size cellulose acetate filter onto the surface of an agar medium such as antibiotic-free CCDA, CSM, or blood-containing medium. Ten to 15 drops of fecal suspension are placed onto the filter, and the plate is incubated at 37°C for 45 to 60 min. The filter is then removed, and the plate is incubated at 37°C under microaerobic conditions, preferably with an atmosphere containing increased hydrogen (for the hydrogen-requiring species). Stool samples containing ~10^5 CFU of *Campylobacter*/ml will be detected with this method, and thus, the filtration method is not as sensitive as primary culture with selective media (39).

Species within the genus *Campylobacter* and *Arcobacter* have different optimal temperatures for growth. The choice of incubation temperature for routine stool cultures, therefore, is critical in determining the spectrum of species that will be isolated. By convention, most laboratories use 42°C as the primary incubation temperature for *Campylobacter*. This temperature allows the growth of *C. jejuni* and *C. coli* on selective media. *C. upsaliensis* also grows well at 42°C but usually is not recovered on selective media. *C. fetus* exhibits variable growth at this temperature and may not be recovered. *Arcobacter* species are not thermophilic and will generally not be recovered at 42°C.

In contrast, most *Campylobacter* and *Arcobacter* species grow well at 37°C. Selective media, such as Skirrow medium, were devised for use at 42°C and have poor selective properties at 37°C, whereas CCDA and CSM show good selective properties at 37°C (26). Plates should be incubated for a minimum of 72 h before being reported as negative. It has been reported that incubation of CCDA medium for 5 to 6 days increases the yield of *C. jejuni* and *C. coli* compared with that obtained after 2 days of incubation (28).

Because of the expense of including several types of media and the filtration method in the initial workup for campylobacters, a practical approach is to use a single medium for isolation of thermophilic *Campylobacter* spp., such as Campy-CVA or CCDA (or equivalent) incubated at 42°C, in the workup for acute bacterial gastroenteritis. If the primary culture workup is unrevealing and if a patient has persistent diarrhea, cultures for non-*C. jejuni* and non-*C. coli* species may be appropriate. Additional stool samples should be plated on multiple selective media (e.g., CCDA and Campy-CVA), processed by the filtration method as well, and incubated at 37°C under microaerobic conditions with increased hydrogen.

IDENTIFICATION

The identification of campylobacters is made difficult because of their complex and rapidly evolving taxonomy, fastidious growth requirements, and biochemical inertness (Table 2). These problems have resulted in a proliferation of phenotypic and genotypic methods for identifying members of this group (93).

TABLE 2 Useful phenotypic properties of *Campylobacter* and *Arcobacter* species[a]

Organism	Catalase	H_2 required	Urease	H_2S (TSI)	Hippurate hydrolysis	Indoxyl acetate hydrolysis	Aryl sulfatase	Selenite reduction	Growth in 1% glycine
C. jejuni subsp. *jejuni*	+	−	−	−	+	+	V	V	+
C. jejuni subsp. *doylei*	V	−	−	−	V	+	−	−	+
C. coli	+	−	−	V	−	+	−	+	+
C. fetus subsp. *fetus*	+	−	−	−	−	−	−	V	+
C. fetus subsp. *venerealis*	V	−	−	−	−	−	−	V	V
C. lari	+	−	V	−	−	−	−	V	+
C. upsaliensis	−	−	−	−	−	+	−	+	+
C. hyointestinalis subsp. *hyointestinalis*	+	V	−	+	−	−	−	+	+
C. hyointestinalis subsp. *lawsonii*	+	V	+	+[b]	−	−	−	+	V
C. lanienae	+	−	−	−	−	−	ND	+	V
C. sputorum[b] bv. sputorum	−	+	−	+	−	−	+	V	+
C. sputorum bv. faecalis	+	+	−	+	−	−	+	V	+
C. sputorum bv. paraureolyticus	−	+	+	+	−	−	+	V	+
C. helveticus	−	−	−	−	−	+	ND	−	V
C. hominis	−	+[c]	ND	−	−	−	ND	−	+
C. mucosalis	−	+	−	+	−	−	−	V	V
C. concisus	−	+	−	V	−	−	+	V	V
C. curvus	−	+	−	V	V	V	+	−	+
C. rectus	V	+	−	−	−	+	+	−	+
C. showae	+	+	−	−	−	V	+	−	V
C. gracilis[c]	V	ND	−	−	−	V	ND	−	+
A. cryaerophilus	V	−	−	−	−	+	−	−	V
A. butzleri	V	−	−	−	−	+	−	−	+
A. nitrofigilis	+	−	+	−	−	+	−	ND	−
A. skirrowii	+	−	−	−	−	+	−	ND	V
B. ureolyticus	V	+	+	−	−	−	ND	−	+

[a] Adapted from references 29, 60, 67, 71, 105, 117, 129, 131, and 133. +, positive reaction; −, negative reaction; V, variable reaction; ND, not determined; TSI, triple sugar iron agar.
[b] Strains of *C. sputorum* and *C. hyointestinalis* subsp. *lawsonii* normally produce large amounts of H_2S in triple sugar iron agar (67).
[c] Anaerobic growth only.

Campylobacter spp. and *Arcobacter* spp.

Depending on the medium used, *Campylobacter* colonies may have different appearances. In general, *Campylobacter* spp. produce gray, flat, irregular, and spreading colonies. Spreading along the streak line is commonly seen, particularly on freshly prepared media. As the moisture content decreases, the organisms may form round, convex, and glistening colonies with little spreading observed. Thus, proper storage of media to ensure correct moisture content is important for optimal isolation and recognition of *Campylobacter* spp. Hemolysis on blood agar is not observed. *Arcobacter* colonies are morphologically similar to *Campylobacter* colonies (129, 133).

The Gram stain appearance of arcobacters may differ from that of typical campylobacters. *A. butzleri* is only slightly curved, and *A. cryaerophilus* tends to be much more helical in appearance than campylobacters. Commercial systems for identification of *Campylobacter* species were not found to be more accurate than conventional tests (52). Unfortunately, *Campylobacter* species are difficult to differentiate from *Arcobacter* species based on phenotypic tests. However, an aerotolerant species (i.e., one that grows under aerobic conditions) that grows on MacConkey agar (under microaerobic conditions) may be presumptively identified as an *Arcobacter* species. The failure to grow on MacConkey agar, however, does not rule out an *Arcobacter* species.

C. jejuni and *C. coli*

For initial analysis, a Gram stain examination of the colony should be performed along with an oxidase test. Oxidase-positive colonies exhibiting a characteristic Gram stain appearance (e.g., gram-negative, curved to S-shaped rods) isolated from selective media incubated at 42°C under microaerobic conditions can be reliably reported as *Campylobacter* spp., and only hippurate hydrolysis testing is recommended (Fig. 1). Hydrolysis of sodium hippurate is the major test for distinguishing *C. jejuni* (and also *C. jejuni* subsp. *doylei*) from other *Campylobacter* species. *C. jejuni,* the most common *Campylobacter* species, is relatively easy to identify phenotypically; strains isolated on selective media that grow at 42°C, are oxidase positive, show characteristic microscopic morphology, and give a positive result with hippurate hydrolysis should be reported as *C. jejuni* subsp. *jejuni,* and for routine clinical purposes, no other tests need to be performed. Methods for the hippurate hydrolysis test are described elsewhere (73). A large inoculum (i.e., full loop) should be used in performing this test. Occasional strains of *C. jejuni* may be hippurate negative, making them more difficult to identify. Gas-liquid chromatography for detecting benzoic acid (liberated through hydrolysis of sodium hippurate) is the most sensitive assay for hippurate hydrolysis and can be used for more definitive determination. Molecular detection of the *hipO* (hippuricase) gene or other *C. jejuni*-specific markers (see Table 3) by PCR may be useful for identifying phenotypically negative isolates (43). Except in hippuricase activity, which *C. coli* is lacking, *C. coli* and *C. jejuni* are similar biochemically (Table 2). Thus, molecular methods are needed to accurately identify *C. coli.* Tests of susceptibility (inhibition) or resistance of *Campylobacter* spp. to nalidixic acid and cephalothin have routinely been used as an aid for species identification. However, with the increasing prevalence of fluoroquinolone resistance in these species, these disk identification assays can no longer be relied upon.

For species other than *C. jejuni,* phenotypic characterization is more problematic. An algorithm for identification of the thermophilic *Campylobacter* spp. is shown in Fig. 1. The most useful tests for initial identification include those for growth at 25, 37, and 42°C; catalase; hippurate hydrolysis (73); indoxyl acetate hydrolysis (74); and production of H_2S (8). Indoxyl acetate hydrolysis is useful for differentiating some species of thermophilic *Campylobacter*. The disk method is rapid (5 to 30 min) and easy to perform. Disks are prepared by making a 20% solution of indoxyl acetate in acetone and adding 25 μl to a blank paper disk (0.6 cm). Dry the disks at room temperature and store them at 4°C in a brown tube with desiccant. Indoxyl acetate disks are also available ready made from commercial sources. Place a large loopful of growth from a plate onto the indoxyl acetate disk and add a drop of sterile distilled water. Hydrolysis of indoxyl acetate is indicated by the appearance of dark blue or blue-green. Weakly positive strains show pale blue in 10 to 30 min. Absence of color change is indicative of a negative reaction.

Additional tests can be performed to aid in the identification of *Campylobacter* spp. (Fig. 1). To obtain consistent and reproducible results, a standardized suspension and inoculum should be used for performing phenotypic tests. For growth temperature and oxygen tolerance studies, a suspension of the organism in heart infusion broth or tryptic soy broth to the turbidity of a McFarland standard of 1 should be used. A fiber-tipped swab dipped in the broth suspension should be used to make a single streak across the plate (Mueller-Hinton agar with 5% sheep blood is a suitable medium) and the plate should be incubated at the desired temperature and/or under the appropriate atmospheric conditions (8, 82).

Several commercial systems have been developed to aid in the identification of *Campylobacter* spp. to the genus level. Two immunologic reagents are currently available in the United States for culture identification, INDX Campy-JCL (Hardy Diagnostics, Santa Maria, Calif., and Fisher Scientific, Hampton, N.H.) and Dry Spot campylobacter test kit (Remel). INDX Campy-JCL was previously evaluated and does not differentiate between *C. jejuni* and *C. coli* (86). The Dry Spot campylobacter latex test is reported by the manufacturer to identify, but not differentiate among, *C. jejuni, C. coli, C. lari,* and *C. upsaliensis,* with variable results for *C. fetus* subsp. *fetus* (Oxoid USA; http://www.oxoid.com). A DNA probe (Accuprobe; Gen-Probe Inc., San Diego, Calif.) directed against *Campylobacter* rRNA sequences identifies *Campylobacter* species to the genus level and detects *C. jejuni* subsp. *jejuni, C. jejuni* subsp. *doylei, C. coli,* and *C. lari* (106, 124). However, the probe also hybridized with 2 of 17 *C. hyointestinalis* strains (106). Thus, these methods may be useful for confirming the identities of *Campylobacter* species to the genus level if other tests are not conclusive. However, cross-reactivity in these tests with closely related taxa and/or more newly described species needs to be determined.

Because many species of *Campylobacter* and *Arcobacter* are difficult to identify by phenotypic testing, tests for detection of species-specific sequences via PCR have been developed. *C. jejuni, C. coli,* and other *Campylobacter* and *Arcobacter* species have been reported to be reliably differentiated based on polymorphism in the *ceuE* gene (37), a GTPase gene (136), a 16S rRNA gene (75), a 23S rRNA gene (50), and the *glyA* gene (4). Table 3 lists some of the more commonly used published PCR assays for the identification of *C. jejuni* and *C. coli.* Recently published evaluations of some of these assays highlight the importance of validating their sensitivities and specificities (15, 94). In addition, it has been reported that the use of heated lysates rather than purified DNA may in some cases not always provide a suitable reaction template for these PCR assays (80, 94). As false

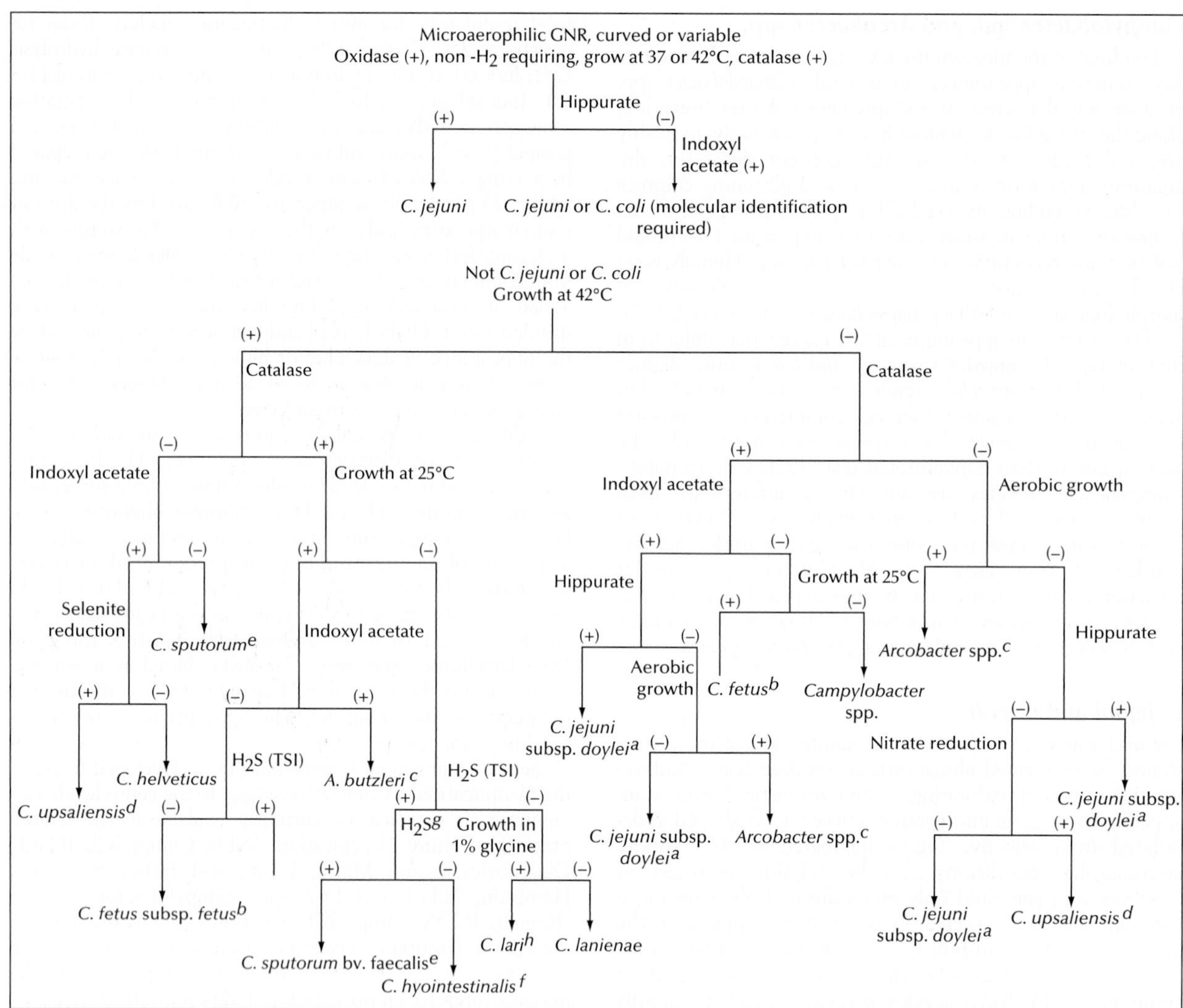

FIGURE 1 Practical algorithm for identifying *Campylobacter* and *Arcobacter* spp. that do not require increased hydrogen for primary isolation in the clinical laboratory. GNR, gram-negative rods; TSI, triple sugar iron agar. [a]*C. jejuni* subsp. *doylei* produces variable results in the catalase and hippurate tests. [b]Strains of *C. fetus* subsp. *fetus* can be variable for growth at 42°C. [c]*A. butzleri* is variable for growth at 42°C and produces variable results in the catalase test. *A. cryaerophilus* produces variable results in the catalase test. [d]*C. upsaliensis* is variable for growth at 42°C. [e]Results for the catalase test are biovar dependent; *C. sputorum* bv. faecalis is catalase positive. Some strains of *C. sputorum* may grow better in environments with increased hydrogen concentration. [f]*C. hyointestinalis* grows under microaerophilic conditions, but some strains require additional hydrogen (66). [g]Rapid H_2S test (69). [h]Urease-positive *C. lari* strains are referred to as the urease-positive thermophilic campylobacter group.

negatives or nonspecifically amplified product(s) have been noted for some of the *C. jejuni*-specific assays, a second PCR targeting another *C. jejuni*-specific gene may be necessary in some instances.

TYPING SYSTEMS

Typing systems for *Campylobacter* epidemiologic studies vary in complexities and abilities to discriminate among strains. Common phenotypic methods that have been applied include biotyping, phage typing, and serotyping (89, 100). The most frequently used system is serotyping. The heat-labile serotyping scheme originally described by Lior et al. (70) can detect over 100 serotypes of *C. jejuni*, *C. coli*, and *C. lari*. Uncharacterized bacterial surface antigens and, in some serotypes, flagellar antigens are the serodeterminants for this serotyping system (3). The heat-stable (HS) serotyping scheme described by Penner and Hennessy (101) detects 60 types of *C. jejuni* and *C. coli* (100). Initially thought to detect lipopolysaccharide antigenic determinants, the HS system has been shown to detect a *Campylobacter* capsular polysaccharide (55). Serotyping is performed in only a few reference laboratories worldwide because of the time and expense needed to maintain quality antisera. A serotyping reagent kit is also commercially available (Denka Seiken USA Inc., Campbell, Calif.).

TABLE 3 Differentiation of *C. jejuni* and *C. coli* by PCR

Species	Target gene	Primers[a]	Reference
C. jejuni	Unknown	F, 5′-CAT CTT CCC TAG TCA AGC CT-3′ R, 5′-AAG ATA TGG CTC TAG CAA GAC-3′	134
	hipO	F, 5′-GAA GAG GGT TTG GGT GGT-3′ R, 5′-AGC TAG CTT CGC ATA ATA ACT TG-3′	68
	mapA	F, 5′-ATG TTT AAA AAA TTT TTG-3′ R, 5′-AAG TTC AGA GAT TAA ACT AG-3′	119
C. coli	Unknown	F, 5′-AGG CAA GGG AGC CTT TAA TC-3′ R, 5′-TAT CCC TAT CTA CAA ATT CGC-3′	134
	ceuE	F, 5′-ATG AAA AAA TAT TTA GTT TTT GCA-3′ R, 5′-ATT TTA TTA TTT GTA GCA GCG-3′	37
	Putative aspartokinase gene	F, 5′-GGT ATG ATT TCT ACA AAG CGA G-3′ R, 5′-ATA AAA GAC TAT CGT CGC GTG-3′	68

[a] F, forward primer; R, reverse primer.

The limitations of phenotypic subtyping methods and the rapid growth of molecular biology techniques in the 1990s led to the development of a range of molecular biology-based subtyping methods, such as restriction endonuclease analysis, ribotyping, PCR-based techniques, pulsed-field gel electrophoresis of macrorestricted chromosomal DNA (PFGE), and amplified fragment length polymorphism (89, 100). The development of a rapid one-day standardized PFGE protocol (108), which is used by participants of the PulseNet national surveillance network for foodborne pathogens (http://www.cdc.gov/pulsenet), has facilitated the use of the PFGE approach for investigations of campylobacteriosis outbreaks (92). However, interpretation of data can be difficult since genomic rearrangements can lead to changes in PFGE profiles (31). Advances in DNA sequencing technology have provided a means to investigate strain variation at the nucleotide level and have led to the emergence of DNA sequencing-based subtyping systems such as multilocus sequence typing (22). In addition, the generation of *Campylobacter* whole-genome sequences has led the way for the development of a new technique, genomotyping based on microarray technology (61). At present, no method alone is adequate for all applications, and a combination of methods such as serotyping and molecular methods should be used for reliably determining strain relatedness and for studying the epidemiology of *Campylobacter* infections (89).

SEROLOGIC TESTS

Serum immunoglobulin G (IgG), IgM, and IgA levels rise in response to infection, but elevated serum and fecal IgA levels appear during the first few weeks of infection and then fall rapidly (10, 123). Serum antibody assays vary in both sensitivity and specificity for detecting *Campylobacter* infection, and test performance appears to be population dependent. Patients with *Campylobacter* infection may have false-positive legionella antibody tests (14). Serologic testing appears to be useful for epidemiologic investigations and is not recommended for routine diagnosis (122).

ANTIMICROBIAL SUSCEPTIBILITY

C. jejuni and *C. coli* have variable susceptibilities to a variety of antimicrobial agents, including macrolides, fluoroquinolones, aminoglycosides, chloramphenicol, nitrofurantoin, and tetracycline (http://www.cdc.gov/NARMS) (11). Most isolates are not susceptible to cephalosporins and penicillins (11). Azithromycin and erythromycin are drugs of choice for treating *C. jejuni* gastrointestinal infections, and for susceptible organisms, ciprofloxacin or norfloxacin may also be used (35). Early therapy of susceptible *Campylobacter* infection with erythromycin or ciprofloxacin is effective in eliminating the organism from stools and may also reduce the duration of symptoms associated with infection (11).

C. jejuni is generally susceptible to erythromycin, with resistance rates of less than 5% (27). Rates of erythromycin resistance in *C. coli* vary considerably, with up to 80% of strains showing resistance in some studies (27). Although ciprofloxacin has been effective in treating *Campylobacter* infections, the emergence of ciprofloxacin resistance during therapy has been reported (104). Several in vitro studies now show significant rates of resistance to fluoroquinolones (27, 58, 87). Individuals infected with fluoroquinolone-resistant *C. jejuni* have been shown to have diarrhea for a longer duration, and thus, routine testing of isolates may be indicated (88). *C. jejuni* and *C. coli* may also produce a β-lactamase that appears to be active against amoxicillin, ampicillin, and ticarcillin; this enzyme has been reported to be inhibited by clavulanic acid but not sulbactam or tazobactam (62).

Parenteral therapy is used to treat systemic *C. fetus* infections; drugs used include erythromycin, ampicillin, aminoglycosides, and chloramphenicol, depending upon the type of infection (11). *C. gracilis* is generally susceptible to a variety of antimicrobial agents, including amoxicillin-clavulanate, cefoxitin, ceftriaxone, clindamycin, metronidazole, and piperacillin-tazobactam (80).

Agar dilution is the method recognized by the Clinical and Laboratory Standards Institute (formerly NCCLS) for testing *Campylobacter* spp., with published quality control ranges for several antimicrobial agents (18, 78). A broth microdilution method with published quality control ranges for several antimicrobial agents was also recently approved by the Clinical and Laboratory Standards Institute (79). The E test (PDM Epsilometer; AB Biodisk, Solna, Sweden) using Mueller-Hinton agar with 5% sheep blood compares favorably with the agar dilution method (7).

EVALUATION, INTERPRETATION, AND REPORTING OF RESULTS

Campylobacter species, including the common thermophilic species *C. jejuni* and *C. coli,* should be sought in all diarrheic stools submitted to the laboratory for routine culture. Except for epidemiological purposes, cultures of formed stools should not be performed. Isolation of *Campylobacter* from a patient with acute diarrhea is usually significant since the carrier rate in developed countries is quite low; however, in developing countries, isolation might be more difficult to interpret, especially in the presence of other enteric pathogens. In acute infection, there is usually a high number of organisms in the stool; however, the quantity of organisms is not related to the severity of infection, nor is it indicative of a carrier state. Gram stain analysis of fecal samples for organisms with typical *Campylobacter* morphology is a highly sensitive and specific test that is currently underutilized; it should be performed for rapid preliminary diagnosis of *Campylobacter* infection. Other species, such as *C. fetus* subsp. *fetus* and *C. upsaliensis*, may be important causes of diarrhea and are not isolated on routine selective media. Special methods including alternative incubation techniques are required as described in this chapter and should be performed by special request. Oxidase-positive, curved, gram-negative rods that are hippurate hydrolysis positive should be reported as *C. jejuni* without further workup. The importance of identifying other species will depend upon the clinical circumstances, but identification tests should always be performed on isolates from blood or other sterile sites since results may influence antimicrobial therapy decisions. Given that fluoroquinolone resistance is present in a significant proportion of *C. jejuni* isolates, fluoroquinolone susceptibility testing is suggested for patients who are receiving or being considered for therapy of gastroenteritis. Susceptibility testing should be performed on all isolates from sterile clinical sites.

Use of trade names is for identification only and does not imply endorsement by the Public Health Service or by the U.S. Department of Health and Human Services.

REFERENCES

1. **Abbott, S. L., M. Waddington, D. Lindquist, J. Ware, W. Cheung, J. Ely, and J. M. Janda.** 2005. Description of *Campylobacter curvus* and *C. curvus*-like strains associated with sporadic episodes of bloody gastroenteritis and Brainerd's diarrhea. *J. Clin. Microbiol.* **43:**585–588.
2. **Aho, M., M. Kauppi, and J. Hirn.** 1988. The stability of small number of campylobacteria in four different transport media. *Acta Vet. Scand.* **29:**437–442.
3. **Alm, R. A., P. Guerry, M. E. Power, H. Lior, and T. J. Trust.** 1991. Analysis of the role of flagella in the heat-labile Lior serotyping scheme of thermophilic campylobacters by mutant allele exchange. *J. Clin. Microbiol.* **29:** 2438–2445.
4. **Al Rashid, S. T., I. Dakuna, H. Louie, D. Ng, P. Vandamme, W. Johnson, and V. L. Chan.** 2000. Identification of *Campylobacter jejuni, C. coli, C. lari, C. upsaliensis, Arcobacter butzleri,* and *A. butzleri*-like species based on the *glyA* gene. *J. Clin. Microbiol.* **38:** 1488–1494.
5. **Anderson, K. F., J. A. Kiehlbauch, D. C. Anderson, H. M. McClure, and I. K. Wachsmuth.** 1993. *Arcobacter (Campylobacter) butzleri*-associated diarrheal illness in a nonhuman primate. *Infect. Immun.* **61:**2220–2223.
6. **Aspinall, S. T., D. R. Wareing, P. G. Hayward, and D. N. Hutchinson.** 1996. A comparison of a new selective medium (CAT) with membrane filtration for the isolation of thermophilic campylobacters including Campylobacter upsaliensis. *J. Appl. Bacteriol.* **80:**645–650.
7. **Baker, C. N.** 1992. The E-Test and *Campylobacter jejuni. Diagn. Microbiol. Infect. Dis.* **15:**469–472.
8. **Barrett, T. J., C. M. Patton, and G. K. Morris.** 1988. Differentiation of *Campylobacter* species using phenotypic characterization. *Lab. Med.* **19:**96–102.
9. **Black, R. E., M. M. Levine, M. L. Clements, T. P. Hughs, and M. J. Blaser.** 1988. Experimental *Campylobacter jejuni* infections in humans. *J. Infect. Dis.* **157:**472–480.
10. **Black, R. E., D. Perlman, M. L. Clements, M. M. Levine, and M. J. Blaser.** 1992. Human volunteer studies with *Campylobacter jejuni*, p. 207–215. *In* I. Nachamkin, M. J. Blaser, and L. S. Tompkins (ed.), Campylobacter jejuni: *Current Status and Future Trends.* American Society for Microbiology, Washington, D.C.
11. **Blaser, M. J., and B. M. Allos.** 2005. *Campylobacter jejuni* and related species, p. 2548–2557. *In* G. L. Mandell, J. E. Bennett, and R. Dolin (ed.), *Principles and Practice of Infectious Diseases.* Elsevier Churchill Livingstone, Philadelphia, Pa.
12. **Bolton, F.** 2001. Methods for isolation of *Campylobacter* from humans, animals, food and water, p. 87–93. *In* World Health Organization, *The Increasing Incidence of Human Campylobacteriosis: Report and Proceedings of a WHO Consultation of Experts.* World Health Organzation, Geneva, Switzerland.
13. **Bolton, F. J., and L. Robertson.** 1982. A selective medium for isolating *Campylobacter jejuni/coli. J. Clin. Pathol.* **35:** 462–467.
14. **Boswell, T. C. J., and G. Kudesia.** 1992. Serological cross-reactions between *Legionella pneumophila* and *Campylobacter* in the indirect fluorescent antibody test. *Epidemiol. Infect.* **109:**291–295.
15. **Burnett, T. A., A. H. M. P. Kuhnert, and S. P. Djordjevic.** 2002. *Campylobacter jejuni* and *Campylobacter coli* isolates from poultry and humans using six PCR-based assays. *FEMS Microbiol. Lett.* **216:**201–209.
16. **Cary, S. G., and E. B. Blair.** 1964. New transport medium for shipment of clinical specimens. I. Fecal specimens. *J. Bacteriol.* **88:**96–98.
17. **Centers for Disease Control and Prevention.** 2004. Preliminary FoodNet data on the incidence of infection with pathogens transmitted commonly through food—selected sites, United States, 2003. *Morb. Mortal. Wkly. Rep.* **53:**338–343.
18. **Clinical and Laboratory Standards Institute.** 2005. *Performance Standards for Antimicrobial Susceptibility Testing, Fifteenth Informational Supplement.* M100-S15. Clinical and Laboratory Standards Institute, Wayne, Pa.
19. **Colmegna, I., R. Cuchacovich, and L. R. Espinoza.** 2004. HLA-B27-associated reactive arthritis: pathogenetic and clinical considerations. *Clin. Microbiol. Rev.* **17:**348–369.
20. **de Boer, E., J. J. H. C. Tilburg, D. L. Woodward, H. Lior, and W. M. Johnson.** 1996. A selective medium for the isolation of *Arcobacter* from meats. *Lett. Appl. Microbiol.* **23:**64–66.
21. **Dediste, A., O. Vandenberg, L. Vlaes, A. Ebraert, N. Douat, P. Bahwere, and J.-P. Butzler.** 2003. Evaluation of the ProSpecT microplate assay for detecton of *Campylobacter:* a routine laboratory perspective. *Clin. Microbiol. Infect.* **9:**1085–1090.
22. **Dingle, K. E., F. M. Colles, D. R. A. Wareing, R. Ure, A. J. Fox, F. E. Bolton, H. J. Bootsma, R. J. L. Willems, R. Urwin, and M. C. J. Maiden.** 2001. Multilocus sequence typing system for *Campylobacter jejuni. J. Clin. Microbiol.* **39:**14–23.
23. **Donachie, S. P., J. P. Bowman, S. L. W. On, and M. Alam.** 2005. *Arcobacter halophilus* sp. nov., the first obligate halophile in the genus *Arcobacter. Int. J. Syst. Evol. Microbiol.* **55:**1271–1277.

24. **Edmonds, P., C. M. Patton, P. M. Griffin, T. J. Barrett, G. P. Schmid, C. N. Baker, M. A. Lambert, and D. J. Brenner.** 1987. *Campylobacter hyointestinalis* associated with human gastrointestinal disease in the United States. *J. Clin. Microbiol.* **25:**685–691.
25. **Endtz, H. P., C. W. Ang, N. Van Den Braak, A. Luijendijk, B. C. Jacobs, P. de Man, J. M. van Duin, A. van Belkum, and H. A. Verbrugh.** 2000. Evaluation of a new commercial immunoassay for rapid detection of *Campylobacter jejuni* in stool samples. *Eur. J. Clin. Microbiol. Infect. Dis.* **19:**794–797.
26. **Endtz, H. P., G. J. Ruijs, A. H. Zwinderman, T. van der Reijden, M. Biever, and R. P. Mouton.** 1991. Comparison of six media, including a semisolid agar, for the isolation of various *Campylobacter* species from stool specimens. *J. Clin. Microbiol.* **29:**1007–1010.
27. **Engberg, J., F. M. Aarestrup, D. E. Taylor, P. Gerner-Smidt, and I. Nachamkin.** 2001. Quinolone and macrolide resistance in *Campylobacter jejuni* and *C. coli:* resistance mechanisms and trends in human isolates. *Emerg. Infect. Dis.* **7:**24–34.
28. **Engberg, J., S. L. W. On, C. S. Harrington, and P. Gerner-Smidt.** 2000. Prevalence of *Campylobacter, Arcobacter, Helicobacter*, and *Sutterella* spp. in human fecal samples as estimated by a reevaluation of isolation methods for *Campylobacter*. *J. Clin. Microbiol.* **38:**286–291.
29. **Etoh, Y., F. E. Dewhirst, B. J. Paster, A. Yamamoto, and N. Goto.** 1993. *Campylobacter showae* sp. nov., isolated from the human oral cavity. *Int. J. Syst. Bacteriol.* **43:**631–639.
30. **Figura, N., P. Guglielmetti, A. Zanchi, N. Partini, D. Armellini, P. F. Bayeli, M. Bugnoli, and S. Verdiani.** 1993. Two cases of *Campylobacter mucosalis* enteritis in children. *J. Clin. Microbiol.* **31:**727–728.
31. **Fitzgerald, C., A. Sails, and B. Swaminathan.** 2005. Genetic techniques: molecular subtyping methods, p. 271–293. *In* T. McMeekin (ed.), *Detecting Pathogens in Food.* Woodhouse Publishing, Cambridge, United Kingdom.
32. **Foster, G., B. Holmes, A. G. Steigerwalt, P. A. Lawson, P. Thorne, D. E. Byrer, H. M. Ross, J. Xerry, P. M. Thompson, and M. D. Collins.** 2005. *Campylobacter insulaenigrae* sp. nov., isolated from marine mammals. *Int. J. Syst. Evol. Microbiol.* **54:**2369–2373.
33. **Friedman, C. R., R. M. Hoekstra, M. Samuel, R. Marcus, J. Bender, B. Shiferaw, S. Reddy, S. Ajuja, D. L. Helfrick, F. Hardnett, M. Carter, B. Anderson, and R. V. Tauxe.** 2004. Risk factors for sporadic *Campylobacter* infection in the United States. A case-control study in FoodNet sites. *Clin. Infect. Dis.* **38**(Suppl. 3)**:**285–296.
34. **Friedman, C. R., J. Neimann, H. C. Wegener, and R. V. Tauxe.** 2000. Epidemiology of *Campylobacter jejuni* infections in the United States and other industrialized nations, p. 121–138. *In* I. Nachamkin and M. J. Blaser (ed.), Campylobacter, 2nd ed. ASM Press, Washington, D.C.
35. **Gilbert, D. N., R. C. Moellering, Jr., and M. A. Sande.** 2000. *The Sanford Guide to Antimicrobial Therapy.* Antimicrobial Therapy, Inc., Hyde Park, Vt.
36. **Gilbert, M., P. C. R. Godschalk, C. T. Parker, H. P. Endtz, and W. W. Wakarchuk.** 2005. Genetic basis for the variation in the lipooligosaccharide outer core of *Campylobacter jejuni* and possible association of glycotransferase genes with post-infectious neuropathies, p. 219–248. *In* J. M. Ketley and M. E. Konkel (ed.), Campylobacter: *Molecular and Cellular Biology.* Horizon Bioscience, Norfolk, United Kingdom.
37. **Gonzalez, I., K. A. Grant, P. T. Richardson, S. F. Park, and M. D. Collins.** 1997. Specific identification of the enteropathogens *Campylobacter jejuni* and *Campylobacter coli* by using a PCR test based on the *ceuE* gene encoding a putative virulence determinant. *J. Clin. Micriobol.* **35:**759–763.
38. **Goossens, H., M. De Boeck, H. Coignau, L. Vlaes, C. Van den Borre, and J.-P. Butzler.** 1986. Modified selective medium for isolation of *Campylobacter* spp. from feces: comparison with Preston medium, a blood-free medium, and a filtration system. *J. Clin. Microbiol.* **24:**840–843.
39. **Goossens, H., L. Vlaes, M. De Boeck, B. Pot, K. Kersters, J. Levy, P. de Mol, J. P. Butzler, and P. Vandamme.** 1990. Is "*Campylobacter upsaliensis*" an unrecognised cause of human diarrhoea? *Lancet* **335:**584–586.
40. **Guerrant, R. L., T. Van Gilder, T. S. Steiner, N. M. Thielman, L. Slutsker, R. V. Tauxe, T. Hennessy, P. M. Griffin, H. L. DuPont, R. B. Sack, P. I. Tarr, M. Neill, I. Nachamkin, L. B. Reller, M. T. Osterholm, M. L. Bennish, and L. K. Pickering.** 2001. Practice guidelines for managing infectious diarrhea. *Clin. Infect. Dis.* **32:**331–351.
41. **Gun-Monro, J., R. P. Rennie, J. H. Thornley, H. L. Richardson, D. Hodge, and J. Lynch.** 1987. Laboratory and clinical evaluation of isolation media for *Campylobacter jejuni*. *J. Clin. Microbiol.* **25:**2274–2277.
42. **Han, X. Y., J. J. Tarrand, and D. C. Rice.** 2005. Oral *Campylobacter* species involved in extraoral abscess: a report of three cases. *J. Clin. Microbiol.* **43:**2513–2515.
43. **Hani, E., and V. L. Chan.** 1995. Expression and characterization of *Campylobacter jejuni* benzoylglycine amidohydrolase (hippuricase) gene in *Escherichia coli*. *J. Bacteriol.* **177:**2396–2402.
44. **Harrington, P., J. Archer, J. P. Davis, D. R. Croft, and J. K. Varma.** 2002. Outbreak of *Campylobacter jejuni* infections associated with drinking unpasteurized milk procured through a cow-leasing program, Wisconsin, 2001. *Morb. Mortal. Wkly. Rep.* **51:**548–549.
45. **Helms, M., P. Vastrup, P. Gerner-Smidt, and K. Molbak.** 2003. Short and long term mortality associated with foodborne bacterial gastrointestinal infections: registry based study. *Br. Med. J.* **326:**1–5.
46. **Hindiyeh, M., S. Jense, S. Hohmann, H. Benett, C. Edwards, W. Aldeen, A. Croft, J. Daly, S. Mottice, and K. C. Carroll.** 2000. Rapid detection of *Campylobacter jejuni* in stool specimens by an enzyme immunoassay and surveillance for *Campylobacter upsaliensis* in the greater Salt Lake City area. *J. Clin. Microbiol.* **38:**3076–3079.
47. **Hines, J., and I. Nachamkin.** 1996. Effective use of the clinical microbiology laboratory for diagnosing diarrheal diseases. *Clin. Infect. Dis.* **23:**1292–1301.
48. **Houf, K., S. L. W. On, T. Coenye, J. Mast, J. Van Hoof, and P. Vandamme.** 2005. *Arcobacter cibarius* sp. nov., isolated from broiler carcasses. *Int. J. Syst. Evol. Microbiol.* **55:**713–717.
49. **Hu, L., and D. J. Kopecko.** 2005. Invasion, p. 369–383. *In* J. M. Ketley and M. E. Konkel (ed.), Campylobacter: *Molecular and Cellular Biology.* Horizon Bioscience, Norfolk, United Kingdom.
50. **Hurtado, A., and R. J. Owen.** 1997. A molecular scheme based on 23S rRNA gene polymorphisms for rapid identification of *Campylobacter* and *Arcobacter* species. *J. Clin. Microbiol.* **35:**2401–2404.
51. **Hutchinson, D. N., and F. J. Bolton.** 1984. Improved blood free selective medium for the isolation of *Campylobacter jejuni* from faecal specimens. *J. Clin. Pathol.* **37:**956–957.
52. **Huysmans, M. B., J. D. Turnidge, and J. H. Williams.** 1995. Evaluation of API Campy in comparison with conventional methods for identification of thermophilic campylobacters. *J. Clin. Microbiol.* **33:**3345–3346.
53. **Jagannathan, A., and C. Penn.** 2005. Motility, p. 331–347. *In* J. M. Ketley and M. E. Konkel (ed.), Campylobacter: *Molecular and Cellular Biology.* Horizon Bioscience, Norfolk, United Kingdom.
54. **Johnson, C. C., and S. M. Finegold.** 1987. Uncommonly encountered motile, anaerobic gram-negative bacilli associated with infection. *Rev. Infect. Dis.* **9:**1150–1162.

55. **Karlyshev, A. V., D. Linton, N. A. Gregson, A. J. Lastovica, and B. W. Wren.** 2000. Genetic and biochemical evidence of a *Campylobacter jejuni* capsular polysaccharide that accounts for Penner serotype specificity. *Mol. Microbiol.* **35:**529–541.
56. **Karmali, M. A., and P. C. Fleming.** 1979. Campylobacter enteritis in children. *J. Pediatr.* **94:**527–533.
57. **Karmali, M. A., A. E. Simor, M. Roscoe, P. C. Flemming, S. S. Smith, and J. Lane.** 1986. Evaluation of a blood-free, charcoal-based, selective medium for the isolation of *Campylobacter* organisms from feces. *J. Clin. Microbiol.* **23:**456–459.
58. **Kassenborg, H. D., K. E. Smith, D. J. Vugia, T. Rabatsky-Ehr, M. R. Bates, M. A. Carter, N. B. Dumas, M. P. Cassidy, N. Marano, R. V. Tauxe, and F. J. Angulo.** 2004. Fluoroquinolone-resistant *Campylobacter* infections: eating poultry outside of the home and foreign travel are risk factors. *Clin. Infect. Dis.* **38**(Suppl. 3):279–284.
59. **Kasten, M. J., F. Allerberger, and J. P. Anhalt.** 1991. *Campylobacter* bacteremia: clinical experience with three different blood culture systems at Mayo Clinic 1984–1990. *Infection* **19:**88–90.
60. **Kiehlbauch, J. A., D. J. Brenner, M. A. Nicholson, C. N. Baker, C. M. Patton, A. G. Steigerwalt, and I. K. Wachsmuth.** 1991. *Campylobacter butzleri* sp. nov. isolated from humans and animals with diarrheal illness. *J. Clin. Microbiol.* **29:**376–385.
61. **Klena, J. D., and M. E. Konkel.** 2005. Methods for epidemiologic analysis of *Campylobacter jejuni*, p. 165–179. *In* J. M. Ketley and M. E. Konkel (ed.), Campylobacter: *Molecular and Cellular Biology.* Horizon Bioscience, Norfolk, United Kingdom.
62. **Lachance, N., C. Gaudreau, F. Lamothe, and L. A. Larivière.** 1991. Role of the β-lactamase of *Campylobacter jejuni* in resistance to beta-lactam agents. *Antimicrob. Agents Chemother.* **35:**813–818.
63. **Lara-Tejero, M., and J. E. Galan.** 2002. Cytolethal distending toxin: limited damage as a strategy to modulate cellular functions. *Trends Microbiol.* **10:**147–152.
64. **Larsen, J. C., and P. Guerry.** 2005. Plasmids of *Campylobacter jejuni* 81-176, p. 181–192. *In* J. M. Ketley and M. E. Konkel (ed.), Campylobacter: *Molecular and Cellular Biology.* Horizon Bioscience, Norfolk, Unied Kingdom.
65. **Lastovica, A. J., E. Le Roux, and J. L. Penner.** 1989. "*Campylobacter upsaliensis*": isolated from blood cultures of pediatric patients. *J. Clin. Microbiol.* **27:**657–659.
66. **Lastovica, A., J., and M. B. Skirrow.** 2000. Clinical significance of *Campylobacter* and related species other than *Campylobacter jejuni*, p. 89–121. *In* I. Nachamkin and M. J. Blaser (ed.), Campylobacter, 2nd ed. ASM Press, Washington, D.C.
67. **Lawson, A. J., S. L. W. On, J. M. J. Logan, and J. Stanley.** 2001. *Campylobacter hominis* sp. nov., from the human gastrointestinal tract. *Int. J. Syst. Evol. Microbiol.* **51:**651–660.
68. **Linton, D., A. J. Lawson, R. J. Owen, and J. Stanley.** 1997. PCR detection, identification to species level, and fingerprinting of *Campylobacter jejuni* and *Campylobacter coli* direct from diarrheic samples. *J. Clin. Microbiol.* **35:** 2568–2572.
69. **Lior, H.** 1984. New extended biotyping scheme for *Campylobacter jejuni, Campylobacter coli*, and "*Campylobacter laridis.*" *J. Clin. Microbiol.* **20:**636–640.
70. **Lior, H., D. L. Woodward, J. A. Edgar, L. J. Laroche, and P. Gill.** 1982. Serotyping of *Campylobacter jejuni* by slide agglutination based on heat-labile antigenic factors. *J. Clin. Microbiol.* **15:**761–768.
71. **Logan, J. M. J., A. Burnens, D. Linton, A. J. Lawson, and J. Stanley.** 2000. *Campylobacter lanienae* sp. nov., a new species isolated from workers in an abattoir. *Int. J. Syst. Evol. Microbiol.* **50:**865–872.
72. **Luechtefeld, N. W., L. B. Reller, M. J. Blaser, and W.-L. L. Wang.** 1982. Comparison of atmospheres of incubation for primary isolation of *Campylobacter fetus* subsp. *jejuni* from animal specimens: 5% oxygen versus candle jar. *J. Clin. Microbiol.* **15:**53–57.
73. **MacFaddin, J. F.** 2000. Hippurate hydrolysis test, p. 188–204. *In* J. F. MacFaddin (ed.), *Biochemical Tests for Identification of Medical Bacteria.* Lippincott Williams & Wilkins, Philadelphia, Pa.
74. **MacFaddin, J. F.** 2000. Indoxyl substrate hydrolysis tests, p. 233–238. *In* J. F. MacFaddin (ed.), *Biochemical Tests for Identification of Medical Bacteria.* Lippincott Williams & Wilkins, Philadelphia, Pa.
75. **Marshall, S. M., P. L. Melito, D. L. Woodward, W. M. Johnson, F. G. Rodgers, and M. R. Mulvey.** 1999. Rapid identification of *Campylobacter, Arcobacter*, and *Helicobacter* isolates by PCR-restriction fragment length polymorphism analysis of the 16S rRNA gene. *J. Clin. Microbiol.* **37:**4158–4160.
76. **Martin, W. T., C. M. Patton, G. K. Morris, M. E. Potter, and N. D. Puhr.** 1983. Selective enrichment broth for isolation of *Campylobacter jejuni. J. Clin. Microbiol.* **17:** 853–855.
77. **McClung, C. R., D. G. Patriquin, and R. E. Davis.** 1983. *Campylobacter nitrofigilis* sp. nov., a nitrogen-fixing bacterium associated with roots of *Spartina alterniflora* Loisel. *Int. J. Syst. Bacteriol.* **33:**605–612.
78. **McDermott, P. F., S. M. Bodeis, F. M. Aarestrup, S. Brown, M. Traczewski, P. I. Fedorka-Cray, M. Wallace, I. A. Critchley, C. Thornsberry, S. Graff, R. Flamm, J. Beyer, D. Shortridge, L. J. Piddock, V. Ricci, M. M. Johnson, R. N. Jones, B. Reller, S. Mirrett, J. Aldrobi, R. Rennie, C. Brosnikoff, L. Turnbull, G. Stein, S. Schooley, R. A. Hanson, and R. D. Walker.** 2005. Development of a standardized susceptibility test for *Campylobacter* with quality-control ranges for ciprofloxacin, doxycycline, erythromycin, gentamicin and meropenem. *Microb. Drug Resist.* **10:**124–131.
79. **McDermott, P. F., S. M. Bodeis-Jones, T. R. Fritsche, R. N. Jones, R. D. Walker, and the Campylobacter Susceptibility Testing Group.** 2005. Broth microdilution susceptibility testing of *Campylobacter jejuni* and the determination of quality control ranges for fourteen antimicrobial agents. *J. Clin. Microbiol.* **43:**6136–6138.
80. **Mohran, Z. S., R. R. Arthur, B. A. Oyofo, L. F. Peruski, M. O. Wasfy, T. F. Ismail, and J. R. Murphy.** 1998. Differentiation of *Campylobacter* isolates on the basis of sensitivity to boiling in water as measured by PCR-detectable DNA. *Appl. Environ. Microbiol.* **64:**363–365.
81. **Molitoris, E., H. M. Wexler, and S. M. Finegold.** 1997. Sources and antimicrobial susceptibilities of *Campylobacter gracilis* and *Sutterella wadsworthensis. Clin. Infect. Dis.* **25S:**S264–S265.
82. **Morris, G. K., and C. M. Patton.** 1985. *Campylobacter*, p. 302–308. *In* E. Lennette, A. Balows, W. J. Hausler, Jr., and H. J. Shadomy (ed.), *Manual of Clinical Microbiology.* American Society for Microbiology, Washington, D.C.
83. **Nachamkin, I.** 2001. *Campylobacter jejuni*, p. 179–192. *In* M. P. Doyle, L. R. Beuchat, and T. J. Montville (ed.), *Food Microbiology: Fundamentals and Frontiers.* ASM Press, Washington, D.C.
84. **Nachamkin, I.** 1997. Microbiologic approaches for studying *Campylobacter* in patients with Guillain-Barré syndrome. *J. Infect. Dis.* **176**(Suppl. 2):S106–S114.
85. **Nachamkin, I., B. M. Allos, and T. W. Ho.** 1998. *Campylobacter* and Guillain-Barré syndrome. *Clin. Microbiol. Rev.* **11:**555–567.
86. **Nachamkin, I., and S. Barbagallo.** 1990. Culture confirmation of *Campylobacter* spp. by latex agglutination. *J. Clin. Microbiol.* **28:**817–818.

87. **Nachamkin, I., B. S. Ung, and M. Li.** 2002. Increasing fluoroquinolone resistance in *Campylobacter jejuni*, Pennsylvania, USA, 1982–2001. *Emerg. Infect. Dis.* **8:** 1501–1503.
88. **Nelson, J. M., K. E. Smith, D. J. Vugia, T. Rabatsky-Ehr, S. D. Segler, H. D. Kassenborg, S. M. Zansky, K. Joyce, N. Marano, R. M. Koekstra, and F. J. Angulo.** 2004. Prolonged diarrhea due to ciprofloxacin-resistant *Campylobacter* infection. *J. Infect. Dis.* **190:**1150–1157.
89. **Newell, D. G., J. A. Frost, B. Duim, J. A. Wagenaar, R. H. Madden, J. van der Plas, and S. L. W. On.** 2000. New developments in the subtyping of *Campylobacter* species, p. 27–44. *In* I. Nachamkin and M. J. Blaser (ed.), Campylobacter, 2nd ed. ASM Press, Washington, D.C.
90. **Ng, L.-K., D. E. Taylor, and M. E. Stiles.** 1988. Characterization of freshly isolated *Campylobacter coli* strains and suitability of selective media for their growth. *J. Clin. Microbiol.* **26:**518–523.
91. **Oberhelman, R. A., and D. N. Taylor.** 2000. *Campylobacter* infections in developing countries, p. 139–153. *In* I. Nachamkin and M. J. Blaser (ed.), Campylobacter, 2nd ed. ASM Press, Washington, D.C.
92. **Olsen, S. J., G. R. Hansen, L. Bartlett, C. Fitzgerald, A. Sonder, R. Manjrekar, T. Riggs, J. Kim, R. Flahart, G. Pezzino, and D. L. Swerdlow.** 2001. An outbreak of *Campylobacter jejuni* infections associated with food handler contamination: the use of pulsed-field gel electrophoresis. *J. Infect. Dis.* **183:**164–167.
93. **On, S. L.** 1996. Identification methods for campylobacters, helicobacters, and related organisms. *Clin. Microbiol. Rev.* **9:**405–422.
94. **On, S. L., and P. J. Jordon.** 2003. Evaluation of 11 PCR assays for species-level identification of *Campylobacter jejuni* and *Campylobacter coli*. *J. Clin. Microbiol.* **41:**330–336.
95. **On, S. L. W.** 2001. Taxonomy of *Campylobacter*, *Arcobacter*, *Helicobacter* and related bacteria: current status, future prospects and immediate concerns. *J. Appl. Microbiol.* **90:**1S–15S.
96. **On, S. L. W.** 1994. Confirmation of human *Campylobacter concisus* isolates misidentified as *Campylobacter mucosalis* and suggestions for improved differentiation between the two species. *J. Clin. Microbiol.* **32:**2305–2306.
97. **On, S. L. W., H. I. Atabay, J. E. L. Corry, C. S. Harrington, and P. Vandamme.** 1998. Emended description of *Campylobacter sputorum* and revision of its infrasubspecific (biovar) divisions, including *C. sputorum* biovar paraureolyticus, a urease-producing variant from cattle and humans. *Int. J. Syst. Bacteriol.* **48:**195–206.
98. **Paisley, J. W., S. Mirrett, B. A. Lauer, M. Roe, and L. B. Reller.** 1982. Dark-field microscopy of human feces for presumptive diagnosis of *Campylobacter fetus* subsp. *jejuni* enteritis. *J. Clin. Microbiol.* **15:**61–63.
99. **Park, C. H., D. L. Hixon, A. S. Polhemus, C. B. Ferguson, S. L. Hall, C. C. Risheim, and C. B. Cook.** 1983. A rapid diagnosis of campylobacter enteritis by direct smear examination. *Am. J. Clin. Pathol.* **80:**388–390.
100. **Patton, C. M., and I. K. Wachsmuth.** 1992. Typing schemes: are current methods useful? p. 110–128. *In* I. Nachamkin, M. J. Blaser, and L. S. Tompkins (ed.), Campylobacter jejuni: *Current Status and Future Trends*. American Society for Microbiology, Washington, D.C.
101. **Penner, J. L., and J. N. Hennessy.** 1980. Passive hemagglutination technique for serotyping *Campylobacter fetus* subsp. *jejuni* on the basis of soluble heat-stable antigens. *J. Clin. Microbiol.* **12:**732–737.
102. **Perlman, D. M., N. M. Ampel, R. B. Schifman, D. L. Cohn, C. M. Patton, M. L. Aguirre, W.-L. L. Wang, and M. J. Blaser.** 1988. Persistent *Campylobacter jejuni* infections in patients infected with human immunodeficiency virus (HIV). *Ann. Intern. Med.* **108:**540–546.
103. **Persson, S., and K. E. Olsen.** 2005. Multiplex PCR for identification of *Campylobacter coli* and *Campylobacter jejuni* from pure cultures and directly on stool samples. *J. Med. Microbiol.* **54:**1043–1047.
104. **Petruccelli, B. P., G. S. Murphy, J. L. Sanchez, S. Walz, R. DeFraites, J. Gelnett, R. L. Haberberger, P. Echeverria, and D. N. Taylor.** 1992. Treatment of traveler's diarrhea with ciprofloxacin and loperamide. *J. Infect. Dis.* **165:**557–560.
105. **Popovic-Uroic, T., C. M. Patton, M. A. Nicholson, and J. A. Kiehlbauch.** 1990. Evaluation of the indoxyl acetate hydrolysis test for rapid differentiation of *Campylobacter*, *Helicobacter*, and *Wolinella* species. *J. Clin. Microbiol.* **28:**2335–2339.
106. **Popovic-Uroic, T., C. M. Patton, I. K. Wachsmuth, and P. Roeder.** 1991. Evaluation of an oligonucleotide probe for identification of *Campylobacter* species. *Lab. Med.* **22:** 533–539.
107. **Rams, T. E., D. Feik, and J. Slots.** 1993. *Campylobacter rectus* in human periodontitis. *Oral Microbiol. Immun.* **8:**230–235.
108. **Ribot, E. M., C. Fitzgerald, K. Kubota, B. Swaminathan, and T. J. Barrett.** 2001. Rapid pulsed-field gel electrophoresis protocol for subtyping *Campylobacter jejuni*. *J. Clin. Microbiol.* **39:**1889–1894.
109. **Rubin, S. J., and M. Woodard.** 1983. Enhanced isolation of *Campylobacter jejuni* by cold enrichment in Campy-thio broth. *J. Clin. Microbiol.* **18:**1008–1010.
110. **Samuel, M. C., D. J. Vugia, S. Shallow, R. Marcus, S. Segler, T. McGivern, H. Kassenborg, K. Reilly, M. Kennedy, F. Angulo, and R. V. Tauxe.** 2004. Epidemiology of sporadic *Campylobacter* infection in the United States and declining trend in incidence, FoodNet 1996–1999. *Clin. Infect. Dis.* **38**(Suppl. 3)**:**165–174.
111. **Sazie, E. S. M., and A. E. Titus.** 1982. Rapid diagnosis of *Campylobacter* enteritis. *Ann. Intern. Med.* **96:**62–63.
112. **Skirrow, M. B.** 1994. Diseases due to *Campylobacter*, *Helicobacter* and related bacteria. *J. Comp. Pathol.* **111:**113–149.
113. **Skirrow, M. B.** 1977. *Campylobacter* enteritis: a "new" disease. *Br. Med. J.* **ii:**9–11.
114. **Skirrow, M. B., and M. J. Blaser.** 2000. Clinical aspects of *Campylobacter* infection, p. 69–88. *In* I. Nachamkin and M. J. Blaser (ed.), Campylobacter, 2nd ed. ASM Press, Washington, D.C.
115. **Skirrow, M. B., D. M. Jones, E. Sutcliffe, and J. Benjamin.** 1993. *Campylobacter* bacteremia in England and Wales, 1981–1991. *Epidemiol. Infect.* **110:**567–573.
116. **Spiegel, C. A., and G. Telford.** 1984. Isolation of *Wolinella recta* and *Actinomyces viscosus* from an actinomycotic chest wall mass. *J. Clin. Microbiol.* **20:**1187–1189.
117. **Stanley, J., A. P. Burnens, D. Linton, S. L. W. On, M. Costas, and R. J. Owen.** 1992. *Campylobacter helveticus* sp. nov., a new thermophilic species from domestic animals: characterization, and cloning of a species-specific DNA probe. *J. Gen. Microbiol.* **138:**2293–2303.
118. **Steele, T. W., and R. J. Owen.** 1988. *Campylobacter jejuni* subspecies *doylei* (subsp. nov.), a subspecies of nitrate-negative campylobacters isolated from human clinical specimens. *Int. J. Syst. Bacteriol.* **38:**316–318.
119. **Stucki, U., J. Frey, J. Nicolet, and A. P. Burnens.** 1995. Identification of *Campylobacter jejuni* on the basis of a species-specific gene that encodes a membrane protein. *J. Clin. Microbiol.* **33:**855–859.
120. **Szymanski, C. M., S. Goon, B. Allan, and P. Guerry.** 2005. Protein glycosylation in *Campylobacter*, p. 259–273. *In* J. M. Ketley and M. E. Konkel (ed.), Campylobacter: *Molecular and Cellular Biology*. Horizon Bioscience, Norfolk, United Kingdom.
121. **Tauxe, R. V., C. M. Patton, P. Edmonds, T. J. Barrett, D. J. Brenner, and P. A. Blake.** 1985. Illness associated

with *Campylobacter laridis*, a newly recognized *Campylobacter* species. *J. Clin. Microbiol.* **21:**222–225.

122. **Taylor, B. V., J. Williamson, J. Luck, D. Coleman, D. Jones, and A. McGregor.** 2004. Sensitivity and specificity of serology in determining recent acute *Campylobacter* infection. *Intern. Med. J.* **34:**250–258.

123. **Taylor, D. N., D. M. Perlman, P. D. Echeverria, U. Lexomboon, and M. J. Blaser.** 1993. Campylobacter immunity and quantitative excretion rates in Thai children. *J. Infect. Dis.* **168:**754–758.

124. **Tenover, F. C., L. Carlson, S. Barbagallo, and I. Nachamkin.** 1990. DNA probe culture confirmation assay for identification of thermophilic *Campylobacter* species. *J. Clin. Microbiol.* **28:**1284–1287.

125. **Thompson, J. S., D. S. Hodge, D. E. Smith, and Y. A. Yong.** 1990. Use of tri-gas incubator for routine culture of *Campylobacter* species from fecal specimens. *J. Clin. Microbiol.* **28:**2802–2803.

126. **Thompson, S. A., and M. J. Blaser.** 2000. Pathogenesis of *Campylobacter fetus* infections, p. 321–347. *In* I. Nachamkin and M. J. Blaser (ed.), Campylobacter, 2nd ed. ASM Press, Washington, D.C.

127. **Tolcin, R., M. M. LaSalvia, B. A. Kirkley, E. A. Vetter, F. Cockerill, and G. W. Procop.** 2000. Evaluation of the Alexon-Trend ProSpecT *Campylobacter* microplate assay. *J. Clin. Microbiol.* **38:**3853–3855.

128. **Valenstein, P., M. Pfaller, and M. Yungbluth.** 1996. The use and abuse of routine stool microbiology: a College of American Pathologists Q-probes study of 601 institutions. *Arch. Pathol. Lab. Med.* **120:**206–211.

129. **Vandamme, P.** 2000. Taxonomy of the family *Campylobacteraceae*, p. 3–26. *In* I. Nachamkin and M. J. Blaser (ed.), Campylobacter, 2nd ed. ASM Press, Washington, D.C.

130. **Vandamme, P., M. I. Daneshvar, F. E. Dewhirst, B. J. Paster, K. Kersters, H. Goossens, and C. W. Moss.** 1995. Chemotaxonomic analyses of *Bacteroides gracilis* and *Bacteroides ureolyticus* and reclassification of *B. gracilis* as *Campylobacter gracilis* comb. nov. *Int. J. Syst. Bacteriol.* **45:**145–152.

131. **Vandamme, P., and J. De Ley.** 1991. Proposal for a new family, *Campylobacteraceae*. *Int. J. Syst. Bacteriol.* **41:**451–455.

132. **Vandamme, P., E. Falsen, B. Pot, B. Hoste, K. Kersters, and J. De Ley.** 1989. Identification of EF group 22 campylobacters from gastroenteritis cases as *Campylobacter concisus*. *J. Clin. Microbiol.* **27:**1775–1781.

133. **Vandamme, P., M. Vancanneyt, B. Pot, L. Mels, B. Hoste, D. Dewettinck, L. Vlaes, C. Van den Borre, R. Higgins, and J. Hommez.** 1992. Polyphasic taxonomic study of the emended genus *Arcobacter* with *Arcobacter butzleri* comb. nov. and *Arcobacter skirrowii* sp. nov., an aerotolerant bacterium isolated from veterinary specimens. *Int. J. Syst. Bacteriol.* **42:**344–356.

134. **Vandamme, P., L. J. VanDoorn, S. T. Alrashid, W. G. V. Quint, J. VanderPlas, V. L. Chan, and S. L. W. On.** 1997. *Campylobacter hyoilei* Alderton et al. 1995 and *Campylobacter coli* Veron and Chatelain 1973 are subjective synonyms. *Int. J. Syst. Bacteriol.* **47:**1055–1060.

135. **Vandenberg, O., A. Dediste, K. Houf, S. Ibekwem, H. Souayah, S. Cadranel, N. Douat, G. Zissis, J.-P. Butzler, and P. Vandamme.** 2004. *Arcobacter* species in humans. *Emerg. Infect. Dis.* **10:**1863–1867.

136. **van Doorn, L. J., A. V. Van Haperen, A. Burnens, M. Huysmans, P. Vandamme, B. A. J. Giesendorf, M. J. Blaser, and W. G. V. Quint.** 1999. Rapid identification of thermotolerant *Campylobacter jejuni*, *Campylobacter coli*, *Campylobacter lari*, and *Campylobacter upsaliensis* from various geographic regions by a GTPase-based PCR-reverse hybridization assay. *J. Clin. Microbiol.* **37:**1790–1796.

137. **Van Etterijck, R., J. Breynaert, H. Revets, T. Devreker, Y. Vandenplas, P. Vandamme, and S. Lauwers.** 1996. Isolation of *Campylobacter concisus* from feces of children with and without diarrhea. *J. Clin. Microbiol.* **34:**2304–2306.

138. **Wang, H., and D. R. Murdoch.** 2004. Detection of *Campylobacter* species in faecal samples by direct gram stain microscopy. *Pathology* **36:**343–344.

139. **Wang, W.-L. L., and M. J. Blaser.** 1986. Detection of pathogenic *Campylobacter* species in blood culture systems. *J. Clin. Microbiol.* **23:**709–714.

140. **Wang, W.-L. L., L. B. Reller, B. Smallwood, N. W. Luechtefeld, and M. J. Blaser.** 1983. Evaluation of transport media for *Campylobacter jejuni* in human fecal specimens. *J. Clin. Microbiol.* **18:**803–807.

141. **Wasfy, M., B. Oyofo, A. Elgindy, and A. Churilla.** 1995. Comparison of preservation media for storage of stool samples. *J. Clin. Microbiol.* **33:**2176–2178.

142. **Wassenaar, T. M.** 1997. Toxin production by *Campylobacter* spp. *Clin. Microbiol. Rev.* **10:**466–476.

143. **Wesley, I. V.** 1994. *Arcobacter* infections, p. 181–190. *In* G. W. Beran (ed.), *CRC Handbook of Zoonosis*. CRC Press, Boca Raton, Fla.

144. **Wexler, H. M., D. Reeves, P. H. Summanen, E. Molitoris, M. McTeague, J. Duncan, K. H. Wilson, and S. M. Finegold.** 1996. *Sutterella wadsworthensis* gen. nov., sp. nov., bile-resistant microaerophilic *Campylobacter gracilis*-like clinical isolates. *Int. J. Syst. Bacteriol.* **46:**252–258.

145. **Willison, H. J.** 2005. The immunobiology of Guillain-Barre syndromes. *J. Peripher. Nerv. Syst.* **10:**94–112.

*Helicobacter**

JAMES G. FOX AND FRANCIS MEGRAUD

60

TAXONOMY

Gastric spiral-shaped bacteria have been observed in animals and humans for more than 100 years. The first recorded observations of gastric spiral-shaped bacteria in animals were made by Rappin in 1881 and Bizzozero in 1893. In 1896, Salomon noted spiral bacteria in the stomachs of dogs, cats, and Norway rats (152), but the first observation in humans was made by Krienitz in 1906 (80). In 1982, *Campylobacter pyloridis* (later known as *Helicobacter pylori*) was successfully cultured from stomach biopsy specimens from human patients with gastritis (178). Subsequently, other spiral gram-negative bacteria have been observed in and isolated from the gastrointestinal tracts of mammals such as cats, dogs, ferrets, sea mammals, and rodents (37).

Initially, many spiral gram-negative bacteria isolated from the mammalian gastrointestinal tract were grouped as campylobacters. This classification was based on similar microscopic and ultrastructural morphologies, common microaerobic growth requirements, and similar ecologic niches (Table 1). However, partial sequencing of 16S rRNA genes provided evidence that *Helicobacter pylori* belonged in a different genus (148). The genus *Helicobacter* was formally distinguished from other gram-negative curved rods (e.g., *Campylobacter*) following extensive analysis of enzymatic activities, fatty acid profiles, growth characteristics, and nucleic acid hybridization profiles, 16S rRNA sequence analysis, and most recently, 23S rRNA analysis (20, 51, 124, 133, 173). Sequencing of the *H. pylori* (1, 169) and *Helicobacter hepaticus* (164) genomes has emphasized differences but also similarities between *Campylobacter* and *Helicobacter* organisms.

DESCRIPTION OF THE GENUS

The genus *Helicobacter* comprises 23 species formally validated by international rules of nomenclature (21, 124, 125), with at least a dozen species awaiting validation or considered to be candidate species. Four of the latter, *Helicobacter cetorum*, isolated from stomachs of cetaceans; *Helicobacter winghamensis*, isolated from diarrheic patients; and *Helicobacter marmotae* and *Helicobacter mastomyrinus*, isolated from intestines and livers of rodents, have been formally named (but not validated by the *International Journal of Systematic and Evolutionary Microbiology*) and are listed in Table 1 (44, 64, 105, 157). The genus includes spiral or curved bacilli ranging from 0.3 to 1.0 μm in width and 1.5 to 10.0 μm in length. Helicobacters are gram-negative, non-spore-forming rods that may form spheroid or coccoid bodies if they are cultured for a prolonged period or if growth conditions are not optimal (Fig. 1A and B). These bacteria are motile and usually possess either single or multiple bipolar sheathed flagella (Table 1). *H. pylori* isolates, in contrast to those of other *Helicobacter* species, have multiple monopolar sheathed flagella. Several helicobacters (*Helicobacter pullorum, Helicobacter rodentium, Helicobacter mesocricatorum, Helicobacter canadensis,* and *H. winghamensis*) have unsheathed flagella like those of the campylobacters. The animal gastric helicobacters, *Helicobacter bizzozeronii, Helicobacter felis,* and *Helicobacter salomonis,* as well as the human-animal gastric pathogen "*Helicobacter heilmannii*" (formerly *Gastrospirillum hominis*), have distinctive, tightly spiraled morphologies under light and transmission electron microscopy (Fig. 1C). *H. pylori* can be induced in liquid culture to assume the morphology of "*H. heilmannii*," so these distinctions may not be absolute in vivo (33, 127).

Helicobacters are microaerobic and possess respiratory metabolic capabilities. Successful cultivation of these organisms requires a humid atmosphere maintained at 37°C with reduced levels of oxygen (5 to 10%) and increased levels of carbon dioxide (5 to 12%). Atmospheric hydrogen (as much as 5 to 10%) either is required or stimulates the growth of these organisms. Most *Helicobacter* species grow poorly, if at all, in routine aerobic atmospheres. Several helicobacters, including *H. felis* (88), *H. hepaticus* (40), and *H. rodentium* (156), can grow both anaerobically and microaerobically. Interestingly, *Helicobacter ganmani*, a rodent enteric organism, requires anaerobic conditions for growth (146).

Several biochemical and genetic criteria distinguish this genus, although significant intragenus variation exists with respect to each trait (Table 1). All helicobacters are oxidase positive and appear to be relatively inert with respect to carbohydrate pathways as determined by conventional methods. Nuclear magnetic resonance spectroscopy (65) and genomic (1) studies have revealed the existence of carbohydrate catabolic pathways in *H. pylori* (65). Comparative genomic analysis of *H. pylori* supports the presence of important catabolic pathways such as the pentose phosphate shunt, the Entner-Doudoroff pathway, glycolysis, and an

*This chapter contains information presented in chapter 58 by James Versalovic and James G. Fox in the eighth edition of this Manual.

TABLE 1 Habitats and phenotypic characteristics of *Helicobacter* species[a]

Helicobacter taxon	Source(s)	Primary site(s)	Catalase production	Nitrate reduction	Alkaline phosphatase	Urease	Indoxyl acetate hydrolysis	γ-Glutamyl transferase	Growth		Resistance to[b]:		Flagella
									At 42°C	With 1% glycine	Nalidixic acid	Cephalothin	
Human													
H. bizzozeronii[c]	Human, cat, dog, primate	Stomach	+	+	+	+	+	+	+	−	R	S	Bipolar
H. canis	Human, cat, dog	Intestine	−	−	+	−	+	+	+	−	S	I	Bipolar
H. canadensis	Human, goose	Intestine	+	+/−	−	−	+	−	+	+	R	R	Mono/bipolar
H. cinaedi	Human, hamster, macaque, fox, rat, dog	Intestine	+	+	−	−	−	−	−	+	S	I	Bipolar
H. fennelliae	Human	Intestine	+	−	+	−	+	−	−	+	S	S	Bipolar
H. pullorum	Human, chicken	Intestine	+	+	−	−	−	ND[d]	+	−	R	S	Monopolar
H. pylori	Human	Stomach	+	−	+	+	−	+	−	−	R	S	Monopolar
Helicobacter sp. strain flexispira taxon 8[e]	Human, dog, sheep, mouse	Intestine	+/−	−	−	+	−	+	+	−	R	R	Bipolar
H. winghamensis	Human	Intestine	−	−	−	−	+	ND	−	+	R	R	Bipolar
Nonhuman													
H. acinonychis	Cheetah	Stomach	+	−	+	+	−	+	−	−	R	S	Bipolar
H. aurati	Hamster	Stomach, intestine	+	−	−	+	+	+	+	−	S	R	Bipolar
H. bilis	Mouse, dog, rat	Intestine, liver	+	+	−	+	−	+	+	+	R	R	Bipolar
H. cetorum	Dolphin, whale	Stomach	+	−	−	+	−	+	+	ND	I	S	Bipolar
H. cholecystus	Hamster	Liver	+	+	+	−	−	−	+	+	I	R	Monopolar
H. felis	Cat, dog	Stomach	+	+	+	+	−	+	+	−	R	S	Bipolar
H. ganmani	Mouse	Intestine	+	+	−	−	−	ND	−	−	R	S	Bipolar
H. hepaticus	Mouse	Intestine, liver	+	+	−	+	+	−	−	+	R	R	Bipolar
H. marmotae	Woodchuck, cat	Intestine, liver	+	−	+	+	−	−	+	+	R	R	Bipolar
H. mastomyrinus	Mastomys, mouse	Intestine, liver	+	−	−	+	−	−	+	+	R	R	Bipolar
H. mesocricetorum	Hamster	Intestine	+	+	+	−	ND	−	+	−	S	R	Bipolar
H. muridarum	Mouse, rat	Intestine	+	−	+	+	+	+	−	−	R	R	Bipolar
H. mustelae	Ferret, mink	Stomach	+	+	+	+	+	+	+	−	S	R	Bipolar
H. pametensis	Bird, pig	Intestine	+	+	+	−	−	−	+	+	S	S	Peritrichous
H. rodentium	Mouse	Intestine	+	+	−	−	−	−	+	+	R	R	Bipolar
H. salomonis	Dog	Stomach	+	+	+	+	+	+	−	ND	R	S	Bipolar
H. typhlonius	Mouse	Intestine	+	+	−	−	−	−	+	+	S	R	Bipolar
H. trogontum	Rat	Intestine	+	+	−	+	−	+	+	ND	R	R	Bipolar

[a] Data are from references 21, 38, 40, 42, 43, 61, 69, 105, 133, 156, 160, 161, 173, 176, and 180. All *Helicobacter* species are oxidase positive and lack the ability to oxidize or ferment carbohydrates in routine reactions.

[b] Resistance is determined by disk diffusion. Isolates are incubated for several days at 37°C on blood-containing medium containing 30-μg antibiotic disks. Microaerobic conditions are typically used, and exact incubation times vary among organisms. Resistance (R) is defined as the complete absence of an inhibition zone, whereas intermediate (I; zones usually <15 mm in diameter) and susceptible (S; zones usually >20 mm in diameter) isolates have visible inhibition zones of various sizes.

[c] Likely the same as "*H. heilmannii*." "*H. heilmannii*" (formerly *Gastrospirillum hominis*) has the same phenotype as that listed here for *H. bizzozeronii*. Only a single "*H. heilmannii*" strain has been isolated by culture (4), and thus "*H. heilmanii*" has not been included in Table 1.

[d] ND, not determined.

[e] Formerly regarded as "*Flexispira rappini*," now subgrouped into 10 taxa (21).

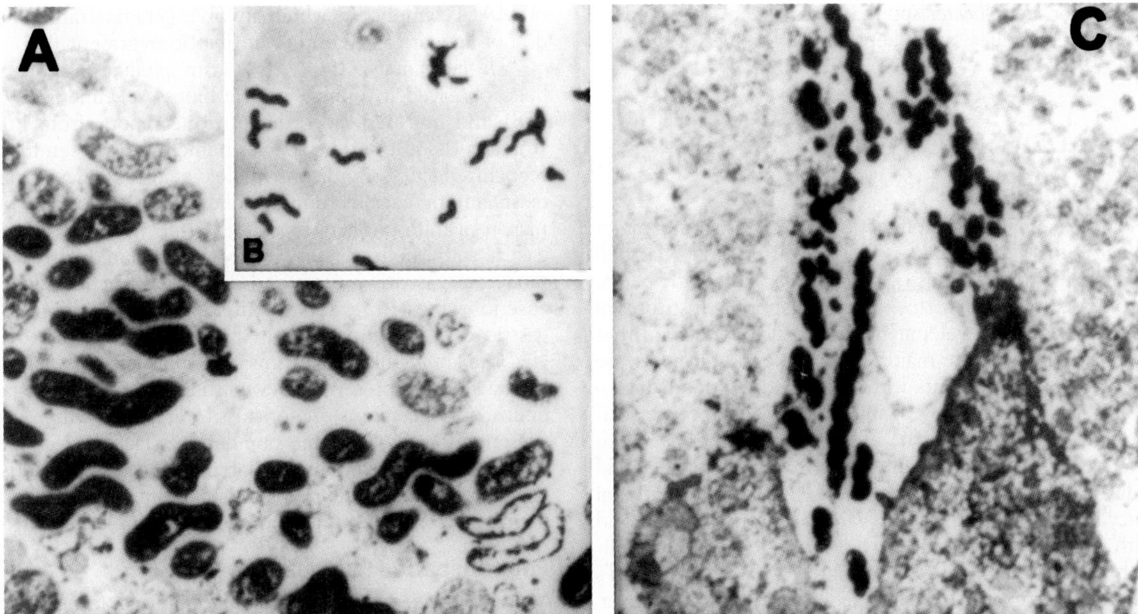

FIGURE 1 Microscopic morphology of *H. pylori* and "*H. heilmanni.*" (A) Transmission electron micrograph of a gastric biopsy specimen from an *H. pylori*-infected individual. (B) Phase-contrast micrograph of *H. pylori.* (C) Transmission electron micrograph of bacteria resembling "*H. heilmannii*" in the gastric pits of an infected cat. Adapted from reference 43 with permission.

altered noncylic version of the Krebs reaction sequence (97). Members of the genus *Helicobacter* have G+C contents ranging from 30 to 48 mol% (180), similar to those of the campylobacters.

NATURAL HABITATS

Helicobacter species have been isolated from the gastrointestinal and hepatobiliary tracts of mammals and birds (Table 1). In this chapter, we will refer to gastric (stomach) and enterohepatic (intestine and liver or bile) helicobacters in order to distinguish these organisms according to their preferred niche(s) in the gastrointestinal tract. Gastric helicobacters possess several unifying features, including phylogenetic clustering (56) and urease activity, and most have the ability to form discrete colonies on plated media (176). Gastric helicobacters inhabit primarily the stomach either within or beneath the mucus gel layer adjacent to the epithelium and rarely invade the bloodstream (in contrast to enterohepatic helicobacters). Recent data suggest that *H. pylori* may on occasion be located intracellularly (121, 154). *H. pylori* colonizes the cardia, corpus, and antrum (distal portion) of the human stomach. Gastric helicobacters may also be found transiently in areas of gastric metaplasia of the proximal small intestine (duodenum), gastric juice (vomitus), saliva, and feces.

The reservoir of *H. pylori* is essentially the human stomach, and *H. pylori* can be considered the gastric helicobacter of humans (103). However, *H. pylori* strains have been isolated occasionally from animals (cats and nonhuman primates), which were most likely infected by humans because of either close cohabitation with humans or, in the case of cats, inadvertent exposure to *H. pylori* while being maintained in a vivarium (26, 60). Conversely, "*H. heilmannii*" is an inhabitant of the stomachs of pigs, cats, dogs, wild rats, and nonhuman primates, and infection with this organism is considered to have zoonotic potential (162).

The route of transmission of *H. pylori* from one human stomach to another human stomach has not been definitely identified. There is evidence for both oral-oral and fecal-oral transmission. Fecal-oral transmission implies (i) that *H. pylori* must survive gut passage (25) which apparently occurs mainly in the case of a short transit time (diarrhea) (131), (ii) that fecal hygiene is not optimal, and (iii) that the water supply is not treated properly. These conditions usually exist in developing countries, making likely that fecal-oral transmission occurs in this context. The rationale for oral-oral transmission relies on the presence of *H. pylori* in gastric juice which has been regurgitated, thus allowing *H. pylori* to temporarily colonize the oral cavity. There are reports of isolation of *H. pylori* from dental plaque and saliva (52, 77, 131). Indeed, a recent 6-year prospective study demonstrated that dental professionals are at greater risk of being infected with *H. pylori* than are controls (98). *H. pylori* could then be transmitted to another subject via the oral-oral route. Another possibility is via vomitus since *H. pylori* can remain viable in this biological medium for hours (7, 131). In any case, the oral-oral route of transmission is probably less efficient than the fecal-oral one. This fact contributes to the lower *H. pylori* prevalence in developed countries. Transmission appears to be most frequent in intrafamilial settings during childhood and accounts for a maximum of two-thirds of the cases; however, in a third of the cases, children are infected while their parents are not (24).

In contrast to the gastric helicobacters, enterohepatic helicobacters inhabit the lower bowels and hepatobiliary tracts of mammals and birds. In humans, enterohepatic helicobacters *(H. canadensis, Helicobacter canis, Helicobacter cinaedi, Helicobacter fennelliae, "Helicobacter rappini," H. pullorum, and H. winghamensis)* have been isolated from rectal swabs and feces and in some cases from blood and other extraintestinal sites (13, 105, 160, 161). Several of these as well as other *Helicobacter* spp. have also been identified by molecular techniques in the hepatobiliary tissues of humans (6, 37, 39).

CLINICAL SIGNIFICANCE

Gastric Helicobacters

H. pylori is the main cause of peptic ulcer disease and a major risk factor for gastric cancer (165). Warren and Marshall (178) first proposed the association of *H. pylori* with peptic ulcer disease. In February 1994, the U.S. National Institutes of Health Consensus Development Conference concluded that *H. pylori* infection is the major cause of peptic ulcer disease and stated that all patients with confirmed peptic ulcer disease associated with *H. pylori* infection should receive antimicrobial treatment (113). This statement has been systematically repeated in all consensus conferences held worldwide since then (89). In June 1994, the International Agency for Research on Cancer Working Group of the World Health Organization identified *H. pylori* as a group I, or definite, human carcinogen. Approximately 50% of the world's population is estimated to be infected with *H. pylori*. However, there is a large difference in the prevalences of *H. pylori* infection among developing and developed countries (140, 181). In developing countries, the infection occurs very early in life and most of the children are infected by the age of 10. The prevalence remains in the range of 80 to 90% for all adult age groups in developing countries. In developed countries, a progressive increase in prevalence is observed, from a low percentage of infection in children to 40 to 50% infection rates in the older age groups. This is not the consequence of a progressive acquisition of the infection but rather the result of a cohort effect (8). Indeed, the majority of subjects acquire the infection in childhood, and the infection persists lifelong. Thus, if the oldest individuals have a higher *H. pylori* infection prevalence, it is because the risk of becoming infected was higher when they were children.

Individuals infected with *H. pylori* may develop acute gastritis (abdominal pain, nausea, and vomiting) within 2 weeks following infection. *H. pylori* establishes a chronic infection in the majority of infected people, represented by chronic gastritis of different types. Prominent mucosal inflammation in chronic active gastritis is often evident in the antrum (antral predominant gastritis), predisposing to hyperacidity and duodenal ulcer disease. Many patients infected with *H. pylori* have recurrent abdominal symptoms (nonulcer dyspepsia) without ulcer disease, and there appears to be a clinical benefit in eradicating *H. pylori* in these patients (108). Inflammation of the duodenum (duodenitis) often occurs with *H. pylori* infection, and duodenal ulcers develop in as many as 16% of infected individuals. *H. pylori* infection has been associated with the majority of duodenal and gastric ulcers (3). *H. pylori*-associated multifocal atrophic pangastritis or atrophic corpus-predominant gastritis results from long-standing infection and is characterized by glandular atrophy, intestinal metaplasia, and sparse inflammatory cells, pathophysiological features which manifest in the patient as low acidity and an increased risk of gastric carcinoma (28, 62). *H. pylori* infection is an independent risk factor for the development of atrophic gastritis, gastric ulcer disease (166), gastric adenocarcinomas (118, 129), and gastric mucosa-associated lymphoid tissue (MALT) lymphomas (32). Gastric MALT lymphoma, a rare stomach cancer, is caused by *H. pylori* infection. Indeed, it is the only cancer which can be cured by antibiotics (15, 183). However, advanced cases of MALT lymphoma which involve genetic translocations do not appear to respond to antibiotic treatment (2).

"*H. heilmannii*" (formerly *Gastrospirillum hominis*) has been observed in human gastric biopsy specimens (29, 67, 158) and cultured, according to one report, from human stomach tissue (4). The species name has not been formally recognized since significant nucleic acid sequence variation exists among various human isolates, resulting in the designation of multiple genotypes (19). Infection with the large gastric spiral helicobacters has been associated with mild to moderate gastritis in cats and dogs (119), peptic ulcer disease in swine (143), and gastritis, peptic ulcer disease, and gastric MALT lymphomas in humans (66, 67, 111, 170). "*H. heilmannii*"-like organisms are relatively uncommon in humans, being present in fewer than 1% of human gastric endoscopy specimens, in contrast to *H. pylori*, which can be present in >90% in some populations. *Helicobacter* species have been observed in and isolated from the stomach tissues of other mammals, including cats, dogs, ferrets, rodents, sea mammals, and nonhuman primates (Table 1).

Enterohepatic Helicobacters

Multiple species, including *H. cinaedi* and *H. fennelliae*, have been implicated as causes of human gastroenteritis and bacteremia, particularly in immunocompromised individuals (54, 86, 144). Cases of human gastroenteritis have also been associated with infection with *H. canadensis* (38), *H. canis* (161), *H. pullorum* (43, 160), and *H. winghamensis* (105). *Helicobacter* sp. strain flexispira organisms have been divided into 10 taxonomic taxa (21). *Helicobacter* sp. strain flexispira taxon 8 includes clinically relevant isolates that have been implicated in cases of human gastroenteritis (5, 149) and bacteremia (21). In contrast to *H. pylori*, *H. cinaedi* has been identified in the blood of multiple patients with febrile bacteremia and has been associated with multifocal cellulitis or monoarticular arthritis in a subset of infected individuals (12, 75). *H. cinaedi* (previously identified in some reports as *Helicobacter* sp. strain Mainz) (174) was cultured from the blood and joint fluid of a human immunodeficiency virus type 1-infected male with septic arthritis and recurrent fever (69). *H. fennelliae* has occasionally been isolated from human blood (115) and was associated with septic shock in a non-human immunodeficiency virus type 1-infected individual (68). Presumably, these bacteremia-associated helicobacters invaded the bloodstream via colonization of the human lower gastrointestinal tract.

Enterohepatic *Helicobacter* species have been detected in the human hepatobiliary tract by using molecular methods. In Chilean patients with chronic cholecystitis, *Helicobacter bilis* and *H. pullorum* were detected in gallbladder tissue and bile specimens (39). *Helicobacter* spp. have been identified in liver specimens from patients with primary sclerosing cholangitis (117), cholangiocarcinoma (116), and hepatocellular carcinoma (6, 116) and most recently in livers (with cirrhosis and hepatocellular carcinoma) of patients with hepatitis C viral infections (147) by genus-specific PCR amplification and partial DNA sequencing. The pathogenic significance of *Helicobacter* species DNA demonstrated by PCR amplification is not clear since helicobacters have not been cultured from the human hepatobiliary tract.

Several other species of enterohepatic helicobacters have not been isolated to date from human specimens, even though they cause significant diseases in other mammals (Table 1). In addition to the intestine, enterohepatic helicobacters colonize and cause inflammation in the mammalian hepatobiliary tract. For example, the isolation of *H. cinaedi* from the colon and liver of a 2-year-old rhesus monkey (42) and the isolation of *H. canis* from a dog with hepatitis (41) implicate these organisms as possible etiologic agents of chronic hepatitis in nonhuman primates and dogs, respectively. *H. hepaticus* infection is associated with multifocal necrotic hepatitis in several strains of barrier-maintained mice and is responsible for the development of hepatic adenomas and hepatocellular carcinomas in A/JCr mice, $B_6C_3F_1$ mice, and A × B recombinant inbred mice (40, 45, 70). Coinfection with *H. hepaticus* and *H. rodentium* as well as monoinfection with *H. bilis* has also recently been demonstrated to be a critical component in the development of cholesterol gallstones in C57L mice fed a lithogenic diet (99).

COLLECTION, TRANSPORT, AND STORAGE OF SPECIMENS

Blood Specimens

Given that *H. pylori* specifically adheres to the gastric mucosal epithelium and seldom is identified intracellularly in gastric infections, it has rarely been isolated from human blood. In contrast, enterohepatic helicobacters translocate across the intestinal barrier and cause invasive infections. If bacteremia is suspected, peripheral venous blood should be collected in commercially available aerobic and anaerobic blood culture bottles as recommended by the manufacturer. Culture conditions are described in the subsequent section. No comparative studies have been performed with the different culture bottles available commercially. However, detection of these slowly growing bacteria which do not lead to detectable turbidity is linked to careful measurement of optical density in blood being incubated in automated blood equipment.

Feces

Gastric helicobacters *H. pylori* and "*H. heilmannii*" are rarely isolated from human fecal specimens. Experimental administration of a diarrheic compound increases the probability of being able to culture *H. pylori* from stools of *H. pylori*-infected patients (130). In contrast, enterohepatic helicobacters, like campylobacters, can be cultivated routinely from fecal specimens. These organisms are likely to be underisolated due to the primary focus of diagnostic laboratories being directed at the isolation of thermophilic campylobacters (e.g., *Campylobacter jejuni*). Enterohepatic helicobacters grow at 37°C but not uniformly at 42°C, the temperature often used for *Campylobacter* species isolation. Importantly, unlike some campylobacters, enterohepatic helicobacters require 5 to 10% hydrogen for optimum growth. They also may be susceptible to antibiotics present in the primary isolation medium, and they rapidly lose their viability.

Gastric Biopsy Specimens

Gastric biopsy specimens are obtained for the direct diagnosis of *H. pylori* or "*H. heilmannii*" infection. This is achieved by the use of a rapid urease test, impression smears, histopathology, or PCR. Culture of *H. pylori* may be necessary for antimicrobial susceptibility testing, diagnostic confirmation, or molecular fingerprinting in epidemiologic studies. It is stressed, however, that the proper collection, storage, and transport of gastric biopsy specimens are important for successful culture of *H. pylori*.

Although endoscopic features of *H. pylori* infection are considered not to be specific, the new method of confocal laser endomicroscopy has allowed, for the first time, surface microscopy imaging of living tissue during ongoing endoscopy and observation of *H. pylori* (76).

Biopsy specimens are routinely obtained from the antrum and corpus by esophagogastroduodenal endoscopy. The recommended number of biopsy specimens is two from each site for histology (22), one or two from each site for culture, and one from the antrum for a urease test. Biopsy specimens for histology are fixed in buffered formalin before being paraffin embedded.

H. pylori is sensitive to desiccation, ambient atmosphere, and room temperature. Therefore, a transport medium must be used to maintain the viability of the organisms. For short-term transport (less than 4 h), saline may be sufficient; otherwise, a semisolid transport medium maintained at 4°C is preferable. Stuart's transport medium, brucella broth with 20% glycerol, or Portagerm pylori (bioMérieux, Durham, N.C.) can be used for this purpose (45, 54, 115). Transport containers which maintain a temperature below 10°C for up to 16 h (Sarstedt, Nümbrecht, Germany) can be used to send biopsy specimens by mail. If culture of *H. pylori* is not possible within 24 h, it is recommended to freeze the biopsy specimen at −70°C in a tube without any medium and to transport it in dry ice. This method has proved to be efficient.

For long-term storage, the recommendation is to freeze freshly isolated cultures at −70°C in glycerol-containing media. Strains can then be recovered decades apart (59). Short-term maintenance is possible for 1 week in glycerol-containing medium at 4°C; 81% of isolates remained viable in one study (59).

Gastric Juice

Gastric juice can be obtained by aspiration after the introduction of a nasogastric tube, but it is easier to collect this fluid with the so-called string test. This test (Enterotest; HDC, San Jose, Calif.) consists of swallowing a capsule fixed to a string. After 30 min, the capsule dissolves and the string is removed. The distal portion of the string, which is impregnated with gastric juice, is cut and introduced into a transport medium. The impregnated material can then be used for culture or PCR (137). Recently, a novel device has been designed for the rapid recovery of gastric epithelia and mucus. It consists of an extendable orogastric brush contained within a plastic tube which is swallowed by the patient. Once the tube is in the stomach lumen, the brush is extended and brushed across the mucosa. It is then retracted into the protective sleeve and withdrawn from the patient. The material from the brush can then be used for culture of *H. pylori* (53).

DIRECT EXAMINATION AND DETECTION

Fecal *H. pylori* Antigen Detection

An enzyme-linked immunosorbent assay (ELISA) can be used to detect *H. pylori* antigens in stools and has been approved in the United States by the Food and Drug Administration. The first commercially available reagent, named Premier platinum HpSA (Meridian, Cincinnati, Ohio), consisting of a polyclonal antibody fixed on microwells, proved to be sensitive and specific in a multicenter study performed in Europe (171). A systematic review of published data including results of 89 studies (10,858 patients) confirmed the value of HpSA as a diagnostic tool for pretreatment (sensitivity, 91%; specificity, 93%) as well as for follow-up posttreatment (47).

A new generation of antigen stool tests using a monoclonal antibody directed against *H. pylori* catalase has also been developed (Amplified-IDEA-HpStar; DaKo, Glostrup, Denmark). This test ensures consistent quality of the reagents and improved reproducibility (94). Monoclonal antibodies have also been used to develop an immunoenzymatic rapid test (Immunocard STAT HpSA; Meridian) (91). The most reliable test is the ELISA laboratory test using monoclonal antibodies (sensitivity, 96%; specificity, 97%). Rapid antigen stool tests using monoclonal antibodies are very promising but need further evaluation.

Some aspects with an impact on the reliability of stool antigen-based assays, such as the influence of the frequency of bowel movements, have not been studied in detail. In principle, a short transit time should favor retrieval of unaltered antigens unless there is an excessive dilution factor, and constipation may lead to antigen degradation. Experimentally, tests performed on spiked stool specimens showed decreased sensitivity after a 24-h delay (110). Antigen stool tests may be well suited for children, from whom it is common to obtain stools, in contrast to adults, who usually prefer another type of test, e.g., the urea breath test (UBT). Although these tests have been found to be quite specific, it will be interesting to ascertain whether enterohepatic helicobacters sometimes present in stools could also be detected and possibly interfere with the interpretation of test results. Up to this point, it has been considered unnecessary to screen stool specimens for enterohepatic helicobacters given the low number of reported enterohepatic helicobacter cases. However, the recent identification of enterohepatic helicobacters in appreciable numbers of samples from diarrheic and nondiarrheic individuals may require a reevaluation of their impact on *H. pylori* stool antigen assays (14, 58).

Gastric Biopsies

Smear Evaluation

Imprint cytology specimens do not require overnight formalin fixation and provide a rapid adjunct to histopathologic examination of gastric biopsy specimens. After biopsy specimens are collected with forceps, imprints are made by pressing a needle against the tissue on a glass slide or by simply rubbing the tissue over the slide. Cytology specimens may be prepared immediately following biopsy by staining the imprints with a rapid Giemsa or Gram stain, and *H. pylori* or "*H. heilmannii*" organisms may be directly visualized. This approach has been demonstrated to match or outperform conventional histology in multiple studies (17, 107, 132). When imprint smears were used, 30 of 32 biopsy specimens with positive *H. pylori* cultures yielded visible organisms by Gram staining (132). "*H. heilmannii*" organisms were detected in 11 of 100 patients with dyspepsia by imprint cytology. Imprint cytology may be more sensitive than histology for detection of this organism (17). Direct fecal smears, like fecal cultures, lack utility for the detection of *H. pylori*.

Urease Testing

H. pylori produces large amounts of extracellular urease which can be detected within hours following introduction of gastric biopsy tissue into a urea-containing medium. Urease catalyzes the hydrolysis of urea into ammonia and carbamate. The net effect of ammonia production is to increase local pH. Biopsy samples are placed in an agar gel or on a paper strip containing a pH indicator. If organisms are present in sufficient numbers in the antral biopsy sample, a color change will occur as a result of urea breakdown and ammonia production by *H. pylori* urease. Commercial rapid urease tests include the agar gel-based tests (e.g., CLOtest [Kimberly-Clark, Neenah, Wis.] and Hp*fast* [GI Supply, Camp Hill, Pa.]) and paper strip tests (e.g., PyloriTek [BARD, Murray Hill, N.J.]) (142, 184). These tests can be used in the endoscopy ward. Detection sensitivity may approach 90%, but this depends on the *H. pylori* density in mucosal biopsy specimens and the number of biopsy specimens sampled. At least one fresh biopsy specimen from the gastric angle or antrum should be submitted for rapid urease testing. The sensitivity of rapid urease testing is maximized if specimens are obtained from the gastric angle (182) and multiple specimens are obtained (100). Agar gel-based tests have their optimal sensitivity after a 24-h incubation, whereas strip tests are optimal within an hour, making them truly rapid tests. The specificities of the urease tests are usually excellent. Agar gel-based rapid urease assays represent a cost-effective and widely used approach to screen biopsy tissue for *H. pylori* infection.

The urease broth tests commonly used in the laboratory are not optimized to have sensitivities equivalent to those of commercially available kits.

Histology

The standard hematoxylin and eosin tissue staining technique is not sufficient to accurately detect *H. pylori*. Various special stains, including Giemsa and the modified Steiner silver, must be used (141). The Warthin Starry stain can also be used but necessitates trained histology personnel to perform the technique. The sensitivity for discerning the presence or absence of *H. pylori* in gastric tissue depends on the quality of the samples and is very much observer dependent. Although the specificity is usually adequate, the presence of bacteria with atypical morphologies may result in misinterpretations. Under optimal conditions, however, histological diagnosis can have a sensitivity and specificity of 95%. Immunohistological staining with specific *H. pylori* antibodies can also improve specificity. More recently, fluorescence in situ hybridization with species-specific 16S rRNA probes (Createogen GmbH, Augsburg, Germany) has been proposed for the detection of *H. pylori* (150) and "*H. heilmannii*" (170) in human gastric biopsy specimens. *H. pylori* and "*H. heilmannii*" can be further distinguished by their respective morphologies in gastric biopsy specimens (Fig. 1).

DNA Amplification

Since rapid urease testing, histologic examination, and culture yield high sensitivities and specificities for the diagnosis of *H. pylori* infection, PCR amplification of *H. pylori* DNA in gastric biopsy specimens may not be cost-effective as a primary diagnostic strategy. Standard PCR methods which specifically detect *H. pylori* in gastric biopsy specimens have been developed and include different target genes such as 23S rRNA (93), *glmM* (92), and *vacA* (175). In a comparative study of five different target sequences, with culture of *H. pylori* as the "gold standard," the method using the *glmM* gene had the best accuracy (92). Development of real-time PCR assays based on the fluorescent resonance energy transfer method may have increased diagnostic utility because of the assays' improved sensitivities and ease of performance and the ability to detect macrolide resistance by using the same assay (see "Antibiotic Susceptibilities"). Species-specific PCR assays have been developed for other helicobacters such as *H. pullorum*

(14) and *H. hepaticus* (145). However, no PCR-based tests for enterohepatic helicobacters are commercially available at this time.

CULTURE AND ISOLATION PROCEDURES

Gastric Helicobacters

Although *H. pylori* can be routinely isolated by culture from human gastric biopsy samples, *H. pylori* infection is usually diagnosed by nonculture methods such as histology, serology, or urease testing. However, the increasing prevalence of antimicrobial resistance (27) has stimulated efforts to culture organisms for antimicrobial susceptibility testing.

For *H. pylori* culture, it is recommended to grind the gastric biopsy specimens to provide a higher yield of bacteria. This can be performed with an electric grinder and probes. However, if PCR has to be performed, disposable grinders are recommended to avoid contamination.

The biopsy suspension must be plated rapidly onto fresh media. Various agar media can be used, including brain heart infusion, brucella agar, Columbia agar, Wilkins Chalgren agar, and Trypticase soy agar supplemented with 10% blood or serum. Cyclodextrin can also be used to improve growth (123). Ideally, more than one medium should be used, one selective and one nonselective. For selectivity, Skirrow's supplement or Dent's supplement gives satisfactory results.

Incubation must be performed at 37°C in a humid microaerobic atmosphere (5% O_2, 10% CO_2, and 85% N_2) which is achieved by using a special incubator or jars. An apparatus which creates the proper atmosphere and ensures that the jar is airtight can be used (Anoxomat; MART Microbiology B.V., Lichentwoorde, The Netherlands). Another alternative is to use commercial gas-generating sachets in jars (CampyPak Plus [BD Diagnostics Systems, Sparks, Md.] and Anaxopack-Campylo [Remel, Lenexa, Kans.]). The presence of hydrogen in the atmosphere enhances growth. Smooth, circular colonies may appear after 3 days of incubation, but the plates must be kept for 10 days before concluding that the culture attempt has a negative result.

Currently, only one "*H. heilmannii*" strain has been cultured from a human gastric biopsy specimen after 7 days on a nonselective medium containing 7% lysed horse blood in a 5% O_2 and 10% CO_2 atmosphere (4).

Enterohepatic Helicobacters

Selective, enriched media and a microaerobic atmosphere are essential for the cultivation of helicobacters from feces or rectal swabs. *H. canadensis*, *H. canis*, *H. cinaedi*, *H. fennelliae*, *H. pullorum*, *Helicobacter* sp. strain flexispira taxon 8, and *H. winghamensis* have been isolated from humans with gastroenteritis (37). Fresh stool specimens should be plated directly onto selective media and incubated for a minimum of 5 days (5 to 7 days) at 37°C in a microaerobic atmosphere. We recommend selective CVA medium (Columbia agar base with 5% sheep blood and cefoperazone, vancomycin, and amphotericin B; Remel) and a defined microaerobic atmosphere in partially evacuated anaerobic jars (5 to 10% carbon dioxide, 5 to 10% hydrogen, 5 to 10% oxygen, and 80% N_2) for the successful isolation of most enterohepatic helicobacters from human as well as animal feces (37, 174). Commercial gas-generating sachets (e.g., CampyPak Plus [BD Diagnostic Systems]) have been used to isolate enterohepatic helicobacters, but because of increased atmospheric hydrogen requirements, the amount of hydrogen may be inadequate in such systems (37). Alternatively, *H. winghamensis* was isolated from human stool on nonselective Mueller-Hinton agar supplemented with 10% sheep blood in a defined microaerobic atmosphere as described above (105). Some authors from South Africa recommend a special protocol that allows the primary isolation of multiple species (84, 85). It must be cautioned, however, that most laboratories do not use the high H_2 level (40%) involved in this approach because of its flammable nature.

Blood culture isolates have been detected in aerobic and anaerobic bottles (usually aerobic bottles only) by using routine media with prolonged incubation (minimum of 6 days) in automated instruments such as the BACTEC (Becton Dickinson, Franklin Lakes, N.J.) (12) and the BacT/Alert (bioMérieux) systems (126). Identifying enterohepatic helicobacters in blood cultures may require special stains. The authors of a multicenter study, which included 22 *H. cinaedi* blood isolates, noted that these thin, gull-shaped organisms were generally not visible upon Gram staining and required acridine orange staining, dark-field microscopy, or Giemsa staining for visualization (75). A modified Gram stain with carbol (0.5% [wt/vol]) or basic fuchsin (0.1% [wt/vol]) as the counterstain is also recommended for detection. Instrument-positive blood cultures should be stained with acridine orange if Gram staining is negative.

Nonselective, blood-enriched media are preferred for the isolation of helicobacters from primary blood culture media and sterile body fluids. *H. cinaedi* isolates from positive blood cultures have been cultivated in 2 to 3 days at 37°C on nonselective blood media (e.g., brucella or Columbia agar base with 5% horse or sheep blood) in a microaerobic atmosphere (e.g., CampyPak Plus [BD Diagnostic Systems] or partially evacuated jars with defined microaerobic atmospheres as described above). Supplementation of atmospheric hydrogen (5 to 10%) permitted successful culture of *H. cinaedi* in microaerobic conditions (174). Supplementation of atmospheric hydrogen occurs by the addition of gas-generating sachets to closed containers or, ideally, by direct supplementation with gas tanks containing 5 to 10% hydrogen (37). The only documented examples of *Helicobacter* species cultivation from nonblood sterile body fluids include the isolation of *H. cinaedi* from cerebrospinal fluid in nonselective Trypticase soy broth (126) and that of *Helicobacter* sp. strain Mainz (reclassified as *H. cinaedi*) from joint fluid on nonselective blood agar at 37°C (69, 174).

IDENTIFICATION

Helicobacters yield various colony phenotypes on blood agar, ranging from discrete, gray, and translucent colonies of *H. pylori* and selected gastric helicobacters to various swarming phenotypes of intestinal helicobacters and some gastric helicobacters (e.g., *H. felis*). Enterohepatic helicobacters yield a swarming phenotype with a thin film (e.g., *H. cinaedi and H. fennelliae*) or a thick, mucoid film similar to that of campylobacters (e.g., *H. pullorum and H. canadensis*). Helicobacters have a characteristic morphology visualized by light microscopy that resembles that of other gram-negative spiral or curved bacteria (Fig. 1; Table 1). These organisms usually appear faint by conventional Gram staining and may require counterstaining with carbol fuchsin (0.5% [wt/vol]) for enhanced visualization. Most helicobacter isolates are motile if observed by phase-contrast microscopy. Helicobacters are routinely tested for oxidase, catalase, and urease activities (Table 1). All helicobacters are oxidase positive. Most *Helicobacter* species, including *H. pylori*, are catalase positive (Table 1).

Gastric Helicobacters

The morphologies of helicobacters observed in gastric biopsy specimens may differ markedly from those observed in a Gram-stained preparation of cultured organisms. For example, *H. pylori* usually appears as a curved or straight rod in culture, whereas stained tissue biopsy samples usually reveal a helical or more strikingly curved appearance. "*H. heilmannii*" (likely identical to *H. bizzozeronii;* Table 1) is usually distinguished from *H. pylori* by its larger size and more pronounced helical morphology in gastric biopsy specimens (Fig. 1) (67). Because *H. felis* cannot be distinguished from "*H. heilmannii*" or *H. bizzozeronii* by light microscopy in human gastric biopsy specimens, *H. felis* must be cultured or identified by electron microscopy (46, 87).

H. pylori infection is diagnosed by microscopic morphology (Gram or Giemsa staining) and the presence of catalase, oxidase, and urease activities from primary culture. *H. cineadi* also has been identified by DNA analysis in gastric biopsy samples that were urease negative (136). *C. jejuni*, another urease-negative relative of *H. pylori* (151), or the rare *C. jejuni* subspecies *doylei* can also be found in the stomach, highlighting the importance of performing biochemical tests. Rapid urease, indoxyl acetate hydrolysis, and hippurate hydrolysis tests distinguish *H. pylori* from *C. jejuni* (chapter 59) (139). Commercial tests for urease (Christensen's urea agar slant; Remel or BBL Microbiology Systems), indoxyl acetate (Remel), and hippurate hydrolysis (Remel) are available and convenient for rapid identification of cultured specimens. In a study of 400 clinical isolates, all *H. pylori* isolates were positive for cytochrome oxidase, catalase, and urease activities (Table 1).

Enterohepatic Helicobacters

The enterohepatic helicobacters possess several distinguishing biochemical characteristics. Most intestinal helicobacters isolated from humans, such as *H. canadensis*, *H. cinaedi*, *H. fennelliae*, and *H. pullorum*, lack urease activity. Distinguishing catalase-positive, urease-negative helicobacters from the enteric campylobacters (e.g., *C. jejuni*) may be especially challenging. Unlike *C. jejuni* and *Campylobacter coli*, *H. cinaedi* and *H. fennelliae* do not survive at 42°C and *H. cinaedi* does not hydrolyze indoxyl acetate (Table 1) (139). Indoxyl acetate hydrolysis distinguishes *C. jejuni* and *C. coli* from *H. pullorum* (Table 1). *H. pullorum* is distinguished from *Campylobacter lari* only by its resistance to nalidixic acid. A nalidixic acid-resistant *C. lari* isolate would require species-specific PCR of 16S rRNA target sequences (160) for differentiation from *H. pullorum*. *H. canadensis* was initially characterized as a separate cluster of *H. pullorum*-like isolates capable of hydrolyzing indoxyl acetate and resistant to nalidixic acid (38). Unlike most other helicobacters, *H. canis* is catalase negative and urease negative. To distinguish *H. canis* from catalase-negative campylobacters, the nitrate reduction and indoxyl acetate hydrolysis tests may be useful (Table 1). It is important to note that diarrheic or nondiarrheic stool specimens may be cocolonized with multiple *Helicobacter* spp. and *Campylobacter* spp., making a complete diagnostic evaluation challenging (84, 85, 155).

NONINVASIVE TESTS

In addition to the detection in stool samples of *H. pylori* antigens by immunoenzymatic techniques and of *H. pylori* DNA by real-time PCR as previously mentioned, there are two other noninvasive approaches that can be utilized for the diagnosis of *H. pylori* infection: the detection of specific antibodies in serum, saliva, and urine, and the UBT.

UBT

The UBT has been developed specifically for *H. pylori* detection (79). It is based on an important feature of this bacterium, production of a large amount of urease. A solution containing isotopically labeled urea is ingested by the patient. If *H. pylori* is present in the stomach, the labeled urea is broken down into labeled CO_2 and ammonia; the labeled CO_2 is then absorbed into the bloodstream and exhaled in the breath of the patient being tested.

This test comprises either a carbon radioactive isotope (^{14}C) or a nonradioactive natural isotope (^{13}C). Both types of the test have been approved by the U.S. Food and Drug Administration for the diagnosis of *H. pylori* infection. $^{14}CO_2$ can be detected by a scintillation counter 20 min after ingestion, whereas for $^{13}CO_2$, the $^{13}C/^{12}C$ ratio is determined before and 30 min after ingestion by a gas isotope ratio mass spectrometer or an infrared spectrometer. The result is then expressed as a δ value between 0 and 30 min. The standardized ^{13}C-UBT must be performed on a subject after an overnight fast. A test meal consisting of citric acid makes this test more sensitive by delaying gastric emptying but also possibly by increasing urease activity (23). An initial breath sample is then obtained by blowing into a tube with a straw. Subsequently, a 75-mg dose of ^{13}C-urea is ingested. The patient must remain inactive, with no smoking, eating, or drinking, and 30 min later, a second breath sample is obtained. If an infrared spectrometer is used, a larger amount of exhaled air must be obtained by blowing into a special balloon. The cutoff used to define a positive result is usually a δ of 4.5‰.

With regard to the ^{14}C-UBT, there has been an ongoing effort to develop an assay which would allow a decrease in the dose of radioactive isotope administered. The test can now be performed with only 1 μCi contained in a capsule (138). The cutoff to define a positive result is usually 2% of the administered dose at 20 min. In contrast to the ^{13}C-UBT, the ^{14}C-UBT cannot be used for children and pregnant women. Furthermore, its use is not allowed in certain countries. The limitation on the ^{13}C-UBT is the availability of a spectrometer, but specimens can be sent by mail.

The UBT is considered to be the best noninvasive test for patient follow-up after *H. pylori* eradication, and its use has been consistently recommended in consensus conferences (96). UBTs have reproducibly proved highly accurate with a high degree of reliability in all the studies performed (sensitivity and specificity in the range of 95%). Importantly, the results are not influenced by transport conditions (tubes of breath air can be transported and stored for weeks at room temperature) and the measurement is observer independent.

Antibody Detection

Serologic testing represents a primary screening method for the diagnosis of *H. pylori* infection. Pooled *H. pylori* antigens of high-molecular-weight surface-associated proteins, acid extracts, or whole-cell lysates (sonicates) are used in most serologic assays. Various cytosolic and cell surface-associated proteins represent immunodominant antigens recognized by serum antibodies of infected individuals (78). Infection with *H. pylori* results in a local and systemic humoral response to multiple antigens (78, 168). In contrast to serum immunoglobulin M (IgM) levels, serum IgA and IgG levels persist for months and years and correlate with active infection in untreated individuals (11, 112, 163). Only a small percentage of individuals do not have detectable systemic seroconversion following infection (100). Anti-*H. pylori* serum IgG levels are more consistently elevated than serum IgA levels. Consequently, serum IgG immunoassays yield greater sensitivities and specificities than serum IgA assays (82).

Commercial ELISA kits detecting anti-*H. pylori* IgG in serum are the serologic tests of choice for the primary screening of patients with uncomplicated infections (82). These recommended ELISA-based tests include HM-CAP (Enteric Products, Westbury, N.Y.), *H. pylori* IgG ELISA (Wampole Laboratories, Cranbury, N.J.), Premier (Meridian), and Pyloriset EIA-GIII (Orion, Espoo, Finland) (109). Overall, the median sensitivity and specificity for all commercially available *H. pylori* serology kits are 92 and 83%, respectively (82). Performance varies significantly among commercial serologic kits, with top performers exceeding 90% in sensitivity and specificity and bottom performers failing to reach 90% in sensitivity or 80% in specificity (82). However, the determined specificity of serology may be incorrectly low in some comparative studies where the gold standard used has poor sensitivity. ELISA serologic testing has the lowest cost per correct diagnosis, but overall accuracy is lower than that of stool antigen testing or UBT (172). Patients infected with "*H. heilmannii*" are usually negative by anti-*H. pylori* IgG assays (67). Serum IgA immunoassays may be used as second-line tests for assessing equivocal or possibly false-negative anti-*H. pylori* serum IgG results. The key advantage of serum IgA studies is that follow-up testing may be performed with the same serum sample. In one study, more than 7% of samples with a negative serum IgG result were found to possess detectable anti-*H. pylori* serum IgA levels when patients had symptoms consistent with *H. pylori* infection (71). With sensitivities of 39 to 82%, serum IgA assays lack the requisite sensitivity to serve as primary screening tests but may be useful in cases when infection is strongly suspected and the serum IgG result is negative or equivocal. Another alternative diagnostic approach is to perform immunoblotting for equivocal specimens.

Although serum IgG assays remain the tests of choice for screening patient sera, whole-blood immunoassays are being used with increasing frequency in physicians' offices and point-of-care testing protocols. Qualitative point-of-care immunoassays produce rapid results (4 to 10 min) with heparinized whole blood or capillary blood specimens. The major drawback of these rapid whole-blood immunoassays is their low sensitivities (usually 80 to 90%) despite specificities comparable to those of laboratory-based serum enzyme immunoassays (30, 31). Concerns regarding interoffice variability with point-of-care whole-blood assays have been raised. Negative results must be confirmed by laboratory ELISA-based serum IgG testing, fecal antigen testing, or UBT.

Sustained immunoglobulin responses to multiple antigens of *H. cinaedi* and *H. fennelliae* have been documented (35). Little is known about the nature of immunoglobulin class and subclass responses following infection with *H. cinaedi* and *H. fennelliae*. No commercial serologic assays have been developed to monitor infection with *H. cinaedi* or other enterohepatic helicobacters.

Detection of *H. pylori* Antibodies in Urine

Specific *H. pylori* IgG antibodies are detected in urine at low concentrations. An ELISA allowing their detection has been developed (Urinelisa; Otsuka,Tokuchima, Japan) as well as a rapid immunoenzymatic test (Rapirun; Otsuka) (73, 90). A pooled sensitivity and a specificity of 92.3 and 89.7%, respectively, have been reported. While the accuracy is not dependent on the pH or the presence of bacteriuria, it may be influenced by a large amount of total IgG. Urine samples cannot be frozen because it would lead to protein precipitation. The test must be performed on fresh samples, or a preservative must be added. These tests, although very attractive because of their noninvasive nature, have not achieved the optimal sensitivity required for routine use.

Detection of *H. pylori* Antibodies in Saliva

Salivary antibodies are secreted during the immune response to infectious agents (134). A commercial kit has been developed to detect *H. pylori*-specific IgG in saliva (Helisal; Provalis, Deeside, United Kingdom). Saliva can be collected by having the patient spit into a tube, but better results are obtained using a special device (OraSure; OraSure Technologies, Inc., Bethlehem, Pa.) designed to obtain gingival transudate enriched with IgG (95). However, this assay also suffers from insufficient sensitivity.

ANTIBIOTIC SUSCEPTIBILITIES

The standard regimen to eradicate *H. pylori* consists of a macrolide (e.g., clarithromycin), a β-lactam (amoxicillin), and a proton pump inhibitor (e.g., omeprazole, lansoprazole, pantoprazole, rabeprozole, or esomeprazole). The antisecretory drug is prescribed to increase the stomach pH in order for the antibiotics to be effective. Acid antisecretories also reduce pain and accelerate ulcer healing. This regimen is recommended to last for 10 days in the United States and 7 days in other countries.

Other alternatives include (i) a triple therapy in which a nitroimidazole (e.g., metronidazole) is used instead of amoxicillin, (ii) bismuth-based therapy with bismuth salts, tetracycline, and metronidazole, and (iii) a quadruple therapy in which a proton pump inhibitor is added to the bismuth-based regimen; all of these therapies are prescribed for 7 to 14 days.

The main cause of failure to eradicate *H. pylori* with the standard antimicrobial regimen is macrolide resistance (104). The eradication rate decreases by 70% (from 88 to 18%) when the strain is resistant versus susceptible (102). This finding should stimulate routine susceptibility testing with clarithromycin. In the case of resistance, clarithromycin must be replaced with an alternate antibiotic. Using metronidazole with amoxicillin and a proton pump inhibitor for 14 days is an alternative (83), but metronidazole resistance also decreases the success rate by 25%. Other antibiotics, e.g., levofloxacin, rifabutin, and furazolidone, may also be used in association with amoxicillin (101).

The prevalence of resistance parallels the use of drugs worldwide (102, 128). For clarithromycin the resistance rate is between 0 and 20%, for metronidazole it is between 10 and 80%, and for fluoroquinolones it is between 0 and 20%. Resistance to amoxicillin and tetracycline is rarely found.

Various susceptibility testing methods such as broth microdilution, disk diffusion, the E test, and agar dilution have been used to assess antimicrobial resistance in *H. pylori* (18, 57, 63). The Clinical and Laboratory Standards Institute (CLSI) made the recommendation of an agar dilution method for testing of *H. pylori* susceptibility to clarithromycin (114). Mueller-Hinton agar base with 5% aged sheep blood and incubation for 72 h at 35°C were selected by the CLSI for susceptibility testing by agar dilution (see chapter 75). Resistance in vitro to clarithromycin by *H. pylori* is clinically relevant, and a MIC breakpoint of 1 μg per ml is recommended by the CLSI

(114). If an agar diffusion method is used, an inhibitory zone of less than 17 mm around an erythromycin disk indicates a resistant strain (55). In contrast to that for clarithromycin, in vitro susceptibility testing for metronidazole has not been standardized, although elevated MICs (>8 μg/ml) have been correlated with treatment failures (9). Given that resistance in *H. pylori* is the consequence of chromosomal mutations, molecular tests have been developed especially for the most important antibiotic, clarithromycin. Point mutations at two sites of the 23S rRNA gene which inhibit macrolide binding are essentially involved (16, 120, 177). A number of methods have been developed for their detection. One of the most widely used is PCR-restriction fragment polymorphism (135, 167, 177). Real-time PCR using the fluorescent resonance energy transfer principle has been developed which allows the detection of both *H. pylori* and its resistance to clarithromycin directly from gastric biopsy specimens. The assay has excellent sensitivity (122) and has been used as well to detect *H. pylori* from stools (153). The same approach has been used to ascertain resistance to fluoroquinolones (48). In contrast, multiple null mutations in the NADPH nitroreductase gene (*rdxA*) are the primary molecular bases for metronidazole resistance in *H. pylori* (50, 72, 81, 106), leading to the inability of cells to reduce and activate nitroimidazole compounds intracellularly.

Eradication of "*H. heilmannii*" by antimicrobial therapy also results in the resolution of gastritis and peptic ulcer disease (49, 66, 67) as well as "*H. heilmannii*"-associated primary low-grade MALT lymphoma (111). Antibiotic susceptibility testing has been described only for multiple isolates from a single patient (4). "*H. heilmannii*" isolates were susceptible to amoxicillin, ciprofloxacin, erythromycin, and tetracycline and resistant to nalidixic acid and metronidazole (4). "*H. heilmannii*" infections have been successfully treated with bismuth alone and with combination therapies that included amoxicillin, metronidazole, and omeprazole (4, 66, 67).

Bacteremias due to intestinal helicobacters in immunocompromised patients require drug combinations in prolonged intravenous treatment regimens, often including aminoglycosides. *Helicobacter* sp. strain flexispira taxon 8 bacteremias require multiagent regimens including aminoglycosides such as amikacin (159) and gentamicin (179) for the clearance of infections. Effective therapy for *H. cinaedi* infection has included ciprofloxacin, gentamicin, or tetracycline for at least 2 to 3 weeks (12, 75, 126). In vitro susceptibility testing of *H. cinaedi* (34, 74, 75) appears to be meaningful, and resistance in vitro has been correlated with treatment failures in patients medicated with erythromycin (12) or ciprofloxacin (75). Relatively limited therapeutic experience is available for *H. fennelliae* infections. Gentamicin (115) and ampicillin-sulbactam (68) have been used successfully to treat bacteremia caused by *H. fennelliae*. Neither in vitro susceptibility testing data nor treatment recommendations have been reported for cases of gastroenteritis caused by *H. canis, H. pullorum, H. canadensis,* or *H. winghamensis*. CLSI recommendations are not available for antimicrobial susceptibility testing of helicobacter organisms other than *H. pylori*.

INTERPRETATION AND REPORTING OF RESULTS

Noninvasive tests are recommended only for patients younger than 50 years and without "alarm" symptoms. The best screening test is the UBT, but the *H. pylori* fecal antigen test or ELISA-based IgG serology can also be used. Rapid whole-blood test results must be confirmed by a laboratory-based ELISA or another test.

Patients with alarm symptoms (36) such as old age, weight loss, or gastrointestinal bleeding should undergo esophagogastroduodenal endoscopy. Rapid urease testing of gastric biopsy specimens can be used to assess *H. pylori* infection status. If results are positive, they can be reported as "positive and consistent with *H. pylori* infection." Histology of gastric biopsy specimens must be interpreted by an experienced pathologist. Routine hematoxylin and eosin staining indicates the nature of gastritis or the presence of gastric adenocarcinoma or gastric MALT lymphoma. *H. pylori* organisms may be visible with Gram staining of impression smears or the use of special stains such as Giemsa or modified Steiner stain. "*H. heilmannii*" infection must be diagnosed by bacterial morphology in gastric biopsy specimens, since this organism is rarely cultured.

In order to perform antimicrobial susceptibility testing, bacteriologic culture of *H. pylori* from gastric biopsy specimens is recommended. Successful culture of *H. pylori* from biopsy specimens may be reported if organisms have the typical gram-negative morphology and are cytochrome oxidase, catalase, and urease positive. Primary biopsy specimen cultures should be incubated at least 7 days prior to a report of a negative result. Susceptibility testing for clarithromycin should be performed by using the NCCLS (CSLI) reference method (114) or a substantially equivalent method. Molecular resistance testing (mutation detection) can be used as an alternative to detect the presence of discrete mutations conferring macrolide resistance (135).

It is necessary to perform a follow-up after an eradication treatment. A delay of at least 4 to 6 weeks after antibiotic treatment is completed must be observed. The method universally recommended is the UBT because it is noninvasive and has high sensitivity. The stool test may also be used but not serology unless it is possible to test at the same time both the serum obtained before treatment and the serum obtained 6 months after treatment. A decreased antibody titer of more than 25% must be observed to claim that the antibiotic treatment has been successful in eradicating *H. pylori* (10).

Enterohepatic helicobacters such as *H. cinaedi* and *H. fennelliae* must be isolated by microbiologic culture from blood or feces for a definitive diagnosis of infection. If the laboratory isolate is negative for the Gram stain, microscopic morphology may be assessed by using a modified Gram stain, Giemsa stain, acridine orange stain, or dark-field microscopy. Appropriate biochemical tests must be performed (Table 1). Enterohepatic helicobacters are typically urease negative and may be easily confused with campylobacters. Even with supplemental tests, the distinctions can be difficult without genotypic tests such as species-specific PCR amplification or targeted DNA sequencing.

REFERENCES

1. **Alm, R. A., L. S. Ling, D. T. Moir, B. L. King, E. D. Brown, P. C. Doig, D. R. Smith, B. Noonan, B. C. Guild, B. L. deJonge, G. Carmel, P. J. Tummino, A. Caruso, M. Uria-Nickelsen, D. M. Mills, C. Ives, R. Gibson, D. Merberg, S. D. Mills, Q. Jiang, D. E. Taylor, G. F. Vovis, and T. J. Trust.** 1999. Genomic-sequence comparison of two unrelated isolates of the human gastric pathogen *Helicobacter pylori*. *Nature* **397:**176–180.
2. **Alpen, B., A. Neubauer, J. Dierlamm, P. Marynen, C. Thiede, E. Bayerdorfer, and M. Stolte.** 2000.

Translocation t(11;18) absent in early gastric marginal zone B-cell lymphoma of MALT type responding to eradication of *Helicobacter pylori* infection. *Blood* **95:**4014–4015.

3. **Anand, B. S., and D. Y. Graham.** 1999. Ulcer and gastritis. *Endoscopy* **31:**215–225.
4. **Andersen, L. P., K. Boye, J. Blom, S. Holck, A. Norgaard, and L. Elsborg.** 1999. Characterization of a culturable "*Gastrospirillum hominis*" *(Helicobacter heilmannii)* strain isolated from human gastric mucosa. *J. Clin. Microbiol.* **37:**1069–1076.
5. **Archer, J. R., S. Romero, A. E. Ritchie, M. E. Hamacher, B. M. Steiner, J. H. Bryner, and R. F. Schell.** 1988. Characterization of an unclassified microaerophilic bacterium associated with gastroenteritis. *J. Clin. Microbiol.* **26:**101–105.
6. **Avenaud, P., A. Marais, L. Monteiro, B. Le Bail, P. Bioulac Sage, C. Balabaud, and F. Megraud.** 2000. Detection of *Helicobacter* species in the liver of patients with and without primary liver carcinoma. *Cancer* **89:**1431–1439.
7. **Axon, A. T.** 1995. Is *Helicobacter pylori* transmitted by the gastro-oral route? *Aliment. Pharmacol. Ther.* **9:**585–588.
8. **Banatvala, N., K. Mayo, F. Megraud, R. Jennings, J. J. Deeks, and R. A. Feldman.** 1993. The cohort effect and *Helicobacter pylori*. *J. Infect. Dis.* **168:**219–221.
9. **Bazzoli, F., D. Berretti, L. De Luca, G. Nicolini, P. Pozzato, S. Fossi, and M. Zagari.** 1999. What can be learnt from the new data about antibiotic resistance? Are there any practical clinical consequences of *Helicobacter pylori* antibiotic resistance? *Eur. J. Gastroenterol. Hepatol.* **11** (Suppl. 2)**:**S39–S45.
10. **Bergey, B., P. Marchildon, J. Peacock, and F. Megraud.** 2003. What is the role of serology in assessing *Helicobacter pylori* eradication? *Aliment. Pharmacol. Ther.* **18:**635–639.
11. **Blecker, U., S. Lanciers, B. Hauser, D. I. Mehta, and Y. Vandenplas.** 1995. Serology as a valid screening test for *Helicobacter pylori* infection in asymptomatic subjects. *Arch. Pathol. Lab. Med.* **119:**30–32.
12. **Burman, W. J., D. L. Cohn, R. R. Reves, and M. L. Wilson.** 1995. Multifocal cellulitis and monoarticular arthritis as manifestations of *Helicobacter cinaedi* bacteremia. *Clin. Infect. Dis.* **20:**564–570.
13. **Burnens, A. P., J. Stanley, U. B. Schaad, and J. Nicolet.** 1993. Novel *Campylobacter*-like organism resembling *Helicobacter fennelliae* isolated from a boy with gastroenteritis and from dogs. *J. Clin. Microbiol.* **31:**1916–1917.
14. **Ceelen, L., A. Decostere, G. Verschraegen, R. Ducatelle, and F. Haesebrouck.** 2005. Prevalence of *Helicobacter pullorum* among patients with gastrointestinal disease and clinically healthy persons. *J. Clin. Microbiol.* **43:**2984–2986.
15. **Chen, L. T., J. T. Lin, J. J. Tai, G. H. Chen, H. Z. Yeh, S. S. Yang, H. P. Wang, S. H. Kuo, B. S. Sheu, C. M. Jan, W. M. Wang, T. E. Wang, C. W. Wu, C. L. Chen, I. J. Su, J. Whang-Peng, and A. L. Cheng.** 2005. Long-term results of anti-*Helicobacter pylori* therapy in early-stage gastric high-grade transformed MALT lymphoma. *J. Natl. Cancer Inst.* **97:**1345–1353.
16. **Debets-Ossenkopp, Y. J., M. Sparrius, J. G. Kusters, J. J. Kolkman, and C. M. Vandenbroucke-Grauls.** 1996. Mechanism of clarithromycin resistance in clinical isolates of *Helicobacter pylori*. *FEMS Microbiol. Lett.* **142:**37–42.
17. **Debongnie, J. C., J. Mairesse, M. Donnay, and X. Dekoninck.** 1994. Touch cytology. A quick, simple, sensitive screening test in the diagnosis of infections of the gastrointestinal mucosa. *Arch. Pathol. Lab. Med.* **118:**1115–1118.
18. **DeCross, A. J., B. J. Marshall, R. W. McCallum, S. R. Hoffman, L. J. Barrett, and R. L. Guerrant.** 1993. Metronidazole susceptibility testing for *Helicobacter pylori*: comparison of disk, broth, and agar dilution methods and their clinical relevance. *J. Clin. Microbiol.* **31:**1971–1974.
19. **De Groote, D., R. Ducatelle, and F. Haesebrouck.** 2000. Helicobacters of possible zoonotic origin: a review. *Acta Gastroenterol. Belg.* **63:**380–387.
20. **Dewhirst, F. D., Z. Shen, L. Stokes, M. Scimeca, and J. G. Fox.** 2005. Discordant 16S rRNA and 23S rRNA phylogenies for the genus *Helicobacter*: implications for phylogenetic inference and systematics. *J. Bacteriol.* **187:**6106–6118.
21. **Dewhirst, F. E., J. G. Fox, E. N. Mendes, B. J. Paster, C. E. Gates, C. A. Kirkbride, and K. A. Eaton.** 2000. '*Flexispira rappini*' strains represent at least 10 Helicobacter taxa. *Int. J. Syst. Evol. Microbiol.* **50**(Pt. 5)**:**1781–1787.
22. **Dixon, M. F., R. M. Genta, J. H. Yardley, and P. Correa.** 1996. Classification and grading of gastritis. The updated Sydney System. International Workshop on the Histopathology of Gastritis, Houston 1994. *Am. J. Surg. Pathol.* **20:**1161–1181.
23. **Dominguez-Munoz, J. E., A. Leodolter, T. Sauerbruch, and P. Malfertheiner.** 1997. A citric acid solution is an optimal test drink in the 13C-urea breath test for the diagnosis of *Helicobacter pylori* infection. *Gut* **40:**459–462.
24. **Dominici, P., S. Bellentani, A. R. Di Biase, G. Saccoccio, A. Le Rose, F. Masutti, L. Viola, F. Balli, C. Tiribelli, R. Grilli, M. Fusillo, and E. Grossi.** 1999. Familial clustering of *Helicobacter pylori* infection: population based study. *Br. Med. J.* **319:**537–540.
25. **Dore, M. P., M. S. Osato, H. M. Malaty, and D. Y. Graham.** 2000. Characterization of a culture method to recover *Helicobacter pylori* from the feces of infected patients. *Helicobacter* **5:**165–168.
26. **Dubois, A., N. Fiala, L. M. Heman-Ackah, E. S. Drazek, A. Tarnawski, W. N. Fishbein, G. I. Perez-Perez, and M. J. Blaser.** 1994. Natural gastric infection with *Helicobacter pylori* in monkeys: a model for spiral bacteria infection in humans. *Gastroenterology* **106:**1405–1417.
27. **Duck, W. M., J. Sobel, J. M. Pruckler, Q. Song, D. Swerdlow, C. Friedman, A. Sulka, B. Swaminathan, T. Taylor, M. Hoekstra, P. Griffin, D. Smoot, R. Peek, D. C. Metz, P. B. Bloom, S. Goldschmidt, J. Parsonnet, G. Triadafilopoulos, G. I. Perez-Perez, N. Vakil, P. Ernst, S. Czinn, D. Dunne, and B. D. Gold.** 2004. Antimicrobial resistance incidence and risk factors among *Helicobacter pylori*-infected persons, United States. *Emerg. Infect. Dis.* **10:**1088–1094.
28. **El-Omar, E. M., K. Oien, A. El-Nujumi, D. Gillen, A. Wirz, S. Dahill, C. Williams, J. E. Ardill, and K. E. McColl.** 1997. *Helicobacter pylori* infection and chronic gastric acid hyposecretion. *Gastroenterology* **113:**15–24.
29. **Engstrand, L., A. M. Nguyen, D. Y. Graham, and F. A. el-Zaatari.** 1992. Reverse transcription and polymerase chain reaction amplification of rRNA for detection of *Helicobacter* species. *J. Clin. Microbiol.* **30:**2295–2301.
30. **European *Helicobacter pylori* Study Group.** 1997. Current European concepts in the management of *Helicobacter pylori* infection. The Maastricht Consensus Report. *Gut* **41:**8–13.
31. **Faigel, D. O., N. Magaret, C. Corless, D. A. Lieberman, and M. B. Fennerty.** 2000. Evaluation of rapid antibody tests for the diagnosis of *Helicobacter pylori* infection. *Am. J. Gastroenterol.* **95:**72–77.
32. **Farinha, P., and R. D. Gascoyne.** 2005. *Helicobacter pylori* and MALT lymphoma. *Gastroenterology* **128:**1579–1605.
33. **Fawcett, P. T., K. M. Gibney, and K. M. Vinette.** 1999. *Helicobacter pylori* can be induced to assume the morphology of *Helicobacter heilmannii*. *J. Clin. Microbiol.* **37:** 1045–1048.
34. **Flores, B. M., C. L. Fennell, K. K. Holmes, and W. E. Stamm.** 1985. In vitro susceptibilities of *Campylobacter*-like organisms to twenty antimicrobial agents. *Antimicrob. Agents Chemother.* **28:**188–191.

35. **Flores, B. M., C. L. Fennell, and W. E. Stamm.** 1989. Characterization of *Campylobacter cinaedi* and *C. fennelliae* antigens and analysis of the human immune response. *J. Infect. Dis.* **159:**635–640.
36. **Ford, A. C., M. Qume, P. Moayyedi, N. L. Arents, A. T. Lassen, R. F. Logan, K. E. McColl, P. Myres, and B. C. Delaney.** 2005. *Helicobacter pylori* "test and treat" or endoscopy for managing dyspepsia: an individual patient data meta-analysis. *Gastroenterology* **128:**1838–1844.
37. **Fox, J. G.** 2002. The non-*H. pylori* helicobacters: their expanding role in gastrointestinal and systemic diseases. *Gut* **50:**273–283.
38. **Fox, J. G., C. C. Chien, F. E. Dewhirst, B. J. Paster, Z. Shen, P. L. Melito, D. L. Woodward, and F. G. Rodgers.** 2000. *Helicobacter canadensis* sp. nov. isolated from humans with diarrhea as an example of an emerging pathogen. *J. Clin. Microbiol.* **38:**2546–2549.
39. **Fox, J. G., F. E. Dewhirst, Z. Shen, Y. Feng, N. S. Taylor, B. J. Paster, R. L. Ericson, C. N. Lau, P. Correa, J. C. Araya, and I. Roa.** 1998. Hepatic *Helicobacter* species identified in bile and gallbladder tissue from Chileans with chronic cholecystitis. *Gastroenterology* **114:**755–763.
40. **Fox, J. G., F. E. Dewhirst, J. G. Tully, B. J. Paster, L. Yan, N. S. Taylor, M. J. Collins, Jr., P. L. Gorelick, and J. M. Ward.** 1994. *Helicobacter hepaticus* sp. nov., a microaerophilic bacterium isolated from livers and intestinal mucosal scrapings from mice. *J. Clin. Microbiol.* **32:**1238–1245.
41. **Fox, J. G., R. Drolet, R. Higgins, S. Messier, L. Yan, B. E. Coleman, B. J. Paster, and F. E. Dewhirst.** 1996. *Helicobacter canis* isolated from a dog liver with multifocal necrotizing hepatitis. *J. Clin. Microbiol.* **34:**2479–2482.
42. **Fox, J. G., L. Handt, B. J. Sheppard, S. Xu, F. E. Dewhirst, S. Motzel, and H. Klein.** 2001. Isolation of *Helicobacter cinaedi* from the colon, liver, and mesenteric lymph node of a rhesus monkey with chronic colitis and hepatitis. *J. Clin. Microbiol.* **39:**1580–1585.
43. **Fox, J. G., and A. Lee.** 1997. The role of *Helicobacter* species in newly recognized gastrointestinal tract diseases of animals. *Lab. Anim. Sci.* **47:**222–255.
44. **Fox, J. G., Z. Shen, S. Xu, Y. Feng, C. A. Dangler, F. E. Dewhirst, B. J. Paster, and J. M. Cullen.** 2002. *Helicobacter marmotae* sp. nov. isolated from livers of woodchucks and intestines of cats. *J. Clin. Microbiol.* **40:**2513–2519.
45. **Fox, J. G., L. Yan, B. Shames, J. Campbell, J. C. Murphy, and X. Li.** 1996. Persistent hepatitis and enterocolitis in germfree mice infected with *Helicobacter hepaticus*. *Infect. Immun.* **64:**3673–3681.
46. **Germani, Y., C. Dauga, P. Duval, M. Huerre, M. Levy, G. Pialoux, P. Sansonetti, and P. A. Grimont.** 1997. Strategy for the detection of *Helicobacter* species by amplification of 16S rRNA genes and identification of *H. felis* in a human gastric biopsy. *Res. Microbiol.* **148:**315–326.
47. **Gisbert, J. P., and J. M. Pajares.** 2004. Stool antigen test for the diagnosis of *Helicobacter pylori* infection: a systematic review. *Helicobacter* **9:**347–368.
48. **Glocker, E., and M. Kist.** 2004. Rapid detection of point mutations in the *gyrA* gene of *Helicobacter pylori* conferring resistance to ciprofloxacin by a fluorescence resonance energy transfer-based real-time PCR approach. *J. Clin. Microbiol.* **42:**2241–2246.
49. **Goddard, A. F., R. P. Logan, J. C. Atherton, D. Jenkins, and R. C. Spiller.** 1997. Healing of duodenal ulcer after eradication of *Helicobacter heilmannii*. *Lancet* **349:**1815–1816.
50. **Goodwin, A., D. Kersulyte, G. Sisson, S. J. Veldhuyzen van Zanten, D. E. Berg, and P. S. Hoffman.** 1998. Metronidazole resistance in *Helicobacter pylori* is due to null mutations in a gene (rdxA) that encodes an oxygen-insensitive NADPH nitroreductase. *Mol. Microbiol.* **28:**383–393.
51. **Goodwin, C., T. Armstrong, T. Chilvers, M. Peters, M. J. Collins, L. Sly, W. McConnell, and W. Harper.** 1989. Transfer of *Campylobacter pylori* and *Campylobacter mustelae* to Helicobacter gen. nov. as *Helicobacter pylori* comb. nov. and *Helicobacter mustelae* comb. nov., respectively. *Int. J. Syst. Bacteriol.* **39:**397–405.
52. **Goosen, C., J. Theron, M. Ntsala, F. F. Maree, A. Olckers, S. J. Botha, A. J. Lastovica, and S. W. van der Merwe.** 2002. Evaluation of a novel heminested PCR assay based on the phosphoglucosamine mutase gene for detection of *Helicobacter pylori* in saliva and dental plaque. *J. Clin. Microbiol.* **40:**205–209.
53. **Graham, D. Y., M. Kudo, R. Reddy, and A. R. Opekun.** 2005. Practical rapid, minimally invasive, reliable nonendoscopic method to obtain *Helicobacter pylori* for culture. *Helicobacter* **10:**1–3.
54. **Grayson, M. L., W. Tee, and B. Dwyer.** 1989. Gastroenteritis associated with *Campylobacter cinaedi*. *Med. J. Aust.* **150:**214–215.
55. **Grignon, B., J. Tankovic, F. Megraud, Y. Glupczynski, M. O. Husson, M. C. Conroy, J. P. Emond, J. Loulergue, J. Raymond, and J. L. Fauchere.** 2002. Validation of diffusion methods for macrolide susceptibility testing of *Helicobacter pylori*. *Microb. Drug Resist.* **8:**61–66.
56. **Gueneau, P., and S. Loiseaux-De Goer.** 2002. Helicobacter: molecular phylogeny and the origin of gastric colonization in the genus. *Infect. Genet. Evol.* **1:**215–223.
57. **Hachem, C. Y., J. E. Clarridge, R. Reddy, R. Flamm, D. G. Evans, S. K. Tanaka, and D. Y. Graham.** 1996. Antimicrobial susceptibility testing of *Helicobacter pylori*. Comparison of E-test, broth microdilution, and disk diffusion for ampicillin, clarithromycin, and metronidazole. *Diagn. Microbiol. Infect. Dis.* **24:**37–41.
58. **Haggerty, T. D., S. Perry, L. Sanchez, G. Perez-Perez, and J. Parsonnet.** 2005. Significance of transiently positive enzyme-linked immunosorbent assay results in detection of *Helicobacter pylori* in stool samples from children. *J. Clin. Microbiol.* **43:**2220–2223.
59. **Han, S. W., R. Flamm, C. Y. Hachem, H. Y. Kim, J. E. Clarridge, D. G. Evans, J. Beyer, J. Drnec, and D. Y. Graham.** 1995. Transport and storage of *Helicobacter pylori* from gastric mucosal biopsies and clinical isolates. *Eur. J. Clin. Microbiol. Infect. Dis.* **14:**349–352.
60. **Handt, L. K., J. G. Fox, F. E. Dewhirst, G. J. Fraser, B. J. Paster, L. L. Yan, H. Rozmiarek, R. Rufo, and I. H. Stalis.** 1994. *Helicobacter pylori* isolated from the domestic cat: public health implications. *Infect. Immun.* **62:**2367–2374.
61. **Hanninen, M. L., I. Happonen, S. Saari, and K. Jalava.** 1996. Culture and characteristics of *Helicobacter bizzozeronii*, a new canine gastric *Helicobacter* sp. *Int. J. Syst. Bacteriol.* **46:**160–166.
62. **Hansson, L. E., O. Nyren, A. W. Hsing, R. Bergstrom, S. Josefsson, W. H. Chow, J. F. Fraumeni, Jr., and H. O. Adami.** 1996. The risk of stomach cancer in patients with gastric or duodenal ulcer disease. *N. Engl. J. Med.* **335:**242–249.
63. **Hardy, D. J., C. W. Hanson, D. M. Hensey, J. M. Beyer, and P. B. Fernandes.** 1988. Susceptibility of *Campylobacter pylori* to macrolides and fluoroquinolones. *J. Antimicrob. Chemother.* **22:**631–636.
64. **Harper, C. G., Y. Feng, S. Xu, N. S. Taylor, M. Kinsel, F. E. Dewhirst, B. J. Paster, M. Greenwell, G. Levine, A. Rogers, and J. G. Fox.** 2002. *Helicobacter cetorum* sp. nov., a urease-positive *Helicobacter* species isolated from dolphins and whales. *J. Clin. Microbiol.* **40:**4536–4543.
65. **Hazell, S. L., and G. L. Mendz.** 1997. How *Helicobacter pylori* works: an overview of the metabolism of *Helicobacter pylori*. *Helicobacter* **2:**1–12.

66. **Heilmann, K. L., and F. Borchard.** 1991. Gastritis due to spiral shaped bacteria other than *Helicobacter pylori:* clinical, histological, and ultrastructural findings. *Gut* **32:**137–140.
67. **Hilzenrat, N., E. Lamoureux, I. Weintrub, E. Alpert, M. Lichter, and L. Alpert.** 1995. *Helicobacter heilmannii*-like spiral bacteria in gastric mucosal biopsies. Prevalence and clinical significance. *Arch. Pathol. Lab. Med.* **119:**1149–1153.
68. **Hsueh, P. R., L. J. Teng, C. C. Hung, Y. C. Chen, P. C. Yang, S. W. Ho, and K. T. Luh.** 1999. Septic shock due to *Helicobacter fennelliae* in a non-human immunodeficiency virus-infected heterosexual patient. *J. Clin. Microbiol.* **37:**2084–2086.
69. **Husmann, M., C. Gries, P. Jehnichen, T. Woelfel, G. Gerken, W. Ludwig, and S. Bhakdi.** 1994. *Helicobacter* sp. strain Mainz isolated from an AIDS patient with septic arthritis: case report and nonradioactive analysis of 16S rRNA sequence. *J. Clin. Microbiol.* **32:**3037–3039.
70. **Ihrig, M., M. D. Schrenzel, and J. G. Fox.** 1999. Differential susceptibility to hepatic inflammation and proliferation in AXB recombinant inbred mice chronically infected with *Helicobacter hepaticus*. *Am. J. Pathol.* **155:**571–582.
71. **Jaskowski, T. D., T. B. Martins, H. R. Hill, and C. M. Litwin.** 1997. Immunoglobulin A antibodies to *Helicobacter pylori*. *J. Clin. Microbiol.* **35:**2999–3000.
72. **Jenks, P. J., R. L. Ferrero, and A. Labigne.** 1999. The role of the rdxA gene in the evolution of metronidazole resistance in *Helicobacter pylori*. *J. Antimicrob. Chemother.* **43:** 753–758.
73. **Katsuragi, K., A. Noda, T. Tachikawa, A. Azuma, F. Mukai, K. Murakami, T. Fujioka, M. Kato, and M. Asaka.** 1998. Highly sensitive urine-based enzyme-linked immunosorbent assay for detection of antibody to *Helicobacter pylori*. *Helicobacter* **3:**289–295.
74. **Kiehlbauch, J. A., D. J. Brenner, D. N. Cameron, A. G. Steigerwalt, J. M. Makowski, C. N. Baker, C. M. Patton, and I. K. Wachsmuth.** 1995. Genotypic and phenotypic characterization of *Helicobacter cinaedi* and *Helicobacter fennelliae* strains isolated from humans and animals. *J. Clin. Microbiol.* **33:**2940–2947.
75. **Kiehlbauch, J. A., R. V. Tauxe, C. N. Baker, and I. K. Wachsmuth.** 1994. *Helicobacter cinaedi*-associated bacteremia and cellulitis in immunocompromised patients. *Ann. Intern. Med.* **121:**90–93.
76. **Kiesslich, R., M. Goetz, J. Burg, M. Stolte, E. Siegel, M. J. Maeurer, S. Thomas, D. Strand, P. R. Galle, and M. F. Neurath.** 2005. Diagnosing *Helicobacter pylori in vivo* by confocal laser endoscopy. *Gastroenterology* **128:** 2119–2123.
77. **Kignel, S., F. de Almeida Pina, E. A. Andre, M. P. Alves Mayer, and E. G. Birman.** 2005. Occurrence of *Helicobacter pylori* in dental plaque and saliva of dyspeptic patients. *Oral Dis.* **11:**17–21.
78. **Kimmel, B., A. Bosserhoff, R. Frank, R. Gross, W. Goebel, and D. Beier.** 2000. Identification of immunodominant antigens from *Helicobacter pylori* and evaluation of their reactivities with sera from patients with different gastroduodenal pathologies. *Infect. Immun.* **68:** 915–920.
79. **Klein, P. D., H. M. Malaty, R. F. Martin, K. S. Graham, R. M. Genta, and D. Y. Graham.** 1996. Noninvasive detection of *Helicobacter pylori* infection in clinical practice: the 13C urea breath test. *Am. J. Gastroenterol.* **91:**690–694.
80. **Krienitz, W.** 1906. Ueber das auftreten von spirochäten verschiedener from in mageninhalt bei carcinoma ventriculi. *Dtsch. Med. Wochenschr.* **28:**672.
81. **Kwon, D. H., J. A. Pena, M. S. Osato, J. G. Fox, D. Y. Graham, and J. Versalovic.** 2000. Frameshift mutations in rdxA and metronidazole resistance in North American *Helicobacter pylori* isolates. *J. Antimicrob. Chemother.* **46:** 793–796.
82. **Laheij, R. J., H. Straatman, J. B. Jansen, and A. L. Verbeek.** 1998. Evaluation of commercially available *Helicobacter pylori* serology kits: a review. *J. Clin. Microbiol.* **36:**2803–2809.
83. **Lamouliatte, H., F. Megraud, J. C. Delchier, J. F. Bretagne, A. Courillon-Mallet, J. D. De Korwin, J. L. Fauchere, A. Labigne, J. F. Flejou, and P. Barthelemy.** 2003. Second-line treatment for failure to eradicate *Helicobacter pylori:* a randomized trial comparing four treatment strategies. *Aliment. Pharmacol. Ther.* **18:**791–797.
84. **Lastovica, A. J., and E. le Roux.** 2000. Efficient isolation of campylobacteria from stools. *J. Clin. Microbiol.* **38:** 2798–2799.
85. **Lastovica, A. J., and M. B. Skirrow.** 2000. Clinical significance of *Campylobacter* and related species other than *Campylobacter jejuni* and *C. coli*, p. 89–120. *In* I. Nachamkin and M. J. Blaser (ed.), *Campylobacter*, 2nd ed. ASM Press, Washington, D.C.
86. **Laughon, B. E., A. A. Vernon, D. A. Druckman, R. Fox, T. C. Quinn, B. F. Polk, and J. G. Bartlett.** 1988. Recovery of *Campylobacter* species from homosexual men. *J. Infect. Dis.* **158:**464–467.
87. **Lavelle, J. P., S. Landas, F. A. Mitros, and J. L. Conklin.** 1994. Acute gastritis associated with spiral organisms from cats. *Dig. Dis. Sci.* **39:**744–750.
88. **Lee, A., S. L. Hazell, J. O'Rourke, and S. Kouprach.** 1988. Isolation of a spiral-shaped bacterium from the cat stomach. *Infect. Immun.* **56:**2843–2850.
89. **Lee, J., and C. O'Morain.** 1997. Who should be treated for *Helicobacter pylori* infection? A review of consensus conferences and guidelines. *Gastroenterology* **113:**S99–S106.
90. **Leodolter, A., D. Vaira, F. Bazzoli, K. Schutze, A. Hirschl, F. Megraud, and P. Malfertheiner.** 2003. European multicentre validation trial of two new non-invasive tests for the detection of *Helicobacter pylori* antibodies: urine-based ELISA and rapid urine test. *Aliment. Pharmacol. Ther.* **18:**927–931.
91. **Leodolter, A., K. Wolle, U. Peitz, A. Schaffranke, T. Wex, and P. Malfertheiner.** 2004. Evaluation of a near-patient fecal antigen test for the assessment of *Helicobacter pylori* status. *Diagn. Microbiol. Infect. Dis.* **48:**145–147.
92. **Lu, J. J., C. L. Perng, R. Y. Shyu, C. H. Chen, Q. Lou, S. K. Chong, and C. H. Lee.** 1999. Comparison of five PCR methods for detection of *Helicobacter pylori* DNA in gastric tissues. *J. Clin. Microbiol.* **37:**772–774.
93. **Maeda, S., H. Yoshida, K. Ogura, F. Kanai, Y. Shiratori, and M. Omata.** 1998. *Helicobacter pylori* specific nested PCR assay for the detection of 23S rRNA mutation associated with clarithromycin resistance. *Gut* **43:**317–321.
94. **Makristathis, A., W. Barousch, E. Pasching, C. Binder, C. Kuderna, P. Apfalter, M. L. Rotter, and A. M. Hirschl.** 2000. Two enzyme immunoassays and PCR for detection of *Helicobacter pylori* in stool specimens from pediatric patients before and after eradication therapy. *J. Clin. Microbiol.* **38:**3710–3714.
95. **Malaty, H. M., N. D. Logan, D. Y. Graham, J. E. Ramchatesingh, and S. G. Reddy.** 2000. *Helicobacter pylori* infection in asymptomatic children: comparison of diagnostic tests. *Helicobacter* **5:**155–159.
96. **Malfertheiner, P., F. Megraud, C. O'Morain, A. P. Hungin, R. Jones, A. Axon, D. Y. Graham, and G. Tytgat.** 2002. Current concepts in the management of *Helicobacter pylori* infection—the Maastricht 2-2000 Consensus Report. *Aliment. Pharmacol. Ther.* **16:**167–180.
97. **Marais, A., G. L. Mendz, S. L. Hazell, and F. Megraud.** 1999. Metabolism and genetics of *Helicobacter pylori:* the genome era. *Microbiol. Mol. Biol. Rev.* **63:**642–674.

98. **Matsuda, R., and T. Morizane.** 2005. *Helicobacter pylori* infection in dental professionals: a 6-year prospective study. *Helicobacter* **10:**307–311.
99. **Maurer, K. J., M. M. Ihrig, A. B. Rogers, V. Ng, G. Bouchard, M. R. Leonard, M. C. Carey, and J. G. Fox.** 2005. Identification of cholelithogenic enterohepatic *Helicobacter* species and their role in murine cholesterol gallstone formation. *Gastroenterology* **128:**1023–1033.
100. **Megraud, F.** 1996. Advantages and disadvantages of current diagnostic tests for the detection of *Helicobacter pylori*. *Scand. J. Gastroenterol. Suppl.* **215:**57–62.
101. **Megraud, F.** 2004. Basis for the management of drug-resistant *Helicobacter pylori* infection. *Drugs* **64:**1893–1904.
102. **Megraud, F.** 2004. *H. pylori* antibiotic resistance: prevalence, importance, and advances in testing. *Gut* **53:**1374–1384.
103. **Megraud, F., and N. Broutet.** 2000. Have we found the source of *Helicobacter pylori*? *Aliment. Pharmacol. Ther.* **14:**7–12.
104. **Megraud, F., and H. Lamouliatte.** 2003. The treatment of refractory *Helicobacter pylori* infection. *Aliment. Pharmacol. Ther.* **17:**1333–1343.
105. **Melito, P. L., C. Munro, P. R. Chipman, D. L. Woodward, T. F. Booth, and F. G. Rodgers.** 2001. *Helicobacter winghamensis* sp. nov., a novel *Helicobacter* sp. isolated from patients with gastroenteritis. *J. Clin. Microbiol.* **39:**2412–2417.
106. **Mendz, G. L., and F. Megraud.** 2002. Is the molecular basis of metronidazole resistance in microaerophilic organisms understood? *Trends Microbiol.* **10:**370–375.
107. **Misra, S. P., M. Dwivedi, V. Misra, and S. C. Gupta.** 1993. Imprint cytology—a cheap, rapid and effective method for diagnosing *Helicobacter pylori*. *Postgrad. Med. J.* **69:**291–295.
108. **Moayyedi, P., J. Deeks, N. J. Talley, B. Delaney, and D. Forman.** 2003. An update of the Cochrane systematic review of *Helicobacter pylori* eradication therapy in nonulcer dyspepsia: resolving the discrepancy between systematic reviews. *Am. J. Gastroenterol.* **98:**2621–2626.
109. **Monteiro, L., A. de Mascarel, A. M. Sarrasqueta, B. Bergey, C. Barberis, P. Talby, D. Roux, L. Shouler, D. Goldfain, H. Lamouliatte, and F. Megraud.** 2001. Diagnosis of *Helicobacter pylori* infection: noninvasive methods compared to invasive methods and evaluation of two new tests. *Am. J. Gastroenterol.* **96:**353–358.
110. **Monteiro, L., N. Gras, R. Vidal, J. Cabrita, and F. Megraud.** 2001. Detection of *Helicobacter pylori* DNA in human feces by PCR: DNA stability and removal of inhibitors. *J. Microbiol. Methods* **45:**89–94.
111. **Morgner, A., N. Lehn, L. P. Andersen, C. Thiede, M. Bennedsen, K. Trebesius, B. Neubauer, A. Neubauer, M. Stolte, and E. Bayerdorffer.** 2000. *Helicobacter heilmannii*-associated primary gastric low-grade MALT lymphoma: complete remission after curing the infection. *Gastroenterology* **118:**821–828.
112. **Morris, A. J., M. R. Ali, G. I. Nicholson, G. I. Perez-Perez, and M. J. Blaser.** 1991. Long-term follow-up of voluntary ingestion of *Helicobacter pylori*. *Ann. Intern. Med.* **114:**662–663.
113. **National Institutes of Health Consensus Conference.** 1994. *Helicobacter pylori* in peptic ulcer disease. National Institutes of Health Consensus Development Panel on *Helicobacter pylori* in Peptic Ulcer Disease. *JAMA* **272:**65–69.
114. **NCCLS.** 2002. *Performance Standards for Antimicrobial Susceptibility Testing: 12th Informational Supplement.* NCCLS, Wayne, Pa.
115. **Ng, V. L., W. K. Hadley, C. L. Fennell, B. M. Flores, and W. E. Stamm.** 1987. Successive bacteremias with "*Campylobacter cinaedi*" and "*Campylobacter fennelliae*" in a bisexual male. *J. Clin. Microbiol.* **25:**2008–2009.
116. **Nilsson, H. O., R. Mulchandani, K. G. Tranberg, U. Stenram, and T. Wadstrom.** 2001. *Helicobacter* species identified in liver from patients with cholangiocarcinoma and hepatocellular carcinoma. *Gastroenterology* **120:** 323–324.
117. **Nilsson, H. O., J. Taneera, M. Castedal, E. Glatz, R. Olsson, and T. Wadstrom.** 2000. Identification of *Helicobacter pylori* and other *Helicobacter* species by PCR, hybridization, and partial DNA sequencing in human liver samples from patients with primary sclerosing cholangitis or primary biliary cirrhosis. *J. Clin. Microbiol.* **38:**1072–1076.
118. **Nomura, A., G. N. Stemmermann, P. H. Chyou, I. Kato, G. I. Perez-Perez, and M. J. Blaser.** 1991. *Helicobacter pylori* infection and gastric carcinoma among Japanese Americans in Hawaii. *N. Engl. J. Med.* **325:**1132–1136.
119. **Norris, C. R., S. L. Marks, K. A. Eaton, S. Z. Torabian, R. J. Munn, and J. V. Solnick.** 1999. Healthy cats are commonly colonized with "*Helicobacter heilmannii*" that is associated with minimal gastritis. *J. Clin. Microbiol.* **37:**189–194.
120. **Occhialini, A., M. Urdaci, F. Doucet-Populaire, C. M. Bebear, H. Lamouliatte, and F. Megraud.** 1997. Macrolide resistance in *Helicobacter pylori*: rapid detection of point mutations and assays of macrolide binding to ribosomes. *Antimicrob. Agents Chemother.* **41:**2724–2728.
121. **Oh, J. D., S. M. Karam, and J. I. Gordon.** 2005. Intracellular *Helicobacter pylori* in gastric epithelial progenitors. *Proc. Natl. Acad. Sci.* USA **102:**5186–5191.
122. **Oleastro, M., A. Menard, A. Santos, H. Lamouliatte, L. Monteiro, P. Barthelemy, and F. Megraud.** 2003. Real-time PCR assay for rapid and accurate detection of point mutations conferring resistance to clarithromycin in *Helicobacter pylori*. *J. Clin. Microbiol.* **41:**397–402.
123. **Olivieri, R., M. Bugnoli, D. Armellini, S. Bianciardi, R. Rappuoli, P. F. Bayeli, L. Abate, E. Esposito, L. de Gregorio, J. Aziz, C. Basagni, and N. Figura.** 1993. Growth of *Helicobacter pylori* in media containing cyclodextrins. *J. Clin. Microbiol.* **31:**160–162.
124. **On, S. L.** 2001. Taxonomy of *Campylobacter*, *Arcobacter*, *Helicobacter* and related bacteria: current status, future prospects and immediate concerns. *Symp. Ser. Soc. Appl. Microbiol.* **30:**1S–15S.
125. **On, S. L. W., A. Lee, J. L. O'Rourke, F. E. Dewhirst, B. J. Paster, J. G. Fox, and P. Vandamme.** 2005. Genus I. *Helicobacter*, p. 1169–1189. *In* D. J. Brenner, N. R. Krieg, J. T. Staley, and G. Garrity (ed.), *Bergey's Manual of Systematic Bacteriology*, 2nd ed. Springer, New York, N.Y.
126. **Orlicek, S. L., D. F. Welch, and T. L. Kuhls.** 1993. Septicemia and meningitis caused by *Helicobacter cinaedi* in a neonate. *J. Clin. Microbiol.* **31:**569–571.
127. **O'Rourke, J. L., J. V. Solnick, B. A. Neilan, K. Seidel, R. Hayter, L. M. Hansen, and A. Lee.** 2004. Description of '*Candidatus Helicobacter heilmannii*' based on DNA sequence analysis of 16S rRNA and urease genes. *Int. J. Syst. Evol. Microbiol.* **54:**2203–2211.
128. **Osato, M. S., R. Reddy, S. G. Reddy, R. L. Penland, H. M. Malaty, and D. Y. Graham.** 2001. Pattern of primary resistance of *Helicobacter pylori* to metronidazole or clarithromycin in the United States. *Arch. Intern. Med.* **161:**1217–1220.
129. **Parsonnet, J., G. D. Friedman, D. P. Vandersteen, Y. Chang, J. H. Vogelman, N. Orentreich, and R. K. Sibley.** 1991. *Helicobacter pylori* infection and the risk of gastric carcinoma. *N. Engl. J. Med.* **325:**1127–1131.
130. **Parsonnet, J., M. Replogle, S. Yang, and R. Hiatt.** 1997. Seroprevalence of CagA-positive strains among

Helicobacter pylori-infected, healthy young adults. *J. Infect. Dis.* **175:**1240–1242.

131. **Parsonnet, J., H. Shmuely, and T. Haggerty.** 1999. Fecal and oral shedding of *Helicobacter pylori* from healthy infected adults. *JAMA* **282:**2240–2245.
132. **Parsonnet, J., K. Welch, C. Compton, R. Strauss, T. Wang, P. Kelsey, and M. J. Ferraro.** 1988. Simple microbiologic detection of *Campylobacter pylori. J. Clin. Microbiol.* **26:**948–949.
133. **Paster, B. J., A. Lee, J. G. Fox, F. E. Dewhirst, L. A. Tordoff, G. J. Fraser, J. L. O'Rourke, N. S. Taylor, and R. Ferrero.** 1991. Phylogeny of *Helicobacter felis* sp. nov., *Helicobacter mustelae*, and related bacteria. *Int. J. Syst. Bacteriol.* **41:**31–38.
134. **Patel, P., M. A. Mendall, S. Khulusi, N. Molineaux, J. Levy, J. D. Maxwell, and T. C. Northfield.** 1994. Salivary antibodies to *Helicobacter pylori:* screening dyspeptic patients before endoscopy. *Lancet* **344:**511–512.
135. **Pena, J. A., J. G. Fox, M. J. Ferraro, and J. Versalovic.** 2001. Molecular resistance testing of *Helicobacter pylori* in gastric biopsies. *Arch. Pathol. Lab. Med.* **125:**493–497.
136. **Pena, J. A., K. McNeil, J. G. Fox, and J. Versalovic.** 2002. Molecular evidence of *Helicobacter cinaedi* organisms in human gastric biopsy specimens. *J. Clin. Microbiol.* **40:**1511–1513.
137. **Perez-Trallero, E., and M. Montes.** 2000. String test for *Helicobacter pylori*. *J. Clin. Microbiol.* **38:**4303.
138. **Peura, D. A., D. J. Pambianco, K. R. Dye, C. Lind, H. F. Frierson, S. R. Hoffman, M. J. Combs, E. Guilfoyle, and B. J. Marshall.** 1996. Microdose 14C-urea breath test offers diagnosis of *Helicobacter pylori* in 10 minutes. *Am. J. Gastroenterol.* **91:**233–238.
139. **Popovic-Uroic, T., C. M. Patton, M. A. Nicholson, and J. A. Kiehlbauch.** 1990. Evaluation of the indoxyl acetate hydrolysis test for rapid differentiation of *Campylobacter, Helicobacter*, and *Wolinella* species. *J. Clin. Microbiol.* **28:**2335–2339.
140. **Pounder, R. E., and D. Ng.** 1995. The prevalence of *Helicobacter pylori* infection in different countries. *Aliment. Pharmacol. Ther.* **9:**33–39.
141. **Powers, C. N.** 1998. Diagnosis of infectious diseases: a cytopathologist's perspective. *Clin. Microbiol. Rev.* **11:** 341–365.
142. **Puetz, T., N. Vakil, S. Phadnis, B. Dunn, and J. Robinson.** 1997. The PyloriTek test and the CLO test: accuracy and incremental cost analysis. *Am. J. Gastroenterol.* **92:**254–257.
143. **Queiroz, D. M., G. A. Rocha, E. N. Mendes, S. B. De Moura, A. M. De Oliveira, and D. Miranda.** 1996. Association between Helicobacter and gastric ulcer disease of the pars esophagea in swine. *Gastroenterology* **111:**19–27.
144. **Quinn, T. C., S. E. Goodell, C. Fennell, S. P. Wang, M. D. Schuffler, K. K. Holmes, and W. E. Stamm.** 1984. Infections with *Campylobacter jejuni* and *Campylobacter*-like organisms in homosexual men. *Ann. Intern. Med.* **101:**187–192.
145. **Riley, L. K., C. L. Franklin, R. R. Hook, Jr., and C. Besch-Williford.** 1996. Identification of murine helicobacters by PCR and restriction enzyme analyses. *J. Clin. Microbiol.* **34:**942–946.
146. **Robertson, B. R., J. L. O'Rourke, P. Vandamme, S. L. On, and A. Lee.** 2001. *Helicobacter ganmani* sp. nov., a urease-negative anaerobe isolated from the intestines of laboratory mice. *Int. J. Syst. Evol. Microbiol.* **51:**1881–1889.
147. **Rocha, M., P. Avenaud, A. Menard, B. Le Bail, C. Balabaud, P. Bioulac-Sage, D. M. de Magalhaes Queiroz, and F. Megraud.** 2005. Association of *Helicobacter* species with hepatitis C cirrhosis with or without hepatocellular carcinoma. *Gut* **54:**396–401.
148. **Romaniuk, P. J., B. Zoltowska, T. J. Trust, D. J. Lane, G. J. Olsen, N. R. Pace, and D. A. Stahl.** 1987. *Campylobacter pylori*, the spiral bacterium associated with human gastritis, is not a true *Campylobacter* sp. *J. Bacteriol.* **169:**2137–2141.
149. **Romero, S., J. R. Archer, M. E. Hamacher, S. M. Bologna, and R. F. Schell.** 1988. Case report of an unclassified microaerophilic bacterium associated with gastroenteritis. *J. Clin. Microbiol.* **26:**142–143.
150. **Russmann, H., V. A. Kempf, S. Koletzko, J. Heesemann, and I. B. Autenrieth.** 2001. Comparison of fluorescent in situ hybridization and conventional culturing for detection of *Helicobacter pylori* in gastric biopsy specimens. *J. Clin. Microbiol.* **39:**304–308.
151. **Sahay, P., A. P. West, D. Birkenhead, and P. M. Hawkey.** 1995. *Campylobacter jejuni* in the stomach. *J. Med. Microbiol.* **43:**75–77.
152. **Salomon, H.** 1898. Uber das Spirillum des Saugetiermagens und sein Verhalten zu den Belegzellen. *Bakteriol. Parasitenkd. Infektkrankh. Hyg. Abt.* **19:**438–442.
153. **Schabereiter-Gurtner, C., A. M. Hirschl, B. Dragosics, P. Hufnagl, S. Puz, Z. Kovach, M. Rotter, and A. Makristathis.** 2004. Novel real-time PCR assay for detection of *Helicobacter pylori* infection and simultaneous clarithromycin susceptibility testing of stool and biopsy specimens. *J. Clin. Microbiol.* **42:**4512–4518.
154. **Semino-Mora, C., S. Q. Doi, A. Marty, V. Simko, I. Carlstedt, and A. Dubois.** 2003. Intracellular and interstitial expression of *Helicobacter pylori* virulence genes in gastric precancerous intestinal metaplasia and adenocarcinoma. *J. Infect. Dis.* **187:**1165–1177.
155. **Shen, Z., Y. Feng, F. E. Dewhirst, and J. G. Fox.** 2001. Coinfection of enteric *Helicobacter* spp. and *Campylobacter* spp. in cats. *J. Clin. Microbiol.* **39:**2166–2172.
156. **Shen, Z., J. G. Fox, F. E. Dewhirst, B. J. Paster, C. J. Foltz, L. Yan, B. Shames, and L. Perry.** 1997. *Helicobacter rodentium* sp. nov., a urease-negative *Helicobacter* species isolated from laboratory mice. *Int. J. Syst. Bacteriol.* **47:**627–634.
157. **Shen, Z., S. Xu, F. E. Dewhirst, B. J. Paster, J. A. Pena, I. M. Modlin, M. Kidd, and J. G. Fox.** 2005. A novel enterohepatic *Helicobacter* species '*Helicobacter mastomyrinus*' isolated from the liver and intestine of rodents. *Helicobacter* **10:**59–70.
158. **Solnick, J. V., J. O'Rourke, A. Lee, B. J. Paster, F. E. Dewhirst, and L. S. Tompkins.** 1993. An uncultured gastric spiral organism is a newly identified Helicobacter in humans. *J. Infect. Dis.* **168:**379–385.
159. **Sorlin, P., P. Vandamme, J. Nortier, B. Hoste, C. Rossi, S. Pavlof, and M. J. Struelens.** 1999. Recurrent "*Flexispira rappini*" bacteremia in an adult patient undergoing hemodialysis: case report. *J. Clin. Microbiol.* **37:**1319–1323.
160. **Stanley, J., D. Linton, A. P. Burnens, F. E. Dewhirst, S. L. On, A. Porter, R. J. Owen, and M. Costas.** 1994. *Helicobacter pullorum* sp. nov.—genotype and phenotype of a new species isolated from poultry and from human patients with gastroenteritis. *Microbiology* **140:**3441–3449.
161. **Stanley, J., D. Linton, A. P. Burnens, F. E. Dewhirst, R. J. Owen, A. Porter, S. L. On, and M. Costas.** 1993. *Helicobacter canis* sp. nov., a new species from dogs: an integrated study of phenotype and genotype. *J. Gen. Microbiol.* **139:**2495–2504.
162. **Stolte, M., E. Wellens, B. Bethke, M. Ritter, and H. Eidt.** 1994. *Helicobacter heilmannii* (formerly *Gastrospirillum hominis*) gastritis: an infection transmitted by animals? *Scand. J. Gastroenterol.* **29:**1061–1064.
163. **Storskrubb, T., P. Aro, J. Ronkainen, M. Vieth, M. Stolte, K. Wreiber, L. Engstrand, H. Nyhlin, E. Bolling-Sternevald, N. J. Talley, and L. Agreus.** 2005. A negative

Helicobacter pylori serology test is more reliable for exclusion of premalignant gastric conditions than a negative test for current *H. pylori* infection: a report on histology and *H. pylori* detection in the general adult population. *Scand. J. Gastroenterol.* **40:**302–311.

164. **Suerbaum, S., C. Josenhans, T. Sterzenbach, B. Drescher, P. Brandt, M. Bell, M. Droge, B. Fartmann, H. P. Fischer, Z. Ge, A. Horster, R. Holland, K. Klein, J. Konig, L. Macko, G. L. Mendz, G. Nyakatura, D. B. Schauer, Z. Shen, J. Weber, M. Frosch, and J. G. Fox.** 2003. The complete genome sequence of the carcinogenic bacterium *Helicobacter hepaticus*. *Proc. Natl. Acad. Sci. USA* **100:**7901–7906.
165. **Suerbaum, S., and P. Michetti.** 2002. *Helicobacter pylori* infection. *N. Engl. J. Med.* **347:**1175–1186.
166. **Sung, J. J., S. C. Chung, T. K. Ling, M. Y. Yung, V. K. Leung, E. K. Ng, M. K. Li, A. F. Cheng, and A. K. Li.** 1995. Antibacterial treatment of gastric ulcers associated with *Helicobacter pylori*. *N. Engl. J. Med.* **332:**139–142.
167. **Szczebara, F., L. Dhaenens, P. Vincent, and M. O. Husson.** 1997. Evaluation of rapid molecular methods for detection of clarithromycin resistance in *Helicobacter pylori*. *Eur. J. Clin. Microbiol. Infect. Dis.* **16:**162–164.
168. **Tinnert, A., A. Mattsson, I. Bolin, J. Dalenback, A. Hamlet, and A. M. Svennerholm.** 1997. Local and systemic immune responses in humans against *Helicobacter pylori* antigens from homologous and heterologous strains. *Microb. Pathog.* **23:**285–296.
169. **Tomb, J. F., O. White, A. R. Kerlavage, R. A. Clayton, G. G. Sutton, R. D. Fleischmann, K. A. Ketchum, H. P. Klenk, S. Gill, B. A. Dougherty, K. Nelson, J. Quackenbush, L. Zhou, E. F. Kirkness, S. Peterson, B. Loftus, D. Richardson, R. Dodson, H. G. Khalak, A. Glodek, K. McKenney, L. M. Fitzegerald, N. Lee, M. D. Adams, E. K. Hickey, D. E. Berg, J. D. Gocayne, T. R. Utterback, J. D. Peterson, J. M. Kelley, M. D. Cotton, J. M. Weidman, C. Fujii, C. Bowman, L. Watthey, E. Wallin, W. S. Hayes, M. Borodovsky, P. D. Karp, H. O. Smith, C. M. Fraser, and J. C. Venter.** 1997. The complete genome sequence of the gastric pathogen *Helicobacter pylori*. *Nature* **388:**539–547.
170. **Trebesius, K., K. Adler, M. Vieth, M. Stolte, and R. Haas.** 2001. Specific detection and prevalence of *Helicobacter heilmannii*-like organisms in the human gastric mucosa by fluorescent in situ hybridization and partial 16S ribosomal DNA sequencing. *J. Clin. Microbiol.* **39:** 1510–1516.
171. **Vaira, D., P. Malfertheiner, F. Megraud, A. T. Axon, M. Deltenre, A. M. Hirschl, G. Gasbarrini, C. O'Morain, J. M. Garcia, M. Quina, G. N. Tytgat, et al.** 1999. Diagnosis of *Helicobacter pylori* infection with a new noninvasive antigen-based assay. *Lancet* **354:**30–33.
172. **Vakil, N., D. Rhew, A. Soll, and J. J. Ofman.** 2000. The cost-effectiveness of diagnostic testing strategies for *Helicobacter pylori*. *Am. J. Gastroenterol.* **95:**1691–1698.
173. **Vandamme, P., E. Falsen, R. Rossau, B. Hoste, P. Segers, R. Tytgat, and J. De Ley.** 1991. Revision of *Campylobacter*, *Helicobacter*, and *Wolinella* taxonomy: emendation of generic descriptions and proposal of *Arcobacter* gen. nov. *Int. J. Syst. Bacteriol.* **41:**88–103.
174. **Vandamme, P., C. S. Harrington, K. Jalava, and S. L. On.** 2000. Misidentifying helicobacters: the *Helicobacter cinaedi* example. *J. Clin. Microbiol.* **38:**2261–2266.
175. **van Doorn, L. J., C. Figueiredo, R. Sanna, A. Plaisier, P. Schneeberger, W. de Boer, and W. Quint.** 1998. Clinical relevance of the *cagA*, *vacA*, and *iceA* status of *Helicobacter pylori*. *Gastroenterology* **115:**58–66.
176. **Versalovic, J., and J. G. Fox.** 2001. Helicobacter pylori: *Molecular and Cellular Biology*, p.15–28. Horizon Scientific Press, Wymondham, United Kingdom.
177. **Versalovic, J., D. Shortridge, K. Kibler, M. V. Griffy, J. Beyer, R. K. Flamm, S. K. Tanaka, D. Y. Graham, and M. F. Go.** 1996. Mutations in 23S rRNA are associated with clarithromycin resistance in *Helicobacter pylori*. *Antimicrob. Agents Chemother.* **40:**477–480.
178. **Warren, J. R., and B. J. Marshall.** 1983. Unidentified curved bacilli on gastric epithelium in active chronic gastritis. *Lancet* **i:**1273–1275.
179. **Weir, S., B. Cuccherini, A. M. Whitney, M. L. Ray, J. P. MacGregor, A. Steigerwalt, M. I. Daneshvar, R. Weyant, B. Wray, J. Steele, W. Strober, and V. J. Gill.** 1999. Recurrent bacteremia caused by a "*Flexispira*"-like organism in a patient with X-linked (Bruton's) agammaglobulinemia. *J. Clin. Microbiol.* **37:**2439–2445.
180. **Whary, M. T., and J. G. Fox.** 2004. Natural and experimental *Helicobacter* infections. *Comp. Med.* **54:**128–158.
181. **Whary, M. T., N. Sundina, L. E. Bravo, P. Correa, F. Quinones, F. Caro, and J. G. Fox.** 2005. Intestinal helminthiasis in Colombian children promotes a Th2 response to *Helicobacter pylori:* possible implications for gastric carcinogenesis. *Cancer Epidemiol. Biomarkers Prev.* **14:**1464–1469.
182. **Woo, J. S., H. M. el-Zimaity, R. M. Genta, M. M. Yousfi, and D. Y. Graham.** 1996. The best gastric site for obtaining a positive rapid urease test. *Helicobacter* **1:**256–259.
183. **Wundisch, T., C. Thiede, A. Morgner, A. Dempfle, A. Gunther, H. Liu, H. Ye, M. Q. Du, T. D. Kim, E. Bayerdorffer, M. Stolte, and A. Neubauer.** 2005. Long-term follow-up of gastric MALT lymphoma after *Helicobacter pylori* eradication. *J. Clin. Oncol.* **23:**8018–8024.
184. **Yousfi, M. M., H. M. El-Zimaity, R. A. Cole, R. M. Genta, and D. Y. Graham.** 1997. Comparison of agar gel (CLOtest) or reagent strip (PyloriTek) rapid urease tests for detection of *Helicobacter pylori* infection. *Am. J. Gastroenterol.* **92:**997–999.

Leptospira

PAUL N. LEVETT

61

TAXONOMY

Serologic Classification

The genus *Leptospira* is comprised of spiral-shaped bacteria with hooked ends (32). This genus, along with the genera *Leptonema* and *Turneriella,* makes up the family *Leptospiraceae* within the order *Spirochaetales* and class "*Spirochaetes*" of the recently proposed phylum *Spirochaetes* (26). The genus was formerly divided into two species, *Leptospira interrogans,* comprising all pathogenic strains, and *Leptospira biflexa,* containing the saprophytic strains isolated from the environment (24, 32). *L. biflexa* and *L. interrogans* were differentiated by a number of biochemical tests (32).

Leptospires are divided into serovars defined by agglutination after cross-absorption with homologous antigen (17, 32, 34). Serovars are considered distinct if more than 10% of the homologous titer remains in at least one of the two antisera on repeated testing (31). Over 60 serovars of *L. biflexa* sensu lato and more than 200 serovars of *L. interrogans* sensu lato are recognized. Serovars that are antigenically related have traditionally been grouped into serogroups (34). Serogroups have no taxonomic standing, but the concept has proved useful for epidemiological understanding, particularly when interpreting the serological results from the microscopic agglutination test (MAT). The serogroups of *L. interrogans* sensu lato and some common serovars are shown in Table 1.

Genotypic Classification

The phenotypic classification of leptospires was replaced by a genotypic one, in which 17 genomospecies include all serovars of *Leptospira* (8, 53, 55, 80). Table 2 lists all species of *Leptospira*. DNA hybridization studies have also confirmed the taxonomic status of the monospecific genera *Leptonema* (8, 54) and *Turneriella* (38). The genetically defined species of *Leptospira* do not correspond to the previous two species (*L. interrogans* sensu lato and *L. biflexa* sensu lato), and both pathogenic and nonpathogenic serovars occur within some species (35). Neither serogroup nor serovar reliably predicts the true species of *Leptospira*. Moreover, genetic heterogeneity resulting from horizontal transfer of genes coding for cell surface antigens occurs within serovars (8, 25), resulting in strains of some serovars being classified in multiple species (Table 3). In addition, the phenotypic characteristics formerly used to differentiate *L. interrogans* sensu lato from *L. biflexa* sensu lato do not differentiate the genetically defined species (8, 80). Both *L. interrogans* and *L. biflexa* are retained as specific names in the genomic classification, and in this chapter, specific names refer to the genetically defined species, including *L. interrogans* sensu stricto and *L. biflexa* sensu stricto.

The molecular classification of leptospires requires the identification of both species and serovar of each isolate. Identification of *Leptospira* species is readily accomplished by 16S rRNA gene sequencing, and sequences are available in GenBank (R. E. Morey and P. N. Levett, unpublished data). Phylogenetic analysis of 16S rRNA gene sequences demonstrates three clades of leptospires, representing pathogens, saprophytes, and a group of species of uncertain pathogenicity (Fig. 1). Serovar identification is discussed below.

The concept of serogroups has no application in the taxonomy of *Leptospira* but remains a convenient tool for serologists.

DESCRIPTION OF THE FAMILY

Leptospires are tightly coiled spirochaetes, usually 0.1 μm by 6 to 20 μm. The helical conformation is right-handed, while the amplitude is approximately 0.1 to 0.15 μm and the wavelength is approximately 0.5 μm (23). The cells have pointed ends, either or both of which are usually bent into a distinctive hook (Fig. 2). Two axial filaments (periplasmic flagella), with polar insertions, are located in the periplasmic space. Leptospires exhibit two distinct forms of movement, either translational (rapid back-and-forth movements) or rotational (spinning rapidly about the long axis of the cell) (27). Morphologically, all leptospires are indistinguishable.

Leptospires are obligate aerobes with an optimum growth temperature of 28 to 30°C. The optimum pH for growth is 7.2 to 7.6. They produce both catalase and oxidase. They grow in simple media enriched with vitamins (vitamins B_2 and B_{12} are growth factors), long-chain fatty acids, and ammonium salts (32).

EPIDEMIOLOGY AND TRANSMISSION

Leptospires are ubiquitous, either free-living in water or associated with renal infection of animals. Leptospirosis is

TABLE 1 Serogroups and selected serovars of *Leptospira interrogans* sensu lato

Serogroup	Serovars
Icterohaemorrhagiae	Copenhageni
	Icterohaemorrhagiae
	Lai
Hebdomadis	Hebdomadis
	Jules
Autumnalis	Autumnalis
	Bim
	Fortbragg
Pyrogenes	Pyrogenes
Bataviae	Bataviae
Grippotyphosa	Canalzonae
	Grippotyphosa
	Ratnapura
Canicola	Canicola
Australis	Australis
	Bratislava
	Lora
Pomona	Pomona
Javanica	Javanica
Sejroe	Sejroe
	Hardjo
Panama	Mangus
	Panama
Cynopteri	Cynopteri
Djasiman	Djasiman
Sarmin	Sarmin
Mini	Mini
	Georgia
Tarassovi	Tarassovi
Ballum	Arborea
	Ballum
Celledoni	Celledoni
Louisiana	Lanka
	Louisiana
Ranarum	Ranarum
Manhao	Manhao
Shermani	Shermani
Hurstbridge	Hurstbridge

TABLE 2 Genospecies of *Leptospira*[a]

Species
L. alexanderi[b]
L. biflexa[c]
L.borgpetersenii[b]
L. broomii
L. fainei
L. inadai
L. interrogans[b]
L. kirschneri[b]
L. meyeri[b]
L. noguchii[b]
L. santarosai[b]
L. weilii[b]
L. wolbachii[c]

[a] Based on data reported by Brenner et al. (8), Ramadass et al. (55), Levett et al. (37a), and Pérolat et al. (53).

[b] These species constitute the clade of pathogenic *Leptospira* species.

[c] Currently only nonpathogenic strains of these species are known.

TABLE 3 Leptospiral serovars found in multiple species[a]

Serovar	Species
Bataviae	*L. interrogans, L. santarosai*
Bulgarica	*L. interrogans, L. kirschneri*
Grippotyphosa	*L. kirschneri, L. interrogans*
Hardjo	*L. borgpetersenii, L. interrogans, L. meyeri*
Icterohaemorrhagiae	*L. interrogans, L. inadai*
Kremastos	*L. interrogans, L. santarosai*
Mwogolo	*L. kirschneri, L. interrogans*
Paidjan	*L. kirschneri, L. interrogans*
Pomona	*L. interrogans, L. noguchii*
Pyrogenes	*L. interrogans, L. santarosai*
Szwajizak	*L. interrogans, L. santarosai*
Valbuzzi	*L. interrogans, L. kirschneri*

[a] Based on data reported by Brenner et al. (8) and by Feresu et al. (25).

presumed to be the most widespread zoonosis in the world (78). The source of infection in humans is usually either direct or indirect contact with the urine of an infected animal. The incidence is very much higher in warm-climate countries than in temperate regions, due mainly to the longer survival of leptospires in the environment under warm, humid conditions. The disease is seasonal, with the peak incidence occurring in summer or fall in temperate regions, where temperature is the limiting factor in survival of leptospires, and during rainy seasons in warm-climate regions, where rapid desiccation would otherwise prevent survival.

Animals, including humans, can be divided into maintenance hosts or accidental (incidental) hosts. A maintenance host is defined as a species in which infection is endemic, usually transferred from animal to animal by direct contact. Infection is usually acquired at an early age, and the prevalence of chronic excretion in the urine increases with the age of the animal. Other animals (such as humans) may become infected by indirect contact with the maintenance host. Animals may be maintenance hosts of some serovars but incidental hosts of others, infection with which may cause severe or fatal disease. The most important maintenance hosts are small mammals, which may transfer infection to domestic farm animals, dogs, and humans. Different rodent species may be reservoirs of distinct serovars, but rats are generally maintenance hosts for serovars of the serogroup Icterohaemorrhagiae, and mice are generally maintenance hosts for serogroup Ballum serovars. Domestic animals are also maintenance hosts; dairy cattle may harbor serovars Hardjo and Pomona; pigs may harbor Pomona, Tarassovi, or Bratislava; and dogs may harbor Canicola. Distinct variations in maintenance hosts and the serovars they carry occur throughout the world, and these associations may change over time.

Knowledge of the prevalent serovars and their maintenance hosts is essential in understanding the epidemiology of the disease. For example, canine leptospirosis is increasing in the northeastern regions of North America. Very few cases have been diagnosed by culture, but serology suggests that they are caused largely by serovar Grippotyphosa (9, 73). Epidemiological evidence implicates raccoons and possibly skunks as the reservoir. Cases are clustered particularly in newly suburbanized areas (73). Canine vaccine composition has been changed to include serovars Grippotyphosa and Pomona as a result of this change in epidemiology.

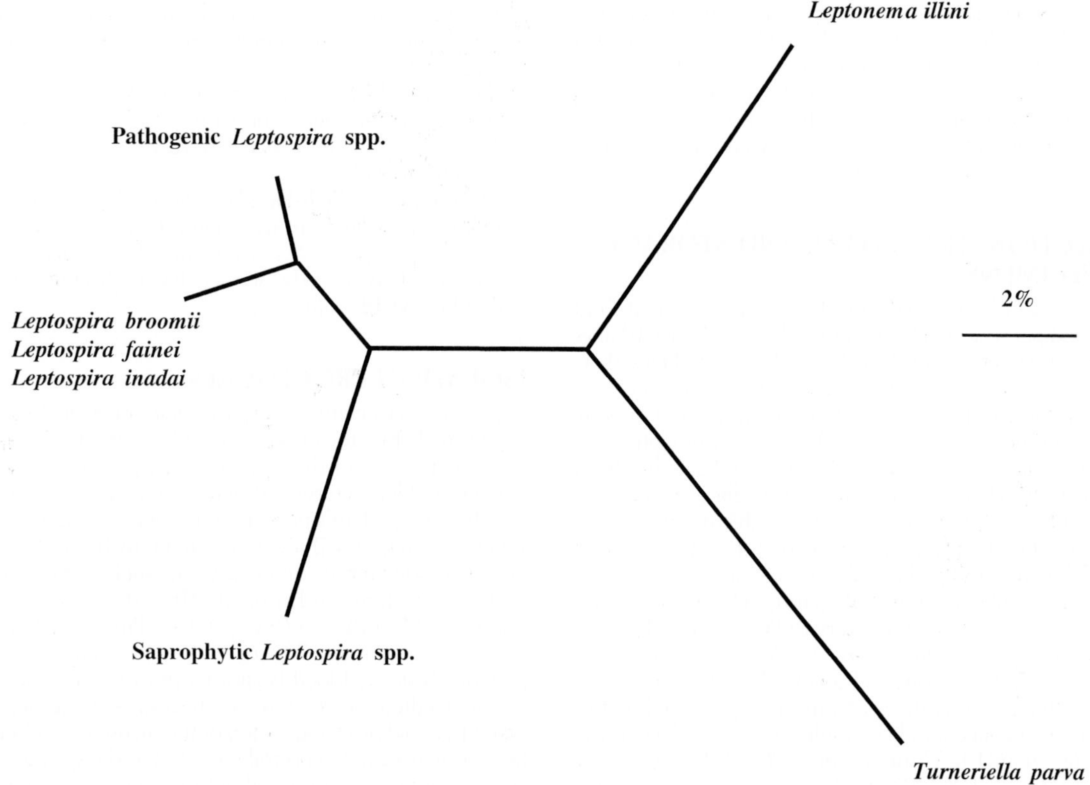

FIGURE 1 Phylogenetic relationships between the genera of the *Leptospiraceae*, based on 16S rRNA gene sequences. The scale bar represents a 2% difference in sequence.

Human infections may be acquired through occupational, recreational, or avocational exposures. Occupation is a significant risk factor for humans. Direct contact with infected animals accounts for most infections in farmers, veterinarians, abattoir workers, rodent control workers, and people in other occupations which require contact with animals, while indirect contact is important for sewer workers, miners, soldiers, septic tank cleaners, fish farmers, rice field workers, and sugar cane cutters. Livestock farming is a major occupational risk factor throughout the world. The highest risk is associated with dairy farming and is associated with serovar Hardjo and in particular with milking of dairy cattle. There is a significant risk associated with recreational exposures occurring in water sports (46, 59).

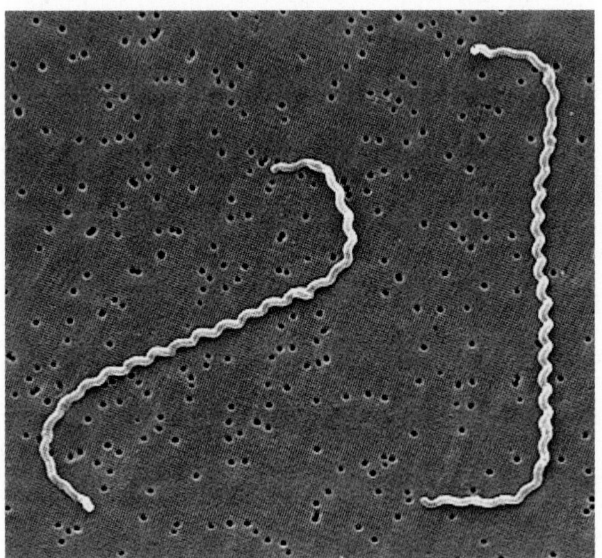

FIGURE 2 Scanning electron micrograph of leptospiral cells bound to a 0.2-μm-pore-size filter. Magnification, approximately ×3,500. Public Health Image Library.

CLINICAL SIGNIFICANCE

The usual portal of entry is through abrasions or cuts in the skin or via the conjunctiva. The great majority of infections are either subclinical or of very mild severity, and most patients will probably not seek, or be brought to, medical attention. The clinical presentation of leptospirosis is biphasic, with a septicemic phase lasting about a week, followed by the immune phase, characterized by antibody production and excretion of leptospires in the urine. Most of the complications of leptospirosis are associated with localization of leptospires within the tissues during the immune phase and thus occur during the second week of the illness.

The overwhelming majority of the recognized cases present with a febrile illness of sudden onset, the symptoms of which include chills, headache, myalgia, abdominal pain, and conjunctival suffusion. Aseptic meningitis may be found in ≤25% of all leptospirosis cases. Between 5 and 10% of all patients with leptospirosis have the icteric form of the disease (Weil's disease), in which the clinical course is often very rapidly progressive. In addition to jaundice, patients with icteric leptospirosis may develop acute renal failure, pulmonary hemorrhage, and cardiac arrythmias. Severe cases often present late in the course of the disease, and this contributes to the high mortality rate, which ranges between 5 and 15%.

COLLECTION, TRANSPORT, AND STORAGE OF SPECIMENS

Leptospires can be isolated from blood, cerebrospinal fluid (CSF), and peritoneal dialysate fluids during the first 10 days of illness. Specimens should be collected before antibiotic therapy is initiated and while the patient is febrile. Under optimal conditions, 1 or 2 drops of blood are inoculated directly into culture medium at the bedside. Survival of leptospires in commercial blood culture media for several days has been reported (51). There are no transport media available, but blood can be collected and shipped at ambient temperature in tubes containing heparin, oxalate, or citrate (23). Citrate or EDTA-containing tubes are optimal for detection by PCR, whereas tubes containing heparin, sodium polyanethol sulfonate, or saponin are inhibitory to PCRs (39, 62).

Urine can be cultured after the first week of illness. Specimens should be collected aseptically into sterile containers without preservatives and must be processed within a short time of collection; best results are obtained when the delay is less than 1 h. Urine specimens for PCR testing may be stabilized in DNA/RNA Protect containers (Sierra Diagnostics, Sonora, Calif.), allowing for transport over long distances (39).

DIRECT EXAMINATION

Microscopy

Leptospires may be visualized in clinical material by dark-field microscopy (×100 and ×400 magnifications) or by immunofluorescence or light microscopy after appropriate staining. Dark-field microscopic examination of body fluids such as blood, urine, CSF, or dialysate fluid is both insensitive and lacking in specificity (3, 72, 76). Approximately 10^4 leptospires/ml are necessary for one cell per field to be visible by dark-field microscopy (69). Direct dark-field microscopy of blood is also subject to misinterpretation of fibrin or protein threads, which may demonstrate Brownian motion (23, 69, 76). Leptospires in tissues were first visualized by silver staining (63), and the Warthin-Starry stain is widely used for histologic examination. More recently, immunohistochemical methods have been applied (70, 81, 82). Immunohistochemical staining can be performed at the Centers for Disease Control and Prevention, Atlanta, Ga. (contact Sherif Zaki at szaki@cdc.gov).

Antigen Detection

Antigen detection is generally regarded as insensitive. An assay for detection of antigen in urine has been described (58) but has not been evaluated widely. There are no commercial antigen detection assays.

Nucleic Acid Techniques

Several primer pairs for conventional PCR detection of leptospires have been described (35). However, only two methods have been subject to extensive clinical evaluation (11, 44). Both methods were found to be more sensitive than culture, and leptospiral DNA has been amplified from serum, urine, aqueous humor, CSF, and tissues obtained at autopsy (10).

Real-time PCR assays have been developed, targeting either 16S rRNA genes or pathogenic-specific sequences (39, 45, 49, 62). These assays have yet to be evaluated in large clinical studies.

A limitation of PCR-based diagnosis of leptospirosis is the inability of most PCR assays to identify the infecting serovar. While this is not significant for individual patient management, the identity of the serovar has both epidemiological and public health value.

ISOLATION PROCEDURES

Leptospiremia occurs during the first stage of the disease, beginning before the onset of symptoms, and has usually finished by the end of the first week of the acute illness (43). Therefore, blood cultures should be taken as soon as possible after the patient's presentation. One or 2 drops of blood (approximately 50 μl) are inoculated into 10 ml of semisolid oleic acid-albumin medium (20, 33), such as Ellinghausen-McCullough-Johnson-Harris (EMJH) (Difco Laboratories, Sparks, Md.) or PLM-5 (Intergen Co., Purchase, N.Y.), containing 0.1% agar and 200 μg of 5-fluorouracil per ml, at the patient's bedside. Blood is allowed to drop onto the surface of the medium; mixing is not necessary. Care should be taken to avoid overinoculation of the medium, as blood contains inhibitors of leptospiral growth. For the greatest recovery rate, multiple cultures should be performed, but this is rarely possible. Inoculation of media with further 10-fold dilutions of blood samples may increase recovery (64). Survival of leptospires in commercial blood culture media for up to a week has been reported (51). Since the organism does not grow in conventional media, positive signals in automated systems are most unlikely. However, if a diagnosis of leptospirosis is suspected after the collection of conventional blood cultures, it is possible to detect leptospires by using PCR assays. There is insufficient experience to show the value of subculture from blood cultures into leptospira culture media, but this should be attempted if possible.

Other samples that may be cultured during the first week of illness include CSF and peritoneal dialysate. Urine cultures may yield growth from the beginning of the second week of symptomatic illness. Survival of leptospires in voided human urine is limited, so urine should be processed immediately, by neutralization of pH with sodium bicarbonate followed by centrifugation. After centrifugation in 15-ml tubes for 30 min at 1,500 × g, the sediment is resuspended in 1 ml of phosphate-buffered saline and 1 or 2 drops are inoculated into semisolid EMJH medium containing 5-fluorouracil as described above.

Cultures in EMJH are incubated in sealed bottles at 28 to 30°C and examined weekly by dark-field microscopy for up to 13 weeks before being discarded. Growth often develops in a discrete band, several millimeters below the surface of the medium, known as a Dinger's ring. Cultures that show growth of other bacteria may be passed through a 0.2- or 0.45-μm-pore-size filter before subculture into fresh medium.

IDENTIFICATION

Isolated leptospires are identified either by serological methods or, more recently, by molecular techniques. Traditional methods relied on cross-agglutinin absorption (17). The number of laboratories that can perform these identification methods is very small. The use of panels of monoclonal antibodies allows laboratories which can perform the MAT to identify isolates of frequently encountered serovars with relative rapidity (66). Monoclonal antibodies are available from the WHO/OIE Leptospirosis Reference Laboratory at the Royal Tropical Institute, Amsterdam, The Netherlands. The molecular-method-based taxonomy of *Leptospira* necessitates the identification of isolates to both species and serovar. Species identification is most practically determined by 16S rRNA gene sequencing (Morey and Levett, unpublished). Sequences of some species differ by only a few bases along the entire length of the 16S rRNA gene, so for accurate identification a full-length sequence is necessary.

Typing Procedures

Because of the difficulties associated with serological identification of leptospiral isolates, there has been great interest in molecular methods for identification and subtyping (29, 66). Methods employed have included digestion of chromosomal DNA by restriction endonucleases, restriction fragment length polymorphisms, ribotyping, pulsed-field gel electrophoresis, and a number of PCR-based approaches (35). The most widely applicable molecular method for identification of serovars is pulsed-field gel electrophoresis (29, 30). This approach has been standardized, using the PulseNet model (R. Galloway and P. N. Levett, *Abstr. Int. Conf. Emerg. Infect. Dis.*, abstr. 214, 2004).

More recently, sequence-based methods such as amplified fragment length polymorphism (AFLP) and variable-number tandem-repeat methods have been developed for the study of leptospiral epidemiology (42, 71). The use of multilocus sequence typing is being investigated. The application of these powerful tools will lead to greater understanding of leptospiral epidemiology at a population level.

SEROLOGICAL TESTS

Most cases of leptospirosis are diagnosed by serology. Antibodies are detectable in the blood approximately 5 to 7 days after the onset of symptoms. The definitive serologic investigation in leptospirosis remains the MAT, in which patients' sera are reacted with live or killed antigen suspensions of leptospiral serovars. After incubation, the serum-antigen mixtures are examined microscopically for agglutination and the titers are determined. The MAT is a complex test to control, perform, and interpret (68), the use of which is limited to regional or national reference laboratories. Protocols for performing the MAT have been described in detail (2, 21, 64). An international proficiency testing scheme under the auspices of the International Leptospirosis Society has stimulated improvement in the performance of the MAT by participating laboratories (14). The range of antigens used should include serovars representative of all serogroups (21, 68) and locally common serovars (67). Titers of antibody to local isolates are often higher than titers of antibody to laboratory stock strains of serovars within the same serogroup. The wide range of antigens is used in order to detect infections with uncommon, or previously undetected, serovars. The test is read by dark-field microscopy. The end point is the highest dilution of serum in which 50% agglutination occurs. Because of the difficulty in detecting the titer at which 50% of the leptospires are agglutinated, the end point is determined by the presence of approximately 50% free, unagglutinated leptospires, by comparison with the control suspension (21). Considerable effort is required to reduce the subjective effect of observer variation, even within laboratories.

Interpretation of the MAT is complicated by the high degree of cross-reaction that occurs between different serogroups, especially in acute-phase samples. Paradoxical reactions, in which the highest titers detected are those of antibody to a serogroup unrelated to the infecting one, are also common (35). The broad cross-reactivity in the acute phase, followed by relative serogroup specificity in convalescent-phase samples, results from the detection in the MAT of both immunoglobulin M (IgM) and IgG antibodies and the presence of several common antigens among leptospires (1, 13, 40).

Paired sera are required to confirm a diagnosis with certainty. A fourfold or greater rise in titer between paired sera confirms the diagnosis, regardless of the interval between samples. The interval between first and second samples depends very much on the delay between onset of symptoms and presentation of the patient. If symptoms typical of leptospirosis are present, an interval of 3 to 5 days may be adequate to detect rising titers. However, if the patient presents earlier in the course of the disease, or if the date of onset is not known precisely, then an interval of 10 to 14 days between samples is more appropriate. Less often, seroconversion does not occur with such rapidity, and a longer interval between samples (or repeated sampling) is necessary. MAT serology is insensitive, particularly with early acute-phase specimens (4, 7, 15). Moreover, patients with fulminant leptospirosis may die before seroconversion occurs (11, 15, 56).

A presumptive diagnosis can be made by detection of a single elevated titer in association with an acute febrile illness. The magnitude of such a titer is dependent upon the background level of exposure in the population, and hence the seroprevalence. In the current CDC case definition, a titer of ≥200 in a patient with a clinically compatible illness is used to indicate a probable case (12).

Titers following acute infection may be extremely high (≥25,600) and may take months, or even years, to fall to low levels (3, 6, 16, 41, 57). Thus, in a high-incidence population, a low cutoff titer for presumptive diagnosis is inappropriate and will generate many false-positive diagnoses. In areas of endemicity a single titer of ≥800 in symptomatic patients is generally indicative of leptospirosis (22), but titers as high as ≥1,600 have been recommended (2). Rarely, seroconversion may be delayed for many weeks after recovery, and longer serological follow-up will be necessary to confirm the diagnosis.

Formalized antigens have been used in the MAT in order to overcome some of the difficulties associated with the use of live antigens. Titers obtained with these antigens are somewhat lower, and more cross-reactions are detected (21, 50). Agglutination of formalized antigens is qualitatively different from that seen with live antigens (2). However, for laboratories without the staff or expertise to maintain live antigens, formalized and lyophilized antigens may represent an alternative. These antigens are not available commercially but may be obtained from WHO Collaborating Centers.

The MAT is the most appropriate test to employ in epidemiological serosurveys, since it can be applied to sera from any animal species and because the range of antigens utilized can be expanded or decreased as required. It is usual to use a titer of ≥100 as evidence of past exposure (21). Contrary to a widely held belief, the MAT is a serogroup-specific assay. However, conclusions about infecting serovars cannot be drawn without isolates; at best the MAT data can give a general impression of which serogroups are present within a population (36).

Because of the complexity of the MAT, rapid screening tests for leptospiral antibodies in acute infection have been developed. Traditional methods based upon agglutination have largely been superseded by IgM detection assays. IgM antibodies become detectable during the first week of illness, allowing the diagnosis to be confirmed and treatment to be initiated while it is likely to be most effective. IgM detection has repeatedly been shown to be more sensitive than MAT when the first specimen is taken early in the acute phase of the illness (15, 56, 75). IgM dipstick assays have been shown to be as sensitive as microtiter plate IgM-enzyme-linked immunosorbent assays (5, 28, 37). Other rapid assays include a latex agglutination assay (61) and a lateral-flow assay (60). Commercial IgM dipstick and latex agglutination assays are available from PanBio, Baltimore, Md., and bioMerieux, Durham, N.C., respectively.

ANTIBIOTIC SUSCEPTIBILITIES

Leptospires are susceptible to many antimicrobial agents, including β-lactams, macrolides, tetracyclines, fluoroquinolones, and streptomycin. Problems in the determination of susceptibility include the long incubation time required (19), the use of media containing serum (48, 79), and the difficulty in quantifying growth accurately. These constraints limited the development of rapid, standardized methods for susceptibility testing. However, broth microdilution methods that have facilitated the testing of larger numbers of isolates against a wide range of antimicrobial agents have been described recently (47, 74). Such studies will lead to the identification of potential new agents for inclusion in clinical trials.

Penicillin and doxycycline are both effective for treatment of leptospirosis and remain the drugs of choice (18); recent clinical studies have shown that expanded-spectrum cephalosporins may be equally effective (52, 65).

EVALUATION, INTERPRETATION, AND REPORTING OF RESULTS

A diagnosis of leptospirosis can be made by isolation of the organism or by amplification of leptospiral DNA from blood, urine, or other specimens; by demonstration of leptospires in tissues by immunohistochemical staining; or by detection of a fourfold or greater rise in titers between acute- and convalescent-phase serum samples tested by the same methodology at the same time. In populations and/or regions where leptospirosis is not endemic, MAT titers of ≥200 in a single specimen obtained after the onset of symptoms are suggestive but not diagnostic of acute or recent leptospirosis. A titer of ≥800 in the presence of compatible symptoms is strong evidence of recent or current leptospirosis (21). Delayed seroconversions are common. Assays that detect IgM antibodies give presumptive evidence of recent exposure to leptospirosis but require confirmation, since IgM titers are persistent (16). Cross-reactive antibodies, sometimes with significant seroconversion, are associated with syphilis, relapsing fever, Lyme disease, and legionellosis (5). Negative test results in the presence of compatible symptoms do not rule out the diagnosis of leptospirosis, and further samples should be examined. The isolation of leptospires, the demonstration of leptospiral DNA by molecular methods, or the detection of leptospires in tissues by immunohistochemistry confirms the diagnosis and differentiates between current infection and past exposure, which may not be clearly differentiated by serology.

Despite recent advances in molecular detection and characterization of leptospires and in the development of rapid serologic tests, there are still relatively few laboratories throughout the world with the appropriate capabilities for *Leptospira* diagnostics. Additional information regarding leptospirosis and diagnostic centers of expertise (77) is available for downloading from the International Leptospirosis Society website (http://www.med.monash.edu.au/microbiology/staff/adler/ilspage.htm).

REFERENCES

1. **Adler, B., and S. Faine.** 1978. The antibodies involved in the human immune response to leptospiral infection. *J. Med. Microbiol.* **11:**387–400.
2. **Alexander, A. D.** 1986. Serological diagnosis of leptospirosis, p. 435–439. *In* N. R. Rose, H. Friedman, and J. L. Fahey (ed.), *Manual of Clinical Laboratory Immunology,* 3rd ed., American Society for Microbiology, Washington, D.C.
3. **Alston, J. M., and J. C. Broom.** 1958. *Leptospirosis in Man and Animals.* E. & S. Livingstone, Edinburgh, United Kingdom.
4. **Appassakij, H., K. Silpapojakul, R. Wansit, and J. Woodtayakorn.** 1995. Evaluation of the immunofluorescent antibody test for the diagnosis of human leptospirosis. *Am. J. Trop. Med. Hyg.* **52:**340–343.
5. **Bajani, M. D., D. A. Ashford, S. L. Bragg, C. W. Woods, T. Aye, R. A. Spiegel, B. D. Plikaytis, B. A. Perkins, M. Phelan, P. N. Levett, and R. S. Weyant.** 2003. Evaluation of four commercially available rapid serologic tests for diagnosis of leptospirosis. *J. Clin. Microbiol.* **41:**803–809.
6. **Blackmore, D. K., L. M. Schollum, and K. M. Moriarty.** 1984. The magnitude and duration of titres of leptospiral agglutinins in human sera. *N. Z. Med. J.* **97:**83–86.
7. **Brandão, A. P., E. D. Camargo, E. D. da Silva, M. V. Silva, and R. V. Abrão.** 1998. Macroscopic agglutination test for rapid diagnosis of human leptospirosis. *J. Clin. Microbiol.* **36:**3138–3142.
8. **Brenner, D. J., A. F. Kaufmann, K. R. Sulzer, A. G. Steigerwalt, F. C. Rogers, and R. S. Weyant.** 1999. Further determination of DNA relatedness between serogroups and serovars in the family Leptospiraceae with a proposal for *Leptospira alexanderi* sp. nov. and four new *Leptospira* genomospecies. *Int. J. Syst. Bacteriol.* **49:**839–858.
9. **Brown, C. A., A. W. Roberts, M. A. Miller, D. A. David, S. A. Brown, C. A. Bolin, J. Jarecki-Black, C. E. Greene, and D. Miller-Liebl.** 1996. *Leptospira interrogans* serovar *grippotyphosa* infection in dogs. *J. Am. Vet. Med. Assoc.* **209:**1265–1267.
10. **Brown, P. D., D. G. Carrington, C. Gravekamp, H. van de Kemp, C. N. Edwards, S. R. Jones, P. R. Prussia, S. Garriques, W. J. Terpstra, and P. N. Levett.** 2003. Direct detection of leptospiral material in human postmortem samples. *Res. Microbiol.* **154:**581–586.
11. **Brown, P. D., C. Gravekamp, D. G. Carrington, H. Van de Kemp, R. A. Hartskeerl, C. N. Edwards, C. O. R. Everard, W. J. Terpstra, and P. N. Levett.** 1995. Evaluation of the polymerase chain reaction for early diagnosis of leptospirosis. *J. Med. Microbiol.* **43:**110–114.
12. **Centers for Disease Control and Prevention.** 1997. Case definitions for infectious conditions under public health surveillance. *Morb. Mortal. Wkly. Rep.* **46**(RR-10)**:**49.
13. **Chapman, A. J., B. Adler, and S. Faine.** 1987. Genus-specific antigens in *Leptospira* revealed by immunoblotting. *Zentbl. Bakteriol.* **264:**279–283.
14. **Chappel, R. J., M. G. Goris, M. F. Palmer, and R. A. Hartskeerl.** 2004. Impact of proficiency testing on results of the microscopic agglutination test for diagnosis of leptospirosis. *J. Clin. Microbiol.* **42:**5484–5488.

15. **Cumberland, P. C., C. O. R. Everard, and P. N. Levett.** 1999. Assessment of the efficacy of the IgM enzyme-linked immunosorbent assay (ELISA) and microscopic agglutination test (MAT) in the diagnosis of acute leptospirosis. *Am. J. Trop. Med. Hyg.* **61:**731–734.
16. **Cumberland, P. C., C. O. R. Everard, J. G. Wheeler, and P. N. Levett.** 2001. Persistence of anti-leptospiral IgM, IgG and agglutinating antibodies in patients presenting with acute febrile illness in Barbados 1979–1989. *Eur. J. Epidemiol.* **17:**601–608.
17. **Dikken, H., and E. Kmety.** 1978. Serological typing methods of leptospires, p. 259–307. *In* T. Bergan and J. R. Norris (ed.), *Methods in Microbiology,* vol. 11. Academic Press, London, United Kingdom.
18. **Edwards, C. N., and P. N. Levett.** 2004. Prevention and treatment of leptospirosis. *Expert. Rev. Anti-Infect. Ther.* **2:**293–298.
19. **Ellinghausen, H. C.** 1983. Growth, cultural characteristics, and antibacterial sensitivity of *Leptospira interrogans* serovar *hardjo. Cornell Vet.* **73:**225–239.
20. **Ellinghausen, H. C., and W. G. McCullough.** 1965. Nutrition of *Leptospira pomona* and growth of 13 other serotypes: fractionation of oleic albumin complex and a medium of bovine albumin and polysorbate 80. *Am. J. Vet. Res.* **26:**45–51.
21. **Faine, S.** 1982. *Guidelines for the Control of Leptospirosis.* World Health Organization, Geneva, Switzerland.
22. **Faine, S.** 1988. Leptospirosis, p. 344–352. *In* A. Balows, W. J. Hausler, M. Ohashi, and A. Turano (ed.), *Laboratory Diagnosis of Infectious Diseases. Principles and Practice,* vol. 1. Springer-Verlag, New York, N.Y.
23. **Faine, S., B. Adler, C. Bolin, and P. Perolat.** 1999. *Leptospira* and leptospirosis, 2nd ed. MedSci, Melbourne, Australia.
24. **Faine, S., and N. D. Stallman.** 1982. Amended descriptions of the genus *Leptospira* Noguchi 1917 and the species *L. interrogans* (Stimson 1907) Wenyon 1926 and *L. biflexa* (Wolbach and Binger 1914) Noguchi 1918. *Int. J. Syst. Bacteriol.* **32:**461–463.
25. **Feresu, S. B., C. A. Bolin, H. van de Kemp, and H. Korver.** 1999. Identification of a serogroup Bataviae *Leptospira* strain isolated from an ox in Zimbabwe. *Zentbl. Bakteriol.* **289:**19–29.
26. **Garrity, G. M., and J. G. Holt.** 2001. The road map to the Manual, p. 119–166. *In* D. R. Boone, R. W. Castenholtz, and G. M. Garrity (ed.), *Bergey's Manual of Systematic Bacteriology,* 2nd ed., vol. 1. Springer-Verlag, New York, N.Y.
27. **Goldstein, S. F., and N. W. Charon.** 1988. Motility of the spirochete *Leptospira. Cell Motil. Cytoskeleton* **9:**101–110.
28. **Gussenhoven, G. C., M. A. W. G. van der Hoorn, M. G. A. Goris, W. J. Terpstra, R. A. Hartskeerl, B. W. Mol, C. W. van Ingen, and H. L. Smits.** 1997. LEPTO dipstick, a dipstick assay for detection of *Leptospira*-specific immunoglobulin M antibodies in human sera. *J. Clin. Microbiol.* **35:**92–97.
29. **Herrmann, J. L.** 1993. Genomic techniques for identification of *Leptospira* strains. *Pathol. Biol.* **41:**943–950.
30. **Herrmann, J. L., E. Bellenger, P. Perolat, G. Baranton, and I. Saint Girons.** 1992. Pulsed-field gel electrophoresis of *Not*I digests of leptospiral DNA: a new rapid method of serovar identification. *J. Clin. Microbiol.* **30:**1696–1702.
31. **International Committee on Systematic Bacteriology Subcommittee on the Taxonomy of *Leptospira*.** 1987. Minutes of the meeting, 5 and 6 September 1986, Manchester, England. *Int. J. Syst. Bacteriol.* **37:**472–473.
32. **Johnson, R. C., and S. Faine.** 1984. *Leptospira,* p. 62–67. *In* N. R. Krieg and J. G. Holt (ed.), *Bergey's Manual of Systematic Bacteriology,* vol. 1. Williams & Wilkins, Baltimore, Md.
33. **Johnson, R. C., and V. G. Harris.** 1967. Differentiation of pathogenic and saprophytic leptospires. 1. Growth at low temperatures. *J. Bacteriol.* **94:**27–31.
34. **Kmety, E., and H. Dikken.** 1993. *Classification of the Species* Leptospira interrogans *and History of Its Serovars.* University Press Groningen, Groningen, The Netherlands.
35. **Levett, P. N.** 2001. Leptospirosis. *Clin. Microbiol. Rev.* **14:**296–326.
36. **Levett, P. N.** 2003. Usefulness of serologic analysis as a predictor of the infecting serovar in patients with severe leptospirosis. *Clin. Infect. Dis.* **36:**447–452.
37. **Levett, P. N., S. L. Branch, C. U. Whittington, C. N. Edwards, and H. Paxton.** 2001. Two methods for rapid serological diagnosis of acute leptospirosis. *Clin. Diagn. Lab. Immunol.* **8:**349–351.

37a. **Levett, P. N., R. E. Morey, R. L. Galloway, and A. G. Steigerwalt.** 2006. *Leptospira broomii* sp. nov., isolated from humans with leptospirosis. *Int. J. Syst. Evol. Microbiol.* **56:** 671–673.

38. **Levett, P. N., R. E. Morey, R. Galloway, A. G. Steigerwalt, and W. A. Ellis.** 2005. Reclassification of *Leptospira parva* Hovind-Hougen *et al.,* 1982 as *Turneriella parva* gen. nov., comb. nov. *Int. J. Syst. Evol. Microbiol.* **55:**1497–1499.
39. **Levett, P. N., R. E. Morey, R. L. Galloway, D. E. Turner, A. G. Steigerwalt, and L. W. Mayer.** 2005. Detection of pathogenic leptospires by real-time quantitative PCR. *J. Med. Microbiol.* **54:**45–49.
40. **Lin, M., O. Surujballi, K. Nielsen, S. Nadin-Davis, and G. Randall.** 1997. Identification of a 35-kilodalton serovar-cross-reactive flagellar protein, FlaB, from *Leptospira interrogans* by N-terminal sequencing, gene cloning, and sequence analysis. *Infect. Immun.* **65:**4355–4359.
41. **Lupidi, R., M. Cinco, D. Balanzin, E. Delprete, and P. E. Varaldo.** 1991. Serological follow-up of patients in a localized outbreak of leptospirosis. *J. Clin. Microbiol.* **29:**805–809.
42. **Majed, Z., E. Bellenger, D. Postic, C. Pourcel, G. Baranton, and M. Picardeau.** 2005. Identification of variable-number tandem-repeat loci in *Leptospira interrogans* sensu stricto. *J. Clin. Microbiol.* **43:**539–545.
43. **McCrumb, F. R., J. L. Stockard, C. R. Robinson, L. H. Turner, D. G. Levis, C. W. Maisey, M. F. Kelleher, C. A. Gleiser, and J. E. Smadel.** 1957. Leptospirosis in Malaya. I. Sporadic cases among military and civilian personnel. *Am. J. Trop. Med. Hyg.* **6:**238–256.
44. **Merien, F., G. Baranton, and P. Pérolat.** 1995. Comparison of polymerase chain reaction with microagglutination test and culture for diagnosis of leptospirosis. *J. Infect. Dis.* **172:**281–285.
45. **Merien, F., D. Portnoi, P. Bourhy, F. Charavay, A. Berlioz-Arthaud, and G. Baranton.** 2005. A rapid and quantitative method for the detection of *Leptospira* species in human leptospirosis. *FEMS Microbiol. Lett.* **249:**139–147.
46. **Morgan, J., S. L. Bornstein, A. M. Karpati, M. Bruce, C. A. Bolin, C. C. Austin, C. W. Woods, J. Lingappa, C. Langkop, B. Davis, D. R. Graham, M. Proctor, D. A. Ashford, M. Bajani, S. L. Bragg, K. Shutt, B. A. Perkins, and J. W. Tappero.** 2002. Outbreak of Leptospirosis among Triathlon participants and community residents in Springfield, Illinois, 1998. *Clin. Infect. Dis.* **34:**1593–1599.
47. **Murray, C. K., and D. R. Hospenthal.** 2004. Broth microdilution susceptibility testing for *Leptospira* spp. *Antimicrob. Agents Chemother.* **48:**1548–1552.
48. **Oie, S., K. Hironaga, A. Koshiro, H. Konishi, and Z. Yoshii.** 1983. In vitro susceptibilities of five *Leptospira* strains to 16 antimicrobial agents. *Antimicrob. Agents Chemother.* **24:**905–908.

49. **Palaniappan, R. U., Y. F. Chang, C. F. Chang, M. J. Pan, C. W. Yang, P. Harpending, S. P. McDonough, E. Dubovi, T. Divers, J. Qu, and B. Roe.** 2005. Evaluation of *lig*-based conventional and real time PCR for the detection of pathogenic leptospires. *Mol. Cell. Probes* **19:**111–117.
50. **Palmer, M. F., S. A. Waitkins, and S. W. Wanyangu.** 1987. A comparison of live and formalised leptospiral microscopic agglutination test. *Zentbl. Bakteriol.* **265:** 151–159.
51. **Palmer, M. F., and W. J. Zochowski.** 2000. Survival of leptospires in commercial blood culture systems revisited. *J. Clin. Pathol.* **53:**713–714.
52. **Panaphut, T., S. Domrongkitchaiporn, A. Vibhagool, B. Thinkamrop, and W. Susaengrat.** 2003. Ceftriaxone compared with sodium penicillin G for treatment of severe leptospirosis. *Clin. Infect. Dis.* **36:**1507–1513.
53. **Pérolat, P., R. J. Chappel, B. Adler, G. Baranton, D. M. Bulach, M. L. Billinghurst, M. Letocart, F. Merien, and M. S. Serrano.** 1998. *Leptospira fainei* sp. nov., isolated from pigs in Australia. *Int. J. Syst. Bacteriol.* **48:**851–858.
54. **Ramadass, P., B. D. W. Jarvis, R. J. Corner, M. Cinco, and R. B. Marshall.** 1990. DNA relatedness among strains of *Leptospira biflexa*. *Int. J. Syst. Bacteriol.* **40:**231–235.
55. **Ramadass, P., B. D. W. Jarvis, R. J. Corner, D. Penny, and R. B. Marshall.** 1992. Genetic characterization of pathogenic *Leptospira* species by DNA hybridization. *Int. J. Syst. Bacteriol.* **42:**215–219.
56. **Ribeiro, M. A., C. S. N. Assis, and E. C. Romero.** 1994. Serodiagnosis of human leptospirosis employing immunodominant antigen. *Serodiagn. Immunother. Infect. Dis.* **6:**140–144.
57. **Romero, E. C., C. R. Caly, and P. H. Yasuda.** 1998. The persistence of leptospiral agglutinins titers in human sera diagnosed by the microscopic agglutination test. *Rev. Inst. Med. Trop. Sao Paulo* **40:**183–184.
58. **Saengjaruk, P., W. Chaicumpa, G. Watt, G. Bunyaraksyotin, V. Wuthiekanun, P. Tapchaisri, C. Sittinont, T. Panaphut, K. Tomanakan, Y. Sakolvaree, M. Chongsa-Nguan, Y. Mahakunkijcharoen, T. Kalambaheti, P. Naigowit, M. A. Wambangco, H. Kurazono, and H. Hayashi.** 2002. Diagnosis of human leptospirosis by monoclonal antibody-based antigen detection in urine. *J. Clin. Microbiol.* **40:**480–489.
59. **Sejvar, J., E. Bancroft, K. Winthrop, J. Bettinger, M. Bajani, S. Bragg, K. Shutt, R. Kaiser, N. Marano, T. Popovic, J. Tappero, D. Ashford, L. Mascola, D. Vugia, B. Perkins, and N. Rosenstein.** 2003. Leptospirosis in "Eco-Challenge" athletes, Malaysian Borneo, 2000. *Emerg. Infect. Dis.* **9:**702–707.
60. **Smits, H. L., C. K. Eapen, S. Sugathan, M. Kuriakose, M. H. Gasem, C. Yersin, D. Sasaki, B. Pujianto, M. Vestering, T. H. Abdoel, and G. C. Gussenhoven.** 2001. Lateral-flow assay for rapid serodiagnosis of human leptospirosis. *Clin. Diagn. Lab. Immunol.* **8:**166–169.
61. **Smits, H. L., M. A. van Der Hoorn, M. G. Goris, G. C. Gussenhoven, C. Yersin, D. M. Sasaki, W. J. Terpstra, and R. A. Hartskeerl.** 2000. Simple latex agglutination assay for rapid serodiagnosis of human leptospirosis. *J. Clin. Microbiol.* **38:**1272–1275.
62. **Smythe, L. D., I. L. Smith, G. A. Smith, M. F. Dohnt, M. L. Symonds, L. J. Barnett, and D. B. McKay.** 2002. A quantitative PCR (TaqMan) assay for pathogenic *Leptospira* spp. *BMC Infect. Dis.* **2:**13.
63. **Stimson, A. M.** 1907. Note on an organism found in yellow-fever tissue. *Public Health Rep.* **22:**541.
64. **Sulzer, C. R., and W. L. Jones.** 1978. *Leptospirosis: Methods in Laboratory Diagnosis.* U.S. Department of Health, Education and Welfare, Atlanta, Ga.
65. **Suputtamongkol, Y., K. Niwattayakul, C. Suttinont, K. Losuwanaluk, R. Limpaiboon, W. Chierakul, V. Wuthiekanun, S. Triengrim, M. Chenchittikul, and N. J. White.** 2004. An open, randomized, controlled trial of penicillin, doxycycline, and cefotaxime for patients with severe leptospirosis. *Clin. Infect. Dis.* **39:**1417–1424.
66. **Terpstra, W. J.** 1992. Typing leptospira from the perspective of a reference laboratory. *Acta Leiden.* **60:**79–87.
67. **Torten, M.** 1979. Leptospirosis, p. 363–420. *In* H. E. Stoenner, M. Torten, and W. Kaplan (ed.), *CRC Handbook Series in Zoonoses. Section A: Bacterial, Rickettsial and Mycotic Diseases,* vol. I. CRC Press, Boca Raton, Fla.
68. **Turner, L. H.** 1968. Leptospirosis II. Serology. *Trans. R. Soc. Trop. Med. Hyg.* **62:**880–889.
69. **Turner, L. H.** 1970. Leptospirosis III. Maintenance, isolation and demonstration of leptospires. *Trans. R. Soc. Trop. Med. Hyg.* **64:**623–646.
70. **Uip, D. E., V. Amato Neto, and M. S. Duarte.** 1992. Diagnóstico precoce da leptospirose por demonstração de antígenos através de exame imuno-histoquímino em músculo da panturrilha. *Rev. Inst. Med. Trop. Sao Paulo* **34:** 375–381.
71. **Vijayachari, P., N. Ahmed, A. P. Sugunan, S. Ghousunnissa, K. R. Rao, S. E. Hasnain, and S. C. Sehgal.** 2004. Use of fluorescent amplified fragment length polymorphism for molecular epidemiology of leptospirosis in India. *J. Clin. Microbiol.* **42:**3575–3580.
72. **Vijayachari, P., A. P. Sugunan, T. Umapathi, and S. C. Sehgal.** 2001. Evaluation of darkground microscopy as a rapid diagnostic procedure in leptospirosis. *Indian J. Med. Res.* **114:**54–58.
73. **Ward, M. P., L. F. Guptill, A. Prahl, and C. C. Wu.** 2004. Serovar-specific prevalence and risk factors for leptospirosis among dogs: 90 cases (1997–2002). *J. Am. Vet. Med. Assoc.* **224:**1958–1963.
74. **Whittington, C. U., and P. N. Levett.** 2001. Development of rapid, microtiter-based antimicrobial susceptibility testing of *Leptospira* species. *Am. J. Trop. Med. Hyg.* **65** (Suppl.)**:**434.
75. **Winslow, W. E., D. J. Merry, M. L. Pirc, and P. L. Devine.** 1997. Evaluation of a commercial enzyme-linked immunosorbent assay for detection of immunoglobulin M antibody in diagnosis of human leptospiral infection. *J. Clin. Microbiol.* **35:**1938–1942.
76. **Wolff, J. W.** 1954. The laboratory diagnosis of leptospirosis. C. C. Thomas, Springfield, Ill.
77. **World Health Organization.** 2003. *Human Leptopirosis: Guidance for Diagnosis, Surveillance and Control.* World Health Organization, Geneva, Switzerland.
78. **World Health Organization.** 1999. Leptospirosis worldwide, 1999. *Wkly. Epidemiol. Rec.* **74:**237–242.
79. **Wylie, J. A. H., and E. Vincent.** 1947. The sensitivity of organisms of the genus *Leptospira* to penicillin and streptomycin. *J. Pathol. Bacteriol.* **59:**247–254.
80. **Yasuda, P. H., A. G. Steigerwalt, K. R. Sulzer, A. F. Kaufmann, F. Rogers, and D. J. Brenner.** 1987. Deoxyribonucleic acid relatedness between serogroups and serovars in the family *Leptospiraceae* with proposals for seven new *Leptospira* species. *Int. J. Syst. Bacteriol.* **37:**407–415.
81. **Zaki, S. R., W.-J. Shieh, and The Epidemic Working Group.** 1996. Leptospirosis associated with outbreak of acute febrile illness and pulmonary haemorrhage, Nicaragua, 1995. *Lancet* **347:**535.
82. **Zaki, S. R., and R. A. Spiegel.** 1998. Leptospirosis, p. 73–92. *In* A. M. Nelson and C. R. Horsburgh (ed.), *Pathology of Emerging Infections 2.* American Society for Microbiology, Washington, D.C.

Borrelia

BETTINA WILSKE, BARBARA J. B. JOHNSON, AND MARTIN E. SCHRIEFER

62

TAXONOMY

Bacteria of the genus *Borrelia* belong to the order *Spirochaetales*, which encompasses the families *Spirochaetaceae* and *Leptospiraceae*. *Borrelia* and *Treponema* are the two genera of the family *Spirochaetaceae* that cause human disease. The type species of the genus *Borrelia* is *Borrelia anserina*, which causes borreliosis in birds. Based on 16S rRNA sequence analyses, spirochetes form a distinct entity (division D) within the eubacterial kingdom. They are neither gram positive nor gram negative. In case of the spirochetes, morphological criteria and DNA data produce concordant phylogenies, a rare trait in other bacterial groups.

DESCRIPTION OF THE GENUS

Common Characteristics

Borreliae are similar in length (8 to 30 μm) but wider (0.2 to 0.5 μm) than the two other human-pathogenic spirochetes, the treponemes and the leptospires (Fig. 1) (10). They are highly motile organisms, with corkscrew and oscillating motility. In contrast to the exoflagella of other bacteria, the flagella of spirochetes are endoflagella. The endoflagella of borreliae (7 to 20 per terminus) are localized beneath the outer membrane and insert subterminally at both ends of the protoplasmic cylinder. The protoplasmic cylinder consists of a peptidoglycan layer and an inner membrane which encloses the internal components of the cell (10). If cultivable, borreliae grow slowly under microaerophilic (9) or anaerobic (86) conditions. They require *N*-acetylglucosamine and long-chain saturated and unsaturated fatty acids and produce lactic acid through glucose fermentation (57).

Species Diversity

The causative agent of Lyme disease was first described by Burgdorfer et al. in the early 1980s (18) and named *Borrelia burgdorferi* (58). Studies published since 1992 have divided *B. burgdorferi* sensu lato into three human-pathogenic species—*B. burgdorferi* sensu stricto, *B. afzelii*, and *B. garinii* (8, 19)—and eight other species (Table 1) (108). In North America, *B. burgdorferi* sensu stricto is the only human-pathogenic species, whereas all three species have been isolated from humans in Europe. There is a strong prevalence of *B. afzelii* among human skin isolates from Europe, whereas isolates from cerebrospinal fluid (CSF) in Europe are most commonly *B. garinii* (Table 2) (19, 35, 94, 117). Studies using *ospA* PCR have shown that the strains causing Lyme arthritis are heterogeneous (Table 2) (34, 106) and not limited to *B. burgdorferi* sensu stricto. A few studies have reported the detection of other *Borrelia* species (*B. valaisiana, B. spielmanii,* and *B. lusitaniae*) in patient samples in Europe (24, 90, 91, 107). Similarly, *B. lonestari*, a species carried by a hard tick but genetically more closely related to the relapsing fever spirochetes, has been implicated in at least one case of erythema migrans (EM) (53).

The relapsing fever borreliae *B. turicatae, B. parkeri,* and *B. hermsii* are transmitted by distinct soft-bodied ticks (*Ornithordoros* species), but they may be a single species because their DNA-DNA similarity is greater than 70%. The species status of other cultivable borreliae, such as *B. anserina, B. crocidurae, B. recurrentis,* and *B. coriaceae,* has been supported by greater DNA-DNA dissimilarity findings (27, 57).

The Genome

The genome of the borreliae is composed of a small linear chromosome of approximately 1,000 kb, which is unusual among bacteria, and both linear and circular plasmids. Also atypical of most bacteria, borreliae have a low G+C content, approximately 30 mol%. The complete nucleotide sequence of the chromosome and 21 plasmids (9 circular and 12 linear) has been published for the type strain, *B. burgdorferi* B31 (20, 40). A total of 59% of the chromosomal open reading frames (ORFs) have homologs in other bacterial species; in contrast, homologs have been identified for only one-third of the plasmid ORFs. The genome encodes a basic set of proteins for DNA replication, transcription, and energy metabolism but, interestingly, lacks most cellular biosynthetic pathways. Of some surprise is the tremendous number (>150) of genes that encode putative lipoproteins, suggesting an essential role for these molecules in the life cycle of the spirochete. Recent genome analysis of another Lyme disease spirochete, *B. garinii* (strain PBi), revealed that most of the chromosome is conserved (92.7% identity on the DNA as well as the amino acid level) in the two species. Furthermore, two colinear plasmids (lp54 and cp26) seem to belong to the basic genome inventory of the *Borrelia* species that cause Lyme disease. However, the authors did not find counterparts of the *B. burgdorferi* plasmids lp36 and lp38 or their respective gene repertoires in the *B. garinii* genome (41).

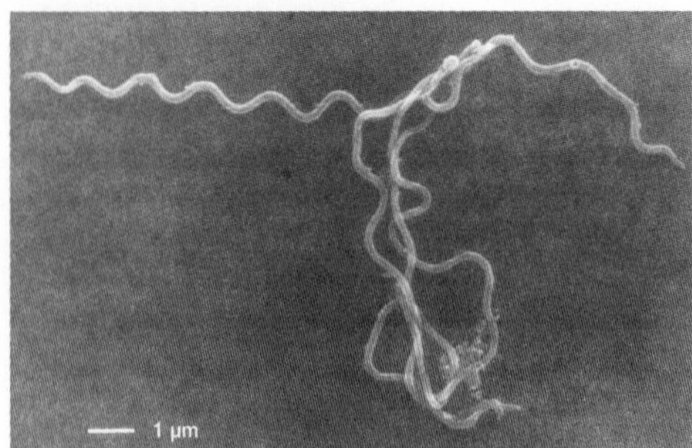

FIGURE 1 *B. burgdorferi* seen by scanning electron microscopy (provided by Gerhard Wanner, Munich, Germany).

Whole-genome microarray analysis revealed that a total of 215 ORFs, 136 of which are plasmid borne, were differentially expressed at 23 and 35°C. These findings highlight the potential importance of plasmid-borne genes in the adaptation of *B. burgdorferi* sensu lato to mammal hosts and tick vectors (74).

The linear plasmids of *B. hermsii* and *B. turicatae* contain genes encoding outer membrane lipoproteins, called variable major proteins (Vmp). These genes are silent except when they are translocated to an expression site immediately adjacent to one of the linear plasmid telomeres. Antigenic variation of Vmp-like proteins due to recombination of *vls* (Vmp-like small) gene sequence cassettes has also been described for *B. burgdorferi*. These *vls* genes have highly variable regions, as well as highly conserved sequences which encode immunogenic epitopes important for serodiagnosis (70, 123).

The large linear plasmid lp54 encodes two major outer surface proteins, OspA and OspB, which are tandemly arrayed in one operon (13). The first gene detected on a circular plasmid (cp26) was the gene encoding OspC, another major outer surface protein of *B. burgdorferi* (95, 118). Sequence analysis of the *ospC* genes from different strains suggested that gene exchange might play a role in diversity and immune evasion of Lyme disease borreliae (54).

EPIDEMIOLOGY AND TRANSMISSION

The ecological components that maintain *Borrelia* species in nature are quite diverse and spread throughout the world (Table 1).

Relapsing Fever Borreliae

Most relapsing fever borreliae are transmitted by soft-bodied ticks of the genus *Ornithodoros* (Fig. 2). The exception is *B. recurrentis,* which is vectored by the human body louse *(Pediculus humanus humanus)*. Infection in this human-specific ectoparasite is limited to the hemolymph, and spirochetes are not passed transovarially to louse progeny. Thus, humans serve as the sole reservoir of *B. recurrentis*. *B. duttonii* is vectored by the soft tick *Ornithodoros moubata,* and as is the case for *B. recurrentis,* humans serve as the only known reservoir. Notably, these human-adapted borreliae are very closely related genetically (27). The remaining relapsing fever *Borrelia* species are transmitted by other *Ornithodoros* ticks and have wild-animal reservoirs, mostly rodents (Table 1). The soft ticks feed rapidly, within 10 to 45 min, and mostly at night.

B. burgdorferi sensu lato

The Lyme disease borreliae of *B. burgdorferi* sensu lato are transmitted by hard-bodied ticks (genus *Ixodes*) (Fig. 2). *Ixodes* species feed on three different hosts depending on the developmental stage of the tick (51). The larvae and nymphs feed primarily on small rodents, whereas adult ticks feed on a variety of mammals (deer, raccoons, domestic and wild carnivores, larger domestic animals, and birds). The feeding period of *Ixodes* ticks is rather long (several days to over a week) and contributes to their geographic dispersal along with the movement of the host. Birds, particularly migratory seabirds, can transport the ticks *(Ixodes uriae)* over very long distances and thus distribute borreliae (especially *B. garinii*) worldwide (75). There appears to be an association between *B. afzelii* and small rodents and *B. garinii* and birds, likely due to different serum sensitivities of the borreliae (51) mediated by complement regulator-acquiring surface proteins (65). In unfed ticks, *B. burgdorferi* sensu lato lives in the midgut. During the blood meal from humans or mice, transcriptional changes (e.g., a switch from OspA to OspC expression) are induced in the borreliae that lead to their migration to the salivary glands (37, 100).

The role of OspC for dissemination in the tick is controversial, but its expression is required for mouse infection (38, 44, 76). Invasion from the *Ixodes scapularis* midgut takes >36 h (28). For *Ixodes ricinus,* however, spirochete migration within the tick and transmission to the mammalian host have been observed with ticks feeding for as few as 17 h (60).

CLINICAL SIGNIFICANCE

Relapsing Fever

Relapsing fever is an infectious disease with an acute onset of clinical signs and symptoms including high fever, shaking chills, severe headache, nausea, myalgias, and severe malaise. Initial physical findings often are conjunctival effusion, petechiae, and diffuse abdominal tenderness. Fever attacks of 3 to 7 days are interspersed with afebrile periods of days to weeks. More detailed descriptions have been published elsewhere for louse-borne relapsing fever (88) and tick-borne relapsing fever in North America (32, 33).

Louse-borne relapsing fever is, in general, more severe than tick-borne relapsing fever, but the number of febrile attacks is often fewer. In tick-borne relapsing fever up to 13 febrile attacks have been reported, and a rash is more often reported than in louse-borne relapsing fever (28 versus 8%). Splenomegaly, hepatomegaly, and jaundice are observed in 77, 66, and 36% of louse-borne relapsing fever cases, whereas these signs are reported in only 41, 17, and 7% of tick-borne relapsing fever cases. In louse-borne relapsing fever, 34% of the patients have respiratory symptoms and 30% have central nervous system involvement; in patients with tick-borne relapsing fever, these figures are 16 and 9%, respectively (59). Complications leading to death (mortality rate of up to 40% in louse-borne relapsing fever) are acute heart and hepatic failure and cerebral hemorrhage. Disease severity increases with compromising conditions common in many areas of endemicity. During pregnancy, relapsing fever may also lead to congenital infection and fetal death.

Lyme Borreliosis

Lyme borreliosis can be defined by early localized, early disseminated, and late-stage manifestations similar to the three stages of syphilis (104). The natural course of untreated *B. burgdorferi* infections varies considerably, and clinical manifestations can occur alone or in various combinations (102, 104, 105, 109). In the majority of cases the infection is self-limiting, but in rare

TABLE 1 Characteristics of arthropod-borne borreliae[a]

Borrelia sp.	Arthropod vector	Animal reservoir	Geographic distribution	Disease
Relapsing fever borreliae				
B. recurrentis	*Pediculus humanus humanus*	Humans	Worldwide	Louse-borne (epidemic) relapsing fever
B. duttonii	*O. moubata*	Humans	Central, eastern, and southern Africa	Tick-borne (endemic) relapsing fever
B. hispanica	*Ornithodoros erraticus*	Rodents	Spain, Portugal, Morocco, Algeria, Tunisia	Hispano-African tick-borne relapsing fever
B. crocidurae, B. merionesi, B. microti, B. dipodilli	*O. erraticus*	Rodents	Morocco, Libya, Egypt, Turkey, Senegal, Kenya	North African tick-borne relapsing fever
B. persica	*Ornithodoros tholozani*	Rodents	Western China, Kashmir, Iraq, Egypt, former USSR, India	Asiatic-African tick-borne relapsing fever
B. caucasica	*Ornithodoros verrucosus*	Rodents	Caucasus to Iraq	Caucasian tick-borne relapsing fever
B. hermsii	*Ornithodoros hermsi*	Rodents	Western United States	American tick-borne relapsing fever
B. turicatae	*Ornithodoros turicata*	Rodents	Southwestern United States	American tick-borne relapsing fever
B. parkeri	*Ornithodoros parkeri*	Rodents	Western United States	American tick-borne relapsing fever
B. mazzottii	*Ornithodoros talajé*	Rodents	Southern United States, Mexico, Central and South America	American tick-borne relapsing fever
B. venezuelensis	*Ornithodoros rudis (Ornithodoros venezuelensis)*	Rodents	Central and South America	American tick-borne relapsing fever
B. burgdorferi sensu lato				
B. burgdorferi	*Ixodes scapularis*	Rodents	Eastern and midwestern United States	Lyme borreliosis
	Ixodes pacificus	Rodents	Western United States	Lyme borreliosis
	I. ricinus	Rodents	Europe	Lyme borreliosis
B. garinii	*I. ricinus, Ixodes persulcatus*	Rodents	Europe, Asia	Lyme borreliosis
	I. uriae	Seabirds	Bipolar	?
B. afzelii	*I. ricinus, I. persulcatus*	Rodents	Europe, Asia	Lyme borreliosis
B. spielmanii	*I. ricinus*	Rodents	Europe	Lyme borreliosis (few cases)
B. japonica	*Ixodes ovatus*	Rodents	Japan	?
B. andersonii	*Ixodes dentatus*	Rabbits	United States	?
B. bissettii	*I. scapularis, I. pacificus*	Rodents	United States	?
B. tanukii	*Ixodes tanukii, I. ovatus*	Rodents	Japan	?
B. turdi	*Ixodes turdus*	?	Japan	?
B. sinica	*I. ovatus*		China	?
B. valaisiana	*I. ricinus*	?	Europe, Asia	?
B. lusitaniae	*I. ricinus*	?	Europe, North Africa	Lyme borreliosis (one case)
Other borreliae				
B. lonestari	*Amblyomma americanum*	?	United States	?
B. miyamotoi	*I. persulcatus*	Rodents	Japan	?
B. theileri	*Rhipicephalus, Boophilus* spp.	Cattle, horses, sheep	South Africa, Australia, North America, Europe	Bovine borreliosis
B. coriaceae	*O. coriaceus*	Deer?	Western United States	Epizootic bovine abortion?
B. anserina	*Argas* spp.	Fowl	Worldwide	Avian borreliosis

[a] Modified from reference 119a.

TABLE 2 Distribution of species of *B. burgdorferi* sensu lato in European isolates from CSF, skin, and synovial fluid specimens[a]

Species	% Distribution[b]		
	CSF (n = 78)	Skin (n = 560)	Synovial fluid (n = 20)
B. burgdorferi sensu stricto	12	1	33
B. afzelii	17	88	29
B. garinii	71	10	38

[a] Data from references 34, 94, 106, and 113.

[b] *B. burgdorferi* sensu lato species identifications from CSF and skin are based on culture; species identification from synovial fluid samples is based on *ospA* PCR results. Culture isolates from synovial fluid are too few to estimate *Borrelia* species distribution.

cases, *B. burgdorferi* may persist and chronic disease manifestations may develop.

EM at the site of the infectious tick bite is the most common manifestation of early (stage I) Lyme borreliosis and occurs in 60 to 90% of patients. The center of the expanding annular lesion often fades to produce a bull's-eye appearance. However, the extension, color intensity, and duration of EM vary considerably. General symptoms such as fever, myalgia, headache, and, rarely, meningismus may accompany the primary EM.

In some patients, hematogenous dissemination of spirochetes to other organs and tissues occurs within days to weeks of infection (stage II). Patients often feel quite ill and may present with fatigue, headache, fever, malaise, arthralgia, and myalgia. Multiple (secondary) erythemata are common in the United States but uncommon in Europe. Neurologic structures, including the meninges, brain, spinal cord, peripheral nerves, and nerve roots, are also potential sites of early disseminated infection. In the United States, 15 to 20% of untreated patients develop neurologic signs, most commonly facial nerve palsy (unilateral or bilateral), meningitis, and radiculoneuropathy. CSF findings in cases of Lyme meningitis almost always include a mononuclear pleocytosis (10 to 1,000 cells/μl) and elevated protein concentration. Meningitis, or even facial palsy without meningismus, is more common among children than adults. Severe encephalitis is occasionally observed in stage II. Bannwarth's syndrome is the most common neurologic manifestation of early, disseminated Lyme borreliosis in Europe. The syndrome is characterized initially by intense, migratory or focal, radicular pain, particularly at night, and by cranial nerve palsy. Pareses of the extremities and the trunk are less frequent. Further clinical manifestations of stage II may include Lyme carditis, most often with atrioventricular conduction blocks, and ophthalmic involvement. Borrelial lymphocytoma, a reddish to livid swelling of the skin in typical locations such as the earlobe, nipple, or scrotum, is manifested among some patients in Europe.

Lyme arthritis and acrodermatitis chronica atrophicans (ACA), occurring months to years after the initial infection, are the most common manifestations of late (stage III) disease. Lyme arthritis can be monoarticular or oligoarticular, typically affecting the knee, and usually takes an intermittent course. Patients with ACA initially develop an infiltrative stage, followed by alterations characteristic of the atrophic stage: creased skin with livid discolorations and plastic protrusion of vessels. ACA is observed almost exclusively in Europe, a finding highly correlated with *B. afzelii* infections. Chronic neuroborreliosis is a very rare manifestation of late (stage III) disease. Parapareses and tetrapareses are its most common symptoms. Examination of the CSF reveals a marked elevation of protein concentration with a low to moderate increase of cells in the CSF. The detection of intrathecally produced specific antibodies is currently regarded as the best marker of chronic neuroborreliosis, although there may be less frequent production of intrathecal antibodies in U.S. patients.

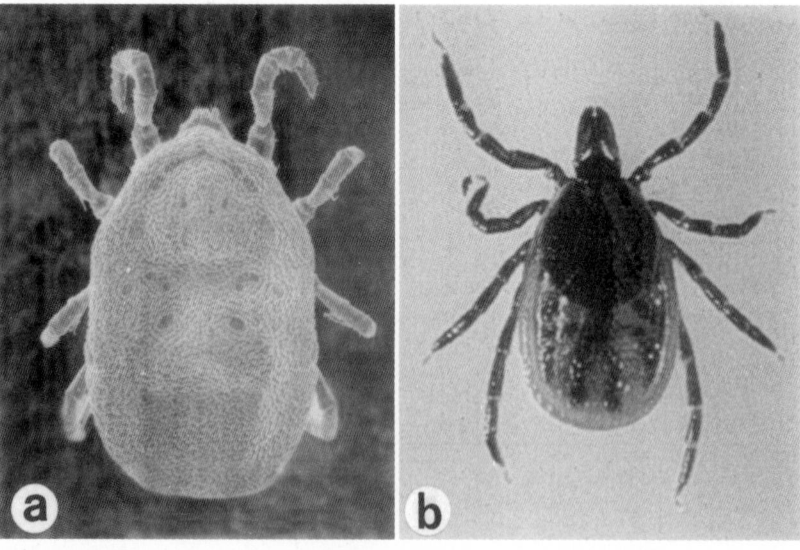

FIGURE 2 Two genera of ticks are vectors for relapsing fever and Lyme borreliosis: *Ornithodoros* (a) and *Ixodes* (b).

Early manifestations of Lyme borreliosis are observed most frequently in the spring, summer, and autumn, coinciding with tick activity. Late manifestations do not show a seasonal pattern.

COLLECTION, TRANSPORT, AND STORAGE OF SPECIMENS

Specimens for laboratory confirmation of Lyme borreliosis are presented in Table 3.

Blood and Serum

For relapsing fever, blood is the specimen of choice. During febrile attacks, borreliae may be easily detected by dark-field or bright-field microscopy of a wet-mount blood sample or a stained blood smear, respectively (see "Direct Examination," "Microscopy"). At this time, the spirochetemia may reach 10^6 to 10^8 cells ml^{-1} (57). Blood from acutely ill patients is also the best source for culture confirmation (26, 27). However, the spirochetemia diminishes with each successive relapse, and visualization or culture isolation of borreliae is often unsuccessful during afebrile periods. In contrast to relapsing fever, spirochetemia in Lyme borreliosis patients is below the level of microscopic detection. Culture and PCR of blood samples generally are not recommended, since the yields are low (43). Even when large blood volumes are cultivated, positive cultures have been derived from only 50% of patients with EM (121).

Serum is suitable for indirect (antibody) evidence of *Borrelia* exposure. Specific antibody detection tests are the most widely utilized tests for laboratory confirmation of Lyme borreliosis. Serodiagnosis of relapsing fever is performed only in a few specialized laboratories.

CSF

In suspected neuroborreliosis patients, CSF (along with serum drawn at the same time) should be obtained for determination of cell counts-cell differentials, protein content, and intrathecal immunoglobulin (immunoglobulin M [IgM] and IgG) synthesis. Laboratory confirmation of neuroborreliosis is most readily achieved by demonstration of *Borrelia*-specific, intrathecal (CSF/serum antibody index) antibody production (see "Serological Tests"). For culture or PCR, however, detection rates are only about 20% (68). Positive PCR results in CSF also seem to correlate inversely with duration of neurologic disease. Among neuroborreliosis patients, 7 of 14 (50%) with a disease duration of less than 2 weeks had a positive PCR result, compared with only 2 of 16 (13%) patients in whom the illness duration was greater than 2 weeks (P = 0.045) (68).

Synovial Fluid or Synovial Biopsy Specimens

Investigation of synovial fluid or a synovial biopsy specimen by PCR may be useful in special circumstances where Lyme arthritis is suspected (73). Culture is usually negative, with few exceptions. Due to the high protein permeability of the synovium, synovial fluid and serum display roughly equivalent antibody titers. Thus, it is sufficient to monitor antibody in serum.

Skin Biopsy Specimens

Skin biopsy samples are the best sources for isolation of *B. burgdorferi;* spirochetes can be isolated in most untreated cases of EM and acrodermatitis (Table 4). In cases of EM, culture success is highest (up to 86%) with biopsy samples taken close to (4 mm inside) the expanding border of the lesion (12), although this is primarily a technique for research, not for routine diagnosis. There are indications that the number of spirochetes in the skin is rather low or unevenly distributed, since an increase in the sensitivity is observed if more than one biopsy sample is investigated (124). Without treatment, *B. burgdorferi* sensu lato can persist for long periods in the skin, as shown by isolation from a 10-year-old acrodermatitis lesion (6). Biopsy samples (taken after thorough disinfection of the skin) should be sent in a small amount of sterile saline or Barbour-Stoenner-Kelly (BSK) medium (with or without rifampin) as soon as possible to the microbiological laboratory.

Other Materials

Ticks are often tested for borreliae as part of epidemiological studies to assess risk to human populations in a given geographic area. Although specialized laboratories offer diagnostic services for individual ticks, detection of spirochetes

TABLE 3 Specimen types used for the diagnosis of Lyme borreliosis

Clinical manifestation	Specimens for: Direct pathogen detection (culture, PCR)	Specimens for: Antibody detection
Stage I (early/localized; days through weeks after tick bite)		
EM	Skin biopsy	Serum
Stage II (early/disseminated; weeks through months after tick bite)		
Multiple erythemata	Skin biopsy	Serum
Borrelial lymphocytoma	Skin biopsy	Serum
Lyme carditis	Endomyocardial biopsy	Serum
Neuroborreliosis	CSF	Paired serum/CSF[a]
Stage III (late/persistent; months through years after tick bite)		
Arthritis	Synovial fluid, synovial biopsy	Serum
ACA	Skin biopsy	Serum
Chronic neuroborreliosis	CSF	Paired serum/CSF[a]

[a] From the same day for AI determination.

TABLE 4 Sensitivity of methods for pathogen detection (PCR and culture) in Lyme borreliosis

Specimen	Sensitivity
Skin (EM, acrodermatitis)	50–70% when using culture or PCR
CSF (neuroborreliosis, stage II)	10–30% when using culture or PCR[a]
Synovial fluid[b] (Lyme arthritis)	50–70% when using PCR (culture is rarely positive)

[a] Up to 50% in patients with disease duration of less than 2 weeks, compared with only 13% in patients for whom the illness duration was greater than 2 weeks.
[b] Higher sensitivity of direct pathogen detection from synovial biopsy specimen.

within ticks by PCR or other methods has not been shown to provide clinically useful information.

General Remarks for Collection and Transport

For culture, collection and preparation of specimens under sterile conditions are of utmost importance. Body fluids should be transported without any additives, and biopsy specimens should be placed in a small quantity of sterile saline or suitable culture medium (see "Isolation Procedures"). Samples should reach the laboratory as quickly as possible (within 2 to 4 h). Before specimens are collected and transported, the laboratory should be contacted so that details of methodology can be agreed upon. If postal transport is unavoidable, overnight delivery is recommended.

DIRECT EXAMINATION

Microscopy

Direct microscopic visualization of borreliae in clinical samples is applicable only to cases of relapsing fever. During acute phases, spirochetemia often reaches 10^6 to 10^8 borreliae/ml and motile spirochetes can be visualized by dark-field microscopy from wet preparations made from a drop of blood. This simple confirmatory test is often overlooked because of the increasingly common use of automated differential blood counts. Spirochetes can be visualized by stained (e.g., Giemsa) thin- or thick-drop films (Fig. 3). Detection of low-level spirochetemias may be assisted by a microhematocrit concentration technique. The hematocrit capillary is filled 75% with citrated blood and centrifuged for 2 min. The buffy coat is then examined directly under the microscope at ×400 to ×1,000 (119a). Failure to observe spirochetes does not rule out disease, and culture isolation (see "Isolation Procedures") may be considered. In Lyme borreliosis, spirochete numbers in patient blood or other tissues are below the level of microscopic detection and microscopy is best applied to the monitoring of borrelial growth in cultured tissues or fluids.

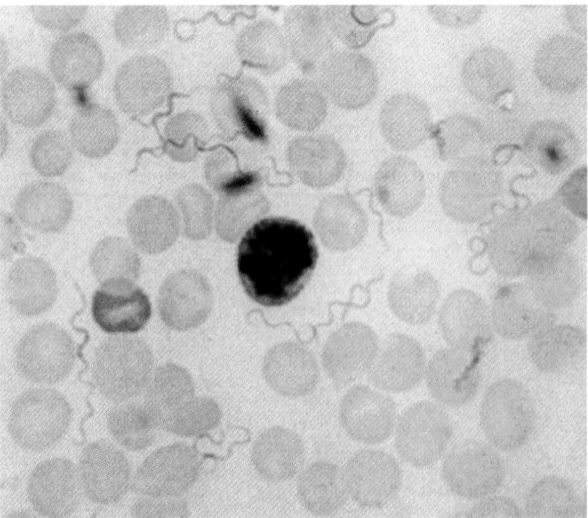

FIGURE 3 *B. hermsii* in a thin smear of rodent blood (Giemsa stain). Magnification, ×1,000.

Antigen Detection

Enzyme-linked immunosorbent assay (ELISA) and immunoblotting have been used for the detection of borrelial antigen in body fluids, including CSF and urine (25, 52). However, a commercial assay for antigen in urine was shown to lack reproducibility, and its use is not recommended (64).

Nucleic Acid Detection Techniques

Nucleic acid amplification techniques (NAT) should be restricted to experienced and specialized laboratories (92). For patients with suspected exposure outside of North America, it is imperative that selected NAT targets sensitively detect all human-pathogenic species. Species identification of amplification products is preferable (120).

Under circumstances where antibody detection and culture isolation fail to provide case confirmation, NAT can serve as a separate adjunct to clinical diagnosis. A variety of chromosomal and plasmid targets for NAT have been developed (for reviews, see references 3, 31, and 96). For PCR, an analytical sensitivity of approximately 10 to 20 borreliae per test sample has been demonstrated. Test sensitivities for both NAT and culture are greater with tissue specimens than with body fluids, except for synovial fluid, with which NAT is superior. Sensitivities of 96% (73) and 86% (14) were reported for NAT from synovial fluid from American patients with Lyme arthritis. European authors found NAT sensitivities ranging between 50 and 70% (34, 87, 106). Patients with Lyme arthritis are nearly always seropositive, so PCR of synovial samples is not used as a primary diagnostic technique. A positive PCR result after antibiotic therapy is of uncertain significance, since the presence of *B. burgdorferi* DNA does not necessarily mean that spirochetes are viable.

From skin biopsy and CSF specimens, NAT demonstrated diagnostic sensitivities of approximately 60 and 20%, respectively (15, 35, 68). A prospective study of PCR and culture detection of *B. burgdorferi* in EM biopsy samples from Slovenian patients showed comparable sensitivities (36% for culture in modified Kelly medium Preac-Mursic [MKP] medium, 24% for culture in BSK II medium, 25% for PCR, 54% with at least one positive test, and 6% with all three tests positive) (82). PCR targeting *ospA*, a plasmid-borne gene, is more sensitive than flagellin PCR, which uses a chromosomal target (79, 124). Borreliae may shed blebs containing plasmids, leading to target imbalance.

PCR amplification of *B. burgdorferi* sequences from urine has been described (89, 96) but is not recommended. Although *Borrelia*-specific DNA was demonstrated in over 70% of skin biopsy samples from patients with florid EM, parallel testing of urine samples was uniformly negative (15).

ISOLATION PROCEDURES

Many Lyme and relapsing fever borreliae are successfully cultured in artificial media. However, for diagnostic purposes, culturing is a slow, time-consuming method characterized by low sensitivity, especially from body fluids of patients with Lyme borreliosis (Table 4). For these reasons culture attempts are most often limited to research applications and performed by reference laboratories (e.g., the National Reference Center for Borreliae in Germany and the Centers for Disease Control and Prevention [CDC] in the United States).

Several media (modified Kelly medium, e.g., BSK II, BSK-H, or MKP) (9, 83, 86) are capable of supporting growth of borreliae. A commercial preparation of BSK-H is available from Sigma Chemical Co., St. Louis, Mo. It is important to verify the quality of each lot of medium by growing a reference strain from a small inoculum (<10 cells). Optimum growth (the generation time of *B. burgdorferi* is about 7 to 20 h) in these media is obtained at 30 to 33°C under microaerophilic conditions. Positive cultures from EM and synovial biopsy or fluid samples (blood and CSF) may be obtained in as few as 4 days, but most isolates require several weeks of incubation and negative cultures should be monitored by dark-field microscopy for at least 6 weeks, with blind passage into fresh medium every 2 weeks.

IDENTIFICATION

Molecular Techniques

Relapsing fever borreliae have been typed on the basis of DNA-DNA reassociation analysis and flagellin gene analysis (27, 57). *B. burgdorferi* has an arrangement of its rRNA genes (a single *rrs* and tandemly repeated *rrl* and *rrf* genes) which distinguishes it from the relapsing fever borreliae (which have single copies of each) (101). Sequencing of 5S-23S intergenic spacers is useful in typing borreliae. A number of molecular genetic methods, including pulsed-field gel electrophoresis of large restriction fragments (11), PCR, and sequence analysis or restriction fragment length polymorphism of the 16S rRNA/16S ribosomal DNA and of the 5S-23S intergenic spacer region (69, 84), have been described for species differentiation (summarized in reference 108). Analysis of certain protein-encoding genes, especially *ospA* and *ospC*, has also been utilized for *B. burgdorferi* sensu lato species identifications (35, 116, 117). However, in most cases, diagnosis and effective management of individual patients are independent of species determinations beyond the Lyme disease and relapsing fever groupings.

Immunological Techniques

Antibody responses to GlpQ, an antigen expressed by relapsing fever species but not Lyme borreliosis species, have been used to discriminate the two infections (100, 119a). For *B. burgdorferi* sensu lato, a serotyping method using monoclonal antibodies to OspA has been established. Eight different serotypes have been described among the pathogenic species for Europe, which has implications for OspA vaccine development (112, 117). Phenotypic analysis of OspC revealed 15 different serotypes (113). Some species-specific monoclonal antibodies have also been described.

SEROLOGICAL TESTS

Borrelia Antigens and Human Humoral Immune Response

In Lyme borreliosis the early antibody response is largely IgM and mainly directed against the outer membrane-associated OspC, p39 (BmpA), and p35 (BBK32, fibronectin-binding protein) and the flagellum subunits p37 (FlaA) and p41 (FlaB) (1, 4, 36, 49, 114).

The level of IgM antibody to most spirochetal antigens peaks within the first weeks of infection. However, IgM antibodies are often detected many months after effective treatment and cure (1). The IgG response increases and broadens slowly over the first weeks of disease. Among the reactive antigens to which there is an early IgG response are p35 (BBK32), p37 (FlaA), p41 (FlaB), OspC, and VlsE (1, 4, 66, 70, 77). During early disseminated (stage II) disease, IgG levels increase and reactivity against p39 (BmpA), DbpA (decorin binding protein), and p58 often appears (49) (Table 5). The late-stage immune response (stage III) is characterized by IgG antibodies to a wide variety of antigens (30, 49). Approximately 80% of the sera from European patients with late disease (arthritis and ACA) react with

TABLE 5 Reactivity of IgG antibodies with recombinant *Borrelia* proteins (DbpA, VlsE, and p58) in the line immunoblot[a]

Diagnosis	No. of sera	No. (%) of sera with reactivity							
		DbpA				VlsE			p58
		PBi (*B. garinii*)	PBr (*B. garinii*)	PKo (*B. afzelii*)	B31 (*B. burgdorferi*)	At least one DbpA[b]	PBi (*B. garinii*)	PKa2 (*B. burgdorferi*)	PBi (*B. garinii*)
EM[c]	15	0 (0.0)	2 (13.3)	4 (26.7)	1 (6.7)	5 (33.3)	12 (80.0)	6 (40.0)	1 (6.7)
Neuroborreliosis	50	19 (38.0)	20 (40.0)	17 (34.0)	6 (12.0)	39 (78.0)	44 (88.0)	41 (82.0)	27 (54.0)
Acrodermatitis	10	1 (10.0)	0 (0.0)	8 (80.0)	1 (10.0)	8 (80.0)	10 (100.0)	10 (100.0)	10 (100.0)
Arthritis	10	7 (70.0)	1 (10.0)	9 (90.0)	2 (20.0)	10 (100.0)	10 (100.0)	9 (90.0)	9 (90.0)
Controls	110	2 (1.8)	2 (1.8)	0 (0.0)	0 (0.0)	4 (3.6)	1 (0.9)	0 (0.0)	1 (0.9)

[a] Modified from reference 42.
[b] The combination of DbpA proteins from different strains (PBi, PBr, PKo, and B31) results in considerable increase of sensitivity in neuroborreliosis.
[c] Disease duration of >2 weeks.

p14, Osp17 (DbpA), p21 (not OspC), p30, p39, p43, p58, and p83/100 (homolog of p93) of *B. afzelii* strain PKo. Interestingly, IgG antibodies against OspC are detected in only 20% of these patients (49). The frequency of IgG reactivity to OspC in American patients with late disease is higher (48%) (30).

OspA is downregulated at the time of initial infection in the mammalian host. This explains why antibodies against OspA are rarely observed in patients with early disease. Among American patients with late disease, 42% were reactive to OspA (30), in contrast to 5 to 7% among European patients (49, 114). Notably, OspA antibodies are quite common in a special group of patients from the United States who suffer from therapy-refractory forms of Lyme arthritis (4). Subsequently it was shown that patients with Lyme borreliosis have a strong IgG response against a conserved epitope (C6 peptide derived from the IR6 region of VlsE) or the whole recombinant VlsE, which appears earlier during disease than immune responses to other borrelial antigens. This was observed in both American and European patients (7, 70, 97). Differences in VlsE reactivity were observed using VlsE proteins derived from different strains (42). Notably, VlsE from a *B. garinii* strain was more reactive for detection of IgM antibodies than VlsE proteins from *B. burgdorferi* sensu lato or *B. afzelii* strains.

Two-Step Approach in Serodiagnosis

For serodiagnosis of Lyme borreliosis, a two-step approach is recommended by the Association of State and Territorial Public Health Laboratory Directors (ASTPHLD) and the CDC (21, 55): "All serum specimens submitted for Lyme disease testing should be evaluated in a two-step process, in which the first step is a sensitive serological test, such as an enzyme immunoassay (EIA) or immunofluorescence assay (IFA). All specimens found to be positive or equivocal by a sensitive EIA or IFA should be tested by a standardized immunoblot procedure. Specimens found to be negative should not be tested further" (21). This procedure is also recommended in the MiQ Lyme borreliosis standard published by the German expert group on the diagnosis of Lyme borreliosis of the German Society for Hygiene and Microbiology (DGHM) (Fig. 4) (120). The concept of a two-step approach, which aims at increasing the predictive value of a positive result with each step, requires that the tests be performed in succession (56, 120). Omitting the first step, a quantitative assay, and proceeding directly with qualitative immunoblots reduces the specificity of the procedure.

IFA

For the IFA, borreliae fixed on glass slides are used as the antigen. IFA for serodiagnosis of relapsing fever, however, is challenging since expression of the major membrane proteins is variable. The specificity of IFA serodiagnosis for Lyme disease may be improved by adsorption of sera with *Treponema phagedenis* sonicate (IFA-ABS) (120). For the IgM test, pretreatment of the sera with anti-IgG-immune serum is recommended to avoid false-positive test results due to rheumatoid factor as well as false-negative results due to high IgG antibody levels. As in all antibody detection assays, it is important to verify

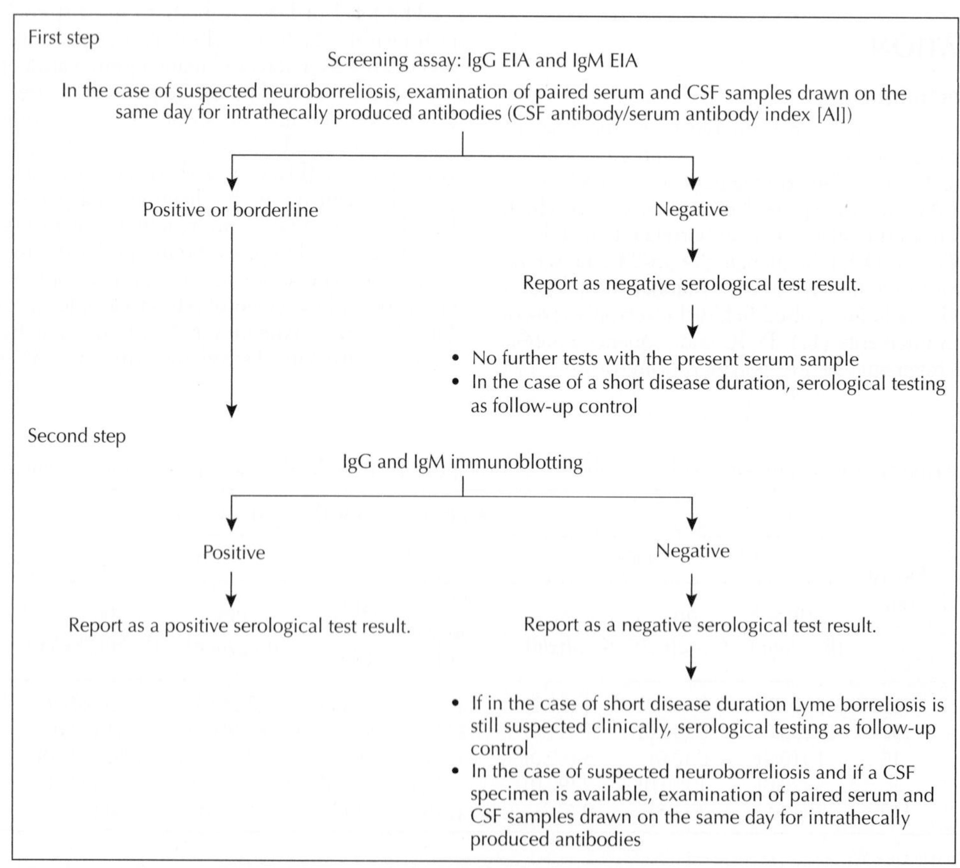

FIGURE 4 Two-step approach for serodiagnosis.

expression of OspC within the antigen source cultures. Although IFA is relatively easy to perform, it is not easy to standardize, and evaluation of test results requires expertise not always available in the routine laboratory. In general, antibody titers of ≥64 and ≥256 are regarded as positive in the IFA-ABS and unadsorbed IFA, respectively. Sera from patients with syphilis are often positive in the unadsorbed assay and are rarely positive in the IFA-ABS (120).

EIA

Different modifications of the EIA have been used for the diagnosis of Lyme borreliosis. In the indirect EIA, antigen is used to coat the plates, followed by incubation with patient serum, enzyme-labeled anti-IgM or anti-IgG, and the EIA substrate. Capture IgM-EIA (μ-capture EIA) has been specially designed to avoid false-positive reactivity due to rheumatoid factor (48). Rheumatoid factor false-positive reactivity can also be overcome by pretreatment of the sera with anti-IgG (114). EIA has the advantage of objective measurement, quantification, and high throughput. Many different antigen preparations have been used, including whole-cell sonicates (93), isolated flagella (46), detergent extracts (114), recombinant antigens (61, 67, 114), and synthetic peptides (70). Use of crude antigen preparations, such as whole-cell sonicates, often results in unacceptable specificity. Improved tests which utilize enriched, specific, or recombinant antigens are now widely used. Tests using an octyl β-D-glucopyranoside detergent extract and Reiter treponeme absorbent, isolated flagella, recombinant VlsE, or the C6 peptide of VlsE are commercially available (Dade-Behring, Marburg, Germany; Dakopatts, Copenhagen, Denmark; Diasorin, Turin, Italy; and Immunetics, Boston, Mass.). Since VlsE is not present in relevant amounts in cultivated borreliae, recombinant VlsE has been added to whole-cell extracts to increase sensitivity in some products (Dade-Behring).

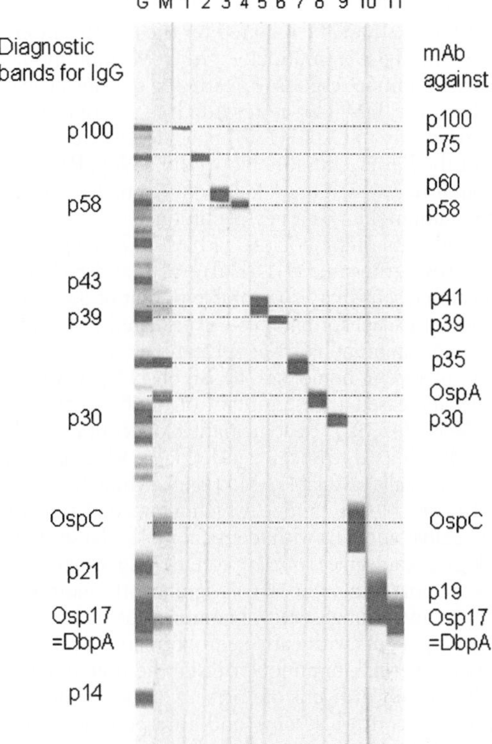

FIGURE 5 Whole-cell immunoblot for identification of diagnostic bands with monoclonal antibodies (mAb). The antigen used is *B. afzelii* strain PKo. Lane G, IgG blot from patient with late disease; lane M, IgM blot from patient with early disease; lanes 1 to 11, different monoclonal antibodies against the respective reactive proteins. (Modified from reference 49.)

Immunoblotting

Western immunoblotting enables assessment of the humoral immune response to individual protein antigens as resolved by sodium dodecyl sulfate-polyacrylamide gel electrophoresis (SDS-PAGE). The Western immunoblot is regarded as a supplementary (United States) or confirmatory (Europe) assay. This implies that it should be employed only when a screening assay is reactive (positive or indeterminate, sometimes called equivocal). Antigen preparations for Western immunoblotting include whole-cell lysates or recombinant antigen mixtures that are transferred after SDS-PAGE to blot membranes.

The advantage of the whole-cell lysate immunoblot is that antibodies against a large number (~50) of antigens can be detected. Herein also lies a significant challenge to the diagnostic laboratorian—discerning reactivity between specific and nonspecific or cross-reactive antigens that may not be clearly resolved from each other. Thus, reliable identification of the immunoreactive bands is imperative, i.e., by use of monoclonal antibodies (Fig. 5) (120). Immunoblotting for Lyme borreliosis is considered technically complex, and in order to realize its maximal performance and utility, standardization and careful quality control must be used.

Numerous immunoblot tests which use antigens of various strains or genospecies of *B. burgdorferi* sensu lato are commercially available. The ASTPHLD and the CDC, as well as the DGHM, have published recommendations for interpretation of the *Borrelia* immunoblot (21, 120). In the United States, immunoblot interpretation rules have been recommended which refer to detection of antibody against whole-cell antigens of specific *B. burgdorferi* sensu stricto strains (30, 36). The IgM immunoblot is interpreted as positive if ≥2 bands of the following proteins are reactive: OspC, 39 kDa (BmpA), and 41 kDa (FlaB). The IgG blot is interpreted as positive if ≥5 bands of the following proteins are reactive: OspC and 18, 28, 30, 39 (BmpA), 41 (FlaB), 45, 58, 66, and 93 kDa. If the immunoblot is used within the first 4 weeks of disease onset (early, stage I or II), both IgM and IgG immunoblots should be performed. A positive IgM immunoblot alone should not be used in determining infection in persons with illness duration of >1 month because the likelihood of a false-positive test for current infection is high for these individuals.

Interpretation of the antibody response among European patients is complicated by the risk of infection with different *Borrelia* species. In addition, immunoblot studies have shown that the immune response of European patients, compared with American patients, is restricted to a narrower spectrum of *Borrelia* proteins (29). Interpretive rules defined in a species- and strain-specific manner have been determined (49) and independently corroborated (62). *B. afzelii* strain PKo is preferred to PBi *(B. garinii)* and PKa2 *(B. burgdorferi* sensu stricto) strains because it permits a two-band criterion for the IgG test: at least two bands positive for p14, Osp17 (DbpA), p21, OspC, p30, p39 (BmpA), p43, p58, and p83/100 (Fig. 5) (120). According to the general Deutsches Institut für Normung (DIN) recommendations on the immunoblot (DIN 58967, Part 40), at least a two-band criterion should be required for the positive interpretation of the IgG immunoblot. In IgM immunoblots, a detectable immune response is restricted to only a few bands. Therefore, the IgM blot is regarded as positive if there is strong reactivity to OspC (120). Specific DIN recommendations for the *Borrelia* immunoblot (DIN 58969, Part 44) have been published which include new antigens (i.e., VlsE) and the line immunoblot as a new technique.

Recombinant immunoblots with Osp17 (DbpA), OspC, p39 (BmpA), truncated p41 (FlaB), p58, and p83/100 have demonstrated sensitivity comparable to that of the whole-cell immunoblot except for patients with isolated EM (115). The recombinant immunoblot was substantially improved by the addition of several homologs of VlsE and DbpA, which considerably increased the sensitivity of antibody detection in early disease (42, 97). Recombinant blots containing DbpA, OspC, p39 (BmpA), truncated p41 (FlaB), VlsE, and p83/100 are commercially available (Mikrogen, Munich, Germany). Using the line blot technique, which allows detection of antibodies against antigens with identical molecular weights (i.e., homologs of the same *Borrelia* protein) (Fig. 6 and Table 5), the recombinant immunoblot is significantly more sensitive than the conventional sonicate immunoblot (i.e., 91.7 versus 68.8%) for patients with early neuroborreliosis (42).

For commercial immunoblot tests, the user should verify that all relevant antigens are present (must be detected by the positive control serum) and interpretation rules are established in defined patient and control populations. In immunoblot evaluation, a scored band must have an intensity equal to or greater than that of the cutoff control. Commercial Western immunoblot test kits licensed by the FDA are available from five different manufacturers. Current listings of 510K, FDA-approved serodiagnostic assays for Lyme disease can be found at http://www.accessdata.fda.gov/scripts/cdrh/cfdocs/cfPMN/pmn.cfm under product code LSR.

Detection of Intrathecally Produced (CSF) Antibodies

Detection of the intrathecal *Borrelia*-specific immune response is one of the most valuable tools for the diagnosis of neuroborreliosis. Methods taking into account potential dysfunction of the blood-CSF barrier, a common finding in neuroborreliosis, are required for accurate assessment of intrathecal antibody production. Since the permeability of the blood-CSF barrier may change rapidly in inflammatory diseases like acute neuroborreliosis, CSF and serum must be obtained at the same time. Long-used procedures for detection of specific intrathecal antibody production in the diagnosis of neurosyphilis have been modified for the diagnosis of neuroborreliosis (47, 103, 119). The most frequently used method is the determination of the CSF/serum antibody index (specific antibody index [AI]).

This method requires measuring the specific antibodies in the blood and in the CSF by means of a calibrated standard curve and determination of a quotient from the antibody units and the IgG concentrations in CSF and serum:

$$\mathrm{AI} = \frac{\text{EIA units in CSF} \times \text{total IgG in serum}}{\text{EIA units in serum} \times \text{total IgG in CSF}}$$

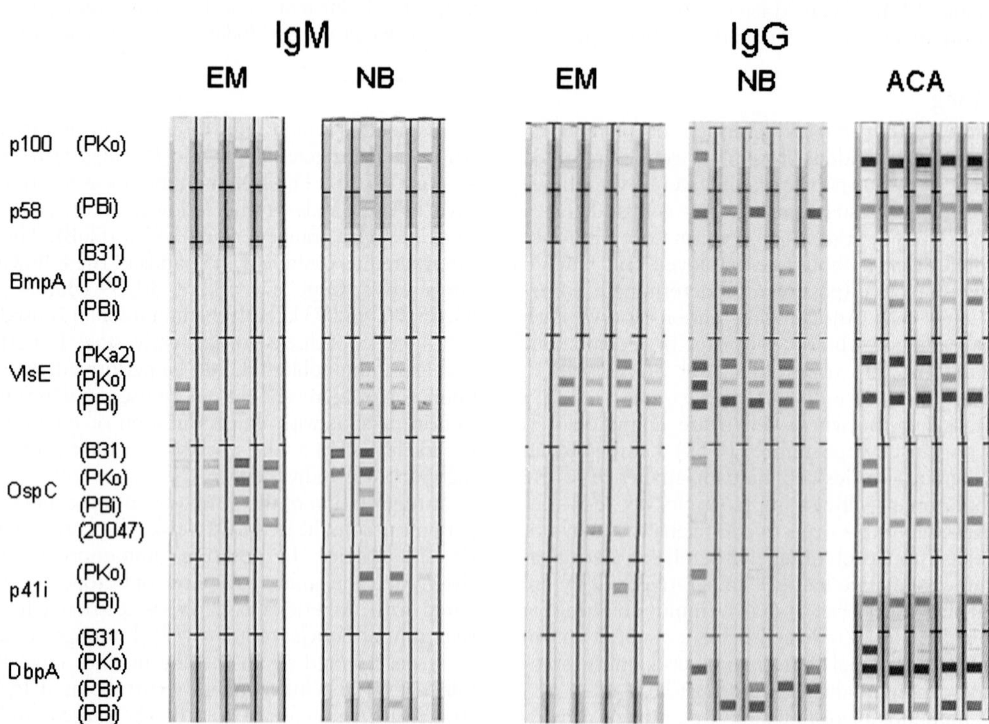

FIGURE 6 Recombinant line immunoblot. Shown are representative IgG blots and IgM blots of patient and control sera. Strains of the following species are shown: *B. burgdorferi* sensu stricto B31 and PKa2, *B. afzelii* PKo, *B. garinii* OspA type 3 (PBr), *B. garinii* OspA type 4 (PBi), and *B. garinii* unknown OspA type (20047). Sera were obtained from patients with EM, early neuroborreliosis (NB), and ACA. (Modified from reference 42.)

For the determination of the AI, EIAs allowing quantitative measurement are suitable (119). The total IgG concentrations of serum and CSF are determined by nephelometry. Alternatively, both serum and CSF can be used for EIA after adjustment to identical concentrations of total IgG (e.g., 1 mg/ dl) and the index is calculated using a simplified formula:

$$AI = \frac{\text{EIA units in CSF}}{\text{EIA units in serum}}$$

By calculating the AI, CSF and serum are compared with regard to the portion of pathogen-specific IgG antibodies in the total IgG content. An AI of ≥2.0 is considered significantly elevated (71, 120). Lower indices (e.g., ≥1.3) are also considered significant by some investigators. However, there is a higher risk of false-positive results due to technical imprecision of measurement of immunoglobulin levels and antibody titers. False-positive AI results are likely with neurosyphilis patients when tested with whole-cell or flagellum sonicates in EIA. Here EIAs with *T. phagedenis* adsorption (Dade-Behring) or recombinant antigens not cross-reacting with *Treponema pallidum* can be helpful for differential diagnosis. Other suitable methods for determination of intrathecal antibody production are the μ- or γ-capture EIA (Dakopatts) (47) and the IgG-matched immunoblot (119). The latter allows comparison of the antibody spectrum (against various *Borrelia* proteins) in serum and in CSF and thus permits conclusions as to the specificity of the intrathecal antibody response.

For cases of neuroborreliosis, intrathecally produced antibody increases dramatically over time. Antibody was detected in only 17% in the first week. Detection rates increased to 80 to 90% of cases between 8 and 41 days after onset of disease and up to 100% of cases after 41 days after onset (47). In a study with children, cases were reported where only the IgM antibody test performed on CSF showed a positive result and no specific antibodies were detected in serum samples taken at the same time (23).

Vaccination and Its Impact on Serology

In the United States, an OspA vaccine (LYMErix) against Lyme borreliosis was licensed for use in humans. In 2002, the producer withdrew the LYMErix vaccine from the market for commercial reasons. Although the OspA vaccine is no longer commercially available, it is still necessary to differentiate between antibodies induced by vaccine and natural infection. Appropriate EIAs include tests lacking the respective vaccine protein, i.e., such as those based on recombinant antigens or peptides or an OspA-deficient mutant strain. Confounding Western immunoblot reactivity that is often observed among OspA vaccine recipients to molecular weight antigens other than p31 is due to fragments of OspA (or cross-reactive OspB) that migrate independently of the intact molecule during SDS-PAGE. Despite concerns, the experienced Lyme borreliosis laboratorian is most often able to distinguish OspA vaccination from early infection using the standard two-test paradigm (2). However, the recent availability of commercial recombinant immunoblots simplifies serodiagnosis in vaccinated individuals.

Controversial Methods

A variety of diagnostic approaches have been developed as alternatives or adjuncts to the more widely practiced methods described above. T-lymphocyte proliferation assays have been used in various scientific studies to investigate the human T-cell response to *Borrelia* antigens (63). However, T-lymphocyte proliferation assays cannot be recommended as diagnostic tests due to their cumbersome nature and concerns about their specificity and standardization (22, 50, 111, 125). Antigen detection tests also are not recommended, as discussed above.

Detection of *B. burgdorferi*-specific antibodies in immune complexes has been proposed to be superior for serodiagnosis of acute Lyme disease (98) and as a marker of active infection (17). Recent work demonstrates that test results for antibodies precipitated from serum as immune complexes are highly correlated with ELISA results obtained using unprocessed serum and are not more likely to reflect active infection than standard serology (72). Transformation of *B. burgdorferi* into spheroplasts (L-forms) in vitro in response to deprivation of serum or culture in CSF has been observed (5, 16). When visualized under a microscope, spheroplasts sometimes appear to be enclosed in a sac, so they have also been called "cysts." If apparently pure L-forms are injected into mice, they are infectious (45). The clinical and diagnostic significance of L-forms has not been demonstrated but warrants further study. There are commercial tests offered that purport to specifically detect cell wall-deficient or "cystic" forms of *B. burgdorferi* by IFA (U.S. patent 6,838,247) and culture (81), but they have not been validated with appropriate controls and are not recommended.

ANTIMICROBIAL SUSCEPTIBILITIES

The antimicrobial susceptibility of *Borrelia* species has been studied intensively in vitro (57, 85). Standard methods for the determination of the minimal bactericidal concentration have not been established. However, there is general agreement on the in vitro susceptibility of borreliae to antimicrobials, as follows. *B. burgdorferi* sensu lato is sensitive to macrolides, tetracyclines, semisynthetic penicillins, and the late second- and third-generation (expanded- and broad-spectrum) cephalosporins; moderately sensitive to penicillin G and chloramphenicol; and resistant to trimethoprim, sulfomethoxazole, rifampin, the aminoglycosides, and the quinolones (57). No significant differences between the Lyme disease borreliae and relapsing fever borreliae (*B. hermsii* and *B. turicatae*) were found with regard to penicillin G, amoxicillin, ceftriaxone, erythromycin, azithromycin, doxycycline, or tetracycline (57). There is no indication for routine antimicrobial susceptibility testing in either Lyme disease or relapsing fever.

Recommendations for Antibiotic Therapy

All clinical manifestations of *B. burgdorferi* infection should be treated with antibiotics. The antibiotic, dosage, duration, and route of application depend on the clinical picture and the stage of the disease (110, 122). In cases of solitary EM, oral treatment with doxycycline, amoxicillin, or cefuroxime axetil is recommended. Disseminated infections require parenteral treatment (ceftriaxone, cefotaxime, or high-dose treatment with penicillin G). In acrodermatitis, the same antibiotics and daily doses are recommended as in EM. In arthritis, oral treatment with doxycycline may be tried first, but in cases of poor therapeutic response, patients should be treated intravenously with cephalosporins or penicillin G. Intravenous cephalosporins or penicillin G is also recommended for stage III neuroborreliosis.

INTERPRETATION AND REPORTING OF RESULTS

General Aspects

Clinical criteria (case history and clinical findings) are decisive factors in the diagnosis and ordering of microbiological laboratory testing. The predictive value of laboratory tests is directly related to the pretest probability. It should be kept in mind that the lower the probability of the clinical diagnosis, the lower the predictive value of a positive test result. For example, a negative serological result has a high negative predictive value for Lyme arthritis, since nearly all cases are seropositive. Whether or not a positive test corresponds with the patient's presentation is a question that can only be answered by the clinician, e.g., by means of clinical case definitions applied to the various manifestations of Lyme borreliosis. Therefore, the laboratory report should not contain any therapy recommendations.

Serological Report

The serological report should contain the following points:

1. Recording of individual test results. Results of the first assay, generally an EIA, are reported as positive, indeterminate, or negative. The immunoblot results are reported as positive or negative. In the case of a positive result, the reactive diagnostic bands may be reported (120). Caution against overinterpretation of minimally reactive blots must be emphasized (e.g., IgG reactivity against p41 is expected in approximately 50% of healthy adults in the United States and Europe and is excluded from the European scoring criteria).
2. Assessment of the final result of the two-step approach regarding its immunodiagnostic significance (e.g., whether specific antibodies have been detected or not)
3. Assessment of serological findings as to the stage of the immune response, as far as test results allow pertinent statements to this effect (see below)
4. Recommendations for further reasonable diagnostic methods (PCR or culture) or for serological follow-up, if indicated

Patterns of Serological Results in Various Stages of Lyme Borreliosis

Antibody tests performed in the early stage of Lyme borreliosis may show a negative or an indeterminate result (Table 6), often due to insufficient time for the full evolution of the immune response. In some cases, seroconversion does not occur until after initiation of treatment. Serological testing of patients with EM alone is not recommended because of the low predictive value of a negative result and the highly characteristic presentation of most rashes. In the presence of a positive clinical correlation and inadequate response to therapy, serology may be warranted up to 6 weeks after onset of disease. During early-stage Lyme borreliosis, detection of IgM is consistent with an active infection. A robust IgG response in the absence of IgM may indicate an anamnestic response to reinfection except with VlsE and C6 peptide assays, where the IgG response is early and predominant (7). Usually only a few bands are detected by immunoblotting in early disease (IgG and IgM) (Fig. 6). In late disease, a positive test for IgG antibodies is mandatory for seroconfirmation. In many cases, IgM antibodies are absent. In principle, an IgM test is not useful for establishing the diagnosis of late disease. The absence of IgG rules out the diagnosis of late Lyme disease even in the presence of IgM. False-positive IgM results due to a polyclonal B-cell activation immune response in the context of herpesvirus infections or autoimmune diseases and rheumatoid disorders also need to be considered. In many cases the origin of such IgM findings remains unclear. The IgG immunoblot usually shows a broad band pattern (Fig. 6). However, positive IgG findings with a broad band pattern in the immunoblot are also compatible with past, asymptomatic, spontaneously resolved, or treated infections. Such result patterns are often found for members of high-risk groups with frequent tick exposure (for example, forest workers) who do not show any clinical manifestations.

In neuroborreliosis, apart from the serum findings, the detection of pathogen-specific, intrathecally produced antibodies is of utmost importance for the diagnosis. An elevated AI is more common in European patients than in U.S. patients, possibly owing to infection with *B. garinii* in Europe. In most cases, determination of the IgG AI will be sufficient. Neuroborreliosis in children is a notable exception to the rule because only the IgM AI may be positive, particularly in cases where disease duration has been short. In the latter circumstances, positive CSF findings may precede positive serology. Therefore, examination of paired serum and CSF specimens is mandatory in such cases. Since a positive AI may be detectable years after treatment and cure, repeated testing is not appropriate for monitoring therapy success. Diagnosis of chronic neuroborreliosis is based on demonstration of a positive AI. Detection of antibodies against *B. burgdorferi* in the serum alone is not sufficient, and direct detection of the pathogen by culture or NAT is rarely successful.

TABLE 6 Sensitivity of antibody detection methods in the diagnosis of Lyme disease

Stage	Sensitivity	Remarks
I	20–50%	Predominance of IgM
II	70–90%	Presence of IgM and IgG; in cases of long disease duration, predominance of IgG
III	Nearly 100%[a]	Usually only IgG

[a] Negative only for patients with a very short duration of symptoms.

Influence of Antimicrobial Therapy on Serodiagnosis

Clinicians are often tempted to order repeated posttreatment serologies in an effort to correlate cure and decreasing antibody titers. However, IgG antibodies against *B. burgdorferi* (especially those against whole-cell antigens) persist for a long time even after successful therapy. Significant titer changes can only be expected several months after the end of therapy; in cases of late manifestations, even years may elapse. Moreover, a decrease in antibody titer does not rule out persistence of the pathogen. Since there is practically no indication for follow-up serological tests, therapeutic success should be based on clinical criteria. A fourfold decline in titer of antibody to VlsE peptide C6 was shown to be an indicator of successful therapy for acute Lyme disease (80) but was not demonstrated for late disease (78) or posttreatment Lyme disease syndrome (39).

Sources of Error in Serodiagnosis

False results, both negative and positive, can occur from the test itself or the nature of the immune response. Seronegative results within the first days of disease are the norm. In Europe, differences between the test antigen and the species causing infection may also contribute to seronegative findings. Deficiencies in diagnostic antigen expression will compromise the sensitivity of tests (important diagnostic antigens such as OspC and DbpA are often not expressed in cultivated borreliae, and VlsE is poorly expressed in vitro). The high background reactivity of many first-generation whole-cell-based assays often results in lower specificity and therefore frequent false-positive results. Cross-reactivity with treponemes can be largely avoided by use of Reiter treponeme adsorbent, although syphilis serology should be performed in cases where treponeme exposure cannot be ruled out. Second- and third-generation assays with improved sensitivity and specificity are preferable to the first-generation tests. Notably, the development of tests based on VlsE has considerably improved serodiagnosis in early disease. Nonetheless, critical assessment of pretest risk factors, clinical history, and presentation will provide the best guidance for laboratory test use and minimize false test outcomes of current and future diagnostic tests.

REFERENCES

1. **Aguero-Rosenfeld, M. E., J. Nowakowski, S. Bittker, D. Cooper, R. B. Nadelman, and G. P. Wormser.** 1996. Evolution of the serologic response to *Borrelia burgdorferi* in treated patients with culture-confirmed erythema migrans. *J. Clin. Microbiol.* **34:**1–9.
2. **Aguero-Rosenfeld, M. E., J. Roberge, C. A. Carbonaro, J. Nowakowski, R. B. Nadelman, and G. P. Wormser.** 1999. Effects of OspA vaccination on Lyme disease serologic testing. *J. Clin. Microbiol.* **37:**3718–3721.
3. **Aguero-Rosenfeld, M. E., G. Wang, I. Schwartz, and G. P. Wormser.** 2005. Diagnosis of Lyme borreliosis. *Clin. Microbiol. Rev.* **18:**484–509.
4. **Akin, E., G. L. McHugh, R. A. Flavell, E. Fikrig, and A. C. Steere.** 1999. The immunoglobulin (IgG) antibody response to OspA and OspB correlates with severe and prolonged Lyme arthritis and the IgG response to P35 correlates with mild and brief arthritis. *Infect. Immun.* **67:**173–181.
5. **Alban, P. S., P. W. Johnson, and D. R. Nelson.** 2000. Serum-starvation-induced changes in protein synthesis and morphology of *Borrelia burgdorferi. Microbiology* **146** (Pt. 1)**:**119–127.
6. **Asbrink, E., and A. Hovmark.** 1988. Early and late cutaneous manifestations in Ixodes-borne borreliosis (erythema migrans borreliosis, Lyme borreliosis). *Ann. N. Y. Acad. Sci.* **539:**4–15.
7. **Bacon, R. M., B. J. Biggerstaff, M. E. Schriefer, R. D. Gilmore, Jr., M. T. Philipp, A. C. Steere, G. P. Wormser, A. R. Marques, and B. J. Johnson.** 2003. Serodiagnosis of Lyme disease by kinetic enzyme-linked immunosorbent assay using recombinant VlsE1 or peptide antigens of *Borrelia burgdorferi* compared with 2-tiered testing using whole-cell lysates. *J. Infect. Dis.* **187:**1187–1199.
8. **Baranton, G., D. Postic, G. Saint, I. P. Boerlin, J. C. Piffaretti, M. Assous, and P. A. Grimont.** 1992. Delineation of *Borrelia burgdorferi* sensu stricto, *Borrelia garinii* sp. nov., and group VS461 associated with Lyme borreliosis. *Int. J. Syst. Bacteriol.* **42:**378–383.
9. **Barbour, A. G.** 1984. Isolation and cultivation of Lyme disease spirochetes. *Yale J. Biol. Med.* **57:**521–525.
10. **Barbour, A. G., and S. F. Hayes.** 1986. Biology of *Borrelia* species. *Microbiol. Rev.* **50:**381–400.
11. **Belfaiza, J., D. Postic, E. Bellenger, G. Baranton, and I. S. Girons.** 1993. Genomic fingerprinting of *Borrelia burgdorferi* sensu lato by pulsed-field gel electrophoresis. *J. Clin. Microbiol.* **31:**2873–2877.
12. **Berger, B. W., R. C. Johnson, C. Kodner, and L. Coleman.** 1992. Cultivation of *Borrelia burgdorferi* from erythema migrans lesions and perilesional skin. *J. Clin. Microbiol.* **30:**359–361.
13. **Bergstrom, S., V. G. Bundoc, and A. G. Barbour.** 1989. Molecular analysis of linear plasmid-encoded major surface proteins, OspA and OspB, of the Lyme disease spirochaete *Borrelia burgdorferi. Mol. Microbiol.* **3:**479–486.
14. **Bradley, J. F., R. C. Johnson, and J. L. Goodman.** 1994. The persistence of spirochetal nucleic acids in active Lyme arthritis. *Ann. Intern. Med.* **120:**487–489.
15. **Brettschneider, S., H. Bruckbauer, N. Klugbauer, and H. Hofmann.** 1998. Diagnostic value of PCR for detection of *Borrelia burgdorferi* in skin biopsy and urine samples from patients with skin borreliosis. *J. Clin. Microbiol.* **36:**2658–2665.
16. **Brorson, O., and S. H. Brorson.** 1998. In vitro conversion of *Borrelia burgdorferi* to cystic forms in spinal fluid, and transformation to mobile spirochetes by incubation in BSK-H medium. *Infection* **26:**144–150.
17. **Brunner, M., and L. H. Sigal.** 2001. Use of serum immune complexes in a new test that accurately confirms early Lyme disease and active infection with *Borrelia burgdorferi. J. Clin. Microbiol.* **39:**3213–3221.
18. **Burgdorfer, W., A. G. Barbour, S. F. Hayes, J. L. Benach, E. Grunwaldt, and J. P. Davis.** 1982. Lyme disease—a tick-borne spirochetosis? *Science* **216:**1317–1319.
19. **Canica, M. M., F. Nato, L. du Merle, J. C. Mazie, G. Baranton, and D. Postic.** 1993. Monoclonal antibodies for identification of *Borrelia afzelii* sp. nov. associated with late cutaneous manifestations of Lyme borreliosis. *Scand. J. Infect. Dis.* **25:**441–448.
20. **Casjens, S., N. Palmer, R. van Vugt, W. M. Huang, B. Stevenson, P. Rosa, R. Lathigra, G. Sutton, J. Peterson, R. J. Dodson, D. Haft, E. Hickey, M. Gwinn, O. White, and C. M. Fraser.** 2000. A bacterial genome in flux: the twelve linear and nine circular extrachromosomal DNAs in an infectious isolate of the Lyme disease spirochete *Borrelia burgdorferi. Mol. Microbiol.* **35:**490–516.
21. **Centers for Disease Control and Prevention.** 1995. Recommendations for test performance and interpretation from the Second National Conference on Serologic Diagnosis of Lyme Disease. *Morb. Mortal. Wkly. Rep.* **44:**590.
22. **Centers for Disease Control and Prevention.** 2005. Caution regarding testing for Lyme disease. *Morb. Mortal. Wkly. Rep.* **54:**125.
23. **Christen, H. J., F. Hanefeld, H. Eiffert, and R. Thomssen.** 1993. Epidemiology and clinical manifestations of Lyme borreliosis in childhood. A prospective multicentre study with special regard to neuroborreliosis. *Acta Paediatr. Suppl.* **386:**1–75.
24. **Collares-Pereira, M., S. Couceiro, I. Franca, K. Kurtenbach, S. M. Schafer, L. Vitorino, L. Goncalves, S. Baptista, M. L. Vieira, and C. Cunha.** 2004. First isolation of *Borrelia lusitaniae* from a human patient. *J. Clin. Microbiol.* **42:**1316–1318.
25. **Coyle, P. K., S. E. Schutzer, A. L. Belman, L. B. Krupp, and Z. Dheng.** 1992. Cerebrospinal fluid immunologic parameters in neurologic Lyme disease, p. 31–44. *In* S. E. Schutzer (ed.), *Lyme Disease: Molecular and Immunologic Approaches.* Cold Spring Harbor Laboratory Press, Cold Spring Harbor, N.Y.
26. **Cutler, S. J., D. Fekade, K. Hussein, K. A. Knox, A. Melka, K. Cann, A. R. Emilianus, D. A. Warrell, and D. J. Wright.** 1994. Successful in-vitro cultivation of *Borrelia recurrentis. Lancet* **343:**242.
27. **Cutler, S. J., J. Moss, M. Fukunaga, D. J. Wright, D. Fekade, and D. Warrell.** 1997. *Borrelia recurrentis* characterization and comparison with relapsing-fever, Lyme-associated, and other *Borrelia* spp. *Int. J. Syst. Bacteriol.* **47:**958–968.
28. **de Silva, A. M., and E. Fikrig.** 1995. Growth and migration of *Borrelia burgdorferi* in *Ixodes* ticks during blood feeding. *Am. J. Trop. Med. Hyg.* **53:**397–404.
29. **Dressler, F., R. Ackermann, and A. C. Steere.** 1994. Antibody responses to the three genomic groups of *Borrelia burgdorferi* in European Lyme borreliosis. *J. Infect. Dis.* **169:**313–318.
30. **Dressler, F., J. A. Whalen, B. N. Reinhardt, and A. C. Steere.** 1993. Western blotting in the serodiagnosis of Lyme disease. *J. Infect. Dis.* **167:**392–400.
31. **Dumler, J. S.** 2001. Molecular diagnosis of Lyme disease: review and meta-analysis. *Mol. Diagn.* **6:**1–11.

32. **Dworkin, M. S., T. G. Schwan, and D. E. Anderson, Jr.** 2002. Tick-borne relapsing fever in North America. *Med. Clin. N. Am.* **86:**417–433, viii–ix.
33. **Dworkin, M. S., P. C. Shoemaker, C. L. Fritz, M. E. Dowell, and D. E. Anderson, Jr.** 2002. The epidemiology of tick-borne relapsing fever in the United States. *Am. J. Trop. Med. Hyg.* **66:**753–758.
34. **Eiffert, H., A. Karsten, R. Thomssen, and H. J. Christen.** 1998. Characterization of *Borrelia burgdorferi* strains in Lyme arthritis. *Scand. J. Infect. Dis.* **30:**265–268.
35. **Eiffert, H., A. Ohlenbusch, H. J. Christen, R. Thomssen, A. Spielman, and F. R. Matuschka.** 1995. Nondifferentiation between Lyme disease spirochetes from vector ticks and human cerebrospinal fluid. *J. Infect. Dis.* **171:**476–479.
36. **Engstrom, S. M., E. Shoop, and R. C. Johnson.** 1995. Immunoblot interpretation criteria for serodiagnosis of early Lyme disease. *J. Clin. Microbiol.* **33:**419–427.
37. **Fingerle, V., G. Liegl, U. Munderloh, and B. Wilske.** 1998. Expression of outer surface proteins A and C of *Borrelia burgdorferi* in *Ixodes ricinus* ticks removed from humans. *Med. Microbiol. Immunol.* **187:**121–126.
38. **Fingerle, V., S. Rauser, B. Hammer, O. Kahl, C. Heimerl, U. Schulte-Spechtel, L. Gern, and B. Wilske.** 2002. Dynamics of dissemination and outer surface protein expression of different European *Borrelia burgdorferi* sensu lato strains in artificially infected *Ixodes ricinus* nymphs. *J. Clin. Microbiol.* **40:**1456–1463.
39. **Fleming, R. V., A. R. Marques, M. S. Klempner, C. H. Schmid, L. G. Dally, D. S. Martin, and M. T. Philipp.** 2004. Pre-treatment and post-treatment assessment of the C(6) test in patients with persistent symptoms and a history of Lyme borreliosis. *Eur. J. Clin. Microbiol. Infect. Dis.* **23:**615–618.
40. **Fraser, C. M., S. Casjens, W. M. Huang, G. G. Sutton, R. Clayton, R. Lathigra, O. White, K. A. Ketchum, R. Dodson, E. K. Hickey, M. Gwinn, B. Dougherty, J. F. Tomb, R. D. Fleischmann, D. Richardson, J. Peterson, A. R. Kerlavage, J. Quackenbush, S. Salzberg, M. Hanson, R. van Vugt, N. Palmer, M. D. Adams, J. Gocayne, J. Weidman, T. Utterback, L. Watthey, L. McDonald, P. Artiach, C. Bowman, S. Garland, C. Fuji, M. D. Cotton, K. Horst, K. Roberts, B. Hatch, H. O. Smith, and J. C. Venter.** 1997. Genomic sequence of a Lyme disease spirochaete, *Borrelia burgdorferi*. *Nature* **390:**580–586.
41. **Glöckner, G., R. Lehmann, A. Romualdi, S. Pradella, U. Schulte-Spechtel, M. Schilhabel, B. Wilske, J. Suhnel, and M. Platzer.** 2004. Comparative analysis of the *Borrelia garinii* genome. *Nucleic Acids Res.* **32:**6038–6046.
42. **Goettner, G., U. Schulte-Spechtel, R. Hillermann, G. Liegl, B. Wilske, and V. Fingerle.** 2005. Improvement of Lyme borreliosis serodiagnosis by a newly developed recombinant IgG and IgM line immunoblot and addition of VlsE and DbpA homologues. *J. Clin. Microbiol.* **43:**3602–3609.
43. **Goodman, J. L., J. F. Bradley, A. E. Ross, P. Goellner, A. Lagus, B. Vitale, B. W. Berger, S. Luger, and R. C. Johnson.** 1995. Bloodstream invasion in early Lyme disease: results from a prospective, controlled, blinded study using the polymerase chain reaction. *Am. J. Med.* **99:**6–12.
44. **Grimm, D., K. Tilly, R. Byram, P. E. Stewart, J. G. Krum, D. M. Bueschel, T. G. Schwan, P. F. Policastro, A. F. Elias, and P. A. Rosa.** 2004. Outer-surface protein C of the Lyme disease spirochete: a protein induced in ticks for infection of mammals. *Proc. Natl. Acad. Sci. USA* **101:**3142–3147.
45. **Gruntar, I., T. Malovrh, R. Murgia, and M. Cinco.** 2001. Conversion of *Borrelia garinii* cystic forms to motile spirochetes in vivo. *APMIS* **109:**383–388.
46. **Hansen, K., P. Hindersson, and N. S. Pedersen.** 1988. Measurement of antibodies to the *Borrelia burgdorferi* flagellum improves serodiagnosis in Lyme disease. *J. Clin. Microbiol.* **26:**338–346.
47. **Hansen, K., and A. M. Lebech.** 1991. Lyme neuroborreliosis: a new sensitive diagnostic assay for intrathecal synthesis of *Borrelia burgdorferi*—specific immunoglobulin G, A, and M. *Ann. Neurol.* **30:**197–205.
48. **Hansen, K., K. Pii, and A. M. Lebech.** 1991. Improved immunoglobulin M serodiagnosis in Lyme borreliosis by using a μ-capture enzyme-linked immunosorbent assay with biotinylated *Borrelia burgdorferi* flagella. *J. Clin. Microbiol.* **29:**166–173.
49. **Hauser, U., G. Lehnert, R. Lobentanzer, and B. Wilske.** 1997. Interpretation criteria for standardized Western blots for three European species of *Borrelia burgdorferi* sensu lato. *J. Clin. Microbiol.* **35:**1433–1444.
50. **Horowitz, H. W., C. S. Pavia, S. Bittker, G. Forseter, D. Cooper, R. B. Nadelman, D. Byrne, R. C. Johnson, and G. P. Wormser.** 1994. Sustained cellular immune responses to *Borrelia burgdorferi*: lack of correlation with clinical presentation and serology. *Clin. Diagn. Lab. Immunol.* **1:**373–378.
51. **Humair, P., and L. Gern.** 2000. The wild hidden face of Lyme borreliosis in Europe. *Microbes Infect.* **2:**915–922.
52. **Hyde, F. W., R. C. Johnson, T. J. White, and C. E. Shelburne.** 1989. Detection of antigens in urine of mice and humans infected with *Borrelia burgdorferi*, etiologic agent of Lyme disease. *J. Clin. Microbiol.* **27:**58–61.
53. **James, A. M., D. Liveris, G. P. Wormser, I. Schwartz, M. A. Montecalvo, and B. J. Johnson.** 2001. *Borrelia lonestari* infection after a bite by an *Amblyomma americanum* tick. *J. Infect. Dis.* **183:**1810–1814.
54. **Jauris-Heipke, S., G. Liegl, V. Preac-Mursic, D. Rössler, E. Schwab, E. Soutschek, G. Will, and B. Wilske.** 1995. Molecular analysis of genes encoding outer surface protein C (OspC) of *Borrelia burgdorferi* sensu lato: relationship to *ospA* genotype and evidence of lateral gene exchange of *ospC*. *J. Clin. Microbiol.* **33:**1860–1866.
55. **Johnson, B. J.** 2006. Lyme disease: serologic assays for antibodies to *Borrelia burgdorferi*, p. 493–500. *In* B. Detrick, R. G. Hamilton, and J. D. Folds (ed.), *Manual of Molecular and Clinical Laboratory Immunology,* 7th ed. ASM Press, Washington, D.C.
56. **Johnson, B. J., K. E. Robbins, R. E. Bailey, B. L. Cao, S. L. Sviat, R. B. Craven, L. W. Mayer, and D. T. Dennis.** 1996. Serodiagnosis of Lyme disease: accuracy of a two-step approach using a flagella-based ELISA and immunoblotting. *J. Infect. Dis.* **174:**346–353.
57. **Johnson, R. C.** 1998. *Borrelia*, p. 1277–1286. *In* L. H. Collier and W. W. Topley (ed.), *Topley & Wilson's Microbiology and Microbial Infections.* Arnold, London, Great Britain.
58. **Johnson, R. C., G. P. Schmid, F. W. Hyde, A. G. Steigerwalt, and D. J. Brenner.** 1984. *Borrelia burgdorferi* sp. nov.: etiologic agent of Lyme disease. *Int. J. Syst. Bacteriol.* **34:**496–497.
59. **Johnson, W. D., Jr.** 1995. *Borrelia* species (relapsing fever), p. 2141–2143. *In* G. L. Mandell, J. E. Bennett, and R. Dolin (ed.), *Mandell, Douglas and Bennett's Principles and Practice of Infectious Diseases.* Churchill Livingstone, New York, N.Y.
60. **Kahl, O., C. Janetzki-Mittmann, J. S. Gray, R. Jonas, J. Stein, and R. de Boer.** 1998. Risk of infection with *Borrelia burgdorferi* sensu lato for a host in relation to the duration of nymphal Ixodes ricinus feeding and the method of tick removal. *Zentbl. Bakteriol.* **287:**41–52.
61. **Kaiser, R., and S. Rauer.** 1999. Advantage of recombinant borrelial proteins for serodiagnosis of neuroborreliosis. *J. Med. Microbiol.* **48:**5–10.
62. **Kaiser, R., and S. Rauer.** 1999. Serodiagnosis of neuroborreliosis: comparison of reliability of three confirmatory assays. *Infection* **27:**177–182.
63. **Kalish, R. S., J. A. Wood, W. Golde, R. Bernard, L. E. Davis, R. C. Grimson, P. K. Coyle, and B. J. Luft.** 2003. Human T lymphocyte response to *Borrelia burgdorferi* infection: no correlation between human leukocyte function

antigen type 1 peptide response and clinical status. *J. Infect. Dis.* **187:**102–108.

64. **Klempner, M. S., C. H. Schmid, L. Hu, A. C. Steere, G. Johnson, B. McCloud, R. Noring, and A. Weinstein.** 2001. Intralaboratory reliability of serologic and urine testing for Lyme disease. *Am. J. Med.* **110:**217–219.
65. **Kraiczy, P., J. Hellwage, C. Skerka, H. Becker, M. Kirschfink, M. M. Simon, V. Brade, P. F. Zipfel, and R. Wallich.** 2004. Complement resistance of *Borrelia burgdorferi* correlates with the expression of BbCRASP-1, a novel linear plasmid-encoded surface protein that interacts with human factor H and FHL-1 and is unrelated to Erp proteins. *J. Biol. Chem.* **279:**2421–2429.
66. **Lahdenne, P., J. Panelius, H. Saxen, T. Heikkila, H. Sillanpaa, M. Peltomaa, M. Arnez, H. I. Huppertz, and I. J. Seppala.** 2003. Improved serodiagnosis of erythema migrans using novel recombinant borrelial BBK32 antigens. *J. Med. Microbiol.* **52:**563–567.
67. **Lawrenz, M. B., J. M. Hardham, R. T. Owens, J. Nowakowski, A. C. Steere, G. P. Wormser, and S. J. Norris.** 1999. Human antibody responses to VlsE antigenic variation protein of *Borrelia burgdorferi*. *J. Clin. Microbiol.* **37:**3997–4004.
68. **Lebech, A. M., K. Hansen, F. Brandrup, O. Clemmensen, and L. Halkier-Sorensen.** 2000. Diagnostic value of PCR for detection of *Borrelia burgdorferi* DNA in clinical specimens from patients with erythema migrans and Lyme neuroborreliosis. *Mol. Diagn.* **5:**139–150.
69. **Le Fleche, A., D. Postic, K. Girardet, O. Peter, and G. Baranton.** 1997. Characterization of *Borrelia lusitaniae* sp. nov. by 16S ribosomal DNA sequence analysis. *Int. J. Syst. Bacteriol.* **47:**921–925.
70. **Liang, F. T., E. Aberer, M. Cinco, L. Gern, C. M. Hu, Y. N. Lobet, M. Ruscio, P. E. Voet, Jr., V. E. Weynants, and M. T. Philipp.** 2000. Antigenic conservation of an immunodominant invariable region of the VlsE lipoprotein among European pathogenic genospecies of *Borrelia burgdorferi* SL. *J. Infect. Dis.* **182:**1455–1462.
71. **Luft, B. J., C. R. Steinman, H. C. Neimark, B. Muralidhar, T. Rush, M. F. Finkel, M. Kunkel, and R. J. Dattwyler.** 1992. Invasion of the central nervous system by *Borrelia burgdorferi* in acute disseminated infection. *JAMA* **267:**1364–1367.
72. **Marques, A. R., R. L. Hornung, L. Dally, and M. T. Philipp.** 2005. Detection of immune complexes is not independent of detection of antibodies in Lyme disease patients and does not confirm active infection with *Borrelia burgdorferi*. *Clin. Diagn. Lab. Immunol.* **12:**1036–1040.
73. **Nocton, J. J., F. Dressler, B. J. Rutledge, P. N. Rys, D. H. Persing, and A. C. Steere.** 1994. Detection of *Borrelia burgdorferi* DNA by polymerase chain reaction in synovial fluid from patients with Lyme arthritis. *N. Engl. J. Med.* **330:**229–234.
74. **Ojaimi, C., C. Brooks, S. Casjens, P. Rosa, A. Elias, A. Barbour, A. Jasinskas, J. Benach, L. Katona, J. Radolf, M. Caimano, J. Skare, K. Swingle, D. Akins, and I. Schwartz.** 2003. Profiling of temperature-induced changes in *Borrelia burgdorferi* gene expression by using whole genome arrays. *Infect. Immun.* **71:**1689–1705.
75. **Olsen, B., D. C. Duffy, T. G. Jaenson, A. Gylfe, J. Bonnedahl, and S. Bergstrom.** 1995. Transhemispheric exchange of Lyme disease spirochetes by seabirds. *J. Clin. Microbiol.* **33:**3270–3274.
76. **Pal, U., X. Yang, M. Chen, L. K. Bockenstedt, J. F. Anderson, R. A. Flavell, M. V. Norgard, and E. Fikrig.** 2004. OspC facilitates *Borrelia burgdorferi* invasion of Ixodes scapularis salivary glands. *J. Clin. Investig.* **113:**220–230.
77. **Panelius, J., P. Lahdenne, H. Saxen, S. A. Carlsson, T. Heikkila, M. Peltomaa, A. Lauhio, and I. Seppala.** 2003. Diagnosis of Lyme neuroborreliosis with antibodies to recombinant proteins DbpA, BBK32, and OspC, and VlsE IR6 peptide. *J. Neurol.* **250:**1318–1327.
78. **Peltomaa, M., G. McHugh, and A. C. Steere.** 2003. Persistence of the antibody response to the VlsE sixth invariant region (IR6) peptide of *Borrelia burgdorferi* after successful antibiotic treatment of Lyme disease. *J. Infect. Dis.* **187:**1178–1186.
79. **Persing, D. H., B. J. Rutledge, P. N. Rys, D. S. Podzorski, P. D. Mitchell, K. D. Reed, B. Liu, E. Fikrig, and S. E. Malawista.** 1994. Target imbalance: disparity of *Borrelia burgdorferi* genetic material in synovial fluid from Lyme arthritis patients. *J. Infect. Dis.* **169:**668–672.
80. **Philipp, M. T., A. R. Marques, P. T. Fawcett, L. G. Dally, and D. S. Martin.** 2003. C6 test as an indicator of therapy outcome for patients with localized or disseminated Lyme borreliosis. *J. Clin. Microbiol.* **41:**4955–4960.
81. **Phillips, S. E., L. H. Mattman, D. Hulinska, and H. Moayad.** 1998. A proposal for the reliable culture of *Borrelia burgdorferi* from patients with chronic Lyme disease, even from those previously aggressively treated. *Infection* **26:**364–367.
82. **Picken, M. M., R. N. Picken, D. Han, Y. Cheng, E. Ruzic-Sabljic, J. Cimperman, V. Maraspin, S. Lotric-Furlan, and F. Strle.** 1997. A two year prospective study to compare culture and polymerase chain reaction amplification for the detection and diagnosis of Lyme borreliosis. *Mol. Pathol.* **50:**186–193.
83. **Pollack, R. J., S. R. Telford III, and A. Spielman.** 1993. Standardization of medium for culturing Lyme disease spirochetes. *J. Clin. Microbiol.* **31:**1251–1255.
84. **Postic, D., M. V. Assous, P. A. Grimont, and G. Baranton.** 1994. Diversity of *Borrelia burgdorferi* sensu lato evidenced by restriction fragment length polymorphism of rrf (5S)-rrl (23S) intergenic spacer amplicons. *Int. J. Syst. Bacteriol.* **44:**743–752.
85. **Preac-Mursic, V.** 1993. Antibiotic susceptibility of *Borrelia burgdorferi*, in vitro and in vivo, p. 301–311. *In* K. Weber and W. Burgdorfer (ed.), *Aspects of Lyme Borreliosis.* Springer Verlag, Berlin, Germany.
86. **Preac-Mursic, V., B. Wilske, and S. Reinhardt.** 1991. Culture of *Borrelia burgdorferi* on six solid media. *Eur. J. Clin. Microbiol. Infect. Dis.* **10:**1076–1079.
87. **Priem, S., M. G. Rittig, T. Kamradt, G. R. Burmester, and A. Krause.** 1997. An optimized PCR leads to rapid and highly sensitive detection of *Borrelia burgdorferi* in patients with Lyme borreliosis. *J. Clin. Microbiol.* **35:**685–690.
88. **Ramos, J. M., E. Malmierca, F. Reyes, W. Wolde, A. Galata, A. Tesfamariam, and M. Gorgolas.** 2004. Characteristics of louse-borne relapsing fever in Ethiopian children and adults. *Ann. Trop. Med. Parasitol.* **98:**191–196.
89. **Rauter, C., M. Mueller, I. Diterich, S. Zeller, D. Hassler, T. Meergans, and T. Hartung.** 2005. Critical evaluation of urine-based PCR assay for diagnosis of Lyme borreliosis. *Clin. Diagn. Lab. Immunol.* **12:**910–917.
90. **Richter, D., D. Postic, N. Sertour, I. Livey, F.-R. Matuschka, and G. Baranton.** 2006. Delineation of *Borrelia burgdorferi* sensu lato species by multilocus sequence analysis and confirmation of the delineation of *B. spielmanii* sp. nov. *Int. J. Syst. Evol. Microbiol.* **56:**873–881.
91. **Rijpkema, S. G., D. J. Tazelaar, M. J. Molkenboer, G. T. Noordhoek, G. Plantinga, L. M. Schouls, and J. F. Schellekens.** 1997. Detection of *Borrelia afzelii*, *Borrelia burgdorferi* sensu stricto, *Borrelia garinii* and group VS116 by PCR in skin biopsies of patients with erythema migrans and acrodermatitis chronica atrophicans. *Clin. Microbiol. Infect.* **3:**109–116.
92. **Roth, A., H. Mauch, and U. B. Göbel.** 1997. MIQ 1, Nukleinsäureamplifikationstechniken. *In Qualitätsstandards in der Mikrobiologisch-Infektiologischen Diagnostik.* Gustav Fischer Verlag, Stuttgart, Germany.

93. **Russell, H., J. S. Sampson, G. P. Schmid, H. W. Wilkinson, and B. Plikaytis.** 1984. Enzyme-linked immunosorbent assay and indirect immunofluorescence assay for Lyme disease. *J. Infect. Dis.* **149:**465–470.

94. **Ruzic-Sabljic, E., V. Maraspin, S. Lotric-Furlan, T. Jurca, M. Logar, A. Pikelj-Pecnik, and F. Strle.** 2002. Characterization of *Borrelia burgdorferi* sensu lato strains isolated from human material in Slovenia. *Wien. Klin. Wochenschr.* **114:**544–550.

95. **Sadziene, A., B. Wilske, M. S. Ferdows, and A. G. Barbour.** 1993. The cryptic *ospC* gene of *Borrelia burgdorferi* B31 is located on a circular plasmid. *Infect. Immun.* **61:**2192–2195.

96. **Schmidt, B. L.** 1997. PCR in laboratory diagnosis of human *Borrelia burgdorferi* infections. *Clin. Microbiol. Rev.* **10:**185–201.

97. **Schulte-Spechtel, U., G. Lehnert, G. Liegl, V. Fingerle, C. Heimerl, B. J. Johnson, and B. Wilske.** 2003. Significant improvement of the recombinant *Borrelia*-specific immunoglobulin G immunoblot test by addition of VlsE and a DbpA homologue derived from *Borrelia garinii* for diagnosis of early neuroborreliosis. *J. Clin. Microbiol.* **41:**1299–1303.

98. **Schutzer, S. E., P. K. Coyle, P. Reid, and B. Holland.** 1999. *Borrelia burgdorferi*-specific immune complexes in acute Lyme disease. *JAMA* **282:**1942–1946.

99. **Schwan, T. G., J. Piesman, W. T. Golde, M. C. Dolan, and P. A. Rosa.** 1995. Induction of an outer surface protein on *Borrelia burgdorferi* during tick feeding. *Proc. Natl. Acad. Sci. USA* **92:**2909–2913.

100. **Schwan, T. G., M. E. Schrumpf, B. J. Hinnebusch, D. E. Anderson, Jr., and M. E. Konkel.** 1996. GlpQ: an antigen for serological discrimination between relapsing fever and Lyme borreliosis. *J. Clin. Microbiol.* **34:**2483–2492.

101. **Schwartz, J. J., A. Gazumyan, and I. Schwartz.** 1992. rRNA gene organization in the Lyme disease spirochete, *Borrelia burgdorferi*. *J. Bacteriol.* **174:**3757–3765.

102. **Stanek, G., and F. Strle.** 2003. Lyme borreliosis. *Lancet* **362:**1639–1647.

103. **Steere, A. C., V. P. Berardi, K. E. Weeks, E. L. Logigian, and R. Ackermann.** 1990. Evaluation of the intrathecal antibody response to *Borrelia burgdorferi* as a diagnostic test for Lyme neuroborreliosis. *J. Infect. Dis.* **161:**1203–1209.

104. **Steere, A. C., J. Coburn, and L. Glickstein.** 2004. The emergence of Lyme disease. *J. Clin. Investig.* **113:**1093–1101.

105. **Steere, A. C., and L. Glickstein.** 2004. Elucidation of Lyme arthritis. *Nat. Rev. Immunol.* **4:**143–152.

106. **Vasiliu, V., P. Herzer, D. Rössler, G. Lehnert, and B. Wilske.** 1998. Heterogeneity of *Borrelia burgdorferi* sensu lato demonstrated by an *ospA*-type-specific PCR in synovial fluid from patients with Lyme arthritis. *Med. Microbiol. Immunol.* **187:**97–102.

107. **Wang, G., A. P. van Dam, and J. Dankert.** 1999. Phenotypic and genetic characterization of a novel *Borrelia burgdorferi* sensu lato isolate from a patient with lyme borreliosis. *J. Clin. Microbiol.* **37:**3025–3028.

108. **Wang, G., A. P. van Dam, I. Schwartz, and J. Dankert.** 1999. Molecular typing of *Borrelia burgdorferi* sensu lato: taxonomic, epidemiological, and clinical implications. *Clin. Microbiol. Rev.* **12:**633–653.

109. **Weber, K., and W. Burgdorfer.** 1993. *Aspects of Lyme Borreliosis*. Springer Verlag, Berlin, Germany.

110. **Weber, K., and H. W. Pfister.** 1994. Clinical management of Lyme borreliosis. *Lancet* **343:**1017–1020.

111. **Wilske, B.** 2005. Epidemiology and diagnosis of Lyme borreliosis. *Ann. Med.* **37:**568–579.

112. **Wilske, B., U. Busch, H. Eiffert, V. Fingerle, H. W. Pfister, D. Rössler, and V. Preac-Mursic.** 1996. Diversity of OspA and OspC among cerebrospinal fluid isolates of *Borrelia burgdorferi* sensu lato from patients with neuroborreliosis in Germany. *Med. Microbiol. Immunol.* **184:**195–201.

113. **Wilske, B., U. Busch, V. Fingerle, S. Jauris-Heipke, V. Preac Mursic, D. Rössler, and G. Will.** 1996. Immunological and molecular variability of OspA and OspC. Implications for *Borrelia* vaccine development. *Infection* **24:**208–212.

114. **Wilske, B., V. Fingerle, P. Herzer, A. Hofmann, G. Lehnert, H. Peters, H. W. Pfister, V. Preac-Mursic, E. Soutschek, and K. Weber.** 1993. Recombinant immunoblot in the serodiagnosis of Lyme borreliosis. Comparison with indirect immunofluorescence and enzyme-linked immunosorbent assay. *Med. Microbiol. Immunol.* **182:**255–270.

115. **Wilske, B., C. Habermann, V. Fingerle, B. Hillenbrand, S. Jauris-Heipke, G. Lehnert, I. Pradel, D. Rössler, and U. Schulte-Spechtel.** 1999. An improved recombinant IgG immunoblot for serodiagnosis of Lyme borreliosis. *Med. Microbiol. Immunol.* **188:**139–144.

116. **Wilske, B., S. Jauris-Heipke, R. Lobentanzer, I. Pradel, V. Preac-Mursic, D. Rössler, E. Soutschek, and R. C. Johnson.** 1995. Phenotypic analysis of outer surface protein C (OspC) of *Borrelia burgdorferi* sensu lato by monoclonal antibodies: relationship to genospecies and OspA serotype. *J. Clin. Microbiol.* **33:**103–109.

117. **Wilske, B., V. Preac-Mursic, U. B. Göbel, B. Graf, S. Jauris, E. Soutschek, E. Schwab, and G. Zumstein.** 1993. An OspA serotyping system for *Borrelia burgdorferi* based on reactivity with monoclonal antibodies and OspA sequence analysis. *J. Clin. Microbiol.* **31:**340–350.

118. **Wilske, B., V. Preac-Mursic, S. Jauris, A. Hofmann, I. Pradel, E. Soutschek, E. Schwab, G. Will, and G. Wanner.** 1993. Immunological and molecular polymorphisms of OspC, an immunodominant major outer surface protein of *Borrelia burgdorferi*. *Infect. Immun.* **61:**2182–2191.

119. **Wilske, B., G. Schierz, V. Preac-Mursic, K. von Busch, R. Kuhbeck, H. W. Pfister, and K. Einhäupl.** 1986. Intrathecal production of specific antibodies against *Borrelia burgdorferi* in patients with lymphocytic meningoradiculitis (Bannwarth's syndrome). *J. Infect. Dis.* **153:**304–314.

119a. **Wilske, B., and M. Schriefer.** 2003. *Borrelia*, p. 937–954. *In* P. R. Murray, E. J. Baron, J. H. Jorgensen, M. A. Pfaller, and R. H. Yolken (ed.), *Manual of Clinical Microbiology*. ASM Press, 8th ed. Washington, D.C.

120. **Wilske, B., L. Zöller, V. Brade, H. Eiffert, U. B. Göbel, G. Stanek, and H. W. Pfister.** 2000. MIQ 12, Lyme-Borreliose, p. 1–59. *In* H. Mauch and R. Lütticken (ed.), *Qualitätsstandards in der Mikrobiologisch-Infektiologischen Diagnostik*. Urban & Fischer Verlag, Munich, Germany.

121. **Wormser, G. P., S. Bittker, D. Cooper, J. Nowakowski, R. B. Nadelman, and C. Pavia.** 2000. Comparison of the yields of blood cultures using serum or plasma from patients with early Lyme disease. *J. Clin. Microbiol.* **38:**1648–1650.

122. **Wormser, G. P., R. B. Nadelman, R. J. Dattwyler, D. T. Dennis, E. D. Shapiro, A. C. Steere, T. J. Rush, D. W. Rahn, P. K. Coyle, D. H. Persing, D. Fish, and B. J. Luft.** 2000. Practice guidelines for the treatment of Lyme disease. The Infectious Diseases Society of America. *Clin. Infect. Dis.* **31**(Suppl. 1)**:**1–14.

123. **Zhang, J. R., J. M. Hardham, A. G. Barbour, and S. J. Norris.** 1997. Antigenic variation in Lyme disease borreliae by promiscuous recombination of VMP-like sequence cassettes. *Cell* **89:**275–285.

124. **Zore, A., E. Ruzic-Sabljic, V. Maraspin, J. Cimperman, S. Lotric-Furlan, A. Pikelj, T. Jurca, M. Logar, and F. Strle.** 2002. Sensitivity of culture and polymerase chain reaction for the etiologic diagnosis of erythema migrans. *Wien. Klin. Wochenschr.* **114:**606–609.

125. **Zoschke, D. C., A. A. Skemp, and D. L. Defosse.** 1991. Lymphoproliferative responses to *Borrelia burgdorferi* in Lyme disease. *Ann. Intern. Med.* **114:**285–289.

Treponema and Other Human Host-Associated Spirochetes*

VICTORIA POPE, STEVEN J. NORRIS, AND ROBERT E. JOHNSON

63

TAXONOMY

The genus *Treponema* (order *Spirochaetales*, family *Spirochaetaceae*) includes four invasive human pathogens (Table 1) and a rabbit pathogen, a large number of oral spirochetes found in the gingival crevices in humans and other animals, and a few commensal skin organisms. The ecologic diversity of this genus was revealed recently by the discovery that *Treponema* species are also associated with bovine digital dermatitis, severe virulent ovine foot rot, and the normal gut flora of termites (25, 40, 119). In 1984, the genus taxonomy was restructured so that the species *Treponema pallidum* includes three of the human pathogens: *T. pallidum* subsp. *pallidum* (venereal syphilis), *T. pallidum* subsp. *endemicum* (endemic syphilis), and *T. pallidum* subsp. *pertenue* (yaws) (113). T. *carateum* (pinta) remains a separate species due to the lack of genetic information. The pathogenic treponemes in this group are very closely related, to the extent that they are distinguished primarily by their patterns of pathogenesis in humans and experimentally infected animals. They are morphologically indistinguishable and, where examined, have >95% DNA homology by hybridization (30), a high degree of sequence identity of known genes (84, 85), nearly identical protein profiles (see reference 90 for a review), and shared reactivity with monoclonal antibodies (82). There may be some subspecies differences, as well as differences between *T. pallidum* and *T. paraluiscuniculi*, a rabbit pathogen, in the flanking-region sequences of the 15.5-kDa lipoprotein gene (17). In addition, differences in the *tpr* and *arp* genes have been used for the molecular subtyping of *T. pallidum* strains (18, 19, 98); this approach has been shown to be useful in epidemiologic studies (100, 117). According to structure, host dependence, protein content, and DNA sequence similarities (17), *T. paraluiscuniculi* appears to be closely related to the human pathogens; however, it causes venereal spirochetosis of rabbits and is not known to cause human disease. *Brachyspira aalborgi* and *Brachyspira* (formerly *Serpulina*) *pilosicoli* are recently described human intestinal spirochetes. Because of the distinctive nature of invasive treponemal pathogens, oral spirochetes, and intestinal spirochetes, these three groups are discussed separately below.

In contrast to the close relationship among the human pathogens, *T. pallidum* subsp. *pallidum* has <5% DNA homology by hybridization with other spirochetes such as *T. phagedenis*, *T. refringens*, and *B. hyodysenteriae* (30). However, 16S rRNA gene sequence similarities indicate an evolutionary relationship between the members of the genus *Treponema* (93). The sequence of the 1.13×10^6-bp *T. pallidum* subsp. *pallidum* Nichols genome was published in 1998 (36), and sequencing of the 2.8×10^6-bp *T. denticola* genome was published in 2004 (112). Although the *T. denticola* genome is much larger, the predicted gene content indicates that both organisms have very limited metabolic capabilities; for example, energy production appears to be limited to glycolysis, and the pathways for synthesis of fatty acids and most amino acids are absent. Many of the additional genes in *T. denticola* are transport systems and degradative proteinases and hydrolases, consistent with a high scavenging activity for acquiring nutrients in the dense biofilm of dental plaque (36, 112).

SPIROCHETES ASSOCIATED WITH HUMAN TREPONEMATOSES

Description

T. pallidum subsp. *pallidum* (*T. pallidum*) and related human pathogens are spirochetes ~0.18 μm in diameter and ranging in length from 6 to 20 μm (Fig. 1). These organisms are coiled into regular helices (6 to 14 per cell) with a wavelength of 1.1 μm and an amplitude of ~0.3 μm (Fig. 1). The ends are pointed and lack the hook shape characteristic of some commensal human spirochetes. Suspensions of *T. pallidum* are best visualized by dark-field microscopy, although the bacterium can also be seen by phase-contrast microscopy. Unstained organisms are not visible by standard bright-field microscopy because of the small cell diameter. Fresh preparations of the organism exhibit rapid rotation about the axis (the characteristic corkscrew motility) due to the action of flagella inserted in both ends and extending down the cell body within the periplasmic space (Fig. 1). Flexing and reversal of rotation can occur also, but translational motion is not observed unless *T. pallidum* is in a viscous medium. The human treponemal pathogens (Table 1) cannot be distinguished at either the light or electron microscopy level. Because the diameter of the treponemes is less than 1 μm, Gram stain cannot be used to visualize any of the pathogenic *Treponema*.

*This chapter contains information presented in chapter 61 by Steven J. Norris, Victoria Pope, Robert E. Johnson, and Sandra A. Larsen in the eighth edition of this Manual.

TABLE 1 Characteristics of the human treponematoses[a]

Organism	Disease	Distribution	Predominant age of onset	Transmission	Congenital infection
T. pallidum subsp. *pallidum*	Venereal syphilis	Worldwide	Adolescents, adults	Sexual contact	Yes
T. pallidum subsp. *pertenue*	Yaws (frambesia, pian)	Tropical areas, Africa, South America, Caribbean, Indonesia	Children	Skin contact	No
T. pallidum subsp. *endemicum*	Endemic syphilis (bejel, dichuchwa)	Arid areas, Africa, Middle East	Children to adults	Mucous membrane	Rarely
T. carateum	Pinta (carate, cute)	Semi-arid, warm areas, Central and South America	Children, adolescents	Skin contact	No

[a] Data from references 2, 28, 29, 95, and 122.

Natural Habitat

The *T. pallidum* subspecies and *T. carateum* are obligate parasites of humans and are not known to have any animal or environmental reservoirs. Venereal syphilis has a worldwide distribution, with the incidence varying widely according to geographic location and socioeconomic groups (Table 1). Endemic syphilis is restricted to desert and temperate regions of North Africa and the Middle East. Yaws occurs most commonly in tropical or desert regions of Africa, South America, and Indonesia. Pinta is found primarily in tropical areas of Central and South America.

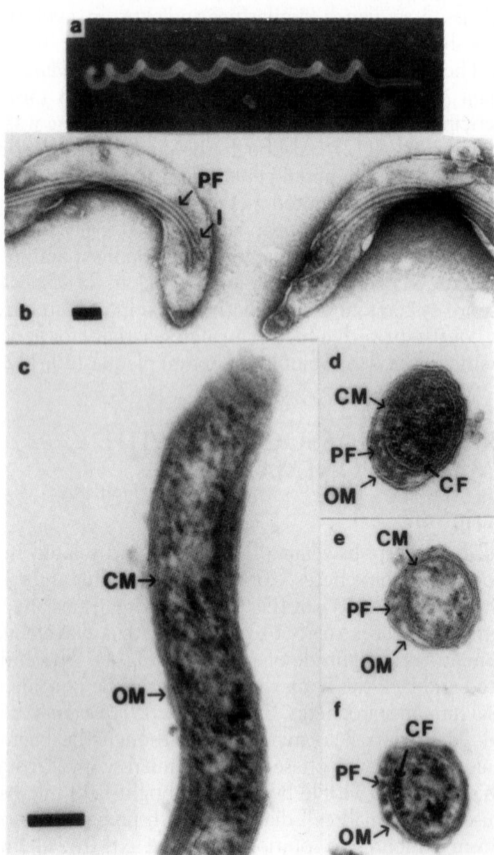

FIGURE 1 Morphology of *T. pallidum*. (a) Scanning electron micrograph showing spiral shape. (b) Negatively stained view of the tips of two organisms. Note the insertion points (I) of periplasmic flagella (PF) near the ends. (c to f) Electron micrographs of ultrathin sections, showing the outer membrane (OM), the cytoplasmic membrane (CM), periplasmic flagella (PF), and the location of the cytoplasmic filaments (CF). Bars, 0.1 μm. Reprinted from reference 88 with permission of Springer NL.

Clinical Significance

Syphilis is still a common sexually transmitted disease in many areas of the world, despite the availability of effective therapy. In 1999, the World Health Organization (WHO) estimated that the worldwide annual incidence of sexually acquired syphilis was 12 million cases (125). In the United States, 34,270 cases were reported in 2003, including 7,177 cases of primary and secondary syphilis and 413 cases of congenital syphilis in infants younger than 1 year. Rates of reported syphilis cases declined rapidly during the 1990s (Fig. 2), but transmission has persisted in certain areas, especially the Southeastern United States. In 1999, to address the increasingly focused occurrence of syphilis, the U.S. Centers for Disease Control and Prevention (CDC), in collaboration with other federal partners, launched "The National Plan to Eliminate Syphilis in the United States" using a combination of improved surveillance, strengthened community involvement, rapid outbreak response, expanded clinical and laboratory services, and enhanced health promotion (http://www.cdc.gov/stopsyphilis/Plan.pdf). The year 2010 target is 0.2 cases of primary and secondary syphilis per 100,000 population, whereas there were 2.5 cases per 100,000 population in 2003.

The male/female ratio of case rates increased from 1.6 in 1999 to 5.3 in 2003 (16). This increase in the rate of primary and secondary cases among men relative to women in the United States, along with reports from localities of outbreaks of syphilis and of high-risk sexual behavior among men who have sex with men (MSM) (24, 94), reflects an increase in sexually transmitted disease (STD) risk behavior among some MSM. Of particular concern is the high prevalence of human immunodeficiency virus (HIV) infection among syphilis cases reported in these outbreak reports and summarized in recent reviews (8, 20). Because of the increase in syphilis among MSM and because the evidence is strong that syphilis increases susceptibility to HIV infection and transmissibility of HIV infection (11, 35), federal agencies and medical organizations representing HIV care providers recommend screening for syphilis and other sexually transmitted infections among MSM (1, 13, 16).

The prevalence of nonvenereal treponematoses is uncertain due to inadequate surveillance, but in 1998 the WHO

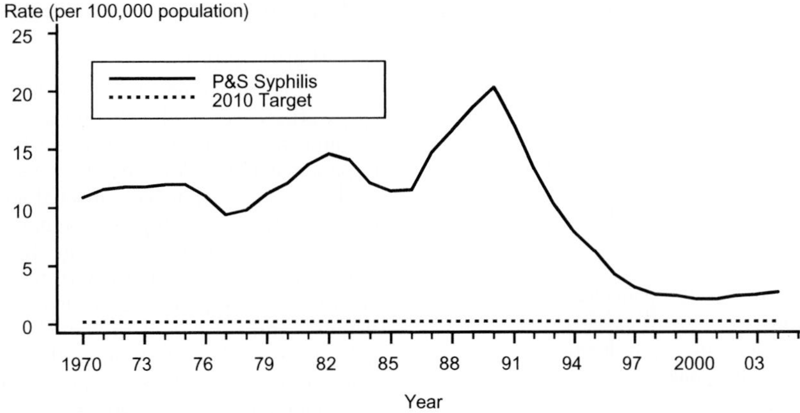

FIGURE 2 Rates of reported primary and secondary syphilis cases per 100,000 population in the United States, 1970 to 2004. The objective of ≤0.2 cases per 100,000 by the year 2010 is indicated (16).

estimated that there were 2.6 million active cases worldwide and 460,000 new cases per year (124).

Transmission of *T. pallidum* occurs through direct contact with active lesions. The transmission of *T. pallidum* subsp. *pallidum* infection, the cause of venereal syphilis, usually occurs consequent to contact of an uninfected individual with the anogenital lesions of an infected individual during sexual intercourse. Transplacental infection of the fetus also occurs in infected pregnant women.

Venereal syphilis exhibits a wide variety of clinical manifestations (Table 2). Early syphilis, defined as syphilis of <1-year duration, is itself subdivided into primary, secondary, and early latent stages. The primary stage is characterized by the appearance of one or more 0.3- to 2.0-cm indurated lesions, called chancres, which typically become encrusted or ulcerated. The lesions occur at the point of organism entry after a 10- to 90-day incubation period. The most common characteristic of secondary syphilis is the presence of skin and mucous membrane lesions. Skin lesions may be macular, papular, follicular, papulosquamous, or pustular. So-called "nickel and dime" macular lesions on the palms of the hands, soles of the feet, and other locations are a common presentation. Raised lesions called condylomata lata may occur in moist intertriginous areas, and erosions called mucous patches may appear on mucosa, such as in the mouth. Neurologic symptoms and signs can also occur during secondary-stage syphilis, and, less commonly, disease manifestations involving other organ systems. Secondary syphilis manifestations do not appear until 6 weeks to 6 months after infection. Primary and secondary syphilis manifestations may overlap, but each resolves spontaneously within a few weeks of its onset.

Numerous treponemes are often present in the ulcers of primary syphilis and the moist intertriginous and mucosal lesions of secondary syphilis. Transmission occurs as a consequence of contact with these primary- and secondary-stage lesions. Nonvenereal transmission is rare. Individuals with venereal syphilis are no longer infectious after healing of secondary syphilis lesions. However, relapses of secondary syphilis can occur in about 25% of untreated patients during the first year of infection (38).

Approximately one-third of untreated patients may develop tertiary or late syphilis following an extended period (usually years to decades) of latency during which clinical symptoms of syphilis are absent (38). The manifestations of late syphilis consist of several characteristic conditions of the central nervous system, disease of the aortic valve and thoracic aorta, and a chronic inflammatory lesion called a gumma, which usually involves the skin or bone but may occur in any organ (122). The cardiovascular and gummatous forms of syphilis are now rarely encountered, presumably because of effective therapy of early syphilis and antimicrobial therapy administered for other infections.

Viable *T. pallidum* is present in the cerebrospinal fluid (CSF) of patients with the primary and secondary stages of syphilis, indicating that central nervous system infection occurs very early in the course of disease (104). Neurologic manifestations, including syphilitic meningitis, may occur as early as 3 months postinfection; thus, neurosyphilis should not be considered solely a late manifestation of the disease (48).

Numerous case reports indicate that HIV infection may result in an increased severity of early syphilis and a poor response to therapy (103), although the results of prospective therapy trials suggest that HIV infection does not markedly affect the natural history of syphilis in most instances of coinfection (104, 106).

Congenital syphilis results from the transmission of *T. pallidum* across the placenta during pregnancy. Early congenital syphilis tends to occur when the mother has early syphilis during the course of pregnancy and may result in stillbirth or fulminant infection of the newborn (Table 2). Late manifestations of congenital syphilis are the outcome of chronic, untreated infection and can result in multiple stigmata (Table 2) that are often not obvious until the second decade of life.

Yaws, endemic syphilis, and pinta were common infections in areas of endemicity prior to the WHO eradication program beginning in 1948; in the early 1950s, it was estimated that 200 million people were exposed to yaws during their lifetimes (95). Nowadays, areas where the diseases are endemic are more restricted, but decreased surveillance has led to an increase in the incidence of yaws in many areas (2). Transmission of endemic treponematoses occurs through direct contact with early lesions or with contaminated fingers or drinking or eating utensils. Yaws and endemic syphilis commonly are transmitted among children (2 to 15 years of age), whereas pinta usually has a later onset (ages 15 to 30 years). Many of the manifestations of yaws and endemic syphilis are similar to those of venereal syphilis (Table 2); the lesions of pinta appear to be restricted to the skin. Congenital transmission of the endemic treponematoses is rare.

TABLE 2 Common manifestations of treponematoses

Venereal syphilis (*T. pallidum* subsp. *pallidum*)
- Primary (local): 10 to 90 days postinfection (avg, 21 days)
  - Chancre (single or multiple, skin or mucous membranes)
  - Regional lymphadenopathy
- Secondary (disseminated): 6 wk–6 mo postinfection
  - Multiple secondary lesions (skin or mucous membranes)
  - Generalized lymphadenopathy, fever, malaise
  - Condylomata lata
  - Alopecia
  - Asymptomatic or symptomatic CNS[a] involvement (syphilitic meningitis)
- Latent (early, ≤1-yr duration; late, >1-yr duration)
  - Reactive serologic tests for syphilis
  - Asymptomatic
- Tertiary (late, chronic): months to years postinfection
  - Gummatous (monocytic infiltrates, tissue destruction, any organ)
  - Cardiovascular (aortic aneurysm)
  - Late forms of neurosyphilis (paresis, tabes dorsalis, optic atrophy)
- Congenital
  - Early (onset, <2 years): fulminant, disseminated infection, mucocutaneous lesions, osteochondritis, anemia, hepatosplenomegaly, CNS involvement; may result in stillbirth
  - Late (persistence, >2 years): interstitial keratitis, bone and tooth deformities, cutaneous fissures (rhagades), eighth-nerve deafness, neurosyphilis, other tertiary manifestations

Yaws (*T. pallidum* subsp. *pertenue*)
- Early: onset 9–90 days postinfection (avg, 21 days)
  - Primary lesion (mother yaw): papular, nontender, often pruritic, crusted, or ulcerated
  - Disseminated lesions (daughter yaws): often resemble primary lesion, or varied appearance
  - Malaise, fever, lymphadenopathy
  - Osteitis, periostitis, other bone and joint manifestations
- Latent: positive serologic tests, no other signs of infection
- Late: 10% of patients
  - Destructive lesions of bone and cartilage (e.g., ulcerative rhinopharyngitis)
  - Hyperkeratotic skin lesions

Endemic syphilis (*T. pallidum* subsp. *endemicum*)
- Early
  - Primary: mucosal or cutaneous lesion usually not detected
  - Secondary: multiple oropharyngeal, cutaneous lesions
  - Generalized lymphadenopathy
  - Periostitis
- Latent: positive serologic tests, no other signs of infection
- Late: destructive skin, bone, and cartilage lesions

Pinta (*T. carateum*): restricted to skin
- Early
  - Initial lesion: hyperkeratotic, pigmented papule or plaque
  - Disseminated skin lesions (pintids)
  - Regional lymphadenopathy
- Late: pigmentary changes in skin (hyper- and hypopigmentation)

[a] CNS, central nervous system.

Collection, Transport, and Storage of Specimens

Blood and Serum

When collecting, preparing, and examining specimens, health care workers need to observe universal safety precautions (60). Serum is the specimen of choice for both nontreponemal and treponemal tests. However, the rapid plasma reagin (RPR) card test and toluidine red unheated serum test (TRUST) also may be performed with plasma samples. The technician must check the product insert to be sure that the plasma sample has not been stored for longer than the recommended storage time and that the blood was collected in the specified anticoagulant. Plasma cannot be used in the Venereal Disease Research Laboratory (VDRL) test, since the sample must be heated before testing, and plasma cannot be used in the fluorescent treponemal antibody absorption (FTA-ABS) test but can be used in other treponemal tests for syphilis such as the *Treponema pallidum* particle agglutination (TP-PA) test. Serum or plasma samples that are to be tested at a later date or shipped to another site for testing should be transferred to another properly labeled tube to prevent contamination by hemoglobin, which can interfere with the interpretation of the test results. Serum does not have to be removed from serum separator tubes. If samples are frozen prior to shipping, they should be shipped on dry ice. There is no evidence that shipping at ambient temperature is detrimental to the sample if care has been taken to avoid possible microbial contamination.

When screening for congenital syphilis, the CDC recommends testing of the mother's serum rather than cord blood. Studies comparing the reactivity of the mother's serum, cord blood, and infant's serum found that the maternal sample is the best indicator that a neonate was at risk of infection, followed by neonatal serum, with cord blood being the least reactive (21, 102). Infant's serum is the specimen of choice for the immunoglobulin M (IgM)-specific tests since cord blood specimen can be contaminated by maternal blood.

Blood collected in EDTA can be used for PCR of *T. pallidum*, but the sample must be refrigerated immediately and shipped as soon as possible on ice by overnight carrier to the testing facility if PCR is not done in-house.

CSF

Care must be taken when collecting CSF to ensure that no blood contaminates the samples. Even amounts that are too small to visibly contaminate the CSF may result in a false-positive test for neurosyphilis if the patient has detectable antibodies in the blood. When samples are to be sent to another laboratory for testing in the VDRL-CSF or FTA-ABS CSF test, shipping on ice is preferred but shipping at ambient temperature is acceptable. If CSF is being sent to the testing facility for PCR, the sample must be frozen as soon as possible after collection and shipped on dry ice to maintain the frozen state.

Tissue and Lesion Samples

Specimens collected from the active epidermal and mucosal lesions of primary, secondary, and early congenital syphilis are most useful, because the lesions tend to contain large concentrations of treponemes. The site should be cleansed and gently abraded with sterile gauze and saline until a serous exudate appears. A specimen for dark-field microscopy is collected on a glass slide and covered with a coverslip; a specimen for direct fluorescent antibody for *T. pallidum* (DFA-TP) examination of serous fluids is collected on a slide and then air dried. The specimen should consist of serous fluid free of erythrocytes, other organisms, and tissue debris. Tissue specimens for a modification of the DFA-TP for tissue (DFAT-TP) or immunohistochemistry (IHC) should be from formalin-fixed, paraffin-embedded sections cut 3 μm thick. Several sections should be sent to the testing facility. Detection of *T. pallidum* in tissues or exudates provides a definitive diagnosis of syphilis.

Tissue or ulcer fluid sample specimens for PCR detection of *T. pallidum* DNA should be frozen immediately after collection and shipped on dry ice if the PCR is being done at another laboratory. However, check with the testing laboratory prior to sending the sample to determine what their protocol requires.

Direct Detection of *Treponema pallidum*

General Principles

Treponemes are not readily detectable with common laboratory stains but can be visualized using dark-field microscopy, DFA-TP, or IHC methods (43, 96). Currently, dark-field microscopy and DFA-TP tests are commonly used to detect *T. pallidum* in primary- or secondary-lesion exudates, while the DFAT-TP (60) and IHC are used for tissue sections. Because of the technical challenges of dark-field microscopy, DFA-TP is recommended for all but the most experienced laboratories. PCR has been introduced as a method for detecting *T. pallidum* infection (as described subsequently) but is not widely available at present.

Continuous in vitro culture of *Treponema pallidum* has not been achieved, but limited multiplication of *T. pallidum* subsp. *pallidum* has been obtained over a 10- to 20-day period in a complex tissue culture system (31, 89). Direct culture of *T. pallidum* from clinical specimens has not been accomplished, and this procedure continues to be limited to the research laboratory setting.

Dark-Field Microscopy

Dark-field microscopy (60) is appropriate for samples from genital or skin lesion exudates. When dark-field microscopy is used, the presence of morphologically similar, nonpathogenic spirochetes within and near the genitalia requires that *T. pallidum* be viewed in its "living state" in order to distinguish its characteristic morphology and motility. It is essential that exudates be examined as soon as possible (ideally within 20 min) to ensure retention of motility. *T. pallidum* is very sensitive to exposure to oxygen, heat, nonphysiologic pH, and desiccation. Wet mounts need to be thoroughly examined using a systematic scan of the entire slide before deciding that a wet mount is negative for treponemes. Because it is difficult or impossible to differentiate *T. pallidum* from other parasitic spirochetes of the gastrointestinal tract by using dark-field microscopy, this method should be used only for genital or skin lesions.

DFA and IHC

Examination of samples from lesions can be done using the DFA-TP test (60). Lesion samples for DFA-TP are air dried onto slides and therefore do not require cell viability or immediate examination. Either labeled polyclonal anti-*T. pallidum* antibody (ViroStat, Portland, Maine) or labeled monoclonal antibody (CDC, Atlanta, Ga.) can be used. Care must be taken in interpretation of the result when polyclonal antibodies are used because they are not specific for pathogenic treponemes. Polyclonal antibodies can be preabsorbed with whole Reiter treponemes prior to use to increase the specificity. Samples for DFA-TP can also be sent to the Syphilis Serology Reference Laboratory at the CDC for testing.

Tissue sections can be stained using either the IHC stain (43, 96) or the DFAT-TP test (60), as the two methods use the same specific antibody for detection. Any tissue can be used, but most frequently tissues for paraffin-embedded sections are collected from the brain, gastrointestinal tract, placenta, umbilical cord (Fig. 3), or skin. Often DFAT-TP or IHC is used to diagnose late-stage or congenital syphilis, although organism concentrations tend to be low during late adult syphilis, in asymptomatic or late congenital syphilis, and in resolving lesions of early syphilis. For tissue, IHC may offer an advantage since a fluorescent microscope is not needed and the counterstain is hematoxylin, which allows tissue structure to be observed simultaneously with the observation of treponemes (43, 96).

PCR

The newest technique for direct detection of *T. pallidum* is PCR (42, 54, 64, 85, 86, 97, 109, 123, 129). PCR as a tool for detecting *T. pallidum* is used by only a few laboratories and is considered an experimental procedure for syphilis diagnosis. However, the PCR test is available at the CDC for patients with suspected neurosyphilis (i.e., reactive serum serology, abnormal CSF or neurologic findings, and a history of syphilis) or for patients with genital ulcer disease. The test also appears useful in detecting congenital syphilis, with sensitivity approaching the "gold standard" of rabbit infectivity testing for amniotic fluid samples (42, 47, 109).

The sample source for PCR is controversial (87). Studies have found whole blood to be a useful sample (58, 68, 117) even for incubating syphilis and latent syphilis (68). Lesion samples are also useful (98, 100, 117) and may be positive for *T. pallidum* by PCR when they are negative by dark-field microscopy or DFA-TP (100). The appropriateness of serum and CSF as sample sources for PCR is still under consideration (87, 123), although CSF has been used to help determine invasion of the central nervous system by *T. pallidum* (104). Contamination with extraneous DNA from other specimens, storage, and transport of the sample prior to testing may seriously affect the results (123).

Methods using PCR and DNA amplification techniques can distinguish various strains of *T. pallidum* subsp. *pallidum* (98). These techniques are being used in some research laboratories to help determine the epidemiology of syphilis outbreaks (100, 117).

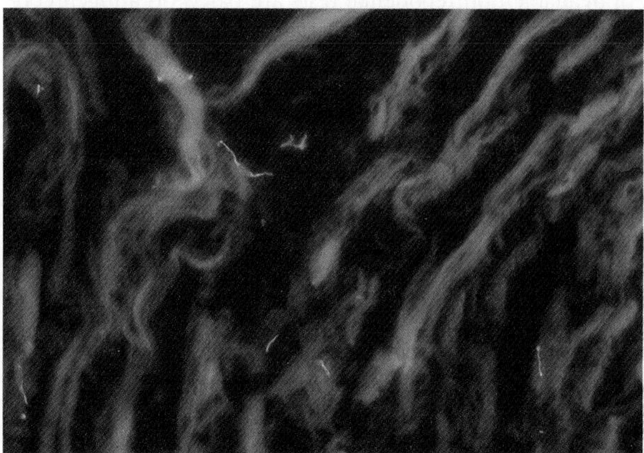

FIGURE 3 DFAT-TP of an umbilical cord section from a baby with congenital syphilis.

Serologic Tests

General Principles

Humoral antibodies produced in response to *T. pallidum* infection become detectable in the primary stage, increase in concentration during the secondary stage, and decline during latent infection. Antibody detection tests supplement the direct organism detection methods used for the diagnosis of primary and secondary syphilis and are the only practical methods of diagnosis during latent and late syphilis.

Serologic tests for syphilis are divided into nontreponemal and treponemal types. Nontreponemal tests detect so-called reaginic antibodies that react with lipoidal particles containing the phospholipid cardiolipin. These tests are commonly used for screening and are widely available, inexpensive, convenient to perform on large numbers of specimens, and useful for determining the efficacy of treatment. Limitations of the nontreponemal serologic tests include a lack of sensitivity in early primary syphilis and in late syphilis and the possibilities of false-positive results or a prozone reaction (false-negative result due to a high ratio of antibody to antigen). Treponemal tests use *T. pallidum* subsp. *pallidum* or its derivatives (e.g., recombinant proteins) as the antigen and detect anti-*T. pallidum* antibodies. In the United States, treponemal tests have been used primarily to verify reactivity in the nontreponemal tests or to confirm a clinical impression of late syphilis in which the nontreponemal test is nonreactive. However, treponemal tests such as the enzyme immunoassay (EIA) are increasingly being used to screen for syphilis. The advantages are lower cost, increased specificity and sensitivity, objective interpretation of results, and hard copies of the results generated by the EIA reader. Rapid treponemal tests, which are available internationally but not in the United States at this time, offer the advantages of specificity and rapid results, usually within 20 min. Although treponemal tests are useful for screening, they cannot be used to monitor treatment or reinfection because 85% of persons successfully treated for syphilis have test results that remain reactive for years, if not for a lifetime. Therefore, a combination of a nontreponemal test with a treponemal test is used to diagnose sexually acquired syphilis. Treponemal tests that detect IgM may be helpful in the diagnosis of congenital syphilis in the neonate. The utility of IgM-based tests to diagnose early adult syphilis or reinfection has not been fully evaluated.

Nontreponemal Tests

All available nontreponemal tests are based on antigen containing measured amounts of cardiolipin, cholesterol, and sufficient purified lecithin to produce standard reactivity (61). The nontreponemal (reagin) tests measure IgM and IgG antibodies to cardiolipin and other lipids released from damaged host cells or from treponemes (5, 70). Antilipoidal antibodies can be produced not only as a consequence of treponemal infections but also during autoimmune diseases, pregnancy, nontreponemal diseases of an acute and chronic nature in which tissue damage occurs, and other conditions (Table 3).

The standard nontreponemal tests use flocculation of lipoidal particles (antigen) to indicate reactivity. The test antigen is mixed with the patient's serum on a solid matrix by rotating at a specific speed for a specified number of minutes before reading the results. The antigen-antibody flocculant is too small to visualize without magnification unless a colored reagent (e.g., carbon particles) is added. The VDRL and unheated serum reagin (USR) tests are flocculation tests requiring microscopic examination, whereas reactions in the RPR test and TRUST can be read without magnification, because of the addition of colored particles that get caught in the antigen-antibody lattice. All of the nontreponemal tests have approximately the same sensitivity and specificity (Table 4).

TABLE 3 Causes of false-positive reactions in serologic tests for syphilis[a]

Disease or condition	Type of test affected	
	Nontreponemal test	Treponemal test
Autoimmune disease	Yes	Yes
Malaria	Yes	No
Recent immunizations	Yes	No
Dermatologic diseases	Yes	Yes
Cardiovascular disease	Yes	Yes
Tuberculosis	Yes	No
Leprosy	Yes	Yes
Intravenous drug abuse	Yes	No
Viral infections	Yes	No
Febrile illness	Yes	Yes
Pregnancy	Yes	No
HIV	Yes	No
Other STDs	Yes	No
Age	No	Yes
Multiple blood transfusions	Yes	No
Lyme disease	No	Yes
Endemic treponematoses	Yes	Yes
Transient unknown causes	Yes	Yes
Technical errors	Yes	Yes

[a] Data from references 7, 50, 61, and 66.

Any of these nontreponemal tests can be performed as a quantitative test by preparing serial twofold dilutions of the patient's serum to reach an endpoint titer. Qualitative nontreponemal tests are used to screen for possible syphilitic infection. Quantitative nontreponemal tests establish a baseline of reactivity from which change can be measured following treatment. The baseline serum sample should be drawn on the day that treatment is begun, and the same test that is used in the initial testing should be used to monitor treatment (32, 33, 34, 111). If early syphilis has been adequately treated, titers are usually nondetectable after 3 years.

The VDRL-CSF test is a modification of the VDRL test that permits detection and titer determination of reaginic antibody in CSF. Preparation of the antigen and the patient specimen differs from that of the serum VDRL test, so care should be taken to follow the appropriate procedures (60). The VDRL-CSF test is the only nontreponemal test standardized for use with CSF specimens.

Treponemal Tests

The greatest value of the treponemal tests is in distinguishing true- and false-positive nontreponemal test results and in establishing the diagnosis of late latent or late syphilis. Problems arise when these tests are used as screening procedures, because treponemal tests generally remain reactive for life following adequate treatment for syphilis and about 1% of the general population has false-positive results unrelated to past syphilis treatment. However, a reactive treponemal test result on a sample that is also reactive in a nontreponemal test is highly specific for treponemal infection. The most commonly used treponemal tests in the United States are the

TABLE 4 Sensitivity and specificity of serologic tests for syphilis

Stage	Sensitivity (%)[a]				Specificity (%) (nonsyphilis)
	Primary	Secondary	Latent	Late	
Nontreponemal tests					
VDRL	78 (74–87)	100	95 (88–100)	71 (37–94)	98 (96–99)
RPR card	86 (77–100)	100	98 (95–100)	73	98 (93–99)
USR	80 (72–88)	100	95 (88–100)		99
TRUST	85 (77–86)	100	98 (95–100)		99 (98–99)
Treponemal tests					
FTA-ABS	84 (70–100)	100	100	96	97 (94–100)
FTA-ABS DS	80 (69–90)	100	100		98 (97–100)
TP-PA	88 (86–100)	100	100		96 (95–100)
IgG EIA	92 (88–97)[b]	100	99 (96–100)	100	99 (98–100)

[a] Ranges of CDC studies are given in parentheses.
[b] Ranges of various studies.

TP-PA and the EIA tests. The number of laboratories that provide the FTA-ABS test is dwindling due to the technical difficulties of performing the test, the complexity of the test, and the lack of laboratory personnel experienced in fluorescence microscopy. As a result, the test is not discussed here, but Larsen et al. (60) give a description of the procedure.

If used appropriately as confirmatory tests, the treponemal tests have few limitations. They vary in their sensitivity for the detection of early primary syphilis and in the late stages of syphilis (Table 4). A treponemal test result should be obtained if late or late latent syphilis is suspected and the nontreponemal test result is nonreactive. The laboratory should be informed that late syphilis is suspected; otherwise, according to laboratory policy, a treponemal test may not be performed when the nontreponemal test result is nonreactive. Treponemal tests are generally 100% reactive in secondary and latent syphilis. Again, these findings should be interpreted in the light of treatment history.

TP-PA Test

The *Treponema pallidum* particle agglutination (TP-PA) test (Fujirebio Diagnostics, Inc., Malvern, Pa.) (60) has replaced the microhemagglutination assay for antibodies to *Treponema pallidum*. Instead of erythrocytes, the test uses gelatin particles sensitized with *T. pallidum* subsp. *pallidum* antigens. There is no separate absorbing step; therefore, the test is simpler to set up and requires less preparation time. The serum sample is diluted in the microtiter plate. Sensitized gelatin particles are added to the 1:40 serum dilution, making a final serum dilution of 1:80. Anti-*T. pallidum* antibodies in the serum react with the sensitized particles, forming a mat of agglutinated particles in the microtiter plate. Unsensitized particles, included as a control for nonspecific reactivity, are added to the 1:20 serum dilution (final dilution, 1:40).

Results are reported as reactive, nonreactive, or inconclusive. Reactive results are reported for a range of agglutination patterns, from a definite large ring with a rough multiform outer margin and peripheral agglutination (1+) to a smooth mat of agglutinated particles covering the entire bottom of the well (4+). Nonreactive results are reported when a definite compact button, with or without a very small hole in its center, forms in the center of the well. A button of unagglutinated particles having a small hole in the center is initially read as "±," and the test should be repeated. If the same pattern is again observed, then the report should be "nonreactive." Because the TP-PA test uses gelatin particles rather than sheep erythrocytes, which were used as the antigen carrier in the microhemagglutination assay for antibodies to *T. pallidum*, nonspecific agglutination of the unsensitized particles only rarely occurs. The sources for error with the TP-PA are usually associated with the use of dusty or improper plates, pipetting errors, or vibrations in the laboratory.

Enzyme Immunoassay

Several tests using the EIA format have been developed for the diagnosis of syphilis. In the United States the Captia Syphilis-G test (Trinity Biotech, Dublin, Ireland; BioRad, Richmond, Calif.; and Wampole Laboratories, Princeton, N.J.) (60, 62, 81, 110) has been cleared by the Food and Drug Administration (FDA) for use as either a confirmatory test or a screening test, while the Trep-Chek test (Phoenix Bio-Tech Corp., Mississauga, Ontario, Canada; and Sigma Chemical Company, St. Louis, Mo.) has been cleared by the FDA for use as a confirmatory test for syphilis. Initial evaluations of these EIA tests have found all to have sensitivities and specificities similar to those of the other treponemal tests (62, 81, 99, 127) (Table 4). A comparison of nine EIAs using either *T. pallidum* sonicates or recombinant antigens revealed that several EIAs had sensitivities similar to that of the IgM FTA-ABS test in the analysis of primary syphilis specimens (110). The actual procedures of the tests are very similar. An aliquot of diluted patient sample is added to a well in the plate. After an incubation period, the plate is washed and an enzyme-labeled conjugate is added. After a second incubation and wash, a substrate is added. The presence of antitreponemal antibodies is indicated by a color change that can be read spectrophotometrically or visually. Obtaining results from a spectrophotometric microplate reader has the advantages of objective interpretation and a printout of the results.

The Captia Syphilis-M test (Trinity Biotech, BioRad, and Wampole Laboratories) and the Trep-Chek M test (Phoenix Bio-Tech) are based on the use of anti-human IgM antibody to capture IgM in the patient's serum, followed by the use of a purified *T. pallidum* antigen to detect IgM anti-*T. pallidum* antibodies in the patient's serum (51). The IgM EIA is most useful in the diagnosis of congenital syphilis. One study found that the IgM capture EIA was more sensitive than the FTA-ABS 19S IgM test in detecting probable cases of congenital syphilis (116). Another study found the IgM EIA to be equal in sensitivity to the IgM Western blot for the detection of neonatal congenital syphilis but less sensitive in delayed-onset congenital syphilis (9). The usefulness of the IgM EIA tests in adult onset syphilis has not been fully determined.

Another EIA test format being increasingly used is the Western blot for *T. pallidum* (12, 37, 60, 67). This test is performed as an experimental test in several laboratories in the United States. However, the MarBlot test (Trinity Biotech) is available outside the United States. The test uses IgG conjugate and appears to be at least as sensitive and specific as the FTA-ABS tests, and efforts have been made to standardize the procedure (37). To date, many investigators agree that the detection of antibodies to the immunodeterminants of 15.5, 17, 44.5, and 47 kDa appears to be diagnostic for acquired syphilis (90). The Western blot for *T. pallidum* has value as a diagnostic test for congenital syphilis, when an IgM-specific conjugate is used (9, 27, 63, 108, 109). The IgM Western blot for congenital syphilis appears to have greater specificity and sensitivity than the IgM EIA.

Rapid Tests

A number of rapid tests are currently on the market outside the United States, with more under development. The tests currently available in rapid-test format are treponemal tests. These tests have several advantages over currently used treponemal tests. They can all be performed within 30 min, some can use whole blood, including finger-stick specimens, as the sample, and no specialized equipment is necessary. Most of the tests on the market use a lateral-flow immunochromatographic strip methodology and follow a similar format. A nitrocellulose strip has a small filter pad at each end. One pad contains the anti-Ig antibodies, antibodies against the control strip, and an indicator such as colloidal gold. The second pad at the opposite end serves to help draw the sample through the strip. The sample (serum, plasma, or whole blood) is placed on the end of the strip that contains the antibodies and conjugate. For some tests, a buffer is added to aid in the migration of the sample up the strip. After a specified time, usually 15 to 30 min, the reaction has taken place. If two lines are present, the sample is considered positive or reactive. If only the control line is visible, the sample in nonreactive. If the control line is not visible, the results are invalid and the test needs to be repeated.

Most rapid tests have not been evaluated in studies published in peer-reviewed journals. The WHO is undertaking an evaluation of selected rapid syphilis tests to encourage the use of tests with acceptable performance in resource-poor settings. Results of the initial laboratory-based WHO evaluation of six rapid tests can be viewed at http://www.who.int/std_diagnostics. In this study, the range of reported sensitivity when using serum samples was 93.6 to 98.4% and specificity was 92.5 to 97.3%.

Interpretation and Reporting of Results

Qualitative results for the microscopic tests (the VDRL test and USR test) are reported as reactive, weakly reactive, or nonreactive. Qualitative results for the macroscopic tests (the RPR card test and TRUST) are reported as reactive (regardless of the degree of reactivity) or nonreactive. Quantitative results may be reported as the reciprocal of the dilution, for example, 4 dils, a titer of 4, or R4 rather than a 1:4 dilution. The endpoint reported is the last dilution giving a fully reactive, not weakly reactive, result. Titers for the same serum specimen may differ two- to fourfold when tested using microscopic versus macroscopic nontreponemal tests, due in part to the exclusion of weakly reactive results in the titer determination for the VDRL and USR tests. This variability underscores the need to use the same test in monitoring treatment efficacy in each patient.

Prozone reactions occur in 1 to 2% of patients with secondary syphilis, due to the high levels of antibodies. Any undiluted serum sample exhibiting a weakly reactive, atypical, or, on rare occasions, "rough negative" reaction should be diluted as in the quantitative assay. In samples exhibiting a prozone effect, reactivity increases and then decreases as the endpoint titer is approached.

Nontreponemal test results must be interpreted according to the stage of syphilis suspected as well as the population being tested and should be confirmed using a treponemal test, since the proportion of positive screening tests that are false positive increases with decreasing prevalence of syphilis. Approximately 30% of those with early primary syphilis have nonreactive nontreponemal test results on the initial visit (Table 4). In secondary syphilis, nearly all patients have nontreponemal test endpoint titers of $\geq$8. For patients with atypical lesions and/or nontreponemal test titers of $<$8, the nontreponemal tests should be repeated and a confirmatory treponemal test should be performed. Even without treatment, the nontreponemal test may be weakly reactive or even nonreactive in the late stages of syphilis.

In congenital syphilis, a paradigm commonly used in the past was that the infant was infected with *T. pallidum* if the infant's nontreponemal test titer at delivery was higher than the mother's titer. However, a lower titer in the infant's serum than in the mother's does not rule out congenital syphilis. Examination of serum sample pairs from mothers and infants with congenital syphilis indicated that only 22% of the infants had a titer higher than that of the mother (116). Passively transferred IgG antibodies reactive in nontreponemal or treponemal tests should be catabolized and undetectable among noninfected infants between the ages of 12 and 18 months.

In any form of syphilis, patients should be monitored to ensure that treatment is effective, i.e., that signs and symptoms have resolved, and that the titer of the quantitative nontreponemal test has declined fourfold, which indicates cure (32, 34, 111). A rise in titer following treatment establishes treatment failure or reinfection. For most patients treated in early syphilis, the titers decline until little or no reaction is detected after 3 years (32, 60, 61, 105). Patients who are treated in the latent or late stage and patients who have had multiple episodes of syphilis may show a more gradual decline in titer (33, 104). A low titer persists in approximately 50% of these patients after 2 years (33). As far as can be determined, this persistent seropositivity does not signify treatment failure or reinfection, and these patients are likely to remain serofast even if they are retreated (33). Recent studies indicate that HIV infection may delay the decline in antibody titer detected by nontreponemal tests for syphilis in patients with primary or secondary syphilis (104). The prognostic significance of this finding is unknown, since only 1 of 101 HIV-positive patients experienced clinical treatment failure during a 1-year posttreatment observation period. A delayed decline in antibody titer was not associated with detection of *T. pallidum* in CSF, and enhanced therapy did not appear to prevent the delay (104).

Diagnostic Criteria for Venereal Syphilis

For the laboratory diagnosis of syphilis, each stage has a particular testing requirement (Table 5) (14). In the United States, the traditional testing scheme is direct microscopic examination of lesion exudates, if present, followed by a

TABLE 5 Criteria for diagnosis of syphilis[a]

- Early syphilis
  - Primary
    - Confirmed (requires 1 *and* 2)
      1. One or more chancres (ulcers)
      2. Direct microscopic identification of *T. pallidum* in clinical specimens (dark field or DFA-TP)
    - Probable (requires 1 *and* either 2 or 3)
      1. A clinically compatible case with one or more chancres
      2. Reactive nontreponemal test and no previous history of syphilis
      3. For persons with a history of syphilis, a fourfold increase in titer on a quantitative nontreponemal test when results of past tests are compared with the most recent test results.
  - Secondary
    - Confirmed
      - Direct microscopic identification of *T. pallidum* in clinical specimens (dark field or DFA-TP)
    - Probable (requires 1 *and* either 2 or 3)
      1. Skin or mucous membrane lesions typical of secondary syphilis
         - a. Macular, papular, follicular, papulosquamous, or pustular
         - b. Condylomata lata (anogenital region or mouth)
         - c. Mucous patches (oropharynx or cervix)
      2. Reactive nontreponemal test titer of ≥4 and no history of syphilis
      3. For persons with a history of syphilis, a fourfold increase in the most recent nontreponemal test titer when compared with previous test results.
  - Early latent
    - Probable (requires 1 *and* either 2 or 3 *and* 4, 5, or 6)
      1. Absence of signs and symptoms of syphilis
      2. No past diagnosis of syphilis and reactive nontreponemal and treponemal test results
      3. A history of syphilis therapy and a current nontreponemal test titer demonstrating fourfold or greater increase from the last nontreponemal test titer (obtained ≤1 yr ago)
      4. A history of symptoms consistent with primary or secondary syphilis during the previous 12 mo
      5. A history of sexual exposure to a partner who had confirmed or probable early syphilis (documented independently as duration of ≤1 yr)
      6. Documented seroconversion or fourfold or greater increase in titer of a nontreponemal test during the previous 12 mo

- Late latent or latent of unknown duration
  - Probable (requires 1 *and* either 2 or 3 *and* 4)
    1. Absence of signs and symptoms
    2. No past diagnosis of syphilis and reactive nontreponemal and treponemal test results; if a reactive treponemal screening test is followed by a nonreactive nontreponemal test, a second, different treponemal test is also reactive.
    3. A history of syphilis therapy and a current nontreponemal test titer demonstrating fourfold or greater increase from the last nontreponemal test titer (obtained >1 yr ago)
    4. No evidence of having acquired the disease within the preceding 12 mo

- Late syphilis
  - Benign (gummatous) and cardiovascular
    - Confirmed (requires 1 *and* 2)
      1. Clinically compatible case
      2. Observation by direct microscopic examination of treponemes in tissue sections by DFAT-TP or detection by other methods (e.g., PCR)
    - Probable (requires 1, 2, *and* 3)
      1. Clinically compatible case
      2. A reactive serum treponemal test
      3. No known history of treatment for syphilis
  - Neurosyphilis
    - Confirmed (requires 1, 2, *and* either 3 or 4)
      1. Clinical signs consistent with neurosyphilis
      2. A reactive serum treponemal test
      3. A reactive VDRL-CSF on a spinal fluid sample
      4. Identification of *T. pallidum* in CSF or tissue by microscopic examination or equivalent methods
    - Probable (requires 1, 2, *and* 3)
      1. Clinical signs consistent with neurosyphilis
      2. A reactive serum treponemal test
      3. Elevated CSF protein or leukocyte count in the absence of other known causes

- Neonatal congenital syphilis
  - Confirmed (requires 1 *and* 2)
    1. Clinically compatible case
    2. Demonstration of *T. pallidum* by direct microscopic examination of specimens from lesions, placenta, umbilical cord, nasal discharge, or autopsy material
  - Probable (requires 1, 2, *and* 3)
    1. Infant born to a mother who had untreated or inadequately[b] treated syphilis at delivery, regardless of findings in the infant
    2. An infant with a reactive treponemal test result
    3. One of the following additional criteria:
       - a. Clinical sign or symptom of congenital syphilis on physical examination
       - b. Abnormal CSF finding without other cause
       - c. Reactive VDRL-CSF test result
       - d. Reactive IgM antibody test specific for syphilis
  - Syphilitic stillbirth
    1. A fetal death that occurs after a 20-week gestation or in which the fetus weighs >500 g
    2. Mother had untreated or inadequately[b] treated syphilis at delivery

[a] Adapted from reference 14.
[b] Nonpenicillin therapy or penicillin given less than 30 days before delivery.

nontreponemal test which, if reactive, is confirmed with a treponemal test (Fig. 4). In recent years, EIAs have been used for screening followed by an RPR or other nontreponemal test. This approach may eliminate many false-positive reactions due to nonspecific nontreponemal test reactivity (Table 3); however, as the rates of syphilis decline, there will be an increasing proportion of reactive results from persons with previously treated syphilis or with false-positive treponemal test results. In addition, the low sensitivity of nontreponemal tests in detecting long-duration infection is an important disadvantage to their use as confirmatory tests. The use of modified serologic screening procedures for syphilis requires careful consideration of the sensitivity and specificity of both the screening and confirmatory steps, as well as the population being tested.

There has been no reliable test for detecting incubating syphilis. However, PCR for the detection of *T. pallidum* DNA may be of some value. There is evidence that DNA can be detected in the blood of persons with incubating syphilis (68) or early syphilis, including the early latent stage (68, 117).

During the primary stage of syphilis, dark-field microscopy and the DFA-TP test (60) are the methods of choice for definitive diagnosis. DFA-TP should be used for specimens from perirectal or oral ulcers because of the inability to distinguish digestive system spirochetes from *T. pallidum* by dark-field microscopy. If the chancre is starting to heal or the patient has used either topical or systemic antibiotics, the number of treponemes may be too small to be detected or they may be nonmotile or degraded. Humoral antibodies, as detected by the current serologic tests for syphilis, usually appear 1 to 4 weeks after the chancre(s) has formed. Thus, a reactive serologic test result may be expected if the chancre is healing. Conversion to reactivity of a serologic test for syphilis or a rise in nontreponemal test titer over 1 to 2 weeks supports a diagnosis of syphilis even if a dark-field or DFA microscopic examination is negative.

By the secondary stage of syphilis, the organism has invaded every organ of the body and virtually all body fluids. All serologic tests for syphilis are usually reactive, and treponemes may be found in moist lesions.

Nontreponemal and treponemal serologic tests are consistently reactive in the early latent stage, but the patient is asymptomatic. Nontreponemal tests may become nonreactive in late latent syphilis. A reactive treponemal test in a patient with a nonreactive nontreponemal test and a history of syphilis should be confirmed by a different treponemal test. A diagnosis of early versus late latent syphilis is made by documentation of onset of infection within or prior to the past year as indicated by (i) seroconversion; (ii) symptoms of primary or secondary syphilis; or (iii) a sex partner documented to have primary, secondary, or early latent syphilis. In the absence of such documentation, the diagnosis is "latent syphilis of unknown duration."

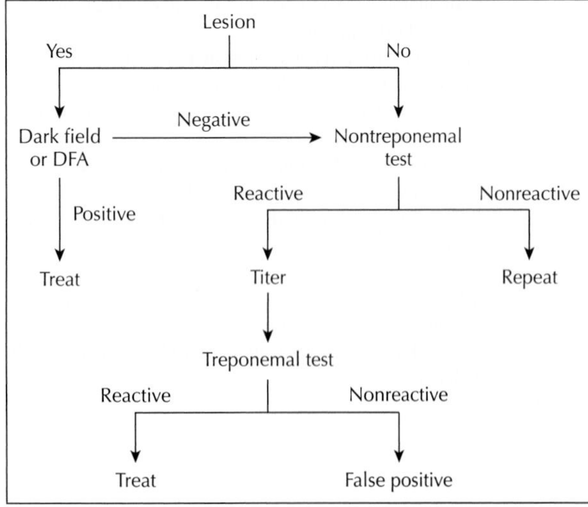

FIGURE 4 Routine screening scheme for early syphilis in the United States.

Neurosyphilis may take many forms (48). Syphilitic meningitis typically occurs during early syphilis. Meningovascular syphilis most often occurs earlier (4 to 7 years) than the classic forms of late neurosyphilis (paresis and tabes dorsalis) (48). The diagnosis of neurosyphilis is based on a combination of clinical and laboratory test criteria (Table 5). CSF examination should include the VDRL-CSF slide test and total protein and leukocyte counts. The VDRL-CSF test is considered to have high specificity but low sensitivity for neurosyphilis (48). Thus, a nonreactive VDRL-CSF test result does not rule out neurosyphilis. The FTA-ABS CSF test appears to have high sensitivity but low specificity for neurosyphilis (52). The FTA-ABS CSF test could be used to rule out neurosyphilis, especially among HIV-infected individuals who commonly have modestly elevated CSF protein and leukocyte counts in the absence of syphilis infection (69). The utility of the EIA or TP-PA in diagnosing neurosyphilis has not been adequately determined, although preliminary evaluations indicate that TP-PA may also be useful. Large-scale studies need to be carried out and the results published before any recommendations can be made. Whether CSF examination is indicated in early syphilis, especially for patients with HIV coinfection, has been controversial. CSF abnormalities and *T. pallidum* can be detected in the CSF of a substantial minority of patients with secondary syphilis (69, 104), but most such patients resolve their CSF abnormalities and appear to clear the CSF of organisms with standard therapy. A relationship between CSF abnormalities or detection of treponemes in the CSF of patients with early syphilis and the development of clinically evident neurosyphilis through enhanced therapy has not been established (69, 80, 104). Thus, routine CSF examination is not considered necessary during early syphilis in the absence of neurologic or ophthalmologic signs or for HIV-infected patients with late latent syphilis or syphilis of unknown duration (15). A nontreponemal serologic test titer of $\geq$32 or, among HIV-infected patients, a CD4 count of $\leq$350 has been associated with an increased frequency of CSF abnormalities in patients with late latent syphilis or syphilis of unknown duration (69), and some experts recommend CSF examination for this group of patients (15).

Late or tertiary syphilis is a chronic, progressive disease, and symptoms may not be evident until 10 to 20 years after the initial infection. Although rare, earlier onset of late or tertiary syphilis has been reported for individuals coinfected with HIV (55). Approximately 71% of patients with late-stage syphilis have reactive nontreponemal tests; however, treponemal tests are almost always reactive and may be the only basis for diagnosis (Table 5). Benign (gummatous) syphilis consists of granuloma-like lesions (gummas) containing lymphocytes and macrophages but few if any detectable spirochetes. Diagnosis of cardiovascular syphilis is made on the basis of findings that indicate aortic insufficiency or thoracic aortic aneurysm, reactive treponemal test results, and no known history of treatment of syphilis. Late forms of neurosyphilis include paresis (infection of the brain parenchyma, resulting in behavioral changes including psychoses), tabes dorsalis (ataxia, paresthesias, and other manifestations resulting from posterior spinal cord and dorsal root ganglia degeneration), and optic atrophy (122).

The choice and interpretation of serologic tests for the diagnosis of syphilis are the same for HIV-infected and uninfected patients, but additional considerations apply to HIV-infected individuals (39, 53, 80, 104). The titers of nontreponemal serologic test results may be higher for patients coinfected with HIV than for those without coexistent HIV infection. The number of primary chancres may be increased (106), and case reports indicate that the course of *T. pallidum* infection may be more rapid and more virulent in a small proportion of HIV-infected individuals. Also, patients with advanced HIV immunodeficiency may become falsely seronegative for syphilis (41, 46).

Diagnostic Criteria for Congenital Syphilis

A primary stage does not occur in congenital syphilis, because the organisms directly enter the fetal circulation (128). Treponemes or the effects thereof are detectable in almost every tissue of the infant. Currently, the diagnosis of neonatal congenital syphilis depends on a combination of results from physical, radiographic, serologic, and direct microscopic examinations as well as maternal clinical history (Table 5). Clinical signs of early congenital syphilis include hepatosplenomegaly, cutaneous lesions, osteochondritis, and snuffles (nasal discharge containing large numbers of *T. pallidum*) (56, 122). Roughly one-half of live-born neonates with congenital syphilis have normal physical findings at the time of birth. If the infant is not treated, other stigmata that may develop later in life include tooth and bone malformations, deafness, blindness, and learning disabilities (Table 2).

Definitive diagnosis is based on the identification of spirochetes in tissues, lesion exudates, or secretions by dark-field examination, DFA-TP, PCR, or other means (Table 5). The standard serologic tests for syphilis, which detect reactive IgG as well as other isotypes, may reflect antibodies passively transferred from the mother to the infant rather than IgM antibodies produced by an infected fetus during gestation. IgM-specific treponemal antibody tests are available and may be useful in the diagnosis of congenital syphilis (see "Serologic Tests" above). In stillbirths, diagnosis of congenital syphilis is made by detection of the treponemes in the tissues (101).

Diagnostic Criteria for Endemic Treponematoses

Serologic tests for syphilis are uniformly reactive with yaws, pinta, and nonvenereal endemic syphilis (bejel) (6, 83, 95). Therefore, patient history, the clinical appearance and anatomic locations of the lesions, the mode of transmission, and the age of the individual are the only criteria that can be used to diagnose these infections as separate entities (6) (Table 1). PCR may be useful in distinguishing these infections in a research setting (17).

Yaws, pinta, and nonvenereal syphilis are often contracted during childhood, but the nontreponemal test titers in affected individuals may remain reactive in adulthood, presenting a dilemma in the diagnosis of subsequent cases of venereal syphilis. Adults from geographic regions in which endemic treponematoses were virtually eliminated by mass campaigns in the 1950s and 1960s would be expected to have nontreponemal test titers of <8 (3). Therefore, any titer of ≥8 for adults from these regions is probably indicative of venereal syphilis. Likewise, titers of ≥8 for children indicate a possible resurgence of yaws in the populations of these areas (2).

Treatment and Antimicrobial Susceptibilities

The CDC has published recommendations for the treatment of syphilis (15) based, in part, on detailed reviews of the literature (4, 103). Routine antimicrobial susceptibility testing of *T. pallidum* is not practical due to the lack of a suitable in vitro culture system, although a number of methods have been applied to the determination of antibiotic sensitivity in the research laboratory (88). *T. pallidum* strains appear to be uniformly susceptible to penicillin and other β-lactams. Penicillin regimens have been the mainstay of syphilis therapy since their introduction in the 1940s. Because treatment with benzathine penicillin as recommended for early syphilis yields low levels of penicillin in the central nervous system, the current recommendations include multiple doses of aqueous or procaine penicillin G for the treatment of neurosyphilis. Ceftriaxone, amoxicillin, and ampicillin are active against *T. pallidum* in vitro and also appear to be effective in the treatment of early syphilis. Ceftriaxone has a long half-life in serum and reaches high levels in the central nervous system. However, multiple doses are required, and there is a 3 to 7% risk of adverse reactions in individuals who are allergic to penicillin; in addition, the data on efficacy in patients are limited. Therefore, the use of ceftriaxone as an alternative therapy for syphilis is recommended only when better-established regimens are contraindicated.

Tetracycline has long been the second-line drug recommended for treatment of syphilis in patients allergic to penicillin. However, the in vitro activity of tetracycline against *T. pallidum* is markedly lower than the activity of penicillin and, in limited comparative trials, treatment failure appears to be more common with tetracycline. Doxycycline has been considered equivalent to tetracycline in recent treatment recommendations. In vitro studies indicate that quinolone compounds have low antimicrobial activity against *T. pallidum* (88).

Azithromycin has been used as a single dose treatment for syphilis contacts in some settings. However, recent findings indicate that a high rate of treatment failures can occur with this regimen (65). The mechanism appears to be a single base pair change in the 23S rRNA genes that confers resistance to erythromycin, azithromycin, and other macrolides (65). This mutation was present in 13, 22, 11, and 88% of clinical specimens from Seattle, San Francisco, Baltimore, and Dublin, Ireland, respectively (65). Therefore, use of macrolides for the treatment of syphilis or syphilis exposure is not recommended.

OTHER HUMAN HOST-ASSOCIATED SPIROCHETES

In addition to *T. pallidum* and related pathogens, a number of anaerobic treponemes and other spirochetes are parasites of humans. These include groups of spirochetes found in the oral cavity (particularly the gingival crevices), in sebaceous secretions in the genital region, and in the colon and rectum (Table 6). In general, these spirochetes are considered commensal organisms. However, there is evidence that spirochetes are involved in gingivitis and periodontal disease and that overgrowth of intestinal spirochetes may correlate with the occurrence of diarrhea or other bowel disorders.

Oral Spirochetes

A variety of spirochetes inhabit supragingival and subgingival plaque in humans; only a small proportion of these have been cultured in vitro and characterized (22, 26, 92). Those that have been cultivated and identified to the species level are within the genus *Treponema* (Table 6). They are spiral-shaped

TABLE 6 Other human host-associated spirochetes

Type	Habitat	Species
Oral spirochetes	Dental plaque in gingival crevices	*Treponema amylovorum* *Treponema denticola* *Treponema lecithinolyticum* *Treponema maltophilum* *Treponema medium* *Treponema parvum* *Treponema pectinovorum* *Treponema putidum* *Treponema skoliodontum* *Treponema socranskii* *Treponema vincentii*
Skin-associated spirochetes	Sebaceous secretions in genital region	*Treponema minutum* *Treponema phagedenis* *Treponema refringens*
Intestinal spirochetes	Colon, rectum, feces	*Brachyspira aalborgi* *Brachyspira pilosicoli*

organisms ranging from 0.15 to 0.30 μm in diameter and from 5 to 16 μm in length (with lengths being variable within each species). Although the species differ from one another slightly in terms of cell diameter and helical configuration, it is generally not possible to identify them on morphologic grounds; genotypic characteristics and biochemical parameters such as growth requirements, carbohydrate fermentation, and enzymatic activities are used to identify species (115).

The oral spirochetes listed in Table 6 are difficult to isolate from healthy gingiva. However, they increase both in prevalence and in number of organisms present in patients with gingivitis or periodontal disease, an inflammation of gum tissue that frequently precedes bone resorption and subsequent tooth loss. Treponemes are detected in the subgingival plaque of 88 to 97% of patients with periodontal disease (77). *T. socranskii* is the most common isolate in patients without periodontal disease, followed by *T. denticola* and *T. pectinovorum*. These organisms are isolated from a greater proportion of patients with periodontal disease than patients without the disease (77, 114, 115). Recent studies using PCR amplification of 16S rRNA gene sequences have revealed that oral spirochetes are a heterogeneous group, consisting of up to 60 different species and as yet uncultured "phylotypes" (26, 92); as many as 23 phylotypes of treponemes have been identified in the lesions of individual patients (23). All of the oral spirochetes clearly fall under the genus *Treponema* (93). Up to 415 cultured and uncultured bacterial species have been identified in human subgingival plaque (92), but treponemes represent one of the most prevalent groups (78, 79). Although it is difficult to establish a causal relationship in polymicrobial infections such as periodontitis, oral spirochetes are almost certainly involved in its etiology.

The isolation and characterization of oral spirochetes require special media and strict anaerobic conditions (75, 76, 113, 114, 115, 126) and are restricted primarily to research laboratories. At present, there is insufficient evidence linking particular oral spirochetes to pathogenic conditions to warrant their detection and identification for diagnostic purposes.

Nonpathogenic Spirochetes of the Genital Region

T. phagedenis, *T. refringens*, and *T. minutum* are treponemal species that inhabit the smegma (sebaceous secretions and desquamated epithelial cells) found beneath the prepuce and in other epithelial folds of the genital region. *T. phagedenis* and *T. refringens* are 0.20 to 0.25 μm in diameter, whereas *T. minutum* tends to be smaller in diameter (0.15 to 0.20 μm). Although *T. phagedenis* and *T. refringens* have been shown to have ≤5% homology with *T. pallidum* by DNA-DNA hybridization (30), comparison of 16S rRNA sequences indicates that they are related to the pathogenic treponemes. These harmless members of the normal flora could potentially be misidentified as *T. pallidum* in dark-field microscopy preparations from skin sites. Careful cleansing of the site as described in reference 60 obviates this possibility. Also, the DFA-TP test (60) is specific for pathogenic treponemes and can be used with specimens potentially contaminated with other organisms. The skin-associated treponemes may be collected with sterile moistened swabs and placed in anaerobic transport medium or directly into selective medium. They are readily cultured in peptone-yeast extract-glucose medium or in thioglycolate medium with 10% heat-inactivated rabbit serum under anaerobic conditions at 37°C (75).

Intestinal Spirochetes

The presence of spirochetes in the colon, rectum, and feces of humans has been recognized for more than 100 years (107). Since the description of "human intestinal spirochetosis" in 1967 (45), there has been a resurgence in interest in the possible involvement of intestinal spirochetes in diarrhea and other gastrointestinal diseases (44), as well as in the apparently high prevalence of these organisms in homosexual males and HIV-infected individuals (107).

Morphologically, most human intestinal spirochetes are relatively short (3 to 6 μm on average) and are 0.2 to 0.4 μm in diameter with one to two helices per cell. Longer cells may also be present. They have pointed ends and four to six periplasmic flagella attached subterminally in a single row at each end of the cell. The human intestinal spirochetes identified thus far fall into two species: *Brachyspira* (formerly *Serpulina*) *pilosicoli* and *Brachyspira aalborgi*. *B. pilosicoli* was initially named *Serpulina pilosicoli* (120, 121); however, this and other *Serpulina* species (e.g., *B. hyodysenteriae*, a cause of swine dysentery) were reclassified as *Brachyspira* based on phenotypic characteristics, rRNA gene sequence analysis, and DNA hybridization studies (91). *B. pilosicoli* has a broad range of natural hosts, including swine, mice, rats, dogs, and chickens. *B. aalborgi* (49) is genetically and phenotypically distinct from *B. pilosicoli* (57, 120), and thus far has been identified only in humans. Recent 16S rRNA gene analyses indicate that *B. aalborgi* can be subdivided into four different clusters or lineages, but it is not known whether this heterogeneity is associated with phenotypic differences (74).

B. pilosicoli and *B. aalborgi* are obligate anaerobes but grow in a variety of media containing blood. Until recently, *B. aalborgi* had been cultured on only one occasion (resulting in the type strain), leading to the conclusion that it was rare relative to *B. pilosicoli*. However, recent PCR analyses of human colonic biopsy specimens indicate that *B. aalborgi* is a common cause of human intestinal spirochetosis (59, 71, 72). In two series of histologically diagnosed cases of intestinal spirochetosis from Australia, Norway, and the United States, *B. aalborgi* sequences were detected in 62.5 and 82.5% of the cases, whereas *B. pilosicoli* sequences were detected in only 0 and 14.3% (72, 73). In 2000, Kraaz et al. (59) isolated a second strain of *B. aalborgi* by using a selective medium consisting of tryptose soy agar with 10% bovine blood, 400 μg of spectinomycin per ml, and 5 μg of polymyxin per ml. They found that a selective medium commonly used for the culture of intestinal spirochetes inhibited the growth of this strain, presumably due to the inclusion of vancomycin and colistin.

When observed in association with rectal or colonic tissue, these organisms are typically attached by the tip to the apical surface of the columnar epithelial cells. Although the spirochetes can form a dense layer visible by light microscopy (using hematoxylin-and-eosin- or silver-staining techniques), signs of tissue damage or inflammation are usually absent.

A clear association between intestinal spirochetes and disease has not been established (107). Spirochetes can be present in healthy individuals as well as in those with diarrhea or other gastrointestinal symptoms. In the early 1900s, several studies examined the presence of spirochetes in human stool specimens by light microscopy. In those studies, involving more than 100 patients, the proportion of subjects with spirochetes ranged from 3.3 to 61%. Recent examinations of rectal biopsy specimens from heterosexual patients by light and electron microscopy or culture have indicated the presence of spirochetes in 1.9 to 6.9% of subjects, and helical organisms were also found to be associated with normal and inflamed appendixes. Higher proportions of homosexual males have been reported to have intestinal spirochetes. At present, there is no clear evidence for an association between intestinal spirochetosis and HIV infection.

B. pilosicoli was isolated from routine anaerobic cultures of blood from seven critically ill patients, including those with stroke, ethylene glycol intoxication, severe arteriopathy, peritonitis, and myeloma (118). The clinical significance and cause-and-effect relationship of *B. pilosicoli* bacteremia and life-threatening illness remain to be determined.

Colonic or rectal biopsy samples can serve as a source of material for culture, histologic examination for spirochetes, or PCR; fresh stool specimens or rectal swabs may also be examined by dark-field microscopy for the presence of spirochetes (107). Positive samples can be cultured under anaerobic conditions at 37°C in the presence of 5 to 10% CO_2 by being streaked onto Trypticase soy agar medium with 5 to 10% defibrinated horse or calf blood and 400 μg of spectinomycin per ml (with or without 5 μg of polymyxin B per ml) to inhibit the growth of other bacteria. After 5 to 14 days of incubation, growth appears as a thin film or as discrete, pinpoint colonies. Longer culture intervals may be required for *B. aalborgi*. Weak beta-hemolysis is typically observed. In the isolation of *Brachyspira* from anaerobic blood cultures, automated detection was not obtained uniformly and required a minimum of 5.6 to 14.9 days (depending on the strain); however, the organisms could be subcultured and observed by dark-field microscopy (10, 118). An alternative method of detection is PCR, using rRNA and/or NADH oxidase *(nox)* gene sequences as targets (59, 71); this approach can also be adapted for use with fixed, paraffin-embedded tissue specimens (71) or with human feces (73).

No commercial kits or serologic procedures for detection of human intestinal spirochetosis are available, and no data on antimicrobial susceptibility or treatment have been reported. Clearly, more information is needed to establish the potential medical importance of these organisms.

REFERENCES

1. **Aberg, J. A., J. E. Gallant, J. Anderson, J. M. Oleske, H. Libman, J. S. Currier, V. E. Stone, and J. E. Kaplan.** 2004. Primary care guidelines for the management of persons infected with human immunodeficiency virus: recommendations of the HIV Medicine Association of the Infectious Diseases Society of America. *Clin. Infect. Dis.* **39:**609–629.
2. **Antal, G. M., S. A. Lukehart, and A. Z. Mehaus.** 2002. The endemic treponematoses. *Microbes Infect.* **4:**83–94.
3. **Antal, G. M., and G. Causse.** 1985. The control of endemic treponematoses. *Rev. Infect. Dis.* **7**(Suppl. 2)**:** S220–S226.
4. **Augenbraun, M. H., and R. Rolfs.** 1999. Treatment of syphilis, 1998: nonpregnant adults. *Clin. Infect. Dis.* **28** (Suppl. 1)**:**S21–S28.
5. **Belisle, J. T., M. E. Brandt, J. D. Radolf, and M. V. Norgard.** 1994. Fatty acids of *Treponema pallidum* and *Borrelia burgdorferi* lipoproteins. *J. Bacteriol.* **176:**2151–2157.
6. **Benenson, A. S.** 1990. Pinta, p. 323–324; Nonvenereal endemic syphilis, p. 425–426; and Yaws, p. 483–486. *In* A. S. Benenson (ed.), *Control of Communicable Diseases in Man,* 15th ed. American Public Health Association, Washington, D.C.
7. **Birnbaum, N. R., R. H. Goldschmidt, and W. O. Buffett.** 1999. Resolving the common clinical dilemmas of syphilis. *Am. Fam. Physician* **59:**2233–2240.
8. **Blocker, M. E., W. C. Levine, and M. E. St. Louis.** 2000. HIV prevalence in patients with syphilis, United States. *Sex. Transm. Dis.* **27:**53–59.
9. **Bromberg, K., S. Rawstron, and G. Tannis.** 1993. Diagnosis of congenital syphilis by combining *Treponema pallidum*-specific IgM detection with immunofluorescent antigen detection for *T. pallidum*. *J. Infect. Dis.* **168:**238–242.
10. **Brooke, C. J., K. R. Margawani, A. K. Pearson, T. V. Riley, I. D. Robertson, and D. J. Hampson.** 2000. Evaluation of blood culture systems for detection of the intestinal spirochaete *Brachyspira (Serpulina) pilosicoli* in human blood. *J. Med. Microbiol.* **49:**1031–1036.
11. **Buchacz, K., P. Patel, M. Taylor, P. R. Kerndt, R. H. Byers, S. D. Holmberg, and J. D. Klausner.** 2004. Syphilis increases HIV viral load and decreases CD4 cell counts in HIV-infected patients with new syphilis infections. *AIDS* **18:**2075–2079.
12. **Byrne, R. E., S. Laske, M. Bell, D. Larson, J. Phillips, and J. Todd.** 1992. Evaluation of a *Treponema pallidum* Western immunoblot assay as a confirmatory test for syphilis. *J. Clin. Microbiol.* **30:**115–122.
13. **Calonge, N. and U. S. Preventive Services Task Force.** 2004. Screening for syphilis infection: recommendation statement. *Ann. Fam. Med.* **2:**362–365.(Erratum, **2:**517.)
14. **Centers for Disease Control and Prevention.** 1997. Conditions under public health surveillance. *Morb. Mortal. Wkly. Rep.* **46:**34–37.
15. **Centers for Disease Control and Prevention.** 2002. 2002 Sexually transmitted diseases treatment guidelines. *Morb. Mortal. Wkly. Rep.* **51**(RR-6)**:**18–29.
16. **Centers for Disease Control and Prevention.** 2004. *Sexually Transmitted Disease Surveillance, 2003,* p. 27–36, 110–133. U.S. Department of Health and Human Services. Atlanta, Ga.
17. **Centurion-Lara, A., C. Castro, R. Castillo, J. M. Shaffer, W. C. Van Voorhis, and S. A. Lukehart.** 1998. The flanking region sequences of the 15-kDa lipoprotein gene differentiate pathogenic treponemes. *J. Infect. Dis.* **177:**1036–1040.
18. **Centurion-Lara, A., C. Godornes, C. Castro, W. C. Van Voorhis, and S. A. Lukehart.** 2000. The *tprK* gene is heterogeneous among *Treponema pallidum* strains and has multiple alleles. *Infect. Immun.* **68:**824–831.
19. **Centurion-Lara, A., E. S. Sun, L. K. Barrett, C. Castro, S. A. Lukehart, and W. C. Van Voorhis.** 2000. Multiple alleles of *Treponema pallidum* repeat gene D in *Treponema pallidum* isolates. *J. Bacteriol.* **182:**2332–2335.
20. **Chesson, H. W., J. D. Heffelfinger, R. F. Voigt, and D. Collins.** 2005. Estimates of primary and secondary syphilis rates in persons with HIV in the United States, 2002. *Sex. Transm. Dis.* **32:**265–269.

21. **Chhabra, R. S., L. P. Brion, M. Castro, L. Freundlich, and J. H. Glaser.** 1993. Comparison of maternal sera, cord blood, and neonatal sera for detecting presumptive congenital syphilis: relationship with maternal treatment. *Pediatrics* **91:**88–91.
22. **Choi, B. K., B. J. Paster, F. E. Dewhirst, and U. B. Göbel.** 1994. Diversity of cultivable and uncultivable oral spirochetes from a patient with severe destructive periodontitis. *Infect. Immun.* **62:**1889–1895.
23. **Choi, B. K., C. Wyss, and U. B. Göbel.** 1996. Phylogenetic analysis of pathogen-related oral spirochetes. *J. Clin. Microbiol.* **34:**1922–1925.
24. **Ciesielski, C. A.** 2003. Sexually transmitted diseases in men who have sex with men: an epidemiologic review. *Curr. Infect. Dis. Rep.* **5:**145–152.
25. **Demirkan, I., S. D. Carter, C. Winstanley, K. D. Bruce, N. M. McNair, M. Woodside, and C. A. Hart.** 2001. Isolation and characterisation of a novel spirochaete from severe virulent ovine foot rot. *J. Med. Microbiol.* **50:** 1061–1068.
26. **Dewhirst, F., M. Tamer, E. R. E. Ericson, C. N. Lau, V. A. Levanos, S. K. Boches, J. L. Galvin, and B. J. Paster.** 2000. The diversity of periodontal spirochetes by 16S rRNA analysis. *Oral Microbiol. Immunol.* **15:**196–202.
27. **Dobson, S. R. M., L. H. Taber, and R. E. Baughn.** 1988. Recognition of *Treponema pallidum* antigens by IgM and IgG antibodies in congenitally infected newborns and their mothers. *J. Infect. Dis.* **157:**903–910.
28. **Engelkens, H. J. H., J. Judanarso, A. P. Oranje, V. D. Vuzevski, P. L. A. Niemel, J. J. van der Sluis, and E. Stolz.** 1991. Endemic treponematoses. I. Yaws. *Int. J. Dermatol.* **30:**77–83.
29. **Engelkens, H. J. H., P. L. A. Niemel, J. J. van der Sluis, A. Meheus, and E. Stolz.** 1991. Endemic treponematoses. II. Pinta and endemic syphilis. *Int. J. Dermatol.* **30:**231–238.
30. **Fieldsteel, A. H.** 1983. Genetics, p. 39–54. *In* R. F. Schell and D. M. Musher (ed.), *Pathogenesis and Immunology of Treponemal Infection.* Marcel Dekker, Inc., New York, N.Y.
31. **Fieldsteel, A. H., D. L. Cox, and R. A. Moeckli.** 1981. Cultivation of virulent *Treponema pallidum* in tissue culture. *Infect. Immun.* **32:**908–915.
32. **Fiumara, N. J.** 1978. Treatment of early latent syphilis of less than one year's duration. *Sex. Transm. Dis.* **5:**85–88.
33. **Fiumara, N. J.** 1979. Serologic responses to treatment of 128 patients with late latent syphilis. *Sex. Transm. Dis.* **6:**243–246.
34. **Fiumara, N. J.** 1980. Treatment of primary and secondary syphilis; serological response. *JAMA* **243:**2500–2502.
35. **Fleming, D. T., and J. N. Wasserheit.** 1999. From epidemiological synergy to public health policy and practice: the contribution of other sexually transmitted diseases to sexual transmission of HIV infection. *Sex. Transm. Dis.* **75:**3–17.
36. **Fraser, C. M., S. J. Norris, G. M. Weinstock, et al.** 1998. Complete genome sequence of *Treponema pallidum*, the syphilis spirochete. *Science* **281:**375–388.
37. **George, R. W., V. Pope, and S. A. Larsen.** 1991. Use of the Western blot for the diagnosis of syphilis. *Clin. Immunol. Newsl.* **8:**124–128.
38. **Gjestland, T.** 1955. The Oslo study of untreated syphilis: an epidemiologic investigation of the natural course of syphilis infection based upon a re-study of the Boeck-Bruusgaard material. *Acta Dermatovenereol.* **35:**1–368.
39. **Gourevitch, M. N., P. A. Selwyn, D. Davenny, D. Buono, E. E. Schoenbaum, R. S. Klein, and F. H. Friedland.** 1993. Effects of HIV infection on the serologic manifestation and response to treatment of syphilis in intravenous drug users. *Ann. Intern. Med.* **118:**350–355.
40. **Graber, J. R., J. R. Leadbetter, and J. A. Breznak.** 2004. Description of *Treponema azotonutricium* sp. nov. and *Treponema primitia* sp. nov., the first spirochetes isolated from termite guts. *Appl. Environ. Microbiol.* **70:**1315–1320.
41. **Gregory, N., M. Sanchez, and M. R. Buchness.** 1990. The spectrum of syphilis in patients with human immunodeficiency virus infection. *J. Am. Acad. Dermatol.* **22:** 1061–1067.
42. **Grimprel, E., P. J. Sanchez, G. D. Wendel, J. M. Burstain, G. H. McCracken, Jr., J. D. Radolf, and M. V. Norgard.** 1991. Use of polymerase chain reaction and rabbit infectivity testing to detect *Treponema pallidum* in amniotic fluid, fetal and neonatal sera, and cerebrospinal fluid. *J. Clin. Microbiol.* **29:**1711–1718.
43. **Guarner, J., K. Southwick, P. Greer, J. Bartlett, M. Fears, A. Santander, S. Blanco, V. Pope, W. Levine, and S. Zaki.** 2000. Testing umbilical cords for funisitis due to *Treponema pallidum* infection, Bolivia. *Emerg. Infect. Dis.* **6:**487–492.
44. **Hampson, D. J., and T. B. E. Stanton (ed.).** 1996. *Intestinal Spirochetes in Domestic Animals and Humans.* CAB International, Wallingford, England.
45. **Harland, W. A., and F. D. Lee.** 1967. Intestinal spirochaetosis. *Br. Med. J.* **3:**718–719.
46. **Hicks, C. B., P. M. Benson, G. P. Lupton, and E. C. Tramont.** 1987. Seronegative secondary syphilis in a patient infected with the human immunodeficiency virus (HIV) with Kaposi sarcoma. *Ann. Intern. Med.* **107:**492–495.
47. **Hollier, L. M., T. W. Harstad, P. J. Sanchez, D. M. Twickler, and G. D. Wendel, Jr.** 2001. Fetal syphilis: clinical and laboratory characteristics. *Obstet. Gynecol.* **97:**947–953.
48. **Hook, E. W., III, and C. M. Marra.** 1992. Acquired syphilis in adults. *N. Engl. J. Med.* **326:**1060–1069.
49. **Hovind-Hougen, K., A. Birch-Andersen, R. Henrik-Nielsen, M. Orholm, J. O. Pedersen, P. S. Teglbjaerg, and E. H. Thaysen.** 1982. Intestinal spirochetosis: morphological characterization and cultivation of the spirochete *Brachyspira aalborgi* gen. nov., sp. nov. *J. Clin. Microbiol.* **16:**1127–1136.
50. **Hunter, E. F., H. Russell, C. E. Farshy, J. S. Sampson, and S. A. Larsen.** 1986. Evaluation of sera from patients with Lyme disease in the fluorescent treponemal antibody-absorption tests for syphilis. *Sex. Transm. Dis.* **13:**232–236.
51. **Ijsselmuiden, O. E., J. J. van der Sluis, A. Mulder, E. Stolz, K. P. Bolton, and R. V. W. van Eijk.** 1989. An IgM capture enzyme-linked immunosorbent assay to detect IgM antibodies to treponemes in patients with syphilis. *Genitourin. Med.* **65:**79–83.
52. **Jaffe, H. W., S. A. Larsen, M. Peters, D. F. Jove, B. Lopez, and A. L. Schroeter.** 1978. Tests for treponemal antibody in CSF. *Arch. Intern. Med.* **138:**252–255.
53. **Janier, M., C. Chastang, E. Spindler, S. Strazzi, C. Rabian, A. Marcelli, and P. Morel.** 1999. A prospective study of the influence of HIV status on seroreversion of serologic tests for syphilis. *Dermatology* **198:**362–369.
54. **Jethwa, H. S., J. L. Schmitz, G. G. Dallabetta, F. F. Behets, I. Hoffman, H. Hamilton, G. Lule, M. Cohen, and J. D. Folds.** 1995. Comparison of molecular and microscopic techniques for detection of *Treponema pallidum* in genital ulcers. *J. Clin. Microbiol.* **33:**180–183.
55. **Johns, D. R., M. Tierney, and D. Felsenstein.** 1987. Alteration in the natural history of neurosyphilis by concurrent infection with the human immunodeficiency virus. *N. Engl. J. Med.* **316:**1569–1572.
56. **Kaufman, R. E., O. G. Jones, J. H. Blount, and P. J. Wiesner.** 1977. Questionnaire survey of reported early congenital syphilis, problems in diagnosis, prevention and treatment. *Sex. Transm. Dis.* **4:**135–139.
57. **Koopman, M. B. H., A. Käsbohrer, G. Beckmann, B. A. M. van der Zeijst, and J. G. K. Kusters.** 1993. Genetic similarity of intestinal spirochetes from humans and various animal species. *J. Clin. Microbiol.* **31:**711–716.

58. **Kouznetsov, A. V., P. Weisenseel, P. Trommler, S. Multhaup, and J. C. Prinz.** 2005. Detection of the 47-kilodalton membrane immunogen gene of *Treponema pallidum* in various tissue sources of patients with syphilis. *Diagn. Microbiol. Infect. Dis.* **51:**143–145.
59. **Kraaz, W., B. Pettersson, U. Thunberg, L. Engstrand, and C. Fellstrom.** 2000. *Brachyspira aalborgi* infection diagnosed by culture and 16S ribosomal DNA sequencing using human colonic biopsy specimens. *J. Clin. Microbiol.* **38:**3555–3560.
60. **Larsen, S. A., V. Pope, R. E. Johnson, and E. J. Kennedy, (ed.).** 1998. *A Manual of Tests for Syphilis,* 9th ed. American Public Health Association, Washington, D.C.
61. **Larsen, S. A., and B. M. Steiner.** 1995. Laboratory diagnosis and interpretation of tests for syphilis. *Clin. Microbiol. Rev.* **8:**1–21.
62. **Lefèvre, J. C., M. A. Bertrand, and R. Bauriaud.** 1990. Evaluation of the Captia enzyme immunoassays for detection of immunoglobulins G and M to *Treponema pallidum* in syphilis. *J. Clin. Microbiol.* **28:**1704–1707.
63. **Lewis, L. L., L. H. Taber, and R. E. Baughn.** 1990. Evaluation of immunoglobulin M Western blot analysis in the diagnosis of congenital syphilis. *J. Clin. Microbiol.* **28:**296–302.
64. **Liu, H., B. Rodes, C.-Y. Chen, and B. Steiner.** 2001. New tests for syphilis: rational design of a PCR method for detection of *Treponema pallidum* in clinical specimens using regions of the DNA polymerase I gene. *J. Clin. Microbiol.* **39:**1941–1946.
65. **Lukehart, S. A., C. Godornes, B. J. Molini, P. Sonnett, S. Hopkins, F. Mulcahy, J. Engelman, S. J. Mitchell, A. M. Rompalo, C. M. Marra, and J. D. Klausner.** 2004. Macrolide resistance in *Treponema pallidum* in the United States and Ireland. *N. Engl. J. Med.* **351:**154–158.
66. **Magnarelli, L. A., J. N. Miller, J. F. Anderson, and G. R. Riviere.** 1990. Cross-reactivity of nonspecific treponemal antibody in serologic tests for Lyme disease. *J. Clin. Microbiol.* **28:**1276–1279.
67. **Marangoni, A., V. Sambri, A. Olmo, A. D'Antuono, M. Negosanti, and R. Cevenini.** 1999. IgG western blot as a confirmatory test in early syphilis. *Zentbl. Bakteriol.* **289:**125–133.
68. **Marfin, A. A., H. Liu, M. Y. Sutton, B. Steiner, A. Pillay, and L. E. Markowitz.** 2001. Amplification of the DNA polymerase I gene of *Treponema pallidum* from whole blood of persons with syphilis. *Diagn. Microbiol. Infect. Dis.* **40:**163–166.
69. **Marra, C. M., C. L. Maxwell, S. L. Smith, S. A. Lukehart, A. M. Rompalo, M. Eaton, B. P. Stoner, M. Augenbraun, D. E. Barker, J. J. Corbet, M. Zajackowski, C. Raines, J. Nerad, J. Kee, and S. H. Barnett.** 2004. Cerebrospinal fluid abnormalities in patients with syphilis: association with clinical and laboratory features. *J. Infect. Dis.* **189:**369–376.
70. **Matthews, H. M., T. K. Yang, and H. M. Jenkin.** 1979. Unique lipid composition of *Treponema pallidum* (Nichols virulent strain). *Infect. Immun.* **24:**713–719.
71. **Mikosza, A. S., T. La, C. J. Brooke, C. F. Lindboe, P. B. Ward, R. G. Heine, J. G. Guccion, W. B. de Boer, and D. J. Hampson.** 1999. PCR amplification from fixed tissue indicates frequent involvement of *Brachyspira aalborgi* in human intestinal spirochetosis. *J. Clin. Microbiol.* **37:**2093–2098.
72. **Mikosza, A. S., T. La, W. B. de Boer, and D. J. Hampson.** 2001. Comparative prevalences of *Brachyspira aalborgi* and *Brachyspira (Serpulina) pilosicoli* as etiologic agents of histologically identified intestinal spirochetosis in Australia. *J. Clin. Microbiol.* **39:**347–350.
73. **Mikosza, A. S., T. La, K. R. Margawani, C. J. Brooke, and D. J. Hampson.** 2001. PCR detection of *Brachyspira aalborgi* and *Brachyspira pilosicoli* in human faeces. *FEMS Microbiol. Lett.* **197:**167–170.
74. **Mikosza, A. S., M. A. Munshi, and D. J. Hampson.** 2004. Analysis of genetic variation in *Brachyspira aalborgii* and related spirochaetes determined by partial sequencing of the 16S rRNA and NADH oxidase genes. *J. Med. Microbiol.* **53:**333–339.
75. **Miller, J. N., R. M. Smibert, and S. J. Norris.** 1992. The genus *Treponema,* p. 3537–3559. *In* A. Balows, H. G. Trouper, M. Dworkin, W. Harder, and K.-H. Schiefer (ed.), *The Prokaryotes. A Handbook on the Biology of Bacteria, Ecophysiology, Isolation, Identifications, and Applications,* 2nd ed. Springer-Verlag, Inc., New York, N.Y.
76. **Moore, L. V. H., W. E. C. Moore, E. P. Cato, R. M. Smibert, J. A. Burmeister, A. M. Best, and R. R. Ranney.** 1987. Bacteriology of human gingivitis. *J. Dent. Res.* **66:**989–995.
77. **Moore, W. E., and L. V. Moore.** 1994. The bacteria of periodontal diseases. *Periodontol. 2000* **5:**66–77.
78. **Moter, A., C. Hoenig, B. Choi, B. Riep, and U. Göbel.** 1998. Molecular epidemiology of oral treponemes associated with periodontal disease. *J. Clin. Microbiol.* **36:**1399–1403.
79. **Mullaly, B., B. Dace, C. Shelburne, L. Wolff, and W. Coulter.** 2000. Prevalence of periodontal pathogens in localized and generalized forms of early-onset periodontitis. *J. Periodontal Res.* **35:**232–241.
80. **Musher, D. M.** 1991. Syphilis, neurosyphilis, penicillin, and AIDS. *J. Infect. Dis.* **163:**1201–1206.
81. **Nayar, R., and J. M. Campos.** 1993. Evaluation of the DCL Syphilis-G enzyme immunoassay test kit for the serologic diagnosis of syphilis. *Am. J. Clin. Pathol.* **99:**282–285.
82. **Noordhoek, G. T., A. Cockayne, L. M. Schouls, R. H. Meloen, E. Stolz, and J. D. A. van Embden.** 1990. A new attempt to distinguish serologically the subspecies of *Treponema pallidum* causing syphilis and yaws. *J. Clin. Microbiol.* **28:**1600–1607.
83. **Noordhoek, G. T., H. J. H. Engelkens, J. Judanarso, J. van der Stek, G. N. M. Aelbers, J. J. van der Sluis, J. D. A. van Embden, and E. Stolz.** 1991. Yaws in West Sumatra, Indonesia: clinical manifestations, serological findings, and characterisation of new *Treponema* isolates by DNA probes. *Eur. J. Clin. Microbiol. Infect. Dis.* **10:**12–19.
84. **Noordhoek, G. T., P. W. M. Hermans, A. N. Paul, L. M. Schouls, J. J. van der Sluis, and J. D. A. van Embden.** 1989. *Treponema pallidum* subspecies *pallidum* (Nichols) and *Treponema pallidum* subspecies *pertenue* (CDC 2575) differ in at least one nucleotide: comparison of two homologous antigens. *Microb. Pathog.* **6:**29–42.
85. **Noordhoek, G. T., B. Wieles, J. J. van der Sluis, and J. D. A. van Embden.** 1990. Polymerase chain reaction and synthetic DNA probes—a means of distinguishing the causative agents of syphilis and yaws? *Infect. Immun.* **58:**2011–2013.
86. **Noordhoek, G. T., E. C. Wolters, M. E. J. De Jonge, and J. D. A. van Embden.** 1991. Detection by polymerase chain reaction of *Treponema pallidum* DNA in cerebrospinal fluid from neurosyphilis patients before and after antibiotic treatment. *J. Clin. Microbiol.* **29:**1976–1984.
87. **Norgard, M. V.** 1993. Clinical and diagnostic issues of acquired and congenital syphilis encompassed in the current syphilis epidemic. *Curr. Opin. Infect. Dis.* **6:**9–16.
88. **Norris, S. J., D. L. Cox, and G. M. Weinstock.** 2001. Biology of *Treponema pallidum*: correlation of functional activities with genome sequence data. *J. Mol. Microbiol. Biotechnol.* **3:**37–62.
89. **Norris, S. J., and D. G. Edmondson.** 1987. Factors affecting the multiplication and subculture of *Treponema pallidum* subsp. *pallidum* in a tissue culture system. *Infect. Immun.* **53:**534–539.
90. **Norris, S. J., and *Treponema pallidum* Polypeptide Research Group.** 1993. Polypeptides of *Treponema pallidum*: progress toward understanding their structural, functional, and immunologic roles. *Microbiol. Rev.* **57:**750–779.

91. **Ochiai, S., Y. Adachi, and K. Mori.** 1997. Unification of the genera *Serpulina* and *Brachyspira*, and proposals of *Brachyspira hyodysenteriae* comb. nov., *Brachyspira innocens* comb. nov. and *Brachyspira pilosicoli* comb. nov. *Microbiol. Immunol.* **41:**445–452.
92. **Paster, B., S. Boches, J. Galvin, R. Ericson, C. Lau, V. Levanos, A. Sahasrabudhe, and F. Dewhirst.** 2001. Bacterial diversity in human subgingival plaque. *J. Bacteriol.* **183:**3770–3783.
93. **Paster, B., and F. Dewhirst.** 2000. Phylogenetic foundation of spirochetes. *J. Mol. Microbiol. Biotechnol.* **2:**341–344.
94. **Paz-Bailey, G., A. Meyers, S. Blank. J. Brown, S. Rubin, J. Braxton, A. Zaidi, J. Schafzin, S. Weigl, and L. E. Markowitz.** 2004. A case-control study of syphilis among men who have sex with men in New York City: association with HIV infection. *Sex. Transm. Dis.* **31:**581–587.
95. **Perine, P. L., D. R. Hopkins, P. L. A. Niemel, R. K. St. John, G. Causse, and G. M. Antal.** 1984. *Handbook of Endemic Treponematoses: Yaws, Endemic Syphilis, and Pinta.* World Health Organization, Geneva, Switzerland.
96. **Phelps, R. G., J. Knispel, E. S. Tu, G. Cernainu, and M. Saruk.** 2000. Immunoperoxidase technique for detecting spirochetes in tissue sections: comparison with other methods. *Int. J. Dermatol.* **39:**609–613.
97. **Pietravalle, M., F. Pimpinelli, A. Maini, E. Capoluongo, C. Felici, L. D'Auria, A. Di Carlo, and F. Ameglio.** 1999. Diagnostic relevance of polymerase chain reaction technology for *T. pallidum* in subjects with syphilis in different phases of infection. *Microbiologia* **22:**99–104.
98. **Pillay, A., H. Liu, C. Y. Chen, B. Holloway, W. Sturm, B. Steiner, and S. A. Morse.** 1998. Molecular subtyping of *Treponema pallidum* subspecies pallidum. *Sex. Transm. Dis.* **25:**408–414.
99. **Pope, V., M. B. Fears, W. E. Morrill, A. Castro, and S. E. Kikkert.** 2000. Comparison of the Serodia *Treponema pallidum* particle agglutination, Captia Syphilis-G, and SpiroTek Reagin II tests with standard test techniques for diagnosis of syphilis. *J. Clin. Microbiol.* **38:**2543–2545.
100. **Pope, V., K. Fox, H. Liu, A. A. Marfin, P. Leone, A. C. Seña, J. Chapin, M B. Fears, and L. Markowitz.** 2005. Molecular subtyping of *Treponema pallidum* from North and South Carolina. *J. Clin. Microbiol.* **43:**3743–3746.
101. **Rawstron, S. A., and K. Romberg.** 1991. Comparison of maternal and newborn serologic tests for syphilis. *Am. J. Dis. Child.* **145:**1383–1388.
102. **Rawstron, S. A., J. Vetrano, G. Tannis, and K. Bromberg.** 1997. Congenital syphilis: detection of *Treponema pallidum* in stillborns. *Clin. Infect. Dis.* **24:**24–27.
103. **Rolfs, R. T.** 1995. Treatment of syphilis, 1993. *Clin. Infect. Dis.* **20**(Suppl.)**:**S23–S38.
104. **Rolfs, R. T., M. R. Joesoef, E. F. Hendershot, A. M. Rompalo, M. H. Augenbraun, M. Chiu, G. Bolan, S. C. Johnson, P. French, E. Steen, J. D. Radolf, S. Larsen, and The Syphilis and HIV Study Group.** 1997. A randomized trial of enhanced therapy for early syphilis in patients with and without human immunodeficiency virus infection. *N. Engl. J. Med.* **337:**307–314.
105. **Romanowski, B., R. Sutherland, F. H. Fick, D. Mooney, and E. J. Love.** 1991. Serologic response to treatment of infectious syphilis. *Ann. Intern. Med.* **114:**1005–1009.
106. **Rompalo, A. M., M. R. Joesoef, J. A. O'Donnell, M. Augenbraun, W. Brady, J. D. Radolf, R. Johnson, R. T. Rolfs, and the Syphilis and HIV Study Group.** 2001. Clinical manifestations of early syphilis by HIV status and gender: results of the Syphilis and HIV study. *Sex. Transm. Dis.* **28:**158–165.
107. **Ruane, P. J., M. M. Nakata, J. F. Reinhardt, and W. L. George.** 1989. Spirochete-like organisms in the human gastrointestinal tract. *Rev. Infect. Dis.* **11:**184–196.
108. **Sanchez, P. J., G. H. McCracken, G. D. Wendel, K. Olson, N. Threlkeid, and M. V. Norgard.** 1989. Molecular analysis of the fetal IgM response to *Treponema pallidum* antigens: implications for improved serodiagnosis of congenital syphilis. *J. Infect. Dis.* **159:**508–517.
109. **Sanchez, P. J., G. D. Wendel, Jr., E. Grimprel, M. Goldberg, M. Hall, O. Arencibia-Mireles, J. D. Radolf, and M. V. Norgard.** 1993. Evaluation of molecular methodologies and rabbit infectivity testing for the diagnosis of congenital syphilis and neonatal central nervous system invasion by *Treponema pallidum*. *J. Infect. Dis.* **167:**148–157.
110. **Schmidt, B. L., M. Edjlalipour, and A. Luger.** 2000. Comparative evaluation of nine different enzyme-linked immunosorbent assays for determination of antibodies against *Treponema pallidum* in patients with primary syphilis. *J. Clin. Microbiol.* **38:**1279–1282.
111. **Schroeter, A. L., J. B. Lucas, E. V. Price, and V. H. Falcone.** 1973. Treatment of early syphilis and reactivity of serologic tests. *JAMA* **221:**471–476.
112. **Seshadri, R., G. S. A. Meyers, H. Tettelin, J. A Eisen, J. F. Heidelberg, R. J. Dodson, T. M. Davidsen, R. T. DeBoy, D. E. Fouts, D. H. Haft, J. Selengut, Q. Ren, L. M. Brinkac, R. Madupu, J. Kolonay, S. A. Durkin, S. C. Daughert, J. Shetty, A. Shvartsbeyn, E. Gebregeorgis, K. Greer, G. Tsegaye, J. Malek, B. Ayodeji, S. Shatsman, M. P. McLeod, D. Smajs, J. K. Howell, S. Pal, A. Amin, P. Vashisth, T. Z. McNeill, O. Xiang, E. Sodergren, E. Baca, G. M. Weinstock, S. J. Norris, C. M. Fraser, and I. Paulsen.** 2004. Comparison of the genome of the oral pathogen *Treponema denticola* with other spirochete genomes. *Proc. Natl. Acad. Sci. USA* **101:**5646–5651.
113. **Smibert, R. M.** 1984. Genus III: *Treponema* Schaudinn 1905, 1728^{AL}, p. 49–57. *In* N. R. Kreig and J. G. Holt (ed.), *Bergey's Manual of Systematic Bacteriology,* vol. 1. The Williams & Wilkins Co., Baltimore, Md.
114. **Smibert, R. M., and J. A. Burmeister.** 1983. *Treponema pectinovorum* sp. nov. isolated from humans with periodontitis. *Int. J. Syst. Bacteriol.* **33:**852–856.
115. **Smibert, R. M., J. L. Johnson, and R. R. Ranney.** 1984. *Treponema socranskii* sp. nov., *Treponema socranskii* subsp. *socranskii* subsp. nov., *Treponema socranskii* subsp. *buccale* subsp. nov., and *Treponema socranskii* subsp. *paredis* subsp. nov. isolated from the human periodontia. *Int. J. Syst. Bacteriol.* **34:**457–462.
116. **Stoll, B. J., F. K. Lee, S. A. Larsen, E. Hale, D. Schwartz, R. J. Rice, R. Ashby, R. Holmes, and A. J. Nahmias.** 1993. Improved serodiagnosis of congenital syphilis with combined assay approach. *J. Infect. Dis.* **167:**1093–1099.
117. **Sutton, M. Y., H. Liu, B. Steiner, A. Pillay, T. Mickey, L. Finelli, S. Morse, L. E. Markowitz, and M. E. St. Louis.** 2001. Molecular subtyping of *Treponema pallidum* in an Arizona County with increasing syphilis morbidity: use of specimens from ulcers and blood. *J. Infect. Dis.* **183:**1601–1606.
118. **Trott, D. J., N. S. Jensen, I. Saint Girons, S. L. Oxberry, T. B. Stanton, D. Lindquist, and D. J. Hampson.** 1997. Identification and characterization of *Serpulina pilosicoli* isolates recovered from the blood of critically ill patients. *J. Clin. Microbiol.* **35:**482–485.
119. **Trott, D. J., M. R. Moeller, R. L. Zuerner, J. P. Goff, W. R. Waters, D. P. Alt, R. L. Walker, and M. J. Wannemuehler.** 2003. Characterization of *Treponema phagendenis*-like spirochetes isolated from papillomatous digital dermatitis lesion in dairy cattle. *J. Clin. Microbiol.* **41:**2522–2529.
120. **Trott, D. J., T. B. Stanton, N. S. Jensen, G. E. Duhamel, J. L. Johnson, and D. J. Hampson.** 1996. *Serpulina pilosicoli* sp. nov., the agent of porcine intestinal spirochetosis. *Int. J. Syst. Bacteriol.* **46:**206–215.

121. **Trott, D. J., T. B. Stanton, N. S. Jensen, and D. J. Hampson.** 1996. Phenotypic characteristics of *Serpulina pilosicoli* the agent of intestinal spirochaetosis. *FEMS Microbiol. Lett.* **142:**209–214.
122. **U.S. Public Health Service.** 1968. *Syphilis: a Synopsis.* U.S. Government Printing Office, Washington, D.C.
123. **Wicher, K., G. T. Noordhoek, F. Abbruscato, and V. Wicher.** 1992. Detection of *Treponema pallidum* in early syphilis by DNA amplification. *J. Clin. Microbiol.* **30:**497–500.
124. **World Health Organization.** 1998. *The Health Report 1998—Life in the 21st Century; a Vision for All.* World Health Organization, Geneva Switzerland.
125. **World Health Organization.** 2001. *Global Prevalence and Incidence of Selected Curable Sexually Transmitted Diseases: Overview and Estimates.* WHO/HIV_AIDS/2001.02. World Health Organization, New York, N.Y.
126. **Wyss, C. , B. K. Choi, P. Schüpbach, B. Guggenheim, and U. B. Göbel.** 1996. *Treponema maltophilum* sp. nov., a small oral spirochete isolated from human periodontal lesions. *Int. J. Syst. Bacteriol.* **46:**745–752.
127. **Young, H. A. M., A. McMillan, and J. Patterson.** 1992. Enzyme immunoassay for antitreponemal IgG: screening or confirmatory test? *J. Clin. Pathol.* **45:**37–41.
128. **Zenker, P. N., and S. M. Berman.** 1990. Congenital syphilis: reporting and reality. *Am. J. Public Health* **80:**271–272.
129. **Zoechling, N., E. M. Schluepen, H. P. Soyer, H. Kerl, and M. Volkenandt.** 1997. Molecular detection of *Treponema pallidum* in secondary and tertiary syphilis. *Br. J. Dermatol.* **136:**683–686.

Mycoplasma and *Ureaplasma**

KEN B. WAITES AND DAVID TAYLOR-ROBINSON

64

TAXONOMY

Bacteria commonly referred to as mycoplasmas ("fungus form") are included within the class *Mollicutes* ("soft skin"), which comprises 4 orders, 5 families, 8 genera, and almost 200 known species, as shown in Table 1. New species, found mainly in animals, are being identified on a frequent basis. Table 2 lists 16 species isolated from humans on multiple occasions, excluding species of animal origin that have been detected in humans from time to time, usually in immunosuppressed hosts, but that are generally considered to be transient colonizers. *Mycoplasma amphoriforme* is the most recent species to have been recognized, having been recovered from the respiratory tracts of several patients with antibody deficiencies and chronic bronchitis or bronchiectasis (121). Mollicutes are eubacteria that have evolved from clostridium-like gram-positive cells by gene deletion. The availability of species-specific PCR technology is ameliorating difficulties of both culture and identification for fastidious mollicutes. Therefore, additional noncultivable, and thus presently unknown, species are likely to be discovered.

DESCRIPTION OF *MOLLICUTES*

It should be noted that the term "mycoplasma" is often used in a trivial way to refer to any members of the class *Mollicutes*, irrespective of whether they actually belong to the genus *Mycoplasma*. It is more accurate to refer to members of the class as mollicutes and to organisms within the individual genera as mycoplasmas, ureaplasmas, and acholeplasmas, etc. Mollicutes are smaller than conventional bacteria, in cellular dimensions as well as genome size, making them the smallest free-living organisms known. Mycoplasmas and ureaplasmas associated with humans have forms ranging from coccoid cells of about 0.2 to 0.3 μm diameter, as in the case of *Ureaplasma* spp. and *Mycoplasma hominis* (87), to tapered rods of 1 to 2 μm in length and 0.1 to 0.2 μm in width in the case of *M. pneumoniae* and *M. penetrans* (122). Mollicutes are contained by a trilayered cell membrane and do not possess a cell wall. The permanent lack of a cell wall barrier makes the mollicutes unique among prokaryotes and differentiates them from bacterial L forms for which the lack of the cell wall is but a temporary reflection of environmental conditions. Lack of a cell wall also renders these organisms insensitive to the activity of beta-lactam antimicrobials, prevents them from staining by Gram stain, and is largely responsible for their pleomorphic form. The extremely small genome (<600 kb in the case of *M. genitalium*) and limited biosynthetic capabilities explain the parasitic or saprophytic existence of these organisms, their sensitivity to environmental conditions, and their fastidious growth requirements, which can complicate cultural detection. Mollicutes require enriched growth medium supplemented with nucleic acid precursors. Except for acholeplasmas, asteroleplasmas, and mesoplasmas, mollicutes require sterols in growth media, supplied by the addition of serum. Growth rates in culture media vary among individual species, with generation times of approximately 1 h for *Ureaplasma* spp., 6 h for *M. pneumoniae*, and 16 h for *M. genitalium* (54).

Typical mycoplasmal colonies vary from 15 to ≥300 μm in diameter. Colonies of some species, such as *M. hominis*, often exhibit a "fried-egg" appearance owing to the contrast between deeper growth in the center of the colony and more shallow growth at the periphery (Fig. 1), and other species, such as *M. pneumoniae*, produce spherical colonies (Fig. 2). Whereas colonies of mycoplasmal species may be observed with the naked eye, those produced by ureaplasmas are typically 15 to 60 μm in diameter and require low-power microscopic magnification for visualization (Fig. 3).

Mycoplasmas and ureaplasmas of human origin can be classified according to whether they ferment glucose, utilize arginine, or hydrolyze urea (Table 2). Except for hydrolysis of urea, which is unique for ureaplasmas, these biochemical features are not sufficient for species distinction. Anaeroplasmas and asteroleplasmas, which occur in ruminants, are strictly anaerobic and oxygen sensitive, whereas most other mollicutes are facultative anaerobes.

Attachment of *M. pneumoniae* to host cells in the respiratory tracts of humans is a prerequisite for colonization and infection. Cytadherence, mediated by the P1 adhesin and other accessory proteins, is followed by induction of ciliostasis, chronic inflammation, and cytotoxicity mediated by hydrogen peroxide, which also acts as a hemolysin. *M. pneumoniae* stimulates B and T lymphocytes and induces formation of autoantibodies which react with a variety of host tissues and the I antigen on erythrocytes, which is responsible for production of cold agglutinins (117). *M. genitalium* also possesses a terminal

*This chapter contains information presented in chapter 62 by Ken B. Waites, Yasuko Rikihisa, and David Taylor-Robinson in the eighth edition of this Manual.

TABLE 1 Classification and some distinguishing features of mollicutes

Classification of class *Mollicutes*	Distinguishing features			
	Sterol required	Genome size (kbp)	G+C content of DNA (mol%)	Other
Order I: *Mycoplasmatales*				
Family I: *Mycoplasmataceae*				
Genus I: *Mycoplasma* (120 species)[a]	Yes	580–1,350	23–40	
Genus II: *Ureaplasma* (7 species)[b]	Yes	730–1,170	25–32	Urea metabolized
Order II: *Entomoplasmatales*				
Family I: *Entomoplasmataceae*				
Genus I: *Entomoplasma* (6 species)	Yes	790–1,140	27–29	
Genus II: *Mesoplasma* (11 species)	No	870–1,100	27–30	Requires 0.04% Tween 80
Family II: *Spiroplasmataceae*				
Genus I: *Spiroplasma* (34 species)	Yes	940–2,200	25–30	Helical structure
Order III: *Acholeplasmatales*[c]				
Family I: *Acholeplasmataceae*				
Genus I: *Acholeplasma* (15 species)	No	1,500–1,650	27–36	
Order IV: *Anaeroplasmatales*				
Family I: *Anaeroplasmataceae*				Obligate anaerobes
Genus I: *Anaeroplasma* (4 species)	Yes	1,500–1,600	29–33	
Genus II: *Asteroleplasma* (1 species)	No	1,500	40	
Phytoplasma[c] (17 candidatus species designations)	Unknown	530–1,350	23–29	Noncultivable

[a] The genus *Mycoplasma* includes cell wall-less uncultivated parasitic bacteria, classified into six candidatus species designations, that attach to the surfaces of erythrocytes and also occur free in the plasma. These bacteria were previously classified in the genera *Haemobartonella* and *Eperythrozoon*. Their G+C contents and sterol requirements are unknown.

[b] *U. urealyticum* and *U. parvum*, formerly considered biovars of *U. urealyticum*, are now classified as two separate species and are the only ureaplasmas of human origin.

[c] Phytoplasmas are uncultivable mollicutes of plants and insects genetically related to the *Acholeplasmatales*, but they have not been assigned individual genus and species designations.

structure, the MgPa adhesin, which facilitates its attachment to epithelial cells (48). Factors involved in *Ureaplasma* and *M. hominis* attachment have not been characterized to the same extent as those involved in *M. pneumoniae* attachment, and *Ureaplasma* spp. and *M. hominis* do not have prominent attachment organelles. Henrich et al. (46) demonstrated the presence of the variable adherence-associated antigen (Vaa) that is believed to be a major adhesin of *M. hominis* and may also assist in evasion of host immune responses through antigenic variation. Ureaplasmas also attach to a variety of cell

TABLE 2 Primary sites of colonization by and metabolism characteristics and pathogenicity of mollicutes of human origin[a]

Species	Primary site of colonization		Metabolism of:		Pathogenicity
	Respiratory tract	Genitourinary tract	Glucose	Arginine	
M. salivarium	+	−	−	+	−
M. orale	+	−	−	+	−
M. buccale	+	−	−	+	−
M. faucium	+	−	−	+	−
M. lipophilum	+	−	−	+	−
M. amphoriforme[b]	?+	−	+	−	?
M. pneumoniae	+	−	+	−	+
M. hominis	+	+	−	+	+
M. genitalium[c]	?+	+	+	−	+
M. fermentans	+	+	+	+	+
M. primatum	−	+	−	+	−
M. spermatophilum	−	+	−	+	−
M. pirum	?	?	+	+	−
M. penetrans	−	+	+	+	?
Ureaplasma spp.[d]	+	+	−	−	+
A. laidlawii	+	−	+	−	−

[a] Symbols: +, positive for trait; −, negative for trait;?, unknown.

[b] All nine isolates reported to date have been from the lower respiratory tract, but no other sites have been sampled.

[c] The organism has been found in the oropharynx, but whether that is a common or primary location is not known.

[d] Metabolize urea.

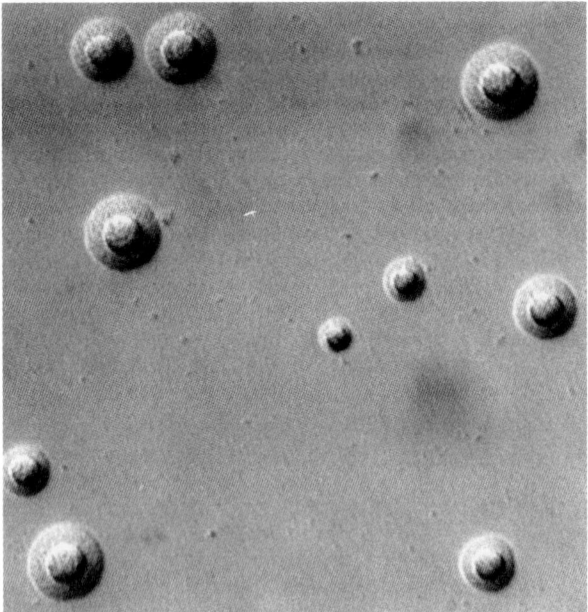

FIGURE 1 Fried-egg-type colonies of *M. hominis* of up to 110 μm in diameter. Magnification, ×132.

types, with attachment mediated by adhesin proteins expressed on the surface of the bacterial cell. The multiple-banded (MB) antigen contains serotype-specific and cross-reactive epitopes and is a prominent antigen recognized during human ureaplasmal infections (116). Ureaplasmas are known to produce immunoglobulin A (IgA) protease which may be associated with disease production, and they release ammonia through urealytic activity (116).

EPIDEMIOLOGY AND TRANSMISSION

Mollicutes are common in practically all mammalian species, as well as many other vertebrates in which they have been sought. Although most mollicutes have species-specific host-organism associations, some mycoplasmas and acholeplasmas of animal origin occur in a wide variety of different animal hosts. Mollicutes in the genera *Spiroplasma, Mesoplasma, Entomoplasma,* and *Acholeplasma* can be isolated from insects and plants.

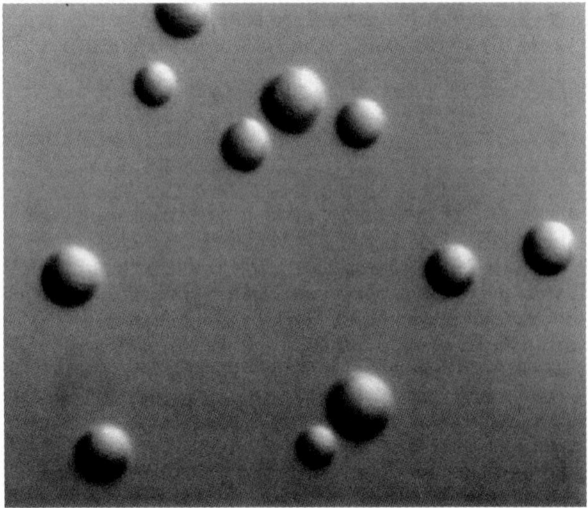

FIGURE 2 Spherical colonies of *M. pneumoniae* of up to 100 μm in diameter. Magnification, ×126.

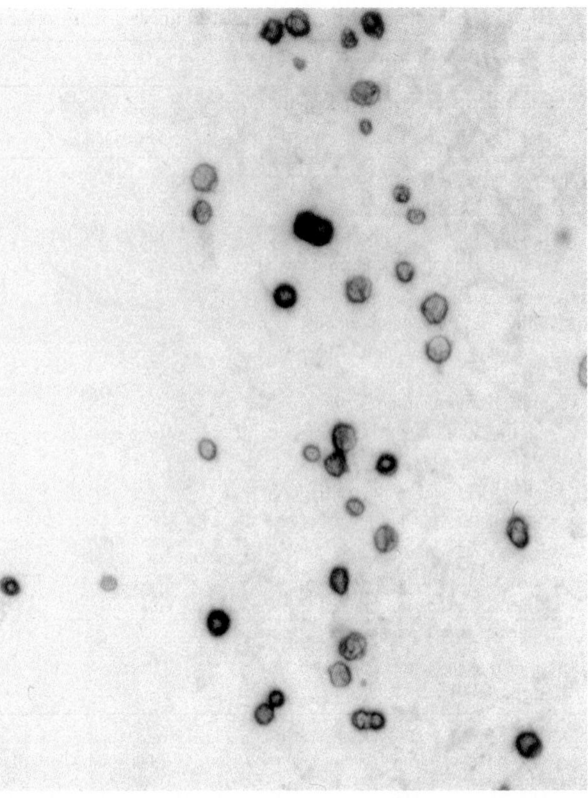

FIGURE 3 Granular, brown, urease-positive colonies of *Ureaplasma* species of 15 to 60 μm in diameter from a vaginal specimen growing on A 8 agar. Magnification, ×100.

In humans, mycoplasmas and ureaplasmas are mucosally associated, residing predominantly in the respiratory or urogenital tract. They rarely penetrate the submucosa, except in cases of immunosuppression or instrumentation, when they may invade the bloodstream and disseminate to many different organs and tissues throughout the body. Many mollicutes exist as commensals in the oropharynx (*M. salivarium, M. orale, M. buccale, M. faucium, M. lipophilum,* and *Acholeplasma laidlawii*) and have been associated with invasive disease only in very rare circumstances. *M. fermentans* has been detected by culture, and more recently by means of PCR assays, in various body sites, including the urogenital tract, throat, lower respiratory tract, and other body locations, including joints (116), but its primary site of colonization and its true disease potential are incompletely understood. Oral commensal mycoplasmas may occasionally spread to the lower respiratory tract and can cause diagnostic confusion with *M. pneumoniae* infection. Frequent occurrence of pathogenic species such as *M. hominis* and ureaplasmas in the lower urogenital tract in healthy men and women has complicated complete understanding of these species' disease-producing capabilities. *M. primatum, M. spermatophilum,* and *Acholeplasma oculi* have been detected in the urogenital tract but have not been associated with disease. PCR assays have demonstrated the frequent occurrence of *M. genitalium* in the urogenital tract in men with urethritis and in lower and upper genital tract sites in women and of *M. penetrans* in urine of homosexual males with human immunodeficiency virus infection (51, 116). Although mycoplasmas are generally considered to be extracellular organisms, intracellular localization is now appreciated for *M. fermentans, M. penetrans, M. genitalium,* and *M. pneumoniae* (11, 28). Intracellular localization may be responsible for protecting the organisms from antibodies and antibiotics, as well as contributing to disease chronicity and difficulty in cultivation in some cases. Variation in surface antigens of *M. hominis* and *Ureaplasma* spp. may be related to the persistence of these organisms at invasive sites. In humans, mycoplasmas and ureaplasmas may be transmitted by direct contact between hosts, e.g., venereally through genital-genital or oral-genital contact and vertically from mother to offspring either at birth or in utero; by respiratory aerosols or fomites in the case of *M. pneumoniae;* or even by nosocomial acquisition through transplanted tissues.

CLINICAL SIGNIFICANCE

Respiratory Infections

M. pneumoniae was first identified and described in the early 1960s. It causes approximately 20% of all community-acquired pneumonias in the general population and up to 50% of pneumonias in certain confined groups (117). Although *M. pneumoniae* has long been associated with pneumonias in school-aged children, adolescents, and young adults, in recent years this organism has also been shown to occur endemically and occasionally epidemically in older persons, as well as children under 5 years of age (117). The most typical clinical syndrome is tracheobronchitis, often accompanied by upper respiratory tract manifestations such as acute pharyngitis. Pneumonia develops in about one-third of persons who are infected. The incubation period is generally 2 to 3 weeks, and spreading throughout households is common. The organism may persist in the respiratory tract for several months after initial infection and sometimes for years in hypogammaglobulinemic patients, possibly because the organism attaches strongly to and invades epithelial cells. Disease tends not to be seasonal, subclinical infections are common, and the disease is ordinarily mild. However, severe infections requiring hospitalization and even resulting in death are known to occur (117).

Extrapulmonary complications of *M. pneumoniae* infections may include meningoencephalitis, ascending paralysis, transverse myelitis, Bell's palsy, pericarditis, hemolytic anemia, arthritis, and mucocutaneous lesions (98, 117). An autoimmune response is thought to play a role in some extrapulmonary complications. However, *M. pneumoniae* has been isolated directly from cerebrospinal, pericardial, and synovial fluids, as well as other extrapulmonary sites, and additional evidence of direct invasion by this organism has been documented by the use of the PCR assay (98). Clinical manifestations are not sufficiently unique to allow differentiation from infections caused by other common bacteria, particularly *Chlamydophila pneumoniae.* Recent data from animal models as well as clinical studies have suggested a potential role for *M. pneumoniae* and *C. pneumoniae* as etiologic or exacerbating factors in bronchial asthma (73), but additional clinical studies are required to determine the ultimate significance of these preliminary findings.

M. fermentans has been recovered from the throats of children with pneumonia, some of whom had no other etiologic agent identified, but the frequency of its occurrence in healthy children is not known (101). It has been detected in adults with an acute influenza-like illness (65) and in bronchoalveolar lavage fluids, peripheral blood lymphocytes, and bone marrow from patients with AIDS and respiratory disease (3, 4). It is apparent that respiratory infection with *M. fermentans* is not necessarily linked with immunodeficiency, but this organism may also behave as an opportunistic respiratory pathogen.

Very little is known about *M. amphoriforme* beyond what has been described in the initial reports of its detection in the lower respiratory tract by culture and/or PCR in a series of patients with antibody deficiencies and chronic bronchitis or bronchiectasis (121). Its biochemical reactivity, colonial appearance, and growth characteristics are similar to those of *M. pneumoniae,* but it is distinct genetically. Repeated isolations over time and clinical improvement after antimicrobial therapy which resulted in the elimination of the mycoplasma suggest a possible pathogenic role, but more work must be done to determine the extent of disease that may be due to this organism.

Genitourinary Infections

Ureaplasma spp. and *M. hominis* can be isolated from the lower genital tract in many healthy, sexually active adults, but there is evidence that these organisms play etiologic roles in some genital tract diseases. Results of human and animal inoculation studies and observations of immunocompromised persons are supportive of ureaplasmas being a cause of nonchlamydial, nongonococcal urethritis (NGU) in men, with further evidence supplied by therapeutic and serologic studies (31, 69, 99, 101). Since the identification of two distinct biovars of *Ureaplasma urealyticum,* biovar 2 *(U. urealyticum)* has been implicated in NGU whereas biovar 1 *(U. parvum)* has not been implicated in this manner (31). Evidence that *M. hominis* causes NGU is lacking. *M. genitalium* has been detected by PCR technology significantly more often in urethral specimens from men with acute NGU than from those without urethritis (51–54) and is now considered to be one of the causes of the disease. *M. genitalium*-positive men have been found to have symptomatic urethritis significantly more often than those infected with *Chlamydia trachomatis* (43). Antibody responses have been detected in some men with acute disease, and *M. genitalium* has also produced urethritis in nonhuman primates (101). *M. genitalium* also may be a rare cause of conjunctivitis associated with urethritis (13). *M. fermentans, M. penetrans,* and *M. pirum* were not detected in the urethras of men with urethritis by PCR assays, suggesting that these organisms are unlikely to have a pathogenic role in this condition (30). In women, there is no evidence that *M. hominis* is a cause of the urethral syndrome, but ureaplasmas may be involved (96).

M. hominis and *Ureaplasma* spp. have not been detected by culture of prostatic biopsy samples from patients with chronic abacterial prostatitis (32), and *M. genitalium* has been found rarely by using a PCR assay (61). In contrast, ureaplasmas have been recovered from an epididymal aspirate from a patient suffering from nonchlamydial, nongonococcal acute epididymo-orchitis accompanied by a specific antibody response (50) and may be an infrequent cause of the disease. *Ureaplasma* spp. produce urease and induce crystallization of struvite and calcium phosphates in urine in vitro and calculi in animal models (109). In addition, ureaplasmas have been found in urinary calculi of patients with infection-type stones more frequently than in those of patients with metabolic-type stones, suggesting a possible causal association (45). *M. hominis* has been isolated from the upper urinary tract only in patients with symptoms of acute pyelonephritis, often with an antibody response, and may cause about 5% of cases of such disease (106). Obstruction or instrumentation of the urinary tract may be a predisposing factor. Ureaplasmas have not been associated in the same way.

Mollicutes do not cause vaginitis but are among various microorganisms that proliferate in patients with bacterial vaginosis (BV). Some studies suggest that *M. hominis* may contribute independently to BV, but evidence is lacking for an independent association of ureaplasmas with BV (116). BV may lead to pelvic inflammatory disease, and *M. hominis* has been isolated from the endometria and fallopian tubes of about 10% of women with salpingitis diagnosed by laparoscopy and accompanied by a specific antibody response (109). The significance of this mycoplasma is difficult to assess in an individual case when several microorganisms are present. Nevertheless, serologic evidence suggests that *M. hominis* may be an independent factor in tubal-factor infertility (7). *Ureaplasma* spp. have been isolated directly from affected fallopian tubes, but not alone. This finding, together with the negative results of serologic tests, studies of inoculation of nonhuman primates, and fallopian tube organ cultures (101), does not support a causal relationship for ureaplasmas in pelvic inflammatory disease. *M. genitalium,* however, may play a role as indicated by its significant association with cervicitis (42, 108) and endometritis (26). In addition, there is serologic evidence that this mycoplasma causes some cases of tubal infertility (24). That ureaplasmas may cause infertility remains speculative (99, 100).

Ureaplasmas have been isolated from internal organs of spontaneously aborted fetuses and from stillborn and premature infants more often than from fetuses from induced abortions or normal full-term infants (116). The results from some serologic and therapeutic studies have also supported a role for these organisms in fetal morbidity (21). BV is a possible confounding factor which must be considered in the association between ureaplasmas in the chorioamnion and low birth weight. Ureaplasmas at this site are directly associated with inflammation (41) and may invade the amniotic sac early in pregnancy in the presence of intact fetal membranes, causing persistent infection and adverse pregnancy outcome (19).

The notion that *M. hominis* causes fever in some women after abortion or after normal delivery is based on its isolation from the blood of about 10% of such women but not from that of afebrile women who have had abortions or that of healthy pregnant women (99). In addition, antibody responses have been detected in about half of febrile aborting women but in few of those who remain afebrile (99). Similar observations have been made for the isolation of *Ureaplasma* spp. which may be responsible for some cases of postpartum endometritis (22). It is possible that ureaplasmas play a causal role in some cases of spontaneous abortion and premature birth through elaboration of phospholipases and stimulation of cytokines which are secreted in response to the presence of the microorganisms in amniotic fluid (116). There is no evidence that *M. genitalium* is a cause of preterm labor or abortion (66, 78).

Neonatal Infections

Colonization of infants by genital mycoplasmas may occur by ascension from the lower genital tract of the mother at the time of delivery or in utero earlier in gestation and may be transient and without sequelae. The rate of vertical transmission may be 18 to 55% among infants born to colonized mothers (116). *Ureaplasma* spp. and *M. hominis* may be isolated from neonates born to mothers with intact membranes and delivered by cesarean section (116). Congenital pneumonia, bacteremia, progression to chronic lung disease of prematurity with the development of inflammatory cytokines in tracheal aspirates, and even death have occurred in very-low-birth-weight infants due to ureaplasmal infection of the lower respiratory tract (116). A meta-analysis of the literature accumulated since the 1980s supports the association of ureaplasmal infection with the development of chronic lung disease (93), but so far there has been no evidence of a reduction in the incidence of chronic lung disease or death when preterm infants have been treated with erythromycin. Both *M. hominis* and *Ureaplasma* spp. have been isolated from maternal and umbilical cord blood, as well as the blood of neonates. Both species can also invade the cerebrospinal fluid of neonates (116). Either mild, subclinical meningitis without sequelae or neurological damage with permanent handicaps may ensue. The frequency of colonization of healthy full-term infants declines after 3 months of age, and fewer than 10% of older children and sexually inexperienced adults are colonized with genital mycoplasmas (116). Vertical transmission of *M. genitalium* from mother to neonate has been reported (67), but its significance in neonates is unknown.

Routine screening of neonates for genital mycoplasmas is not clinically justified based on the available evidence that many healthy neonates may be colonized without consequence. However, if there is clinical, radiological, or laboratory evidence of pneumonia, meningitis, or overall instability, particularly in preterm neonates in whom there are no obvious alternative etiologies, infection with *M. hominis* or *Ureaplasma* spp. should be considered.

Systemic Infections and Immunosuppressed Hosts

Extrapulmonary and extragenital mycoplasmal infections probably occur more often than currently recognized. *M. hominis* is alone among pathogenic mycoplasmas of human origin which may occasionally be detected in routine bacteriologic cultures, so there have been many instances of accidental discovery when mycoplasmas were not specifically sought. Mollicutes can cause invasive disease of the joints as a result of dissemination from the genital or respiratory tract in immunosuppressed persons, especially individuals with hypogammaglobulinemia (109). Mycoplasmas should always be considered early in attempting to diagnose septic arthritis in the setting of congenital antibody deficiency. *M. hominis* bacteremia has been demonstrated after renal transplantation (89), trauma, and genitourinary manipulations, and *M. hominis* has also been found in brain abscesses, osteomyelitis lesions (74), and wound infections, having been isolated, for example, on numerous occasions from sternal wounds in recipients of heart or lung transplants (101). Numerous species, including *M. fermentans, M. salivarium,* and *Ureaplasma* spp., have been detected by culture and/or PCR in synovial fluids of persons with rheumatoid arthritis and other arthritides, although the precise contribution of these organisms to these disease conditions is still uncertain (57, 91, 92). The significance of *M. fermentans* and other mycoplasmas in persons infected with the human immunodeficiency virus, with or without AIDS, has received a great deal of attention. However, the notion that *M. fermentans* is important in AIDS disease progression lacks firm support (109). Despite the fact that mycoplasmas, in particular *M. fermentans,* once received considerable notoriety as possible agents of Gulf War syndrome, there is no credible evidence supporting such an association or causal role (109).

COLLECTION, TRANSPORT, AND STORAGE OF SPECIMENS

Specimen Type and Collection

Body fluids appropriate for mycoplasmal culture or detection by noncultural methods include blood, synovial fluid, amniotic fluid, cerebrospinal fluid, urine, prostatic secretions, semen, wound aspirates, sputum, pleural fluid, bronchoalveolar lavage fluid, and other tracheobronchial secretions, depending on the clinical condition and organisms of interest. Swabs from the nasopharynx, cervix or vagina, wounds, and urethra are also acceptable. Tissue from biopsy or autopsy, including placenta and endometrium tissue, bone chips, and urinary calculi, can also be used. When swabs are used, care must be taken to sample the desired site vigorously to obtain as many cells as possible since mycoplasmas are cell associated. The use of urine specimens may sometimes prove more sensitive than that of urethral swabs for detection of fastidious mycoplasmas such as *M. genitalium* by PCR (52). If determination of the localization of mycoplasmas in the genitourinary tract is desired, urine specimens can be obtained at various stages during urination or after prostatic massage. Care should be taken to avoid collection of specimens that are contaminated by lubricants or antiseptics commonly used in gynecologic practice. Calcium alginate, Dacron, or polyester swabs with aluminum or plastic shafts are preferred. Wooden-shaft cotton swabs should be avoided because of potential inhibitory effects. Swabs should always be removed from specimens before transportation to the laboratory.

Successful isolation of mycoplasmas from blood can be achieved by inoculating blood, free of anticoagulant, into liquid mycoplasmal growth media at the bedside in a 1:10 ratio, using as much blood as possible (at least 10 ml for adults). Mycoplasmas are inhibited by sodium polyanethol sulfonate, the anticoagulant used in most commercial blood culture media, but the inhibitory effect can be overcome by the addition of gelatin (1% [wt/vol]) (83). Use of commercial blood culture media with or without automated blood culture instruments is not recommended for detection of mycoplasmas. None of the newer continuously monitored, nonradiometric, automated blood culture systems will flag bottles containing *M. hominis,* even when additional metabolic substrate and gelatin are added. The organism may survive in these media for several days, however (111).

Transport and Storage

Mycoplasmas are extremely sensitive to adverse environmental conditions, particularly drying and heat. Specimens should be inoculated at the bedside whenever possible by using appropriate transport and/or culture media. Specific mycoplasma media such as SP4 and Shepard's 10 B broths and 2 SP (10% heat-inactivated fetal calf serum with 0.2 M sucrose in 0.02 M phosphate buffer, pH 7.2) are acceptable transport media and can also be used for sample preparation for PCR assays. Other media available commercially for transport and storage of specimens are Stuart's medium, Trypticase soy broth with 0.5% bovine serum albumin, and Mycotrans (Irvine Scientific, Irvine, Calif.). A3B broth (Remel, Inc., Lenexa, Kans.) is available as a transport medium, whereas Remel arginine broth and 10 B and SP4 transport broths also serve as growth media. Liquid specimens do not require special transport media if cultures can be inoculated within 1 h, provided that the specimens are protected from evaporation. Tissues can be placed in a sterile container which can be tightly closed and delivered to the laboratory immediately. Otherwise, tissue specimens should be placed in transport media if delay in culture inoculation is anticipated. Specimens should be refrigerated if immediate transportation to the laboratory is not possible. If specimens must be shipped and/or if the storage time prior to processing is likely to exceed 24 h, the specimen in transport medium should be frozen at −70°C to prevent loss of viability and to minimize bacterial overgrowth. Mollicutes can be stored for long periods in appropriate growth or transport media at −80°C or in liquid nitrogen. Frozen specimens can be shipped with dry ice to a reference laboratory if necessary. Storage at −20°C is deleterious to detection, even by nonculture methods. When frozen specimens are to be examined, they should be thawed rapidly in a water bath at 37°C.

DIRECT EXAMINATION

Microscopy

Mycoplasmas, like chlamydiae and rickettsiae, cannot be clearly visualized by routine light microscopy. Lack of a cell wall precludes visualization of mycoplasmas by Gram staining, but this procedure may prove useful to exclude contaminating bacteria. *M. hominis* may occasionally appear as pinpoint colonies on bacteriologic media, and the lack of a Gram stain reaction by these colonies gives a clue as to their possible mycoplasmal identity, warranting further, more specific evaluation and subculture to mycoplasmal media. A DNA fluorochrome stain such as Hoechst 33258 (ICN Biomedicals, Costa Mesa, Calif.) or acridine orange stain may be useful when applied to body fluids such as amniotic fluid after cytocentrifugation but is not specific for mycoplasmas.

Antigen Detection

Although culture is appropriate for species which can be isolated easily and rapidly from clinical specimens, such as *M. hominis* and *Ureaplasma* spp., it is not ideal for detection of fastidious and/or extremely slow growing organisms such as *M. genitalium* and, to a considerable degree, *M. pneumoniae.* Therefore, alternate non-culture-based methods of detection should be employed even if culture is attempted for these organisms. Rapid methods for antigenic detection of *M. pneumoniae* have been developed, but these techniques are hampered by low sensitivity and cross-reactivity with other commensal mycoplasmas, and they cannot be recommended for diagnostic purposes.

Nucleic Acid Detection Techniques

DNA hybridization techniques for the diagnosis of *M. pneumoniae* infection were developed in the early 1980s. Because probes are relatively insensitive, the more recently available amplification techniques such as the PCR assay have supplanted them, and none are sold commercially in the United States or the United Kingdom.

PCR systems have been developed for all of the clinically important mollicute species that infect humans. Some examples of gene targets used in PCR assays include 16S rRNA (52, 58, 69, 80, 92, 125); other repetitive sequences such as the insertion-like elements of *M. fermentans* (120); the P1 adhesin gene (29, 55, 85), ATPase operon gene (12), and *tuf* gene of *M. pneumoniae* (68); *gap* in *M. hominis* (8); and the MgPa adhesin gene (29, 56) and *gyrA* (15) of *M. genitalium*. Urease genes (14, 124) and the multiple-band antigen gene (59, 82) have been used as targets in *Ureaplasma* spp. Real-time PCR assays have been described for *M. pneumoniae* (72), *M. genitalium* (53, 58, 95), *M. hominis* (8), and *Ureaplasma* spp. (71). For slowly growing organisms such as *M. pneumoniae,* and especially for extremely fastidious species for which optimum cultivation techniques are not established, such as *M. genitalium* and *M. fermentans,* the use of PCR assays may be the only practical means of detecting their presence in clinical material. The sensitivity of PCR is very high, corresponding to a single organism when purified DNA is used. Other advantages are the potential ability to complete the procedure in 1 day, the requirement for only one specimen containing organisms that do not have to be viable, and the ability to detect nucleic acids in preserved tissues.

Comparison of the PCR technique with culture and/or serology, in the case of *M. pneumoniae,* has yielded varied results that are not always in agreement, and large-scale experience with this procedure is still limited. Positive PCR results for *M. pneumoniae* from culture-negative persons without evidence of respiratory disease suggest inadequate assay specificity, persistence of the organism after infection, or existence of the organism in asymptomatic carriers. Positive PCR results from serologically negative persons may be due to an inadequate immune response or to the collection of specimens before specific antibody synthesis could occur. Negative PCR results in cases of culture- or serologic-test-proven infections raise the possibility of inhibitors or other technical problems with the assay. If mycoplasmacidal antibiotics have been administered, PCR results may be negative even though serology is positive. There is some evidence suggesting that PCR inhibition may occur more commonly with nasopharyngeal specimens than throat swabs being assayed for *M. pneumoniae* (35, 86). Commercial reagents available for purification of nucleic acid can be helpful in overcoming PCR inhibition.

In addition to the PCR assays mentioned above, there have been descriptions of multiplex PCR assays to detect *M. genitalium* and other urogenital pathogens (70), a PCR-microtiter plate hybridization assay (125), and a microwell-plate-based PCR assay for large-scale screening for this mycoplasma (38). Since PCR-based assays are the mainstay for diagnosis of *M. genitalium* infection, it is essential that the procedure employed be stringently controlled and carefully monitored. Ideally, positive PCR assays should be confirmed by using a second unrelated target gene. Strong associations between serology and PCR results for *M. genitalium* have been described previously (119), but the analytic sensitivity of a single PCR assay for *M. genitalium* was questioned by Baseman et al. (10), who reported that 61% of culture-positive women tested negative by PCR, despite apparently good quality control parameters for the assay. Assuming that culture positivity was not due to cross contamination, this finding highlights the fact that reduced sensitivity of a single PCR assay may be related to the quality of the specimen or the presence of inhibitors.

PCR technology appears to be less valuable for routine diagnostic purposes in the case of infections with the more rapidly growing and relatively easily cultivable organisms, such as *M. hominis* and *Ureaplasma* spp., but this method can be valuable in clinical studies of ureaplasmal infections. The newest PCR-based techniques permit identification of *Ureaplasma* species as well as limited serotype determination (33, 59, 60, 82). In addition, real-time PCRs that differentiate between *U. urealyticum* and *U. parvum* have been described previously (71).

PCR is also a good tool for identification of an unknown mycoplasma previously obtained by culture. It can be used for characterization of strains within a species and for detection of a specific feature, such as the presence of an antibiotic resistance determinant. Presently, PCR detection for mycoplasmas and most other microorganisms of clinical significance is still too expensive and complex to be carried out routinely in most clinical microbiology laboratories. Some drawbacks must still be corrected, such as the problem of contamination and the presence of inhibitors. Development of commercial PCR kits may bring about better standardization of the technique, and if available at a reasonable cost, PCR could become a major method for the diagnosis of mycoplasmal and ureaplasmal infections.

ISOLATION PROCEDURES

Biosafety Considerations

M. pneumoniae, M. hominis, and ureaplasmas are considered to be category 2 pathogens. Work with these microorganisms and other mycoplasmas of human origin can be undertaken on the laboratory bench and/or in a class 2 safety cabinet.

Growth Media and Inoculation

Growth of mycoplasmas and ureaplasmas pathogenic for humans requires the presence of serum, growth factors such as yeast extract, and a metabolic substrate. No single formulation is ideal for all pertinent species due to different properties, optimum pHs, and substrate requirements. SP4 broth and agar (pH 7.5) are the best media overall and can be used for both *M. pneumoniae* and *M. hominis*, provided that arginine is added for the latter. Shepard's 10 B broth (pH 6.0) can be used for *M. hominis* and *Ureaplasma* spp., with A 8 as the corresponding solid medium. Penicillin G or a broad-spectrum semisynthetic penicillin should be added to minimize bacterial overgrowth. Addition of a pH indicator, such as phenol red, is important for detection because mycoplasmas usually do not produce turbidity in broth culture owing to their small cell size. Compositions of these media are provided elsewhere (110).

Lack of commercially prepared media in the past has effectively prevented many laboratories from offering on-site mycoplasma detection. For self-prepared media, quality control is crucial for each of the main components. These controls must consist of the quantitative growth of a mycoplasma strain(s) in two media that differ only in the component to be tested. New lots or batches of broth are considered satisfactory if the numbers of organisms that grow are within 1 10-fold dilution of the reference batch. Agar plates should ideally support growth of at least 90% of the colonies that are supported by the reference media. Sterility of commercially purchased medium components, such as horse serum, must be confirmed prior to their use. If a reference laboratory is to be used for mycoplasma testing, inquiry should be made as to whether the medium used is self-prepared or purchased from a manufacturer and there should also be verification of the type of quality control procedures performed. Quality control test organisms should include type strains and low-passage-number clinical isolates of the species of interest. For testing of ureaplasmas, it is recommended to include at least one representative from each of the two species. Testing inhibitory properties of media against growth of various other organisms likely present in specimens from nonsterile sites may also be worthwhile to prevent loss of mycoplasmas due to overgrowth of contaminating organisms.

Specimens should always be mixed well before inoculation of media, fluids should be centrifuged (600 × *g* for 15 min), and the pellet should be inoculated. Urine can be filtered through a 0.45-μm-pore-size filter if bacterial contamination is suspected. Furthermore, it is wise to mince, not grind, tissues in broth prior to diluting. Serial dilution of specimens in broth to at least 10^{-3} with subculture of each dilution onto agar is an extremely important step in the cultivation process since it will help overcome possible interference by antibiotics, antibodies, and other inhibitors, including bacteria, that may be present in clinical specimens. Omission of this critical dilution step may be one reason why some laboratories have difficulty in recovering the organisms. Dilution also helps to overcome the problem of rapid decline in culture viability, which is particularly common with ureaplasmas, and it also provides information about the number of organisms present.

Incubation Conditions and Subcultures

Broths should be incubated at 37°C under atmospheric conditions. Agar plates yield the best growth if they are incubated in an atmosphere of room air supplemented with 5 to 10% CO_2 or in an anaerobic environment of 95% N_2 plus 5% CO_2. A candle jar or anaerobe jar with a GasPak catalyst is adequate if dedicated incubators are not available. The relatively rapid growth rates of *M. hominis* and *Ureaplasma* spp. make identification of most positive cultures possible within 2 to 4 days, whereas *M. pneumoniae* usually requires 21 days or more. Several mycoplasmal species of human origin can produce similar biochemical reactions, and identification can be accomplished only by using specific tests once the organisms are isolated. All broths that have changed color should be subcultured into a fresh tube of the corresponding broth (0.1 ml into 0.9 ml) and onto agar (0.02 ml). Subcultures must be performed soon after the color change occurs, particularly if the organism is a *Ureaplasma* species, because the culture can lose viability within a few hours. Subculture also increases the diagnostic yield since some strains may not grow sufficiently from the original specimen inoculated initially onto solid media. Blind subculture periodically during incubation may improve the yield of *M. pneumoniae* and other mycoplasmas since a color change may not always be evident, even if growth occurs. Cultures should be incubated for at least 7 days before being designated negative for genital mycoplasmas and 4 weeks for *M. pneumoniae*. The growth rate of *M. fermentans* is similar to that of *M. pneumoniae*. However, for *M. fermentans*, *M. genitalium*, mycoplasmas of human origin other than *M. pneumoniae* and *M. hominis*, and *Ureaplasma* spp., cultivation conditions are not well established. Due to the advent of PCR assays for use in research and reference laboratories, the need to refine culture techniques for these slowly growing and fastidious organisms is less critical and cultivation methods for them will not be discussed.

Development of Colonies

Broth cultures for *Ureaplasma* spp. should be examined for color change resulting from hydrolysis of urea twice daily for up to 7 days because of the rapid decline in viability of these organisms in culture. This timing is less critical for *Mycoplasma* spp., for which once-daily inspection of broth cultures is sufficient. Agar plates should be examined by using a stereomicroscope at a magnification of ×20 to 60 daily for *Ureaplasma* spp., at 1- to 3-day intervals for *M. hominis*, and every 3 to 5 days for *M. pneumoniae* and other more slowly growing species. *Ureaplasma* colonies (Fig. 3) can be identified on A 8 agar by urease production in the presence of a $CaCl_2$ indicator contained in the medium. The larger *M. hominis* colonies are urease negative and often have the typical fried-egg appearance (Fig. 1). Other species, such as *M. pneumoniae* and *M. genitalium*, will produce much smaller spherical colonies which may or may not demonstrate the fried-egg appearance (Fig. 2). Methylene blue stain applied directly to the agar plate to turn the colonies blue is sometimes useful if there is uncertainty about whether or not mycoplasmal colonies are present. *M. hominis* is the only pathogenic mycoplasma of humans cultivable on bacteriologic media such as chocolate agar and blood agar. However, the pinpoint translucent colonies are easily overlooked and routine bacterial cultures may be discarded before the time needed for *M. hominis* colonies to develop, which may be 4 days or more in some cases. Occurrence of suspicious colonies warrants subculture to appropriate mycoplasma media.

Commercial Media and Culture Kits

In response to the growing desires of many independent or hospital-based clinical laboratories to offer mycoplasmal culturing on-site, numerous companies have developed various transport and growth medium systems. A variety of kits for detection, quantitation, identification, and antimicrobial susceptibility testing of *Ureaplasma* spp. and *M. hominis* from urogenital specimens are available in several European countries but not in the United States. A more complete description of these commercial kits sold in Europe is provided elsewhere (118).

Mycoscreen GU (Irvine Scientific) is a broth-based culture system for screening clinical specimens for genital mycoplasmas. Vials showing evidence of growth as indicated by color change must be subcultured to the Mycotrim GU Triphasic flask system, Mycotrim GU agar, or other solid medium for isolation and identification. A comparable system, Mycotrim RS, has been adapted for detection of *M. pneumoniae* in respiratory specimens. Remel, Inc., has developed several formulations of transport and growth media, including 10 B broth, A 7 agar, A 8 agar, SP4 broth, and SP4 agar.

Some kits and other commercial products and media have been evaluated to a limited degree by independent investigators (1, 16, 23, 25, 81, 94, 123). Commercial products and kits may be of particular value if the need to detect mycoplasmas arises infrequently in laboratories which do not specialize in mycoplasma detection, but users should be aware of the potential limitations of existing products. If commercially prepared media are to be utilized, it is advisable that laboratories perform internal quality control tests.

IDENTIFICATION

Even though the numerous large-colony mycoplasmal species which may be isolated from humans cannot be identified based on colonial morphology or a particular biochemical profile, the body site of origin and rate of growth, in conjunction with biochemical features, give some clues. Biochemical properties such as glucose, arginine, or urea hydrolysis are determined based on color change in the absence of turbidity in the appropriate broth. Utilization of glucose by a mycoplasma in SP4 broth will produce an acidic shift (red to yellow), whereas utilization of arginine will produce a change from red to deeper red in this broth in the presence of the phenol red pH indicator. Urea or arginine hydrolysis in 10 B broth causes an alkaline shift from orange to deep red. Thus, a slowly growing glycolytic organism grown from the respiratory tract that produces spherical colonies on SP4 agar after approximately 5 to 20 days of incubation and exhibits hemolytic activity and hemadsorption with guinea pig erythrocytes is most likely to be *M. pneumoniae*. An alkaline color change which occurs after overnight incubation without turbidity in 10 B broth containing urea is almost certainly due to *Ureaplasma* spp., whereas a urogenital specimen that produces an alkaline reaction within 24 to 72 h in broth supplemented with arginine is likely to contain *M. hominis*. Examination of colonial morphology is sufficient to identify *Ureaplasma* spp., and it is important to keep in mind that these organisms often coexist with *M. hominis* in urogenital specimens.

In order to identify a large-colony mycoplasma completely to the species level, a number of different techniques are available, although they are more appropriate for a reference laboratory than for a hospital microbiology laboratory because of their complexity and the lack of commercial availability of the reagents required. PCR appears to be the best overall choice for mycoplasma species identification since it is much simpler to perform than other methods and it does not require immunologic reagents that may not be readily available. The PCR assay is also less subjective to interpretion than some of the other methods such as epi-immunofluorescence.

TYPING SYSTEMS

Several methods for typing of mollicutes have been described previously and used as a means to study epidemiology in the case of *M. pneumoniae* and differential pathogenicity in the case of the 2 genomic clusters and 14 serotypes of *Ureaplasma* spp. Typing methods have been much less extensively evaluated for other human mycoplasmal species.

Techniques employed initially to serotype ureaplasmas from clinical specimens have included use of polyclonal antibodies (39), immunofluorescence (76), immunoperoxidase (84), and agar growth inhibition (103, 110). Results of earlier studies have been varied and inconsistent due to the inefficient and imprecise methods available, the occurrence of multiple cross-reactions, and the fact that many persons may harbor more than one serotype in their urogenital tracts in the presence or absence of disease. Development of monoclonal antibodies enabled identification of MB antigens responsible for ureaplasma serotype specificity on the cell surface (126). PCR-based assays enabled the more accurate characterization of the two genomic clusters of *Ureaplasma* spp. that led to their designation as two separate species. Pulsed-field gel electrophoresis has been applied to *Ureaplasma* spp. to determine the sizes of the genomes (77, 88), and preliminary information suggests that pulsed-field gel electrophoresis can distinguish among the majority of the 14 *Ureaplasma* serotypes and detect differences within serotypes (K. B. Waites, unpublished data).

Restriction fragment length polymorphism, multilocus sequence typing, Western blotting, two-dimensional gel electrophoresis, and PCR assays have been used to characterize *M. pneumoniae* clinical isolates (27, 34, 37, 49, 79, 90). Most evaluations have determined that there are two genomic groups or subtypes distinguishable by analysis of the P1 adhesin gene, ORF6 gene, P65 gene, and typical DNA restriction fragment pattern. Typing of human mycoplasmas or ureaplasmas for diagnostic or epidemiological purposes is not recommended, and the methods are unavailable except in specialized research or reference laboratories.

SEROLOGIC TESTS

M. pneumoniae Respiratory Disease

Historically, serology has been the most common laboratory means for diagnosis of *M. pneumoniae* respiratory tract infections. Although culture and PCR are also used to detect the presence of *M. pneumoniae* in respiratory specimens, persistence of the organism for variable lengths of time following acute infection makes it difficult in some cases to assess the significance of a positive culture or PCR assay without additional confirmatory tests such as seroconversion.

M. pneumoniae has both lipid and protein antigens which elicit antibody responses that can be detected after about 1 week of illness and peak at 3 to 6 weeks, followed by a gradual decline, allowing the application of several different types of serologic assays based on different antigens and technologies. Serology is a very useful epidemiologic tool in circumstances where the likelihood of mycoplasmal disease is high, but it is less suited for assessment of individual patients in a timely manner. Its main disadvantage is the need for both acute- and convalescent-phase paired sera collected 2 to 3 weeks apart that are tested simultaneously for IgM and IgG to confirm seroconversion. This is especially important for adults over 40 years of age who may not mount an IgM response, presumably because of reinfection (117). Moreover, IgM antibodies can sometimes persist for several weeks to months, making it risky to base diagnosis of acute infection on a single assay for IgM (117). Antibody production may also be delayed in some infections or even absent if the patient is immunosuppressed. False-negative tests for IgM can also occur if serum is collected too soon after the onset of illness. Since *M. pneumoniae* is a mucosal pathogen, IgA is typically produced early in the course of infection. Measurement of IgA in serum may therefore be a better approach for diagnosis of acute infection because of IgA's rapid rise and decline, but very few commercial assays include reagents for IgA detection.

Complement fixation (CF) was the primary method for serologic testing for *M. pneumoniae* in the past. Although CF measures mainly the early IgM response, the test does not differentiate among antibody classes. Cross-reactions with other organisms, most notably *M. genitalium* (63), are well recognized, and false-positive results due to cross-reactive autoantibodies induced by acute inflammation from other unrelated causes may occur. In most clinical laboratories, CF has been replaced by alternative techniques. Table 3 summarizes various assays used to detect *M. pneumoniae* infection in the United States. More detailed descriptions of individual assay kits are available in other reference texts (see, e.g., reference 118).

Immunofluorescent-antibody (IFA) assays, direct and indirect hemagglutination using IgM capture, and other particle agglutination antibody assays (PAs) have been developed to detect antibody to *M. pneumoniae* (5, 40, 62). IFA assays consist of *M. pneumoniae* antigen affixed to microscope slides and measure IgM and IgG separately. This type of assay is technically simple to perform but is subjective in interpretation and requires a fluorescent microscope, and the presence of *M. pneumoniae*-specific IgG may interfere with IgM results (5). Qualitative and semiquantitative PAs using either latex beads or gelatin that detect IgM and IgG simultaneously can be technically easy to perform, but they do not offer any significant advantages over enzyme immunoassays (EIAs). Though commonly used in some countries because of their ease and simplicity of performance, PAs have not been widely used for serologic diagnosis of *M. pneumoniae* infections in the United States.

EIAs, developed in the 1970s, have become the most widely used methods for detection of *M. pneumoniae* antibody in the United States. All are classified as having either moderate or high complexity according to the Clinical Laboratory Improvement Amendments. They may be qualitative or quantitative and may or may not require specialized

TABLE 3 Examples of test kits sold in the United States for detection of serum antibodies to *M. pneumoniae* in serum[a]

Product name	Manufacturer	Antibody(ies) measured	Assay format and description	No. of tests/kit	Specimen throughput	Assay time	
						Start to finish	Hands on
M. pneumoniae antibody (MP) test system	Zeus Scientific, Inc., Branchburg, N.J.	IgM and IgG separately	Indirect immunofluorescence assay available as a slurry of *M. pneumoniae* antigenic substrate or a Crown Titer of *M. pneumoniae* colonies affixed to microscope slides	100	Each slide contains 10 wells	2.5 h	30 min
ETI-MP IgM or IgG	Savyon Diagnostics, Ltd., Ashdod, Israel	IgM and IgG separately	EIA using a 96-well microtiter plate coated with a membrane preparation containing *M. pneumoniae* P1 protein	192	Strips of 8 wells	2.5 h	15–20 min
Immuno*Card*	Meridian Diagnostics, Cincinnati, Ohio	IgM only	Qualitative, membrane-based EIA in a single-sample-card format consisting of a test port containing *M. pneumoniae* antigen and a control port containing immobilized human IgM	30	1 specimen per card	12 min	10 min
M. pneumoniae IgG-IgM antibody test system	Remel, Inc., Lenexa, Kans.	IgM and IgG simultaneously	Qualitative, membrane-based enzyme immunobinding assay consisting of a single sample test containing inactivated *M. pneumoniae* cytadhesin protein	10 or 40	1 specimen per card	10 min	2–3 min
Mycoplasma IgG and IgM enzyme-linked immunosorbent assay system	Zeus Scientific, Inc.	IgM and IgG separately	Qualitative EIA with multiwell break-away strips containing partially purified inactivated *M. pneumoniae*	96	Strips of 8 wells	50 min	5–10 min
GenBio Immuno-WELL *M. pneumoniae* IgM or IgG	Alexon-Trend Inc., Ramsey, Minn.	IgM and IgG separately	EIA using a 96-well microtiter plate coated with purified glycolipid antigen from *M. pneumoniae* (strain FH; ATCC 15531)	96	Strips of 8 wells	IgG, 2.35 h; IgM, 2.75 h	15–20 min

[a] This table does not include all commercially available test kits sold in the United States for serologic diagnosis of *M. pneumoniae* infections. It provides descriptions of tests representing various formats and is limited to those products that have been evaluated in independent studies.

equipment. EIAs are more sensitive than CF or culture, have good specificity, and can be performed with very small volumes of serum. The need for acute- and convalescent-phase sera has remained the obvious limitation for prompt point-of-care diagnosis. However, a membrane-based EIA specific for IgM, the Immuno*Card* (Meridian Diagnostics, Cincinnati, Ohio), has been developed for rapidly detecting an acute *M. pneumoniae* infection by using a single serum specimen. The Immuno*Card* has the advantages of being technically much simpler and quicker (10 min) to perform than other types of assays. It has proved highly reliable for children but has the potential disadvantage of a lack of sensitivity for detection of *M. pneumoniae* infections in some adults in whom the IgM response may be minimal. The Remel EIA is another rapid point-of-care qualitative serologic assay that detects both IgM and IgG simultaneously in an easy-to-read format without the need for any instrumentation. This test has shown good sensitivity and specificity compared to other EIAs, IFA assays, and CF tests. Several comparison studies have been performed, individually evaluating each of the EIA kits listed in Table 3 and several others (5, 6, 9, 40, 62, 97, 104, 105). The best commercial EIA for individual patient diagnosis depends on the age of the patient being tested, the timing of serum collection, the availability of paired sera, the equipment available, and the experience of the laboratory personnel who will perform the test. However, maintaining a large variety of different assays within one laboratory is not practical or cost-effective. According to a recent study (97), the rapid Remel and Meridian tests are better able to detect seropositive samples than the plate type EIAs. Among the latter assays, the Zeus and Savyon kits were more sensitive than the GenBio assay.

Cold agglutinins, detected by agglutination of type O, Rh-negative erythrocytes at 4°C, occur in association with *M. pneumoniae* infection in about 50% of cases (20). Titers of 64 to 128 or a fourfold or greater rise in titer suggests a recent *M. pneumoniae* infection, but the test is nonspecific. Detection of cold agglutinins is not recommended for serologic diagnosis of *M. pneumoniae* infection.

Infections Due to Genital Mycoplasmas

Serologic tests for *M. hominis* and *Ureaplasma* spp. using the techniques of microimmunofluorescence, metabolism inhibition, and EIA have been described previously (17, 18, 64, 102, 103). A microimmunofluorescence assay for *M. genitalium* has also been developed (44) and has been shown to detect antibody responses in men with NGU (99) and women with salpingitis (75). This method is rapid, gives reproducible results, and is quite sensitive and specific, with less cross-reactivity with *M. pneumoniae* than is seen with other methods. A sensitive and specific serologic assay for *M. genitalium* using lipid-associated membrane proteins as antigens has also been developed, and this technique has been used in combination with Western immunoblotting to assess immunoreactivities of women regarded as being culture positive for *M. genitalium* (10). No serologic tests for genital mycoplasmas have been standardized and made commercially available for diagnostic use in the United States. Therefore, they cannot be recommended for routine diagnostic purposes.

ANTIBIOTIC SUSCEPTIBILITIES

Methods Used for Testing

Several methods of susceptibility testing used for conventional bacteria have been employed for testing of mycoplasmas. Agar dilution has been used extensively as a reference method (12, 51, 64). It has the advantages that the end point is relatively stable over time, the inoculum size does not have a great effect, and the method allows detection of mixed cultures readily. However, this technique is not practical for testing small numbers of strains or occasional isolates which may be encountered in diagnostic laboratories. Agar disk diffusion is not useful for testing mycoplasmas since there has been no correlation between inhibitory zones and MICs, and the relatively slow growth of some of these organisms further limits this technology. Broth microdilution to determine MICs is the most practical and widely used method. It is economical and allows several antimicrobials to be tested on the same microtiter plate, but it has numerous disadvantages in that preparation of antimicrobial dilutions is labor-intensive and the end point tends to shift over time. Limited comparisons of agar dilution and broth microdilution indicate that the two methods provide similar results for various antimicrobials tested against *Ureaplasma* spp. and *M. hominis* (47, 115).

Studies using the E test (AB BIODISK, Solna, Sweden) agar gradient diffusion technique for detection of tetracycline resistance in *M. hominis* yielded results comparable to those of broth microdilution (113). Additional comparative studies have also validated this method for determination of in vitro susceptibilities of *M. hominis* to fluoroquinolones (112) and susceptibilities of ureaplasmas to various antimicrobials (36). The E test has the advantages that agar-based testing is relatively simple to perform, the end point does not shift over time, the inoculum size does not have a large effect, and the method can easily be adapted for testing of single isolates.

There are no universally accepted standards for pH, media, incubation conditions, or duration of incubation for performing mycoplasmal or ureaplasmal susceptibility tests. No MIC breakpoints specific for these organisms are endorsed by any regulatory agency. Lack of specific guidelines for susceptibility testing methods, quality control reference MIC ranges, and interpretation of results has led to diverse and often inconsistent susceptibility profiles, especially for the genital mycoplasmas.

MIC assays must include control strains for validation purposes. A control strain may be a commercially purchased type strain or a well-studied clinical isolate for which MIC values are reproducible. An inoculum of 10^4 to 10^5 CFU/ml has been recommended as the optimum inoculum for broth-based testing (110, 114). Nonstandardized conditions at a low pH (6.0) can affect MICs, especially those of macrolides, but such conditions may be required for adequate growth of *Ureaplasma* spp. Step-by-step procedures for performance of in vitro susceptibility tests for mycoplasmas and ureaplasmas of human origin have been published previously (114). Bactericidal activity can be tested directly from the wells in broth microdilution MIC assays by removing the mixture of organisms and antibiotic, diluting it to subinhibitory concentrations in fresh medium, and observing for a color change as evidence of growth (110, 114).

Although some reference laboratories have adopted MIC breakpoints for other bacteria for use in interpretation of MICs when testing mycoplasmas, this practice should be used with caution, and it may be preferable merely to report MICs and allow clinicians to draw their own conclusions about the suitability of a particular agent for use in the treatment of a specific infection. Tetracycline-resistant *M. hominis* and *Ureaplasma* spp. can usually be distinguished by broth- or agar-based methods since MICs for the resistant strains are generally 2 to ≥64 μg/ml (113, 116).

Commercial MIC panels in kits have been available in Europe for several years. Details on these products are provided in reference texts (118).

Susceptibility Profiles and Antimicrobial Resistance

The availability of information on in vitro susceptibilities is greatest for *M. pneumoniae, M. hominis,* and *Ureaplasma* spp., but in some recent studies the activities of numerous antimicrobials against *M. fermentans* and *M. genitalium* have been evaluated. Though incompletely studied, *M. genitalium* has susceptibilities generally similar to those of *M. pneumoniae,* and *M. fermentans* has susceptibilities generally similar to those of *M. hominis,* with some exceptions. A comparison of MICs of several antimicrobial agents is shown in Table 4.

Susceptibility Testing and Treatment of Mycoplasmal Infections

Mollicutes are innately resistant to all beta-lactams. Sulfonamides, trimethoprim, and rifampicin are also inactive. Resistance to macrolides and lincosamides is variable according to species, with *M. hominis* being resistant to erythromycin but susceptible to clindamycin. For *Ureaplasma* spp., the reverse is true. Newer macrolides, azalides, and ketolides have shown in vitro activity comparable to that of erythromycin against *M. pneumoniae.*

M. pneumoniae is susceptible to newer fluoroquinolones, tetracyclines, and macrolides so that susceptibility testing has not been recommended except for the in vitro evaluation of new and previously untested agents. However, a recent study from Japan found that macrolide resistance in *M. pneumoniae* due to transition mutations in domain V on the 23S rRNA gene occurred in approximately 6% of 195 clinical isolates from patients with acute respiratory infections (75a). The clinical significance of this resistance is uncertain, but it suggests the need to monitor clinical isolates. Tetracycline resistance has been well documented in recent years for both *M. hominis* and *Ureaplasma* spp. and is mediated by the *tet*(M) determinant which codes for a protein

TABLE 4 Ranges of MICs of various antimicrobials for *M. pneumoniae*, *M. hominis*, *M. fermentans*, *M. genitalium*, and *Ureaplasma* spp.[a]

Antimicrobial	MIC (μg/ml) for:				
	M. pneumoniae	*M. hominis*	*M. genitalium*	*M. fermentans*	*Ureaplasma* spp.
Tetracycline	0.63–0.25	0.2–2[b]	≤0.01–0.05	0.1–1	0.05–2[b]
Doxycycline	0.02–0.5	0.1–2[b]	≤0.01–0.3	0.05–1	0.02–1[b]
Tigecycline	0.06–0.25	0.125–0.5	ND	ND	1–16
Erythromycin	≤0.004–0.06	32–>1,000	≤0.01	0.5–64	0.02–16
Roxithromycin	≤0.01	>16	0.01	32–64	0.1–2
Dirithromycin	≤0.015–0.5	>64	≤0.015–0.125	≥64	0.25–4
Clarithromycin	≤0.004–0.125	16–>256	≤0.01	1–64	≤0.004–2
Azithromycin	≤0.004–0.01	4–64	≤0.01	≤0.003–0.05	0.5–4
Josamycin	≤0.01–0.03	0.05–2	0.01–0.03	0.1–0.5	0.03–4
Clindamycin	≤0.008–2	≤0.008–2	0.2–1	0.01–0.25	0.2–64
Lincomycin	4–8	0.2–1	1–8	ND	8–256
Pristinamycin	0.02–0.05	0.1–0.5	≤0.01–0.02	ND	0.1–1
Spiramycin	≤0.015–0.25	32–>64	0.125–1	2–4	4–32
Telithromycin	≤0.008–0.06	2–32	≤0.015	0.06–0.25	≤0.015–0.25
Cethromycin	≤0.001–0.016	≤0.008–0.031	ND	≤0.008	≤0.008–0.031
Chloramphenicol	2	2–25	ND	0.5–10	0.4–8
Gentamicin	4	2–16	ND	0.25–>500	0.1–13
Ciprofloxacin	0.5–2	0.1–4	2	0.02–>64	0.1–16
Ofloxacin	0.05–2	0.1–64	1–2	0.02–25	0.2–25
Levofloxacin	0.5–1	0.1–2	0.5–1	0.05–1	0.2–2
Sparfloxacin	≤0.008–0.5	≤0.008–0.1	0.05–0.1	≤0.01–0.05	0.003–1
Gatifloxacin	0.031–1	0.016–0.25	0.125	≤0.008–0.25	0.125–2
Moxifloxacin	0.06–0.125	0.06–0.125	0.03–0.06	≤0.015–0.06	0.125–1
Garenoxacin	≤0.008–0.125	≤0.008–0.063	0.06–0.125	≤0.008–0.015	0.016–1
Gemifloxacin	0.05–0.125	0.0025–0.01	0.05–0.125	0.001–0.01	0.03–0.5
Rifampin	>8	>1,000	ND	25–>50	>1,000
Quinupristin-dalfopristin	0.008–0.06	0.03–8	0.05	0.1–0.5	0.03–0.5
Linezolid	≥64	2–8	ND	ND	>64

[a] Data were compiled from multiple published studies in which different methodologies, and often different antimicrobial concentrations, were used. ND, no data available.
[b] Tetracycline-susceptible strains only. MICs for isolates carrying *tet*(M) are generally 2 to >64 μg/ml.

that binds to the ribosomes, protecting them from the actions of this type of drug. The extent to which tetracycline resistance occurs in genital mycoplasmas varies geographically and according to prior antimicrobial exposure in different populations but may approach 40 to 50%. Information about tetracycline resistance in *M. genitalium* does not exist, but *M. genitalium*-positive men with NGU and women with cervicitis may respond better to azithromycin than they do to a tetracycline, possibly because of the lower MICs. There are very little outcome data documented in a controlled setting with microbiological studies to demonstrate the efficacy of antimicrobial treatment of *M. genitalium* infections. Such information is needed in view of the growing importance of this mycoplasma in sexually transmitted disease. Other agents such as streptogramins, aminoglycosides, and chloramphenicol may show in vitro activity against some mollicute species. Though data are very limited, oxazolidinones such as linezolid appear to be inactive against mycoplasmas.

Extragenital infections, often in immunocompromised hosts, may be caused by multidrug-resistant mycoplasmas and ureaplasmas, making guidance of chemotherapy by in vitro susceptibility tests important in this clinical setting. Eradication of infection under these circumstances can be extremely difficult, requiring prolonged therapy, even when the organisms are susceptible to the expected agents. This difficulty highlights the facts that mollicutes are inhibited but not killed by most commonly used bacteriostatic antimicrobial agents in concentrations achievable in vivo and that a functioning immune system plays an integral part in their eradication. Fluoroquinolones such as levofloxacin, moxifloxacin, and gatifloxacin tend to have greater in vitro activity against mollicutes than older drugs such as ciprofloxacin, but resistant strains have been reported (116). Treatment of mycoplasmal and ureaplasmal infections has been reviewed elsewhere (98, 116, 117).

EVALUATION, INTERPRETATION, AND REPORTING OF RESULTS

Tests offered through diagnostic microbiology laboratories should focus on the species known to cause human disease and for which cultivation techniques are best defined. Unusual organisms, or those for which cultivation conditions are not established, may be detectable by PCR technology offered through a few specialized research or reference laboratories. Such organisms should be sought only after consultation with clinicians and personnel from the reference laboratory. Except for *Ureaplasma* spp., which can be identified by urease production and distinct colonial morphology, until species identification can be confirmed, a preliminary report of "large-colony *Mycoplasma* species" is appropriate. In many instances, as in culturing of specimens from the lower genital tract, this information may be sufficient. Isolates from normally sterile sites and/or from immunosuppressed persons should be identified to the species level.

M. pneumoniae

Detection of *M. pneumoniae* in culture is time-consuming and not overly sensitive. However, isolation of the organism from respiratory tract specimens is clinically significant in most instances and should be correlated with the presence of clinical respiratory disease since a small proportion of asymptomatic carriers may exist. Detection by PCR is becoming more widely available through reference laboratories, but a positive result must still be correlated with clinical events. Reliable serology remains critical for accurate diagnosis of acute *M. pneumoniae* respiratory disease. Detection of IgG and IgM antibodies by EIA is the method of choice. A fourfold rise in antibody titer between acute- and convalescent-phase sera is considered diagnostic of acute infection. For children, adolescents, and young adults, a single positive IgM result obtained by using appropriate immunoglobulin class-specific reagents may be considered diagnostic of acute infection in most but not necessarily all cases because of the possibility of prolonged IgM elevation. Mild respiratory infections due to *M. pneumoniae* do not merit a costly and time-consuming microbiological work-up since empiric treatment will be effective in most instances.

M. hominis

M. hominis can be detected in culture within a few days. It may occasionally be discovered in routine bacteriologic media from appropriate clinical material, but such detection should not be relied upon. Its isolation in any quantity from normally sterile body fluids or tissues is significantly associated with disease, but quantitation of organisms may be of value in other circumstances. When mycoplasmas are detected in nonsterile sites such as the female lower genital tract in numbers exceeding 10^5 organisms, the mycoplasmas are most likely to be associated with BV.

Ureaplasma Species

Ureaplasma species can be detected in culture within 24 to 48 h. The characteristic colonial morphology and urease production are sufficient for identification at the genus level. Isolation in any quantity from normally sterile body fluids or tissues is significantly associated with disease. The detection of fewer than 10^4 organisms in the male urethra is unlikely to be significant. Whether this is true for each species now designated within the genus, i.e., *U. urealyticum* and *U. parvum*, is not clear. Distinguishing between the two species of *Ureaplasma* by PCR may become more important in view of possible differences in pathogenicities in some circumstances (2, 31, 33).

M. genitalium

Growing evidence for the role of *M. genitalium* as a urogenital pathogen has generated interest in the development of diagnostic methods for its detection, though no molecular biology-based assays for direct detection or serology test kits are sold commercially. Even though cultivation techniques for *M. genitalium* have been described previously (10, 54, 107), relatively few clinical isolates have actually been obtained since the initial description of this mycoplasma in the early 1980s. Slow growth, requiring 6 weeks or longer even in enriched SP4 media, and poor sensitivity make culture impractical. The potential importance of this organism in sexually transmitted urogenital infections underscores the need for improved and standardized methods for its detection. At present, noncommercial, nonstandardized PCR-based assays are all that are available. Results of these assays should be used with caution if they are adapted and employed for diagnostic purposes. When *M. genitalium* is detected in clinical specimens from a urogenital tract site such as the male urethra or the female cervix in persons with clinical evidence of urethritis or cervicitis, it should be considered medically significant.

REFERENCES

1. **Abele-Horn, M., C. Blendinger, C. Becher, P. Emmerling, and G. Ruckdeschel.** 1996. Evaluation of commercial kits for quantitative identification and tests on antibiotic susceptibility of genital mycoplasmas. *Zentbl. Bakteriol.* **284:**540–549.
2. **Abele-Horn, M., C. Wolff, P. Dressel, F. Pfaff, and A. Zimmermann.** 1997. Association of *Ureaplasma urealyticum* biovars with clinical outcome for neonates, obstetric patients, and gynecological patients with pelvic inflammatory disease. *J. Clin. Microbiol.* **35:**1199–1202.
3. **Ainsworth, J. G., J. Clarke, R. Goldin, and D. Taylor-Robinson.** 2000. Disseminated *Mycoplasma fermentans* in AIDS patients: several case reports. *Int. J. STD AIDS* **11:**751–755.
4. **Ainsworth, J. G., J. Clarke, M. Lipman, D. Mitchell, and D. Taylor-Robinson.** 2000. Detection of *Mycoplasma fermentans* in broncho-alveolar lavage fluid specimens from AIDS patients with lower respiratory tract infection. *HIV Med.* **1:**219–223.
5. **Alexander, T. S., L. D. Gray, J. A. Kraft, D. S. Leland, M. T. Nikaido, and D. H. Willis.** 1996. Performance of Meridian ImmunoCard *Mycoplasma* test in a multicenter clinical trial. *J. Clin. Microbiol.* **34:**1180–1183.
6. **Aubert, G., B. Pozzetto, O. G. Gaudin, J. Hafid, A. D. Mbida, and A. Ros.** 1992. Evaluation of five commercial tests: complement fixation, microparticle agglutination, indirect immunofluorescence, enzyme-linked immunosorbent assay and latex agglutination, in comparison to immunoblotting for *Mycoplasma pneumoniae* serology. *Ann. Biol. Clin.* (Paris) **50:**593–597.
7. **Baczynska, A., H. Friis Svenstrup, J. Fedder, S. Birkelund, and G. Christiansen.** 2005. The use of enzyme-linked immunosorbent assay for detection of *Mycoplasma hominis* antibodies in infertile women serum samples. *Hum. Reprod.* **20:**1277–1285.
8. **Baczynska, A., H. F. Svenstrup, J. Fedder, S. Birkelund, and G. Christiansen.** 2004. Development of real-time PCR for detection of *Mycoplasma hominis*. *BMC Microbiol.* **4:**35.
9. **Barker, C. E., M. Sillis, and T. G. Wreghitt.** 1990. Evaluation of Serodia Myco II particle agglutination test for detecting *Mycoplasma pneumoniae* antibody: comparison with mu-capture ELISA and indirect immunofluorescence. *J. Clin. Pathol.* **43:**163–165.
10. **Baseman, J. B., M. Cagle, J. E. Korte, C. Herrera, W. G. Rasmussen, J. G. Baseman, R. Shain, and J. M. Piper.** 2004. Diagnostic assessment of *Mycoplasma genitalium* in culture-positive women. *J. Clin. Microbiol.* **42:**203–211.
11. **Baseman, J. B., and J. G. Tully.** 1997. Mycoplasmas: sophisticated, reemerging, and burdened by their notoriety. *Emerg. Infect. Dis.* **3:**21–32.
12. **Bernet, C., M. Garret, B. de Barbeyrac, C. Bebear, and J. Bonnet.** 1989. Detection of *Mycoplasma pneumoniae* by using the polymerase chain reaction. *J. Clin. Microbiol.* **27:**2492–2496.
13. **Bjornelius, E., J. S. Jensen, and P. Lidbrink.** 2 September 2004, posting date. Conjunctivitis associated with *Mycoplasma genitalium* infection. *Clin. Infect. Dis.* **39:**e67–e69. [Online.] http://www.journals.uchicago.edu/CID/Journal/contentsv39n7.html.

14. **Blanchard, A., J. Hentschel, L. Duffy, K. Baldus, and G. H. Cassell.** 1993. Detection of *Ureaplasma urealyticum* by polymerase chain reaction in the urogenital tract of adults, in amniotic fluid, and in the respiratory tract of newborns. *Clin. Infect. Dis.* **17**(Suppl. 1):S148–S153.
15. **Blaylock, M. W., O. Musatovova, J. G. Baseman, and J. B. Baseman.** 2004. Determination of infectious load of *Mycoplasma genitalium* in clinical samples of human vaginal cells. *J. Clin. Microbiol.* **42:**746–752.
16. **Broitman, N. L., C. M. Floyd, C. A. Johnson, L. M. de la Maza, and E. M. Peterson.** 1992. Comparison of commercially available media for detection and isolation of *Ureaplasma urealyticum* and *Mycoplasma hominis*. *J. Clin. Microbiol.* **30:**1335–1337.
17. **Brown, M. B., G. H. Cassell, W. M. McCormack, and J. K. Davis.** 1987. Measurement of antibody to *Mycoplasma hominis* by an enzyme-linked immunoassay and detection of class-specific antibody responses in women with postpartum fever. *Am. J. Obstet. Gynecol.* **156:**701–708.
18. **Brown, M. B., G. H. Cassell, D. Taylor-Robinson, and M. C. Shepard.** 1983. Measurement of antibody to *Ureaplasma urealyticum* by an enzyme-linked immunosorbent assay and detection of antibody responses in patients with nongonococcal urethritis. *J. Clin. Microbiol.* **17:**288–295.
19. **Cassell, G. H., R. O. Davis, K. B. Waites, M. B. Brown, P. A. Marriott, S. Stagno, and J. K. Davis.** 1983. Isolation of *Mycoplasma hominis* and *Ureaplasma urealyticum* from amniotic fluid at 16–20 weeks of gestation: potential effect on outcome of pregnancy. *Sex. Transm. Dis.* **10:**294–302.
20. **Cassell, G. H., G. Gambill, and L. B. Duffy.** 1996. ELISA in respiratory infections of humans, p. 123–136. *In* J. G. Tully and S. Razin (ed.), *Molecular and Diagnostic Procedures in Diagnostic Mycoplasmology.* Academic Press, New York, N.Y.
21. **Cassell, G. H., K. B. Waites, and D. T. Crouse.** 2001. Mycoplasmal infections, p. 733–767. *In* J. S. Remington and J. O. Klein (ed.), *Infectious Diseases of the Fetus and Newborn Infant,* 5th ed. W. B. Saunders Co., Inc., Philadelphia, Pa.
22. **Chaim, W., S. Horowitz, J. B. David, F. Ingel, B. Evinson, and M. Mazor.** 2003. *Ureaplasma urealyticum* in the development of postpartum endometritis. *Eur. J. Obstet. Gynecol. Reprod. Biol.* **109:**145–148.
23. **Cheah, F. C., T. P. Anderson, B. A. Darlow, and D. R. Murdoch.** 2005. Comparison of the *Mycoplasma* Duo test with PCR for detection of ureaplasma species in endotracheal aspirates from premature infants. *J. Clin. Microbiol.* **43:**509–510.
24. **Clausen, H. F., J. Fedder, M. Drasbek, P. K. Nielsen, B. Toft, H. J. Ingerslev, S. Birkelund, and G. Christiansen.** 2001. Serological investigation of *Mycoplasma genitalium* in infertile women. *Hum. Reprod.* **16:**1866–1874.
25. **Clegg, A., M. Passey, M. Yoannes, and A. Michael.** 1997. High rates of genital mycoplasma infection in the highlands of Papua New Guinea determined both by culture and by a commercial detection kit. *J. Clin. Microbiol.* **35:**197–200.
26. **Cohen, C. R., L. E. Manhart, E. A. Bukusi, S. Astete, R. C. Brunham, K. K. Holmes, S. K. Sinei, J. J. Bwayo, and P. A. Totten.** 2002. Association between *Mycoplasma genitalium* and acute endometritis. *Lancet* **359:**765–766.
27. **Cousin-Allery, A., A. Charron, B. de Barbeyrac, G. Fremy, J. Skov Jensen, H. Renaudin, and C. Bebear.** 2000. Molecular typing of *Mycoplasma pneumoniae* strains by PCR-based methods and pulsed-field gel electrophoresis. Application to French and Danish isolates. *Epidemiol. Infect.* **124:**103–111.
28. **Dallo, S. F., and J. B. Baseman.** 2000. Intracellular DNA replication and long-term survival of pathogenic mycoplasmas. *Microb. Pathog.* **29:**301–309.
29. **de Barbeyrac, B., C. Bernet-Poggi, F. Febrer, H. Renaudin, M. Dupon, and C. Bebear.** 1993. Detection of *Mycoplasma pneumoniae* and *Mycoplasma genitalium* in clinical samples by polymerase chain reaction. *Clin. Infect. Dis.* **17**(Suppl. 1): S83–S89.
30. **Deguchi, T., C. B. Gilroy, and D. Taylor-Robinson.** 1996. Failure to detect *Mycoplasma fermentans*, *Mycoplasma penetrans*, or *Mycoplasma pirum* in the urethra of patients with acute nongonococcal urethritis. *Eur. J. Clin. Microbiol. Infect. Dis.* **15:**169–171.
31. **Deguchi, T., T. Yoshida, T. Miyazawa, M. Yasuda, M. Tamaki, H. Ishiko, and S. Maeda.** 2004. Association of *Ureaplasma urealyticum* (biovar 2) with nongonococcal urethritis. *Sex. Transm. Dis.* **31:**192–195.
32. **Doble, A., B. J. Thomas, P. M. Furr, M. M. Walker, J. R. W. Harris, R. O. Witherow, and D. Taylor-Robinson.** 1989. A search for infectious agents in chronic abacterial prostatitis using ultrasound guided biopsy. *Br. J. Urol.* **64:**297–301.
33. **Domingues, D., L. T. Tavira, A. Duarte, A. Sanca, E. Prieto, and F. Exposto.** 2002. *Ureaplasma urealyticum* biovar determination in women attending a family planning clinic in Guine-Bissau, using polymerase chain reaction of the multiple-banded antigen gene. *J. Clin. Lab. Anal.* **16:**71–75.
34. **Dorigo-Zetsma, J. W., J. Dankert, and S. A. Zaat.** 2000. Genotyping of *Mycoplasma pneumoniae* clinical isolates reveals eight P1 subtypes within two genomic groups. *J. Clin. Microbiol.* **38:**965–970.
35. **Dorigo-Zetsma, J. W., R. P. Verkooyen, H. P. van Helden, H. van der Nat, and J. M. van den Bosch.** 2001. Molecular detection of *Mycoplasma pneumoniae* in adults with community-acquired pneumonia requiring hospitalization. *J. Clin. Microbiol.* **39:**1184–1186.
36. **Dosa, E., E. Nagy, W. Falk, I. Szoke, and U. Ballies.** 1999. Evaluation of the Etest for susceptibility testing of *Mycoplasma hominis* and *Ureaplasma urealyticum*. *J. Antimicrob. Chemother.* **43:**575–578.
37. **Dumke, R., I. Catrein, E. Pirkil, R. Herrmann, and E. Jacobs.** 2003. Subtyping of *Mycoplasma pneumoniae* isolates based on extended genome sequencing and on expression profiles. *Int. J. Med. Microbiol.* **292:**513–525.
38. **Dutro, S. M., J. K. Hebb, C. A. Garin, J. P. Hughes, G. E. Kenny, and P. A. Totten.** 2003. Development and performance of a microwell-plate-based polymerase chain reaction assay for *Mycoplasma genitalium*. *Sex. Transm. Dis.* **30:**756–763.
39. **Echahidi, F., G. Muyldermans, S. Lauwers, and A. Naessens.** 2000. Development of monoclonal antibodies against *Ureaplasma urealyticum* serotypes and their use for serotyping clinical isolates. *Clin. Diagn. Lab. Immunol.* **7:**563–567.
40. **Echevarria, J. M., P. Leon, P. Balfagon, J. A. Lopez, and M. V. Fernandez.** 1990. Diagnosis of *Mycoplasma pneumoniae* infection by microparticle agglutination and antibody-capture enzyme-immunoassay. *Eur. J. Clin. Microbiol. Infect. Dis.* **9:**217–220.
41. **Eschenbach, D. A.** 1993. *Ureaplasma urealyticum* and premature birth. *Clin. Infect. Dis.* **17**(Suppl. 1):S100–S106.
42. **Falk, L., H. Fredlund, and J. S. Jensen.** 2005. Signs and symptoms of urethritis and cervicitis among women with or without *Mycoplasma genitalium* or *Chlamydia trachomatis* infection. *Sex. Transm. Infect.* **81:**73–78.
43. **Falk, L., H. Fredlund, and J. S. Jensen.** 2004. Symptomatic urethritis is more prevalent in men infected with *Mycoplasma genitalium* than with *Chlamydia trachomatis*. *Sex. Transm. Infect.* **80:**289–293.
44. **Furr, P. M., and D. Taylor-Robinson.** 1984. Microimmunofluorescence technique for detection of antibody to *Mycoplasma genitalium*. *J. Clin. Pathol.* **37:**1072–1074.
45. **Grenabo, L., H. Hedelin, and S. Pettersson.** 1988. Urinary infection stones caused by *Ureaplasma urealyticum*: a review. *Scand. J. Infect. Dis. Suppl.* **53:**46–49.

46. **Henrich, B., R. C. Feldmann, and U. Hadding.** 1993. Cytoadhesins of *Mycoplasma hominis*. *Infect. Immun.* **61:** 2945–2951.
47. **Hilliard, N. J., L. B. Duffy, D. M. Crabb, and K. B. Waites.** 2005. In vitro comparison of agar and microbroth dilution methods for determination of MICs for *Mycoplasma hominis*. *J. Microbiol. Methods* **60:**285–288.
48. **Hu, P. C., U. Schaper, A. M. Collier, W. A. Clyde, Jr., M. Horikawa, Y. S. Huang, and M. F. Barile.** 1987. A *Mycoplasma genitalium* protein resembling the *Mycoplasma pneumoniae* attachment protein. *Infect. Immun.* **55:**1126–1131.
49. **Jacobs, E., A. Pilatschek, B. Gerstenecker, K. Oberle, and W. Bredt.** 1990. Immunodominant epitopes of the adhesin of *Mycoplasma pneumoniae*. *J. Clin. Microbiol.* **28:** 1194–1197.
50. **Jalil, N., A. Doble, C. Gilchrist, and D. Taylor-Robinson.** 1988. Infection of the epididymis by *Ureaplasma urealyticum*. *Genitourin. Med.* **64:**367–368.
51. **Jensen, J. S.** 2004. *Mycoplasma genitalium:* the aetiological agent of urethritis and other sexually transmitted diseases. *J. Eur. Acad. Dermatol. Venereol.* **18:**1–11.
52. **Jensen, J. S., E. Bjornelius, B. Dohn, and P. Lidbrink.** 2004. Comparison of first void urine and urogenital swab specimens for detection of *Mycoplasma genitalium* and *Chlamydia trachomatis* by polymerase chain reaction in patients attending a sexually transmitted disease clinic. *Sex. Transm. Dis.* **31:** 499–507.
53. **Jensen, J. S., E. Bjornelius, B. Dohn, and P. Lidbrink.** 2004. Use of TaqMan 5′ nuclease real-time PCR for quantitative detection of *Mycoplasma genitalium* DNA in males with and without urethritis who were attendees at a sexually transmitted disease clinic. *J. Clin. Microbiol.* **42:**683–692.
54. **Jensen, J. S., H. T. Hansen, and K. Lind.** 1996. Isolation of *Mycoplasma genitalium* strains from the male urethra. *J. Clin. Microbiol.* **34:**286–291.
55. **Jensen, J. S., J. Sondergard-Andersen, S. A. Uldum, and K. Lind.** 1989. Detection of *Mycoplasma pneumoniae* in simulated clinical samples by polymerase chain reaction. Brief report. *APMIS* **97:**1046–1048.
56. **Jensen, J. S., S. A. Uldum, J. Sondergard-Andersen, J. Vuust, and K. Lind.** 1991. Polymerase chain reaction for detection of *Mycoplasma genitalium* in clinical samples. *J. Clin. Microbiol.* **29:**46–50.
57. **Johnson, S., D. Sidebottom, F. Bruckner, and D. Collins.** 2000. Identification of *Mycoplasma fermentans* in synovial fluid samples from arthritis patients with inflammatory disease. *J. Clin. Microbiol.* **38:**90–93.
58. **Jurstrand, M., J. S. Jensen, H. Fredlund, L. Falk, and P. Molling.** 2005. Detection of *Mycoplasma genitalium* in urogenital specimens by real-time PCR and by conventional PCR assay. *J. Med. Microbiol.* **54:**23–29.
59. **Knox, C. L., and P. Timms.** 1998. Comparison of PCR, nested PCR, and random amplified polymorphic DNA PCR for detection and typing of *Ureaplasma urealyticum* in specimens from pregnant women. *J. Clin. Microbiol.* **36:**3032–3039.
60. **Kong, F., Z. Ma, G. James, S. Gordon, and G. L. Gilbert.** 2000. Molecular genotyping of human *Ureaplasma* species based on multiple-banded antigen (MBA) gene sequences. *Int. J. Syst. Evol. Microbiol.* **50**(Pt. 5)**:**1921–1929.
61. **Krieger, J. N., D. E. Riley, M. C. Roberts, and R. E. Berger.** 1996. Prokaryotic DNA sequences in patients with chronic idiopathic prostatitis. *J. Clin. Microbiol.* **34:** 3120–3128.
62. **Lieberman, D., S. Horowitz, O. Horovitz, F. Schlaeffer, and A. Porath.** 1995. Microparticle agglutination versus antibody-capture enzyme immunoassay for diagnosis of community-acquired *Mycoplasma pneumoniae* pneumonia. *Eur. J. Clin. Microbiol. Infect. Dis.* **14:**577–584.
63. **Lind, K.** 1982. Serological cross-reactions between "*Mycoplasma genitalium*" and *M. pneumoniae*. *Lancet* **ii:**1158–1159.
64. **Lo, S. C., R. Y. Wang, T. Grandinetti, N. Zou, C. L. Haley, M. M. Hayes, D. J. Wear, and J. W. Shih.** 2003. *Mycoplasma hominis* lipid-associated membrane protein antigens for effective detection of *M. hominis*-specific antibodies in humans. *Clin. Infect. Dis.* **36:**1246–1253.
65. **Lo, S. C., D. J. Wear, S. L. Green, P. G. Jones, and J. F. Legier.** 1993. Adult respiratory distress syndrome with or without systemic disease associated with infections due to *Mycoplasma fermentans*. *Clin. Infect. Dis.* **17**(Suppl. 1)**:** S259–S263.
66. **Lu, G. C., J. R. Schwebke, L. B. Duffy, G. H. Cassell, J. C. Hauth, W. W. Andrews, and R. L. Goldenberg.** 2001. Midtrimester vaginal *Mycoplasma genitalium* in women with subsequent spontaneous preterm birth. *Am. J. Obstet. Gynecol.* **185:**163–165.
67. **Luki, N., P. Lebel, M. Boucher, B. Doray, J. Turgeon, and R. Brousseau.** 1998. Comparison of polymerase chain reaction assay with culture for detection of genital mycoplasmas in perinatal infections. *Eur. J. Clin. Microbiol. Infect. Dis.* **17:** 255–263.
68. **Luneberg, E., J. S. Jensen, and M. Frosch.** 1993. Detection of *Mycoplasma pneumoniae* by polymerase chain reaction and nonradioactive hybridization in microtiter plates. *J. Clin. Microbiol.* **31:**1088–1094.
69. **Maeda, S., T. Deguchi, H. Ishiko, T. Matsumoto, S. Naito, H. Kumon, T. Tsukamoto, S. Onodera, and S. Kamidono.** 2004. Detection of *Mycoplasma genitalium*, *Mycoplasma hominis*, *Ureaplasma parvum* (biovar 1) and *Ureaplasma urealyticum* (biovar 2) in patients with non-gonococcal urethritis using polymerase chain reaction-microtiter plate hybridization. *Int. J. Urol.* **11:**750–754.
70. **Mahony, J. B., D. Jang, S. Chong, K. Luinstra, J. Sellors, M. Tyndall, and M. Chernesky.** 1997. Detection of *Chlamydia trachomatis*, *Neisseria gonorrhoeae*, *Ureaplasma urealyticum*, and *Mycoplasma genitalium* in first-void urine specimens by multiplex polymerase chain reaction. *Mol. Diagn.* **2:**161–168.
71. **Mallard, K., K. Schopfer, and T. Bodmer.** 2005. Development of real-time PCR for the differential detection and quantification of *Ureaplasma urealyticum* and *Ureaplasma parvum*. *J. Microbiol. Methods* **60:**13–19.
72. **Maltezou, H. C., B. La-Scola, H. Astra, I. Constantopoulou, V. Vlahou, D. A. Kafetzis, A. G. Constantopoulos, and D. Raoult.** 2004. *Mycoplasma pneumoniae* and *Legionella pneumophila* in community-acquired lower respiratory tract infections among hospitalized children: diagnosis by real time PCR. *Scand. J. Infect. Dis.* **36:**639–642.
73. **Martin, R. J., M. Kraft, H. W. Chu, E. A. Berns, and G. H. Cassell.** 2001. A link between chronic asthma and chronic infection. *J. Allergy Clin. Immunol.* **107:**595–601.
74. **Meyer, R. D., and W. Clough.** 1993. Extragenital *Mycoplasma hominis* infections in adults: emphasis on immunosuppression. *Clin. Infect. Dis.* **17**(Suppl. 1)**:**S243–S249.
75. **Moller, B. R., D. Taylor-Robinson, and P. M. Furr.** 1984. Serological evidence implicating *Mycoplasma genitalium* in pelvic inflammatory disease. *Lancet* **i:**1102–1103.

75a. **Morozumi, M., K. Hasegawa, R. Kobayashi, N. Inoue, S. Iwata, H. Kuroki, N. Kawamura, E. Nakayama, T. Tajima, K. Shimizu, and K. Ubukata.** 2005. Emergence of macrolide-resistant *Mycoplasma pneumoniae* with a 23S rRNA gene mutation. *Antimicrob. Agents Chemother.* **49:**2302–2306.

76. **Naessens, A., W. Foulon, J. Breynaert, and S. Lauwers.** 1988. Serotypes of *Ureaplasma urealyticum* isolated from normal pregnant women and patients with pregnancy complications. *J. Clin. Microbiol.* **26:**319–322.

77. **Neimark, H. C., and C. S. Lange.** 1990. Pulse-field electrophoresis indicates full-length *Mycoplasma* chromosomes range widely in size. *Nucleic Acids Res.* **18:**5443–5448.
78. **Oakeshott, P., P. Hay, D. Taylor-Robinson, S. Hay, B. Dohn, S. Kerry, and J. S. Jensen.** 2004. Prevalence of *Mycoplasma genitalium* in early pregnancy and relationship between its presence and pregnancy outcome. *BJOG* **111:** 1464–1467.
79. **Ovyn, C., D. van Strijp, M. Ieven, D. Ursi, B. van Gemen, and H. Goossens.** 1996. Typing of *Mycoplasma pneumoniae* by nucleic acid sequence-based amplification, NASBA. *Mol. Cell. Probes* **10:**319–324.
80. **Perni, S. C., S. Vardhana, I. Korneeva, S. L. Tuttle, L. R. Paraskevas, S. T. Chasen, R. B. Kalish, and S. S. Witkin.** 2004. *Mycoplasma hominis* and *Ureaplasma urealyticum* in midtrimester amniotic fluid: association with amniotic fluid cytokine levels and pregnancy outcome. *Am. J. Obstet. Gynecol.* **191:**1382–1386.
81. **Phillips, L. E., K. H. Goodrich, R. M. Turner, and S. Faro.** 1986. Isolation of *Mycoplasma* species and *Ureaplasma urealyticum* from obstetrical and gynecological patients by using commercially available medium formulations. *J. Clin. Microbiol.* **24:**377–379.
82. **Pitcher, D., M. Sillis, and J. A. Robertson.** 2001. Simple method for determining biovar and serovar types of *Ureaplasma urealyticum* clinical isolates using PCR-single-strand conformation polymorphism analysis. *J. Clin. Microbiol.* **39:**1840–1844.
83. **Pratt, B. C.** 1991. Recovery of *Mycoplasma hominis* from blood culture media. *Med. Lab. Sci.* **48:**350.
84. **Quinn, P. A., L. U. Arshoff, and H. C. Li.** 1981. Serotyping of *Ureaplasma urealyticum* by immunoperoxidase assay. *J. Clin. Microbiol.* **13:**670–676.
85. **Ramirez, J. A., S. Ahkee, A. Tolentino, R. D. Miller, and J. T. Summersgill.** 1996. Diagnosis of *Legionella pneumophila*, *Mycoplasma pneumoniae*, or *Chlamydia pneumoniae* lower respiratory infection using the polymerase chain reaction on a single throat swab specimen. *Diagn. Microbiol. Infect. Dis.* **24:**7–14.
86. **Reznikov, M., T. K. Blackmore, J. J. Finlay-Jones, and D. L. Gordon.** 1995. Comparison of nasopharyngeal aspirates and throat swab specimens in a polymerase chain reaction-based test for *Mycoplasma pneumoniae*. *Eur. J. Clin. Microbiol. Infect. Dis.* **14:**58–61.
87. **Robertson, J. A., M. Alfa, and E. S. Boatman.** 1983. Morphology of the cells and colonies of *Mycoplasma hominis*. *Sex. Transm. Dis.* **10:**232–239.
88. **Robertson, J. A., L. E. Pyle, G. W. Stemke, and L. R. Finch.** 1990. Human ureaplasmas show diverse genome sizes by pulsed-field electrophoresis. *Nucleic Acids Res.* **18:**1451–1455.
89. **Rohner, P., I. Schnyder, B. Ninet, J. Schrenzel, D. Lew, T. Ramla, J. Garbino, and V. Jacomo.** 2004. Severe *Mycoplasma hominis* infections in two renal transplant patients. *Eur. J. Clin. Microbiol. Infect. Dis.* **23:**203–204.
90. **Sasaki, T., T. Kenri, N. Okazaki, M. Iseki, R. Yamashita, M. Shintani, Y. Sasaki, and M. Yayoshi.** 1996. Epidemiological study of *Mycoplasma pneumoniae* infections in Japan based on PCR-restriction fragment length polymorphism of the P1 cytadhesin gene. *J. Clin. Microbiol.* **34:** 447–449.
91. **Schaeverbeke, T., C. B. Gilroy, C. Bebear, J. Dehais, and D. Taylor-Robinson.** 1996. *Mycoplasma fermentans*, but not *M. penetrans*, detected by PCR assays in synovium from patients with rheumatoid arthritis and other rheumatic disorders. *J. Clin. Pathol.* **49:**824–828.
92. **Schaeverbeke, T., H. Renaudin, M. Clerc, L. Lequen, J. P. Vernhes, B. De Barbeyrac, B. Bannwarth, C. Bebear, and J. Dehais.** 1997. Systematic detection of mycoplasmas by culture and polymerase chain reaction (PCR) procedures in 209 synovial fluid samples. *Br. J. Rheumatol.* **36:**310–314.
93. **Schelonka, R. L., B. Katz, K. B. Waites, and D. Benjamin.** 2005. A critical appraisal of the role of *Ureaplasma* and development of bronchopulmonary dysplasia using metaanalytic techniques. *Pediatr. Infect. Dis.* **24:**1033–1039.
94. **Sillis, M.** 1993. Genital mycoplasmas revisited—an evaluation of a new culture medium. *Br. J. Biomed. Sci.* **50:**89–91.
95. **Simms, I., K. Eastick, H. Mallinson, K. Thomas, R. Gokhale, P. Hay, A. Herring, and P. A. Rogers.** 2003. Associations between *Mycoplasma genitalium*, *Chlamydia trachomatis* and pelvic inflammatory disease. *J. Clin. Pathol.* **56:**616–618.
96. **Stamm, W. E., K. Running, J. Hale, and K. K. Holmes.** 1983. Etiologic role of *Mycoplasma hominis* and *Ureaplasma urealyticum* in women with the acute urethral syndrome. *Sex. Transm. Dis.* **10:**318–322.
97. **Talkington, D. F., S. Shott, M. T. Fallon, S. B. Schwartz, and W. L. Thacker.** 2004. Analysis of eight commercial enzyme immunoassay tests for detection of antibodies to *Mycoplasma pneumoniae* in human serum. *Clin. Diagn. Lab. Immunol.* **11:**862–867.
98. **Talkington, D. F., K. B. Waites, S. B. Schwartz, and R. E. Besser.** 2001. Emerging from obscurity: understanding pulmonary and extrapulmonary syndromes, pathogenesis, and epidemiology of human *Mycoplasma pneumoniae* infections, p. 57–84. *In* W. M. Scheld, W. A. Craig, and J. M. Hughes (ed.), *Emerging Infections 5*. American Society for Microbiology, Washington, D.C.
99. **Taylor-Robinson, D.** 1989. Genital mycoplasma infections. *Clin. Lab. Med.* **9:**501–523.
100. **Taylor-Robinson, D.** 1986. Evaluation of the role of *Ureaplasma urealyticum* in infertility. *Pediatr. Infect. Dis.* **5:**S262–S265.
101. **Taylor-Robinson, D.** 1996. Infections due to species of *Mycoplasma* and *Ureaplasma:* an update. *Clin. Infect. Dis.* **23:**671–684.
102. **Taylor-Robinson, D.** 1983. Metabolism inhibition test, p. 411–417. *In* J. G. Tully and S. Razin (ed.), *Methods in Mycoplasmology*, vol. 1. Academic Press, New York, N.Y.
103. **Taylor-Robinson, D., and C. W. Csonka.** 1981. Laboratory and clinical aspects of mycoplasmal infections of the human genitourinary tract, p. 151–186. *In* J. W. Harris (ed.), *Recent Advances in Sexually Transmitted Diseases*, no. 2. Churchill Livingstone, Ltd., Edinburgh, United Kingdom.
104. **Thacker, W. L., and D. F. Talkington.** 2000. Analysis of complement fixation and commercial enzyme immunoassays for detection of antibodies to *Mycoplasma pneumoniae* in human serum. *Clin. Diagn. Lab. Immunol.* **7:**778–780.
105. **Thacker, W. L., and D. F. Talkington.** 1995. Comparison of two rapid commercial tests with complement fixation for serologic diagnosis of *Mycoplasma pneumoniae* infections. *J. Clin. Microbiol.* **33:**1212–1214.
106. **Thomsen, A. C.** 1978. Mycoplasmas in human pyelonephritis: demonstration of antibodies in serum and urine. *J. Clin. Microbiol.* **8:**197–202.
107. **Tully, J. G., D. Taylor-Robinson, D. L. Rose, R. M. Cole, and J. M. Bove.** 1983. *Mycoplasma genitalium*, a new species from the human urogenital tract. *Int. J. Syst. Bacteriol.* **33:**387–396.
108. **Uno, M., T. Deguchi, H. Komeda, M. Hayasaki, M. Iida, M. Nagatani, and Y. Kawada.** 1997. *Mycoplasma genitalium* in the cervices of Japanese women. *Sex. Transm. Dis.* **24:**284–286.
109. **Waites, K., and D. Talkington.** 2005. New developments in human diseases due to mycoplasmas, p. 289–354. *In*

A. Blanchard and G. Browning (ed.), *Mycoplasmas: Pathogenesis, Molecular Biology, and Emerging Strategies for Control.* Horizon Scientific Press, Norwich, United Kingdom.

110. **Waites, K. B., C. M. Bebear, J. A. Robertson, D. F. Talkington, and G. E. Kenny (ed.).** 2001. *Cumitech 34, Laboratory Diagnosis of Mycoplasmal Infections.* American Society for Microbiology, Washington, D.C.

111. **Waites, K. B., and K. C. Canupp.** 2001. Evaluation of BacT/ALERT system for detection of *Mycoplasma hominis* in simulated blood cultures. *J. Clin. Microbiol.* **39:**4328–4331.

112. **Waites, K. B., K. C. Canupp, and G. E. Kenny.** 1999. In vitro susceptibilities of *Mycoplasma hominis* to six fluoroquinolones as determined by E test. *Antimicrob. Agents Chemother.* **43:**2571–2573.

113. **Waites, K. B., D. M. Crabb, L. B. Duffy, and G. H. Cassell.** 1997. Evaluation of the Etest for detection of tetracycline resistance in *Mycoplasma hominis. Diagn. Microbiol. Infect. Dis.* **27:**117–122.

114. **Waites, K. B., L. B. Duffy, S. Schwartz, and D. F. Talkington.** 2004. *Mycoplasma* and *Ureaplasma,* p. 3.15.1–3.15.17. *In* H. Isenberg (ed.), *Clinical Microbiology Procedures Handbook,* 2nd ed. ASM Press, Washington, D.C.

115. **Waites, K. B., T. A. Figarola, T. Schmid, D. M. Crabb, L. B. Duffy, and J. W. Simecka.** 1991. Comparison of agar versus broth dilution techniques for determining antibiotic susceptibilities of *Ureaplasma urealyticum. Diagn. Microbiol. Infect. Dis.* **14:**265–271.

116. **Waites, K. B., B. Katz, and R. L. Schelonka.** 2005. Mycoplasmas and ureaplasmas as neonatal pathogens. *Clin. Microbiol. Rev.* **18:**757–789.

117. **Waites, K. B., and D. F. Talkington.** 2004. *Mycoplasma pneumoniae* and its role as a human pathogen. *Clin. Microbiol. Rev.* **17:**697–728.

118. **Waites, K. B., D. F. Talkington, and C. M. Bebear.** 2002. Mycoplasmas, p. 201–224. *In* A. L. Truant (ed.), *Manual of Commercial Methods in Clinical Microbiology.* American Society for Microbiology, Washington, D.C.

119. **Wang, R. Y., T. Grandinetti, J. W. Shih, S. H. Weiss, C. L. Haley, M. M. Hayes, and S. C. Lo.** 1997. *Mycoplasma genitalium* infection and host antibody immune response in patients infected by HIV, patients attending STD clinics and in healthy blood donors. *FEMS Immunol. Med. Microbiol.* **19:**237–245.

120. **Wang, R. Y., W. S. Hu, M. S. Dawson, J. W. Shih, and S. C. Lo.** 1992. Selective detection of *Mycoplasma fermentans* by polymerase chain reaction and by using a nucleotide sequence within the insertion sequence-like element. *J. Clin. Microbiol.* **30:**245–248.

121. **Webster, D., H. Windsor, C. Ling, D. Windsor, and D. Pitcher.** 2003. Chronic bronchitis in immunocompromised patients: association with a novel *Mycoplasma* species. *Eur. J. Clin. Microbiol. Infect.* **22:**530–534.

122. **Wilson, M. H., and A. M. Collier.** 1976. Ultrastructural study of *Mycoplasma pneumoniae* in organ culture. *J. Bacteriol.* **125:**332–339.

123. **Wood, J. C., R. M. Lu, E. M. Peterson, and L. M. de la Maza.** 1985. Evaluation of Mycotrim-GU for isolation of *Mycoplasma* species and *Ureaplasma urealyticum. J. Clin. Microbiol.* **22:**789–792.

124. **Yoon, B. H., R. Romero, J. H. Lim, S. S. Shim, J. S. Hong, J. Y. Shim, and J. K. Jun.** 2003. The clinical significance of detecting *Ureaplasma urealyticum* by the polymerase chain reaction in the amniotic fluid of patients with preterm labor. *Am. J. Obstet. Gynecol.* **189:**919–924.

125. **Yoshida, T., S. Maeda, T. Deguchi, T. Miyazawa, and H. Ishiko.** 2003. Rapid detection of *Mycoplasma genitalium, Mycoplasma hominis, Ureaplasma parvum,* and *Ureaplasma urealyticum* organisms in genitourinary samples by PCR-microtiter plate hybridization assay. *J. Clin. Microbiol.* **41:**1850–1855.

126. **Zheng, X., L. J. Teng, H. L. Watson, J. I. Glass, A. Blanchard, and G. H. Cassell.** 1995. Small repeating units within the *Ureaplasma urealyticum* MB antigen gene encode serovar specificity and are associated with antigen size variation. *Infect. Immun.* **63:**891–898.

Chlamydia and *Chlamydophila**

ANDREAS ESSIG

65

TAXONOMY AND NOMENCLATURE

Chlamydia and *Chlamydophila* are nonmotile, obligate intracellular prokaryotic pathogens characterized by a unique biphasic developmental cycle bearing two chlamydial forms that differ essentially in terms of morphology and function. According to the *Approved List of Bacterial Names,* published in 1980, the *Chlamydiaceae* contained one genus with just two species, *Chlamydia trachomatis* and *Chlamydia psittaci,* which were separated by their capability to accumulate glycogen in inclusions (Fig. 1A) and their susceptibility to sulfadiazine. In the 1990s, the application of DNA-based classification methods contributed to the recognition of the emerging human pathogen *Chlamydia pneumoniae* (35) and of *Chlamydia pecorum* (31), a pathogen of ruminants, as new species of the *Chlamydiaceae*. Phylogenetic analyses of the 16S and 23S rRNA genes were the rationale for the proposal of an emended description of the order *Chlamydiales,* and a revised taxonomy of the family *Chlamydiaceae* in 1999 (25). According to this proposal, members of the order *Chlamydiales* are obligately intracellular bacteria that have the unique chlamydia-like developmental cycle and more than 80% sequence identity with chlamydial 16S rRNA genes and/or 23S rRNA genes. The emended order now includes four families: *Chlamydiaceae, Parachlamydiaceae, Simkaniaceae* (49), and *Waddliaceae* (87).

Early divergence of *C. trachomatis*-like strains in the *Chlamydiaceae* was postulated on the basis of sequence data from the ribosomal genes and supported by other data such as genome size, glycogen production, and *ompA* sequence analysis. This led to the proposal to divide the family *Chlamydiaceae* into two genera, *Chlamydia* and *Chlamydophila* (25). As a consequence *Chlamydia pneumoniae, Chlamydia psittaci,* and *Chlamydia pecorum* were placed into the new genus *Chlamydophila*. However, the newly proposed nomenclature was controversial. The division into two genera was especially objected to by experts in the field who argued that the new genus designations ignore the unique, highly conserved biology shared by these organisms that was recognized when they were in a single genus (92). Although the new taxonomy was validly published, the ongoing debate resulted in simultaneous use of the former and the new nomenclature in the literature.

*This chapter contains material presented in chapter 63 by James B. Mahony, Brian K. Coombes, and Max A. Chernesky in the eighth edition of this Manual.

DESCRIPTION OF THE *CHLAMYDIACEAE*

The *Chlamydiaceae* contain the known human pathogens *C. trachomatis, C. pneumoniae,* and *C. psittaci* as well as organisms such as *C. abortus* and *C. felis* that have been only rarely associated with human infections. Members of the *Chlamydiaceae* show less than 10% overall 16S rRNA gene diversity and less than 10% overall 23S rRNA gene diversity. The 16S rRNA gene of the *C. abortus* strain B 577 (accession no. D85709) has been suggested as a consensus sequence for the family (25). The genome sizes of the *Chlamydiaceae* range from 1.0 to 1.24 Mbp with a G+C content of about 40%.

The cell wall harbors a common lipopolysaccharide (LPS) that differs from LPS of other bacteria in its relatively low endotoxic activity. This has been related to its lipid A, which has unusual long-chain fatty acids (12). Accounting for about 60% of the protein mass, the 40-kDa chlamydial major outer membrane protein (MOMP), encoded by the *ompA* gene, is an important structural component of the organisms' outer membrane. The variable domains (VD1 through 4) lead to multiple *C. trachomatis* serovars associated with different clinical manifestations of oculogenital infections. In contrast, *C. pneumoniae* isolates possess a strikingly high MOMP homology (45) and serovars of *C. pneumoniae* have not been described. The 60-kDa cysteine-rich OMP 2 (OmcB) is also highly conserved and could account for the osmotic stability of elementary bodies (EBs) by forming a disulfide–cross-links network with the periplasmic MOMP domains and other proteins (26). OmcB binds heparin, and this may be related to mammalian host cell adhesion and entry (102).

The unique developmental cycle differentiates chlamydiae from all other bacteria, leading to important consequences in laboratory diagnosis, clinical course, and antibiotic therapy. So-called EBs of chlamydiae infect eukaryotic host cells and can survive for only a limited period of time outside the host cell. Once inside the host cell, they differentiate to metabolically active reticulate bodies (RB) that multiply by binary fission (Fig. 1D) within vacuoles that are continuously growing and that develop into large intracytoplasmic inclusions (Fig. 1C). Reticulate bodies reorganize back to EBs at the end of the chlamydial developmental cycle (Fig. 1D). After 48 to 72 h, hundreds of EBs are released from the host cell to perpetuate the infectious cycle. Genomic transcriptional analysis of the chlamydial developmental cycle revealed

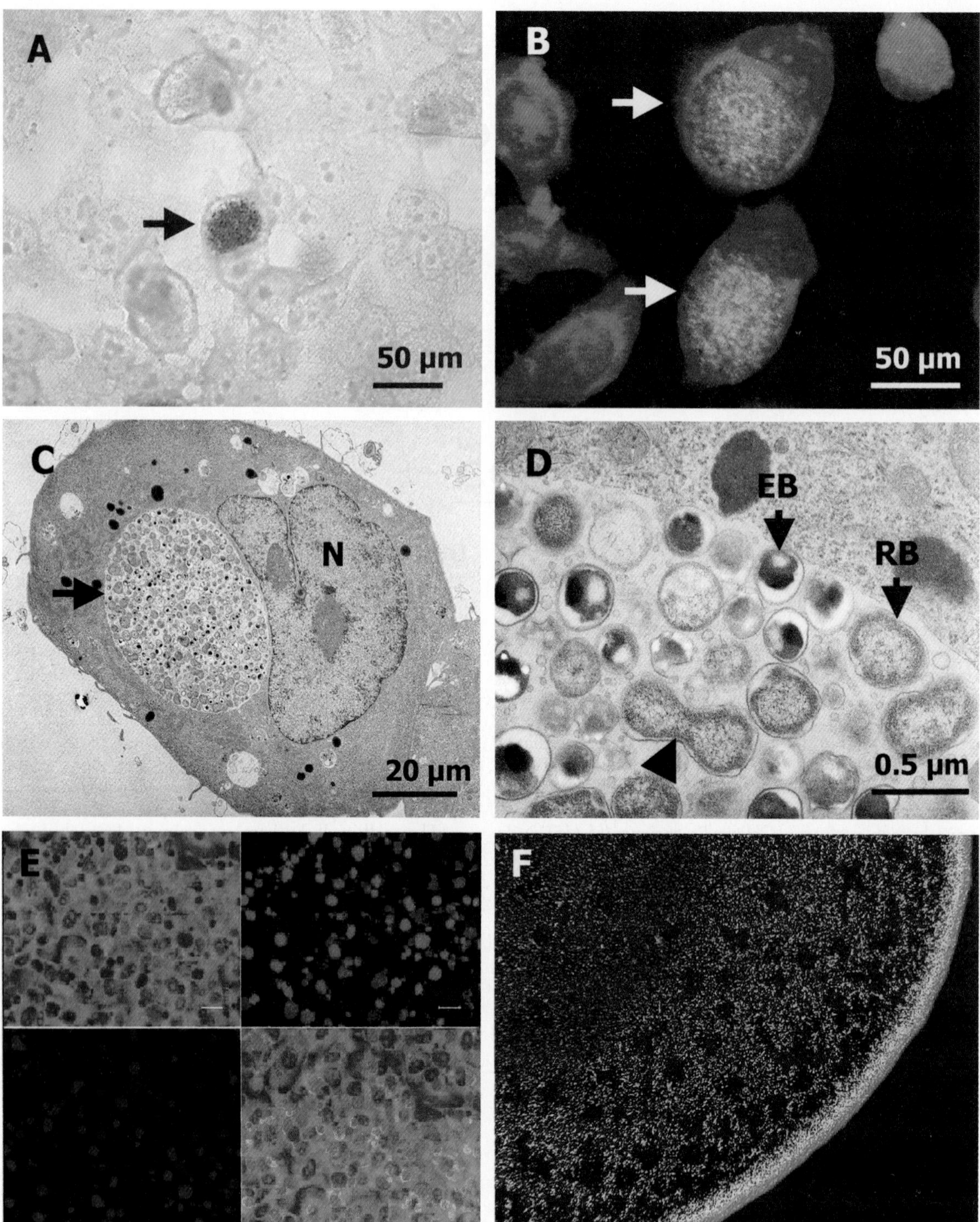

FIGURE 1 Identification of *C. trachomatis* by staining intracytoplasmic inclusions with iodine (A) and an FITC-conjugated monoclonal antibody directed at the MOMP (B). Transmission electron microscopy of a *C. pneumoniae*-infected cell shows an intracytoplasmic inclusion impressing the cell nucleus (C) and filled with EBs and RBs (D) at 60 h postinfection; the arrowhead shows a dividing RB. Identification of culture-grown *C. pneumoniae* by fluorescence in situ hybridization using rRNA targeted oligonucleotide probes (E). Simultaneous use of a Cy5-labeled probe that targets a chlamydial 16S rRNA sequence common to all members of the *Chlamydiaceae* (blue) and a Cy3-labeled probe specific for *C. pneumoniae* (red). Due to the overlap of colors, *C. pneumoniae* appears purple in the composite image; host cells are counterstained by a 5(6)-carboxyfluorescein-*N*-hydroxysuccinimide ester (FLUOS)-labeled eukaryotic probe (green). IgG-MIF image (magnification, ×400) showing bright homogeneous fluorescence of *C. pneumoniae* EBs at a serum dilution of 1:512 (F). (Photographs courtesy of Sonja Maier, Sven Poppert, and Ulrike Simnacher, Department of Medical Microbiology and Hygiene, University of Ulm; and Matthias Horn, Division of Microbial Ecology, University of Vienna.)

a small subset of genes that control the differentiation stages of the cycle and have evolutionary origins in eukaryotic lineages (6).

Evidence is accumulating that factors including gamma interferon, antibiotics, and nutrient deprivation may drive chlamydiae into a state of persistence. Persistent chlamydial forms are morphologically characterized by aberrant enlarged RBs located within small intracellular inclusions that are arrested in a viable but noninfectious state (40). It was proposed that persistence is an alternative life cycle used by chlamydiae to avoid the host immune response (5). As a consequence, chronic infections have been attributed to chlamydial persistence (20). However, the clinical significance of chlamydial persistence is still a matter of debate because diagnostic tools to detect persistence in the human host are lacking.

The chlamydiae can elicit the induction of apoptosis under some circumstances and actively inhibit apoptosis under others (27, 29, 75, 116). This points to an important strategy that chlamydiae have evolved to promote their survival through the modulation of programmed cell death pathways in infected host cells.

Sequence information is now available for *C. trachomatis* (101), *C. pneumoniae* (51, 96), *C. caviae* (83), *C. abortus*, and a *Chlamydia*-like endosymbiont of *Acanthamoeba* (41). Genome analysis of this environmental chlamydial strain showed that about 700 million years ago the last common ancestor of pathogenic and symbiotic chlamydiae was already adapted to intracellular survival in early eukaryotes and contained many virulence factors found in modern pathogenic chlamydiae, including a type III secretion system (41). Comparison of the *C. pneumoniae* genome with the *C. trachomatis* genome has provided an understanding of the common biological processes required for infection and survival in mammalian cells. Prominent comparative findings include expansion of a novel family of 21 sequence-variant OMPs, conservation of a type-III secretion virulence system, three serine/threonine protein kinases and a pair of paralogous phospholipase D-like proteins, additional purine and biotin biosynthetic capability, a homologue for aromatic amino acid (tryptophan) hydroxylase, and the loss of tryptophan biosynthesis genes (51).

CLINICAL SIGNIFICANCE, EPIDEMIOLOGY, AND TRANSMISSION

C. trachomatis

Based on the antigenic reactivity of the MOMP, *C. trachomatis* is currently divided into 18 serovars. Serovars A, B, Ba, and C can be isolated from patients with clinical trachoma in areas of endemicity in poor countries in Africa, the Middle East, Asia, and South America. Acute manifestations of trachoma primarily include a follicular keratoconjunctivitis, while late-stage manifestations include tarsoconjunctival scarring with trichiasis, entropium, and subsequent loss of vision (97). According to estimates of the World Health Organization (WHO), approximately 1.3 million people in the world suffer from preventable blindness due to trachoma. Trachoma is transmitted under poor hygienic conditions between members of the same family or between families with shared facilities via discharges from the eyes of infected patients. Flies feeding from the mucopurulent eye discharges of infected and weakened humans may carry the organisms on their legs from one person to another across relatively long distances.

The *C. trachomatis* serovars D through K including the serovars Da and Ia and the genovariant Ja are associated with genital tract disease and are among the most common sexually transmitted bacterial organisms in industrialized countries. According to surveillance data of the Centers for Disease Control and Prevention (CDC), these organisms are responsible for approximately 1 million reported infections in 2004 in the United States and typically cause nongonococcal urethritis in men and cervicitis in women. Infection of the urethra and the lower genital tract may cause dysuria, whitish or clear urethral or mucopurulent vaginal discharge, and postcoital bleeding. Urethritis and the rarer manifestations proctitis and conjunctivitis are observed in both men and women. The bulk of infections are asymptomatic and therefore remain undetected (77). This may result in ascending infections such as epididymitis in men and endometritis, salpingitis, pelvic inflammatory disease, and perihepatitis (Fitz-Hugh-Curtis Syndrome) in women. Manifestations of upper genital infection in women are irregular uterine bleeding, pelvic discomfort, or abdominal pain. Salpingitis may lead to tubal scarring and therefore to severe reproductive complications such as tubal-factor infertility and ectopic pregnancy. Tubal-factor infertility attributable to *C. trachomatis* is the most frequent form of infection-induced infertility. *C. trachomatis*-infected pregnant women may transmit the organisms during delivery to the infants, who are therefore at risk to develop conjunctivitis and/or pneumonia. Sequelae of *C. trachomatis* infection in both men and women may involve HLA-B27-associated reactive arthritis, presenting most frequently as an acute asymmetric oligoarthritis with or without enthesiopathic and extramusculoskeletal symptoms (19, 121). The young age of sexually active people is strongly associated with infection. Additionally, sex workers, persons with a new sex partner, or persons who have had several sex partners are at increased risk of infection. Screening women who are at risk for *C. trachomatis* infection can prevent serious complications such as pelvic inflammatory disease (93). Consequently, screening programs have been established in some European countries and the United States to identify and treat infections of asymptomatic individuals and their partners.

The *C. trachomatis* serovars L1, L2, L2a, and L3 including the newly identified variant L2b cause lymphogranuloma venereum (LGV), a systemic sexually transmitted disease that is endemic in parts of Africa, Asia, South America, and the Caribbean but rare in industrialized countries. However, recent reports about outbreaks in Europe and the United States show that health care providers should be vigilant for LGV (73, 99), especially among men who have sex with men. The primary lesion, a small, painless papule that tends to ulcerate at the site of inoculation, often escapes attention. Proctitis is more common in people who practice receptive anal intercourse, and elevated white blood cell counts in anorectal smear specimens may predict LGV in these patients (110). Ulcer formation may favor transmission of human immunodeficiency virus and other sexually transmitted and bloodborne diseases. The cardinal feature of LGV is the presence of painful inguinal and/or femoral lymphadenopathy (82). Complications of LGV include development of coalescing fluctuant lymph nodes (buboes) that result in discharging sinuses and fistula formation. If untreated, fibrosis can lead to lymphatic obstruction causing elephantiasis of the genitalia.

C. pneumoniae

C. pneumoniae causes infections of the upper and lower respiratory tract such as sinusitis, pharyngitis, bronchitis, and pneumonia (54). *C. pneumoniae* was identified as the causative agent in 10 to 15% of cases of community-acquired pneumonia in adults (57) as well as in children (81). However, data from studies yielding prevalence rates under 1% for *C. pneumoniae* pose the question whether its role in community-acquired pneumonia is overestimated (104). Severe and life-threatening *C. pneumoniae* infections have been described in patients with acute leukemia and treatment-induced neutropenia (38). Chronic infection with *C. pneumoniae* was reported among patients with chronic obstructive pulmonary disease and may also play a role in the natural history of asthma, including exacerbations. The clinical symptoms of *C. pneumoniae* infection are nonspecific and do not differ significantly from those caused by other atypical organisms such as viruses and *Mycoplasma pneumoniae*. Persistent cough seems not to be strongly associated with *C. pneumoniae* (115). Primary infection occurs mainly in school-age children, while reinfection has been observed in adults. Seroprevalence rates from 40 to 70% show that *C. pneumoniae* is a widely spread organism in industrialized as well as developing countries.

Atherosclerosis has been recognized as a chronic inflammatory disease of the artery vessel wall (86). The role of *C. pneumoniae* in the etiology of atherosclerosis has been discussed since 1988, when Saikku and coworkers presented serological evidence of an association of *C. pneumoniae* with coronary heart disease and acute myocardial infarction (88). In subsequent studies, the organisms were identified in atherosclerotic lesions of patients by culture, PCR, immunohistochemistry, and transmission electron microscopy; however, the discrepancies of study results (120) including those of animal studies and the failure of large-scale treatment studies (14, 36, 74) have raised skepticism about the organism's role in atherosclerosis (44). In addition, a heterogeneous spectrum of extrapulmonary diseases has been linked to *C. pneumoniae* including multiple sclerosis (100), Alzheimer's disease (3), and chronic fatigue syndrome (17); however, a causal relationship between these diseases and *C. pneumoniae* infection has not been substantiated.

C. psittaci

Psittacine birds and a wide range of other avian species may act as natural reservoirs for *C. psittaci*. In the recently proposed new *Chlamydophila psittaci* taxon (25), only the avian chlamydial strains previously designated *Chlamydia psittaci* are retained. Persons at risk for infection with *C. psittaci* include mainly those who have contact with pet birds and those who are employed in the poultry industry or in slaughterhouses. Infectious forms of the organisms are shed from symptomatic and from apparently healthy birds and may remain viable for several months. *C. psittaci* can be readily transmitted to humans following inhalation of aerosols from nasal discharges and from infectious fecal or feather dust. Symptomatic *C. psittaci* infection in humans may present as a severe chronic pneumonia (24), although mild illness and asymptomatic infections in persons exposed to infected birds have also been observed (70). Typical symptoms include fever, chills, muscular aches and pains, severe headache, hepato- and/or splenomegaly, and gastrointestinal symptoms. Cardiac complications may involve endocarditis and myocarditis. Fatal cases were common in the preantibiotic era. Due to quarantine of imported birds and improved veterinary-hygienic measures, outbreaks and sporadic cases of psittacosis are rarely observed nowadays.

C. abortus

Chlamydiae associated with ruminant abortion and formerly contained within the *Chlamydia psittaci* taxon were transferred to a new species: *Chlamydophila abortus* (114). *C. abortus* has been acknowledged as a cause of abortion and fetal loss in sheep and has also been broadly detected in calves (46). There are a number of reports of pregnant women who have had spontaneous abortions following exposure to animals infected with *C. abortus* (80, 117). The incidence of this animal-acquired infection is not known, but sheep and goats during the birthing season represent a potential risk to pregnant women. Obstetricians should consider this diagnosis along with early antibiotic treatment and cesarean section delivery in the context of the patient's case history.

Environmental Chlamydiae

The host range of chlamydiae was further broadened with the discovery of *Chlamydia*-related endosymbionts in free-living amoebae (1, 18, 30). The so-called environmental chlamydiae that have been placed in the family *Parachlamydiaceae* share the chlamydial developmental cycle and represent an evolutionary early-diverging sister of the pathogenic chlamydiae (41). Environmental chlamydiae were discussed as potential emerging pathogens; however, clinical evidence for their importance in human infection is still pending. *Simkania negevensis*, currently the only member of the *Simkaniaceae*, is a recently discovered *Chlamydia*-like intracellular agent which has been associated with respiratory infections in infants (49). The natural host of *Simkania* is not known; however, the organisms were successfully grown in various cell lines as well as in free-living amoebae and were identified in drinking water and in reclaimed wastewater (50).

COLLECTION, TRANSPORT, AND STORAGE

General Comments

Since chlamydiae are obligate intracellular pathogens, the objective of specimen collection should usually be to include the host cells that harbor the organisms (8). Outside their host, chlamydiae survive only briefly, and efforts must be undertaken to maintain the organisms' viability for successful culture. Commercial diagnostic nonculture assays do not require the presence of viable chlamydiae in the specimen; nevertheless, the instructions of the manufacturers given in the package insert should be followed for appropriate collection, transport, and storage of specimens. This includes the use of swabs and transport media specified by the manufacturer.

For successful culture of chlamydiae, the time between collection and processing of the specimens in the laboratory should be minimized while keeping specimens cold (4 to 8°C). Specimens should be forwarded to the laboratory within 24 h in a special chlamydial transport medium such as 2-sucrose phosphate or sucrose phosphate glutamate supplemented with fetal calf serum (5 to 10%), gentamicin (10 μg/ml), vancomycin (25 to 100 μg/ml), and amphotericin B (2 μg/ml) or nystatin (25 U/ml). Tetracyclines, macrolides, and penicillins cannot be used in the transport media since they have activity against chlamydiae. If specimens cannot be processed within 24 h, storage at −70°C in transport media is acceptable. Specimens for culture should not be stored at −20°C or in frost-free freezers. To test the adequacy of specimen transport, periodic transport of specimens with known numbers of inclusion-forming units should be conducted. Swab specimens should be collected on swabs with a Dacron tip and an aluminum or plastic shaft. Swab tips made of calcium alginate and swabs with wooden shafts may inhibit the growth of chlamydiae. It is recommended to check new lots of swabs that are used to collect specimens for culture of chlamydiae for possible inhibition of chlamydial growth (21, 47).

C. trachomatis

The type and anatomical site of specimen collection for laboratory diagnosis of *C. trachomatis* infection depend on both the clinical picture and the laboratory test selection as comprehensively reviewed elsewhere (8, 47, 60, 97). Noninvasively collected specimens such as first-void urine (FVU; first 10 to 30 ml of urine) and vulvovaginal swab specimens are excellent for diagnosis of *C. trachomatis* genital tract infection by nucleic acid amplification techniques (NAATs). Sensitivity and specificity of NAATs for *C. trachomatis* on noninvasively collected specimens are similar to those obtained on samples collected directly from the cervix or urethra (90, 94, 111, 112). Patients and clinicians may prefer self-sampling to the standard collection methods (42, 85). FVU specimens should be obtained at least 2 h after the last micturition. Ambient-temperature storage of fresh unprocessed urine should not exceed 24 h to avoid denaturation of chlamydial DNA. Subsequent processing of the urine specimens for NAAT varies depending on the manufacturers' instructions. Both urine and (self-collected) vulvovaginal specimens are not recommended for testing by culture and nonamplification assays such as enzyme immunoassay (EIA), direct fluorescence assay (DFA), and nucleic acid hybridization (NAH) because of their relatively low sensitivity (47).

Traditional sites for specimen collection in *C. trachomatis* genital tract infection involve the endocervix in females and the urethra in males. Proficient specimen collection including vaginal speculum examination in females is required to obtain appropriate samples that contain sufficient columnar or squamocolumnar cells. Purulent discharges have to be cleaned before a swab is inserted 1 to 2 cm into the cervical os past the squamocolumnar junction, rotated more than two times, and removed without touching the vaginal mucosa (8). Urethral specimens from males are collected by placing a dry swab 3 to 4 cm into the urethra and rotating prior to removal. Urination prior to specimen collection may reduce test sensitivity by washing out infected columnar cells. *C. trachomatis* also infects the female urethra, and recovery rates may be improved by collecting a specimen from the urethra as well as from the cervix and sending both to the laboratory. In women with salpingitis, samples may be collected by needle aspiration of the involved fallopian tube. Endometrial specimens have also yielded chlamydiae. Further appropriate sites include the conjunctiva in chlamydial eye infection (trachoma, inclusion conjunctivitis, and newborn conjunctivitis) and the nasopharynx and deeper respiratory tract of infants in newborn pneumonia. For men who have sex with men, screening of rectal and pharyngeal specimens is recommended since early reports support the utility of commercial NAATs as a screening test for this population (53, 59). In cases of suspected LGV, ulcer swabs, aspirates of bubo fluid, and rectal or urethral swabs should be collected in transport medium. Buboes of LGV may contain only small amounts of thin milky fluid, and it may be necessary to inject 2 to 5 ml of sterile saline to obtain any fluid by aspiration (60).

C. pneumoniae

The optimal sites for specimen collection in *C. pneumoniae* infection are poorly defined. Respiratory specimens from which the organisms were cultured include sputum, bronchoalveolar lavage fluid, nasopharyngeal aspirates, throat washings, and throat swabs (tonsil area). Swab specimens should be collected using a Dacron tip and an aluminum or plastic shaft (21) and placed immediately in transport medium. Specimens need to be kept at 4 to 8°C in chlamydial transport medium, since the organisms are inactivated rapidly at room temperature. Rapid freezing or freezing and thawing of specimens should be avoided (54). Liquid specimens are collected in transport medium at a specimen-to-medium ratio of 1:2 (21). Testing of vascular tissue specimens and blood samples, except for research studies, is of questionable value.

C. psittaci

C. psittaci strains seem to be the most stable organisms among the pathogenic chlamydiae. Nevertheless, specimens should be collected in chlamydial transport medium. Appropriate specimens include sputum, bronchoalveolar lavage fluid, pleural fluid, blood, and tissue biopsy specimens from various anatomical sites.

DIRECT EXAMINATION

NAAT

C. trachomatis

Due to their high sensitivity and specificity, NAATs are the tests of choice for diagnosis of genital *C. trachomatis* infections in routine clinical laboratories. NAATs can be used to detect *C. trachomatis* without a pelvic examination or intraurethral swab specimen by testing self- or clinician-collected vaginal swabs or urine, respectively (16, 42, 90, 94, 111, 112). This facilitates the establishment of screening programs in asymptomatic individuals and may enhance the compliance for testing asymptomatic contact persons of infected individuals. Increasing experience is available for the use of NAATs in conjunctival, oropharyngeal, and rectal samples (53, 59) and in LGV (73, 105). For research studies of trachoma patients, NAATs have been recommended as the "gold standard"; however, the commercial assays presently available are too expensive and too complex for use in national trachoma programs (97). In many evaluations, NAATs detected 20 to 30% more positive specimens than could be detected by earlier technologies. However, NAATs are not a perfect gold standard. An expansion of the gold standard has evolved as multiple specimens from each patient have been tested by more than one FDA-cleared NAAT, enabling the gold standard to be redefined for identification of an infected patient. An infected-patient gold standard for evaluation of new diagnostic tests for *C. trachomatis* infection has been recently proposed consisting of (i) two NAATs different from the test under evaluation; (ii) three samples from each patient including cervical swabs, male urethral swabs, and urine from both men and women; and (iii) two positive results among the three samples (65).

Licensed NAATs for detection of *C. trachomatis* include (in the order of their introduction) the PCR-based Roche Amplicor (Roche Diagnostics, Basel, Switzerland), the APTIMA transcription-mediated amplification (Gen-Probe, Inc., San Diego, Calif.) and the BD ProbeTec strand displacement amplification (SDA) (Becton Dickinson and Company, Diagnostic Systems, Franklin Lakes, N.J.). The formerly frequently used Abbott LCx ligase chain reaction was withdrawn from the commercial market by the manufacturer in 2003. Both the PCR and SDA assay amplify nucleotide sequences of the 7.5-kbp cryptic plasmid of *C. trachomatis*, which is present in an average copy number of about four plasmids per chromosome in EBs and up to seven plasmids per chromosome in replicating RBs (78). *C. trachomatis* strains that do not harbor the cryptic plasmid have been sporadically isolated from urethral specimens (28, 103). The transcription-mediated amplification-based assays target specific sequences of the 23S rRNA, which is also present in multiple copies. Each of the three commercially available NAAT systems offers the option for combination testing of *C. trachomatis* and *Neisseria gonorrhoeae* in the same specimen.

Considering the multiplicity of target sites for the amplification procedures being used, NAATs should be able to produce a positive signal from less than one EB; however, the actual sensitivity in clinical specimens is lower because of sampling variability and inhibition of amplification. Since inhibitor problems of NAATs can be reduced by dilution of specimens, heating, freeze-thaw cycles, or overnight storage at 4°C, the use of internal inhibitor controls of the amplification assays (as supplied by the manufacturers of PCR and SDA) is helpful for identification of clinical specimens containing inhibitory factors (62). All these assays are highly specific if problems with cross-contamination, labeling errors, and mistakes in specimen collection can be avoided. Confirmatory testing of positive specimens is recommended if a low positive predictive value can be expected (<90%) or if a false-positive result would have serious psychosocial or legal consequences (47).

Clinical evaluations of the NAATs have shown that they are more sensitive than culture and other nonculture methods including microscopy, antigen detection, and nucleic acid hybridization assays. As a consequence, less sensitive diagnostic tests cannot be used to confirm positive results of the more sensitive NAAT assays (47). Even among NAATs, the assays employed for confirmatory testing should have equivalent sensitivities (89). Concerns regarding consistency of test performance and reproducibility are a matter of ongoing debate. Mishandling of specimens can lead to incorrect results. Therefore, laboratory implementation of NAATs requires close attention to quality control measures such as manufacturer- or expert-based training of laboratory staff, participation in proficiency testing programs, and standard operating procedures based on the manufacturers' instructions in the package inserts (47).

In settings where resources are limited, including developing countries, the concept of pooling to detect *C. trachomatis* by NAATs has proved to be a simple, accurate, and cost-effective procedure compared to individual testing (58). Specimen pools may consist of aliquots from five processed specimens (FVU or genital swab) combined into one amplification tube. Subsequent testing of individual samples is required only if the pooled sample gives a positive result. Following this strategy, considerable savings of reagent costs can be obtained, especially in low-prevalence populations.

C. pneumoniae

A vast number of PCR-based protocols using different formats and target genes have been developed in research laboratories for detection of *C. pneumoniae* in both respiratory and nonrespiratory samples. However, the lack of a reliable gold standard for *C. pneumoniae* infection has made it difficult to evaluate the published protocols thoroughly. Broad application of NAATs for diagnosis of *C. pneumoniae* infection has been hampered because many PCR protocols are not reliable or robust enough to provide reproducible results in routine clinical laboratories. Even in specialized laboratories, there seems to be a substantial interlaboratory variation in the performance of *C. pneumoniae* NAATs, and the need for standardization of these assays has been recognized (21). Subsequently, specific recommendations for standardizing *C. pneumoniae* PCR assays were made, and it was suggested to compare the performance of newly developed PCR protocols with at least one of four recommended assays that target the *PSTI* fragment (13), the *ompA* gene (109), or the 16S rRNA gene (32, 61). However, all of these assays must be considered research tools (21), because commercial FDA-cleared assays are currently not available. Real-time PCR technology provides promising results that warrant further evaluation of this approach for detection of *C. pneumoniae* infection (2, 55, 84, 108).

C. psittaci

NAATs could be helpful for detection of avian *C. psittaci* strains from clinical samples since culture of these organisms is dangerous and requires biosafety level 3 (BSL-3) facilities. Some PCR-based assays have been developed for diagnosis of human ornithosis (24, 61, 67, 109). Due to the rarity of the disease, the performance characteristics of these assays have been only poorly evaluated in clinical specimens.

NAH

Two NAH tests are commercially available for detection of *C. trachomatis*. The Gen-Probe PACE 2 test (Gen-Probe Inc.) hybridizes to a species-specific sequence of chlamydial 16S rRNA that is present in a high copy number in replicating chlamydiae. Available data suggest that it is about as sensitive as the better antigen detection and cell culture methods and is relatively specific. However, it was shown that commercial NAATs improved the detection of infections in women by 17 to 38% compared to PACE 2 (9). The second NAH test, the Digene Hybrid Capture II, is a nucleic acid probe-signal amplification assay (Digene Corp., Gaithersburg, Md.) that uses RNA hybridization probes for DNA sequences encoding both genomic and cryptic plasmid sequences of *C. trachomatis*. This assay was shown to reach the sensitivity of a commercial NAAT when cervical specimens were investigated (113). NAHs are considered highly robust test methods for detection of *C. trachomatis*. NAH tests have been recommended for endocervical swabs or urethral swabs from men when a NAAT is not available or not economical. As is the case with other non-NAATs, NAH tests have not been recommended for use in noninvasive-collection specimens such as urine and vulvovaginal swabs (47). Both NAH systems also offer a test format that enables detection of *C. trachomatis* and *N. gonorrhoeae* in a single specimen.

DFA

The presence of typical intracytoplasmic inclusions in epithelial cells of the conjunctiva, urethra, or cervix of infected patients can be demonstrated when air-dried smears are fixed on a slide with absolute methanol and stained with Giemsa. Cytological testing was particularly useful in diagnosing acute inclusion conjunctivitis of the newborn, but the more sensitive immunofluorescence procedures have largely replaced this method. DFAs use fluorescein isothiocyanate (FITC)-conjugated monoclonal antibodies that are directed at a *C. trachomatis*-specific epitope of the MOMP (*Chlamydia CEL;* Cellabs, Brookvale, Australia; Pathfinder; Bio-Rad Laboratories, Redmond, Wash.). DFAs are based on detecting EBs in smears, although staining of inclusions can also succeed if intact infected host cells are collected. Checking for the presence of columnar cells allows assessment of the adequacy of the sample. The procedure offers rapid diagnosis, taking only 30 min to perform, making DFA tests useful especially for laboratories that test only a limited number of specimens. However, this method requires an experienced microscopist who can distinguish between fluorescing chlamydial particles and nonspecific fluorescence. The DFA test has approximately 75 to 85% sensitivity and 98 to 99% specificity compared with culture and a lower sensitivity than NAATs (11, 72). DFA tests may be another alternative for testing endocervical swabs from females or urethral swabs from males when a NAAT is not available or not economical. In addition, DFAs have been recommended for use with conjunctival specimens and for testing of individuals with possible rectal and pharyngeal exposure to *C. trachomatis*, if a *C. trachomatis* MOMP-specific stain is used (47). Nontrachomatis chlamydial conjunctivitis should be considered if DFA testing reveals the presence of chlamydial LPS but not *C. trachomatis*-specific MOMP.

EIA

EIA-based tests for detection of *C. trachomatis* use either monoclonal or polyclonal antibodies to detect chlamydial LPS, which is more soluble than MOMP. Although they can theoretically detect all chlamydiae, EIAs have not been well evaluated for the diagnosis of infections with *C. pneumoniae* or *C. psittaci*. The performance characteristics of EIAs for laboratory diagnosis of *C. trachomatis* have been reviewed comprehensively elsewhere (8). Using cultures as reference standards, the sensitivities of EIAs applied to endocervical swabs were in a range from 62 to 72% (72). Although in single studies specificities of >99% have been reported, EIA methods that detect chlamydial LPS harbor a risk for false-positive results caused by cross-reaction with LPS of other microorganisms. Therefore, a positive EIA screening test should be verified, especially in low-prevalence populations (47). To overcome logistical and economic challenges associated with confirmatory testing, a blocking antibody format has been introduced, increasing the test specifity of some EIAs to about 99.5%. EIAs are not recommended for testing of noninvasively collected specimens such as urine and vulvovaginal swabs. EIAs are preferred in laboratories where cost is a major factor and large numbers of specimens require bulk processing, but results should note the low sensitivity of this method compared to that of NAATs.

Rapid or point-of-care tests designed for office- or clinic-based settings have been developed that provide test results in less than 30 min for *C. trachomatis* infection in women. Similar to EIAs, they also use antibodies against chlamydial LPS with the potential to yield false-positive results due to cross-reaction with other gram-negative bacteria. Point-of-care tests have not been recommended in laboratory settings because sensitivity and specificity are lower, quality controls are less rigorous, and costs are higher than for tests designed for laboratory use (47).

ISOLATION PROCEDURES

Biosafety Considerations

C. pneumoniae and *C. trachomatis* are BSL-2 organisms, whereas *C. psittaci* is a BSL-3 organism. Transmission of the organisms from patient specimens or infected cell cultures may occur through aerosols, splashes onto the mucous membranes of the eyes, and hand-to-face actions. In recent years, fewer laboratory-acquired infections have been reported probably due to the common usage of class II biosafety cabinets in laboratories that work with *Chlamydia*-infected cell cultures. Use of a class II biosafety cabinet protects laboratory staff from exposure to aerosols as well as specimens and cell cultures from contamination. Further important means for preventing laboratory-acquired infection include the use of gloves, alcohol-based hand disinfectants, safety centrifuge caps, and face protection, if appropriate. Laboratory infections with *C. trachomatis* usually manifest as follicular conjunctivitis. The LGV strains are more invasive, and severe cases of laboratory-associated pneumonia and lymphadenitis are reported. *C. psittaci* must be considered a potentially dangerous organism, requiring appropriate BSL-3 facilities. Laboratory-acquired *C. pneumoniae* infections might be underestimated since the mild clinical course may not prompt infected laboratory workers to seek medical attention.

Specimen Processing

Ocular and Genital Tract Specimens

For culture of chlamydiae from ocular and genital tract sites, only swabs that are rapidly forwarded to the laboratory in a special chlamydial transport medium are acceptable (see above). Specimens to be assayed by commercial EIA, DFA, NAH, or NAAT should be processed as directed by the manufacturer.

Bubo Pus

To prepare bubo pus, the aspirate fluid of fluctuant lymph nodes is ground and then suspended in nutrient broth or cell culture medium to at least 20% by weight. Even when the pus is not viscous, dilution is advisable. The material should be tested for bacterial contaminants and inoculated onto monolayer cultures of McCoy or HeLa 229 cells.

Blood

Blood samples may be helpful for diagnosis of *C. psittaci* endocarditis (95). The blood clot should be ground, and cell culture medium should be added to make a 10% solution. The suspension is inoculated directly into cell culture by using serial dilutions (from 1:2 to 1:10), since the concentrated material may be toxic to the cells. Collection in EDTA-treated tubes may be appropriate if fractionated blood is to be investigated. Processing of peripheral blood mononuclear cells (PBMCs) for detection of *C. pneumoniae* in cardiovascular patients should be confined to clinical trials. Protocols for isolation and processing of PBMCs have been published elsewhere (10).

Sputum, Throat Washings, and Other Secretions from the Respiratory Tract

Sputum and other respiratory samples are suspended in antibiotic-containing transport medium or cell culture medium at a ratio of specimen to medium of 1:2 to 1:10 depending on specimen consistency. Specimens are homogenized by adding sterile glass beads to the sample and vigorous vortexing for 1 to 2 min in a tightly stoppered container. Extracts should be centrifuged for 20 to 30 min at $100 \times g$ to remove coarse material before the supernatant fluid is inoculated onto cell monolayers. Serial dilutions may be required if the inoculum is toxic to cells.

Fecal Samples

Human rectal swabs for *C. trachomatis* and avian material for *C. psittaci* are suspended in chlamydial transport medium or antibiotic-containing cell culture medium. The suspension is shaken thoroughly and centrifuged at 300 × *g* for 10 min, and the supernatant is removed. It may be further diluted (1:2 and 1:20) with medium before being inoculated into cell culture. Rectal swabs for commercial NAAT are processed in accordance with the corresponding protocol of the manufacturer.

Tissue Samples

Frozen tissue is thawed in a refrigerator at 4°C. The specimen is weighed, minced with sterile scissors or a scalpel, and ground with a mortar and pestle or homogenizer. A volume of cell culture medium required to make a 10 to 20% suspension is added, and the suspension is thoroughly mixed. For tissue specimens, serial dilutions (1:10 to 1:100) are often required for inoculation to prevent toxicity.

Isolation

Cell culture was considered the gold standard for diagnosis of genital *C. trachomatis* infection because its sensitivity and specificity were thought to be close to 100%. Problems associated with cell culture isolation of chlamydiae including technical complexity and long turnaround time and stringent requirements related to collection, transport, and storage of specimens have driven the development of commercially available noncultural methods that have found widespread application in many routine laboratories. With the advent of antigen detection methods, it became clear that the sensitivity of culture was substantially lower than previously thought, most probably due to the presence of nonviable chlamydiae that died during transport and processing. Culture for detection of chlamydiae in clinical specimens is generally now performed only in specialized laboratories (8). Culture is strongly recommended in treatment failures (when a viable isolate is needed for susceptibility testing) and in cases related to possible sexual assault for medicolegal reasons (47).

Historically, chlamydiae were cultivated in the yolk sac of embryonated eggs. The yolk sac method (for details, see reference 91) is still used for preparing antigens for the microimmunofluorescence test (MIF). For isolation of chlamydiae from clinical specimens, appropriately collected and transported samples are inoculated onto preformed cell monolayers. A number of susceptible permanent cell lines, including McCoy, HeLa 229, HEp-2, HL, BGMK, Vero, and L cells, have been used. Clinical samples are centrifuged onto monolayers to enhance infection. Strains of *C. psittaci* and LGV biovars are capable of serial growth in cell culture without centrifugation. Cultures are incubated for 48 to 72 h in the presence of the host cell protein synthesis inhibitor cycloheximide. McCoy and HeLa 229 cells are most commonly used for *C. trachomatis*. HL and HEp-2 cells seem to be more sensitive for recovery of the fastidious *C. pneumoniae* from clinical specimens. Visualization of cell culture-grown chlamydiae is achieved by immunostaining of inoculated cell monolayers for intracytoplasmic inclusions. A positive culture shows one or more typical intracellular inclusions (Fig. 1B).

Cell culture methods may vary among laboratories. Host cells are plated either onto 12-mm glass coverslips contained in 15-mm-diameter (1 dram [1 dram = 3.697 ml]) disposable glass vials (shell vial method) or in 6-, 12-, or 24-well tissue culture plates. The cells are seeded in concentrations of 1×10^5 to 2×10^5 cells/ml to give a healthy and confluent monolayer after 24 to 48 h of incubation. For optimal results, cell monolayers should be inoculated with patient specimens within 24 h after reaching confluency. Clinical specimens are thoroughly vortexed with glass beads in tightly closed screw-cap vials to facilitate release of chlamydiae before inoculation. The cell culture medium of the cell monolayers to be inoculated is discarded and replaced by a volume of 0.2 to 2 ml of the vortexed specimen. The inoculated specimen is centrifuged onto the cell monolayers at 900 to 3,000 × *g* for 1 h at 22 to 35°C. Cells are incubated at 35°C for 1 to 2 h to allow uptake of chlamydiae before the medium is replaced with chlamydial isolation medium consisting of the cell culture medium supplemented with fetal calf serum (10%), L-glutamine (2 mM), cycloheximide (1 to 2 μg/ml), gentamicin (10 μg/ml), vancomycin (25 μg/ml), and amphotericin B (2 μg/ml). Cultures are incubated at 35°C in 5% CO_2 for 48 to 72 h. Then, one coverslip per specimen is removed for immunostaining of inoculated monolayers. Both cell detritus and toxic effects of the inoculum may make it difficult to read slides. Dilution of cell-rich material (bubo pus, sputum, tissue samples, and rectal swabs) and blind performance of subpassages can be helpful for microscopic interpretation of slides.

If a blind subpassage or passage of positive material is to be performed, the corresponding cell monolayers of duplicate wells are scraped and disrupted by vortexing with glass beads. Cell debris of harvested material is removed by low-speed centrifugation (300 × *g*) for 10 min, and the supernatant is passed onto preformed cell monolayers as described above. For *C. pneumoniae,* most laboratories agree that at least two passages are needed to maximize the recovery of the organisms from respiratory specimens. Modifications of the standard procedure including use of serum-free culture medium, pretreatment of cell monolayers with polyethylene glycol or diethylaminoethyl-dextran, and extension of culture times have not been sufficiently tested to warrant their routine recommendation (21). Laboratories processing large numbers of specimens may use flat-bottom 48- or 96-well microtiter plates onto which cells are plated directly. Processing and incubation are as described above, but microscopy is modified because cells are stained directly in the well, requiring use of inverted microscopes and long working objectives.

Continuous quality control is important for maintaining a sensitive and specific culture system. Because of its technical complexity, there are multiple opportunities to modify factors in the culture system that may impact the isolation efficiency (97). Therefore, positive controls with a known number of inclusion-forming units should be run routinely to check the sensitivity of the culture system. Negative controls with uninfected human cells may help to evaluate episodes of cross-contamination as a result of handling positive patient specimens or positive controls. Routine testing of cell culture systems for *Mycoplasma* contamination has been recommended because *Mycoplasma* contamination may impair the growth of chlamydiae and may decrease the sensitivity of the culture system (21). In addition, *Mycoplasma* testing should be done with all chlamydial strains handled in the laboratory, since contamination of chlamydial isolates including strains provided by ATCC has been reported (43).

IDENTIFICATION

The basic procedure for detection of isolated chlamydiae involves demonstration of intracytoplasmic inclusions by fluorescent-antibody staining that provides both morphological and immunological identification of chlamydiae. Screening of cultures can be performed with a commercially available FITC-conjugated monoclonal anti-LPS antibody (Pathfinder

Bio-Rad), which recognizes all chlamydiae known to cause infections in humans. Confirmation of positive genital cultures can be done by the use of a *C. trachomatis* MOMP-specific monoclonal antibody (Fig. 1B). For respiratory cultures, a *C. pneumoniae*-specific monoclonal antibody may additionally be appropriate (69). Monoclonal antibodies specific for *C. psittaci* are not commercially available. Using DFA procedures, inclusions of *C. trachomatis*-infected cells are visible at 24 h postinfection. Less expensive but also less sensitive methods that were commonly used before the advent of monoclonal antibodies include Giemsa staining (which needs an experienced and well-trained microscopist for interpretation) and iodine staining for identification of glycogen-containing inclusions that are produced by *C. trachomatis* but not by *C. psittaci* or *C. pneumoniae* (Fig. 1A).

Identification of replicating chlamydiae can also be done by fluorescence in situ hybridization using fluorescently labeled oligonucleotide probes complementary to order-, genus-, and species-specific target sites on the chlamydial 16S rRNA (79). The risk of false-positive signals caused by nonspecific binding of the fluorescent dyes to nontarget organisms or structures of the host cells can be minimized by the simultaneous application of multiple probes with hierarchical specificity labeled with different dyes leading to a characteristic hybridization pattern (Fig. 1E).

TYPING SYSTEMS

Serotyping and genotyping procedures are important tools of epidemiological studies. They are of clinical use if medicolegal issues are involved or if lymphogranuloma venereum is suspected. The most convenient method for serotyping of *C. trachomatis* isolates appears to be the microwell typing system (107), in which inclusions in microtiter plates are stained with pools of monoclonal antibodies (available at Washington Research Foundation, Seattle, Wash.) that recognize serovar- and subspecies-specific epitopes of the MOMP. Genotyping of *C. trachomatis* isolates usually involves either restriction fragment length polymorphism analysis of the MOMP-encoding *ompA* gene or sequence analysis of the variable domains in the *ompA* gene. These variable regions include the peptides responsible for species, serovar, and serogroup specificities. PCR amplification of *ompA* using extracted DNA from patient specimens such as urine or genital samples allows direct genotyping from *C. trachomatis*-positive individuals without isolation of the organisms (4, 48). *ompA* sequencing is currently the only tool to identify all known and additional new genotypes of avian *C. psittaci* strains (34). Different serotypes or genotypes of *C. pneumoniae* have not been described.

SEROLOGICAL TESTS

Serological testing may be helpful in the diagnosis of human ornithosis, lymphogranuloma venereum, neonatal pneumonia caused by *C. trachomatis*, and respiratory *C. pneumoniae* infections. Serological testing for diagnosis of uncomplicated genital infections of the urethra and the lower genital tract as well as for *C. trachomatis* screening in asymptomatic individuals is not recommended (47). Since a reference standard has not been defined, the diagnostic value of some serological assays for detection of chronic or persistent chlamydial infections is difficult to estimate. General problems of chlamydial serodiagnosis arise from the difficulty in obtaining paired serum samples, the high seroprevalence of *C. pneumoniae* in adult populations, and the lack of standardized species-specific test methods. The most commonly used serological assay formats include the complement fixation (CF) test, the MIF test, and the EIA to detect immunoglobulin M (IgM), IgA, IgG, or total classes of antibodies with either family, species, or serotype specificity. Some of these assays have been commercialized and are being used by clinical laboratories, although their performance characteristics have been evaluated only in a limited number of studies. The surface-associated chlamydial macromolecules including the MOMP, OmcB, and LPS may induce a strong antibody response in infected individuals. However, these molecules share common epitopes among the different chlamydial species that make them prone to cross-reactive antibody responses. In an effort to identify species-specific immunoreactive antigens, protein profiles have been described, but interpretation is difficult and Western blot methods using whole chlamydial elementary bodies as antigens are not ready for routine use in clinical laboratories (23).

CF Test

The CF test is based on antibody reactivity to the chlamydial LPS antigen common to all members of the *Chlamydiaceae*. The CF test may be useful in diagnosing LGV in patients who present compatible clinical symptoms. A titer of ≥256 strongly supports the clinical diagnosis, while a titer of <32 rules it out except in the very early stages of the disease (60). In addition, the CF test is useful for diagnosis of psittacosis; however, in the absence of a typical patient history (exposure to birds), *C. pneumoniae* infection should be considered in patients with positive test results. Due to its potential for cross-reactivity and its low sensitivity for reinfection, CF is not recommended for serodiagnosis of *C. pneumoniae* infections (21). The CF test also lacks sensitivity for the diagnosis of trachoma, inclusion conjunctivitis, and uncomplicated genital infections caused by *C. trachomatis*.

MIF Test

The MIF test developed by Wang and Grayston in the early 1970s is still considered the method of choice for serodiagnosis of chlamydial infections. With this procedure, species- and serovar-specific antibody responses in human chlamydial infection can be detected. The MIF test allows quantitative detection of IgM and IgG antibodies that may be helpful in distinguishing recent from past infections.

The MIF is the diagnostic test of choice for *C. trachomatis* pneumonitis in infants because elevated levels of IgM antibodies are regularly associated with disease (8). A single IgM titer of ≥32 may support the diagnosis of neonatal pneumonia caused by *C. trachomatis*. IgG antibodies are less useful because infants may present with typical symptoms when they still have a high level of maternal IgG. In LGV-infected individuals, a MIF IgG titer of ≥128 strongly supports the clinical diagnosis, although invasive genital infection with *C. trachomatis* serovars D through K, such as pelvic inflammatory disease, salpingitis, or epididymitis, can also give rise to high serum titers of antichlamydial antibody (60). The MIF test may be useful in diagnosis of psittacosis and is the serological testing method of choice for diagnosis of acute *C. pneumoniae* infection. Criteria for acute infection of *C. pneumoniae* generally include paired sera demonstrating at least a fourfold rise in titer and single serum samples with IgM titers of ≥16 and/or IgG titers of ≥512. However, single IgG titers of ≥512 should be interpreted with caution because elevated IgG titers may persist for several years in the absence of clinically apparent disease (21). IgG titers in the range of 1:16 to 1:256 are suggestive of past infection.

The usefulness of IgA as a diagnostic marker in acute or chronic *C. pneumoniae* infections has not been substantiated.

The MIF assay is performed using purified formalinized EBs of representative strains or serovars of *C. trachomatis*, *C. psittaci*, and *C. pneumoniae* that are dotted in a specific pattern onto glass slides. MIF antigens are commercially available from the Washington Research Foundation. Serial dilutions of patient sera are placed over the fixed antigen dots and incubated, and bound antibody is detected with fluorescein-conjugated anti-IgG or anti-IgM antibody (Fig. 1F). A more detailed description of the MIF procedure has been summarized elsewhere (118). In addition, recommendations for standardizing the MIF assay in terms of antigen preparation, testing, interpretation of results, and quality assurance should be followed (21).

The MIF assay format is technically demanding, time-consuming, and less useful for higher volume testing. In addition, subjective reading of titers may contribute to intra- and interlaboratory variation in MIF assay results (76). For these reasons, well-trained and experienced laboratory staff are needed. A few standardized kits based on the MIF format have been developed and marketed (Focus Diagnostics, Cypress, Calif.; Labsystems OY, Helsinki, Finland; Savyon Diagnostics Ltd., Ashdod, Israel). Initial studies suggest that their performance characteristics are similar and seem to correspond well to those of the classical MIF method (7, 66). However, at the time of writing, none of these assays are cleared by the FDA for use in the United States for the diagnosis of *C. pneumoniae* or *C. trachomatis* infections.

EIA

To overcome the problems associated with MIF testing, EIAs have been developed that offer a more automated workflow and objective end points for serodiagnosis of chlamydial infections. EIAs based on synthetic peptides from the variable domain 4 (VD4) of the *C. trachomatis* MOMP have been marketed for detection of *C. trachomatis*-specific IgG and IgA antibodies (CT-EIA [Labsystems OY]; SeroCT [Savyon Diagnostics Ltd.]; CT pELISA [Medac, Wedel, Germany]). These assays performed as well as the MIF assay in a few studies (71); however, little is known regarding how long specific antibodies may persist in individuals with resolved infections. For these reasons they cannot reliably differentiate current and past infections. This makes them of little use in *C. trachomatis* infections of the lower genital tract where adequate specimens for direct detection of the organisms can be noninvasively obtained. Further studies are needed to clarify if *C. trachomatis* species-specific antibody tests are convenient tools for diagnosis of upper genital tract infections.

The major antigenic determinants of *C. pneumoniae* that are broadly immunodominant among infected individuals are elusive. Commercial assays designed for specific diagnosis of *C. pneumoniae* infection are based on either whole elementary bodies (Savyon Diagnostics Ltd.) or (to obtain more specificity) on LPS-extracted EB preparations (Labsystems OY and Medac). Most kits have been compared only to MIF (39), but none was evaluated adequately with sera from culture- or PCR-positive patients. Thus, their diagnostic value for acute *C. pneumoniae* infections remains to be determined (21).

ANTIMICROBIAL SUSCEPTIBILITIES AND TREATMENT

Evaluation of antimicrobial resistance and potential clinical treatment failure in chlamydial infection is hampered by the lack of standardized antimicrobial susceptibility tests and the fact that in vitro resistance does not correlate with the patient's clinical outcome (106). For these reasons, antimicrobial susceptibility testing of *Chlamydia* organisms has little clinical utility and is currently performed only in some research laboratories. Antimicrobial susceptibility testing in chlamydiae requires growing the organisms in epithelial cells cultured in medium containing increasing concentrations of antibiotics. Cells are stained with an FITC-labeled anti-chlamydial antibody, and the lowest concentration of antibiotic that inhibits inclusion formation after 48 h of incubation is reported as the MIC (106, 119). The minimum chlamydicidal concentration has been defined as the lowest concentration of antibiotic producing no viable bacterial progeny as determined after passage from antimicrobial-containing medium to antimicrobial-free medium. However, variation of antimicrobial susceptibility results is common because they depend on factors including the cell type used, the inoculum size, and the time between infection and the addition of an antimicrobial.

Tetracyclines, macrolides, fluoroquinolones, and rifampin are commonly used for antibiotic treatment of chlamydial infections. A single dose of azithromycin has been shown to be as effective for the treatment of uncomplicated genital *C. trachomatis* infections in adults as a standard 7-day course of doxycycline (56, 64). Alternative regimens include a 7-day course of erythromycin, ofloxacin, or levofloxacin (15). Cotreatment or testing for chlamydiae should be considered among gonorrhea-infected patients because of the frequency of coinfection. Systemic treatment with erythromycin has been recommended for ophthalmia neonatorum as well as for infant pneumonia caused by *C. trachomatis*. In the treatment of adult inclusion conjunctivitis, a single 1-g azithromycin dose was as effective as a standard 10-day treatment with doxycycline (52). Recommended treatment regimens for both bubonic and anogenital LGV include tetracycline, doxycycline, or erythromycin for 14 days (60). Doxycyline, azithromycin, erythromycin, levofloxacin, and newer macrolides such as clarithromycin and roxithromycin have been recommended for treatment of *C. pneumoniae* infection; however, evidence from clinical trials supporting their use is limited.

Chlamydial resistance to recommended antimicrobial agents appears to be rare and confined to only a few clinical isolates of *C. trachomatis* and has not yet been reported for *C. pneumoniae* or *C. psittaci* infections. Nevertheless, concern has been raised about resistance because recurrent or persistent chlamydial infections were observed in women adequately treated for *C. trachomatis* infection and in a few cases of *C. pneumoniae* infections (37). Treatment failure in genital tract infection has been associated with isolation of *C. trachomatis* variants resistant to tetracyclines, macrolides, or fluoroquinolones (98). Mutations in the 23S rRNA gene have been linked to resistance of clinical *C. trachomatis* isolates to macrolides (68). Resistant clinical isolates demonstrate a heterotypic pattern, in which a small proportion of organisms survive antimicrobial concentrations well above the MIC (106), and most isolates lose their resistance properties after prolonged culture in antibiotic-free medium. However, heterotypic resistance was also identified in *C. trachomatis* strains isolated from patients with single-incident infections (106), suggesting that the results of susceptibility testing may not predict the microbiological efficacy in vivo.

In vitro, chlamydial resistance to fluoroquinolones, macrolides, tetracyclines, and rifampin can be induced with large numbers of organisms cultured in the presence of antimicrobials. In an animal model, persistence of *C. pneumoniae* after antimicrobial therapy has been demonstrated (63). The emergence of *Chlamydia suis* strains isolated from livestock and displaying a chromosomally stable *tet*(C) resistance gene raises the issue of antibiotic use in animal feeds (22).

INTERPRETATION AND REPORTING OF RESULTS

The laboratory diagnosis of chlamydial infections is still challenging; however, commercial NAATs enable the reliable detection of genital *C. trachomatis* infection even from noninvasively obtained specimens. Reporting of test results for chlamydiae should include the type of test used and a clinical interpretation if possible. Apart from presumptive clinical treatment failure, test of cure is recommended for pregnant women because antibiotic treatment regimens for *C. trachomatis* infections during pregnancy may not be highly efficacious. Due to the presence of nonviable bacteria, nonculture tests for *C. trachomatis,* especially NAATs, may remain positive when performed <3 weeks after completion of therapy. In cases of treatment failure and sexual assault, isolation should be attempted and specimens should be forwarded to a specialized laboratory. Sexual partners of infected patients should be notified, examined, and treated for *C. trachomatis*. Patients and their partners should be instructed to abstain from sexual intercourse until therapy is completed.

Interpretation of serological results is particularly challenging in chlamydial infections. A reliable serologic marker for chronic or persistent chlamydial infection is not available. Especially in *C. pneumoniae,* there is poor agreement between the presence of chlamydial antibody and direct markers of current infection, such as culture or PCR (33). Single-point serology for diagnosis of *C. pneumoniae* infection is discouraged, except when specific IgM antibodies are positive. Paired sera should be tested in the same assay on the same day, and seroconversion or a fourfold rise or fall in titer is diagnostic for a recent infection. Obviously, there is a general lack of reliable and standardized assays for laboratory diagnosis of *C. pneumoniae* and this basically hampers the current understanding of the organism's true prevalence and role in respiratory infections as well as in extrapulmonary diseases.

REFERENCES

1. **Amann, R., N. Springer, W. Schonhuber, W. Ludwig, E. N. Schmid, K. D. Muller, and R. Michel.** 1997. Obligate intracellular bacterial parasites of acanthamoebae related to *Chlamydia* spp. *Appl. Environ. Microbiol.* **63:**115–121.
2. **Apfalter, P., W. Barousch, M. Nehr, A. Makristathis, B. Willinger, M. Rotter, and A. M. Hirschl.** 2003. Comparison of a new quantitative *ompA*-based real-time PCR TaqMan assay for detection of *Chlamydia pneumoniae* DNA in respiratory specimens with four conventional PCR assays. *J. Clin. Microbiol.* **41:**592–600.
3. **Balin, B. J., H. C. Gerard, E. J. Arking, D. M. Appelt, P. J. Branigan, J. T. Abrams, J. A. Whittum-Hudson, and A. P. Hudson.** 1998. Identification and localization of *Chlamydia pneumoniae* in the Alzheimer's brain. *Med. Microbiol. Immunol.* **187:**23–42.
4. **Bandea, C. I., K. Kubota, T. M. Brown, P. H. Kilmarx, V. Bhullar, S. Yanpaisarn, P. Chaisilwattana, W. Siriwasin, and C. M. Black.** 2001. Typing of *Chlamydia trachomatis* strains from urine samples by amplification and sequencing the major outer membrane protein gene *(omp1)*. *Sex. Transm. Infect.* **77:**419–422.
5. **Belland, R. J., D. E. Nelson, D. Virok, D. D. Crane, D. Hogan, D. Sturdevant, W. L. Beatty, and H. D. Caldwell.** 2003. Transcriptome analysis of chlamydial growth during IFN-gamma-mediated persistence and reactivation. *Proc. Natl. Acad. Sci. USA* **100:**15971–15976.
6. **Belland, R. J., G. Zhong, D. D. Crane, D. Hogan, D. Sturdevant, J. Sharma, W. L. Beatty, and H. D. Caldwell.** 2003. Genomic transcriptional profiling of the developmental cycle of *Chlamydia trachomatis*. *Proc. Natl. Acad. Sci. USA* **100:**8478–8483.
7. **Bennedsen, M., L. Berthelsen, and I. Lind.** 2002. Performance of three microimmunofluorescence assays for detection of *Chlamydia pneumoniae* immunoglobulin M, G, and A antibodies. *Clin. Diagn. Lab. Immunol.* **9:**833–839.
8. **Black, C. M.** 1997. Current methods of laboratory diagnosis of *Chlamydia trachomatis* infections. *Clin. Microbiol. Rev.* **10:**160–184.
9. **Black, C. M., J. Marrazzo, R. E. Johnson, E. W. Hook III, R. B. Jones, T. A. Green, J. Schachter, W. E. Stamm, G. Bolan, M. E. St. Louis, and D. H. Martin.** 2002. Head-to-head multicenter comparison of DNA probe and nucleic acid amplification tests for *Chlamydia trachomatis* infection in women performed with an improved reference standard. *J. Clin. Microbiol.* **40:**3757–3763.
10. **Boman, J., S. Soderberg, J. Forsberg, L. S. Birgander, A. Allard, K. Persson, E. Jidell, U. Kumlin, P. Juto, A. Waldenstrom, and G. Wadell.** 1998. High prevalence of *Chlamydia pneumoniae* DNA in peripheral blood mononuclear cells in patients with cardiovascular disease and in middle-aged blood donors. *J. Infect. Dis.* **178:**274–277.
11. **Boyadzhyan, B., T. Yashina, J. H. Yatabe, M. Patnaik, and C. S. Hill.** 2004. Comparison of the APTIMA CT and GC assays with the APTIMA combo 2 assay, the Abbott LCx assay, and direct fluorescent-antibody and culture assays for detection of *Chlamydia trachomatis* and *Neisseria gonorrhoeae*. *J. Clin. Microbiol.* **42:**3089–3093.
12. **Brade, H., L. Brade, and F. E. Nano.** 1987. Chemical and serological investigations on the genus-specific lipopolysaccharide epitope of *Chlamydia*. *Proc. Natl. Acad. Sci. USA* **84:**2508–2512.
13. **Campbell, L. A., M. M. Perez, D. J. Hamilton, C. C. Kuo, and J. T. Grayston.** 1992. Detection of *Chlamydia pneumoniae* by polymerase chain reaction. *J. Clin. Microbiol.* **30:**434–439.
14. **Cannon, C. P., E. Braunwald, C. H. McCabe, J. T. Grayston, B. Muhlestein, R. P. Giugliano, R. Cairns, and A. M. Skene.** 2005. Antibiotic treatment of *Chlamydia pneumoniae* after acute coronary syndrome. *N. Engl. J. Med.* **352:**1646–1654.
15. **Centers for Disease Control and Prevention.** 2002. Sexually transmitted diseases treatment guidelines 2002. *Morb. Mortal. Wkly. Rep.* **51**(RR-6)**:**1–77.
16. **Chernesky, M. A., D. H. Martin, E. W. Hook, D. Willis, J. Jordan, S. Wang, J. R. Lane, D. Fuller, and J. Schachter.** 2005. Ability of new APTIMA CT and APTIMA GC assays to detect *Chlamydia trachomatis* and *Neisseria gonorrhoeae* in male urine and urethral swabs. *J. Clin. Microbiol.* **43:**127–131.
17. **Chia, J. K., and L. Y. Chia.** 1999. Chronic *Chlamydia pneumoniae* infection: a treatable cause of chronic fatigue syndrome. *Clin. Infect. Dis.* **29:**452–453.
18. **Collingro, A., S. Poppert, E. Heinz, S. Schmitz-Esser, A. Essig, M. Schweikert, M. Wagner, and M. Horn.** 2005. Recovery of an environmental chlamydia strain from activated sludge by co-cultivation with *Acanthamoeba* sp. *Microbiology* **151:**301–309.
19. **Colmegna, I., R. Cuchacovich, and L. R. Espinoza.** 2004. HLA-B27-associated reactive arthritis: pathogenetic and clinical considerations. *Clin. Microbiol. Rev.* **17:**348-369.

20. **Dean, D., R. J. Suchland, and W. E. Stamm.** 2000. Evidence for long-term cervical persistence of *Chlamydia trachomatis* by omp1 genotyping. *J. Infect. Dis.* **182:**909–916.
21. **Dowell, S. F., R. W. Peeling, J. Boman, G. M. Carlone, B. S. Fields, J. Guarner, M. R. Hammerschlag, L. A. Jackson, C. C. Kuo, M. Maass, T. O. Messmer, D. F. Talkington, M. L. Tondella, and S. R. Zaki.** 2001. Standardizing *Chlamydia pneumoniae* assays: recommendations from the Centers for Disease Control and Prevention (USA) and the Laboratory Centre for Disease Control (Canada). *Clin. Infect. Dis.* **33:**492–503.
22. **Dugan, J., D. D. Rockey, L. Jones, and A. A. Andersen.** 2004. Tetracycline resistance in *Chlamydia suis* mediated by genomic islands inserted into the chlamydial *inv*-like gene. *Antimicrob. Agents Chemother.* **48:**3989–3995.
23. **Essig, A., U. Simnacher, M. Susa, and R. Marre.** 1999. Analysis of the humoral immune response to *Chlamydia pneumoniae* by immunoblotting and immunoprecipitation. *Clin. Diagn. Lab. Immunol.* **6:**819–825.
24. **Essig, A., P. Zucs, M. Susa, G. Wasenauer, U. Mamat, M. Hetzel, U. Vogel, S. Wieshammer, H. Brade, and R. Marre.** 1995. Diagnosis of ornithosis by cell culture and polymerase chain reaction in a patient with chronic pneumonia. *Clin. Infect. Dis.* **21:**1495–1497.
25. **Everett, K. D., R. M. Bush, and A. A. Andersen.** 1999. Emended description of the order *Chlamydiales*, proposal of *Parachlamydiaceae* fam. nov. and *Simkaniaceae* fam. nov., each containing one monotypic genus, revised taxonomy of the family *Chlamydiaceae*, including a new genus and five new species, and standards for the identification of organisms. *Int. J. Syst. Bacteriol.* **49**(Pt. 2)**:**415–440.
26. **Everett, K. D., and T. P. Hatch.** 1995. Architecture of the cell envelope of *Chlamydia psittaci* 6BC. *J. Bacteriol.* **177:**877–882.
27. **Fan, T., H. Lu, H. Hu, L. Shi, G. A. McClarty, D. M. Nance, A. H. Greenberg, and G. Zhong.** 1998. Inhibition of apoptosis in chlamydia-infected cells: blockade of mitochondrial cytochrome c release and caspase activation. *J. Exp. Med.* **187:**487–496.
28. **Farencena, A., M. Comanducci, M. Donati, G. Ratti, and R. Cevenini.** 1997. Characterization of a new isolate of *Chlamydia trachomatis* which lacks the common plasmid and has properties of biovar trachoma. *Infect. Immun.* **65:**2965–2969.
29. **Fischer, S. F., J. Vier, S. Kirschnek, A. Klos, S. Hess, S. Ying, and G. Hacker.** 2004. *Chlamydia* inhibit host cell apoptosis by degradation of proapoptotic BH3-only proteins. *J. Exp. Med.* **200:**905–916.
30. **Fritsche, T. R., M. Horn, M. Wagner, R. P. Herwig, K. H. Schleifer, and R. K. Gautom.** 2000. Phylogenetic diversity among geographically dispersed *Chlamydiales* endosymbionts recovered from clinical and environmental isolates of *Acanthamoeba* spp. *Appl. Environ. Microbiol.* **66:**2613–2619.
31. **Fukushi, H., and K. Hirai.** 1992. Proposal of *Chlamydia pecorum* sp. nov. for *Chlamydia* strains derived from ruminants. *Int. J. Syst. Bacteriol.* **42:**306–308.
32. **Gaydos, C. A., T. C. Quinn, and J. J. Eiden.** 1992. Identification of *Chlamydia pneumoniae* by DNA amplification of the 16S rRNA gene. *J. Clin. Microbiol.* **30:**796–800.
33. **Gaydos, C. A., P. M. Roblin, M. R. Hammerschlag, C. L. Hyman, J. J. Eiden, J. Schachter, and T. C. Quinn.** 1994. Diagnostic utility of PCR-enzyme immunoassay, culture, and serology for detection of *Chlamydia pneumoniae* in symptomatic and asymptomatic patients. *J. Clin. Microbiol.* **32:**903–905.
34. **Geens, T., A. Desplanques, M. Van Loock, B. M. Bonner, E. F. Kaleta, S. Magnino, A. A. Andersen, K. D. Everett, and D. Vanrompay.** 2005. Sequencing of the *Chlamydophila psittaci ompA* gene reveals a new genotype, E/B, and the need for a rapid discriminatory genotyping method. *J. Clin. Microbiol.* **43:**2456–2461.
35. **Grayston, J. T., L. A. Campbell, C. C. Kuo, C. H. Mordhorst, P. Saikku, D. H. Thom, and S. P. Wang.** 1990. A new respiratory tract pathogen: *Chlamydia pneumoniae* strain TWAR. *J. Infect. Dis.* **161:**618–625.
36. **Grayston, J. T., R. A. Kronmal, L. A. Jackson, A. F. Parisi, J. B. Muhlestein, J. D. Cohen, W. J. Rogers, J. R. Crouse, S. L. Borrowdale, E. Schron, and C. Knirsch.** 2005. Azithromycin for the secondary prevention of coronary events. *N. Engl. J. Med.* **352:**1637–1645.
37. **Hammerschlag, M. R., K. Chirgwin, P. M. Roblin, M. Gelling, W. Dumornay, L. Mandel, P. Smith, and J. Schachter.** 1992. Persistent infection with *Chlamydia pneumoniae* following acute respiratory illness. *Clin. Infect. Dis.* **14:**178–182.
38. **Heinemann, M., W. V. Kern, D. Bunjes, R. Marre, and A. Essig.** 2000. Severe *Chlamydia pneumoniae* infection in patients with neutropenia: case reports and literature review. *Clin. Infect. Dis.* **31:**181–184.
39. **Hermann, C., K. Gueinzius, A. Oehme, S. Von Aulock, E. Straube, and T. Hartung.** 2004. Comparison of quantitative and semiquantitative enzyme-linked immunosorbent assays for immunoglobulin G against *Chlamydophila pneumoniae* to a microimmunofluorescence test for use with patients with respiratory tract infections. *J. Clin. Microbiol.* **42:**2476–2479.
40. **Hogan, R. J., S. A. Mathews, S. Mukhopadhyay, J. T. Summersgill, and P. Timms.** 2004. Chlamydial persistence: beyond the biphasic paradigm. *Infect. Immun.* **72:**1843–1855.
41. **Horn, M., A. Collingro, S. Schmitz-Esser, C. L. Beier, U. Purkhold, B. Fartmann, P. Brandt, G. J. Nyakatura, M. Droege, D. Frishman, T. Rattei, H. W. Mewes, and M. Wagner.** 2004. Illuminating the evolutionary history of chlamydiae. *Science* **304:**728–730.
42. **Hsieh, Y. H., M. R. Howell, J. C. Gaydos, K. T. McKee, Jr., T. C. Quinn, and C. A. Gaydos.** 2003. Preference among female Army recruits for use of self-administrated vaginal swabs or urine to screen for *Chlamydia trachomatis* genital infections. *Sex. Transm. Dis.* **30:**769–773.
43. **Huniche, B. S., L. T. Jensen, S. Birkelund, and G. Christiansen.** 1998. *Mycoplasma* contamination of *Chlamydia pneumoniae* isolates. *Scand. J. Infect. Dis.* **30:**181–187.
44. **Ieven, M. M., and V. Y. Hoymans.** 2005. Involvement of *Chlamydia pneumoniae* in atherosclerosis: more evidence for lack of evidence. *J. Clin. Microbiol.* **43:**19–24.
45. **Jantos, C. A., S. Heck, R. Roggendorf, M. Sen-Gupta, and J. H. Hegemann.** 1997. Antigenic and molecular analyses of different *Chlamydia pneumoniae* strains. *J. Clin. Microbiol.* **35:**620–623.
46. **Jee, J., F. J. Degraves, T. Kim, and B. Kaltenboeck.** 2004. High prevalence of natural *Chlamydophila* species infection in calves. *J. Clin. Microbiol.* **42:**5664–5672.
47. **Johnson, R. E., W. J. Newhall, J. R. Papp, J. S. Knapp, C. M. Black, T. L. Gift, R. Steece, L. E. Markowitz, O. J. Devine, C. M. Walsh, S. Wang, D. C. Gunter, K. L. Irwin, S. DeLisle, and S. M. Berman.** 2002. Screening tests to detect *Chlamydia trachomatis* and *Neisseria gonorrhoeae* infections—2002. *MMWR Recomm. Rep.* **51:**1–38.
48. **Jurstrand, M., L. Falk, H. Fredlund, M. Lindberg, P. Olcen, S. Andersson, K. Persson, J. Albert, and A. Backman.** 2001. Characterization of *Chlamydia trachomatis omp1* genotypes among sexually transmitted disease patients in Sweden. *J. Clin. Microbiol.* **39:**3915–3919.
49. **Kahane, S., K. D. Everett, N. Kimmel, and M. G. Friedman.** 1999. *Simkania negevensis* strain ZT: growth, antigenic and genome characteristics. *Int. J. Syst. Bacteriol.* **49**(Pt. 2)**:**815–820.
50. **Kahane, S., N. Platzner, B. Dvoskin, A. Itzhaki, and M. G. Friedman.** 2004. Evidence for the presence of *Simkania*

negevensis in drinking water and in reclaimed wastewater in Israel. *Appl. Environ. Microbiol.* **70:**3346–3351.

51. **Kalman, S., W. Mitchell, R. Marathe, C. Lammel, J. Fan, R. W. Hyman, L. Olinger, J. Grimwood, R. W. Davis, and R. S. Stephens.** 1999. Comparative genomes of *Chlamydia pneumoniae* and *C. trachomatis*. *Nat. Genet.* **21:**385–389.
52. **Katusic, D., I. Petricek, Z. Mandic, I. Petric, J. Salopek-Rabatic, V. Kruzic, K. Oreskovic, J. Sikic, and G. Petricek.** 2003. Azithromycin vs doxycycline in the treatment of inclusion conjunctivitis. *Am. J. Ophthalmol.* **135:** 447–451.
53. **Kent, C. K., J. K. Chaw, W. Wong, S. Liska, S. Gibson, G. Hubbard, and J. D. Klausner.** 2005. Prevalence of rectal, urethral, and pharyngeal chlamydia and gonorrhea detected in 2 clinical settings among men who have sex with men: San Francisco, California, 2003. *Clin. Infect. Dis.* **41:**67–74.
54. **Kuo, C. C., L. A. Jackson, L. A. Campbell, and J. T. Grayston.** 1995. *Chlamydia pneumoniae* (TWAR). *Clin. Microbiol. Rev.* **8:**451–461.
55. **Kuoppa, Y., J. Boman, L. Scott, U. Kumlin, I. Eriksson, and A. Allard.** 2002. Quantitative detection of respiratory *Chlamydia pneumoniae* infection by real-time PCR. *J. Clin. Microbiol.* **40:**2273–2274.
56. **Lau, C. Y., and A. K. Qureshi.** 2002. Azithromycin versus doxycycline for genital chlamydial infections: a meta-analysis of randomized clinical trials. *Sex. Transm. Dis.* **29:**497–502.
57. **Lim, W. S., J. T. Macfarlane, T. C. Boswell, T. G. Harrison, D. Rose, M. Leinonen, and P. Saikku.** 2001. Study of community acquired pneumonia aetiology (SCAPA) in adults admitted to hospital: implications for management guidelines. *Thorax* **56:**296–301.
58. **Lindan, C., M. Mathur, S. Kumta, H. Jerajani, A. Gogate, J. Schachter, and J. Moncada.** 2005. Utility of pooled urine specimens for detection of *Chlamydia trachomatis* and *Neisseria gonorrhoeae* in men attending public sexually transmitted infection clinics in Mumbai, India, by PCR. *J. Clin. Microbiol.* **43:**1674–1677.
59. **Lister, N. A., S. N. Tabrizi, C. K. Fairley, and S. Garland.** 2004. Validation of Roche COBAS Amplicor assay for detection of *Chlamydia trachomatis* in rectal and pharyngeal specimens by an *omp1* PCR assay. *J. Clin. Microbiol.* **42:**239–241.
60. **Mabey, D., and R. W. Peeling.** 2002. Lymphogranuloma venereum. *Sex. Transm. Infect.* **78:**90–92.
61. **Madico, G., T. C. Quinn, J. Boman, and C. A. Gaydos.** 2000. Touchdown enzyme time release-PCR for detection and identification of *Chlamydia trachomatis, C. pneumoniae,* and *C. psittaci* using the 16S and 16S-23S spacer rRNA genes. *J. Clin. Microbiol.* **38:**1085–1093.
62. **Mahony, J., S. Chong, D. Jang, K. Luinstra, M. Faught, D. Dalby, J. Sellors, and M. Chernesky.** 1998. Urine specimens from pregnant and nonpregnant women inhibitory to amplification of *Chlamydia trachomatis* nucleic acid by PCR, ligase chain reaction, and transcription-mediated amplification: identification of urinary substances associated with inhibition and removal of inhibitory activity. *J. Clin. Microbiol.* **36:**3122–3126.
63. **Malinverni, R., C. C. Kuo, L. A. Campbell, and J. T. Grayston.** 1995. Reactivation of *Chlamydia pneumoniae* lung infection in mice by cortisone. *J. Infect. Dis.* **172:**593–594.
64. **Martin, D. H., T. F. Mroczkowski, Z. A. Dalu, J. McCarty, R. B. Jones, S. J. Hopkins, R. B. Johnson, and The Azithromycin for Chlamydial Infections Study Group.** 1992. A controlled trial of a single dose of azithromycin for the treatment of chlamydial urethritis and cervicitis. *N. Engl. J. Med.* **327:**921–925.
65. **Martin, D. H., M. Nsuami, J. Schachter, E. W. Hook III, D. Ferrero, T. C. Quinn, and C. Gaydos.** 2004. Use of multiple nucleic acid amplification tests to define the infected-patient "gold standard" in clinical trials of new diagnostic tests for *Chlamydia trachomatis* infections. *J. Clin. Microbiol.* **42:**4749–4758.
66. **Messmer, T. O., J. Martinez, F. Hassouna, E. R. Zell, W. Harris, S. Dowell, and G. M. Carlone.** 2001. Comparison of two commercial microimmunofluorescence kits and an enzyme immunoassay kit for detection of serum immunoglobulin G antibodies to *Chlamydia pneumoniae*. *Clin. Diagn. Lab. Immunol.* **8:**588–592.
67. **Messmer, T. O., S. K. Skelton, J. F. Moroney, H. Daugharty, and B. S. Fields.** 1997. Application of a nested, multiplex PCR to psittacosis outbreaks. *J. Clin. Microbiol.* **35:**2043–2046.
68. **Misyurina, O. Y., E. V. Chipitsyna, Y. P. Finashutina, V. N. Lazarev, T. A. Akopian, A. M. Savicheva, and V. M. Govorun.** 2004. Mutations in a 23S rRNA gene of *Chlamydia trachomatis* associated with resistance to macrolides. *Antimicrob. Agents Chemother.* **48:**1347–1349.
69. **Montalban, G. S., P. M. Roblin, and M. R. Hammerschlag.** 1994. Performance of three commercially available monoclonal reagents for confirmation of *Chlamydia pneumoniae* in cell culture. *J. Clin. Microbiol.* **32:**1406–1407.
70. **Moroney, J. F., R. Guevara, C. Iverson, F. M. Chen, S. K. Skelton, T. O. Messmer, B. Plikaytis, P. O. Williams, P. Blake, and J. C. Butler.** 1998. Detection of chlamydiosis in a shipment of pet birds, leading to recognition of an outbreak of clinically mild psittacosis in humans. *Clin. Infect. Dis.* **26:**1425–1429.
71. **Morre, S. A., C. Munk, K. Persson, S. Kruger-Kjaer, R. van Dijk, C. J. Meijer, and A. J. van Den Brule.** 2002. Comparison of three commercially available peptide-based immunoglobulin G (IgG) and IgA assays to microimmunofluorescence assay for detection of *Chlamydia trachomatis* antibodies. *J. Clin. Microbiol.* **40:**584–587.
72. **Newhall, W. J., R. E. Johnson, S. DeLisle, D. Fine, A. Hadgu, B. Matsuda, D. Osmond, J. Campbell, and W. E. Stamm.** 1999. Head-to-head evaluation of five chlamydia tests relative to a quality-assured culture standard. *J. Clin. Microbiol.* **37:**681–685.
73. **Nieuwenhuis, R. F., J. M. Ossewaarde, H. M. Gotz, J. Dees, H. B. Thio, M. G. Thomeer, J. C. den Hollander, M. H. Neumann, and W. I. van der Meijden.** 2004. Resurgence of lymphogranuloma venereum in Western Europe: an outbreak of *Chlamydia trachomatis* serovar l2 proctitis in The Netherlands among men who have sex with men. *Clin. Infect. Dis.* **39:**996–1003.
74. **O'Connor, C. M., M. W. Dunne, M. A. Pfeffer, J. B. Muhlestein, L. Yao, S. Gupta, R. J. Benner, M. R. Fisher, and T. D. Cook.** 2003. Azithromycin for the secondary prevention of coronary heart disease events: the WIZARD study: a randomized controlled trial. *JAMA* **290:**1459–1466.
75. **Ojcius, D. M., P. Souque, J. L. Perfettini, and A. Dautry-Varsat.** 1998. Apoptosis of epithelial cells and macrophages due to infection with the obligate intracellular pathogen *Chlamydia psittaci*. *J. Immunol.* **161:**4220–4226.
76. **Peeling, R. W., S. P. Wang, J. T. Grayston, F. Blasi, J. Boman, A. Clad, H. Freidank, C. A. Gaydos, J. Gnarpe, T. Hagiwara, R. B. Jones, J. Orfila, K. Persson, M. Puolakkainen, P. Saikku, and J. Schachter.** 2000. *Chlamydia pneumoniae* serology: interlaboratory variation in microimmunofluorescence assay results. *J. Infect. Dis.* **181**(Suppl. 3)**:**S426–S429.
77. **Peipert, J. F.** 2003. Clinical practice. Genital chlamydial infections. *N. Engl. J. Med.* **349:**2424–2430.
78. **Pickett, M. A., J. S. Everson, P. J. Pead, and I. N. Clarke.** 2005. The plasmids of *Chlamydia trachomatis* and *Chlamydophila pneumoniae* (N16): accurate determination of copy number and the paradoxical effect of plasmid-curing agents. *Microbiology* **151:**893–903.
79. **Poppert, S., A. Essig, R. Marre, M. Wagner, and M. Horn.** 2002. Detection and differentiation of chlamydiae

by fluorescence in situ hybridization. *Appl. Environ. Microbiol.* **68:**4081–4089.

80. **Pospischil, A., R. Thoma, M. Hilbe, P. Grest, and J. O. Gebbers.** 2002. Abortion in woman caused by caprine *Chlamydophila abortus* (*Chlamydia psittaci* serovar 1). *Swiss Med. Wkly.* **132:**64–66.
81. **Principi, N., S. Esposito, F. Blasi, and L. Allegra.** 2001. Role of *Mycoplasma pneumoniae* and *Chlamydia pneumoniae* in children with community-acquired lower respiratory tract infections. *Clin. Infect. Dis.* **32:**1281–1289.
82. **Rampf, J., A. Essig, R. Hinrichs, M. Merkel, K. Scharffetter-Kochanek, and C. Sunderkotter.** 2004. Lymphogranuloma venereum—a rare cause of genital ulcers in central Europe. *Dermatology* **209:**230–232.
83. **Read, T. D., G. S. Myers, R. C. Brunham, W. C. Nelson, I. T. Paulsen, J. Heidelberg, E. Holtzapple, H. Khouri, N. B. Federova, H. A. Carty, L. A. Umayam, D. H. Haft, J. Peterson, M. J. Beanan, O. White, S. L. Salzberg, R. C. Hsia, G. McClarty, R. G. Rank, P. M. Bavoil, and C. M. Fraser.** 2003. Genome sequence of *Chlamydophila caviae* (*Chlamydia psittaci* GPIC): examining the role of niche-specific genes in the evolution of the *Chlamydiaceae*. *Nucleic Acids Res.* **31:**2134–2147.
84. **Reischl, U., N. Lehn, U. Simnacher, R. Marre, and A. Essig.** 2003. Rapid and standardized detection of *Chlamydia pneumoniae* using LightCycler real-time fluorescence PCR. *Eur. J. Clin. Microbiol. Infect. Dis.* **22:**54–57.
85. **Richardson, E., J. W. Sellors, S. Mackinnon, V. Woodcox, M. Howard, D. Jang, T. Karwalajtys, and M. A. Chernesky.** 2003. Prevalence of *Chlamydia trachomatis* infections and specimen collection preference among women, using self-collected vaginal swabs in community settings. *Sex. Transm. Dis.* **30:**880–885.
86. **Ross, R.** 1999. Atherosclerosis—an inflammatory disease. *N. Engl. J. Med.* **340:**115–126.
87. **Rurangirwa, F. R., P. M. Dilbeck, T. B. Crawford, T. C. McGuire, and T. F. McElwain.** 1999. Analysis of the 16S rRNA gene of micro-organism WSU 86-1044 from an aborted bovine foetus reveals that it is a member of the order *Chlamydiales*: proposal of *Waddliaceae* fam. nov., *Waddlia chondrophila* gen. nov., sp. nov. *Int. J. Syst. Bacteriol.* **49**(Pt. 2)**:**577–581.
88. **Saikku, P., M. Leinonen, K. Mattila, M. R. Ekman, M. S. Nieminen, P. H. Makela, J. K. Huttunen, and V. Valtonen.** 1988. Serological evidence of an association of a novel *Chlamydia*, TWAR, with chronic coronary heart disease and acute myocardial infarction. *Lancet* **ii:**983–986.
89. **Schachter, J., E. W. Hook, D. H. Martin, D. Willis, P. Fine, D. Fuller, J. Jordan, W. M. Janda, and M. Chernesky.** 2005. Confirming positive results of nucleic acid amplification tests (NAATs) for *Chlamydia trachomatis*: all NAATs are not created equal. *J. Clin. Microbiol.* **43:**1372–1373.
90. **Schachter, J., W. M. McCormack, M. A. Chernesky, D. H. Martin, B. Van Der Pol, P. A. Rice, E. W. Hook III, W. E. Stamm, T. C. Quinn, and J. M. Chow.** 2003. Vaginal swabs are appropriate specimens for diagnosis of genital tract infection with *Chlamydia trachomatis*. *J. Clin. Microbiol.* **41:**3784–3789.
91. **Schachter, J., and W. E. Stamm.** 1999. *Chlamydia*, p. 795–806. *In* P. R. Murray, E. J. Baron, J. H. Jorgensen, M. A. Pfaller, and R. H. Yolken (ed.), *Manual of Clinical Microbiology,* 7th ed. ASM Press, Washington, D.C.
92. **Schachter, J., R. S. Stephens, P. Timms, C. Kuo, P. M. Bavoil, S. Birkelund, J. Boman, H. Caldwell, L. A. Campbell, M. Chernesky, G. Christiansen, I. N. Clarke, C. Gaydos, J. T. Grayston, T. Hackstadt, R. Hsia, B. Kaltenboeck, M. Leinonnen, D. Ocjius, G. McClarty, J. Orfila, R. Peeling, M. Puolakkainen, T. C. Quinn, R. G. Rank, J. Raulston, G. L. Ridgeway, P. Saikku, W. E. Stamm, D. T. Taylor-Robinson, S. P. Wang, and P. B. Wyrick.** 2001. Radical changes to chlamydial taxonomy are not necessary just yet. *Int. J. Syst. Evol. Microbiol.* **51:**249, 251–253.
93. **Scholes, D., A. Stergachis, F. E. Heidrich, H. Andrilla, K. K. Holmes, and W. E. Stamm.** 1996. Prevention of pelvic inflammatory disease by screening for cervical chlamydial infection. *N. Engl. J. Med.* **334:**1362–1366.
94. **Shafer, M. A., J. Moncada, C. B. Boyer, K. Betsinger, S. D. Flinn, and J. Schachter.** 2003. Comparing first-void urine specimens, self-collected vaginal swabs, and endocervical specimens to detect *Chlamydia trachomatis* and *Neisseria gonorrhoeae* by a nucleic acid amplification test. *J. Clin. Microbiol.* **41:**4395–4399.
95. **Shapiro, D. S., S. C. Kenney, M. Johnson, C. H. Davis, S. T. Knight, and P. B. Wyrick.** 1992. Brief report: *Chlamydia psittaci* endocarditis diagnosed by blood culture. *N. Engl. J. Med.* **326:**1192–1195.
96. **Shirai, M., H. Hirakawa, M. Kimoto, M. Tabuchi, F. Kishi, K. Ouchi, T. Shiba, K. Ishii, M. Hattori, S. Kuhara, and T. Nakazawa.** 2000. Comparison of whole genome sequences of *Chlamydia pneumoniae* J138 from Japan and CWL029 from USA. *Nucleic Acids Res.* **28:**2311–2314.
97. **Solomon, A. W., R. W. Peeling, A. Foster, and D. C. Mabey.** 2004. Diagnosis and assessment of trachoma. *Clin. Microbiol. Rev.* **17:**982–1011.
98. **Somani, J., V. B. Bhullar, K. A. Workowski, C. E. Farshy, and C. M. Black.** 2000. Multiple drug-resistant *Chlamydia trachomatis* associated with clinical treatment failure. *J. Infect. Dis.* **181:**1421–1427.
99. **Spaargaren, J., J. Schachter, J. Moncada, H. J. de Vries, H. S. Fennema, A. S. Pena, R. A. Coutinho, and S. A. Morre.** 2005. Slow epidemic of lymphogranuloma venereum L2b strain. *Emerg. Infect. Dis.* **11:**1787–1788.
100. **Sriram, S., C. W. Stratton, S. Yao, A. Tharp, L. Ding, J. D. Bannan, and W. M. Mitchell.** 1999. *Chlamydia pneumoniae* infection of the central nervous system in multiple sclerosis. *Ann. Neurol.* **46:**6–14.
101. **Stephens, R. S., S. Kalman, C. Lammel, J. Fan, R. Marathe, L. Aravind, W. Mitchell, L. Olinger, R. L. Tatusov, Q. Zhao, E. V. Koonin, and R. W. Davis.** 1998. Genome sequence of an obligate intracellular pathogen of humans: *Chlamydia trachomatis*. *Science* **282:**754–759.
102. **Stephens, R. S., K. Koshiyama, E. Lewis, and A. Kubo.** 2001. Heparin-binding outer membrane protein of chlamydiae. *Mol. Microbiol.* **40:**691–699.
103. **Stothard, D. R., J. A. Williams, B. Van Der Pol, and R. B. Jones.** 1998. Identification of a *Chlamydia trachomatis* serovar E urogenital isolate which lacks the cryptic plasmid. *Infect. Immun.* **66:**6010–6013.
104. **Stralin, K., E. Tornqvist, M. S. Kaltoft, P. Olcen, and H. Holmberg.** 2006. Etiologic diagnosis of adult bacterial pneumonia by culture and PCR applied to respiratory tract samples. *J. Clin. Microbiol.* **44:**643–645.
105. **Sturm, P. D., P. Moodley, K. Govender, L. Bohlken, T. Vanmali, and A. W. Sturm.** 2005. Molecular diagnosis of lymphogranuloma venereum in patients with genital ulcer disease. *J. Clin. Microbiol.* **43:**2973–2975.
106. **Suchland, R. J., W. M. Geisler, and W. E. Stamm.** 2003. Methodologies and cell lines used for antimicrobial susceptibility testing of *Chlamydia* spp. *Antimicrob. Agents Chemother.* **47:**636–642.
107. **Suchland, R. J., and W. E. Stamm.** 1991. Simplified microtiter cell culture method for rapid immunotyping of *Chlamydia trachomatis*. *J. Clin. Microbiol.* **29:**1333–1338.
108. **Tondella, M. L., D. F. Talkington, B. P. Holloway, S. F. Dowell, K. Cowley, M. Soriano-Gabarro, M. S. Elkind, and B. S. Fields.** 2002. Development and evaluation of real-time PCR-based fluorescence assays for detection of *Chlamydia pneumoniae*. *J. Clin. Microbiol.* **40:**575–583.

109. **Tong, C. Y., and M. Sillis.** 1993. Detection of *Chlamydia pneumoniae* and *Chlamydia psittaci* in sputum samples by PCR. *J. Clin. Pathol.* **46:**313–317.

110. **Van der Bij, A. K., J. Spaargaren, S. A. Morre, H. S. Fennema, A. Mindel, R. A. Coutinho, and H. J. de Vries.** 2006. Diagnostic and clinical implications of anorectal lymphogranuloma venereum in men who have sex with men: a retrospective case-control study. *Clin. Infect. Dis.* **42:**186–194.

111. **Van Der Pol, B., D. V. Ferrero, L. Buck-Barrington, E. Hook III, C. Lenderman, T. Quinn, C. A. Gaydos, J. Lovchik, J. Schachter, J. Moncada, G. Hall, M. J. Tuohy, and R. B. Jones.** 2001. Multicenter evaluation of the BDProbeTec ET System for detection of *Chlamydia trachomatis* and *Neisseria gonorrhoeae* in urine specimens, female endocervical swabs, and male urethral swabs. *J. Clin. Microbiol.* **39:**1008–1016.

112. **Van Der Pol, B., T. C. Quinn, C. A. Gaydos, K. Crotchfelt, J. Schachter, J. Moncada, D. Jungkind, D. H. Martin, B. Turner, C. Peyton, and R. B. Jones.** 2000. Multicenter evaluation of the AMPLICOR and automated COBAS AMPLICOR CT/NG tests for detection of *Chlamydia trachomatis*. *J. Clin. Microbiol.* **38:**1105–1112.

113. **Van Der Pol, B., J. A. Williams, N. J. Smith, B. E. Batteiger, A. P. Cullen, H. Erdman, T. Edens, K. Davis, H. Salim-Hammad, V. W. Chou, L. Scearce, J. Blutman, and W. J. Payne.** 2002. Evaluation of the Digene Hybrid Capture II Assay with the Rapid Capture System for detection of *Chlamydia trachomatis* and *Neisseria gonorrhoeae*. *J. Clin. Microbiol.* **40:**3558–3564.

114. **Van Loock, M., D. Vanrompay, B. Herrmann, S. J. Vander, G. Volckaert, B. M. Goddeeris, and K. D. Everett.** 2003. Missing links in the divergence of *Chlamydophila abortus* from *Chlamydophila psittaci*. *Int. J. Syst. Evol. Microbiol.* **53:**761–770.

115. **Wadowsky, R. M., E. A. Castilla, S. Laus, A. Kozy, R. W. Atchison, L. A. Kingsley, J. I. Ward, and D. P. Greenberg.** 2002. Evaluation of *Chlamydia pneumoniae* and *Mycoplasma pneumoniae* as etiologic agents of persistent cough in adolescents and adults. *J. Clin. Microbiol.* **40:**637–640.

116. **Wahl, C., F. Oswald, U. Simnacher, S. Weiss, R. Marre, and A. Essig.** 2001. Survival of *Chlamydia pneumoniae*-infected Mono Mac 6 cells is dependent on NF-kappaB binding activity. *Infect. Immun.* **69:**7039–7045.

117. **Walder, G., H. Hotzel, C. Brezinka, W. Gritsch, R. Tauber, R. Wurzner, and F. Ploner.** 2005. An unusual cause of sepsis during pregnancy: recognizing infection with *Chlamydophila abortus*. *Obstet. Gynecol.* **106:**1215–1217.

118. **Wang, S.** 2000. The microimmunofluorescence test for *Chlamydia pneumoniae* infection: technique and interpretation. *J. Infect. Dis.* **181**(Suppl. 3)**:**S421–S425.

119. **Wang, S. A., J. R. Papp, W. E. Stamm, R. W. Peeling, D. H. Martin, and K. K. Holmes.** 2005. Evaluation of antimicrobial resistance and treatment failures for *Chlamydia trachomatis:* a meeting report. *J. Infect. Dis.* **191:**917–923.

120. **Weiss, S. M., P. M. Roblin, C. A. Gaydos, P. Cummings, D. L. Patton, N. Schulhoff, J. Shani, R. Frankel, K. Penney, T. C. Quinn, M. R. Hammerschlag, and J. Schachter.** 1996. Failure to detect *Chlamydia pneumoniae* in coronary atheromas of patients undergoing atherectomy. *J. Infect. Dis.* **173:**957–962.

121. **Zeidler, H., J. Kuipers, and L. Kohler.** 2004. *Chlamydia*-induced arthritis. *Curr. Opin. Rheumatol.* **16:**380–392.

Rickettsia and *Orientia*

DAVID H. WALKER AND DONALD H. BOUYER

66

TAXONOMY

The family *Rickettsiaceae* comprises two genera of small, obligately intracellular bacteria that reside free within the cytosol, namely, *Rickettsia* and *Orientia*. Although the number and diversity of strains in each genus are similar, the practices of species designation differ remarkably. The second edition of *Bergey's Manual of Systematic Bacteriology* lists 20 validated names of *Rickettsia* species, and others have been proposed (84). *Orientia tsutsugamushi*, the single species of the genus, has 0.8% divergence of the *rrs* (16S rRNA) gene. Similarly, other obligately intracellular bacteria have 0.5% *rrs* divergence within a species (e.g., *Ehrlichia chaffeensis*, *Coxiella burnetii*, and *Chlamydia trachomatis*). A recent proposal of criteria for the limits of divergence of *Rickettsia* species would allow different species to be as closely related as 0.2% divergence for *rrs*, 0.8% for citrate synthetase (*gltA*), 1.2% for outer membrane protein A (*ompA*), 0.8% for outer membrane protein B (*ompB*), and 0.7% for surface protein 4 (*sca4*) (15). There are no common or universal concepts that can be utilized to delineate prokaryotic species as there are with eukaryotes.

The typhus group (TG) and spotted fever group (SFG), defined originally by their distinctive lipopolysaccharide antigens, constitute the genus along with other ancestral species such as *R. bellii* and *R. canadensis*. The TG consists of only two members, *R. prowazekii* and *R. typhi*, whereas the SFG contains bacteria that are generally recognized as human pathogens (*R. rickettsii, R. akari, R. conorii, R. africae, R. sibirica, R. japonica, R. honei, R. felis, R. parkeri, R. slovaca, R. aeschlimannii,* and *R. australis*) as well as a steadily growing list of organisms identified only in arthropods (3, 50, 55, 84). Most of these species of undetermined pathogenicity, including *R. montanensis, R. bellii, R. peacockii,* and *R. rhipicephali,* are much more prevalent in U.S. ticks than is pathogenic *R. rickettsii*. In Europe, *R. helvetica* and *R. massiliae* have been proposed as human-infecting species based on limited evidence (5, 14). SFG isolates from Israel and the Astrakhan region of Russia, which have wider geographic distributions, are genetic variants of *R. conorii*. Similarly, SFG isolates recovered from *Hyalomma* ticks in Inner Mongolia and Africa and from patients in France and Africa have been designated the mongolotimonae strain of *R. sibirica*.

Orientia tsutsugamushi diverges from *Rickettsia* by approximately 10% in the *rrs* gene and differs greatly in its cell wall structure, containing completely unrelated proteins and lacking lipopolysaccharide and peptidoglycan (Table 1). Phylogeny using *groEL* reveals similar genetic diversity for the unispecies genus *Orientia* as for the *Rickettsia* genus, for which some believe that too many species have been created (Fig. 1) (35). *O. tsutsugamushi*, originally classified serologically, has subsequently been analyzed genetically (51). In each geographic area there are several genetic variants, and they differ from the genetic variants in other regions. Clonal evolutionary divergence has produced an enormous number of genotypes. Genetic variants of *O. tsutsugamushi* correspond to particular arthropod hosts in which divergence most likely occurred.

DESCRIPTION OF GENERA

Species of *Rickettsia* are small (0.3 to 0.5 μm by 1 to 2 μm), obligately intracellular bacteria of the *α-Proteobacteria* with a gram-negative cell wall structure that contains lipopolysaccharide, peptidoglycan, a major 135-kDa S-layer protein (OmpB), a 17-kDa lipoprotein, and for SFG rickettsiae a surface-exposed protein (OmpA) containing a variable number of nearly identical tandem repeat units (71). *Rickettsia* organisms have small (1.11 to 1.27 Mb), A+T-rich genomes resulting from reductive evolution with a high proportion (19 to 24%) of noncoding sequence and remarkable synteny (39). The lack of genes for enzymes for sugar metabolism, lipid biosynthesis, nucleotide synthesis, and amino acid synthesis and the presence of genes encoding enzymes for the complete tricarboxylic acid cycle and several copies of ATP/ADP translocase suggest both independent synthesis of ATP and acquisition of host ATP and rickettsial utilization of host sources for nutrition and building blocks. Rickettsiae adhere to the host cell receptor Ku70 by OmpB (and also by OmpA to an unknown receptor for SFG rickettsiae), trigger signaling pathways leading to recruitment and activation of induced phagocytosis, and escape from the phagosome by membranolytic activities of rickettsial phospholipase D and TlyC (36, 37, 82). *O. tsutsugamushi* (0.3 to 0.5 μm by 0.8 to 1.5 μm) has a major surface protein of 54 to 58 kDa as well as 110-, 80-, 47-, 42-, 35-, 28-, and 25-kDa surface proteins but lacks muramic acid, glucosamine, 2-keto-3-deoctulonic acid, and hydroxy fatty acids, suggesting the absence of lipopolysaccharide and peptidoglycan. Compared with *Rickettsia* spp., *Orientia* has a more plastic gram-negative

TABLE 1 Characteristics of *Rickettsia* spp. and *Orientia tsutsugamushi*[a]

Organisms	LPS	PG	OmpA	OmpB	17-kDa lipoprotein	56-kDa protein
SFG	S	+	+	+	+	0
Typhus group	T	+	0	+	+	0
R. canadensis	T	+	+	+	+	0
O. tsutsugamushi	0	0	0	0	0	+

[a] Abbreviations and symbols: LPS, lipopolysaccharide; S, spotted fever group lipopolysaccharide present; T, typhus group lipopolysaccharide present; PG, peptidoglycan; +, present; 0, absent.

cell wall with a thicker outer leaflet and thinner inner leaflet of the outer envelope and does not have a slime layer.

EPIDEMIOLOGY AND TRANSMISSION

Rickettsia spp. reside in an arthropod host (tick, mite, louse, flea, or other insect) for at least a part of their life cycle, during which they are maintained by transovarian transmission and/or cycles involving horizontal transmission to mammalian hosts (38) (Table 2). *Orientia* resides free in the cytosol and is maintained in nature by transovarian transmission in trombiculid mites, which transmit the infection to humans during feeding as the larval stage (Table 2).

CLINICAL SIGNIFICANCE

In addition to Rocky Mountain spotted fever (RMSF), rickettsialpox, murine typhus, flying squirrel-associated *R. prowazekii* infection, flea-borne spotted fever, and *R. parkeri* infection, which are indigenous to the United States, the potential for imported cases is significant for African tick bite fever, boutonneuse fever, murine typhus, and scrub typhus (Table 2) (10, 27, 28, 48, 54, 62, 75, 80). Other rickettsioses, either because of their geographic distribution and the infrequency of travelers' exposure to them or because of their incidence, are unlikely to be imported. RMSF, louse-borne typhus, and scrub typhus are life-threatening illnesses even for young, previously healthy persons. Murine typhus, boutonneuse fever, and North Asian tick typhus can have a fatal outcome in patients who are elderly or have underlying diseases or other risk factors. Although *R. felis, R. africae,* and *R. parkeri* cause milder, usually nonfatal rickettsioses, their importance has increased, with diagnoses over a wide geographic distribution (18, 45, 47, 85).

An average of 7 days after tick bite inoculation of rickettsiae, patients with RMSF develop fever, severe headache, malaise, and myalgia, frequently accompanied by nausea, vomiting, and abdominal pain and sometimes cough (27). A rash typically appears only after 3 to 5 days of illness. Rickettsiae infect endothelial cells, frequently leading to increased vascular permeability and focal hemorrhages (21). In severe cases, noncardiogenic pulmonary edema and rickettsial encephalitis

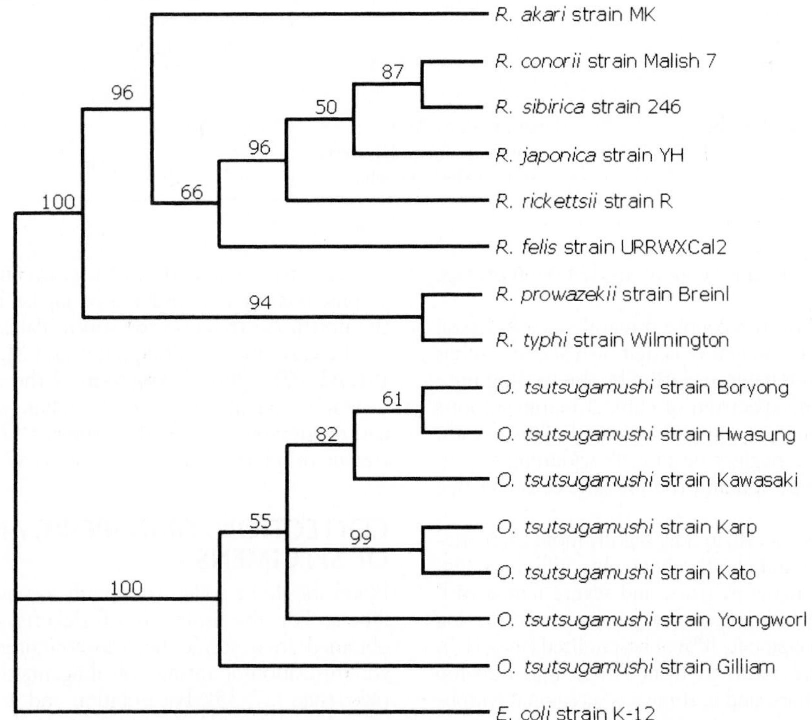

FIGURE 1 Phylogeny of *Rickettsia* and *Orientia* as determined by unweighted maximum parsimony analyses of *groEL* gene sequences prepared by PAUP 4.0 software with *Escherichia coli* as the outgroup. Numerical values on the branches represent the quantity of genetic divergence from the nearest node.

TABLE 2 Etiology, epidemiology, and ecology of rickettsial diseases

Organism	Disease	Geographic distribution	Typical mode of transmission to humans	Natural cycle
Spotted fever group				
R. rickettsii	Rocky Mountain spotted fever	Western Hemisphere	Tick bite	Transovarian in ticks and rodent-tick cycles
R. akari	Rickettsialpox	United States, Ukraine, Croatia, Korea	Mite bite	Transovarian in mites and mite-mouse cycles
R. conorii	Boutonneuse fever	Southern Europe, Africa, Middle East	Tick bite	Transovarian in ticks
R. africae	African tick bite fever	Sub-Saharan Africa, Caribbean	Tick bite	Transovarian in ticks
R. parkeri	American tick bite fever	North and South America	Tick bite	Transovarian in ticks
R. sibirica	North Asian tick typhus	Asia, Europe, Africa	Tick bite	Transovarian in ticks
R. japonica	Japanese spotted fever	Japan	Tick bite	Ticks
R. australis	Queensland tick typhus	Australia	Tick bite	Ticks
R. honei	Flinders Island spotted fever	Australia, Thailand	Tick bite	Transovarian in ticks
R. slovaca	Tick-borne lymphadenopathy	Eurasia	Tick bite	Unknown
R. felis	Flea-borne spotted fever	North and South America, Europe, Africa	Not known	Transovarian in cat fleas
Typhus group				
R. prowazekii	Primary louse-borne typhus	Worldwide	Infected louse feces rubbed into broken skin or mucous membranes or inhaled as aerosol	Human-louse cycle; flying squirrel-flea and/or louse cycle
R. prowazekii	Brill-Zinsser disease	Worldwide	Recrudescence years after primary attack of louse-borne typhus	
R. typhi	Murine typhus	Worldwide	Infected flea feces rubbed into broken skin or mucous membranes or inhaled as an aerosol	Rat-flea cycle; opossum-flea cycle
Scrub typhus group				
O. tsutsugamushi	Scrub typhus	Japan, eastern Asia, northern Australia, west and southwest Pacific	Chigger bite	Transovarian in mites

with coma and seizures are grave conditions that often presage death (74).

Rickettsialpox has been recognized mainly as a nonfatal urban disease with disseminated vesicular rash and an eschar at the location of rickettsial inoculation by the feeding mite (28, 31). The complete spectrum of clinical manifestations of *R. felis* infections has yet to be determined. This disease suffers from diagnostic neglect despite its widening recognized geographic distribution and the prevalence of cat flea exposure (62, 85).

Murine typhus causes a rash in only slightly more than one-half of patients, cough and chest radiographic infiltrates suggesting pneumonia in many patients, and severe illness with seizures, coma, and renal and respiratory failure necessitating intensive care unit admission in 10% of hospitalized cases (10).

Travelers who have returned from Africa and develop fever, one or more eschars, and in some cases regional lymphadenopathy and a maculopapular or vesicular rash are very likely infected with *R. africae* (54).

Rickettsia prowazekii, R. rickettsii, R. typhi, and *R. conorii* are bioterror threats via aerosol exposure to organisms that are stable and infectious at a low dose (72).

Scrub typhus caused by *O. tsutsugamushi* occurs in the geographic area that is bordered by Japan, Korea, and Russia on the north, Australia on the south, Pakistan and Afghanistan on the east, and the Philippines and Micronesia on the west (51, 63, 67). Clinical symptoms of the disease include fever, headache, maculopapular rash, eschar, lymphadenopathy, and central nervous system involvement (24, 58, 65). Without treatment, mortality can reach up to 30% (24).

COLLECTION, TRANSPORT, AND STORAGE OF SPECIMENS

Blood should be collected as early as possible in the course of illness. For the isolation of rickettsiae, blood should be obtained in a sterile heparin-containing vial prior to the administration of antimicrobial agents that are active against rickettsiae (27, 33). For isolation and immunocytologic diagnosis, blood should be stored temporarily at 4°C and processed as promptly as possible. If inoculation of cell culture or animals must be delayed for more than 24 h, plasma, buffy coat, whole blood, or biopsied tissue should be frozen rapidly and stored at −70°C or in liquid nitrogen. EDTA- or sodium citrate-anticoagulated blood collected in the acute state has been used effectively for the diagnosis of murine typhus, epidemic typhus, Japanese spotted fever, scrub typhus and, with lower sensitivity, RMSF and African tick bite fever, by PCR (17, 54, 61, 62, 64, 68, 69). PCR provides a higher diagnostic yield when applied to biopsy specimens of rickettsia-infected lesions, particularly eschars (44, 45). If whole blood, plasma, buffy coat, or tissue cannot be processed for PCR within several days, it should be stored at −20°C or lower.

For serologic diagnosis, blood is collected as early in the course of disease as possible, a second sample is collected after 1 or 2 weeks, and, if a fourfold rise in antibodies has not occurred, a third sample is collected 3 or 4 weeks after onset. The serum may be stored for several days at 4°C but should be stored frozen at −20°C or lower for longer periods to avoid degradation of the antibodies. However, blood samples collected by fingerstick on appropriate blotting paper in remote areas and sent by ordinary mail can be eluted for serologic diagnosis (13).

A 3-mm-diameter punch biopsy specimen of a skin lesion, preferably a maculopapule containing a petechia or the margin of an eschar, should be collected as soon as possible (41, 73). Although treatment should not be delayed, it is best to perform the biopsy prior to the completion of 24 h of treatment with a tetracycline or chloramphenicol. For immunohistologic detection of SFG or TG rickettsiae, the specimen can be snap-frozen for frozen sectioning or fixed in formaldehyde for the preparation of paraffin-embedded sections (21, 28, 41, 73–75, 77). The former approach yields an answer more rapidly, but freezing artifacts distorts the architecture of the tissue, and fixed tissue is more convenient for shipping to a reference laboratory (44). Aseptically collected autopsy tissues, e.g., spleen and lung, are useful for rickettsial isolation, ideally inoculated fresh, or held for 24 h at 4°C or stored frozen at −70°C for longer periods, if the specimen must be shipped to a public health or reference laboratory. Autopsy tissues can also be examined for rickettsiae by immunohistochemistry or PCR.

Body lice *(Pediculus humanus corporis)* removed from patients suspected of having epidemic typhus can be examined for the presence of rickettsiae. Body lice acquire rickettsiae and remain infected for life, thus providing a useful specimen for PCR diagnosis even after a prolonged period of shipping at ambient temperature and humidity, which do not ensure survival of the lice (60).

ISOLATION PROCEDURES

Due to their high infectivity and low dose capability, rickettsial isolation is performed in biosafety level 3 laboratories. Cumbersome historic methods such as inoculation of adult male guinea pigs, mice, or the yolk sac of embryonated chicken eggs have been supplanted by cell culture methods, except for isolation of *O. tsutsugamushi,* which is achieved by intraperitoneal inoculation of mice (27, 33). Vero, L-929, HEL, and MRC5 cells have been used in antibiotic-free media to isolate rickettsiae. The best results reported are achieved with heparin-anticoagulated plasma, buffy coat, or skin lesion biopsy specimen collected prior to administration of antirickettsial therapy.

Samples containing 0.5 ml of triturated clinical material mixed with 0.5 ml of tissue culture medium are inoculated as promptly as possible onto 3.7-ml shell vials with 12-mm-diameter round coverslips having a confluent layer of cells and centrifuged at 700 × *g* for 1 h at room temperature to enhance attachment and entry of rickettsiae into host cells (2, 33). After removal of the inoculum, the shell vials are washed with phosphate-buffered saline and incubated with minimal essential medium containing 10% fetal calf serum in an atmosphere containing 5% CO_2 at 34°C. At 48 and 72 h, a coverslip is examined by Giemsa or Gimenez stain or by immunofluorescence with antibodies against SFG and TG rickettsiae. Detection of four or more organisms is interpreted as a positive result. This method has yielded a diagnosis in 59% of samples from patients with boutonneuse fever who had neither been treated nor developed antibodies to *R. conorii* prior to collection of the sample (33). Rickettsiae were detected at 48 h of growth in 82% of the positive samples. Universal precautions should be exercised, and work should be performed in a laminar flow biosafety hood with use of gloves and gown. Although the quantity of rickettsiae in the cell culture is relatively low, avoidance of aerosol, internal, or contact exposure should be taken as for mycobacteria, fungi, and viruses.

IDENTIFICATION OF *RICKETTSIA* AND *ORIENTIA* ISOLATES

Rickettsiae isolated in cell culture can be identified by indirect immunofluorescence with group-, species-, and strain-specific monoclonal antibodies. In an increasing number of laboratories, rickettsial isolates are identified by molecular methods such as PCR amplification of genes that are genus specific (17-kDa protein, citrate synthase, or OmpB) or SFG specific (OmpA) (57). Determination of DNA sequences identifies unique isolates. *O. tsutsugamushi,* being more distantly related to *Rickettsia* spp., lacks the above cell wall genes but can be identified by PCR of the gene encoding the major immunodominant 56-kDa surface protein.

Identifying the species of rickettsial isolates by microimmunofluorescence serotyping requires intravenous inoculation of mice with rickettsiae on days 0 and 7 and collection of sera on day 10 (49). These high-titer antibodies react with conformational species-specific epitopes of OmpA and OmpB. Antibodies against group-specific lipopolysaccharide develop later in the murine immune response to *Rickettsia.* This rather cumbersome and expensive method requires propagation of large quantities of the isolate and of the prototype strains for immunofluorescence titration as well as for development of the typing sera. Genetic analysis of a larger portion of the genome is currently favored for identification of isolates. An isolate that is known to be a *Rickettsia* should be identified in a biosafety level 3 laboratory, and isolates of *R. rickettsii* and *R. prowazekii* must be handled as required by U.S. federal regulations for select agents.

DIRECT DETECTION OF THE ETIOLOGIC AGENT IN CLINICAL SAMPLES BY IMMUNOLOGIC AND GENETIC METHODS

The diagnoses of RMSF, boutonneuse fever, murine typhus, louse-borne typhus, and rickettsialpox have been established by immunohistochemical detection of rickettsiae in formalin-fixed, paraffin-embedded sections of biopsy specimens of rash and eschar lesions (21, 27, 28, 41, 73, 75, 77) (Fig. 2, left). Monoclonal antibodies that are specific for lipopolysaccharides of either SFG or TG rickettsiae have been used to detect rickettsiae by immunoperoxidase staining (Fig. 2, right). There is no antibody commercially available (75, 76). The sensitivity and specificity of immunohistochemical detection of *R. rickettsii* in cutaneous biopsy specimens are 70 and 100%, respectively (27, 73). Eschar biopsies yield

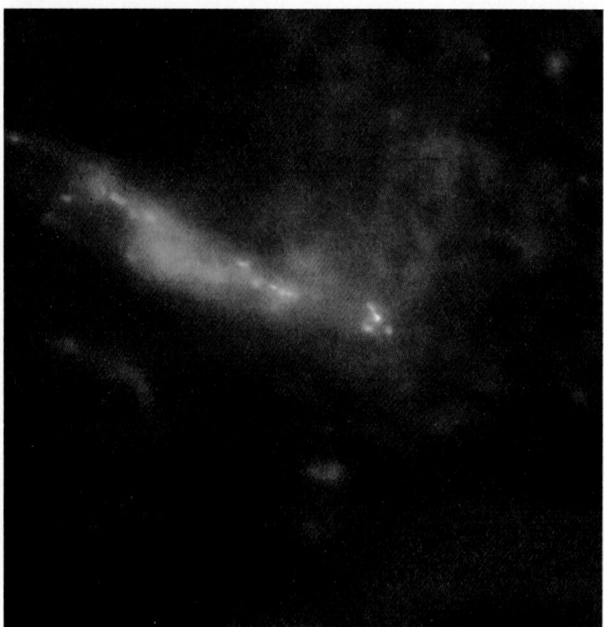

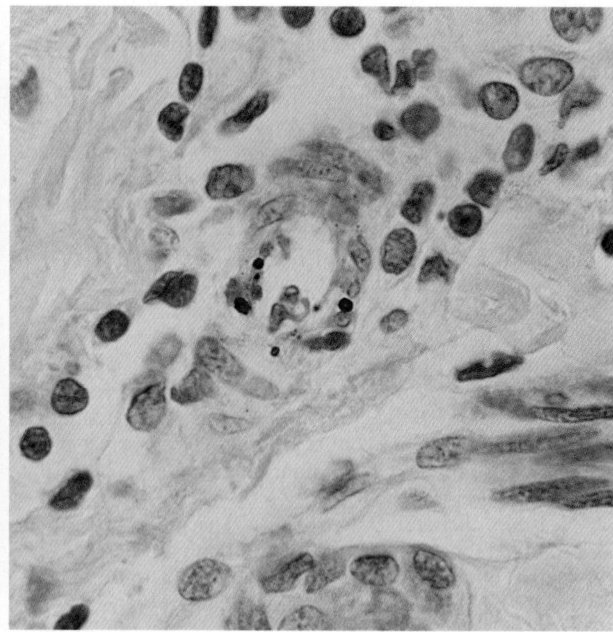

FIGURE 2 (Left) Direct immunofluorescence staining of skin biopsy specimens with anti-SFG *Rickettsia* antibodies facilitates rapid diagnosis. Rickettsiae are present in the vessel wall. (Right) Demonstration of rickettsial organisms in the microvasculature of the dermis in a patient with a history of Rocky Mountain spotted fever. Rickettsiae are seen in the vessel wall. An immunoperoxidase stain, using monoclonal antibodies directed against spotted fever group lipopolysaccharide, was used. Skin biopsy magnification, ×800.

sensitive specimens for the diagnosis of SFG rickettsioses that manifest that lesion and should be considered for diagnostic evaluation in patients suspected to have rickettsialpox, boutonneuse fever, or African tick bite fever.

Immunocytochemical detection of *R. conorii* in circulating endothelial cells has been accomplished by capture of the endothelial cells from blood samples using magnetic beads coated with a monoclonal antibody to a human endothelial cell surface antigen followed by immunofluorescent staining of the intracellular rickettsiae (33). This method has a sensitivity of 50% and a specificity of 94%. Rickettsiae are detected in 56% of untreated patients and in 29% of patients receiving antirickettsial treatment. *O. tsutsugamushi* has been identified using immunohistochemistry in human endothelial cells, macrophages, and cardiac myocytes (42). In situ hybridization has not been reported for the detection of rickettsiae in tissue samples.

PCR has been applied to the amplification of the DNA of *R. rickettsii*, *R. conorii*, *R. japonica*, *R. typhi*, *R. prowazekii*, *R. africae*, *R. felis*, *R. akari*, *R. slovaca*, and *O. tsutsugamushi*, usually from peripheral blood, buffy coat, or plasma, but occasionally from fresh, frozen, or paraffin-embedded tissue or arthropod vectors from patients (8, 12, 17, 44, 54, 59-62, 64, 66, 68–70). Nested PCR applied to skin biopsy specimens, particularly of eschars prior to treatment, has a sensitivity of 78% (16). For all pathogenic *Rickettsia* spp., the 17-kDa lipoprotein gene is the principal target, employing the primers CATTACTTGGTTCTCAATTCGGT and GTTTTATTAGTGGTTACGTAACC, which amplify a 231-bp DNA fragment (62). The *gltA*, *rrs*, and *ompA* genes have also been amplified diagnostically, with the *Rickettsia* being identified through either restriction fragment length polymorphism analysis using AluI and XbaI or sequencing of the PCR product (62). The availability of rickettsial genome sequences offers the possible design of an enormous number of primer sets. The approach of using primer sets on a single occasion to reduce the chances of amplicon contamination and false-positive results seems impractical. With batch processing being done annually, the delay in laboratory results reduces the clinical value (16). The single use of primers requires that their utility and sensitivity be unknown. The potential for amplicon contamination originating from a positive patient sample remains even if there is no positive control. Recent advances in technology such as real-time PCR allow for increased sensitivity in the detection of rickettsiae (12, 32, 43, 59, 70). The advantage of real-time PCR is detection of rickettsial organisms during the early or acute phase of disease before the generation of antibody. The targets for primer design have ranged from housekeeping genes (*gltA*) to antigen genes (*ompA* and *ompB*). The sensitivities for detection vary among primer sets. For example, real-time assays utilizing primer set RR.190.547F (CCTGCCGATAATTATACAGGTTTA) and RR.190.701R (GTTCCGTTAATGGCAGCAT), which generates a product of 154 bp, can detect five copies of rickettsial DNA (12). The primer set CS-5 and CS-6 detects 1 copy of *R. rickettsii* DNA and 10 copies of *R. bellii* DNA. Perhaps the best potential demonstration of real-time PCR as a diagnostic assay was observed in the primers targeting *ompB* and an *ompB* probe (70). For *O. tsutsugamushi*, the 56-kDa protein gene is the usual target of diagnostic PCR (68). The nested 56-kDa gene PCR assay is highly sensitive for the diagnosis of *O. tsutsugamushi* infections during the acute phase of the disease (61). PCR amplification of DNA from blood samples, using primers p34 (TCAAGCTTATTGCTAGTGCAATGTCTGC) and p55 (AGGGATCCCTGCTGCTGTGCTTGCTGCG), which generate a 1,003-bp product, followed by nested PCR with primers p10 (GATCAAGCTTC-

CTCAGCCTACTATAATGCC) and p11 (CTAGGGATCC-CGACAGATGCACTATTAGGC), amplifies a 483-bp product. This assay detects 10 prototype strains of *O. tsutsugamushi* and does not amplify *R. typhi* or *R. honei*. A duplex PCR assay using the *groEL* gene identifies both SFG rickettsiae and *O. tsutsugamushi* (46). Real-time PCR assays utilizing the *Orientia htrA* gene have been applied to diagnosis with clinical samples (24, 66).

Molecular and immunohistochemical diagnostic testing, the most useful methods for establishing a diagnosis during the acute stage of illness when therapeutic decisions are critical, are available at this time, to the best of our knowledge, in only a few reference laboratories including ours. Individual cases for immunohistochemistry may be referred to the following laboratories after contacting the directors for consultation: David H. Walker, M.D., Department of Pathology, University of Texas Medical Branch, 301 University Blvd., Keiller Building, Room 1.116, Galveston, TX 77555-0609, telephone (409) 772-3989, fax (409) 772-1850, e-mail dwalker@utmb.edu; J. Stephen Dumler, M.D., Division of Medical Microbiology, Department of Pathology, The Johns Hopkins Medical Institutions, Meyer B1-193, 600 North Wolfe Street, Baltimore, MD 21287, telephone (410) 955-5077, fax (410) 614-8087, e-mail sdumler@jhmi.edu; and Sherif Zaki, M.D., Ph.D., Department of Pathology, Centers for Disease Control and Prevention, 1600 Clifton Road Mail Stop G32, CDC, Atlanta, GA 30333, telephone (404) 639-3133, e-mail sxz1@cdc.gov.

SEROLOGIC TESTS

For most clinical microbiology laboratories, assays for antibodies to rickettsiae are the only tests performed. This situation is unfortunate for the patient with a life-threatening, acutely incapacitating rickettsial disease because these assays are useful principally for serologic confirmation of the diagnosis in convalescence and usually do not provide information that is helpful in making critical therapeutic decisions during the acute stages of illness. Patients who died of rickettsioses usually had received many antibiotics, none of which had antirickettsial activity owing in part to the lack of laboratory data providing clinical guidance for a rickettsial diagnosis. The earlier a diagnosis is established, the shorter the course of rickettsial illness after an appropriate antirickettsial antibiotic is administered.

Serologic assays for the diagnosis of rickettsial infections include the "gold standard" indirect immunofluorescence assay (IFA), indirect immunoperoxidase assay, latex agglutination, enzyme immunoassay (EIA), *Proteus vulgaris* OX-19 and OX-2 and *Proteus mirabilis* OX-K strain agglutination, line blot, Western immunoblotting, and rapid flow assays (4, 7, 9–11, 19, 22, 25–30, 52, 73, 81, 83). Only a portion of these assays are available as commercial kits or as assays performed in reference laboratories for some, but not all, rickettsial diseases. Other serologic tests such as indirect hemagglutination, microagglutination, and complement fixation are no longer in general use.

The IFA contains all the rickettsial heat-labile protein antigens and group-shared lipopolysaccharide antigen and, thus, provides group-reactive serology. IFA reagents are available commercially for SFG and TG rickettsiae from Panbio, Inc., Baltimore, Md.; Focus Technologies, Cypress, Calif., and bioMerieux, Durham, N.C.; they are also available for *O. tsutsugamushi* from Panbio, Inc. In cases of RMSF, IFA detects antibodies at a diagnostic titer of ≥64, usually in the second week of illness. Effective antirickettsial treatment of RMSF must be initiated by day 5 of illness to avoid a potentially fatal outcome. For boutonneuse fever, a diagnostic IFA titer of ≥40 occurs in 46% of patients between days 5 and 9 of illness, in 90% of patients between 20 and 29 days, and in 100% of patients thereafter. In murine typhus, diagnostic IFA titers are present in 50% of cases by the end of the first week of illness and in nearly all cases by 15 days after onset (10). In areas where particular rickettsial diseases are endemic, a higher diagnostic cutoff titer is required. For example, for the IFA diagnosis of scrub typhus in patients residing in zones of endemicity, an IFA titer to *O. tsutsugamushi* of ≥400 is 96% specific and 48% sensitive, with sensitivity rising from 29% in the first week to 56% in the second week (4). Lowering the diagnostic cutoff titer to 100 raises the sensitivity only to 84% and reduces the specificity to 78%. These considerations are not as important when testing patients who have visited regions of endemicity for only a short period. Each laboratory performing the test should establish its own cutoff titers for the patient population, the microscope and reagents used, and the laboratorian's judgment of the minimal positive signal.

Indirect immunoperoxidase assays for scrub typhus, murine typhus, boutonneuse fever, and presumably other rickettsioses yield results similar to those of IFA when the immunoglobulin G (IgG) diagnostic titer is set at 128 and that of IgM is set at 32 (29). Advantages include the use of a light microscope rather than a fluorescent microscope and the production of a permanent slide result.

Latex agglutination test reagents are available commercially from Panbio, Inc., only for RMSF in the United States. Latex beads coated with an extracted rickettsial protein-carbohydrate complex containing rickettsial lipopolysaccharide are agglutinated mainly by IgM antibodies, with reports of a sensitivity of 71 to 94% and a specificity of 96 to 99% (19). A diagnostic titer of 128 is often detected early in the second week of illness.

EIAs have been developed in various formats including antigens coating microtiter wells or immobilized on nitrocellulose or other sheets for use in the commercial reference laboratory setting. Dot-EIA kits are commercially available as Dip-S-Ticks from Panbio, Inc., for detecting antibodies against *R. rickettsii*, *R. conorii*, *R. typhi*, and *O. tsutsugamushi* (29, 81). No peer-reviewed publications have evaluated the use of the dot-EIA for the diagnosis of RMSF. When compared with an IFA titer of ≥64 for the diagnosis of murine typhus, the dot-EIA showed a sensitivity of 88% and specificity of 91% (29). The dot-EIA for diagnosis of scrub typhus had sensitivities and specificities of only 80 and 77%, respectively, when compared with an IFA cutoff titer of 64, and 89 and 66%, respectively, at an IFA cutoff titer of 128 (81). These SFG rickettsiae and *R. typhi* kits detect cross-reactive antibodies as demonstrated in an outbreak of African tick bite fever by clinical and epidemiologic data. The dot-EIA of *R. conorii* antigen provided early diagnostic evidence of a SFG rickettsiosis. Subsequent analysis revealed poor specificity with a high rate of false-positive results. These assays are diagnostic tools that do not require expensive, specialized equipment, but they suffer from apparent low specificity. Standard EIAs for detecting IgG or IgM antibodies against SFG rickettsiae or *O. tsutsugamushi* are also available from Panbio. The utilization of these tests for paired sera from populations with clinical (fever, headache, or rash) and epidemiologic (tick exposure) features consistent with rickettsiosis would most likely yield useful information. A multitest Dip-S-Ticks EIA for scrub typhus, murine typhus, and leptospirosis was not useful in Thailand, where nearly all patients had antibodies to more than one agent and others had antibodies against an agent that was not the cause of the illness (79). The diagnosis of scrub typhus by detection of antibodies in clinical samples in an IgM capture enzyme-linked immunosorbent assay can be utilized for single serum samples from early-stage infections (22). The performance values of this assay are a sensitivity of 96.3% and a specificity of 99%. A comparison of serologic methods for scrub typhus revealed that EIA containing recombinant p56 of Karp, Kato, and Gilliam strains was most sensitive (100%) and rapid lateral flow assay of antibodies against recombinant Karp p56 had a sensitivity of 86% (22). The latter, which is especially useful in situations with limited laboratory facilities and a low number of specimens, is available from Panbio Ltd., Brisbane, Australia.

The assays that have been most widely used for the diagnosis of rickettsial diseases are agglutination of the OX-19 and OX-2 strains of *Proteus vulgaris* for rickettsioses and the OX-K strain of *Proteus mirabilis* for *O. tsutsugamushi* infections. These assays have poor sensitivity and specificity (26, 73). They should be replaced by more accurate serologic methods such as IFA or EIA. However, there are situations in developing countries where the choice is between the *Proteus* agglutination tests and none at all for the detection of important public health problems such as outbreaks of louse-borne typhus. In fact, the evidence leading to the discovery of Japanese spotted fever and Flinders Island spotted fever included *Proteus* agglutinating antibodies.

Shared antigens of OmpA, OmpB, and group-specific lipopolysaccharide impede establishment of a species-specific diagnosis by serologic methods. The criterion of a fourfold or greater difference in IFA titers between the two suspected agents distinguished infections by *R. prowazekii* and *R. typhi* in only 34% of cases and infections by *R. africae* from those by *R. conorii* in only 26% (34, 54). Western immunoblotting detection of antibodies against OmpA or OmpB of only one *Rickettsia* species has also been proposed as a criterion for species-specific diagnosis. However, it was effective in distinguishing *R. prowazekii* and *R. typhi* infections or *R. africae* and *R. conorii* infections in only one-half of the cases (23, 34, 54). Cumbersome, expensive cross-absorption of sera prior to IFA or Western immunoblotting is more effective in establishing a species-specific diagnosis. However, interpretation of these results requires careful evaluation of the performance of valid controls, the quality and quantity of each antigen preparation, and the potential for the occurrence of infection by an untested, even as yet unrecognized, agent. In the past, knowledge of the geographic origin of the case sufficed to designate the specific diagnosis. However, the increasing number and geographic overlap of rickettsioses challenge the old assumptions.

ANTIMICROBIAL SUSCEPTIBILITY TESTING

Data supporting the use of doxycycline or another tetracycline antibiotic as the drug of choice for the treatment of infections caused by *Rickettsia* spp. and *O. tsutsugamushi* and the use of chloramphenicol as an alternative drug have been derived principally by empiric experience and retrospective case studies (20). In addition to historic studies of the activity of antimicrobial agents against these obligately intracellular bacteria in infected animals and embryonated eggs, studies of the effects of antimicrobial agents in cell culture have supported the consideration of alternative drugs such as fluoroquinolones, josamycin, azithromycin, and clarithromycin. Indeed, several fluoroquinolones, josamycin, and azithromycin have been used successfully for the treatment of boutonneuse fever under certain circumstances but cannot be recommended for more pathogenic rickettsioses (1, 6, 40, 53, 56). Except for cases of scrub typhus in Thailand which have not responded to doxycycline or chloramphenicol but for which azithromycin may be effective, there is little concern regarding rickettsial development of antimicrobial resistance (53, 78). During pregnancy, chloramphenicol has been used to treat RMSF and josamycin for boutonneuse fever. Antimicrobial susceptibility studies of rickettsiae are not routinely performed clinical laboratory tests.

INTERPRETATION AND REPORTING OF RESULTS

When reporting the results of an assay for antibodies in a single serum sample, the laboratorian seldom knows the duration of illness and whether the serum sample is from the acute or the convalescent phase of the disease. For sera that are nonreactive by dot-EIA, by IFA at a dilution of 1:64, by indirect immunoperoxidase assay at a dilution of 1:128, by latex agglutination at a dilution of 1:64, or by Weil Felix *Proteus* agglutination at a titer of 1:160, the laboratory report should state that no antibodies were detected at the particular cutoff dilution, which may differ among some laboratories and some patient populations, that negative results are expected in the acute stage of rickettsial illness, and that a second sample should be submitted to evaluate the possibility of seroconversion if no alternative diagnosis has been established. If paired acute- and convalescent-phase sera separated by an appropriate interval are available, they should be tested simultaneously. It is wise to test for all the rickettsial and ehrlichial agents to which the patient is likely to have been exposed in the United States. SFG rickettsiae, *Ehrlichia chaffeensis*, *Anaplasma phagocytophilum*, and *R. typhi* are the likely agents unless travel to an area where scrub typhus is endemic has occurred. If the paired sera are negative, the report should state that the results do not support the diagnosis of rickettsial infection, but that occasionally antibody synthesis is delayed, particularly in cases with early antirickettsial therapy. If a single serum sample contains an IFA antibody titer of ≥64, an IgM-IFA titer of ≥1:32, an indirect immunoperoxidase antibody titer of ≥128, a latex agglutination titer of ≥64, or a Weil Felix titer of ≥1:320, the laboratory report should state that antibodies reactive with the particular rickettsial antigen were detected at the measured titer, that the result provides supportive evidence for the diagnosis of the rickettsial disease, and that a convalescent-phase sample should be submitted to assess the possibility of seroconversion. If paired sera measured simultaneously show a fourfold or greater rise in titer, the interpretation is stated that the results strongly support the rickettsial diagnosis indicated by the tested antigen. If a significant titer was detected in the acute-phase sample, but no rise or only a single doubling dilution rise was measured, it should be stated that an additional later sample should be tested to evaluate a fourfold rise or fall in titer. The concept that recrudescent typhus could be distinguished from primary louse-borne typhus by the absence of IgM antibodies to *R. prowazekii* and of *Proteus* OX-19 agglutinating antibodies has been challenged (11). The manufacturers of the dot-EIA have recommended the interpretation that strongly reactive samples (three or four dots) may indicate the presence of a specific antibody response and that weakly reactive samples (one or two dots) are infrequent but possible in normal populations. Retesting 2 to 3 weeks later would establish the diagnosis if three or four dots develop in the convalescent serology and should always be performed.

Isolation of a rickettsia from blood or tissue may be interpreted as indicating an etiologic role. The level of identification of the isolate should be stated, whether identified only as to a group containing particular organisms or to the species level.

Immunohistologic and immunocytologic diagnostic interpretation states the method, reactivity of the method (e.g., antibody reactive with SFG rickettsiae), and location of the antigen (e.g., in vascular endothelium and frequently adjacent vascular smooth muscle for *R. rickettsii*). Detection of three or more rickettsiae in vascular endothelium in biopsy specimens or four or more rickettsiae in captured circulating endothelial cells is diagnostic of rickettsial infection.

Interpretation of PCR results should state the target gene, the organisms that would be detected, and the presence or absence of a DNA product of a particular size. If a specific oligonucleotide probe or DNA sequencing confirmed the specificity of the identification, this result should be stated. For negative immunohistologic, immunocytologic, and PCR results, it should always be stated that the failure to detect the agent does not exclude the diagnosis along with data regarding the sensitivity and specificity of the assay in the particular laboratory and the effects of antirickettsial treatment on the sensitivity.

Special efforts should be made to establish the diagnosis of fatal cases including rickettsial isolation, immunohistology, PCR, and serology on samples collected at necropsy.

REFERENCES

1. **Bella, F., B. Font, S. Uriz, T. Munoz, E. Espejo, J. Traveria, J. A. Serrano, and F. Segura.** 1990. Randomized trial of doxycycline versus josamycin for Mediterranean spotted fever. *Antimicrob. Agents Chemother.* **34:**937–938.
2. **Birg, M. L., B. La Scola, V. Roux, P. Brouqui, and D. Raoult.** 1999. Isolation of *Rickettsia prowazekii* from blood by shell vial cell culture. *J. Clin. Microbiol.* **37:**3722–3724.
3. **Bouyer, D. H., J. Stenos, P. Crocquet-Valdes, C. G. Moron, V. L. Popov, J. E. Zavala-Velazquez, L. D. Foil, D. R. Stothard, A. F. Azad, and D. H. Walker.** 2001. *Rickettsia felis:* molecular characterization of a new member of the spotted fever group. *Int. J. Syst. Evol. Microbiol.* **51:**339–347.
4. **Brown, G. W., A. Shirai, C. Rogers, and M. G. Groves.** 1983. Diagnostic criteria for scrub typhus: probability values for immunofluorescent antibody and Proteus OXK agglutinin titers. *Am. J. Trop. Med. Hyg.* **32:**1101–1107.
5. **Cardenosa, N., F. Segura, and D. Raoult.** 2003. Serosurvey among Mediterranean spotted fever patients of a new spotted fever group rickettsial strain (Bar 29). *Eur. J. Epidemiol.* **18:**351–356.
6. **Cascio, A., C. Colomba, D. Di Rosa, L. Salsa, L. di Martino, and L. Titone.** 2001. Efficacy and safety of clarithromycin as treatment for Mediterranean spotted fever in children: a randomized controlled trial. *Clin. Infect. Dis.* **33:**409–411.
7. **Ching, W. M., D. Rowland, Z. Zhang, A. L. Bourgeois, D. Kelly, G. A. Dasch, and P. L. Devine.** 2001. Early diagnosis of scrub typhus with a rapid flow assay using recombinant major outer membrane protein antigen (r56) of *Orientia tsutsugamushi*. *Clin. Diagn. Lab. Immunol.* **8:**409–414.
8. **Choi, Y.-J., W.-J. Jang, J.-H. Kim, J.-S. Ryu, S.-H. Lee, K.-H. Park, H.-S. Paik, Y.-S. Koh, M.-S. Choi, and I.-S. Kim.** 2005. Spotted fever group and typhus group rickettsioses in humans, South Korea. *Emerg. Infect. Dis.* **11:**237–244.
9. **Coleman, R. E., V. Sangkasuwan, N. Suwanabun, C. Eamsila, S. Mungviriya, P. Devine, A. L. Richards, D. Rowland, W.-M. Ching, J. Sattabongkot, and K. Lerdthusnee.** 2002. Comparative evaluation of selected diagnostic assays for the detection of IgG and IgM antibody to *Orientia tsutsugamushi* in Thailand. *Am. J. Trop. Med. Hyg.* **67:**497–503.
10. **Dumler, J., J. P. Taylor, and D. H. Walker.** 1991. Clinical and laboratory features of murine typhus in south Texas, 1980 through 1987. *JAMA* **266:**1365–1370.
11. **Eremeeva, M. E., N. M. Balayeva, and D. Raoult.** 1994. Serological response of patients suffering from primary and recrudescent typhus: comparison of complement fixation reaction, Weil-Felix test, microimmunofluorescence, and immunoblotting. *Clin. Diagn. Lab. Immunol.* **1:**318–324.
12. **Eremeeva, M. E., A. Madan, C. D. Shaw, K. Tang, and G. A. Dasch.** 2005. New perspectives on rickettsial evolution from new genome sequences of *Rickettsia*, particularly *R. canadensis*, and *Orientia tsutsugamushi*. *Ann. N. Y. Acad. Sci.* **1063:**47–63.
13. **Fenollar, F., and D. Raoult.** 1999. Diagnosis of rickettsial diseases using samples dried on blotting paper. *Clin. Diagn. Lab. Immunol.* **6:**483–488.
14. **Fournier, P. E., C. Allombert, Y. Supputamongkol, G. Caruso, P. Brouqui, and D. Raoult.** 2004. Aneruptive fever associated with antibodies to *Rickettsia helvetica* in Europe and Thailand. *J. Clin. Microbiol.* **42:**816–818.
15. **Fournier, P. E., J. S. Dumler, G. Greub, J. Zhang, Y. Wu, and D. Raoult.** 2003. Gene sequence-based criteria for identification of new *Rickettsia* isolates and description of *Rickettsia heilongjiangenis* sp. nov. *J. Clin. Microbiol.* **41:**5456–5465.
16. **Fournier, P. E., and D. Raoult.** 2004. Suicide PCR on skin biopsy specimens for diagnosis of rickettsioses. *J. Clin. Microbiol.* **42:**3428–3434.
17. **Furuya, Y., T. Katayama, Y. Yoshida, and I. Kaiho.** 1995. Specific amplification of *Rickettsia japonica* DNA from clinical specimens by PCR. *J. Clin. Microbiol.* **33:**487–489.
18. **Galvao, M. A. M., C. L. Mafra, C. B. Chamone, S. B. Calic, J. E. Zavala-Velazquez, and D. H. Walker.** 2004. Clinical and laboratory evidence of *Rickettsia felis* infections in Latin America. *Rev. Soc. Bras. Med. Trop.* **37:**237–240.
19. **Hechemy, K. E., R. L. Anacker, R. N. Philip, K. T. Kleeman, J. N. MacCormack, S. J. Sasowski, and E. E. Michaelson.** 1980. Detection of Rocky Mountain spotted fever antibodies by a latex agglutination test. *J. Clin. Microbiol.* **12:**144–150.
20. **Holman, R. C., C. D. Paddock, A. T. Curns, J. W. Krebs, J. H. McQuiston, and J. E. Childs.** 2001. Analysis of risk factors for fatal Rocky Mountain spotted fever: evidence for superiority of tetracyclines for therapy. *J. Infect. Dis.* **184:**1437–1444.
21. **Horney, L. F., and D. H. Walker.** 1988. Meningoencephalitis as a major manifestation of Rocky Mountain spotted fever. *South. Med. J.* **81:**915–918.
22. **Jang, W. J., M. S. Huh, K. H. Park, M. S. Choi, and I. S. Kim.** 2003. Evaluation of an immunoglobulin M capture enzyme-linked immunosorbent assay for diagnosis of *Orientia tsutsugamushi* infection. *Clin. Diagn. Lab. Immunol.* **10:**394–398.
23. **Jensenius, M., P. E. Fournier, S. Vene, S. H. Ringertz, B. Myrvang, and D. Raoult.** 2004. Comparison of immunofluorescence, Western blotting, and cross-adsorption assays for diagnosis of African tick bite fever. *Clin. Diagn. Lab. Immunol.* **11:**786–788.
24. **Jiang, J., T. C. Chan, J. J. Temenak, G. A. Dasch, W. M. Ching, and A. L. Richards.** 2004. Development of a quantitative real-time polymerase chain reaction assay specific for *Orientia tsutsugamushi*. *Am. J. Trop. Med. Hyg.* **70:**351–356.
25. **Jiang, J., K. J. Marienau, L. A. May, H. J. Beecham III, R. Wilkinson, W.-M. Ching, and A. L. Richards.** 2003. Laboratory diagnosis of two scrub typhus outbreaks at Camp Fuji, Japan in 2000 and 2001 by enzyme-linked immunosorbent assay, rapid flow assay, and Western blot assay using outer membrane 56-kD recombinant proteins. *Am. J. Trop. Med. Hyg.* **69:**60–66.

26. **Kaplan, J. E., and L. B. Schonberger.** 1986. The sensitivity of various serologic tests in the diagnosis of Rocky Mountain spotted fever. *Am. J. Trop. Med. Hyg.* **35:**840–844.
27. **Kaplowitz, L. G., J. V. Lange, J. J. Fischer, and D. H. Walker.** 1983. Correlation of rickettsial titers, circulating endotoxin, and clinical features in Rocky Mountain spotted fever. *Arch. Intern. Med.* **143:**1149–1151.
28. **Kass, E. M., W. K. Szaniawski, H. Levy, J. Leach, K. Srinivasan, and C. Rives.** 1994. Rickettsialpox in a New York City hospital, 1980 to 1989. *N. Engl. J. Med.* **331:**1612–1617.
29. **Kelly, D. J., C. T. Chan, H. Paxton, K. Thompson, R. Howard, and G. A. Dasch.** 1995. Comparative evaluation of a commercial enzyme immunoassay for the detection of human antibody to *Rickettsia typhi*. *Clin. Diagn. Lab. Immunol.* **2:**356–360.
30. **Kelly, D. J., P. W. Wong, E. Gan, and G. E. Lewis, Jr.** 1988. Comparative evaluation of the indirect immunoperoxidase test for the serodiagnosis of rickettsial disease. *Am. J. Trop. Med. Hyg.* **38:**400–406.
31. **Krusell, A., J. A. Comer, and D. J. Sexton.** 2002. Rickettsialpox in North Carolina: a case report. *Emerg. Infect. Dis.* **8:**727–728.
32. **Labruna, M. B., T. Whitworth, M. C. Horta, D. H. Bouyer, J. W. McBride, A. Pinter, V. Popov, S. M. Gennari, and D. H. Walker.** 2004. *Rickettsia* species infecting *Amblyomma cooperi* ticks from an area in the state of Sao Paulo, Brazil, where Brazilian spotted fever is endemic. *J. Clin. Microbiol.* **42:**90–98.
33. **La Scola, B., and D. Raoult.** 1996. Diagnosis of Mediterranean spotted fever by cultivation of *Rickettsia conorii* from blood and skin samples using the centrifugation-shell vial technique and by detection of *R. conorii* in circulating endothelial cells: a 6-year follow-up. *J. Clin. Microbiol.* **34:**2722–2727.
34. **La Scola, B., L. Rydkina, J. B. Ndihokubwayo, S. Vene, and D. Raoult.** 2000. Serological differentiation of murine typhus and epidemic typhus using cross-adsorption and Western blotting. *Clin. Diagn. Lab. Immunol.* **7:**612–616.
35. **Lee, J.-H., H.-S. Park, W.-J. Jang, S.-E. Koh, J.-M. Kim, S.-K. Shim, M.-Y. Park, Y.-W. Kim, B.-J. Kim, Y.-H. Kook, K.-H. Park, and S.-H. Lee.** 2003. Differentiation of rickettsiae by *groEL* gene analysis. *J. Clin. Microbiol.* **41:**2952–2960.
36. **Martinez, J. J., S. Seveau, E. Veiga, S. Matsuyama, and P. Cossart.** 2005. Ku70, a component of DNA-dependent protein kinase, is a mammalian receptor for *Rickettsia conorii*. *Cell* **123:**1013–1023.
37. **Martinez, J. J. and P. Cossart.** 2004. Early signaling events involved in the entry of *Rickettsia conorii* into mammalian cells. *J. Cell Sci.* **117:**5097–5106.
38. **McDade, J. E., C. C. Shepard, M. A. Redus, V. F. Newhouse, and J. D. Smith.** 1980. Evidence of *Rickettsia prowazekii* infections in the United States. *Am. J. Trop. Med. Hyg.* **29:**277–284.
39. **McLeod, M. P., X. Qin, S. E. Karpathy, J. Gioia, S. K. Highlander, G. E. Fox, T. Z. McNeill, J. Jiang, D. Muzny, L. S. Jacob, A. C. Hawes, E. Sodergren, R. Gill, J. Hume, M. Morgan, G. Fan, A. A. Amin, R. A. Gibbs, C. Hong, X.-Y. Yu, D. H. Walker, and G. M. Weinstock.** 2004. Complete genome sequence of *Rickettsia typhi* and comparison with sequences of other rickettsiae. *J. Bacteriol.* **186:**5842–5855.
40. **Meloni, G., and T. Meloni.** 1996. Azithromycin vs. doxycycline for Mediterranean spotted fever. *Pediatr. Infect. Dis. J.* **15:**1042–1044.
41. **Montenegro, M. R., S. Mansueto, B. C. Hegarty, and D. H. Walker.** 1983. The histology of "taches noires" of boutonneuse fever and demonstration of *Rickettsia conorii* in them by immunofluorescence. *Virchows Arch.* **400:**309–317.
42. **Moron, C. L., H. M. Feng, D. J. Wear, and D. H. Walker.** 2000. Identification of the target cells of *Orientia tsutsugamushi* in human cases of scrub typhus. *Mod. Pathol.* **14:**752–759.
43. **Ndip, L. M., E. B. Fokam, D. H. Bouyer, R. N. Ndip, V. P. Titanji, D. H. Walker, and J. W. McBride.** 2004. Detection of *Rickettsia africae* in patients and ticks along the coastal region of Cameroon. *Am. J. Trop. Med. Hyg.* **71:**363–366.
44. **Ono, A., K. Nakamura, S. Higuchi, Y. Miwa, K. Nakamura, T. Tsunoda, H. Kuwabara, Y. Furuya, K. Dobashi, and M. Mori.** 2002. Successful diagnosis using scab for PCR specimen in Tsutsugamushi disease. *Intern. Med.* **41:**408–411.
45. **Paddock, C. D., J. W. Sumner, J. A. Comer, S. R. Zaki, C. S. Goldsmith, J. Goddard, S. L. McLellan, C. L. Tamminga, and C. A. Ohl.** 2004. *Rickettsia parkeri:* a newly recognized cause of spotted fever rickettsiosis in the United States. *Clin. Infect. Dis.* **38:**805–811.
46. **Park, H. S., J. H. Lee, E. J. Jeong, J. E. Kim, S. J. Hong, T. K. Park, T. Y. Kim, W. J. Jang, K. H. Park, B. J. Kim, Y. H. Kook, and S. H. Lee.** 2005. Rapid and simple identification of *Orientia tsutsugamushi* from other group rickettsiae by duplex PCR assay using GroEL gene. *Microbiol. Immunol.* **49:**545–549.
47. **Parola, P., R. S. Miller, P. McDaniel, S. R. Telford III, J.-M. Rolain, C. Wongsrichanalai, and D. Raoult.** 2003. Emerging rickettsioses of the Thai-Myanmar border. *Emerg. Infect. Dis.* **9:**592–595.
48. **Parola, P., D. Vogelaers, C. Roure, F. Janbon, and D. Raoult.** 1998. Murine typhus in travelers returning from Indonesia. *Emerg. Infect. Dis.* **4:**677–680.
49. **Philip, R. N., E. A. Casper, W. Burgdorfer, R. K. Gerloff, L. E. Hughes, and E. J. Bell.** 1978. Serologic typing of rickettsiae of the spotted fever group by microimmunofluorescence. *J. Immunol.* **121:**1961–1968.
50. **Pretorius, A.-M., and R. J. Birtles.** 2002. *Rickettsia aeschlimannii:* a new pathogenic spotted fever group rickettsia, South Africa. *Emerg. Infect. Dis.* **8:**874.
51. **Qiang, Y., A. Tamura, H. Urakami, Y. Makisaka, S. Koyama, M. Fukuhara, and T. Kadosaka.** 2003. Phylogenetic characterization of *Orientia tsutsugamushi* isolated in Taiwan according to the sequence homologies of 56-kDa type-specific antigen genes. *Microbiol. Immunol.* **47:**577–583.
52. **Raoult, D., and G. A. Dasch.** 1989. Line blot and Western blot immunoassays for diagnosis of Mediterranean spotted fever. *J. Clin. Microbiol.* **27:**2073–2079.
53. **Raoult, D., and M. Drancourt.** 1991. Antimicrobial therapy of rickettsial diseases. *Antimicrob. Agents Chemother.* **35:**2457–2462.
54. **Raoult, D., P.-E. Fournier, F. Fenollar, M. Jensenius, T. Prioe, J. J. De Pina, G. Caruso, N. Jones, H. Laferl, J. E. Rosenblatt, and T. J. Marrie.** 2001. *Rickettsia africae*, a tick-borne pathogen in travelers to sub-Saharan Africa. *N. Engl. J. Med.* **344:**1501–1510.
55. **Raoult, D., A. Lakos, F. Fenollar, J. Beytout, P. Brouqui, and P.-E. Fournier.** 2002. Spotless rickettsiosis caused by *Rickettsia slovaca* and associated with *Dermacentor* ticks. *Clin. Infect. Dis.* **34:**1331–1336.
56. **Raoult, D., and M. Maurin.** 2002. *Rickettsia* species, p. 913–921. *In* V. L. Yu, R. Webber, and D. Raoult (ed.), *Antimicrobial Therapy and Vaccines*, 2nd ed. Apple Trees Production, LLC., New York, N.Y.
57. **Regnery, R. L., C. L. Spruill, and B. D. Plikaytis.** 1991. Genotypic identification of rickettsiae and estimation of intraspecies sequence divergence for portions of two rickettsial genes. *J. Bacteriol.* **173:**1576–1589.
58. **Richards, A. L., O. C. Teik, J. L. Lockman, E. Rahardjo, and F. S. Wignall.** 1997. Scrub typhus in an American living in Jakarta, Indonesia. *Infect. Dis. Clin. Pract.* **6:**268–273.
59. **Rolain, J. M., L. Stuhl, M. Maurin, and D. Raoult.** 2002. Evaluation of antibiotic susceptibilities of three rickettsial species including *Rickettsia felis* by a quantitative PCR DNA assay. *Antimicrob. Agents Chemother.* **46:**2747–2751.

60. **Roux, V., and D. Raoult.** 1999. Body lice as tools for diagnosis and surveillance of reemerging diseases. *J. Clin. Microbiol.* **37:**596–599.
61. **Saisongkorh, W., M. Chenchittikul, and K. Silpapojakul.** 2004. Evaluation of nested PCR for the diagnosis of scrub typhus among patients with acute pyrexia of unknown origin. *Trans. R. Soc. Trop. Med. Hyg.* **98:**360–366.
62. **Schriefer, M. E., J. B. Sacci, Jr., J. S. Dumler, M. G. Bullen, and A. F. Azad.** 1994. Identification of a novel rickettsial infection in a patient diagnosed with murine typhus. *J. Clin. Microbiol.* **32:**949–954.
63. **Seong, S.-Y., M.-S. Choi, and I.-S. Kim.** 2001. *Orientia tsutsugamushi* infection: overview and immune responses. *Microbes Infect.* **3:**11–21.
64. **Sexton, D. J., S. S. Kanj, K. Wilson, G. R. Corey, B. C. Hegarty, M. G. Levy, and E. B. Breitschwerdt.** 1994. The use of a polymerase chain reaction as a diagnostic test for Rocky Mountain spotted fever. *Am. J. Trop. Med. Hyg.* **50:**59–63.
65. **Silpapojakul, K.** 1997. Scrub typhus in the Western Pacific region. *Ann. Acad. Med. Singapore* **26:**794–800.
66. **Singhsilarak, T., W. Leowattana, S. Looareesuwan, V. Wongchotigul, J. Jiang, A. L. Richards, and G. Watt.** 2005. Short report: detection of *Orientia tsutsugamushi* in clinical samples by quantitative real-time polymerase chain reaction. *Am. J. Trop. Med. Hyg.* **72:**640–641.
67. **Sirisanthana, V., T. Puthanakit, and T. Sirisanthana.** 2003. Epidemiologic, clinical and laboratory features of scrub typhus in thirty Thai children. *Pediatr. Infect. Dis.* **22:**341–345.
68. **Sugita, Y., Y. Yamakawa, K. Takahashi, T. Nagatani, K. Okuda, and H. Nakajima.** 1993. A polymerase chain reaction system for rapid diagnosis of scrub typhus within six hours. *Am. J. Trop. Med. Hyg.* **49:**636–640.
69. **Tzianabos, T., B. E. Anderson, and J. E. McDade.** 1989. Detection of *Rickettsia rickettsii* DNA in clinical specimens by using polymerase chain reaction technology. *J. Clin. Microbiol.* **27:**2866–2868.
70. **Valbuena, G., W. Bradford, and D. H. Walker.** 2003. Expression analysis of the T-cell-targeting chemokines CXCL9 and CXCL10 in mice and humans with endothelial infections caused by rickettsiae of the spotted fever group. *Am. J. Pathol.* **163:**1357–1369.
71. **Vishwanath, S.** 1991. Antigenic relationships among the rickettsiae of the spotted fever and typhus groups. *FEMS Microbiol. Lett.* **81:**341–344.
72. **Walker, D. H.** 2003. Principles of the malicious use of infectious agents to create terror: reasons for concern for organisms of the genus *Rickettsia*. *Ann. N. Y. Acad. Sci.* **990:**739–742.
73. **Walker, D. H., M. S. Burday, and J. D. Folds.** 1980. Laboratory diagnosis of Rocky Mountain spotted fever. *South. Med. J.* **73:**1443–1447.
74. **Walker, D. H., C. G. Crawford, and B. G. Cain.** 1980. Rickettsial infection of pulmonary microcirculation: the basis for interstitial pneumonitis in Rocky Mountain spotted fever. *Hum. Pathol.* **11:**263–272.
75. **Walker, D. H., H.-M. Feng, S. Ladner, A. N. Billings, S. R. Zaki, D. J. Wear, and B. Hightower.** 1997. Immunohistochemical diagnosis of typhus rickettsioses using an anti-lipopolysaccharide monoclonal antibody. *Mod. Pathol.* **10:**1038–1042.
76. **Walker, D. H., S. D. Hudnall, W. K. Szaniawski, and H. M. Feng.** 1999. Monoclonal antibody-based immunohistochemical diagnosis of rickettsialpox: the macrophage is the principal target. *Mod. Pathol.* **12:**529–533.
77. **Walker, D. H., F. M. Parks, T. G. Betz, J. P. Taylor, and J. W. Muehlberger.** 1989. Histopathology and immunohistologic demonstration of the distribution of *Rickettsia typhi* in fatal murine typhus. *Am. J. Clin. Pathol.* **91:**720–724.
78. **Watt, G., C. Chouriyagune, R. Ruangweerayud, P. Watcharapichat, D. Phulsuksombati, K. Jongsakul, P. Teja-Isavadharm, D. Bhodhidatta, K. D. Corcoran, G. A. Dasch, and D. Strickman.** 1996. Scrub typhus infections poorly responsive to antibiotics in northern Thailand. *Lancet* **348:**86–89.
79. **Watt, G., K. Jongsakul, R. Ruangvirayuth, P. Kantipong, and K. Silpapojakul.** 2005. Short report: prospective evaluation of a multi-test strip for the diagnoses of scrub and murine typhus, leptospirosis, dengue fever, and *Salmonella typhi* infection. *Am. J. Trop. Med. Hyg.* **72:**10–12.
80. **Watt, G., and D. Strickman.** 1994. Life-threatening scrub typhus in a traveler returning from Thailand. *Clin. Infect. Dis.* **18:**624–626.
81. **Weddle, J. R., T.-C. Chan, K. Thompson, H. Paxton, D. J. Kelly, G. Dasch, and D. Strickman.** 1995. Effectiveness of a dot-blot immunoassay of anti-*Rickettsia tsutsugamushi* antibodies for serologic analysis of scrub typhus. *Am. J. Trop. Med. Hyg.* **53:**43–46.
82. **Whitworth, T., V. L. Popov X. J. Yu, D. H. Walker, and D. H. Bouyer.** 2005. Expression of *Rickettsia prowazekii pld* or *tlyC* gene in *Salmonella enterica* serovar Typhimurium mediates phagosomal escape. *Infect. Immun.* **73:**6668–6673.
83. **Wilkinson, R., D. Rowland, and W. M. Ching.** 2003. Development of an improved rapid lateral flow assay for the detection of *Orientia tsutsugamushi*-specific IgG/IgM antibodies. *Ann. N. Y. Acad. Sci.* **990:**386–390.
84. **Yu, X. J., and D. H. Walker.** 2005. Family I. Rickettsiaceae, p. 96–116. *In* G. M. Garrity (ed.), *Bergey's Manual of Systematic Bacteriology*, 2nd ed., vol 2. Williams & Wilkins, Baltimore, Md.
85. **Zavala-Velazquez, J. E., J. A. Ruiz-Sosa, R. A. Sanchez-Elias, G. Becerra-Carmona, and D. H. Walker.** 2000. *Rickettsia felis* rickettsiosis in Yucatan. *Lancet* **356:**1079–1080.

Ehrlichia, Anaplasma, and Related Intracellular Bacteria*

JUAN P. OLANO AND MARIA E. AGUERO-ROSENFELD

67

TAXONOMY

Members of the genus *Ehrlichia* and *Anaplasma* have become important agents of human disease. Together with a number of other pathogens in several genera, they are obligate intracellular bacteria currently placed in the *Proteobacteria* phylum, section alpha, order *Rickettsiales* and family *Anaplasmataceae*. While most closely related to the genera *Rickettsia* and *Orientia*, organisms classically considered ehrlichiae could be divided into four major clades. Taxonomic classification of this group of bacteria (Fig. 1) is largely based upon sequence analysis of 16S rRNA genes and *groESL* operons (50). This classification has been further supported by sequence analysis of the citrate synthase *(gltA)*, the β-subunit of RNA polymerase *(rpoB)*, FtsZ protein *(ftsZ)*, and rRNA genes (73–75, 83, 94, 132). The phylogenetic approach is further supported by serologic cross-reactions, comparisons among major immunodominant surface proteins, and the cellular tropisms of these bacteria (46, 77). All members of the tribes *Ehrlichieae* and *Wolbachieae* are included in the family *Anaplasmataceae* with elimination of the tribe structure of the family *Rickettsiaceae*. Current and former denominations of these bacteria associated with human and veterinary infections are found in Table 1. All tick-borne bacteria of *Anaplasmataceae* are grouped within two closely related genera, *Ehrlichia* and *Anaplasma*. The former members of the *Ehrlichia phagocytophila* group that include the species *Ehrlichia equi* and the bacterium formerly known as human granulocytic ehrlichiosis (HGE) agent were merged into a single species within the genus *Anaplasma* as *A. phagocytophilum*. Although minor sequence differences in the 16S rRNA gene exist between the former members of the *E. phagocytophila* group, it seems that such differences are related to their biological and ecological differences (34, 95, 128). Genetic variants of *A. phagocytophilum* have been reported in ticks and mammals in the Northeast United States and Europe (95, 128). Recently, a new agent closely related to *Ehrlichia ruminantium* has been found in *Ixodes ricinus* ticks removed from asymptomatic individuals in Northern Italy. This agent has been proposed as "*Candidatus* Ehrlichia walkerii" (27, 82, 123).

While *Ehrlichia* species infect predominantly leukocytes of humans and other mammals, *Anaplasma* species infect bone marrow-derived cells of all lineages in different animal hosts. *Neorickettsia* species infect predominantly mononuclear phagocytes and occasionally enterocytes in mammalian hosts. The genus *Aegyptianella* is currently listed as incerta sedis. *Wolbachia* spp. are "endocytosymbionts" of insects and helminths that are transmitted only by transovarial and transstadial (between stages of development) passage.

DESCRIPTION OF THE GENERA

Ehrlichia and *Anaplasma* spp. are obligate intracellular gram-negative bacteria that propagate and reside in cytoplasmic membrane-lined vacuoles in bone marrow-derived cells including granulocytes, monocytes, erythrocytes, and platelets, and for *E. ruminantium*, also within endothelial cells (118, 137, 141). Infection of endothelial cells is not surprising since both hematopoietic and endothelial cells are derived from a common ancestor, the hemangioblast that gives rise to angioblasts (endothelial precursor cells) and the hematopoietic stem cells. In fact, angioblasts share several cell surface markers with the hematopoietic stem cells and some of those markers are retained down to the endothelial differentiation (116).

For the genera *Ehrlichia* and *Anaplasma*, organisms are transmitted by tick bite, whereas organisms in the genera *Wolbachia* and *Neorickettsia* are not. Individual small (0.2- to 0.4-μm) dense forms of bacterial cells resembling chlamydial elementary bodies have been described, as have larger forms (0.8 to 1.5 μm) resembling reticulate bodies (113). Both are capable of binary fission, and a developmental cycle has not been demonstrated. After a few days, the elementary bodies dividing in the phagosome form an initial pleomorphic inclusion that matures into a microscopic colony known as a morula. *Neorickettsia sennetsu* grows as bacterial cells that may maintain their individual vacuolar membranes when they undergo binary fission, and thus an intracellular inclusion may not be identified by light microscopy. Cell lysis is a feature of the infectious process and leads to the release of cell-free bacteria that can infect other competent cells (22). Unlike *Rickettsia*, members of the genera *Ehrlichia* and *Anaplasma* do not show thickening of either leaflet of the outer membrane and the outer membrane appears to be more ruffled in *A. phagocytophilum* than in *N. sennetsu* or *Ehrlichia chaffeensis* (118). By transmission electron microscopy, *Ehrlichia* and *Anaplasma* spp. do not appear to contain significant amounts of peptidoglycan, a fact confirmed by the absence of genes

*This chapter contains information presented in chapter 65 by Maria E. Aguero-Rosenfeld and J. Stephen Dumler in the eighth edition of this Manual.

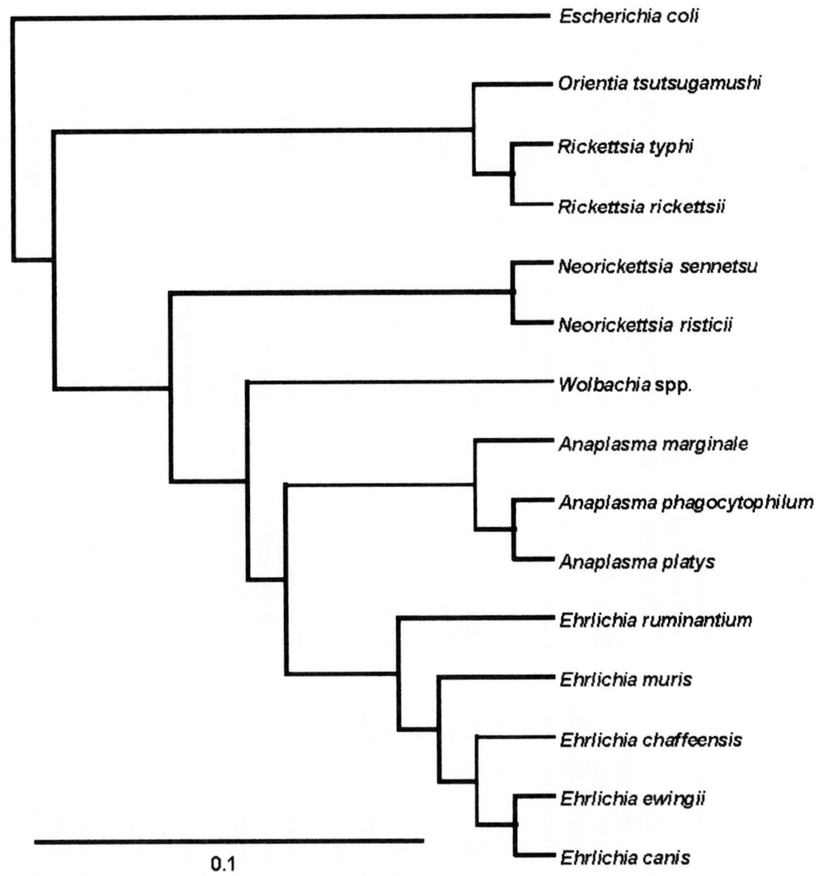

FIGURE 1 Neighbor-joining phylogenetic tree inferred from 16S ribosomal RNA gene sequences of selected *Ehrlichia, Anaplasma, Neorickettsia,* and *Wolbachia* spp. *Escherichia coli* is used as an outgroup. The bar represents the estimated number of substitutions per site.

necessary for the synthesis of this cell wall component on the full genome sequences currently available for *Anaplasma marginale* and *E. ruminantium* (20, 40). The genome size of *N. sennetsu* is approximately 800 kb, whereas those of *E. chaffeensis* and *E. ruminantium* are 1,200 kb, and those of *A. phagocytophilum* and *A. marginale* are 1,500 and 1,200 kb, respectively. With the availability of five full genomic sequences (*A. marginale* and *E. ruminantium, E. chaffeensis, Ehrlichia canis,* and *A. phagocytophilum*), certain themes have emerged including the low G+C content seen in other endosymbionts (*A. marginale* is the exception; it contains more G+C than any other intracellular bacterium) and a large proportion of noncoding sequences that have resulted from both reductive evolution due to their intracellular niche and ongoing sequence duplication events. Many of the genes for the glycolytic pathway are absent (142). Carbon sources are proline and glutamate. All enzymes for Krebs cycle are present, as well as the enzymes necessary for purine and pyrimidine metabolism, in contrast to rickettsiae, which lack such enzymes. ATP synthesis is possible since they possess the ATP synthase complex and other enzymes of the aerobic respiration chain. However, ATP/ADP translocases are not present, in contrast to the *Rickettsia* genus. Genes for type IV secretion systems are present as in other α-proteobacteria and most likely represent virulence genes (100). A surprising feature of the genomes is the presence of a large number of pseudogenes that are the product of sequence duplication events rather than reductive evolution seen in other intracellular bacteria (20). The active duplication of tandemly repeated sequences probably counteracts the reductive evolution to create new genes and therefore increase antigenic diversity as a mechanism of survival.

A. marginale and *Aegyptianella* spp. are intraerythrocytic bacteria of ruminants and birds, amphibians, or reptiles, respectively. These organisms also reside in small membrane-bound inclusions (18) and are not known to be associated with human disease.

EPIDEMIOLOGY AND TRANSMISSION

Ehrlichia and *Anaplasma* spp. are zoonotic agents that are transmitted to animals and humans most frequently after a tick bite or possibly by ingestion of fish infested by *Neorickettsia*-infected flukes. *Wolbachia* spp. are symbionts of a broad range of arthropods and helminths. Thus, most species have the potential for vertebrate and invertebrate life stages (Table 1). Based on a recent publication, transovarial transmission in ticks does not appear to occur, and thus, *Ehrlichia* and *Anaplasma* species depend upon high levels of bacteremia and in some cases persistent infection for enzootic maintenance (86). Transstadial and interstadial transmission in ticks allows ehrlichiae to be acquired from blood meals on naturally infected animals by the immature stages of ticks (larvae and nymphs), which can transmit the ehrlichiae to other mammalian hosts after molting to the next stage (nymph or adult).

TABLE 1 Selected features of *Ehrlichia, Anaplasma, Neorickettsia,* and *Aegyptianella* species of human and veterinary interest

Organism name	Former denomination(s)	Vector	Disease[a]	Hosts developing disease	Infected cells	Reservoir host
Anaplasma phagocytophilum	*Ehrlichia equi*	*Ixodes persulcatus* group	EGE	Horses	Granulocytes	Deer, sheep
	Ehrlichia phagocytophila HGE agent		Tick-borne fever HGA	Ruminants Humans, dogs		White-footed mice
Anaplasma marginale, A. centrale, A. ovis		Several tick species	Ruminant anaplasmosis	Cattle (sheep, goats)	Erythrocytes	Ruminants, wild cervids?
Anaplasma platys	*Ehrlichia platys*	*Rhipicephalus sanguineus*? *Amblyomma* spp.?	Canine cyclic thrombocytopenia	Dogs	Platelets	Ruminants?
Anaplasma bovis	*Ehrlichia bovis*	*Rhipicephalus appendiculatus* *Amblyomma variegatum*	Bovine ehrlichiosis	Cattle	Mononuclear leukocytes	Ruminants? Rabbits?
Ehrlichia chaffeensis		*Amblyomma americanum* *Dermacentor variabilis*	HME	Humans Dogs	Mononuclear leukocytes	White-tailed deer Domestic dogs Others?
Ehrlichia ewingii		*Amblyomma americanum*	CGE Ehrlichiosis ewingii	Dogs Humans	Granulocytes	Canids?
Ehrlichia canis		*Rhipicephalus sanguineus*	CME	Dogs Humans?	Mononuclear leukocytes	Canids
Ehrlichia ruminantium	*Cowdria ruminantium*	*Amblyomma* species	Cowdriosis (heartwater)	Domestic and wild ruminants	Granulocytes Endothelial cells	Ruminants
Ehrlichia muris		*Haemaphysalis flava*	Not named	Laboratory mice	Mononuclear leukocytes	Not known
Neorickettsia sennetsu	*Ehrlichia sennetsu*	Unknown; possibly acquired by ingestion	Sennetsu fever	Humans	Mononuclear leukocytes	Fluke-infested fish?
Neorickettsia risticii	*Ehrlichia risticii*	Ingestion of fluke-infested insects	Potomac horse fever	Horses	Mononuclear leukocytes	*Juga* spp. flukes
Neorickettsia helminthoeca		Ingestion of fluke-infested salmonid fish	Salmon poisoning disease	Dogs, bears	Mononuclear leukocytes	Fluke-infested fish
Aegyptianella spp. (genus and species incertae sedis)		*Amblyomma* spp.	Not known	Birds, amphibians, reptiles	Erythrocytes	Not known

[a] EGE, equine granulocytic ehrlichiosis (anaplasmosis); CGE, canine granulocytic ehrlichiosis; CME, canine monocytic ehrlichiosis.

Humans are only inadvertently infected and represent an end stage host for ehrlichiae. Natural maintenance of tick-borne ehrlichiae depends on the presence of appropriate tick vectors and mammalian hosts in the local environment (6, 87, 117, 135).

Natural reservoirs that are known to exist for *E. chaffeensis* involve both white-tailed deer *(Odocoileus virginianus)* and domestic dogs, and perhaps other animals that host *Ambylomma americanum* ticks (43, 85). Other minor reservoirs include opossums, raccoons, voles, coyotes, and goats (104). White-tailed deer also serve as a reservoir of *Ehrlichia ewingii* and of another ehrlichial agent closely related to *Anaplasma platys,* the white-tailed deer agent, which has not yet been associated with human disease (8). The identities of the major reservoirs for *A. phagocytophilum* are incompletely investigated, although small mammals, especially the white-footed mouse *(Peromyscus leucopus)* in the eastern United States, and other small mammals such as chipmunks *(Tamias striatus)* and voles *(Clethrionomys gapperi)* are naturally infected and are frequent hosts of the immature stages of *Ixodes scapularis* (135, 139). The role of white-footed mice as a reservoir of *A. phagocytophilum* in nature has been questioned, since immunity that develops after infection may render them temporarily host incompetent (84). Persistent or prolonged infection of animal reservoirs is essential for maintenance of zoonotic pathogens. Mice infected with *Borrelia burgdorferi* remain infected for many months, essential for continuous transmission to different stages of developing *I. scapularis* ticks (56). In Europe, red deer, sheep, cattle, and goats are persistently infected and serve as reservoirs of *A. phagocytophilum.* The reservoir for *N. sennetsu* is not known; however, epidemiological data suggest that consumption of raw fish was associated with sennetsu fever. Other species of *Neorickettsia* seem to have a complex transmission process involving trematode stages. *Neorickettsia risticii,* the agent of Potomac horse fever, appears to be transmitted to horses by accidental ingestion of insects carrying *N. risticii*-infected cercariae (89). Similarly, *Neorickettsia helminthoeca* infects dogs through ingestion of trematode-infested fish.

Over 20 species of ticks have been identified in the transmission of *A. marginale* worldwide (81). Other modes of transmission such as accidental inoculation of infected erythrocytes or blood-sucking insects have also been reported for *A. marginale.* Tick vectors also appear to be important in the transmission of members of the genus *Aegyptianella* to birds and amphibians (71).

CLINICAL SIGNIFICANCE

Human Diseases

HME

The causative agent of human monocytotropic ehrlichiosis (HME) is *E. chaffeensis,* a monocytotropic ehrlichia that was first identified as a human pathogen in a patient with a severe febrile illness after tick bites in 1986 (91). More than 1,300 cases of HME have been identified by the CDC between 1999 and 2004 (32, 33, 59); however, serologic data compiled at a major commercial laboratory that performs serologic testing for *E. chaffeensis* comprise more than 722 diagnostic serologic results between 1992 and 1995 alone, suggesting that HME occurs much more frequently than is reported (137). In another study based on a commercial laboratory, between 1997 and 1998, a total of 486 cases were diagnosed serologically (101). Passive and active case identification has revealed that clinically apparent HME occurs as frequently as or more frequently than Rocky Mountain spotted fever in Oklahoma, Georgia, Maryland, Tennessee, and North Carolina (127, 137). In fact, a 3-year prospective study conducted in Cape Girardeau, Mo., revealed an incidence between 2 and 4.7 per 100,000 population, a figure that is almost 1 order of magnitude higher than the one obtained by passive surveillance (102). Most cases are identified in the south central and southeastern United States, but increasingly infections have been identified in the mid-Atlantic region as well. Prospective evaluation of individuals with high rates of tick exposure shows that approximately 75% of seroconversions with antibody to *E. chaffeensis* are subclinical (57). Recent reports from Latin America, Africa, Europe, and Asia seem to indicate that *E. chaffeensis,* or closely related microorganisms, is also found in those localities (24, 39, 60, 120, 143). *E. chaffeensis* nucleotide sequences were found in different tick species from different regions of China, using PCR to amplify ehrlichial 16S rRNA genes (30).

The median incubation period for HME is 9 days, and two of every three patients are males; the median age is 44 years (57, 104). Patients typically present with high fever (97%), headache (81%), malaise (84%), and myalgia (40 to 60%), usually without other specific physical findings. Manifestations of gastrointestinal involvement (nausea, vomiting, and diarrhea), respiratory involvement (cough or pulmonary infiltrates), and joint pain are rare. Central nervous system involvement (stiff neck, confusion) and meningitis have been described (127). Rash patterns are variable in character, distribution, and temporal appearance. It could be petechial, macular, maculopapular, and erythematous (103, 104). Rash frequency is higher in the pediatric population and is present in up to 67% of cases (124). In spite of the nonspecific clinical symptoms and signs, laboratory findings are abnormal in at least 86% of patients, including leukopenia (60 to 74%) with lymphopenia and neutropenia, thrombocytopenia (70 to 90%), and increased serum aspartate transaminase activities (80 to 90%). Severe complications include a toxic shock-like syndrome with multiorgan failure, meningoencephalitis, diffuse alveolar damage associated with adult respiratory distress syndrome, and fulminant infections in patients immunocompromised by human immunodeficiency virus (HIV), high-dose corticosteroids, or organ transplantation (55, 93, 106, 107, 122). The case fatality rate of approximately 2 to 3% would be higher if effective antimicrobial therapy were not available. Fatal disease has been described most frequently in males, older patients, and those immunocompromised and with debilitating illnesses.

HGA, Formerly Known as Human Granulocytic Ehrlichiosis

The causative agent of human granulocytotropic anaplasmosis (HGA) is *A. phagocytophilum,* causing an illness identical to that of the formerly named *E. equi* and *E. phagocytophila* in horses and ruminants, respectively (58, 90). HGA was first identified in 1990 in a patient from Wisconsin after tick bites in an area where *E. chaffeensis* and its tick vector do not exist (11). Although the most frequent mode of transmission is through the bite of an infected *Ixodes* tick, other modalities of infection are likely to exist; perinatal transmission has been reported (68). Transmission by accidental inoculation of infected blood or by transfusion is probably rare but should also be considered.

As for HME, HGA is not a reportable illness in most states; thus, the true incidence and prevalence of the infection are unknown. However, prospective passive case collection in northwestern Wisconsin during 1990 through 1995 revealed a yearly incidence rate of 16 cases per 100,000 population, with peak rates identified as high as 58 cases per 100,000 population in some counties in 1995 (13). Between 1999 and 2004 over 2,000 cases have been reported nationwide (32, 33, 59). The highest annual incidence rates were in the Northeast and upper Midwest states. Infected patients have been identified in many other states as well as in several European and Asian countries (9, 17, 21, 23, 41, 65, 79, 110, 112, 115, 137). Subclinical infection is probably the norm, as nearly 14 and 11% of the population assessed in northwestern Wisconsin and Westchester County, N.Y., respectively, have antibodies indicative of prior infection (2, 12). The tick vectors for HME and HGA coexist in the mid-Atlantic, southern New England states, and in the southern Midwest. Thus, both diseases can occur in these areas (41). Furthermore, human ehrlichioses, including HME, HGA, and *E. ewingii* infections, are clinically undistinguishable.

HGA has a median incubation period of 5 to 11 days after *Ixodes* spp. tick bites and occurs in patients with a median age of 43 to 60 years (1, 3, 13). Twice as many men as women have the illness (14). Patients present with high fever, myalgias, headache, and malaise, with gastrointestinal, respiratory, musculoskeletal, or central nervous system involvement in fewer patients. Rash is observed in less than 11% of patients. Leukopenia with lymphopenia, thrombocytopenia, and increased serum aspartate transaminase activities are present in most patients during early stages of the disease. The hematological abnormalities may normalize before antimicrobial treatment, and lymphocytosis with atypical lymphocytes has been observed after the first week of infection (14, 70). Severe complications of HGA include a septic shock-like illness with multiorgan failure, adult respiratory distress syndrome, and opportunistic infections (13, 62, 70, 138); meningitis has not been documented with HGA. At least six deaths have been associated with HGA; at least three of those patients had opportunistic infections including *Candida* esophagitis, *Cryptococcus* pneumonia, invasive pulmonary aspergillosis, and herpes esophagitis (13, 62, 138).

Ehrlichiosis Ewingii

The association of *E. ewingii* with human disease was first demonstrated by detection of its DNA in the blood of patients presenting with clinical and routine laboratory findings indistinguishable from HME in Missouri (29). The main vector is also the Lone star tick (*A. americanum*), and therefore, the distribution of the disease is similar to that of HME. Evidence of *E. ewingii* in *Dermacentor variabilis* ticks has also been documented (145, 149). White-tailed deer are also reservoirs for this bacterium, and recent epidemiological studies suggest that dogs might also play a role as such (8, 149). Ehrlichiosis ewingii seems to affect mostly immunosuppressed patients including patients with HIV. Although clinical descriptions exist for only a few patients, it has not been reported as a cause of death and patients coinfected with HIV and *E. ewingii* seem to have a milder disease than those patients coinfected with HIV and *E. chaffeensis* (29, 105). In dogs, *E. ewingii* is responsible for canine granulocytotropic ehrlichiosis.

Sennetsu Ehrlichiosis (Neorickettsiosis)

Named after the Japanese term for glandular fever, *N. sennetsu* was first isolated from patients with suspected infectious mononucleosis in 1953 (97). Rarely identified now, patients develop a self-limited febrile illness with chills, headache, malaise, sore throat, anorexia, and generalized lymphadenopathy. Cases were identified only in Japan and possibly Malaysia. Laboratory findings include early leukopenia and atypical lymphocytes in the peripheral blood during early convalescence. No fatalities or severe complications have been reported.

Other Human Ehrlichioses

In 1996, an *E. canis*-like agent was isolated from the blood of an asymptomatic man from Venezuela who had morulae in peripheral blood monocytes. Serological investigations in children with febrile illness and healthy adults exposed to dogs with canine ehrlichiosis in that geographic area showed antibodies in two healthy individuals reacting with the Venezuelan agent (Venezuelan human ehrlichia), *E. chaffeensis*, *E. canis*, and *Ehrlichia muris*. Comparison of the 16S rRNA gene of the Venezuelan human ehrlichia agent with two strains of *E. canis* showed one or two base differences (111). Two additional cases were identified by real-time PCR in patients from Cape Girardeau, Mo., as part of a prospective study performed between 1997 and 1999. In fact, one of the cases was a dual infection caused by *E. chaffeensis* and *E. canis* (J. P. Olano and J. W. McBride, unpublished data).

While *Wolbachia* spp. are not known to be directly pathogenic for humans or animals, emerging experimental evidence indicates a potential role for the intracellular bacterial components ("symbionts") of such helminths as *Brugia malayi*, *Onchocerca volvulus*, and *Wuchereria bancrofti* as potentiators of the inflammatory reactions that are considered significant parts of the pathogenesis of the parasite infection (66, 134).

Animal Diseases

Members of *Ehrlichia, Anaplasma, Neorickettsia,* and *Aegyptianella* and related genera were known as veterinary pathogens long before they were recognized as human pathogens. Work in this area by dedicated veterinary microbiologists has contributed tremendously to the recognition and understanding of the diseases they cause in humans.

Canine Ehrlichiosis

Several agents produce infections in dogs, as shown in Table 1, which include canine monocytic ehrlichiosis caused by *E. canis* and *E. chaffeensis*, granulocytic ehrlichiosis caused by *E. ewingii*, granulocytic anaplasmosis caused by *A. phagocytophilum*, and canine cyclic thrombocytopenia caused by *A. platys* (53, 54, 118, 129). *Neorickettsia helminthoeca*, agent of salmon poisoning disease, also causes infection in dogs; it infects mononuclear cells and is acquired after ingesting salmonid fish encysted with a fluke harboring the organism (118).

Equine Ehrlichiosis

Potomac horse fever is a febrile gastrointestinal disease of horses caused by *N. risticii*, which infects monocytes (67), and is acquired through a complex aquatic ecosystem where infected insects seem to be implicated (89).

Equine granulocytic ehrlichiosis caused by *A. phagocytophilum*, formerly *E. equi*, is a seasonal disease first described in 1969. Although it has been described as occurring mostly in the foothills of Northern California (88), it also occurs in other regions of the United States and Europe. It causes a self-limiting disease in horses, which is similar to HGA in humans (15) and appears to be transmitted in California through the bite of infected *Ixodes pacificus* ticks. Tick-borne fever of ruminants is caused by the granulocytotropic *A. phagocytophilum*, formerly *E. phagocytophila*, and is transmitted via the bite of infected *I. ricinus* ticks in Europe (58).

Anaplasmosis of Ruminants

A. marginale is the etiologic agent of bovine anaplasmosis, the most prevalent tick-borne disease of cattle worldwide. Mechanical transmission by biting flies and other insects may also occur. Organisms develop as an intraerythrocytic inclusion and can produce severe anemia, weight loss, abortion, and sometimes death. A feature of this infection is the persistent low-level bacteremia even after clinical recovery; therefore, infected animals become a reservoir for transmission to other animals. This feature is shared with the related *A. phagocytophilum* infections of deer and *A. platys* infection of dogs. Antigenic variation has been postulated to play a role in the persistence of *A. marginale* infection and transmission (108).

Aegyptianella Infection of Birds and Amphibians

Members of the genus *Aegyptianella* infect erythrocytes of different animal species throughout the world. The type species is *Aegyptianella pullorum* of birds. Other species such as *A. bacterifera* have been associated with infections in amphibians. *A. botuliformis,* which infects helmeted guineafowls in Africa, appears to be transmitted through the bite of infected *Amblyomma* species (71). Based on 16S rRNA and *groEL* gene sequencing, *A. pullorum* is most closely related to *Anaplasma* spp.

Heartwater (Cowdriosis)

Ehrlichia (Cowdria) ruminantium is an intracellular bacterium that infects neutrophils and endothelial cells of cattle, sheep, goats, and certain wildlife species (118). Heartwater is an acute disease that can cause mortality rates up to 90% in susceptible ruminants. It occurs most frequently in sub-Saharan Africa and in the islands of the Atlantic and Indian Oceans and the Caribbean Sea and is transmitted by *Amblyomma* tick vectors.

COLLECTION, TRANSPORT, AND STORAGE OF SPECIMENS

EDTA- or acid-citrate-dextrose-anticoagulated blood or cerebrospinal fluid (CSF) and serum should be obtained for diagnosis or confirmation of HME or HGA. Currently, there are three methods for diagnosis during the acute phase of illness, when ehrlichiae are likely to be present in circulating peripheral blood or CSF leukocytes: PCR amplification of *Ehrlichia* or *Anaplasma* species nucleic acids, detection of morulae in the cytoplasm of infected leukocytes by nonspecific Romanowsky stains (e.g., Giemsa or Wright) or by specific immunocytologic or immunohistologic stains using *E. chaffeensis* or *A. phagocytophilum* antibodies, and culture of *Ehrlichia* or *Anaplasma* species from blood or CSF. EDTA-anticoagulated blood is the most useful specimen for most tests and should be obtained during the acute phase of illness (1, 61, 103).

Samples for PCR should be tested promptly, but if the blood is maintained at 4°C, it may still be possible to amplify nucleic acids several days to a week or more later. If delays beyond several days are anticipated, the blood should be frozen at –20°C until used. There is less experience with collection and storage of CSF for PCR, but it is expected that similar conditions will yield appropriate results. PCR using serum or plasma is far less sensitive than PCR using samples that contain infected leukocytes.

Peripheral blood buffy coat smears or cytocentrifuged preparations of CSF cells should be prepared within several hours of obtaining the samples since leukocytes degenerate rapidly. Once prepared, air-dried blood smears and cytocentrifuged CSF preparations are stable at room temperature for months or years.

The culture conditions for *Ehrlichia* and *Anaplasma* species are still being optimized. Currently the preferred specimen for culture is peripheral blood. Samples should be obtained by sterile venipuncture or lumbar puncture and submitted as soon as possible to the laboratory that is to attempt culture. Usually, this requires overnight courier service since culture is currently performed only in a few public health and research laboratories. Samples to be cultured should be maintained at approximately 4°C during shipping; it is important to avoid freezing, which is likely to reduce the content of viable ehrlichiae. Success rates in culturing *A. phagocytophilum* are far better than those for *E. chaffeensis.* The time elapsed between collection of the blood sample and inoculation in cell lines appears to be especially critical for *E. chaffeensis* isolation. EDTA-anticoagulated blood stored for up to 18 days at 4°C has also been successfully used to culture *A. phagocytophilum* in vitro (78). After cultivation, ehrlichia-infected cells may be stored in a frozen state at −80°C for several months or in liquid nitrogen for longer periods. Storage of infected cells is best accomplished when more than 50 to 90% of the host cells are infected and is achieved by suspension of at least 10^6 cells per ml in tissue culture medium that contains 10% dimethyl sulfoxide (DMSO) and at least 30% fetal bovine serum.

LABORATORY CONFIRMATION OF *EHRLICHIA CHAFFEENSIS*

Direct Examination

Microscopy by Romanowsky Staining of Peripheral Blood

Patients with suspected HME should have Romanowsky-stained (Giemsa or Wright stain) peripheral blood or buffy coat leukocytes examined for the presence of ehrlichial morulae. This method is very insensitive, identifying up to 29% (2 of 7) of culture-confirmed *E. chaffeensis*-infected patients (127). Ordinarily *E. chaffeensis* organisms are detected predominantly in monocytes, and their detection seems to correlate with severity of infection. When present, ehrlichial morulae are small (1- to 3-μm diameter) round-to-oval clusters of bacteria that stain basophilic to amphophilic with Romanowsky stains (Fig. 4). These clusters are present in the cytoplasm and have a stippled appearance owing to individual bacteria within the vacuole. Detection of morulae is more common in immunocompromised patients. Numbers of infected cells range from 0.2 to 10%, suggesting that up to 500 cells should be examined in suspicious cases.

Antigen Detection by Immunohistology

Immunohistologic methods may be used to identify *E. chaffeensis* within human tissues, including bone marrow, liver, and spleen. An immunohistologic study of bone marrow, however, detected *E. chaffeensis* in only 40% of specimens obtained during the active infection (48). Most immunohistologic studies have been performed using polyclonal antibodies that react with other *Ehrlichia* species. A monoclonal antibody may specifically detect *E. chaffeensis* in human tissues (150). Unfortunately, commercial sources for direct immunohistologic detection of *E. chaffeensis* are not currently available.

Nucleic Acid Detection Techniques

The most widely used nucleic acid amplification test is PCR amplification of *E. chaffeensis* nucleic acids from clinical samples by using the HE1/HE3 primer set (7, 52, 126). This primer pair amplifies a 389-bp fragment of the 16S rRNA gene

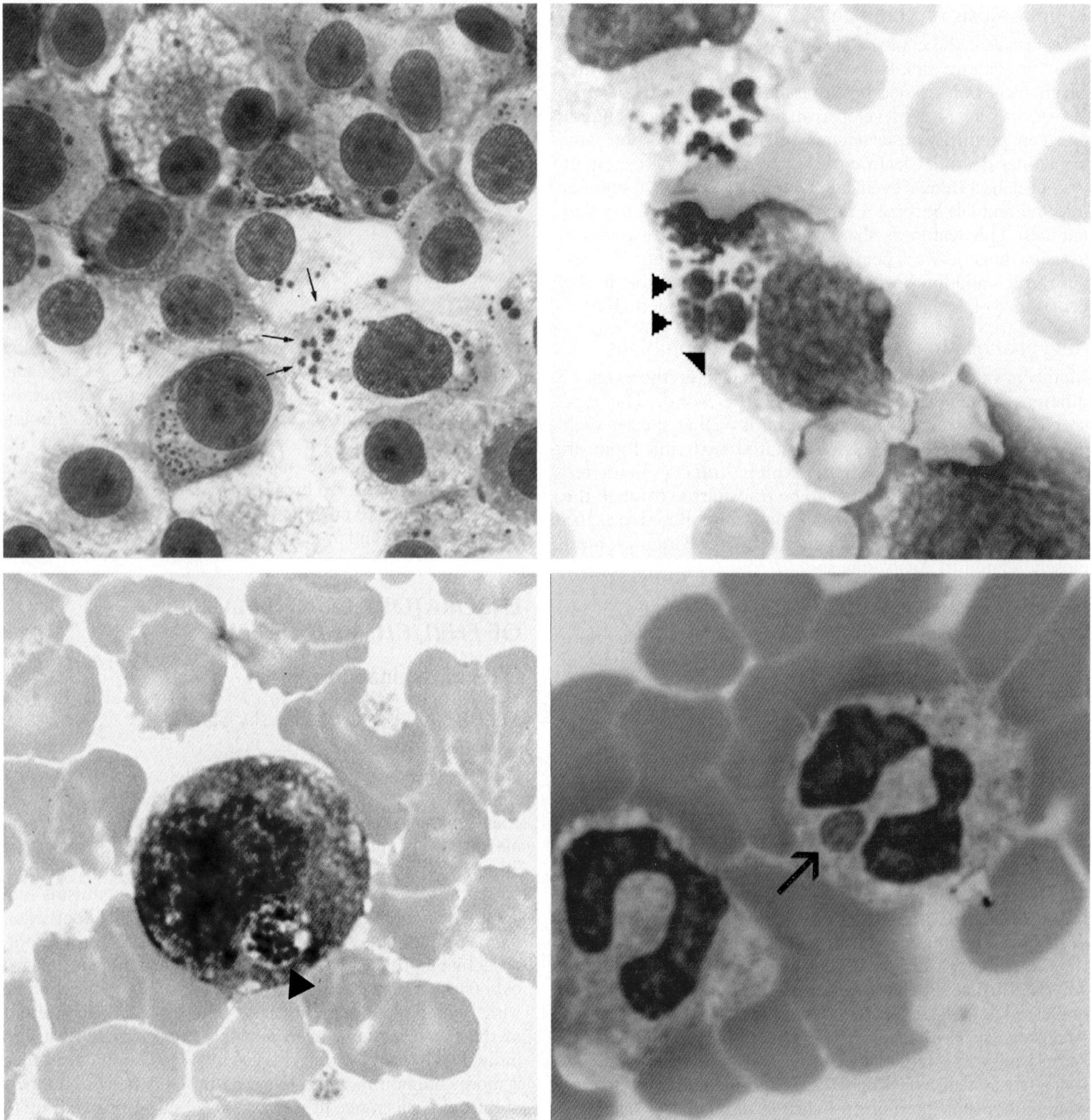

FIGURE 2 (top left) *E. chaffeensis* cultured in the canine histiocyte cell line, DH82. Note the presence of basophilic, stippled, intracytoplasmic inclusions approximately 2 to 3 μm in diameter (arrows). The smaller intracytoplasmic granules may also be ehrlichial morulae (Romanowsky [Leukostat] stain; original magnification, ×1,000).

FIGURE 3 (top right) *A. phagocytophilum* cultured in the human promyelocytic cell line HL-60 from the blood of an infected patient. Note the presence of multiple basophilic, stippled, intracytoplasmic inclusions (arrowheads) in an HL-60 cell (Wright stain; original magnification, ×1,000).

FIGURE 4 (bottom) *E. chaffeensis* (A [left]) and *A. phagocytophilum* (B [right]) in peripheral blood leukocytes. Note that the *E. chaffeensis* morula (arrowhead) is present in a monocyte (A) and that *A. phagocytophilum* morula (arrow) is present in a neutrophil (B) (Wright stain; original magnification, ×1,000).

sequences. The product may be detected by simple nucleic acid staining (e.g., ethidium bromide) after agarose gel electrophoresis or by Southern hybridization of the amplified products, using an internal probe that is reported to increase analytical sensitivity (38). A clinical evaluation of *E. chaffeensis* PCR using the HE1/HE3 system showed a sensitivity of 79 to 100% compared with detection of *E. chaffeensis* or *E. canis* antibodies in convalescence; however, *E. chaffeensis* nucleic acids were frequently detected in patients who never developed antibodies, a finding of uncertain significance given the high degree of analytical specificity demonstrated with this system (7, 126). Similar results occur when using a nested PCR that employs broad-range "*Ehrlichia* genus" primers in an initial step followed by PCR with the HE1/HE3 primer pair (80). A nested PCR assay with broad-range 16S rRNA primers (8F and 1448R) followed by a second (nested) reaction with primers 15F and 208R on whole blood yielded similar results to culture in another study (127). Other targets for PCR that have not been fully evaluated for clinical sensitivity or specificity include the *groESL* operon, a variable-length PCR target of unknown significance that is present in *E. chaffeensis* (105, 127, 131), the 120-kDa antigen gene that encodes an immunodominant antigen with tandemly repeated subunits that may vary among *E. chaffeensis* isolates, the quinolinate synthase A gene, *nadA*, and the p28 multigene family (105, 136, 152, 153). In a prospective study, the overall PCR sensitivity and specificity were 56 and 100%, respectively, using the 16S rRNA subunit, *nadA*, and 120-kDa protein genes (102). However, in this study several blood samples had high titers of antiehrlichial antibodies by indirect fluorescent-antibody (IFA) and were in the late phases of the disease, suggesting that the sensitivity was decreased due to lower numbers of circulating ehrlichiae. When sensitivity was calculated based on seroconversion rates, it increased to 84%. Posttest probabilities for a positive and negative PCR result were 96 and 11.1%, respectively. Posttest probabilities take into account a clinical case definition and therefore are most useful when used in the appropriate clinical setting (102).

Real-time multicolor PCR and real-time multiplex reverse transcriptase PCR assays have been developed recently with extremely high analytical sensitivity and specificity comparable to that of nested PCR assays (45, 125). Advantages of this technique include a lower risk of contamination, greater speed, lower cost, and a multicolor and multiplexing format allowing detection of multiple ehrlichial pathogens at the same time.

Isolation Procedures

E. chaffeensis has been isolated from peripheral blood of more than 30 patients with HME, and an *E. canis*-like organism was isolated only once from an asymptomatic human (42, 107, 111, 127). The most frequently used cell for primary isolation is the canine histiocytic cell line, DH82; however, *E. chaffeensis* has been successfully cultivated in other cells including the human macrophage-like THP-1 cells, the fibroblast-like HEL-22 cells, Vero cells, and HL-60 cells (human promyelocytic cell line differentiated to monocytic pathway), among others (63). Isolation may be successful even when infected leukocytes are not observed on examination of peripheral blood (127). The usual format for isolation involves direct inoculation of leukocyte fractions or, less optimally, whole blood into flasks with a confluent layer of adherent cells or into flasks that contain approximately 2×10^5 to 1×10^6 nonadherent cells per ml of tissue culture medium. Macrophage-like cells that are highly phagocytic may be adversely affected by the presence of numerous erythrocytes; thus, it is recommended that either (i) leukocytes be fractionated from erythrocytes by density gradient centrifugation (e.g., Ficoll-Paque), (ii) leukocytes be harvested after erythrocyte lysis (hypotonic lysis, $NHCl_4$ lysis, etc.), or (iii) cell confluency be reestablished after cultivation with erythrocyte-containing samples by addition of uninfected host cells. Since *E. chaffeensis* may be present in a very small proportion of peripheral blood leukocytes, it is usually advisable to inoculate cultures with as many peripheral blood leukocytes as possible. This may be difficult owing to leukopenia that often accompanies HME. A method using 2 to 3 ml of EDTA-anticoagulated blood, diluted in 2 volumes of sterile Hanks' balanced salt solution, followed by Histopaque (Sigma, St. Louis, Mo.) gradient separation of leukocytes gave a high yield of isolation in a study of the use of culture to diagnose HME (127).

The blood mononuclear cells are resuspended in a 2-ml volume of tissue culture medium supplemented with 5% fetal bovine serum and allowed to interact with adherent host cells in a 25-cm^2 flask for 3 h, usually enhanced by incubation with rocking at 37°C in 5% CO_2. The inoculum is removed if significant erythrocyte contamination is present and the monolayer is replenished with 5 ml of fresh tissue culture medium. Since *Ehrlichia* species are bacteria, antibiotics in the medium must be avoided. The generation time of *E. chaffeensis* is approximately 19 h (19), and thus, cultures must be maintained to allow a slow logarithmic or stable growth phase to avoid the host cells outgrowing the ehrlichiae.

Identification

The presence of infected cells is determined by sampling the medium (DH82 cells and THP-1 cells) or by lightly scraping part of the monolayer. Aliquots of the culture are cytocentrifuged, followed by Romanowsky or immunofluorescent stains, and cells are examined for the presence of intracytoplasmic morulae or *E. chaffeensis* antigen (Fig. 2). Culture may require 1 month or more but has been achieved in as short a time as a few days (42, 47, 127). Confirmation of the infectious agent is currently best achieved by PCR amplification using species-specific primers (5).

Serologic Tests

The majority of cases of HME are diagnosed by retrospective serologic confirmation, and serology is the most sensitive method for diagnostic confirmation. The most widely used test is the IFA test, which utilizes ehrlichia-infected cells fixed to glass slides. Ehrlichial antigens may be difficult to prepare and are available mostly through public health and research laboratories, although commercial production and distribution are now available. Commercial sources of IFA serodiagnostic kits include Focus Technologies (Cypress, Calif.) and PanBio Diagnostics (Columbia, Md.). Immunoblot procedures are becoming increasingly popular because of the perception of increased specificity (25, 35, 146).

Currently, there is little standardization for any method of ehrlichial serology, and cutoff titers are dependent on validation in individual laboratories that perform these assays. The algorithm for serologic testing by IFA includes an initial screen at a dilution of 1:64 or 1:80 for antibodies to *E. chaffeensis*. Reactive samples are then titrated.

Ehrlichia chaffeensis IFA

E. chaffeensis antibodies are detected by IFA using *E. chaffeensis* Arkansas strain-infected DH82 canine macrophage-like cells. Sera are serially diluted starting at a dilution of 1:64. The presence of antibodies is detected after incubation with fluorescein isothiocyanate-conjugated anti-human immunoglobulins. A positive reaction is detected by the fluorescent demonstration of typical intracytoplasmic ehrlichial morula morphology. It is important to identify the appropriate proportion of infected cells as determined by a positive control serum and the appropriate morphology for each antigen preparation to preclude false-positive interpretations. Prescreening for autoantibodies or routine removal of rheumatoid factors lessens the risk of misinterpretation due to antibodies reactive with cellular components including nuclear or cytoplasmic antigens. A fourfold increase or decrease in antibody titer, with a peak titer or a single convalescent titer of ≥64 for a patient with a consistent clinical history, supports the diagnosis of HME. Antibody titers may be detected in a small proportion of subjects without HME owing to the presence of antigens that are highly conserved among bacterial species, including heat shock proteins (44, 146). Acute-phase sera should be obtained at the time of presentation with acute illness, and convalescent sera are best obtained 3 to 6 weeks later (44).

The sensitivity and specificity of the IFA for *E. chaffeensis* infections in the convalescent phase are not known but are assumed to be high because of a high degree of correlation of the presence of *E. chaffeensis* antibodies and characteristic clinical findings (57). In the early phases of the disease, IFA testing is not sensitive when compared to PCR (37). A systematic evaluation of the usefulness of immunoglobulin M (IgM) testing is not available, although a preliminary evaluation based on nine culture-confirmed cases suggests that it might be slightly more sensitive than IgG for the diagnosis of HME during the acute phase (37). Previously, the serologically cross-reactive *E. canis* was used as a surrogate antigen; however, this serodiagnostic assay has a lower sensitivity than that obtained using *E. chaffeensis*, and its use should be discouraged (7). The role of immunoblots in diagnosis is not well established; however, many patients with *E. chaffeensis* infection can be differentiated from patients with HGA by the demonstration of antibodies reactive with one or more of the 22-, 28-, 29-, 46-, 54-, or 120-kDa antigens of *E. chaffeensis* (25, 35). A recombinant 120-kDa protein that has been applied in a dot blot method appears to offer a sensitive and specific serologic confirmation tool (151). Antibodies to *E. chaffeensis* have also been detected in patients diagnosed with Rocky Mountain spotted fever, Q fever, brucellosis, Lyme disease, and Epstein-Barr virus infections, suggesting that false-positive reactions do occur (44, 146). Antigenic diversity among isolates of *E. chaffeensis* is well described (36) but may not affect the detection of the polyclonal antibody response that is generated with human infection. Several reports have characterized patients with HME without antibody responses, even long after onset (52, 121, 127). However, in the few cases in which *E. chaffeensis* infection has been most clearly proven by cultivation of the agent, most patients who survived developed clear serologic reactions detected by IFA methods in convalescence (36, 42, 47, 105, 127). Hypothetical reasons for false-negative results include infection by antigenically diverse strains (unproven) and abrogation of antibody response by early therapy (127).

LABORATORY CONFIRMATION OF *ANAPLASMA PHAGOCYTOPHILUM*

Direct Examination

Microscopy by Romanowsky Staining of Peripheral Blood

Examination of Romanowsky-stained (Giemsa or Wright stain) peripheral blood or buffy coat leukocytes for the presence of ehrlichial morulae is highly valuable in the diagnosis of HGA. Usually, 800 to 1,000 granulocytes are examined under ×500 to ×1,000 magnification for the presence of morulae (1, 3, 13). Since most patients presenting with positive smears have less than 1% of infected granulocytes and usually have leukopenia, buffy coat preparations have a higher yield than peripheral smears. Infection rates as high as 40% of peripheral granulocytes have been described (11). As for HME, the presence of detectable infected granulocytes in peripheral blood seems to correlate with the severity of infection (3, 11, 13). The sensitivity of the buffy coat smear examination in the acute phase of HGA is approximately 60% (14). When present, ehrlichial morulae are small (1- to 3-μm diameter) round-to-oval clusters of bacteria that stain basophilic to amphophilic with Romanowsky stains (Fig. 4). These clusters are present in the cytoplasm of neutrophils or eosinophils and have a stippled appearance owing to individual bacteria within the vacuole.

Immunohistology for Antigen Detection

Immunohistologic methods may also be used to identify *A. phagocytophilum* within human tissues, including bone marrow, liver, and spleen.

Nucleic Acid Detection Techniques

Multiple PCR assays for detection of *A. phagocytophilum* nucleic acids have been published (51, 96, 130). Most utilize regions of the 16S rRNA gene that are relatively specific as targets for amplification. The most frequently applied and evaluated method employs the primer set ge9f and ge10r, which amplifies a 919-bp fragment, most often used as a single stage reaction, with or without a hybridization probe to enhance sensitivity (34, 51). A popular alternative is the use of nested PCR with an outer set of primers that anneal to and amplify eubacterial 16S rRNA genes, followed by an internal PCR with *A. phagocytophilum*-specific primers (96, 126). PCR amplification of the *groESL* region by use of a nested reaction has also been useful to detect ehrlichial DNA in blood during the acute phase. Primers HS1 and HS6 are used in the primary reaction followed by primers HS43 and HS45. The size of the amplified product distinguishes *E. chaffeensis* from *A. phagocytophilum* (528 versus 480 bp, respectively) (130). The analytical sensitivity and specificity of several published primer sets were evaluated by Massung and Slater (96) by using DNA extracted from serial dilutions of *A. phagocytophilum*-infected HL-60 cells. Specificity was evaluated using DNA extracted from cultures of *E. chaffeensis, Rickettsia rickettsii*, and *Bartonella henselae*. The primer sets with the greatest sensitivity and specificity were those used in a nested reaction to amplify the 16S RNA gene, ge3a-ge10 and ge9-ge2, and those amplifying the *msp2* gene, msp2-3f-msp2-3r (96). Both PCR assays detected as few as 0.25 infected HL-60 cell. Most recently a multiplex assay to detect *Ehrlichia* and *Anaplasma* spp. by real-time reverse transcriptase-PCR was developed and evaluated in peripheral blood of dogs suspected of ehrlichiosis (125). The assay has a sensitivity of 100 16S rRNA transcripts, which corresponds to about one infected cell in a test sample, can detect single or multiple infections, and has the potential for automation.

Isolation Procedures

A. phagocytophilum has been successfully cultivated more often from human patients than has *E. chaffeensis, E. canis*, or *N. sennetsu* owing to the higher quantity of organisms that are present in peripheral blood in many infected patients (1). More than 65 isolates have been cultured from infected patients at a single medical center in the United States. Although HGA has been described in Europe and Asia, no human isolates of *A. phagocytophilum* have been reported yet in any locality outside the United States. Few animal isolates, however, have been cultured in Europe (16, 144). Isolation is best achieved in the human promyelocytic cell line HL-60 (61) and has also been accomplished when ehrlichiae are not observed in peripheral blood smears. The optimal conditions for recovery of these bacteria have not been conclusively determined, but cultivation in HL-60 cells has been achieved with or without the presence of granulocyte-differentiating chemicals (e.g., DMSO or retinoic acid) (64). Because erythrocytes do not adversely affect the HL-60 cells, direct inoculation of EDTA-anticoagulated blood is effective. Fractionation of blood into leukocytes by preparation of buffy coat or by isolation of granulocyte fractions by density gradient centrifugation is also effective (119). Ordinarily, approximately 100 to 500 μl of EDTA-anticoagulated blood containing approximately between 10^2 and 10^4 infected granulocytes is inoculated into a total of approximately 100-fold more uninfected HL-60 cells that are in the exponential growth phase and are subsequently maintained at a concentration between 2×10^5 and 1×10^6 cells per ml of tissue culture medium.

Identification

Cultures are examined every 2 to 3 days by Romanowsky staining of cytocentrifuged preparations of 20 to 50 μl of culture suspensions. Ehrlichial morulae appear as small aggregates of basophilic bacteria in the cytoplasm of the HL-60 cells (Fig. 3). Since HL-60 cells may contain a variety of cytoplasmic granules, immunocytology can be very helpful for the inexperienced laboratorian. Unfortunately, immunohistological reagents are currently not commercially available. Cultures usually require between 5 and 10 days of cultivation before morulae are clearly identified, but infected cells may be detected as early as 3 days postinoculation. Time to detection of organisms in culture correlates with the amount of bacteria present in blood at the time of culture inoculation (78). Definitive identification is achieved by PCR amplification using species-specific primers (34, 60, 109) or by sequence analysis of 16S rRNA genes that have been amplified by universal eubacterial PCR (34). The exact length of incubation before cultures are considered negative is still unknown, but they should be kept for at least 14 days, with the cell density being maintained at about 2×10^5/ml.

Serologic Tests

A. phagocytophilum IFA

A. phagocytophilum is a single species that now includes three previously distinct organisms, *E. phagocytophila, E. equi,* and the former HGE agent (15, 34, 61). Thus, IFA serologic testing is performed using any of these antigens (46, 72, 140). Previously, most testing was performed using neutrophils obtained from the blood of animals experimentally infected with *E. phagocytophila* or *E. equi* (11, 46, 90). Currently, the preferred method for testing human sera is the use of a human isolate propagated in the human HL-60 promyelocyte cell line (4, 41, 72, 114). It is now well demonstrated that antigenic diversity exists among *A. phagocytophilum* isolates, but it is unlikely that such diversity affects detection under clinical circumstances (10, 140). Interpretation of immunofluorescent patterns is similar to that for *E. chaffeensis* and requires an experienced microscopist. IFA kits are currently available from Focus Technologies and PanBio Diagnostics.

Sera should be screened at a single dilution (1:64 or 1:80), and the presence of antibodies is determined after incubation with fluorescein isothiocyanate-conjugated anti-human IgG/IgM. If specimens test reactive, they are serially diluted to determine the end point titer. A serologic confirmation of the diagnosis is achieved when a fourfold rise in titer is demonstrated in convalescence with a minimum titer of 80, or when a single antibody titer of ≥80 is demonstrated in a patient with typical clinical features of HGA (3, 13). Approximately 25 to 45% of infected patients have antibodies at the time of presentation (3, 4, 13); however, up to 11 to 14% of the population possesses antibodies in some highly endemic regions, rendering this early serologic information less useful (2, 12). The typical response during acute infection is a rapid rise (within 2 weeks of onset) in antibody levels reaching high titers (≥640) within the first month (4). In a treated cohort of patients whose diagnosis of HGA was confirmed by culture, the antibody titers declined gradually over the next few months and about one-half of the patients had detectable antibodies by IFA 1 year after infection (4). However, many patients have antibodies detectable for months to years after initial infection (14).

The sensitivity and specificity of the HGA serologic tests are both believed to be high because of good correlation between typical clinical cases and serologic reactions to *A. phagocytophilum* group antigens (3, 4, 13). HGA serology had a sensitivity of 91.3% in a group of 24 culture-confirmed patients (4) and a median sensitivity of 95% among a group of 28 patients diagnosed by culture, PCR, or the presence of morulae in blood smears (140). IgM testing appears to be a useful tool for identification of recent infection, although the sensitivity may not be as high as that for IgG testing (140). Although enzyme-linked immunosorbent assays (ELISA) and immunoblots have been described (46, 114), they are not routinely used in the serology of HGA. Immunoblots may be used to differentiate among *A. phagocytophilum* and *E. chaffeensis* infections by demonstration of a major *A. phagocytophilum* antigen of approximately 44 kDa in sera of HGA patients (46, 72, 146). Cross-reactivity between *E. chaffeensis* and *A. phagocytophilum* group has been observed in IFA. Under those circumstances, testing with both antigens often shows higher titers with antigens of the homologous infecting agent (3, 140).

False-positive reactions have been observed in patients with other rickettsial infections, Q fever, and Epstein-Barr virus infections. Many patients with HGA develop antibodies that react with *B. burgdorferi* by ELISA and demonstrate diagnostic IgG or IgM immunoblots (148). Although some patients have been confirmed by culture to have concurrent infection with *A. phagocytophilum* and *B. burgdorferi,* the statistical probability that this mechanism accounts for most of these concurrent positive serologic results is very low (99, 146). Another explanation is the exposure to the various tick-borne agents at different times rather than by a single tick bite. The most frequent scenario is the presence of antibodies to the various agents in individuals living in areas of high endemicity (12, 92). Autoantibodies to platelets and other leukocyte components can cause false-positive IFA tests (147).

Other immunoassays employing recombinant p44 antigens have been developed and show promise as alternative tests to IFA (133, 154). Antigens of 42 to 49 kDa are immunodominant in *A. phagocytophilum* infection and are encoded by a multigene family (31, 98) similar to the major surface proteins (*msp*) of *A. marginale* (108).

ANTIMICROBIAL SUSCEPTIBILITIES

Routine antimicrobial susceptibility testing of *Ehrlichia* or *Anaplasma* species isolates is unnecessary. These bacteria are maintained enzootically by transmission among ticks and feral mammalian reservoir hosts (6, 85, 109, 135, 139). The level of exposure of such vertebrate and invertebrate hosts to antimicrobial selection factors is very low, and thus antimicrobial resistance is very unlikely. Most patients with either HME or HGA become afebrile and have clinical improvement within 48 h of therapy with a tetracycline antibiotic, including doxycycline, the drug of choice (13, 57). Retrospective analysis of patients with HME has shown a significant degree of efficacy for tetracyclines or chloramphenicol compared with other broad-spectrum antimicrobials (57). With in vitro studies, tetracycline antibiotics are uniformly bactericidal for *Ehrlichia* and *Anaplasma* species, whereas the MICs of chloramphenicol cannot be safely achieved in humans with HME or HGA (26, 69, 80). In contrast, the most frequently used antibiotics for patients who have had recent tick bites, amoxicillin and ceftriaxone, and broad-spectrum antibiotics that might be prescribed for undifferentiated fever such as other cephalosporins, aminoglycosides, and macrolides are not effective for inhibition of ehrlichial growth in vitro. The rifamycins (rifampin and rifabutin) can achieve effective inhibition or killing of *Ehrlichia* and *Anaplasma* species in vitro, and the fluoroquinolones (ofloxacin, levofloxacin, and trovafloxacin) have very low MICs for human isolates of *A. phagocytophilum* (69, 80). Rifampin has been successfully used to treat HGA during pregnancy and appears to be a useful alternative for patients who cannot receive tetracyclines (28). A recent publication describes a method to evaluate in vitro susceptibility testing by real-time PCR, showing *E. chaffeensis* to be susceptible to doxycycline and rifampin and to have partial susceptibility to the fluoroquinolones. Resistance to macrolides, cotrimoxazole, and beta-lactam compounds was confirmed (19).

Whereas persistent infections with *Ehrlichia* and *Anaplasma* species may occur frequently in naturally and experimentally infected animals even after treatment with tetracycline (58, 76), persistence of ehrlichiae in humans has rarely been documented (49, 121). Therapy is usually highly effective at eliminating ehrlichiae from the blood of infected humans.

INTERPRETATION AND REPORTING OF RESULTS

The current algorithm for identification and confirmation of infections by *Ehrlichia* and *Anaplasma* species requires a complete evaluation of the history, physical examination, and laboratory results that will suggest the diagnosis. Before specific tests for etiologic determination are attempted, a decision concerning therapy should be made since delays may lead to increased morbidity and perhaps mortality. At the time of acute illness and prior to institution of antiehrlichial therapy, EDTA-anticoagulated blood should be obtained for PCR amplification of *E. chaffeensis* and *A. phagocytophilum* and considered for the possibility of in vitro cultivation. A peripheral blood or buffy coat smear should be examined for the presence of morulae that would confirm the presumptive diagnosis. Serum should be obtained and tested for antibodies to *E. chaffeensis* or *A. phagocytophilum*, with an aliquot saved for repeat testing when a convalescent serum is obtained 2 to 4 weeks later.

The presence of intracytoplasmic inclusions within a leukocyte in peripheral blood might be due to the presence of overlying platelets, Döhle bodies, toxic granulations, nuclear fragments, Auer rods in blasts, other bacteria, yeasts, inorganic materials, or granules of normal large granular lymphocytes or granulocytes. If the typical morphology of an *Ehrlichia* or *Anaplasma* spp. morula is observed, an assessment as to the hematopoietic lineage and the percentage of cells that contain morulae should be made and reported.

A positive PCR result should be reported as such, indicating the presence of *E. chaffeensis* or *A. phagocytophilum* DNA present, and it should be made clear that a positive PCR is not equivalent to the culture of ehrlichiae from blood. Laboratories that use a broad-range PCR to identify *Ehrlichia* or *Anaplasma* spp. DNA in blood may also detect *E. ewingii* infection that may mimic either HME or HGA (29).

IFA serologic results should be reported as the titer of antibodies determined to be reactive with *E. chaffeensis* or *A. phagocytophilum*, including the positive cutoff values determined in the laboratory. An interpretation should indicate whether the titers are considered "significant" or "positive" based upon a fourfold increase or decrease or as single high-titered serum. It should be remembered that infections with *E. ewingii* would yield serologic patterns considered diagnostic of *E. chaffeensis* that are difficult to differentiate even with immunoblot methods. Immunoblot analyses should provide information about antibodies that react with specific antigens considered unique or diagnostic of infection with a single species of *Ehrlichia* or *Anaplasma*.

Human ehrlichioses became nationally notifiable in 1999, but not all states report these diseases. For the purpose of surveillance, the Council of State and Territorial Epidemiologists (CSTE) and the CDC developed a case definition that was amended in 2000 to include ehrlichioses other than HME and HGA (http://www.cste.org/ps/2000/2000-id-03.htm). According to this definition, a case presenting with compatible clinical and routine laboratory abnormalities described above could be classified as confirmed or probable based on specific laboratory findings. A confirmed HME or HGA case is supported by (i) a fourfold change in antibody titer to *E. chaffeensis* or *A. phagocytophilum* antigen, respectively, by IFA in paired serum samples; or (ii) positive PCR and confirmation of *E. chaffeensis* or *A. phagocytophilum* DNA, respectively; or (iii) identification of morulae in leukocytes, and a positive IFA titer to *E. chaffeensis* or *A. phagocytophilum* antigen, respectively (based on a cutoff established by the laboratory performing the assay); or (iv) immunostaining of *E. chaffeensis* or *A. phagocytophilum* antigen, respectively, in a biopsy or autopsy sample; or (v) culture of *E. chaffeensis* or *A. phagocytophilum*, respectively, from a clinical sample. The diagnosis of other human ehrlichiosis or ehrlichiosis caused by an unspecified agent is supported by (i) demonstration of a fourfold change in antibody titer to more than one *Ehrlichia* or *Anaplasma* sp. by IFA in paired serum samples, in which the dominant reactivity cannot be determined; or (ii) identification of an *Ehrlichia* or *Anaplasma* sp. other than *E. chaffeensis* or *A. phagocytophilum* by PCR, immunostaining, or culture. According to the CSTE case definition, a probable HME or HGA case is that with a clinically compatible illness with either a single positive IFA titer (based on the cutoff established by the laboratory performing the assay) or the visualization of morulae in leukocytes.

REFERENCES

1. **Aguero-Rosenfeld, M. E.** 2002. Diagnosis of human granulocytic ehrlichiosis: state of art. *Vector Borne Zoonotic Dis.* **2**:233–239.
2. **Aguero-Rosenfeld, M. E., L. Donnarumma, L. Zentmaier, J. Jacob, M. Frey, R. Noto, C. A. Carbonaro, and G. P. Wormser.** 2002. Seroprevalence of antibodies that react with *Anaplasma phagocytophila*, the agent of human granulocytic ehrlichiosis, in different populations in Westchester County, New York. *J. Clin. Microbiol.* **40**:2612–2615.

3. **Aguero-Rosenfeld, M. E., H. W. Horowitz, G. P. Wormser, D. F. McKenna, J. Nowakowski, J. Munoz, and J. S. Dumler.** 1996. Human granulocytic ehrlichiosis (HGE): a case series from a single medical center in New York State. *Ann. Intern. Med.* **125:**904–908.
4. **Aguero-Rosenfeld, M. E., F. Kalantarpour, M. Baluch, H. W. Horowitz, D. F. McKenna, J. T. Raffalli, T.-C. Hsieh, J. Wu, J. S. Dumler, and G. P. Wormser.** 2000. Serology of culture-confirmed cases of human granulocytic ehrlichiosis. *J. Clin. Microbiol.* **38:**635–638.
5. **Anderson, B. E., J. E. Dawson, D. C. Jones, and K. H. Wilson.** 1991. *Ehrlichia chaffeensis,* a new species associated with human ehrlichiosis. *J. Clin. Microbiol.* **29:**2838–2842.
6. **Anderson, B. E., K. G. Sims, J. G. Olson, J. E. Childs, J. F. Piesman, C. M. Happ, G. O. Maupin, and B. J. B. Johnson.** 1993. *Amblyomma americanum*: a potential vector of human ehrlichiosis. *Am. J. Trop. Med. Hyg.* **49:**239–244.
7. **Anderson, B. E., J. W. Sumner, J. E. Dawson, T. Tzianabos, C. R. Greene, J. G. Olson, D. B. Fishbein, M. Olsen-Rasmussen, B. P. Hollowau, E. H. George, and A. F. Azad.** 1992. Detection of the etiologic agent of human ehrlichiosis by polymerase chain reaction. *J. Clin. Microbiol.* **30:**775–780.
8. **Arens, M. Q., A. M. Liddell, G. Buening, M. Gaudreault-Keener, J. W. Sumner, J. A. Comer, R. S. Buller, and G. A. Storch.** 2003. Detection of *Ehrlichia* sp. in the blood of wild white-tailed deer in Missouri by PCR assay and serologic analysis. *J. Clin. Microbiol.* **41:**1263–1265.
9. **Arnez, M., M. Petrovec, S. Lotric-Furlan, T. A. Zupanc, and F. Strle.** 2001. First European pediatric case of human granulocytic ehrlichiosis. *J. Clin. Microbiol.* **39:**4591–4592.
10. **Asanovich, K. M., J. S. Bakken, J. E. Madigan, M. Aguero-Rosenfeld, G. P. Wormser, and J. S. Dumler.** 1997. Antigenic diversity of granulocytic *Ehrlichia* isolates from humans in Wisconsin and New York and a horse from California. *J. Infect. Dis.* **176:**1029–1034.
11. **Bakken, J. S., J. S. Dumler, S.-M. Chen, M. R. Eckman, L. L. Van Etta, and D. H. Walker.** 1994. Human granulocytic ehrlichiosis in the upper Midwest United States. A new species emerging? *JAMA* **272:**212–218.
12. **Bakken, J. S., P. Goellner, M. Van Etten, D. Z. Boyle, O. L. Swonger, S. Mattson, J. Krueth, R. L. Tilden, K. Asanovich, J. Walls, and J. S. Dumler.** 1998. Seroprevalence of human granulocytic ehrlichiosis among permanent residents of northwestern Wisconsin. *Clin. Infect. Dis.* **27:** 1491–1496.
13. **Bakken, J. S., J. Krueth, C. Wilson-Nordskog, R. L. Tilden, K. Asanovich, and J. S. Dumler.** 1996. Clinical and laboratory characteristics of human granulocytic ehrlichiosis. *JAMA* **275:**199–205.
14. **Bakken, J. S., M. E. Aguero-Rosenfeld, R. L. Tilden, G. P. Wormser, H. W. Horowitz, J. T. Raffalli, M. Baluch, D. Riddell, J. J. Walls, and J. S. Dumler.** 2001. Serial measurements of hematologic counts during the active phase of human granulocytic ehrlichiosis. *Clin. Infect. Dis.* **32:**862–870.
15. **Barlough, J. E., J. E. Madigan, E. DeRock, J. S. Dumler, and J. S. Bakken.** 1995. Protection against *Ehrlichia equi* is conferred by prior infection with the human granulocytotropic ehrlichia (HGE agent). *J. Clin. Microbiol.* **33:**3333–3334.
16. **Bjoersdorff, A., B. Bagert, R. F. Massung, A. Gusa, and I. Eliasson.** 2002. Isolation and characterization of two European strains of *Ehrlichia phagocytophila* of equine origin. *Clin. Diagn. Lab. Immunol.* **9:**341–343.
17. **Blanco, J. R., and J. A. Oteo.** 2002. Human granulocytic ehrlichiosis in Europe. *Clin. Microbiol. Infect.* **8:**763–772.
18. **Blouin, E. F., and K. M. Kocan.** 1998. Morphology and development of *Anaplasma marginale (Rickettsiales: Anaplasmataceae)* in cultured *Ixodes scapularis* (Acari: *Ixodidae*) cells. *J. Med. Entomol.* **35:**788–797.
19. **Branger, S., J. M. Rolain, and D. Raoult.** 2004. Evaluation of antibiotic susceptibilities of *Ehrlichia canis, Ehrlichia chaffeensis,* and *Anaplasma phagocytophilum* by real-time PCR. *Antimicrob. Agents Chemother.* **48:**4822–4828.
20. **Brayton, K. A., L. S. Kappmeyer, D. R. Herndon, et al.** 2005. Complete genome sequencing of *Anaplasma marginale* reveals that the surface is skewed to two superfamilies of outer membrane proteins. *Proc. Natl. Acad. Sci. USA* **102:**844–849.
21. **Brouqui, P., F. Bacellar, G. Baranton, R. J. Birtles, A. Bjoersdorff, J. R. Blanco, G. Caruso, M. Cinco, P. E. Fournier, E. Francavilla, M. Jensenius, J. Kazar, H. Laferl, A. Lakos, S. Lotric Furlan, M. Maurin, J. A. Oteo, P. Parola, C. Perez-Eid, O. Peter, D. Postic, D. Raoult, A. Tellez, Y. Tselentis, and B. Wilske.** 2004. Guidelines for the diagnosis of tick-borne bacterial diseases in Europe. *Clin. Microbiol. Infect.* **10:**1108–1132.
22. **Brouqui, P., M. L. Birg, and D. Raoult.** 1994. Cytopathic effect, plaque formation, and lysis of *Ehrlichia chaffeensis* grown on continuous cell lines. *Infect. Immun.* **62:**405–411.
23. **Brouqui, P., J. S. Dumler, R. Lienhard, M. Brossard, and D. Raoult.** 1995. Human granulocytic ehrlichiosis in Europe. *Lancet* **346:**782–783.
24. **Brouqui, P., C. Le Cam, P. J. Kelly, et al.** 1994. Serologic evidence for human ehrlichiosis in Africa. *Eur. J. Epidemiol.* **10:**695–698.
25. **Brouqui, P., C. Lecam, J. Olson, and D. Raoult.** 1994. Serologic diagnosis of human monocytic ehrlichiosis by immunoblot analysis. *Clin. Diagn. Lab. Immunol.* **1:**645–649.
26. **Brouqui, P., and D. Raoult.** 1992. In vitro antibiotic susceptibility of the newly recognized agent of ehrlichiosis in humans, *Ehrlichia chaffeensis. Antimicrob. Agents Chemother.* **36:**2799–2803.
27. **Brouqui, P., Y. O. Sanogo, G. Caruso, F. Merola, and D. Raoult.** 2003. *Candidatus Ehrlichia walkerii:* a new *Ehrlichia* detected in *Ixodes ricinus* tick collected from asymptomatic humans in Northern Italy. *Ann. N. Y. Acad. Sci.* **990:**134–140.
28. **Buitrago, M. I, J. W. IJdo, P. Rinaudo, H. Simon, J. Copel, J. Gadbaw, R. Heimer, E. Fikrig, and F. J. Bia.** 1998. Human granulocytic ehrlichiosis during pregnancy treated successfully with rifampin. *Clin. Infect. Dis.* **27:**213–215.
29. **Buller, R. S., M. Arens, S. P. Hmiel, C. D. Paddock, J. W. Sumner, Y. Rikihisa, A. Unver, M. Gaudreault-Keener, F. A. Manian, A. M. Liddell, N. Schmulewitz, and G. A. Storch.** 1999. *Ehrlichia ewingii,* a newly recognized agent of human ehrlichiosis. *N. Engl. J. Med.* **341:**148–155.
30. **Cao, W. C., Y. M. Gao, P. H. Zhang, et al.** 2000. Identification of *Ehrlichia chaffeensis* by nested PCR in ticks from Southern China. *J. Clin. Microbiol.* **38:**2778–2780.
31. **Caspersen, K., J.-H. Park, S. Patil, and J. S. Dumler.** 2002. Genetic variability and stability of *Anaplasma phagocytophila msp2 (p44)*. *Infect. Immun.* **70:**1230–1234.
32. **Centers for Disease Control and Prevention.** 2005. Summary of provisional cases of selected notifiable diseases, United States 2004. *Morb. Mortal. Wkly. Rep.* **53:**1213.
33. **Centers for Disease Control and Prevention.** 2005. Summary of notifiable diseases, United States, 2003. *Morb. Mortal. Wkly. Rep.* **52:**16, 20, 27, 72.
34. **Chen, S. M., J. S. Dumler, J. S. Bakken, and D. H. Walker.** 1994. Identification of a granulocytotropic *Ehrlichia* species as the etiologic agent of human disease. *J. Clin. Microbiol.* **32:**589–595.
35. **Chen, S. M., J. S. Dumler, H.-M. Feng, and D. H. Walker.** 1994. Identification of the antigenic constituents of *Ehrlichia chaffeensis. Am. J. Trop. Med. Hyg.* **50:**52–58.
36. **Chen, S. M., X. J. Yu, V. L. Popov, E. L. Westerman, F. G. Hamilton, and D. H. Walker.** 1997. Genetic and antigenic diversity of *Ehrlichia chaffeensis:* comparative analysis of a novel human strain from Oklahoma and previously isolated strains. *J. Infect. Dis.* **175:**856–863.

37. **Childs, J. E., J. W. Sumner, W. L. Nicholson, R. F. Massung, S. M. Standaert, and C. D. Paddock.** 1999. Outcome of diagnostic tests using samples from patients with culture-proven human monocytic ehrlichiosis: implications for surveillance. *J. Clin. Microbiol.* **37:**2997–3000.
38. **Chu, F. K.** 1998. Rapid and sensitive PCR-based detection and differentiation of aetiologic agents of human granulocytotropic and monocytotropic ehrlichiosis. *Mol. Cell. Probes* **12:**93–99.
39. **Cinco, M., F. Barbone, M. Grazia Ciufolini, et al.** 2004. Seroprevalence of tick-borne infections in forestry rangers from northeastern Italy. *Clin. Microbiol. Infect.* **10:**1056–1061.
40. **Collins, N. E., J. Liebenberg, E. P. de Villiers, et al.** 2005. The genome of the heartwater agent *Ehrlichia ruminantium* contains multiple tandem repeats of actively variable copy number. *Proc. Natl. Acad. Sci. USA* **102:**838–843.
41. **Comer, J. A., W. L. Nicholson, J. G. Olson, and J. E. Childs.** 1999. Serologic testing for human granulocytic ehrlichiosis at a National Referral Center. *J. Clin. Microbiol.* **37:**558–564.
42. **Dawson, J. E., B. E. Anderson, D. B. Fishbein, J. L. Sanchez, C. S. Goldsmith, K. H. Wilson, and C. W. Duntley.** 1991. Isolation and characterization of an *Ehrlichia* from a patient diagnosed with human ehrlichiosis. *J. Clin. Microbiol.* **29:**2741–2745.
43. **Dawson, J. E., and S. A. Ewing.** 1992. Susceptibility of dogs to infection with *Ehrlichia chaffeensis*, the causative agent of human ehrlichiosis. *Am. J. Vet. Res.* **53:**1322–1327.
44. **Dawson, J. E., D. B. Fishbein, T. R. Eng, M. A. Redus, and N. R. Greene.** 1990. Diagnosis of human ehrlichiosis with the indirect fluorescent antibody test: kinetics and specificity. *J. Infect. Dis.* **162:**91–95.
45. **Doyle, K. C., M. B. Labruna., E. B. Breitschwerdt, Y. W. Tang, R. E. Corstvet, B. C. Hegarty, K. C. Bloch, P. Li, D. H. Walker, and J. W. McBride.** 2005. Detection of medically important *Ehrlichia* by quantitative multicolor Taqman real-time polymerase chain reaction of the *dsb* gene. *J. Mol. Diagn.* **7:**504–510.
46. **Dumler, J. S., K. M. Asanovich, J. S. Bakken, P. Richter, R. Kimsey, and J. E. Madigan.** 1995. Serologic cross-reaction among *Ehrlichia equi, Ehrlichia phagocytophila,* and human granulocytic ehrlichia. *J. Clin. Microbiol.* **33:**1098–1103.
47. **Dumler, J. S., S. M. Chen, K. Asanovich, E. Trigiani, V. L. Popov, and D. H. Walker.** 1995. Isolation and characterization of a new strain of *Ehrlichia chaffeensis* from a patient with nearly fatal monocytic ehrlichiosis. *J. Clin. Microbiol.* **33:**1704–1711.
48. **Dumler, J. S., J. E. Dawson, and D. H. Walker.** 1993. Human ehrlichiosis: hematopathology and immunohistologic detection of *Ehrlichia chaffeensis. Hum. Pathol.* **24:**391–396.
49. **Dumler, J. S., W. L. Sutker, and D. H. Walker.** 1993. Persistent infection with *Ehrlichia chaffeensis. Clin. Infect. Dis.* **17:**903–905.
50. **Dumler, J. S., A. F. Barbet, C. P. J. Bekker, G. A. Dasch, G. H. Palmer, S. C. Ray Y. Rikihisa, and F. R. Rurangirwa.** 2001. Reorganization of genera in the families *Rickettsiaceae* and *Anaplasmataceae* in the order *Rickettsiales:* unification of some species of *Ehrlichia* with *Anaplasma, Cowdria* with *Ehrlichia,* and *Ehrlichia* with *Neorickettsia,* designation of six new species combinations and designation of *Ehrlichia equi* and "HGE agent" as subjective synonyms of *Ehrlichia phagocytophila. Int. J. Syst. Evol. Bacteriol.* **51:**2145–2165.
51. **Edelman, D. C., and J. S. Dumler.** 1996. Evaluation of an improved PCR diagnostic assay for human granulocytic ehrlichiosis. *Mol. Diagn.* **1:**41–49.
52. **Everett, E. D., K. A. Evans, R. B. Henry, and G. McDonald.** 1994. Human ehrlichiosis in adults after tick exposure: diagnosis using polymerase chain reaction. *Ann. Intern. Med.* **120:**730–735.
53. **Egenvall, A., B. N. Bonnett, A. Gunnarsson, A. Hedhammar, M. Shoukri, S. Bornstein, and K. Artursson.** 2000. Seroprevalence of granulocytic *Ehrlichia* spp. and *Borrelia burgdorferi* sensu lato in Swedish dogs 1991–94. *Scand. J. Infect. Dis.* **32:**19–25.
54. **Ewing, S. A., W. R. Roberson, R. G. Buckner, and C. S. Hayat.** 1971. A new strain of *Ehrlichia canis. J. Am. Vet. Med. Assoc.* **159:**1771–1774.
55. **Fichtenbaum, C. J., L. R. Peterson, and G. J. Weil.** 1993. Ehrlichiosis presenting as a life-threatening illness with features of the toxic shock syndrome. *Am. J. Med.* **95:**351–357.
56. **Fish, D.** 1995. Environmental risk and prevention of Lyme disease. *Am. J. Med.* **98:**2S–8S.
57. **Fishbein, D. B., J. E. Dawson, and L. E. Robinson.** 1994. Human ehrlichiosis in the United States, 1985 to 1990. *Ann. Intern. Med.* **120:**736–743.
58. **Foggie, A.** 1951. Studies on the infectious agent of tick-borne fever in sheep. *J. Pathol. Bacteriol.* **63:**1–15.
59. **Gardner, S. L., R. C. Holman, J. W. Krebs, R. Berkelman, and J. E. Childs.** 2003. National surveillance for the human ehrlichioses in the United States, 1997–2001, and proposed methods of data quality. *Ann. N. Y. Acad. Sci.* **990:**80–89.
60. **Gongora-Biachi, R. A., J. Zavala-Velazquez, C. J. Castro-Sansores, and P. Gonzalez-Martinez.** 1999. First case of human ehrlichiosis in Mexico. *Emerg. Infect. Dis.* **5:**481.
61. **Goodman, J. L., C. Nelson, B. Vitale, J. S. Dumler, J. E. Madigan, T. J. Kurtti, and U. G. Munderloh.** 1996. Direct cultivation of the causative agent of human granulocytic ehrlichiosis. *N. Engl. J. Med.* **334:**209–215.
62. **Hardalo, C., V. Quagliarello, and J. S. Dumler.** 1995. Human granulocytic ehrlichiosis in Connecticut: report of a fatal case. *Clin. Infect. Dis.* **21:**910–914.
63. **Heimer, R., D. Tisdale, and J. E. Dawson.** 1998. A single tissue culture system for the propagation of the agents of the human ehrlichiosis. *Am. J. Trop. Hyg.* **58:**812–815.
64. **Heimer, R., A. Van Andel, G. P. Wormser, and M. L. Wilson.** 1997. Propagation of granulocytic *Ehrlichia* spp. from human and equine sources in HL-60 cells induced to differentiate into functional granulocytes. *J. Clin. Microbiol.* **35:**923–927.
65. **Heo, E.-J., J.-H. Park, J.-R. Koo, M.-S. Park, M.-Y. Park, J. S. Dumler, and J.-S. Chae.** 2002. Serologic and molecular detection of *Ehrlichia chaffeensis* and *Anaplasma phagocytophila* (human granulocytic ehrlichiosis agent) in Korean patients. *J. Clin. Microbiol.* **40:**3082–3085.
66. **Hise, A. G., I. Gillette-Fergusson, and E. Pearlman.** 2004. The role of endosymbiotic *Wolbachia* bacteria in filarial disease. *Cell. Microbiol.* **6:**97–104.
67. **Holland, C. J., E. Weiss, W. Burgdorfer, A. I. Cole, and I. Kakoma.** 1985. *Ehrlichia risticii* sp. nov.: etiologic agent of equine monocytic ehrlichiosis (synonym, Potomac horse fever). *Int. J. Syst. Bacteriol.* **35:**524–526.
68. **Horowitz, H. W., E. Kilchevsky, S. Haber, M. Aguero-Rosenfeld, R. Kranwinkel, E. K. James, S. J. Wong, F. Chu, D. Liveris, and I. Schwartz.** 1998. Perinatal transmission of the agent of human granulocytic ehrlichiosis. *N. Engl. J. Med.* **339:**375–378.
69. **Horowitz, H. W., T.-C. Hsieh, M. E. Aguero-Rosenfeld, F. Kalantarpour, I. Chowdhury, G. P. Wormser, and J. Wu.** 2001. Antimicrobial susceptibility of *Ehrlichia phagocytophila. Antimicrob. Agents Chemother.* **45:**786–788.
70. **Hossain, D., M. E. Aguero-Rosenfeld, H. W. Horowitz, J. M. Wu, T.-C. Hsieh, N. Sachdeva, S. J. Peterson, J. S. Dumler, and G. P. Wormser.** 1999. Clinical and laboratory evolution of a culture-confirmed case of human granulocytic ehrlichiosis. *Conn. Med.* **63:**265–270.
71. **Huchzermeyer, F. W., I. G. Horak, J. F. Putterill, and R. A. Earle.** 1992. Description of *Aegyptianella botuliformis* n. sp.

(Rickettsiales: Anaplasmataceae) from the helmeted guineafowl, *Numida meleagris. Onderstepoort J. Vet. Res.* **59:**97–101.

72. **IJdo, J. W., Y. Zhang, E. Hodzic, L. A. Magnarelli, M. L. Wilson, S. R. Telford III, S. W. Barthold, and E. Fikrig.** 1997. The early humoral response in human granulocytic ehrlichiosis. *J. Infect. Dis.* **176:**687–692.
73. **Inokuma, H., P. Brouqui, M. Drancourt, and D. Raoult.** 2001. Citrate synthase gene sequence: a new tool for phylogenetic analysis and identification of *Ehrlichia. J. Clin. Microbiol.* **39:**3031–3039.
74. **Inokuma, H., K. Fujii, M. Okuda, T. Onishi, J.-P. Beaufils, D. Raoult, and P. Brouqui.** 2002. Determination of the nucleotide sequences of heat shock operon *groESL* and the citrate synthase gene *(gltA)* of *Anaplasma (Ehrlichia) platys* for phylogenetic and diagnostic studies. *Clin. Diagn. Lab. Immunol.* **9:**1132–1136.
75. **Inokuma, H., Y. Terada, T. Kamio, D. Raoult, and P. Brouqui.** 2001. Analysis of the 16S RNA gene sequence of *Anaplasma centrale* and its phylogenetic relatedness to other *Ehrlichiae. Clin. Diagn. Lab. Immunol.* **8:**241–244.
76. **Iqbal, Z., and Y. Rikihisa.** 1994. Reisolation of *Ehrlichia canis* from blood and tissues of dogs after doxycycline treatment. *J. Clin. Microbiol.* **32:**1644–1649.
77. **Jongejan, F., L. A. Wassink, M. J. C. Thielemans, N. M. Perie, and G. Uilenberg.** 1989. Serotypes in *Cowdria ruminantium* and their relationship with *Ehrlichia phagocytophila* determined by immunofluorescence. *Vet. Microbiol.* **21:**31–40.
78. **Kalantarpour, F., I. Chowdhury, G. P. Wormser, and M. E. Aguero-Rosenfeld.** 2000. Survival of the human granulocytic (HGE) agent under refrigeration conditions. *J. Clin. Microbiol.* **38:**2398–2399.
79. **Karlsson, U., A. Bjoersdorff, R. Massung, and B. Christensson.** 2001. Human granulocytic ehrlichiosis—a clinical case in Scandinavia. *Scand. J. Infect. Dis.* **33:**73–74.
80. **Klein, M. B., C. M. Nelson, and J. L. Goodman.** 1997. Antibiotic susceptibility of the newly cultivated agent of human granulocytic ehrlichiosis: promising activity of quinolones and rifamycins. *Antimicrob. Agents Chemother.* **41:**76–79.
81. **Kocan, K. M.** 1995. Targeting ticks for control of selected hemoparasitic diseases of cattle. *Vet. Parasitol.* **57:**121–151.
82. **Koutaro, M., A. S. Santos, J. S. Dumler, and P. Brouqui.** 2005. Distribution of *Ehrlichia walkeri* in *Ixodes ricinus* (Acari: *Ixodidae)* from the northern part of Italy. *J. Med. Entomol.* **42:**82–85.
83. **Lee, K. N., I. Padmalayam, B. Baumstark, S. L. Baker, and R. F. Massung.** 2003. Characterization of the *ftsZ* gene from *Ehrlichia chaffeensis, Anaplasma phagocytophilum, Rickettsia rickettsii,* and use as a differential PCR target. *DNA Cell Biol.* **22:**179–186.
84. **Levin, M. L., and D. Fish.** 2000. Immunity reduces reservoir host competence of *Peromyscus leucopus* for *Ehrlichia phagocytophila. Infect. Immun.* **68:**1514–1518.
85. **Lockhart, J. M., W. R. Davidson, D. E. Stallknecht, J. E. Dawson, and E. W. Howerth.** 1997. Isolation of *Ehrlichia chaffeensis* from wild white-tailed deer *(Odocoileus virginianus)* confirms their role as natural reservoir hosts. *J. Clin. Microbiol.* **35:**1681–1686.
86. **Long, S. W., X. Zhang, J. Zhang, R. P. Ruble, P. Teel, and X. J. Yu.** 2003. Evaluation of transovarial transmission and transmissibility of *Ehrlichia chaffeensis (Rickettsiales: Anaplasmataceae)* in *Amblyomma americanum* (Acari: *Ixodidae). J. Med. Entomol.* **40:**1000–1004.
87. **MacLeod, J. R., and W. S. Gordon.** 1993. Studies in tick-borne fever of sheep. Transmission by the tick, *Ixodes ricinus,* with a description of the disease produced. *Parasitology* **25:**273–285.
88. **Madigan, J. E., and D. Gribble.** 1987. Equine ehrlichiosis in northern California: 49 cases (1968–1981). *J. Am. Vet. Med. Assoc.* **190:**445–448.
89. **Madigan, J. E., N. Pusterla, E. Johnson, J.-S. Chae, J. Berger Pusterla, E. DeRock, and S. P. Lawler.** 2000. Transmission of *Ehrlichia risticii,* the agent of Potomac horse fever, using naturally infected aquatic insects and helminth vectors: preliminary report. *Equine Vet. J.* **32:**275–279.
90. **Madigan, J. E., P. J. Richter, R. B. Kimsey, J. E. Barlough, J. S. Bakken, and J. S. Dumler.** 1995. Transmission and passage in horses of the agent of human granulocytic ehrlichiosis. *J. Infect. Dis.* **172:**1141–1144.
91. **Maeda, K., N. Markowitz, R. C. Hawley, M. Ristic, D. Cox, and J. McDade.** 1987. Human infection with *Ehrlichia canis,* a leukocytic rickettsia. *N. Engl. J. Med.* **316:**853–856.
92. **Magnarelli, L. A., J. S. Dumler, and J. F. Anderson.** 1995. Coexistence of antibodies to tick-borne pathogens of babesiosis, ehrlichiosis, and Lyme borreliosis in human sera. *J. Clin. Microbiol.* **33:**3054–3057.
93. **Marty, A. M., J. S. Dumler, G. Imes, H. P. Brusman, L. L. Smrkovski, and D. M. Frisman.** 1995. Ehrlichiosis mimicking thrombotic thrombocytopenic purpura. Case report and pathological correlation. *Hum. Pathol.* **26:**920–925.
94. **Massung, R. F., K. Lee, M. Mauel, and A. Gusa.** 2002. Characterization of the rRNA genes of *Ehrlichia chaffeensis* and *Anaplasma phagocytophila. DNA Cell Biol.* **21:**587–596.
95. **Massung, R. F., M. J. Mauel, J. H. Owens, N. Allan, J. W. Courtney, K. C. Stafford, and T. N. Mather.** 2002. Genetic variants of *Ehrlichia phagocytophila,* Rhode Island and Connecticut. *Emerg. Infect. Dis.* **8:**467–472.
96. **Massung, R. F., and K. G. Slater.** 2003. Comparison of PCR assays for detection of the agent of human granulocytic ehrlichiosis, *Anaplasma phagocytophilum. J. Clin. Microbiol.* **41:**717–722.
97. **Misao, T., and Y. Kobayashi.** 1954. Studies on infectious mononucleosis. I. Isolation of etiologic agent from blood, bone marrow, and lymph node of a patient with infectious mononucleosis by using mice. *Tokyo Iji Shinshi* **71:**683–686.
98. **Murphy, C. I., J. R. Storey, J. Recchia, L. A. Doros-Richert, C. Gingrich-Baker, K. Munroe, J. S. Bakken, R. T. Coughlin, and G. A. Beltz.** 1998. Major antigenic proteins of the agent of human granulocytic ehrlichiosis are encoded by members of a multigene family. *Infect. Immun.* **66:**3711–3718.
99. **Nadelman, R. B., H. W. Horowitz, T.-C. Hsieh, J. M. Wu, M. Aguero-Rosenfeld, L. Schwartz, J. Nowakowski, S. Varde, and G. P. Wormser.** 1997. Simultaneous human granulocytic ehrlichiosis and Lyme borreliosis. *N. Engl. J. Med.* **337:**27–30.
100. **Ohashi, N., N. Zhi, Q. Lin, and Y. Rikihisa.** 2002. Characterization and transcriptional analysis of gene clusters for a type IV secretion machinery in human granulocytic and monocytic ehrlichiosis agents. *Infect. Immun.* **70:**2128–2138.
101. **Olano, J. P., W. Hogrefe, B. Seaton, and D. H. Walker.** 2003. Clinical manifestations, epidemiology, and laboratory diagnosis of human monocytotropic ehrlichiosis in a commercial laboratory setting. *Clin. Diagn. Lab. Immunol.* **10:**891–896.
102. **Olano, J. P., E. Masters, W. Hogrefe, and D. H. Walker.** 2003. Human monocytotropic ehrlichiosis, Missouri. *Emerg. Infect. Dis.* **9:**1579–1586.
103. **Olano, J. P., and D. H. Walker.** 2002. Human ehrlichioses. *Med. Clin. N. Am.* **86:**375–392.
104. **Paddock, C. D., and J. E. Childs.** 2003. *Ehrlichia chaffeensis:* a prototypical emerging pathogen. *Clin. Microbiol. Rev.* **16:**37–64.
105. **Paddock, C. D., S. M. Folk, G. M. Shore, L. J. Machado, M. M. Huycke, L. N. Slater, A. M. Lidell, R. S. Buller, G. A. Storch, T. P. Monson, D. Rimland,**

J. W. Sumner, J. Singleton, K. C. Bloch, Y.-W. Tang, S. M. Standaert, and J. E. Childs. 2001. Infections with *Ehrlichia chaffeensis* and *Ehrlichia ewingii* in persons coinfected with human immunodeficiency virus. *Clin. Infect. Dis.* **33:**1586–1594.

106. **Paddock, C. D., D. P. Suchard, K. L. Grumbach, W. K. Hadley, R. L. Kerschmann, N. W. Abbey, J. E. Dawson, B. E. Anderson, K. G. Sims, J. S. Dumler, and B. G. Herndier.** 1993. Fatal seronegative ehrlichiosis in a patient with HIV infection. *N. Engl. J. Med.* **329:**1164–1167.
107. **Paddock, C. D., J. W. Sumner, G. M. Shore, D. C. Bartley, R. C. Elie, J. G. McQuade, C. R. Martin, C. S. Goldsmith, and J. E. Childs.** 1997. Isolation and characterization of *Ehrlichia chaffeensis* strains from patients with fatal ehrlichiosis. *J. Clin. Microbiol.* **35:**2496–2502.
108. **Palmer, G. H., W. C. Brown, and F. R. Rurangirwa.** 2000. Antigenic variation in the persistence and transmission of the ehrlichia *Anaplasma marginale*. *Microbes Infect.* **2:**167–176.
109. **Pancholi, P., C. P. Kolbert, P. D. Mitchell, K. D. Reed, J. S. Dumler, J. S. Bakken, S. R. Telford III, and D. H. Persing.** 1995. *Ixodes dammini* as a potential vector of human granulocytic ehrlichiosis. *J. Infect. Dis.* **172:** 1007–1012.
110. **Park, J.-H., E.-J. Heo, K.-S. Choi, J. S. Dumler, and J.-S. Chae.** 2003. Detection of antibodies to *Anaplasma phagocytophilum* and *Ehrlichia chaffeensis* antigens in sera of Korean patients by Western immunoblotting and indirect immunofluorescence assays. *Clin. Diagn. Lab. Immunol.* **10:**1059–1064.
111. **Perez, M., Y. Rikihisa, and B. Wen.** 1996. *Ehrlichia canis*-like agent isolated from a man in Venezuela: antigenic and genetic characterization. *J. Clin. Microbiol.* **34:**2133–2139.
112. **Petrovec, M., S. L. Furlan, T. A. Zupanc, F. Strle, P. Brouqui, V. Roux, and J. S. Dumler.** 1997. Human disease in Europe caused by a granulocytic *Ehrlichia*. *J. Clin. Microbiol.* **35:**1556–1559.
113. **Popov, V. L., S.-M. Chen, H.-M. Feng, and D. H. Walker.** 1995. Ultrastructural variation of cultured *Ehrlichia chaffeensis*. *J. Med. Microbiol.* **43:**411–421.
114. **Ravyn, M. D., J. L. Goodman, C. B. Kodner, D. K. Westad, L. A. Coleman, S. M. Engstrom, C. M. Nelson, and R. C. Johnson.** 1998. Immunodiagnosis of human granulocytic ehrlichiosis by using culture-derived human isolates. *J. Clin. Microbiol.* **36:**1480–1488.
115. **Remy, V., Y. Hansmann, S. De Martino, D. Christmann, and P. Brouqui.** 2003. Human anaplasmosis presenting as atypical pneumonitis in France. *Clin. Infect. Dis.* **37:**846–848.
116. **Reyes, M., A. Dudek, B. Jahagirdar, L. Koodie, P. H. Marker, and C. M. Verfaillie.** 2002. Origin of endothelial progenitors in human postnatal bone marrow. *J. Clin. Investig.* **109:**337–346.
117. **Richter, P. J., R. B. Kimsey, J. E. Madigan, et al.** 1996. *Ixodes pacificus* as a vector of *Ehrlichia equi*. *J. Med. Entomol.* **33:**1–5.
118. **Rikihisa, Y.** 1991. The tribe *Ehrlichieae* and ehrlichial diseases. *Clin. Microbiol. Rev.* **4:**286–308.
119. **Rikihisa, Y., N. Zhi, G. P. Wormser, B. Wen, H. W. Horowitz, and K. E. Hechemy.** 1997. Ultrastructural and antigenic characterization of a granulocytic ehrlichiosis agent directly isolated and stably cultivated from a patient in New York State. *J. Infect. Dis.* **175:**210–213.
120. **Ripoll, C. M., C. E. Remondegui, G. Ordonez, et al.** 1999. Evidence of rickettsial spotted fever and ehrlichial infections in a subtropical territory of Jujuy, Argentina. *Am. J. Trop. Med. Hyg.* **61:**350–354.
121. **Roland, W. E., G. McDonald, C. W. Cauldwell, and E. D. Everett.** 1995. Ehrlichiosis—a cause of prolonged fever. *Clin. Infect. Dis.* **20:**821–825.
122. **Safdar, N., R. B. Love, and D. Maki.** 2002. Severe *Ehrlichia chaffeensis* infection in a lung transplant recipient: a review of ehrlichiosis in the immunocompromised patient. *Emerg. Infect. Dis.* **8:**320–323.
123. **Sanogo, Y. O., P. Parola, S. Shpynov, J. L. Camicas, P. Brouqui, G. Caruso, and D. Raoult.** 2003. Genetic diversity of bacterial agents detected in ticks removed from asymptomatic patients in Northern Italy. *Ann. N. Y. Acad. Sci.* **990:**182–190.
124. **Schutze, G. E., and R. F. Jacobs.** 1997. Human monocytic ehrlichiosis in children. *Pediatrics* **100:**E10.
125. **Sirigireddy, K. R., and R. R. Ganta.** 2005. Multiplex detection of *Ehrlichia* and *Anaplasma* species pathogens in peripheral blood by real-time reverse transcriptase-polymerase chain reaction. *J. Mol. Diagn.* **7:**308–316.
126. **Standaert, S. M., J. E. Dawson, W. Schaffner, J. E. Childs, K. L. Biggie, J. Singleton, Jr., R. R. Gerhardt, M. L. Knight, and R. H. Hutcheson.** 1995. Ehrlichiosis in a golf-oriented retirement community. *N. Engl. J. Med.* **333:**420–425.
127. **Standaert, S. M., T. Yu, M. A. Scott, J. E. Childs, C. D. Paddock, W. L. Nicholson, J. Singleton, Jr., and M. J. Blaser.** 2000. Primary isolation of *Ehrlichia chaffeensis* from patients with febrile illnesses: clinical and molecular characteristics. *J. Infect. Dis.* **181:**1082–1088.
128. **Stuen, S., I. Van De Pol, K. Bergstrom, and L. M. Schouls.** 2002. Identification of *Anaplasma phagocytophila* (formerly *Ehrlichia phagocytophila*) variants in blood from sheep in Norway. *J. Clin. Microbiol.* **40:**3192–3197.
129. **Suksawat, J., B. C. Hegarty, and E. B. Breitschwerdt.** 2000. Seroprevalence of *Ehrlichia canis, Ehrlichia equi,* and *Ehrlichia risticii* in sick dogs from North Carolina and Virginia. *J. Vet. Intern. Med.* **14:**50–55.
130. **Sumner, J. W., W. L. Nicholson, and R. F. Massung.** 1997. PCR amplification and comparison of nucleotide sequences from the *groESL* heat shock operon of *Ehrlichia* species. *J. Clin Microbiol.* **35:**2087–2092.
131. **Sumner, J. W., K. G. Sims, D. C. Jones, and B. E. Anderson.** 1993. *Ehrlichia chaffeensis* expresses an immunoreactive protein homologous to the *Escherichia coli* GroEL protein. *Infect. Immun.* **61:**3536–3539.
132. **Taillardat-Bisch, A.-V., D. Raoult, and M. Drancourt.** 2003. RNA polymerase β-subunit-based phylogeny of *Ehrlichia* spp., *Anaplasma* spp., *Neorickettsia* spp. and *Wolbachia pipientis*. *Int. J. Syst. Evol. Microbiol.* **53:**455–458.
133. **Tajima, T., N. Zhi, Q. Lin, Y. Rikihisa, H. W. Horowitz, J. T. Raffalli, G. P. Wormser, and K. E. Hechemy.** 2000. Comparison of two recombinant major outer membrane proteins of the human granulocytic ehrlichiosis agent for use in an enzyme-linked immunosorbent assay. *Clin. Diagn. Lab. Immunol.* **7:**652–657.
134. **Taylor, M. J.** 2003. *Wolbachia* in the inflammatory pathogenesis of human filariasis. *Ann. N. Y. Acad. Sci.* **990:**444–449.
135. **Telford, S. R., III, J. E. Dawson, P. Katavolos, C. K. Warner, C. P. Kolbert, and D. H. Persing.** 1996. Perpetuation of the agent of human granulocytic ehrlichiosis in a deer tick-rodent cycle. *Proc. Natl. Acad. Sci. USA* **93:**6209–6214.
136. **Wagner, E. R., W. G. Bremer, Y. Rikihisa, et al.** 2004. Development of a p28-based PCR assay for *Ehrlichia chaffeensis*. *Mol. Cell. Probes* **18:**111–116.
137. **Walker, D. H., and J. S. Dumler.** 1996. Emergence of ehrlichioses as human health problems. *Emerg. Infect. Dis.* **2:**18–29.
138. **Walker, D. H., and J. S. Dumler.** 1997. Human monocytic and granulocytic ehrlichioses. Discovery and diagnosis of emerging tick-borne infections and the critical role of the pathologist. *Arch. Pathol. Lab. Med.* **121:**785–791.
139. **Walls, J. J., B. Greig, D. S. Neitzel, and J. S. Dumler.** 1997. Natural infection of small mammal species in

Minnesota with the agent of human granulocytic ehrlichiosis. *J. Clin. Microbiol.* **35:**853–855.

140. **Walls, J. J., M. E. Aguero-Rosenfeld, J. S. Bakken, J. L. Goodman, D. Hossain, R. C. Johnson, and J. S. Dumler.** 1999. Inter- and intralaboratory comparison of *Ehrlichia equi* and human granulocytic ehrlichiosis (HGE) agent strains for serodiagnosis of HGE by the immunofluorescent-antibody test. *J. Clin. Microbiol.* **37:**2968–2973.
141. **Weiss, E., and J. W. Moulder.** 1984. The Rickettsias and Chlamydias, p. 687–739. *In* N. R. Krieg and J. G. Holt (ed.), *Bergey's Manual of Determinative Bacteriology,* vol. 1. Williams and Wilkins, Baltimore, Md.
142. **Weiss, E., J. C. Williams, G. A. Dasch, and Y.-H Kang.** 1989. Energy metabolism of monocytic *Ehrlichia. Proc. Natl. Acad. Sci. USA* **86:**1674–1678.
143. **Wen, B., R. Jian, Y. Zhang, and R. Chen.** 2002. Simultaneous detection of *Anaplasma marginale* and a new *Ehrlichia* species closely related to *Ehrlichia chaffeensis* by sequence analyses of 16S ribosomal DNA in *Boophilus microplus* ticks from Tibet. *J. Clin. Microbiol.* **40:**3286–3290.
144. **Woldehiwet, Z., B. K. Horrocks, H. Scaife, G. Ross, U. G. Munderloh, K. Bown, S. W. Edwards, and C. A. Hart.** 2002. Cultivation of an ovine strain of *Ehrlichia phagocytophila* in tick cell cultures. *J. Comp. Pathol.* **127:**142–149.
145. **Wolf, L., T. McPherson, B. Harrison, B. Engber, A. Anderson, and P. Whitt.** 2000. Prevalence of *Ehrlichia ewingii* in *Amblyomma americanum* in North Carolina. *J. Clin. Microbiol.* **38:**2795.
146. **Wong, S. J., G. S. Brady, and J. S. Dumler.** 1997. Serological responses to *Ehrlichia equi, Ehrlichia chaffeensis,* and *Borrelia burgdorferi* in patients from New York State. *J. Clin. Microbiol.* **35:**2198–2205.
147. **Wong, S. J., and J. A. Thomas.** 1998. Cytoplasmic, nuclear, and platelet autoantibodies in human granulocytic ehrlichiosis patients. *J. Clin. Microbiol.* **36:**1959–1963.
148. **Wormser, G. P., H. W. Horowitz, J. Nowakowski, D. McKenna, J. S. Dumler, S. Varde, I. Schwartz, C. Carbonaro, and M. Aguero-Rosenfeld.** 1997. Positive Lyme disease serology in patients with clinical and laboratory evidence of human granulocytic ehrlichiosis. *Am. J. Clin. Pathol.* **107:**142–147.
149. **Yabsley, M. J., A. S. Varela, C. M. Tate, V. G. Dugan, D. E. Stallknecht, S. E. Little, and W. R. Davidson.** 2002. *Ehrlichia ewingii* infection in white-tailed deer *(Odocoileus virginianus). Emerg. Infect. Dis.* **8:**668–671.
150. **Yu, X., P. Brouqui, J. S. Dumler, and D. Raoult.** 1993. Detection of *Ehrlichia chaffeensis* in human tissue by using a species-specific monoclonal antibody. *J. Clin. Microbiol.* **31:**3284–3288.
151. **Yu, X.-J., P. Crocquet-Valdes, L. C. Cullman, and D. H. Walker.** 1996. The recombinant 120-kilodalton protein of *Ehrlichia chaffeensis,* a potential diagnostic tool. *J. Clin. Microbiol.* **34:**2853–2855.
152. **Yu, X.-J., P. Crocquet-Valdes, and D. H. Walker.** 1997. Cloning and sequencing of the gene for a 120-kDa immunodominant protein of *Ehrlichia chaffeensis. Gene* **184:**149–154.
153. **Yu, X., J. F. Piesman, J. G. Olson, and D. H. Walker.** 1997. Geographic distribution of different genetic types of *Ehrlichia chaffeensis. Am. J. Trop. Med. Hyg.* **56:**679–680.
154. **Zhi, N., N. Ohashi, Y. Rikihisa, H. W. Horowitz, G. P. Wormser, and K. E. Hechemy.** 1998. Cloning and expression of the 44-kilodalton major outer membrane protein gene of the human granulocytic ehrlichiosis agent and application of the recombinant protein to serodiagnosis. *J. Clin. Microbiol.* **36:**1666–1673.

Coxiella

PHILIPPE BROUQUI, THOMAS MARRIE, AND DIDIER RAOULT

68

TAXONOMY

Coxiella burnetii is the only species of the genus and has been placed in the γ subdivision of the class *Proteobacteria,* close to *Rickettsiella grylli, Legionella* spp., and *Francisella* spp., on the basis of comparison of the 16S rRNA-encoding gene sequences.

DESCRIPTION OF THE GENUS

C. burnetii, the organism responsible for Q fever, is a pleomorphic coccobacillus with a gram-negative cell wall (4). It is an obligate intracellular microorganism measuring 0.2 by 0.7 μm. It does not stain with Gram stain but does stain with Gimenez stain. *C. burnetii* undergoes a developmental cycle in which there is a large-cell and a small-cell variant (59). The small-cell variant attaches to the host cell (usually a macrophage) and is ingested. *C. burnetii* develops within the phagolysosome, where the acid pH activates its metabolic enzymes. Following maturation to the large-cell variant, sporogenesis begins (59). Spore formation explains why *C. burnetii* is so successful as a pathogen. It can survive for up to 10 months at 15 to 20°C, for more than 1 month on meat in cold storage, and for more than 40 months in skim milk at room temperature (12). *C. burnetii* was shown to survive in free-living amoebae, suggesting a possible mechanism to explain the survival and resistance of the pathogen in the environment (Fig. 1) (47).

C. burnetii undergoes phase variation akin to the smooth-to-rough transition of lipopolysaccharides (LPS) of gram-negative bacteria (91). In nature and in laboratory animals, it exists in the phase I state, in which the organisms react with late-convalescent-phase (45 days) guinea pig sera and only slightly with early-convalescent-phase (21 days) sera (91). Apparently phase II LPS is a deletion mutant of phase I LPS (96), of which the fitness, in vitro, is superior to that of phase I. After numerous passages in cell culture or embryonated eggs, truncation of the LPS occurs, yielding the antigenic form, phase II.

EPIDEMIOLOGY AND TRANSMISSION

Q fever is a worldwide zoonosis. *C. burnetii* has been identified in arthropods, fish, birds, rodents, marsupials, and livestock (3). Indeed, it naturally infects more than 40 species (including 12 genera) of ticks on five continents (4). Lice, mites, and parasitic flukes are also infected (64). Bandicoots, rats, rabbits, mice, porcupines, hedgehogs, tortoises, cattle, sheep, goats, dogs, swine, cats, camels, buffaloes, baboons, leopards, hyenas, chickens, ducks, geese, turkeys, pigeons, bats, and shrews have all been infected with this microorganism (43, 64).

The extreme infectivity of *C. burnetii* results in large outbreaks and makes it a potential bioweapon. The major route of transmission of Q fever to humans is by inhalation of dust particles contaminated with parturient fluids. The organism can stick on wool and dust and can be spread by the wind to distant places. Cases of Q fever have occurred miles away from the lambing site in the direction in which the winds blew (8, 93, 95). Ingestion of milk and milk products is a risk factor for transmission of Q fever (25). Raw milk from cows was considered a risk factor for Q fever in California, and the decrease in the prevalence of Q fever in this state could be partly related to cessation of the practice of drinking raw milk. However, the consumption of goat cheese made from raw as well as pasteurized milk was reported as a risk factor (25, 35). In experimental animal models, the route of infection (aerosol or intraperitoneal) has been shown to determine the specific organs that are involved (lung and liver, respectively) (45). Sexually transmitted Q fever has been suggested, but this route needs to be confirmed (61).

The current understanding of the natural history of Q fever is that a nonimmune patient comes into contact with *C. burnetii,* which causes a primary infection that could be asymptomatic or symptomatic (76). The symptomatic primary infection is acute Q fever. The spontaneous evolution of acute infection is usually a complete recovery in the normal host. In immunocompromised hosts, *C. burnetii* can multiply despite an antibody response following primary infection (symptomatic or not). In these cases, because the immune system is unable to control the infection, chronic infection develops. This hypothesis is supported by all available data from human beings as well as from animal models (75). Preliminary data support that the inoculum size, the route of infection, host factors, and the specific strain all contribute to the clinical expression (e.g., pneumonia versus hepatitis) of acute infection (75, 88).

The immune control of Q fever is T-cell dependent, but it does not lead to *C. burnetii* eradication, and immunosuppression can induce relapse of infection in apparently cured patients or laboratory animals (85, 86). *C. burnetii* DNA can be found in apparently cured people as well as in the dental pulp of experimentally infected and cured guinea pigs (1).

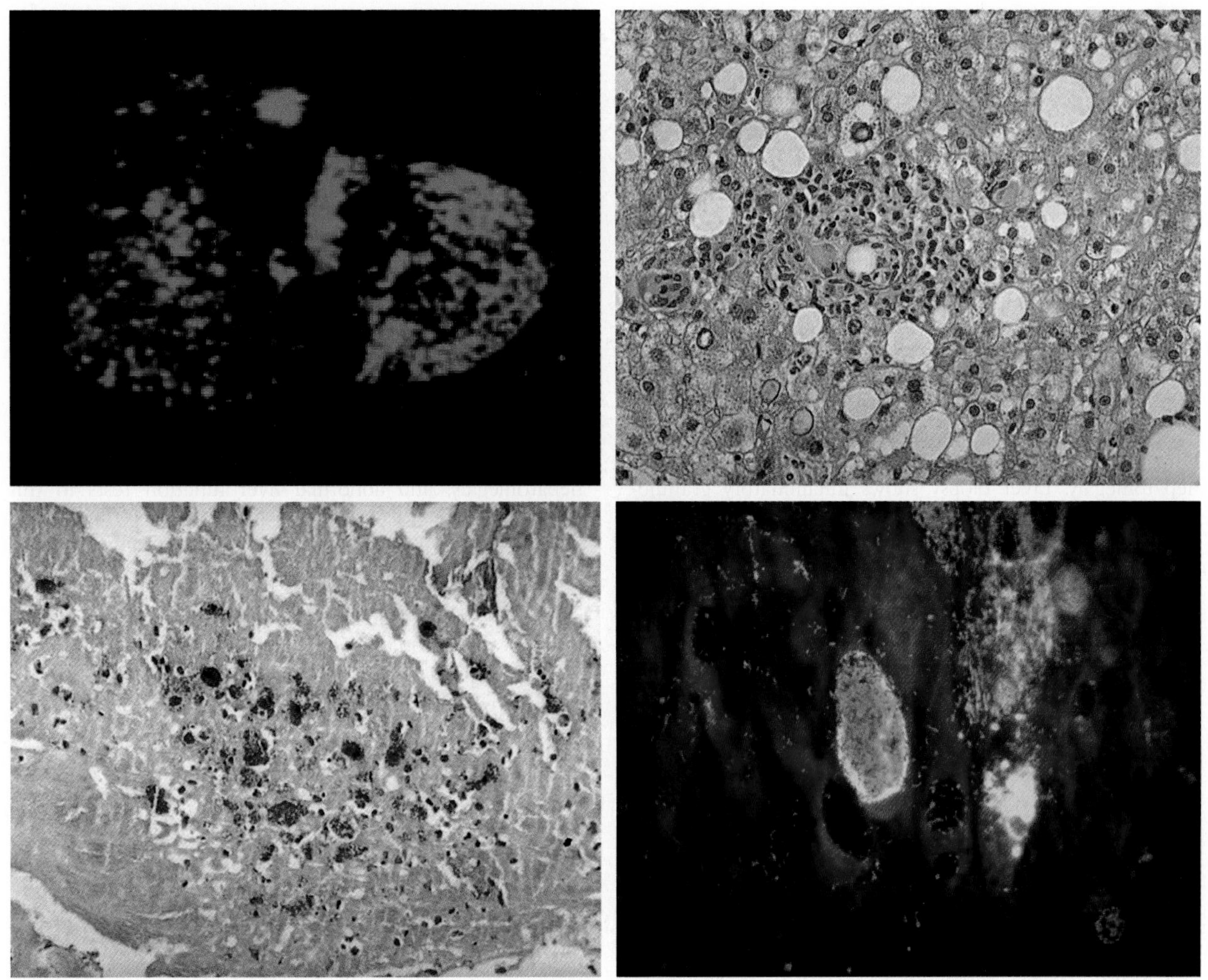

FIGURE 1 (top left) *Coxiella burnetii* in amoebae. Direct fluorescent-antibody stain with anti-*C. burnetii* monoclonal antibodies. Confocal microscopy. Magnification, ×1,000. (Courtesy of B. La Scola, Marseille, France.)

FIGURE 2 (top right) Hematoxylin and eosin stain of liver biopsy in a patient with acute Q fever. Doughnut ring granuloma. Magnification, ×400. (Courtesy of H. Lepidi, Marseille, France.)

FIGURE 3 (bottom left) Alkaline phosphatase immunohistochemistry on the heart valve from a patient with chronic Q fever endocarditis. *C. burnetii* microorganisms are stained pink within mononuclear cells. Magnification, ×400.

FIGURE 4 (bottom right) Identification of *C. burnetii* in shell vial culture at day 6 by the use of specific monoclonal antibody-based direct fluorescent-antibody test. Magnification, ×1,000.

Therefore, patients with acute Q fever who become immunocompromised or who have cardiac valve lesions are particularly at risk to develop chronic infection and especially endocarditis (19, 77).

Following primary infection, 60% of patients seroconvert without clinical manifestations and only 2% need to be hospitalized. A chronic infection develops in less than 1% of acutely infected patients and is often associated with a subtle and unique immune defect (58). Interleukin 10 (IL-10) seems to play a key role in the evolution of chronic infection (36).

Among children with Q fever, boys and girls are equally represented whereas men are 2.45 times more frequently infected than women (54). This has been suggested to be related to occupational exposure, although the protective role of 17β estradiol has been clearly demonstrated in a mouse model (48).

Since 30 to 50% of patients with Q fever and a valve lesion may develop Q fever endocarditis in the 2 years postinfection (19), echocardiography is recommended to detect such lesions as bicuspid aortic valve and minimal valvular leaks in all patients with acute Q fever (18).

CLINICAL SIGNIFICANCE

Acute Q Fever

The onset is usually abrupt, and patients present with high fever (91%), headaches (51%), myalgias (37%), arthralgias

(29%), and cough (34%), less frequently a rash (11%) or a meningeal syndrome (4%). Laboratory investigations show thrombocytopenia (35%), elevated liver enzymes (62%), and an elevated erythrocyte sedimentation rate (55%). The chest radiograph is abnormal in 27% of patients (77). The clinical presentation varies from country to country without clear explanation as to which one of the three major manifestations, i.e., isolated fever, hepatitis, or pneumonia, dominates.

Clinically isolated fever, without pneumonia or hepatitis, is usually associated with severe headache, and in some patients it persists long enough to meet the criteria for fever of unknown etiology. Pneumonia is the major clinical presentation of Q fever in Nova Scotia (Canada), the Basque country (Spain), and in the United Kingdom. Hepatitis is the most common form worldwide including France and Australia. Usually, increased liver enzymes suggest hepatitis; however, a few patients present with jaundice and/or hepatomegaly. Liver biopsy shows inflammatory granulomas, typically organized in the form of a "doughnut"; i.e., the granuloma contains a central lipid vacuole surrounded by a fibrinoid ring (58) (Fig. 2). Neurological manifestations of Q fever occur in 2% or more of cases and include meningitis, meningoencephalitis, peripheral neuropathy, and myelitis (5). Cardiac involvement occurs in 2% of acutely ill patients. This includes myocarditis (29), which led to death in two of the eight patients reported to date (29), and pericarditis, which is frequent but nonspecific (50). Among 204 patients with pericardial effusions, 10 (5%) were diagnosed as having Q fever by systematic testing (49). Other atypical presentations of acute Q fever have been reported such as acute acalculous cholecystitis (81) and isolated lymphadenitis from which *C. burnetii* has been cultured (26). Moreover, as *C. burnetii* occurs worldwide, it has been reported as a cause of fever in travelers returning from tropical countries (65) and may be associated with concurrent malaria (10).

Chronic fatigue following acute Q fever has been described in Australia and the United Kingdom (2, 66). It was reported that 20% of patients with post-Q-fever fatigue syndrome have moderate cytokine dysregulation (66). Q fever in immunocompromised hosts has been reported in patients with cancer (68) as well as in those with human immunodeficiency virus infection (52, 74). Q fever, when contracted during pregnancy, can result in abortion or neonatal death and in premature birth or low birth weight (71). About 4% of parturients in an area where Q fever is endemic have evidence of previous exposure to *C. burnetii*, and this correlates with adverse pregnancy outcomes (44). Twenty-three cases of Q fever during pregnancy have been reported (90). Most of these patients had complications including fetal or newborn death (11 cases) and premature birth (7 cases); only five patients had a normal pregnancy. One-half of the patients develop a serological profile of chronic Q fever during pregnancy, and, as in other mammals, *C. burnetii* can be isolated from the milk, the placenta, and the vaginal discharge. Multiple premature births have been reported in such cases (90), and these patients are subject to relapses during subsequent pregnancies. Patients with a valve lesion, an arterial aneurysm, or a prosthesis who have an episode of acute Q fever are at very high risk for chronic infection (77). Of acutely infected patients with a preexisting valvulopathy, 38% develop endocarditis within 2 years (19). In Greek children acute Q fever accounts for 3% of fever with unknown etiology (53). Children are less frequently symptomatic than adults and have milder disease, mostly pneumonitis (54). Chronic infection has rarely been reported, and when it occurs it manifests as endocarditis and osteomyelitis (11).

Chronic Q Fever

The major clinical form of chronic Q fever is endocarditis. At least 800 cases have been reported since 1949. In France, Q fever causes 5% of endocarditis cases with an estimated prevalence of $1/10^6$ inhabitants per year, which is close to what has been observed in Israel and Switzerland. In the largest published series of blood-culture-negative endocarditis, Q fever represented one-half (48%) of the etiologies, another 28% being due to *Bartonella* spp. and only 1% due to other fastidious growing microbes (38). The clinical presentation of patients with Q fever endocarditis varies according to the delays in diagnosis (70). A better knowledge of the disease has led to a significant reduction in this delay, explaining the decrease in the prevalence of heart failure, hepatomegaly, and abnormal liver function tests in this group of patients (37). Patients are usually afebrile or have low-grade intermittent fever.

Echocardiography is frequently inconclusive and fails to identify vegetations so that the diagnosis of endocarditis can easily be missed. A clue to the diagnosis is the presence of a known valve lesion and unexplained illness (fever, hepatitis, weakness, digital clubbing, weight loss, stroke, or renal insufficiency), an elevated erythrocyte sedimentation rate, increased serum transaminase levels, or thrombocytopenia. In such cases, positive Q fever serology complements the diagnosis made using modified Duke Criteria (27). Vascular infection is the second most commonly identified site of chronic Q fever. We have diagnosed 25 cases in our laboratory (28, 77), and 6 more were reported from other centers including England, the United States, Switzerland, and Australia (16, 17, 21, 60). Other manifestations of chronic Q fever include osteomyelitis (13), chronic hepatitis diagnosed in patients with alcoholism (77), pseudotumor of the spleen, pseudotumor of the lung, and infection of a ventriculoperitoneal drain (51). Recently, a case of vasculitis and pulmonary amyloidosis (41) following acute Q fever and resulting in the death of the patient was reported.

COLLECTION, TRANSPORT, AND STORAGE OF SPECIMENS

Biosafety level 2 practice and facilities are recommended for nonpropagative laboratory procedures including serological examination and staining of impression smears. Biosafety level 3 practice and facilities are recommended for activities involving inoculation, incubation, and harvesting of cell cultures, the necropsy of infected animals, and the manipulation of infected tissues (14). Although *C. burnetii* can be isolated from blood and a variety of tissues, this biosafety level is not feasible in most laboratories. Since the organism can withstand very harsh environmental conditions, it is unlikely that it will die during transport to a suitable laboratory. Blood should be collected in tubes containing EDTA or sodium citrate (heparin interferes with PCR), and the leukocyte layer should be saved for PCR. Solid specimens should be frozen at −80°C until they are cultured. Most laboratories depend on serological techniques to diagnose *C. burnetii* infection. For the diagnosis of acute Q fever, it is best that acute- and convalescent-phase serum samples collected 2 to 4 weeks apart be tested. Serum samples from patients with Q fever present no hazard to laboratory workers when handled using standard biosafety level 2 precautions.

LABORATORY DIAGNOSIS

Direct Examination

Antigen Detection

C. burnetii can be identified in tissues by a direct immunofluorescence technique. This is of limited utility for the routine diagnosis of *C. burnetii* since, with the exception of heart valve tissue from patients with Q fever endocarditis (9), tissue specimens from patients with acute Q fever are not generally submitted to the laboratory. The main reason for this is that the illness is mild to moderate in severity and death is extremely unusual. However, patients with Q fever endocarditis do have large numbers of *C. burnetii* organisms in the affected valvular tissue. These can be demonstrated by direct immunofluorescence (73) or electron microscopy. Other techniques that can be used to detect *C. burnetii* in tissues include immunohistology (9) (Fig. 3) and capture enzyme-linked immunosorbent assays (ELISAs) or enzyme-linked immunofluorescence assays (92).

Nucleic Acid Detection Techniques

PCR has successfully been used to detect DNA in cell cultures and clinical samples (89). Several genes have then been used to generate specific primers including 16S rRNA, 23S rRNA genes, superoxide dismutase, plasmid-based sequences, and the transposase encoding IS*111* multicopy insertion sequence gene (30). LightCycler nested PCR (LCN-PCR) using the IS*111* multicopy gene has been reported to be very sensitive. Because this is a closed glass capillary system, it does not pose more contamination risk than standard real-time PCR. It allows molecular detection of *C. burnetii* in sera from patients with Q fever endocarditis or vascular infection as well as in acute-phase sera of patients with acute Q fever (10, 20). LCN-PCR is particularly useful for early seronegative acute Q fever patients, but lacks sensitivity after 4 weeks of disease evolution. Thus, it is suggested that this test be added to serology in the first 2 weeks after the onset of symptoms to improve early diagnosis and in the 2 weeks following the onset of symptoms in the remaining seronegative patients only if suspicion of Q fever is high (31). Consequently, a positive PCR in a late-convalescent-phase serum should be carefully interpreted with the help of other conventional diagnostic methods and clinical data (84). LCN-PCR is also valuable for patients with phase I antibody titers between 800 and 6,400. In this range a positive PCR is correlated with chronic infection. For patients with chronic infection who have a higher level of antibody, the PCR is usually negative. Identification of *C. burnetii* at the strain level has been made possible with the use of a multispacer typing method allowing definition of three monophyletic groups among 158 isolates from all over the world (33). More recently a LightCycler PCR assay using hydrolysis probes has been used to detect *C. burnetii* in sera from patients with malaria (10).

Isolation Procedures and Identification

Isolation of *C. burnetii* must be done only in a biosafety level 3 containment facility due to its extreme infectivity. This microorganism can be isolated by inoculation of specimens into conventional cell cultures (e.g., Vero cells) (69), embryonated egg yolk sacs (63), or laboratory animals, such as mice or guinea pigs (39). The spleen of the inoculated animal is the most useful organ for the recovery of *C. burnetii*. Ground spleen extracts (0.2 to 0.5 ml of a 10% suspension) should be inoculated into embryonated eggs, which die 7 to 9 days later. These methods are used infrequently, but inoculation of animals remains helpful when the organism must be isolated from tissues contaminated with multiple bacteria or in order to obtain phase I *C. burnetii* antigens from phase II cells. The adaptation of a viral shell vial culture system using a human embryonic lung fibroblast (HEL cells) has improved the isolation of intracellular bacteria, especially *C. burnetii* (55, 69, 78). Plasma and buffy coat layers from heparinized blood are diluted 1:2 with Eagle's minimal essential medium (EMEM). Tissue specimens are homogenized in sterile phosphate-buffered saline (PBS) and diluted 1:2 in EMEM. Shell vials containing 12-mm-diameter round glass coverslips are seeded with 50,000 human embryonic lung cells in 1 ml of EMEM containing 10% fetal calf serum. The cells are incubated for 3 days at 37°C in an atmosphere containing 5% CO_2 until the monolayer is confluent. Then 1 ml of each homogenized specimen is placed into each of three shell vials. A 1-h centrifugation step (700 × *g* at 23°C) enhances the attachment and penetration of the bacteria into the cells. The supernatant is removed, and the monolayer is washed twice with PBS. Then 1 ml of EMEM containing 10% fetal calf serum is added to each vial. After an incubation period of 6 days, *C. burnetii* organisms are visualized as short rods by microscopic examination after staining with the Gimenez stain. Briefly, the infected cell smear is covered with carbol basic fuchsin (100 ml of 10% [wt/vol] basic fuchsin in 95% ethanol added to 250 ml of 4% [vol/vol] aqueous phenol and to 650 ml of distilled water) and allowed to stand 1 to 2 min. The smear is then washed in tap water and covered with malachite green solution (0.8% aqueous malachite green oxalate) for 6 to 9 s, washed again, and air dried (32). Confirmation of the presence of *C. burnetii* within the cells is performed by an indirect immunofluorescence assay with polyclonal or monoclonal anti-*C. burnetii* antibodies (Fig. 4) (69, 78). Positive cultures are passaged in cells several times to establish the isolated strain.

Serologic Tests

The microagglutination test (24, 64), the complement fixation test (22), the indirect immunofluorescent antibody (IFA) test (22, 62), and ELISA (97) have been used for the serological diagnosis of *C. burnetii* infection. With experimentally infected guinea pigs, ELISA is more sensitive than the IFA test. Antibodies against phase I whole cells are detected by day 9 with ELISA, by day 16 with the IFA test, and by day 20 with the complement fixation test. A commercial ELISA test (PanBio *Coxiella burnetii* immunoglobulin M [IgM] ELISA; QFM-200, Brisbane, Australia) has also been used for the serological diagnosis of acute Q fever, especially for the detection of IgM antibodies (23). However, the ELISA for the diagnosis of Q fever has not been standardized, rendering comparison of titers from laboratory to laboratory impossible. There are no accepted criteria for the diagnosis of acute versus chronic Q fever by this test. The complement fixation test is not as sensitive as the IFA test. Serum samples from about 20% of patients with acute Q fever are anticomplementary. A prozone phenomenon may be present in serum samples from some patients with chronic Q fever. This could result in a false-negative test result unless the laboratory is aware of this possibility.

The IFA test is the serological test of choice for the diagnosis of both acute and chronic Q fever. It is carried out by the procedure of Philip et al. (67) with purified whole-cell antigens at a concentration of 200 μg/ml. Both phase I and phase II antigens are used. Each antigen (phase I and II cells) is spotted onto slides, air dried, and fixed in acetone for 15 min at room temperature (approximately 20°C). Serum dilutions are added to each antigen spot and incubated in a moist chamber for 1 h at room temperature. Slides are then rinsed three times with PBS before being incubated with a fluorescein isothiocyanate-conjugated anti-human polyvalent (α, γ, or μ chain-specific) immunoglobulin or anti-IgG-, anti-IgA-, or anti-IgM-specific immunoglobulin and incubated for 30 min at 37°C in a moist chamber. The slides are then washed in PBS, rinsed in distilled water, and dried. Coverslips are mounted onto the slides with glycerol mounting medium. The slides are immediately read using a microscope with a UV light source at a magnification of ×400. The end point is the highest dilution showing whole-cell fluorescence. This method can be used to determine IgG, IgM, and IgA antibody fractions to phase I and phase II. However, test results can be confounded by the presence of rheumatoid factor. Thus, rheumatoid factor absorbent is used to remove IgG before the determination of IgM and IgA (94). The choice of negative cutoff titer depends upon the source and purity of the antigen and the amount of background antigen stimulation in the population to be studied. We use 1:50 dilution as our first positive dilution (94). Others have used a 1:8 dilution. An IFA diagnostic kit (Q Fever IFA IgG, Focus Diagnostics, Inc., Cypress, Calif.) is commercially available.

The antigenic variation of *C. burnetii* is extremely useful in differentiating acute and chronic illness. In acute Q fever, antibodies to phase II antigens predominate, and their titer is higher than the phase I antibody titer. IgM antibodies appear usually at about the same time as IgG. On the other hand, in chronic forms of the disease, such as endocarditis, high-titer anti-phase I antibodies are detected uniformly. For the diagnosis of acute Q fever, cutoff values of anti-phase II IgG antibody of 200 or greater and of anti-phase II IgM antibody of 50 or greater are mandatory. For the diagnosis of chronic Q fever endocarditis, a titer of anti-phase I IgG of 800 or greater has been shown to raise the posttest probability to 98% (94).

ANTIMICROBIAL SUSCEPTIBILITIES

Antibiotic susceptibility testing of *C. burnetii* is difficult since this organism cannot be grown in axenic medium and methods are not standardized; therefore, susceptibility testing should be conducted only in appropriately experienced laboratories. Three models of infection have been used: animals, chick embryos, and cell culture; but only the last system is used today.

A shell vial assay with HEL cells for assessment of the bacteriostatic effects of antibiotics against *C. burnetii* has been developed (78). With this system, amikacin and amoxicillin were not effective and ceftriaxone and fusidic acid were inconsistently active, while cotrimoxazole, rifampin, doxycycline, tetracycline, minocycline, and clarithromycin (58) as well as sparfloxacin and the quinolones PD 127,391 and PD 131,628 (40) were bacteriostatic. By the same technique, moxifloxacin demonstrated better activity than ofloxacin and pefloxacin (82), and telithromycin showed better activity than erythromycin, with MICs of 1 μg/ml and 8 μg/ml, respectively (83). When P388D$_1$ and L929 cell multiplication was inhibited with cycloheximide during antibiotic challenges, pefloxacin, rifampin, and doxycycline (69) as well as clarithromycin (58) were bacteriostatic.

Lack of bactericidal activity was related to antibiotic inactivation by the low pH of the phagolysosomes in which *C. burnetii* multiplied. It has been subsequently shown that the addition of chloroquine, a lysosomotropic alkalinizing agent, to antibiotics improved the activities of doxycycline and pefloxacin, which then became bactericidal (57). Real-time quantitative PCR has been reported to be a faster and reliable technique for antimicrobial susceptibility testing of *C. burnetii*-infected cells (6, 7).

INTERPRETATION AND REPORTING OF RESULTS

The diagnosis of Q fever is currently based on serology. In acute Q fever, seroconversion usually is detected 7 to 15 days after the onset of clinical symptoms. Approximately 90% of patients have detectable antibodies by the third week. IFA antibody titers reach their maximum levels 4 to 8 weeks after the onset of disease and then decrease gradually during the ensuing 12 months (34). IgM titers declined to undetectable levels after 10 to 17 weeks (15, 22). In blood culture-negative endocarditis, the sensitivity and the posttest probability of having Q fever in a single-step serological assay with an 800-titer cutoff were 100 and 99.5%, respectively (80). Thus, in chronic Q fever a single serum sample is diagnostic. Consequently it has been suggested to modify the Duke criteria for the diagnosis of endocarditis and proposed that a single-serum *C. burnetii* phase I IgG antibody titer of 800 or a single positive blood culture for *C. burnetii* be considered major criteria for endocarditis (27). Serum samples from patients with Q fever endocarditis may cross-react with *Bartonella* spp., but cross-reaction is weak and differences in titers allow easy differentiation (46). For patients with a serological diagnosis of *Bartonella* endocarditis, the patient's sera should also be assayed for *C. burnetii* antibodies. Cross-reaction with other antigens is distinctly unusual.

The persistence of high levels of anti-phase I antibodies despite appropriate treatment, or the reappearance of such antibodies, should raise the suspicion of possible chronic Q fever. Patients with valvular or vascular abnormalities, those who are immunocompromised, and pregnant women should have repeated *C. burnetii* serology tests if they have a medical history of acute Q fever or a prolonged and unexplained febrile episode. In uncertain cases, a PCR performed with blood may help to determine if the patient is convalescent (negative) or infected (positive).

The follow-up of patients treated for chronic Q fever also should be done serologically. During therapy, serologic testing should be performed once monthly for 6 months and every 3 months thereafter. The levels of antibodies decrease very slowly, but this decrease correlates with the serum doxycycline level and a 2-dilution decrease for anti-phase I IgG and IgA is associated with cure. When the antibodies are initially present, IgM antibodies disappear first, and then IgA antibodies disappear; but IgG titers remain positive for years (79). Antimicrobial treatment can be stopped after 18 months to 3 years if the anti-phase I IgG titer by IFA is below 400 and IgA anti-phase I is undetectable (72).

REFERENCES

1. **Aboudharam, G., M. Drancourt, and D. Raoult.** 2004. Culture of *C. burnetii* from the dental pulp of experimentally infected guinea pigs. *Microb. Pathog.* **36:**349–350.
2. **Ayres, J. G., N. Flint, E. G. Smith, W. S. Tunnicliffe, T. J. Fletcher, K. Hammond, D. Ward, and B. P. Marmion.** 1998. Post-infection fatigue syndrome following Q fever. *Q. J. Med.* **91:**105–123.
3. **Babudieri, B.** 1959. Q fever: a zoonosis. *Adv. Vet. Sci. Comp. Med.* **5:**82–182.

4. **Baca, O. G., and D. Paretsky.** 1983. Q fever and *Coxiella burnetii:* a model for host-parasite interactions. *Microbiol. Rev.* **47:**127–149.
5. **Bernit, E., J. Pouget, F. Janbon, H. Dutronc, P. Martinez, P. Brouqui, and D. Raoult.** 2002. Neurological involvement in acute Q fever—a report of 29 cases and review of the literature. *Arch. Intern. Med.* **162:**693–700.
6. **Boulos, A., J. M. Rolain, M. Maurin, and D. Raoult.** 2004. Measurement of the antibiotic susceptibility of *Coxiella burnetii* using real time PCR. *Int. J. Antimicrob. Agents* **23:**169–174.
7. **Brennan, R. E., and J. E. Samuel.** 2003. Evaluation of *Coxiella burnetii* antibiotic susceptibilities by real-time PCR assay. *J. Clin. Microbiol.* **41:**1869–1874.
8. **Brouqui, P., S. Badiaga, and D. Raoult.** 2004. Q fever outbreak in homeless shelter. *Emerg. Infect. Dis.* **10:**1297–1299.
9. **Brouqui, P., J. S. Dumler, and D. Raoult.** 1994. Immunohistologic demonstration of *Coxiella burnetii* in the valves of patients with Q fever endocarditis. *Am. J. Med.* **97:**451–458.
10. **Brouqui, P., J. M. Rolain, C. Foucault, and D. Raoult.** 2005. Q fever and *Plasmodium falciparum* malaria co-infection in a patient returning from the Comoros Archipelago. *Am. J. Trop. Med. Hyg.* **73:**1028–1030.
11. **Chevalier, P., F. Vandenesch, P. Brouqui, G. Kirkorian, A. Tabib, J. Etienne, D. Raoult, R. Loire, and P. Touboul.** 1997. Fulminant myocardial failure in a previously healthy young man. *Circulation* **95:**1654–1657.
12. **Christie, A. B.** 1980. Q fever, p. 800. *In* A. B. Christie (ed.), *Infectious Diseases: Epidemiology and Clinical Practice.* Churchill Livingstone, New York, N.Y.
13. **Cottalorda, J., J. L. Jouve, G. Bollini, P. Touzet, A. Poujol, F. Kelberine, and D. Raoult.** 1995. Osteoarticular infection due to *Coxiella burnetii* in children. *J. Pediatr. Orthoped. Part B* **4:**219–221.
14. **Craven, R. B., M. L. Eberhard, T. Folks, B. Kay, R. C. Knudsen, B. W. J. Mathy, C. J. Peters, M. A. Tipple, J. E. Bennett, D. Hackstadt, D. E. Wilson, J. Crane, P. J. Gerone, T. Hamm, D. L. Hunt, P. Jahrling, and T. Kost.** 2005. *Biosafety in Microbiological and Biochemical Laboratories,* p. 149–150. HHS Publication, CDC/NIH. Government Printing Office, Washington, D.C.
15. **Dupuis, G., O. Peter, M. Peacock, W. Burgdorfer, and E. Haller.** 1985. Immunoglobulin responses in acute Q fever. *J. Clin. Microbiol.* **22:**484–487.
16. **Duroux-Vouilloz, C., G. Praz, P. Francioli, and O. Peter.** 1998. Fièvre Q avec endocardite: présentation clinique et suivi sérologique de 21 patients. *Schweiz. Med. Wochenschr.* **128:**521–527.
17. **Ellis, M. E., C. C. Smith, and M. A. Moffat.** 1983. Chronic or fatal Q-fever infection: a review of 16 patients seen in North-East Scotland (1967–80). *Q. J. Med.* **52:**54–66.
18. **Fenollar, F, F. Thuny, B. Xeridat, H. Lepidi, and D. Raoult.** 2006. Endocarditis following acute Q fever in patient with previously undiagnosed valvulopathies. *Clin. Infect. Dis.* **42:**818–821.
19. **Fenollar, F., P. E. Fournier, M. P. Carrieri, G. Habib, T. Messana, and D. Raoult.** 2001. Risk factors and prevention of Q fever endocarditis. *Clin. Infect. Dis.* **33:**312–316.
20. **Fenollar, F., P. E. Fournier, and D. Raoult.** 2004. Molecular detection of *Coxiella burnetti* in the sera of patients with Q fever endocarditis or vascular infection. *J. Clin. Microbiol.* **42:**4919–4924.
21. **Fergusson, R. J., T. R. D. Shaw, A. H. Kitchin, M. B. Matthews, J. M. Inglis, and J. F. Peutherer.** 1985. Subclinical chronic Q fever. *Q. J. Med* **57:**669–676.
22. **Field, P. R., J. G. Hunt, and A. M. Murphy.** 1983. Detection and persistence of specific IgM antibody to *Coxiella burnetii* by enzyme-linked immunosorbent assay: a comparison with immunofluorescence and complement fixation tests. *J. Infect. Dis.* **148:**477–487.
23. **Field, P. R., J. L. Mitchell, A. Santiago, D. J. Dickeson, S. W. Chan, D. W. T. Ho, A. M. Murphy, A. J. Cuzzubbo, and P. L. Devine.** 2000. Comparison of a commercial enzyme-linked immunosorbent assay with immunofluorescence and complement fixation tests for detection of *Coxiella burnetii* (Q fever) immunoglobulin M. *J. Clin. Microbiol.* **38:**1645–1647.
24. **Fiset, P., R. A. Ormsbee, R. Silberman, M. Peacock, and S. H. Spielman.** 1969. A microagglutination technique for detection and measurement of rickettsial antibodies. *Acta Virol.* **13:**60–66.
25. **Fishbein, D. B., and D. Raoult.** 1992. A cluster of *Coxiella burnetii* infections associated with exposure to vaccinated goats and their unpasteurized dairy products. *Am. J. Trop. Med. Hyg.* **47:**35–40.
26. **Foucault, C., H. Lepidi, J. F. Poujet-Abadie, B. Granel, F. Roblot, T. Ariga, and D. Raoult.** 2004. Q fever and lymphadenopathy: report of four new cases and review. *Eur. J. Clin. Microbiol. Infect. Dis.* **23:**759–764.
27. **Fournier, P. E., J. P. Casalta, G. Habib, T. Messana, and D. Raoult.** 1996. Modification of the diagnostic criteria proposed by the Duke Endocarditis Service to permit improved diagnosis of Q fever endocarditis. *Am. J. Med.* **100:**629–633.
28. **Fournier, P. E., J. P. Casalta, P. Piquet, P. Tournigand, A. Branchereau, and D. Raoult.** 1998. *Coxiella burnetii* infection of aneurysms or vascular grafts: report of seven cases and review. *Clin. Infect. Dis.* **26:**116–121.
29. **Fournier, P. E., J. Etienne, J. R. Harle, G. Habib, and D. Raoult.** 2001. Myocarditis, a rare but severe manifestation of Q fever: report of 8 cases and review of the literature. *Clin. Infect. Dis.* **32:**1440–1447.
30. **Fournier, P. E., T. J. Marrie, and D. Raoult.** 1998. Diagnosis of Q fever. *J. Clin. Microbiol.* **36:**1823–1834.
31. **Fournier, P. E., and D. Raoult.** 2003. Comparison of PCR and serology assays for early diagnosis of acute Q fever. *J. Clin. Microbiol.* **41:**5094–5098.
32. **Gimenez, D. F.** 1965. Gram staining of *Coxiella burnetii. J. Bacteriol.* **90:**834–835.
33. **Glazunova, O., V. Roux, O. Freylikman, Z. Sekeyova, G. Fournous, J. Tyczka, N. Tokarevich, E. Kovacava, T. J. Marrie, and D. Raoult.** 2005. *Coxiella burnetii* genotyping. *Emerg. Infect. Dis.* **11:**1211–1217.
34. **Guigno, D., B. Coupland, E. G. Smith, I. D. Farrell, U. Desselberger, and E. O. Caul.** 1992. Primary humoral antibody response to *Coxiella burnetii,* the causative agent of Q fever. *J. Clin. Microbiol.* **30:**1958–1967.
35. **Hatchette, T. F., R. C. Hudson, W. M. Scheld, N. A. Campbell, J. E. Hatchette, S. Ratnam, D. Raoult, C. Donovan, and T. J. Marrie.** 2001. Goat-associated Q fever: a new disease in Newfoundland. *Emerg. Infect. Dis* **7:** 413–419.
36. **Honstettre, A. L., G. V. Imbert, E. Ghigo, F. R. Gouriet, C. Capo, D. Raoult, and J. L. Mege.** 2003. Dysregulation of cytokines in acute Q fever: role of interleukin-10 and tumor necrosis factor in chronic evolution of Q fever. *J. Infect. Dis.* **187:**956–962.
37. **Houpikian, P., G. Habib, T. Mesana, and D. Raoult.** 2002. Changing clinical presentation of Q fever endocarditis. *Clin. Infect. Dis.* **34:**E28–E31.
38. **Houpikian, P., and D. Raoult.** 2005. Blood culture-negative endocarditis in a reference center—etiologic diagnosis of 348 cases. *Medicine* **84:**162–173.
39. **Huebner, R. J., G. A. Hottle, and E. B. Robinson.** 1948. Action of streptomycin in experimental infection with Q fever. *Public Health Rep.* **63:**357–362.
40. **Jabarit-Aldighieri, N., H. Torres, and D. Raoult.** 1992. Susceptibility of *R. conorii, R. rickettsii,* and *C. burnetii* to CI-960 (PD 127,391), PD 131,628, pefloxacin, ofloxacin, and ciprofloxacin. *Antimicrob. Agents Chemother.* **36:**2529–2532.

41. **Kayser, K., M. Wiebel, V. Schulz, and H. J. Gabius.** 1995. Necrotizing bronchitis, angiitis, and amyloidosis associated with chronic Q fever. *Respiration* **62:**114–116.
42. Reference deleted.
43. **Lang, G. H.** 1990. Coxiellosis (Q fever) in animals, p. 23–48. *In* T. J. Marrie (ed.), *Q Fever, the Disease*. CRC press, Boca Raton, Fla.
44. **Langley, J. M., T. J. Marrie, J. C. Leblanc, A. Almudevar, L. Resch, and D. Raoult.** 2003. *Coxiella burnetii* seropositivity in parturient women is associated with adverse pregnancy outcomes. *Am. J. Obstet. Gynecol.* **189:**228–232.
45. **La Scola, B., H. Lepidi, and D. Raoult.** 1997. Pathologic changes during acute Q fever: influence of the route of infection and inoculum size in infected guinea pigs. *Infect. Immun.* **65:**2443–2447.
46. **La Scola, B., T. J. Marrie, H. Lepidi, D. Janigan, A. Stein, and D. Raoult.** 1996. Influence of the route of infection on pathologic changes during acute Q fever in animal models, p. 489–496. *In* J. Kazar and R. Toman (ed.), *Rickettsiae and Rickettsial Diseases*. Veda, Bratislava, Slovakia.
47. **La Scola, B., and D. Raoult.** 2001. Survival of *Coxiella burnetii* within free-living amoebae *Acanthamoeba castellanii*. *Clin. Microbiol. Infect.* **7:**75–79.
48. **Leone, M., A. Honstettre, H. Lepidi, C. Capo, F. Bayard, D. Raoult, and J. L. Mege.** 2004. Effect of sex on Coxiella burnetii infection: protective role of 17 beta-estradiol. *J. Infect. Dis.* **189:**339–345.
49. **Levy, P. Y., R. Corey, P. Berger, G. Habib, J. L. Bonnet, S. Levy, T. Messana, P. Djiane, Y. Frances, C. Botta, P. DeMicco, H. Dumon, O. Mundler, J. J. Chomel, and D. Raoult.** 2003. Etiologic diagnosis of 204 pericardial effusions. *Medicine* **82:**385–391.
50. **Levy, P. Y., and D. Raoult.** 1999. *Coxiella burnetii* pericarditis: a report of 15 cases and review. *Clin. Infect. Dis.* **29:**393–397.
51. **Lohuis, P. J. F. M., P. C. Ligtenberg, R. J. A. Diepersloot, and M. de Graaf.** 1994. Q fever in a patient with a ventriculo-peritoneal drain. Case report and short review of the literature. *Neth. J. Med.* **44:**60–64.
52. **Madariaga, M. G., J. Pulvirenti, M. Sekosan, C. D. Paddock, and S. R. Zaki.** 2004. Q fever endocarditis in HIV-infected patient. *Emerg. Infect. Dis.* **10:**501–504.
53. **Maltezou, H. C., I. Constantopoulou, C. Kallergi, V. Vlahou, D. Georgakopoulos, D. A. Kafetzis, and D. Raoult.** 2004. Q fever in children in Greece. *Am. J. Trop. Med. Hyg.* **70:**540–544.
54. **Maltezou, H. C., and D. Raoult.** 2002. Q fever in children. *Lancet Infect. Dis.* **2:**686–691.
55. **Marrero, M., and D. Raoult.** 1989. Centrifugation-shell vial technique for rapid detection of Mediterranean spotted fever rickettsia in blood culture. *Am. J. Trop. Med. Hyg.* **40:**197–199.
56. Reference deleted.
57. **Maurin, M., A. Benoliel, P. Bongrand, and D. Raoult.** 1992. Phagolysosomal alkalinization and the bactericidal effect of antibiotics: the *Coxiella burnetii* paradigm. *J. Infect. Dis.* **166:**1097–1102.
58. **Maurin, M., and D. Raoult.** 1999. Q fever. *Clin. Microbiol. Rev.* **12:**518–553.
59. **McCaul, T. F., and J. C. Williams.** 1981. Developmental cycle of *Coxiella burnetii*: structure and morphogenesis of vegetative and sporogenic differentiations. *J. Bacteriol.* **147:**1063–1076.
60. **Mejia, A., B. Toursarkissian, R. T. Hagino, J. G. Myers, and M. T. Sykes.** 2000. Primary aortoduodenal fistula and Q fever: an underrecognized association? *Ann. Vasc. Surg.* **14:**271–273.
61. **Milazzo, A., R. Hall, P. A. Storm, R. J. Harris, W. Winslow, and B. P. Marmion.** 2001. Sexually transmitted Q fever. *Clin. Infect . Dis.* **33:**399–402.
62. **Murphy, A. M., and P. R. Field.** 1970. The persistence of complement-fixing antibodies to Q-fever *(Coxiella burnetii)* after infection. *Med. J. Australia* **1:**1148–1150.
63. **Ormsbee, R. A.** 1952. The growth of *Coxiella burnetii* in embryonated eggs. *J. Bacteriol.* **63:**73.
64. **Ormsbee, R. A.** 1965. Q fever rickettsia, p. 1144–1160. *In* F. L. Horsfall and I. Tamm (ed.), *Viral and Rickettsial Infections of Man*. J. P. Lippincott, Philadelphia, Pa.
65. **Parola, P., G. Soula, P. Gazin, C. Foucault, J. Delmont, and P. Brouqui.** 2006. Fever in travelers returning from tropical areas: prospective observational study of 613 cases hospitalised in Marseilles, France 1999–2003. *Travel Med. Infect. Dis.* **4:**61–70.
66. **Penttila, I. A., R. J. Harris, P. Storm, D. Haynes, D. A. Worswick, and B. P. Marmion.** 1998. Cytokine dysregulation in the post-Q-fever fatigue syndrome. *Q. J. Med.* **91:**549–560.
67. **Philip, R. N., E. A. Casper, R. A. Ormsbee, M. G. Peacock, and W. Burgdorfer.** 1976. Microimmunofluorescence test for the serological study of Rocky Mountain spotted fever and typhus. *J. Clin. Microbiol.* **3:**51–61.
68. **Raoult, D., P. Brouqui, B. Marchou, and J. A. Gastaut.** 1992. Acute and chronic Q fever in patients with cancer. *Clin. Infect. Dis.* **14:**127–130.
69. **Raoult, D., M. Drancourt, and G. Vestris.** 1990. Bactericidal effect of doxycycline associated with lysosomotropic agents on *Coxiella burnetii* in P388D1 cells. *Antimicrob. Agents Chemother.* **34:**1512–1514.
70. **Raoult, D., J. Etienne, P. Massip, S. Iaocono, M. A. Prince, P. Beaurain, S. Benichou, J. C. Auvergnat, P. Mathieu, and P. Bachet.** 1987. Q fever endocarditis in the south of France. *J. Infect. Dis.* **155:**570–573.
71. **Raoult, D., F. Fenollar, and A. Stein.** 2002. Q fever during pregnancy—diagnosis, treatment, and follow-up. *Arch. Intern. Med.* **162:**701–704.
72. **Raoult, D., P. Houpikian, H. Tissot-Dupont, J. M. Riss, J. Arditi-Djiane, and P. Brouqui.** 1999. Treatment of Q fever endocarditis: comparison of two regimens containing doxycycline and ofloxacin or hydroxychloroquine. *Arch. Intern. Med.* **159:**167–173.
73. **Raoult, D., J. C. Laurent, and M. Mutillod.** 1994. Monoclonal antibodies to *Coxiella burnetii* for antigenic detection in cell cultures and in paraffin-embedded tissues. *Am. J. Clin. Pathol.* **101:**318–320.
74. **Raoult, D., P. Y. Levy, H. T. Dupont, C. Chicheportiche, C. Tamalet, J. A. Gastaut, and J. Salducci.** 1993. Q fever and HIV infection. *AIDS* **7:**81–86.
75. **Raoult, D., T. J. Marrie, and J. L. Mege.** 2005. Natural history and pathophysiology of Q fever. *Lancet Infect. Dis.* **5:**219–226.
76. **Raoult, D., J. L. Mege, and T. J. Marrie.** 2001. Q fever: queries remaining after decades of research, p. 29–56. *In* M. Scheld, W. A. Craig, and J. M. Hughes (ed.), *Emerging Infections 5*. ASM Press, Washington, D.C.
77. **Raoult, D., H. Tissot-Dupont, C. Foucault, J. Gouvernet, P. E. Fournier, E. Bernit, A. Stein, M. Nesri, J. R. Harle, and P. J. Weiller.** 2000. Q fever 1985–1998—clinical and epidemiologic features of 1,383 infections. *Medicine* **79:**109–123.
78. **Raoult, D., H. Torres, and M. Drancourt.** 1991. Shell-vial assay: evaluation of a new technique for determining antibiotic susceptibility, tested in 13 isolates of *Coxiella burnetii*. *Antimicrob. Agents Chemother.* **35:**2070–2077.
79. **Rolain, J. M., A. Boulos, M. N. Mallet, and D. Raoult.** 2005. Correlation between ratio of serum doxycycline concentration to MIC and rapid decline of antibody levels during treatment of Q fever endocarditis. *Antimicrob. Agents Chemother.* **49:**2673–2676.
80. **Rolain, J. M., C. Lecam, and D. Raoult.** 2003. Simplified serological diagnosis of endocarditis due to *Coxiella burnetii* and *Bartonella*. *Clin. Diagn. Lab. Immunol.* **10:**1147–1148.
81. **Rolain, J. M., H. Lepidi, J. R. Harle, T. Allegre, E. D. Dorval, Z. Khayat, and D. Raoult.** 2003. Acute acalculous cholecystitis associated with Q fever: report of seven cases

and review of the literature. *Eur. J. Clin. Microbiol. Infect. Dis.* **22:**222–227.

82. **Rolain, J. M., M. Maurin, and D. Raoult.** 2001. Bacteriostatic and bactericidal activities of moxifloxacin against *Coxiella burnetii. Antimicrob. Agents Chemother.* **45:**301–302.
83. **Rolain, J. M., M. Maurin, A. Bryskier, and D. Raoult.** 2000. In vitro activities of telithromycin (HMR 3647) against *Rickettsia rickettsii, Rickettsia conorii, Rickettsia africae, Rickettsia typhi, Rickettsia prowazekii, Coxiella burnetii, Bartonella henselae, Bartonella quintana, Bartonella bacilliformis,* and *Ehrlichia chaffeensis. Antimicrob. Agents Chemother.* **44:**1391–1393.
84. **Rolain, J. M., and D. Raoult.** 2005. Molecular detection of *Coxiella burnetii* in blood and sera during Q fever. *Q. J. Med.* **98:**615–617.
85. **Sidwell, R. W., B. D. Thorpe, and L. P. Gebhardt.** 1964. Studies of latent Q fever infections. I. Effects of whole body X irradiation upon latently infected guinea pigs, white mice and deer mice. *Am. J. Hyg.* **79:**113–124.
86. **Sidwell, R. W., B. D. Thorpe, and L. P. Gebhardt.** 1964. Studies of latent Q fever infections. II. Effects of multiple cortisone injections. *Am. J. Hyg.* **79:**320–327.
87. Reference deleted.
88. **Stein, A., C. Louveau, H. Lepidi, F. Ricci, P. Baylac, B. Davoust, and D. Raoult.** 2005. Q fever pneumonia: virulence of *Coxiella burnetii* pathovars in a murine model of aerosol infection. *Infect. Immun.* **73:**2469–2477.
89. **Stein, A., and D. Raoult.** 1992. A simple method for amplification of DNA from paraffin-embedded tissues. *Nucleic Acids Res.* **20:**5237–5238.
90. **Stein, A., and D. Raoult.** 1998. Q fever during pregnancy: a public health problem in southern France. *Clin. Infect. Dis.* **27:**592–596.
91. **Stoker, M. G. P., and P. Fiset.** 1956. Phase variation of the Nine Mile and other strains of *Rickettsia burnetii. Can. J. Microbiol.* **2:**310–321.
92. **Thiele, D., M. Karo, and H. Krauss.** 1992. Monoclonal antibody based capture ELISA/ELIFA for detection of *Coxiella burnetii* in clinical specimens. *Eur. J. Epidemiol.* **8:**568–574.
93. **Tissot-Dupont, H., M. A. Amadei, M. Nezri, and D. Raoult.** 2004. Wind in November, Q fever in December. *Emerg. Infect. Dis.* **10:**1264–1269.
94. **Tissot-Dupont, H., X. Thirion, and D. Raoult.** 1994. Q fever serology: cutoff determination for microimmunofluorescence. *Clin. Diagn. Lab. Immunol.* **1:**189–196.
95. **Tissot-Dupont, H., S. Torres, M. Nezri, and D. Raoult.** 1999. Hyperendemic focus of Q fever related to sheep and wind. *Am. J. Epidemiol.* **150:**67–74.
96. **Vodkin, M. H., and J. C. Williams.** 1986. Overlapping deletion in two spontaneous phase variants of *Coxiella burnetii. J. Gen. Microbiol.* **132:**2587–2594.
97. **Waag, D., J. Chulay, T. Marrie, M. England, and J. Williams.** 1995. Validation of an enzyme immunoassay for serodiagnosis of acute Q fever. *Eur. J. Clin. Microbiol. Infect. Dis.* **14:**421–427.

Tropheryma

DIDIER RAOULT, FLORENCE FENOLLAR, AND DAVID RELMAN

69

Tropheryma whipplei is the bacterial agent of Whipple's disease and was described for the first time in 1907 by an American pathologist, George Hoyt Whipple (44). The clinical manifestations of this disease are diverse, protean, and nonspecific (19, 33). Due to the varied manifestations of the disease, the differential diagnosis is large, sometimes leading to a delayed diagnosis. Without treatment, the natural evolution of the disease is always fatal. The recent isolation of *T. whipplei* has opened new perspectives for the management of the disease (36).

TAXONOMY

In 1991, Wilson et al. sequenced a fragment of 16S rRNA gene from tissue of a patient with Whipple's disease (45). This partial sequence suggested a bacterium related to the *Actinomyces* clade. In 1992, Relman et al. described a nearly complete bacterial 16S rRNA gene sequence that was detected in five patients with Whipple's disease but not in a group of controls (39). The inferred phylogeny of the presumed causative agent suggested that the organism is an actinomycete and a member of the phylum *Actinobacteria*. The bacterium was originally named "*Tropheryma whippelii,*" but this was subsequently revised to *Tropheryma whipplei*, following its cultivation and phenotypic characterization, in order to accommodate the nomenclature rules of the International Society of Systematic Bacteriology (25).

DESCRIPTION OF THE GENOME

The entire genomes of two different strains of *T. whipplei* have been sequenced (2, 38). Sequencing of *T. whipplei* Twist revealed a 927,303-bp genome which carries 808 predicted protein-coding genes and with a GC content of 47% (38). Sequencing of *T. whipplei* TW08/27 revealed a 925,938-bp genome which carries 784 predicted protein-coding genes and with a GC content of 46.3% (2). *T. whipplei* possesses a unique circular chromosome and is the only known reduced-genome species (<1 Mb) within the *Actinobacteria* (2, 38). The genomic sequences of the two strains are nearly (>99%) identical at the nucleotide sequence level, encoding quasi-identical gene complements. This specific genome includes apparent deficiencies in energy metabolism and amino acids synthesis, suggesting a requirement of external nutrients. Alignment of the two genome sequences reveals a large chromosomal inversion, the extremities of which are located within two paralogous genes (2). These genes belong to a large family of predicted cell surface proteins defined by the presence of a common repeat highly conserved at the nucleotide level. The repeats appear to trigger genome fragment rearrangements in *T. whipplei*, potentially resulting in the expression of different subsets of cell surface proteins (2). This phenomenon might represent a new mechanism for evasion of the host's immune response during the course of this chronic disease.

NATURAL HABITAT

The source of *T. whipplei* and its transmission are presently unknown. The bacterium seems to be present in the environment. Studies based on PCR have shown the presence of *T. whipplei* DNA in effluent from sewage plants (30) and in human stools and saliva (10, 11, 23), and it has been speculated that *T. whipplei* is acquired via the oral route (19). Different studies have been performed to establish the presence of *T. whipplei* DNA in people without Whipple's disease in saliva, duodenal biopsy specimens, gastric liquids, and stools (11, 12, 41). However, the data should be analyzed with caution because they are based on "home-brew PCR" and have not been independently confirmed (10, 15, 31). It has been suggested that *T. whipplei* may have a specific geographic and racial distribution, with a predominance in Caucasians and in Central Europe (10).

CLINICAL FEATURES OF WHIPPLE'S DISEASE

The most common clinical presentation of Whipple's disease is an association of diarrhea, arthralgias, and lymphadenopathy, but all organs may be affected (17, 33). Many cases are associated with long-standing, relapsing and remitting arthralgias. As many as 15% of patients lack gastrointestinal symptoms throughout their illness (42), and small-bowel biopsies may be normal (34). It is therefore not surprising that in many of these atypical cases the diagnosis may not be made for some time and may be entirely missed until it is demonstrated at necropsy. The main clinical manifestations of Whipple's disease are summarized in Table 1.

TABLE 1 Clinical manifestations of Whipple's disease

Manifestations
Classic manifestations
Diarrhea
Arthralgias
Weight loss
Abdominal pain
Lymphadenopathy
Cutaneous pigmentation
Fever of unknown origin
CNS involvements
Cognitive impairment
Ophthalmoplegia
Myoclonic signs
Hypothalamic involvement
Cerebellar involvement
Abnormal ocular movements
Ophthalmologic manifestations
Uveitis
Cardiovascular manifestations
Blood culture-negative endocarditis
Pericarditis
Myocarditis

COLLECTION, TRANSPORT, AND STORAGE OF SPECIMENS

When Whipple's disease is suspected, saliva and stools for PCR and blood for PCR and immunohistochemistry are easy to sample and test. Saliva and stools are not considered useful samples by some authors (11, 12, 41). However, we have never obtained a positive PCR assay from these samples from people without a final diagnosis of Whipple's disease, except in one case (our unpublished data) (15). Small-bowel endoscopic biopsies should also be sampled systematically in suspected cases of Whipple's disease, even in the absence of intestinal symptoms. Several biopsies must be sampled from the duodenum and jejunum because the lesions can be focal and sparse (19). In cases of suspected Whipple's endocarditis, the excised cardiac valve should be tested by periodic acid-Schiff (PAS) staining, PCR, and immunohistochemistry. In cases of suspected neurologic Whipple's disease, cerebrospinal fluid (CSF) should be sampled as well as saliva, stools, blood, and small-bowel mucosa. If these investigations are not diagnostic, another disease site should be sampled based on associated signs and symptoms (lymph node, synovial biopsy, liver, cardiac valve, or vitreous fluid). If all these examinations are negative and accessible lesions are observed on brain magnetic resonance imaging, a stereotaxic biopsy should be performed for PCR and immunohistochemistry. Finally, if a diagnosis of Whipple's disease is established, even in the absence of neurologic signs, CSF should be systematically sampled and tested by PCR due to the common, subclinical involvement of the central nervous system (CNS) in this disease (6, 43). For PCR and culture, fresh samples should be frozen at −80°C and transported in dry ice. For PAS staining and immunohistochemistry, all the samples should be fixed in 10% formalin and transported at room temperature.

DIRECT EXAMINATION

Electronic Microscopy

Electron microscopy has been reported to demonstrate typical bacteria in macrophages from all kinds of tissues (Table 2) (19). Electron microscopy is not a practical tool for the diagnosis of the disease.

PAS Staining

The histological study of small-bowel biopsy specimens by use of PAS staining was the first tool for the diagnosis of Whipple's disease and is still considered an important and sometimes definitive diagnostic criterion (Table 2). The criterion is based on the observation of (i) diastase-resistant, magenta-stained inclusions within macrophages of the lamina propria and (ii) lymphatic dilatation. This PAS staining pattern, which has long been considered pathognomonic of Whipple's disease, is found in other diseases (19, 33). The presence of noncaseous granulomas composed of epithelioid cells may be observed in lymphatic tissues, the gastrointestinal tract, liver, or lung in Whipple's disease. These granulomas are often PAS negative (10, 19, 33). Depending on clinical manifestations, other tissues may be appropriate for PAS staining to establish the diagnosis of Whipple's disease, such as lymph node, synovium, cardiac valve, brain, or CSF (10, 19, 33).

Immunohistochemistry

The culture of *T. whipplei* has made possible the generation of polyclonal antibodies directed against the bacterium (27, 29) and an immunohistochemical diagnosis of Whipple's

TABLE 2 Diagnostic tools for the diagnosis of Whipple's disease

Technique	Sample(s)	Advantage	Disadvantage
Electron microscopy	Small-bowel tissue; all other kinds of tissues; body fluids	None	Not available in all laboratories; laborious
PAS staining	Small-bowel tissue; all other kinds of tissues; body fluids	Available in all laboratories; can be used on archival samples	Low specificity
Nucleic acid amplification	Blood; saliva; stools; small-bowel tissue; all other kinds of tissues; body fluids	Available in some laboratories	Specificity variable depending on sample type and laboratory
Immunodetection	Blood; small-bowel tissue; all other kinds of tissues; body fluids	Good specificity; can be used on archival samples	Noncommercialized antibodies
Culture	Blood; small-bowel tissue; all other kinds of tissues; body fluids	New strain isolation	Specific technology; long time required for the primary isolation
Serology	Serum	Simple procedure	Presently experimental

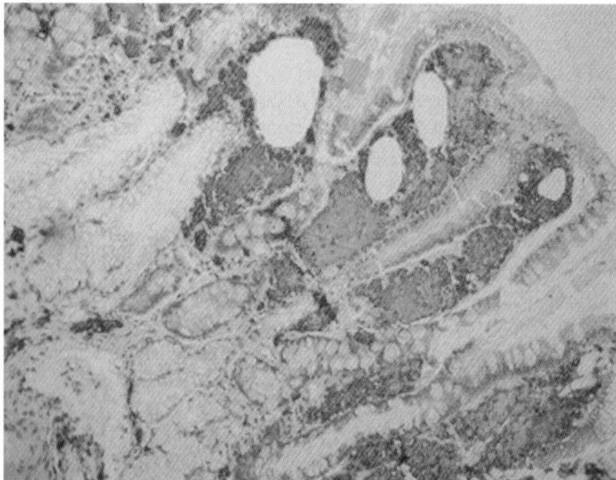

FIGURE 1 Immunohistochemistry performed on duodenal biopsies using rabbit polyclonal antibodies specifically directed against *Tropheryma whipplei*. Original magnification, ×100. Courtesy of Hubert Lepidi.

disease (26–28, 37). This technique has been performed on various kinds of tissues (duodenum, lymph node, brain, and cardiac valve), on body fluids such as aqueous humor, and on blood monocytes (1, 8, 9, 26, 27, 36, 37). This technique provides direct visualization of the bacilli in macrophages (Fig. 1) and offers increased sensitivity and specificity over the traditional PAS staining method (Table 2). It can also be used retrospectively on fixed samples (9).

Molecular Detection

PCR assays can be performed with a variety of tissue types (e.g., intestinal mucosa, lymph nodes, cardiac valves, and brain) and body fluids (CSF, blood, and saliva [Table 2]) (18). DNA extraction is a key step: different protocols have been proposed, involving phenol-chloroform-ethanol purification, chaotropic lysis, Chelex suspension, or a QIAamp DNA binding column (18). Some authors have also used digestion buffer before DNA extraction (18). These protocols can be applied to paraffin-embedded samples, as well as fresh samples. PCR amplification of the 16S rRNA gene was the first molecular tool for the diagnosis of Whipple's disease (39). As with all PCR assays, it is critical to include positive and negative controls (including water and DNA extracted from controls tissues). For each assay, the positive and negative controls must be, respectively, positive and negative to validate the results. Recently, a PCR assay targeting the 16S-23S intergenic region by using a real-time PCR apparatus has been successful for the diagnosis of Whipple's disease (15). This technique offers the advantages of reduced time for PCR analysis and lowered risk of contamination. The availability of the genome has also offered the possibility of selecting DNA targets in a more rational and informed manner. A real-time PCR assay targeting repeated sequences of *T. whipplei* significantly enhanced PCR assay sensitivity without altering its specificity, when compared to regular PCR (16). When amplified product is detected, the identification of the *T. whipplei* sequence should be confirmed by sequencing or hybridization. A problem with nonstandardized PCR assays is DNA contamination. In addition to general recommendations for avoiding contamination, we believe that when positive results from PAS staining or immunohistochemistry are not obtained in parallel with a positive PCR result (especially from blood, CSF, saliva, and stools), it is imperative to obtain confirmation of the diagnosis by using a different sample type tested with a different procedure (e.g., using a different DNA target to reduce the likelihood of false-positive PCR results).

Isolation Procedure

The cultivation of *T. whipplei* from various samples can be achieved with cell culture techniques and human fibroblasts (Table 2) (8, 14, 25, 32, 36, 37). Based on this technique, isolates have been obtained from cardiac valve, duodenal biopsy tissue, blood, aqueous humor, CSF, adenopathy, and synovial fluid (14, 32). Among them, 17 isolates (1 from a duodenal biopsy, 2 from cardiac valves, 7 from CSF, 4 from a blood sample, 2 from lymph node, and 1 from synovial fluid) have been established in serial cultures (2, 14, 32) (our unpublished data). In our experience, the delay before primary detection of *T. whipplei* from clinical samples is approximately 30 days (14), but it may be shorter (32). The cultivation of *T. whipplei* from contaminated specimen types such as intestinal biopsy specimens requires the use of drugs such as colistin, amphotericin B, cephalothin, or ciprofloxacin. *T. whipplei* genome analysis indicates deficiencies in amino acid biosynthetic pathways. As a consequence, the missing amino acids must be obtained from the environment. This information has allowed the design of a medium supplemented with amino acids, in which *T. whipplei* grows axenically (40). By use of this technique, two strains of *T. whipplei* from CSF, two strains from blood, one strain from synovial fluid, one strain from adenopathy, and one strain from cardiac valve have been isolated and established in parallel to cell culture (our unpublished data).

Identification

Every 15 days for 180 days of culture, the culture medium is changed, and before the medium is replaced 100 μl of the supernatant is obtained for centrifugation and stained by immunofluorescence using anti-*T. whipplei* polyclonal rabbit antibodies to detect bacterial growth. In parallel, a PCR assay is performed to confirm the growth and the identification. Confirmation of isolates as *T. whipplei* must be systematically obtained by specific PCR assay and amplicon sequencing or hybridization.

SEROLOGIC TESTING

The culture of *T. whipplei* has led to the development of serologic tests for this disease. However, serologic testing for Whipple's disease is not currently available (Table 2) (33, 35, 36).

ANTIMICROBIAL SUSCEPTIBILITIES

A study of the susceptibilities of three strains of *T. whipplei* to antibiotics in cell culture has indicated that doxycycline, macrolides, ketolides, aminoglycosides, penicillin, rifampin, teicoplanin, chloramphenicol, and trimethoprim-sulfamethoxazole are active against this organism, with MICs ranging from 0.25 to 2 μg/ml (4). Vancomycin was somewhat active with a MIC of 10 μg/ml. Cephalosporins (including ceftriaxone), colimycin, aztreonam, and fluoroquinolones are not active. Variability in the susceptibility of imipenem is also observed. A combination of doxycycline and hydroxychloroquine has been shown to be bactericidal in vitro because *T. whipplei* resides in acidic vacuoles of host cells (4, 22). The antibiotic susceptibilities of these three

TABLE 3 Strategy for interpretation of results depending on sample type and diagnostic technique[a]

Sample(s)	PAS	IHC	PCR	Confirmed diagnosis
Small bowel	+	− or NA	− or NA	No
Lymph nodes,	+	NA	+	Yes
cardiac valve, brain,	− or NA	+	+	Yes
other biopsy	− or NA	− or NA	+	Yes (?)
specimens	− or NA	+	− or NA	Yes (?)
CSF, blood	+	− or NA	− or NA	No
	+	− or NA	+	Yes
	− or NA	+	+	Yes
	− or NA	− or NA	+	?[b]
Saliva, stools	NA	NA	+	Predictive value depending on the laboratory

[a]Abbreviations and symbols: IHC, immunohistochemistry; NA, not available; −, negative; +, positive.
[b]Needs to be confirmed on a second sample, using a second DNA target if possible.

strains grown in axenic medium have also been studied (3). The active compounds on axenic medium are sulfamethoxazole, doxycycline, macrolides, penicillin G, streptomycin, rifampin, chloramphenicol, thiamphenicol, teicoplanin, vancomycin, amoxicillin, gentamicin, aztreonam, levofloxacin, and ceftriaxone, with MICs ranging from 0.06 to 1 μg/ml. Trimethoprim is not effective in vitro as predicted from genomic analysis (5).

INTERPRETATION OF RESULTS

A strategy for interpretation of diagnostic test results based on sample type and technique is summarized in Table 3. When a patient presents with "typical" features of Whipple's disease, including diarrhea, malabsorption, lymphadenopathy, and/or arthralgias, the diagnosis should be suspected. For cases of Whipple's disease without intestinal symptoms, such as Whipple's disease endocarditis and isolated neurologic disease, the diagnosis is more difficult. One of the main problems is the interpretation of an isolated positive PCR. These results must always be confirmed with a second specimen, such as blood or CSF, ideally using a different procedure and/or different DNA target. In these cases, the presence of a positive PCR from saliva or stool may be useful in confirming the diagnosis of Whipple's disease.

TREATMENT

Presently, the recommended treatment is an oral regimen of trimethoprim and sulfamethoxazole administered from 1 to 2 years. Many recommend that this regimen be preceded with treatment for 14 days consisting of intramuscular streptomycin and intravenous benzyl penicillin (penicillin G) (7, 13, 20, 21, 24). Based on recent data from in vitro assays, a therapeutic regimen that includes a combination of doxycycline and hydroxychloroquine to eradicate intracellular organisms is now suggested. Moreover, high doses of sulfamethoxazole in association with doxycycline and hydroxychloroquine may improve the treatment of CNS disease and reduce the likelihood of relapse. Clinical trials are now needed to confirm this strategy.

REFERENCES

1. **Baisden, B. L., H. Lepidi, D. Raoult, P. Argani, J. H. Yardley, and J. S. Dumler.** 2002. Diagnosis of Whipple disease by immunohistochemical analysis. A sensitive and specific method for the detection of *Tropheryma whipplei* (the Whipple Bacillus) in paraffin-embedded tissue. *Am. J. Clin. Pathol.* **118:**742–748.
2. **Bentley, S. D., M. Maiwald, L. D. Murphy, M. J. Pallen, C. A. Yeats, L. G. Dover, H. T. Nobertczak, G. S. Besra, M. A. Quail, D. E. Harris, A. von Herbay, A. Goble, S. Rutter, R. Squares, S. Squares, B. G. Barrell, J. Parkhill, and D. A. Relman.** 2003. Sequencing and analysis of the genome of the Whipple's disease bacterium *Tropheryma whipplei*. *Lancet* **361:**637–644.
3. **Boulos, A., J. M. Rolain, M. N. Mallet, and D. Raoult.** 2005. Molecular evaluation of antibiotic susceptibility against *Tropheryma whipplei* in axenic medium. *J. Antimicrob. Chem.* **2:**178–181.
4. **Boulos, A., J. M. Rolain, and D. Raoult.** 2004. Antibiotic susceptibility of *Tropheryma whipplei* in MRC5 cells. *Antimicrob. Agents Chemother.* **48:**747–752.
5. **Cannon, W. R.** 2003. Whipple's disease, genomics and drug therapy. *Lancet* **361:**1916.
6. **Dearment, M. C., T. A. Woodward, D. M. Menke, P. W. Brazis, L. W. Bancroft, and S. T. Persellin.** 2003. Whipple's disease with destructive arthritis, abdominal lymphadenopathy, and central nervous system involvement. *J. Rheumatol.* **30:**1347–1350.
7. **Dobbins, W. O., III.** 1987. *Whipple's Disease.* Chorles C Thomas, Springfield, Ill.
8. **Drancourt, M., B. Bodaghi, P. Le Hoang, H. Lepidi, F. Fenollar, M. Birg, J. Lelièvre, and D. Raoult.** 2003. Culture of *Tropheryma whipplei* from the vitreous fluid of a patient presenting with unilateral uveitis. *Ann. Intern. Med.* **139:**1046–1047.
9. **Dumler, J. S., B. L. Baisden, J. H. Yardley, and D. Raoult.** 2003. Immunodetection of *Tropheryma whipplei* in intestinal tissues of Dr. Whipple's 1907 patient. *N. Engl. J. Med.* **348:**1411–1412.
10. **Dutly, F., and M. Altwegg.** 2001. Whipple's disease and "*Tropheryma whippelii.*" *Clin. Microbiol. Rev.* **14:**561–583.
11. **Dutly, F., H. P. Hinrikson, T. Seidel, S. Morgenegg, M. Altwegg, and P. Bauerfeind.** 2000. *Tropheryma whippelii*

DNA in saliva of patients without Whipple's disease. *Infection* **28:**219–222.

12. **Ehrbar, H., P. Bauerfeind, F. Dutly, H. Koelz, and M. Altwegg.** 1999. PCR-positive tests for *Tropheryma whippelii* in patients without Whipple's disease. *Lancet* **353:**2214.
13. **Fantry, G., and S. James.** 1995. Whipple's disease. *Dig. Dis.* **13:**108–118.
14. **Fenollar, F., M. Birg, V. Gauduchon, and D. Raoult.** 2003. Culture of *Tropheryma whipplei* from human samples: a 3-year experience (1999 to 2002). *J. Clin. Microbiol.* **41:**3816–3822.
15. **Fenollar, F., P. Fournier, R. Gerolami, H. Lepidi, C. Poyart, and D. Raoult.** 2002. Quantitative detection of *Tropheryma whipplei* DNA by real-time PCR. *J. Clin. Microbiol.* **40:**1119–1120.
16. **Fenollar, F., P. Fournier, C. Robert, and D. Raoult.** 2004. Genome selected repeated sequences increase the sensitivity of PCR detection of *Tropheryma whipplei*. *J. Clin. Microbiol.* **42:**401–403.
17. **Fenollar, F., H. Lepidi, and D. Raoult.** 2001. Whipple's endocarditis: review of the literature and comparisons with Q fever, *Bartonella* infection, and blood culture-positive endocarditis. *Clin. Infect. Dis.* **33:**1309–1316.
18. **Fenollar, F., and D. Raoult.** 2001. Molecular techniques in Whipple's disease. *Expert Rev. Mol. Diagn.* **1:**299–309.
19. **Fenollar, F., and D. Raoult.** 2001. Whipple's disease. *Clin. Diagn. Lab. Immunol.* **8:**1–8.
20. **Feurle, G., and T. Marth.** 1994. An evaluation of antimicrobial treatment for Whipple's disease. Tetracyline versus trimethoprim-sulfamethoxazole. *Dig. Dis. Sci.* **39:** 1642–1648.
21. **Fleming, J., R. Wiesner, and R. Shorter.** 1988. Whipple's disease: clinical, biochemical, and histopathologic features and assessment of treatment in 19 patients. *Mayo Clin. Proc.* **63:**539–551.
22. **Ghigo, E., C. Capo, M. Aurouze, J. Gorvel, D. Raoult, and J. Mege.** 2002. The survival of *Tropheryma whipplei*, the agent of Whipple's disease, requires phagosome acidification. *Infect. Immun.* **70:**1501–1506.
23. **Gross, M., C. Jung, and W. Zoller.** 1999. Detection of *Tropheryma whippelii* (Whipple's disease) in faeces. *Ital. J. Gastroenterol.* **31:**70–72.
24. **Keinath, R., D. Merrell, R. Vlietstra, and W. I. Dobbins.** 1985. Antibiotic treatment and relapse in Whipple's disease. *Gastroenterology* **88:**1867–1873.
25. **La Scola, B., F. Fenollar, P. Fournier, M. Altwegg, M. Mallet, and D. Raoult.** 2001. Description of *Tropheryma whipplei* gen. nov., sp. nov., the Whipple's disease bacillus. *Int. J. Syst. Evol. Microbiol* **51:**1471–1479.
26. **Lepidi, H., N. Costedoat, J. Piette, J. Harlé, and D. Raoult.** 2002. Immunohistological detection of *Tropheryma whipplei* (Whipple bacillus) in lymph nodes. *Am. J. Med.* **113:**334–336.
27. **Lepidi, H., F. Fenollar, R. Gerolami, J. Mege, M. Bonzi, M. Chappuis, J. Sahel, and D. Raoult.** 2003. Whipple's disease: immunospecific and quantitative immunohistochemical study of intestinal biopsies. *Human Pathol.* **34:** 589–596.
28. **Lepidi, H., F. Fenollar, J. S. Dumler, V. Gauduchon, L. Chalabreysse, A. Bammert, M. F. Bonzi, F. Thivolet-Bejui, F. Vandenesch, and D. Raoult.** 2004. Cardiac valves in patients with Whipple endocarditis: microbiological, molecular, quantitative histologic, and immunohistochemical studies of 5 patients. *J. Infect. Dis.* **190:**935–945.
29. **Liang, Z., B. La Scola, and D. Raoult.** 2002. Monoclonal antibodies to immunodominant epitope of *Tropheryma whipplei*. *Clin. Diagn. Lab. Immunol.* **9:**156–159.
30. **Maiwald, M., F. Schuhmacher, H. Ditton, and A. von Herbay.** 1998. Environmental occurrence of the Whipple's disease bacterium *(Tropheryma whippelii)*. *Appl. Environ. Microbiol.* **64:**760–762.
31. **Maiwald, M., A. von Herbay, D. Persing, P. Mitchell, M. Abdelmalek, J. Thorvilson, D. Fredricks, and D. Relman.** 2001. *Tropheryma whippelii* DNA is rare in the intestinal mucosa of patients without other evidence of Whipple disease. *Ann. Intern. Med.* **134:**115–119.
32. **Maiwald, M., A. von Herbay, D. N. Fredricks, C. C. Ouverney, J. C. Kosek, and D. A. Relman.** 2003. Cultivation of *Tropheryma whipplei* from cerebrospinal fluid. *J. Infect. Dis.* **188:**801–808.
33. **Marth, T., and D. Raoult.** 2003. Whipple's disease. *Lancet* **361:**239–246.
34. **Misbah, S. A., A. Aslam, and C. Costello.** 2004. Whipple's disease. *Lancet* **363:**654–656.
35. **Morgenegg, S., F. Dutly, and M. Altwegg.** 2000. Cloning and sequencing of a part of the heat shock protein 65 (hsp65) gene of "*Tropheryma whippelii*" and its use for the detection of "*T. whippelii*" in clinical specimens by PCR. *J. Clin. Microbiol.* **38:**2248–2253.
36. **Raoult, D., M. Birg, B. La Scola, P. Fournier, M. Enea, H. Lepidi, V. Roux, J. Piette, F. Vandenesch, D. Vital-Durand, and T. Marrie.** 2000. Cultivation of the bacillus of Whipple's disease. *N. Engl. J.* Med. **342:**620–625.
37. **Raoult, D., B. La Scola, P. Lecocq, H. Lepidi, and P. Fournier.** 2001. Culture and immunological detection of *Tropheryma whippelii* from the duodenum of a patient with Whipple disease. *JAMA* **285:**1039–1043.
38. **Raoult, D., H. Ogata, S. Audic, C. Robert, K. Suhre, M. Drancourt, and J. Claverie.** 2003. *Tropheryma whipplei* Twist: a human pathogenic Actinobacteria with a reduced genome. *Genome Res.* **13:**1800–1809.
39. **Relman, D. A., T. M. Schmidt, R. P. MacDermott, and S. Falkow.** 1992. Identification of the uncultured bacillus of Whipple's disease. *N. Engl. J. Med.* **327:**293–301.
40. **Renesto, P., N. Crapoulet, H. Ogata, B. La Scola, G. Vestris, J. Claverie, and D. Raoult.** 2003. Genome-based design of a cell-free culture medium for *Tropheryma whipplei*. *Lancet* **362:**447–449.
41. **Street, S., H. Donoghue, and G. Neild.** 1999. *Tropheryma whippelii* DNA in saliva of healthy people. *Lancet* **354:**1178–1179.
42. **Vital-Durand, D., C. Lecomte, P. Cathebras, H. Rousset, and P. Godeau.** 1997. Whipple's disease—clinical review of 52 cases. The SNFMI Research Group on Whipple Disease. Societe Nationale Francaise de Medecine Interne. *Medicine* **76:**170–184.
43. **von Herbay, A., H. Ditton, F. Schuhmacher, and M. Maiwald.** 1997. Whipple's disease: staging and monitoring by cytology and polymerase chain reaction analysis of cerebral fluid. *Gastroenterology* **113:**434–441.
44. **Whipple, G.** 1907. A hitherto undescribed disease characterized anatomically by deposits of fat and fatty acids in the intestinal and mesenteric lymphatic tissues. *Bull. Johns Hopkins Hosp.* **18:**382–393.
45. **Wilson, K., R. Blitchington, R. Frothingham, and J. Wilson.** 1991. Phylogeny of the Whipple's-disease associated bacterium. *Lancet* **338:**474–475.

ANTIBACTERIAL AGENTS AND SUSCEPTIBILITY TEST METHODS

V

VOLUME EDITOR
JAMES H. JORGENSEN

SECTION EDITORS
MARY JANE FERRARO AND
JOHN D. TURNIDGE

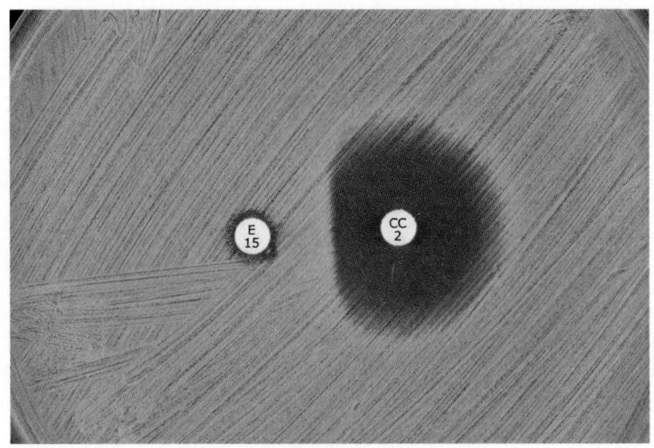

D-zone test (J. Jorgensen, University of Texas).

Antibacterial Agents

JOSEPH D. C. YAO AND ROBERT C. MOELLERING, JR.

70

Antimicrobial chemotherapy has played a vital role in the treatment of human infectious diseases in the 20th century. Since the discovery of penicillin in the 1920s, literally hundreds of antimicrobial agents have been developed or synthesized, and dozens of these are currently available for clinical use. While the broad number and variety of agents available provide a great deal of flexibility for the clinician in the use of these agents, the sheer numbers available and the continuing development of agents make it difficult for clinicians to keep up with progress in the field. Similarly, this variety presents significant challenges for the clinical microbiologist, who must decide which agents are appropriate for inclusion in routine and specialized susceptibility testing.

This chapter provides an overview of the antibacterial agents currently marketed in the United States, with major emphasis on their mechanisms of action, spectra of activity, important pharmacological parameters, and toxicities. Antibiotics that have fallen into disuse or remained investigational are mentioned only briefly.

PENICILLINS

The penicillins (Table 1) are a group of natural and semisynthetic antibiotics containing the chemical nucleus 6-aminopenicillanic acid, which consists of a β-lactam ring fused to a thiazolidine ring (Fig. 1a). The naturally occurring compounds are produced by a number of *Penicillium* spp. The penicillins differ from one another in the substitution at position 6, where changes in the side chain may modify the pharmacokinetic and antibacterial properties of the drug.

Mechanism of Action

The major antibacterial action of penicillins is derived from their ability to inhibit a number of bacterial enzymes, namely, penicillin-binding proteins (PBPs), that are essential for peptidoglycan synthesis (358). This ability to inhibit bacterial cell wall enzymes such as the transpeptidases usually confers on the penicillins bactericidal activity against gram-positive bacteria. The bactericidal activity of the penicillins is often related to their ability to trigger membrane-associated autolytic enzymes that destroy the cell wall. Other minor mechanisms of action include inhibition of bacterial endopeptidase and glycosidase, enzymes involved in bacterial cell growth. There is also recent evidence suggesting that penicillins may inhibit RNA synthesis in some bacteria, causing death without cell lysis, but the significance of these observations remains to be proven (223).

Pharmacology

Oral absorption differs markedly among the penicillins. As a natural congener of penicillin G, penicillin V resists gastric acid inactivation and is better absorbed from the gastrointestinal tract than is penicillin G. Amoxicillin is a semisynthetic analog of ampicillin and has greater gastrointestinal absorption than ampicillin (95 versus 40% absorption). Bacampicillin is an ampicillin ester that is absorbed considerably better from the gastrointestinal tract than is ampicillin or amoxicillin. This ester is inactive until naturally occurring esterases in the intestinal mucosa and serum hydrolyze them to release the parent compound, ampicillin, into the serum. The isoxazolyl penicillins, such as oxacillin, cloxacillin, dicloxacillin, and nafcillin, are acid stable and are also absorbed from the gastrointestinal tract (140), in contradistinction to certain other antistaphylococcal penicillins, such as methicillin, which are not acid resistant and cannot be given via the oral route.

Repository forms of penicillin G, available in procaine or benzathine, delay absorption from an intramuscular depot. Procaine penicillin G provides detectable levels for 12 to 24 h, suitable for treatment of uncomplicated pneumococcal pneumonia and gonorrhea due to fully susceptible organisms. Benzathine penicillin G achieves very low levels in blood for prolonged periods (3 to 4 weeks) and is useful for the therapy of syphilis and for prophylaxis of streptococcal pharyngitis and rheumatic fever.

Penicillins are well distributed to many body compartments, including the lungs, liver, kidneys, muscle, bone, and placenta. Penetration into the eye, brain, cerebrospinal fluid (CSF), and prostate is poor in the absence of inflammation. These drugs are metabolized to a small degree and are rapidly excreted, essentially unchanged, via the kidneys. With average half-lives of 0.5 to 1.5 h, they are usually administered every 4 to 6 h to maintain effective levels in blood. The renal tubular excretion of penicillins can be blocked by probenecid, thus prolonging their half-lives in serum.

Dosage reduction of most penicillins is necessary only in severe renal insufficiency (creatinine clearance of ≤10 ml/min). Dosages of all penicillins except nafcillin and the isoxazolyl penicillins are adjusted for hemodialysis. Peritoneal dialysis requires dosage reduction for carbenicillin and ticarcillin.

TABLE 1 Penicillins

Natural
  Benzylpenicillin (penicillin G)
  Phenoxymethyl penicillin (penicillin V)

Semisynthetic
  Penicillinase resistant
    Methicillin
    Nafcillin
    Cloxacillin
    Dicloxacillin
    Oxacillin
  Extended spectrum
    Aminopenicillins
      Ampicillin
      Amoxicillin
      Bacampicillin
      Pivampicillin
    Carboxypenicillins
      Carbenicillin
      Ticarcillin
    Ureidopenicillins
      Azlocillin
      Mezlocillin
      Piperacillin

Penicillin + β-lactamase inhibitor combinations
  Ampicillin-sulbactam
  Ticarcillin-clavulanate
  Amoxicillin-clavulanate
  Piperacillin-tazobactam

Spectrum of Activity

The penicillins have activity against most gram-positive and many gram-negative and anaerobic organisms. Penicillin G is very effective against penicillin-susceptible *Staphylococcus aureus, Streptococcus pneumoniae, Streptococcus pyogenes,* viridans group streptococci, *Streptococcus bovis, Neisseria gonorrhoeae, Neisseria meningitidis, Pasteurella multocida,* anaerobic cocci, *Clostridium* spp., *Fusobacterium* spp., *Prevotella* spp., and *Porphyromonas* spp. However, the occurrence of penicillin-resistant pneumococci has recently been increasing worldwide (190). Penicillin is the drug of choice for syphilis and *Actinomyces* infections. Penicillin V has a spectrum of activity similar to that of penicillin G except that it is less active against *N. gonorrhoeae.* Penicillinase-resistant penicillins, of which methicillin is the prototype, are primarily effective against penicillinase-producing staphylococci (115). The agents are at least 25 times more active than other penicillins against penicillinase-positive staphylococci. Although they are also active against *S. pneumoniae* and *S. pyogenes,* their MICs for these organisms are higher than those of penicillin G. They are not active against enterococci, members of the family *Enterobacteriaceae, Pseudomonas* spp., or members of the *Bacteroides fragilis* group.

Ampicillin and amoxicillin have spectra of activity similar to that of penicillin G, but they are more active against enterococci and *Listeria monocytogenes.* Although they are also more active against *Haemophilus influenzae* and *Haemophilus parainfluenzae,* up to 35% of *H. influenzae* isolates are resistant, usually because of β-lactamase production. *Salmonella* and *Shigella* spp., including *Salmonella enterica* serovar Typhi, and many strains of *Escherichia coli* and *Proteus mirabilis* are susceptible to these agents. Ampicillin is more effective against shigellae, whereas amoxicillin is more effective against salmonellae. Both of these agents are degraded by β-lactamase and are inactive against many *Enterobacteriaceae* and *Pseudomonas* spp.

The carboxypenicillins and ureidopenicillins have increased activity against gram-negative bacteria that are resistant to ampicillin. Although these drugs are susceptible to staphylococcal penicillinase, they are more stable against hydrolysis by the β-lactamases of *Enterobacteriaceae* and *Pseudomonas aeruginosa.* Carbenicillin and ticarcillin are relatively active against streptococci as well as against *Haemophilus* spp., *Neisseria* spp., and a variety of anaerobes (124). They inhibit *Enterobacteriaceae* but are inactive against *Klebsiella* spp. Although carboxypenicillins are not particularly active against the enterococci, they may act synergistically with aminoglycosides against these organisms.

The ureidopenicillins have greater in vitro activity against streptococci and enterococci than do the carboxypenicillins, and they inhibit more than 75% of *Klebsiella* spp. (87, 343). They have excellent activity against many *Enterobacteriaceae* and anaerobic bacteria, including members of the *B. fragilis* group. On a weight basis, their activities in decreasing order of potency against *P. aeruginosa* are as follows: piperacillin, azlocillin > mezlocillin, ticarcillin > carbenicillin (66). These agents also act synergistically with aminoglycosides against *P. aeruginosa.*

Adverse Effects

Common reactions to penicillins include allergic skin rashes, diarrhea, and drug fever. Severe anaphylactic reactions, which can be fatal, may occur in previously sensitized patients rechallenged with penicillins, but fortunately, such reactions are quite rare. At high doses (usually $>30 \times 10^6$ U/day), penicillin G can cause myoclonic twitching and seizures due to central nervous system toxicity. All of the penicillins may cause interstitial nephritis on an allergic basis, but methicillin is more likely than the other penicillins to cause this complication. Hepatitis has been associated with prolonged use of oxacillin. High-dose carbenicillin can result in sodium overload and hypokalemia. Neutropenia may occur with any of the penicillins. Thrombocytopenia and Coombs-positive hemolytic anemia are rare complications of penicillin therapy. Bleeding tendencies due to interference with platelet function can occur with the use of carboxypenicillins and ureidopenicillins (105). Although pseudomembranous colitis has been associated with all the penicillins, it occurs more frequently with ampicillin (19).

CEPHALOSPORINS

Cephalosporins are derivatives of the fermentation products of *Cephalosporium acremonium* (also designated *Acremonium chrysogenum*). They contain a 7-aminocephalosporanic acid nucleus, which consists of a β-lactam ring fused to a dihydrothiazine ring (Fig. lb). Various substitutions at positions 3 and 7 alter their antibacterial activities and pharmacokinetic properties. The addition of a methoxy group at position 7 of the β-lactam ring results in a new group of compounds called cephamycins, which are highly resistant to a variety of β-lactamases.

Mechanism of Action

Similar to the penicillins, cephalosporins act by binding to PBPs of susceptible organisms, thereby interfering with

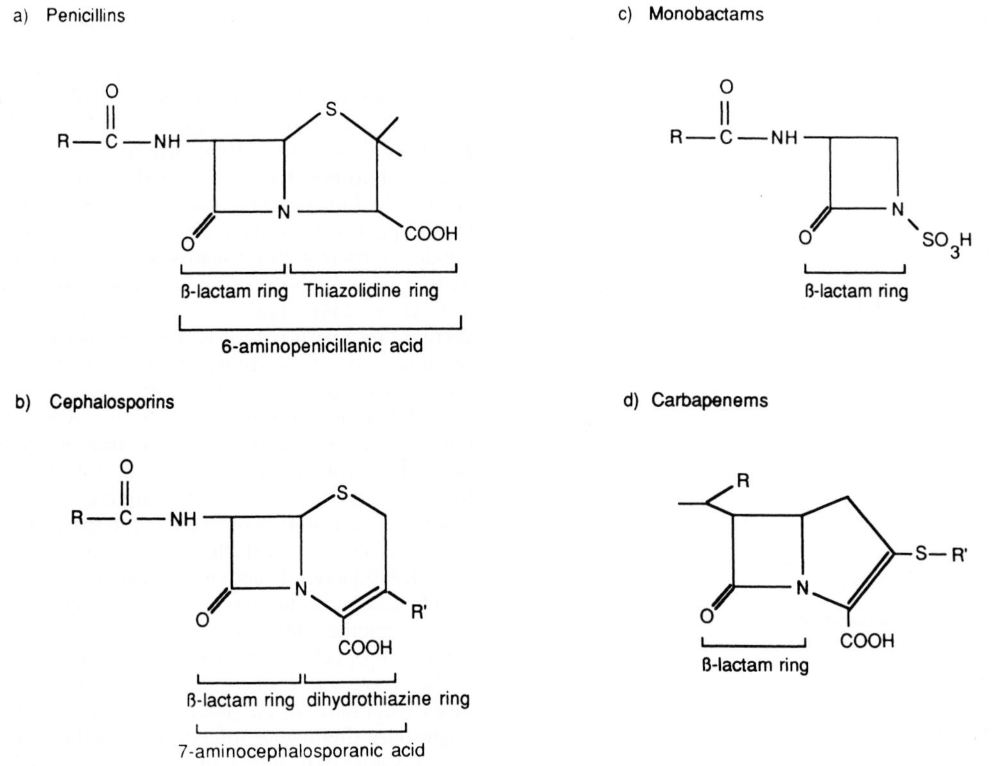

a) Penicillins

R—C(=O)—NH

ß-lactam ring Thiazolidine ring

6-aminopenicillanic acid

b) Cephalosporins

ß-lactam ring dihydrothiazine ring

7-aminocephalosporanic acid

c) Monobactams

ß-lactam ring

d) Carbapenems

ß-lactam ring

FIGURE 1 Chemical structures of β-lactam antibiotics.

synthesis of peptidoglycan of the bacterial cell wall. In addition, these β-lactam agents may produce bactericidal effects by triggering autolytic enzymes in the cell envelope (358).

Pharmacology

Most cephalosporins require parenteral administration, but a growing number are available in oral form. Cephalexin, cephradine, cefadroxil, cefaclor, cefuroxime axetil, cefprozil, loracarbef, cefdinir, cefditoren pivoxil, cefixime, cefpodoxime proxetil, and ceftibuten are given orally and have good gastrointestinal absorption (60 to 90% of the oral dose). Cefuroxime axetil is an acetoxyethyl ester of cefuroxime, and it is deesterified at the intestinal mucosa and absorbed into the bloodstream as cefuroxime. Cefditoren pivoxil and cefpodoxime proxetil are prodrugs that are absorbed and hydrolyzed by esterases in vivo to release the active drugs, cefditoren and cefpodoxime, respectively. Relatively high concentrations of these agents are attained across the placenta and in synovial, pleural, pericardial, and peritoneal fluids. Levels in bile are usually high, especially with cefoperazone, which is excreted mainly in the bile. Ceftizoxime, cefotaxime, ceftriaxone, cefoperazone, moxalactam, and cefepime enter well into the CSF and are useful for the treatment of meningitis. Cefuroxime penetrates inflamed meninges, but levels in CSF are inadequate in providing bactericidal activity against susceptible bacteria.

Cephalothin, cephapirin, and cefotaxime are converted to the desacetyl forms before excretion. All cephalosporins except cefoperazone are excreted primarily by the kidneys, and for these drugs, dosage adjustments are necessary in patients with renal insufficiency (creatinine clearance of <50 ml/min). Like that of the penicillins, the renal excretion of cephalosporins, except for ceftriaxone, is impeded by probenecid. In general, these agents are removed by hemodialysis but not by peritoneal dialysis. Of the cephalosporins, cefonicid and ceftriaxone have the longest elimination half-lives, at 4.5 and 8 h, respectively, permitting once- or twice-daily drug administration in the treatment of serious infections.

Spectrum of Activity

Cephalosporins are classified by a well-accepted but somewhat arbitrary scheme of grouping by generations based on general features of their antibacterial activity (Table 2). The first-generation (narrow-spectrum) drugs, exemplified by cephalothin and cefazolin, have good activity against gram-positive organisms and relatively modest activity against gram-negative organisms. They are active against penicillin-susceptible and -resistant *S. aureus* as well as *S. pneumoniae*, *S. pyogenes*, and other aerobic and anaerobic streptococci. Methicillin-resistant *S. aureus*, *Staphylococcus epidermidis*, and enterococci are resistant. Some *Enterobacteriaceae*, including many strains of *E. coli*, *Klebsiella* spp., and *P. mirabilis*, are susceptible. *Pseudomonas* spp. (including *P. aeruginosa*), many *Proteus* spp., and *Serratia* and *Enterobacter* spp. are resistant. These agents are active against penicillin-susceptible anaerobes except members of the *B. fragilis* group. They have only modest activity against *H. influenzae*.

The second-generation (expanded-spectrum) cephalosporins are stable against certain β-lactamases found in gram-negative bacteria and, as a result, have increased activity against gram-negative organisms. The agents are more active than narrow-spectrum drugs against *E. coli*, *Klebsiella* spp., and *Proteus* spp. Their activity also extends to cover some *Enterobacter* and *Serratia* strains, and they have good activity against *Haemophilus* spp., *Neisseria* spp., and many anaerobes.

TABLE 2 Cephalosporins

Narrow spectrum (first generation)
Cefadroxil
Cefazolin
Cephalexin
Cephaloridine
Cephalothin
Cephapirin
Cephradine
Expanded spectrum (second generation)
Cefaclor
Cefamandole
Cefonicid
Ceforanide
Cefuroxime
Cefprozil
Loracarbef
Cefmetazole
Cefotetan
Cefoxitin
Broad spectrum (third generation)
Cefdinir
Cefditoren
Cefixime
Cefoperazone
Cefotaxime
Cefpodoxime
Ceftazidime
Ceftibuten
Ceftizoxime
Ceftriaxone
Extended spectrum (fourth generation)
Cefepime
Cefpirome

Cefaclor, cefuroxime, cefamandole, cefonicid, and cefprozil are active against ampicillin-resistant *H. influenzae* and *Moraxella catarrhalis* (334). However, cefamandole exhibits a significant inoculum effect and is not suitable for treating life-threatening infections due to *H. influenzae.* Ceforanide and cefonicid have spectra of antibacterial activities similar to that of cefamandole, but they are less active than cefamandole against gram-positive cocci. Loracarbef belongs to a new class of cephalosporin derivatives known as carbacephems in which the sulfur atom of the dihydrothiazine ring is replaced by a methylene group to form a tetrahydropyridine ring (67). Since this structural modification of the cephalosporin nucleus is minor, loracarbef is considered a cephalosporin. Its spectrum of antibacterial activity is very similar to those of cefaclor, cefuroxime, and cefprozil. None of the expanded-spectrum agents is active against *Pseudomonas* spp.

Cefoxitin, cefotetan, and cefmetazole belong to a unique group of expanded-spectrum cephalosporins that have marked activity against anaerobes, including members of the *B. fragilis* group (175, 364). Cefotetan is two to four times less active than cefoxitin and cefmetazole against gram-positive cocci, but it is more potent than these two drugs against susceptible *Enterobacteriaceae.* The three drugs are equally active against *H. influenzae, M. catarrhalis,* and *N. gonorrhoeae,* including penicillin-resistant strains. While these drugs are comparable in their activities against the *B. fragilis* group, cefoxitin is the most active against *Prevotella* spp., *Porphyromonas* spp., and gram-positive anaerobic cocci. Cefotetan and cefmetazole have the advantage of more prolonged half-lives in serum.

Third-generation (broad-spectrum) cephalosporins are generally less active than the narrow-spectrum agents against gram-positive cocci, but they are much more active against the *Enterobacteriaceae* and *P. aeruginosa.* Their potent broad spectra of activity against gram-negative organisms are due to their stability against β-lactamases and their ability to pass through the outer cell envelopes of gram-negative rods (104, 254). There are two subgroups among these agents: those with potent activity against *P. aeruginosa* (ceftazidime and cefoperazone) and those without such activity (ceftizoxime, cefotaxime, and ceftriaxone).

Cefotaxime inhibits more than 90% of strains of *Enterobacteriaceae,* including those resistant to aminoglycosides. The MIC_{90}s for strains of *E. coli, Proteus* spp., and *Klebsiella* spp. tested are <0.5 μg/ml. Its activity against strains of *Serratia marcescens, Enterobacter cloacae,* and *Acinetobacter* spp. is variable, and it is inactive against *P. aeruginosa.* It has moderate activity against anaerobes but is inferior to cefoxitin and cefotetan against most of these isolates.

Ceftizoxime and ceftriaxone have spectra of activity similar to that of cefotaxime, with a few exceptions. Ceftriaxone is the most active agent against penicillinase-positive or -negative strains of *N. gonorrhoeae* (108). It is effective as single-dose therapy for infections caused by these organisms (51). Because of its long half-life in serum (the longest of the currently available cephalosporins), ceftriaxone is used frequently in outpatient antibiotic therapy of serious infections, including Lyme disease (229).

Cefoperazone is less active than cefotaxime against many *Enterobacteriaceae* and gram-positive cocci. However, it has activity against *P. aeruginosa,* with an MIC_{50} of ≤16 μg/ml. Its activity against anaerobes is similar to that of cefotaxime (177). Ceftazidime has potent activity against *P. aeruginosa,* with an MIC_{90} of <8 μg/ml (248). It is more active than the ureidopenicillins against these strains. This agent has activity similar to that of cefotaxime against the *Enterobacteriaceae* but is not as active against gram-positive cocci. It has little activity against gram-negative anaerobes.

Cefdinir (63), cefditoren (173, 178), cefixime (15), cefpodoxime (116, 298), and ceftibuten (177, 376) are extended-spectrum oral cephalosporins that are more stable than the narrow- and expanded-spectrum oral cephalosporins against gram-negative bacterial β-lactamases. Compared with the earlier cephalosporins, the newer drugs are equally active against streptococci (MIC_{90}s ≤ 0.06 μg/ml) but less active against methicillin-susceptible staphylococci (MIC_{90}s = 2 μg/ml). While they have potent activities similar to that of ceftizoxime against many *Enterobacteriaceae, H. influenzae, M. catarrhalis,* and *N. gonorrhoeae* (including β-lactamase-producing strains), they are inactive against *Pseudomonas, Enterobacter, Serratia,* and *Morganella* spp. and anaerobes. None of the currently available cephalosporins is clinically useful against enterococci.

Cefepime is a so-called fourth-generation (extended-spectrum) cephalosporin approved for clinical use in the United States. Cefepime and cefpirome (formerly HR 810), which is currently undergoing clinical evaluations, have the unique features of reduced affinity for and increased stability against the Bush class I β-lactamases. Therefore, these agents are active against stably derepressed class I β-lactamase mutants of *Enterobacteriaceae* and *P. aeruginosa.* In addition, cefepime and cefpirome penetrate well through the outer membrane of gram-negative bacteria, due to a quaternary nitrogen substitution that makes them zwitterions (net neutral charge). They are more active in vitro than cefotaxime and ceftriaxone against some *Enterobacteriaceae, Proteus, Providencia, Morganella,* and *Citrobacter* (MIC_{90}s ≤ 0.1 μg/ml) (126, 180, 301). Cefepime has activity comparable to that of ceftazidime against *P. aeruginosa,* with MIC_{90}s of ≤4 μg/ml, and it is active against some ceftazidime-resistant strains (279). Against staphylococci (MIC_{90}s ≤ 2 μg/ml) and streptococci (MIC_{90}s ≤ 0.12 μg/ml), the activities of this group of drugs are comparable to those of the narrow-spectrum cephalosporins (126, 180). However, they are not active clinically against enterococci or anaerobes.

Adverse Effects

Cephalosporins are generally very well tolerated. The most common side effects are diarrhea and hypersensitivity reactions such as rash, drug fever, and serum sickness. Cross-reactions with these drugs occur in only 3 to 7% of penicillin-allergic patients (186). Other infrequent side effects include pseudomembranous colitis, elevated serum creatinine and transaminase levels, leukopenia, thrombocytopenia, and Coombs-positive hemolytic anemia. These abnormalities are usually mild and reversible. Prolonged use of ceftriaxone has been associated with formation of gallbladder sludge, which usually resolves after the drug is discontinued (304), and, rarely, cholecystitis.

Disulfiram-like reactions have been described to occur in patients receiving cefamandole, cefotetan, and cefoperazone. This reaction is attributed to the *N*-methylthiotetrazole side chains of these antibiotics, which are similar to the chemical structure of disulfiram. Hypoprothrombinemia and bleeding tendencies have been observed with these cephalosporins. Causes of the coagulopathy included (i) alteration to healthy gut flora by the antibiotics, thus inhibiting the synthesis of vitamin K and its precursors, and (ii) the *N*-methylthiotetrazole side chain, which inhibits the vitamin K-dependent carboxylase enzyme responsible for converting clotting factors II, VII, IX, and X to their active forms and also prevents regeneration of active vitamin K from its inactive form (302).

OTHER β-LACTAM ANTIBIOTICS

■ Monobactams

Aztreonam is the only monobactam antibiotic currently in clinical use. The monobactams are β-lactams with various side chains affixed to a monocyclic nucleus (Fig. 1c).

Mechanism of Action

Aztreonam binds primarily to PBP 3 of gram-negative aerobes, including *P. aeruginosa,* thereby disrupting bacterial cell wall synthesis. It is not hydrolyzed by most commonly occurring plasmid-mediated and chromosomally mediated β-lactamases, and it does not induce the production of these enzymes (42).

Pharmacology

Given intravenously, aztreonam is widely distributed to body tissues and fluids. Average serum drug concentrations exceed the MIC_{90}s for most *Enterobacteriaceae* four to eight times for 8 h and are inhibitory to *P. aeruginosa* for 4 h. Aztreonam crosses inflamed meninges in sufficient amount to be potentially therapeutic for meningitis caused by susceptible organisms. Its half-life in serum is about 1.7 h, and it is excreted mainly unchanged by the kidney. Dosage modification is necessary for patients with renal failure. The drug is removed by both hemodialysis and peritoneal dialysis.

Spectrum of Activity

The antibacterial activity of aztreonam is limited to aerobic gram-negative rods, inhibiting most *Enterobacteriaceae, Neisseria* spp., and *Haemophilus* spp., with MIC_{90}s of ≤0.5 μg/ml (17, 332). It has significant activity against *Enterobacter* spp. and *S. marcescens,* with most strains being inhibited at ≤16 μg/ml. However, many *Acinetobacter* spp., *Burkholderia cepacia,* and *Stenotrophomonas maltophilia* are resistant. It shows in vitro synergism when combined with aminoglycosides against 30 to 60% of aztreonam-susceptible organisms, including *P. aeruginosa* and aminoglycoside-resistant gram-negative rods (41). Bacterial tolerance and inoculum effect are generally not seen with this agent. Aztreonam is not active against gram-positive bacteria or anaerobes.

Adverse Effects

Aztreonam is generally a safe agent, with a toxicity profile similar to those of other β-lactam drugs. Nausea, diarrhea, skin rash, eosinophilia, mild elevation of serum transaminase levels, and transiently elevated serum creatinine levels have occurred. It has minimal cross-reactivity with other β-lactams and can be used safely in patients allergic to penicillins or cephalosporins (303). Hematologic abnormalities have not been reported.

■ Carbapenems

Carbapenems are a unique class of β-lactam agents with the widest spectrum of antibacterial activity of the currently available antibiotics. Structurally, they differ from other β-lactams in having a hydroxyethyl side chain in *trans* configuration at position 6 and lacking a sulfur or oxygen atom in the bicyclic nucleus (Fig. 1d). The unique stereochemistry of the hydroxyethyl side chain confers stability against β-lactamases. Imipenem (*N*-formimidoyl thienamycin), a semisynthetic derivative of thienamycin produced by *Streptomyces* spp., meropenem, and ertapenem are the carbapenems currently available for clinical use (20, 259). Other members of this class currently undergoing preclinical evaluation or clinical trials include biapenem, doripenem, faropenem, and panipenem.

Mechanism of Action

Carbapenems bind to PBP 1 and PBP 2 of gram-negative and gram-positive bacteria, causing cell elongation and lysis (318). They are stable against most plasmid-mediated or chromosomally mediated β-lactamases except those produced by *S. maltophilia* and some strains of *B. fragilis* (249). Bacterial resistance arises from production of carbapenemases (metallo-β-lactamases) capable of hydrolyzing the carbapenem nucleus and from alteration of the porin channels in the bacterial cell wall, reducing the permeability of the drugs.

Pharmacology

After intravenous administration, the carbapenems distribute widely in the body but undergo no significant biliary excretion. Imipenem is metabolized and inactivated in the kidneys by a dehydropeptidase I (DHP-I) enzyme found in the brush border of proximal renal tubular cells. To achieve adequate concentrations in serum and urine, a DHP inhibitor, cilastatin, was developed; it is combined with imipenem in a 1:1 dosage ratio for clinical use. Cilastatin has no antibacterial activity, nor does it alter the activity of imipenem. It has a renal protective effect by preventing excessive accumulation of potentially toxic imipenem metabolites in the renal tubular cells. Meropenem, ertapenem, faropenem, and biapenem contain a β-methyl group substitution at position C-1 of the bicyclic nucleus resulting in increased stability against inactivation by human renal DHP-I. These agents do not require concomitant administration of a DHP-I inhibitor.

The pharmacokinetics of imipenem and meropenem are very similar, with elimination half-lives in serum of about 1 h. Peak concentrations of the drugs in serum are about 25 to 35 μg/ml and 55 to 70 μg/ml following 0.5- and 1-g doses, respectively. These drugs penetrate inflamed meninges well, with drug levels of 0.5 to 6 μg/ml in the CSF (68, 259). Ertapenem is highly (>95%) bound to human plasma proteins, with poor penetration into the CSF. Its relatively long plasma half-life of 4 h allows for once-daily dosing frequency. The peak concentration in serum of 155 μg/ml is reached following a single intravenous dose of 1 g (256). Dosage adjustment of these carbapenem drugs is necessary for creatinine clearance of ≤30 ml/min. These agents, including cilastatin, are effectively removed by hemodialysis.

Spectrum of Activity

In general, all the carbapenems have similar antibacterial potencies, with minor differences. They have excellent in vitro activity against aerobic gram-positive species: staphylococci (penicillin-susceptible and -resistant isolates); viridans group streptococci; group A, B, C, and G streptococci; *Bacillus* spp.; and *L. monocytogenes.* Imipenem is two to four times more active than meropenem and ertapenem against streptococci and staphylococci, but methicillin-resistant staphylococci are usually resistant to all carbapenems. Although the MICs of carbapenems for penicillin-resistant pneumococci are elevated (MIC_{90}s of 0.25 to 2 μg/ml), many strains remain susceptible to these drugs, with imipenem being most potent (265). Ertapenem has poor activity against *Enterococcus faecalis,* but these isolates are inhibited by other carbapenems at ≤4 μg/ml. However, *Enterococcus faecium* strains are usually resistant.

More than 90% of *Enterobacteriaceae,* including those resistant to other β-lactams and aminoglycosides (254), are susceptible to carbapenems, with the following decreasing order of activity: doripenem, ertapenem, meropenem > biapenem > faropenem, imipenem (89, 97, 124, 157, 179, 215, 259, 362). These agents are highly active against clinical isolates of extended-spectrum β-lactamase-producing *Klebsiella pneumoniae* and *E. coli,* with MIC_{90}s of 0.015 to 0.125 μg/ml (193, 205). Most *Enterobacter* spp., *Citrobacter* spp., and *Serratia* spp. are inhibited by ≤2 μg/ml. Although ertapenem is inactive against *Acinetobacter* and *Pseudomonas,* it is 5- to 10-fold more active than other carbapenems against fastidious gram-negative bacteria such as *Haemophilus, Moraxella, Neisseria,* and *Pasteurella.* Most strains of *P. aeruginosa* are inhibited by other carbapenems at 4 to 8 μg/ml, with meropenem as the most potent agent, including against imipenem-resistant strains (123, 157, 204, 275). While they inhibit *B. cepacia* and *Pseudomonas stutzeri,* carbapenems are inactive against *S. maltophilia* (83). Emergence of resistant *Pseudomonas* spp. has been observed during therapy with imipenem (373). The drug may show in vitro antagonism when combined with broad-spectrum cephalosporins or extended-spectrum penicillins as a result of its ability to induce class I β-lactamase production (249).

Carbapenems are the most potent β-lactams against anaerobes, with activities comparable to those of clindamycin and metronidazole. The MIC_{90}s for anaerobic gram-positive cocci, *Clostridium,* the *B. fragilis* group, *Fusobacterium, Porphyromonas,* and *Prevotella* are ≤4 μg/ml (133, 214, 275, 363, 366, 368). This class of drugs is also active in vitro against *Actinomyces, Nocardia,* and atypical mycobacteria (25, 72, 84, 97, 133).

Adverse Effects

The side effects of carbapenems are similar to those of other β-lactam antibiotics. Nausea, vomiting, and diarrhea occur in up to 5% of patients, usually associated with parenteral administration of ertapenem and imipenem. Pseudomembranous colitis can occur with carbapenems. Allergic reactions such as drug fever, skin rashes, and urticaria are seen in about 3% of patients. Cross-reactivity with other β-lactam agents is possible but has not been fully studied. Seizures of unclear etiology have occurred in up to 1% of patients receiving ertapenem and imipenem, particularly in the elderly age group and in patients with renal insufficiency or underlying neurologic disorders. Meropenem has not been associated with seizures. Reversible elevation of serum transaminases, leukopenia, and thrombocytopenia have been described for carbapenems, but no coagulopathy has been reported.

β-LACTAMASE INHIBITORS

Clavulanic Acid

Clavulanic acid is a naturally occurring, weak antimicrobial agent found initially in cultures of *Streptomyces clavuligerus* (252). It inhibits β-lactamases from staphylococci and many gram-negative bacteria. This agent acts primarily as a "suicide inhibitor" by forming an irreversible acyl enzyme complex with the β-lactamase, leading to loss of activity of the enzyme.

Clavulanic acid acts synergistically with various penicillins and cephalosporins against β-lactamase-producing staphylococci, klebsiellae, *H. influenzae, M. catarrhalis, N. gonorrhoeae, E. coli, Proteus* spp., the *B. fragilis* group, *Prevotella* spp., and *Porphyromonas* spp. (12, 114, 124). Plasmid-mediated TEM β-lactamases present in ceftazidime-resistant strains of *K. pneumoniae* and *E. coli* are inactivated by this drug (169). However, the inducible β-lactamases (chromosomal class I) of *Enterobacter, Citrobacter, Proteus, Acinetobacter, Serratia,* and *Pseudomonas* spp. are not inhibited by clavulanic acid (191). The combination of clavulanic acid with ampicillin, amoxicillin, or ticarcillin is active in vitro against *Mycobacterium tuberculosis,* which is known to produce β-lactamases (73, 380).

In the United States, clavulanic acid is available for clinical use in combination with oral amoxicillin at dosage ratios of 1:2, 1:4, 1:7, and 1:16 and in a 1:15 or 1:30 parenteral combination with ticarcillin. Intravenous combinations of clavulanic acid and amoxicillin at ratios of 1:5 and 1:10 are also used outside of North America. The pharmacological parameters of amoxicillin and ticarcillin are not significantly altered when either drug is combined with clavulanic acid. Amoxicillin-clavulanate is moderately well absorbed from the gastrointestinal tract, with a half-life in serum of about 1 h for each component. One-third of a dose is metabolized, while the remainder is excreted unchanged in the urine. The drug is widely distributed to various body tissues and fluids, but it penetrates uninflamed meninges very poorly.

Adverse reactions are similar to those reported for amoxicillin or ticarcillin used alone. Nausea, vomiting, abdominal cramps, and diarrhea occur in 5 to 10% of patients taking amoxicillin-clavulanate. The incidence of allergic skin reactions is similar to that with ampicillin alone.

Sulbactam

Sulbactam is a semisynthetic 6-desaminopenicillin sulfone with weak antibacterial activity (5). It functions as an effective inhibitor of certain plasmid-mediated and chromosomally mediated β-lactamases of *S. aureus*, many *Enterobacteriaceae*, *H. influenzae*, *M. catarrhalis*, *Neisseria* spp., *Legionella* spp., the *B. fragilis* group, *Prevotella* spp., *Porphyromonas* spp., and *Mycobacterium* spp. (122, 237). Sulbactam alone is active against *N. gonorrhoeae*, *N. meningitidis*, some *Acinetobacter* spp., and *B. cepacia* (170, 239). It acts synergistically with penicillins and cephalosporins against organisms that are otherwise resistant to the β-lactam drugs because of the production of β-lactamases. A combination of sulbactam (8 μg/ml) and ampicillin (16 μg/ml) inhibits most strains of staphylococci, *Klebsiella* spp., *E. coli*, *H. influenzae*, *M. catarrhalis*, *Neisseria* spp., the *B. fragilis* group, *Prevotella* spp., and *Porphyromonas* spp. that are ampicillin resistant (284, 365). Like clavulanic acid, sulbactam does not inhibit the β-lactamases of *Enterobacter*, *Citrobacter*, *Providencia*, indole-positive *Proteus*, *Pseudomonas* spp., or *S. maltophilia*.

For clinical use, sulbactam is combined with ampicillin as a parenteral preparation in a 1:2 ratio. The pharmacological properties of the drugs are not affected by each other in this combination. Ampicillin-sulbactam penetrates well into body tissues and fluids, including peritoneal and blister fluids. It enters the CSF in the presence of inflamed meninges. Like ampicillin, sulbactam has a half-life in serum of 1 h, and 85% of the drug is excreted unchanged via the kidneys. Since clearances of sulbactam and ampicillin are affected similarly in patients with impaired renal function, dosage adjustments are similar for the two drugs.

The most common side effects of the ampicillin-sulbactam combination have been nausea, diarrhea, and skin rash. Transient eosinophilia and transaminasemia have been reported. Adverse reactions attributed to ampicillin may also occur with the use of ampicillin-sulbactam.

Tazobactam

Tazobactam (formerly YTR 830) is a penicillanic acid sulfone derivative structurally related to sulbactam. Like clavulanic acid and sulbactam, tazobactam acts as a suicidal β-lactamase inhibitor and binds to bacterial PBP 1 or PBP 2 (239). Despite having very poor intrinsic antibacterial activity by itself, it is comparable to clavulanate and sulbactam in lowering the MICs up to 20-fold for many organisms when combined with various β-lactams against β-lactamase-producing organisms. Tazobactam actively inhibits the β-lactamases of staphylococci, *H. influenzae*, *N. gonorrhoeae*, *E. coli*, the *B. fragilis* group, *Prevotella* spp., and *Porphyromonas* spp. (3, 145, 194). It also has activity against the class I β-lactamases of *Acinetobacter*, *Citrobacter*, *Proteus*, *Providencia*, and *Morganella* spp., but it remains inactive against those of *Enterobacter* spp., *Pseudomonas* spp., *S. maltophilia*, and some *Klebsiella* spp. (191, 194, 239). Of the penicillin–β-lactamase inhibitor combinations, piperacillin-tazobactam is the one most active (two- to eightfold-lower MICs) against β-lactamase-producing aerobic and anaerobic gram-negative rods (99, 194).

Available as a 1:8 ratio dosage combination with piperacillin, tazobactam is administered parenterally. The two drugs do not affect each other's metabolism or pharmacokinetics. High concentrations of both agents are achieved in the intestinal mucosa, lungs, and skin, with relatively poor distribution to muscle, fat, the prostate, and CSF (in the absence of inflamed meninges). With a half-life in serum of about 1 h, elimination of tazobactam is mainly via the renal route and is not affected by hepatic failure (316). Major adverse effects of the piperacillin-tazobactam combination are similar to those of piperacillin alone, such as diarrhea, skin rash, and allergic reactions. Mild elevation in serum transaminase levels may be encountered in about 10% of patients.

AMINOGLYCOSIDES AND AMINOCYCLITOLS

Since the first aminoglycoside (aminoglycosidic aminocyclitol), streptomycin, was introduced in 1944, this class of antibiotic has played a vital role in the treatment of serious infections with gram-negative organisms. Among the unique features of the aminoglycosides is the bactericidal activity against aerobic gram-negative rods (including *Pseudomonas* spp.), activity against *M. tuberculosis*, and relatively low incidence of bacterial resistance. The currently available aminoglycosides are derived from *Micromonospora* spp. (gentamicin, sisomicin, and netilmicin) or from *Streptomyces* spp. (streptomycin, neomycin, kanamycin, tobramycin, and paromomycin). The difference in origin of these compounds accounts for the differences of their suffixes, "micin" versus "mycin." Streptomycin, neomycin, kanamycin, tobramycin, and gentamicin are naturally occurring aminoglycosides, whereas amikacin and netilmicin are semisynthetic derivatives of kanamycin and sisomicin, respectively. Structurally, each of these aminoglycosides contains two or more amino sugars linked by glycosidic bonds to an aminocyclitol ring nucleus.

Spectinomycin is an aminocyclitol antibiotic isolated from *Streptomyces spectabilis*. Although it contains an aminocyclitol nucleus, it is not strictly an aminoglycoside because it does not contain an amino sugar or a glycosidic bond.

Mechanism of Action

Aminoglycosides are bactericidal agents that inhibit bacterial protein synthesis by binding irreversibly to the bacterial 30S ribosomal subunit. The aminoglycoside-bound bacterial ribosomes then become unavailable for translation of mRNA during protein synthesis, thereby leading to cell death (79). The aminoglycosides also cause misreading of the genetic code, with resultant production of nonsense proteins. To reach the intracellular ribosomal binding targets, an aerobic energy-dependent process is necessary to enable successful penetration of the bacterial inner cell membrane by the aminoglycosides. Bacterial uptake of these agents is facilitated by inhibitors of bacterial cell wall synthesis such as β-lactams and vancomycin. This interaction forms the basis of antibacterial synergism between aminoglycosides and β-lactam antibiotics (81, 130). There are three known mechanisms of bacterial resistance to aminoglycosides: (i) decreased intracellular accumulation of the antibiotic by altering the outer membrane permeability, decreasing inner membrane transport, or active efflux; (ii) modification of the target site by mutation in the ribosomal proteins or 16S RNA; and (iii) enzymatic modification of the drug (the most common mechanism present).

Spectinomycin acts similarly to the aminoglycosides by binding to the 30S ribosomal subunits and inhibiting protein synthesis. However, it does not cause misreading of the mRNA and is not bactericidal.

Pharmacology

All aminoglycosides have similar pharmacological properties. Gastrointestinal absorption of these agents is unpredictable and always low. Because of its severe toxicity with systemic administration, neomycin is available only for oral and topical use. After intravenous administration, aminoglycosides are freely distributed in the extracellular space but penetrate poorly into the CSF, vitreous fluid of the eye, biliary tract, prostate, and tracheobronchial secretions, even in the presence of inflammation.

In adults with normal renal function, the aminoglycosides have half-lives in serum of about 2 to 3 h. They are primarily excreted, essentially unchanged, via the kidneys. There is considerable variation in the elimination of aminoglycosides among individuals, especially in patients with impaired renal function. Monitoring of serum aminoglycoside levels in these patients is essential for providing adequate therapy and reducing toxicity. With their features of concentration-dependent killing and prolonged postantibiotic effect, aminoglycosides may be administered once daily to achieve maximum bactericidal activity at high concentrations in serum without increased risk of toxicities (21). In renal failure, the drugs accumulate and dosage reductions are necessary. Aminoglycosides are substantially removed by hemodialysis and to a lesser extent by peritoneal dialysis.

Spectrum of Activity

Aminoglycoside antibiotics are active primarily against aerobic gram-negative rods and *S. aureus*. As a group, they are particularly potent against the *Enterobacteriaceae*, *P. aeruginosa*, and *Acinetobacter* spp. Certain differences in antimicrobial spectra among the various aminoglycosides do exist. Kanamycin is limited in its spectrum because of the common resistance of *P. aeruginosa* and frequent occurrence of plasmid-mediated inactivating enzymes among other gram-negative bacilli (79). It is now used occasionally as a "second-line" drug in combination with other antibiotics for the therapy of mycobacterial infections (350, 351). Similarly, widespread resistance among *Enterobacteriaceae* has limited the usefulness of streptomycin. As a single agent, streptomycin is used in the therapy of infections due to *Francisella tularensis* (tularemia) and *Yersinia pestis* (plague) (219). It is often used in conjunction with tetracycline for the treatment of brucellosis. It has the greatest in vitro activity of the aminoglycosides against *M. tuberculosis*. It may also be used in combination with penicillin or vancomycin for the treatment of infective endocarditis due to viridans group streptococci or enterococci, provided that the organisms do not possess high-level ribosomal or enzymatic resistance to streptomycin (356, 357, 371, 372).

Although gentamicin and tobramycin have very similar antibacterial activity profiles, gentamicin is more active in vitro against *Serratia* spp., whereas tobramycin is more active against *P. aeruginosa* (247). However, these minor differences have not been correlated with greater efficacy of one agent over the other. For the most part, gentamicin and tobramycin are susceptible to inactivation by the same modifying enzymes produced by resistant bacteria, except that in contrast to gentamicin, tobramycin can be inactivated by 6-acetyltransferase and 4′-adenyltransferase and has variable susceptibility to 3-acetyltransferase. Netilmicin and amikacin are resistant to many of these aminoglycoside-modifying enzymes and therefore are active against most *Enterobacteriaceae* that are resistant to gentamicin and tobramycin (242). Netilmicin is intrinsically less active than gentamicin and tobramycin against *P. aeruginosa*, and most gentamicin-resistant *Serratia*, *Proteus*, *Providencia*, and *Pseudomonas* isolates are also usually resistant to netilmicin (121). Amikacin is often used as the aminoglycoside of choice when gentamicin and tobramycin resistances are prevalent. In addition, amikacin is active against many *Mycobacterium* spp. (350, 351). Aminoglycosides are only moderately active against *Haemophilus* and *Neisseria* spp. Of the agents active against *Bartonella* spp., aminoglycosides are the only drugs consistently bactericidal toward this group of organisms (218, 219).

Although active against staphylococci, aminoglycosides are not recommended as single agents for the treatment of staphylococcal infections. Gentamicin is often combined with a penicillin or vancomycin for synergy in the treatment of serious infections due to staphylococci, enterococci, or viridans group streptococci (356, 357, 371). The aminoglycosides are not active against anaerobes.

Paromomycin is an aminoglycoside notable for its amebicidal and antihelminthic effects, and it is used clinically for the treatment of intestinal amebiasis and tapeworm infections (228). It has modest antibacterial activity against gram-positive cocci and *Enterobacteriaceae*, but *P. aeruginosa* isolates are generally resistant.

Spectinomycin is used primarily for uncomplicated anogenital infections due to *N. gonorrhoeae* (354), including β-lactamase-producing strains, and gonococci are rarely resistant to this drug (108). It is useful in patients with penicillin allergy. Spectinomycin is ineffective for pharyngeal gonococcal infections, syphilis, or chlamydial infections.

Adverse Effects

Considerable intrinsic toxicity, mainly in the form of nephrotoxicity and auditory or vestibular toxicity, is characteristic of all of the aminoglycosides. The nephrotoxic potential varies among the aminoglycosides, with neomycin being the most toxic and streptomycin the least. This effect is usually reversible when the drug is discontinued. The presence of hypotension, prolonged duration of therapy, preexisting renal insufficiency, and possibly excessive trough serum aminoglycoside concentrations increase the risk of nephrotoxicity.

All aminoglycosides are capable of causing damage to the eighth cranial nerve in humans. Vestibular toxicity is more frequently associated with streptomycin, gentamicin, and tobramycin, whereas auditory toxicity is more typical of kanamycin and amikacin. This frequently irreversible side effect may occur even after discontinuation of the drug and is cumulative with repeated courses of the agent. The ototoxicity is a result of selective destruction of the hair cells in the cochlea. Clinically detectable auditory and vestibular dysfunction has been reported to occur in 3 to 5% of patients receiving gentamicin, tobramycin, or amikacin who underwent audiometric testing (106).

Neuromuscular paralysis, which is usually reversible, can occur after rapid intravenous infusion of aminoglycosides. This phenomenon occurs particularly in the setting of myasthenia gravis or concurrent use of succinylcholine during anesthesia. Other minor adverse reactions include local pain and allergic skin rashes. No known serious adverse reactions have been reported for spectinomycin.

QUINOLONES

Quinolones belong to a group of potent antibiotics biochemically related to nalidixic acid, which was developed initially as a urinary antiseptic. Nalidixic acid and its early analogs, oxolinic acid and cinoxacin, have limited clinical applications as a result of the widespread emergence of bacterial resistance. Newer quinolones have been synthesized by modifying the original two-ring quinolone (or naphthyridone) nucleus with different side chain substitutions (10). These new agents, also known as fluoroquinolones, each contain a fluorine atom attached to the nucleus at position 6. Cinoxacin, enoxacin, norfloxacin, lomefloxacin, ciprofloxacin, ofloxacin, levofloxacin, sparfloxacin, trovafloxacin, gatifloxacin, gemifloxacin, and moxifloxacin are currently available for clinical use in the United States. Temafloxacin and grepafloxacin have been withdrawn from clinical use due to toxicities. Garenoxacin and sitafloxacin are currently undergoing clinical investigation in the United States. Several closely related fluoroquinolones (enrofloxacin and sarafloxacin) are approved for agricultural and veterinary use in the United States and elsewhere.

Mechanism of Action

The primary bacterial target of the quinolones is DNA gyrase, a type II DNA topoisomerase enzyme essential for DNA replication, recombination, and repair (150). Newer fluoroquinolones also inhibit DNA topoisomerase IV. The DNA gyrase A subunit is the main target of quinolones in gram-negative bacteria, whereas topoisomerase IV is the primary target in gram-positive bacteria. Inhibition of these bacterial enzyme targets causes relaxation or decatenation of the supercoiled DNA, leading to termination of chromosomal replication and interference with cell division and gene expression. By inhibiting bacterial DNA synthesis, these agents are bactericidal. However, the antibacterial activity of quinolones is reduced in the presence of low pH, urine, and divalent cations (Mg^{2+} and Ca^{2+}).

Bacterial resistance to quinolones may occur by one or more of the following mechanisms: single-step chromosomal mutations in the structural genes for DNA gyrase and topoisomerase IV, mutations in the regulatory genes governing bacterial outer membrane permeability to the drug, and expression or overexpression of energy-dependent efflux pumps that can actively remove drugs from the bacterial cell (148, 267). Transferable plasmid-mediated resistance to nalidixic acid and fluoroquinolones can also occur in *Enterobacteriaceae* by acquisition of a resistance gene encoding a protein which inhibits the binding of quinolones to bacterial DNA gyrase (168, 234, 258). In addition, a transferable aminoglycoside acetyltransferase [AAC(6′).1B] has been shown to confer low-level resistance to ciprofloxacin (284a).

Pharmacology

Fluoroquinolones are generally well absorbed from the gastrointestinal tract, with the exception of norfloxacin. The oral bioavailability varies from 60 to 95% for the various fluoroquinolones (325, 375). After oral administration, concentrations in serum peak in 1 to 2 h. The presence of food does not significantly alter the absorption of these drugs. However, coadministration with iron- or zinc-containing multivitamins or with antacids containing aluminum, magnesium, or calcium substantially reduces the gastrointestinal absorption and subsequent peak concentrations of quinolones in serum. The degree of serum protein binding is generally low, ranging from 8% for ofloxacin to 75% for trovafloxacin. The prolonged elimination half-lives of fluoroquinolones, ranging from 3.5 h for ciprofloxacin to 20 h for sparfloxacin, allow for twice- or once-daily dosing (139, 237, 338). Ciprofloxacin, ofloxacin, levofloxacin, trovafloxacin, gatifloxacin, and moxifloxacin are also available for intravenous use. The intravenous formulation of trovafloxacin is prepared as alatrofloxacin mesylate, which is a prodrug of trovafloxacin and is rapidly hydrolyzed in vivo to yield the active drug.

Quinolones have good penetration into the lungs, kidneys, muscle, bone, intestinal wall, and extravascular body fluids. Concentrations in the prostate are about twice those in the serum, and concentrations 25 to 100 times above peak concentrations in serum are achieved in the urine. In the presence of meningeal inflammation, only ofloxacin, levofloxacin, trovafloxacin, gatifloxacin, and moxifloxacin achieve concentrations of >1 μg/ml in the CSF (212, 222). Quinolones penetrate well into phagocytes, such that concentrations within neutrophils and macrophages are as high as 14 times those in serum (340). This feature accounts for their excellent in vivo activity against such intracellular pathogens as *Brucella, Listeria, Salmonella,* and *Mycobacterium* spp.

Trovafloxacin and pefloxacin are metabolized mainly by the liver to form glucuronide conjugates, and pefloxacin is converted into norfloxacin in vivo. Ofloxacin exhibits little or no in vivo metabolism, and it is excreted mainly (90%) via the kidneys. The other quinolones are cleared by both the hepatic and renal routes in various proportions, with elimination primarily via the kidneys. This renal elimination is blocked by probenecid. Small amounts of these drugs are also excreted in the bile.

Hepatic insufficiency prolongs the elimination half-lives of pefloxacin and trovafloxacin, whereas the clearance of other fluoroquinolones is significantly diminished in the presence of renal failure. All of these drugs are only partially removed by hemodialysis ($<15\%$) and are minimally affected by peritoneal dialysis because of their marked extravascular penetration, as reflected in their very large volumes of distribution.

Spectrum of Activity

Quinolones may be categorized into groups with similar spectra of antibacterial activity (Table 3), analogous to the classification of cephalosporins (10). The narrow-spectrum quinolones are inactive against gram-positive cocci, and their clinical utility is limited by widespread prevalence and rapid emergence of bacterial resistance. Broad-spectrum (second-generation) fluoroquinolones are active against both gram-positive and gram-negative bacteria (237, 335,

TABLE 3 Quinolones

Narrow spectrum (first generation)
Cinoxacin
Nalidixic acid
Oxolinic acid
Broad spectrum (second generation)
Ciprofloxacin
Enoxacin
Fleroxacin[a]
Levofloxacin
Lomefloxacin
Norfloxacin
Ofloxacin
Pefloxacin[a]
Rufloxacin[a]
Expanded spectrum (third generation)
Sparfloxacin
Tosufloxacin[a]
Extended spectrum (fourth generation)
Gatifloxacin
Garenoxacin[a]
Gemifloxacin
Moxifloxacin
Sitafloxacin[a]
Trovafloxacin

[a] Not licensed for clinical use in the United States.

346, 378). Increased activity against gram-positive cocci and favorable pharmacodynamic properties (high ratios of area under the curve from 0 to 24 h to MIC) are major features of the newer fluoroquinolones (third and fourth generations), with potencies two- to eightfold greater than those of broad-spectrum agents (9, 23, 37, 62, 64, 75, 82, 217, 271). MIC_{90}s for methicillin-susceptible and -resistant *S. aureus* and coagulase-negative staphylococci are in the range of 0.03 to 1 μg/ml, while methicillin-resistant staphylococci are becoming increasingly resistant to these agents. Although potency against enterococci is lower, gatifloxacin is two- to fourfold (MIC_{90}s of 0.25 to 0.5 μg/ml) and gemifloxacin and moxifloxacin are four- to eightfold (MIC_{90}s of 0.03 to 0.25 μg/ml) more active than levofloxacin against multidrug-resistant *S. pneumoniae*.

In contrast to earlier drugs of this class, many of the expanded- and extended-spectrum quinolones possess potent activity against anaerobes, including members of the *B. fragilis* group and *Clostridium difficile* (57, 95, 257, 317). The relative activities of these newer drugs against all anaerobes in decreasing order of potency are as follows: sitafloxacin > garenoxacin > gatifloxacin, trovafloxacin > moxifloxacin, tosufloxacin. The more active of these agents inhibit *the B. fragilis* group, *Prevotella, Porphyromonas, Fusobacterium, Clostridium,* and anaerobic gram-positive cocci at concentrations of 0.06 to 2 μg/ml. However, increasing fluoroquinolone resistance has emerged among *Bacteroides* spp. since the introduction of the newer drugs (28, 131, 314).

The fluoroquinolones possess excellent activity in vivo against *Enterobacteriaceae, P. aeruginosa, Citrobacter* spp., *Serratia* spp., *Acinetobacter* spp., *H. influenzae*, and gram-negative cocci such as *N. gonorrhoeae, N. meningitidis*, and *M. catarrhalis* (23, 27, 29, 62, 64, 82, 217, 344). Enteropathogenic gram-negative rods such as *Salmonella, Shigella, Yersinia enterocolitica, Vibrio* spp., *Aeromonas* spp., *Plesiomonas* spp., *Campylobacter jejuni*, and enteroinvasive and enterotoxigenic *E. coli* are all susceptible to the quinolones (98, 378). Clinical studies have shown these drugs to be effective in the prophylaxis and treatment of infectious diarrheas. However, reduced susceptibility and resistance to quinolones have emerged in clinical isolates of *Salmonella, Shigella*, and *Campylobacter* spp. (100, 163). *Legionella* spp. are susceptible to these agents, with MICs of most fluoroquinolones of 0.12 to 1.0 μg/ml for these organisms (29, 37, 82, 94). Fluoroquinolones are the first class of oral antibiotics with outstanding potency against *P. aeruginosa*. Ciprofloxacin and trovafloxacin are the most active among these drugs against *P. aeruginosa*, with MIC_{90}s of 0.5 to 1 μg/ml. However, *Burkholderia* spp. and *S. maltophilia* are variably resistant to quinolones (344)

The fluoroquinolones, especially ciprofloxacin, levofloxacin, ofloxacin, and sparfloxacin, are active in vitro against *M. tuberculosis*, the *Mycobacterium fortuitum* group, *Mycobacterium chelonae, Mycobacterium kansasii*, and *Mycobacterium xenopi* (80, 335, 383). Their activity against *Mycobacterium avium* complex is fair to poor. They also exhibit activity against *Chlamydia trachomatis, Chlamydophila pneumoniae*, and *Mycoplasma hominis*, with MIC_{90}s of 0.1 to 1 μg/ml, but are less potent against *Ureaplasma urealyticum* (98, 187). Ciprofloxacin and pefloxacin have been shown to inhibit *Rickettsia conorii, Rickettsia rickettsii*, and *Coxiella burnetii* (281, 282, 382). The broad-spectrum fluoroquinolones also possess potent activity against *Bartonella* spp. (218) and *Brucella melitensis* (101). Although quinolones possess in vitro activity against *Plasmodium falciparum* at achievable concentrations in serum, they are relatively ineffective when used clinically for the treatment of malaria. *Nocardia* spp. are relatively resistant to the quinolones (25, 84).

No significant inoculum effect has been observed among the bacteria susceptible to quinolones. Combinations of quinolones with (β-lactam drugs or aminoglycosides are usually indifferent or additive in their effects against gram-negative and gram-positive bacteria and mycobacteria (378). However, bactericidal activities of quinolones can be antagonized by rifampin or chloramphenicol.

Adverse Effects

Gastrointestinal symptoms, occurring in up to 10% of patients as nausea, vomiting, abdominal discomfort, and diarrhea, are the most common side effects (11, 202, 319). However, *C. difficile* colitis occurs infrequently with the use of quinolones. Headaches, fatigue, insomnia, dizziness, agitation, and, rarely, seizures can occur. These adverse neurologic effects are usually associated with high dosages in elderly patients or concurrent use of nonsteroidal anti-inflammatory drugs.

Allergic reactions are uncommon and often manifest as rash, urticaria, and generalized pruritus. Dose-related photosensitivity occurs most frequently in patients on fleroxacin, sparfloxacin, and lomefloxacin. Prolongation of the QT interval has also occurred with sparfloxacin and grepafloxacin. Rare laboratory abnormalities occurring during fluoroquinolone therapy include elevations in serum transaminases, eosinophilia, leukopenia, and thrombocytopenia. Trovafloxacin is rarely used because it results in rare occurrences of liver dysfunction or failure. Gatifloxacin can cause hypoglycemia and hyperglycemia, and its use is contraindicated in diabetic patients.

Enoxacin and, to a lesser extent, ciprofloxacin and pefloxacin increase the levels of theophylline and caffeine in serum as a result of decreased hepatic clearance (11, 277, 369). Other reported drug interactions include augmentation of the anticoagulant effects of warfarin by ciprofloxacin, norfloxacin, and ofloxacin and an increase in serum cyclosporine levels with ciprofloxacin (277).

Although irreversible cartilage erosions and skeletal abnormalities were observed in studies of quinolone toxicity in animals (11), such effects have not yet been documented clinically. However, quinolones are generally contraindicated for use in patients less than 18 years old and in pregnant or nursing mothers. Tendinitis and tendon rupture, mainly involving the Achilles tendon, have occurred with the use of fluoroquinolones, most frequently with pefloxacin and ciprofloxacin (188).

MACROLIDES

Macrolides have been in use since the early 1950s, with erythromycin as the prototypical antibiotic of this class for over 30 years (355). Their chemical structures consist of a macrocyclic lactone ring attached to two sugar moieties, desosamine and cladinose. They differ from each other in the size (14 to 16 atoms) and substitution pattern of the lactone ring. Erythromycin is a naturally occurring 14-membered-ring macrolide derived from *Streptomyces erythraeus*, and other natural analogs include oleandomycin, spiramycin, and josamycin. Clarithromycin and dirithromycin are 14-membered-ring semisynthetic macrolides, while azithromycin is a 15-membered-ring derivative also known as an azalide, with a nitrogen atom incorporated in its lactone ring. These new macrolides offer significant advantages over erythromycin because of expanded antimicrobial spectra, improved pharmacokinetic parameters, and less frequent adverse effects and drug interactions. Roxithromycin, flurithromycin, and rokitamycin are new macrolides available for clinical use currently in Europe, Asia, and South America (189).

Mechanism of Action

Macrolides are generally bacteriostatic agents that inhibit bacterial RNA-dependent protein synthesis. They may be bactericidal at high drug concentrations and against a small inoculum of bacteria. They bind reversibly to the 23S rRNA of the 50S ribosomal subunits of susceptible organisms, thereby blocking the translocation reaction of polypeptide chain elongation (342). The presence of *erm* gene-encoded rRNA methylases that modify the 23S rRNA target-binding site is the primary mechanism of macrolide resistance and confers macrolide-lincosamide-streptogramin B (MLS_B) coresistance (93). Other less common mechanisms of resistance to macrolides include production of macrolide-inactivating enzymes (esterases, phosphorylases, and glycosidases), *mef* gene-encoded active efflux of drug, and mutations in 23S rRNA and ribosomal proteins (197).

Pharmacology

Erythromycin is available in various topical, parenteral (lactobionate and gluceptate), and oral (base stearate, ethylsuccinate, and estolate) preparations. While clarithromycin and dirithromycin are available only in oral forms, azithromycin is formulated for oral and intravenous administration. When administered orally, erythromycin base is rapidly inactivated by gastric acid, whereas the newer macrolides are stable against acid degradation. Intestinal absorption of erythromycin (except for the estolate form) and azithromycin is reduced up to 50% in the presence of food. Peak levels in serum of 2 to 3, 1 to 2, 0.2 to 0.6, and 0.4 μg/ml are reached at 3 h after oral doses of erythromycin (500 mg), clarithromycin (250 mg), dirithromycin (500 mg), and azithromycin (500 mg), respectively. Much higher concentrations of erythromycin are achieved with intravenous infusion. Tissue distributions of macrolides are excellent, with concentrations in various tissues 10- to 100-fold higher than that in serum (370). The high concentrations reached rapidly within neutrophils and macrophages account for their potent activity against intracellular pathogens (305). They penetrate poorly into the brain and CSF, but they do cross the placenta and are excreted in breast milk.

Erythromycin, clarithromycin, and dirithromycin are metabolized by the liver and primarily excreted in the bile. Azithromycin is excreted largely unchanged in the bile. Clarithromycin exhibits first-pass metabolism, producing a microbiologically active 14-hydroxy derivative that is two to four times more potent than the parent drug against some organisms. Following gastrointestinal absorption, dirithromycin is rapidly converted by nonenzymatic hydrolysis to erythromycylamine, an active derivative with microbiological activity similar to that of its parent compound. Erythromycin, clarithromycin, 14-hydroxy clarithromycin, azithromycin, and dirithromycin have terminal half-lives in serum of 1.5, 5, 8.5, 41, and 44 h, respectively. Because of its exceptionally high tissue penetration, azithromycin has a half-life in tissue of 2 to 4 days (305). Dosage adjustment of clarithromycin is necessary for patients with moderate to severe renal failure (creatinine clearance of <30 ml/min). Except for clarithromycin, macrolides are removed minimally by hemodialysis or peritoneal dialysis.

Spectrum of Activity

Macrolides are relatively broad-spectrum antibiotics, with activity against gram-positive and some gram-negative bacteria, mycoplasmas, chlamydiae, treponemes, and rickettsiae (148, 305, 370). Erythromycin shows good activity against staphylococci and streptococci, including *S. pneumoniae*, but emergence of resistance among these isolates (especially group A streptococci) is a problem in certain parts of the world (55, 190). Erythromycin and dirithromycin exhibit similar in vitro antibacterial activities (22). Clarithromycin is two- to fourfold more active than the other macrolides, and azithromycin is less active than erythromycin against most staphylococci and streptococci (16). These drugs are bactericidal against susceptible strains of streptococci but bacteriostatic toward staphylococci and enterococci. Erythromycin-resistant strains display cross-resistance to these drugs, and methicillin-resistant staphylococci and many enterococci are resistant to all macrolides. These drugs are also active against *Corynebacterium* spp., *L. monocytogenes*, and *Actinomyces israelii* (16).

The antibacterial activity of macrolides against gram-negative rods is influenced by pH, with increasing potency (lower MICs) as the pH rises to 8.5. *H. influenzae* and *M. catarrhalis* are more susceptible to azithromycin (MIC_{90} of 0.5 μg/ml) than to other macrolides (8- to 16-fold-higher MIC_{90}s) (206, 250, 273). However, additive (and possibly synergistic) activity between clarithromycin and its 14-hydroxy metabolite reduces the MIC of clarithromycin for *H. influenzae* two- to fourfold (251). Clarithromycin is the most active drug in this class against *C. pneumoniae* (MIC_{90} of 0.25 μg/ml) and *Legionella* isolates (MIC_{90} of 0.25 μg/ml) (16). All four macrolides are equally potent against *Bordetella pertussis* and *Mycoplasma pneumoniae*, and erythromycin has long been established as the drug of choice for therapy of infections due to these pathogens and *Legionella* spp. Macrolides are active against *Campylobacter* spp., *Helicobacter pylori, P. multocida, N. meningitidis,* and *Borrelia burgdorferi* (16, 225, 273, 341). Unlike other macrolides, azithromycin is also active in vitro against *E. coli, Shigella* spp., *Salmonella* spp., and *Y. enterocolitica* (206, 250).

Macrolide antibiotics are effective in vitro against many pathogens that cause sexually transmitted diseases. *N. gonorrhoeae, Haemophilus ducreyi, C. trachomatis,* and *U. urealyticum* are all susceptible, but only azithromycin is active against *M. hominis* (16, 206). Erythromycin may be used for the treatment of gonorrhea and syphilis in patients who cannot tolerate penicillin G (51), but data on the new macrolides for these indications are limited. Azithromycin is effective as an alternative to tetracyclines for the treatment of genital chlamydial infections (320). As a group, macrolides are among the most potent agents inhibitory toward *Bartonella* spp. (218).

The macrolides have good activity against anaerobic bacteria such as the *B. fragilis* group, *Fusobacterium* spp., *Prevotella* spp., *Porphyromonas* spp., *Propionibacterium acnes,* and anaerobic gram-positive cocci, with MIC_{90}s of 1 to 4 μg/ml (16). Except for dirithromycin, they are active against most *Clostridium* spp., especially *Clostridium perfringens*, with most strains inhibited at ≤1 μg/ml. For this reason, erythromycin is commonly used preoperatively with or without neomycin as oral bowel preparations.

Atypical mycobacteria are more susceptible than *M. tuberculosis* to macrolide antibiotics (206, 251). The MIC_{90}s of clarithromycin and azithromycin for *M. avium* complex are in the range of 2 to 4 μg/ml, allowing additive or synergistic killing activity of these organisms within infected macrophages when these drugs are combined with other antimycobacterial drugs (16). Erythromycin is used occasionally to treat infections due to *Mycobacterium scrofulaceum*, *M. kansasii*, and *M. chelonae* (236, 350) and in combination with ampicillin against *Nocardia asteroides* (113).

Spiramycin and the new macrolides offer comparable in vitro activity against *Toxoplasma gondii*, and they are effective in the treatment of toxoplasmosis (228). Although spiramycin has been used to treat cryptosporidiosis, the therapeutic efficacy remains to be proven (77).

Adverse Effects

The incidence of serious side effects related to the use of erythromycin is relatively low. Gastrointestinal irritation, such as abdominal cramps, nausea, vomiting, and diarrhea, is common with oral administration and can occur when the drug is given intravenously. These side effects occur less frequently with dirithromycin, clarithromycin, and azithromycin. Thrombophlebitis is associated with intravenous infusion, but it can be avoided by dilution of the dose in a large volume of fluid and by slow infusion. Hypersensitivity reactions may include skin rash, fever, and eosinophilia. Cholestatic hepatitis occurring in adults has frequently been associated with the estolate form but has also been reported with other forms of erythromycin (329) and azithromycin (7). For this reason, erythromycin estolate is no longer recommended for use in adults.

Reversible hearing loss may occur with the use of large doses and very high concentrations of erythromycin in serum (≥4 g/day), usually in elderly patients with renal insufficiency (40, 152). Ototoxicity has also been reported with high doses of clarithromycin and azithromycin used to treat *M. avium* complex infections. Pseudomembranous colitis and superinfection of the gastrointestinal tract or vagina with *Candida* spp. or gram-negative rods occur rarely. Concurrent erythromycin therapy increases the levels of theophylline, cyclosporine, and digoxin in serum by interfering with their hepatic metabolism (345). It also increases the anticoagulant effect of warfarin. To date, no clinically significant interactions have been observed between these drugs and dirithromycin, clarithromycin, or azithromycin. However, cardiac arrhythmias have occurred during concurrent use of terfenadine with erythromycin or clarithromycin.

KETOLIDES

Ketolides are semisynthetic derivatives of erythromycin A, having a ketone group instead of an L-cladinose moiety at the 3 position on the erythronolide A ring. This modification of the chemical structure results in increased stability in acid media, noninducibility of MLS_B resistance, and enhanced activity against gram-positive cocci. The ketolides currently under clinical development also have a substituted carbamate link between carbon atoms 11 and 12 in the macrolide nucleus. This modification enables them to retain activity against bacteria whose ribosomes have been methylated at position A2058 as a result of acquired methylase genes (1). Telithromycin is the first and only ketolide approved for clinical use in the United States. Other ketolides, including cethromycin (ABT-773), are undergoing preclinical and clinical studies.

Mechanism of Action

Like the macrolide antibiotics, ketolides inhibit the translation function in susceptible organisms at the level of the 50S ribosomal subunit. Specifically, ketolides interact with the bacterial 23S rRNA at domains II and V of the peptidyltransferase site (147). These drugs are also able to inhibit the formation of the 30S ribosomal unit. Although ketolides do not induce MLS_B resistance, staphylococci with constitutively expressed MLS_B resistance encoded by *erm* genes are resistant to telithromycin. Although these drugs do not appear to be affected by efflux, mutations occurring in 23S rRNA and ribosomal proteins L4 and L22 can lead to in vitro resistance to ketolides (154). This class of drugs has a low potential to select for resistance or induce cross-resistance among other MLS_B antimicrobials.

Pharmacology

Telithromycin is administered orally as a once-daily dose of 800 mg, with rapid gastrointestinal absorption yielding a mean peak concentration in plasma of 2 μg/ml in 1 to 2 h and steady state in 2 days. A mean trough concentration in plasma of 0.07 μg/ml is attained at 24 h after dosing (246). The oral bioavailability of 57% is unaffected by food ingestion. With about 70% of the drug protein bound, telithromycin exhibits biphasic elimination from plasma with initial and terminal half-lives of 2 to 3 h and 9 to 10 h, respectively. The drug penetrates well into bronchopulmonary, tonsillar, and sinus tissues and middle ear fluid, and it is accumulated by polymorphonuclear neutrophils with an intracellular/plasma concentration ratio of >500 at 24 h. Hepatic metabolism with elimination via feces (~80%) is the main route of excretion, and <15% of the administered dose is eliminated in the urine. Dosage adjustments are not necessary in patients with renal or hepatic impairment (86).

Spectrum of Activity

Ketolides possess a good spectrum of potent activity against respiratory pathogens as well as intracellular bacteria, and telithromycin is designed specifically for the treatment of community-acquired respiratory tract infections. It is more active than macrolides against *S. pneumoniae* isolates, irrespective of penicillin susceptibility, with an MIC_{90} of ≤1 μg/ml for telithromycin, and 90% of penicillin-resistant strains are inhibited at 0.25 μg/ml (102, 110, 183, 210). Almost all macrolide-resistant strains of pneumococci are inhibited at ≤0.5 μg/ml, regardless of the underlying mechanism of macrolide resistance. Telithromycin is more active than erythromycin and clarithromycin and as potent as azithromycin against *H. influenzae* (MIC_{90}s of 2 to 4 μg/ml) and *M. catarrhalis* (MIC_{90}s of 0.06 to 0.125 μg/ml). The activity of telithromycin is unaffected by β-lactamase production in these strains, but the MICs are increased twofold in the presence of 5% CO_2. A significant postantibiotic effect may be observed for up to 9 h with this drug against the major respiratory pathogens (86).

Telithromycin is also active against staphylococci, with MIC_{90}s of 0.125 to 0.25 μg/ml for *S. aureus* and coagulase-negative staphylococci, regardless of the susceptibility to oxacillin. However, isolates harboring the constitutive MLS_B mechanism of resistance are resistant to ketolides. Enterococci without underlying resistance to macrolides and clindamycin are susceptible to telithromycin, with MIC_{90}s of 0.125 μg/ml for *E. faecalis* and *E. faecium*. Higher MIC_{90}s (4 to 8 μg/ml) are observed with erythromycin- or clindamycin-resistant enterococci (306). Telithromycin displays good in vitro activity against beta-hemolytic streptococci and viridans group streptococci, regardless of their susceptibility to penicillin G, with all isolates inhibited at ≤0.5 μg/ml. While streptococcal isolates with the *mefA* gene-mediated drug efflux mechanism of resistance to erythromycin remain susceptible to telithromycin, MICs are higher (2 to 16 μg/ml) among the strains with inducible or constitutive *erm* gene-mediated resistance to erythromycin. Other gram-positive cocci, such as *Pediococcus, Leuconostoc, Stomatococcus,* and *Rhodococcus equi*, are susceptible to telithromycin, with MIC_{90}s of 0.03 to 0.25 μg/ml.

This drug is also very active against gram-positive rods, inhibiting *Corynebacterium* (including *C. diphtheriae* and *C. jeikeium*), *Listeria, Lactobacillus, Actinomyces,* and *Erysipelothrix* at concentrations of ≤0.125 μg/ml (306). Telithromycin is inhibitory (MIC_{90}s of 0.125 to 0.5 μg/ml) to *Peptostreptococcus* spp., *Prevotella* spp., *Porphyromonas* spp., *Bilophila* spp., and *C. perfringens,* but it is not active against other *Clostridium* spp., *Fusobacterium* spp., or the *B. fragilis* group (367). This drug has poor activity against other gram-negative rods, including the *Enterobacteriaceae, Acinetobacter* spp., *P. aeruginosa,* and *B. burgdorferi* (166).

Intracellular pathogens, such as *Legionella, Mycoplasma, Chlamydia,* and *Chlamydophila* are highly susceptible to telithromycin, with MIC_{90}s of 0.004 to 0.25 μg/ml (110). *Rickettsia* spp., *Bartonella* spp., *C. burnetii,* and *F. tularensis* are also susceptible to this agent. Telithromycin is comparable to the macrolides in its activity against mycobacteria, with an MIC_{90} of 4 μg/ml for *M. chelonae* and *M. avium* complex, and it is not active against *M. tuberculosis, Mycobacterium bovis,* and other atypical mycobacteria (111).

Adverse Effects

Telithromycin is well tolerated by all patient populations, with gastrointestinal symptoms, such as diarrhea (15%), nausea (9%), vomiting, and dizziness, as the most frequent adverse effects (8). Occurrence of *C. difficile*-associated diarrhea has not been reported in clinical trial studies. While elevation of serum transaminase levels is found in <10% of patients, rare cases of severe hepatotoxicity can occur (60). Since ketolides are substrates and inhibitors of the hepatic cytochrome P450 CYP3A4 isoenzyme pathway, their potential to lengthen the QT interval is augmented by concomitant administration of other CYP3A4 inhibitors, such as ketoconazole and itraconazole (24).

TETRACYCLINES AND GLYCYLCYCLINES

Tetracyclines are broad-spectrum bacteriostatic antibiotics with the hydronaphthacene nucleus, which contains four fused rings. The congeners form three groups based on their duration of action. Chlortetracycline, oxytetracycline, and tetracycline are short-acting drugs, demeclocycline and methacycline are intermediate-acting drugs, and doxycycline and minocycline are long-acting drugs. Glycylcyclines are a group of semisynthetic tetracycline derivatives containing a glycylamido substitution at position 9, and tigecycline (formerly GAR-936, and a 9-*t*-butylglycylamido analog of minocycline) is the first in this class of drugs available for clinical use.

Mechanism of Action

Tetracyclines and glycylcyclines act against susceptible microorganisms by inhibiting protein synthesis. They enter bacteria by an energy-dependent process and bind reversibly to the 30S ribosomal subunits, preventing the attachment of aminoacyl-tRNA to the ribosomal acceptor A-site in the RNA-ribosome complex (56). Resistance to tetracyclines occurs among clinical isolates as a result of active efflux of the drug from the cell, an altered ribosomal target site that prevents binding of the drug (ribosomal protection), or production of modifying enzymes that inactivate the drug. With stearic hindrance from the bulky side group at position 9, glycylcyclines are unaffected by bacterial ribosomal protection proteins and evade the efflux pumps present in tetracycline-resistant strains. These drugs also have higher binding affinity for the bacterial ribosomes than tetracyclines. Reduced susceptibility to tigecycline has been found among clinical and laboratory-derived strains of *P. mirabilis, Morganella morganii, Klebsiella pneumoniae, P. aeruginosa,* and *S. aureus* possessing multicomponent efflux pumps (220, 294) and in some *Bacteroides* spp. with the *tet*(X) gene-mediated monooxygenase enzyme that degrades tetracyclines (238).

Pharmacology

Tetracyclines are incompletely absorbed from the gastrointestinal tract, but their absorption is improved in the fasting state. Ingestion of food, especially dairy products, and other substances such as antacids and iron preparations impairs the absorption of these drugs. Less interference with absorption by foods occurs with doxycycline and minocycline. These long-acting tetracyclines are more readily absorbed, and therefore, lower doses are required. Peak concentrations in serum of 3 to 5 μg/ml are reached in 2 h after standard oral dosages. Intravenous preparations are available, and peak concentrations in serum of 10 to 20 μg/ml are reached in 1 h after intravenous administration. Tetracyclines are usually bacteriostatic at these clinically achievable concentrations in serum.

Tissue penetration of these drugs is excellent, but levels in CSF are low even in the presence of meningeal inflammation. Tetracyclines cross the placenta and are incorporated into fetal bone and teeth. They are excreted in high concentrations in human milk. Therefore, tetracyclines are not advised for pregnant or lactating women. Minocycline, the most lipophilic tetracycline at physiological pH, reaches relatively high concentrations in saliva and tears, making it an ideal antibiotic to eradicate the meningococcal carrier state (146, 158).

Tetracyclines are metabolized by the liver and concentrated in the bile. Biliary concentrations of tetracyclines are three to five times higher than concurrent levels in plasma, with significant drug accumulation in the blood of patients with hepatic insufficiency or biliary obstruction. These drugs are excreted primarily in the urine except for doxycycline, which is excreted primarily (90%) as an inactive conjugate via the biliary tract in the feces. Renal failure prolongs the half-lives of the tetracyclines except doxycycline. Therefore, doxycycline is considered the tetracycline of choice for extrarenal infections in the presence of renal failure.

Tigecycline is administered as an intravenous formulation because of limited oral bioavailability. With multiple doses of 50 mg infused every 12 h, the peak concentration in serum is ~0.8 μg/ml (227). Despite having plasma protein binding of 80%, the drug has a rapid and wide distribution into tissues, with highest levels in bone and bone marrow. Although drug levels of >1 μg/ml can be achieved in CSF in a rabbit model of meningitis, penetration into human CSF with or without meningitis remains unknown (260). It is eliminated primarily by the liver via glucuronidation and biliary excretion of unchanged drug, and the mean elimination half-life is 36 h. With <30% of the drug excreted unchanged in the urine, dosage adjustment is not required for renal insufficiency, hemodialysis, or mild to moderate hepatic dysfunction.

Spectrum of Activity

All tetracyclines have similar antimicrobial spectra, with activity against many gram-positive and gram-negative bacteria, mycoplasmas, chlamydiae, rickettsiae, and some protozoa. Many gram-positive aerobic cocci, including *S. aureus, S. pyogenes,* and *S. pneumoniae,* are susceptible at concentrations achievable in serum. However, tetracycline-resistant strains of *S. pneumoniae* are common (190). Although many *E. coli* isolates are susceptible to tetracyclines, pseudomonads and many *Enterobacteriaceae* are resistant. *Shigella* and *Salmonella* spp. are increasingly resistant to these agents (54). Tetracyclines are used mainly for the treatment of acute, uncomplicated urinary tract infections due to *E. coli* (161) and as effective prophylactic therapy for traveler's diarrhea caused by enterotoxigenic *E. coli* (117). With activity against *Burkholderia pseudomallei, Brucella* spp., *Vibrio* spp., and *Mycobacterium marinum* (351), they have been used successfully in the treatment of infections due to these bacteria. Their efficacy in the therapy of cholera is diminishing owing to the emergence of resistant *Vibrio cholerae* isolates (381). Minocycline is active against *Nocardia* spp. (84). Many anaerobic bacteria, including members of the *B. fragilis* group and *Actinomyces* spp., are susceptible to tetracyclines (265).

These drugs are useful in the treatment of urethritis and acute pelvic inflammatory diseases caused by *N. gonorrhoeae, C. trachomatis, U. urealyticum,* and *M. hominis*. Resistance to tetracyclines among *N. gonorrhoeae* strains is increasing (108). The drugs are effective for the treatment of other chlamydial infections (psittacosis, lymphogranuloma venereum, and trachoma) (51). Other infections responsive to tetracyclines include granuloma inguinale, chancroid, relapsing fever, and tularemia. Tetracyclines are the drugs of choice for treating rickettsial infections (Rocky Mountain spotted fever, endemic and scrub typhus, and Q fever). Many pathogenic spirochetes, including *Treponema pallidum* and *B. burgdorferi,* are susceptible (51, 229, 243). Protozoa such as *P. falciparum* and *Entamoeba histolytica* are also inhibited by these drugs (228, 263).

Due to its potent and wide-spectrum activity against gram-positive, gram-negative, and anaerobic organisms, tigecycline is useful for treatment of complicated skin and skin structure infections, intra-abdominal infections, and nosocomial infections due to multidrug-resistant pathogens except *P. aeruginosa* (32, 119, 156, 167, 260, 264). All staphylococci, including methicillin-resistant and vancomycin-intermediate strains, are inhibited at $\leq$1 μg/ml. Vancomycin-susceptible and -resistant enterococci typically show MIC_{90}s of 0.25 to 0.5 μg/ml, and *E. faecium* and *E. faecalis* are inhibited equally well by this drug. However, tigecycline exhibits no bactericidal activity (minimum bactericidal concentration at which 90% of strains tested are killed [MBC_{90}] > 32 μg/ml) against staphylococci and enterococci in time-kill studies. Viridans group streptococci, beta-hemolytic streptococci, and multidrug-resistant pneumococci are highly susceptible, with MIC_{90}s ranging from $\leq$0.25 to 0.5 μg/ml. The drug is also very active against the *Enterobacteriaceae* and nonfermentative gram-negative rods, including strains producing extended-spectrum β-lactamases, with MIC_{90}s of $\leq$2 μg/ml. Of note is its potent inhibition of multidrug-resistant *Acinetobacter baumannii* and *S. maltophilia* (MIC_{90}s of 2 μg/ml). Among fastidious respiratory tract pathogens, MIC_{90}s are 0.5 and 1 μg/ml for *H. influenzae* and *M. catarrhalis,* respectively. *Proteus, Morganella,* and *Providencia* spp. and *P. aeruginosa* are generally resistant (MIC_{90}s of >16 μg/ml). Tigecycline is also active against most *B. fragilis* group isolates (MIC_{90} = 8 μg/ml), *Peptostreptococcus* spp. (MIC_{90} = 4 μg/ml), *Clostridium* spp. (MIC_{90} = 0.5 μg/ml), *Prevotella* spp., *Propionibacterium* spp., and *Fusobacterium* spp.

Compared to tetracyclines, tigecycline exhibits more potent activity against *M. pneumoniae, M. hominis, C. pneumoniae,* and *C. trachomatis,* with MIC_{90}s in the range of 0.125 to 0.5 μg/ml. It is less active toward *U. urealyticum* and *Legionella* spp., with MIC_{90}s of 8 μg/ml. Rapidly growing mycobacteria, including *Mycobacterium abscessus, M. chelonae,* and the *M. fortuitum* group, are 4- to 11-fold more susceptible (MIC_{90}s of $\leq$0.25 μg/ml) to this drug than to tetracyclines (347). However, slowly growing nontuberculous mycobacteria, such as *M. kansasii, M. marinum,* and *M. xenopi,* are less susceptible to tigecycline than to minocycline.

Susceptibility testing with tigecycline should be done using freshly prepared media or media containing a biocatalytic oxygen-reducing reagent (e.g., Oxyrase), because the drug is prone to oxidative degradation. Testing using aged broth media (prepared >12 h prior to inoculation) yielded MIC results that are generally 1 to 2 dilutions higher than those obtained using fresh media (34, 162).

Adverse Effects

Tetracyclines have irritative effects on the upper gastrointestinal tract, producing esophageal ulcerations, nausea, vomiting, and epigastric distress. Alterations in the enteric flora occur with the use of tetracyclines, often resulting in diarrhea, and pseudomembranous colitis can develop with prolonged use. Hypersensitivity reactions are unusual, generally manifesting themselves as urticaria, fixed drug eruptions, morbilliform rashes, and anaphylaxis. Cross-reactivity among tetracyclines is the rule. Photosensitivity reactions consist of an erythematous rash on areas exposed to sunlight and can occur with all analogs, especially demeclocycline (120).

Minocycline has been known to cause vertigo, and benign intracranial hypertension (pseudotumor cerebri) has been described with many of the analogs (352). Tetracycline can aggravate preexisting renal failure by inhibiting protein synthesis, increasing the azotemia from amino acid metabolism. Tetracyclines cause depression of bone growth, permanent discoloration of the teeth, and enamel hypoplasia when given during tooth and skeletal development (143). Therefore, these drugs are usually avoided in childhood (<8 years of age) and during pregnancy.

Tigecycline is generally well tolerated, with nausea, vomiting, headache, and diarrhea reported as the most common side effects. Due to adverse effects similar to those of tetracyclines on bone and tooth development, use of this drug is contraindicated in pregnant women, nursing mothers, and those <18 years of age. It may also show cross-hypersensitivity to tetracyclines (385).

LINCOSAMIDES

The lincosamide antibiotics include lincomycin, which was initially isolated from *Streptomyces lincolnensis,* and clindamycin, which is a chemical modification of lincomycin. The chemical structure of each drug consists of an amino acid linked to an amino sugar. Compared with lincomycin, clindamycin has increased antibacterial activity and improved absorption after oral administration (224). Both drugs are available for parenteral and oral use, but lincomycin is rarely used now in the United States.

Mechanism of Action

Lincosamides bind to the 50S ribosomal subunits of susceptible bacteria and prevent elongation of peptide chains by interfering with peptidyl transfer, thereby suppressing protein synthesis. The ribosomal binding sites are the same as or closely related to those that bind macrolides, streptogramins, and chloramphenicol (197, 342). Lincosamides can be bactericidal or bacteriostatic, depending on the drug concentration, bacterial species, and inoculum of bacteria.

Pharmacology

About 90% of an oral clindamycin dose is absorbed from the gastrointestinal tract, with no interference from the ingestion of food. A single oral dose of 150 mg yields a peak concentration in serum of 2 to 3 μg/ml in 1 h. Peak levels in serum of 10 to 12 μg/ml are obtained at 1 h after a 600-mg intravenous dose. Therapeutic serum drug levels are maintained for 6 to 9 h after these dosages (199, 224).

Clindamycin distributes well into bone, the lungs, pleural fluid, and bile, but it penetrates poorly into CSF, even with meningitis. It readily crosses the placenta and enters fetal tissues. Clindamycin is actively concentrated in neutrophils and macrophages.

The normal half-life of clindamycin is 2.4 h. Most of the drug is metabolized by the liver and excreted in an inactive form in the urine. Its half-life is prolonged by severe liver dysfunction, necessitating dosage reduction in patients with severe liver disease. Although the serum drug levels are increased in patients with severe renal failure, dose modification is not essential. The drug is not removed significantly by hemodialysis or peritoneal dialysis.

Spectrum of Activity

Lincosamides have a broad spectrum of activity against the aerobic gram-positive cocci and anaerobes. Clindamycin is more potent than lincomycin against methicillin-susceptible *Staphylococcus* spp., *S. pneumoniae,* and group A and viridans group streptococci (199, 224). The MIC_{90}s are in the range of 0.01 to 0.1 μg/ml for these strains. However, resistance to clindamycin has emerged in clinical isolates of these bacteria that are also resistant to erythromycin (55). The prevalence of clindamycin-resistant *S. aureus* may be 15 to 20% in some institutions. Enterococci are uniformly resistant to the lincosamides. All of the *Enterobacteriaceae* are resistant to lincosamides.

Clindamycin is one of the most active antibiotics available against anaerobes, including members of the *B. fragilis* group and *C. perfringens,* with MIC_{90}s of ≤2 μg/ml (18, 199). However, clindamycin resistance (which appears to be increasing) is found in 10 to 15% of *B. fragilis* group organisms, 15 to 20% of *Prevotella* and *Porphyromonas* spp., 10 to 20% of clostridial species, 10% of peptococci, and most *Fusobacterium varium* strains (2, 314). Clindamycin has been used successfully as single-agent therapy for actinomycosis (287), babesiosis (228, 377), and malaria (200). It is also effective in combination with pyrimethamine for toxoplasma encephalitis (76, 286) and in combination with primaquine for *Pneumocystis jirovecii* pneumonia (336).

Adverse Effects

Clindamycin-associated diarrhea occurs in up to 20% of patients, and use of this drug has been associated with pseudomembranous colitis caused by toxin-producing *C. difficile* (19). This complication is not dose related and may occur after oral or parenteral therapy. Prompt cessation of the antibiotic in conjunction with oral vancomycin, metronidazole, or bacitracin therapy is effective in reversing this complication.

Other uncommon side effects include skin rashes, fever, and reversible elevation of serum transaminases. Clindamycin can block neuromuscular transmission and may potentiate the action of neuromuscular blocking agents during anesthesia.

GLYCOPEPTIDES AND LIPOPEPTIDES

Vancomycin, a bactericidal antibiotic obtained from *Streptomyces orientalis*, is the only glycopeptide marketed for clinical use in the United States. Initially introduced for its efficacy against penicillin-resistant staphylococci, it has become most useful against methicillin-resistant staphylococci and in patients allergic to penicillins or cephalosporins. Teicoplanin (formerly teichomycin A), a new complex glycopeptide chemically related to vancomycin (315), is currently available for clinical use in most countries of the world except the United States. Dalbavancin, oritavancin, and telavancin are semisynthetic lipoglycopeptides (glycopeptide derivatives with hydrophobic substituents) currently at various stages of clinical development (185, 262). Daptomycin is a unique, naturally occurring cyclic lipopeptide antibiotic found among the fermentation by-products of *Streptomyces roseosporus* and has potent activity against gram-positive bacteria. Ramoplanin is an investigational semisynthetic lipoglycodepsipeptide with a spectrum of activity similar to those of the glycopeptides (103), but systemic toxicity limits its clinical trials only to oral administration and topical application.

Mechanism of Action

Glycopeptides inhibit peptidoglycan synthesis in the bacterial cell wall by complexing with the D-alanyl-D-alanine portion of the cell wall precursor (244). Resistance to vancomycin and teicoplanin can occur by one of two mechanisms: (i) the presence of a complex series of bacterial cytoplasmic enzymes in vancomycin-resistant enterococci synthesizing abnormal peptidoglycan precursors terminating in D-Ala-D-lactate residues (instead of D-Ala-D-Ala), thereby markedly lowering the binding affinity with the glycopeptides (52), or (ii) increased accumulation of peptidoglycan precursors (murein monomers) resulting in a thickened cell wall with "trapping" of drug molecules, thereby preventing further diffusion of drug into the inner part of cell wall layers of vancomycin-intermediate *S. aureus* (69, 70, 153).

Daptomycin binds irreversibly to the cytoplasmic membrane of susceptible bacteria via a calcium ion-dependent insertion of the hydrophobic tail of the molecule and causes membrane depolarization, resulting in release of potassium ions and disruption of cellular ion concentration gradients (44, 311). The end effect is cell death without cell lysis, providing potent bactericidal activity of this drug. It is unable to penetrate the outer membrane of gram-negative bacteria. Resistance to daptomycin has occurred in enterococci (208, 297) and *S. aureus* (151, 312), possibly due to the physical barrier of a thickened bacterial cell wall similar to those found in vancomycin-intermediate *S. aureus* or to other mechanisms, such as alteration of the charge of the outer cell envelope (71).

Ramoplanin acts by binding to a lipid II intermediate present in the cell membrane of gram-positive organisms and inhibiting bacterial transglycosylase (PBP 1b), an enzyme essential for peptidoglycan synthesis. With this unique mechanism of action, this drug is bactericidal against vancomycin-resistant enterococci and staphylococci.

Pharmacology

Vancomycin and teicoplanin can be administered orally or parenterally. After oral administration, the drugs are poorly absorbed, and high concentrations in stools are achieved, accounting for their efficacy in treating pseudomembranous colitis (109). Desirable peak and trough levels in serum of 20 to 50 μg/ml and 5 to 15 μg/ml, respectively, are obtained after a 1-g intravenous dose of vancomycin every 12 h in healthy subjects (296). Similar serum drug concentrations are reached with intravenous teicoplanin, which has the advantage of a longer serum half-life and which can be administered once daily. Therapeutic levels of both drugs are achieved in synovial, ascitic, pericardial, and pleural fluids, with variable penetration into the CSF only in the presence of inflamed meninges (144, 234).

Vancomycin and teicoplanin have half-lives in serum of 6 and 45 h, respectively, in patients with healthy renal function, and they are eliminated from the body by glomerular filtration. In severe renal insufficiency, their excretion is prolonged to about 9 days, and they are not removed by hemodialysis or peritoneal dialysis.

Intravenous infusion of daptomycin at 6 mg/kg of body weight results in peak and trough concentrations of 82 and 6 μg/ml, respectively, in serum. About 90% of the drug is bound to plasma proteins, with limited metabolism. Despite its wide distribution into various body sites and tissues, daptomycin shows poor penetration into the CSF and alveolar space, where it is bound by surfactant, precluding its use for the treatment of meningitis and pneumonia (323). Its elimination half-life is 9 h, and 80% of the drug excreted via the kidneys, with two-thirds as intact drug (299). The dosing interval is increased to every 48 h when creatinine clearance is ≤30 ml/min.

Without systemic absorption or intestinal degradation of the drug, ramoplanin administered orally at dosages of 200 and 400 mg twice daily reaches high concentrations in the stool, with mean minimum drug levels of ~460 and ~760 μg/g in the feces, respectively. This feature enables the drug to be developed for clinical trials in treatment of *C. difficile*-associated diarrhea and gastrointestinal decolonization to prevent nosocomial bacteremia due to vancomycin-resistant enterococci.

Spectrum of Activity

Glycopeptides and lipopeptides are active mainly against aerobic and anaerobic gram-positive organisms, including methicillin-susceptible and -resistant staphylococci, streptococci, enterococci, *Corynebacterium* spp., *Bacillus* spp., *L. monocytogenes, Clostridium* spp., and *Actinomyces* spp. The MICs of vancomycin for *S. aureus, S. epidermidis,* streptococci, and enterococci are typically in the range of 0.25 to 2 μg/ml (176). The bactericidal activity varies, with MBCs 20-fold higher than MICs for viridans group streptococci. These agents are essentially bacteriostatic against enterococci and staphylococci. Teicoplanin (138, 141, 211), ramoplanin (65), and daptomycin (14, 211, 374) are two- to fourfold more active than vancomycin against these gram-positive cocci. Resistance to vancomycin has emerged among clinical isolates of enterococci (52) and staphylococci (153). Cross-resistance with teicoplanin is variable in these strains, but most are susceptible to daptomycin and ramoplanin (172), with MICs of ≤2 μg/ml. Other naturally vancomycin-resistant gram-positive organisms, such as *Leuconostoc, Lactobacillus,* and *Pediococcus* spp., are susceptible to ramoplanin (65, 172, 293).

Vancomycin is useful in the prevention and treatment of endocarditis due to gram-positive bacteria in patients who are allergic to penicillin (74, 371). It is the drug of choice for treating *C. jeikeium* infections (128) and is useful for *Chryseobacterium meningosepticum* meningitis (144) and antibiotic-associated *C. difficile* colitis (19, 109).

The glycopeptides and lipopeptides are not active against gram-negative organisms or mycobacteria. They show no cross-resistance with other unrelated antibiotics. They act synergistically with aminoglycosides or rifampin against staphylococci, streptococci, and enterococci (240, 337, 356, 357), and they are bactericidal with aminoglycosides against *Listeria* spp.

Daptomycin exhibits concentration-dependent bactericidal activity in vitro against most gram-positive bacteria in their growing and stationary phases (295). The MIC_{90}s for multidrug-resistant isolates of staphylococci (including vancomycin-intermediate *S. aureus*), pneumococci, and streptococci are ≤1 μg/ml (182, 327, 328). Vancomycin-susceptible and -resistant enterococci are inhibited equally at an MIC_{90} of ≤4 μg/ml (182, 327). The drug is active (MIC_{90}s of ≤2 μg/ml) against *Listeria, Corynebacterium* spp., *Propionibacterium* spp., *C. difficile, C. perfringens,* and peptostreptococci (134). While *Leuconostoc, Pediococcus,* and *Lactobacillus* are susceptible, other *Clostridium* spp., *Actinomyces,* and *Eubacterium* showed MIC_{90}s in the range of 4 to 16 μg/ml. Since optimal in vitro activity of daptomycin depends on the calcium ion concentration in the growth medium, media used for susceptibility testing with this drug should contain the recommended calcium concentration of 50 μg/ml. Current E-test strips of daptomycin used in the drug gradient diffusion method are manufactured with added calcium. Inconsistent results have been observed with the disk diffusion method, and the agar dilution method has not been validated for testing this drug.

Adverse Effects

The most frequent side effects of vancomycin are fever, chills, and phlebitis at the site of infusion. Rapid or bolus infusion of vancomycin causes tingling and flushing of the face, neck, and thorax, known as the red man syndrome, as a result of histamine release by basophils and mast cells (278). This phenomenon is not due to allergic hypersensitivity. Allergic maculopapular or diffuse erythematous rashes can occur in up to 5% of patients. Reversible leukopenia or eosinophilia can rarely develop with glycopeptide use.

Hearing loss due to ototoxicity has been described occasionally for patients in whom serum vancomycin concentrations exceed 50 μg/ml, but it is hard to find unequivocal evidence of vancomycin ototoxicity in humans or animals (40). Vancomycin-induced nephrotoxicity has been rare since the recent availability of highly purified vancomycin preparations. However, the risk of nephrotoxicity increases during combination therapy with vancomycin and aminoglycosides.

Teicoplanin is generally well tolerated and does not produce the red man syndrome or nephrotoxicity. It does cause irritation at the site of intravenous infusion, and ototoxicity has been reported (78).

Common adverse reactions of daptomycin include diarrhea, rash, dizziness, and dyspnea. Elevated serum creatinine phosphokinase levels, myalgias, and reversible myopathy can occur (4, 45), but these adverse effects are significantly reduced with lower dosages and once-daily dosing.

STREPTOGRAMINS

Streptogramins are natural cyclic peptides produced by *Streptomyces* spp. They are a unique class of antibiotics in which each member of the class is a combination of at least two structurally unrelated components, group A and B streptogramins, acting synergistically against susceptible bacteria (269). Group A streptogramins are polyunsaturated macrolactones consisting of lactam and lactone linkages with an oxazole ring, and the main compounds in this group are pristinamycin II_A and pristinamycin II_B. Group B streptogramins are cyclic hexadepsipeptides, with pristinamycin I_A and pristinamycin I_C as the principal compounds. Quinupristin-dalfopristin is the first injectable streptogramin antibiotic combination developed for clinical use in the United States. It is a 30:70 mixture of the semisynthetic streptogramins quinupristin and dalfopristin, which are water-soluble derivatives of pristinamycin I_A and pristinamycin II_A, respectively.

Mechanism of Action

The streptogramins exert a synergistic bactericidal effect on susceptible organisms by inhibiting bacterial protein synthesis. They enter bacterial cells via passive diffusion and then bind specifically and irreversibly to the 50S subunits of the 70S bacterial ribosomes. Binding of group A streptogramins to the ribosome induces a conformational change in the ribosome which increases its affinity for group B compounds. Group A streptogramins prevent peptide bond formation during the chain elongation step, while group B components cause release of the incomplete peptide chains from the 50S ribosomal subunit (342).

Acquired bacterial resistance to the streptogramins, which may be chromosomal or plasmid mediated, is mainly due to modification of the drug target by methylation of the bacterial 23S rRNA, resulting in resistance to all macrolides, lincosamides, and group B streptogramins (MLS_B resistance phenotype), but not to group A streptogramins. Mutations in the L22 ribosomal protein gene (*rplV*), active efflux of group A and B streptogramins, and drug inactivation by streptogramin A acetylase and streptogramin B hydrolase have been described.

Pharmacokinetics

Quinupristin-dalfopristin is administered intravenously, with distribution into most tissues. Both components are highly protein bound (70 to 90%) and rapidly cleared from plasma via biliary excretion by hepatic conjugation processes (209). Less than 20% of the administered drug combination is excreted in the urine. Following intravenous doses of 7.5 mg/kg, peak concentrations in serum of quinupristin and dalfopristin reach 2.7 and 7.2 μg/ml, respectively, with elimination half-lives of 1 and 0.75 h. The two components penetrate and accumulate in macrophages, and the ratio of peak in vitro cellular and extracellular concentrations is 50:35. The drug combination does not cross the noninflamed blood-brain barrier or placenta to any significant degree. Dosage adjustment is needed for patients with renal insufficiency (creatinine clearance of <30 min/min), and the drug combination is removed in modest amounts by dialysis.

Spectrum of Activity

Streptogramins are active mainly against gram-positive bacteria, with modest activities against selected gram-negative and anaerobic pathogens. Quinupristin-dalfopristin has potent bactericidal activity against methicillin-susceptible and -resistant *S. aureus*, coagulase-negative staphylococci, and streptococci, with MIC_{90}s of ≤1 μg/ml and MBCs within two- to fourfold of the MICs (31, 112). Staphylococci and streptococci, including *S. pneumoniae*, that are resistant to β-lactam drugs, macrolides, and fluoroquinolones usually remain susceptible to quinupristin-dalfopristin. While most *E. faecium* strains (MIC_{90}s of ≤4 μg/ml) are susceptible, *E. faecalis* is intrinsically resistant (MIC_{90}s ≥32 μg/ml) to the drug combination because of active efflux of dalfopristin. Although it is not bactericidal against enterococci, quinupristin-dalfopristin inhibits vancomycin-resistant *E. faecium* (VanA or VanB phenotype), including multidrug-resistant strains, at MIC_{90}s of ≤2 μg/ml (209). This drug combination has been a significant addition to the current therapeutic options for serious multidrug-resistant gram-positive bacterial infections (195, 201, 235, 270). *N. meningitidis, N. gonorrhoeae, M. pneumoniae, C. pneumoniae*, and *Legionella pneumophila* are all highly susceptible to the drug (MIC_{90}s of ≤2 μg/ml). Quinupristin-dalfopristin is also active against *M. catarrhalis* and *H. influenzae*, with MIC_{90}s of ≤4 μg/ml. *Enterobacteriaceae* and other nonfermenting gram-negative rods are resistant.

Among the anaerobes, *C. perfringens* and *C. difficile* are the most susceptible (MIC_{90}s of 0.25 μg/ml). Quinupristin-dalfopristin is active against the *B. fragilis* group (MIC_{90} of 4 μg/ml) as well as other anaerobic bacteria, including *Prevotella, Porphyromonas, Fusobacterium, P. acnes, Lactobacillus*, and peptostreptococci, with MIC_{90}s of 2 to 4 μg/ml.

Adverse Effects

Phlebitis at the site of intravenous infusion is the major local adverse reaction, and the incidence and severity are dose and concentration related (209, 292). The most common systemic side effects that may lead to discontinuation of therapy are arthralgias and myalgia, both of which are reversible on discontinuation of the combination (235, 280). Elevated levels of serum transaminases and cutaneous reactions such as itching, burning, and erythema of the face, neck, or upper body have also been reported.

OXAZOLIDINONES

Oxazolidinones are a unique group of synthetic antibiotics originally discovered in the 1970s (216). Linezolid is currently the only oxazolidinone available for clinical use (233), while other analogs are undergoing preclinical development.

Mechanism of Action

The oxazolidinones inhibit bacterial protein synthesis by preventing the formation of a functional initiation complex consisting of $tRNA^{fMet}$, mRNA, initiation factors, and the ribosome (330). Linezolid binds to the domain V region of 23S rRNA in the 50S ribosomal subunit, thereby distorting the binding site for $tRNA^{fMet}$ and inhibiting formation of a functional 70S initiation complex, thus preventing initiation of mRNA translation. In this regard, this class of antibiotics is unique, without cross-resistance with other antibiotics that also inhibit ribosomal protein synthesis. Resistance to linezolid has occurred in clinical isolates of methicillin-resistant *S. aureus*, vancomycin-resistant enterococci, and pneumococci as a result of point mutations in genes encoding the 23S rRNA (30, 231) or L4 ribosomal protein (379). Oxazolidinones are generally inactive against gram-negative bacteria because of endogenous efflux pumps present in these organisms (330).

Pharmacology

Linezolid is available in oral and parenteral forms. Rapid and extensive absorption occurs after oral administration (>95% bioavailability), reaching maximum concentrations in serum of 15 to 20 μg/ml within 2 h after an oral dose of 600 mg. The drug is metabolized primarily in the liver, and the elimination half-life is about 5 h. With 30% of the drug being protein bound, it is well distributed in all body tissues, including the CSF. The drug is eliminated via the kidneys, with 30% being excreted unchanged in the urine. No dose adjustment is necessary in patients with renal insufficiency or mild to moderate hepatic impairment, while 20% of a dose is removed by hemodialysis (213).

Spectrum of Activity

As a group, oxazolidinones have various activities against most gram-positive bacteria and mycobacteria. Linezolid has excellent activity against staphylococci (including methicillin-resistant strains), streptococci, and multidrug-resistant enterococci, with MIC_{90}s ranging from 1 to 4 μg/ml (61, 203,

386). The MIC_{90}s are in the range of 0.5 to 2 μg/ml for pneumococci. Although the antibacterial effect of linezolid is generally bacteriostatic, the drug is bactericidal against most strains of staphylococci and pneumococci. Other bacteria that are inhibited by linezolid include *Actinomyces* spp., *Bacillus cereus, Corynebacterium* spp., *Leuconostoc* spp., *Pediococcus* spp., *R. equi, L. monocytogenes, Clostridium* spp., and gram-positive anaerobic cocci (134). Both slowly and rapidly growing *Mycobacterium* spp. and *Nocardia* spp. are also susceptible to linezolid, with MIC_{90}s of ≤8 μg/ml (38, 39, 348). Linezolid is an important therapeutic option for skin and soft tissue infections (149, 360), respiratory tract infections (290), and infections due to methicillin-resistant staphylococci (309, 326) and vancomycin-resistant enterococci (272, 276).

Adverse Effects

The most common drug-related adverse events (≤5% incidence) are diarrhea, headache, and nausea (118, 291). Prolonged use of linezolid (usually for >28 days) has led to rare optic neuropathy (198), peripheral neuropathy (36), and myelosuppression, including anemia, leukopenia, thrombocytopenia, and pancytopenia that are reversible upon discontinuation of therapy (6, 129). As a mild nonselective inhibitor of monoamine oxidase, linezolid can interact with adrenergic or serotonergic drugs, and rare cases of serotonin syndrome have been reported with concomitant use of selective serotonin reuptake inhibitor drugs (26, 181).

SULFONAMIDES AND TRIMETHOPRIM (TMP)

Sulfonamides were the first effective systemic antimicrobial agents used in the United States during the 1930s. They are derived from sulfanilamide, which shares chemical similarities with *para*-aminobenzoic acid, a factor essential for bacterial folic acid synthesis. Various substitutions at the sulfonyl radical attached to the benzene ring nucleus enhance the antibacterial activity and also determine the pharmacological properties of the drug.

TMP is a pyrimidine analog that inhibits the enzyme dihydrofolate reductase, interfering with folic acid metabolism, subsequent pyrimidine synthesis, and one-carbon fragment metabolism in the bacteria. Since TMP and sulfonamides block the bacterial folic acid metabolic pathway at different sites, they potentiate the antibacterial activity of one another and act synergistically against a wide variety of organisms. Such a combination, TMP-sulfamethoxazole (TMP-SMX), also called co-trimoxazole, was introduced clinically in 1968 and has proven to be very effective in the treatment of many infections (289, 300).

Mechanism of Action

Sulfonamides competitively inhibit bacterial modification of *para*-aminobenzoic acid into dihydrofolate, whereas TMP inhibits bacterial dihydrofolate reductase. This sequential inhibition of folate metabolism ultimately prevents the synthesis of bacterial DNA (155). Since mammalian cells do not synthesize folic acid, human purine synthesis is not affected significantly by sulfonamides or TMP. The antibacterial effect of these agents may be reduced in patients receiving high doses of folinic acid.

Pharmacology

Sulfonamides are usually administered in the oral and topical forms; the intravenous preparations (sulfadiazine and sulfisoxazole) are rarely used. The sulfonamides vary in their durations of action. Thus, sulfamethizole and sulfisoxazole are short-acting compounds, sulfadiazine and SMX are intermediate-acting compounds, and sulfadoxine is a long-acting compound. Mafenide acetate (Sulfamylon cream) and silver sulfadiazine are applied topically to burn patients and have significant percutaneous absorption. Sulfacetamide is available as an ophthalmic preparation, and various combinations of other sulfonamides are available orally (triple sulfa, or trisulfapyrimidine) or as vaginal creams or suppositories.

The orally administered sulfonamides are absorbed rapidly and completely from the gastrointestinal tract. They are metabolized in the liver by acetylation and glucuronidation and are excreted by the kidneys as free drug and inactive metabolites. Sulfonamides compete for bilirubin-binding sites on plasma albumin and increase levels of unconjugated bilirubin in blood. For this reason they should not be given to neonates, in whom increased serum bilirubin levels may cause kernicterus.

Sulfonamides are well distributed throughout the body, with levels in the CSF and synovial, pleural, and peritoneal fluids about 80% of concentrations in serum. They readily cross the placenta and enter the fetal circulation. Sulfonamides may be used in renal failure, but the drugs may accumulate during prolonged therapy as a result of reduced renal excretion.

TMP is available only for oral use and is absorbed almost completely from the gastrointestinal tract. After the usual 100-mg dose, peak levels in serum reach 1 μg/ml in 1 to 4 h. This drug distributes widely in body tissues, including the kidneys, lungs, and prostate, and in body fluids (267). Concentrations in CSF are about 40% of levels in serum. Its half-life in serum is about 10 h in healthy subjects and is prolonged in those with renal insufficiency. Up to 80% of a dose is excreted unchanged in the urine by tubular secretion; the remaining fraction is excreted as inactive metabolites by the kidneys or in the bile.

A fixed combination of TMP-SMX in a dose ratio of 1:5 is available for oral and intravenous use. An intravenous dose of 160 mg of TMP with 800 mg of SMX produces average peak levels in serum of 3.4 and 47.3 μg/ml, respectively, in 1 h. Similar peak levels are reached at 2 to 4 h after the same dose is taken orally. Widely distributed in the body, both drugs reach therapeutic levels in the CSF (40% of levels in serum). Excretion is primarily by the kidneys; dosage reduction is necessary in patients with creatinine clearances of ≤30 ml/min. Both TMP and SMX are removed by hemodialysis and partially by peritoneal dialysis.

Spectrum of Activity

Sulfonamides are inhibitory to a variety of gram-positive and gram-negative bacteria, actinomycetes, chlamydiae, toxoplasmas, and plasmodia. Their in vitro antimicrobial activities are irregular, being strongly influenced by inoculum size and composition of the test media. Susceptibility testing endpoints are often difficult to determine because of the presence of hazy growth within zones of inhibition in disk diffusion tests and because of the phenomenon of "trailing" in dilution tests. Sulfadiazine and sulfisoxazole are effective for rheumatic fever prophylaxis, but they are not useful in treating established group A beta-hemolytic streptococcal pharyngitis. These drugs may be used for prophylaxis of close contacts of patients with meningitis due to sulfonamide-susceptible *N. meningitidis*. Sulfisoxazole can be used to treat chlamydial urethritis, and sulfacetamide ophthalmic solution is effective for trachoma and inclusion conjunctivitis.

Sulfadiazine in combination with pyrimethamine has been used successfully to treat toxoplasmosis, and sulfadoxine combined with pyrimethamine (Fansidar) is effective in the prophylaxis and therapy of *P. falciparum* malaria (228, 230). Sulfonamides are active against *N. asteroides* (84), and they show moderate activity against *M. kansasii*, the *M. fortuitum* group, *M. marinum*, and *M. scrofulaceum* (285). Other uses of sulfonamides include therapy of melioidosis, dermatitis herpetiformis, lymphogranuloma venereum, and chancroid.

Among the gram-negative rods, *E. coli* strains were initially susceptible to the sulfonamides, especially at levels achievable in the urine. Therefore, these drugs have been used primarily in the treatment of first-episode acute urinary tract infections due to *E. coli*. However, increasing bacterial resistance has limited their efficacy in recent years. *S. marcescens*, *P. aeruginosa*, enterococci, and anaerobes are usually resistant to the sulfonamides.

TMP is active in vitro against many gram-positive cocci and most gram-negative rods. *P. aeruginosa*, most anaerobes, *M. pneumoniae*, and mycobacteria are resistant. The MIC varies considerably with the test media used. Like the sulfonamides, TMP is used primarily in the therapy of uncomplicated and recurrent urinary tract infections due to susceptible organisms (161). However, the prevalence of TMP-resistant *Enterobacteriaceae* is increasing (135).

Combinations of TMP with other agents, such as rifampin, polymyxins, and aminoglycosides, have demonstrated in vitro synergistic activity against various gram-negative rods. TMP combined with dapsone is effective in the treatment of *P. jirovecii* pneumonia in immunocompromised patients.

Many gram-positive cocci, including staphylococci and streptococci, and most gram-negative rods except *P. aeruginosa* are susceptible to TMP-SMX (43). However, 10 to 50% of strains of *S. pneumoniae* are resistant in many parts of the world (190). The drug combination has variable bactericidal effects on enterococci in vitro, depending on the test media used for susceptibility testing (245). Unlike many bacteria that can utilize only thymidine for growth, enterococci can use thymidine, thymine, exogenous folinic acid, dihydrofolate, and tetrahydrofolate, resulting in higher MICs (25- to 50-fold increase) on media containing these compounds (241). This fact also explains the ineffectiveness of TMP-SMX against enterococci in vivo.

With good activity against *M. catarrhalis* and *H. influenzae*, including β-lactamase-producing strains, TMP-SMX is useful for the therapy of acute otitis media, sinusitis, acute bronchitis, and pneumonia. It has shown excellent results in the prophylaxis and therapy of acute and chronic urinary tract infections (161, 321). It is an effective alternative therapy for uncomplicated urogenital gonorrhea, including cases caused by penicillinase-producing *N. gonorrhoeae* (51). It can also be used for the treatment of chancroid, but resistance to TMP-SMX in *H. ducreyi* is increasing. The drug combination is also useful in treating infections due to salmonellae, shigellae, enteropathogenic *E. coli*, and *Y. enterocolitica* (243). It has been used successfully for prophylaxis and treatment of traveler's diarrhea (90), but resistance to TMP-SMX in *Shigella* spp. and *E. coli* now severely limits its usefulness in many parts of the world.

Other microorganisms susceptible to TMP-SMX include *Brucella* spp., *B. pseudomallei*, *B. cepacia*, *S. maltophilia*, *M. kansasii*, *M. marinum*, and *M. scrofulaceum*. *M. tuberculosis* and *M. chelonae* are generally resistant. It is a valuable antibiotic for the treatment of *N. asteroides* infections (349), *B. cepacia* and *S. maltophilia* bacteremia, *L. monocytogenes* meningitis, gastroenteritis due to *Isospora belli* and *Cyclospora* spp. (228, 266), and Whipple's disease. In immunocompromised hosts (e.g., those with leukemia or AIDS and organ transplant recipients), TMP-SMX is effective for the prophylaxis and treatment of *P. jirovecii* pneumonia (49, 50, 384).

Adverse Effects

Sulfonamides are known to cause nausea, vomiting, headache, and fever. Hypersensitivity reactions can occur as rashes, vasculitis, erythema nodosum, erythema multiforme, and Stevens-Johnson syndrome (46). Very high doses of less-water-soluble sulfonamides such as sulfadiazine may result in crystalluria, with renal tubular deposits of sulfonamide crystals. Bone marrow toxicity with anemia, leukopenia, or thrombocytopenia can occur. Sulfonamides should be avoided in patients with glucose-6-phosphate dehydrogenase deficiency because of associated hemolytic anemia. Sulfonamides also potentiate the effects of warfarin, phenytoin, and oral hypoglycemic agents.

In general, TMP is well tolerated. With prolonged use, megaloblastic anemia, neutropenia, and thrombocytopenia can develop, especially in folate-deficient patients. Adverse reactions to TMP-SMX due to either the TMP or, more commonly, the SMX component can occur. Mild gastrointestinal symptoms and allergic skin rashes occur in about 3% of patients (196). Megaloblastic bone marrow changes with leukopenia, thrombocytopenia, or granulocytopenia may develop, usually in patients with preexisting folate deficiency. Nephrotoxicity usually occurs in patients with underlying renal dysfunction. Patients with AIDS have a much higher frequency of adverse reactions (as much as 70%) (137).

POLYPEPTIDES

■ Polymyxins

Polymyxins are a group of related cyclic basic polypeptides originally derived from *Bacillus polymyxa*. They have limited spectra of antimicrobial activity and significant toxicity. Only polymyxins B and E (colistin) are available for therapeutic use in humans.

Mechanism of Action

Acting like detergents or surfactants, members of this group of antibiotics interact with the phospholipids of the bacterial cell membrane, thereby increasing cell permeability and disrupting osmotic integrity. This process results in leakage of intracellular constituents, leading to cell death. The bactericidal action is reduced in the presence of calcium, which interferes with the attachment of drugs to the cell membrane.

Pharmacology

The polymyxins are usually administered via the parenteral, oral, or topical route. They are not significantly absorbed when given orally or topically, and intramuscular injections can be painful. Peak concentrations in serum of 5 μg/ml are obtained with a total daily dose of intravenous polymyxin B at 2.5 mg (25,000 U)/kg of body weight. Colistin sulfate is given orally for local antibacterial effect in the gut, while colistimethate sodium, a sulfomethyl derivative of colistin, is used for intravenous or intramuscular injections. The half-life of polymyxin B in serum is about 6 to 7 h, and that of colistin is 2 to 4 h. They do not penetrate well into pleural fluid, synovial fluid, or CSF, even in the presence of inflammation. Excretion is mostly via the kidneys by glomerular filtration. Levels in serum and toxicity are increased in states of renal insufficiency. These drugs are not removed by hemodialysis, but small amounts can be removed by peritoneal dialysis.

Polymyxin is often used topically as 0.1% polymyxin in combination with bacitracin or neomycin for treatment of skin, mucous membrane, eye, and ear infections. It is poorly absorbed from these surfaces. When the drug is used for irrigation of serous or wound cavities, systemic absorption can be significant enough to produce toxicity.

Spectrum of Activity

Polymyxins are active only against gram-negative rods, especially *Pseudomonas* spp. The MIC_{90}s for *Pseudomonas* spp., including *P. aeruginosa,* are <8 μg/ml. *Proteus, Providencia, Serratia,* and *Neisseria* isolates are usually resistant. Emergence of resistance during therapy is rare, and there is no cross-resistance with other antibiotics. Polymyxins B and E have identical antimicrobial spectra and show complete cross-resistance to one another.

The combination of polymyxins with TMP-SMX may be synergistic in the treatment of serious infection due to multiply resistant *Serratia* spp., *P. aeruginosa, B. cepacia,* and *S. maltophilia* (83, 288). The polymyxins are usually reserved for serious, life-threatening *Pseudomonas* or gram-negative rod infections caused by organisms resistant to all other antibiotics. Aerosolized polymyxins have been used successfully to treat *P. aeruginosa* colonization or respiratory infections in patients with cystic fibrosis or bronchiectasis (107).

Adverse Effects

Neurotoxicity and nephrotoxicity are the two major side effects of polymyxins. Paresthesia with flushing, dizziness, vertigo, ataxia, slurred speech, drowsiness, or mental confusion occurs when levels in serum exceed 1 to 2 μg/ml. Polymyxins also have a curare-like effect that can block neuromuscular transmission. Dose-related renal dysfunction occurs in about 20% of patients receiving appropriate therapeutic dosages. Allergic reactions such as fever and skin rashes are rare, but urticaria and shock after rapid intravenous infusion have occurred.

■ Bacitracin

Originally isolated from *Bacillus licheniformis* (formerly *Bacillus subtilis*), bacitracin is a peptide antibiotic consisting of peptide-linked amino acids. Although it was introduced initially for the systemic treatment of severe staphylococcal infections, it is now mainly restricted to topical use because of its systemic toxicity.

Mechanism of Action

Bacitracin inhibits dephosphorylation of a lipid pyrophosphate, a step essential for bacterial cell wall synthesis. It also disrupts the bacterial cytoplastic membrane.

Pharmacology

Bacitracin is often used in various topical preparations, such as creams, ointments, antibiotic sprays and powders, and solutions for wound irrigation or bladder instillation. When used as a topical antibiotic, no significant amount of bacitracin is absorbed systemically. Large doses used to irrigate serous cavities may be associated with systemic toxicity.

Spectrum of Activity

The drug is active mainly against gram-positive bacteria, especially staphylococci and group A beta-hemolytic streptococci. However, group C and G streptococci are less susceptible, and group B streptococci are resistant (113). *Neisseria* spp. are also susceptible, but gram-negative rods are resistant. Bacitracin is often combined with neomycin, polymyxin B, or both in topical preparations to provide broad-spectrum antibacterial coverage. Orally administered bacitracin is effective in treating antibiotic-associated *C. difficile* colitis (88).

Adverse Effects

Systemic administration of bacitracin results in significant nephrotoxicity. Side effects are rare when the drug is given orally or applied topically. The drug is nonirritating to skin and mucous membranes. Allergic skin sensitization is rare.

CHLORAMPHENICOL

Chloramphenicol is a unique antibiotic originally derived from *Streptomyces venezuelae*. It contains a nitrobenzene ring. It is a highly effective, broad-spectrum antimicrobial agent with specific indications for use in seriously ill patients. Thiamphenicol is an analog of chloramphenicol with a similar spectrum of antimicrobial activity (253). Only chloramphenicol is available for clinical use in the United States.

Mechanism of Action

The drug is a bacteriostatic agent that inhibits protein synthesis by binding reversibly to the peptidyltransferase component of the 50S ribosomal subunit and preventing the transpeptidation process of peptide chain elongation. At therapeutic concentrations achievable in serum, it can be bactericidal against common meningeal pathogens such as *S. pneumoniae, N. meningitidis,* and *H. influenzae* (212, 253). Bacterial resistance occurs with plasmid-mediated, *cat* gene-encoded production of chloramphenicol acetyltransferase enzyme, which inactivates the drug (308).

Pharmacology

Chloramphenicol is available for topical, oral, or parenteral use. It is not absorbed in any significant amount when applied topically, but it is rapidly and completely absorbed from the gastrointestinal tract. After an oral or intravenous dose of 1 g, peak concentrations in serum at 2 h can reach 10 to 15 μg/ml. It diffuses well into many tissues and body fluids, including CSF, where levels are generally 30 to 50% of concentrations in serum even without meningeal inflammation (313). The antibiotic readily crosses the placental barrier and is present in human milk.

Chloramphenicol is metabolized and inactivated by glucuronidation in the liver, with a half-life of 4 h in adults. The active drug (5 to 10%) and its inactive metabolites are excreted by the kidneys. Careful monitoring of serum chloramphenicol levels, maintaining peak concentrations in serum in the therapeutic range of 10 to 20 μg/ml, is useful for ensuring therapeutic efficacy and reduced toxicity. Patients with hepatic failure have high levels of active drug in serum owing to a prolonged half-life. Dosage modification is not necessary in the presence of renal insufficiency, since the metabolites are not as toxic as the active drug. Levels in serum are not affected by hemodialysis or peritoneal dialysis.

Spectrum of Activity

Chloramphenicol is very active against many gram-positive and gram-negative bacteria, chlamydiae, mycoplasmas, and rickettsiae. MIC_{90}s for most gram-positive aerobic and anaerobic cocci are ≤12.5 μg/ml (253). However, the drug is usually inactive against methicillin-resistant *S. aureus* and *S. epidermidis* and is variably active against enterococci. *N.*

meningitidis, *H. influenzae* (ampicillin-resistant and -susceptible strains), and most *Enterobacteriaceae* are susceptible. Its activity against *Serratia* and *Enterobacter* isolates is variable, and *Pseudomonas* spp. are usually resistant. Salmonellae, including *S. enterica* serovar Typhi, are also susceptible, but resistant isolates are being encountered with increasing frequency (54).

Chloramphenicol has excellent activity against anaerobic bacteria, including members of the *B. fragilis* group. Almost all of these isolates are inhibited at concentrations of ≤10 μg/ml (2, 314). It is also active against *Rickettsia* spp. and *C. burnetii*.

Adverse Effects

Bone marrow toxicity is the major complication of chloramphenicol use. This side effect may occur as either dose-related bone marrow suppression or idiosyncratic aplastic anemia. Reversible bone marrow depression with anemia, leukopenia, and thrombocytopenia occurs as a result of a direct pharmacological effect of the drug on hematopoiesis. High doses (>4 g/day), prolonged therapy, and excessively high levels in serum (>20 μg/ml) predispose patients to develop this type of complication. The second form of bone marrow toxicity is a rare but usually fatal complication that manifests as aplastic anemia. This response is not dose related, and the precise mechanism is unknown. It can occur weeks to months after the use of chloramphenicol, and it can develop after the use of oral, intravenous, or topical preparations.

Gray baby syndrome, characterized by vomiting, abdominal distention, cyanosis, hypothermia, and circulatory collapse, may occur in premature infants and neonates. This toxicity results from the immature hepatic function of neonates, which impairs hepatic inactivation of the drug. Reversible optic neuritis causing decreased visual acuity has been reported for patients receiving prolonged therapy. Chloramphenicol can occasionally cause hypersensitivity reactions, including skin rashes, drug fevers, and anaphylaxis. It potentiates the action of warfarin, phenytoin, and oral hypoglycemic agents by competitive inhibition of hepatic microsomal enzymes.

METRONIDAZOLE

Metronidazole is a 5-nitroimidazole derivative that was first introduced in 1959 for the treatment of *Trichomonas vaginalis* infections. It now has an important therapeutic role in the treatment of infections due to anaerobic bacteria and certain protozoan parasites. Tinidazole, a second-generation 5-nitroimidazole compound, is approved in the United States for treatment of trichomoniasis, giardiasis, and amebiasis.

Mechanism of Action

Metronidazole owes its bactericidal activity to the nitro group of its chemical structure. After the drug gains entry into the cells of susceptible organisms, the nitro group is reduced by a nitroreductase enzyme in the cytoplasm, generating certain short-lived, highly cytotoxic intermediate compounds, free radicals, that disrupt host DNA (96). Resistance to nitroimidazoles may be due to decreased uptake of the drug or inducible production of 5-nitroimidazole reductase enzyme that can scavenge the free-radical intermediates (207).

Pharmacology

Metronidazole can be administered via the topical, oral, or intravenous route. It is absorbed rapidly and almost completely when given orally. Peak levels in serum of 6 μg/ml are obtained 1 h after an oral dose of 250 mg. Intravenous doses of 7.5 mg/kg result in peak concentrations in serum of 20 to 25 μg/ml. The drug has a half-life in serum of 8 h. Therapeutic levels are achieved in all body tissues and fluids, including abscess cavities and CSF, even without meningeal inflammation. The drug crosses the placenta and is secreted in breast milk. It is metabolized mainly in the liver, and 60 to 80% is excreted by the kidneys. With impaired hepatic function, plasma clearance of metronidazole is delayed and dosage adjustments are necessary. The pharmacokinetics are minimally affected by renal insufficiency. Metronidazole and its metabolites are removed completely by dialysis.

Spectrum of Activity

Metronidazole exhibits potent activity against almost all anaerobic bacteria, including the *B. fragilis* group and *Fusobacterium* and *Clostridium* spp. (18). It is the only antimicrobial agent with consistent bactericidal activity against members of the *B. fragilis* group. However, the susceptibility of gram-positive anaerobic cocci is somewhat variable, with MIC_{90}s of 16 μg/ml for these organisms. Most strains of the genera *Actinomyces*, *Arachnia*, and *Propionibacterium* are resistant. Frequencies of metronidazole-resistant *B. fragilis* group isolates (MICs of >16 μg/ml) in the range of 2 to 5% have been reported from various institutions (2, 314). Tinidazole is somewhat more potent than metronidazole in its antianaerobe activities (58, 174). Nitroimidazoles have no activity against aerobic bacteria, including the *Enterobacteriaceae*.

The drug is effective in the treatment of antibiotic-associated colitis caused by *C. difficile* (19, 53), with efficacy equivalent to that of oral vancomycin for this indication (333). It is also useful in combination with an aminoglycoside for treating polymicrobial soft tissue infections and mixed aerobic-anaerobic intra-abdominal and pelvic infections.

Metronidazole and tinidazole are active against the protozoa *T. vaginalis*, *Giardia lamblia*, and *E. histolytica*. It is the drug of choice for the treatment of trichomoniasis, giardiasis, and intestinal and invasive amebiasis, including amebic liver abscess (127, 228, 331).

Adverse Effects

Metronidazole is generally well tolerated, and adverse side effects are uncommon. It can cause mild gastrointestinal symptoms such as nausea, abdominal cramps, and diarrhea. An unpleasant, metallic taste may be experienced with oral therapy. Metronidazole can potentiate the effect of warfarin and prolong the prothrombin time.

Although metronidazole is carcinogenic in mice and rats, there is no evidence for carcinogenicity in humans. However, use of this agent in pregnancy, especially during the first trimester, and in nursing mothers should be avoided.

RIFAMYCINS

Rifamycins are a group of macrocyclic compounds produced by the mold *Streptomyces mediterranei*. Rifampin, also known as rifampicin and a semisynthetic antibiotic derived from rifamycin B, was the first of this class of drugs introduced for clinical use in 1968 as an effective antituberculous drug. A closely related compound, rifabutin, a derivative of rifamycin S, is another potent antimycobacterial agent, especially against *M. avium* complex (261). Rifaximin, a derivative of rifampin, possesses an additional pyridoimidazole ring and is a nonabsorbed oral drug used for therapy of uncomplicated traveler's diarrhea.

Mechanism of Action

Rifamycins exert their bactericidal effects by forming a stable complex with bacterial DNA-dependent RNA polymerase, preventing the chain initiation process of DNA transcription (359). Mammalian RNA synthesis is not affected, because the mammalian enzyme is much less sensitive to the drug. Rifampin-resistant isolates possess an altered RNA polymerase enzyme that arises easily from single-step mutations during monotherapy with rifampin.

Pharmacology

Rifampin is well absorbed after oral administration, reaching peak concentrations in serum of 5 to 10 μg/ml in 2 to 4 h following a 600-mg dose. A parenteral preparation is also available. Rifampin is deacetylated in the liver to an active metabolite and excreted in the bile, and it undergoes enterohepatic circulation. The normal half-life in serum varies from 1.5 to 5 h. The drug distributes well to almost all body tissues and fluids, reaching concentrations equal to or exceeding that in serum. Levels in CSF are highest in the presence of inflamed meninges. It is able to enter phagocytes and kill living intracellular organisms (215), and it crosses the placenta. About 30 to 40% of the drug is excreted in the urine, and it does not accumulate in patients with impaired renal function. Hemodialysis and peritoneal dialysis do not eliminate the drug. Dosage adjustments are necessary for patients with severe hepatic dysfunction.

Due to an additional pyridoimidazole ring in its chemical structure, rifaximin is largely unabsorbed after oral administration, with >99% of the drug present in the stool and <1% of an oral dose detectable in plasma of both healthy volunteers and persons with damaged intestinal mucosa (164). Average fecal concentrations of drug reach 8,000 μg/g on the third day of therapy at a dosage of 400 mg orally twice daily (171).

Spectrum of Activity

In addition to its well-known antimycobacterial effects (59), rifampin has a wide spectrum of antimicrobial activity. It is bactericidal against gram-positive cocci such as staphylococci (including methicillin-resistant strains), streptococci, and anaerobic cocci, with MICs in the range of 0.01 to 0.5 μg/ml. It remains an important adjunct in combination therapy of serious and chronic staphylococcal infections (340). However, it is bacteriostatic against enterococci, with usual MICs of <16 μg/ml (240).

N. gonorrhoeae, *N. meningitidis*, and *H. influenzae*, including β-lactamase-producing strains, are susceptible to rifampin, which is used frequently in the prophylaxis of meningococcal and *H. influenzae* type b meningitis (146). MICs for *Enterobacteriaceae* are ≤12 μg/ml, while MICs for *S. marcescens* and *P. aeruginosa* are higher (240). Besides fluoroquinolones, rifampin is one of the most active agents against *L. pneumophila* and other *Legionella* spp., with MICs of ≤0.03 μg/ml. Because of its ability to enter phagocytes, rifampin inhibits the growth of *Brucella* spp. and *C. burnetii* intracellularly (282), and it is used frequently in combination therapy of infections due to these organisms. Although *Chlamydia* spp. are very susceptible to rifampin in vitro, resistance emerges rapidly when rifampin is used alone.

Rifaximin has broad-spectrum inhibitory activity against enteric bacterial pathogens, including enterotoxigenic and enteroaggregative strains of *E. coli*, *Aeromonas*, *Shigella*, and *Salmonella*, with MIC_{90}s ranging from 4 to 16 μg/ml (136, 164, 310). Although it is less active against *C. jejuni* (MIC_{90} of 512 μg/ml), *Y. enterocolitica* (MIC_{90} of 128 μg/ml), *C. difficile* (MIC_{90} of 128 μg/ml), and *H. pylori* (MIC_{50} of 4 μg/ml), concentrations of rifaximin achieved in the intestinal lumen are >10-fold higher than the MICs of the drug for these pathogens. This drug has been used successfully to treat and prevent uncomplicated traveler's diarrhea (91, 92, 324).

Adverse Effects

Rifampin has many side effects, including gastrointestinal discomfort and hypersensitivity reactions, such as drug fever, skin rashes, and eosinophilia. It produces a harmless, orange-red coloration of saliva, tears, urine, and sweat. In up to 20% of patients, an influenza-like syndrome with fever, chills, arthralgias, and myalgias may develop after several months of intermittent therapy (142). This immunologic reaction may be associated with hemolytic anemia, thrombocytopenia, and renal failure. Rifampin-induced hepatitis occurs in <1% of patients and is more frequent during concurrent isoniazid therapy for tuberculosis. As a result of its ability to induce human hepatic cytochrome P450 enzyme, rifampin has clinically significant interactions with many drugs, such as antagonizing the effect of oral contraceptives and diminishing the anticoagulant activity of warfarin.

Headache, nausea, abdominal pain, and fatigue are the most frequent side effects reported for rifaximin. Rare hypersensitivity reactions, including allergic dermatitis, rash, angioneurotic edema, urticaria, and pruritus, can occur with rifaximin, which is contraindicated in those who are allergic to rifampin (164). However, unlike rifampin, rifaximin does not cause clinically relevant interactions with drugs because of the lack of systemic absorption of this drug.

NITROFURANTOIN

Nitrofurantoin belongs to a class of compounds consisting of a primary nitro group joined to a heterocyclic ring. Its role in human therapeutics is limited to treatment of urinary tract infections (161).

Mechanism of Action

The mechanism of action of nitrofurantoin is not fully understood, but highly reactive electrophilic intermediates of the drug activated by bacterial reductases were found to bind nonspecifically to bacterial ribosomal proteins and inhibit inducible synthesis of essential bacterial enzymes, causing complete cessation of protein synthesis and damage to bacterial DNA and RNA (221). However, inhibition of bacterial protein synthesis can occur in the absence of reductive activation of the drug (226). Despite over 30 years of clinical use, there is no emergence of clinically significant bacterial resistance to this drug.

Pharmacology

The drug is available in microcrystalline (Furadantin) and macrocrystalline (Macrodantin) forms. It is administered orally and is well absorbed from the gastrointestinal tract. Very low levels of the drug are achieved in serum and most body tissues after usual oral doses. With a half-life in serum of about 20 min, two-thirds of the drug is rapidly metabolized and inactivated in various tissues. The remaining one-third is excreted unchanged into the urine. An average dose of nitrofurantoin yields a concentration in urine of 50 to 250 μg/ml in patients with healthy renal function. In alkaline urine, more of the drug is dissociated into the ionized form, with lowered antibacterial activity. Nitrofurantoin accumulates in the sera of patients with creatinine clearances of <60 ml/min. The drug is removed by hemodialysis. The risk of systemic toxicity increases in the presence of severe uremia. It is contraindicated in patients with significant renal impairment and hepatic failure.

Spectrum of Activity

Nitrofurantoin has a broad spectrum of activity against gram-positive and gram-negative bacteria, particularly the common urinary tract pathogens. It is active against gram-positive cocci, such as *S. aureus, S. epidermidis, Staphylococcus saprophyticus,* and *E. faecalis*, with MICs in the range of 4 to 25 μg/ml (159). *S. pneumoniae, S. pyogenes,* and *Corynebacterium* spp. are also susceptible, but they rarely cause urinary tract infections. Over 90% of *E. coli* isolates and many coliform bacteria are susceptible to nitrofurantoin at MICs of <32 μg/ml. However, only one-third of *Enterobacter* and *Klebsiella* isolates are susceptible. *Pseudomonas* and most *Proteus* spp. are resistant. Susceptible organisms rarely become resistant to this drug during therapy.

Adverse Effects

Gastrointestinal irritation, with anorexia, nausea, and vomiting, is the most common side effect. Diarrhea and abdominal cramps may occur. Hypersensitivity reactions, such as drug fever, chills, arthralgia, skin rashes, and a lupus-like syndrome, have been observed (160). Pulmonary reactions are the most common serious side effects associated with nitrofurantoin use. Acute pneumonitis with fever, cough, dyspnea, eosinophilia, and pulmonary infiltrates present on chest radiographs can occur after a few days of therapy (160). This immunologically mediated reaction is more common in elderly patients and is rapidly reversible after cessation of therapy. Chronic pulmonary reactions with interstitial pneumonitis leading to irreversible pulmonary fibrosis can occur in patients on continuous therapy for 6 months or more (232).

Peripheral polyneuropathy is a serious side effect that occurs more often in patients with renal failure. Hemolytic anemia, megaloblastic anemia, and bone marrow suppression with leukopenia can occur. Rare hepatotoxic reactions, such as cholestatic jaundice and chronic active hepatitis, have been reported (307).

FOSFOMYCIN

Fosfomycin, first isolated from cultures of *Streptomyces* spp. in 1969, is a phosphonic acid derivative originally named phosphonomycin (322). In the United States, it is used as single-dose therapy for uncomplicated urinary tract infections due to susceptible organisms (161).

Mechanism of Action

Fosfomycin is bactericidal by inhibiting pyruvyl transferase, a bacterial cytoplasmic enzyme that catalyzes the formation of uridine diphosphate-*N*-acetylmuramic acid during the first step of peptidoglycan synthesis (184). There is little cross-resistance between fosfomycin and other antibacterial agents, most likely because it differs from other agents in its chemical structure and site of action. Rare resistance to fosfomycin can occur by two mechanisms: (i) mutations of the structural or regulatory genes for the bacterial proteins that transport the drug into the cell or (ii) plasmid-mediated production of a drug-inactivating enzyme (255).

Pharmacology

Originally formulated as sodium and calcium salts for oral and intravenous use, fosfomycin is available in the United States as an oral, water-soluble tromethamine salt. Following oral administration, it is rapidly absorbed and converted to the free acid, fosfomycin. With markedly improved oral bioavailability (35 to 40%), fosfomycin has a mean elimination half-life of 5.5 h, and it is primarily excreted unchanged in the urine (268). Following a single oral dose of 3 g, peak concentrations in serum (range, 22 to 32 μg/ml) are achieved within 2 h after administration, with peak urinary concentrations (1,000 to 4,400 μg/ml) occurring within 4 h and remaining high (>128 μg/ml) for 24 to 48 h, sufficient to inhibit most urinary tract pathogens. Peak urinary concentrations are reached later and are lowered when the drug is administered with food or antiperistaltic agents. In patients with renal impairment (creatinine clearance of <30 ml/min), peak serum fosfomycin concentrations are increased, with decreased urinary elimination and reduced urinary concentrations of the drug.

While not bound to plasma protein, it is widely distributed in various body fluids and tissues, including the kidneys, prostate, and seminal vesicles, from which it is cleared slowly. Although it crosses the placental barrier, the drug can be used safely during pregnancy if clearly needed.

Spectrum of Activity

Fosfomycin has a broad spectrum of activity against most gram-positive and gram-negative bacteria isolated from patients with lower urinary tract infections. *E. coli, Serratia, Klebsiella, Citrobacter, Enterobacter, S. aureus,* and enterococci are generally inhibited by fosfomycin at concentrations of <64 μg/ml (13, 268, 322). Fosfomycin is bactericidal at concentrations that are similar to the MICs, at ≤2-fold differences. It is more active than TMP and nalidixic acid, while similar to norfloxacin and co-trimoxazole, in its activity against these organisms (13). At a breakpoint concentration of ≤128 mg/ml, 60, 20, and 80% of isolates of *Pseudomonas* spp., *M. morganii,* and *S. saprophyticus*, respectively, are susceptible to fosfomycin (274). In multiple-dose use, bacterial resistance to fosfomycin emerges rapidly, and it can be chromosomal or, more rarely, plasmid mediated. However, cross-resistance with other antimicrobials has been uncommon (283).

The in vitro activity of fosfomycin is affected by test medium and conditions (268, 274). Fosfomycin has much greater in vitro activity, and closer correlation with in vivo activity, when the test medium is supplemented with glucose-6-phosphate at 25 μg/ml, which is recommended for susceptibility testing with the agar and broth dilution methods. The disk diffusion testing method utilizes disks containing 200 μg of fosfomycin tromethamine and 50 or 100 μg of glucose-6-phosphate.

Adverse Effects

Mild, self-limiting gastrointestinal disturbances, mainly diarrhea, are the most frequent side effects (3 to 5%). Other minor adverse events include headaches, dizziness, rash, and vaginitis.

METHENAMINE

Methenamine is a tertiary amine with properties of a monoacidic base; it is used as a urinary antiseptic. To be activated, it is combined chemically with a poorly metabolized acid and administered as the mandelate (Mandelamine) or hippurate (Hiprex or Urex) salt.

Mechanism of Action

Methenamine has no antibacterial action by itself, but it is converted at acid pH to ammonia and formaldehyde, which provides the antiseptic action. This hydrolytic process occurs in the urine, and an effective bacteriostatic concentration of formaldehyde is reached at a urine pH of <5.5. Since the serum is at physiological pH, formaldehyde is not released while methenamine circulates in the body.

Pharmacology

The agent is well absorbed from the gastrointestinal tract and is rapidly excreted in the urine. The elimination half-life of methenamine is about 4 h. At a urinary pH of 5.0, about 20% of methenamine excreted in the urine is hydrolyzed to formaldehyde and ammonia. Bactericidal levels (>20 mg/ml) of formaldehyde are generated in the bladder urine at 2 h after oral administration and may be maintained for at least 6 h or until the patient voids (192). The mandelate and hippurate moieties are also rapidly excreted in the urine in active, unchanged forms by glomerular filtration and tubular secretion. The agent is contraindicated in patients with hepatic insufficiency because of the ammonia produced.

Spectrum of Activity

With the liberation of enough formaldehyde into the urine, methenamine is essentially active against all gram-positive and gram-negative bacteria and also against fungi (192). However, it is not effective for treating urinary tract infections due to urea-splitting organisms such as *Proteus* and *Morganella*, which can convert urea to ammonium hydroxide, thereby preventing the hydrolysis of methenamine to formaldehyde. Combination with acetohydroxamic acid, a urease inhibitor, has been suggested for treating these infections by *Proteus* and *Morganella*. Since bacteria and fungi do not become resistant to formaldehyde, emergence of resistance to methenamine is not a problem.

Methenamine is not useful for acute urinary tract infections. It has been used successfully as prophylactic therapy for recurrent bacteriuria, particularly infections caused by highly resistant gram-negative rods or yeasts. It is also effective as prolonged suppressive therapy for chronic bacteriuria in the absence of structural abnormalities of the urinary tract.

Adverse Effects

Methenamine and its acid salts are generally well tolerated. Some patients may develop nausea, vomiting, abdominal cramps, and diarrhea. High doses or prolonged administration of the drug can cause urinary tract irritation by the free formaldehyde, resulting in urinary frequency, dysuria, albuminuria, and hematuria. Skin rashes may also occur. To avoid precipitation of urate crystals in the urine, methenamine salts should not be used in patients with gout or hyperuricemia.

MUPIROCIN

Mupirocin, formerly pseudomonic acid A, is a topical antibacterial agent derived from the fermentation products of *Pseudomonas fluorescens* (125). It contains a unique 9-hydroxynonanoic acid moiety in its chemical structure, and it inhibits isoleucyl-tRNA synthetase, resulting in cessation of bacterial protein synthesis (165). Low-level resistance (MICs of 4 to 256 μg/ml) results from an altered synthetase enzyme due to mutations in the bacterial chromosomal *ileS* gene, whereas high-level, transferable resistance (MIC of ≥512 μg/ml) is mediated by the *mupA* gene, which encodes an entirely different synthetase.

Originally developed for the topical treatment of superficial soft tissue infections, particularly those due to staphylococci, mupirocin is available as a 2% ointment or cream in the United States. After topical application, <1% of the drug is absorbed systemically, with no detectable levels in the urine or feces. Penetration into deeper dermal layers of the skin is increased with traumatized skin or use of occlusive dressings. The drug is highly protein bound (95%), and its activity is lowered in the presence of serum. It is most active at moderately acid pH, with no inoculum effect (353). Mupirocin is slowly metabolized in the skin to the inactive monic acid.

It has excellent in vitro activity, primarily against the gram-positive cocci. *S. aureus*, including methicillin-resistant strains, and coagulase-negative staphylococci are uniformly very susceptible, with MIC_{90}s of <0.5 μg/ml (47). Emergence of resistant strains of staphylococci can occur with widespread use of mupirocin (33, 35, 339). Most streptococci (including *S. pneumoniae*, beta-hemolytic streptococci of groups A, B, C, and G, and viridans group streptococci) are inhibited by concentrations of ≤1 μg/ml. Resistant bacteria include enterococci, *Corynebacterium* spp., *Erysipelothrix* spp., *P. acnes*, gram-positive anaerobes, and most gram-negative bacteria. However, *H. influenzae, N. gonorrhoeae, N. meningitidis, M. catarrhalis, B. pertussis*, and *P. multocida* are quite susceptible, with MICs in the range of 0.02 to 0.025 μg/ml. There is no cross-resistance between mupirocin and other major groups of antibiotics. Clinically, mupirocin is efficacious in the therapy of superficial skin infections, such as impetigo, folliculitis, and burn wound infections, that are caused by staphylococci or streptococci (132). Although this drug has been used successfully to eradicate nasal carriage of *S. aureus*, including methicillin-resistant strains (48, 85), it may not prevent nosocomial *S. aureus* infections (361).

No systemic toxic effects have been reported with mupirocin. Local irritation, such as burning, stinging, itch, and rash, which may be due to the polyethylene glycol base in the vehicle ointment, may occur.

APPENDIX

Approximate Concentrations of Antibacterial Agents in Serum

The concentrations of antimicrobial agents listed below are approximations taken from various reports and publications. Several factors can influence the level of antimicrobial agent in individual patients, including inherent differences in the patients themselves, their physical condition, the dosages, and the routes of administration. The values can also be influenced by the assay methods used to obtain them. Therefore, these concentrations should be used only as approximate values, and clinicians should use their knowledge of the patient and the drugs, the recommendations from U.S. Food and Drug Administration-approved package inserts, or other reputable sources in planning their therapeutic regimens.

Antimicrobial agent	Serum half-life (h)	Unit dose	Average peak level in serum (µg/ml)[a]		
			p.o.	i.m.	i.v.[b]
Amikacin	2–2.5	7.5 mg/kg		15–20	20–40
Amoxicillin	1	500 mg	6–8		
Amoxicillin-clavulanate	1.3 / 1.0	250/125 mg	3.3 (Amox)		
			1.5 (Clav)		
		500/125 mg	6.5 (Amox)		
			1.8 (Clav)		
		875/125 mg	11.6 (Amox)		
			2.2 (Clav)		
		1,000/62.5 mg	17 (Amox)		
			2.1 (Clav)		
Ampicillin	1.1	500 mg	2.5–5	8–10	
		1 g			40
Ampicillin-sulbactam	1.1/1.0	3 g			120 (Amp)
					60 (Sulb)
		1.5 g			18 (Amp)
					13 (Sulb)
Azithromycin	48	500 mg	0.4		3.5
Azlocillin	1	2 g			130
Aztreonam	1.7	1 g		45	90–160
Bacampicillin	1.1	800 mg	13		
Carbenicillin	1.1	1 g		20–30	150
Carbenicillin indanyl sodium	1.1	764 mg	10		
Cefaclor	0.6	500 mg	16		
Cefadroxil	1.5	500 mg	10		
Cefamandole	0.5–1	1 g		20–36	90–140
Cefazolin	1.8	1 g		65	185
Cefepime	2	1 g		30	82
Cefdinir	1.7	300 mg	1.6		
Cefditoren	1.6	200 mg	3.1		
		400 mg	4.4		
Cefixime	3–4	400 mg	3.5		
Cefmetazole	1.5	1 g			70
Cefonicid	4	1 g		98	220
Cefoperazone	2	1 g		65–75	153
Ceforanide	3	1 g		70	125
Cefotaxime	1	1 g		20	40–45
Cefotetan	3–4.5	1 g		50–80	160
Cefoxitin	1	1 g		20–25	55–110
Cefpirome	2	1 g		45	85
Cefpodoxime	2.5	200 mg	2.3		
Cefprozil	1.5	500 mg	10.5		
Ceftazidime	2	1 g		40	70
Ceftibuten	2.5	400 mg	15		
Ceftizoxime	1.5	1 g		39	80–90
Ceftriaxone	6–9	500 mg		40–45	
		1 g			150
Cefuroxime	1.5	750 mg		27	50
Cefuroxime axetil	1.5	500 mg	9		
Cephalexin	0.9	500 mg	18		
Cephalothin	0.6	1 g			30–60
Cephapirin	0.6	1 g			40–70
Cephradine	0.8	500 mg	16		
Chloramphenicol	4	1 g	10–18		10–15
Chlortetracycline	6–9	500 mg	2–4	12	
Cinoxacin	1–1.5	500 mg	15		
Ciprofloxacin	5–6	400 mg			4.5
		500 mg	3.0		
		500 mg XR[c]	1.6		
		750 mg	4.0		
		1,000 mg XR	3.1		

(Continued on next page)

Antimicrobial agent	Serum half-life (h)	Unit dose	Average peak level in serum (μg/ml)[a]		
			p.o.	i.m.	i.v.[b]
Clarithromycin	5–7	250 mg	1–2		
		500 mg	3–4		
		1,000 mg XR	2–3		
Clinafloxacin	5.2	200 mg	1.5		
Clindamycin	2.5	300 mg	3	6	
		600 mg			10–12
Cloxacillin	0.5	500 mg	10		
Colistimethate sodium	2–4.5	150 mg		5–6	
Daptomycin	9	4 mg/kg			70
		6 mg/kg			82
Demeclocycline	12	300 mg	1–2		
Dicloxacillin	0.5–0.7	500 mg	15		
Dirithromycin	40	500 mg	0.5		
Doxycycline	18–22	100 mg	2.5		4
Enoxacin	4–6	400 mg	3–5		
Ertapenem	4	1 g		70	155
Erythromycin	1.5	500 mg	2–3		
		1 g			10
Fleroxacin	12	400 mg	5		7–8
Fosfomycin	5.7	3 g	25		
		50 mg/kg			275
Fusidic acid	13–19	500 mg	25–30		50
Gatifloxacin	7	400 mg	4		4.5
Gemifloxacin	7–8	320 mg	1.8		
Gentamicin	2–3	1.5 mg/kg	4–6		4–8
Imipenem	1	500 mg			25–35
Kanamycin	2.2–3	7.5 mg/kg		20–25	
Levofloxacin	6–8	500 mg	5.5		6.5
		750 mg	8.5		12
Lincomycin	5	500 mg	3.5		
		600 mg		10	16–21
Linezolid	5	600 mg	15		15
Lomefloxacin	6.5	400 mg	3		
Loracarbef	1	400 mg	14		
Meropenem	1	500 mg			25–35
Methicillin	0.5	1 g	15		60
Metronidazole	8	500 mg	12		20–25
Mezlocillin	1	1 g			15
		3 g			260
Minocycline	14–16	100 mg	1		
Moxifloxacin	12	400 mg	4.5		4.5
Nafcillin	0.5	500 mg			5–8
		1 g			20–40
Nalidixic acid	1.5	1 g	20–50		
Netilmicin	2.5	2 mg/kg		5–7	6–8
Nitrofurantoin	0.3	100 mg	<2		
Norfloxacin	3.3	400 mg	1.5		
Ofloxacin	5	400 mg	4		
Ornidazole	13	500 mg	10		20
Oxacillin	0.5	500 mg	4–6	14–16	
		1 g			40
Oxytetracycline	9	500 mg	1–2		
Pefloxacin	10	400 mg	3		5.5
Penicillin G	0.5	500 mg		1.5–2.5	
Aqueous		1 × 10⁶ U		8–10	10
Benzathine		1.2 × 10⁶ U		0.1–0.15	
Procaine		1.2 × 10⁶ U	3		
Penicillin V	0.5	500 mg	3–5		
Piperacillin	1.1	2 g			36
		4 g			240

(Continued on next page)

Antimicrobial agent	Serum half-life (h)	Unit dose	Average peak level in serum (μg/ml)[a]		
			p.o.	i.m.	i.v.[b]
Piperacillin-tazobactam	1.1/1.0	3.375 g			242 (Pip) 24 (Tazo)
		4.5 g			298 (Pip) 34 (Tazo)
Pivampicillin	0.5–1	350 mg	2		
Polymyxin B	6–7	2.5 mg/kg		5	
Quinupristin-dalfopristin	1/0.75	7.5 mg/kg			3 (Q) 7.5 (D)
Rifampin	2–5	600 mg	7–9		10
Sparfloxacin	20	200 mg	1.1		
Spectinomycin	1–2	2 g		100	
Spiramycin	3.8	2 g	3		
Streptomycin	2–3	1 g		25–50	
Sulfadiazine	17	2 g	100–150		
Sulfadoxine	150–200	1 g	50–75		
Sulfamethizole	4–7	2 g	60		
SMX	10–12	1 g	40		
Sulfisoxazole	5–7	2 g	170		
Teicoplanin	45	200 mg		7	
		400 mg			20–40
Telithromycin	9–10	800 mg	2		
Tetracycline	8	500 mg	4		8
Ticarcillin	1.2	1 g		20–30	
		3 g			190
Ticarcillin-clavulanate	1.2/1.0	3.1 g			330 (Ticar) 8 (Clav)
Tigecycline	36	50 mg			0.8
Tinidazole	12–14	2 g	48		
Tobramycin	2–2.8	1.5 mg/kg		4–6	4–8
TMP	10–12	100 mg	1		
TMP-SMX		160/800 mg	3 (TMP) 46 (SMX)		9 (TMP) 106 (SMX)
Trovafloxacin (alatrofloxacin i.v.)	11	300 mg			4.5
Vancomycin	6	500 mg			20–40

[a] p.o., oral; i.m., intramuscular; i.v., intravenous.
[b] At 30 min following intravenous infusion.
[c] XR, extended-release formulation.

REFERENCES

1. **Ackermann, G., and A. C. Rodloff.** 2003. Drugs of the 21st century: telithromycin (HMR 3647)—the first ketolide. *J. Antimicrob. Chemother.* **51:**497–511.
2. **Aldridge, K. E., D. Ashcraft, K. Cambre, C. L. Pierson, S. G. Jenkins, and J. E. Rosenblatt.** 2001. Multicenter survey of the changing in vitro antimicrobial susceptibilities of clinical isolates of *Bacteroides fragilis* group, *Prevotella*, *Fusobacterium*, *Porphyromonas*, and *Peptostreptococcus* species. *Antimicrob. Agents Chemother.* **45:**1238–1243.
3. **Appelbaum, P. C., M. R. Jacobs, S. K. Spangler, and S. Yamabe.** 1986. Comparative activity of beta-lactamase inhibitors YTR 830, clavulanate, and sulbactam combined with beta-lactams against beta-lactamase-producing anaerobes. *Antimicrob. Agents Chemother.* **30:**789–791.
4. **Arbeit, R. D., D. Maki, F. P. Tally, E. Campanaro, B. I. Eisenstein, and the Daptomycin 98-01 and 99-01 Investigators.** 2004. The safety and efficacy of daptomycin for the treatment of complicated skin and skin-structure infections. *Clin. Infect. Dis.* **38:**1673–1681.
5. **Aswapokee, N., and H. C. Neu.** 1978. A sulfone beta-lactam compound which acts as a beta-lactamase inhibitor. *J. Antibiot.* (Tokyo) **31:**1238–1244.
6. **Attassi, K., E. Hershberger, R. Alam, and M. J. Zervos.** 2002. Thrombocytopenia associated with linezolid therapy. *Clin. Infect. Dis.* **34:**695–698.
7. **Baciewicz, A. M., A. Al-Nimr, and P. Whelan.** 2005. Azithromycin-induced hepatoxicity. *Am. J. Med.* **118:** 1438–1439.
8. **Balfour, J. A., and D. P. Figgitt.** 2001. Telithromycin. *Drugs* **61:**815–829.
9. **Balfour, J. A., and L. R. Wiseman.** 1999. Moxifloxacin. *Drugs* **57:**363–373.
10. **Ball, P.** 2000. Quinolone generations: natural history or natural selection? *J. Antimicrob. Chemother.* **46**(Suppl. 1):17–24.
11. **Ball, P., L. Mandell, Y. Niki, and G. Tillotson.** 1999. Comparative tolerability of the newer fluoroquinolone antibacterials. *Drug Saf.* **21:**407–421.
12. **Bansal, M. B., S. K. Chuah, and H. Thadepalli.** 1985. In vitro activity and in vivo evaluation of ticarcillin plus

clavulanic acid against aerobic and anaerobic bacteria. *Am. J. Med.* **79:**33–38.

13. **Barry, A. L., and S. D. Brown.** 1995. Antibacterial spectrum of fosfomycin trometamol. *J. Antimicrob. Chemother.* **35:**228–230.
14. **Barry, A. L., P. C. Fuchs, and S. D. Brown.** 2001. In vitro activities of daptomycin against 2,789 clinical isolates from 11 North American medical centers. *Antimicrob. Agents Chemother.* **45:**1919–1922.
15. **Barry, A. L., and R. N. Jones.** 1987. Cefixime: spectrum of antibacterial activity against 16,016 clinical isolates. *Pediatr. Infect. Dis. J.* **6:**954–957.
16. **Barry, A. L., R. N. Jones, and C. Thornsberry.** 1988. In vitro activities of azithromycin (CP 62,993), clarithromycin (A-56268; TE-031), erythromycin, roxithromycin, and clindamycin. *Antimicrob. Agents Chemother.* **32:**752–754.
17. **Barry, A. L., C. Thornsberry, R. N. Jones, and T. L. Gavan.** 1985. Aztreonam: antibacterial activity, beta-lactamase stability, and interpretive standards and quality control guidelines for disk-diffusion susceptibility tests. *Rev. Infect. Dis.* **7**(Suppl. 4)**:**S594–S604.
18. **Bartlett, J. G.** 1982. Anti-anaerobic antibacterial agents. *Lancet* **ii:**478–481.
19. **Bartlett, J. G.** 1992. Antibiotic-associated diarrhea. *Clin. Infect. Dis.* **15:**573–581.
20. **Barza, M.** 1985. Imipenem: first of a new class of beta-lactam antibiotics. *Ann. Intern. Med.* **103:**552–560.
21. **Bates, R. D., and M. C. Nahata.** 1994. Once-daily administration of aminoglycosides. *Ann. Pharmacother.* **28:**757–766.
22. **Bauernfeind, A.** 1993. In-vitro activity of dirithromycin in comparison with other new and established macrolides. *J. Antimicrob. Chemother.* **31**(Suppl. C)**:**39–49.
23. **Bauernfeind, A.** 1997. Comparison of the antibacterial activities of the quinolones Bay 12-8039, gatifloxacin (AM 1155), trovafloxacin, clinafloxacin, levofloxacin and ciprofloxacin. *J. Antimicrob. Chemother.* **40:**639–651.
24. **Bearden, D. T., M. M. Neuhauser, and K. W. Garey.** 2001. Telithromycin: an oral ketolide for respiratory infections. *Pharmacotherapy* **21:**1204–1222.
25. **Berkey, P., D. Moore, and K. Rolston.** 1988. In vitro susceptibilities of *Nocardia* species to newer antimicrobial agents. *Antimicrob. Agents Chemother.* **32:**1078–1079.
26. **Bernard, L., R. Stern, D. Lew, and P. Hoffmeyer.** 2003. Serotonin syndrome after concomitant treatment with linezolid and citalopram. *Clin. Infect. Dis.* **36:**1197.
27. **Beskid, G., and B. L. Prosser.** 1993. A multicenter study on the comparative in vitro activity of fleroxacin and three other quinolones: an interim report from 27 centers. *Am. J. Med.* **94**(Suppl. 3A)**:**2S–8S.
28. **Betriu, C., I. Rodriguez-Avial, M. Gomez, E. Culebras, and J. J. Picazo.** 2005. Changing patterns of fluoroquinolone resistance among *Bacteroides fragilis* group organisms over a 6-year period (1997–2002). *Diagn. Microbiol. Infect. Dis.* **53:**221–223.
29. **Blondeau, J. M.** 1999. A review of the comparative in-vitro activities of 12 antimicrobial agents, with a focus on five new respiratory quinolones. *J. Antimicrob. Chemother.* **43**(Suppl. B)**:**1–11.
30. **Bonora, M. G., M. Solbiati, E. Stepan, A. Zorzi, A. Luzzani, M. R. Catania, and R. Fontana.** 2006. Emergence of linezolid resistance in the vancomycin-resistant *Enterococcus faecium* multilocus sequence typing C1 epidemic lineage. *J. Clin. Microbiol.* **44:**1153–1155.
31. **Bouanchaud, D. H.** 1997. In-vitro and in-vivo antibacterial activity of quinupristin/dalfopristin. *J. Antimicrob. Chemother.* **39**(Suppl. A)**:**15–21.
32. **Bouchillon, S. K., D. J. Hoban, B. M. Johnson, J. L. Johnson, A. Hsiung, and M. J. Dowzicky.** 2005. In vitro activity of tigecycline against 3989 Gram-negative and Gram-positive clinical isolates from the United States Tigecycline Evaluation and Surveillance Trial (TEST Program; 2004). *Diagn. Microbiol. Infect. Dis.* **52:**173–179.
33. **Boyce, J. M.** 1996. Preventing staphylococcal infections by eradicating nasal carriage of *Staphylococcus aureus*: proceeding with caution. *Infect. Control Hosp. Epidemiol.* **17:**775–779.
34. **Bradford, P. A., P. J. Petersen, M. Young, C. H. Jones, M. Tischler, and J. O'Connell.** 2005. Tigecycline MIC testing by broth dilution requires use of fresh medium or addition of the biocatalytic oxygen-reducing reagent oxyrase to standardize the test method. *Antimicrob. Agents Chemother.* **49:**3903–3909.
35. **Bradley, S. F., M. A. Ramsey, T. M. Morton, and C. A. Kauffman.** 1995. Mupirocin resistance: clinical and molecular epidemiology. *Infect. Control Hosp. Epidemiol.* **16:**354–358.
36. **Bressler, A. M., S. M. Zimmer, J. L. Gilmore, and J. Somani.** 2004. Peripheral neuropathy associated with prolonged use of linezolid. *Lancet Infect. Dis.* **4:**528–531.
37. **Brighty, K. E., and T. D. Gootz.** 1997. The chemistry and biological profile of trovafloxacin. *J. Antimicrob. Chemother.* **39**(Suppl. B)**:**1–14.
38. **Brown-Elliott, B. A., C. J. Crist, L. B. Mann, R. W. Wilson, and R. J. Wallace, Jr.** 2003. In vitro activity of linezolid against slowly growing nontuberculous mycobacteria. *Antimicrob. Agents Chemother.* **47:**1736–1738.
39. **Brown-Elliott, B. A., S. C. Ward, C. J. Crist, L. B. Mann, R. W. Wilson, and R. J. Wallace, Jr.** 2001. In vitro activities of linezolid against multiple *Nocardia* species. *Antimicrob. Agents Chemother.* **45:**1295–1297.
40. **Brummett, R. E., and K. E. Fox.** 1989. Vancomycin- and erythromycin-induced hearing loss in humans. *Antimicrob. Agents Chemother.* **33:**791–796.
41. **Buesing, M. A., and J. H. Jorgensen.** 1984. In vitro activity of aztreonam in combination with newer beta-lactams and amikacin against multiply resistant gram-negative bacilli. *Antimicrob. Agents Chemother.* **25:**283–285.
42. **Bush, K., J. S. Freudenberger, and R. B. Sykes.** 1982. Interaction of azthreonam and related monobactams with beta-lactamases from gram-negative bacteria. *Antimicrob. Agents Chemother.* **22:**414–420.
43. **Bushby, S. R.** 1973. Trimethoprim-sulfamethoxazole: in vitro microbiological aspects. *J. Infect. Dis.* **128**(Suppl.)**:**442–462.
44. **Canepari, P., M. Boaretti, M. del Mar Lleo, and G. Satta.** 1990. Lipoteichoic acid as a new target for activity of antibiotics: mode of action of daptomycin (LY146032). *Antimicrob. Agents Chemother.* **34:**1220–1226.
45. **Carpenter, C. F., and H. F. Chambers.** 2004. Daptomycin: another novel agent for treating infections due to drug-resistant gram-positive pathogens. *Clin. Infect. Dis.* **38:** 994–1000.
46. **Carroll, O. M., P. A. Bryan, and R. J. Robinson.** 1966. Stevens-Johnson syndrome associated with long-acting sulfonamides. *JAMA* **195:**691–693.
47. **Casewell, M. W., and R. L. Hill.** 1985. In-vitro activity of mupirocin (pseudomonic acid) against clinical isolates of *Staphylococcus aureus*. *J. Antimicrob. Chemother.* **15:**523–531.
48. **Casewell, M. W., and R. L. Hill.** 1986. Elimination of nasal carriage of *Staphylococcus aureus* with mupirocin (pseudomonic acid): a controlled trial. *J. Antimicrob. Chemother.* **17:**365–372.
49. **Centers for Disease Control and Prevention.** 2004. Treating opportunistic infections among HIV-exposed and infected children: recommendations from CDC, the National Institutes of Health, and the Infectious Diseases Society of America. *Morb. Mortal. Wkly. Rep.* **53**(RR-14)**:**1–92.
50. **Centers for Disease Control and Prevention.** 2004. Treating opportunistic infections among HIV-infected adults and adolescents: recommendations from CDC, the National Institutes of Health, and the Infectious Diseases Society of America. *Morb. Mortal. Wkly. Rep.* **53**(RR-15)**:**1–112.

51. **Centers for Disease Control and Prevention.** 2006. Sexually transmitted diseases treatment guidelines—2006. *Morb. Mortal. Wkly. Rep.* **55**(RR-11):1–93.
52. **Cetinkaya, Y., P. Falk, and C. G. Mayhall.** 2000. Vancomycin-resistant enterococci. *Clin. Microbiol. Rev.* **13:**686–707.
53. **Cherry, R. D., D. Portnoy, M. Jabbari, D. S. Daly, D. G. Kinnear, and C. A. Goresky.** 1982. Metronidazole: an alternate therapy for antibiotic-associated colitis. *Gastroenterology* **82:**849–851.
54. **Cherubin, C. E.** 1981. Antibiotic resistance of *Salmonella* in Europe and the United States. *Rev. Infect. Dis.* **3:**1105–1126.
55. **Cherubin, C. E., and D. B. Azabache.** 1992. While nearly no one was watching: the rise of erythromycin and clindamycin resistance in *Streptococcus pneumoniae* and *Streptococcus pyogenes*. *Antimicrobic Newsl.* **8:**37–44.
56. **Chopra, I., and M. Roberts.** 2001. Tetracycline antibiotics: mode of action, applications, molecular biology, and epidemiology of bacterial resistance. *Microbiol. Mol Biol. Rev.* **65:**232–260.
57. **Chow, A. W., N. Cheng, and K. H. Bartlett.** 1985. In vitro susceptibility of *Clostridium difficile* to new beta-lactam and quinolone antibiotics. *Antimicrob. Agents Chemother.* **28:**842–844.
58. **Citron, D. M., K. L. Tyrrell, H. Fernandez, C. V. Merriam, and E. J. C. Goldstein.** 2005. In vitro activities of tinidazole and metronidazole against *Clostridium difficile, Prevotella bivia* and *Bacteroides fragilis*. *Anaerobe* **11:**315–317.
59. **Clark, J., and A. Wallace.** 1967. The susceptibility of mycobacteria to rifamide and rifampicin. *Tubercle* **48:**144–148.
60. **Clay, K. D., J. S. Hanson, S. D. Pope, R. W. Rissmiller, P. P. Purdum, and P. M. Banks.** 2006. Severe hepatotoxicity of telithromycin: three case reports and literature review. *Ann. Intern. Med.* **144:**E1–E6.
61. **Clemett, D., and A. Markham.** 2000. Linezolid. *Drugs* **59:**815–827.
62. **Cohen, M. A., M. D. Huband, J. W. Gage, S. L. Yoder, G. E. Roland, and S. J. Gracheck.** 1997. In-vitro activity of clinafloxacin, trovafloxacin, and ciprofloxacin. *J. Antimicrob. Chemother.* **40:**205–211.
63. **Cohen, M. A., E. T. Joannides, G. E. Roland, M. A. Meservey, M. D. Huband, M. A. Shapiro, J. C. Sesnie, and C. L. Heifetz.** 1994. In vitro evaluation of cefdinir (FK482), a new oral cephalosporin with enhanced antistaphylococcal activity and beta-lactamase stability. *Diagn. Microbiol. Infect. Dis.* **18:**31–39.
64. **Cohen, M. A., S. L. Yoder, and G. H. Talbot.** 1996. Sparfloxacin worldwide in vitro literature: isolate data available through 1994. *Diagn. Microbiol. Infect. Dis.* **25:**53–64.
65. **Collins, L. A., G. M. Eliopoulos, C. B. Wennersten, M. J. Ferraro, and R. C. Moellering, Jr.** 1993. In vitro activity of ramoplanin against vancomycin-resistant gram-positive organisms. *Antimicrob. Agents Chemother.* **37:**1364–1366.
66. **Coppens, L., and J. Klastersky.** 1979. Comparative study of anti-*Pseudomonas* activity of azlocillin, mezlocillin, and ticarcillin. *Antimicrob. Agents Chemother.* **15:**396–399.
67. **Copper, R. D.** 1992. The carbacephems: a new beta-lactam antibiotic class. *Am. J. Med.* **92**(Suppl. 6A)**:**2S–6S.
68. **Craig, W. A.** 1997. The pharmacology of meropenem, a new carbapenem antibiotic. *Clin. Infect. Dis.* **24**(Suppl. 2)**:**S266–S275.
69. **Cui, L., A. Iwamoto, J.-Q. Lian, H.-M. Neoh, T. Maruyama, Y. Horikawa, and K. Hiramatsu.** 2006. Novel mechanism of antibiotic resistance originating in vancomycin-intermediate *Staphylococcus aureus*. *Antimicrob. Agents Chemother.* **50:**428–438.
70. **Cui, L., X. Ma, K. Sato, K. Okuma, F. C. Tenover, E. M. Mamizuka, C. G. Gemmell, M.-N. Kim, M.-C. Ploy, N. El Solh, V. Ferraz, and K. Hiramatsu.** 2003. Cell wall thickening is a common feature of vancomycin resistance in *Staphylococcus aureus*. *J. Clin. Microbiol.* **41:**5–14.
71. **Cui, L., E. Tominaga, H.-M. Neoh, and K. Hiramatsu.** 2006. Correlation between reduced daptomycin susceptibility and vancomycin resistance in vancomycin-intermediate *Staphylococcus aureus*. *Antimicrob. Agents Chemother.* **50:**1079–1082.
72. **Cynamon, M. H., and G. S. Palmer.** 1982. In vitro susceptibility of *Mycobacterium fortuitum* to *N*-formimidoyl thienamycin and several cephamycins. *Antimicrob. Agents Chemother.* **22:**1079–1081.
73. **Cynamon, M. H., and G. S. Palmer.** 1983. In vitro activity of amoxicillin in combination with clavulanic acid against *Mycobacterium tuberculosis*. *Antimicrob. Agents Chemother.* **24:**429–431.
74. **Dajani, A. S., K. A. Taubert, W. Wilson, A. F. Bolger, A. Bayer, P. Ferrieri, M. H. Gewitz, S. T. Shulman, S. Nouri, J. W. Newburger, C. Hutto, T. J. Pallasch, T. W. Gage, M. E. Levison, G. Peter, and G. Zuccaro, Jr.** 1997. Prevention of bacterial endocarditis: recommendations by the American Heart Association. *JAMA* **277:**1794–1801.
75. **Dalhoff, A., and F.-J. Schmitz.** 2003. In vitro antibacterial activity and pharmacodynamics of new quinolones. *Eur. J. Clin. Microbiol. Infect. Dis.* **22:**203–221.
76. **Dannemann, B., J. A. McCutchan, D. Israelski, D. Antoniskis, C. Leport, B. Luft, J. Nussbaum, N. Clumeck, P. Morlat, J. Chiu, J. L. Vilde, P. Haseltine, J. Leedom, J. Remington, M. Orellana, D. Feigal, A. Bartok, and the California Collaborative Treatment Group.** 1992. Treatment of toxoplasmic encephalitis in patients with AIDS: a randomized trial comparing pyrimethamine plus clindamycin to pyrimethamine plus sulfadiazine. *Ann. Intern. Med.* **116:**33–43.
77. **Davey, P., J.-C. Pechere, and D. Speller.** 1988. Spiramycin reassessed. *J. Antimicrob. Chemother.* **22**(Suppl. B)**:**1–213.
78. **Davey, P. G., and A. H. Williams.** 1991. A review of the safety profile of teicoplanin. *J. Antimicrob. Chemother.* **27**(Suppl. B)**:**69–73.
79. **Davies, J. E.** 1983. Resistance to aminoglycosides: mechanisms and frequency. *Rev. Infect. Dis.* **5**(Suppl. 2)**:** S261–S267.
80. **Davies, S., P. D. Sparham, and R. C. Spencer.** 1987. Comparative in-vitro activity of five fluoroquinolones against mycobacteria. *J. Antimicrob. Chemother.* **19:**605–609.
81. **Davis, B. D.** 1982. Bactericidal synergism between beta-lactams and aminoglycosides: mechanism and possible therapeutic implications. *Rev. Infect. Dis.* **4:**237–245.
82. **Davis, R., and H. M. Bryson.** 1994. Levofloxacin: a review of its antibacterial activity, pharmacokinetics and therapeutic efficacy. *Drugs* **47:**677–700.
83. **Denton, M., and K. G. Kerr.** 1998. Microbiological and clinical aspects of infection associated with *Stenotrophomonas maltophilia*. *Clin. Microbiol. Rev.* **11:**57–80.
84. **Dewsnup, D. H., and D. N. Wright.** 1984. In vitro susceptibility of *Nocardia asteroides* to 25 antimicrobial agents. *Antimicrob. Agents Chemother.* **25:**165–167.
85. **Doebbeling, B. N., D. L. Breneman, H. C. Neu, R. Aly, B. G. Yangco, H. P. Holley, Jr., R. J. Marsh, M. A. Pfaller, J. E. McGowan, Jr., B. E. Scully, D. R. Reagan, R. P. Wenzel, and the Mupirocin Collaborative Study Group.** 1993. Elimination of *Staphylococcus aureus* nasal carriage in health care workers: analysis of six clinical trials with calcium mupirocin ointment. *Clin. Infect. Dis.* **17:**466–474.
86. **Drusano, G.** 2001. Pharmacodynamic and pharmacokinetic considerations in antimicrobial selection: focus on telithromycin. *Clin. Microbiol. Infect.* **7**(Suppl. 3)**:**24–29.
87. **Drusano, G. L., S. C. Schimpff, and W. L. Hewitt.** 1984. The acylampicillins: mezlocillin, piperacillin, and azlocillin. *Rev. Infect. Dis.* **6:**13–32.

88. **Dudley, M. N., J. C. McLaughlin, G. Carrington, J. Frick, C. H. Nightingale, and R. Quintiliani.** 1986. Oral bacitracin vs vancomycin therapy for *Clostridium difficile*-induced diarrhea: a randomized double-blind trial. *Arch. Intern. Med.* **146:**1101–1104.
89. **du Plessis, M., T. P. Capper, and K. P. Klugman.** 2002. In vitro activity of faropenem against respiratory pathogens. *J. Antimicrob. Chemother.* **49:**573–584.
90. **DuPont, H. L.** 2005. Travelers' diarrhea: antimicrobial therapy and chemoprevention. *Nat. Clin. Pract. Gastroenterol. Hepatol.* **2:**191–198.
91. **DuPont, H. L., Z. D. Jiang, C. D. Ericsson, J. A. Adachi, J. J. Mathewson, M. W. DuPont, E. Palazzini, L. M. Riopel, D. Ashley, and F. Martinez-Sandoval.** 2001. Rifaximin versus ciprofloxacin for the treatment of traveler's diarrhea: a randomized, double-blind clinical trial. *Clin. Infect. Dis.* **33:**1807–1815.
92. **DuPont, H. L., Z. D. Jiang, P. C. Okhuysen, C. D. Ericsson, F. J. de la Cabada, S. Ke, M. W. DuPont, and F. Martinez-Sandoval.** 2005. A randomized, double-blind, placebo-controlled trial of rifaximin to prevent travelers' diarrhea. *Ann. Intern. Med.* **142:**805–812.
93. **Eady, E. A., J. I. Ross, and J. H. Cove.** 1990. Multiple mechanisms of erythromycin resistance. *J. Antimicrob. Chemother.* **26:**461–465.
94. **Edelstein, P. H., E. A. Gaudet, and M. A. Edelstein.** 1989. In vitro activity of lomefloxacin (NY-198 or SC 47111), ciprofloxacin, and erythromycin against 100 clinical *Legionella* strains. *Diagn. Microbiol. Infect. Dis.* **12**(Suppl. 3)**:** 93S–95S.
95. **Ednie, L. M., M. R. Jacobs, and P. C. Appelbaum.** 1998. Activities of gatifloxacin compared to those of seven other agents against anaerobic organisms. *Antimicrob. Agents Chemother.* **42:**2459–2462.
96. **Edwards, D. I.** 1993. Nitroimidazole drugs: action and resistance mechanisms. I. Mechanisms of action. *J. Antimicrob. Chemother.* **31:**9–20.
97. **Edwards, J. R.** 1995. Meropenem: a microbiological overview. *J. Antimicrob. Chemother.* **36**(Suppl. A)**:**1–17.
98. **Eliopoulos, G. M., and C. T. Eliopoulos.** 1993. Activity in vitro of the quinolones, p. 161–193. *In* D. C. Hooper and J. S. Wolfson (ed.), *Quinolone Antimicrobial Agents*, 2nd ed. American Society for Microbiology, Washington, D.C.
99. **Eliopoulos, G. M., K. Klimm, M. J. Ferraro, G. A. Jacoby, and R. C. Moellering, Jr.** 1989. Comparative in vitro activity of piperacillin combined with the beta-lactamase inhibitor tazobactam (YTR 830). *Diagn. Microbiol. Infect. Dis.* **12:**481–488.
100. **Engberg, J., F. M. Aarestrup, D. E. Taylor, P. Gerner-Smidt, and I. Nachamkin.** 2001. Quinolone and macrolide resistance in *Campylobacter jejuni* and *C. coli*: resistance mechanisms and trends in human isolates. *Emerg. Infect. Dis.* **7:**24–34.
101. **Falagas, M. E., and I. A. Bliziotis.** 2006. Quinolones for treatment of human brucellosis: critical review of the evidence from microbiological and clinical studies. *Antimicrob. Agents Chemother.* **50:**22–33.
102. **Farrell, D. J., and D. Felmingham.** 2004. Activities of telithromycin against 13,874 *Streptococcus pneumoniae* isolates collected between 1999 and 2003. *Antimicrob. Agents Chemother.* **48:**1882–1884.
103. **Farver, D. K., D. D. Hedge, and S. C. Lee.** 2005. Ramoplanin: a lipoglycodepsipeptide antibiotic. *Ann. Pharmacother.* **39:**863–868.
104. **Fass, R. J.** 1983. Comparative in vitro activities of third-generation cephalosporins. *Arch. Intern. Med.* **143:** 1743–1745.
105. **Fass, R. J., E. A. Copelan, J. T. Brandt, M. L. Moeschberger, and J. J. Ashton.** 1987. Platelet-mediated bleeding caused by broad-spectrum penicillins. *J. Infect. Dis.* **155:**1242–1248.
106. **Fee, W. E., Jr.** 1980. Aminoglycoside ototoxicity in the human. *Laryngoscope* **90**(Suppl. 24)**:**1–19.
107. **Feeley, T. W., G. C. Du Moulin, J. Hedley-Whyte, L. S. Bushnell, J. P. Gilbert, and D. S. Feingold.** 1975. Aerosol polymyxin and pneumonia in seriously ill patients. *N. Engl. J. Med.* **293:**471–475.
108. **Fekete, T.** 1993. Antimicrobial susceptibility testing of *Neisseria gonorrhoeae* and implications for epidemiology and therapy. *Clin. Microbiol. Rev.* **6:**22–33.
109. **Fekety, R., J. Silva, B. Buggy, and H. G. Deery.** 1984. Treatment of antibiotic-associated colitis with vancomycin. *J. Antimicrob. Chemother.* **14**(Suppl. D)**:**97–102.
110. **Felmingham, D.** 2001. Microbiological profile of telithromycin, the first ketolide antimicrobial. *Clin. Microbiol. Infect.* **7**(Suppl. 3)**:**2–10.
111. **Fernandez-Roblas, R., J. Esteban, F. Cabria, J. C. Lopez, M. S. Jimenez, and F. Soriano.** 2000. In vitro susceptibilities of rapidly growing mycobacteria to telithromycin (HMR 3647) and seven other antimicrobials. *Antimicrob. Agents Chemother.* **44:**181–182.
112. **Finch, R. G.** 1996. Antibacterial activity of quinupristin/dalfopristin: rationale for clinical use. *Drugs* **51**(Suppl. 1)**:** 31–37.
113. **Finland, M., C. Garner, C. Wilcox, and L. D. Sabath.** 1976. Susceptibility of beta-hemolytic streptococci to 65 antibacterial agents. *Antimicrob. Agents Chemother.* **9:**11–19.
114. **Finlay, J., L. Miller, and J. A. Poupard.** 2003. A review of the antimicrobial activity of clavulanate. *J. Antimicrob. Chemother.* **52:**18–23.
115. **Ford, C. W., J. C. Hamel, D. Stapert, J. K. Moerman, D. K. Hutchinson, M. R. Barbachyn, and G. E. Zurenko.** 1997. Oxazolidinones: new antibacterial agents. *Trends Microbiol.* **5:**196–200.
116. **Frampton, J. E., R. N. Brogden, H. D. Langtry, and M. M. Buckley.** 1992. Cefpodoxime proxetil: a review of its antibacterial activity, pharmacokinetic properties and therapeutic potential. *Drugs* **44:**889–917.
117. **Freeman, L. D., D. R. Hooper, D. F. Lathen, D. P. Nelson, W. O. Harrison, and D. S. Anderson.** 1983. Brief prophylaxis with doxycycline for the prevention of traveler's diarrhea. *Gastroenterology* **84:**276–280.
118. **French, G.** 2003. Safety and tolerability of linezolid. *J. Antimicrob. Chemother.* **51**(Suppl. S2)**:**ii45–ii53.
119. **Fritsche, T. R., J. T. Kirby, and R. N. Jones.** 2004. In vitro activity of tigecycline (GAR-936) tested against 11,859 recent clinical isolates associated with community-acquired respiratory tract and gram-positive cutaneous infections. *Diagn. Microbiol. Infect. Dis.* **49:**201–209.
120. **Frost, P., G. D. Weinstein, and E. C. Gomez.** 1972. Phototoxic potential of minocycline and doxycycline. *Arch. Dermatol.* **105:**681–683.
121. **Fu, K. P., and H. C. Neu.** 1976. In vitro study of netilmicin compared with other aminoglycosides. *Antimicrob. Agents Chemother.* **10:**526–534.
122. **Fu, K. P., and H. C. Neu.** 1979. Comparative inhibition of beta-lactamases by novel beta-lactam compounds. *Antimicrob. Agents Chemother.* **15:**171–176.
123. **Fuchs, P. C., A. L. Barry, and S. D. Brown.** 2001. In vitro activities of ertapenem (MK-0826) against clinical bacterial isolates from 11 North American medical centers. *Antimicrob. Agents Chemother.* **45:**1915–1918.
124. **Fuchs, P. C., A. L. Barry, C. Thornsberry, and R. N. Jones.** 1984. In vitro activity of ticarcillin plus clavulanic acid against 632 clinical isolates. *Antimicrob. Agents Chemother.* **25:**392–394.
125. **Fuller, A. T., G. Mellows, M. Woolford, G. T. Banks, K. D. Barrow, and E. B. Chain.** 1971. Pseudomonic acid: an

antibiotic produced by *Pseudomonas fluorescens*. *Nature* **234:**416–417.
126. **Fung-Tomc, J. C.** 1997. Fourth-generation cephalosporins. *Clin. Microbiol. Newsl.* **19:**129–136.
127. **Gardner, T. B., and D. R. Hill.** 2001. Treatment of giardiasis. *Clin. Microbiol. Rev.* **14:**114–128.
128. **Geraci, J. E., and W. R. Wilson.** 1981. Vancomycin therapy for infective endocarditis. *Rev. Infect. Dis.* **3**(Suppl.): S250–S258.
129. **Gerson, S. L., S. L. Kaplan, J. B. Bruss, V. Le, F. M. Arellano, B. Hafkin, and D. J. Kuter.** 2002. Hematologic effects of linezolid: summary of clinical experience. *Antimicrob. Agents Chemother.* **46:**2723–2726.
130. **Giamarellou, H.** 1986. Aminoglycosides plus beta-lactams against gram-negative organisms: evaluation of in vitro synergy and chemical interactions. *Am. J. Med.* **80:**126–137.
131. **Golan, Y., L. A. McDermott, N. V. Jacobus, E. J. C. Goldstein, S. Finegold, L. J. Harrell, D. W. Hecht, S. G. Jenkins, C. Pierson, R. Venezia, J. Rihs, P. Iannini, S. L. Gorbach, and D. R. Snydman.** 2003. Emergence of fluoroquinolone resistance among *Bacteroides* species. *J. Antimicrob. Chemother* **52:**208–213.
132. **Goldfarb, J., D. Crenshaw, J. O'Horo, E. Lemon, and J. L. Blumer.** 1988. Randomized clinical trial of topical mupirocin versus oral erythromycin for impetigo. *Antimicrob. Agents Chemother.* **32:**1780–1783.
133. **Goldstein, E. J., D. M. Citron, C. Vreni Merriam, Y. Warren, and K. L. Tyrrell.** 2000. Comparative In vitro activities of ertapenem (MK-0826) against 1,001 anaerobes isolated from human intra-abdominal infections. *Antimicrob. Agents Chemother.* **44:**2389–2394.
134. **Goldstein, E. J., D. M. Citron, C. Vreni Merriam, Y. A. Warren, K. L. Tyrrell, and H. T. Fernandez.** 2003. In vitro activities of daptomycin, vancomycin, quinupristin-dalfopristin, linezolid, and five other antimicrobials against 307 gram-positive anaerobic and 31 *Corynebacterium* clinical isolates. *Antimicrob. Agents Chemother.* **47:**337–341.
135. **Goldstein, F. W., B. Papadopoulou, and J. F. Acar.** 1986. The changing pattern of trimethoprim resistance in Paris, with a review of worldwide experience. *Rev. Infect. Dis.* **8:**725–737.
136. **Gomi, H., Z. D. Jiang, J. A. Adachi, D. Ashley, B. Lowe, M. P. Verenkar, R. Steffen, and H. L. DuPont.** 2001. In vitro antimicrobial susceptibility testing of bacterial enteropathogens causing traveler's diarrhea in four geographic regions. *Antimicrob. Agents Chemother.* **45:**212–216.
137. **Gordin, F. M., G. L. Simon, C. B. Wofsy, and J. Mills.** 1984. Adverse reactions to trimethoprim-sulfamethoxazole in patients with the acquired immunodeficiency syndrome. *Ann. Intern. Med.* **100:**495–499.
138. **Gorzynski, E. A., D. Amsterdam, T. R. Beam, Jr., and C. Rotstein.** 1989. Comparative in vitro activities of teicoplanin, vancomycin, oxacillin, and other antimicrobial agents against bacteremic isolates of gram-positive cocci. *Antimicrob. Agents Chemother.* **33:**2019–2022.
139. **Grasela, D. M.** 2000. Clinical pharmacology of gatifloxacin, a new fluoroquinolone. *Clin. Infect. Dis.* **31**(Suppl. 2):S51–S58.
140. **Gravenkemper, C. F., J. V. Bennett, J. L. Brodie, and W. M. Kirby.** 1965. Dicloxacillin: in vitro and pharmacologic comparisons with oxacillin and cloxacillin. *Arch. Intern. Med.* **116:**340–345.
141. **Greenwood, D.** 1988. Microbiological properties of teicoplanin. *J. Antimicrob. Chemother.* **21**(Suppl. A):1–13.
142. **Grosset, J., and S. Leventis.** 1983. Adverse effects of rifampin. *Rev. Infect. Dis.* **5**(Suppl. 3):S440–S450.
143. **Grossman, E. R., A. Walchek, and H. Freedman.** 1971. Tetracyclines and permanent teeth: the relation between dose and tooth color. *Pediatrics* **47:**567–570.
144. **Gump, D. W.** 1981. Vancomycin for treatment of bacterial meningitis. *Rev. Infect. Dis.* **3**(Suppl.):S289–S292.
145. **Gutmann, L., M. D. Kitzis, S. Yamabe, and J. F. Acar.** 1986. Comparative evaluation of a new beta-lactamase inhibitor, YTR 830, combined with different beta-lactam antibiotics against bacteria harboring known beta-lactamases. *Antimicrob. Agents Chemother.* **29:**955–957.
146. **Guttler, R. B., G. W. Counts, C. K. Avent, and H. N. Beaty.** 1971. Effect of rifampin and minocycline on meningococcal carrier rates. *J. Infect. Dis.* **124:**199–205.
147. **Hansen, L. H., P. Mauvais, and S. Douthwaite.** 1999. The macrolide-ketolide antibiotic binding site is formed by structures in domains II and V of 23S ribosomal RNA. *Mol. Microbiol.* **31:**623–631.
148. **Hardy, D. J., D. M. Hensey, J. M. Beyer, C. Vojtko, E. J. McDonald, and P. B. Fernandes.** 1988. Comparative in vitro activities of new 14-, 15-, and 16-membered macrolides. *Antimicrob. Agents Chemother.* **32:**1710–1719.
149. **Hau, T.** 2002. Efficacy and safety of linezolid in the treatment of skin and soft tissue infections. *Eur. J. Clin. Microbiol. Infect. Dis.* **21:**491–498.
150. **Hawkey, P. M.** 2003. Mechanisms of quinolone action and microbial response. *J. Antimicrob. Chemother.* **51**(Suppl. 1): 29–35.
151. **Hayden, M. K., K. Rezai, R. A. Hayes, K. Lolans, J. P. Quinn, and R. A. Weinstein.** 2005. Development of daptomycin resistance in vivo in methicillin-resistant *Staphylococcus aureus*. *J. Clin. Microbiol.* **43:**5285–5287.
152. **Haydon, R. C., J. W. Thelin, and W. E. Davis.** 1984. Erythromycin ototoxicity: analysis and conclusions based on 22 case reports. *Otolaryngol. Head Neck Surg.* **92:**678–684.
153. **Hiramatsu, K.** 2001. Vancomycin-resistant *Staphylococcus aureus*: a new model of antibiotic resistance. *Lancet. Infect. Dis.* **1:**147–155.
154. **Hisanaga, T., D. J. Hoban, and G. G. Zhanel.** 2005. Mechanisms of resistance to telithromycin in *Streptococcus pneumoniae*. *J. Antimicrob. Chemother.* **56:**447–450.
155. **Hitchings, G. H.** 1973. Mechanism of action of trimethoprim-sulfamethoxazole. *J. Infect. Dis.* **128**(Suppl.)**:**433–436.
156. **Hoban, D. J., S. K. Bouchillon, B. M. Johnson, J. L. Johnson, and M. J. Dowzicky.** 2005. In vitro activity of tigecycline against 6792 Gram-negative and Gram-positive clinical isolates from the global Tigecycline Evaluation and Surveillance Trial (TEST Program, 2004). *Diagn. Microbiol. Infect. Dis.* **52:**215–227.
157. **Hoban, D. J., R. N. Jones, N. Yamane, R. Frei, A. Trilla, and A. C. Pignatari.** 1993. In vitro activity of three carbapenem antibiotics: comparative studies with biapenem (L-627), imipenem, and meropenem against aerobic pathogens isolated worldwide. *Diagn. Microbiol. Infect. Dis.* **17:**299–305.
158. **Hoeprich, P. D., and D. M. Warshauer.** 1974. Entry of four tetracyclines into saliva and tears. *Antimicrob. Agents Chemother.* **5:**330–336.
159. **Hof, H., O. Zak, E. Schweizer, and A. Denzler.** 1984. Antibacterial activities of nitrothiazole derivatives. *J. Antimicrob. Chemother.* **14:**31–39.
160. **Holmberg, L., G. Boman, L. E. Bottiger, B. Eriksson, R. Spross, and A. Wessling.** 1980. Adverse reactions to nitrofurantoin: analysis of 921 reports. *Am. J. Med.* **69:**733–738.
161. **Hooton, T. M., and W. E. Stamm.** 1997. Diagnosis and treatment of uncomplicated urinary tract infection. *Infect. Dis. Clin. N. Am.* **11:**551–581.
162. **Hope, R., M. Warner, S. Mushtaq, M. E. Ward, T. Parsons, and D. M. Livermore.** 2005. Effect of medium type, age and aeration on the MICs of tigecycline and classical tetracyclines. *J. Antimicrob. Chemother.* **56:**1042–1046.
163. **Horiuchi, S., Y. Inagaki, N. Yamamoto, N. Okamura, Y. Imagawa, and R. Nakaya.** 1993. Reduced susceptibilities of *Shigella sonnei* strains isolated from patients with dysentery

to fluoroquinolones. *Antimicrob. Agents Chemother.* **37:** 2486–2489.

164. **Huang, D. B., and H. L. DuPont.** 2005. Rifaximin: a novel antimicrobial for enteric infections. *J. Infect.* **50:**97–106.
165. **Hughes, J., and G. Mellows.** 1978. Inhibition of isoleucyl-transfer ribonucleic acid synthetase in *Escherichia coli* by pseudomonic acid. *Biochem. J.* **176:**305–318.
166. **Hunfeld, K.-P., T. A. Wichelhaus, R. Rodel, G. Acker, V. Brade, and P. Kraiczy.** 2004. Comparison of in vitro activities of ketolides, macrolides, and an azalide against the spirochete *Borrelia burgdorferi*. *Antimicrob. Agents Chemother.* **48:**344–347.
167. **Jacobus, N. V., L. A. McDermott, R. Ruthazer, and D. R. Snydman.** 2004. In vitro activities of tigecycline against the *Bacteroides fragilis* group. *Antimicrob. Agents Chemother.* **48:**1034–1036.
168. **Jacoby, G. A., N. Chow, and K. B. Waites.** 2003. Prevalence of plasmid-mediated quinolone resistance. *Antimicrob. Agents Chemother.* **47:**559–562.
169. **Jacoby, G. A., and L. S. Munoz-Price.** 2005. The new beta-lactamases. *N. Engl. J. Med.* **352:**380–391.
170. **Jacoby, G. A., and L. Sutton.** 1989. *Pseudomonas cepacia* susceptibility to sulbactam. *Antimicrob. Agents Chemother.* **33:**583–584.
171. **Jiang, Z. D., S. Ke, E. Palazzini, L. Riopel, and H. Dupont.** 2000. In vitro activity and fecal concentration of rifaximin after oral administration. *Antimicrob. Agents Chemother.* **44:**2205–2206.
172. **Johnson, A. P., A. H. Uttley, N. Woodford, and R. C. George.** 1990. Resistance to vancomycin and teicoplanin: an emerging clinical problem. *Clin. Microbiol. Rev.* **3:** 280–291.
173. **Johnson, D. M., D. J. Biedenbach, M. L. Beach, M. A. Pfaller, and R. N. Jones.** 2000. Antimicrobial activity and in vitro susceptibility test development for cefditoren against *Haemophilus influenzae*, *Moraxella catarrhalis*, and *Streptococcus* species. *Diagn. Microbiol. Infect. Dis.* **37:**99–105.
174. **Jokipii, A. M. M., and L. Jokipii.** 1987. Comparative activity of metronidazole and tinidazole against *Clostridium difficile* and *Peptostreptococcus anaerobius*. *Antimicrob. Agents Chemother.* **31:**183–186.
175. **Jones, R. N.** 1989. Review of the in-vitro spectrum and characteristics of cefmetazole (CS-1170). *J. Antimicrob. Chemother.* **23**(Suppl. D)**:**1–12.
176. **Jones, R. N.** 2006. Microbiological features of vancomycin in the 21st century: minimum inhibitory concentration creep, bactericidal/static activity, and applied breakpoints to predict clinical outcomes or detect resistant strains. *Clin. Infect. Dis.* **42**(Suppl. 1)**:**S13–S24.
177. **Jones, R. N., and A. L. Barry.** 1983. Cefoperazone: a review of its antimicrobial spectrum, beta-lactamase stability, enzyme inhibition, and other in vitro characteristics. *Rev. Infect. Dis.* **5**(Suppl. 1)**:**S108–S126.
178. **Jones, R. N., D. J. Biedenbach, and D. M. Johnson.** 2000. Cefditoren activity against nearly 1,000 non-fastidious bacterial isolates and the development of in vitro susceptibility test methods. *Diagn. Microbiol. Infect. Dis.* **37:**143–146.
179. **Jones, R. N., H. K. Huynh, D. J. Biedenbach, T. R. Fritsche, and H. S. Sader.** 2004. Doripenem (S-4661), a novel carbapenem: comparative activity against contemporary pathogens including bactericidal action and preliminary in vitro methods evaluations. *J. Antimicrob. Chemother.* **54:**144–154.
180. **Jones, R. N., M. A. Pfaller, S. D. Allen, E. H. Gerlach, P. C. Fuchs, and K. E. Aldridge.** 1991. Antimicrobial activity of cefpirome: an update compared to five third-generation cephalosporins against nearly 6000 recent clinical isolates from five medical centers. *Diagn. Microbiol. Infect. Dis.* **14:**361–364.
181. **Jones, S. L., E. Athan, and D. O'Brien.** 2004. Serotonin syndrome due to co-administration of linezolid and venlafaxine. *J. Antimicrob. Chemother.* **54:**289–290.
182. **Jorgensen, J. H., S. A. Crawford, C. C. Kelly, and J. E. Patterson.** 2003. In vitro activity of daptomycin against vancomycin-resistant enterococci of various Van types and comparison of susceptibility testing methods. *Antimicrob. Agents Chemother.* **47:**3760–3763.
183. **Jorgensen, J. H., S. A. Crawford, M. L. McElmeel, and C. G. Whitney.** 2004. Activities of cethromycin and telithromycin against recent North American isolates of *Streptococcus penumoniae*. *Antimicrob. Agents Chemother.* **48:**605–607.
184. **Kahan, F. M., J. S. Kahan, P. J. Cassidy, and H. Kropp.** 1974. The mechanism of action of fosfomycin (phosphonomycin). *Ann. N. Y. Acad. Sci.* **235:**364–386.
185. **Kahne, D., C. Leimkuhler, W. Lu, and C. Walsh.** 2005. Glycopeptide and lipoglycopeptide antibiotics. *Chem. Rev.* **105:**425–448.
186. **Kelkar, P. S., and J. T. Li.** 2001. Cephalosporin allergy. *N. Engl. J. Med.* **345:**804–809.
187. **Kenny, G. E., T. M. Hooton, M. C. Roberts, F. D. Cartwright, and J. Hoyt.** 1989. Susceptibilities of genital mycoplasmas to the newer quinolones as determined by the agar dilution method. *Antimicrob. Agents Chemother.* **33:**103–107.
188. **Khaliq, Y., and G. G. Zhanel.** 2003. Fluoroquinolone-associated tendinopathy: a critical review of the literature. *Clin. Infect. Dis.* **36:**1404–1410.
189. **Kirst, H. A., and G. D. Sides.** 1989. New directions for macrolide antibiotics: structural modifications and in vitro activity. *Antimicrob. Agents Chemother.* **33:** 1413–1418.
190. **Klugman, K. P.** 1990. Pneumococcal resistance to antibiotics. *Clin. Microbiol. Rev.* **3:**171–196.
191. **Knapp, C. C., J. Sierra-Madero, and J. A. Washington.** 1989. Activity of ticarcillin/clavulanate and piperacillin/tazobactam (YTR 830; CL-298,741) against clinical isolates and against mutants derepressed for class I beta-lactamase. *Diagn. Microbiol. Infect. Dis.* **12:**511–515.
192. **Knight, V., J. W. Draper, E. A. Brady, and C. A. Attmore.** 1952. Methenamine mandelate: antimicrobial activity, absorption and excretion. *Antibiot. Chemother.* **2:**615–635.
193. **Kohler, J., K. L. Dorso, K. Young, G. G. Hammond, H. Rosen, H. Kropp, and L. L. Silver.** 1999. In vitro activities of the potent, broad-spectrum carbapenem MK-0826 (L-749,345) against broad-spectrum beta-lactamase- and extended-spectrum beta-lactamase-producing *Klebsiella pneumoniae* and *Escherichia coli* clinical isolates. *Antimicrob. Agents Chemother.* **43:**1170–1176.
194. **Kuck, N. A., N. V. Jacobus, P. J. Petersen, W. J. Weiss, and R. T. Testa.** 1989. Comparative in vitro and in vivo activities of piperacillin combined with the beta-lactamase inhibitors tazobactam, clavulanic acid, and sulbactam. *Antimicrob. Agents Chemother.* **33:**1964–1969.
195. **Lamb, H. M., D. P. Figgitt, and D. Faulds.** 1999. Quinupristin/dalfopristin: a review of its use in the management of serious gram-positive infections. *Drugs* **58:** 1061–1097.
196. **Lawson, D. H., and B. J. Paice.** 1982. Adverse reactions to trimethoprim-sulfamethoxazole. *Rev. Infect. Dis.* **4:**429–433.
197. **Leclercq, R.** 2002. Mechanisms of resistance to macrolides and lincosamides: nature of the resistance elements and their clinical implications. *Clin. Infect. Dis.* **34:**482–492.
198. **Lee, E., S. Burger, J. Shah, C. Melton, M. Mullen, F. Warren, and R. Press.** 2003. Linezolid-associated toxic optic neuropathy: a report of 2 cases. *Clin. Infect. Dis.* **37:**1389–1391.

199. **Leigh, D. A.** 1981. Antibacterial activity and pharmacokinetics of clindamycin. *J. Antimicrob. Chemother.* **7**(Suppl. A): 3–9.
200. **Lell, B., and P. G. Kremsner.** 2002. Clindamycin as an antimalarial drug: review of clinical trials. *Antimicrob. Agents Chemother.* **46:**2315–2320.
201. **Linden, P. K., R. C. Moellering, Jr., C. A. Wood, S. J. Rehm, J. Flaherty, F. Bompart, and G. H. Talbot.** 2001. Treatment of vancomycin-resistant *Enterococcus faecium* infections with quinupristin/dalfopristin. *Clin. Infect. Dis.* **33:**1816–1823.
202. **Lipsky, B. A., and C. A. Baker.** 1999. Fluoroquinolone toxicity profiles: a review focusing on newer agents. *Clin. Infect. Dis.* **28:**352–364.
203. **Livermore, D. M.** 2003. Linezolid in vitro: mechanism and antibacterial spectrum. *J. Antimicrob. Chemother.* **51**(Suppl. 2):ii9–ii16.
204. **Livermore, D. M., M. W. Carter, S. Bagel, B. Wiedemann, F. Baquero, E. Loza, H. P. Endtz, N. van Den Braak, C. J. Fernandes, L. Fernandes, N. Frimodt-Moller, L. S. Rasmussen, H. Giamarellou, E. Giamarellos-Bourboulis, V. Jarlier, J. Nguyen, C. E. Nord, M. J. Struelens, C. Nonhoff, J. Turnidge, J. Bell, R. Zbinden, S. Pfister, L. Mixson, and D. L. Shungu.** 2001. In vitro activities of ertapenem (MK-0826) against recent clinical bacteria collected in Europe and Australia. *Antimicrob. Agents Chemother.* **45:**1860–1867.
205. **Livermore, D. M., K. J. Oakton, M. W. Carter, and M. Warner.** 2001. Activity of ertapenem (MK-0826) versus *Enterobacteriaceae* with potent beta-lactamases. *Antimicrob. Agents Chemother.* **45:**2831–2837.
206. **Lode, H., K. Borner, P. Koeppe, and T. Schaberg.** 1996. Azithromycin: review of key chemical, pharmacokinetic and microbiological features. *J. Antimicrob. Chemother.* **37** (Suppl. C):1–8.
207. **Lofmark, S., H. Fang, M. Hedberg, and C. Edlund.** 2005. Inducible metronidazole resistance and *nim* genes in clinical *Bacteroides fragilis* group isolates. *Antimicrob. Agents Chemother.* **49:**1253–1256.
208. **Long, J. K., T. K. Choueiri, G. S. Hall, R. K. Avery, and M. A. Sekeres.** 2005. Daptomycin-resistant *Enterococcus faecium* in a patient with acute myeloid leukemia. *Mayo Clin. Proc.* **80:**1215–1216.
209. **Low, D. E.** 1995. Quinupristin/dalfopristin: spectrum of activity, pharmacokinetics, and initial clinical experience. *Microb. Drug Resist.* **1:**223–234.
210. **Low, D. E., S. Brown, and D. Felmingham.** 2004. Clinical and bacteriological efficacy of the ketolide telithromycin against isolates of key respiratory pathogens: a pooled analysis of phase III studies. *Clin. Microbiol. Infect.* **10:**27–36.
211. **Low, D. E., A. McGeer, and R. Poon.** 1989. Activities of daptomycin and teicoplanin against *Staphylococcus haemolyticus* and *Staphylococcus epidermidis*, including evaluation of susceptibility testing recommendations. *Antimicrob. Agents Chemother.* **33:**585–588.
212. **Lutsar, I., G. H. McCracken, Jr., and I. R. Friedland.** 1998. Antibiotic pharmacodynamics in cerebrospinal fluid. *Clin. Infect. Dis.* **27:**1117–1127.
213. **MacGowan, A. P.** 2003. Pharmacokinetic and pharmacodynamic profile of linezolid in healthy volunteers and patients with Gram-positive infections. *J. Antimicrob. Chemother.* **51**(Suppl. S2):ii17–ii25.
214. **Malanoski, G. J., L. Collins, C. Wennersten, R. C. Moellering, Jr., and G. M. Eliopoulos.** 1993. In vitro activity of biapenem against clinical isolates of gram-positive and gram-negative bacteria. *Antimicrob. Agents Chemother.* **37:**2009–2016.
215. **Mandell, G. L.** 1983. The antimicrobial activity of rifampin: emphasis on the relation to phagocytes. *Rev. Infect. Dis.* **5**(Suppl. 3):S463–S467.
216. **Marchese, A., and G. C. Schito.** 2001. The oxazolidinones as a new family of antimicrobial agent. *Clin. Microbiol. Infect.* **7**(Suppl. 4):66–74.
217. **Marco, F., R. N. Jones, D. J. Hoban, A. C. Pignatari, N. Yamane, and R. Frei.** 1994. In-vitro activity of OPC-17116 against more than 6,000 consecutive clinical isolates: a multicentre international study. *J. Antimicrob. Chemother.* **33:**647–654.
218. **Maurin, M., S. Gasquet, C. Ducco, and D. Raoult.** 1995. MICs of 28 antibiotic compounds for 14 *Bartonella* (formerly *Rochalimaea*) isolates. *Antimicrob. Agents Chemother.* **39:**2387–2391.
219. **Maurin, M., and D. Raoult.** 2001. Use of aminoglycosides in treatment of infections due to intracellular bacteria. *Antimicrob. Agents Chemother.* **45:**2977–2986.
220. **McAleese, F., P. Petersen, A. Ruzin, P. M. Dunman, E. Murphy, S. J. Projan, and P. A. Bradford.** 2005. A novel MATE family efflux pump contributes to the reduced susceptibility of laboratory-derived *Staphylococcus aureus* mutants to tigecycline. *Antimicrob. Agents Chemother.* **49:**1865–1871.
221. **McCalla, D. R.** 1977. Biological effects of nitrofurans. *J. Antimicrob. Chemother.* **3:**517–520.
222. **McCracken, G. H., Jr.** 2000. Pharmacodynamics of gatifloxacin in experimental models of pneumococcal meningitis. *Clin. Infect. Dis.* **31**(Suppl. 2):S45–S50.
223. **McDowell, T. D., and K. E. Reed.** 1989. Mechanism of penicillin killing in the absence of bacterial lysis. *Antimicrob. Agents Chemother.* **33:**1680–1685.
224. **McGehee, R. F., Jr., C. B. Smith, C. Wilcox, and M. Finland.** 1968. Comparative studies of antibacterial activity in vitro and absorption and excretion of lincomycin and clinimycin. *Am. J. Med. Sci.* **256:**279–292.
225. **McNulty, C. A., J. Dent, and R. Wise.** 1985. Susceptibility of clinical isolates of *Campylobacter pyloridis* to 11 antimicrobial agents. *Antimicrob. Agents Chemother.* **28:**837–838.
226. **McOsker, C. C., and P. M. Fitzpatrick.** 1994. Nitrofurantoin: mechanism of action and implications for resistance development in common uropathogens. *J. Antimicrob. Chemother.* **33**(Suppl. A):23–30.
227. **Meagher, A. K., P. G. Ambrose, T. H. Grasela, and E. J. Ellis-Grosse.** 2005. Pharmacokinetic/pharmacodynamic profile for tigecycline—a new glycylcycline antimicrobial agent. *Diagn. Microbiol. Infect. Dis.* **52:**165–171.
228. **Medical Letter on Drugs and Therapeutics.** 2004. Drugs for parasitic infections. *Med. Lett. Drugs Ther.* **46:**1–12.
229. **Medical Letter on Drugs and Therapeutics.** 2005. Treatment of Lyme disease. *Med. Lett. Drugs Ther.* **47:**41–43.
230. **Medical Letter on Drugs and Therapeutics.** 2005. Prevention of malaria. *Med. Lett. Drugs Ther.* **47:**100–102.
231. **Meka, V. G., and H. S. Gold.** 2004. Antimicrobial resistance to linezolid. *Clin. Infect. Dis.* **39:**1010–1015.
232. **Mendez, J. L., H. F. Nadrous, T. E. Hartman, and J. H. Ryu.** 2005. Chronic nitrofurantoin-induced lung disease. *Mayo Clin. Proc.* **80:**1298–1302.
233. **Moellering, R. C.** 2003. Linezolid: the first oxazolidinone antimicrobial. *Ann. Intern. Med.* **138:**135–142.
234. **Moellering, R. C., Jr.** 1984. Pharmacokinetics of vancomycin. *J. Antimicrob. Chemother.* **14**(Suppl. D):43–52.
235. **Moellering, R. C., P. K. Linden, J. Reinhardt, E. A. Blumberg, F. Bompart, and G. H. Talbot for the Synercid Emergency-Use Study Group.** 1999. The efficacy and safety of quinupristin/dalfopristin for the treatment of infections caused by vancomycin-resistant *Enterococcus faecium*. *J. Antimicrob. Chemother.* **44:**251–261.
236. **Molavi, A., and L. Weinstein.** 1971. In-vitro activity of erythromycin against atypical mycobacteria. *J. Infect. Dis.* **123:**216–219.
237. **Monk, J. P., and D. M. Campoli-Richards.** 1987. Ofloxacin: a review of its antibacterial activity, pharmacokinetic properties and therapeutic use. *Drugs* **33:**346–391.

238. **Moore, I. F., D. W. Hughes, and G. D. Wright.** 2005. Tigecycline is modified by the flavin-dependent monooxygenase TetX. *Biochemistry* **44:**11829–11835.
239. **Moosdeen, F., J. D. Williams, and S. Yamabe.** 1988. Antibacterial characteristics of YTR 830, a sulfone beta-lactamase inhibitor, compared with those of clavulanic acid and sulbactam. *Antimicrob. Agents Chemother.* **32:**925–927.
240. **Morris, A. B., R. B. Brown, and M. Sands.** 1993. Use of rifampin in nonstaphylococcal, nonmycobacterial disease. *Antimicrob. Agents Chemother.* **37:**1–7.
241. **Murray, B. E.** 1990. The life and times of the *Enterococcus*. *Clin. Microbiol. Rev.* **3:**46–65.
242. **Muscato, J. J., D. W. Wilbur, J. J. Stout, and R. A. Fahrlender.** 1991. An evaluation of the susceptibility patterns of gram-negative organisms isolated in cancer centres with aminoglycoside usage. *J. Antimicrob. Chemother.* **27**(Suppl. C)**:**1–7.
243. **Nadelman, R. B., S. W. Luger, E. Frank, M. Wisniewski, J. J. Collins, and G. P. Wormser.** 1992. Comparison of cefuroxime axetil and doxycycline in the treatment of early Lyme disease. *Ann. Intern. Med.* **117:**273–280.
244. **Nagarajan, R.** 1991. Antibacterial activities and modes of action of vancomycin and related glycopeptides. *Antimicrob. Agents Chemother.* **35:**605–609.
245. **Najjar, A., and B. E. Murray.** 1987. Failure to demonstrate a consistent in vitro bactericidal effect of trimethoprim-sulfamethoxazole against enterococci. *Antimicrob. Agents Chemother.* **31:**808–810.
246. **Namour, F., D. H. Wessels, M. H. Pascual, D. Reynolds, E. Sultan, and B. Lenfant.** 2001. Pharmacokinetics of the new ketolide telithromycin (HMR 3647) administered in ascending single and multiple doses. *Antimicrob. Agents Chemother.* **45:**170–175.
247. **Neu, H. C.** 1976. Tobramycin: an overview. *J. Infect. Dis.* **134**(Suppl.)**:**S3–S19.
248. **Neu, H. C.** 1982. The new beta-lactamase-stable cephalosporins. *Ann. Intern. Med.* **97:**408–419.
249. **Neu, H. C.** 1985. Carbapenems: special properties contributing to their activity. *Am. J. Med.* **78**(Suppl. 6A)**:**33–40.
250. **Neu, H. C.** 1991. Clinical microbiology of azithromycin. *Am. J. Med.* **91**(Suppl. 3A)**:**12S–18S.
251. **Neu, H. C.** 1991. The development of macrolides: clarithromycin in perspective. *J. Antimicrob. Chemother.* **27**(Suppl. A)**:**1–9.
252. **Neu, H. C., and K. P. Fu.** 1978. Clavulanic acid, a novel inhibitor of beta-lactamases. *Antimicrob. Agents Chemother.* **14:**650–655.
253. **Neu, H. C., and K. P. Fu.** 1980. In vitro activity of chloramphenicol and thiamphenicol analogs. *Antimicrob. Agents Chemother.* **18:**311–316.
254. **Neu, H. C., and P. Labthavikul.** 1982. Comparative in vitro activity of *N*-formimidoyl thienamycin against gram-positive and gram-negative aerobic and anaerobic species and its beta-lactamase stability. *Antimicrob. Agents Chemother.* **21:**180–187.
255. **Nilsson, A. I., O. G. Berg, O. Aspevall, G. Kahlmeter, and D. I. Andersson.** 2003. Biological costs and mechanisms of fosfomycin resistance in *Escherichia coli*. *Antimicrob. Agents Chemother.* **47:**2850–2858.
256. **Nix, D. E., A. K. Majumdar, and M. J. DiNubile.** 2004. Pharmacokinetics and pharmacodynamics of ertapenem: an overview for clinicians. *J. Antimicrob. Chemother.* **53**(Suppl. 2)**:**ii23–ii28.
257. **Nord, C. E.** 1996. In vitro activity of quinolones and other antimicrobial agents against anaerobic bacteria. *Clin. Infect. Dis.* **23**(Suppl. 1)**:**S15–S18.
258. **Nordmann, P., and L. Poirel.** 2005. Emergence of plasmid-mediated resistance to quinolones in *Enterobacteriaceae*. *J. Antimicrob. Chemother.* **56:**463–469.
259. **Norrby, S. R., K. L. Faulkner, and P. A. Newell.** 1997. Differentiating meropenem and imipenem/cilastatin. *Infect. Dis. Clin. Pract.* **6:**291–303.
260. **Noskin, G. A.** 2005. Tigecycline: a new glycylcycline for treatment of serious infections. *Clin. Infect. Dis.* **41**(Suppl. 5)**:**S303–S314.
261. **O'Brien, R. J., M. A. Lyle, and D. E. Snider, Jr.** 1987. Rifabutin (ansamycin LM 427): a new rifamycin-S derivative for the treatment of mycobacterial diseases. *Rev. Infect. Dis.* **9:**519–530.
262. **Pace, J. L., and G. Yang.** 2006. Glycopeptides: update on an old successful antibiotic class. *Biochem. Pharmacol.* **71:**968–980.
263. **Pang, L. W., N. Limsomwong, E. F. Boudreau, and P. Singharaj.** 1987. Doxycycline prophylaxis for falciparum malaria. *Lancet* **i:**1161–1164.
264. **Pankey, G. A.** 2005. Tigecycline. *J. Antimicrob. Chemother.* **56:**470–480.
265. **Pankuch, G. A., T. A. Davies, M. R. Jacobs, and P. C. Appelbaum.** 2002. Antipneumococcal activity of ertapenem (MK-0826) compared to those of other agents. *Antimicrob. Agents Chemother.* **46:**42–46.
266. **Pape, J. W., R. I. Verdier, and W. D. Johnson, Jr.** 1989. Treatment and prophylaxis of *Isospora belli* infection in patients with the acquired immunodeficiency syndrome. *N. Engl. J. Med.* **320:**1044–1047.
267. **Patel, R. B., and P. G. Welling.** 1980. Clinical pharmacokinetics of co-trimoxazole (trimethoprim-sulphamethoxazole). *Clin. Pharmacokinet.* **5:**405–423.
268. **Patel, S. S., J. A. Balfour, and H. M. Bryson.** 1997. Fosfomycin tromethamine: a review of its antibacterial activity, pharmacokinetic properties and therapeutic efficacy as a single-dose oral treatment for acute uncomplicated lower urinary tract infections. *Drugs* **53:**637–656.
269. **Pechere, J. C.** 1996. Streptogramins: a unique class of antibiotics. *Drugs* **51**(Suppl. 1)**:**13–19.
270. **Pechere, J. C.** 1999. Current and future management of infections due to methicillin-resistant staphylococci infections: the role of quinupristin/dalfopristin. *J. Antimicrob. Chemother.* **44**(Suppl. A)**:**11–18.
271. **Perry, C. M., J. A. Barman Balfour, and H. M. Lamb.** 1999. Gatifloxacin. *Drugs* **58:**683–696.
272. **Perry, C. M., and B. Jarvis.** 2001. Linezolid: a review of its use in the management of serious gram-positive infections. *Drugs* **61:**525–551.
273. **Peters, D. H., H. A. Friedel, and D. McTavish.** 1992. Azithromycin: a review of its antimicrobial activity, pharmacokinetic properties and clinical efficacy. *Drugs* **44:**750–799.
274. **Pfaller, M. A., A. L. Barry, and P. C. Fuchs.** 1993. Evaluation of disk susceptibility testing of fosfomycin tromethamine. *Diagn. Microbiol. Infect. Dis.* **17:**67–70.
275. **Pitkin, D. H., W. Sheikh, and H. L. Nadler.** 1997. Comparative in vitro activity of meropenem versus other extended-spectrum antimicrobials against randomly chosen and selected resistant clinical isolates tested in 26 North American centers. *Clin. Infect. Dis.* **24**(Suppl. 2)**:**S238–S248.
276. **Plouffe, J. F.** 2000. Emerging therapies for serious gram-positive bacterial infections: a focus on linezolid. *Clin. Infect. Dis.* **31**(Suppl. 4)**:**S144–S149.
277. **Polk, R. E.** 1989. Drug-drug interactions with ciprofloxacin and other fluoroquinolones. *Am. J. Med.* **87**(Suppl. 5A)**:**76S–81S.
278. **Polk, R. E., D. P. Healy, L. B. Schwartz, D. T. Rock, M. L. Garson, and K. Roller.** 1988. Vancomycin and the red-man syndrome: pharmacodynamics of histamine release. *J. Infect. Dis.* **157:**502–507.
279. **Qadri, S. M., B. A. Cunha, Y. Ueno, F. Abumustafa, H. Imambaccus, D. D. Tullo, and P. Domenico.** 1995. Activity of cefepime against nosocomial blood culture isolates. *J. Antimicrob. Chemother.* **36:**531–536.

280. **Raad, I., R. Hachem, H. Hanna, E. Girgawy, K. Rolston, E. Whimbey, R. Husni, and G. Bodey.** 2001. Treatment of vancomycin-resistant enterococcal infections in the immunocompromised host: quinupristin-dalfopristin in combination with minocycline. *Antimicrob. Agents Chemother.* **45:**3202–3204.

281. **Raoult, D., P. Roussellier, V. Galicher, R. Perez, and J. Tamalet.** 1986. In vitro susceptibility of *Rickettsia conorii* to ciprofloxacin as determined by suppressing lethality in chicken embryos and by plaque assay. *Antimicrob. Agents Chemother.* **29:**424–425.

282. **Raoult, D., H. Torres, and M. Drancourt.** 1991. Shell-vial assay: evaluation of a new technique for determining antibiotic susceptibility, tested in 13 isolates of *Coxiella burnetii. Antimicrob. Agents Chemother.* **35:**2070–2077.

283. **Reeves, D. S.** 1994. Fosfomycin trometamol. *J. Antimicrob. Chemother.* **34:**853–858.

284. **Retsema, J. A., A. R. English, A. Girard, J. E. Lynch, M. Anderson, L. Brennan, C. Cimochowski, J. Faiella, W. Norcia, and P. Sawyer.** 1986. Sulbactam/ampicillin: in vitro spectrum, potency, and activity in models of acute infection. *Rev. Infect. Dis.* **8**(Suppl. 5):S528–S534.

284a. **Robicsek, A., J. Strahilevitz, G. A. Jacoby, M. Macielag, D. Abbanat, C. H. Park, K. Bush, and D. C. Hooper.** 2006. Fluoroquinolone-modifying enzyme: a new adaptation of a common aminoglycoside acetyltransferase. *Nat. Med.* **12:**83–88.

285. **Rodloff, A. C.** 1982. In-vitro susceptibility test of non-tuberculous mycobacteria to sulphamethoxazole, trimethoprim, and combinations of both. *J. Antimicrob. Chemother.* **9:**195–199.

286. **Rolston, K. V., and J. Hoy.** 1987. Role of clindamycin in the treatment of central nervous system toxoplasmosis. *Am. J. Med.* **83:**551–554.

287. **Rose, H. D., and M. W. Rytel.** 1972. Actinomycosis treated with clindamycin. *JAMA* **221:**1052.

288. **Rosenblatt, J. E., and P. R. Stewart.** 1974. Combined activity of sulfamethoxazole, trimethoprim, and polymyxin B against gram-negative bacilli. *Antimicrob. Agents Chemother.* **6:**84–92.

289. **Rubin, R. H., and M. N. Swartz.** 1980. Trimethoprim-sulfamethoxazole. *N. Engl. J. Med.* **303:**426–432.

290. **Rubinstein, E., S. Cammarata, T. Oliphant, and R. Wunderink.** 2001. Linezolid (PNU-100766) versus vancomycin in the treatment of hospitalized patients with nosocomial pneumonia: a randomized, double-blind, multicenter study. *Clin. Infect. Dis.* **32:**402–412.

291. **Rubinstein, E., R. Isturiz, H. C. Standiford, L. G. Smith, T. H. Oliphant, S. Cammarata, B. Hafkin, V. Le, and J. Remington.** 2003. Worldwide assessment of linezolid's clinical safety and tolerability: comparator-controlled phase III studies. *Antimicrob. Agents Chemother.* **47:**1824–1831.

292. **Rubinstein, E., P. Prokocimer, and G. H. Talbot.** 1999. Safety and tolerability of quinupristin/dalfopristin: administration guidelines. *J. Antimicrob. Chemother.* **44**(Suppl. A):37–46.

293. **Ruoff, K. L., D. R. Kuritzkes, J. S. Wolfson, and M. J. Ferraro.** 1988. Vancomycin-resistant gram-positive bacteria isolated from human sources. *J. Clin. Microbiol.* **26:**2064–2068.

294. **Ruzin, A., M. A. Visalli, D. Keeney, and P. A. Bradford.** 2005. Influence of transcriptional activator RamA on expression of multidrug efflux pump AcrAB and tigecycline susceptibility in *Klebsiella pneumoniae. Antimicrob. Agents Chemother.* **49:**1017–1022.

295. **Rybak, M. J.** 2006. The efficacy and safety of daptomycin: first in a new class of antibiotics for gram-positive bacteria. *Clin. Microbiol. Infect.* **12**(Suppl. 1):24–32.

296. **Rybak, M. J.** 2006. The pharmacokinetic and pharmacodynamic properties of vancomycin. *Clin. Infect. Dis.* **42**(Suppl. 1):S35–S39.

297. **Sabol, K., J. E. Patterson, J. S. Lewis, A. Owens, J. Cadena, and J. H. Jorgensen.** 2005. Emergence of daptomycin resistance in *Enterococcus faecium* during daptomycin therapy. *Antimicrob. Agents Chemother.* **49:**1664–1665.

298. **Sader, H. S., R. N. Jones, J. A. Washington, P. R. Murray, E. H. Gerlach, S. D. Allen, and M. E. Erwin.** 1993. In vitro activity of cefpodoxime compared with other oral cephalosporins tested against 5,556 recent clinical isolates from five medical centers. *Diagn. Microbiol. Infect. Dis.* **17:**143–150.

299. **Safdar, N., D. Andes, and W. A. Craig.** 2004. In vivo pharmacodynamic activity of daptomycin. *Antimicrob. Agents Chemother.* **48:**63–68.

300. **Salter, A. J.** 1982. Trimethoprim-sulfamethoxazole: an assessment of more than 12 years of use. *Rev. Infect. Dis.* **4:**196–236.

301. **Sanders, C. C.** 1993. Cefepime: the next generation? *Clin. Infect. Dis.* **17:**369–379.

302. **Sattler, F. R., M. R. Weitekamp, and J. O. Ballard.** 1986. Potential for bleeding with the new beta-lactam antibiotics. *Ann. Intern. Med.* **105:**924–931.

303. **Saxon, A., A. Hassner, E. A. Swabb, B. Wheeler, and N. F. Adkinson, Jr.** 1984. Lack of cross-reactivity between aztreonam, a monobactam antibiotic, and penicillin in penicillin-allergic subjects. *J. Infect. Dis.* **149:**16–22.

304. **Schaad, U. B., J. Wedgwood-Krucko, and H. Tschaeppeler.** 1988. Reversible ceftriaxone-associated biliary pseudolithiasis in children. *Lancet* **ii:**1411–1413.

305. **Schentag, J. J., and C. H. Ballow.** 1991. Tissue-directed pharmacokinetics. *Am. J. Med.* **91**(Suppl. 3A):5S–11S.

306. **Schulin, T., C. B. Wennersten, R. C. Moellering, Jr., and G. M. Eliopoulos.** 1998. In-vitro activity of the new ketolide antibiotic HMR 3647 against gram-positive bacteria. *J. Antimicrob. Chemother.* **42:**297–301.

307. **Sharp, J. R., K. G. Ishak, and H. J. Zimmerman.** 1980. Chronic active hepatitis and severe hepatic necrosis associated with nitrofurantoin. *Ann. Intern. Med.* **92:**14–19.

308. **Shaw, W. V.** 1984. Bacterial resistance to chloramphenicol. *Br. Med. Bull.* **40:**36–41.

309. **Shorr, A. F., M. J. Kunkel, and M. Kollef.** 2005. Linezolid versus vancomycin in *Staphylococcus aureus* bacteremia: pooled analysis of randomized studies. *J. Antimicrob. Chemother.* **56:**923–929.

310. **Sierra, J. M., J. Ruiz, M. M. Navia, M. Vargas, and J. Vila.** 2001. In vitro activity of rifaximin against enteropathogens producing traveler's diarrhea. *Antimicrob. Agents Chemother.* **45:**643–644.

311. **Silverman, J. A., N. G. Perlmutter, and H. M. Shapiro.** 2003. Correlation of daptomycin bactericidal activity and membrane depolarization in *Staphylococcus aureus. Antimicrob. Agents Chemother.* **47:**2538–2544.

312. **Skiest, D. J.** 2006. Treatment failure resulting from resistance of *Staphylococcus aureus* to daptomycin. *J. Clin. Microbiol.* **44:**655–656.

313. **Smith, A. L., and A. Weber.** 1983. Pharmacology of chloramphenicol. *Pediatr. Clin. N. Am.* **30:**209–236.

314. **Snydman, D. R., N. V. Jacobus, L. A. McDermott, R. Ruthazer, E. J. Goldstein, S. M. Finegold, L. J. Harrell, D. W. Hecht, S. G. Jenkins, C. Pierson, R. Venezia, J. Rihs, and S. L. Gorbach.** 2002. National survey on the susceptibility of *Bacteroides fragilis* group: report and analysis of trends for 1997–2000. *Clin. Infect. Dis.* **35**(Suppl. 1):S126–S134.

315. **Somma, S., L. Gastaldo, and A. Corti.** 1984. Teicoplanin, a new antibiotic from *Actinoplanes teichomyceticus* nov. sp. *Antimicrob. Agents Chemother.* **26:**917–923.

316. **Sorgel, F., and M. Kinzig.** 1993. The chemistry, pharmacokinetics and tissue distribution of piperacillin/tazobactam. *J. Antimicrob. Chemother.* **31**(Suppl. A):39–60.
317. **Spangler, S. K., M. R. Jacobs, and P. C. Appelbaum.** 1996. Susceptibility of anaerobic bacteria to trovafloxacin: comparison with other quinolones and non-quinolone antibiotics. *Infect. Dis. Clin. Pract.* **5**(Suppl. 3):S101–S109.
318. **Spratt, B. G., V. Jobanputra, and W. Zimmermann.** 1977. Binding of thienamycin and clavulanic acid to the penicillin-binding proteins of *Escherichia coli* K-12. *Antimicrob. Agents Chemother.* **12:**406–409.
319. **Stahlmann, R., and H. Lode.** 1999. Toxicity of quinolones. *Drugs* **58**(Suppl. 2):37–42.
320. **Stamm, W. E.** 1991. Azithromycin in the treatment of uncomplicated genital chlamydial infections. *Am. J. Med.* **91**(Suppl. 3A):19S–22S.
321. **Stapleton, A., and W. E. Stamm.** 1997. Prevention of urinary tract infection. *Infect. Dis. Clin. N. Am.* **11:**719–733.
322. **Stapley, E. O., D. Hendlin, J. M. Mata, M. Jackson, H. Wallick, S. Hernandez, S. Mochales, S. A. Currie, and R. M. Miller.** 1969. Phosphonomycin. Discovery and in vitro biological characterization. *Antimicrob. Agents Chemother.* **9:**284–290.
323. **Steenbergen, J. N., J. Alder, G. M. Thorne, and F. P. Tally.** 2005. Daptomycin: a lipopeptide antibiotic for the treatment of serious gram-positive infections. *J. Antimicrob. Chemother.* **55:**283–288.
324. **Steffen, R., D. A. Sack, L. Riopel, Z. D. Jiang, M. Sturchler, C. D. Ericsson, B. Lowe, P. Waiyaki, M. White, and H. L. DuPont.** 2003. Therapy of travelers' diarrhea with rifaximin on various continents. *Am. J. Gastroenterol.* **98:**1073–1078.
325. **Stein, G. E.** 1996. Pharmacokinetics and pharmacodynamics of newer fluoroquinolones. *Clin. Infect. Dis.* **23**(Suppl. 1):S19–S24.
326. **Stevens, D. L., D. Herr, H. Lampiris, J. L. Hunt, D. H. Batts, and B. Hafkin.** 2002. Linezolid versus vancomycin for the treatment of methicillin-resistant *Staphylococcus aureus* infections. *Clin. Infect. Dis.* **34:**1481–1490.
327. **Streit, J. M., R. N. Jones, and H. S. Sader.** 2004. Daptomycin activity and spectrum: a worldwide sample of 6737 clinical gram-positive organisms. *J. Antimicrob. Chemother.* **53:**669–674.
328. **Streit, J. M., J. N. Steenbergen, G. M. Thorne, J. Alder, and R. N. Jones.** 2005. Daptomycin tested against 915 bloodstream isolates of viridans group streptococci (eight species) and *Streptococcus bovis*. *J. Antimicrob. Chemother.* **55:**574–578.
329. **Sullivan, D., M. E. Csuka, and B. Blanchard.** 1980. Erythromycin ethylsuccinate hepatotoxicity. *JAMA* **243:**1074.
330. **Swaney, S. M., H. Aoki, M. C. Ganoza, and D. L. Shinabarger.** 1998. The oxazolidinone linezolid inhibits initiation of protein synthesis in bacteria. *Antimicrob. Agents Chemother.* **42:**3251–3255.
331. **Swedberg, J., J. F. Steiner, F. Deiss, S. Steiner, and D. A. Driggers.** 1985. Comparison of single-dose vs one-week course of metronidazole for symptomatic bacterial vaginosis. *JAMA* **254:**1046–1049.
332. **Sykes, R. B., and D. P. Bonner.** 1985. Aztreonam: the first monobactam. *Am. J. Med.* **78**(Suppl. 2A):2–10.
333. **Teasley, D. G., D. N. Gerding, M. M. Olson, L. R. Peterson, R. L. Gebhard, M. J. Schwartz, and J. T. Lee, Jr.** 1983. Prospective randomised trial of metronidazole versus vancomycin for *Clostridium difficile*-associated diarrhoea and colitis. *Lancet* **ii:**1043–1046.
334. **Thornsberry, C.** 1992. Review of the in vitro antibacterial activity of cefprozil, a new oral cephalosporin. *Clin. Infect. Dis.* **14**(Suppl. 2):S189–S194.
335. **Todd, P. A., and D. Faulds.** 1991. Ofloxacin: a reappraisal of its antimicrobial activity, pharmacology and therapeutic use. *Drugs* **42:**825–876.
336. **Toma, E., S. Fournier, M. Dumont, P. Bolduc, and H. Deschamps.** 1993. Clindamycin/primaquine versus trimethoprim-sulfamethoxazole as primary therapy for *Pneumocystis carinii* pneumonia in AIDS: a randomized, double-blind pilot trial. *Clin. Infect. Dis.* **17:**178–184.
337. **Tuazon, C. U., and H. Miller.** 1984. Comparative in vitro activities of teichomycin and vancomycin alone and in combination with rifampin and aminoglycosides against staphylococci and enterococci. *Antimicrob. Agents Chemother.* **25:** 411–412.
338. **Turnidge, J.** 1999. Pharmacokinetics and pharmacodynamics of fluoroquinolones. *Drugs* **58**(Suppl. 2):29–36.
339. **Upton, A., S. Lang, and H. Heffernan.** 2003. Mupirocin and *Staphylococcus aureus*: a recent paradigm of emerging antibiotic resistance. *J. Antimicrob. Chemother.* **51:**613–617.
340. **Van der Auwera, P., T. Matsumoto, and M. Husson.** 1988. Intraphagocytic penetration of antibiotics. *J. Antimicrob. Chemother.* **22:**185–192.
341. **Vanhoof, R., B. Gordts, R. Dierickx, H. Coignau, and J. P. Butzler.** 1980. Bacteriostatic and bactericidal activities of 24 antimicrobial agents against *Campylobacter fetus* subsp. *jejuni*. *Antimicrob. Agents Chemother.* **18:** 118–121.
342. **Vannuffel, P., and C. Cocito.** 1996. Mechanism of action of streptogramins and macrolides. *Drugs* **51**(Suppl. 1): 20–30.
343. **Verbist, L.** 1979. Comparison of the activities of the new ureidopenicillins piperacillin, mezlocillin, azlocillin, and Bay k 4999 against gram-negative organisms. *Antimicrob. Agents Chemother.* **16:**115–119.
344. **Visalli, M. A., S. Bajaksouzian, M. R. Jacobs, and P. C. Appelbaum.** 1997. Comparative activity of trovafloxacin, alone and in combination with other agents, against gram-negative nonfermentative rods. *Antimicrob. Agents Chemother.* **41:**1475–1481.
345. **von Rosenstiel, N. A., and D. Adam.** 1995. Macrolide antibacterials: drug interactions of clinical significance. *Drug Saf.* **13:**105–122.
346. **Wadworth, A. N., and K. L. Goa.** 1991. Lomefloxacin: a review of its antibacterial activity, pharmacokinetic properties and therapeutic use. *Drugs* **42:**1018–1060.
347. **Wallace, R. J., Jr., B. A. Brown-Elliott, C. J. Crist, L. Mann, and R. W. Wilson.** 2002. Comparison of the in vitro activity of the glycylcycline tigecycline (formerly GAR-936) with those of tetracycline, minocycline, and doxycycline against isolates of nontuberculous mycobacteria. *Antimicrob. Agents Chemother.* **46:**3164–3167.
348. **Wallace, R. J., Jr., B. A. Brown-Elliott, S. C. Ward, C. J. Crist, L. B. Mann, and R. W. Wilson.** 2001. Activities of linezolid against rapidly growing mycobacteria. *Antimicrob. Agents Chemother.* **45:**764–767.
349. **Wallace, R. J., Jr., E. J. Septimus, T. W. Williams, Jr., R. H. Conklin, T. K. Satterwhite, M. B. Bushby, and D. C. Hollowell.** 1982. Use of trimethoprim-sulfamethoxazole for treatment of infections due to *Nocardia*. *Rev. Infect. Dis.* **4:**315–325.
350. **Wallace, R. J., Jr., J. M. Swenson, V. A. Silcox, and M. G. Bullen.** 1985. Treatment of nonpulmonary infections due to *Mycobacterium fortuitum* and *Mycobacterium chelonei* on the basis of in vitro susceptibilities. *J. Infect. Dis.* **152:**500–514.
351. **Wallace, R. J., Jr., and K. Wiss.** 1981. Susceptibility of *Mycobacterium marinum* to tetracyclines and aminoglycosides. *Antimicrob. Agents Chemother.* **20:**610–612.
352. **Walters, B. N., and S. S. Gubbay.** 1981. Tetracycline and benign intracranial hypertension: report of five cases. *Br. Med. J.* **282:**19–20.

353. **Ward, A., and D. M. Campoli-Richards.** 1986. Mupirocin: a review of its antibacterial activity, pharmacokinetic properties and therapeutic use. *Drugs* **32:**425–444.
354. **Ward, M. E.** 1977. The bactericidal action of spectinomycin on *Neisseria gonorrhoeae*. *J. Antimicrob. Chemother.* **3:**323–329.
355. **Washington, J. A., II, and W. R. Wilson.** 1985. Erythromycin: a microbial and clinical perspective after 30 years of clinical use. *Mayo Clin. Proc.* **60:**189–203.
356. **Watanakunakorn, C., and C. Bakie.** 1973. Synergism of vancomycin-gentamicin and vancomycin-streptomycin against enterococci. *Antimicrob. Agents Chemother.* **4:**120–124.
357. **Watanakunakorn, C., and J. C. Tisone.** 1982. Synergism between vancomycin and gentamicin or tobramycin for methicillin-susceptible and methicillin-resistant *Staphylococcus aureus* strains. *Antimicrob. Agents Chemother.* **22:**903–905.
358. **Waxman, D. J., and J. L. Strominger.** 1983. Penicillin-binding proteins and the mechanism of action of beta-lactam antibiotics. *Annu. Rev. Biochem.* **52:**825–869.
359. **Wehrli, W.** 1983. Rifampin: mechanisms of action and resistance. *Rev. Infect. Dis.* **5**(Suppl. 3)**:**S407–S411.
360. **Weigelt, J., K. Itani, D. Stevens, W. Lau, M. Dryden, and C. Knirsch for the Linezolid CCSTI Study Group.** 2005. Linezolid versus vancomycin in treatment of complicated skin and soft tissue infections. *Antimicrob. Agents Chemother.* **49:**2260–2266.
361. **Wertheim, H. F., M. C. Vos, A. Ott, A. Voss, J. A. Kluytmans, C. M. Vandenbroucke-Grauls, M. H. Meester, P. H. van Keulen, and H. A. Verbrugh.** 2004. Mupirocin prophylaxis against nosocomial *Staphylococcus aureus* infections in nonsurgical patients: a randomized study. *Ann. Intern. Med.* **140:**419–425.
362. **Wexler, H. M.** 2004. In vitro activity of ertapenem: review of recent studies. *J. Antimicrob. Chemother.* **53**(Suppl. 2)**:** ii11–ii21.
363. **Wexler, H. M., A. E. Engel, D. Glass, and C. Li.** 2005. In vitro activities of doripenem and comparator agents against 364 anaerobic clinical isolates. *Antimicrob. Agents Chemother.* **49:**4413–4417.
364. **Wexler, H. M., and S. M. Finegold.** 1988. In vitro activity of cefotetan compared with that of other antimicrobial agents against anaerobic bacteria. *Antimicrob. Agents Chemother.* **32:**601–604.
365. **Wexler, H. M., B. Harris, W. T. Carter, and S. M. Finegold.** 1985. In vitro efficacy of sulbactam combined with ampicillin against anaerobic bacteria. *Antimicrob. Agents Chemother.* **27:**876–878.
366. **Wexler, H. M., D. Molitoris, and S. M. Finegold.** 2000. In vitro activities of MK-826 (L-749,345) against 363 strains of anaerobic bacteria. *Antimicrob. Agents Chemother.* **44:**2222–2224.
367. **Wexler, H. M., E. Molitoris, D. Molitoris, and S. M. Finegold.** 2001. In vitro activity of telithromycin (HMR 3647) against 502 strains of anaerobic bacteria. *J. Antimicrob. Chemother.* **47:**467–469.
368. **Wexler, H. M., D. Molitoris, S. St. John, A. Vu, E. K. Read, and S. M. Finegold.** 2002. In vitro activities of faropenem against 579 strains of anaerobic bacteria. *Antimicrob. Agents Chemother.* **46:**3669–3675.
369. **Wijnands, W. J., and T. B. Vree.** 1988. Interaction between the fluoroquinolones and the bronchodilator theophylline. *J. Antimicrob. Chemother.* **22**(Suppl. C)**:**109–114.
370. **Williams, J. D., and A. M. Sefton.** 1993. Comparison of macrolide antibiotics. *J. Antimicrob. Chemother.* **31**(Suppl. C)**:** 11–26.
371. **Wilson, W. R., A. W. Karchmer, A. S. Dajani, K. A. Taubert, A. Bayer, D. Kaye, A. L. Bisno, P. Ferrieri, S. T. Shulman, and D. T. Durack.** 1995. Antibiotic treatment of adults with infective endocarditis due to streptococci, enterococci, staphylococci, and HACEK microorganisms. *JAMA* **274:**1706–1713.
372. **Wilson, W. R., R. L. Thompson, C. J. Wilkowske, J. A. Washington, E. R. Giuliani, and J. E. Geraci.** 1981. Short-term therapy for streptococcal infective endocarditis: combined intramuscular administration of penicillin and streptomycin. *JAMA* **245:**360–363.
373. **Winston, D. J., M. A. McGrattan, and R. W. Busuttil.** 1984. Imipenem therapy of *Pseudomonas aeruginosa* and other serious bacterial infections. *Antimicrob. Agents Chemother.* **26:**673–677.
374. **Wise, R., J. M. Andrews, and J. P. Ashby.** 2001. Activity of daptomycin against gram-positive pathogens: a comparison with other agents and the determination of a tentative breakpoint. *J. Antimicrob. Chemother.* **48:**563–567.
375. **Wise, R., D. Lister, C. A. McNulty, D. Griggs, and J. M. Andrews.** 1986. The comparative pharmacokinetics of five quinolones. *J. Antimicrob. Chemother.* **18**(Suppl. D)**:**71–81.
376. **Wiseman, L. R., and J. A. Balfour.** 1994. Ceftibuten: a review of its antibacterial activity, pharmacokinetic properties and clinical efficacy. *Drugs* **47:**784–808.
377. **Wittner, M., K. S. Rowin, H. B. Tanowitz, J. F. Hobbs, S. Saltzman, B. Wenz, R. Hirsch, E. Chisholm, and G. R. Healy.** 1982. Successful chemotherapy of transfusion babesiosis. *Ann. Intern. Med.* **96:**601–604.
378. **Wolfson, J. S., and D. C. Hooper.** 1989. Fluoroquinolone antimicrobial agents. *Clin. Microbiol. Rev.* **2:**378–424.
379. **Wolter, N., A. M. Smith, D. J. Farrell, W. Schaffner, M. Moore, C. G. Whitney, J. H. Jorgensen, and K. P. Klugman.** 2005. Novel mechanism of resistance to oxazolidinones, macrolides, and chloramphenicol in ribosomal protein L4 of the pneumococcus. *Antimicrob. Agents Chemother.* **49:**3554–3557.
380. **Wong, C. S., G. S. Palmer, and M. H. Cynamon.** 1988. In-vitro susceptibility of *Mycobacterium tuberculosis*, *Mycobacterium bovis* and *Mycobacterium kansasii* to amoxycillin and ticarcillin in combination with clavulanic acid. *J. Antimicrob. Chemother.* **22:**863–866.
381. **World Health Organization.** 1993. *Guidelines for Cholera Control.* World Health Organization, Geneva, Switzerland.
382. **Yeaman, M. R., L. A. Mitscher, and O. G. Baca.** 1987. In vitro susceptibility of *Coxiella burnetii* to antibiotics, including several quinolones. *Antimicrob. Agents Chemother.* **31:**1079–1084.
383. **Young, L. S., O. G. Berlin, and C. B. Inderlied.** 1987. Activity of ciprofloxacin and other fluorinated quinolones against mycobacteria. *Am. J. Med.* **82**(Suppl. 4A)**:** 23S–26S.
384. **Young, L. S., and J. Hindler.** 1987. Use of trimethoprim-sulfamethoxazole singly and in combination with other antibiotics in immunocompromised patients. *Rev. Infect. Dis.* **9**(Suppl. 2)**:**S177–S183.
385. **Zhanel, G. G., K. Homenuik, K. Nichol, A. Noreddin, L. Vercaigne, J. Embil, A. Gin, J. A. Karlowsky, and D. J. Hoban.** 2004. The glycylcyclines: a comparative review with the tetracyclines. *Drugs* **64:**63–88.
386. **Zurenko, G. E., B. H. Yagi, R. D. Schaadt, J. W. Allison, J. O. Kilburn, S. E. Glickman, D. K. Hutchinson, M. R. Barbachyn, and S. J. Brickner.** 1996. In vitro activities of U-100592 and U-100766, novel oxazolidinone antibacterial agents. *Antimicrob. Agents Chemother.* **40:**839–845.

Mechanisms of Resistance to Antibacterial Agents*

LOUIS B. RICE AND ROBERT A. BONOMO

71

GENERAL CONCEPTS, INOCULUM EFFECTS, AND TOLERANCE

In considering the growing problem of antimicrobial resistance in bacteria, it is worth remembering that resistance is neither a new phenomenon nor unexpected in an environment in which potent antimicrobial agents are used. The diversity of the microbial world and the relatively specific activities of our antimicrobial agents virtually ensure widespread resistance among bacteria. In many cases, this resistance is recognized when an antibiotic is first tested for development. For example, it is not considered a problem or threat that *Escherichia coli* is resistant to vancomycin. We simply understand that *E. coli* is not among vancomycin's spectrum of activity and avoid using vancomycin when *E. coli* infection is known or highly suspected (i.e. *E. coli*, has natural or primary resistance to vancomycin). Conversely, the increasing resistance of *E. coli* to ciprofloxacin represents an important problem, since we frequently use the fluoroquinolone class of antimicrobial agents to treat infections in which *E. coli* is likely to be involved. So when we speak of the problem of resistance, we must recognize that most problems result from expression of resistance by bacteria that are intrinsically susceptible to the antibiotic in question (i.e, acquired resistance).

It is also important to recognize that resistance as a clinical entity is essentially a relative phenomenon, in many ways a problem only indirectly related to the microbiologic techniques often used to detect it. For example, it is possible to incorporate enough ticarcillin into an agar plate to inhibit an ampicillin-resistant strain of *Enterococcus faecium* (in many cases this requires about 10,000 μg/ml). So in one sense, ampicillin-resistant *E. faecium* isolates are susceptible to high concentrations of ticarcillin. However, such concentrations cannot be achieved at the site of infection, so ampicillin-resistant *E. faecium* strains are not considered susceptible to ticarcillin. It is the responsibility of the Clinical and Laboratory Standards Institute (formerly the National Committee for Clinical Laboratory Standards), the U.S. Food and Drug Administration, and other standard-setting bodies in different countries to make determinations on susceptible, intermediate, and resistant breakpoints for new antimicrobial agents, considering factors of in vitro susceptibility, pharmacokinetics, and pharmacodynamics. These issues become very important in treating meningitis, in which relatively minor increases in the MIC of penicillin for *Streptococcus pneumoniae* can foil treatment, but in many cases are less relevant in the treatment of simple urinary tract infections, given the tendency of many antibiotics to concentrate in the urine.

The relativity of resistance is no better exemplified than by considerations of susceptibility in bacterial strains that exhibit significant inoculum effects, such as those resistant by virtue of producing β-lactamase. β-Lactamase-mediated resistance results from a chemical interaction in which the β-lactamase molecule binds to the β-lactam antibiotic in a manner that ultimately results in the hydrolysis of the critical β-lactam ring structure (Fig. 1). The rapidity and efficiency with which binding and hydrolysis proceed are dependent upon the affinity with which the β-lactamase molecule binds the antibiotic and the efficiency of the subsequent hydrolysis. High affinity and rapid hydrolysis mean that the cell wall synthesis machinery (penicillin binding proteins, or PBPs) can be defended with few β-lactamase molecules compared to the number of β-lactam molecules likely to be present in the vicinity of the PBPs. Low affinity and slow hydrolysis mean that more β-lactamase molecules are necessary for effective resistance but also that resistance can be more easily overcome by adding more antibiotic molecules. Increasing the inoculum of organisms in a solution with a fixed concentration of β-lactam antibiotic has the effect of increasing the number of β-lactamase molecules and can in some instances result in clinically important levels of resistance. The MIC for a *Klebsiella pneumoniae* strain that produces extended-spectrum β-lactamase TEM-26, for example, may be 1 μg of cefotaxime/ml with a standard inoculum (ca. 10^5 CFU/ml). However, when the inoculum is increased to 10^7 CFU/ml, the MIC increases to greater than 256 μg/ml (210). This type of resistance is likely to be important in treating a large-inoculum infection such as pneumonia. The existence of inoculum effects has led to the common practice of considering all *K. pneumoniae* strains that are resistant to ceftazidime to be resistant to all cephalosporins (excepting the cephamycins), regardless of in vitro susceptibility test results using the standard inoculum.

A second, more amorphous and difficult-to-evaluate concept in considering antimicrobial resistance is that of

* This chapter contains information presented in chapter 68, by Louis B. Rice, Daniel Sahm, and Robert A. Bonomo in the eighth edition of this Manual.

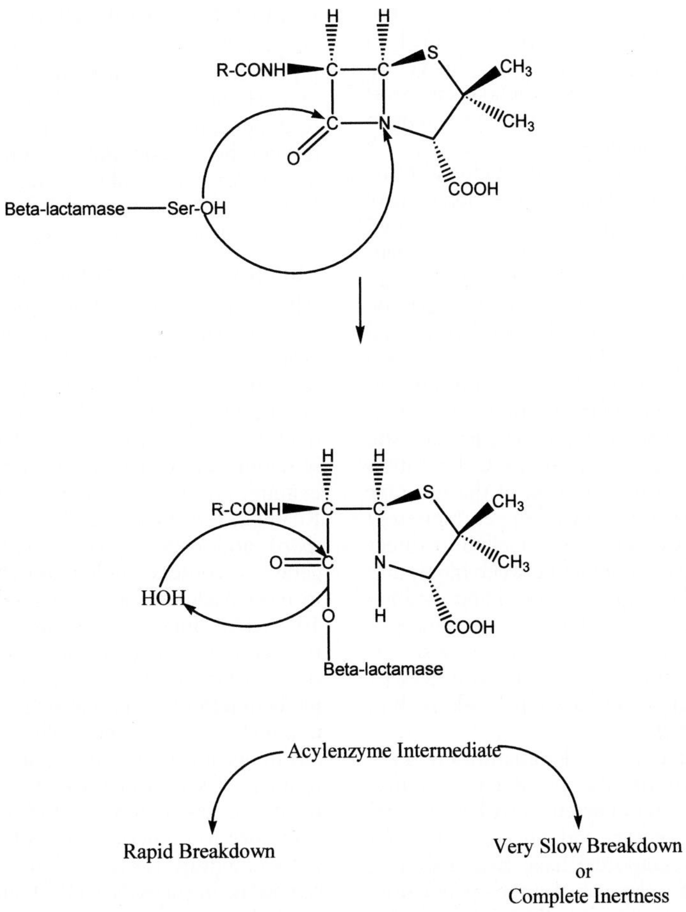

FIGURE 1 Penicillin-interactive, active-site serine peptidases and their reactions with β-lactam carbonyl donors. Modified from reference 87 with permission of Annual Reviews (http://www.annualreviews.org).

tolerance, or resistance to killing at antimicrobial concentrations sufficient to inhibit further growth. Tolerance is an unimportant concept for the treatment of most infections, since for therapeutic success it is usually sufficient to inhibit further growth of bacteria (bacteriostatic activity), allowing the patient's immune defenses to kill the growth-inhibited organisms and clean up the debris. In some instances, however, antimicrobial killing of the bacteria (bactericidal activity) is required to yield a high percentage of treatment success. Instances in which bactericidal activity is preferred include cases of endocarditis, meningitis, and osteomyelitis, in which the immune system has limited access to the infection site. They also include circumstances in which the immune system is severely compromised, such as it is in patients undergoing high-dose chemotherapy for hematologic malignancies. In these instances, antibiotics that are primarily bacteriostatic, such as the tetracyclines and the macrolides, are considered poor choices for therapy whereas β-lactam antibiotics, which are primarily bactericidal, are preferred. Some bacteria are naturally tolerant to β-lactam antibiotics. Bactericidal activity against enterococci, for example, requires two agents, one active against cell wall synthesis and an aminoglycoside (154). Recognition of this bactericidal synergism has raised cure rates for enterococcal endocarditis from about 40 to 70% or greater (207). Unfortunately, expression of aminoglycoside-modifying enzymes (AMEs) negates the synergism and appears to decrease the cure rates for enterococcal endocarditis. Although some level of tolerance to β-lactam antibiotics can be demonstrated for several different bacterial species, the impact on the treatment of clinical infections appears to be less dramatic than for enterococci.

Emergence and Spread of Antibiotic Resistance

The emergence of antimicrobial resistance phenotypes is inevitably linked to the clinical (or other) use of the antimicrobial agent against which resistance is directed. One reason for this association is trivial—we do not generally test for resistance to antibiotics that are not in clinical use. The second reason is that nature abhors a vacuum, so when an effective antibiotic eliminates susceptible flora, resistant varieties soon fill the niche. Once a resistance phenotype has emerged within a previously susceptible species, the rapidity and efficiency with which it spreads are impacted by a host of different factors, including the degree of resistance expressed, the ability of the organism to tolerate the resistance mechanism, linkage to other genes, the site of primary colonization, and others. The rapidity and completeness of resistance gene spread are often unpredictable. For example, the staphylococcal β-lactamase gene (conferring resistance to penicillin) was first described shortly after the introduction of penicillin into clinical use and is now almost universally present within staphylococci in the hospital and the community. It was not until the early 1980s that this gene was described in *Enterococcus*, and it has never spread widely in this genus. The reverse appears to be true with the vancomycin resistance genes, which are found widely in *E. faecium* but remain exceedingly rare in *Staphylococcus aureus.*

An important cause of the spread of antimicrobial resistance is the failure to adhere to appropriate infection control techniques, both within and outside the hospital. It is well established that strains of methicillin-resistant *S. aureus* (MRSA) within individual hospitals, and even within entire cities, are often clonally related, as determined by genetic techniques such as pulsed-field gel electrophoresis and staphylococcal protein A typing (211). The spread of these problematic pathogens has been attributed to transmission from patient to patient, presumably by transiently or persistently colonized health care workers (228). The primary site of *S. aureus* colonization is the anterior nares. Colonization of the nares facilitates aerosol transmission of the resistant bacteria, particularly during periods of viral upper respiratory infection in the colonized worker. It also facilitates direct transmission, given the frequent contact between hands and noses in many people and the frequently poor hand-washing practices of health care workers. The clinical consequences of patient colonization can be significant. Studies have shown a correlation between patient colonization with MRSA and subsequent infection during periods of high risk, such as the postoperative period (184).

Although antibiotic resistance is predominantly a nosocomial problem, resistant bacteria are also spread in the community setting. Sites in which resistant bacteria have been known to spread include day care centers and nursing homes (1, 274). Penicillin-resistant pneumococci have been found to colonize as many as 25% of a day care center's population. Transmission probably reaches its peak in the winter months, when viral upper respiratory infections are prevalent. The prevalence of viral upper respiratory tract infections works in two ways to increase transmission: (i) it probably increases the inoculum of resistant organisms being spread by those already colonized (see above-mentioned references for *S. aureus* colonization), and (ii) it makes those who are not colonized more likely to become colonized because of the increased likelihood that they will be receiving antimicrobial therapy. Nursing homes are predisposed to resistance for a variety of reasons, including the debilitated state of much of their populations, frequent movement back and forth to tertiary care hospitals, and frequent use of antimicrobial agents in an effort to ward off infections that will necessitate hospital admissions.

A final important source for the emergence and spread of antibiotic-resistant bacteria is nonhuman niches in which antibiotics are used. It is now well established that antimicrobial use in food animals is associated with both resistance in bacterial species that contaminate food and infect humans, primarily *Salmonella* and *Campylobacter* species, and the transfer of resistance determinants to human counterparts, such as *Enterococcus* (69). Compelling evidence also exists that high rates of ciprofloxacin resistance in *E. coli* can be associated with the use of fluoroquinolones in poultry (64). Finally, the European outbreak of vancomycin-resistant enterococci with the *vanA* determinant was almost certainly fueled by the use of avoparcin (a glycopeptide antibiotic) as a growth promoter in food animals (266). Data are also emerging that the use of antibiotics to promote growth of animals is often expensive and unnecessary, which has prompted many stakeholders in this issue to outline specific instances in which such antimicrobial use will be permitted.

Genetic Bases of Resistance

Acquired antimicrobial resistance results from biochemical processes that are encoded by bacterial genes. A general list of mechanisms of resistance is presented in Table 1. In order to understand the biochemical processes, it is useful to first discuss the genetic underpinnings of resistance and its evolution. Antimicrobial resistance arises by (i) mutation of cellular genes, (ii) acquisition of exogenous resistance genes, or (iii) mutation of acquired genes.

Mutation of Cellular Genes

All antibiotics have targets, which are often (but not always) proteins with important functional responsibilities in cell growth or maintenance. Cellular genes encode these proteins. Interactions between antibiotics and target proteins are often quite specific, and changing a single amino acid, frequently as a result of a single base change in the gene, can sometimes alter these interactions. Perhaps the most familiar example of this mechanism is resistance to rifampin. Rifampin targets the cellular RNA polymerase (encoded by *rpoB*), and a single point mutation in the RNA polymerase gene may confer complete resistance. These mutations occur in most bacterial species at a relatively high frequency (ca. 10^{-8}/CFU). Incubating enough cells with inhibitory concentrations of rifampin will eliminate susceptible cells and allow the resistant mutants to proliferate. The rifampin in the medium is not actually causing resistance but rather selecting mutants that occur naturally but which have no selective advantage for survival in the absence of rifampin in the environment. Other examples of mutational resistance include resistance to streptomycin through ribosomal mutation (63), resistance to fluoroquinolones through mutations of cellular topoisomerases (144), and resistance to linezolid through mutations in the rRNA (197), among others.

Resistance mutations may also be found in genes that regulate cellular processes. Perhaps the most completely studied example of regulatory mutation resulting in resistance is the derepression of the chromosomal β-lactamase of *Enterobacter* spp. (111). Mutations in a cellular amidase gene (designated *ampD*) result in the buildup of a cell wall breakdown product that has the effect of dramatically increasing expression of a chromosomal β-lactamase gene (*ampC*). Other examples of regulatory changes include the down-regulation of expression of the porin OmpD2 in *Pseudomonas aeruginosa* associated with resistance to imipenem (134) and the insertion of an insertion sequence (IS element) upstream of a chromosomal carbapenemase gene conferring imipenem resistance on *Bacteroides fragilis* (188).

Whether mutational resistance is likely to persist will depend in some measure on whether the resistance mutation is tolerable to the cell. For example, although decreased expression of OMPD2 appears to be readily achievable for *P. aeruginosa,* the fact that the resistant strains have not spread widely in the nearly 20 years of carbapenem use probably reflects the fact that this porin has functions that are beneficial to the bacterium, favoring reexpression of the porin once the imipenem threat has been dissipated. Similarly, intermediate levels of susceptibility to vancomycin in *S. aureus* have thus far been attributed to marked changes in the composition of the cell wall (231). These changes are unlikely to be favored in an environment free of vancomycin, since *S. aureus* likely "decided" a long time ago the optimal size and composition of its cell wall. The deleterious effects of acquiring resistance are often referred to as the fitness cost.

Disadvantageous resistance mutations do not always disappear. Although initial point mutations in the *rpoB* gene

TABLE 1 Common associations of resistance mechanisms

Antibiotic class	Resistance type	Resistance mechanism	Common example
Aminoglycosides	Decreased uptake	Changes in outer membrane permeability	*P. aeruginosa*
	Enzymatic modification (AMEs)	Phosphotransferase	Wide range of enteric gram-negative bacteria
		Adenyltransferase	Wide range of enteric gram-negative bacteria
		Acetyltransferase	Wide range of enteric gram-negative bacteria
		Bifunctional enzyme	*aac(6′)-aph(2″)* in *S. aureus, E. faecium,* and *E. faecalis*
ß-Lactams	Altered PBP(s)	PBP2a (additional PBP)	*mecA* in *S. aureus* and coagulase-negative staphylococci
		PBP2x, PBP2b, PBP1a (acquired from other streptococci by transformation)	*S. pneumoniae*
		PBP5 (point mutation)	*E. faecium*
	Enzymatic degradation (β-lactamases)	Ambler class A	TEM-1 in *E. coli, H. influenzae,* and *N. gonorrhoeae*
			SHV-1 in *K. pneumoniae*
			K1 (OXY-1) in *Klebsiella oxytoca*
			ESBLs (TEM-3+, SHV-2+, and CTX-M types) in *K. pneumoniae* and *E. coli*
			BRO-1 in *Moraxella catarrhalis*
			PC1 in *S. aureus*
			PSE-1 in *P. aeruginosa*
			ß-lactamases of *C. koseri* and *P. vulgaris*
		Ambler class B	L-1 in *Stenotrophomonas maltophilia*
			CcrA in *Bacteroides fragilis*
		Ambler class C	AmpC in *E. cloacae* and *Citrobacter freundii,* and similar enzymes in *Serratia marcescens, Morganella morganii, Providencia stuartii,* and *P. rettgeri*
		Ambler class D	OXA-1 in *E. coli*
Chloramphenicol	Enzymatic degradation	CATs	CAT in *S. pneumoniae*
	Efflux	Membrane transporters	*cmlA* and *flo*-encoded efflux in *E. coli* and *Salmonella* spp.
Glycopeptides	Altered target	Altered peptidoglycan cross-link target (D-Ala–D-Ala to D-Ala–D-Lac or D-Ala–D-Ser) encoded by complex gene cluster	VanA gene cluster in *E. faecium, E. faecalis,* and *S. aureus;* VanB gene cluster in *E. faecium* and *E. faecalis*
	Target overproduction	Excess peptidoglycan	Glycopeptide-intermediate strains of *S. aureus* and *Staphylococcus haemolyticus*
Oxazolidinones	Altered target	Mutation leading to reduced binding to active site	G2576U mutation in rRNA in *E. faecium* and *S. aureus*
Macrolides-lincosamides-streptogramin B	Altered target	Ribosomal active-site methylation with reduced binding	*erm*-encoded methylases in *S. aureus, S. pneumoniae,* and *Streptococcus pyogenes*
Macrolides	Efflux	Mef efflux pump	*mef*-encoded efflux in *S. pneumoniae* and *Streptococcus pyogenes; msrA* in *S. aureus*
Streptogramin A	Enzymatic degradation	Acetyltransferases	*vat*(A)-, *vat*(B)-, and *vat*(C)-encoded enzymes in *S. aureus*
			vat(D)- and *vat*(E)-encoded enzymes in *E. faecium*
Quinolones	Altered target	Mutation leading to reduced binding to active site(s) (quinolone resistance-determining region)	Mutations in *gyrA* in enteric gram-negative bacteria and *S. aureus*
			Mutations in *gyrA* and *parC* in *S. pneumoniae*

(Continued on next page)

TABLE 1 Common associations of resistance mechanisms *(Continued)*

Antibiotic class	Resistance type	Resistance mechanism	Common example
	Efflux	New membrane transporters	NorA in *S. aureus*
	Protection from DNA binding	Acquired protection protein	*qnr* gene and variants
	Enzymatic modification	Mutated aminoglycoside acetyltransferase	*aac(6')-Ib* variant in *E. coli*
Rifampin	Altered target	Mutations leading to reduced binding to RNA polymerase	Mutations in *rpoB* in *S. aureus* and *Mycobacterium tuberculosis*
Tetracyclines	Efflux	New membrane transporters	*tet* genes encoding efflux proteins in gram-positive bacteria (mainly group 2) and gram-negative bacteria (mainly group 1)
	Altered target	Production of proteins that bind to the ribosome and alter the conformation of the active site (ribosomal protection proteins)	*tet*(M) in a variety of gram-positive bacteria
Sulfonamides	Altered target	Mutation or recombination of genes encoding DHPS	Found in a wide range of species, e.g., *E. coli, S. aureus,* and *S. pneumoniae*
		Acquisition of new, low-affinity DHPS genes	*sul*I and *sul*II in enteric gram-negative bacteria
Trimethoprim	Altered target	Mutations in gene encoding DHFR	*S. aureus, S. pneumoniae,* and *H. influenzae*
		Acquisition of new, low-affinity DHFR genes	*dhfr*I and *dhfr*II encoded, found in a wide range of species
	Overproduction of target	Promoter mutation leading to overproduction of DHFR	*E. coli*

that confer rifampin resistance on *Salmonella enterica* serovar Enteritidis appear to decrease the fitness of the organism for survival in vivo, persistence in a live host is frequently associated with compensatory mutations that at least partially restore fitness to the strain while retaining the resistance (rather than mutating back to susceptibility) (22). Similarly, transfer of mutated *pbp5* into *E. faecium* strains is often associated with decreases in the expression of ampicillin resistance, but growth on increased concentrations of ampicillin easily yields colonies that grow well at higher concentrations (209). Similar findings have been reported for *S. aureus* strains transformed with the *mecA* gene encoding methicillin resistance (156). In summary, although mutational resistance often confers a fitness cost, subsequent adaptations may make the expression of resistance less costly.

Acquisition of Resistance Genes

If resistance is not achievable through mutation, threatened bacterial species have little choice but to look elsewhere for resistance determinants. They are aided in this effort by the fact that most antimicrobial agents are natural products or derivatives of natural products. Therefore, resistance genes for most antibiotics must exist in the microbial world, either in the species that produce the antibiotic or within species that live in the same ecological niche as the antibiotic producers (54). The challenge for susceptible human pathogens is to find and acquire these resistance determinants. To assist in this acquisition, bacteria have evolved a range of mechanisms that promote gene exchange. Perhaps the simplest of these techniques is natural transformation, referring to the ability of some bacterial species to absorb naked DNA molecules from the environment under the appropriate circumstances (92). Once taken up by the susceptible bacterium, these foreign pieces of DNA enter the bacterial chromosome by recombining across regions of sufficient homology. In some cases, functional genes result from this recombination. If the acquired gene encodes a protein that is less susceptible to inhibition than the native protein, a reduction in susceptibility may result. Perhaps the best-studied example of the formation of these "mosaic" genes to confer resistance is penicillin and cephalosporin resistance in *Streptococcus pneumoniae* (92). A variety of mosaic PBP (*pbp*) genes in resistant strains have been described previously, with the level and degree of resistance determined by the number and nature of gene recombinations. Mosaic topoisomerase genes in fluoroquinolone-resistant transformable bacteria have also been described previously (55).

Most bacteria are incapable of natural transformation and so have developed other mechanisms for acquiring useful genetic determinants. A commonly employed mechanism for genetic exchange is the transfer of conjugative plasmids. These extrachromosomal replicative DNA forms may carry a variety of important genes. Some plasmids are relatively narrow in their host range, and others transfer into and replicate within several different species. Transfer frequencies can be very high, as in the F factor of *E. coli* (virtual complete transfer in 1 h) and the pheromone-responsive plasmids found in *Enterococcus faecalis* (ca. 10^{-1}

transconjugant/recipient CFU in 24 h), or more modest, as observed with the broad-host-range enterococcal plasmids such as pAMß1 one (10^{-7} to 10^{-6} transconjugants/recipient CFU in 24 h) (32). Having entered into a new genus on broad-host-range plasmids, resistance determinants can readily transfer onto more frequently transferable plasmids to increase their movement through the new genus. In the first case of true vancomycin-resistant *S. aureus* described in the literature, it appears that vancomycin resistance transposon Tn*1546* entered into *S. aureus* from *E. faecalis* on a broad-host-range plasmid and then transposed into a conjugative plasmid native to the staphylococcus (79, 268). Plasmids may also integrate into the chromosomes of the recipient strains, potentially increasing the stability of the genetic information they carry.

Bacteria also take advantage of bacterial viruses (bacteriophages) for genetic exchange. These discreet packages deliver to uninfected cells quantities of DNA approximating the sizes of their genomes (in most cases roughly 40 kb). Designed to incorporate their own genomes into the manufactured phage head, they sometimes incorporate bits of chromosomal DNA adjacent to the phage integration site (specialized transduction) and other times incorporate an appropriately sized plasmid or chromosomal DNA segment unrelated to the integrated phage genome (generalized transduction). Since the staphylococcal ß-lactamase gene is frequently identified on nonconjugative plasmids of approximately 35 to 40 kb and since bacteriophages in staphylococci have been well described for decades, it has been speculated that the high prevalence of β-lactamase production in staphylococci has resulted from the bacteriophage-mediated transfer of these plasmids. Bacteriophages have also been implicated in the transfer of virulence determinants (71).

Nonreplicative mobile elements known as transposons have also been implicated in the transfer of resistance genes (204). Transposons encode their own ability to transfer between replicons (autonomously replicating DNA segments). In some cases, the transposons themselves encode conjugation functions, which allow them to transfer from bacterial chromosome to bacterial chromosome. The best characterized of these conjugative transposons is Tn*916*, an 18-kb element originally identified in *E. faecalis* but which has a very broad host range (205). Tn*916* encodes resistance to tetracycline and minocycline through the *tet*(M) resistance gene. Many different Tn*916*-like transposons have now been identified in enterococci and beyond, and some of them, such as Tn*1545* from *S. pneumoniae*, possess additional resistance genes (conferring resistance to erythromycin and kanamycin) (205). Some investigators have suggested that the conjugation events associated with Tn*916*-like transposons are akin to cell fusion events, in which portions of the genome distinct from those adjacent to the inserted transposon can exchange via homologous recombination (249). Transposons with structural similarity to Tn*916* have been implicated in the transfer of vancomycin resistance between *E. faecium* strains (37).

Transposons lacking conjugative functions may also transfer between strains. The most common mechanism through which this transfer is presumed to occur is either transient or more permanent integration into transferable plasmids. Among the more common classes of nonconjugative transposons are the Tn*3* family of elements (including Tn*917* conferring erythromycin resistance, and Tn*1546*, conferring VanA-type vancomycin resistance) (11, 223) and the composite elements formed by mobile IS elements flanking resistance genes (including Tn*4001*, conferring high-level gentamicin resistance in many gram-positive species) (81).

The precise origin of resistance genes is often difficult to discern, but in some cases it is at least possible to determine that acquired resistance determinants originated in other genera. The VanB-type vancomycin resistance gene in enterococci, for example, has a G+C content of nearly 50% (67). The enterococcal genome, in contrast, has an approximately 35 to 38% G+C content. These differences virtually confirm the origin of the *vanB* determinant in a genus other than *Enterococcus*. The likely origin appears to be streptomycetes, probably species that manufacture glycopeptide antibiotics, with entry into enterococci facilitated by the incorporation of these resistance operons into transposons.

It is worth noting at this point that any concept of the bacterial genome as a fixed entity is untenable. Comparisons of *E. coli* genomes reveal striking differences between enteropathogenic and uropathogenic strains, with the different regions constituting "pathogenicity islands" that confer specific virulence traits that give the strains their clinical profiles (95, 270). Data emanating from a comparative study of 36 *S. aureus* genomes indicate that 22% of the genome is dispensable, with many of the variable regions constituting presumed pathogenicity islands and regions of antimicrobial resistance (78). Finally, it is estimated that 25% of the genome of *E. faecalis* strain V583 was acquired from outside the genus (183).

Mutation of Acquired Genes

As bacteria have responded to the challenge of antimicrobial agents, so have we responded to the challenge of antibiotic resistance. Our typical response to the appearance of antimicrobial resistance has been a concerted effort to develop novel antimicrobial agents that will be active against resistant strains. The emergence of β-lactamase-mediated resistance to antibiotics is an instructive example of this interplay. Ampicillin was developed as the first penicillin with clinically significant activity against gram-negative rods, primarily *E. coli*. Within a few years of the clinical introduction of ampicillin, strains of *E. coli* were described that were resistant to this antibiotic by virtue of production of a plasmid-mediated β-lactamase designated TEM (named after the patient from whom the resistant strain was isolated). *S. aureus* expressed a similar β-lactamase, prompting a concerted effort on the part of the pharmaceutical industry to develop β-lactam antibiotics resistant to hydrolysis. Among the more successful compounds that were developed were methicillin, with activity against β-lactamase-producing *S. aureus;* the cephalosporins and carbapenems, with widespread activity against many β-lactamase-producing species; and the β-lactamase inhibitors, which restored the activity of β-lactams susceptible to hydrolysis.

The most successful and widely developed class of β-lactamase-resistant β-lactam antibiotics is the cephalosporins. So many of these agents have been developed for clinical use that they were frequently lumped into "generations" to facilitate remembrance of their spectra of activity. The extended-spectrum (previously referred to as third-generation), cephalosporins cefotaxime, ceftizoxime, ceftriaxone, and ceftazidime are particularly potent antibiotics that are resistant to hydrolysis by the original TEM enzyme. Unfortunately, increasing clinical use of these agents, particularly ceftazidime, has been associated with the emergence of resistant gram-negative rods, particularly *K. pneumoniae* (114). Molecular analysis of these resistant strains revealed that the resistance is mediated by β-lactamases and that many of these β-lactamases are derived from the native TEM enzyme through one or more point mutations in the bla_{TEM} gene.

Biochemical Mechanisms of Resistance

Modification of the Antibiotic

Many antibiotic-modifying enzymes have been described previously, including the β-lactamases, the AMEs, and chloramphenicol acetyltransferases (CATs). Although these enzymes are in many cases acquired, some are intrinsic to certain genera. For example, chromosomally encoded β-lactamases are intrinsic to almost all gram-negative rods. Expression of these enzymes is often only at very low levels, conferring resistance to only very susceptible β-lactams, as in the case of *K. pneumoniae* resistance to ampicillin through expression of the chromosomally expressed SHV-1 enzyme (208), or to no β-lactams at all, as in the case of wild-type *E. coli* strains. In some bacterial genera (notably *Enterobacter* and *Pseudomonas*), chromosomally expressed β-lactamases are under regulatory control, with derangements in these regulatory mechanisms resulting in high-level, broad-spectrum β-lactam resistance (112). In some instances, AMEs are intrinsic to bacterial species as well, as in the cases of the chromosomally expressed acetyltransferases of *Providencia stuartii* and *Serratia marcescens* (203, 224).

Modifying enzymes in general confer high levels of resistance to the antibiotics against which they have activity. Expression of the TEM-1 β-lactamase by *E. coli,* for example, can increase the MIC of ampicillin from 8 to >10,000 μg/ml. Similarly, expression of the bifunctional aminoglycoside resistance enzyme in *E. faecalis* raises the MIC of gentamicin from 32 to 64 μg/ml to >2,000 μg/ml. As effective as these mechanisms are, however, some antibiotics appear to be immune to inactivating enzymes. Vancomycin has been in clinical use since 1958, yet there are still no examples of vancomycin-modifying enzymes in bacteria.

Modification of the Target Molecule

Since antibiotic interaction with target molecules is generally quite specific, minor alterations of the target molecule can have important effects on antibiotic binding. Numerous examples exist of antibiotic target modification as a mechanism of resistance, including the many erythromycin ribosomal methylases that confer resistance to the macrolide-lincosamide-streptogramin B classes of antibiotics (269). Modifications of PBPs can affect the affinities of these molecules for β-lactam antibiotics, as noted above for *S. pneumoniae,* and especially for ampicillin-resistant *E. faecium* through mutations in PBP5 (92, 209). Modification of PBPs seems to be a favored mechanism of β-lactam resistance in gram-positive bacteria, whereas β-lactamase production is favored in gram-negative rods. Although the reason for this difference is unknown, it is interesting that β-lactamases produced by gram-positive bacteria diffuse into the external medium once produced whereas those produced by gram-negative rods are kept within the periplasmic space by the outer membrane. The ability to concentrate β-lactamases enhances their efficacy and may help explain the preference for this mechanism among gram-negative rods.

Other important examples of target modifications include the altered cell wall precursors that confer resistance to glycopeptide antibiotics; mutated DNA gyrase and topoisomerase IV, conferring resistance to fluoroquinolone antimicrobial agents; ribosomal protection mechanisms conferring resistance to tetracyclines; and RNA polymerase mutations conferring resistance to rifampin. The degree of resistance conferred by target modifications is variable and may be dependent upon the ability of the mutated target to perform its normal function. Mutations in PBPs of *S. pneumoniae,* for example, confer a relatively low level of resistance (although one that is significant in the treatment of meningitis) (92), whereas VanA-type vancomycin resistance mutations confer a very high level of resistance to vancomycin on enterococci (12).

Restricted Access to the Target

It is axiomatic that an antibiotic must reach its target in order to be effective. Therefore, for targets for which barriers must be crossed by the antibiotic, strengthening of these barriers can be a highly effective mechanism of resistance. All gram-negative bacteria have an outer membrane that must be traversed before the cytoplasmic membrane can be reached. Reductions in the quantities of known or presumed porins (channels for movement of materials across the outer membrane) have been documented as important contributors to resistance to imipenem in *P. aeruginosa*, cefepime in *Enterobacter cloacae*, and cefoxitin and ceftazidime in *K. pneumoniae* (129, 134, 145). In most instances, this restricted entry must be in combination with the production of an at least moderately active β-lactamase to confer high-level resistance. Barriers to entry can also exist in the cytoplasmic membrane. Movement of aminoglycosides across the cytoplasmic membrane is an oxygen-dependent process, so these antibiotics are inactive in anaerobic environments (and hence against strictly anaerobic species) (127).

Efflux Pumps

Among the most active areas of research in antimicrobial resistance is the identification and characterization of pumps that efflux one or more antibiotic classes from the bacterial cell. Several classes of pumps in gram-positive and/or gram-negative bacteria have been described previously. The pumps may be quite selective, or they may have broad substrate specificities. The majority of these pumps are located in the cytoplasmic membrane and use proton motive force to drive drug efflux. The major families of efflux transporters are (i) the major facilitator superfamily, which includes QacA and NorA/Bmr of gram-positive bacteria and EmrB of *E. coli;* (ii) the small multidrug-resistance family, including Smr of *S. aureus* and EmrE of *E. coli;* and (iii) the resistance-nodulation-cell division (RND) family, including AcrAB-TolC of *E. coli* and MexAB-OprM of *P. aeruginosa.* The structure of the AcrAB-TolC RND-type efflux pump is shown in Fig. 2. Deciphering the crystal structure of this pump was a major achievement (157). Among other things, it revealed that there is a periplasmic opening in the pump that can allow passage of molecules, explaining the previously confusing observation that RND pumps include β-lactam antibiotics (which do not enter the cytoplasm) among their substrates. In some instances, combinations of different types of pumps can result in higher levels of resistance than are achieved by the activity of a single pump alone (128).

Attribution of resistance to a specific mechanism may be difficult when more than one mechanism is involved. For example, resistance to imipenem in *P. aeruginosa* is contributed to by reduced access (through down-regulation of OmpD2) and production of AmpC β-lactamase (134). Neither mechanism alone is sufficient to yield clinically significant levels of resistance, yet both are required for high levels of resistance to result.

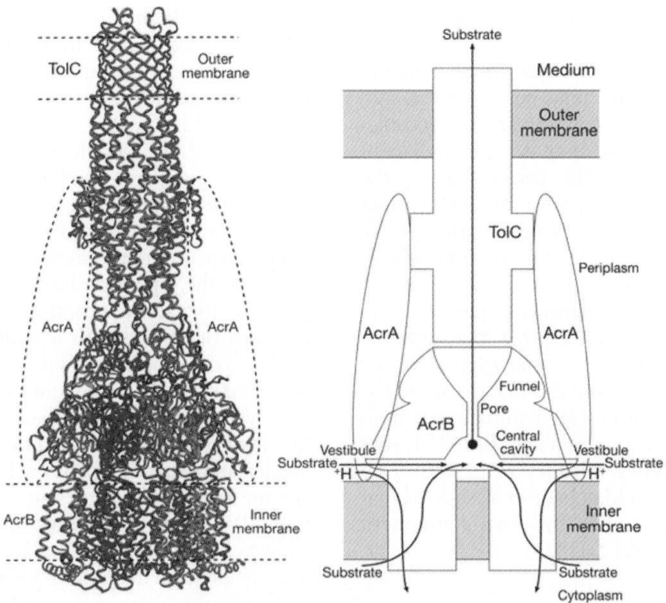

FIGURE 2 Representation of the crystal structure of the AcrAB-TolC three-component resistance nodulation-cell division-multidrug efflux pump. On the left are the three components of the pumps as they link the cytoplasmic (inner) membrane to the outer membrane. The periplasmic linker protein (AcrA) is shown only in outline to allow visualization of the linkage between AcrB and TolC. On the right, an outline of the pump shown at the left is presented, detailing the functional regions of the pump. Reprinted from reference 157 with permission of the publisher.

RESISTANCE MECHANISMS FOR DIFFERENT ANTIMICROBIAL CLASSES

Aminoglycoside Resistance

In explaining resistance to aminoglycosides (amikacin, gentamicin, kanamycin, neomycin, netilmicin, paromomycin, streptomycin, and tobramycin), we will first explain how aminoglycosides reach their targets in bacterial cells and then review their mechanism of action. The clinical indications for aminoglycoside therapy will also be summarized.

The aminoglycosides contain an aminocyclitol ring (streptidine or 2-deoxystrepamine) and two or more amino sugars linked by glycosidic bonds. They are hydrophilic antibiotics whose antimicrobial activity is concentration dependent. They are particularly active against aerobic, gram-negative rods. As a class, these agents have other highly desirable qualities: they are rapidly bactericidal, demonstrate a "postantibiotic" effect, and exhibit predictable pharmacodynamics.

Mechanism of Action of Aminoglycosides

Aminoglycosides have unique effects on protein translation in prokaryotes. These effects may explain why aminoglycosides are bactericidal whereas most other antibiotics that target the ribosome (chloramphenicol, macrolides, and tetracyclines) are bacteriostatic.

First, aminoglycosides penetrate bacteria by three main steps. The positively charged aminoglycosides bind to the negatively charged bacterial cell. Next, in an energy-dependent process driven by the membrane-bound electron transport system present only in aerobic bacteria, a small fraction of the aminoglycosides that are attached to the bacterium are taken into the cell.

Once inside the cell, the principal target of aminoglycoside action is the 30S subunit of the ribosome. The molecular details of aminoglycoside binding to the ribosome are unique. Gentamicin attaches to the highly conserved tRNA acceptor A site of the *E. coli* 16S rRNA (152). This binding prevents the elongation of the growing peptide chain by causing misreading or premature termination of peptide synthesis. By interfering with the translation of mRNA, protein production is altered, aberrant proteins are synthesized and inserted into the cell membrane, cell permeability is increased, more aminoglycosides are taken up into the cell, and cell death ensues.

Mistranslated proteins may also affect the bacterial cell. Paromomycin increases the error rate of protein translation by allowing the incorporation of the wrong tRNAs (the missense substitution rate of amino acids at specified positions in proteins is 1 in 3,000). Spectinomycin, a nonaminoglycoside aminocyclitol, inhibits translocation of the peptidyl-tRNA from the A site to the P site. Streptomycin also makes the ribosome error prone by allowing the binding of different tRNAs (39). Resistance to aminoglycosides can occur through four mechanisms: (i) loss of cell permeability (decreased uptake); (ii) alterations in the ribosome that prevent binding; (iii) expulsion by efflux pumps; and (iv) enzymatic inactivation by AMEs.

Resistance Due to Decreased Uptake and Altered Electrical Potential, Divalent Cations, and Efflux

It is well known that bacterial respiration generates an electrical potential across the membrane. Hence, anaerobes and facultative anaerobes (e.g., enterococci and certain small-colony variants of staphylococci) do not allow movement of aminoglycosides across their cell membranes. This intrinsic resistance confers low-level cross-resistance to all aminoglycosides.

Studies of *P. aeruginosa* and *E. coli* indicate that movement across the outer membrane may be due to a self-promoted uptake mechanism. The cationic aminoglycosides displace divalent cations (e.g., Mg^{2+}) that bridge adjacent lipopolysaccharide molecules, thereby permeabilizing the outer membrane and allowing the entry of aminoglycosides (118). Consistent with this model, divalent cations have long been known to antagonize the activity of aminoglycosides against gram-negative bacteria (35).

Recent data indicate that *P. aeruginosa* possesses an inducible RND-type pump (MexXY-OprM) that effluxes aminoglycosides (115, 141). In *E. coli*, aminoglycosides are captured from both the periplasm and the cytoplasm by the AcrD multidrug efflux transporter (2). Evaluating a multidrug-resistant strain, *Acinetobacter baumanii* BM4454, that was resistant to aminoglycosides, Magnet et al. found an RND-type efflux pump (139), and Marchand et al. showed that the pump was under stringent control by a two-component regulatory and sensor system, *adeRS* (142).

Modification of the Ribosome

Bacterial cells have multiple copies of the rRNA genes. Mutations that affect aminoglycoside binding to the ribosome include alterations in ribosomal proteins and 16S rRNA and enzymatic methylation of the rRNA. Ribosomal mutations have been demonstrated to confer resistance to spectinomycin and streptomycin (258) and more recently to other aminoglycosides as well (148). The newly identified 16S rRNA methylases (RmtA, RmtB, and ArmA) in gram-negative rods have been noted as emerging problems (280). The first such novel enzyme was found in *K. pneumoniae* BM4536 and designated *armA* ("aminoglycoside resistance methylase A") (82, 83).

Aminoglycoside-Modifying Enzymes

As that of β-lactamases (see below), inactivation of aminoglycosides by AMEs is the most important mechanism in terms of frequency and level of resistance (15). AMEs are believed to originate from *Actinomycetes* that synthesize these antibiotics (*Streptomyces* and *Micromonospora* spp.). It is also possible that AMEs originated from enzymes involved in normal cellular respiration (housekeeping functions) (202). These enzymes are phosphotransferases (APHs), nucleotidyltransferases or adenyltransferases (ANTs), and acetyltransferases (AACs). AMEs covalently modify specific amino or hydroxyl groups, resulting in aminoglycosides that bind poorly (higher K_ms, lower affinities) to the ribosome. AMEs can be passed from one bacterium to another by mobile genetic elements. These resistance determinants are frequently carried on specialized genetic elements called integrons (225, 273).

Sites of AME modification of aminoglycosides are identified by a standard numbering system. The streptidine or 2-deoxystreptamine nucleus forms the center for the numbering scheme (from 2-deoxystreptamine derive all aminoglycosides except streptomycin and spectinomycin). The first sugar moiety at the 4 position has positions numbered with a single prime (1′ to 6′); the second sugar moiety at the 6 position gets positions numbered with a double prime (1″ to 6″). Hence, AAC(6′) acetylates an amino group at the 6′ position (via an acetyltransferase) on the amino sugar attached to the 4 position (Fig. 3). Each AME class consists of numerous enzymes that can modify different OH or NH_2 groups. These classes are divided into subclasses. In each subclass, there are different enzyme types that are designated by a roman numeral, e.g., AAC(3)-I. Isoenzymes are also described and are designated by a lowercase letter "a" or "b," etc. These isoenzymes are functionally identical and confer identical resistance phenotypes.

Currently, there are seven major phosphotransferases [APH(3′), APH(2″), APH(3″), APH(6), APH(9), APH(4), and APH(7″)], four nucleotidyltransferases [ANT(6), ANT(3″), ANT(4′), and ANT(2″)], and four acetyltransferases [AAC(2′), AAC(6), AAC(1), and AAC(3)]. A bifunctional AME also exists that is able to acetylate and phosphorylate AAC(6)-APH(2″). This enzyme is found in *Staphylococcus*, *Streptococcus*, and *Enterococcus* species and is responsible for high-level resistance to aminoglycosides (70). The gene *aac(6′)-aph(2″)* that encodes the synthesis of this enzyme is present on Tn*4001*-like transposons which are inserted both into plasmids and into the chromosomes of aminoglycoside-resistant isolates. Most health care-associated MRSA strains express this enzyme.

Resistance to β-Lactam Antibiotics

Penicillin-Binding Protein-Mediated Resistance

β-Lactam antibiotics act by inhibiting the PBPs, the transpeptidases that manufacture peptidoglycan. The specific functions of different PBPs have been identified for some bacteria, but the precise ways in which they interact with one another and with cell wall precursors remain largely a mystery. Some are clearly essential for cell viability (generally the high-molecular-weight transpeptidases and their partner transglycosylases), whereas others appear to be dispensable, with

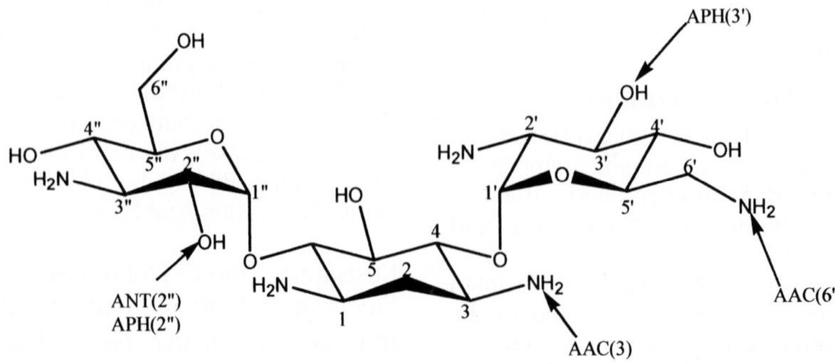

FIGURE 3 Sites of modification on kanamycin B by various AMEs. The arrows point to the sites of modification by the specific enzymes, namely, acetyltransferases, phosphotransferases, and nucleotidyltransferases. Reprinted from reference 125 with permission.

no apparent deleterious effects on cellular structure or function resulting from their absence (most commonly the low-molecular-weight carboxypeptidases). It has long been suspected that some PBPs are redundant and can serve the functions of others. For example, *E. faecium* strains in which all of the PBPs except low-affinity PBP5 are saturated grow normally, implying that PBP5 can perform all of the penicillin-inhibiting functions required for cell wall synthesis (276). On the other hand, *E. faecium* strains in which *pbp5* has been deleted grow normally as well, implying that the other PBPs can provide all of these functions (209).

PBPs are all members of a larger family of serine peptidases that includes most of the β-lactamases. PBPs and β-lactamases interact with β-lactam molecules (which themselves are structural analogues of the peptidyl-D-alanyl-D-alanine termini of peptidoglycan precursors) by catalytically disrupting the β-lactam bond, resulting in a serine-ester-linked acyl-enzyme derivative (Fig. 1). In the case of β-lactamases, a water molecule then hydrolyzes the ester linkage of the acyl-enzyme intermediate, releasing the irreversibly damaged penicilloyl (or cephalosporyl) moiety and regenerating the active enzyme. PBP-β-lactam acyl-enzyme derivatives are in general less accommodating of nucleophilic attack by the water molecule, resulting in persistence of the covalent bond and inactivation of the PBP. The stability of this interaction allows identification of these proteins by binding to radiolabeled penicillin and is the genesis of their designation as "penicillin binding proteins."

Inhibition of PBPs interrupts cell wall synthesis, which by itself should inhibit cell growth rather than kill the cell. However, the interaction of β-lactam molecules with PBPs triggers the activity of cell wall-degrading molecules known as autolysins, which rupture the cell, leading to cell death (248). The extent to which these autolytic enzymes are activated correlates in most cases with the killing activity of a β-lactam against a particular bacterial strain.

Some bacterial species are intrinsically resistant to some β-lactam antibiotics by virtue of decreased PBP affinity. For example, enterococci are resistant to clinically achievable levels of cephalosporin antibiotics because of the presence of low-affinity PBP5. Similar low affinities are demonstrated for the semisynthetic antistaphylococcal penicillins nafcillin and oxacillin, as well as for the antipseudomonal penicillins carbenicillin and ticarcillin. Ampicillin, mezlocillin, and piperacillin bind enterococcal PBP5 with diminished affinity, resulting in MICs that are higher than those for streptococci. These concentrations are within the achievable range in human serum.

PBP-mediated resistance for normally susceptible bacteria takes several forms, including (i) overproduction of a PBP, (ii) acquisition of a foreign PBP with low affinity, (iii) recombination of a susceptible PBP with more resistant varieties, and (iv) generation of point mutations within PBPs that lower affinities for the β-lactam antibiotic.

PBP Overexpression

Increased expression of a PBP as a mechanism of conferring resistance is relatively uncommon. Clear examples of settings in which increased quantities of a PBP are associated with resistance include the increased levels of methicillin resistance found in *S. aureus* strains overexpressing PBP4 (99) and increased levels of penicillin resistance in *E. faecium* strains that overexpress PBP5 (209). The existence of this mechanism serves as a reminder that, like that of β-lactamases, susceptibility or resistance depends on the number of β-lactam molecules relative to the number of targets. Increasing the number of target molecules can, under the correct circumstances, result in resistance. Imipenem's effectiveness against *E. coli* has been partially attributed to the fact that its primary target is PBP2, which is present in roughly 200 copies, in contrast to PBP3, estimated to be present in 2,000 copies.

Acquisition of Foreign PBPs

Acquisition of a foreign PBP as a mechanism of resistance is best exemplified by the expression of methicillin resistance in *S. aureus* strains by virtue of the expression of PBP2a, a low-affinity PBP not native to *S. aureus* (42). Structural analysis of PBP2a suggests that it possesses both transglycosylase and transpeptidase domains. However, it is not clear that the transglycosylase domain is functional. In fact, the transglycosylase domain from PBP2 is required for proper functioning of PBP2a (187). PBP2a confers resistance to all β-lactam antibiotics, although it is bound relatively well by ampicillin (43). The fact that virtually all MRSA strains express β-lactamase limits the utility of ampicillin, but in vitro and animal studies suggest that combinations of ampicillin with β-lactamase inhibitors may be effective (43). To date, there are no clinical data in humans to support using these combinations to treat MRSA infections.

The origin of the *mecA* gene (which encodes PBP2a) is unknown. A *mecA* homologue has been identified in *Staphylococcus sciuri*, a staphylococcal species associated with rodents and primitive mammals (50). The deduced amino acid sequences of the two product enzymes exhibit 88% similarity across the entire proteins and 91% identity within the transpeptidase domain. *Staphylococcus sciuri* strains are not methicillin resistant, however, which may owe to the lack of an effective promoter upstream of the gene (279).

Expression of methicillin resistance in *S. aureus* is commonly under regulatory control, either by the product of the upstream *mecI* gene or *in trans* by the homologous *blaI* gene that regulates the expression of β-lactamase (the promoter regions of *mecA* and the *blaZ* β-lactamase genes are similar) (91). The *mecI* and *blaI* repressors are in turn controlled by the *mecR1* and *blaR1* sensor-transducers, although the precise mechanism of this interaction is incompletely understood. The efficiency of induction varies with the mechanism (*blaR1-blaI*-mediated induction is faster), leading to difficulties in detecting the methicillin resistance phenotype. In fact, only a small minority of a resistant population may express high levels of resistance. Several techniques are used in the laboratory to bring out the resistance (e.g., prolonged incubation or an increase of salt in the media), and more recently techniques have been developed to bypass phenotypic expression in favor of directly identifying the *mecA* gene or directly detecting the PBP2a protein.

Expression of PBP2a-mediated resistance to β-lactams in *S. aureus* is also influenced by the expression of other genetic loci called *fem* ("factors essential for methicillin resistance") or *aux* ("auxiliary") genes (42). *fem* and *aux* genes were first identified by transposon mutagenesis of MRSA to look for insertions that would reduce the expression of resistance. Many *fem* and *aux* factors have now been identified, and all are involved in the formation of the staphylococcal cell wall (42). These data indicate that minor perturbations of the normal processes prevent PBP2a from functioning, suggesting that it has a restricted substrate specificity.

The *mecA* gene is located within a larger (ca. 21 to 67 kb) region of the chromosome known as the staphylococcal cassette chromosome *mec* (SCC*mec*) region (110). It has now been conclusively demonstrated that SCC*mec* is a mobile element, with mobility conferred by the presence of the *ccrA* and *ccrB* genes. The basic elements of SCC*mec* are the *mecR1-mecI-pbp2a* region and *ccrA* (Fig. 4). In recent community-acquired *S. aureus* isolates, little else is included in the SCC*mec* complex (173). Hence, the SCC*mec* regions in these isolates are relatively small (20 to 30 kb) and the isolates themselves tend to be resistant only to β-lactams. Nosocomial isolates have larger SCC*mec* regions, owing to the accumulation over time of integrated plasmids or transposons that contribute to the multiresistance of these isolates (110). Although the SCC*mec* element has never been shown to be transferable in vitro, compelling data have emerged from the study of clinical isolates indicating that the type IV SCC*mec* element has been recently acquired (72). It is intriguing that these data are being found now that the smaller SCC*mec* elements are more prevalent. Since they fall below the 40 kb typical of the staphylococcal bacteriophage, it is conceivable that SCC*mec* type IV is transferable by transduction. The large sizes of SCC*mec* types I to III preclude this sort of transfer, providing a rationale for the prominence of person-to-person spread of MRSA in the hospital rather than the spread of the resistance determinant from strain to strain. Transfer of the *mec* region between staphylococcal strains has never been conclusively documented. The spread of MRSA within institutions is therefore largely due to the transmission of resistant organisms from patient to patient, probably on the hands of transiently colonized health care workers (228). Single strains have spread through entire hospitals and even cities (211). Recent data indicate that *mecA* stabilities differ among different *S. aureus* clones (119), suggesting one potential explanation for the limited lineages within which the resistance determinant has been found.

Resistance Mutations by Recombination with Foreign DNA

Resistance through recombination between PBPs of native, susceptible species and those of less susceptible species is a phenomenon largely restricted to species that are capable of natural transformation or of taking up of naked DNA from the environment. Prominent among these species are *S. pneumoniae*, viridans group streptococci, *Neisseria gonorrhoeae*, and *Neisseria meningitidis* (92). *S. pneumoniae* contains six PBPs (1a, 1b, 2a, 2b, 2x, and 3), all of which are subject to recombination with foreign PBPs taken up by transformation. In most cases, resistant *pbp*

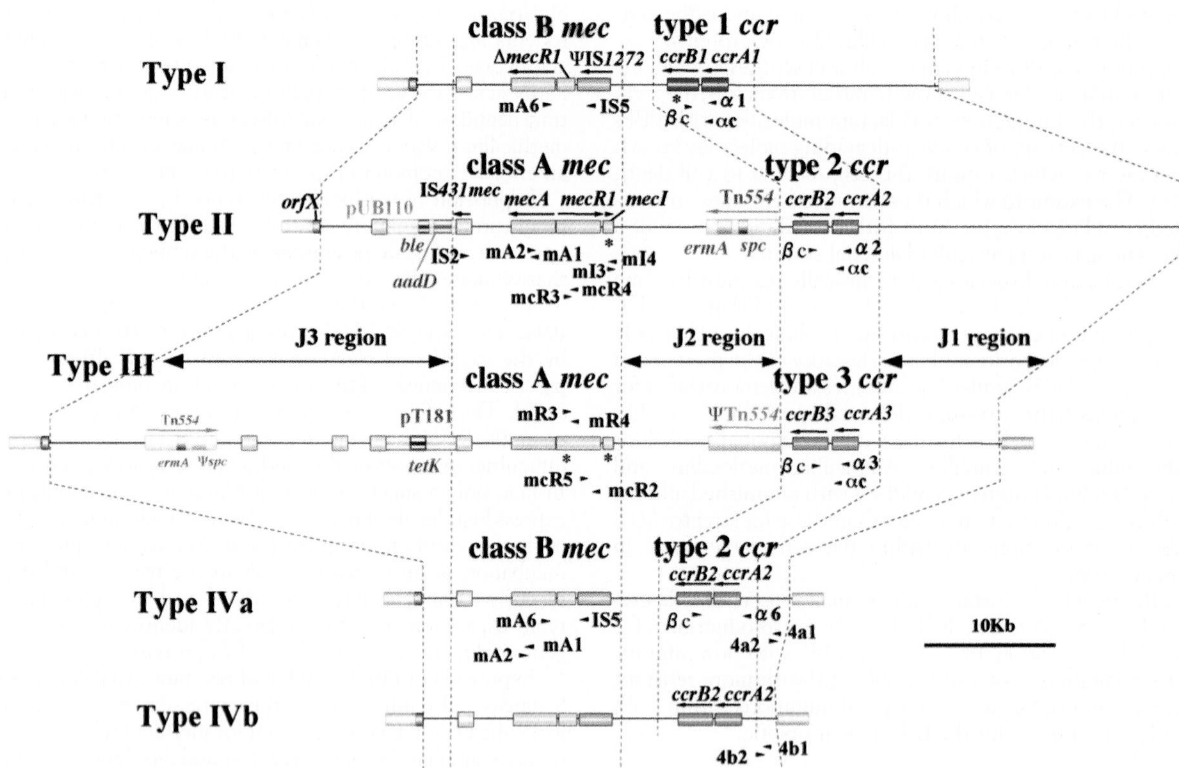

FIGURE 4 Four (of five currently described) SCC*mec* types. Types I, II, and III are found predominantly in health care-associated MRSA, whereas type IV is commonly found in the more susceptible community-associated MRSA around the world. The individual classes of *mec* regions are indicated, as are the variants of the *ccrA* and *ccrB* genes that confer mobility. IS elements and integrated transposons are also indicated. J, or junkyard, regions indicate areas that are not components of the basic SCC*mec*. Antimicrobial resistance genes found within the integrated transposons or plasmids are indicated below the lines, whereas the names of the integrated transposons or plasmids are indicated above the lines. Type V SCC*mec*, recently described, is slightly larger than the type IV elements, reflecting the inclusion of three genes of a putative restriction-modification system. Reprinted from reference 173.

genes demonstrate mosaic patterns (individual segments of foreign *pbp* genes integrated with the native *pbp* gene) with the foreign DNA from the less-penicillin-susceptible viridans group streptococci (92). In fact, genetic exchange appears to be common among these closely related species, with mosaic patterns demonstrable even in PBPs from susceptible *Streptococcus mitis* strains (7). Penicillin resistance in *S. pneumoniae* can be established by alterations in PBP2x, PBP2b, or PBP1a, whereas alterations in PBP2x or PBP1a are required for cephalosporin resistance (17). Penicillin resistance in *S. pneumoniae* has been reported for some time, with cephalosporin resistance emerging more recently, most commonly in strains already resistant to penicillin. However, strains resistant to cephalosporins but susceptible to penicillin have also been reported (234). High-level resistance (≥2 μg/ml) usually implies modification of more than one PBP, sometimes with several mosaic regions in each one (17).

Like that of PBP2a-mediated resistance to methicillin in *S. aureus*, expression of penicillin and cephalosporin resistance in *S. pneumoniae* is dependent on the proper functioning of auxiliary genes. The *fib* locus of *S. pneumoniae* (*fibA* and *fibB*) is analogous to *femA* and *femB* in *S. aureus*. It is involved in the formation of interpeptide bridges, and inactivation of the *fib* locus is associated with reduction of cross-linked muropeptides and loss of penicillin resistance even in the presence of low-affinity mosaic PBPs (265). The *murM-murN* operon encodes enzymes involved in the biosynthesis of branched, structured cell wall muropeptides commonly found in penicillin-resistant pneumococci (74). Inactivation of *murM-murN* results in the loss of branched-chain muropeptides as well as the loss of penicillin resistance.

Among gram-negative species, *Neisseria* species are well known to be naturally transformable. It is therefore not entirely surprising that strains of both *N. gonorrhoeae* and *N. meningitidis* have been described in which mosaic PBP genes are associated with decreased susceptibility to penicillin (92). Similar to those in *S. pneumoniae*, the resistant portions of the PBP genes have been acquired from closely related commensal *Neisseria* species that are more resistant to penicillin (239). Although penicillin resistance in *N. meningitidis* remains extremely rare, both β-lactamase-mediated resistance and PBP-mediated resistance to β-lactams in *N. gonorrhoeae* are quite common.

Generation of Point Mutations

The final mechanism of PBP-mediated β-lactam resistance is the generation of point mutations within the *pbp* genes that result in lower affinity for the β-lactam in question. This form of mutational resistance is seen most commonly in PBP5 of *E. faecium* strains, raising MICs of penicillin from 4 to 16 μg/ml to as high as >1,000 μg/ml. Strains with high-level penicillin resistance now represent the majority of clinical *E. faecium* isolates in the United States (218). These mutations further reduce the affinities for cephalosporins and other β-lactams with lower affinities for the nonmutated version, leading to an increase in resistance that may have implications for the likelihood that antibiotic use will promote colonization with multiresistant *E. faecium* (57). Most of the mutations occur in the vicinity of one or more of several conserved boxes important for β-lactam binding (216). A systematic study of several common mutations of PBP5 has revealed that resistance increases with an increasing number of mutations, with some loci conferring higher levels of resistance than others (206). Among those in gram-negative species, point mutations of the *ftsI* gene of *Haemophilus influenzae* (encoding the transpeptidase domain[s] of PBP3a and/or PBP3b) have been associated with non-β-lactamase-mediated resistance to ampicillin and cephalosporins (255). Although mutations within PBP4 have also been noted in this species, it is not clear that these have a significant impact on β-lactam susceptibility.

β-Lactamase-Mediated Resistance

Classification of β-Lactamases

Two schemes are currently used to classify β-lactamases: the Ambler classification system and the Bush-Medeiros-Jacoby classification system (6, 33, 34). The Ambler classification separates β-lactamases into four distinct classes based on similarities in amino acid sequences. Classes A, C, and D are serine β-lactamases, whereas class B enzymes are metallo-β-lactamases that require zinc for activity (see above). The Bush-Medeiros-Jacoby scheme classifies β-lactamases according to functional similarities (substrate and inhibitor profiles). There are four categories and multiple subgroups in the Bush-Medeiros-Jacoby system (groups 1, 2, 2a, 2b, 2br, 2d, 2be, 2c, 2f, 3, and 3a, etc.) (34). A comparison of the two classification systems is summarized in Table 2. In the discussions that ensue, we will refer to both classification systems.

TABLE 2 ß-lactamase classification

Bush-Jacoby-Medeiros system	Major subgroups	Ambler system	Main attributes
Group 1 cephalosporinases		C (cephalosporinases)	Usually chromosomal; resistance to all ß-lactams except carbapenems; not inhibited by clavulanate
Group 2 penicillinases (clavulanic acid susceptible)	2a	A (serine ß-lactamases)	Staphylococcal penicillinases
	2b	A	Broad-spectrum: TEM-1, TEM-2, SHV-1
	2be	A	Extended-spectrum: TEM and SHV variants, predominantly
	2br	A	Inhibitor-resistant TEM
	2c	A	Carbenicillin hydrolyzing
	2e	A	Cephalosporinases inhibited by clavulanate
	2f	A	Carbapenemases inhibited by clavulanate
	2d	D (oxacillin hydrolyzing)	Oxacillin-hydrolyzing (OXA)
Group 3 metallo-β-lactamase	3a	B (metalloenzymes)	Zinc-dependent carbapenemases
	3b	B	
	3c	B	
Group 4		Not classified	Miscellaneous enzymes, most not yet sequenced

At the time of this writing, 533 β-lactamases have been reported (Karen Bush, personal communication). These include 64 group 1 chromosomal cephalosporinases and 415 group 2 β-lactamases (these are penicillinases that are usually inhibited by clavulanic acid). The group 2be β-lactamases consist of 213 extended-spectrum β-lactamases (ESBLs). As will be discussed below, ESBLs in gram-negative bacteria confer resistance to ceftazidime and other extended-spectrum cephalosporins and are susceptible to inhibition by clavulanic acid. Twenty-nine inhibitor-resistant β-lactamases (resistant to clavulanic acid inactivation; group 2br) have been found, and 12 carbapenemases have been described previously. There are 45 group 3 enzymes (metallo-β-lactamases), and fewer than a dozen β-lactamases that are still unclassified (group 4).

β-Lactamase Mechanism

β-Lactamases are members of a superfamily of active-site serine proteases (147). The mechanism of hydrolysis of β-lactams by β-lactamases has been best studied with TEM-1. TEM-1 β-lactamase disrupts the amide bond of a β-lactam in a two-step reaction. First, the negatively charged carboxylate group of the β-lactam antibiotic is attracted to the active site by the enzyme's positively charged residues. There, the β-lactam is properly positioned, participating in key hydrogen bonding interactions with the enzyme (122). Next, the β-lactam is acylated (Fig. 1). A conserved serine, Ser70, in the active site of TEM-1 serves as the reactive nucleophile in this acylation reaction. Recent ultrahigh-resolution X-ray crystallography studies of TEM-1 (0.85 Å) indicate that Glu166, acting through the catalytic water, activates Ser70 for nucleophilic attack of the β-lactam ring. Then, a strategically positioned water molecule is activated by a general base (e.g., again Glu166). This water molecule deacylates the β-lactam and regenerates the active β-lactamase. This symmetric mechanism is also supported by the ultrahigh-resolution structure (0.90 Å) of another common class A β-lactamase, SHV-2, found in *K. pneumoniae* (170).

β-Lactamase Processing

Generally speaking, β-lactamases are secreted into the periplasmic space in gram-negative bacteria and into the surrounding medium by gram-positive bacteria. Membrane-associated enzymes (in *Bacillus licheniformis, Bacillus cereus,* and *Bacteroides vulgatus*) have been reported rarely. β-Lactamases are synthesized as precursor proteins. As that in other bacteria, the export of proteins into the periplasmic space is mediated by an amino-terminal signal peptide. After transport, the signal peptide of the β-lactamase is cleaved by a processing enzyme, signal peptidase I.

Genetic Environment of β-Lactamases

β-Lactamases can be chromosome-, plasmid-, or transposon- expressed enzymes that are produced in a constitutive or inducible manner. An increasing number of β-lactamases have been found that are carried on integrons. Integrons are genetic elements of variable lengths that contain a 5′ conserved integrase gene *(int)*, mobile antibiotic resistance genes (called cassettes), and an integration site for the gene cassette, *attI* (att, "attachment"). To date, five distinct integron classes have been found to be associated with cassettes that contain antibiotic resistance genes. Three main classes of integrons (classes 1, 2, and 3) have been identified in gram-negative bacteria. Integrons capture antibiotic resistance gene cassettes by using a site-specific recombination mechanism. In the class 1 integrons, the 3′ conserved segment includes two open reading frames of known function: *qacEΔ1*, a deletion derivative of the antiseptic resistance gene *qacE*, and *sulI*, a sulfonamide resistance gene (Fig. 5). As integrons carry multiple resistance determinants and can be readily mobilized, their impact on antibiotic resistance is significant. In the words of Hall and Collis, "integrons thus act both as natural cloning systems and as expression vectors" (93). The capture and spread of antibiotic resistance determinants by integrons underlie the rapid evolution of multiple-antibiotic resistance among diverse gram-negative clinical isolates (213). It should be noted that gene cassettes are mobile and can also exist in free circular form. However, these cassettes do not include all functions required for their mobility. Cassettes are formally part of the integron only when they are integrated at the integron-receptor site. The genes within the cassette do not have promoters.

Integrons are an important source of the spread of *bla* genes. Integrons carrying β-lactamases encompassing Ambler classes A, B, and D have been found in *Acinetobacter baumannii, P. aeruginosa,* and other species of gram-negative bacteria (271). The β-lactamases carried on integrons are VEB-1, VEB-2, GES-1, GES-2, IBI-1, CTX-M-2, CTX-M-9, PSE-1, and numerous OXA β-lactamases (163, 190, 191). OXA and metallo-β-lactamases that confer resistance to carbapenems (IMP-1 to IMP-4 and IMP-8 to IMP-12, VIM-1, VIM-2, and GIM-1) are also included among integron-carried β-lactamases (41, 271).

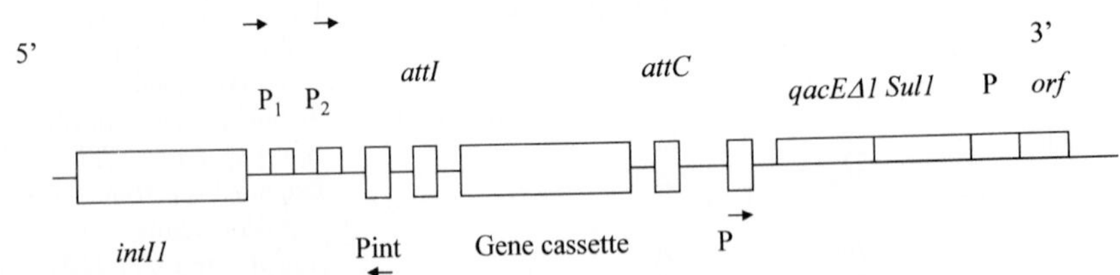

FIGURE 5 Simplified representation of a class 1 integron. P_1, promoter for the gene cassette; P_2, second promoter; Pint, promoter for the integrase; *attI*, integration site; *attC*, sequence in the gene cassette recognized by the integrase; *qacEΔ1*, partially deleted gene that encodes quaternary ammonium compound resistance; *SulI*, gene for sulfonamide resistance; P, promoter; *orf*, open reading frame. As pictured, integrons contain components of a site-specific recombination system that recognizes and captures mobile gene cassettes. Gene cassettes can be antibiotic resistance genes followed by a repeat sequence called a 59-bp element (59be) or *attC*. Cassette-free integrons exist in which the *int* and *sul* regions are contiguous.

Class A β-Lactamases (Bush Group 2b Penicillinases)

Class A β-lactamases possess four important structural motifs that create a complex hydrogen bonding network to fix the β-lactam in the substrate binding pocket. Residues Ser70-Xaa-Xaa-Lys73, Ser130-Asp131-Asn132 (SDN loop), and Lys/Arg234-Thr/Ser235-Gly236 define the conserved residues critical for β-lactam binding and hydrolysis (122). The Ω loop (amino acids Arg164 to Asn179) is unique in class A β-lactamases. A highly conserved Glu166 residue that functions as a general base (electron donor) in the catalytic process is located in the Ω loop. The salt bridge formed between Arg164 and Asn179 defines the limits, or neck, of the Ω loop.

The two commonly encountered class A β-lactamases found in *Enterobacteriaceae* are designated TEM-1 and SHV-1. TEM-1 and SHV-1 β-lactamases are primarily penicillinases with diminished activity against cephalosporin substrates. These two families of β-lactamases have received considerable attention over the past two decades since they are the progenitors of the ESBLs and the inhibitor-resistant TEM β-lactamases now common in many hospitals.

Bush group 2be. ESBLs are generally class A β-lactamases that have expanded or changed substrate profiles as a result of amino acid substitutions. Normally, extended-spectrum cephalosporins are very poor substrates for hydrolysis by Bush group 2b enzymes (high K_ms and low k_{cat}s). Extended-spectrum cephalosporins are extremely potent β-lactams. Mutations at critical amino acids expand the spectra of these enzymes and allow the hydrolysis of extended-spectrum cephalosporins (185). In most cases, ESBL mutations render the enzymes more susceptible to inhibition by mechanism-based inactivators (clavulanic acid, sulbactam, and tazobactam). It is unclear why this increased susceptibility occurs. The impact of enteric gram-negative rods possessing ESBLs on the choice of empiric and definitive antimicrobial therapy has been substantial (123, 135, 178, 180, 181).

Among the TEM family enzymes, five amino acid residues appear to be most important for conferring the ESBL phenotype: Gly238 and Ala237 (located on the b3 β-pleated sheet), Arg164 and Asp179 (located on the neck of the Ω loop), and Asp104 (located directly across from G238 and A237 at the opening of the active-site cavity (122, 200). Of note, the replacement of Gly to Ser, Ala, or Asp at the Ambler position 238 is a common mutation in both TEM and SHV ESBLs (http://www.lahey.org/studies/webt.html).

Non-TEM, non-SHV ESBLs. Among the non-TEM, non-SHV ESBLs, the CTX-M β-lactamases are the most prevalent. They can be divided into distinct clusters (see http://www.lahey.org/studies/webt.html). Unlike most (but not all) TEM- and SHV-derived ESBLs, CTX-M β-lactamases hydrolyze cefotaxime and cetriaxone better than they do ceftazidime. It appears that CTX-M enzymes are more readily inhibited by tazobactam than they are by clavulanic acid. The first CTX-M type β-lactamase (MEN-1) was described nearly a decade ago. There are now nearly 60 members of this family.

CTX-M β-lactamases are commonly found in *K. pneumoniae, E. coli,* typhoidal and nontyphoidal *Salmonella, Shigella* spp., *Citrobacter freundii, Enterobacter* spp., and *Serratia marcescens* (121, 126, 179). The chromosome-carried β-lactamase of *Kluyvera ascorbata* is a probable progenitor of some plasmid-carried CTX-M enzymes (121). Other CTX-M β-lactamases may derive from *Kluyvera georgiana* (174). A recent comprehensive review delineates the lineage of many CTX-M enzymes resulting from *Kluyvera* spp. (25). Of note, different genetic elements may be involved in the mobilization of $bla_{CTX\text{-}M}$ genes.

Many other clinically important non-TEM, non-SHV ESBLs have been described previously (K1, GES-1, PER-1, PER-2, VEB-1, BES-1, IBI-1, IBI-2, and OXA type) (28, 29, 193).

Structural biology of ESBLs. Important insights have emerged from the study of a number of atomic structures of class A ESBL enzymes. The common theme that emerges is that the active site is selectively remodeled and expanded to accommodate the bulky R1 side chain of extended-spectrum cephalosporin. Although the details of this modification are different for many of the ESBLs, the remodeling comes at a price. Many of these ESBLs are not as catalytically efficient as are the wild-type progenitors against certain substrates. With the expanded substrate spectrum, one uniformly observes decreases in MICs of penicillin and in k_{cat}/K_m ratios. In addition, these enzymes are less stable under proteolysis and heat. The structures of Toho-1, TEM-52, TEM-64, the Gly238Ala ESBL in TEM, SHV-2, and K1 β-lactamases all reveal insights into why expanded-spectrum cephalosporins fit into the active site (45, 108, 109, 170, 175, 229, 251, 264).

Serine carbapenemases of Bush group 2f or class A type. In the past, β-lactamases able to hydrolyze carbapenems were rare. It is regrettable that this is no longer the case. Representatives of these carbapenemases are Sme-1, Sme-2, NMC-A, IMI-1, GES-2, and KPC-1, KPC-2, and KPC-3 (191, 281). Class A carbapenemases hydrolyze imipenem but are not resistant to clavulanic acid inhibition. $bla_{NMC\text{-}A}$ and $bla_{IMI\text{-}1}$ are chromosomally located genes in *E. cloacae* and are induced by cefoxitin and imipenem (168, 201). $bla_{NMC\text{-}A}$ is regulated by a LysR-type regulatory protein (160). It is felt that $bla_{IMI\text{-}1}$ is regulated in the same manner (201). $bla_{Sme\text{-}1}$ is a chromosomally located gene encoding serine carbapenemase of class A in *E. cloacae* and *Serratia marcescens.*

A notable increase in bacteria expressing class A carbapenamases has occurred in the United States. Numerous studies are revealing that KPC ("*Klebsiella pneumonia* carbapenemase") β-lactamases are becoming endemic in East Coast cities. First found in *K. pneumoniae,* these β-lactamases have been detected in *Salmonella enterica* serotype Cubana, *Klebsiella oxytoca,* and *Enterobacter* spp. strain MS 412 (106, 153, 281, 282). $bla_{KPC\text{-}1}$ is located on a nonconjugative plasmid (281), and $bla_{KPC\text{-}2}$ in *Salmonella* and *Klebsiella oxytoca* was isolated from conjugative plasmids (153, 282). The plasmid carrying $bla_{KPC\text{-}3}$ from New York was also transferable by conjugation (278).

Detection of KPC β-lactamases may be a problem for clinical laboratories because of the positive ESBL confirmation tests (clavulanate-potentiated activities of ceftriaxone, ceftazidime, cefepime, and aztreonam). To improve detection of KPC-expressing *K. pneumoniae,* careful inoculum preparation for broth-based susceptibility methods must be carried out to avoid underinoculation. Investigators in this area have found that resistant isolates are readily detected by agar-based methods but not by broth methods (31). Bratu et al. have also advised that using ertapenem or meropenem will improve detection (31).

Among these serine carbapenemases exists a notable curiosity. $bla_{GES\text{-}2}$ is a plasmid-carried β-lactamase gene found in *P. aeruginosa* (194). bla_{GES-2} is a point mutation mutant of the clavulanic acid-inhibited ESBL gene bla_{GES-1} (a non-TEM, non-SHV ESBL gene). It is curious that GES-1 is an ESBL and that a single point mutation (Gly → Asp at position 170 in the Ω loop) can add an imipenemase activity to GES-2. The OXA carbapenemases will be discussed subsequently.

Inhibitor-resistant class A β-lactamases: Bush group 2br. Amino acid mutations within TEM and SHV that confer resistance to inhibition by β-lactamase inhibitors have also been characterized at the following amino acid positions: Met69, Ser130, Arg244, Arg275, and Asn276 (26, 56, 68, 196, 220, 242, 247, 257, 260). Most inhibitor-resistant β-lactamases are variants of the TEM-1 enzyme, with only two descriptions of clinical isolates expressing SHV β-lactamases that are resistant to inhibitors (SHV-10 and SHV-49) known at the time of this writing (59, 196). It is possible that the frequency of inhibitor-resistant β-lactamases in TEM and SHV family enzymes is underestimated, since many laboratories in the United States do not identify the corresponding strains routinely (120). Cephalosporins or high-dose piperacillin-tazobactam may be effective for the treatment of infection with *E. coli* strains expressing some inhibitor-resistant β-lactamases.

Mutants of TEM β-lactamases are being recovered that maintain the ESBL phenotype but also demonstrate inhibitor resistance. These are referred to as complex mutants of TEM (CMTs). There are now four identified CMTs (73, 164, 192, 232). It is still unknown how these enzymes will impact empirical treatment. At this time, clinical microbiology laboratories do not have the resources to detect such complex phenotypes.

Class B β-Lactamases (Bush Group 3 Enzymes)

In contrast to the serine-dependent β-lactamases (those of classes A, C, and D), class B β-lactamases are metalloenzymes. These enzymes contain an αββα motif with a central β sandwich and two α helices on each side. As such, class B β-lactamases require zinc or another heavy metal for catalysis and their activities are inhibited by chelating agents (EDTA). The zinc atom is held in place by three histidines and a water molecule. Some metallo-β-lactamases contain a second Zn binding site. These two sites function separately, with the primary Zn binding site assisted by the secondary site. A coordinated water molecule also serves a critical role in catalysis (263).

With few exceptions (see below), class B β-lactamases confer resistance to a wide range of β-lactam compounds, including cephamycins and carbapenems. The class B β-lactamases are resistant to inactivation by clavulanate, sulbactam, and tazobactam. Aztreonam, a monobactam, may act as an inhibitor, but there are metallo-β-lactamases that hydrolyze aztreonam. Of note, isolates expressing VIM-2 can be susceptible to aztreonam (189).

Class B β-lactamases can be grouped into three different subclasses (B1, B2, and B3). Amino acid positions can be assigned according to a specific numbering system, designated BBL, that is based upon structural alignment (84). Although the genes encoding metallo-β-lactamases show very little primary structure sequence identity (17 to 37%), the three-dimensional structures of the known metallo-β-lactamases appear similar (36, 48, 238, 256).

Because of the metal ion, the catalytic pathway for metallo-β-lactamases does not involve an acyl-enzyme intermediate as it does for class A and C β-lactamases. The catalytic pathway for class B also incorporates a hydrolytic water molecule (the bridging water molecule) that possesses enhanced nucleophilicity due to the proximity to the metal ion. The zinc ions coordinate two water molecules. The addition of the hydroxide to the carbonyl carbon of the β-lactam leads to the formation of a transient, noncovalent reaction intermediate.

The majority of metallo-β-lactamases are chromosomally encoded, and their expression may be constitutive or inducible. The metallo-β-lactamases of *Bacillus cereus, Stenotrophomonas maltophilia, Aeromonas hydrophilia,* and *Aeromonas jandaei* are inducible. In *Aeromonas jandaei,* regulation of the metallo-β-lactamase appears to involve two-component-signal transduction systems (4).

The metallo-β-lactamases of the VIM and IMP types are becoming increasingly important as threats to our antimicrobial armamentarium. These metallo-β-lactamases are broad-spectrum enzymes, are active against most β-lactams, including carbapenems, and have been found in various gram-negative clinical isolates mostly in the Far East and the Mediterranean regions. bla_{VIM} is an integron-borne metallo-β-lactamase gene that is usually found in *P. aeruginosa* isolates. bla_{VIM-2} has now spread to more than 20 countries. The majority of metallo-β-lactamase genes are mobilized on integrons, transposons, and mobile common regions (263). At the time of this writing, there are 13 VIM and 18 IMP types identified. Like VIM metallo-β-lactamase genes, IMP metallo-β-lactamase genes are widespread. IMP metallo-β-lactamase genes have been found as parts of integrons in the following bacteria: *P. aeruginosa, Pseudomonas putida, Serratia marcescens, Pseudomonas stutzeri, Acinetobacter baumannii, Pseudomonas fluorescens, K. pneumoniae, Klebsiella oxytoca, Enterobacter aerogenes, Achromobacter xylosoxidans,* and *E. coli* (263).

As stated above, the atomic structures of a number of class B β-lactamases have been solved (36, 48, 84, 85). The structures are being used to design novel inhibitors of class B β-lactamases.

Class C β-Lactamases

Ambler class C (Bush-Jacoby-Medeiros group 1) chromosomally encoded β-lactamases are produced to a greater or lesser degree by almost all gram-negative bacteria (*Salmonella* and *Klebsiella* being the only known exceptions). Chromosomally encoded (and inducible) enzymes are particularly important in clinical isolates of *Citrobacter freundii, Enterobacter aerogenes, E. cloacae, Morganella morganii, P. aeruginosa,* and *Serratia marcescens.* Although class C β-lactamases hydrolyze cephalosporins (including extended-spectrum cephalosporins) more effectively than they do penicillins, it should be kept in mind that these enzymes have great efficiencies for the hydrolysis of penicillins (the K_ms are very low). Most class C enzymes are resistant to inhibition by clavulanate, sulbactam, and tazobactam.

Class C β-lactamases have larger active-site cavities than class A enzymes, which may allow them to bind the bulky extended-spectrum cephalosporins (oxyimino-β-lactams) (51, 136). It is claimed that this conformational expansion and flexibility facilitate hydrolysis of oxyimino-β-lactams by making the acyl-enzyme intermediate more open to attack by water (51, 136, 151).

The important structural elements described for class A enzymes are also present in class C β-lactamases. The active-site serine (Ser64) is located near the N terminus of a long helix and is followed on the next helix turn by a lysine (Ser64-Xaa-Xaa-Lys67). The second element contains a Tyr-Xaa-Asn (Tyr150) or Ser-Xaa-Asn pattern corresponding to the Ser130-Asp131-Asn132 loop of class A β-lactamases.

The opposite side of the active site is marked by Lys315/Arg/His-Thr/Ser-Gly corresponding to the KTG motif of class A enzymes.

Class C cephalosporinases acylate β-lactams in the same manner that class A enzymes do. First, the catalytic Ser64 attacks the β-lactam carbonyl carbon and the acyl-enzyme forms. The approaches of the activated water molecule are different between AmpC and class A enzymes (for class C, the approach is from the β-face). This difference implies that the deacylation mechanism is distinct. Unlike that of class A enzymes, the ring amine of the acyl-enzyme of class C facilitates deacylation. This substrate-assisted catalysis distinguishes class C from class A. In examination of the catalytic mechanism, a Glu166 equivalent in class C β-lactamases is not readily apparent; this role may be filled by the tyrosine (Tyr150) in the Tyr-Xaa-Asn motif.

The first class C β-lactamase structure determined was that of the AmpC cephalosporinase of *Citrobacter freundii* by Oefner et al. (171). Determination of the structures of the P99 β-lactamase of *E. cloacae,* AmpC β-lactamase from *E. coli,* and *E. cloacae* GC1 and *E. cloacae* 908R β-lactamases has ensued (51, 137; http://www.rcsb.org). The GC1 β-lactamase of *E. cloacae* has improved hydrolytic activity for oxyimino-β-lactam antibiotics because of a tripepetide insertion in the Ω loop (tandem repeat Ala211-Val212-Arg213). In a strict sense this is a class C ESBL. As a result of this addition, the opening of the active-site binding cavity is wider and the substrate spectrum has expanded (51).

In the clinically important class C enzyme-producing gram-negative rods, β-lactamase production is normally repressed. The details of the repression have been mostly elucidated for *Enterobacter* spp. (111). Repression and activation are closely linked to the processes of cell wall synthesis and breakdown. The molecule that serves as both the repressor and the activator of *ampC* transcription is AmpR, a transcriptional regulator of the LysR family. AmpR is present as a repressor by virtue of its interaction with UDP-MurNac-pentapeptide, a peptidoglycan precursor molecule. In this form AmpR is incapable of activating *ampC* and in fact serves as a repressor of *ampR* expression. In the setting of high concentrations of cell wall breakdown product anhydro-MurNAc-tripeptide (or anhydro-MurNac-pentapeptide), however, UDP-MurNAc-pentapeptide is displaced from its site in AmpR, resulting in the conversion of AmpR into an activator of *ampC* transcription.

Increases in *ampC* expression may result from the action of β-lactam antibiotics, certain of which cause the release of significant quantities of anhydro-MurNAc-tripeptide and/or -pentapeptide from the peptidoglycan. This anhydro-UDP-MurNAc-tripeptide enters the cell through a channel (AmpG) and overwhelms the recycling ability of the cytosolic amidase (AmpD) specific for recycling of muropeptides. Under these circumstances (induction), β-lactamase is produced only as long as the antibiotic is present in the medium.

Constitutive high-level production of AmpC β-lactamase most commonly results from a mutation in the *ampD* gene, reducing the quantity of (or eliminating) AmpD from the cytoplasm. Under these circumstances, a constant high level of anhydro-MurNAc-tripeptide is present in the cytoplasm, and AmpR serves as a constitutive activator of *ampC* transcription. Constitutive production can also result from deletion of *ampR,* but in this circumstance β-lactamase production is generally at a low level.

The widespread dissemination of *ampC*-type β-lactamase genes on transferable plasmids is a continuing challenge. These plasmid-carried AmpC cephalosporinases are separated into four general groups. Group 1 plasmid-carried AmpC cephalosporinases consist of those that originated from the chromosomally encoded AmpC of *Citrobacter freundii* (BIL-1, CMY-2, LAT-1, and LAT-2). Members of group 2 are related to the chromosomally encoded cephalosporinase of *E. cloacae* (MIR-1 and ACT-1); group 3 β-lactamases belong to the AmpC group of *P. aeruginosa* (CMY-1, FOX-1, and MOX-1), and group 4 enzymes belong to the CMY-1 β-lactamases (CMY-1 cluster). Plasmid-mediated class C β-lactamases have been identified in many gram-negative bacteria from all parts of the world. Host strains harboring these enzymes include *K. pneumoniae, Enterobacter aerogenes, S. enterica* serotypes Enteritidis and Senftenberg, *E. coli, Proteus mirabilis, Morganella morganii,* and *Klebsiella oxytoca.* The loss of porin proteins in clinical isolates with plasmid-carried AmpC enzymes may result in resistance to carbapenems (30, 240).

Class D β-Lactamases

The OXA-type (oxacillin-hydrolyzing) β-lactamases have been most commonly identified in *Enterobacteriaceae, Acinetobacter* spp., and *P. aeruginosa* (161). OXA enzymes confer resistance to a wide variety of penicillins. They are only weakly inhibited by clavulanic acid but are inhibited by sodium chloride (NaCl). Overall, the amino acid identities between class D and class A or class C β-lactamases are less than 20%. The frequent location of class D genes on mobile genetic elements (plasmids or integrons) facilitates spread (162, 190, 261).

Several OXA β-lactamases (OXA-11 and OXA-14 to OXA-20) are associated with an ESBL phenotype. These OXA types have been found exclusively in *P. aeruginosa.* A comparison of the crystal structure of the OXA-10 β-lactamase with that of the class C enzyme from *E. cloacae* P99 and that of the class A TEM-1 enzyme from *E. coli* shows that the class D and class A enzymes share a common fold pattern (α helices and β-pleated sheets), although the distributions of secondary-structure elements are different. A remarkable feature is the nearly perfect symmetry of all atoms that constitute the catalytic machinery for acylation (Ser67, Lys70, Ser115, and Lys205 in OXA-10 and Ser70, Lys73, Ser130, and Lys234 in TEM-1). There seems to be an extension of the substrate binding site (tripeptide strand) in OXA-10. The role of the peptide extension is not known. The oxyanion hole is provided by the main-chain nitrogen atoms of Ser67 and Phe208. In class D the same residue (Lys70) is involved in acylation and deacylation (149, 176).

OXA enzymes are assuming greater importance due to the ability of members of this class to hydrolyze carbapenems. The first description of a serine carbapenemase in *Acinetebacter baumannii* was that of ARI-1 (OXA-23) in 1985 (182). Although OXA carbapenemases hydrolyze imipenem inefficiently, their presence in an organism with an active efflux pump or a porin mutation may confer clinically significant levels of resistance (101). It is notable that *Acinetobacter baumannii* isolates possess a chromosomally encoded oxacillinase, OXA-69, that confers very low level imipenem resistance. The OXA-69 gene is ubiquitous in *Acinetobacter baumannii* and is referred to as a housekeeping gene (100).

Resistance to Chloramphenicol

Acetyltransferases

Chloramphenicol is a broad-spectrum antimicrobial agent whose use has waned in recent years due to well-characterized hematologic toxicity and a wealth of less toxic therapeutic options. The most common mechanism of resistance to chloramphenicol is the elaboration of CATs. A large number of CAT genes have been reported, and these determinants generally confer extremely high levels of resistance on the organisms expressing them. Substantial structural similarities exist among the different CAT variants, although their nucleotide sequences may be quite divergent (159). Relationships among the different CATs have been described in detail in a recent review by Schwarz and colleagues (222). Chloramphenicol contains two hydroxyl groups that are acetylated in a reaction catalyzed by CAT in which acetyl coenzyme A serves as the acyl donor. Initial acetylation occurs at the C-3 hydroxyl group to give 3-acetoxy-chloramphenicol (226). Following nonenzymatic rearrangement into 1-acetoxy-chloramphenicol and reacetylation, the 1,3-diacetoxy-chloramphenicol product is formed. Neither the mono- nor the diacetoxy derivatives are able to bind to the 50S ribosomal subunit and inhibit prokaryotic peptidyltransferase (226).

CATs are generally divided into two types: type A (classical) CATs and type B (xenobiotic) CATs (222). Five structurally similar type A CATs (A, B, C, D, and that expressed by the prototypic plasmid pC194) in *S. aureus* have been described previously (77). The *cat* genes encoding these enzymes are commonly located on small, multicopy plasmids, and expression is inducible through a translational attenuation mechanism (222). *E. faecalis* and *S. pneumoniae* also express inducible CAT genes that are similar to the type D gene of *S. aureus*. Two CAT genes encoding constitutive CAT expression in *Clostridium perfringens* have been described previously. *catP* is generally found within transposon Tn*4451*, whereas *catQ* (nearly identical to *catD* of *Clostridium difficile*) is chromosomal (222).

Three types of type A CATs (I, II, and III) have been identified in gram-negative bacteria. The widely prevalent type I enzymes are distinguished by their ability to bind and inhibit (without acetylation) the activity of fusidic acid (19). These enzymes are frequently found associated with transposon Tn9 or related elements. Type II CATs are notable for their sensitivity to inhibition by thiol-reactive agents and for their association with *H. influenzae* (158). Most knowledge of the structural features of the type A CAT enzymes comes from the study of the type III enzyme, for which the tertiary structure is known at high resolution (159). The structural determinants of binding for each substrate are also known for this enzyme.

Type B (xenobiotic) acetyltransferases (159) are structurally unrelated to classic CATs, and those that have been demonstrated to acetylate chloramphenicol confer only low levels of chloramphenicol resistance even when the genes are present in high copy numbers. Their natural substrate is likely something other than chloramphenicol, explaining their limited ability to acetylate this antibiotic. First described in *Agrobacter tumefaciens*, they have now been identified in a wide range of species (222). Included among this class of agents are the virginiamycin acetyltransferases found in *S. aureus* and *E. faecium* (see "Resistance to Macrolides" below). In fact, although they are members of this class, the *vat* gene products do not confer resistance to chloramphenicol nor have they been demonstrated to be able to acetylate chloramphenicol in vitro (159). They are, however, quite adept at acetylating streptogramins. The crystal structures of two trimeric type B CATs have been determined previously (18, 198).

Decreased Accumulation of Chloramphenicol

It is now well recognized that chloramphenicol serves as a substrate for many of the multidrug-resistance efflux pumps that exist in gram-positive and gram-negative bacteria, including those found in *E. coli, P. aeruginosa, Bacillus subtilis*, and *S. aureus* (165). In addition, there are efflux systems that are specific for chloramphenicol. The first chloramphenicol-specific efflux gene to be described was *cmlA* within the In4 integron of Tn*1696* (21). *cmlA* encodes an efflux mechanism that uses chloramphenicol but not florfenicol (a chloramphenicol derivative licensed for use in animals in 1996 in the United States for the treatment of bovine respiratory pathogens) as a substrate. Gram-negative bacteria also express efflux genes specific for both chloramphenicol and florfenicol (flo_{Pp} and flo_{St}). These resistance genes are being reported with increasing frequency from animal-derived *E. coli* and *Salmonella* isolates (24, 272). In fact, the chloramphenicol resistance expressed by multiresistant *S. enterica* serotype Typhimurium DT104 is most commonly encoded by flo_{St} (24), emphasizing again the potential negative impact of using similar antimicrobial agents in humans and animals.

Resistance to Glycopeptides

Glycopeptide antibiotics (vancomycin and teicoplanin) inhibit cell wall synthesis by binding to the pentapeptide peptidoglycan precursor molecule as it exits the cytoplasmic membrane. This binding prevents the cross-linking (transpeptidation) of peptidoglycan precursors necessary for the formation of normal, stable cell walls. The large size of the glycopeptide molecules also appears to inhibit the other major peptidoglycan linkage reaction (transglycosylation) by steric hindrance. The specific moiety bound by vancomycin is the terminal D-alanyl-D-alanine of the pentapeptide. The vast majority of bacteria that have been studied have peptidoglycan precursors that are pentapeptides terminating in D-Ala-D-Ala and therefore are theoretically susceptible to vancomycin. However, the large size of the vancomycin molecule exceeds the exclusion limits of the porins in gram-negative-bacterium outer membranes, so vancomycin cannot access the target in these species. Hence, vancomycin is active only against bacteria lacking outer membranes, which are predominantly gram positive.

Acquired resistance to vancomycin in gram-positive bacteria comes in three varieties largely defined by the species in association with which they have been described: (i) altered precursor formation in enterococci, (ii) mutational cell wall changes in staphylococci, and (iii) tolerance in pneumococci. The importance of the first type of resistance is characterized more by its prevalence than by the importance of the species as causes of infection, whereas the other two types of resistance are defined more by the importance of the species involved than by their prevalence.

To date, six varieties of enterococcal glycopeptide resistance have been described (corresponding to VanA through VanE and VanG). Of these, the most clinically important are VanA and VanB (12). VanA and VanB are encoded by similar operons in which three genes (*vanH, vanA*, and *vanX* or $vanH_B$, *vanB*, and $vanX_B$) are required for the expression of resistance (12). Two other genes (*vanY* and *vanZ* or $vanY_B$ and *vanW*) serve to amplify resistance but are not required for its expression (8, 9), and two more genes (*vanS* and *vanR* or $vanS_B$ and $vanR_B$) regulate the transcription of the three essential genes (10, 66). The ultimate purpose of these genes is to alter the structure of the pentapeptide precursor from terminating in D-alanyl-D-alanine to terminating in D-alanine-D-lactate and in so doing to reduce the binding affinity of vancomycin for its target (roughly 1,000 fold). Since the terminal amino acid is cleaved off of the pentapeptide in the transpeptidation reaction, the final composition of the cell wall is indistinguishable from that in strains lacking the resistance determinant.

VanA enterococci are phenotypically resistant to vancomycin and teicoplanin, whereas VanB strains are resistant to vancomycin but appear to be susceptible to teicoplanin. This susceptibility results from the fact that teicoplanin does not induce expression of resistance (66). Once the VanB operon is expressed, however, resistance to teicoplanin results. Consequently, teicoplanin has been disappointing as a therapy for infections caused by VanB enterococci, since mutations in the VanB regulatory apparatus resulting in either inducibility by teicoplanin or constitutive expression occur readily during therapy (13, 96, 117).

Both VanA and VanB operons are carried by transposons. The VanA operon is found exclusively within transposon Tn*1546*, a 10.4-kb Tn*3* family element that is presumed to disseminate among enterococci by integrating into conjugative plasmids (11). The genes of the VanA operon are highly conserved in their sequences among different strains, but the restriction maps of the operons and of Tn*1546* often differ markedly among clinical strains (53). These differences result from insertions of a variety of IS elements with or without subsequent deletions of parts of the mobile element and have been used by some investigators to establish lineages of strains within defined clinical settings. The VanB operon is most commonly carried on transposons designated Tn*5382* or Tn*1549* (37, 86). It is likely that Tn*5382* and Tn*1549* are identical. These transposons exhibit significant homology to prototype enterococcal conjugative transposon Tn*916*. In contrast to the *vanA* gene, *vanB* has three allelic variants (*vanB1*, *vanB2*, and *vanB3*). The *vanB2* gene is associated with Tn*5382*.

The overwhelming majority of clinical vancomycin-resistant strains are *E. faecium*, a predilection that remains unexplained (218). In the United States, the vast majority of *E. faecium* strains that are resistant to vancomycin also express high levels of resistance to ampicillin, thereby negating the two most effective and reliable antienterococcal agents. In some strains, this linkage is actually physical, with insertion of Tn*5382* immediately downstream of the *pbp5* gene resulting in high-level ampicillin resistance (37). These two determinants transfer between enterococcal chromosomes together through mechanisms that are yet to be determined.

The origins of the vancomycin resistance determinants are obscure, but it is clear from sequence comparisons that they did not develop within the enterococci (see above). Their entry into enterococci, markedly delayed considering that vancomycin was introduced into clinical use in 1958, was likely facilitated by the administration of high concentrations of glycopeptides to mammalian gastrointestinal tracts. In Europe, this exposure occurred largely in the gastrointestinal tracts of food animals that were fed the glycopeptide avoparcin as a growth promoter (266). Evidence is now quite convincing that the animal strains transferred to the European human population through the food chain (237). In the United States, where glycopeptides were never used in animal feeds, the exchange event likely occurred in the gastrointestinal tracts of hospital patients who were given vancomycin orally to treat real or presumed *Clostridium difficile*-associated diarrhea. The U.S. *E. faecium* strains were likely highly adapted to the hospital environment through acquisition of antibiotic resistance and virulence determinants. These differences in origin may explain why vancomycin-resistant infections in European hospitals are quite rare, despite sometimes heavy colonization of the community population, whereas vancomycin-resistant infections in the United States now constitute more than 25% of all enterococcal infections acquired in the hospital, despite no compelling evidence of colonization in the community at all. Emerging data indicate that many of the vancomycin-resistant strains isolated from outbreaks of clinical infection belong to a specific clonal group, suggesting that some vancomycin-resistant *E. faecium* strains are particularly likely to disseminate and cause clinical infections (275). Thankfully, the VanA and VanB operons have remained restricted to *E. faecalis* and *E. faecium*, with few exceptions. Despite in vitro transfer of the VanA determinant to *S. aureus* (167), and at least three instances in which VanA-expressing *S. aureus* isolates have been recovered from clinical samples (41a), vancomycin-resistant *S. aureus* remains exceedingly rare. In all cases, resistance has been conferred by the VanA operon and in one well-characterized case transfer appears to have been facilitated by the presence of Tn*1546* on a broad-host-range plasmid in *E. faecalis*, with transposition of Tn*1546* to a staphylococcal plasmid once entry into the staphylococcus occurred (79, 268).

The VanC operon is intrinsic to the cell wall synthesis machinery of minor enterococcal species *Enterococcus casseliflavus* (including the biotype formerly classified as *Enterococcus flavescens*) and *Enterococcus gallinarum* (60, 262). The peptidoglycan precursor in VanC strains terminates in D-alanine-D-serine, reducing vancomycin affinity about sevenfold and resulting in low levels of resistance. Precursors terminate in D-alanine-D-serine in strains of *E. faecalis* with VanE (76), whereas in VanD-expressing *E. faecium* it terminates in D-alanine-D-lactate. The failure to observe dissemination of VanD may be explained in part by the fact that the VanX equivalent enzyme in *E. faecium* BM4339 appears to be ineffective in an enterococcal background. Resistance is expressed in BM4339 because that strain lacks a functional cellular ligase (*ddl*) gene, eliminating the need for VanX activity to express resistance (40).

Mutational resistance to glycopeptides in *S. aureus* is a rare clinical entity that most commonly takes the form of reduced susceptibility rather than frank resistance. For resistant strains, alternately called vancomycin-intermediate *S. aureus* or GISA (glycopeptide-intermediate *S. aureus*), MICs of vancomycin are in the 4- to 8-μg/ml range (133). However, within these cultures are smaller populations of cells that express higher levels of resistance. Animal studies suggest that the level of resistance expressed by GISA strains will reduce the effectiveness of vancomycin therapy (47).

The exact mechanism of glycopeptide resistance in GISA strains remains incompletely understood (27). One consistent finding is a thickened cell wall with increased numbers of unlinked precursors and abnormal septum formation (52). Consistent with this phenotype is the fact that all clinically isolated GISA strains studied have virtually undetectable quantities of PBP4, a low-molecular-weight PBP associated with peptidoglycan cross-linking (75). Restoration of PBP4 on a high-copy-number plasmid restores cross-linking and vancomycin susceptibility to these strains. Preliminary work suggests that a range of genes may be involved in the expression of vancomycin resistance, that the phenotype may be due to different genetic mutations in different strains, and that vancomycin-resistant mutants may evolve from strains that are hypermutators (14). It has been suggested that vancomycin resistance results from the absorption of most of the vancomycin by the unlinked precursors (false vancomycin targets) before it can arrive at its true target, the peptidoglycan precursors attached to lipid II as they emerge from the cytoplasmic membrane (104). Further work will be required before we understand the details of vancomycin resistance in these rare but troublesome strains.

Glycopeptide resistance in coagulase-negative species of staphylococci has also been reported. In contrast to that in *S. aureus*, resistance in *Staphylococcus haemolyticus* has been associated with changes in the compositions of the cross-links of the peptidoglycan (20). The mechanism by which this would lead to vancomycin resistance is unknown.

Vancomycin is, in general, a less bactericidal antibiotic than are the β-lactams. Evidence for the importance of this observation can be found in several studies. The bacteremia associated with *S. aureus* endocarditis, for example, takes roughly twice as much time to clear with vancomycin treatment as with treatment with β-lactam oxacillin (131). Recent clinical data also suggest that vancomycin treatment is associated with higher rates of failure and relapse than nafcillin treatment of bacteremia due to methicillin-susceptible *S. aureus* (44). Reports of vancomycin tolerance in *S. pneumoniae* first appeared in 1990 (253). *S. pneumoniae* is the most common cause of bacterial meningitis in most patient populations, and bactericidal therapy is optimal for treatment of this condition. At least one case of presumed recrudescence of meningitis after treatment of a case of vancomycin-tolerant pneumococcal meningitis has been reported (98). Tolerance appears to involve mutations within an operon *(vex123)* encoding an ABC transporter, but the mechanism by which this occurs remains undefined (90). Recent work suggests that tolerance may be more common in clinical pneumococcal isolates than was previously believed, that tolerance is associated with antibiotic resistance, and that vancomycin-tolerant strains are more likely to be tolerant to other classes of antimicrobial agents as well (212). Further work will be required before we understand the true importance of pneumococcal tolerance for the treatment of clinical infections.

Resistance to Linezolid

The oxazolidinone antibiotic linezolid inhibits bacterial protein synthesis by interacting with the N-formylmethionyl-tRNA-ribosome-mRNA ternary complex commonly referred to as the initiation complex (230). Linezolid exerts excellent bacteriostatic activity against a wide range of gram-positive pathogens, including methicillin-resistant staphylococci and multiresistant enterococci. Clinical use of this agent has been associated with the emergence of resistant strains, most commonly after prolonged therapy of infections with difficult-to-eradicate bacteria. Resistance in both *E. faecium* and *S. aureus* has now been described, and there are suggestions that the rate of emergence of resistance in *E. faecium* may be significant. Analysis of linezolid-resistant enterococcal laboratory mutants suggests that resistance is associated with a G2576U (*E. coli* numbering scheme) point mutation in the 23S rRNA, although mutations at other positions may also contribute to resistance (197). A G2576U mutation has been described in resistant clinical isolates of *E. faecium* and in the analogous position of the 23S ribosomal subunit of a resistant *S. aureus* isolate (88, 252). Since the 23S subunit genes exist in multiple copies in different bacteria (four in *E. faecalis* and six in *E. faecium*), it has been suggested that more than one copy of the genes must be mutated to confer resistance. This in fact appears to be the case, with strains having a higher percentage of mutated 23S genes expressing greater levels of resistance (143). Multiple mutated gene copies do not arise independently, however. Once the first gene is mutated, subsequent copies can be mutated through recombination with the resistant gene (138). In this fashion, persistent selective pressure exerted by linezolid can lead to rapid development of high-level (MIC, >128 μg/ml) resistance. Despite this potential and the increasing use of linezolid in clinical settings, rates of resistance to this antimicrobial agent remain very low.

Resistance to Macrolides

Erythromycin (the first macrolide) was initially isolated from *Streptomyces erythreus*, a soil organism found in the Philippines. There are currently four macrolides in common use: erythromycin, clarithromycin, azithromycin, and roxithromycin. Macrolides inhibit protein synthesis in susceptible organisms by binding reversibly to the peptidyl-tRNA binding region of the 50S ribosomal subunit, inhibiting translocation of a newly synthesized peptidyl-tRNA molecule from the acceptor site on the ribosome to the peptidyl (or donor site). Erythromycin does not bind to mammalian ribosomes. Most gram-negative organisms are resistant to erythromycin because entry of erythromycin into the cell is restricted.

Resistance to macrolides occurs through several mechanisms. Among the more important of these mechanisms is methylation of the ribosome, preventing erythromycin binding (269). This methylation is most commonly accomplished by different *erm* ("erythromycin ribosomal methylase") genes. Methylated ribosomes confer resistance to macrolides, the related lincosamides (clindamycin and lincomycin), and streptogramin B (MLS_B resistance). Many *erm* genes have been described previously, such as *erm*(A) and the related *erm*(TR) and *erm*(B) and the related *erm*(AM), and resistance is frequently inducible by macrolides but not by clindamycin ($iMLS_B$). In some strains, *erm*-type resistance is expressed constitutively ($cMLS_B$), resulting in resistance to clindamycin as well.

The second major mechanism of resistance to macrolides is through expression of efflux pumps encoded by *mef* genes (Mef in gram-positive bacteria and AcrAB-TolC in *H. influenzae* and *E. coli*) (284). The efflux pumps confer resistance to the macrolides but not to clindamycin, hence the phenotypic description of this resistance type as M type. *mef* genes have been studied most extensively in *S. pneumoniae* [*mef*(E)] and *Streptococcus pyogenes* [*mef*(A)], but similar genes in a variety of gram-positive genera have been described. The prevalence of *mef*-mediated resistance versus that mediated by MLS_B-type mechanisms in *S. pneumoniae* varies in different parts of the world. Minor mechanisms of resistance to macrolides include esterases that hydrolyze the antibiotics and point mutations within the genes for the 50S ribosomal subunit.

Resistance to Ketolides

Ketolides belong to a new class of semisynthetic 14-membered-ring macrolides, which differ from erythromycin by having a 3-keto group instead of the neutral sugar L-cladinose. Ketolides bind to an additional site on the bacterial ribosome, increasing their binding affinities relative to those of other macrolides (58). Telithromycin, a ketolide, is uniformly and highly active against pneumococci (regardless of their susceptibility or resistance to erythromycin and/or penicillin), erythromycin-susceptible *Streptococcus pyogenes*, and erythromycin-resistant *Streptococcus pyogenes* strains of the M phenotype or the $iMLS_B$ or $cMLS_B$ phenotype [in which resistance is mediated by a methylase encoded by the *erm*(TR) gene] (16). Ketolides are less active against erythromycin-resistant *Streptococcus pyogenes* strains with the $cMLS_B$ phenotype or the $iMLS_A$ subtype [in which resistance is mediated by a methylase encoded by the *erm*(AM) gene], these strains ranging in phenotypes from the upper limits of susceptibility to resistant. Methicillin-resistant staphylococci, which commonly express a $cMLS_B$ phenotype, are not susceptible to telithromycin (16).

Resistance to Quinupristin-Dalfopristin

Quinupristin-dalfopristin is a mixture of semisynthetic streptogramins A and B licensed in Europe and the United States. A related streptogramin A and B combination, virginiamycin, has been used for years as a growth promoter in animal feed. Resistance to these mixtures can result from resistance to streptogramin A alone, was first described in staphylococci, and was conferred by genes encoding streptogramin A acetyltransferases [*vat*(A), *vat*(B), and *vat*(C)] or ATP binding efflux genes [*vga*(A) and *vga*(B)]. Quinupristin-dalfopristin's excellent activities against *E. faecium* and MRSA make it an attractive alternative for the treatment of multiresistant *E. faecium* and health care-associated infections with methicillin-resistant staphylococci, especially since the combination retains in vitro activity against streptogramin B-resistant strains. Two acetyltransferase-encoding resistance genes have now been described that confer resistance to quinupristin-dalfopristin in *E. faecium* strains—*vat*(D) [previously *sat*(A)] and *vat*(E) [previously *sat*(G)]. In most cases, these resistance genes are found along with an *erm* resistance gene (236), suggesting that resistance to both streptogramin A and B may be necessary to confer clinically significant levels of resistance to quinupristin-dalfopristin in *E. faecium*. The presence of these resistance genes on transferable plasmids suggests that the potential for their spread within the genus is significant. Although quinupristin-dalfopristin remains active against the majority of human *E. faecium* strains, the use of virginiamycin in animal feeds has been associated with high percentages of resistance in isolates derived from animals (97). In many cases, the known mechanisms of resistance to quinupristin-dalfopristin are not present in these isolates (97), indicating that there is still much to be learned about resistance to quinupristin-dalfopristin in *E. faecium*.

Metronidazole Resistance

Metronidazole is a member of the nitroimidazole family of bactericidal antimicrobials. The 5-nitroimidazole molecule is a prodrug whose activation depends upon reduction of the nitro group in the absence of oxygen. An exception to this rule occurs in *Helicobacter pylori*, where the RdxA protein reduces metronidazole in a microaerophilic environment (259). The nitro group of metronidazole accepts a single electron from electron transport proteins (ferredoxins) in bacteria, yielding a toxic radical anion. Metronidazole's activity appears to result in DNA damage and cell death (62). Resistance to metronidazole is rare. Decreased uptake and/or a reduced rate of reduction is believed to be responsible for metronidazole resistance in some cases (61). Five *Bacteroides* genes, *nimA* to *nimE*, have been implicated in resistance to 5-metronidazole antibiotics. Analysis of the NimA-susceptible and -resistant *Bacteroides* strains and recent crystal structure analysis suggest that the enzyme utilizes pyruvate for a two-electron reaction resulting in an amine that prevents the formation of the toxic anion radical (38, 130). Expression of *nim* genes varies depending on the positioning of a variety of IS elements that supply active promoters (235).

Resistance to Nitrofurantoin

The antibiotics nitrofurazone and nitrofurantoin are used in the treatment of genitourinary infections and as topical antibacterial agents. Nitrofurazone is used primarily as a topical antiseptic (89). Nitrofurantoin, 1-[(5-nitrofurfurylidene)amino]hydantoin, is a synthetic antibacterial agent used primarily in the treatment of urinary tract infections. The mechanisms of action of nitrofurazone and nitrofurantoin have not been fully elucidated. Investigators have reported that the ability of nitrofurantoin to kill bacteria correlates with the presence of bacterial nitroreductases which convert nitrofurantoin into highly reactive electrophilic intermediates (150). These intermediates are believed to attack bacterial ribosomal proteins nonspecifically, causing complete inhibition of protein synthesis. In *E. coli*, nitroreductases are type I oxygen-insensitive enzymes encoded by the *nfnA* (*nfsA*) and the *nfnB* (*nfsB*) genes. Strains of bacteria that are resistant to nitrofurantoin have been shown to possess diminished nitroreductase activity (199). Resistance to nitrofurantoin from reduced nitroreductase activity seems to be present in other genera as well.

Resistance to Polymyxin B and Polymyxin E (Colistin)

Clinical and scientific interest in the cationic polypeptides colistin (polymyxin E) and polymyxin B is increasing. Although they were first used in the early 1960s, these agents are now viewed as the last-line therapeutic option for multidrug-resistant gram-negative-bacterium infections. As a chemical class, the polymyxins are polycationic peptide antibiotics isolated from *Bacillus polymyxa* (116). These polypeptide antibiotics exert their bactericidal activity by binding to the gram-negative-bacterium cell membrane and disrupting its permeability, resulting in leakage of intracellular components. They also disrupt bacterial biofilm formation. In mechanistic terms, polymyxin binds to phosphorylated head groups of lipid A. Hence, by disrupting cell membranes, these agents become rapidly bactericidal against certain gram-negative bacteria (244, 254).

Not all gram-negative bacteria are susceptible to polymyxins. Organisms that are resistant to polymyxins have cell walls that prevent access of the drug to the cell membrane. In general, polymyxins are bactericidal against *P. aeruginosa*, *Acinetobacter* spp., some *Proteus mirabilis* strains, and some strains of *Serratia marcescens*. *Proteus* spp., *Providentia* spp., *Neisseria* spp., and gram-positive bacteria are resistant to polymyxins (244, 254).

Polymyxin-resistant mutants and bacteria exhibit a modified lipopolysaccharide. In *E. coli*, *S. enterica* serotype Typhimurium, and many other pathogenic gram-negative bacteria, modification of the phosphate groups of lipid A confers resistance to polymyxin and cationic antimicrobial peptides. Lipopolysaccharide modifications that include alteration of the fatty acid content of lipid A, phosphoethanolamine addition to the core and lipid A head groups, and 4-amino-4-deoxy-L-arabinose (Ara4N) addition to the core and lipid A regions have been well studied (254). Recent evidence also implicates the presence of the MtrC-MtrD-MtrE efflux pump and lipid A modification as well as the type IV pilin secretion system to modulate levels of polymyxin resistance in *N. meningitidis* (254).

Concerns exist about the reliability and reproducibility of susceptibility testing methods for polymyxins. A recent article addresses the urgent need for quality control ranges for susceptibility determination (116).

Resistance to Quinolones

The fluoroquinolones are among the most widely used antimicrobial agents in both hospital and community settings.

Quinolone antibiotics all act by directly inhibiting DNA synthesis. Their targets include two type II topoisomerases, DNA gyrase and topoisomerase IV. These two enzymes are structurally related in that both exist as tetramers composed of two different subunits (GyrA and GyrB of DNA gyrase; ParC and ParE of topoisomerase IV). DNA gyrase maintains the negative supercoiling of DNA, whereas topoisomerase IV separates interlocked daughter DNA strands formed during replication, facilitating segregation into daughter cells. Fluoroquinolones bind to the topoisomerase-DNA complexes and disrupt various cellular processes involving DNA (such as those involving the replication fork, transcription of RNA, and DNA helicase) (102, 227, 277). The end result is cellular death through unclear mechanisms.

The affinities of fluoroquinolones for the two targets vary, explaining to some degree the differing potencies of the various agents against different bacterial species. The enzyme for which a particular fluoroquinolone exerts the greatest affinity is referred to as the primary target (5, 23, 177). In general, the primary target of fluoroquinolones in gram-negative bacteria is DNA gyrase, whereas in gram-positive bacteria it is topoisomerase IV.

Alterations in Target Enzymes

The most common mechanism of clinically significant levels of fluoroquinolone resistance is through alterations of the topoisomerase enzymes. These alterations are created by spontaneous mutations that occur within the respective genes. In GyrA and ParC, resistance-associated mutations are often localized to a region in the amino termini of the enzymes that contains the active-site tyrosine that is covalently linked to the broken DNA strand. This 130-bp region of *gyrA* has been referred to as the quinolone resistance-determining region. X-ray crystallographic studies of a fragment of the GyrA enzyme suggest that these mutations are clustered in three dimensions, lending support to the hypothesis that the region constitutes a part of the quinolone binding site (155). Particularly frequent sites for resistance-associated mutations are Ser83 and Asp87 of DNA gyrase and Ser79 and Asp83 of ParC (186).

Experimental data suggest that point mutations occur singly in roughly 1 in 10^6 to 10^9 cells. The level of resistance conferred by a single point mutation in the primary target enzyme depends upon the reduction of enzyme affinity created by the mutation, as well as the affinity of the fluoroquinolone for the secondary target. In this scenario, it is expected that fluoroquinolones exhibiting strong affinity for both target enzymes would be less likely to be associated with the emergence of resistant strains, since the retained activity against the secondary target would be enough to inhibit the bacterium even in the presence of a primary target mutation. Fluoroquinolone-species combinations for which single mutations result in significantly higher MICs (such as ciprofloxacin and *S. aureus* or *P. aeruginosa*) would be expected to readily select out resistant mutants in the clinical setting (and have [49]).

Most highly resistant strains exhibit more than one mutation in both the GyrA and ParC enzymes, a phenomenon that can be reproduced in the laboratory by serial passage of strains on progressively higher concentrations of fluoroquinolones. It is noteworthy in this context that fluoroquinolone resistance conferred by enzyme mutations is essentially class resistance. In other words, the activities of all fluoroquinolones are impacted by mutations that result in resistance. Therefore, while single point mutations that confer resistance to one fluoroquinolone may not result in MICs of another that represent clinical resistance, the MICs of the second fluoroquinolone will inevitably be increased. In the setting of such preexisting mutations, the second fluoroquinolone could then select out an additional mutation that would result in clinically significant levels of resistance. This reasoning has led to the recommendation that the most potent and broadly active fluoroquinolone should always be used first, to prevent the emergence of resistance. The wisdom of this recommendation remains to be tested.

Mutations in GyrB and ParE are far less common than those in their companion subunits and tend to cluster in the middle portion of the subunit (105). A clear understanding of the impact these mutations have on enzyme structure or function will await detailed crystallographic studies of enzyme-fluoroquinolone complexes.

Resistance Due to Decreased Intracellular Accumulation

Fluoroquinolones penetrate the outer membranes of gram-negative bacteria through porins, and so the absence of specific porins can impact the level of susceptibility. However, their ability to diffuse through outer and cytoplasmic membranes is sufficient to retain activity against strains lacking solely porins (166). More important in reducing intracellular accumulation of fluoroquinolones is the expression of multidrug-resistance pumps (186). Several such pumps have been identified in human pathogenic bacteria. Resistance results when the expression of pumps is increased due to mutations within the regulatory genes (285). By themselves, pumps generally confer only a low level of resistance to fluoroquinolones. However, their expression may amplify the level of resistance conferred by point mutations within the topoisomerase genes. By so doing, they may increase the risk that a given fluoroquinolone will select out resistant mutants through single point mutations.

In the past few years, plasmid-mediated and transferable resistance to fluoroquinolones has been recognized in a variety of gram-negative-bacterium species. This resistance is conferred by the product of the *qnr* gene and its homologues (113, 169). The mechanism underlying the resistance is protection of the DNA from quinolone binding (250). In general, only low levels of resistance are conferred by this mechanism, but as with other accessory mechanisms, the presence of Qnr can facilitate the clinical emergence of strains resistant by virtue of point mutations in the topoisomerase genes. The prevalence of this mechanism appears to be increasing, which may be explained partly by the frequent presence of *qnr* within complex *sul*I-type integrons (169).

Resistance to Rifampin

Rifampin is particularly active against gram-positive bacteria and mycobacteria. It acts by inhibiting bacterial DNA-dependent RNA polymerase. Point mutations in the chromosomal *rpoB* gene confer resistance to rifampin (267). The frequency with which these point mutations occur precludes using rifampin as a single agent for the treatment of bacterial infections.

Resistance to Tetracyclines

The tetracyclines are a group of bacteriostatic antibiotics that act by inhibiting attachment of aminoacyl-tRNA to the ribosome acceptor site, thereby preventing elongation of the peptide chains of nascent proteins (221). In order to gain access to the bacterial ribosome, tetracyclines need to enter the cell. In *E. coli* and presumably in other gram-negative bacteria, they enter the periplasmic space through outer membrane porins

OmpC and OmpF, probably chelated to magnesium ions (221). Once in the periplasmic space, the weakly lipophilic tetracycline molecule dissociates from the magnesium ion and crosses into the cell by diffusing through the lipid bilayer in an energy-dependent process. Once inside the cell, tetracycline-ion complexes bind to the ribosome at a single, high affinity binding site on the 30S subunit, blocking access of the aminoacyl-tRNA to the ribosome acceptor site. Although high affinity, binding of tetracycline to the ribosome is reversible (46).

Tetracyclines are broad-spectrum and effective antimicrobial agents. Unfortunately, widespread use of tetracyclines to treat clinical infections and to promote growth in livestock has been associated with the emergence and dissemination of a variety of resistance determinants. As a consequence, the number of infections for which tetracyclines are considered recommended first-line therapy has been limited for many years (217). The vast majority of tetracycline resistance determinants fall into one of two classes: (i) efflux or (ii) ribosomal protection. The designations of the different resistance determinants and their classes can be found in detail in an excellent review of tetracyclines by Chopra and Roberts (46). Initial designations of tetracycline resistance determinants used the prefix *tet* or *otr* with letters (A, for example) designating the different determinants. Since the number of resistance determinants now exceeds the number of letters in the alphabet, a system using numbers has been devised (132).

Tetracycline efflux proteins are all membrane associated and members of the major facilitator superfamily of proteins. They expel tetracycline from the cell by exchanging a proton for a tetracycline-cation complex. In general, the efflux proteins confer resistance to tetracyclines but tend to spare minocycline (46). The single exception to this rule is the gram-negative-bacterium Tet(B) protein that confers resistance to both tetracycline and minocycline. The efflux proteins have been divided into six groups based on amino acid identity. Group 1 consists of Tet efflux proteins that are found primarily in gram-negative species [with the exception of Tet(Z)], whereas group 2 [consisting only of Tet(K) and Tet(L)] is found primarily in gram-positive species. Groups 3 through 6 are small groups consisting of one or two efflux proteins each.

Ribosome protection proteins account for the other major mechanism of tetracycline resistance. These proteins exhibit homology to elongation factors EF-Tu and EF-G and exhibit ribosome-dependent GTPase activity (219). They act by binding to the ribosome, thereby changing its conformation and inhibiting binding of tetracycline. Tet(M) and Tet(O) are the best characterized of these proteins. Ribosome protection proteins are widespread in bacteria, in many cases as a result of the incorporation of the corresponding genes into broad-host-range conjugative transposons.

Both efflux proteins and ribosome protection proteins are regulated in ways such that their expression is increased in the presence of tetracyclines. The gram-negative-bacterium efflux proteins are regulated by repressors that are divergently transcribed relative to the efflux proteins (103). Binding of a repressor to tetracycline changes the conformation of the repressor so that it can no longer bind to the operator region, resulting in increased transcription of both the efflux protein and the repressor genes. The gram-positive-bacterium efflux genes are not associated with specific protein repressors, but sequence analysis suggests that these determinants may be regulated by mechanisms similar to translational attenuation. Study of this area has been limited (241). Transcription of ribosome protection genes is augmented by growth in the presence of tetracycline.

Intrinsic mechanisms of tetracycline resistance exist in many if not all gram-negative bacteria. Among the best characterized of these systems is the *mar* ("multiple antibiotic resistance") operon (3). This locus consists of a repressor (MarR) that represses transcription of *marA*, which encodes a transcriptional activator of a variety of genes. Overexpression of MarA results in decreased expression of OmpF, a porin through which tetracycline enters the periplasmic space, and increased expression of multidrug efflux pump AcrAB, a member of the resistance-nodulation-cell division family of efflux proteins that includes tetracyclines among its substrates. Several similar pump systems have been identified in *P. aeruginosa* and other gram-negative bacteria (195). As our knowledge of the genomes of different bacterial species becomes more complete, we will no doubt discover several other pump systems that impact levels of susceptibility to tetracyclines and other antibiotics.

The remarkable diversity of species within which tetracycline resistance determinants are found owes much to the inclusion of these resistance genes within broad-host-range transferable genetic elements. These include transferable plasmids in gram-negative species, where *tet* genes may be found included within integrons, and conjugative transposons. Among the best studied of the conjugative transposons is the Tn*916* family, originally described in *E. faecalis* (205). The complete sequence of Tn*916* has been determined and is remarkable for its dearth of restriction enzyme digestion sites [except in the region of the *tet*(M) gene, which appears to be a late arrival to the element] (172). This lack of restriction sites likely facilitates the entry of this transposon into a variety of different bacterial species. Transfer of Tn*916*-like elements from enterococci into many other species has been demonstrated in vitro and in animal models, and the remnants of Tn*916*-like sequences in *N. gonorrhoeae* are impressive testimony to the ability of these elements to travel widely (205). Transfer of Tn*916*-like elements, which is increased after exposure to tetracycline, has also been suggested to facilitate transfer of unlinked genes, further amplifying the risks of overexposure to tetracycline in the environment.

Resistance to Tigecycline

The recent licensing of the glycylcycline tigecycline offers a broad-spectrum antimicrobial alternative for treating infections due to resistant pathogens, including MRSA and ESBL-producing *K. pneumoniae.* Tigecycline's broad spectrum of antimicrobial activity is due to its resistance to the common efflux or ribosome protection mechanisms that confer resistance to older tetracyclines. Some bacterial species, notably *P. aeruginosa* and *Proteus* spp., are intrinsically resistant to tigecycline because they express RND-type efflux pumps that effectively extrude the antibiotic (214). Resistance to tigecycline in other gram-negative species has also been reported, generally resulting from activation of normally repressed AcrAB-type RND efflux pumps (215). Determination of the ultimate importance of these pump activations for clinical resistance to tigecycline will await more extensive clinical use.

Resistance to Trimethoprim-Sulfamethoxazole

Biosynthesis of several amino acids and purines depends upon the availability of tetrahydrofolate. With few exceptions, bacteria are unable to absorb preformed folic acid and hence rely upon their ability to synthesize it. Sulfamethoxazole and trimethoprim are inhibitors of two enzymes (dihydropteroic acid synthase [DHPS] and dihydrofolate reductase [DHFR], respectively) that act sequentially in the manufacture of tetrahydrofolate. It is thought that the two inhibitors act synergistically to inhibit folate synthesis, although the mechanism for possible synergism (since sequential blockage of a fully inhibited pathway should not augment resistance) is not clear.

Intrinsic Resistance

Trimethoprim-sulfamethoxazole is a remarkably broad spectrum antimicrobial agent. Intrinsic resistance is relatively rare and may occur through decreased access to the target enzymes (*P. aeruginosa*) (245), low affinity for DHFR enzymes (*Neisseria* spp., *Clostridium* spp., *Brucella* spp., *Bacteroides* spp., *Moraxella catarrhalis,* and *Nocardia* spp.) (246) or the ability to absorb exogenous folate (*Enterococcus* spp. and *Lactobacillus* spp.) (283) or thymine (*Enterococcus* spp.) (94). The decreased access to the target enzyme in *P. aeruginosa* appears to be the result of both a permeability barrier and active efflux from the cell (124, 146). The percentage contribution of each of these mechanisms to resistance remains unclear.

Acquired Resistance to Trimethoprim

Mutational resistance to trimethoprim has been described for several species and involves promoter mutations leading to overproduction of DHFR (in *E. coli*), point mutations within the *dhfr* gene leading to resistance (in *S. aureus and S. pneumoniae*) or both mechanisms (in *H. influenzae*) (107). More common is the acquisition of low-affinity-associated *dhfr* genes, of which approximately 20 have been described previously (107). Expression of *dhfr*I and variant *dhfr*II genes, which are most commonly found on plasmids in gram-negative bacteria, increases resistance to levels greatly exceeding clinically achievable concentrations of the drug.

Acquired Resistance to Sulfonamides

Point mutations or small insertions of DNA segments within chromosomal *dhps* genes conferring resistance to sulfonamides have been reported for many different species (65, 107). More extensive changes within *dhps* genes resulting in resistance have been reported for *N. meningitidis* and *Streptococcus pyogenes.* In these instances, the extensive changes have suggested acquisition of at least some parts of the *dhps* genes from other species via transformation and recombination (233, 243). Plasmid-mediated, transferable resistance to sulfonamides has been reported for gram-negative bacteria (107). In contrast to the diversity in *dhfr* genes, only two acquired low-affinity *dhps* genes (*sul*I and *sul*II) have been described. Genes conferring resistance to sulfonamides are frequently incorporated into multiresistance integrons, which are themselves frequently integrated into transferable plasmids. The transferability of these resistance plasmids and the frequent association with other resistance genes explain in part the widespread nature and persistence of resistance to sulfonamides. One trimethoprim-sulfamethoxazole-resistant *E. coli* strain was reported to have spread widely in the United States, causing urinary tract infections in young women in at least two states (140), although more recent data suggest that this widespread prevalence may owe more to the parallel emergence of related strains than to the direct spread of an outbreak isolate (80).

REFERENCES

1. **Adcock, P. M., P. Pastor, F. Medley, J. E. Patterson, and T. V. Murphy.** 1998. Methicillin-resistant *Staphylococcus aureus* in two child care centers. *J. Infect. Dis.* **178:**577–580.
2. **Aires, J. R., and H. Nikaido.** 2005. Aminoglycosides are captured from both periplasm and cytoplasm by the AcrD multidrug efflux transporter of *Escherichia coli. J. Bacteriol.* **187:**1923–1929.
3. **Alekshun, M. N., and S. B. Levy.** 1997. Regulation of chromosomally mediated multiple antibiotic resistance: the *mar* regulon. *Antimicrob. Agents Chemother.* **41:**2067–2075.
4. **Alksne, L. E., and B. A. Rasmussen.** 1997. Expression of the AsbA1, OXA-12, and AsbM1 ß-lactamases in *Aeromonas jandaei* AER 14 is coordinated by a two-component regulon. *J. Bacteriol.* **179:**2006–2013.
5. **Alovero, F. L., X. S. Pan, J. E. Morris, R. H. Manzo, and L. M. Fisher.** 2000. Engineering the specificity of antibacterial fluoroquinolones: benzenesulfonamide modifications at C-7 of ciprofloxacin change its primary target in *Streptococcus pneumoniae* from topoisomerase IV to gyrase. *Antimicrob. Agents Chemother.* **44:**320–325.
6. **Ambler, R. P.** 1980. The structure of ß-lactamases. *Philos. Trans. R. Soc. Lond. B* **289:**321–331.
7. **Amoroso, A., D. Demares, M. Mollerach, G. Gutkind, and J. Coyette.** 2001. All detectable high-molecular-mass penicillin-binding proteins are modified in a high-level beta-lactam-resistant clinical isolate of *Streptococcus mitis. Antimicrob. Agents Chemother.* **45:**2075–2081.
8. **Arthur, M., F. Depardieu, C. Molinas, P. Reynolds, and P. Courvalin.** 1995. The *vanZ* gene of Tn*1546* from *Enterococcus faecium* BM4147 confers resistance to teicoplanin. *Gene* **154:**87–92.
9. **Arthur, M., C. Molinas, and P. Courvalin.** 1992. Sequence of the *vanY* gene required for production of a vancomycin-inducible D,D-carboxypeptidase in *Enterococcus faecium* BM4147. *Gene* **120:**111–114.
10. **Arthur, M., C. Molinas, and P. Courvalin.** 1992. The VanS-VanR two-component regulatory system controls synthesis of depsipeptide peptidoglycan precursors in *Enterococcus faecium* 4147. *J. Bacteriol.* **174:**2582–2591.
11. **Arthur, M., C. Molinas, F. Depardieu, and P. Courvalin.** 1993. Characterization of Tn*1546*, a Tn*3*-related transposon conferring glycopeptide resistance by synthesis of depsipeptide peptidoglycan precursors in *Enterococcus faecium* BM4147. *J. Bacteriol.* **175:**117–127.
12. **Arthur, M., P. Reynolds, and P. Courvalin.** 1996. Glycopeptide resistance in enterococci. *Trends Microbiol.* **4:**401–407.
13. **Aslangul, E., M. Baptista, B. Fantin, F. Depardieu, M. Arthur, P. Courvalin, and C. Carbon.** 1997. Selection of glycopeptide-resistant mutants of VanB-type *Enterococcus faecalis* BM4281 in vitro and in experimental endocarditis. *J. Infect. Dis.* **175:**598–605.
14. **Avison, M. B., P. M. Bennett, R. A. Howe, and T. R. Walsh.** 2002. Preliminary analysis of the genetic basis for vancomycin resistance in *Staphylococcus aureus* strain Mu50. *J. Antimicrob. Chemother.* **49:**255–260.
15. **Azucena, E., and S. Mobashery.** 2001. Aminoglycoside-modifying enzymes: mechanisms of catalytic processes and inhibition. *Drug Resist. Updat.* **4:**106–117.
16. **Balfour, J. A., and D. P. Figgitt.** 2001. Telithromycin. *Drugs* **61:**815–829.
17. **Barcus, V. A., K. Ghanekar, M. Yeo, T. J. Coffey, and C. G. Dowson.** 1995. Genetics of high level penicillin resistance in clinical isolates of Streptococcus pneumoniae. *FEMS Microbiol. Lett.* **126:**299–303.
18. **Beaman, T. W., M. Sugantino, and S. L. Roderick.** 1998. Structure of the hexapeptide xenobiotic acetyltransferase from *Pseudomonas aeruginosa. Biochemistry* **37:**6689–6696.
19. **Bennett, A. D., and W. V. Shaw.** 1983. Resistance to fusidic acid in *Escherichia coli* mediated by the type I variant of chloramphenicol acetyltransferase. A plasmid-encoded mechanism involving antibiotic binding. *Biochem. J.* **215:**29–38.

20. **Billot-Klein, D., L. Gutmann, D. Bryant, D. Bell, J. van Heijenoort, J. Grewal, and D. M. Shlaes.** 1996. Peptidoglycan synthesis and structure in *Staphylococcus haemolyticus* expressing increasing levels of resistance to glycopeptide antibiotics. *J. Bacteriol.* **178:**4696–4703.
21. **Bissonnette, L., S. Champetier, J. P. Buisson, and P. H. Roy.** 1991. Characterization of the nonenzymatic chloramphenicol resistance (*cmlA*) gene of the In4 integron of Tn*1696*: similarity of the product to transmembrane transport proteins. *J. Bacteriol.* **173:**4493–4502.
22. **Bjorkman, J., I. Nagaev, O. G. Berg, D. Hughes, and D. I. Andersson.** 2000. Effects of environment on compensatory mutations to ameliorate costs of antibiotic resistance. *Science* **287:**1479–1482.
23. **Blanche, F., B. Cameron, F. X. Bernard, L. Maton, B. Manse, L. Ferrero, N. Ratet, C. Lecoq, A. Goniot, D. Bisch, and J. Crouzet.** 1996. Differential behaviors of *Staphylococcus aureus* and *Escherichia coli* type II DNA topoisomerases. *Antimicrob. Agents Chemother.* **40:**2714–2720.
24. **Bolton, L. F., L. C. Kelley, M. D. Lee, P. J. Fedorka-Cray, and J. J. Maurer.** 1999. Detection of multidrug-resistant *Salmonella enterica* serotype Typhimurium DT104 based on a gene which confers cross-resistance to florfenicol and chloramphenicol. *J. Clin. Microbiol.* **37:**1348–1351.
25. **Bonnet, R.** 2004. Growing group of extended-spectrum beta-lactamases: the CTX-M enzymes. *Antimicrob. Agents Chemother.* **48:**1–14.
26. **Bonomo, R. A., C. G. Dawes, J. R. Knox, and D. M. Shlaes.** 1995. Beta-lactamase mutations far from the active site influence inhibitor binding. *Biochim. Biophys. Acta* **1247:**121–125.
27. **Boyle-Vavra, S., H. Labischinski, C. C. Ebert, K. Ehlert, and R. S. Daum. 2001.** A spectrum of changes occurs in peptidoglycan composition of glycopeptide-intermediate clinical *Staphylococcus aureus* isolates. *Antimicrob. Agents Chemother.* **45:**280–287.
28. **Bradford, P. A.** 2001. Extended-spectrum beta-lactamases in the 21st century: characterization, epidemiology, and detection of this important resistance threat. *Clin. Microbiol. Rev.* **14:**933–951.
29. **Bradford, P. A.** 2001. What's new in beta-lactamases? *Curr. Infect. Dis. Rep.* **3:**13–19.
30. **Bradford, P. A., C. Urban, N. Mariano, S. J. Projan, J. J. Rahal, and K. Bush.** 1997. Imipenem resistance in *Klebsiella pneumoniae* is associated with the combination of ACT-1, a plasmid-mediated AmpC beta-lactamase, and the loss of an outer membrane protein. *Antimicrob. Agents Chemother.* **41:**563–569.
31. **Bratu, S., M. Mooty, S. Nichani, D. Landman, C. Gullans, B. Pettinato, U. Karumudi, P. Tolaney, and J. Quale.** 2005. Emergence of KPC-possessing *Klebsiella pneumoniae* in Brooklyn, New York: epidemiology and recommendations for detection. *Antimicrob. Agents Chemother.* **49:**3018–3020.
32. **Bruand, C., L. Chatelier, S. D. Ehrlich, and L. Janniere.** 1993. A fourth class of theta-replicating plasmids: the pAMß1 family from Gram-positive bacteria. *Proc. Natl. Acad. Sci. USA* **90:**11668–11672.
33. **Bush, K.** 2001. New beta-lactamases in gram-negative bacteria: diversity and impact on the selection of antimicrobial therapy. *Clin. Infect. Dis.* **32:**1085–1089.
34. **Bush, K., G. A. Jacoby, and A. A. Medeiros.** 1995. A functional classification scheme for beta-lactamases and its correlation with molecular structure. *Antimicrob. Agents Chemother.* **39:**1211–1233.
35. **Campbell, B. D., and R. J. Kadner.** 1980. Relation of aerobiosis and ionic strength to the uptake of dihydrostreptomycin in *Escherichia coli. Biochim. Biophys. Acta* **593:**1–10.
36. **Carfi, A., S. Pares, E. Duee, M. Galleni, C. Duez, J. M. Frere, and O. Dideberg.** 1995. The 3-D structure of a zinc metallo-ß-lactamase from *Bacillus cereus* reveals a new type of protein fold. *EMBO J.* **14:**4914–4921.
37. **Carias, L. L., S. D. Rudin, C. J. Donskey, and L. B. Rice.** 1998. Genetic linkage and cotransfer of a novel, *vanB*-containing transposon (Tn*5382*) and a low-affinity penicillin-binding protein 5 gene in a clinical vancomycin-resistant *Enterococcus faecium* isolate. *J. Bacteriol.* **180:**4426–4434.
38. **Carlier, J. P., N. Sellier, M. N. Rager, and G. Reysset.** 1997. Metabolism of a 5-nitroimidazole in susceptible and resistant isogenic strains of *Bacteroides fragilis. Antimicrob. Agents Chemother.* **41:**1495–1499.
39. **Carter, A. P., W. M. Clemons, D. E. Brodersen, R. J. Morgan-Warren, B. T. Wimberly, and V. Ramakrishnan.** 2000. Functional insights from the structure of the 30S ribosomal subunit and its interactions with antibiotics. *Nature* **407:**340–348.
40. **Casadewall, B., P. E. Reynolds, and P. Courvalin.** 2001. Regulation of expression of the *vanD* glycopeptide resistance gene cluster from *Enterococcus faecium* BM4339. *J. Bacteriol.* **183:**3436–3446.
41. **Castanheira, M., M. A. Toleman, R. N. Jones, F. J. Schmidt, and T. R. Walsh.** 2004. Molecular characterization of a beta-lactamase gene, blaGIM-1, encoding a new subclass of metallo-beta-lactamase. *Antimicrob. Agents Chemother.* **48:**4654–4661.

41a. **Centers for Disease Control and Prevention.** 2004. Vancomycin-resistant *Staphylococcus aureus*—New York, 2004. *Morb. Mortal. Wkly. Rep.* **53:**322–323.

42. **Chambers, H. F.** 1997. Methicillin resistance in staphylococci: molecular and biochemical basis and clinical implications. *Clin. Microbiol. Rev.* **10:**781–791.
43. **Chambers, H. F., M. Sachdeva, and S. Kennedy.** 1990. Binding affinity for penicillin-binding protein 2a correlates with in vivo activity of beta-lactam antibiotics against methicillin-resistant *Staphylococcus aureus. J. Infect. Dis.* **162:** 705–710.
44. **Chang, F. Y., J. E. Peacock, Jr., D. M. Musher, P. Triplett, B. B. MacDonald, J. M. Mylotte, A. O'Donnell, M. M. Wagener, and V. L. Yu.** 2003. *Staphylococcus aureus* bacteremia: recurrence and the impact of antibiotic treatment in a prospective multicenter study. *Medicine (Baltimore)* **82:**333–339.
45. **Chen, Y., J. Delmas, J. Sirot, B. Shoichet, and R. Bonnet.** 2005. Atomic resolution structures of CTX-M beta-lactamases: extended spectrum activities from increased mobility and decreased stability. *J. Mol. Biol.* **348:**349–362.
46. **Chopra, I., and M. Roberts.** 2001. Tetracycline antibiotics: mode of action, applications, molecular biology, and epidemiology of bacterial resistance. *Microbiol. Mol. Biol. Rev.* **65:**232–260.
47. **Climo, M. W., R. L. Patron, and G. L. Archer.** 1999. Combinations of vancomycin and beta-lactams are synergistic against staphylococci with reduced susceptibilities to vancomycin. *Antimicrob. Agents Chemother.* **43:**1747–1753.
48. **Concha, N. O., C. A. Janson, P. Rowling, S. Pearson, C. A. Cheever, B. P. Clarke, C. Lewis, M. Galleni, J. M. Frere, D. J. Payne, J. H. Bateson, and S. S. Abdel-Meguid.** 2000. Crystal structure of the IMP-1 metallo ß-lactamase from *Pseudomonas aeruginosa* and its complex with a mercaptocarboxylate inhibitor: binding determinants of a potent, broad-spectrum inhibitor. *Biochemistry* **39:**4288–4298.
49. **Coronado, V. G., J. R. Edwards, D. H. Culver, R. P. Gaynes, and the National Nosocomial Infections Surveillance System.** 1995. Ciprofloxacin resistance among nosocomial *Pseudomonas aeruginosa* and *Staphylococcus aureus* in the United States. *Infect. Control Hosp. Epidemiol.* **16:**71–75.

50. **Couto, I., H. de Lencastre, E. Severina, W. Kloos, J. A. Webster, R. J. Hubner, I. S. Sanches, and A. Tomasz.** 1996. Ubiquitous presence of a *mecA* homologue in natural isolates of *Staphylococcus sciuri*. *Microb. Drug Resist.* **2:**377–391.
51. **Crichlow, G. V., A. P. Kuzin, M. Nukaga, K. Mayama, T. Sawai, and J. R. Knox.** 1999. Structure of the extended-spectrum class C beta-lactamase of *Enterobacter cloacae* GC1, a natural mutant with a tandem tripeptide insertion. *Biochemistry* **38:**10256–10261.
52. **Cui, L., X. Ma, K. Sato, K. Okuma, F. C. Tenover, E. M. Mamizuka, C. G. Gemmell, M. N. Kim, M. C. Ploy, N. El-Solh, V. Ferraz, and K. Hiramatsu.** 2003. Cell wall thickening is a common feature of vancomycin resistance in *Staphylococcus aureus*. *J. Clin. Microbiol.* **41:**5–14.
53. **Darini, A. L., M. F. Palepou, and N. Woodford.** 2000. Effects of the movement of insertion sequences on the structure of VanA glycopeptide resistance elements in *Enterococcus faecium*. *Antimicrob. Agents Chemother.* **44:** 1362–1364.
54. **D'Costa, V. M., K. M. McGrann, D. W. Hughes, and G. D. Wright.** 2006. Sampling the antibiotic resistome. *Science* **311:**374–377.
55. **de la Campa, A. G., L. Balsalobre, C. Ardanuy, A. Fenoll, E. Perez-Trallero, and J. Linares.** 2004. Fluoroquinolone resistance in penicillin-resistant *Streptococcus pneumoniae* clones, Spain. *Emerg. Infect. Dis.* **10:**1751–1759.
56. **Delaire, M., R. Labia, J. P. Samama, and J. M. Masson.** 1992. Site-directed mutagenesis at the active site of *Escherichia coli* TEM-1 beta-lactamase. Suicide inhibitor-resistant mutants reveal the role of arginine 244 and methionine 69 in catalysis. *J. Biol. Chem.* **267:**20600–20606.
57. **Donskey, C. J., J. A. Hanrahan, R. A. Hutton, and L. B. Rice.** 2000. Effect of parenteral antibiotic administration on establishment of colonization with vancomycin-resistant *Enterococcus faecium* in the mouse gastrointestinal tract. *J. Infect. Dis.* **181:**1830–1833.
58. **Douthwaite, S., L. H. Hansen, and P. Mauvais.** 2000. Macrolide-ketolide inhibition of MLS-resistant ribosomes is improved by alternative drug interaction with domain II of 23S rRNA. *Mol. Microbiol.* **36:**183–193.
59. **Dubois, V., L. Poirel, C. Arpin, L. Coulange, C. Bebear, P. Nordmann, and C. Quentin.** 2004. SHV-49, a novel inhibitor-resistant beta-lactamase in a clinical isolate of *Klebsiella pneumoniae*. *Antimicrob. Agents Chemother.* **48:** 4466–4469.
60. **Dutka-Malen, S., B. Blaimont, G. Wauters, and P. Courvalin.** 1994. Emergence of high-level resistance to glycopeptides in *Enterococcus gallinarum* and *Enterococcus casseliflavus*. *Antimicrob. Agents Chemother.* **38:**1675–1677.
61. **Edwards, D. I.** 1993. Nitroimidazole drugs—action and resistance mechanisms. I. Mechanisms of action. *J. Antimicrob. Chemother.* **31:**9–20.
62. **Edwards, D. I.** 1993. Nitroimidazole drugs—action and resistance mechanisms. II. Mechanisms of resistance. *J. Antimicrob. Chemother.* **31:**201–210.
63. **Eliopoulos, G. M., B. F. Farber, B. E. Murray, C. Wennersten, and R. Moellering, Jr.** 1984. Ribosomal resistance of clinical enterococcal isolates to streptomycin. *Antimicrob. Agents Chemother.* **25:**398–399.
64. **Ena, J., M. M. Lopez-Perezagua, C. Martinez-Peinado, M. A. Cia-Barrio, and I. Ruiz-Lopez.** 1998. Emergence of ciprofloxacin resistance in *Escherichia coli* isolates after widespread use of fluoroquinolones. *Diagn. Microbiol. Infect. Dis.* **30:**103–107.
65. **Enne, V. I., A. King, D. M. Livermore, and L. M. Hall.** 2002. Sulfonamide resistance in *Haemophilus influenzae* mediated by acquisition of *sul2* or a short insertion in chromosomal *folP*. *Antimicrob. Agents Chemother.* **46:**1934–1939.
66. **Evers, S., and R. Courvalin.** 1996. Regulation of VanB-type vancomycin resistance gene expression by the VanSB-VanRB two-component regulatory system in *Enterococcus faecalis* V583. *J. Bacteriol.* **178:**1302–1309.
67. **Evers, S., D. F. Sahm, and P. Courvalin.** 1993. The *vanB* gene of vancomycin-resistant *Enterococcus faecalis* V583 is structurally-related to genes encoding D-ala:D-ala ligases and glycopeptide-resistance proteins VanA and VanC. *Gene* **124:**143–144.
68. **Farzaneh, S., E. B. Chaibi, J. Peduzzi, M. Barthelemy, R. Labia, J. Blazquez, and F. Baquero.** 1996. Implication of Ile-69 and Thr-182 residues in kinetic characteristics of IRT-3 (TEM-32) beta-lactamase. *Antimicrob. Agents Chemother.* **40:**2434–2436.
69. **Ferber, D.** 2000. Antibiotic resistance. Superbugs on the hoof? *Science* **288:**792–794.
70. **Ferretti, J. J., K. S. Gilmore, and P. Courvalin.** 1986. Nucleotide sequence of the gene specifying the bifunctional 6′-aminoglycoside acetyltransferase-2″ aminoglycoside phosphotransferase enzyme in *Streptococcus faecalis* and identification and cloning of the gene regions specifying the two activities. *J. Bacteriol.* **167:**631–638.
71. **Ferretti, J. J., W. M. McShan, D. Ajdic, D. J. Savic, G. Savic, K. Lyon, C. Primeaux, S. Sezate, A. N. Suvorov, S. Kenton, H. S. Lai, S. P. Lin, Y. Qian, H. G. Jia, F. Z. Najar, Q. Ren, H. Zhu, L. Song, J. White, X. Yuan, S. W. Clifton, B. A. Roe, and R. McLaughlin.** 2001. Complete genome sequence of an M1 strain of *Streptococcus pyogenes*. *Proc. Natl. Acad. Sci. USA* **98:**4658–4663.
72. **Fey, P. D., B. Said-Salim, M. E. Rupp, S. H. Hinrichs, D. J. Boxrud, C. C. Davis, B. N. Kreiswirth, and P. M. Schlievert.** 2003. Comparative molecular analysis of community- or hospital-acquired methicillin-resistant *Staphylococcus aureus*. *Antimicrob. Agents Chemother.* **47:**196–203.
73. **Fiett, J., A. Palucha, B. Miaczynska, M. Stankiewicz, H. Przondo-Mordarska, W. Hryniewicz, and M. Gniadkowski.** 2000. A novel complex mutant beta-lactamase, TEM-68, identified in a *Klebsiella pneumoniae* isolate from an outbreak of extended-spectrum beta-lactamase-producing *Klebsiellae*. *Antimicrob. Agents Chemother.* **44:**1499–1505.
74. **Filipe, S. R., and A. Tomasz.** 2000. Inhibition of the expression of penicillin resistance in *Streptococcus pneumoniae* by inactivation of cell wall muropeptide branching genes. *Proc. Natl. Acad. Sci. USA* **97:**4891–4896.
75. **Finan, J. E., G. L. Archer, M. J. Pucci, and M. W. Climo.** 2001. Role of penicillin-binding protein 4 in expression of vancomycin resistance among clinical isolates of oxacillin-resistant *Staphylococcus aureus*. *Antimicrob. Agents Chemother.* **45:**3070–3075.
76. **Fines, M., B. Perichon, P. Reynolds, D. F. Sahm, and P. Courvalin.** 1999. VanE, a new type of acquired glycopeptide resistance in *Enterococcus faecalis* BM4405. *Antimicrob. Agents Chemother.* **43:**2161–2164.
77. **Fitton, J. E., and W. V. Shaw.** 1979. Comparison of chloramphenicol acetyltransferase variants in staphylococci. Purification, inhibitor studies and N-terminal sequences. *Biochem. J.* **177:**575–582.
78. **Fitzgerald, J. R., D. E. Sturdevant, S. M. Mackie, S. R. Gill, and J. M. Musser.** 2001. Evolutionary genomics of *Staphylococcus aureus:* insights into the origin of methicillin-resistant strains and the toxic shock syndrome epidemic. *Proc. Natl. Acad. Sci. USA* **98:**8821–8826.
79. **Flannagan, S. E., J. W. Chow, S. M. Donabedian, W. J. Brown, M. B. Perri, M. J. Zervos, Y. Ozawa, and D. B. Clewell.** 2003. Plasmid content of a vancomycin-resistant *Enterococcus faecalis* isolate from a patient also colonized by *Staphylococcus aureus* with a VanA phenotype. *Antimicrob. Agents Chemother.* **47:**3954–3959.

80. **France, A. M., K. M. Kugeler, A. Freeman, C. A. Zalewski, M. Blahna, L. Zhang, C. F. Marrs, and B. Foxman.** 2005. Clonal groups and the spread of resistance to trimethoprim-sulfamethoxazole in uropathogenic *Escherichia coli*. *Clin. Infect. Dis.* **40:**1101–1107.
81. **Galas, D. J., and M. Chandler.** 1989. Bacterial insertion sequences, p. 109–162. *In* D. E. Berg and M. M. Howe (ed.), *Mobile DNA*. American Society for Microbiology, Washington, D.C.
82. **Galimand, M., P. Courvalin, and T. Lambert.** 2003. Plasmid-mediated high-level resistance to aminoglycosides in *Enterobacteriaceae* due to 16S rRNA methylation. *Antimicrob. Agents Chemother.* **47:**2565–2571.
83. **Galimand, M., S. Sabtcheva, P. Courvalin, and T. Lambert.** 2005. Worldwide-disseminated *armA* aminoglycoside resistance methylase gene is borne by composite transposon Tn*1548*. *Antimicrob. Agents Chemother.* **49:**2949–2953.
84. **Galleni, M., J. Lamotte-Brasseur, G. M. Rossolini, J. Spencer, O. Dideberg, and J. M. Frere.** 2001. Standard numbering scheme for class B beta-lactamases. *Antimicrob. Agents Chemother.* **45:**660–663.
85. **Garau, G., C. Bebrone, C. Anne, M. Galleni, J. M. Frere, and O. Dideberg.** 2005. A metallo-beta-lactamase enzyme in action: crystal structures of the monozinc carbapenemase CphA and its complex with biapenem. *J. Mol. Biol.* **345:**785–795.
86. **Garnier, F., S. Taourit, P. Glaser, P. Courvalin, and M. Galimand.** 2000. Characterization of transposon Tn*1549*, conferring VanB-type resistance in Enterococcus spp. *Microbiology* **146:**1481–1489.
87. **Ghuysen, J. M.** 1991. Serine ß-lactamases and penicillin-binding proteins. *Annu. Rev. Microbiol.* **45:**37–67.
88. **Gonzales, R. D., P. C. Schreckenberger, M. B. Graham, S. Kelkar, K. DenBesten, and J. P. Quinn.** 2001. Infections due to vancomycin-resistant *Enterococcus faecium* resistant to linezolid. *Lancet* **357:**1179.
89. **Guay, D. R.** 2001. An update on the role of nitrofurans in the management of urinary tract infections. *Drugs* **61:** 353–364.
90. **Haas, W., J. Sublett, D. Kaushal, and E. I. Tuomanen.** 2004. Revising the role of the pneumococcal *vex-vncRS* locus in vancomycin tolerance. *J. Bacteriol.* **186:**8463–8471.
91. **Hackbarth, C. J., and H. F. Chambers.** 1993. *blaI* and *blaR1* regulate ß-lactamase and PBP 2a production in methicillin-resistant *Staphylococcus aureus*. *Antimicrob. Agents Chemother.* **37:**1144–1149.
92. **Hakenbeck, R., and J. Coyette.** 1998. Resistant penicillin-binding proteins. *Cell. Mol. Life. Sci.* **54:**332–340.
93. **Hall, R. M., and C. M. Collis.** 1995. Mobile gene cassettes and integrons: capture and spread of genes by site-specific recombination. *Mol. Microbiol.* **15:**593–600.
94. **Hamilton-Miller, J. M.** 1988. Reversal of activity of trimethoprim against gram-positive cocci by thymidine, thymine and 'folates'. *J. Antimicrob. Chemother.* **22:**35–39.
95. **Hayashi, T., K. Makino, M. Ohnishi, K. Kurokawa, K. Ishii, K. Yokoyama, C. G. Han, E. Ohtsubo, K. Nakayama, T. Murata, M. Tanaka, T. Tobe, T. Iida, H. Takami, T. Honda, C. Sasakawa, N. Ogasawara, T. Yasunaga, S. Kuhara, T. Shiba, M. Hattori, and H. Shinagawa.** 2001. Complete genome sequence of enterohemorrhagic *Escherichia coli* O157:H7 and genomic comparison with a laboratory strain K-12. *DNA Res.* **8:**11–22.
96. **Hayden, M. K., G. M. Trenholm, J. E. Schultz, and D. F. Sahm.** 1993. In vivo development of teicoplanin resistance in a VanB *Enterococcus faecium* isolate. *J. Infect. Dis.* **167:** 1224–1227.
97. **Hayes, J. R., D. D. Wagner, L. L. English, L. E. Carr, and S. W. Joseph.** 2005. Distribution of streptogramin resistance determinants among *Enterococcus faecium* from a poultry production environment of the USA. *J. Antimicrob. Chemother.* **55:**123–126.
98. **Henriques Normark, B., R. Novak, A. Ortqvist, G. Kallenius, E. Tuomanen, and S. Normark.** 2001. Clinical isolates of *Streptococcus pneumoniae* that exhibit tolerance of vancomycin. *Clin. Infect. Dis.* **32:**552–558.
99. **Henze, U. U., and B. Berger-Bachi.** 1995. *Staphylococcus aureus* penicillin-binding protein 4 and intrinsic beta-lactam resistance. *Antimicrob. Agents Chemother.* **39:**2415–2422.
100. **Heritier, C., L. Poirel, P. E. Fournier, J. M. Claverie, D. Raoult, and P. Nordmann.** 2005. Characterization of the naturally occurring oxacillinase of *Acinetobacter baumannii*. *Antimicrob. Agents Chemother.* **49:**4174–4179.
101. **Heritier, C., L. Poirel, T. Lambert, and P. Nordmann.** 2005. Contribution of acquired carbapenem-hydrolyzing oxacillinases to carbapenem resistance in *Acinetobacter baumannii*. *Antimicrob. Agents Chemother.* **49:**3198–3202.
102. **Hiasa, H., D. O. Yousef, and K. J. Marians. 1996.** DNA strand cleavage is required for replication fork arrest by a frozen topoisomerase-quinolone-DNA ternary complex. *J. Biol. Chem.* **271:**26424–26429.
103. **Hillen, W., and C. Berens.** 1994. Mechanisms underlying expression of Tn*10* encoded tetracycline resistance. *Annu. Rev. Microbiol.* **48:**345–369.
104. **Hiramatsu, K.** 1998. Vancomycin resistance in staphylococci. *Drug Resist. Updat.* **1:**135–150.
105. **Hooper, D. C.** 2001. Emerging mechanisms of fluoroquinolone resistance. *Emerg. Infect. Dis.* **7:**337–341.
106. **Hossain, A., M. J. Ferraro, R. M. Pino, R. B. Dew III, E. S. Moland, T. J. Lockhart, K. S. Thomson, R. V. Goering, and N. D. Hanson.** 2004. Plasmid-mediated carbapenem-hydrolyzing enzyme KPC-2 in an *Enterobacter* sp. *Antimicrob. Agents Chemother*. **48:**4438–4440.
107. **Huovinen, P.** 2001. Resistance to trimethoprim-sulfamethoxazole. *Clin. Infect. Dis.* **32:**1608–1614.
108. **Ibuka, A., A. Taguchi, M. Ishiguro, S. Fushinobu, Y. Ishii, S. Kamitori, K. Okuyama, K. Yamaguchi, M. Konno, and H. Matsuzawa.** 1999. Crystal structure of the E166A mutant of extended-spectrum beta-lactamase Toho-1 at 1.8 A resolution. *J. Mol. Biol.* **285:**2079–2087.
109. **Ibuka, A. S., Y. Ishii, M. Galleni, M. Ishiguro, K. Yamaguchi, J. M. Frere, H. Matsuzawa, and H. Sakai.** 2003. Crystal structure of extended-spectrum beta-lactamase Toho-1: insights into the molecular mechanism for catalytic reaction and substrate specificity expansion. *Biochemistry* **42:**10634–10643.
110. **Ito, T., Y. Katayama, K. Asada, N. Mori, K. Tsutsumimoto, C. Tiensasitorn, and K. Hiramatsu.** 2001. Structural comparison of three types of staphylococcal cassette chromosome *mec* integrated in the chromosome in methicillin-resistant *Staphylococcus aureus*. *Antimicrob. Agents Chemother.* **45:**1323–1336.
111. **Jacobs, C., J.-M. Frere, and S. Normark.** 1997. Cytosolic intermediates for cell wall biosynthesis and degradation control inducible ß-lactam resistance in gram-negative bacteria. *Cell* **88:**823–832.
112. **Jacobs, C., B. Joris, M. Jamin, K. Klarsov, J. Van Beeumen, D. Mengin-Lecreuix, J. van Heijenoort, J. T. Park, S. Normark, and J.-M. Frère.** 1995. AmpD, essential for both ß-lactamase regulation and cell wall recycling, is a novel cytosolic *N*-acetylmuramyl-L-alanine amidase. *Mol. Microbiol.* **15:**553–559.
113. **Jacoby, G. A.** 2005. Mechanisms of resistance to quinolones. *Clin. Infect. Dis.* **41**(Suppl. 2):S120-S126.
114. **Jacoby, G. A., and A. A. Medeiros.** 1991. More extended-spectrum ß-lactamases. *Antimicrob. Agents Chemother.* **35:**1697–1704.
115. **Jeannot, K., M. L. Sobel, F. El Garch, K. Poole, and P. Plesiat.** 2005. Induction of the MexXY efflux pump in

Pseudomonas aeruginosa is dependent on drug-ribosome interaction. *J. Bacteriol.* **187:**5341–5346.

116. **Jones, R. N., T. R. Anderegg, and J. M. Swenson.** 2005. Quality control guidelines for testing gram-negative control strains with polymyxin B and colistin (polymyxin E) by standardized methods. *J. Clin. Microbiol.* **43:**925–927.
117. **Kaatz, G. W., S. M. Seo, N. J. Dorman, and S. A. Lerner.** 1990. Emergence of teicoplanin resistance during therapy of *Staphylococcus aureus* endocarditis. *J. Infect. Dis.* **162:**103–108.
118. **Kadurugamuwa, J. L., J. S. Lam, and T. J. Beveridge.** 1993. Interaction of gentamicin with the A band and B band lipopolysaccharides of *Pseudomonas aeruginosa* and its possible lethal effect. *Antimicrob. Agents Chemother.* **37:**715–721.
119. **Katayama, Y., D. A. Robinson, M. C. Enright, and H. F. Chambers.** 2005. Genetic background affects stability of *mecA* in *Staphylococcus aureus. J. Clin. Microbiol.* **43:**2380–2383.
120. **Kaye, K. S., H. S. Gold, M. J. Schwaber, L. Venkataraman, Y. Qi, P. C. De Girolami, M. H. Samore, G. Anderson, J. K. Rasheed, and F. C. Tenover.** 2004. Variety of beta-lactamases produced by amoxicillin-clavulanate-resistant *Escherichia coli* isolated in the northeastern United States. *Antimicrob. Agents Chemother.* **48:**1520–1525.
121. **Kim, J., Y. M. Lim, Y. S. Jeong, and S. Y. Seol.** 2005. Occurrence of CTX-M-3, CTX-M-15, CTX-M-14, and CTX-M-9 extended-spectrum beta-lactamases in *Enterobacteriaceae* clinical isolates in Korea. *Antimicrob. Agents Chemother.* **49:**1572–1575.
122. **Knox, J. R.** 1995. Extended-spectrum and inhibitor-resistant TEM-type beta-lactamases: mutations, specificity, and three-dimensional structure. *Antimicrob. Agents Chemother.* **39:**2593–2601.
123. **Ko, W. C., D. L. Paterson, A. J. Sagnimeni, D. S. Hansen, A. Von Gottberg, S. Mohapatra, J. M. Casellas, H. Goossens, L. Mulazimoglu, G. Trenholme, K. P. Klugman, J. G. McCormack, and V. L. Yu.** 2002. Community-acquired *Klebsiella pneumoniae* bacteremia: global differences in clinical patterns. *Emerg. Infect. Dis.* **8:**160–166.
124. **Kohler, T., M. Kok, M. Michea-Hamzehpour, P. Plesiat, N. Gotoh, T. Nishino, L. K. Curty, and J. C. Pechere.** 1996. Multidrug efflux in intrinsic resistance to trimethoprim and sulfamethoxazole in *Pseudomonas aeruginosa. Antimicrob. Agents Chemother.* **40:**2288–2290.
125. **Kotra, L. P., J. Haddad, and S. Mobashery.** 2000. Aminoglycosides: perspectives on mechanisms of action and resistance and strategies to counter resistance. *Antimicrob. Agents Chemother.* **44:**3249–3256.
126. **Lartigue, M. F., L. Poirel, J. W. Decousser, and P. Nordmann.** 2005. Multidrug-resistant *Shigella sonnei* and *Salmonella enterica* Serotype typhimurium isolates producing CTX-M beta-lactamases as causes of community-acquired infection in France. *Clin. Infect. Dis.* **40:**1069–1070.
127. **Leclerq, R., S. Dutka-Malen, A. Brisson-Noel, C. Molinas, E. Derlot, M. Arthur, J. Duval, and P. Courvalin.** 1992. Resistance of enterococci to aminoglycosides and glycopeptides. *Clin. Infect. Dis.* **15:**495–501.
128. **Lee, A., W. Mao, M. S. Warren, A. Mistry, K. Hoshino, R. Okumura, H. Ishida, and O. Lomovskaya.** 2000. Interplay between efflux pumps may provide either additive or multiplicative effects on drug resistance. *J. Bacteriol.* **182:**3142–3150.
129. **Lee, E. H., M. H. Nicolas, M. D. Kitzis, G. Pialoux, E. Collatz, and L. Gutmann.** 1991. Association of two resistance mechanisms in a clinical isolate of *Enterobacter cloacae* with high-level resistance to imipenem. *Antimicrob. Agents Chemother.* **35:**1093–1098.
130. **Leiros, H. K., S. Kozielski-Stuhrmann, U. Kapp, L. Terradot, G. A. Leonard, and S. M. McSweeney.** 2004. Structural basis of 5-nitroimidazole antibiotic resistance: the crystal structure of NimA from *Deinococcus radiodurans. J. Biol. Chem.* **279:**55840–55849.
131. **Levine, D. P., B. S. Fromm, and B. R. Reddy.** 1991. Slow response to vancomycin or vancomycin plus rifampin in methicillin-resistant *Staphylococcus aureus* endocarditis. *Ann. Intern. Med.* **115:**674–680.
132. **Levy, S. B., L. M. McMurry, T. M. Barbosa, V. Burdett, P. Courvalin, W. Hillen, M. C. Roberts, J. I. Rood, and D. E. Taylor.** 1999. Nomenclature for new tetracycline resistance determinants. *Antimicrob. Agents Chemother.* **43:**1523–1524.
133. **Linares, J.** 2001. The VISA/GISA problem: therapeutic implications. *Clin. Microbiol. Infect.* **7:**8–15.
134. **Livermore, D. M.** 1992. Interplay of impermeability and chromosomal β-lactamase activity in imipenem-resistant *Pseudomonas aeruginosa. Antimicrob. Agents Chemother.* **36:**2046–2048.
135. **Livermore, D. M., D. F. Brown, J. P. Quinn, Y. Carmeli, D. L. Paterson, and V. L. Yu.** 2004. Should third-generation cephalosporins be avoided against AmpC-inducible *Enterobacteriaceae? Clin. Microbiol. Infect.* **10:**84–85.
136. **Lobkovsky, E., E. M. Billings, P. C. Moews, J. Rahil, R. F. Pratt, and J. R. Knox.** 1994. Crystallographic structure of a phosphonate derivative of the *Enterobacter cloacae* P99 cephalosporinase: mechanistic interpretation of a beta-lactamase transition-state analog. *Biochemistry* **33:**6762–6772.
137. **Lobkovsky, E., P. C. Moews, H. Liu, H. Zhao, J. M. Frere, and J. R. Knox.** 1993. Evolution of an enzyme activity: crystallographic structure at 2-A resolution of cephalosporinase from the *ampC* gene of *Enterobacter cloacae* P99 and comparison with a class A penicillinase. *Proc. Natl. Acad. Sci. USA* **90:**11257–11261.
138. **Lobritz, M., R. Hutton-Thomas, S. Marshall, and L. B. Rice.** 2003. Recombination proficiency influences frequency and locus of mutational resistance to linezolid in *Enterococcus faecalis. Antimicrob. Agents Chemother.* **47:**3318–3320.
139. **Magnet, S., P. Courvalin, and T. Lambert.** 2001. Resistance-nodulation-cell division-type efflux pump involved in aminoglycoside resistance in *Acinetobacter baumannii* strain BM4454. *Antimicrob. Agents Chemother.* **45:**3375–3380.
140. **Manges, A. R., J. R. Johnson, B. Foxman, T. T. O'Bryan, K. E. Fullerton, and L. W. Riley.** 2001. Widespread distribution of urinary tract infections caused by a multidrug-resistant *Escherichia coli* clonal group. *N. Engl. J. Med.* **345:**1007–1013.
141. **Mao, W., M. S. Warren, A. Lee, A. Mistry, and O. Lomovskaya.** 2001. MexXY-OprM efflux pump is required for antagonism of aminoglycosides by divalent cations in *Pseudomonas aeruginosa. Antimicrob. Agents Chemother.* **45:**2001–2007.
142. **Marchand, I., L. Damier-Piolle, P. Courvalin, and T. Lambert.** 2004. Expression of the RND-type efflux pump AdeABC in *Acinetobacter baumannii* is regulated by the AdeRS two-component system. *Antimicrob. Agents Chemother.* **48:**3298–3304.
143. **Marshall, S. H., C. J. Donskey, R. Hutton-Thomas, R. A. Salata, and L. B. Rice.** 2002. Gene dosage and linezolid resistance in *Enterococcus faecium* and *Enterococcus faecalis. Antimicrob. Agents Chemother.* **46:**3334–3336.
144. **Martinez, J. L., A. Alonso, J. M. Gomez-Gomez, and F. Baquero.** 1998. Quinolone resistance by mutations in chromosomal gyrase genes. Just the tip of the iceberg? *J. Antimicrob. Chemother.* **42:**683–688.

145. **Martinez-Martinez, L., S. Hernandez-Alles, S. Alberti, J. M. Tomas, V. J. Benedi, and G. A. Jacoby.** 1996. In vivo selection of porin-deficient mutants of *Klebsiella pneumoniae* with increased resistance to cefoxitin and expanded-spectrum cephalosporins. *Antimicrob. Agents Chemother.* **40:**342–348.
146. **Maseda, H., H. Yoneyama, and T. Nakae.** 2000. Assignment of the substrate-selective subunits of the MexEF-OprN multidrug efflux pump of *Pseudomonas aeruginosa. Antimicrob. Agents Chemother.* **44:**658–664.
147. **Matagne, A., J. Lamotte-Brasseur, and J. M. Frere.** 1998. Catalytic properties of class A beta-lactamases: efficiency and diversity. *Biochem. J.* **330:**581–598.
148. **Maus, C. E., B. B. Plikaytis, and T. M. Shinnick.** 2005. Molecular analysis of cross-resistance to capreomycin, kanamycin, amikacin, and viomycin in *Mycobacterium tuberculosis. Antimicrob. Agents Chemother.* **49:**3192–3197.
149. **Maveyraud, L., D. Golemi, L. P. Kotra, S. Tranier, S. Vakulenko, S. Mobashery, and J. P. Samama.** 2000. Insights into class D beta-lactamases are revealed by the crystal structure of the OXA10 enzyme from *Pseudomonas aeruginosa. Structure* **8:**1289–1298.
150. **McOsker, C. C., and P. M. Fitzpatrick.** 1994. Nitrofurantoin: mechanism of action and implications for resistance development in common uropathogens. *J. Antimicrob. Chemother.* **33**(Suppl. A)**:**23–30.
151. **Minasov, G., X. Wang, and B. K. Shoichet.** 2002. An ultrahigh resolution structure of TEM-1 beta-lactamase suggests a role for Glu166 as the general base in acylation. *J. Am. Chem. Soc.* **124:**5333–5340.
152. **Mingeot-Leclercq, M. P., Y. Glupczynski, and P. M. Tulkens.** 1999. Aminoglycosides: activity and resistance. *Antimicrob. Agents Chemother.* **43:**727–737.
153. **Miriagou, V., L. S. Tzouvelekis, S. Rossiter, E. Tzelepi, F. J. Angulo, and J. M. Whichard.** 2003. Imipenem resistance in a *Salmonella* clinical strain due to plasmid-mediated class A carbapenemase KPC-2. *Antimicrob. Agents Chemother.* **47:**1297–1300.
154. **Moellering, R. C., and A. N. Weinberg.** 1971. Studies on antibiotic synergism against enterococci. II. Effect of various antibiotics on the uptake of 14^{C}-labelled streptomycin by enterococci. *J. Clin. Investig.* **50:**2580–2584.
155. **Morais Cabral, J. H., A. P. Jackson, C. V. Smith, N. Shikotra, A. Maxwell, and R. C. Liddington.** 1997. Crystal structure of the breakage-reunion domain of DNA gyrase. *Nature* **388:**903–906.
156. **Murakami, K., and A. Tomasz.** 1989. Involvement of multiple genetic determinants in high-level methicillin resistance in *Staphylococcus aureus. J. Bacteriol.* **171:**874–879.
157. **Murakami, S., R. Nakashima, E. Yamashita, and A. Yamaguchi.** 2002. Crystal structure of bacterial multidrug efflux transporter AcrB. *Nature* **419:**587–593.
158. **Murray, I. A., J. V. Martinez-Suarez, T. J. Close, and W. V. Shaw.** 1990. Nucleotide sequences of genes encoding the type II chloramphenicol acetyltransferases of *Escherichia coli* and *Haemophilus influenzae,* which are sensitive to inhibition by thiol-reactive reagents. *Biochem. J.* **272:**505–510.
159. **Murray, I. A., and W. V. Shaw.** 1997. O-Acetyltransferases for chloramphenicol and other natural products. *Antimicrob. Agents Chemother.* **41:**1–6.
160. **Naas, T., and P. Nordmann.** 1994. Analysis of a carbapenem-hydrolyzing class A beta-lactamase from *Enterobacter cloacae* and of its LysR-type regulatory protein. *Proc. Natl. Acad. Sci.* USA **91:**7693–7697.
161. **Naas, T., and P. Nordmann.** 1999. OXA-type beta-lactamases. *Curr. Pharm. Des.* **5:**865–879.
162. **Navia, M. M., J. Ruiz, and J. Vila.** 2002. Characterization of an integron carrying a new class D beta-lactamase (OXA-37) in Acinetobacter baumannii. *Microb. Drug. Resist.* **8:**261–265.
163. **Navia, M. M., J. Ruiz, and J. Vila.** 2004. Molecular characterization of the integrons in *Shigella* strains isolated from patients with traveler's diarrhea. *Diagn. Microbiol. Infect. Dis.* **48:**175–179.
164. **Neuwirth, C., S. Madec, E. Siebor, A. Pechinot, J. M. Duez, M. Pruneaux, M. Fouchereau-Peron, A. Kazmierczak, and R. Labia.** 2001. TEM-89 beta-lactamase produced by a *Proteus mirabilis* clinical isolate: new complex mutant (CMT 3) with mutations in both TEM-59 (IRT-17) and TEM-3. *Antimicrob. Agents Chemother.* **45:**3591–3594.
165. **Nikaido, H.** 1998. Multiple antibiotic resistance and efflux. *Curr. Opin. Microbiol.* **1:**516–523.
166. **Nikaido, H., and D. G. Thanassi.** 1993. Penetration of lipophilic agents with multiple protonation sites into bacterial cells: tetracyclines and fluoroquinolones as examples. *Antimicrob. Agents Chemother.* **37:**1393–1399.
167. **Noble, W. C., Z. Virani, and R. G. A. Gee.** 1992. Co-transfer of vancomycin and other resistance genes from *Enterococcus faecalis* NCTC 12201 to *Staphylococcus aureus. FEMS Microbiol. Lett.* **93:**195–198.
168. **Nordmann, P., S. Mariotte, T. Naas, R. Labia, and M. H. Nicolas.** 1993. Biochemical properties of a carbapenem-hydrolyzing beta-lactamase from *Enterobacter cloacae* and cloning of the gene into *Escherichia coli. Antimicrob. Agents Chemother.* **37:**939–946.
169. **Nordmann, P., and L. Poirel.** 2005. Emergence of plasmid-mediated resistance to quinolones in *Enterobacteriaceae. J. Antimicrob. Chemother.* **56:**463–469.
170. **Nukaga, M., K. Mayama, A. M. Hujer, R. A. Bonomo, and J. R. Knox.** 2003. Ultrahigh resolution structure of a class A beta-lactamase: on the mechanism and specificity of the extended-spectrum SHV-2 enzyme. *J. Mol. Biol.* **328:**289–301.
171. **Oefner, C., A. D'Arcy, J. J. Daly, K. Gubernator, R. L. Charnas, I. Heinze, C. Hubschwerlen, and F. K. Winkler.** 1990. Refined crystal structure of beta-lactamase from *Citrobacter freundii* indicates a mechanism for beta-lactam hydrolysis. *Nature* **343:**284–288.
172. **Oggioni, M. R., C. G. Dowson, J. M. Smith, R. Provvedi, and G. Pozzi.** 1996. The tetracycline resistance gene *tet*(M) exhibits mosaic structure. *Plasmid* **35:**156–163.
173. **Okuma, K., K. Iwakawa, J. D. Turnidge, W. B. Grubb, J. M. Bell, F. G. O'Brien, G. W. Coombs, J. W. Pearman, F. C. Tenover, M. Kapi, C. Tiensasitorn, T. Ito, and K. Hiramatsu.** 2002. Dissemination of new methicillin-resistant *Staphylococcus aureus* clones in the community. *J. Clin. Microbiol.* **40:**4289–4294.
174. **Olson, A. B., M. Silverman, D. A. Boyd, A. McGeer, B. M. Willey, V. Pong-Porter, N. Daneman, and M. R. Mulvey.** 2005. Identification of a progenitor of the CTX-M-9 group of extended-spectrum beta-lactamases from *Kluyvera georgiana* isolated in Guyana. *Antimicrob. Agents Chemother.* **49:**2112–2115.
175. **Orencia, M. C., J. S. Yoon, J. E. Ness, W. P. Stemmer, and R. C. Stevens.** 2001. Predicting the emergence of antibiotic resistance by directed evolution and structural analysis. *Nat. Struct. Biol.* **8:**238–242.
176. **Paetzel, M., F. Danel, L. de Castro, S. C. Mosimann, M. G. Page, and N. C. Strynadka.** 2000. Crystal structure of the class D beta-lactamase OXA-10. *Nat. Struct. Biol.* **7:**918–925.
177. **Pan, X. S., and L. M. Fisher.** 1999. *Streptococcus pneumoniae* DNA gyrase and topoisomerase IV: overexpression, purification, and differential inhibition by fluoroquinolones. *Antimicrob. Agents Chemother.* **43:**1129–1136.

178. **Paterson, D. L.** 2001. Extended-spectrum beta-lactamases: the European experience. *Curr. Opin. Infect. Dis.* **14:**697–701.
179. **Paterson, D. L., K. M. Hujer, A. M. Hujer, B. Yeiser, M. D. Bonomo, L. B. Rice, and R. A. Bonomo.** 2003. Extended-spectrum beta-lactamases in *Klebsiella pneumoniae* bloodstream isolates from seven countries: dominance and widespread prevalence of SHV- and CTX-M-type beta-lactamases. *Antimicrob. Agents Chemother.* **47:**3554–3560.
180. **Paterson, D. L., W. C. Ko, A. Von Gottberg, S. Mohapatra, J. M. Casellas, H. Goossens, L. Mulazimoglu, G. Trenholme, K. P. Klugman, R. A. Bonomo, L. B. Rice, M. M. Wagener, J. G. McCormack, and V. L. Yu.** 2004. Antibiotic therapy for *Klebsiella pneumoniae* bacteremia: implications of production of extended-spectrum beta-lactamases. *Clin. Infect. Dis.* **39:**31–37.
181. **Paterson, D. L., W. C. Ko, A. Von Gottberg, S. Mohapatra, J. M. Casellas, H. Goossens, L. Mulazimoglu, G. Trenholme, K. P. Klugman, R. A. Bonomo, L. B. Rice, M. M. Wagener, J. G. McCormack, and V. L. Yu.** 2004. International prospective study of *Klebsiella preumoniae* bacteremia: implications of extended-spectrum beta-lactamase production in nosocomial infections. *Ann. Intern. Med.* **140:**26–32.
182. **Paton, R., R. S. Miles, J. Hood, and S. G. B. Amyes.** 1993. ARI-1: ß-lactamase-mediated imipenem resistance in *Acinetobacter baumannii. Int. J. Antimicrob. Agents* **2:**81–88.
183. **Paulsen, I. T., L. Banerjei, G. S. Myers, K. E. Nelson, R. Seshadri, T. D. Read, D. E. Fouts, J. A. Eisen, S. R. Gill, J. F. Heidelberg, H. Tettelin, R. J. Dodson, L. Umayam, L. Brinkac, M. Beanan, S. Daugherty, R. T. DeBoy, S. Durkin, J. Kolonay, R. Madupu, W. Nelson, J. Vamathevan, B. Tran, J. Upton, T. Hansen, J. Shetty, H. Khouri, T. Utterback, D. Radune, K. A. Ketchum, B. A. Dougherty, and C. M. Fraser.** 2003. Role of mobile DNA in the evolution of vancomycin-resistant *Enterococcus faecalis. Science* **299:**2071–2074.
184. **Perl, T. M., J. J. Cullen, R. P. Wenzel, M. B. Zimmerman, M. A. Pfaller, D. Sheppard, J. Twombley, P. P. French, and L. A. Herwaldt.** 2002. Intranasal mupirocin to prevent postoperative *Staphylococcus aureus* infections. *N. Engl. J. Med.* **346:**1871–1877.
185. **Phillipon, A., R. Labia, and G. A. Jacoby.** 1989. Extended-spectrum ß-lactamases. *Antimicrob. Agents Chemother.* **33:**1131–1136.
186. **Piddock, L. J.** 1999. Mechanisms of fluoroquinolone resistance: an update, 1994–1998. *Drugs* **58:**11–18.
187. **Pinho, M. G., H. de Lencastre, and A. Tomasz.** 2001. An acquired and a native penicillin-binding protein cooperate in building the cell wall of drug-resistant staphylococci. *Proc. Natl. Acad. Sci. USA.* **98:**10886–10891.
188. **Podglajen, I., J. Breuil, A. Rohaut, C. Monsempes, and E. Collatz.** 2001. Multiple mobile promoter regions for the rare carbapenem resistance gene of *Bacteroides fragilis. J. Bacteriol.* **183:**3531–3535.
189. **Poirel, L., L. Collet, and P. Nordmann.** 2000. Carbapenem-hydrolyzing metallo-beta-lactamase from a nosocomial isolate of *Pseudomonas aeruginosa* in France. *Emerg. Infect. Dis.* **6:**84–85.
190. **Poirel, L., P. Gerome, C. De Champs, J. Stephanazzi, T. Naas, and P. Nordmann.** 2002. Integron-located oxa-32 gene cassette encoding an extended-spectrum variant of OXA-2 beta-lactamase from *Pseudomonas aeruginosa. Antimicrob. Agents Chemother*. **46:**566–569.
191. **Poirel, L., D. Girlich, T. Naas, and P. Nordmann.** 2001. OXA-28, an extended-spectrum variant of OXA-10 beta-lactamase from *Pseudomonas aeruginosa* and its plasmid- and integron-located gene. *Antimicrob. Agents Chemother.* **45:**447–453.
192. **Poirel, L., H. Mammeri, and P. Nordmann.** 2004. TEM-121, a novel complex mutant of TEM-type beta-lactamase from *Enterobacter aerogenes. Antimicrob. Agents Chemother.* **48:**4528–4531.
193. **Poirel, L., T. Naas, M. Guibert, E. B. Chaibi, R. Labia, and P. Nordmann.** 1999. Molecular and biochemical characterization of VEB-1, a novel class A extended-spectrum beta-lactamase encoded by an *Escherichia coli* integron gene. *Antimicrob. Agents Chemother.* **43:**573–581.
194. **Poirel, L., G. F. Weldhagen, T. Naas, C. De Champs, M. G. Dove, and P. Nordmann.** 2001. GES-2, a class A beta-lactamase from *Pseudomonas aeruginosa* with increased hydrolysis of imipenem. *Antimicrob. Agents Chemother.* **45:**2598–2603.
195. **Poole, K., K. Krebes, C. McNally, and S. Neshat.** 1993. Multiple antibiotic resistance in *Pseudomonas aeruginosa:* evidence for involvement of an efflux operon. *J. Bacteriol.* **175:**7363–7372.
196. **Prinarakis, E. E., V. Miriagou, E. Tzelepi, M. Gazouli, and L. S. Tzouvelekis.** 1997. Emergence of an inhibitor-resistant beta-lactamase (SHV-10) derived from an SHV-5 variant. *Antimicrob. Agents Chemother.* **41:**838–840.
197. **Prystowsky, J., F. Siddiqui, J. Chosay, D. L. Shinabarger, J. Millichap, L. R. Peterson, and G. A. Noskin.** 2001. Resistance to linezolid: characterization of mutations in rRNA and comparison of their occurrences in vancomycin-resistant enterococci. *Antimicrob. Agents Chemother.* **45:**2154–2156.
198. **Qiu, W., R. Shi, M. L. Lu, M. Zhou, P. H. Roy, J. Lapointe, and S. X. Lin.** 2004. Crystal structure of chloramphenicol acetyltransferase B2 encoded by the multiresistance transposon Tn2424. *Proteins* **57:**858–861.
199. **Race, P. R., A. L. Lovering, R. M. Green, A. Ossor, S. A. White, P. F. Searle, C. J. Wrighton, and E. I. Hyde.** 2005. Structural and mechanistic studies of *Escherichia coli* nitroreductase with the antibiotic nitrofurazone. Reversed binding orientations in different redox states of the enzyme. *J. Biol. Chem.* **280:**13256–13264.
200. **Raquet, X., J. Lamotte-Brasseur, E. Fonze, S. Goussard, P. Courvalin, and J. M. Frere.** 1994. TEM beta-lactamase mutants hydrolysing third-generation cephalosporins. A kinetic and molecular modelling analysis. *J. Mol. Biol.* **244:**625–639.
201. **Rasmussen, B. A., K. Bush, D. Keeney, Y. Yang, R. Hare, C. O'Gara, and A. A. Medeiros.** 1996. Characterization of IMI-1 beta-lactamase, a class A carbapenem-hydrolyzing enzyme from *Enterobacter cloacae. Antimicrob. Agents Chemother.* **40:**2080–2086.
202. **Rather, P. N.** 1998. Origins of aminoglycoside modifying enzymes. *Drug Resist. Updat.* **1:**285–291.
203. **Rather, P. N., E. Orosz, K. J. Shaw, R. Hare, and G. Miller.** 1993. Characterization and transcriptional regulation of the 2′-*N*-acetyltransferase gene from *Providencia stuartii. J. Bacteriol.* **175:**6492–6498.
204. **Rice, L. B.** 2000. Bacterial monopolists: the bundling and dissemination of antimicrobial resistance genes in gram-positive bacteria. *Clin. Infect. Dis.* **31:**762–769.
205. **Rice, L. B.** 1998. Tn*916*-family conjugative transposons and dissemination of antimicrobial resistance determinants. *Antimicrob. Agents Chemother.* **42:**1871–1877.
206. **Rice, L. B., S. Bellais, L. L. Carias, R. Hutton-Thomas, R. A. Bonomo, P. Caspers, M. G. Page, and L. Gutmann.** 2004. Impact of specific *pbp5* mutations on expression of beta-lactam resistance in *Enterococcus faecium. Antimicrob. Agents Chemother.* **48:**3028–3032.
207. **Rice, L. B., S. B. Calderwood, G. M. Eliopoulos, B. F. Farber, and A. W. Karchmer.** 1991. Enterococcal endocarditis: a comparison of native and prosthetic valve disease. *Rev. Infect. Dis.* **13:**1–7.

208. **Rice, L. B., L. L. Carias, A. M. Hujer, M. Bonafede, R. Hutton, C. Hoyen, and R. A. Bonomo.** 2000. High-level expression of chromosomally encoded SHV-1 ß-lactamase and an outer membrane protein change confer resistance to ceftazidime and piperacillin-tazobactam in a clinical isolate of *Klebsiella pneumoniae*. *Antimicrob. Agents Chemother.* **44:**362–367.
209. **Rice, L. B., L. L. Carias, R. Hutton-Thomas, F. Sifaoui, L. Gutmann, and S. D. Rudin.** 2001. Penicillin-binding protein 5 and expression of ampicillin resistance in *Enterococcus faecium*. *Antimicrob. Agents Chemother.* **45:**1480–1486.
210. **Rice, L. B., J. D. C. Yao, K. Klimm, G. M. Eliopoulos, and R. C. Moellering, Jr.** 1991. Efficacy of different ß-lactams against an extended spectrum ß-lactamase-producing *Klebsiella pneumoniae* strain in the rat intra-abdominal abscess model. *Antimicrob. Agents Chemother.* **35:**1243–1244.
211. **Roberts, R. B., A. de Lancastre, W. Eisner, E. P. Severina, B. Shopsin, B. N. Kreiswirth, A. Tomasz, and the MRSA Collaborative Study Group.** 1998. Molecular epidemiology of methicillin-resistant *Staphylococcus aureus* in 12 New York hospitals. *J. Infect. Dis.* **178:**164–171.
212. **Rodriguez, C. A., R. Atkinson, W. Bitar, C. G. Whitney, K. M. Edwards, L. Mitchell, J. Li, J. Sublett, C. S. Li, T. Liu, P. J. Chesney, and E. I. Tuomanen.** 2004. Tolerance to vancomycin in pneumococci: detection with a molecular marker and assessment of clinical impact. *J. Infect. Dis.* **190:**1481–1487.
213. **Rowe-Magnus, D. A., A. M. Guerout, and D. Mazel.** 2002. Bacterial resistance evolution by recruitment of super-integron gene cassettes. *Mol. Microbiol.* **43:**1657–1669.
214. **Ruzin, A., D. Keeney, and P. A. Bradford.** 2005. AcrAB efflux pump plays a role in decreased susceptibility to tigecycline in *Morganella morganii*. *Antimicrob. Agents Chemother.* **49:**791–793.
215. **Ruzin, A., M. A. Visalli, D. Keeney, and P. A. Bradford.** 2005. Influence of transcriptional activator RamA on expression of multidrug efflux pump AcrAB and tigecycline susceptibility in *Klebsiella pneumoniae*. *Antimicrob. Agents Chemother.* **49:**1017–1022.
216. **Rybkine, T., J.-L. Mainardi, W. Sougakoff, E. Collatz, and L. Gutmann.** 1998. Penicillin-binding protein 5 sequence alterations in clinical isolates of *Enterococcus faecium* with different levels of ß-lactam resistance. *J. Infect. Dis.* **178:**159–163.
217. **Sabath, L. D.** 1969. Drug resistance of bacteria. *N. Engl. J. Med.* **280:**91–94.
218. **Sahm, D. F., M. K. Marsilio, and G. Piazza.** 1999. Antimicrobial resistance in key bloodstream bacterial isolates: electronic surveillance with The Surveillance Network Database—USA. *Clin. Infect. Dis.* **29:**259–263.
219. **Sanchez-Pescador, R., J. T. Brown, M. Roberts, and M. S. Urdea.** 1988. Homology of the TetM with translational elongation factors: implications for potential modes of tetM-conferred tetracycline resistance. *Nucleic Acids Res.* **16:**1218.
220. **Saves, I., O. Burlet-Schiltz, P. Swaren, F. Lefevre, J. M. Masson, J. C. Prome, and J. P. Samama.** 1995. The asparagine to aspartic acid substitution at position 276 of TEM-35 and TEM-36 is involved in the beta-lactamase resistance to clavulanic acid. *J. Biol. Chem.* **270:**18240–18245.
221. **Schnappinger, D., and W. Hillen.** 1996. Tetracyclines: antibiotic action, uptake, and resistance mechanisms. *Arch. Microbiol.* **165:**359–369.
222. **Schwarz, S., C. Kehrenberg, B. Doublet, and A. Cloeckaert.** 2004. Molecular basis of bacterial resistance to chloramphenicol and florfenicol. *FEMS. Microbiol. Rev.* **28:**519–542.
223. **Shaw, J. H., and D. B. Clewell.** 1985. Complete nucleotide sequence of macrolide-lincosamide-streptogramin B resistance transposon Tn*917* in *Streptococcus faecalis*. *J. Bacteriol.* **164:**782–796.
224. **Shaw, K. J., P. Rather, F. Sabatelli, P. Mann, H. Munayyer, R. Mierzwa, G. Petrikkos, R. S. Hare, G. H. Miller, P. Bennett, and P. Downey.** 1992. Characterization of the chromosomal *aac(6')-Ic* gene from *Serratia marcescens*. *Antimicrob. Agents Chemother.* **36:**1447–1455.
225. **Shaw, K. J., P. N. Rather, R. S. Hare, and G. H. Miller.** 1993. Molecular genetics of aminoglycoside resistance genes and familial relationships of the aminoglycoside-modifying enzymes. *Microbiol. Rev.* **57:**138–163.
226. **Shaw, W. V.** 1983. Chloramphenicol acetyltransferase: enzymology and molecular biology. *Crit. Rev. Biochem.* **14:**1–46.
227. **Shea, M. E., and H. Hiasa.** 1999. Interactions between DNA helicases and frozen topoisomerase IV-quinolone-DNA ternary complexes. *J. Biol. Chem.* **274:**22747–22754.
228. **Sherertz, R. J., D. R. Reagan, K. D. Hampton, K. L. Robertson, S. A. Streed, H. M. Hoen, R. Thomas, and J. M. Gwaltney, Jr.** 1996. A cloud adult: the *Staphylococcus aureus*-virus interaction revisited. *Ann. Intern. Med.* **124:** 539–547.
229. **Shimamura, T., A. Ibuka, S. Fushinobu, T. Wakagi, M. Ishiguro, Y. Ishii, and H. Matsuzawa.** 2002. Acyl-intermediate structures of the extended-spectrum class A beta-lactamase, Toho-1, in complex with cefotaxime, cephalothin, and benzylpenicillin. *J. Biol. Chem.* **277:** 46601–46608.
230. **Shinabarger, D. L., K. R. Marotti, R. W. Murray, A. H. Lin, E. P. Melchior, S. M. Swaney, D. S. Dunyak, W. F. Demyan, and J. M. Buysse.** 1997. Mechanism of action of oxazolidinones: effects of linezolid and eperezolid on translation reactions. *Antimicrob. Agents Chemother.* **41:** 2132–2136.
231. **Sieradzki, K., R. B. Roberts, S. W. Haber, and A. Tomasz.** 1999. The development of vancomycin resistance in a patient with methicillin-resistant *Staphylococcus aureus* infection. *N. Engl. J. Med.* **340:**517–523.
232. **Sirot, D., C. Recule, E. B. Chaibi, L. Bret, J. Croize, C. Chanal-Claris, R. Labia, and J. Sirot.** 1997. A complex mutant of TEM-1 beta-lactamase with mutations encountered in both IRT-4 and extended-spectrum TEM-15, produced by an *Escherichia coli* clinical isolate. *Antimicrob. Agents Chemother.* **41:**1322–1325.
233. **Skold, O.** 2000. Sulfonamide resistance: mechanisms and trends. *Drug Resist. Updat.* **3:**155–160.
234. **Smith, A. M., R. F. Botha, H. J. Koornhof, and K. P. Klugman.** 2001. Emergence of a pneumococcal clone with cephalosporin resistance and penicillin susceptibility. *Antimicrob. Agents Chemother.* **45:**2648–2650.
235. **Soki, J., M. Gal, J. S. Brazier, V. O. Rotimi, E. Urban, E. Nagy, and B. I. Duerden.** 2005. Molecular investigation of genetic elements contributing to metronidazole resistance in *Bacteroides* strains. *J. Antimicrob. Chemother.* **57:**212–220.
236. **Soltani, M., D. Beighton, J. Philpott-Howard, and N. Woodford. 2000.** Mechanisms of resistance to quinupristin-dalfopristin among isolates of *Enterococcus faecium* from animals, raw meat, and hospital patients in Western Europe. *Antimicrob. Agents Chemother.* **44:**433–436.
237. **Sorensen, T. L., M. Blom, D. L. Monnet, N. Frimodt-Moller, R. L. Poulsen, and F. Espersen.** 2001. Transient intestinal carriage after ingestion of antibiotic-resistant *Enterococcus faecium* from chicken and pork. *N. Engl. J. Med.* **345:**1161–1166.
238. **Spencer, J., A. R. Clarke, and T. R. Walsh.** 2001. Novel mechanism of hydrolysis of therapeutic beta-lactams by

Stenotrophomonas maltophilia L1 metallo-beta-lactamase. *J. Biol. Chem.* **276:**33638–33644.

239. **Spratt, B. G., Q.-Y. Zhang, D. M. Jones, A. Hutchison, J. A. Brannigan, and C. G. Dowson.** 1989. Recruitment of a penicillin-binding protein gene from *Neisseria flavescens* during the emergence of penicillin resistance in *Neisseria meningitidis*. *Proc. Natl. Acad. Sci. USA* **86:**8988–8992.
240. **Stapleton, P. D., K. P. Shannon, and G. L. French.** 1999. Carbapenem resistance in *Escherichia coli* associated with plasmid-determined CMY-4 ß-lactamase production and loss of an outer membrane protein. *Antimicrob. Agents Chemother.* **43:**1206–1210.
241. **Su, Y. A., P. He, and D. B. Clewell.** 1992. Characterization of the *tet*M determinant of Tn*916*: evidence for regulation by transcriptional attenuation. *Antimicrob. Agents Chemother.* **36:**769–778.
242. **Swaren, P., D. Golemi, S. Cabantous, A. Bulychev, L. Maveyraud, S. Mobashery, and J. P. Samama.** 1999. X-ray structure of the Asn276Asp variant of the *Escherichia coli* TEM-1 beta-lactamase: direct observation of electrostatic modulation in resistance to inactivation by clavulanic acid. *Biochemistry* **38:**9570–9576.
243. **Swedberg, G., S. Ringertz, and O. Skold.** 1998. Sulfonamide resistance in *Streptococcus pyogenes* is associated with differences in the amino acid sequence of its chromosomal dihydropteroate synthase. *Antimicrob. Agents Chemother.* **42:**1062–1067.
244. **Tam, V. H., A. N. Schilling, G. Vo, S. Kabbara, A. L. Kwa, N. P. Wiederhold, and R. E. Lewis.** 2005. Pharmacodynamics of polymyxin B against *Pseudomonas aeruginosa*. *Antimicrob. Agents Chemother.* **49:**3624–3630.
245. **Then, R. L.** 1982. Mechanisms of resistance to trimethoprim, the sulfonamides, and trimethoprim-sulfamethoxazole. *Rev. Infect. Dis.* **4:**261–269.
246. **Then, R. L., and P. Angehrn.** 1979. Low trimethoprim susceptibility of anaerobic bacteria due to insensitive dihydrofolate reductases. *Antimicrob. Agents Chemother.* **15:**1–6.
247. **Thomson, C. J., and S. G. Amyes.** 1992. TRC-1: emergence of a clavulanic acid-resistant TEM beta-lactamase in a clinical strain. *FEMS Microbiol. Lett.* **70:**113–117.
248. **Tomasz, A.** 1983. Murein hydrolases: enzymes in search of a physiologic function. *In* R. Hackenbeck, J. Holtje, and H. Labischinski (ed.), *The Target of Penicillin.* Walter de Gruyter, Berlin, Germany.
249. **Torres, O. R., R. Z. Korman, S. A. Zahler, and G. M. Dunny.** 1991. The conjugative transposon Tn*925*: enhancement of conjugal transfer by tetracycline in *Enterococcus faecalis* and mobilization of chromosomal genes in both *Bacillus subtilis* and *E. faecalis*. *Mol. Gen. Genet.* **225:**395–400.
250. **Tran, J. H., G. A. Jacoby, and D. C. Hooper.** 2005. Interaction of the plasmid-encoded quinolone resistance protein Qnr with *Escherichia coli* DNA gyrase. *Antimicrob. Agents Chemother.* **49:**118–125.
251. **Tranier, S., A. T. Bouthors, L. Maveyraud, V. Guillet, W. Sougakoff, and J. P. Samama.** 2000. The high resolution crystal structure for class A beta-lactamase PER-1 reveals the bases for its increase in breadth of activity. *J. Biol. Chem.* **275:**28075–28082.
252. **Tsiodras, S., H. S. Gold, G. Sakoulas, G. M. Eliopoulos, C. Wennersten, L. Venkataraman, R. C. Moellering, Jr., and M. J. Ferraro.** 2001. Linezolid resistance in a clinical isolate of *Staphylococcus aureus*. *Lancet* **358:**207–208.
253. **Tuomanen, E., and A. Tomasz.** 1990. Mechanism of phenotypic tolerance of nongrowing pneumococci to beta-lactam antibiotics. *Scand. J. Infect. Dis. Suppl.* **74:**102–112.
254. **Tzeng, Y. L., K. D. Ambrose, S. Zughaier, X. Zhou, Y. K. Miller, W. M. Shafer, and D. S. Stephens.** 2005. Cationic antimicrobial peptide resistance in *Neisseria meningitidis*. *J. Bacteriol.* **187:**5387–5396.
255. **Ubukata, K., Y. Shibasaki, K. Yamamoto, N. Chiba, K. Hasegawa, Y. Takeuchi, K. Sunakawa, M. Inoue, and M. Konno.** 2001. Association of amino acid substitutions in penicillin-binding protein 3 with beta-lactam resistance in beta-lactamase-negative ampicillin-resistant *Haemophilus influenzae*. *Antimicrob. Agents Chemother.* **45:**1693–1699.
256. **Ullah, J. H., T. R. Walsh, I. A. Taylor, D. C. Emery, C. S. Verma, S. J. Gamblin, and J. Spencer.** 1998. The crystal structure of the L1 metallo-ß-lactamase from *Stenotrophomonas maltophilia* at 1.7 A resolution. *J. Mol. Biol.* **284:**125–136.
257. **Vakulenko, S. B., B. Geryk, L. P. Kotra, S. Mobashery, and S. A. Lerner.** 1998. Selection and characterization of beta-lactam-beta-lactamase inactivator-resistant mutants following PCR mutagenesis of the TEM-1 beta-lactamase gene. *Antimicrob. Agents Chemother.* **42:**1542–1548.
258. **Vakulenko, S. B., and S. Mobashery.** 2003. Versatility of aminoglycosides and prospects for their future. *Clin. Microbiol. Rev.* **16:**430–450.
259. **van der Wouden, E. J., J. C. Thijs, J. G. Kusters, A. A. van Zwet, and J. H. Kleibeuker.** 2001. Mechanism and clinical significance of metronidazole resistance in *Helicobacter pylori*. *Scand. J. Gastroenterol. Suppl.* **2001:**10–14.
260. **Vedel, G., A. Bellaouaj, L. Gilly, R. Labia, A. Phillipon, P. Nevot, and G. Paul.** 1992. Clinical isolates of *Escherichia coli* producing TRI ß-lactamases: novel TEM enzymes conferring resistance to ß-lactamase inhibitors. *J. Antimicrob. Chemother.* **30:**449–462.
261. **Vila, J., M. Navia, J. Ruiz, and C. Casals.** 1997. Cloning and nucleotide sequence analysis of a gene encoding an OXA-derived beta-lactamase in *Acinetobacter baumannii*. *Antimicrob. Agents Chemother.* **41:**2757–2759.
262. **Vincent, S., P. Minkler, B. Bincziewski, L. Etter, and D. M. Shlaes.** 1992. Vancomycin resistance in *Enterococcus gallinarum*. *Antimicrob. Agents Chemother.* **36:**1392–1399.
263. **Walsh, T. R., M. A. Toleman, L. Poirel, and P. Nordmann.** 2005. Metallo-beta-lactamases: the quiet before the storm? *Clin. Microbiol. Rev.* **18:**306–325.
264. **Wang, X., G. Minasov, and B. K. Shoichet.** 2002. Evolution of an antibiotic resistance enzyme constrained by stability and activity trade-offs. *J. Mol. Biol.* **320:**85–95.
265. **Weber, B., K. Ehlert, A. Diehl, P. Reichmann, H. Labischinski, and R. Hakenbeck.** 2000. The fib locus in *Streptococcus pneumoniae* is required for peptidoglycan crosslinking and PBP-mediated beta-lactam resistance. *FEMS Microbiol. Lett.* **188:**81–85.
266. **Wegener, H. C., F. M. Aarestrup, L. B. Jensen, A. M. Hammerum, and F. Bager.** 1999. Use of antimicrobial growth promoters in food animals and *Enterococcus faecium* resistance to therapeutic antimicrobial drugs in Europe. *Emerg. Infect. Dis.* **5:**329–335.
267. **Wehrli, W.** 1983. Rifampin: mechanisms of action and resistance. *Rev. Infect. Dis.* **5**(Suppl. 3)**:**S407–S411.
268. **Weigel, L. M., D. B. Clewell, S. R. Gill, N. C. Clark, L. K. McDougal, S. E. Flannagan, J. F. Kolonay, J. Shetty, G. E. Killgore, and F. C. Tenover.** 2003. Genetic analysis of a high-level vancomycin-resistant isolate of *Staphylococcus aureus*. *Science* **302:**1569–1571.
269. **Weisblum, B.** 1995. Erythromycin resistance by ribosome modification. *Antimicrob. Agents Chemother.* **39:**577–585.
270. **Welch, R. A., V. Burland, G. Plunkett III, P. Redford, P. Roesch, D. Rasko, E. L. Buckles, S. R. Liou, A. Boutin, J. Hackett, D. Stroud, G. F. Mayhew, D. J. Rose, S. Zhou, D. C. Schwartz, N. T. Perna, H. L. Mobley, M. S. Donnenberg, and F. R. Blattner.** 2002. Extensive mosaic structure revealed by the complete

genome sequence of uropathogenic *Escherichia coli. Proc. Natl. Acad. Sci. USA* **99:**17020–17024.

271. **Weldhagen, G. F.** 2004. Integrons and beta-lactamases—a novel perspective on resistance. *Int. J. Antimicrob. Agents* **23:**556–562.
272. **White, D. G., C. Hudson, J. J. Maurer, S. Ayers, S. Zhao, M. D. Lee, L. Bolton, T. Foley, and J. Sherwood.** 2000. Characterization of chloramphenicol and florfenicol resistance in *Escherichia coli* associated with bovine diarrhea. *J. Clin. Microbiol.* **38:**4593–4598.
273. **White, P. A., C. J. McIver, and W. D. Rawlinson.** 2001. Integrons and gene cassettes in the enterobacteriaceae. *Antimicrob. Agents Chemother.* **45:**2658–2661.
274. **Wiener, J., J. P. Quinn, P. A. Bradford, R. V. Goering, C. Nathan, K. Bush, and R. A. Weinstein.** 1999. Multiple antibiotic-resistant *Klebsiella* and *Escherichia coli* in nursing homes. *JAMA* **281:**517–523.
275. **Willems, R. J., J. Top, M. van Santen, D. A. Robinson, T. M. Coque, F. Baquero, H. Grundmann, and M. J. Bonten.** 2005. Global spread of vancomycin-resistant *Enterococcus faecium* from distinct nosocomial genetic complex. *Emerg. Infect. Dis.* **11:**821–828.
276. **Williamson, R., C. LaBouguenec, L. Gutmann, and T. Horaud.** 1985. One or two low affinity penicillin-binding proteins may be responsible for the range of susceptibility of *Enterococcus faecium* to penicillin. *J. Gen. Microbiol.* **131:**1933–1940.
277. **Willmott, C. J., S. E. Critchlow, I. C. Eperon, and A. Maxwell.** 1994. The complex of DNA gyrase and quinolone drugs with DNA forms a barrier to transcription by RNA polymerase. *J. Mol. Biol.* **242:**351–363.
278. **Woodford, N., P. M. Tierno, Jr., K. Young, L. Tysall, M. F. Palepou, E. Ward, R. E. Painter, D. F. Suber, D. Shungu, L. L. Silver, K. Inglima, J. Kornblum, and D. M. Livermore.** 2004. Outbreak of *Klebsiella pneumoniae* producing a new carbapenem-hydrolyzing class A beta-lactamase, KPC-3, in a New York medical center. *Antimicrob. Agents Chemother.* **48:**4793–4799.
279. **Wu, S. W., H. de Lencastre, and A. Tomasz.** 2001. Recruitment of the *mecA* gene homologue of *Staphylococcus sciuri* into a resistance determinant and expression of the resistant phenotype in *Staphylococcus aureus. J. Bacteriol.* **183:**2417–2424.
280. **Yamane, K., J. Wachino, Y. Doi, H. Kurokawa, and Y. Arakawa.** 2005. Global spread of multiple aminoglycoside resistance genes. *Emerg. Infect. Dis.* **11:**951–953.
281. **Yigit, H., A. M. Queenan, G. J. Anderson, A. Domenech-Sanchez, J. W. Biddle, C. D. Steward, S. Alberti, K. Bush, and F. C. Tenover.** 2001. Novel carbapenem-hydrolyzing beta-lactamase, KPC-1, from a carbapenem-resistant strain of *Klebsiella pneumoniae. Antimicrob. Agents Chemother.* **45:**1151–1161.
282. **Yigit, H., A. M. Queenan, J. K. Rasheed, J. W. Biddle, A. Domenech-Sanchez, S. Alberti, K. Bush, and F. C. Tenover.** 2003. Carbapenem-resistant strain of *Klebsiella oxytoca* harboring carbapenem-hydrolyzing beta-lactamase KPC-2. *Antimicrob. Agents Chemother.* **47:**3881–3889.
283. **Zervos, M. J., and D. R. Schaberg.** 1985. Reversal of in vitro susceptibility of enterococci to trimethoprim-sulfamethoxazole by folinic acid. *Antimicrob. Agents Chemother.* **28:**446–448.
284. **Zhong, P., and V. D. Shortridge.** 2000. The role of efflux in macrolide resistance. *Drug. Resist. Updat.* **3:**325–329.
285. **Ziha-Zarifi, I., C. Llanes, T. Kohler, J. C. Pechere, and P. Plesiat.** 1999. In vivo emergence of multidrug-resistant mutants of *Pseudomonas aeruginosa* overexpressing the active efflux system MexA-MexB-OprM. *Antimicrob. Agents Chemother.* **43:**287–291.

Susceptibility Test Methods: General Considerations

JOHN D. TURNIDGE, MARY JANE FERRARO, AND JAMES H. JORGENSEN

72

Determination of the antimicrobial susceptibilities of significant bacterial isolates is one of the principal functions of the clinical microbiology laboratory. From the physician's pragmatic point of view, the results of susceptibility tests are often considered as important as or more important than the identification of the pathogen involved. This is particularly true in an era of increasing antimicrobial resistance in which treatment options are at times limited to newer, more costly antibacterial agents. As a result, the laboratory must give high priority not only to producing technically accurate data but also to reporting those data to physicians in an easily interpretable manner.

The main objective of susceptibility testing is to predict the outcome of treatment with the antimicrobial agents tested. The implication of the result "susceptible" is that there is a high probability that the patient will respond to treatment with the appropriate dosage regimen for that antimicrobial agent. The result "resistant" implies that treatment with the agent is likely to fail. One group has coined the term "90-60 rule," that is, for many infections we can expect treatment success about 90% of the time when the organism tests as "susceptible" to that treatment and success may still occur in around 60% of cases when the organism tests as "resistant" to the agent used (36). The 60% response rate to ineffective antimicrobials is said to reflect the natural response to many bacterial infections in the immunologically normal host (31).

Most test methods also include an "intermediate" category of susceptibility, which can have several meanings. With agents that can be safely administered at higher doses, this category may imply that higher doses may be required to ensure efficacy or that the agent may prove efficacious if it is normally concentrated in an infected body fluid, e.g., urine. Conversely, for body compartments where drug penetration is restricted even in the presence of inflammation (e.g., subarachnoid space containing cerebrospinal fluid), it suggests that extreme caution should be taken in the use of the agent. It may also represent a buffer zone that prevents strains with borderline susceptibilities from being incorrectly categorized as resistant.

A further aim of susceptibility testing is to guide the clinician in the selection of the most appropriate agent for a particular clinical problem. In most clinical settings, susceptibility test results are usually obtained 24 to 48 h or more after the patient has been given empirical treatment. The test results may confirm the susceptibility of the organism to the drug initially prescribed or may indicate resistance, in which case alternative therapy will likely be required. The report describing the susceptibility testing results should provide the clinician with alternative agents to which the organism is susceptible. These alternatives also may be useful if the patient subsequently develops an adverse reaction to the initial antimicrobial agent. There is a growing emphasis from the professional societies and managed care organizations on the use of susceptibility test results to direct therapy toward the most narrow-spectrum, least expensive agent to which the pathogen should respond. This is particularly true for hospitalized patients, in whom the rate of antimicrobial resistance tends to be higher, and it is easier to make therapeutic changes for inpatients than for outpatients. This makes the accuracy of susceptibility testing even more critical for effective patient care.

The clinical microbiology laboratory should perform susceptibility testing only with pathogens for which well-standardized methods are available and pathogens whose resistance is known or suspected to be a clinical problem; susceptibility testing should not be performed on normal flora or colonizing organisms. Currently, routine susceptibility testing methods are best standardized for the common aerobic and facultative bacteria and systemic antibacterial agents. For some uncommon or fastidious bacteria and for topical antibacterial agents, simple routine test methods have not been standardized. Taking into account this limitation, the Clinical and Laboratory Standards Institute (CLSI; formerly the NCCLS) has recently released recommendations on how some of these bacteria may be tested and the results interpreted (10). With some pathogens (e.g., *Mycobacterium tuberculosis* and invasive fungi), routine testing is important for patient management, but testing is best performed by specialized laboratories in which test volumes are sufficient to maintain technical proficiency and where unusual results are likely to be recognized. Susceptibility testing methods for certain other pathogens (e.g., mycoplasmas, chlamydiae, legionellae, spirochetes, viruses, protozoa, and helminths) may not be well established at present and/or are limited to a few specialty laboratories. A number of choices exist in antibacterial susceptibility testing with respect to methodology and selection of agents for routine testing.

SELECTING AN ANTIMICROBIAL SUSCEPTIBILITY TESTING METHOD

Clinical microbiology laboratories can choose from among several conventional or novel methods for performance of routine antibacterial susceptibility testing. These include the broth microdilution, disk diffusion, antimicrobial gradient, and automated instrument methods. In recent years there has been a trend toward the use of commercial broth microdilution and automated instrument methods instead of the disk diffusion procedure. However, there may be renewed interest in the disk diffusion test because of its inherent flexibility in drug selection, ability to respond quickly to changes in interpretive breakpoints, and low cost. The availability of numerous antibacterial agents and the diversity of antimicrobial agent formularies at different institutions have made it difficult for manufacturers of commercial test systems to provide standard test panels that fit everyone's needs. Thus, the inherent flexibility in drug selection that is provided by the disk diffusion test is an undeniable asset of the method. The test is also one of the most established and best proven of all susceptibility tests and continues to be updated and refined through frequent (usually annual) CLSI publications (12, 13). Furthermore, the qualitative interpretive category results of susceptible, intermediate, and resistant provided by the disk test are readily understood by clinicians. Instrumentation is now available for reading and interpreting inhibition zone diameters, as well as storing this information, and may reduce interobserver reading errors (28, 32).

Advantages of the microdilution and agar gradient diffusion methods include the generation of a quantitative result (i.e., an MIC) rather than a category result, the ability to test accurately some anaerobic or fastidious species that may not be tested by the disk diffusion method (6, 8, 11, 22, 25), and the ancillary benefits of computer systems that accompany many of the microdilution and automated systems (22). Indeed, computerized data management systems are very important in laboratories that may have limited or inflexible laboratory information systems. However, an MIC method should not be chosen on the basis that MICs are routinely more useful to physicians. There is no clear evidence that MICs are more relevant than susceptibility category results to the selection of appropriate antibacterial therapy for most infections (17).

A laboratory may choose to perform rapid, automated antibacterial susceptibility testing in order to generate results faster than manual methods can generate them. The provision of susceptibility results 1 day sooner than that provided by conventional methods seems a logical advance in patient care. Two studies have demonstrated both the clinical and economic benefits derived from the use of rapid susceptibility testing and reporting (2, 19), while a further study has not shown such a benefit (4). However, rapid susceptibility testing results may not have substantial impact unless the laboratory uses more aggressive means of communication to make physicians aware of the results (43). This may be because physicians have come to expect antimicrobial susceptibility testing results approximately 48 h after the submission of a specimen or because the results, although generated more rapidly, are still not available soon enough to assist with the initial selection of antimicrobial therapy.

A previously cited shortcoming of rapid susceptibility testing methods was the failure to detect some inducible or subtle resistance mechanisms (21, 28, 41, 42). However, the instruments most notorious for such problems are no longer marketed and the manufacturers of the remaining instruments have made substantial efforts to correct earlier problems (29, 35, 39, 44) or to extend testing to include fastidious organisms (24). It is important to emphasize that accuracy should not be sacrificed in an effort to generate a rapid susceptibility testing result.

SELECTING ANTIBACTERIAL AGENTS FOR ROUTINE TESTING

The laboratory has the responsibility to test and report on the antimicrobial agents that are most appropriate for the organism isolated, the site of infection, and the clinical practice setting in which the laboratory functions. The battery of antimicrobial agents routinely tested and reported on by the laboratory will depend on the characteristics of the patients under care in the institution and the likelihood of encountering highly resistant organisms (23). A laboratory serving a tertiary-care medical center, which specializes in the care of immunosuppressed patients, may need to test routinely agents that are broader in spectrum than those tested by a laboratory that supports a primary-care outpatient practice in which antibiotic-resistant organisms are less commonly encountered.

When a laboratory's routine susceptibility testing batteries are determined, several principles should be followed. First, the antimicrobial agents that are included in the institution's formulary and that physicians prescribe on a daily basis should be tested. Second, the species tested strongly influences the choice of antimicrobial agents for testing. The CLSI publishes tables that list the antimicrobial agents appropriate for testing against various groups of aerobic and fastidious bacteria (13). The guidelines indicate the drugs that are most appropriate for testing against each organism group and for treatment based upon the specimen source (e.g., cerebrospinal fluid, blood, urine, or feces). The lists also include a few agents that may be tested as surrogates for other agents because of the greater ability of a particular agent to detect resistance to closely related drugs (e.g., the use of the cefoxitin disk test to predict overall β-lactam resistance in staphylococci) (13). This initial list of agents must be tailored to an individual institution's specific needs through discussions with infectious disease physicians, pharmacists, and committees concerned with infection control and the institutional formulary (23).

A third important step in defining routine testing batteries is ascertaining the availability of specific antimicrobial agents for testing by the laboratory's routine testing methodology. Certain methods (e.g., the disk diffusion, gradient diffusion, and in-house-prepared broth and agar dilution methods) allow the greatest flexibility in the selection of test batteries. In contrast, some commercial systems may have less flexibility or delays in adding the latest antimicrobial agents approved for clinical use. However, practicality limits the maximum number of drugs that can be tested simultaneously with an isolate by any susceptibility testing method. For example, a maximum of 12 disks can be placed on a 150-mm-diameter Mueller-Hinton agar plate and a similar number can ordinarily be accommodated in a microdilution panel if full concentration ranges of each agent are to be included for routine determination of MICs. Some commercial test panels attempt to resolve this problem by testing a larger array of antimicrobial agents, although in a very limited concentration range (perhaps two to four dilutions for each agent).

ESTABLISHING SUSCEPTIBILITY BREAKPOINTS

There is general agreement that the MIC is the most basic laboratory measurement of the activity of an antimicrobial agent against an organism. It is defined as the lowest concentration that will inhibit the growth of a test organism over a defined interval related to the organism's growth rate, most commonly 18 to 24 h. The MIC is the fundamental measurement that forms the basis of most susceptibility testing methods and against which the levels of drug achieved in human body fluids may be compared to determine breakpoints for defining susceptibility.

The conventional technique for measuring the MIC involves exposing the test organism to a series of twofold dilutions of the antimicrobial agent in a suitable culture system, e.g., broth or agar for bacteria. The twofold dilution scheme was originally used because of the convenience of preparing dilutions from a single starting concentration in broth or agar dilution methods. Subsequently, this system proved to be meaningful because an antibiotic's MICs for a single bacterial species in the absence of resistance mechanisms have a statistically normal distribution when plotted on a logarithmic scale. This provides investigators with the opportunity to examine the distributions of MICs for bacterial populations and distinguish strains for which MICs are abnormally high (potentially resistant strains) from those for which MICs are normal (susceptible strains) (26).

MIC measurements are influenced in vitro by a number of factors, including the composition of the medium, the size of the inoculum, the duration of incubation, and the presence of resistant subpopulations of the organism. The in vitro test conditions also do not encompass other factors that can have an influence on in vivo antimicrobial activity. These include sub-MIC effects, postantibiotic effects, protein binding, effects on organism virulence or toxin production, variations in redox potential at sites of infection, and the pharmacokinetic changes resulting from different drug levels in blood and at the site of infection over time. Nevertheless, if determined under standardized conditions, MIC measurements provide a fixed reference point for the setting of pharmacodynamic breakpoints with the power to predict efficacy in vivo. Pharmacological breakpoints can be applied directly to routine dilution testing methods that generate MICs, such as broth microdilution, agar dilution, gradient methods, and some automated instruments. They also provide reference values for deriving breakpoints for disk diffusion methods. Breakpoints (or interpretative criteria) are the values that determine the categories of susceptible, intermediate, and resistant. The approach to setting breakpoints varies by organization or regulatory body, but with few exceptions it is based on the agent's MICs. Depending on the approach taken, up to four sources of data can be examined in establishing breakpoints.

MIC Distributions

Examination of MIC distributions can indicate the range of MICs for a population of strains that lack any known mechanisms of resistance to the particular drug. These distributions may aid in the recognition of new resistance mechanisms by highlighting strains for which the MICs fall outside the normal distribution. However, the distributions of MICs have limited direct application since they vary between species, and for some strains for which the MICs are outside the normal range, the MICs may be below clinically derived breakpoints. Such strains may or may not respond to treatment. An example of the latter point is the fact that the penicillin MICs for some β-lactamase-producing organisms and the expanded-spectrum cephalosporin MICs for extended-spectrum β-lactamase-producing gram-negative bacilli may be relatively low but do not translate to reliable clinical efficacy. Indeed, knowledge of the presence of specific resistance mechanisms that inactivate compounds of a particular drug class is very useful in deriving microbiological breakpoints.

Pharmacokinetics and Pharmacodynamics

Pharmacokinetics examines the absorption, distribution, accumulation, and elimination (metabolism and excretion) of a drug in the body over time. These parameters are usually determined with healthy volunteers. A drug's MICs can be compared with the concentration of the drug achievable in blood or other body fluids (e.g., cerebrospinal fluid). In the past, breakpoints were chosen generally such that the MICs for susceptible pathogens would be exceeded by the drug level for most or all of the dosing interval. Newer data now considered when establishing breakpoints include pharmacodynamic calculations. Pharmacodynamics is the study of the time course of drug action against the microorganism. For antimicrobial agents, the desired action is pathogen eradication. In vitro pharmacodynamic studies have revealed that agents fall into three classes: those with principally time-dependent antimicrobial action and no or short postantibiotic effects, those with time-dependent action and long postantibiotic effects, and those with prominent concentration-dependent action (17). For drugs with time-dependent action and no or short postantibiotic effects, the critical determinant of bacterial killing in vivo is the percentage of time in a dosing interval that the drug concentration is above the MIC. For the other two classes, the important determinant is the ratio of the area under the concentration-time curve to the MIC and/or the ratio of the peak concentration to the MIC. For β-lactams, short-acting macrolides, and clindamycin, the relevant measure is the percentage of time that the drug concentration is above the MIC, and the ratio of the area under the concentration-time curve or of the peak concentration to the MIC is the relevant parameter for aminoglycosides, long-acting macrolides, tetracyclines, glycopeptides, and fluoroquinolones (18). These values can be used to calculate the maximum MICs or breakpoints that would allow the achievement of optimum efficacy with standard drug dosing schedules.

Clinical and Bacteriological Response Rates

During clinical trials, the clinical and/or bacteriologic eradication response rates of organisms for which the MICs of new antimicrobial agents have been determined give an indication of the relevance of breakpoints selected by using the MIC distributions and the pharmacokinetic-pharmacodynamic properties of the drug. Response rates of at least 80% may be expected for organisms classified as susceptible, although the rates may be lower depending on the site and type of infection. While in some countries breakpoints are determined primarily from clinical and bacteriological response rates, the CLSI evaluates clinical and bacteriological response rates in conjunction with population distributions and pharmacokinetics and pharmacodynamics in establishing the breakpoints in an attempt to provide the best correlation between in vitro test results and clinical outcome (7).

Inhibition Zone Diameter Distributions for Disk Diffusion Methods

Once the MIC breakpoints are selected, disk diffusion breakpoints can be chosen by plotting the inhibition zone diameters against the MICs derived from the testing of a large number of strains of various species. A statistical approach that uses the linear regression formula may be used to calculate the appropriate zone diameter intercepts for the predetermined MIC breakpoints. An alternative, pragmatic approach to deriving disk diffusion breakpoints is the use of the error rate-bounded method, in which the zone diameter criteria are selected on the basis of the minimization of the disk interpretive errors, especially the very major errors (5, 34) (Fig. 1). Newer statistical techniques are being studied to improve correlation with MICs (16). The newest CLSI approach focuses on the rate of interpretive errors near the proposed breakpoint versus those with MICs more than a single $\log_2$ dilution from the MIC breakpoints (7). The concept is that errors that occur with isolates for which MICs are very close to the MIC breakpoints are less of a concern than errors that occur with more highly resistant or susceptible strains.

Breakpoints derived by professional groups or regulatory bodies in various countries are often quite similar. For instance, there are a small number of breakpoint discrepancies between the CLSI and the U.S. Food and Drug Administration, which are under review by both groups. Also, there can be notable differences in the breakpoints used in different countries or regions for the same agents. The reasons for the differences may be that certain countries use different dosages or administration intervals for some drugs. In addition, some countries are more conservative in assessing the susceptibility to antimicrobial agents and place greater emphasis on the detection of emerging resistance, noted primarily by examination of microorganism population distributions. Technical factors such as the inoculum density, atmosphere of incubation, and test medium can also affect MICs and zone diameters, thereby justifying different interpretive criteria in some countries. These technical differences are summarized in chapter 73 of this Manual. Two non-U.S. methods minimize or avoid the use of an intermediate category of susceptibility based on the rationale that such results are of little value to the clinician (3, 31). The lack of a buffer between susceptible and resistant categories can result in higher rates of incorrect categorization. It may be safer for a laboratory to employ a method that uses an intermediate category or, if not, to report intermediate results as resistant.

Information on a range of international susceptibility testing methods and/or breakpoints can be downloaded or purchased from the following websites: the CLSI website at http://www.clsi.org; the European Committee on Antimicrobial Susceptibility Testing website at http://www.eucast.org; the British Society for Antimicrobial Chemotherapy website at http://www.bsac.org.uk; the Société Française de Microbiologie website at http://www.sfm.asso.fr/; the Deutsches Institut für Normung website at http://www.beuth.de/; the Swedish Reference Group for Antibiotics website at http://www.srga.org; a website featuring the Danish commercial disk diffusion method at http://www.rosco.dk; and a website featuring the Australian calibrated dichotomous sensitivity (CDS) disk diffusion method at http://www.med.unsw.edu.au/pathology-cds/.

FUTURE DIRECTIONS AND NEEDS IN ANTIMICROBIAL SUSCEPTIBILITY TESTING

Antimicrobial resistance is becoming widespread among a variety of clinically significant bacterial species (40, 45). Therefore, the microbiology laboratory plays a key role in the patient management process by providing accurate data on which physicians can base therapy decisions. Susceptibility testing results, however, are also used by investigators in surveillance studies and by infection control practitioners to detect and control the spread of antibiotic-resistant organisms (9, 38). Surveillance can be performed at the laboratory, local, regional, national, and international levels through direct interchange of data from laboratory information systems to centralized databases (37). Thus, the

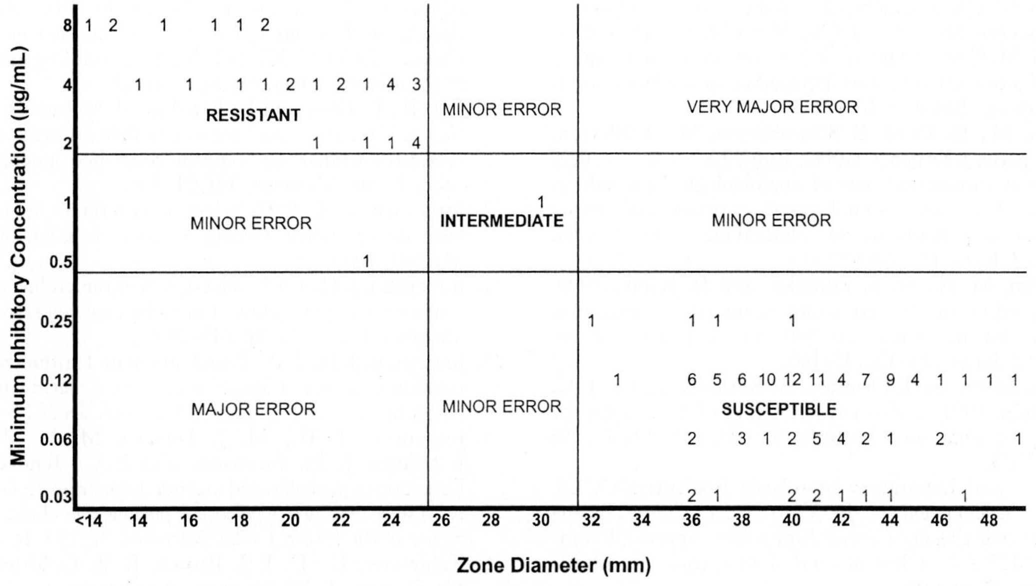

FIGURE 1 Comparison of zone diameters with MICs of a hypothetical antimicrobial agent.

accuracy of stored results becomes almost as important as the accuracy of test performance and interpretation.

To meet these challenges and responsibilities, clinical microbiologists must continuously assess and update their susceptibility testing strategies. The first priority is to use accurate and reliable methods, whether they are conventional or perhaps newer molecular methods. Then, careful monitoring of test performance with well-characterized control strains that challenge the capability of the testing methods becomes essential. Today, laboratories must use a variety of testing methods, each tailored specifically to a particular species or group of organisms. It is not likely that a single method, whether conventional or commercial, will be optimal for all antimicrobial agents, organisms, and resistance mechanisms. This will require increased education and training for clinical microbiologists in the future. Some assistance may be sought from the computer-based "expert" systems that allow a rapid and accurate view of antimicrobial susceptibility profiles and recognition of potentially aberrant results or novel resistance mechanisms (15, 39). Rapid progress is also being made on molecular methods that are starting to have practical application in the routine clinical laboratory (1, 30, 33; chapter 78).

More effective means of conveying critical antimicrobial susceptibility testing information to clinicians in a time frame that allows efficient and effective management of patients and in a format that is unambiguous to clinicians in various practice specialties are still needed. Clinical microbiologists should become more proactive in the reporting of antimicrobial susceptibility results and in cross-linking that information to other databases (e.g., those for pharmacy prescriptions) to ensure that patients receive the most efficacious cost-effective therapy.

REFERENCES

1. **Allaouchiche, B., H. Jaumain, G. Zambardi, D. Chassard, and J. Freney.** 1999. Clinical impact of rapid oxacillin susceptibility testing using a PCR assay in *Staphylococcus aureus* bacteraemia. *J. Infect.* **39:**198–204.
2. **Barenfanger, J., C. Drake, and G. Kacich.** 1999. Clinical and financial benefits of rapid identification and antimicrobial susceptibility testing. *J. Clin. Microbiol.* **37:**1415–1418.
3. **Bell, S. M.** 1988. Additions and modifications to the range of antibiotics tested by the CDS method of antibiotic sensitivity testing. *Pathology* **20:**303–304.
4. **Bruins, M., H. Oord, P. Bloembergen, M. Wolfhagen, A. Casparie, J. Degener, and G. Ruijs.** 2005. Lack of effect of shorter turnaround time of microbiological procedures on clinical outcomes: a randomised controlled trial among hospitalised patients in the Netherlands. *Eur. J. Clin. Microbiol. Infect. Dis.* **24:**305–313.
5. **Brunden, M. N., G. E. Zurenko, and B. Kapik.** 1992. Modification of the error-rate bounded classification scheme for use with two MIC break points. *Diagn. Microbiol. Infect. Dis.* **15:**135–140.
6. **Citron, D. M., M. I. Ostoravi, A. Karlsson, and E. J. C. Goldstein.** 1991. Evaluation of the E test for susceptibility testing of anaerobic bacteria. *J. Clin. Microbiol.* **29:**2197–2203.
7. **Clinical and Laboratory Standards Institute/NCCLS.** 2001. *Development of In Vitro Susceptibility Testing Criteria and Quality Control Parameters.* Approved standard M23-A2. Clinical and Laboratory Standards Institute, Wayne, Pa.
8. **Clinical and Laboratory Standards Institute/NCCLS.** 2001. *Methods for Antimicrobial Susceptibility Testing of Anaerobic Bacteria.* Approved standard M11-A5. Clinical and Laboratory Standards Institute, Wayne, Pa.
9. **Clinical and Laboratory Standards Institute/NCCLS.** 2005. *Analysis and Presentation of Cumulative Antimicrobial Susceptibility Test Data.* Approved guideline M39-A2. Clinical and Laboratory Standards Institute, Wayne, Pa.
10. **Clinical and Laboratory Standards Institute/NCCLS.** 2005. *Methods for Antimicrobial Dilution and Disk Susceptibility Testing of Infrequently-Isolated or Fastidious Bacteria.* Proposed guideline M45-P. Clinical and Laboratory Standards Institute, Wayne, Pa.
11. **Clinical and Laboratory Standards Institute/NCCLS.** 2006. *Methods for Dilution Antimicrobial Susceptibility Tests for Bacteria That Grow Aerobically.* Approved standard M7-A6. Clinical and Laboratory Standards Institute, Wayne, Pa.
12. **Clinical and Laboratory Standards Institute/NCCLS.** 2006. *Performance Standards for Antimicrobial Disk Susceptibility Tests.* Approved standard M2-A8. Clinical and Laboratory Standards Institute, Wayne, Pa.
13. **Clinical and Laboratory Standards Institute/NCCLS.** 2006. *Performance Standards for Antimicrobial Susceptibility Testing.* Supplement M100-S16. Clinical and Laboratory Standards Institute, Wayne, Pa.
14. Reference deleted.
15. **Courvalin, P.** 1992. Interpretive reading of antimicrobial susceptibility tests. *ASM News* **58:**368–375.
16. **Craig, B. A.** 2000. Modeling approach to diameter breakpoint determination. *Diagn. Microbiol. Infect. Dis.* **36:**193–202.
17. **Craig, W. A.** 2002. Pharmacodynamics of antimicrobials: general concepts and applications, p. 1–22. *In* C. H. Nightingale, T. Murakawa, and P. G. Ambrose (ed.), *Antimicrobial Pharmacodynamics in Theory and Clinical Practice.* Marcel Dekker, New York, N.Y.
18. **Craig, W. A.** 1998. Pharmacokinetic/pharmacodynamic parameters: rationale for antibacterial dosing of mice and men. *Clin. Infect. Dis.* **26:**1–10.
19. **Doern, G. V., R. Vautour, M. Gaudet, and B. Levy.** 1994. Clinical impact of rapid in vitro antimicrobial susceptibility testing and bacterial identification. *J. Clin. Microbiol.* **32:**1757–1762.
20. **International Organization for Standardization.** 2006. *Susceptibility Testing of Infectious Agents and Evaluation of Performance of Antimicrobial Susceptibility Devices,* part 1. *Reference Method for Testing the In Vitro Activity of Antimicrobial Agents against Bacteria Involved in Infectious Diseases.* ISO/DIS 20776-1. International Organization for Standardization, Geneva, Switzerland.
21. **Jett, B., L. Free, and D. F. Sahm.** 1996. Factors influencing the Vitek gram-positive susceptibility system's detection of *vanB*-encoded vancomycin resistance among enterococci. *J. Clin. Microbiol.* **34:**701–706.
22. **Jorgensen, J. H.** 1993. Selection criteria for an antimicrobial susceptibility testing system. *J. Clin. Microbiol.* **31:**2841–2844.
23. **Jorgensen, J. H.** 1993. Selection of antimicrobial agents for routine testing in a clinical microbiology laboratory. *Diagn. Microbiol. Infect. Dis.* **16:**245–249.
24. **Jorgensen, J. H.** 2000. Rapid automated antimicrobial susceptibility testing of *Streptococcus pneumoniae* by use of the bioMerieux VITEK 2. *J. Clin. Microbiol.* **38:**2814–2818.
25. **Jorgensen, J. H., M. J. Ferraro, M. L. McElmeel, J. Spargo, J. M. Swenson, and F. C. Tenover.** 1994. Detection of penicillin and extended-spectrum cephalosporin resistance among *Streptococcus pneumoniae* clinical isolates by use of the E test. *J. Clin. Microbiol.* **32:**159–163.
26. **Kahlmeter, G., D. F. J. Brown, F. W. Goldstein, A. P. MacGowan, J. W. Mouton, A. Österland, A. Rodloff, M. Steinbakk, P. Urbanskova, and A. Vatopoulos.** 2003. European harmonization of MIC breakpoints for

antimicrobial susceptibility testing of bacteria. *J. Antimicrob. Chemother.* **52:**145–148.

27. **Katsanis, G. P., J. Spargo, M. J. Ferraro, L. Sutton, and G. A. Jacoby.** 1994. Detection of *Klebsiella pneumoniae* and *Escherichia coli* strains producing extended-spectrum β-lactamases. *J. Clin. Microbiol.* **32:**691–696.
28. **Korgenski, E. K., and J. A. Daly.** 1998. Evaluation of the BIOMIC video reader system for determining interpretive categories of isolates on the basis of disk diffusion susceptibility results. *J. Clin. Microbiol.* **36:**302–304.
29. **Ling, T. K. W., P. C. Tam, Z. K. Liu, and A. F. B. Cheng.** 2001. Evaluation of VITEK 2 rapid identification and susceptibility testing system against gram-negative clinical isolates. *J. Clin. Microbiol.* **39:**2964–2966.
30. **Louie, L., S. O. Matsumura, E. Choi, M. Louie, and A. E. Simor.** 2000. Evaluation of three rapid methods for detection of methicillin resistance in *Staphylococcus aureus*. *J. Clin. Microbiol.* **38:**2170–2173.
31. **MacGowan, A. P., and R. Wise.** 2001. Establishing MIC breakpoints and the interpretation of in vitro susceptibility tests. *J. Antimicrob. Chemother.* **48**(Suppl. S1)**:**17–28.
32. **Madeiros, A., and J. Crellin.** 2000. Evaluation of the Sirscan automated zone reader in a clinical microbiology laboratory. *J. Clin. Microbiol.* **38:**1688–1693.
33. **Martineau, F., F. J. Picard, L. Grenier, P. H. Roy, M. Ouellette, and M. G. Bergeron.** 2000. Multiplex PCR assays for the detection of clinically relevant antibiotic resistance genes in staphylococci isolated from patients infected after cardiac surgery. The ESPRIT Trial. *J. Antimicrob. Chemother.* **46:**527–534.
34. **Metzler, D. M., and R. M. DeHaan.** 1974. Susceptibility tests of anaerobic bacteria: statistical and clinical considerations. *J. Infect. Dis.* **130:**588–594.
35. **Nadler, H. L., C. Dolan, L. Mele, and S. R. Kurtz.** 1985. Accuracy and reproducibility of the AutoMicrobic System Gram-Negative General Susceptibility-Plus card for testing selected challenge organisms. *J. Clin. Microbiol.* **22:**355–360.
36. **Rex, J. H., and M. A. Pfaller.** 2002. Has antifungal susceptibility testing come of age? *Clin. Infect. Dis.* **35:**982–989.
37. **Sahm, D. F., J. A. Karlowsky, L. J. Kelly, I. A. Critchley, M. E. Jones, C. Thornsberry, Y. Mauriz, and J. Kahn.** 2001. Need for annual surveillance of antimicrobial resistance in *Streptococcus pneumoniae* in the United States: 2-year longitudinal analysis. *Antimicrob. Agents Chemother.* **45:**1037–1042.
38. **Sahm, D. F., and F. C. Tenover.** 1997. Surveillance for the emergence and dissemination of antimicrobial resistance in bacteria, p. 767–785. *In* F. C. Tenover and J. E. McGowan (ed.), *Infectious Disease Clinics of North America*, vol. 11, no. 4. *Antimicrobial Resistance.* The W. B. Saunders Co., Philadelphia, Pa.
39. **Sanders, C. C., M. Peyret, E. S. Moland, S. J. Cavalieri, C. Shubert, K. S. Thomson, J.-M. Boeufgras, and W. E. Sanders, Jr.** 2001. Potential impact of the VITEK 2 system and the Advanced Expert System on the clinical laboratory of a university-based hospital. *J. Clin. Microbiol.* **39:** 2379–2385.
40. **Tenover, F. C.** 2001. Development and spread of bacterial resistance to antimicrobial agents. An overview. *Clin. Infect. Dis.* **15**(Suppl.)**:**S108–S115.
41. **Tenover, F. C., J. M. Swenson, C. O'Hara, and S. A. Stocker.** 1995. Ability of commercial and reference antimicrobial susceptibility testing methods to detect vancomycin resistance in enterococci. *J. Clin. Microbiol.* **33:**1524–1527.
42. **Tenover, F. C., J. Tokars, J. Swenson, S. Paul, K. Splitalny, and W. Jarvis.** 1993. Ability of clinical laboratories to detect antimicrobial-resistant enterococci. *J. Clin. Microbiol.* **31:**1695–1699.
43. **Trenholme, G. M., R. L. Kaplan, P. H. Karahusis, T. Stine, J. Fuhrer, W. Landau, and S. Levin.** 1989. Clinical impact of rapid identification and susceptibility testing of bacterial blood culture isolates. *J. Clin. Microbiol.* **27:** 1342–1345.
44. **Washington, J. A., C. C. Knapp, and C. C. Sanders.** 1988. Accuracy of microdilution and the AutoMicrobic System in detection of β-lactam resistance in gram-negative bacterial mutants with derepressed β-lactamase. *Rev. Infect. Dis.* **10:**824–829.
45. **Williams, R. M.** 2001. Globalization of antimicrobial resistance: epidemiological challenges. *Clin. Infect. Dis.* **15**(Suppl.)**:**S116–S117.

Susceptibility Test Methods: Dilution and Disk Diffusion Methods

JAMES H. JORGENSEN AND JOHN D. TURNIDGE

73

A number of methods can be used to perform antimicrobial susceptibility tests in a clinical laboratory setting or for research purposes, such as assessing the activities of new antimicrobial agents. Susceptibility testing can be performed reliably by using broth or agar dilution tests or agar diffusion methods. The choice of methodology to be used in individual laboratories may be based on factors such as relative ease of performance, cost, flexibility in selection of drugs for testing, use of automated or semiautomated devices to facilitate testing, and the perceived accuracy of the methodology (54, 55, 57). A misconception has existed regarding the clinical relevance of determining and routinely reporting MICs versus the interpretive category results (i.e., susceptible, intermediate, or resistant) that are derived using the disk diffusion method. This misconception may have been based on the assumption that the dilution test is the inherently more accurate of the two methods. Since there is a direct relationship between the sizes of the zones of inhibition and the MICs with most drugs and since MICs and zone diameters for reference strains have similar interlaboratory and intralaboratory reproducibilities, there is little objective evidence that one method is more accurate than the other with the majority of common, rapidly growing bacteria (29, 55). While an MIC may be perceived as more accurate than a result from a disk test, the MIC generated using the standard doubling-dilution series may be a concentration somewhere between the concentration inhibiting the organism and the next lower concentration tested (i.e., usually 1 $\log_2$ dilution lower). For example, an organism may grow in the presence of an antimicrobial agent at a concentration of 4 μg/ml but not at 8 μg/ml. The actual MIC could be anywhere between 4 and 8 μg/ml. Despite our statement that MICs are not inherently more accurate, there are some species with resistance mechanisms that may not be reliably detected by standard disk testing (e.g., vancomycin-intermediate *Staphylococcus aureus*) (47, 80), some species for which the standard disk test is not well calibrated (e.g., *Stenotrophomonas maltophilia* and *Burkholderia cepacia*), some species for which no disk test standards exist (e.g., *Corynebacterium* spp. and *Bacillus* spp.) (24), a few drugs that do not appear to diffuse well in agar (e.g., colistin, polymyxin B, and daptomycin) (43, 44), and some species with mechanisms of diminished susceptibility for which MICs are needed to guide selection of therapy and appropriate dosing (e.g., penicillin- and cephalosporin-intermediate *Streptococcus pneumoniae*) (29, 58). However, there are a few instances in which disk testing may provide superior detection of some resistance mechanisms, e.g., use of the cefoxitin disk test to screen for *mecA*-mediated oxacillin resistance in staphylococci (78) and disk approximation testing to detect inducible clindamycin resistance in staphylococci and streptococci (61).

There may also be the misconception that physicians prefer a quantitative (MIC) result rather than a report of a susceptibility category. To the contrary, few physicians other than those who specialize in infectious diseases have the training or experience to reliably interpret MICs. For that reason, the laboratory is obliged to provide a category interpretation (susceptible, intermediate, or resistant) with each MIC result in order to avoid potential misinterpretation of the data (25). There may be only a limited number of specific clinical indications for determining MICs to assist in patient management. These include primarily testing of isolates from patients with endocarditis or osteomyelitis (29). At this time, the pharmacodynamic principles that relate to the importance of the levels of antibiotic in serum or body fluid in relation to the MIC for an organism are useful in determining interpretive breakpoints but are not generally used to optimize therapy of individual patients (30). For research purposes, MICs are useful for evaluating relative degrees of susceptibility of bacteria to various antimicrobial agents and for ranking the activities of drugs against various species. For clinical laboratory purposes, however, the decision as to whether to perform dilution or disk diffusion testing is usually based on logistical reasons, including ease of performance of a method, its cost, and factors such as selection of a system that can provide identification of common bacteria in addition to susceptibility testing (57). Several commercial systems are now available for performing susceptibility testing; however, a major challenge posed by such systems is the relative inflexibility of standard panels of antimicrobial agents that can be tested. The inability to match precisely an institution's antimicrobial agent formulary with drugs readily available in commercial systems has led some laboratories to adopt or retain the highly flexible disk diffusion test for routine use (56).

The selection of antibacterial agents for testing is complicated by the large number of agents available today and the diversity of institutional formularies. Some of these compounds, however, exhibit similar if not identical activities in vitro, so that in some cases, one compound can be tested as a surrogate to represent one or more closely related compounds. Such extrapolations, which have generally been agreed upon internationally, are listed in Table 1. Use of these drug surrogates can substantially reduce the number of agents required for testing and in some cases provide necessary flexibility in adapting commercial test systems for routine use in a variety of institutions. For instance, the susceptibility of *Staphylococcus* spp. to oxacillin (or cefoxitin) can be extrapolated to apply to all currently available penicillinase-stable penicillins, cephalosporins, and carbapenems. It is thus unnecessary to test any of the agents in these chemical classes, with the exception of the beta-lactamase-labile compounds (e.g., penicillin, ampicillin, amoxicillin, and piperacillin) represented by penicillin itself (25, 26). Other extrapolations are possible, especially if there is demonstrated susceptibility to a less potent member of the chemical class of antimicrobial agent.

It is important that the microbiologist work with the hospital formulary committee to ensure that the antibacterial agents being tested in the laboratory reflect those in the institution's current formulary (56). Failure to do so can contribute to antibiotic misuse (36). Guidelines for the selection of antibacterial agents to be tested routinely are published annually by the Clinical and Laboratory Standards Institute (CLSI; formerly called the NCCLS) (27) and are summarized in Table 2. While this listing is sometimes regarded rigidly as the standard for selecting the agents that must be tested, it is a list of agents that should be considered for routine testing only, and many variables go into the decision as to which agents should be tested in any particular setting (56). The CLSI also cautions that the decision about testing and reporting of some agents selectively should be made by the clinical microbiologist in conjunction with the infectious disease practitioners, the pharmacy, and/or the infection control committees (25, 26, 27).

DILUTION METHODS

Broth or agar dilution susceptibility testing methods are used to determine the minimal concentration, usually in micrograms per milliliter, of an antimicrobial agent required to inhibit or kill a microorganism. Antimicrobial agents are usually tested at $\log_2$ (twofold) serial dilutions, and the lowest concentration that inhibits visible growth of an organism is regarded as the MIC. The concentration range used may vary with the drug, the organism being tested, and the site of infection. Ranges should encompass the concentrations defining the interpretive categories (i.e., susceptible, intermediate, and resistant) and also the ranges that include the expected MICs for quality control reference strains. Other dilution methods include those that test a single concentration or a selected few concentrations of antimicrobial agents (i.e., breakpoint susceptibility tests and single-drug-concentration screens; see below).

Dilution methods offer flexibility in the sense that the standard medium used to test frequently encountered organisms (e.g., staphylococci, enterococci, members of the family *Enterobacteriaceae,* and *Pseudomonas aeruginosa*) may be supplemented or even replaced with another medium to allow accurate testing of certain fastidious bacterial species that may not be reliably tested by disk diffusion. Dilution methods are also readily adaptable to automated test systems.

DILUTION TESTING: AGAR METHOD

Dilution of Antimicrobial Agents

The solvents and diluents needed to prepare stock solutions of most commonly used antimicrobial agents are listed in the CLSI document on dilution testing (25).

TABLE 1 Antibacterial susceptibility results that may be extrapolated from other test results

Test drug (result)	Organism(s)	Drugs for which result can be extrapolated
Penicillin G	*Staphylococcus* spp., *Neisseria gonorrhoeae*	Phenoxymethylpenicillin, phenethicillin, ampicillin, amoxicillin, bacampicillin, cyclacillin, hetacillin, carbenicillin, mezlocillin, azlocillin, ticarcillin, piperacillin
Ampicillin	All	Amoxicillin, bacampicillin, cyclacillin, hetacillin
Ampicillin	*Enterococcus* spp.	Penicillin
Oxacillin	*Staphylococcus* spp.	All penicillins including antistaphylococcal penicillins, all cephalosporins, all beta-lactamase inhibitor combinations, all carbapenems, loracarbef
Cephalothin	*Enterobacteriaceae*	Cephapirin, cephradine, cephalexin, cefaclor, and cefadroxil but not other cephalosporins
Erythromycin	Gram-positive cocci	Azithromycin, clarithromycin, dirithromycin, roxithromyxin
Clindamycin	All	Lincomycin
Tetracycline	All (except *Staphylococcus*, *Enterococcus*, and *Acinetobacter* spp.)	Doxycycline, minocycline chlortetracycline, demeclocycline, oxytetracycline, methacycline
Sulfisoxazole	All	All sulfonamides
Cephalothin or cefazolin (susceptible)	*Enterobacteriaceae*	Susceptibility to broad-spectrum cephalosporins

TABLE 2 Antimicrobial agents recommended for routine dilution and disk diffusion susceptibility testing[a]

Antimicrobial agent	Group[b] recommended for testing with:						
	Enterobacteriaceae	*Pseudomonas* spp. and other non-*Enterobacteriaceae*[c]	*Acinetobacter* spp.[c]	*Burkholderia cepacia*[c]	*Stenotrophomonas maltophilia*[c]	Staphylococci	Enterococci
Penicillins							
Penicillin G						A	A[e]
Ampicillin	A						A[d,e]
Oxacillin[f] or methicillin						A	
Ticarcillin[d]	B	A	B				
Mezlocillin[d]	B	A	B				
Piperacillin[d]	B	A	B				
Ampicillin-sulbactam	B		B				
Amoxicillin-clavulanic acid	B						
Piperacillin-tazobactam	B	B	B				
Ticarcillin-clavulanic acid	B	B[g]	B	B	B		
Cephalosporins							
Cephalothin	A[h]						
Cefazolin	A						
Cefamandole	B						
Cefonicid	B						
Cefuroxime	B						
Cefmetazole	B						
Cefoperazone	B	B					
Cefoxitin	B						
Cefotetan	B						
Cefotaxime	B		B				
Ceftriaxone	B		B				
Ceftizoxime	B	U					
Ceftazidime	C	A	A	B	B		
Cefepime	B	B	B				
Other beta-lactams							
Ertapenem	B						
Imipenem	B	B	A				
Meropenem	B	B	A	B			
Aztreonam	C	B					
Aminogylcosides[h]							
Gentamicin	A	A	B			C	C[i]
Netilmicin	C	C					
Tobramycin	C	B	B				
Amikacin	B	B	B				
Streptomycin							C[i]

Macrolides							
Azithromycin						B	
Clarithromycin						B	
Erythromycin						B	C
Quinolones							
Ciprofloxacin	B	B	B			C	U
Gatifloxacin	U		B			C	
Levofloxacin	B	U	B	B	B	C	U
Lomefloxacin	U	U				U	
Moxifloxacin						C	
Norfloxacin	U	U				U	U
Ofloxacin	U	U				C	
Miscellaneous							
Chloramphenicol	C	C		B	B	C	C
Clindamycin						B	
Daptomycin						B	B
Doxycline			B				
Linezolid						B	B
Minocycline			B	B	B		
Nitrofurantoin	U					U	U
Polymyxin			C				
Quinupristin-dalfopristin						C	B
Rifampin						C	C
Sulfisoxazole	U					U	
Tetracycline	C	U[j]	B[j]			C	U
Telithromycin						B	
Trimethoprim-sulfamethoxazole	B	B	B	A	A	B	
Trimethoprim	U					U	
Vancomycin						B	B[e]

[a] Modified from the CLSI informational supplement (27) with permission. Current standards and supplements to them may be obtained from the CLSI, 940 West Valley Rd., Suite 1400, Wayne, PA 19087-1898.

[b] Group A comprises primary drugs to be tested and reported, group B comprises those to be tested as primary drugs but reported selectively, group C comprises supplemental drugs to be reported selectively, and group U comprises drugs to be tested with urinary isolates only.

[c] Some agents should be tested only by using an MIC method and not by using disk diffusion. See the latest CLSI standards for specific examples.

[d] Results of tests with penicillin apply to other penicillins (e.g., ampicillin, amoxicillin, carboxypenicillins, and ureidopenicillins) against beta-lactamase-negative enterococci.

[e] Combination therapy consisting of penicillin, ampicillin, or vancomycin and an aminoglycoside is recommended.

[f] Staphylococci resistant to the penicillinase-resistant penicillins should also be considered resistant to penicillins, beta-lactam-beta-lactamase-inactivating combinations, cephalosporins, and carbapenems.

[g] Ticarcillin-clavulanic acid or piperacillin-tazobactam should not be considered a therapeutic alternative for *P. aeruginosa* isolates resistant to carboxy- or ureidopenicillins.

[h] Cephalothin test results may also be used to represent those for cephapirin, cephradine, cephalexin, cefaclor, cefadroxil, and cefazolin (except against the *Enterobacteriaceae*). Cefuroxime, cefixime, cefpodoxime, cefprozil, ceftibuten, and loracarbef may be tested separately on a supplemental basis because their activities may be greater than those of cephalothin or cefazolin against the *Enterobacteriaceae*.

[i] For use of aminoglycosides to screen enterococci for synergy resistance, see the section "Breakpoint Susceptibility Tests" and "Resistance Screens."

[j] Doxycycline or minocycline may be tested on a supplemental basis because of their greater activities against some nonfermentative gram-negative bacilli and staphylococci.

Preparation, Supplementation, and Storage of Media

Mueller-Hinton agar is the recommended medium for testing most commonly encountered aerobic and facultatively anaerobic bacteria (25). The dehydrated agar base is commercially available and should be prepared as described by the manufacturer. Before sterilization, the molten agar is usually distributed into screw-cap tubes in exact aliquots sufficient to dilute the desired antimicrobial concentrations 10-fold. Tubes of agar, one for each drug concentration to be tested, are sterilized by autoclaving at 121°C for 15 min, and the agar is allowed to equilibrate to 48 to 50°C in a preheated water bath. Once the agar has equilibrated, the appropriate volume of antimicrobial agent is added, the tube contents are mixed by gentle inversion and poured into 100-mm-diameter round or square sterile plastic petri plates set on a level surface, and the agar is allowed to solidify. For growth controls, plates containing drug-free agar are also prepared. All plates should be filled to a depth of 3 to 4 mm (20 to 25 ml of agar per round plate and 30 ml per square plate), and the pH of each batch should be checked to confirm the acceptable pH range of 7.2 to 7.4 (25).

After sterilization and temperature equilibration of the molten agar, any necessary supplements are aseptically added to the Mueller-Hinton agar at the time of addition of the drug solutions. For testing of streptococci, supplementation with 5% defibrinated sheep or horse blood is recommended (25). However, sheep blood supplementation may antagonize the activities of sulfonamide and trimethoprim against some organisms (11). The presence of blood also affects results with novobiocin and nafcillin as well as the in vitro activities of cephalosporins against enterococci (15, 73); therefore, blood supplementation should not be used unless necessary for bacterial growth (see chapter 75 for acceptable methods for testing of fastidious bacterial species). Performance standards for Mueller-Hinton agar have been defined sufficiently such that calcium and magnesium supplementation is unnecessary (22). The agar should be supplemented with 2% NaCl for testing of oxacillin against staphylococci (49).

Once prepared, plates should be sealed in plastic bags and stored at 4 to 8°C. In general, they should be used within 5 days of preparation or as long as the MICs for control strains that are tested routinely are within the acceptable ranges. However, certain agents are sufficiently labile that plates may not be stored prior to use, e.g., carbapenems, cefaclor, and clavulanic acid. Before inoculation, plates that have been stored under refrigeration should be allowed to equilibrate to room temperature and the agar surface should be dry.

Inoculation Procedures

Variations in inoculum size may substantially affect MICs; therefore, careful inoculum standardization is required to obtain accurate results. The recommended final inoculum for agar dilution is 10^4 CFU per spot (25). This may be achieved in either of two ways. Four or five colonies are picked from overnight growth cultures on agar-based medium and inoculated into 4 to 5 ml of suitable broth that will support good growth (usually tryptic soy broth). Broths are incubated at 35°C until visibly turbid, and then the suspension is diluted until it matches the turbidity of a 0.5 McFarland, barium sulfate ($BaSO_4$), or latex particle turbidity standard (ca. 10^8 CFU/ml). The 0.5 McFarland standard may be purchased or the barium sulfate standard may be prepared as described in the CLSI document (25). The accuracy of the standard should be verified by using a spectrophotometer with a 1-cm light path; for the 0.5 McFarland standard, the absorbance at 625 nm should be 0.08 to 0.13 (25). An alternative inoculum standardization method, one that is preferred by many microbiologists, utilizes direct suspension of colonies from overnight growth cultures on a nonselective agar medium in saline or broth to a turbidity that matches the 0.5 McFarland standard. This approach eliminates the time needed for growing the inoculum in broth (25). In either case, normal saline or sterile broth is used to make a 1:10 dilution of the suspension to give an adjusted concentration of 10^7 CFU/ml (25).

Once the adjusted bacterial inoculum suspension is prepared, inoculation of the antimicrobial agent plates should be accomplished within 30 min, since longer delays may lead to changes in inoculum size. By using a pipette, a calibrated loop, or, more commonly, an inoculum-replicating device, 0.001 to 0.002 ml (1 to 2 μl) of the 10^7-CFU/ml suspension is delivered to the agar surface, resulting in the final desired inoculum of approximately 10^4 CFU per spot. For convenience, use of a replicator is preferred, because consistent inoculum volumes for up to 36 different isolates are simultaneously delivered (25, 76). To use this device, an aliquot of the adjusted inoculum for each isolate is pipetted into the appropriate well of an inoculum seed plate and a multiprong inoculator is used to pick up and gently transfer 1 to 2 μl from the wells to the agar surfaces. Replicators are also available that deliver only 0.1 to 0.2 μl per spot and that do not require the 0.5 McFarland standard suspension to be diluted prior to delivery to the agar surface (25). The surfaces of the agar plates must be dry before inoculation, which should begin with the lowest drug concentration. To check for viability of each test isolate and also as an added check for purity, control plates that do not contain drugs are inoculated last. Finally, plates should be clearly marked so that the locations of the different isolates being tested on each plate are known.

Incubation

Inoculated plates are allowed to stand for several minutes until the inoculum drops have been completely absorbed by the medium; then they are inverted and incubated in air at 35°C for 16 to 20 h before results are read. To facilitate detection of vancomycin-resistant enterococci and methicillin-resistant or vancomycin-resistant or -intermediate staphylococci, plates containing vancomycin or oxacillin should be incubated for a full 24 h before results are read (25). Incubation should not be carried out in the presence of an increased CO_2 concentration unless a fastidious organism is being tested (see chapter 75).

Interpretation and Reporting of Results

Before reading and recording the results obtained with clinical isolates, those obtained with applicable quality control strains tested at the same time should be checked to ensure that their values are within the acceptable ranges (see "Quality Control" below) and the drug-free control plates should be examined for isolate viability and purity. Endpoints for each antimicrobial agent are best determined by placing plates on a dark background and examining them for the lowest concentration that inhibits visible growth, which is recorded as the MIC. A single colony or a faint haze left by the initial inoculum should not be regarded as growth. If two or more colonies persist at antimicrobial concentrations beyond an otherwise obvious endpoint or if there is no growth at lower concentrations but there is growth at higher concentrations, the isolate should be subcultured to confirm purity and the test should be repeated. Substances that may antagonize the antibacterial activities of sulfonamides and trimethoprim may be carried over with the inoculum and cause "trailing," or less definite endpoints (11,

15). Therefore, the MICs of these antimicrobial agents should be interpreted as the endpoints at which 80% or more diminution of growth occurs. Although much less pronounced, trailing endpoints may also occur for some organisms with bacteriostatic agents such as chloramphenicol, the tetracyclines, linezolid, and quinupristin-dalfopristin (25).

The MIC of each antimicrobial agent is usually recorded in micrograms per milliliter, although in Europe and in the international standard reference method, the values are expressed as milligrams per liter (39, 40, 50). These quantitative results should be reported with the appropriate corresponding interpretive category (susceptible, intermediate, or resistant), or the interpretive category may be reported alone. The MIC interpretive standards for these susceptibility categories, as currently recommended by the CLSI (25), are provided in Table 3. For detailed instructions concerning the

TABLE 3 Interpretive standards for dilution and disk diffusion susceptibility testing[a]

Antimicrobial agent and organism	MIC (μg/ml)			Zone diam (mm)		
	Susceptible	Intermediate	Resistant	Susceptible	Intermediate	Resistant
Penicillins						
Penicillin G						
Staphylococci[b]	≤0.12		≥0.25	≥29		≤28
Enterococci[c]	≤8		≥16	≥15		≤14
Methicillin[d]	≤8		≥16	≥14	10–13	≤9
Oxacillin[d]						
S. aureus	≤2		≥4	≥13	11–12	≤10
Coagulase-negative staphylococci	≤0.25		≥0.5	≥18		≤17
Ampicillin						
Enterobacteriaceae	≤8	16	≥32	≥17	14–16	≤13
Staphylococci	≤0.25		≥0.5	≥29		≤28
Enterococci[c]	≤8		≥16	≥17		≤16
Amoxicillin-clavulanic acid						
Staphylococci	≤4/2		≥8/4	≥20		≤19
Other organisms	≤8/4	16/8	≥32/16	≥18	14–17	≤13
Ampicillin-sulbactam	≤8/4	16/8	≥32/16	≥15	12–14	≤11
Azlocillin	≤64		≥128	≥18		≤17
P. aeruginosa						
Carbenicillin						
P. aeruginosa	≤128	256	≥512	≥17	14–16	≤13
Other gram-negative bacilli	≤16	32	≥64	≥23	20–22	≤19
Mecillinam	≤8	16	≥32	≥15	12–14	≤11
Mezlocillin						
P. aeruginosa	≤64		≥128	≥16		≤15
Other gram-negative bacilli	≤16	32–64	≥128	≥21	18–20	≤17
Piperacillin						
P. aeruginosa	≤64		≥128	≥18		≤17
Other gram-negative bacilli	≤16	32–64	≥128	≥21	18–20	≤17
Piperacillin-tazobactam						
P. aeruginosa	≤64/4		≥128/4	≥18		≤17
Other gram-negative bacilli	≤16/4	32/4–64/4	≥128/4	≥21	18–20	≤17
Staphylococci	≤8/4		≥16/4	≥18		≤17
Ticarcillin						
P. aeruginosa	≤64		≥128	≥15		≤14
Other gram-negative bacilli	≤16	32–64	≥128	≥20	15–19	≤14
Ticarcillin-clavulanic acid						
P. aeruginosa	≤64/2		≥128/2	≥15		≤14
Other gram-negative bacilli	≤16/2	32/2–64/2	≥128/2	≥20	15–19	≤14
Staphylococci	≤8/2		≥16/2	≥23		≤22

(Continued on next page)

TABLE 3 Interpretive standards for dilution and disk diffusion susceptibility testing[a] *(Continued)*

Antimicrobial agent and organism	MIC (μg/ml)			Zone diam (mm)		
	Susceptible	Intermediate	Resistant	Susceptible	Intermediate	Resistant
Cephalosporins						
Cefaclor	<8	16	≥32	≥18	15–17	≤14
Cefamandole	≤8	16	≥32	≥18	15–17	≤14
Cefazolin	≤8	16	≥32	≥18	15–17	≤14
Cefepime	≤8	16	≥32	≥18	15–17	≤14
Cefetamet	≤4	8	≥16	≥18	15–17	≤14
Cefixime	≤1	2	≥4	≥19	16–18	≤15
Cefmetazole	≤16	32	≥64	≥16	13–15	≤12
Cefonicid	≤8	16	≥32	≥18	15–17	≤14
Cefoperazone	≤16	32	≥64	≥21	16–20	≤15
Cefotaxime	≤8	16–32	≥64	≥23	15–22	≤14
Cefotetan	≤16	32	≥64	≥16	13–15	≤12
Cefoxitin	≤8	16	≥32	≥18	15–17	≤14
Cefpodoxime	≤2	4	≥8	≥21	18–20	≤17
Cefprozil	≤8	16	≥32	≥18	15–17	≤14
Ceftazidime	≤8	16	≥32	≥18	15–17	<14
Ceftibuten	≤8	16	≥32	≥21	18–20	≤17
Ceftizoxime	≤8	16–32	≥64	≥20	15–19	≤14
Ceftriaxone	≤8	16–32	≥64	≥21	14–20	≤13
Cefuroxime axetil	≤4	8–16	≥32	≥23	15–22	≤14
Cefuroxime sodium	≤8	16	≥32	≥18	15–17	≤14
Cephalothin	≤8	16	≥32	≥18	15–17	≤14
Loracarbef	≤8	16	≥32	≥18	15–17	≤14
Moxalactam	≤8	16–32	≥64	≥23	15–22	≤14
Other beta-lactams						
Aztreonam	≤8	16	≥32	≥22	16–21	≤15
Ertapenem	≤2	4	≥8	≥19	14–18	≤15
Imipenem	≤4	8	≥16	≥16	14–15	≤13
Meropenem	≤4	8	≥16	≥16	14–15	≤13
Aminoglycosides						
Amikacin	≤16	32	≥64	≥17	15–16	≤14
Gentamicin	≤4	8	≥16	≥15	13–14	≤12
Enterococci (high-level resistance)	≤500		>500	≥10	7–9	6
Netilmicin	≤8	16	≥32	≥15	13–14	≤12
Tobramycin	≤4	8	≥16	≥15	13–14	≤12
Streptomycin						
Enterococci (high-level resistance)						
Broth microdilution method	≤1,000		>1,000			
Agar-based method	≤2,000		>2,000	≥10	7–9	6
Glycopeptides						
Teicoplanin	≤8	16	≥32	≥14	11–13	≤10
Vancomycin						
Enterococci	≤4	8–16	≥32	≥17	15–16	≤14
S. aureus	≤2	4–8	≥16	≥15	Determine MIC if ≤14	
Coagulase-negative staphylococci	≤4	8–16	≥32	≥15	Determine MIC if ≤14	
Lipopeptide						
Daptomycin						
Enterococci	≤4					
Staphylococci	≤1					

(Continued on next page)

TABLE 3 *(Continued)*

Antimicrobial agent and organism	MIC (μg/ml)			Zone diam (mm)		
	Susceptible	Intermediate	Resistant	Susceptible	Intermediate	Resistant
Macrolides						
Azithromycin	≤2	4	≥8	≥18	14–17	≤13
Clarithromycin	≤2	4	≥8	≥18	14–17	≤13
Dirithromycin	≤2	4	≥8	≥19	16–18	≤15
Erythromycin	≤0.5	1–4	≥8	≥23	14–22	≤13
Ketolide						
Telithromycin	≤1	2	≥4	≥22	17–21	≤18
Quinolones						
Ciprofloxacin	≤1	2	≥4	≥21	16–20	≤15
Enoxacin	≤2	4	≥8	≥18	15–17	≤14
Fleroxacin	≤2	4	≥8	≥19	16–18	≤15
Gatifloxacin	≤2	4	≥8	≥18	15–17	≥14
Levofloxacin	≤2	4	≥8	≥17	14–16	≤13
Lomefloxacin	≤2	4	≥8	≥22	19–21	≤18
Moxifloxacin	≤0.5	1	≥2	≥24	19–23	≤20
Nalidixic acid[e]	≤8	16	≥32	≥19	14–18	≤13
Norfloxacin[e]	≤4	8	≥16	≥17	13–16	≤12
Ofloxacin	≤2	4	≥8	≥16	13–15	≥12
Sparfloxacin	≤0.5	1	≥2	≥19	16–18	≤15
Tetracyclines						
Doxycycline	≤4	8	≥16	≥16	13–15	≤12
Minocycline	≤4	8	≥16	≥19	15–18	≤14
Tetracycline	≤4	8	≥16	≥19	15–18	≤14
Other						
Chloramphenicol	≤8	16	≥32	≥18	13–17	≤12
Clindamycin	≤0.5	1–2	≥4	≥21	15–20	≤14
Colistin	≤2		≥4			
Fosfomycin	≤64	128	≥256	≥16	13–15	≤12
Linezolid						
Enterococci	≤2	4	≥8	≥23	19–22	≤20
Staphylococci	≤2			≥21		
Nitrofurantoin	≤32	64	≥128	≥17	15–16	≤14
Polymyxin	≤2		≥4			
Quinupristin-dalfopristin	≤1	2	≥4	≥19	16–18	≤15
Rifampin	≤1	2	≥4	≥20	17–19	≤16
Sulfonamide	≤256		≥512	≥17	13–16	≤12
Trimethoprim[e]	≤8		≥16	≥16	11–15	≤10
Trimethoprim-sulfamethoxazole	≤2/38		≥4/76	≥16	11–15	≤10

[a] Adapted from CLSI data (27) with permission. The interpretive data are valid only if the methodologies in documents M2-A8 (26) and M7-A6 (25) are followed. Breakpoints for some agents apply only to certain genera or species. The CLSI frequently updates the interpretive tables through new editions of the standards and supplements to them. Users should refer to the most recent editions. The current standards and supplements to them may be obtained from the CLSI, 940 West Valley Rd., Suite 1400, Wayne, PA 19087-1898.

[b] Penicillin should be used as the class representative for all penicillins (e.g., ampicillin, amoxicillin, mezlocillin, piperacillin, and ticarcillin). Isolates for which MICs are ≤0.03 μg of penicillin per ml generally do not produce beta-lactamase, whereas those for which MICs are ≥0.25 μg/ml do and should be regarded as resistant to penicillins. Isolates for which MICs of penicillin are 0.06 or 0.12 μg/ml should be tested for beta-lactamase.

[c] Therapy for serious enterococcal infections requires high doses of penicillin or ampicillin in combination with an aminoglycoside. Vancomycin may be substituted for the penicillin in instances of penicillin hypersensitivity or of penicillin or ampicillin resistance.

[d] Oxacillin or methicillin may be tested; however, oxacillin is preferred because of its greater stability in vitro. The results from the testing of oxacillin apply also to other penicillinase-resistant penicillins. Oxacillin-resistant staphylococci should be considered resistant to all penicillins, cephalosporins, carbacephems, carbapenems, and beta-lactam–beta-lactamase inhibitor combinations. Disk testing with cefoxitin is the most sensitive and specific method for phenotypic detection of *mecA*-mediated oxacillin resistance in staphylococci (27, 78).

[e] For the treatment of urinary tract infections only.

use of these criteria and categories, the latest CLSI standards for dilution testing methods should be consulted (27). Note that the interpretive standards for most of the penicillin class drugs vary with the organism being tested. In an attempt to minimize confusion regarding different breakpoints that may apply to individual species, the CLSI has divided the interpretive breakpoint tables into a number of different tables for the various organism groups (25).

The three interpretive categories are defined as follows. Susceptible indicates that an infection caused by the tested microorganism may be appropriately treated with the usually recommended dose of antibiotic. Intermediate indicates that the isolate may be inhibited by attainable concentrations of certain drugs (e.g., the beta-lactams) if higher dosages can be used safely or if the infection involves a body site indicating that the drug is physiologically concentrated (e.g., the urinary tract). The intermediate category also serves as a buffer zone that prevents slight technical artifacts from causing major interpretive discrepancies. Resistant isolates are not inhibited by the concentration of antimicrobial agent normally achievable with the recommended dose and/or yield results that fall within a range indicating that specific resistance mechanisms are likely to be present (25).

Advantages and Disadvantages

Dilution testing by the agar method is a well-standardized, reliable susceptibility testing technique that may be used as a reference for evaluating other testing methods. In addition, the simultaneous testing of a large number of isolates with a few drugs is efficient (such as when new agents are evaluated in the pharmaceutical industry), and microbial contamination or population heterogeneity is more readily detected by the agar method than by broth methods. The agar dilution method has been considered the reference test method in many areas of Europe (39), while broth microdilution has been much more widely used for research and clinical purposes in North America (55) and is now considered the international reference method for determining MICs (50). The major disadvantages of the agar method are associated with the time-consuming and labor-intensive tasks of preparing the plates, especially if the number of different antimicrobial agents to be tested for each isolate is high or if only a few isolates are to be tested.

DILUTION TESTING: BROTH METHODS

The general approaches for broth methods include broth macrodilution, in which the broth volume for each antimicrobial concentration is ≥1.0 ml (usually 2 ml) contained in test tubes, and broth microdilution, in which antimicrobial dilutions are most often in 0.1-ml volumes in wells of microdilution trays.

Broth Macrodilution Methods

Dilution of Antimicrobial Agents

Stock solutions are prepared as discussed in the CLSI document on dilution testing (25) and are the same as those used for agar dilution tests. As in the agar method, the actual volumes used for the dilutions would be proportionally increased according to the number of tests being prepared, with a minimum of 1.0 ml needed for each drug concentration. Because addition of the inoculum results in a 1:2 dilution of each concentration, all final drug concentrations must be prepared at twice the actual desired testing concentration (see "Inoculation Procedures" below).

Preparation, Supplementation, and Storage of Media

Cation-adjusted Mueller-Hinton broth (CAMHB) is recommended for routine testing of commonly encountered nonfastidious organisms (25). Adjustment of the cations Ca^{2+} (20 to 25 mg/liter) and Mg^{2+} (10 to 12.5 mg/liter) is required to ensure acceptable results when *P. aeruginosa* isolates are tested with aminoglycosides and when tetracycline is tested with other bacteria (9). However, for convenience and consistency, cation adjustment of Mueller-Hinton broth is now recommended for testing of all species and antimicrobial agents (25). Some manufacturers provide Mueller-Hinton broth that already has appropriate concentrations of divalent cations, so the cation content of commercial dehydrated media must be ascertained and care must be taken to supplement the broth with the appropriate cation levels. If adjustment is necessary, it can be accomplished by the addition of suitable volumes of filter-sterilized, chilled $CaCl_2$ stock (3.68 g of $CaCl_2 \cdot 2H_2O$ dissolved in 100 ml of deionized water for a concentration of 10 mg of Ca^{2+} per ml) and $MgCl_2$ stock (8.36 g of $MgCl_2 \cdot 6H_2O$ in 100 ml of deionized water for a concentration of 10 mg of Mg^{2+} per ml) to the cooled broth (25). Insufficient cation concentrations result in increased aminoglycoside activity (32), and excess cation content results in decreased aminoglycoside activity against *P. aeruginosa* (7, 32). For testing of daptomycin, the calcium level of the test medium must be increased to 50 mg/liter to achieve reliable MICs (25, 43). While the effects of inappropriate calcium and magnesium ion contents are well recognized, other ions, including zinc and manganese, may adversely affect the activities of some drugs, e.g., carbapenems (31). The CLSI has initiated a consensus standard for manufacturers of Mueller-Hinton broth that attempts to specify all known factors that determine performance of the medium (23). Reliable detection of staphylococcal resistance to oxacillin requires that the CAMHB used for testing that agent be supplemented with 2% NaCl (25, 83).

To minimize evaporation and deterioration of antimicrobial agents, tubes should be tightly capped and stored at 4 to 8°C until needed. With most agents, the dilutions should be used within 5 days of preparation or as long as quality control ranges are maintained (see "Quality Control" below). As in agar dilution testing, certain beta-lactam agents are too labile for prolonged storage at final test concentrations.

Inoculation Procedures

The recommended final inoculum is 5×10^5 CFU/ml. Isolates are inoculated into a broth that will support good growth (such as tryptic soy broth) and incubated until turbid. The turbidity is adjusted to match that of a 0.5 McFarland standard (approximately 10^8 CFU/ml). Alternatively, four or five colonies from overnight growth cultures on a nonselective agar plate may be directly suspended in broth to match the turbidity of the McFarland standard (25). This alternative is preferred for testing of oxacillin against staphylococci (25). A portion of the standardized suspension is diluted approximately 1:100 (10^6 CFU/ml) with broth or saline. When 1 ml of this dilution is added to each tube containing 1 ml of the drug diluted in CAMHB, a final inoculum of 5×10^5 CFU/ml is achieved. Broth not containing an antimicrobial agent is inoculated as a control for organism viability (growth control). All tubes should be inoculated within 30 min of inoculum preparation, and an aliquot of the inoculum should be plated to check for purity.

Incubation

Tubes are incubated in air at 35°C for 16 to 20 h before MICs are determined. Incubation should be extended to a full 24 h for the detection of vancomycin-resistant enterococci and oxacillin-resistant or vancomycin-resistant or -intermediate staphylococci (25). An atmosphere with increased CO_2 should not be used.

Interpretation and Reporting of Results

Before MICs for the test strains are read and recorded, the growth controls should be examined for viability, inoculum subcultures should be checked for contamination, and appropriate MICs obtained with the quality control strains should be confirmed (see "Quality Control" below). Growth or lack thereof in the antimicrobial agent-containing tubes is best determined by comparison with the growth control. Generally, growth is indicated by turbidity, a single sedimented button of ≥2 mm in diameter, or several buttons with smaller diameters. As with the agar method, trailing endpoints may be seen when trimethoprim or sulfonamides are tested, and the concentration at which 80% or greater diminution of growth, compared with that of the growth control, occurs should be recorded as the MIC (25). Other interpretation problems include the "skipped tube" phenomenon, in which growth is not observed at one concentration but is observed at lower and higher drug concentrations. Most authorities suggest that when this occurs, the skipped tube should be ignored and the concentration that finally inhibits growth at serially higher concentrations should be recorded as the MIC. If more than one skipped tube occurs or if there is growth at higher antimicrobial concentrations but not at lower ones, the results should not be reported and the test for that drug should be repeated.

The lowest concentration that completely inhibits visible growth of the organism as detected by the unaided eye is recorded as the MIC. The CLSI MIC interpretive standards in effect as of the date of this writing (27) for the susceptibility categories are provided in Table 3. The definitions of and comments concerning these categories that were given for the agar method also pertain to the broth macrodilution method.

Advantages and Disadvantages

The broth macrodilution method is a well-standardized and reliable method that may be useful for research purposes or for testing of one drug with a bacterial isolate. However, because of the laborious nature of the procedure and the availability of more convenient dilution systems (e.g., microdilution), this procedure is generally not useful for routine susceptibility testing in most clinical microbiology laboratories.

Broth Microdilution Method

The convenience afforded by the availability of dilution susceptibility testing in microdilution trays has led to the widespread use of broth microdilution methods. In fact, the broth microdilution method is now considered the international reference susceptibility testing method (50). The disposable plastic trays, containing a panel of several antimicrobial agents to be tested simultaneously, may be prepared in-house or obtained commercially either frozen or freeze-dried. When commercial systems are used, the manufacturers' recommendations concerning storage, inoculation, incubation, and interpretation should be followed. The primary focus of this section will be the in-house preparation and use of broth microdilution panels. However, most of the principles and practices discussed here are pertinent to the broth microdilution method regardless of the source of the antibiotic panels.

Dilution of Antimicrobial Agents

Antimicrobial stock solutions are prepared as outlined in the CLSI document on dilution testing (25). The dilution scheme for preparing broth microdilution panels is the same as that described for agar and broth microdilution methods. Automated dispensing systems for preparation of microdilution panels use tubes that contain from 10 to 200 ml or more of broth containing each antimicrobial concentration. From the master tube dilutions, aliquots of 0.05 or 0.1 ml are simultaneously dispensed into the corresponding wells of each broth microdilution tray by using a mechanized dispenser. If 0.05-ml volumes are dispensed, allowances must be made for the 1:2 dilution of the final drug concentration that will occur when the 0.05 ml of inoculum is added (see "Inoculation Procedures" below). When 0.1-ml aliquots are dispensed, the volume of inoculum normally used is sufficiently small (≤0.005 ml) that adjustments in the antimicrobial dilution scheme are not needed. As a general rule, when the inoculum volume is less than 10% of the broth volume in the well, dilution of the antimicrobial concentration by the inoculum does not have to be taken into account (25).

Preparation, Supplementation, and Storage of Media

CAMHB is the recommended medium for broth microdilution testing of nonfastidious organisms and should be prepared as discussed above for the broth macrodilution method. Also, supplementation of the broth with 2% NaCl is required for detection of oxacillin-resistant staphylococci (25). After the antimicrobial dilutions have been dispensed into the plastic trays, the panels are stacked in groups of 5 to 10, with a tray lid or an empty tray placed on top to minimize contamination and evaporation. Each stack is sealed in a plastic bag and frozen immediately at −20°C or, preferably, at −60°C or colder. At −20°C, preservation is ensured for at least 6 weeks with most drugs, but the shelf life may be extended to months if the trays are stored at −60 to −70°C. Care must be taken in storing highly labile compounds such as cefaclor, clavulanic acid, and carbapenems, which may lose potency during storage. If thawed, panels must be used or discarded but not refrozen, since freeze-thaw cycles cause substantial deterioration of beta-lactam antibiotics. For this reason, −20°C household type freezers with self-defrosting units must not be used.

Inoculation Procedures

As with the macrodilution procedure, the final desired inoculum concentration is 5×10^5 CFU/ml. The isolates may be grown in broth to match the turbidity of a 0.5 McFarland standard (ca. 1×10^8 to 2×10^8 CFU/ml), or a suspension of that density can be made from colonies grown overnight on a nonselective agar medium (8), which is the method preferred for detecting oxacillin-resistant staphylococci (25). For broth microdilution procedures that require 0.001- to 0.005-ml volumes to inoculate wells containing 0.1 ml of broth, a portion of the 0.5 McFarland standard suspension is diluted 1:10 (10^7 CFU/ml) in sterile saline or broth. Multipoint metal or disposable plastic inoculum replicators designed to collect and deliver appropriate volumes are used to transfer the inoculum from the diluted suspension to the wells of the broth microdilution tray, resulting in further dilutions ranging from 1:20 to 1:50. Final inoculum concentrations should be 4×10^5 to 6×10^5 CFU/ml (4×10^4 to 6×10^4 CFU per well). For protocols that use an inoculum volume of 0.05 ml to inoculate 0.05 ml of broth, a 1:100 dilution of a 0.5 McFarland standard suspension (ca. 10^6 CFU/ml) is used. When the inoculum is added to the wells, the 1:2 dilution of the 10^6-CFU/ml inoculum results in a final inoculum concentration of 5×10^5 CFU/ml (5×10^4 CFU per well) and also halves the antibiotic concentration in each well. Special care should be taken to confirm the inoculum density on a periodic basis to ensure that the appropriate density of inoculum is achieved. Moreover, slight deviations from the initial 1:10 dilution described above may be necessary to provide the target inoculum density with some species or organism groups. Insufficient inoculum can be a significant problem with inducible resistance mechanisms of some organisms and may not be recognized as a problem based on the MICs obtained for the very susceptible quality control strains.

Broth microdilution trays should be inoculated within 30 min of inoculum preparation, and an aliquot should be subcultured to check the purity of the isolates. Finally, one well of each panel not containing an antimicrobial agent should be inoculated and used as a growth control, and a second uninoculated well serves as a sterility control.

Incubation

After inoculation, each tray should be covered with plastic tape, sealed in a plastic bag, or tightly fitted with a lid or an empty tray to prevent evaporation during incubation. Trays are incubated in ambient air at 35°C for 16 to 20 h before results are read and should not be incubated in stacks of more than four trays for uniform temperature distribution. The incubator should be kept sufficiently humid to avoid evaporation but not so humid that condensation results in contamination problems. A full 24 h of incubation is recommended for the detection of vancomycin-resistant enterococci and oxacillin-resistant or vancomycin-resistant or -intermediate staphylococci (25). Incubation in an atmosphere with increased CO_2 should not be used with nonfastidious organisms.

Interpretation and Reporting of Results

Before MICs for the clinical isolates are read and recorded, the growth control wells should be examined for organism viability and the inoculum purity should be checked. The appropriateness of the MICs obtained for the quality control strains should be confirmed if tests of these strains were set up simultaneously with those of clinical isolates (see "Quality Control" below). Various viewing devices are available and should be used to facilitate examination of the broth microdilution wells for growth. The simplest and most reliable method is the use of a parabolic magnifying mirror and tray stand that allow clear visual inspection of the undersides of the microdilution trays. Growth is best determined by comparison with that in the growth control well and generally is indicated by turbidity throughout the well or by buttons, single or multiple, in the well bottom. The occurrence of trailing endpoints with trimethoprim or sulfonamides should be ignored, and the MIC endpoint should be based on ≥80% growth inhibition. Results for drugs with more than one skipped well should not be reported, as with the broth macrodilution test.

The CLSI MIC interpretive criteria (27) for susceptibility categories are given in Table 3. It should be noted that these values are published each year and only the most recent tables should be used for interpretation of results. The definitions of the interpretive categories and the comments concerning the use of these standards for agar and broth macrodilution methods are also applicable to broth microdilution methods.

Advantages and Disadvantages

The broth microdilution method represents a standardized reference method for susceptibility testing. Inoculation and reading procedures allow relatively convenient simultaneous testing of several antimicrobial agents with individual isolates. Because few laboratories have the facilities required for preparation of broth microdilution trays, several sources of commercially prepared antibiotic panels are available today. Such products provide trays with wells containing prepared antimicrobial dilutions either frozen or freeze-dried. Trays with frozen dilutions must be stored frozen in the laboratory, whereas dried panels can be stored at room temperature. Most of these products are accompanied by multipoint inoculating devices, or multichannel pipetters. Results of testing may be determined by visual examination or by use of semiautomated or automated instrumentation.

Breakpoint Susceptibility Tests

Breakpoint susceptibility testing refers to methods by which antimicrobial agents are tested only at the specific concentrations necessary for differentiating between the interpretive categories of susceptible, intermediate, and resistant rather than in a range of five or more doubling-dilution concentrations used to determine MICs. When two drug concentrations are selected adjacent to the breakpoints defining the intermediate and resistant categories, any one of the interpretive categories may be determined. Growth at both concentrations indicates resistance, growth at only the lower concentration signifies an intermediate result, and no growth at either concentration indicates susceptibility.

Like full-range dilution testing, breakpoint methods require the use of appropriately adjusted and supplemented Mueller-Hinton broth or agar. In addition, the standard inoculation, incubation, and interpretation procedures recommended for the full-range dilution methods should be followed.

Considering the limited range of drug concentrations tested, a greater number and variety of antimicrobial agents can be incorporated into a broth microdilution panel for breakpoint testing than into panels designed for full-range dilution testing (37). However, convenient quality control procedures to ensure that appropriate concentrations of each antimicrobial agent are present are lacking for breakpoint panels. One possible approach is to use one organism for which the modal MIC is equal to or no less than one doubling dilution less than the lower or lowest concentration tested and a second organism for which the modal MIC is equal to or no more than one doubling dilution greater than the higher or highest concentration tested (25). One of these two quality control organisms should provide on-scale results (25). Despite the theoretical soundness of this approach, routine quality control of breakpoint panels is difficult and not readily accomplished in the clinical laboratory.

Resistance Screens

In some circumstances, testing a single drug concentration may be a reliable and convenient method for detecting antimicrobial resistance. The most clinically useful resistance screens are those for resistance to oxacillin in *S. aureus*, resistance of *Enterococcus* spp. and *Staphylococcus* spp. to vancomycin, and high-level resistance to gentamicin and streptomycin in enterococci (25). These practical and reliable methods are described in chapter 74 of this Manual.

Gradient Diffusion Method

The E test (AB Biodisk, Solna, Sweden) is a commercial method for quantitative antimicrobial susceptibility testing that incorporates a preformed antimicrobial gradient applied to one side of a plastic strip to provide drug diffusion into an agar medium. The test is performed in a manner similar to disk diffusion testing, in that a 0.5 McFarland standard suspension of a test isolate is generally swabbed onto the agar surface for inoculation. Following incubation, the MIC is read directly from a scale on the top of the E-test strip at the point where the ellipse of organism growth inhibition intercepts the strip. Several strips, each containing a different antimicrobial agent, can be placed radially on the surface of a large round Mueller-Hinton agar plate, or they can be placed in opposing directions on large rectangular plates. MICs determined by this method generally agree well with MICs generated by standard broth or agar dilution methods (6, 48, 54). The E test combines the simplicity and flexibility of the disk diffusion test with the ability to determine MICs of up to five antimicrobial agents on a single large agar plate. However, E-test strips are much more expensive than the paper disks used for diffusion testing. Strengths of the E-test method include the simplicity of the procedure itself and the ability to determine an MIC of an infrequently tested drug and to test fastidious or anaerobic bacteria by applying the strips onto specialized enriched media (see chapters 75 and 76 of this Manual).

QUALITY CONTROL

Quality control recommendations are designed for evaluation of the precision and accuracy of test procedures, monitoring of reagent performance, and evaluation of the performance of the individuals who are conducting the tests.

Reference Strains

A critical element in accomplishing the goals of quality control is the selection and use of reference bacterial strains that are genetically stable and for which MICs are in the midrange of MICs of each antimicrobial agent tested (25). That is, the dilutions in a series should ideally encompass at least two concentration increments above and below the previously established MIC for the reference strain. If there are four or fewer dilutions in a series or if nonconsecutive dilutions are tested (e.g., in breakpoint susceptibility testing), quality control for the correct interpretive category only rather than actual MIC ranges may be accomplished. *Escherichia coli* ATCC 25922, *P. aeruginosa* ATCC 27853, *Enterococcus faecalis* ATCC 29212, and *S. aureus* ATCC 29213 are the recommended reference strains for both agar and broth dilution methods (25). The beta-lactamase-producing strain *E. coli* ATCC 35218 is recommended only for penicillin–beta-lactamase inhibitor combinations (25). These organisms may be obtained from the American Type Culture Collection or other reliable commercial sources. For proper storage and subculture procedures, the recommendations of either the CLSI (25) or the commercial provider should be followed.

MIC Ranges

The acceptable quality control MIC ranges for the various reference strains are given in the CLSI document on dilution testing (25). Updates of these MIC ranges are published annually (27) and should be readily available in each clinical laboratory. An out-of-control result is defined as an MIC not within the acceptable range of values. Certain out-of-control results can be directly related to the medium used for testing. High MICs of gentamicin for *P. aeruginosa* ATCC 27853 suggest an inappropriately high divalent cation content or excessively low pH of the Mueller-Hinton medium, and low MICs indicate an insufficient divalent cation concentration or elevated pH. Although trimethoprim-sulfamethoxazole is not recommended for therapy of *Enterococcus faecalis* infections, results obtained with the ATCC 29212 strain can be useful for detecting excessive amounts of substances such as thymidine that interfere with the in vitro activity of antifolate drugs. Trimethoprim-sulfamethoxazole MICs of >0.5 to 9.5 μg/ml indicate the presence of such interfering substances (25).

Batch and Lot Quality Control

Representative plates, panels, or trays from each new reagent batch if prepared in-house or from each new lot if obtained from a commercial source should be subjected to quality control and sterility testing. MICs obtained by testing reference quality control strains should be within acceptable CLSI ranges (27). If such accuracy is not achieved, the batch or lot should be rejected or patient results obtained with the antimicrobial agent(s) in question should not be reported (see below). Similarly, if selected uninoculated plates or trays fail the sterility check after incubation, the batch or lot should be rejected. In addition to these formal quality control procedures that use reference strains, careful review of susceptibility results obtained during daily testing of clinical isolates is important to identify aberrant or unusual susceptibility patterns possibly indicative of reagent or technical problems.

Quality Control Frequency

In addition to batch and lot testing, quality control tests should be performed daily, or at least every day that the plates or trays are being used to test clinical isolates. When quality control is performed on each day of testing, performance is considered satisfactory if no more than 3 out of 30 consecutive results for each drug-reference strain combination are outside the acceptable limits. If this frequency is exceeded, the laboratory must perform corrective action to determine the source of the error and to correct it as described below. However, if daily quality control testing does not reveal an excessive rate of errors, daily testing may be replaced by weekly testing as outlined below (25, 27).

To convert to a weekly quality control testing interval, each drug-reference strain combination is tested for 20 or 30 consecutive testing days to obtain a total of 20 to 30 MICs for each combination. If no more than 1 of 20 or 3 of 30 MICs per combination are outside the accuracy range, weekly testing may replace daily testing. During weekly testing, a single MIC outside the acceptable range requires that daily testing be performed for five consecutive days unless there is an obvious source of error (e.g., contamination, use of an incorrect reference strain or an incorrect inoculum density, testing of an incorrect antimicrobial agent, or use of an incorrect atmosphere for incubation). In such a circumstance, the quality control test need be repeated only once. If no obvious source of error is noted, but all five MICs for a problem drug-organism combination are within the accuracy range, weekly testing may be resumed. If one or more of the five MICs for the problem drug-organism combination are outside the accuracy range, daily testing must be initiated and further means to resolve the problem must be pursued. Returning to weekly testing requires again documenting 20 or 30 consecutive days with no more than one or three MICs outside the accuracy range. If more than the acceptable number of MICs for organism-drug combinations are outside the accuracy range, daily quality control testing must be continued while the problem is being resolved (25, 27).

DISK DIFFUSION TESTING

The disk diffusion method of susceptibility testing allows categorization of most bacterial isolates as susceptible, intermediate, or resistant to a variety of antimicrobial agents. To perform the test, commercially prepared filter paper disks impregnated with a specified single concentration of an antimicrobial agent are applied to the surface of an agar medium that has been inoculated with the test organism. The drug in the disk diffuses through the agar. As the distance from the disk increases, the concentration of the antimicrobial agent decreases logarithmically, creating a gradient of drug concentrations in the agar medium surrounding each disk. Concomitant with the diffusion of the drug, the bacteria that were inoculated onto the surface and are not inhibited by the concentration of the antimicrobial agent continue to multiply until a lawn of growth is visible. In areas where the concentration of the drug is inhibitory, no growth occurs, forming a zone of inhibition around each disk.

The disk diffusion procedure has been standardized primarily for testing common, rapidly growing bacteria (10, 26). This method should not be used to evaluate antimicrobial susceptibilities of bacteria that show marked strain-to-strain variability in growth rates, e.g., some fastidious or anaerobic bacteria. The test, however, has been modified to allow reliable testing of certain fastidious bacteria (discussed in chapter 75 of this Manual).

The diameter of the zone of inhibition is influenced by the rate of diffusion of the antimicrobial agent through the agar, which may vary among different drugs depending upon the size of the drug molecule and its hydrophilicity. The zone size, however, is inversely proportional to the logarithm of the MIC, measured as discussed earlier in this chapter. Criteria currently recommended for interpreting zone diameters and MIC results for commonly used antimicrobial agents are listed in Table 3 and published annually by the CLSI (27).

Establishing Zone-of-Inhibition Diameter Interpretive Criteria

The first step in determining interpretive criteria for the disk diffusion test is selection of MIC breakpoints that define susceptibility and resistance categories for each antimicrobial agent. Zone-of-inhibition diameters that correspond to these breakpoints are initially established by testing 300 or more bacterial isolates by both dilution and disk diffusion methods and correlating zone-of-inhibition diameters and MICs determined for each drug tested (21). Isolates tested should include not only those commonly encountered in clinical laboratories but also those with resistance mechanisms pertinent to the class of antimicrobial agent being tested (21). Organisms evaluated should be those most likely to be tested with the antimicrobial agent in question. The data from these studies are analyzed by preparing a scattergram of values (see the example in chapter 72). By convention, each MIC (log_2 scale) is plotted on the *y* axis, and the corresponding zone-of-inhibition diameter (arithmetic scale) is plotted on the *x* axis. Regression analysis can be performed, and a straight regression line showing the best fit is drawn. From this line, an approximation of the MIC can be inferred from any zone-of-inhibition diameter. For antimicrobial agents to which isolates are either susceptible or resistant and only infrequently intermediate, regression analysis is not valid. In such cases, the data are plotted as a scattergram and the interpretive standards are selected so as to allow optimal separation of resistant and susceptible populations (19, 21, 67). This approach, often called the error-rate-bounded method, may also be employed to minimize interpretive errors that can ensue from strictly applying the linear regression formula to a data set (21).

Antimicrobial Agent Disks

The amounts of antimicrobial agents in the disks used for agar diffusion testing are standardized, and in the United States, only a single disk for each drug is recommended (54). The optimal amount of an antimicrobial agent per disk is determined early in the development of a new drug by testing disks with several different drug contents that can be evaluated by using scattergrams and regression lines (21). The most desirable concentration of a drug per disk is that which produces a zone-of-inhibition diameter of at least 10 mm with resistant isolates and a zone diameter of no larger than 30 mm with susceptible isolates.

Commercially prepared antimicrobial disks usually are supplied in separate containers, each with a desiccant. They must not be used beyond the specified expiration date and should be stored under refrigeration (2 to 8°C) or frozen in a non-frost-free freezer at −20°C or colder until needed. Disks containing a beta-lactam agent should always be stored frozen to ensure that they retain their potency, although a small supply may be stored in the refrigerator for up to 1 week. Unopened disk containers should be removed from the refrigerator or freezer 1 to 2 h before use. This allows the disks to equilibrate to room temperature before the container is opened, thus minimizing the amount of condensation that will occur when warm air contacts the cold disks. A commercially available, mechanical disk-dispensing apparatus can be used and should be fitted with a tight cover, supplied with an adequate desiccant, stored in the refrigerator when not in use, and warmed to room temperature before being opened.

Agar Medium

The recommended medium for disk diffusion testing in the United States is Mueller-Hinton agar (26). This unsupplemented medium has been selected by the CLSI for several reasons: (i) it demonstrates good batch-to-batch reproducibility for susceptibility testing; (ii) it is low in sulfonamide, trimethoprim, and tetracycline inhibitors; (iii) it supports the growth of most nonfastidious bacterial pathogens; and (iv) years of data and clinical experience regarding its performance have been accrued. Fastidious bacteria, such as *Haemophilus* species, *Neisseria gonorrhoeae, Neisseria meningitidis,* and streptococci, do not grow satisfactorily on unsupplemented Mueller-Hinton agar but can be tested by the disk method by using supplemented or modified test media as discussed in chapter 75 of this Manual.

Plates of Mueller-Hinton agar may be purchased, or the agar may be prepared from a commercially available dehydrated base according to the manufacturer's directions. If the agar is prepared, only formulations that have been tested according to and have met acceptance limits recommended by the CLSI should be used (22). The prepared medium is autoclaved and immediately placed in a 45 to 50°C water bath. When cool, it is poured into round plastic flat-bottomed petri dishes on a level surface to give a uniform depth of about 4 mm (60 to 70 ml of medium for 150-mm-diameter plates and 25 to 30 ml for 100-mm-diameter plates) and allowed to cool to room temperature. Agar deeper than 4 mm may cause false resistance results (excessively small zones), whereas agar less than 4 mm deep may be associated with excessively large zones and false susceptibility.

Each batch of Mueller-Hinton agar should be checked when the medium is prepared to ensure that the pH is between 7.2 and 7.4 at room temperature, which means that the pH must be measured after the medium has solidified. This can be done by allowing a small amount of agar to solidify around the tip of a pH electrode in a beaker or a cup, by macerating a sufficient amount of agar in neutral distilled water, or by using a properly calibrated surface electrode. A pH outside the range of 7.2 to 7.4 may adversely affect susceptibility test results. If the pH is too low, drugs such as the aminoglycosides, macrolides, and fluoroquinolones will appear to lose potency whereas others (for example, the penicillins and tetracyclines) may appear to have excessive activity. The opposite effects are possible if the pH is too high.

Freshly prepared plates may be used the same day or stored in a refrigerator (2 to 8°C); if refrigerated, they should be wrapped in plastic to minimize evaporation. Just before use, if excess moisture is visible on the surface, plates should be placed in an incubator (35°C) or, with lids ajar, in a laminar-flow hood at room temperature until the moisture evaporates (usually 10 to 30 min). At the time the medium is to be inoculated, no droplets of moisture should be visible on its surface or on the petri dish cover.

Various components of or supplements to Mueller-Hinton medium may affect susceptibility test results; therefore, appropriate quality control procedures (see "Quality Control" below) must be performed and zone diameters must be within acceptable limits. For example, media containing excessive amounts of thymidine or thymine can reverse the inhibitory effects of sulfonamides and trimethoprim, causing zones of growth inhibition to be smaller or less distinct. Organisms may therefore appear to be resistant to these drugs when in fact they are not. Variation in the concentrations of divalent cations, primarily calcium and magnesium, affects results of aminoglycoside and tetracycline tests with *P. aeruginosa* isolates (26). A cation content that is too high reduces zone sizes, whereas a cation content that is too low has the opposite effect. Sheep blood should not be added to Mueller-Hinton medium for testing of nonfastidious organisms, because the blood can significantly alter the zone diameters with several agents and bacterial species (15).

Inoculation Procedure

To ensure reproducibility of disk diffusion susceptibility test results, the inoculum must be standardized (10, 26). The inoculum may be prepared by the growth method or by direct suspension from colonies on the agar plate, as described above for dilution testing.

When trimethoprim-sulfamethoxazole is tested by the direct inoculum suspension method, colonies from blood agar medium may carry over enough trimethoprim or sulfonamide antagonists to produce a haze of growth inside the zones of inhibition with susceptible isolates.

The Mueller-Hinton agar plate should be inoculated within 15 min after the inoculum suspension has been adjusted. A sterile cotton swab is dipped into the suspension, rotated several times, and gently pressed onto the inside wall of the tube above the fluid level to remove excess inoculum from the swab. The swab is then streaked over the entire surface of the agar plate three times, with the plate rotated approximately 60° each time to ensure even distribution of the inoculum. A final sweep of the swab is made around the agar rim. The lid may be left ajar for 3 to 5 min but no longer than 15 min to allow any excess surface moisture to be absorbed before the drug-impregnated disks are applied.

Antimicrobial Disks

Within 15 min after the plates are inoculated, selected antimicrobial agent disks are distributed evenly onto the surface, with at least 24 mm (center to center) between them. Disks are placed individually with sterile forceps or more commonly with a mechanical dispensing apparatus and then gently pressed down onto the agar surface to provide uniform contact. No more than 12 disks should be placed onto one 150-mm-diameter plate and no more than 5 disks should be placed onto a 100-mm-diameter plate to avoid overlapping zones. Some of the antimicrobial agent in the disk diffuses almost immediately; therefore, once a disk contacts the agar surface, the disk should not be moved.

Incubation

No longer than 15 min after disks are applied, the plates are inverted and incubated at 35°C in ambient air. A delay of more than 15 min before incubation permits excess prediffusion of the antimicrobial agents. The interpretive standards for nonfastidious bacteria are based on results of test samples incubated in ambient air, and the zone-of-inhibition diameters for some drugs, such as the aminoglycosides, macrolides, and tetracyclines, are significantly altered by CO_2; therefore, plates should not be incubated in atmospheres with increased CO_2. Testing isolates of some fastidious bacteria, however, requires incubation in 5% CO_2, and zone diameter criteria for those species have been established on that basis (see chapter 75 of this Manual).

Interpretation and Reporting of Results

Each plate is examined after incubation for 16 to 18 h for all nonfastidious bacterial isolates except staphylococci and enterococci, which must be incubated for a full 24 h to allow detection of resistance to oxacillin and vancomycin (26). If plates are inoculated correctly, the diameters of the zones of inhibition are uniformly circular and the lawns of growth are confluent. Growth that consists of individual isolated colonies indicates that the inoculum was too light, and the test must be repeated. The diameters of the zones of complete inhibition, including the diameter of the disk, are measured to the nearest whole millimeter with calipers or a ruler. With unsupplemented Mueller-Hinton agar, the measuring device is held on the back of the inverted petri dish, which is illuminated with reflected light located a few inches above a black, nonreflecting background.

The zone margin is the area where no obvious growth is visible. When isolates of staphylococci or enterococci are tested, any discernible growth (especially a haze of pinpoint colonies) within the zone of inhibition around the oxacillin disk (for staphylococci) or vancomycin disk (for enterococci) is indicative of resistance. For other bacteria, discrete colonies growing within a clear zone of inhibition may indicate testing of a mixed culture that should be subcultured, reidentified, and retested. However, the presence of colonies within a zone of inhibition may also indicate selection of high-frequency mutants indicative of eventual resistance to that agent, e.g., *Enterobacter* spp. with penicillins and cephalosporins. With *Proteus* species, if a thin film of swarming growth is visible in an otherwise obvious zone of inhibition, the margin of heavy growth is measured and the film is disregarded. With trimethoprim, the sulfonamides, and combinations of the two agents, antagonists in the medium may allow some minimal growth; therefore, the zone diameter is measured at the obvious margin, and slight growth (20% or less of the lawn of growth) is disregarded.

The zone diameters measured around each disk are interpreted on the basis of guidelines published by the CLSI, and the organisms are reported as susceptible, intermediate, or resistant to the antimicrobial agents tested (Table 3) (27). The clinical interpretation of the categories of susceptible, intermediate, and resistant has already been provided above under "Dilution Methods." Computer programs are available that accompany some automated zone size reading devices to allow MICs to be derived from the linear regression equation with selected antimicrobial agents and bacterial isolates (14, 63) (see also chapter 17).

Advantages and Disadvantages

The disk diffusion test has several advantages: (i) it is technically simple to perform and very reproducible, (ii) the reagents are relatively inexpensive, (iii) it does not require any special equipment, (iv) it provides susceptibility category results that are easily understood by clinicians, and (v) it is flexible regarding selection of antimicrobial agents for testing. The primary limitation of the disk diffusion test is the spectrum of organisms for which it has been standardized. There have not been adequate studies to develop reliable interpretive standards for disk testing of bacteria not listed in the CLSI disk diffusion document (26) or the recently developed CLSI guideline for infrequently isolated or fastidious bacteria (24). It is also important to note that only certain drugs have been validated for disk diffusion testing of *Stenotrophomonas maltophilia* and *Burkholderia cepacia* (27). The disk test is inadequate for detection of vancomycin-intermediate *S. aureus* (26, 80, 81), does not detect daptomycin resistance in staphylococci and enterococci (45, 72) or colistin resistance in gram-negative bacilli (44), and in the past was reported to have difficulties in the detection of oxacillin-heteroresistant staphylococci (33, 60) and enterococci with low-level (VanB-type) vancomycin resistance (71, 81). A potential disadvantage of disk diffusion susceptibility testing is that it provides only a qualitative result and a quantitative result indicating the degree of susceptibility (MIC) may be needed in some cases, e.g., those involving penicillin and cephalosporin susceptibilities of *S. pneumoniae* and certain viridans group streptococci (see chapter 75 of this Manual).

Quality Control

The goals of a quality control program for disk diffusion are to monitor the precision and accuracy of the procedure, the performance of the reagents (medium and disks), and the performance of persons who do the testing and read, interpret, and report results. To best achieve these goals, reference strains are selected for their genetic stability and their usefulness in the disk diffusion test.

Reference Strains

Reference strains recommended by the CLSI for quality control of the disk diffusion procedure when nonfastidious bacteria are tested are *E. coli* ATCC 25922, *P. aeruginosa* ATCC 27853, *S. aureus* ATCC 25923 (not the same strain used for quality control of MIC tests), *Enterococcus faecalis* ATCC 29212, and *E. coli* ATCC 35218 (27, 28). *E. coli* ATCC 35218 is recommended as a control only for beta-lactamase inhibitor combinations containing clavulanic acid, sulbactam, or tazobactam. *Enterococcus faecalis* ATCC 29212 can be used to ensure that the levels of inhibitors of trimethoprim or sulfonamides in Mueller-Hinton agar do not exceed acceptable limits and can also be used to control disks containing a high concentration of gentamicin or streptomycin (see chapter 74 of this Manual).

The reference strains listed above should be obtained from a reliable source, and stock cultures should be maintained in such a way that viability is ensured and the opportunity for selection of resistant variants is minimal (28). The procedures for maintaining and storing working stock cultures are described in the CLSI standard (26). If an unexplained result indicates that the inherent susceptibility of the strain has been altered, a fresh subculture of that organism should be obtained.

Zone-of-Inhibition Diameter Ranges

The ranges of zone diameters for reference strains used to monitor performance of the disk diffusion test are updated frequently and published annually; therefore, readers should refer to the most recent CLSI document for this information (27). Generally, results of 1 in every 20 tests in a series of tests might be out of the accepted limits. If a second result falls outside the stated limits, corrective action must be taken. The action taken and the results of that action must be documented.

Frequency of Testing

Each new batch or lot of Mueller-Hinton agar must be tested with the reference strains listed above before the medium is released for use with clinical specimens, and quality control must be done before a new lot of antimicrobial disks is introduced. Appropriate reference strains also should be tested each day that the disk diffusion test is performed. The frequency of testing, however, may be reduced if satisfactory performance is documented for 20 or 30 consecutive days of testing: for each combination of drug and reference strain, no more than 1 of 20 or 3 of 30 zone-of-inhibition diameters may be outside the accepted limits published by the CLSI (27). When this criterion is fulfilled, each reference strain need be tested only once per week and any time a reagent component of the test is changed. However, if a zone-of-inhibition diameter falls outside the acceptable control limits, corrective action must be taken. If the problem appears to be caused by an obvious error such as use of the wrong disk or the wrong reference strain, contamination of the reference strain, or incubation in an incorrect atmosphere, repeating the test with the appropriate parameter is acceptable. However, if a cause of the error is not obvious, quality control must be performed daily for a period that will allow discovery of the source of the aberrant result and documentation of how the problem was resolved. This may be accomplished by the same approach described above under "Quality Control" in "Dilution Methods."

Special Disk Tests

Two specialized applications of the disk test are described in detail in chapter 74. In brief, disk testing with cefoxitin is now the preferred method for detection of *mecA*-mediated oxacillin resistance in both *S. aureus* and coagulase-negative staphylococcal species (26, 27, 78). Cefoxitin serves as a surrogate marker for the principal mechanism of oxacillin resistance in staphylococci and provides more reliable results than oxacillin itself. Secondly, inducible clindamycin resistance is not reliably detected by standard dilution or disk diffusion susceptibility testing without induction of the expression of *erm*-mediated macrolide-lincosamide-streptogramin B resistance in staphylococci and hemolytic streptococci (61). Such strains can be accurately detected only by induction of resistance expression by exposure to a macrolide. A disk approximation test in which erythromycin and clindamycin disks are placed in close proximity allows recognition of inducible resistance by truncating the clindamycin zone and giving rise to a positive "D-zone test" (27, 42). When recognized through disk approximation testing, such strains should be reported as resistant to clindamycin (27, 61). A similar approach may be taken by incorporating a subinhibitory concentration of erythromycin into broth or agar dilution tests with clindamycin, although this approach is not as convenient as the use of the disk approximation method.

ANTIBACTERIAL SUSCEPTIBILITY TESTING METHODS THAT MAY BE USED OUTSIDE OF THE UNITED STATES

The CLSI is best known for developing laboratory testing standards for use in the United States, including those for antimicrobial susceptibility testing (25, 26, 27). The CLSI standards are recognized as U.S. national standards by the American National Standards Institute and by federal regulations, including the Clinical Laboratory Improvement Amendments (46), and as standard reference procedures by the Food and Drug Administration. However, the CLSI procedures are also used by an increasing number of laboratories outside of the United States, including countries in North and South America and in several areas of Europe, Asia, and Australasia. Some countries have national standards or professional committees comprising their own expert microbiologists that establish methods of susceptibility testing for their countries and interpretive criteria for those tests that may or may not be the same as those of the CLSI (17, 41), as described further in chapter 72.

Several variations on dilution and diffusion methods are used for routine susceptibility testing outside the United States (Table 4). Most non-U.S. methods are specific to individual countries, having developed and evolved locally over many years. Many of the non-U.S. methods differ from the CLSI procedures in the choice of media, inoculum preparation procedures, and, for diffusion methods, disk contents. There are also some variations between these methods in breakpoints and the approaches to establishing the breakpoints (41, 69). Variation in test methods can cause considerable confusion in laboratories, especially if both CLSI and non-CLSI methods are used for different organisms. Thus, it is important that any method should be followed in all its detail for valid application of specific breakpoints.

In the past, there have been limited efforts at harmonizing breakpoints internationally (88, 89). The Europeans through the European Society of Clinical Microbiology and Infectious Diseases have formed the European Union Committee on Antimicrobial Susceptibility Testing (EUCAST). EUCAST has defined reference agar and broth microdilution MIC methods (39, 40) for use in Europe. One encouraging prospect for the future is the establishment for the first time of a global standard reference MIC susceptibility method (broth microdilution) developed through the International Organization for Standards (ISO; Geneva, Switzerland) (50) in concert with the European Committee on Standardization (Brussels, Belgium). The global reference method is in essence the CLSI and EUCAST broth microdilution methods with a few differences harmonized in the ISO standard (50). This will hopefully provide a degree of international standardization for reference MIC determinations and allow a benchmark for assessment of the performance of commercial devices for susceptibility testing. In a second document, the ISO has established criteria for acceptable performance of susceptibility testing devices (51).

International Dilution Methods

Both broth and agar dilution methods have been developed in countries outside the United States. In the past, methods using a limited range of concentrations (often one or two), or so-called breakpoint methods, have been advocated (87). They are the standard form of susceptibility testing advocated by the Japanese Society for Chemotherapy (52, 53) and as an alternative to disk diffusion testing by the British Society for Antimicrobial Chemotherapy (BSAC) (1, 16). Reasonably current published methods and standards include those of the BSAC (1; see also http://www.bsac.org.uk), the Société Française de Microbiologie (CA-SFM; http://www.sfm.asso.fr), the Deutsches Institut für Normung (DIN; documents are available through http://www.beuth.de), and the Swedish Reference Group for Antibiotics (SRGA; http://www.srga.org).

Breakpoint methods may be popular in larger laboratories because large numbers of isolates can be tested cost-effectively using replicators and the methods provide susceptibility category (i.e., qualitative) endpoints. Optical readers are available to facilitate reading of agar dilution plates (e.g., Mastascanelite; Mast Laboratories, Bootle, United Kingdom; see http://www.mastascan.com). However, there are considerable difficulties with quality control, including the lack of

TABLE 4 Non-U.S. disk diffusion methods for susceptibility testing

Method (reference)	Country	Society	Agar medium	Comments
BSAC (2)	United Kingdom	BSAC	Iso-Sensitest	
CA-SFM (65)	France	CA-SFM	Mueller-Hinton	Similar to CLSI
DIN (34, 35)	Germany	DIN	Mueller-Hinton	
SRGA (68, 70)	Sweden	SRGA	Iso-Sensitest or Mueller-Hinton	
Neo-sensitabs	Denmark		Mueller-Hinton	Uses antimicrobials incorporated into compressed tablets rather than paper disks. Size of tablets results in substantially larger zones than conventional 6-mm-diam disks.
Calibrated dichotomous sensitivity (12, 13)	Australia		Sensitest	Dichotomous (no intermediate category). Disk strengths chosen to give annular radius of inhibition of ~6 mm where possible.

appropriate control strains for which the MICs are near the breakpoints and the complexity of quantifying drug concentrations prior to use (64). In addition, problems have been reported in the past with the use of Iso-Sensitest agar (3, 84) and with the incorporation of inhibitors to prevent swarming of *Proteus* spp., such as *p*-nitrophenylglycerol (85), or increased agar content for the same purpose (86). In turn, the choice of Mueller-Hinton by the CLSI has been criticized for not providing luxuriant growth of all organisms (88), suggesting that there is no absolutely ideal medium. As the best-studied, most widely used medium for susceptibility testing, Mueller-Hinton broth was chosen for the ISO reference method (50).

International Diffusion Methods

A wide variety of diffusion methods have been developed in different countries over the years. They are quite diverse in their approaches. Almost all have been maintained primarily because of the widespread popularity of disk testing. None appear to offer any major advantage over the modified Kirby-Bauer method (10) advocated by the CLSI (26). As pointed out above, disk methods are inexpensive and flexible and may become more popular through the use of zone readers and interconnected computers for interpretation of zone diameters (4, 63).

The previously recommended BSAC standard diffusion methods and the comparative and Stokes' methods differed from other diffusion methods in that susceptibility categorization was achieved by comparison with a control strain rather than by reference to a defined set of zone diameters (16). This technique attracted criticism because it was not based upon or derived from correlations with MICs (18) and has now been replaced by a correlated diffusion method (2) which is now well developed and kept up-to-date (http://www.bsac.org.uk/susceptibility_testing.cfm). For the new BSAC method, Iso-Sensitest (Oxoid, Basingstoke, United Kingdom) is the recommended agar, supplemented for fastidious bacteria with whole defibrinated horse blood with or without NAD. Mueller-Hinton supplemented with 5% sodium chloride is recommended for the detection of methicillin and oxacillin resistance in staphylococci. The inoculum is prepared to produce semiconfluent growth only, rather than the confluent growth lawn used in the CLSI method. One important change in the newer British method is the elimination of an intermediate category for most organism-antimicrobial agent combinations (62).

Since 1980, the CA-SFM has put considerable effort into standardization of susceptibility testing, including regular updates with breakpoints for new drugs that are published frequently (65; see also http://www.sfm.asso.fr). Like the CLSI, the CA-SFM has selected Mueller-Hinton as the test medium. For diffusion testing, plates can be inoculated by flooding as well as swabbing. In most other aspects, this method resembles that of the CLSI, including the use of control organisms and the choice of disk strength. The CA-SFM provides zone diameter breakpoints for drugs available in France and elsewhere that are not approved for clinical use in the United States, e.g., fusidic acid and pristinamycin (65).

The German standards organization, DIN, published acceptable methods for diffusion susceptibility testing as early as 1979, with irregular updates since then (34, 35). They too use Mueller Hinton agar but will tolerate the use of other media provided that the MIC-zone diameter relationships have been determined for those media. Like the CA-SFM method, the DIN method has much in common with the CLSI method.

The SRGA (68, 77) method uses Iso-Sensitest, although the SRGA also accepts Mueller-Hinton as an alternative. The SRGA system is based on the methodology developed by the original International Collaborative Study (38) that was the first to provide a sound theoretical basis to diffusion susceptibility testing. The breakpoints for susceptibility were restructured in 1981 into the more conventional susceptible, intermediate, and resistant categories (77) and are updated regularly (70).

A method developed by a commercial firm in Denmark differs technically if not in principle from the other methods. This method employs so-called Neo-sensitabs that are compressed tablets 9 mm in diameter into which the antibiotic has been incorporated (Rosco Diagnostica, Taarstrup, Denmark; http://www.rosco.dk). The method and the interpretive zone diameter criteria are updated and published by the manufacturer periodically. Not only are the tablets larger and thicker than conventional 6-mm-diameter paper disks, they usually contain larger amounts of antibiotic, resulting in significantly larger zones of inhibition with most drugs. This has the disadvantage of reducing the number of tablets that can be put on a single plate and still produce readable zones. However, the system does have the advantage that the tablets can be stored at room temperature for up to 4 years, obviating the need for storage under refrigeration or freezing. This is an obvious benefit for laboratories in developing countries where reliable refrigeration and power can be a problem.

A diffusion method developed in Australia in 1975 (12, 13) and still widely used in that country has a number of unique features. The calibrated dichotomous sensitivity method employs Sensitest agar and an unusual method for inoculum preparation and is unique in defining just two categories of susceptibility: susceptible and resistant. In order to simplify test result reading, each new drug is calibrated against the MIC breakpoint to yield wherever possible a zone diameter of 18 mm. This is achieved by adjusting disk strengths, which in most cases are substantially lower than those used with other methods. The lack of an intermediate category, which increases the risk of serious interpretive errors (e.g., susceptible instead of resistant), the absence of some common drugs from the test range, and some unusual use of surrogate drugs for testing have restricted the adoption of this method outside of Australia. The interpretative criteria are updated regularly and can be found on the Web (http://www.med.unsw.edu.au/pathology-cds/).

Non-CLSI Breakpoints

Each international method has, of necessity, had to develop its own breakpoints because of differences in media, inocula, and, in the case of disk diffusion methods, disk strengths. In addition, some non-U.S. organizations have developed specialized methods for setting breakpoints. The BSAC has developed a formula based on maximum blood concentrations, protein binding, and elimination half-life. This is now integrated with other considerations including pharmacodynamics and clinical outcome data (69). The Japanese Society for Chemotherapy uses both a formula and a comparison with favorable outcome in clinical studies where the MICs for the pathogens have been determined (5, 52, 53, 74, 75). The Spanish Society for Chemotherapy has also published breakpoints which tend to be more conservative as they are based primarily on MIC distributions (66). EUCAST has recently set about the task of establishing breakpoints for Europe (see http://www.eucast.org). A feature of the program has been the collation of large amounts of MIC data to establish wild-type strain distributions and cutoff values as a prelude to formal breakpoint setting (59). EUCAST integrates wild-type strain distributions and pharmacokinetic-pharmacodynamic information in a manner similar to that used recently by the CLSI. As dosages used in Europe can be different from those used in the United States, some breakpoints will differ from those set by the CLSI. Most other groups have set breakpoints without major reference to pharmacokinetics or pharmacodynamics.

COMMON SOURCES OF ERROR IN ANTIBACTERIAL SUSCEPTIBILITY TESTING

Potential sources of error in antibacterial susceptibility testing may be categorized as those that relate to the test system and its components, those associated with the test procedure, those peculiar to certain organism and drug combinations, and those that relate to reporting (34, 60). The most common sources of error encountered in clinical microbiology laboratories are reviewed in the following paragraphs.

Various components of the susceptibility test system may be a source of error. First, the system itself may have limitations regarding the organisms that should be tested. For example, the disk diffusion method should be used only to test rapidly growing bacterial pathogens that have consistent growth rates (those for which interpretive criteria have been developed and published by the CLSI). Second, the medium used may be a source of error if it fails to conform to recommended composition and performance. Factors common to both agar-based and broth-based systems are the pH of the medium, which for Mueller-Hinton agar or broth should be between 7.2 and 7.4, and its cation content. The concentration of magnesium and calcium in the broth medium should be that recommended by the CLSI to ensure reliable results. For detection of oxacillin resistance in staphylococci by testing of oxacillin, it is essential that the proper amount of sodium chloride be included in the agar or broth used for dilution testing. For agar dilution and disk diffusion, the Mueller-Hinton agar should be 3 to 4 mm deep. Third, the components of the system (antimicrobial disks, agar plates, and trays) must be stored properly, and they should not be used beyond the stated expiration dates.

Steps in the susceptibility test procedure that may be a source of error if they are not performed correctly include inoculum preparation, incubation (conditions and duration), endpoint interpretation, and performance of appropriate quality control. The inoculum must be pure, and it must contain an adequate density of bacteria. With rare exceptions, all systems should be incubated in ambient air at 35°C. The incubation time, however, varies. For conventional dilution and disk diffusion systems, incubation for 16 to 20 h and 16 to 18 h, respectively, is recommended except in tests of staphylococci with oxacillin and vancomycin and enterococci with vancomycin, in which systems must be incubated for a full 24 h (25, 26, 82). The endpoints for all susceptibility tests must be measured accurately, following guidelines published by the CLSI (25, 26). If endpoints are interpreted by an instrument, the reliability of that instrument must be monitored. Moreover, with all susceptibility test systems, appropriate reference strains must be tested at regular intervals, any problems that occur must be thoroughly investigated, and corrective action must be well documented.

Testing of certain antimicrobial agents with some bacteria may yield misleading results, because in vitro results do not necessarily correlate with in vivo activity. Examples include narrow- and expanded-spectrum cephalosporins and aminoglycosides tested with *Salmonella* spp. and *Shigella* spp.; all beta-lactam agents except the penicillinase-resistant penicillins (oxacillin, nafcillin, methicillin, or cefoxitin as a surrogate marker) tested with oxacillin-resistant staphylococci; cephalosporins, aminoglycosides (except concentrations used to detect high-level resistance), clindamycin, and trimethoprim-sulfamethoxazole tested with enterococci; and cephalosporins tested with *Listeria* spp. (25, 26, 27). Therefore, for these combinations of organisms and drugs, results should not be reported. Other potential problems associated with reporting are possible transcriptional errors for laboratories that use a manual recording and reporting system and possible errors in transmission of data for laboratories in which an automated susceptibility test system is interfaced with the laboratory and/or hospital information system.

PROBLEM ORGANISMS AND RESISTANCE MECHANISMS

The dilution and diffusion methods described in this chapter have been developed through careful studies and standardized by national professional organizations and diagnostic device manufacturers. Despite this, there are still some organisms for which methods have not yet been standardized (e.g., corynebacteria and some fastidious bacteria in the case of disk testing) or which fail to provide reliable results with some of the standard tests (e.g., *Stenotrophomonas maltophilia* and *Burkholderia cepacia* in the case of disk diffusion testing of some drugs). Certain other organisms may possess resistance mechanisms that are inducible (VanB-type resistance in some enterococci, ampC beta-lactamase in some gram-negative species) or that result in subtle phenotypic expression under standard inoculum and test conditions (e.g., inducible clindamycin resistance in staphylococci and some streptococci; extended-spectrum beta-lactamases in some gram-negative bacilli). Reliable detection of these subtle resistance traits may require the use of different or modified test methods that are outlined in chapter 74 of this Manual. The CLSI adopted revised MIC and disk diffusion breakpoints for testing coagulase-negative staphylococci with oxacillin in an attempt to avoid errors of false susceptibility (25, 26, 27, 79, 90). However, testing of cefoxitin with both *S. aureus* and coagulase-negative species has more recently been recommended by the CLSI as the simplest and most reliable method for detection of *mecA*-mediated oxacillin resistance (27, 78). The screening tests for detection of extended-spectrum beta-lactamases by using cefpodoxime have been expanded by the CLSI to include testing of *Proteus mirabilis* in addition to *E. coli* and *Klebsiella* spp. (27). There has not previously been uniform agreement regarding what level of accuracy is acceptable when selecting a testing method or system for performing antimicrobial susceptibility testing (55). Recently, general guidelines for acceptable performance (e.g., rates of essential agreement and category agreement) have been developed through an international consensus effort (ISO) (51). However, it is important to keep in mind that new resistance mechanisms or decreases in susceptibility to important therapeutic agents can arise at any time to challenge our methods of susceptibility testing, e.g., in the case of vancomycin-resistant or -intermediate *S. aureus* (20, 47, 80, 81). Thus, susceptibility testing methods must continue to evolve and develop over time as new challenges are presented.

REFERENCES

1. **Andrews, J. M.** 2001. Determination of minimum inhibitory concentrations. *J. Antimicrob. Chemother.* **48**(Suppl. S1):5–16.

2. **Andrews, J. M., for the BSAC Working Party in Susceptibility Testing.** 2001. BSAC standardized disc susceptibility testing method. *J. Antimicrob. Chemother.* **48** (Suppl. S1):43–57.
3. **Andrews, J. M., J. P. Ashby, and R. Wise.** 1990. Problems with Iso-Sensitest agar. *J. Antimicrob. Chemother.* **26:**596–597.
4. **Andrews, J. M., F. J. Boswell, and R. Wise.** 2000. Evaluation of the Oxoid Aura image system for measuring zones of inhibition with the disc diffusion technique. *J. Antimicrob. Chemother*. **46:**535–540.
5. **Arakawa, S., T. Matsui, S. Kamidono, Y. Kawada, H. Kumon, K. Hirai, T. Hirose, T. Matsumoto, K. Yamaguchi, T. Yoshida, K. Watanabe, K. Ueno, A. Saito, and T. Teranishi.** 1998. Derivation of a calculation formula for breakpoints of antimicrobial agents in urinary tract infections. *J. Infect. Chemother.* **4:**97–106.
6. **Baker, C. N., S. A. Stocker, D. H. Culver, and C. Thornsberry.** 1991. Comparison of the E test to agar dilution, broth microdilution, and agar diffusion susceptibility testing techniques by using a special challenge set of bacteria. *J. Clin. Microbiol.* **29:**533–538.
7. **Barry, A. L.** 1991. Procedures and theoretical considerations for testing antimicrobial agents in agar media, p. 1–16. *In* V. Lorian (ed.), *Antibiotics in Laboratory Medicine,* 3rd ed. The Williams & Wilkins Co., Baltimore, Md.
8. **Barry, A. L., R. E. Badal, and R. W. Hawkinson.** 1983. Influence of inoculum growth phase on microdilution susceptibility tests. *J. Clin. Microbiol.* **18:**645–651.
9. **Barry, A. L., L. B. Reller, G. H. Miller, J. A. Washington, F. D. Schoenknecht, L. R. Peterson, R. S. Hare, and C. Knapp.** 1992. Revision of standards for adjusting the cation content of Mueller-Hinton broth for testing susceptibility of *Pseudomonas aeruginosa* to aminoglycosides. *J. Clin. Microbiol.* **30:**585–589.
10. **Bauer, A. W., W. M. M. Kirby, J. C. Sherris, and M. Turck.** 1966. Antibiotic susceptibility testing by standardized single disk method. *Am. J. Clin. Pathol.* **45:**493–496.
11. **Bauer, A. W., and J. C. Sherris.** 1964. The determination of sulfonamide susceptibility of bacteria. *Chemotherapia* **9:**1–19.
12. **Bell, S. M.** 1975. The CDS method of antibiotic sensitivity testing (Calibrated Dichotomous Sensitivity test). *Pathology* **7**(Suppl.)**:**1–48.
13. **Bell, S. M.** 1988. Additions and modifications to the range of antibiotics tested by the CDS method of antibiotic sensitivity testing. *Pathology* **20:**303–304.
14. **Berk, I., and P. M. Tierno, Jr.** 1996. Comparison of efficacy and cost-effectiveness of BIOMIC VIDEO and Vitek antimicrobial susceptibility test systems for use in the clinical microbiology laboratory. *J. Clin. Microbiol.* **34:**1980–1984.
15. **Brenner, V. C., and J. C. Sherris.** 1972. Influence of different media and bloods on the results of diffusion antibiotic susceptibility tests. *Antimicrob. Agents Chemother.* **1:**116–122.
16. **British Society for Antimicrobial Chemotherapy.** 1991. Report of the working party on antibiotic sensitivity testing of the British Society for Antimicrobial Chemotherapy: a guide to sensitivity testing. *J. Antimicrob. Chemother.* **27** (Suppl. D)**:**1–50.
17. **Brown, D. F. J.** 1994. Developments in antimicrobial susceptibility testing. *Rev. Med. Microbiol.* **5:**65–75.
18. **Brown, D. F. J.** 1990. The comparative method for antimicrobial susceptibility testing—time for a change? *J. Antimicrob. Chemother.* **25:**307–312.
19. **Brunden, M. N., G. E. Zurenko, and B. Kapik.** 1992. Modification of the error-bounded classification scheme for use with two MIC breakpoints. *Diagn. Microbiol. Infect. Dis.* **15:**135–140.
20. **Centers for Disease Control and Prevention.** 2004. Brief report: vancomycin-resistant *Staphylocccus aureus*—New York, 2004. *Morb. Mortal. Wkly. Rep.* **53:**322–323.
21. **Clinical and Laboratory Standards Institute/NCCLS.** 2001. *Development of In Vitro Susceptibility Testing Criteria and Quality Control Parameters.* Approved standard M23-A2. Clinical and Laboratory Standards Institute, Wayne, Pa.
22. **Clinical and Laboratory Standards Institute/NCCLS.** 1996. *Evaluating Production Lots of Dehydrated Mueller-Hinton Agar.* Approved standard M6-A. Clinical and Laboratory Standards Institute, Wayne, Pa.
23. **Clinical and Laboratory Standards Institute/NCCLS.** 2001. *Evaluation of Lots of Dehydrated Mueller-Hinton Broth for Antimicrobial Susceptibility Testing.* Proposed standard M32-P. Clinical and Laboratory Standards Institute, Wayne, Pa.
24. **Clinical and Laboratory Standards Institute/NCCLS.** 2005. *Methods for Antimicrobial Dilution and Disk Susceptibility Testing of Infrequently-Isolated or Fastidious Bacteria.* Proposed guideline M45-P. Clinical and Laboratory Standards Institute, Wayne, Pa.
25. **Clinical and Laboratory Standards Institute/NCCLS.** 2006. *Methods for Dilution Antimicrobial Susceptibility Tests for Bacteria That Grow Aerobically.* Approved standard M7-A6. Clinical and Laboratory Standards Institute, Wayne, Pa.
26. **Clinical and Laboratory Standards Institute/NCCLS.** 2006. *Performance Standards for Antimicrobial Disk Susceptibility Tests.* Approved standard M2-A8. Clinical and Laboratory Standards Institute, Wayne, Pa.
27. **Clinical and Laboratory Standards Institute/NCCLS.** 2006. *Performance Standards for Antimicrobial Susceptibility Testing.* Supplement M100-S16. Clinical and Laboratory Standards Institute, Wayne, Pa.
28. **Coyle, M. B., M. F. Lampe, C. L. Aitkin, P. Feigl, and J. C. Sherris.** 1976. Reproducibility of control strains for antibiotic susceptibility testing. *Antimicrob. Agents Chemother.* **10:**436–440.
29. **Craig, W. A.** 1993. Qualitative susceptibility tests versus quantitative MIC tests. *Diagn. Microbiol. Infect. Dis.* **16:** 231–236.
30. **Craig, W. A.** 1998. Pharmacokinetic/pharmacodynamic parameters for antibacterial dosing of mice and men. *Clin. Infect. Dis.* **26:**1–12.
31. **Daly, J. S., R. A. Dodge, R. H. Glew, D. T. Soja, B. A. DeLuca, and S. Hebert.** 1997. Effect of zinc concentration in Mueller-Hinton agar on susceptibility of *Pseudomonas aeruginosa* to imipenem. *J. Clin. Microbiol.* **35:**1027–1029.
32. **D'Amato, R. F., C. Thornsberry, C. N. Baker, and L. A. Kirven.** 1975. Effect of calcium and magnesium ions on the susceptibility of *Pseudomonas* species to tetracycline, gentamicin, polymyxin B, and carbenicillin. *Antimicrob. Agents Chemother.* **7:**596–600.
33. **De Lencastre, H., A. M. Sa Figueiredo, C. Urban, J. Rahal, and A. Tomasz.** 1991. Multiple mechanisms of methicillin resistance and improved methods for detection in clinical isolates of *Staphylococcus aureus*. *Antimicrob. Agents Chemother.* **35:**632–639.
34. **Deutches Institut für Normung.** 2002. *Susceptibility Testing of Pathogens to Antimicrobial Agents, Part 3. Agar Diffusion Test.* DIN 58940-3. Beuth Verlag, Berlin, Germany.
35. **Deutches Institut für Normung.** 2003. *Susceptibility Testing of Pathogens to Antimicrobial Agents, Part 6. Determination of the Minimum Inhibitory Concentration (MIC) with the Agar Dilution Method.* DIN 58940-6. Beuth Verlag, Berlin, Germany.
36. **Diekema, D. J., K. Lee, P. Raney, L. A. Herwaldt, G. V. Doern, and F. C. Tenover.** 2004. Accuracy and appropriateness of antimicrobial susceptibility test reporting for bacteria isolated from blood cultures. *J. Clin. Microbiol.* **42:**2258–2260.
37. **Doern, G. V.** 1987. Breakpoint susceptibility testing. *Clin. Microbiol. Newsl.* **9:**81–84.
38. **Ericsson, J. M., and J. C. Sherris.** 1971. Antibiotic sensitivity testing. Report of an international collaborative study. *Acta Pathol. Microbiol. Scan. Sect. B Suppl.* **217:**1–90.

39. **European Committee for Antimicrobial Susceptibility Testing.** 2000. Determination of minimum inhibitory concentration (MICs) of antibacterial agents by agar dilution. European Committee for Antimicrobial Susceptibility Testing definitive document. *Clin. Microbiol. Infect.* **6:**509–515.
40. **European Committee for Antimicrobial Susceptibility Testing.** 2003. Determination of minimum inhibitory concentration (MICs) of antibacterial agents by broth dilution. *Clin. Microbiol. Infect.* **9:**1–7.
41. **Ferraro, M. J.** 2001. Should we reevaluate antibiotic breakpoints? *Clin. Infect. Dis.* **33**(Suppl. 3)**:**S227–S229.
42. **Fiebelkorn, K. R., S. A. Crawford, M. L. McElmeel, and J. H. Jorgensen.** 2003. Practical disk diffusion method for detection of inducible clindamycin resistance in *Staphylococcus aureus* and coagulase-negative staphylococci. *J. Clin. Microbiol.* **41:**4740–4744.
43. **Fuchs, P. C., A. L. Barry, and S. D. Brown.** 2000. Daptomycin susceptibility tests: interpretive criteria, quality control and effect of calcium on in vitro tests. *Diagn. Microbiol. Infect. Dis.* **38:**51–58.
44. **Gales, A. C., A. O. Reis, and R. N. Jones.** 2001. Contemporary assessment of antimicrobial susceptibility testing methods for polymyxin B and colistin: review of available interpretive criteria and quality control guidelines. *J. Clin. Microbiol.* **39:**183–190.
45. **Hayden, M. K., K. Rezai, K. R. A. Hayes, K. Lolans, J. P. Quinn, and R. A. Weinstein.** 2005. Development of daptomycin resistance in vivo in methicillin-resistant *Staphylococcus aureus*. *J. Clin. Microbiol.* **43:**5285–5287.
46. **Health Care Financing Administration.** 1992. Clinical laboratory improvement amendments of 1988, final rule. *Fed. Regist.* **57:**7137–7186.
47. **Hiramatsu, K., H. Hanaki, T. Ino, K. Yabuta, T. Oguri, and F. C. Tenover.** 1997. Methicillin-resistant *Staphylococcus aureus* clinical strain with reduced vancomycin susceptibility. *J. Antimicrob. Chemother.* **40:**135–136.
48. **Huang, M., P. N. Baker, S. Banerjee, and F. C. Tenover.** 1992. Accuracy of the E test for determining antimicrobial susceptibilities of staphylococci, enterococci, *Campylobacter jejuni,* and gram-negative bacteria resistant to antimicrobial agents. *J. Clin. Microbiol.* **30:**3243–3248.
49. **Huang, M. B., E. T. Gay, C. N. Baker, S. N. Banerjee, and F. C. Tenover.** 1993. Two percent sodium chloride is required for susceptibility testing of staphylococci with oxacillin when using agar-based dilution methods. *J. Clin. Microbiol.* **31:**2683–2688.
50. **International Organization for Standardization.** 2006. *Susceptibility Testing of Infectious Agents and Evaluation of Performance of Antimicrobial Susceptibility Devices, Part 1. Reference Method for Testing the in vitro Activity of Antimicrobial Agents against Bacteria Involved in Infectious Diseases.* ISO/DIS 20776-1. International Organization for Standardization, Geneva, Switzerland.
51. **International Organization for Standardization.** 2006. *Susceptibility Testing of Infectious Agents and Evaluation of Performance of Antimicrobial Susceptibility Devices, Part 2. Evaluation of Performance of Antimicrobial Susceptibility Test Devices.* ISO/DIS 20776-2. International Organization for Standardization, Geneva, Switzerland.
52. **Japanese Society for Chemotherapy.** 1990. Report of the Committee for Japanese Standards for Antimicrobial Susceptibility Testing for Bacteria. *Chemotherapy* **38:**102–105. (In Japanese.)
53. **Japanese Society for Chemotherapy.** 1993. Report of the Committee for Japanese Standards for Antimicrobial Susceptibility Testing for Bacteria. *Chemotherapy* **41:**183–189. (In Japanese.)
54. **Jones, R. N.** 2001. Method preferences and test accuracy of antimicrobial susceptibility testing: updates from the College of American Pathologists Microbiology Surveys Program. *Arch. Pathol. Lab. Med.* **10:**1285–1289.
55. **Jorgensen, J. H.** 1993. Selection criteria for an antimicrobial susceptibility testing system. *J. Clin. Microbiol.* **31:**2841–2844.
56. **Jorgensen, J. H.** 1993. Selection of antimicrobial agents for routine testing in a clinical microbiology laboratory. *Diagn. Microbiol. Infect. Dis.* **16:**245–249.
57. **Jorgensen, J. H., and M. J. Ferraro.** 1998. Antimicrobial susceptibility testing: general principles and contemporary practices. *Clin. Infect. Dis.* **26:**973–980.
58. **Jorgensen, J. H., and M. J. Ferraro.** 2000. Antimicrobial susceptibility testing: special needs for fastidious organisms and difficult-to-detect resistance mechanisms. *Clin. Infect. Dis.* **30:**799–808.
59. **Kahlmeter, G., D. F. J. Brown, F. W. Goldstein, A. P. MacGowan, J. W. Mouton, A. Österland, A. Rodloff, M. Steinbakk, P. Urbaskova, and A. Vatopoulos.** 2003. European harmonization of MIC breakpoints for antimicrobial susceptibility testing of bacteria. *J. Antimicrob. Chemother.* **52:**145–148.
60. **Kiehlbauch, J. A., G. E. Hannett, M. Salfinger, W. Archinal, C. Monserrat, and C. Carlyn.** 2000. Use of the National Committee for Clinical Laboratory Standards guidelines for disk diffusion susceptibility testing in New York State laboratories. *J. Clin. Microbiol.* **38:**3341–3348.
61. **Lewis, J. S., II, and J. H. Jorgensen.** 2005. Inducible clindamycin resistance in staphylococci: should clinicians and microbiologists be concerned? *Clin. Infect. Dis.* **40:** 280–285.
62. **MacGowan, A. P., and R. Wise.** 2001. Establishing MIC breakpoints and the interpretation of in vitro susceptibility tests. *J. Antimicrob. Chemother.* **48**(Suppl. S1)**:**17–28.
63. **Madeiros, A., and J. Crellin.** 2000. Evaluation of the Sirscan automated zone reader in a clinical microbiology laboratory. *J. Clin. Microbiol.* **38:**1688–1693.
64. **McDermott, S. N., and T. F. Hartley.** 1989. New datum handling methods for the quality control of antimicrobial solutions and plates used in the antimicrobial susceptibility test. *J. Clin. Microbiol.* **27:**1814–1825.
65. **Members of the SFM Antibiogram Committee.** 2003. Comité de l'Antibiogramme de la Société Française de Microbiologie report 2003. *Int. J. Antimicrob. Agents* **21:**364–391.
66. **Mesa Española de Normalización de la Sensibilidad y Resistancia a los Antimicrobianos.** 2000. Recommendations from MENSURA for selection of antimicrobial agents for susceptibility testing and criteria for the interpretation of antibiograms. *Rev. Esp. Quimioter.* **13:**73–86.
67. **Metzler, C., and R. M. DeHaan.** 1974. Susceptibility tests of anaerobic bacteria: statistical and clinical considerations. *J. Infect. Dis.* **130:**588–594.
68. **Olsson-Liljequist, B., P. Larson, M. Walder, and H. Miorner.** 1997. Antimicrobial susceptibility testing in Sweden. III. Methodology for susceptibility testing. *Scand. J. Infect. Dis.* **Suppl. 105:**13–23.
69. **Phillips, I.** 2001. Reevaluation of antibiotic breakpoints. *Clin. Infect. Dis.* **33**(Suppl. 3)**:**S230–S232.
70. **Ringertz, S., B. Olsson-Liljequist, G. Kahlmeter, and G. Kronvall.** 1997. Antimicrobial susceptibility testing in Sweden. II. Species-related zone diameter breakpoints to avoid interpretive errors and guard against unrecognized evolution of resistance. *Scand. J. Infect. Dis.* **Suppl. 105:**8–12.
71. **Rosenberg, J., F. C. Tenover, J. Wong, W. Jarvis, and D. J. Vugia.** 1997. Are clinical laboratories in California accurately reporting vancomycin-resistant enterococci? *J. Clin. Microbiol.* **35:**2526–2530.
72. **Sabol, K., J. E. Patterson, J. S. Lewis II, A. Owens, J. Cadena, and J. H. Jorgensen.** 2005. Emergence of

daptomycin resistance in *Enterococcus faecium* during daptomycin therapy. *Antimicrob. Agents Chemother.* **49:**1664–1665.

73. **Sahm, D. F., C. N. Baker, R. N. Jones, and C. Thornsberry.** 1984. Influence of growth medium on the in vitro activities of second- and third-generation cephalosporins against *Streptococcus faecalis*. *J. Clin. Microbiol.* **20:**561–567.
74. **Saito, A.** 1995. Clinical breakpoints for antimicrobial agents in pulmonary infections and sepsis: report of the Committee for Japanese Standards for Antimicrobial Susceptibility Testing of Bacteria. *J. Infect. Chemother.* **1:**83–88.
75. **Saito, A., T. Inamatsu, J. Okada, T. Oguri, H. Kanno, N. Kusano, H. Kumon, K. Yamaguchi, A. Watanabe, and K. Watanabe.** 1999. Clinical breakpoints in pulmonary infections and sepsis: new antimicrobial agents and supplemental information for some agents already released. *J. Infect. Chemother.* **5:**223–226.
76. **Steers, E., E. L. Foltz, and B. S. Graves.** 1959. An inocula replicating apparatus for routine testing of bacterial susceptibility to antibiotics. *Antibiot. Chemother.* **9:**307–311.
77. **Swedish Reference Group for Antibiotics.** 1981. A revised system for antibiotic sensitivity testing. *Scand. J. Infect. Dis.* **13:**148–152.
78. **Swenson, J. M., F. C. Tenover, and the Cefoxitin Disk Study Group.** 2005. Results of disk diffusion testing with cefoxitin correlate with presence of *mecA* in *Staphylococcus* spp. *J. Clin. Microbiol.* **43:**3818–3823.
79. **Tenover, F. C., R. N. Jones, J. M. Swenson, B. Zimmer, S. McAllister, and J. H. Jorgensen.** 1999. Methods for improved detection of oxacillin resistance in coagulase-negative staphylococci: results of a multicenter study. *J. Clin. Microbiol.* **37:**4051–4058.
80. **Tenover, F. C., M. V. Lancaster, B. C. Hill, C. D. Steward, S. A. Stocker, G. A. Hancock, C. M. O'Hara, S. K. McAllister, N. C. Clark, and K. Hiramatsu.** 1998. Characterization of staphylococci with reduced susceptibilities to vancomycin and other glycopepetides. *J. Clin. Microbiol.* **36:**1020–1027.
81. **Tenover, F. C., and L. C. McDonald.** 2005. Vancomycin-resistant staphylococci and enterococci: epidemiology and control. *Curr. Opin. Infect. Dis.* **18:**300–305.
82. **Tenover, F. C., J. M. Swenson, C. M. O'Hara, and S. A. Stocker.** 1995. Ability of commercial and reference antimicrobial susceptibility testing methods to detect vancomycin resistance in enterococci. *J. Clin. Microbiol.* **33:**1524–1527.
83. **Thornsberry, C., and L. K. McDougal.** 1983. Successful use of broth microdilution in susceptibility tests for methicillin-resistant (heteroresistant) staphylococci. *J. Clin. Microbiol.* **18:**1084–1091.
84. **Toohey, M., G. Francis, and N. Stingemore.** 1990. Variation in Iso-Sensitest agar affecting β-lactam testing. *Newsl. Antimicrob. Spec. Interest Group Aust. Soc. Microbiol.* **1**(6)**:**6–8.
85. **Ward, P. B., S. Palladino, J. C. Looker, and P. Feddema.** 1993. P-Nitrophenylglycerol in susceptibility testing media alters the MICs of antimicrobials for *Pseudomonas aeruginosa*. *J. Antimicrob. Chemother.* **31:**489–496.
86. **Ward, P. B., S. Palladino, B. McLaren, R. J. Rathur, and J. C. Looker.** 1993 The effect of increased agar concentration in susceptibility testing media on MICs of antimicrobials for Gram-negative bacilli. *J. Antimicrob. Chemother.* **31:**1005–1007.
87. **Wheat, P. F.** 1989. The agar-dilution susceptibility technique: past and present. *Clin. Microbiol. Newsl.* **11:**164–166.
88. **Williams, J. D.** 1990. Prospects for standardisation of methods and guidelines for disc susceptibility testing. *Eur. J. Clin. Microbiol. Infect. Dis.* **9:**496–501.
89. **Wise, R., and I. Phillips.** 2000. Towards a common susceptibility testing method? *J. Antimicrob. Chemother.* **45:** 919–920.
90. **York, M. K., L. Gibbs, F. Chehab, and G. F. Brooks.** 1996. Comparison of PCR detection of *mecA* with standard susceptibility testing methods to determine methicillin resistance in coagulase-negative staphylococci. *J. Clin. Microbiol.* **34:**249–253.

Special Phenotypic Methods for Detecting Antibacterial Resistance*

JANA M. SWENSON, JEAN B. PATEL, AND JAMES H. JORGENSEN

74

Special phenotypic tests for detecting antibacterial resistance range from the rapid and simple spot β-lactamase test to the more time-consuming and complex minimal bactericidal concentration (MBC) assays. These tests may either supplement or replace traditional testing methods depending on the organism and the assay. This chapter describes tests for detection of high-level aminoglycoside resistance and acquired vancomycin resistance in enterococci; tests for detection of inducible clindamycin resistance in streptococci; tests for detection of oxacillin, vancomycin, and inducible clindamycin resistance in staphylococci; tests for detection of β-lactamases in multiple organisms; and tests for determination of bactericidal activity.

Quality control information is given for all of the tests in each section; however, guidelines for the frequency of quality control testing are not provided, because they have not been determined and may vary depending on laboratory circumstances. A practical approach would be to perform quality control testing each day clinical isolates are tested or less frequently (e.g., weekly) once a laboratory has thoroughly documented that less frequent quality control testing can validate the reliability of the procedures. However, the College of American Pathologists recommends that quality control testing be done daily on β-lactamase tests. Quality control tests should be performed each time new lots of material are put into use.

TESTS TO DETECT RESISTANCE IN ENTEROCOCCI

Systemic enterococcal infections, such as endocarditis, are commonly treated with a cell wall-active agent (either a β-lactam drug or a glycopeptide such as vancomycin) and an aminoglycoside (usually gentamicin or streptomycin). These agents act synergistically to enhance killing (175). However, when an enterococcal strain is resistant to the cell wall-active agent or has high-level resistance (HLR) to the aminoglycoside, there is no synergism and combination therapy does not provide a bactericidal effect (129). Because of this, it is important to determine the susceptibility to both the aminoglycoside and the cell wall-active agent individually in order to predict the likelihood of synergy. Methods for detection of aminoglycoside and vancomycin resistance are discussed here. A discussion of methods for detection of high-level penicillin and ampicillin resistance was included in the last edition of this Manual.

Detection of High-Level Resistance to Aminoglycosides

Because aminoglycosides have poor activity against enterococci (MICs range from 8 to 256 μg/ml), they cannot be used as single agents for therapy (75, 129). This intrinsic, moderate-level resistance is due to poor uptake of the aminoglycoside by the cell (129). Acquired aminoglycoside resistance in enterococci is due either to mutations resulting in decreased binding of the agent to the ribosome, as occurs with streptomycin (called ribosomal resistance), or, more commonly, to the acquisition of new genes that encode enzymes that modify aminoglycosides (called acquired resistance). Acquired aminoglycoside resistance usually corresponds to MICs that are significantly above the concentrations normally tested in routine susceptibility tests, e.g., ≥2,000 μg/ml for streptomycin and ≥500 μg/ml for gentamicin, and is designated HLR (129) (see also chapters 30 and 71).

Synergy between an aminoglycoside and a cell wall-active agent can be determined directly by performing complex time-kill studies (101) or can be predicted by using less cumbersome screening tests. Gentamicin and streptomycin are the only two agents that should be tested on a routine basis. All enterococcal isolates that are resistant to gentamicin are considered resistant to tobramycin and amikacin as well. Resistance to streptomycin is mediated by a different resistance mechanism, and consequently, streptomycin resistance must be determined separately from gentamicin resistance. Isolates of *Enterococcus faecium* are intrinsically resistant to the synergistic actions of amikacin, kanamycin, tobramycin, and netilmicin with cell wall-active agents, irrespective of in vitro testing results for HLR (125). *E. faecalis* strains that are susceptible to gentamicin may be resistant to kanamycin and amikacin. In vitro tests with amikacin cannot reliably predict HLR to amikacin in *E. faecalis,* but kanamycin may be used to predict HLR to amikacin and kanamycin (161), although optimal methods for testing have not been determined. The genes for two additional

* This chapter contains information presented in chapter 74 by Jana M. Swenson, Janet Fick Hindler, and James H. Jorgensen in the eighth edition of this Manual.

enzymes that mediate gentamicin resistance have been described, *aph2″-(Ic)* and *aph2″-(Id)*, (28, 199), neither of which is detected using the screening methods described below since their presence seems to lead to intermediate, not high-level, resistance. Only time-kill or molecular studies can detect the presence of these enzymes. Methods for detection of HLR to aminoglycosides are summarized in Table 1 and discussed below.

Agar Dilution Screening Method

Agar plates are prepared with brain heart infusion (BHI) agar supplemented with 500 μg of gentamicin per ml or 2,000 μg of streptomycin per ml. The plates are inoculated by spotting 10 μl of a suspension that is equivalent to a 0.5 McFarland standard prepared from growth on an 18- to 24-h agar plate, giving a final inoculum of 10^6 CFU per spot. The plates are incubated for a full 24 h in ambient air. The presence of more than one colony or a haze of growth should be read as resistant. For streptomycin, the plates should be reincubated for an additional 24 h if there is no growth at 24 h. Mueller-Hinton agar (MHA), MHA plus 5% sheep blood, or dextrose phosphate agar may be substituted for BHI agar, but because growth is better on BHI agar, this is the preferred medium. Commercially prepared agar screen plates are available and have performed well (61, 157, 158). Kanamycin agar screen tests have not been as extensively evaluated and are not standardized, but it has been reported that for determining HLR to both amikacin and kanamycin in *E. faecalis*, kanamycin at 2,000 μg/ml in BHI agar can be used (161).

Broth Microdilution Screening Method

Broth dilution tests are prepared using a single well or a tube containing BHI broth supplemented with 500 μg of gentamicin per ml or 1,000 μg of streptomycin per ml. The final inoculum concentration is that recommended for routine broth microdilution testing, i.e., 5×10^5 CFU/ml. The plates are incubated for 24 h in ambient air. For streptomycin, the plates should be reincubated for an additional 24 h if there is no growth at 24 h. Any growth is interpreted as denoting resistance.

The recommended streptomycin concentration for use in the broth microdilution screen is one-half that used in the agar dilution screen test. Because this test is often included as part of a routine gram-positive MIC panel, the inoculum is that commonly used in broth microdilution testing (5×10^5 CFU/ml). The total number of cells tested in the agar dilution screening procedure (10^6 CFU/spot) is 20-fold larger than that normally used in the broth microdilution test (5×10^4 CFU/0.1-ml well). In order to provide a test that uses a low inoculum and at the same time maximizes the detection of HLR to streptomycin, it was necessary to lower the concentration recommended for testing streptomycin from 2,000 to 1,000 μg/ml in the broth microdilution test. Because of poorer growth and the lower inoculum, Mueller-Hinton broth is inadequate for use in the broth microdilution screen test (183). The performance of other aminoglycosides in this test has not been evaluated.

Disk Diffusion Screening Method

The standard disk diffusion procedure (37) described in chapter 73 (with unsupplemented MHA) is used, except that special high-content disks (gentamicin at 120 μg and streptomycin at 300 μg) are required (162). Zones are measured after 18 to 24 h of incubation in ambient air at 35°C. Isolates for which the zone diameters are ≥10 mm are categorized as susceptible. The absence of a zone of inhibition corresponds to the presence of HLR. Strains for which the zones of inhibition are 7 to 9 mm usually display HLR, but a few are strains for which the MICs are only moderately elevated (183). Therefore, strains for which the zone diameters are 7 to 9 mm should be tested by either the standard agar or the broth microdilution screen method to determine susceptibility or resistance. High-content gentamicin and streptomycin disks are available commercially.

Quality Control

For both gentamicin and streptomycin, *E. faecalis* ATCC 29212 is used as the susceptible control and *E. faecalis* ATCC 51299 is used as the resistant control strain (182).

TABLE 1 Screening methods for detecting vancomycin and high-level aminoglycoside resistance in enterococci

Parameter	Screening procedure			
	Vancomycin agar dilution	Aminoglycoside agar dilution	Aminoglycoside broth microdilution	Aminoglycoside disk diffusion
Medium	BHI agar	BHI agar	BHI broth	MHA
Inoculum	10^5–10^6 CFU/spot	10^6 CFU/spot	5×10^4 CFU/0.1ml	0.5 McFarland[a]
Incubation (h)	24	24[b]	24[b]	18–24
Drug concn				
Gentamicin	NA	500 μg/ml	500 μg/ml	120 μg/disk
Streptomycin	NA	2,000 μg/ml	1,000 μg/ml	300 μg/disk
Vancomycin	6 μg/ml	NA[c]	NA	NA
Endpoint	>1 colony	>1 colony	Any growth	6 mm = resistant, 7–9 mm = inconclusive,[d] ≥10 mm = susceptible

[a] CLSI disk diffusion method (37).
[b] If streptomycin is negative at 24 h, reincubate for an additional 24 h.
[c] NA, not applicable.
[d] If the zone is 7 to 9 mm, the test is inconclusive, and an agar or broth microdilution test should be performed to confirm susceptibility or resistance.

Only *E. faecalis* ATCC 29212 is used for control of disk diffusion tests. The expected quality control limits are 16 to 23 mm for gentamicin (120-μg) disks and 14 to 20 mm for streptomycin (300-μg) disks (38).

Detection of Vancomycin Resistance in Enterococci

As defined by the Clinical and Laboratory Standards Institute (CLSI, formerly NCCLS), the MIC interpretive criteria for vancomycin are ≤4 μg/ml for susceptible, 8 to 16 μg/ml for intermediate, and ≥32 μg/ml for resistant. The three most common phenotypes of resistance are (i) high-level vancomycin resistance (MICs, ≥64 μg/ml) with accompanying teicoplanin resistance (MICs, ≥16 μg/ml) (VanA phenotype); (ii) moderate- to high-level vancomycin resistance (MICs, 16 to 512 μg/ml), most commonly without teicoplanin resistance (VanB phenotype); and (iii) intrinsic low-level resistance associated with *Enterococcus gallinarum* and *Enterococcus casseliflavus* (MICs, 2 to 32 μg/ml) (VanC phenotype) (107, 108). Both the VanA and VanB phenotypes are most commonly seen in *E. faecalis* and *E. faecium* but have been found in other species (107). Three additional genotypes have been described recently, *vanD* (137, 144), *vanE* (60), and *van*G (122). The VanD-type resistance, resulting in HLR to vancomycin (MICs, ≥64 μg/ml) and variable resistance to teicoplanin, has been found only in *E. faecium*. The VanE-type resistance, found in *E. faecalis*, exhibits intermediate vancomycin MICs (16 μg/ml), and the organism remains susceptible to teicoplanin. The VanG phenotype is similar to the VanD phenotype.

Many methods commonly used by clinical laboratories, including disk diffusion and the Vitek Legacy and MicroScan systems, have traditionally had problems detecting low-level vancomycin resistance (both VanB and VanC types) (52, 136, 159, 160, 185, 193, 211). However, systems continue to improve (27, 64, 81, 90, 193, 202) and the newer Vitek 2 and Phoenix systems perform very well for the detection of vancomycin resistance in enterococci (1, 50, 54, 177, 202). Disk diffusion testing requires 24 h of incubation and examination of zones under transmitted light.

The vancomycin agar screening test first described by Willey et al. (211) was adopted by the CLSI in 1993 (29, 181) (Table 1). The sensitivity and specificity levels of 96 to 99% and 100%, respectively, were noted at that time. Commercially prepared plates also perform well (52, 61, 204). However, there may still be some confusion among clinical laboratorians about the characterization of susceptibility or resistance for the *van*C-containing enterococci, *E. gallinarum* and *E. casseliflavus*, because their growth is variable on the agar screen plate. Both of these species intrinsically contain a *van*C gene, but the MICs of vancomycin for them range from 2 to 32 μg/ml (107). Whether the presence of this gene is associated with therapeutic failures is not known. Since the vancomycin MICs for these strains are often >4 μg/ml, the strains are likely to grow on the agar screen plates, where a higher inoculum and a richer medium may promote growth (61, 157, 181). Most strains of *van*C-containing enterococci are motile at 30°C; *E. casseliflavus* is typically yellow pigmented. These characteristics have been used to distinguish *van*C-containing enterococci from other species (14, 61, 62). However, some *E. gallinarum* and *E. casseliflavus* strains may be nonmotile. Because of this, a better test to differentiate them from *E. faecalis* and *E. faecium* is fermentation of 1% methyl-α-D-glucopyranoside (MGP). All *van*C-containing enterococci acidify MGP, whereas *E. faecium* and *E. faecalis* do not (149) (see also chapter 30).

Vancomycin Agar Screen Test

Agar plates are prepared with BHI agar supplemented with 6 μg of vancomycin per ml (BHI-V6). Using growth from an 18- to 24-h agar plate, make a suspension equivalent in turbidity to a 0.5 McFarland standard and inoculate the plates by spotting 1 to 10 μl or swabbing an area 10 to 15 mm in diameter. The final inoculum is 10^5 to 10^6 CFU per spot. After inoculation, incubate the plates for a full 24 h in ambient air at 35°C. The presence of more than one colony or a haze of growth indicates resistance.

Quality Control

For quality control, *E. faecalis* ATCC 29212 (no growth, i.e., susceptible) and *E. faecalis* ATCC 51299 (growth, i.e., resistant) should be tested (182). Plates made with BHI agars from certain manufacturers may allow light growth of *E. faecalis* ATCC 29212, especially if the higher inoculum (10 μl) is used or the plates are held longer than 24 h.

Reporting Resistance in Enterococci

For any serious enterococcal infection, results of the screen for HLR to gentamicin and streptomycin should be reported in concert with the results of the testing of the cell wall-active agent (penicillin, ampicillin, or vancomycin), because synergy would not be expected if any one of the agents reported is resistant. Helpful suggestions on reporting the results of enterococcal tests are given by Hindler and Sahm (75).

TESTS TO DETECT RESISTANCE IN STAPHYLOCOCCI

Detection of Oxacillin Resistance in Staphylococci

Strains of *Staphylococcus aureus* resistant to oxacillin are still referred to as MRSA (for methicillin-resistant *S. aureus*). Even though methicillin is no longer available, the acronym "MRSA" has persisted and therefore will also be used here. MIC interpretive criteria recommended by the CLSI for oxacillin and *S. aureus* are ≤2 μg/ml for susceptible and ≥4 μg/ml for resistant (38). At least three different resistance mechanisms contribute to oxacillin resistance in *S. aureus:* (i) production of a supplemental penicillin-binding protein (PBP), PBP 2a, encoded by a chromosomal *mecA* gene; (ii) inactivation of the drug by increased production of β-lactamase; and (iii) production of modified intrinsic PBPs (MOD-SA) with altered affinity for the drug (23, 25, 42, 69, 197). Studies to determine the prevalence of the different resistance mechanisms have not been done; however, it is assumed that the last two occur only rarely. Strains that possess *mecA* (the classic resistance) are either heterogeneous or homogeneous in their expression of resistance. With homogeneous expression, virtually all cells express resistance when tested by standard in vitro test methods. However, testing of a heteroresistant isolate results in some cells that appear to be susceptible and others that appear to be resistant. Often only 1 in 10^4 to 1 in 10^8 *mecA*-positive cells in the test population expresses resistance (71, 156, 198). Heterogeneous expression occasionally results in MICs that appear to be borderline, i.e., oxacillin MICs of 2 to 8 μg/ml, and consequently, the isolates may be misinterpreted as susceptible (MICs ≤2 μg/ml) (164). Isolates that have classic resistance are usually resistant to other agents such as erythromycin, clindamycin, chloramphenicol, tetracycline, trimethoprim-sulfamethoxazole, older fluoroquinolones, or aminoglycosides. However, some MRSA isolates, such as those described in community-associated infections (referred to as CA-MRSA), are not multiply resistant (18, 138, 216). Resistance mediated by β-lactamase or the presence of modified PBPs (MOD-SA) also results in borderline resistance. β-Lactamase-mediated resistance can usually be distinguished from the classic type (*mecA* positive) of resistance or MOD-SA resistance by the addition of a β-lactamase inhibitor (e.g., clavulanic acid) to the oxacillin MIC test, which lowers the MIC by 2 dilutions or more. Isolates that are resistant by either the β-lactamase or the MOD-SA mechanism usually do not have multiple drug resistance, similar to CA-MRSA.

Reference dilution methods recommended by the CLSI are generally reliable for detection of oxacillin resistance in *S. aureus,* and since lowering of the MIC breakpoints for coagulase-negative staphylococci in 1999 (32), the sensitivity of detection in that group has improved. However, recent studies have found that correlation of these interpretive criteria with the presence or absence of *mecA* is optimal only for *S. epidermidis, S. haemolyticus,* and, possibly, *S. hominis* (66, 80, 115). For other species of coagulase-negative staphylococci (e.g., *S. saprophyticus* and *S. lugdunensis*) the new breakpoints tended to be less specific, i.e., many *mecA*-negative strains were categorized as resistant by disk and MIC methods (59, 80, 115, 121, 150). In 2005, the CLSI revised the staphylococcus tables to group *S. lugdunensis* strains with *S. aureus,* which has helped to resolve some of these problems (35). More recently, it was shown (J. Swenson, unpublished data) that there are still *mecA*-negative *S. lugdunensis* strains categorized as oxacillin resistant by disk diffusion using the 1-μg oxacillin disk (a major interpretive error). Because of this, the CLSI now recommends that testing of *S. lugdunensis* by disk diffusion be done using cefoxitin as a surrogate for oxacillin (see below); oxacillin interpretive criteria for *S. lugdunensis* no longer appear in CLSI M100 tables for staphylococci (38).

Despite continued improvements in reference testing methods with oxacillin, other phenotypic tests have been studied. The use of cefoxitin has recently been highlighted by many investigators as an excellent surrogate for use in detecting *mecA*-mediated resistance in staphylococci. Special phenotypic methods using cefoxitin as well as other methods are discussed below.

Detection Using Cefoxitin as a Surrogate for Oxacillin

Within the past several years, there have been multiple reports of the use of cefoxitin as a surrogate marker for detection of *mecA*-mediated oxacillin resistance. Cefoxitin is a more potent inducer of the *mecA* regulatory system than are other penicillins (123). Following recent studies including a multilaboratory study (187), the CLSI has adopted a cefoxitin disk diffusion method that is equal in sensitivity and specificity to oxacillin disk diffusion for detecting *mecA*-mediated resistance in *S. aureus*. For coagulase-negative staphylococci, the cefoxitin disk diffusion test is equal in sensitivity but greater in specificity when compared to disk diffusion with oxacillin (37). The major drawback of the test is the failure to detect *mecA*-positive strains of *S. simulans* (187).

The cefoxitin disk test is performed using the routine disk diffusion procedure, except that modified interpretive criteria are used: for *S. aureus,* results of ≤19 mm are reported as oxacillin resistant and results of ≥20 mm are considered oxacillin susceptible; for coagulase-negative staphylococci, ≤24 mm is resistant and ≥25 mm is susceptible. The test is easy to read using reflected light and does not require careful examination of the disk diffusion zones for light growth or small colonies. The use of cefoxitin in an agar dilution screen similar to the oxacillin salt-agar screen has also been investigated (58, 187) and warrants further study.

Oxacillin-Salt Agar Screening Test

Although the oxacillin-salt agar screen test has been widely used, recent studies have questioned its sensitivity, especially for heterogeneously resistant strains (17). It is less sensitive than the cefoxitin disk diffusion test (16, 57, 188). The oxacillin-salt agar screen test cannot be used for detecting oxacillin resistance in coagulase-negative staphylococci because it uses 6 μg of oxacillin per ml (190). Consequently, the CLSI eliminated recommendations for using the agar screen to test coagulase-negative staphylococci.

Test Method

MHA supplemented with 4% sodium chloride and 6 μg of oxacillin per ml is used for the agar screen method recommended by the CLSI (36, 37). Plates containing methicillin are not recommended. For the test, inoculum suspensions are prepared by selecting colonies from overnight growth on a nonselective agar plate. The colonies are transferred to broth (e.g., tryptic soy broth) or saline to produce a suspension that matches the turbidity of a 0.5 McFarland standard. This suspension is used to inoculate the oxacillin agar screen plate by either (i) dipping a cotton swab into the test suspension, expressing the excess liquid from the swab, and inoculating an area 10 to 15 mm in diameter (or streaking the swab onto a quadrant of the agar surface) or (ii) spotting an area 10 to 15 mm in diameter with a 1-μl loop that has been dipped in the suspension (186). Test plates are incubated for a full 24 h at 35°C (no higher) in ambient air and examined for growth of more than one colony, which indicates resistance. Once again, the test is currently not recommended for coagulase-negative staphylococci (36, 37).

Quality Control

S. aureus ATCC 29213 (oxacillin susceptible) and *S. aureus* ATCC 43300 (oxacillin resistant) are the recommended quality control strains.

Other Tests for Detection of Oxacillin Resistance in Staphylococci

Several commercial rapid methods that detect oxacillin resistance in staphylococci are available. They include latex agglutination tests that detect the presence of PBP 2a, the MRSA-Screen test (Denka-Seikin Co., Ltd., Tokyo, Japan), the PBP 2′ latex agglutination test (Oxoid Limited, Basingstoke, United Kingdom), the Mastalex test (Mast Diagnostics, Bootle, United Kingdom) (11), and the Slidex MRSA Detection test (bioMérieux, Marcy l'Etoile, France). Only the first two tests have been cleared by the U.S. Food and Drug Administration (FDA). The MRSA-Screen test, cleared for use only with *S. aureus,* has been widely evaluated and has high sensitivity and specificity for that species (17, 116, 164, 188, 203, 205, 214). Detection of resistance in coagulase-negative staphylococci by the MRSA-Screen test has been less successful, requiring either induction, an increased inoculum, or an increased agglutination time for adequate sensitivity (77, 79, 115, 213). The Oxoid PBP 2′ latex agglutination test was approved by the FDA for testing both *S. aureus* and coagulase-negative staphylococci, the latter requiring induction with oxacillin or cefoxitin. Although not extensively evaluated, its use for same-day reporting of MRSA from blood cultures has been described (119). When confirmation of the presence of the *mecA* gene is required, besides these commercial rapid methods, molecular analysis may also be performed by standard PCR methods (see chapter 16).

Limitations of Methods for Detection of Oxacillin Resistance

Growth of an *S. aureus* isolate on an oxacillin agar screen plate generally means that the isolate is *mecA* positive. When performed properly, the oxacillin agar screen method detects most *mecA*-positive *S. aureus* strains. Occasionally a heteroresistant *mecA*-positive strain is not detected; this may be due in part to a low frequency of resistance expression (17, 153) or to lot-to-lot or manufacturer-to-manufacturer variation in the test medium (74, 76). When the oxacillin agar screen test was compared directly to the use of cefoxitin by disk diffusion, investigators found increased sensitivity in detecting *mecA*-mediated resistance by using cefoxitin disk diffusion, although the statistical significance of this finding was not determined (16, 207).

The oxacillin agar screen test generally does not detect borderline-resistant strains, whether caused by *mecA*-mediated heteroresistance or by the other mechanisms responsible for borderline resistance. Although MOD-SA isolates, particularly those associated with MICs of ≥8 μg/ml, may grow on agar screen plates (186), isolates with borderline resistance due to β-lactamase are usually associated with oxacillin MICs of ≤4 μg/ml and do not usually grow on the screen plates. Cefoxitin disk diffusion testing performs well for detection of borderline resistance caused by *mecA* (57, 187) but does not detect other types of borderline resistance. MOD-SA strains which do not contain *mecA* are categorized as susceptible by cefoxitin disk diffusion despite the oxacillin MIC that they express (187). Since borderline resistance caused by β-lactamase or MOD-SA is infrequently encountered in clinical specimens of *S. aureus*, the possibility of their presence minimally affects the utility of these tests. Testing by a dilution method may also fail to detect extremely heteroresistant, *mecA*-positive *S. aureus* strains (164), which often have borderline resistance. However, if dilution testing is performed so that oxacillin MICs below 2 μg/ml can be detected, MIC testing can be used to discern isolates with borderline resistance, i.e., those with oxacillin MICs of 2 to 8 μg/ml.

Reporting Results

The CLSI recommends that oxacillin-resistant staphylococci be reported as resistant to all β-lactam agents, including penicillins, cephems (i.e., all cephalosporins, including cephamycins), β-lactam/β-lactamase inhibitor combination agents, and carbapenems. These agents are clinically ineffective against oxacillin-resistant staphylococcal infections, even though they may demonstrate in vitro activity (36, 37). Consequently, an isolate that grows on the oxacillin agar screen plate or demonstrates a cefoxitin zone diameter in the resistant range should be considered resistant to these agents as well as to all penicillinase-stable penicillins. Isolates of *S. aureus* that appear oxacillin resistant by an alternative test method but fail to grow on the agar screen plate are probably borderline resistant and lack *mecA* (102, 127, 153). Much less is known about borderline resistance than about *mecA*-positive resistance because there have been few clinical studies (120); however, in animal model studies, isolates with β-lactamase-mediated resistance appear to be effectively treated with β-lactam agents (24, 25, 143, 194). If a phenotypically oxacillin-resistant *S. aureus* strain is isolated from a seriously ill patient and it does not contain *mecA*, this information should be conveyed to the patient's physician. The incidence of phenotypically susceptible *mecA*-positive strains of *S. aureus* is not known. However, should phenotypically susceptible strains be isolated from serious infections in patients with a history of MRSA infection, confirmation by one of the rapid molecular methods such as detection of PBP 2a by latex agglutination should be considered (154, 163, 164).

Detection of Vancomycin Resistance in Staphylococci

Vancomycin resistance in staphylococci is a rapidly evolving subject. Previously, vancomycin-intermediate (MIC of 8 to 16 μg/ml) *S. aureus* (VISA) and *Staphylococcus* species other than *S. aureus* (VISS) were identified and characterized (174). In addition, *S. aureus* strains with reduced susceptibility to vancomycin (MIC, 4 μg/ml) were described and were associated with the same risk factors as VISA (63). More recently, vancomycin-resistant *S. aureus* (VRSA) strains with *vanA*-mediated resistance (MICs, 32 to 1,024 μg/ml) were isolated from four patients in the United States (20–22; T. Madhavan, D. Sievery, J. Rudrik, J. Torresan, and D. Schulman, *Abstr. 43rd IDSA Ann. Meet.*, abstr. 1073, 2005). Until January 2006, the CLSI interpretive criteria for vancomycin and *S. aureus* were as follows: ≤4 μg/ml, susceptible; 8 to 16 μg/ml, intermediate; and ≥32 μg/ml, resistant. As of January 2006, the susceptible category is ≤2 μg/ml, 4 to 8 μg/ml is intermediate, and ≥16 μg/ml is resistant (38). It is important to note that the CLSI interpretive criteria for vancomycin susceptibility in coagulase negative staphylococci (CoNS) were not changed and thus are different from the criteria for *S. aureus*. No *van* gene-mediated vancomycin resistance has been reported for CoNS, but there are reports of isolates with elevated vancomycin MICs (3, 47, 103, 165, 169, 206).

Some routine susceptibility testing methods fail to detect vancomycin-intermediate or vancomycin-resistant staphylococci (191; R. B. Carey, J. B. Patel, S. McAllister, A. Thompson, P. Raney, F. C. Tenover, C. Ginocchio, D. Bopp, N. Dumas, and D. Kohlerschmidt, *Abstr. 44th Intersci. Conf. Antimicrob. Agents Chemother.*, abstr. D-66, 2004; Madhavan et al., Abstr. 43rd IDSA Ann. Meet.). The CLSI reference broth microdilution method and E test are reliable for detection of VISA and VRSA. However, the disk diffusion test cannot detect VISA or VISS because these isolates produce zone sizes within the susceptible range (≥15 mm). In contrast, the disk diffusion test does detect VRSA. An evaluation of automated susceptibility testing systems revealed that not all systems were able to detect one or more VRSA (Carey et al., 44th ICAAC). Some manufacturers of automated susceptibility testing have made adjustments in their testing systems to address this problem.

The BHI-V6 screen agar, used to detect vancomycin-resistant enterococci, was evaluated for detection of vancomycin-intermediate or -resistant staphylococci in two studies (191; R. B. Carey, D. Lonsway, S. McAllister, J. Patel, P. Raney, and A. Thompson, unpublished data). In both studies, all isolates for which the vancomycin MICs were ≥8 μg/ml grew on the screen agar. Isolates for which the MICs were 4 μg/ml demonstrated variable growth. In both studies, the agar was inoculated with a suspension of organism equal to a 0.5 McFarland standard. In the study by Tenover et al., the plates were inoculated using a 10-μl drop from a calibrated pipette. Carey et al. evaluated the amount and method of inoculum delivery. Delivery of a 10-μl drop from a calibrated pipette was the most sensitive method, demonstrating confluent growth at 24 h for all isolates with MICs ≥8 μg/ml. Inoculation of the agar using a swab immersed in the inoculum and then expressed also resulted in growth of isolates for which the MICs were 8 μg/ml, although for some isolates the growth was a haze or isolated colonies. Other inoculation methods, 10 μl delivered by calibrated loop, 1 μl delivered by calibrated pipette, and 10 μl of a suspension prepared using the Prompt Inoculation System-D (3M Company, St. Paul, Minn.), all demonstrated significantly less sensitivity. In both studies, isolates with a vancomycin MIC ≤2 μg/ml did not grow on commercially prepared media. These studies demonstrate that the BHI-V6 agar is a sensitive method for detection of staphylococci for which the vancomycin MICs are ≥8 μg/ml, using either the 10-μl drop or swab inoculation methods. Additional studies with more isolates are needed to evaluate this agar for detection of *S. aureus* isolates for which the MICs are 4 μg/ml.

Although reduced susceptibility to vancomycin can occur in both *S. aureus* and CoNS, the occurrence in *S. aureus* is more concerning because this species is more frequently a cause of serious infection. It is for this reason that the Centers for Disease Control and Prevention recommended use of the screen agar for detection of *S. aureus* with reduced susceptibility to vancomycin (22). This recommendation is for laboratories that may miss these isolates when using their primary susceptibility testing method. However, some laboratories may consider limiting this testing to methicillin-resistant *S. aureus* strains since these are the isolates most likely to develop reduced susceptibility to vancomycin. Use of the BHI-V6 agar for *S. aureus* is described in the CLSI documents (36, 37).

Test Method

The recommended method for inoculating the agar is a 10-μl drop of a 0.5 McFarland suspension delivered with a micropipette. Alternatively, a swab can be used to spot an area 10 to 15 mm in diameter. The agar plate should be read after 24 h of incubation and carefully examined with transmitted light. Greater than one colony of growth or a light film of growth is considered positive (36, 37).

Quality Control

As mentioned above, the BHI-V6 plate is the same screening agar used to detect vancomycin-resistant enterococci (VRE) and the same quality control strains recommended for the VRE test can also be used for the *S. aureus* test (38). These strains are vancomycin-susceptible *E. faecalis* ATCC 29212 and *vanB*-mediated, vancomycin-resistant *E. faecalis* ATCC 51299. Since the amount of inoculum applied for the VRE test (1 to 10 μl of a 0.5 McFarland suspension) spans the recommended inoculum for the *S. aureus* test, a laboratory that uses this medium for both purposes need perform quality control only once, either daily or weekly.

Reporting Results

Growth of *S. aureus* on the BHI-V6 agar is presumptive for either VISA or VRSA (36, 37) (http://www.cdc.gov/ncidod/dhqp/ar_visavrsa_algo.html). Additional testing is needed to confirm vancomycin resistance. First, the identity and purity of the isolate should be confirmed. Then, the MIC of the isolate should be determined using a validated method. For many laboratories the most available method is the E test. It is recommended that any *S. aureus* isolate for which the vancomycin MIC is ≥4 μg/ml be sent to a reference laboratory for confirmation. In the United States, several states request that VISA and/or VRSA be reported to the public health authority.

Detection of Inducible Clindamycin Resistance by Use of the D-Zone Test

Although erythromycin and clindamycin are in separate antimicrobial agent classes, macrolides and lincosamides, respectively, their mechanisms of action (inhibition of protein synthesis) and mechanisms of resistance are similar. The two main mechanisms of resistance are (i) an efflux pump and (ii) a methylase enzyme that alters the ribosomal binding site of the antimicrobial agents. The first type, which confers resistance to macrolides only (designated M-type, for macrolide), is mediated in staphylococci by *msrA*. The second type, which confers resistance to macrolides, lincosamides, and streptogramin B agents (designated MLS_B type, for macrolide-lincosamide-streptogramin B), is mediated by an *erm* gene. In staphylococci, the MLS_B-type resistance can be either constitutive or inducible; if inducible, the isolate appears to be susceptible to the lincosamide (i.e., clindamycin) when using routine testing methods, unless induced by a macrolide (i.e., erythromycin). It is important to determine if resistance (whether inducible or constitutive) to clindamycin exists when it is being considered for therapy. Detailed explanation of these resistance mechanisms can be found in chapter 71.

Phenotypically, if an isolate has M-type resistance it is resistant to erythromycin but susceptible to clindamycin. If an isolate has MLS_B-type resistance, then it is erythromycin resistant and may be susceptible or resistant to clindamycin because it is either constitutive or inducible to that drug. In strains that are erythromycin resistant but clindamycin susceptible, it is important to determine if inducible clindamycin resistance exists (and an *erm* gene is present) or if the strain remains clindamycin susceptible (and an efflux gene is present).

Test Method

Detection of inducible clindamycin resistance can be easily accomplished using a disk diffusion procedure by placing a 15-μg erythromycin disk adjacent to a 2-μg clindamycin disk and looking for a flattening of the clindamycin zone, which looks like the letter D and is therefore referred to as a D zone. For laboratories that are already performing disk diffusion, this may be done by placing the disks from 15 to 26 mm apart (55) with the other disks tested on an MHA plate. Some disk dispensers may position disks more than 26 mm apart even if the disks are placed in adjacent positions. Therefore, because dispensers may vary and the distance is critical, the distance should be verified before being adopted as a standard procedure. Placing the disks 15 to 20 mm, rather than 26 mm, apart may make the test easier to interpret (179, 215), although to accomplish this the disks must be placed on the plates by hand instead of with a disk dispenser. For laboratories that routinely perform antimicrobial susceptibility methods other than disk diffusion, Jorgensen et al. have shown that the test can be performed on a standard blood agar plate used for purity checks (94) by streaking one-third of the plate for confluent growth and then streaking for isolation on the rest of the plate. In that study, the investigators showed that dilutions of the 0.5 McFarland inoculum of up to 1:250 can be used. The disks are placed 15 mm apart on the portion of the plate where confluent growth would occur. In a later study, it was determined that the BBL Prompt system (BD, Sparks, Md.) should not be used to inoculate the purity plate for D-zone determination (215). In that study, the investigators suggested that no more than a 1:20 dilution of a 0.5 McFarland suspension should be used to inoculate the purity plate. However, if the Prompt inoculum wand was used directly to inoculate the plate, it may have delivered inadequate inoculum. More recently the Prompt System was successfully used for this purpose (J. F. Hindler and D. A. Bruckner, *Abstr. 105th Gen. Meet. Am. Soc. Microbiol.*, abstr. C-325, 2005) by transferring inoculum from the Prompt reservoir tray, using a 10-μl loop, and streaking one-third of the plate to obtain confluent growth. For either method, organisms that show a blunting or flattening of the clindamycin zone are considered D-zone test positive; those that show no flattening are D-zone test negative.

Quality Control and Quality Assessment

Two strains have been designated for quality assessment purposes (i.e., for training, competency assessment, or test evaluation): *S. aureus* BAA-977, which contains inducible *ermA*-mediated resistance; and *S. aureus* BAA-976, which contains *msrA*-mediated resistance to erythromycin only. *S. aureus* ATCC 25923 should be used as the routine quality control strain for daily or weekly quality control testing of clindamycin and erythromycin disks using MHA. If the test is performed as part of the purity check procedure, the CLSI recommends that the disk content should be verified using *S. aureus* ATCC 25923 on MHA (38). However, this would require that laboratories that do not do disk diffusion routinely would have to have a supply of MHA plates on hand for quality control purposes only. An alternative to this would be to use the two quality assessment strains, BAA-977 and BAA-976, as quality control organisms at daily or weekly intervals based on CLSI recommendations when using the purity plate method.

Reporting Results

The incidence of inducible clindamycin resistance in staphylococci can be highly variable, both by geographic area and by organism group (i.e., hospital-associated MRSA, community-associated MRSA, and coagulase-negative staphylococci). The CLSI now recommends that isolates that are D-zone test positive should be reported as clindamycin resistant (36, 37). However, there is some controversy about this, given that clindamycin has been effective in some situations where inducible resistance was demonstrated (112). As a conservative approach, the CLSI has suggested that inducibly clindamycin-resistant strains could be reported as resistant with a comment stating, "This isolate is presumed to be resistant based on detection of inducible clindamycin resistance. Clindamycin may still be effective in some patients." If the test is not offered routinely, it should be available by request for cases where clindamycin is being considered for therapy (36, 37).

TESTS TO DETECT RESISTANCE IN STREPTOCOCCI

Oxacillin Disk Screen Test for Detection of Penicillin Resistance in Pneumococci

A screening test in which a 1-μg oxacillin disk is used to detect penicillin resistance in pneumococci was first described following an outbreak caused by *Streptococcus pneumoniae* resistant to multiple antimicrobial agents in South Africa in the 1970s (45, 82, 184). Since then, this test has been used extensively and shown to be highly sensitive but not specific for detection of penicillin-nonsusceptible pneumococci (46). Strains identified as nonsusceptible by this method may be penicillin susceptible, intermediate, or resistant. Penicillin MIC tests must be performed with any strain that produces a zone diameter of ≤19 mm to determine if it is resistant (46). MIC tests rather than the oxacillin disk screen should be used routinely on strains isolated from cerebrospinal fluid and blood.

Detection of Inducible Clindamycin Resistance by Use of the D-Zone Test

The importance of determining erythromycin and clindamycin resistance phenotypes and the detection of inducible clindamycin resistance follows the same logic as that described for staphylococci (see "Detection of Inducible Clindamycin Resistance by Use of the D-Zone Test" above); however, the gene responsible for the M phenotype (i.e., erythromycin resistance and clindamycin susceptibility) in streptococci is *mef*(A). The MLS_B phenotype exists in isolates of beta-hemolytic streptococci, *S. pneumoniae,* and viridans group streptococci; however, in pneumococci and viridans streptococci it is usually the constitutive type and only rarely inducible (128, 201). Therefore, inducible clindamycin resistance needs to be determined only in isolates of beta-hemolytic streptococci.

Test Method

Detection of inducible clindamycin resistance in beta-hemolytic streptococci can be accomplished using a disk diffusion procedure similar to that for staphylococci by placing a 15-μg erythromycin disk adjacent to a 2-μg clindamycin disk and looking for a flattening of the clindamycin zone, which looks like the letter D and is therefore referred to as a D zone. For laboratories that are already performing disk diffusion, the disks must be placed by hand at a distance of 12 mm from each other (151) on an MHA plate with 5% sheep blood along with other disks being tested. A disk dispenser cannot be used to place the two disks since they must not be farther away than 12 mm (151). For laboratories that routinely perform other antimicrobial susceptibility methods, the purity plate method suggested by Jorgensen et al. can also be performed on a standard blood agar plate used for purity checks (94, 151) by streaking one-third of the plate for confluent growth and then streaking for isolation on the rest of the plate. The disks are then placed 12 mm apart on the portion of the plate where confluent growth would occur. Only the use of a 0.5 McFarland suspension has been evaluated for inoculation of the purity plate (151). For either method, organisms that show a blunting or flattening of the clindamycin zone are considered D-zone test positive; those that show no flattening are D-zone test negative.

Quality Control and Quality Assessment

Two strains have been designated for quality assessment (i.e., for training, competency assessment, or test evaluation) of the D-zone test: *S. aureus* BAA-977, which contains inducible *ermA*-mediated resistance to clindamycin, and *S. aureus* BAA-976, which contains *msrA*-mediated resistance to erythromycin only. *S. pneumoniae* ATCC 49619 should be used as the routine quality control strain for daily or weekly quality control testing of clindamycin and erythromycin disks, using MHA with 5% sheep blood. If the test is performed as part of the purity check procedure, ideally the disk content should be verified using *S. pneumoniae* ATCC 49619 on MHA with 5% sheep blood. However, this would require that laboratories that do not do disk diffusion routinely would have to have a supply of MHA with 5% sheep blood on hand for quality control purposes only. An alternative to this would be to use the two quality assessment strains, BAA-977 and BAA-976, as quality control organisms at daily or weekly intervals based on CLSI recommendations when using the purity plate method.

Reporting Results

The incidence of inducible clindamycin resistance in beta-hemolytic streptococci can be highly variable, both by geographic area and organism group (44, 106). However, when inducible clindamycin resistance is detected, the CLSI recommends that, as for staphylococci, isolates shown to be D-zone test positive should be reported as clindamycin resistant. As a conservative approach, the CLSI has suggested that inducibly clindamycin-resistant strains could be reported as resistant with a comment stating, "This isolate is presumed to be resistant based on detection of inducible clindamycin resistance. Clindamycin may still be effective in some patients." If the test is not offered routinely, it should be available by request for cases where clindamycin is being considered for therapy.

DETECTION OF ENZYMES MEDIATING RESISTANCE

β-Lactamase Tests

In the clinical laboratory, β-lactamase tests must be used only when they can provide clinically useful information, and the definitions of positive or negative reactions must not be extended beyond their intended meanings. For example, a β-lactamase-positive result for a *Neisseria gonorrhoeae* isolate means that the isolate is resistant to penicillin but does not imply that the isolate is resistant to the extended-spectrum cephalosporin group of β-lactam agents. Similarly, direct β-lactamase tests for members of the family *Enterobacteriaceae* or for *Pseudomonas* spp. (all of which produce a variety of β-lactamases that result in various susceptibilities to β-lactam agents) have little clinical value and should not be used for these species. A list of the organisms for which β-lactamase tests are useful is given in Table 2.

Direct Tests for β-Lactamase Activity

In the direct β-lactamase test, a positive reaction indicates that the isolate is resistant to the β-lactam agents noted in Table 2, but a negative reaction is inconclusive. For example, most ampicillin-resistant *Haemophilus influenzae* isolates produce β-lactamase, which can be detected by direct β-lactamase tests; however, rare strains are ampicillin resistant but β-lactamase negative (8, 46, 56). For the latter, conventional disk diffusion or dilution tests are needed to detect the resistance (see chapter 73). Three direct β-lactamase assays, the acidimetric, iodometric, and chromogenic methods, have been widely used (73, 110). Each method involves testing bacteria grown on nonselective media, and the results are available within 1 to 60 min. The acidimetric and iodometric methods use a colorimetric indicator to detect the presence of penicilloic acid in the reaction vessel following β-lactamase hydrolysis of penicillin. In the acidimetric method, the substrates are citrate-buffered penicillin and a phenol red indicator. A decreasing pH associated with the presence of penicilloic acid results in a color change from red (negative result) to yellow (positive result) (53). The substrates in the iodometric test are phosphate-buffered penicillin plus a starch-iodine complex. Penicilloic acid, if present, reduces the iodine and prevents it from combining with starch, resulting in a colorless reaction (positive); a bluish purple color corresponds to a negative result (15).

The chromogenic cephalosporin nitrocefin can be used in a test tube assay (135) but has been incorporated into

TABLE 2 Bacteria for which β-lactamase tests have been used in the clinical laboratory

Species	Method(s) commonly used	Predicted resistance[a]
Bacteroides spp. and other gram-negative anaerobes, except *B. fragilis* group	Direct β-lactamase tests[b]	Penicillins[c]
Enterococcus spp.	Direct β-lactamase tests	Penicillins[c]
Haemophilus influenzae	Direct β-lactamase tests	Penicillins[c]
Moraxella catarrhalis	Direct β-lactamase tests (nitrocefin only)	Penicillins[c]
Neisseria gonorrhoeae	Direct β-lactamase tests	Penicillins[c]
Staphylococcus spp.	Direct β-lactamase tests with prior induction	Penicillins[c]
Escherichia coli	NCCLS ESBL screening and confirmation tests	Penicillins, cephems, and aztreonam
Klebsiella pneumoniae and *K. oxytoca*	NCCLS ESBL screening and confirmation tests	Penicillins, cephems, and aztreonam

[a] A positive result indicates resistance; however, a negative result is inconclusive, since other resistance mechanisms may occur.

[b] Includes chromogenic cephalosporin, acidimetric, and iodometric tests.

[c] A positive result indicates resistance to all penicillinase-labile penicillins, including amoxicillin, ampicillin, azlocillin, carbenicillin, mezlocillin, piperacillin, and ticarcillin.

several filter paper-type disk or strip products that are commercially available and widely used in clinical laboratories. β-Lactamase hydrolysis of the chromogenic cephalosporin molecule causes an electron shift that results in a colored product (135). Although the acidimetric and iodometric methods have varied in performance, perhaps due in part to lack of experience with these methods, the chromogenic method has been reliable in detecting β-lactamases produced by all of the organisms indicated in Table 2 (92, 134).

The colorimetric β-lactamase tests rely on visualization of a colored product that presumably results from β-lactamase destruction of the substrate β-lactam molecule. However, these tests are not 100% specific, and other substances may yield colored end points. Serum may cause a colored reaction with the nitrocefin test (135), and, if reagents are not stored properly, spontaneous degradation of penicillin may produce false-positive acidimetric or iodometric β-lactamase reactions.

While some bacteria (e.g., *H. influenzae, N. gonorrhoeae,* and enterococci) constitutively produce β-lactamase, others (e.g., staphylococci) may produce detectable amounts of enzyme only after exposure to an inducing agent, which is generally a β-lactam (48). If staphylococci produce a positive β-lactamase result without induction, the results can be reported. However, if no β-lactamase is detected, then the test must be performed with cells that have been exposed to an inducing agent before a negative result is reported. This can be done by testing organisms that have been grown in the presence of subinhibitory concentrations of a β-lactam agent (e.g., 0.25 μg of cefoxitin per ml) in a broth or agar system. Alternatively, growth from around the periphery of the zone surrounding a β-lactam disk (e.g., a 1-μg oxacillin or 30-μg cefoxitin disk) can be tested. A positive result may take longer to develop for staphylococci than for other organisms, and the test should not be considered negative until it has been allowed to react for at least 60 min.

β-Lactamase testing by the chromogenic nitrocefin method with anaerobic gram-negative bacilli other than those from the *Bacteroides fragilis* group may be performed prior to susceptibility testing (33). Members of the *B. fragilis* group characteristically produce β-lactamase, and they should be considered penicillin resistant. As with aerobes, resistance to β-lactam drugs is not always mediated by β-lactamase production (e.g., in some strains of *Bacteroides distasonis* and *B. fragilis*) (2, 33, 83).

The *S. aureus* strains recommended by the CLSI for quality control of routine disk diffusion and dilution tests (36–38) can be used for quality control of β-lactamase tests. *S. aureus* ATCC 25923 is β-lactamase negative, whereas *S. aureus* ATCC 29213 is β-lactamase positive.

Tests for Extended-Spectrum β-Lactamases

The genes generally responsible for β-lactamase-mediated ampicillin resistance in *Escherichia coli, Klebsiella* spp., *Proteus mirabilis,* and some other genera of the family *Enterobacteriaceae* can undergo simple point mutations that result in the production of novel β-lactamases that are capable of hydrolyzing extended-spectrum cephalosporins (e.g., cefotaxime, ceftriaxone, ceftizoxime, and ceftazidime) and aztreonam, as well as older β-lactam drugs. These enzymes are referred to as extended-spectrum β-lactamases (ESBLs) (9, 12, 85, 113, 147, 196) and are discussed in chapter 71. More than 200 different types of ESBLs have been noted to occur in several gram-negative species and are associated with a variety of in vitro antimicrobial susceptibility profiles (12, 196; http://www.lahey.org/Studies/).

The in vitro susceptibility results obtained with an isolate that produces ESBLs often defy typical "hierarchy" rules of β-lactam (particularly cephem) activity. Sometimes the more narrow spectrum cephems (particularly the cephamycins, such as cefoxitin or cefotetan) are more active than broad-spectrum agents (26, 126). Several reports suggest that ESBL-producing isolates should be considered resistant to all extended-spectrum penicillins, cephalosporins, and monobactams even if they appear to be susceptible to these agents in vitro (139, 140, 173). The β-lactamase-stable carbapenems (ertapenem, imipenem, meropenem) are active in vitro (4, 84, 91, 148, 171, 172, 212) and appear to be clinically effective against ESBL producers (88, 124, 139, 142). Some ESBL-producing isolates are susceptible to β-lactam/β-lactamase inhibitor combination agents in vitro, but the effectiveness of these agents in vivo is uncertain, particularly if there is a high concentration of organisms at the infection site (86). The genes that code for production of ESBLs are often linked to other resistance genes, so that ESBL-producing isolates are often multiply resistant (e.g., resistant to aminoglycosides and trimethoprim-sulfamethoxazole) (96).

Routine disk diffusion and MIC tests using traditional breakpoints may not always identify isolates that produce ESBLs (87, 89, 96, 126). Thus, the CLSI has developed MIC and disk diffusion screening breakpoints for aztreonam, cefotaxime, cefpodoxime, ceftazidime, and ceftriaxone for *E. coli, Klebsiella oxytoca,* and *Klebsiella pneumoniae* and, more recently, for cefpodoxime, ceftazidime, and cefotaxime for *Proteus mirabilis* that aid in detecting ESBL-producing isolates (38) of those species. ESBL-producing clinical isolates may demonstrate high-level resistance to one or more of the screening drugs (88, 96, 114, 124, 171, 210). Thus, the sensitivity of the screen test increases when more than one screening drug is used (51, 126, 212). Cefpodoxime is most likely to detect isolates producing ESBLs, but this agent lacks specificity, particularly for *E. coli* (65, 126, 195). However, the CLSI has modified the screening breakpoints for cefpodoxime for *E. coli* and *Klebsiella* spp. in order to increase the specificity with a minimal effect on the sensitivity (34). Only cefpodoxime, cefotaxime, and ceftazidime have been validated for use with *P. mirabilis* (38).

Unlike inducible AmpC β-lactamases, ESBLs are inhibited by clavulanic acid, and this property is used in laboratory tests to identify ESBLs in the clinical laboratory. These tests are based on enhanced activity when a β-lactam (usually ceftazidime or cefotaxime) is tested with clavulanic acid compared to the activity when the β-lactam is tested alone. The CLSI describes standard disk diffusion and broth microdilution MIC tests to be used as phenotypic confirmatory tests for the presence of ESBLs in *E. coli, K. oxytoca, K. pneumoniae,* and *P. mirabilis.* For broth microdilution, cefotaxime and ceftazidime are tested with and without 4 μg of clavulanic acid per ml. A decrease in the MIC of ≥3 dilutions for the agents tested in combination with clavulanic acid compared to the values obtained for the agents tested alone indicates the presence of an ESBL. For disk diffusion, the same agents incorporated into disks with and without 10 μg of clavulanic acid are tested. An increase in the zone diameter of ≥5 mm for either of the disks with clavulanic acid indicates the presence of an ESBL. *K. pneumoniae* ATCC 700603 should be included for quality control purposes; accepted ranges are given in the current CLSI M100 tables (38). Isolates of *E. coli, Klebsiella* spp., and *P. mirabilis* confirmed to be ESBL producers should be reported as resistant to penicillins (not including β-lactam/β-lactamase inhibitor combinations), cephalosporins (which excludes the cephamycins, cefoxitin and cefotetan), and aztreonam (36–38). For screen-positive strains that do not show a clavulanic acid effect, there are insufficient data to justify modifying reports at present; these isolates should be reported as they test. One of the limitations of the phenotypic confirmatory test is that some ESBL-producing strains may demonstrate a negative confirmatory test result, which may occur as a result of decreased porin production, hyperproduction of a TEM-1 or SHV-1 β-lactamase, production of additional β-lactamases (e.g., AmpC) that are not inhibited by clavulanic acid, or a combination of these (12, 196). Steward et al. (180) showed in a recent study that cefepime with and without clavulanic acid is superior to the current confirmatory test agents (both cefotaxime and ceftazidime with and without clavulanic acid) in detection of ESBLs in some strains that have multiple β-lactam resistance mechanisms. The CLSI has not addressed the utility of the screening or phenotypic confirmatory tests for detecting ESBLs in members of the family *Enterobacteriaceae* other than *E. coli*, *Klebsiella* spp., and *P. mirabilis*. In theory, however, they should detect ESBLs in other genera that are normally susceptible to extended-spectrum cephalosporins.

Typically, screening for and confirmation of ESBL production is a two-step process; however, there are several FDA-cleared commercial products that incorporate a confirmatory test on a primary susceptibility test panel. The laboratory's ability to detect and report the presence of ESBLs in a timely manner will likely affect the selection of appropriate therapy for patients with infections caused by ESBL-producing strains. Consequently every laboratory should have a procedure to address the detection of ESBLs (105, 140, 148, 173, 192). There is some debate as to the significance of ESBLs in isolates from noninvasive infections, such as uncomplicated urinary tract infections (51, 141). However, regardless of the source, ESBL-producing isolates are important from an infection control perspective.

Tests for Detection of Plasmid-Mediated AmpC-Type β-Lactamases

Inducible AmpC-type β-lactamases occur on the chromosome of several gram-negative bacilli such as *Enterobacter cloacae*, *Citrobacter freundii*, *Serratia marcescens*, and *Pseudomonas aeruginosa* (113). These enzymes confer resistance to a wide spectrum of β-lactams, and they are resistant to the commonly used β-lactamase inhibitors (see details in chapter 71). AmpC-type β-lactamases may be located on transmissible plasmids in several bacterial species that lack an inducible chromosomal enzyme, including *E. coli*, *Klebsiella* spp., *Salmonella* spp., and *P. mirabilis* (146). These plasmids often carry resistant determinants for multiple classes of antimicrobial agents. AmpC-type enzymes in porin-deficient strains can result in carbapenem resistance (10, 176). Therefore, detection of plasmid-mediated AmpC-type enzymes may be important for treatment decisions, infection control, and epidemiological investigations (19, 131, 132).

Isolates with a plasmid-mediated AmpC-type enzyme are usually resistant to cephamycins (e.g., cefoxitin and cefotetan), which is a useful phenotypic marker for the β-lactamase. However, loss of a porin can also result in cephamycin resistance (72), so a more specific test is necessary. Several tests have been proposed for detecting this type of resistance. Two assays, the modified three-dimensional extract test and the cefoxitin-agar medium-based assay, are too labor-intensive for routine use in the clinical laboratory (39, 133). The more promising assay is a disk diffusion assay similar to the CLSI disk diffusion confirmatory test for ESBL detection. This test incorporates 20 μg of β-lactamase inhibitor, 48-1220 or LN-2-128, into a 30-μg cefotetan disk. In one study (7), a 4-mm reduction in zone size around the disk with cefotetan plus 48-1220 when compared to the zone size around the disk with cefotetan only correlated well with the presence of a plasmid-mediated AmpC-type enzyme in isolates of *Klebsiella* spp. and *E. coli*. Although this test holds promise for phenotypic detection of AmpC β-lactamases, these β-lactamase inhibitors are not commercially available so the test cannot yet be used by clinical laboratories.

DETERMINATION OF BACTERICIDAL ACTIVITIES OF ANTIMICROBIAL AGENTS

Most in vitro susceptibility test methods measure the abilities of antimicrobial agents to inhibit the growth of bacteria. It is also possible to assess the ability of a drug to provide a bactericidal effect on an isolate or group of isolates. This may be useful in managing serious infections that require bactericidal action for optimal efficacy such as endocarditis and osteomyelitis (152), for immunosuppressed patients (170), and to study the pharmacodynamic properties of new or established antimicrobial agents or drug combinations (6, 111, 178). The tests most often performed include determination of the MBC, serum bactericidal titers (SBT), and kinetic time-kill assays. Even in the most sophisticated clinical laboratories serving large tertiary-care medical centers, determinations of bactericidal activity probably account for fewer than 1% of all susceptibility tests performed. Thus, these are highly specialized tests performed for very limited indications.

Tests of bactericidal activity are primarily used for selection and monitoring of therapy for patients with infective endocarditis (41, 93, 145, 152, 155, 167, 168, 208), osteomyelitis (93, 130, 145, 152, 209), meningitis (145, 155, 166), or for neutropenic cancer patients (97, 100, 170). These tests may be favored by certain physicians or specialty groups (e.g., infectious disease specialists) for the management of their patients' very complicated infections but do not represent standard care in most medical centers. Data in support of the use of bactericidal activity determinations for patient management are limited, and early studies were often performed using nonstandardized methods (41, 93, 117, 167, 189). Prior reviews have highlighted the technical problems and lack of expert consensus for interpreting the results of bactericidal determinations (117, 118, 152). The perception that the tests are not reproducible may have stifled the development of consensus criteria for when and how these tests can best be applied. The lack of standardization of the specific assays has been addressed by the CLSI through the publication of standard methods for determining bactericidal activity (30, 31). This section discusses bactericidal testing in a clinical laboratory setting and reflects the consensus standards developed by the CLSI.

Clinical Use of Bactericidal Testing

For those who favor the use of bactericidal tests for management of serious infections, a typical sequence is to first determine the MICs and MBCs of a limited number of agents that could be used to treat the patient in order to select the agent with the most favorable (i.e., lowest) MBC relative to the safely achievable levels of the drug. Determination of the MBC provides an opportunity to detect possible tolerance of the patient's isolate to drugs that would normally be considered bactericidal against the species being tested and might result in clinical failure (43, 70, 78, 130, 200). Once one or more drugs have been selected on the basis of the MIC and MBC results and the patient has been started on standard doses of the agent(s), the second step is to assess the bactericidal activity achieved in the patient by performance of the serum bactericidal test(s). The goal is to ensure that the dosage regimen provides sufficient bactericidal activity in that patient's blood or, possibly, cerebrospinal fluid. The body fluid (usually serum) is serially diluted and inoculated with the patient's infecting organism. The SBT test result is expressed as a titer indicating the dilution of serum or body fluid that is bactericidal; a higher titer indicates better activity. If the SBT is deemed to be too low, it may be possible to alter the dosage regimen or to select an alternative regimen in an effort to avoid a poor therapeutic outcome (152, 208, 209). Performance of the SBT test can also provide an assessment of the effectiveness of drug combinations intended to provide a synergistic effect in order to treat a highly resistant bacterial isolate or an organism not killed by single-agent therapy (e.g., *Enterococcus* spp.) (30).

Performance of bactericidal tests requires considerable technical proficiency on the part of the laboratory and a highly informed and experienced clinician to make use of the data. The interpretation of the SBT must take into account knowledge of the key pharmacodynamic property of the antimicrobial agent (i.e., concentration-dependent versus time-dependent killing activity), the location and severity of the infection, the pathogenic potential of the infecting organism, and the potential toxicity and cost of the treatment regimen. Bactericidal testing should not be performed unless there is close communication between the clinical microbiologist and the requesting clinician. Potential pitfalls include selecting potentially more toxic or expensive drugs on the basis of a low MIC or MBC (unless the physician is very knowledgeable about various classes of antimicrobial agents) and raising antibiotic levels to potentially toxic levels in order to achieve a higher or more favorable SBT. Therefore, laboratories should undertake bactericidal testing only after thorough discussions with their clinician customers.

Determination of the MBC

There are several basic requirements for standardized determination of the MBC. The test may be performed by either the tube broth macrodilution method or the broth microdilution procedure. A detailed description of the methods can be found in the CLSI document that deals specifically with bactericidal tests (31). In brief, the test usually uses standard cation-adjusted Mueller-Hinton broth (with lysed horse blood supplementation if needed for fastidious organisms) dispensed in 1-ml aliquots in glass tubes (13 by 100 mm) or in 0.1-ml volumes in plastic microdilution trays. A significant component in performance of the MBC test is the inoculum preparation and inoculation procedure. An actively growing (log-phase) inoculum is used (31, 189) rather than an inoculum that is allowed to grow to the stationary phase or fresh colonies suspended in broth or saline, as for a standard MIC test (36). Use of a log-phase inoculum is necessary to accurately assess the bactericidal properties of drugs that require actively growing cells to exert a bactericidal effect. In addition, it is important to dispense the standardized inoculum suspension below the meniscus of the broth carefully in each tube or well to prevent splashing that can lead to organisms sticking to the wall of the tube or well above the meniscus rather than being in contact with the drug in the test medium (31). If splashing or aerosolization of the inoculum occurs, viable organisms recovered at the time of the final subculture may represent bacteria that were not sufficiently exposed to the drug during the course of the test and thus would give the erroneous perception that the drug was not bactericidal (31, 98, 189).

After determination of the MIC following incubation at 35°C, quantitative subcultures (usually 0.01 ml) are performed at 24 h (following vortexing or shaking at 20 h) with samples from each tube or well with concentrations at and above the MIC of the drug being tested. The aliquots are streaked across the entire surface of a plate containing a standard growth medium (e.g., sheep blood agar). By transferring a small sample volume and spreading it across the entire plate, possible carryover effects of the antibiotic are minimized. In order to calculate the degree of killing at each antibiotic concentration, it is necessary that colony counts be performed on the positive control tube or well at the time of initial inoculation of the MIC test. As in the standard MIC procedure, the target inoculum density is 5×10^5 CFU/ml (31, 36). After the subculture plates are incubated for 24 to 48 h, any visible colonies are counted on each subculture plate. The standard definition of the MBC is the reduction of the initial inoculum by $\geq$99.9% (3 logs) (31). In practice, it is advisable to correct for pipetting error and to account for the Poisson distribution of bacterial cells in a liquid by using statistically derived rejection value tables (31). The tables define the number of colonies that can be tolerated based on the initial inoculum density of each test. If the number of colonies on a particular plate exceeds the rejection value for that test, the antibiotic did not achieve the strict definition of a bactericidal effect at that given concentration of the drug. It is then hoped that the next higher concentration of the drug will have fewer surviving colonies to fulfill the definition of a bactericidal effect. The MBC of an antibiotic should be reported in micrograms per milliliter in the same manner as the MIC is reported. A given MBC test should be considered invalid if there is evidence of contamination of the inoculum or the subcultured tubes or wells, if there is no growth in the positive control well or tube or there is growth in the sterility well or tube, or if there are several skipped dilutions in the MIC portion of the test (31, 67).

Assessment of Bactericidal Activity by the Time-Kill Method

Measuring the rate of bactericidal activity by time-kill analysis provides the opportunity to assess the speed with which killing may occur at a given antibiotic concentration. It is a more laborious approach than determination of the MBC and thus may be best reserved for research purposes. It is also possible to assess the activities of drugs in combination in order to recognize synergistic, indifferent, or antagonistic effects of two or more drugs tested together (31, 99, 104). This approach appears to correlate better with in vivo studies of combined drug effects than the alternative checkerboard titration method (5, 13, 40). The details of performance of the time-kill test have been defined in the CLSI guideline (31). Many of the same critical factors that affect the outcome of the MBC test apply to the performance of time-kill assays, e.g., preparation of an actively growing inoculum and use of quantitative subcultures from antibiotic-containing tubes. The time-kill method requires that multiple samples be removed at various times (e.g., 0, 4, 8, 12, and 24 h) for colony counts, and thus, the volume of medium for each antibiotic concentration tested is usually ≥10 ml contained in a glass test tube or flask (31). A given antibiotic is often tested at more than one concentration that relates to the previously determined MIC of that agent (e.g., the MIC, two times the MIC, or four times the MIC). When high concentrations (four or more times the MIC) of a drug are tested by the time-kill method, it is necessary to demonstrate that antibiotic carryover has not falsely diminished the number of colonies on subculture plates (31). The results of a time-kill assay are frequently depicted graphically by plotting the colony counts of each antibiotic and concentration tested over time (Fig. 1). A bactericidal effect is again defined as ≥99.9% killing at a specified time (31). When drugs are tested in combination by the time-kill method, synergy is often defined as a ≥2 log decrease in the number of CFU achieved with a drug combination compared to that achieved with the most active drug tested alone (31).

Performance of the Serum Bactericidal Test

The determinations of the serum inhibitory and bactericidal titers are performed in a manner analogous to the MIC and MBC procedures, except that the patient's serum, rather than preweighed and prediluted concentrations of the drug, is used as the source of antibiotic. A guideline that describes the details of the serum bactericidal test has been published by the CLSI (30). The principal steps in performing the test include (i) obtaining one or more blood samples from the patient at specified intervals; (ii) preparing twofold dilutions of the patient's serum in pooled and pretested human serum in glass tubes or plastic microdilution trays; (iii) inoculating each tube or well with a standardized, actively growing inoculum (as described above for the MBC test) of the patient's own infecting organism in an appropriate growth medium (usually cation-adjusted Mueller-Hinton broth); and (iv) incubating for 20 to 24 h (30). Pooled human serum is recommended as the diluent of the patient's serum in each tube or well in order to make protein binding consistent throughout the range of serum dilutions, especially for drugs that are highly protein bound. The pretesting of the pooled human serum includes screening for human immunodeficiency virus type 1 and hepatitis B and C viruses, for antibiotic activity, and for optical clarity (30). In addition, the pooled serum should be heat inactivated immediately prior to use, and the pH should be adjusted to the correct range of 7.2 to 7.4 (30). An alternative to the laborious serum preparation step just described is the creation of a serum ultrafiltrate that precludes the need for a serum diluent (30, 109).

The blood samples for testing are usually obtained from the patient shortly after the antibiotic is administered, at the time of the presumed peak level in serum (usually 30 to

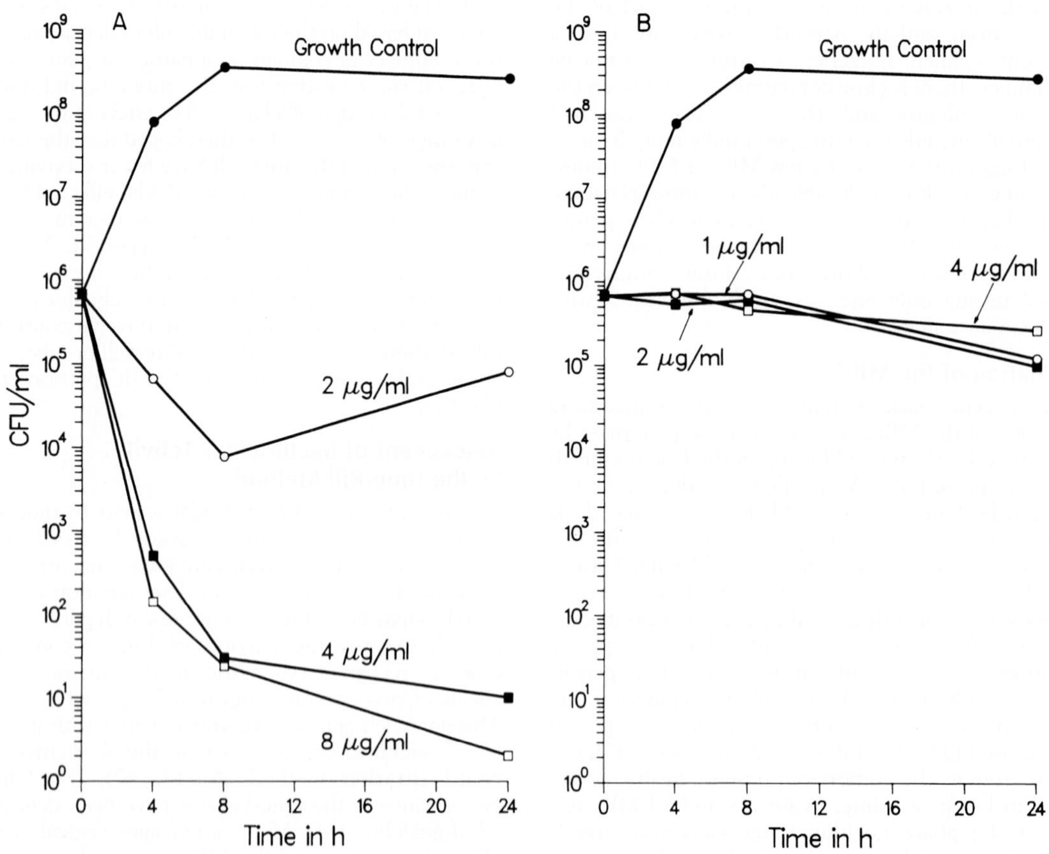

FIGURE 1 Results of time-kill assay of an *Enterococcus faecium* isolate. (A) Daptomycin tested at the MIC (2 µg/ml) and at two and four times the MIC, demonstrating a bactericidal effect at two and four times the MIC. (B) Vancomycin tested at the MIC (1 µg/ml) and at two and four times the MIC, without evidence of a bactericidal effect. Reproduced from reference 95 with permission.

60 min after administration), and often immediately prior to administration of the next drug dose (trough level) (30). The end points of the test are indicated by the highest dilution (titer) of the patient's serum sample that prevents visible growth following the incubation period (serum inhibitory titer). Similar to the MBC determination, quantitative subcultures are performed from each dilution of the patient's serum that has prevented visible growth. The SBT is defined as that dilution (titer) that provides a ≥99.9% reduction of the original inoculum of the test based upon the standard rejection value tables (30). Thus, the results of the test are reported as dilutions (the titer) of the patient's serum rather than as a drug concentration (in micrograms per milliliter) as in the MIC and MBC tests.

Interpreting the Results of Bactericidal Determinations

The interpretation of the results of the bactericidal determinations described above has not received the same degree of critical scrutiny or level of consensus standards that have been achieved for interpretation of MICs. However, a few general statements can be made. A favorable MBC would typically be the same as or perhaps 1 or 2 dilutions greater than the MIC of agents that are normally considered bactericidal (e.g., β-lactams, glycopeptides-lipopeptides, aminoglycosides, and fluoroquinolones). A principal rationale for performing MBC or kinetic time-kill studies would be to detect an isolate that is not effectively killed by a typically bactericidal drug. This failure to exert a bactericidal effect is often described as tolerance and is defined as an MBC ≥32-fold the MIC of a particular agent (31, 70). Failure to achieve at least a 3-$\log_{10}$ reduction of CFU in the kinetic time-kill assay could likewise signify a tolerant strain (31).

Results of the serum bactericidal test that reflect a high titer of antibacterial activity in the serum suggest that the patient has been dosed adequately, has not experienced abnormal elimination of the antibiotic, and does not have a tolerant bacterial isolate. This perception can be quantified by comparing the peak and trough titers obtained with those that have been shown to correlate with rapid organism eradication in collaborative studies (152, 208, 209). For rapid clearance of bacteremia and optimal time to sterilization of cardiac vegetations in endocarditis, a peak SBT of ≥1:64 and a trough SBT of ≥1:32 should be achieved whenever possible (152, 208). However, lower bactericidal titers do not necessarily signify a poor clinical outcome. In patients with chronic osteomyelitis, limited data have suggested that peak SBTs of ≥1:16 and trough SBTs of ≥1:4 predict clinical cure, while titers as low as 1:2 at the trough have been shown to be satisfactory in acute osteomyelitis (152, 209). Titers of ≥1:8 have generally (80% of cases) been associated with satisfactory outcomes for cancer chemotherapy patients (100).

Limitations of Bactericidal Determinations

As stated earlier, clinical microbiologists and infectious disease specialists are not uniformly convinced of the importance of bactericidal determinations as a routine part of even highly complicated bacterial infections. Part of the controversy over the use of these tests may stem from the fact that the procedures themselves have only rather recently been standardized to a significant degree. Indeed, there are still several procedural steps in these tests that can be difficult to control (Table 3), not the least of which are the critical steps of inoculum preparation and dispensing and the final step of accurately counting the surviving bacteria. Despite full attention to the critical details of these test procedures, confusing results may still occur in the form of the skip tube phenomenon (67) or trailing bactericidal end points due to persisters (31). Persisters are thought to represent a fraction of the bacterial population and occasionally exceed 0.1% of the population due to metabolically inactive cells not effectively eradicated during the test (68). A point of occasional concern is the paradoxical or Eagle effect, in which a bactericidal effect can be demonstrated at a relatively low drug concentration, but cells are found not to be killed at very high drug concentrations relative to the MIC (31). This phenomenon has been attributed to secondary effects of some cell wall-active agents on intracellular processes such as protein synthesis, thereby slowing the growth rate and preventing the drug's principal effect on cell wall synthesis of rapidly growing cells (49). A major contribution of the CLSI guidelines is the provision of suggested quality control measures, including established MBC ranges for commonly used control organisms (31, 36). Despite these vigorous efforts to standardize these determinations, it is likely that bactericidal tests will continue to be a subject of discussion and be performed at relatively few institutions for purposes of patient management.

TABLE 3 Technical factors that are critical for reliable determination of MBCs and SBTs and potential pitfalls in those procedure steps

Procedure step	Potential pitfall
Preparation of an actively growing, log-phase inoculum	Use of stationary-phase inoculum will increase the percentage of persisters and potentially result in false tolerance with antibiotics that require rapidly growing cells to exert a bactericidal effect
Delivery of the inoculum aliquot below the meniscus of the broth	Splashing of the inoculum suspension onto the wall of the tube or microdilution well will prevent some cells from contact with the antibiotic and lead to an inaccurate number of colonies upon final subculture
Quantitative subculture of tubes or wells containing drug concentrations at the MIC or higher following incubation	Subculture of too large a volume may cause the problem of antibiotic carryover and persistent inhibition; subculture of an insufficient volume precludes accurate counting of surviving organisms
Determination of ≥99.9% reduction in CFU/ml	Inaccurate pipetting or failure to compensate for pipetting error or Poisson distribution of bacteria will compromise calculation of the bactericidal end point
Failure to account for protein binding in the SBT test	SBT may be falsely elevated with drugs that are highly protein bound (e.g, >90%)

REFERENCES

1. **Abele-Horn, M., L. Hommers, R. Trabold, and M. Frosch.** 2006. Validation of VITEK 2 version 4.01 software for detection, identification, and classification of glycopeptide-resistant enterococci. *J. Clin. Microbiol.* **44:**71–76.
2. **Aldridge, K. E., D. Ashcraft, K. Cambre, C. L. Pierson, S. G. Jenkins, and J. E. Rosenblatt.** 2001. Multicenter survey of the changing in vitro antimicrobial susceptibilities of clinical isolates of *Bacteroides fragilis* group, *Prevotella, Fusobacterium, Porphyromonas,* and *Peptostreptococcus* species. *Antimicrob. Agents Chemother.* **45:**1238–1242.
3. **Aubert, G., S. Passot, F. Lucht, and G. Dorche.** 1990. Selection of vancomycin- and teicoplanin-resistant *Staphylococcus haemolyticus* during teicoplanin treatment of *S. epidermidis* infection. *J. Antimicrob. Chemother.* **25:** 491–493.
4. **Babini, G. S., and D. M. Livermore.** 2000. Antimicrobial resistance amongst *Klebsiella* spp. collected from intensive care units in Southern and Western Europe in 1997–1998. *J. Antimicrob. Chemother.* **45:**183–189.
5. **Bayer, A. S., and J. O. Morrison.** 1984. Disparity between timed-kill and checkerboard methods for determination of in vitro bactericidal interactions of vancomycin plus rifampin versus methicillin-susceptible and -resistant *Staphylococcus aureus. Antimicrob. Agents Chemother.* **26:** 220–223.
6. **Bergeret, M., and J. Raymond.** 1999. In vitro bactericidal activity of cefpirome and cefamandole in combination with glycopeptides against methicillin-resistant *Staphylococcus aureus. J. Antimicrob. Chemother.* **43:**291–294.
7. **Black, J. A., K. S. Thomson, and J. D. D. Pitout.** 2004. Use of β-lactamase inhibitors in disk tests to detect plasmid-mediated AmpC β-lactamases. *J. Clin. Microbiol.* **42:**2203–2206.
8. **Blondeau, J. M., D. Vaughan, R. Laskowski, and S. Borsos.** 2001. Susceptibility of Canadian isolates of *Haemophilus influenzae, Moraxella catarrhalis* and *Streptococcus pneumoniae* to oral antimicrobial agents. *Int. J. Antimicrob. Agents* **17:**457–464.
9. **Bonnet, R., C. De Champs, D. Sirot, C. Chanal, R. Labia, and J. Sirot.** 1999. Diversity of TEM mutants in *Proteus mirabilis. Antimicrob. Agents Chemother.* **43:** 2671–2677.
10. **Bradford, P. A., C. Urban, N. Mariano, S. J. Projan, J. J. Rahal, and K. Bush.** 1997. Imipenem resistance in *Klebsiella pneumoniae* is associated with the combination of ACT-1, a plasmid-mediated AmpC β-lactamase, and the loss of an outer membrane protein. *Antimicrob. Agents Chemother.* **41:**563–569.
11. **Brown, D. F., and E. Walpole.** 2001. Evaluation of the Mastalex latex agglutination test for methicillin resistance in *Staphylococcus aureus* grown on different screening media. *J. Antimicrob. Chemother.* **47:**187–189.
12. **Bush, K.** 2001. New β-lactamases in gram-negative bacteria: diversity and impact on the selection of antimicrobial therapy. *Clin. Infect. Dis.* **32:**1085–1089.
13. **Cappelletty, D. M., and M. J. Rybak.** 1996. Comparison of methodologies for synergism testing of drug combinations against resistant strains of *Pseudomonas aeruginosa. Antimicrob. Agents Chemother.* **40:**677–683.
14. **Cartwright, C. P., F. Stock, G. A. Fahle, and V. J. Gill.** 1995. Comparison of pigment production and motility tests with PCR for reliable identification of intrinsically vancomycin-resistant enterococci. *J. Clin. Microbiol.* **33:** 1931–1933.
15. **Catlin, B. W.** 1975. Iodometric detection of *Haemophilus influenzae* β-lactamase: rapid presumptive test for ampicillin resistance. *Antimicrob. Agents Chemother.* **7:** 265–270.
16. **Cauwelier, B., B. Gordts, P. Descheemaecker, and H. Van Landuyt.** 2004. Evaluation of a disk diffusion method with cefoxitin (30 μg) for detection of methicillin-resistant *Staphylococcus aureus. Eur. J. Clin. Microbiol. Infect. Dis.* **23:**389–392.
17. **Cavassini, M., A. Wenger, K. Jaton, D. S. Blanc, and J. Bille.** 1999. Evaluation of MRSA-Screen, a simple anti-PBP 2a slide latex agglutination kit, for rapid detection of methicillin resistance in *Staphylococcus aureus. J. Clin. Microbiol.* **37:**1591–1594.
18. **Centers for Disease Control and Prevention.** 1999. Four pediatric deaths from community-acquired methicillin-resistant *Staphylococcus aureus*—Minnesota and North Dakota, 1997–1999. *Morb. Mortal. Wkly. Rep.* **48:**707–710.
19. **Centers for Disease Control and Prevention.** 2002. Outbreak of multidrug-resistant *Salmonella* Newport—United States, January–April 2002. *Morb. Mortal. Wkly. Rep.* **51:**545–548.
20. **Centers for Disease Control and Prevention.** 2002. Public health dispatch: vancomycin-resistant *Staphylococcus aureus*—Pennsylvania, 2002. *Morb. Mortal. Wkly. Rep.* **51:**302.
21. **Centers for Disease Control and Prevention.** 2002. *Staphylococcus aureus* resistant to vancomycin—United States, 2002. *Morb. Mortal. Wkly. Rep.* **51:**565–567.
22. **Centers for Disease Control and Prevention.** 2004. Brief report: vancomycin-resistant *Staphylococcus aureus*—New York, 2004. *Morb. Mortal. Wkly. Rep.* **53:**322–323.
23. **Chambers, H. F.** 1997. Methicillin resistance in staphylococci: molecular and biochemical basis and clinical implications. *Clin. Microbiol. Rev.* **10:**781–791.
24. **Chambers, H. F., G. Archer, and M. Matsuhashi.** 1989. Low-level methicillin resistance in *Staphylococcus aureus. Antimicrob. Agents Chemother.* **33:**424–428.
25. **Chambers, H. F., and C. J. Hackbarth.** 1992. Methicillin-resistant *Staphylococcus aureus:* genetics and mechanisms of resistance, p. 21–35. *In* M. T. Cafferkey (ed.), *Methicillin-Resistant* Staphylococcus aureus: *Clinical Management and Laboratory Aspects.* Marcel Dekker, Inc., New York, N.Y.
26. **Chanal-Claris, C., D. Sirot, L. Bret, P. Chatron, R. Labia, and J. Sirot.** 1997. Novel extended-spectrum TEM-type β-lactamase from an *Escherichia coli* isolate resistant to ceftazidime and susceptible to cephalothin. *Antimicrob. Agents Chemother.* **41:**715–716.
27. **Chen, Y., S. A. Marshall, P. Winokur, S. Coffman, W. Wilke, P. Murray, C. Spiegel, M. A. Pfaller, G. V. Doern, and R. N. Jones.** 1998. Use of molecular and reference susceptibility testing methods in a multicenter evaluation of MicroScan dried overnight gram-positive MIC panels for detection of vancomycin and high-level aminoglycoside resistances in enterococci. *J. Clin. Microbiol.* **36:**2996–3001.
28. **Chow, J. W., M. J. Zervos, S. A. Lerner, L. A. Thal, S. Donabedian, D. Jaworski, S. Tsai, K. Shaw, and D. B. Clewell.** 1997. A novel gentamicin resistance gene in enterococcus. *Antimicrob. Agents Chemother.* **41:**511–514.
29. **Clinical and Laboratory Standards Institute/NCCLS.** 1993. *Methods for Dilution Antimicrobial Susceptibility Tests for Bacteria That Grow Aerobically. Approved Standard M7-A3.* Clinical and Laboratory Standards Institute, Villanova, Pa.
30. **Clinical and Laboratory Standards Institute/NCCLS.** 1999. *Methodology for the Serum Bactericidal Test. Document M21-A.* Clinical and Laboratory Standards Institute, Wayne, Pa.
31. **Clinical and Laboratory Standards Institute/NCCLS.** 1999. *Methods for Determining Bactericidal Activity of Antimicrobial Agents. Document M26-A.* Clinical and Laboratory Standards Institute, Wayne, Pa.
32. **Clinical and Laboratory Standards Institute/NCCLS.** 1999. *Performance Standards for Antimicrobial Susceptibility*

Testing; Ninth Informational Supplement, M100-S9. Clinical and Laboratory Standards Institute, Wayne, Pa.

33. **Clinical and Laboratory Standards Institute/NCCLS.** 2001. *Methods for Antimicrobial Susceptibility Testing of Anaerobic Bacteria; Approved Standard—Sixth Edition. NCCLS Document M11-A6.* Clinical and Laboratory Standards Institute, Wayne, Pa.
34. **Clinical and Laboratory Standards Institute/NCCLS.** 2002. *Performance Standards for Antimicrobial Susceptibility Testing; Twelfth Informational Supplement. NCCLS Document M100-S12.* Clinical and Laboratory Standards Institute, Wayne, Pa.
35. **Clinical and Laboratory Standards Institute/NCCLS.** 2005. *Performance Standards for Antimicrobial Susceptibility Testing: Fifteenth Information Supplement. CLSI Document M100-S15.* Clinical and Laboratory Standards Institute, Wayne, Pa.
36. **Clinical and Laboratory Standards Institute/NCCLS.** 2006. *Methods for Dilution Antimicrobial Susceptibility Tests for Bacteria That Grow Aerobically; Approved Standard—Sixth Edition. CLSI Document M7-A7.* Clinical and Laboratory Standards Institute, Wayne, Pa.
37. **Clinical and Laboratory Standards Institute/NCCLS.** 2006. *Performance Standards for Antimicrobial Disk Susceptibility Tests; Approved Standard—Eighth Edition. CLSI Document M2-A9.* Clinical and Laboratory Standards Institute, Wayne, Pa.
38. **Clinical and Laboratory Standards Institute/NCCLS.** 2006. *Performance Standards for Antimicrobial Susceptibility Testing: Sixteenth Informational Supplement. CLSI Document M100-S16,* 16th ed. Clinical and Laboratory Standards Institute, Wayne, Pa.
39. **Coudron, P. E., E. S. Moland, and K. S. Thomson.** 2000. Occurrence and detection of AmpC β-lactamases among *Escherichia coli, Klebsiella pneumoniae,* and *Proteus mirabilis* isolates at a veterans medical center. *J. Clin. Microbiol.* **38:**1791–1796.
40. **D'Alessandri, R. M., D. J. McNeely, and R. M. Kluge.** 1998. Antibiotic synergy and antagonism against clinical isolates of *Klebsiella* species. *Antimicrob. Agents Chemother.* **10:**889–892.
41. **DeGirolami, P. C., and G. Eliopoulos.** 1987. Antimicrobial susceptibility tests and their role in therapeutic drug monitoring. *Clin. Lab. Med.* **7:**499–513.
42. **De Lencastre, H., S. A. Figueiredo, C. Urban, J. Rahal, and A. Tomasz.** 1991. Multiple mechanisms of methicillin resistance and improved methods for detection in clinical isolates of *Staphylococcus aureus. Antimicrob. Agents Chemother.* **35:**632–639.
43. **Denny, A. E., L. R. Peterson, D. N. Gerding, and W. H. Hall.** 1979. Serious staphylococcal infections with strains tolerant to bactericidal antibiotics. *Ann. Intern. Med.* **139:**1026–1031.
44. **Desjardins, M., K. L. Delgaty, K. Ramotar, C. Seetaram, and B. Toye.** 2004. Prevalence and mechanisms of erythromycin resistance in group A and group B *Streptococcus:* implications for reporting susceptibility results. *J. Clin. Microbiol.* **42:**5620–5623.
45. **Dixon, J. M., A. E. Lipinski, and M. E. Graham.** 1977. Detection and prevalence of pneumococci with increased resistance to penicillin. *Can. Med. Assoc. J.* **117:**1159–1161.
46. **Doern, G. V., A. Brueggemann, and G. Pierce.** 1997. Assessment of the oxacillin disk screening test for determining penicillin resistance in *Streptococcus pneumoniae. Eur. J. Clin. Microbiol. Infect. Dis.* **16:**311–314.
47. **Dunne, W. M., Jr., H. Quershi, H. Pervez, and D. A. Nafziger.** 2001. *Staphylococcus epidermidis* with intermediate resistance to vancomycin: elusive phenotype or laboratory artifact? *Clin. Infect. Dis.* **33:**135–137.
48. **Dyke, J. W.** 1979. β-lactamases of *Staphylococcus aureus,* p. 291–310. *In* J. M. Hamilton-Miller (ed.), *β-lactamases.* Academic Press, Ltd., London, United Kingdom.
49. **Eagle, H., and A. D. Musselman.** 1948. The rate of bacterial action of penicillin in vitro as a function of its concentration and its paradoxically reduced activity at high concentrations against certain organisms. *J. Exp. Med.* **88:**131.
50. **Eisner, A., G. Gorkiewicz, G. Feierl, E. Leitner, J. Kofer, H. H. Kessler, and E. Marth.** 2005. Identification of glycopeptide-resistant enterococci by VITEK 2 system and conventional and real-time polymerase chain reaction. *Diagn. Microbiol. Infect. Dis.* **53:**17–21.
51. **Emery, C. L., and L. A. Weymouth.** 1997. Detection and clinical significance of extended-spectrum β-lactamases in a tertiary-care medical center. *J. Clin. Microbiol.* **35:**2061–2067.
52. **Endtz, H. P., N. Van Den Braak, A. Van Belkum, W. H. Groessens, D. Kreft, A. B. Stroebel, and H. A. Verbrugh.** 1998. Comparison of eight methods to detect vancomycin resistance in enterococci. *J. Clin. Microbiol.* **36:**592–594.
53. **Escamilla, J.** 1976. Susceptibility of *Haemophilus influenza* to ampicillin as determined by use of a modified, one-minute β-lactamase test. *Antimicrob. Agents Chemother.* **9:**196–198.
54. **Fahr, A., U. Eigner, M. Armbrust, A. Caganic, G. Dettori, C. Chezzi, L. Bertoncini, M. Benecchi, and M. G. Menozzi.** 2003. Two-center collaborative evaluation of the performance of the BD Phoenix automated microbiology system for identification and antimicrobial susceptibility testing of *Enterococcus* spp. and *Staphylococcus* spp. *J. Clin. Microbiol.* **41:**1135–1142.
55. **Feibelkorn, K. R., S. A. Crawford, M. L. McElmeel, and J. H. Jorgensen.** 2003. Practical disk diffusion method for detection of inducible clindamycin resistance in *Staphylococcus aureus* and coagulase-negative staphylococci. *J. Clin. Microbiol.* **41:**4740–4744.
56. **Felmingham, D., and R. N. Gruneberg.** 2000. The Alexander Project 1996–1997: latest susceptibility data from this international study of bacterial pathogens from community-acquired lower respiratory tract infections. *J. Antimicrob. Chemother.* **45:**191–203.
57. **Felten, A., B. Grandry, P. H. Lagrange, and I. Casin.** 2002. Evaluation of three techniques for detection of low-level methicillin-resistant *Staphylococcus aureus* (MRSA): a disk diffusion method with cefoxitin and moxalactam, the Vitek 2 system, and the MRSA-Screen latex agglutination test. *J. Clin. Microbiol.* **40:**2766–2771.
58. **Fernandes, C. J., L. A. Fernandes, P. Collignon, and the Australian Group on Antimicrobial Resistance.** 2005. Cefoxitin resistance as a surrogate marker for the detection of methicillin-resistant *Staphylococcus aureus. J. Antimicrob. Chemother.* **55:**506–510.
59. **Ferreira, R. B. R., N. L. P. Iorio, K. L. Malvar, A. P. F. Nunes, L. S. Fonseca, C. C. R. Bastos, and K. R. N. Santos.** 2003. Coagulase-negative staphylococci: comparison of phenotypic and genotypic oxacillin susceptibility tests and evaluation of the agar screening test by using different concentrations of oxacillin. *J. Clin. Microbiol.* **41:**3609–3614.
60. **Fines, M., B. Perichon, P. Reynolds, D. F. Sahm, and P. Courvalin.** 1999. VanE, a new type of acquired glycopeptide resistance in *Enterococcus faecalis* BM4405. *Antimicrob. Agents Chemother.* **43:**2161–2164.
61. **Free, L., and D. Sahm.** 1995. Investigation of the reformulated Remel Synergy Quad plate for detection of high-level aminoglycoside and vancomycin resistance in enterococci. *J. Clin. Microbiol.* **33:**1643–1645.
62. **Freeman, C., A. Robinson, B. Cooper, M. Mazens-Sullivan, R. Quintiliani, Jr., and C. Nightingale.** 1995. In vitro antimicrobial susceptibility of glycopeptide-resistant enterococci. *Diagn. Microbiol. Infect. Dis.* **21:**47–50.

63. **Fridkin, S. K., J. Hageman, L. K. McDougal, J. Mohammed, W. R. Jarvis, T. M. Perl, F. C. Tenover, and Vancomycin-Intermediate Staphylococcus aureus Epidemiology Study Group.** 2003. Epidemiological and microbiological characterization of infections caused by *Staphylococcus aureus* with reduced susceptibility to vancomycin, United States, 1997–2001. *Clin. Infect. Dis.* **36:**429–439.
64. **Garcia-Garrote, F., E. Cercenado, and E. Bouza.** 2000. Evaluation of a new system, VITEK 2, for identification and antimicrobial susceptibility testing of enterococci. *J. Clin. Microbiol.* **38:**2108–2111.
65. **Gibb, A. P., and M. Crichton.** 2000. Cefpodoxime screening of *Escherichia coli* and *Klebsiella* spp. by Vitek for detection of organisms producing extended-spectrum β-lactamases. *Diagn. Microbiol. Infect. Dis.* **38:**255–257.
66. **Gradelski, E., L. Valera, L. Aleksunes, D. Bonner, and J. Fung-Tomc.** 2001. Correlation between genotype and phenotype categorization of staphylococci based on methicillin susceptibility and resistance. *J. Clin. Microbiol.* **39:** 2961–2963.
67. **Gresser-Burns, M. E., C. J. Shanholtzer, L. R. Peterson, and D. N. Gerding.** 1987. Occurrence and reproducibility of the "skip" phenomenon in bactericidal testing of *Staphylococcus aureus*. *Diagn. Microbiol. Infect. Dis.* **6:** 335–342.
68. **Gunnison, J. B., M. A. Fraher, and E. Jawetz.** 1963. Persistence of *Staphylococcus aureus* in penicillin in vitro. *J. Gen. Microbiol.* **34:**335–349.
69. **Hackbarth, C. J., and H. F. Chambers.** 1989. Methicillin-resistant staphylococci: genetics and mechanisms of resistance. *Antimicrob. Agents Chemother.* **33:**991–994.
70. **Handwerger, S., and A. Tomasz.** 1985. Antibiotic tolerance among clinical isolates of bacteria. *Rev. Infect. Dis.* **7:**368–386.
71. **Hartman, B. J., and A. Tomasz.** 1986. Expression of methicillin resistance in heterogeneous strains of *Staphylococcus aureus*. *Antimicrob. Agents Chemother.* **29:** 85–92.
72. **Hernandez-Alles, S., M. Conejo, A. Pascual, J. M. Tomas, V. J. Benedi, and L. Martinez-Martinez.** 2000. Relationship between outer membrane alterations and susceptibility to antimicrobial agents in isogenic strains of *Klebsiella pneumoniae*. *J. Antimicrob. Chemother.* **46:**273–277.
73. **Hindler, J.** 1997. Antimicrobial susceptibility tests, p. 105–154. *In* H. D. Isenberg (ed.), *Essential Procedures in Clinical Microbiology*. American Society for Microbiology, Washington, D.C.
74. **Hindler, J. A., and C. B. Inderlied.** 1985. Effect of source of Mueller-Hinton agar and resistance frequency on the detection of methicillin-resistant *Staphylococcus aureus*. *J. Clin. Microbiol.* **21:**205–210.
75. **Hindler, J. A., and D. F. Sahm.** 1992. Controversies and confusion regarding antimicrobial susceptibility testing of enterococci. *Antimicrob. Newsl.* **8:**65–74.
76. **Hindler, J. A., and N. L. Warner.** 1984. Effect of source of Mueller-Hinton agar on detection of oxacillin resistance in *Staphylococcus aureus* using a screening methodology. *J. Clin. Microbiol.* **25:**734–735.
77. **Horstkotte, M. A., J. K.-M. Knobloch, H. Rohde, and D. Mack.** 2001. Rapid detection of methicillin resistance in coagulase-negative staphylococci by a penicillin-binding protein 2a-specific latex agglutination test. *J. Clin. Microbiol.* **39:**3700–3702.
78. **Hunter, T. H.** 1950. Speculations on the mechanism of cure of endocarditis. *JAMA* **144:**527.
79. **Hussain, Z., L. Stoakes, S. Garrow, S. Longo, V. Fitzgerald, and R. Lannigan.** 2000. Rapid detection of mecA-positive and mecA-negative coagulase-negative staphylococci by an anti-penicillin binding protein 2a slide latex agglutination test. *J. Clin. Microbiol.* **38:**2051–2054.
80. **Hussain, Z., L. Stoakes, V. Massey, D. Diagre, V. Fitzgerald, S. El Sayed, and R. Lannigan.** 2000. Correlation of oxacillin MIC with *mecA* gene carriage in coagulase-negative staphylococci. *J. Clin. Microbiol.* **38:** 752–754.
81. **Iwen, P. C., D. M. Kelley, J. Linder, and S. H. Hinrichs.** 1996. Revised approach for identification and detection of ampicillin and vancomycin resistance in *Enterococcus* species by using MicroScan panels. *J. Clin. Microbiol.* **34:** 1779–1783.
82. **Jacobs, M. R., H. J. Koornhof, R. M. Robins-Browne, C. M. Stevenson, Z. A. Vermaak, I. Freiman, G. B. Miller, M. A. Witcomb, M. Isaacson, J. I. Ward, and R. Austrian.** 1978. Emergence of multiply resistant pneumococci. *N. Engl. J. Med.* **299:**735–740.
83. **Jacobs, M. R., S. K. Spangler, and P. C. Appelbaum.** 1992. β-Lactamase production and susceptibility of US and European anaerobic gram-negative bacilli to β-lactams and other agents. *Eur. J. Clin. Microbiol. Infect. Dis.* **11:** 1081–1093.
84. **Jacoby, G., P. Han, and J. Tran.** 1997. Comparative in vitro activities of carbapenem L-749,345 and other antimicrobials against multiresistant gram-negative clinical pathogens. *Antimicrob. Agents Chemother.* **41:**1830–1831.
85. **Jacoby, G., A. A. Medeiros, T. F. O'Brien, M. E. Pinto, and J. Jiang.** 1989. Broad-spectrum transmissible β-lactamases. *N. Engl. J. Med.* **319:**723–724.
86. **Jacoby, G. A.** 1998. Epidemiology of extended-spectrum β-lactamases. *Clin. Infect. Dis.* **27:**81–83.
87. **Jacoby, G. A., and P. Han.** 1996. Detection of extended-spectrum β-lactamases in clinical isolates of *Klebsiella pneumoniae* and *Escherichia coli*. *J. Clin. Microbiol.* **34:**908–911.
88. **Jacoby, G. A., and A. A. Medeiros.** 1991. More extended-spectrum β-lactamases. *Antimicrob. Agents Chemother.* **35:**1697–1704.
89. **Jarlier, V., M. H. Nicolas, G. Fournier, and A. Philippon.** 1988. Extended broad-spectrum β-lactamases conferring transferable resistance to newer β-lactam agents in Enterobacteriaceae: hospital prevalence and susceptibility patterns. *Rev. Infect. Dis.* **10:**867–878.
90. **Jett, B., L. Free, and D. F. Sahm.** 1996. Factors influencing the Vitek gram-positive susceptibility system's detection of *vanB*-encoded vancomycin resistance among enterococci. *J. Clin. Microbiol.* **34:**701–706.
91. **Jones, R. N.** 2001. Resistance patterns among nosocomial pathogens: trends over the past few years. *Chest* **119:** 397S–404S.
92. **Jones, R. N., D. C. Edson, and CAP Microbiology Resource Committee of the College of American Pathologists.** 1991. Antimicrobial susceptibility testing trends and accuracy in the United States. *Arch. Pathol. Lab. Med.* **115:**429–436.
93. **Jordan, G. W., and M. M. Kawachi.** 1981. Analysis of serum bactericidal activity in endocarditis, osteomyelitis, and other bacterial infections. *Medicine* **60:**49–61.
94. **Jorgensen, J. H., S. A. Crawford, M. L. McElmeel, and K. R. Feibelkorn.** 2004. Detection of inducible clindamycin resistance of staphylococci in correlation with performance of automated broth susceptibility testing. *J. Clin. Microbiol.* **42:**1800–1802.
95. **Jorgensen, J. H., L. A. Maher, and J. S. Redding.** 1987. In vitro activity of LY146032 (daptomycin) against selected aerobic bacteria. *Eur. J. Clin. Microbiol.* **6:**91–96.
96. **Katsanis, G. P., J. Spargo, M. J. Ferraro, L. Sutton, and G. A. Jacoby.** 1994. Detection of *Klebsiella pneumoniae* and *Escherichia coli* strains producing extended-spectrum β-lactamases. *J. Clin. Microbiol.* **32:**691–696.

97. **Kiehn, T. E., P. D. Ellner, and D. Budzko.** 1989. Role of the microbiology laboratory in care of the immunosuppressed patient. *Rev. Infect. Dis.* **11**(Suppl. 7): S1706–S1710.
98. **Kim, K. S., and B. F. Anthony.** 1981. Importance of bacterial growth phase in determining minimum bactericidal concentrations of penicillin and methicillin. *Antimicrob. Agents Chemother.* **19:**1075–1077.
99. **King, T. C., D. Schlessinger, and D. J. Krogstad.** 1981. The assessment of antimicrobial combinations. *J. Infect. Dis.* **129:**193.
100. **Klastersky, J., D. Daneau, G. Swings, and D. Weerts.** 1974. Antibacterial activity in serum and urine as a therapeutic guide in bacterial infections. *J. Infect. Dis.* **129:** 187–193.
101. **Knapp, C., and J. A. Moody.** 1992. Tests to assess bactericidal activity, p. 5.16.1–5.16.33. *In* H. D. Isenberg (ed.), *Clinical Microbiology Procedures Handbook.* American Society for Microbiology, Washington, D.C.
102. **Knapp, C. C., M. D. Ludwig, J. A. Washington, and H. F. Chambers.** 1996. Evaluation of Vitek GPS-SA card for testing of oxacillin against borderline-susceptible staphylococci that lack *mec. J. Clin. Microbiol.* **34:** 1603–1605.
103. **Krcmery, V., Jr., J. Trupl, L. Drgona, J. Lacka, E. Kukuckova, and E. Oravcova.** 1996. Nosocomial bacteremia due to vancomycin-resistant *Staphylococcus epidermidis* in four patients with cancer, neutropenia, and previous treatment with vancomycin. *Eur. J. Clin. Microbiol. Infect. Dis.* **15:**259–261.
104. **Krogstad, D. J., and R. C. Moellering, Jr.** 1998. Antimicrobial combinations, p. 537–599. *In* V. Lorian (ed.), *Antibiotics in Laboratory Medicine.* Williams and Wilkins, Baltimore, Md.
105. **Lautenbach, E., J. B. Patel, W. B. Bilker, P. H. Edelstein, and N. O. Fishman.** 2001. Extended-spectrum β-lactamase-producing *Escherichia coli* and *Klebsiella pneumoniae:* risk factors for infection and impact of resistance on outcomes. *Clin. Infect. Dis.* **32:**1162–1171.
106. **Leclercq, R.** 2002. Mechanisms of resistance to macrolides and lincosamides: nature of the resistance elements and their clinical implications. *Clin. Infect. Dis.* **34:**482–492.
107. **Leclercq, R., and P. Courvalin.** 1997. Resistance to glycopeptides in enterococci. *Clin. Infect. Dis.* **24:**545–556.
108. **Leclercq, R., S. Dutka-Malen, J. Duval, and P. Courvalin.** 1992. Vancomycin resistance gene *vanC* is specific to *Enterococcus gallinarum. Antimicrob. Agents Chemother.* **36:** 2005–2008.
109. **Leggett, J. E., S. A. Wolz, and W. A. Craig.** 1989. Use of serum ultrafiltrate in the serum dilution test. *J. Infect. Dis.* **160:**616–623.
110. **Leitch, C., and S. Boonlayangoor.** 1992. β-Lactamase tests, p. 5.3.1–5.3.8. *In* H. D. Isenberg (ed.), *Clinical Microbiology Procedures Handbook.* American Society for Microbiology, Washington, D.C.
111. **Lemmen, S. W., S. Zolldann, S. Klik, R. Lutticken, K. Kummerer, and H. Haffner.** 2004. Serum bactericidal activity of piperacillin-tazobactam against *Staphylococcus aureus,* piperacillin-susceptible and piperacillin-resistant *Escherichia coli* and *Pseudomonas aeruginosa. Chemotherapy* **50:**27–30.
112. **Lewis, J. S., II, and J. H. Jorgensen.** 2005. Inducible clindamycin resistance in staphylococci: should clinicians and microbiologists be concerned? *Clin. Infect. Dis.* **40:**280–285.
113. **Livermore, D. M.** 1995. β-Lactamases in laboratory and clinical resistance. *Clin. Microbiol. Rev.* **8:**557–584.
114. **Livermore, D. M., and M. Yuan.** 1996. Antibiotic resistance and production of extended-spectrum β-lactamases amongst *Klebsiella* spp. from intensive care units in Europe. *J. Antimicrob. Chemother.* **38:**409–424.
115. **Louie, L., A. Majury, J. Goodfellow, M. Louie, and A. E. Simor.** 2001. Evaluation of a latex agglutination test (MRSA-Screen) for detection of oxacillin resistance in coagulase-negative staphylococci. *J. Clin. Microbiol.* **39:**4149–4151.
116. **Louie, L., S. O. Matsumura, E. Choi, M. Louie, and A. E. Simor.** 2000. Evaluation of three rapid methods for detection of methicillin resistance in *Staphylococcus aureus. J. Clin. Microbiol.* **38:**2170–2173.
117. **MacGowan, A., C. McMullin, P. James, K. Bowker, D. Reeves, and L. White.** 1997. External quality assessment of the serum bactericidal test: results of a methodology/interpretation questionnaire. *J. Antimicrob. Chemother.* **39:** 277–284.
118. **MacLowry, J. D.** 1989. Perspective. The serum dilution test. *J. Infect. Dis.* **160:**624–626.
119. **Marlowe, E. M., A. Linscott, J. M. Kanatani, and D. A. Bruckner.** 2002. Practical therapeutic applications of the Oxoid PBP2' latex agglutination test for the rapid identification of methicillin-resistant *Staphylococcus aureus* in blood cultures. *Am. J. Clin. Pathol.* **118:**287–291.
120. **Massanari, R. M., M. A. Pfaller, D. S. Wakesfield, G. T. Hammons, L. A. McNut, R. F. Woolson, and C. M. Helms.** 1988. Implications of acquired oxacillin resistance in management and control of *Staphylococcus aureus* infections. *J. Infect. Dis.* **158:**701–709.
121. **Mateo, M., J. R. Maestre, L. Aguilar, F. Cafini, P. Puente, P. Sanchez, L. Alou, M. J. Gimenez, and J. Prieto.** 2005. Genotypic versus phenotypic characterization, with respect to susceptibility and identification, of 17 clinical isolates of *Staphylococcus lugdunensis. J. Antimicrob. Chemother.* **56:**287–291.
122. **McKessar, S., A. Berry, J. Bell, J. Turnidge, and J. C. Paton.** 2001. Genetic characterization of vanG, a novel vancomycin resistance locus in *Enterococcus faecalis. Antimicrob. Agents Chemother.* **44:**3224–3228.
123. **McKinney, T. K., V. K. Sharma, W. A. Craig, and G. L. Archer.** 2001. Transcription of the gene mediating methicillin resistance in *Staphylococcus aureus (mecA)* is corepressed but not coinduced by cognate *mecA* and beta-lactamase regulators. *J. Bacteriol.* **183:**6862–6868.
124. **Meyer, K. S., C. Urban, J. A. Eagan, B. J. Berger, and J. J. Rahal.** 1993. Nosocomial outbreak of *Klebsiella* infection resistant to late-generation cephalosporins. *Ann. Intern. Med.* **119:**353–358.
125. **Moellering, R. C., Jr., O. M. Koraeniowski, M. A. Sande, and C. B. Wennersten.** 1979. Species-specific resistance to antimicrobial synergism in *Streptococcus faecium* and *Streptococcus faecalis. J. Infect. Dis.* **140:** 203–208.
126. **Moland, E. S., C. C. Sanders, and K. S. Thomson.** 1998. Can results obtained with commercially available MicroScan microdilution panels serve as an indicator of β-lactamase production among *Escherichia coli* and *Klebsiella* isolates with hidden resistance to expanded-spectrum cephalosporins and aztreonam? *J. Clin. Microbiol.* **36:**2575–2579.
127. **Montanari, M. P., O. Massidda, M. Mingoia, and P. E. Varalco.** 1996. Borderline susceptibility to methicillin in *Staphylococcus aureus:* a new mechanism of resistance? *Microb. Drug Resist.* **2:**257–260.
128. **Montanari, M. P., M. Mingoia, I. Cochetti, and P. E. Varaldo.** 2003. Phenotypes and genotypes of erythromycin-resistant pneumococci in Italy. *J. Clin. Microbiol.* **41:** 428–431.
129. **Murray, B. E.** 1990. The life and times of the enterococcus. *Clin. Microbiol. Rev.* **3:**46–65.

130. **Musher, D. M., and R. Fletcher.** 1982. Tolerant *Staphylococcus aureus* causing vertebral osteomyelitis. *Ann. Intern. Med.* **93:**796–800.
131. **M'Zali, F. H., J. Heritage, D. M. Gascoyne-Binzi, M. Denton, N. J. Todd, and P. M. Hawkey.** 1997. Transcontinental importation into the UK of *Escherichia coli* expressing a plasmid-mediated AmpC-type β-lactamase exposed during an outbreak of SHV-5 extended-spectrum β-lactamase in a Leeds hospital. *J. Antimicrob. Chemother.* **40:**823–831.
132. **Nadjar, D., M. Rouveau, C. Verdet, J. L. Donay, J. L. Herrmann, P. H. Lagrange, A. Philippon, and G. Arlet.** 2000. Outbreak of *Klebsiella pneumoniae* producing transferable AmpC-type β-lactamase (ACC-1) originating from *Hafnia alvei*. *FEMS Microbiol. Lett.* **187:**35–40.
133. **Nasim, K., S. Elsayed, J. D. D. Pitout, J. Conly, D. L. Church, and D. B. Gregson.** 2004. New method for laboratory detection of AmpC β-lactamases in *Escherichia coli* and *Klebsiella pneumoniae*. *J. Clin. Microbiol.* **42:** 4799–4802.
134. **Neumann, M. A., D. F. Sahm, C. Thornsberry, and J. E. McGowan, Jr.** 1991. *Cumitech 6A, New Developments in Antimicrobial Agent Susceptibility Testing: a Practical Guide*. American Society for Microbiology, Washington, D.C.
135. **O'Callaghan, C. H., A. Morris, S. M. Kirby, and A. H. Shingler.** 1972. Novel method for detection of β-lactamases by using a chromogenic cephalosporin substrate. *Antimicrob. Agents Chemother.* **1:**283–288.
136. **Okabe, T., K. Oana, Y. Kawakami, M. Yamaguchi, Y. Takahashi, Y. Okimura, T. Honda, and T. Katsuyama.** 2000. Limitations of Vitek GPS-418 cards in exact detection of vancomycin-resistant enterococci with the *vanB* genotype. *J. Clin. Microbiol.* **38:**2409–2411.
137. **Ostrowsky, B., N. C. Clark, C. Thauvin-Eliopoulos, L. Venkataraman, M. Samore, F. C. Tenover, G. M. Eliopoulos, R. C. Moellering, Jr., and H. S. Gold.** 1999. A cluster of VanD vancomycin-resistant *Enterococcus faecium:* molecular characterization and epidemiology. *J. Infect. Dis.* **180:**1177–1185.
138. **Palavecino, E.** 2004. Community-acquired methicillin-resistant *Staphylococcus aureus* infections. *Clin. Lab. Med.* **24:**403–418.
139. **Paterson, D. L.** 2000. Recommendation for treatment of severe infections caused by Enterobacteriaceae producing extended-spectrum β-lactamases (ESBLs). *Clin. Microbiol. Infect.* **6:**460–463.
140. **Paterson, D. L., W. C. Ko, A. Von Gottberg, J. M. Casellas, L. Mulazimoglu, K. P. Klugman, R. A. Bonomo, L. B. Rice, J. G. McCormack, and V. L. Yu.** 2001. Outcome of cephalosporin treatment for serious infections due to apparently susceptible organisms producing extended-spectrum β-lactamases: implications for the clinical microbiology laboratory. *J. Clin. Microbiol.* **39:** 2206–2212.
141. **Paterson, D. L., N. Singh, J. D. Rihs, C. Squier, B. L. Rihs, and R. R. Muder.** 2001. Control of an outbreak of infection due to extended-spectrum β-lactamase-producing *Escherichia coli* in a liver transplantation unit. *Clin. Infect. Dis.* **33:**126–128.
142. **Patterson, J. E.** 2000. Extended-spectrum β-lactamases. *Semin. Respir. Infect.* **15:**299–307.
143. **Pefanis, A., C. Thauvin-Eliopoulos, G. Eliopoulos, and R. C. Moellering, Jr.** 1993. Activity of ampicillin-sulbactam and oxacillin in experimental endocarditis caused by β-lactamase-hyperproducing *Staphylococcus aureus*. *Antimicrob. Agents Chemother.* **37:**507–511.
144. **Perichon, B., P. Reynolds, and P. Courvalin.** 1997. VanD-type glycopeptide-resistant *Enterococcus faecium* BM4339. *Antimicrob. Agents Chemother.* **41:**2016–2018.
145. **Peterson, L. R., and C. J. Shanholtzer.** 1992. Tests for bactericidal effects of antimicrobial agents: technical performance and clinical relevance. *Clin. Microbiol. Rev.* **5:**420–432.
146. **Philippon, A., G. Arlet, and G. A. Jacoby.** 2002. Plasmid-determined AmpC-type β-lactamases. *Antimicrob. Agents Chemother.* **46:**1–11.
147. **Philippon, A., R. Labia, and G. Jacoby.** 1989. Extended-spectrum β-lactamases. *Antimicrob. Agents Chemother.* **33:**1131–1136.
148. **Quinn, J. P.** 1994. Clinical significance of extended-spectrum β-lactamases. *Eur. J. Clin. Microbiol. Infect. Dis.* **13:**39–42.
149. **Ramotar, K., W. Woods, L. Larocque, and B. Toye.** 2000. Comparison of phenotype methods to identify enterococci intrinsically resistant to vancomycin (vanC VRE). *Diagn. Microbiol. Infect. Dis.* **36:**119–124.
150. **Ramotar, K., W. Woods, and B. Toye.** 2001. Oxacillin susceptibility testing of *Staphylococcus saprophyticus* using disk diffusion, agar dilution, broth microdilution, and the Vitek GPS-105 card. *Diagn. Microbiol. Infect. Dis.* **40:** 203–205.
151. **Raney, P. M., F. C. Tenover, R. B. Carey, J. E. McGowan, Jr., and J. B. Patel.** Investigation of inducible clindamycin and telithromycin resistance in isolates of β-hemolytic streptococci. *Diagn. Microbiol. Infect. Dis.*, in press.
152. **Reller, L. B.** 1986. The serum bactericidal test. *Rev. Infect. Dis.* **8:**803–808.
153. **Resende, C. A., and A. M. Figueiredo.** 1997. Discrimination of methicillin-resistant *Staphylococcus aureus* from borderline-resistant and susceptible isolates by different methods. *J. Med. Microbiol.* **46:**145–149.
154. **Roghmann, M.** 2000. Predicting methicillin resistance and the effect of inadequate empiric therapy on survival in patients with *Staphylococcus aureus* bacteremia. *Ann. Intern. Med.* **160:**1001–1004.
155. **Rosenblatt, J. E.** 1987. Laboratory tests used to guide antimicrobial therapy. *Mayo Clin. Proc.* **62:**799–805.
156. **Sabath, L.** 1977. Chemical and physical factors influencing methicillin resistance of *Staphylococcus aureus* and *Staphylococcus epidermidis*. *J. Antimicrob. Chemother.* **3:** 47–51.
157. **Sahm, D. F., S. Boonlayangoor, P. C. Iwen, J. L. Baade, and G. L. Woods.** 1991. Factors influencing determination of high-level aminoglycoside resistance in *Enterococcus faecalis*. *J. Clin. Microbiol.* **29:**1934–1939.
158. **Sahm, D. F., S. Boonlayangoor, and J. E. Schulz.** 1991. Detection of high-level aminoglycoside resistance in enterococci other than *Enterococcus faecalis*. *J. Clin. Microbiol.* **29:**2595–2598.
159. **Sahm, D. F., J. Kissinger, M. S. Gilmore, P. R. Murray, R. Mulder, J. Solliday, and B. Clarke.** 1989. In vitro susceptibility studies of vancomycin-resistant *Enterococcus faecalis*. *Antimicrob. Agents Chemother.* **33:**1588–1591.
160. **Sahm, D. F., and L. Olsen.** 1990. In vitro detection of enterococcal vancomycin resistance. *Antimicrob. Agents Chemother.* **34:**1846–1848.
161. **Sahm, D. F., and C. Torres.** 1988. Effects of medium and inoculum variations on screening for high-level aminoglycoside resistance in *Enterococcus faecalis*. *J. Clin. Microbiol.* **26:**250–256.
162. **Sahm, D. F., and C. Torres.** 1988. High-content aminoglycoside disks for determining aminoglycoside-penicillin synergy against *Enterococcus faecalis*. *J. Clin. Microbiol.* **26:**257–260.
163. **Sakoulas, G., P. DeGirolami, and H. S. Gold.** 2001. Methicillin-susceptible *Staphylococcus aureus*: believe it, or not. *Ann. Intern. Med.* **161:**1237–1238.

164. **Sakoulas, G., H. S. Gold, L. Venkataraman, P. DeGirolami, G. M. Eliopoulos, and Q. Qian.** 2001. Methicillin-resistant *Staphylococcus aureus:* comparison of susceptibility testing methods and analysis of *mecA*-positive susceptible strains. *J. Clin. Microbiol.* **39:** 3946–3951.

165. **Sanyal, D., A. P. Johnson, R. C. George, B. D. Cookson, and A. J. Williams.** 1991. Peritonitis due to vancomycin-resistant *Staphylococcus epidermidis*. *Lancet* **337:**54.

166. **Scheld, W. M., and M. A. Sande.** 1983. Bactericidal versus bacteriostatic antibiotic therapy of experimental pneumococcal meningitis in rabbits. *J. Clin. Investig.* **71:** 411–419.

167. **Schlichter, J. G., and H. MacLean.** 1947. A method for determining the effective therapeutic level in the treatment of subacute bacterial endocarditis with penicillin: a preliminary report. *Am. Heart J.* **34:**209–211.

168. **Schlichter, J. G., H. MacLean, and A. Milzer.** 1949. Effective penicillin therapy in subacute bacterial endocarditis and other chronic infections. *Am. J. Med. Sci.* **217:**600–608.

169. **Schwalbe, R. S., J. T. Stapleton, and P. H. Gilligan.** 1987. Emergence of vancomycin resistance in coagulase-negative staphylococci. *N. Engl. J. Med.* **316:**927–931.

170. **Sculier, J. P., and J. Klastersky.** 1984. Significance of serum bactericidal activity in gram-negative bacillary bacteremia in patients with and without granulocytopenia. *Am. J. Med.* **76:**429–435.

171. **Shehabi, A. A., A. Mahafzah, I. Baadran, F. A. Qadar, and N. Dajani.** 2000. High incidence of *Klebsiella pneumoniae* clinical isolates to extended-spectrum *β*-lactam drugs in intensive care units. *Diagn. Microbiol. Infect. Dis.* **36:** 53–56.

172. **Sirot, D.** 1995. Extended-spectrum plasmid-mediated *β*-lactamases. *J. Antimicrob. Chemother.* **36:**19–34.

173. **Siu, L. K., P. L. Lu, P. R. Hsueh, F. M. Lin, S. C. Chang, K. T. Luh, M. Ho, and C. Y. Lee.** 1999. Bacteremia due to extended-spectrum *β*-lactamase-producing *Escherichia coli* and *Klebsiella pneumoniae* in a pediatric oncology ward: clinical features and identification of different plasmids carrying both SHV-5 and TEM-1 genes. *J. Clin. Microbiol.* **37:**4020–4027.

174. **Srinivasan, A., J. D. Dick, and T. M. Perl.** 2002. Vancomycin resistance in staphylococci. *Clin. Microbiol. Rev.* **15:**430–438.

175. **Standiford, H. D., J. B. deMaine, and W. M. Kirby.** 1970. Antibiotic synergism of enterococci. *Arch. Intern. Med.* **126:**255–259.

176. **Stapleton, P. D., K. P. Shannon, and G. L. French.** 1999. Carbapenem resistance in *Escherichia coli* associated with plasmid-determined CMY-4 *β*-lactamase production and loss of an outer membrane protein. *Antimicrob. Agents Chemother.* **43:**1206–1210.

177. **Stefaniuk, E., A. Baraniak, M. Gniadkowski, and K. Hryniewicz.** 2003. Evaluation of the BD Phoenix automated identification and susceptibility testing system in clinical microbiology laboratory practice. *Eur. J. Clin. Microbiol. Infect. Dis.* **22:**479–485.

178. **Stein, G. E., S. Schooley, and G. W. Kaatz.** 2003. Serum bactericidal activity of the methoxyfluoroquinolones gatifloxacin and moxifloxacin against clinical isolates of *Staphylococcus* species: are the susceptibility breakpoints too high? *Clin. Infect. Dis.* **37:**1392–1395.

179. **Steward, C. D., P. M. Raney, A. K. Morrell, P. P. Williams, L. K. McDougal, L. Jevitt, J. E. McGowan, Jr., and F. C. Tenover.** 2005. Testing for inducible clindamycin resistance in erythromycin-resistant isolates of *Staphylococcus aureus*. *J. Clin. Microbiol.* **43:**1716–1721.

180. **Steward, C. D., J. K. Rasheed, S. K. Hubert, J. W. Biddle, P. Raney, G. J. Anderson, P. P. Williams, K. L. Brittain, A. Oliver, J. E. McGowan, Jr., and F. C. Tenover.** 2001. Characterization of clinical isolates of *Klebsiella pneumoniae* from 19 laboratories using the National Committee for Clinical Laboratory Standards extended-spectrum *β*-lactamase detection methods. *J. Clin. Microbiol.* **39:**2864–2872.

181. **Swenson, J. M., N. Clark, M. J. Ferraro, D. F. Sahm, G. Doern, M. A. Pfaller, L. B. Reller, M. P. Weinstein, R. J. Zabransky, and F. C. Tenover.** 1994. Development of a standardized screening method for detection of vancomycin-resistant enterococci. *J. Clin. Microbiol.* **32:**1700–1704.

182. **Swenson, J. M., N. C. Clark, D. F. Sahm, M. J. Ferraro, G. Doern, J. Hindler, J. H. Jorgensen, M. A. Pfaller, L. B. Reller, M. P. Weinstein, R. J. Zabransky, and F. C. Tenover.** 1995. Molecular characterization and multilaboratory evaluation of *Enterococcus faecalis* ATCC 51299 and quality control of screening tests for vancomycin and high-level aminoglycoside resistance in enterococci. *J. Clin. Microbiol.* **33:**3019–3021.

183. **Swenson, J. M., M. J. Ferraro, D. Sahm, N. C. Clark, D. Culver, F. C. Tenover, and the National Committee for Clinical Laboratory Standards Study Group on Enterococci.** 1995. Multilaboratory evaluation of screening methods for detection of high-level aminoglycoside resistance in enterococci. *J. Clin. Microbiol.* **33:**3008–3018.

184. **Swenson, J. M., B. C. Hill, and C. Thornsberry.** 1986. Screening pneumococci for penicillin resistance. *J. Clin. Microbiol.* **24:**749–752.

185. **Swenson, J. M., B. C. Hill, and C. Thornsberry.** 1989. Problems with the disk diffusion test for detection of vancomycin resistance in enterococci. *J. Clin. Microbiol.* **27:** 2140–2142. (Erratum, **28:**403, 1990.)

186. **Swenson, J. M., J. Spargo, F. C. Tenover, and M. J. Ferraro.** 2001. Optimal inoculation methods and quality control for the NCCLS oxacillin agar screen test for detection of oxacillin resistance in *Staphylococcus aureus*. *J. Clin. Microbiol.* **39:**3781–3784.

187. **Swenson, J. M., F. C. Tenover, and the Cefoxitin Disk Study Group.** 2005. Results of disk diffusion testing with cefoxitin correlate with presence of *mecA* in *Staphylococcus* spp. *J. Clin. Microbiol.* **43:**3818–3823.

188. **Swenson, J. M., P. P. Williams, G. Killgore, C. M. O'Hara, and F. C. Tenover.** 2001. Performance of eight methods, including two new rapid methods, for detection of oxacillin resistance in a challenge set of *Staphylococcus aureus* organisms. *J. Clin. Microbiol.* **39:**3785–3788.

189. **Taylor, P. C., F. D. Schoenknecht, J. C. Sherris, and E. C. Linner.** 1983. Determination of minimum bactericidal concentrations of oxacillin for *Staphylococcus aureus:* influence and significance of technical factors. *Antimicrob. Agents Chemother.* **23:**142–150.

190. **Tenover, F. C., R. N. Jones, J. M. Swenson, B. Zimmer, S. McAllister, and J. H. Jorgensen.** 1999. Methods for improved detection of oxacillin resistance in coagulase-negative staphylococci: results of a multicenter study. *J. Clin. Microbiol.* **37:**4051–4058.

191. **Tenover, F. C., M. V. Lancaster, B. C. Hill, C. D. Steward, S. A. Stocker, G. A. Hancock, C. M. O'Hara, N. C. Clark, and K. Hiramatsu.** 1998. Characterization of staphylococci with reduced susceptibility to vancomycin and other glycopeptides. *J. Clin. Microbiol.* **36:**1020–1027.

192. **Tenover, F. C., M. J. Mohammed, T. S. Gorton, and Z. F. Dembek.** 1999. Detection and reporting of organisms producing extended-spectrum *β*-lactamases: survey of laboratories in Connecticut. *J. Clin. Microbiol.* **37:** 4065–4070.

193. **Tenover, F. C., J. M. Swenson, C. M. O'Hara, and S. A. Stocker.** 1995. Ability of commercial and reference antimicrobial susceptibility testing methods to detect vancomycin resistance in enterococci. *J. Clin. Microbiol.* **33:**1524–1527.
194. **Thauvin-Eliopoulos, E., L. B. Rice, G. M. Eliopoulos, and R. C. Moellering, Jr.** 1990. Efficacy of oxacillin and ampicillin-sulbactam combination in experimental endocarditis caused by β-lactamase-hyperproducing *Staphylococcus aureus*. *Antimicrob. Agents Chemother.* **34:**728–732.
195. **Thomson, K. S.** 2001. Controversies about extended-spectrum and AmpC β-lactamases. *Emerg. Infect. Dis.* **7:**333–336.
196. **Thomson, K. S., and E. Smith Moland.** 2000. Version 2000: the new β-lactamases of gram-negative bacteria at the dawn of the new millennium. *Microbes Infect.* **2:**1225–1235.
197. **Tomasz, A., H. B. Drugeon, H. M. de Lencastre, D. Jabes, L. McDougal, and J. Bille.** 1989. New mechanism for methicillin resistance in *Staphylococcus aureus:* clinical isolates that lack the PBP 2a gene and contain modified penicillin-binding proteins with modified penicillin-binding capacity. *Antimicrob. Agents Chemother.* **33:** 1869–1874.
198. **Tomasz, A., S. Nachman, and H. Leaf.** 1991. Stable classes of phenotypic expression in methicillin-resistant clinical isolates of staphylococci. *Antimicrob. Agents Chemother.* **35:**124–129.
199. **Tsai, S., M. J. Zervos, D. B. Clewell, S. Donabedian, D. F. Sahm, and J. W. Chow.** 1998. A new high-level gentamicin resistance gene, aph(2")-Id, in *Enterococcus* spp. *Antimicrob. Agents Chemother.* **42:**1229–1232.
200. **Tuomanen, E., D. T. Durack, and A. Tomasz.** 1986. Antibiotic tolerance among clinical isolates of bacteria. *Antimicrob. Agents Chemother.* **30:**521–527.
201. **Uh, Y., D. H. Shin, I. H. Jang, G. Y. Hwang, M. K. Lee, K. J. Yoon, and H. Y. Kim.** 2004. Antimicrobial susceptibility patterns and macrolide resistance genes of viridans group streptococci from blood cultures in Korea. *J. Antimicrob. Chemother.* **53:**1095–1097.
202. **van den Braak, N., W. Goessens, A. van Belkum, H. Verbrugh, and H. Endtz.** 2001. Accuracy of the VITEK 2 system to detect glycopeptide resistance in enterococci. *J. Clin. Microbiol.* **39:**351–353.
203. **van Griethuysen, A., M. Pouw, N. van Leeuwen, M. Heck, P. Willemse, A. Buiting, and J. Kluytmans.** 1999. Rapid slide latex agglutination test for detection of methicillin resistance in *Staphylococcus aureus*. *J. Clin. Microbiol.* **37:**2789–2792.
204. **Van Horn, K. G., C. A. Gedris, K. M. Rodney, and J. B. Mitchell.** 1996. Evaluation of commercial vancomycin agar screen plates for detection of vancomycin-resistant enterococci. *J. Clin. Microbiol.* **34:**2042–2044.
205. **van Leeuwen, W. B., C. van Pelt, A. Luijendijk, H. A. Verbrugh, and W. H. F. Goessens.** 1999. Rapid detection of methicillin resistance in *Staphylococcus aureus* isolates by the MRSA-Screen latex agglutination test. *J. Clin. Microbiol.* **37:**3029–3030.
206. **Veach, L. A., M. A. Pfaller, M. Barrett, F. P. Koontz, and R. P. Wenzel.** 1990. Vancomycin resistance in *Staphylococcus haemolyticus* causing colonization and bloodstream infection. *J. Clin. Microbiol.* **28:**2064–2068.
207. **Velasco, D., M. del Mar Tomas, M. Cartelle, A. Becceiro, A. Perez, F. Molina, R. Moure, R. Villanueva, and G. Bou.** 2005. Evaluation of different methods for detecting methicillin (oxacillin) resistance in *Staphylococcus aureus*. *J. Antimicrob. Chemother.* **55:**379–382.
208. **Weinstein, M. P., C. W. Stratton, A. Ackley, H. B. Hawley, P. A. Robinson, B. D. Fisher, D. V. Alcid, D. S. Stevens, and L. B. Reller.** 1985. Multicenter collaborative evaluation of a standardized bactericidal test as a prognostic indicator in infective endocarditis. *Am. J. Med.* **78:**262–269.
209. **Weinstein, M. P., C. W. Stratton, H. B. Hawley, A. Ackley, and L. B. Reller.** 1987. Multicenter collaborative evaluation of a standardized serum bactericidal test as a predictor of therapeutic efficacy in acute and chronic osteomyelitis. *Am. J. Med.* **83:**218–222.
210. **Wiener, J., J. P. Quinn, P. A. Bradford, R. V. Goering, C. Nathan, K. Bush, and R. A. Weinstein.** 1999. Multiple antibiotic-resistant *Klebsiella* and *Escherichia coli* in nursing homes. *JAMA* **281:**517–523.
211. **Willey, B. M., B. N. Kreiswirth, A. E. Simor, G. Williams, S. R. Scriver, A. Phillips, and D. E. Low.** 1992. Detection of vancomycin resistance in *Enterococcus* species. *J. Clin. Microbiol.* **30:**1621–1624.
212. **Winokur, P. L., R. Canton, J. M. Casellas, and N. Legakis.** 2001. Variations in the prevalence of strains expressing an extended-spectrum β-lactamase phenotype and characterization of isolates from Europe, the Americas, and the Western Pacific region. *Clin. Infect. Dis.* **32:**94–103.
213. **Yamazumi, T., I. Furuta, D. Diekema, M. A. Pfaller, and R. N. Jones.** 2001. Comparison of the Vitek gram-positive susceptibility 106 card, the MRSA-Screen latex agglutination test, and *mecA* analysis for detecting oxacillin resistance in a geographically diverse collection of clinical isolates of coagulase-negative staphylococci. *J. Clin. Microbiol.* **39:**3623–3626.
214. **Yamazumi, T., S. A. Marshall, W. W. Wilke, D. J. Diekema, M. A. Pfaller, and R. N. Jones.** 2001. Comparison of the Vitek gram-positive susceptibility 106 card and the MRSA-Screen latex agglutination test for determining oxacillin resistance in clinical bloodstream isolates of *Staphylococcus aureus*. *J. Clin. Microbiol.* **39:**53–56.
215. **Zelazny, A. M., M. J. Ferraro, A. Glennen, J. F. Hindler, L. M. Mann, S. Munro, P. R. Murray, L. B. Reller, F. C. Tenover, and J. H. Jorgensen.** 2005. Selection of strains for quality assessment of the disk induction method for detection of inducible clindamycin resistance in staphylococci: a CLSI collaborative study. *J. Clin. Microbiol.* **43:**2613–2615.
216. **Zetola, N., J. S. Francis, E. L. Nuermberger, and W. R. Bishai.** 2005. Community-acquired meticillin-resistant *Staphylococcus aureus:* an emerging threat. *Lancet Infect. Dis.* **5:**275–286.

Susceptibility Test Methods: Fastidious Bacteria*

JANET FICK HINDLER AND JEAN B. PATEL

75

Most fastidious bacteria do not grow satisfactorily in standard in vitro susceptibility test systems that use unsupplemented media. For certain fastidious species that are more frequently encountered, such as *Haemophilus influenzae, Neisseria gonorrhoeae, Streptococcus pneumoniae, Neisseria meningitidis,* and other *Streptococcus* spp., slight modifications have been made to standard Clinical and Laboratory Standards Institute (CLSI), formerly NCCLS, disk diffusion and MIC methods to allow reliable testing of these bacteria. The modifications generally involve the use of a test medium with added nutrients and sometimes extended incubation times and/or incubation in an atmosphere with increased levels of CO_2 (Table 1). Specific zone diameter and MIC interpretive criteria have been developed by CLSI for these bacteria, as have acceptable ranges for recommended quality control (QC) strains. CLSI also describes a standard MIC method for testing *Helicobacter pylori* by using an agar dilution procedure. Standard MIC methods for testing potential agents of bioterrorism to include *Bacillus anthracis, Yersinia pestis, Burkholderia mallei, Burkholderia pseudomallei, Francisella tularensis,* and *Brucella* spp. have been developed, and conditions for testing these are listed in Table 2 (41). Most recently, CLSI has published a proposed guideline for testing infrequently isolated or fastidious bacteria including *Abiotrophia* spp., *Granulicatella* spp., *Aeromonas* spp., *Plesiomonas* spp., *Bacillus* spp. (not *B. anthracis*), *Campylobacter jejuni/coli, Corynebacterium* spp., *Erysipelothrix rhusiopathiae,* the HACEK group, *Lactobacillus* spp., *Leuconostoc* spp., *Listeria monocytogenes, Moraxella catarrhalis, Pasteurella* spp., *Pediococcus* spp., *Vibrio* spp., (not *V. cholerae*) (38). Interpretive criteria for these organisms were primarily adapted from those for organisms included in CLSI standards (41), taking into consideration information in the literature and the experiences of authors of the guideline. This is in contrast to the extensive microbiological, clinical, and pharmacodynamic databases normally used for development of interpretive criteria that appear in CLSI standards. The classification of M45 as a guideline rather than a standard was based on this fact. A summary of the testing conditions for these organisms appears in Table 3.

*This chapter contains information presented in chapter 71 by Janet Fick Hindler and Jana M. Swenson in the eighth edition of this Manual.

There are no specific recommendations for other fastidious bacteria such as *Bordetella* spp. and *Legionella* spp. This is because in part (i) infections caused by these bacteria usually respond to drugs of choice, (ii) isolates are infrequently encountered, and (iii) isolates are often difficult to grow and special media are required.

In addition to conventional MIC test methods (e.g., agar dilution or broth dilution methods), the E-test MIC determination method (AB Biodisk, Solna, Sweden) has been used to test many types of fastidious bacteria. The E-test approach allows placement of strips on special media and the use of various incubation conditions. The limitations of this method include its cost and lack of clearance by the U.S. Food and Drug Administration (FDA) for testing many less commonly encountered fastidious bacteria. Prior to use of the E test for clinical testing in the United States, the FDA clearance status for the particular organism-antimicrobial agent combination should be known. If FDA clearance has not been granted, the results should be interpreted with caution and should be qualified on the patient report.

This chapter summarizes the standard methods recommended by CLSI for antimicrobial susceptibility testing of *Streptococcus* spp. (including *S. pneumoniae*), *H. influenzae, N. gonorrhoeae, N. meningitidis,* and *H. pylori.* The standards for testing potential agents of bioterrorism are also discussed. Methods for testing the infrequently isolated or fastidious bacteria included in the new CLSI M45 guideline are summarized. The incidence of resistance, test methods, and indications for testing and the reporting of results are provided.

S. PNEUMONIAE

Incidence of Resistance

Since it was first reported in 1967, penicillin resistance in pneumococci has been steadily increasing worldwide (15, 62, 63, 114, 216). Interpretive criteria for penicillin and *S. pneumoniae* were originally developed for isolates associated with meningitis and are defined by the CLSI as follows: susceptible, ≤0.06 μg/ml; intermediate, 0.12 to 1 μg/ml; and resistant, ≥2 μg/ml (41). Infections outside the central nervous system, such as pulmonary infections, due to strains for which penicillin MICs are in the intermediate range may be treatable with penicillin (62, 146). It has been suggested

TABLE 1 Disk diffusion and MIC testing conditions and recommended QC strains for select fastidious bacteria

Organism(s)	Method	Medium[a]	Inoculum source[b]	Incubation atmosphere[c]	Incubation length (h)	Recommended QC strain(s)
S. pneumoniae and *Streptococcus* spp.	Disk diffusion	MHA + 5% sheep blood	18–20-h growth (from SBA)	5–7% CO_2	20–24	*S. pneumoniae* ATCC 49619
	Broth microdilution	CAMHB-LHB	18–20-h growth (from SBA)	Ambient air	20–24	*S. pneumoniae* ATCC 49619
H. influenzae and *Haemophilus parainfluenzae*	Disk diffusion	HTM agar	20–24-h growth (from CHOC)	5–7% CO_2	16–18	*H. influenzae* ATCC 49247, *H. influenzae* ATCC 49766[d]
	Broth microdilution	HTM broth	20–24-h growth (from CHOC)	Ambient air	20–24	*H. influenzae* ATCC 49247, *H. influenzae* ATCC 49766[d]
N. gonorrhoeae	Disk diffusion	GC agar base + supplement	20–24-h growth (from CHOC)	5–7% CO_2	20–24	*N. gonorrhoeae* ATCC 49226
	Agar dilution	GC agar base + supplement	20–24-h growth (from CHOC)	5–7% CO_2	20–24	*N. gonorrhoeae* ATCC 49226
N. meningitidis	Disk diffusion	MHA + 5% sheep blood	20–24-h growth (from CHOC)	5–7% CO_2	20–24	*S. pneumoniae* ATCC 49619
	Broth microdilution	CAMHB-LHB	20–24-h growth (from CHOC)	5–7% CO_2	20–24	*S. pneumoniae* ATCC 49619
	Agar dilution	MHA + 5% sheep blood	20–24-h growth (from CHOC)	5–7% CO_2	20–24	*S. pneumoniae* ATCC 49619
H. pylori	Agar dilution	MHA + 5% aged (≥2-wk-old) sheep blood	72-h growth (from SBA)[e]	Microaerobic; produced by gas-generating system for campylobacters	~72	*H. pylori* ATCC 43504

[a] HTM, GC agar base, and CAMHB-LHB are defined in the text.

[b] Inoculum suspension is in Mueller-Hinton broth or 0.9% NaCl standardized to a 0.5 McFarland standard for disk diffusion. For broth dilution, final organism concentration is 5×10^5 CFU/ml; for agar dilution, final organism concentration is 10^4 CFU/spot; CHOC, chocolate agar; SBA, sheep blood agar.

[c] Incubation temperature, 35°C.

[d] In addition, *H. influenzae* ATCC 10211 can be used to assess growth-supporting capabilities of HTM. *H. influenzae* ATCC 49766 is used for QC of select cephalosporins (e.g., cefaclor, cefamandole, and cefuroxime).

[e] Suspension is in 0.9% NaCl standardized to a 2.0 McFarland standard.

that penicillin MIC interpretive criteria be revised to reflect this (68, 89, 146). The rates for strains not susceptible to penicillin exceed 50% in some parts of the world (15, 99, 104), and in a recent U.S. survey (25), most of the strains not susceptible to penicillin demonstrated high-level resistance (MICs ≥2 μg/ml) rather than intermediate resistance (21.2% versus 14.2%). Some of the highest penicillin resistance rates occur in Asia, where 16.2% of the isolates were reported to be intermediately resistant and 44.1% were highly resistant in 2001–2002 (104). Strains of pneumococci that are susceptible to penicillin generally are susceptible to other β-lactam agents; however, as the penicillin MIC increases, the MICs of other β-lactam agents increase also (25, 99, 114, 160). Pneumococcal strains resistant to cefotaxime or ceftriaxone were not reported until the early 1990s (23, 179), and current rates of resistance to the extended-spectrum cephalosporins vary by location (15, 99, 104, 160). In a recent international survey of over 21,000 isolates, 96.5% of all isolates were susceptible to ceftriaxone (MIC, ≤1.0 μg/ml) whereas among isolates not susceptible to penicillin (MIC, ≥0.12 μg/ml), 89.1% were susceptible to ceftriaxone (160).

Resistance has been described for all classes of antimicrobial agents that are usually considered for treating pneumococcal infections, except for the glycopeptides and linezolid (15, 25, 63, 99, 104, 120, 160). In a recent U.S. survey (24), 31% of isolates were macrolide resistant. Resistance to macrolides in Asian-Pacific countries is much higher, exceeding 75% in some areas (104). Erythromycin MICs for pneumococci with macrolide-lincosamide-streptogramin B (MLS)-type resistance (encoded by the *ermB* gene) are usually ≥64 μg/ml, and clindamycin MICs are ≥8 μg/ml, whereas for isolates of the M phenotype (encoded by the *mefA* gene), erythromycin MICs are in the range of 1 to 32 μg/ml and clindamycin MICs are ≤0.25 μg/ml (54, 99). Susceptibility and resistance to azithromycin, clarithromycin, and dirithromycin among *S. pneumoniae* isolates can be predicted by testing erythromycin (41). Telithromycin, a ketolide, is considerably more active than macrolides against *S. pneumoniae,* with fewer than 1% of isolates showing resistance in recent North American studies (25, 52, 114).

Resistance rates for trimethoprim-sulfamethoxazole (TMP-SMX) range from 35 to 47% in the United States and are similar to those outside the United States (15, 25, 104). Resistance rates for fluoroquinolones remain low (24, 25, 104, 114); however, a higher prevalence of resistance to fluoroquinolones has been shown in other countries (92, 212). Resistance has only been rarely reported for linezolid (6, 25), and resistance rates for quinupristin-dalfopristin are <1% (6, 54) among *S. pneumoniae* strains. Resistance to tigecycline has not been described (69).

Multidrug resistance in *S. pneumoniae* is defined as resistance to three or more antimicrobial classes, commonly penicillins, TMP-SMX, and macrolides (114, 120). As many

TABLE 2 Broth microdilution MIC testing conditions, recommended QC strains, and drugs recommended for testing potential agents of bioterrorism

Organism(s)	Medium[a]	Inoculum source[b]	Incubation atmosphere[c]	Incubation length (h)	Recommended QC strain(s)	Drugs recommended for testing
B. anthracis	CAMHB	16–18-h growth (from SBA)	Ambient air	16–20	*Escherichia coli* ATCC 25922, *S. aureus* ATCC 29213	Ciprofloxacin, doxycycline, penicillin, tetracycline
Brucella spp.	Brucella broth, pH adjusted to 7.1 ± 0.1	48-h growth (from SBA)	Ambient air	48	*E. coli* ATCC 25922, *S. pneumoniae* ATCC 49619	Doxycycline, gentamicin, tetracycline, TMP-SMX, streptomycin
B. mallei, *B. pseudomallei*	CAMHB	16–18-h growth (from SBA)	Ambient air	16–20	*E. coli* ATCC 25922, *E. coli* ATCC 35218, *P. aeruginosa* ATCC 27853	Amoxicillin-clavulanic acid, ceftazidime, doxycycline, imipenem, tetracycline, TMP-SMX (*B. pseudomallei* only)
F. tularensis	CAMHB with 2% defined growth supplement, pH adjusted to 7.3 ± 0.1	24-h growth (from CHOC)	Ambient air	48	*E. coli* ATCC 25922, *S. aureus* ATCC 29213, *P. aeruginosa* ATCC 27853	Chloramphenicol, ciprofloxacin, doxycycline, gentamicin, levofloxacin, streptomycin, tetracycline
Y. pestis	CAMHB	24-h growth (from SBA)	Ambient air	24[d]	*E. coli* ATCC 25922	Chloramphenicol, ciprofloxacin, doxycycline, gentamicin, streptomycin, tetracycline, TMP-SMX

[a] CAMHB, cation-adjusted Mueller-Hinton broth.
[b] Inoculum suspension is in CAMHB standardized to a 0.5 McFarland standard. Final organism concentration is 5×10^5 CFU/ml. CHOC, chocolate agar; SBA, sheep blood agar.
[c] Incubation temperature, 35°C.
[d] If unacceptable growth in the control well, reincubate for an additional 24 h.

as 25% of *S. pneumoniae* isolates in the United States have been reported to be multidrug resistant, and rates are higher in other countries (15, 104, 120).

Reference Test Methods

CLSI describes both a broth microdilution method and a disk diffusion method for the testing of pneumococci (39-41). Details of these procedures are listed in Table 1. The broth microdilution method may be used to test all of the antimicrobial agents recommended by CLSI for pneumococci. With the exception of the oxacillin disk screening test for penicillin susceptibility, the disk diffusion method does not work for testing the β-lactam agents, including the cephalosporins (40, 41, 188). When used to predict penicillin susceptibility, oxacillin disk diffusion zone diameters of ≥20 mm indicate that the isolate is susceptible to penicillin (41). However, strains with zone diameters of ≤19 mm cannot be readily categorized as resistant, since a strain with an oxacillin zone diameter of ≤19 mm may be penicillin susceptible, intermediate, or resistant (53) when the actual penicillin MIC for the strain is determined. Therefore, if the oxacillin screen test is used without follow-up MIC testing for strains with zones of ≤19 mm, the potential for overstating penicillin resistance is high.

Commercial Methods for Testing

Several options are available for determining MICs of various antimicrobial agents for pneumococci. The E-test method has been extensively evaluated, and a recent evaluation was performed by Tenover et al. (191). All drugs recommended by CLSI for testing against pneumococci except clindamycin and telithromycin have been cleared by the FDA for testing by the E test. The accuracy of the E test has been reported to be >90% for most relevant drugs;

TABLE 3 Disk diffusion and MIC testing conditions, recommended QC strains, and agents to consider for primary testing for infrequently isolated or less common fastidious bacteria

Organism(s)	Method	Medium[a]	Inoculum source[b]	Incubation atmosphere[c]	Incubation length (h)	Recommended QC strain(s)	Agents to consider for primary testing
Abiotrophia spp., *Granulicatella* spp.	Broth microdilution	CAMHB-LHB[c] +0.001% pyridoxal HCl	20–24-h growth, from CHOC containing cysteine	Ambient air	20–24	*S. pneumoniae* ATCC 49619	Cefotaxime or ceftriaxone, penicillin, vancomycin
Aeromonas hydrophila complex, *Plesiomonas shigelloides*	Broth microdilution	CAMHB	16–18-h growth (from SBA)	Ambient air	16–20	*E. coli* ATCC 25922, *E. coli* ATCC 35218[d]	Amoxicillin-clavulanic acid, broad-spectrum or extended-spectrum cephalosporins, fluoroquinolones, TMP-SMX
	Disk diffusion	MHA	16–18-h growth (from SBA)	Ambient air	16–18	*E. coli* ATCC 25922, *E. coli* ATCC 35218	
Bacillus spp. (not *B. anthracis*)	Broth microdilution	CAMHB	16–18-h growth (from SBA)	Ambient air	16–20	*S. aureus* ATCC 29213	Clindamycin, gentamicin (for combined therapy, vancomycin)
C. jejuni, *C. coli*	Broth microdilution	CAMHB-LHB	24–48-h growth (from SBA)	10% CO_2, 5% O_2, 85% N_2 (microaerobic)	48 at 36°C or 24 at 42°C	*C. jejuni* ATCC 33560	Ciprofloxacin, erythromycin
Corynebacterium spp.	Broth microdilution	CAMHB-LHB	24–48 h growth, (from SBA or CHOC)	Ambient air	48	*S. pneumoniae* ATCC 49619	Erythromycin, gentamicin, penicillin, vancomycin
E. rhusiopathiae	Broth microdilution	CAMHB-LHB	18–24-h growth (from SBA)	Ambient air	20–24	*S. pneumoniae* ATCC 49619	Penicillin or ampicillin
HACEK group	Broth microdilution	CAMHB-LHB	24–48-h growth, (from CHOC)	Ambient air	24–48	*S. pneumoniae* ATCC 49619, *E. coli* ATCC 35218	Ampicillin, amoxicillin-clavulanic acid, ceftriaxone or cefotaxime, ciprofloxacin or levofloxacin, imipenem, TMP-SMX

Lactobacillus spp.	Broth microdilution	CAMHB-LHB	18–24-h growth (from SBA)	Ambient air	20–24	*S. pneumoniae* ATCC 49619	Penicillin or ampicillin, gentamicin (for combined therapy)
Leuconostoc spp.	Broth microdilution	CAMHB-LHB	18–24-h growth (from SBA)	Ambient air	20–24	*S. pneumoniae* ATCC 49619	Penicillin or ampicillin
L. monocytogenes	Broth microdilution	CAMHB-LHB	18–24-h growth (from SBA)	Ambient air	20–24	*S. pneumoniae* ATCC 49619	Penicillin or ampicillin, TMP-SMX
M. catarrhalis	Broth microdilution	CAMHB	18–24-h growth (from SBA)	Ambient air	20–24	*S. aureus* ATCC 29213, *E. coli* ATCC 35218	Amoxicillin-clavulanic acid, cefaclor or cefuroxime, TMP-SMX
Pasteurella spp.	Broth microdilution	CAMHB-LHB	18–24-h growth (from SBA)	Ambient air	18–24	*S. pneumoniae* ATCC 49619, *E. coli* ATCC 35218	β-Lactam/β-lactamase inhibitor combinations, cephalosporins, fluoroquinolones, macrolides, penicillins, tetracyclines, TMP-SMX
	Disk diffusion	MHA with 5% sheep blood	18–24-h growth (from SBA)	Ambient air	18–24	*S. pneumoniae* ATCC 49619, *E. coli* ATCC 35218, *S. aureus* ATCC 25923 (disk diffusion)	
Pediococcus spp.	Broth microdilution	CAMHB-LHB	18–24-h growth (from SBA)	Ambient air	20–24	*S. pneumoniae* ATCC 49619	Penicillin, gentamicin (for combined therapy)
Vibrio spp. (not *V. cholerae*)[e]	Broth microdilution	CAMHB	16–18-h growth (from SBA)	Ambient air	16–20	*E. coli* ATCC 25922, *E. coli* ATCC 35218	Cefotaxime, ceftazidime
	Disk diffusion	MHA	16–18-h growth (from SBA)	Ambient air	16–18	*E. coli* ATCC 25922, *E. coli* ATCC 35218	Tetracycline, fluoroquinolones

[a] CAMHB-LHB and MHA are defined in the text.
[b] Suspension is in Mueller-Hinton broth or 0.9% NaCl standardized to a 0.5 McFarland standard for disk diffusion. For broth dilution, final organism concentration is 5 × 10^5 CFU/ml. CHOC, chocolate agar; SBA, sheep blood agar.
[c] Incubation temperature, 35°C (except for *C. jejuni* and *C. coli*).
[d] *E. coli* ATCC 35218 is used for quality control when testing β-lactam/β-lactamase inhibitor combination drugs.
[e] For halophilic species, prepare inoculum in 0.85% NaCl (normal saline).

however, the number of minor errors with penicillin is relatively high. E-test penicillin MICs are slightly lower than those determined by reference broth microdilution (110). Since the E test uses incubation in CO_2, the MICs of the macrolides and ketolides tend to be 1 to 2 dilutions higher than those by the broth tests, in which incubation is done in ambient air (21). This is because these agents are less active at lower pH, which occurs with CO_2 incubation.

Other commercially available FDA-cleared panels or systems specifically designed for testing pneumococci include MicroScan (Dade Behring MicroScan Inc., West Sacramento, Calif.), Phoenix (BD Diagnostic Systems, Sparks, Md.), Sensititre (Trek Diagnostic Systems, Inc, Westlake, Ohio), and Vitek 2 (bioMerieux, Inc., Hazelwood, Mo.). The Pasco, MicroScan MICroSTREP, Sensititre, and Vitek 2 systems have been evaluated and found to produce MICs that are comparable to those obtained with the CLSI broth microdilution reference method (83, 107, 108, 142).

Strategies for Testing and Reporting of Results

CLSI stipulates that *S. pneumoniae* isolates from cerebrospinal fluid (CSF) be routinely tested by a reliable MIC method to determine susceptibilities to penicillin and cefotaxime or ceftriaxone, and meropenem should be added if it is on the institution's formulary. In addition, vancomycin should be tested by either an MIC or a disk diffusion method (41). Along with penicillin, CLSI recommends primary testing and reporting of erythromycin and TMP-SMX for isolates from non-CSF sources. Both drugs can be tested by either an MIC or a disk diffusion method. However, in communities where penicillin resistance is high and resistance to other agents is likely, MIC testing of penicillin, cefotaxime or ceftriaxone, meropenem, vancomycin, and one representative each of the macrolide, fluoroquinolone, and tetracycline classes would be appropriate for testing of strains isolated from non-CSF sources. Other drugs that might warrant testing if being considered for treatment of infections other than meningitis include cefepime, clindamycin, and telithromycin. Infections, such as pneumonia, caused by strains for which the MICs of penicillin are in the intermediate range may be treatable with penicillin or an extended-spectrum cephalosporin if maximal doses are used (68, 89, 146), and it may be appropriate to include a comment to this effect on the patient report. CLSI standards include a second set of nonmeningitis MIC breakpoints for cefotaxime and ceftriaxone that apply to infections other than meningitis (41). For CSF isolates, only interpretations using the original meningitis breakpoints should be reported; for isolates from other sites, both meningitis and nonmeningitis interpretations should be reported (41).

The oxacillin screening procedure should be used only for isolates from patients with non-life-threatening infections. If the zone diameter is ≤19 mm, at a minimum the MICs of penicillin and an extended-spectrum cephalosporin should then be determined (41).

STREPTOCOCCI OTHER THAN PNEUMOCOCCI

Incidence of Resistance

Because there are significant differences in susceptibility of β-lactam agents in viridans group versus beta-hemolytic streptococci, there are separate ampicillin, penicillin, cefotaxime, ceftriaxone, and cefepime interpretive criteria for the two organism groups. As defined by CLSI (41), the members of the viridans group include strains identified as *Streptococcus mitis, S. oralis, S. sanguinis, S. salivarius, S. intermedius, S. constellatus, S. mutans,* and *S. bovis,* as well as the small-colony-forming beta-hemolytic strains with group A, C, F, or G antigens (the *S. anginosus* group, which was previously called *S. milleri*). The beta-hemolytic group includes the large-colony-forming pyogenic strains with group A (*S. pyogenes*), C, or G antigens and strains with group B (*S. agalactiae*) antigen.

Although beta-hemolytic streptococci have been uniformly susceptible to penicillin, two reports have described penicillin MICs of 0.25 to 0.5 μg/ml for group B streptococci (17) and group C streptococci (194). The clinical significance of these elevated MICs is not known. High-level aminoglycoside resistance has been described for group B streptococci (26). The MLS-type macrolide resistance due to *erm* genes in beta-hemolytic streptococci may be either inducible or constitutive (45). If the resistance is inducible, the strains will be resistant to erythromycin (and the other 14- and 15-membered macrolides) but appear to be susceptible to clindamycin unless resistance is induced. Resistance rates for erythromycin vary for group A streptococci and were recently reported to be as high as 32% in parts of California (213). In a large Canadian study conducted in 2002–2003, the predominant mechanism for erythromycin resistance in group A streptococcus was *mefA* whereas that in group B streptococcus was *erm* (47). Resistance rates among streptococci vary for tetracyclines and are low for fluoroquinolones (6, 25, 69). In several recent large surveillance studies, resistance was not observed for daptomycin (101), linezolid, or quinupristin-dalfopristin (6, 69).

Penicillin resistance in viridans group streptococci has been described, and resistance rates can be >50% (2, 69), particularly for *S. mitis* and *S. sanguinis*. Ahmed et al. noted 67.5% penicillin resistance among 40 blood culture isolates from bacteremic children with cancer (2). Resistance has been described for some viridans group isolates for macrolides, lincosamides, tetracyclines, quinupristin-dalfopristin, and fluoroquinolones (2, 3, 69, 195). Single reports of resistance to vancomycin have been noted for *S. bovis* (161) and for *S. mitis* (124), and resistance to linezolid has been reported on at least one occasion (172). In a recent study, all 92 viridans group streptococci selected to represent more resistant strains were susceptible to daptomycin (101). High-level aminoglycoside resistance has been described for viridans group streptococci (95).

Reference Test Methods

Studies by CLSI to determine interpretive criteria for both MIC and disk diffusion testing have resulted in breakpoints for streptococci that were initially published in 1995. Penicillin and select cephalosporin breakpoints were subsequently modified as mentioned above. Details for MIC and disk diffusion tests are described in Table 1. The disk diffusion test may be used to determine the penicillin susceptibility of beta-hemolytic streptococci; however, it is unreliable and should not be used for viridans group streptococci. Other agents may be tested by either the MIC or the disk method. Aminoglycoside MICs of >1,000 μg/ml for streptococci (207) have been described; however, there are no published methods for screening for high-level aminoglycoside resistance in streptococci.

Susceptibility testing of members of the genera *Abiotrophia* and *Granulicatella* (formerly known as "nutritionally deficient streptococci") are included in the new CLSI M45 document as described below. Recent CLSI standards describe a disk approximation test for inducible resistance to clindamycin in beta-hemolytic streptococci whereby erythromycin is used to induce resistance to clindamycin. Mueller-Hinton agar (MHA) supplemented with 5% sheep blood is inoculated as for a disk diffusion test, and a 15-μg erythromycin disk and a 2-μg clindamycin disk are placed approximately 12 mm apart on the agar surface. The plate is incubated at 35°C overnight, and flattening of the clindamycin zone indicates inducible clindamycin resistance (41).

Commercial Test Methods

There have been few reports of evaluations of commercial susceptibility test systems for streptococci other than pneumococci, although it might be expected that systems capable of testing pneumococci would also perform adequately for other streptococci. The MicroScan and Phoenix systems are cleared by the FDA for the testing of *Streptococcus* spp. The Vitek 2 system is FDA cleared for testing of group B streptococci. The E test has not been extensively evaluated but does appear to be a possible alternative to the reference methods for testing *Streptococcus* spp. (106, 173).

Strategies for Testing and Reporting of Results

Routine testing of β-hemolytic streptococci is unnecessary since there have been only sporadic reports of decreased susceptibility to penicillin, primarily in group B streptococci (17, 194). However, if erythromycin is being used to treat infections caused by group A streptococci and treatment failure is suspected, testing might be considered. Similarly, if erythromycin is being considered for prophylaxis of pregnant women who are highly allergic to penicillin, in an effort to prevent perinatal group B streptococcal disease, testing should be done. If clindamycin is being considered for β-hemolytic streptococci that test clindamycin susceptible and erythromycin resistant, the determination of inducible clindamycin resistance should be considered. For viridans group streptococci, penicillin MICs should be determined for strains isolated from blood, especially for patients with infective endocarditis. Disk diffusion is not reliable for testing penicillin in viridans group streptococci (10).

H. INFLUENZAE

Incidence of Resistance

Ampicillin resistance in *H. influenzae* is most commonly mediated by a plasmid-borne β-lactamase, TEM-1 being the most common enzyme. The incidence of β-lactamase-producing *H. influenzae* organisms ranges from 5% to nearly 40% in various geographic areas (15, 25, 63, 100, 105, 183, 217). Recently, a decrease in β-lactamase-producing isolates has been documented in North America (90). Ampicillin resistance can result from altered penicillin-binding proteins in β-lactamase-negative, ampicillin-resistant (BLNAR) strains, but this mechanism of resistance appears to be uncommon. In a recent survey, Brown and Rybak noted that 0.4% of 3,296 isolates from throughout the United States were BLNAR (25). Among 395 isolates collected from patients with meningitis during 1999 through 2002 in Japan, 13.9% were shown to be BLNAR (86). However, in a respiratory surveillance study conducted during a similar time in Japan, only one BLNAR strain among 281 isolates was found (98). Compared with β-lactamase-producing or ampicillin-susceptible *H. influenzae,* BLNAR isolates are less susceptible to amoxicillin-clavulanic acid and to various cephalosporins such as cefaclor, cefuroxime, cefixime, and cefotaxime (13). Use of a 2-μg rather than a 10-μg ampicillin disk and a 1/2 μg rather than a 10/30 μg amoxicillin-clavulanic acid disk with the standard CLSI disk diffusion method has been suggested as a method to better identify BLNAR strains (115).

Resistance among *H. influenzae* isolates to broad-spectrum oral cephalosporins (e.g., cefixime and cefpodoxime) and to extended-spectrum cephalosporins (e.g., cefotaxime) is rare (217). Resistance to expanded-spectrum cephalosporins (e.g., cefuroxime) is uncommon, <3% in a recent survey (102). The narrower-spectrum, β-lactamase-labile cephalosporins (e.g., loracarbef and cefprozil) are less active, with resistance rates ranging from 3 to nearly 30% (25, 102, 105, 183, 217).

Resistance to TMP-SMX among *H. influenzae* organisms occurs in approximately 20% of isolates from North America (93, 100, 102, 217), but resistance rates as high as 60% have been noted in other parts of the world including Southeast Asia (64). Resistance to tetracyclines is <3% (25, 102, 217), and resistance to fluoroquinolones is rare (25, 60, 93). Although erythromycin has not been considered a drug of choice for the treatment of infections caused by *H. influenzae,* some of the newer macrolides are more active than erythromycin and may be effective as treatment. Less than 2% of isolates examined in various studies were resistant to azithromycin; however, clarithromycin resistance rates approached 20% (25, 98, 100, 102, 105, 183, 217). Telithromycin is highly active against *H. influenzae* with resistance rates of approximately 1% (25, 98, 217).

Reference Test Methods

β-Lactamase production in *H. influenzae* can easily be detected by the chromogenic cephalosporin, acidometric, or iodometric β-lactamase test methods (see chapter 74).

CLSI has developed broth microdilution MIC and disk diffusion methods for testing *H. influenzae,* and these methods can also be used to test *H. parainfluenzae*. Testing of the more unusual *Haemophilus* spp. including *H. aphrophilus, H. paraphrophilus,* and *H. segnis* are now addressed in the new CLSI M45 document. Specific variables related to each of the methods for testing *H. influenzae* and *H. parainfluenzae* are listed in Table 1. *Haemophilus* test medium (HTM) is recommended and consists of a Mueller-Hinton base, 15 μg of hematin per ml, 15 μg of NAD per ml, and 5 mg of yeast extract per ml. Cation-adjusted Mueller-Hinton broth (CAMHB) is used with the components listed above for the preparation of HTM broth, which also contains 0.2 IU of thymidine phosphorylase per ml. Although HTM agar is transparent, some investigators have reported difficulties in measuring zones and poor growth of some strains (88, 141). Broth microdilution tests with HTM generally give clearer endpoints. The problems most often noted with both the disk diffusion and the broth microdilution methods are equivocal endpoints with BLNAR strains with several β-lactams. Because of this, CLSI recommends that BLNAR strains (which are best detected by tests with ampicillin) be considered resistant to amoxicillin-clavulanic acid, ampicillin-sulbactam, cefaclor, cefamandole, cefetamet, cefonicid, cefprozil, cefuroxime, loracarbef, and piperacillin-tazobactam and that the activities of these agents against BLNAR strains not be tested (41).

Commercial Test Methods

Currently, the only FDA-cleared broth microdilution system for testing *Haemophilus* spp. is Sensititre. The E test has been cleared by the FDA for testing *H. influenzae* with most drugs that would be used for treating *Haemophilus* infections, and results with E test have been shown to be comparable to those obtained by CLSI reference methods (111).

Strategies for Testing and Reporting of Results

β-Lactamase testing will detect the most common type of clinically significant resistance in *H. influenzae*. β-Lactamase-positive isolates are ampicillin and amoxicillin resistant. To detect BLNAR strains, an ampicillin disk diffusion or MIC test is required. However, since the incidence of BLNAR is low in many geographic areas, such tests may not be routinely needed, and for practical purposes, a negative β-lactamase test result translates into ampicillin susceptibility. Frequently, the β-lactamase test is the only test routinely performed with clinical isolates. Because of increasing resistance to TMP-SMX, testing should be considered and CLSI recommends that this agent be tested and reported routinely (41). Other oral agents that might be considered, such as amoxicillin-clavulanic acid, the oral cephalosporins, newer macrolides, and quinolones, are predictably active against *H. influenzae* and are often prescribed empirically. Consequently, routine testing of these drugs is generally not useful. However, these and other agents may be tested for surveillance or epidemiological purposes (41).

N. GONORRHOEAE

Incidence of Resistance

During the past 2 decades, increasing rates of penicillin and tetracycline resistance among *N. gonorrhoeae* isolates have led to recommending ceftriaxone, cefixime, ciprofloxacin, ofloxacin, or levofloxacin as the primary agents for uncomplicated gonorrhea instead of penicillin or tetracycline (30). Penicillin resistance is due to the production of a plasmid-associated TEM-1 type β-lactamase (penicillinase-producing *N. gonorrhoeae* [PPNG]) or to mutations in chromosomal genes that result in altered penicillin-binding proteins or diminished outer membrane permeability (chromosomally mediated resistant *N. gonorrhoeae* [CMRNG]). The activities of other β-lactams against PPNG are generally unaltered; however, CMRNG may show decreased susceptibility to other β-lactams (49). Tetracycline resistance in *N. gonorrhoeae* can be plasmid- or chromosomally mediated, with plasmid-mediated resistance resulting in a higher level of resistance.

The Gonococcal Isolate Surveillance Program, which tests urethral isolates from male clients visiting sexually transmitted disease clinics throughout the United States, reported that 16.4% of 6,552 isolates were resistant to penicillin or tetracycline or both in 2003. The incidence of PPNG peaked at 11.0% in 1991 and was only 1% in 2003. The incidence of tetracycline resistance has remained fairly stable and was 3.7% in 2003. All 6,552 isolates tested in 2003 were susceptible to ceftriaxone and cefixime; however, there appears to be a subtle shift towards higher MICs for both these agents. Nevertheless, only 4 isolates had elevated ceftriaxone MICs of 0.5 μg/ml and 45 isolates had elevated cefixime MICs of 0.5 to 2.0 μg/ml (29).

Fluoroquinolone resistance has become widespread throughout Asia and is increasing in the United States. In a study of 115 isolates of *N. gonorrhoeae* from female sex workers in the Philippines, 49% of isolates had ciprofloxacin MICs of ≥4 μg/ml and 63% of isolates had MICs ≥1 μg/ml (8). In Japan in 2002, 70% of 87 *N. gonorrhoeae* isolates from males with urethritis were ciprofloxacin resistant and only 1 isolate produced β-lactamase (177). The Gonococcal Antimicrobial Susceptibility Program conducted by the World Health Organization noted that ciprofloxacin resistance rates for gonococci from patients in India in 2001 varied from 10.6 to 100% among 10 regions studied (165). In the 2003 Gonococcal Isolate Surveillance Program study, 0.9% of the isolates exhibited intermediate susceptibility and 4.1% were resistant to ciprofloxacin (29). Newman et al. noted that 17% of isolates from 117 patients seen at a public sexually transmitted disease clinic in Hawaii in 2001 were ciprofloxacin resistant (150).

Reference Test Methods

Routine β-lactamase tests readily detect PPNG and can reliably be performed by either the chromogenic cephalosporin, acidimetric, or iodometric method.

CLSI recommends the use of GC agar base for disk diffusion and agar dilution MIC testing. For both tests, a 1% defined growth supplement must be added; however, in agar dilution tests with imipenem and with clavulanate, the growth supplement must be free of cysteine to avoid inhibition of the activities of these two agents (39-41). The agar dilution method is preferred to the broth dilution method for MIC testing because *N. gonorrhoeae* has a tendency to autolyse in liquid media. For other details of testing, see Table 1.

Commercial Test Methods

The only commercial method currently available for susceptibility testing of *N. gonorrhoeae* is E test, which has been shown to produce results comparable to those of conventional reference agar dilution methods (18).

Strategies for Testing and Reporting Results

Generally, there is no need for routine clinical laboratories to perform antimicrobial susceptibility tests with *N. gonorrhoeae* unless there are unusual circumstances. These might include the patient's intolerance to the drugs of choice, treatment failure (assuming that compliance was not an issue), or a disseminated gonococcal infection. Additionally, if fluoroquinolone resistance is noted in a particular geographic area, testing may be warranted if fluoroquinolones are being prescribed. Some laboratories may perform β-lactamase tests for all isolates if β-lactamase results are requested by the local public health departments for epidemiological purposes. However, many public health departments have eliminated this requirement. Surveillance for established and emerging resistance for *N. gonorrhoeae* is generally performed by designated state and local public health agencies.

N. MENINGITIDIS

Incidence of Resistance

Increasing numbers of β-lactamase-negative *N. meningitidis* isolates from the United States and elsewhere have reduced susceptibility to penicillin (MICs, 0.12 to 1.0 μg/ml), although the frequency of these isolates in different regions varies widely (85, 167, 200).

A study of 400 *N. meningitidis* isolates obtained in 1998 and 1999 in Spain showed that 37% of them had penicillin MICs of 0.12 to 1.0 μg/ml (200). In a study of 53 invasive isolates collected in 1998–99 in the United States, 30.2% had penicillin MICs of 0.12 to 0.25 μg/ml (167). There have been two recent reports from Europe of *N. meningitidis* isolates with penicillin MICs of 1.5 μg/ml and 2.0 μg/ml; E test was used for testing the first isolate, and agar dilution was used for the second (59, 80). The clinical significance of isolates for which penicillin MICs are elevated is uncertain, and penicillin remains the drug of choice for the treatment of meningococcal disease (74, 138). Many infections caused by isolates with reduced susceptibility to penicillin have successfully been treated with high doses of penicillin (186, 208); however, rare reports cited clinical failure (meningitis) when a lower than recommended dose of penicillin was used (198). The broad-spectrum cephalosporins (e.g., ceftriaxone) remain highly active against isolates with elevated penicillin MICs (85, 164, 167, 200). In the 1980s, four isolates of β-lactamase-producing *N. meningitidis* were reported (20, 50, 67), and one isolate was reported in 1996 (201); additional isolates have not been noted.

Regarding agents used for prophylaxis, resistance to sulfonamides occurs frequently, and resistance to rifampin has been documented on several occasions (109, 164, 171, 200). There are two reports of *N. meningitidis* isolated from CSF with decreased susceptibility to ciprofloxacin (MIC, 0.12 and 0.25 μg/ml), one from Australia and another from Spain; however, *N. meningitidis* is typically very susceptible to this agent (MIC, ≤0.03 μg/ml) (4, 178).

Strategies for Testing and Reporting of Results

CLSI recently published standards for susceptibility testing of *N. meningitidis* that utilizes either the broth microdilution method and CAMHB with 2 to 5% lysed horse blood (CAMHB-LHB) or the agar dilution method and MHA with 5% sheep blood, both with incubation in 5% CO_2 (41, 109). Interpretive criteria are listed for agents such as penicillin, cefotaxime, and ceftriaxone, which might be prescribed for treating a meningococcal infection. In addition, interpretive criteria are listed for agents such as ciprofloxacin and rifampin, which might be used for prophylaxis of meningococcal case contacts. CLSI also approved a disk diffusion method for testing *N. meningitidis* which utilizes MHA with 5% sheep blood and CO_2 incubation. As with MIC tests, interpretive criteria are listed for several therapeutic and prophylactic agents. Unfortunately, these do not include breakpoints for ampicillin and penicillin, as results obtained with these agents were unreliable (41). Several investigators have examined modified penicillin disk diffusion methods by using 2- and 10-IU penicillin disks and 1-μg oxacillin disks and also determined that these cannot reliably distinguish *N. meningitidis* isolates that are susceptible from those that have decreased ampicillin and penicillin susceptibility (19, 27, 157). Therefore, disk diffusion testing should not be used for these drugs.

Because of the lack of clinical failures with the drugs of choice for the treatment of meningococcal infections, susceptibility testing is not warranted in most situations (170, 171). Although the E test has not yet been cleared by the FDA for testing *N. meningitidis,* several studies have shown it to be reliable for testing meningococci and to perform best by using MHA with 5% sheep blood incubated in CO_2 (1, 136, 155, 157, 199). However, in a 14-lab study, Vazquez et al. noted some difficulties in obtaining reliable results for rifampin with E test (199).

H. PYLORI

Incidence of Resistance

The rates of resistance for *H. pylori* vary considerably among the agents recommended for therapy (e.g., amoxicillin, clarithromycin, metronidazole, and tetracycline), with resistance to metronidazole being highest. Using the CLSI reference method, Osato et al. reported approximately 35% resistance to metronidazole among 3,193 isolates in the United States (152). In a Korean study that used similar methodologies, 40.6% of 652 isolates were metronidazole resistant (118); however, a study in Japan reported only 12.4% metronidazole resistance among 388 isolates but noted significant differences from various geographic areas (116). Clarithromycin resistance rates were lower, with approximately 11% resistance in the U.S. study and 5.9 and 12.9% resistance observed in the Korean and Japanese studies, respectively. The incidence of resistance to tetracycline and amoxicillin is currently very low (118, 126, 152). Kim et al. recently identified discordant susceptibility results for clarithromycin, metronidazole, and tetracycline when testing multiple isolates from different locations in the stomach of individual patients (117). A similar finding was reported by Osato et al. (151) for metronidazole susceptibility. These results suggest that resistant isolates are not evenly distributed throughout the stomach and susceptibility results for isolates from a single biopsy may not be representative of the entire population.

Reference Test Method

CLSI describes an agar dilution MIC method for testing *H. pylori*. The test medium is MHA supplemented with aged (≥2-week-old) sheep blood. The inoculum is prepared from 72-h-old growth on a blood agar plate to obtain a final concentration of bacteria approximating 10^5 CFU/spot. Incubation is for 3 days at 35°C in a microaerobic atmosphere produced by a gas-generating system typically used for campylobacters. *H. pylori* ATCC 43504 has been designated as a QC strain, and currently there are only interpretive criteria for clarithromycin. Other antimicrobial agents that have been studied and for which there are CLSI QC ranges include amoxicillin, metronidazole, telithromycin, and tetracycline (41).

Commercial Test Methods

Although no commercial methods are FDA cleared for antimicrobial susceptibility testing of *H. pylori,* several investigators have examined the E test. In one study the percent agreement (i.e., results within ±1 doubling dilution) between E test and agar dilution was 84.6% for amoxicillin, 94.1% for clarithromycin, 89.9% for metronidazole, and 89.1% for tetracycline (159). In a multilaboratory study, laboratories correctly identified clarithromycin- and metronidazole-susceptible and -resistant strains 93% of the time using E test (16). However, two studies reported significant discrepancies for metronidazole susceptibility by agar dilution and E test (139, 151). All of these E-test evaluations report differences in methods for agar dilution and E test, such as media, inoculum, and incubation conditions, which may account for the different results.

Strategies for Testing and Reporting of Results

Because of growth requirements and complex antimicrobial susceptibility testing recommendations, testing of *H. pylori* is not practical for the routine clinical laboratory. However, because of the significant resistance noted for metronidazole and clarithromycin, testing may be required in select situations, in which case a reliable reference laboratory should be used. Although there are currently no CLSI interpretive criteria for metronidazole, investigators have used an MIC of >8 μg/ml for resistance (118, 126, 151, 152).

POTENTIAL BACTERIAL AGENTS OF BIOTERRORISM

Several bacterial agents are identified as potential agents of bioterrorism by the Centers for Disease Control and Prevention (http://www.bt.cdc.gov/agent/index.asp). These include *Bacillus anthracis, Yersinia pestis, Francisella tularensis, Burkholderia mallei, Burkholderia pseudomallei,* and *Brucella* spp. Until recently, standardized antimicrobial susceptibility testing methods and interpretive criteria did not exist for any of these bacteria. The antimicrobial susceptibility patterns for most of them are predictable, so susceptibility testing of naturally occurring isolates is often not necessary. However, it is possible for antimicrobial resistance to spontaneously occur among these organisms and, in the case of a bioterrorism event, there is the possibility of engineered resistance. To detect any possible resistance, standardized broth microdilution susceptibility testing methods and interpretive criteria were established and published by CLSI (41).

Acquired resistance to antimicrobial agents commonly used for treatment of infections caused by *B. anthracis, Y. pestis, F. tularensis, B. mallei, B. pseudomallei,* and *Brucella* spp. is rare. Isolates of *B. anthracis* may contain inducible β-lactamases, which can confer resistance to penicillins and cephalosporins (32, 56, 130). Because of this potential resistance, penicillin is recommended for anthrax prophylaxis only when the organism burden would be low and this recommendation is limited to young children and pregnant women who should not receive other prophylaxis therapies such as fluoroquinolones and tetracyclines (28). Laboratory-generated fluoroquinolone resistance in *B. anthracis* was reported, but fluoroquinolone resistance in clinical isolates has not been reported (34, 163). There are reports of two spontaneously occurring drug-resistant *Y. pestis* isolates recovered in Madagascar (71, 81). Both isolates acquired conjugative plasmids. In one isolate, the plasmid carried resistant determinants for ampicillin, chloramphenicol, tetracycline, kanamycin, streptomycin, and sulfonamide. In the other isolate, the plasmid conferred resistance to streptomycin. Susceptibility studies of *B. pseudomallei* and *B. mallei* indicate that most isolates are susceptible to amoxicillin-clavulanic acid, ceftazidime, imipenem, tetracycline, doxycycline, and TMP-SMX, using CLSI interpretive criteria (192). However, some isolates of *B. pseudomallei* have elevated ceftazidime MICs (i.e., MIC $\geq$8 μg/ml) (97, 192). Clinical isolates of *Brucella* spp. with reduced susceptibility to rifampin and TMP-SMX have been reported (14, 119, 140). In these studies, the susceptibility testing methods used were either not clearly defined or different from the methods currently recommended by CLSI. Also, resistant isolates were not characterized for resistance determinants or mutations. Therefore, the definition of resistance to rifampin or TMP-SMX among *Brucella* spp. is unclear. Isolates of *F. tularensis* demonstrate β-lactamase activity, and they are resistant to β-lactams including cephalosporins and carbapenems (12, 96). Resistance to aminoglycosides, tetracyclines, fluoroquinolones, and chloramphenicol has not been reported.

B. anthracis, B. mallei, B. pseudomallei, and Y. pestis demonstrate sufficient growth with commonly used broth microdilution MIC testing medium and incubation conditions (Table 2). However, the recommended testing medium for *F. tularensis* is CAMHB with 2% of a defined growth supplement. This is the same cysteine-containing defined growth supplement that is added to GC agar base for susceptibility testing of *Neisseria gonorrhoeae*. The supplement is commercially available from two manufacturers: IsoVitalex Enrichment (BD Diagnostics, Franklin Lakes, N.J.) and XV Factor Enrichment (PML Microbiologicals, Wilsonville, Oreg.). Some isolates of *Brucella* spp., particularly isolates of *B. abortus,* require CO_2 incubation. Studies are under way to determine if incubation in CO_2 significantly changes MIC values for antimicrobial agents that should be tested such as aminoglycosides, tetracyclines, or TMP-SMX. For the slower-growing organisms, *F. tularensis, Y. pestis,* and *Brucella* spp., 48 h of incubation may be needed to achieve sufficient growth.

There are few studies comparing alternative susceptibility testing methods to the standard CLSI reference broth microdilution methods. One study compared E test to broth microdilution for testing *B. anthracis* (143). In this study, E-test MICs were within a single doubling dilution of the broth microdilution MICs for ceftriaxone, chloramphenicol, ciprofloxacin, clindamycin, erythromycin, rifampin, tetracycline, and vancomycin, but not for penicillin. Penicillin MIC values for E test tended to be lower than those obtained by broth microdilution. A similar trend for penicillin MICs was noted for *B. anthracis* in a study comparing E test to agar dilution (197). These results suggest that E test is acceptable for susceptibility testing of *B. anthracis* with antimicrobial agents other than penicillin. Similar studies are needed to establish alternative methods for the other potential agents of bioterrorism so that testing is available in more laboratories.

Susceptibility testing of potential agents of bioterrorism raises safety concerns for clinical microbiology laboratories. All of the above-mentioned organisms require at least biosafety level (BSL) 2 practices, containment, and facilities. BSL 3 conditions are recommended for activities with a high potential for aerosol production (166). Since the inoculum preparation for susceptibility testing has the potential for aerosol production, all susceptibility testing procedures must be performed in a BSL 3 facility. Laboratories without BSL 3 facilities should send isolates to an appropriately equipped reference laboratory that has select agent clearance status, such as that at reference laboratories within the Laboratory Response Network and at the Centers for Disease Control and Prevention (http://www.cdc.gov/od/sap/ and http://www.bt.cdc.gov/lrn/biological.asp).

ABIOTROPHIA SPECIES AND *GRANULICATELLA* SPECIES

For *Abiotrophia* spp. and *Granulicatella* spp., resistance has been reported to agents from several different antimicrobial classes including penicillins, cephalosporins, carbapenems, macrolides, lincosamides, fluoroquinolones, and tetracyclines. In a study of 20 blood isolates by Murray et al., resistant rates for specific agents were as follows: penicillin, 5%; cefotaxime, 35%; cefepime, 47%; meropenem, 10%; erythromycin, 30%; clindamycin, 5%; and tetracycline, 10% (145). These results are consistent with those previously reported (73, 196). Murray et al. also noted a levofloxacin-resistant *Abiotrophia elegans* (currently known as *Granulicatella elegans*) which was isolated from a patient who had received 10 days of levofloxacin prophylaxis (145). Little is known about mechanisms of resistance in these bacteria. There is one report of an *Abiotrophia defectiva* isolate with a conjugative, Tn*916*-like, transposon, Tn*3872* (162). The transposon carried *ermB* and *tetM* resistance determinants, which conferred resistance to erythromycin and tetracycline, respectively. This finding demonstrates, that these bacteria are able to acquire and transfer mobile genetic elements which confer antimicrobial resistance.

Because *Abiotrophia* spp. and *Granulicatella* spp. are fastidious, it is recommended that these be tested in CAMHB-LHB supplemented with 0.001% pyridoxal hydrochloride and incubated in CO_2 (Table 3) (38, 193). In a report by Namdari et al., a procedure for adding pyridoxal to an inoculum prepared with the Prompt system and a MicroScan dried gram-positive panel is described (147). It should be noted that susceptibility testing of aminoglycosides against *Abiotrophia* spp. and *Granulicatella* spp. is not recommended even though aminoglycosides are commonly used in combination therapy with an agent active against the cell wall, such as penicillin or vancomycin, for treating serious infections caused by these organisms. Since the aminoglycoside acts synergistically with the agent, in vitro susceptibility to aminoglycosides does not predict in vivo susceptibility (22).

AEROMONAS HYDROPHILA COMPLEX (*A. CAVIAE, A. HYDROPHILA, A. JANDAEI, A. SCHUBERTII,* AND *A. VERONII*) AND *PLESIOMONAS SHIGELLOIDES*

Aeromonas spp. are typically resistant to ampicillin, show variable results with β-lactam/β-lactamase inhibitor combinations, and are resistant to narrow-spectrum cephalosporins (122, 154, 203, 204). Inducible β-lactamases in *Aeromonas* spp. have been noted, and resistance may emerge during therapy with a β-lactam agent (123). A recent study showed that all 18 isolates from patients with traveler's diarrhea were susceptible to cefotaxime and ciprofloxacin and were variably resistant to chloramphenicol, tetracycline, and TMP-SMX (204). In Taiwan, where *Aeromonas* spp. are frequently encountered, results from 234 isolates in 1996 demonstrated that most isolates were susceptible to expanded-spectrum cephalosporins, fluoroquinolones, and aminoglycosides and approximately one-half of the isolates were susceptible to tetracycline and TMP-SMX. These authors remarked that there appeared to be species differences and *A. sobria* was more susceptible than either *A. hydrophila* or *A. caviae* (122). Similar results were noted by Vila et al. from Spain in 2002 (203).

Plesiomonas spp. are typically resistant to ampicillin and other penicillins including piperacillin and susceptible to β-lactamase inhibitor combinations and several other classes of antimicrobial agents (37, 78, 113, 185). However, Stock and Wiedemann noted ceftazidime resistance for 20 of 52 human isolates when an inoculum of 10^6 CFU/ml was used with a standard CLSI broth microdilution method. In another study, these same authors saw considerable variations in MICs when different media and inoculum concentrations from 10^4 to 10^7 were used to test 30 different β-lactams (184).

Although *Aeromonas* spp. and *Plesiomonas shigelloides* cause diarrheal disease, otherwise healthy individuals with diarrhea due to these bacteria usually recover spontaneously without treatment (78, 203) and routine antimicrobial susceptibility testing of isolates from fecal specimens is not recommended (38). However, both genera can cause a variety of other infections where treatment may be necessary (9, 78, 122, 123, 185, 204). Consequently, for isolates from extraintestinal sources, antimicrobial susceptibility testing may be warranted. These organisms share growth characteristics similar to those of *Enterobacteriaceae,* which led CLSI to recommend broth microdilution MIC testing using a method similar to that used for *Enterobacteriaceae*.

BACILLUS SPECIES

Bacillus spp. other than *B. anthracis* are common contaminants in the clinical laboratory, but these bacteria can cause serious disease. Since the susceptibility profiles of *Bacillus* spp. are quite variable, susceptibility testing should be considered when *Bacillus* spp. are isolated from normally sterile body sites. Isolates of *Bacillus* spp. can have β-lactamases that confer resistance to penicillins and possibly cephalosporins (174). *B. cereus* is the most common species found in clinical specimens, and most of these isolates are resistant to penicillin and extended-spectrum cephalosporins, although penicillin resistance does not always predict cephalosporin resistance (197, 205). Penicillin and cephalosporin resistance also occurs in other species of *Bacillus,* but it is less common. Resistance to several other agents has been reported. These agents include aminoglycosides, erythromycin, clindamycin, chloramphenicol, tetracycline, fluoroquinolones, TMP-SMX, and vancomycin. Resistance to carbapenems has not been reported for *Bacillus* spp. (197, 205; F. Cockerill, unpublished data).

Standard susceptibility testing methods for nonfastidious bacteria can be used for testing *Bacillus* spp. CLSI provides guidelines for broth microdilution testing (Table 3) (38). Agar dilution and E-test methods using MHA were compared in a study by Turnbull et al. (197). In both studies E-test MICs were similar to agar dilution MICs for several agents including cefotaxime, ciprofloxacin, erythromycin, gentamicin, penicillin, tetracycline, and vancomycin. Two commercial β-lactamase tests, Nitrocefin (Oxoid, Basingstoke, England) and Intralactam strips (Mast Diagnostics, Merseyside, United Kingdom) were evaluated in a study by Andrews and Wise (7); both tests failed to detect β-lactamase activity in four of five penicillin-resistant isolates of *B. cereus*. Therefore, β-lactamase testing is not recommended for predicting penicillin susceptibility in *Bacillus* spp.

C. JEJUNI

Resistance to macrolides and fluoroquinolones, the drugs of choice for treating gastrointestinal infections caused by *C. jejuni* and *C. coli,* is being reported with increasing frequency for human and animal isolates. The National Antimicrobial Resistance Monitoring System noted no ciprofloxacin resistance among *C. jejuni* human isolates in 1990, but a resistance rate of 12% occurred in 1997 and this increased to 18% in 2001. Erythromycin resistance was 1% in 1997 and 2% in 2001 (82). Smith et al. examined nearly 5,000 *C. jejuni* isolates from feces of Minnesota residents and noted an increase in the incidence of ciprofloxacin resistance from 1.3% in 1992 to 10.2% in 1998 (180). Of 537 *C. jejuni* isolates from human fecal specimens obtained during 1997 and 1998 in Spain, 75% were resistant to ciprofloxacin and 3.2% were resistant to erythromycin (175). A recent study noted that patients with invasive illness due to resistant isolates were more likely to have adverse effects than those infected with susceptible isolates (91). Resistance among animal isolates, which may subsequently be transmitted to humans, has been associated with the addition of macrolides and fluoroquinolones to animal food as growth-promoting agents (57).

Because of the increasing incidence of resistance, testing of isolates from individual patients with severe illness or prolonged symptoms may be warranted or isolates might be tested for epidemiologic purposes. Susceptibility testing by broth microdilution in CAMHB-LHB and incubation in a campylobacter environment (Table 3) is suggested. Agar dilution using MHA supplemented with 5% sheep blood has been shown to be satisfactory and is listed as an alternative method by the CLSI (41). Disk diffusion methods have been used successfully by some investigators (72, 175), although CLSI has not yet identified a reliable disk diffusion method. The E test correlated well with agar dilution in a study by Baker when ciprofloxacin, erythromycin, and tetracycline were tested (11), and Hayward et al. had similar success when testing gatifloxacin (87).

CORYNEBACTERIUM SPECIES

The many *Corynebacterium* spp. may exhibit a variety of susceptibility profiles. Most isolates of *C. amycolatum*, *C. jeikeium*, and *C. urealyticum* are multiresistant to antimicrobial agents that are often considered for therapy of gram-positive infections, including penicillins, cephalosporins, macrolides, aminoglycosides, quinolones, tetracyclines, and clindamycin. These species remain susceptible to teicoplanin and vancomycin. Considerable variation in activities of antimicrobial agents occurs with the various other species of *Corynebacterium*, and many strains may be highly susceptible (70, 127, 158, 169, 182, 206). Virtually all isolates of *C. urealyticum* are resistant to quinolones, which has important implications for empiric therapy for urinary tract infections due to this species (65). Significant antimicrobial resistance remains rare for *C. diphtheriae*, and penicillin resistance has not been reported to date (58). However, among 15 isolates from Vietnamese children with diphtheria, 4 were resistant to erythromycin (121), and 5 of 410 isolates from around the world tested by Engler et al. showed reduced susceptibility to macrolides and ketolides (58).

Growth characteristics among the *Corynebacterium* spp. may vary, and previous studies have used a variety of methods, media, and incubation conditions for antimicrobial susceptibility testing. Prior to the publication of CLSI M45, the absence of interpretive criteria specifically for *Corynebacterium* spp. led to inconsistencies in interpreting results when CLSI interpretive criteria for other gram-positive organisms (e.g., streptococci and staphylococci) were applied (58, 70, 127, 206). CLSI recommends broth microdilution with CAMHB-LHB and incubation in ambient air (Table 3). Some strains grow satisfactorily after 24 h of incubation, but others need 48 h. The 48 h is particularly important for detecting resistance to β-lactams, and it is recommended, if growth is not satisfactory or if an isolate appears susceptible to β-lactams at 24 h, that the test be reincubated and final results be read after 48 h of incubation (38). Currently, disk diffusion testing of *Corynebacterium* spp. is not recommended by CLSI. Several investigators have used E test satisfactorily for testing *Corynebacterium* spp. (215), and Engler et al. used E test to confirm the reduced susceptibility to macrolides and ketolides that was initially identified by agar dilution testing of *C. diphtheriae* (58). Susceptibility testing of *Corynebacterium* spp. is warranted when the organisms are isolated from normally sterile sites.

ERYSIPELOTHRIX RHUSIOPATHIAE

Erysipelothrix rhusiopathiae is an intrinsically vancomycin-resistant gram-positive bacillus. Other agents that have little to no activity against isolates of this species are aminoglycosides and TMP-SMX. Antimicrobial susceptibility studies of isolates from a number of sources have shown all isolates of *E. rhusiopathiae* to be susceptible to penicillins, cephalosporins, carbapenems, and fluoroquinolones (66, 79, 189, 202, 209). Resistance to clindamycin, erythromycin, and tetracycline does occur. In one study of 214 isolates from pigs and swine in Japan the occurrence of resistance was as follows: erythromycin, 2%; clindamycin, 1%; and tetracycline, 53% (209). The tetracycline-resistant isolates were positive for *tet*M (210).

Isolates of *E. rhusiopathiae* are slightly fastidious, so CAMHB-LHB is recommended for broth microdilution MIC testing (38). There are also reports of agar dilution using either MHA supplemented with 5% horse blood or unsupplemented MHA (66, 189, 209).

HACEK GROUP

There are limited antimicrobial susceptibility test data on the HACEK organisms (i.e., *Haemophilus*, *Actinobacillus*, *Cardiobacterium*, *Eikenella*, and *Kingella* spp.) in part because these organisms are infrequently encountered and often difficult to grow. Members of HACEK are susceptible to extended-spectrum cephalosporins and fluoroquinolones and are often susceptible in vitro to ampicillin and penicillin (10, 43, 61, 125). Occasional isolates of *Cardiobacterium hominis*, *Eikenella corrodens*, and *Kingella* spp. produce β-lactamase (75, 128, 132, 181); however, β-lactamase production in *Actinobacillus actinomycetemcomitans* has not been documented (133, 156). Recent American Heart Association recommendations for treatment of patients with endocarditis caused by HACEK organisms suggest that because of difficulties in performing antimicrobial susceptibility testing and potential failure to identify ampicillin-resistant strains, HACEK organisms should be considered ampicillin resistant and ampicillin should not be used for patients with endocarditis due to HACEK organisms (10).

Broth microdilution with CAMHB-LHB can be used for testing HACEK organisms. Some isolates may require 48 h of incubation to obtain adequate growth as evidenced by substantial turbidity in the positive growth control well. Some isolates may not grow satisfactorily in CAMHB-LHB. Susceptibility testing may be warranted for isolates from normally sterile sites, and β-lactamase testing should be performed on HACEK isolates (38).

LACTOBACILLUS, PEDIOCOCCUS, AND *LEUCONOSTOC* SPECIES

Lactobacillus spp., *Pediococcus* spp., and *Leuconostoc* spp. are intrinsically vancomycin-resistant gram-positive bacteria. It is important to note that some species of *Lactobacillus* are vancomycin susceptible; they include *L. gasseri*, *L. delbrueckii*, *L. casei*, *L. paracasei*, *and L. acidophilus* (46). Isolates of all three genera are susceptible to penicillin, ampicillin, and amoxicillin (42, 44, 187, 211), but their susceptibility to cephalosporins is variable. For example, in one study the ceftriaxone MIC ranges were as follows: *Leuconostoc*, ≤0.25 to 128 μg/ml ($n = 47$); *Pediococcus*, ≤0.25 to 16 μg/ml ($n = 24$); and *Lactobacillus*, 1 to >128 μg/ml ($n = 13$) (187). Most isolates are susceptible to carbapenems, but isolates with elevated imipenem MICs (>0.5 μg/ml) have been reported for all three genera (42, 76, 187, 211). There is one report of an imipenem therapeutic failure for a central nervous system infection due to *Leuconostoc* with an imipenem MIC of 4 μg/ml (48). Ciprofloxacin has little activity for all three genera. In a report by Swenson et al. (187) the ciprofloxacin MIC_{90} of *Leuconostoc* and *Lactobacillus* isolates was 4 μg/ml, and for *Pediococcus* the MIC_{90} was 16 μg/ml. Isolates of *Lactobacillus* and *Leuconostoc* are susceptible to clindamycin and erythromycin, but isolates of *Pediococcus* can be resistant to both agents (187, 211). Gentamicin, which may be used in combination therapy, has good activity against isolates of all three genera. In one study, the MIC_{90} was 0.5 μg/ml for *Lactobacillus* and *Leuconostoc* and 2 μg/ml for *Pediococcus* (187).

The medium recommended by CLSI for broth microdilution testing of *Lactobacillus* spp., *Pediococcus* spp., and *Leuconostoc* spp. is CAMHB-LHB (Table 3). There are several reports of susceptibility testing by agar dilution using either unsupplemented MHA or MHA with 5% sheep blood (42, 44, 76). If testing by agar dilution, incubation in air with 5% CO_2 may be necessary to achieve sufficient growth.

L. MONOCYTOGENES

Clinical isolates of *L. monocytogenes* remain susceptible to the drugs of choice including ampicillin (or penicillin) and TMP-SMX. With the exception of occasional resistance to tetracyclines (31), *L. monocytogenes* is typically susceptible in vitro to other agents active against gram-positive bacteria, including chloramphenicol, vancomycin, and macrolides (84, 135, 137, 176); however, these have not proved to be as useful in vivo as the aforementioned agents (94, 103). Although *L. monocytogenes* may appear susceptible to cephalosporins in vitro, these agents are not effective clinically.

Listeria infections are generally treated empirically, and antimicrobial susceptibility testing is usually not necessary. Only criteria for susceptibility (MIC, ≤2.0 μg/ml) are listed for ampicillin and penicillin in CLSI guidelines because clinical isolates of *L. monocytogenes* have not been noted to have results other than those indicating susceptibility (38). *L. monocytogenes* is not truly fastidious, and testing in Mueller-Hinton broth without the blood supplement has been done satisfactorily (137). However, CLSI recommends using CAMHB-LHB. It is important to remember that cephalosporins should not be tested or reported for *L. monocytogenes* as these results might indicate false susceptibility (5). This cautionary note is emphasized in CLSI documents (38) and illustrates why it is inappropriate to indiscriminately report susceptibility results for any agent without knowing if it would be a reasonable therapeutic option. Because cephalosporins are frequently used empirically for the treatment of meningitis, the laboratory should quickly communicate smear or culture findings suspicious for *Listeria* whenever they occur.

M. CATARRHALIS

More than 90% of *M. catarrhalis* isolates produce β-lactamase (15, 63, 93, 100, 102, 183, 217) and are resistant to amoxicillin, ampicillin, and penicillin. These isolates remain susceptible to amoxicillin-clavulanic acid, which is often prescribed for *M. catarrhalis* infections. Most clinical isolates produce one of two types of chromosomally mediated β-lactamases: BRO-1 or BRO-2 (112, 148, 168). BRO-1-producing strains are 10-fold or more prevalent than BRO-2-producing strains, and ampicillin and penicillin MICs for BRO-1 strains appear to be higher (e.g., ≥4.0 μg/ml) than those for BRO-2 strains (e.g., ≤0.5 μg/ml) (51, 112, 168). Because of the low MICs for the latter strains, their clinical significance in response to β-lactamase-labile penicillins is questionable. Resistance rates for TMP-SMX are low in most studies (69, 93, 217); however, Johnson et al. reported over 10% resistance in isolates from Latin America (102). Resistance to the other recommended drugs for treating *M. catarrhalis* infections remains less than 1% (63, 69, 93, 102, 183, 217).

Only the chromogenic cephalosporin method has reliably detected the β-lactamases produced by *M. catarrhalis* (55). Routine β-lactamase testing may not be necessary because of the high incidence of β-lactamase-positive strains. Nevertheless, some advocate reporting of β-lactamase results to highlight the fact that this pathogen is generally unresponsive to some agents (e.g., amoxicillin) commonly prescribed for the treatment of respiratory tract infections. MIC testing without β-lactamase testing can be problematic as there is some overlap in ampicillin and amoxicillin MICs in β-lactamase-positive and -negative strains (168). Since *M. catarrhalis* typically responds to the drugs of choice, testing beyond the β-lactamase test is rarely indicated (38). CLSI document M45-P addresses MIC testing of *M. catarrhalis*, and the recommended test medium is CAMHB (Table 3). Despite the lack of disk diffusion testing recommendations, Doern and Tubert (55) demonstrated that disk diffusion interpretive criteria for nonfastidious bacteria published by NCCLS in 1984 appear to be satisfactory, at least as they pertain to the susceptible category for amoxicillin-clavulanic acid, cephalothin, chloramphenicol, erythromycin, tetracycline, and TMP-SMX (149). However, because of the absence of frank resistance to these agents among the 74 clinical isolates examined, the investigators were unable to make definitive recommendations pertaining to disk diffusion testing.

PASTEURELLA SPECIES

Human isolates of *Pasteurella* spp. are generally susceptible to penicillin with MICs ≤0.5 μg/ml (36, 77, 144); however, β-lactamase production in an isolate from a respiratory tract infection has been documented. β-Lactamase was detected with the nitrocefin-impregnated disk method, and the isolate had an amoxicillin MIC of 8 μg/ml and an amoxicillin-clavulanic acid MIC of 0.25 μg/ml (131). *Pasteurella* spp. are generally very susceptible to many other antimicrobial agents, and no resistance has been documented for parenteral cephalosporins, quinolones, tetracyclines, chloramphenicol, or TMP-SMX (36, 77, 144). Resistance to erythromycin can occur, and there is at least one report of failure of erythromycin to cure a cat bite victim who went on to develop meningitis (129).

Broth microdilution and disk diffusion methods are described by CLSI for testing *Pasteurella* spp. (Table 3). Due to the absence of nonsusceptible strains, there are only susceptible interpretive criteria for agents that might be tested, with the exception of erythromycin. Susceptibility testing may be warranted for isolates from normally sterile sites, and β-lactamase testing should be done on these isolates as well as those from respiratory sources (38). Testing of isolates from bite wounds is not necessary since bite wound infections are generally treated empirically with agents that would cover a variety of organisms likely to be implicated in the infection.

VIBRIO SPECIES (NOT *V. CHOLERAE*)

The non-cholera *Vibrio* spp. are generally susceptible to most antimicrobial agents, including newer cephalosporins, aminoglycosides, fluoroquinolones, and tetracyclines; however, as with other organisms, resistance to one or more of these can occur (33, 35, 134, 153, 190). One study noted ampicillin resistance for 5 of 6 environmental isolates of *Vibrio vulnificus* (214), but Chuang et al. recently reported that all 42 clinical isolates of *V. vulnificus* were ampicillin susceptible (35). Chuang et al. also demonstrated synergistic killing of *V. vulnificus* with a combination of minocycline and cefotaxime (35), and this finding has contributed to current recommendations for treating *V. vulnificus* infections with doxycycline and ceftazidime (74).

Although the non-cholera *Vibrio* spp. cause diarrheal disease, otherwise healthy individuals with diarrhea due to these bacteria usually recover spontaneously without treatment. When *Vibrio* spp. are isolated from sources associated with serious infections, antimicrobial susceptibility testing of them is warranted (33, 134). CLSI suggests use of broth microdilution or disk diffusion. For testing of these halophilic organisms, some have suggested use of MHA containing 1% NaCl. However, CLSI recommends preparation of the inoculum suspension in 0.85% NaCl solution for both disk diffusion and broth microdilution MIC testing with unsupplemented MHA or CAMHB, respectively (38).

CONCLUSION

Infections caused by many of the fastidious bacteria discussed in this chapter are treated empirically as these bacteria are often susceptible to the drugs of choice. Consequently, susceptibility testing is infrequently needed. In certain circumstances testing may be warranted, such as when there appears to be clinical failure, patient intolerance to the drug(s) of choice, or serious infections for which there are several appropriate drugs that might be prescribed. Additionally, susceptibility testing may aid in species identification (e.g., differentiating *C. jeikeium* from other *Corynebacterium* species). If a physician seems unsure about requesting antimicrobial susceptibility testing on a fastidious organism, he/she should be encouraged to seek assistance from an infectious diseases clinician or pharmacist.

The E test has been examined for testing a variety of fastidious bacteria. For the less common species, many of the data generated have been obtained from comparisons with nonstandardized in vitro test methods with limited examination of the clinical correlation of the results. Consequently, the results for E test should be interpreted with caution in the clinical setting. Requests for susceptibility testing of fastidious bacteria are often for isolates associated with serious infections, and MIC results are likely to be more useful than qualitative results. The disk diffusion test should be used only for bacteria for which there are CLSI interpretive criteria. It is important for laboratory workers to maintain an awareness of the methods available for testing fastidious bacteria and their strengths and limitations. If testing must be performed, it should be done by a laboratory familiar with these limitations.

REFERENCES

1. **Abadi, F. J., D. E. Yakubu, and T. H. Pennington.** 1995. Antimicrobial susceptibility of penicillin-sensitive and penicillin-resistant meningococci. *J. Antimicrob. Chemother.* **35:**687–690.
2. **Ahmed, R., T. Hassall, B. Morland, and J. Gray.** 2003. Viridans streptococcus bacteremia in children on chemotherapy for cancer: an underestimated problem. *Pediatr. Hematol. Oncol.* **20:**439–444.
3. **Alcaide, F., J. Liñares, R. Pallares, J. Carratala, M. A. Benitez, F. Gudiol, and R. Martin.** 1995. In vitro activities of 22 beta-lactam antibiotics against penicillin-resistant and penicillin-susceptible viridans group streptococci isolated from blood. *Antimicrob. Agents Chemother.* **39:**2243–2247.
4. **Alcala, B., C. Salcedo, L. de la Fuente, L. Arreaza, M. J. Uria, R. Abad, R. Enriquez, J. A. Vazquez, M. Motge, and J. de Batlle.** 2004. *Neisseria meningitidis* showing decreased susceptibility to ciprofloxacin: first report in Spain. *J. Antimicrob. Chemother.* **53:**409.
5. **Allerberger, F. J., and M. P. Dierich.** 1992. Listeriosis and cephalosporins. *Clin. Infect. Dis.* **15:**177–178.
6. **Anderegg, T. R., H. S. Sader, T. R. Fritsche, J. E. Ross, and R. N. Jones.** 2005. Trends in linezolid susceptibility patterns: report from the 2002–2003 worldwide Zyvox Annual Appraisal of Potency and Spectrum (ZAAPS) Program. *Int. J. Antimicrob. Agents* **26:**13–21.
7. **Andrews, J. M., and R. Wise.** 2002. Susceptibility testing of *Bacillus* species. *J. Antimicrob. Chemother.* **49:**1040–1042.
8. **Aplasca De Los Reyes, M. R., V. Pato-Mesola, J. D. Klausner, R. Manalastas, T. Wi, C. U. Tuazon, G. Dallabetta, W. L. Whittington, and K. K. Holmes.** 2001. A randomized trial of ciprofloxacin versus cefixime for treatment of gonorrhea after rapid emergence of gonococcal ciprofloxacin resistance in The Philippines. *Clin. Infect. Dis.* **32:**1313–1318.
9. **Avison, M. B., P. M. Bennett, and T. R. Walsh.** 2000. beta-Lactamase expression in *Plesiomonas shigelloides*. *J. Antimicrob. Chemother.* **45:**877–880.
10. **Baddour, L. M., W. R. Wilson, A. S. Bayer, V. G. Fowler, Jr., A. F. Bolger, M. E. Levison, P. Ferrieri, M. A. Gerber, L. Y. Tani, M. H. Gewitz, D. C. Tong, J. M. Steckelberg, R. S. Baltimore, S. T. Shulman, J. C. Burns, D. A. Falace, J. W. Newburger, T. J. Pallasch, M. Takahashi, and K. A. Taubert.** 2005. Infective endocarditis: diagnosis, antimicrobial therapy, and management of complications: a statement for healthcare professionals from the Committee on Rheumatic Fever, Endocarditis, and Kawasaki Disease, Council on Cardiovascular Disease in the Young, and the Councils on Clinical Cardiology, Stroke, and Cardiovascular Surgery and Anesthesia, American Heart Association: endorsed by the Infectious Diseases Society of America. *Circulation* **111:**e394–e434.
11. **Baker, C. N.** 1992. The E-Test and *Campylobacter jejuni*. *Diagn. Microbiol. Infect. Dis.* **15:**469–472.
12. **Baker, C. N., D. G. Hollis, and C. Thornsberry.** 1985. Antimicrobial susceptibility testing of *Francisella tularensis* with a modified Mueller-Hinton broth. *J. Clin. Microbiol.* **22:**212–215.
13. **Barry, A. L., P. C. Fuchs, and M. A. Pfaller.** 1993. Susceptibilities of β-lactamase-producing and -nonproducing ampicillin-resistant strains of *Haemophilus influenzae* to ceftibuten, cefaclor, cefuroxime, cefixime, cefotaxime, and amoxicillin/clavulanic acid. *Antimicrob. Agents Chemother.* **37:**14–18.
14. **Baykam, N., H. Esener, O. Ergonul, S. Eren, A. K. Celikbas, and B. Dokuzoguz.** 2004. In vitro antimicrobial susceptibility of *Brucella* species. *Int. J. Antimicrob. Agents* **23:**405–407.
15. **Beekmann, S. E., K. P. Heilmann, S. S. Richter, J. Garcia-de-Lomas, and G. V. Doern.** 2005. Antimicrobial resistance in *Streptococcus pneumoniae, Haemophilus influenzae, Moraxella catarrhalis* and group A beta-haemolytic streptococci in 2002–2003. Results of the multinational GRASP Surveillance Program. *Int. J. Antimicrob. Agents* **25:**148–156.
16. **Best, L. M., D. J. Haldane, M. Keelan, D. E. Taylor, A. B. Thomson, V. Loo, C. A. Fallone, P. Lyn, F. M. Smaill, R. Hunt, C. Gaudreau, J. Kennedy, M. Alfa, R. Pelletier, and S. J. Veldhuyzen Van Zanten.** 2003. Multilaboratory

comparison of proficiencies in susceptibility testing of *Helicobacter pylori* and correlation between agar dilution and E test methods. *Antimicrob. Agents Chemother.* **47:**3138–3144.

17. **Betriu, C., M. Gomez, A. Sanchez, A. Cruceyra, J. Romero, and J. J. Picazo.** 1994. Antibiotic resistance and penicillin tolerance in clinical isolates of group B streptococci. *Antimicrob. Agents Chemother.* **38:**2183–2186.
18. **Biedenbach, D. J., and R. N. Jones.** 1996. Comparative assessment of E test for testing susceptibilities of *Neisseria gonorrhoeae* to penicillin, tetracycline, ceftriaxone, cefotaxime, and ciprofloxacin: investigation using 510(k) review criteria, recommended by the Food and Drug Administration. *J. Clin. Microbiol.* **34:**3214–3217.
19. **Block, C., Y. Davidson, and N. Keller.** 1998. Unreliability of disc diffusion test for screening for reduced penicillin susceptibility in *Neisseria meningitidis*. *J. Clin. Microbiol.* **36:** 3103–3104.
20. **Botha, P.** 1988. Penicillin-resistant *Neisseria meningitidis* in southern Africa. *Lancet* **i:**54.
21. **Bouchillon, S. K., J. L. Johnson, D. J. Hoban, T. M. Stevens, and B. M. Johnson.** 2005. Impact of carbon dioxide on the susceptibility of key respiratory tract pathogens to telithromycin and azithromycin. *J. Antimicrob. Chemother.* **56:**224–227.
22. **Bouvet, A., A. C. Cremieux, A. Contrepois, J. M. Vallois, C. Lamesch, and C. Carbon.** 1985. Comparison of penicillin and vancomycin, individually and in combination with gentamicin and amikacin, in the treatment of experimental endocarditis induced by nutritionally variant streptococci. *Antimicrob. Agents Chemother.* **28:**607–611.
23. **Bradley, J. S., and J. D. Connor.** 1991. Ceftriaxone failure in meningitis caused by *Streptococcus pneumoniae* with reduced susceptibility to beta-lactam antibiotics. *Pediatr. Infect. Dis. J.* **10:**871–873.
24. **Brown, S. D., D. J. Farrell, and I. Morrissey.** 2004. Prevalence and molecular analysis of macrolide and fluoroquinolone resistance among isolates of *Streptococcus pneumoniae* collected during the 2000–2001 PROTEKT US Study. *J. Clin. Microbiol.* **42:**4980–4987.
25. **Brown, S. D., and M. J. Rybak.** 2004. Antimicrobial susceptibility of *Streptococcus pneumoniae, Streptococcus pyogenes* and *Haemophilus influenzae* collected from patients across the USA, in 2001–2002, as part of the PROTEKT US study. *J. Antimicrob. Chemother.* **54**(Suppl. 1)**:**i7–15.
26. **Buu-Hoi, A., C. Le Bouguenec, and T. Horaud.** 1990. High-level chromosomal gentamicin resistance in *Streptococcus agalactiae* (group B). *Antimicrob. Agents Chemother.* **34:**985–988.
27. **Campos, J., G. Trujillo, T. Seuba, and A. Rodriguez.** 1992. Discriminative criteria for *Neisseria meningitidis* isolates that are moderately susceptible to penicillin and ampicillin. *Antimicrob. Agents Chemother.* **36:**1028–1031.
28. **Centers for Disease Control and Prevention.** 2001. Update: interim recommendations for antimicrobial prophylaxis for children and breastfeeding mothers and treatment of children with anthrax. *Morb. Mortal. Wkly. Rep.* **50:**1014–1016.
29. **Centers for Disease Control and Prevention.** 2004. *Sexually Transmitted Disease Surveillance 2003 Supplement: Gonococcal Isolate Surveillance Project (GISP) Annual Report—2003.* U.S. Department of Health and Human Services, Public Health Services, Atlanta, Ga.
30. **Centers for Disease Control and Prevention.** 2002. Sexually transmitted diseases treatment guidelines. *Morb. Mortal. Wkly. Rep.* **51**(No. RR-6)**:**1–80.
31. **Charpentier, E., and P. Courvalin.** 1999. Antibiotic resistance in *Listeria* spp. *Antimicrob. Agents Chemother.* **43:** 2103–2108.
32. **Chen, Y., J. Succi, F. C. Tenover, and T. M. Koehler.** 2003. Beta-lactamase genes of the penicillin-susceptible *Bacillus anthracis* Sterne strain. *J. Bacteriol.* **185:**823–830.
33. **Chiang, S. R., and Y. C. Chuang.** 2003. *Vibrio vulnificus* infection: clinical manifestations, pathogenesis, and antimicrobial therapy. *J. Microbiol. Immunol. Infect.* **36:**81–88.
34. **Choe, C. H., S. S. Bouhaouala, I. Brook, T. B. Elliot, and G. B. Knudson.** 2000. In vitro development of resistance to ofloxacin and doxycycline in *Bacillus anthracis* Sterne. *Antimicrob. Agents Chemother.* **44:**1766.
35. **Chuang, Y. C., J. W. Liu, W. C. Ko, K. Y. Lin, J. J. Wu, and K. Y. Huang.** 1997. In vitro synergism between cefotaxime and minocycline against *Vibrio vulnificus*. *Antimicrob. Agents Chemother.* **41:**2214–2217.
36. **Citron, D. M., Y. A. Warren, H. T. Fernandez, M. A. Goldstein, K. L. Tyrrell, and E. J. Goldstein.** 2005. Broth microdilution and disk diffusion tests for susceptibility testing of *Pasteurella* species isolated from human clinical specimens. *J. Clin. Microbiol.* **43:**2485–2488.
37. **Clark, R. B., P. D. Lister, L. Arneson-Rotert, and J. M. Janda.** 1990. In vitro susceptibilities of *Plesiomonas shigelloides* to 24 antibiotics and antibiotic-beta-lactamase-inhibitor combinations. *Antimicrob. Agents Chemother.* **34:** 159–160.
38. **Clinical and Laboratory Standards Institute/NCCLS.** 2005. *Methods for Antimicrobial Dilution and Disk Susceptibility Testing of Infrequently-Isolated or Fastidious Bacteria.* Proposed guideline M45-P. CLSI, Wayne, Pa.
39. **Clinical and Laboratory Standards Institute/NCCLS.** 2006. *Methods for Dilution Antimicrobial Susceptibility Tests for Bacteria That Grow Aerobically,* 7th ed. Approved standard M7-A7. CLSI, Wayne, Pa.
40. **Clinical and Laboratory Standards Institute/NCCLS.** 2006. *Performance Standards for Antimicrobial Disk Susceptibility Tests,* 9th ed. Approved standard M2-A9. CLSI, Wayne, Pa.
41. **Clinical and Laboratory Standards Institute/NCCLS.** 2006. *Performance Standards for Antimicrobial Susceptibility Testing.* Sixteenth informational supplement. M100-S16. CLSI, Wayne, Pa.
42. **Collins, L. A., G. J. Malanoski, G. M. Eliopoulos, C. B. Wennersten, M. J. Ferraro, and R. C. Moellering, Jr.** 1993. In vitro activity of RP59500, an injectable streptogramin antibiotic, against vancomycin-resistant gram-positive organisms. *Antimicrob. Agents Chemother.* **37:**598–601.
43. **Cormican, M. G., and R. N. Jones.** 1995. Antimicrobial activity of cefotaxime tested against infrequently isolated pathogenic species (unusual pathogens). *Diagn. Microbiol. Infect. Dis.* **22:**43–48.
44. **de la Maza, L., K. L. Ruoff, and M. J. Ferraro.** 1989. In vitro activities of daptomycin and other antimicrobial agents against vancomycin-resistant gram-positive bacteria. *Antimicrob. Agents Chemother.* **33:**1383–1384.
45. **De Mouy, D., J. Cavallo, R. LeClercq, R. Fabre, and T. A.-B. Network.** 2001. Antibiotic susceptibility and mechanisms of erythromycin resistance in clinical isolates of *Streptococcus agalactiae*: French multicenter study. *Antimicrob. Agents Chemother.* **45:**2400–2402.
46. **Delgado, S., A. B. Florez, and B. Mayo.** 2005. Antibiotic susceptibility of *Lactobacillus* and *Bifidobacterium* species from the human gastrointestinal tract. *Curr. Microbiol.* **50:** 202–207.
47. **Desjardins, M., K. L. Delgaty, K. Ramotar, C. Seetaram, and B. Toye.** 2004. Prevalence and mechanisms of erythromycin resistance in group A and group B *Streptococcus*: implications for reporting susceptibility results. *J. Clin. Microbiol.* **42:**5620–5623.
48. **Deye, G., J. Lewis, J. Patterson, and J. Jorgensen.** 2003. A case of *Leuconostoc* ventriculitis with resistance to carbapenem antibiotics. *Clin. Infect. Dis.* **37:**869–870.
49. **Dillon, J., and K. H. Yeung.** 1989. Beta-lactamase plasmids and chromosomally-mediated antibiotic resistance in pathogenic *Neisseria* species. *Clin. Microbiol. Rev.* **2**(Suppl.)**:** S125–S133.

50. **Dillon, J. R., M. Pauze, and K. H. Yeung.** 1983. Spread of penicillinase-producing and transfer plasmids from the gonococcus to *Neisseria meningitidis*. *Lancet* **i:**779–781.
51. **Doern, G. V.** 1986. *Branhamella catarrhalis*, an emerging human pathogen. *Diagn. Microbiol. Infect. Dis.* **4:**191–201.
52. **Doern, G. V., and S. D. Brown.** 2004. Antimicrobial susceptibility among community-acquired respiratory tract pathogens in the USA: data from PROTEKT US 2000-01. *J. Infect.* **48:**56–65.
53. **Doern, G. V., A. Brueggemann, and G. Pierce.** 1997. Assessment of the oxacillin disk screening test for determining penicillin resistance in *Streptococcus pneumoniae*. *Eur. J. Clin. Microbiol. Infect. Dis.* **16:**311–314.
54. **Doern, G. V., K. P. Heilmann, H. K. Huyni, P. R. Rhomberg, S. L. Coffman, and A. B. Brueggemann.** 2001. Antimicrobial resistance among clinical isolates of *Streptococcus pneumoniae* in the United States during 1999–2000, including a comparison of resistance rates since 1994–1995. *Antimicrob. Agents Chemother.* **45:**1721–1729.
55. **Doern, G. V., and T. A. Tubert.** 1987. Detection of β-lactamase activity among clinical isolates of *Branhamella catarrhalis* with six different β-lactamase assays. *J. Clin. Microbiol.* **25:**1380–1383.
56. **Doganay, M., and N. Aydin.** 1991. Antimicrobial susceptibility of *Bacillus anthracis*. *Scand. J. Infect. Dis.* **23:** 333–335.
57. **Engberg, J., F. M. Aarestrup, D. E. Taylor, P. Gerner-Smidt, and I. Nachamkin.** 2001. Quinolone and macrolide resistance in *Campylobacter jejuni* and *C. coli*: resistance mechanisms and trends in human isolates. *Emerg. Infect. Dis.* **7:**24–34.
58. **Engler, K. H., M. Warner, and R. C. George.** 2001. In vitro activity of ketolides HMR 3004 and HMR 3647 and seven other antimicrobial agents against *Corynebacterium diphtheriae*. *J. Antimicrob. Chemother.* **47:**27–31.
59. **Fangio, P., L. Desbouchages, J. C. Lacherade, B. De Jonghe, J. P. Terville, M. Leneveu, and H. Outin.** 2005. *Neisseria meningitidis* C:2b:P1.2,5 with decreased susceptibility to penicillin isolated from a patient with meningitis and purpura fulminans. *Eur. J. Clin. Microbiol. Infect. Dis.* **24:**140–141.
60. **Farrell, D. J., I. Morrissey, S. Bakker, S. Buckridge, and D. Felmingham.** 2005. Global distribution of TEM-1 and ROB-1 {beta}-lactamases in *Haemophilus influenzae*. *J. Antimicrob. Chemother.* **56:**773–776.
61. **Feder, H. M., Jr., J. C. Roberts, J. C. Salazar, H. B. Leopold, and O. Toro-Salazar.** 2003. HACEK endocarditis in infants and children: two cases and a literature review. *Pediatr. Infect. Dis. J.* **22:**557–562.
62. **Feldman, C.** 2004. Clinical relevance of antimicrobial resistance in the management of pneumococcal community-acquired pneumonia. *J. Lab. Clin. Med.* **143:**269–283.
63. **Felmingham, D.** 2004. Comparative antimicrobial susceptibility of respiratory tract pathogens. *Chemotherapy* **50** (Suppl. 1)**:**3–10.
64. **Felmingham, D., and R. N. Gruneberg.** 2000. The Alexander Project 1996-1997: latest susceptibility data from this international study of bacterial pathogens from community-acquired lower respiratory tract infections. *J. Antimicrob. Chemother.* **45:**191–203.
65. **Fernandez-Natal, I., J. Guerra, M. Alcoba, F. Cachon, and F. Soriano.** 2001. Bacteremia caused by multiply resistant *Corynebacterium urealyticum:* six case reports and review. *Eur. J. Clin. Microbiol. Infect. Dis.* **20:**514–517.
66. **Fidalgo, S. G., C. J. Longbottom, and T. V. Rjley.** 2002. Susceptibility of *Erysipelothrix rhusiopathiae* to antimicrobial agents and home disinfectants. *Pathology* **34:**462–465.
67. **Fontanals, D., V. Pineda, I. Pons, and J. C. Rojo.** 1989. Penicillin-resistant beta-lactamase-producing *Neisseria meningitidis* in Spain. *Eur. J. Clin. Microbiol. Infect. Dis.* **8:**90–91.
68. **Friedland, I. R.** 1995. Comparison of the response to antimicrobial therapy of penicillin-resistant and penicillin-susceptible pneumococcal disease. *Ped. Infect. Dis. J.* **14:**885–890.
69. **Fritsche, T. R., J. T. Kirby, and R. N. Jones.** 2004. In vitro activity of tigecycline (GAR-936) tested against 11,859 recent clinical isolates associated with community-acquired respiratory tract and gram-positive cutaneous infections. *Diagn. Microbiol. Infect. Dis.* **49:**201–209.
70. **Funke, G., V. Punter, and A. von Graevenitz.** 1996. Antimicrobial susceptibility patterns of some recently established coryneform bacteria. *Antimicrob. Agents Chemother.* **40:**2874–2878.
71. **Galimand, M., A. Guiyoule, G. Gerbaud, B. Rasoamanana, S. Chanteau, E. Carniel, and P. Courvalin.** 1997. Multidrug resistance in *Yersinia pestis* mediated by a transferable plasmid. *N. Engl. J. Med.* **337:**677–680.
72. **Gaudreau, C., and H. Gilbert.** 1997. Comparison of disc diffusion and agar dilution methods for antibiotic susceptibility testing of *Campylobacter jejuni* subsp. *jejuni* and *Campylobacter coli*. *J. Antimicrob. Chemother.* **39:**707–712.
73. **Gephart, J. F., and J. A. Washington, 2nd.** 1982. Antimicrobial susceptibilities of nutritionally variant streptococci. *J. Infect. Dis.* **146:**536–539.
74. **Gilbert, D. N., R. C. Moellering, Jr., G. M. Eliopoulos, and M. A. Sande.** 2005. *The Sanford Guide to Antimicrobial Therapy*, 35th ed. Antimicrobial Therapy, Inc., Hyde Park, Vt.
75. **Goldstein, E. J., D. M. Citron, C. V. Merriam, Y. A. Warren, K. L. Tyrrell, and H. Fernandez.** 2002. In vitro activities of a new des-fluoroquinolone, BMS 284756, and seven other antimicrobial agents against 151 isolates of *Eikenella corrodens*. *Antimicrob. Agents Chemother.* **46:**1141–1143.
76. **Goldstein, E. J., D. M. Citron, C. V. Merriam, Y. A. Warren, K. L. Tyrrell, and H. T. Fernandez.** 2003. In vitro activities of daptomycin, vancomycin, quinupristin-dalfopristin, linezolid, and five other antimicrobials against 307 gram-positive anaerobic and 31 *Corynebacterium* clinical isolates. *Antimicrob. Agents Chemother.* **47:**337–341.
77. **Goldstein, E. J., D. M. Citron, C. V. Merriam, Y. A. Warren, K. L. Tyrrell, and H. T. Fernandez.** 2002. In vitro activities of garenoxacin (BMS-284756) against 170 clinical isolates of nine *Pasteurella* species. *Antimicrob. Agents Chemother.* **46:**3068–3070.
78. **Gonzalez-Rey, C., S. B. Svenson, L. Bravo, A. Siitonen, V. Pasquale, S. Dumontet, I. Ciznar, and K. Krovacek.** 2004. Serotypes and antimicrobial susceptibility of *Plesiomonas shigelloides* isolates from humans, animals and aquatic environments in different countries. *Comp. Immunol. Microbiol. Infect. Dis.* **27:**129–139.
79. **Gorby, G. L., and J. E. Peacock, Jr.** 1988. *Erysipelothrix rhusiopathiae* endocarditis: microbiologic, epidemiologic, and clinical features of an occupational disease. *Rev. Infect. Dis.* **10:**317–325.
80. **Grzybowska, W., S. Tyski, L. Berthelsen, and I. Lind.** 2001. Cluster analysis of *Neisseria meningitidis* type 22 strains isolated in Poland. *Eur. J. Clin. Microbiol. Infect. Dis.* **20:**243–247.
81. **Guiyoule, A., G. Gerbaud, C. Buchrieser, M. Galimand, L. Rahalison, S. Chanteau, P. Courvalin, and E. Carniel.** 2001. Transferable plasmid-mediated resistance to streptomycin in a clinical isolate of *Yersinia pestis*. *Emerg. Infect. Dis.* **7:**43–48.
82. **Gupta, A., J. M. Nelson, T. J. Barrett, R. V. Tauxe, S. P. Rossiter, C. R. Friedman, K. W. Joyce, K. E. Smith, T. F. Jones, M. A. Hawkins, B. Shiferaw, J. L. Beebe, D. J. Vugia, T. Rabatsky-Ehr, J. A. Benson, T. P. Root, and F. J. Angulo.** 2004. Antimicrobial resistance among *Campylobacter* strains, United States, 1997–2001. *Emerg. Infect. Dis.* **10:**1102–1109.
83. **Guthrie, L., S. Banks, W. Setiawan, and K. B. Waites.** 1999. Comparison of MicroScan MICroSTREP, PASCO,

and Sensititre MIC panels for determining antimicrobial susceptibilities of *Streptococcus pneumoniae*. *Diagn. Microbiol. Infect. Dis.* **33**:267–273.

84. **Hansen, J. M., P. Gerner-Smidt, and B. Bruun.** 2005. Antibiotic susceptibility of *Listeria monocytogenes* in Denmark 1958-2001. *APMIS* **113**:31–36.
85. **Hansman, D., S. Wati, A. Lawrence, and J. Turnidge.** 2004. Have South Australian isolates of *Neisseria meningitidis* become less susceptible to penicillin, rifampicin and other drugs? A study of strains isolated over three decades, 1971–1999. *Pathology* **36**:160–165.
86. **Hasegawa, K., N. Chiba, R. Kobayashi, S. Y. Murayama, S. Iwata, K. Sunakawa, and K. Ubukata.** 2004. Rapidly increasing prevalence of beta-lactamase-nonproducing, ampicillin-resistant *Haemophilus influenzae* type b in patients with meningitis. *Antimicrob. Agents Chemother.* **48**: 1509–1514.
87. **Hayward, C. L., M. E. Erwin, M. S. Barrett, and R. N. Jones.** 1999. Comparative antimicrobial activity of gatifloxacin tested against *Campylobacter jejuni* including fluoroquinolone-resistant clinical isolates. *Diagn. Microbiol. Infect. Dis.* **34**:99–102.
88. **Heelan, J. S., D. Chesney, and G. Guadagno.** 1992. Investigation of ampicillin-intermediate strains of *Haemophilus influenzae* by using the disk diffusion procedure and current National Committee for Clinical Laboratory Standards guidelines. *J. Clin. Microbiol.* **30**:1674–1677.
89. **Heffelfinger, J. D., S. F. Dowell, J. H. Jorgensen, K. P. Klugman, L. R. Mabry, D. M. Musher, J. F. Plouffe, A. Rakowsky, A. Schuchat, C. G. Whitney, and The Drug-Resistant *Streptococcus pneumoniae* Therapeutic Working Group.** 2000. Management of community-acquired pneumonia in the era of pneumococcal resistance. *Arch. Intern. Med.* **160**:1399–1408.
90. **Heilmann, K. P., C. L. Rice, A. L. Miller, N. J. Miller, S. E. Beekmann, M. A. Pfaller, S. S. Richter, and G. V. Doern.** 2005. Decreasing prevalence of beta-lactamase production among respiratory tract isolates of *Haemophilus influenzae* in the United States. *Antimicrob. Agents Chemother.* **49**:2561–2564.
91. **Helms, M., J. Simonsen, K. E. Olsen, and K. Molbak.** 2005. Adverse health events associated with antimicrobial drug resistance in *Campylobacter* species: a registry-based cohort study. *J. Infect. Dis.* **191**:1050–1055.
92. **Ho, P. L., R. W. Yung, D. N. Tsang, T. L. Que, M. Ho, W. H. Seto, T. K. Ng, W. C. Yam, and W. W. Ng.** 2001. Increasing resistance of *Streptococcus pneumoniae* to fluoroquinolones: results of a Hong Kong multicentre study in 2000. *J. Antimicrob. Chemother.* **48**:659–665.
93. **Hoban, D. J., S. K. Bouchillon, J. L. Johnson, G. G. Zhanel, D. L. Butler, K. A. Saunders, L. A. Miller, and J. A. Poupard.** 2003. Comparative in vitro potency of amoxycillin-clavulanic acid and four oral agents against recent North American clinical isolates from a global surveillance study. *Int. J. Antimicrob. Agents* **21**:425–433.
94. **Hof, H.** 2003. Listeriosis: therapeutic options. *FEMS Immunol. Med. Microbiol.* **35**:203–205.
95. **Horodniceanu, T., A. Buu-Hoi, A. Delbos, and G. Bieth.** 1982. High-level aminoglycoside resistance in Group A, B, C, D (*Streptococcus bovis*), and viridans streptococci. *Antimicrob. Agents Chemother.* **21**:176–179.
96. **Ikaheimo, I., H. Syrjala, J. Karhukorpi, R. Schildt, and M. Koskela.** 2000. In vitro antibiotic susceptibility of *Francisella tularensis* isolated from humans and animals. *J. Antimicrob. Chemother.* **46**:287–290.
97. **Inglis, T. J. J., F. Rodrigues, P. Rigby, R. Norton, and B. J. Currie.** 2004. Comparison of the susceptibilities of *Burkholderia pseudomallei* to meropenem and ceftazidime by conventional and intracellular methods. *Antimicrob. Agents Chemother.* **48**:2999–3005.
98. **Inoue, M., N. Y. Lee, S. W. Hong, K. Lee, and D. Felmingham.** 2004. PROTEKT 1999–2000: a multicentre study of the antibiotic susceptibility of respiratory tract pathogens in Hong Kong, Japan and South Korea. *Int. J. Antimicrob. Agents* **23**:44–51.
99. **Jacobs, M. R.** 2004. *Streptococcus pneumoniae:* epidemiology and patterns of resistance. *Am. J. Med.* **117**(Suppl. 3A):3S–15S.
100. **Jacobs, M. R., S. Bajaksouzian, A. Windau, C. E. Good, G. Lin, G. A. Pankuch, and P. C. Appelbaum.** 2004. Susceptibility of *Streptococcus pneumoniae, Haemophilus influenzae,* and *Moraxella catarrhalis* to 17 oral antimicrobial agents based on pharmacodynamic parameters: 1998–2001 U S Surveillance Study. *Clin. Lab Med.* **24**: 503–530.
101. **Johnson, A. P., S. Mushtaq, M. Warner, and D. M. Livermore.** 2004. Activity of daptomycin against multiresistant Gram-positive bacteria including enterococci and *Staphylococcus aureus* resistant to linezolid. *Int. J. Antimicrob. Agents* **24**:315–319.
102. **Johnson, D. M., H. S. Sader, T. R. Fritsche, D. J. Biedenbach, and R. N. Jones.** 2003. Susceptibility trends of *Haemophilus influenzae* and *Moraxella catarrhalis* against orally administered antimicrobial agents: five-year report from the SENTRY Antimicrobial Surveillance Program. *Diagn. Microbiol. Infect. Dis.* **47**:373–376.
103. **Jones, E. M., and A. P. MacGowan.** 1995. Antimicrobial chemotherapy of human infection due to *Listeria monocytogenes*. *Eur. J. Clin. Microbiol. Infect. Dis.* **14**:165–175.
104. **Jones, M. E., R. S. Blosser-Middleton, C. Thornsberry, J. A. Karlowsky, and D. F. Sahm.** 2003. The activity of levofloxacin and other antimicrobials against clinical isolates of *Streptococcus pneumoniae* collected worldwide during 1999–2002. *Diagn. Microbiol. Infect. Dis.* **47**: 579–586.
105. **Jones, M. E., J. A. Karlowsky, D. C. Draghi, C. Thornsberry, D. F. Sahm, and J. S. Bradley.** 2004. Rates of antimicrobial resistance among common bacterial pathogens causing respiratory, blood, urine, and skin and soft tissue infections in pediatric patients. *Eur. J. Clin. Microbiol. Infect. Dis.* **23**:445–455.
106. **Jones, R., D. Johnson, M. Erwin, M. Beach, D. Biedenbach, and M. Pfaller.** 1999. Comparative antimicrobial activity of gatifloxacin tested against *Streptococcus* spp. including quality control guidelines and Etest method validation. *Diagn. Microbiol. Infect. Dis.* **34**:91–98.
107. **Jorgensen, J., M. McElmeel, and S. Crawford.** 1998. Evaluation of the Dade MicroScan MICroSTREP antimicrobial susceptibility testing panel with selected *Streptococcus pneumoniae* challenge strains and recent clinical isolates. *J. Clin. Microbiol.* **36**:788–791.
108. **Jorgensen, J. H., A. L. Barry, M. M. Traczewski, D. F. Sahm, M. L. McElmeel, and S. A. Crawford.** 2000. Rapid automated antimicrobial susceptibility testing of *Streptococcus pneumoniae* by use of the bioMerieux Vitek 2. *J. Clin. Microbiol.* **38**:2814–2818.
109. **Jorgensen, J. H., S. A. Crawford, and K. R. Fiebelkorn.** 2005. Susceptibility of *Neisseria meningitidis* to 16 antimicrobial agents and characterization of resistance mechanisms affecting some agents. *J. Clin. Microbiol.* **43**: 3162–3171.
110. **Jorgensen, J. H., M. J. Ferraro, M. L. McElmeel, J. Spargo, J. M. Swenson, and F. C. Tenover.** 1994. Detection of penicillin and extended-spectrum cephalosporin resistance among *Streptococcus pneumoniae* clinical isolates by use of the E Test. *J. Clin. Microbiol.* **32**:159–163.
111. **Jorgensen, J. H., A. W. Howell, and L. A. Maher.** 1991. Quantitative antimicrobial susceptibility testing of *Haemophilus influenzae* and *Streptococcus pneumoniae* by using the E test. *J. Clin. Microbiol.* **29**:109–114.

112. **Kadry, A. A., S. I. Fouda, N. A. Elkhizzi, and A. M. Shibl.** 2003. Correlation between susceptibility and BRO type enzyme of *Moraxella catarrhalis* strains. *Int. J. Antimicrob. Agents* **22:**532–536.
113. **Kain, K. C., and M. T. Kelly.** 1989. Antimicrobial susceptibility of *Plesiomonas shigelloides* from patients with diarrhea. *Antimicrob. Agents Chemother.* **33:**1609–1610.
114. **Karchmer, A. W.** 2004. Increased antibiotic resistance in respiratory tract pathogens: PROTEKT US—an update. *Clin. Infect. Dis.* **39**(Suppl. 3)**:**S142–S150.
115. **Karpanoja, P., A. Nissinen, P. Huovinen, and H. Sarkkinen.** 2004. Disc diffusion susceptibility testing of *Haemophilus influenzae* by NCCLS methodology using low-strength ampicillin and co-amoxiclav discs. *J. Antimicrob. Chemother.* **53:**660–663.
116. **Kato, M., Y. Yamaoka, J. J. Kim, R. Reddy, M. Asaka, K. Kashima, M. S. Osato, F. A. El-Zaatari, D. Y. Graham, and D. H. Kwon.** 2000. Regional differences in metronidazole resistance and increasing clarithromycin resistance among *Helicobacter pylori* isolates from Japan. *Antimicrob. Agents Chemother.* **44:**2214–2216.
117. **Kim, J. J., J. G. Kim, and D. H. Kwon.** 2003. Mixed-infection of antibiotic susceptible and resistant *Helicobacter pylori* isolates in a single patient and underestimation of antimicrobial susceptibility testing. *Helicobacter* **8:**202–206.
118. **Kim, J. J., R. Reddy, M. Lee, J. G. Kim, F. A. El-Zaatari, M. S. Osato, D. Y. Graham, and D. H. Kwon.** 2001. Analysis of metronidazole, clarithromycin and tetracycline resistance of *Helicobacter pylori* isolates from Korea. *J. Antimicrob. Chemother.* **47:**459–461.
119. **Kinsara, A., A. Al-Mowallad, and A. O. Osoba.** 1999. Increasing resistance of *Brucellae* to co-trimoxazole. *Antimicrob. Agents Chemother.* **43:**1531.
120. **Klugman, K. P., D. E. Low, J. Metlay, J.-C. Pechere, and K. Weiss.** 2004. Community-acquired pneumonia: new management strategies for evolving pathogens and antimicrobial susceptibilities. *Int. J. Antimicrob. Agents* **24:**411–422.
121. **Kneen, R., N. G. Pham, T. Solomon, T. M. Tran, T. T. Nguyen, B. L. Tran, J. Wain, N. P. Day, T. H. Tran, C. M. Parry, and N. J. White.** 1998. Penicillin vs. erythromycin in the treatment of diphtheria. *Clin. Infect. Dis.* **27:**845–850.
122. **Ko, W., K. Yu, C. Liu, C. Huang, H. Leu, and Y. Chuang.** 1996. Increasing antibiotic resistance in clinical isolates of *Aeromonas* strains in Taiwan. *Antimicrob. Agents Chemother.* **40:**1260–1262.
123. **Ko, W.-C., H.-M. Wu, T.-C. Chang, J.-J. Yan, and J.-J. Wu.** 1998. Inducible beta-lactam resistance in *Aeromonas hydrophila:* therapeutic challenge for antimicrobial therapy. *J. Clin. Microbiol.* **36:**3188–3192.
124. **Krcmery, V., Jr., S. Spanik, and J. Trupl.** 1996. First report of vancomycin-resistant *Streptococcus mitis* bacteremia in a leukemic patient after prophylaxis with quinolones and during treatment with vancomycin. *J. Chemother.* **8:**325–326.
125. **Kugler, K. C., D. J. Biedenbach, and R. N. Jones.** 1999. Determination of the antimicrobial activity of 29 clinically important compounds tested against fastidious HACEK group organisms. *Diagn. Microbiol. Infect. Dis.* **34:**73–76.
126. **Kusters, J. G., and E. J. Kuipers.** 2001. Antibiotic resistance of *Helicobacter pylori. Symp. Ser. Soc. Appl. Microbiol.* **2001:**134S–144S.
127. **Lagrou, K., J. Verhaegen, M. Janssens, G. Wauters, and L. Verbist.** 1998. Prospective study of catalase-positive coryneform organisms in clinical specimens: identification, clinical relevance, and antibiotic susceptibility. *Diagn. Microbiol. Infect. Dis.* **30:**7–15.
128. **Le Quellec, A., D. Bessis, C. Perez, and A. J. Ciurana.** 1994. Endocarditis due to beta-lactamase-producing *Cardiobacterium hominis. Clin. Infect. Dis.* **19:**994–995.
129. **Levin, J. M., and D. A. Talan.** 1990. Erythromycin failure with subsequent *Pasteurella multocida* meningitis and septic arthritis in a cat-bite victim. *Ann. Emerg. Med.* **19:**1458–1461.
130. **Lightfoot, N. F., R. J. D. Scott, and P. C. B. Turnbull.** 1990. Antimicrobial susceptibility of *Bacillus anthracis. Salisbury Med. Bull.* **68**(Suppl.)**:**95–98.
131. **Lion, C., A. Lozniewski, V. Rosner, and M. Weber.** 1999. Lung abscess due to beta-lactamase-producing *Pasteurella multocida. Clin. Infect. Dis.* **29:**1345–1346.
132. **Lu, P. L., P. R. Hsueh, C. C. Hung, L. J. Teng, T. N. Jang, and K. T. Luh.** 2000. Infective endocarditis complicated with progressive heart failure due to beta-lactamase-producing *Cardiobacterium hominis. J. Clin. Microbiol.* **38:**2015–2017.
133. **Madinier, I. M., T. B. Fosse, C. Hitzig, Y. Charbit, and L. R. Hannoun.** 1999. Resistance profile survey of 50 periodontal strains of *Actinobacillus actinomycetemcomitans. J. Periodontol.* **70:**888–892.
134. **Maluping, R. P., C. R. Lavilla-Pitogo, A. DePaola, J. M. Janda, K. Krovacek, and C. Greko.** 2005. Antimicrobial susceptibility of *Aeromonas* spp., *Vibrio* spp. and *Plesiomonas shigelloides* isolated in the Philippines and Thailand. *Int. J. Antimicrob. Agents* **25:**348–350.
135. **Marco, F., M. Almela, J. Nolla-Salas, P. Coll, I. Gasser, M. D. Ferrer, and M. de Simon.** 2000. In vitro activities of 22 antimicrobial agents against *Listeria monocytogenes* strains isolated in Barcelona, Spain. *Diagn. Microbiol. Infect. Dis.* **38:**259–261.
136. **Marshall, S. A., P. R. Rhomberg, and R. N. Jones.** 1997. Comparative evaluation of E test for susceptibility testing *Neisseria meningitidis* with eight antimicrobial agents. An investigation using U.S. Food and Drug Administration regulatory criteria. *Diagn. Microbiol. Infect. Dis.* **27:**93–97.
137. **Martinez-Martinez, L., P. Joyanes, A. I. Suarez, and E. J. Perea.** 2001. Activities of gemifloxacin and five other antimicrobial agents against *Listeria monocytogenes* and coryneform bacteria isolated from clinical samples. *Antimicrob. Agents Chemother.* **45:**2390–2392.
138. **Medical Letter.** 2004. Choice of antibacterial drugs, p. 13–26. *In* M. Abramowicz (ed.), *The Medical Letter,* vol. 2. The Medical Letter, Inc., New Rochelle, N.Y.
139. **Megraud, F., N. Lehn, T. Lind, E. Bayerdorffer, C. O'Morain, R. Spiller, P. Unge, S. V. van Zanten, M. Wrangstadh, and C. F. Burman.** 1999. Antimicrobial susceptibility testing of *Helicobacter pylori* in a large multicenter trial: the MACH 2 study. *Antimicrob. Agents Chemother.* **43:**2747–2752.
140. **Memish, Z., M. W. Mah, S. Al Mahmoud, M. Al Shaalan, and M. Y. Khan.** 2000. *Brucella* bacteraemia: clinical and laboratory observations in 160 patients. *J. Infect.* **40:**59–63.
141. **Mendelman, P. M., E. A. Wiley, T. L. Stull, C. Clausen, D. O. Chaffin, and O. Onay.** 1990. Problems with current recommendations for susceptibility testing of *Haemophilus influenzae. Antimicrob. Agents Chemother.* **34:**1480–1484.
142. **Mohammed, J. M., and F. C. Tenover.** 2000. Evaluation of the PASCO Strep Plus broth microdilution antimicrobial susceptibility panels for testing *Streptococcus pneumoniae* and other streptococcal species. *J. Clin. Microbiol.* **38:**1713–1716.
143. **Mohammed, M. J., C. K. Marston, T. Popovic, R. S. Weyant, and F. C. Tenover.** 2002. Antimicrobial susceptibility testing of *Bacillus anthracis:* comparison of results obtained by using the National Committee for Clinical Laboratory Standards broth microdilution reference and

E test agar gradient diffusion methods. *J. Clin. Microbiol.* **40:**1902–1907.

144. **Mortensen, J. E., O. Giger, and G. L. Rodgers.** 1998. In vitro activity of oral antimicrobial agents against clinical isolates of *Pasteurella multocida*. *Diagn. Microbiol. Infect. Dis.* **30:**99–102.
145. **Murray, C. K., E. A. Walter, S. Crawford, M. L. McElmeel, and J. H. Jorgensen.** 2001. *Abiotrophia* bacteremia in a patient with neutropenic fever and antimicrobial susceptibility testing of *Abiotrophia* isolates. *Clin. Infect. Dis.* **32:**E140–E142.
146. **Musher, D. M., J. G. Bartlett, and G. V. Doern.** 2001. A fresh look at the definition of susceptibility of *Streptococcus pneumoniae* to beta-lactam antibiotics. *Arch. Intern. Med.* **161:**2538–2544.
147. **Namdari, H., K. Kintner, B. A. Jackson, S. Namdari, J. L. Hughes, R. R. Peairs, and D. J. Savage.** 1999. *Abiotrophia* species as a cause of endophthalmitis following cataract extraction. *J. Clin. Microbiol.* **37:**1564–1566.
148. **Nash, D. R., R. J. Wallace, Jr., V. A. Steingrube, and P. A. Shurin.** 1986. Isoelectric focusing of β-lactamases from sputum and middle ear isolates of *Branhamella catarrhalis* recovered in the United States. *Drugs* **31:**48–54.
149. **National Committee for Clinical Laboratory Standards.** 1984. *Performance Standards for Antimicrobial Disk Susceptibility Tests,* 3rd ed. Approved standard M2-A3. NCCLS, Villanova, Pa.
150. **Newman, L. M., S. A. Wang, R. G. Ohye, N. O'Connor, M. V. Lee, and H. S. Weinstock.** 2004. The epidemiology of fluoroquinolone-resistant *Neisseria gonorrhoeae* in Hawaii, 2001. *Clin. Infect. Dis.* **38:**649–654.
151. **Osato, M. S., R. Reddy, S. G. Reddy, R. L. Penland, and D. Y. Graham.** 2001. Comparison of the E test and the NCCLS-approved agar dilution method to detect metronidazole and clarithromycin resistant *Helicobacter pylori*. *Int. J. Antimicrob. Agents* **17:**39–44.
152. **Osato, M. S., R. Reddy, S. G. Reddy, R. L. Penland, H. M. Malaty, and D. Y. Graham.** 2001. Pattern of primary resistance of *Helicobacter pylori* to metronidazole or clarithromycin in the United States. *Arch. Intern. Med.* **161:**1217–1220.
153. **Ottaviani, D., I. Bacchiocchi, L. Masini, F. Leoni, A. Carraturo, M. Giammarioli, and G. Sbaraglia.** 2001. Antimicrobial susceptibility of potentially pathogenic halophilic vibrios isolated from seafood. *Int. J. Antimicrob. Agents* **18:**135–140.
154. **Overman, T. L., and J. M. Janda.** 1999. Antimicrobial susceptibility patterns of *Aeromonas jandaei, A. schubertii, A. trota,* and *A. veronii* biotype *veronii*. *J. Clin. Microbiol.* **37:**706–708.
155. **Pascual, A., P. Joyanes, L. Martinez-Martinez, A. I. Suarez, and E. J. Perea.** 1996. Comparison of broth microdilution and E-test for susceptibility testing of *Neisseria meningitidis*. *J. Clin. Microbiol.* **34:**588–591.
156. **Paturel, L., J. P. Casalta, G. Habib, M. Nezri, and D. Raoult.** 2004. *Actinobacillus actinomycetemcomitans* endocarditis. *Clin. Microbiol. Infect.* **10:**98–118.
157. **Perez-Trallero, E., N. Gomez, and J. M. Garcia-Arenzana.** 1994. E test as susceptibility test for evaluation of *Neisseria meningitidis* isolates. *J. Clin. Microbiol.* **32:**2341–2342.
158. **Philippon, A., and F. Bimet.** 1990. In vitro susceptibility of *Corynebacterium* group D2 and *Corynebacterium jeikeium* to twelve antibiotics. *Eur. J. Clin. Microbiol. Infect. Dis.* **9:**892–895.
159. **Piccolomini, R., G. Di Bonaventura, G. Catamo, F. Carbone, and M. Neri.** 1997. Comparative evaluation of the E test, agar dilution, and broth microdilution for testing susceptibilities of *Helicobacter pylori* strains to 20 antimicrobial agents. *J. Clin. Microbiol.* **35:**1842–1846.
160. **Pottumarthy, S., T. R. Fritsche, and R. N. Jones.** 2005. Comparative activity of oral and parenteral cephalosporins tested against multidrug-resistant *Streptococcus pneumoniae:* report from the SENTRY Antimicrobial Surveillance Program (1997–2003). *Diagn. Microbiol. Infect. Dis.* **51:** 147–150.
161. **Poyart, C., C. Pierre, G. Quesne, B. Pron, P. Berche, and P. Trieu-Cuot.** 1997. Emergence of vancomycin resistance in the genus *Streptococcus:* characterization of a VAN-B transferable determinant in *Streptococcus bovis*. *Antimicrob. Agents Chemother.* **41:**24–29.
162. **Poyart, C., G. Quesne, P. Acar, P. Berche, and P. Trieu-Cuot.** 2000. Characterization of the Tn*916*-like transposon Tn*3872* in a strain of *Abiotrophia defectiva (Streptococcus defectivus)* causing sequential episodes of endocarditis in a child. *Antimicrob. Agents Chemother.* **44:**790–793.
163. **Price, L. B., A. Vogler, T. Pearson, J. D. Busch, J. M. Schupp, and P. Keim.** 2003. In vitro selection and characterization of *Bacillus anthracis* mutants with high-level resistance to ciprofloxacin. *Antimicrob. Agents Chemother.* **47:**2362–2365.
164. **Rainbow, J., E. Cebelinski, J. Bartkus, A. Glennen, D. Boxrud, and R. Lynfield.** 2005. Rifampin-resistant meningococcal disease. *Emerg. Infect. Dis.* **11:**977–979.
165. **Ray, K., M. Bala, S. Kumari, and J. P. Narain.** 2005. Antimicrobial resistance of *Neisseria gonorrhoeae* in selected World Health Organization Southeast Asia Region countries: an overview. *Sex. Transm. Dis.* **32:**178–184.
166. **Richmond, J. Y., and R. W. McKinney (ed.).** 1999. *Biosafety in Microbiological and Biomedical Laboratories,* 4th ed. U.S. Government Printing Office, Washington, D.C.
167. **Richter, S. S., K. A. Gordon, P. R. Rhomberg, M. A. Pfaller, and R. N. Jones.** 2001. *Neisseria meningitidis* with decreased susceptibility to penicillin: report from the SENTRY antimicrobial surveillance program, North America, 1998–99. *Diagn. Microbiol. Infect. Dis.* **41:**83–88.
168. **Richter, S. S., P. L. Winokur, A. B. Brueggemann, H. K. Huynh, P. R. Rhomberg, E. M. Wingert, and G. V. Doern.** 2000. Molecular characterization of the beta-lactamases from clinical isolates of *Moraxella (Branhamella) catarrhalis* obtained from 24 U.S. medical centers during 1994–1995 and 1997–1998. *Antimicrob. Agents Chemother.* **44:**444–446.
169. **Riegel, P., R. Ruimy, R. Christen, and H. Monteil.** 1996. Species identities and antimicrobial susceptibilities of corynebacteria isolated from various clinical sources. *Eur. J. Clin. Microbiol. Infect. Dis.* **15:**657–662.
170. **Rosenstein, N. E., B. A. Perkins, D. S. Stephens, T. Popovic, and J. M. Hughes.** 2001. Meningococcal disease. *N. Engl. J. Med.* **344:**1378–1388.
171. **Rosenstein, N. E., S. A. Stocker, T. Popovic, F. C. Tenover, and B. A. Perkins.** 2000. Antimicrobial resistance of *Neisseria meningitidis* in the United States, 1997. The Active Bacterial Core Surveillance (ABCs) Team. *Clin. Infect. Dis.* **30:**212–213.
172. **Ross, J. E., T. R. Anderegg, H. S. Sader, T. R. Fritsche, and R. N. Jones.** 2005. Trends in linezolid susceptibility patterns in 2002: report from the worldwide Zyvox Annual Appraisal of Potency and Spectrum Program. *Diagn. Microbiol. Infect. Dis.* **52:**53–58.
173. **Rosser, S. J., M. J. Alfa, S. Hoban, J. Kennedy, and G. K. Harding.** 1999. E Test versus agar dilution for antimicrobial susceptibility testing of viridans group streptococci. *J. Clin. Microbiol.* **37:**26–30.
174. **Sabath, L. D., and E. P. Abraham.** 1965. Cephalosporinase and penicillinase activity of *Bacillus cereus*. *Antimicrob. Agents Chemother.* **5:**392–397.
175. **Saenz, Y., M. Zarazaga, M. Lantero, M. J. Gastanares, F. Baquero, and C. Torres.** 2000. Antibiotic resistance in

Campylobacter strains isolated from animals, foods, and humans in Spain in 1997–1998. *Antimicrob. Agents Chemother.* **44:**267–271.

176. **Safdar, A., and D. Armstrong.** 2003. Antimicrobial activities against 84 *Listeria monocytogenes* isolates from patients with systemic listeriosis at a comprehensive cancer center (1955–1997). *J. Clin. Microbiol.* **41:**483–485.
177. **Shigemura, K., H. Okada, T. Shirakawa, K. Tanaka, S. Arakawa, S. Kinoshita, A. Gotoh, and S. Kamidono.** 2004. Susceptibilities of *Neisseria gonorrhoeae* to fluoroquinolones and other antimicrobial agents in Hyogo and Osaka, Japan. *Sex. Transm. Infect.* **80:**105–107.
178. **Shultz, T. R., J. W. Tapsall, P. A. White, and P. J. Newton.** 2000. An invasive isolate of *Neisseria meningitidis* showing decreased susceptibility to quinolones. *Antimicrob. Agents Chemother.* **44:**1116.
179. **Sloas, M. M., F. F. Barrett, P. J. Chesney, B. K. English, B. C. Hill, F. C. Tenover, and R. J. Leggiadro.** 1992. Cephalosporin treatment failure in penicillin- and cephalosporin-resistant *Streptococcus pneumoniae* meningitis. *Pediatr. Infect. Dis. J.* **11:**662–666.
180. **Smith, K. E., J. M. Besser, C. W. Hedberg, F. T. Leano, J. B. Bender, J. H. Wicklund, B. P. Johnson, K. A. Moore, and M. T. Osterholm.** 1999. Quinolone-resistant *Campylobacter jejuni* infections in Minnesota, 1992–1998. Investigation Team. *N. Engl. J. Med.* **340:**1525–1532.
181. **Sordillo, E. M., M. Rendel, R. Sood, J. Belinfanti, O. Murray, and D. Brook.** 1993. Septicemia due to beta-lactamase-positive *Kingella kingae*. *Clin. Infect. Dis.* **17:**818–819.
182. **Soriano, F., R. Fernandez-Roblas, R. Calvo, and G. Garcia-Calvo.** 1998. In vitro susceptibilities of aerobic and facultative non-spore-forming gram-positive bacilli to HMR 3647 (RU 66647) and 14 other antimicrobials. *Antimicrob. Agents Chemother.* **42:**1028–1033.
183. **Soriano, F., J. J. Granizo, P. Coronel, M. Gimeno, E. Rodenas, M. Gracia, C. Garcia, R. Fernandez-Roblas, J. Esteban, and I. Gadea.** 2004. Antimicrobial susceptibility of *Haemophilus influenzae, Haemophilus parainfluenzae* and *Moraxella catarrhalis* isolated from adult patients with respiratory tract infections in four southern European countries. The ARISE project. *Int. J. Antimicrob. Agents* **23:**296–299.
184. **Stock, I., and B. Wiedemann.** 2001. beta-Lactam-susceptibility patterns of *Plesiomonas shigelloides* strains: importance of inoculum and medium. *Scand. J. Infect. Dis.* **33:**692–696.
185. **Stock, I., and B. Wiedemann.** 2001. Natural antimicrobial susceptibilities of *Plesiomonas shigelloides* strains. *J. Antimicrob. Chemother.* **48:**803–811.
186. **Sutcliffe, E. M., D. M. Jones, S. El-Sheikh, and A. Percival.** 1988. Penicillin-insensitive meningococci in the UK. *Lancet* **i:**657–658.
187. **Swenson, J. M., R. R. Facklam, and C. Thornsberry.** 1990. Antimicrobial susceptibility of vancomycin-resistant *Leuconostoc, Pediococcus,* and *Lactobacillus* species. *Antimicrob. Agents Chemother.* **34:**543–549.
188. **Swenson, J. M., B. C. Hill, and C. Thornsberry.** 1986. Screening pneumococci for penicillin resistance. *J. Clin. Microbiol.* **24:**749–752.
189. **Takahashi, T., T. Sawada, M. Muramatsu, Y. Tamura, T. Fujisawa, Y. Benno, and T. Mitsuoka.** 1987. Serotype, antimicrobial susceptibility, and pathogenicity of *Erysipelothrix rhusiopathiae* isolates from tonsils of apparently healthy slaughter pigs. *J. Clin. Microbiol.* **25:**536–539.
190. **Tang, H. J., M. C. Chang, W. C. Ko, K. Y. Huang, C. L. Lee, and Y. C. Chuang.** 2002. In vitro and in vivo activities of newer fluoroquinolones against *Vibrio vulnificus*. *Antimicrob. Agents Chemother.* **46:**3580–3584.
191. **Tenover, F. C., C. N. Baker, and J. M. Swenson.** 1996. Evaluation of commercial methods for determining antimicrobial susceptibility of *Streptococcus pneumoniae*. *J. Clin. Microbiol.* **34:**10–14.
192. **Thibault, F. M., E. Hernandez, D. R. Vidal, M. Girardet, and J.-D. Cavallo.** 2004. Antibiotic susceptibility of 65 isolates of *Burkholderia pseudomallei* and *Burkholderia mallei* to 35 antimicrobial agents. *J. Antimicrob. Chemother.* **54:**1134–1138.
193. **Thornsberry, C., J. M. Swenson, C. N. Baker, L. K. McDougal, S. A. Stocker, and B. C. Hill.** 1988. Methods for determining susceptibility of fastidious and unusual pathogens to selected antimicrobial agents. *Diagn. Microbiol. Infect. Dis.* **9:**139–153.
194. **Traub, W. H., and B. Leonhard.** 1997. Comparative susceptibility of clinical group A, B, C, F, and G β-hemolytic streptococcal isolates to 24 antimicrobial drugs. *Chemotherapy* **43:**10–20.
195. **Tuohy, M., and J. Washington.** 1997. Antimicrobial susceptibility of viridans group streptococci. *Diagn. Microbiol. Infect. Dis.* **29:**277–280.
196. **Tuohy, M. J., G. W. Procop, and J. A. Washington.** 2000. Antimicrobial susceptibility of *Abiotrophia adiacens* and *Abiotrophia defectiva*. *Diagn. Microbiol. Infect. Dis.* **38:**189–191.
197. **Turnbull, P. C. B., N. M. Sirianni, C. I. LeBron, M. N. Samaan, F. N. Sutton, A. E. Reyes, and L. F. Peruski, Jr.** 2004. MICs of selected antibiotics for *Bacillus anthracis, Bacillus cereus, Bacillus thuringiensis,* and *Bacillus mycoides* from a range of clinical and environmental sources as determined by the E test. *J. Clin. Microbiol.* **42:**3626–3634.
198. **Turner, P. C., K. W. Southern, N. J. Spencer, and H. Pullen.** 1990. Treatment failure in meningococcal meningitis. *Lancet* **335:**732–733.
199. **Vazquez, J. A., L. Arreaza, C. Block, I. Ehrhard, S. J. Gray, S. Heuberger, S. Hoffmann, P. Kriz, P. Nicolas, P. Olcen, A. Skoczynska, L. Spanjaard, P. Stefanelli, M.-K. Taha, and G. Tzanakaki.** 2003. Interlaboratory comparison of agar dilution and Etest methods for determining the MICs of antibiotics used in management of *Neisseria meningitidis* infections. *Antimicrob. Agents Chemother.* **47:**3430–3434.
200. **Vazquez, J. A., S. Berron, M. J. Gimenez, L. de la Fuente, and L. Aguilar.** 2001. In vitro susceptibility of *Neisseria meningitidis* isolates to gemifloxacin and ten other antimicrobial agents. *Eur. J. Clin. Microbiol. Infect. Dis.* **20:**150–151.
201. **Vazquez, J. A., A. M. Enriquez, L. De la Fuente, S. Berron, and M. Baquero.** 1996. Isolation of a strain of beta-lactamase-producing *Neisseria meningitidis* in Spain. *Eur. J. Clin. Microbiol. Infect. Dis.* **15:**181–182.
202. **Venditti, M., V. Gelfusa, A. Tarasi, C. Brandimarte, and P. Serra.** 1990. Antimicrobial susceptibilities of *Erysipelothrix rhusiopathiae*. *Antimicrob. Agents Chemother.* **34:**2038–2040.
203. **Vila, J., F. Marco, L. Soler, M. Chacon, and M. J. Figueras.** 2002. In vitro antimicrobial susceptibility of clinical isolates of *Aeromonas caviae, Aeromonas hydrophila* and *Aeromonas veronii* biotype *sobria*. *J. Antimicrob. Chemother.* **49:**701–702.
204. **Vila, J., J. Ruiz, F. Gallardo, M. Vargas, L. Soler, M. J. Figueras, and J. Gascon.** 2003. *Aeromonas* spp. and traveler's diarrhea: clinical features and antimicrobial resistance. *Emerg. Infect. Dis.* **9:**552–555.
205. **Weber, D. J., S. M. Saviteer, W. A. Rutala, and C. A. Thomann.** 1988. In vitro susceptibility of *Bacillus* spp. to selected antimicrobial agents. *Antimicrob. Agents Chemother.* **32:**642–645.
206. **Weiss, K., M. Laverdiere, and R. Rivest.** 1996. Comparison of antimicrobial susceptibilities of *Corynebacterium* species by broth microdilution and disk diffusion methods. *Antimicrob. Agents Chemother.* **40:**930–933.
207. **Wilson, W. R., A. W. Karchmer, A. S. Dajani, K. A. Taubert, A. Bayer, D. Kaye, A. L. Bisno, P. Ferrieri,**

S. T. Shulman, and D. T. Durack. 1995. Antibiotic treatment of adults with infective endocarditis due to streptococci, enterococci, staphylococci, and HACEK microorganisms. *JAMA* **274:**1706–1713.

208. **Woods, C. R., A. L. Smith, B. L. Wasilauskas, J. Campos, and L. B. Givner.** 1994. Invasive disease caused by *Neisseria meningitidis* relatively resistant to penicillin in North Carolina. *J. Infect. Dis.* **170:**453–456.
209. **Yamamoto, K., M. Kijima, H. Yoshimura, and T. Takahashi.** 2001. Antimicrobial susceptibilities of *Erysipelothrix rhusiopathiae* isolated from pigs with swine erysipelas in Japan, 1988–1998. *J. Vet. Med. B* **48:**115–126.
210. **Yamamoto, K., Y. Sasaki, Y. Ogikubo, N. Noguchi, M. Sasatsu, and T. Takahashi.** 2001. Identification of the tetracycline resistance gene, *tet*(M), in *Erysipelothrix rhusiopathiae*. *J. Vet. Med. B* **48:**293–301.
211. **Yamane, N., and R. N. Jones.** 1991. In vitro activity of 43 antimicrobial agents tested against ampicillin-resistant enterococci and gram-positive species resistant to vancomycin. *Diagn. Microbiol. Infect. Dis.* **14:**337–345.
212. **Yokota, S., K. Sato, O. Kuwahara, S. Habadera, N. Tsukamoto, H. Ohuchi, H. Akizawa, T. Himi, and N. Fujii.** 2002. Fluoroquinolone-resistant *Streptococcus pneumoniae* strains occur frequently in elderly patients in Japan. *Antimicrob. Agents Chemother.* **46:**3311–3315.
213. **York, M., L. Gibbs, F. Perdreau-Remington, and G. F. Brooks.** 1999. Characterization of antimicrobial resistance in *Streptococcus pyogenes* isolates from the San Francisco Bay area of Northern California. *J. Clin. Microbiol.* **37:**1727–1731.
214. **Zanetti, S., T. Spanu, A. Deriu, L. Romano, L. A. Sechi, and G. Fadda.** 2001. In vitro susceptibility of *Vibrio* spp. isolated from the environment. *Int. J. Antimicrob. Agents* **17:**407–409.
215. **Zapardiel, J., E. Nieto, M. I. Gegundez, I. Gadea, and F. Soriano.** 1994. Problems in minimum inhibitory concentration determinations in coryneform organisms. Comparison of an agar dilution and the E test. *Diagn. Microbiol. Infect. Dis.* **19:**171–173.
216. **Zhanel, G. G., L. Palatnick, K. A. Nichol, T. Bellyou, D. E. Low, and D. J. Hoban.** 2003. Antimicrobial resistance in respiratory tract *Streptococcus pneumoniae* isolates: results of the Canadian Respiratory Organism Susceptibility Study, 1997 to 2002. *Antimicrob. Agents Chemother.* **47:**1867–1874.
217. **Zhanel, G. G., L. Palatnick, K. A. Nichol, D. E. Low, and D. J. Hoban.** 2003. Antimicrobial resistance in *Haemophilus influenzae* and *Moraxella catarrhalis* respiratory tract isolates: results of the Canadian Respiratory Organism Susceptibility Study, 1997 to 2002. *Antimicrob. Agents Chemother.* **47:**1875–1881.

Susceptibility Test Methods: Anaerobic Bacteria

DIANE M. CITRON AND DAVID W. HECHT

76

The importance of anaerobes as the cause of significant infections, as well as the benefits of specific antimicrobial treatment and prophylaxis against anaerobic bacteria, is well recognized (24, 26). In general, performance of antimicrobial susceptibility testing is viewed as a necessity for effective guidance of antimicrobial therapy. However, when and how susceptibility testing of anaerobes should be performed has been the subject of debate, due in part to several confounding factors and misconceptions (6, 22, 25, 83). For example, specimens obtained from most infections involving anaerobes are polymicrobic, making recovery and identification of individual isolates slow and causing antimicrobial susceptibility results to be unacceptably delayed so that a consistent impact on individual clinical outcomes is difficult to achieve. For the clinician, the combination of surgical management and use of empiric broad-spectrum antimicrobial therapy has limited the correlation of potential antimicrobial resistance with outcome. Such observations have led many laboratories away from the performance of susceptibility testing. However, there is substantial evidence that antimicrobial resistance is significant among many anaerobes worldwide and that inappropriate therapy can result in poor clinical responses and increased mortality (59, 67, 69). Antimicrobial susceptibility data have also revealed significant differences among individual hospitals on a regional and local basis, suggesting that one medical center's patterns are not applicable to organisms from other institutions (45, 72, 73). Thus, the need for susceptibility testing of anaerobes is considerably more important now than in the past.

If possible, individual hospitals should establish patterns of resistance for some anaerobes on a periodic basis, with individual patient isolates being tested as needed to assist in patient care. For surveillance purposes, the testing of 75 to 100 isolates representing anaerobes with known resistance, such as members of the *Bacteroides fragilis* group, *Prevotella* spp., *Fusobacterium* spp., and *Clostridium* spp., should be considered. Preferably, 30 isolates should be from the *B. fragilis* group, and at least 10 of each of the other genera should be tested. Alternatively, cumulative susceptibility results from individual patient isolates should be included in the hospital antibiogram. Antimicrobial agents to be tested should generally be based upon the hospital's formulary, although one agent from each antimicrobial class should be included, even if it is not on the hospital formulary, to detect resistance. These data would be important as part of the cumulative susceptibility report if the formulary were changed and could aid in the choice of empiric therapy. For individual patient management, susceptibility should be performed when (i) selecting an active agent is critical for disease management, (ii) there is consideration for long-term therapy, (iii) anaerobes are isolated from specific body sites (e.g., blood, brain, bone, or joint), or (iv) there is the failure of a usual regimen (Table 1).

This chapter describes currently available methodologies and their interpretation for susceptibility testing of anaerobes. The Clinical Laboratory Standards Institute (CLSI, formerly NCCLS) anaerobe working group has established an agar dilution reference method using brucella blood agar as the testing medium (15–17). This method is not considered simple or economical to perform but will serve as the method to which other more practical methods can be compared (Table 2). At present, alternative testing methods include the limited agar dilution, broth microdilution (for the *B. fragilis* group), and the E test. β-Lactamase testing provides very limited data but can be useful if penicillin therapy is being considered. Broth disk elution and disk diffusion tests are not considered appropriate for anaerobic susceptibility testing because their results do not correlate with those of the agar dilution reference method (14).

CURRENT PATTERNS OF ANTIBIOTIC RESISTANCE

Susceptibility testing of anaerobes has not been routinely performed at most hospitals (39). As a result, most of the published literature reporting susceptibility of anaerobes is generated by reference laboratories testing a limited number of isolates from one or more medical centers (1–3, 31, 37, 44, 45, 72, 73). Over the last decade, significant variations in susceptibility results for anaerobes have been reported from different countries, geographic locations within countries, and even hospitals within the same cities (45, 47, 53, 54, 56, 72, 79). Of particular note, the incidence of clindamycin resistance has increased from <10 to >40% for the *B. fragilis* group at some hospitals (45, 73), while resistance to cephalosporins and cephamycins is also rising (45, 72–74, 79). Some differences in susceptibility results among various reports may be accounted for by the use of different testing methods, lack of uniformity in interpretive breakpoints among countries, and clustering of MICs at the breakpoint for some species with

TABLE 1 Indications for susceptibility testing of anaerobic bacteria

Indication	Examples[a]
Surveillance	
Annual monitoring of isolates at individual medical centers	*B. fragilis* group, *Prevotella* spp., *Fusobacterium* spp., *Clostridium* spp., *B. wadsworthia*
Clinical	
Known resistance of a particular species	*B. fragilis* (clindamycin, cephamycins, piperacillin, fluoroquinolones); *Prevotella* spp. and *Fusobacterium* spp. (penicillin, clindamycin)
Failure of a usual therapeutic regimen	Any anaerobe
Pivotal role of antimicrobial agent in clinical outcome	*B. fragilis* group (osteomyelitis, joint infection)
Need for long-term therapy	*B. fragilis* group, *Prevotella* spp. (osteomyelitis, endocarditis, brain abscess, liver abscess, lung abscess)
Infections of specific body sites	Any anaerobe (brain abscess, endocarditis, prosthetic devices or graft, bacteremia)

[a] Examples only, and not intended as all-inclusive. See the text for specific recommendations.

some antimicrobial agent combinations (4, 42). Regardless, it is clear from recent publications that resistance to many classes of antimicrobial agents among anaerobes is increasing, and clinicians and laboratories can no longer assume susceptibility of anaerobes to these agents without testing. Further, neither national nor even local data from other institutions are sufficient to predict susceptibility of anaerobes to antimicrobial agents at one's own hospital (45, 72, 73). A general outline of current resistance patterns for anaerobic bacteria is provided below (40).

Gram-Negative Bacilli and Cocci

B. fragilis Group

Among the 13 members of the *B. fragilis* group, *B. fragilis* is generally the most susceptible, although greater than 95% of all species are resistant to penicillin and ampicillin. The carboxy- and ureidopenicillins, ticarcillin, and mezlocillin are somewhat more active than penicillin, but <50% of isolates are susceptible (2, 9, 79). Piperacillin is the most active of the ureidopenicillins against the *B. fragilis* group, although susceptibility has fallen from approximately 90 to 70% over the last 8 to 10 years (2, 41, 72, 73). The isoxazolyl penicillins, such as oxacillin and nafcillin, are not active against these organisms. The principal mechanism of resistance to penicillins is β-lactamase production. Thus, β-lactam–β-lactamase inhibitor combinations, such as ampicillin-sulbactam, amoxicillin-clavulanic acid, ticarcillin-clavulanic acid, and piperacillin-tazobactam, are active against nearly all strains of *B. fragilis* group, with <2% resistance reported in most studies (3, 9, 41, 44, 47, 53, 72, 73, 79).

Among the cephalosporins and cephamycins, cefoxitin remains very active against members of the *B. fragilis* group, with 80 to 90% of isolates susceptible. Cefotetan demonstrates activity against *B. fragilis* similar to that of cefoxitin, but it is much less active against the other members of the *B. fragilis* group (2). With the exception of ceftizoxime, broad-spectrum cephalosporins generally have poor activity against most members of the *B. fragilis* group, inhibiting <50% of isolates (73). Susceptibility to ceftizoxime varies widely among published studies (60 to 90%), probably due to differences in testing methods (4). Narrow-spectrum cephalosporins, such as cefazolin, are not active against members of the *B. fragilis* group.

A marked decrease in susceptibility to clindamycin among *Bacteroides* spp. has become widely recognized worldwide, as noted above (1, 3, 9, 44, 45, 47, 53, 72, 73, 79). The clindamycin resistance determinants include several *erm* genes that are frequently located on transferable plasmids and are often linked to transferable tetracycline resistance (65, 82). Among other agents, chloramphenicol, metronidazole, and carbapenems (imipenem, ertapenem, and meropenem) are nearly uniformly active against all members of the *B. fragilis* group in the United States (2, 36, 72), although imipenem-resistant strains have been reported from Japan, the United States, Hungary, Kuwait, and other countries (5, 63, 75). Of note, imipenem resistance is mediated by a zinc metalloenzyme that confers resistance to all current β-lactam and β-lactam–β-lactamase inhibitor combination agents and has

TABLE 2 Methods for susceptibility testing of anaerobic bacteria

Method	Medium	Inoculum	Incubation time (h)	Advantages	Disadvantages
Agar dilution[a]	Brucella blood agar	10^5 cells/spot	48	Reference method, multiple isolates tested/antibiotic	Labor intensive, expensive
Broth microdilution[b]	Supplemented brucella broth	10^6 cells/ml (10^5/well)	48	Economical, commercial panels available, multiple antibiotics/isolate	Limited shelf life of frozen panels, poor growth by some strains
E test	Brucella blood agar	0.5 McFarland, swab plate	24–48	Precise MIC value, convenient for individual patient isolates	Expensive for surveillance use

[a] Media are commercially available.
[b] Frozen panels available from PML Microbiologicals, Inc. (Wilsonville, Oreg.); lyophilized panels are available from Trek Diagnostic Systems.

been reported to be transferable (64, 75). Of more concern, however, strains resistant to metronidazole in France have been reported, associated with a transferable plasmid (64), and in recent years, additional resistant strains carrying *nim* genes have been reported in Washington state, the United Kingdom, and other countries in Europe (27, 55, 70). *nim* genes encode a nitroimidazole reductase which converts nitroimidazoles to aminoimidazole, preventing the formation of the active toxic nitroso residue (11). Among fluoroquinolone agents, trovafloxacin (a trifluoronaphthyridone) had excellent activity against most members of the *B. fragilis* group; however, it is no longer marketed in most countries, including the United States (15, 43, 44, 46, 71, 72). Other fluoroquinolones such as moxifloxacin, recently approved by the FDA for skin structure infections and intra-abdominal infections, and gatifloxacin also exhibit good activity against a broad range of anaerobes (9, 23, 48, 71). Resistance to fluoroquinolones in *Bacteroides* and other anaerobes is increasing with the widespread use of this class of antimicrobial agents (29, 61, 72; D. M. Citron, *Abstr. 45th Intersci. Conf. Antimicrob. Agents Chemother.*, abstr. E-1440, 2005). Tigecycline, a glycylcycline derivative of minocycline, was recently approved by the FDA for intra-abdominal and skin and soft tissue infections. Although breakpoints for anaerobes have not yet been defined by CLSI, several studies describe its activity against anaerobic organisms (10, 49).

Prevotella and *Porphyromonas*

Recent taxonomic changes for this group of anaerobes are provided in reference 51. In general, data on the susceptibility of these organisms (mostly former *Bacteroides* species) are more limited than those of the *B. fragilis* group. Overall, both genera are more susceptible than the *B. fragilis* group. Currently, about 50% of *Prevotella* spp. are resistant to penicillin and ampicillin due to β-lactamase production, with susceptibility to piperacillin, cefoxitin, and cefotetan ranging from 70 to 90% in most published studies (30, 35, 44, 53, 57). Eight percent of *Porphyromonas* strains were reported to produce β-lactamase in a survey from Japan (78), as were 17% of strains recovered from serious pelvic infections (62). Susceptibility of *Porphyromonas* isolates is rarely reported separately in most published literature from the United States, but β-lactamase production is considered rare at present (36). As in the case of the *B. fragilis* group, both genera are nearly uniformly susceptible to carbapenems, metronidazole, and chloramphenicol, although clindamycin resistance has been observed in a small percentage of strains (36).

Other Gram-Negative Bacilli

Penicillin resistance among isolates of the genus *Fusobacterium* has been observed; *Fusobacterium nucleatum* strains from saliva in infants show increasing rates of β-lactamase production related to age, day care attendance, and exposure to antimicrobial agents (60), and a β-lactamase-producing strain was responsible in a case of fatal sepsis in a compromised patient (38). In general, >90% of *Fusobacterium* spp. are susceptible to cephalosporins and cephamycins (36, 50, 53, 81). *Campylobacter rectus* and *Campylobacter curvus* (formerly *Wolinella*) vary in their susceptibility to β-lactams but remain very susceptible to chloramphenicol, metronidazole, and clindamycin (81). *Bilophila wadsworthia* is a gram-negative anaerobe from the gastrointestinal tract that frequently produces β-lactamase and therefore is resistant to penicillin and ampicillin. High MIC_{90} values are also seen when testing piperacillin, with values clustering near the breakpoints. *B. wadsworthia* is susceptible to clindamycin, cefoxitin, β-lactam–β-lactamase inhibitor combinations, carbapenems, and metronidazole (7). *Campylobacter gracilis* (formerly *Bacteroides gracilis*) was previously considered to be resistant to many β-lactam agents. However, data suggest that when properly identified and tested, this organism is susceptible to most agents tested, including β-lactam–β-lactamase inhibitor combinations, cefoxitin, and clindamycin (58). In fact, a newly described but more resistant organism, *Sutterella wadsworthensis*, was often isolated from the same samples and identified as *C. gracilis*. *S. wadsworthensis* may demonstrate resistance to clindamycin, piperacillin, and/or metronidazole (58).

Gram-Positive Bacilli and Cocci

Non-Spore-Forming Gram-Positive Bacilli

The *Eubacterium* group, *Actinomyces*, *Propionibacterium*, and *Bifidobacterium* are usually susceptible to β-lactam agents, including the penicillins, cephalosporins and cephamycins, carbapenems, and β-lactam–β-lactamase inhibitor combinations. *Lactobacillus* spp. are variably susceptible to cephalosporins and may be inhibited effectively only by penicillin (36). Vancomycin is active against all *Propionibacterium* spp., *Actinomyces* spp., *Eubacterium* spp., peptostreptococci, and some *Lactobacillus* spp., but *Lactobacillus casei* and several other species are usually resistant (36). The newer antimicrobial agents such as linezolid, daptomycin, dalbavancin, telavancin, and ramoplanin with activity against gram-positive aerobic organisms also exhibit excellent in vitro activity against most anaerobic gram-positive species (8, 12, 32–34). Most non-spore-forming gram-positive anaerobes are resistant to metronidazole.

Spore-Forming Gram-Positive Bacilli

Clostridium perfringens is generally very susceptible to most antianaerobic agents and to fluoroquinolones (9, 44, 46). However, non-perfringens *Clostridium* spp. and *Clostridium difficile* have variable susceptibility (19, 35–37, 44, 66, 79). Drugs to which resistance among non-perfringens species is observed include clindamycin, fluoroquinolones, and β-lactams; however, chloramphenicol and metronidazole remain active. *C. difficile* may be resistant to many β-lactams, including cephalosporins, fluoroquinolones, and clindamycin, but retains susceptibility to metronidazole and vancomycin, while *Clostridium innocuum* has vancomycin MICs of 8 to 32 μg/ml (35–37, 66).

Gram-Positive Cocci

At present, only *Peptococcus niger* remains in this genus, and several of the species in the genus *Peptostreptococcus* have been reclassified into other genera (76). In general, these organisms are highly susceptible to all β-lactams, β-lactam–β-lactamase inhibitors, cephalosporins, carbapenems, chloramphenicol, and metronidazole (36, 46, 53, 66, 79, 81). Fluoroquinolone resistance is increasing among the species isolated from skin and soft tissue infections (Citron, 45th ICAAC), and some strains may be resistant to clindamycin. Occasionally, microaerophilic streptococci including *Abiotrophia* and *Granulicatella* species are initially identified as *Peptostreptococcus* spp. and reported to be resistant to metronidazole. The presumptive identification of a metronidazole-resistant *Peptostreptococcus* sp. should prompt further identification of the organism because such isolates are rare. The *nimB* gene coding for metronidazole resistance has been demonstrated in two highly resistant strains of *Finegoldia magna*, although it appears to be prevalent in susceptible strains of other gram-positive cocci as well (80).

DESCRIPTION OF TEST METHODS

Agar Dilution

Media

The recommended medium is supplemented brucella blood agar, which supports the growth of essentially all anaerobes (17). Brucella base agar is supplemented with hemin (5 μg/ml) and vitamin K_1 (1 μg/ml) prior to autoclaving and 5% defibrinated or laked sheep blood after cooling to 48 to 50°C. To prepare hemin stock solution (5 mg/ml), dissolve 0.5 g of hemin in 10 ml of 1 N NaOH and bring to a 100-ml volume with distilled water. Sterilize by autoclaving at 121°C for 15 min. Add 1 ml of agar per liter. The stock solution may be stored at 4 to 8°C for 1 month. Vitamin K_1 stock solution (10 mg/ml) is prepared by mixing 0.2 ml of Vitamin K_1 (3-phytyl menadione) with 20 ml of 95% ethanol, and it is added to the agar base to achieve a final concentration of 1 μg/ml prior to autoclaving. The stock solution can be stored for up to 6 months at 4°C in a dark bottle. Lysed (laked) sheep blood is prepared by a single cycle of alternate freezing and thawing and does not require clarification by centrifugation. Laked blood may be stored at –20°C for up to 6 months.

The agar is dispensed in 17-ml volumes in test tubes prior to autoclaving. After autoclaving, these tubes may be stored at 4 to 8°C for up to 1 month. On the day of the test, the agar is melted by heating and then cooled in a water bath to 48 to 50°C. Laked blood (1 ml) and the antimicrobial dilutions (2 ml) are added, and after mixing by gently inverting the tubes twice, the plates are poured. After they have solidified, the plates are dried in the incubator by inverting them with the lids ajar for 45 min. The CLSI recommends that plates not be stored any longer than 7 days in closed containers at 4 to 8°C. However, for research and precise evaluation purposes, storage for no longer than 72 h is recommended. Due to instability, plates containing imipenem (but not meropenem and ertapenem) or clavulanic acid must be used on the day of preparation.

Inoculum Preparation

The inoculum may be prepared by suspending colonies taken from a 24- to 72-h brucella blood agar plate into brucella broth or other clear broth medium to a density equal to the 0.5 McFarland standard. Alternatively, the initial suspension may be prepared by inoculating five or more colonies into enriched thioglycolate or other broth medium that supports good growth and by incubating for 4 to 24 h to obtain adequate turbidity (dilution may be required) (17). Equivalence to a 0.5 McFarland standard can be measured visually or by using a colorimeter or a simple photometer device (e.g., Vitek, Hazelwood, Mo.; Microscan, West Sacramento, Calif.; Trek Diagnostic Systems, Inc., Cleveland, Ohio). Although it is more accurate than visual inspection, the use of different broth media can affect photometer readings, requiring the user to verify the size of the inoculum by performing colony counts. Species with large cells, such as *C. perfringens,* require fewer cells to achieve this turbidity and will show correspondingly lower colony counts, while the converse is true for organisms with smaller cells, such as *Veillonella* or *Micromonas micros.*

The organism suspensions are dispensed by pipette into the wells of the replicator head (32 to 36 wells) and applied to the plates with a multipronged replicator device that delivers approximately 0.001 ml per spot (10^5 CFU). The drug-free control plates are inoculated first, followed by the antimicrobial plates, starting with the lowest drug concentration. The plates should be marked to ensure proper orientation.

Contamination by aerobic bacteria during the inoculation procedure can be detected by inoculating drug-free plates and incubating them in an aerobic environment. If using thioglycolate or other agar-containing broth media for inoculum preparation, an additional control plate may be inoculated and refrigerated to distinguish the inoculum residue that occurs at the time of setting up the MIC testing plates. Agar dilution plates can be inoculated in an aerobic environment, although the exposure time prior to incubation should be minimized. After stamping the plates, the inoculation spots should absorb for 10 to 15 min into the medium, at which time the plates are stacked upside down (to prevent condensation from falling on spots) and immediately placed into an anaerobic environment for incubation.

Incubation Conditions

An anaerobic chamber or anaerobic jars equipped with disposable hydrogen/carbon dioxide generators and palladium-coated catalyst pellets or ascorbic acid envelopes are recommended for incubating agar dilution plates. The incubation atmosphere should contain approximately 5% CO_2, and an indicator of anaerobiasis should be included. Incubation is at 35 to 37°C for 44 to 48 h (17).

Interpretation of Results

Since 1993, the CLSI has defined the endpoint for agar dilution testing as the concentration at which the change from the growth control is the most marked (14). This change is defined as no growth or lighter growth, a haze, multiple tiny colonies, or one to several normal-sized colonies. The technologist should take care to discern a few colonies that may be present as the result of a "splash" from a resistant neighboring isolate from the few colonies that precede full growth of the strain. Endpoints can be difficult to interpret when testing some gram-negative organisms with β-lactams, particularly ceftizoxime and piperacillin. This is especially problematic with many strains of fusobacteria that produce L forms that appear as transparent hazes in the presence of even very high concentrations of β-lactam agents. The current CLSI document for susceptibility testing of anaerobes now includes a color figure illustrating the endpoints described above and should be utilized as an additional guide when using this test method (17). It is important to compare the drug-containing plates to the drug-free control plate when reading the tests, because spots of different species of anaerobic bacteria can have very different appearances, ranging from mucoid-opaque, as with the *B. fragilis* group, to gray-transparent, as with *Bacteroides ureolyticus*.

The interpretation of MIC results should be done according to criteria recommended by the CLSI (Table 3) (17). In 1993, an intermediate category was established for anaerobic bacteria (14). For many antimicrobial agents used against anaerobes, a significant percentage of strains have susceptibility test endpoints that cluster at or near the suggested breakpoints. In the twofold-dilution method, the degree of acceptable variation of endpoints (usually plus or minus 1 twofold dilution) does not permit adequate distinction of the qualitative categories. If an intermediate value is determined for any anaerobe, the CLSI recommends maximum dosages of the antimicrobial agent for therapy. With such dosages, it is believed that organisms with susceptible or intermediate endpoints are amenable to therapy. This recommendation is predicated upon the presumed surgical intervention that frequently accompanies infections involving these organisms.

TABLE 3 Interpretive categories for MICs for anaerobic bacteria[a]

Antimicrobial agent	MIC (μg/ml)		
	Susceptible	Intermediate	Resistant
Amoxicillin-clavulanic acid	≤4/2	8/4	≥16/8
Ampicillin[b]	≤0.5	1	≥2
Ampicillin-sulbactam	≤8/4	16/8	≥32/16
Cefotetan	≤16	32	≥64
Cefoxitin	≤16	32	≥64
Chloramphenicol	≤8	16	≥32
Clindamycin	≤2	4	≥8
Ertapenem	≤4	8	≥16
Imipenem	≤4	8	≥16
Metronidazole	≤8	16	≥32
Meropenem	≤4	8	≥16
Penicillin[b]	≤0.5	1	≥2
Piperacillin	≤32	64	≥128
Piperacillin-tazobactam	≤32/4	64/4	≥128/4
Tetracycline	≤4	8	≥16
Ticarcillin-clavulanic acid	≤32/2	64/2	≥128/2
Trovafloxacin	≤2	4	≥8

[a] Adapted from reference 17 with permission of the publisher.
[b] Members of the *B. fragilis* group are presumed to be resistant. Other gram-negative anaerobes may be screened for β-lactamase activity by using a chromogenic cephalosporin test if penicillin therapy is contemplated. Higher levels in blood are achievable; infection with non-β-lactamase-producing organisms with higher MICs might be treatable.

Broth Microdilution Test

The broth microdilution procedure has been validated by CLSI for testing only members of the *B. fragilis* group. Other, more-oxygen-sensitive anaerobes did not grow consistently when inoculated on the bench. Testing in an anaerobic chamber using reduced MIC trays may improve growth and make this method suitable for other species of anaerobes. The anaerobe working group of CLSI is evaluating additional antimicrobial agents and other species for correlation of the broth microdilution method to the reference standard.

Media

Brucella broth supplemented with hemin (5 μg/ml), vitamin K_1 (1 μg/ml), and lysed horse blood (5%) is the recommended medium. Microdilution trays may be prepared fresh, frozen after preparation, or purchased commercially as lyophilized or frozen panels. Following the manufacturer's recommendations for storage of commercially prepared panels is recommended, whereas in-house-prepared trays may be kept at −70°C for up to 6 months if stored in sealed plastic bags. Antimicrobial agents should be diluted according to the scheme described by the CLSI (17) and prepared in large volumes, 15 to 100 ml, depending on the device used to simultaneously dispense aliquots of 0.1 ml per well into the standard 96-well panels. If the inoculum is to be added by pipette, the antimicrobial solutions are prepared at twice the desired concentration and the wells are filled with 0.05 ml, after which 0.05 ml of inoculum is added to each well for a final volume of 0.1 ml. Final volumes of less than 0.1 ml are not recommended for testing anaerobes due to loss of liquid by evaporation. Inoculum effects may be exaggerated when smaller volumes are used.

Inoculum Preparation

Inoculum preparation is similar to that of the agar dilution procedure. Organisms may be suspended into a clear broth to equal the turbidity of the 0.5 McFarland standard, or the isolate can be grown in a supplemented thioglycolate or other broth that supports growth of the organism for 4 to 24 h and then diluted to the turbidity of the 0.5 McFarland standard (approximately 1.5×10^8 CFU/ml). The final concentration of the organism is 1×10^6 to 2×10^6 CFU/ml (10^5 CFU/well). Depending on the method of tray inoculation, the dilution technique will differ. If 10 μl is added to each well, then the 0.5 McFarland suspension is diluted 1:10. If 50 μl is added, then the 0.5 McFarland suspension is diluted 1:50. If a lyophilized tray is used, the 0.5 McFarland suspension is diluted 1:100.

Inoculation Procedure

Frozen trays should be brought to room temperature prior to inoculation. The inoculation can be accomplished by using a disposable, hand-held, 96-prong inoculator, a mechanized dispenser, or a multichannel pipettor, depending on the preparation method of the panel, within 15 min after inocula are prepared. While the members of the *B. fragilis* group are relatively oxygen tolerant, reducing the trays in an oxygen-free environment prior to inoculation (2 to 4 h) may enhance the growth of certain fastidious anaerobes and reduce the "edge" effect of outer rows being reduced more rapidly than inner wells (52). Trays should be reduced prior to inoculation if metronidazole is to be tested, since the antimicrobial activity of metronidazole is dependent on the formation of an active intermediate that requires a reduced atmosphere (52). False resistance can occur with nonfastidious, rapidly growing strains that produce significant growth before metronidazole is reduced to its active form. Control wells should include a well with broth but no drug (growth control) and an uninoculated well as a sterility check. This well may also be used as a negative control well for visual comparison with growth in inoculated wells. Alternatively, an uninoculated tray may be incubated as a sterility check, especially if the trays are prepared in-house.

It is advisable to perform a colony count and a purity check of the inoculum. This is accomplished by removing 10 μl from the growth control well, diluting it into 10 ml of saline (1:100), and spreading 0.1 ml onto the surface of a nonselective blood agar plate for anaerobic incubation. The presence of 100 to 200 colonies indicates an inoculum of 1×10^6 to 2×10^6 CFU/ml. A small amount of the growth control well can be inoculated onto a quadrant of a blood agar plate for aerobic incubation to detect aerobic contamination.

Incubation Conditions

Trays are most conveniently incubated in an anaerobic chamber for 40 to 48 h. Alternatively, they can be placed into large anaerobic jars, regular anaerobic jars laid on their side, or anaerobic pouches with the appropriate anaerobic gas generator. No more than four trays should be stacked on top of each other to ensure uniformity of heating and gas exchange. Trays should not be sealed with sealing tape (unless perforated) if set up on the bench, as this will decrease the rate of diffusion of anaerobic gases to the inoculum and may result in poor growth or false resistance to metronidazole.

Interpretation of Results

The plates may be examined with reflective light by using a viewing device, such as a stand with a magnifying mirror. Broth microdilution MIC determinations require criteria similar to those for the agar dilution procedure for reading endpoints: the concentration at which the most significant reduction in growth is observed is interpreted as the MIC. Similar to that of agar dilution, this decrease in growth may include a tiny, gradually diminishing button of growth, with trailing endpoints also being observed (17). If the growth in the drug-free growth control well is poor, the test should not be read. At this time, breakpoints for broth microdilution are similar to those for agar dilution (17).

E Test

The E test (AB BIODISK, Solna, Sweden) has been used more frequently for testing anaerobic organisms in recent years, primarily because of its convenience. Several studies have demonstrated its utility and indicate that results correlate well with the CLSI reference approved agar dilution method (13, 68). Rosenblatt has noted that some strains of *Prevotella* and *Bacteroides* spp. show very major errors (false susceptibility) with penicillin and ceftriaxone; however, a β-lactamase test would provide the correct result in these instances. In addition, false resistance to metronidazole among anaerobes has been reported when using the E test. This phenomenon can be the result of test conditions and medium quality and is generally eliminated if test plates are reduced in an anaerobic atmosphere overnight prior to their use (18).

Procedure

The E test consists of plastic strips coated with a gradient of antimicrobial on one side and an MIC interpretive scale on the other side. The method consists of streaking to confluence (three directions) a 0.5 to 1 McFarland standard of the test organism on a 150-mm-diameter supplemented brucella blood agar plate. Up to six E-test strips can be applied to the surface of the plate in a radial fashion with the lowest concentration toward the center. If large plates are not available, two strips, one on each half, may be placed on a standard-size plate with the high concentrations of the strips opposite each other. Following 24 to 48 h of anaerobic incubation, an elliptical zone of inhibition is formed. MICs are read at the point of intersection of the ellipse with the interpretive scale of MICs.

Validation for most antimicrobial agents recommended for testing of anaerobes has been confirmed for the E test (68). The complete list of FDA-approved antimicrobial agents for anaerobe testing is found in the E-test package insert. The E test provides a flexible and simple procedure that is well suited for individual isolate testing in smaller laboratories or for those labs that do not perform batch testing of anaerobe susceptibility. Its main drawback is the relatively high cost for each strip. This can be alleviated somewhat by limiting the number of antimicrobial agents being tested to a few relevant drugs from the hospital's formulary.

β-Lactamase Testing

β-Lactamase testing of anaerobes can be performed as described by the CLSI (17). Two easily performed methods include a nitrocefin disk assay (Cefinase; BD Diagnostics Systems, Sparks, Md.) and the S1 chromogenic cephalosporin disk (International BioClinical, Inc., Portland, Oreg.). Both tests should be performed according to the manufacturers' directions. Hydrolysis of the β-lactam ring by β-lactamases causes a color change on the disks from yellow to red. Most reactions occur within 5 to 10 min, but some β-lactamase-positive strains of *Bacteroides* spp. may react more slowly (up to 30 min) (21). When testing *Bilophila wadsworthia*, 1% pyruvate should be added to the testing growth medium for consistent results (77).

β-Lactamase testing has limited utility in detecting resistance to certain β-lactam agents among anaerobes. While a chromogenic cephalosporin test is simple and quick and generally detects β-lactamases produced by species of *Prevotella, Porphyromonas, Bacteroides,* and other anaerobes, resistance to β-lactam drugs is not always mediated by β-lactamase production (e.g., some strains of *Bacteroides distasonis* and *B. fragilis* are resistant because of alterations of penicillin-binding proteins) (20, 28). Therefore, β-lactamase test results are limited in their clinical application. A positive test does, however, provide clinically relevant information quickly in some situations and can predict resistance to penicillin G and ampicillin.

QUALITY CONTROL

A quality control program is designed to monitor the accuracy and precision of a susceptibility test procedure, the performance of reagents and equipment, and the performance of persons who conduct the tests. Quality control must be performed to demonstrate that any new medium used adequately supports the growth of the test organisms and that antimicrobial agents have not deteriorated during shipping or storage. These tests must be a part of any testing program using any of the methods described above. Ideally, the quality control strain(s) that most closely resembles the tested organism(s) should be included. The recommended quality control strains are *B. fragilis* ATCC 25285, *Bacteroides thetaiotaomicron* ATCC 29741, and *Eubacterium lentum* ATCC 43055. The CLSI is currently evaluating a nontoxigenic strain of *C. difficile* (ATCC 700057) for replacement of the *E. lentum* strain. Two quality control strains should be used for each assessment when using the agar dilution procedure. When testing an individual strain using broth microdilution or E test, one quality control strain should be included. Expected values for quality control strains are published by the CLSI (17). For some antimicrobial agent-quality control organism combinations, no quality control ranges are recommended because of the difficulty in reading of endpoints.

CONCLUSIONS

Increasing antimicrobial resistance among anaerobes has become a significant problem in recent years, underscoring the need for more antimicrobial susceptibility testing. Current methodologies allow for accurate surveillance or individual isolate testing by most laboratories. Future studies comparing broth microdilution to the reference agar method and the anticipated development of an improved microdilution system will result in better standardization of the more user-friendly method and possibly more widespread commercial availability.

REFERENCES

1. **Aldridge, K. E.** 2002. Ertapenem (MK-0826), a new carbapenem: comparative in vitro activity against clinically significant anaerobes. *Diagn. Microbiol. Infect. Dis.* **44:**181–186.
2. **Aldridge, K. E., D. Ashcraft, K. Cambre, C. L. Pierson, S. G. Jenkins, and J. E. Rosenblatt.** 2001. Multicenter survey of the changing in vitro antimicrobial susceptibilities of clinical isolates of *Bacteroides fragilis* group, *Prevotella, Fusobacterium, Porphyromonas,* and *Peptostreptococcus* species. *Antimicrob. Agents Chemother.* **45:**1238–1243.
3. **Aldridge, K. E., D. Ashcraft, M. O'Brien, and C. V. Sanders.** 2003. Bacteremia due to *Bacteroides fragilis* group:

distribution of species, beta-lactamase production, and antimicrobial susceptibility patterns. *Antimicrob. Agents Chemother.* **47:**148–153.

4. **Aldridge, K. E., and D. D. Schiro.** 1994. Major methodology-dependent discordant susceptibility results for *Bacteroides fragilis* group isolates but not other anaerobes. *Diagn. Microbiol. Infect.* Dis. **20:**135–142.
5. **Bandoh, K., K. Ueno, K. Watanabe, and N. Kato.** 1993. Susceptibility patterns and resistance to imipenem in the *Bacteroides fragilis* group species in Japan: a 4-year study. *Clin. Infect. Dis.* **16:**S382–S386.
6. **Baron, E. J., D. M. Citron, and H. M. Wexler.** 1990. Son of anaerobic susceptibility testing—revisited. *Clin. Microbiol. Newsl.* **12:**69–70.
7. **Baron, E. J., G. Ropers, P. Summanen, and R. J. Courcol.** 1993. Bactericidal activity of selected antimicrobial agents against *Bilophila wadsworthia* and *Bacteroides gracilis*. *Clin. Infect. Dis.* **16:**S339–S343.
8. **Behra-Miellet, J., L. Calvet, and L. Dubreuil.** 2003. Activity of linezolid against anaerobic bacteria. *Int. J. Antimicrob. Agents* **22:**28–34.
9. **Behra-Miellet, J., L. Dubreuil, and E. Jumas-Bilak.** 2002. Antianaerobic activity of moxifloxacin compared with that of ofloxacin, ciprofloxacin, clindamycin, metronidazole and beta-lactams. *Int. J. Antimicrob. Agents* **20:**366–374.
10. **Betriu, C., E. Culebras, M. Gomez, I. Rodriguez-Avial, and J. J. Picazo.** 2005. In vitro activity of tigecycline against *Bacteroides* species. *J. Antimicrob. Chemother.* **56:**349–352.
11. **Carlier, J. P., N. Sellier, M. N. Rager, and G. Reysset.** 1997. Metabolism of a 5-nitroimidazole in susceptible and resistant isogenic strains of *Bacteroides fragilis*. *Antimicrob. Agents Chemother.* **41:**1495–1499.
12. **Citron, D. M., C. V. Merriam, K. L. Tyrrell, Y. A. Warren, H. Fernandez, and E. J. Goldstein.** 2003. In vitro activities of ramoplanin, teicoplanin, vancomycin, linezolid, bacitracin, and four other antimicrobials against intestinal anaerobic bacteria. *Antimicrob. Agents Chemother.* **47:**2334–2338.
13. **Citron, D. M., M. I. Ostovari, A. Karlsson, and E. J. Goldstein.** 1991. Evaluation of the E test for susceptibility testing of anaerobic bacteria. *J. Clin. Microbiol.* **29:** 2197–2203.
14. **Clinical and Laboratory Standards Institute.** 1993. *Methods for Antimicrobial Susceptibility Testing of Anaerobic Bacteria,* 3rd ed. *Approved Standard M11-A3.* National Committee for Clinical Laboratory Standards, Villanova, Pa.
15. **Clinical and Laboratory Standards Institute.** 1997. *Methods for Antimicrobial Susceptibility Testing of Anaerobic Bacteria,* 4th ed. *Approved Standard M11-A4.* National Committee for Clinical Laboratory Standards, Wayne, Pa.
16. **Clinical and Laboratory Standards Institute.** 2001. *Methods for Antimicrobial Susceptibility Testing of Anaerobic Bacteria,* 5th ed. *Approved Standard M11-A5.* National Committee for Clinical Laboratory Standards, Wayne, Pa.
17. **Clinical and Laboratory Standards Institute/NCCLS.** 2004. *Methods for Antimicrobial Susceptibility Testing of Anaerobic Bacteria. Approved Standard M11-A6.* Clinical and Laboratory Standards Institute, Wayne, Pa.
18. **Cormican, M. G., M. E. Erwin, and R. N. Jones.** 1996. False resistance to metronidazole by E-test among anaerobic bacteria investigations of contributing test conditions and medium quality. *Diagn. Microbiol. Infect.* Dis. **24:**117–119.
19. **Credito, K. L., and P. C. Appelbaum.** 2004. Activity of OPT-80, a novel macrocycle, compared with those of eight other agents against selected anaerobic species. *Antimicrob. Agents Chemother.* **48:**4430–4434.
20. **Cuchural, G. J., S. Hurlbut, M. H. Malamy, and F. P. Tally.** 1988. Permeability to beta-lactams in *Bacteroides fragilis*. *J. Antimicrob. Chemother.* **22:**785–790.
21. **Doern, G. V., R. N. Jones, E. H. Gerlach, J. A. Washington, D. J. Biedenbach, A. Brueggemann, M. E. Erwin, C. Knapp, and J. Raymond.** 1995. Multicenter clinical laboratory evaluation of a beta-lactamase disk assay employing a novel chromogenic cephalosporin, S1. *J. Clin. Microbiol.* **33:**1665–1667.
22. **Dougherty, S. H.** 1997. Antimicrobial culture and susceptibility testing has little value for routine management of secondary bacterial peritonitis. *Clin. Infect. Dis.* **25:** S258–S261.
23. **Ednie, L. M., M. R. Jacobs, and P. C. Appelbaum.** 1998. Activities of gatifloxacin compared to those of seven other agents against anaerobic organisms. *Antimicrob. Agents Chemother.* **42:**2459–2462.
24. **Finegold, S. M.** 1989. Therapy of anaerobic infections, p. 793–818. *In* S. M. Finegold and W. L. George (ed.), *Anaerobic Infections in Humans*. Academic Press, Orlando, Fla.
25. **Finegold, S. M.** 1997. Perspective on susceptibility testing of anaerobic bacteria. *Clin. Infect. Dis.* **25:**S251–S253.
26. **Finegold, S. M., and E. J. Goldstein.** 1993. Proceedings of the 1st North American Congress on Anaerobic Bacteria and Anaerobic Infections, July 1992. *Clin. Infect. Dis.* **16**(Suppl. 4):S159–S457.
27. **Gal, M., and J. S. Brazier.** 2004. Metronidazole resistance in *Bacteroides* spp. carrying *nim* genes and the selection of slow-growing metronidazole-resistant mutants. *J. Antimicrob. Chemother.* **54:**109–116.
28. **Georgopapadakou, N. H.** 1993. Penicillin-binding proteins and bacterial resistance to beta-lactams. *Antimicrob. Agents Chemother.* **37:**2045–2053.
29. **Golan, Y., L. A. McDermott, N. V. Jacobus, E. J. Goldstein, S. Finegold, L. J. Harrell, D. W. Hecht, S. G. Jenkins, C. Pierson, R. Venezia, J. Rihs, P. Iannini, S. L. Gorbach, and D. R. Snydman.** 2003. Emergence of fluoroquinolone resistance among *Bacteroides* species. *J. Antimicrob. Chemother.* **52:**208–213.
30. **Goldstein, E. J., and D. M. Citron.** 1993. Comparative susceptibilities of 173 aerobic and anaerobic bite wound isolates to sparfloxacin, temafloxacin, clarithromycin, and older agents. *Antimicrob. Agents Chemother.* **37:**1150–1153.
31. **Goldstein, E. J., D. M. Citron, C. V. Merriam, Y. Warren, and K. Tyrrell.** 1999. Activities of telithromycin (HMR 3647, RU 66647) compared to those of erythromycin, azithromycin, clarithromycin, roxithromycin, and other antimicrobial agents against unusual anaerobes. *Antimicrob. Agents Chemother.* **43:**2801–2805.
32. **Goldstein, E. J., D. M. Citron, C. V. Merriam, Y. Warren, K. Tyrrell, and H. T. Fernandez.** 2003. In vitro activities of dalbavancin and nine comparator agents against anaerobic gram-positive species and corynebacteria. *Antimicrob. Agents Chemother.* **47:**1968–1971.
33. **Goldstein, E. J., D. M. Citron, C. V. Merriam, Y. A. Warren, K. L. Tyrrell, and H. T. Fernandez.** 2004. In vitro activities of the new semisynthetic glycopeptide telavancin (TD-6424), vancomycin, daptomycin, linezolid, and four comparator agents against anaerobic gram-positive species and Corynebacterium spp. *Antimicrob. Agents Chemother.* **48:**2149–2152.
34. **Goldstein, E. J., D. M. Citron, C. V. Merriam, Y. A. Warren, K. L. Tyrrell, and H. T. Fernandez.** 2003. In vitro activities of daptomycin, vancomycin, quinupristin-dalfopristin, linezolid, and five other antimicrobials against 307 gram-positive anaerobic and 31 *Corynebacterium* clinical isolates. *Antimicrob. Agents Chemother.* **47:**337–341.
35. **Goldstein, E. J., D. M. Citron, M. C. Vreni, K. Tyrrell, and Y. Warren.** 1999. Activities of gemifloxacin (SB 265805, LB20304) compared to those of other oral antimicrobial agents against unusual anaerobes. *Antimicrob. Agents Chemother.* **43:**2726–2730.

36. **Goldstein, E. J., D. M. Citron, M. C. Vreni, Y. Warren, and K. L. Tyrrell.** 2000. Comparative in vitro activities of ertapenem (MK-0826) against 1,001 anaerobes isolated from human intra-abdominal infections. *Antimicrob. Agents Chemother.* **44:**2389–2394.
37. **Goldstein, E. J., D. M. Citron, Y. Warren, K. Tyrrell, and C. V. Merriam.** 1999. In vitro activity of gemifloxacin (SB 265805) against anaerobes. *Antimicrob. Agents Chemother.* **43:**2231–2235.
38. **Goldstein, E. J., P. H. Summanen, D. M. Citron, M. H. Rosove, and S. M. Finegold.** 1995. Fatal sepsis due to a beta-lactamase-producing strain of *Fusobacterium nucleatum* subspecies *polymorphum*. *Clin. Infect. Dis.* **20:**797–800.
39. **Goldstein, E. J. C., D. M. Citron, R. J. Goldman, M. C. Claros, and S. Hunt-Gerrado.** 1995. United States national hospital survey of anaerobic culture and susceptibility methods, II. *Anaerobe* **1:**309–314.
40. **Hecht, D. W.** 2004. Prevalence of antibiotic resistance in anaerobic bacteria: worrisome developments. *Clin. Infect. Dis.* **39:**92–97.
41. **Hecht, D. W., and L. Lederer.** 1995. Effect of choice of medium on the results of in vitro susceptibility testing of eight antibiotics against the *Bacteroides fragilis* group. *Clin. Infect. Dis.* **20:**S346–S349.
42. **Hecht, D. W., L. Lederer, and J. R. Osmolski.** 1995. Susceptibility results for the *Bacteroides fragilis* group: comparison of the broth microdilution and agar dilution methods. *Clin. Infect. Dis.* **20:**S342–S345.
43. **Hecht, D. W., and J. R. Osmolski.** 1996. Comparison of activities of trovafloxacin (CP-99,219) and five other agents against 585 anaerobes with use of three media. *Clin. Infect. Dis.* **23:**S44–S50.
44. **Hecht, D. W., and J. R. Osmolski.** 2003. Activities of garenoxacin (BMS-284756) and other agents against anaerobic clinical isolates. *Antimicrob. Agents Chemother.* **47:**910–916.
45. **Hecht, D. W., J. R. Osmolski, and J. P. O'Keefe.** 1993. Variation in the susceptibility of *Bacteroides fragilis* group isolates from six Chicago hospitals. *Clin. Infect. Dis.* **16:** S357–S360.
46. **Hecht, D. W., and H. M. Wexler.** 1996. In vitro susceptibility of anaerobes to quinolones in the United States. *Clin. Infect. Dis.* **23:**S2–S8.
47. **Hedberg, M., and C. E. Nord.** 2003. Antimicrobial susceptibility of Bacteroides fragilis group isolates in Europe. *Clin. Microbiol. Infect.* **9:**475–488.
48. **Hoellman, D. B., L. M. Kelly, M. R. Jacobs, and P. C. Appelbaum.** 2001. Comparative antianaerobic activity of BMS 284756. *Antimicrob .Agents Chemother.* **45:**589–592.
49. **Jacobus, N. V., L. A. McDermott, R. Ruthazer, and D. R. Snydman.** 2004. In vitro activities of tigecycline against the *Bacteroides fragilis* group. *Antimicrob. Agents Chemother.* **48:** 1034–1036.
50. **Johnson, C. C.** 1993. Susceptibility of anaerobic bacteria to beta-lactam antibiotics in the United States. *Clin. Infect. Dis.* **16:**S371–S376.
51. **Jousimies-Somer, H., and P. Summanen.** 2002. Recent taxonomic changes and terminology update of clinically significant anaerobic gram-negative bacteria (excluding spirochetes). *Clin. Infect. Dis.* **35:**S17–S21.
52. **Jousimies-Somer, H. R., P. Summanen, D. M. Citron, E. J. Baron, H. M. Wexler, and S. M. Finegold.** 2002. *Wadsworth-KTL Anaerobic Bacteriology Manual*. Star Publishing, Belmont, Calif.
53. **Koeth, L. M., C. E. Good, P. C. Appelbaum, E. J. Goldstein, A. C. Rodloff, M. Claros, and L. J. Dubreuil.** 2004. Surveillance of susceptibility patterns in 1,297 European and US anaerobic and capnophilic isolates to co-amoxiclav and five other antimicrobial agents. *J. Antimicrob. Chemother.* **53:**1039–1044.
54. **Labbe, A. C., A. M. Bourgault, J. Vincelette, P. L. Turgeon, and F. Lamothe.** 1999. Trends in antimicrobial resistance among clinical isolates of the *Bacteroides fragilis* group from 1992 to 1997 in Montreal, Canada. *Antimicrob. Agents Chemother.* **43:**2517–2519.
55. **Lofmark, S., H. Fang, M. Hedberg, and C. Edlund.** 2005. Inducible metronidazole resistance and nim genes in clinical *Bacteroides fragilis* group isolates. *Antimicrob. Agents Chemother.* **49:**1253–1256.
56. **Lubbe, M. M., P. L. Botha, and L. J. Chalkley.** 1999. Comparative activity of eighteen antimicrobial agents against anaerobic bacteria isolated in South Africa. *Eur. J. Clin. Microbiol. Infect. Dis.* **18:**46–54.
57. **Matto, J., S. Asikainen, M. L. Vaisanen, B. Von Troil-Linden, E. Kononen, M. Saarela, K. Salminen, S. M. Finegold, and H. Jousimies-Somer.** 1999. Beta-lactamase production in *Prevotella intermedia*, *Prevotella nigrescens*, and *Prevotella pallens* genotypes and in vitro susceptibilities to selected antimicrobial agents. *Antimicrob. Agents Chemother.* **43:**2383–2388.
58. **Molitoris, E., H. M. Wexler, and S. M. Finegold.** 1997. Sources and antimicrobial susceptibilities of *Campylobacter gracilis* and *Sutterella wadsworthensis*. *Clin. Infect. Dis.* **25:**S264–S265.
59. **Nguyen, M. H., V. L. Yu, A. J. Morris, L. McDermott, M. W. Wagener, L. Harrell, and D. R. Snydman.** 2000. Antimicrobial resistance and clinical outcome of *Bacteroides* bacteremia: findings of a multicenter prospective observational trial. *Clin. Infect. Dis.* **30:**870–876.
60. **Nyfors, S., E. Kononen, R. Syrjanen, E. Komulainen, and H. Jousimies-Somer.** 2003. Emergence of penicillin resistance among *Fusobacterium nucleatum* populations of commensal oral flora during early childhood. *J. Antimicrob. Chemother.* **51:**107–112.
61. **Oh, H., A. N. El, T. Davies, P. C. Appelbaum, and C. Edlund.** 2001. gyrA mutations associated with quinolone resistance in *Bacteroides fragilis* group strains. *Antimicrob. Agents Chemother.* **45:**1977–1981.
62. **Pelak, B. A., D. M. Citron, M. Motyl, E. J. Goldstein, G. L. Woods, and H. Teppler.** 2002. Comparative in vitro activities of ertapenem against bacterial pathogens from patients with acute pelvic infection. *J.Antimicrob. Chemother.* **50:**735–741.
63. **Podglajen, I., J. Breuil, and E. Collatz.** 1994. Insertion of a novel DNA sequence, 1S1186, upstream of the silent carbapenemase gene *cfiA*, promotes expression of carbapenem resistance in clinical isolates of *Bacteroides fragilis*. *Mol. Microbiol.* **12:**105–114.
64. **Reysset, G., A. Haggoud, W. J. Su, and M. Sebald.** 1992. Genetic and molecular analysis of pIP417 and pIP419: *Bacteroides* plasmids encoding 5-nitroimidazole resistance. *Plasmid* **27:**181–190.
65. **Roberts, M. C., J. Sutcliffe, P. Courvalin, L. B. Jensen, J. Rood, and H. Seppala.** 1999. Nomenclature for macrolide and macrolide-lincosamide-streptogramin B resistance determinants. *Antimicrob. Agents Chemother.* **43:**2823–2830.
66. **Rosenblatt, J.** 1989. Antimicrobic susceptibility of anaerobic bacteria, p. 715–727. *In* S. M. Finegold and W. L. George (ed.), *Anaerobic Infections in Humans*. Academic Press, San Diego, Calif.
67. **Rosenblatt, J. E., and I. Brook.** 1993. Clinical relevance of susceptibility testing of anaerobic bacteria. *Clin. Infect. Dis.* **16:**S446–S448.
68. **Rosenblatt, J. E., and D. R. Gustafson.** 1995. Evaluation of the Etest for susceptibility testing of anaerobic bacteria. *Diagn. Microbiol. Infect. Dis.* **22:**279–284.
69. **Salonen, J. H., E. Eerola, and O. Meurman.** 1998. Clinical significance and outcome of anaerobic bacteremia. *Clin. Infect. Dis.* **26:**1413–1417.
70. **Schapiro, J. M., R. Gupta, E. Stefansson, F. C. Fang, and A. P. Limaye.** 2004. Isolation of metronidazole-resistant

Bacteroides fragilis carrying the *nimA* nitroreductase gene from a patient in Washington State. *J. Clin. Microbiol.* **42:**4127–4129.

71. **Snydman, D. R., N. V. Jacobus, L. A. McDermott, R. Ruthazer, E. Goldstein, S. Finegold, L. Harrell, D. W. Hecht, S. Jenkins, C. Pierson, R. Venezia, J. Rihs, and S. L. Gorbach.** 2002. In vitro activities of newer quinolones against bacteroides group organisms. *Antimicrob. Agents Chemother.* **46:**3276–3279.
72. **Snydman, D. R., N. V. Jacobus, L. A. McDermott, R. Ruthazer, E. J. Goldstein, S. M. Finegold, L. J. Harrell, D. W. Hecht, S. G. Jenkins, C. Pierson, R. Venezia, J. Rihs, and S. L. Gorbach.** 2002. National survey on the susceptibility of *Bacteroides fragilis* Group: report and analysis of trends for 1997-2000. *Clin. Infect. Dis.* **35:** S126–S134.
73. **Snydman, D. R., N. V. Jacobus, L. A. McDermott, S. Supran, G. J. Cuchural, Jr., S. Finegold, L. Harrell, D. W. Hecht, P. Iannini, S. Jenkins, C. Pierson, J. Rihs, and S. L. Gorbach.** 1999. Multicenter study of in vitro susceptibility of the *Bacteroides fragilis* group, 1995 to 1996, with comparison of resistance trends from 1990 to 1996. *Antimicrob. Agents Chemother.* **43:**2417–2422.
74. **Snydman, D. R., L. McDermott, G. J. Cuchural, Jr., D. W. Hecht, P. B. Iannini, L. J. Harrell, S. G. Jenkins, J. P. O'Keefe, C. L. Pierson, J. D. Rihs, V. L. Yu, S. M. Finegold, and S. L. Gorbach.** 1996. Analysis of trends in antimicrobial resistance patterns among clinical isolates of *Bacteroides fragilis* group species from 1990 to 1994. *Clin. Infect. Dis.* **23:**S54–S65.
75. **Soki, J., E. Fodor, D. W. Hecht, R. Edwards, V. O. Rotimi, I. Kerekes, E. Urban, and E. Nagy.** 2004. Molecular characterization of imipenem-resistant, *cfiA*-positive *Bacteroides fragilis* isolates from the USA, Hungary and Kuwait. *J. Med. Microbiol.* **53:**413–419.
76. **Song, Y., C. Liu, M. McTeague, and S. M. Finegold.** 2003. 16S ribosomal DNA sequence-based analysis of clinically significant gram-positive anaerobic cocci. *J. Clin. Microbiol.* **41:**1363–1369.
77. **Summanen, P., H. M. Wexler, and S. M. Finegold.** 1992. Antimicrobial susceptibility testing of *Bilophila wadsworthia* by using triphenyltetrazolium chloride to facilitate endpoint determination. *Antimicrob. Agents Chemother.* **36:**1658–1664.
78. **Tanaka, K., C. Kawamura, K. Fukui, H. Kato, N. Kato, T. Nakamura, K. Watanabe, and K. Ueno.** 1999. Antimicrobial susceptibility and beta-lactamase production of *Prevotella* spp. and *Porphyromonas* spp. *Anaerobe* **5:**461–463.
79. **Teng, L. J., P. R. Hsueh, J. C. Tsai, S. J. Liaw, S. W. Ho, and K. T. Luh.** 2002. High incidence of cefoxitin and clindamycin resistance among anaerobes in Taiwan. *Antimicrob. Agents Chemother.* **46:**2908–2913.
80. **Theron, M. M., M. N. Janse van Rensburg, and L. J. Chalkley.** 2004. Nitroimidazole resistance genes *(nimB)* in anaerobic Gram-positive cocci (previously *Peptostreptococcus* spp.). *J. Antimicrob. Chemother.* **54:**240–242.
81. **Wexler, H. M., D. Molitoris, S. St. John, A. Vu, E. K. Read, and S. M. Finegold.** 2002. In vitro activities of faropenem against 579 strains of anaerobic bacteria. *Antimicrob. Agents Chemother.* **46:**3669–3675.
82. **Whittle, G., N. B. Shoemaker, and A. A. Salyers.** 2002. The role of Bacteroides conjugative transposons in the dissemination of antibiotic resistance genes. *Cell. Mol. Life Sci.* **59:**2044–2054.
83. **Wilson, S. E., and J. Huh.** 1997. In defense of routine antimicrobial susceptibility testing of operative site flora in patients with peritonitis. *Clin. Infect. Dis.* **25:**S254–S257.

Susceptibility Test Methods: Mycobacteria, *Nocardia*, and Other Actinomycetes*

GAIL L. WOODS, NANCY G. WARREN, AND CLARK B. INDERLIED

77

In his review article entitled "The White Plague," M. F. Perutz recounted that Cardinal Richelieu (1585 to 1642), Heinrich Heine (1797 to 1856), Frédéric Chopin (1810 to 1849), Anton Chekhov (1860 to 1904), Franz Kafka (1883 to 1924), George Orwell (1903 to 1950), and Eleanor Roosevelt (1884 to 1962) all had a common fate (112). Each of them died of tuberculosis. For many of these famous cases, it is unknown if the disease was only poorly understood or if management of the disease was simply inadequate or even inappropriate. For some, effective antimicrobial agents for the treatment of tuberculosis had not been discovered or were discovered too late. Streptomycin and *p*-aminosalicylic acid were not introduced until the late 1940s, and isoniazid, ethambutol, and rifampin were not used to treat tuberculosis until 1952, 1961, and 1968, respectively. Therefore, it is also possible that the more contemporary of these patients were early victims of antimicrobial resistance. In the same article, Professor Perutz related the response of the Nobel laureate Gerhard Domagk (1895 to 1964) to Otto Warburg's (1883 to 1970) comment that Domagk "deserved monuments in each valley and every mountain." Domagk, who in 1935 discovered Prontosil (a precursor of sulfanilamide), Conteben (thiosemicarbzone), and Neoteben (isonicotinic acid hydrazide), replied to Warburg that "no one is interested any longer in diseases that can be cured." Domagk could not have anticipated the extent to which antibiotic resistance would come to complicate the chemotherapy of all infectious diseases, especially tuberculosis.

ANTIMICROBIAL AGENTS

Although a variety of antimicrobial agents are available for the treatment of mycobacterial diseases, not all agents are suitable for treating all types of infections. Furthermore, in the face of antimicrobial resistance, the choice of alternative therapies can be problematic and clinical experience becomes a prevailing factor. For other uncommon mycobacterial infections, the physician is not infrequently faced with a dilemma in choosing a treatment regimen because of a lack of clinical precedence or unclear efficacy. The situation is confounded further by the need to treat mycobacterial infections with a combination of agents to improve efficacy, to prevent resistance, or to overcome intrinsic resistance (34).

The antimicrobial agents that are used in the treatment of mycobacterial infections are discussed below and, for the most commonly encountered species, the primary agents are summarized in Table 1 (75, 160). For tuberculosis, first-line drugs are those usually used to treat uncomplicated cases. The Clinical and Laboratory Standards Institute (CLSI, formerly National Committee for Clinical Laboratory Standards [NCCLS]) document on drug susceptibility testing of mycobacteria (28) currently recommends that first-line testing include ethambutol (EMB), rifampin (RMP), two levels of isoniazid (INH), and pyrazinamide (PZA). In the United States, streptomycin (SM) has been moved from first-line to second-line testing (28). Second-line drugs are those used when first-line therapy fails or is inappropriate. These agents are often accompanied by more severe side effects.

Drug resistance in *Mycobacterium tuberculosis* occurs randomly and at a low frequency and is usually a result of single-step mutations. There are two types of drug resistance seen in *M. tuberculosis:* primary and acquired. Primary drug resistance occurs when drug-resistant organisms are found in a previously untreated person. Acquired resistance, the most common form of resistance, can emerge against any of the antituberculosis agents during chemotherapy (111).

Antibiotic resistance in bacteria can occur by a number of mechanisms (summarized for *M. tuberculosis* in Table 2). Five of these categories are found in mycobacteria: decreased uptake of drug such as seen in dormant acid-fast bacilli; drug inactivation by production of β-lactamases; increased efflux as seen in fluoroquinolone resistance; alteration of the target as described below with RMP and INH; and reduced pro-drug-activating enzymes as exhibited in PZA resistance (157).

Isoniazid

Isoniazid (INH) (isonicotinic acid hydrazide), a synthetic antimicrobial agent introduced in 1952 for the treatment of tuberculosis, is remarkably specific and potently bactericidal for tubercle bacilli. INH has comparatively low toxicity and is active against virtually all wild-type strains of *M. tuberculosis.* The mechanism of action of INH occurs in three steps: (i) activation of the drug, (ii) binding of the "active" form to the target(s) of inhibition, and (iii) exertion of an inhibitory effect. In turn, the mechanism of INH resistance can involve alterations in each of these steps, alone or in combination. While the mechanism of INH activation is not completely resolved, it is likely that the process involves an oxidation

*This chapter contains information presented in chapter 73 by Clark B. Inderlied and Gaby E. Pfyffer in the eighth edition of this Manual.

TABLE 1 Antimicrobial agents recommended for primary treatment of common mycobacterial infections

Mycobacterium species	Site of infection: antimicrobial agents
M. tuberculosis complex[a]	Any site: isoniazid + rifampin + ethambutol + pyrazinamide
M. avium complex	Pulmonary: clarithromycin (or azithromycin) + rifampin + ethambutol; disseminated: clarithromycin (or azithromycin) + ethambutol ± rifabutin
M. kansasii	Pulmonary: isoniazid + rifampin + ethambutol
M. abscessus, M. chelonae, M. fortuitum[b]	Nonpulmonary: clarithromycin (if susceptible) + ≥1 other drug, based on susceptibility test results
M. abscessus[c]	Pulmonary: multidrug regimen, based on susceptibility test results, that includes clarithromycin
M. marinum	Clarithromycin, doxycycline or minocycline, trimethoprim-sulfamethoxazole, or rifampin + ethambutol

[a] Almost all (>95%) *M. bovis* isolates are resistant to pyrazinamide.
[b] Surgical debridement often is important for successful therapy.
[c] Currently there are no drug regimens of proven efficacy. Antimicrobial therapy may provide symptomatic improvement and disease regression. Surgical resection of limited disease (if possible) and multidrug therapy are optimal.

reaction catalyzed by a catalase-peroxidase encoded by the *katG* gene (182). The oxidized form of INH can then covalently bind to the nicotinamide moiety of NAD(H) to form INH-NAD(H) adducts, which in turn compete with NAD(H) for binding to an enoyl-acyl carrier protein reductase encoded by the *inhA* gene (76).

The primary effect of INH is on mycolic acid synthesis, as evidenced by the increased fragility of the mycobacterial cell, increased intracellular viscosity, decreased cellular hydrophobicity, and loss of acid fastness of INH-resistant isolates (169). The mycolic acids are produced by the fatty acid synthesis (FAS) I and II enzyme systems. It is the FAS II system that synthesizes the long-chain mycolic acids that are species specific. Activated INH targets one of the FASII enzymes, the enoyl-acyl carrier protein (ACP) reductase of InhA. However, InhA is not the only target, because activated INH also targets the fatty acid elongation enzyme ketoacyl-ACP synthase A or KasA. In addition, INH appears to interfere with NAD metabolism, energy metabolism, and macromolecular synthesis (36, 170, 171).

The mechanism of action of INH correlates with the known mechanisms of INH resistance. Banerjee et al. (6) reported that INH and ethionamide resistance in *M. tuberculosis* correlated with a missense mutation in the *inhA* gene. Other studies showed that *katG* mutations account for 30 to 60% of INH resistance (65, 101) and that *inhA* mutations confer a low level of INH resistance that may not always be clinically significant (89). Mutations in two other genes may confer some INH resistance: the *ahpC* gene, which encodes an alkyl hydroperoxide reductase subunit (38, 80, 142, 168, 181), and the *kasA* gene, which encodes the previously mentioned KasA enzyme (90). The degree to which mutations in *ahpC* and *kasA* contribute to INH resistance is not clear, although the role of *ahpC* appears to be minor. In aggregate, however, mutations in these four genes (*katG, inhA, ahpC,* and *kasA*) may account for ~90% of INH resistance (Table 2) (39, 149).

INH is active only against replicating tubercle bacilli in the presence of oxygen; slowly replicating bacilli in the caseous lesions are not readily killed by INH, and dormant bacilli under anaerobic conditions are unlikely to be affected. INH resistance develops rapidly when patients are given monotherapy, and the frequency of INH resistance within a population of tubercle bacilli ranges from 10^{-5} to 10^{-6} (33). Wild-type isolates of *M. tuberculosis* are inhibited by INH at concentrations of <0.2 μg/ml (93). Other slowly growing mycobacteria, such as *M. kansasii* and *M. xenopi*, are inhibited by 1 to 5 μg/ml. Most other nontuberculous mycobacteria, including the *M. avium* complex (MAC), *M. marinum*, and all rapidly growing mycobacteria, are resistant to INH.

TABLE 2 Mechanisms of drug resistance in *Mycobacterium tuberculosis*[a]

Antimicrobial agent	Gene involved	Target	Mechanism of action
RMP	*rpoB*	β Subunit of RNA polymerase	Inhibits transcription
INH	*katG*	Catalase-peroxidase	Inhibits mycolic acid biosynthesis; other multiple effects on DNA, lipids, carbohydrates, and NAD metabolism
	inhA[b]	EnvM analog 3-ketoacyl-acyl carrier protein reductase analog	
	kasA[b]	B-Keroacyl ACP synthase	
	ahpC[b]	Subunit of alkyl hydroperoxide reductase	
EMB	*embB*	Arabinosyltransferase	Inhibits arbinogalactan synthesis
SM	*rpsL*	Ribosomal protein S12	Inhibits protein synthesis
		16S rRNA	Inhibits protein synthesis
PZA	*pncA*	Pyrazinamidase	Acidifies cytoplasm and de-energizes membrane
Ethionamide	*inhA*		Inhibits mycolic acid biosynthesis
Fluoroquinolones	*gyrA*	DNA gyrase A subunit	Inhibits DNA gyrase
Amikacin, kanamycin	*rrs*	16S rRNA	Inhibits protein synthesis

[a] Adapted from reference 157.
[b] Mechanism of action statement similar to that of *katG*.

INH is well absorbed when administered orally or intramuscularly; it is distributed throughout the body, and the levels in cerebrospinal fluid (CSF) may equal the levels in plasma in patients with meningeal inflammation or 20% of the levels in plasma in patients without inflammation (160). INH is metabolized in the liver and intestines, primarily by acetylation by an *N*-acetyltransferase, which can vary significantly from person to person. However, the acetylator phenotype of an individual does not appear to influence either the efficacy of INH or the risk of hepatotoxicity. Adverse drug reactions include infrequent, age-related hepatitis and, less frequently, peripheral neuropathy, hypersensitivity reactions such as fever and rash, and arthralgias.

Rifampin

Rifampin (RMP) (rifampicin) was introduced in 1968 as a potent antituberculosis agent. It affects intracellular, slowly replicating bacilli in caseous lesions as well as the actively replicating bacilli in open cavities. RMP is active against a wide variety of non-acid-fast bacteria and several other slowly growing mycobacteria, notably *M. leprae, M. kansasii, M. xenopi,* and *M. marinum,* but has variable activity in vitro against MAC and is inactive against the rapidly growing mycobacteria. It easily diffuses through the mycobacterial cell membrane due to its lipophilic nature and binds to the bacterial RNA polymerase, thus inhibiting RNA synthesis (156). RMP inhibits the prokaryotic DNA-dependent RNA polymerase by binding to the β subunit at the presumed catalytic center of the enzyme. The mammalian RNA polymerase is inhibited by RMP only at significantly higher concentrations than is the prokaryotic enzyme. The RNA polymerase of MAC isolates appears to be susceptible to RMP; therefore, the primary mechanism of intrinsic resistance is most probably impermeability.

Telenti et al. (150) first showed that RMP resistance correlated with changes, primarily amino acid substitutions, within a conserved region of the *rpoB* gene that encodes the β subunit of the *M. tuberculosis* RNA polymerase. Subsequent studies showed that >96% of RMP resistance could be attributed to mutations within an 81-bp region of the *rpoB* gene (103). Rifamycin resistance that is due to mutations outside this "hot spot" are rare, but such mutations appear to cluster at codon 176 at the beginning of the *rpoB* gene (62). In two strains of *M. avium* with high MIC values, missense mutations were detected, but in two other strains, no mutations were detected. This agrees with the observations of Guerrero et al. (54), who showed that mutations in the *rpoB* gene in *M. avium* and *M. intracellulare* are rare and that high RMP MIC values most probably are a reflection of impermeability to the drug.

RMP is well absorbed from the gastrointestinal tract, and peak concentrations of 5 to 10 μg/ml are reached 1 to 2 h after an oral dose of 600 mg; concentrations in CSF reach 50% of the levels in plasma in patients with meningeal inflammation. RMP is available in combination with INH as a single capsule (Rifamate) containing 300 mg of RMP and 150 mg of INH and in combination with INH and pyrazinamide as a single capsule (Rifater). An RMP concentration of 0.5 μg/ml is bactericidal for wild-type isolates of *M. tuberculosis.* Adverse drug reactions include hepatotoxicity, gastrointestinal and hypersensitivity reactions, and a red-orange discoloration of urine, tears, other body fluids, and soft contact lenses. RMP also induces increased hepatic metabolism of several other drugs, including methadone and birth control pills. Of particular concern is the interaction of RMP and, to a somewhat lesser degree, rifabutin with protease inhibitors (saquinavir, ritonavir, and indinavir), which leads to enhanced hepatic metabolism and may result in subtherapeutic levels of the antiviral agents (9).

Rifabutin and Rifapentine

Rifabutin (ansamycin), a spiropiperidyl rifamycin, and rifapentine, a cyclopentyl rifamycin, have potent in vitro activity against *M. tuberculosis*. Rifabutin also is very active against MAC (64, 129). The mode of action and mechanism of resistance of both drugs appear to be identical to those of RMP; however, approximately 30% of RMP-resistant *M. tuberculosis* isolates are susceptible to rifabutin and rifapentine. The latter observation correlates with certain specific mutations in the *rpoB* gene (14). Yang et al. (178) analyzed clinical strains of *M. tuberculosis* for cross-resistance to rifamycins. Alterations at codons 513 and 531 correlate with resistance to RMP, rifabutin, and rifalazil (KRM-1648). Point mutations at codons 516 and 529, deletion at codon 518, and insertion at codon 514 influence susceptibility to RMP but not to rifabutin or KM-1648, while alteration at codons 515, 521, and 533 did not influence susceptibility to RMP, rifabutin, and KR-1648 (178). These findings were confirmed by analyzing recombinant *M. tuberculosis* clones containing plasmids with specific mutations (166). As with RMP, both rifabutin and rifapentine are metabolized to the corresponding biologically active 25-desacetyl metabolite. Rifabutin decreases the incidence of disseminated MAC disease in human immunodeficiency virus (HIV)-infected patients when used as a prophylactic agent, and it is approved for that indication (87, 107). The role of rifabutin as a therapeutic agent for MAC disease is unclear, but there may be a significant dose effect (73). In addition to being more active than RMP on a weight basis, rifabutin has a long elimination half-life in humans and concentrates in tissues, notably lung tissues, where the levels are 10-fold higher than in serum. This may account for the reported effectiveness of rifabutin in the therapy of MAC pulmonary infections.

Rifabutin is absorbed from the gastrointestinal tract and reaches peak levels of 0.5 μg/ml in serum about 4 h after a 300-mg dose. Adverse drug reactions with rifabutin are similar to those observed with RMP, including the above-mentioned important adverse interactions with antiretroviral agents (9). Some unique rifabutin toxicities include leukopenia, thrombocytopenia, arthralgias, and uveitis when coadministered with clarithromycin.

Rifapentine was approved by the U.S. Food and Drug Administration (FDA) for the treatment of tuberculosis in 1998 (5). In a study of 722 patients, 361 received rifapentine plus INH, PZA, and EMB while the remaining patients received RMP in place of rifapentine along with the other drugs (5). In the intensive phase of the study, rifapentine was administered twice a week while RMP was administered daily. In the continuation phase, rifapentine and INH were administered once a week and RMP and INH were administered twice a week. Sputum conversion was somewhat higher in the rifapentine group than in the RMP group: 87 and 81%, respectively. However, relapse was somewhat higher in the rifapentine group than in the RMP group: 10 and 5%, respectively. Rifapentine reaches a peak concentration of 15 μg/ml in serum 5 to 6 h after a 600-mg dose, with a half-life of about 13 h.

Pyrazinamide

Pyrazinamide (PZA) is a synthetic derivative (pyrazine analog) of nicotinamide and, in combination with INH, is rapidly bactericidal for replicating and nonreplicating forms of *M. tuberculosis,* with an average MIC of 20 μg/ml (157). PZA is totally inactive against other *Mycobacterium* species, including M. *bovis*, MAC, and the rapidly growing mycobacteria. PZA is active only at an acidic pH; therefore, the pH of the growth medium must be adjusted for accurate measurements of the in vitro activity of the drug. It is most likely that PZA is active only in the acidic milieu of the phagolysosome and, depending on the concentration achieved at the site of the infection, may be bacteriostatic or bactericidal. PZA is hydrolyzed in the liver to the active metabolite pyrazinoic acid, and although the mechanism of action of PZA is unknown, its activity depends on this conversion. M. *tuberculosis* produces a pyrazinamidase, and most strains of PZA-resistant M. *tuberculosis* lack this enzyme; however, some PZA-resistant isolates retain enzyme activity, suggesting that there are other mechanisms of resistance such as drug efflux (183, 184).

The lack of pyrazinamidase activity and its correlation with PZA resistance have been associated with mutations in the *pncA* gene that encodes the enzyme (135, 136, 143). Indeed, it now appears that 72 to 97% of PZA resistance can be attributed to mutations in the *pncA* gene (Table 2). Data from one study suggest that this correlation can be used to distinguish between M. *tuberculosis* and M. *bovis* (134); however, PZA-susceptible M. *bovis* isolates, although uncommon, have been described.

PZA is well absorbed from the gastrointestinal tract and widely distributed throughout the body, with maximum levels in serum of approximately 45 μg/ml 1 to 4 h following an oral dose of 1 g (20 to 25 mg/kg of body weight). Hepatotoxicity occurs in a small number of patients; photosensitivity and rash are rare. Gout is an important contraindication because of the hyperuricemia associated with PZA therapy. PZA therapy is usually discontinued after the first 2 months of short-course treatment for tuberculosis, whereas INH and RMP treatment is continued for an additional 4 months.

Ethambutol

Ethambutol (EMB) [dextro-2,2-(ethylenediimino)-di-1-butanol-dihydrochloride] is a synthetic antituberculosis compound that was introduced in 1961. The MIC values of EMB tested against wild-type isolates of M. *tuberculosis* range from 1 to 5 μg/ml, but the activity of the drug against other slowly growing nontuberculous mycobacteria is more variable. The drug is active only against growing bacilli and has no activity against nongrowing mycobacteria. The primary mechanism of action of EMB is bacteriostatic inhibition of cell wall synthesis, while evidence points to a specific effect on arabinogalactan synthesis (147). The frequency of mutation to EMB resistance in M. *tuberculosis* is on the order of 10^{-5}, and there is evidence that EMB resistance in M. *tuberculosis* correlates with a specific mutation (at codon 306) in the *embB* gene, which encodes an arabinosyltransferase (144). Mutations in this codon have been associated with MIC values of 20 to 40 μg/ml for several EMB-resistant isolates of M. *tuberculosis* (1). While mutations in the *embB* gene result in high-level resistance in M. *tuberculosis*, this mutation accounts for only 70% of resistant strains; thus, other gene mutations are likely to play an additional role (157). Although many MAC isolates have high EMB MIC values, combinations of EMB and other agents, notably quinolones and macrolides, are synergistic (66, 78), and it has been shown that the MIC value does not correlate with clinical response (141). It appears that EMB affects the permeability of the MAC cell wall and perhaps increases the intracellular concentration of the other potentially more active drugs (67).

Peak concentrations of EMB in serum are 5 μg/ml 2 to 4 h after a 25-mg/kg dose. The most important adverse effect associated with EMB is decreased visual acuity due to optic neuritis that is related to both the dose and duration of treatment. EMB is not recommended for the treatment of children too young to be monitored for changes in vision unless no other drug is appropriate because of resistance. The effects on vision are generally reversible when the drug is discontinued.

Aminoglycosides

The aminoglycosides that are used for the treatment of tuberculosis and other mycobacterial infections include streptomycin (SM), kanamycin (a glycoside of 2-deoxystreptamine), and amikacin, which is a derivative of kanamycin. In addition, tobramycin is active against M. *chelonae*, and capreomycin and viomycin, basic peptide antibiotics with a mechanism of action similar to that of the aminoglycosides, are active against M. *tuberculosis* and certain other species of mycobacteria. Gentamicin is inactive against mycobacteria at the usual concentrations attained in serum.

The primary mechanism of action of the aminoglycosides is inhibition of the post- to pretranslocation step of protein synthesis by blocking the binding of the aminoacyl-tRNA (e-type binding). Viomycin also blocks aminoacyl-tRNA translocation, and viomycin resistance crosses to capreomycin, suggesting that the mechanism of action is the same. SM MIC values for wild-type isolates of M. *tuberculosis* are usually well below the peak concentration in serum of 25 to 50 μg/ml 1 to 2 h after a 1-g intramuscular dose. Amikacin is the most potent of the aminoglycosides. There is comparatively little clinical experience with amikacin in the treatment of tuberculosis because the drug is expensive and inconvenient to administer, but amikacin often is used in combination with one or more other agents for treatment of serious infections caused by rapidly growing mycobacteria. Amikacin also is active against MAC; the majority of isolates have an MIC of <32 μg/ml, which approaches the maximum concentration in serum. In an early uncontrolled trial of disseminated MAC in HIV-infected patients, amikacin was shown to be the active component of a multiple-drug regimen (26). In that trial, treatment was associated with a positive microbiological and clinical response, but the clinical utility of amikacin for disseminated MAC is uncertain (4). The drug may be useful in an "induction" regimen to clear a bacteremia.

The molecular basis of SM resistance (Table 2) in M. *tuberculosis* results from mutations in the gene that encodes ribosomal protein S12 or from mutations in the 16S rRNA region, which is structurally linked to the S12 protein in the assembled ribosome (47, 81, 104). Finken et al. (47) showed that mutations in the *rpsL* gene coding for the S12 protein were present in 20 of 38 SM-resistant strains and that there was a mutation in the *ssr* gene, encoding 16S rRNA, in 9 strains. Nair et al. (104) determined the nucleotide sequence of the *rpsL* gene and showed that SM resistance, in a small number of isolates, appeared to be a result of point mutations at codon 43 of this gene, a site of SM resistance in *Escherichia coli*. Adverse drug reactions associated with aminoglycosides and peptide antibiotics include hearing loss, tinnitis, loss of balance, and renal failure.

Cycloserine

D-Cycloserine (4-amino-3-isooxazolidinone) is an analog of D-alanine that inhibits the synthesis of D-alanyl-D-alanine, an essential component of the mycobacterial cell wall. Cycloserine is active against all mycobacteria as well as several other types of bacteria. Although it is one of the secondary drugs for treatment of tuberculosis, in vitro susceptibility testing is not recommended due to technical problems with the test (28, 113). Peak levels in serum of 20 to 40 μg/ml are achieved 4 h following an oral dose of 250 mg. The drug is widely distributed through the body, including the CSF. There are significant adverse drug reactions associated with cycloserine treatment, notably peripheral neuropathy and central nervous system dysfunction including seizures and psychotic disturbances.

Ethionamide

Ethionamide (2-ethyl-pyridine-4-carbonic acid thioamide) is a derivative of isonicotinic acid and, like INH, blocks mycolic acid synthesis. However, isolates of *M. tuberculosis* that are resistant to high concentrations of INH are susceptible to ethionamide, suggesting that the site of action may be different from that of INH. However, mutations in the *inhA* gene have been associated with ethionamide resistance (6). The average MIC for *M. tuberculosis* is 0.6 to 2.5 μg/ml, and levels of 2 to 20 μg/ml in serum are achieved 3 to 4 h following an oral dose of 0.5 to 1 g. Side effects associated with ethionamide include gastrointestinal irritation with nausea, vomiting, and cramps and neurologic symptoms.

Dapsone

Dapsone (diaminodiphenyl sulfone) is a synthetic compound that was shown to be active against *M. leprae* in the early 1940s. Dapsone is an antifolate that, like other inhibitors of folic acid synthesis, exerts primarily a bacteriostatic effect and is only weakly bactericidal. Dapsone is administered orally and is well absorbed and distributed throughout the body. Levels in tissue are approximately 2 μg/ml following a 200-mg dose. The drug has a long half-life in serum, of 10 to 50 h depending on the individual patient. Common adverse drug reactions include nausea, vomiting, anorexia, and methemaglobinemia; hematuria, rash, pruritus, and fever also can occur. Traditionally, dapsone is used in combination with RMP and clofazimine for the treatment of leprosy. Acedapsone is a diacetylated form of dapsone with an extraordinarily long half-life of 46 days; as a result, this drug is administered infrequently (e.g., five injections per year), with peak concentrations in tissue occurring 20 to 35 days after administration. Acedapsone is relatively inactive against *M. leprae*, but in vivo it is deacetylated to the parent compound.

Macrolides and Ketolides

Azithromycin and clarithromycin are the most important agents in the treatment of all forms of MAC disease and are effective and approved prophylactic agents for preventing disseminated MAC disease in HIV-infected persons (58, 117, 180). These drugs also are useful in the treatment of disease caused by *M. marinum*, *M. haemophilum*, *M. kansasii*, *M. simiae*, and rapidly growing mycobacteria other than *M. fortuitum*. Indeed, they are viewed as potential cornerstones in the treatment of nontuberculous mycobacterial infections (4). Azithromycin, an azalide (a subclass of macrolides), and clarithromycin are structurally similar to erythromycin and have modifications that improve their acid stability and increase their potency, half-life, achievable concentrations in tissue, and bioavailability without causing toxicity. These macrolides are bacteriostatic agents and inhibit the growth of microorganisms by binding to the 50S subunit of the prokaryotic ribosome, blocking protein synthesis at the peptidyltransferase step. Meier et al. (92) showed that both clarithromycin- and azithromycin-resistant mutants of *M. intracellulare* have a single-base mutation at adenine-2058 in the 23S rRNA gene, a site of mutation or methylation that has been associated with macrolide resistance in other bacteria (106). The same genetic basis for macrolide resistance was found in *M. chelonae* and *M. abscessus* (158).

The in vitro activity of azithromycin against MAC appears to be quite modest, with MIC values 32- to 64-fold above the maximum concentration in serum (74). The remarkable ability of azithromycin to concentrate in tissues most likely accounts for its therapeutic activity in animal studies and humans (76, 83). Azithromycin is rapidly absorbed from the gastrointestinal tract and widely distributed throughout the body. It has a terminal half-life of 68 h. The peak concentration in serum following a 500-mg dose is 0.4 to 0.6 μg/ml; however, the drug concentrates in tissues to high levels. In a small study with humans, the levels of azithromycin in polymorphonuclear neutrophils were nearly 1,000-fold higher than the levels in serum (3, 133).

Clarithromycin inhibits 90% of MAC isolates with MIC values of 0.25 to 0.5 μg/ml when measured by a radiometric broth macrodilution method at a neutral to slightly alkaline pH (the activities of all macrolides are strongly influenced by pH). Peak levels in serum of 2 to 3 μg/ml are achieved 5 to 6 h following a 500-mg dose; the concentrations in tissue are 4 to 5 times greater than the concentrations in serum, and the concentration in macrophages is 20 to 30 times greater. The elimination half-life is 5 to 7 h following a 500-mg dose twice a day.

The ketolides are semisynthetic derivatives of erythromycin with structural changes that improved antimicrobial activity and pharmacokinetics. Telithromycin, a ketolide licensed in the United States and Europe, is active against mycobacteria in vitro but has not been evaluated in a clinical trial in humans (46, 121).

Quinolones

Ciprofloxacin, ofloxacin, levofloxacin, gatifloxacin, and moxifloxacin are fluorinated carboxyquinolones with good in vitro activity against multidrug-resistant and pansusceptible *M. tuberculosis* (15, 70, 75). MIC values of ciprofloxacin and ofloxacin against susceptible isolates of *M. tuberculosis* range from 0.25 to 3 μg/ml and from 0.5 to 2.5 μg/ml, respectively. Measurements of the early bactericidal activity of ciprofloxacin in patients with pulmonary tuberculosis suggested that the drug is effective at a high dosage (1,000 mg/day) (140). Fluoroquinolones have variable activity against MAC (179). Most *M. fortuitum* group isolates are susceptible to ciprofloxacin (currently the class representative for fluoroquinolones), whereas activity against *M. abscessus* and *M. chelonae* is more variable.

The CLSI recommends that ofloxacin be included as the class representative for fluoroquinolones in the panel of secondary antituberculosis drugs (28). The suggested susceptibility breakpoint is 2 μg/ml for the agar proportion method (28). However, levofloxacin (the L-isomer of ofloxacin) is nearly twice as active against *M. tuberculosis* as ofloxacin in vitro. For this reason, protocols for susceptibility testing of levofloxacin are desirable. Data from a recent study support susceptibility breakpoints of 2 μg/ml for BACTEC TB460 and BACTEC MGIT 960 and 1 μg/ml for agar proportion (132).

The mechanism of action of all fluorinated quinolones is inhibition of DNA synthesis as a result of binding to the DNA gyrase (bacterial topoisomerase II) (123). Although this is the presumed mechanism of action in mycobacteria, fewer studies have been performed with mycobacteria than with other microorganisms. Takiff et al. (148) showed that quinolone resistance in *M. tuberculosis* can be ascribed to mutations in the *gyrA* and *gyrB* genes, which encode the DNA gyrase subunits (Table 2). In *M. tuberculosis,* fluoroquinolones function by binding to the bacterial enzyme-DNA complex, with suggested mechanisms being strand-breakage, SOS-mediated autolysis, and replication blockage. When combined with various first-line antimycobacterial drugs, fluoroquinolones have shown greater reductions in CFUs within infected macrophages than the individual drugs alone. While there are no reports of cross-resistance between quinolones and other classes of antimycobacterial agents, there is cross-resistance within the quinolone class, such that reduced susceptibility to one quinolone may likely confer reduced efficacy to all quinolones (51).

Recently, moxifloxacin has received attention as being useful in the treatment of tuberculosis, especially multidrug cases. Although slightly delayed in the first few days of response, the antimycobacterial effect of moxifloxacin appears to be similar to that of INH after 5 days of treatment (119). The newer quinolones (sparfloxacin, gatifloxacin, and moxifloxacin) have lower MICs than levofloxicin, ciprofloxacin, and ofloxacin. Treatment studies with mice have shown moxifloxacin has the most bactericidal efficacy against *M. tuberculosis,* followed by sparfloxacin, levofloxicin, and ofloxacin (in that order). Against *M. tuberculosis,* moxifloxacin has a reported MIC of 0.12 to 0.5 μg/ml (51).

Ciprofloxacin is well absorbed from the gastrointestinal tract and is rapidly distributed throughout the body. Maximum concentrations in serum of 2.4 or 4.3 μg/ml are achieved 1 to 2 h after an oral dose of 500 or 750 mg, respectively. The elimination half-life of ciprofloxacin is 4 h in subjects with normal renal function. Maximum ofloxacin concentrations in serum are achieved 1 to 2 h after an oral dose. Following a single 400-mg dose, the concentration of ofloxacin in serum is 2.9 μg/ml; after a steady-state dose, it is 4.6 μg/ml. The maximum concentration of levofloxacin in serum is approximately twice that of ofloxacin at the same dosage. The efficacy of fluoroquinolones in the treatment of pulmonary tuberculosis may relate, in part, to the observation that these quinolones concentrate in lung tissue to levels at least four times greater than the concentration in serum. Adverse effects with ciprofloxacin and other fluoroquinolones may be less severe than with the other secondary agents (12).

p-Aminosalicylic Acid

p-Aminosalicylic acid (PAS) is an antifolate that is active against *M. tuberculosis* but inactive against most other mycobacteria. There is some evidence that PAS also may affect iron transport in *M. tuberculosis* and salicylic acid metabolism. The average MIC for susceptible isolates of *M. tuberculosis* is 1 μg/ml, and peak levels of 7 to 8 μg/ml are achieved in serum 1 to 2 h after a 4-g dose. PAS is incompletely absorbed in the gastrointestinal tract and is associated with significant gastrointestinal side effects; in combination with the need for large dosages (10 to 12 g/day), this leads to frequent problems with treatment adherence.

Clofazimine

Clofazimine [3-(*p*-chloroanilino)-10-(*p*-chlorophenyl)-2, 10-dihydro-2-isopropyliminophenazine] is a substituted iminophenazine, bright red dye. It has weak bactericidal activity against *M. leprae* but is used in combination with RMP and dapsone as a conventional treatment regimen for leprosy. However, it may take up to 50 days of treatment before there is evidence of tissue antimicrobial activity, which may influence the length of time before there is a clinical response in the treatment of leprosy. Clofazimine has good in vitro activity against MAC, but despite this, it appears to offer little in the treatment of disseminated MAC (137). Indeed, treatment regimens that contained clofazimine have been associated with higher mortality than those that did not (24). The drug also has good in vitro activity against *M. tuberculosis,* but there is little or no information on the in vivo activity.

The mechanism of action of clofazimine is unknown; however, it is highly lipophilic and binds preferentially to mycobacterial DNA. The absorption of clofazimine following an oral dose is variable and ranges from 45 to 60%. The average concentrations in serum are 0.7 to 1.0 μg/ml following a dose of 100 to 300 mg. The half-life is extraordinarily long (estimated to be 70 days), and the drug tends to be deposited in fatty tissues and cells of the reticuloendothelial system. Adverse drug reactions are limited primarily to a pink or red discoloration of the skin, conjunctiva, cornea, and body fluids and gastrointestinal intolerance including pain, diarrhea, nausea, and vomiting.

Amithiozone

Amithiozone (Thiacetazone, Tibione, or Panthrone) is a thiosemicarbazole that is active against *M. tuberculosis,* with an average MIC for wild-type strains of 1 μg/ml. Resistance develops quickly when monotherapy is given. Peak levels in serum of 1 to 4 μg/ml are achieved 1 to 2 h following an oral dose of 150 mg. Adverse drug reactions are gastrointestinal irritation and bone marrow suppression, and hepatotoxicity can occur in patients receiving concomitant INH. Additionally, there appears to be an association of Stevens-Johnson syndrome and severe epidermal necrolysis in HIV-infected patients with tuberculosis treated by regimens containing amithiozone (42, 53). Consequently, the World Health Organization recommends that amithiozone not be used to treat patients known or suspected to be infected with HIV (109). Amithiozone is not available in the United States and is not used in Europe because of the adverse effects, but it has been used successfully in combination with INH for the treatment of tuberculosis in some African countries, where adverse effects are believed to be less severe.

M. TUBERCULOSIS COMPLEX

Drug Resistance

In the early 1960s, the World Health Organization organized two meetings that led to the description of reliable criteria and techniques for testing mycobacteria for resistance to antituberculosis drugs (20, 21). The critical proportion for resistance on Löwenstein-Jensen slants varied according to the drug, e.g., 1% for INH and RMP and 10% for SM, EMB, PZA, ethionamide, kanamycin, and cycloserine. However, based on the experience of Russel and Middlebrook with 7H10 agar (128), the Centers for Disease Control and Prevention (CDC) recommended Middlebrook 7H10 agar and 1% as the critical proportion for all drugs (85).

Resistance is fundamentally a phenomenon linked to large initial bacterial populations. In pulmonary tuberculosis, the greatest populations are those prevailing in cavities, which can contain 10^7 to 10^9 organisms, whereas the populations found in hard caseous foci, the most common type of lesion, generally do not exceed 10^2 to 10^4 organisms (19). The greater frequency of resistance during treatment of cavitary tuberculosis was shown as early as 1949 (68, 69). David at CDC (33) demonstrated the probability distribution of drug-resistant mutants and in a fluctuation test showed that *M. tuberculosis* spontaneously mutated to resistance to INH, SM,

EMB, and RMP. The average mutation rates for INH, SM, EMB, and RMP were calculated to be 3×10^{-8}, 3×10^{-8}, 1×10^{-7}, and 2×10^{-10} mutation per bacterium per generation, respectively. Thus, the mutation rate for resistance to two drugs is theoretically less than 10^{-15}. Implicit in all the studies of the genetic basis of antimicrobial resistance in *M. tuberculosis* is that the multiple-drug-resistance (MDR) phenotype (minimally defined as simultaneous resistance to INH and RMP) is the result of accumulative mutations rather than the acquisition of an MDR transfer factor (103).

Special-Population Hypothesis

According to the generally accepted theory, resistance appearing during drug treatment is due to selection and multiplication of the resistant mutants preexisting in the tubercle bacillus population of the host. Inasmuch as the susceptible bacilli are the predominant part of the population, initial killing involves a greater number of microorganisms. The consequence is a sharp fall in the population of bacilli during the initial period of treatment. The rise due to multiplication of the resistant mutants occurs later. This "fall-and-rise" phenomenon, as demonstrated in the patient's sputum, was described in the late 1940s (32, 120). In 1979, Mitchison (97) suggested the "special-populations" hypothesis to explain the action of the major antituberculous drugs against the various subpopulations of tubercle bacilli (Fig. 1). The subpopulations include (i) rapidly growing bacilli in the pulmonary lesions; (ii) bacilli that grow in short metabolic spurts and that might be susceptible to RMP but not INH; (iii) bacilli that reside in the acidic environment

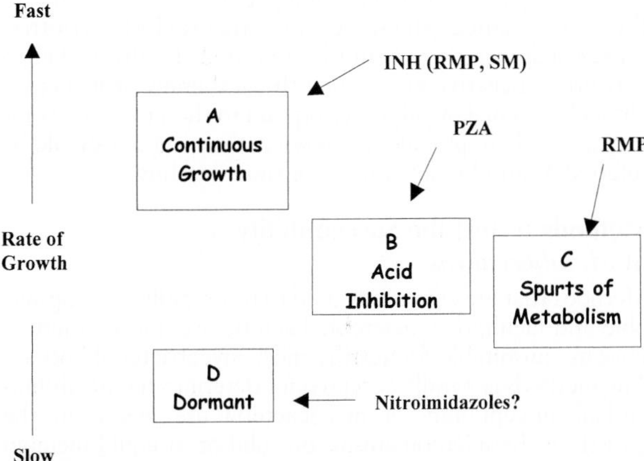

FIGURE 1 Schematic representation of the special-populations hypothesis of Mitchison (98). The model accounts for the action of antimycobacterial agents on different populations of *M. tuberculosis* bacilli in various sites in the infected host. (A) INH, RMP, and SM are active primarily against bacilli in a continuous state of growth, which are the majority population at the start of treatment. (B) PZA is active only against bacilli within the acidic early caseous lesions that develop within the first 2 months of chemotherapy (98). (C) The comparatively rapid bactericidal activity of RMP is important for the eradication of bacilli that grow for short periods (not long enough to be affected by INH). (D) Some tubercle bacilli may be sequestered in lesions in a metabolically inactive and dormant state; however, there is evidence that these dormant bacilli may actually be in an anaerobic state and susceptible to nitroimidazoles such as metronidazole (165). (Reprinted from reference 98 with permission of Oxford University Press.)

of the caseous lesions; and (iv) dormant, nonreplicating bacilli. The hypothesis was developed to explain in part the basis of the early bactericidal activity and the later sterilizing activity of antituberculosis agents. Each drug in the conventional multiple-drug treatment regimen for tuberculosis is more or less effective in eradicating tubercle bacilli within each of these special populations. Thus, the use of multiple drugs in the treatment of tuberculosis is aimed at both preventing drug resistance and achieving a maximum therapeutic effect. Figure 1 depicts the special-populations hypothesis, as presented by Mitchison in 1992 (98) in his Garrod lecture, altered to include a reference to the observation by Wayne and Sramek (165) that dormant *M. tuberculosis* is susceptible to nitroimidazoles. This study was based on the assumption that dormant tubercle bacilli are in an anaerobic metabolic state and therefore would be susceptible to agents such as metronidazole.

Critical Concentrations

The criteria for defining drug-resistant *M. tuberculosis* were established on an empirical basis, i.e., that there is a certain proportion of drug-resistant mutants above which therapeutic success is less likely to be realized. The procedures used to perform drug susceptibility tests and the criteria for interpreting the results take into account two factors: (i) the critical proportion of drug-resistant mutants and (ii) the critical concentration of the drug in the test medium. On the basis of clinical and bacteriologic studies, the significant proportion of bacilli resistant to an antituberculosis drug, above which a clinical response is unlikely, was generally set at 1%. The critical concentration of a drug is the concentration that inhibits the growth of most cells within the population of a wild-type strain of tubercle bacilli without appreciably affecting the growth of the resistant mutant cells that might be present. In other words, if the proportion of tubercle bacilli that are resistant to the critical concentration of a drug exceeds 1%, it is unlikely that the use of that drug will lead to a therapeutic success. It should be noted that this concentration may not have a direct relationship to the peak level of the drug in serum. The critical concentrations of antituberculosis drugs, in different media, are given in Table 3 (28, 82).

Low versus High Critical Concentrations

On occasion, both the agar proportion and BACTEC 460TB methods may indicate that an *M. tuberculosis* isolate is resistant to INH, EMB, or SM at the low critical concentration of the drug (Table 3) but susceptible to the same drug at the high concentration. Indeed, it is unclear if testing the low concentration of EMB has any merit, especially because recent evidence indicates that mutations in the *embB* gene are associated only with resistance at the high concentration (1, 144). Similar studies have not been performed with SM; however, the merit of testing SM at the low concentration must be questioned. If the low concentration of the drug only were tested, the report of "resistant" could potentially mislead a clinician to believe that the drug has no value in the treatment of tuberculosis. On the other hand, low-level resistance to INH may be suggestive of resistance to ethionamide (157). Therefore, it is important to test both concentrations of INH or, if only the low concentration is tested, to reflex test the higher concentration when an isolate is resistant to the lower concentration, recognizing that there is not uniform consensus regarding the clinical relevance of the results of testing at a higher concentration when two concentrations are used (28). The clinician should be alerted that when an isolate is resistant to the low concentration but susceptible to the high concentration, therapeutic effect may be achieved with an

TABLE 3 Critical concentrations of antimycobacterial agents to test against *M. tuberculosis* by radiometric (BACTEC 460TB) or agar proportion methods

Antimicrobial agent	Typical MIC (μg/ml) for susceptible strains	Concn in serum (μg/ml)[e]	Medium and concn (μg/ml)[f]					
			BACTEC 460TB 12B low	BACTEC 460TB 12B high	7H10 low	7H10 high	7H11 low	7H11 high
Primary agents								
INH	0.05–0.2	7	0.1	0.4	0.2	1	0.2	1
RMP	0.5	10	2		1		1	
PZA[a]	20	45	100		NR[i]	NR	NR	
EMB	1–5	2–5	2.5[g]	7.5	5	10	7.5	
Secondary agents								
SM	8	25–50	2[g]	6	2	10	2	10
Capreomycin	1–50	30	1.25[h]		10		10	
Kanamycin[b]	5	14–29	5[h]		5		6	
Ethionamide	0.6–2.5	2–20	1.25[h]		5		10	
PAS	1	7.5	4[h]		2		8	
Rifabutin[c]	0.06–8	0.2–0.5	0.5[h]		0.5/1/2		0.5	
Ofloxacin[d]	0.5–2.5	3–11	2[h]		2		2	

[a] PZA tested at pH 6 in BACTEC 12B medium.
[b] Kanamycin is the class representative for amikacin.
[c] RMP-susceptible versus RMP-resistant isolates; about 30% of RMP-resistant isolates are rifabutin susceptible.
[d] Ofloxacin is the class representative for fluoroquinolones.
[e] Concentrations in serum 1 to 4 h after administration of the usual dosage.
[f] Unless otherwise stated, the concentrations shown are from references 28, 63, and 106.
[g] Woodley (172) showed that 2.5 μg of EMB per ml and 2.0 μg of SM per ml tested against susceptible and resistant isolates agreed with the 7H10 proportion method 97 to 99 and 100%, respectively.
[h] According to reference 113.
[i] NR, no recommendation.

adjustment in dosage (e.g., INH). The CLSI recommends that the following comment be appended to the results:

> These results indicate low-level resistance to INH. Experts believe that patients infected with strains exhibiting this level of INH resistance may benefit from continuing therapy with INH. A specialist in the treatment of tuberculosis should be consulted concerning the appropriate therapeutic regimen and dosages (28).

Extent of Service

In the United States, mycobacteriology laboratories can be classified by the levels or extents of services provided based on criteria proposed by CDC and the American Thoracic Society (ATS). In general, the criteria emphasize the importance of the number of specimens processed, the expertise of the laboratory staff, and the cost-effectiveness of the procedures and protocols (61, 85). The ATS recognizes three levels of service (levels I, II, and III), ranging from specimen referral, to identification and drug susceptibility testing of *M. tuberculosis*, to identification of other mycobacteria. It is recommended that a laboratory should perform susceptibility testing only if the laboratory is capable of identifying the isolate to species and if it regularly performs susceptibility tests on that type of isolate (e.g., at least 10 tests per week). Because certain drugs are tested infrequently (e.g., cycloserine or amikacin), must be prepared from reference powders (e.g., rifabutin or ciprofloxacin), or are problematic (e.g., cycloserine [113]), second-line drug testing should be referred to a laboratory with specific expertise in testing these agents.

When To Perform Susceptibility Tests

The approved CLSI standard on susceptibility testing of mycobacteria (28) states that the first isolate of *M. tuberculosis* obtained from each patient should be tested. This ensures the most effective treatment for a patient and contributes to the surveillance database for tuberculosis control. Susceptibility testing should be repeated if cultures fail to convert to negative after 3 months of therapy or if there is clinical evidence of failure to respond to therapy. If a laboratory is unable to provide this service, then isolates should be referred to another laboratory for timely testing.

Methods To Test the Susceptibility of *M. tuberculosis*

Methods that are commonly used to test rapidly growing aerobic and facultative anaerobic bacteria are, for a variety of reasons, unsuitable for testing most mycobacterial species. The methods generally accepted for determining the antimicrobial susceptibility of mycobacteria are based on the growth of the microorganisms on solid or in liquid medium containing a specified concentration of a single drug. In the past, four growth-based methods have been described: the proportion method, the radiometric or BACTEC 460TB (Becton Dickinson Microbiology Systems, Sparks, Md.) method (a modified proportion method), the absolute-concentration method, and the resistance ratio method (56, 63, 75, 138). Only the agar proportion, BACTEC 460TB, and the commercial nonradiometric broth systems are discussed further in this chapter; the last two are described elsewhere (63). These nonradiometric methods, either manual or fully automated, have been created mainly to overcome the safety and regulatory principles associated with radiolabeled substrates. They include VersaTREK (formerly called the ESP Culture System II; Trek Diagnostic Systems, Inc., Cleveland, Ohio) (176), the Mycobacteria Growth Indicator Tube (MGIT; Becton Dickinson) (57, 115), automated MGIT 960 (Becton Dickinson), and the MB/BacT ALERT 3D (Bio-Mérieux, Durham, N.C.) (118). Descriptions of luciferase reporter mycobacteriophages (125) and molecular beacons (86) await further review of broader testing at this time.

Based on the current CLSI guidelines (28), a rapid susceptibility testing method should be used in conjunction with rapid methods of primary culture and identification to allow the earliest possible detection of resistance. The recommended rapid broth methods for susceptibility testing of *M. tuberculosis* are commercial systems that have been cleared by the FDA. At present, three such FDA-approved systems are available, i.e., the BACTEC 460TB, the ESP Culture System II, and, more recently, BACTEC MGIT 960. Most importantly, any such rapid method utilized should have been previously demonstrated to generate results that correlate with those obtained with the standardized agar proportion method. Optimally, susceptibility results for *M. tuberculosis* should be reported within 28 days of receipt of the specimen in the laboratory (13, 152). There are no commercially available broth systems cleared by the FDA for testing nontuberculous mycobacteria.

Source of Inoculum for Susceptibility Testing

The source of the inoculum for a susceptibility test may be either a smear-positive specimen (direct method) or growth from a primary culture or subculture (indirect method). The direct method is used when antimicrobial resistance is known or suspected. However, the indirect method is considered the standard method for inoculum preparation, and results of the direct method are usually confirmed by subsequent testing by the indirect method. With both the direct and the indirect methods, the inoculum must be a pure culture and careful attention must be given to avoid over- or underinoculation.

For the direct method, the inoculum is either a digested, decontaminated clinical specimen or an untreated, normally sterile body fluid, in which acid-fast bacilli are seen in stained smears. To ensure adequate but not excessive growth in the direct susceptibility test on solid medium, specimens are diluted according to the number of organisms observed in the stained smear of the clinical specimen. A typical dilution scheme is shown in Table 4. Theoretically, this type of inoculum is more representative of the population of the tubercle bacilli in a particular lesion in the host. It is prudent to include an undiluted inoculum if the smear-positive specimen is from a patient who is receiving antimicrobial therapy, because a significant proportion of the bacilli seen on the smear may be nonviable. The direct susceptibility test has two major advantages. First, results can be reported within 3 weeks from the time of specimen receipt in the laboratory for a majority of smear-positive specimens. Second, the proportion of resistant bacteria better represents the patient's bacterial population. Use of the direct method may be warranted in situations where there is a high prevalence of drug resistance (49). However, cost can become a critical factor when there is a high incidence of smear-positive specimens containing nontuberculous mycobacteria. Also, it is not possible to accurately calibrate the inoculum, which may result in insufficient or excessive growth on drug-free quadrants. In addition, if contaminants grow, results are not interpretable. The rate of failure for direct susceptibility testing can reach 15% or more, necessitating retesting by the indirect method. The direct method is not recommended for routine use with the BACTEC 460TB or any of the newer, nonradiometric, liquid-medium-based procedures at this time.

TABLE 4 Guidelines for selection of the dilution of a specimen concentrate prior to inoculation of 7H10 medium for susceptibility testing using the direct method

Dilutions to test[a]	No. of acid-fast bacilli observed with:	
	Carbol fuchsin stain	Fluorochrome stain
Undiluted, 10^{-2}	0	<25
10^{-1}, 10^{-2}	1–10	25–250
10^{-2}, 10^{-3}	>10	>250

[a] Dilutions of concentrated specimen are prepared based on the number of bacilli observed in the initial acid-fast smear. Sterile distilled water is used to prepare the dilutions; the carbol fuchsin stain is examined with the oil immersion objective (1,000×), and the fluorochrome stain is examined with the high-dry objective (450×). If the patient is receiving therapy, not all bacilli observed in the smear may be viable; therefore, the undiluted specimen should be tested as well as the appropriate dilution based on the microscopic criteria given in this table.

For the indirect method, the source of the inoculum is a pure subculture, usually from the primary isolation media. Careful attention should be paid to the selection of colony types so that the final inoculum is representative of all types present to ensure that there is a balance of potentially resistant and susceptible bacilli. The source of inoculum for the liquid medium-based susceptibility testing can be growth on a solid medium or in broth. When using turbid growth in a liquid medium (such as Middlebrook 7H9 broth, BACTEC 12B, MGIT, MB/BacT, or VersaTREK), it is important to do a purity check because a mixed culture (tubercle bacilli and nontuberculous organisms) can give rise to apparent resistance.

Media Used for Susceptibility Testing

Although a variety of media have been used for drug susceptibility testing of slowly growing mycobacteria, including Middlebrook 7H10 or 7H11 agar and Löwenstein-Jensen media, there is considerable variability in the results. Egg-based media are unsuitable for susceptibility testing, not only because of uncertainty about the potency of the drugs after inspissation but also because phospholipids, proteins, and certain amino acids present in the medium affect some drugs. In an effort to provide uniformity in the testing of mycobacteria, CDC (85) and CLSI (28) recommend that Middlebrook 7H10 agar supplemented with oleic acid-albumin-dextrose-catalase (OADC) be used as the standard medium for susceptibility testing of slowly growing mycobacteria by the agar proportion method. A majority of *M. tuberculosis* clinical isolates grow on this medium, and under a dissecting microscope, the transparency of 7H10 agar facilitates the recognition of mixed mycobacterial species or the presence of contaminants. Occasionally, there is insufficient growth of drug-resistant strains of *M. tuberculosis* on 7H10 medium for the test to be valid. With these isolates, 7H11 medium may be substituted for 7H10 agar, but it is necessary to use higher concentrations of some drugs, as shown in Table 3 (59, 75). At present there is no standard formulation for Middlebrook 7H10 agar or OADC (such as there is for Mueller-Hinton medium), and it has been demonstrated that quality control of the medium, especially the OADC supplement, is critical (55).

The medium used for studies with mycobacteria in the BACTEC 460TB instrument is an enriched Middlebrook 7H9 broth containing 4 μCi of [^{14}C] palmitic acid per vial, which is referred to as 7H12 or BACTEC 12B medium.

Drugs Used for Susceptibility Testing

Antimicrobial agents for susceptibility testing (reference powders) can be obtained directly from the manufacturer or from commercial sources. In the United States, most antimicrobial agents are also available from U.S. Pharmacopoeial

Convention, Inc., Reference Standards Order Department, 12601 Twinbrook Parkway, Rockville, MD 20852. The reference powder should be accompanied by information about its assay potency (in micrograms per milligram), expiration date, and lot number, as well as the stability and solubility of the agent. Preparations formulated for therapeutic use in humans or animals should not be used. Unopened vials of powders should be stored as specified by the manufacturer, and opened containers should be stored in a desiccator at the recommended temperature. Stock solutions of most agents at 1,000 μg/ml or greater remain stable for at least 6 months at –20°C and for 1 year at –70 to –80°C. Directions provided by the drug manufacturer should be followed in addition to these general recommendations. Paper disks impregnated with standardized amounts of the primary and secondary drugs are available from commercial sources for use in the disk elution modification of the proportion method. Use of these disks obviates errors in weighing and dilution, as well as errors in labeling, because the disks are coded with the drug name and concentration. This technique provides results equivalent to those obtained with solutions prepared from reference powders. Quality control (QC) testing should be performed with each new batch of antimicrobial agent.

Agar Proportion Method

The agar proportion method for susceptibility testing of slowly growing mycobacteria was developed in the early 1960s by G. Canetti (19, 21). The method was modified and standardized in the United States and has been considered the standard method of drug testing for *M. tuberculosis* complex to all drugs except PZA in the United States and many European countries for many years. The preferred medium for the proportion test is Middlebrook 7H10 agar. Drugs can either be prepared from reference powders (agar diffusion) or be added as drug-impregnated disks (disk elution) (56). With regard to testing PZA, the BACTEC 460TB is considered the reference method (28).

Inoculum and Incubation

The inoculum can be prepared by the direct or indirect method. When the direct method is used, cultures should be examined weekly for 3 weeks, and even though mature colonies may appear on control media in less than 3 weeks, a report of "susceptible" should not be submitted until week 3. Resistant strains of *M. tuberculosis* complex may be slow to produce visible growth because of metabolic differences compared with susceptible wild-type isolates. If cultures are incubated beyond 3 weeks, degradation of the antimicrobial compound may permit the appearance of colonies of organisms that were susceptible to the initial concentration of the drug. Because the controls are inoculated with a processed specimen, isolated colonies should also be examined for colony morphology and pigmentation differences, as well as for the presence of mixed species of mycobacteria or contaminants. Small colonies of rapid growers, as well as the rough, dry colonies of some MAC strains, are similar in appearance to *M. tuberculosis* colonies on 7H10 agar. Also, rapidly growing mycobacteria may be slow to develop on primary isolation media and rapidly growing mycobacteria will appear as MDR when tested against primary antituberculosis agents. For a test to be valid, the control must show good growth (at least 50 to 150 colonies). Susceptibility testing results must never be reported without a preliminary identification.

When using the indirect method, a sufficient number of colonies must be selected to make a suspension that is equivalent to a 1.0 McFarland standard or, if there is insufficient growth, a sufficient number should be subcultured into Dubos Tween-albumin broth and incubated at 35 to 37°C until the turbidity matches a 1.0 McFarland standard. The suspension should not contain clumps of organisms. The actual number of CFU per milliliter is likely to vary from suspension to suspension, so that two dilutions (usually 10^{-2} and 10^{-4}) of the suspension must be used to inoculate two sets of media. If the source of the inoculum is old or if there is scant growth, 10^{-1} and 10^{-3} dilutions should be used or the isolate should be subcultured in broth. QC strains should be tested at dilutions of 10^{-2} and 10^{-4}. Quadrant plates are commonly used for the agar proportion method, and 0.1 ml (about 3 drops from a Pasteur pipette) of each dilution of the inoculum is placed into each quadrant, using 1 dilution per set of plates. The plates are allowed to dry thoroughly after inoculation, placed in individual CO_2-permeable polyethylene bags (clear sandwich bags), and incubated at 35 to 37°C in 5 to 10% CO_2 in air. The plates must be protected from light during storage and incubation to prevent the formation of formaldehyde from the medium ingredients. To check strains for purity, blood agar and 7H10 agar plates are inoculated with 1 or 2 drops of the suspension and streaked for isolation.

Reading, Interpreting, and Reporting Results

Purity control plates are examined for contamination after 1 to 2 days; the 7H10 plate should be examined throughout the incubation period, and the blood agar plate should be examined for 1 week. Once the "no-drug" control quadrant of the test isolate or control strain shows at least 50 to 150 colonies, the plates can be read and interpreted. If there are fewer than 50 colonies in the no-drug quadrant by 3 weeks, the test is repeated. Use of the designations 1+ to 4+ to report the amount of growth is discouraged. This grading scheme may be helpful, however, for in-house evaluation of appropriate inoculum size. The reference agar proportion method employs a percentage calculation to detect resistance or susceptibility. The number of colonies observed in each quadrant is reported as a percentage of the number of colonies in the no-drug control quadrant. If the percentage of colonies exceeds 1%, the isolate should be reported as resistant to that drug at the concentration tested. The percentage of resistant colonies can be used as an indicator of therapeutic efficacy and should immediately be reported to the physician, along with the drug concentration and test method.

Microcolonies may be observed when using the agar proportion method, especially when testing against EMB. Several possibilities may account for the presence of microcolonies: growth of susceptible organisms in the presence of degraded drug, true resistance, or partial resistance. One study reported that most strains that had microcolonies in the EMB quadrant had EMB-susceptible results when tested with the BACTEC 460 method (J. Ridderhof, I. George, and W. Gross, *Abstr. Intersci. Conf. Antimicrob. Agents Chemother., 1999*, abstr. 865, 1999). The significance of microcolonies is unknown, and each laboratory should determine how to best report these findings, based on its own in-house experience.

Quality Control

M. tuberculosis H37Rv (ATCC 27294), which is susceptible to all primary and secondary antituberculosis drugs, is recommended for QC. Strains of *M. tuberculosis* that are resistant to INH, RMP, and/or other drugs are available from the American Type Culture Collection; however, these strains are resistant to high concentrations of the respective drugs and are not ideal for QC testing. Ideally, a strain of *M. tuberculosis* that shows resistance at or near the cutoff values of a particular drug should be used for QC. A number of strains used in the Centers for Disease Control and Prevention's Model Performance Evaluation Program offer these characteristics. Also, for safety considerations, it is not advisable to use a single *M. tuberculosis* strain that is resistant to more than two drugs (28). Aliquots of suspensions of QC strains of *M. tuberculosis,* adjusted to match a 1.0 McFarland standard in 7H9 broth, can be stored at −70°C for up to 6 months. QC testing should be performed with each new batch of medium or antimicrobial agent, and media should be checked for sterility and shown to support adequate growth. Guthertz et al. (55) demonstrated the importance of controlling for all components of 7H10 agar including lots of Middlebrook 7H10 agar, glycerol, and especially OADC. The issue of which QC results should be available before releasing patient test results is discussed below.

BACTEC 460TB Method

Although nonradiometric systems are cleared by the FDA for susceptibility testing of *M. tuberculosis* to primary drugs, the BACTEC 460TB method continues to be important in drug testing. Mycobacteria easily grow in the BACTEC 12B medium containing [^{14}C]palmitic acid. This compound is metabolized, resulting in the production of $^{14}CO_2$; therefore, growth or inhibition of growth in BACTEC 12B medium is measured as changes in the growth-dependent production of CO_2. The instrument quantitatively detects the amount of $^{14}CO_2$ released, expressed in terms of a growth index (GI), and then automatically replaces the headspace with 5 to 10% unlabeled CO_2 in air, thereby maintaining the recommended CO_2 atmosphere. The rate and amount of $^{14}CO_2$ produced are directly proportional to the rate and amount of growth.

The BACTEC 460TB system can be used to test all primary drugs (RMP, INH, PZA, and EMB), as well as the secondary drugs including the newer quinolones and rifamycins (113). The rapid availability of results with the BACTEC 460TB procedure may take precedence over cost considerations. Irrespective of its rapidity, it is prudent to consider the limitations of the BACTEC 460TB method. In some clinical situations, the method might be best considered a screening test, because it does not allow an estimate of the percentage of resistant bacilli and is vulnerable to major errors (false susceptibility or resistance) due to the use of mixed populations of mycobacterial species. Indeed, when an MDR isolate of *M. tuberculosis* is detected for the first time by the BACTEC 460TB method, the identity of the isolate should be confirmed and the presence of a contaminant or mixed culture should be ruled out before secondary agents are tested. While the importance of promptly reporting an MDR isolate of *M. tuberculosis* cannot be overstated, the consequences of a false report of multiple resistance must be recognized as well (108). Clinician concerns about discrepancies between susceptibility test results and clinical response or status must be communicated back to the laboratory as part of an effective quality assurance program.

Three of the primary drugs (INH, RMP, and EMB) and SM are available as lyophilized powders in the BACTEC SIRE kit, designed specifically for use with 12B medium and the BACTEC 460TB instrument. Alternatively, stock solutions of these agents can be prepared from reference powders. Lyophilized vials of PZA are also available for the pH 6.0 modified BACTEC PZA test medium. The secondary drugs must be prepared from reference powders. Critical concentrations for most of these drugs have been established, and the results of the radiometric and proportion methods correlate well (113).

Inoculum and Incubation

The source of inoculum for susceptibility testing should be fresh growth of actively growing bacilli. If growth from a primary BACTEC 12B vial is used for the inoculum, the daily GI reading should be at least 500 or, even better, between 800 and 900. The higher the GI, the shorter the period until the control vial reaches >30 and the earlier the test results can be interpreted. If the primary vial is past the GI peak or if the vial was kept at room temperature for more than 2 days, a fresh 12B vial should be inoculated. Other types of broth culture (Dubos, Middlebrook 7H9, Septichek AFB, VersaTREK Myco, MGIT, or MB/BacT medium) can be used as a source of inoculum; however, it is necessary to ensure that the broth culture is not contaminated or not mixed with other mycobacterial species. A variety of procedures may be used for mycobacterial purity checks (28). After the inoculum is thoroughly mixed to break up clumps, the turbidity should be adjusted to match a 0.5 McFarland standard rather than a 1.0 McFarland standard. This inoculum is then used to inoculate the drug-containing vials. A control vial (without drugs) is inoculated with a 1:100 dilution of the inoculum. All dilutions should be prepared with diluting fluid or distilled water, but not a broth or other substrate-containing medium. Additionally an undiluted control may be used to monitor the growth kinetics of the inoculum and also can serve as a source of inoculum if a test must be repeated.

Also, fresh growth on any solid media may serve as an inoculum source. It is important to harvest several (5 to 10) colonies in order to ensure a representative sample of growth (harvesting from only 2 or 3 single colonies is inadequate), and it is very important to thoroughly homogenize the inoculum in a tube containing 3 to 5 ml of diluting fluid and glass beads. After being vortexed for 1 to 2 min, the tube is left to stand undisturbed for 30 min to allow larger particles to settle, and then the top half of the supernatant is transferred into a new tube. The turbidity is adjusted to match a 0.5 McFarland standard, and this suspension is used to inoculate the drug-containing vials. Blood agar and 7H10 plates are inoculated with a few drops of the inoculum suspension to check for purity.

As safety precautions, disposable tuberculin syringes with a permanently attached needle should be used; rubber gloves, N95 mask, and a gown must be worn; and all steps involving the preparation of inocula and inoculation of vials should be performed in a class II or III biological safety cabinet.

Prior to inoculation, BACTEC 12B vials must be prerun in the BACTEC 460TB instrument to establish a gas phase of 5% CO_2 in air in the headspace of the vial; any vial with an initial GI of 20 must be rejected. Each prerun vial is inoculated with 0.1 ml of the adjusted suspension of the test or QC isolate, and the vials are incubated at 37 ± 1°C (the temperature of incubation is critical) in the dark.

Reading, Interpreting, and Reporting Results

Vials are read on the BACTEC 460TB instrument at intervals of 24 ± 1 h for a minimum of 4 days and until the control vial reaches a GI of 30. For laboratories with limited weekend coverage, an alternative schedule is to inoculate the vials on Friday and first read them on Monday (60). The Monday reading is disregarded, because it reflects 2 days of CO_2 production, and the vials are read daily for at least 3 days (5 days total). Batch testing is discouraged unless the susceptibility test can be started during the same week that the isolate is identified to species, i.e., identified as *M. tuberculosis* complex. In those situations, to avoid any delay, the isolate should be sent to a reference laboratory that works 7 days a week.

When the GI of the control is 30 after a minimum of 4 days, the difference in GI from one day to the next, designated the ΔGI, should be interpreted as follows:

ΔGI of control > ΔGI of drug = susceptible

ΔGI of control < ΔGI of drug = resistant

If the GI is 500 and >500 on the next reading, the isolate should be considered resistant to that drug regardless of the ΔGI (it is necessary to check that the GI of the control was not >30 in less than 3 days to exclude overinoculation). Continued incubation for a few days may allow one to resolve borderline results, but the incubation should not be extended beyond 3 days after the control vial is positive. Susceptibility test results should never be reported without identification of the isolate as *M. tuberculosis* complex or *M. tuberculosis*, especially when the isolate is resistant to a drug(s). Usually, BACTEC 460TB results are straightforward; however, if the ΔGIs are close (within 10%), a preliminary report should be issued and the test should be repeated. Secondary drugs should be tested if the isolate is resistant to RMP or any two primary drugs (28). Use of the term "borderline," as recommended by the BACTEC manufacturer, is not encouraged, because the definition of this term is unclear and may mislead the clinician into believing that a drug has no use in the treatment of tuberculosis. Susceptibility test results should be reported without delay. The report should include the test method, the name of the drug, the concentration tested, and the result (susceptible or resistant). It is not possible to report the percent resistance by using the BACTEC 460TB method. Drug resistance should be reported by telephone and/or fax to the requesting physician, the infection control program, and the local tuberculosis control program, and a follow-up hard-copy report should be submitted. It is prudent to confirm the receipt of a fax report in lieu of direct communication with the physician or public health official.

Quality Control

Reference strains with known susceptibility patterns should be tested with each new batch of drug and BACTEC 12B medium. In addition, QC tests should be performed at least once a week in laboratories that perform tests daily or weekly or when a patient isolate is tested if tests are performed less frequently. The H37Rv strain of *M. tuberculosis* (ATCC 27294), which is susceptible to all standard antituberculosis agents, is commonly used for QC. Mutants of H37Rv selected for in vitro resistance to single or multiple drugs are also available; however, these strains are resistant to very high concentrations and are not particularly suitable for QC purposes. In addition, reporting the test results for a patient isolate should not be delayed because of the pending test results for a resistant QC strain. Suspensions of QC strains may be prepared in BACTEC diluting solution and frozen at −70°C in 1-ml test samples for up to 6 months (138). A single tube is thawed for QC testing, and the same procedure as that for clinical isolates is used. At present, there is no published consensus on which QC results should be available before the test results on a patient isolate may be released. However, it seems reasonable that the QC test results for medium components be available and acceptable, as well as the results for the "susceptible" QC strain (e.g., ATCC 27294).

Testing PZA

Reliable testing of PZA by the radiometric method is different from testing by the BACTEC 460TB method for the other primary drugs (96), because PZA activity is best measured at pH 5.5 rather than pH 6.8, the usual pH of the growth medium. However, most strains of *M. tuberculosis* grow poorly at pH 5.5 and some fail to grow altogether. As a compromise between testing at the pH for optimum PZA activity and testing at the pH for optimum growth, Salfinger et al. (131) recommended that PZA be tested at pH 5.9 ± 0.1. In addition, to accurately and reliably test PZA, several other adjustments to the standard radiometric method are made. (i) To prepare the inoculum, each isolate must be subcultured in a fresh BACTEC 12B vial supplemented with BACTEC reconstituting fluid, which is an aqueous solution of polyoxyethylene stearate (POES) (139). The isolate is tested daily, and once the GI is 300 to 500, this culture is used for susceptibility testing. Alternatively, a 1:10 dilution of the inoculum (GI = 999 or 0.5 McFarland standard) used for testing the other primary drugs is used and the suspension is vigorously homogenized before use. (ii) Either the lyophilized PZA is reconstituted with POES or PZA reference powder is dissolved in POES to achieve a final concentration of 100 μg/ml, the critical concentration for the BACTEC method, which is equivalent to 25 to 50 μg/ml (used in the proportion method) (138). (iii) A special BACTEC 12B medium at pH 6.0 supplemented with POES is used to test PZA. (iv) The PZA-containing vial and the control vial are inoculated with the same suspension; i.e., the inoculum for the control vial should not be diluted. (v) The vials are tested daily until the control vial reaches a GI of 200; if the GI fails to reach 200 within 14 days, the test is uninterpretable. (vi) The isolate is considered susceptible to PZA if the GI of the PZA vial is <10% of the GI of the control vial. If the GIs of the test and control vials are very close, the result is considered borderline and the test must be repeated. (vii) In addition to the use of H37Rv (PZA susceptible) for QC testing, *M. bovis* BCG (PZA resistant) can be used as a control for PZA resistance. If an isolate tests resistant to PZA, especially if it is resistant to PZA alone, it should be identified to the species level, because *M. bovis* and *M. bovis* BCG are PZA resistant whereas almost all *M. tuberculosis* isolates are PZA susceptible. This is especially important if the laboratory identifies isolates only to the level of the *M. tuberculosis* complex. Some *M. tuberculosis* isolates grow poorly at pH 6.0 (130), and other isolates may be inhibited by the POES supplement (95).

VersaTREK

VersaTREK (fomerly called ESP Culture System II; Trek Diagnostic Systems, Inc.) is a fully automated, continuously monitoring system for growth and detection of mycobacteria (176), which allows testing of the susceptibility of *M. tuberculosis* to major primary drugs (i.e., INH, RMP, EMB, and PZA) as well as the secondary agent SM. The VersaTREK technology is based on detection of pressure changes (gas production or gas consumption due to microbial growth) within the headspace above the broth culture medium in a sealed bottle. The culture medium consists of a Middlebrook 7H9 broth, which has been enriched with glycerol and Casitone, and contains a cellulose sponge. Before the medium is inoculated with a test strain, growth and antibiotic supplements must be added.

Inoculum and Incubation

VersaTREK Myco antibiotics are supplied as lyophilate by the manufacturer. Preparation of the bottles requires the addition of 1.0 ml of antibiotic solution. The final concentrations in the Myco bottles are as follows: INH, 0.1 μg/ml; RMP, 1.0 μg/ml; EMB, 5.0 μg/ml; and SM, 8.0 μg/ml. INH and EMB can be tested at higher concentrations (0.4 and 8.0 μg/ml, respectively). For the inoculation of organisms into the VersaTREK Myco bottles, 0.5 ml of a 1:10 dilution from a McFarland standard of 1 must be added to the drug-containing bottles. The inoculum can be prepared from either solid (e.g., Löwenstein-Jensen) or liquid (e.g., VersaTREK Myco) medium. Cultures are kept in the instrument at 35°C, and growth is automatically monitored.

Reading, Interpreting, and Reporting Results

At the end of the specified incubation period, as determined by the drug-free control bottle for each isolate that is tested, the isolate is manually determined to be susceptible or resistant to a drug. If the control bottle (without drugs) signals positive, the time to detection is calculated. Drug-containing bottles are monitored for another 3 days after the control bottle has turned positive. Results are interpreted according to the following rules: a strain is considered resistant if the time of detection is the same time as or up to 3 days after that for the control bottle; a strain is considered susceptible if no growth occurs in the drug-containing bottle or if the time of detection is more than 3 days after that for the control bottle. The few studies demonstrate good agreement of the VersaTREK (formerly called ESP Culture System II) with the BACTEC 460TB and the agar proportion method and detection times, which are very comparable to those obtained by the radiometric method (10, 126, 176).

Quality Control

Each new VersaTREK Myco Susceptibility Kit and/or lots of medium and growth supplement should be tested with strains of *M. tuberculosis* appropriate for QC. A pansusceptible strain of *M. tuberculosis* should be included with each testing run (28).

MGIT (Manual and Automated MGIT 960) Systems

In 1995, the MGIT was introduced for the growth and detection of mycobacteria from clinical specimens (57, 115). Each MGIT tube contains modified Middlebrook 7H9 broth, and in the bottom is a fluorescence-quenching-based oxygen sensor (silicon rubber impregnated with a ruthenium pentahydrate). The fluorescent compound is sensitive to the presence of oxygen dissolved in the medium. The fluorescence of the indicator is quenched in the presence of oxygen, but fluorescence increases as soon as actively respiring microorganisms utilize the dissolved oxygen. Fluorescence is detected using a 365-nm UV transilluminator. The MGIT system is available as a manual system or a fully automated, continuously monitoring system called BACTEC MGIT 960. Apart from using nonradiometric medium, it frees the technician from using syringes. In addition to detecting and monitoring growth, the system can be used for testing of susceptibility to INH, RMP, EMB, PZA, and SM. Fluorescence of the drug-containing tubes is compared with that of the drug-free growth control tube. When using the instrument, the ratio of relative growth between the drug-containing tube and the growth control tube is determined by software algorithms. If the relative growth in the drug tube equals or exceeds that in the growth control tube, the organism is considered resistant to the drug; if the relative growth is less than that in the growth control tube, the organism is considered susceptible.

Five drugs (INH, RMP, EMB, PZA, and SM) are designed specifically for use with the BACTEC MGIT 960 instrument. Stock solutions of these drugs also can be prepared from reference powders. Lyophilized vials of PZA are available for testing susceptibility based on an adapted protocol utilizing BACTEC MGIT 960 PZA medium at pH 5.9. Similar to the BACTEC 460TB procedure, the BACTEC MGIT 960 employs a two-tier test, with the first tier comprising the four SIRE drugs being tested at drug concentrations equivalent to the critical concentrations of the agar proportion method (i.e., SM, 1.0 μg/ml; INH, 0.1 μg/ml; RMP, 1.0 μg/ml; and EMB, 5.0 μg/ml). If there is resistance to INH, EMB, and/or SM, a second test that involves a higher concentration of the drug(s) (SM, 4.0 μg/ml; INH, 0.4 μg/ml; and EMB, 7.5 μg/ml) may be used. There appears to be good correlation between the MGIT and the BACTEC 460TB system or the agar proportion method (8, 114, 127). The time to results is comparable to that for the radiometric technique. A multicenter report suggests that an overall correlation between the BACTEC 460 and the agar proportion method could be achieved with amikacin, kanamycin, and ofloxacin; however, inconsistent results in both methods were obtained with cycloserine (113). A recent report validated the use of BACTEC 460 and MGIT 960 for testing the susceptibility of *M. tuberculosis*, including multidrug-resistant strains, to levofloxacin (132).

Inoculum and Incubation

Inoculum (0.5 ml) for drug susceptibility testing may be prepared from either liquid or solid media. To ensure viability of the colonies, accuracy of results, and reproducibility of dilutions, strict adherence to the guidelines of the manufacturer is imperative. Prior to inoculating the AST tubes, 0.8 ml of the BACTEC MGIT 960 drug susceptibility testing supplement (OADC) and 100 μl of the drug solution (INH, RMP, or EMB) are added to the MGIT. With a liquid source of inoculum, the MGIT must nominally be used no sooner than the day following the instrument's positivity (day 1) and no later than 5 days following the day of the instrument's positivity. If it is older, the isolate must first be subcultured again. With solid media, the isolate can be used no longer than 14 days after the first appearance of colonies on the plate or slant.

If growth from a primary MGIT is taken for susceptibility testing, the suspension can immediately be used for testing. Appropriate dilutions (1:5) have been made for day 3 through 5 positive MGIT 960 tubes prior to inoculation of the drug set to avoid overinoculation. When working with a solid medium source, inoculum preparation includes vortexing with glass beads and two specified settling times to ensure homogeneity of the final cell suspension. The suspension has to be adjusted to a McFarland standard of 0.5 equivalent and then diluted 1:5 before inoculation of the MGIT 960 AST set. For the growth control tube, 100 μl of a positive MGIT 960 broth is pipetted into 10 ml of sterile saline to prepare a 1:100 dilution of the growth suspension. From this suspension, 0.5 ml is inoculated into a fresh MGIT without drug. Cultures are kept at 35°C, and growth is automatically monitored.

Reading, Interpreting, and Reporting Results

Drug results are listed automatically on the data report form (S, susceptible; R, resistant; X, invalid result), together with growth units and time to result. As with all drug susceptibility testing, the report should indicate the method used and the concentration of drug tested. Interpretive comments, such as those suggested by the CLSI (28), should be considered.

Quality Control

Reference strains with known susceptibility patterns should be tested with each new batch of drug and MGIT medium and included with each test run (28).

Testing PZA

PZA can reliably be tested by using the novel BACTEC MGIT PZA tube, which contains 7 ml of MGIT broth, modified with a reduced pH (114). Inocula can be prepared either from MGIT medium or from solid medium, such as Löwenstein-Jensen medium. Prior to inoculating the PZA set tubes, 0.8 ml of MGIT PZA supplement and 100 μl of PZA solution (100 μg/ml) are added. MGIT cultures are used no sooner than the day following the instrument's positivity (day 1) and no later than 5 days following the day of positivity. On days 1 and 2 following positivity, the inoculum is used undiluted, while on days 3 to 5, suspensions are diluted 1:5 with sterile saline. Then 0.5 ml is inoculated into the MGIT PZA tubes. The growth control tube is inoculated with 0.5 ml of a 1:10 dilution of the respective suspension. Cultures grown on Löwenstein-Jensen medium are used no later than 14 days after the first colonies appear on the slant. To ensure homogeneity, a suspension adjusted to a McFarland standard of 0.5 equivalent is prepared by using glass beads and then diluted 1:5 prior to inoculation of the MGIT PZA set. All inoculated PZA sets must be loaded into the instrument within 8 h of inoculation. Again, using predefined algorithms, readings are automatically interpreted by the instrument. In contrast to BACTEC 460TB, the PZA "borderline" category no longer exists with this method.

MB/BacT ALERT 3D

The MB/BacT ALERT 3D System (bioMerieux), a fully automated, nonradiometric system, can also be used for mycobacterial culture susceptibility testing of *M. tuberculosis* outside the United States (118). With this technology, carbon dioxide is released into the medium by actively metabolizing microorganisms and is detected by a gas-permeable sensor containing an indicator embedded at the bottom of the culture bottles. Color changes are monitored by a reflectometric detection unit, and data are compiled by an internal database management system.

Inoculum and Incubation

Following the instructions of the manufacturer, the MB/BacT process bottles containing a modified Middlebrook 7H9 medium (with casein, bovine serum albumin, and catalase) are supplemented with the following final drug concentrations: INH, 1 μg/ml; RMP, 1 μg/ml; SM, 1 μg/ml; and EMB, 2 μg/ml. Subsequently, bottles are inoculated with 0.5 ml of a suspension of *M. tuberculosis* adjusted to a McFarland standard of 2. Two bottles without drugs serve as growth controls, one inoculated with 0.5 ml of the cell suspension adjusted to a McFarland standard of 2 (control 1) and one with 0.5 ml of the cell suspension (McFarland standard of 2) diluted 1:100 (control 2).

Reading, Interpreting, and Reporting Results

At the time that the MB/BacT System recognizes growth in the control 2 bottle, testing is terminated and the growth status of the bottles containing the drugs is determined. An isolate is considered resistant if the drug-containing bottle is positive before or on the same day as the corresponding diluted control bottle (control 2). Susceptibility is defined as the drug-containing bottle remaining negative or becoming positive later than the control 2 bottle. On the basis of preliminary studies, there is excellent agreement of the MB/BacT results with susceptibility data generated by the agar proportion method and BACTEC 460TB (18, 40, 118), in particular for INH and RMP. The manufacturer increased the EMB concentration to 2.5 μg/ml in order to improve the correlation with the results of the agar proportion method (138). The time necessary to determine the susceptibility patterns of *M. tuberculosis* is within what has been observed for the BACTEC 460TB System.

Quality Control

Reference strains with known susceptibility patterns should be tested with each new batch of drug and MB/BacT medium, and with each test run (28).

M. AVIUM COMPLEX

Clinical Significance

MAC is commonly isolated from a variety of clinical specimens and in many clinical laboratories is the most frequently encountered *Mycobacterium* species. Isolation of MAC from blood or other sterile sites is almost always clinically significant and is especially important in HIV-infected patients with profound CD4 T-cell lymphocytopenia, i.e., ≤75 CD4 T lymphocytes per μl. Although disseminated MAC infection remains a complication in HIV-infected patients, the incidence has dramatically decreased due to the introduction of effective prophylaxis and immune system restoration associated with the use of highly active antiretroviral therapy. Also, disseminated MAC disease still occurs in patients who fail to respond to antiretroviral treatment because of drug resistance, drug intolerance, or lack of compliance. In many of these patients, MAC infection represents a relapse of MAC disease rather than a new infection. MAC is also a cause of chronic pulmonary lung disease and is the leading cause of lung disease due to nontuberculous mycobacteria in the United States. The incidence of MAC lung disease has been steadily increasing in patients with underlying bronchiectasis, chronic obstructive pulmonary disease, or cystic fibrosis. Nevertheless, the detection of MAC in respiratory or gastrointestinal tract specimens can be difficult to interpret, especially in patients who are not clearly at risk for MAC disease. Clinical, histopathologic, and/or radiologic evidence of MAC disease, repeated isolation of MAC, increasing numbers of bacilli in sequential specimens, or the absence of other identifiable causes of signs and symptoms are important factors to consider in assessing the clinical significance of MAC isolates.

Drug Resistance

Most MAC isolates are intrinsically resistant to INH and PZA, and these antimicrobial agents play no role in the treatment of MAC infection (4). The intrinsic resistance to INH most likely is due to a lack of a complete antimicrobial effect (7, 91). Cell-free in vitro studies have shown that certain drug targets (e.g., ribosomes, ribosomal subunits, and RNA polymerase) bind the corresponding drugs (e.g., macrolides, aminoglycosides, and rifamycins) and that the target functions are inhibited, yet many of these compounds are ineffective against whole cells. MAC isolates have variable MIC values to aminoglycosides (amikacin, kanamycin, and SM) and rifamycins (RMP and rifabutin), and one or both of these agents are often used in combination with other drugs for treatment of MAC disease.

Correlation between in vitro MAC susceptibility test results and clinical response has been demonstrated in a controlled clinical trial only with azithromycin and clarithromycin (23). Although wild-type MAC isolates are uniformly susceptible to macrolides, resistance develops quickly with macrolide monotherapy and may eventually develop with combination therapy. An analysis of macrolide-resistant MAC isolates showed that over 95% of clinically significant macrolide resistance in MAC is a consequence of mutations in the V-domain of the 23S rRNA gene (92, 106). Therefore, clinically significant macrolide resistance can be defined as a clarithromycin MIC of ≥32 μg/ml or an azithromycin MIC of ≥256 μg/ml (75, 106). Predicting in vivo susceptibility is always less reliable; however, a positive clinical and microbiological response is expected if the MIC values of clarithromycin and azithromycin are ≤4 and ≤32 μg/ml, respectively. Clarithromycin and azithromycin are approved by the FDA for the treatment of MAC disease, but either agent must be combined with at least one and often two additional agents, commonly EMB and RMP (24). Clarithromycin, azithromycin, and rifabutin are approved as prophylactic agents for disseminated MAC infection in HIV-infected patients; however, their mechanism of action as prophylactic agents is unclear.

When To Perform Susceptibility Tests

Universally accepted guidelines regarding indications for susceptibility testing of MAC do not exist. However, testing should be considered for clinically significant isolates from patients on prior macrolide therapy, from patients who become bacteremic while on macrolide preventive therapy, and from patients who relapse while on macrolide therapy. Testing initial isolates from blood or tissue of patients with disseminated disease or respiratory samples from patients with pulmonary disease to establish baseline values also may be valuable. Susceptibility testing should be repeated after 3 months for patients with disseminated disease and after 6 months for patients with chronic pulmonary disease if the patient does not improve clinically and remains culture positive.

Test Methods

Broth microdilution and macrodilution and agar dilution methods that measure, in a quantitative manner, the in vitro activity of antimycobacterial agents against MAC have been described. In Europe, an agar dilution method with Mueller-Hinton agar supplemented with OADC is used; however, in the United States, there is consensus that both radiometric broth macrodilution and broth microdilution methods are accurate and reliable and that agar-based methods should not be used. The current recommendations of the CLSI Subcommittee on Antimycobacterial Susceptibility Testing indicate that susceptibility testing for MAC should be restricted to clarithromycin or azithromycin (28). Clarithromycin results predict those of azithromycin; therefore, testing both agents is not necessary. BACTEC 12B medium can be used for macrodilution testing, and either Middlebrook 7H9 broth with casein or Mueller-Hinton broth supplemented with OADC or OAD is acceptable for microdilution tests. The concentration ranges of clarithromycin and azithromycin to test are shown in Table 5.

The issue of pH remains somewhat controversial. One view is that testing at pH 7.2 to 7.4 is potentially misleading because MAC isolates tend to grow more slowly, and some fail to grow, at this pH. Thus, MIC values measured in this pH range may reflect synergy between a suboptimal pH for growth and inhibitory drug activity (72; S. Beaty, S. Siddiqi, and M. Gnacek, *Abstr. 92nd Gen. Meet. Am. Soc. Microbiol. 1992,* abstr. U-102, 1992). Also, BACTEC 12B medium is unstable at pH 7.2 to 7.4 because of the poor buffering capacity of the medium at pH values above 7.2. In addition, the intracellular environment of MAC-infected macrophages is pH 6.0 to 6.5, which suggests that macrolides should be tested under the mildly acidic, more clinically relevant conditions. Although MAC can block phagolysosome fusion, the intracellular pH remains in the range of pH 6.0 to 6.5 (110, 122, 146). Blocking phagolysosome fusion prevents a drop to pH 5.0 or lower but does not result in an increase in the intracellular pH to 7.2 to 7.4. The CLSI does not make a specific recommendation but states that pH 6.8 and 7.4 are both acceptable, providing that the recommended interpretive criteria are followed (Table 5). Data from a multicenter study (175) showed that testing in broth at either pH is satisfactory, supporting the CLSI view.

Inoculum and Incubation

Currently there are no specific recommendations regarding inoculum preparation. The options include the use of "seed" BACTEC vials (subcultures of fresh growth) for the radiometric method or the preparation of a suspension of mycobacteria taken directly from an agar plate or a broth culture for microdilution. However, if possible, only transparent colony types should be tested because this variant generally is more virulent and more resistant to antimicrobial agents than the opaque variant. The inoculum should be between 10^4 and 10^5 CFU/ml for the radiometric broth macrodilution test and approximately 5×10^5 CFU/ml for the broth microdilution test. Tween 80 or other surfactants should not be used to disperse clumps of bacilli because of the potential synergistic effect of the surfactant activity of Tween 80 and antimicrobial agents.

Incubation is at 37°C. For the radiometric test, incubation should not extend beyond 10 days, and the "no-drug" control should not exceed a GI of 999 in less than 4 days. For broth microdilution, trays are incubated for 7 to14 days. The endpoint for the radiometric test is defined by the GI value for the inoculum diluted 1:100, whereas the endpoint for the broth microdilution assay is visible turbidity.

TABLE 5 Susceptibility testing of clarithromycin and azithromycin against M. *avium* complex[a]

Antimicrobial agent	Concn range (μg/ml) for:		pH	Interpretive criteria			QC (M. *avium* ATCC 700898)	
	BACTEC	Microtiter		Susceptible (μg/ml)	Intermediate (μg/ml)	Resistant (μg/ml)	Concn range (μg/ml)	Expected endpoints (μg/ml)
Clarithromycin	2–64 or 4, 16, and 64	1–64	6.8	≤16	32	≥64	1, 2, and 4	1–4
Clarithromycin	2–64 or 4, 8, and 32	2–64	7.3–7.4	≤4	8–16	≥32	0.5, 1, and 2	0.5–2
Azithromycin	16–512 or 32, 128, and 512	NR[b]	6.8	≤128	256	≥512	8, 16, and 32	8–32

[a] Data from reference 28.
[b] NR, no recommendation.

Reporting Results

When testing clarithromycin or azithromycin, both the MIC value and an interpretation, based on the pH of the medium and the breakpoints listed in Table 5, should be reported (28). Because untreated wild strains of MAC rarely, if ever, are intermediate or resistant to macrolides, the CLSI subcommittee recommends that laboratories confirm such results by repeat testing (28). A confirmed intermediate result may suggest that the patient has a mixed population of MAC organisms and should be monitored for emerging resistance. Testing agents other than the macrolides (e.g., amikacin, ciprofloxacin, or moxifloxacin) should be restricted to situations in which the clinician has extensive experience in the use of these agents in the treatment of MAC disease or for research purposes. Testing EMB or RMP should be discouraged because MIC values do not necessarily correlate with clinical response and, therefore, could be misleading. If drugs other than macrolides are tested, only the MIC values should be reported without an interpretation. However, it is important to recognize that disseminated MAC disease is principally an infection of macrophages in the blood, bone marrow, spleen, and other tissues. Thus, clinical effectiveness is likely to relate to both potent activity and the ability of drugs to accumulate in cells and tissues to levels above the MIC for the infecting microorganism.

OTHER SLOWLY GROWING MYCOBACTERIA

In the mid-1980s, Woods and Washington (177) reviewed the nontuberculous mycobacterioses and concluded that no clear recommendations could be made for treatment of these infections and that the need for susceptibility testing was difficult or impossible to assess. Now, many years later, the situation has not appreciably changed. Nevertheless, for certain species of nontuberculous mycobacteria, there has been an accumulation of information and experience that can be the basis for some recommendations (28). Susceptibility testing is often helpful with these less frequently encountered species because of the paucity of information about treatment options, and in vitro results provide some rational basis for guiding treatment (52). Furthermore, baseline information may be useful if there is a microbiologic relapse. However, the vagaries of testing and interpretation of results mandate that the testing be performed in an experienced laboratory and, to better ensure consistency of results, that follow-up testing be performed by the same laboratory.

M. kansasii

Isolates of *M. kansasii* from patients not previously treated with RMP are predictably susceptible to RMP, and patients have been successfully treated with RMP, INH, and EMB, with or without SM (4). However, resistance to RMP can develop during therapy, and a patient's history of RMP therapy may be unknown or unclear. Therefore, CLSI recommends that all initial isolates of *M. kansasii* be tested for susceptibility to rifampin only, by agar proportion, as described for *M. tuberculosis,* or a broth-based method that yields comparable results (28). Susceptibility testing should be repeated if cultures remain positive after 3 months of appropriate therapy.

Untreated wild strains of *M. kansasii* are susceptible to the critical concentrations of RMP and EMB used to test *M. tuberculosis* (discussed earlier in the chapter) but are resistant to the critical concentration of INH (0.2 μg/ml by agar proportion) and show variable susceptibility to the higher concentration (1.0 μg/ml). Despite these in vitro results, INH appears clinically active. Therefore, because in vitro results do not correlate with clinical outcome, testing susceptibility of *M. kansasii* to INH should not be done. Isolates of *M. kansasii* that are resistant to RMP (MIC ≥ 1 μg/ml) should be tested against the following secondary drugs: rifabutin, EMB, SM, clarithromycin, amikacin, ciprofloxacin (as the class representative for the older fluoroquinolones), trimethoprim-sulfamethoxazole or sulfamethoxazole, and moxifloxacin. Unfortunately, however, for most of these agents data regarding both concentrations to be tested and optimal testing conditions are limited. Tentative testing and interpretive guidelines for these agents are shown in Table 6 (28).

M. marinum

Routine susceptibility testing of *M. marinum* is not recommended and should be discouraged. Isolates are consistently susceptible to several clinically useful antimicrobial agents, including RMP, EMB, doxycycline (or minocycline), trimethoprim-sulfamethoxazole, and clarithromycin (28). Additionally, the risk of acquired mutational resistance to one or more of these agents is extremely low. Successful treatment may require surgical excision or debridement as well as antimicrobial therapy. However, if a patient fails to respond clinically after several months of appropriate therapy and remains culture positive, susceptibility testing of *M. marinum* should be considered. Agar proportion, agar disk elution, and broth microdilution have been used, but there are insufficient data to recommend any one method. Drugs suggested by CLSI to test are RMP, EMB, clarithromycin (the class agent for newer macrolides), amikacin, and sulfamethoxazole or trimethoprim-sulfamethoxazole (28).

M. haemophilum

M. haemophilum is an opportunistic pathogen in immunocompromised patients, and there is some correlation between susceptibility test results and clinical efficacy, although virtually all treatment regimens examined included combinations of agents (145). Wild-type isolates of *M. haemophilum* appear to be susceptible to quinolones, rifamycins, clarithromycin, and azithromycin and resistant to PZA and EMB; they are likely to be resistant to INH and SM (11, 145).

M. xenopi, M. szulgai, and *M. malmoense*

In vitro susceptibility test results for *M. xenopi, M. szulgai,* and *M. malmoense* may be helpful because of the paucity of

TABLE 6 Tentative breakpoint concentrations for antimicrobial agents that might be tested against *M. kansasii* and selected slowly growing mycobacteria other than *M. tuberculosis*[a]

Antimicrobial agent	Resistance breakpoint (μg/ml)
RMP	1–2
Rifabutin	0.5–2
EMB	5
INH[b]	5
SM	10
Clarithromycin	32
Amikacin	10
Ciprofloxacin	2
Trimethoprim-sulfamethoxazole	2/38

[a] Data from reference 28.
[b] Not recommended for testing *M. kansasii.*

information about the susceptibility patterns of these species. For example, susceptibility testing has been reported to be important to the management of infections caused by M. *xenopi* (153), but an earlier report indicated that the correlation between susceptibility test results and therapeutic response was inconsistent (177). Pulmonary infections by these three species have been successfully treated with INH, EMB, and RMP, and data from at least one report indicated that clarithromycin was effective in the treatment of M. *xenopi* infections (4). Candidate drugs for testing with these species are the same as for M. *kansasii* (Table 6). The test method should be either the BACTEC radiometric, broth microdilution, or agar proportion; however, there may be advantages to defining the in vitro susceptibility in terms of an MIC. Extrapolation of the M. *tuberculosis* "critical concentrations" to these species of mycobacteria may be misleading, because there is some evidence that infections caused by these species can be successfully treated with higher concentrations of INH, SM, and EMB than might be used for M. *tuberculosis* (4).

M. gordonae

Testing M. *gordonae* is inappropriate because isolates almost always represent contaminants; M. *gordonae* rarely causes actual disease (164). Before testing M. *gordonae* isolates, one should ask whether there is convincing evidence that the isolate is playing a role in the disease process. Until these questions are answered in the affirmative, susceptibility testing is inappropriate because the results could be misleading and the patient may be misdiagnosed and inappropriately treated.

The most prudent approach to the testing of slowly growing mycobacteria other than M. *tuberculosis* complex is to restrict it to reference laboratories with extensive experience working with these species. Interpretation of the susceptibility test results requires good communication between the laboratory and the clinician.

RAPIDLY GROWING MYCOBACTERIA

Clinical Significance

Rapidly growing mycobacteria are defined as acid-fast bacilli that form visible colonies from a dilute inoculum on a solid medium within 5 to 7 days. It is important to note that this definition does not necessarily apply to the original culture of a patient's specimen. Although there are over 30 species of rapidly growing mycobacteria, most human disease is caused by M. *abscessus*, M. *chelonae*, or M. *fortuitum* group (17). These three species/groups are important causes of skin and soft tissue infections, especially following penetrating trauma with possible soil or water contamination. They also cause nosocomial infections (e.g., catheter-related bacteremia and wound infections following augmentation mammaplasty or cardiac bypass surgery), and M. *abscessus* can cause pulmonary disease, especially in patients with cystic fibrosis. Disseminated disease is uncommon and is usually associated with cellular immune deficiency, particularly that due to corticosteroid therapy, although it is rare in HIV-infected patients. Several other rapidly growing mycobacteria are infrequent to rare causes of disease in humans, including M. *mucogenicum*, M. *immunogenum*, M. *neoaurum*, M. *mageritense*, M. *smegmatis*, M. *goodii*, and M. *wolinskyi* (17, 161, 162), and at least two species are animal pathogens (51). Clinical isolates of rapidly growing mycobacteria should be identified to species, because the antimicrobial susceptibility patterns differ for the different species. For example, M. *abscessus* and M. *chelonae* are always resistant to trimethoprim-sulfamethoxazole, whereas M. *fortuitum* group virtually always is susceptible.

Susceptibility testing should be performed for any clinically significant, rapidly growing mycobacteria. This includes isolates from blood, sterile body fluids, tissue, and material collected from skin and soft tissue lesions, and multiple isolates from sputum (or other respiratory specimens). The recovery of rapidly growing mycobacteria from sputum or other respiratory specimens is more difficult to interpret, because frequently these isolates are not clinically significant. However, the repeated isolation of a rapidly growing mycobacterium from a respiratory specimen, especially one that is smear positive for acid-fast bacilli, is highly suggestive of true pulmonary disease. In patients with wound infections, debridement and excision of the infected tissue are frequently necessary adjuncts to antimicrobial therapy, although cutaneous infections occasionally resolve spontaneously with neither surgical intervention nor antimicrobial therapy (159).

Methods

Broth microdilution is recommended for susceptibility testing of the *Mycobacterium fortuitum* group, *Mycobacterium chelonae*, and *Mycobacterium abscessus* and, theoretically, also should be appropriate for testing other clinically significant, rapidly growing mycobacteria, although data to support this are not currently available (28). The E test has been evaluated for testing rapidly growing mycobacteria, but the method did not yield results comparable to those of broth microdilution (173) and, therefore, cannot be recommended at this time. As mentioned earlier, for optimal interpretation of MIC results, isolates should be identified to the species level. If cultures (from any site except respiratory) are positive after 6 months of appropriate antimicrobial therapy, susceptibility testing should be repeated, and the species identity should be confirmed.

Broth Microdilution Method

The broth microdilution method for testing rapidly growing mycobacteria is essentially a modification of the CLSI standard method for non-acid-fast organisms that grow aerobically (27); it has been described in detail by Brown et al. (16). Antimicrobial agents (and concentrations in serial twofold dilutions) that should be tested are amikacin (1 to 128 μg/ml), cefoxitin (2 to 256 μg/ml), ciprofloxacin (0.125 to 16 μg/ml), clarithromycin (0.06 to 64 μg/ml), doxycycline (or minocycline) (0.25 to 32 μg/ml), imipenem (1 to 64 μg/ml), and sulfamethoxazole (or trimethoprim-sulfamethoxazole) (1 to 64 μg/ml). Additionally, for isolates of M. *chelonae* only, tobramycin (1 to 32 μg/ml) should be tested. Testing linezolid and one of the newer fluoroquinolones (e.g., moxifloxacin) also should be considered. Commercially manufactured broth microdilution panels are available (Trek Diagnostic Systems). Alternatively, broth microdilution plates can be prepared by the method described by Brown et al. (16); once prepared, the plates can be sealed in plastic bags and stored at −70°C for up to 6 months.

Inoculum

Fresh growth is prepared by inoculating a blood agar plate with the test organism and incubating the plate at 30°C for 72 h. The current recommendation is to prepare the inoculum by collecting growth from the blood agar plate with a sterile cotton swab and making a suspension in sterile distilled water that is equivalent to the density of 0.5 McFarland turbidity standard. The final inoculum should be approximately 5×10^5 CFU/ml or 5×10^4 CFU/100 μl/well of a microtiter plate. The purity of the inoculum should be checked for each isolate, and periodically the size of the inoculum should be verified by quantitative plate culture.

Incubation and Reading

The microtiter plates are sealed and incubated for 3 to 5 days at 30°C in air. Plates must not be incubated beyond 5 days because of drug instability. If there is not sufficient growth after 5 days of incubation to interpret the results, the test should be repeated. Three days typically is sufficient for *M. fortuitum* complex; *M. chelonae* and *M. abscessus* usually require 4 days (occasionally 5 days). The MIC is defined as the lowest concentration of antimicrobial agent that completely inhibits visible growth. As with other types of bacteria, "trailing" is common when testing sulfonamides, and the MICs of these agents should be read at approximately 80% inhibition of growth. Trailing also is often seen with isolates of *M. fortuitum* group and clarithromycin; when this occurs, the endpoint is read at the end of the trailing.

Reporting Results

MIC values and an interpretation, based on the breakpoints for the rapidly growing mycobacteria listed in Table 7 (28), are reported for each drug, with the following exceptions. Imipenem results should not be reported for *M. chelonae* or *M. abscessus*. This recommendation is based on data from a multicenter evaluation (174), which showed that imipenem MIC values for these two species (which usually are at the resistance breakpoint of 8 to16 μg/ml) were not reproducible, resulting in major category changes of susceptibility. As previously indicated, tobramycin results should be reported only for *M. chelonae*. Because tobramycin is the aminoglycoside of choice for *M. chelonae* infections, amikacin results need be reported only if the isolate of *M. chelonae* is tobramycin resistant.

Quality Control

The QC strain recommended for monitoring test performance and for verifying the concentration of antimicrobial agents is *M. peregrinum* ATCC 700686. *Staphylococcus aureus* ATCC 29213 is an acceptable alternative. QC tests should be performed on each new batch of test plates and once each week or each time testing is performed. Currently, interlaboratory proficiency testing available for testing rapidly growing mycobacteria is limited. Therefore, laboratories are encouraged to submit isolates to reference laboratories with extensive experience in testing these mycobacteria for confirmatory tests in lieu of a formal proficiency test program.

Alternative Susceptibility Testing Methods

In the last decade, drug susceptibility testing of mycobacteria has become a very dynamic field, spawning many new technologies that may prove successful in a clinical laboratory. They all comply with the CDC goal that susceptibility test results be available within a mean of 28 days from the time the specimen arrives in the laboratory (13). Some of these techniques are based on improved methods for measuring inhibition of growth, while others are based on molecular assays for both analytes that correlate with growth or direct detection of mutations associated with resistance (2). Methods that distinguish viable from nonviable tubercle bacilli include tetrazolium dye reduction (29, 48, 102), flow cytometry (99), and a particle-counting immunoassay to quantify mycobacterial antigen (41). Jacobs et al. (77) described a method based on the use of a luciferase reporter mycobacteriophage. The premise was that viable mycobacteria support the infection and multiplication of phages, whereas inhibited or killed mycobacteria do not. Therefore, mycobacteria susceptible to INH or RMP supported the phage infection and expressed luciferase. When exposed to INH or RMP, the cells were killed and no light was produced. This assay was modified to allow easy detection of the emitted light with a Polaroid film box (also known as the "Bronx box") (125). Cooksey et al. (30) introduced the luciferase gene into *M. tuberculosis* H37Ra by electroporation of a plasmid containing the luciferase gene linked to the *hsp60* promoter. The results of a broth microtiter assay with the luciferase-H37Ra strain were comparable to the results of a conventional broth microdilution assay. Cangelosi et al. (22) described an alternative approach based on the measurement of the precursor rRNA. In this assay, *M. tuberculosis* nucleic acid is probed with specific pre-16S rRNA stem sequences in the presence or absence of drugs that have a direct or indirect effect on rRNA synthesis. Responses to RMP and ciprofloxacin were

TABLE 7 Antimicrobial agents to test against rapidly growing mycobacteria by broth microdilution method[a]

Antimicrobial agent	Concn range (μg/ml)	MIC (μg/ml) for:			QC concn range (μg/ml) for:	
		Susceptible strains	Intermediate strains	Resistant strains	*M. peregrinum* ATCC 700686[g]	*S. aureus* ATCC 29213[g]
Amikacin[b]	1–128	≤16	32	≥64	≤1–4	1–4
Cefoxitin	2–256	≤16	32–64	≥128	16–32	1–4
Ciprofloxacin	0.125–16	≤1	2	≥4	≤0.125–0.5	0.125–0.5
Clarithromycin[c]	0.06–64	≤2	4	≥8	≤0.06–0.5	0.125–0.5
Doxycycline[d]	0.25–32	≤1	2–8	≥16	≤0.125–0.5	0.125–0.5
Imipenem[e]	1–64	≤4	8	≥16	2–16	
Sulfamethoxazole	1–64	≤32		≥64	≤1–4	32–128
Tobramycin[f]	1–32	≤4	8	≥16	4–8	0.125–1

[a] Table and footnotes are adapted from reference 28.

[b] An amikacin MIC of ≥64 μg/ml for *M. abscessus* is unusual and must be confirmed.

[c] Class agent for all newer macrolides. *M. chelonae* and *M. abscessus* should be read at 3 days but not more than 4 days. Trailing across a breakpoint should be interpreted as resistance with *M. fortuitum*.

[d] Doxycycline and minocycline are interchangeable.

[e] Do not report for *M. chelonae* or *M. abscessus*. An imipenem MIC of ≥8 μg/ml for *M. fortuitum* is unusual and should be confirmed.

[f] Report results only for *M. chelonae*.

[g] Expected range for QC purposes. Potencies of drug preparations also can be tested with *E. coli* ATCC 25922 and *Pseudomonas aeruginosa* ATCC 27853 and compared with expected ranges as described in CLSI document M7 (27).

detected within 24 and 48 h, respectively. Detectable pre-rRNA was depleted in susceptible cells but remained abundant in resistant cells. The ability of RMP to block the lytic cell cycle of bacteriophage D29 within susceptible *M. tuberculosis* and hence the production of plaques on a lawn has led to another bacteriophage-based assay for susceptibility testing of *M. tuberculosis* to a variety of drugs (43, 44).

Mutations in genes that encode targets of antimycobacterial agents (Table 2) can be detected by a variety of methods. A particular focus of such studies has been RMP resistance because of the pivotal role of RMP in the treatment of tuberculosis and other mycobacterial infections and the conserved nature of the genetic basis for resistance (>96% of RMP resistance correlates with mutations in an 81-bp segment of the *rpoB* gene). The methods used to detect *rpoB* mutations include PCR amplification of the target sequence and detection by DNA sequencing (71, 79, 150; V. Sintchenko, P. J. Jelfs, W. K. Chew, and G. L. Gilbert, Letter, *J. Antimicrob. Chemother.* **44**:294–295, 1999), the line probe assay (31, 37, 88), single-strand conformation polymorphism (45, 151), dideoxy fingerprinting (45), the mismatch RNA-RNA protection assay (105), the heteroduplex generator assay (167), the use of molecular beacons synthesized from modified oligonucleotides (86, 116), and PCR–enzyme-linked immunosorbent assay (50). Similar approaches have been developed for detecting mutations involved in INH (124), EMB and RMP (163), and PZA (35, 100) resistance. Torres et al. (154) have proposed real-time PCR coupled to fluorescence detection for a rapid detection of RMP and INH resistance associated with mutations in *M. tuberculosis*. DNA microarray technology described for mycobacterial identification has also been applied to the efficient detection of mutations associated with resistance to TB drugs (94, 155). Undoubtedly, the application of these assays for routine use in the clinical mycobacteriology laboratory is likely to require technical simplification or automation as well as outcome analysis to justify the anticipated increased costs compared with conventional approaches. Indeed, even if these goals are achieved, it is likely that there are many more mutations to be discovered before antimicrobial resistance in *M. tuberculosis* and other mycobacteria can reliably be detected by molecular assays.

NOCARDIA AND OTHER AEROBIC ACTINOMYCETES

Clinical Significance

Nocardia spp. and other aerobic actinomycetes (*Actinomadura, Rhodococcus, Gordonia, Tsukamurella,* and *Streptomyces* spp.) can cause serious disease in healthy hosts, and infections by these microorganisms in immunocompromised hosts can be systemic and life threatening (84). Combination antimicrobial therapy for several months is often necessary to achieve a positive outcome. In vitro susceptibility testing may be of great value in guiding treatment and monitoring for resistance.

Testing Method

The antimicrobial agents that are recommended for primary and secondary in vitro susceptibility testing are listed in Table 8. The broth microdilution method described for rapidly growing mycobacteria is recommended for testing *Nocardia* and other aerobic actinomycetes (28). The inoculum should

TABLE 8 Antimicrobial agents to test against *Nocardia* and other aerobic actinomycetes[a]

Antimicrobial agent	Concn range (μg/ml)	MIC (μg/ml) for:			QC concn (μg/ml) for[e]:	
		Susceptible strains	Intermediate strains	Resistant strains	*S. aureus* ATCC 29213	*E. coli* ATCC 35218
Primary						
Amikacin[b]	1–16	≤8		≥16	1–4	
Amoxicillin-clavulanic acid	2/1–32/16	≤8/4	16/8	≥32/16	0.12/0.06–0.5/0.25	4/2–16/8
Ceftriaxone	4–64	≤8	16–32	≥64	1–8	
Ciprofloxacin	0.25–4	≤1	2	≥4	0.12–0.5	
Clarithromycin[c]	0.5–8	≤2	4	≥8	0.12–0.5	
Imipenem	1–16	≤4	8	≥16	0.016–0.06	
Linezolid[d]	0.5–8	≤8			1–4	
Minocycline[b]	0.5–8	≤1	2–4	≥8	0.06–0.5	
Sulfamethoxazole[b]	4–64	≤32		≥64	32–128	
or						
Trimethoprim-sulfamethoxazole	0.25/4.75–4/76	≤2/38		≥4/76	≤0.5/9.5	
Tobramycin	1–16	≤4	8	≥16	0.12–1	
Secondary						
Cefepime	2–32	≤8	16	≥32	1–4	
Cefotaxime	4–64	≤8	16–32	≥64	1–4	
Doxycycline	0.5–8	≤1	2–4	≥8	0.12–1	
Gentamicin	1–16	≤4	8	≥16	0.12–1	

[a] Table and footnotes are adapted from reference 28.
[b] The breakpoints for these antimicrobial agents are different from the current CLSI recommendations for organisms that grow aerobically.
[c] Used as a class agent for newer macrolides.
[d] Proposed breakpoint. No *Nocardia* isolates with linezolid MICs of >8 μg/ml have been reported.
[e] At present there are no standard quality control strains of *Nocardia* or other aerobic actinomycetes. These standard *S. aureus* and *E. coli* strains should be used for QC of the concentration of antimicrobial agents.

be prepared as a suspension of microorganisms harvested from a blood agar plate that was incubated for 1 to 3 days at 37°C in air. Some species may require incubation for up to 5 days in order to have sufficient growth. Presently there are no standard strains available for QC, but standard strains of *S. aureus* and *E. coli* can be used for QC of the drug preparations.

Reporting of Results

MIC values and an interpretation, based on the breakpoints for *Nocardia* spp. and other aerobic actinomycetes listed in Table 8 (28), are reported for each drug. The interpretive criteria recommended for the aerobic actinomycetes by the CLSI in document M24-A for amikacin, minocycline, and sulfamethoxazole are different from the criteria for rapidly growing aerobic bacteria recommended by the CLSI in document M7-A5 (27).

REFERENCES

1. **Alcaide, F., G. E. Pfyffer, and A. Telenti.** 1997. Role of *embB* in natural and acquired resistance to ethambutol in mycobacteria. *Antimicrob. Agents Chemother.* **41:**2270–2273.
2. **Alcaide, F., and A. Telenti.** 1997. Molecular techniques in the diagnosis of drug-resistant tuberculosis. *Ann. Acad. Med. Singapore* **26:**647–650.
3. **Amsden, G. W.** 1996. Erythromycin, clarithromycin, and azithromycin: are the differences real? *Clin. Ther.* **18:**56–72.
4. **Anonymous.** 1997. Diagnosis and treatment of disease caused by nontuberculous mycobacteria. *Am. J. Respir. Crit. Care Med.* **156:**S1–S25.
5. **Anonymous.** 1998. *Priftin (Rifapentine) Prescribing Information.* Hoechst Marion Roussel, Inc., Kansas City, Mo.
6. **Banerjee, A., E. Dubnau, A. Quemard, V. Balasubramanian, K. S. Um, T. Wilson, D. Collins, G. de Lisle, and W. R. Jacobs, Jr.** 1994. *inhA*, a gene encoding a target for isoniazid and ethionamide in *Mycobacterium tuberculosis. Science* **263:**227–230.
7. **Barry, C. E., III, and K. Mdluli.** 1996. Drug sensitivity and environmental adaptation of mycobacterial cell wall components. *Trends Microbiol.* **4:**275–281.
8. **Bémer, P., F. Palicova, S. Rüsch-Gerdes, S. H. Siddiqi, H. B. Drugeon, and G. E. Pfyffer.** 2002. Multicenter evaluation of fully-automated BACTEC Mycobacteria Growth Indicator Tube 960 System for susceptibility testing of *Mycobacterium tuberculosis. J. Clin. Microbiol.* **40:**150–154.
9. **Benson, C.** 1997. Critical drug interactions with agents used for prophylaxis and treatment of *Mycobacterium avium* infections. *Am. J. Med.* **102:**32–36.
10. **Bergmann, J. S., and G. L. Woods.** 1998. Evaluation of the ESP culture system II for testing susceptibilities of *Mycobacterium tuberculosis* isolates to four primary antituberculous drugs. *J. Clin. Microbiol.* **36:**2940–2943.
11. **Bernard, E. M., F. F. Edwards, T. E. Kiehn, S. T. Brown, and D. Armstrong.** 1993. Activities of antimicrobial agents against clinical isolates of *Mycobacterium haemophilum. Antimicrob. Agents Chemother.* **37:**2323–2326.
12. **Berning, S. E., L. Madsen, M. D. Iseman, and C. A. Peloquin.** 1995. Long-term safety of ofloxacin and ciprofloxacin in the treatment of mycobacterial infections. *Am. J. Respir. Crit. Care Med.* **151:**2006–2009.
13. **Bird, B. R., M. M. Denniston, R. E. Huebner, and R. C. Good.** 1996. Changing practices in mycobacteriology: a follow-up survey of state and territorial public health laboratories. *J. Clin. Microbiol.* **34:**554–559.
14. **Bodmer, T., G. Zurcher, P. Imboden, and A. Telenti.** 1995. Mutation position and type of substitution in the beta-subunit of the RNA polymerase influence in-vitro activity of rifamycins in rifampicin-resistant *Mycobacterium tuberculosis. J. Antimicrob. Chemother.* **35:**345–348.
15. **Bozeman, L., W. Burman, B. Metchock, L. Welch, M. Weiner, and the Tuberculosis Trials Consortium.** 2005. Fluoroquinolone susceptibility among *Mycobacterium tuberculosis* isolates from the United States and Canada. *J. Infect. Dis.* **40:**386–391.
16. **Brown, B. A., J. M. Swenson, and R. J. Wallace, Jr.** 1992. Broth microdilution test for rapidly growing mycobacteria, p. 5.11.1–5.11.10. *In* H. D. Isenberg (ed.), *Clinical Microbiology Procedures Handbook*, vol. 1. American Society for Microbiology, Washington, D.C.
17. **Brown-Elliott, B. A., and R. J. Wallace, Jr.** 2002. Clinical and taxonomic status of pathogenic nonpigmented or late-pigmenting rapidly growing mycobacteria. *Clin. Microbiol. Rev.* **15:**716–746.
18. **Brunello, F., and R. Fontana.** 2000. Reliability of the MB/BacT system for testing susceptibility of *Mycobacterium tuberculosis* complex isolates to antituberculous drugs. *J. Clin. Microbiol.* **38:**872–873.
19. **Canetti, G.** 1965. Present aspects of bacterial resistance in tuberculosis. *Am. Rev. Respir. Dis.* **92:**687–702.
20. **Canetti, G., W. Fox, A. Khomenko, H. T. Mahler, N. K. Menon, D. A. Mitchison, N. Rist, and N. A. Smelev.** 1969. Advances in techniques of testing mycobacterial drug sensitivity, and the use of sensitivity tests in tuberculosis control programs. *Bull. W. H. O.* **41:**21–43.
21. **Canetti, G., S. Froman, J. Grosset, P. Hauduroy, M. Lagerova, H. T. Mahler, G. Meissner, D. A. Mitchison, and L. Sula.** 1963. Mycobacteria: laboratory methods for testing drug sensitivity and resistance. *Bull. W. H. O.* **29:**565–578.
22. **Cangelosi, G. A., W. H. Brabant, T. B. Britschgi, and C. K. Wallis.** 1996. Detection of rifampin- and ciprofloxacin-resistant *Mycobacterium tuberculosis* by using species-specific assays for precursor rRNA. *Antimicrob. Agents Chemother.* **40:**1790–1795.
23. **Chaisson, R. E., C. A. Benson, M. P. Dube, L. B. Heifets, J. A. Korvick, S. Elkin, T. Smith, J. C. Craft, F. R. Sattler, and the AIDS Clinical Trials Group Protocol 157 Study Team.** 1994. Clarithromycin therapy for bacteremic *Mycobacterium avium* complex disease. *Ann. Intern. Med.* **121:**905–911.
24. **Chaisson, R. E., P. Keiser, M. Pierce, W. J. Fessel, J. Ruskin, C. Lahart, C. A. Benson, K. Meek, N. Siepman, and J. C. Craft.** 1997. Clarithromycin and ethambutol with or without clofazimine for the treatment of bacteremic *Mycobacterium avium* complex disease in patients with HIV infection. *AIDS* **11:**311–317.
25. **Chen, C. H., J. F. Shih, P. J. Lindholm-Levy, and L. B. Heifets.** 1989. Minimal inhibitory concentrations of rifabutin, ciprofloxacin, and ofloxacin against *Mycobacterium tuberculosis* isolated before treatment of patients in Taiwan. *Am. Rev. Respir. Dis.* **140:**987–989.
26. **Chiu, J., J. Nussbaum, S. Bozette, J. G. Tilles, L. S. Young, J. Leedom, P. N. R. Heseltine, and J. A. McCutchan.** 1990. Treatment of disseminated *Mycobacterium avium* complex infection in AIDS with amikacin, ethambutol, rifampin, and ciprofloxacin. *Ann. Intern. Med.* **113:**358–361.
27. **Clinical and Laboratory Standards Institute/NCCLS.** 2000. *Methods for Dilution Antimicrobial Susceptibility Tests for Bacteria That Grow Aerobically; Approved Standard—Fifth Edition.* CLSI/NCCLS document M7-A5. Clinical and Laboratory Standards Institute/NCCLS, Wayne, Pa.
28. **Clinical and Laboratory Standards Institute/NCCLS.** 2003. *Susceptibility Testing of Mycobacteria, Nocardiae, and Other Aerobic Actinomycetes; Approved Standard.* CLSI/NCCLS document M24-A. Clinical and Laboratory Standards Institute/NCCLS, Wayne, Pa.
29. **Collins, L., and S. G. Franzblau.** 1997. Microplate alamar blue assay versus BACTEC 460 system for high-throughput screening of compounds against *Mycobacterium tuberculosis*

and *Mycobacterium avium*. *Antimicrob. Agents Chemother.* **41:**1004–1009.

30. **Cooksey, R. C., J. T. Crawford, W. R. Jacobs, Jr., and T. M. Shinnick.** 1993. A rapid method for screening antimicrobial agents for activities against a strain of *Mycobacterium tuberculosis* expressing firefly luciferase. *Antimicrob. Agents Chemother.* **37:**1348–1352.
31. **Cooksey, R. C., G. P. Morlock, S. Glickman, and J. T. Crawford.** 1997. Evaluation of a line probe assay kit for characterization of *rpoB* mutations in rifampin-resistant *Mycobacterium tuberculosis* isolates from New York City. *J. Clin. Microbiol.* **35:**1281–1283.
32. **Crofton, J., and D. A. Mitchison.** 1948. Streptomycin resistance in pulmonary tuberculosis. *Br. Med. J.* **2:**1009–1015.
33. **David, H. L.** 1970. Probability distribution of drug-resistant mutants in unselected populations of *Mycobacterium tuberculosis*. *Appl. Microbiol.* **20:**810–814.
34. **Davidson, P. D.** 1987. Drug resistance and the selection of therapy for tuberculosis. *Am. Rev. Respir. Dis.* **136:**255–257.
35. **Davies, A. P., O. J. Billington, T. D. McHugh, D. A. Mitchison, and S. H. Gillespie.** 2000. Comparison of phenotypic and genotypic methods for pyrazinamide susceptibility testing with *Mycobacterium tuberculosis*. *J. Clin. Microbiol.* **38:**3686–3688.
36. **Davis, W. B., and M. M. Weber.** 1977. Specificity of isoniazid on growth inhibition and competition for an oxidized nicotiniamide adenine dinucleotide regulatory site on the electron transport pathway in *Mycobacterium phlei*. *Antimicrob. Agents Chemother.* **12:**213–218.
37. **De Beenhouwer, H., Z. Lhiang, G. Jannes, W. Mijs, L. Machtelinckx, R. Rossau, H. Traore, and F. Portaels.** 1995. Rapid detection of rifampicin resistance in sputum and biopsy specimens from tuberculosis patients by PCR and line probe assay. *Tubercle Lung Dis.* **76:**425–430.
38. **Deretic, V., W. Philipp, S. Dhandayuthapani, M. H. Mudd, R. Curcic, T. Garbe, B. Heym, L. E. Via, and S. T. Cole.** 1995. *Mycobacterium tuberculosis* is a natural mutant with an inactivated oxidative-stress regulatory gene: implications for sensitivity to isoniazid. *Mol. Microbiol.* **17:**889–900.
39. **Dhandayuthapani, S., M. Mudd, and V. Deretic.** 1997. Interactions of OxyR with the promoter region of the *oxyR* and *ahpC* genes from *Mycobacterium leprae* and *Mycobacterium tuberculosis*. *J. Bacteriol.* **179:**2401–2409.
40. **Diaz-Infantes, M. S., M. J. Ruiz-Serrano, L. Martinez-Sanchez, A. Ortega, and E. Bouza.** 2000. Evaluation of the MB/BacT Mycobacterium Detection System for susceptibility testing of *Mycobacterium tuberculosis*. *J. Clin. Microbiol.* **38:**1988–1989.
41. **Drowart, A., C. L. Cambiaso, K. Huygen, E. Serruys, F. Portaels, E. Jann, and J. P. Van Vooren.** 1997. Detection of rifampicin and isoniazid resistances of *Mycobacterium tuberculosis* strains by particle counting immunoassay (PACIA). *Int. J. Tubercle Lung Dis.* **1:**284–288.
42. **Dukes, C. S., J. Sugarman, J. P. Cegielski, G. J. Lallinger, and D. H. Mwakyusa.** 1992. Severe cutaneous hypersensitivity reactions during treatment of tuberculosis in patients with HIV infection in Tanzania. *Trop. Geogr. Med.* **44:**308–311.
43. **Eltringham, I. J., F. A. Drobniewski, J. A. Mangan, P. D. Butcher, and S. M. Wilson.** 1999. Evaluation of reverse transcription-PCR and a bacteriophage-based assay for rapid phenotypic detection of rifampin resistance in clinical isolates of *Mycobacterium tuberculosis*. *J. Clin. Microbiol.* **37:**3524–3527.
44. **Eltringham, I. J., S. M. Wilson, and F. A. Drobniewski.** 1999. Evaluation of a bacteriophage-based assay (phage amplified biologically assay) as a rapid screen for resistance to isoniazid, ethambutol, streptomycin, pyrazinamide, and ciprofloxacin among clinical isolates of *Mycobacterium tuberculosis*. *J. Clin. Microbiol.* **37:**3528–3532.
45. **Felmlee, T. A., Q. Liu, A. C. Whelen, D. Williams, S. S. Sommer, and D. H. Persing.** 1995. Genotypic detection of *Mycobacterium tuberculosis* rifampin resistance: comparison of single-strand conformation polymorphism and dideoxy fingerprinting. *J. Clin. Microbiol.* **33:**1617–1623.
46. **Fernandez-Roblas, R., J. Esteban, F. Cabria, J. C. Lopez, M. S. Jimenez, and F. Soriano.** 2000 In vitro susceptibilities of rapidly growing mycobacteria to telithromycin (HMR 3647) and seven other antimicrobials. *Antimicrob. Agents Chemother.* **44:**181–182.
47. **Finken, M., P. Kirschner, A. Meier, A. Wrede, and E. C. Böttger.** 1993. Molecular basis of streptomycin resistance in *Mycobacterium tuberculosis:* alterations of the ribosomal protein S12 gene and point mutations within a functional 16S ribosomal RNA pseudoknot. *Mol. Microbiol.* **9:**1239–1246.
48. **Franzblau, S. G., R. S. Witzig, J. C. McLaughlin, P. Torres, G. Madico, A. Hernandez, M. T. Degnan, M. B. Cook, V. K. Quenzer, R. M. Ferguson, and R. H. Gilman.** 1998. Rapid, low-technology MIC determination with clinical *Mycobacterium tuberculosis* isolates by using the microplate Alamar Blue assay. *J. Clin. Microbiol.* **36:**362–366.
49. **Frieden, T. R., T. Sterling, A. Pablos-Mendez, J. O. Kilburn, G. M. Cauthen, and S. W. Doolery.** 1993. The emergence of drug-resistant tuberculosis in New York City. *N. Engl. J. Med.* **328:**521–526.
50. **Garcia, L., M. Alonso-Sanz, M. J. Rebollo, J. C. Tercero, and F. Chaves.** 2001. Mutations in the *rpoB* gene of rifampin-resistant *Mycobacterium tuberculosis* isolates in Spain and their rapid detection by PCR-enzyme-linked immunosorbent assay. *J. Clin. Microbiol.* **39:**1813–1818.
51. **Ginsburg, A. S., J. H. Grosset, and W. R. Bishai.** 2003. Fluoroquinolones, tuberculosis, and resistance. *Lancet Infect. Dis.* **3:**432–442.
52. **Good, R. C.** 1985. Opportunistic pathogens in the genus *Mycobacterium*. *Annu. Rev. Microbiol.* **39:**347–369.
53. **Grosset, J. H.** 1992. Treatment of tuberculosis in HIV infection. *Tubercle Lung Dis.* **73:**378–383.
54. **Guerrero, C., L. Stockman, F. Marchesi, T. Bodmer, G. D. Roberts, and A. Telenti.** 1994. Evaluation of the *rpoB* gene in rifampicin-susceptible and resistant *Mycobacterium avium* and *Mycobacterium intracellulare*. *J. Antimicrob. Chemother.* **33:**661–663.
55. **Guthertz, L. S., M. E. Griffith, E. G. Ford, J. M. Janda, and T. F. Midura.** 1988. Quality control of individual components used in Middlebrook 7H10 medium for mycobacterial susceptibility testing. *J. Clin. Microbiol.* **26:**2338–2342.
56. **Hacek, D.** 1992. Modified proportion agar dilution test for slowly growing mycobacteria, p. 5.13.1–5.13.15. *In* H. D. Isenberg (ed.), *Clinical Microbiology Procedures Handbook*, vol. 1. American Society for Microbiology, Washington, D.C.
57. **Hanna, B. A., A. Ebrahimzadeh, L. B. Elliott, M. A. Morgan, S. M. Novak, S. Rüsch-Gerdes, M. Acio, D. F. Dunbar, T. M. Holmes, C. H. Rexer, C. Savthyakumar, and A. M. Vannier.** 1999. Multicenter evaluation of the BACTEC MGIT 960 system for recovery of mycobacteria. *J. Clin. Microbiol.* **37:**748–752.
58. **Havlir, D. V., M. P. Dube, F. R. Sattler, D. N. Forthal, C. A. Kemper, M. W. Dunne, D. M. Parenti, J. P. Lavelle, A. White, M. D. Witt, S. A. Bozzette, J. A. McCutchan, and the California Collaborative Treatment Group.** 1996. Prophylaxis against disseminated *Mycobacterium avium* complex with weekly azithromycin, daily rifabutin, or both. *N. Engl. J. Med.* **335:**392–398.
59. **Hawkins, J. E.** 1984. Drug susceptibility testing, p. 177–193. *In* G. P. Kubica and L. G. Wayne (ed.), *The Mycobacteria: a Sourcebook*, part A. Marcel Dekker, Inc., New York, N.Y.
60. **Hawkins, J. E.** 1986. Non-weekend schedule for BACTEC susceptibility testing of *Mycobacterium tuberculosis*. *J. Clin. Microbiol.* **23:**934–937.

61. **Hawkins, J. E., R. C. Good, G. P. Kubica, P. R. Gangadharam, H. M. Gruft, and K. D. Stottmeier.** 1983. The levels of service concept in mycobacteriology. *Am. Thorac. Soc. News* **9:**19–25.
62. **Heep, M., B. Brandstätter, U. Rieger, N. Lehn, E. Richter, S. Rüsch-Gerdes, and S. Niemann.** 2001. Frequency of *rpoB* mutations inside and outside the cluster I region in rifampin-resistant clinical *Mycobacterium tuberculosis* isolates. *J. Clin. Microbiol.* **39:**107–110.
63. **Heifets, L. B.** 1991. *Drug Susceptibility in the Chemotherapy of Mycobacterial Infections,* p. 212. CRC Press, Inc., Boca Raton, Fla.
64. **Heifets, L. B., M. D. Iseman, P. J. Lindholm-Levy, and W. Kanes.** 1985. Determination of ansamycin MICs for *Mycobacterium avium* complex in liquid medium by radiometric and conventional methods. *Antimicrob. Agents Chemother.* **28:**570–575.
65. **Heym, B., Y. Zhang, S. Poulet, D. Young, and S. T. Cole.** 1993. Characterization of the *katG* gene encoding a catalase-peroxidase required for isoniazid susceptibility of *Mycobacterium tuberculosis. J. Bacteriol.* **175:**4255–4259.
66. **Hoffner, S. E., M. Kratz, B. Olsson-Liljequist, S. B. Svenson, and G. Källenius.** 1989. In-vitro synergistic activity between ethambutol and fluorinated quinolones against *Mycobacterium avium* complex. *J. Antimicrob. Chemother.* **24:**317–324.
67. **Hoffner, S. E., S. B. Svenson, and A. E. Beezer.** 1990. Microcalorimetric studies of the initial interaction between antimycobacterial drugs and *Mycobacterium avium. J. Antimicrob. Chemother.* **25:**353–359.
68. **Howard, W. L., F. Maresh, E. E. Mueller, S. A. Yanitelli, and G. F. Woodruff.** 1949. The role of pulmonary cavitation in the development of bacterial resistance to streptomycin. *Am. Rev. Tuberc.* **59:**391–401.
69. **Howlett, H. S., J. B. O'Connor, J. F. Sadusk, J. E. Swift, and F. A. Beardsley.** 1949. Sensitivity of tubercle bacilli to streptomycin: the influence of various factors upon the emergence of resistant strains. *Am. Rev. Tuberc.* **59:**402–414.
70. **Hu, Y., A. R. Coates, and D. A. Mitchison.** 2003. Sterilizing activities of fluoroquinolones against rifampin-tolerant populations of *Mycobacterium tuberculosis. Antimicrob. Agents Chemother.* **47:**653–657.
71. **Hunt, J. M., G. D. Roberts, L. Stockman, T. A. Felmlee, and D. H. Persing.** 1994. Detection of a genetic locus encoding resistance to rifampin in mycobacterial cultures and in clinical specimens. *Diagn. Microbiol. Infect. Dis.* **18:**219–227.
72. **Inderlied, C. B.** 1994. Antimycobacterial susceptibility testing: present practices and future trends. *Eur. J. Clin. Micrbiol. Infect. Dis.* **13:**980–993.
73. **Inderlied, C. B., C. A. Kemper, and L. E. M. Bermudez.** 1993. The *Mycobacterium avium* complex. *Clin. Microbiol. Rev.* **6:**266–310.
74. **Inderlied, C. B., P. T. Kolonski, M. Wu, and L. S. Young.** 1989. In vitro and in vivo activity of azithromycin (CP 62,993) against the *Mycobacterium avium* complex. *J. Infect. Dis.* **159:**994–997.
75. **Inderlied, C. B., and K. A. Nash.** 1996. Antimycobacterial agents: in vitro susceptibility testing, spectra of activity, mechanisms of action and resistance, and assays for activity in biologic fluids, p. 127–175. *In* V. Lorian (ed.), *Antibiotics in Laboratory Medicine,* 4th ed. The Williams & Wilkins Co., Baltimore, Md.
76. **Inderlied, C. B., and K. A. Nash.** 2005. *In* V. Lorian (ed.), *Antibiotics in Laboratory Medicine,* p. 179. Lippincott Williams & Wilkins, Philadelphia, Pa.
77. **Jacobs, W. R., Jr., R. G. Barletta, R. Udani, J. Chan, G. Kalkut, G. Sosne, T. Kieser, G. J. Sarkis, G. F. Hatfull, and B. R. Bloom.** 1993. Rapid assessment of drug susceptibilities of *Mycobacterium tuberculosis* by means of luciferase reporter phages. *Science* **260:**819–822.
78. **Källenius, G., S. G. Svenson, and S. E. Hoffner.** 1989. Ethambutol: a key for *Mycobacterium avium* complex chemotherapy. *Am. Rev. Respir. Dis.* **140:**264.
79. **Kapur, V., L. L. Li, S. Iordanescu, M. R. Hamrick, A. Wanger, B. N. Kreiswirth, and J. M. Musser.** 1994. Characterization by automated DNA sequencing of mutations in the gene *(rpoB)* encoding the RNA polymerase beta subunit in rifampin-resistant *Mycobacterium tuberculosis* strains from New York City and Texas. *J. Clin. Microbiol.* **32:**1095–1098.
80. **Kelley, C. L., D. A. Rouse, and S. L. Morris.** 1997. Analysis of *ahpC* gene mutations in isoniazid-resistant clinical isolates of *Mycobacterium tuberculosis. Antimicrob. Agents Chemother.* **41:**2057–2058.
81. **Kenney, T. J., and G. Churchward.** 1994. Cloning and sequence analysis of the *rpsL* and *rpsG* genes of *Mycobacterium smegmatis* and characterization of mutations causing resistance to streptomycin. *J. Bacteriol.* **176:**6153–6156.
82. **Kent, P. T., and G. P. Kubica.** 1985. *Public Health Mycobacteriology—a Guide for the Level III Laboratory.* U.S. Department of Health and Human Services, Centers for Disease Control, Atlanta, Ga.
83. **Koletar S. L., A. J. Berry, M. H. Cynamon, J. Jacobson, J. S. Currier, R. R. MacGregor, M. W. Dunne, and O. J. Williams.** 1999. Azithromycin as treatment for disseminated *Mycobacterium avium* complex in AIDS patients. *Antimicrob. Agents Chemother.* **43:**2869–2872.
84. **Kontoyiannis, D. P., K. Ruoff, and D. C. Hooper.** 1998. *Nocardia* bacteremia. Report of 4 cases and review of the literature. *Medicine* **77:**255–267.
85. **Kubica, G. P., and W. E. Dye.** 1967. *Laboratory Methods for Clinical and Public Health Mycobacteriology.* U.S. Government Printing Office, Washington, D.C.
86. **Lin, S. Y., W. Probert, M. Lo, and E. Desmond.** 2004. Rapid detection of isoniazid and rifampin resistance mutations in *Mycobacterium tuberculosis* complex from cultures or smear-positive sputa by use of molecular beacons. *J. Clin. Microbiol.* **42:**4204–4208.
87. **Masur, H.** 1993. Recommendations on prophylaxis and therapy for disseminated *Mycobacterium avium* complex disease in patients infected with the human-immunodeficiency-virus. *N. Engl. J. Med.* **329:**898–904.
88. **McNerney, R., P. Kiepiela, K. S. Bishop, P. M. Nye, and N. G. Stocker.** 2001. Rapid screening of *Mycobacterium tuberculosis* for susceptibility to rifampin and streptomycin. *Int. J. Tuberc. Lung Dis.* **4:**69–75.
89. **Mdluli, K., D. R. Sherman, M. J. Hickey, B. N. Kreiswirth, S. Morris, C. K. Stover, and C. Barry III.** 1996. Biochemical and genetic data suggest that InhA is not the primary target for activated isoniazid in *Mycobacterium tuberculosis. J. Infect. Dis.* **174:**1085–1090.
90. **Mdluli, K., R. A. Slayden, Y. Zhu, S. Ramaswamy, X. Pan, D. Mead, D. D. Crane, J. M. Musser, and C. E. Barry III.** 1998. Inhibition of a *Mycobacterium tuberculosis*-ketoacyl ACP synthase by isoniazid. *Science* **280:**1607–1610.
91. **Mdluli, K., J. Swanson, E. Fischer, R. E. Lee, and C. E. Barry III.** 1998. Mechanisms involved in the intrinsic isoniazid resistance of *Mycobacterium avium. Mol. Microbiol.* **27:**1223–1233.
92. **Meier, A., P. Kirschner, B. Springer, V. A. Steingrube, B. A. Brown, R. J. Wallace, Jr., and E. C. Böttger.** 1994. Identification of mutations in 23S rRNA gene of clarithromycin-resistant *Mycobacterium intracellulare. Antimicrob. Agents Chemother.* **38:**381–384.
93. **Miesel, L., D. A. Rozwarski, J. C. Sacchettini, and W. R. Jacobs, Jr.** 1998. Mechanisms for isoniazid action and resistance. *Novartis Found. Symp.* **217:**209–221.
94. **Mikhailovich, V. M., S. A. Lapa, D. A. Gryadunov, B. N. Strizhkov, A. Y. Sobolev, O. L. Skotnikova, O. A. I. Rtuganova, A. M. Moroz, V. I. Litvinov, L. K. Shipina,**

M. A. Vladimirskii, L. N. Chernousova, V. V. Erokhin, and A. D. Mirzabekov. 2001. Detection of rifampicin-resistant *Mycobacterium tuberculosis* strains by hybridization polymerase chain reaction on a specialized TB-microchip. *Bull. Exp. Biol. Med.* **131:**94–98.

95. **Miller, M. A., L. Thibert, F. Desjardins, S. H. Siddiqi, and A. Dascal.** 1996. Growth inhibition of *Mycobacterium tuberculosis* by polyoxyethylene stearate present in the BACTEC pyrazinamide susceptibility test. *J. Clin. Microbiol.* **34:**84–86.
96. **Miller, M. A., L. Thibert, F. Desjardins, S. H. Siddiqi, and A. Dascal.** 1995. Testing of susceptibility of *Mycobacterium tuberculosis* to pyrazinamide: comparison of Bactec method with pyrazinamidase assay. *J. Clin. Microbiol.* **33:**2468–2470.
97. **Mitchison, D. A.** 1979. Basic mechanisms of chemotherapy. *Chest* **76**(Suppl.)**:**771–781.
98. **Mitchison, D. A.** 1992. The Garrod Lecture. Understanding the chemotherapy of tuberculosis-current problems. *J. Antimicrob. Chemother.* **29:**477–493.
99. **Moore, A. V., S. M. Kirk, S. M. Callister, G. H. Mazurek, and R. F. Schell.** 1999. Safe determination of susceptibility of *Mycobacterium tuberculosis* to antimycobacterial agents by flow cytometry. *J. Clin. Microbiol.* **37:**479–483.
100. **Morlock, G. P., J. T. Crawford, W. R. Butler, S. E. Brim, D. Sikes, G. H. Mazurek, C. L. Woodley, and R. C. Cooksey.** 2000. Phenotypic characterization of *pncA* mutants of *Mycobacterium tuberculosis*. *Antimicrob. Agents Chemother.* **44:**2291–2295.
101. **Morris, S., G. H. Bai, P. Suffys, L. Portillo-Gomez, M. Fairchok, and D. Rouse.** 1995. Molecular mechanisms of multiple drug resistance in clinical isolates of *Mycobacterium tuberculosis*. *J. Infect. Dis.* **171:**954–960.
102. **Mshana, R. N., G. Tadesse, G. Abate, and H. Miorner.** 1998. Use of 3-(4,5-dimethylthiazol-2-yl)-2,5-diphenyl tetrazolium bromide for rapid detection of rifampin-resistant *Mycobacterium tuberculosis*. *J. Clin. Microbiol.* **36:**1214–1219.
103. **Musser, J. M.** 1995. Antimicrobial agent resistance in mycobacteria: molecular genetic insights. *Clin. Microbiol. Rev.* **8:**496–514.
104. **Nair, J., D. A. Rouse, G. H. Bai, and S. L. Morris.** 1993. The *rpsL* gene and streptomycin resistance in single and multiple drug-resistant strains of *Mycobacterium tuberculosis*. *Mol. Microbiol.* **10:**521–527.
105. **Nash, K. A., A. Gaytan, and C. B. Inderlied.** 1997. Detection of rifampin resistance in *Mycobacterium tuberculosis* by use of a rapid, simple, and specific RNA/RNA mismatch assay. *J. Infect. Dis.* **176:**533–536.
106. **Nash, K. A., and C. B. Inderlied.** 1995. Genetic basis of macrolide resistance in *Mycobacterium avium* isolated from patients with disseminated disease. *Antimicrob. Agents Chemother.* **39:**2625–2630.
107. **Nightingale, S. D., W. D. Cameron, F. M. Gordin, P. M. Sullam, D. L. Cohn, R. E. Chaisson, L. J. Eron, P. D. Saprti, B. Bihari, D. L. Kaufman, J. J. Stern, D. D. Pearce, W. G. Weinberg, A. LaMarca, and F. P. Siegel.** 1993. Two controlled trials of rifabutin prophylaxis against *Mycobacterium avium* complex infection in AIDS. *N. Engl. J. Med.* **329:**828–833.
108. **Nitta, A. T., P. T. Davidson, M. L. de Koning, and R. J. Kilman.** 1996. Misdiagnosis of multidrug-resistant tuberculosis possibly due to laboratory-related errors. *JAMA* **276:**1980–1983.
109. **Nunn, P., J. Porter, and P. Winstanley.** 1993. Thiacetazone—avoid like poison or use with care. *Trans. R. Soc. Trop. Med. Hyg.* **87:**578–582.
110. **Oh, Y. K., and R. M. Straubinger.** 1996. Intracellular fate of *Mycobacterium avium:* use of dual-label spectrofluorometry to investigate the influence of bacterial viability and opsonization on phagosomal pH and phagosome-lysosome interaction. *Infect. Immun.* **64:**319–325.
111. **Parsons, L. M., A. Somoskovi, R. Urbanczik, and M. Salfinger.** 2004. Laboratory diagnostic aspects of drug resistant tuberculosis. *Front. Biosci.* **9:**2086–2105.
112. **Perutz, M. F.** 1994. The white plague. *N. Y. Rev. Books* **XLI:**35–39.
113. **Pfyffer, G. E., D. A. Bonato, A. Ebrahimzadeh, W. Gross, J. Hotaling, J. Kornblum, A. Laszlo, G. Roberts, M. Salfinger, F. Wittwer, and S. Siddiqi.** 1999. Multicenter laboratory validation of susceptibility testing of *Mycobacterium tuberculosis* against classical second-line and newer antimicrobial drugs by using the radiometric BACTEC 460 technique and the proportion method with solid media. *J. Clin. Microbiol.* **37:**3179–3186.
114. **Pfyffer, G. E., F. Palicova, and S. Rüsch-Gerdes.** 2002. Testing of susceptibility of *Mycobacterium tuberculosis* to pyrazinamide with the nonradiometric BACTEC MGIT 960 system. *J. Clin. Microbiol.* **40:**1670–1674.
115. **Pfyffer, G. E., H. M. Welscher, P. Kissling, C. Cieslak, M. J. Casal, J. Gutierrez, and S. Rüsch-Gerdes.** 1997. Comparison of the Mycobacteria Growth Indicator Tube (MGIT) with radiometric and solid culture for recovery of acid-fast bacilli. *J. Clin. Microbiol.* **35:**364–368.
116. **Piatek, A. S., A. Telenti, M. R. Murray, H. El-Hajj, W. R. Jacobs, Jr., F. R. Kramer, and D. Alland.** 2000. Genotypic analysis of *Mycobacterium tuberculosis* in two distinct populations using molecular beacons: implications for rapid susceptibility testing. *Antimicrob. Agents Chemother.* **44:**103–110.
117. **Pierce, M., S. Crampton, D. Henry, L. Heifets, A. LaMarca, M. Montecalvo, G. P. Wormser, H. Jablonowski, J. Jemsek, M. Cynamon, B. G. Yangco, G. Notario, and J. C. Craft.** 1996. A randomized trial of clarithromycin as prophylaxis against disseminated *Mycobacterium avium* complex infection in patients with advanced acquired immunodeficiency syndrome. *N. Engl. J. Med.* **335:**384–391.
118. **Piersimoni, C., C. Scarparo, A. Callegaro, C. P. Tosi, D. Nista, S. Bornigia, M. Scagnelli, A. Rigon, G. Ruggiero, and A. Goglio.** 2001. Comparison of MB/BacT Alert 3D system with radiometric BACTEC system and Lowenstein-Jensen medium for recovery and identification of mycobacteria from clinical specimens: a multicenter study. *J. Clin. Microbiol.* **39:**651–657.
119. **Pletz, M. W., A. DeRoux, A. Roth, K. H. Neumann, H. Mauch, and H. Lode.** 2004. Early bactericidal activity of moxifloxacin in treatment of pulmonary tuberculosis: a prospective, randomized study. *Antimicrob. Agents Chemother.* **48:**780–782.
120. **Pyle, M.** 1947. Relative number of resistant tubercle bacilli in sputa of patients before and during treatment with streptomycin. *Proc. Mayo Clin.* **22:**465–473.
121. **Rastogi, N., K. S. Goh, M. Berchel, and A. Bryskier.** 2000. In vitro activities of the ketolides telithromycin (HMR 3647) and HMR 3004 compared to those of clarithromycin against slowly growing mycobacteria at pHs 6.8 and 7.4. *Antimicrob. Agents Chemother.* **44:**2848–2852.
122. **Rathman, M., M. D. Sjaastad, and S. Falkow.** 1996. Acidification of phagosomes containing *Salmonella typhimurium* in murine macrophages. *Infect. Immun.* **64:**2765–2773.
123. **Revel Viravau, V., Q. C. Truong, N. Moreau, V. Jarlier, and W. Sougakoff.** 1996. Sequence analysis, purification, and study of inhibition by 4-quinolones of the DNA gyrase from *Mycobacterium smegmatis*. *Antimicrob. Agents Chemother.* **40:**2054–2061.
124. **Rinder, H., K. Feldmann, E. Tortoli, J. Grosset, M. Casal, E. Richter, M. Rifai, V. Jarlier, M. Vaquero, S. Rüsch-Gerdes, E. Cambau, J. Gutierrez, and T. Loscher.** 1999. Culture-independent prediction of isoniazid resistance in *Mycobacterium tuberculosis* by *katG* gene analysis directly from sputum samples. *Mol. Diagn.* **4:**145–152.

125. **Riska, P. F., Y. Su, S. Bardarov, L. Freundlich, G. Sarkis, G. Hatfull, C. Carriere, V. Kumar, J. Chan, and W. R. Jacobs, Jr.** 1999. Rapid film-based determination of antibiotic susceptibilities of *Mycobacterium tuberculosis* strains by using a luciferase reporter phage and the Bronx Box. *J. Clin. Microbiol.* **37:**1144–1149.
126. **Ruiz, P., F. J. Zerolo, and M. J. Casal.** 2000. Comparison of susceptibility testing of *Mycobacterium tuberculosis* using the ESP culture system II with that using the BACTEC method. *J. Clin. Microbiol.* **38:**4663–4664.
127. **Rüsch-Gerdes, S., C. Domehl, G. Nardi, M. R. Gismondo, H. M. Welscher, and G. E. Pfyffer.** 1999. Multicenter evaluation of the mycobacteria growth indicator tube for testing susceptibility of *Mycobacterium tuberculosis* to first-line drugs. *J. Clin. Microbiol.* **37:**45–48.
128. **Russel, W. R., and G. Middlebrook.** 1961. *Chemotherapy of Tuberculosis.* Charles C. Thomas, Springfield, Ill.
129. **Saito, H., K. Sato, and H. Tomioka.** 1988. Comparative in vitro and in vivo activity of rifabutin and rifampicin against *Mycobacterium avium* complex. *Tubercle* **69:**187–192.
130. **Salfinger, M., and L. B. Heifets.** 1988. Determination of pyrazinamide MICs for *Mycobacterium tuberculosis* at different pHs by the radiometric method. *Antimicrob. Agents Chemother.* **32:**1002–1004.
131. **Salfinger, M., L. B. Reller, B. Demchuk, and Z. T. Johnson.** 1989. Rapid radiometric method for pyrazinamide susceptibility testing of *M. tuberculosis. Res. Microbiol.* **140:**301–309.
132. **Sanders, C. A., R. R. Nieda, and E. P. Desmond.** 2004. Validation of the use of Middlebrook 7H10 agar, BACTEC MGIT 960, and BACTEC 460 12B media for testing the susceptibility of *Mycobacterium tuberculosis* to levofloxacin. *J. Clin. Microbiol.* **42:**5225–5228.
133. **Schentag, J. J., and C. H. Ballow.** 1991. Tissue-directed pharmacokinetics. *Am. J. Med.* **91:**5S–11S.
134. **Scorpio, A., D. Collins, D. Whipple, D. Cave, J. Bates, and Y. Zhang.** 1997. Rapid differentiation of bovine and human tubercle bacilli based on a characteristic mutation in the bovine pyrazinamidase gene. *J. Clin. Microbiol.* **35:**106–110.
135. **Scorpio, A., P. Lindholm Levy, L. Heifets, R. Gilman, S. Siddiqi, M. Cynamon, and Y. Zhang.** 1997. Characterization of *pncA* mutations in pyrazinamide-resistant *Mycobacterium tuberculosis. Antimicrob. Agents Chemother.* **41:**540–543.
136. **Scorpio, A., and Y. Zhang.** 1996. Mutations in *pncA*, a gene encoding pyrazinamidase/nicotinamidase, cause resistance to the antituberculous drug pyrazinamide in tubercle bacillus. *Nat. Med.* **2:**662–667.
137. **Shafran, S. D., J. Singer, D. P. Zarowny, P. Phillips, I. Salit, S. L. Walmsley, I. W. Fong, M. J. Gill, A. R. Rachlis, R. G. Lalonde, M. M. Fanning, C. M. Tsoukas, and the Canadian HIV Trials Network Protocol 010 Study Group.** 1996. A comparison of two regimens for the treatment of *Mycobacterium avium* complex bacteremia in AIDS: rifabutin, ethambutol, and clarithromycin versus rifampin, ethambutol, clofazimine, and ciprofloxacin. *N. Engl. J. Med.* **335:**377–383.
138. **Siddiqi, S. H.** 1992. Radiometric (Bactec) tests for slowly growing mycobacteria, p. 5.14.1–5.14.25. *In* H. D. Isenberg (ed.), *Clinical Microbiology Procedures Handbook,* vol. 1. American Society for Microbiology, Washington, D.C.
139. **Siddiqi, S. H., J. P. Libonati, M. E. Carter, N. M. Hooper, J. F. Baker, C. C. Hwangbo, and L. E. Warfel.** 1988. Enhancement of mycobacterial growth in Middlebrook 7H12 medium by polyoxyethylene stearate. *Curr. Microbiol.* **17:**105–110.
140. **Sirgel, F. A., F. J. Botha, D. P. Parkin, B. W. Van de Wal, R. Schall, P. R. Donald, and D. A. Mitchison.** 1997. The early bactericidal activity of ciprofloxacin in patients with pulmonary tuberculosis. *Am. J. Respir. Crit. Care Med.* **156:**901–905.
141. **Sison, J. P., Y. Yao, C. A. Kemper, J. R. Hamilton, E. Brummer, D. A. Stevens, and S. C. Deresinski.** 1996. Treatment of *Mycobacterium avium* complex infection: do the results of in vitro susceptibility tests predict therapeutic outcome in humans? *J. Infect. Dis.* **173:**677–683.
142. **Sreevatsan, S., X. Pan, Y. Zhang, V. Deretic, and J. M. Musser.** 1997. Analysis of the *oxyR-ahpC* region in isoniazid-resistant and -susceptible *Mycobacterium tuberculosis* complex organisms recovered from diseased humans and animals in diverse localities. *Antimicrob. Agents Chemother.* **41:**600–606.
143. **Sreevatsan, S., X. Pan, Y. Zhang, B. N. Kreiswirth, and J. M. Musser.** 1997. Mutations associated with pyrazinamide resistance in *pncA* of *Mycobacterium tuberculosis* complex organisms. *Antimicrob. Agents Chemother.* **41:**636–640.
144. **Sreevatsan, S., K. E. Stockbauer, X. Pan, B. N. Kreiswirth, S. L. Moghazeh, W. Jacobs, Jr., A. Telenti, and J. M. Musser.** 1997. Ethambutol resistance in *Mycobacterium tuberculosis:* critical role of *embB* mutations. *Antimicrob. Agents Chemother.* **41:**1677–1681.
145. **Straus, W. L., S. M. Ostroff, D. B. Jernigan, T. E. Kiehn, E. M. Sordillo, D. Armstrong, N. Boone, N. Schneider, J. O. Kilburn, V. A. Silcox, V. LaBombardi, and R. C. Good.** 1994. Clinical and epidemiologic characteristics of *Mycobacterium haemophilum,* an emerging pathogen in immunocompromised patients. *Ann. Intern. Med.* **120:**118–125.
146. **Sturgill-Koszycki, S., P. H. Schlesinger, P. Chakraborty, P. L. Haddix, H. L. Collins, A. K. Fok, R. D. Allen, S. L. Gluck, J. Heuser, and D. G. Russell.** 1994. Lack of acidification in *Mycobacterium* phagosomes produced by exclusion of the vesicular proton-ATPase. *Science* **263:**678–681.
147. **Takayama, K., and J. O. Kilburn.** 1989. Inhibition of synthesis of arabinogalactan by ethambutol in *Mycobacterium smegmatis. Antimicrob. Agents Chemother.* **33:**1493–1499.
148. **Takiff, H. E., L. Salazar, C. Guerrero, W. Philipp, W. M. Huang, B. Kreiswirth, S. T. Cole, W. Jacobs, Jr., and A. Telenti.** 1994. Cloning and nucleotide sequence of *Mycobacterium tuberculosis gyrA* and *gyrB* genes and detection of quinolone resistance mutations. *Antimicrob. Agents Chemother.* **38:**773–780.
149. **Telenti, A., N. Honore, C. Bernasconi, J. March, A. Ortega, B. Heym, H. E. Takiff, and S. T. Cole.** 1997. Genotypic assessment of isoniazid and rifampin resistance in *Mycobacterium tuberculosis:* a blind study at reference laboratory level. *J. Clin. Microbiol.* **35:**719–723.
150. **Telenti, A., P. Imboden, F. Marchesi, D. Lowrie, S. Cole, M. J. Colston, L. Matter, K. Schopfer, and T. Bodmer.** 1993. Detection of rifampin-resistance mutations in *Mycobacterium tuberculosis. Lancet* **341:**647–650.
151. **Telenti, A., P. Imboden, F. Marchesi, T. Schmidheini, and T. Bodmer.** 1993. Direct, automated detection of rifampin-resistant *Mycobacterium tuberculosis* by polymerase chain reaction and single-strand conformation polymorphism analysis. *Antimicrob. Agents Chemother.* **37:**2054–2058.
152. **Tenover, F. C., J. T. Crawford, R. E. Huebner, L. J. Geiter, C. R. Horsburgh, and R. C. Good.** 1993. The resurgence of tuberculosis: is your laboratory ready? *J. Clin. Microbiol.* **31:**767–770.
153. **Terashima, T., F. Sakamaki, N. Hasegawa, M. Kanazawa, and T. Kawashiro.** 1994. Pulmonary infection due to *Mycobacterium xenopi. Intern. Med.* **33:**536–539.
154. **Torres, M. J., A. Criado, J. C. Palomares, and J. Aznar.** 2000. Use of real-time PCR and fluorimetry for rapid detection of rifampin and isoniazid resistance-associated mutations in *Mycobacterium tuberculosis. J. Clin. Microbiol.* **38:**3194–3199.

155. **Troesch, A., H. Nguyen, C. G. Miyada, S. Desvarenne, T. R. Gingeras, P. M. Kaplan, P. Cros, and C. Mabilat.** 1999. Mycobacterium species identification and rifampin resistance testing with high-density DNA probe arrays. *J. Clin. Microbiol.* **37:**49–55.
156. **Vernon, A. A.** 2003. Rifamycin antibiotics, with focus on newer agents, p. 759–771. *In* W. M. Rom and S. M. Garay (ed.), *Tuberculosis,* 2nd ed. Lippincott Williams and Wilkins, New York, N.Y.
157. **Wade, M. M., and Y. Zang.** 2004. Mechanisms of drug resistance in Mycobacterium tuberculosis. *Front. Biosci.* **9:**975–994.
158. **Wallace, R., Jr., A. Meier, B. A. Brown, Y. Zhang, P. Sander, G. O. Onyi, and E. C. Böttger.** 1996. Genetic basis for clarithromycin resistance among isolates of *Mycobacterium chelonae* and *Mycobacterium abscessus. Antimicrob. Agents Chemother.* **40:**1676–1681.
159. **Wallace, R. J., Jr.** 1989. The clinical presentation, diagnosis, and therapy of cutaneous and pulmonary infections due to the rapidly growing mycobacteria, *M. fortuitum* and *M. chelonae. Clin. Chest Med.* **10:**419–429.
160. **Wallace, R. J., Jr., and D. E. Griffith.** 2005. Antimycobacterial agents, p. 350–360. *In* G. L. Mandell, R. G. Douglas, Jr., and J. E. Bennett (ed.), *Principles and Practices of Infectious Diseases,* 6th ed. Elsevier Churchill Livingstone, Inc., Philadelphia, Pa.
161. **Wallace, R. J., Jr., J. M. Musser, S. I. Hull, V. A. Silcox, L. C. Steele, G. D. Forrester, A. Labidi, and R. K. Selander.** 1989. Diversity and sources of rapidly growing mycobacteria associated with infections following cardiac surgery. *J. Infect. Dis.* **159:**708–716.
162. **Wallace, R. J., Jr., D. R. Nash, M. Tsukamura, Z. M. Blacklock, and V. A. Silcox.** 1988. Human disease due to *Mycobacterium smegmatis. J. Infect. Dis.* **158:**52–59.
163. **Watterson, S. A., S. M. Wilson, M. D. Yates, and F. A. Drobniewski.** 1998. Comparison of three molecular assays for rapid detection of rifampin resistance in *Mycobacterium tuberculosis. J. Clin. Microbiol.* **36:**1969–1973.
164. **Wayne, L. G., and H. A. Sramek.** 1992. Agents of newly recognized or infrequently encountered mycobacterial diseases. *Clin. Microbiol. Rev.* **5:**1–25.
165. **Wayne, L. G., and H. A. Sramek.** 1994. Metronidazole is bactericidal to dormant cells of *Mycobacterium tuberculosis. Antimicrob. Agents Chemother.* **38:**2054–2058.
166. **Williams, D. L., L. Spring, L. Collins, L. P. Miller, L. B. Heifets, P. R. Gangadharam, and T. P. Gillis.** 1998. Contribution of *rpoB* mutations to development of rifamycin cross-resistance in *Mycobacterium tuberculosis. Antimicrob. Agents Chemother.* **42:**1853–1857.
167. **Williams, D. L., L. Spring, T. P. Gillis, M. Salfinger, and D. H. Persing.** 1998. Evaluation of a polymerase chain reaction-based universal heteroduplex generator assay for direct detection of rifampin susceptibility of *Mycobacterium tuberculosis* from sputum specimens. *Clin. Infect. Dis.* **26:**446–450.
168. **Wilson, T. M., and D. M. Collins.** 1996. *ahpC,* a gene involved in isoniazid resistance of the *Mycobacterium tuberculosis* complex. *Mol. Microbiol.* **19:**1025–1034.
169. **Winder, F. G.** 1982. Mode of action of the antimycobacterial agents and associated aspects of the molecular biology of the mycobacteria, p. 353–438. *In* C. Ratledge and J. Stanford (ed.), *The Biology of the Mycobacteria,* vol. 1. *Physiology, Identification and Classification.* Academic Press, Inc., New York, N.Y.
170. **Winder, F. G., and P. B. Collins.** 1969. The effect of isoniazid on nicotinamide nucleotide concentrations in tubercle bacilli. *Am. Rev. Respir. Dis.* **100:**101–103.
171. **Winder, F. G., and P. B. Collins.** 1968. The effect of isoniazid on nicotinamide nucleotide levels in *Mycobacterium bovis* strain BCG. *Am. Rev. Respir. Dis.* **97:**719–720.
172. **Woodley, C. L.** 1986. Evaluation of streptomycin and ethambutol concentrations for susceptibility testing of *Mycobacterium tuberculosis* by radiometric and conventional procedures. *J. Clin. Microbiol.* **23:**385–386.
173. **Woods, G. L., J. S. Bergmann, F. G. Witebsky, G. A. Fahle, B. Boulet, M. Plaunt, B. A. Brown, R. J. Wallace, Jr., and A. Wanger.** 2000. Multisite reproducibility of Etest for susceptibility testing of *Mycobacterium abscessus, Mycobacterium chelonae,* and *Mycobacterium fortuitum. J. Clin. Microbiol.* **38:**656–661.
174. **Woods, G. L., J. S. Bergmann, F. G. Witebsky, G. A. Fahle, A. Wanger, B. Boulet, M. Plaunt, B. A. Brown, and R. J. Wallace, Jr.** 1999. Multisite reproducibility of results obtained by the broth microdilution method for susceptibility testing of *Mycobacterium abscessus, Mycobacterium chelonae,* and *Mycobacterium fortuitum. J. Clin. Microbiol.* **37:**1676–1682.
175. **Woods, G. L., N. Williams-Bouver, R. J. Wallace, Jr., B. A. Brown-Elliot, F. G. Witebsky, P. S. Conville, M. Plaunt, G. Hall, P. Aralar, and C. Inderlied.** 2003. Multisite reproducibility of results obtained by two broth dilution methods for susceptibility testing of *Mycobacterium avium* complex. *J. Clin. Microbiol.* **41:**627–631.
176. **Woods, G. L., G. Fish, M. Plaunt, and T. Murphy.** 1997. Clinical evaluation of difco ESP culture system II for growth and detection of mycobacteria. *J. Clin. Microbiol.* **35:**121–124.
177. **Woods, G. L., and J. A. Washington III.** 1987. Mycobacteria other than *Mycobacterium tuberculosis:* review of microbiologic and clinical aspects. *Rev. Infect. Dis.* **9:**275–294.
178. **Yang, B., H. Koga, H. Ohno, K. Ogawa, M. Fukuda, Y. Hirakata, S. Maesaki, K. Tomono, T. Tashiro, and S. Kohno.** 1998. Relationship between antimycobacterial activities of rifampicin, rifabutin and KRM-1648 and *rpoB* mutations of *Mycobacterium tuberculosis. J. Antimicrob. Chemother.* **42:**621–628. (Erratum, **43:**613, 1999.)
179. **Young, L. S., O. G. Berlin, and C. B. Inderlied.** 1987. Activity of ciprofloxacin and other fluorinated quinolones against mycobacteria. *Am. J. Med.* **82:**23–26.
180. **Young, L. S., L. Wiviott, M. Wu, P. Kolonoski, R. Bolan, and C. B. Inderlied.** 1991. Azithromycin for treatment of *Mycobacterium avium-intracellulare* complex infection in patients with AIDS. *Lancet* **338:**1107–1109.
181. **Zhang, Y., S. Dhandayuthapani, and V. Deretic.** 1996. Molecular basis for the exquisite sensitivity of *Mycobacterium tuberculosis* to isoniazid. *Proc. Natl. Acad. Sci. USA* **93:** 13212–13216.
182. **Zhang, Y., B. Heym, B. Allen, D. Young, and S. Cole.** 1992. The catalase-peroxidase gene and isoniazid resistance of *Mycobacterium tuberculosis. Nature* **358:**591–593.
183. **Zhang, Y., and D. Mitchison.** 2003. The curious characteristics of pyrazinamide: a review. *Int. J. Tuberc. Lung Dis.* **7:**6–21.
184. **Zhang, Y., A. Scorpio, H. Nikaido, and Z. Sun.** 1999. Role of acid pH and deficient efflux of pyrazinoic acid in unique susceptibility of *Mycobacterium tuberculosis* to pyrazinamide. *J. Bacteriol.* **181:**2044–2049.

Detection and Characterization of Antimicrobial Resistance Genes in Pathogenic Bacteria

J. KAMILE RASHEED, FRANKLIN COCKERILL, AND FRED C. TENOVER

78

For the last several years, innovative new technologies for clinical microbiology laboratories have focused on decreasing the time required to detect pathogenic microorganisms directly in clinical samples. However, the dramatic increase in multidrug resistance among a plethora of bacterial genera has necessitated the development of tests specifically designed to detect resistant strains, particularly to guide infection control efforts in health care facilities. Rapid tests that identify patients colonized or infected with organisms, such as methicillin-resistant *Staphylococcus aureus* (MRSA) and vancomycin-resistant enterococci, can save infection control programs thousands of dollars each year by permitting isolation rooms to be utilized more effectively than would otherwise be the case (208, 247). Yet, multidrug resistance is not an issue just among health care-associated pathogens. Multidrug-resistant *Salmonella* species (258) and pneumococci (123) are among the community-associated pathogens that pose therapeutic challenges.

A wide variety of DNA probes and PCR assays focused on the detection of acquired resistance genes have been described over the last two decades (42, 229). Within the last few years, reports of several novel methods of detecting resistance genotypes have appeared in the literature. These include real-time PCR assays with molecular beacons, peptide-nucleic acid fluorescent in situ hybridization probes, microarrays, and pyrosequencing methods. In addition, sets of PCR primers designated analyte-specific reagents (ASRs) are available commercially. This chapter will focus specifically on genotypic methods for detecting and characterizing antimicrobial-resistant bacterial pathogens. Molecular methods for characterizing viruses and fungi are covered elsewhere in this Manual.

RATIONALE FOR USING GENETIC TESTS TO DETECT RESISTANCE GENES

There are four major reasons to use genetic tests to identify antimicrobial resistance genes or mutations associated with resistance. First, genetic methods can be used to detect resistance genes, or mutations that are associated with resistance, in organisms directly in clinical specimens. These results may be used to guide therapy or to decide whether to place a patient in a hospital isolation room.

Second, genetic methods can arbitrate MIC results that are at or near the breakpoint for resistance for bacterial species. For example, isolates of *S. aureus* for which the oxacillin MICs are between 2 and 8 μg/ml (borderline resistant) may contain the *mecA* (methicillin) resistance gene determinant or may represent a falsely resistant result from an automated susceptibility testing method (76, 222). A test indicating the absence of *mecA* in an isolate of *S. aureus* suggests that a physician could use an antimicrobial agent other than vancomycin to treat the infection.

Third, genetic tests are more accurate than analysis of resistance phenotypes for monitoring the epidemiologic spread of a particular resistance gene in a hospital or community setting. For example, tracking the spread of the *vanA* vancomycin resistance gene in enterococci or *S. aureus* with PCR assays has been helpful in documenting the spread of multiresistant enterococci in Europe (1, 83) and vancomycin-resistant *S. aureus* (VRSA) in the United States (33).

Fourth, genetic tests can be used as the "gold standard" for resistance tests in evaluating the accuracy of new susceptibility testing methods (54, 221).

However, there are several potential pitfalls associated with using genetic tests to detect resistant organisms. These include the lack of expression of resistance genes that are detected (28), the problem of mixed or normal flora that may contain resistance genes (such as *vanB* in *Clostridium* species in fecal samples) (14, 15), mutations in target organisms that alter sequences used for PCR primers and lead to false-negative results, and the emergence of novel resistance genes that are not detected by existing genetic assays. Each of these factors can affect the sensitivity or specificity of molecular assays (42).

GENETIC TESTS FOR RESISTANCE GENES AND DNA SEQUENCING STRATEGIES TO DETECT MUTATIONS ASSOCIATED WITH RESISTANCE

General Guidelines

The ideal genetic test targets nucleic acid sequences within the open reading frame (or coding region) of the resistance gene and avoids sequences outside of the gene that may contain insertion elements or promoter sequences that may be present in susceptible strains or strains with other types of resistance genes. Among the primers that have been described for studying antibacterial resistance are those directed to β-lactamase genes and the genes that encode resistance to aminocyclitols, aminoglycosides, chloramphenicol, glycopeptides, isoniazid, macrolides, mupirocin, oxazolidinones, quinolones, rifampin, sulfonamides, tetracyclines, and trimethoprim. Examples of PCR primers that target resistance genes or mutations associated with resistance are shown in Table 1. In addition, multiplex PCR assays for the detection of aminoglycoside resistance genes in enterococci, plasmid-carried *ampC* genes in *Enterobacteriaceae,* and glycopeptide resistance genes in enterococci and staphylococci are shown in Table 2. The tables are not meant to be exhaustive but rather give an indication of the types of assays that have been described previously. Appropriate specificity controls (organisms that have a similar resistance pattern but contain resistance genes other than the target gene) should always be included in all reactions using these primers. Examples of DNA probes that can be used to detect resistance genes have been described in previous editions of this Manual (229).

DNA Sequencing

DNA sequence analysis has been particularly helpful for identifying point mutations associated with resistance to fluoroquinolones (54, 86, 104), extended-spectrum β-lactamases (19, 183, 184), oxazolidinones (257), and antimycobacterial drugs (139, 224). There are a number of mutations associated with resistance to isoniazid, rifampin, and streptomycin (10, 69, 266). Unfortunately, additional genetic loci associated with resistance must also be involved since only 60 to 90% of resistance can be explained by these loci, although pyrosequencing assays have improved detection (10, 266). Other novel pyrosequencing assays that target mutations associated with resistance, such as changes in rRNA sequences associated with linezolid resistance, can provide high-throughput results in a few hours (205).

In-House Assays and ASRs

Utilization of home-brew PCR assays for detecting resistance genes or implementing assays reported in the literature in a clinical microbiology laboratory has always been a problem. In-house validation of research protocols can be time-consuming. Yet, many of these assays provide significant advances in turnaround time or cost-effectiveness over those of traditional test methods. A recent advancement is the availability of ASRs. In the United States, reagents for nucleic acid amplification-based technologies may be available from manufacturers in the form of ASRs. ASRs are produced under "good manufacturing practices"; however, unlike Food and Drug Administration (FDA)-cleared diagnostic kits, the clinical utility of the ASRs does not have to be validated in prospective multisite trials before marketing. The process of making materials available through ASRs has its advantages and drawbacks. Because time-consuming clinical trials are obviated, the ASRs can be available to clinical laboratories much sooner than diagnostic kits. From the manufacturers' perspective, the process allows a product to be evaluated by a number of users to ensure optimal performance. Therefore, if optimization of an ASR is indicated, this can be accomplished before time-consuming and costly clinical trials are undertaken for an FDA-approved kit version. A major drawback of ASRs, in contrast to FDA-approved kits, is that FDA guidelines prohibit the provision of testing protocols for the ASRs by the manufacturer. Manufacturers can only refer customers to protocols published in the medical literature or to scientists or practitioners who have established working protocols in their laboratories. Another drawback of ASRs relates to the extent of verification required by certifying agencies before tests can be implemented in clinical practice. For example, the Clinical Laboratory Improvement Amendments of 1988 require a more extensive verification process for ASRs than for FDA-approved kits (44). The FDA requires laboratories to add a disclaimer on reports for tests that use ASRs. The mandatory language for this disclaimer is, "This test was developed and its performance characteristics determined by the (laboratory name). It has not been cleared or approved by the U. S. FDA" (45).

SPECIFIC APPLICATIONS

The following sections review applications of molecular diagnostic methods for specific classes of resistance determinants.

AMINOGLYCOSIDE RESISTANCE GENES

The diversity of known aminoglycoside resistance genes, which are common in both gram-positive and gram-negative organisms (173, 201, 260), continues to expand with the recognition of additional acetyltransferases, adenylyltransferases, and phosphotransferases. Unfortunately, the lack of consensus sequences among the acetyltransferase and adenylyltransferase genes prohibits detection of multiple determinants with a single PCR primer set (201), making it difficult to use amplification-based tests to predict aminoglycoside resistance, especially in gram-negative organisms. However, multiplex assays for high-level gentamicin resistance in enterococci (Table 2) are available to predict the effectiveness of combination therapy (synergy) with aminoglycosides and cell wall-active agents (116, 239). Among the newer aminoglycoside resistance genes reported to be found in gram-negative organisms is the *armA* resistance determinant (75, 82, 261).

DETECTING GENES ASSOCIATED WITH RESISTANCE TO β-LACTAM DRUGS

Oxacillin Resistance in Staphylococci

Detection of oxacillin resistance in staphylococci, which is mediated primarily by the *mecA* determinant (32), by phenotypic methods continues to be a problem (222), particularly with coagulase-negative staphylococci (228). A *mecA* PCR assay can differentiate those isolates that are borderline resistant to oxacillin due to the modification of penicillin binding proteins (PBPs; the so-called MOD strains) or the production of large quantities of β-lactamase from isolates that are resistant due to the presence of the *mecA* determinant (132). The rare strains of *S. aureus* that are resistant to oxacillin by virtue of containing modified PBPs with reduced affinity for oxacillin may be misclassified as oxacillin susceptible by the *mecA* gene test since these strains are truly oxacillin resistant but do not contain the *mecA* gene (231, 247). A latex agglutination assay to identify the *mecA* gene product, i.e., PBP 2a, can be used for isolated colonies of *S. aureus* (28, 99, 241). These tests provide an alternative to phenotypic tests for the clinical microbiology laboratory, presuming that the caveats of their use are understood.

An increasing body of evidence demonstrates that identification and isolation of hospitalized patients who are nasal carriers of MRSA can reduce the incidence of health care-associated infections caused by these organisms and can reduce costs (161). Therefore, emphasis has been placed on the importance of active microbiology surveillance programs for the detection of nasal carriers of MRSA in the health care

TABLE 1 PCR assays for antimicrobial resistance genes

Antimicrobial agent and gene	Primers (5′ → 3′)	Product size	Use	Reference(s)
Aminoglycosides				
Aminoglycoside-modifying enzymes				
aac(6′)-Ia	ATG AAT TAT CAA ATT GTG TTA CTC TTT GAT TAA ACT	558 bp	Detection, probe	168[a]
aac(6′)-Ic	CTA CGA TTA CGT CAA CGG CTG C TTG CTT CGC CCA CTC CTG CAC C	130 bp	Detection	91[b]
aac(3)-Ia	ACC TAC TCC CAA CAT CAG CC ATA TAG ATC TCA CTA CGC GC	169 bp	Detection	240[c]
aac(3)-Ic	GAT GAT CTC TAC TCA AAC C TTA GGC AGC AGG TTG AGG	472 bp	Cloning, sequencing	188
aac(3)-IV	GTT ACA CCG GAC CTT GGA AAC GGC ATT GAG CGT CAG	675 bp	Detection	88
aphA-3	GGG ACC ACC TAT GAT GTG GAA CG CAG GCT TGA TCC CCA GTA AGT C	595 bp	Detection	80
aph(3′)-VIa	ATA CAG AGA CCA CAT ACA GT GGA CAA TCA ATA ATA GCA AT	235 bp	Detection	245
aad(2″)-Ia	ATG TTA CGC AGC AGG GCA GTC G CGT CAG ATC AAT ATC ATC GTG C	188 bp	Detection	242
aac(6′)-Ie-aph(2″)-Ia	GAG CAA TAA GGG CAT ACC AAA AAT C CCG TGC ATT TGT CTT AAA AAA CTG G	485 bp	Detection	108
aac(6′)-Iih	GGA TAG CGG ATG ATT ATC A TAA GAG TTT AAT GAA TAA TTA	856 bp	Sequencing	55
aph(2″)-Ib	TAT GGA TCC ATG GTT AAC TTG GAC GCT GAG ATT AAG CTT CCT GCT AAA ATA TAA ACA TCT CTG CT	920 bp	Detection	108
aph(3′)-IIIa	GGC TAA AAT GAG AAT ATC ACC GG CTT TAA AAA ATC ATA CAG CTC GCG	523 bp	Detection	217, 239
ant(4′)-Ia	CAA ACT GCT AAA TCG GTA GAA GCC GGA AAG TTG ACC AGA CAT TAC GAA CT	294 bp	Detection	217, 239
aadA	TGA TTT GCT GGT TAC GGT GAC CGC TAT GTT CTC TTG CTT TTG	284 bp	Detection, probe	38
aadE	ACT GGC TTA ATC AAT TTG GG GCC TTT CCG CCA CCT CAC CG	597 bp	Detection, probe	38
aad-6	AGA AGA TGT AAT AAT ATA G CTG TAA TCA CTG TTC CCG CCT	978 bp	Detection	118
strA-strB	TAT CTG CGA TTG GAC CCT CTG CAT TGC TCA TCA TTT GAT CGG CT	519 bp	Detection	216
16S rRNA methylases				
armA	AGG TTG TTT CCA TTT CTG AG TCT CTT CCA TTC CCT TCT CC	590 bp	Detection, sequencing	260
rmtA	CTA GCG TCC ATC CTT TCC TC TTT GCT TCC ATG CCC TTG CC	635 bp	Detection	264
rmtB	ATG AAC ATC AAC GAT GCC CT CCT TCT GAT TGG CTT ATC CA	769 bp	Detection, sequencing, probe	261
Spectinomycin				
rrs (Neisseria meningitidis, N. gonorrhoeae)	CTT ACC TGG TCT TGA CA CGA TTA CTA GCG ATT CC	373 bp	Sequencing	74
β-lactams				
mecA	TGG CTA TCG TGT CAC AAT CG CTG GAA CTT GTT GAG CAG AG	310 bp	Detection	243
bla_{SHV}	GCC GGG TTA TTC TTA TTT GTC GC TCT TTC CGA TGC CGC CGC CAG TCA	1,017 bp	Sequencing	148

(Continued on next page)

TABLE 1 *(Continued)*

Antimicrobial agent and gene	Primers (5′ → 3′)	Product size	Use	Reference(s)
bla_{SHV}	GGT TAT GCG TTA TAT TCG CC ATC TTT CGC TCC AGC TGT TC	275 bp	Probe[d]	184[e]
bla_{SHV}	GGT TAT GCG TTA TAT TCG CC TTA GCG TTG CCA GTG CTC	867 bp	Detection	184
bla_{TEM}	ATG AGT ATT CAA CAT TTC CG TTA CTG TCA TGC CAT CC	351 bp	Detection, probe	183
bla_{TEM}	ATG AGT ATT CAA CAT TTC CG CTG ACA GTT ACC AAT GCT TA	867 bp	Detection	184
bla_{CTX-M}	CGC TTT GCG ATG TGC AG ACC GCG ATA TCG TTG GT	550 bp	Detection, probe	19
$bla_{CTX-M-2}$	ATG ATG ACT CAG AGC ATT CG TTA TTG CAT CAG AAA CCG TG	884 bp	Detection	167
$bla_{CTX-M-9}$	GTG ACA AAG AGA GTG CAA CGG ATG ATT CTC GCC GCT GAA GCC	857 bp	Detection	194
$bla_{CTX-M-10}$	GCT GAT GAG CGC TTT GCG TTA CAA ACC GTT GGT GAC G	684 bp	Detection	150
bla_{GES-1}	ATG CGC TTC ATT CAC GCA C CTA TTT GTC CGT GCT CAG G	864 bp	Probe[d]	170
$bla_{GES/IBC}$	GTT TTG CAA TGT GCT CAA CG TGC CAT AGC AAT AGG CGT AG	371 bp	Detection, sequencing	249
bla_{PER-1}	ATG AAT GTC ATT ATA AAA GC AAT TTG GGC TTA GGG CAA GAA A	926 bp	Detection, probe	238
bla_{PER-2}	CGC TTC TGC TCT GCT GAT GGC AGC TTC TTT AAC GCC	469 bp	Detection	16
bla_{PSE}	ACC GTA TTG AGC CTG ATT TA ATT GAA GCC TGT GTT TGA GC	321 bp	Detection	17[f]
bla_{ROB-1}	TGT TTG CAA TCG CTG CC TTA TCG TAC ACT TTC CA	400 bp	Detection	107
bla_{TLA-1}	TCT CAG CGC AAA TCC GCG CTA TTT CCC ATC CTT AAC TAG	974 bp	Detection	4
bla_{VEB-1}	CGA CTT CCA TTT CCC GAT GC GGA CTC TGC AAC AAA TAC GC	643 bp	Detection	141
bla_{KPC}	TGT CAC TGT ATC GCC GTC TAT TTT TCC GAG ATG GGT GAC	331 bp	Detection	262
bla_{KPC-2}	GCT ACA CCT AGC TCC ACC TTC ACA GTG GTT GGT AAT CCA TGC	989 bp	Sequencing	137
bla_{IMI-1}	ATA GCC ATC TTG TTT AGC TC TCT GCG ATT ACT TTA TCC TC	818 bp	Probe[d]	12
bla_{NmcA}	TGC AGC TTA ATT ATT TTC AGA TTA G ATT TTT TTC ATG ATG AAG TTA AGC C	2,122 bp	Sequencing	175[g]
bla_{SME-1}	AAC GGC TTC ATT TTT GTT TAG GCT TCC GCA ATA GTT TTA TCA	830 bp	Detection	180
bla_{IMP}	CTA CCG CAG CAG AGT CTT TG AAC CAG TTT TGC CTT ACC AT	587 bp	Detection	200
bla_{VIM}	TCT ACA TGA CCG CGT CTG TC TGT GCT TTG ACA ACG TTC GC	748 bp	Detection	171
bla_{VIM}	AGT GGT GAG TAT CCG ACA G ATG AAA GTG CGT GGA GAC	261 bp	Detection, probe	77
bla_{SPM-1}	CCT ACA ATC TAA CGG CGA CC TCG CCG TGT CCA GGT ATA AC	649 bp	Detection	195
ampC (promoter, *Escherichia coli*)	GAT CGT TCT GCC GCT GTG GGG CAG CAA ATG TGG AGC AA	271 bp	Sequencing	30
bla_{ACC}	AAC AGC CTC AGC AGC CGG TTA TTC GCC GCA ATC ATC CCT AGC	346 bp	Detection	163[h]
bla_{ACT-1}	ATT CGT ATG CTG GAT CTC GCC ACC CAT GAC CCA GTT CGC CAT ATC CTG	396 bp	Detection	48
bla_{DHA}	CCG TCA CTC ACA CAC GGA AGG CGT ATC CGC AGG GGC CTG TTC	1,199 bp	Detection, sequencing	136[i]
bla_{FOX}	TGT GGA CGG CAT TAT CCA G AAA GCG CGT AAC CGG ATT G	868 bp	Detection, sequencing	138

(Continued on next page)

TABLE 1 PCR assays for antimicrobial resistance genes *(Continued)*

Antimicrobial agent and gene	Primers (5′ → 3′)	Product size	Use	Reference(s)
bla$_{OXA-1}$	CCA AAG ACG TGG ATG GTT AAA TTC GAC CCC AAG TT	540 bp	Detection	207
bla$_{OXA-2}$	TTC AAG CCA AAG GCA CGA TAG TCC GAG TTG ACT GCC GGG TTG	703 bp	Detection	214
bla$_{OXA-10}$	CGT GCT TTG TAA AAG TAG CAG CAT GAT TTT GGT GGG AAT GG	652 bp	Detection	214
bla$_{OXA-1}$ group	TTT TCT GTT GTT TGG GTT TC TTT CTT GGC TTT TAT GCT TG	447 bp	Detection	17
bla$_{OXA-2}$ group	AAG AAA CGC TAC TCG CCT GC CCA CTC AAC CCA TCC TAC CC	486 bp	Detection	17
bla$_{OXA-10}$ group	TCA ACA AAT CGC CAG AGA AG TCC CAC ACC AGA AAA ACC AG	276 bp	Detection	17
bla$_{OXA-23}$	CCT CAG GTG TGC TGG TTA TTC CCC AAC CAG TCT TTC CAA AA	513 bp	Detection	29
bla$_{OXA-24}$	TTC CCC TAA CAT GAA TTT GT GTA CTA ATC AAA GTT GTG AA	1,020 bp	Detection, sequencing	20
Chloramphenicol/ florfenicol				
catA1	CCA CCG TTG ATA TAT CCC CCT GCC ACT CAT CGC AGT	623 bp	Detection	87
cmlA	TGT CAT TTA CGG CAT ACT CG ATC AGG CAT CCC ATT CCC AT	456 bp	Detection	88
flo	CAC GTT GAG CCT CTA TAT GG ATG CAG AAG TAG AAC GCG AC	869 bp	Detection	144
Glycopeptides				
vanA	GCT ATT CAG CTG TAC TC CAG CGG CCA TCA TAC GG	783 bp	Detection	196[j]
vanA	GGG AAA ACG ACA ATT GC GTA CAA TGC GGC CGT TA	732 bp	Detection	65
vanB	CGC CAT ATT CTC CCC GGA TAG AAG CCC TCT GCA TCC AAG CAC	667 bp	Detection	120
vanC1	GAA AGA CAA CAG GAA GAC CGC ATC GCA TCA CAA GCA CCA ATC	796 bp	Detection	37
vanC2/3	CGG GGA AGA TGG CAG TAT CGC AGG GAC GGT GAT TTT	484 bp	Detection	110
vanC3	GCC TTT ACT TAT TGT TCC GCT TGT TCT TTG ACC TTA	224 bp	Detection	39
vanD	TAA GGC GCT TGC ATA TAC CG TGC AGC CAA GTA TCC GGT AA	461 bp	Detection	165
vanE	TGT GGT ATC GGA GCT GCA G GTC GAT TCT CGC TAA TCC	513 bp	Detection, probe	68
vanG	CGG TTG TGC CGT ACT TGG C GGG TAA AGC CAT AGT CTG GGG C	811 bp	Detection	134
Macrolides, lincosamides, and streptogramins				
ermA	CTT CGA TAG TTT ATT AAT ATT AGT TCT AAA AAG CAT GTA AAA GAA	645 bp	Detection	219
ermA (ermTR)	AGA AGG TTA TAA TGA AAC AGA A GGC ATG ACA TAA ACC TTC AT	212 bp	Detection	186
ermB	GAA AAG GTA CTC AAC CAA ATA AGT AAC GGT ACT TAA ATT GTT TAC	639 bp	Detection	219
ermC	TCA AAA CAT AAT ATA GAT AAA GCT AAT ATT GTT TAA ATC GTC AAT	642 bp	Detection	219
ermF	GCA GAC AGG CGC AAG CAG CAA ACC ACG TTC CCA TGA GTG GTA TGG	606 bp	Detection	191

(Continued on next page)

TABLE 1 *(Continued)*

Antimicrobial agent and gene	Primers (5′ → 3′)	Product size	Use	Reference(s)
ermG	AGG GAA AGG TCA TTT TAC TGC CCC TAC CTA TAA CTA AAC ATT	664 bp	Detection	186
mefA/mefE	AGT ATC ATT AAT CAC TAG TGC TTC TTC TGG TAC TAA AAG TGG	348 bp	Detection	219
mefA	GAC CAA AAG CCA CAT TGT GGA CCT CCT GTC TAT AAT CGC ATG	1,431 bp	Restriction enzyme analysis	154
mefE	CTA TGC GAT TTT GGG ACC TG GAA AGC CCC ATT ATT GCA CA	801 bp	Detection	128
ereA	AGT CGG CGG TTA TTT CAT TGC TCC CTC ATT TTC ATT TA	746 bp	Detection	204
ereB	CGG ATA AAG AAG CAC TAC AC AAC GAC CTC AGA TAC AGA TG	788 bp	Detection	204
mphA	AAC TGT ACG CAC TTG C GGT ACT CTT CGT TAC C	837 bp	Detection	219
msrA/msrB	GTC AAA AAC TGC TAA CAC AAG AAT AAT ACT GCT AAC GAT AAT	343 bp	Detection	204
smp	AAA TTG TTT AAA AAG AAA TC TTT GAA CCA TAA TAT TCA TC	616 bp	Detection, probe	220
vat	CAA TGA CCA TGG ACC TGA TC AGC ATT TCG ATA TCT CC	615 bp	Detection	6
vatB	CCT GAT CCA AAT AGC ATA TAT CC CTA AAT CAG AGC TAC AAA GTG	601 bp	Detection	5
satG (vatE)	CTA TAC CTG ACG CAA ATG C GGT TCA AAT CTT GGT CCG	511 bp	Detection	250
vga	TCT AAT GGT ACA GGA AAG ACA ACG ATC GTG AGA TAC AAA GAT TAT	399 bp	Detection	219
linA/linA′	GTA GAT GTA TTA ACT GGA A GAA AAA GAA GTT GAG CTT C	325 bp	Detection, probe	147
linB	CCT ACC TAT TGT TTG TGG AA ATA ACG TTA CTC TCC TAT TC	944 bp	Detection	22
Mupirocin				
Isoleucyl-tRNA synthetase (IRS) gene	CCA TGC CTT ACC AGT TGA ATT GGA TCC CCG AGC ACT ATC CGA	1.65 kb	Probe[d]	81
mupA	CCC ATG GCT TAC CAG TTG A CCA TGG AGC ACT ATC CGA A	1.65 kb	Detection, probe	182
mupA	TGA CAA TAG AAA AGG ACA GG CTC TAA TTC AAC TGG TAA GCC	190 bp	Detection	157
ileS-2	GTT TAT CTT CTG ATG CTG AG CCC CAG TTA CAC CGA TAT AA	237 bp	Detection	149
Quinolones				
gyrA (Mycobacterium tuberculosis)	CAG CTA CAT CGA CTA TGC GA GGG CTT CGG TGT ACC TCA T	320 bp	Sequencing	109
gyrA (Acinetobacter baumannii)	AAA TCT GCC CGT GTC GTT GGT GCC ATA CCT ACG GCG ATA CC	343 bp	Sequencing	244
gyrA (E. coli)	ACG TAC TAG GCA ATG ACT GG AGA AGT CGC CGT CGA TAG AAC	190 bp	Sequencing	66[k]
gyrA (S. pneumoniae)	TTC TCT ACG GAA TGA ATG GAT ATC ACG AAG CAT TTC CAG	272 bp	Sequencing	104
gyrB (S. pneumoniae)	TTC TCC GAT TTC CTC ATG AGA AGG GTA CGA ATG TGG	458 bp	Sequencing	158
parC (S. pneumoniae)	TGG GTT GAA GCC GGT TCA CAA GAC CGT TGG TTC TTT C	361 bp	Sequencing	104
parE (S. pneumoniae)	CCA ATC TAA GAA TCC TG GCA ATA TAG ACA TGA CC	357 bp	Sequencing	166
qnrA	TCA GCA AGA GGA TTT CTC A GGC AGC ACT ATT ACT CCC A	627 bp	Detection	193

(Continued on next page)

TABLE 1 PCR assays for antimicrobial resistance genes *(Continued)*

Antimicrobial agent and gene	Primers (5′ → 3′)	Product size	Use	Reference(s)
qnr	CCG TAT GGA TAT TAT TGA TAA AG CTA ATC CGG CAG CAC TAT TA	661 bp	Detection	126
Sulfonamides				
sulA	AGC CAA TCA TGC AAA GAC AG ATT TTC CGC TTC ATC AGC CAG	916 bp	Sequencing	131
sulI	CTT CGA TGA GAG CCG GCG GC GCA AGG CGG AAA CCC GCG CC	437 bp	Detection	88
Dihyropteroate synthase (DHPS) gene *(Pneumocystis carinii)*	TTA CTC CTG ATT CTT TTT TCG ATG GG GCC TTA ATT GCT TGT TCT GCA ACC	259 bp	SSCP[l] assay	125
Tetracycline				
tet(A)	GTA ATT CTG AGC ACT GT CCT GGA CAA CAT TGC TT	954 bp	Probe[d]	92[m]
tet(B)	CAG TGC TGT TGT TGT CAT TAA GCT TGG AAT ACT GAG TGT AA	528 bp	Detection, sequencing	191
tet(E)	GTG ATG ATG GCA CTG GT TGC TGT ACA TCG CTC TT	1,196 bp	Probe[d]	73[n]
tet(G)	GCT CGG TGG TAT CTC TGC TC AGC AAC AGA ATC GGG AAC AC	468 bp	Detection	144
tet(K)	GTA GGA TCT GCT GCA TTC CC CAC TAT TAC CTA TTG TCG C	552 bp	Detection	118
tet(L)	GGA TCG ATA GTA GCC ATG GG GTA TCC CAC CAA TGT AGC CG	516 bp	Detection	118
tet(M)	GAA CTC GAA CAA GAG GAA AGC ATG GAA GCC CAG AAA GGA T	741 bp	Detection	152
tet(O)	AAC TTA GGC ATT CTG GCT CAC TCC CAC TGT TCC ATA TCG TCA	519 bp	Detection	152
tetA(P)	CAC AGA TTG TAT GGG GAT TAG G CAT TTA TAG AAA GCA CAG TAG C	764 bp	Detection, sequencing	124
tet(Q)	ATT GCG GAA GTG GAG CGG AC GCC GGA CGG AGG ATT TGA GA	814 bp	Detection	151
tet(S)	CGC TAC ATT TGC GAG ACT CAG GGC TCT CAT ACT GAA TGC CAC	569 bp	Detection	118
tet(T)	CAG TGG GAA TAT AAG GAC ACG TC CAA GCC TTC TCT ACA GCA TC	644 bp	Detection	118
tet(V)	GAC AAC GGC ATG AAC GTT CGC GAG CAT GTT C	405 bp	Detection	60
tet(W)	GAG AGC CTG CTA TAT GCC AGC GGG CGT ATC CAC AAT GTT AAC	168 bp	Detection	8
tet(39)	CTC CTT CTC TAT TGT GGC TA CAC TAA TAC CTC TGG ACA TCA	711 bp	Detection	2
Trimethoprim				
dhfrVIII	CTA ACG GCG CTA TCT TCG TGA ACA ACG TAT GAA TTC TTC CAT GCC ATT CTG CTC GTA G	300 bp	Detection	218
dfr1	ACG GAT CCT GGC TGT TGG TTG GAC GC CGG AAT TCA CCT TCC GGC TCG ATG TC	254 bp	Detection	79
dfr9	ATG AAT TCC CGT GGC ATG AAC CAG AAG AT ATG GAT CCT TCA GTA ATG GTC GGG ACC TC	399 bp	Detection	79
dfrA	CCC TGC TAT TAA AGC ACC CAT GAC CAG ATA ACT C	262 bp	Detection, sequencing	52
dfrA1	GTG AAA CTA TCA CTA ATG G TTA ACC CTT TTG CCA GAT TT	474 bp	Detection, RFLP[o] analysis	143[p]
dfrA14	GAG CAG CTI[q] CTI TTI AAA GC TTA GCC CTT TII CCA ATT TT	393 bp	Detection	143[r]
dfrA7	TTG AAA ATT TCA TTG ATT T TTA GCC TTT TTT CCA AAT CT	474 bp	Detection	143[s]

(Continued on next page)

TABLE 1 *(Continued)*

Antimicrobial agent and gene	Primers (5′ → 3′)	Product size	Use	Reference(s)
dfrB1	GAT CAC GTG CGC AAG AAA TC AAG CGC AGC CAC AGG ATA AAT	141 bp	Detection	143[t]
dfrA12	GGT GS[u]G CAG AAG ATT TTT CGC TGG GAA GAA GGC GTC ACC CTC	309 bp	Detection	143[v]
Ethambutol				
embB (*M. tuberculosis*)	ACG CTG AAA CTG CTG GCG AT ACA GAC TGG CGT CGC TGA CA	400 bp	SSCP[l] assay	3
Pyrazinamide				
pncA (*M. tuberculosis*)	GCT GGT CAT GTT CGC GAT CG CAG GAG CTG CAA ACC AAC TCG	673 bp	Sequencing	212
Rifampin				
rpoB (*M. tuberculosis*)	GGG AGC GGA TGA CCA CCC A GCG GTA CGG CGT TTC GAT GAA C	350 bp	Sequencing	109
rpoB (Mycobacteria)	CCA CCC AGG ACG TGG AGG CGA TCA CAC AGT GCG ACG GGT GCA CGT CGC GGA CCT	224 bp	Sequencing	43
Streptomycin				
rpsL (*M. tuberculosis*)	GGC CGA CAA ACA GAA CGT GTT CAC CAA CTG GGT GAC	501 bp	Sequencing	211
rrs (*M. tuberculosis*)	TTG GCC ATG CTC TTG ATG CCC TGC ACA CAG GCC ACA AGG GA	1,140 bp	Sequencing	135
rrs (Mycobacteria)	GAT GAC GGC CTT CGG GTT GT TCT AGT CTG CCC GTA TCG CC	238 bp	Sequencing (530 loop)	94
rrs (Mycobacteria)	GTA GTC CAC GCC GTA AAC GG AGG CCA CAA GGG AAC GCC TA	238 bp	Sequencing (912–915 domain)	94
Isoniazid				
katG	GAA ACA GCG GCG CTG GAT CGT GTT GTC CCA TTT CGT CGG GG	209 bp	SSCP[l] assay	226
katG	TTT CGG CGC ATG GCC ATG A ACA GCC ACC GAG CAC GAC	894 bp	Sequencing, RFLP[o] analysis	90
inhA	TCG ACG GCC GGC ATG G CCG GTC CGC CGA ACG	905 bp	Sequencing	109
ahpC	ATG CAT TGT CCG CTT TGA TG TTC TAT ACT CAT TGA TT	588 bp	Sequencing	112

[a] This reference also describes primer sets for the detection of *aac(6′)-Ib, aac(6′)-Id, aac(6′)-If, aac(6′)-Ig*, and *aac(6′)-Ih*.
[b] This reference also describes primer sets for the detection of *aac(6′)-Id, aac(6′)-Ie, aac(6′)-Ig, aac(6′)-Ih, aac(6′)-Ii, aac(6′)-Ij, aac(6′)-Il*, and *aac(6′)-IIb*.
[c] This reference also describes primer sets for the detection of *aac(3)-IIa, aac(3)-IIIa, aac(3)-IVa, aad(4′)-Ia, aac(6′)-aph(2″)*, and *aph(3′)-IIIa*.
[d] This primer set is used in this reference for the synthesis of an intragenic probe and not for direct detection.
[e] This reference also describes primer sets for the detection and sequencing of bla_{SHV} and the detection of bla_{TEM}.
[f] This primer set amplifies genes encoding PSE-1, PSE-4, and CARB-3.
[g] This primer set amplifies both the *nmcA* structural gene and its regulatory gene, *nmcR*.
[h] This primer set is one of six that comprise a multiplex PCR method for the detection of members of six families of plasmid-mediated *ampC* β-lactamase genes.
[i] This reference also describes primer sets for the detection and/or sequencing of bla_{FOX}, bla_{CMY}, and bla_{ACT-1}.
[j] This reference also describes primer sets for the detection of *vanB, vanC1*, and *vanC2*.
[k] This reference also describes primer sets for the DNA sequencing of *parC* and *parE* of *E. coli*.
[l] SSCP, single-strand conformational polymorphism.
[m] This reference also describes primer sets for the synthesis of probes for *tet*(C), *tet*(D), *tet*(E), *tet*(G), *tet*(H), and *tet*(M).
[n] This reference also describes primer sets for the synthesis of probes for *tet*(A), *tet*(B), *tet*(C), *tet*(D), and *tet*(G).
[o] RFLP, restriction fragment length polymorphism.
[p] This primer set also amplifies *dfrA5, dfrA15, dfrA15b, dfrA16*, and *dfrA16b*.
[q] I, inosine (International Union of Biochemistry [IUB] codes for DNA bases).
[r] This primer set also amplifies *dfrA1, dfrA5, dfrA6, dfrA15*, and *dfrA16*.
[s] This primer set also amplifies *dfrA17*.
[t] This primer set also amplifies *dfrB2 and dfrB3*.
[u] S, G, or C (International Union of Biochemistry [IUB] codes for DNA bases).
[v] This primer set also amplifies *dfrA13*.

TABLE 2 Multiplex PCR assays for detection of antimicrobial resistance genes

Antimicrobial agent organisms and genes	Product size (bp)	Reference
Aminoglycosides (enterococci)		
aac(6′)-Ie-aph(2″)-Ia	348	239
aph(2″)-Ib	867	
aph(2″)-Ic	444	
aph(2″)-Id	641	
aph(3′)-IIIa	523	
ant(4′)-Ia	294	
aac(6′)-Ii	410	116
aac(6′)-aph(2″)	675	
ant(4′)-Ia	266	
ant(6)-Ia	563	
ant(9)-Ia	476	
aph(2″)-Ic	837	
aph(3′)-IIIa	354	
β-Lactams (*Enterobacteriaceae*)		
$bla_{MOX-1-2}$, bla_{CMY-1}, $bla_{CMY-8-11}$	520	163[a]
$bla_{LAT-1-4}$, $bla_{CMY-2-7}$, bla_{BIL-1}	462	
$bla_{DHA-1-2}$	405	
bla_{ACC}	346	
bla_{MIR-1}, bla_{ACT-1}	302	
$bla_{FOX-1–5b}$	190	
Glycopeptides (enterococci and staphylococci)		
vanA	732	59
vanB	647	
vanC1/2	815/827	
vanD	500	
vanE	430	
vanG	941	
ddl (Enterococcus faecalis)	475	
ddl (E. faecium)	1,091	
nuc (S. aureus)	218	
Staphylococcus epidermidis gene fragment	125[b]	

[a] This reference describes primers for the detection of genes within six plasmid-mediated *ampC*-specific gene families in the *Enterobacteriaceae*.
[b] This PCR product is amplified with primers complementary to a chromosomal fragment specific for *S. epidermidis*.

setting. Conventional culture-based methods for detection of MRSA from nasal swabs frequently require ≥48 h before a final report can be issued. Various studies have evaluated molecular methods that detect nasal carriers of MRSA more rapidly than conventional culture-based methods (96, 161, 247). For example, Warren and colleagues demonstrated the utility of a commercially available real-time PCR method for identifying MRSA directly from nasal swabs (247). This testing method anchors one primer in *orfX*, which is unique to the *S. aureus* chromosome, and the second in the staphylococcal chromosomal cassette carrying the *mecA* gene (SCCmec), which is adjacent to *orfX* (96). These investigators showed that this assay is as sensitive as a direct plating culture method; final results were available within 2 h versus 48 to 72 h for results from culture.

β-Lactam Resistance in Pneumococci

Resistance to penicillin, extended-spectrum cephalosporins, and other antimicrobial agents in pneumococci has become a global problem (123, 133). Resistance to β-lactams develops when pneumococcal PBPs are remodeled through the acquisition of chromosomal DNA from other pneumococci or other streptococcal species (46, 63). Although remodeling is not a random process, it has been difficult to develop PCR primers that accurately differentiate strains with low-level penicillin resistance from those with high-level resistance. Using primers for the *pbp2b* gene, Ubukata et al. (236) attempted to resolve this issue. In their assay, the lack of product in the presence of amplification controls suggests that the *pbp2b* gene had been remodeled and therefore mediates resistance. However, such an assay does not reliably indicate which strains could be treated with penicillin versus an extended-spectrum cephalosporin, as might be desirable for an assay to be used in a clinical laboratory, but may be used as a screening tool for analyzing large groups of strains for resistance. A study by du Plessis et al. (64) also attempted to identify penicillin-resistant pneumococci directly in cerebrospinal fluid by using PCR primers directed to *pbp2b* sequences. This method was modestly successful in identifying isolates with altered PBPs associated with penicillin resistance.

β-Lactamase Genes in Gram-Negative Organisms

A variety of PCR primer sets have been developed to detect the genes encoding the TEM, SHV, OXA, CTX-M, GES, and AmpC (e.g., CMY-2, DHA-1, and MIR-1) β-lactamases and the metallo-β-lactamases (e.g., VIM-1 and SPM-1) present in gram-negative organisms (Tables 1 and 2).

Health care-associated infections caused by *Klebsiella pneumoniae, K. oxytoca* (7, 72, 198, 214), and other *Enterobacteriaceae* that produce extended-spectrum β-lactamases (49, 129) and other enzymes capable of hydrolyzing cefotaxime, ceftriaxone, ceftazidime, cefepime, and aztreonam are increasing in the United States and around the world (7, 18, 23, 78, 103, 122, 160, 253). More important are the emerging KPC-type carbapenemases that mediate resistance to imipenem, meropenem, and ertapenem (24, 27, 95, 140, 256, 262, 263). Resistance mediated by these determinants may be missed by automated methods (26). Other carbapenemases, including NmcA, Sme-1, IMI-1, and GES-2 and IMP-, VIM-, and some class D OXA-type enzymes (142, 145, 175, 185, 200, 203, 246), present in *Enterobacteriaceae, Acinetobacter* species, and *Pseudomonas* species continue to mediate resistance to imipenem and, in most cases, meropenem. Phenotypically, it can be difficult to differentiate resistance caused by a carbapenemase from resistance mediated by an AmpC-type enzyme in a strain with decreased permeability to carbapenems due to down-regulation of one or more porins (25, 102, 169). Thus, PCR assays directed to AmpC β-lactamases (163) and carbapenemase genes (Table 1) can be useful in differentiating the two mechanisms. This differentiation may be facilitated by the findings in a recent report describing a multiplex PCR method for the detection of plasmid-mediated AmpC β-lactamases (Table 2) (163) and specific inhibition of these enzymes by boronic acid compounds (47, 259).

CHLORAMPHENICOL RESISTANCE

Genes encoding chloramphenicol acetyltransferases are present in both gram-negative and gram-positive organisms and mediate resistance to chloramphenicol (199, 202). PCR primers capable of detecting the *cat* genes present in streptococci and enterococci have been described previously (232). Primers to detect the *catA*1 and *cmlA* genes, both of which mediate chloramphenicol resistance in *Salmonella* species (87, 88), have also been reported previously.

RESISTANCE TO VANCOMYCIN AND OTHER GLYCOPEPTIDES

Acquired vancomycin resistance was first noted in enterococci (117, 187, 237) but has subsequently been documented in a variety of other pathogens (14, 15, 159, 176, 177, 215), including *S. aureus* (31, 33, 248). Glycopeptide resistance is mediated by several different determinants, including *vanA, vanB, vanC, vanD, vanE,* and *vanG* (11, 50, 57, 68, 134, 155, 164, 196). The *vanA* determinant has spread via conjugation from enterococcal donors to five independent isolates of *S. aureus* in the United States (33, 230, 248; Centers for Disease Control and Prevention, unpublished data). Molecular analysis of the transposons involved has shown differences among the first four isolates examined (40; Centers for Disease Control and Prevention, unpublished data). The first VRSA isolate from Michigan and the fourth VRSA isolate (also from Michigan) demonstrate a classic Tn*1546* structure; the others contain insertion sequences but also show deletions at the 5′ end of the transposon (40). PCR assays can differentiate the three unique *vanB* genes, designated *vanB1, vanB2,* and *vanB3* (51, 120), and the three *vanC* genes, *vanC1, vanC2,* and *vanC3* (39). Subtypes of *vanD,* including *vanD1, vanD2, vanD3,* and *vanD4,* also exist, but differentiation via PCR is difficult (21, 53). PCR has been used to detect *vanA* and *vanB* in enterococci in fecal samples to aid infection control efforts (156, 197). Furthermore, a multiplex PCR method has been developed for the simultaneous detection of the *van* alphabet (*vanA, vanB, vanC, vanD, vanE,* and *vanG*) and identification of the most clinically relevant enterococci and staphylococci at the species level (Table 2) (59). Commercial ASRs have become available for the direct and rapid detection of *vanA* and *vanB* genes in perirectal swab samples by using real-time PCR. A recent report indicated enhanced sensitivity and a significant reduction in the time to results (3.5 versus ≥72 h) for one ASR assay compared with those for vancomycin-containing agar plates (208). False-positive results may potentially occur with any assay intended to detect *vanB* genes in enterococci due to the occasional presence of these genes in anaerobic bacteria (14, 15, 62). However, as *van* genes from these organisms could potentially be transferred to enterococci, it may still be important from the infection control perspective to identify them, although this issue remains controversial. Genotypic detection of vancomycin-intermediate *S. aureus* strains has yet to be accomplished via molecular methods.

MACROLIDE, LINCOSAMIDE, AND STREPTOGRAMIN RESISTANCE

Resistance to macrolides, lincosamides (such as clindamycin), and streptogramins can be mediated by a variety of *erm* genes including *ermA* and *ermA* (subclass *ermTR*), *ermB*, and *ermC*. On the other hand, *msrA,* which is primarily in staphylococci, mediates resistance only to macrolides and streptogramins and the macrolide efflux gene *mefA*, found in streptococci and pneumococci, confers resistance to 14- and 15-membered macrolides only (36, 70, 154, 174, 192, 254, 255). Roberts et al. (192) proposed that *mefA* and *mefE,* which show high levels of DNA homology, be considered a single class. However, others suggest that, in spite of the high degree of relatedness of the genes, a distinction between them should be maintained because of significant differences that exist between them (114). A real-time PCR assay which can distinguish *mefA* and *mefE* has been described previously (115). Pneumococci containing both *ermB* and *mefA* are being identified with increasing frequency (67). Many community-associated MRSA isolates are erythromycin resistant and clindamycin susceptible and contain *msrA* (111). PCR assays can differentiate *msrA* from *erm* genes (113, 213). Mutations in 23S rRNA and ribosomal protein L4 mutations in pneumococci have also been shown to mediate macrolide resistance and can be detected through traditional PCR or pyrosequencing assays (58, 89, 223).

Mechanisms active against both the streptogramin A and streptogramin B components of quinupristin-dalfopristin are necessary to result in a resistance phenotype. Several of the loci previously classified as *sat* genes have been reclassified as *vat* genes (93, 192, 250, 251). For example, *vatD* is the former *satA* and *vatE* is the former *satG*. Resistance to the streptogramin B component is mediated by the lactonases *vgb* and *vgbB* or the *ermB* methylase. In staphylococci, in particular, many of these genes are clustered together.

MUPIROCIN RESISTANCE

Mupirocin is an antistaphylococcal agent that is used to reduce nasal carriage of staphylococci among infected patients and hospital personnel. A PCR assay that can detect high-level mupirocin resistance has been described previously (81). However, the practical value of the assay has not been assessed in a clinical laboratory setting.

OXAZOLIDINONE RESISTANCE

Resistance to the oxazolidinone, or linezolid, among staphylococci and enterococci has been described previously (13, 234, 252, 255). Mutations in 23S rRNA, usually at position 2576, are responsible for the resistance phenotype (178). Detection of the G2576T mutations in enterococci can be accomplished by using a simple PCR assay followed by restriction fragment length polymorphism analysis of the products. Alternatively, the mutation can be detected by using pyrosequencing (205, 257).

QUINOLONE RESISTANCE

There are two major mechanisms of quinolone resistance: (i) alteration of the target sites, the organism's gyrase (*gyrA* and *gyrB*), and topoisomerase (*parC* and *parE*) (66, 100, 224, 225, 233) and (ii) active efflux of the drug out of the cell (56, 66, 100, 162), which limits access of the drug to the target site. Resistance is usually associated with point mutations in the *gyr* or *par* loci. Since DNA probes, in most cases, are not sufficiently sensitive to detect these changes, investigators have used PCR coupled with direct sequencing of the amplification products to identify changes in the nucleotide sequences of the *gyrA*, *gyrB*, *parC*, and *parE* genes (86, 104, 109, 244). The primers, however, appear to be species specific (Table 1). Low-level fluoroquinolone resistance mediated by the novel resistance genes of the *qnr* family (100, 106, 146, 172), which are frequently plasmid carried, can be detected via PCR (101, 126, 193).

SULFONAMIDE RESISTANCE

There are three major sulfonamide resistance genes, *sulI*, *sulII*, and *sulIII*. All three have been cloned and sequenced, and PCR assays for each gene have been described (85, 98, 181). Interestingly, the *sul* genes are often associated with transposable DNA elements, such as Tn*21* and small, multicopy plasmids (84, 98), that can shuttle multiple resistance genes from organism to organism. Thus, the *sul* genes can serve as indicators of multidrug resistance in gram-negative organisms.

TETRACYCLINE RESISTANCE

Tetracycline resistance is widespread among the bacterial kingdom (35, 121, 190). PCR assays have been developed for the *tet*(A), *tet*(B), *tet*(C), *tet*(D), *tet*(E), *tet*(F), *tet*(H), *tet*(K), *tet*(L), *tet*(M), *tet*(N), *tet*(O), *tet*(Q), *tet*(S), *tet*(U), and *tet*(V) determinants (34, 60, 61, 71, 73, 92, 127, 130, 189, 209, 210, 265). Multiple alleles of several of these determinants exist. For example, there are six *tet*(M) alleles present in *Streptococcus pneumoniae,* designated *tet*(M)1 through *tet*(M)6, that have been differentiated through restriction analysis of PCR fragments (61). Such epidemiologic studies using genotyping of resistance determinants contribute to our understanding of resistance transfer and evolution. Primers for the *tet*(M), *tet*(O), and *tet*(Q) determinants are useful for detecting tetracycline resistance genes directly in periodontal samples (151, 152), where the presence of resistant organisms may indicate those patients who are likely to fail therapy with tetracycline (127). Multiple types of the *tet*(M) gene also have been recognized through sequence analysis (153).

TRIMETHOPRIM RESISTANCE

The number of genes capable of mediating trimethoprim resistance in bacteria continues to expand (9, 97, 98, 119, 206). DNA probes have proven to be powerful tools for detecting and classifying novel trimethoprim resistance genes (called *dhfr*) (9, 105, 179). However, because consensus sequences common to all the *dhfr* genes have not been identified, PCR primers that could simplify the detection of this family of genes have not been developed, although PCR primers for some individual genes have been developed (52, 88, 119, 218).

GUIDELINES FOR USING GENETIC TESTS

PCR assays in which the products are visualized on agarose gels are rapidly being replaced by real-time PCR assays using fluorescent resonance energy transfer probes or molecular beacons for detection of amplification products. These closed systems are more efficient and less prone to overall contamination than traditional PCR assays. The critical issue with PCR assays of any sort, however, is the reliability of results. The need for quality control measures, including controls for the presence of inhibitory substances, cannot be stressed enough, especially for detection of genes directly in clinical specimens. The temperatures used in PCR assays optimized for use with purified DNA or DNA from bacterial isolates obtained in pure culture may not be stringent enough to avoid false-positive results when used with clinical samples, such as blood and cerebrospinal fluid, where considerably more nonspecific priming can occur (227). Using control reactions containing no template DNA to identify nonspecific products due to contamination of *Taq* polymerase with DNA, such as provided by cloning vector DNA, is critical (227, 235).

One should never assume that PCR primers reported in the literature have undergone rigorous testing. Rather, primer sets should be thoroughly tested for specificity, self-complementarity, and dimer formation before use. According to the Clinical Laboratory Improvement Amendments of 1988, validation of DNA probe and PCR tests by the clinical laboratory in which they are to be used is mandatory before they can be used for analysis of clinical specimens. Methods for validation are published by the Clinical and Laboratory Standards Institute (41).

Studies to determine the reservoirs of resistance genes and routes of resistance gene transfer in hospitals and community settings are still needed. Such studies would also help to determine the frequency with which organisms carry resistance genes that are not expressed. Although still considered experimental, many of the PCR methods for detecting resistance genes described herein are already having a positive effect on guiding therapy early in the course of infection and making the treatment of infectious diseases less empiric.

REFERENCES

1. **Aarestrup, F. M., P. Ahrens, M. Madsen, L. V. Pallesen, R. L. Poulsen, and H. Westh.** 1996. Glycopeptide susceptibility among Danish *Enterococcus faecium* and *Enterococcus faecalis* isolates of animal and human origin and PCR identification of genes within the VanA cluster. *Antimicrob. Agents Chemother.* **40:**1938–1940.
2. **Agersø, Y., and L. Guardabassi.** 2005. Identification of Tet 39, a novel class of tetracycline resistance determinant in *Acinetobacter* spp. of environmental and clinical origin. *J. Antimicrob. Chemother.* **55:**566–569.
3. **Alcaide, F., G. E. Pfyffer, and A. Telenti.** 1997. Role of *embB* in natural and acquired resistance to ethambutol in mycobacteria. *Antimicrob. Agents Chemother.* **41:**2270–2273.
4. **Alcantar-Curiel, D., J. C. Tinoco, C. Gayosso, A. Carlos, C. Daza, M. C. Perez-Prado, L. Salcido, J. I. Santos, and**

C. M. Alpuche-Aranda. 2004. Nosocomial bacteremia and urinary tract infections caused by extended-spectrum β-lactamase-producing *Klebsiella pneumoniae* with plasmids carrying both SHV-5 and TLA-1 genes. *Clin. Infect. Dis.* **38:**1067–1074.

5. **Allignet, J., and N. El Solh.** 1995. Diversity among the gram-positive acetyltransferases inactivating streptogramin A and structurally related compounds and characterization of a new staphylococcal determinant, *vatB*. *Antimicrob. Agents Chemother.* **39:**2027–2036.
6. **Allignet, J., V. Loncle, C. Simenel, M. Delepierre, and N. El Solh.** 1993. Sequence of a staphylococcal gene, *vat*, encoding an acetyltransferase inactivating the A-type compounds of virginiamycin-like antibiotics. *Gene* **130:**91–98.
7. **Alvarez, M., J. H. Tran, N. Chow, and G. A. Jacoby.** 2004. Epidemiology of conjugative plasmid-mediated AmpC β-lactamases in the United States. *Antimicrob. Agents Chemother.* **48:**533–537.
8. **Aminov, R. I., N. Garrigues-Jeanjean, and R. I. Mackie.** 2001. Molecular ecology of tetracycline resistance: development and validation of primers for detection of tetracycline resistance genes encoding ribosomal protection proteins. *Appl. Environ. Microbiol.* **67:**22–32.
9. **Amyes, S. G. B., and K. J. Towner.** 1990. Trimethoprim resistance: epidemiology and molecular aspects. *J. Med. Microbiol.* **31:**1–19.
10. **Arnold, C., L. Westland, G. Mowat, A. Underwood, J. Magee, and S. Gharbia.** 2005. Single-nucleotide polymorphism-based differentiation and drug resistance detection in *Mycobacterium tuberculosis* from isolates or directly from sputum. *Clin. Microbiol. Infect.* **11:**122–130.
11. **Arthur, M., and R. Quintiliani, Jr.** 2001. Regulation of VanA- and VanB-type glycopeptide resistance in enterococci. *Antimicrob. Agents Chemother.* **45:**375–381.
12. **Aubron, C., L. Poirel, R. J. Ash, and P. Nordmann.** 2005. Carbapenemase-producing *Enterobacteriaceae*, U.S. rivers. *Emerg. Infect. Dis.* **11:**260–264.
13. **Auckland, C., L. Teare, F. Cooke, M. E. Kaufmann, M. Warner, G. Jones, K. Bamford, H. Ayles, and A. P. Johnson.** 2002. Linezolid-resistant enterococci: report of the first isolates in the United Kingdom. *J. Antimicrob. Chemother.* **50:**743–746.
14. **Ballard, S. A., E. A. Grabsch, P. D. R. Johnson, and M. L. Grayson.** 2005. Comparison of three PCR primer sets for identification of *vanB* gene carriage in feces and correlation with carriage of vancomycin-resistant enterococci: interference by *vanB*-containing anaerobic bacilli. *Antimicrob. Agents Chemother.* **49:**77–81.
15. **Ballard, S. A., K. K. Pertile, M. Lim, P. D. R. Johnson, and M. L. Grayson.** 2005. Molecular characterization of *vanB* elements in naturally occurring gut anaerobes. *Antimicrob. Agents Chemother.* **49:**1688–1694.
16. **Bauernfeind, A., I. Stemplinger, R. Jungwirth, P. Mangold, S. Amann, E. Akalin, Ö. Ang, C. Bal, and J. M. Casellas.** 1996. Characterization of β-lactamase gene bla_{PER-2}, which encodes an extended-spectrum class A β-lactamase. *Antimicrob. Agents Chemother.* **40:**616–620.
17. **Bert, F., C. Branger, and N. Lambert-Zechovsky.** 2002. Identification of PSE and OXA β-lactamase genes in *Pseudomonas aeruginosa* using PCR-restriction fragment length polymorphism. *J. Antimicrob. Chemother.* **50:**11–18.
18. **Bonnet, R.** 2004. Growing group of extended-spectrum β-lactamases: the CTX-M enzymes. *Antimicrob. Agents Chemother.* **48:**1–14.
19. **Bonnet, R., C. Dutour, J. L. M. Sampaio, C. Chanal, D. Sirot, R. Labia, C. De Champs, and J. Sirot.** 2001. Novel cefotaximase (CTX-M-16) with increased catalytic efficiency due to substitution Asp-240 → Gly. *Antimicrob. Agents Chemother.* **45:**2269–2275.
20. **Bou, G., A. Oliver, and J. Martínez-Beltrán.** 2000. OXA-24, a novel class D β-lactamase with carbapenemase activity in an *Acinetobacter baumannii* clinical strain. *Antimicrob. Agents Chemother.* **44:**1556–1561.
21. **Boyd, D. A., J. Conly, H. Dedier, G. Peters, L. Robertson, E. Slater, and M. R. Mulvey.** 2000. Molecular characterization of the *vanD* gene cluster and a novel insertion element in a vancomycin-resistant enterococcus isolated in Canada. *J. Clin. Microbiol.* **38:**2392–2394.
22. **Bozdogan, B., L. Berrezouga, M.-S. Kuo, D. A. Yurek, K. A. Farley, B. J. Stockman, and R. Leclercq.** 1999. A new resistance gene, *linB*, conferring resistance to lincosamides by nucleotidylation in *Enterococcus faecium* HM1025. *Antimicrob. Agents Chemother.* **43:**925–929.
23. **Bradford, P. A.** 2001. Extended-spectrum β-lactamases in the 21st century: characterization, epidemiology, and detection of this important resistance threat. *Clin. Microbiol. Rev.* **14:**933–951.
24. **Bradford, P. A., S. Bratu, C. Urban, M. Visalli, N. Mariano, D. Landman, J. J. Rahal, S. Brooks, S. Cebular, and J. Quale.** 2004. Emergence of carbapenem-resistant *Klebsiella* species possessing the class A carbapenem-hydrolyzing KPC-2 and inhibitor-resistant TEM-30 β-lactamases in New York City. *Clin. Infect. Dis.* **39:**55–60.
25. **Bradford, P. A., C. Urban, N. Mariano, S. J. Projan, J. J. Rahal, and K. Bush.** 1997. Imipenem resistance in *Klebsiella pneumoniae* is associated with the combination of ACT-1, a plasmid-mediated AmpC β-lactamase, and the loss of an outer membrane protein. *Antimicrob. Agents Chemother.* **41:**563–569.
26. **Bratu, S., M. Mooty, S. Nichani, D. Landman, C. Gullans, B. Pettinato, U. Karumudi, P. Tolaney, and J. Quale.** 2005. Emergence of KPC-possessing *Klebsiella pneumoniae* in Brooklyn, New York: epidemiology and recommendations for detection. *Antimicrob. Agents Chemother.* **49:**3018–3020.
27. **Bratu, S., P. Tolaney, U. Karumudi, J. Quale, M. Mooty, S. Nichani, and D. Landman.** 2005. Carbapenemase-producing *Klebsiella pneumoniae* in Brooklyn, NY: molecular epidemiology and *in vitro* activity of polymyxin B and other agents. *J. Antimicrob. Chemother.* **56:**128–132.
28. **Bressler, A. M., T. Williams, E. E. Culler, W. Zhu, D. Lonsway, J. B. Patel, and F. S. Nolte.** 2005. Correlation of penicillin binding protein 2a detection with oxacillin resistance in *Staphylococcus aureus* and discovery of a novel penicillin binding protein 2a mutation. *J. Clin. Microbiol.* **43:**4541–4544.
29. **Brown, S., H. K. Young, and S. G. B. Amyes.** 2005. Characterisation of OXA-51, a novel class D carbapenemase found in genetically unrelated clinical strains of *Acinetobacter baumannii* from Argentina. *Clin. Microbiol. Infect.* **11:**15–23.
30. **Caroff, N., E. Espaze, D. Gautreau, H. Richet, and A. Reynaud.** 2000. Analysis of the effects of −42 and −32 *ampC* promoter mutations in clinical isolates of *Escherichia coli* hyperproducing AmpC. *J. Antimicrob. Chemother.* **45:**783–788.
31. **Centers for Disease Control and Prevention.** 2004. Vancomycin-resistant *Staphylococcus aureus*—New York, 2004. *Morb. Mortal. Wkly. Rep.* **53:**322–323.
32. **Chambers, H. F.** 1988. Methicillin-resistant staphylococci. *Clin. Microbiol. Rev.* **1:**173–186.
33. **Chang, S., D. M. Sievert, J. C. Hageman, M. L. Boulton, F. C. Tenover, F. P. Downes, S. Shah, J. T. Rudrik, G. R. Pupp, W. J. Brown, D. Cardo, and S. K. Fridkin.** 2003. Infection with vancomycin-resistant *Staphylococcus aureus* containing the *vanA* resistance gene. *N. Engl. J. Med.* **348:**1342–1347.
34. **Charpentier, E., G. Gerbaud, and P. Courvalin.** 1993. Characterization of a new class of tetracycline-resistance

gene *tet*(S) in *Listeria monocytogenes* BM4210. *Gene* **131:**27–34.

35. **Chopra, I., and M. Roberts.** 2001. Tetracycline antibiotics: mode of action, applications, molecular biology, and epidemiology of bacterial resistance. *Microbiol. Mol. Biol. Rev.* **65:**232–260.
36. **Clancy, J., J. Petitpas, F. Dib-Hajj, W. Yuan, M. Cronan, A. V. Kamath, J. Bergeron, and J. A. Retsema.** 1996. Molecular cloning and functional analysis of a novel macrolide-resistance determinant, *mefA*, from *Streptococcus pyogenes*. *Mol. Microbiol.* **22:**867–879.
37. **Clark, N. C., R. C. Cooksey, B. C. Hill, J. M. Swenson, and F. C. Tenover.** 1993. Characterization of glycopeptide-resistant enterococci from U.S. hospitals. *Antimicrob. Agents Chemother.* **37:**2311–2317.
38. **Clark, N. C., Ö. Olsvik, J. M. Swenson, C. A. Spiegel, and F. C. Tenover.** 1999. Detection of a streptomycin/spectinomycin adenylyltransferase gene *(aadA)* in *Enterococcus faecalis*. *Antimicrob. Agents Chemother.* **43:**157–160.
39. **Clark, N. C., L. M. Teixeira, R. R. Facklam, and F. C. Tenover.** 1998. Detection and differentiation of *vanC-1*, *vanC-2*, and *vanC-3* glycopeptide resistance genes in enterococci. *J. Clin. Microbiol.* **36:**2294–2297.
40. **Clark, N. C., L. M. Weigel, J. B. Patel, and F. C. Tenover.** 2005. Comparison of Tn*1546*-like elements in vancomycin-resistant *Staphylococcus aureus* isolates from Michigan and Pennsylvania. *Antimicrob. Agents Chemother.* **49:**470–472.
41. **Clinical and Laboratory Standards Institute/NCCLS.** 2005. *Molecular Diagnostic Methods for Infectious Diseases. Proposed Guideline,* 2nd ed. MM3-P2. Clinical and Laboratory Standards Institute, Wayne, Pa.
42. **Cockerill, F. R., III.** 1999. Genetic methods for assessing antimicrobial resistance. *Antimicrob. Agents Chemother.* **43:** 199–212.
43. **Cockerill, F. R., III, D. E. Williams, K. D. Eisenach, B. C. Kline, L. K. Miller, L. Stockman, J. Voyles, G. M. Caron, S. K. Bundy, G. D. Roberts, W. R. Wilson, A. C. Whelen, J. M. Hunt, and D. H. Persing.** 1996. Prospective evaluation of the utility of molecular techniques for diagnosing nosocomial transmission of multidrug-resistant tuberculosis. *Mayo Clin. Proc.* **71:**221–229.
44. **Code of Federal Regulations.** 2003. 42 CFR 493. U.S. Government Printing Office, Washington, D.C.
45. **Code of Federal Regulations.** 2004. Restrictions on the sale, distribution and use of analyte specific reagents. Title 21, CFR part 809.30. U.S. Government Printing Office, Washington, D.C.
46. **Coffey, T. J., C. G. Dowson, M. Daniels, J. Zhou, C. Martin, B. G. Spratt, and J. M. Musser.** 1991. Horizontal transfer of multiple penicillin-binding protein genes, and capsular biosynthetic genes, in natural populations of *Streptococcus pneumoniae*. *Mol. Microbiol.* **5:**2255–2260.
47. **Coudron, P. E.** 2005. Inhibitor-based methods for detection of plasmid-mediated AmpC β-lactamases in *Klebsiella* spp., *Escherichia coli*, and *Proteus mirabilis*. *J. Clin. Microbiol.* **43:**4163–4167.
48. **Coudron, P. E., N. D. Hanson, and M. W. Climo.** 2003. Occurrence of extended-spectrum and AmpC beta-lactamases in bloodstream isolates of *Klebsiella pneumoniae*: isolates harbor plasmid-mediated FOX-5 and ACT-1 AmpC beta-lactamases. *J. Clin. Microbiol.* **41:**772–777.
49. **Coudron, P. E., E. S. Moland, and C. C. Sanders.** 1997. Occurrence and detection of extended-spectrum β-lactamases in members of the family *Enterobacteriaceae* at a veterans medical center: seek and you may find. *J. Clin. Microbiol.* **35:**2593–2597.
50. **Courvalin, P.** 2005. Genetics of glycopeptide resistance in Gram-positive pathogens. *Int. J. Med. Microbiol.* **294:** 479–486.
51. **Dahl, K. H., G. S. Simonsen, Ø. Olsvik, and A. Sundsfjord.** 1999. Heterogeneity in the *vanB* gene cluster of genomically diverse clinical strains of vancomycin-resistant enterococci. *Antimicrob. Agents Chemother.* **43:** 1105–1110.
52. **Dale, G. E., H. Langen, M. G. P. Page, R. L. Then, and D. Stuber.** 1995. Cloning and characterization of a novel, plasmid-encoded trimethoprim-resistant dihydrofolate reductase from *Staphylococcus haemolyticus* MUR313. *Antimicrob. Agents Chemother.* **39:**1920–1924.
53. **Dalla Costa, L. M., P. E. Reynolds, H. A. Souza, D. C. Souza, M.-F. I. Palepou, and N. Woodford.** 2000. Characterization of a divergent *vanD*-type resistance element from the first glycopeptide-resistant strain of *Enterococcus faecium* isolated in Brazil. *Antimicrob. Agents Chemother.* **44:**3444–3446.
54. **Deguchi, T., M. Yasuda, M. Asano, K. Tada, H. Iwata, H. Komeda, T. Ezaki, I. Saito, and Y. Kawada.** 1995. DNA gyrase mutations in quinolone-resistant clinical isolates of *Neisseria gonorrhoeae*. *Antimicrob. Agents Chemother.* **39:**561–563.
55. **del Campo, R., J. C. Galán, C. Tenorio, P. Ruiz-Gargajosa, M. Zarazaga, C. Torres, and F. Baquero.** 2005. New *aac(6')-I* genes in *Enterococcus hirae* and *Enterococcus durans*: effect on β-lactam/aminoglycoside synergy. *J. Antimicrob. Chemother.* **55:**1053–1055.
56. **del Mar Tavío, M., J. Vila, J. Ruiz, J. Ruiz, A. M. Martín-Sánchez, and M. T. Jiménez de Anta.** 1999. Mechanisms involved in the development of resistance to fluoroquinolones in *Escherichia coli* isolates. *J. Antimicrob. Chemother.* **44:**735–742.
57. **Depardieu, F., M. G. Bonora, P. E. Reynolds, and P. Courvalin.** 2003. The *vanG* glycopeptide resistance operon from *Enterococcus faecalis* revisited. *Mol. Microbiol.* **50:** 931–948.
58. **Depardieu, F., and P. Courvalin.** 2001. Mutation in 23S rRNA responsible for resistance to 16-membered macrolides and streptogramins in *Streptococcus pneumoniae*. *Antimicrob. Agents Chemother.* **45:**319–323.
59. **Depardieu, F., B. Perichon, and P. Courvalin.** 2004. Detection of the *van* alphabet and identification of enterococci and staphylococci at the species level by multiplex PCR. *J. Clin. Microbiol.* **42:**5857–5860.
60. **De Rossi, E., M. C. J. Blokpoel, R. Cantoni, M. Branzoni, G. Riccardi, D. B. Young, K. A. L. De Smet, and O. Ciferri.** 1998. Molecular cloning and functional analysis of a novel tetracycline resistance determinant, *tet*(V), from *Mycobacterium smegmatis*. *Antimicrob. Agents Chemother.* **42:**1931–1937.
61. **Doherty, N., K. Trzcinski, P. Pickerill, P. Zawadzki, and C. G. Dowson.** 2000. Genetic diversity of the *tet*(M) gene in tetracycline-resistant clonal lineages of *Streptococcus pneumoniae*. *Antimicrob. Agents Chemother.* **44:**2979–2984.
62. **Domingo, M.-C., A. Huletsky, A. Bernal, R. Giroux, D. K. Boudreau, F. J. Picard, and M. G. Bergeron.** 2005. Characterization of a Tn*5382*-like transposon containing the *vanB2* gene cluster in a *Clostridium* strain isolated from human faeces. *J. Antimicrob. Chemother.* **55:**466–474.
63. **Dowson, C. G., A. Hutchison, and B. G. Spratt.** 1989. Extensive re-modelling of the transpeptidase domain of penicillin-binding protein 2B of a penicillin-resistant South African isolate of *Streptococcus pneumoniae*. *Mol. Microbiol.* **3:**95–102.
64. **du Plessis, M., A. M. Smith, and K. P. Klugman.** 1998. Rapid detection of penicillin-resistant *Streptococcus pneumoniae* in cerebrospinal fluid by a seminested-PCR strategy. *J. Clin. Microbiol.* **36:**453–457.
65. **Dutka-Malen, S., S. Evers, and P. Courvalin.** 1995. Detection of glycopeptide resistance genotypes and

identification to the species level of clinically relevant enterococci by PCR. *J. Clin. Microbiol.* **33:**24–27.

66. **Everett, M. J., Y. F. Jin, V. Ricci, and L. J. V. Piddock.** 1996. Contributions of individual mechanisms to fluoroquinolone resistance in 36 *Escherichia coli* strains isolated from humans and animals. *Antimicrob. Agents Chemother.* **40:**2380–2386.
67. **Farrell, D. J., S. G. Jenkins, S. D. Brown, M. Patel, B. S. Lavin, and K. P. Klugman.** 2005. Emergence and spread of *Streptococcus pneumoniae* with *erm*(B) and *mef*(A) resistance. *Emerg. Infect. Dis.* **11:**851–858.
68. **Fines, M., B. Perichon, P. Reynolds, D. F. Sahm, and P. Courvalin.** 1999. VanE, a new type of acquired glycopeptide resistance in *Enterococcus faecalis* BM4405. *Antimicrob. Agents Chemother.* **43:**2161–2164.
69. **Finken, M., P. Kirschner, A. Meier, A. Wrede, and E. C. Böttger.** 1993. Molecular basis of streptomycin resistance in *Mycobacterium tuberculosis:* alterations of the ribosomal protein S12 gene and point mutations within a functional 16S ribosomal RNA pseudoknot. *Mol. Microbiol.* **9:**1239–1246.
70. **Fitoussi, F., C. Loukil, I. Gros, O. Clermont, P. Mariani, S. Bonacorsi, I. Le Thomas, D. Deforche, and E. Bingen.** 2001. Mechanisms of macrolide resistance in clinical group B streptococci isolated in France. *Antimicrob. Agents Chemother.* **45:**1889–1891.
71. **Fletcher, H. M., and F. L. Macrina.** 1991. Molecular survey of clindamycin and tetracycline resistance determinants in *Bacteroides* species. *Antimicrob. Agents Chemother.* **35:**2415–2418.
72. **Fournier, B., and P. H. Roy.** 1997. Variability of chromosomally encoded β-lactamases from *Klebsiella oxytoca. Antimicrob. Agents Chemother.* **41:**1641–1648.
73. **Frech, G., and S. Schwarz.** 2000. Molecular analysis of tetracycline resistance in *Salmonella enterica* subsp. *enterica* serovars Typhimurium, Enteritidis, Dublin, Choleraesuis, Hadar and Saintpaul: construction and application of specific gene probes. *J. Appl. Microbiol.* **89:**633–641.
74. **Galimand, M., G. Gerbaud, and P. Courvalin.** 2000. Spectinomycin resistance in *Neisseria* spp. due to mutations in 16S rRNA. *Antimicrob. Agents Chemother.* **44:**1365–1366.
75. **Galimand, M., S. Sabtcheva, P. Courvalin, and T. Lambert.** 2005. Worldwide disseminated *armA* aminoglycoside resis tance methylase gene is borne by a composite transposon *Tn1548*. *Antimicrob. Agents Chemother.* **49:** 2949–2953.
76. **Geha, D. J., J. R. Uhl, C. A. Gustaferro, and D. H. Persing.** 1994. Multiplex PCR for identification of methicillin-resistant staphylococci in the clinical laboratory. *J. Clin. Microbiol.* **32:**1768–1772.
77. **Giakkoupi, P., A. Xanthaki, M. Kanelopoulou, A. Vlahaki, V. Miriagou, S. Kontou, E. Papafraggas, H. Malamou-Lada, L. S. Tzouvelekis, N. J. Legakis, and A. C. Vatopoulos.** 2003. VIM-1 metallo-β-lactamase-producing *Klebsiella pneumoniae* strains in Greek hospitals. *J. Clin. Microbiol.* **41:**3893–3896.
78. **Giamarellou, H.** 2005. Multidrug resistance in Gram-negative bacteria that produce extended-spectrum β-lactamases (ESBLs). *Clin. Microbiol. Infect.* **11**(Suppl. 4)**:**1–16.
79. **Gibreel, A., and O. Sköld.** 1998. High-level resistance to trimethoprim in clinical isolates of *Campylobacter jejuni* by acquisition of foreign genes *(dfr1* and *dfr9)* expressing drug-insensitive dihydrofolate reductases. *Antimicrob. Agents Chemother.* **42:**3059–3064.
80. **Gibreel, A., O. Sköld, and D. E. Taylor.** 2004. Characterization of plasmid-mediated *aphA-3* kanamycin resistance in *Campylobacter jejuni*. *Microb. Drug Resist.* **10:**98–105.
81. **Gilbart, J., C. R. Perry, and B. Slocombe.** 1993. High-level mupirocin resistance in *Staphylococcus aureus:* evidence for two distinct isoleucyl-tRNA synthetases. *Antimicrob. Agents Chemother.* **37:**32–38.
82. **González-Zorn, B., T. Teshager, M. Casas, M. C. Porrero, M. A. Moreno, P. Courvalin, and L. Domínguez.** 2005. *armA* and aminoglycoside resistance in *Escherichia coli*. *Emerg. Infect. Dis.* **11:**954–956.
83. **Gordts, B., H. Van Landuyt, M. Ieven, P. Vandamme, and H. Goossens.** 1995. Vancomycin-resistant enterococci colonizing the intestinal tracts of hospitalized patients. *J. Clin. Microbiol.* **33:**2842–2846.
84. **Grape, M., A. Farra, G. Kronvall, and L. Sundström.** 2005. Integrons and gene cassettes in clinical isolates of co-trimoxazole-resistant Gram-negative bacteria. *Clin. Microbiol. Infect.* **11:**185–192.
85. **Grape, M., L. Sundström, and G. Kronvall.** 2003. Sulphonamide resistance gene *sul3* found in *Escherichia coli* isolates from human sources. *J. Antimicrob. Chemother.* **52:** 1022–1024.
86. **Griggs, D. J., K. Gensberg, and L. J. V. Piddock.** 1996. Mutations in *gyrA* gene of quinolone-resistant salmonella serotypes isolated from humans and animals. *Antimicrob. Agents Chemother.* **40:**1009–1013.
87. **Guerra, B., E. Junker, A. Miko, R. Helmuth, and M. C. Mendoza.** 2004. Characterization and localization of drug resistance determinants in multidrug-resistant, integron-carrying *Salmonella enterica* serotype Typhimurium strains. *Microb. Drug Resist.* **10:**83–91.
88. **Guerra, B., S. M. Soto, J. M. Argüelles, and M. C. Mendoza.** 2001. Multidrug resistance is mediated by large plasmids carrying a class 1 integron in the emergent *Salmonella enterica* serotype [4, 5,12:i:−]. *Antimicrob. Agents Chemother.* **45:**1305–1308.
89. **Haanperä, M., P. Huovinen, and J. Jalava.** 2005. Detection and quantification of macrolide resistance mutations at positions 2058 and 2059 of the 23S rRNA gene by pyrosequencing. *Antimicrob. Agents Chemother.* **49:**457–460.
90. **Haas, W. H., K. Schilke, J. Brand, B. Amthor, K. Weyer, P. B. Fourie, G. Bretzel, V. Sticht-Groh, and H. J. Bremer.** 1997. Molecular analysis of *katG* gene mutations in strains of *Mycobacterium tuberculosis* complex from Africa. *Antimicrob. Agents Chemother.* **41:**1601–1603.
91. **Hannecart-Pokorni, E., F. Depuydt, L. De Wit, E. Van Bossuyt, J. Content, and R. Vanhoof.** 1997. Characterization of the 6′-*N*-aminoglycoside acetyltransferase gene *aac(6′)-Il* associated with a *sulI*-type integron. *Antimicrob. Agents Chemother.* **41:**314–318.
92. **Hansen, L. M., P. C. Blanchard, and D. C. Hirsh.** 1996. Distribution of *tet*(H) among *Pasteurella* isolates from the United States and Canada. *Antimicrob. Agents Chemother.* **40:**1558–1560.
93. **Haroche, J., J. Allignet, S. Aubert, A. E. Van Den Bogaard, and N. El Solh.** 2000. *satG*, conferring resistance to streptogramin A, is widely distributed in *Enterococcus faecium* strains but not in staphylococci. *Antimicrob. Agents Chemother.* **44:**190–191.
94. **Honoré, N., and S. T. Cole.** 1994. Streptomycin resistance in mycobacteria. *Antimicrob. Agents Chemother.* **38:** 238–242.
95. **Hossain, A., M. J. Ferraro, R. M. Pino, R. B. Dew III, E. S. Moland, T. J. Lockhart, K. S. Thomson, R. V. Goering, and N. D. Hanson.** 2004. Plasmid-mediated carbapenem-hydrolyzing enzyme KPC-2 in an *Enterobacter* sp. *Antimicrob. Agents Chemother.* **48:**4438–4440.
96. **Huletsky, A., R. Giroux, V. Rossbach, M. Gagnon, M. Vaillancourt, M. Bernier, F. Gagnon, K. Truchon, M. Bastien, F. J. Picard, A. Van Belkum, M. Ouellette, P. H. Roy, and M. G. Bergeron.** 2004. New real-time PCR assay for rapid detection of methicillin-resistant *Staphylococcus aureus* directly from specimens containing a mixture of staphylococci. *J. Clin. Microbiol.* **42:**1875–1884.

97. **Huovinen, P.** 2001. Resistance to trimethoprim-sulfamethoxazole. *Clin. Infect. Dis.* **32:**1608–1614.
98. **Huovinen, P., L. Sundström, G. Swedberg, and O. Sköld.** 1995. Trimethoprim and sulfonamide resistance. *Antimicrob. Agents Chemother.* **39:**279–289.
99. **Hussain, Z., L. Stoakes, S. Garrow, S. Longo, V. Fitzgerald, and R. Lannigan.** 2000. Rapid detection of *mecA*-positive and *mecA*-negative coagulase-negative staphylococci by an anti-penicillin binding protein 2a slide latex agglutination test. *J. Clin. Microbiol.* **38:**2051–2054.
100. **Jacoby, G. A.** 2005. Mechanisms of resistance to quinolones. *Clin. Infect. Dis.* **41:**S120–S126.
101. **Jacoby, G. A., N. Chow, and K. B. Waites.** 2003. Prevalence of plasmid-mediated quinolone resistance. *Antimicrob. Agents Chemother.* **47:**559–562.
102. **Jacoby, G. A., D. M. Mills, and N. Chow.** 2004. Role of β-lactamases and porins in resistance to ertapenem and other β-lactams in *Klebsiella pneumoniae*. *Antimicrob. Agents Chemother.* **48:**3203–3206.
103. **Jacoby, G. A., and L. S. Munoz-Price.** 2005. The new β-lactamases. *N. Engl. J. Med.* **352:**380–391.
104. **Janoir, C., V. Zeller, M.-D. Kitzis, N. J. Moreau, and L. Gutmann.** 1996. High-level fluoroquinolone resistance in *Streptococcus pneumoniae* requires mutations in *parC* and *gyrA*. *Antimicrob. Agents Chemother.* **40:**2760–2764.
105. **Jansson, C., A. Franklin, and O. Sköld.** 1992. Spread of a newly found trimethoprim resistance gene, *dhfrIX*, among porcine isolates and human pathogens. *Antimicrob. Agents Chemother.* **36:**2704–2708.
106. **Jonas, D., K. Biehler, D. Hartung, B. Spitzmüller, and F. D. Daschner.** 2005. Plasmid-mediated quinolone resistance in isolates obtained in German intensive care units. *Antimicrob. Agents Chemother.* **49:**773–775.
107. **Juteau, J.-M., M. Sirois, A. A. Medeiros, and R. C. Levesque.** 1991. Molecular distribution of ROB-1 β-lactamase in *Actinobacillus pleuropneumoniae*. *Antimicrob. Agents Chemother.* **35:**1397–1402.
108. **Kao, S. J., I. You, D. B. Clewell, S. M. Donabedian, M. J. Zervos, J. Petrin, K. J. Shaw, and J. W. Chow.** 2000. Detection of the high-level aminoglycoside resistance gene *aph(2″)-Ib* in *Enterococcus faecium*. *Antimicrob. Agents Chemother.* **44:**2876–2879.
109. **Kapur, V., L.-L. Li, M. R. Hamrick, B. B. Plikaytis, T. M. Shinnick, A. Telenti, W. R. Jacobs, Jr., A. Banerjee, S. Cole, K. Y. Yuen, J. E. Clarridge III, B. N. Kreiswirth, and J. M. Musser.** 1995. Rapid *Mycobacterium* species assignment and unambiguous identification of mutations associated with antimicrobial resistance in *Mycobacterium tuberculosis* by automated DNA sequencing. *Arch. Pathol. Lab. Med.* **119:**131–138.
110. **Kariyama, R., R. Mitsuhata, J. W. Chow, D. B. Clewell, and H. Kumon.** 2000. Simple and reliable multiplex PCR assay for surveillance isolates of vancomycin-resistant enterococci. *J. Clin. Microbiol.* **38:**3092–3095.
111. **Kazakova, S. V., J. C. Hageman, M. Matava, A. Srinivasan, L. Phelan, B. Garfinkel, T. Boo, S. McAllister, J. Anderson, B. Jensen, D. Dodson, D. Lonsway, L. K. McDougal, M. Arduino, V. J. Fraser, G. Killgore, F. C. Tenover, S. Cody, and D. B. Jernigan.** 2005. A clone of methicillin-resistant *Staphylococcus aureus* among professional football players. *N. Engl. J. Med.* **352:**468–475.
112. **Kelley, C. L., D. A. Rouse, and S. L. Morris.** 1997. Analysis of *ahpC* gene mutations in isoniazid-resistant clinical isolates of *Mycobacterium tuberculosis*. *Antimicrob. Agents Chemother.* **41:**2057–2058.
113. **Kim, H. B., B. Lee, H.-C. Jang, S. H. Kim, C. I. Kang, Y. J. Choi, S. W. Park, B. S. Kim, E.-C. Kim, M.-D. Oh, and K. W. Choe.** 2004. A high frequency of macrolide-lincosamide-streptogramin resistance determinants in *Staphylococcus aureus* isolated in South Korea. *Microb. Drug Resist.* **10:**248–254.
114. **Klaassen, C. H. W., and J. W. Mouton.** 2005. Molecular detection of the macrolide efflux gene: to discriminate or not to discriminate between *mef*(A) and *mef*(E). *Antimicrob. Agents Chemother.* **49:**1271–1278.
115. **Klomberg, D. M., H. A. de Valk, J. W. Mouton, and C. H. W. Klaassen.** 2005. Rapid and reliable real-time PCR assay for detection of the macrolide efflux gene and subsequent discrimination between its distinct subclasses *mef*(A) and *mef*(E). *J. Microbiol. Methods* **60:**269–273.
116. **Kobayashi, N., M. Alam, Y. Nishimoto, S. Urasawa, N. Uehara, and N. Watanabe.** 2001. Distribution of aminoglycoside resistance genes in recent clinical isolates of *Enterococcus faecalis, Enterococcus faecium* and *Enterococcus avium*. *Epidemiol. Infect.* **126:**197–204.
117. **Leclercq, R., E. Derlot, J. Duval, and P. Courvalin.** 1988. Plasmid-mediated resistance to vancomycin and teicoplanin in *Enterococcus faecium*. *N. Engl. J. Med.* **319:**157–161.
118. **Leclercq, R., C. Huet, M. Picherot, P. Trieu-Cuot, and C. Poyart.** 2005. Genetic basis of antibiotic resistance in clinical isolates of *Streptococcus gallolyticus (Streptococcus bovis)*. *Antimicrob. Agents Chemother.* **49:**1646–1648.
119. **Lee, J. C., J. Y. Oh, J. W. Cho, J. C. Park, J. M. Kim, S. Y. Seol, and D. T. Cho.** 2001. The prevalence of trimethoprim-resistance-conferring dihydrofolate reductase genes in urinary isolates of *Escherichia coli* in Korea. *J. Antimicrob. Chemother.* **47:**599–604.
120. **Lee, W. G., J. A. Jernigan, J. K. Rasheed, G. J. Anderson, and F. C. Tenover.** 2001. Possible horizontal transfer of the *vanB2* gene among genetically diverse strains of vancomycin-resistant *Enterococcus faecium* in a Korean hospital. *J. Clin. Microbiol.* **39:**1165–1168.
121. **Levy, S. B., L. M. McMurry, T. M. Barbosa, V. Burdett, P. Courvalin, W. Hillen, M. C. Roberts, J. I. Rood, and D. E. Taylor.** 1999. Nomenclature for new tetracycline resistance determinants. *Antimicrob. Agents Chemother.* **43:**1523–1524.
122. **Livermore, D. M., and P. M. Hawkey.** 2005. CTX-M: changing the face of ESBLs in the UK. *J. Antimicrob. Chemother.* **56:**451–454.
123. **Low, D. E.** 2005. Changing trends in antimicrobial-resistant pneumococci: it's not all bad news. *Clin. Infect. Dis.* **41:**228–233.
124. **Lyras, D., and J. I. Rood.** 1996. Genetic organization and distribution of tetracycline resistance determinants in *Clostridium perfringens*. *Antimicrob. Agents Chemother.* **40:**2500–2504.
125. **Ma, L., and J. A. Kovacs.** 2001. Rapid detection of mutations in the human-derived *Pneumocystis carinii* dihydropteroate synthase gene associated with sulfa resistance. *Antimicrob. Agents Chemother.* **45:**776–780.
126. **Mammeri, H., M. Van De Loo, L. Poirel, L. Martinez-Martinez, and P. Nordmann.** 2005. Emergence of plasmid-mediated quinolone resistance in *Escherichia coli* in Europe. *Antimicrob. Agents Chemother.* **49:**71–76.
127. **Manch-Citron, J. N., G. H. Lopez, A. Dey, J. W. Rapley, S. R. MacNeill, and C. M. Cobb.** 2000. PCR monitoring for tetracycline resistance genes in subgingival plaque following site-specific periodontal therapy: a preliminary report. *J. Clin. Periodontol.* **27:**437–446.
128. **Marchandin, H., H. Jean-Pierre, E. Jumas-Bilak, L. Isson, B. Drouillard, H. Darbas, and C. Carriere.** 2001. Distribution of macrolide resistance genes *erm*(B) and *mef*(A) among 160 penicillin-intermediate clinical isolates of *Streptococcus pneumoniae* isolated in southern France. *Pathol. Biol.* **49:**522–527.
129. **Mariotte, S., P. Nordmann, and M. H. Nicolas.** 1994. Extended-spectrum β-lactamase in *Proteus mirabilis*. *J. Antimicrob. Chemother.* **33:**925–935.

130. **Martin, P., P. Trieu-Cuot, and P. Courvalin.** 1986. Nucleotide sequence of the *tet*M tetracycline resistance determinant of the streptococcal conjugative shuttle transposon Tn*1545*. *Nucleic Acids Res.* **14:**7047–7058.
131. **Maskell, J. P., A. M. Sefton, and L. M. C. Hall.** 1997. Mechanism of sulfonamide resistance in clinical isolates of *Streptococcus pneumoniae*. *Antimicrob. Agents Chemother.* **41:**2121–2126.
132. **Massanari, R. M., M. A. Pfaller, D. S. Wakefield, G. T. Hammons, L.-A. McNutt, R. F. Woolson, and C. M. Helms.** 1988. Implications of acquired oxacillin resistance in the management and control of *Staphylococcus aureus* infections. *J. Infect. Dis.* **158:**702–709.
133. **McDougal, L. K., J. K. Rasheed, J. W. Biddle, and F. C. Tenover.** 1995. Identification of multiple clones of extended-spectrum cephalosporin-resistant *Streptococcus pneumoniae* isolates in the United States. *Antimicrob. Agents Chemother.* **39:**2282–2288.
134. **McKessar, S. J., A. M. Berry, J. M. Bell, J. D. Turnidge, and J. C. Paton.** 2000. Genetic characterization of *van*G, a novel vancomycin resistance locus of *Enterococcus faecalis*. *Antimicrob. Agents Chemother.* **44:**3224–3228.
135. **Meier, A., P. Kirschner, F.-C. Bange, U. Vogel, and E. C. Böttger.** 1994. Genetic alterations in streptomycin-resistant *Mycobacterium tuberculosis:* mapping of mutations conferring resistance. *Antimicrob. Agents Chemother.* **38:**228–233.
136. **Moland, E. S., J. A. Black, J. Ourada, M. D. Reisbig, N. D. Hanson, and K. S. Thomson.** 2002. Occurrence of newer β-lactamases in *Klebsiella pneumoniae* isolates from 24 U.S. hospitals. *Antimicrob. Agents Chemother.* **46:**3837–3842.
137. **Moland, E. S., N. D. Hanson, V. L. Herrera, J. A. Black, T. J. Lockhart, A. Hossain, J. A. Johnson, R. V. Goering, and K. S. Thomson.** 2003. Plasmid-mediated, carbapenem-hydrolysing β-lactamase, KPC-2, in *Klebsiella pneumoniae* isolates. *J. Antimicrob. Chemother.* **51:**711–714.
138. **Mulvey, M. R., E. Bryce, D. A. Boyd, M. Ofner-Agostini, A. M. Land, A. E. Simor, S. Paton, the Canadian Hospital Epidemiology Committee, the Canadian Nosocomial Infection Surveillance Program, and Health Canada.** 2005. Molecular characterization of cefoxitin-resistant *Escherichia coli* from Canadian hospitals. *Antimicrob. Agents Chemother.* **49:**358–365.
139. **Musser, J. M., V. Kapur, D. L. Williams, B. N. Kreiswirth, D. van Soolingen, and J. D. A. van Embden.** 1996. Characterization of the catalase-peroxidase gene (*katG*) and *inhA* locus in isoniazid-resistant and -susceptible strains of *Mycobacterium tuberculosis* by automated DNA sequencing: restricted array of mutations associated with drug resistance. *J. Infect. Dis.* **173:**196–202.
140. **Naas, T., P. Nordmann, G. Vedel, and C. Poyart.** 2005. Plasmid-mediated carbapenem-hydrolyzing β-lactamase KPC in a *Klebsiella pneumoniae* isolate from France. *Antimicrob. Agents Chemother.* **49:**4423–4424.
141. **Naas, T., L. Poirel, A. Karim, and P. Nordmann.** 1999. Molecular characterization of In50, a class 1 integron encoding the gene for the extended-spectrum β-lactamase VEB-1 in *Pseudomonas aeruginosa*. *FEMS Microbiol. Lett.* **176:**411–419.
142. **Naas, T., L. Vandel, W. Sougakoff, D. M. Livermore, and P. Nordmann.** 1994. Cloning and sequence analysis of the gene for a carbapenem-hydrolyzing Class A β-lactamase, Sme-1, from *Serratia marcescens* S6. *Antimicrob. Agents Chemother.* **38:**1262–1270.
143. **Navia, M. M., J. Ruiz, J. Sanchez-Cespedes, and J. Vila.** 2003. Detection of dihydrofolate reductase genes by PCR and RFLP. *Diagn. Microbiol. Infect. Dis.* **46:**295–298.
144. **Ng, L.-K., M. R. Mulvey, I. Martin, G. A. Peters, and W. Johnson.** 1999. Genetic characterization of antimicrobial resistance in Canadian isolates of *Salmonella* serovar Typhimurium DT104. *Antimicrob. Agents Chemother.* **43:** 3018–3021.
145. **Nordmann, P., and L. Poirel.** 2002. Emerging carbapenemases in Gram-negative aerobes. *Clin. Microbiol. Infect.* **8:**321–331.
146. **Nordmann, P., and L. Poirel.** 2005. Emergence of plasmid-mediated resistance to quinolones in Enterobacteriaceae. *J. Antimicrob. Chemother.* **56:**463–469.
147. **Novotna, G., V. Adamkova, J. Janata, O. Melter, and J. Spizek.** 2005. Prevalence of resistance mechanisms against macrolides and lincosamides in methicillin-resistant coagulase-negative staphylococci in the Czech Republic and occurrence of an undefined mechanism of resistance to lincosamides. *Antimicrob. Agents Chemother.* **49:**3586–3589.
148. **Nüesch-Inderbinen, M. T., H. Hächler, and F. H. Kayser.** 1996. Detection of genes coding for extended-spectrum SHV beta-lactamases in clinical isolates by a molecular genetic method, and comparison with the E Test. *Eur. J. Clin. Microbiol. Infect. Dis.* **15:**398–402.
149. **Nunes, E. L., K. R. dos Santos, P. J. Mondino, M. Bastos, and M. Giambiagi-deMarval.** 1999. Detection of *ileS-2* gene encoding mupirocin resistance in methicillin-resistant *Staphylococcus aureus* by multiplex PCR. *Diagn. Microbiol. Infect. Dis.* **34:**77–81.
150. **Oliver, A., J. C. Pérez-Díaz, T. M. Coque, F. Baquero, and R. Cantón.** 2001. Nucleotide sequence and characterization of a novel cefotaxime-hydrolyzing β-lactamase (CTX-M-10) isolated in Spain. *Antimicrob. Agents Chemother.* **45:**616–620.
151. **Olsvik, B., M. J. Flynn, F. C. Tenover, J. Slots, and I. Olsen.** 1996. Tetracycline resistance in *Prevotella* isolates from periodontally diseased patients is due to the *tet*(Q) gene. *Oral Microbiol. Immunol.* **11:**304–308.
152. **Olsvik, B., I. Olsen, and F. C. Tenover.** 1995. Detection of *tet*(M) and *tet*(O) using the polymerase chain reaction in bacteria isolated from patients with periodontal disease. *Oral Microbiol. Immunol.* **10:**87–92.
153. **Olsvik, B., F. C. Tenover, I. Olsen, and J. K. Rasheed.** 1996. Three subtypes of the *tet*(M) gene identified in bacterial isolates from periodontal pockets. *Oral Microbiol. Immunol.* **11:**299–303.
154. **Oster, P., A. Zanchi, S. Cresti, M. Lattanzi, F. Montagnani, C. Cellesi, and G. M. Rossolini.** 1999. Patterns of macrolide resistance determinants among community-acquired *Streptococcus pneumoniae* isolates over a 5-year period of decreased macrolide susceptibility rates. *Antimicrob. Agents Chemother.* **43:**2510–2512.
155. **Ostrowsky, B. E., N. C. Clark, C. Thauvin-Eliopoulos, L. Venkataraman, M. H. Samore, F. C. Tenover, G. M. Eliopoulos, R. C. Moellering, Jr., and H. S. Gold.** 1999. A cluster of VanD vancomycin-resistant *Enterococcus faecium:* molecular characterization and clinical epidemiology. *J. Infect. Dis.* **180:**1177–1185.
156. **Padiglione, A. A., E. A. Grabsch, D. Olden, M. Hellard, M. I. Sinclair, C. K. Fairley, and M. L. Grayson.** 2000. Fecal colonization with vancomycin-resistant enterococci in Australia. *Emerg. Infect. Dis.* **6:**534–536.
157. **Palepou, M.-F., A. P. Johnson, B. D. Cookson, H. Beattie, A. Charlett, and N. Woodford.** 1998. Evaluation of disc diffusion and Etest for determining the susceptibility of *Staphylococcus aureus* to mupirocin. *J. Antimicrob. Chemother.* **42:**577–583.
158. **Pan, X.-S., J. Ambler, S. Mehtar, and L. M. Fisher.** 1996. Involvement of topoisomerase IV and DNA gyrase as ciprofloxacin targets in *Streptococcus pneumoniae*. *Antimicrob. Agents Chemother.* **40:**2321–2326.
159. **Patel, R.** 1999. Enterococcal-type glycopeptide resistance genes in non-enterococcal organisms. *FEMS Microbiol. Lett.* **185:**1–7.
160. **Paterson, D. L., K. M. Hujer, A. M. Hujer, B. Yeiser, M. D. Bonomo, L. B. Rice, R. A. Bonomo, and the**

International Klebsiella Study Group. 2003. Extended-spectrum β-lactamases in *Klebsiella pneumoniae* bloodstream isolates from seven countries: dominance and widespread prevalence of SHV- and CTX-M-type β-lactamases. *Antimicrob. Agents Chemother.* **47:**3554–3560.

161. **Paule, S. M., A. C. Pasquariello, D. M. Hacek, A. G. Fisher, R. B. Thomson, Jr., K. L. Kaul, and L. R. Peterson.** 2005. Direct detection of *Staphylococcus aureus* from adult and neonate nasal swab specimens using real-time polymerase chain reaction. *J. Mol. Diagn.* **6:**191–196.

162. **Paulsen, I. T., M. H. Brown, and R. A. Skurray.** 1996. Proton-dependent multidrug efflux systems. *Microbiol. Rev.* **60:**575–608.

163. **Pérez-Pérez, F. J., and N. D. Hanson.** 2002. Detection of plasmid-mediated AmpC β-lactamase genes in clinical isolates by using multiplex PCR. *J. Clin. Microbiol.* **40:** 2153–2162.

164. **Perichon, B., B. Casadewall, P. Reynolds, and P. Courvalin.** 2000. Glycopeptide-resistant *Enterococcus faecium* BM4416 is a VanD-type strain with an impaired D-alanine:D-alanine ligase. *Antimicrob. Agents Chemother.* **44:**1346–1348.

165. **Perichon, B., P. Reynolds, and P. Courvalin.** 1997. VanD-type glycopeptide-resistant *Enterococcus faecium* BM4339. *Antimicrob. Agents Chemother.* **41:**2016–2018.

166. **Perichon, B., J. Tankovic, and P. Courvalin.** 1997. Characterization of a mutation in the *parE* gene that confers fluoroquinolone resistance in *Streptococcus pneumoniae*. *Antimicrob. Agents Chemother.* **41:**1166–1167.

167. **Petroni, A., A. Corso, R. Melano, M. L. Cacace, A. M. Bru, A. Rossi, and M. Galas.** 2002. Plasmidic extended-spectrum β-lactamases in *Vibrio cholerae* O1 El Tor isolates in Argentina. *Antimicrob. Agents Chemother.* **46:**1462–1468.

168. **Ploy, M.-C., H. Giamarellou, P. Bourlioux, P. Courvalin, and T. Lambert.** 1994. Detection of *aac(6')-I* genes in amikacin-resistant *Acinetobacter* spp. by PCR. *Antimicrob. Agents Chemother.* **38:**2925–2928.

169. **Poirel, L., C. Héritier, C. Spicq, and P. Nordmann.** 2004. In vivo acquisition of high-level resistance to imipenem in *Escherichia coli*. *J. Clin. Microbiol.* **42:** 3831–3833.

170. **Poirel, L., I. Le Thomas, T. Naas, A. Karim, and P. Nordmann.** 2000. Biochemical sequence analyses of GES-1, a novel class A extended-spectrum β-lactamase, and the class 1 integron In52 from *Klebsiella pneumoniae*. *Antimicrob. Agents Chemother.* **44:**622–632.

171. **Poirel, L., T. Naas, D. Nicolas, L. Collet, S. Bellais, J.-D. Cavallo, and P. Nordmann.** 2000. Characterization of VIM-2, a carbapenem-hydrolyzing metallo-β-lactamase and its plasmid- and integron-borne gene from a *Pseudomonas aeruginosa* clinical isolate in France. *Antimicrob. Agents Chemother.* **44:**891–897.

172. **Poirel, L., J.-M. Rodriguez-Martinez, H. Mammeri, A. Liard, and P. Nordmann.** 2005. Origin of plasmid-mediated quinolone resistance determinant QnrA. *Antimicrob. Agents Chemother.* **49:**3523–3525.

173. **Poole, K.** 2005. Aminoglycoside resistance in *Pseudomonas aeruginosa*. *Antimicrob. Agents Chemother.* **49:**479–487.

174. **Poole, K.** 2005. Efflux-mediated antimicrobial resistance. *J. Antimicrob. Chemother.* **56:**20–51.

175. **Pottumarthy, S., E. S. Moland, S. Juretschko, S. R. Swanzy, K. S. Thomson, and T. R. Fritsche.** 2003. NmcA carbapenem-hydrolyzing enzyme in *Enterobacter cloacae* in North America. *Emerg. Infect. Dis.* **9:**999–1002.

176. **Power, E. G. M., Y. H. Abdulla, H. G. Talsania, W. Spice, S. Aathithan, and G. L. French.** 1995. *vanA* genes in vancomycin-resistant clinical isolates of *Oerskovia turbata* and *Arcanobacterium (Corynebacterium) haemolyticum*. *J. Antimicrob. Chemother.* **36:**595–606.

177. **Poyart, C., C. Pierre, G. Quesne, B. Pron, P. Berche, and P. Trieu-Cu.** 1997. Emergence of vancomycin resistance in the genus *Streptococcus*: characterization of a *vanB* transferable determinant in *Streptococcus bovis*. *Antimicrob. Agents Chemother.* **41:**24–29.

178. **Prystowsky, J., F. Siddiqui, J. Chosay, D. L. Sinabarger, J. Millichap, L. R. Peterson, and G. A. Noskin.** 2001. Resistance to linezolid: characterization of mutations in rRNA and comparison of their occurrences in vancomycin-resistant enterococci. *Antimicrob. Agents Chemother.* **45:**2154–2156.

179. **Pulkkinen, L., P. Huovinen, E. Vuorio, and P. Toivanen.** 1984. Characterization of trimethoprim resistance by use of probes specific for transposon Tn7. *Antimicrob. Agents Chemother.* **26:**82–86.

180. **Queenan, A. M., C. Torres-Viera, H. S. Gold, Y. Carmeli, G. M. Eliopoulos, R. C. Moellering, Jr., J. P. Quinn, J. Hindler, A. A. Medeiros, and K. Bush.** 2000. SME-type carbapenem-hydrolyzing class A β-lactamases from geographically diverse *Serratia marcescens* strains. *Antimicrob. Agents Chemother.* **44:**3035–3039.

181. **Rådström, P., G. Swedberg, and O. Sköld.** 1991. Genetic analyses of sulfonamide resistance and its dissemination in gram-negative bacteria illustrate new aspects of R plasmid evolution. *Antimicrob. Agents Chemother.* **35:**1840–1848.

182. **Ramsey, M. A., S. F. Bradley, C. A. Kauffman, and T. M. Morton.** 1996. Identification of chromosomal location of *mupA* gene, encoding low-level mupirocin resistance in staphylococcal isolates. *Antimicrob. Agents Chemother.* **40:** 2820–2823.

183. **Rasheed, J. K., G. J. Anderson, H. Yigit, A. M. Queenan, A. Doménech-Sánchez, J. M. Swenson, J. W. Biddle, M. J. Ferraro, G. A. Jacoby, and F. C. Tenover.** 2000. Characterization of the extended-spectrum β-lactamase reference strain, *Klebsiella pneumoniae* K6 (ATCC 700603), which produces the novel enzyme SHV-18. *Antimicrob. Agents Chemother.* **44:**2382–2388.

184. **Rasheed, J. K., C. Jay, B. Metchock, F. Berkowitz, L. Weigel, J. Crellin, C. Steward, B. Hill, A. A. Medeiros, and F. C. Tenover.** 1997. Evolution of extended-spectrum β-lactam resistance (SHV-8) in a strain of *Escherichia coli* during multiple episodes of bacteremia. *Antimicrob. Agents Chemother.* **41:**647–653.

185. **Rasmussen, B. A., K. Bush, D. Keeney, Y. Yang, R. Hare, C. O'Gara, and A. A. Medeiros.** 1996. Characterization of IMI-1 β-lactamase, a class A carbapenem-hydrolyzing enzyme from *Enterobacter cloacae*. *Antimicrob. Agents Chemother.* **40:**2080–2086.

186. **Reig, M., J.-C. Galan, F. Baquero, and J. C. Perez-Diaz.** 2001. Macrolide resistance in *Peptostreptococcus* spp. mediated by *ermTR*: possible source of macrolide-lincosamide-streptogramin B resistance in *Streptococcus pyogenes*. *Antimicrob. Agents Chemother.* **45:**630–632.

187. **Reynolds, P. E., and P. Courvalin.** 2005. Vancomycin resistance in enterococci due to synthesis of precursors terminating in D-alanyl-D-serine. *Antimicrob. Agents Chemother.* **49:**21–25.

188. **Riccio, M. L., J.-D. Docquier, E. Dell'Amico, F. Luzzaro, G. Amicosante, and G. M. Rossolini.** 2003. Novel 3-*N*-aminoglycoside acetyltransferase gene, *aac(3)-Ic*, from a *Pseudomonas aeruginosa* integron. *Antimicrob. Agents Chemother.* **47:**1746–1748.

189. **Ridenhour, M. B., H. M. Fletcher, J. E. Mortensen, and L. Daneo-Moore.** 1996. A novel tetracycline-resistant determinant, *tet*(U), is encoded on the plasmid pKQ10 in *Enterococcus faecium*. *Plasmid* **35:**71–80.

190. **Roberts, M. C.** 2005. Update on acquired tetracycline resistance genes. *FEMS Microbiol. Lett.* **245:**195–203.

191. **Roberts, M. C., W. O. Chung, and D. E. Roe.** 1996. Characterization of tetracycline and erythromycin resistance determinants in *Treponema denticola*. *Antimicrob. Agents Chemother.* **40:**1690–1694.

192. **Roberts, M. C., J. Sutcliffe, P. Courvalin, L. B. Jensen, J. Rood, and H. Seppala.** 1999. Nomenclature for macrolide and macrolide-lincosamide-streptogramin B resistance determinants. *Antimicrob. Agents Chemother.* **43:**2823–2830.
193. **Robicsek, A., D. F. Sahm, J. Strahilevitz, G. A. Jacoby, and D. C. Hooper.** 2005. Broader distribution of plasmid-mediated quinolone resistance in the United States. *Antimicrob. Agents Chemother.* **49:**3001–3003.
194. **Sabaté, M., R. Tarragó, F. Navarro, E. Miró, C. Vergés, J. Barbé, and G. Prats.** 2000. Cloning and sequence of the gene encoding a novel cefotaxime-hydrolyzing β-lactamase (CTX-M-9) from *Escherichia coli* in Spain. *Antimicrob. Agents Chemother.* **44:**1970–1973.
195. **Sader, H. S., A. O. Reis, S. Silbert, and A. C. Gales.** 2005. IMPs, VIMs and SPMs: the diversity of metallo-β-lactamases produced by carbapenem-resistant *Pseudomonas aeruginosa* in a Brazilian hospital. *Clin. Microbiol. Infect.* **11:** 73–76.
196. **Sahm, D. F., L. Free, and S. Handwerger.** 1995. Inducible and constitutive expression of *vanC-1*-encoded resistance to vancomycin in *Enterococcus gallinarum*. *Antimicrob. Agents Chemother.* **39:**1480–1484.
197. **Satake, S., N. Clark, D. Rimland, F. S. Nolte, and F. C. Tenover.** 1997. Detection of vancomycin-resistant enterococci in fecal samples by PCR. *J. Clin. Microbiol.* **35:** 2325–2330.
198. **Saurina, G., J. M. Quale, V. M. Manikal, E. Oydna, and D. Landman.** 2000. Antimicrobial resistance in *Enterobacteriaceae* in Brooklyn, NY: epidemiology and relation to antibiotic usage patterns. *J. Antimicrob. Chemother.* **45:**895–898.
199. **Schwarz, S., C. Kehrenberg, B. Doublet, and A. Cloeckaert.** 2004. Molecular basis of bacterial resistance to chloramphenicol and florfenicol. *FEMS Microbiol. Rev.* **28:**519–542.
200. **Senda, K., Y. Arakawa, S. Ichiyama, K. Nakashima, H. Ito, S. Ohsuka, K. Shimokata, N. Kato, and M. Ohta.** 1996. PCR detection of metallo-β-lactamase gene (bla_{IMP}) in gram-negative rods resistant to broad-spectrum β-lactams. *J. Clin. Microbiol.* **34:**2909–2913.
201. **Shaw, K. J., P. N. Rather, R. S. Hare, and G. H. Miller.** 1993. Molecular genetics of aminoglycoside resistance genes and familial relationships of the aminoglycoside-modifying enzymes. *Microbiol. Rev.* **57:**138–163.
202. **Shaw, W. V.** 1983. Chloramphenicol acetyltransferase: enzymology and molecular biology. *Crit. Rev. Biochem.* **14:**1–46.
203. **Shibata, N., Y. Doi, K. Yamane, T. Yagi, H. Kurokawa, K. Shibayama, H. Kato, K. Kai, and Y. Arakawa.** 2003. PCR typing of genetic determinants for metallo-β-lactamases and integrases carried by gram-negative bacteria isolated in Japan, with focus on the class 3 integron. *J. Clin. Microbiol.* **41:**5407–5413.
204. **Shortridge, V. D., R. K. Flamm, N. Ramer, J. Beyer, and S. K. Tanaka.** 1996. Novel mechanism of macrolide resistance in *Streptococcus pneumoniae*. *Diagn. Microbiol. Infect. Dis.* **26:**73–78.
205. **Sinclair, A., C. Arnold, and N. Woodford.** 2003. Rapid detection and estimation by pyrosequencing of 23S rRNA genes with a single nucleotide polymorphism conferring linezolid resistance in enterococci. *Antimicrob. Agents Chemother.* **47:**3620–3622.
206. **Singh, K. V., R. R. Reves, L. K. Pickering, and B. E. Murray.** 1992. Identification by DNA sequence analysis of a new plasmid-encoded trimethoprim resistance gene in fecal *Escherichia coli* isolates from children in day-care centers. *Antimicrob. Agents Chemother.* **36:**1720–1726.
207. **Siu, L. K., J. Y. C. Lo, K. Y. Yuen, P. Y. Chau, M. H. Ng, and P. L. Ho.** 2000. β-lactamases in *Shigella flexneri* isolates from Hong Kong and Shanghai and a novel OXA-1-like β-lactamase, OXA-30. *Antimicrob. Agents Chemother.* **44:**2034–2038.
208. **Sloan, L. M., J. R. Uhl, E. A. Vetter, C. D. Schleck, W. S. Harmsen, J. Manahan, R. L. Thompson, J. E. Rosenblatt, and F. R. Cockerill III.** 2004. Comparison of the Roche LightCycler *vanA/vanB* detection assay and culture for detection of vancomycin-resistant enterococci from perianal swabs. *J. Clin. Microbiol.* **42:**2636–2643.
209. **Sougakoff, W., B. Papadopoulou, P. Nordmann, and P. Courvalin.** 1987. Nucleotide sequence and distribution of gene *tet*O encoding tetracycline resistance in *Campylobacter coli*. *FEMS Microbiol. Lett.* **44:**153–159.
210. **Speer, B. S., N. B. Shoemaker, and A. A. Salyers.** 1992. Bacterial resistance to tetracycline: mechanisms, transfer, and clinical significance. *Clin. Microbiol. Rev.* **5:**387–399.
211. **Sreevatsan, S., X. Pan, K. E. Stockbauer, D. L. Williams, B. N. Kreiswirth, and J. M. Musser.** 1996. Characterization of *rpsL* and *rrs* mutations in streptomycin-resistant *Mycobacterium tuberculosis* isolates from diverse geographic localities. *Antimicrob. Agents Chemother.* **40:**1024–1026.
212. **Sreevatsan, S., X. Pan, Y. Zhang, B. N. Kreiswirth, and J. M. Musser.** 1997. Mutations associated with pyrazinamide resistance in *pncA* of *Mycobacterium tuberculosis* complex organisms. *Antimicrob. Agents Chemother.* **41:** 636–640.
213. **Steward, C. D., P. M. Raney, A. K. Morrell, P. P. Williams, L. K. McDougal, L. Jevitt, J. E. McGowan, Jr., and F. C. Tenover.** 2005. Testing for induction of clindamycin resistance in erythromycin-resistant isolates of *Staphylococcus aureus*. *J. Clin. Microbiol.* **43:**1716–1721.
214. **Steward, C. D., J. K. Rasheed, S. K. Hubert, J. W. Biddle, P. M. Raney, G. J. Anderson, P. P. Williams, K. L. Brittain, A. Oliver, J. E. McGowan, Jr., and F. C. Tenover.** 2001. Characterization of clinical isolates of *Klebsiella pneumoniae* from 19 laboratories using the National Committee for Clinical Laboratory Standards extended-spectrum β-lactamase detection methods. *J. Clin. Microbiol.* **39:**2864–2872.
215. **Stinear, T. P., D. C. Olden, P. D. R. Johnson, J. K. Davies, and M. L. Grayson.** 2001. Enterococcal *vanB* resistance locus in anaerobic bacteria in human faeces. *Lancet* **357:**855–856.
216. **Sunde, M., and M. Norström.** 2005. The genetic background for streptomycin resistance in *Escherichia coli* influences the distribution of MICs. *J. Antimicrob. Chemother.* **56:**87–90.
217. **Sundsfjord, A., G. S. Simonsen, B. C. Haldorsen, H. Haaheim, S.-O. Hjelmevoll, P. Littauer, and K. H. Dahl.** 2004. Genetic methods for detection of antimicrobial resistance. *APMIS* **112:**815–837.
218. **Sundström, L., C. Jansson, K. Bremer, E. Heikkilä, B. Olsson-Liljequist, and O. Sköld.** 1995. A new *dhfrVIII* trimethoprim-resistance gene, flanked by *IS26*, whose product is remote from other dihydrofolate reductases in parsimony analysis. *Gene* **154:**7–14.
219. **Sutcliffe, J., T. Grebe, A. Tait-Kamradt, and L. Wondrack.** 1996. Detection of erythromycin-resistant determinants by PCR. *Antimicrob. Agents Chemother.* **40:** 2562–2566.
220. **Sutcliffe, J., A. Tait-Kamradt, and L. Wondrack.** 1996. *Streptococcus pneumoniae* and *Streptococcus pyogenes* resistant to macrolides but sensitive to clindamycin: a common resistance pattern mediated by an efflux system. *Antimicrob. Agents Chemother.* **40:**1817–1824.
221. **Swenson, J. M., M. J. Ferraro, D. F. Sahm, N. C. Clark, D. H. Culver, F. C. Tenover, and the National Committee for Clinical Laboratory Standards Study Group on Enterococci.** 1995. Multilaboratory evaluation of screening methods for detection of high-level aminoglycoside resistance in enterococci. *J. Clin. Microbiol.* **33:**3008–3018.

222. **Swenson, J. M., P. P. Williams, G. Killgore, C. M. O'Hara, and F. C. Tenover.** 2001. Performance of eight methods, including two new rapid methods, for detection of oxacillin resistance in a challenge set of *Staphylococcus aureus* organisms. *J. Clin. Microbiol.* **39:**3785–3788.
223. **Tait-Kamradt, A., J. Davies, M. Cronan, M. R. Jacobs, P. C. Appelbaum, and J. Sutcliffe.** 2000. Mutations in 23S rRNA and ribosomal protein L4 account for resistance in pneumococcal strains selected in vitro by macrolide passage. *Antimicrob. Agents Chemother.* **44:**2118–2125.
224. **Takiff, H. E., L. Salazar, C. Guerrero, W. Philipp, W. M. Huang, B. Kreiswirth, S. T. Cole, W. R. Jacobs, Jr., and A. Telenti.** 1994. Cloning and nucleotide sequence of *Mycobacterium tuberculosis gyrA* and *gyrB* genes and detection of quinolone resistance mutations. *Antimicrob. Agents Chemother.* **38:**773–780.
225. **Tankovic, J., B. Perichon, J. Duval, and P. Courvalin.** 1996. Contribution of mutations in *gyrA* and *parC* genes to fluoroquinolone resistance of mutants of *Streptococcus pneumoniae* obtained in vivo and in vitro. *Antimicrob. Agents Chemother.* **40:**2505–2510.
226. **Telenti, A., N. Honoré, C. Bernasconi, J. March, A. Ortega, B. Heym, H. E. Takiff, and S. T. Cole.** 1997. Genotypic assessment of isoniazid and rifampin resistance in *Mycobacterium tuberculosis:* a blind study at reference laboratory level. *J. Clin. Microbiol.* **35:**719–723.
227. **Tenover, F. C., M. B. Huang, J. K. Rasheed, and D. H. Persing.** 1994. Development of PCR assays to detect ampicillin resistance genes in cerebrospinal fluid samples containing *Haemophilus influenzae. J. Clin. Microbiol.* **32:**2729–2737.
228. **Tenover, F. C., R. N. Jones, J. M. Swenson, B. Zimmer, S. McAllister, J. H. Jorgensen, and the NCCLS Staphylococcus Working Group.** 1999. Methods for improved detection of oxacillin resistance in coagulase-negative staphylococci: results of a multicenter study. *J. Clin. Microbiol.* **37:**4051–4058.
229. **Tenover, F. C., and J. K. Rasheed.** 1999. Genetic methods for detecting antibacterial and antiviral resistance genes, p. 1578–1592. *In* P. R. Murray, E. J. Baron, M. A. Pfaller, F. C. Tenover, and R. H. Yolken (ed.), *Manual of Clinical Microbiology*, 7th ed. American Society for Microbiology, Washington, D.C.
230. **Tenover, F. C., L. M. Weigel, P. C. Appelbaum, L. K. McDougal, J. Chaitram, S. McAllister, N. Clark, G. Killgore, C. M. O'Hara, L. Jevitt, J. B. Patel, and B. Bozdogan.** 2004. Vancomycin-resistant *Staphylococcus aureus* isolate from a patient in Pennsylvania. *Antimicrob. Agents Chemother.* **48:**275–280.
231. **Tomasz, A., H. B. Drugeon, H. M. De Lencastre, D. Jabes, L. McDougal, and J. Bille.** 1989. New mechanism for methicillin resistance in *Staphylococcus aureus:* clinical isolates that lack the PBP 2a gene and contain normal penicillin-binding proteins with modified penicillin-binding capacity. *Antimicrob. Agents Chemother.* **33:** 1869–1874.
232. **Trieu-Cuot, P., G. De Cespédès, F. Bentorcha, F. Delbos, E. Gaspar, and T. Horaud.** 1993. Study of heterogeneity of chloramphenicol acetyltransferase (CAT) genes in streptococci and enterococci by polymerase chain reaction: characterization of a new CAT determinant. *Antimicrob. Agents Chemother.* **37:**2593–2598.
233. **Truong, Q. C., J.-C. Nguyen Van, D. Shlaes, L. Gutmann, and N. J. Moreau.** 1997. A novel, double mutation in DNA gyrase A of *Escherichia coli* conferring resistance to quinolone antibiotics. *Antimicrob. Agents Chemother.* **41:**85–90.
234. **Tsiodras, S., H. S. Gold, G. Sakoulas, G. M. Eliopoulos, C. Wennersten, L. Venkataraman, and R. C. Moellering, Jr.** 2001. Linezolid resistance in a clinical isolate of *Staphylococcus aureus. Lancet* **358:**207–208.
235. **Tyler, K. D., G. Wang, S. D. Tyler, and W. M. Johnson.** 1997. Factors affecting reliability and reproducibility of amplification-based DNA fingerprinting of representative bacterial pathogens. *J. Clin. Microbiol.* **35:**339–346.
236. **Ubukata, K., Y. Asahi, A. Yamane, and M. Konno.** 1996. Combinational detection of autolysin and penicillin-binding protein 2B genes of *Streptococcus pneumoniae* by PCR. *J. Clin. Microbiol.* **34:**592–596.
237. **Uttley, A. H. C., C. H. Collins, J. Naidoo, and R. C. George.** 1988. Vancomycin-resistant enterococci. *Lancet* **i:**57–58.
238. **Vahaboglu, H., L. M. C. Hall, L. Mulazimoglu, S. Dodanli, I. Yildirim, and D. M. Livermore.** 1995. Resistance to extended-spectrum cephalosporins, caused by PER-1 β-lactamase, in *Salmonella typhimurium* from Istanbul, Turkey. *J. Med. Microbiol.* **43:**294–299.
239. **Vakulenko, S. B., S. M. Donabedian, A. M. Voskresenskiy, M. J. Zervos, S. A. Lerner, and J. W. Chow.** 2003. Multiplex PCR for detection of aminoglycoside resistance genes in enterococci. *Antimicrob. Agents Chemother.* **47:**1423–1426.
240. **Van de Klundert, J. A. M., and J. S. Vliegenthart.** 1993. PCR detection of genes coding for aminoglycoside-modifying enzymes, p. 547–552. *In* D. H. Persing, T. F. Smith, F. C. Tenover, and T. J. White (ed.), *Diagnostic Molecular Microbiology: Principles and Applications*. American Society for Microbiology, Washington, D.C.
241. **Van Griethuysen, A., M. Pouw, N. Van Leeuwen, M. Heck, P. Willemse, A. Buiting, and J. Kluytmans.** 1999. Rapid slide latex agglutination test for detection of methicillin resistance in *Staphylococcus aureus*. *J. Clin. Microbiol.* **37:**2789–2792.
242. **Vanhoof, R., J. Content, E. Van Bossuyt, L. Dewit, and E. Hannecart-Pokorni.** 1992. Identification of the *aadB* gene coding for the aminoglycoside-2″-O-nucleotidyltransferase, ANT(2″), by means of the polymerase chain reaction. *J. Antimicrob. Chemother.* **29:**365–374.
243. **Vannuffel, P., J. Gigi, H. Ezzedine, B. Vandercam, M. Delmee, G. Wauters, and J.-L. Gala.** 1995. Specific detection of methicillin-resistant *Staphylococcus* species by multiplex PCR. *J. Clin. Microbiol.* **33:**2864–2867.
244. **Vila, J., J. Ruiz, P. Goni, A. Marcos, and T. J. De Anta.** 1995. Mutation in the *gyrA* gene of quinolone-resistant clinical isolates of *Acinetobacter baumannii. Antimicrob. Agents Chemother.* **39:**1201–1203.
245. **Vila, J., J. Ruiz, M. Navia, B. Becerril, I. Garcia, S. Perea, I. Lopez-Hernandez, I. Alamo, F. Ballester, A. M. Planes, J. Martinez-Beltran, and T. J. De Anta.** 1999. Spread of amikacin resistance in *Acinetobacter baumannii* strains isolated in Spain due to an epidemic strain. *J. Clin. Microbiol.* **37:**758–761.
246. **Walsh, T. R., M. A. Toleman, L. Poirel, and P. Nordmann.** 2005. Metallo-β-lactamases: the quiet before the storm? *Clin. Microbiol. Rev.* **18:**306–325.
247. **Warren, D. K., R. S. Liao, L. R. Merz, M. Eveland, and W. M. Dunne, Jr.** 2004. Detection of methicillin-resistant *Staphylococcus aureus* directly from nasal swab specimens by a real-time PCR assay. *J. Clin. Microbiol.* **42:**5578–5581.
248. **Weigel, L. M., D. B. Clewell, S. R. Gill, N. C. Clark, L. K. McDougal, S. E. Flannagan, J. F. Kolonay, J. Shetty, G. E. Killgore, and F. C. Tenover.** 2003. Genetic analysis of a high-level vancomycin-resistant isolate of *Staphylococcus aureus. Science* **302:**1569–1571.
249. **Weldhagen, G. F., and A. Prinsloo.** 2004. Molecular detection of GES-2 extended spectrum β-lactamase producing *Pseudomonas aeruginosa* in Pretoria, South Africa. *Int. J. Antimicrob. Agents* **24:**35–38.

250. **Werner, G., B. Hildebrandt, I. Klare, and W. Witte.** 2000. Linkage of determinants for streptogramin A, macrolide-lincosamide-streptogramin B, and chloramphenicol resistance on a conjugative plasmid in *Enterococcus faecium* and dissemination of this cluster among streptogramin-resistant enterococci. *Int. J. Med. Microbiol.* **290:**543–548.
251. **Werner, G., and W. Witte.** 1999. Characterization of a new enterococcal gene, *sat*G, encoding a putative acetyltransferase conferring resistance to streptogramin A compounds. *Antimicrob. Agents Chemother.* **43:**1813–1814.
252. **Wilson, P., J. A. Andrews, R. Charlesworth, R. Walesby, M. Singer, D. J. Farrell, and M. Robbins.** 2003. Linezolid resistance in clinical isolates of *Staphylococcus aureus*. *J. Antimicrob. Chemother.* **51:**186–188.
253. **Winokur, P. L., R. Canton, J. M. Casellas, and N. J. Legakis.** 2001. Variations in the prevalence of strains expressing an extended-spectrum β-lactamase phenotype and characterization of isolates from Europe, the Americas, and the Western Pacific region. *Clin. Infect. Dis.* **32**(Suppl. 2)**:**S94–S103.
254. **Wondrack, L., M. Massa, B. V. Yang, and J. Sutcliffe.** 1996. Clinical strain of *Staphylococcus aureus* inactivates and causes efflux of macrolides. *Antimicrob. Agents Chemother.* **40:**992–998.
255. **Woodford, N.** 2005. Biological counterstrike: antibiotic resistance mechanisms of Gram-positive cocci. *Clin. Microbiol. Infect.* **11**(Suppl. 3)**:**2–21.
256. **Woodford, N., P. M. Tierno, Jr., K. Young, L. Tysall, M.-F. I. Palepou, E. Ward, R. E. Painter, D. F. Suber, D. Shungu, L. L. Silver, K. Inglima, J. Kornblum, and D. M. Livermore.** 2004. Outbreak of *Klebsiella pneumoniae* producing a new carbapenem-hydrolyzing class A β-lactamase, KPC-3, in a New York medical center. *Antimicrob. Agents Chemother.* **48:**4793–4799.
257. **Woodford, N., L. Tysall, C. Auckland, M. W. Stockdale, A. J. Lawson, R. A. Walker, and D. M. Livermore.** 2002. Detection of oxazolidinone-resistant *Enterococcus faecalis* and *Enterococcus faecium* strains by real-time PCR and PCR-restriction fragment length polymorphism analysis. *J. Clin. Microbiol.* **40:**4298–4300.
258. **Wright, J. G., L. A. Tengelsen, K. E. Smith, J. B. Bender, R. K. Frank, J. H. Grendon, D. H. Rice, A. M. B. Thiessen, C. J. Gilbertson, S. Sivapalasingam, T. J. Barrett, T. E. Besser, D. D. Hancock, and F. J. Angulo.** 2005. Multidrug-resistant *Salmonella* Typhimurium in four animal facilities. *Emerg. Infect. Dis.* **11:**1235–1241.
259. **Yagi, T., J.-I. Wachino, H. Kurokawa, S. Suzuki, K. Yamane, Y. Doi, N. Shibata, H. Kato, K. Shibayama, and Y. Arakawa.** 2005. Practical methods using boronic acid compounds for identification of class C β-lactamase-producing *Klebsiella pneumoniae* and *Escherichia coli*. *J. Clin. Microbiol.* **43:**2551–2558.
260. **Yamane, K., J.-I. Wachino, Y. Doi, H. Kurokawa, and Y. Arakawa.** 2005. Global spread of multiple aminoglycoside resistance genes. *Emerg. Infect. Dis.* **11:**951–953.
261. **Yan, J.-J., J.-J. Wu, W.-C. Ko, S.-H. Tsai, C.-L. Chuang, H.-M. Wu, Y.-J. Lu, and J.-D. Li.** 2004. Plasmid-mediated 16S rRNA methylases conferring high-level aminoglycoside resistance in *Escherichia coli* and *Klebsiella pneumoniae* isolates from two Taiwanese hospitals. *J. Antimicrob. Chemother.* **54:**1007–1012.
262. **Yigit, H., A. M. Queenan, G. J. Anderson, A. Doménech-Sánchez, J. W. Biddle, C. D. Steward, S. Albertí, K. Bush, and F. C. Tenover.** 2001. Novel carbapenem-hydrolyzing β-lactamase, KPC-1, from a carbapenem-resistant strain of *Klebsiella pneumoniae*. *Antimicrob. Agents Chemother.* **45:**1151–1161.
263. **Yigit, H., A. M. Queenan, J. K. Rasheed, J. W. Biddle, A. Domenech-Sanchez, S. Alberti, K. Bush, and F. C. Tenover.** 2003. Carbapenem-resistant strain of *Klebsiella oxytoca* harboring carbapenem-hydrolyzing β-lactamase KPC-2. *Antimicrob. Agents Chemother.* **47:**3881–3889.
264. **Yokoyama, K., Y. Doi, K. Yamane, H. Kurokawa, N. Shibata, K. Shibayama, T. Yagi, H. Kato, and Y. Arakawa.** 2003. Acquisition of 16S rRNA methylase gene in *Pseudomonas*. *Lancet* **362:**1888–1893.
265. **Zhao, J., and T. Aoki.** 1992. Nucleotide sequence analysis of the class G tetracycline resistance determinant from *Vibrio anguillarum*. *Microbiol. Immunol.* **36:**1051–1060.
266. **Zhao, J.-R., Y.-J. Bai, Y. Wang, Q.-H. Zhang, M. Luo, and X.-J. Yan.** 2005. Development of a pyrosequencing approach for rapid screening of rifampin, isoniazid and ethambutol-resistant *Mycobacterium tuberculosis*. *Int. J. Tuberc. Lung Dis.* **9:**328–332.

Author Index

Volume 1 comprises pages 1–1268; volume 2 comprises pages 1269–2256.

Subject Index

Volume 1 comprises pages 1–1268; volume 2 comprises pages 1269–2256.